## CONSONANTS

| | | |
|---|---|---|
| **b** as in **b**aby | **k** as in **k**eep, a**c**tion, **c**atara**c**t | **t** as in **t**ake |
| **ch** as in **ch**urch | **l** as in **l**ie | **th** as in **th**ing |
| **d** as in **d**o | **m** as in **m**ake | **v** as in **v**ein |
| **dh** as in rhy**th**m, **th**is, mo**th**er | **n** as in **n**o | **w** as in **w**e |
| **f** as in **f**all | **p** as in **p**ain | **y** as in **y**es |
| **g** as in **g**o | **r** as in **r**ed | **z** as in **z**oo |
| **h** as in **h**ouse | **s** as in **s**o | **zh** as in trea**s**ure, a**z**ure |
| **j** as in **j**oin | **sh** as in **sh**oe | |

*A stressed syllable is indicated by an accent mark ( ΄ ) following the syllable.* A word may contain more than one stressed syllable, for example, **periangitis** [per´ē-an-jī´tis].

## Word Origins

*Information about a word's origins is called its* **etymology.** Many of the defined words in this dictionary have Greek or Latin origins. Some have roots in another language, such as Anglo-Saxon, a precursor of English. A word's etymology will appear in brackets at the end of the definition. For example, the following information accompanies the entry *spore:* [G. *sporos,* seed]. The *G* indicates that the word is of Greek origin. An *L* would indicate Latin origin and an *A.S.* would signal Anglo-Saxon origin.

Etymologies are your shortcut to learning more words with less effort. For example, if you have learned that the prefix *oto-* means *ear,* you will have little difficulty figuring out what *otocyst* means the first time you see that word.

In the A-Z section of the dictionary, building blocks like *peri-* and *-itis* are marked with this symbol: △. Hundreds of these building blocks are also listed in alphabetical order in an appendix, Medical Prefixes, Suffixes, and Combining Forms.

*The acronym* **TA,** *in brackets, follows the pronunciation of certain Latin words or terms, for example,* **acinus.** TA indicates that a term derives from the *Terminologia Anatomica,* a universal system of anatomical terminology in Latin.

---

## Parts of a Definition

| | | |
|---|---|---|
| building blocks | **rho·do-, rhod-** rosy, red color. [G. *rhodon,* rose] | pronunciation |
| headword | **rhy·thm** (ridh´ŭm) **1.** measured time or motion; the regular alteration of two or more different or opposite states. **2.** | multiple definitions, numbered |
| synonym | SYN rhythm method (1). **3.** regular occurrence of an electrical event in the electroencephalogram. SEE ALSO wave. | cross-reference to a related term |
| etymology | [G. *rhythmos*] | |
| synonym cross-reference to a specific definition | **Ri·vi·nus ca·nals** (ri-vē´nus) SEE major sublingual duct, minor sublingual ducts. | cross-reference |

*Note. Examples have been modified for demonstration purposes.*

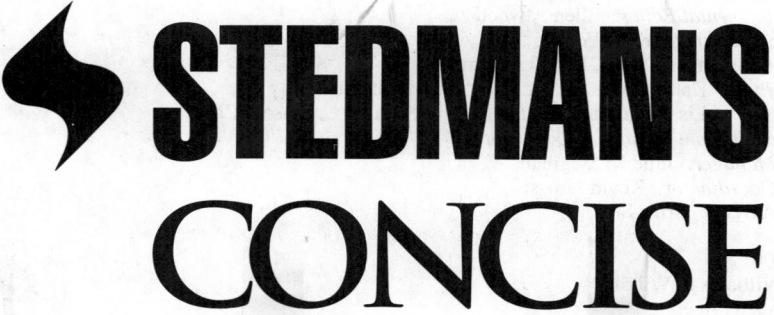

# STEDMAN'S CONCISE

## MEDICAL DICTIONARY
## FOR THE HEALTH
## PROFESSIONS

**ILLUSTRATED
4TH EDITION**

EDITOR

## John H. Dirckx, M.D.
Director, University of Dayton
Student Health Center
Dayton, Ohio

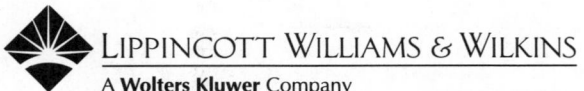

LIPPINCOTT WILLIAMS & WILKINS
A **Wolters Kluwer** Company

Philadelphia • Baltimore • New York • London
Buenos Aires • Hong Kong • Sydney • Tokyo

*Publisher*: Elizabeth Haigh
*Chief Editor & Lexicographer*: John H. Dirckx, M.D.
*Project Editor*: Beverly Wolpert
*Senior Managing Editor*: Vincent Ercolano
*Senior Developmental Editor*: Ellen Atwood
*Senior Online Editor*: Barbara Ferretti
*Art Direction*: Jonathan Dimes, Jennifer Clements
*Associate Editors*: Kathy Cadle, Kari Chairet, Trista DiPaula,
      Lisa Fahnestock, Will Howard, Kathryn C. Mason, CMT
*Software Development Manager*: Dave Horne
*Production Manager*: Julie K. Stegman
*Production Coordinator*: Kevin Iarossi
*Production Adviser*: Brian Smith

Copyright 2001
Lippincott Williams & Wilkins
351 W. Camden Street
Baltimore, MD 21201-2436 USA

Database design by Lexi-Comp, Inc., Hudson, OH
Printed in the United States of America by Quebecor World, Versailles, KY

First Edition 1987
Second Edition 1994
Third Edition 1997

**Library of Congress Cataloging-in-Publication Data**

Stedman's concise medical dictionary for the health professions : illustrated.—4th ed / editor, John H. Dirckx.
  p. ; cm.
 Includes bibliographical references and index.
 ISBN 0-7817-3012-0
 1. Medicine—Dictionaries. I. Title: Concise medical dictionary for the health professions.
II. Title: Medical dictionary for the health professions. III. Stedman, Thomas Lathrop,
1853–1938. IV. Dirckx, John H., 1938–
 [DNLM: 1. Medicine—Dictionary—English. W 13 S8125 2001]
R121 .S8 2001
610′.3—dc21               2001016460

# Contents

# A Message from the Publisher

F eaturing more than 48,000 entries and hundreds of illustrations, *Stedman's Concise Medical Dictionary for the Health Professions, Illustrated 4th Edition*, gives students, educators, and practitioners access to the core language of medicine and the health professions. A compact counterpart to the more general *Stedman's Medical Dictionary, Stedman's Concise* meets the quick-reference needs of students and practitioners throughout the health professions, with particular emphasis on athletic training and athletic therapy, audiology, clinical laboratory sciences, dental assisting, dental hygiene, emergency medical services, exercise science, health information management, massage therapy, medical assisting, medical terminology, nursing, nutrition, occupational therapy, pharmacy and pharmacy technology, physical therapy, radiography and radiologic technology, respiratory therapy, speech-language pathology, and veterinary medicine.

This new edition offers pronunciations for every defined term, plus new and revised images, tables, and appendices. It also features expanded international content, including for the first time British spellings and contributions from a total of nine Canadian consultants in nursing, nutrition, athletic therapy, medical transcription, and other medical specialties. Students, educators, and practitioners in nursing, massage therapy, emergency medical services, and the veterinary field will also find a new emphasis on the vocabulary of their respective professions. The dictionary's chief editor and lexicographer, John H. Dirckx, M.D., has also attached usage notes to many of the definitions. In these "microessays," Dr. Dirckx provides guidelines on the proper usage of commonly misused or misunderstood terms such as *prostate* and *septum*.

## Health Professions Consultants

To expand and refresh the content of *Stedman's Concise,* we nearly doubled the number of consultants, from 17 to 32, representing more than two dozen fields. Well regarded as both scholars and practitioners, these consultants evaluated the terms and definitions in the preceding edition, added new content, and made revisions.

In all, the consultants provided approximately 1,000 new terms and definitions. The new *Concise* was further enriched by the inclusion of more than 5,000 entries from *Stedman's Medical Dictionary, 27th Edition*.

## More Color—More Illustrations

This new edition offers more than 350 photographs, radiographs, and illustrations, most in full color. Our 32 consultants provided detailed guidance as we selected these images. The art program features images from two award-winning sources, medical illustrator Neil Hardy and A.D.A.M.®, the medical education software company. The A.D.A.M.® art is showcased in a quick-reference, 32-page anatomical atlas. This edition of the *Concise* also includes a full-color insert containing about 90 illustrations depicting imaging technologies and diagnostic techniques.

In the front pages of the book, the Illustrations Index gives the page number of every image in the *Concise*. In the A–Z section, an icon next to an entry—a white "i" in a blue square (■)—indicates that a term and its definition are illustrated, either at the entry itself or in the inserts or appendices.

## Expanded and Revised Appendices

Nearly three dozen appendices round out this new edition. These include lists, scales, tables, and more than 30 labeled images that provide fast access to information that students, educators, and practitioners need in the classroom, laboratory, and clinic. A table of contents appears on the first page of the appendix section.

## Acknowledgments

We at Lippincott Williams & Wilkins are grateful, first and foremost, to John H. Dirckx—physician and etymologist—for the erudition, experience, and irrepressible love of language he has brought to his service as chief editor and lexicographer of *Stedman's Concise Medical Dictionary for the Health Professions, Illustrated 4th Edition*. We extend special thanks to Elizabeth Haigh, our Publisher, for her vision, leadership, and sure instincts for the needs of *Concise* users, and to Vincent Ercolano, Senior Managing Editor, for the benefits of his experience with the third edition and his managerial expertise. Thanks to the collegiality and unflagging commitment to quality of Ellen Atwood, Senior Developmental Editor; Dave Horne, Software Development Manager; Barbara Ferretti, Senior Online Editor; Julie K. Stegman, Production Manager; Kevin Iarossi, Production Coordinator; and Brian Smith, Production Adviser, this fourth edition represents a new level of excellence and relevance for students, educators, and practitioners. Without the hard work and fine efforts of our associate editors, Kathy Cadle, Kari Chairet, Trista DiPaula, Lisa Fahnestock, Will Howard, and Kathryn Mason, CMT, this dictionary would not have been possible. Likewise, the art program would not have been possible without the discerning, conscientious art direction provided by Jennifer Clements and Jonathan Dimes.

We thank our consultants in the medical specialties for writing and revising the thousands of entries in this and other Stedman's dictionaries. We are grateful, as well, to our health professions consultants, who reviewed, revised, and contributed new content to *Stedman's Concise*.

Finally, we warmly and respectfully honor the memory of the late Barbara Werner, who was Chief Copyeditor of this edition of *Stedman's Concise* in its early stages. In recent years, there has hardly been a Stedman's publication that has not been graced—and strengthened—by her intellectual sophistication, rigorous approach to her profession, and professional and personal fellowship.

## Your Medical Word Resource Publisher

We strive to provide students, practitioners, and educators with the most up-to-date and accurate medical language references. We welcome your suggestions for improvements, changes, corrections, and additions—whatever makes it possible for this Stedman's product to serve you better.

Beverly Wolpert
Project Editor
*Stedman's Concise Medical Dictionary*
*for the Health Professions, Illustrated 4th Edition*
Lippincott Williams & Wilkins
Baltimore, Maryland

# Editor's Preface

When this book left the bindery, it was the latest addition to a family of medical dictionaries that can trace its lineage further back than any other in any language.

The first edition of Dunglison's *New Dictionary of Medical Science and Literature* appeared in 1833, just five years after the first edition of Noah Webster's *American Dictionary of the English Language*. Robley Dunglison, M.D. (1789–1869), a native of England, was professor of medicine at the University of Virginia and served as personal physician to presidents Jefferson, Madison, Monroe, and Jackson.

Dunglison's medical dictionary passed through 19 editions during his lifetime, after which his son, Richard J. Dunglison, assumed the editorship. The last edition of the dictionary to bear the Dunglison name, the 23rd, was edited in 1903 by Thomas Lathrop Stedman (1853–1938). Dr. Stedman then made a thorough revision of the work, and the first edition of *Stedman's Medical Dictionary* was published in 1911. Since then, new editions of *Stedman's* have been issued at intervals of two to eight years, the 27th having appeared in 2000.

Meanwhile, auxiliary versions have broadened the audience and enhanced the accessibility of the work. During the 1980s, *Stedman's* became the first American medical dictionary to practice database publishing, with electronic storage, retrieval, updating, and composition. In 1994, as a by-product of this technology, the 24th edition was made available in electronic form, and since then the *Stedman's* database has generated a long series of word books and electronic versions on disk and CD.

The first edition of *Stedman's Concise Medical Dictionary,* designed specially for students and practitioners in the allied health professions, appeared in 1987 as *Stedman's Pocket Medical Dictionary*. Although derived from the same database as the full-scale dictionary, *Stedman's Concise* contains supplemental material provided by a panel of consultants in a variety of health professions. For this fourth edition, *Stedman's* has assembled the largest group of consultants ever, including representatives of four previously unincluded disciplines: emergency medical services, massage therapy, medical transcription, and nursing.

## Some Departures from Traditional Practice

Even the most lucid dictionary entry is useless to readers if they cannot find it. And that is exactly what can happen if you are looking for the *Babinski reflex* in a work that lists it as *test, Babinski,* or if you are in search of *Kimmelstiel-Wilson disease* in a dictionary that calls it *syndrome, Kimmelstiel-Wilson.*

This newest edition of *Stedman's Concise Medical Dictionary* makes a bold departure from traditional practice by forsaking this sometimes confusing entry-subentry format. That means that each term consisting of a phrase instead of a single word, such as *colloid goiter, eosinophilic pneumonia,* and *persistent chronic hepatitis,* has been entered alphabetically according to the first word in that phrase.

Also new to this edition are a number of terms pertaining to alternative and complementary medicine. While their inclusion does not imply an endorsement of these concepts or methods, it does constitute recognition that they have become a part of modern practice and that terms referring to them now appear in clinical reports and medical literature.

This volume, like the 27th edition of *Stedman's Medical Dictionary,* incorporates *Terminologia Anatomica* (TA), the latest revision of international anatomic nomenclature, promulgated in 1997 to replace *Nomina Anatomica* (NA). Important as it is to make the most recent version of such terminology accessible to readers, however, one must recognize that older terms will continue to be used for decades to come. Hence, for example, we have retained the time-honored phrase *gray matter* as well as the far less familiar alternative *gray substance,* recommended by the compilers of TA as an English equivalent of *substantia grisea.*

## Consistency: A Safeguard Against Ambiguity

In 1841, Ralph Waldo Emerson wrote: "A foolish consistency is the hobgoblin of little minds." That cavalier remark has often been quoted in a reproachful tone against editors and lexicographers who strive for maximum uniformity and standardization of language.

But before judging too harshly of this zeal for conformity, one ought to remember that eliminating senseless and confusing diversity of language is one of the principal functions of a dictionary. The sheer bulk of medical material published each day, the increasing reliance on electronic ways of handling it, and the challenge of making it accessible by means of key words all demand safeguards against ambiguity.

As an example of our heightened efforts to eliminate divergence of form that does not parallel divergence of sense, the term *disk* is spelled throughout *Stedman's Concise* with *k,* whether it refers to a germinal, intercalated, intervertebral, or optic disk. Neither etymologic considerations nor modern usage can justify keeping the alternative spelling *disc* in service, much less distinguishing it semantically from the term spelled *disk.*

Another kind of standardization, initiated in the 27th edition of *Stedman's Medical Dictionary* in response to a widespread trend among physicians and medical editors, is an across-the-board elimination of the possessive form with *'s* in eponyms such as *Alzheimer disease* and *Ewing sarcoma.* Besides doing away with inconsistencies, this step simplifies typography and reduces confusion over the spelling of names that end in *s,* such as *Graves, Homans,* and *Langerhans.* It should also appease those who object that, since Addison neither invented nor suffered from the disease he described, it isn't proper to call it *Addison's* disease.

## Thanks and Acknowledgments

I am deeply grateful to all our consultants for their contributions not only to the content of this dictionary but to its overall tone and quality. Indeed, the term *consultant* scarcely does justice to the breadth and value of their work. It is my pleasure to acknowledge the smooth guidance of Beverly Wolpert, the multifarious managerial skills of Vincent Ercolano, and the patient and meticulous editing of Ellen Atwood and Barbara Ferretti.

Lastly, a word of tribute and solemn farewell to Barbara Werner, whose creative editorial labors during recent years have left their mark on all the Stedman's publications, and whose sudden death in 2000 interrupted her work on this dictionary.

*John H. Dirckx, M.D., has been director of the Student Health Center at the University of Dayton (Ohio) since 1968. His lifelong interest in and study of language have given rise to several books and numerous articles related to medical terminology. He has served as a Stedman's consultant since 1994, and edited the previous (third) edition of* Stedman's Concise Medical Dictionary for the Health Professions (*1997*).

# Consultants in the Health Professions

**Lynn Bookalam, MSc, CAT(C)**
Sports Medicine Clinic Coordinator/Head Therapist, Athletics Department,
Lecturer, Department of Physical Education, McGill University, Montreal, QC,
Canada

**Athletic Therapy,
British English Medical
Terminology**

**Malissa Martin, EdD, ATC, CSCS**
Associate Professor, Athletic Training Education Program Director, Department
of Health, Physical Education, Recreation and Safety, Middle Tennessee State
University, Murfreesboro, TN, USA

**Athletic Training**

**Nicholas M. Hipskind, PhD, CCC-A**
Associate Professor of Audiology, Department of Speech and Hearing Sciences,
Associate Dean, University Division, Indiana University, Bloomington, IN, USA

**Audiology**

**Réal J. Gaboriault, PhD**
Research Director, Canadian Touch Research Centre; Director, Kiné-Concept
Institute, Montreal, QC, Canada

**Biotechnology, British
English Medical
Terminology**

**Ljubisa Terzic, MD, FYAN**
Professor of Anatomy and Dean, Canadian College of Massage and
Hydrotherapy, Toronto, ON, Canada

**Cardiology, British
English Medical
Terminology**

**Susan Cockayne, PhD, CLS(NCA)**
Associate Professor, Department of Microbiology, Brigham Young University,
Provo, UT, USA

**Clinical Laboratory
Sciences, Bacteriology,
Mycology**

**Dorothea M. Cavallucci, MS, CDA, EFDA, RDH**
Assistant Dean of Academic Affairs, Program Director of Dental Assisting,
Associate Professor of Dental Assisting and Dental Hygiene, Harcum College,
Bryn Mawr, PA, USA

**Dental Assisting**

**Robin Sylvis, RDH, MS**
Associate Professor and Clinic Director, Dental Hygiene Program, Chairperson,
Science Department, Harcum College, Bryn Mawr, PA, USA

**Dental Hygiene**

**John T. Mayhall, DDS, PhD**
Professor and Head, Oral Anatomy, Faculty of Dentistry, University of Toronto,
Toronto, ON, Canada

**Dentistry, British
English Medical
Terminology**

**Keith L. Moore, PhD, FRSM, FIAC**
Professor of Anatomy and Cell Biology, Faculty of Medicine, University of
Toronto, Toronto, ON, Canada; Member, Federative Committee on Anatomical
Terminology, International Federation of Associations of Anatomists

**Embryology, British
English Medical
Terminology**

**Bruce J. Walz, PhD, NREMT-P**
Associate Professor and Chair, Department of Emergency Health Services,
University of Maryland Baltimore County, Baltimore, MD, USA

**Emergency Medical
Services**

**John H. McDonald, PhD**
Associate Professor, Department of Biological Sciences, University of
Delaware, Newark, DE, USA

**Evolutionary Genetics
Molecular Evolution**

**William D. McArdle, PhD**
Emeritus Professor, Department of Family, Nutrition, and Exercise Sciences,
Queens College, Flushing, NY, USA

**Exercise Science**

**Sara J. Wellman, AS, RHIT**
Associate Faculty, Department of Health Information Management, Indiana
University Northwest, Gary, IN, USA

**Health Information
Management**

**Ruth Werner, LMT, NCTMB**
Faculty, Myotherapy College of Utah, Salt Lake City, UT, USA, and Ogden
Institute of Massage Therapy, Ogden, UT, USA

**Massage Therapy**

**Julie Hosley, RN, CMA**
Program Director, Medical Assisting, Carteret Community College, Morehead
City, NC, USA

**Medical Assisting**

**Marjorie Canfield Willis, CMA-AC**
Professor of Allied Health, Director, Medical Assisting Program, Director,
Medical Transcription Program, School of Allied Health Professions, Orange
Coast College, Costa Mesa, CA, USA

**Medical Terminology**

**Kim Koppin**
Program Development Officer, School of Continuing Education, Loyalist
College, Belleville, ON, Canada

**Medical Transcription,
British English Medical
Terminology**

**Pamela S. Harrmann, RN, BS, CCRN**
Intensive Care Nurse, Des Moines, IA, USA

**Nursing**

**Joanne Profetto-McGrath, RN, BScN, BA, MEd, PhD**
Assistant Professor, Faculty of Nursing, University of Alberta, Edmonton,
AB, Canada

**Nursing, British English
Medical Terminology**

**Wanda H. Howell, PhD, RD, CNSD**
Associate Professor and Director, Didactic Program in Dietetics, Department
of Nutritional Sciences, University of Arizona, Tucson, AZ, USA

**Nutrition**

**Susan Crawford, PhD, RD**
Research Associate and Adjunct Professor, Gerontology Research Centre,
Simon Fraser University, Vancouver, BC, Canada

**Nutrition, British English
Medical Terminology**

**Reba L. Anderson, PhD, OTR, FAOTA**                Occupational Therapy
Professor Emeritus, Nova Southeastern University, Ft. Lauderdale, FL, USA

**Jennie Q. Lou, MD, MSc, OTR**                Occupational Therapy
Assistant Professor of Occupational Therapy, Associate Professor of Public
Health, College of Allied Health, Health Professions Division, Nova
Southeastern University, Ft. Lauderdale, FL, USA

**W. Steven Pray, RPh, PhD**                Pharmacy and Pharmacy Technology
Professor of Nonprescription Products and Devices, School of Pharmacy,
Southwestern Oklahoma State University, Weatherford, OK, USA

**Susan Sullivan Glenney, MS, PT**                Physical Therapy
Assistant Professor of Physical Therapy, University of Hartford, West Hartford,
CT, USA

**Rose Sgarlat Myers, PT, PhD**                Physical Therapy
Consultant, Physical Therapy Education, Myers Associates, Earlysville, VA,
USA

**Gail E. Orr, RN, BA**                Psychology, British English Medical Terminology
Program Development Officer, Professor of Health and Social Sciences,
School of Continuing Education, Loyalist College, Belleville, ON, Canada

**Michael E. Madden, PhD, RT(R)(CT)(MR)(ARRT)**                Radiography and Radiologic Technology
Director, Medical Diagnostic Imaging Programs, Fort Hays State University,
Hays, KS, USA

**Robert L. Chatburn, RRT, FAARC**                Respiratory Therapy
Associate Professor, Department of Pediatrics, Case Western Reserve
University, Cleveland, OH, USA; Director, Respiratory Care Department,
University Hospitals of Cleveland, Cleveland, OH, USA

**Amy B. Wohlert, PhD, CCC-SLP**                Speech-Language Pathology
Professor and Chair, Department of Speech and Hearing Sciences, University of
New Mexico, Albuquerque, NM, USA

**Linda L. Merrill, RVT**                Veterinary Medicine
Senior Veterinary Technician, Seattle Veterinary Associates, Seattle, WA, USA

# Consultants to the Stedman's Dictionaries

**Edward D. Miller, MD**                                    Anesthesiology

The Frances Watt Baker, MD, and Lenox D. Baker, Jr., MD, Dean of the
Medical Faculty, Chief Executive Officer, Johns Hopkins Medicine, Johns
Hopkins School of Medicine, Baltimore, MD, USA

**Patricia Charache, MD**                                  Bacteriology

Professor of Pathology, Medicine, and Oncology, Departments of Pathology
and Medicine, Johns Hopkins Medical Institutions, Baltimore, MD, USA

**R. Donald Allison, PhD**                                 Biochemistry

Associate Scientist, Department of Biochemistry and Molecular Biology,
University of Florida College of Medicine, Gainesville, FL, USA

**Douglas R. Bacon, MD, MA**                               Biography and Eponyms

Associate Professor and Vice Chairman for Education, Department of
Anesthesiology, State University of New York at Buffalo; Chief of
Anesthesiology Service, Buffalo VA Medical Center, Buffalo, NY, USA

**Sheldon M. Schuster, PhD**                               Biotechnology

Professor, Biochemistry and Molecular Biology, Program Director,
Biotechnology Program, University of Florida, Gainesville, FL, USA

**David H. Spodick, MD, DSc**                              Cardiology

Professor of Medicine, University of Massachusetts Medical School,
Worcester, MA, USA; Lecturer in Medicine, Tufts University School of
Medicine; Lecturer in Medicine, Boston University School of Medicine,
Boston, MA, USA; Director of Clinical Cardiology and Director of
Cardiovascular Fellowship Training, St. Vincent Hospital, Worcester, MA, USA

**George S. Schuster, DDS, MS, PhD**                        Dentistry

Ione and Arthur Merritt Professor, Chairman, Department of Oral Biology and
Maxillofacial Pathology, Medical College of Georgia, School of Dentistry,
Augusta, GA, USA

**Colin Wood, MD**                                         Dermatology

Professor Emeritus of Pathology, University of Maryland School of Medicine,
Baltimore, MD, USA

**Kathleen K. Sulik, PhD**                                 Embryology

Professor, Department of Cell Biology and Anatomy, University of North
Carolina, Chapel Hill, NC, USA

**Philip M. Buttaravoli, MD, FACEP**                       Emergency Medicine

Medical Director, Emergency Department, Palm Beach Gardens Medical
Center, Palm Beach Gardens, FL, USA

**John H. Dirckx, MD**
Director, University of Dayton Health Center, Dayton, OH, USA

**Etymologies and High-Profile Terms**

**J. Patrick O'Leary, MD**
The Isidore Cohn, Jr., Professor and Chairman of Surgery, Louisiana State University Medical School, New Orleans, LA, USA

**General Surgery**

**Clair A. Francomano, MD**
Clinical Director, National Human Genome Research Institute, National Institutes of Health, Bethesda, MD, USA

**Genetics**

**Arthur F. Dalley II, PhD**
Professor of Cell Biology, Director of Gross Anatomy, Department of Cell Biology, Vanderbilt University School of Medicine, Nashville, TN, USA; President, American Association of Clinical Anatomists

**Gross Anatomy**

**David N. Menton, PhD**
Associate Professor of Anatomy, Washington University School of Medicine, St. Louis, MO, USA

**Histology**

**Stanley S. Lefkowitz, PhD**
Professor, Department of Microbiology and Immunology, Texas Tech University Health Sciences Center, Lubbock, TX, USA

**Immunology and Virology**

**Alfred Jay Bollet, MD**
Clinical Professor of Medicine, Yale University School of Medicine, New Haven, CT, USA

**Internal Medicine**

**John M. Last, MD, FRACP, FRCPC**
Professor Emeritus, Department of Epidemiology and Community Medicine, University of Ottawa, Ottawa, ON, Canada

**Medical Statistics and Epidemiology**

**John Bennett, MD**
Head, Clinical Mycology Section, Laboratory of Clinical Investigation, National Institute of Allergy and Infectious Diseases, Bethesda, MD, USA

**Mycology**

**Duane E. Haines, PhD**
Professor of Anatomy, Chairman, Department of Anatomy, University of Mississippi Medical Center, Jackson, MS, USA

**Neuroanatomy**

**Asa J. Wilbourn, MD**
Director, EMG Laboratory, Cleveland Clinic Foundation; Clinical Professor of Neurology, Case Western Reserve University School of Medicine, Cleveland, OH, USA

**Neurology**

**Richard Prayson, MD**
Department of Anatomic Pathology, Cleveland Clinic Foundation, Cleveland, OH, USA

**Neuropathology**

**Iain Kalfas, MD**                                            **Neurosurgery**
Department of Neurosurgery, Cleveland Clinic Foundation, Cleveland, OH, USA

**Thomas W. Filardo, MD**                                      **New Terms Editor**
Physician-Consultant, Evendale, OH, USA

**Martin L. Nusynowitz, MD**                                   **Nuclear Medicine**
Professor, Radiology, Internal Medicine, and Pathology, University of Texas
Medical Branch at Galveston, Galveston, TX, USA

**Sharon T. Phelan, MD**                                       **Obstetrics and**
Associate Professor, Department of Obstetrics and Gynecology, University of      **Gynecology**
Alabama at Birmingham, Birmingham, AL, USA

**Barbara A. Conley, MD**                                      **Oncology**
Senior Investigator, Clinical Investigations Branch, Cancer Therapy Evaluation
Program, National Cancer Institute, Rockville, MD, USA

**John B. Kerrison, MD**                                       **Ophthalmology**
Assistant Chief of Service, Wilmer Eye Institute, Johns Hopkins Hospital,
Baltimore, MD, USA

**Joseph D. Zuckerman, MD**                                    **Orthopedics**
Walter A. L. Thompson Professor of Orthopaedic Surgery, New York University
School of Medicine; Chairman, NYU-Hospital for Joint Diseases, Department of
Orthopaedic Surgery, New York, NY, USA

**James B. Snow, Jr., MD, FACS**                               **Otorhinolaryngology**
Former Director, National Institute on Deafness and Other Communication
Disorders, National Institutes of Health, Bethesda, MD; Professor Emeritus of
Otorhinolaryngology, University of Pennsylvania School of Medicine,
Philadelphia, PA, USA

**David G. Bostwick, MD**                                      **Pathology**
Consultant and Professor of Pathology and Urology, Mayo Clinic and Mayo
Medical School, Rochester, MN, USA

**Steven I. Gutman, MD, MBA**                                  **Pathology, Hematology,**
Director, Division of Clinical Laboratory Devices, Division of Clinical          **and Laboratory**
Laboratory Devices, U.S. Food and Drug Administration, Rockville, MD, USA        **Medicine/Stains and**
                                                               **Procedures**

**David E. Hall, MD**                                          **Pediatrics**
Clinical Associate Professor of Pediatrics, Emory University School of Medicine,
Scottish Rite Children's Medical Center, Atlanta, GA, USA

**Arthur Raines, PhD**
Professor Emeritus of Pharmacology and Neurology, Department of
Pharmacology, Georgetown University Medical Center, Washington, DC, USA

**Pharmacology and Toxicology**

**David B. Young, PhD**
Professor, Physiology and Biophysics, University of Mississippi Medical Center,
Jackson, MS, USA

**Physiology**

**John B. Mulliken, MD**
Associate Professor of Surgery, Harvard Medical School; Director Craniofacial
Centre, Children's Hospital, Boston, MA, USA

**Plastic and Reconstructive Surgery**

**Douglas D. Woodruff, MD**
Private Practice, Baltimore, MD, USA

**Psychiatry/Psychology**

**John A. Day, Jr., MD, FCCP**
Attending Physician, Division of Pulmonary and Critical Care, St. Vincent
Hospital and University of Massachusetts Memorial Health Care; Assistant
Professor of Medicine, University of Massachusetts Medical School, Worcester,
MA, USA

**Pulmonary Diseases**

**Paul J. Friedman, MD**
Professor of Radiology and Chief of Thoracic Radiology, School of Medicine,
University of California, San Diego, CA, USA

**Radiology**

**Ronald B. Ponn, MD**
Assistant Clinical Professor and Associate Section Chief of Cardiothoracic
Surgery, Yale University School of Medicine and Yale-New Haven Hospital,
New Haven, CT, USA

**Thoracic Surgery**

**Lynne S. Garcia, MS, MT(ASCP), CLS(NCA), F(AAM)**
Department of Pathology and Laboratory Medicine, UCLA Medical Center,
Los Angeles, CA, USA

**Tropical Medicine/ Parasitology**

**David A. Bloom, MD**
Chief, Pediatric Urology, Professor of Surgery, University of Michigan and
Mott Children's Hospital, Ann Arbor, MI, USA

**Urology and Urologic Surgery**

**Michael J. Burridge, BVM&S, MPVM, PhD**
Professor, Department of Pathobiology, College of Veterinary Medicine,
University of Florida, Gainesville, FL, USA

**Veterinary Medicine**

# Illustrations Index

The Illustrations Index provides a quick way to find any image in *Stedman's Concise*. The page number accompanying each term listed below tells you where to find an illustration of that term. A page number preceded by the letter *A* indicates that the image can be found in the first color insert, the 32-page anatomical atlas. A page number preceded by the letter *B* indicates that the image can be found in the second color insert, a 16-page section dedicated to diagnostic medicine and imaging techniques. A page number preceded by *APP* indicates that the image appears in the appendices. When you look up a word in the A-Z section, you can tell if it is illustrated—either at the word itself or in the inserts or appendices—if it is accompanied by this symbol: 🖻 .

# Illustration Sources

Courtesy of Acuson Corporation, Mountain View, CA (Doppler ultrasonography, echocardiogram, echocardiography).

Courtesy of Advanced Technology Laboratory, Bothell, WA (sonography).

From Aehlert, B. *Aehlert's EMT Basic Study Guide*. Baltimore: Lippincott Williams & Wilkins, 1998 (burns).

Courtesy of American Academy of Dermatology, Schaumburg, IL ( bulla, cherry angioma, crust, erosion, fissure, keloid, macule, nodule, papule, patch, plaque, pustule, scale, telangiectasia, tumor, ulcer, vesicle, wheal).

Courtesy of American Cancer Society, Inc., Atlanta, GA (malignant melanoma).

Courtesy of *American Journal of Human Genetics,* 56:746–747, 1995 (symbols).

Courtesy of Baschat A, MD, Center for Advanced Fetal Care, University of Maryland School of Medicine, Baltimore, MD (Doppler flow sonogram).

Courtesy of Bennett, J, PhD, National Institutes of Health, Bethesda, MD (brain).

From Bickley LS, Hoecklelman RA. *Bates' Guide to Physical Examination and History Taking* (7th ed). Baltimore: Lippincott Williams & Wilkins, 1999 (vitiligo).

From Boyd, SH. *Boyd's Introduction to the Study of Disease* (11th ed.). Philadelphia: Lea & Febiger, 1992 (lobar pneumonia).

From Brant WE, Helms CA. *Fundamentals of Diagnostic Radiology* (2nd ed.). Baltimore: Lippincott Williams & Wilkins, 1999 (carpal tunnel syndrome, classic breast carcinoma, CT scan, intestinal obstruction, mammography, normal radiograph, right-sided pneumothorax, upper gastrointestinal series).

Courtesy of Burdick Corporation, Milton, WI (electrocardiography).

Courtesy of Cavallucci D, BS, CDA, EFDA, RDH, Harcum College, Bryn Mawr, PA (film—bitewing, occlusal, periapical).

Courtesy of Chatburn RL, RRT, FAARC (mechanical ventilation algorithms).

From Cormack DH, PhD. *Essential Histology*. Philadelphia: Lippincott-Raven, 1997 (microtubules).

Adapted from Crawford JD, Terry ME, Rourke GM. *Pediatrics* 5: 785, fig. 1, 1950 (West body surface nomogram-young child/infant).

From Daffner RH. *Clinical Radiology: The Essentials* (2nd ed.). Baltimore: Lippincott Williams & Wilkins, 1998 (cholelithiasis, gout, herniated nucleus pulposus, multiple sclerosis, rheumatoid arthritis, spondylosis).

Courtesy of Day JA, MD, University of Massachusetts Medical School, Worcester, MA (adult respiratory distress syndrome, interstitial lung disease).

From DuBois EF. *Basal Metabolism in Health and Disease*. Philadelphia: Lea & Febiger, 1936. Copyright 1920 by WM Boothby & RB Sandiford (DuBois body surface nomogram—adult/child).

From Eisenberg RL, Dennis CA, May CR. *Radiographic Positioning* (2nd ed.). Boston: Little, Brown, 1995 (abduction vs. adduction, anatomic planes, body part terminology, eversion vs. inversion, flexion vs. extension, radiographic positions, radiographic projections, supination vs. pronation).

Adapted from Erhardt R. *Developmental Hand Dysfunction* (2nd ed.). San Antonio, TX: Therapy Skill Builders, 1994 (pinch and grasp development).

From Eroschenko VP. *Di Fiore's Atlas of Histology with Functional Correlations* (8th ed.). Baltimore: Lippincott Williams & Wilkins, 1996 (lung).

From Feinsilver SH, Fein A. *A Textbook on Bronchoscopy*. Baltimore: Lippincott Williams & Wilkins, 1995 (amyloidosis, bronchus, carcinoma, carina, granuloma, metastasis of melanoma, trachea, vocal fold).

From Gartner LP, Hiatt JL. *Color Atlas of Histology* (3rd ed.). Baltimore: Lippincott Williams & Wilkins, 1999 (basophil, eosinophil, monocyte, neutrophil).

Courtesy of General Electric Medical Systems, Milwaukee, WI (gamma camera, magnetic resonance imaging, positron emission tomography).

From Goodheart HP, MD. *A Photo Guide of Common Skin Disorders: Diagnosis and Management*. Baltimore: Lippincott Williams & Wilkins, 1999 (acanthosis nigricans, cyst, dermatomyositis, ecchymoses, excoriation, lichenification, morpheaform basal cell carcinoma, neurofibroma, nodular basal cell carcinoma, scabies, ulcerated basal cell carcinoma).

Courtesy of Hawke M, MD, Toronto, Canada (cholesteatoma, otitis externa, otitis media, tympanic membrane, tympanosclerosis).

From Henretig FM, MD, King C, MD. *Textbook of Pediatric Emergency Procedures*. Baltimore: Lippincott Williams & Wilkins, 1997 (dislocation—radiograph).

Adapted from Hipskind N, PhD, Indiana University, Bloomington, IN (pure tone audiogram).

Courtesy of Hoag Memorial Presbyterian Hospital, Newport Beach, CA (bone scan).

Adapted from *Journal of Parenteral and Enteral Nutrition,* 17(4): 1SA-52SA, July-Aug. 1993 (clinical decision algorithm: route of nutrition support).

Adapted from Klein MD, Ossman NH, Tracy B. *Normal Development Copybook*. San Antonio, TX: Therapy Skill Builders, 1991 (developmental milestones).

From Koneman EW, Allen SD, Janda WM, Schreckenberger PC, Winn WC, Jr. *Color Atlas and Textbook of Diagnostic Microbiology* (5th ed.). Philadelphia: Lippincott Williams & Wilkins, 1997 (*Ascaris lumbricoides, Enterobius, Plasmodium malariae*).

From Langlais RP, Miller CS. *Color Atlas of Common Oral Diseases* (2nd ed.). Baltimore: Lippincott Williams & Wilkins, 1998 (herpes simplex).

From Langland OE, Langlais RP. *Principles of Dental Imaging*. Baltimore: Lippincott Williams & Wilkins, 1997 (apical granuloma, apical periodontal cyst).

Courtesy of Laurence J, Underwood R, Mission Viejo, CA (syphilis).

Adapted from Martin FN. *Introduction to Audiology* (5th ed.). Englewood Cliffs, NJ: Prentice Hall, 1994 (tympanogram).

From McArdle WD, Katch FI, Katch VL. *Essentials of Exercise Physiology*. Baltimore: Lippincott Williams & Wilkins, 1994 (intravenous urography).

From McClatchey KD. *Clinical Laboratory Medicine*. Baltimore: Lippincott Williams & Wilkins, 1994 (gonococci, Heinz-Ehrlich bodies).

From McKenzie SB, Clare N, Burns C, Larson L, Metz J. *Textbook of Hematology* (2nd ed.). Baltimore: Lippincott Williams & Wilkins, 1996 (anisocytosis, hemolytic anemia, macrocytosis, microcytosis, microtic anemia, Philadelphia chromosome, poikilocytosis, rouleaux, sickle cell anemia, thalassemia).

From MediClip, Clinical Cardiopulmonary. Baltimore: Lippincott Williams & Wilkins, 1997 (ECG-lead placement).

From Ming SC, Goldman H. *Pathology of the Gastrointestinal Tract* (2nd ed.). Baltimore: Lippincott Williams & Wilkins, 1998 (benign tumor of the stomach, ulcerative squamous cell carcinoma).

Courtesy of Minister of Public Works & Government Services Canada (Canada's Food Guide to Healthy Eating—nutrition rainbow).

Courtesy of Mission Hospital Regional Medical Center, Mission Viejo, CA (colon polypectomy, esophageal varices, sonogram).

From Neville BW, Damm DD, White DK. *Color Atlas of Clinical Oral Pathology* (2nd ed.). Baltimore: Lippincott Williams & Wilkins, 1998 (candidiasis, leukoplakia).

Courtesy of Newport Diagnostic Center, Newport Beach, CA (brain with Alzheimer disease vs. normal brain).

Courtesy of Olympus America, Inc., Melville, NY (colonoscope).

Courtesy of Orange Coast College, Costa Mesa, CA (barium enema, echocardiogram).

Courtesy of Phillips Medical Systems, Shelton, CT (computed tomography—apparatus).

From Pray WS. *Nonprescription Product Therapeutics*. Baltimore: Lippincott Williams & Wilkins, 1999 (female pattern alopecia, male pattern alopecia).

From Rassner G, trans. Burgdorf WHC. *Atlas of Dermatology* (3rd ed.). Philadelphia: Lea & Febiger, 1994 (actinic keratoses, angiosarcoma, basal cell carcinoma, Bowen disease, cavernous hemangioma, condyloma acuminatum, dermatitis herpetiformis, impetigo, lentigo maligna, lupus erythematosus, nodular basal cell carcinoma, paronychia, Peutz-Jeghers syndrome, purpura fulminans, pyogenic granuloma, scleroderma, seborrheic keratoses, superficial basal cell carcinoma, varicosis).

From *Roche Lexikon Medizin* (3rd ed.). Munich, Germany: Urban & Schwarzenberg, 1993 (angioneurotic edema, arteriography, blood cells, bronchiogenic carcinoma, cataract, cerebral hemorrhage, coloboma, diabetic retinopathy, diverticulosis, elephantiasis, erythrocytes, heart, herpes zoster, hyphema, keratoacanthoma, laryngeal carcinoma, lymphocyte, mastoiditis, mycosis fungoides, oligodendrocyte, Paget disease, papilledema, pernicious anemia, placenta, retinal tear, rosacea, splenomegaly, staphylococci, streptococci, sympathetic trunk, tinea pedis, ulcerative colitis, yeast).

From Rosdahl DB. *Textbook of Basic Nursing* (7th ed.). Philadelphia: Lippincott Williams & Wilkins, 1999 (auscultation, ulcer).

From Sanders CV, Nesbitt LT, Jr. *The Skin and Infection: A Color Atlas and Text*. Baltimore: Lippincott Williams & Wilkins, 1995 (AIDS, genital herpes, Kaposi sarcoma, lepromatous leprosy, Lyme disease, *Pthirus pubis*, tinea corporis, toxic epidermal necrolysis, varicella).

Courtesy of Scheie Eye Institute, Philadelphia, PA (fundus of eye, retinal detachment).

Courtesy of Skin Cancer Foundation, New York, NY (basal cell carcinoma, squamous cell carcinoma).

From Sun T. *Parasitic Disorders: Pathology, Diagnosis, and Management* (2nd ed.). Baltimore: Lippincott Williams & Wilkins, 1998 (*Entamoeba histolytica*).

Courtesy of U.S. Department of Agriculture, U.S. Department of Health & Human Services (Food Guide Pyramid).

Adapted from U.S. Department of Agriculture, U.S. Department of Health & Human Services, *Nutrition and Your Health: Dietary Guidelines for Americans* (5th ed.), 2000 (body mass index).

Courtesy of Wang F, MD, Orange, CA (ventilation-perfusion scan).

Courtesy of Welch Allyn, Inc., Skaneateles Falls, NY (exostosis, foreign body, glaucomatous, ophthalmoscope, ophthalmoscopy, otomycosis, otoscope, otoscopy, perforation).

From Willis MC. *Medical Terminology: The Language of Health Care*. Baltimore: Lippincott Williams & Wilkins, 1996 (lesions, rhythm).

From Yochum TR, Rowe LJ. *Essentials of Skeletal Radiology* (2nd ed.). Baltimore: Lippincott Williams & Wilkins, 1996 (cephalometric film, exostosis, myositis ossificans).

# Artwork Credits

Artwork in this edition of *Stedman's Concise Medical Dictionary for the Health Professions, Illustrated 4th Edition,* was created or adapted by the following individuals (see Illustration Sources for sources of adaptations):

All artwork in the anatomy insert, **imagery© 1999 adam.com**™. All rights reserved.

**Mary Anna Barratt-Dimes,** Parkton, MD: pure tone audiogram, route of nutrition support, tympanogram.

**Kimberly M. Battista,** Baltimore, MD: burns.

**Susan Caldwell,** Pikesville, MD: Apgar score.

**Duckwall Productions,** Baltimore, MD: osteoarthritis.

**Neil O. Hardy,** Westport, CT: abdominal regions, alveolar abscess, amniocentesis, aneurysm, antibody, arteriole, artery, asthma, atrioventricular valve, auditory ossicles, bacteria, Bárány caloric test, biopsy, bone, brain, bronchus, bronchoscopy, capillary, caries, cerebral cortex, closed chest massage, clubbing, cochlea, colonoscope, colostomy, coronary artery, cranial nerves, deciduous dentition, decubitus ulcer, dental implant, dermatomes, DNA, ear, electrocardiography, electroencephalography, embolism, enterostomy, epidural hematoma, epithelium, eye, facial nerves, Foley catheter, fracture, glaucoma, gustation, Heimlich maneuver, human immunodeficiency virus, hyperopia, hyphema, ileostomy, incisions, inguinal hernia, injection, innervation of the hand and wrist, intervertebral disc herniation, intestine, islet of Langerhans, joints, kidney, larynx, LeFort fracture, lung, magnetic resonance imaging, meniscal tears, metered-dose inhaler, mitochondrion, mouth, muscle fiber, myopia, nephrolithiasis, neuroglia, neuron, nutrient absorption, nystagmus, obesity, olfaction, orbit, otitis externa, otitis media, pancreas, percutaneous transluminal angioplasty, percussion, peripheral pulse, permanent dentition, polyp, postural drainage, pulmonary circulation, quadrants, respiration, retina, scoliosis, sonography, spinal curvatures, spirometry, splenomegaly, spondylolisthesis, swallowing, talipes cavus and t. planus, temporomandibular joint, tooth, total parenteral nutrition, *Toxicodendron,* tracheostomy, varicosis, vascular stent, venous valves, ventricles, vision, wound.

**Tim Hengst,** Thousand Oaks, CA: pelvic spaces.

**Mark Miller,** Liberty, MO: ECG-lead placements.

**Siri Mills,** Munich, Germany: heart, sympathetic trunk.

**Michael Schenk,** Jackson MS: bomb calorimeter, developmental milestones, finger, hiatal hernia, human calorimeter, mastication, pinch and grasp development, rigidity, skinfold measurement.

**Mikki Senkarik,** San Antonio, TX: abduction vs. adduction, anatomic planes, body part terminology, colonoscopy, esophagoduodenoscopy, eversion vs. inversion, flexion vs. extension, radiographic positions, radiographic projections, supination vs. pronation.

# A

α (al′fa) SEE alpha.

**A 1.** adenine; alanine. **2.** as a subscript, refers to alveolar gas. **3.** symbol (usually capitalized italic) for absorbance. **4.** symbol for adenosine or adenylic acid in polynucleotides; alanine in polypeptides; first substrate in a multisubstrate enzyme-catalyzed reaction.

**°A** degree absolute; replaced by K (kelvin).

**Å** angstrom.

**A⁻** anion.

**A** absorbance.

**a 1.** ante; area; asymmetric; artery;  auris. **2.** atto-. **3.** as a subscript, refers to systemic arterial blood.

***a*** specific absorption coefficient; absorptivity.

△**a-, an-** not, without, -less; equivalent to L. *in-* and E. *un-*. [G. not, un-; usually *an-* before a vowel]

**AA, aa** amino acid; aminoacyl.

**AAA** abdominal aortic aneurysm; commonly, procedure for surgical correction of an AAA.

**AAC** augmentative and alternative communication.

**A-aO₂ dif·fer·ence** the difference or gradient between the partial pressure of oxygen in the alveolar spaces and that in arterial blood. Normally less than 10 mmHg, it is increased with large right-to-left cardiac or vascular shunts. SEE alveolar air equation. SYN alveolar-arterial oxygen tension difference.

**Aar·on sign** (ar′ŏn) in acute appendicitis, a referred pain or feeling of distress in the epigastrium or precordial region on continuous firm pressure over the McBurney point.

**AASH** adrenal androgen-stimulating hormone.

**Ab** antibody.

△**ab-, abs- 1.** from, away from, off. **2.** prefix applied to electrical units in the CGS-electromagnetic system to distinguish them from units in the CGS-electrostatic system (prefix stat-) and those in the metric system or SI system (no prefix). [L. *ab*, from; usually *abs-* before c, q, and t; often *a-* before m, p, or v]

**A·bad·ie sign of ta·bes dor·sa·lis** (ah-bah-dē′) insensibility to pressure over the tendo achillis.

**ab·am·pere** (ab-am′pēr) electromagnetic unit of current equal to 10 absolute amperes; a current that exerts a force of $2\pi$ dynes on a unit magnetic pole at the center of a circle of wire 1 cm in radius.

**A bands** the dark-staining anisotropic cross striations in the myofibrils of muscle fibers, comprising regions of overlapping thick (myosin) and thin (actin) filaments.

**abap·i·cal** (ă-bap′i-kăl) opposite the apex.

**abar·og·no·sis** (ā-bar′og-nō′sis) loss of ability to appreciate the weight of objects held in the hand, or to differentiate objects of different weights. When the primary senses are intact, abarognosis is caused by a lesion of the contralateral parietal lobe. [G. *a-* priv. + *baros*, weight, + *gnōsis*, knowledge]

**aba·sia** (ă-bā′zē-ă) inability to walk. SEE gait. [G. *a-* priv. + *basis*, step]

**aba·sia-asta·sia** SEE astasia-abasia.

**aba·sia tre·pi·dans** abasia due to trembling of the lower limbs.

**aba·sic, abatic** (ă-bā′sik, ă-bat′ik) **1.** affected by, or associated with, abasia. **2.** refers to loss of pyrimidine sites in DNA.

**ab·ax·i·al, ab·ax·ile** (ab-ak′sē-ăl, ab-ak′sīl) **1.** lying outside the axis of any body or part. **2.** situated at the opposite extremity of the axis of a part.

**Ab·bott ar·tery** (ab′ot) an anomalous artery arising from the posteromedial proximal descending aorta, important during coarctation repair.

**Ab·bott meth·od** (ab′ot) a method of treatment of scoliosis by use of a series of plaster jackets applied after partial correction of the curvature by external force.

**Ab·bott stain for spores** (ab′ot) spores are stained blue with alkaline methylene blue; bodies of the bacilli become pink with eosin counterstain.

**Ab·bott tube** (ab′ot) SYN Miller-Abbott tube.

**ab·cix·i·mab** monoclonal antibody with antithrombotic properties used for the prevention and treatment of arterial occlusive disorders.

**ab·do·men** (ab-dō′men, ab′dō-men) the part of the trunk that lies between the thorax and the pelvis; considered by some anatomists to include the pelvis (abdominopelvic cavity). It includes the greater part of the abdominal cavity (cavitas abdominis [TA]), and is divided by arbitrary planes into nine regions. SEE ALSO abdominal regions. SYN venter (1). [L. *abdomen*, etym. uncertain]

**ab·dom·i·nal** (ab-dom′i-năl) relating to the abdomen.

**ab·dom·i·nal an·gi·na, an·gi·na ab·do·mi·nis** intermittent abdominal pain, frequently occurring at a fixed time after eating, caused by inadequacy of the mesenteric circulation from arteriosclerosis or other arterial disease. SYN intestinal angina.

**ab·dom·i·nal au·ra** epileptic aura characterized by abdominal discomfort, including nausea, malaise, pain, and hunger; some phenomena reflect ictal autonomic dysfunction. SEE ALSO aura (1).

**ab·dom·i·nal cav·i·ty** the space bounded by the abdominal walls, the diaphragm, and the pelvis; it usually is arbitrarily separated from the pelvic cavity by a plane across the superior aperture of the pelvis; however, it may include the pelvis with the abdomen (see abdominopelvic cavity); within the cavitas lie the greater part of the organs of digestion, the spleen, the kidneys, and the suprarenal glands. SYN enterocele (2).

**ab·dom·i·nal guard·ing** a spasm of abdominal wall muscles, detected on palpation, to protect inflamed abdominal viscera from pressure; usually a result of inflammation of the peritoneal surface as in appendicitis, diverticulitis, or generalized peritonitis.

**ab·dom·i·nal her·nia** a hernia protruding through or into any part of the abdominal wall. SYN laparocele.

**ab·dom·i·nal hys·ter·ec·to·my** removal of the uterus through an incision in the abdominal wall. SYN abdominohysterectomy.

**ab·dom·i·nal hys·ter·ot·o·my** transabdominal incision into the uterus. Also called abdominohysterotomy; celiohysterotomy; laparohysterotomy; laparouterotomy. SYN abdominohysterotomy.

**ab·dom·i·nal os·ti·um of uter·ine tube** the fimbriated or ovarian extremity of an oviduct.

**ab·dom·i·nal pad** SYN laparotomy pad.

**ab·dom·i·nal preg·nan·cy** the implantation and development of a fertilized ovum in the peritoneal cavity, usually following early rupture of a tubal pregnancy; very rarely, primary implantation may occur in the peritoneal cavity. SYN abdominocyesis (1).

**ab·dom·i·nal pres·sure** pressure surrounding the bladder; estimated from rectal, gastric, or intraperitoneal pressure.

**ab·dom·i·nal re·gions** the topographical subdivisions of the abdomen; based on subdividing the abdomen by the transpyloric, transtubercular and midinguinal planes; including the right and left hypochondriac, right and left lateral, right and left inguinal, and the unpaired epigastric, umbilical and pubic regions. See this page.

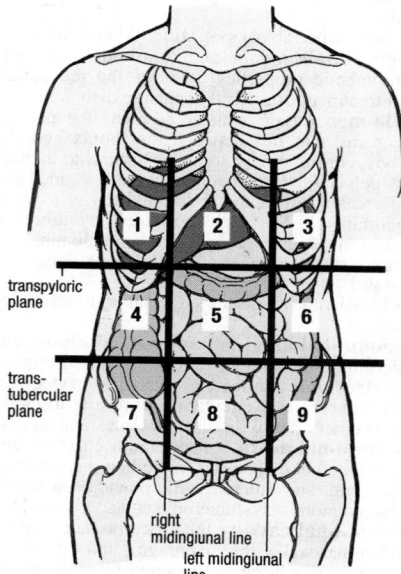

transpyloric plane

trans-tubercular plane

right midingiunal line

left midingiunal line

**abdominal regions:** (1) right hypochondriac, (2) epigastric, (3) left hypochondriac, (4) right lateral (lumbar), (5) umbilical, (6) left lateral (lumbar), (7) right iliac, (8) hypogastric (suprapubic), (9) left iliac

**ab·dom·i·nal res·pi·ra·tion** breathing effected mainly by the action of the diaphragm.

**ab·dom·i·nal sec·tion** SYN celiotomy.

**ab·dom·i·nal tes·tis** testis that has never descended from its retroperitoneal/abdominal origin through the internal inguinal ring.

**ab·dom·i·no-, ab·dom·in-** the abdomen, abdominal. [L. *abdomen, abdominis*]

**ab·dom·i·no·cen·te·sis** (ab-dom'i-nō-sen-tē'sis) paracentesis of the abdomen. [abdomino- + G. *kentēsis,* puncture]

**ab·dom·i·no·cy·e·sis** (ab-dom'i-nō-sī-ē'sis) **1.** SYN abdominal pregnancy. **2.** SYN secondary abdominal pregnancy. [abdomino- + G. *kyēsis,* pregnancy]

**ab·dom·i·no·cys·tic** (ab-dom-i-nō-sis'tik) SYN abdominovesical. [abdomino- + G. *kystis,* bladder]

**ab·dom·i·no·gen·i·tal** (ab-dom'i-nō-gen'i-tăl) relating to the abdomen and the genital organs.

**ab·dom·i·no·hys·ter·ec·to·my** (ab-dom'i-nō-his-ter-ek'tō-mē) SYN abdominal hysterectomy.

**ab·dom·i·no·hys·ter·ot·o·my** (ab-dom'i-nō-his-ter-ot'ō-mē) SYN abdominal hysterotomy.

**ab·dom·i·no·pel·vic** (ab-dom'i-nō-pel'vik) relating to the abdomen and pelvis, especially the combined abdominal and pelvic cavities.

**ab·dom·i·no·per·i·ne·al** (ab-dom'i-nō-pār-i-nē'ăl) relating to both abdomen and perineum.

**ab·dom·i·no·per·i·ne·al re·sec·tion** a surgical cancer treatment involving resection of the lower sigmoid colon, rectum, anus, and surrounding skin, and formation of a sigmoid colostomy; performed as a synchronous or sequential transabdominal and perineal procedure.

**ab·dom·i·no·plas·ty** (ab-dom'i-nō-plas-tē) an operation performed on the abdominal wall for esthetic purposes. [abdomino- + G. *plastos,* formed]

**ab·dom·i·nos·co·py** (ab-dom-i-nos'kŏ-pē) SYN peritoneoscopy. [abdomino- + G. *skopeō,* to examine]

**ab·dom·i·no·scro·tal** (ab-dom'i-nō-skrō'tăl) relating to the abdomen and the scrotum.

**ab·dom·i·no·tho·rac·ic** (ab-dom'i-nō-thō-ras'ik) relating to both abdomen and thorax.

**ab·dom·i·no·tho·rac·ic arch** a bell-shaped line defined by the lower end of the sternum and the costal arches on each side, constituting a boundary line between the anterolateral portions of the thoracic and abdominal walls.

**ab·dom·i·no·vag·i·nal** (ab-dom'i-nō-vaj'i-năl) relating to both abdomen and vagina.

**ab·dom·i·no·ves·i·cal** (ab-dom'i-nō-ves'i-kăl) relating to the abdomen and urinary bladder, or to the abdomen and gallbladder. SYN abdominocystic.

**ab·duce** (ab-doos') SYN abduct.

**ab·du·cens** (ab-doo'senz) SYN abducent (1). [L.]

**ab·du·cens nerve** SYN abducent nerve [CN VI].

**ab·du·cens oc·u·li** SYN lateral rectus muscle.

**ab·du·cent** (ab-doo'sent) **1.** abducting; drawing away, especially away from the median plane. SYN abducens. **2.** SYN abducent nerve [CN VI]. [L. *abducens*]

**ab·du·cent nerve [CN VI]** a small motor nerve supplying the lateral rectus muscle of the eye; its origin is in the dorsal part of the tegmentum of the pons just below the surface of the rhomboid fossa, and it emerges from the brain in the fissure between the medulla oblongata and the posterior border of the pons (medullopontine sulcus); it enters the dura of the clivus and passes through the cavernous sinus, entering the orbit through the superior orbital fissure. SYN nervus abducens [CN VI] [TA], abducens nerve, abducent (2), sixth cranial nerve [CN VI].

**ab·duct** (ab-dŭkt') to move away from the median plane. SYN abduce.

**ab·duc·tion** (ab-dŭk'shŭn) **1.** movement of a body part away from the median plane (of the body, in the case of limbs; of the hand or foot, in the case of digits). **2.** monocular rotation (duction) of the eye toward the temple. **3.** a position resulting from such movement. Cf. adduction. See page APP 90. [L. *abductio*]

**ab·duc·tor** (ab-dŭk'ter, ab-duk'tōr) a muscle that draws a part away from the median plane; or, in the case of the digits, away from the normal axis of the middle finger or the second toe.

**ab·duc·tor di·gi·ti mi·ni·mi mus·cle of foot**

*origin*, lateral and medial processes of calcaneal tuberosity; *insertion*, lateral side of proximal phalanx of fifth toe; *action*, abducts and flexes little toe; *nerve supply*, lateral plantar nerve.

**ab·duc·tor di·gi·ti mi·ni·mi mus·cle of hand** *origin*, pisiform bone and pisohamate ligament; *insertion*, medial side of base of proximal phalanx of the little finger; *action*, abducts and flexes little finger; *nerve supply*, ulnar.

**ab·duc·tor hal·lu·cis mus·cle** *origin*, medial process of calcaneal tuberosity, flexor retinaculum, and plantar aponeurosis; *insertion*, medial side of proximal phalanx of great toe; *action*, abducts great toe; *nerve supply*, medial plantar. SYN musculus abductor hallucis [TA].

**ab·duc·tor spas·mod·ic dys·pho·nia** a breathy form of spasmodic dysphonia caused by excessive and long vocal cord opening for voiceless phonemes extending into vowels.

**Ab·egg rule** (ă′beg) the tendency of the sum of the maximum positive and maximum negative valence of a particular element to equal 8; e.g., C may have a valence of +4 and −4, O of +6 and −2.

**A·bell-Ken·dall meth·od** (ā′bel-ken′dăl) a standard method for estimation of total serum cholesterol that avoids interference by bilirubin, protein, and hemoglobin.

**ab·er·rant** (ab-er′ant) **1.** wandering off; said of certain ducts, vessels, or nerves deviating from the normal course or pattern. **2.** differing from the normal; in botany or zoology, said of certain atypical individuals in a species. **3.** SYN ectopic (1). [L. *aberrans*]

**ab·er·rant goi·ter** enlargement of a supernumerary thyroid gland.

**ab·er·ra·tion** (ab-er-ā′shŭn) **1.** deviating from the normal course or pattern. **2.** deviant development or growth. SEE ALSO chromosome aberration. [L. *aberratio*]

**abe·ta·lip·o·pro·tein·e·mia** (ā-bā′tă-lip′ō-prō′tēn-ē′mē-ă) a disorder characterized by an absence from plasma of low density lipoproteins that migrate electrophoretically as beta globulins, presence of acanthocytes in blood, retinal pigmentary degeneration, malabsorption, engorgement of upper intestinal absorptive cells with dietary triglycerides, and neuromuscular abnormalities; autosomal recessive inheritance. [G. *a-*, priv., + β, + lipoprotein + *-emia*, blood]

**ABG** arterial blood gas; air-bone gap.

**abi·ot·ic** (ā-b-ī-ot′ik) **1.** incompatible with life. **2.** without life.

**ab·i·ot·ro·phy** (ab-ē-ot′rō-fē) an age-dependent manifestation of a genetically determined trait that has been latent from the time of conception. [G. *a-* priv. + *bios*, life, + *trophē*, nourishment]

**abl** an oncogene found in the Abelson strain of mouse leukemia virus and involved in the Philadelphia chromosome translocation in chronic granulocytic leukemia.

**ab·late** (ab-lāt′) to remove, or to destroy the function of. [L. *ab-latus*, pp. *ab-latus*, to take away]

**ab·la·tion** (ab-lā′shŭn) removal of a body part or the destruction of its function, as by a surgical procedure, morbid process, or noxious substance. [L. see ablate]

**ABN** advance beneficiary notice.

**ab·ner·val, ab·neu·ral** (ab-ner′văl, ab-noor′ăl) **1.** away from a nerve or neural axis. **2.** denoting specifically a current of electricity passing through a muscular fiber in a direction away from the point of entrance of the nerve fiber.

**ab·nor·mal·i·ty** (ab-nōr-mal′i-tē) **1.** the state or quality of being abnormal. **2.** an anomaly, deformity, malformation, impairment, or dysfunction.

**ab·nor·mal oc·clu·sion** an arrangement of the teeth which is not considered to be within the normal range of variation.

**ab·nor·mal ST seg·ment** SYN isoelectric period.

**ABO he·mo·lyt·ic dis·ease of the newborn** erythroblastosis fetalis due to maternal-fetal incompatibility with respect to an antigen of the ABO blood group; the fetus possesses A or B antigen which is lacking in the mother, and the mother produces immune antibody which causes hemolysis of fetal erythrocytes.

**ab·o·rad, ab·o·ral** (ab-ō′rad, ab-ō′-răl) in a direction away from the mouth; opposite of orad. [L. *ab*, from, + *os* (*or-*), mouth]

**abort** (ă-bōrt′) **1.** to give birth to an embryo or fetus before it is viable. **2.** to arrest a disease in its earliest stages. **3.** to arrest in growth or development; to cause to remain rudimentary. **4.** to remove products of conception prior to viability. [L. *aborior*, to fail at onset]

**a·bort·ed sys·to·le** a loss of the systolic beat in the radial pulse through weakness of the ventricular contraction.

**abor·ti·fa·cient** (ă-bōr-ti-fā′shent) **1.** producing abortion. SYN abortive (3). **2.** an agent that produces abortion. [L. *abortus*, abortion, + *facio*, to make]

**abor·tion** (ă-bōr′shŭn) **1.** expulsion from the uterus of an embryo or fetus prior to the stage of viability (20 weeks' gestation or fetal weight <500 g). A distinction made between abortion and premature birth: premature infants are those born after the stage of viability but prior to 37 weeks. Abortion may be either spontaneous (occurring from natural causes) or induced (artificial or therapeutic). **2.** the arrest of any action or process before its normal completion.

**abor·tion·ist** (ă-bōr′shŭn-ist) one who interrupts a pregnancy.

**abor·tive** (ă-bōr′tiv) **1.** not reaching completion; said of a disease subsiding before it has completed its course. **2.** SYN rudimentary. **3.** SYN abortifacient (1). [L. *abortivus*]

**a·bor·tive trans·duc·tion** transduction in which the genetic fragment from the donor bacterium is not integrated in the genome of the recipient bacterium, and, when the latter divides, is transmitted to only one of the daughter cells.

**abor·tus** (ă-bōr′tŭs) any product (or all products) of an abortion. [L.]

**ABP** androgen binding protein.

**ABR** auditory brainstem response.

**abra·chia** (ă-brā′kē-ă) congenital absence of arms. SEE amelia. [G. *a-* priv. + *brachiōn*, arm]

**abra·chi·o·ceph·a·ly, abra·chi·o·ce·pha·lia** (ă-brā′kē-ō-sef′ă-lē, ă-brā′kē-ō-se-fā′lē-ă) congenital absence of arms and head. [G. *a-* priv. + *brachiōn*, arm, + *kephalē*, head]

**abrade** (ă-brād′) **1.** to wear away by mechanical action. **2.** to scrape away the surface layer from a part. [L. *ab-rado*, pp. *-rasus*, to scrape off]

**a·brad·ed wound** SYN abrasion (1).

**A·brams heart re·flex** (ā′brămz) a contraction of the myocardium when the skin of the precordial region is irritated.

**abra·sion** (ă-brā′zhŭn) **1.** an excoriation, or circumscribed removal of the superficial layers of skin or mucous membrane. SYN abraded wound. **2.** a scraping away of a portion of the surface. **3.** DENTISTRY the pathological grinding or wearing away of tooth substance by incorrect tooth-brushing methods, foreign objects, bruxism, or similar causes. SYN grinding. Cf. attrition. [SEE abrade]

**abra·sive** (a-brā′siv) **1.** causing abrasion. **2.** any material used to produce abrasions. **3.** a substance used in dentistry for abrading, grinding, or polishing.

**abra·sive·ness** (ă-brā′siv-nes) **1.** that property of a substance which causes surface wear by friction. **2.** the quality of being able to scratch or wear away another material.

**ab·re·ac·tion** (ab-rē-ak′shŭn) in freudian psycho-analysis, an emotional release or catharsis associated with the recollection of previously repressed unpleasant experiences.

**ab·rup·tio pla·cen·tae** (ab-rŭp′shē-ō pla-sen′tē) premature detachment of a normally situated placenta.

**ab·scess** (ab′ses) **1.** a circumscribed collection of purulent exudate appearing in an acute or chronic localized infection, caused by tissue destruction and frequently associated with swelling and other signs of inflammation. **2.** a cavity formed by liquefactive necrosis within solid tissue. [L. *abscessus,* a going away]

**ab·scis·sion** (ab-si′shŭn) cutting away. [L. *abscindo,* pp. -*scissus,* to cut away from]

**ab·sco·pal** (ab-skō′păl, ab-skop′ăl) denoting the effect that irradiation of a tissue has on remote nonirradiated tissue. [ab- + G. *skopos,* target, + -al]

**ab·sco·pal ef·fect** a reaction produced following irradiation but occurring outside the zone of actual radiation absorption.

**ab·sence** (ab′sens) paroxysmal attacks of impaired consciousness, occasionally accompanied by spasm or twitching of cephalic muscles, which usually can be brought on by hyperventilation. [L. *absentia*]

**ab·sence sei·zure** a brief seizure characterized by arrest of activity and occasionally clonic movements. There is loss of consciousness or slowing of thought. The EEG typically shows generalized spike wave discharges greater than 2.5 Hz. More prolonged absence seizures may have automatisms.

**Ab·sid·ia** (ab-sid′ē-ă) a genus of fungi commonly found in nature. Thermophilic species survive in compost piles at temperatures exceeding 45°C and may cause zygomycosis in humans.

**ab·so·lute hu·mid·i·ty** the mass of water vapor actually present per unit volume of gas or air.

**ab·so·lute hy·per·o·pia** manifest hyperopia that cannot be overcome by an effort of accommodation.

**ab·so·lute leu·ko·cy·to·sis** an actual increase in the total number of leukocytes in the blood, as distinguished from a relative increase (such as that observed in dehydration).

**ab·so·lute scale** SYN Kelvin scale.

**ab·so·lute tem·per·a·ture (T)** temperature reckoned in kelvins from absolute zero.

**ab·so·lute u·nit** a unit whose value is constant regardless of place or time and not dependent on gravitation.

**ab·so·lute ze·ro** the lowest possible temperature, that at which the form of translational motion constituting heat is assumed no longer to exist, determined as −273.15°C or 0 Kelvin.

**ab·sorb** (ab-sōrb′) **1.** to take in by absorption. **2.** to reduce the intensity of transmitted light. [L. *ab-sorbeo,* pp. -*sorptus,* to suck in]

**ab·sorb·a·ble gel·a·tin film** a sterile, non-antigenic, absorbable, water-insoluble sheet of gelatin prepared by drying a gelatin-formaldehyde solution on plates; used in the closure and repair of defects in membranes such as the dura mater or the pleura; it undergoes absorption over a period of 1 to 6 months.

**ab·sor·bance (A, A), ab·sor·ban·cy, ab·sorb·en·cy** (ab-sōr′bans, ab-sōr′ban-sē, ab-sōr′ben-sē) SPECTROPHOTOMETRY, 2 minus the log of the percentage transmittance of light. SYN extinction (2), optic density, optical density.

**ab·sorb·an·cy in·dex 1.** SYN specific absorption coefficient. **2.** SYN molar absorption coefficient.

**ab·sorbed dose** the amount of energy absorbed per unit mass of irradiated material at the target site; RADIATION THERAPY the former unit for absorbed dose is the rad; the current (SI) unit is the gray.

**ab·sor·bent** (ab-sōr′bent) **1.** having the power to absorb, soak up, or take into itself a gas, liquid, light rays, or heat. SYN absorptive. **2.** any substance possessing such power. **3.** material (usually caustic) for removal of carbon dioxide from circuits in which rebreathing occurs; e.g., anesthesia equipment.

**ab·sorp·tion** (ab-sōrp′shŭn) **1.** the taking in, incorporation, or reception of gases, liquids, light, or heat. Cf. adsorption. **2.** RADIOLOGY the uptake of energy from radiation by the tissue or medium through which it passes. **3.** MEDICAL PHYSICS the number of disintegrations per second of a radio-nuclide. Radioactivity. Unit (SI): becquerel. [L. *absorptio,* fr. *absorbeo,* to swallow]

**ab·sorp·tion chro·ma·tog·ra·phy** SYN chromatography.

**ab·sorp·tion co·ef·fi·cient 1.** the milliliters of a gas at standard temperature and pressure that will saturate 100 ml of liquid; **2.** the amount of light absorbed in passing through 1 cm of a 1 molar solution of a given substance, expressed as a constant in Beer-Lambert law; **3.** X-RAY a measure of the rate of decrease of intensity of a beam in its passage through a substance, resulting from a combination of scattering and conversion to other forms of energy.

**ab·sorp·tion lines** the dark lines in the solar spectrum due to absorption by the solar and the earth's atmosphere.

**ab·sorp·tion spec·trum** the spectrum observed after light has passed through, and been partially absorbed by, a solution or translucent substance; many molecular groupings have characteristic light absorption patterns, which can be used for detection and quantitative assay.

**ab·sorp·tive** (ab-sōrp′tiv) SYN absorbent (1).

**ab·sorp·tiv·i·ty (a)** (ab-sōrp-tiv′i-tē) **1.** SYN specific absorption coefficient. **2.** SYN molar absorption coefficient.

**ab·sti·nence** (ab′sti-nens) refraining from the use of certain articles of diet, alcoholic beverages, illegal drugs, or from sexual intercourse. [L. *abs-tineo,* to hold back, fr. *teneo,* to hold]

**ab·stract** (ab′strakt) **1.** a preparation made by evaporating a fluid extract to a powder and triturating with milk sugar. **2.** a condensation or summary of a scientific or literary article or address. [L. *abs-traho,* pp. *-tractus,* to draw away]

**ab•strac•tion** (ab-strak′shŭn) **1.** distillation or separation of the volatile constituents of a substance. **2.** exclusive mental concentration. **3.** the making of an abstract from the crude drug. **4.** malocclusion in which the teeth or associated structures are lower than their normal occlusal plane. **5.** the process of selecting a certain aspect of a concept from the whole. [L. *abs-traho,* pp. *-tractus,* to draw away]

**ab•stract think•ing** thinking in terms of concepts and general principles (e.g., perceiving a table and a chair as furniture), as contrasted with concrete thinking.

**ab•ter•mi•nal** (ab-ter′mi-năl) in a direction away from the end and toward the center; denoting the course of an electrical current in a muscle. [L. *ab,* from, + *terminus,* end]

**abu•lia** (ă-boo′lē-ă) **1.** loss or impairment of the ability to perform voluntary actions or to make decisions. **2.** reduction in speech, movement, thought, and emotional reaction; a common result of bilateral frontal lobe disease. [G. *a-* priv. + *boulē,* will]

**abu•lic** (ă-boo′lik) relating to, or suffering from, abulia.

**abuse** (ă-byus′) **1.** misuse, wrong use, especially excessive use, of anything. **2.** injurious, harmful, or offensive treatment, as in child abuse or sexual abuse

**abut•ment** (ă-bŭt′ment) DENTISTRY a natural tooth or implanted tooth substitute, used for the support or anchorage of a fixed or removable prosthesis.

**AC** alternating current; ante cibum.

**Ac** actinium; acetyl.

**a.c.** ante cibum.

**AC/A** accommodative covergence-accommodation *ratio.*

**acal•cu•lia** (ā′kal-kyu′lē-a) a form of aphasia characterized by the inability to perform simple mathematical problems; found with lesions of the cerebral hemispheres, and often an early sign of dementia. [G. *a-* priv. + L. *calculo,* to reckon]

**acan•tha** (ă-kan′thă) **1.** a spine or spinous process. **2.** the spinous process of a vertebra. [G. *akantha,* a thorn]

**acan•tha•me•bi•a•sis** (ă-kan′thă-mē-bī′ă-sis) infection by free-living soil amebae of the genus *Acanthamoeba* that may result in a necrotizing dermal or tissue invasion, or a fulminating and usually fatal primary amebic meningoencephalitis.

*Acan•tha•moe•ba* **me•di•um** nonnutrient agar plates with an *E. coli* overlay used to detect the presence of *Acanthamoeba* or *Naegleria* from tissue or soil samples.

**acan•tha•moe•bi•a•sis [Br.]** SEE acanthamebiasis.

**acan•thes•the•sia** (ă-kan-thes-thē′zē-ă) paresthesia in which there is the sensation of a pinprick. [G. *akantha,* thorn, + *aisthēsis,* sensation]

**acan•thi•on** (ă-kan′thē-on) the tip of the anterior nasal spine. [G. *akantha,* thorn]

♻**acantho-** a spinous process; spiny, thorny. [G. *akantha,* a thorn, the backbone, the spine, fr. *akē,* a point, + *anthos,* a flower]

**acan•tho•cyte** (ă-kan′thō-sīt) an erythrocyte characterized by spiny cytoplasmic projections. SYN acanthrocyte. [acantho- + G. *kytos,* cell]

**acan•tho•cy•to•sis** (ă-kan′thō-sī-tō′sis) a rare condition in which the majority of erythrocytes are acanthocytes; a regular feature of abetalipoproteinemia. SYN acanthrocytosis.

**acan•thoid** (ă-kan′thoyd) spine-shaped.

**ac•an•thol•y•sis** (ak-an-thol′i-sis) separation of individual epidermal keratinocytes from their neighbors, as in conditions such as pemphigus vulgaris and Darier disease. [acantho- + G. *lysis,* loosening]

**ac•an•tho•ma** (ak-an-thō′mă) a tumor formed by proliferation of epithelial squamous cells. SEE ALSO keratoacanthoma. [acantho- + G. *-oma,* tumor]

**acan•tho•me•a•tal line** an imaginary line between the acanthion and the external auditory meatus; used for radiographic positioning of the skull.

**acan•thor•rhex•is** (ă-kan-thō-rek′sĭs) rupture of the intercellular bridges of the prickle cell layer of the epidermis, as in contact-type dermatitis. SEE spongiosis. [acantho + G. *rhexis,* rupture]

**ac•an•tho•sis** (ak-an-thō′sis) an increase in the thickness of the stratum spinosum of the epidermis. [acantho- + G. *-osis,* condition]

◧**ac•an•tho•sis ni•gri•cans** an eruption of velvet warty benign growths and hyperpigmentation occurring in the skin of the axillae, neck, anogenital area, and groins; in adults, may be associated with internal malignancy, endocrine disorders, or obesity; a benign (juvenile) type occurs in children. See page B4. [L. fr. *niger,* black]

**ac•an•thot•ic** (ak-an-thot′ik) pertaining to or characteristic of acanthosis.

**acan•thro•cyte** (a-kan′thrō-sīt) SYN acanthocyte.

**acan•thro•cy•to•sis** (ă-kan′thrō-sī-tō′sis) SYN acanthocytosis.

**acap•nia** (ă-kap′nē-ă) absence of carbon dioxide in the blood; sometimes used erroneously for hypocapnia. [G. *a-* priv. + *kapnos,* smoke]

**acar•dia** (ā-kar′dē-ă) congenital absence of the heart; a condition sometimes occurring in monozygotic twins or in the smaller of conjoined twins when its partner monopolizes the placental blood supply. [G. *a-* priv. + *kardia,* heart]

**ac•a•ri•a•sis** (ak-ar-ī′ă-sis) any disease caused by mites, usually a skin infestation. SEE mange. SYN acaridiasis, acarinosis.

**acar•i•cide** (ă-kar′i-sīd) an agent that kills acarines; commonly used to denote chemicals that kill ticks. [Mod. L. *acarus,* a mite, fr. G. *akari* + L. *caedo,* to cut, kill]

**ac•a•rid** (ak′ă-rid) a general term for a member of the family Acaridae or for a mite. [G. *akari,* mite]

**Acar•i•dae** (ă-kar′i-dē) a family of the order Acarina, a large group of exceptionally small mites, usually 0.5 mm or less, abundant in dried fruits and meats, grain, meal, and flour; frequently a cause of severe dermatitis among persons hypersensitized by frequent handling of infested products.

**ac•ar•i•di•a•sis** (ak′ar-i-dī′ă-sis) SYN acariasis.

**Ac•a•ri•na** (ak-ă-rī′nă) an order of Arachnida that includes the mites and ticks. [G. *akari,* a mite]

**ac•a•rine** (ak′ă-rīn) a member of the order Acarina.

**ac•ar•i•no•sis** (ak′ă-ri-nō′sis, ă-kar′i-nō′sis) SYN acariasis.

**ac·a·ro·der·ma·ti·tis** (ak′ă-rō-der-mă-tī′tis) a skin inflammation or eruption produced by a mite. [G. *akari*, mite, + *derma* (*dermat-*), skin]

**ac·a·ro·pho·bia** (ak′ă-rō-fō′bē-ă) morbid fear of small parasites, small particles, or itching. [G. *akari*, mite, + *phobos*, fear]

**Ac·a·rus** (ak′ă-rŭs) a genus of mites of the family Acaridae. [G. *akari*, mite]

**Ac·a·rus sca·bi·ei** former term for *Sarcoptes scabiei*.

**acar·y·ote** (ă-kar′ē-ōt) SYN akaryocyte.

**ac·cel·er·ant** (ak-sel′er-ant) SYN accelerator.

**ac·cel·er·a·tion-de·cel·er·a·tion in·ju·ry** SYN whiplash injury.

**ac·cel·er·a·tor** (ak-sel′er-ā-ter) **1.** anything that increases rapidity of action or function. **2.** PHYSIOLOGY a nerve, muscle, or substance that quickens movement or response. **3.** a catalytic agent used to hasten a chemical reaction. **4.** NUCLEAR PHYSICS a device that accelerates charged particles (e.g., protons) to high speed in order to produce nuclear reactions in a target, often for the production of radionuclides or for radiation therapy. SYN accelerant. [L. *accelerans*, pres. p. of *ac-celero*, to hasten, fr. *celer*, swift]

**ac·cel·er·a·tor fac·tor** SYN factor V.

**ac·cel·er·a·tor fi·bers** postganglionic sympathetic nerve fibers originating in the superior, middle, and inferior cervical ganglia of the sympathetic trunk, conveying nervous impulses to the heart that increase the rapidity and force of the cardiac pulsations.

**ac·cel·er·a·tor glob·u·lin (AcG, ac-g)** globulin in serum that promotes the conversion of prothrombin to thrombin in the presence of thromboplastin and ionized calcium. SEE factor V, serum accelerator globulin.

**ac·cel·er·a·tor nerves** certain of the cardiopulmonary splanchnic nerves establishing the sympathetic innervation of the heart; originating from ganglion cells of the superior, middle, and inferior cervical ganglion of the sympathetic trunk, the unmyelinated efferent fibers of the accelerator nerves stimulate an increase in the heart rate.

**ac·cen·tu·a·tor** (ak-sent′yu-ā-ter) a substance, such as aniline, the presence of which allows a combination between a tissue or histologic element and a stain that might otherwise be impossible. [L. *accentus*, accent, fr. *cano*, to sing]

**ac·cep·tor** (ak-sep′ter) a compound that will take up a chemical group (e.g., an amine group, a methyl group, a carbamoyl group) from another compound (the donor). [L. *ac-cipio*, pp. *-ceptus*, to accept]

**ac·cess** (ak′ses) a way or means of approach or admittance. DENTISTRY **1.** the space required for visualization and for manipulation of instruments to remove decay and prepare a tooth for restoration. **2.** the opening in the crown of a tooth required to allow adequate admittance to the pulp space to clean, shape, and seal the root canal(s). [L. *accessus*]

**ac·ces·so·ry** (ak-ses′ō-rē) ANATOMY denoting a muscle, nerve, gland, etc., that is auxiliary or supernumerary to some similar, generally more important structure. [L. *accessorius*, fr. *ac-cedo*, pp. *-cessus*, to move toward]

**ac·ces·so·ry ad·re·nal** an island of cortical tissue separate from the adrenal gland, usually found in the retroperitoneal tissues, kidney, or genital organs. SYN adrenal rest.

**ac·ces·so·ry cell** SYN antigen-presenting cell.

**ac·ces·so·ry ce·phal·ic vein** a variable vein that passes along the radial border of the forearm to join the cephalic vein near the elbow. SYN vena cephalica accessoria [TA].

**ac·ces·so·ry gland** a small mass of glandular structure, detached from but lying near another and larger gland, to which it is similar in structure and probably in function.

**ac·ces·so·ry hem·i·az·y·gos vein** formed by the union of the fourth to seventh left posterior intercostal veins, passes along the side of the bodies of the fifth, sixth, and seventh thoracic vertebrae, then crosses the midline behind the aorta, esophagus, and thoracic duct, and empties into the azygos vein, sometimes in common with the hemiazygos vein. SYN vena hemiazygos accessoria [TA].

**ac·ces·so·ry lig·a·ments** ligaments about a joint that are in addition to the articular capsule. They may lie within, or on the outside of the latter.

**ac·ces·so·ry mol·e·cules** cell surface adhesion molecules on T cells that are involved in binding of one cell to another cell or in signal transduction.

**ac·ces·so·ry nerve [CN XI]** arises by two sets of roots: the presumed cranial, emerging from the side of the medulla, and spinal, emerging from the ventrolateral part of the first five cervical segments of the spinal cord; these roots unite to form the accessory nerve trunk, which divides into two branches, internal and external; the internal branch, carrying fibers of the cranial root, unites with the vagus in the jugular foramen and supplies the muscles of the pharynx, larynx, and soft palate; the external branch continues independently through the jugular foramen to supply the sternocleidomastoid and trapezius muscles. While the accessory nerve was originally believed to have cranial and spinal roots, it is now the general view that the so-called cranial root is actually a portion of the vagus nerve. SYN nervus accessorius [CN XI] [TA], eleventh cranial nerve [CN XI].

**ac·ces·so·ry nip·ple** a supernumerary nipple occurring on the mammary line.

**ac·ces·so·ry ob·tu·ra·tor ar·tery** term applied to the anastomosis of the pubic branch of the inferior epigastric artery with the pubic branch of the obturator artery when it contributes a significant supply through the obturator canal. SYN arteria obturatoria accessoria [TA].

**ac·ces·so·ry or·gans of the eye** the eyelids, with lashes and eyebrows, lacrimal apparatus, conjunctival sac, and extrinsic muscles of the eyeball.

**ac·ces·so·ry pan·cre·at·ic duct** the excretory duct of the head of the pancreas, one branch of which joins the pancreatic duct, the other opening independently into the duodenum at the lesser duodenal papilla. SYN ductus pancreaticus accessorius [TA], Santorini canal, Santorini duct.

**ac·ces·so·ry phren·ic nerves** accessory nerve strands that arise from the fifth cervical nerve, often as branches of the nerve to the subclavius, passing downward to join the phrenic nerve. SYN nervi phrenici accessorii [TA].

**ac·ces·so·ry spleen** one of the small globular masses of splenic tissue occasionally found in the region of the spleen, in one of the peritoneal folds or elsewhere. SYN lien accessorius.

**ac·ces·so·ry symp·tom** a symptom that usually but not always accompanies a certain disease, as distinguished from a pathognomonic symptom. SYN concomitant symptom.

**ac·ces·so·ry ver·te·bral vein** a vein that accompanies the vertebral vein but passes through the foramen of the transverse process of the seventh cervical vertebra and opens independently into the brachiocephalic vein. SYN vena vertebralis accessoria [TA].

**ac·ci·dent** (ak'si-dent) an unanticipated but often predictable event leading to injury, e.g., in traffic, industry, or a domestic setting, or such an event developing in the course of a disease. [L. *ac-cido*, to happen]

**ac·ci·den·tal hy·po·ther·mia** unintentional decrease in body temperature, especially in the newborn, infants, and elderly, particularly during operations.

**ac·ci·den·tal my·i·a·sis** gastrointestinal myiasis from ingestion of contaminated food.

**ac·ci·den·tal par·a·site** SYN incidental parasite.

**ac·cli·ma·ti·sa·tion [Br.]** SEE acclimatization.

**ac·cli·ma·ti·za·tion, ac·cli·ma·tion** (ă-klī-mă-ti-zā'shŭn, ak-lǐ-mā'shŭn) physiological adaptation to a variation in environmental factors such as temperature, climate, or altitude.

**ac·com·mo·dat·ing re·sis·tance** in isokinetic testing or training, application of a counterforce to muscle action so as to regulate the speed of contraction.

**ac·com·mo·da·tion** (ă-kom'ŏ-dā'shŭn) **1.** the act or state of adjustment or adaptation; especially change in the shape of the ocular lens for various focal distances. **2.** SENSORIMOTOR THEORY the alteration of schemata or cognitive expectations to conform with experience. [L. *ac-commodo*, pp. *-atus*, to adapt, fr. *modus*, a measure]

**ac·com·mo·da·tion re·flex** increased convexity of the lens, due to contraction of the ciliary muscle and relaxation of the suspensory ligament, to maintain a distinct retinal image.

**ac·com·mo·da·tive** (ă-kom'ŏ-dā-tiv) relating to accommodation.

**ac·com·mo·da·tive as·the·no·pia** asthenopia due to errors of refraction and excessive contraction of the ciliary muscle.

**ac·com·mo·da·tive con·ver·gence-ac·com·mo·da·tion ra·ti·o (AC/A)** the amount of convergence (measured in prism diopters of convergence) divided by the amount of accommodation (measured in diopters) required to direct both eyes upon an object.

**ac·com·mo·da·tive in·suf·fi·cien·cy** a lack of appropriate accommodation for near focus.

**ac·cor·di·on graft** a skin graft in which multiple slits have been made, so it can be stretched to cover a large area.

**ac·cou·cheur's hand** position of the hand in tetany or in muscular dystrophy; the fingers are flexed at the metacarpophalangeal joints and extended at the phalangeal joints, with the thumb flexed and adducted into the palm; in resemblance to the position of the physician's hand in making a vaginal examination. SYN obstetric hand, obstetrical hand.

**ac·cre·tio cor·dis** (ă-krē'shē-ō kōr'dis) adhesion of the pericardium to adjacent extracardiac structures.

**ac·cre·tion** (ă-krē'shŭn) **1.** increase by addition to the periphery of material of the same nature as that already present; e.g., the manner of growth of crystals. **2.** DENTISTRY foreign material (usually plaque or calculus) collecting on the surface of a tooth or in a cavity. **3.** a growing together. [L. *accretio*, fr. *ad*, to, + *crescere*, to grow]

**ac·cre·tion·ary growth** growth by an increase of intercellular material.

**ac·cur·a·cy** (ak'kyu-ră-sē) the degree to which a measurement represents the true value of the attribute that is being measured. In the laboratory accuracy of a test is determined when possible by comparing results from the test in question with results generated from an established reference method.

**ACE** angiotensin-converting enzyme.

**A cells** alpha cells of pancreas or of anterior lobe of hypophysis. SYN alpha cells (3).

**acel·lu·lar** (ā-sel'yu-ler) **1.** devoid of cells. **2.** a term applied to unicellular organisms that do not become multicellular and are complete within a single cell unit. [G. *a-* priv. + L. *cellula*, a small chamber]

**acen·tric** (ā-sen'trik) lacking a center. CYTOGENETICS denoting a chromosome fragment without a centromere. [G. *a-* priv. + *kentron*, center]

**a·ce·phal·gic mi·graine** a classic migraine episode in which the teichopsia is not followed by a headache.

**ace·pha·lia, aceph·a·lism** (ă-se-fā'lē-ă, ă-sef'ă-lizm) SYN acephaly.

**aceph·a·lo·car·dia** (ă-sef'ă-lō-kar'dē-ă) absence of head and heart in a parasitic twin. [G. *a-* priv. + *kephalē*, head, + *kardia*, heart]

**aceph·a·lo·chei·ria, a·ceph·a·lo·chi·ri·a** (ă-sef'ă-lō-kī'rē-ă) congenital absence of head and hands. [G. *a-* priv. + *kephalē*, head, + *cheir*, hand]

**aceph·a·lo·gas·ter·ia** (ă-sef'ă-lō-gas-tēr'ē-ă) congenital absence of head, thorax, and abdomen in a parasitic twin with pelvis and lower limbs only.

**aceph·a·lo·po·dia** (ă-sef'ă-lō-pō'dē-ă) congenital absence of head and feet. [G. *a-* priv. + *kephalē*, head, + *pous*, foot]

**aceph·a·lo·sto·mia** (ă-sef'ă-lō-stō'mē-ă) congenital absence of the greater part of the head with, however, the presence of a mouthlike opening. [G. *a-* priv. + *kephalē*, head, + *stoma*, mouth]

**aceph·a·lo·tho·ra·cia** (ă-sef'ă-lō-thōr-ā'sē-ă) congenital absence of head and thorax. [G. *a-* priv. + *kephalē*, head, + *thorax*, chest]

**aceph·a·lous** (ă-sef'ă-lŭs) headless.

**aceph·a·lus** (ă-sef'ă-lŭs) a headless fetus. [G. *a-* priv. + *kephalē*, head]

**aceph·a·ly** (ă-sef'ă-lē) congenital absence of the head. SYN acephalia, acephalism. [G. *a-* priv. + *kephalē*, head]

△**acet-, aceto-** combining forms denoting the two-carbon fragment of acetic acid.

**ac·e·tab·u·la** (as-ĕ-tab'yu-lă) plural of acetabulum.

**ac·e·tab·u·lar** (as-e-tab'yu-lăr) relating to the acetabulum.

**ac·e·tab·u·lar fos·sa** a depressed area in the floor of the acetabulum superior to the acetabular notch. SYN fossa acetabuli [TA].

**ac·e·tab·u·lec·to·my** (as'ĕ-tab-yu-lek'tō-mē) excision of the acetabulum. [acetabulum + G. *ektomē*, excision]

**ac·e·tab·u·lo·plas·ty** (as-ĕ-tab′yu-lō-plas-tē) any operation aimed at restoring the acetabulum to as near a normal state as possible. [acetabulum + G. *plastos,* formed]

**ac·e·tab·u·lum,** pl. **ac·e·tab·u·la** (as-ĕ-tab′yu-lŭm, as-ĕ-tab′yu-lă) [TA] a cup-shaped depression on the external surface of the hip bone, with which the head of the femur articulates. SYN cotyloid cavity. [L. vinegar cup]

**ac·e·tal** (as′e-tal) product of the addition of 2 moles of alcohol to one of an aldehyde. SEE ALSO hemiacetal, hemiketal, ketal.

**ac·e·tate** (as′e-tāt) a salt or ester of acetic acid.

**ac·e·tate-CoA ligase** SYN acetyl-CoA ligase.

**ac·e·tate thi·o·ki·nase** SYN acetyl-CoA ligase.

**ac·e·to·ac·e·tate** (as′e-tō-as′e-tāt) a salt or ion of acetoacetic acid. A ketone body formed in ketogenesis.

**ac·e·to·a·ce·tic ac·id** (as′e-tō-a-sē′tik as′id) one of the ketone bodies, formed in excess and appearing in the urine in starvation or diabetic acidosis. SYN diacetic acid.

**ac·e·to·a·ce·tyl-CoA** (as′e-tō-a-sē′til) intermediate in the oxidation of fatty acids and in the formation of ketone bodies; also formed from two molecules of acetyl-CoA; major role is condensation with acetyl-CoA to form the important β-hydroxy-β-methylglutaryl-CoA.

**ac·e·to·a·ce·tyl-CoA thi·o·lase** SYN acetyl-CoA acetyltransferase.

**ac·e·tone** (as′e-tōn) a colorless, volatile, inflammable liquid; small amounts are found in normal urine, but larger quantities occur in urine and blood of diabetic persons, sometimes imparting an ethereal odor to the urine and breath. Used as a solvent in some pharmaceutical and commercial preparations.

**ac·e·tone bod·y** SYN ketone body.

**ac·e·ton·e·mia** (as′ĕ-tō-nē′mē-ă) the presence of acetone or acetone bodies in relatively large amounts in the blood. [acetone + G. *haima,* blood]

**ac·e·to·nu·ria** (as′e-tō-nyur′ē-ă) excretion in the urine of large amounts of acetone. [acetone + G. *ouron,* urine]

**ace·to·whit·en·ing** (ă-sē′tō-hwīt′en-ing) blanching of skin or mucous membranes after application of 3–5% acetic acid solution, a sign of increased cellular protein and increased nuclear density; used particularly on genital skin and mucous membranes, including the uterine cervix, to identify zones of squamous cell change for biopsy and condyloma acuminatum for treatment. SYN cervicoscopy, visual inspection with acetic acid. [acetic acid + whitening]

**ace·tyl (Ac)** (as′e-til) the radical $CH_3CO–$; an acetic acid molecule from which the hydroxyl group has been removed.

**ace·tyl-ac·ti·vat·ing en·zyme** SYN acetyl-CoA ligase.

**acet·y·lase** (a-set′il-ās) any enzyme catalyzing acetylation or deacetylation, as in the formation of *N*-acetylglutamate from glutamate plus acetyl-CoA, or the reverse; acetylases are usually called acetyltransferases.

**acet·y·la·tion** (a-set-i-lā′shŭn) formation of an acetyl derivative.

**ace·tyl·cho·line (ACH, Ach)** (as-e-til-kō′lēn) (2-acetoxyethyl)trimethylammonium ion; the neurotransmitter substance at cholinergic synapses, which causes cardiac inhibition, vasodila-

tion, gastrointestinal peristalsis, and other parasympathetic effects.

**ace·tyl-CoA** condensation product of coenzyme A and acetic acid, symbolized as $CoAS~COCH_3$; intermediate in transfer of two-carbon fragment, notably in its entrance into the tricarboxylic acid cycle and in fatty acid synthesis.

**ace·tyl-CoA ace·tyl·trans·fer·ase** an acetyltransferase forming acetoacetyl-CoA from two molecules of acetyl-CoA, releasing one CoA. A key step in ketogenesis and sterol synthesis. SYN acetoacetyl-CoA thiolase, acetyl-CoA thiolase.

**ace·tyl-CoA li·gase** a ligase that catalyzes the reaction of acetate and CoA and ATP to form AMP, pyrophosphate, and acetyl-CoA. A key step in the activation of acetate. SYN acetate thiokinase, acetate-CoA ligase, acetyl-activating enzyme, acetyl-CoA synthetase.

**ace·tyl-CoA syn·the·tase** SYN acetyl-CoA ligase.

**ace·tyl-CoA thi·o·lase** SYN acetyl-CoA acetyltransferase.

**ace·tyl·trans·fer·ase** (as′e-til-trans′fer-ās) any enzyme transferring acetyl groups from one compound to another. SEE ALSO choline acetyltransferase. SYN transacetylase.

**AcG, ac-g** accelerator globulin.

**ACH, Ach** acetylcholine.

**A chain 1.** a polypeptide component of insulin containing 21 amino acyl residues; insulin is formed by the linkage of an A chain to a B chain; **2.** in general, one of the polypeptides in a multiprotein complex.

**acha·la·sia** (ak-ă-lā′zē-ă) failure to relax; referring especially to visceral openings such as the pylorus, cardia, or any other sphincter muscles. [G. *a-* priv. + *chalasis,* a slackening]

**ach·a·la·sia of the car·dia** SYN esophageal achalasia.

**ach·a·la·sia of the up·per sphinc·ter** SYN cricopharyngeal achalasia.

**ache** (āk) a dull, poorly localized pain, usually one of less than severe intensity.

**achei·ria** (ă-kī′rē-ă) **1.** congenital absence of one or both hands. **2.** anesthesia in, with loss of the sense of possession of, one or both hands. **3.** a form of dyscheiria in which the patient is unable to tell on which side of the body a stimulus has been applied. [G. *a- priv.* + *cheir,* hand]

**achei·rop·o·dy, achi·rop·o·dy** (ă-kī-rop′ō-dē) congenital absence of the hands and feet; autosomal recessive inheritance. [G. *a-* priv. + *cheir,* hand, + *podos,* foot]

**achei·rous, achi·rous** (ă-kī′rŭs) characterized by or relating to acheiria (1).

**achieve·ment age** the relationship between the chronologic age and the age of achievement, as established by standard achievement tests.

**achieve·ment quo·tient** a ratio, percentile rating, or related quotient denoting the amount a child has learned in relation to peers of the same age or level of education.

**achieve·ment test** a standardized test used to measure acquired learning, in contrast to an intelligence test, which is an index of potential learning ability.

**Achil·les re·flex, Achil·les ten·don re·flex** a contraction of the calf muscles when the tendo calcaneus is sharply struck. SYN ankle reflex, triceps surae reflex.

**Achil·les ten·don** (ă-kil′ēz) SYN tendo calcaneus.

**achil·lo·bur·si·tis** (ă-kil'ō-ber-sī'tis) inflammation of a bursa in proximity to the tendo calcaneus. SYN retrocalcaneobursitis.

**achil·lo·dyn·ia** (ă-kil-ō-din'ē-ă) pain due to inflammation of the bursa between the calcaneus and the tendo calcaneus (achillobursitis). [Achilles (tendon) + G. *odynē*, pain]

**ach·il·lor·rha·phy** (ă-kil-ōr'ă-fē) suture of the tendo calcaneus. [Achilles (tendon) + G. *rhaphē*, a sewing]

**ach·il·lot·o·my** (ă-kil-ot'ō-mē) division of the tendo calcaneus. [Achilles (tendon) + G. *tomē*, incision]

**achlor·hy·dria** (ā-klōr-hī'drē-ă) absence of hydrochloric acid from the gastric juice. [G. *a-* priv. + chlorhydric (acid)]

**achlor·o·phyl·lous** (ā-klōr-ōf'ĭ-lŭs) without chlorophyll, as in fungi.

**acho·lia** (ă-kō'lē-ă) suppressed or absent secretion of bile. [G. *a-* priv. + *cholē*, bile]

**achol·ic** (ă-kol'ik) without bile, as in acholic (pale) stools.

**achol·u·ria** (ā-kol-yur'-ē-ă) absence of bile pigments from the urine in certain cases of jaundice. [G. *a-* priv. + *cholē*, bile, + *ouron*, urine]

**achol·u·ric** (ā-kōl-yu'rik) without bile in the urine.

**achol·u·ric jaun·dice** jaundice with excessive amounts of unconjugated bilirubin in the plasma and without bile pigments in the urine.

**achon·dro·gen·e·sis** (ā-kon-drō-jen'ē-sis) dwarfism accompanied by various bone aplasias of all four limbs, a normal or enlarged skull, and a short trunk with delayed ossification of the lower spine. [G. *a-* priv. + *chondros*, cartilage, + *genesis*, origin]

**achon·dro·gen·e·sis type IA** achondrogenesis with hypervascular cartilage and hypercellular bone; uncertain inheritance pattern. SYN Houston-Harris syndrome.

**achon·dro·gen·e·sis type IB** achondrogenesis with severely disorganized intracartilaginous ossification; autosomal recessive inheritance, caused by mutation in the diastrophic dysplasia sulfate transporter gene (DTDST) on chromosome 5q. SYN Parenti-Fraccaro syndrome.

**achon·dro·gen·e·sis type II** achondrogenesis with autosomal dominant inheritance, caused by mutation in the collagen type II gene (COL2A1) on chromosome 12q. SYN Langer-Saldino syndrome.

**achon·dro·pla·sia** (ā-kon-drō-plā'zē-ă) a type of chondrodystrophy characterized by an abnormality in conversion of cartilage into bone, predominantly affecting long bones, in which epiphysial growth is retarded and ceases early, resulting in dwarfism apparent at birth, with short limbs but normal trunk. SYN achondroplastic dwarfism. [G. *a-* priv. + *chondros*, cartilage, + *plasis*, a molding]

**achon·dro·plas·tic** (ă-kon-drō-plas'tik) relating to or characterized by achondroplasia.

**achon·dro·plas·tic dwarf·ism** SYN achondroplasia.

**achres·tic a·ne·mia** a form of chronic progressive macrocytic anemia that can be fatal in which the changes in bone marrow and circulating blood closely resemble those of pernicious anemia, but in which there is only transient or no response to therapy with vitamin B$_{12}$; glossitis, gastrointestinal disturbances, central nervous system disease, and pyrexia are not observed, and there is only little bleeding or hemolysis. [G. *a-* priv. + *chrēsis*, a using]

**achro·ma·cyte** (ă-krō'mă-sīt) SYN achromocyte.

**ach·ro·mat·ic** (ak-rō-mat'ik) 1. colorless. 2. not staining readily. 3. refracting light without chromatic aberration. [G. *a-* priv. + *chrōma*, color]

**ach·ro·mat·ic lens** a compound lens made of two or more lenses having different indices of refraction, so correlated as to minimize chromatic aberration.

**ach·ro·mat·ic ob·jec·tive** an objective that is corrected for two colors chromatically, and one color spherically.

**ach·ro·mat·ic vi·sion** SYN achromatopsia.

**achro·ma·tism** (ă-krō'mă-tizm) 1. the quality of being achromatic. 2. the annulment of chromatic aberration by combining glasses of different refractive indices and different dispersion.

**achro·mat·o·cyte** (ā-krō-mat'ō-sīt) SYN achromocyte.

**achro·mat·o·phil** (ă-krō-mat'ō-fil) 1. not being colored by histologic or bacteriologic stains. SYN achromophilic, achromophilous. 2. a cell or tissue that cannot be stained in the usual way. SYN achromophil. [G. *a-* priv. + *chrōma*, color, + *philos*, fond]

**achro·ma·top·sia, achro·ma·top·sy** (ă-krō-mă-top'sē-ă, ă-krō'mă-top-sē) a severe congenital deficiency in color perception, often associated with nystagmus and reduced visual acuity. SYN achromatic vision, monochromatism (2). [G. *a-* priv. + *chrōma*, color, + *opsis*, vision]

**achro·ma·tous** (ă-krō'mă-tŭs) colorless.

**achro·ma·tu·ria** (ā-krō-mă-tyu'rē-ă) the passage of colorless or very pale urine. [G. *a-* priv. + *chrōma*, color, + *ouron*, urine]

**achro·mia** (ă-krō'mē-ă) 1. depigmentation; absence or loss of natural pigmentation of the skin and iris. SEE ALSO depigmentation. 2. inability of a cell or tissue to be colored by one or more biologic stains [G. *a-* priv. + *chrōma*, color]

**achro·mic** (ā-krō'mik) colorless.

*Achrom·o·bacter* (a'krō-mō-bak'ter) a Gram-negative bacterial genus of uncertain clinical significance, closely related to members of the *Alcaligenes* and *Ochrobactrum* species.

**achro·mo·cyte** (ă-krō'mō-sīt) a hypochromic, crescent-shaped erythrocyte, probably resulting from artifactual rupture of a red cell. SYN achromacyte, achromatocyte, ghost corpuscle, phantom corpuscle, Ponfick shadow, shadow (3), Traube corpuscle. [G. *a-* priv. + *chrōma*, color, + *kytos*, hollow (cell)]

**achro·mo·phil** (ă-krō'mō-fil) SYN achromatophil.

**achro·mo·phil·ic, achro·moph·i·lous** (ā-krō-mō-fil'ik, ā-krō-mof'i-lŭs) SYN achromatophil (1).

**achy·lia** (ă-kī'lē-ă) 1. absence of gastric juice or other digestive secretions. 2. absence of chyle. [G. *a-* priv. + *chylos*, juice]

**achy·lous** (ă-kī'lŭs) 1. lacking in gastric juice or other digestive secretions. 2. having no chyle. [G. *achylos*, without juice]

**ac·id** (as'id) 1. a compound yielding a hydrogen ion in a polar solvent (e.g., in water); acids form salts by replacing all or part of the ionizable hydrogen with an electropositive element or radical. 2. in popular language, any chemical compound that has a sour taste (given by the hydrogen ion). 3. sour; sharp to the taste. 4. relating to acid; giving an acid reaction. [L. *acidus*, sour]

**ac·id-ash di·et** SYN alkaline-ash diet.

**ac·id-base bal·ance** the normal balance between acid and base in the blood plasma, expressed in the hydrogen ion concentration or pH, resulting from the relative amounts of acidic and basic materials ingested and produced by body metabolism, compared to the relative amounts of acidic and basic materials excreted from the body and consumed by body metabolism; the normal state of acid-base balance is not one of neutrality, with equal concentrations of hydrogen and hydroxyl ions, but a more alkaline state with a certain excess of hydroxyl ions.

**ac·id cell** SYN parietal cell.

**ac·i·de·mia** (as-i-d-ē′mē-ă) an increase in the H-ion concentration of the blood or a fall below normal in pH, despite shifts in bicarbonate concentration. [acid + G. *haima*, blood]

**ac·id-fast** (as′id-fast) denoting bacteria that are not decolorized by acid-alcohol after having been stained with dyes such as basic fuchsin; e.g., the mycobacteria and a few nocardiae.

**ac·id fuch·sin** [CI 42685] a mixture of sulfonated salts of rosanilin and pararosanilin; used as an indicator dye and for staining of cytoplasm and collagen.

**a·ci·dic dyes** dyes which ionize in solution to produce negatively charged ions or anions; they consist of sodium salts of phenols and carboxylic acid dyes; their solutions tend to be neutral or slightly alkaline; examples are eosin and aniline blue.

**a·cid·i·fied se·rum test** lysis of the patient's red cells in acidified fresh serum, specific for paroxysmal nocturnal hemoglobinuria. SYN Ham test.

**acid·i·fy** (a-sid′i-fī) 1. to render acid. 2. to become acid.

**ac·id in·di·ges·tion** indigestion resulting from hyperchlorhydria; often used by the laity as a synonym for pyrosis.

**acid·i·ty** (a-sid′i-tē) 1. the state of being acid. 2. the acid content of a fluid.

**ac·i·do·phil, ac·i·do·phile** (ă-sid′ō-fil, ă-sid′ō-fīl) 1. SYN acidophilic. 2. one of the acid-staining cells of the anterior pituitary. 3. a microorganism that grows well in a highly acid medium. [acid + G. *philos*, fond]

**ac·i·do·phil ad·e·no·ma** a tumor of the adenohypophysis in which cell cytoplasm stains with acid dyes; often growth-hormone producing. SYN eosinophil adenoma.

**ac·i·do·phil·ic** (as′i-dō-fil′ik, ă-sid′ō-fil-ik) having an affinity for acid dyes; denoting a cell or tissue element that stains with an acid dye, such as eosin. SYN acidophil (1), acidophile, oxychromatic.

**ac·i·do·sis** (as-i-dō′sis) a pathologic state characterized by an increase in the concentration of hydrogen ions in the arterial blood above the normal level, 40 nmol/L, or pH 7.4; may be caused by an accumulation of carbon dioxide or acidic products of metabolism, or by a decrease in the concentration of alkaline compounds. [acid + G. -*ōsis*, condition]

**ac·id per·fu·sion test** SYN Bernstein test.

**ac·id phos·pha·tase** a phosphatase with an optimum pH of less than 7.0, notably present in the prostate gland.

**ac·id stain** a dye in which the anion is the colored component of the dye molecule, e.g., sodium eosinate (eosin).

**ac·id sul·fate** SYN bisulfate.

**ac·id tide** a temporary increase in the acidity of the urine occurring during fasting.

**acid·u·lous** (a-sid′yu-lŭs) acid or sour.

**ac·i·du·ria** (as-i-dyu′rē-ă) 1. excretion of an acid urine. 2. excretion of an abnormal amount of any specified acid. Individual types of aciduria are prefixed by the specific acid; e.g., aminoaciduria, ketoaciduria. [acid + G. *ouron*, urine]

**ac·i·du·ric** (as-i-dyu′rik) pertaining to bacteria that tolerate an acid environment. [acid + L. *duro*, to endure]

**ac·i·nar** (as′i-nar) pertaining to the acinus. SYN acinic.

**ac·i·nar cell** any secreting cell lining an acinus, especially applied to the cells of the pancreas that furnish pancreatic juice and enzymes to distinguish them from the cells of ducts and the islets of Langerhans. SYN acinous cell.

**ac·i·ni** (as′i-nī) plural of acinus.

**acin·ic** (a-sin′ik) SYN acinar.

**acin·ic cell ad·e·no·car·ci·no·ma** an adenocarcinoma arising from secreting cells of a racemose gland, particularly the salivary glands.

**acin·i·form** (a-sin′i-fŏrm) SYN acinous. [L. *acinus*, grape, + *forma*, shape]

**ac·i·ni·tis** (as-in-ī′tis) inflammation of an acinus.

**ac·i·nose** (as′i-nōs) SYN acinous.

**ac·i·no·tu·bu·lar gland** SYN tubuloacinar gland.

**ac·i·nous** (as′i-nŭs) resembling an acinus or grape-shaped structure. SYN aciniform, acinose.

**ac·i·nous cell** SYN acinar cell.

**ac·i·nous gland** a gland in which the secretory unit(s) has a grapelike shape and a very small lumen; e.g., the exocrine part of the pancreas.

**a-c interval** the interval between the onset of the a wave and that of the c wave of the jugular pulse.

**ac·i·nus**, gen. and pl. **ac·i·ni** (as′i-nŭs, as′i-nī) [TA] one of the minute grape-shaped secretory portions of an acinous gland. Some authorities use the terms acinus and alveolus interchangeably, whereas others differentiate them by the constricted openings of the acinus into the excretory duct. [L. berry, grape]

**ac·la·sis** (ak′lă-sis) a state of continuity between normal and abnormal tissue. [G. *a-* priv. + *klasis*, a breaking away, a fragment]

**ac·mes·the·sia** (ak-mes-thē′zē-ă) 1. sensitivity to pinprick. 2. a cutaneous sensation of a sharp point. [G. *acmē*, point, + *aisthēsis*, sensation]

**ac·ne** (ak′nē) an inflammatory follicular, papular, and pustular eruption involving the pilosebaceous apparatus. [probably a corruption (or copyist's error) of G. *akmē*, point of efflorescence]

**ac·ne con·glo·ba·ta** severe cystic acne, characterized by cystic lesions, abscesses, communicating sinuses, and thickened, nodular scars; usually sparing the face.

**ac·ne cos·me·ti·ca** low-grade, non-inflammatory acne lesions from repeated application of comedogenic agents in cosmetics.

**ac·ne er·y·the·ma·to·sa** SYN rosacea.

**ac·ne·form, ac·ne·i·form** (ak′nē-fŏrm, ak-nē′i-fŏrm) resembling acne.

**ac·ne ful·mi·nans** (ak′nē ful′mi-nanz) severe scarring acne in teenaged males, which may be associated with fever, polyarthralgia, crusted ulcerative lesions, weight loss, and anemia. [L. *fulmen, fulminis*, thunder, lightning]

**ac·ne in·du·ra·ta** deeply seated acne, with large

papules and pustules, large scars, and hypertrophic scars.

**ac·ne ke·loid** a chronic eruption of fibrous papules which develop at the site of follicular lesions, usually on the back of the neck at the hairline. SYN dermatitis papillaris capillitii, folliculitis keloidalis.

**ac·ne ke·ra·to·sa** an eruption of papules consisting of horny plugs projecting from the hair follicles, accompanied by inflammation.

**ac·ne me·di·ca·men·to·sa** acne caused or exacerbated by drugs.

**ac·ne ne·crot·i·ca miliaris** SYN acne varioliformis.

**ac·ne pa·pu·lo·sa** acne vulgaris in which papular lesions predominate.

**ac·ne punc·ta·ta** acne with black comedones.

**ac·ne pus·tu·lo·sa** acne vulgaris in which pustular lesions predominate.

**ac·ne ro·sa·cea** SYN rosacea.

**ac·ne va·ri·o·li·for·mis** a pyogenic infection involving follicles occurring chiefly on the forehead and temples, followed by scar formation. SYN acne necrotica miliaris.

**ac·ne vul·ga·ris** an eruption, predominantly of the face, upper back, and chest, composed of comedones, cysts, papules, and pustules on an inflammatory base; the condition occurs in a majority of cases during puberty and adolescence, due to androgenic stimulation of sebum secretion, with plugging of follicles by keratinization, associated with proliferation of *Propionibacterium acnes*.

**cis-ac·o·nit·ic ac·id** (sis-ak-ō-nit′ik as′-id) dehydration product of citric acid; an intermediate in the tricarboxylic acid cycle.

**aco·rea** (ă-kō′rē-ă) congenital absence of the pupil of the eye. [G. *a-* priv. + *korē,* pupil]

**A·cos·ta dis·ease** (ah-cōs′tah) SYN altitude sickness.

⚠ **-acou·sis 1.** suffix referring to hearing and the ability to hear. **2.** SYN hearing. SEE audio-, audition.

**acous·tic** (ă-koos′tik) pertaining to hearing and the perception of sound. [Gr. *akoustikos*]

**a·cous·ti·cal sur·round** SYN sound field.

**a·cous·tic me·a·tus 1.** external: auditory canal; the passage leading inward through the tympanic portion of the temporal bone, from the auricle to the membrana tympani; **2.** internal: a canal running through the petrous portion of the temporal bone, giving passage to the facial and vestibulocochlear nerves and to the labyrinthine artery and veins. SYN meatus acusticus.

**a·cous·tic nerve** SYN vestibulocochlear nerve [CN VIII].

**a·cous·tic neu·ro·ma, a·cous·tic neu·ri·le·mo·ma** a benign tumor arising from Schwann cells of the auditory nerve (8th cranial nerve).

**a·cous·tic ra·di·a·tion** the fibers that pass from the medial geniculate body to the transverse temporal gyri of the cerebral cortex by way of the sublentiform part of the internal capsule. SYN radiatio acustica [TA].

**a·cous·tic re·flex** contraction of the stapedius muscle in response to intense sound, increasing impedance of the middle ear and thereby protecting the inner ear from the sound. SYN stapedial reflex.

**a·cous·tic re·flex thres·hold (ART)** lowest

sound intensity required to elicit contraction of the stapedius muscle in the middle ear.

**acous·tics** (ă-koos′tiks) the science concerned with sounds and their perception. [G. *akoustikos,* relating to hearing]

**a·cous·tic stim·u·la·tion test** a test for fetal well-being through use of an acoustic device to stimulate the fetus and cause acceleration of fetal heart rate.

**a·cous·tic trau·ma hearing loss** sensory hearing loss due to exposure to high-intensity noise.

**ACP** acyl carrier protein.

**ac·quired** (ă-kwīrd′) denoting a disease, condition, or abnormality that is not inherited. [L. *acquiro* (*adq-*), to obtain, fr. *quaero,* to seek]

**ac·quired cen·tric** SYN centric occlusion.

**ac·quired char·ac·ter** a character developed in a plant or animal as a result of environmental influences during the individual's life.

**ac·quired drives** SYN secondary drives.

**ac·quired ep·i·lep·tic a·pha·sia** SYN Landau-Kleffner syndrome.

**ac·quired hy·per·lip·o·pro·tein·e·mia** nonfamilial hyperlipoproteinemia that develops as a consequence of some primary disease, such as thyroid deficiency.

**ac·quired im·mu·ni·ty** resistance resulting from previous exposure of the individual in question to an infectious agent or antigen; it may be *active,* as a result of naturally acquired infection or vaccination; or *passive,* being acquired from transfer of antibodies from another person or from an animal, either from mother to fetus or by inoculation.

**ac·quired im·mu·no·de·fi·cien·cy syn·drome** SYN AIDS.

**ac·quired ne·vus** a melanocytic nevus that is not visible at birth, but appears in childhood or adult life.

**ac·quired tox·o·plas·mo·sis in a·dults** a form of toxoplasmosis that may result in fever, encephalomyelitis, chorioretinopathy, maculopapular rash, arthralgia, myalgia, myocarditis, and pneumonitis; a lymphadenopathic form seems to be more prevalent in adults, and such persons may manifest fever, lymphadenopathy, malaise, and headache, a form frequently found in patients with AIDS.

**ac·qui·si·tion** (ak-wi-zish′ŭn) PSYCHOLOGY the empirical demonstration of an increase in the strength of the conditioned response in successive trials of pairing the conditioned and unconditioned stimuli.

**ac·ral** (ak′răl) relating to or affecting the peripheral parts, e.g., limbs, fingers, ears, etc. [G. *akron,* extremity]

**Acra·nia** (ā-krā′nē-ă) a group of the phylum Chordata whose members possess a notochord, gill slits, and nerve cord but no vertebrae, ribs, or skull; e.g., *Amphioxus,* tunicates, and acorn worms. [G. *a-* priv. + *kranion,* skull]

**acra·nia** (ā-krā′nē-ă) complete or partial absence of a skull; associated with anencephaly. [G. *a-* priv. + *kranion,* skull]

**acra·ni·al** (ā-krā′nē-ăl) having no cranium; relating to acrania or an acranius.

**Ac·re·mo·ni·um** (ak-rĕ-mō′nē-ŭm) a genus of fungi (family Moniliaceae, order Moniliales) that causes keratomycosis and eumycotic mycetoma; produces the antibiotic cephalosporin.

**ac·ri·dine orange** (ak′ri-dēn aw′renj) [CI 46005]

10-azaanthracene; a basic fluorescent dye useful as a metachromatic stain for nucleic acids; also used in screening cervical smears for abnormal and malignant cells.

△**acro-** Combining form meaning: **1.** extremity, tip, end, peak, topmost. **2.** extreme. [G. *akron*, highest point, extremity; *akros*, topmost, outermost, inmost, extreme, tip]

**ac·ro·ag·no·sis** (ak'rō-ag-nō'sis) loss or impairment of the sensory recognition of a limb. Absence of acrognosis.

**ac·ro·an·es·the·sia** (ak'rō-an-es-thē'zē-ă) anesthesia of one or more of the extremities. [acro- + G. *an-* priv. + *aisthēsis* sensation]

**ac·ro·a·tax·ia** (ak'rō-ă-tak'sē-ă) ataxia affecting the distal portion of the extremities, i.e., hands and fingers, feet, and toes. Cf. proximoataxia. [acro- + ataxia]

**ac·ro·blast** (ak'rō-blast) component of the developing spermatid composed of numerous Golgi elements; it contains the proacrosomal granules. [acro- + G. *blastos*, germ]

**ac·ro·brach·y·ceph·a·ly** (ak'rō-brak-i-sef'ă-lē) type of craniosynostosis with premature closure of the coronal suture. [acro- + G. *brachys*, short, + *kephalē*, head]

**ac·ro·cen·tric** (ak-rō-sen'trik) having the centromere close to one end; said of a normal chromosome. [acro- + G. *kentron*, center]

**ac·ro·cen·tric chro·mo·some** a chromosome with the centromere placed very close to one end so that the short arm is very small, often with a satellite.

**ac·ro·ce·phal·ic** (ak-rō-se-fal'ik) SYN oxycephalic.

**ac·ro·ceph·a·lo·syn·dac·ty·ly** (ak'rō-sef'ă-lō-sin-dak'ti-lē) a group of congenital syndromes characterized by peaking of the cranium and fusion or webbing of digits. [acrocephaly + G. *syn*, together, + *daktylos*, finger]

**ac·ro·ceph·a·lous** (ak-rō-sef'ă-lŭs) SYN oxycephalic.

**ac·ro·ceph·a·ly, ac·ro·ce·pha·lia** (ak'rō-sef'ă-lē, ak-rō-se-fā'lē-ă) SYN oxycephaly. [acro- + G. *kephalē*, head]

**ac·ro·chor·don** (ak-rō-kōr'don) SYN skin tag. [acro- + G. *chordē*, cord]

**ac·ro·cy·a·no·sis** (ak'rō-sī-ă-nō'sis) a circulatory disorder in which the hands, and less commonly the feet, are persistently cold and blue; some forms are related to Raynaud phenomenon. SYN Crocq disease, Raynaud sign. [acro- + G. *kyanos*, blue, + *-osis*, condition]

**ac·ro·cy·a·not·ic** (ak'rō-sī-ă-not'ik) characterized by acrocyanosis.

**ac·ro·der·ma·ti·tis** (ak'rō-der-mă-tī'tis) inflammation of the skin of the extremities. [acro- + G. *derma*, skin, + *-itis*, inflammation]

**ac·ro·der·ma·ti·tis chron·i·ca a·troph·i·cans** a late skin manifestation of Lyme disease, appearing first on the feet, hands, elbows, or knees, and composed of indurated, erythematous plaques that become atrophic.

**ac·ro·der·ma·ti·tis con·tin·u·a** SYN pustulosis palmaris et plantaris.

**ac·ro·der·ma·ti·tis per·stans** SYN pustulosis palmaris et plantaris.

**ac·ro·der·ma·to·sis** (ak'rō-der-mă-tō'sis) any cutaneous affection involving the more distal portions of the extremities. [acro- + G. *derma*, skin, + *-osis*, condition]

**ac·ro·dyn·ia** (ak-rō-din'ē-ă) **1.** pain in peripheral or acral parts of the body. **2.** a syndrome caused almost exclusively by mercury poisoning: in children, characterized by erythema of the extremities, chest, and nose, polyneuritis, and gastrointestinal symptoms; in adults, by anorexia, photophobia, sweating, and tachycardia. SYN dermatopolyneuritis, erythredema, Feer disease, pink disease, Swift disease. [acro- + G. *odynē*, pain]

**ac·ro·es·the·sia** (ak'ro-es-thē'zē-ă) **1.** an extreme degree of hyperesthesia. **2.** hyperesthesia of one or more of the extremities. [acro- + G. *aisthēsis*, sensation]

**ac·rog·no·sis** (ak-rog-nō'sis) cenesthesia, or normal sensory perception, of the extremities. [acro- + G. *gnōsis*, knowledge]

**ac·ro·ker·a·to·sis** (ak'rō-ker-ă-tō'sis) nodular overgrowth of the horny layer of the skin on the fingers and toes, and occasionally on the ear and nose. [acro- + G. *keras*, horn, + *-osis*, condition]

**ac·ro·me·gal·ic** (ak'rō-mĕ-gal'ik) pertaining to or characterized by acromegaly.

**ac·ro·meg·a·ly** (ak-rō-meg'ă-lē) a disorder marked by progressive enlargement of the head, face, hands, and feet, due to excessive secretion of somatotropin; organomegaly and metabolic disorders occur; diabetes mellitus may develop. [acro- + G. *megas*, large]

**ac·ro·mel·al·gia** (ak-rō-mel-al'jē-ă) SEE erythromelalgia. [acro- + G. *melos*, limb, + *algos*, pain]

**ac·ro·me·lia** (ak-rō-mē'lē-ă) SYN acromesomelia.

**ac·ro·mel·ic** (ak-rō-mel'ik) affecting the terminal part of a limb. [acro- + G. *melos*, limb]

**ac·ro·mes·o·me·lia** (ak'rō-mē-sō-mē'lē-ă) a form of dwarfism in which shortening is striking in the most distal segment of the limbs; autosomal recessive inheritance. SYN acromelia. [acro- + G. *melos*, limb, + *ia*, condition]

**ac·ro·mes·o·mel·ic dwarfism** a form of short-limb dwarfism characterized by pug-nose and shortening particularly striking in the distal segment of the limbs, i.e., the forearms and lower legs, fingers and toes; autosomal recessive inheritance.

**ac·ro·met·a·gen·e·sis** (ak'rō-met-ă-jen'ĕ-sis) abnormal growth of the limbs resulting in deformity. [acro- + G. *meta*, beyond, + *genesis*, origin]

**acro·mi·al** (ă-krō'mē-ăl) relating to the acromion.

**a·cro·mi·al an·gle** the prominent angle at the junction of the posterior and lateral borders of the acromion. SYN angulus acromii [TA].

**a·cro·mi·al pro·cess** SYN acromion.

**acro·mi·o·cla·vic·u·lar** (ă-krō'mē-ō-kla-vik'yu-lăr) relating to the acromion and the clavicle; denoting the articulation and ligaments between the clavicle and the acromion of the scapula. SYN scapuloclavicular (1).

**a·cro·mi·o·cla·vic·u·lar joint** a plane synovial joint between the acromial end of the clavicle and the medial margin of the acromion.

**acro·mi·o·cor·a·coid** (ă-krō-mē-ō-kōr'ă-koyd) SYN coracoacromial.

**acro·mi·o·hu·mer·al** (ă-krō'mē-ō-hyu'mer-ăl) relating to the acromion and the humerus.

**acro·mi·on** (ă-krō'mē-on) the lateral end of the spine of the scapula, which projects as a broad flattened process overhanging the glenoid fossa; it articulates with the clavicle and gives attachment to part of the deltoid and trapezius muscles.

SYN acromial process. [G. *akrōmion*, fr. *akron*, tip, + *ōmos*, shoulder]

**acro·mi·o·scap·u·lar** (ă-krō′mē-ō-skap′yu-lăr) relating to both the acromion and body of the scapula.

**acro·mi·o·tho·rac·ic** (ă-krō′mē-ō-thō-ras′ik) SYN thoracoacromial.

**a·cro·mi·o·tho·rac·ic ar·tery** SYN thoracoacromial artery.

**ac·ro·my·o·to·nia, ac·ro·my·ot·o·nus** (ak′rō-mī-ō-tō′nē-ă, ak-rō-mī-ot′ō-nŭs) myotonia affecting the extremities only, resulting in spastic deformity of the hand or foot. [acro- + G. *mys*, muscle, + *tonos*, tension]

**ac·ro·os·te·ol·y·sis** (ak′rō-os-tē-ol′i-sis) congenital condition manifested by palmar and plantar ulcerating lesions with osteolysis involving distal phalanges of the fingers and toes. [acro- + G. *osteon*, bone, + *lysis*, loosening]

**ac·ro·par·es·the·sia** (ak′rō-par-es-thēs′ē-a) **1.** paresthesia of one or more of the extremities. **2.** nocturnal paresthesia involving the hands, most often of middle-aged women; formerly attributed to a lesion in the thoracic outlet, but now known to be a classic symptom of carpal tunnel syndrome. [acro- + paresthesia]

**ac·ro·pho·bia** (ak-rō-fō′bē-ă) morbid fear of heights. [acro- + G. *phobos*, fear]

**ac·ro·pus·tu·lo·sis** (ak′rō-pŭs-tyu-lō′sis) pustular eruptions of the hands and feet, often a form of psoriasis. [acro- + pustulosis]

**ac·ro·scle·ro·sis, ac·ro·scle·ro·der·ma** (ak′rō-sklē-rō′sis, ak′rō-sklēr-ō-der′mă) stiffness and tightness of the skin of the fingers, with atrophy of the soft tissue and osteoporosis of the distal phalanges of the hands and feet; a limited form of progressive systemic sclerosis occurring with Raynaud phenomenon. SEE CREST syndrome. SYN sclerodactyly, sclerodactylia.

**ac·ro·sin** (ak′rō-sin) a serine proteinase in spermatozoa similar in specificity to trypsin.

**ac·ro·so·mal cap** a collapsed membranous vesicle that covers the anterior part of the nucleus of the spermatid, derived from the acrosomal granule. SYN head cap.

**ac·ro·so·mal gran·ule** the single glycoprotein-rich granule within an acrosomal vesicle, which results from the coalescence of proacrosomal granules.

**ac·ro·so·mal ves·i·cle** a vesicle derived from the Golgi apparatus during spermiogenesis; together with the acrosomal granule within, it spreads in a thin layer over the pole of the nucleus to form the acrosomal cap.

**ac·ro·some** (ak′rō-sōm) a cap-like organelle that surrounds the anterior two-thirds of the nucleus of a sperm cell. Within this cap are enzymes that are thought to facilitate entry of the spermatozoon into the oocyte. [acro- + G. *soma*, body]

**acrot·ic** (ă-krot′ik) marked by weakness or absence of the pulse; pulseless. [G. *a-* priv. + *krotos*, a striking]

**ac·ro·tism** (ak′rō-tizm) absence or imperceptibility of the pulse. [G. *a-* priv. + *krotos*, a striking]

**ACT** activated clotting time.

**ACTH** adrenocorticotropic hormone.

**ACTH-pro·duc·ing ad·e·no·ma** a pituitary tumor composed of corticotrophs that produce ACTH, often a basophilic adenoma; may give rise to Cushing disease or Nelson syndrome.

**ac·tin** (ak′tin) one of the protein components into which actomyosin can be split; it can exist in a fibrous form (F-actin) or a globular form (G-actin).

**ac·tin fil·a·ment** one of the contractile elements in muscular fibers and other cells; in skeletal muscle, the actin filaments are about 5 nm wide and 100 μm long, and attach to the transverse Z filaments.

**ac·tin·ic** (ak-tin′ik) relating to the chemically active rays of the electromagnetic spectrum particularly to sunlight. [G. *aktis* (*aktin-*), a ray]

**ac·tin·ic der·ma·ti·tis** SYN photodermatitis.

**ac·tin·ic gran·u·lo·ma** an annular eruption on sun-exposed skin which microscopically shows phagocytosis of dermal elastic fibers by giant cells and histiocytes. SYN Miescher granuloma.

**⊟ac·tin·ic ker·a·to·sis** a premalignant warty lesion occurring on the sun-exposed skin of the face or hands in aged light-skinned persons; hyperkeratosis may form a cutaneous horn, and squamous cell carcinoma of low-grade malignancy may develop in a small proportion of untreated patients. See page B6.

**ac·tin·ides** (ak′tin-īdz) those elements with atomic numbers 89 to 103, corresponding to the lanthanides in the Periodic Table. [*actinium*, first element of the series]

**ac·tin·i·um (Ac)** (ak-tin′ē-ŭm) an element, atomic no. 89, atomic wt. 227.05; it possesses no stable isotopes and exists in nature only as a disintegration product of uranium and thorium. [G. *aktis*, a ray]

**△actino-** combining form meaning a ray, as of light; applied to any form of radiation or to any structure with radiating parts. SEE ALSO radio-. [G. *aktis*, *aktinos*, a ray of light, a beam.]

*Ac·ti·no·ba·cil·lus* (ak′tin-ō-bă-sil′lŭs) a genus of nonmotile, nonsporeforming, aerobic, facultatively anaerobic bacteria (family Brucellaceae) containing Gram-negative rods interspersed with coccal elements. The metabolism of these bacteria is fermentative. They are pathogenic to animals. The type species is *Actinobacillus lignieresii*. [actino- + L. *bacillus*, little rod]

*Ac·ti·no·ba·cil·lus ac·ti·no·my·ce·tem·co·mi·tans* a species of doubtful taxonomic position; frequently associated with human periodontal disease as well as subacute and chronic endocarditis; occurs with actinomycetes in actinomycotic lesions.

**ac·ti·no·der·ma·ti·tis** (ak′ti-nō-der-mă-tī′tis) SYN photodermatitis.

*Ac·ti·no·mad·u·ra* (ak′ti-nō-mad′yu-ră) a genus of aerobic, Gram-positive, non-acid-fast fungi whose filaments fragment into spores. *Actinomadura pelletieri* is an agent of mycetoma. [actino- + *Madura*, India]

*Ac·ti·no·ma·du·ra la·tin·a* a species of bacteria associated with mycetoma in South America.

*Ac·ti·no·ma·du·ra pel·let·i·er·i* SEE *Actinomadura latina*.

*Ac·ti·no·my·ces* (ak′ti-nō-mī′sēz) a genus of slow-growing, nonmotile, nonsporeforming, anaerobic to facultatively anaerobic bacteria (family Actinomycetaceae) containing Gram-positive, irregularly staining filaments. These organisms can cause chronic suppurative infection in humans. The type species is *Actinomyces bovis*. [actino- + G. *mykēs*, fungus]

*Ac·ti·no·my·ces bo·vis* a species of bacteria causing actinomycosis in cattle; infection in humans is not established; it is the type species of its genus.

**Ac·ti·no·my·ces is·rae·li·i** a species of bacteria causing human actinomycosis and, occasionally, infections in cattle.

**Ac·ti·no·my·ce·ta·ce·ae** (ak'ti-nō-mī'sē-tā'sē-ē) a family of nonsporeforming, nonmotile, facultatively anaerobic bacteria (order Actinomycetales) containing Gram-positive, non-acid-fast, predominantly diphtheroid cells which tend to form branched filaments. This family contains the genera *Actinomyces* (type genus), *Arachnia, Bacterionema, Bifidobacterium,* and *Rothia*.

**Ac·ti·no·my·ce·ta·les** (ak'ti-nō-mī'sē-tā'lēz) an order of bacteria consisting of moldlike, rod-shaped, clubbed or filamentous forms with tendency to branching; it includes the families Mycobacteriaceae, Actinomycetaceae, Streptomycetaceae, and Nocardiaceae.

**ac·ti·no·my·cetes** (ak'ti-nō-mī-sē'tēz) a term used to refer to members of the genus *Actinomyces;* sometimes improperly used to refer to any member of the family Actinomycetaceae or order Actinomycetales.

**ac·ti·no·my·ce·to·ma** (ak'tin-ō-mī-set-ō'ma) mycetoma caused by higher bacteria. Cf. eumycetoma.

**ac·ti·no·my·co·ma** (ak'ti-nō-mī-kō'mǎ) a swelling caused by an actinomycete. SEE mycetoma. [actino- + G. *mykēs,* fungus, + *-oma,* tumor]

**ac·ti·no·my·co·sis** (ak'ti-nō-mī-kō'sis) a disease primarily of cattle and humans caused by *Actinomyces bovis* in cattle and by *A. israelii* and *Arachnia propionica* in humans. These actinomycetes are part of the normal bacterial flora of the mouth and pharynx, but they may produce chronic destructive abscesses or granulomas which eventually discharge a viscid pus containing minute yellowish granules (sulfur granules). In humans, the disease commonly affects the cervicofacial area, abdomen, or thorax. [actino- + G. *mykēs,* fungus, + *-osis,* condition]

**ac·ti·no·my·cot·ic** (ak'ti-nō-mī-kot'ik) relating to actinomycosis.

**ac·ti·no·ther·a·py** (ak'ti-nō-thār'ă-pē) DERMATOLOGY ultraviolet light therapy.

**ac·tion** (ak'shŭn) **1.** the performance of any function, the manner of such performance, or its result. **2.** the exertion of any force or power, physical, chemical, or mental. [L. *actio,* from *ago,* pp. *actus,* to do]

**ac·tion cur·rent** an electrical current induced in muscle fibers when they are effectively stimulated; normally it is followed by contraction.

**ac·tion po·ten·tial** the change in membrane potential occurring in nerve, muscle, or other excitable tissue when excitation occurs.

**ac·ti·vat·ed clot·ting time (ACT)** the most common test used for coagulation time in cardiovascular surgery.

**ac·ti·vat·ed par·tial throm·bo·plas·tin time (aPTT)** the time needed for plasma to form a fibrin clot following the addition of calcium and a phospholipid reagent; used to evaluate the intrinsic clotting system.

**ac·ti·va·tion** (ak-ti-vā'shŭn) **1.** the act of rendering active. **2.** an increase in the energy content of an atom or molecule, through the raising of temperature, absorption of light photons, or other means. **3.** techniques of stimulating the brain by light, sound, electricity, or chemical agents, in order to elicit abnormal activity in the electroencephalogram. **4.** stimulation of peripheral nerve fibers to the point that action potentials are initiated. **5.** stimulation of cell division in an oocyte by fertilization or by artificial means. **6.** the act of making radioactive.

**ac·ti·va·tor** (ak'ti-vā-ter) **1.** a substance that renders another substance, or catalyst, active, or that accelerates a process or reaction. **2.** the fragment, produced by chemical cleavage of a proactivator, that induces the enzymic activity of another substance. **3.** an apparatus for making substances radioactive. **4.** a removable type of myofunctional orthodontic appliance that acts as a passive transmitter of force, produced by the function of the activated muscles, to the teeth and alveolar process that are in contact with it.

**ac·tive an·a·phy·lax·is** reaction following inoculation of antigen in a subject previously sensitized to the specific antigen, in contrast to passive anaphylaxis.

**ac·tive chron·ic hep·a·ti·tis** hepatitis with chronic portal inflammation and progressive hepatic degeneration; an autoimmune sequela to hepatitis B or C. SYN posthepatitic cirrhosis.

**ac·tive con·ges·tion** congestion due to an increased flow of arterial blood to a part of the body or organ.

**ac·tive cool-down** SYN active recovery.

**ac·tive hy·per·e·mia** hyperemia due to an increased afflux of arterial blood into dilated capillaries. SYN fluxionary hyperemia.

**ac·tive im·mu·ni·ty** SEE acquired immunity.

**ac·tive meth·yl** a methyl group attached to a quaternary ammonium ion or a tertiary sulfonium ion that can take part in transmethylation reactions.

**ac·tive prin·ci·ple** a constituent of a drug, usually an alkaloid or glycoside, upon the presence of which the characteristic therapeutic action of the substance largely depends.

**ac·tive re·cov·ery** exercising with gradually diminishing intensity immediately after a bout of vigorous exercise; facilitates lactate removal by maintaining blood flow in muscles during recovery. SYN active cool-down, tapering-off.

**ac·tive re·pres·sor** a repressor that combines directly with an operator gene to repress the operator and its structural genes, thus repressing protein synthesis; an active repressor may be repressed by an inducer, with resulting protein synthesis; a homeostatic mechanism for regulation of inducible enzyme systems.

**ac·tive site** that portion of an enzyme molecule at which the actual reaction proceeds; one or more residues or atoms in a spatial arrangement that permits interaction with the substrate.

**ac·tive splint** SYN dynamic splint.

**ac·tive trans·port** the passage of ions or molecules across a cell membrane, not by passive diffusion but by an energy-consuming process against an electrochemical gradient.

**ac·tiv·in** (ak'ti-vin) placental hormone that reaches maximum levels in maternal serum during labor. [active + -in]

**ac·tiv·i·ties of dai·ly liv·ing (ADL)** activities that an average person performs routinely in the course of a day, such as bathing, dressing, and meal preparation. An inability to perform these renders one dependent on others, resulting in a self-care deficit. A major goal of occupational therapy is to enable the client to perform activities of daily living.

**ac·tiv·i·ties of dai·ly liv·ing scale** a scale to score physical activity and its limitations, based on answers to simple questions about mobility, self-care, grooming, etc; widely used in geriatrics, rheumatology, etc.

**ac·tiv·i·ty** (ak-tiv′i-tē) **1.** in electroencephalography, the presence of neurogenic electrical energy. **2.** in physical chemistry, an ideal concentration for which the law of mass action will apply perfectly; the ratio of the activity to the true concentration is the activity coefficient (γ), which becomes 1.00 at infinite dilution. **3.** for enzymes, the amount of substrate consumed (or product formed) in a given time under given conditions; turnover number. **4.** the number of nuclear transformations (disintegrations) in a given quantity of a material per unit time. Units: curie (Ci), millicurie (mCi), becquerel (Bq), megabecquerel (MBq). SEE ALSO radioactivity.

**ac·tiv·i·ty ad·ap·ta·tion** the process that changes an aspect of an activity to make successful performance possible and thus to accomplish a particular therapeutic goal.

**ac·tiv·i·ty a·nal·y·sis** the process of examining an activity or movement pattern in order to distinguish its component parts. SYN biomechanical analysis.

**ac·tiv·i·ty co·ef·fi·cient** (γ) SEE activity (2).

**ac·tiv·i·ty grad·ing** changing incrementally the process, tools, materials, or environment of a given activity in order to increase or decrease performance demands gradually, and in order ultimately to ensure best performance. SYN sport-specific training.

**ac·tiv·i·ty group** a group designed to assist individuals who share common concerns or problems related to the acquisition or maintenance of performance components and occupational skills.

**ac·tiv·i·ty pat·tern a·nal·y·sis** any method of determining the type, amount, and organization of activity that occupies the lives of individuals on a recurring basis.

**ac·tiv·i·ty syn·the·sis** the process of combining component parts of the human and nonhuman environment so as to design an activity suitable for evaluation or intervention.

**ac·to·my·o·sin** (ak′tō-mī′ō-sin) a protein complex composed of actin and myosin; the essential contractile substance of muscle fiber.

**ac·tu·al cau·tery** a cautery acting directly through heat and not by chemical means.

**acu·i·ty** (ă-kyu′i-tē) sharpness, clearness, distinctness. **2.** severity. [thr. Fr., fr. L. *acuo*, pp. *acutus*, sharpen]

**acu·le·ate** (ă-kyu′lē-āt) pointed; covered with sharp spines. [L. *aculeatus*, pointed, fr. *acus*, needle]

**acu·men·tin** (ak-yu-men′tin) a neutrophil and macrophage motility protein that links to the actin molecule to control filament length.

**acu·mi·nate** (ă-kyu′mi-nāt) pointed; tapering to a point. [L. *acumino*, pp. *-atus*, to sharpen]

**acu·pres·sure** (ak′yu-pre′sher) application of pressure in sites used for acupuncture with therapeutic intent.

**acu·punc·ture** (ak-yu-punk′cher) puncture with long, fine needles: **1.** an ancient Asian system of healing. **2.** more recently, acupuncture anesthesia or analgesia. [L. *acus*, needle, + puncture]

**acu·punc·ture an·es·the·sia** percutaneous insertion of, and stimulation by, needles placed in critical areas of the body to produce loss of sensation in another area.

**a·cute** (ă-kyut′) **1.** referring to a disease: brief, not chronic; sometimes loosely used to mean severe. **2.** referring to treatment or exposure: brief, intense, short-term; sometimes specifically referring to brief exposure of high intensity. [L. *acutus*, sharp]

**a·cute ab·do·men** any serious acute intra-abdominal condition (such as appendicitis) attended by pain, tenderness, and muscular rigidity, and for which emergency surgery must be considered. SYN surgical abdomen.

**a·cute a·dre·no·cor·ti·cal in·suf·fi·cien·cy** severe adrenocortical insufficiency when an illness or trauma causes an increased demand for adrenocortical hormones in a patient with adrenal insufficiency. SYN addisonian crisis, adrenal crisis.

**a·cute Af·ri·can sleep·ing sick·ness** (af′-ri-kăn) SYN Rhodesian trypanosomiasis.

**a·cute an·te·ri·or po·li·o·my·e·li·tis** inflammation of the anterior cornua of the spinal cord; an acute infectious disease caused by the poliomyelitis virus and marked by fever, pains, and gastroenteric disturbances, followed by a flaccid paralysis of one or more muscular groups, and later by atrophy.

**a·cute as·cend·ing pa·ral·y·sis** a paralysis of rapid course beginning in the legs and involving progressively the trunk, arms, and neck, ending sometimes in death in from one to three weeks.

**a·cute bul·bar po·li·o·my·e·li·tis** poliomyelitis virus infection affecting nerve cells in the medulla oblongata and producing paralysis of the lower motor cranial nerves.

**a·cute care hos·pi·tal** a hospital where inpatients have an average length of stay of 30 days or less.

**a·cute com·pres·sion tri·ad** the rising venous pressure, falling arterial pressure, and decreased heart sounds of pericardial tamponade. SYN Beck triad.

**a·cute con·ta·gious con·junc·ti·vi·tis** acute conjunctivitis marked by intense hyperemia and profuse mucopurulent discharge. SYN pinkeye (1).

**a·cute dis·sem·i·nat·ed en·ceph·a·lo·my·e·li·tis** an acute demyelinating disorder of the central nervous system, in which focal demyelination is present throughout the brain and spinal cord. This process is common to postinfectious, postexanthem, and postvaccinal encephalomyelitis.

**a·cute ep·i·dem·ic leu·ko·en·ceph·a·li·tis** a disease characterized by acute onset of fever, followed by convulsions, delirium, and coma, and associated with perivascular demyelination and hemorrhagic foci in the central nervous system. SYN Strümpell disease (2).

**a·cute ful·mi·nat·ing me·nin·go·coc·ce·mia** rapidly systemic infection with *Neisseria meningitidis*, usually without meningitis, characterized by rash, usually petechial or purpuric, high fever, and hypotension. May lead to death within hours.

**a·cute hem·or·rhag·ic con·junc·ti·vi·tis** specific acute endemic conjunctivitis with eyelid swelling, tearing, conjunctival hemorrhages, and follicles; usually caused by Enterovirus type 70.

**a·cute hem·or·rhag·ic pan·cre·a·ti·tis** an

acute inflammation of the pancreas accompanied by the formation of necrotic areas and hemorrhages into the substance of the gland; clinically marked by sudden severe abdominal pain, nausea, fever, and leukocytosis; areas of fat necrosis are present on the surface of the pancreas and in the omentum due to the action of the escaped pancreatic enzyme (trypsin and lipase).

a•cute id•i•o•path•ic pol•y•neu•ri•tis a neurological syndrome, probably an immune-mediated disorder, often a sequela of certain virus infections, marked by paresthesia of the limbs and muscular weakness or a flaccid paralysis; the characteristic laboratory finding is increased protein in the cerebrospinal fluid without increase in cell count.

a•cute in•flam•ma•tion any inflammation that has a fairly rapid onset, quickly becomes severe, usually manifested for only a few days; characterized histopathologically by edema, hyperemia, and infiltrates of polymorphonuclear leukocytes.

a•cute in•flam•ma•tory de•my•e•li•nat•ing pol•y•ra•dic•u•lo•neu•rop•a•thy the classic type of Guillain-Barré syndrome, in which the predominant type of underlying nerve fiber pathology is demyelination. SEE ALSO acute motor axonal neuropathy.

a•cute in•ter•mit•tent por•phyr•ia, a•cute por•phyr•i•a SYN intermittent acute porphyria.

a•cute iso•lat•ed my•o•car•di•tis an acute interstitial myocarditis of unknown cause, the endocardium and pericardium being unaffected. SYN Fiedler myocarditis.

a•cute lym•pho•cy•tic leu•ke•mi•a (ALL) SEE lymphocytic leukemia.

a•cute ma•lar•ia a form of malaria consisting of a chill accompanied and followed by fever with its attendant general symptoms, and terminating in a sweating stage; the paroxysms, caused by release of merozoites from infected cells, recur every 48 hours in tertian (vivax or ovale) malaria, every 72 hours in quartan (malariae) malaria, and at indefinite but frequent intervals, usually about 48 hours, in malignant tertian (falciparum) malaria.

a•cute mas•sive liv•er ne•cro•sis a lesion in which there is extensive and rapid death of parenchymal cells of the liver, sometimes with fatty degeneration; the necrosis may result from fulminant viral infection or chemical poisoning; associated with jaundice.

a•cute mo•tor ax•o•nal neu•rop•a•thy an acute, pure motor axon-degenerating type of polyradiculoneuropathy, a variant of Guillain-Barré syndrome; seen principally in a seasonal pattern (spring or summer) among children in rural China following epidemics of diarrhea caused by *Campylobacter jejuni*.

a•cute mul•ti•fo•cal plac•oid pig•ment ep•i•the•li•op•a•thy an acute disease manifested by rapid loss of vision, and multifocal, cream-colored placoid lesions of the retinal pigment epithelium; resolves with restoration of vision.

a•cute nec•ro•tiz•ing en•ceph•a•li•tis an acute form of encephalitis, characterized by destruction of brain parenchyma.

a•cute nec•ro•tiz•ing hem•or•rhag•ic en•ceph•a•lo•my•e•li•tis a fulminating demyelinating disorder of the central nervous system that affects mainly children and young adults. Almost always preceded by a respiratory infection, char-

acterized by the abrupt onset of fever, headache, confusion, and nuchal rigidity, soon followed by focal seizures, hemiplegia, or quadriplegia, brainstem findings, and coma. SYN Hurst disease.

a•cute nec•ro•tiz•ing ul•cer•a•tive gin•gi•vi•tis (ANUG) SEE necrotizing ulcerative gingivitis.

a•cute phase re•ac•tion refers to the changes in synthesis on certain proteins within the serum during an inflammatory response; this response provides rapid protection for the host against microorganisms via nonspecific defense mechanisms. SYN acute phase response.

a•cute phase res•ponse SYN acute phase reaction.

a•cute pro•my•e•lo•cyt•ic leu•ke•mia leukemia presenting as a severe bleeding disorder, with infiltration of the bone marrow by abnormal promyelocytes and myelocytes, a low plasma fibrinogen, and defective coagulation.

a•cute pul•mo•nary al•ve•o•li•tis acute inflammation involving formation of exudate in pulmonary alveoli and impaired gas exchange; may result in necrosis with hemorrhage into the lungs; occurs in Goodpasture syndrome, in association with glomerulonephritis.

a•cute res•pi•ra•to•ry fail•ure (ARF) loss of pulmonary function either acute or chronic that results in hypoxemia or hypercarbia.

a•cute ret•i•nal ne•cro•sis (ARN) a viral syndrome occurring in immunocompetent patients, characterized by peripheral retinal destruction that becomes circumferential and leads to retinal detachment.

a•cute rhi•ni•tis an acute catarrhal inflammation of the mucous membrane of the nose, marked by sneezing, lacrimation, and a profuse secretion of watery mucus; usually associated with infection by one of the common cold viruses. SYN coryza.

a•cute sen•sor•y-mo•tor ax•o•nal neu•rop•a•thy an acute axon-degenerating polyradiculoneuropathy that affects both motor and sensory fibers; a variant of Guillain-Barré syndrome.

a•cute sit•u•a•tion•al re•ac•tion SYN stress reaction.

a•cute try•pan•o•so•mi•a•sis SYN Rhodesian trypanosomiasis.

a•cute tu•ber•cu•lo•sis a rapidly fatal disease due to the general dissemination of tubercle bacilli in the blood, resulting in the formation of miliary tubercles in various organs and tissues, and producing symptoms of profound toxemia. SYN disseminated tuberculosis.

a•cute yel•low at•ro•phy of the liv•er a lesion in which there is extensive and rapid death of parenchymal cells of the liver, sometimes with fatty degeneration; may result from fulminant viral infection or chemical poisoning; associated with jaundice. SYN Rokitansky disease.

acy•a•not•ic (ă-sī-ă-not′ik) characterized by absence of cyanosis.

a•cy•clic com•pound an organic compound in which the chain does not form a ring. SYN open chain compound.

ac•yl (as′il) an organic radical derived from an organic acid by the removal of the carboxylic hydroxyl group.

ac•yl•am•i•dase (as-il-am′i-dās) SYN amidase.

ac•yl car•ri•er pro•tein (ACP) one of the proteins of the complex in cytoplasm that contains all of the enzymes required to convert acetyl-CoA (and, in certain cases, butyryl-CoA or propionyl-CoA) and malonyl-CoA to palmitic acid. This complex is tightly bound together in mammalian tissues and in yeast, but that from *Escherichia coli* is readily dissociated. The ACP thus isolated is a heat-stable protein with a molecular weight of about 10,000. It contains a free –SH that binds the acyl intermediates in the synthesis of fatty acids as thioesters. This –SH group is part of a 4′-phosphopantetheine, added to the apoprotein by ACP phosphodiesterase, which thus plays the same role that it does in coenzyme A. ACP is involved in every step of the fatty acid synthetic process.

**ac·yl-CoA** condensation product of a carboxylic acid and coenzyme A; metabolic intermediate of importance, notably in the oxidation and synthesis of fat.

**ac·yl-CoA de·hy·dro·gen·ase (NADPH)** enzyme catalyzing the reversible reduction of enoyl-CoA derivatives of chain length 4–16, with NADPH as the hydrogen donor, forming acyl-CoA and NADP⁺.

**ac·yl·trans·fer·ase** (as-il-trans′fer-ās) [EC class 2.3] an enzyme catalyzing the transfer of an acyl group from an acyl-CoA to any of various acceptors. SYN transacylases.

**acys·tia** (ā-sis′tē-ă) congenital absence of the urinary bladder. [G. *a-* priv. + *kystis,* bladder]

△**ad-** prefix denoting increase, adherence, to, toward; near; very. [L. *ad,* to, toward;]

△**-ad** in anatomical nomenclature, -ward; toward or in the direction of the part indicated by the main portion of the word. [L. *ad,* to]

**ADA** Americans with Disabilities Act.

**adac·ty·lous** (ā-dak′tĭ-lŭs) without fingers or toes.

**adac·ty·ly** (ā-dak′ti-lē) congenital absence of digits (fingers or toes). [G. *a-* priv. + *daktylos,* digit]

**ad·am·site (DM)** (ad′ăm-sīt) a vomiting agent that has been used in military training and in riot control. [Roger *Adams,* Am. chemist]

**Ad·ams-Stokes dis·ease** (ad′ămz-stōks) SYN Adams-Stokes syndrome.

**Ad·ams-Stokes syn·drome** (ad′ămz-stōks) a syndrome characterized by slow or absent pulse, vertigo, syncope, convulsions, and sometimes Cheyne-Stokes respiration; usually as a result of advanced A-V block or sick sinus syndrome. SYN Adams-Stokes disease, Morgagni disease, Spens syndrome, Stokes-Adams syndrome.

**ad·an·so·ni·an clas·si·fi·ca·tion** (ad′ăn-sō′nē-ăn) the classification of organisms based on giving equal weight to every character of the organism; this principle has its greatest application in numerical taxonomy. [M. *Adanson*]

**ad·ap·ta·tion** (ad-ap-tā′shŭn) **1.** preferential survival of members of a species because of a phenotype that gives them an enhanced capacity to withstand the environment. **2.** an advantageous change in function or constitution of an organ or tissue to meet new conditions. **3.** adjustment of the sensitivity of the retina to light intensity. **4.** a property of certain sensory receptors that modifies the response to repeated or continued stimuli at constant intensity. **5.** the fitting, condensing, or contouring of a restorative material, foil, or shell to a tooth or cast so as to be in close contact. **6.** the dynamic process wherein the thoughts, feelings, behavior, and biophysiologic mechanisms of the individual continually change to adjust to a

constantly changing environment. **7.** a homeostatic response. [L. *ad-apto,* pp. *-atus,* to adjust]

**adapt·er, adap·tor** (a-dap′ter, a-dap′ter) **1.** a connecting part, joining two pieces of apparatus. **2.** a converter of electric current to a desired form.

**adap·tive be·hav·ior scales** a behavioral assessment device to quantify the levels of skills of mentally retarded and developmentally delayed individuals in interacting with the environment; consists of three developmentally related factors: 1) personal self-sufficiency, e.g., eating, dressing; 2) community self-sufficiency, e.g., shopping, communicating; 3) personal and social responsibility, e.g., use of leisure time, job performance. SEE intelligence.

**a·dap·tive hy·per·tro·phy** thickening of the walls of a hollow organ, like the urinary bladder, when there is obstruction to outflow.

**ad·ap·tom·e·ter** (ad-ap-tom′ĕ-ter) a device for determining the course of retinal dark adaptation and for measuring the minimum light threshold.

**ADD** attention deficit disorder.

**ad·dict** (ad′ikt) a person who is habituated to a substance or practice, especially one considered harmful or illegal.

**ad·dic·tion** (ă-dik′shŭn) habitual psychological and physiological dependence on a substance or practice that is beyond voluntary control. [L. *ad-dico,* pp. *-dictus,* consent, fr. *ad-* + *dico,* to say]

**Ad·di·son ane·mia** (ad′ĭ-son) SYN pernicious anemia.

**Ad·di·son dis·ease** (ad′ĭ-son) SYN chronic adrenocortical insufficiency.

**ad·di·so·ni·an cri·sis** (ad′ĭ-sō′nē-ăn) SYN acute adrenocortical insufficiency.

**ad·di·tive** (ad′i-tiv) **1.** a substance not naturally a part of a material (e.g., food) but deliberately added to fulfill some specific purpose (e.g., preservation). **2.** tending to add or be added; denoting addition. **3.** in quantitative studies (e.g., genetics, epidemiology, physiology, statistics), having the property that the total combined effect of two or more factors equals the sum of their individual effects in isolation. Cf. synergism.

**ad·di·tive ef·fect** an effect wherein two or more substances or actions used in combination produce a total effect the same as the arithmetic sum of the individual effects.

**ad·dres·sin** (ad-res′in) a molecule on the surface of a cell that serves as a homing device to direct another molecule to a specific location. [address, fr. O.Fr. *adresser,* to direct, fr. L.L. *addirectiare,* fr. L. *ad,* to, + *directus,* straight, direct, + -in]

**ad·dres·in li·gands** ligands on cells for specific homing receptors on lymphocytes.

**ad·duct** (a-dŭkt′) to draw toward the median plane. [L. *ad-duco,* pp. *-ductus,* to bring toward]

■**ad·duc·tion** (ă-dŭk′shŭn) **1.** movement of a body part toward the median plane (of the body, in the case of limbs; of the hand or foot, in the case of digits). **2.** monocular rotation (duction) of the eye toward the nose. **3.** a position resulting from such movement. Cf. abduction. See page APP 90.

**ad·duc·tor** (ă-dŭk′ter) a muscle that draws a part toward the median plane; or, in the case of the digits, toward the normal axis of the middle finger or the second toe.

**ad·duc·tor bre·vis mus·cle** *origin,* superior ramus of pubis; *insertion,* upper third of medial lip of linea aspera; *action,* adducts thigh; *nerve sup-*

*ply*, obturator. SYN musculus adductor brevis [TA], short adductor muscle.

**ad·duc·tor ca·nal** the space in the middle third of the thigh between the vastus medialis and adductor muscles, converted into a canal by the overlying sartorius muscle. It gives passage to the femoral vessels and saphenous nerve, ending at the adductor hiatus. SYN canalis adductorius [TA], Hunter canal.

**ad·duc·tor hal·lu·cis mus·cle** *origin*, by two heads, the transverse head from the capsules of the lateral four metatarsophalangeal joints and the oblique head from the lateral cuneiform and bases of the third and fourth metatarsal bones; *insertion*, lateral side of base of proximal phalanx of great toe; *action*, adducts great toe; *nerve supply*, lateral plantar. SYN musculus adductor hallucis [TA].

**ad·duc·tor lon·gus mus·cle** *origin*, symphysis and crest of pubis; *insertion*, middle third of medial lip of linea aspera; *action*, adducts thigh; *nerve supply*, obturator. SYN musculus adductor longus [TA], long adductor muscle.

**ad·duc·tor mag·nus mus·cle** *origin*, ischial tuberosity and ischiopubic ramus; *insertion*, linea aspera and adductor tubercle of femur; *action*, adducts and extends thigh; *nerve supply*, obturator and sciatic. SYN musculus adductor magnus [TA], great adductor muscle.

**ad·duc·tor pol·li·cis mus·cle** *origin*, by two heads, the transverse head from the shaft of the third metacarpal and the oblique head from the front of the base of the second metacarpal, the trapezoid and capitate bones; *insertion*, medial side of base of proximal phalanx of thumb; *action*, adducts thumb; *nerve supply*, ulnar. SYN musculus adductor pollicis [TA].

**ad·duc·tor spas·mod·ic dys·pho·nia** a form of spasmodic dysphonia in which excessive closure of the vocal cords affects the initiation and maintenance of phonation.

**Ade** adenine.

**aden·drit·ic, aden·dric** (ā-den-drit′ik, ā-den′drik) without dendrites. [G., *a-* priv. + *dendron*, tree]

**ad·e·nec·to·my** (ad-ĕ-nek′tō-mē) excision of a gland. [aden- + G. *ektomē*, excision]

**ad·e·nec·to·pia** (ad′ĕ-nek-tō′pē-ă) presence of a gland other than in its normal anatomical position. [aden- + G. *ek*, out of, + *topos*, place]

**aden·i·form** (ă-den′i-fōrm) SYN adenoid (1).

**ad·e·nine (A, Ade)** (ad′ĕ-nēn) one of the two major purines (the other being guanine) found in both RNA and DNA, and also in various free nucleotides.

**ad·e·nine de·ox·y·ri·bo·nu·cle·o·tide** SYN deoxyadenylic acid.

**ad·e·nine nu·cle·o·tide** SYN adenylic acid.

**ad·e·ni·tis** (ad-ĕ-nī′tis) inflammation of a lymph node or of a gland. [aden- + G. *-itis*, inflammation]

**ad·e·ni·za·tion** (ad-ĕ-nī-zā′shŭn) conversion into a glandlike structure.

△**ad·e·no-, aden-** combining forms denoting gland, glandular; corresponds to L. *glandul-*, *glandi-*. [G. *adēn, adenos* a gland]

**ad·e·no·ac·an·tho·ma** (ad′ĕ-nō-ak-an-thō′mă) a malignant neoplasm consisting chiefly of glandular epithelium (adenocarcinoma), usually well differentiated, with foci of metaplasia to squa-

mous (or epidermoid) neoplastic cells. SYN adenoid squamous cell carcinoma.

**ad·e·no·blast** (ad′ĕ-nō-blast) a proliferating embryonic cell with the potential to form glandular parenchyma. [adeno- + G. *blastos*, germ]

**ad·e·no·car·ci·no·ma** (ad′ĕ-nō-kar-si-nō′mă) a malignant neoplasm of epithelial cells in glandular or glandlike pattern.

**ad·e·no·car·ci·no·ma in Bar·rett e·soph·a·gus** (bar′it) an adenocarcinoma arising in the esophagus that has become lined with columnar cells (Barrett mucosa).

**ad·e·no·cel·lu·li·tis** (ad′ĕ-nō-sel-yu-lī′tis) inflammation of a gland, usually a lymph node, and of the adjacent connective tissue.

**ad·e·no·chon·dro·ma** (ad′ĕ-nō-kon-drō′mă) SYN pulmonary hamartoma. [adeno- + G. *chondros*, cartilage, + *-oma*, tumor]

**ad·e·no·cys·to·ma** (ad′ĕ-nō-sis-tō′mă) adenoma in which the neoplastic glandular epithelium forms cysts.

**ad·e·no·cyte** (ad′ĕ-nō-sīt) a secretory cell of a gland. [adeno- + G. *kytos*, a hollow (cell)]

**ad·e·no·fi·bro·ma** (ad′ĕ-nō-fī-brō′mă) a benign neoplasm composed of glandular and fibrous tissues, with a relatively large proportion of glands.

**ad·e·no·fi·bro·my·o·ma** (ad′ĕ-nō-fī′brō-mī-ō′mă) SYN adenomatoid tumor.

**ad·e·no·fi·bro·sis** (ad′ĕ-nō-fī-brō′sis) SYN sclerosing adenosis.

**ad·e·nog·en·ous** (ad-ĕ-noj′en-ŭs) having an origin from glandular tissue.

**ad·e·no·hy·po·phy·si·al** (ad′ĕ-nō-hī-pō-fiz′ē-ăl) relating to the adenohypophysis.

**ad·e·no·hy·poph·y·sis** (ad′ĕ-nō-hī-pof′i-sis) the anterior pituitary gland. It consists of the distal part, intermediate part, and infundibular part. SEE ALSO hypophysis. SYN lobus anterior hypophyseos [TA], anterior lobe of hypophysis.

**ad·e·no·hy·poph·y·si·tis** (ad′ĕ-nō-hī-pof-ĭ-sī′tis) inflammatory reaction or sepsis affecting the anterior pituitary gland, often related to pregnancy.

**ad·e·noid** (ad′ĕ-noyd) **1.** glandlike; of glandular appearance. SYN adeniform, lymphoid (2). **2.** SEE adenoids. [adeno- + G. *eidos*, appearance]

**ad·e·noi·dal·pha·ryn·ge·al-con·junc·ti·val vi·rus** SYN adenovirus.

**ad·e·noid cys·tic car·cin·o·ma** a histologic type of carcinoma characterized by round, glandlike spaces or cysts bordered by layers of epithelial cells without intervening stroma, forming a pattern like a slice of Swiss cheese; perineural invasion and hematogenous metastasis are common; occurs most commonly in salivary glands. SYN cylindromatous carcinoma.

**ad·e·noid·ec·to·my** (ad′ĕ-noy-dek′tō-mē) an operation for the removal of adenoid growths in the nasopharynx. [adenoid + G. *ektomē*, excision]

**ad·e·noid fa·ci·es** the open-mouthed and often dull appearance in children with adenoid hypertrophy, associated with a pinched nose.

**ad·e·noid·i·tis** (ad′ĕ-noy-dī′tis) inflammation of nasopharyngeal lymphoid tissue.

**ad·e·noids** (ad′ĕ-noydz) **1.** a normal collection of unencapsulated lymphoid tissue in the nasopharynx. Also called pharyngeal tonsils. **2.** common terminology for the large (normal) pharyngeal tonsils of children. [G. *adēn*, gland, + *-eidos*, resemblance]

**ad·e·noid squa·mous cell car·cin·o·ma** SYN adenoacanthoma.

**ad·e·noid tis·sue** SYN lymphatic tissue.

**ad·e·no·li·po·ma** (ad'ĕ-nō-li-pō'mă) a benign neoplasm composed of glandular and adipose tissues. [G. *adēn*, gland, + *lipos*, fat, + *-oma*, tumor]

**ad·e·no·lip·o·ma·to·sis** (ad'ĕ-nō-lip'ō-mă-tō'sis) a condition characterized by development of multiple adenolipomas.

**ad·e·no·ma** (ad-ĕ-nō'mă) an ordinarily benign neoplasm of epithelial tissue in which the tumor cells form glands or glandlike structures in the stroma; usually well circumscribed, tending to compress rather than infiltrate or invade adjacent tissue. [adeno- + G. *-oma*, tumor]

**ad·e·no·ma·toid** (ad-ĕ-nō'mă-toyd) resembling an adenoma.

**ad·e·no·ma·toid o·don·to·gen·ic tu·mor** a benign epithelial odontogenic tumor appearing radiographically as a well-circumscribed, radiolucent-radiopaque lesion usually surrounding the crown of an impacted tooth in an adolescent or young adult; characterized histologically by columnar cells organized in a ductlike configuration interspersed with spindle-shaped cells and amyloidlike deposition that gradually undergoes dystrophic calcification. SYN ameloblastic adenomatoid tumor.

**ad·e·no·ma·toid tu·mor** a small benign tumor of the epididymis or female genital tract, consisting of fibrous tissue enclosing glandlike spaces lined by mesothelial cells. SYN adenofibromyoma, Recklinghausen tumor.

**ad·e·no·ma·to·sis** (ad'ĕ-nō-mă-tō'sis) a condition characterized by multiple glandular overgrowths.

**ad·e·nom·a·tous** (ad-ĕ-nō'mă-tŭs) relating to an adenoma, and to some types of glandular hyperplasia.

**ad·e·no·ma·tous goi·ter** an enlargement of the thyroid gland due to the growth of one or more encapsulated adenomas or multiple nonencapsulated colloid nodules within its substance.

**ad·e·no·ma·tous hy·per·pla·sia** SYN complex endometrial hyperplasia.

**ad·e·no·ma·tous pol·yp** a polyp that consists of benign neoplastic tissue derived from glandular epithelium.

**ad·e·no·ma·tous pol·y·po·sis co·li** SYN familial adenomatous polyposis.

**ad·e·no·mere** (ad'ĕ-nō-mēr) structural unit in the parenchyma of a developing gland that becomes the functional portion of the organ. [adeno- + G. *meros*, part]

**ad·e·no·my·o·ma** (ad'ĕ-nō-mī-ō'mă) a benign neoplasm of muscle (usually smooth muscle) with glandular elements; occurs most frequently in uterus and uterine ligaments. [G. *adēn*, gland, + *mys*, muscle, + *-oma*, tumor]

**ad·e·no·my·o·sis** (ad'ĕ-nō-mī-ō'sis) the ectopic occurrence or diffuse implantation of adenomatous tissue in muscle (usually smooth muscle). [G. *adēn*, gland, + *mys*, muscle, + *-osis* condition]

**ad·e·nop·a·thy** (ad-ĕ-nop'ă-thē) swelling or morbid enlargement of the lymph nodes. [adeno- + G. *pathos*, suffering]

**ad·e·no·sal·pin·gi·tis** (ad'ĕ-nō-sal-pin-jī'tis) SYN salpingitis isthmica nodosa.

**ad·e·no·sar·co·ma** (ad'ĕ-nō-sar-kō'mă) a malignant neoplasm arising simultaneously or consecutively in mesodermal tissue and glandular epithelium of the same part.

**aden·o·sine (Ado)** (ă-den'ō-sēn) a condensation product of adenine and D-ribose; a nucleoside found among the hydrolysis products of all nucleic acids and of the various adenine nucleotides.

**aden·o·sine 3',5'-cy·clic mon·o·phos·phate (cAMP)** an activator of phosphorylase kinase and an effector of other enzymes, formed in muscle from ATP by adenylate cyclase and broken down to 5'-AMP by a phosphodiesterase; sometimes referred to as the "second messenger." A related compound (2',3') is also known. SYN cyclic AMP.

**aden·o·sine 5'-di·phos·phate (ADP)** a condensation product of adenosine with pyrophosphoric acid, formed from ATP by the hydrolysis of the terminal phosphate group of the latter compound.

**aden·o·sine di·phos·phate** SEE adenosine 5'-diphosphate.

**aden·o·sine mon·o·phos·phate (AMP)** adenosine-5'-monophosphate. SEE adenylic acid.

**aden·o·sine phos·phate** specifically, adenosine 3'- or 5'-phosphate. SEE adenylic acid.

**aden·o·sine 5'-phos·pho·sul·fate (APS)** an intermediate in the formation of PAPS (active sulfate).

**ad·e·no·sine tri·phos·pha·tase (ATPase)** (a-den'ō-sēn-trī-fos'fă-tās) an enzyme in muscle (myosin) and elsewhere that catalyzes the release of the terminal phosphate group of adenosine 5'-triphosphate.

**aden·o·sine 5'-tri·phos·phate (ATP)** adenosine (5) pyrophosphate; adenosine with triphosphoric acid esterfied at its 5' position; immediate precursors of adenine nucleotides in RNA. The primary energy currency of a cell.

**ad·e·no·sis** (ad-ĕ-nō'sis) a rarely used term for a more or less generalized glandular disease.

**ad·e·not·o·my** (ad-ĕ-not'ō-mē) incision of a gland. [adeno- + G. *tomē*, a cutting]

**ad·e·no·ton·sil·lec·to·my** (ad'ĕ-nō-ton-si-lek'tō-mē) operative removal of tonsils and adenoids.

**Ad·e·no·vi·ri·dae** (ad'ĕ-nō-vir'i-dē) a family of double-stranded DNA viruses, commonly known as adenoviruses, that develop in the nuclei of infected cells in mammals and birds.

**ad·e·no·vi·rus** (ad'ĕ-nō-vī'rŭs) adenoidal-pharyngeal-conjunctival or A-P-C virus; any virus of the family Adenoviridae. More than 40 types are known to infect man causing upper respiratory symptoms, acute respiratory disease, conjunctivitis, gastroenteritis, hemorrhagic cystitis, and serous infections in neonates. SYN adenoidal-pharyngeal-conjunctival virus. [G. *adēn*, gland, + virus]

**ad·e·nyl** (ad'e-nil) the radical or ion of adenine.

**aden·y·late** (a-den'i-lāt) salt or ester of adenylic acid.

**aden·y·late cy·clase** an enzyme acting on ATP to form 3',5'-cyclic AMP plus pyrophosphate. A crucial step in the regulation and formation of second messengers. SYN 3',5'-cyclic AMP synthetase.

**aden·y·late ki·nase** adenylic acid kinase; a phosphotransferase that catalyzes the reversible phosphorylation of a molecule of ADP by MgADP, yielding MgATP and AMP.

**ad·e·nyl·ic ac·id** (ad-e-nil'ik as'id) a condensation product of adenosine and phosphoric acid; a nucleotide found among the hydrolysis products of all nucleic acids. SEE ALSO AMP. SYN adenine nucleotide.

**a•deps**, gen. **adi•pis** (ad'eps, ad'i-pis) denoting fat or adipose tissue. [L. lard, fat]

**a•deps la•nae** the greasy substance obtained from the wool of the sheep *Ovis aries* (family Bovidae). Used as an emollient base for creams and ointments. [L. fat of wool]

**ad•e•quate stim•u•lus** a stimulus to which a particular receptor responds effectively and that gives rise to a characteristic sensation; e.g., light and sound waves that stimulate, respectively, visual and auditory receptors.

**ader•mia** (ă-der'mē-ă) congenital defect or absence of skin. [G. *a-* priv. + *derma*, skin]

**ader•mo•gen•e•sis** (ă-der-mō-jen'ĕ-sis) failure or imperfection in the regeneration of the skin, especially the imperfect repair of a cutaneous defect. [G. *a-* priv. + *derma*, skin, + *genesis*, origin]

**ADH** alcohol dehydrogenase.

**ADHD** attention deficit hyperactivity disorder.

**ad•her•ence** (ad-hēr'ens) **1.** the act or quality of sticking to something. SEE ALSO adhesion. **2.** the extent to which a patient continues treatment under limited supervision. Cf. compliance (2), maintenance. [L. *adhaereo*, to stick to]

**ad•hes•i•ol•y•sis** (ad-hēz-ē-ol'ĭ-sis) severing of adhesive band(s); done by laparoscopy or laparotomy. [adhesion + lysis]

**ad•he•sion** (ad-hē'zhŭn) **1.** the adhering or uniting of two surfaces or parts, especially the union of the opposing surfaces of a wound. SYN conglutination (1). **2.** in the pleural cavity, inflammatory bands that connect opposing serous surfaces. **3.** mutual attraction of unlike molecules. **4.** molecular attraction between the surfaces of bodies in contact. [L. *adhaesio*,, fr. *adhaereo*, to stick to]

**ad•he•sion mol•e•cules** molecules that are involved in T helper-accessory cell, T helper-B cell, and T cytotoxic-target cell interactions.

**ad•he•si•ot•o•my** (ad-hē-sē-ot'ō-mē) surgical section or lysis of adhesions.

**ad•he•sive** (ad-hē'siv) **1.** relating to, or having the characteristics of, an adhesion. **2.** any material that adheres to a surface or causes adherence between surfaces.

**ad•he•sive ab•sor•bent dress•ing** a sterile individual dressing consisting of a plain absorbent compress affixed to a film of fabric coated with a pressure-sensitive adhesive.

**ad•he•sive ban•dage** a dressing of plain absorbent gauze affixed to plastic or fabric coated with a pressure-sensitive adhesive.

**ad•he•sive cap•su•li•tis** a condition in which there is limitation of motion in a joint due to inflammatory thickening of the capsule, a common cause of stiffness in the shoulder.

**ad•he•sive oti•tis** inflammation of the middle ear caused by prolonged auditory tube dysfunction resulting in permanent retraction of the eardrum and obliteration of the middle ear space.

**ad•he•sive per•i•car•di•tis** pericarditis with adhesions between the two pericardial layers, between the pericardium and heart, or between the pericardium and neighboring structures.

**ad•he•sive per•i•to•ni•tis** a form of peritonitis in which a fibrinous exudate occurs, matting together the intestines and various other organs.

**ad•he•sive pleu•ri•sy** SYN dry pleurisy.

**ad•he•sive vag•i•ni•tis** inflammation of vaginal

mucosa with adhesions of the vaginal walls to each other.

**a•di•a•ba•tic** (ā-dē-ă-bă'tik) referring to a thermodynamic process in which there is no gain or loss of heat between the system and its surroundings. [G. *adiabatos*, impassable, fr. *a* priv. + *diabainō*, to go through]

**ad•i•ad•o•cho•ki•ne•sis** (ă-dī'ă-dō-kō-kin-ē'sis) inability to perform rapid alternating movements, a sign of cerebellar dysfunction. Cf. diadochokinesia. [G. *a-* priv. + *diadochos*, successive, + *kinēsis*, movement]

**adi•a•pho•re•sis** (ā'dī-ă-fō-rē'sis) SYN anhidrosis. [G. *a-* priv. + *diaphorēsis*, perspiration]

**adi•a•pho•ria** (ā-dī-ă-fō'rē-ă) failure to respond to stimulation after a series of previously applied stimuli. [G. *a-* priv. + *dia*, through, + *phoros*, bearing]

**Adie syn•drome, Adie pu•pil** (ā'dē) an idiopathic postganglionic denervation of the parasympathetically innervated intraocular muscles, usually complicated by signs of aberrant regeneration of these nerves: a weak light reaction with segmental palsy of iris sphincter, a strong, slow near response. Deep tendon reflexes are often asymmetrically reduced. SEE ALSO tonic pupil. SYN Holmes-Adie pupil, Holmes-Adie syndrome, pupillotonic pseudostrabismus.

△**adip-, adi•po-** fat, fatty. Corresponds to G. lip-, lipo-. SEE ALSO adipo-. [L. *adeps, adipis*, soft animal fat, lard, grease]

**adi•pis** (ad'i-pis) gen. of adeps.

**ad•i•po•cel•lu•lar** (ad'i-pō-sel'yu-ler) relating to both fatty and cellular tissues, or to connective tissue with many fat cells.

**ad•i•po•cer•a•tous** (ad-i-pō-ser'ă-tŭs) relating to adipocere. SYN lipoceratous.

**ad•i•po•cere** (ad'i-pō-sēr) a fatty substance of waxy consistency into which dead animal tissues (as those of a corpse) are sometimes converted when kept from the air under certain conditions of temperature. SYN lipocere. [adipo- + L. *cera*, wax]

**ad•i•po•cyte** (ad'i-pō-sīt) SYN fat cell.

**ad•i•po•gen•e•sis** (ad'i-pō-jen'ĕ-sis) SYN lipogenesis.

**ad•i•po•gen•ic, ad•i•pog•e•nous** (ad'i-pō-jen'ik, ad-i-poj'ĕ-nŭs) SYN lipogenic.

**ad•i•poid** (ad'i-poyd) SYN lipoid. [adipo- + G. *eidos*, resemblance]

**ad•i•po•ki•net•ic** (ad'i-pō-ki-net'ik) denoting a substance or factor that causes mobilization of stored lipid. [adipo- + G. *kinēsis*, movement]

**ad•i•po•ki•nin, ad•i•po•ki•net•ic hor•mone** (ad-i-pō-kī'nin) an anterior pituitary hormone that causes mobilization of fat from adipose tissue.

**ad•i•pose** (ad'i-pōs) denoting fat.

**ad•i•pose cell** SYN fat cell.

**ad•i•pose de•gen•er•a•tion** SYN fatty degeneration.

**ad•i•pose fos•sae** subcutaneous spaces containing accumulations of fat in the breast.

**ad•i•pose in•fil•tra•tion** growth of normal adult fat cells in sites where they are not usually present.

**ad•i•pose tis•sue** a connective tissue consisting chiefly of fat cells surrounded by reticular fibers and arranged in lobular groups or along the course of one of the smaller blood vessels. SYN fat (1).

**ad·i·po·sis** (ad-i-pō'sis) excessive local or general accumulation of fat in the body. SYN lipomatosis, liposis (1), steatosis (1). [adipo- + G. *-osis*, condition]

**ad·i·po·sis car·di·ac·a** SYN fatty heart (2).

**ad·i·pos·i·ty** (ad-i-pos'i-tē) 1. SYN obesity. 2. excessive accumulation of lipids in a site or organ.

**ad·i·po·so·gen·i·tal dys·tro·phy** SYN dystrophia adiposogenitalis.

**ad·i·po·su·ria** (ad'i-pō-syu'rē-ă) SYN lipuria. [adipo- + G. *ouron,* urine]

**ad·i·tus,** pl. **ad·i·tus** (ad'i-tŭs) [TA] SYN aperture, inlet. [L. access, fr. *ad-eo,* pp. *-itus,* go to]

**ad·just·ment dis·or·der** 1. a class of mental and behavioral disorders in which the development of symptoms is related to the presence of some environmental stressor or life event and is expected to remit when the stress ceases; 2. a disorder whose essential feature is a maladaptive reaction to an identifiable psychological stress, or stressors, that occurs within weeks of the onset of the stressors and persists for up to six months.

**ad·ju·vant** (ad'joo-vănt) 1. a substance added to a drug product formulation that affects the action of the active ingredient in a predictable way. 2. in immunology, a vehicle used to enhance antigenicity; e.g., a suspension of minerals (alum, aluminum hydroxide, or phosphate) on which antigen is adsorbed; or water-in-oil emulsion in which antigen solution is emulsified in mineral oil (Freund incomplete adjuvant), sometimes with the inclusion of killed mycobacteria (Freund complete adjuvant) to further enhance antigenicity (inhibits degradation of antigen and/or causes influx of macrophages). 3. additional therapy given to enhance or extend primary therapy's effect, as in chemotherapy's addition to a surgical regimen. 4. a treatment added to a curative treatment to prevent recurrence of clinical cancer from microscopic residual disease. [L. *ad-juvo,* pres. p. *-juvans,* to give aid to]

**ADL** activities of daily living. SEE activities of daily living scale.

**ad lib.** l. *ad libitum,* freely, as desired.

**ad·mit·tance** (ad-mit'ans) SYN immittance.

**ad·mit·ting phys·i·cian** physician who formally and legally accepts a patient for admission to a health care facility.

**ad·mix·ture** (ad-miks'cher) a product of mixing.

**ad·neu·ral, ad·ner·val** (ad-noor'ăl, ad-ner'văl) 1. lying near a nerve. 2. in the direction of a nerve; said of an electric current passing through muscular tissue toward the point of entrance of the nerve.

**ad·nexa,** sing. **ad·nex·um** (ad-nek'să, ad-nek'sŭm) parts accessory to an organ or structure, especially the uterus. SEE ALSO appendage. SYN annexa. [L. connected parts]

**ad·nex·al** (ad-nek'săl) relating to the adnexa. SYN annexal.

**ad·nex·al ad·e·no·ma** an adenoma arising in, or forming structures resembling, skin appendages.

**ad·nex·um** (ad-nek'sŭm) singular of adnexa.

**Ado** adenosine.

**ad·o·les·cence** (ad-ō-les'ens) the period of life beginning with puberty and ending with physical maturity. [L. *adolescentia*]

**ad·o·les·cent** (ad-ō-les'ent) 1. pertaining to adolescence. 2. an individual in that stage of development.

**ad·o·les·cent med·i·cine** the branch of medicine concerned with the treatment of youth in the approximate age range of 13 to 21 years. SYN hebiatrics.

**adop·tive im·mu·no·ther·a·py** passive transfer of immunity from an immune donor through inoculation of sensitized lymphocytes, transfer factor, immune RNA, or antibodies in serum or gamma globulin.

**ADP** adenosine 5'-diphosphate.

**ADR** adverse drug reaction.

**ad·re·nal** (ă-drē'năl) 1. near or upon the kidney; denoting the suprarenal (adrenal) gland. 2. a suprarenal gland or separate tissue or product thereof. SEE ALSO suprarenal. [L. *ad,* to, + *ren,* kidney]

**ad·re·nal an·dro·gen-stim·u·lat·ing hor·mone (AASH)** a putative pituitary hormone that may be responsible for increased secretion of adrenal androgens at the time of puberty.

**ad·re·nal cor·ti·cal car·ci·no·ma** a carcinoma arising in the adrenal cortex that may cause virilism or Cushing syndrome.

**ad·re·nal cri·sis** SYN acute adrenocortical insufficiency.

**ad·re·nal·ec·to·my** (ă-drē-năl-ek'tō-mē) removal of one or both adrenal glands. [adrenal + G. *ektomē,* excision]

**ad·re·nal gland** SYN suprarenal gland.

**ad·re·nal hy·per·ten·sion** hypertension due to an adrenal medullary pheochromocytoma or to hyperactivity or functioning tumor of the adrenal cortex.

**ad·ren·a·line** SYN epinephrine.

**adre·nal·i·tis** (ă-drē-năl-ī'tis) inflammation of the adrenal gland.

**adre·na·lop·a·thy** (ă-drē-nă-lop'ă-thē) any pathologic condition of the adrenal glands. SYN adrenopathy. [adrenal + G. *pathos,* suffering]

**ad·re·nal rest** SYN accessory adrenal.

**ad·re·ner·gic** (ad-rĕ-ner'jik) 1. relating to nerve cells or fibers of the autonomic nervous system that employ norepinephrine as their neurotransmitter. Cf. cholinergic. 2. relating to drugs that mimic the actions of the sympathetic nervous system. SEE α-adrenergic receptors, β-adrenergic receptors. [adren- + G. *ergon,* work]

**ad·re·ner·gic block·ade** selective inhibition by a drug of the responses of effector cells to adrenergic sympathetic nerve impulses (sympatholytic) and to epinephrine and related amines (adrenolytic).

**ad·re·ner·gic block·ing a·gent** a compound that selectively blocks or inhibits responses to sympathetic adrenergic nerve activity (sympatholytic agent) and to epinephrine, norepinephrine, and other adrenergic amines (adrenolytic agent); two distinct classes exist, α- and β-adrenergic receptor blocking agents.

**α-ad·re·ner·gic block·ing a·gent** an agent that competitively blocks α-adrenergic receptors; used in the treatment of hypertension. SYN α-adrenoceptor antagonist.

**β-ad·re·ner·gic block·ing a·gent** a class of drugs that compete with β-adrenergic agonists for available receptor sites; some compete for both $\beta_1$ and $\beta_2$ receptors (e.g., propranolol) while others are primarily either $\beta_1$ (e.g., metoprolol) or $\beta_2$ blockers; used in the treatment of a variety of cardiovascular diseases where β-adrenergic blockade is desirable. SYN beta-blocker.

**ad·re·ner·gic bron·cho·di·la·tors** a class of sympathomimetic antiasthma drugs that act by stimulating receptors in the bronchi and other organs; they are classified into three groups: α-adrenergic, $β_1$-adrenergic, and $β_2$-adrenergic bronchodilators.

**ad·re·ner·gic fi·bers** nerve fibers that transmit nervous impulses to other nerve cells (or smooth muscle or gland cells) by the medium of the adrenaline-like transmitter substance norepinephrine (noradrenaline).

**ad·re·ner·gic neu·ro·nal block·ing a·gent** a drug that prevents the release of norepinephrine from sympathetic nerve terminals.

**ad·re·ner·gic re·cep·tor** reactive components of effector tissues, most of which are innervated by the sympathetic nervous system. Such receptors can be activated by norepinephrine, epinephrine, and adrenergic drugs; receptor activation results in a change in effector tissue function, such as contraction of arteriolar muscles or relaxation of bronchial muscles. SYN adrenoreceptor.

**α-ad·re·ner·gic re·cep·tors** adrenergic receptors in effector tissues capable of selective activation by methoxamine and blockade by phenoxybenzamine. Their activation results in physiological responses such as increased peripheral vascular resistance, mydriasis, and contraction of pilomotor muscles.

**β-ad·re·ner·gic re·cep·tors** adrenergic receptors in effector tissues capable of selective activation by isoproterenol and blockade by propranolol. Their activation results in physiological responses such as increases in cardiac rate and force of contraction ($β_1$), and relaxation of bronchial and vascular smooth muscle ($β_2$).

**adren·ic** (ă-drē′nik) relating to the suprarenal gland.

△**adre·no-, adre·nal-, adren-** relating to the adrenal gland. [L. *ad*, to, near, + *renes*, the kidneys, + -o- + -*alis*, pertaining to]

**adre·no·cep·tive** (ă-drēn-ō-sep′tiv) referring to chemical sites in effectors with which the adrenergic mediator unites. Cf. cholinoceptive.

**α-adre·no·cep·tor an·tag·o·nist** SYN α-adrenergic blocking agent.

**adre·no·cor·ti·cal** (ă-drē-nō-kōr′ti-kăl) pertaining to the cortex of the adrenal gland.

**adre·no·cor·ti·cal in·suf·fi·cien·cy** loss, to varying degrees, of adrenocortical function. SYN hypocorticoidism.

**adre·no·cor·ti·co·mi·met·ic** (ă-drē′nō-kōr′ti-kō-mi-met′ik) mimicking or producing effects similar to adrenocortical function. [adrenal + cortex + G. *mimētikos*, imitating]

**adre·no·cor·ti·co·tro·pic hor·mone (ACTH)** the hormone of the anterior lobe of the hypophysis which governs the nutrition and growth of the adrenal cortex, stimulates it to functional activity, and also possesses extraadrenal adipokinetic activity. SYN adrenotropin, corticotropin (1).

**adre·no·cor·ti·co·tro·pic re·leas·ing fac·tor** hormone produced by the hypothalamus that causes the pituitary to secrete adrenocorticotropic hormone.

**adre·no·gen·ic, adre·nog·e·nous** (ă-drē-nō-jen′ik, a-drē-noj′ē-nŭs) of adrenal origin. [adreno- + G. -*gen*, producing]

**adre·no·gen·i·tal syn·drome** generic designation for a group of disorders caused by adrenocortical hyperplasia or malignant tumors and

characterized by masculinization of women, feminization of men, or precocious sexual development of children; representative of excessive or abnormal secretory patterns of adrenocortical steroids, especially those with androgenic or estrogenic effects.

**adre·no·lyt·ic** (ă-drēn-ō-lit′ik) denoting antagonism to or inhibition or blockade of the action of epinephrine, norepinephrine, and related sympathomimetics. SEE ALSO adrenergic blocking agent. [adreno- + G. *lysis*, loosening, dissolution]

**ad·re·no·med·ul·lary hor·mones** hormones produced by the adrenal medulla, particularly the catecholamines epinephrine and norepinephrine.

**adre·no·meg·a·ly** (ă-drē-nō-meg′ă-lē) enlargement of the adrenal glands. [adreno- + G. *megas*, big]

**adre·no·mi·met·ic** (ă-drē′nō-mi-met′ik) having an action similar to that of the compounds epinephrine and norepinephrine; a term proposed to replace the less specific term, sympathomimetic. Cf. adrenergic, cholinomimetic. [adreno- + G. *mimētikos*, imitative]

**adre·no·mi·met·ic am·ine** SYN sympathomimetic amine.

**adre·no·my·e·lo·neu·rop·a·thy** (ad-rē′nō-mī′e-lō-noo-rop′ă-thē) a disorder of adult males, consisting of long-standing adrenal insufficiency, hypogonadism, progressive myelopathy, peripheral neuropathy, and sphincter disturbances; considered a variant of adrenoleukodystrophy. [adreno- + G. *myelos*, medulla, + *neuron*, nerve, + *pathos*, suffering]

**adre·nop·a·thy** (ă-drē-nop′ă-thē) SYN adrenalopathy.

**adre·no·pause** decrease in function of adrenal glands with increasing age, analogous to menopause.

**adre·no·re·cep·tor** (ă-drē′nō-rē-sep′ter) SYN adrenergic receptor.

**adre·no·tro·pin** (ă-drē-nō-trō′pin) SYN adrenocorticotropic hormone.

**Ad·son test** (ad′son) a test for thoracic outlet syndrome; the patient is seated, with head extended and turned to the side of the lesion; with deep inspiration there is a diminution or total loss of radial pulse on the affected side. Not all patients with a positive Adson test have thoracic outlet syndrome.

**ad·sorb** (ad-sōrb′) to take up by adsorption. [L. *ad*, to, + *sorbeo*, to suck in]

**ad·sorb·ent** (ad-sōr′bent) **1.** a solid substance with the property of attaching other substances to its surface without covalent bonding. **2.** an antigen or antibody used in immune adsorption.

**ad·sorp·tion** (ad-sōrp′shŭn) the property of a solid substance to attract and hold to its surface a gas, liquid, or a substance in solution or in suspension. Cf. absorption. [L. *ad*, to, + *sorbeo*, to suck up]

**ad·sorp·tion the·o·ry of nar·co·sis** that a drug becomes concentrated at the surface of the cell as a result of adsorption, and thus alters permeability and metabolism.

**ad·ter·mi·nal** (ad-ter′mi-năl) in a direction toward the nerve endings, muscular insertions, or the extremity of any structure.

**adult** (ă-dŭlt′) fully grown and physically mature. [L. *adultus*, grown up fr. *adolesco*, to grow up]

**adul·ter·ant** (ă-dŭl′ter-ănt) an impurity; an additive that is considered to have an undesirable effect or to dilute the active material so as to reduce its therapeutic or monetary value.

**adul·ter·a·tion** (ă-dul-ter-ā′shŭn) the alteration of any substance by the deliberate addition of a component not ordinarily part of that substance; usually used to imply that the substance is debased as a result.

**adult foveo·mac·ular ret·i·nal dys·tro·phy** an autosomal dominant disorder presenting in the fifth decade with a mild decrease in vision and subfoveal, round yellow lesion with a central hyperpigmented spot.

**adult lac·tase de·fi·cien·cy** onset of lactase deficiency, with resulting milk intolerance and malabsorption, in adulthood. Inherited forms may not be manifested until adulthood; any process that damages the intestinal lining cells can cause lactase deficiency in adults.

**adult pseu·do·hy·per·tro·phic mus·cu·lar dys·tro·phy** muscular dystrophy of late onset, often in the second or third decade, with relatively mild course.

🔢 **adult res·pi·ra·to·ry dis·tress syn·drome (ARDS)** acute lung injury from a variety of causes, characterized by interstitial and/or alveolar edema and hemorrhage as well as perivascular pulmonary edema associated with hyaline membrane, proliferation of collagen fibers, and swollen epithelium with increased pinocytosis. See page B13. SYN wet lung (2), white lung.

**adult rick·ets** SYN osteomalacia.

**adult T-cell leu·ke·mia (ATL)** SYN adult T-cell lymphoma.

**adult T-cell lym·pho·ma (ATL)** an acute or subacute disease associated with a human T-cell virus, with lymphadenopathy, hepatosplenomegaly, skin lesions, peripheral blood involvement, and hypercalcemia. SYN adult T-cell leukemia.

**ad·vance ben·e·fic·i·ary no·tice (ABN)** document signed by or on behalf of a patient that authorizes a care provider to bill the patient for services Medicare may decline to cover. SYN notice of noncoverage.

**ad·vance dir·ec·tive** a legal document with written instructions signed by the patient (or the patient's next of kin if the patient cannot sign) as to what type of care measures and services are or are not to be provided to prolong life in the event of a life-threatening illness. SYN durable power of attorney (1).

**ad·vanced life sup·port** definitive emergency medical care that includes defibrillation, airway management, and use of drugs and medications. Cf. basic life support.

**ad·vanced mul·ti·ple-beam equal·i·za·tion ra·di·og·ra·phy (AMBER)** a variant of scanning equalization radiography using several x-ray beams.

**ad·vance·ment** (ad-vans′ment) surgical procedure in which a ligamentous or partially tendinous insertion or a skin flap is partially severed or released from its attachment and sutured to a more distal point.

**ad·vance·ment flap** SYN bipedicle flap.

**ad·ven·ti·tia** (ad-ven-tish′ă) the outermost connective tissue covering of any organ, vessel, or other structure not covered by a serosa. SYN tunica adventitia [TA]. [L. *adventicius,* coming from abroad, foreign, fr. *ad,* to + *venio,* to come]

**ad·ven·ti·tial** (ad-ven-tish′ăl) relating to the outer coat or adventitia of a blood vessel or other structure. SYN adventitious (3).

**ad·ven·ti·tial cell** SYN pericyte.

**ad·ven·ti·tial neu·ri·tis** inflammation of the sheath of a nerve. SEE ALSO perineuritis.

**ad·ven·ti·tious** (ad-ven-tish′ŭs) **1.** arising from an external source or occurring in an unusual place or manner. SEE ALSO extrinsic. **2.** occurring accidentally or spontaneously, as opposed to natural causes or hereditary. **3.** SYN adventitial.

**ad·ven·ti·tious cyst** SYN pseudocyst (1).

**ad·ven·ti·tious lung sounds** breath sounds that are not normally heard, and that fall into one of two categories: (1) continuous: musical-type sounds with a persistent pitch (for example, wheezes, rhonchi); (2) discontinuous: intermittent, crackling, or bubbling sounds (rales).

**ad·verse drug re·ac·tion (ADR), ad·verse drug event** any noxious, unintended, and undesired effect of a drug after its administration for prophylaxis, diagnosis, or therapy.

**ad·verse re·ac·tion** any undesirable or unwanted consequence of a preventive, diagnostic, or therapeutic procedure or regimen.

**ady·nam·ic il·e·us** obstruction of the bowel due to paralysis of the bowel wall, usually as a result of localized or generalized peritonitis or shock. SYN paralytic ileus.

⚠ **ae-** for words so beginning and not found here, see under e-.

**A-E am·pu·ta·tion** *a*bove-the-*e*lbow amputation.

**Ae·des** (ā-ē′dēz) a widespread genus of small mosquitoes frequently found in tropical and subtropical regions; various species are vectors for yellow fever, dengue, and other human diseases. [G. *aēdēs,* unpleasant, unfriendly]

**Ae·des at·lan·tic·us** mosquitoes in the family Culicidae known to transmit viruses that cause dengue, yellow fever, and encephalitis.

**Ae·des dor·sal·is** mosquito species that is a secondary or suspected vector of Western equine encephalitis.

**Ae·des mel·an·im·on** mosquito species that is a vector of Western equine encephalitis and California group encephalitis.

**Ae·des mitchel·lae** mosquito species that is a secondary or suspected vector of Eastern equine encephalitis.

**Ae·des nigro·mac·u·lis** mosquito species that is a secondary or suspected vector of Western equine encephalitis and California group encephalitis.

**Ae·des tae·nio·rhyn·chus** mosquito species that is a vector of Venezuelan equine encephalitis and a secondary or suspected vector of California group encephalitis.

**Ae·des tri·ser·i·atus** mosquito species that is a vector of California group encephalitis.

**Ae·des triv·it·ta·tus** mosquito species that is a vector of California group encephalitis.

**Ae·des vex·ans** mosquito species that is a vector of California group encephalitis and a secondary or suspected vector of Eastern equine encephalitis.

**ae·quor·in** (ēk′wōr-in) a luminescent protein isolated from the jellyfish *Aequorea* which emits blue light in the presence of even minute amounts of calcium ion; injected intracellularly, it is used to measure free calcium ion transients within cells. SEE ALSO fura-2.

△**aer-, aero-** the air, a gas; aerial, gassy. [G. *aēr* (L. *aer*), air]

**aer•ate** (ār′āte) **1.** to supply (blood) with oxygen. **2.** to expose to the circulation of air for purification. **3.** to supply or charge (liquid) with a gas, especially carbon dioxide.

**aer•ation** (ār-ā′shŭn) the process of charging a liquid with air or gas; especially the transfer of oxygen to the blood in the lungs.

**aer•i•al sick•ness** SYN altitude sickness.

**aer•obe** (ār′ōb) **1.** an organism that can live and grow in the presence of oxygen. **2.** an organism that can use oxygen as a final electron acceptor in a respiratory chain. [aero- + G. *bios*, life]

**aer•o•bic** (ār-ō′bik) **1.** living in air. **2.** relating to an aerobe. SYN aerophilic, aerophilous.

**aer•o•bic cap•ac•i•ty** SYN maximal oxygen consumption.

**aer•o•bic pow•er** SYN maximal oxygen consumption.

**aer•o•bic res•pi•ra•tion** a form of respiration in which molecular oxygen is consumed and carbon dioxide and water are produced.

**aer•o•bics** (ār-ō′bĭks) a program of physical conditioning based on sustained, strenuous exercise and intended to improve cardiovascular and respiratory fitness.

**aer•o•bic sys•tem** the combination of physiologic (pulmonary, cardiovascular, muscular) and biochemical (aerobic glycolysis, citric acid cycle, electron transport chain) functions normally used in performing physical work.

**aer•o•bi•o•sis** (ār-ō-bī-ō′sis) existence in an atmosphere containing oxygen. [aero- + G. *biōsis*, mode of living]

**aer•o•bi•ot•ic** (ār-ō-bī-ot′ik) relating to aerobiosis.

**aer•o•cele** (ār′ō-sēl) distention of a small natural cavity with gas. [aero- + G. *kēlē*, tumor]

**aer•o•col•pos** (ār-ō-kol′pos) distention of the vagina with gas. [aero- + G. *kolpos*, lap, hollow]

**aer•o•don•tal•gia** (ār′ō-don-tal′jē-ă) dental pain caused by either increased or reduced atmospheric pressure. [aero- + G. *odous*, tooth, + *algos*, pain]

**aer•o•dy•nam•ics** (ār′ō-dī-nam′iks) the study of air and other gases in motion, the forces that set them in motion, and the results of such motion. [aero- + G. *dynamis*, force]

**aer•o•dy•nam•ic the•o•ry** generally accepted theory that the vibration of the vocal folds in phonation is produced by the flow of exhaled air past lightly approximated vocal folds; opposed to the now untenable concept that vocal fold motion in phonation results from contraction of the intrinsic muscles of the larynx at the frequency of the vocal fold vibration.

**aer•o•gas•tral•gia** (ār′ō-gas-tral′jē-ă) pain due to distention of the stomach by swallowed air. [aero- + G. *gastēr*, stomach, + *algos*, pain]

**aer•o•genic, aer•o•genous** (ār-ō-jen′ik) gasforming.

*Aer•o•mon•as* (ār-ō-mō′nas) a genus of aerobic, facultatively anaerobic bacteria (family Vibrionaceae) containing gram-negative, rod-shaped to coccoid cells that occur singly or in pairs or in clumps of chains; motile cells ordinarily possess a single, polar flagellum; some species are nonmotile. The metabolism of these organisms is both respiratory and fermentative. These bacteria are found in water and sewage; some are patho-genic to fresh water and marine animals. The type species is *Aeromonas hydrophila*.

**aer•o•pha•gia, aer•oph•a•gy** (ār-ō-fā′jē-ă, ār-of′ă-jē) an abnormal swallowing of air as seen in crib-biting and wind-sucking. [aero- + G. *phagō*, to eat]

**aer•o•phil, aer•o•phile** (ār′ō-fil, ār′ō-fīl) **1.** airloving. **2.** an aerobic organism (aerobe), especially an obligate aerobe. [aero- + G. *philos*, fond]

**aer•o•phil•ic, aer•oph•i•lous** (ār-ō-fil′ik, ār-of′i-lŭs) SYN aerobic.

**aer•o•pho•bia** (ār-ō-fō′bē-ă) morbid dread of fresh air or of air in motion. [aero- + G. *phobos*, fear]

**aer•o•pi•e•so•ther•a•py** (ār′ō-pī-ē′sō-thār′ă-pē) treatment of disease by compressed (or rarified) air. [aero- + G. *piesis*, pressure, + *therapeia*, medical treatment]

**aer•o•si•nus•i•tis** (ār-ō-sī-nŭ-sī′tis) inflammation of the paranasal sinuses caused by pressure difference within the sinus relative to ambient pressure, secondary to obstruction of the sinus orifice, sometimes due to high altitude flying or by descent from high altitude. SYN barosinusitis.

**aer•o•sol** (ār′ō-sol) **1.** liquid or particulate matter dispersed in air in the form of a fine mist for therapeutic, insecticidal, or other purposes. **2.** a product that is packaged under pressure and contains therapeutically or chemically active ingredients intended for topical application, inhalation, or introduction into body orifices. [aero- + solution]

**aer•o•sol gen•er•a•tor** a device for producing airborne suspensions of small particles for inhalation therapy or experimental work.

**aer•o•sphere** (ār′ō-sfēr) the lower portion of the earth's atmosphere, containing sufficient oxygen to support life. [aero- + sphere]

**aer•o•tax•is** (ār-ō-tak′sis) movement or an organism with respect to a supply or air or oxygen. [aero- + G. *taxis*, orderly arrangement]

**aer•o•ti•tis me•dia** (ār-ō-tī′tis mē′dē-ă) an acute or chronic inflammation of the middle ear caused by a reduction in pressure in the tympanic cavity relative to ambient pressure, secondary to auditory tube obstruction; often occurs on descent from high altitude. SYN barotitis media. [aero- + G. *ous*, ear, + *-itis*, inflammation]

**aer•o•tol•er•ant** (ār-ō-tŏl′ĕr-ănt) able to survive in the presence of oxygen; said of some anaerobic microorganisms. [aero- + tolerant]

**aer•o•trop•ism** (ār-ŏt′ro-pizm) movement of an organism with respect to a supply of air or oxygen. [aero- + tropism]

**aes•cu•la•pi•an** (es-kyu-lā′pē-an) relating to Aesculapius, the art of medicine, or a medical practitioner. [L. *Aesculapius*, G. *Asklēpios*, the god of medicine]

**aes•the•sia [Br.]** SEE perception.

**aes•the•si•o-** SEE esthesio-.

**aes•the•si•o•me•ter [Br.]** SEE esthesiometer.

**aes•the•si•o•neu•ro•sis [Br.]** any sensory neurosis; e.g., anesthesia, hyperesthesia, paraesthesia.

**aes•the•si•o•phys•i•ol•o•gy [Br.]** SEE esthesiophysiology.

**aes•the•sod•ic [Br.]** SYN esthesiodic.

**aes•tiv•al [Br.]** SEE estival.

**aes•ti•va•tion [Br.]** SEE estivation.

**aet•i•o•log•ic [Br.]** SEE etiologic.

**aet•i•o•log•ic•al [Br.]** SEE etiologic.

**aet·i·o·log·y** [Br.] SEE etiology.

**AFA fix·a·tive** a combination of alcohol, formalin, and acetic acid used for the fixation of nematodes, trematodes, and cestodes.

**AFB** acid-fast bacillus.

**afe·brile** (ā-feb′ril) SYN apyretic.

**afe·tal** (ă-fē′tăl) without relation to a fetus or intrauterine life.

**af·fect** (af′fekt) the emotional feeling, tone, and mood attached to a thought, including its external manifestations. [L. *affectus*, state of mind, fr. *afficio*, to have influence on]

**af·fec·tion** (ă-fek′shŭn) 1. a moderate feeling of tenderness, caring, or love. 2. an abnormal condition of body or mind. [L. *affectio*, fr. *af-ficio*, to affect, influence]

**af·fec·tive** (af-fek′tiv) pertaining to mood, emotion, feeling, sensibility, or a mental state.

**af·fec·tive dis·or·der** a mental disorder characterized by a disturbance in mood.

**af·fec·tive per·son·al·i·ty** a chronic behavioral pattern in an enduring disturbance of feelings or mood expressed as a form of depression and related emotional features that color the whole of the psychic life.

**af·fec·tive psy·cho·sis** psychosis with predominant affective features.

**af·fer·ent** (af′er-ent) inflowing; conducting toward a center, denoting certain arteries, veins, lymphatics, and nerves. Opposite of efferent. SYN centripetal (1). [L. *afferens*, fr. *af-fero*, to bring to]

**af·fer·ent fi·bers** those that convey impulses to a ganglion or to a nerve center in the brain or spinal cord.

**af·fer·ent glo·mer·u·lar ar·te·ri·ole** a branch of an interlobular artery of the kidney that conveys blood to the glomerulus. SYN arteriola glomerularis afferens [TA].

**af·fer·ent lym·phat·ic** a lymphatic vessel entering, or bringing lymph to, a node.

**af·fer·ent nerve** a nerve conveying impulses from the periphery to the central nervous system. SYN centripetal nerve.

**af·fer·ent ves·sel** any artery conveying blood to a part.

**af·fin·i·ty** (ă-fin′i-tē) 1. CHEMISTRY the force that impels certain atoms to unite with certain others. 2. selective staining of a tissue by a dye. 3. the strength of binding between a Fab site of an antibody and an antigenic determinant. [L. *affinis*, neighboring, fr. *ad*, to, + *finis*, end, boundary]

**A fi·bers** myelinated nerve fibers in somatic nerves, measuring 1 to 22 μm in diameter, conducting nerve impulses at a rate of 6 to 120 m/sec.

**afi·bril·lar** (ā-fī′bri-ler) denoting a biological structure that does not contain fibrils.

**afi·brin·o·gen·e·mia** (ā-fī′brin-ō-jĕ-nē′mē-ă) the absence of fibrinogen in the plasma. SEE ALSO hypofibrinogenemia.

**Afip·i·a** (ă-fip′ē-ă) a genus of Gram-negative, oxidase-positive, motile, nonfermenting bacteria that have been placed in the class Proteobacteria. They are morphologically variable, appearing as rods or filaments that may stain poorly. Over 10 species have been identified, one of which was formerly thought to be the cause of catscratch disease. Their current pathogenic role is uncertain. The type strain is *A. felis*.

**AFORMED phe·nom·e·non** as induced pulsus alternans progresses, a state in which alternating heart depolarizations fail to eject any blood, thus allowing longer diastolic filling; the subsequent beat is then able to produce a significant ejection; at high rates the cardiac minute volume and blood pressure may appear normal. [*A*lternating *f*ailure *o*f *r*esponse, *m*echanical, to *e*lectrical *d*epolarization]

**AFP** α-fetoprotein.

**Af·ri·can sleep·ing sick·ness** (af′ri-kăn) SEE Gambian trypanosomiasis, Rhodesian trypanosomiasis.

**Af·ri·can tick-bite fe·ver** (af′ri-kăn) a febrile disease caused by the bacterium *Rickettsia africae* in southern Africa and characterized by taches noires at the sites of bites by infected *Amblyomma* ticks and lymphadenopathy.

**Af·ri·can try·pan·o·so·mi·a·sis** (af′ri-kăn) a serious endemic disease in tropical Africa, of two types: Gambian or West African trypanosomiasis and Rhodesian or East African trypanosomiasis.

**af·ter·birth** (af′ter-berth) the placenta and membranes that are extruded from the uterus after birth. SYN secundines.

**af·ter·im·age** (af′ter-im′ij) persistence of a visual response after cessation of the stimulus.

**af·ter·im·pres·sion** (af′ter-im-presh′ŭn) SYN aftersensation.

**af·ter·load** (af′ter-lōd) 1. the arrangement of a muscle so that, in shortening, it lifts a weight from an adjustable support or otherwise does work against a constant opposing force to which it is not exposed at rest. 2. the load or force thus encountered in shortening.

**af·ter·load·ing ra·di·a·tion** method of administering radiation that involves initial placement of local catheters with later installation of the radiation source.

**af·ter·pains** (af′ter-pānz) painful cramplike contractions of the uterus occurring after childbirth.

**af·ter·per·cep·tion** (af′ter-per-sep′shŭn) subjective persistence of a stimulus after its cessation. Cf. palinopsia.

**af·ter·po·ten·tial** (af′ter-pō-ten′shăl) the small change in electrical potential in a stimulated nerve that follows the main, or spike, potential; it consists of an initial negative deflection followed by a positive deflection in the oscillograph record.

**af·ter·sen·sa·tion** (af′ter-sen-sā′shŭn) subjective persistence of sensation after cessation of stimulus. SYN afterimpression.

**af·ter·sound** (af′ter-sownd) subjective persistence of an auditory stimulus after cessation of the stimulus.

**af·ter·taste** (af′ter-tāst) subjective persistence of a gustatory stimulus after contact with the stimulating substance has ceased.

**afunc·tion·al oc·clu·sion** a malocclusion which does not permit normal function of the dentition.

**Ag** 1. silver (argentum). 2. antigen.

**ag·a·lac·tia, ag·a·lac·to·sis** (ā-gal-ak′shē-ă, ā-gal-ak-tō′sis) absence of milk in the breasts after childbirth. [G. *a*- priv. + *gala* (*galakt*-), milk]

**aga·lac·tor·rhea** (ā-ga-lak-tō-rē′ă) absence of the secretion or flow of breast milk. [G. *a*- priv. + *gala*, milk, + *rhoia*, a flow]

**ag·a·lac·tous** (ā-gal-ak′tŭs) relating to agalactia, or to the diminution or absence of breast milk.

**ag·am·ic, ag·a·mous** (ā-gam′ik, ag′ă-mŭs) denoting nonsexual reproduction, as by fission or budding.

**agam·ma·glob·u·lin·e·mia** (ā-gam′ă-glob′yu-li-nē′mē-ă) absence of, or extremely low levels of, the gamma fraction of serum globulin; sometimes used loosely to denote absence of immunoglobulins in general. SEE ALSO hypogammaglobulinemia.

**agan·gli·on·ic** (ā-gang-glē-on′ik) without ganglia.

**agan·gli·o·no·sis** (ā-gang′glē-ō-nō′sis) the state of being without ganglia; e.g., absence of ganglion cells from the myenteric plexus as a characteristic of congenital megacolon. [G. ā- priv. + ganglion + -osis, condition]

**agar** (ah′gar) a complex polysaccharide (a sulfated galactan) derived from seaweed (various red algae); used as a solidifying agent in culture media; it has the valuable property of melting at 100°C, but not solidifying until 49°C. [Bengalese]

**agas·tric** (ā-gas′trik) without stomach or digestive tract. [G. a- priv. + gastēr, belly]

**AGC** automatic gain control.

**AGCUS** atypical glandular cells of undetermined significance.

**age** (āj) **1.** the period that has elapsed since birth. **2.** one of the periods into which human life is divided, distinguished by physical evolution, equilibrium, and involution; e.g., the seven ages of man are: infancy, childhood, adolescence, maturity, middle life, senescence, and senility. **3.** to grow old; to gradually develop changes in structure that are not due to preventable disease or trauma and that are associated with decreased functional capacity and an increased probability of death. **4.** to cause artificially the appearance characteristic of one who has lived long or of a thing that has existed for a long time. **5.** DENTISTRY to heat an alloy for amalgam so as to make it set more slowly, increase strength, reduce flow, and have a longer shelf life. Aging occurs by relieving internal strains. [F. âge, L. aetas]

**agen·e·sis** (ā-jen′ĕ-sis) absence or failure of formation of any part. [G. a- priv. + genesis, production]

**agen·i·tal·ism** (ā-jen′i-tal-izm) congenital absence of genitalia.

**agen·o·so·mia** (ā-gen-ō-sō′mē-ă) markedly defective formation or absence of the genitalia in a fetus; usually accompanied by protrusion of the abdominal viscera through an incomplete abdominal wall. [G. a- priv. + genos, sex, + soma, body]

**agent** (ā′jent) **1.** an active force or substance capable of producing an effect. **2.** a disease, a factor such as a microorganism, chemical substance, or a form of radiation the presence or absence of which (as in deficiency diseases) results in disease or more advanced disease. [L. ago, pres. p. agens (agent-), to perform]

**ageu·sia** (ā-goo′sē-ă) loss of the sense of taste. [G. a- priv. + geusis, taste]

**ag·glu·ti·nant** (ă-gloo′ti-nant) a substance that holds parts together or causes agglutination. [L. ad, to, + gluten, glue]

**ag·glu·ti·na·tion** (ă-gloo-ti-nā′shŭn) **1.** the process by which suspended bacteria, cells, or other particles are caused to adhere and form clumps; similar to precipitation, but the particles are larger and are in suspension rather than being in

solution. For specific agglutination reactions in the various blood groups, see Blood Groups appendix. **2.** adhesion of the surfaces of a wound. [L. ad, to, + gluten, glue]

**ag·glu·ti·na·tive** (ă-gloo′ti-nă-tiv) causing, or able to cause, agglutination.

**ag·glu·ti·nin** (ă-gloo′ti-nin) **1.** an antibody that causes clumping or agglutination of the bacteria or other cells which either stimulate the formation of the agglutinin, or contain immunologically similar, reactive antigen. **2.** a substance, other than a specific agglutinating antibody, that causes organic particles to agglutinate.

**ag·glu·tin·o·gen** (ă-gloo-tin′ō-jen) an antigenic substance that stimulates the formation of specific agglutinin, which, under certain conditions, causes agglutination of cells that contain the antigen or particles coated with the antigen. SYN agglutogen. [agglutinin + G. -gen, production]

**ag·glu·tin·o·gen·ic** (ă-gloo′tin-ō-jen′ik) capable of causing the production of an agglutinin. SYN agglutogenic.

**ag·glu·tin·o·phil·ic** (ă-gloo′tin-ō-fil′ik) readily undergoing agglutination. [agglutination + G. phileō, to love]

**ag·glu·to·gen** (ă-gloo′tō-jen) SYN agglutinogen.

**ag·glu·to·gen·ic** (ă-gloo-tō-jen′ik) SYN agglutinogenic.

**ag·gre·can** (ag′gre-kan) candidate gene for otosclerosis located at 15q25 to q26.

**ag·gre·gate** (ag′rĕ-gāt) **1.** to unite or come together in a mass or cluster. **2.** the total of individual units making up a mass or cluster. [L. aggrego, pp. -atus, to add to, fr. grex (greg-), a flock]

**ag·gre·ga·tion** (ag-rĕ-gā′shŭn) a crowded mass of independent but similar units; a cluster.

**ag·gres·sion** (ă-gresh′ŭn) a domineering, forceful, or assaultive verbal or physical action toward another person as the motor component of anger, hostility, or rage. [L. aggressio, fr. aggredior, to accost, attack]

**ag·gres·sive** (ă-gres′iv) **1.** denoting aggression. **2.** denoting a competitive forcefulness or invasiveness, as of a behavioral pattern, a pathogenic organism, or a disease process.

**ag·gres·sive an·gi·o·myx·o·ma** locally invasive, but nonmetastasizing tumor of genital organs in young women.

**ag·ing** (ā′jing) **1.** the process of growing old, especially by failure of replacement of cells in sufficient number to maintain full functional capacity; particularly affects cells (e.g., neurons) incapable of mitotic division. **2.** the gradual deterioration of a mature organism resulting from time-dependent, irreversible changes in structure. **3.** in the cardiovascular system, the progressive replacement of functional cell types by fibrous connective tissue. **4.** a demographic term, meaning an increase over time in the proportion of older persons in the population.

**ag·i·tat·ed de·pres·sion** depression with excitement and restlessness.

**aglos·so·sto·mia** (ā-glos-ō-stō′mē-ă) congenital absence of the tongue, with a malformed (usually closed) mouth. [G. a- priv. + glōssa, tongue, + stoma, mouth]

**a·glu·ti·tion** (ā-gloo-tish′ŭn) SYN dysphagia.

**agly·cos·u·ria** (ā-glī-kō-syu′rē-ă) absence of carbohydrate in the urine.

**agly·cos·u·ric** (ă-glī-kō-syu′rik) relating to aglycosuria.

**ag·na·thia** (ag-nā′thē-ă) congenital absence of the lower jaw, usually accompanied by approximation of the ears. SEE ALSO otocephaly, synotia. [G. *a-* priv. + *gnathos,* jaw]

**ag·na·thous** (ag′nā-thŭs) relating to agnathia.

**ag·no·gen·ic** (ag-nō-jen′ik) SYN idiopathic. [G. *a-* priv. + *gnosis,* knowledge, + *genesis,* origin]

**ag·no·sia** (ag-nō′zē-ă) impairment of ability to recognize, or comprehend the meaning of, various sensory stimuli, not attributable to disorders of the primary receptors or general intellect; agnosias are receptive defects caused by lesions in various portions of the cerebrum. [G. ignorance; from *a-* priv. + *gnōsis,* knowledge]

△**-agogue, -agog** leading, promoting, stimulating; a promoter or stimulant of. [G. *agōgos,* leading forth, fr. *agō,* to lead.]

**agom·pho·sis, ag·om·phi·a·sis** (ag-om-fō′sis, ag-om-fī′ă-sis) SYN anodontia. [G. *a-* priv. + *gomphos,* peg, bolt]

**ago·nad·al** (ā-gon′ă-dăl) denoting the absence of gonads (testes or ovaries).

**ag·o·nist** (ag′on-ist) **1.** denoting a muscle in a state of contraction, with reference to its opposing muscle, or antagonist. **2.** a drug capable of combining with receptors to initiate drug actions; it possesses affinity and intrinsic activity. [G. *agōn,* a contest]

**ag·o·ra·pho·bia** (ag′ōr-ă-fō′bē-ă) a mental disorder characterized by an irrational fear of leaving the familiar setting of home, or venturing into the open; often associated with panic attacks. [G. *agora,* marketplace, + *phobos,* fear]

**ag·or·a·pho·bic** (ă-gōr-ă-fō′bik) relating to or characteristic of agoraphobia.

△**-agra** sudden onslaught of acute pain. [G. *agra,* a hunting, a catching, a trap]

**agram·ma·tism** (ă-gram′ă-tizm) a form of aphasia characterized by a reduced ability to understand or produce most grammatical markers, usually related to severe expressive aphasia.

**a·gran·u·lar en·do·plas·mic re·tic·u·lum** endoplasmic reticulum that is lacking in ribosomal granules; involved in synthesis of complex lipids and fatty acids, detoxification of drugs, carbohydrate synthesis, and sequestering of $Ca^{++}$.

**agran·u·lo·cyte** (ā-gran′yu-lō-sīt) a nongranular leukocyte. [G. *a-* priv. + L. *granulum,* granule, + G. *kytos,* cell]

**agran·u·lo·cy·to·sis** (ā-gran′yu-lō-sī-tō′sis) an acute condition characterized by pronounced leukopenia; infected ulcers are likely to develop in the throat, intestinal tract, and other mucous membranes, as well as in the skin.

**agran·u·lo·plas·tic** (ā-gran′yu-lō-plas′tik) incapable of forming nongranular cells, and incapable of forming granular cells. [G. *a-* priv. + L. *granulum,* granule, + G. *plastikos,* formative]

**agraph·ia** (ă-graf′ē-ă) inability to write properly in the absence of abnormalities of the limb; often accompanies aphasia and alexia; caused by lesions in various portions of the cerebrum. SYN anorthography, logagraphia. [G. *a-* priv. + *graphō,* to write]

**agraph·ic** (ă-graf′ik) relating to or marked by agraphia.

**agre·tope** (ag-rē′tōp) that part of a processed antigen that binds to the major histocompatibility complex molecule. [*a*ntigen + *re*striction + *-tope*]

**AGUS** atypical glandular cells of undetermined significance. SEE ALSO Bethesda system.

**agy·ria** (ā-jī′rē-ă) congenital lack or underdevelopment of the convolutional pattern of the cerebral cortex. SYN lissencephalia. [G. *a-* priv. + *gyros,* circle]

**AH con·duc·tion time** SEE atrioventricular conduction.

**AHF** antihemophilic factor A.

**AH in·ter·val** the time from the initial rapid deflection of the atrial wave to the initial rapid deflection of the His bundle (H) potential; it approximates the conduction time through the AV node (normally 50–120 msec).

**Ahu·ma·da-del Cas·ti·llo syn·drome** (ah-oomah′ahah del kas-tē′yō) unphysiologic lactation and amenorrhea not following pregnancy characterized by hyperprolactinemia and a pituitary adenoma.

**Ai·car·di syn·drome** (ĕ-kahr-dē′) an X-linked dominant disorder with lethality in hemizygous males; characterized by agenesis of corpus callosum, chorioretinal abnormality with "holes," cleft lip with or without cleft palate, seizures, and characteristic EEG changes.

**AID** artificial insemination donor.

🔲**AIDS** (ādz) a syndrome of the immune system characterized by opportunistic diseases, including candidiasis, *Pneumocystis carinii* pneumonia, oral hairy leukoplakia, herpes zoster, Kaposi sarcoma, toxoplasmosis, isosporiasis, cryptococcosis, non-Hodgkin lymphoma, and tuberculosis. The syndrome is caused by the human immunodeficiency virus (HIV-1, HIV-2), which is transmitted by body fluids (notably blood and semen) through sexual contact, sharing of contaminated needles (by IV drug abusers), accidental needle sticks, contact with contaminated blood, or transfusion of contaminated blood or blood products. Hallmark of the immunodeficiency is depletion of T4$^+$ helper/inducer lymphocytes, primarily the result of selective tropism of the virus for the lymphocytes. See page B3. SYN acquired immunodeficiency syndrome.

**AIH** artificial insemination (homologous).

**ai·lu·ro·pho·bia** (ī′loo-rō-fō′bē-ă) morbid fear of or aversion to cats. [G. *ailouros,* cat, + *phobos,* fear]

**AIR** 5-aminoimidazole ribose 5′phosphate; 5-aminoimidazole ribotide.

**air** (ār) **1.** a mixture of odorless gases found in the atmosphere in the following approximate percentages: oxygen, 20.95; nitrogen, 78.08; argon 0.93; carbon dioxide, 0.03; other gases, 0.01. **2.** SYN ventilate. [G. *aēr;* L. *aer*]

**air a·bra·sion** the use of abrasive particles such as aluminum oxide under high pressure to abrade and sometimes remove dentin and enamel.

**air-bone gap (ABG)** an abnormal condition in which the auditory threshold for an air-conducted test tone is higher than that for a bone-conducted test tone of the same frequency. SEE ALSO conductive hearing loss.

**Air·bras·ive** (ār-brā′sive) a dental device designed for polishing teeth, powered by air and water pressure, that delivers a stream of specially processed sodium bicarbonate slurry mixture through a handpiece nozzle.

**air bron·cho·gram** radiographic appearance of an air-filled bronchus surrounded by fluid-filled airspaces.

**air cells 1.** SYN pulmonary alveolus. **2.** air-containing spaces in the skull.

**air·con·di·tion·er lung** an extrinsic allergic alveolitis caused by forced air contaminated by thermophilic actinomycetes and other organisms.

**air con·duc·tion** in relation to hearing, the transmission of sound to the inner ear through the external auditory canal and the structures of the middle ear.

**air con·trast en·e·ma** a double contrast enema in which air is introduced after coating of the colon with a dense barium suspension for radiographic study. SYN double contrast enema.

**air em·bo·lism** embolism that occurs when air enters a blood vessel, usually a vein, as a result of trauma, surgery, or deliberate injection; a large air embolism can cause lethal derangement of cardiac function.

**air hun·ger** extremely deep ventilation such as occurs in patients with acidosis attempting to increase ventilation of alveoli and exhale more carbon dioxide. SEE ALSO Kussmaul respiration.

**air med·i·cal trans·port** the transport of patients by aircraft, either from the scene of a medical or trauma incident or an interfacility transport utilizing aircraft, most often helicopter.

**air·plane splint** a complicated splint that holds the arm in abduction at about shoulder level with the forearm midway in flexion, generally with an axillary strut for support.

**air pol·lu·tion** contamination of air by smoke, particulate matter, and harmful gases, mainly oxides of carbon, sulfur, and nitrogen, as from automobile exhausts, industrial emissions, and burning rubbish. SEE ALSO smog.

**air·port ma·lar·i·a** malaria inadvertently imported by transport of an infected anopheline mosquito on an airplane.

**air sick·ness** a form of motion sickness caused by flying in an airplane.

**air splint** a plastic splint inflated by air used to immobilize part or all of an extremity.

**air·trap·ping** (ār-trap′ing) slow or incomplete emptying of air from all or part of a lung on expiration; implies obstruction of regional airways or emphysema.

**air ves·i·cles** SYN pulmonary alveolus.

**air·way** (ār′wā) **1.** any part of the respiratory tract through which air passes during breathing. **2.** in anesthesia or resuscitation, a device for correcting obstruction to breathing, especially an oropharyngeal, nasopharyngeal, or endotracheal airway, or tracheotomy tube.

**air·way a·nat·o·my** the tracheobronchial structure, similar to an inverted tree, containing three types of airways: cartilaginous airways (trachea, main stem bronchi, and approximately five generations of small bronchi); membranous bronchioles (approximately eight generations of non-cartilaginous airways); and respiratory bronchioles (approximately five generations of gas-exchange or alveolar ducts).

**air·way man·age·ment** assistance given to a patient in maintaining a patent airway, with or without intubation.

**air·way ob·struc·tion** a type of respiratory dysfunction that produces reduced airflow, usually on expiration; the obstruction can be localized (for example, tumor, stricture, foreign body) or generalized (for example, emphysema, asthma).

**air·way re·sis·tance** PHYSIOLOGY the resistance to flow of gases during ventilation due to obstruction or turbulent flow in the upper and lower airways; to be differentiated during inhalation from resistance to inflation due to decreases in pulmonary or thoracic compliance.

**Airy disk** (ā′rē) the image of a circular blur formed by a distant point source of light on the retina because of diffraction by the edge of the pupillary aperture where the diameter of the image decreases as the aperture increases.

**A-K am·pu·ta·tion** *above*-the-*k*nee amputation.

**ak·a·mu·shi dis·ease** (ak-ah-moo′shē di-zēz′) SYN tsutsugamushi disease.

**akar·y·o·cyte, akar·y·ote** (ā-kar′ē-ō-sīt, ā-kar′ē-ōt) a cell without a nucleus, such as the erythrocyte. SYN acaryote. [G. *a*- priv. + *karyon*, kernel, + *kytos*, a hollow (cell)]

**a·ka·thi·sia** (ak-ă-thiz′ē-ă) a syndrome characterized by an inability to remain in a sitting posture, with motor restlessness and a feeling of muscular quivering; may appear as a side effect of antipsychotic and neuroleptic medication. [G. *a*- priv. + *kathisis*, a sitting]

**aker·a·to·sis** (ă-ker-ă-tō′sis) deficiency or absence of the horny layer of the epidermis.

**Ak·er·lund de·for·mi·ty** (ak′ĕr-lung) indentation (incisura) with niche of duodenal cap as seen radiologically.

**aki·ne·sia, aki·ne·sis** (ā-ki-nē′sē-ă, ā-ki-nē′sis) absence or loss of the power of voluntary movement, due to an extrapyramidal disorder. [G. *a*- priv. + *kinēsis*, movement]

**akin·es·the·sia** (ā-kin′es-thē′zē-ă) inability to perceive movement or position. [G. *a*- priv. + *kinēsis*, motion, + *aisthēsis*, sensation]

**aki·net·ic, aki·ne·sic** (ā-ki-net′ik, ā-ki-nē′sik) relating to or suffering from akinesia.

**a·ki·net·ic mu·tism** subacute or chronic state of altered consciousness, in which the patient appears alert intermittently, but is not responsive, although the descending motor pathways appear intact; due to lesions of various cerebral structures.

**Al** aluminum.

**ALA** δ-aminolevulinic acid. Cf. Ala.

**Ala** alanine or its mono- or diradical.

**ala**, gen. and pl. **alae** (ā′lă, ā′lē) **1.** SYN wing. **2.** pronounced, longitudinal cuticular ridges in nematodes, usually found in larval stages (*Ascaris lumbricoides*), although occasionally present in adult worm (*Enterobius vermicularis*). [L. wing]

**alact·acid ox·y·gen debt, alac·tic ox·y·gen debt** rapid phase of recovery oxygen consumption used to replenish intramuscular high-energy phosphates (ATP and PCr) used in the final phase of exercise; also reflects energy cost of slightly elevated level of physiologic dynamics (e.g., heart rate, breathing rate) as recovery progresses.

**Al·a·gille syn·drome** (ah-lah-zhēl′) an autosomal dominant syndrome that becomes apparent in childhood and is associated with jaundice due to a paucity of intrahepatic bile ducts; characteristics include a narrow face and pointed chin, broad forehead, long, straight nose, deep-set eyes, posterior embryotoxon in the eye, cardiovascular abnormalities, vertebral defects, and nephropathy.

**ala·lia** (ā-lā′lē-ă) mutism; inability to speak. SEE aphonia. [G. *a*- priv. + *lalia*, talking]

**a·la mi·nor os·sis sphe·noi·dalis** [TA] SYN lesser wing of sphenoid bone.

**A·land Is·land al·bi·nism** (ah'lahnt ī'land) SYN ocular albinism 2.

**al·a·nine (A, Ala)** (al'ă-nēn) 2-aminopropionic acid; α-aminopropionic acid; one of the amino acids widely occurring in proteins.

**al·a·nine a·mi·no·trans·fer·ase (ALT)** (al'ă-nēn ă-mē'nō-trans'fer-āz) an enzyme transferring amino groups from L-alanine to 2-ketoglutarate, or the reverse (from L-glutamate to pyruvate); serum concentration is increased in viral hepatitis and myocardial infarction. SYN glutamic-pyruvic transaminase, serum glutamic-pyruvic transaminase.

**al·a·nine-glu·cose cy·cle** alanine, synthesized in muscle from glucose-derived pyruvate, travels from the blood to the liver, which converts the alanine to glucose and urea. The liver releases glucose back into the blood to transport to muscle as an energy substrate.

**ala of nose** the outer wall of each nostril.

**Al·an·son am·pu·ta·tion** (al'ăn-sŏn) a circular amputation, the stump shaped like a cone.

**al·a·nyl** (al'ă-nil) the acyl radical of alanine.

**a·lar** (ā'lăr) **1.** relating to a wing; winged. **2.** SYN axillary. **3.** relating to the wings (alae) of such structures as the nose, sphenoid, sacrum, etc.

**ALARA** acronym for a philosophy of use of radiation based on using dosages *as* low *as* reasonably *a*chievable to attain the desired diagnostic, therapeutic, or other goal.

**a·lar lam·i·na of neu·ral tube** the dorsal division of the lateral walls of the neural tube; alar plate of neural tube.

**a·larm re·ac·tion** the various phenomena, e.g., stimulated endocrine activity, which the body exhibits as an adaptive response to injury or stress; first phase of the general adaptation syndrome.

**a·lar plate of neu·ral tube** SYN alar lamina of neural tube.

**a·lar spine** SYN sphenoidal spine.

**a·lar·yn·ge·al speech** production of speech using a sound source other than the larynx, as in esophageal speech or use of an artificial larynx. SEE esophageal speech. SEE ALSO artificial larynx.

**al·ba** (al'bă) SYN white matter. [fem. of L. *albus*, white]

**Al·bar·ran test** (ahl-bah-rhan') a test for renal insufficiency wherein the drinking of large quantities of water will cause a proportionate increase in the volume of urine if the kidneys are sound, but not if the epithelium of the secreting tubules is damaged.

**Al·bert su·ture** (al'bert) a modified Czerny suture, the first row of stitches passing through the entire thickness of the wall of the gut.

**al·bi·cans**, pl. **al·bi·can·tia** (al'bi-kanz, al'bi-kan'tē-ă) **1.** SYN white. **2.** SYN corpus albicans. [L.]

**al·bi·du·ria** (al-bi-dyu'rē-ă) the passing of pale or white urine of low specific gravity, as in chyluria. SYN albinuria. [L. *albidus*, whitish, + G. *ouron*, urine]

**Al·bi·ni nod·ules** (ahl-bē'nē) any of several minute fibrous nodules on the margins of the mitral and tricuspid valves of the heart, sometimes present in the neonate and representing fetal tissue rests.

**al·bi·nism** (al'bi-nizm) a group of inherited (usually autosomal recessive) disorders with deficiency or absence of pigment in the skin, hair, and eyes, or eyes only, due to an abnormality in production of melanin. SEE ocular albinism, piebaldism. [albino + ism]

**al·bi·no** (al-bī'nō) an individual with albinism. [Pg., little white one, fr. *albo*, white, fr. L. *albus* + *-ino*, dim. suffix]

**al·bi·no rats** rats with white fur and pink eyes; used extensively in laboratory experiments.

**al·bi·not·ic** (al-bi-not'ik) pertaining to albinism.

**al·bi·nu·ria** (al-bi-nyu'rē-ă) SYN albiduria.

**Al·bright dis·ease** (awl'brīt) SYN McCune-Albright syndrome.

**Al·bright he·red·i·tary os·te·o·dys·tro·phy** (awl'brīt) an inherited form of hyperparathyroidism associated with ectopic calcification and ossification and skeletal defects, notably small fourth metacarpals; intelligence may be normal or subnormal. Inheritance is heterogeneous; the autosomal form is caused by mutation in the guanine nucleotide-binding protein gene (GNAS1) on 20q. There are also the recessive and X-linked forms. SEE ALSO pseudohypoparathyroidism. SYN Albright syndrome (2).

**Al·bright syn·drome** (awl'brīt) **1.** SYN McCune-Albright syndrome. **2.** SYN Albright hereditary osteodystrophy.

**al·bu·gin·ea** (al-byu-jin'ē-ă) a white fibrous tissue layer, such as the tunica albuginea. SEE tunica albuginea. [L. *albugineus*, fr. *albugo*, white spot]

**al·bu·men** (al-byu'men) SYN ovalbumin. SEE ALSO albumin.

**al·bu·min** (al-byu'min) a type of simple protein, varieties of which are widely distributed throughout the tissues and fluids of plants and animals; albumin is soluble in pure water, precipitated from solution by strong acids, and coagulably by heat in acid or neutral solution. [L. *albumen* (*-min-*), the white of egg]

**al·bu·min-glob·u·lin ra·tio** the ratio of albumin to globulin in the serum or in the urine in kidney disease; the normal ratio in the serum is approximately 1.55.

**al·bu·mi·noid** (al-byu'min-oyd) **1.** resembling albumin. **2.** any protein. **3.** a simple type of protein, insoluble in neutral solvents, present in horny and cartilaginous tissues and in the lens of the eye; e.g., keratin, elastin, collagen. SYN scleroprotein.

**al·bu·min·ous** (al-byu'min-ŭs) relating to, containing, or consisting of albumin.

**al·bu·min·ur·ia** (al-byu-min-yu'rē-ă) presence of protein in urine, chiefly albumin but also globulin; usually indicative of disease, but sometimes resulting from a temporary or transient dysfunction. SYN proteinuria (2). [albumin + G. *ouron*, urine]

**al·bu·min·ur·ic** (al-byu-mi-nyu'rik) relating to or characterized by albuminuria.

**al·cap·ton** (al-kap'tŏn) SYN homogentisic acid.

**al·cap·ton·u·ria, al·kap·ton·u·ria** (al-kap-tō-nyu'rē-ă) excretion of homogentisic acid (alkapton) in the urine due to congenital lack of the enzyme homogentisate 1,2-dioxygenase; urine turns dark if allowed to stand; may recur and subside at irregular intervals; arthritis and ochronosis are late complications. [alkapton + G. *ouron*, urine]

**al·co·hol** (al'kō-hol) **1.** one of a series of organic chemical compounds in which a hydrogen (H) attached to carbon is replaced by a hydroxyl (OH); alcohols react with acids to form esters and with alkali metals to form alcoholates. **2.** ethanol, $C_2H_5OH$, made from carbohydrates by fermentation and synthetically from ethylene or acetylene. It has been used in beverages and as a solvent, vehicle, and preservative; medicinally, it is used externally as a rubefacient, coolant, and disinfectant, and internally as an analgesic, stomachic, and sedative. SYN ethanol, ethyl alcohol. **3.** the azeotropic mixture of $CH_3CH_2OH$ and water (92.3% by weight of ethanol). [Ar. *al*, the, + *kohl*, fine antimonial powder, the term being applied first to a fine powder, then to anything impalpable (spirit)]

**al·co·hol am·nes·tic syn·drome** an amnestic syndrome resulting from alcoholism; alcoholic "blackouts." Cf. Korsakoff syndrome.

**al·co·hol de·hy·dro·gen·ase (ADH)** (al′ko-hol dē-hī-droj′en-ās) an oxidoreductase that reversibly converts an alcohol to an aldehyde (or ketone) with $NAD^+$ as the H acceptor. For example, ethanol + $NAD^+$ ↔ acetaldehyde + NADH. Plays an important role in alcoholism.

**al·co·hol-gly·cer·in fix·a·tive** alcohol (70%) with 5% glycerin; suitable for most nematodes.

**al·co·hol·ic** (al-kō-hol′ik) **1.** relating to, containing, or produced by alcohol. **2.** one who suffers from alcoholism. **3.** one who abuses or is dependent upon alcohol.

**al·co·hol·ic cir·rho·sis** cirrhosis that frequently develops in chronic alcoholism, characterized in an early stage by enlargement of the liver due to fatty change with mild fibrosis, and later by Laënnec cirrhosis with contraction of the liver.

**al·co·hol·ism** (al′kō-hol-izm) chronic alcohol abuse, dependence, or addiction; chronic excessive drinking of alcoholic beverages resulting in impairment of health and/or social or occupational functioning, and increasing adaptation to the effects of alcohol requiring increasing doses to achieve and sustain a desired effect.

**al·co·hol·y·sis** (al-kō-hol′ĭ-sis) splitting of a chemical bond with the addition of the elements of alcohol at the point of splitting. [alcohol + G. *lysis*, dissolution]

**ALD** assistive listening device.

**al·de·hyde** (al′dĕ-hīd) a compound containing the radical —CH=O, reducible to an alcohol (—CH₂OH), oxidizable to a carboxylic acid (—COOH); e.g., acetaldehyde.

**Al·der anom·a·ly** (ahl′der) coarse azurophilic granulation of leukocytes, especially granulocytes, which may be associated with gargoylism and Morquio disease.

**al·do·pen·tose** (al-dō-pen′tōs) a monosaccharide with five carbon atoms, of which one is a (potential) aldehyde group; e.g., ribose.

**al·dose** (al′dōs) a monosaccharide potentially containing the characteristic group of the aldehydes, —CHO; a polyhydroxyaldehyde.

**al·dos·ter·one** (al-dos′ter-ōn) a hormone produced by the adrenal cortex; its major action is to facilitate potassium exchange for sodium in the distal renal tubule, causing sodium reabsorption and potassium and hydrogen loss; the principal mineralocorticoid.

**al·dos·ter·one an·tag·o·nist** an agent that opposes the action of the adrenal hormone aldosterone on renal tubular mineralocorticoid retention; these agents, e.g., spironolactone, are useful in

treating the hypertension of primary hyperaldosteronism, or the sodium retention of secondary hyperaldosteronism.

**al·do·ste·ron·ism** (al-dos′ter-on-izm) a disorder caused by excessive secretion of aldosterone. SYN hyperaldosteronism.

**alec·i·thal** (ă-les′i-thal) without yolk; denoting oocytes (ova) with little or no deutoplasm. [G. *a*-priv. + *lekithos*, yolk]

**Alep·po boil** (ă-lĕp′ō) the lesion occurring in cutaneous leishmaniasis. SEE cutaneous leishmaniasis.

**aleu·ke·mia** (ā-loo-kē′mē-ă) **1.** literally, a lack of leukocytes in the blood. The term is generally used to indicate varieties of leukemic disease in which the white blood cell count in circulating blood is normal or even less than normal (i.e., no leukocytosis), but a few young leukocytes are observed; sometimes used more restrictedly for unusual instances of leukemia with no leukocytosis and no young forms in the blood. **2.** leukemic changes in bone marrow associated with a subnormal number of leukocytes in the blood. SEE ALSO subleukemic leukemia. [G. *a*- priv. + *leukos*, white, + *haima*, blood]

**aleu·ke·mic** (ā-loo-kē′mik) pertaining to aleukemia.

**aleu·ke·mic leu·ke·mia** leukemia in which abnormal (or leukemic) cells are absent in the peripheral blood.

**aleu·ke·moid** (ā-loo-kē′moyd) resembling aleukemia symptomatically.

**aleu·kia** (ā-loo′kē-ă) absence or extremely decreased number of leukocytes in the circulating blood; sometimes also termed aleukemic myelosis. [G. *a*- priv. + *leukos*, white]

**aleu·ko·cyt·ic** (ā-loo-kō-sit′ik) manifesting absence or extremely reduced numbers of leukocytes in blood or lesions.

**aleu·ko·cy·to·sis** (ā-loo-kō-sī-tō′sis) absence or great reduction of white blood cells in the circulating blood, or the lack of leukocytes in an anatomical lesion. [G. *a*- priv. + *leukos*, white, + *kytos*, a hollow (cell)]

**Al·ex·an·der dis·ease** (al-eg-zan′der) a rare, fatal central nervous system degenerative disease of infants, characterized by psychomotor retardation, seizures, and paralysis; megaloencephaly is associated with widespread leukodystrophic changes, especially in the frontal lobes.

**Al·ex·an·der hear·ing im·pair·ment** (al-eg-zan′der) high frequency deafness due to membranous cochlear dysplasia.

**Al·ex·an·der law** (al-eg-zan′der) states that a jerky nystagmus becomes worse when gazing in the direction of the fast component.

**alex·ia** (ă-lek′sē-ă) an inability to comprehend the meaning of written or printed words and sentences, caused by a cerebral lesion. Also called **optical alexia, sensory alexia,** or **visual alexia,** in distinction to **motor alexia** (anarthria), in which there is loss of the power to read aloud although the significance of what is written or printed is understood. SYN text blindness, word blindness, visual aphasia (1). [G. *a*- priv. + *lexis*, a word or phrase]

**alex·ic** (ă-lek′sik) pertaining to alexia.

**alex·i·thy·mia** (ă-lek-si-thī′mē-ă) difficulty in recognizing and describing one's emotions, defining them in terms of somatic sensations or behavioral reactions. [G. *a-* priv. + *lexis,* word, + *-thymia,* feelings, passion]

**al•gae** (al'jē) a division of eukaryotic, photosynthetic, nonflowering organisms that includes many seaweeds. [pl. of L. *alga,* seaweed]

**al•gal** (al'găl) resembling or pertaining to algae.

△**al•ge-, al•ge•si-, al•gio-, al•go-** pain; corresponds to L. dolor-. [G. *algos,* a pain]

**al•ge•sia** (al-jē'zē-ă) SYN algesthesia. [G. *algēsis,* a sense of pain]

**al•ge•sic** (al-jēz-ik) **1.** painful; related to or causing pain. **2.** relating to hypersensitivity to pain. SYN algetic.

**al•ge•sim•e•ter** (al-jē-sim'ĕ-ter) SYN algesiometer.

**al•ge•si•o•gen•ic** (al-jē'zē-ō-jen'ik) pain-producing. SYN algogenic. [G. *algēsis,* sense of pain, + *-gen,* production]

**al•ge•si•om•e•ter** (al-jē-zē-om'ĕ-ter) an instrument for measuring the degree of sensitivity to a painful stimulus. SYN algesimeter, algometer, odynometer. [G. *algēsis,* sense of pain, + *metron,* measure]

**al•ges•the•sia, al•ges•the•sis** (al-jes-thē'zē-ă, al-jes-thē'sis) **1.** the appreciation of pain. **2.** hypersensitivity to pain. SYN algesia. [G. *algos,* pain, + *aisthēsis,* sensation]

**al•get•ic** (al-jet'ik) SYN algesic.

△**-al•gia** pain, painful condition. [G. *algos,* a pain]

**al•gid stage** the stage of collapse in cholera.

**al•go•gen•ic** (al-gō-jen'ik) SYN algesiogenic.

**al•go•lag•nia** (al-gō-lag'nē-ă) form of sexual perversion in which the infliction or the experiencing of pain increases the pleasure of the sexual act or causes sexual pleasure independent of the act; includes both sadism (active algolagnia) and masochism (passive algolagnia). SYN algophilia (2). [algo- + G. *lagneia,* lust]

**al•gom•e•ter** (al-gom'ĕ-ter) SYN algesiometer. [algo- + G. *metron,* measure]

**al•go•phil•ia** (al-gō-fil'ē-ă) **1.** pleasure experienced in the thought of pain in others or in oneself. **2.** SYN algolagnia. [algo- + G. *phileō,* to love]

**al•go•pho•bia** (al-gō-fō'bē-ă) abnormal fear of or sensitiveness to pain. [algo- + G. *phobos,* fear]

**al•go•rithm** (al'gō-ridhm) a process consisting of steps, each depending on the outcome of the previous one. In clinical medicine, a step-by-step protocol for management of a health care problem; in computed tomography, the formulas used for calculation of the final image from the x-ray transmission data. [Mediev. L. *algorismus,* after Muhammad ibn-Musa *al-Khwarizmi,* Arabian mathematician, + G. *arithmos,* number]

**al•go•vas•cu•lar** (al-gō-vas'kyu-lăr) relating to changes in the lumen of the blood vessels occurring under the influence of pain. [G. *algos,* pain]

**alien•a•tion** (ā-lē-en-ā'shŭn) a condition characterized by lack of meaningful relationships with others, sometimes resulting in depersonalization and estrangement from others. [L. *alieno,* pp. *-atus,* to make strange]

**ali•e•nia** (ā-li-ē'nē-ă) congenital absence of the spleen. [G. *a-* priv. + L. *lien,* spleen]

**al•i•form** (al'i-fōrm) wing-shaped. [L. *ala,* + *forma,* shape]

**align•ment** (ă-līn'ment) **1.** the longitudinal position of a bone or limb. **2.** DENTISTRY the arrangement of the teeth in relation to the supporting structures and the adjacent and opposing dentitions.

**align•ment curve** the line passing through the center of the teeth laterally in the direction of the curve of the dental arch.

**al•i•men•ta•ry** (al-i-men'ter-ē) relating to food or nutrition. [L. *alimentarius,* fr. *alimentum,* nourishment]

**al•i•men•ta•ry ca•nal** SYN digestive tract.

**al•i•men•ta•ry gly•cos•ur•ia** glycosuria developing after the ingestion of a moderate amount of sugar or starch because the rate of intestinal absorption exceeds the capacity of the liver and the other tissues to remove the glucose, thus allowing blood glucose levels to become high enough for renal excretion to occur.

**al•i•men•ta•ry hy•per•in•su•lin•ism** elevated levels of insulin in the plasma following ingestion of meals by individuals with abnormally rapid gastric emptying.

**al•i•men•ta•ry li•pe•mia** relatively transient lipemia occurring after the ingestion of foods with a large content of fat.

**al•i•men•ta•ry pen•to•su•ria** the urinary excretion of L-arabinose and L-xylose, as the result of the excessive ingestion of fruits containing these pentoses.

**al•i•men•ta•ry tract** SYN digestive tract.

**al•i•men•ta•tion** (al-i-men-tā'shŭn) providing nourishment. SEE ALSO feeding.

**al•i•na•sal** (al'i-nā'săl) relating to the wings of the nose (alae nasi), or flaring portions of the nostrils. [L. *ala,* + *nasus,* nose]

**al•i•phat•ic** (al-i-fat'ik) denoting the acyclic carbon compounds, most of which belong to the fatty acid series. [G. *aleiphar (aleiphat-),* fat, oil]

**al•i•phat•ic ac•ids** the acids of nonaromatic hydrocarbons (e.g., acetic, propionic, butyric acids); the so-called fatty acids of the formula R–COOH, where R is a nonaromatic (aliphatic) hydrocarbon.

**al•i•quant** (al'ĭ-kwant) in chemistry and immunology, pertaining to a portion that results from dividing the whole in a manner that some is left after the aliquants (equal in volume or weight) have been apportioned.

**al•i•quot** (al'i-kwot) in chemistry and immunology, pertaining to a portion of the whole; loosely, any one of two or more samples of something, of the same volume or weight. [L. a few, several]

**al•i•sphe•noid** (al-i-sfē'noyd) relating to the greater wing of the sphenoid bone. [L. *ala,* + *sphēn,* wedge]

**aliz•a•rin** (ă-liz'ă-rin) [CI 58000] 1,2-dihydroxyanthraquinone; a red dye that occurs in the root of madder as orange needles, slightly soluble in water; used by the ancients as a dye. Now made synthetically from anthracene and used in the manufacture of dyes, e.g., alizarin blue, alizarin orange, "Turkey red." As an indicator, it is yellow below pH 5.5 and red above pH 6.8; other modified alizarins have other colors and change color at other pH values.

**al•ka•lae•mia [Br.]** SEE alkalemia.

**al•ka•le•mia** (al-kă-lē'mē-ă) a decrease in H-ion concentration of the blood or a rise in pH, irrespective of alterations in the level of bicarbonate ion. [alkali + G. *haima,* blood]

**al•ka•les•cent** (al-ka-les'ent) **1.** slightly alkaline. **2.** becoming alkaline.

**al•ka•li,** pl. **al•ka•lis, al•ka•lies** (al'kă-lī, al-kă-līz) **1.** a strongly basic substance yielding hydroxide ions (OH⁻) in solution; e.g., sodium hydroxide, potassium hydroxide. **2.** SYN base (3). **3.** SYN alkali metal. [Ar., *al*, the, + *qalīy*, soda ash]

**al•ka•li met•al** an alkali of the family Li, Na, K, Rb, Cs, and Fr, all of which have highly ionized hydroxides. SYN alkali (3).

**al•ka•line** (al′kǎ-līn) relating to or having the reaction of an alkali.

**al•ka•line-ash di•et** a diet consisting mainly of fruits, vegetables, and milk which, when catabolized, leave an alkaline residue to be excreted in the urine. SYN acid-ash diet.

**al•ka•line earth el•e•ments** those elements in the family Be, Mg, Ca, Sr, Ba, and Ra, the hydroxides of which are highly ionized and hence alkaline in water solution.

**al•ka•line earths** SEE alkaline earth elements.

**al•ka•line phos•pha•tase** a phosphatase with an optimum pH of above 7.0 present in many tissues; low levels of this enzyme are seen in cases of hypophosphatasia.

**al•ka•line tide** a period of urinary neutrality or even alkalinity after meals due to withdrawal of hydrogen ion for the purpose of secretion of the highly acid gastric juice.

**al•ka•lin•i•ty** (al-kǎ-lin′i-tē) the state of being alkaline.

**al•ka•li•nu•ria** (al′kǎ-li-nyu′rē-ǎ) the passage of alkaline urine. SYN alkaluria. [alkaline + G. *ouron*, urine]

**al•ka•li re•serve** the sum total of the basic ions (mainly bicarbonates) of the blood and other body fluids which, acting as buffers, maintain the normal pH of the blood.

**al•ka•loid** (al′kǎ-loyd) originally, any one of hundreds of plant products distinguished by alkaline (basic) reactions, but now restricted to heterocyclic nitrogen-containing and often complex structures possessing pharmacologic activity; their trivial names usually end in -ine (e.g., morphine, atropine, colchicine). Alkaloids are synthesized by plants and are found in the leaf, bark, seed, or other parts, usually constituting the active principle of the crude drug; they are a loosely defined group, but may be classified according to the chemical structure of their main nucleus. For medicinal purposes, due to improved water solubility, the salts of alkaloids are usually used. SEE ALSO individual alkaloid or alkaloid class.

**al•ka•lo•sis** (al-kǎ-lō′sis) a disorder characterized by H-ion loss or base excess in body fluids (metabolic alkalosis), or caused by $CO_2$ loss due to hyperventilation (respiratory alkalosis).

**al•ka•lot•ic** (al-kǎ-lot′ik) relating to alkalosis.

**al•ka•lu•ria** (al-kǎ-lyu′rē-ǎ) SYN alkalinuria.

**al•kane** (al′kān) the general term for a saturated acyclic hydrocarbon; e.g., propane, butane.

**al•kap•ton** (al-kap′tŏn) SYN homogentisic acid. [alkali + G. *kaptō*, to suck up greedily]

**al•kene** (al′kēn) an acyclic hydrocarbon containing one or more double bonds; e.g., ethene, propene. SYN olefin.

**al•ke•nyl** (al′ken-il) the radical of an alkene.

**al•kide** (al′kīd) SYN alkyl (2).

**al•kyl** (al′kil) **1.** a hydrocarbon radical of the general formula $C_nH_{2n+1}$. **2.** a compound, such as tetraethyl lead, in which a metal is combined with alkyl radicals. SYN alkide.

**al•kyl•a•tion** (al′ki-lā′shŭn) substitution of an al-

kyl radical for a hydrogen atom; e.g., introduction of a side chain into an aromatic compound.

**ALL** acute lymphocytic leukemia.

**al•la•ches•the•sia** (al′ǎ-kes-thē′zē-ǎ) a condition in which a tactile sensation is referred to a point other than that to which the stimulus is applied. [G. *allachē*, elsewhere, + *aisthēsis*, sensation]

**al•laes•the•sia [Br.]** SYN allocheiria.

△**al•lan•to-, al•lant-** allantois; allantoid; sausage. [G. *allas, allantos*, sausage]

**al•lan•to•cho•ri•on** (ă-lan-tō-kōr′ē-on) extraembryonic membrane formed by the fusion of the allantois and chorion.

**al•lan•to•ic** (ă-lan-tō′ik) relating to the allantois.

**al•lan•to•ic flu•id** the fluid within the allantoic cavity.

**al•lan•to•ic stalk** the narrow connection between the intraembryonic portion of the allantois and the extraembryonic allantoic vesicle.

**al•lan•to•ic ves•i•cle** the hollow portion of the allantois.

**al•lan•toid** (ă-lan′toyd) **1.** sausage-shaped. **2.** relating to, or resembling, the allantois. [allanto- + G. *eidos*, appearance]

**al•lan•toid mem•brane** SYN allantois.

**al•lan•toid•o•an•gi•op•a•gous twins** unequal monochorial twins with fusion of their allantoic vessels within the placenta; the lesser twin is essentially a parasite on the placental circulation of the larger twin.

**al•lan•to•in•u•ria** (ă-lan′tō-in-yu′rē-ǎ) the urinary excretion of allantoin; normal in most mammals, abnormal in humans. [allantoin + G. *ouron*, urine]

**al•lan•to•is** (ă-lan′tō-is) a fetal membrane developing from the hindgut (or yolk sac, in humans). In humans it is vestigial; externally, in mammals, it contributes to the formation of the umbilical cord and placenta. SYN allantoid membrane. [allanto- + G. *eidos*, appearance]

**al•lele** (ă-lēl′) any one of a series of two or more different genes that may occupy the same locus on a specific chromosome. As autosomal chromosomes are paired, each autosomal gene is represented twice in normal somatic cells. If the same allele occupies both units of the locus, the individual or cell is homozygous for this allele If the alleles are different, the individual or cell is heterozygous for both alleles. SEE ALSO DNA markers. SYN allelomorph. [G. *allēlōn*, reciprocally]

**al•le•lic** (ă-lē′lik) relating to an allele.

**al•le•lic gene** SEE allele, dominance of traits.

**al•le•lo•morph** (ă-lē′lŏ-mōrf) SYN allele. [G. *allēlōn*, reciprocally, + *morphē*, shape]

**al•le•lo•tax•is, al•le•lo•taxy** (ă-lēl-ō-taks′is, ă-lēl-ō-taks′ē) development of an organ from a number of embryonal structures or tissues. [G. *allēlōn*, reciprocally, + *taxis*, an arranging]

**Al•len cog•ni•tive lev•el scale** (al′ĕn) a leather-lacing task used in occupational therapy to assess a client's level of cognitive function.

**Al•len test** (al′ĕn) a test for radial or ulnar patency; either the radial or ulnar artery is digitally compressed by the examiner after blood has been forced out of the hand by clenching it into a fist; failure of the blood to diffuse into the hand when opened indicates that the artery not compressed is occluded. [Edgar Van Nuys Allen]

**al•ler•gen** (al′er-jen) term for an incitant of altered reactivity (allergy), an antigenic substance. [allergy + G. *-gen,* producing]

**al·ler·gen·ic** (al-er-jen'ik) SYN antigenic.

**al·ler·gen·ic ex·tract** extract (usually containing protein) from various sources, e.g., food, bacteria, pollen, and the like, suspected of in stimulating manifestations of allergy; may be used for skin testing or desensitization. SYN allergic extract.

**al·ler·gic** (ă-ler'jik) relating to any response stimulated by an allergen.

**al·ler·gic con·junc·ti·vi·tis** SYN vernal conjunctivitis.

**al·ler·gic con·tact der·ma·ti·tis** a delayed type IV allergic reaction of the skin with varying degrees of erythema, edema, and vesiculation resulting from cutaneous contact with a specific allergen. SYN contact allergy.

**al·ler·gic ec·ze·ma** macular, papular, or vesicular eruption due to an allergic reaction.

**al·ler·gic ex·tract** SYN allergenic extract.

**al·ler·gic pur·pu·ra** nonthrombocytopenic purpura due to sensitization to foods, drugs, and insect bites. SYN anaphylactoid purpura (1).

**al·ler·gic re·ac·tion** a local or general reaction of an organism following contact with a specific allergen to which it has been previously exposed and sensitized.

**al·ler·gic rhi·ni·tis** rhinitis associated with hay fever.

**al·ler·gic sa·lute** (ă-ler'jik sal-oot') a characteristic wiping or rubbing of the nose with a transverse or upward movement of the hand, as seen in children with allergic rhinitis.

**al·ler·gist** (al'er-jist) one who specializes in the treatment of allergies.

**al·ler·gol·ogy** (al-er-gol'ō-gē) the science concerned with allergic conditions.

**al·ler·gy** (al'er-jē) **1.** hypersensitivity caused by exposure to a particular antigen (allergen) resulting in a marked increase in reactivity to that antigen upon subsequent exposure sometimes resulting in harmful consequences. SEE ALSO allergic reaction, anaphylaxis, immune. **2.** that branch of medicine concerned with the study, diagnosis, and treatment of allergic manifestations. **3.** an acquired hypersensitivity to certain drugs and biologic materials. [G. *allos,* other, + *ergon,* work]

**al·lied health pro·fes·sion·al** an individual trained to perform services in the care of patients; includes a variety of therapy technicians (e.g., pulmonary), radiology technicians, physical therapists, etc.

**al·li·ga·tor for·ceps** a long forceps with a small hinged jaw on the end.

**all or none law** SYN Bowditch law.

△**al·lo-** **1.** other; differing from the normal or usual. **2.** chemical prefix formerly used with amino acids whenever their side chain contained an asymmetric carbon; for example, the alloisoleucines and allothreonines. [G. *allos,* other]

**al·lo·an·ti·body** (al-ō-an'ti-bod-ē) an antibody specific for an alloantigen. Isoantibody is sometimes used in this sense.

**al·lo·an·ti·gen** (al-ō-an'ti-jen) an antigen that occurs in some, but not in other members of the same species. Isoantigen is sometimes used in this sense.

**al·lo·chei·ria, al·lo·chi·ria** (al-ō-kī'rē-ă, al-ō-kī'rē-ă) a form of allachesthesia in which the sensa-

tion of a stimulus in one limb is referred to the contralateral limb. SYN allaesthesia, Bamberger sign (2). [allo- + G. *cheir,* hand]

**al·lo·cor·tex** (al'ō-kōr'teks) O. Vogt's term denoting several regions of the cerebral cortex, in particular the olfactory cortex and the hippocampus, characterized by fewer cell layers than the isocortex; SEE ALSO cerebral cortex. SYN heterotypic cortex. [allo- + L. *cortex,* bark (cortex)]

**al·lo·dip·loid** (al-ō-dip'loyd) SEE alloploid.

**al·lo·dyn·ia** (al-ō-din'ē-ă) condition in which ordinarily nonpainful stimuli evoke pain. [allo- + G. *odynē,* pain]

**al·lo·e·rot·ic** (al'ō-ĕ-rot'ik) pertaining to or characterized by alloerotism. SYN heteroerotic.

**al·lo·er·o·tism** (al-ō-ĕr'ŏ-tizm) sexual attraction toward another person. Cf. autoerotism. SYN heteroerotism. [allo- + G. *erōs,* love]

**al·lo·ge·ne·ic graft** SYN allograft.

**al·lo·graft** (al'ō-graft) a graft transplanted between genetically nonidentical individuals of the same species. SYN allogeneic graft, homologous graft, homoplastic graft.

**al·lo·graft re·jec·tion** (al'lō-graft rē-jek-shŭn) the rejection of tissue transplanted between two genetically different individuals of the same species. Rejection is caused by T lymphocytes responding to the foreign major histocompatibility complex of the graft. SYN homograft.

**al·lo·ker·a·to·plas·ty** (al-ō-ker'ă-tō-plas-tē) replacement of opaque corneal tissue with a transparent prosthesis, usually plastic.

**al·lo·la·lia** (al-ō-lā'lē-ă) any speech defect, especially one caused by a cerebral disorder. [allo- + G. *lalia,* talking]

**al·lom·er·ism** (ă-lom'er-izm) the state of differing in chemical composition but having the same crystalline form. [allo- + G. *meros,* part]

**al·lo·mor·phism** (al-ō-mōr'fizm) **1.** change of shape in cells due to mechanical causes, such as flattening from pressure, or to progressive metaplasia, such as the change of bile duct cells into liver cells. **2.** the state of being similar in chemical composition but differing in form (especially crystalline). [allo- + G. *morphē,* form]

**al·lo·path·ic** (al-ō-path'ik) relating to allopathy.

**al·lop·a·thy** (al-op'ă-thē) a therapeutic system in which a disease is treated by producing a second condition that is incompatible with or antagonistic to the first. Cf. homeopathy. SYN heteropathy (2). [allo- + G. *pathos,* suffering]

**al·lo·plast** (al'ō-plast) **1.** a graft of an inert metal or plastic material. **2.** a relatively inert foreign body used for implantation into tissues. [allo- + G. *plastos,* formed]

**al·lo·plas·ty** (al'ō-plas-tē) repair of defects by allotransplantation.

**al·lo·ploid** (al'ō-ployd) relating to a hybrid individual or cell with two or more sets of chromosomes derived from two different ancestral species. [allo- + -ploid]

**al·lo·ploi·dy** (al-ō-ploy'dē) the condition of being alloploid.

**al·lo·pol·y·ploid** (al-ō-pol'i-ployd) an alloploid having three or more haploid sets of chromosomes. [allo- + polyploid]

**al·lo·pol·y·ploi·dy** (al-ō-pol'i-ploy-dē) the condition of being allopolyploid.

**al·lo·psy·chic** (al-ō-sī'kik) denoting the mental processes in their relation to the outer world. [allo- + G. *psychē,* mind]

**al·lo·rhyth·mia** (al-ŏ-rith'mē-ă) an irregularity in the cardiac rhythm that repeats itself any number of times. [allo- + G. *rhythmos*, rhythm]

**al·lo·rhyth·mic** (al-ō-ridh'mik) relating to or characterized by allorhythmia.

**al·lo·some** (al'ō-sōm) one of the chromosomes differing in appearance or behavior from the autosomes and sometimes unequally distributed among the germ cells. SYN heterochromosome, heterotypical chromosome. [allo- + G. *sōma, body*]

**al·lo·ste·ric** (al-ō-stăr'ik) pertaining to or characterized by allosterism.

**al·lo·ste·ric site** postulated as the place on an enzyme, other than the active site, where a compound, which may be the ultimate product of the biosynthetic pathway involving the enzyme, may bind and influence the activity of the enzyme by changing the enzyme's conformation.

**al·lo·ster·ism, al·lo·ste·ry** (ă-los'ter-izm, ă-los'ter-ē) the influencing of an enzyme activity, or the binding of a ligand to a protein, by a change in the conformation of the protein, brought about by the binding of a substrate or other effector at a site (allosteric site) other than the active site of the protein. Cf. hysteresis.

**al·lo·tope** (al'ō-tōp) the antigenic determinant of an allotype. [allo- + -tope]

**al·lo·trans·plan·ta·tion** (al'ō-tranz-plan-ta'shŭn) transplantation of an allograft.

**al·lo·trope** (al'ō-trōp) an element in one of the allotropic forms that it may assume. [allo- + G. *tropos*, a turning]

**al·lo·tro·pic** (al-ō-trop'ik) **1.** relating to allotropism. **2.** denoting a type of personality characterized by a preoccupation with the reactions of others.

**al·lot·ro·pism, al·lot·ro·py** (ă-lot'rŏ-pizm, ă-lot'rŏ-pē) the existence of certain elements, in several forms differing in physical properties; e.g., carbon black, graphite, and diamond are all pure carbon. [allo- + G. *tropos*, a turning]

**al·lo·type** (al'ō-tīp) any one of the genetically determined antigenic differences within a given class of immunoglobulin that occur among members of the same species. SEE ALSO antibody. [allo- + G. *typos*, model]

**al·lo·typ·ic** (al-ō-tip'ik) pertaining to an allotype.

**al·low·ance** (a'lau-antz) **1.** permission. **2.** a portion allotted.

**al·lox·u·re·mia** (al-oks-yu-rē'mē-ă) the presence of purine bases in the blood. [alloxan + G. *haima*, blood]

**al·lox·u·ria** (al-oks-yu'rē-ă) the presence of purine bodies in the urine. [alloxan + G. *ouron*, urine]

**al·loy** (al'oy) a substance composed of a mixture of two or more metals.

**Al·mei·da dis·ease** (ahl-mā'dah) SYN paracoccidioidomycosis.

**alo·gia** (ā-lō'jē-ă) **1.** SYN aphasia. **2.** inability to speak due to mental deficiency or an episode of dementia. [G. *a-* priv. + *logos*, speech]

**al·o·pe·cia** (al-ō-pē'shē-ă) absense or loss of hair. SYN baldness. [G. *alōpekia*, a disease like fox mange, fr. *alōpēx*, a fox]

**al·o·pe·cia ad·na·ta** underdevelopment of the eyelashes. SEE ALSO alopecia congenitalis. SYN madarosis.

**al·o·pe·cia ar·e·a·ta** a condition of undetermined etiology characterized by circumscribed,

nonscarring, usually asymmetrical areas of baldness on the scalp, eyebrows, and beard area. SYN alopecia circumscripta.

**al·o·pe·cia ca·pi·tis to·ta·lis** SYN alopecia totalis.

**al·o·pe·cia cir·cum·scrip·ta** SYN alopecia areata.

**al·o·pe·cia con·ge·ni·ta·lis** absence of all hair at birth, associated with psychomotor epilepsy.

**al·o·pe·cia he·re·di·ta·ria** SYN androgenic alopecia.

**al·o·pe·cia mar·gi·na·lis** hair loss at the hair line, a condition most commonly seen in blacks; commonly transient and caused by chronic traction, although long-continued traction may cause permanent alopecia.

**al·o·pe·cia me·di·ca·men·to·sa** diffuse hair loss, most notably of the scalp, caused by administration of various types of drugs.

**al·o·pe·cia pit·y·ro·des** a loss of hair, of the body as well as of the scalp, accompanied by an abundant branlike desquamation.

**al·o·pe·cia symp·to·ma·ti·ca** alopecia occurring in the course of various constitutional or local diseases, or following prolonged febrile illness.

**al·o·pe·cia to·ta·lis** total loss of hair of the scalp either within a very short period of time or from progression of localized alopecia, especially alopecia areata. Cf. alopecia universalis. SYN alopecia capitis totalis.

**al·o·pe·cia uni·ver·sa·lis** total loss of hair from all parts of the body. Cf. alopecia totalis.

**al·o·pe·cic** (al-ō-pē'sik) relating to alopecia.

**al·pha** (α) (al'fă) **1.** first letter of the Greek alphabet; used as a classifier in the nomenclature of many sciences. **2.** Bunsen solubility coefficient. **3.** CHEMISTRY denotes the first in a series, a position immediately adjacent to a carboxyl group, the first of a series of closely related compounds, an aromatic substituent on an aliphatic chain, or the direction of a chemical bond away from the viewer. **4.** alpha particle. **5.** CHEMISTRY symbol for angle of optical rotation; degree of dissociation. For terms with the prefix α, see the specific term.

**al·pha an·gle 1.** the angle between the visual and optic axes as they cross at the nodal point of the eye; **2.** the angle between the visual line and the major axis of the corneal ellipse.

**al·pha cells 1.** acidophil cells that constitute about 35% of the cells of the anterior lobe of the hypophysis; there are two varieties: one elaborates somatotropic hormone; the other mammotropic hormone; **2.** cells of the islets of Langerhans that secrete glucagon. **3.** SYN A cells.

**al·pha fi·bers** large somatic motor or proprioceptive nerve fibers conducting impulses at rates near 100 m/sec.

**al·pha gran·ule** a granule of an alpha cell that was named as the first of several kinds or because it was acidophilic.

**Al·pha·her·pes·vir·inae** (al'fa-her'pēz-vir'i-nē) a subfamily of Herpesviridae containing Simplexvirus and Varicellavirus.

**al·pha par·ti·cle (al·pha)** a particle consisting of two neutrons and two protons, with a positive charge ($2e^+$); emitted energetically from the nuclei of unstable isotopes of high atomic number (elements of mass number from 82 up); identical to the helium nucleus.

**al•pha rhythm 1.** a wave pattern in the encephalogram in the frequency band of 8 to 13 Hz; **2.** the posterior dominant 8–13 Hz rhythm in the awake, relaxed person with closed eyes. SYN alpha wave.

**Al•pha•vi•rus** (al′fă-vī-rŭs) one of the genera of the family Togaviridae that was formerly classified as part of the "group A" arboviruses and includes the viruses that cause eastern equine, western equine, and Venezuelan encephalitis.

**al•pha wave** SYN alpha rhythm.

**Al•port syn•drome** (al′port) a genetically heterogeneous disorder characterized by nephritis associated with microscopic hematuria and slow progressive renal failure, sensorineural hearing loss, and ocular abnormalities such as lenticonus and maculopathy; autosomal dominant, autosomal recessive, and X-linked recessive forms exist. The X-linked form is caused by mutation in the collagen type IV alpha-5 gene (COL4A5) on chromosome Xq; the autosomal recessive form is due to mutation in the collagen type IV alpha-3 gene (COL4A3) or alpha-4 gene (COL4A4) on 2q.

**ALS** amyotrophic lateral sclerosis; antilymphocyte serum.

**Al•ström syn•drome** (ahl′strerm) retinal degeneration with nystagmus and loss of central vision, associated with obesity in childhood; sensorineural hearing loss and diabetes mellitus usually occur after age 10; autosomal recessive inheritance.

**ALT** alanine aminotransferase.

**ALT:AST ra•tio** the ratio of serum alanine aminotransferase to serum aspartate aminotransferase; elevated serum levels of both enzymes characterize hepatic disease; when both levels are abnormally elevated and the ALT:AST ratio is greater than 1.0, severe hepatic necrosis or alcoholic hepatic disease is likely; when the ratio is less than 1.0, an acute nonalcoholic hepatic condition is favored.

**Al•te•mei•er operation** (ahl′tĕ-mī-er) an operation for rectal prolapse that involves a sleeve resection of the prolapsed rectum and colon with a primary anastomosis performed transanally.

**al•ter•nans** (awl-ter′nanz) alternating; often used substantively for alternation of the heart, either electrical or mechanical. Alternating; used as a noun in the sense of pulsus alternans. [L.]

**al•ter•nate cov•er test** a test to detect phoria or strabismus; attention is directed to a small fixation object, and one eye is covered for several seconds; then the cover is moved quickly to the other eye; if the eye moves when it is uncovered, a strabismus or phoria is present.

**al•ter•nat•ing cur•rent (AC)** electric current that reverses direction (positive-negative polarity) many times each second (with each rotation of the armature of the dynamo generating the current).

**al•ter•nat•ing pulse** mechanical alternation, a pulse regular in time but with alternate beats stronger and weaker, often detectable only with the sphygmomanometer and usually indicating serious myocardial disease. SYN pulsus alternans.

**al•ter•nat•ing trem•or** a form of hyperkinesia characterized by regular, symmetrical, to-and-fro movements (at about 4 per second) that are produced by patterned, alternating contraction of muscles and their antagonists.

**al•ter•na•tion** (awl-ter-nā′shŭn) the occurrence of two things or phases in succession and recurrently; used interchangeably with alternans.

**al•ter•na•tive med•i•cine** a term used by practitioners of Western medicine for methods of healing, some ancient and widely practiced, that are not firmly based on accepted scientific principles and may be of limited known effectiveness. Examples of alternative practices include acupuncture and acupressure, homeopathy, osteopathy, chiropractic, massage, hypnosis, megavitamin therapy, pulse diagnosis, tongue diagnosis, iridology, rolfing, faith healing, and prayer. SYN complementary medicine.

**al•ter•na•tive splic•ing** different ways of assembling exons to produce different mature mRNAs.

**al•ti•tude sick•ness** a syndrome caused by low inspired oxygen pressure (as at high altitude) and characterized by nausea, headache, dyspnea, malaise, and insomnia; in severe instances, pulmonary edema and adult respiratory distress syndrome can occur; SYN Acosta disease, mountain sickness. SYN aerial sickness.

**Alt•mann an•i•lin-ac•id fuch•sin stain** (ahlt′mahn) a mixture of picric acid, anilin, and acid fuchsin which stains mitochondria crimson against a yellow background.

**Alt•mann fix•a•tive** (ahlt′mahn) a bichromate-osmic acid fixative.

**alu•mi•no•sis** (ă-loo-min-ō′sis) a pneumoconiosis caused by inhalation of aluminum particles.

**alu•mi•num (Al)** (ă-loo′min-ŭm) a white silvery metal of very light weight; atomic no. 13, atomic wt. 26.981539. Many salts and compounds are used in medicine and dentistry. [L. alumen, alum]

**al•vei** (al′vē-ī) plural of alveus.

**al•ve•o•al•gia** (al′vē-ō-al′jē-ă) a postoperative complication of tooth extraction in which the blood clot in the socket disintegrates, resulting in focal osteomyelitis and severe pain. SYN alveolalgia. [alveolus + G. algos, pain]

**al•ve•o•lal•gia** (al′vē-ō-lal′jē-ă) SYN alveoalgia.

**al•ve•o•lar** (al-vē′ō-lăr) relating to an alveolus.

**al•ve•o•lar ab•scess** an abscess situated within the alveolar process of the jaws, most often caused by extension of infection from an adjacent nonvital tooth. See page 36. SYN dental abscess, dentoalveolar abscess.

**al•ve•o•lar air** SYN alveolar gas.

**al•ve•o•lar air equa•tion** an equation that calculates an approximation of alveolar oxygen tension if the fractional concentration of inspired oxygen, arterial carbon dioxide tension, and respiratory exchange ratio (that is, carbon dioxide production divided by oxygen consumption) are known.

**al•ve•o•lar-ar•te•ri•al ox•y•gen dif•fer•ence** the gradient between the partial pressure of oxygen in the alveolar spaces and the arterial blood: $P_{(A-a)}O_2$. Normally in young adults this value is less than 20 mmHg.

**al•ve•o•lar-ar•te•ri•al ox•y•gen ten•sion dif•fer•ence** SYN A-aO$_2$ difference.

**al•ve•o•lar ca•nals of max•il•la** canals in the body of the maxilla that transmit nerves and vessels from the alveolar foramina to the maxillary teeth.

**al•ve•o•lar-cap•il•lary mem•brane** the alveolar epithelium, interstitial space, and the capillary endothelium barrier that gases must cross in respiration; it is approximately 1 micron thick in

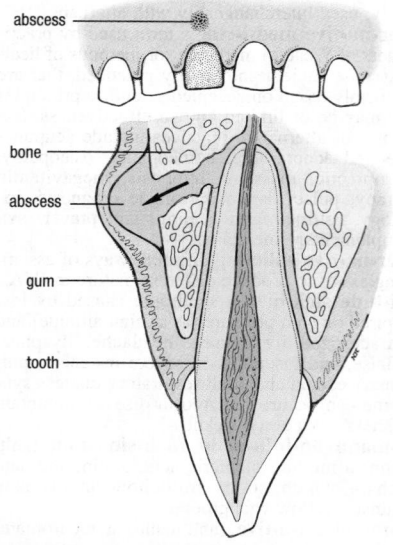

**alveolar abscess:** sagittal section

Labels on figure: abscess, bone, abscess, gum, tooth

healthy individuals and normally represents only a minimal obstacle to gas diffusion.

**al·ve·o·lar cell** any of the cells lining the alveoli of the lung, including the squamous alveolar cells, the great alveolar cells, and the alveolar macrophages.

**al·ve·o·lar cell car·ci·no·ma** SYN bronchiolar carcinoma. SYN bronchiolar adenocarcinoma, bronchoalveolar carcinoma.

**al·ve·o·lar dead space** the difference between physiologic dead space and anatomical dead space; it represents that part of the physiologic dead space resulting from ventilation of relatively underperfused or nonperfused alveoli; it differs specifically in being placed so as to fill and empty in parallel with functional alveoli, rather than being interposed in the conducting tubes between functional alveoli and the external environment.

**al·ve·o·lar duct 1.** the part of the respiratory passages distal to the respiratory bronchiole; from it arise alveolar sacs and alveoli; **2.** the smallest of the intralobular ducts in the mammary gland, into which the secretory alveoli open. SYN ductulus alveolaris.

**al·ve·o·lar gas** (al-vē′ō-lăr) gas symbol subscript A; the gas in the pulmonary alveoli, where $O_2$-$CO_2$ exchange with pulmonary capillary blood occurs. SYN alveolar air.

**al·ve·o·lar gin·gi·va** gingival tissue applied to the alveolar bone.

**al·ve·o·lar gland** a gland in which the secretory unit(s) has a saclike form and an obvious lumen; e.g., the active mammary gland.

**al·ve·o·lar mac·ro·phage** a vigorously phagocytic macrophage on the epithelial surface of lung alveoli where it ingests inhaled particulate matter. SYN coniophage, dust cell.

**al·ve·o·lar point** SYN prosthion.

**al·ve·o·lar pores** openings in the interalveolar septa of the lung that permit air flow between adjacent alveoli.

**al·ve·o·lar sac** terminal dilation of the alveolar ducts that give rise to alveoli in the lung; a small air chamber in the pulmonary tissue from which the pulmonary alveoli project like bays and into which an alveolar duct opens; SYN sacculus alveolaris [TA].

**al·ve·o·lar soft part sar·co·ma** a malignant tumor formed of a reticular stroma of connective tissue enclosing aggregates of large round or polygonal cells; occurs in subcutaneous and fibromuscular tissues.

**al·ve·o·lar ven·ti·la·tion (VA)** the volume of gas expired from the alveoli to the outside of the body per minute; calculated as the respiratory frequency (f) multiplied by the difference between tidal volume and the dead space ($V_T - V_D$); units: ml/min BTPS.

**al·ve·o·lec·to·my** (al′vē-ō-lek′tō-mē) surgical excision of a portion of the dentoalveolar process at the time of tooth removal to facilitate a dental prosthesis. [alveolus + G. *ektomē*, excision]

**al·ve·o·li** (al-vē′ō-lī) plural of alveolus.

**al·ve·o·lin·gual** (al′vē-o-ling′gwăl) SYN alveolo-lingual.

**al·ve·o·li pul·mo·nis** SYN pulmonary alveolus.

**al·ve·o·li·tis** (al′vē-ō-lī′tis) **1.** inflammation of alveoli. **2.** inflammation of a tooth socket.

**al·ve·o·lo-** an alveolus, the alveolar process; alveolar. [L. *alveolus*, a concave vessel, a bowl, a basin, fr. *alveus*, a trough, + -*olus*, small, little; akin to *alvus*, the belly, the womb]

**al·ve·o·lo·cap·il·lary block** the presence of material that impairs the diffusion of gases between the air in the alveolar spaces and the blood in alveolar capillaries; block can be caused by edema, cellular infiltration, fibrosis, or tumor, and results in undersaturation of peripheral arterial blood with oxygen.

**al·ve·o·lo·cla·sia** (al-vē′ō-lō-klā′zē-ă) destruction of the alveolus. [alveolo- + G. *klasis*, breaking]

**al·ve·o·lo·den·tal** (al-vē′ō-lō-den′tăl) relating to the alveoli and the teeth.

**al·ve·o·lo·den·tal lig·a·ment** SYN periodontal ligament.

**al·ve·o·lo·den·tal mem·brane** SYN periodontal ligament.

**al·ve·o·lo·la·bi·al** (al-vē′ō-lō-lā′bē-ăl) relating to the labial or vestibular (outer) surface of the alveolar process of the upper or lower jaw.

**al·ve·o·lo·lin·gual** (al-vē′ō-lō-ling′gwăl) relating to the lingual (inner) surface of the alveolar process of the lower jaw. SYN alveolingual.

**al·ve·o·lo·pal·a·tal** (al-vē′ō-lō-pal′ă-tăl) relating to the palatal surface of the alveolar process of the upper jaw.

**al·ve·o·lo·plas·ty** (al-vē′ō-lō-plas-tē) surgical preparation of the alveolar ridges for the reception of dentures; shaping and smoothing of socket margins after extraction of teeth with subsequent suturing to insure optimal healing. SYN alveoplasty. [alveolo- + G. *plassō*, to form]

**al·ve·o·lot·o·my** (al-vē′ō-lō-lot′ō-mē) surgical opening into a dental alveolus to allow drainage of pus from a periapical or other intraosseous abscess. [alveolo- + G. *tomē*, incision]

**al·ve·o·lus**, gen. and pl. **al·ve·o·li** (al-vē′ō-lŭs, al-vē′ō-lī) [TA] a small cell, cavity, or socket. **1.** SYN pulmonary alveolus. **2.** one of the terminal secretory portions of an alveolar or racemose gland. **3.** one of the honeycomb pits in the wall of the stomach. **4.** SYN tooth socket. [L. dim. of *alveus,* trough, hollow sac, cavity]

**al·ve·o·plas·ty** (al′vē-ō-plas-tē) SYN alveolo-plasty.

**al·ve·us** (al′vē-ŭs, al′vē-ī) a channel or trough. [L. tray, trough, cavity, fr. *alvus,* belly]

**alym·pho·cy·to·sis** (ā-lim′fō-sī-tō′sis) absence or great reduction of lymphocytes.

**alym·pho·pla·sia** (ā-lim-fō-plā′zē-ă) aplasia or hypoplasia of lymphoid tissue.

ℹ️ **Alz·heim·er dis·ease, Alz·heim·er de·men·tia** (awlz′hī-měr) progressive mental deterioration manifested by loss of memory, ability to calculate, and visual-spatial orientation; confusion; disorientation. Begins in late middle life and results in death in 5–10 years. The brain is atrophic; histologically, there is distortion of the intracellular neurofibrils (neurofibrillary tangles) and senile plaques composed of granular or filamentous argentophilic masses with an amyloid core; the most common degenerative brain disorder. See page B12. SYN presenile dementia (2), dementia presenilis, primary senile dementia.

**Alz·heim·er scle·ro·sis** (awlz′hī-měr) hyaline degeneration of the medium and smaller blood vessels of the brain.

**al·zyme** (al′zīm) union of antibody and enzyme to form a hybrid catalytic molecule.

**Am** americium.

**am** ammeter.

**am·a·crine** (am′ă-krīn) **1.** a cell or structure lacking a long, fibrous process. **2.** denoting such a cell or structure. [G. *a-* priv. + *makros,* long, + *is* (*in-*), fiber]

**am·al·gam** (ă-mal′gam) an alloy of an element or a metal with mercury. In dentistry, primarily of two types: silver-tin alloy, containing small amounts of copper, zinc and perhaps other metals, and a second type containing more copper (12 to 30% by weight); they are used for restoring teeth and making dies. [G. *malagma,* a soft mass]

**am·al·gam tat·too** a bluish-black or gray macular lesion of the oral mucous membrane caused by accidental implantation of silver amalgam into the tissue during tooth restoration or extraction.

**Am·a·ni·ta** (am-ă-nī′tă) a genus of fungi, many members of which are highly poisonous. [G. *amanitai,* fungi]

**Am·a·ni·ta mus·ca·ria** a toxic species of mushroom with yellow to red pileus and white gills; it contains muscarine, which produces psychosis-like states and other symptoms.

**Am·a·ni·ta phal·loi·des** a species containing poisonous principles, including phalloidin and amanitin, that cause gastroenteritis, hepatic necrosis, and renal necrosis.

**amas·tia** (ă-mas′tē-ă) absence of the breasts. SYN amazia. [G. *a-* priv. + *mastos,* breast]

**amas·ti·gote** (ă-mas′ti-gōt) SYN Leishman-Donovan body. [G. *a-* priv. + *mastix,* whip]

**am·au·ro·sis** (am-aw-rō′sis) blindness, especially that occurring without apparent change in the eye itself, as from a brain lesion. [G. *amauros,* dark, obscure, + *-osis,* condition]

**am·au·ro·sis fu·gax** transient blindness that may result from carotid artery insufficiency, retinal artery embolus, or centrifugal force (visual blackout in flight).

**am·au·rot·ic** (am-aw-rot′ik) relating to or suffering from amaurosis.

**am·au·rot·ic cat eye** a yellow reflex from the pupil in cases of retinoblastoma or pseudoglioma.

**am·au·rot·ic pu·pil** pupil in an eye that is blind because of ocular or optic nerve disease; this pupil will not contract to light except when the normal fellow eye is stimulated with light.

**ama·zia** (ă-mā′zē-ă) SYN amastia.

**am·ba·geu·sia** (am-bă-gyu′sē-ă) loss of taste from both sides of the tongue. [L. *ambo,* both, + G. *a-* priv. + *geusis,* taste]

**AMBER** (am′ber) advanced multiple-beam equalization radiography.

**am·ber co·don** the termination codon UAG.

△**am·bi-** around; on all (both) sides; both, double; corresponds to G. *amphi-.* [L., around, about, akin to *ambo,* both]

**am·bi·dex·ter·i·ty** (am-bi-deks-ter′i-tē) the ability to use both hands with equal ease.

**am·bi·dex·trous** (am-bi-deks′trŭs) having equal facility in the use of both hands.

**am·bi·ent** (am′bē-ent) surrounding, encompassing; pertaining to the environment in which an organism or apparatus functions. [L. *ambiens,* going around]

**am·bi·gu·i·ty** (am-bi-gyu′ĭ-tē) condition of being ambiguous; uncertainty.

**am·big·u·ous ex·ter·nal gen·i·ta·lia** external genitalia not clearly of either sex; most commonly designates external genitalia that are incompletely masculinized.

**am·big·u·ous gen·i·ta·lia** SYN genital ambiguity.

**am·bi·lat·er·al** (am-bi-lat′er-ăl) relating to both sides. [ambi- + L. *latus,* side]

**am·bi·le·vous** (am-bi-lē′vŭs) awkwardness in the use of both hands. [ambi- + L. *laevus,* left]

**am·bi·sex·u·al** (am-bi-seks′yu-ăl) **1.** denoting sexual characteristics found in both sexes, e.g., breasts, pubic hair. **2.** slang term for bisexual.

**am·biv·a·lence** (am-biv′ă-lens) the coexistence of antithetical attitudes or emotions toward a given person or thing, or idea, as in the simultaneous feeling and expression of love and hate toward the same person. [ambi- + L. *valentia,* strength]

**am·biv·a·lent** (am-biv′ă-lent) relating to or characterized by ambivalence.

△**am·bly-** dullness, dimness; blunt, dull, dim, dimmed. [G. *amblys,* blunt, dulled; faint, dim]

**am·bly·a·phia** (am-bli-ā′fē-ă) diminution in tactile sensibility. [ambly- + G. *haphē,* touch]

**am·bly·geus·tia** (am-bli-gyus′tē-ă) a diminution in the sense of taste. [ambly- + G. *geusis,* taste]

**am·bly·o·gen·ic** (am′blē-ō-jen′ic) inducing amblyopia. [amblyopia + -genic]

**am·bly·o·gen·ic per·i·od** period during early visual development when the visual neurosensory system is vulnerable to developing amblyopia from blurred retinal image formation, bilateral cortical suppression (as in strabismic amblyopia), or both.

**Am·bly·om·ma** (am-blē-om′ă) a genus of hard ticks characterized by eyes, festoons, and deeply imbedded ventral plates near the festoons in males. [ambly- + G. *omma,* eye, vision]

**am·bly·o·pia** (am-blē-ō′pē-ă) visual impairment not due to an ocular lesion and not fully correctable by an artificial lens. [G. *amblyōpia*, dimness of vision, fr. *amblys* dull, + *ōps*, eye]

**am·bly·o·pic** (am-blē-ō′pik) relating to, or suffering from, amblyopia.

**am·bly·o·scope** (am′blē-ō-skōp) a reflecting stereoscope used to evaluate or simulate binocular vision. SEE ALSO haploscope. [amblyopia + G. *skopeō*, to view]

**am·bo·cep·tor** (am′bō-sep-tŏr) complement-fixing antibody; now used chiefly to denote the anti-sheep erythrocyte antibody used in the hemolytic system of complement-fixation tests. [ambo- + L. *capio*, to take]

**Am·bu bag** proprietary name for a self-reinflating bag with nonrebreathing valves to provide positive pressure ventilation during resuscitation with oxygen or air.

**am·bu·lance** (am′byu-lans) a vehicle used to transport sick or injured persons to a treatment facility. [Fr., fr. (*hôpital*), *ambulant*, mobile hospital]

**am·bu·lance ser·vice** SYN emergency medical service.

**am·bu·la·tion** (am-byu-lā′shŭn) the activity of moving or walking about. [L. *ambulo*, to walk]

**am·bu·la·to·ry, am·bu·lant** (am′byu-lă-tōr-ē, am′byu-lant) walking about or able to walk about; denoting a patient who is not confined to bed or hospital as a result of disease or surgery. [L. *ambulans*, walking]

**am·bu·la·to·ry care** medical or surgical health care provided during an episode of care that lasts less than 24 hours and from which the patient goes home; outpatient rather than inpatient care.

**am·bu·la·to·ry pa·tient group (APG)** a classification of patients by surgical procedure into categories for the purpose of determining reimbursement of health care costs, based on the premise that treatment of similar procedures would generate similar costs.

**Am·bu·la·to·ry Pay·ment Clas·si·fi·ca·tion group (APC)** outpatient services grouped according to similarity of resource costs and clinical indications.

**am·bu·la·to·ry sur·gery** operative procedures performed on patients who are admitted to and discharged from a hospital on the same day. SYN outpatient surgery.

**ame·ba**, pl. **ame·bae, ame·bas** (ă-mē′bă, ă-mē′ bē, ă-mē′băs) common name for *Amoeba* and similar naked, lobose, sarcodine protozoa.

**am·e·bi·a·sis** (ă-mē-bī′ă-sis) infection with *Entamoeba histolytica* or other pathogenic amebas. [ameba + G. *-iasis*, condition]

**ame·bic** (ă-mē′bik) relating to, resembling, or caused by amebas.

**ame·bic ab·scess** an area of liquefaction necrosis of the liver or other organ containing amebae, often following amebic dysentery. SYN tropical abscess.

**ame·bic co·li·tis** inflammation of the colon in amebiasis.

**ame·bic dys·en·tery** diarrhea resulting from ulcerative inflammation of the colon, caused chiefly by infection with *Entamoeba histolytica*; may be associated with amebic infection of other organs.

**ame·bic gran·u·lo·ma** SYN ameboma.

**ame·bi·ci·dal** (ă-mē-bi-sī′dăl) destructive to amebas.

**ame·bi·cide** (ă-mē′bi-sīd) any agent that causes

the destruction of amebas. [ameba + L. *caedo*, to kill]

**ame·bi·form** (ă-mē′bi-fōrm) of the shape or appearance of an ameba. [ameba + L. *forma*, shape]

**ame·bo·cyte** (ă-mē′bō-sīt) 1. a wandering cell found in invertebrates. 2. an *in vitro* tissue culture leukocyte. [ameba, + *kytos*, cell]

**ame·boid** (ă-mē′boyd) 1. resembling an ameba in appearance or characteristics. 2. of irregular outline with peripheral projections; denoting the outline of a form of colony in plate culture. [ameba + G. *eidos*, appearance]

**ame·boid cell** a cell such as a leukocyte, having ameboid movements, with a power of locomotion. SYN wandering cell.

**ame·boid move·ment** the form of movement characteristic of the protoplasm of leukocytes, amebae, and other unicellular organisms; it involves the massing of the protoplasm at a point where surface pressure is least and its extrusion in the form of a pseudopod; the protoplasm may return to the body of the cell, resulting in the retraction of the pseudopod, or the entire mass may flow into the latter and thereby result in locomotion of the cell.

**am·e·bo·ma** (ă-mē-bō′mă) a nodular, tumor-like focus of proliferative inflammation sometimes developing in chronic amebiasis, especially in the wall of the colon. SYN amebic granuloma. [ameba + G. *-oma*, tumor]

**am·e·bu·ria** (am-ē-byu′rē-ă) the presence of amebas in the urine. [ameba + G. *ouron*, urine]

**ame·lia** (ă-mē′lē-ă) congenital absence of a limb or limbs. [G. *a-* priv. + *melos*, a limb]

**am·e·lo·blast** (ă-mel′ō-blast) one of the columnar epithelial cells of the inner layer of the enamel organ of a developing tooth, concerned with the formation of enamel. [Early E. *amel*, enamel, + G. *blastos*, germ]

**am·e·lo·blas·tic ad·e·no·ma·toid tu·mor** SYN adenomatoid odontogenic tumor.

**am·e·lo·blas·tic fi·bro·ma** a benign mixed odontogenic tumor characterized by neoplastic proliferation of both epithelial and mesenchymal components of the tooth bud without the production of dental hard tissue; presents clinically as a slow-growing painless radiolucency occurring most commonly in the mandible of children and adolescents.

**am·e·lo·blas·tic fi·bro·sar·co·ma** a rapidly growing, painful, destructive, radiolucent odontogenic tumor that usually arises through malignant change in the mesenchymal component of a pre-existing ameloblastic fibroma. SYN ameloblastic sarcoma.

**am·e·lo·blas·tic lay·er** the internal layer of the enamel organ. SYN enamel layer.

**am·e·lo·blas·tic odon·to·ma** a benign mixed odontogenic tumor composed of an undifferentiated component histologically identical to an ameloblastoma and a well differentiated component identical to an odontoma.

**am·e·lo·blas·tic sar·co·ma** SYN ameloblastic fibrosarcoma.

**am·e·lo·blas·to·ma** (am′ĕ-lō-blas-tō′mă) a benign odontogenic epithelial neoplasm; it behaves as a slowly growing expansile radiolucent tumor, occurs most commonly in the posterior regions of the mandible, and has a marked tendency to recur if inadequately excised. [ameloblast + G. *-oma*, tumor]

**am·e·lo·den·tin·al** (am′ĕ-lō-den′ti-năl) SYN dentinoenamel.

**am·e·lo·gen·e·sis** (am′ĕ-lō-jen′ĕ-sis) the deposition and maturation of enamel. SYN enamelogenesis.

**am·e·lo·gen·in** (am′el-ō-jen-in) any of several proteins that form much of the organic matrix during the early development of tooth enamel. [amelogenesis + -in]

**amen·or·rhea** (ā-men-ō-rē′ă) absence or abnormal cessation of the menses. [G. *a*- priv. + *mēn,* month, + *rhoia,* flow]

**amen·or·rhea-ga·lac·tor·rhea syn·drome** unphysiologic lactation from endocrinological causes or from a pituitary tumor.

**amen·or·rhe·al, amen·or·rhe·ic** (ā-men-ō-rē′ăl, ā-men-ō-rē′ik) relating to, accompanied by, or due to amenorrhea.

**amen·tia** (ă-men′shē-ă) SYN dementia. [L. madness, fr. *ab,* from, + *mens,* mind]

**amen·ti·al** (ā-men′shē-al) pertaining to amentia.

**Amer·i·can Law In·sti·tute rule** a test of criminal responsibility (1962): "a person is not responsible for criminal conduct if at the time of such conduct as a result of mental disease or defect he lacks substantial capacity either to appreciate the wrongfulness of his conduct or to conform his conduct to the requirements of law."

**Amer·i·can leish·man·i·a·sis** SYN mucocutaneous leishmaniasis.

**Amer·i·can Man·u·al Al·pha·bet** specific hand and finger positions used to represent each of the letters of the alphabet, used in conjunction with American Sign Language and other sign languages. SEE ALSO augmentative and alternative communication, fingerspelling, sign language.

**Amer·i·can Na·tion·al Stand·ards In·sti·tute (ANSI)** organization that sets standards for physical measures in the United States.

**Amer·i·can Sign Lan·guage (ASL)** the manual sign and gesture language used by the deaf community in the United States. It is a language distinct from English, with its own grammar and syntax, but no written form.

**Amer·i·cans with Dis·a·bil·i·ties Act** federal legislation (Public Law 101-336, enacted in 1990) guaranteeing persons with disabilities equal access to employment, education, public accommodations, transportation, telecommunications, and government services at all levels.

**am·er·i·ci·um (Am)** (am′ĕ-ris′ē-ŭm) an element obtained by the bombardment of uranium with neutrons or β decay of plutoniums 241, 242, and 243; atomic no. 95; atomic weight 243.06. [241]Am (half-life of 432.2 years) has been used in the diagnosis of bone disorders. [243]Am has a half-life of 7370 years. [the Americas]

**Ames test** (āmz) a screening test for possible carcinogens using strains of *Salmonella typhimurium* that are unable to synthesize histidine; if the test substance produces mutations that regain the ability to synthesize histidine, the substance is carcinogenic.

**ame·tria** (ā-mē′trē-ă) congenital absence of the uterus. [G. *a*- priv. + *mētra,* uterus]

**am·e·tro·pia** (am-ĕ-trō′pē-ă) the optic condition in which there is an error of refraction so that with the eye at rest the retina is not in conjugate focus with light rays from distant objects, i.e., only less distant objects are focused on the retina.

[G. *ametros,* disproportionate, fr. *a*- priv. + *metron,* measure, + *ōps,* eye]

**am·e·tro·pic** (am-ĕ-trō′pik) relating to, or suffering from, ametropia.

△**-am·ic** chemical suffix denoting the replacement of one COOH group of a dicarboxylic acid by a carboxamide group (—CONH₂); applied only to trivial names (e.g., succinamic acid).

**ami·cro·bic** (ā-mī-krō′bik) not microbic; not related to or caused by microorganisms.

**am·i·dase** (am′i-dās) an enzyme that catalyzes the hydrolysis of monocarboxylic amides to free acid plus NH₃; ω-amidase acts on amides such as α-ketoglutaramic acid and α-ketosuccinamic acid. SYN acylamidase.

**am·i·das·es** SYN amidohydrolase.

**am·ide** (am′īd, am′id) a substance formally derived from ammonia through the substitution of one or more of the hydrogen atoms by acyl groups, R—CO—NH₂, or from a carboxylic acid by replacement of a carboxylic OH by NH₂. Replacement of one hydrogen atom constitutes a **primary amide**; that of two hydrogen atoms, a **secondary amide**; and that of three atoms, a **tertiary amide**.

**am·i·dine** (am′i-dēn) the monovalent radical —C(NH)-NH₂.

△**ami·do-** prefix denoting the amide radical, R-CO-NH- or R-SO₂-NH-, etc. [am(monia) + -id(e) + -o-]

**ami·do·hy·dro·lase** (am′i-dō-hī′drō-lās) [EC class 3.5.1 and 3.5.2] an enzyme hydrolyzing C-N bonds of amides and cyclic amides; e.g., asparaginase, barbiturase, urease, amidase. SYN amidases, deamidase, deamidizing enzyme.

**amim·ia** (ā-mim′ē-a) **1.** inability to express ideas by nonverbal communication, such as gestures or signs. **2.** asymbolia; the inability to comprehend the meaning of gestures, signs, symbols, or pantomime. [G. *a*- priv. + *minos,* a mimic]

**am·i·nate** (am′i-nāt) to combine with ammonia.

**amine** (ă-mēn′, am′in) a substance derived from ammonia by the replacement of one or more of the hydrogen atoms by hydrocarbon or other radicals. The substitution of one hydrogen atom constitutes a **primary amine**, e.g., NH₂CH₃; that of two atoms, a **secondary amine**, e.g., NH(CH₃)₂; that of three atoms, a **tertiary amine**, e.g., N(CH₃)₃; and that of four atoms, a **quaternary ammonium ion**, e.g., ⁺N( CH₃)₄, a positively charged ion isolated only in association with a negative ion. The amines form salts with acids.

**amine ox·i·dase (fla·vin-con·tain·ing)** an oxidoreductase containing flavin and oxidizing amines with the aid of O₂ and water to aldehydes or ketones with the release of NH₃ and H₂O₂. Acted upon by antidepressants.

△**amino-** prefix denoting a compound containing the radical, —NH₂. [am(monia) + in(e) + -o-]

**ami·no ac·id (AA, aa)** (ă-mē′nō as′id) an organic acid in which one of the hydrogen atoms on a carbon atom has been replaced by NH₂. Usually refers to an aminocarboxylic acid. However, taurine is also an amino acid. SEE ALSO α-amino acid.

**α-ami·no ac·id** typically, an amino acid of the general formula R-CHNH₂-COOH (i.e., the NH₂ in the α position); the L forms of these are the hydrolysis products of proteins.

**ami·no ac·id de·hy·dro·gen·ase** enzyme catalyzing the oxidative deamination of amino acids to the corresponding oxo (keto) acids. Cf. amino acid oxidase.

**ami·no·ac·i·de·mia** (am′i-nō-as-id-ē-mē-ă) the presence of excessive amounts of specific amino acids in the blood. [amino acid + G. *haima,* blood]

**ami·no ac·id ox·i·dase** flavoenzyme oxidizing, with $O_2$ and $H_2O$, either L- or D-amino acids specifically, to the corresponding 2-keto acids, $NH_3$ and $H_2O_2$. Cf. amino acid dehydrogenase.

**ami·no·ac·i·du·ria** (am′i-nō-as-i-dyu′rē-ă) excretion of amino acids in the urine, especially in excessive amounts. [amino acid + G. *ouron,* urine]

**ami·no·ac·yl (AA, aa)** (ă-mē′nō-as′il) the radical formed from an amino acid by removal of OH from a COOH group.

**ami·no·ac·yl·ase** (ă-mē′nō-as′i-lās) an enzyme catalyzing hydrolysis of a wide variety of *N*-acyl amino acids to the corresponding amino acid and an acid anion.

***p*-ami·no·ben·zo·ic acid (PABA)** (păr′a-ă-mē′nō-ben-zō′ik as′id) a factor in the vitamin B complex, a part of all folic acids and required for its formation; neutralizes the bacteriostatic effects of the sulfonamides since it furnishes an essential growth factor for bacteria, with the use of which sulfonamides interfere; used as an ultraviolet screen in lotions and creams.

**γ-ami·no·bu·tyr·ic ac·id (GABA)** (gam-mah-ă-mē′nō-byu-tēr′ik as′id) 4-aminobutyric acid; a constituent of the central nervous system; quantitatively the principal inhibitory neurotransmitter. Used in the treatment of a number of disorders (e.g., epilepsy).

**δ-ami·no·bu·tyr·ic ac·id aminotransferase** an enzyme catalyzing the reversible transfer of an amino group from δ-aminobutyric acid to 2-oxoglutarate, thus forming a L-glutamic acid and succinate semialdehyde. An important step in the catabolism of δ-aminobutyric acid.

**5-ami·no·im·id·az·ole ri·bose 5′phos·phate (AIR)** (fīv-ă-mē′nō-im-id-az′ōl rī-bōs-fīv-fos-făt) 5-amino-1-β-D-ribofuranosylimidazole 5′-phosphate; an intermediate in the biosynthesis of purines. SYN 5-aminoimidazole ribotide.

**5-a·mi·no·i·mid·a·zole ri·bo·tide (AIR)** SYN 5-aminoimidazole ribose 5′phosphate.

**δ-ami·no·lev·u·lin·ic ac·id (ALA)** (ă-mē′nō-lev-yu-lin′ik as′id) an acid formed by δ-aminolevulinate synthase from glycine and succinyl-coenzyme A; a precursor of porphobilinogen, hence an important intermediate in the biosynthesis of hematin. ALA levels are elevated in cases of lead poisoning.

**am·i·nol·y·sis** (am-i-nol′i-sis) replacement of a halogen in an alkyl or aryl molecule by an amine radical, with elimination of hydrogen halide.

**ami·no·pep·ti·dae** (ă-mē′nō-pep′ti-dās) [EC subgroup 3.4.11] enzyme catalyzing the breakdown of a peptide, removing the amino acid at the amino end of the chain (i.e., an exopeptidase); found in intestinal secretions.

**ami·no·pep·ti·dase (cy·to·sol)** an enzyme of broad specificity, containing zinc, and catalyzing the hydrolysis of the N-terminal amino acid of a peptide (i.e., an exopeptidase).

**ami·no·pep·ti·dase (mi·cro·som·al)** an aminopeptidase of broad specificity, but preferring alanine and discriminating against proline.

**am·i·noph·er·ase** (am-i-nof′er-ās) SYN aminotransferase.

**α-ami·no·suc·cin·ic ac·id** (al-fa-ă-mē′nō-sŭksin′ik as′id) SYN aspartic acid.

**ami·no·ter·mi·nal** the α-$NH_2$ group or the aminoacyl residue containing it at one end of a peptide or protein (usually at left as written).

**ami·no·trans·fer·ase** (ă-mē′nō-trans′fer-ā) [EC sub-group 2.6.1] enzyme transferring amino groups between an amino acid to (usually) a 2-keto acid. SYN aminopherase, transaminases.

**am·i·nu·ria** (am-i-nyu′rē-ă) excretion of amines in the urine. [amine + G. *ouron,* urine]

**ami·to·sis** (am-i-tō′sis) direct division of the nucleus and cell, without the complicated changes in the nucleus that occur in the ordinary process of cell reproduction. SYN direct nuclear division, Remak nuclear division. [G. *a-* priv. + mitosis]

**ami·tot·ic** (am-i-tot′ik) relating to or marked by amitosis.

**am·me·ter (am)** (am′mē-ter) an instrument for measuring strength of electric current in amperes.

**am·mo·ne·mia, am·mo·ni·e·mia** (am-ō-nē-ē′mē-ă) the presence of ammonia or some of its compounds in the blood, thought to be formed from the decomposition of urea; it usually results in subnormal temperature, weak pulse, gastroenteric symptoms, and coma. [ammonia + G. *haima,* blood]

**Am·mon horn** (am′mon) one of the two interlocking gyri composing the hippocampus, the other being the dentate gyrus. Based on cytoarchitectural features, Ammon horn can be divided into region I (regio I cornus ammonis [TA]), region II (regio II cornus ammonis [TA]), region III (regio III cornus ammonis [TA]) and region IV (regio IV cornus ammonis [TA]). SYN cornu ammonis [TA]. [G. *Ammōn,* the Egyptian deity *Amūn*]

**am·mo·nia-ly·ase** (ă-mō′nē-ă-lī′ās) enzyme removing ammonia or an amino compound nonhydrolytically by rupture of a C—N bond leaving a double bond.

△**am·mo·ni·o-** combining form indicating an ammonium group.

**am·mo·ni·um** (ă-mō′nē-ŭm) the ion, $NH_4^+$, formed by combination of $NH_3$ and $H^+$; behaves as a univalent metal in forming ammonium compounds.

**am·mo·ni·u·ria** (ă-mō-nē-yu′rē-ă) excretion of urine that contains an excessive amount of ammonia. [ammonia + G. *ouron,* urine]

**am·mo·nol·y·sis** (ă-mō-nol′i-sis) the breaking of a chemical bond with the addition of the elements of ammonia ($NH_2$ and H) at the point of breakage. [ammonia + G. *lysis,* dissolution]

**am·ne·sia** (am-nē′zē-ă) a disturbance in the memory of information stored in long-term memory, in contrast to short-term memory, manifested by total or partial inability to recall past experiences. [G. *amnēsia,* forgetfulness]

**am·ne·si·ac** (am-nē′sē-ak) one suffering from amnesia.

**am·ne·sic** (am-nē′sik) relating to or characterized by amnesia. SYN amnestic (1).

**am·nes·tic** (am-nes′tik) **1.** SYN amnesic. **2.** an agent causing amnesia. **3.** a disorder in which the essential feature is an impairment of the memory function.

**am·nes·tic apha·sia, am·ne·sic apha·sia** SYN nominal aphasia.

**am·nes·tic syn·drome 1.** SYN Korsakoff syn-drome. **2.** an organic brain syndrome with short term (but not immediate) memory disturbance, regardless of the etiology.

△**am·ni·o-** the amnion. [G. *amnion*]

⚕**am·ni·o·cen·te·sis** (am′nē-ō-sen-tē′sis) trans-abdominal aspiration of fluid from the amniotic sac for diagnostic purposes. See this page. [amnio- + G. *kentēsis*, puncture]

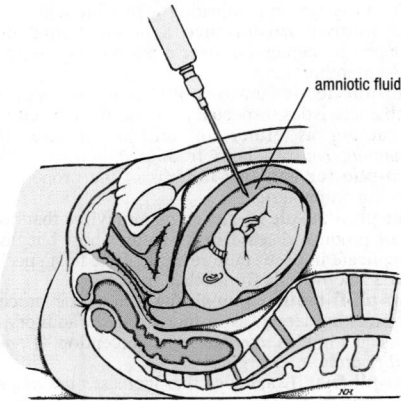

amniotic fluid

**amniocentesis**

**am·ni·o·cho·ri·al, am·ni·o·cho·ri·on·ic** (am′nē-ō-kōr′ē-ăl, am′nē-ō-kōr-ē-on′ik) relating to both amnion and chorion.

**am·ni·o·gen·e·sis** (am′nē-ō-jen′ĕ-sis) formation of the amnion. [amnio- + G. *genesis*, production]

**am·ni·o·hook** (am′nē-ō-huk′) instrument de-signed to tear a hole in the amnionic sac without injuring the fetus.

**am·ni·o·in·fu·sion** (am′nē-ō-in-fyu′zhun) infu-sion of warmed saline through an intrauterine catheter during labor, for umbilical cord compro-mise due to low volume of amnionic fluid, or for thick meconium in labor.

**am·ni·o·ma** (am-nē-ō′mă) broad flat tumor of the skin resulting from antenatal adhesion of the am-nion. [amnio- + G. *-oma*, tumor]

**am·ni·on** (am′nē-on) innermost of the extraem-bryonic membranes enveloping the embryo in utero and containing the amniotic fluid; it con-sists of an internal embryonic layer with its ecto-dermal component, and an external somatic mes-odermal component; in the later stages of preg-nancy the amnion expands and partially fuses to the inner wall of the chorionic vesicle; derived from the trophoblast cells. [G. the membrane around the fetus, fr. *amnios*, lamb]

**am·ni·on·ic, am·ni·ot·ic** (am-nē-on′ik, am-nē-ot′ik) relating to the amnion.

**am·ni·on·ic am·pu·ta·tion** SYN congenital am-putation.

**am·ni·on·ic band, am·ni·ot·ic band** strand of amniotic tissue adherent to the embryo or fetus, which can cause constriction of embryonic limbs. SEE ALSO congenital amputation. SYN amnionic band syndrome, anular band, constriction ring (2), Simonart bands (1), Simonart ligaments.

**am·ni·on·ic band syn·drome** SYN amnionic band.

**am·ni·on·ic cor·pus·cle** SYN corpus amylaceum.

**am·ni·on·ic flu·id, am·ni·ot·ic flu·id** a liquid within the amniotic sac that surrounds the fetus and protects it from mechanical injury. SYN li-quor amnii.

**am·ni·on·ic flu·id em·bo·lism** obstruction and constriction of pulmonary blood vessels by amni-otic fluid entering the maternal circulation, caus-ing obstetric shock. SEE ALSO amnionic fluid syn-drome.

**am·ni·on·ic flu·id in·dex** the sum of the diame-ters of the largest vertical pocket of amnionic fluid in each of the four quadrants of the uterus as obtained by ultrasound; a measure of fluid volume during pregnancy.

**am·ni·on·ic flu·id syn·drome** pulmonary em-bolic phenomena thought to be due to infusion of amniotic fluid containing epithelial squames into maternal blood vessels; shock ensues and sudden death may occur. SEE amnionic fluid embolism.

**am·ni·o·ni·tis** (am′nē-ō-nī′tis) inflammation re-sulting from infection of the amniotic sac, which, in turn, usually results from premature rupture of the membranes (a condition often associated with neonatal infection). [amnion + G. *-itis*, inflamma-tion]

**am·ni·on no·do·sum** nodules in the amnion that consist of typical stratified squamous epithelium. SYN squamous metaplasia of amnion.

**am·ni·or·rhea** (am-nē-ō-rē′ă) escape of amniotic fluid. [amnio- + G. *rhoia*, flow]

**am·ni·or·rhex·is** (am-nē-ō-rek′sis) rupture of the amniotic membrane. [amnio- + G. *rhēxis*, rup-ture]

**am·ni·o·scope** (am′nē-ō-skōp) an endoscope for studying amniotic fluid through the intact amni-otic sac.

**am·ni·os·co·py** (am-nē-os′kŏ-pē) examination of the amniotic fluid in the lowest part of the amni-otic sac by means of an endoscope introduced through the cervical canal. [amnio- + G. *skopeō*, to view]

**am·ni·o·tome** (am′nē-ō-tōm) an instrument for puncturing the fetal membranes. [amnio- + G. *tomē*, cutting]

**am·ni·ot·o·my** (am-nē-ot′ō-mē) artificial rupture of the fetal membranes as a means of inducing or expediting labor.

**A-mode** in diagnostic ultrasound, a one-dimen-sional presentation of a reflected sound wave in which echo amplitude (A) is displayed along the vertical axis and time of rebound (depth) along the horizontal axis; the echo information is pre-sented from interfaces along a single line in the direction of the sound beam.

*Amoe·ba* (ă-mē′bă) a genus of naked, lobose, pseudopod-forming protozoa of the class Sarco-dina (or Rhizopoda), that are abundant soil-dwellers, especially in rich organic debris, and are also commonly found as parasites. The typi-cal amebic parasites of man are now placed in the genera *Entamoeba*, *Endolimax*, and *Ioda-moeba*. [Mod. L. fr. G. *amoibē* change]

**amoe·ba [Br.]** SEE ameba.

**amoe·ba·pore** (ă-mē′ba-pōr) an active peptide released from *Entamoeba histolytica* that can in-sert ion channels into liposomes and possesses cytolytic and bactericidal activities. [amoeba + G. *poros*, passageway]

**Amoe·bi·da** (ă-mē'bĭ-dă) an order of ameboid protozoa, distinguished by possession of mitochondria and lack of a flagellate phase; most species are free-living, but some are parasites of human beings or animals; *Entamoeba* is an important human pathogen.

**amoe·bo·cyte [Br.]** SEE amebocyte.

**amoe·boid [Br.]** SEE ameboid.

**amorph** (ā'mōrf) an allele that has no phenotypically recognizable product and therefore its existence can be inferred on molecular evidence only. [G. *a-* neg. + *morphē*, form, shape]

**amor·phia, amor·phism** (ă-mōr'fē-ă, ă-mōr'-fizm) condition of being amorphous (1). [G. *a-* priv. + *morphē*, form]

**amor·phous** (ă-mōr'fŭs) **1.** without definite shape or visible differentiation in structure. **2.** not crystallized.

**amor·phous se·le·ni·um plate** SYN selenium plate.

**amor·phous sil·i·con** light-sensitive material used in digital radiography and fluoroscopy.

**AMP** adenosine monophosphate; specifically, the 5'-monophosphate unless modified by a numerical prefix. SEE adenylic acid.

**Am·père** (ahm-pār'), André Marie, French physicist, 1775–1836. SEE ampere.

**am·pere (A)** (am-pēr') **1.** the practical unit of electrical current; the absolute, practical ampere originally was defined as having the value of 1/10 of the electromagnetic unit (see abampere and coulomb. **2.** legal definition: the current that, flowing for 1 second, will deposit 1.118 mg of silver from silver nitrate solution. **3.** scientific (SI) definition: the current that, if maintained in two straight parallel conductors of infinite length and of negligible circular cross-sections and placed 1 m apart in a vacuum, produces between them a force of $2 \times 10^{-7}$ N/m of length. [A. *Ampère*]

**Am·père pos·tu·late** (am'pēr) SYN Avogadro law.

△**amph-** SEE amphi-, ampho-.

△**am·phi-** on both sides, surrounding, double; corresponds to L. *ambi-*. [G. *amphi*, *amphi-*, on both sides, about, around]

**am·phi·ar·thro·di·al** (am'fi-ar-thrō'dē-ăl) relating to a symphysis (1) (amphiarthrosis).

**am·phi·as·ter** (am-fi-as'ter) the double-star figure formed by the two astrospheres and their connecting spindle fibers during mitosis. [amphi- + G. *astēr*, star]

**am·phi·bol·ic fis·tu·la, am·phib·o·lous fis··tu·la** a complete anal fistula opening both externally and internally.

**am·phi·cen·tric** (am-fi-sen'trik) centering at both ends, said of a rete mirabile that begins when a vessel breaks up into a number of branches and ends as the branches join again to reconstitute the vessel. [amphi- + G. *kentron*, center]

**am·phid** (am'fid) in the nervous system of nematodes, a pair of laterally placed minute receptor organs in the cephalic or cervical region. [amphi- + -id]

△**am·pho-** on both sides, surrounding, double. [G. *amphō*, both]

**am·pho·cyte** (am'fō-sīt) SYN amphophil (2).

**am·pho·phil, am·pho·phile** (am'fō-fil, am'fō-fīl) **1.** having an affinity for both acid and basic dyes. SYN amphophilic, amphophilous. **2.** a cell that stains readily with either acid or basic dyes. SYN amphocyte. [ampho- + G. *philos*, fond]

**am·pho·phil·ic, am·phoph·i·lous** (am-fō-fil'ik, am-fof'i-lŭs) SYN amphophil (1).

**am·phor·ic** (am-fōr'ik) denoting a hollow sound heard on percussion and auscultation of the thorax over a pulmonary cavity or pneumothorax. [G. *amphora*, a jar]

**am·phor·ic rale** sound heard through the stethoscope associated with the movement of fluid in a lung cavity communicating with a bronchus.

**am·phor·ic res·o·nance** a hollow sound produced by percussing over a pulmonary cavity or pneumothorax.

**am·pho·ter·ic** (am-fō-tār'ik) having two opposite characteristics, especially having the capacity of reacting as either an acid or a base. [G. *amphoteroi* (pl.), both, fr. *amphō*, both]

**am·pho·ter·ism** (am-fō-ter'izm) the property of being amphoteric.

**am·pho·tro·pic vi·rus** an oncornavirus that does not produce disease in its natural host but does replicate in tissue culture cells of the host species and also in cells from other species.

**am·pli·fi·ca·tion** (am'pli-fi-kă'shŭn) the process of making larger, as in increasing an auditory or visual stimulus to enhance its perception. [L. *amplificatio*, an enlarging]

**am·pli·fi·er 1.** a device that increases the magnification of a microscope. **2.** an electronic apparatus that increases the strength of input signals.

**am·pli·tude of ac·com·mo·da·tion** the difference in refractivity of the eye at rest and when fully accommodated.

**am·poule [Br.]** SEE ampule.

**am·pule** (am'pyul) a hermetically sealed container, usually made of glass, containing a sterile medicinal solution, or powder to be made up in solution, to be used for subcutaneous, intramuscular, or intravenous injection.

**am·pul·la,** gen. and pl. **am·pul·lae** (am-pul'lă, am-pul'l-ē) [TA] a saccular dilation of a canal or duct. [L. a two-handled bottle]

**am·pul·la of duc·tus def·er·ens** the dilation of the ductus deferens where it approaches its contralateral partner just before it is joined by the duct of the seminal vesicle. SYN ampulla ductus deferentis [TA].

**am·pul·la duc·tus de·fe·ren·tis** [TA] SYN ampulla of ductus deferens.

**am·pul·la mem·bra·na·cea** SYN membranous ampullae of the semicircular ducts.

**am·pul·lar** (am-pul'ăr) relating in any sense to an ampulla.

**am·pul·lar preg·nan·cy** tubal pregnancy situated near the midportion of the oviduct.

**am·pul·la·ry crest** an elevation on the inner surface of the ampulla of each semicircular duct; filaments of the vestibular nerve pass through the crista to reach hair cells on its surface; the hair cells are capped by the cupula, a gelatinous protein-polysaccharide mass.

**am·pul·la of the sem·i·cir·cu·lar ducts** a nearly spherical enlargement of one end of each of the three semicircular ducts, anterior, posterior, and lateral, where they connect with the utricle. Each contains a neuroepithelial crista ampullaris.

**am·pul·la tu·bae uter·in·ae** [TA] SYN ampulla of uterine tube.

**am·pul·la of uter·ine tube** the wide portion of

the uterine (fallopian) tube near the fimbriated extremity; it has a complexly folded mucosa with a columnar epithelium of mostly ciliated cells among which are secretory cells. SYN ampulla tubae uterinae [TA].

**am·pul·li·tis** (am-pul-lī'tis) inflammation of any ampulla, especially of the dilated extremity of the vas deferens or of the ampulla of Vater. [ampulla + G. *itis*, inflammation]

**am·pu·ta·tion** (am-pyu-tā'shŭn) **1.** the cutting off of a limb or part of a limb, the breast, or other projecting part. SYN congenital amputation. **2.** in dentistry, removal of the root of a tooth, or of the pulp, or of a nerve root or ganglion; a modifying adjective is therefore used (pulp amputation; root amputation). [L. *amputatio,* fr. *am-puto,* pp. *-atus,* to cut around, prune]

**am·pu·ta·tion in con·ti·nu·i·ty** amputation through a segment of a limb, not at a joint.

**am·pu·ta·tion neu·ro·ma** SYN traumatic neuroma.

**am·pu·tee** (am'pyu-tē) a person with an amputated limb or part of limb.

**Am·sel cri·ter·i·a** (am'sel) criteria for clinical diagnosis of bacterial vaginosis; the diagnosis is made if three of the following four criteria are positive: homogeneous discharge, pH ≥ 4.8, presence of clue cells, and amine odor with the application of KOH to the discharge.

**Ams·ler chart** (ams'ler) a 10-cm square divided into 5-mm squares upon which an individual may project a defect in the central visual field.

**amu** atomic mass unit.

**amu·sia** (ā-myu'zē-ă) a form of aphasia characterized by an inability to produce or recognize music. [G. *a-* priv. + *mousa,* music]

**Amus·sat val·vu·la** (ah-moo-sah') SYN posterior urethral valves.

**amy·e·lia** (ā-mī-ē'lē-ă) congenital absence of the spinal cord, found in association with anencephaly. [G. *a-* priv. + *myelos,* marrow]

**amy·el·ic** (ā-mī-ē'lik) SYN amyelous.

**amy·e·li·nat·ed** (ā-mī'ĕ-li-nā'ted) SYN unmyelinated.

**amy·e·li·na·tion** (ā-mī'ĕ-li-nā'shŭn) failure of formation of myelin sheath of a nerve.

**amy·e·lin·ic** (ā-mī'ĕ-lin'ik) SYN unmyelinated.

**amy·e·lo·ic, amy·e·lon·ic** (ā-mī-ĕ-lō'ik, ā-mī-ĕ-lon'ik) **1.** SYN amyelous. **2.** in hematology, sometimes used to indicate the absence of bone marrow or the lack of functional participation of bone marrow in hemopoiesis. [G. *a-* priv. + *myelos,* marrow]

**amy·e·lous** (ā-mī'ĕ-lŭs) without spinal cord. SYN amyelic, amyelonic (1), amyelonic.

**amyg·da·la,** gen. and pl. **amyg·da·lae** (ă-mig'dă-lă, ă-mig'dă-lē) denoting the cerebellar tonsil, as well as the lymphatic tonsils (pharyngeal, palatine, lingual, laryngeal, and tubal). [L. fr. G. *amygdalē,* almond; in Mediev. & Mod. L., a tonsil]

**amyg·da·loid** (ă-mig'dă-loyd) resembling an almond or a tonsil. [amygdala + G. *eidos,* appearance]

**amyg·da·loid body** a rounded mass of gray matter in the temporal lobe internal to the cortex of the uncus and immediately anterior to the inferior horn of the lateral ventricle; its major afferents are olfactory and its efferent connections are with the hypothalamus and mediodorsal nucleus of the thalamus and it is also reciprocally associated

with the cortex of the temporal lobe; it is subdivided into two major nuclear groups, basolateral and corticormedial.

**amyg·dal·ose** (ā-mig'dal-ōs) SYN gentiobiose.

**am·yl** (ā'mil) the radical formed from a pentane, $C_5H_{12}$, by removal of one H. Several isomeric forms exist. SYN pentyl (1).

△**amyl- 1.** SEE amylo-. **2.** pentyl- SEE amyl.

**am·y·la·ceous** (am'i-lā'shŭs) starchy.

**am·y·lase** (am'il-ās) one of a group of amylolytic enzymes that cleave starch, glycogen, and related 1,4-α-glucans.

**am·y·lase-cre·at·i·nine clear·ance ra·tio** a test for the diagnosis of acute pancreatitis; it is determined by measuring amylase and creatinine in serum and urine.

**am·y·la·su·ria** (am-i-lā-syu'rē-ă) the excretion of amylase (sometimes termed diastase) in the urine, especially increased amounts in acute pancreatitis. SYN diastasuria.

**am·y·lin** (am'i-lin) the cellulose of starch; the insoluble envelope of starch grains.

△**am·y·lo-** starch, of polysaccharide nature or origin. [G. *amylon,* unmilled; starch, fr. *a-* + *mylē,* a mill]

**am·y·lo·gen·e·sis** (am-i-lō-jen'ĕ-sis) biosynthesis of starch. [amylo- + G. *genesis,* production]

**am·y·lo·gen·ic** (am-i-lō-jen'ik) relating to amylogenesis.

**am·y·loid** (am'i-loyd) **1.** any of a group of chemically diverse proteins that appears microscopically homogeneous, but is composed of linear nonbranching aggregated fibrils arranged in sheets when seen under the electron microscope; it stains dark brown with iodine, produces a characteristic green color in polarized light after staining with Congo red, is metachromatic with either methyl violet (pink-red) or crystal violet (purple-red), and fluoresces yellow after thioflavine T staining; amyloid occurs characteristically as pathologic extracellular deposits (amyloidosis), especially in association with reticuloendothelial tissue; the chemical nature of the proteinaceous fibrils is dependent upon the underlying disease process. **2.** resembling or containing starch. [amylo- + G. *eidos,* resemblance]

**am·y·loid de·gen·er·a·tion** infiltration of amyloid between cells and fibers of tissues and organs. SYN waxy degeneration (1).

**am·y·loid kid·ney** a kidney in which amyloidosis has occurred, usually in association with some chronic illness such as multiple myeloma, tuberculosis, osteomyelitis, or other chronic suppurative inflammation. SYN waxy kidney.

**am·y·loid ne·phro·sis 1.** SYN renal amyloidosis. **2.** nephrotic syndrome due to deposition of amyloid in the kidney.

**am·y·loi·do·sis** (am'i-loy-dō'sis) **1.** a disease characterized by extracellular accumulation of amyloid in various organs and tissues of the body; may be primary or secondary. **2.** the process of deposition of amyloid protein. [amyloid + G. *-osis,* condition]

**am·y·loi·do·sis of ag·ing** characterized by deposition of Congo-red-staining material, derived from a variety of proteins, especially in nervous tissue, myocardium and pancreas. Associated with Alzheimer disease; intractable congestive heart failure may result.

**am·y·loid tu·mor** SYN nodular amyloidosis.

**am·y·lol·y·sis** (am-i-lol'i-sis) hydrolysis of starch

into soluble products. [amylo- + G. *lysis,* dissolution]

**am•y•lo•lyt•ic** (am-i-lō-lit′ik) relating to amylolysis.

**am•y•lo•pec•tin** (am-i-lō-pek′tin) a branched-chain polyglucose (glucan) in starch containing both 1,4 and 1,6 linkages. Cf. amylose.

**am•y•lor′rhea** (am′i-lō-rē′ă) passage of undigested starch in the stools, implying a deficiency of amylase activity in the intestine. [amylo- + G. *rhoia,* flow]

**am•y•lose** (am′i-lōs) an unbranched polyglucose (glucan) in starch, similar to cellulose, containing $\alpha(1 \to 4)$ linkages. Cf. amylopectin.

**am•y•lo•su•ria, am•y•lu•ria** (am′i-lō-syu′rē-ă, am-i-lyu′rē-ă) excretion of starch in the urine.

**amy•o•es•the•sia, amy•o•es•the•sis** (ā-mī′ō-es-thē′zē-ă, ā-mī′ō-es-thē′sis) absence of muscle sensation. [G. *a-* priv. + *mys,* muscle, + *aisthēsis,* perception]

**amy•o•sta•sia** (ā-mī-ō-stā′zē-ă) difficulty in standing, due to muscular tremor or incoordination. [G. *a-* priv. + *mys,* muscle, + *stasis,* standing]

**amy•o•stat•ic** (ā-mī-ō-stat′ik) showing muscular tremors.

**amy•os•the•nia** (ā-mī′os-thē′nē-ă) muscular weakness. [G. *a-* priv. + *mys,* muscle, + *sthenos,* strength]

**amy•os•then•ic** (ā-mī-os-then′ik) relating to or causing muscular weakness.

**amy•o•taxy, amy•o•tax•ia** (ā-mī′ō-tak-sē, ā-mī-ō-tak′sē-ă) muscular ataxia. [G. *a-* priv. + *mys,* muscle, + *taxis,* order]

**amy•o•to•nia** (ā-mī-ō-tō′nē-ă) generalized absence of muscle tone, usually associated with flabby musculature and an increased range of passive movement at joints. [G. *a-* priv. + *mys,* muscle, + *tonos,* tone]

**amy•o•to•nia con•gen•i•ta 1.** atonic pseudoparalysis of congenital origin (neither familial nor hereditary), observed especially in infants and characterized by absence of tone in muscles innervated by the spinal nerves. SYN myatonia congenita. **2.** an indefinite term for a number of congenital neuromuscular disorders that cause generalized myotonia in young children and have a benign course. SYN Oppenheim disease.

**amy•o•tro•phic** (ā-mī-ō-trō′fik) relating to muscular atrophy.

**amy•o•tro•phic lat•er•al scle•ro•sis (ALS)** a disease of the motor tracts of the lateral columns and anterior horns of the spinal cord, causing progressive muscular atrophy, increased reflexes, fibrillary twitching, and spastic irritability of muscles; associated with a defect in superoxide dismutase. SYN Aran-Duchenne disease, Charcot disease, Cruveilhier disease, Duchenne-Aran disease, Lou Gehrig disease, progressive muscular atrophy.

**amy•ot•ro•phy** (ā-mī-ot′rō-fē) muscular wasting or atrophy. [G. *a-* priv. + *mys,* muscle, + *trophē,* nourishment]

**amyx•or•rhea** (ā-mik-sō-rē′ă) absence of the normal secretion of mucus. [G. *a-* priv. + *myxa,* mucus, + *rhoia,* flow]

**ANA** antinuclear antibody.

△**ana-** prefix: up, toward, apart; not to be confused with *an-* (a form of the prefix *a-,* without, used before a vowel). [G. *ana,* up]

**an•a•bi•o•sis** (an′ă-bī-ō′sis) resuscitation after apparent death. [G. a reviving, fr. *ana,* again, + *biōsis,* life]

**an•a•bi•ot•ic cell** cell that is capable of resuscitation after apparent death; the existence of anabiotic tumor cells is postulated to explain the recurrence of a cancer after a very long symptomless period following operation.

**an•a•bol•ic** (an-ă-bol′ik) relating to or promoting anabolism.

**an•a•bol•ic ste•roid** prescription drug abused by some athletes to increase muscle mass; functions in a manner similar to that of the chief male hormone, testosterone. Masculinizing effects are minimized by synthetically manipulating chemical structure to emphasize tissue-building, nitrogen-retaining processes. SEE ALSO ergogenic aid. SYN androgenic steroid.

**anab•o•lism** (a-nab′ō-lizm) **1.** the building up in the body of complex chemical compounds from simpler compounds (e.g., proteins from amino acids), usually with the use of energy. Cf. catabolism, metabolism. **2.** the sum of synthetic metabolic reactions. [G. *anabolē,* a raising up]

**anab•o•lite** (ă-nab′ō-līt) any substance formed as a result of anabolic processes.

**an•a•cid•i•ty** (an-ă-sid′i-tē) absence of acidity; used especially to denote absence of hydrochloric acid in the gastric juice.

**anac•la•sis** (ă-nak′lă-sis) **1.** reflection of light or sound. **2.** refraction of the ocular media. [G. a bending back, reflection]

**an•a•clit•ic** (an-ă-klit′ik) leaning or depending upon; in psychoanalysis, relating to the dependence of the infant on the mother or mother substitute. SEE anaclitic depression. [G. *ana,* toward, + *klinō,* to lean]

**an•a•clit•ic de•pres•sion** impairment of an infant's physical, social, and intellectual development following separation from its mother or from a mothering surrogate; characterized by listlessness, withdrawal, and anorexia.

**an•a•crot•ic, an•a•di•crot•ic** (an-ă-krot′ik, an-ă-dī-krot′ik) referring to the upstroke or ascending limb of the arterial pulse tracing.

**an•a•crot•ic pulse, an•a•di•crot•ic pulse** a pulse wave showing one or more notches or indentations on its rising limb that are sometimes detectable by palpation.

**anac•ro•tism** (ă-nak′rō-tizm) peculiarity of the pulse wave. SEE anacrotic pulse. SYN anadicrotism. [G. *ana,* up, + *krotos,* a beat]

**an•a•cu•sis** (an′ă-koo′sis) absence of the ability to perceive sound. SYN anakusis. [G. *an-* priv. + *akousis,* hearing]

**an•a•di•cro•tism** (an-ă-dik′rō-tizm) SYN anacrotism. [G. *ana,* up, + *di-krotos,* double beating]

**an•ad•re•nal•ism** (an-ă-drē′năl-izm) complete lack of adrenal function.

**an•a•dro•mous** (an-a-drō′mus) migrating from ocean water to fresh water to spawn; some such fish harbor human pathogens. SEE ALSO catadromous.

**an•aer•obe** (an′ăr-ōb, an-ār′ōb) a microorganism that can live and grow in the absence of oxygen. [G. *an-* priv. + *aēr,* air, + *bios,* life]

**an•aer•o•bic, an•aer•o•bi•ot•ic** (an-ār-ō′bik, an-ār-ō-bī-ŏt′ik) relating to an anaerobe; living without oxygen.

**an•aer•o•bic pow•er** maximal power (work per unit time) developed during all-out, short-term physical effort; reflects energy-output capacity of intramuscular high-energy phosphates (ATP and PCr) and anaerobic glycolysis.

**an•aer•o•bic res•pi•ra•tion** a form of respiration in which molecular oxygen is not consumed; e.g., nitrate respiration, sulfate respiration.

**an•aer•o•bi•o•sis** (an-ār-ō-bī-ō′sis) existence in an oxygen-free atmosphere. [G. *an-* priv. + *aēr,* air, + *biōsis,* way of living]

**An•aer•o•bo•plasma** (an-ār-ō′bō-plaz′ma) an order in the class Molicutes that is oxygen-sensitive. A role in human disease has not been defined.

**an•aer•o•gen•ic** (an-ār-ō-jen′ik) not producing gas. [G. *an-* priv. + *aēr,* air, + *-gen,* producing]

**an•a•gen** (an′ă-jen) growth phase of the hair cycle, lasting about 3 to 6 years in human scalp hair. [G. *ana,* up, + *-gen,* producing]

**an•a•gen ef•flu•vi•um** sudden diffuse hair shedding with cancer chemotherapy or radiation, usually reversible when treatment ends. SEE ALSO telogen effluvium.

**an•a•ku•sis** (an-ă-koo′sis) SYN anacusis.

**anal** (ā′năl) relating to the anus.

**anal atre•sia, a•tre•si•a ani** congenital absence of an anal opening due to the presence of a membranous septum (persistence of the cloacal membrane) or a complete absence of the anal canal. SYN imperforate anus (1), proctatresia.

**an•al•bu•mi•ne•mia** (an′al-byu-mi-nē′mē-ă) absence of albumin from the serum. [G. *an-* priv. + albumin + G. *haima,* blood]

**anal ca•nal** the terminal portion of the alimentary canal; it extends from the pelvic diaphragm to the anal orifice. SYN canalis analis [TA].

**anal col•umns** a number of vertical ridges in the mucous membrane of the upper half of the anal canal formed as the caliber of the canal is sharply reduced from that of the rectal ampulla. SYN columnae anales [TA], Morgagni columns, rectal columns.

**anal ducts** short ducts lined with simple columnar to stratified columnar epithelium that extend from the valvulae anales to the sinus anales.

**an•a•lep•tic** (an-ă-lep′tik) **1.** strengthening, stimulating, or invigorating. **2.** a restorative remedy. **3.** a central nervous system stimulant, particularly used to denote agents that reverse depressed central nervous system function. [G. *analēptikos,* restorative]

**an•a•lep•tic en•e•ma** an enema of a pint of lukewarm water with one-half teaspoonful of table salt.

**anal fis•sure** a crack or slit in the mucous membrane of the anus.

**anal fis•tu•la** a fistula opening at or near the anus; usually, but not always, opening into the rectum above the internal sphincter.

**an•al•ge•sia** (an-ăl-jē′zē-ă) a neurologic or pharmacologic state in which painful stimuli are so moderated that, though still perceived, they are no longer painful. Cf. anesthesia. [G. insensibility, fr. *an-* priv. + *algēsis,* sensation of pain]

**an•al•ge•sia al•ge•ra** SYN analgesia dolorosa.

**an•al•ge•sia do•lo•ro•sa** spontaneous pain in a body area that lacks sensation. SYN analgesia algera.

**an•al•ge•sic** (an-ăl-jē′zik) **1.** a compound capable of producing analgesia, i.e., one that relieves pain by altering perception of nociceptive stimuli without producing anesthesia or loss of con-

sciousness. **2.** characterized by reduced response to painful stimuli.

**anal•i•ty** (ā-nal′i-tē) referring to the psychic organization derived from, and characteristic of, the freudian anal period of psychosexual development.

**an•al•ler•gic** (an-ă-ler′jik) not allergic.

**an•a•log** (an′ă-log) **1.** one of two organs or parts in different species of animals or plants which differ in structure or development but are similar in function. **2.** a compound that resembles another in structure but is not necessarily an isomer; analogs are often used to block enzymatic reactions by combining with enzymes. SYN analogue. [G. *analogos,* proportionate]

**anal•o•gous** (ă-nal′ō-gŭs) possessing a functional resemblance, but having a different origin or structure.

**an•a•logue** (an′ă-log) SYN analog.

**anal pec•ten** the middle third of the anal canal. SYN pecten analis, pecten (2).

**an•al•pha•lip•o•pro•tein•e•mia** (an-al′fă-lip′ō-prō′tēn-ē′mē-ă) familial high density lipoprotein deficiency; a heritable disorder of lipid metabolism characterized by almost complete absence from plasma of high density lipoproteins, and by storage of cholesterol esters in foam cells, tonsillar enlargement, an orange or yellow-gray color of the pharyngeal and rectal mucosa, hepatosplenomegaly, lymph node enlargement, corneal opacity, and peripheral neuropathy; autosomal recessive inheritance. [G. *an-,* priv., + *alpha,* α, + lipoprotein + *-emia,* blood]

**anal phase** in psychoanalytic personality theory, the stage of psychosexual development, occurring when a child is between 1 and 3 years, during which activities, interests, and concerns center on the anal zone.

**anal pit** SYN proctodeum (1).

**anal plate** the anal portion of the cloacal plate.

**anal re•flex** contraction of the internal sphincter gripping the finger passed into the rectum.

**anal si•nus•es 1.** the grooves between the anal columns; SYN Morgagni sinus (1). **2.** pockets or crypts in the columnar zone of the anal canal between the anocutaneous line and the anorectal line; the sinuses give the mucosa a scalloped appearance.

**anal verge** the transitional zone between the moist, hairless, modified skin of the anal canal and the perianal skin.

**anal•y•sis,** pl. **anal•y•ses** (ă-nal′i-sis, ă-nal′i-sēz) **1.** the breaking up of a chemical compound or mixture into simpler elements; a process by which the composition of a substance is determined. **2.** the examination and study of a whole in terms of its parts. **3.** SEE psychoanalysis. [G. a breaking up, fr. *ana,* up, + *lysis,* a loosening]

**anal•y•sis of var•i•ance (ANOVA)** a statistical technique that isolates and assesses the contribution of categorical independent variables to variation in the mean of a continuous dependent variable.

**an•a•lyst** (an′ă-list) **1.** one who makes analytical determinations. **2.** psychoanalyst.

**an•a•lyte** (an′ă-līt) a material or substance whose presence or concentration in a specimen is determined by analysis.

**an•a•lyt•ic, an•a•lyt•i•cal** (an-ă-lit′ik, an-ă-lit′ik-ăl) **1.** relating to analysis. **2.** relating to psychoanalysis.

**an·a·lyt·i·cal psy·chol·o·gy** SYN jungian psychoanalysis.

**an·a·lyz·er, an·a·lyz·or** (an'ă-līz-er, an'ă-līz-ŏr) **1.** any instrument that performs an analysis. **2.** the prism in a polariscope by means of which the polarized light is examined. **3.** the neural basis of the conditioned reflex; includes all of the sensory side of the reflex arc and its central connections. **4.** a device that electronically determines the frequency and amplitude of a particular channel of an electroencephalogram.

**an·am·ne·sis** (an-am-nē'sis) **1.** the act of remembering. **2.** the medical or developmental history of a patient. [G. *anamnēsis,* recollection]

**an·am·nes·tic** (an-am-nes'tik) **1.** assisting the memory. SYN mnemonic. **2.** relating to the medical history of a patient.

**an·am·nes·tic re·ac·tion** augmented production of an antibody due to previous response of the subject to stimulus by the same antigen.

**an·a·phase** (an'ă-fāz) the stage of mitosis or meiosis in which the chromosomes move from the equatorial plate toward the poles of the cell. In mitosis a full set of daughter chromosomes (46 in humans) moves toward each pole. In the first division of meiosis one member of each homologous pair (23 in humans), consisting of two chromatids united at the centromere, moves toward each pole. In the second division of meiosis the centromere divides, and the two chromatids separate with one moving to each pole. [G. *ana,* up, + *phasis,* appearance]

**an·a·phia** (an-ā'fē-ă, an-af'ē-ă) absence of the sense of touch. [G. *an-* priv. + *haphē,* touch]

**an·aph·ro·di·si·ac** (an'af-rō-diz'ē-ak) **1.** repressing or destroying sexual desire. **2.** an agent that lessens or abolishes sexual desire. [G. *an-* priv. + *aphrodisia,* sexual pleasure]

**an·a·phy·lac·tic** (an'ă-fī-lak'tik) relating to anaphylaxis; manifesting extremely great sensitivity to foreign protein or other material.

**an·a·phy·lac·tic an·ti·body** SYN cytotropic antibody.

**an·a·phy·lac·tic shock** a severe, often fatal form of shock characterized by smooth muscle contraction and capillary dilation initiated by cytotropic (IgE class) antibodies. SEE ALSO anaphylaxis, serum sickness.

**an·a·phy·lac·to·gen** (an'ă-fī-lak'tō-jen) a substance (antigen) capable of rendering an individual susceptible to anaphylaxis; a substance (antigen) that will cause an anaphylactic reaction in such a sensitized individual.

**an·a·phy·lac·to·gen·e·sis** (an'ă-fī-lak-tō-jen'ē-sis) the production of anaphylaxis.

**an·a·phy·lac·to·gen·ic** (an'ă-fī-lak-tō-jen'ik) producing anaphylaxis; pertaining to substances (antigens) that result in an individual becoming susceptible to anaphylaxis.

**an·a·phy·lac·toid** (an'ă-fī-lak'toyd) resembling anaphylaxis. [anaphylaxis + G. *eidos,* resemblance]

**an·a·phy·lac·toid pur·pu·ra 1.** SYN allergic purpura. **2.** SYN Henoch-Schönlein purpura.

**an·a·phy·lac·toid shock** a reaction that is similar to anaphylactic shock, but which does not require the incubation period characteristic of induced sensitivity (anaphylaxis); it is unrelated to antigen-antibody reactions.

**an·a·phyl·a·tox·in, an·a·phyl·o·tox·in** (an'ă-fil-ă-tok'sin, an'ă-fil-ō-tok'sin) **1.** a substance postulated to be the immediate cause of anaphylactic shock and that is assumed to result from the *in vivo* combination of specific antibody and the specific sensitizing material. **2.** the small fragment (C3a) split from the third component (C3) of complement, which produces a local wheal following intracutaneous injection. [anaphylaxis + toxin]

**an·a·phy·lax·is** (an'ă-fī-lak'sis) the immediate, transient kind of immunologic (allergic) reaction characterized by contraction of smooth muscle and dilation of capillaries due to release of pharmacologically active substances (histamine, bradykinin, serotonin, and slow-reacting substance), classically initiated by the combination of antigen (allergen) with mast-cell-fixed, cytophilic antibody (chiefly IgE); the reaction can be initiated, also, by relatively large quantities of serum aggregates (antigen-antibody complexes, and others) that seemingly activate complement leading to production of anaphylatoxin, a reaction sometimes termed "aggregate anaphylaxis." [G. *ana,* away from, back from, + *phylaxis,* protection]

**an·a·pla·sia** (an-ă-plā'sē-ă) loss of structural differentiation, especially as seen in most, but not all, malignant neoplasms. SYN dedifferentiation (2). [G. *ana,* again, + *plasis,* a molding]

**an·a·plas·tic** (an-ă-plas'tik) **1.** relating to anaplasty. **2.** characterized by or pertaining to anaplasia. **3.** growing without form or structure.

**an·a·plas·tic cell 1.** a cell that has reverted to an embryonal state; **2.** an undifferentiated cell, characteristic of malignant neoplasms.

**an·a·plas·to·lo·gy** (an'ă-plas-tol'ō-jē) application of prosthetic materials for construction and/or reconstruction of a missing body part. [G. *ana,* again, + *plastos,* formed]

**an·a·poph·y·sis** (an-ă-pof'i-sis) an accessory spinal process of a vertebra, found especially in the thoracic or lumbar vertebrae. [G. *ana,* back, + *apophysis,* offshoot]

**anap·tic** (ă-nap'tik) relating to anaphia.

**an·a·rith·mia** (an-ă-rith'mē-ă) aphasia characterized by an inability to count or use numbers. [G. *an-* priv. + *arithmos,* number]

**an·ar·thria** (an-ar'thrē-a) loss of the power of articulate speech. SEE ALSO aphasia, alexia, dysarthria. [G. *anarthros,* without joints; (of sound) inarticulate]

**an·a·sar·ca** (an-ă-sar'kă) a generalized infiltration of edema fluid into subcutaneous connective tissue. [G. *ana,* through, + *sarx* (*sark-*), flesh]

**an·a·sar·cous** (an-ă-sar'kŭs) characterized by anasarca.

**an·as·tig·mats** (an-ă-stig'mats) **1.** lenses in which astigmatism is corrected. **2.** lenses in which both astigmatism and field curvature are corrected.

**anas·to·mose** (ă-nas'tō-mōs) **1.** to form one or more open communications with another structure; said of blood vessels and tubular and hollow viscera. USAGE NOTE: Not correctly said of nerves. **2.** to unite surgically by means of an anastomosis; to make a communication between formerly separate structures.

**anas·to·mo·sis,** pl. **anas·to·mo·ses** (ă-nas'tō-mō'sis, ă-nas'tō-mōs-sez) **1.** a natural communication, direct or indirect, between two blood vessels or other tubular structures. USAGE NOTE: Not correctly applied to nerves. SEE communication. **2.** an operative union of two hollow or tubular structures. **3.** an opening created by surgery, trauma, or disease between two or more normally separate spaces or organs. [G. *anastomōsis*, from *anastomoō*, to furnish with a mouth]

**anas•to•mot•ic** (a-nas-tō-mot′ik) pertaining to an anastomosis.

**anas•to•mot•ic branch** a blood vessel that interconnects two neighboring vessels. USAGE NOTE: Not correctly applied to nerves.

**anas•to•mot•ic ul•cer** an ulcer of the jejunum, after gastroenterostomy.

**an•a•tom•ic** (an′ă-tom′ik) **1.** relating to anatomy. **2.** SYN structural. **3.** denoting a strictly morphologic feature distinct from its physiologic or surgical considerations, e.g., anatomic neck of humerus, anatomic dead space, anatomic lobulation of the liver.

**an•a•tom•ic con•ju•gate** measure of pelvic dimension describing the distance between the sacral promontory and the inferior border of the pubic symphysis, measured manually per vaginam or by ultrasonography. It is used to extrapolate the true conjugate.

**an•a•tom•ic crown** the portion of a tooth covered by enamel.

**an•a•tom•i•c dead space** the volume of the conducting airways from the external environment (at the nose and mouth) down to the level at which inspired gas exchanges oxygen and carbon dioxide with pulmonary capillary blood; formerly presumed to extend down to the beginning of alveolar epithelium in the respiratory bronchioles, but more recent evidence indicates that effective gas exchange extends some distance up the thicker-walled conducting airways because of rapid longitudinal mixing. Cf. alveolar dead space, physiologic dead space.

**an•a•tom•ic pa•thol•o•gy** the subspecialty of pathology that pertains to the gross and microscopic study of organs and tissues removed for biopsy or during postmortem examination, and also the interpretation of the results of such study. SYN pathological anatomy.

**an•a•tom•ic snuff•box** (an′ă-tom′ic snŭf′boks) a hollow seen on the radial aspect of the wrist when the thumb is extended fully; it is bounded by the tendon of the extensor pollicis longus posteriorly and of the tendons of the extensor pollicis brevis and abductor pollicis longus anteriorly. The radial artery crosses the floor which is formed by the scaphoid and the trapezium bones.

**an•a•tom•ic tooth** an artificial tooth that duplicates the anatomic form of a natural tooth.

**an•a•tom•ic wart** SYN postmortem wart.

**anat•o•mist** (ă-nat′ŏ-mist) a specialist in the science of anatomy.

**anat•o•my** (ă-nat′ŏ-mē) **1.** the morphologic structure of an organism. **2.** the science of the morphology or structure of organisms. **3.** SYN dissection. **4.** a work describing the form and structure of an organism and its various parts. [G. *anatomē*, dissection, from *ana*, apart, + *tomē*, a cutting]

**an•a•tri•crot•ic** (an′ă-trī-krot′ik) characterized by anatricrotism; denoting a sphygmographic tracing with three waves on the ascending limb.

**an•a•tric•ro•tism** (an′ă-trik′rō-tizm) a condition of the pulse manifested by a triple beat on the ascending limb of the sphygmographic tracing. [G. *ana*, up, + *tri-*, thrice, + *krotos*, beating]

**ANCA** antineutrophil cytoplasmic antibody.

**an•chor•age** (ang′kōr-ij) **1.** operative fixation of loose or prolapsed abdominal or pelvic organs. **2.** the part to which anything is fastened. In dentistry, a tooth or an implanted tooth substitute with which a fixed or removable partial denture, crown, or restoration is retained. **3.** the nature and degree of resistance to displacement offered by an anatomical unit when used for the purpose of effecting tooth movement. [L. *ancora*, fr. G. *ankyra*, anchor]

**an•chor•ing fi•brils** collagen fibrils that insert in to the basal lamina of the epidermis and bind it down to the underlying dermis.

**an•chor splint** a splint used for fracture of the jaw, with wires around teeth and a rod to hold it in place.

**an•cil•lary** (an′si-lār-ē) auxiliary, accessory, or secondary. [L. *ancillaris*, relating to a maidservant]

**an•cil•lary ports** a supplemental entry site to allow insertion of instruments other than the endoscope during endoscopic surgery.

**an•cil•lary ser•vic•es** diagnostic or therapeutic services provided by a physician for inpatients or outpatients as an adjunct to basic medical or surgical services.

**an•cip•i•tal, an•cip•i•tate, an•cip•i•tous** (an-sip′i-tăl, an-sip′i-tāt, an-sip′i-tŭs) two-headed; two-edged. [L. *anceps*, two-headed]

**an•co•nad** (ang′kō-nad) toward the elbow. [G. *ankōn*, elbow, + L. *ad*, to]

**an•co•nal, an•co•ne•al** (ang′kō-năl, ang-kō′nē-ăl) **1.** relating to the elbow (ancon). **2.** relating to the anconeus muscle.

**an•co•ne•us mus•cle** *origin*, back of lateral condyle of humerus; *insertion*, olecranon process and posterior surface of ulna; *action*, extends forearm and abducts ulna in pronation of wrist; *nerve supply*, radial. SYN musculus anconeus [TA].

△**an•cy•lo-** SEE ankylo-.

***An•cy•los•to•ma*** (an-si-los′tō-mă, an-ki-los′tō-mă) a genus of Nematoda, the Old World hookworm, the members of which are parasitic in the duodenum. They attach themselves to the mucous membrane, suck blood, and may cause anemia. The eggs are passed with the feces, and the larvae develop in moist soil to become infectious third-stage (filariform) larvae that enter the human body through the skin and possibly in drinking water; they migrate by the bloodstream to lung alveoli, are carried to bronchi and trachea, swallowed, and passed to the intestine, where they mature. SEE ALSO ancylostomiasis, *Necator*. [G. *ankylos*, curved, hooked, + *stoma*, mouth]

***An•cy•los•to•ma bra•zi•li•ense*** a species characterized by one pair of ventral buccal teeth, normally an intestinal parasite of dogs and cats but also found in humans as a cause of human cutaneous larva migrans.

***An•cy•los•to•ma ca•ni•num*** a species possessing three pairs of ventral teeth in the oral cavity; common in dogs, but also occurring in human skin as a cause of cutaneous larva migrans.

***An•cy•los•to•ma du•o•de•na•le*** the Old World hookworm of humans, a species widespread in temperate areas, in contrast to the more tropical distribution of the New World hookworm, *Necator americanus*. It is the only hookworm found in the U.S.

An•cy•los•to•ma tu•bae•for•me a nematode species found in the cat; cutaneous larva migrans seen in humans.

an•cy•lo•sto•mi•a•sis (an′si-lō-stō-mī′ă-sis, an′ ki-lō-stō-mī′ă-sis) hookworm disease caused by *Ancylostoma duodenale* and characterized by eosinophilia, anemia, emaciation, dyspepsia, and, in children with severe chronic infections, swelling of the abdomen with mental and physical maldevelopment.

an•cy•roid (an′si-royd) shaped like the fluke of an anchor; denoting the cornua of the lateral ventricles of the brain and the coracoid process of the scapula. [G. *ankyra,* anchor, + *eidos,* resemblance]

An•dersch nerve (ahn′dĕrsh) SYN tympanic nerve.

An•der•sen dis•ease (an′der-sen) SYN type 4 glycogenosis.

An•der•son splint (an′der-sŭn) a skeletal traction splint with pins inserted into proximal and distal ends of a fracture; reduction is obtained by an external plate attached to the pins.

An•des vi•rus (an′dēz) a species of Hantavirus in Argentina causing hantavirus pulmonary syndrome.

⚠an•dro- masculine. [G. *anēr, andros,* a male human being]

an•dro•blas•to•ma (an′drō-blas-tō′mă) **1.** a testicular tumor microscopically resembling fetal testis, with varying proportions of tubular and stromal elements; the tubules contain Sertoli cells, which may cause feminization. **2.** SYN arrhenoblastoma. [G. *anēr (andro-),* man, + *blastos,* germ, + *-oma,* tumor]

an•dro•gen (an′drō-jen) generic term for an agent, usually a hormone (e.g., androsterone, testosterone), that stimulates activity of the accessory male sex organs, promotes development of male sex characteristics, or prevents changes in the latter that follow castration; natural androgens are steroids, derivatives of androstane.

an•dro•gen bind•ing pro•tein (ABP) a protein secreted by testicular Sertoli cells along with inhibin and müllerian inhibiting substance. Androgen binding protein probably maintains a high concentration of androgen in the seminiferous tubules.

an•dro•gen•ic al•o•pe•cia gradual decrease of scalp hair density in adults as a result of familial increased susceptibility of hair follicles to androgen secretion following puberty. SEE female pattern alopecia, male pattern alopecia. SYN alopecia hereditaria, patterned alopecia.

an•dro•gen•ic ste•roid SYN anabolic steroid.

an•dro•gen in•sen•si•tiv•ity syn•drome SYN androgen resistance syndromes.

an•dro•gen re•sis•tance syn•dromes a class of disorders associated with 5α-steroid reductase deficiency, testicular feminization, and related disorders. Cf. Reifenstein syndrome, testicular feminization syndrome. SYN androgen insensitivity syndrome.

an•drog•y•nous (an-droj′i-nŭs) pertaining to androgyny.

an•drog•y•ny (an-droj′i-nē) **1.** SYN female pseudohermaphroditism. **2.** having both masculine and feminine characteristics, as in attitudes and behaviors that contain features of stereotyped, culturally sanctioned sexual roles of both male and female. [andro- + G. *gynē,* woman]

an•droid obe•sity central obesity (apple shape) with fat excess primarily in abdominal wall and visceral mesentery; associated with glucose intolerance, diabetes, decreased sex hormone–binding globulin, increased levels of free testosterone, and increased cardiovascular risk.

an•droid pel•vis a masculine or funnel-shaped pelvis.

an•dro•mor•phous (an-drō-mōr′fŭs) having a male form or habitus. [andro- + G. *morphē,* form]

an•dro•pause a postulated decrease in function of male gonads with increasing age, analogous to menopause.

an•dro•pho•bia (an-drō-fō′bē-ă) morbid fear of men, or of the male sex, resulting in avoidance of situations where men are present. [andro- + G. *phobos,* fear]

an•dro•stane (an′drō-stān) the parent hydrocarbon of the androgenic steroids.

an•dro•stane•di•ol (an-drō-stān′dī-ol) 5α-androstane-3β,17β-diol; a steroid metabolite, of which 5β isomers are also known.

an•dro•stane•di•one (an-drō-stān′dī-ōn) 5α-androstane-3,17-dione; a steroid metabolite, of which the 5β isomer is also known.

an•dro•stene (an′drō-stēn) androstane with an unsaturated (i.e., —CH=CH—) bond in the molecule.

an•dro•stene•di•ol (an-drō-stēn′dī-ol) 5-androsten-3β,17β-diol; a steroid metabolite differing from androstanediol by possessing a double bond between C-5 and C-6.

an•dro•stene•di•one (an-drō-stēn′dī-ōn) 4-androstene-3,17-dione; an androgenic steroid of weaker biological potency than testosterone; secreted by the testis, ovary, and adrenal cortex.

an•dro•ste•nol a substance that is a postulated pheromone; it is found in male sweat where it is oxidized to androstenone. In tests, women like the dry musky smell of androstenol, but find androstenone to have a chemical, urinelike odor that is unpleasant; however, ovulating women react neutrally.

an•dros•ter•one (an-dros′ter-ōn) *cis*-androsterone; 3α-hydroxy-5α-androstan-17-one; (3α-hydroxyetioallocholan-17-one; 3-epihydroxyetioallocholan-17-one); a steroid metabolite, found in male urine, having weak androgenic potency. Formed in testes from progesterone.

an•e•cho•ic (an-ĕ-kō′ik) the property of appearing echo-free or without echoes on a sonographic image; a clear cyst appears anechoic. [G. *an-* priv. + echo + ic]

an•e•cho•ic cham•ber a soundproof environment in which reverberation is largely eliminated, for the performance of audiologic testing and research.

Anel meth•od (ah′nel) ligation of an artery immediately above (on the proximal side of) an aneurysm.

ane•mia (ă-nē′mē-ă) any condition in which the number of red blood cells per mm³, the amount of hemoglobin in 100 ml of blood, and/or the volume of packed red blood cells per 100 ml of blood are less than normal; clinically, generally pertaining to the concentration of oxygen-transporting material in a designated volume of blood, in contrast to total quantities as in oligocythemia, oligochromemia, and oligemia. Anemia is frequently manifested by pallor of the skin and mucous membranes, shortness of breath, palpitations of the heart, soft systolic murmurs, lethargy, and fatigability. [G. *anaimia,* fr. *an-* priv. + *haima,* blood]

**ane·mic** (ă-nē′mik) pertaining to or manifesting the various features of anemia.

**ane·mic an·ox·ia** anemic hypoxia in which oxygen is almost completely lacking.

**ane·mic ha·lo** pale, relatively avascular areas in the skin seen around vascular spiders, cherry angiomas, and sometimes in acute macular eruptions.

**ane·mic hy·pox·ia** hypoxia resulting from a decreased concentration of functional hemoglobin or a reduced number of erythrocytes.

**ane·mic in·farct** an infarct in which little or no bleeding into tissue spaces occurs when the blood supply is obstructed. SYN white infarct (1).

**ane·mic mur·mur** a nonvalvular murmur heard on auscultation of the heart and large blood vessels in cases of profound anemia associated mainly with turbulent blood flow due to decreased blood viscosity. SYN hemic murmur.

**an·e·mo·pho·bia** (an′ē-mō-fō′bē-ă) morbid fear of wind. [G. *anemos,* wind, + *phobos,* fear]

**an·en·ce·phal·ic** (an-en-se-fal′ik) relating to anencephaly.

**an·en·ceph·a·ly** (an′en-sef′ă-lē) congenital defective development of the brain, with absence of the bones of the neurocranium and absent or rudimentary cerebral and cerebellar hemispheres, brainstem, and basal ganglia. Cf. meroanencephaly. [G. *an-* priv. + *enkephalos,* brain]

**aneph·ric** (ă-nef′rik) lacking kidneys. [*a-* priv. + G. *nephros,* kidney]

**an·er·ga·sia** (an-er-gā′zē-ă) absence of psychic activity as the result of organic brain disease. [G. *an-* priv. + *ergasia,* work]

**an·er·gas·tic** (an-er-gas′tik) pertaining to or characterized by anergasia.

**an·er·gic** (an-er′jik) relating to, or marked by, anergy.

**an·er·gy** (an′er-jē) **1.** absence of ability to generate a sensitivity reaction in a subject to substances expected to be antigenic (immunogenic, allergenic) in that individual. **2.** lack of energy. [G. *an-* priv. + *energeia,* energy, from *ergon,* work]

**an·e·ryth·ro·pla·sia** (an′ĕ-rith-rō-plā′zē-ă) a condition in which there is no formation of red blood cells. [G. *an-* priv. + erythro(cyte) + G. *plasis,* a molding]

**an·e·ryth·ro·plas·tic** (an′ĕ-rith-rō-plas′tik) pertaining to or characterized by anerythroplasia.

**an·es·the·ki·ne·sia** (an-es′thē-ki-nē′zē-ă) combined sensory and motor paralysis. [G. *an-* priv. + *aisthēsis,* sensation, + *kinēsis,* movement]

**an·es·the·sia** (an′es-thē′zē-ă) **1.** loss of sensation resulting from pharmacologic depression of nerve function or from neurological dysfunction. **2.** broad term for anesthesiology as a clinical specialty. [G. *anaisthēsia,* fr. *an-* priv. + *aisthēsis,* sensation]

**an·es·the·sia do·lo·ro·sa** severe spontaneous pain occurring in an anesthetic area.

**an·es·the·sia rec·ord** a written account of drugs administered, procedures undertaken, and physiologic responses during the course of surgical or obstetrical anesthesia.

**an·es·the·si·ol·o·gist** (an′es-thē-zē-ol′ō-jist) **1.** a physician specializing in anesthesiology. **2.** an

individual with a doctorate degree who is board-certified and legally qualified to administer anesthetics and related techniques. Cf. anesthetist.

**an·es·the·si·ol·o·gy** (an′es-thē-zē-ol′ō-jē) the medical specialty concerned with the pharmacological, physiological, and clinical basis of anesthesia and related fields, including resuscitation, intensive respiratory care, and the management of acute and chronic pain. [anesthesia + G. *logos,* treatise]

**an·es·thet·ic** (an-es-thet′ik) **1.** a compound that reversibly depresses neuronal function, producing loss of ability to perceive pain and/or other sensations. **2.** collective designation for anesthetizing agents administered to an individual at a particular time. **3.** characterized by loss of sensation or capable of producing loss of sensation. **4.** associated with or due to the state of anesthesia.

**an·es·thet·ic depth** the degree of central nervous system depression produced by a general anesthetic agent; a function of potency of the anesthetic and the concentration in which it is administered.

**an·es·thet·ic gas** SEE inhalation anesthetic.

**an·es·thet·ic in·dex** ratio of the number of units of anesthetic required for anesthesia to the number of units of anesthetic required to produce respiratory or cardiovascular failure.

**an·es·thet·ic lep·ro·sy** a form of leprosy chiefly affecting the nerves, marked by hyperesthesia succeeded by anesthesia, and by paralysis, ulceration, and various trophic disturbances, terminating in gangrene and mutilation. SYN Danielssen disease, trophoneurotic leprosy.

**anes·the·tist** (ă-nes′thĕ-tist) one who administers an anesthetic, whether an anesthesiologist, a physician who is not an anesthesiologist, a nurse anesthetist, or an anesthesia assistant.

**anes·the·ti·za·tion** (ă-nes′thĕ-ti-za′shŭn) the act of producing loss of sensation.

**anes·the·tize** (ă-nes′thĕ-tīz) to produce loss of sensation.

**an·es·trus** (an-es′trŭs) the period between two estrus (heat) cycles. [G. *an-* priv. + *oistros,* estrus]

**an·e·to·der·ma** (an-ĕ-tō-der′mă) atrophoderma in which the skin becomes baglike and wrinkled. [G. *anetos,* relaxed, + *derma,* skin]

**an·eu·ploid** (an′yu-ployd) having an abnormal number of chromosomes not an exact multiple of the haploid number, as contrasted with abnormal numbers of complete haploid sets of chromosomes, such as diploid, triploid, etc. [G. *an-* priv. + euploid]

**an·eu·ploi·dy** (an′yu-ploy-dē) state of being aneuploid.

**an·eu·rysm** (an′yu-rizm) **1.** circumscribed dilation of an artery or a cardiac chamber, a direct communication with the lumen, usually due to an acquired or congenital weakness of the wall of the artery or chamber. **2.** circumscribed dilation of a cardiac chamber usually due to an acquired or congenital weakness of the wall of the heart. See page 50. [G. *aneurysma (-mat-),* a dilation, fr. *eurys,* wide]

**an·eu·rys·mal, an·eu·rys·mat·ic** (an-yu-riz′măl, an-yu-riz-mat′ik) relating to an aneurysm.

**an·eu·rys·mal bone cyst** a solitary benign osteolytic lesion expanding a long bone or within a vertebra, consisting of blood-filled spaces, and

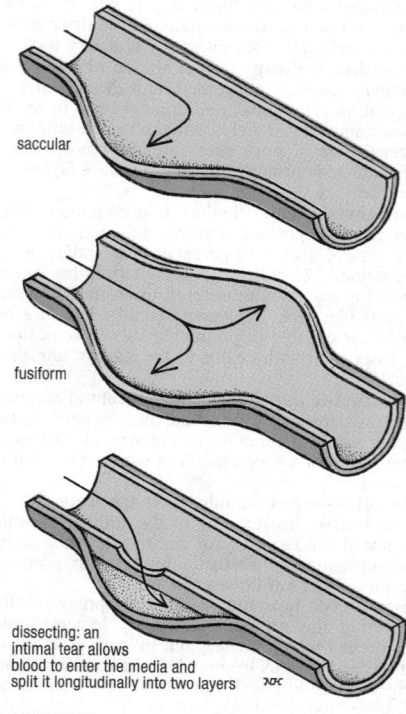

saccular

fusiform

dissecting: an intimal tear allows blood to enter the media and split it longitudinally into two layers

**aneurysm**

separated by fibrous tissue containing multinucleated giant cells; such cysts cause swelling, pain, and tenderness.

**an·eu·rys·mal bru·it** blowing murmur heard over an aneurysm.

**an·eu·rys·mal var·ix** dilation and tortuosity of a vein resulting from an acquired communication with an adjacent artery. SYN Pott aneurysm.

**an·eu·rys·mec·to·my** (an-yu-riz-mek'tō-mē) excision of an aneurysm. [aneurysm + G. *ektomē*, excision]

**an·eu·rys·mo·graph** (an'yu-riz'mōg'răf) demonstration of an aneurysm, usually by means of x-rays and a contrast medium. [aneurysm + G. *graphō*, to write]

**an·eu·rys·mo·plas·ty** (an-yu-riz'mō-plas-tē) repair of an aneurysm by opening the sac and suturing its walls. SEE ALSO aneurysmorrhaphy. SYN endoaneurysmoplasty, endoaneurysmorrhaphy. [aneurysm + G. *plastos*, formed]

**an·eu·rys·mor·rha·phy** (an'yu-riz-mōr'ă-fē) closure by suture of the sac of an aneurysm to restore the normal lumen dimensions. [aneurysm + G. *rhaphē*, suture]

**an·eu·rys·mot·o·my** (an'yu-riz-mot'ō-mē) incision into the sac of an aneurysm. [aneurysm + G. *tomē*, incision]

**ANF** antinuclear factor.

**An·ge·luc·ci syn·drome** (ahn-jĕ-loo'chē) extreme excitability, vasomotor disturbances, and palpitation associated with vernal conjunctivitis.

**an·gel wing** a deformity in which both scapulae project conspicuously. SEE ALSO winged scapula.

**an·gi·ec·ta·sia, an·gi·ec·ta·sis** (an-jē-ek-tā'zē-ă, an-jē-ek'tă-sis) dilation of a lymphatic or blood vessel. [angio- + G. *ektasis*, a stretching]

**an·gi·ec·tat·ic** (an-jē-ek-tat'ik) marked by the presence of dilated blood vessels. [angio- + G. *ektatos*, capable of extension]

**an·gi·ec·to·pia** (an-jē-ek-tō'pē-ă) abnormal location of a blood vessel. [angio- + G. *ektopos*, out of place]

**an·gi·i·tis, an·gi·tis** (an-jē-ī'tis, an-jī'tis) inflammation of a blood vessel (arteritis, phlebitis) or lymphatic vessel (lymphangitis). SYN vasculitis. [angio- + G. -*itis*, inflammation]

**an·gi·na** (an'ji-nă) **1.** a severe, often constricting pain; usually refers to angina pectoris. **2.** old term for a sore throat from any cause. [L. quinsy]

**an·gi·na cru·ris** intermittent claudication of the leg.

**an·gi·na in·ver·sa** SYN Prinzmetal angina.

**an·gi·nal** (an'ji-năl, an-jī'năl) relating to angina in any sense.

**an·gi·na pec·to·ris** paroxysmal severe constricting pain in the chest due to myocardial ischemia; typically radiates from the precordium to one or both shoulders, neck, or jaw; often precipitated by exertion, exposure to cold, or emotional excitement. SYN stenocardia.

**an·gi·ni·form** (an-jin'i-fōrm) resembling angina.

**an·gi·noid** (an'jin-oid) rarely used term for resembling an angina, especially angina pectoris.

**an·gi·nose, an·gi·nous** (an'ji-nōs, an'ji-nŭs) rarely used term for relating to any angina.

**an·gi·nose scar·la·ti·na, scar·la·ti·na an·gi·no·sa** a form of scarlatina in which the throat affection is unusually severe. SYN Fothergill disease (2).

△**an·gio-, an·gi-** blood or lymph vessels; a covering, an enclosure; corresponds to L. *vas-,vaso-, vasculo-*. [G. *angeion*, a vessel or cavity of the body, fr. *angos*, a vessel, vat, bucket, + -*eion*, small, little]

**an·gi·o·blast** (an'jē-ō-blast) **1.** a cell taking part in blood vessel formation. SYN vasoformative cell. **2.** primordial mesenchymal tissue from which embryonic blood cells and vascular endothelium are differentiated. [angio- + G. *blastos*, germ]

**an·gi·o·blas·to·ma** (an'jē-ō-blas-tō'mă) SYN hemangioblastoma.

**an·gi·o·car·di·og·ra·phy** (an'jē-ō-kar-dē-og'răfē) diagnostic X-ray imaging of the heart and great vessels made visible by injection of a radiopaque solution. SEE coronary angiography. [angio- + G. *kardia*, heart, + *graphō*, to write]

**an·gi·o·car·di·o·ki·net·ic, an·gi·o·car·di·o·ci·net·ic** (an'jē-ō-kar'dē-ō-ki-net'ik, an'jē-ō-kar-dē-ō-si-net'ik) causing dilation or contraction in the heart and blood vessels. [angio- + G. *kardia*, heart, + *kinēsis*, movement]

**an·gi·o·car·di·op·a·thy** (an'jē-ō-kar-dē-op'ă-thē) disease affecting both heart and blood vessels. [angio- + G. *kardia*, heart, + *pathos*, disease]

**an·gi·o·dys·pla·sia** (an'jē-ō-dis-plā'zē-ă) degenerative or congenital structural abnormality of the normally distributed vasculature.

**an·gi·o·dys·tro·phy, an·gi·o·dys·tro·phia** (an'jē-ō-dis'trō-fē, an'jē-ō-dis-trō'fē-ă) defective formation or growth associated with marked vascular changes. [angio- + G. *dys-*, bad, + *trophē*, nourishment]

🔟 **an·gi·o·e·de·ma** (an'jē-ō-ĕ-dē'mă) recurrent large circumscribed areas of subcutaneous edema of sudden onset, usually disappearing within 24 hours; seen mainly in young women, frequently as an allergic reaction to foods or drugs. See this page. SYN angioneurotic edema, Bannister disease, giant urticaria.

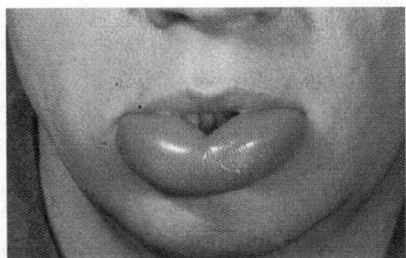

**angioedema:** seen in the lower lip

**an·gi·o·en·do·the·li·o·ma·to·sis** (an'jē-ō-en-dō-thē'lē-ō-mă-tō'sis) proliferation of endothelial cells within blood vessels.

**an·gi·o·fi·bro·ma** (an'jē-ō-fī-brō'mă) SYN telangiectatic fibroma.

**an·gi·o·fi·bro·sis** (an'jē-ō-fī-brō'sis) fibrosis of the walls of blood vessels.

**an·gi·o·gen·e·sis fac·tor** a substance of 2000 to 20,000 MW which is secreted by macrophages and stimulates neovascularization in healing wounds or in the stroma of tumors.

**an·gi·o·gen·ic** (an'jē-ō-jen'ik) **1.** relating to angiogenesis. **2.** of vascular origin.

**an·gi·o·gli·o·ma** (an'jē-ō-glī-ō'mă) a mixed glioma and angioma.

**an·gi·o·gram** (an'jē-ō-gram) radiograph obtained by angiography. [angio- + G. *gramma*, a writing]

**an·gi·o·graph·ic** (an-jē-ō-graf'ik) relating to or utilizing angiography.

**an·gi·og·ra·phy** (an-jē-og'ră-fē) radiography of vessels after the injection of a radiopaque contrast material; usually requires percutaneous insertion of a radiopaque catheter and positioning under fluoroscopic control. SEE ALSO arteriography, venography. [angio- + G. *graphō*, to write]

**an·gi·og·ra·phy cath·e·ter** a thin-walled tube suitable for percutaneous puncture and injection of contrast media for radiography.

**an·gi·oid** (an'jē-oyd) resembling blood vessels; in a branching pattern. [angio- + G. *eidos*, resemblance]

**an·gi·oid streaks** breaks in Bruch membrane visible in the peripapillary fundus oculi, and sometimes mistaken for choroidal vessels. SYN Knapp streaks, Knapp striae.

**an·gi·o·im·mu·no·blas·tic lym·phad·e·nop·a·thy with dys·pro·tein·e·mia** a lymphoproliferative disorder characterized by generalized lymphadenopathy, hepatosplenomegaly, fever, sweats, weight loss, skin lesions, and pruritus with hypergammaglobulinemia; occurs primarily in older adults, often with fatal outcome. Proliferation of B cells, deficiency of T cells has been demonstrated.

**an·gi·o·ker·a·to·ma** (an'jē-ō-ker-ă-tō'mă) a superficial capillary telangiectasis, over which there is a wartlike hyperkeratosis and acanthosis.

SYN telangiectatic wart. [angio- + G. *keras*, horn, + -*ōma*, tumor]

**an·gi·o·ker·a·to·sis** (an'jē-ō-ker-ă-tō'sis) the occurrence of multiple angiokeratomas.

**an·gi·o·ki·ne·sis** (an'jē-ō-ki-nē'sis) SYN vasomotion. [angio- + G. *kinēsis*, movement]

**an·gi·o·ki·net·ic** (an'jē-ō-ki-net'ik) SYN vasomotor. [angio- + G. *kinētikos*, pertaining to movement]

**an·gi·o·lith** (an'jē-ō-lith) an arteriolith or a phlebolith. [angio- + G. *lithos*, stone]

**an·gi·o·lith·ic** (an'jē-ō-lith'ik) relating to an angiolith.

**an·gi·ol·o·gy** (an-jē-ol'ō-jē) the science concerned with the blood vessels and lymphatics in all their relations. [angio- + G. *logos*, treatise, discourse]

**an·gi·o·lu·poid** (an'jē-ō-loo'poyd) a sarcoid-like eruption of the skin in which the granulomatous telangiectatic papules are distributed over the nose and cheeks. [angio- + L. *lupus*, wolf, + G. *eidos*, resemblance]

**an·gi·ol·y·sis** (an-jē-ol'i-sis) obliteration of a blood vessel, such as occurs in the newborn infant after tying of the umbilical cord. [angio- + G. *lysis*, destruction]

**an·gi·o·ma** (an-jē-ō'mă) a swelling or tumor due to proliferation, with or without dilation, of the blood vessels (hemangioma) or lymphatics (lymphangioma). [angio- + G. -*ōma*, tumor]

**an·gi·o·ma ser·pi·gi·no·sum** the presence of rings of red dots on the skin, especially in female children, which tend to widen peripherally, due to dilatation of superficial capillaries. SYN essential telangiectasia (2).

**an·gi·o·ma·toid** (an-jē-ō'mă-toyd) resembling a tumor of vascular origin.

**an·gi·o·ma·to·sis** (an'jē-ō-mă-tō'sis) a condition characterized by multiple angiomas.

**an·gi·o·ma·tous** (an-jē-ō'mă-tŭs) relating to or resembling an angioma.

**an·gi·o·myx·o·ma** (an'jē-ō-miks-ō'mă) a myxoma in which there is an unusually large number of vascular structures.

**an·gi·o·neu·rec·to·my** (an'jē-ō-noo-rek'tō-mē) **1.** excision of the vessels and nerves of a part. [angio- + G. *neuron*, nerve, + *ektomē*, excision] **2.** excision of a segment of the spermatic cord to produce sterility. [angio- + G. *neuron*, nerve, + *ektomē*, excision]

**an·gi·o·neu·rot·ic ede·ma** SYN angioedema.

**an·gi·op·a·thy** (an-jē-op'ă-thē) any disease of the blood vessels or lymphatics. [angio- + G. *pathos*, suffering]

**an·gi·o·phac·o·ma·to·sis, an·gi·o·phak·o·ma·to·sis** (an'jē-ō-fak'ō-mă-tō'sis) the angiomatous phacomatoses: von Hippel-Lindau disease and the Sturge-Weber syndrome.

**an·gi·o·plas·ty** (an'jē-ō-plas-tē) reconstitution or recanalization of a blood vessel; may involve balloon dilation, mechanical stripping of intima, forceful injection of fibrinolytics, or placement of a stent. [angio- + G. *plastos*, formed, shaped]

**an·gi·o·plas·ty bal·loon** a balloon near the tip of an angioplastic catheter, designed to distend narrowed vessels. SEE balloon-tip catheter.

**an·gi·o·poi·e·sis** (an'jē-ō-poy-ē'sis) formation of blood or lymphatic vessels. SYN vasifaction, vasoformation. [angio- + G. *poiesis*, making]

**an·gi·o·poi·et·ic** (an'jē-ō-poy-et'ik) relating to angiopoiesis. SYN vasifactive, vasoformative.

**an·gi·or·rha·phy** (an-jē-ōr′ă-fē) suture repair of any vessel, especially of a blood vessel. [angio- + G. *rhaphē,* a seam]

**an·gi·o·sar·co·ma** (an′jē-ō-sar-kō′mă) a rare malignant neoplasm occurring most often in the breast and skin, and believed to originate from the endothelial cells of blood vessels; microscopically composed of closely packed round or spindle-shaped cells, some of which line small spaces resembling vascular clefts. See page B7.

**an·gi·os·co·py** (an-jē-os′kō-pē) **1.** visualization with a microscope of the passage of substances (e.g., contrast media, radiopaque agents) through capillaries after intravenous injection. **2.** visualization of the interior of blood vessels, especially the pulmonary arteries, using a fiberoptic catheter inserted through a peripheral artery. [angio- + G. *skopeō,* to view]

**an·gi·o·sco·to·ma** (an′jē-ō-skō-tō′mă) ribbon-shaped defect of the visual fields caused by the retinal vessels overlying photoreceptors. [angio- + G. *skotōma,* dizziness, vertigo]

**an·gi·o·sco·tom·e·try** (an′jē-ō-skō-tom′ĕ-trē) the measurement or projection of the angioscotoma pattern.

**an·gi·o·some** composite anatomic vascular territories of skin and underlying muscles, tendons, nerves, and bones, based on segmental or distributing arteries.

**an·gi·o·spasm** (an′jē-ō-spazm) SYN vasospasm.

**an·gi·o·spas·tic** (an′jē-ō-spas′tik) SYN vasospastic.

**an·gi·o·ste·no·sis** (an′jē-ō-stĕ-nō′sis) narrowing of one or more blood vessels. [angio- + G. *stenōsis,* a narrowing]

**an·gi·o·ten·sin** (an-jē-ō-ten′sin) a family of peptides with vasoconstrictive activity, produced by action of renin on angiotensinogen.

**an·gi·o·ten·sin-con·vert·ing en·zyme (ACE)** a hydrolase responsible for the conversion of angiotensin I to the vasoactive angiotensin II by removal of a dipeptide (histidylleucine) from angiotensin I. Drugs that inhibit ACE are used to treat hypertension and congestive heart failure.

**an·gi·o·ten·sin-con·vert·ing en·zyme in·hib·i·tor** a class of drugs used in the treatment of hypertension; they produce a reduction of peripheral arterial resistance, although the exact mechanism of action has not been fully determined; they block the conversion of angiotensin I to angiotensin II, a powerful vasoconstrictor.

**an·gi·o·ten·sin III amide** a synthetic substance closely related to naturally occurring angiotensin II; it is a potent vasopressor useful in certain types of shock and circulatory collapse.

**an·gi·o·ten·sin·o·gen·ase** (an′jē-ō-ten-sin′ŏ-jen-ās) SYN renin.

**an·gi·o·ten·sin re·cep·tor** cell-surface G-protein–coupled receptors that mediate the effects of angiotensin II. Two types are recognized: AT$_1$ and AT$_2$; the former mediates the powerful vascular smooth-muscle contraction responsible for the hypertensive response produced by angiotensin II; the latter is not sufficiently understood to be assigned any physiologic function.

**an·gi·o·ten·sin re·cep·tor block·er** an agent, such as losartan, that bind with angiotensin receptors, thus preventing access of angiotensin II to the receptor and consequently reducing the vasoconstriction produced by this agonist; used in the treatment of hypertension.

**an·gi·ot·o·my** (an-jē-ot′ō-mē) sectioning of a blood vessel, or the creation of an opening into a vessel prior to its repair. [angio- + G. *tomē,* cutting]

**an·gi·o·to·nia** (an′jē-ō-tō′nē-ă) SYN vasotonia.

**an·gi·o·tro·phic** (an′jē-ō-trōf′ik) rarely used term for vasotrophic. [angio- + G. *trophē,* nourishment]

**An·gle** (ang′gl), Edward Hartley, U.S. orthodontist, 1855–1930. SEE Angle classification of malocclusion.

**an·gle** (θ) (ang′gl) the meeting point of two lines or planes; the figure formed by the junction of two lines or planes; the space bounded on two sides by lines or planes that meet. For specific angles, see descriptive term, e.g., axioincisal, distobuccal, labiogingival, linguogingival (2), mesiogingival, proximobuccal, etc. SYN angulus [TA]. [L. *angulus*]

**An·gle clas·si·fi·ca·tion of mal·oc·clu·sion** (ang′gl) a classification of different types of malocclusion, based primarily on the mesiodistal relationship of the permanent molars upon their eruption and locking, and composed of three classes; *Class I:* normal relationship of the jaws, wherein the mesiobuccal cusp of the maxillary first molar occludes in the buccal groove of the mandibular first permanent molar but with crowding and rotation of teeth elsewhere; *Class II:* distal relationship of the mandible, wherein the distobuccal cusp of the maxillary first permanent molar occludes in the buccal groove of the mandibular first molar, and further classified as Division 1, labioversion of maxillary incisor teeth, and Division 2, linguoversion of maxillary central incisors, both of which may be unilateral conditions; *Class III:* mesial relationship of the mandible, wherein the mesiobuccal cusp of the maxillary first molar occludes in the embrasure between the mandibular first and second permanent molars, further classified as a unilateral condition.

**an·gle-clo·sure glau·co·ma** primary glaucoma in which contact of the iris with the peripheral cornea excludes aqueous humor from the trabecular drainage meshwork. SYN narrow-angle glaucoma.

**an·gle of con·ver·gence** the angle that the visual axis makes with the median line when a near object is viewed.

**an·gle of ec·cen·tric·i·ty** in strabismus, the angle between the line of fixation and the line of normal foveal fixation.

**an·gle of i·ris** SYN iridocorneal angle.

**an·gle of jaw** SYN angle of mandible.

**an·gle of man·di·ble** the angle formed by the lower margin of the body and the posterior margin of the ramus of the mandible. SYN angulus mandibulae [TA], angle of jaw.

**an·gle re·ces·sion** tearing of the iris root between the longitudinal and circular ciliary muscles; often leading to glaucoma.

**an·gle of re·tro·ver·sion** the angle formed by a line drawn through the center of the longitudinal axis of the neck and head of the humerus meeting a line drawn along the transverse axis of the condyles, when the base is viewed from above, looking straight down from above the head of the humerus; the normal angle of retroversion of the humerus is between 20° and 40°.

**an·gle of tor·sion** the amount of rotation of a

long bone along its axis or between two axes, measured in degrees.

**Ång·ström** (ang'strĕm), Anders J., Swedish physicist, 1814–1874. SEE angstrom.

**ang·strom (Å)** (ang-strŏm) a unit of wavelength, $10^{-10}$ m, roughly the diameter of an atom; equivalent to 0.1 nm. [A.J. Ångström]

**Ång·ström law** (ang-strŏm) a substance absorbs light of the same wavelength as it emits when luminous.

**Ång·ström unit (Å)** (ang-strŏm) SEE angstrom.

**an·gu·lar ar·tery** the terminal branch of the facial artery; *distribution*, muscles and skin of side of nose; *anastomoses*, lateral nasal, and dorsal artery of nose and palpebrals from the ophthalmic artery, thereby providing an external-internal carotid arterial anastomosis; SYN arteria angularis [TA].

**an·gu·lar chei·li·tis** inflammation and fissuring radiating from the commissures of the mouth. SYN angular stomatitis.

**an·gu·lar cur·va·ture** a gibbous deformity, i.e., a sharp angulation of the spine, occurring in Pott disease. SYN Pott curvature.

**an·gu·lar gy·rus** a folded convolution in the inferior parietal lobule formed by the union of the posterior ends of the superior and middle temporal gyri.

**an·gu·lar spine** SYN sphenoidal spine.

**an·gu·lar sto·ma·ti·tis** SYN angular cheilitis.

**an·gu·lar vein** a short vein at the medial angle of the eye, formed by the supraorbital and supratrochlear veins and continuing as the facial vein.

**an·gu·la·tion** (ang'gyu-lā'shŭn) **1.** formation of an angle; an abnormal angle or bend in an organ. **2.** in orthopedics, a method of describing the alignment of long bones that have been affected by injury or disease; can be described in both anteroposterior and lateral planes.

**an·gu·lus,** gen. and pl. **an·gu·li** (ang'gyu-lŭs, ang'gyu-lī) [TA] SYN angle. [L.]

**an·gu·lus ac·ro·mii** [TA] SYN acromial angle.

**an·gu·lus cos·tae** [TA] SYN costal angle.

**an·gu·lus ir·i·do·cor·ne·a·lis** [TA] SYN iridocorneal angle.

**an·gu·lus man·dib·u·lae** [TA] SYN angle of mandible.

**an·gu·lus pon·to·cer·e·bel·la·ris** [TA] SYN cerebellopontine angle.

**an·gu·lus ster·ni** [TA] SYN sternal angle.

**an·gu·lus sub·pu·bi·cus** [TA] SYN subpubic angle.

**an·he·do·nia** (an-hē-dō'nē-ă) absence of pleasure from the performance of acts that would ordinarily be pleasurable. [G. *an-* priv. + *hedonē*, pleasure]

**an·hi·dro·sis** (an-hǐ-drō'sis) inability to tolerate heat; absence of sweat glands. SYN adiaphoresis. [G. *an-* priv. + *hidrōs*, sweat]

**an·hi·drot·ic** (an-hǐ-drot'ik) **1.** relating to, or characterized by, anhidrosis. **2.** denoting a reduction or absence of sweat glands, characteristic of congenital ectodermal defect and anhidrotic ectodermal dysplasia.

**an·hy·drase** (an-hī'drās) an enzyme that catalyzes the removal of water from a compound; most such enzymes are now known as hydrases, hydrolyases, or dehydratases.

**an·hy·dra·tion** (an-hī-drā'shŭn) SYN dehydration (1).

**an·hy·dride** (an-hī'drīd) an oxide that can combine with water to form an acid or that is derived from an acid by the abstraction of water.

**an·hy·dro-** chemical prefix denoting the removal of water. Cf. pyro- (2). [G. *an-* priv., + *hydōr*, water]

**an·hy·drous** (an-hī'drŭs) containing no water, especially water of crystallization.

**an·ic·ter·ic vi·ral hep·a·ti·tis** a relatively mild hepatitis, without jaundice.

**an·i·lide** (an'i-lid) an *N*-acyl aniline; e.g., acetanilide.

**ani·linc·tion, ani·linc·tus** (ā-ni-lingk'shŭn, ā-ni-lingk'tŭs) SYN anilingus.

**an·i·line** (an'i-lin an'i-lēn) an oily, colorless or brownish liquid, of aromatic odor and acrid taste, that is the parent substance of many synthetic dyes. Aniline is highly toxic and may cause industrial poisoning. [Ar. *an-nil,* indigo]

**ani·lin·gus** (ā-ni-ling'gŭs) sexual stimulation by licking or kissing the anus. SYN anilinction, anilinctus. [L. *anus,* + *lingo,* to lick]

**an·il·ism** (an'i-lizm) chronic aniline poisoning, characterized by nausea, vertigo, muscular weakness, cyanosis, and respiratory and circulatory failure.

**an·i·ma** (an'i-mă) **1.** the soul or spirit. SEE animus (4). **2.** in jungian psychology, the inner self, in contrast to persona; a female archetype in a man. Cf. animus (5). [L. breath, soul]

**an·i·mal** (an'i-măl) **1.** a living, sentient organism that has membranous cell walls, requires oxygen and organic foods, and is capable of voluntary movement, as distinguished from a plant or mineral. **2.** one of the lower animal organisms as distinguished from humans. [L.]

**an·i·mal mod·el** study in a population of laboratory animals that uses conditions of animals analogous to conditions of humans to simulate processes comparable to those that occur in human populations.

**an·i·mal pole** the point in a telolecithal egg opposite the yolk, site of the nucleus and most of the protoplasm; from this region, the polar bodies are extruded during maturation. SYN germinal pole.

**an·i·ma·tion** (an-i-mā'shŭn) **1.** the state of being alive. **2.** liveliness; high spirits. [L. *animo,* pp. *-atus,* to make alive; *anima,* breath, soul]

**an·i·mus** (an'i-mŭs) **1.** an animating or energizing spirit. **2.** intention to do something; disposition. **3.** in psychiatry, a spirit of active hostility or grudge. **4.** the ideal image toward which a person strives. **5.** in jungian psychology, a male archetype in a woman. Cf. anima (2). [L. *animus,* breath, rational soul in man, will]

**AN in·ter·val** the time between onset of the atrial deflection and the nodal potential (normally 40–100 msec).

**an·i·on (A⁻)** (an'ī-on) an ion that carries a negative charge, going therefore to the positively charged anode; in salts, acid radicals are anions.

**an·i·on ex·change** the process by which an anion in a mobile (liquid) phase exchanges with another anion previously bound to a solid, positively charged phase, the latter being an anion exchanger. Anion exchange may also be used chromatographically, to separate anions, and medicinally, to remove an anion (e.g., Cl⁻) from gastric contents or bile acids in the intestine.

**an·i·on-ex·change res·in** SEE anion exchange.

**an·i·on gap** the arithmetical difference between

the concentrations of routinely measured cations ($Na^+$ + $K^+$) and of routinely measured anions ($Cl^-$ + $HCO_3^-$) in plasma or serum; unmeasured anions (phosphate, sulfate, protein, other organic ions) account for the gap, which is increased in metabolic acidosis due to diabetic ketosis, renal failure, or extraneous substances (methanol, salicylate).

**an·i·on·ic neu·tro·phil·ac·ti·vat·ing pep·tide** SYN interleukin-8.

**an·i·rid·ia** (an-i-rid′ē-ă) absence of the iris. Cf. irideremia. [G. *an-* priv. + *irid-* + *-ia*]

**an·is·ei·ko·nia** (an′ī-sī-kō′nē-ă) an ocular condition in which the image of an object in one eye differs in size or shape from the image of the same object in the fellow eye. [G. *anisos,* unequal, + *eikōn,* an image]

△**an·i·so-** unequal, dissimilar, unlike. [G. *anisos,* unequal, fr. *an-,* not, + *isos,* equal]

**an·i·so·ac·com·mo·da·tion** (an-ī′sō-ă-kom-ō-dā′shŭn) variation between the two eyes in accommodation capacity. [aniso- + L. *accommodo,* to adapt]

**an·i·so·chro·mat·ic** (an-ī′sō-krō-mat′ik) not uniformly of one color.

**an·i·so·co·ria** (an-ī-sō-kō′rē-ă) a condition in which the two pupils are not of equal size. [aniso- + G. *korē,* pupil]

∎**an·i·so·cy·to·sis** (an-ī′sō-sī-tō′sis) considerable variation in the size of cells that are normally uniform, especially with reference to red blood cells. See page B2. [aniso- + G. *kytos,* cell, + *-osis,* condition]

**an·i·so·dac·ty·lous** (an-ī′sō-dak′ti-lŭs) relating to anisodactyly.

**an·i·so·dac·ty·ly** (an-ī′sō-dak′ti-lē) unequal length in corresponding fingers. [aniso- + G. *daktylos,* finger]

**an·i·sog·a·my** (an′i-sog′ă-mē) fusion of two gametes unequal in size or form; fertilization as distinguished from isogamy or conjugation. [aniso- + G. *gamos,* marriage]

**an·i·sog·na·thous** (an-i-sog′nă-thŭs) having jaws of unequal size, the upper being wider than the lower. [aniso- + G. *gnathos,* jaw]

**an·i·so·kar·y·o·sis** (an-ī′sō-kar-ē-ō′sis) variation in size of nuclei, greater than the normal range for a tissue. [aniso- + G. *karyon,* nut (nucleus), + *-osis,* condition]

**an·i·so·mas·tia** (an-i-sō-mas′tē-ă) inequality in the size of the breasts. [aniso- + G. *mastos,* breast]

**an·i·so·me·lia** (an-i-sō-mē′lē-ă) a condition of inequality between two paired limbs. [aniso- + G. *melos,* limb]

**an·i·so·me·tro·pia** (an-ī′sō-me-trō′pē-ă) a difference in the refractive power of the two eyes. [aniso- + G. *metron,* measure, + *ōps,* sight]

**an·i·so·me·tro·pic** (an-ī′sō-me-trop′ik) **1.** relating to anisometropia. **2.** having eyes of unequal refractive power.

**an·i·so·pi·e·sis** (an-ī-sō-pī-ē′sis) unequal arterial blood pressure on the two sides of the body. [aniso- + G. *piesis,* pressure]

**an·i·so·sphyg·mia** (an-ī-sō-sfig′mē-ă) difference in volume, force, or time of the pulse in the corresponding arteries on two sides of the body, e.g., the two radials, or femorals. [aniso- + G. *sphygmos,* pulse]

**an·i·sos·then·ic** (an-ī-sos-then′ik) of unequal strength; denoting two muscles or groups of muscles that are either paired or are antagonists. [aniso- + G. *sthenos,* strength]

**an·i·so·ton·ic** (an-ī-sō-ton′ik) not having equal tension; having unequal osmotic pressure. [aniso- + G. *tonus,* tension]

**A·nitsch·kow cell** (ah-nich′kov) SYN cardiac histiocyte.

**A·nitsch·kow my·o·cyte** (ah-nich′kov) SYN cardiac histiocyte.

**an·kle** (ang′kl) **1.** SYN ankle joint. **2.** the region of the ankle joint. **3.** SYN talus.

**an·kle bone** SYN talus.

**an·kle-foot or·tho·sis** an orthosis beginning at the toes, crossing the ankle, and terminating on the calf.

**an·kle joint** a hinge synovial joint between the tibia and fibula above and the talus below. SYN ankle (1), mortise joint, talocrural joint.

**an·kle re·flex** SYN Achilles reflex.

△**an·ky·lo-** bent, crooked, stiff, fused, fixed, closed SEE ALSO ancylo-. [G. *ankylos,* bent, crooked; *ankylōsis,* stiffening of the joints, fr. *ankos,* a bend, a hollow]

**an·ky·lo·glos·sia** (ang′ki-lō-glos′ē-ă) partial or complete fusion of the tongue to the floor of the mouth; abnormal shortness of the frenulum linguae. SYN tongue-tie. [ankylo- + G. *glōssa,* tongue]

**an·ky·lo·poi·et·ic** (ang′ki-lō-poy-et′ik) forming ankylosis.

**an·ky·losed** (ang′ki-lōst) stiffened; bound by adhesions; denoting a joint in a state of ankylosis.

**an·ky·los·ing spon·dy·li·tis** arthritis of the spine, resembling rheumatoid arthritis, that may progress to bony ankylosis with lipping of vertebral margins; the disease is more common in the male, often with the rheumatoid factor absent and the HLA antigen present. There is a striking association with the B27 tissue type and the strong familial aggregation suggests an important genetic factor. SYN rheumatoid spondylitis.

**an·ky·lo·sis** (ang′ki-lō′sis) stiffening or fixation of a joint as the result of a disease process, with fibrous or bony union across the joint. [G. *ankylōsis,* stiffening of a joint]

**an·ky·lot·ic** (ang-ki-lot′ik) characterized by or pertaining to an ankylosis.

**an·la·ge,** pl. **an·la·gen** (ahn′lah-gĕ, ahn′lah-gĕn) **1.** SYN primordium. **2.** in psychoanalysis, genetic predisposition to a given trait or personality characteristic. [Ger. plan, outline]

**an·neal·ing lamp** an alcohol lamp with a soot-free flame used in dentistry to drive off the protective $NH_3$ gas coating from the surface of cohesive gold foil.

**an·nec·tent** (a-nek′tent) connected with; joined. [L. *an-necto,* pres. p. *an-nectens,* to join to]

**an·nexa** (a-nek′să) SYN adnexa.

**an·nex·al** (a-neks-ăl) SYN adnexal.

**an·nu·lo·a·or·tic ec·ta·sia** supravalvular dilation of the aorta involving both its wall and the valve ring, which, however, remains of smaller diameter than the more distal ectatic wall; many cases are related to Marfan syndrome.

**an·nu·lor·rha·phy** (an-yŭ-lōr′ă-fē) closure of a hernial ring by suture. [L. *anulus,* ring, + G. *rhaphē,* seam]

**an·nu·lus** (an′yŭ-lŭs) SYN ring.

**ano·coc·cyg·e·al** (ā-nō-kok-sij′ē-ăl) relating to both anus and coccyx.

**a·no·coc·cyg·e·al nerve** one of several small

nerves arising from the coccygeal plexus, supplying the skin over the coccyx. SYN nervus anococcygeus [TA].

**an•ode** (an′ōd) **1.** the positive pole of a galvanic battery or the electrode connected with it; an electrode toward which negatively charged ions (anions) migrate; a positively charged electrode. **2.** the portion, usually made of tungsten, of an x-ray tube from which x-rays are released by bombardment by cathode rays (electrons). [G. *anodos,* a way up, fr. *ana,* up, + *hodos,* a way]

**an•o•derm** (ā′nō-derm) lining of the anal canal, extending from the dentate line to the anal verge; it is devoid of hair and sebaceous and sweat glands but is richly supplied with tactile and nociceptive (pain, itch) endings innervated by the inferior rectal (pudendal) nerve.

**an•o•don•tia** (an-ō-don′shē-ă) congenital absence of the teeth; developmental, not due to extraction or impaction. SYN agomphosis, agomphiasis. [G. *an-* priv. + *odous,* tooth]

**ano•gen•i•tal** (ā′nō-jen′ĭ-tăl) relating to both the anal and the genital regions.

**a•no•gen•i•tal ra•phe** in the male embryo the line of closure of the genital folds and swellings extending from the anus to the tip of the penis; it is differentiated in the adult into three regions: perineal raphe, scrotal raphe, and penile raphe.

**anom•a•lad** (ă-nom′ă-lad) a malformation together with its subsequently derived structural changes. [SEE *anomaly*]

**a•nom•a•lous com•plex** a complex in the electrocardiogram differing significantly from the physiologic type in the same lead.

**a•nom•a•lous pul•mo•nary ve•nous con•nec•tions, total or partial** connections in which some or all of the pulmonary veins connect to the right atrium or one of its tributaries.

**a•nom•a•lous ret•i•nal cor•re•spon•dence** a condition, frequent in strabismus, in which corresponding retinal points do not have the same visual direction; the fovea of one eye corresponds to an extrafoveal area of the fellow eye.

**anom•a•ly** (ă-nom′ă-lē) deviation from the average or norm; anything that is structurally unusual or irregular or contrary to a general rule, especially a congenital defect. [G. *anōmalia,* irregularity]

**an•o•mer** (an′ŏ-mer) one of two sugar molecules that are epimeric at the hemiacetal or hemiketal carbon atom. SEE ALSO sugars. Cf. epimer.

**ano•mia** (ă-nō′mē-ă) SYN nominal aphasia. [G. *a-* priv. + *ōnoma,* name]

**a•nom•ic a•pha•sia** an aphasia in which the principal deficit is difficulty in naming persons and objects seen, heard, or felt; due to lesions in various portions of the language area. SYN nominal aphasia.

**an•o•nych•ia, an•o•ny•cho•sis** (an-ō-nik′ē-ă, an-ō-nī-kō′sis) absence of the nails. [G. *an-* priv. + *onyx (onych-),* nail]

**anon•y•ma** (ă-non′i-mă) without name; a term formerly applied to the large vessels in the thorax (now called the brachiocephalic trunk and vein) and the hip bone. SYN innominate. [G. *an-* priv. + *onyma,* name]

*Anoph•e•les* (ă-nof′ĕ-lēz) a genus of mosquitoes (family Culicidae, subfamily Anophelinae). The sporogenous cycle of the malarial parasite is passed in the body cavity of female mosquitoes of certain species of this genus. [G. *anophelēs,*

useless, harmful, fr. *an-* priv. + *ōpheleō,* to be of use]

**anoph•e•line** (ă-nof′ĕ-līn) referring to the *Anopheles* mosquito.

**an•oph•thal•mia** (an-of-thal′mē-ă) congenital absence of all tissues of the eyes. [G. *an-* priv. + *ophthalmos,* eye]

**ano•plas•ty** (ā′nō-plas-tē) plastic surgery of the anus. [L. *anus* + G. *plastos,* formed]

**an•or•chia** (an-ōr′kē-ă) SYN anorchism.

**an•or•chism** (an-ōr′kizm) absence of the testes; may be congenital or acquired. SYN anorchia. [G. *an-* priv. + *orchis,* testicle]

**ano•rec•tal** (ā′nō-rek′tăl) relating to both anus and rectum.

**an•o•rec•tic** (an-ō-rek′tic) **1.** relating to, characteristic of, or suffering from anorexia, especially anorexia nervosa. **2.** an agent that causes anorexia. SYN anorexic.

**an•o•rex•ia** (an-ō-rek′sē-ă) diminished appetite; aversion to food. [G. fr. *an-* priv. + *orexis,* appetite]

**an•o•re•xia ath•let•i•ca** continuum of subclinical eating behaviors of athletes who do not meet the criteria for a true eating disorder, but who practice at least one unhealthful method of weight control (e.g., fasting, vomiting, use of diet pills, laxatives, or diuretics).

**an•o•rex•ia ner•vo•sa** a personality disorder manifested by extreme fear of becoming obese and an aversion to eating, usually occurring in young women and often resulting in life-threatening weight loss, accompanied by a disturbance in body image, hyperactivity, and amenorrhea.

**an•o•rex•i•ant** (an-ō-rek′sē-ănt) a drug ("diet pills"), process, or event that leads to anorexia.

**an•o•rex•ic** (an-ō-rek′sik) SYN anorectic.

**an•or•gas•my, an•or•gas•mia** (an-ōr-gaz′mē, an-ōr-gaz′mē-ă) failure to experience an orgasm; may be biogenic (secondary to a physical disorder or medication), psychogenic (secondary to psychological or situational factors), or a combination of the two. [G. *an-* priv. + orgasm + *-ia*]

**an•or•thog•ra•phy** (an-ōr-thog′ră-fē) SYN agraphia. [G. *an-* priv. + *orthos,* straight, + *graphō,* to write]

**ano•scope** (ā′nō-skōp) a short speculum for examining the anal canal and lower rectum.

**ano•sig•moid•os•co•py** (ā′nō-sig-moy-dos′kŏ-pē) endoscopy of the anus, rectum and sigmoid colon.

**an•os•mia** (an-oz′mē-ă) loss of the sense of smell. It may be due to lesion of the olfactory nerve, obstruction of the nasal fossae, or functional, without any apparent causative lesion. [G. *an-* priv. + *osmē,* sense of smell]

**an•os•mic** (an-oz′mik) relating to anosmia.

**ano•sog•no•sia** (ă-nō′sog-nō′sē-ă) ignorance of the presence of disease, specifically of paralysis. Most often seen in patients with non-dominant parietal lobe lesions, who deny their hemiparesis. [G. *a-* priv. + *nosos,* disease, + *gnōsis,* knowledge]

**ano•sog•no•sic** (ă-nō-sog-nō′sik) relating to anosognosia.

**a•no•sog•no•sic ep•i•lep•sy** epilepsy characterized by attacks of which the person is unaware.

**ano•spi•nal** (ā′nō-spī′năl) relating to the anus and the spinal cord.

**an•os•to•sis** (an-os-tō′sis) failure of ossification. [G. *an-* priv. + *osteon,* bone]

**an•o•tia** (an-ō'shē-ă) congenital absence of one or both external ears. [G. *an-* priv. + *ous,* ear]

**ANOVA** analysis of variance.

**ano•ves•i•cal** (ā'nō-ves'i-kăl) relating in any way to both anus and urinary bladder.

**an•ov•u•lar** (an-ov'yu-lăr) absence of discharge of an ovum from the ovary during an ovarian cycle.

**an•ov•u•lar men•stru•a•tion** menstrual bleeding without recent ovulation; also occurs in subhuman primates.

**an•ov•u•la•tion** (an-ov-yu-lā'shŭn) suspension or cessation of ovulation.

**an•ox•e•mia** (an-ok-sē'mē-ă) absence of oxygen in arterial blood; formerly often used to include moderate decrease in oxygen now properly distinguished as hypoxemia. [G. *an-* priv. + oxygen + G. *haima,* blood]

**an•ox•ia** (an-ok'sē-ă) absence or almost complete absence of oxygen from inspired gases, arterial blood, or tissues; to be differentiated from hypoxia. [G. *an-* priv. + oxygen]

**an•ox•ic** (an-ok'sik) denoting or characteristic of anoxia.

**an•ox•ic an•ox•ia** hypoxic hypoxia in which oxygen is almost completely lacking.

**An•rep phe•nom•e•non** (ahn'rep) homeometric autoregulation of the heart whereby cardiac performance improves as the afterload (aortic pressure) is increased.

**an•sa,** gen. and pl. **an•sae** (an'să, an-sē) [TA] any anatomic structure in the form of a loop or an arc. SEE ALSO loop. [L. loop, handle]

**an•sa cer•vi•ca•lis** [TA] a loop in the cervical plexus consisting of fibers from the first three cervical nerves. Fibers from a loop between the C1 and C2 spinal nerves accompany the hypoglossal nerve for a short distance, leaving it as the superior root of the ansa cervicalis. Fibers from a loop between the C2 and C3 spinal nerves form the inferior root of the ansa cervicalis. Most commonly, the roots merge, forming the ansa cervicalis, which gives rise to branches innervating infrahyoid muscles. SYN cervical loop.

**an•sae ner•vo•rum spi•na•li•um** SYN loops of spinal nerves.

**an•sa pe•dun•cu•la•ris** [TA] a complex fiber bundle curving around the medial edge of the internal capsule and connecting the anterior part of the temporal lobe (temporal cortex), amygdala, and olfactory cortex with the mediodorsal nucleus of the thalamus; it enters the thalamus as a component of the inferior thalamic peduncle which also contains a major part of the fibers connecting the mediodorsal nucleus to the orbitofrontal cortex.

**an•sa sub•cla•via** [TA] a nerve cord connecting the middle cervical and stellate sympathetic ganglia, forming a loop around the subclavian artery.

**an•sate** (an'sāt) SYN ansiform.

**an•ser•ine bur•sa** the bursa between the tibial collateral ligament of the knee joint and the tendons of the sartorius, gracilis, and semitendinosus muscles.

**ANSI** American National Standards Institute.

**an•si•form** (an'si-fōrm) in the shape of a loop or arc. SYN ansate. [L. *ansa,* handle, + *forma,* shape]

**an•so•par•a•me•di•an fissure** the fissure separating lobule HVIIA, crus II of the ansiform lob-

ule, from lobule HVIIB, the paramedian lobule, of the posterior lobe of the cerebellum.

**ant** one of the most numerous insects (order Hymenoptera), characterized by an extraordinary development of colonial dwelling and caste specialization.

△**ant-** SEE anti-.

**ant•ac•id** (ant-as'id) **1.** neutralizing an acid. **2.** any agent that reduces or neutralizes acidity, as of the gastric juice or any other secretion.

**an•tag•o•nism** (an-tag'on-izm) **1.** denoting mutual opposition in action between structures, agents, diseases, or physiologic processes. Cf. synergism. **2.** the situation in which the combined effect of two or more factors is smaller than the solitary effect of any one of the factors. SYN mutual resistance. [G. *antagōnisma,* from *anti,* against, + *agōnizomai,* to fight, fr. *agōn,* a contest]

**an•tag•o•nist** (an-tag'ŏ-nist) something opposing or resisting the action of another; any structure, agent, disease, or physiologic process that tends to neutralize or impede some action or effect. Cf. synergist.

**an•tag•o•nis•tic mus•cles** those having opposite functions, the contraction of one tending to "neutralize" that of the other.

**an•tal•gic gait** (ant-al'jik gāt) a limping walk used to avoid pain. [G. *anti-,* against, + *algos,* pain]

△**an•te-** before, in front of (in time or place or order). SEE ALSO pre-, pro- (1). [L. *ante,* before, in front of]

**an•te•brach•i•al** (an'te-brā'kē-ăl) relating to the forearm.

**an•te•bra•chi•um** (an-te-brā'kē-ŭm) [TA] SYN forearm. [ante- + L. *brachium,* arm]

**an•te•ced•ent** (an-te-sē'dent) a precursor. [L. *antecedo,* to go before]

**an•te ci•bum (AC, a.c.)** (an'tē sī'bŭm) before a meal. The plural is ante cibos, before meals. [L.]

**an•te•cu•bi•tal** (an-te-kyu'bi-tăl) in front of the elbow. [ante- + L. *cubitum,* elbow]

**an•te•flex•ion** (an-te-flek'shŭn) a bending forward; a sharp forward curve or angulation; denoting especially the normal forward bend in the uterus at the junction of corpus and cervix uteri.

**an•te•gon•i•al notch** the highest point of the notch or concavity of the lower border of the ramus where it joins the body of the mandible.

**an•te•grade** (an'tĕ-grād) in the direction of normal movement, as in blood flow or peristalsis. [ante- + L. *gradior,* to walk]

**an•te•grade block** SYN anterograde block.

**an•te•grade u•rog•ra•phy** radiography following percutaneous injection of contrast agent with a needle or catheter into the renal calices or pelvis (antegrade pyelography), or into the urinary bladder (antegrade cystography).

**an•te•mor•tem** (an'te-mōr-tem) before death. Cf. postmortem. [ante- + L. *mors* (*mort-*), death]

**an•te•na•tal** (an-te-nā'tăl) SYN prenatal. [ante- + L. *natus,* birth]

**an•te•or•bi•tal [Br.]** SEE antorbital.

**an•te•par•tum** (an'te-par-tŭm) before labor or childbirth. Cf. intrapartum, postpartum. [ante- + L. *pario,* pp. *partus,* to bring forth]

**ant•ep•i•lep•tic [Br.]** . SEE antiepileptic.

**an•te•py•ret•ic** (an'te-pī-ret'ik) before the occurrence of fever; before the period of reaction following shock. [ante- + G. *pyretos,* fever]

🔲**an•te•ri•or** (an-tēr′ē-er) **1.** HUMAN ANATOMY denoting the front surface of the body; often used to indicate the position of one structure relative to another, i.e., situated nearer the front part of the body. SYN ventral (2). **2.** near the head or rostral end of certain embryos. **3.** before, in relation to time or space. See page APP 89. [L.]

**an•ter•i•or amyg•da•loid area** the most rostral portion of the amygdaloid complex composed of scattered cells representing a transition into the more distinctly organized divisions of the amygdala. SYN area amygdaloidea anterior [TA].

**an•ter•i•or apha•sia** SYN expressive aphasia.

**an•ter•i•or ap•pre•hen•sion test 1.** SYN shoulder apprehension sign. **2.** a test of shoulder stability; apprehension with abduction and external rotation of the joint suggests anterior instability. SYN crank test.

**an•te•ri•or au•ric•u•lar mus•cle** *origin*, galea aponeurotica; *insertion*, cartilage of auricle; *action*, draws pinna of ear upward and forward; *nerve supply*, facial. Considered by some to be the anterior part of the temporoparietal muscle. SYN musculus attrahens aurem, musculus attrahens auriculam.

**an•te•ri•or au•ric•u•lar nerves** branches of the auriculotemporal nerve that supply the tragus and upper part of the auricle. SYN nervi auriculares anteriores [TA].

**an•ter•i•or ba•sal seg•men•tal ar•tery** anterior basal branch of superior basal veins of the lower right and left lobes of left and right lungs.

**an•te•ri•or bor•der of tib•ia** the sharp subcutaneous ridge of the tibia that extends from the tuberosity to the anterior part of the medial malleolus. SYN shin (2).

**an•te•ri•or car•di•nal veins** SEE cardinal veins.

**an•te•ri•or ce•re•bral vein** a small vein that parallels the anterior cerebral artery and drains into the basal vein.

**an•te•ri•or cham•ber of eye•ball** the space between the cornea anteriorly and the iris posteriorly, filled with a watery fluid (aqueous humor) and communicating through the pupil with the posterior chamber. SYN camera anterior bulbi oculi [TA].

**an•te•ri•or cil•i•ary ar•tery** one of several arteries derived from muscular branches of the ophthalmic that perforate the anterior part of the sclera and anastomose with posterior ciliary arteries.

**an•te•ri•or clin•oid proc•ess** the posteriorly directed projection that is the medial end of the sphenoidal ridge (lesser wing of sphenoid); it provides attachment for the free edge of the tentorium cerebelli. SYN processus clinoideus anterior [TA].

**an•te•ri•or col•umn** the pronounced, ventrally oriented ridge of gray matter in each half of the spinal cord; it corresponds to the anterior or ventral horn appearing in transverse sections of the cord, and contains the motor neurons innervating the skeletal musculature of the trunk, neck, and extremities. SEE ALSO gray columns.

**an•te•ri•or com•mis•sure** a round bundle of nerve fibers that crosses the midline of the brain near the anterior limit of the third ventricle. It consists of a smaller anterior part, the fibers of which pass in part to the olfactory bulbs, and a larger posterior part, which interconnects the left

and right temporal lobes. SYN praecommissure, precommissure.

**an•ter•i•or com•mis•sure of the lar•ynx** the junction of the vocal cords anteriorly in the larynx.

**an•ter•i•or con•dy•loid fo•ra•men** SYN hypoglossal canal.

**an•ter•i•or cor•ne•al dy•stro•phy** corneal opacification with involvement of the epithelium, basement membrane, or Bowman membrane of the cornea.

**an•ter•i•or cru•ci•ate lig•a•ment** the ligament that extends from the anterior intercondylar area of the tibia to the posterior part of the medial surface of the lateral condyle of the femur. SYN ligamentum cruciatum anterius [TA].

**an•ter•i•or e•las•tic lam•i•na of cor•nea** a homogeneous, acellular tissue layer just beneath the epithelium of the cornea. SYN Bowman membrane, Bowman layer, lamina limitans anterior corneae.

**an•te•ri•or em•bry•o•tox•on** SYN arcus cornealis.

**an•te•ri•or fo•cal point** the point where parallel rays from the retina are focused.

**an•te•ri•or fu•nic•u•lus** anterior white column of spinal cord, a column or bundle of white matter on either side of the anterior median fissure, between that and the anterolateral sulcus.

**an•te•ri•or horn 1.** the anterior or frontal division of the lateral ventricle of the brain, extending forward from Monro interventricular foramen; SEE lateral ventricle. **2.** the anterior or ventral gray column of the spinal cord as appearing in cross section. SEE ALSO gray columns. SYN cornu anterius [TA], praecornu, precornu, ventral horn.

**an•te•ri•or in•ter•cos•tal veins** tributaries to the musculophrenic or internal thoracic veins from the anterior portions of intercostal spaces.

**an•te•ri•or in•ter•os•se•ous nerve** a branch of the median nerve arising in the elbow region, running on interosseous membrane, supplying the flexor pollicis longus, part of flexor digitorum profundus and the pronator quadratus muscles, as well as radiocarpal and intercarpal joints. SYN nervus interosseus antebrachii anterior [TA].

**an•te•ri•or la•bi•al veins** tributaries of the femoral or external pudendal veins draining the mons pubis and anterior labia majora.

**an•te•ri•or lac•ri•mal crest** a vertical ridge on the lateral surface of the frontal process of the maxilla that forms part of the medial rim of the orbit.

**an•te•ri•or lay•er of thor•a•co•lum•bar fas••cia** fascial membrane extending from transverse processes of lumbar vertebrae. SYN fascia musculi quadrati lumborum.

**an•te•ri•or lim•it•ing lay•er of cor•nea** a transparent homogeneous acellular layer, 6 to 9 μm thick, lying between the basal lamina of the outer layer of stratified epithelium and the substantia propria of the cornea; considered to be a basement membrane.

**an•te•ri•or lim•it•ing ring** the periphery of the cornea marking the termination of Descemet membrane and the anterior border of the trabecular meshwork; an important landmark in gonioscopy. SYN Schwalbe ring.

**an•te•ri•or lin•gual gland** one of the small mixed glands deeply placed near the apex of the tongue on each side of the frenulum. SYN apical gland.

**an·te·ri·or lobe of hy·poph·y·sis** SYN adenohypophysis.

**an·ter·i·or me·di·as·ti·nos·co·py** modification of the Chamberlain procedure in which a mediastinoscope is used for exploration of the anterior mediastinum and subaortic regions.

**an·ter·i·or me·nin·ge·al branch of an·ter·i·or eth·moid·al ar·tery** *origin*, anterior ethmoidal; *distribution*, meninges in anterior cranial fossa; *anastomoses*, branches of middle meningeal and meningeal branches of internal carotid and lacrimal.

**an·te·ri·or na·sal spine** a pointed projection at the anterior extremity of the intermaxillary suture; the tip, as seen on a lateral cephalometric radiograph, is used as a cephalometric landmark.

**an·ter·i·or nu·clei of thal·a·mus** collective term for three groups of nerve cells that together form the anterior thalamic tubercle; the anteroventral nerve, a relatively large nerve; the anteromedial nerve; and the anterodorsal nerve, a small (but large-celled) nerve. These nuclei receive the mammillothalamic tract from the mammillary body, and additional afferents by way of the fornix; they project collecively to the cortex of the cingulate and parahippocampal gyrus. SYN nuclei anteriores thalami [TA].

**an·ter·i·or nu·cle·us** SEE anterior horn.

**an·te·ri·or oc·u·lar seg·ment** that portion of the eye comprising the cornea, iris, lens, and their associated chambers and adnexa.

**an·ter·i·or per·fo·rat·ing ar·ter·i·es** *origin*: as part of the anteromedial central arteries arising from the precommunicating part (A1 segment) of the anterior cerebral artery; enters the anterior perforated substance of the cranial base.

**an·te·ri·or pi·tu·i·tary go·nad·o·tro·pin** any gonadotropin of hypophysial origin. SYN pituitary gonadotropic hormone.

**an·te·ri·or pi·tu·i·tar·y-like hor·mone** SYN chorionic gonadotropin.

**an·te·ri·or and pos·te·ri·or su·pe·ri·or pan··cre·at·i·co·du·o·de·nal ar·tery** *origin*, gastroduodenal; one of two arteries, anterior and superior; *distribution*, head of pancreas, duodenum, common bile duct; *anastomoses*, inferior pancreaticoduodenal, splenic.

**an·te·ri·or pyr·a·mid** SYN pyramid of medulla oblongata.

**an·te·ri·or rhi·nos·co·py** inspection of the anterior portion of the nasal cavity with or without the aid of a nasal speculum.

**an·te·ri·or scle·ri·tis** inflammation of the sclera adjacent to the cornea.

**an·ter·i·or seg·men·tal ar·tery** SEE left pulmonary artery, right pulmonary artery.

**an·te·ri·or spi·no·cer·e·bel·lar tract** a bundle of fibers originating in the base of the posterior horn and zona intermedia throughout lumbosacral segments of the spinal cord, crossing to the opposite side and ascending in a peripheral position in the ventral half of the lateral funiculus. In its ascent through the rhombencephalon, the tract curves sharply dorsalward along the rostral border of the trigeminal motor nucleus, entering the cerebellum in a caudal direction over the dorsal surface of the superior cerebellar peduncle, and terminating as mossy fibers in the granular layer of the cortex of the cerebellar vermis. The bundle

conveys proprioceptive and exteroceptive information largely from the opposite lower extremity. SYN Gowers tract.

**an·te·ri·or staph·y·lo·ma** a bulging near the anterior pole of the eyeball. SYN corneal staphyloma.

**an·te·ri·or thor·a·cot·o·my** anterior incision into the chest, usually submammary.

**an·te·ri·or tib·i·al com·part·ment syn·drome** ischemic necrosis of the muscles of the anterior tibial compartment of the leg, presumed due to compression of arteries by swollen muscles following unaccustomed exertion.

**an·te·ri·or tib·i·o·fas·cial mus·cle** separate fibers of the tibialis anterior inserted into the fascia of the dorsum of the foot. SYN musculus tibiofascialis anterior, musculus tibiofascialis anticus.

**an·te·ri·or tooth** any of the incisor and canine teeth.

**an·te·ri·or ver·te·bral vein** the small vein that accompanies the ascending cervical artery; it opens below into the vertebral vein.

**an·ter·i·or ves·ti·bu·lar ar·tery** *origin*: as a terminal branch, with the common cochlear artery, of the labyrinthine artery; *branch*: vestibulocochlear artery; *distribution*: to vestibular ganglion, utricle and (especially the ampullae of the) lateral and posterior semicircular ducts.

△**an·tero-** anterior. [L. *anterior*, more before, earlier, fr. *ante*, before, + -r- -*ior*, more]

**an·ter·o·grade** (an′ter-ō-grād) **1.** moving forward. Cf. antegrade. **2.** extending forward from a particular point in time; used in reference to amnesia. [L. *gradior*, pp. *gressus*, to step, go]

**an·ter·o·grade am·ne·sia** amnesia in reference to events occurring after the trauma or disease that caused the condition.

**an·ter·o·grade block** conduction block of an impulse traveling in its ordinary direction, for example, from the sinoatrial node toward the ventricular myocardium. SYN antegrade block.

**an·ter·o·in·fe·ri·or** (an′ter-ō-in-fēr′ē-er) in front and below.

**an·ter·o·lat·er·al** (an′ter-ō-lat′er-ăl) in front and away from the middle line.

**an·te·ro·lis·the·sis** forward displacement of a vertebral body with respect to the vertebral body immediately below it, due to congenital anomaly, degenerative change, or trauma. SYN spondylolisthesis. [antero- + G. *olisthēsis*, a slipping]

**an·ter·o·me·di·al** (an′ter-ō-mē′dē-ăl) in front and toward the middle line.

**an·ter·o·me·di·an** (an′ter-ō-mē′dē-an) in front and in the central line.

**an·ter·o·pos·te·ri·or** (an′ter-ō-pos-tēr′ē-er) **1.** relating to both front and rear. **2.** in x-ray imaging, describing the direction of the beam through the patient from anterior to posterior.

**an·ter·o·pos·te·ri·or pro·jec·tion** SYN AP projection.

**an·ter·o·su·pe·ri·or** (an′ter-ō-soo-pēr′ē-er) in front and above.

**an·ter·o·ven·tral nu·clei of thal·a·mus** SEE anterior nuclei of thalamus.

**an·te·sys·to·le** (an-te-sis′tō-lē) premature activation of the ventricle, responsible for the pre-excitation syndrome of the Wolff-Parkinson-White or Lown-Ganong-Levine types.

**an·te·ver·sion** (an-tē-ver′zhŭn) forward displacement or turning forward of a body segment. [L. *ante*, before, forward, + *verto, versus*, to turn]

**an·te·vert·ed** (an-te-vert′ed) tilted forward; in a position of anteversion.

**ant·he·lix** (ant′hē-liks, an′thē-liks) SYN antihelix. [anti- + G. *helix,* coil]

**an·thel·min·tic** (ant-hel-min′tik, an-thel-min′tik) **1.** an agent that destroys or expels intestinal worms. SYN helminthagogue. **2.** having the power to destroy or expel intestinal worms. [anti- + G. *helmins,* worm]

**an·thrac·ic** (an-thras′ik) relating to anthrax.

**an·thra·coid** (an′thră-koyd) resembling a carbuncle or cutaneous anthrax. [G. *anthrax,* carbuncle, + *eidos,* resemblance]

**an·thra·co·sil·i·co·sis** (an′thră-kō-sil′i-kō′sis) pneumoconiosis from accumulation of carbon and silica in the lungs from inhaled coal dust; the silica content produces fibrous nodules. SYN coal worker's pneumoconiosis. [anthraco- + silicosis]

**an·thra·co·sis** (an-thră-kō′sis) pneumoconiosis from accumulation of carbon from inhaled smoke or coal dust in the lungs. SYN collier's lung, melanedema, miner's lung (1). [anthraco- + G. *-osis,* condition]

**an·thrax** (an′thraks) a disease in humans caused by infection with *Bacillus anthracis;* marked by hemorrhage and serous effusions in various organs and body cavities and by symptoms of extreme prostration. SYN carbuncle (2). [G. *anthrax* (*anthrak-*), charcoal, coal, a carbuncle]

△**an·thro·po-** human. [G. *anthrōpos,* a human being (of either sex)]

**an·thro·po·cen·tric** (an′thrō-pō-sen′trik) with a human bias, under the assumption that humankind is the central fact of the universe. [anthropo- + G. *kentron,* center]

**an·thro·poid** (an′thrō-poyd) **1.** resembling man in structure and form. **2.** one of the monkeys resembling man; an ape. [G. *anthrōpo-eidēs,* man-like]

**an·thro·poid pel·vis** an apelike pelvis, with a long anteroposterior diameter and a narrow transverse diameter.

**an·thro·pol·o·gy** (an-thrō-pol′ō-jē) the scientific study of human beings with respect to physical features, classification, distribution, and social and cultural relationships. [anthropo- + G. *logos,* treatise]

**an·thro·po·met·ric** (an-thrō-pō-met′rik) relating to anthropometry.

**an·thro·pom·e·try** (an-thrō-pom′ě-trē) the branch of anthropology concerned with comparative measurements of the human body. [anthropo- + G. *metron,* measure]

**an·thro·po·mor·phism** (an′thrō-pō-mōr′fizm) ascription of human shape or qualities to nonhuman creatures or inanimate objects. [anthropo- + G. *morphē,* form]

**an·thro·po·phil·ic** (an′thrō-pō-fil′ik) human-seeking or human-preferring, especially with reference to: 1) bloodsucking arthropods, denoting the preference of a parasite for the human host as a source of blood or tissues over an animal host; and 2) dermatophytic fungi which grow preferentially on humans rather than other animals. [anthropo- + G. *phileō,* to love]

**an·thro·po·zo·o·no·sis** (an′thrō-pō-zō′ō-nō′sis) a zoonosis maintained in nature by animals and transmissible to man; e.g., rabies, brucellosis. [anthropo- + G. *zōon,* animal, + *nosos,* disease]

△**an·ti-** **1.** against, opposing, or, in relation to symptoms and diseases, curative. **2.** prefix denoting an antibody (immunoglobulin) specific for the thing indicated; e.g., antitoxin (antibody specific for a toxin). [G. *anti,* against, opposite, instead of]

**an·ti·ad·ren·er·gic** (an′tē-ad-rě-ner′jik) antagonistic to the action of sympathetic or other adrenergic nerve fibers. SEE ALSO sympatholytic.

**an·ti·ag·glu·ti·nin** (an′tē-ă-gloo′ti-nin) a specific antibody that inhibits or destroys the action of an agglutinin.

**an·ti·an·a·phy·lax·is** (an′tē-an′ă-fī-lak′sis) SYN desensitization (1).

**an·ti·a·ne·mic** (an′tē-ă-nē′mik) pertaining to factors or substances that prevent or correct anemic conditions.

**an·ti·an·ti·body** (an′tē-an′tē-bod-ē) antibody specific for another antibody.

**an·ti·an·ti·tox·in** (an′tē-an-tē-tok′sin) an antiantibody that inhibits or counteracts the effects of an antitoxin.

**an·ti·anx·i·e·ty a·gent** a functional category of drugs useful in the treatment of anxiety and able to reduce anxiety at doses that do not cause excessive sedation (e.g., diazepam). SYN anxiolytic (1).

**an·ti·bac·te·ri·al** (an′tē-bak-tēr′ē-ăl) destructive to or preventing the growth of bacteria.

**an·ti·base·ment mem·brane an·ti·bod·y** autoantibodies to renal glomerular basement membrane antigens.

**an·ti·base·ment mem·brane glo·mer·u·lo·ne·phri·tis** glomerulonephritis resulting from anti-basement membrane antibodies, characterized by smooth linear deposits of IgG and C3 along glomerular capillary walls; includes rapidly progressive glomerulonephritis and glomerulonephritis in Goodpasture syndrome.

**an·ti·base·ment mem·brane ne·phri·tis** glomerulonephritis produced by autologous or heterologous antibodies to the glomerular capillary basement membranes, the latter known as anti-kidney serum nephritis.

**an·ti·bi·o·sis** (an′tē-bī-ō′sis) **1.** an association of two organisms which is detrimental to one of them, in contrast to probiosis. **2.** production of an antibiotic by bacteria or other organisms inhibitory to other living things, especially among soil microbes. [anti- + G. *biōsis,* life]

**an·ti·bi·ot·ic** (an′tē-bī-ot′ik) **1.** relating to antibiosis. **2.** prejudicial to life. **3.** a soluble substance derived from a mold or bacterium that inhibits the growth of other microorganisms. **4.** relating to such an action.

**an·ti·bi·ot·ic en·ter·o·co·li·tis** enterocolitis caused by oral administration of broad spectrum antibiotics, resulting from overgrowth of antibiotic-resistant staphylococci or yeasts and fungi, when the normal fecal Gram-negative organisms are suppressed, resulting in diarrhea or pseudomembranous disease.

**an·ti·body (Ab)** (an′tē-bod-ē) an immunoglobulin molecule with a specific amino acid sequence evoked in man or other animals by an antigen, and characterized by reacting specifically with the antigen in some demonstrable way, antibody and antigen each being defined in terms of the other. It is believed that antibodies may also exist naturally, without being present as a result of the stimulus provided by the introduction of an antigen: 1) in the broad sense any body or substance, soluble or cellular, which is evoked by the stimulus provided by the introduction of antigen and which reacts specifically with antigen in some demonstrable way; 2) one of the classes of globulins (immunoglobulins) present in the blood serum or body fluids of an animal as a result of antigenic stimulus or occurring "naturally." Different genetically inherited determinants, Gm (found on IgG H chains), Am (found on IgA H chains), and Km (found on K-type L chains and formerly called InV), control the antigenicity of the antibody molecule; subclasses are denoted either alphabetically or numerically (e.g., G3mb1 or G3m5). The various classes differ widely in their ability to react in different kinds of serologic tests. SEE ALSO immunoglobulin. See this page.

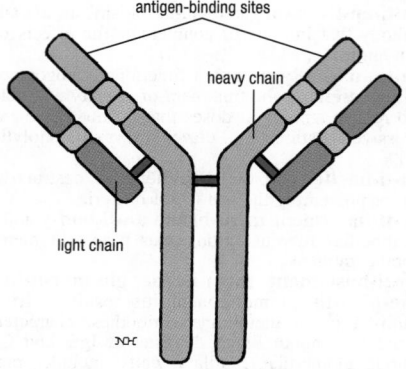

**antibody** (schematic view of an immunoglobulin molecule)

**an·ti·bod·y-com·bin·ing site** SYN paratope.
**an·ti·bod·y ex·cess** in a precipitation test, the presence of antibody in an amount greater than that required to combine with all of the antigen present.
**an·ti·cho·lin·er·gic** (an′tē-kol-i-ner′jik) antagonistic to the action of parasympathetic or other cholinergic nerve fibers (e.g., atropine).
**an·ti·cho·lin·es·ter·ase** (an′tē-kō-lin-es′ter-ās) one of the drugs that inhibit or inactivate acetylcholinesterase, either reversibly (e.g., physostigmine) or irreversibly (e.g., tetraethyl pyrophosphate).
**α₁-an·ti·chy·mo·tryp·sin** (alfa-wun-an′ti-kī′mō-trip-sin) an inhibitor protein of the digestive protease, chymotrypsin.
**an·ti·cli·nal** (an-tē-klī′năl) inclined in opposite directions, as two sides of a pyramid. [anti- + G. *klinō*, to incline]
**an·ti·co·ag·u·lant** (an′tē-kō-ag′yu-lant) 1. preventing coagulation. 2. an agent having such action (e.g., warfarin).
**an·ti·co·don** (an-tē-kō′don) the trinucleotide sequence complementary to a codon found in one loop of a tRNA molecule; e.g., if a codon is A-G-C, its anticodon is U (or T)-C-G. The complementarity principle arises from Watson-Crick base-pairing, in which A is complementary to U (or T) and G is complementary to C. Sometimes called "nodoc."
**an·ti·com·ple·ment** (an-tē-kom′plě-ment) a sub-

stance that combines with a complement and neutralizes its action by preventing its union with an antibody.
**an·ti·con·vul·sant** (an′tē-kon-vŭl′sant) 1. preventing or arresting seizures. 2. an agent having such action.
**an·ti·de·pres·sant** (an′tē-dē-pres′ănt) 1. counteracting depression. 2. an agent used in treating depression.
**an·ti·diar·rhe·al** (an-tē-dī-ă-rē′ăl) counteracting diarrhea.
**an·ti·di·ar·rhoe·al [Br.]** SEE antidiarrheal.
**an·ti·di·u·re·sis** (an′tē-dī-yu-rē′sis) reduction of urinary volume.
**an·ti·di·u·ret·ic** (an′tē-dī-yu-ret′ik) a drug or hormone that reduces urine production by the kidneys.
**an·ti·di·u·ret·ic hor·mone** SYN vasopressin.
**an·ti·dot·al** (an-tē-dō′tăl) relating to or acting as an antidote.
**an·ti·dote** (an′tē-dōt) an agent that neutralizes a poison or counteracts its effects. [G. *antidotos,* fr. *anti,* against, + *dotos,* what is given, fr. *didōmi,* to give]
**an·ti·drom·ic** (an-tē-drom′ik) moving in the direction opposite to normal; said of impulses in nerves and in the conduction system of the heart.
**an·ti·dys·ki·net·ic a·gent** a functional category of drugs with anticholinergic action, used to treat Parkinson disease and some of the acute movement disorders that may be caused by antipsychotic agents.
**an·ti·e·met·ic** (an′tē-ĕ-met′ik) 1. preventing or arresting vomiting. 2. a remedy that tends to control nausea and vomiting. [anti- + G. *emetikos,* emetic]
**an·ti·en·zyme** (an-tē-en′zīm) an agent or principle that retards, inhibits, or destroys the activity of an enzyme; may be an inhibitory enzyme or an antibody to an enzyme.
**an·ti·ep·i·lep·tic** (an-tē-ĕp-ĭ-lĕp′tik) 1. preventing or arresting epilepsy. 2. an agent having such action.
**an·ti·es·tro·gen** (an′tē-es′trō-jen) any substance capable of preventing full expression of the biological effects of estrogenic hormones on responsive tissues.
**an·ti·es·tro·gen·ic** (an-tē-ĕs-trō-jĕn′ik) counteracting or suppressing estrogenic activity.
**an·ti·fe·brile** (an-tē-feb′ril) SYN antipyretic (1). [anti- + L. *febris,* fever]
**an·ti·fi·bri·nol·y·sin** (an′tē-fī-bri-nol′i-sin) SYN antiplasmin.
**an·ti·fi·bri·no·lyt·ic** (an′tē-fī-brin-ō-lit′ik) denoting a substance that decreases the breakdown of fibrin; e.g., aminocaproic acid.
**an·ti·gen (Ag)** (an′ti-jen) any substance that, as a result of coming in contact with appropriate cells, induces a state of sensitivity and/or immune responsiveness after a latent period (days to weeks) and which reacts in a demonstrable way with antibodies and/or immune cells of the sensitized subject *in vivo* or *in vitro.* Modern usage tends to retain the broad meaning of antigen, employing the terms "antigenic determinant" or "determinant group" for the particular chemical group of a molecule that confers antigenic specificity. SEE ALSO hapten. SYN immunogen. [anti(body) + G. *-gen,* producing]
**an·ti·gen-an·ti·bod·y re·ac·tion** the phenomenon, occurring *in vitro* or *in vivo,* of antibody

combining with antigen of the type that stimulated the formation of the antibody, thereby resulting in agglutination, precipitation, complement fixation, greater susceptibility to ingestion and destruction by phagocytes, or neutralization of exotoxin. SEE ALSO skin test.

**an·ti·ge·ne·mia** (an'ti-jĕ-nē'mē-ă) persistence of antigen in circulating blood; e.g., HB_s-antigenemia (presence of hepatitis B virus surface antigen in serum). [antigen + G. *haima,* blood]

**an·ti·gen ex·cess** 1. in a precipitation test, the presence of uncombined antigen above that required to combine with all of the antibody; 2. *in vivo* the resultant antigen-antibody interaction in such an antigen excess may give rise to immune complexes, which have a potential to induce cellular damage.

**an·ti·gen·ic** (an-ti-jen'ik) having the properties of an antigen (allergen). SYN allergenic, immunogenic.

**an·ti·gen·ic de·ter·mi·nant** the particular chemical group of a molecule that determines immunological specificity.

**an·ti·gen·ic drift** the process of "evolutionary" changes in molecular structure of DNA/RNA in microorganisms during their passage from one host to another; it may be due to recombination, deletion, or insertion of genes, point mutations or combinations of these events; it leads to alteration (usually slow and progressive) in the antigenic composition, and therefore in the immunologic responses of individuals and populations to exposure to the microorganism concerned.

**an·ti·ge·nic·i·ty** (an'ti-jĕ-nis'i-tē) the state or property of being antigenic. SYN immunogenicity.

**an·ti·gen·ic shift** mutation, i.e., sudden change in molecular structure of RNA/DNA in microorganisms, especially viruses, which produces new strains of the microorganism; hosts previously exposed to other strains have little or no acquired immunity to the new strain.

**an·ti·gen·ome** the complementary positive RNA strand on which the negative-strand genome of a virus is made.

**an·ti·gen pep·tides** the protein fragments that bind to MHC molecules.

**an·ti·gen-pre·sent·ing cell (APC)** cells that process protein antigens into peptides and present them on their surface in a form that can be recognized by lymphocytes. APCs include Langerhans cells, dendritic cells, macrophages, B cells, and in humans, activated T cells. SYN accessory cell.

**an·ti·gen-sen·si·tive cell** a small lymphocyte that, although not itself an immunologically activated cell, responds to antigenic (immunogenic) stimulus by a process of division and differentiation that results in the production of immunologically activated cells.

**an·ti·gen u·nit** the smallest amount of antigen that, in the presence of specific antiserum, will fix 1 complement unit.

**an·ti·hae·mo·phil·ic [Br.]** SEE antihemophilic.

**an·ti-HB_s** antibody to the hepatitis B surface antigen (HB_sAg).

**an·ti-HB_c** antibody to the hepatitis B core antigen (HB_cAg).

**an·ti·he·lix** (an-tē-hē'liks) an elevated ridge of cartilage anterior and roughly parallel to the posterior portion of the helix of the auricle. SYN anthelix.

**an·ti·hem·ag·glu·ti·nin** (an'tē-hē-mă-gloo'ti-nin) a substance (including antibody) that inhibits or prevents hemagglutination.

**an·ti·he·mo·ly·sin** (an'tē-hē-mol'i-sin, an'tē-hem-ol'i-sin) a substance (including antibody) that inhibits or prevents the effects of hemolysin.

**an·ti·he·mo·lyt·ic** (an'tē-hem-ō-lit'ik) preventing hemolysis.

**an·ti·he·mo·phil·ic** (an-tē-hē-mō-fil'ik) correcting or counteracting the hemorrhagic tendency in hemophilia. [anti- + hemophilic]

**an·ti·he·mo·phil·ic fac·tor A (AHF)** SYN factor VIII.

**an·ti·he·mo·phil·ic glob·u·lin A** SYN factor VIII.

**an·ti·he·mo·phil·ic glob·u·lin B** SYN factor IX.

**an·ti·hem·or·rhag·ic** (an'tē-hem-ō-rāj'ik) arresting hemorrhage. SYN hemostatic (2).

**an·ti·his·ta·mines** (an-tē-his'tă-mēnz) drugs having an action antagonistic to that of histamine; used in the treatment of allergy symptoms.

**an·ti·his·ta·min·ic** (an'tē-his-tă-min'ik) 1. tending to neutralize or antagonize the action of histamine or to inhibit its production in the body. 2. an agent having such an effect, used to relieve the symptoms of allergy.

**an·ti·hor·mone** (an-tē-hōr'mōn) any substance demonstrable in serum that inhibits or prevents the usual effects of certain hormones, e.g., specific antibodies.

**an·ti·hu·man glob·u·lin** serum from a rabbit or other animal previously immunized with purified human globulin to prepare antibodies directed against IgG and complement; used in the direct and indirect Coombs tests. SYN Coombs serum.

**an·ti·hy·per·ten·sive** (an'tē-hī-per-ten'siv) indicating a drug or mode of treatment that reduces the blood pressure of hypertensive individuals.

**an·ti·id·i·o·type an·ti·bod·y, an·ti·id·i·o·type au·to·an·ti·bod·y** an antiantibody, the activity of which is directed specifically against the antigenic determinants (idiotope) of a particular immunoglobulin (antibody) molecule.

**an·ti·in·flam·ma·to·ry** (an'tē-in-flam'ă-tō-rē) reducing inflammation by acting on body responses, without directly antagonizing the causative agent; denoting agents such as glucocorticoids and aspirin.

**anti·leu·ko·tri·ene** (an-tē-loo-ko-trī'ēn) a drug that prevents or alleviates bronchoconstruction in asthma by blocking the production or action of naturally occurring leukotrienes; may also be useful in psoriasis.

**an·ti·lith·ic** (an-tē-lith'ik) 1. preventing the formation of calculi or promoting their dissolution. 2. an agent so acting. [anti- + G. *lithos,* stone]

**an·ti·lym·pho·cyte se·rum (ALS)** antiserum against lymphocytes, used to suppress rejection of grafts or organ transplants.

**an·ti·ly·sin** (an-tē-lī'sin) an antibody that inhibits or prevents the effects of lysin.

**anti-MAG an·ti·bod·y** a specific antibody against myelin-associated glycoprotein; the most important of the specific antibodies against myelin so far identified, present in the majority of patients with IgM-associated polyneuropathies.

**an·ti·mere** (an'ti-mēr) 1. a segment of an animal body formed by planes cutting the axis of the body at right angles. 2. one of the symmetrical parts of a bilateral organism. 3. the right or left half of the body. [anti- + G. *meros,* a part]

a
n

**an·ti·me·tab·o·lite** (an'tē-me-tab'ō-līt) a substance that competes with, replaces, or antagonizes a particular metabolite; e.g., ethionine is an antimetabolite of methionine.

**an·ti·mi·cro·bi·al** (an'tē-mī-krō'bē-ăl) tending to destroy microbes, to prevent their multiplication or growth, or to prevent their pathogenic action.

**an·ti·mon·gol·oid** (an-tē-mon'gō-loyd) the condition in which the lateral portion of the palpebral fissure is lower than the medial portion.

**an·ti·mo·ny (Sb)** (an'ti-mō-nē) a metallic element, atomic no. 51, atomic wt. 121.757, valences 0, −3, +3, +5; used in alloys; toxic and irritating to the skin and mucous membranes. [G. *anti* + *monos*, not found alone]

**an·ti·mu·ta·gen** (an-tē-myu'tă-jen) a factor that reduces or interferes with the mutagenic actions of effects of a substance.

**an·ti·my·cot·ic** (an'tē-mī-kot'ik) antagonistic to fungi. [anti- + G. *mykēs*, fungus]

**an·ti·ne·o·plas·tic** (an'tē-nē-ō-plas'tik) preventing the development, maturation, or spread of neoplastic cells.

**an·ti·neu·tro·phil cy·to·plas·mic an·ti·bod·y (ANCA)** an autoantibody to cytoplasmic constituents of monocytes and neutrophils found in patients with vasculitis.

**an·tin·i·on** (an-tin'ē-on) the space between the eyebrows; the point on the skull opposite the inion. SEE ALSO glabella. [anti- + G. *inion*, nape of the neck]

**an·ti·nu·cle·ar an·ti·bod·y (ANA), an·ti·nu·cle·ar fac·tor (ANF)** an antibody showing an affinity for cell nuclei, demonstrated by exposing a cell substrate to the serum to be tested, followed by exposure to an antihuman-globulin serum; found in the serum of a high proportion of patients with systemic lupus erythematosus, rheumatoid arthritis, and certain collagen diseases, in some of their healthy relatives, and in about 1% of normal individuals.

**an·ti·o·es·tro·gen·ic [Br.]** SEE antiestrogenic.

**an·ti·on·co·gene** (an-tē-on'kō-jēn) a tumor-suppressing gene involved in controlling cellular growth; inactivation of this type of gene leads to deregulated cellular proliferation, as in cancer. SYN tumor suppressor gene (2).

**an·ti·par·a·sit·ic** (an'tē-par-ă-sit'ik) destructive to parasites.

**an·ti·per·i·stal·sis** (an'tē-per-i-stahl'sis) SYN reversed peristalsis.

**an·ti·per·i·stal·tic** (an'tē-per-i-stahl'tik) 1. relating to antiperistalsis. 2. impeding or arresting peristalsis.

**an·ti·per·spi·rant** (an-tē-per'spi-rant) 1. having an inhibitory action upon the secretion of sweat. 2. an agent having such an action (e.g., aluminum chloride).

**an·ti·phlo·gis·tic** (an'tē-flō-jis'tik) 1. older term denoting preventing or relieving inflammation. 2. an agent that reduces inflammation. [anti- + G. *phogistos*, burnt up]

**an·ti·phos·pho·lip·id an·ti·bod·y syn·drome (aPLS, APS)** a tendency for recurrent thrombosis together with recurrent abortion, thrombocytopenia, and neurologic disease, with antibodies against certain negatively charged phospholipids such as cardiolipin, phosphatidylserine, and phosphatidylethanolamine.

**an·ti·plas·min** (an-tē-plaz'min) a substance that inhibits or prevents the effects of plasmin; found in plasma and some tissues, especially the spleen and liver. SYN antifibrinolysin.

α₂ **an·ti·plas·min** (al-fa-too-an-tē-plaz'min) a major protease inhibitor of plasmin and plasminogen, key components of the fibrinolytic system. Also inhibits other serine proteases, including the coagulation contact factors, factor Xa, and thrombin.

**an·ti·pode** (an'ti-pōd) that which is diametrically opposite. [G. *antipous*, with the feet opposite]

**an·ti·port** (an'tē-pōrt) the coupled transport of two different molecules or ions through a membrane in opposite directions by a common carrier mechanism (antiporter). Cf. symport, uniport. [anti- + L. *porto*, to carry]

**an·ti·pro·throm·bin** (an'tē-prō-throm'bin) an anticoagulant that inhibits or prevents the conversion of prothrombin into thrombin; examples are heparin, which is present in various tissues (especially in liver), and dicoumarin, which is isolated from partially decomposed sweet clover.

**an·ti·pru·rit·ic** (an'tē-proo-rit'ik) 1. preventing or relieving itching. 2. an agent that relieves itching.

**an·ti·psy·chot·ic** (an'tē-sī-kot'ik) 1. SYN antipsychotic agent. 2. denoting the actions of such an agent.

**an·ti·psy·chot·ic a·gent** a functional category of neuroleptic drugs that are helpful in the treatment of psychosis and have a capacity to ameliorate thought disorders (e.g., chlorpromazine, haloperidol). SYN antipsychotic (1).

**an·ti·py·ret·ic** (an'tē-pī-ret'ik) 1. reducing fever. SYN antifebrile. 2. an agent that reduces fever (e.g., acetaminophen, aspirin). [anti- + G. *pyretos*, fever]

**an·ti·scor·bu·tic** (an'tē-skōr-byu'tik) 1. preventive or curative of scurvy (scorbutus). 2. a treatment for scurvy (e.g., vitamin C).

**an·ti·se·cre·to·ry** (an'tē-sē-krē'tō-rē) inhibitory to secretion, said of certain drugs that reduce or suppress gastric secretion (e.g., ranitidine, omeprazole).

**an·ti·sep·sis** (an-tē-sep'sis) prevention of infection by inhibiting the growth of infectious agents. SEE ALSO disinfection. [anti- + G. *sēpsis*, putrefaction]

**an·ti·sep·tic** (an-tē-sep'tik) 1. relating to antisepsis. 2. an agent or substance capable of effecting antisepsis.

**an·ti·sep·tic dress·ing** a sterile dressing of gauze impregnated with an antiseptic.

**an·ti·se·rum** (an-tē-sē'rŭm) serum that contains demonstrable antibody or antibodies specific for one or more antigens; may be prepared from the blood of animals inoculated with an antigenic material or from the blood of animals and persons that have been stimulated by natural contact with an antigen (as by an attack of disease). SYN immune serum.

**an·ti·se·rum an·a·phy·lax·is** SYN passive anaphylaxis.

**an·ti·so·cial** (an-tē-sō'shŭl) opposed to the rights of individuals or to the legal norms of society. Cf. asocial.

**an·ti·so·cial per·son·al·i·ty dis·or·der** a personality disorder characterized by a history of continuous and chronic antisocial behavior with disregard for and violation of the rights of others, beginning before the age of 15; early childhood signs include chronic lying, stealing, fighting, and truancy; in adolescence there may be unusu-ally early or aggressive sexual behavior, exces-sive drinking, and use of illicit drugs, such be-havior continuing in adulthood.

**an·ti·spas·mod·ic** (an'tē-spaz-mod'ik) **1.** pre-venting or alleviating muscle spasms (cramps). **2.** an agent that quiets spasm.

**an·ti·strep·to·coc·cic** (an'tē-strep-tō-kok'sik) de-structive to streptococci or antagonistic to their toxins.

**an·ti·tac** (an'tē-tak) monoclonal antibody that recognizes the alpha chain of the IL-2 receptor.

**anti·ter·min·a·tion** a state of bacterial RNA pol-ymerase wherein it is resistant to pause, arrest, or termination signals. SEE ALSO hesitant, overdrive.

**an·ti·tox·ic** (an-tē-tok'sik) neutralizing the action of a poison; specifically, relating to an antitoxin. SEE ALSO antidotal.

**an·ti·tox·in** (an-tē-tok'sin) antibody formed in re-sponse to antigenic poisonous substances of bio-logic origin, such as bacterial exotoxins, phytotoxins, and zootoxins; in general usage, se-rum from humans or animals (usually horses) immunized by injections of the specific toxoid. Antitoxin neutralizes the pharmacologic effects of its specific toxin. [anti- + G. *toxikon,* poison]

**an·ti·tox·in u·nit** a unit expressing the strength or activity of an antitoxin; in general, determined with reference to a preserved standard prepara-tion of antitoxin. SEE ALSO L doses.

**an·ti·trag·i·cus mus·cle** a band of transverse muscular fibers on the outer surface of the anti-tragus, arising from the border of the intertragic notch and inserted into the anthelix and cauda helicis. SYN musculus antitragicus [TA].

**an·ti·tra·gus** (an-tē-trā'gŭs) [TA] a projection of the cartilage of the auricle, in front of the tail of the helix, just above the lobule, and posterior to the tragus from which it is separated by the inter-tragic notch. [G. *anti-tragos,* the eminence of the external ear, fr. *anti,* opposite, + *tragos,* a goat, the tragus]

**an·ti·trep·o·ne·mal** (an'tē-trep-ō-nē'măl) SYN treponemicidal.

**an·ti·tro·pic** (an-tē-trō'pik) similar, bilaterally symmetrical, but in an opposite location (as in a mirror image), e.g., the right thumb in relation to the left thumb.

**an·ti·tryp·sic** (an-tē-trip'sik) SYN antitryptic.

**an·ti·tryp·sin** (an-tē-trip'sin) a substance that blocks the action of trypsin.

**α₁-an·ti·tryp·sin de·fi·cien·cy** absence of a se-rum proteinase inhibitor, which may cause re-lapsing nodular nonsuppurative panniculitis.

**α-1 an·ti·tryp·sin de·fi·cien·cy pan·nic·u·li·tis** painful subcutaneous nodules in severe anti-trypsin deficiency.

**an·ti·tryp·tic** (an-tē-trip'tik) possessing proper-ties of antitrypsin. SYN antitrypsic.

**an·ti·tus·sive** (an-tē-tŭs'iv) **1.** relieving cough. **2.** a cough remedy (e.g., codeine). [anti- + L. *tussis,* cough]

**an·ti·ven·in** (an-tē-ven'in) an antitoxin specific for an animal or insect venom. [anti- + L. *venenum,* poison]

**an·ti·vi·ral** (an-tē-vī'răl) opposing a virus; inter-fering with its replication; weakening or abolish-ing its action.

**an·ti·vi·ral pro·tein (AVP)** a human or animal factor, induced by interferon in virus-infected

cells, which mediates interferon inhibition of virus replication.

**an·ti·vi·ta·min** (an-tē-vī'tă-min) a substance that prevents a vitamin from exerting its typical bio-logical effects. Most antivitamins have chemical structures like those of vitamins and appear to function as competitive antagonists.

**An·ton syn·drome** (ahn'ton) in cortical blind-ness, lack of awareness of being blind.

**ant·orb·i·tal** (ant-or'bĭ-tăl) situated in front of an orbit.

**an·tra** (an'tră) plural of antrum.

**an·tral** (an'trăl) relating to an antrum.

**an·tral fol·li·cle** SYN vesicular ovarian follicle.

**an·tral la·vage** irrigation of the maxillary sinus through its natural ostium or through a puncture of the inferior meatus.

**an·trec·to·my** (an-trek'tō-mē) **1.** removal of the walls of an antrum. **2.** removal of the antrum (distal half) of the stomach. [antrum + G. *ektomē,* excision]

△**an·tro-** an antrum. [L. *antrum,* from G. *antron,* a cave]

**an·tro·du·o·de·nec·to·my** (an'trō-doo-ō-dĕ-nek'tō-mē) surgical removal of the antrum of the stomach and the ulcer-bearing part of the duode-num.

**an·tro·na·sal** (an-trō-nā'săl) relating to a maxil-lary sinus and the corresponding nasal cavity.

**an·tro·scope** (an'trō-skōp) an instrument to aid in the visual examination of any cavity, particularly the antrum of Highmore (maxillary sinus). [antro- + G. *skopeō,* to view]

**an·tros·co·py** (an-tros'kŏ-pē) examination of any cavity, especially of the antrum of Highmore, by means of an antroscope.

**an·tros·to·my** (an-tros'tō-mē) formation of a per-manent opening into any antrum. [antro- + G. *stoma,* mouth]

**an·trot·o·my** (an-trot'ō-mē) incision through the wall of any antrum. [antro- + G. *tomē,* incision]

**an·tro·tym·pan·ic** (an'trō-tim-pan'ik) relating to the mastoid antrum and the tympanic cavity.

**an·trum,** pl. **an·tra** (an'trŭm, an'tră) **1.** any nearly closed cavity, particularly one with bony walls. **2.** SYN pyloric antrum. [L. fr. G. *antron,* a cave]

**An·tyl·lus meth·od** (an-til'ŭs) ligation of the ar-tery above and below an aneurysm, followed by incision into and emptying of the sac.

**ANUG** acute necrotizing ulcerative gingivitis.

**a·nu·lar** (an'yu-lăr) ring-shaped.

**an·u·lar band** SYN amnionic band.

**an·u·lar cat·a·ract** congenital cataract in which a central white membrane replaces the nucleus.

**an·u·lar lip·id** the layer(s) of lipid bound to and/or surrounding an integral membrane pro-tein.

**an·u·lar pla·cen·ta** a placenta in the form of a band encircling the interior of the uterus.

**an·u·lar scle·ri·tis** an often protracted inflamma-tion of the anterior portion of the sclera, forming a ring around the corneoscleral limbus.

**an·u·lar sco·to·ma** a circular scotoma surround-ing the center of the field of vision. SEE ring scotoma.

**an·u·lar staph·y·lo·ma** a staphyloma extending around the periphery of the cornea.

**an·u·lar stric·ture** a ringlike constriction encir-cling the wall of a canal.

**an·u·lar syn·ech·ia** adhesion of the entire pupillary margin of the iris to the capsule of the lens.

**a·nu·lo·plasty** (an'yu-lō-plas-tē) reconstruction of the ring (or anulus) of an incompetent cardiac valve. [L. *anulus,* ring, + G. *plastos,* formed]

**a·nu·lor·rha·phy** (an-yu-lō'ă-fē) closure of a hernial ring by suture. [L. *anulus,* ring, + G. *rhaphē,* seam]

**an·u·lus** (an'yu-lŭs) [TA] SYN ring (1). [L.]

**an·u·lus fi·bro·sus** [TA] **1.** SYN right and left fibrous rings of heart. **2.** SYN anulus fibrosus of intervertebral disk.

**an·u·lus fi·bro·sus dis·ci in·ter·ver·te·bra·lis** [TA] SYN anulus fibrosus of intervertebral disk.

**an·u·lus fi·bro·sus of in·ter·ver·te·bral disk** the ring of fibrocartilage and fibrous tissue forming the circumference of the intervertebral disk; surrounds the nucleus pulposus, which can herniate when the anulus is diseased or injured. SYN anulus fibrosus disci intervertebralis [TA], anulus fibrosus (2) [TA].

**an·u·lus in·gui·na·lis su·per·fi·ci·a·lis** [TA] SYN superficial inguinal ring.

**an·u·lus tym·pa·ni·cus** [TA] SYN tympanic ring.

**an·u·lus um·bi·li·ca·lis** [TA] SYN umbilical ring.

**an·u·lus of Zinn** (tsin) SYN common tendinous ring of extraocular muscles.

**an·u·ria** (an-yu'rē-ă) absence of urine formation.

**an·u·ric** (an-yur'ik) relating to anuria.

**anus,** gen. and pl. **ani** (ā'nŭs, ā'nī) [TA] the lower opening of the digestive tract, lying in the cleft between the buttocks, through which feces are discharged. [L.]

**an·vil** SYN incus.

**anx·i·e·ty** (ang-zī'ĕ-tē) **1.** apprehension of danger and dread accompanied by restlessness, tension, tachycardia, and dyspnea unattached to a clearly identifiable stimulus. **2.** EXPERIMENTAL PSYCHOLOGY a drive or motivational state learned from and thereafter associated with previously neutral cues. [L. *anxietas,* anxiety, fr. *anxius,* distressed, fr. *ango,* to press tight, to torment]

**anx·i·e·ty dis·or·ders** a category of interrelated mental illnesses involving anxiety reactions in response to stress. The types include: 1) generalized anxiety, by far the most prevalent condition, which strikes slightly more females than males, mostly in the 20–35 age group; 2) panic disorder, in which a person suffers repeated panic attacks. Some 2–5 percent of Americans are subject to this ailment, about twice as many women as men; 3) obsessive-compulsive disorder, afflicting 2–3 percent of the U.S. population. About two-thirds of these patients go on to experience a major depressive episode; 4) posttraumatic stress disorder, most frequent among combat veterans or survivors of major physical trauma; and 5) the phobias (e.g., fear of snakes, crowds, confinement, heights, etc.), which on a minor scale affect about one in eight people in the U.S. Drugs that have proven effective against anxiety disorders are beta-blockers, which act on adrenaline receptors; anxiolytics; antidepressants; and serotonergic drugs. Regular exercise has also proved beneficial.

**anx·i·e·ty hys·te·ria** hysteria characterized by manifest anxiety.

**anx·i·e·ty neu·ro·sis** chronic abnormal distress and worry to the point of panic followed by a tendency to avoid or run from the feared situation, associated with overaction of the sympathetic nervous system.

**anx·i·e·ty re·ac·tion** a psychological reaction or experience involving the apprehension of danger accompanied by a feeling of dread and such physical symptoms as an increase in the rate of breathing, sweating, and tachycardia, in the absence of a clearly identifiable fear stimulus; when chronic, it is called generalized anxiety disorder. SEE ALSO panic attack.

**anx·i·o·lyt·ic** (ang'zē-ō-lit'ik) **1.** SYN antianxiety agent. **2.** denoting the actions of such an agent. [anxiety + G. *lysis,* a dissolution or loosening]

***Aon·cho·the·ca*** (ā-on-kō-thē'ka) one of three trichurid nematode genera, commonly referred to as *Capillaria.*

**a·or·ta,** gen. and pl. **a·or·tae** (ā-ōr'tă, ā-ōr'tē) [TA] a large artery which is the main trunk of the systemic arterial system, arising from the left ventricle and ending at the left side of the body of the 4th lumbar vertebra by dividing to form the right and left common iliac arteries. The aorta is made up of the ascending aorta, aortic arch, and descending aorta, which is divided into the thoracic aorta and the abdominal aorta. [Mod. L. fr. G. *aortē,* from *aeirō,* to lift up]

**a·or·tal** (ā-ōr'tăl) SYN aortic.

**a·or·tal·gia** (ā-ōr-tal'jē-ă) pain assumed to be due to aneurysm or other pathologic conditions of the aorta. [aorta + G. *algos,* pain]

**a·or·tic** (ā-ōr'tik) relating to the aorta or the aortic orifice of the left ventricle of the heart. SYN aortal.

**a·or·tic arch 1.** the curved portion between the ascending and descending parts of the aorta; it begins as a continuation of the ascending aorta posterior to the sternal angle, runs posteriorly and slightly to the left as it passes over the root of the left lung, and becomes the descending aorta as it reaches and begins to course along the vertebral column; it gives rise to the brachiocephalic trunk, the left common carotid and left subclavian arteries; **2.** any member of the several pairs of arterial channels encircling the embryonic pharynx in the mesenchyme of the pharyngeal arches (branchial arches in fish); there are potentially six pairs, but in mammals the fifth pair is poorly developed or absent. The first and second pairs are functional only in very young embryos; the third pair is involved in the formation of the carotids; the fourth arch on the left is incorporated in the arch of the aorta; the sixth pair forms the proximal part of the pulmonary arteries.

**a·or·tic arch syn·drome** SYN Takayasu arteritis. SYN Martorell syndrome.

**a·or·tic a·tre·sia** congenital absence of the normal valvular orifice into the aorta.

**a·or·tic bulb** the dilated first part of the aorta containing the aortic semilunar valves and the aortic sinuses. SYN bulbus aortae [TA].

**a·or·tic co·arc·ta·tion** congenital narrowing of the aorta, usually located just distal to the left subclavian artery, causing upper-extremity hypertension, excess left ventricular workload, and diminished blood flow to the lower extremities and abdominal viscera.

**a·or·tic dis·sec·tion** a pathologic process, characterized by splitting of the media layer of the aorta, which leads to formation of a dissecting aneurysm.

**a•or•tic hi•a•tus** the opening in the diaphragm bounded by the two crura, the vertebral column, and the median arcuate ligament, through which pass the aorta and thoracic duct.

**a•or•tic in•suf•fi•cien•cy** SYN aortic regurgitation.

**a•or•tic mur•mur** a murmur produced at the aortic orifice, either obstructive or regurgitant.

**a•or•tic nip•ple** a colloquial term for the radiographic appearance of the left superior intercostal or accessory hemiazygos vein as a bump on the aortic knob.

**a•or•tic notch** the notch in a sphygmographic tracing caused by rebound following closure of the aortic valves.

**a•or•tic or•i•fice** the opening from the left ventricle into the ascending aorta; it is guarded by the aortic valve.

**a•or•tic re•gur•gi•ta•tion** reflux of blood through an incompetent aortic valve into the left ventricle during ventricular diastole. SYN aortic insufficiency, Corrigan disease.

**a•or•tic si•nus** the space between the superior aspect of each cusp of the aortic valve and the dilated portion of the wall of the ascending aorta, immediately above each cusp.

**a•or•tic ste•no•sis** pathologic narrowing of the aortic valve orifice.

▣ **a•or•tic valve** the valve between the left ventricle and the ascending aorta, consisting of three fibrous semilunar cusps (valvules). They are named in accordance with their embryonic derivation: the anteriorly located cusp is the right cusp (above which the right coronary artery arises), the left posteriorly positioned cusp is the left cusp (above which the left coronary artery arises), and the right posteriorly positioned cusp is the posterior or noncoronary cusp. See this page.

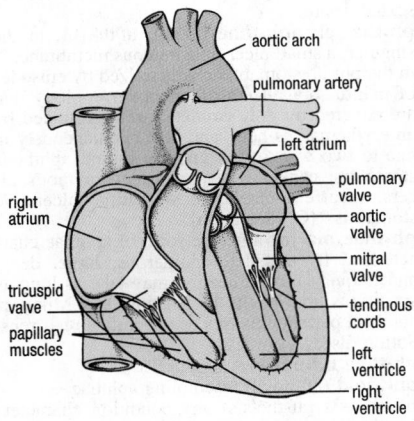

aortic arch

pulmonary artery

left atrium

pulmonary valve

aortic valve

mitral valve

right atrium

tricuspid valve

papillary muscles

tendinous cords

left ventricle

right ventricle

**heart valves:** aortic, pulmonary, tricuspid, and mitral valves

**a•or•tic ves•ti•bule** the anterosuperior portion of the left ventricle of the heart immediately below the aortic orifice, having fibrous walls and affording room for the segments of the closed aortic valve.

**aor•ti•tis** (ā-ōr-tī′tis) inflammation of the aorta.

**aor•to•cor•o•nary** (ā-ōr′tō-kōr′ō-nār-ē) relating to the aorta and the coronary arteries.

**aor•to•gram** (ā-ōr′tō-gram) the image or set of images resulting from aortography.

**aor•tog•ra•phy** (ā-ōr-tog′ră-fē) **1.** radiographic imaging of the aorta and its branches by injection of contrast medium. **2.** imaging of the aorta by ultrasound or magnetic resonance. [aorta + G. *graphō*, to write]

**a•or•to•il•i•ac by•pass** an operation in which a vascular prosthesis is united with the aorta and iliac artery to relieve obstruction of the lower abdominal aorta, its bifurcation, and the proximal iliac branches.

**a•or•to•il•i•ac oc•clu•sive dis•ease** obstruction of the abdominal aorta and its main branches by atherosclerosis.

**aor•top•a•thy** (ā-ōr-top′ă-thē) disease affecting the aorta. [aorta + G. *pathos*, suffering]

**aor•to•plas•ty** (ā-ōr′tō-plas′tē) a procedure for surgical repair of the aorta.

**a•or•to•re•nal by•pass** insertion of a graft of autogenous artery, saphenous vein, or synthetic material between the aorta and the distal renal artery, to circumvent an obstruction of the renal artery.

**aor•tor•rha•phy** (ā-ōr-tōr′ă-fē) suture of the aorta. [aorta + G. *rhaphē*, seam]

**aor•to•scle•ro•sis** (ā-ōr′tō-skler-ō′sis) arteriosclerosis of the aorta.

**aor•tot•o•my** (ā-ōr-tot′ō-mē) incision of the aorta. [aorta + G. *tomē*, a cutting]

**apal•les•the•sia** (ă-pal-es-thē′zē-ă) SYN pallanesthesia. [G. *a-* priv. + *pallo*, to tremble, quiver, + *aisthēsis*, feeling]

**apar•a•lyt•ic** (ā-par′ă-lit′ik) without paralysis; not causing paralysis.

**ap•a•thet•ic** (ap-ă-thet′ik) exhibiting apathy; indifferent.

**ap•a•thism** (ap′ă-thizm) a sluggishness of reaction. Cf. erethism.

**ap•a•thy** (ap′ă-thē) indifference; absence of interest in the environment. Often one of the earliest signs of cerebral disease. [G. *apatheia*, fr. *a-* priv. + *pathos*, suffering]

**ap•a•tite** (ap′ă-tīt) a class of naturally occurring crystalline minerals containing calcium and phosphorus; hydroxyapatite is a component of bones and teeth.

**ap•a•tite cal•cu•lus** a calculus in which the crystalloid component consists of calcium fluorophosphate.

**A-pat•tern es•o•tro•pia** convergent strabismus greater in upward than in downward gaze.

**A-pat•tern ex•o•tro•pia** divergent strabismus greater in downward than in upward gaze.

**APC** Ambulatory Payment Classification group; antigen-presenting cell.

**apel•lous** (ā-pel′ŭs) **1.** without skin. **2.** without foreskin; circumcised. [G. *a-* not + L. *pellis*, skin]

**ape•ri•od•ic** (ā-pēr-ē-od′ik) not occurring periodically.

**aper•i•stal•sis** (ā′per-i-stahl′sis) absence of peristalsis.

**aper•to•gnath•ia** (ă-per-tō-nath′ē-ă) an open bite deformity, a type of malocclusion characterized by premature posterior occlusion and absence of anterior occlusion. [L. *apertus*, open, + G. *gnathos*, jaw]

**A•pert syn•drome** (ah-pār′) disorder characterized by craniosynostosis and syndactyly; mental retardation is a variable feature. SEE ALSO acrocephalosyndactyly.

**ap·er·tu·ra**, pl. **ap·er·tu·rae** (ap-er-tyu'ră, ap-er-tyu'rē) [TA] SYN aperture. [L. fr. *aperio,* pp. *apertus,* to open]

**ap·er·tu·ra la·te·ra·lis ven·tric·u·li quar·ti** [TA] SYN lateral aperture of fourth ventricle.

**ap·er·tu·ra me·di·a·na ven·tric·u·li quar·ti** [TA] SYN median aperture of fourth ventricle.

**ap·er·ture** (ap'er-cher) **1.** an inlet or entrance to a cavity or channel; in anatomy, an open gap or hole. **2.** the diameter of the objective of a microscope. SYN aditus [TA], apertura [TA]. [L. *apertura,* an opening]

**apex**, gen. **ap·i·cis**, pl. **ap·i·ces** (ā'peks, ap'i-sis, ap'i-sēs) [TA] the extremity of a conical or pyramidal structure, such as the heart or the lung. [L. summit or tip]

**apex an·ter·i·or an·gu·la·tion** angulation in the lateral plane in which the apex of the angle is directed anteriorly.

**apex beat** the visible and/or palpable pulsation made by the apex of the left ventricle as it strikes the chest wall in systole; normally in the fifth intercostal space, about 10 cm to the left of the median line. SYN ictus cordis.

**apex·car·di·og·ra·phy** (ā'peks-kar'dē-og-ră-fē) noninvasive graphic recording of cardiac pulsations from the region of the apex, usually of the left ventricle, and resembling the ventricular pressure curve.

**apex·i·fi·ca·tion** (ā-pek'si-fi-kā'shŭn) induced tooth root development or closure of the root apex by hard tissue deposition.

**apex pneu·mo·nia, ap·i·cal pneu·mo·ni·a** pneumonia of the apex or apices.

**apex pos·ter·i·or an·gu·la·tion** angulation in the lateral plane in which the apex of the angle is directed posteriorly.

**APG** ambulatory patient group.

❶ **Ap·gar score** (ap'gahr) evaluation of a newborn infant's physical status by assigning numerical values (0 to 2) to each of 5 criteria: 1) heart rate, 2) respiratory effort, 3) muscle tone, 4) response to stimulation, and 5) skin color; a score of 8 to 10 indicates the best possible condition. See this page.

| Apgar score | | | | |
|---|---|---|---|---|
| after 60 seconds | score | 0 | 1 | 2 |
| heart rate | ...... | absent | under 100 | over 100 |
| respiratory effort | ...... | absent | slow, irregular | good (screams) |
| muscle tone | ...... | limp | good in limbs | active movement |
| reaction to nasal catheter | ...... | none | makes grimaces | coughing or sneezing |
| skin color | ...... | pale | rosy trunk, blue extremities | rosy |
| score | ___ | (total points: 8–10 is normal) | | |

**apha·gia** (ă-fā'jē-ă) inability to eat. [G. *a-* priv. + *phagō,* to eat]

**apha·kia** (ă-fā'kē-ă) absence of the lens of the eye. [G. *a-* priv. + *phakos,* lentil, anything shaped like a lentil]

**apha·kic eye** the eye from which the lens is absent.

**apha·lan·gia** (ā-fă-lan'jē-ă) congenital absence of a digit, or more specifically, absence of one or more of the long bones (phalanges) of a finger or toe. [G. *a-* priv. + phalanx]

**apha·sia** (ă-fā'zē-ă) impaired or absent comprehension or production of, or communication by, speech, writing, or signs; due to an acquired lesion of the dominant cerebral hemisphere. SYN alogia (1), dysphasia, dysphrasia, logagnosia, logamnesia, logasthenia. [G. speechlessness, fr. *a-* priv. + *phasis,* speech]

**apha·si·ac, apha·sic** (ă-fā'zē-ak, ă-fā'sik) relating to or suffering from aphasia. SYN dysphasic.

**apha·si·ol·o·gist** (ă-fā'zē-ol'ŏ-gist) a specialist who deals with speech disorders caused by dysfunction of the language areas of the brain.

**apha·si·ol·o·gy** (ă-fā'zē-ol'ŏ-gē) the science of speech disorders caused by dysfunction of the cerebral language areas.

**apher·e·sis** (ā-fer-e'sis) extraction of certain fluid or cellular elements from withdrawn blood, which is then reinfused into the donor or patient; performed therapeutically to remove harmful elements from the blood, and also to obtain immune globulins. [G. *aphairesis,* withdrawal]

**apho·nia** (ā-fō'nē-ă) loss of the voice as a result of disease or injury to the larynx. [G. *a-* priv. + *phōnē,* voice]

**aphon·ic** (ā-fon'ik) relating to aphonia.

**aphra·sia** (ă-frā'zē-ă) inability to speak, from any cause. [G. *a-* priv. + *phrasis,* speaking]

**aph·ro·dis·i·ac** (af-rō-diz'ē-ak) **1.** increasing sexual desire. **2.** anything that arouses or increases sexual desire.

**aph·tha**, pl. **aph·thae** (af'thă, af'thē) **1.** in the singular, a small ulcer on a mucous membrane. **2.** in the plural, stomatitis characterized by episodes of painful oral ulcers of unknown etiology that are covered by gray exudate, are surrounded by an erythematous halo, and heal spontaneously in one to two weeks. SYN aphthae minor, aphthous stomatitis, canker sores, recurrent aphthous ulcers, recurrent ulcerative stomatitis, ulcerative stomatitis. [G. ulceration]

**aph·thae ma·jor** a severe form of aphthae characterized by unusually numerous, large, deep, and frequent ulcers; healing may take as long as six weeks and results in scarring. SYN Mikulicz aphthae, periadenitis mucosa necrotica recurrens, Sutton disease.

**aph·thae mi·nor** SYN aphtha (2).

**aph·thoid** (af'thoyd) resembling aphthae.

**aph·tho·sis** (af-thō'sis) any condition characterized by the presence of aphthae.

**aph·thous** (af'thŭs) characterized by or relating to aphthae or aphthosis.

**aph·thous sto·ma·ti·tis** SYN aphtha (2).

*Aph·tho·vi·rus* (af'thō-vī'rus) a genus in the family Picornaviridae associated with foot and mouth disease of cattle.

**ap·i·cal** (ap'i-kăl) **1.** relating to the apex or tip of a pyramidal or pointed structure. **2.** situated nearer to the apex of a structure in relation to a specific reference point; opposite of basal.

**ap·i·cal cap** a curved shadow at the apex of one or both hemithoraces on chest x-ray; caused by pleural and pulmonary fibrosis.

**ap·i·cal fo·ra·men of tooth** the opening at the apex of the root of a tooth that gives passage to the nerve and blood vessels.

**ap·i·cal gland** SYN anterior lingual gland.

**ap·i·cal gran·u·lo·ma** SYN periapical granuloma. See this page.

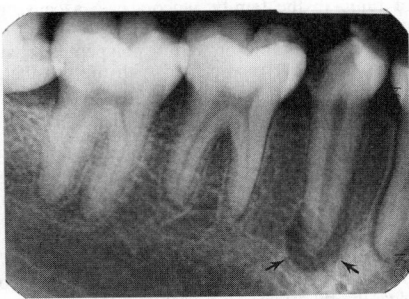

**apical granuloma** (arrows) of nonvital mandibular second premolar

**ap·i·cal per·i·o·don·tal cyst** an inflammatory odontogenic cyst derived histogenetically from Malassez epithelial rests surrounding the root apex of a nonvital tooth. See this page.

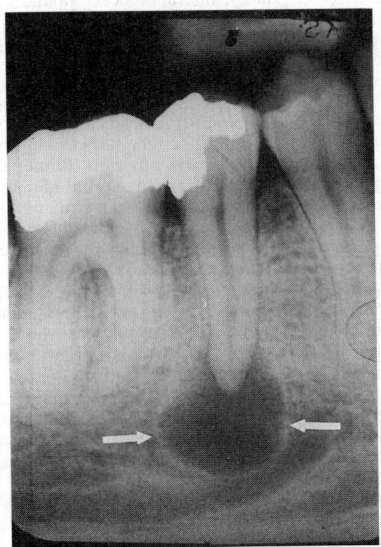

**apical periodontal cyst** (arrows) at roots of mandibular second premolar

**ap·i·cal pulse** a pulse heard directly over the apex of the heart by use of a stethoscope.

**ap·i·cal seg·men·tal ar·tery** SEE left pulmonary artery, right pulmonary artery.

**ap·i·cal seg·men·tal ar·tery of su·per·i·or lo··bar ar·tery of right lung** branch (of the infe-

rior lobar branch) of the right pulmonary artery serving the apical segment of the inferior lobe of the right lung.

**ap·i·cal space** the space between the alveolar wall and the apex of the root of a tooth where an alveolar abscess usually has its origin.

**ap·i·cec·to·my** (ap-i-sek'tō-mē) **1.** opening and exenteration of air cells in the apex of the petrous part of the temporal bone. **2.** in dental surgery, an obsolete synonym for apicoectomy. [L. *apex,* summit or tip, + G. *ektomē,* excision]

**ap·i·ces** (ap'i-sēs) plural of apex.

**ap·i·ci·tis** (ap-i-sī'tis) inflammation of the apex of a structure or organ.

**ap·i·co-** an apex; apical [L. *apex, apicis,* a summit or a tip + -o-]

**ap·i·co·ec·to·my** (ap'i-kō-ek'tō-mē) surgical removal of a dental root apex. SYN root resection. [apico- + G. *ektomē,* excision]

**ap·i·col·y·sis** (ap-i-kol'i-sis) surgical collapse of the upper portion of the lung by the operative detachment of the parietal pleura allowing a medial displacement of the pulmonary apex. [apico- + G. *lysis,* destruction]

**ap·i·cot·o·my** (ap-i-kot'ō-mē) incision into an apical structure. [apico- + G. *tomē,* a cutting]

**ap·la·nat·ic** (ap-la-nat'ik) pertaining to aplanatism, or to an aplanatic lens.

**ap·la·nat·ic lens** a lens designed to correct spherical aberration and coma.

**apla·sia** (ā-plā'zē-ă) **1.** defective development or congenital absence of an organ or tissue. **2.** HEMATOLOGY incomplete, retarded, or defective development, or cessation of the usual regenerative process. [G. *a-* priv. + *plasis,* a molding]

**aplas·tic** (ā-plas'tik, ă-plas'tik) pertaining to aplasia, or conditions characterized by defective regeneration, as in aplastic anemia.

**aplas·tic a·ne·mia** anemia characterized by a greatly decreased formation of erythrocytes and hemoglobin, usually associated with pronounced granulocytopenia and thrombocytopenia, as a result of hypoplastic or aplastic bone marrow. SYN Ehrlich anemia.

**aplas·tic lymph** lymph containing a relatively large number of leukocytes, but comparatively little fibrinogen; such lymph does not form a good clot and manifests only a slight tendency to become organized.

**aPLS** antiphospholipid antibody syndrome.

**ap·nea** (ap'nē-ă) absence of breathing. [G. *apnoia,* want of breath]

**ap·ne·a·hy·pop·nea in·dex** the number of apneic and hypopneic episodes combined per hour of sleep.

**ap·ne·ic** (ap'nē-ik) related to or suffering from apnea.

**ap·ne·ic pause** cessation of air flow for more than 10 seconds. SEE sleep apnea.

**ap·neu·mia** (ap-noo'mē-ă) congenital absence of the lungs. [G. *a-* priv. + *pneumōn,* lung]

**ap·neu·sis, ap·neus·tic breath·ing** (ap-noo'sis) an abnormal respiratory pattern consisting of a pause at full inspiration; cramp caused by a lesion at the mid or caudal pontine level of the brainstem. [G. *a-* priv. + *pneusis,* a breathing, fr. *pneō,* to breathe]

**apo-** combining form meaning, usually, separated from or derived from. [G. *apo,* away from, off; *apo-* becomes *ap-,* especially before a vowel or h]

**ap•o•chro•mat•ic ob•jec•tive** an objective in which chromatic aberration is corrected for three colors and spherical aberration is corrected for two.

**ap•o•crine** (ap′ŏ-krin) denoting a mechanism of glandular secretion in which the apical portion of secretory cells is shed and incorporated into the secretion. SEE ALSO apocrine gland. [G. *apo-krinō*, to separate]

**ap•o•crine ad•e•no•ma** SYN papillary hidradenoma.

**ap•o•crine car•ci•no•ma 1.** a carcinoma composed predominantly of cells with abundant eosinophilic granular cytoplasm, occurring in the breast; **2.** a carcinoma of the apocrine glands.

**ap•o•crine chrom•hi•dro•sis** excretion of colored sweat, usually black, from apocrine glands of the face; due to an abnormal lipochrome content of the secretion.

**ap•o•crine gland** a gland whose secretory product includes an apical portion of the secretory cell such as the secretion of lipid droplets in lactation.

**ap•o•crine hi•dro•cys•to•ma** SYN sudoriferous cyst.

**ap•o•crine met•a•pla•sia** alteration of acinar epithelium of breast tissue to resemble apocrine sweat glands; seen commonly in fibrocystic disease of the breasts.

**apo•dal** (ă-pŏ′dăl) relating to apodia. [G. *a-* priv. + *pous*, foot]

**apo•dia** (ă-pō′dē-ă) congenital absence of feet. [G. *a-* priv. + *pous*, foot]

**ap•o•en•zyme** (ap′ō-en-zīm) the protein portion of an enzyme as contrasted with the nonprotein portion, or coenzyme, or prosthetic portion (if present).

**ap•o•fer•ri•tin** (ap-ō-fer′i-tin) a protein in the intestinal wall that combines with a ferric hydroxide-phosphate compound to form ferritin, the first stage in the absorption of iron.

**apo-2L** SYN TRAIL.

**ap•o•lip•o•pro•tein** (ap′ō-lip-ō-prō′tēn) the protein component of lipoprotein complexes that is a normal constituent of plasma chylomicrons, HDL, LDL, and VLDL in man.

**ap•o•neu•rec•to•my** (ap′ō-noo-rek′tō-mē) excision of an aponeurosis. [aponeurosis + G. *ektomē*, excision]

**ap•o•neu•ro•gen•ic pto•sis** drooping of the eyelid caused by dehiscence of the tendon of the levator muscle.

**ap•o•neu•ror•rha•phy** (ap′ō-noo-rōr′ă-fē) SYN fasciorrhaphy. [aponeurosis + G. *rhaphē*, suture]

**ap•o•neu•ro•sis** (ap′ō-noo-rō′sis), pl. **ap•o•neu•ro•ses** (ap′ō-noo-rō-sēz) a fibrous sheet or flat, expanded tendon, giving attachment to muscular fibers and serving as the means of origin or insertion of a flat muscle; it sometimes serves as a fascia for other muscles. [G. the end of the muscle where it becomes tendon, fr. *apo*, from, + *neuron*, sinew]

**ap•o•neu•ro•si•tis** (ap′ō-noo-rō-sī′tis) inflammation of an aponeurosis.

**ap•o•neu•rot•ic** (ap′ō-noo-rot′ik) relating to an aponeurosis.

**ap•o•neu•rot•ic fi•bro•ma** a calcifying recurrent non-metastasizing but infiltrating fibroma seen most frequently on the palms of young people as a small firm nodule not attached to the overlying skin.

**ap•o•neu•rot•o•my** (ap′ō-noo-rot′ō-mē) incision of an aponeurosis.

**apoph•y•sis**, pl. **apoph•y•ses** (ă-pof′i-sis, ă-pof′i-sēz) an outgrowth or projection, especially one from a bone. A bony process or outgrowth that lacks an independent center of ossification. [G. an offshoot]

**apoph•y•si•tis** (ă-pof-i-sī′tis) inflammation of any apophysis.

**Ap•o•phy•so•my•ces** (ap-ō-fiz-ō-mī′sēz) a genus of fungi in the family Mucoraceae; a cause of mucormycosis.

**ap•o•pro•tein** (ap-ō-prō′tēn) a polypeptide chain (protein) not yet complexed with the prosthetic group that is necessary to form the active holoprotein.

**ap•o•pto•sis** programmed cell death; deletion of individual cells by fragmentation into membrane-bound particles, which are phagocytized by other cells. SYN programmed cell death. [G. a falling or dropping off, fr. *apo*, off, + *ptosis*, a falling]

**ap•o•re•pres•sor** (ap′ō-rē-pres′er) SYN inactive repressor.

**ap•o•stax•is** (ap-ō-staks′is) slight hemorrhage, or bleeding by drops. [G. a trickling down]

**apos•thia** (ă-pos′thē-ă) congenital absence of the prepuce. [G. *a-* priv. + *posthē*, foreskin]

**a•poth•e•car•ies′ weight** a system of weights based upon the weight of a grain of wheat; now superseded by the metric system (based on grams). One grain is the equivalent of 64.8 mg. One scruple contains 20 grains; one dram contains 60 grains; one apothecary ounce contains 8 drams (480 grains); one apothecary pound contains 12 ounces (5760 grains).

**ap•pa•ra•tus** (ap-ă-rā′tŭs) **1.** a collection of instruments adapted for a special purpose. **2.** an instrument made up of several parts. **3.** a group or system of glands, ducts, blood vessels, muscles, or other anatomic structures involved in the performance of some function. SEE ALSO system. [L. equipment. fr. *ap-paro*, pp. *-atus*, to prepare]

**ap•pend•age** (ă-pen′dij) any part, subordinate in function or size, attached to a main structure. SEE ALSO adnexa. SYN appendix (1). [L. *appendix*]

**ap•pend•ag•es of skin** the hair, nails, and sweat, sebaceous, and mammary glands.

**ap•pen•dec•to•my** (ap-pen-dek′tō-mē) surgical removal of the vermiform appendix. SYN appendicectomy. [appendix + G. *ektomē*, excision]

**ap•pen•dic•e•al, ap•pen•di•cal** (ă-pen-dis′ē-ăl, ă-pen′di-kăl) relating to an appendix.

**ap•pen•dic•e•al ab•scess** an intraperitoneal abscess, usually in the right iliac fossa, resulting from extension of infection in acute appendicitis, especially with perforation of the appendix. SYN periappendiceal abscess.

**ap•pen•di•cec•to•my** (ap-pen-di-sek′tō-mē) SYN appendectomy.

**ap•pen•di•ces omentales** [TA] SYN omental appendices.

**ap•pen•di•ci•tis** (ă-pen-di-sī′tis) inflammation of the vermiform appendix. [appendix + G. *-itis*, inflammation]

△**ap•pen•di•co-** an appendix, usually the vermiform appendix. [L. *appendix, appendicis* an appendage, fr. *appendo*, to hang something onto something, fr. *ad-, ap-*, to, onto, + *pendo*, to hang, + *-o-*]

**ap•pen•di•co•lith** (ă-pen′di-kō-lith) a calcified

concretion in the appendix visible on an abdominal radiograph. [appendico- + G. *lithos*, stone]

**ap·pen·di·co·li·thi·a·sis** (ă-pen′di-kō-li-thī′ă-sis) the presence of concretions in the vermiform appendix. [appendico- + G. *lithos*, stone]

**ap·pen·di·col·y·sis** (ă-pen-di-kol′i-sis) an operation for freeing the appendix from adhesions. [appendico- + G. *lysis*, a loosening]

**ap·pen·di·cos·to·my** (ă-pen-di-kos′tō-mē) an operation for opening into the intestine through the tip of the vermiform appendix, previously attached to the anterior abdominal wall. [appendico- + G. *stoma*, mouth]

**ap·pen·dic·u·lar** (ap′en-dik′yu-lăr) **1.** relating to an appendix or appendage. **2.** relating to the limbs, as opposed to axial, which refers to the trunk and head.

**ap·pen·dic·u·lar ar·tery** the branch of the ileocolic artery that descends posterior to the terminal ileum in the mesoappendix to supply the vermiform appendix. SYN arteria appendicularis [TA].

**ap·pen·dic·u·lar mus·cle** one of the skeletal muscles of the limbs.

**ap·pen·dic·u·lar skel·e·ton** the bones of the limbs including the shoulder and pelvic girdles.

**ap·pen·dic·u·lar vein** the tributary of the ileocolic vein that accompanies the appendicular artery.

**ap·pen·dix**, gen. **ap·pen·di·cis**, pl. **ap·pen·di·ces** (ă-pen′diks, ă-pen′di-sis, ă-pen′di-sēs) **1.** SYN appendage. **2.** a wormlike intestinal diverticulum extending from the blind end of the cecum; it varies in length and ends in a blind extremity. [L. appendage, fr. *ap-pendo*, to hang something on]

**ap·pen·dix ep·i·plo·i·ca**, pl. **ap·pen·di·ces ep·i·plo·i·cae** one of a number of little processes or sacs of peritoneum filled with adipose tissue and projecting from the serous coat of the large intestine, except the rectum; they are most evident on the transverse and sigmoid colon, being most numerous along the free tenia.

**ap·pen·dix of tes·tis** a vesicular structure attached to the cephalic pole of the testis; a vestige of the paramesonephric (müllerian) duct.

**ap·pen·dix ver·mi·for·mis** [TA] SYN vermiform appendix.

**ap·per·cep·tion** (ap-er-sep′shŭn) **1.** the final stage of attentive perception in which something is clearly apprehended and thus is relatively prominent in awareness; the full apprehension of any psychic content. **2.** the process of referring the perception of ideas to one's own personality. [L. *ad*, to, + *per- cipio*, pp. *-ceptus*, to take wholly, perceive]

**ap·per·cep·tive** (ap-er-sep′tiv) relating to, involved in, or capable of apperception.

**ap·pe·tite** (ap′ĕ-tīt) a desire or motive derived from a biologic or psychological need for food, water, sex, or affection; a desire or longing to satisfy any conscious physical or mental need. [L. *ad-peto*, pp. *-petitus*, to seek after, desire]

**ap·pla·na·tion** (ap′lan-ā′shŭn) TONOMETRY the flattening of the cornea by pressure. Intraocular pressure is directly proportional to external pressure, and inversely proportional to the area flattened. SEE ALSO applanation tonometer. [L. *ad*, toward, + *planum*, plane]

**ap·pla·na·tion to·nom·e·ter** an instrument for determining ocular tension by application of a small, flat disk to the cornea.

**ap·pla·nom·e·try** (ap-lan-om′ĕ-trē) use of an applanation tonometer.

**ap·ple jel·ly nod·ules** descriptive term for the papular lesions of lupus vulgaris, as they appear on diascopy.

**ap·pli·ance** (ă-plī′ans) a device used to provide function to a part, or for therapeutic purposes. [fr, O. Fr. *aplier*, to apply, fr. L. *applico*, to fold together]

**ap·pli·ca·tor** (ap′li-kā-tōr) a slender rod of wood, flexible metal, or synthetic material, at one end of which is attached a pledget of cotton or other substance for making local applications to any accessible surface. [L. *ap-plico*, to attach to]

**ap·po·si·tion** (ap-ō-zish′ŭn) **1.** the placing in contact of two substances. **2.** the condition of being placed or fitted together. **3.** the relationship of fracture fragments to one another. **4.** the process of thickening of the cell wall. **5.** the deposition of the matrix of the hard dental structures; enamel, dentin, and cementum. [L. *ap-pono*, pp. *-positus*, to place at or to]

**ap·po·si·tion·al growth** growth accomplished by the addition of new layers on those previously formed; e.g., the addition of lamellae in the formation of bone; it is the characteristic mode of growth when rigid materials are involved.

**ap·po·si·tion su·ture** a suture of the skin only. SYN coaptation suture.

**ap·proach** (ă-prōch′) **1.** in psychiatry, a term used to describe how interpersonal relationships are negotiated. **2.** the path or method used to expose the operative field during an operation. [M.E., fr. O. Fr., fr L.L. *appropio*, to come nearer, fr. *ad*, to + *propius*, nearer]

**AP pro·jec·tion** a radiographic study in which x-rays travel from anterior to posterior. SYN anteroposterior projection.

**ap·prox·i·mate** (ă-prok′si-māt) to bring close together. DENTISTRY **1.** proximate, denoting the contact surfaces, either mesial or distal, of two adjacent teeth. **2.** close together; denoting the teeth in the human jaw, as distinguished from the separated teeth in certain of the lower animals. [L. *ad*, to, + *proximus*, nearest]

**ap·prox·i·ma·tion** (ă-prok-si-mā′shŭn) in surgery, bringing tissue edges into desired apposition for suturing.

**ap·prox·i·ma·tion su·ture** a suture that pulls together the deep tissues.

**aprac·tic** (ā-prak′tik) SYN apraxic.

**aprax·ia** (ā-prak′sē-ă) **1.** a disorder of voluntary movement, consisting of impairment in the performance of skilled or purposeful movements, notwithstanding the preservation of comprehension, muscular power, sensibility, and coordination in general; due to acquired cerebral disease. **2.** a psychomotor defect in which the proper use of an object cannot be carried out although the object can be named and its uses described. [G. *a-* priv. + *prattō*, to do]

**aprax·ia of speech** SYN verbal apraxia.

**aprax·ic** (ā-prak′sik) marked by or pertaining to apraxia. SYN apractic.

**aproc·tia** (ā-prok′shē-ă) congenital absence or imperforation of the anus. [G. *a-* priv. + *prōktos*, anus]

**apron·ec·to·my** surgical excision of a redundant and dependent panniculus adiposus of the abdominal wall, which is commonly called an apron.

**ap•ro•so•pia** (ap-rō-sō′pē-ă) congenital absence of most or all of the face, usually associated with other malformations. [G. *a-* priv. + *prosōpon,* face]

**APS** adenosine 5′-phosphosulfate; antiphospholipid antibody syndrome.

**ap•ti•tude test** an occupation-oriented intelligence test used to evaluate a person's abilities, talents, and skills; particularly valuable in vocational counseling.

**aPTT** activated partial thromboplastin time.

**APUD, APUD cells** designation for cells in various organs secreting polypeptide hormones. Cells in this group have certain biochemical characteristics in common: they contain amines, such as catecholamine and 5-hydroxytryptamine, take up precursors of these amines in vivo, and contain amino-acid decarboxylase. [*amine precursor uptake, decarboxylase*]

**apy•ret•ic** (ā-pī-ret′ik) without fever, denoting apyrexia; having a normal body temperature. SYN afebrile.

**apy•rex•ia** (ā-pī-rek′sē-ă) absence of fever. [G. *a-* priv. + *pyrexis,* fever]

**aq.** L. *aqua,* water.

**aq. dest.** L. *aqua destillata,* distilled water.

**aq•ua•gen•ic pru•ri•tus** intense itching produced by brief contact with water at any temperature without visible changes in the skin.

**aq•ua•pho•bia** (ak-wă-fō′bē-ă) morbid fear of water. [L. *aqua,* water, + G. *phobos,* fear]

**aq•ue•duct** (ak′we-dŭkt) a conduit or canal. SYN aqueductus [TA]. [L. *aquaeductus*]

**aq•ue•duc•tus,** pl. **aq•ue•duc•tus** (ak-we-dŭk′tŭs) [TA] SYN aqueduct. [L. fr. *aqua,* water, + *ductus,* a leading, fr. *duco,* pp. *ductus,* to lead]

**aq•ue•duc•tus co•chle•ae** [TA] SYN perilymphatic duct.

**aque•ous** (ak′wē-ŭs, ā′kwē-ŭs) watery; of, like, or containing water.

**aque•ous cham•bers** the combined anterior and posterior chambers of the eye containing the aqueous humor.

**aque•ous hu•mor** the watery fluid that fills the anterior and posterior chambers of the eye. It is secreted by the ciliary processes within the posterior chamber and passes through the the pupil into the anterior chamber where it filters through the trabecular meshwork and is reabsorbed into the venous system at the iridocorneal angle by way of the sinus venosus of the sclera.

**aque•ous phase** the water portion of a system consisting of two liquid phases, one mainly water, the other a liquid immiscible with water (e.g., benzene, ether).

**Ar** argon.

△**ar•ab-** gum arabic; similar gummy substances. [G. *Araps, Arabos,* an Arab]

**arach•nase** (ă-rak′nāz) a positive control plasma for the monitoring of clotting-endpoint coagulation tests used in the detection of circulating lupus anticoagulants: it is a normal plasma that contains a venom extract from the brown recluse spider, *Loxosceles reclusa,* which mimics the presence of a lupus anticoagulant (LA) in a variety of clotting-endpoint tests.

**arach•ne•pho•bia** (ă-rak-nē-fō′bē-ă) morbid fear of spiders. SYN arachnophobia. [G. *arachnē,* spider, + *phobos,* fear]

**Arach•ni•da** (ă-rak′ni-dă) a class of arthropods in the subphylum Chelicerata, consisting of spiders, scorpions, harvestmen, mites, ticks, and allies. [G. *arachnē,* spider]

**arach•nid•ism** (ă-rak′ni-dizm) systemic poisoning following the bite of a spider (especially of the black widow).

**arach•no•dac•ty•ly** (ă-rak-nō-dak′ti-lē) a condition in which the hands and fingers, and often the feet and toes, are abnormally long and slender; a characteristic of Marfan syndrome and kindred hereditary disorders of connective tissue. [G. *arachnē,* spider, + *daktylos,* finger]

**arach•noid** (ă-rak′noyd) a delicate fibrous membrane forming the middle of the three coverings of the central nervous system. Its external surface is closely applied (but not attached) to the internal surface of the dura mater, with only a potential space (subdural space) intervening. Thus, in a spinal puncture, dura mater and arachnoid are penetrated simultaneously as if a single layer. SEE ALSO leptomeninges. SYN arachnoidea mater [TA], arachnoid membrane, arachnoidea, arachnoides. [G. *arachnē,* spider, cobweb, + *eidos,* resemblance]

**arach•noid of brain** SYN cranial arachnoid mater.

**arach•noid cyst** a fluid-filled cyst lined with arachnoid membrane, frequently situated near the lateral aspect of the lateral sulcus; usually congenital in origin.

**arach•noi•dea, arach•noi•des** (ă-rak-noyd′ē-ă, ă-rak-noy′dēz) SYN arachnoid. [Mod. L. *arachnoideus* fr. G. *arachnē,* spider, + *eidos,* resemblance]

**arach•noi•dea ma•ter** [TA] SYN arachnoid.

**arach•noi•dea ma•ter cra•ni•a•lis** [TA] SYN cranial arachnoid mater.

**arach•noi•dea ma•ter encephali** SYN cranial arachnoid mater.

**arach•noid gran•u•la•tions** tufted prolongations of pia-arachnoid, composed of numerous arachnoid villi that penetrate dural venous sinuses and effect transfer of cerebrospinal fluid to the venous system. SYN granulationes arachnoideales [TA], pacchionian bodies.

**arach•noid•i•tis** (ă-rak-noy-dī′tis) inflammation of the arachnoid membrane often with involvement of the subjacent subarachnoid space. SEE ALSO leptomeningitis. [arachnoidea + *-itis,* inflammation]

**arach•noid ma•ter** a delicate fibrous membrane forming the middle of the three coverings of the central nervous system. In life the arachnoid (specifically the arachnoid barrier cell layer) is tenuously attached to the externally adjacent dura mater (specifically the dural border cells) and there is no naturally occurring space at the dura-arachnoid interface. Thus in a spinal puncture dura mater and arachnoid are penetrated simultaneously as if a single layer. Separation of the arachnoid mater from the dura mater (usually through the dural border cell layer) may result from traumatic or pathologic processes creating what is commonly, but incorrectly, called a subdural hematoma. The arachnoid mater is named for the delicate, spiderweb-like filaments that extend from its deep surface, through the CSF of the subarachnoid space, to the pia mater.

**arach•noid mem•brane** SYN arachnoid.

**arach•noid vil•li** tufted prolongations of pia-arachnoid that protrude through the meningeal layer of the dura mater and have a thin limiting membrane; collections of arachnoid villi form arachnoid granulations that lie in venous lacunae at the margin of the superior sagittal sinus; the spongy tissue of the arachnoid villus contains tubules that serve as one-way valves for transfer of cerebrospinal fluid from the subarachnoid space to the venous system. Both arachnoid villi and the granulations formed from them are major sites of fluid transfer. SEE ALSO arachnoid granulations.

**arach·no·pho·bia** (ă-rak-nō-fō′bē-ă) SYN arachnephobia.

**A·ran-Du·chenne dis·ease** (ah′rahn-doo-shen′) SYN amyotrophic lateral sclerosis.

**ar·bor,** pl. **ar·bo·res** (ar′bōr, ar-bō′rēz) in anatomy, a treelike structure with branchings. [L. tree]

**ar·bo·res·cent** (ar-bō-res′ent) SYN dendriform.

**ar·bo·ri·za·tion** (ar′bōr-i-zā′shŭn) **1.** the terminal branching of nerve fibers or blood vessels in a treelike pattern. **2.** the branched pattern formed by a dried smear of cervical mucus, indicating the effect of estrogen unopposed by progesterone.

**ar·bo·rize** (ar′bōr-īz) to spread in a treelike branching pattern.

**ar·bo·vi·rus** (ar′bō-vī′rŭs) a large, heterogeneous group of RNA viruses. There are over 500 species, which have been recovered from arthropods, bats, and rodents. These taxonomically diverse viruses are unified by an epidemiological concept, i.e., transmission between vertebrate hosts by blood-feeding arthropod vectors, such as mosquitoes, ticks, sandflies, and midges. In most instances diseases produced by these viruses are mild and difficult to distinguish from illnesses caused by viruses of other taxonomic groups. Infections may be separated into several clinical syndromes: undifferentiated type fevers (systemic febrile disease), hepatitis, hemorrhagic fevers, and encephalitides. [ar, arthropod, + bo, borne, + virus]

**arc** (ark) **1.** a curved line or segment of a circle. **2.** continuous luminous passage of an electric current in a gas or vacuum between two or more separated carbon or other electrodes. [L. arcus, a bow]

**ar·cade** (ar-kād) an anatomic structure or structures (especially a blood vessel) taking the form of a series of arches. [L. arcus, arc, bow]

**Ar·can·o·bac·te·ri·um** (ar-kă′nō-bac-tēr′ē-ŭm) a genus of nonmotile, facultatively anaerobic bacteria containing Gram-positive slender irregular rods, sometimes showing clubbed ends. These organisms are obligate parasites of the pharynx in farm animals and humans, occasionally causing lesions on the pharynx or skin. The type species is Arcanobacterium haemolyticum.

**arch** any structure resembling a bent bow or an arch; an arc. In anatomy, any vaulted or archlike structure. SYN arcus [TA]. [thru O. Fr. fr. L. arcus, bow]

△**arch-, ar·che-, ar·chi-, ar·cho-** combining forms meaning primitive, or ancestral; also first, or chief, primitive, ancestral, extreme. [G. archē, origin, beginning, + -o-]

**ar·che·o·ki·net·ic** (ar-kē-ō-ki-net′ik) denoting a low and primitive type of motor nerve mechanism, such as is found in the peripheral and the ganglionic nervous systems. Cf. neokinetic, pale-

okinetic. [G. archaios, ancient, + kinētikos, relating to movement]

**ar·che·type** (ar′kē-tīp) **1.** a primitive structural plan from which various modifications have evolved. **2.** JUNGIAN PSYCHOLOGY structural manifestation of the collective unconscious. SYN imago (2). [G. archetypos, pattern, model, fr. archē, beginning, + typtō, to stamp out]

**arch of foot 1.** longitudinalis: consisting of a medial longitudinal arch, including the calcaneus, talus, navicular, three cuneiform bones, and the three medial metatarsals, and a lateral longitudinal arch formed by calcaneus, cuboid and two lateral metatarsals; **2.** transversalis: formed by the proximal parts of the metatarsal bones, the three cuneiform bones, and the cuboid. SYN arcus pedis.

**arch of tho·rac·ic duct** SEE thoracic duct.

**arch·wire** (arch′wīr) a device consisting of a wire conforming to the alveolar or dental arch, used as an anchorage in correcting irregularities in the position of the teeth.

**ar·ci·form** (ar′si-fōrm) SYN arcuate.

**Ar·co·bac·ter** (ar-kō-bak′ter) a genus of bacteria in the family Campylobacteraceae that are Gram-negative, aerotolerant, and able to grow at 15° C. The type strain is Arcobacter butzleri.

**Ar·co·bac·ter butzleri** a bacterial species of Arcobacter found in poultry and meat; has been associated with diarrheal and systemic diseases in humans.

**arc·ta·tion** (ark-tā′shŭn) a narrowing, contraction, stricture, or coarctation. [L. arto (improp. arcto), pp. -atus, to tighten]

**ar·cu·ate** (ar′kyu-āt) denoting a form that is arched or has the shape of a bow. SYN arciform. [L. arcuatus, bowed]

**ar·cu·ate ar·ter·ies of kid·ney** curved arteries at the corticomedullary border, arising from interlobar arteries and giving rise to interlobular arteries. SYN arteriae arcuatae renis [TA].

**ar·cu·ate ar·tery of foot (inconstant)** origin, dorsalis pedis; branches, passes laterally dorsal to the bases of the metatarsals, giving rise to the second, third, and fourth dorsal metatarsal arteries at the level of the medial cuneiform bone. SYN arteria arcuata [TA].

**ar·cu·ate fi·bers** nervous or tendinous fibers passing in the form of an arch from one part to another.

**ar·cu·ate nu·clei** a variable assembly of small cell groups, probably outlying components of the pontine nuclei, on the ventral and medial aspects of the pyramid in the medulla oblongata.

**ar·cu·ate veins of kid·ney** veins that parallel the arcuate arteries, receive blood from interlobular veins and straight venules, and terminate in interlobar veins.

**ar·cu·ate zone** the inner third of the basilar membrane of the cochlear duct extending from the tympanic lip of the osseous spiral lamina to the outer pillar cell of the spiral organ (organ of Corti). SYN zona arcuata, zona tecta.

**ar·cu·a·tion** (ar-kyu-ā′shŭn) a bending or curvature.

**ar·cus** (ar′kŭs) [TA] SYN arch. [L. a bow]

**ar·cus cor·ne·a·lis** an opaque, grayish ring at the periphery of the cornea just within the sclerocorneal junction, of frequent occurrence in the aged; it results from a deposit of fatty granules in, or hyaline degeneration of, the lamellae and cells of the cornea. SYN anterior embryotoxon, geron-toxon.

**ar·cus pal·mar·is** SYN palmar arch.

**ar·cus pal·ma·ris pro·fun·dus** [TA] SYN palmar arch (1).

**ar·cus pal·ma·ris su·per·fi·ci·a·les** [TA] SYN palmar arch (2).

**ar·cus pe·dis** SYN arch of foot.

**ARDS** adult respiratory distress syndrome.

**ar·ea (a),** pl. **ar·e·ae** (ăr′ē-ă, ăr′ē-ē) **1.** any circumscribed surface or space. **2.** all of the part supplied by a given artery or nerve. **3.** a part of an organ having a special function, as the motor area of the brain. SEE ALSO regio, region, space, spatium, zone. [L. a courtyard]

**ar·ea a·myg·da·loi·dea an·ter·i·or** [TA] SYN anterior amygdaloid area.

**ar·ea of car·di·ac dull·ness** a triangular area determined by percussion of the front of the chest; it corresponds to the part of the heart that is not covered by lung tissue.

**ar·ea coch·lea** [TA] SYN cochlear area.

**are·flex·ia** (ā-rē-flek′sē-ă) absence of reflexes.

**Are·na·vi·ri·dae** (ă-rē-nă-vir′i-dē) a family of RNA viruses, many of which are parasites of rodents, that includes lymphocytic choriomeningitis virus, Lassa virus, and the Tacaribe virus complex. [L. *arena* (*harena*), sand]

**Are·na·vi·rus** (ă-rē′nă-vī′rŭs) a genus in the family Arenaviridae that is associated with lymphocytic choriomeningitis and a number of hemorrhagic fevers.

**are·ola,** pl. **are·o·lae** (ă-rē′ō-lă, ă-rē′ō-lē) **1.** any small area. **2.** one of the spaces or interstices in areolar tissue. **3.** SYN areola of breast. **4.** a pigmented, depigmented, or erythematous zone surrounding a papule, pustule, wheal, or cutaneous neoplasm. SYN halo (3). [L. dim. of *area*]

**are·ola of breast** a circular pigmented area surrounding the nipple or papilla mammae; its surface is dotted with little projections corresponding to the areolar glands beneath. SYN areola mammae [TA], areola papillaris, areola (3).

**are·ola mam·mae** [TA] SYN areola of breast.

**are·ola pa·pil·la·ris** SYN areola of breast.

**are·o·lar** (ă-rē′ō-lăr) relating to an areola.

**are·o·lar glands** a number of small mammary glands forming small rounded projections from the surface of the areola of the breast; they enlarge with pregnancy and during lactation secrete a substance presumed to resist chapping. SYN Montgomery follicles.

**are·o·lar tis·sue** loose, irregularly arranged connective tissue that consists of collagenous and elastic fibers, a protein polysaccharide ground substance, and connective tissue cells (fibroblasts, macrophages, mast cells, and sometimes fat cells, plasma cells, leukocytes, and pigment cells).

**are·o·lar ve·nous plex·us** a venous plexus in the areola surrounding the nipple, formed by the mammary veins, and sending its blood to the lateral thoracic vein. SYN Haller circle (2).

**are·ola um·bil·i·ci** a pigmented ring around the umbilicus in the pregnant woman.

**ARF** acute respiratory failure.

**ar·ga·sid** (ar-gas′id) common name for members of the family Argasidae.

**Argas·i·dae** (ar-gas′i-dē) family of ticks, the soft ticks, so called because of their wrinkled appearance that fills out when the tick is engorged with blood. Argasid ticks, chiefly species of *Ornithodoros*, harbor and transmit spirochetes of the genus *Borrelia* that cause relapsing fever in birds and mammals.

**ar·gen·taf·fin, ar·gen·taf·fine** (ar-jen′tă-fin, ar-jen′tă-fēn) pertaining to cells or tissue elements that reduce silver ions in solution, thereby becoming stained brown or black. [L. *argentum,* silver, + *affinitas,* affinity]

**ar·gen·taf·fin cell** cell containing granules that precipitate silver from an ammoniacal silver nitrate solution. SEE ALSO enteroendocrine cells.

**ar·gen·taf·fi·no·ma** (ar′jen-tă-fi-nō′mă, ar′jen-taf-i-nō′mă) SYN carcinoid tumor.

**ar·gen·to·phil, ar·gen·to·phile** (ar-jen′tō-fil, ar-jen′tō-fīl) SYN argyrophil.

**ar·gi·nase** (ar′ji-nās) an enzyme of the liver that catalyzes the hydrolysis of L-arginine to L-ornithine and urea; a key enzyme of the urea cycle.

**ar·gi·nine** (ar′ji-nēn) 2-amino-5-guanidinopentanoic acid; one of the amino acids occurring among the hydrolysis products of proteins, particularly abundant in the basic proteins such as histones and protamines. A dibasic amino acid.

**ar·gi·nine va·so·pres·sin (AVP)** vasopressin containing an arginyl residue in position 8 (as in chickens and most mammals, including humans); porcine vasopressin has a lysyl residue at position 8. All are vasopressors.

**ar·gi·ni·no·suc·cin·ic ac·id** (ar′ji-ni-nō-sŭk-sin′ik as′id) formed as an intermediate in the conversion of L-citrulline to L-arginine in the urea cycle.

**ar·gi·ni·no·suc·cin·ic·ac·i·du·ria** (ar-ji-nin′ō-sŭk-sin′ik-as-i-dyu′rē-ă) an autosomal recessive disorder characterized by excessive urinary excretion of argininosuccinic acid, epilepsy, ataxia, mental retardation, liver disease, and friable, tufted hair; presumed to be the consequence of a deficiency of an enzyme responsible for splitting argininosuccinic acid to arginine and fumaric acid.

**ar·gon (Ar)** (ar′gon) a gaseous element, atomic no. 18, atomic wt. 39.948, present in the dry atmosphere in the proportion of about 0.94%; one of the noble gases. [G. ntr. of *argos,* lazy, inactive, fr. *a-* priv. + *ergon,* work]

**ar·gon la·ser** laser used for ophthalmic procedures, including retinal photocoagulation and trabeculoplasty, consisting of photons in the blue (488 nm) or green (514 nm) spectrum.

**Ar·gyll Ro·bert·son pu·pil** (ahr′gil-ro′bert-sŭn) a form of reflex iridoplegia characterized by miosis, irregular shape, and a loss of the direct and consensual pupillary reflex to light, with normal pupillary constriction to a near vision effort (light-near dissociation); often present in tabetic neurosyphilis.

**ar·gyr·ia, ar·gy·rism** (ar-jir′ē-ă, ar′ji-rizm) a slate-gray or bluish discoloration of the skin and deep tissues, due to the deposit of silver, occurring after medicinal administration of a soluble silver salt. [G. *argyros,* silver]

**ar·gyr·ic** (ar-jir′ik) relating to argyria.

**ar·gyr·o·phil, ar·gyr·o·phile** (ar-ji′rō-fil, ar-ji′rō-fīl) pertaining to tissue elements that are capable of impregnation with silver ions and being made visible after an external reducing agent is used. SYN argentophil, argentophile. [G. *argyros,* silver, + *philos,* fond]

**arhin·ia** (ă-rin′ē-ă) congenital absence of the nose. SYN arrhinia.

**ari•bo•fla•vin•o•sis** (ă-rī′bō-flā-vi-nō′sis) a commonly used term for hyporiboflavinosis.

**ar•is•to•te•lian meth•od** (ă-ris-tō-tē′lē-ăn) a method of study that stresses the relation between a general category and a particular object.

**Ar•is•tot•le a•nom•a•ly** (ar′is-tot′ĕl) when a small object is held between the first and second fingers crossed in such a way that it touches or presses upon skin surfaces that ordinarily are not pressed upon simultaneously by a single object, it is perceived falsely as two.

**a•rith•me•tic mean** the mean calculated by adding a set of values and then dividing the sum by the number of values.

**Arlt op•er•a•tion** (ahrlt) transplantation of the eyelashes back from the edge of the lid in trichiasis.

**arm 1.** the segment of the upper limb between the shoulder and the elbow; colloquially, the whole upper limb. SYN brachio- (1), brachium (1). **2.** an anatomic extension resembling an arm. **3.** a specifically shaped and positioned extension of a removable partial denture framework. [L. *armus,* forequarter of an animal; G. *harmos,* a shoulder joint]

**ar•ma•men•tar•i•um** (ar′mă-men-tār′ē-ŭm) all the therapeutic means available to the health practitioner for professional practice. [L. an arsenal, fr. *armamenta,* implements, tackle, fr. *arma,* armor, arms]

**Arm•i•tage-Doll mod•el** (ar′mi-tazh-dol) a model of carcinogenesis with the premise that the main variable determining change in risk is not age but time.

**ARN** acute retinal necrosis.

**Ar•neth count** (ahr-net′) the percentage distribution of polymorphonuclear neutrophils, based on the number of lobes in the nuclei (from one to five). SEE ALSO Arneth index.

**Ar•neth in•dex** (ahr-net′) an expression based on adding the percentages of polymorphonuclear neutrophils with one or two lobes in their nuclei, plus one-half the percentage with three lobes; the normal value is 60%. SEE ALSO Arneth count.

**Ar•nold body** (ahr′nŏld) a minute fragment or "ghost" resulting from degeneration of an erythrocyte (sometimes mistaken for a blood platelet).

**Ar•nold-Chi•a•ri mal•for•ma•tion** (ar′nŏld kē-ahr′ē) deformity of posterior fossa structures caused by tethering of the spinal cord with caudad traction and displacement of the rhombencephalon; may be accompanied by spina bifida and associated anomalies such as meningomyelocele; weak evidence of autosomal recessive inheritance.

**ar•o•mat•ic** (ar-ō-mat′ik) **1.** having an agreeable, somewhat pungent, spicy odor. **2.** one of a group of vegetable drugs having a fragrant odor and slightly stimulant properties. **3.** SEE cyclic compound. [G. *arōmatikos,* fr. *arōma,* spice, sweet herb]

**ar•o•mat•ic D-amino ac•id de•car•box•yl•ase** an enzyme that catalyzes the decarboxylation of L-dopa to dopamine, of L-tryptophan to tryptamine, and of L-hydroxytryptophan to serotonin; important in the biosynthetic pathway of catecholamines and melanin.

**ar•o•mat•ic am•mo•nia spir•it** a hydroalcoholic solution containing approximately 2% ammonia and 4% ammonium carbonate and the aromatics: lemon oil, lavender oil, and myristica oil. Used

mainly by inhalation to produce reflex stimulation in persons who have fainted or are at risk of syncope.

**ar•o•mat•ic com•pound** SEE cyclic compound.

**ar•o•mat•ic se•ries** all the compounds derived from benzene, or similar cyclic compounds that obey Hückel rule.

**aro•ma•ti•sa•tion [Br.]** SEE aromatization.

**aro•ma•tise [Br.]** SEE aromatize.

**aro•ma•ti•za•tion** (ă-rō-mă-tĭ-zā′shŭn) conversion of a nonaromatic compound to an aromatic compound.

**aro•ma•tize** (ă-rō′mă-tīz) to convert a nonaromatic compound to an aromatic compound.

**ar•rec•tor,** pl. **ar•rec•to•res** (ă-rek′tŏr, ă-rek-tō′ rēz) SYN erector. [L. that which raises, fr. *arrigo,* pp. *-rectus,* to raise up]

**ar•rec•tor mus•cle of hair, ar•rec•tor pi•li mus•cles** bundles of smooth muscle fibers, attached to the deep part of the hair follicles, passing outward alongside the sebaceous glands to the papillary layer of the corium; they act to pull the hairs erect, causing "goose bumps" or "goose flesh" (cutis anserina). SYN musculi arrectores pilorum [TA], erector muscles of hairs.

**ar•rest** (ă-rest′) **1.** to stop, check, or restrain. **2.** a stoppage; interference with, or checking of, the regular course of a disease, a symptom, or the performance of a function. **3.** inhibition of a developmental process, usually at the ultimate stage of development; premature arrest may lead to a congenital abnormality. [O. Fr. *arester,* fr. LL. *adresto,* to stop behind]

**ar•rest of ac•tive phase dys•to•cia** stoppage of further cervical dilation for longer than two hours after labor has entered active phase (generally defined as active contraction with at least 4 cm of cervical dilatation); causes include inadequate uterine contractions and cephalopelvic disproportion.

**ar•rest of des•cent dys•to•cia** failure of fetus to descend after an hour in second stage despite maternal effort; typically due to inadequate maternal effort, fetal malposition, or fetal size.

**ar•rest of la•bor** absence of progress of active labor (as defined by cervical dilation and descent of the presenting part) for two hr or longer.

**ar•rest sig•nal** a DNA sequence that causes arrest of RNA polymerase transcription.

**Ar•rhe•ni•us-Mad•sen the•o•ry** (ă-rē′nē-ŭs-mad-sen) that the reaction of an antigen with its antibody is a reversible reaction, the equilibrium being determined according to the law of mass action by the concentrations of the reacting substances.

**ar•rhe•no•blas•to•ma** (ă-rē′nō-blas-tō′mă) a rare ovarian tumor that produces masculinization and often contains tubules and luteinized cells. SYN androblastoma (2), gynandroblastoma (1). [G. *arrhēn,* male, + *blastos,* germ, + *-ōma,* tumor]

**ar•rhin•ia** (ă-rin′ē-ă) SYN arhinia. [G. *a-* priv. + *rhis* (*rhin-*), nose]

**ar•rhyth•mia** (ă-ridh′mē-ă) loss of rhythm; denoting especially an irregularity of the heartbeat. SEE ALSO dysrhythmia. [G. *a-* priv. + *rhythmos,* rhythm]

**ar•rhyth•mic** (ă-ridh′mik) marked by loss of rhythm; pertaining to arrhythmia.

**ar•rhyth•mo•gen•ic** (ă-ridh-mō-jen′ik) capable of inducing cardiac arrhythmias. [G. *a-* priv. + *rhythmos,* rhythm, + *-gen,* production]

**Ar·ru·ga for·ceps** (ah-roo′gah) forceps for the intracapsular extraction of a cataract.

**ar·se·nic (As)** (ar′sĕ-nik) a metallic element, atomic no. 33, atomic wt. 74.92159; forms a number of poisonous compounds, some of which are used in medicine. [L. *arsenicum*, G. *arsenikon*, fr. Pers. *zarnik*]

**ar·sen·i·cal** (ar-sen′i-kăl) **1.** a drug or agent, the effect of which depends on its arsenic content. **2.** denoting or containing arsenic.

**ART** acoustic reflex threshold.

**ar·te·fact** (ar′tĕ-fakt) SYN artifact.

**ar·te·ria**, gen. and pl. **ar·te·ri·ae** (ar-tēr′ē-ă, ar-tēr′ē-ē) [TA] SYN artery. SEE ALSO branch. [L. from G. *artēria,* the windpipe, later an artery as distinct from a vein]

**ar·te·ria an·gu·la·ris** [TA] SYN angular artery.

**ar·te·ria ap·pen·di·cu·la·ris** [TA] SYN appendicular artery.

**ar·te·ria ar·cu·a·ta** [TA] SYN arcuate artery of foot (inconstant).

**ar·te·ria as·cen·dens** [TA] SYN ascending artery.

**ar·te·ria ax·il·la·ris** [TA] SYN axillary artery.

**ar·te·ria bas·i·la·ris** [TA] SYN basilar artery.

**ar·te·ria bra·chi·a·lis** [TA] SYN brachial artery.

**ar·te·ria buc·ca·lis** [TA] SYN buccal artery.

**ar·te·ria bul·bi pe·nis** [TA] SYN artery of bulb of penis.

**ar·te·ria bul·bi ves·tib·u·li** [TA] SYN artery of bulb of vestibule.

**ar·te·ria ca·na·lis pte·ry·goi·dei** [TA] SYN artery of pterygoid canal.

**ar·te·ria ce·li·aca** SYN celiac trunk.

**ar·te·ria cen·tra·lis ret·i·nae** [TA] SYN central retinal artery.

**ar·te·ria coch·le·a·ris com·mu·nis** [TA] SYN common cochlear artery.

**ar·te·ria cre·ma·ste·ri·ca** [TA] SYN cremasteric artery.

**ar·te·ria cys·ti·ca** [TA] SYN cystic artery.

**ar·te·ria des·cen·dens ge·nus** [TA] SYN descending genicular artery.

**ar·te·ria dor·sa·lis cli·to·ri·dis** [TA] SYN dorsal artery of clitoris.

**ar·te·ria dor·sa·lis pe·nis** [TA] SYN dorsal artery of penis.

**ar·te·ria duc·tus de·fe·ren·tis** [TA] SYN artery to ductus deferens.

**ar·te·ri·ae ar·cu·a·tae re·nis** [TA] SYN arcuate arteries of kidney.

**ar·te·ri·ae a·tri·a·les** SYN atrial arteries.

**ar·te·ri·ae il·e·a·les** [TA] SYN ileal arteries.

**ar·te·ri·ae in·ter·lo·bu·la·res** [TA] SYN interlobular arteries.

**ar·te·ri·ae je·ju·na·les** [TA] SYN jejunal arteries.

**ar·te·ri·ae lum·ba·les** [TA] SYN lumbar artery.

**ar·te·ri·ae pal·pe·bra·les** [TA] SYN palpebral arteries.

**ar·te·ri·ae per·fo·ran·tes** [TA] SYN perforating arteries.

**ar·te·ria ep·i·scle·ra·lis** [TA] SYN episcleral artery.

**ar·te·ri·ae pu·den·dae ex·ter·nae** [TA] SYN external pudendal arteries.

**ar·te·ri·ae sig·moi·de·ae** [TA] SYN sigmoid arteries.

**ar·te·ri·ae ven·tri·cu·lar·es** [TA] SYN ventricular arteries.

**ar·te·ria fa·ci·a·lis** [TA] SYN facial artery.

**ar·te·ria fe·mo·ra·lis** [TA] SYN femoral artery.

**ar·te·ria gas·tro·du·o·de·na·lis** [TA] SYN gastroduodenal artery.

**ar·te·ria hy·a·loi·dea** [TA] SYN hyaloid artery.

**ar·te·ria il·e·o·co·li·ca** [TA] SYN ileocolic artery.

**ar·te·ria il·i·o·lum·ba·lis** [TA] SYN iliolumbar artery.

**ar·te·ria in·fra·or·bi·ta·lis** [TA] SYN infraorbital artery.

**ar·te·ri·al** (ar-tē′rē-ăl) relating to one or more arteries or to the entire system of arteries.

**ar·te·ria la·cri·ma·lis** [TA] SYN lacrimal artery.

**ar·te·ri·al blood** blood that is oxygenated in the lungs, found in the left chambers of the heart and in the arteries, and relatively bright red.

**ar·te·ri·al ca·nal** SYN ductus arteriosus.

**ar·te·ri·al cap·il·lary** a capillary opening from an arteriole or metarteriole.

**ar·te·ri·al cir·cle of cer·e·brum** an anastomotic "circle" of arteries (roughly pentagonal in outline) at the base of the brain, formed, sequentially and in anterior to posterior direction, by the anterior communicating artery, the two anterior cerebral, the two internal carotid, the two posterior communicating, and the two posterior cerebral arteries.

**ar·te·ri·al cone** the left or anterosuperior, smooth-walled portion of the cavity of the right ventricle of the heart, which begins at the supraventricular crest and terminates in the pulmonary trunk. SYN conus arteriosus [TA], infundibulum (4).

**ar·te·ri·al duct** SYN ductus arteriosus.

**ar·te·ri·al for·ceps** a locking forceps with sloping blades for grasping the end of a blood vessel until a ligature is applied.

**ar·te·ria li·e·na·lis** [TA] SYN splenic artery.

**ar·te·ria lig·a·men·ti ter·e·tis uter·i** [TA] SYN artery of round ligament of uterus.

**ar·te·ria lin·gu·la·ris** [TA] SEE left pulmonary artery.

**ar·te·ri·al line** an intra-arterial catheter.

**ar·te·ri·al neph·ro·scle·ro·sis** patchy atrophic scarring of the kidney due to arteriosclerotic narrowing of the lumens of large branches of the renal artery, occurring in old or hypertensive persons and occasionally causing hypertension. SYN arterionephrosclerosis.

**ar·te·ri·al scle·ro·sis** SYN arteriosclerosis.

**ar·te·ri·al spi·der** SYN spider angioma.

**ar·te·ri·al ten·sion** the blood pressure within an artery.

**ar·te·ria lu·so·ria** an aberrant right subclavian artery arising from the descending aorta; it passes posterior to the esophagus, often producing dysphagia.

**ar·te·ria mas·se·te·ri·ca** [TA] SYN masseteric artery.

**ar·te·ria max·il·la·ris** [TA] SYN maxillary artery.

**ar·te·ria me·di·a·na** SYN median artery.

**ar·te·ria men·ta·lis** [TA] SYN mental artery.

**ar·te·ria me·ta·tar·salis plan·tar·is** [TA] SYN plantar metatarsal artery.

**ar·te·ria mus·cu·lo·phre·ni·ca** [TA] SYN musculophrenic artery.

**ar·te·ria nu·tri·cia** [TA] SYN nutrient artery.

**ar·te·ria nu·tri·cia fe·mo·ris** [TA] SYN nutrient artery of femur.

**ar·te·ria nu·tri·cia fi·bu·lae** [TA] SYN nutrient artery of fibula.

**ar·te·ria ob·tu·ra·to·ria** [TA] SYN obturator artery.

**ar·te·ria ob·tu·ra·to·ria ac·ces·so·ria** [TA] SYN accessory obturator artery.

**ar·te·ria oc·ci·pi·ta·lis** [TA] SYN occipital artery.

**ar·te·ria oph·thal·mi·ca** [TA] SYN ophthalmic artery.

**ar·te·ria o·va·ri·ca** [TA] SYN ovarian artery.

**ar·te·ria pe·ri·car·di·a·co·phre·ni·ca** [TA] SYN pericardiacophrenic artery.

**ar·te·ria pe·ri·ne·al·is** [TA] SYN perineal artery.

**ar·te·ria pe·ro·nea** [TA] SYN peroneal artery.

**ar·te·ria pha·ryn·gea as·cen·dens** [TA] SYN ascending pharyngeal artery.

**ar·te·ri·a plan·ta·ris pro·fun·da** [TA] SYN deep plantar artery.

**arteria polaris temporalis** [TA] SYN polar temporal artery.

**ar·te·ria pop·lit·ea** [TA] SYN popliteal artery.

**ar·te·ria pre·pan·cre·a·ti·ca** [TA] SYN prepancreatic artery.

**ar·te·ria pro·fun·da cli·to·r·idis** [TA] SYN deep artery of clitoris.

**ar·te·ria pro·fun·da pe·nis** [TA] SYN deep artery of penis.

**ar·te·ria pte·ry·go·men·in·ge·a·lis** [TA] SYN pterygomeningeal artery.

**ar·te·ria pul·mo·na·lis** SYN pulmonary trunk.

**ar·te·ria qua·dri·gem·in·a·lis** SYN collicular artery.

**ar·te·ria ra·di·a·lis** [TA] SYN radial artery.

**ar·te·ria re·cur·rens ul·na·ris** [TA] SYN recurrent ulnar artery.

**ar·te·ria re·na·lis** [TA] SYN renal artery.

**ar·te·ria sphe·no·pa·la·ti·na** [TA] SYN sphenopalatine artery.

**ar·te·ria sty·lo·mas·toi·dea** [TA] SYN stylomastoid artery.

**ar·te·ria sub·cla·via** [TA] SYN subclavian artery.

**ar·te·ria sub·cos·ta·lis** [TA] SYN subcostal artery.

**ar·te·ria sub·lin·gua·lis** [TA] SYN sublingual artery.

**ar·te·ria sub·men·ta·lis** [TA] SYN submental artery.

**ar·te·ria sub·scap·u·la·ris** [TA] SYN subscapular artery.

**ar·te·ria su·pra·or·bi·ta·lis** [TA] SYN supraorbital artery.

**ar·te·ria su·pra·scap·u·la·ris** [TA] SYN suprascapular artery.

**ar·te·ria su·pra·troch·le·a·ris** [TA] SYN supratrochlear artery.

**ar·te·ria su·ra·lis** [TA] SYN sural artery.

**ar·te·ria tes·ti·cu·la·ris** [TA] SYN testicular artery.

**ar·te·ria tho·ra·co·a·cro·mi·a·lis** [TA] SYN thoracoacromial artery.

**ar·te·ria tho·ra·co·dor·sa·lis** [TA] SYN thoracodorsal artery.

**ar·te·ria trans·ver·sa col·li** [TA] SYN transverse cervical artery.

**ar·te·ria trans·ver·sa fa·ci·ei** [TA] SYN transverse facial artery.

**ar·te·ria ul·na·ris** [TA] SYN ulnar artery.

**ar·te·ria um·bi·li·ca·lis** [TA] SYN umbilical artery.

**ar·te·ria u·re·thra·lis** [TA] SYN urethral artery.

**ar·te·ria u·te·ri·na** [TA] SYN uterine artery.

**ar·te·ria va·gi·na·lis** [TA] SYN vaginal artery.

**ar·te·ria ver·te·bra·lis** [TA] SYN vertebral artery.

**ar·te·ria zy·go·mat·i·co·or·bi·ta·lis** [TA] SYN zygomatico-orbital artery.

**ar·te·ri·ec·to·my** (ar-tēr-ē-ek′tō-mē) excision of part of an artery. [L. *arteria*, artery, + G. *ektomē*, excision]

**ar·te·ries of brain** arteries and arterial branches supplying the brain; they are derived from the cerebral arterial circle and the anterior choroidal artery.

**ar·ter·ies of pe·nis** SEE dorsal artery of penis, deep artery of penis.

△**arterio-, arteri-** artery. [L. *arteria*, fr. G. *artēria*, a windpipe, an artery]

**ar·te·ri·o·cap·il·lary** (ar-tēr′ē-ō-kap′i-lār-ē) relating to both arteries and capillaries.

**ar·te·ri·o·gram** (ar-tēr′ē-ō-gram) radiographic demonstration of an artery after injection of contrast medium. [arterio- + G. *gramma*, something written]

**ar·te·ri·o·graph·ic** (ar-tēr′ē-ō-graf′ik) relating to or utilizing arteriography.

▣**ar·te·ri·og·ra·phy** (ar-tēr-ē-og′ră-fē) visualization of an artery or arteries by x-ray imaging after injection of a radiopaque contrast medium. See this page. [arterio- + G. *graphō*, to write]

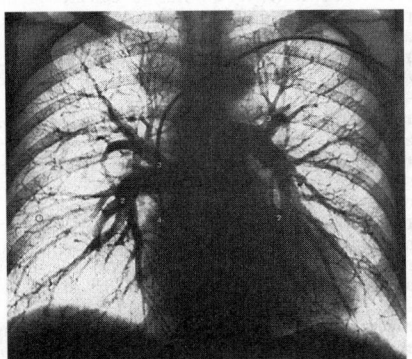

**arteriography:** normal study of the pulmonary arteries

**ar·te·ri·o·la**, pl. **ar·te·ri·o·lae** (ar-tēr-ē-ō′lă, ar-tēr-ē-ō′lē) [TA] SYN arteriole. [Mod. L. dim. of *arteria*, artery]

**ar·te·ri·o·la glo·mer·u·lar·is af·fer·ens** [TA] SYN afferent glomerular arteriole.

**ar·te·ri·o·la glo·mer·u·la·ris ef·fer·ens** [TA] SYN ductus deferens.

**ar·te·ri·o·la ma·cu·la·ris in·fe·ri·or** [TA] SYN inferior macular arteriole.

**ar·te·ri·o·la ma·cu·la·ris su·pe·ri·or** [TA] SYN superior macular arteriole.

**ar·te·ri·o·lar** (ar-ter-ē-ō′lăr) of or pertaining to an arteriole or the arterioles collectively.

**ar·te·ri·o·lar neph·ro·scle·ro·sis** renal scarring due to arteriolar sclerosis resulting from long-standing hypertension; chronic renal failure develops infrequently. SYN arteriolonephrosclerosis.

**ar·te·ri·o·lar net·work** a vascular network formed by anastomoses between minute arteries just before they become capillaries.

**ar·te·ri·ole** (ar-tēr′ē-ōl) a minute artery with a tunica media comprising only one or two layers of smooth muscle cells; a terminal artery continuous with the capillary network. See this page. SYN arteriola [TA].

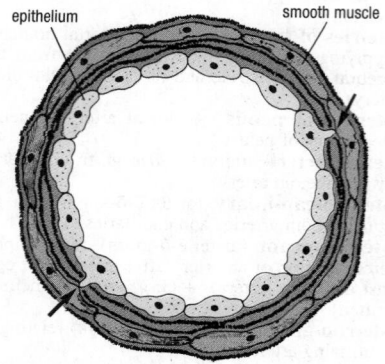

epithelium     smooth muscle

**arteriole:** arrows show points of contact between epithelium and smooth muscle

**ar·te·ri·o·lith** (ar-tēr′ē-ō-lith) a calcareous deposit in an arterial wall or thrombus. [L. *arteria,* artery, + G. *lithos,* a stone]

**ar·ter·i·o·li·tis** (ar-tēr′ē-ō-lī′tis) inflammation of the wall of the arterioles. [L. *arteriola,* arteriole, + G. *-itis,* inflammation]

△**ar·te·ri·o·lo-** the arterioles. [Modern L. *arteriola,* arteriole]

**ar·te·ri·o·lo·ne·cro·sis** (ar-tēr-ē-ō′lō-ně-krō′sis) SYN necrotizing arteriolitis. [L. *arteriola,* arteriole, + G. *nekrōsis,* a killing]

**ar·te·ri·o·lo·neph·ro·scle·ro·sis** (ar-tēr-ē-ō′lō-nef′rō-skler-ō-sis) SYN arteriolar nephrosclerosis.

**ar·te·ri·o·lo·scle·ro·sis** (ar-tēr-ē-ō′lō-skler-ō′sis) arteriosclerosis affecting mainly the arterioles, seen especially in chronic hypertension.

**ar·te·ri·o·mo·tor** (ar-tēr′ē-ō-mō′ter) causing changes in the caliber of an artery; vasomotor with special reference to the arteries.

**ar·te·ri·o·neph·ro·scle·ro·sis** (ar-tēr′ē-ō-nef′rō-skler-ō′sis) SYN arterial nephrosclerosis.

**ar·te·ri·op·a·thy** (ar-tēr-ē-op′ă-thē) any disease of the arteries. [arterio- + G. *pathos,* suffering]

**ar·te·ri·o·plas·ty** (ar-tēr′ē-ō-plas-tē) any operation for the reconstruction of the wall of an artery. [arterio- + G. *plastos,* formed]

**ar·te·ri·o·pres·sor** (ar-tēr′ē-ō-pres′ser) causing increased arterial blood pressure.

**ar·te·ri·or·rha·phy** (ar-tēr-ē-ōr′ă-fē) suture of an artery. [arterio- + G. *rhaphē,* seam]

**ar·te·ri·or·rhex·is** (ar-tēr′ē-ō-rek′sis) rupture of an artery. [arterio- + G. *rhēxis,* rupture]

**ar·te·ri·o·scle·ro·sis** (ar-tēr′ē-ō-skler-ō′sis) hardening of the arteries; types generally recognized are: atherosclerosis, Mönckeberg arteriosclerosis, and arteriolosclerosis. SYN arterial sclerosis. [arterio- + G. *sklērōsis,* hardness]

**ar·te·ri·o·scle·ro·sis ob·lit·er·ans** arteriosclerosis producing narrowing and occlusion of the arterial lumen.

**ar·te·ri·o·scle·rot·ic** (ar-tēr′ē-ō-skler-ot′ik) relating to or affected by arteriosclerosis.

**ar·te·ri·o·scle·rot·ic an·eu·rysm** the most com-

mon type of aneurysm, occurring in the abdominal aorta and other large arteries, primarily in the elderly.

**ar·te·ri·o·spasm** (ar-tēr′ē-ō-spazm) spasm of an artery or arteries.

**ar·te·ri·o·ste·no·sis** (ar-tēr′ē-ō-stě-nō′sis) narrowing of the caliber of an artery, either temporary, through vasoconstriction, or permanent, through arteriosclerosis. [arterio- + G. *stenōsis,* a narrowing]

**ar·te·ri·ot·o·my** (ar-tēr-ē-ot′ō-mē) any surgical incision into the lumen of an artery, e.g., to remove an embolus. [arterio- + G. *tomē,* incision]

**ar·te·ri·o·ve·nous (A-V, AV)** (ar-tēr′ē-ō-vē′nŭs) relating to both an artery and a vein or to both arteries and veins in general; both arterial and venous, as an "arteriovenous (A-V) anastomosis."

**ar·te·ri·o·ve·nous a·nas·to·mo·sis (ava)** vessels through which blood is shunted from arterioles to venules without passing through the capillaries.

**ar·te·ri·o·ve·nous an·eu·rysm 1.** a dilated arteriovenous shunt. **2.** communication between an artery and a vein, sometimes congenital.

**ar·te·ri·o·ve·nous car·bon di·ox·ide dif·fer·ence** the difference in carbon dioxide content (in ml per 100 ml blood) between arterial and venous blood.

**ar·te·ri·o·ve·nous fis·tu·la** an abnormal communication between an artery and a vein, usually resulting in the formation of an arteriovenous aneurysm.

**ar·te·ri·o·ve·nous ox·y·gen dif·fer·ence** the difference in the oxygen content (in ml per 100 ml blood) between arterial and venous blood.

**ar·te·ri·o·ve·nous shunt** the passage of blood directly from arteries to veins, without going through the capillary network.

**ar·te·ri·tis** (ar-ter-ī′tis) inflammation or infection involving an artery or arteries. [L. *arteria,* artery, + G. *-itis,* inflammation]

**ar·te·ri·tis ob·li·te·rans, ob·lit·er·at·ing ar·te·ri·tis** SYN endarteritis obliterans.

**ar·tery** (ar′ter-ē) a relatively thick-walled, muscular blood vessel conveying blood in a direction away from the heart and pulsating with each heartbeat. With the exception of the pulmonary and umbilical arteries, the arteries convey red or aerated blood. See page 77. SYN arteria [TA]. [L. *arteria,* fr. G. *artēria*]

**ar·tery of an·gu·lar gy·rus** the last branch of the terminal part of the middle cerebral artery distributed to parts of the temporal, parietal, and occipital lobes.

**ar·tery of bulb of pe·nis** a branch of the internal pudendal artery which supplies the bulb of the penis including the bulbar urethra. SYN arteria bulbi penis [TA].

**ar·tery of bulb of ves·ti·bule** the branch of the internal pudendal artery in the female that supplies the bulb of the vestibule. SYN arteria bulbi vestibuli [TA].

**ar·tery to duc·tus def·er·ens** *origin,* anterior division of internal iliac, or sometimes superior vesical; *distribution,* ductus deferens, seminal vesicles, testicle, ureter; *anastomoses,* testicular, cremasteric arteries. SYN arteria ductus deferentis [TA].

**ar·tery of the pan·cre·at·ic tail** *origin,* splenic artery near the left gastroepiploic; *distribution,*

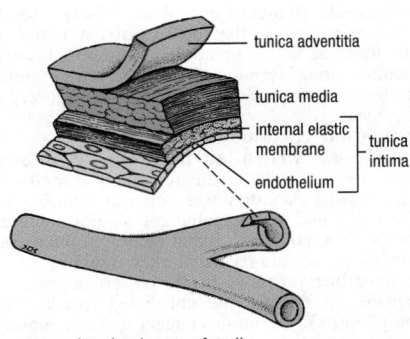

tunica adventitia

tunica media

internal elastic membrane — tunica intima

endothelium

**artery:** showing layers of wall

the tail of the pancreas; *anastomoses*, with other pancreatic arteries.

**ar·tery of pter·y·goid ca·nal** *origin*: usually arises from the third part of the maxillary artery, but frequently from the greater palatine artery, within the pterygopalatine fossa. Passes posteriorly to run through the pterygoid canal with the corresponding nerve, supplying the contents and wall of the canal, the mucous membrane of the upper pharynx, the auditory tube and the tympanic cavity. SYN arteria canalis pterygoidei [TA].

**ar·tery of round lig·a·ment of uter·us** *origin*, inferior epigastric; *distribution*, round ligament of uterus. SYN arteria ligamenti teretis uteri [TA].

**ar·tery to sci·at·ic nerve** *origin*, inferior gluteal; *distribution*, sciatic nerve; *anastomoses*, branches of profunda femoris.

**ar·thral·gia** (ar-thral′jē-ă) pain in a joint, especially one not inflammatory in character. SYN arthrodynia. [G. *arthron*, joint, + *algos*, pain]

**ar·thral·gic** (ar-thral′jik) relating to or affected with arthralgia. SYN arthrodynic.

**ar·threc·to·my** (ar-threk′tō-mē) excision of a joint. [G. *arthron*, joint, + *ektomē*, excision]

**ar·thrit·ic** (ar-thrit′ik) relating to arthritis.

**ar·thrit·ic gen·er·al pseu·do·pa·ral·y·sis** a disease, occurring in arthritic subjects, having symptoms resembling those of general paresis, the lesions of which consist of diffuse changes of a degenerative and noninflammatory character due to intracranial atheroma.

**ar·thri·tis**, pl. **ar·thrit·i·des** (ar-thrī′tis, ar-thrit′ i-dēz) inflammation of a joint or a state characterized by inflammation of joints. SYN articular rheumatism. [G. fr. *arthron*, joint, + *-itis*, inflammation]

**ar·thri·tis de·for·mans** SYN rheumatoid arthritis.

△**ar·thro-, arthr-** a joint, an articulation; corresponds to L. *articul-*. [G. *arthron*, a joint, fr. *arariskō*, to join, to fit together]

**ar·thro·cele** (ar′thrō-sēl) **1.** hernia of the synovial membrane through the capsule of a joint. **2.** any swelling of a joint. [arthro- + G. *kēlē*, hernia, tumor]

**ar·thro·cen·te·sis** (ar′thrō-sen-tē′is) aspiration of fluid from a joint through a needle. [arthro- + G. *kentēsis*, puncture]

**ar·thro·chon·dri·tis** (ar′thrō-kon-drī′tis) inflammation of an articular cartilage. [arthro- + G. *chondros*, cartilage, + *-itis*, inflammation]

**ar·thro·cla·sia** (ar-thrō-klā′zē-ă) forcible break-ing up of adhesions in ankylosis. [arthro- + G. *klasis*, a breaking]

**Arth·ro·der·ma** (ar′thrō-der′mă) a genus of ascomycetous fungi composed of the anamorph genera *Microsporium* and *Trichoderma* species.

**ar·throd·e·sis** (ar-throd′ĕ-sis, ar-thrō-dē′sis) the stiffening of a joint by operative means. SYN artificial ankylosis, syndesis. [arthro- + G. *desis*, a binding together]

**ar·thro·dia** (ar-thrō′dē-ă) SYN plane joint. [G. *arthrōdia*, a gliding joint, fr. *arthron*, joint, + *eidos*, form]

**ar·thro·di·al** (ar-thrō′dē-ăl) relating to arthrodia.

**ar·thro·di·al joint** SYN plane joint.

**ar·thro·dyn·ia** (ar-thrō-din′ē-ă) SYN arthralgia. [arthro- + G. *odynē*, pain]

**ar·thro·dyn·ic** (ar-thrō-din′ik) SYN arthralgic.

**ar·thro·dys·pla·sia** (ar′thrō-dis-plā′zē-ă) hereditary congenital defect of joint development. [arthro- + G. *dys*, bad, + *plasis*, a molding]

**ar·thro·en·dos·co·py** (ar′thrō-en-dos′kŏ-pē) SYN arthroscopy.

**ar·thro·gram** (ar′thrō-gram) roentgenogram of a joint; usually implies the introduction of a contrast agent into the joint capsule. [arthro- + G. *gramma*, a writing]

**ar·throg·ra·phy** (ar-throg′ră-fē) radiography of a joint after injecting one or more contrast media into the joint. [arthro- + G. *graphō*, to describe]

**ar·thro·gry·po·sis** (ar′thrō-gri-pō′sis) congenital defect of the limbs characterized by contractures of joints. [arthro- + G. *gryphōsis*, a crooking]

**ar·thro·gry·po·sis mul·ti·plex con·gen·i·ta** limitation of range of joint motion and contractures present at birth, usually involving multiple joints; a syndrome probably of diverse etiology that may result from changes in spinal cord, muscle, or connective tissue.

**ar·thro·kin·e·mat·ics** (ar-thrō-kin-ĕ-mat′iks) the study of movements between adjoining articular (joint) surfaces. [arthro- + G. *kinēma, kinēmatos*, movement, + *-ics*]

**ar·throl·y·sis** (ar-throl′i-sis) restoration of mobility in stiff and ankylosed joints. [arthro- + G. *lysis*, a loosening]

**ar·throm·e·ter** (ar-throm′ĕ-ter) SYN goniometer (3).

**ar·throm·e·try** (ar-throm′ĕ-trē) measurement of the range of movement in a joint. [arthro- + G. *metron*, measure]

**ar·thro-oph·thal·mop·a·thy** (ar′thrō-of′thal-mop′ă-thē) disease affecting joints and eyes. [arthro- + ophthalmo- + G. *pathos*, suffering]

**ar·thro·path·ia pso·ri·a·ti·ca** SYN psoriatic arthritis.

**ar·throp·a·thy** (ar-throp′ă-thē) any disease affecting a joint. [arthro- + G. *pathos*, suffering]

**ar·thro·plas·ty** (ar′thrō-plas-tē) **1.** creation of an artificial joint to correct ankylosis. **2.** an operation to restore as far as possible the integrity and functional power of a joint. [arthro- + G. *plastos*, formed]

**ar·thro·pneu·mo·ra·di·og·raph·y** (ar′thrō-noo′ mō-rā-dē-og′ra-fē) radiographic examination of a joint after it has been injected with air. [arthro- + pneumo- + radiography]

**ar·thro·pod** (ar′thrō-pod) a member of the phylum Arthropoda. [arthro- + G. *pous*, foot]

**Ar·throp·o·da** (ar-throp′ŏ-dă) a phylum of the Metazoa that includes the classes Crustacea (crabs, shrimps, crayfish, lobsters), Insecta,

Arachnida (spiders, scorpions, mites, ticks), Chilopoda (centipedes), Diplopoda (millipedes), Merostomata (horseshoe crabs), and various other extinct or lesser known groups. Arthropoda forms the largest assemblage of living organisms, 75% insects, of which over a million species are known. [arthro- + G. *pous,* foot]

**ar·thro·po·di·a·sis** (ar'thrō-pō-dī'ă-sis) direct effects of arthropods upon vertebrates, including acariasis, allergy, dermatosis, entomophobia, and actions of contact toxins.

**ar·thro·py·o·sis** (ar'thrō-pī-ō'sis) suppuration in a joint. [arthro- + G. *pyōsis,* suppuration]

**ar·thro·scle·ro·sis** (ar'thrō-skler-ō'sis) stiffness of the joints, especially in the aged. [arthro- + G. *sklērōsis,* hardening]

**ar·thro·scope** (ar'thrō-skōp) an endoscope for examining the interior of a joint.

**ar·thros·co·py** (ar-thros'kŏ-pē) endoscopic examination of the interior of a joint. SYN arthroendoscopy. [arthro- + G. *skopeō,* to view]

**ar·thro·sis** (ar-thrō'sis) 1. SYN joint. [G. *arthrōsis,* a jointing] 2. a degenerative disorder of a joint. [arthro- + G. *-osis,* condition]

**ar·thros·to·my** (ar-thros'tō-mē) establishment of a temporary opening into a joint cavity. [arthro- + G. *stoma,* mouth]

**ar·thro·sy·no·vi·tis** (ar'thrō-sin-ō-vī'tis) inflammation of the synovial membrane of a joint.

**ar·throt·o·my** (ar-throt'ŏ-mē) cutting into a joint. [arthro- + G. *tomē,* a cutting]

**ar·throx·e·sis** (ar-throk'sĕ-sis) removal of diseased tissue from a joint by means of the sharp spoon or other scraping instrument. [arthro- + G. *xesis,* a scraping]

**ar·tic·u·lar** (ar-tik'yu-lăr) relating to a joint.

**ar·tic·u·lar cap·sule** a sac enclosing a joint, formed by an outer fibrous articular capsule and an inner synovial membrane. SYN capsula articularis [TA], joint capsule.

**ar·tic·u·lar car·ti·lage** the cartilage covering the articular surfaces of the bones participating in a synovial joint.

**ar·tic·u·lar cor·pus·cles** encapsulated nerve terminations within joint capsules. SYN corpuscula articularia [TA].

**ar·tic·u·lar crest** SYN intermediate sacral crest.

**ar·tic·u·lar disk** a plate or ring of fibrocartilage attached to the joint capsule and separating the articular surfaces of the bones for a varying distance, sometimes completely; it serves to adapt two articular surfaces that are not entirely congruent.

**ar·ti·cu·la·ris cu·bi·ti mus·cle** the name applied to a small slip of the medial head of the triceps that inserts into the capsule of the elbow joint. SYN musculus articularis cubiti [TA].

**ar·ti·cu·la·ris gen·us mus·cle** *origin,* lower fourth of anterior surface of shaft of femur; *insertion,* suprapatellar bursa of knee joint; *action,* retracts suprapatellar bursa, during extension of knee; *nerve supply,* femoral. SYN musculus articularis genus [TA].

**ar·tic·u·lar la·mel·la** the compact layer of bone on its articular surface that is firmly attached to the overlying articular cartilage.

**ar·tic·u·lar mus·cle** a muscle that inserts directly onto the capsule of a joint, acting to retract the capsule in certain movements.

**ar·tic·u·lar nerve** a branch of a nerve supplying a joint.

**ar·ti·cu·lar pro·cess** one of the bilateral small flat projections on the surfaces of the arches of the vertebae, at the point where the pedicles and laminae join, forming the zygapophysial joint surfaces. SYN processus articularis [TA], zygapophysis.

**ar·tic·u·lar rheu·ma·tism** SYN arthritis.

**ar·tic·u·lar vas·cu·lar net·work of el·bow** vascular networks in the region of the elbow, composed of anastomoses between branches of the radial and middle collateral, superior and inferior ulnar collateral, radial recurrent, interosseous recurrent, and recurrent ulnar arteries.

**ar·tic·u·late** (ar-tik'yu-lit) 1. SYN articulated. 2. capable of distinct and connected speech. (ar-tik'yū-lāt). 3. to join or connect together loosely to allow motion between the parts. 4. to speak distinctly and connectedly. [L. *articulo,* pp. *-atus,* to articulate]

**ar·tic·u·lat·ed** (ar-tik'yu-lā-ted) jointed. SYN articulate (1).

**ar·tic·u·la·tio,** pl. **ar·tic·u·la·ti·o·nes** (ar-tik-ū-lā'shē-ō, ar-tik-ū-lā-shē-ō'nēz) [TA] SYN synovial joint. [L. a forming of vines]

**ar·tic·u·la·tion** (ar-tik-yu-lā'shŭn) 1. SYN joint. 2. a joining or connecting together loosely so as to allow motion between the parts. 3. distinct connected speech or enunciation. 4. in dentistry, the contact relationship of the occlusal surfaces of the teeth during jaw movement. SEE synovial joint.

**ar·tic·u·la·tion dis·or·der** any error in pronunciation including phoneme omissions, substitutions, distortions, and additions.

**ar·tic·u·la·tor** (ar-tik'yu-lā-těr) a mechanical device which represents the temporomandibular joints and jaw members to which maxillary and mandibular casts may be attached.

**ar·tic·u·la·tors** organs of the speech mechanism that form the configurations required for production of meaningful speech sounds, i.e., the teeth, lips, mandible, tongue, velum, and pharynx. SEE ALSO speech mechanism.

**ar·tic·u·la·to·ry a·prax·ia** SYN verbal apraxia.

**ar·ti·fact** (ar'ti-fakt) 1. anything, especially in a histologic specimen or a graphic record, that is caused by the technique used or is not a natural occurrence, but is merely incidental. 2. a skin lesion produced or perpetuated by self-inflicted action, as in dermatitis artefacta. SYN artefact. [L. *ars,* art, + *facio,* pp. *factus,* to make]

**ar·ti·fac·tu·al, ar·ti·fac·ti·tious** (ar-ti-fak'chyu-ăl, ar'ti-fak-tish'ŭs) produced or caused by an artifact.

**ar·ti·fi·cial an·ky·lo·sis** SYN arthrodesis.

**ar·ti·fi·cial heart** a mechanical pump used to replace the function of a damaged heart, either temporarily or as a permanent prosthesis.

**ar·ti·fi·cial in·sem·i·na·tion** the introduction of semen into the vagina other than by coitus.

**ar·ti·fi·cial kid·ney** SYN hemodialyzer.

**ar·ti·fi·cial lar·ynx** mechanical device used to create alaryngeal speech. The most common types are battery powered and provide a buzzing sound source; the vibrating source is placed against the neck or in the oral cavity via a tube, and speech is articulated normally. Pneumatic assistive listening devices use expired air from the trachea to create vibration, which is relayed to the oral cavity by a tube. SYN electrolarynx.

**ar·ti·fi·cial mem·brane rup·ture** rupture of the

membranes induced by use of an amniohook or similar device.

**ar·ti·fi·cial nose** SYN hygroscopic condenser humidifier.

**ar·ti·fi·cial pace·mak·er** any device that substitutes for the normal pacemaker and controls the rhythm of the organ; especially an electronic cardiac pacemaker, which may be implanted in the chest, with electrodes attached to the external cardiac surface, or passed through the venous circulation into the right side of the heart (pervenous pacemaker).

**ar·ti·fi·cial pneu·mo·thor·ax** pneumothorax produced by the injection of air, or a more slowly absorbed gas such as nitrogen, into the pleural space to collapse the lung.

**ar·ti·fi·cial ra·di·o·ac·tiv·i·ty** the radioactivity of isotopes created by the bombardment of naturally occurring isotopes by subatomic particles, or high levels of x- or gamma radiation.

**ar·ti·fi·cial res·pi·ra·tion** SYN artificial ventilation.

**ar·ti·fi·cial se·lec·tion** interference with natural selection by purposeful breeding of animals or plants of specific genotype or phenotype to produce a strain with desired characteristics.

**ar·ti·fi·cial ven·ti·la·tion** application of mechanically or manually generated pressures, usually positive, to gas(es) in or about the airway as a means of producing gas exchange between the lungs and surrounding atmosphere. SYN artificial respiration.

**ar·y·ep·i·glot·tic fold, ar·y·te·no·ep·i·glot··tid·e·an fold** a prominent fold of mucous membrane stretching between the lateral margin of the epiglottis and the arytenoid cartilage on either side; it encloses the aryepiglottic muscle. SYN plica aryepiglottica [TA].

**ar·y·ep·i·glot·tic mus·cle** the fibers of the oblique arytenoid muscle that extend from the summit of the arytenoid cartilage to the side of the epiglottis; *action,* constricts the laryngeal aperture. SYN musculus aryepiglotticus [TA].

**ar·yl** (ar′il) an organic radical derived from an aromatic compound by removing a hydrogen atom.

**ar·yl·sul·fa·tase** (ar-il-sŭl′fă-tās) an enzyme that cleaves phenol sulfates, including cerebroside sulfates (i.e., a phenol sulfate + $H_2O \rightarrow$ a phenol + sulfate anion). Some arylsulfatases are inhibited by sulfate (type II) and some are not (type I). SYN sulfatase (2).

**ar·y·te·noid** (ar-ĭ-tē′noyd) denoting a cartilage (arytenoid cartilage) and muscles (oblique and transverse arytenoid muscles) of the larynx.

**ar·y·te·noid car·ti·lage** one of a pair of small triangular pyramidal laryngeal cartilages that articulate with the lamina of the cricoid cartilage. It gives attachment at its anteriorly directed vocal process to the posterior part of the corresponding vocal ligament and to several muscles at its laterally-directed muscular process. SYN cartilago arytenoidea [TA].

**ar·y·te·noid dis·lo·ca·tion** separation of the cricoarytenoid joint with subluxation of the arytenoid cartilage.

**ar·y·te·noi·dec·to·my** (ar′ĭ-tē-noy-dek′tō-mē) excision of an arytenoid cartilage, usually in bilateral vocal fold paralysis, to improve breathing. [arytenoid + G. *ektomē,* excision]

**ar·yt·e·noi·di·tis** (ă-rĭt′ĕ-noy-dī′tis) inflamma-

tion of an arytenoid cartilage or its mucosal cover.

**ar·y·te·noi·do·pexy** (ar′ĭ-tĕ-noy′dō-pek′sē) fixation by surgery of cartilages or muscles of arytenoids. [arytenoid + G. *pēxis,* fixation]

**A.S.** *auris sinistra* [L.], left ear.

**As** arsenic.

**as·bes·tos** (as-bes′tŏs) product obtained from fibrous hydrated silicates divided into amphiboles and serpentines; it is insoluble and is used to provide tensile strength and moldability, thermal insulation, and resistance to fire, heat, and corrosion; inhalation of asbestos particles can cause asbestosis and cancer of the lung and pleura. [G. unquenchable; so called in the erroneous belief that when heated, it could not be quenched]

**as·bes·tos bod·ies** ferruginous bodies with asbestos fibers as a core; a histologic hallmark of exposure to asbestos.

**as·bes·to·sis** (as-bes-tō′sis) pneumoconiosis due to inhalation of asbestos fibers suspended in the ambient air; sometimes complicated by pleural mesothelioma or bronchogenic carcinoma.

**as·ca·ri·a·sis** (as-kă-rī′ă-sis) disease caused by infection with *Ascaris* or related ascarid nematodes. [G. *askaris,* an intestinal worm, + *-iasis,* condition]

**as·car·i·cide** (as-kar′i-sīd) **1.** causing the death of ascarid nematodes. **2.** an agent having such properties. [ascarid + L. *caedo,* to kill]

*As·ca·ris* (as′kă-ris) a genus of large, heavy-bodied roundworms parasitic in the small intestine; abundant in humans and many other vertebrates. [G. *askaris,* an intestinal worm]

*As·ca·ris lum·bri·coi·des* a large roundworm of humans, one of the commonest human parasites; various symptoms such as restlessness, fever, and diarrhea are attributed to its presence, but usually it causes no definite symptoms. See this page.

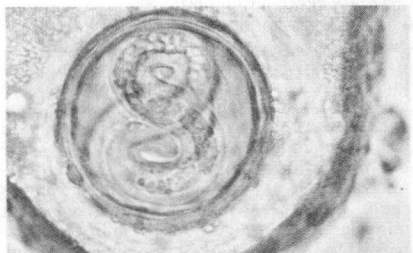

***Ascaris lumbricoides:*** egg containing larvae

**as·cend·ing ar·tery** the branch of the inferior branch of the ileocolic artery that passes superiorly along the ascending colon to communicate with a branch of the right colic artery to supply the ascending colon. SYN arteria ascendens [TA].

**as·cend·ing branch of the in·fe·ri·or mes··en·ter·ic ar·tery** branch of the left colic artery (from inferior mesenteric artery) that passes anteriorly to the left kidney into the transverse mesocolon, where it anastomoses with the middle colic artery. It thus forms an anastomosis between superior and inferior mesenteric arteries, and is a component of the marginal artery (Drummond) of the colon.

**as·cend·ing co·lon** the portion of the colon between the ileocecal orifice and the right colic flexure.

**as·cend·ing de·gen·er·a·tion 1.** retrograde degeneration of an injured nerve fiber; i.e., toward the nerve cell of the fiber; **2.** degeneration cephalad to a spinal cord lesion.

**as·cend·ing lum·bar vein** a paired, vertical vein of the posterior abdominal wall, adjacent and parallel to the vertebral column, posterior to the origin of the psoas major muscle; it connects the common iliac, iliolumbar, and lumbar veins in the paravertebral line, the right vein joining the right subcostal vein to form the azygos vein, the left vein uniting with the left subcostal vein to form the hemiazygos vein.

**as·cend·ing pha·ryn·ge·al ar·tery** *origin,* external carotid; *distribution,* wall of pharynx and soft palate, posterior cranial fossa. SYN arteria pharyngea ascendens [TA].

**as·cer·tain·ment bi·as** systematic failure to represent equally all classes of cases or persons supposed to be represented in a sample.

**Asch·er syn·drome** (ahsh′ĕr) a condition in which a congenital double lip is associated with blepharochalasis and nontoxic thyroid gland enlargement.

**Asch·off bod·ies** (ahsh′of) a form of granulomatous inflammation observed in acute rheumatic carditis.

**as·ci·tes** (ă-sī′tēz) accumulation of serous fluid in the peritoneal cavity. SYN hydroperitoneum, hydroperitonia. [L. fr. G. *askos,* a bag, + *-ites*]

**ascit·ic** (ă-sit′ik) relating to ascites.

**As·co·my·ce·tes** (as′kō-mī-sē′tēz) a class of fungi characterized by the presence of asci and ascospores. Such fungi have generally two distinct reproductive phases, the sexual or perfect stage and the asexual or imperfect stage. *Ajellomyces capsulatum* and *Ajellomyces dermatitidis* are pathogenic members of this class. [G. *askos,* a bag, + *mykēs,* mushroom]

**as·cor·bate** (as-kōr′bāt) a salt or ester of ascorbic acid.

**as·cor·bate ox·i·dase** a copper-containing enzyme that catalyzes the oxidation of L-ascorbic acid with $O_2$ to L-dehydroascorbic acid. Some forms of ascorbate oxidase use $NADP^+$ as well. Used as an antitumor agent.

**ascor·bic ac·id** (as-kōr′bik as′id) 2,3-didehydro-L-*threo*-hexono-1,4-lactone; used in preventing scurvy, as a strong reducing agent, and as an antioxidant in foodstuffs. SYN vitamin C. [G. *a*-priv. + Mod.L. *scorbutus,* scurvy, fr. Germanic]

**ASCUS** atypical squamous cells of undetermined significance.

**△-ase** a termination denoting an enzyme, suffixed to the name of the substance (substrate) upon which the enzyme acts; e.g., phosphatase, lipase, proteinase. May also indicate the reaction catalyzed e.g., decarboxylase, oxidase. [Fr. *(diast)-ase,* an amylase that converts starch to maltose, fr. G. *diastasis,* separation, fr. *dia-,* through, apart, + *stasis,* a standing]

**A·sel·li gland** (ă-sel′ē) a single large lymph node ventral to the abdominal aorta that receives all the lymph from the intestines in many smaller mammals.

**as·e·ma·sia, ase·mia** (as-ĕ-mā′zē-ă, ă-sē′mē-ă) SYN asymbolia. [G. *a*- priv. + *sēmasia,* the giving of a signal, fr. *sēma,* sign]

**asep·sis** (ā-sep′sis) a condition in which living pathogenic organisms are absent; a state of sterility (2). [G. *a*- priv. + *sēpsis,* putrefaction]

**asep·tic** (ā-sep′tik) marked by or relating to asepsis.

**asep·tic ne·cro·sis** death or decay of tissue due to local ischemia in the absence of infection. SYN avascular necrosis.

**asep·tic sur·gery** the performance of an operation with sterilized hands, instruments, etc., and utilizing precautions against the introduction of infectious microorganisms from without.

**asex·u·al** (ā-seks′yu-ăl) **1.** referring to reproduction without nuclear fusion in an organism. **2.** having no sexual desire or interest. [G. *a*- priv. + sexual]

**asex·u·al dwarf·ism** dwarfism in which adult sexual development is deficient.

**asex·u·al gen·er·a·tion** reproduction by fission, gemmation, or in any other way without union of the male and female cell, or conjugation. SEE ALSO parthenogenesis. SYN heterogenesis (2), nonsexual generation.

**asex·u·al re·pro·duc·tion** reproduction other than by union of male and female sex cells.

**Ash·er·man syn·drome** (ash′ĕr-măn) SYN traumatic amenorrhea.

**ash-leaf mac·ule** a hypopigmented, often ash-leaf-shaped macule that is present at birth in many patients with tuberous sclerosis.

**Ash·man phe·nom·e·non** (ash′măn) aberrant ventricular conduction of a beat ending a short cycle that is preceded by a longer cycle most commonly during atrial fibrillation.

**asi·a·lism** (ā-sī′ă-lism) absence of saliva. [G. *a*-priv. + *sialon* saliva + -ism]

**ASL** American Sign Language.

**aso·cial** (ā-sō′shŭl) not social; withdrawn from society; indifferent to social rules or customs; e.g., a recluse, a regressed schizophrenic person, a schizoid personality. Cf. antisocial.

**Asp** aspartic acid or its radical forms.

**as·par·tate** (as-par′tāt) a salt or ester of aspartic acid.

**as·par·tate a·mi·no·trans·fer·ase (AST)** an enzyme catalyzing the reversible transfer of an amine group from L-glutamic acid to oxaloacetic acid, forming α-ketoglutaric acid and L-aspartic acid; a diagnostic aid in viral hepatitis and in myocardial infarction. SYN glutamic-oxaloacetic transaminase, serum glutamic-oxaloacetic transaminase.

**as·par·tic ac·id (Asp)** (as-par′tik as′id) the L-isomer is one of the amino acids occurring in proteins. SYN α-aminosuccinic acid.

**β-as·par·tyl(ace·tyl·glu·cos·a·mine)** (bāt-ĕ-as-par′til-as′e-til-gloo′kō-să-mēn) a compound of *N*-acetylglucosamine and asparagine, linked via the amide nitrogen of the latter and carbon-1 of the former. An important structural linkage in many glycoproteins.

**as·pect** (as′pekt) **1.** the manner of appearance; looks. **2.** the side of an object that is directed in any designated direction. [L. *aspectus,* fr. *a*-*spicio,* pp. *-spectus,* to look at]

**As·per·ger disorder** (ahs′pĕr-gĕr) a pervasive developmental disorder characterized by severe and enduring impairment in social skills and restrictive and repetitive behaviors and interests, leading to impaired social and occupational functioning but without significant delays in language development.

**as•per•gil•lo•ma** (as′per-ji-lō′mă) **1.** an infectious granuloma caused by *Aspergillus*. **2.** a variety of bronchopulmonary aspergillosis; a ball-like mass of *Aspergillus fumigatus* colonizing an existing cavity in the lung. [aspergillus + -*oma*, tumor]

**as•per•gil•lo•sis** (as′per-ji-lō′sis) the presence of *Aspergillus* in the tissues or on a mucous surface of humans and animals, and the symptoms produced thereby.

**As•per•gil•lus** (as-per-jil′ŭs) a genus of fungi that contains many species, a number of them with black, brown, or green spores. A few species are pathogenic for man. [Med. L. a sprinkler, fr. L. *aspergo*, to sprinkle]

**as•phyx•ia** (as-fik′sē-ă) impairment of ventilatory exchange of oxygen and carbon dioxide; combined hypercapnia and hypoxia or anoxia. [G. *a*-priv. + *sphyzō*, to throb]

**as•phyx•i•al** (as-fik′sē-ăl) relating to asphyxia.

**as•phyx•ia li•vi•da** a form of asphyxia neonatorum in which the skin is cyanotic, but the heart is strong and the reflexes are preserved.

**as•phyx•ia ne•o•na•to•rum** asphyxia occurring in the newborn.

**as•phyx•i•ate** (as-fik′sē-āt) to induce asphyxia.

**as•phyx•i•at•ing tho•ra•cic dy•stro•phy** hereditary hypoplasia of the thorax, associated with pelvic skeletal abnormality. SYN Jeune syndrome.

**as•phyx•i•a•tion** (as-fik-sē-ā′shŭn) the production of, or the state of, asphyxia.

**as•pi•rate 1.** (as′pi-rāt) to remove by aspiration. **2.** (as′pi-rit) substance removed by aspiration. [L. *a-spiro*, pp. -*atus*, to breathe on, give the H sound]

**as•pi•ra•tion** (as-pi-rā′shŭn) **1.** removal, by suction, of a gas or fluid from a body cavity, from unusual accumulations, or from a container. **2.** the inspiratory sucking into the airways of fluid or foreign body, as of vomitus. **3.** a surgical technique for cataract, requiring a small corneal incision, severance of the lens capsule, fragmentation of the lens material, and removal with a needle. [L. *aspiratio*, fr. *aspiro*, to breathe on]

**as•pi•ra•tion bi•op•sy** SYN needle biopsy.

**as•pi•ra•tion pneu•mo•nia** bronchopneumonia resulting from the inhalation of foreign material, usually food particles or vomit, into the bronchi; pneumonia developing secondary to the presence in the airways of fluid, blood, saliva, or gastric contents.

**as•pi•ra•tor** (as′pi-rā-ter, as′pi-rā-tōr) an apparatus for removing fluid by aspiration from any of the body cavities; it consists usually of a hollow needle or trocar and cannula, connected by tubing with a container vacuumized by a syringe or reversed air (suction) pump.

**asple•nia** (ā-splē′nē-ă) congenital or surgical absence of the spleen.

**asplen•ic** (ă-splen′ik) having no spleen.

**as•sas•sin bug** (ă-sas′in bŭg) an insect of the family Reduviidae that inflicts irritating, painful bites in animals and man; related to the cone-nosed bugs (triatomines), a vector of American trypanosomiasis. [Fr., fr. It. *assassino*, fr. Ar. *hashshāshin*, those addicted to hashish]

**as•say** (as′sā, ă-sā′) **1.** test of purity; trial. **2.** to examine; to subject to analysis. **3.** the quantitative or qualitative evaluation of a substance for impurities, toxicity, etc; the results of such an evaluation. [M.E., fr. O.Fr. *essaier*, fr. L.L. *ex-agium*, a weighing]

**as•sess•ment** (ă-ses′ment) appraisal, evaluation, or measurement, particularly by objective means. [Fr. *assesser*, fr. L. *assideo*, to assist (in judging)]

**As•séz•at tri•an•gle** (ah-sā-zah′) a triangle formed by lines connecting the nasion with the alveolar and nasal point; used to indicate prognathism in comparative craniology.

**as•sim•i•la•tion** (ă-sim-i-lā′shŭn) **1.** incorporation of digested materials from food into the tissues. **2.** amalgamation and modification of newly perceived information and experiences into the existing cognitive structure. [L. *as-similo*, pp. -*atus*, to make alike]

**as•sim•i•la•tion pel•vis** a deformity in which the transverse processes of the last lumbar vertebra are fused with the sacrum, or the last sacral with the first coccygeal body.

**as•sis•tant** provider of support services to a health professional.

**as•sist-con•trol ven•ti•la•tion 1.** continuous mandatory ventilation. **2.** a mode of mechanical ventilation in which all breaths are mandatory and are either patient or machine triggered, and machine cycled; a minimum breathing rate is set but the patient can trigger breaths at a higher frequency.

**as•sist•ed res•pi•ra•tion** SYN assisted ventilation.

**as•sist•ed ven•ti•la•tion** application of mechanically or manually generated positive pressure to gas(es) in or about the airway during inhalation as a means of augmenting movement of gases into the lungs. SYN assisted respiration.

**as•sis•tive lis•ten•ing de•vice (ALD)** any device that improves sound perception for listeners with hearing impairments; usually applied to devices such as closed-loop FM systems used in addition to or instead of hearing aids.

**as•so•ci•at•ed move•ment** a movement of parts that act together.

**as•so•ci•a•tion** (ă-sō-sē-ā′shŭn) **1.** a connection of persons, things, or ideas by some common factor. **2.** a functional connection of two ideas, events, or psychologic phenomena established through learning or experience. SEE ALSO conditioning. **3.** statistical dependence between two or more events, characteristics, or other variables. **4.** in medical genetics, a grouping of congenital anomalies found together more frequently than otherwise expected; the use of this term implies that the cause is unknown. [L. *as-socio*, pp. -*sociatus*, to join to; *ad* + *socius*, companion]

**as•so•ci•a•tion cor•tex, as•so•ci•a•tion ar•e•as** generic term denoting the large expanses of the cerebral cortex that are not sensory or motor in the customary sense, but are involved in advanced stages of sensory information processing, multisensory integration, or sensorimotor integration. SEE ALSO cerebral cortex.

**as•so•ci•a•tion fi•bers** nerve fibers interconnecting subdivisions of the cerebral cortex of the same hemisphere or different segments of the spinal cord on the same side.

**as•so•ci•a•tion test** a word (stimulus word) is spoken to the subject, who is to reply immediately with another word (reaction word) suggested by the first; used as a diagnostic aid in psychiatry and psychology.

**as•so•ci•a•tive a•pha•sia** SYN conduction aphasia.

**as·sort·a·tive mat·ing** selection of a mate with preference for (or aversion to) a particular genotype, i.e., nonrandom mating.

**as·sort·ment** (ă-sōrt′ment) in genetics, the relationship between nonallelic genetic traits that are transmitted from parent to child more or less independently in accordance with the degree of linkage between the respective loci.

**AST** aspartate aminotransferase.

**asta·sia** (ă-stā′zē-ă) inability, through muscular incoordination, to stand. [G. unsteadiness, from *a*-priv. + *stasis*, standing]

**asta·sia-aba·sia** (ă-stā′zē-ă-ă-bā′zē-ă) inability to stand or walk in a normal manner; the gait is bizarre and often the patient sways and nearly falls, but recovers at the last moment; a symptom of hysteria-conversion reaction. SYN Blocq disease.

**astat·ic** (ā-stat′ik) pertaining to astasia.

**astat·ic sei·zure** seizure causing loss of erect posture.

**as·ta·tine (At)** (as′tă-tēn) an artificial radioactive element of the halogen series; atomic no. 85, atomic wt. 211. [G. *astatos*, unstable]

**aste·a·to·sis** (ă-stē-ă-tō′sis) diminished or arrested secretion of the sebaceous glands. [G. *a*-priv. + *stear* (*steat*-), fat]

**as·ter** (as′ter) SYN astrosphere. [Mod. L. fr. G. *astēr*, a star]

**aster·e·og·no·sis** (ă-stēr-ē-og-nō′sis) SYN tactile agnosia. [G. *a*- priv. + *stereos*, solid + *gnōsis*, knowledge]

**as·te·ri·on** (ăs-tē′rē-on) a craniometric point at the junction of the lambdoid, occipitomastoid, and parietomastoid sutures. [G. *asterios*, starry]

**aster·ix·is** (as-ter-ik′sis) involuntary jerking movements, especially in the hands, due to arrhythmic lapses of sustained posture; seen primarily with metabolic and toxic encephalopathies, especially hepatic encephalopathy. SYN flapping tremor. [G. *a*- priv. + *stērixis*, fixed position]

**aster·nal** (ā-ster′năl) **1.** not related to or connected with the sternum, e.g., asternal rib. **2.** without a sternum. [G. *a*- priv. + *sternon*, chest]

**aster·nia** (ă-ster′nē-ă) congenital absence of the sternum.

**as·ter·oid bod·y 1.** an eosinophilic inclusion resembling a star with delicate radiating lines, occurring in a vacuolated area of cytoplasm of a multinucleated giant cell; **2.** a structure that is characteristic of sporotrichosis when found in the skin or secondary lesions of this mycosis; in tissue, it surrounds the 3- to 5-μm in diameter ovoid yeast of *Sporothrix schenkii*.

**as·ter·oid hy·a·lo·sis** numerous small spherical bodies ("snowball" opacities) in the corpus vitreum, visible ophthalmoscopically; an age change, usually unilateral, and not affecting vision.

**as·the·nia** (as-thē′nē-ă) weakness or debility. [G. *astheneia*, weakness, fr. *a*- priv. + *sthenos*, strength]

**as·then·ic** (as-then′ik) **1.** relating to asthenia. **2.** denoting a thin, delicate body habitus.

**as·the·no·pia** (as-thē-nō′pē-ă) subjective symptoms of ocular fatigue, discomfort, lacrimation, and headaches arising from use of the eyes. SYN eyestrain. [G. *astheneia*, weakness, + *ōps*, eye]

**as·the·nop·ic** (as-thē-nop′ik) relating to or suffering from asthenopia.

**as·the·no·sper·mia** (as-thē-nō-sper′mē-ă) loss or reduction of motility of the spermatozoa, frequently associated with infertility. [G. *astheneia*, weakness, + *sperma*, seed, semen]

**asthe·no·zo·o·sper·mia** (as′thē-nō-zō-ō-sperm′ē-ă) loss or reduction of mobility of the spermatozoa, frequently associated with infertility. [G. *astheneia*, weakness + *zōos*, living, + *sperma*, seed, semen, + -ia]

**asth·ma** (az′mă) an inflammatory disease of the lungs characterized by reversible (in most cases) airway obstruction. Originally, a term used to mean "difficult breathing"; now used to denote bronchial asthma. See this page. SYN reactive airways disease. [G.]

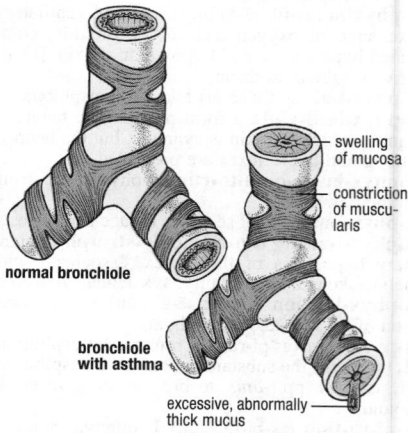

swelling of mucosa

constriction of muscularis

**normal bronchiole**

**bronchiole with asthma**

excessive, abnormally thick mucus

**asthma:** changes in bronchiole during asthma attack

**asth·mat·ic** (az-mat′ik) relating to or suffering from asthma.

**as·tig·mat·ic** (as′tig-mat′ik) relating to or suffering from astigmatism.

**as·tig·mat·ic lens** SYN cylindrical lens.

**astig·ma·tism** (ă-stig′mă-tizm) **1.** a lens or optical system having different refractivity in different meridians. **2.** a condition of unequal curvatures along the different meridians in one or more of the refractive surfaces (cornea, anterior or posterior surface of the lens) of the eye, in consequence of which the rays from a luminous point are not focused at a single point on the retina. SYN astigmia. [G. *a*- priv. + *stigma* (*stigmat*-), a point]

**astig·ma·tom·e·try, as·tig·mom·e·try** (ă-stig-mă-tom′ĕ-trē, as-tig-mom′ĕ-trē) determination of the form and measurement of the degree of astigmatism.

**astig·mia** (ă-stig′mē-ă) SYN astigmatism.

**asto·mia** (ā-stō′mē-ă) congenital absence of a mouth. [G. *a*- priv. + *stoma*, mouth]

**as·trag·a·lar** (as-trag′ă-lar) relating to the astragalus or talus.

**as·trag·a·lec·to·my** (as-trag-ă-lek′tō-mē) removal of the astragalus, or talus. [astragalus, + G. *ektomē*, excision]

**as·tral** (as′trăl) relating to an astrosphere.

**as·trin·gent** (as-trin′jent) **1.** causing contraction of the tissues, arrest of secretion, or control of bleeding. **2.** an agent having these effects. [L. *astringens*]

**as·tro·blast** (as'trō-blast) a primordial cell developing into an astrocyte. [G. *astron,* star, + *blastos,* germ]

**as·tro·blas·to·ma** (as'trō-blas-tō'mă) a relatively poorly differentiated glioma composed of young, immature, neoplastic cells of the astrocytic series, frequently arranged radially with short fibrils terminating on small blood vessels. [astro- + G. *blastos,* germ, + *-oma,* tumor]

**as·tro·cyte** (as'trō-sīt) one of the large neuroglia cells of nervous tissue. SEE ALSO neuroglia. SYN astroglia, macroglia. [G. *astron,* star, + *kytos,* hollow (cell)]

**as·tro·cy·to·ma** (as'trō-sī-tō'mă) a glioma derived from astrocytes; in persons less than 20 years of age, astrocytomas usually arise in a cerebellar hemisphere; in adults, astrocytoma usually occur in the cerebrum, sometimes growing rapidly and invading extensively. [G. *astron,* star, + *kytos,* cell, + *-oma,* tumor]

**as·trog·lia** (as-trog'lē-ă) SYN astrocyte. [G. *astron,* star, + neuroglia]

**as·tro·sphere** (as'trō-sfēr) a set of radiating microtubules extending outward from the cytocentrum and centrosphere of a dividing cell. SYN aster, attraction sphere. [G. *astron,* star, + *sphaira,* ball]

**As·tro·vi·rus** (as'rō-vī'rŭs) a small RNA virus and the only genus in the family Astroviridae; it is associated with diarrhea and is detected in the feces of numerous animals.

**asym·bo·lia** (ā-sim-bō'lē-ă) a form of aphasia in which the significance of signs and symbols is not appreciated. SYN asemasia, asemia. [G. *a-* priv. + *symbolon,* an outward sign]

**asym·met·ric** (ā-sim-et'rik) not symmetrical; denoting a lack of symmetry between two or more like parts.

**asym·met·ric fe·tal growth re·stric·tion** normal fetal head size as a result of preferential shunting of blood to brain, and decreased abdominal circumference from decreased adipose tissue and liver size; probably caused by placental insufficiency.

**asym·me·try** (ā-sim'e-trē) **1.** lack of symmetry; disproportion between two normally similar parts. **2.** significant difference in amplitude or frequency of EEG activity recorded simultaneously from the two sides of the brain.

**asymp·tom·at·ic** (ā'simp-tō-mat'ik) without symptoms, or producing no symptoms.

**asymp·tot·ic** (ā'simp-tot'ik) pertaining to a limiting value, for example of a dependent variable, when the independent variable approaches zero or infinity.

**asyn·cli·tism** (ā-sin'kli-tizm) absence of synclitism or parallelism; may be used, e.g., to refer to the axis of the presenting part of the child and the pelvic planes in childbirth, to the dental arches, or to the planes of the skull. SYN obliquity. [G. *a-* priv. + *syn-klinō,* to incline together]

**asyn·cli·tism of the skull** SYN plagiocephaly.

**asyn·de·sis** (ā-sin'dĕ-sis) **1.** rarely used term for a mental defect in which separate ideas or thoughts cannot be joined into a coherent concept. **2.** a breaking up of the connecting links in language, said to be characteristic of the language disturbance of schizophrenics. [G. *a-* priv. + *syn,* together, + *desis,* binding]

**asyn·ech·ia** (ā-si-nek'ē-ă) discontinuity of structure. [G. *a-* priv. + *synecheia,* continuity]

**asyn·er·gic** (ā'sin-er'jik) characterized by asynergia.

**asyn·er·gy** (ā-sin'er-jē) lack of coordination among various muscle groups during the performance of complex movements, resulting in loss of skill and speed. When severe, results in decomposition of movement, wherein complex motor acts are performed in a series of isolated movements; caused by cerebellar disorders.

**asys·tem·at·ic** (ā'sis-tĕ-mat'ik) not systematic; not relating to one system or set of organs.

**asys·to·le** (ā-sis'tō-lē) absence of contractions of the heart. [G. *a-* priv, + *systolē,* a contracting]

**asys·tol·ic** (ā-sis-tol'ik) **1.** relating to asystole. **2.** not systolic.

**AT** the adenine-thymine hydrogen-bonded base pair observed in double-stranded polynucleotides.

**At** astatine.

**a·tac·tic a·ba·sia, atax·ic a·ba·si·a** difficulty in walking due to ataxia of the legs.

**at·a·vism** (at'ă-vizm) the appearance in an individual of characteristics presumed to have been present in some remote ancestor; reversion to an earlier biological type. [L. *atavus,* a remote ancestor]

**at·a·vis·tic** (at-ă-vis'tik) relating to atavism.

**atax·ia** (ă-tak'sē-ă) an inability to coordinate muscle activity, causing jerkiness, incoordination, and inefficiency of voluntary movement. Most often due to disorders of the cerebellum or the posterior columns of the spinal cord; may involve limbs, head, or trunk. SYN incoordination. [G. *a-*prov. + *taxis,* order]

**atax·i·a·pha·sia** (ă-tak'sē-ă-fā'zē-ă) inability to form connected sentences, although single words may be used intelligibly. [G. *a-* priv. + *taxis,* order, + *phasis,* an affirmation, speech]

**atax·ia tel·an·gi·ec·ta·sia, atax·i·a-tel·an·gi··ec·ta·sia** a slowly progressive multisystem disorder with ataxia appearing with the onset of walking; telangiectases of the conjunctiva and skin; athetosis and nystagmus; and recurrent infections of the respiratory system caused by immunoglobulin deficiencies. Approximately 70% of the patients have an IgA deficiency concomitant with decreased T helper cell function.

**atax·ic** (ă-tak'sik) relating to, marked by, or suffering from ataxia.

**atax·ic dys·ar·thria** dysarthria associated with damage to the cerebellar system, characterized by imprecise consonants, excess and equal stress, inconsistent articulatory errors, and monotony of pitch and volume. SEE ataxia.

**atax·ic gait** SYN cerebellar gait.

**atax·i·o·phe·mia** (ă-tak-sē-ō-fē'mē-ă) incoordination of the muscles concerned in speech production. [G. *a-* priv. + *taxis,* order, + *phēmē,* voice, speech]

**A/T clon·ing** cloning of fragments where the only overhanging (or uncomplemented) ends are the A or T bases; occurs often in use of specific enzymes to cut or make DNA fragments.

△**-ate** termination used as a replacement for "-ic acid" when the acid is neutralized (e.g., sodium acetate) or esterified (e.g., ethyl acetate).

**at·el·ec·ta·sis** (at-ĕ-lek'tă-sis) reduction or absence of air in part or all of a lung, with resulting loss of lung volume. SEE ALSO pulmonary collapse. [G. *ateles*, incomplete, + *ektasis*, extension]

**at·e·lec·ta·sis of the mid·dle ear** reduction in the volume of the middle ear because of eustachian tube obstruction followed by absorption of the oxygen in the middle ear and subsequent retraction of the tympanic membrane medially.

**at·e·lec·tat·ic** (at-ĕ-lek-tat′ik) relating to atelectasis.

**ate·lia** (ă-tē′lē-ă) SYN ateliosis.

**atel·i·o·sis** (ă-tē′lē-ō′sis) incomplete development of the body or any of its parts, as in infantilism and dwarfism. SYN atelia. [G. *ateles*, incomplete, + -*osis*, condition]

**atel·i·ot·ic** (ă-tē-lē-ot′ik) marked by ateliosis.

**athe·lia** (ă-thē-lē-ă) congenital absence of the nipples. [G. *a*- priv. + *thēlē*, nipple]

△**ath·ero-** gruel-like, soft, pasty materials; atheroma, atheromatous. [G. *athērē*, gruel, porridge]

**ath·er·o·em·bo·lism** (ath′er-ō-em′bō-lizm) cholesterol embolism, with or without calcific matter, originating from an atheroma of the aorta or other diseased artery.

**ath·er·o·gen·e·sis** (ath′er-ō-jen′ĕ-sis) formation of atheroma, important in the pathogenesis of arteriosclerosis.

**ath·er·o·gen·ic** (ath-er-ō-jen′ik) having the capacity to initiate, increase, or accelerate the process of atherogenesis.

**ath·er·o·ma** (ath-er-ō′mă) the lipid deposits in the intima of arteries, producing a yellow swelling on the endothelial surface; a characteristic of atherosclerosis. [G. *athērē*, gruel, + -*ōma*, tumor]

**ath·er·om·a·tous** (ath-er-ō′mă-tŭs) relating to or affected by atheroma.

**ath·er·om·a·tous de·gen·er·a·tion** focal accumulation of lipid material (atheroma) in the intima and subintimal portion of arteries, eventually resulting in fibrous thickening or calcification.

**ath·er·o·matous em·bo·lism** SYN cholesterol embolism.

**ath·er·o·scle·ro·sis** (ath′er-ō-skler-ō′sis) arteriosclerosis characterized by irregularly distributed lipid deposits in the intima of large and medium-sized arteries; such deposits provoke fibrosis and calcification. Atherosclerosis is set in motion when cells lining the arteries are damaged as a result of high blood pressure, smoking, toxic substances in the environment, and other agents. Plaques develop when high density lipoproteins accumulate at the site of arterial damage and platelets act to form a fibrous cap over this fatty core. Deposits impede or eventually shut off blood flow.

**ath·er·o·scle·rot·ic** (ath′er-ō-skler-ot′ik) relating to or characterized by atherosclerosis.

**ath·e·toid** (ath′ĕ-toyd) resembling athetosis.

**ath·e·to·sic, ath·e·tot·ic** (ath-ĕ-tō′sik, ath-ĕ-tot′ik) pertaining to, or marked by, athetosis.

**ath·e·to·sis** (ath-ĕ-tō′sis) slow, writhing, involuntary movements of flexion, extension, pronation, and supination of the fingers and hands, and sometimes of the toes and feet. Usually caused by an extrapyramidal lesion. SYN Hammond disease. [G. *athetos*, without position or place]

**ath·lete's foot** SYN tinea pedis.

**ath·lete's heart** nonpathological enlarged heart in athletes reflecting specific adaptation to prolonged training. Manifestations in response to resistance training are thickened left ventricular wall and concentric hypertrophy, and in response to endurance training are enlarged left ventricular cavity and eccentric hypertrophy. SEE hypertrophy.

**ath·le·tic trai·ner, ath·le·tic therapist** one who is skilled in the prevention, evaluation, treatment, and rehabilitation of athletic injuries.

**ath·le·tic train·ing** provision of comprehensive health care services to athletes, including prevent preparation, evaluation of illnesses and injuries, first aid and emergency care, rehabilitation, and other, related services.

**athy·mia** (ā-thī′mē-ă) **1.** absence of affect or emotivity; morbid impassivity. **2.** congenital absence of the thymus, often with associated immunodeficiency. SYN athymism. [G. *a*-priv. + *thymos*, mind, also thymus]

**athy·mism** (ā-thī′mizm) SYN athymia (2).

**athy·roid·ism** (ā-thī′royd-izm) congenital absence of the thyroid gland or suppression or absence of its hormonal secretion. SEE hypothyroidism.

**athy·rot·ic** (ā-thī-rot′ik) relating to athyroidism.

**ATL** adult T-cell leukemia; adult T-cell lymphoma.

**at·lan·tad** (at-lan′tad) in a direction toward the atlas.

**at·lan·tal** (at-lan′tăl) relating to the atlas.

△**at·lan·to-, at·lo-** the atlas (the bone that supports the head). [G. *Atlas, Atlantos*, Atlas, the mythical Titan who supported the heavens on his shoulders]

**at·lan·to·ax·i·al** (at-lan′tō-ak′sē-ăl) pertaining to the atlas and the axis; denoting the joint between the first two cervical vertebrae. SYN atloaxoid.

**at·las** (at′las) first cervical vertebra, articulating with the occipital bone and rotating around the dens of the axis. SYN vertebra C1. [G. *Atlas*, in Greek mythology a Titan who supported the heavens on his shoulders]

**at·lo·ax·oid** (at-lō-ak′soyd) SYN atlantoaxial.

**atm** standard atmosphere.

△**atmo-** prefix denoting steam or vapor; or derived by action of steam or vapor. [G. *atmos*, steam, vapor]

**at·mos·phere** (at′mŏs-fēr) **1.** any gas surrounding a given body; a gaseous medium. **2.** a unit of air pressure. SEE ALSO standard atmosphere. [atmo- + G. *sphaira*, sphere]

**at·om** (at′ŏm) the once ultimate particle of an element, believed to be as indivisible as its name indicates. Discovery of radioactivity demonstrated the existence of subatomic particles, notably protons, neutrons, and electrons, the first two comprising most of the mass of the atomic nucleus. We now know that subatomic particles are further divisible ino hadrons, leptons, and quarks. [G. *atomos*, indivisible, uncut]

**atom·ic** (ă-tom′ik) relating to an atom.

**atom·ic ab·sorp·tion spec·tro·pho·tom·e·try** determination of concentration by the ability of atoms to absorb radiant energy of specific wavelengths.

**atom·ic mass num·ber** the mass of the atom of a particular isotope relative to hydrogen-1 (or to one twelfth the mass of carbon-12), generally very close to the whole number represented by the sum of the protons and neutrons in the atomic nucleus of the isotope; it is not to be confused with the atomic weight of an element, which may include a number of isotopes in natural proportion.

**atom•ic mass u•nit (amu)** a unit of mass by definition equal to $^1/_{12}$ of the mass of an atom of carbon-12, which equals $1.6605402 \times 10^{-27}$ kg; in terms of energy, 1 amu equals 931.49432 MeV. Cf. dalton.

**atom•ic num•ber (Z)** the number of protons in the nucleus of an atom; it indicates the position of the element in the periodic system.

**atom•ic weight (AW, at. wt.)** the mass in grams of 1 mol ($6.02 \times 10^{23}$, atoms) of an atomic species; the mass of an atom of a chemical element in relation to the mass of an atom of carbon-12 ($^{12}$C), which is set equal to 12.000, thus a ratio and therefore dimensionless (although the actual mass, numerically the same, is sometimes expressed in daltons); not necessarily the weight of any individual atom of an element, since most elements are made up of several isotopes of different masses. SEE ALSO molecular weight.

**at•om•iz•er** (at′ŏm-ī-zer) a device used to reduce liquid medication to fine particles in the form of a spray or aerosol; useful in delivering medication to the nose and throat. SEE ALSO nebulizer, vaporizer. [G. *atomos*, indivisible particle]

**aton•ic** (ā-ton′ik) relaxed; without normal tone or tension.

**aton•ic blad•der** a large, dilated, and nonemptying urinary bladder; usually due to disturbance of innervation or to chronic obstruction.

**at•o•ny** (at′ŏ-nē) relaxation, flaccidity, or lack of tone or tension. [G. *atonia,* languor]

**at•o•pen** (at′ō-pen) the excitant causing any form of atopy.

**atop•ic** (ā-top′ik) relating to or marked by atopy. [G. *atopos,* out of place; strange]

**atop•ic al•ler•gy** SEE atopy.

**atop•ic cat•a•ract** a cataract associated with atopic dermatitis.

**atop•ic der•ma•ti•tis** dermatitis characterized by the distinctive phenomena of atopy, including infantile and flexural eczema.

**atop•ic ker•a•to•con•junc•ti•vi•tis** a chronic papillary inflammation of the conjunctiva showing Trantas dots in a patient with a history of hypersensitivity.

*Ato•po•bium* (at-ō-pō′bē-um) an obligatorily anaerobic genus of Gram-positive, non–spore-bearing bacteria that appear as cocci and coccobacilli, sometimes in short chains. The type species is *Atopobium parvulus,* a slow-growing organism forming tiny colonies on standard media, formerly called *Peptostreptococcus parvulus* and *Streptococcus parvulus.*

**atop•og•no•sia, atop•og•no•sis** (ā-top-og-nō′zē-ă, ā-top-og-nō′sis) sensory inattention; inability to locate a sensation properly. Usually caused by a contralateral parietal lobe lesion. [G. *a-* priv. + *topos,* place, + *gnōsis,* knowledge]

**at•o•py** (at′ŏ-pē) a genetically determined state of hypersensitivity to environmental allergens. Type I allergic reaction is associated with the IgE antibody and a group of diseases, principally asthma, hay fever, and atopic dermatitis. [G. *atopia,* strangeness, fr. *a-* priv. + *topos,* a place]

**atox•ic** (ā-tok′sik) not toxic.

**ATP** adenosine 5′-triphosphate.

**ATPase** adenosine triphosphatase.

**ATPS** symbol indicating that a gas volume has been expressed as if it were saturated with water

vapor at the *a*mbient *t*emperature and barometric *p*ressure; the condition of an expired gas equilibrated in a spirometer.

**a•trau•mat•ic su•ture** a suture swaged onto the end of an eyeless needle.

**atre•sia** (ă-trē′zē-ă) congenital absence of a normal opening or normally patent lumen. [G. *a-* priv. + *trēsis,* a hole]

**atret•ic** (ă-tret′ik) relating to atresia. SYN imperforate.

△**at•re•to-** lack of an opening. [G. *atrētos,* imperforate fr. *a-,* not + *trētos,* perforated, fr. *tetrainō, titrēmi,* to bore through, to pierce.]

**atria** (ā′trē-ă) plural of atrium.

**atri•al** (ā′trē-ăl) relating to an atrium.

**atri•al ar•ter•ies** branches of the right and left coronary arteries distributed to the muscle of the atria. SYN arteriae atriales.

**atri•al au•ri•cle** SYN auricle of atrium.

**atri•al cap•ture beat** the cardiac cycle resulting when, after a period of A-V dissociation, the atria regain control of the ventricles; atrial depolarization due to retrograde transmission from a ventricular ectopic beat or an electronically paced ventricular impulse.

**atri•al cha•ot•ic tach•y•car•dia** multifocal origin of tachycardia within the atrium; often confused with atrial fibrillation during physical examination. SYN multifocal atrial tachycardia.

**atri•al com•plex** p wave in the electrocardiogram.

**atri•al dis•so•ci•a•tion** mutually independent beating of the two atria or of parts of the atria.

**atri•al ex•tra•sys•to•le** a premature contraction of the heart arising from an ectopic atrial focus.

**atri•al fi•bril•la•tion, au•ric•u•lar fi•bril•la•tion** fibrillation in which the normal rhythmical contractions of the cardiac atria are replaced by rapid irregular twitchings of the muscular wall; the ventricles respond irregularly to the dysrhythmic bombardment from the atria.

**atri•al flut•ter, au•ric•u•lar flut•ter** rapid regular atrial contractions occurring usually at rates between 250 and 350 per minute and often producing "saw-tooth" waves in the electrocardiogram, particularly leads II, III, and aVF.

**atri•al fu•sion beat** a beat that occurs when the atria are activated in part by the sinus impulse and in part by an ectopic or retrograde impulse from A-V junction or ventricle.

**atri•al sep•tal de•fect** a congenital defect in the interatrial septum between the atria of the heart, due to failure of the foramen primum or foramen secundum to close normally.

**atri•al sep•tos•to•my** establishment of a communication between the two atria of the heart.

**atrich•ia** (ā-trik′ē-ă) absence of hair, congenital or acquired. SYN atrichosis. [G. *a-* priv. + *thrix* (*trich-*), hair]

**atri•cho•sis** (at-ri-kō′sis) SYN atrichia.

**atrich•ous** (at′ri-kŭs) without hair.

△**atrio-** the atrium; atrial. [L. *atrium,* an entrance hall]

**atri•o•meg•a•ly** (ā′trē-ō-meg′ă-lē) enlargement of the atrium. [atrio- + G. *megas,* great]

**atri•o•sep•to•plas•ty** (ā′trē-ō-sep′tō-plas-tē) surgical repair of an atrial septal defect. [atrio- + L. *septum,* partition, + G. *plastos,* formed]

**atri•o•sep•tos•to•my** (ā′trē-ō-sep-tos′tō-mē) establishment of a communication between the two atria of the heart. [atrio- + L. *septum*, partition, + G. *stoma*, mouth]

**atri·o·ven·tric·u·lar** (A-V, AV) (ā'trē-ō-ven-trik'yu-lar) relating to both the atria and the ventricles of the heart, especially to the ordinary, orthograde transmission of conduction or blood flow.

**atri·o·ven·tric·u·lar block** partial or complete block of electric impulses originating in the atrium or sinus node preventing them from reaching the atrioventricular node and ventricles. In first degree A-V block, there is prolongation of A-V conduction time (P-R interval); in second degree AV block, some but not all atrial impulses fail to reach the ventricles, thus some ventricular beats are dropped; in complete A-V block, complete atrioventricular dissociation (2) occurs; no impulses can reach the ventricles despite even a slow ventricular rate (under 45 per minute); atria and ventricles beat independently. SYN block (3).

**atri·o·ven·tric·u·lar bun·dle** the bundle of modified cardiac muscle fibers that begins at the atrioventricular node as the trunk of the atrioventricular bundle and passes through the right atrioventricular fibrous ring to the membranous part of the interventricular septum where the trunk divides into two branches, the right and left crura of the atrioventricular bundle; the two crura ramify in the subendocardium of their respective ventricles. SYN His bundle, Kent bundle (1), ventriculonector.

**atri·o·ven·tric·u·lar ca·nal** the canal in the embryonic heart leading from the common sinuatrial chamber to the ventricle.

**atri·o·ven·tric·u·lar ca·nal cush·ions** a pair of mounds of embryonic connective tissue covered by endothelium, bulging into the embryonic atrioventricular canal; located one dorsally and one ventrally, they grow together and fuse with each other and with the lower edge of the septum primum, dividing the originally single canal into right and left atrioventricular orifices.

**atri·o·ven·tric·u·lar con·duc·tion** forward conduction of the cardiac impulse from atria to ventricles via the A-V node or any bypass tract, represented in the electrocardiogram by the P-R interval. P-H conduction time is from the onset of the P wave to the first high frequency component of the His bundle electrogram (normally 119 ± 38 msec); A-H conduction time is from the onset of the first high frequency component of the atrial electrogram to the first high frequency component of the His bundle electrogram (normally 92 ± 38 msec); P-A conduction time is from the onset of the P wave to the onset of the atrial electrogram (normally 27 ± 18 msec).

**atri·o·ven·tric·u·lar dis·so·ci·a·tion, A-V dis·so·ci·a·tion 1.** any situation in which atria and ventricles are activated and contract independently, as in complete A-V block; **2.** more specifically, the dissociation between atria and ventricles that results from slowing of the atrial pacemaker or acceleration of the ventricular pacemaker at nearly equal (rarely equal) rates, each depolarizing its own chamber, thus interfering with depolarization by the other (interference-dissociation).

**atri·o·ven·tric·u·lar ex·tra·sys·to·le, A-V ex·tra·sys·to·le** an extrasystole arising from the "junctional" tissues, either the A-V node or A-V bundle.

**atri·o·ven·tric·u·lar junc·tion·al bi·gem·i·ny** paired beats, each pair consisting of an A-V nodal extrasystole coupled to a beat of the dominant, usually sinus, rhythm.

**atri·o·ven·tric·u·lar junc·tion·al rhy·thm** the cardiac rhythm when the heart is controlled by the A-V junction (including node); arising in the A-V junction, the impulse ascends to the atria and descends to the ventricles, each at varying speeds depending on site of the pacemaker. SYN AV junctional rhythm.

**atri·o·ven·tric·u·lar no·dal ex·tra·sys·to·le, A-V no·dal ex·tra·sys·to·le** a premature beat arising from the A-V junction and leading to a simultaneous or almost simultaneous contraction of atria and ventricles.

**atri·o·ven·tric·u·lar node** (AV node) a small node of modified cardiac muscle fibers located near the ostium of the coronary sinus; it gives rise to the atrioventricular bundle of the conduction system of the heart.

**atri·o·ven·tric·u·lar sep·tum** the small part of the membranous septum of the heart just above the septal cusp of the tricuspid valve that separates the right atrium from the left ventricle.

**atri·o·ven·tric·u·lar valves** SEE tricuspid valve, mitral valve.

**atri·um,** pl. **atria** (ā'trē-ŭm, ā'trē-ă) [TA] **1.** a chamber or cavity to which are connected several chambers or passageways. **2.** SYN atrium of heart. **3.** that part of the tympanic cavity that lies immediately deep to the eardrum. **4.** in the lung, a subdivision of the alveolar duct from which alveolar sacs open. [L. entrance hall]

**atri·um cor·dis** [TA] SYN atrium of heart.

**atri·um cor·dis dex·trum** [TA] SYN right atrium of heart.

**atri·um cor·dis si·nis·trum** [TA] SYN left atrium of heart.

**atri·um dex·trum cor·dis** SYN right atrium of heart.

**atri·um of heart** the upper chamber of each half of the heart. SYN atrium cordis [TA], atrium (2) [TA].

**atri·um pul·mo·na·le** SYN left atrium of heart.

**atri·um si·nis·trum cor·dis** SYN left atrium of heart.

**atro·phia** (ă-trō'fē-ă) SYN atrophy. [G. fr. a- priv. + *trophē*, nourishment]

**atroph·ic** (ă-trōf'ik) denoting atrophy.

**atroph·ic ex·ca·va·tion** an exaggeration of the normal or physiologic cupping of the optic disk caused by atrophy of the optic nerve.

**atroph·ic gas·tri·tis** chronic gastritis with atrophy of the mucous membrane and destruction of the peptic glands, sometimes associated with pernicious anemia or gastric carcinoma; also applied to gastric atrophy without inflammatory changes.

**atroph·ic rhi·ni·tis** chronic rhinitis with thinning of the mucous membrane; often associated with crusts and foul-smelling discharge.

**atroph·ic vag·i·ni·tis** thinning and atrophy of the vaginal epithelium usually resulting from diminished estrogen stimulation; a common occurrence in postmenopausal women.

**at·ro·phied** (at'rō-fēd) characterized by atrophy.

**at·ro·pho·der·ma** (at'rō-fō-der'mă) atrophy of the skin that may occur either in discrete localized areas or in widespread areas. SEE ALSO anetoderma.

**at·ro·pho·der·ma·to·sis** (at'rō-fō-der-mă-tō'sis)

any cutaneous disorder in which a prominent symptom is skin atrophy.

**at·ro·phy** (at'rō-fē) a wasting of tissues, organs, or the entire body, as from death and reabsorption of cells, diminished cellular proliferation, decreased cellular volume, pressure, ischemia, malnutrition, lessened function, or hormonal changes. SYN atrophia. [G. *atrophia,* fr. *a-* priv. + *trophē,* nourishment]

**at·tached gin·gi·va** that part of the oral mucosa which is firmly bound to the tooth and alveolar process.

**at·tach·ment** (ă-tach'ment) 1. a connection of one part with another. 2. in dentistry, a mechanical device for the fixation and stabilization of a dental prosthesis.

**at·tack** (ă-tak') a sudden illness or an episode or exacerbation of chronic or recurrent illness.

**at·tack rate** a cumulative incidence rate used for particular groups observed for limited periods under special circumstances, such as during an epidemic.

**at·tend·ing phys·i·cian** physician who is formally and legally responsible for a patient's care throughout the stay in a health care facility.

**at·tend·ing staff** physicians and surgeons who are members of a hospital staff and regularly attend their patients at the hospital; may also supervise and teach house staff, fellows, and medical students.

**at·ten·tion def·i·cit dis·or·der (ADD)** a disorder of attention and impulse control with specific DSM criteria, appearing in childhood and sometimes persisting to adulthood. Hyperactivity may be a feature, but is not necessary for the diagnosis. SEE ALSO attention deficit hyperactivity disorder.

**at·ten·tion def·i·cit hy·per·ac·tiv·i·ty dis·or·der (ADHD)** a disorder of childhood and adolescence manifested at home, in school, and in social situations by developmentally inappropriate degrees of inattention, impulsiveness, and hyperactivity; also called hyperactivity or hyperactive child syndrome. SEE ALSO attention deficit disorder.

**at·ten·tion span** the length of time a person can concentrate on a subject.

**at·ten·u·at·ed vi·rus** a variant strain of a pathogenic virus, so modified as to excite the production of protective antibodies, yet not producing the specific disease.

**at·ten·u·a·tion** (ă-ten-yu-ā'shŭn) 1. the act of attenuating. 2. diminution of virulence in a strain of an organism, obtained through selection of variants which occur naturally or through experimental means. 3. loss of energy of a beam of radiant energy due to absorption, scattering, beam divergence, and other causes as the beam propagates through a medium. 4. regulation of termination of transcription; involved in control of gene expression in specific tissues.

**at·ti·cot·o·my** (at-i-kot'ō-mē) operative opening into the tympanic attic. [attic + G. *tomē,* incision]

**at·ti·tude** (at'i-tood) 1. position of the body and limbs. 2. manner of acting. 3. PSYCHOLOGY a predisposition to behave or react in a certain way toward persons, objects, institutions, or issues. [Mediev. L. *aptitudo,* fr. L. *aptus,* fit]

△**at·to- (a)** prefix used in the SI and metric systems to signify one quintillionth ($10^{-18}$). [Danish *atten,* eighteen]

**at·trac·tin** (a-trak'tin) a glycoprotein of T cell origin involved in T cell clustering and monocyte movement.

**at·trac·tion** (ă-trak'shŭn) a property or force by which anything tends to cause something else to approach it. [L. *at-traho,* pp. *-tractus,* to draw toward]

**at·trac·tion sphere** SYN astrosphere.

**at·tri·tion** (ă-trish'ŭn) 1. wearing away by friction or rubbing. 2. in dentistry, physiological loss of tooth structure caused by the abrasive character of food or from bruxism. Cf. abrasion. [L. *attero,* pp. *-tritus,* to rub against, rub away]

**at. wt.** atomic weight.

**atyp·i·cal** (ā-tip'i-kal) not typical; not corresponding to the normal form or type. [G. *a-* priv. + *typikos,* conformed to a type]

**atyp·i·cal an·ti·psy·chot·ic a·gent** a functional category of newer antipsychotic drugs thought to exert their action predominantly via serotonergic blockade.

**atyp·i·cal en·do·me·tri·al hy·per·pla·sia** increase in the number of endometrial glands, which have little, if any, stroma separating them but retain an orderly architecture distinguishing them from adenocarcinoma.

**atyp·i·cal gland·u·lar cells of un·de·ter·mined sig·nif·i·cance (AGUS, AGCUS)** the term in the Bethesda system for reporting cervical and/or vaginal cytologic diagnosis describing cells that show either endometrial or endocervical differentiation and display nuclear atypia that exceeds reactive or reparative changes but lacks definite features of invasive adenocarcinoma. SEE ALSO Bethesda system.

**atyp·i·cal li·po·ma** lipoma, occurring primarily in older men on the posterior neck, shoulders, and back, which is benign but microscopically atypical, containing giant cells with multiple overlapping nuclei forming a circle. SYN pleomorphic lipoma.

**atyp·i·cal mea·sles** unusual clinical manifestation of natural measles infection in persons with waning vaccination immunity, particularly in those who had received formaldehyde-inactivated vaccine; an accelerated allergic reaction characterized by high fever, absence of Koplik spots, a shortened prodromal period, atypical rash, and pneumonia.

**atyp·i·cal my·co·bac·te·ria** species of mycobacteria other than *M. tuberculosis* or *M. bovis* that can cause disease in immunocompromised humans.

**atyp·i·cal pneu·mo·nia** SYN primary atypical pneumonia.

**atyp·i·cal squa·mous cells of un·de·ter·mined sig·nif·i·cance (ASCUS)** the term in the Bethesda system for reporting cervical/vaginal cytologic diagnosis describing cellular abnormalities that are more marked than those attributable to reactive changes but that quantitatively or qualitatively fall short of a definitive diagnosis of squamous intraepithelial lesion (SIL); may reflect a benign or a potentially serious lesion. SEE ALSO Bethesda system, reactive changes.

**atyp·i·cal ver·ru·cous en·do·car·di·tis** SYN Libman-Sacks endocarditis.

**Au** gold (aurum).

**Au·bert phe·nom·e·non** (ow'bert) a phenomenon in which a bright perpendicular line appears to incline to one side when the observer turns the head to the opposite side in a dark room.

**au·dile** (aw'dil) **1.** relating to audition. **2.** denoting the type of mental imagery in which one recalls most readily that which has been heard rather than seen or read. Cf. motile. **3.** SYN auditive.

△**audio-** the sense of hearing. [L. *audio,* to hear]

**au·di·o·an·al·ge·sia** (aw'dē-ō-an-ăl-jē'zē-ă) use of music or sound delivered through earphones to mask pain during dental or surgical procedures.

**au·di·o·gen·ic** (awd'ē-ō-jen'ik) **1.** caused by sound, especially a loud noise. **2.** sound-producing. [audio- + G. *genesis,* production]

**au·di·o·gram** (aw'dē-ō-gram) the graphic record drawn from the results of hearing tests with the audiometer; charts the threshold of hearing at various frequencies against sound intensity in decibels. [audio- + G. *gramma,* a drawing]

**au·di·ol·o·gist** (aw-dē-ol'ō-jist) a specialist in evaluation and rehabilitation of those whose communication disorders center in whole or in part in the hearing function.

**au·di·ol·o·gy** (aw-dē-ol'ō-jē) the study of hearing disorders through the identification and measurement of hearing function loss as well as the rehabilitation of persons with hearing impairments.

**au·di·om·e·ter** (aw-dē-om'ĕ-ter) an electrical instrument for measuring the threshold of hearing for pure tones of frequencies generally varying from 128 to 8000 Hz (recorded in decibels). [audio- + G. *metron,* measure]

**au·di·o·met·ric** (aw'dē-ō-met'rik) related to measurement of hearing levels.

**au·di·om·e·try** (aw-dē-om'ĕ-trē) **1.** the measurement of hearing. **2.** the use of an audiometer. **3.** rapid measurement of the hearing of an individual or a group against a predetermined limit of normality; auditory responses to different frequencies presented at a constant intensity level are tested.

**au·di·o·vi·su·al** (aw'dē-ō-viz'yu-ăl) pertaining to a communication or teaching technique that combines both audible and visible symbols.

**audit** (aw'dit) **1.** a formal review or analysis of a body of data, particularly fiscal accounts. **2.** to perform an audit. [L. *auditus,* a hearing, fr. *audio,* to hear]

**au·di·tion** (aw-dish'ŭn) SYN hearing. [L. *auditio,* a hearing, fr. *audio,* to hear]

**au·di·tive** (aw'di-tiv) one who recalls most readily that which has been heard. SYN audile (3).

**au·di·to·ry** (aw'di-tōr-ē) pertaining to the sense of hearing or to the organs of hearing. [L. *audio,* pp. *auditus,* to hear]

**au·di·to·ry ag·no·sia** inability to recognize sounds, words, or music; caused by a lesion of the auditory cortex of the temporal lobe.

**au·di·to·ry a·pha·sia** an impairment in comprehension of the auditory forms of language and communication, including the ability to write from dictation in the presence of normal hearing. Spontaneous speech, reading, and writing are not affected. SYN word deafness.

**au·di·to·ry ar·ea** SYN auditory cortex.

**au·di·to·ry au·ra** epileptic aura characterized by illusions or hallucinations of sounds. SEE ALSO aura (1).

**au·di·to·ry brain·stem re·sponse (ABR)** a response produced by the auditory nerve and the brainstem to repetitive acoustic stimuli. SYN brainstem evoked response.

**au·di·to·ry brain·stem re·sponse au·di·om·e·try, ABR au·di·om·e·try** an electrophysiologic measure of auditory function utilizing responses produced by the auditory nerve and the brainstem to repetitive acoustic stimuli. SYN brainstem evoked response audiometry, BSER audiometry.

**au·di·to·ry cap·sule** the cartilage that, in the embryo, surrounds the developing otic vesicle and develops into the bony labyrinth of the internal ear.

**au·di·to·ry cor·tex** the region of the cerebral cortex that receives the auditory radiation from the medial geniculate body, a thalamic cell group receiving auditory input from the cochlear nuclei in the rhombencephalon. SYN auditory area.

**au·di·to·ry de·fen·sive·ness** excessive reaction to sound (e.g., because of its volume or novelty).

**au·di·to·ry feed·back** the unwanted sound that occurs in an amplification system when the microphone picks up the sound from the speaker; a major problem in the use of hearing aids.

**au·di·to·ry field** the space included within the limits of hearing of a definite sound, as of a tuning fork.

**au·di·to·ry hairs** cilia on the free surface of the auditory cells.

**au·di·to·ry nerve** SYN cochlear nerve.

**au·di·to·ry neu·ro·path·y** a disorder of hearing in children characterized by sensorineural hearing loss for pure tones, reduced word discrimination disproportionate to the pure-tone loss, normal outer hair cell function as determined by measurement of otoacoustic emissions, and absence or abnormality of auditory brainstem response.

■**au·di·to·ry os·si·cles** the small bones of the middle ear; they are articulated to form a chain for the transmission of sound from the tympanic membrane to the oval window. See this page. SYN ossicula auditus [TA], ear bones.

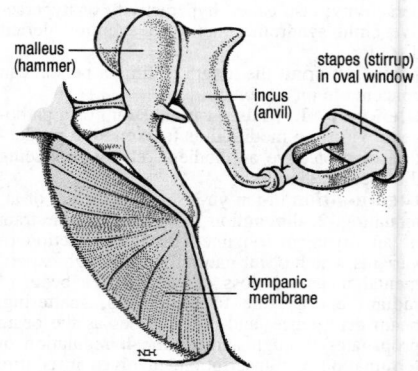

**auditory ossicles:** bones of the inner ear

**au·di·to·ry pits** paired depressions, one on either side of the head of the embryo, marking the location of the future auditory vesicles.

**au·di·to·ry pros·the·sis** generic term for implantable devices to restore sound perception to the deaf, the most common of which is the cochlear implant; a brainstem implant to stimulate the neurons of the cochlear nucleus is under development.

**au·di·to·ry re·cep·tor cells** columnar cells in the epithelium of the organ of Corti, having hairs (stereocilia) on their apical ends.

**au·di·to·ry re·flex** any reflex occurring in response to a sound, e.g., cochleopalpebral reflex.

**au·di·to·ry tube** SYN pharyngotympanic (auditory) tube.

**au·di·to·ry ver·ti·go** SYN Ménière disease.

**au·di·to·ry ves·i·cle** one of the paired sacs of invaginated ectoderm that develop into the membranous labyrinth of the internal ear. SYN otic vesicle.

**Au·en·brug·ger sign** (ow'en-broog-ĕr) an epigastric prominence seen in cases of marked pericardial effusion.

**Au·er bod·ies, Au·er rods** (ow'ĕr) rod-shaped structures of uncertain nature in the cytoplasm of immature myeloid cells, especially myeloblasts, in acute myelocytic leukemia.

**aug·men·ta·tion mam·ma·plas·ty** plastic surgery to enlarge the breast, often by insertion of an implant.

**aug·men·ta·tive and al·ter·na·tive com·mun·i·ca·tion (AAC) 1.** any type of compensation for impaired use of verbal language, including techniques such as gesture systems and devices such as voice amplifiers, picture boards, and computerized instrumentation; SEE ALSO communication board. **2.** the clinical practice of determining appropriate compensatory techniques for inadequate verbal communication, and providing training in the use of those techniques. SYN nonoral communication, nonverbal communication.

**au·ra**, pl. **au·rae** (aw'ră, aw'rē) **1.** subjective symptoms occurring at the onset of a partial epileptic seizure; often characteristic for the brain region involved in the seizure, e.g., visual aura, occipital lobe auditory aura, temporal lobe. **2.** subjective symptoms at the onset of a migraine headache. [L. breeze, odor, gleam of light]

**au·ral** (aw'răl) **1.** relating to the ear (auris). **2.** relating to an aura.

**au·ral re·ha·bil·i·ta·tion** procedures to enhance the communication capacity of persons with hearing impairments, such as auditory training, lip reading, and hearing aid orientation.

△**au·ri-** combining form denoting the ear. SEE ALSO ot-, oto-. [L. *auris*, an ear.]

**au·ri·cle** (aw'ri-kl) **1.** the projecting shell-like structure on the side of the head, constituting, with the external acoustic meatus, the external ear. SYN auricula (1), pinna (1). **2.** SYN auricle of atrium.

**au·ri·cle of atri·um** a small conical ("ear-shaped") pouch projecting from the upper anterior portion of each atrium of the heart, increasing slightly the atrial volume. SYN atrial auricle, auricle (2), auricula (2).

**au·ri·cle he·ma·to·ma** hematoma between the perichondrium and cartilage of the outer ear.

**au·ri·cles of atria** a small conical ("ear-shaped") pouch projecting from the upper anterior portion of each atrium of the heart, increasing slightly the atrial volume. SEE left atrium of heart, right atrium of heart. SYN auricula atrii [TA].

**au·ric·u·la**, pl. **au·ric·u·lae** (aw-rik'yu-lă, aw-rik'yu-lē) **1.** SYN auricle (1). **2.** SYN auricle of atrium. [L. the external ear, dim. of *auris*, ear]

**au·ric·u·la a·trii** [TA] SYN auricles of atria. SEE left atrium of heart, right atrium of heart.

**au·ric·u·lar** (aw-rik'yu-lăr) relating to the ear, or to an auricle in any sense.

**au·ric·u·lar car·ti·lage** the cartilage of the auricle. SYN cartilago auriculae [TA].

**au·ric·u·la·re** (aw-rik'yu-lăr-ē) a craniometric point at the center of the opening of the external acoustic meatus; or, in certain cases, the middle of the upper edge of this opening. SYN auricular point. [L. *auricularis*, pertaining to the ear]

**au·ric·u·lar point** SYN auriculare.

**au·ric·u·lar tu·ber·cle** a small projection from the upper end of the posterior portion of the incurved free margin of the helix. SYN darwinian tubercle.

**au·ric·u·lo·pres·sor re·flex** peripheral vasoconstriction and a rise in blood pressure in response to a fall in pressure in the great veins. SYN Pavlov reflex.

**au·ric·u·lo·tem·po·ral** (aw-rik'yu-lō-tem'pō-răl) relating to the auricle or pinna of the ear and the temporal region.

**au·ric·u·lo·tem·po·ral nerve** a branch of the mandibular, usually arising by two roots embracing the middle meningeal artery; it passes through the parotid gland conveying postsynaptic parasympathetic secretomotor fibers from the otic ganglion, and terminating in the skin of the temple and scalp; also sends branches to the external acoustic meatus, tympanic membrane, and auricle as well as a communicating branch to the facial nerve. SYN nervus auriculotemporalis [TA].

**au·ris**, pl. **au·res** (aw'ris, aw'rēz) [TA] SYN ear. [L.]

**au·ro·pal·pe·bral re·flex** brisk closure of the eyes in reaction to sudden presentation of a loud noise. SYN Moro reflex.

**au·rum** (aw'rŭm) SYN gold. [L.]

**aus·cul·tate, aus·cult** (aws'kŭl-tāt, aws-kŭlt') to perform auscultation.

▪**aus·cul·ta·tion** (aws-kŭl-tā'shŭn) listening to the sounds made by various body structures and functions as a diagnostic method, usually with a stethoscope. See page 90. [L. *ausculto*, pp. *-atus*, to listen to]

**aus·cul·ta·to·ry** (aws-kŭl'tă-tō-rē) relating to auscultation.

**aus·cul·ta·to·ry al·ter·nans** alternation in the intensity of heart sounds or murmurs in the presence of a regular cardiac rhythm.

**aus·cul·ta·to·ry gap** the period during which Korotkoff sounds indicating true systolic pressure fade away and reappear at a lower pressure point; responsible for errors made in recording falsely low systolic blood pressure, especially in hypertensive patients, of up to 25 mmHg, and avoided by pumping the cuff 30 mmHg above palpable systolic pressure.

**aus·cul·ta·to·ry per·cus·sion** auscultation of the chest or other part at the same time that percussion is made, to aid in hearing the sound made by percussion.

**Au·spitz sign** (ow'spitz) a finding typical of psoriasis, in which removal of a scale leads to pinpoint bleeding.

**Aus·tin Flint phe·nom·e·non, Aus·tin Flint mur·mur** (aw'stin flint) the murmur of relative mitral stenosis during significant aortic regurgitation owing to narrowing of the mitral orifice by

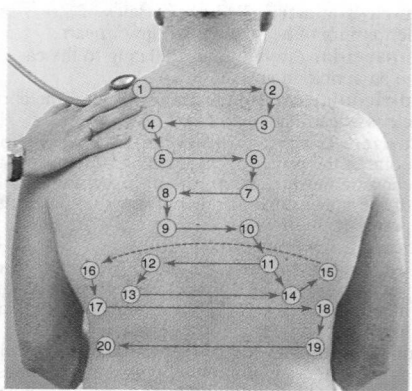

**auscultation of the lungs:** the examiner places the chest-piece of the stethoscope at selected sites on the surface of the thorax while the subject breathes deeply in and out through the mouth

pressure of the aortic regurgitant flow on the anterior mitral leaflet.

**Aus·tra·li·an X dis·ease** (aw-strā'lē-ăn) SYN Murray Valley encephalitis.

**au·thor·i·tar·i·an per·son·al·i·ty** a cluster of personality traits reflecting a desire for security and order, e.g., rigidity, unquestioning obedience, scapegoating, desire for structured lines of authority.

**au·thor·i·ty fig·ure** a real or projected person in a position of power; parents, police, and boss are authority figures to some people; during the transference phase of psychoanalysis, the psychoanalyst becomes an authority figure.

**au·tism** (aw'tizm) a tendency to morbid self-absorption at the expense of regulation by outward reality. [G. *autos,* self]

**au·tis·tic** (aw-tis'tik) pertaining to or characterized by autism.

△**au·to-, aut-** prefixes meaning self, same. [G. *autos,* self]

**au·to·ag·glu·ti·na·tion** (aw'to-ă-gloo-ti-nā'shŭn) **1.** nonspecific agglutination or clumping together of cells (e.g., bacteria, erythrocytes) due to physical-chemical factors. **2.** the agglutination of red blood cells by specific autoantibody present in one's own serum.

**au·to·ag·glu·ti·nin** (aw'tō-ă-gloo'ti-nin) an agglutinating autoantibody.

**au·to·al·ler·gic** (aw'tō-ă-ler'jik) pertaining to autoallergy.

**au·to·al·ler·gy** (aw-tō-al'er-jē) an altered reactivity in which antibodies (autoantibodies) are produced against an individual's own tissues, causing a destructive rather than a protective effect. SYN autoimmunity.

**au·to·an·ti·body** (aw-tō-an'ti-bod-ē) antibody occurring in response to antigenic constituents of the host's tissue, and which reacts with the inciting tissue component.

**au·to·an·ti·gen** (aw-to-an'ti-jen) a "self" antigen; any tissue constituent that evokes an immune response by the host.

**au·to·ca·tal·y·sis** (aw'tō-kă-tal'i-sis) a reaction in which one or more of the products formed acts to catalyze the reaction; beginning slowly, the rate of such a reaction rapidly increases. Cf. chain reaction.

**au·to·cat·a·lyt·ic** (aw'tō-kat-ă-lit'ik) relating to autocatalysis.

**au·toch·thon·ous** (aw-tok'thon-ŭs) **1.** native to the place inhabited; aboriginal. **2.** originating in the place where found; said of a disease originating in the part of the body where found, or of a disease acquired in the place where the patient is. [auto- + G. *chthon,* land, ground, country]

**au·toch·thon·ous i·de·as** thoughts that suddenly burst into awareness as if they are vitally important, often as if they have come from an outside source.

**au·toc·la·sis, au·to·cla·sia** (aw-tok'lă-sis, aw-tō-klă'zē-ă) **1.** a breaking up or rupturing from intrinsic or internal causes. **2.** progressive immunologically induced tissue destruction. [auto- + G. *klasis,* breaking]

**au·to·clave** (aw'tō-klāv) **1.** an apparatus for sterilization by steam under pressure. **2.** to sterilize in an autoclave. [auto- + L. *clavis,* a key, in the sense of self-locking]

**au·to·coid** (aw'tō-koyd) a chemical substance produced by one type of cell that affects the function of different types of cells in the same region, thus functioning as a local hormone or messenger. [G. *autos,* self, + *eidos,* form]

**au·to·crine** (aw'tō-krin) denoting self-stimulation through cellular production of a factor and a specific receptor for it. [auto- + G. *krinō,* to separate]

**au·to·crine hy·poth·e·sis** that tumor cells containing viral oncogenes may have encoded a growth factor, normally produced by other cell types, and thereby produce the factor autonomously, leading to uncontrolled proliferation.

**au·to·cy·to·ly·sin** (aw'tō-sī-tol'i-sin) SYN autolysin.

**au·to·cy·tol·y·sis** (aw'tō-sī-tol'i-sis) SYN autolysis.

**au·to·cy·to·tox·in** (aw'tō-sī-tō-toks'in) a cytotoxic autoantibody.

**au·to·der·mic graft** a skin autograft.

**au·to·di·ges·tion** (aw'tō-dī-jes'chŭn) SYN autolysis.

**au·to·ech·o·la·lia** (aw'tō-ek-ō-lā'lē-ă) a morbid repetition of another person's or one's own words. [auto- + echolalia]

**au·to·e·rot·ic** (aw'tō-ĕ-rot'ik) pertaining to autoerotism.

**au·to·er·o·tism** (aw-tō-ār'ō-tizm) **1.** sexual arousal or gratification using one's own body, as in masturbation. **2.** sexual self-love. SEE ALSO narcissism (1). Cf. alloerotism. [auto- + G. *erōtikos,* relating to love]

**au·to·e·ryth·ro·cyte sen·si·ti·za·tion syn·drome** a condition, usually occurring in women, in which the individual bruises easily (purpura simplex) and the ecchymoses tend to enlarge and involve adjacent tissues, resulting in pain in the affected parts; thought to be a form of localized autosensitization. SYN Gardner-Diamond syndrome.

**au·tog·a·my** (aw-tog'ă-mē) a form of self-fertilization in which fission of the cell nucleus occurs without division of the cell, the two pronuclei so formed reuniting to form the synkaryon; in other cases, the cell body also divides, but the two daughter cells immediately conjugate. [auto- + G. *gamos,* marriage]

**au·to·ge·ne·ic graft** SYN autograft.

**au·tog·e·nous vac·cine** a vaccine made from a culture of the patient's own bacteria.

**au·to·graft** (aw'tō-graft) a tissue or an organ transferred by grafting into a new position in the body of the same individual. SYN autogeneic graft, autologous graft, autoplastic graft, autotransplant. [auto- + A.S. *graef*]

**au·to·hae·mo·ly·sin [Br.]** SEE autohemolysin.

**au·to·hem·ag·glu·ti·na·tion** (aw'tō-hē'mă-glooti-nā'shŭn) autoagglutination of erythrocytes.

**au·to·he·mo·ly·sin** (aw'tō-hē-mol'i-sin) an autoantibody that causes lysis of erythrocytes in the same individual in whose body the lysin is formed.

**au·to·he·mol·y·sis** (aw'tō-hē-mol'i-sis) hemolysis occurring in certain diseases as a result of an autohemolysin.

**au·to·im·mune** (aw-tō-i-myun') arising from and directed against the individual's own tissues, as in autoimmune disease.

**au·to·im·mune dis·ease** any disorder in which loss of function or destruction of normal tissue arises from humoral or cellular immune responses of the individual to his own tissue constituents; may be systemic, as systemic lupus erythematosus, or organ specific, as thyroiditis.

**au·to·im·mune he·mo·lyt·ic a·ne·mia 1.** anemia caused by severe hemolysis in cold hemagglutinin disease; **2.** (warm antibody type) acquired hemolytic anemia due to serum autoantibodies that react with the patient's red blood cells, antigenic specificity being chiefly in the Rh complex; it may be idiopathic or secondary to neoplastic, autoimmune, or other disease.

**au·to·im·mu·ni·ty** (aw'tō-i-myu'ni-tē) IMMUNOLOGY the condition in which one's own tissues are subject to deleterious effects of the immune system, as in autoallergy and in autoimmune disease; immune response against the body's own tissues. SYN autoallergy.

**au·to·im·mu·ni·za·tion** (aw'tō-im'yu-ni-zā' shŭn) induction of autoimmunity.

**au·to·im·mu·no·cy·to·pe·nia** (aw-tō-im'yu-nō-sī-tō-pē'nē-ă) anemia, thrombocytopenia, and leukopenia resulting from cytotoxic autoimmune reactions.

**au·to·in·fec·tion** (aw'tō-in-fek'shŭn) **1.** reinfection by microbes or parasitic organisms on or within the body that have already passed through an infective cycle, such as a succession of boils, or a new infective cycle with production of a new generation of larvae and adults. **2.** self-infection by direct contagion as with parasite eggs passed in the infectious state transmitted by fingernails (anal-oral route). SYN autoreinfection.

**au·to·in·fu·sion** (aw'tō-in-fyu'zhŭn) forcing the blood from the extremities or other areas such as the spleen, as by the application of a bandage or pressure device, to raise the blood pressure and fill the vessels in the vital centers; resorted to after excessive loss of blood or other body fluids. Cf. autotransfusion.

**au·to·in·oc·u·la·tion** (aw'tō-in-ok-yu-lā'shŭn) a secondary infection originating from a focus of infection already present in the body.

**au·to·in·tox·i·cant** (aw'tō-in-toks'i-kant) an endogenous toxic agent that causes autointoxication.

**au·to·in·tox·i·ca·tion** (aw'tō-in-toks-i-kā'shŭn) a disorder resulting from absorption of the waste products of metabolism, decomposed matter from the intestine, or the products of dead and infected tissue as in gangrene. SYN endogenic toxicosis.

**au·to·i·sol·y·sin** (aw'tō-ī-sol'i-sin) an antibody that in the presence of complement causes lysis of cells in the individual in whose body the lysin is formed, as well as in others of the same species.

**au·to·ker·a·to·plas·ty** (aw-tō-ker'ă-tō-plas-tē) grafting of corneal tissue from one eye of a patient to the fellow eye. [auto- + G. *keras,* horn, + *plastos,* formed]

**au·to·ki·ne·sia, au·to·ki·ne·sis** (aw-tō-ki-ne'sē-ă, aw-tō-ki-nē'sis) voluntary movement. [auto- + G. *kinēsis,* movement]

**au·to·ki·net·ic** (aw-tō-kĭ-net'ik) relating to autokinesis.

**au·tol·o·gous** (aw-tol'ŏ-gŭs) **1.** occurring naturally and normally in a certain type of tissue or in a specific structure of the body. **2.** sometimes used to denote a neoplasm derived from cells that occur normally at that site, e.g., a squamous cell carcinoma in the upper esophagus. **3.** TRANSPLANTATION referring to a graft in which the donor and recipient areas are in the same individual. [auto- + G. *logos,* relation]

**au·tol·o·gous graft** SYN autograft.

**au·tol·y·sate** (aw-tol'i-sāt) the mixture of substances resulting from autolysis.

**au·tol·y·sin** (aw-tol'i-sin) an antibody that causes lysis of the cells and tissues in the body of the individual in whom the lysin is formed. SYN autocytolysin.

**au·tol·y·sis** (aw-tol'i-sis) **1.** enzymatic digestion of cells (especially dead or degenerate) by enzymes present within them (autogenous). **2.** destruction of cells as a result of a lysin formed in those cells or others in the same organism. SYN autocytolysis, autodigestion, isophagy. [auto- + G. *lysis,* dissolution]

**au·to·lyt·ic** (aw-tō-lit'ik) pertaining to or causing autolysis.

**au·to·lyt·ic en·zyme** an enzyme capable of causing lysis of the cell forming it.

**au·to·mat·ed dif·fer·en·tial leu·ko·cyte count·er** an instrument using digital imaging or cytochemical techniques to differentiate leukocytes.

**au·to·mat·ed lam·el·lar ker·a·tec·to·my** resection of a disk of corneal tissue using a precise machine to alter the refractive power of the eye.

**au·to·mat·ic au·di·to·ry brain·stem re·sponse** a technique of ABR in which the stimulus modification is programmed on the basis of the electrical responses recorded. The device determines automatically if predetermined thresholds have been achieved. It is useful in newborn hearing screening.

**au·to·mat·ic beat** in contrast to forced beat, an ectopic beat that arises *de novo* and is not precipitated by the preceding beat; thus escaped and parasystolic beats are automatic.

**au·to·mat·ic gain con·trol (AGC)** a feature of some hearing aids that reduces amplification at high-input intensity levels.

**au·to·mat·ic speech** overlearned or low-content language that can be produced with little awareness of meaning, such as consecutive numbers, days of the week, verses, prayers, expletives, or other common expressions. SYN nonpropositional speech.

**au•to•mat•ic trans•port ven•til•a•tor** a positive-pressure ventilator that supports respiration automatically and with less need for adjustment than a standard hospital ventilator; designed for use in an ambulance to ventilate an intubated patient. SEE ALSO ventilator.

**au•tom•a•tism** (aw-tom′ă-tizm) **1.** the state of being independent of the will or of central innervation; applicable, for example, to the heart's action. **2.** an epileptic attack consisting of stereotyped psychic, sensory, or motor phenomena carried out in a state of impaired consciousness and of which the individual usually has no knowledge. **3.** a condition in which an individual is consciously or unconsciously, but involuntarily, compelled to the performance of certain motor or verbal acts, often purposeless and sometimes foolish or harmful. SYN telergy. [G. *automatos*, self-moving, + -in]

**au•to•mo•tor sei•zure** seizure characterized by an automatism predominantly involving the distal limbs.

**au•to•nom•ic** (aw-tō-nom′ik) relating to the autonomic nervous system.

**au•to•no•mic di•vi•sion of ner•vous sys•tem** that part of the nervous system which represents the motor innervation of smooth muscle, cardiac muscle, and gland cells. It consists of two physiologically and anatomically distinct, mutually antagonistic components: the sympathetic and parasympathetic parts. In both of these parts the pathway of innervation consists of a synaptic sequence of two motor neurons, one of which lies in the spinal cord or brainstem as the presynaptic (preganglionic) neuron, the thin but myelinated axon of which (presynaptic (preganglionic) or B fiber) emerges with an outgoing spinal or cranial nerve and synapses with one or more of the postsynaptic (postganglionic or, more strictly, ganglionic) neurons composing the autonomic ganglia; the unmyelinated postsynaptic fibers in turn innervate the smooth muscle, cardiac muscle, or gland cells. The presynaptic neurons of the sympathetic part lie in the intermediolateral cell column of the thoracic and upper two lumbar segments of the spinal gray matter; those of the parasympathetic part compose the visceral motor (visceral efferent) nuclei of the brainstem as well as the lateral column of the second to fourth sacral segments of the spinal cord. The ganglia of the sympathetic part are the paravertebral ganglia of the sympathetic trunk and the lumbar and sacral prevertebral or collateral ganglia; those of the parasympathetic part lie either near the organ to be innervated or as intramural ganglia within the organ itself except in the head, where there are four discrete parasympathetic ganglia (ciliary, otic, pterygopalatine, and submandibular). Impulse transmission from presynaptic to postsynaptic neuron is mediated by acetylcholine in both the sympathetic and parasympathetic parts; transmission from the postsynaptic fiber to the visceral effector tissues is classically said to be by acetylcholine in the parasympathetic part and by noradrenalin in the sympathetic part; recent evidence suggests the existence of further noncholinergic, nonadrenergic classes of postsynaptic fibers. SYN divisio autonomica systema-

tis nervosi peripherici [TA], autonomic nervous system.

**au•to•no•mic dys•re•flex•ia** a syndrome occurring in some persons with spinal cord lesions and resulting from functional impairment of the autonomic nervous system. Symptoms include hypertension, bradycardia, severe headaches, pallor below and flushing above the cord lesion, and convulsions. SYN autonomic hyperreflexia.

**au•to•nom•ic gan•glia** visceral ganglia. SEE autonomic division of nervous system.

**au•to•nom•ic hy•per•re•flex•ia** SYN autonomic dysreflexia.

**au•to•nom•ic im•bal•ance** a lack of balance between sympathetic and parasympathetic nervous systems, especially in relation to vasomotor disturbances. SYN vasomotor imbalance.

**au•to•nom•ic ner•vous sys•tem** SYN autonomic division of nervous system.

**au•to•nom•ic neu•ro•gen•ic blad•der** malfunctioning urinary bladder, secondary to low spinal cord lesions.

**au•to•nom•ic plex•us•es** plexuses of nerves in relation to blood vessels and viscera, the component fibers of which are sympathetic, parasympathetic, and sensory.

**au•to•nom•ic sei•zure** seizure characterized by objectively documented dysfunction of the autonomic nervous system, usually involving cardiovascular, gastrointestinal, or sudomotor functions.

**au•to•nom•ic visceral motor nu•clei** nuclei located in the spinal cord (T1–L2, S2–S4) and in the brainstem (Edinger-Westphal nucleus, superior and inferior salivatory nuclei, dorsal vagal nucleus, and parts of the ambiguus nucleus) from which general visceral efferent preganglionic fibers arise; may be sympathetic (T1–L2) or parasympathetic (craniosacral); hypothalamic nuclei/areas function in concert with autonomic nuclei.

**au•to•nom•o•tro•pic** (aw′tō-nom-ō-trōp′ik) acting on the autonomic nervous system. [autonomic + G. *trepō*, to turn]

**au•to•ox•i•da•tion** (aw′tō-oks-i-dā′shŭn) the direct combination of a substance with molecular oxygen at ordinary temperatures. SYN autoxidation.

**au•to-PEEP** auto-positive-end-expiratory-pressure.

**au•to•pha•gia** (aw-tō-fā′jē-ă) **1.** biting one's own flesh; e.g., as a symptom of Lesch-Nyhan syndrome. **2.** maintenance of the nutrition of the whole body by metabolic consumption of some of the body tissues. **3.** SYN autophagy. [auto- + G. *phagō*, to eat]

**au•to•pha•gic** (aw-tō-fā′jik) relating to or characterized by autophagia.

**au•toph•a•gy** (aw-tof′ă-jē) segregation and disposal of damaged organelles within a cell. SYN autophagia (3). [auto- + G. *phagō*, to eat]

**au•to•plas•tic** (aw′tō-plas-tik) relating to autoplasty.

**au•to•plas•tic graft** SYN autograft.

**au•to•plas•ty** (aw′tō-plas-tē) repair of defects by autotransplantation.

**au•to•pol•y•mer res•in, au•to•po•ly•mer•iz•ing res•in** any resin that can be polymerized by chemical catalysis rather than by the application of heat; used in dentistry for dental restoration, denture repair, and impression trays. SYN cold cure resin, cold-curing resin.

**au·to·pos·i·tive-end-ex·pir·a·to·ry-pres·sure (au·to-PEEP)** developing in the periphery of the lung as a consequence of incomplete emptying of lung units due to inadequate expiratory time. SYN intrinsic PEEP, occult PEEP.

**au·top·sy** (aw'top-sē) an examination of the organs of a dead body to determine the cause of death or to study the pathologic changes present. SYN necropsy. [G. *autopsia,* seeing with one's own eyes]

**au·to·ra·di·o·graph** (aw-tō-rā'dē-ō-graf) image of the distribution and concentration of radioactivity in a tissue or other substance made by placing a photographic emulsion on the surface of, or in close proximity to, the substance.

**au·to·ra·di·og·ra·phy** (aw'tō-rā-dē-og'ră-fē) the process of producing an autoradiograph. SYN radioautography.

**au·to·re·cep·tor** (au'tō-rē-sep-tŏr, au'tō-rē-sep-ter) a site on a neuron that binds the neurotransmitter released by that neuron, which then regulates the neuron's activity. [auto- + receptor]

**au·to·reg·u·la·tion** (aw'tō-reg-yu-lā'shŭn) **1.** the tendency of the blood flow to an organ or part to remain at or return to the same level despite changes in the pressure in the artery which conveys blood to it. **2.** in general, any biologic system equipped with inhibitory feedback systems such that a given change tends to be largely or completely counteracted; e.g., baroreceptor reflexes form a basis for autoregulation of the systemic arterial blood pressure.

**au·to·re·in·fec·tion** (aw'tō-rē-in-fek'shŭn) SYN autoinfection.

**au·to·re·pro·duc·tion** (aw'tō-rē-prō-duk'shŭn) the ability of a gene or virus, or nucleoprotein molecule generally, to bring about the synthesis of another molecule like itself from smaller molecules within the cell.

**au·to·se·rum** (aw-tō-sē'rŭm) serum obtained from the patient's own blood and used in autoserotherapy.

**au·to·site** (aw'tō-sīt) that member of abnormal, unequal conjoined twins that is able to live independently and nourish the other member (parasite) of the pair. [auto- + G. *sitos,* food]

**au·to·so·mal** (aw-tō-sō'măl) pertaining to an autosome.

**au·to·so·mal gene** a gene located on any chromosome other than the sex chromosomes (X or Y).

**au·to·some** (aw'tō-sōm) any chromosome other than a sex chromosome; autosomes normally occur in pairs in somatic cells and singly in gametes. [auto- + G. *sōma,* body]

**au·to·sug·ges·tion** (aw'tō-sŭg-jes'chŭn) **1.** constant dwelling upon an idea or concept, thereby inducing some change in the mental or bodily functions. **2.** reproduction in the brain of impressions previously received which become then the starting point of new acts or ideas.

**au·to·top·ag·no·sia** (aw'tō-top'ag-nō'zē-ă) inability to recognize or to orient any part of one's own body; caused by a parietal lobe lesion. Cf. somatotopagnosis. [auto- + G. *topos,* place, + G. *a-* priv. + gnōsis]

**au·to·tox·ic** (aw-tō-toks'ik) relating to autointoxication.

**au·to·trans·fu·sion** (aw'tō-tranz-fyu'zhŭn) withdrawal and reinjection/transfusion of the patient's own blood. Cf. autoinfusion.

**au·to·trans·plant** (aw-tō-tranz'plant) SYN autograft.

**au·to·trans·plan·ta·tion** (aw'tō-tranz-plan-tā'shŭn) the performance of an autograft.

**au·to·troph** (aw'tō-trōf) a microorganism that uses only inorganic materials as its source of nutrients; carbon dioxide serves as the sole carbon source. [auto- + G. *trophē,* nourishment]

**au·to·tro·phic** (aw-tō-trōf'ik) **1.** self-nourishing. The ability of an organism to produce food from inorganic compounds. **2.** pertaining to an autotroph.

**au·tox·i·da·tion** (aw-tok-si-dā'shŭn) SYN autoxidation.

△**auxano-, auxo-, aux-** increase, e.g., in size, intensity, speed. [G. *auxanō,* to increase]

**aux·an·o·gram** (awk-san'ō-gram) a plate culture of bacteria in which variable conditions are provided in order to determine the effect of these conditions on the growth of the bacteria. [auxano- + G. *gramma,* something written]

**aux·an·o·graph·ic** (awk'san-ō-graf'ik) pertaining to auxanogram or auxanography.

**aux·a·nog·ra·phy** (awk-să-nog'ră-fē) the study, using auxanograms, of the effects of different conditions on the growth of bacteria.

**aux·e·sis** (awk-sē'sis) increase in size, especially as in hypertrophy. [G. increase]

**aux·il·ia·ry** (awk-zil'yă-rē) **1.** functioning in an augmenting capacity; supplementary. **2.** functioning as a subordinate; secondary.

**aux·i·lyt·ic** (awk'si-lit'ik) increasing the destructive power of a lysin, or favoring lysis. [G. *auxō,* to increase, + *lysis,* dissolution]

**aux·o·chrome** (awk'sō-krōm) the chemical group within a dye molecule by which the dye is bound to reactive end groups in tissues. [auxo- + G. *chrōma,* color]

**aux·o·ton·ic** (awk-sō-ton'ik) denoting the condition in which a contracting muscle shortens against an increasing load. Cf. isometric (2), isotonic (3).

**aux·o·troph** (awk'sō-trōf) a mutant microorganism that requires some nutrient that is not required by the organism (prototroph) from which the mutant was derived. [auxo- + G. *trophē,* nourishment]

**aux·o·tro·phic** (awk-sō-trōf'ik) pertaining to an auxotroph.

**A-V, AV** arteriovenous; atrioventricular.

**ava** arteriovenous anastomosis.

**avas·cu·lar** (ā-vas'kyu-ler) without blood or lymphatic vessels.

**avas·cu·lar·i·za·tion** (ā-vas'kyu-lar-ī-zā'shŭn) **1.** expulsion of blood from a part, as by means of an Esmarch tourniquet or arterial compression. **2.** loss of vascularity, as by scarring.

**avas·cu·lar ne·cro·sis** SYN aseptic necrosis.

**AV dif·fer·ence** arteriovenous difference of concentration of a substance.

**A·vel·lis syn·drome** (ah-vel'is) unilateral paralysis of the larynx and velum palati, with contralateral loss of pain and temperature sensibility in the parts below.

**av·er·age** a value that represents or summarizes the relevant features of a set of values; it is usually computed by a mathematical manipulation of the individual values in a set. [M.E. *averays,* loss from damage to ship or cargo, fr. It. *avaris,* fr. Ar. *'awariya,* damaged goods, + damage]

**aver·sion ther·a·py** a form of behavior therapy

that pairs an unpleasant stimulus with undesirable behavior(s) so that the patient learns to avoid the latter.

**aVF, aVL, aVR** augmented electrocardiographic leads from the foot (left), left arm, and right arm, respectively.

**avi·an** (ā′vē-ăn) pertaining to birds. [L. *avis,* bird]

**avi·an leu·ko·sis-sar·co·ma com·plex, avi·an leu·ke·mi·a-sar·co·ma com·plex 1.** a group of transmissible virus-induced diseases of chickens; the agents are closely related viruses (avian leukosis-sarcoma virus) causing proliferation of immature erythroid, myeloid, or lymphoid cells; **2.** a division of the RNA tumor viruses causing the avian leukosis-sarcoma complex of diseases. SYN avian leukosis-sarcoma virus.

**avi·an leu·ko·sis-sar·co·ma vi·rus** SYN avian leukosis-sarcoma complex (2).

**avi·an neu·ro·lym·pho·ma·to·sis vi·rus** the herpesvirus that causes avian lymphomatosis (Marek disease); is distinct from those causing other forms of leukosis. SYN Marek disease virus.

**avid·i·ty** a measure of the binding strength of a multivalent antibody to a multivalent antigen. SEE ALSO affinity.

**AV in·ter·val** the time from the beginning of atrial systole to the beginning of ventricular systole as measured from pressure pulses or cardiac volume curves in animals, or from the electrocardiogram in humans.

**avir·u·lent** (ā-vir′yu-lent) not virulent.

**avi·ta·min·o·sis** (ā-vī′tă-min-ō′sis) properly, hypovitaminosis.

**AV junc·tion** imprecisely defined zone surrounding and including the AV node and the adjacent atrial and ventricular myocardium.

**AV junc·tion·al rhy·thm** SYN atrioventricular junctional rhythm.

**AV node** atrioventricular node.

**Avo·gad·ro con·stant** (ah-vō-gahd′rō) SYN Avogadro number.

**Avo·gad·ro hy·poth·e·sis** (ah-vō-gahd′rō) SYN Avogadro law.

**Avo·gad·ro law** (ah-vō-gahd′rō) equal volumes of gases contain equal numbers of molecules, the conditions of pressure and temperature being the same. SYN Ampère postulate, Avogadro hypothesis, Avogadro postulate.

**Avo·gad·ro num·ber ($N_A$, lambda)** (ah-vō-gahd′rō) the number of molecules in one grammolecular weight (1 mol) of any compound; defined as the number of atoms in 0.0120 kg of pure carbon-12; equivalent to $6.0221367 \times 10^{23}$. SYN Avogadro constant.

**Avo·gad·ro pos·tu·late** (ah-vō-gahd′rō) SYN Avogadro law.

**avoid·ant per·son·al·i·ty** a personality characterized by a hypersensitivity to potential rejection, humiliation, or shame, an unwillingness to enter into relationships without unusually strong guarantees of uncritical acceptance, social withdrawal in spite of a desire for affection and acceptance, and low self-esteem.

**av·oir·du·pois** (av′ĕr-dŭ-poyz′, av-wahr-doo-pwah′) a system of weights in which 16 ounces make a pound, equivalent of 453.59237 g. See Weights and Measures appendix. [Fr. to have weight, corrupted fr. O. Fr. *avoir,* property, + *de, of,* + *pois,* weight]

**av·oir·du·pois weight** a system of weights based on the grain; 7000 grains equal 256 drams, or 16 ounces, or 1 pound.

**AVP** antiviral protein; arginine vasopressin.

**AVPU** prehospital mnemonic for assessment of mental status. Alert; responsive to verbal stimuli; responsive to painful stimuli; and unresponsive.

**avulsed wound** a wound caused by or resulting from avulsion.

**avul·sion** (ă-vŭl′shŭn) a tearing away or forcible separation. Cf. evulsion. [L. *a-vello,* pp. *-vulsus,* to tear away]

**avul·sion frac·ture** a fracture that occurs when a joint capsule, ligament, or muscle insertion of origin is pulled from the bone as a result of a sprain, dislocation, or strong contracture of the muscle against resistance; as the soft tissue is pulled away from the bone, a fragment or fragments of the bone may come away with it.

**AW** atomic weight.

**ax** axis.

**axen·ic** (ā-zen′ik) sterile, denoting especially a pure culture; e.g., a protozoan culture free from bacteria. Also used to denote "germ-free" animals born and raised in a sterile environment. [G. *a-* priv. + *xenos,* foreign]

**ax·es** (ak′sēz) plural of axis.

**ax·es of Fick** (fik) three axes that pass through the center of the eye vertically (Z), horizontally in the coronal plane (X), and horizontally in the sagittal plane (Y). All ocular rotations can be described by rotation along one of these axes.

**ax·i·al** (ak′sē-ăl) **1.** relating to an axis. SYN axialis, axile. **2.** relating to or situated in the central part of the body, in the head and trunk as distinguished from the limbs, e.g., axial skeleton. **3.** DENTISTRY relating to or parallel with the long axis of a tooth. **4.** RADIOLOGY an axial image is one obtained by rotating around the axis of the body, producing a transverse planar image, i.e., a section transverse to the axis.

**ax·i·al an·gle** an angle formed by two surfaces of a body, the line of union of which is parallel with its axis; the axial angles of a tooth are the distobuccal, distolabial, distolingual, mesiobuccal, mesiolabial, and mesiolingual.

**ax·i·al cur·rent** the central rapidly moving portion of the bloodstream in an artery.

**ax·i·al fil·a·ment** the central filament of a flagellum or cilium; with the electron microscope it is seen as a complex of nine peripheral diplomicrotubules and a central pair of microtubules. SYN axoneme (2).

**ax·i·al hy·per·o·pia** hyperopia due to shortening of the anteroposterior diameter of the globe of the eye.

**ax·i·a·lis** SYN axial (1).

**ax·i·al load·ing** loading (application of weight or force) along the long axis of the body.

**ax·i·al mus·cle** one of the skeletal muscles of the trunk or head.

**ax·i·al pat·tern flap** a flap that includes a direct specific artery within its longitudinal axis.

**ax·i·al plate** the primitive streak of an embryo.

**ax·i·al point** SYN nodal point.

**ax·i·al skel·e·ton** articulated bones of head and vertebral column, i.e., head and trunk, as opposed to the appendicular skeleton, the articulated bones of the upper and lower limbs.

**ax·if·u·gal** (ak-sif′yu-găl) extending away from an axis or axon. SYN axofugal. [L. *axis* + *fugio,* to flee from]

**ax·ile** (ak′sīl) SYN axial (1).

**ax·il·la**, gen. and pl. **ax·il·lae** (ak′sil′ă, ak-sil′ē) the space below the shoulder joint, bounded by the pectoralis major anteriorly, the latissimus dorsi posteriorly, the serratus anterior medially, and the humerus laterally; it has a superior opening between the clavicle, scapula, and first rib (cervicoaxillary canal), and an inferior opening covered by the axillary fascia; it contains the axillary artery and vein, the infraclavicular part of the brachial plexus, axillary lymph nodes and vessels, and areolar tissue. SYN axillary cavity. [L.]

**ax·il·lary** (ak′sil-ār-ē) relating to the axilla. SYN alar (2).

**ax·il·lary ar·tery** the continuation of the subclavian artery after crossing the first rib to enter the axilla; becomes the brachial artery upon passing the inferior border of the teres major muscle. It is accompanied by the cords of the brachial plexus, and is enclosed with them and the axillary vein in the axillary sheath as it traverses the axilla. Three parts of the axillary artery are described: proximal, posterior, and distal to the pectoralis minor muscle. *Branches:* 1st part—superior thoracic artery; 2nd part—thoracoacromial arterial trunk, lateral thoracic artery; 3rd part—subscapular artery, anterior and posterior humeral circumflex arteries. SYN arteria axillaris [TA].

**ax·il·lary cav·i·ty** SYN axilla.

**ax·il·lary hair** hair of the armpit.

**ax·il·lary lymph nodes** numerous nodes around the axillary veins which receive the lymphatic drainage from the upper limb, scapular region and pectoral region (including mammary glands); they drain into the subclavian trunk.

**ax·il·lary nerve** arises from the posterior cord of the brachial plexus in the axilla, passes laterally and posteriorly through quadrangular space with the posterior circumflex artery, winding round the surgical neck of the humerus to supply the deltoid and teres minor muscles, terminating as the superior lateral brachial cutaneous nerve. SYN nervus axillaris [TA].

**ax·il·lary thor·a·cot·o·my** lateral thoracotomy placed below the axillary hairline; may be transverse or vertical.

**ax·il·lary vein** a continuation of the basilic and brachial veins running from the lower border of the teres major muscle to the outer border of the first rib where it becomes the subclavian vein.

△**ax·io-** an axis. SEE ALSO axo-. [L. *axis*]

**ax·i·o·plasm** (ak′sē-ō-plazm) SYN axoplasm.

**ax·i·o·ver·sion** (ak′sē-ō-ver′zhŭn) abnormal inclination of the long axis of a tooth.

**ax·ip·e·tal** (ak-sip′ĕ-tăl) SYN centripetal (2). [L. *axis* + *peto*, to seek]

**ax·is** (**ax**), pl. **ax·es** (ak′sis, ak′sēz) **1.** a straight line joining two opposing poles of a spherical body, about which the body may revolve. **2.** the central line of the body or any of its parts. **3.** the vertebral column. **4.** the central nervous system. **5.** the second cervical vertebra. SYN epistropheus, vertebra C2, vertebra dentata. **6.** an artery that divides, immediately upon its origin, into a number of branches, e.g., celiac axis. SEE trunk. [L. axle, axis]

**ax·is de·vi·a·tion** deflection of the electrical axis of the heart to the right or left of the normal. SEE ALSO axis. SYN axis shift.

**ax·is shift** SYN axis deviation.

**ax·is-trac·tion for·ceps** obstetrical forceps provided with a second handle so attached that traction can be made in the line in which the head must move in the axis of the pelvis.

△**axo-** axis; axion. [G. *axōn*, axis]

**ax·o·ax·on·ic** (ak′sō-ak-son′ik) relating to synaptic contact between the axon of one nerve cell and that of another. SEE synapse.

**ax·o·den·drit·ic** (ak′sō-den-drit′ik) pertaining to the synaptic relationship of an axon with a dendrite of another neuron. SEE synapse.

**ax·of·u·gal** (ak-sof′yu-găl) SYN axifugal. [axo- + L. *fugio*, to flee]

**ax·o·lem·ma** (ak′sō-lem′ă) the plasma membrane of the axon. SYN Mauthner sheath. [axo- + G. *lemma*, husk]

**ax·ol·y·sis** (ak-sol′i-sis) destruction or dissolution of a nerve axon. [axo- + G. *lysis*, dissolution]

**ax·on** (ak′son) the single process of a nerve cell that under normal conditions conducts nervous impulses away from the cell body and its remaining processes (dendrites). Axons 0.5 μm thick or over are generally enveloped by a segmented myelin sheath provided by oligodendroglia cells (in brain and spinal cord) or Schwann cells (in peripheral nerves). Nerve cells synaptically transmit impulses to other nerve cells or to effector cells (muscle cells, gland cells) exclusively by way of the synaptic terminals of their axons. [G. *axōn*, axis]

**ax·o·nal** (ak′sō-năl) pertaining to an axon.

**ax·o·neme** (ak′sō-nēm) **1.** the central thread running in the axis of the chromosome. **2.** SYN axial filament. **3.** the distinctive array of microtubules in the core of eukaryotic cilia and flagella comprising a central pair surrounded by a sheaf of nine doublet microtubules. [axo- + G. *nēma*, a thread]

**ax·on hil·lock** the conical area of origin of the axon from the nerve cell body; it contains parallel arrays of microtubules and is devoid of Nissl substance.

**ax·on·og·ra·phy** (ak-sŏ-nog′ră-fē) the recording of electrical changes in axons.

**ax·on·ot·me·sis** (ak-sŏ-nŏt′mē′sis) interruption of the axons of a nerve followed by complete degeneration of the peripheral segment, without severance of the supporting structure of the nerve; such a lesion may result from pinching, crushing, or prolonged pressure. SEE ALSO neurapraxia, neurotmesis. [axon + G. *tmēsis*, a cutting]

**ax·on ter·mi·nals** the somewhat enlarged, often club-shaped endings by which axons make synaptic contacts with other nerve cells or with effector cells (muscle or gland cells). Axon terminals contain neurotransmitters of various kinds, sometimes more than one. SEE ALSO synapse. SYN end-feet, neuropodia, terminal boutons, boutons terminaux.

**ax·op·e·tal** (ak-sop′ĕ-tăl) extending in a direction toward an axon. [axo- + L. *peto*, to seek]

**ax·o·plasm** (ak′sō-plazm) neuroplasm of the axon. SYN axioplasm.

**ax·o·plas·mic trans·port** transport by way of flow of axoplasm toward cell soma (retrograde) or toward axon terminal (anterograde).

**ax·o·so·mat·ic** (ak-sō-sō-mat′ik) relating to the synaptic relationship of an axon with a nerve cell body. SEE synapse. [axo- + G. *sōma*, body]

**Ayer·za syn·drome** (ah-yār′sah) sclerosis of the

pulmonary arteries in chronic cor pulmonale; associated with severe cyanosis, it is a condition resembling polycythemia vera but resulting from primary pulmonary arteriosclerosis or primary pulmonary hypertension and characterized by plexiform lesions of arterioles.

**aze•o•trope** (ā-zē′ō-trōp) a mixture of two or more liquids that boils without change in proportion of the liquids, either in the liquid or the vapor phase. [G. *a*- priv. + *zeō*, to boil, + *tropos*, a turning]

**aze•o•tro•pic** (ā-zē-ō-trōp′ik) denoting or characteristic of an azeotrope.

**az•i•do•thy•mi•dine (AZT)** (az′i-dō-thī′mi-dēn) SEE AZT.

△**azo-** prefix denoting the presence in a molecule of the group ≡C–N=N–C≡. Cf. diazo-. [Fr. *azote*, nitrogen]

**az•ole** (az′ōl) SYN pyrrole.

**azoo•sper•mia** (ā-zō-ō-sper′mē-ă) absence of living spermatozoa in the semen; failure of spermatogenesis. [G. *a*- priv. + *zōon*, animal, + *sperma*, seed]

**az•o•pro•tein** (az-ō-prō′tēn) any of the modified proteins produced by treatment with diazonium derivatives of various aromatic amines; used to elicit antibody formation and demonstrate antibody specificity.

**az•o•tae•mia [Br.]** SYN uremia.

**az•o•te•mia** (āz-ō-tē′mē-ă) SYN uremia. [azo- (azote) + G. *haima*, blood]

**az•o•tem•ic** (āz-ō-tēm′ik) relating to azotemia.

**azo•tu•ria** (āz-ō-tyur′ē-ă) an increased elimination of urea in the urine. [azo- (azote) + G. *ouron*, urine]

**AZT** azidothymidine; a thymidine analogue that is an inhibitor of replication of HIV virus *in vitro* and is used in the management of AIDS.

**az•ure** (azh′yur) a term for a group of basic blue methylthionine or phenothiazine dyes; used as biological stains, especially in blood and nuclear stains.

**az•ure lu•nul•es of nails** bluish nonblanching discoloration of the lunules of all the fingernails, in hepatolenticular degeneration.

**az•u•res•in** (azh′yu-res′in) a complex of azure A and carbacrylic resin; used as an indicator for the detection of gastric achlorhydria without intubation.

**az•u•ro•phil, az•u•ro•phile** (azh′yu-rō-fil, azh′ yu-rō-fīl) staining readily with an azure dye, denoting especially the hyperchromatin and reddish purple granules of certain blood cells. [azure + G. *philos*, fond]

**azy•go•gram** (az′i-gō-gram) radiographic demonstration of the azygos venous system after injection of contrast medium. [azygos + G. *gramma*, a writing]

**azy•gog•ra•phy** (az′i-gog′ră-fē) radiography of the azygos venous system after injection of contrast medium.

**az•y•gos** (āz′ī-gos) **1.** an unpaired (azygous) anatomic structure. **2.** SYN azygos vein. [G. *a*- priv. + *zygon*, a yoke]

**az•y•gos lobe of right lung** a small accessory lobe sometimes formed above the hilum of the right lung; separated from the rest of the upper lobe by a deep groove lodging the azygos vein.

**az•y•gos vein** arises from the merger of the right ascending lumbar vein with the right subcostal vein and often a communication with the inferior vena cava; ascends through the aortic hiatus of the diaphragm or its right crus; it runs along the right side of the thoracic vertebral bodies in the posterior mediastinum, and terminates by arching anteriorly over the root of the right lung to enter the posterior aspect of the superior vena cava. SYN azygos (2).

**az•y•gous** (āz′ī-gŭs) unpaired; single. [G. *azygos*]

# B

β (bā′ta) beta. SEE beta.
β– symbol for electron.
β⁺ positron.
**B 1.** boron; aspartic acid; bromouridine; second substrate in a multisubstrate enzyme-catalyzed reaction. **2.** as a subscript, refers to barometric pressure.
**b 1.** as a subscript, refers to blood. **2.** bis [L.], twice.
**Ba** barium.
*Ba•be•sia* (bă-bē′zē-ă) the economically most important genus of the family Babesiidae; characterized by multiplication in host red blood cells to form pairs and tetrads; it causes babesiosis (piroplasmosis) in most types of domestic animals, and two species cause disease in splenectomized or normal people; vectors are ixodid or argasid ticks. [V. *Babès*]
*Ba•be•sia mi•cro•ti* a malaria-like protozoan naturally parasitizing certain rodents; a number of human cases have been reported from Nantucket and Martha's Vineyard islands and nearby coastal New England. The local tick vector is *Ixodes scapularis*, whose numbers and infection levels have greatly increased in recent years with the increase in the deer population, which serves as an abundant blood source for *I. scapularis*. SEE ALSO *Borrelia burgdorferi*.
**ba•be•si•o•sis** (bă-bē′zē-ō′sis) a disease caused by infection with a species of *Babesia*, the infection being transmitted by ticks. In animals, the disease is characterized by fever, malaise, listlessness, severe anemia, and hemoglobulinuria; the death rate frequently is higher in adult than in young animals.
**Babès nodes** (bah′besh) collections of lymphocytes in the central nervous system found in rabies.
**Ba•bin•ski phe•nom•e•non** (bă-bin′skē) SYN Babinski sign (1).
**Ba•bin•ski sign** (bă-bin′skē) **1.** extension of the great toe and abduction of the other toes instead of the normal flexion reflex to plantar stimulation, considered indicative of pyramidal tract involvement ("positive" Babinski); SYN Babinski phenomenon, paradoxical extensor reflex. **2.** in hemiplegia, weakness of the platysma muscle on the affected side, as is evident in such actions as blowing or opening the mouth; **3.** when the patient is lying supine with arms crossed on the front of the chest, and attempts to assume the sitting posture, the thigh on the side of an *organic* paralysis is flexed and the heel raised, whereas the limb on the sound side remains flat; **4.** in hemiplegia, the forearm on the affected side turns to a pronated position when placed in a position of supination.
**Ba•bin•ski syn•drome** (bă-bin′skē) the combination of cardiac, arterial, and central nervous system manifestations of late syphilis.
**ba•by** (bā′bē) an infant; a newborn child.
**ba•by tooth** SYN deciduous tooth.
**bac•cate** (bak′āt) berry-like. [L. *bacca*, berry]
**bac•ci•form** (bak′sĭ-fōrm) berry-shaped. [L. *bacca*, berry]
**Ba•cil•la•ce•ae** (bă-si-lā′sē-ē) a family of aerobic or facultatively anaerobic, sporeforming, ordinarily motile bacteria (order Eubacteriales) containing Gram-positive rods. Some species are

pathogenic. Ordinarily two genera, *Bacillus* and *Clostridium*, are included. The type genus is *Bacillus*.
**ba•cil•lar, bac•il•la•ry** (bas′i-lar, bas′i-lā-rē) shaped like a rod; consisting of rods or rodlike elements.
**bac•il•la•ry an•gi•o•ma•to•sis** an infection of immunocompromised patients by a newly recognized Rickettsial species *Bartonella henselae*, characterized by fever and granulomatous cutaneous nodules, and peliosis hepatis in some cases. Skin biopsy shows vascular proliferation and infiltration of vessel walls by neutrophils and clumps of organisms seen with Warthin-Starry silver staining.
**bac•il•la•ry dys•en•tery** infection with *Shigella dysenteriae*, *S. flexneri*, or other organisms.
**ba•cil•le Cal•mette-Gué•rin** (bah-sēl′ kahl-met′ ga-ră′) an attenuated strain of *Mycobacterium bovis* used in the preparation of BCG vaccine, which is used for immunization against tuberculosis and in cancer chemotherapy. [Fr.]
**bac•il•le•mia** (bas-i-lē′mē-ă) the presence of rod-shaped bacteria in the circulating blood. [bacillus + G. *haima*, blood]
**ba•cil•li** (bă-sil′ī) plural of bacillus.
**ba•cil•li•form** (ba-sil′i-fōrm) rod-shaped. [L. *bacillus*, a rod, + *forma*, form]
**ba•cil•lin** (ba-sil′in) an antibiotic substance produced by *Bacillus subtilis*.
**bac•il•lo•sis** (bas-i-lō′sis) a general infection with bacilli.
**bac•il•lu•ria** (bas-i-lyu′rē-ă) the presence of bacilli in the urine. [bacillus + G. *ouron*, urine]
*Ba•cil•lus* (ba-sil′ŭs) a genus of aerobic or facultatively anaerobic, sporeforming, ordinarily motile bacteria (family Bacillaceae) containing Gram-positive rods. Motile cells are peritrichous; spores are thick-walled and stain poorly with Gram stain; these organisms are chemoheterotrophic and are found primarily in soil. A few species are animal pathogens; some species evoke antibody production. The type species is *Bacillus subtilis*. [L. dim. of *baculus*, rod, staff]
**ba•cil•lus**, pl. **ba•cil•li** (ba-sil′ŭs, bă-sil′ī) **1.** a vernacular term used to refer to any member of the genus *Bacillus*. **2.** term formerly used to refer to any rod-shaped bacterium. [L. dim. of *baculus*, a rod, staff]
*Ba•cil•lus ce•re•us* a species that causes an emetic type and a diarrheal type of food poisoning in humans, and can cause infections in humans and other mammals.
*Ba•cil•lus cir•cu•lans* a bacterial species found in soil that has been incriminated in human infections including septicemia, mixed abscess infections, and wound infections.
*Ba•cil•lus pu•mi•lis* a usually saprophytic species of bacteria that has been associated with food poisoning and rarely with abscess or bowel fistula formation.
*Ba•cil•lus sphae•ri•cus* a species that is an insect pathogen and that has been associated with human and other mammalian infections, especially in compromised hosts.
**back•ache** (bak′āk) nonspecific term used to describe back pain; generally refers to pain below the cervical level.
**back•board splint** a board splint with slots for

fixation by straps; shorter ones are used for neck injuries, longer ones for back injuries.

**back·bone** (bak'bōn) SYN vertebral column.

**back·cross** (bak'kros) mating of an individual heterozygous at one or more loci to an individual homozygous at the same loci.

**back-ex·trap·o·la·tion** a process to determine the onset of exhalation during the forced expiratory vital capacity maneuver; excessive back extrapolation volume (usually expressed as a percentage of the forced vital capacity) is an indication of hesitation or false starting.

**back·flow** the reversal of the normal flow of a current. SEE ALSO regurgitation.

**back·ground ra·di·a·tion** irradiation from environmental sources, including the earth's crust, the atmosphere, cosmic rays, and ingested radionuclides in the body.

**back pres·sure** pressure exerted upstream in the circulation as a result of obstruction to forward flow, as when congestion in the pulmonary circulation results from stenosis of the mitral valve or failure of the left ventricle.

**back·pro·jec·tion** (bak'prō-jek'shŭn) in computed tomography or other imaging techniques requiring reconstruction from multiple projections, an algorithm for calculating the contribution of each voxel of the structure to the measured ray data, in order to generate an image; the oldest and simplest method of image reconstruction.

**back table pro·ce·dure** procedure performed on an organ that has been removed from a patient before it is replaced.

**back·track·ing** the backwards movement of RNA polymerase along the DNA template to a state more stable than that encountered when some base pairs disrupt the attachment of the 3' end from the active transcription site.

**back·ward heart fail·ure** a concept that maintains that the phenomena of congestive heart failure result from passive engorgement of the veins caused by a "backward" rise in pressure proximal to the failing cardiac chambers. Cf. forward heart failure.

**Ba·con a·no·scope** (bā'kŏn) an instrument resembling a rectal speculum, with a long slit on one side and a light source opposite.

**bac·te·re·mia** (bak-tēr-ē'mē-ă) the presence of viable bacteria in the circulating blood; may be transient following trauma such as dental or other iatrogenic manipulation or may be persistent or recurrent as a result of infection. SYN bacteriemia. [bacteria + G. *haima*, blood]

**bac·te·ria** (bak-tēr'ē-ă) plural of bacterium. See this page.

**bac·te·ri·al** (bak-tēr'ē-ăl) relating to bacteria.

**bac·te·ri·al cap·sule** a layer of slime of variable composition which covers the surface of some bacteria; capsulated cells of pathogenic bacteria are usually more virulent than cells without capsules because the former are more resistant to phagocytic action.

**bac·te·ri·al end·ar·te·ri·tis** implantation and growth of bacteria with formation of vegetations on the arterial wall, such as may occur in a patent ductus arteriosus or arteriovenous fistula.

**bac·te·ri·al en·do·car·di·tis** endocarditis caused by the direct invasion of bacteria and leading to deformity and destruction of the valve leaflets.

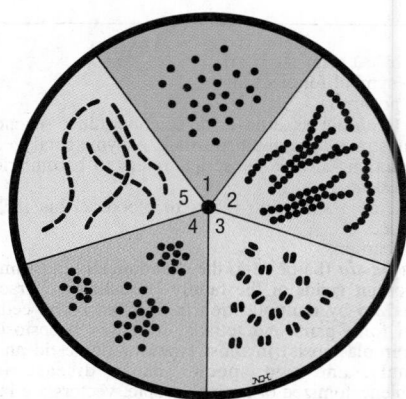

**bacteria:** (1) cocci, (2) streptococci, (3) diplococci, (4) staphylococci, (5) bacilli

Two types are acute bacterial endocarditis and subacute bacterial endocarditis.

**bac·te·ri·al food poi·son·ing** a term commonly used to refer to conditions limited to enteritis or gastroenteritis (excluding the enteric fevers and the dysenteries) caused by bacterial multiplication per se or by a soluble bacterial exotoxin.

**bac·te·ri·al plaque** DENTISTRY a mass of filamentous microorganisms and large variety of smaller forms attached to the surface of a tooth which, depending on bacterial activity and environmental factors, may give rise to caries, calculus, or inflammatory changes in adjacent tissue. SYN dental plaque (2).

**bac·te·ri·al trans·lo·ca·tion** the movement of bacteria or bacterial products across the intestinal membrane to emerge either in the lymphatics or the visceral circulation.

**bac·te·ri·al vag·in·o·sis** infection of the vagina apparently caused by *Gardnerella vaginalis* and other anaerobes. Characterized by excessive, sometimes malodorous, discharge.

**bac·te·ri·al vi·rus** a virus which "infects" bacteria; a bacteriophage.

**bac·te·ri·cid·al** (bak-tēr'i-sī'dăl) causing the death of bacteria. Cf. bacteriostatic. SYN bactericidal.

**bac·te·ri·cide** (bak-tēr'i-sīd) an agent that destroys bacteria. SYN bacteriocide. [bacteria + L. *caedo*, to kill]

**bac·ter·id** (bak'ter-id) **1.** a recurrent or persistent eruption of discrete sterile pustules of the palms and soles, thought to be an allergic response to bacterial infection at a remote site. **2.** a dissemination of a previously localized bacterial skin infection. [bacteria + -*id* (1)]

**bac·te·ri·e·mia** (bak-tēr-ē-ē'mē-ă) SYN bacteremia.

△**bac·te·rio-, bac·te·ri-** bacteria. [see bacterium]

**bac·te·ri·o·cid·al** (bak-tēr'ē-ō-sī'dăl) SYN bactericidal.

**bac·ter·i·o·cide** (bak-tēr'ē-ō-sīd) SYN bactericide.

**bac·te·ri·o·cid·in** (bak-tēr'ē-ō-sī'din) antibody having bactericidal activity.

**bac·te·ri·o·cin·o·gen·ic plas·mids** bacterial plasmids responsible for the elaboration of bacteriocins. SYN bacteriocinogens.

**bac·te·ri·o·cin·o·gens** (bak-tēr′ē-ō-sin′ō-jenz) SYN bacteriocinogenic plasmids.

**bac·te·ri·o·cins** (bak-tēr′ē-ō-sinz) proteins produced by certain bacteria that exert a lethal effect on closely related bacteria; in general, bacteriocins have a narrower range of activity than antibiotics do and are more potent.

**bac·te·ri·o·gen·ic** (bak-tēr′ē-ō-jen′ik) caused by bacteria.

**bac·te·ri·o·gen·ic ag·glu·ti·na·tion** the clumping of erythrocytes as a result of effects of bacteria or their products.

**bac·te·ri·o·log·ic, bac·te·ri·o·log·i·cal** (bak′ tēr-ē-ō-loj′ik, bak′tēr-ē-ō-loj′i-kăl) relating to bacteria or to bacteriology.

**bac·te·ri·ol·o·gist** (bak′ter-ē-ol′ŏ-jist) one who primarily studies or works with bacteria.

**bac·te·ri·ol·o·gy** (bak-tēr-ē-ol′ŏ-jē) the branch of science concerned with the study of bacteria. [bacterio- + G. *logos,* study]

**bac·te·ri·o·ly·sin** (bak-tēr-ē-ol′i-sin) specific antibody that combines with bacterial cells (i.e., antigen) and, in the presence of complement, causes lysis or dissolution of the cells.

**bac·te·ri·ol·y·sis** (bak-tēr-ē-ol′i-sis) the dissolution of bacteria, e.g., by means of hypotonic solutions or by specific antibody and complement. [bacterio- + G. *lysis,* dissolution]

**bac·te·ri·o·lyt·ic** (bak-tēr-ē-ō-lit′ik) pertaining to lytic destruction of bacteria; manifesting the ability to cause dissolution of bacterial cells.

**bac·te·ri·o·pexy** (bak-tēr′ē-ō-pek-sē) immobilization of bacteria by phagocytic cells. [bacterio- + G. *pēxis,* fixation]

**bac·te·ri·o·phage** (bak-tēr′ē-ō-fāj) a virus with specific affinity for bacteria. Bacteriophages have been found in essentially all groups of bacteria; like other viruses they contain either RNA or DNA (but never both) and vary in structure from simple to complex; their relationships to host bacteria are specific and may be genetically intimate. Bacteriophages are named after the bacterial species, group, or strain for which they are specific, e.g., corynebacteriophage, coliphage. SEE ALSO coliphage. SYN phage. [bacterio- + G. *phagō,* to eat]

**bac·te·ri·op·so·nin** (bak-tēr-ē-op′sō-nin) an opsonin acting upon bacteria.

**bac·te·ri·o·sis** (bak-tēr-ē-ō′sis) a localized or generalized bacterial infection.

**bac·te·ri·o·stat·ic** (bak-tēr′ē-ō-stat′ik) inhibiting or retarding the growth of bacteria.

**bac·te·ri·um,** pl. **bac·te·ria** (bak-tēr′ē-ŭm, bak-tēr′ē-ă) a unicellular prokaryotic microorganism that usually multiplies by cell division and has a cell wall that provides a constancy of form; may be aerobic or anaerobic, motile or nonmotile, and free-living, saprophytic, parasitic, or pathogenic. SEE ALSO Cyanobacteria. [Mod. L. fr. G. *baktēr-ion,* dim. of *baktron,* a staff]

**bac·te·ri·u·ria** (bak-tēr-ē-yu′rē-ă) the presence of bacteria in the urine.

***Bac·te·roi·des*** (bak-ter-oy′dēz) a genus that includes many species of obligate anaerobic, nonsporeforming bacteria (family Bacteroidaceae) containing Gram-negative rods. Both motile and nonmotile species occur; motile cells are peritrichous. Some species ferment carbohydrates and produce combinations of succinic, lactic, acetic, formic, or propionic acids, sometimes with short-chained alcohols; butyric acid is not a major product. Those species which do not ferment carbohydrates produce from peptone either trace to moderate amounts of succinic, formic, acetic, and lactic acids or major amounts of acetic and butyric acids with moderate amounts of alcohols and isovaleric, propionic, and isobutyric acids. They are part of the normal flora of the intestinal tract and to a lesser degree, the respiratory, and urogenital cavities of humans and animals; many species formerly classified as *Bacteroides* have been reclassified as belonging to the genus *Prevotella.* Many species can be pathogenic. The type species is *Bacteroides fragilis.* [G. *bacterion* + *eidos,* form]

***Bac·te·roi·des ca·pil·lo·sus*** a species isolated from human cysts and wounds, the mouth, and feces.

***Bac·te·roi·des di·siens*** a species isolated from abdominal and urogenital infections, and from the mouth.

***Bac·te·roi·des dis·tas·on·is*** bacterial species that is part of the normal human fecal flora; an occasional cause of intraabdominal infections.

***Bac·te·roi·des frag·i·lis*** a species that is one of the predominant organisms in the lower intestinal tract of man and other animals; also found in specimens from appendicitis, peritonitis, rectal abscesses, pilonidal cysts, surgical wounds, and lesions of the urogenital tract; it is the type species of the genus *Bacteroides.*

***Bac·te·roi·des mel·a·nin·o·ge·ni·cus*** SYN *Prevotella melaninogenica.*

***Bac·te·roi·des o·ris*** a species isolated from the gingival crevice, systemic infections, face, neck, and chest abscesses, wound drainages, and blood and various bodily fluids.

***Bac·te·roi·des splanch·ni·cus*** a species in the indole positive group, found in normal human colonic flora, and occasionally in human specimens with unique metabolic properties that include production of large amounts of N-butyric acid; it appears to be closely related to the genus *Porphyromonas.*

***Bac·te·roi·des the·ta·i·o·ta·mi·cron*** a species implicated in intra-abdominal infections.

**BAER** brainstem auditory evoked response. SEE evoked response.

**Ba·er law** (bār) the general organ characteristics found in all members of a group appear earlier in embryogenesis than the special organ characteristics that distinguish specific members of the group; this law is the predecessor of the recapitulation theory.

**Ba·er·mann con·cen·tra·tion** (bār′mahn) preparation that relies on the principle that active nematode larvae will migrate from a fresh fecal specimen through several layers of gauze into tap water, from which the larvae can be recovered by centrifugation.

**Bae·yer the·o·ry** (bā′yer) theory that carbon bonds are set at fixed angles (109° 28′) and that those carbon rings are most stable that least distort those angles; for this reason, planar rings composed of five or six carbon atoms (e.g., cyclopentane, benzene) are more common than rings containing less than five or more than six carbon atoms.

**bag** a pouch, sac, or receptacle. [A.S. *baelg*]

**bag·as·so·sis** (bag-ă-sō′sis) extrinsic allergic alveolitis following exposure to sugar cane fiber (bagasse); variously attributed to inhalation of spores of soil fungi and, particularly, thermophilic actinomycetes.

**bag-valve-mask de•vice, bag-mask de•vice** a hand-powered positive-pressure ventilation device consisting of a mask, one-way valve, and self-inflating bag; may be attached to an endotracheal or tracheostomy tube.

**bag of wa•ters** colloquialism for the amniotic sac and contained amniotic fluid.

**Bail•lar•ger lines, Bail•lar•ger bands** (bī-yahr-zhā′) two laminae of white fibers that course parallel to the surface of the cerebral cortex and are visible as the stria of the internal pyramidal layer in cortical layer V (outer line) and the stria of the internal granular layer in cortical layer IV (inner line); the line of Gennari in the calcarine cortex represents the outer of these lines

**Bail•li•art oph•thal•mo•dy•na•mom•e•ter** (bī-yē-ar′) an instrument used to measure the blood pressure of the central retinal artery; of value in diagnosing occlusion of the proximal carotid artery.

**Ba•ker ac•id he•ma•te•in** (bā′kĕr) an acidic solution of oxidized hematoxylin used on frozen sections for staining phospholipids.

**Ba•ker cyst** (bā′kĕr) a collection of synovial fluid which has escaped from the knee joint or a bursa and formed a new synovial-fluid lined sac in the popliteal space; seen in degenerative or other joint diseases that produce increased amounts of synovial fluid.

**Ba•ker pyr•i•dine ex•trac•tion** (bā′kĕr) hot pyridine treatment, used to extract phospholipids from tissues in histochemical staining of this material.

**bak•er's itch** an eruption on the hands and arms of bakers due to an allergic reaction to flour or other substances handled, or to the grain itch mite.

**BAL** bronchoalveolar lavage.

**Bal•a•muth a•que•ous egg yolk in•fu•sion me•di•um** (bal′ă-moot) used to detect the presence of intestinal amebae, primarily *Entamoeba histolytica.*

**Bal•a•muth•ia** (bal-ă-moo′thē-ă) a genus of free-living ameba that causes granulomatous amebic encephalitis.

**bal•ance** (bal′ans) **1.** an apparatus for weighing; e.g., scales. **2.** the normal state of action and reaction between two or more parts or organs of the body. **3.** quantities, concentrations, and proportionate amounts of bodily constituents. **4.** the difference between intake and utilization, storage, or excretion of a substance by the body. SEE ALSO equilibrium. [L. *bi-*, twice, + *lanx*, dish, scale]

**bal•anced an•es•the•sia** a technique of general anesthesia based on the concept that administration of a mixture of small amounts of several neuronal depressants summates the advantages, but not the disadvantages, of, the individual components of the mixture.

**bal•anced di•et** a diet containing the essential nutrients with a reasonable ration of all the major food groups.

**bal•anced oc•clu•sion** the simultaneous contacting of the upper and lower teeth on the right and left and in the anterior and posterior occlusal areas in centric and eccentric positions within the functional range.

**bal•anced pol•y•mor•phism** a unilocal trait in which two alleles are maintained at stable frequencies because the heterozygote is more fit than either of the homozygotes. SEE ALSO overdominance.

**bal•anced trans•lo•ca•tion** translocation of the long arm of an acrocentric chromosome to another chromosome; an individual with a balanced translocation has a normal diploid genome and is clinically normal but has a chromosome count of 45 and as a result of asymmetrical meiosis may have children lacking the genes on the translocated segment or have them in trisomy.

**bal•anc•ing side** the segment of the dentition that is opposite the direction in which the lower jaw is being moved.

**bal•anc•ing side con•dyle** DENTISTRY the mandibular condyle on the side away from which the mandible moves in a lateral excursion.

**ba•lan•ic** (ba-lan′ik) relating to the glans penis or glans clitoridis. [G. *balanos,* acorn, glans]

**bal•a•ni•tis** (bal-ă-nī′tis) inflammation of the glans penis or clitoris. [G. *balanos,* acorn, glans, + *-itis,* inflammation]

△**balano-, balan-** glans penis. [G. *balanos,* acorn, glans]

**bal•a•no•plas•ty** (bal′an-ō-plas-tē) surgical reconstruction of the glans penis. [balano- + G. *plastos,* formed]

**bal•a•no•pos•thi•tis** (bal′an-ō-pos-thī′tis) inflammation of the glans penis and overlying prepuce. [balano- + G. *posthē,* prepuce, + *-itis,* inflammation]

**bal•an•ti•di•a•sis** (bal′an-ti-dī′ă-sis) a disease caused by the presence of *Balantidium coli* in the large intestine; characterized by diarrhea, dysentery, and occasionally ulceration.

**Ba•lan•ti•di•um** (bal-an-tid′ē-ŭm) a genus of ciliates (family Balantidiidae) found in the digestive tract of vertebrates and invertebrates. [G. *balantidion,* dim of *ballantion,* a bag]

**Ba•lan•ti•di•um co•li** a very large parasitic ciliate species, usually 50 to 80 μm in length, reaching up to 200 μm in pigs, found in the cecum or large intestine, swimming actively in the lumen; usually harmless in man but may invade and ulcerate the intestinal wall, producing a colitis resembling amebic dysentery.

**bald•ness** (bawld′nes) SYN alopecia.

**Ba•lint syn•drome** (bah-lēnt′) an entity characterized by optic ataxia and simultanagnosia. This difficulty in applying the visual system to a visual task is usually due to damage to the superior temporal-occipital areas in both hemispheres.

**Bal•kan frame, Bal•kan splint** (bawl′kăn) an overhead frame, supported on uprights attached to the bedposts or to a separate stand, from which a splinted limb is slung in the treatment of fracture or joint disease.

**ball 1.** a round mass. SEE bezoar. **2.** in veterinary medicine, a large pill or bolus.

**Bal•lance sign** (bal′ăns) the presence of a dull percussion note in both flanks, constant on the left side but shifting with change of position on the right, said to indicate ruptured spleen; the dullness is due to the presence of fluid blood on the right side but coagulated blood on the left.

**ball-and-sock•et joint** a multiaxial synovial joint in which a more or less extensive sphere on the head of one bone fits into a rounded cavity in the other bone. SYN cotyloid joint, enarthrodial joint, enarthrosis, spheroid joint.

**bal·lis·mus** (bal-iz′mŭs) a type of involuntary movement affecting the proximal limb musculature, manifested as jerking, flinging movements of the extremity; caused by a lesion of or near the contralateral subthalamic nucleus. Usually only one side of the body is involved, resulting in hemiballismus. [G. *ballismos,* a jumping about]

**bal·loon** (bă-loon) **1.** an inflatable spherical or ovoid device used to retain tubes or catheters in, or provide support to, various body structures. **2.** a distensible device used to stretch or occlude a stenotic viscus or blood vessel. **3.** to distend a body cavity with a gas or fluid to facilitate its examination, dilate a structure, or occlude its lumen. [Fr. *ballon,* fr. It. *ballone,* fr. *balla,* ball, fr. Germanic]

**bal·loon·sep·tos·to·my** (bă-lūn′sep-tos′tō-mē) creation of an artificial interatrial septal defect by cardiac catheterization during which an inflated balloon is pulled across the interatrial septum through the foramen ovale; used in cases of transposition of the great vessels and tricuspid atresia.

**bal·loon-tip cath·e·ter 1.** a single- or double-lumen tube with a balloon at its tip that can be inflated or deflated without removal after installation; the balloon may be inflated to facilitate the passage of the tube through a blood vessel (propelled by the bloodstream) or to occlude the vessel in which the tube alone would allow free flow; such catheters are used to enter the pulmonary artery to facilitate hemodynamic measurements. SEE ALSO Swan-Ganz catheter. **2.** a tube with an inflatable balloon at its tip used to enter arteries and then removed while inflated to withdraw clots (embolectomy catheter) **3.** SYN Fogarty catheter.

**Ball op·er·a·tion** (bal) division of the sensory nerve trunks supplying the anus, for relief of pruritus ani.

**bal·lot·able pa·tel·la** (ba-lŏt′abl pă-tel′ă) a condition in which the patella can be balloted because of an effusion of blood or fluid in the capsule of the knee joint. SYN floating patella.

**bal·lotte·ment** (bal-ot-maw′) maneuver used in physical examination to estimate the size, shape, or consistency of an organ not near the surface, particularly when there is ascites, by a rhythmic, thrusting motion of the hand or fingers similar to that involved in bouncing a ball. [Fr. *balloter,* to toss up]

**ball and soc·ket a·but·ment** an abutment connected to a fixed partial denture by a ball and socket-shaped nonrigid connector.

**ball valve** any of a variety of prosthetic cardiac valves consisting of a ball within a retaining cage affixed to the orifice; when appropriately sized, used in aortic, mitral, or tricuspid position.

**balm** (bawlm) **1.** an ointment, especially a fragrant one. **2.** a soothing application. [L. *balsamum,* fr. G. *balsamon,* the balsam tree]

**BALT** bronchus-associated lymphoid tissue.

**Bam·ber·ger dis·ease** (bahm′bĕr-gĕr) **1.** SYN saltatory spasm. **2.** SYN polyserositis.

**Bam·ber·ger-Ma·rie dis·ease** (bahm′bĕr-gĕr-mah-rē′) SYN hypertrophic pulmonary osteoarthropathy.

**Bam·ber·ger-Pins-E·wart sign** (bahm′bĕr-ger-pins-yu′wart) SYN Bamberger sign.

**Bam·ber·ger sign** (bahm′bĕr-gĕr) **1.** jugular pulse in tricuspid insufficiency; **2.** SYN allocheiria. **3.** dullness on percussion at the angle of the scapula, clearing up as the patient leans forward, indicating pericarditis with effusion. SYN Bamberger-Pins-Ewart sign.

**bam·boo hair** hair with regularly spaced nodules along the shaft caused by intermittent fractures with invagination of the distal hair into the proximal portion, with intervening lengths of normal hair, giving the appearance of bamboo; seen in Netherton syndrome. SYN trichorrhexis invaginata.

**bam·boo spine** RADIOLOGY the appearance of the thoracic or lumbar spine with ankylosing spondylitis.

**ba·na·na sign** the abnormal curvature of the cerebellum noted on ultrasound imaging in a fetus with Arnold-Chiari malformation.

**band 1.** any appliance or part of an apparatus that encircles or binds a part of the body. SEE ALSO zone. **2.** any ribbon-shaped or cordlike anatomic structure that encircles or binds another structure or that connects two or more parts. SEE fascia, line, linea, stria, tenia. **3.** a narrow strip containing one or more macromolecules (on occasions, small molecules) detected in electrophoresis or certain types of chromatography.

**ban·dage** (ban′dij) **1.** a piece of cloth or other material, of varying shape and size, applied to a body part to provide compression, protect from external contamination, prevent drying, absorb drainage, prevent motion, and retain surgical dressings. **2.** to cover a body part by application of a bandage.

**ban·dage con·tact lens** a contact lens placed on the cornea to cover a defect.

**band cell** any cell of the granulocytic (leukocytic) series that has a nucleus that could be described as a curved or coiled band, no matter how marked the indentation, if it does not completely segment the nucleus into lobes connected by a filament. SYN stab cell, staff cell.

**band·ing** the process of differential staining of chromosomes to reveal characteristic patterns of bands that permit identification of individual chromosomes and recognition of missing segments; each of the 22 pairs of human chromosomes and the X and Y chromosomes has an identifying banding pattern.

**Ban·dl ring** (bahn-dĕl) SYN pathologic retraction ring.

**band-shaped ker·a·top·a·thy** a horizontal, gray, interpalpebral opacity of the cornea in hypercalcemia, chronic iridocyclitis, and Still disease.

**Bang ba·cil·lus** (bahng) SYN *Brucella abortus.*

**Ban·kart le·sion** avulsion or damage to the anterior lip of the glenoid fossa as the humerus slides forward in an anterior dislocation.

**Ban·nis·ter dis·ease** (ban′is-ter) SYN angioedema.

**Bann·warth syn·drome** neurologic manifestations of Lyme disease, also called chronic lymphocytic meningitis and tick-borne meningopolyneuritis.

**bar 1.** a unit of pressure equal to 1 megadyne ($10^6$ dyne) per cm$^2$ in the CGS system, 0.9869233 atmosphere, or $10^5$ Pa (N/m$^2$) in the SI system. **2.** a metal segment of greater length than width that serves to connect two or more parts of a removable partial denture. **3.** a segment of tissue or bone that unites two or more similar structures.

**bar·aes·the·sia [Br.]** SYN pressure sense.

**bar·ag·no·sis** (bar-ag-nō'sis) loss of ability to appreciate the weight of objects held in the hand, or to differentiate objects of different weights. When the primary senses are intact, caused by a lesion of the contralateral parietal lobe. [G. *baros*, weight + *a-* priv., + *gnōsis*, a knowing]

**Bá·rá·ny ca·lor·ic test** (bah'rah-nē) a test for vestibular function, made by irrigating the external auditory meatus with either hot or cold water; this normally causes stimulation of the vestibular apparatus, resulting in nystagmus and past-pointing; in vestibular disease, the response may be reduced or absent. See this page. SYN caloric test.

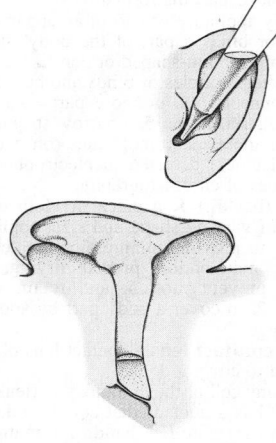

**Bárány caloric test:** for vestibular function

**Bá·rá·ny sign** (bah'rah-nē) in cases of ear disease, in which the vestibule is healthy, injection into the external auditory canal of water below the body temperature will cause rotatory nystagmus toward the opposite side; when the injected fluid is above the body temperature the nystagmus will be toward the injected side; if the labyrinth is diseased or nonfunctional there may be diminished or absent nystagmus.

**bar·ber's itch** SYN tinea barbae.

**bar·ber's pi·lo·ni·dal si·nus** pilonidal sinus occurring in barbers, usually in the web between the fingers, due to the burying of exogenous hairs by the alternate loosening and tightening of tissues of the hand by the manipulation of scissors.

**bar·bi·tu·rism** (bar'bi-chyur-izm) chronic poisoning by any of the derivatives of barbituric acid; symptoms include cutaneous eruption, chills, fever, and headache.

**bar·bo·tage** (bar-bō-tahzh') a method of spinal anesthesia in which a portion of the anesthetic solution is injected into the cerebrospinal fluid, which is then aspirated back into the syringe and reinjected. [Fr. *barboter*, to dabble]

**bare lym·pho·cyte syn·drome** absence of HLA antigens on peripheral mononuclear cells, which may result in immunodeficiency.

**bar·es·the·sia** (bar-es-thē'zē-ă) SYN pressure sense. [G. *baros*, weight, + *aisthēsis*, sensation]

**bar·es·the·si·om·e·ter** (bar'es-thē'zē-om'ĕ-ter) an instrument for measuring the pressure sense. [G. *baros*, weight, + *aisthēsis*, sensation, + *metron*, measure]

**bar·i·at·ric** (bar-ē-at'rik) relating to bariatrics.

**bar·i·at·rics** (bar-ē-at'riks) that branch of medicine concerned with the management of obesity. [G. *baros*, weight, + *iatreia*, medical treatment]

**bar·i·um (Ba)** (ba'rē-ŭm, bā'rē-ŭm) a metallic, alkaline, divalent earth element; atomic no. 56, atomic wt. 137.327. Salts are often used in diagnosis. [G. *barys*, heavy]

**bar·i·um en·e·ma (BE)** a type of contrast enema; administration of barium, a radiopaque medium, for radiographic and fluoroscopic study of the lower intestinal tract. See this page.

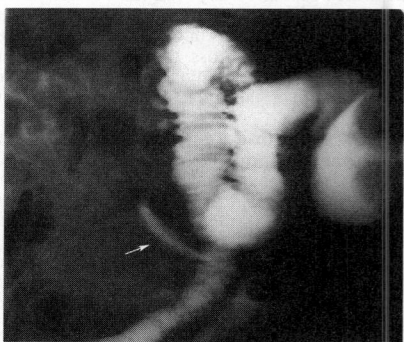

**barium enema:** radiograph of colon showing ruptured diverticulum (arrow)

**bar·i·um swal·low** oral administration of barium sulfate suspension for radiographic investigation of the hypopharynx and esophagus.

**Bar·kan mem·brane** (bahr'kăn) a theoretical tissue covering the trabecular meshwork; thought to obstruct aqueous humor outflow and be responsible for congenital glaucoma.

**Bar·kan op·er·a·tion** (bahr'kăn) goniotomy for congenital glaucoma under direct observation of the anterior chamber angle.

**Bark·man re·flex** (bahrk'mahn) contraction of the ipsilateral rectus muscle in response to a stimulus applied to the skin below a nipple.

**Bar·low dis·ease** (bahr'lō) SYN infantile scurvy.

**Bar·low ma·neu·ver** (bahr'lō) test for hip instability, with dislocation occurring with flexion, adduction, and posterior force.

**Bar·mah For·est virus** (băr'mă) a species of Alphavirus that has caused outbreaks of polyarthritis in humans in Australia; transmitted by mosquitoes. [the virus was first isolated from mosquitoes collected at the Barmah Forest in southeastern Australia in 1974]

**Barnes curve** (barnz) a curve corresponding in general with Carus curve, being the segment of a circle whose center is the promontory of the sacrum.

**Barnes zone** (barnz) the lower fourth of the pregnant uterus, attachment of the placenta to any part of which may cause dangerous hemorrhage.

**baro-** weight, pressure. [G. *baros*, weight]

**bar·o·cep·tor** (bar'ō-sep-ter) SYN baroreceptor.

**bar·og·no·sis** (bar'og-nō'sis) ability to appreciate

the weight of objects, or to differentiate objects of different weights. [G. *baros*, weight, + *gnōsis*, knowledge]

**bar·o·met·ric pres·sure (Pb)** the absolute pressure of the ambient atmosphere, varying with weather, altitude, etc.; expressed in millibars (meteorology) or mmHg or torr (respiratory physiology); at sea level, one atmosphere (atm, 760 mmHg or torr) is equivalent to: 14.69595 lb/sq in, 1013.25 millibars, $1013.25 \times 10^6$ dynes/cm$^2$, and, in SI units, 101,325 pascals (Pa).

**bar·o·phil·ic** (bar'ō-fil'ik) thriving under high environmental pressure; applied to microorganisms. [G. *baros*, weight, + *phileō*, to love]

**bar·o·re·cep·tor** (bar'ō-rē-sep'ter) **1.** in general, any sensor of pressure changes. **2.** sensory nerve ending in the cardiac atria, vena cava, aortic arch, and carotid sinus, sensitive to stretching of the wall resulting from increased pressure from within, and functioning as the receptor of central reflex mechanisms that tend to reduce that pressure. SYN baroceptor, pressoreceptor. [G. *baros,* weight, + receptor]

**bar·o·re·flex** (bar-ō-rē'fleks) a reflex triggered by stimulation of a baroreceptor.

**bar·o·si·nus·i·tis** (bar'ō-sī-nus-ī'tis) SYN aerosinusitis. [G. *baros,* weight, pressure, + sinusitis]

**bar·o·stat** (bar'ō-stat) a pressure-regulating device or structure. [G., *baros*, weight, pressure, + *statos*, made to stand]

**bar·o·tax·is** (bar-ō-tak'sis) reaction of living tissue to changes in pressure. [G. *baros,* weight, + *taxis,* order]

**bar·o·ti·tis me·dia** (bar-ō-tī'tis mē'dē-ă) SYN aerotitis media.

**bar·o·trau·ma** (bar'ō-traw'mă) **1.** injury to the middle ear or paranasal sinuses, resulting from imbalance between ambient pressure and that within the affected cavity. **2.** lung injury that occurs when a patient is on a ventilator and is subjected to excessive airway pressure (pulmonary barotrauma). [G. *baros,* weight, + trauma]

**Bar·ra·quer meth·od** (bah-rah-kār') SYN zonulolysis.

**Barr chro·ma·tin bod·y** (bahr) SYN sex chromatin.

**bar·rel chest** a chest with increased anteroposterior diameter, seen in emphysema.

**bar·rel dis·tor·tion** irregular image produced when peripheral magnification is greater than axial magnification. SEE Petzval surface.

**Barré sign** (bah-rā') a hemiplegic placed in the prone position with the limbs flexed at the knees is unable to maintain the flexed position on the side of the lesion but extends the leg.

**Bar·rett ep·i·the·li·um** (bar'et) columnar esophageal epithelium seen in Barrett syndrome.

**Bar·rett syn·drome, Bar·rett esoph·a·gus, Bar·rett met·a·pla·si·a** (bar'et) chronic peptic ulceration of the lower esophagus, which is lined by columnar epithelium, resembling the mucosa of the gastric cardia, acquired as a result of longstanding chronic esophagitis; esophageal stricture with reflux, and adenocarcinoma, also have been reported.

**bar·ri·er** (bar'ē-er) **1.** an obstacle or impediment. **2.** PSYCHIATRY a conflictual agent that blocks behavior that could help resolve a personal struggle. [M.E., fr. O.Fr. *barriere,* fr. L.L. *barraria*]

**bar·ri·er con·tra·cep·tive** a mechanical device designed to prevent spermatozoa from penetrat-

ing the cervical os; usually used in combination with a spermicidal agent, i.e., vaginal diaphragm.

**Barth her·nia** (bahrt) a loop of intestine between a persistent vitelline duct and the abdominal wall.

**Bar·tho·lin ab·scess** (bahr'tō-lin) an abscess of the vulvovaginal gland.

**Bar·tho·lin cyst** (bahr'tō-lin) a cyst arising from the major vestibular gland or its ducts.

**Bar·tho·lin cys·tec·to·my** (bahr'tō-lin) removal of a cyst of a major vestibular gland.

**Bar·tho·lin gland** (bahr'tō-lin) SYN greater vestibular gland.

**bar·tho·lin·i·tis** (bar-thō-lin-ī'tis) inflammation of a vulvovaginal (Bartholin) gland.

**Barth syn·drome** (bahrt) an X-linked syndrome characterized by poor growth, neutropenia, cardiomyopathy, and excess excretion of 3-methylglutaconic acid in the urine; some patients also show skeletal muscle weakness.

**Bar·ton ban·dage** (bahr'tŏn) a figure-of-8 bandage supporting the mandible below and anteriorly; used in mandibular fracture.

*Bar·ton·el·la* (bar-to-nel'ă) a genus of bacteria closely resembling *Rickettsia* in staining properties, morphology, and mode of transmission between hosts. Organisms usually reside extracellularly in arthropod hosts and intracellularly in mammalian hosts. The type of species is *Rochalimaea quintana*. [A. L. *Barton*]

*Bar·ton·el·la ba·cil·li·for·mis* a species found in the blood, lymph nodes, spleen, and liver in Oroya fever and in blood and eruptive elements in verruga peruana.

**Bar·ton·el·la·ceae** (bar-ton-el-ā'sē-ē) a family of bacteria that currently includes the genus *Bartonella*. On the basis of S16 rRNA studies, the former genera of *Rochalimaea* and *Grahamella* have been merged with the genus *Bartonella*, retaining their species names.

*Bar·ton·el·la hen·sel·ae* a recently recognized species, formerly classified as a riskettsialike organism in the genus *Rochalimaea;* causes bacillary angiomatosis, particularly in immunocompromised persons, and a form of cat-scratch disease.

**bar·ton·el·lo·sis** (bar-tō-nel-ō'sis) a disease, endemic in certain valleys of the Andes in Peru, Chile, Ecuador, Bolivia, and Colombia, caused by *Bartonella bacilliformis*, which is transmitted by the bite of the nocturnally biting sandfly, *Phlebotomus verrucarum;* occurs in three forms: 1) Oroya fever; 2) verruca peruana; 3) a combination or sequence of these.

**Bar·ton for·ceps** (bahr'tŏn) an obstetrical forceps with one fixed curved blade and a hinged anterior blade for application to a high transverse head.

**Bar·ton frac·ture** (bahr'tŏn) fracture of the distal radius with volar subluxation or dislocation of the radiocarpal joint.

**Bart syn·drome** (bahrt) a form of epidermolysis bullosa with blistering of the extremities and intertriginous areas, congenital localized absence of skin, erosions of the mouth, and dystrophic nails; there is often spontaneous improvement with no residual scarring; autosomal dominant inheritance, caused by mutation in the collagen type VII gene (COL7A1) on chromosome 3p.

**Bart·ter syn·drome** (bahr'tĕr) a disorder due to a defect in active chloride reabsorption in the loop of Henle; characterized by primary juxta-glomerular cell hyperplasia with secondary hyperaldosteronism, hypokalemic alkalosis, hypercalciuria, elevated renin or angiotensin levels, normal or low blood pressure, and growth retardation; edema is absent. Autosomal recessive inheritance, caused by mutation in either the Na-K-2Cl cotransporter gene (SLC12A1) on chromosome 15q or the K(+) channel gene (KCNJ1) on 11q.

⚠**bar·y·to-** prefix indicating the presence of barium in a mineral.

**ba·sad** (bā′sad) in a direction toward the base of any object or structure.

**ba·sal** (bā′săl) **1.** situated nearer the base of a pyramid-shaped organ in relation to a specific reference point; opposite of apical. **2.** in dentistry, denoting the floor of a cavity in the grinding surface of a tooth. **3.** denoting a standard or reference state of a function, as a basis for comparison.

**ba·sal an·es·the·sia** parenteral administration of one or more sedatives to produce a state of depressed consciousness short of a general anesthesia.

**ba·sal bod·y** an elongated centriolar structure situated at the base of each cilium at the apical margin of a cell. SYN basal granule.

**ba·sal cell** a cell of the deepest layer of stratified epithelium.

🔲**ba·sal cell car·ci·no·ma, ba·sal cell ep·i·the·li·o·ma** a slow-growing, invasive, but usually non-metastasizing neoplasm of the epidermis or hair follicles, most commonly arising in sun-damaged skin of the elderly and fair-skinned. See this page and B7.

**ba·sal cell ne·vus** a hereditary disease noted in infancy or adolescence, characterized by lesions of the eyelids, nose, cheeks, neck, and axillae, appearing as flesh-colored papules histologically indistinguishable from basal cell epithelioma; the lesions usually remain benign, but in some cases malignant change occurs.

**ba·sal cell ne·vus syn·drome** a syndrome of myriad basal cell nevi with development of basal cell carcinomas in adult life, odontogenic keratocysts, erythematous pitting of the palms and soles, calcification of the cerebral falx, and frequently skeletal anomalies, particularly ribs that are bifid or broadened anteriorly; autosomal dominant inheritance. SYN Gorlin syndrome.

**ba·sal en·ceph·a·lo·cele** a defect in the skull floor with the herniation of brain tissue sometimes associated with coloboma of optic nerve.

**ba·sal gan·glia** large masses of gray matter at the base of the cerebral hemisphere: the striate body (caudate and lentiform nuclei) and cell groups associated with the striate body, such as the subthalamic nucleus and substantia nigra.

**ba·sal gran·ule** SYN basal body.

**ba·sal joint re·flex** opposition and adduction of the thumb with flexion at its metacarpophalangeal joint and extension at its interphalangeal joint, when firm passive flexion of the third, fourth, or fifth finger is made; the reflex is pres-

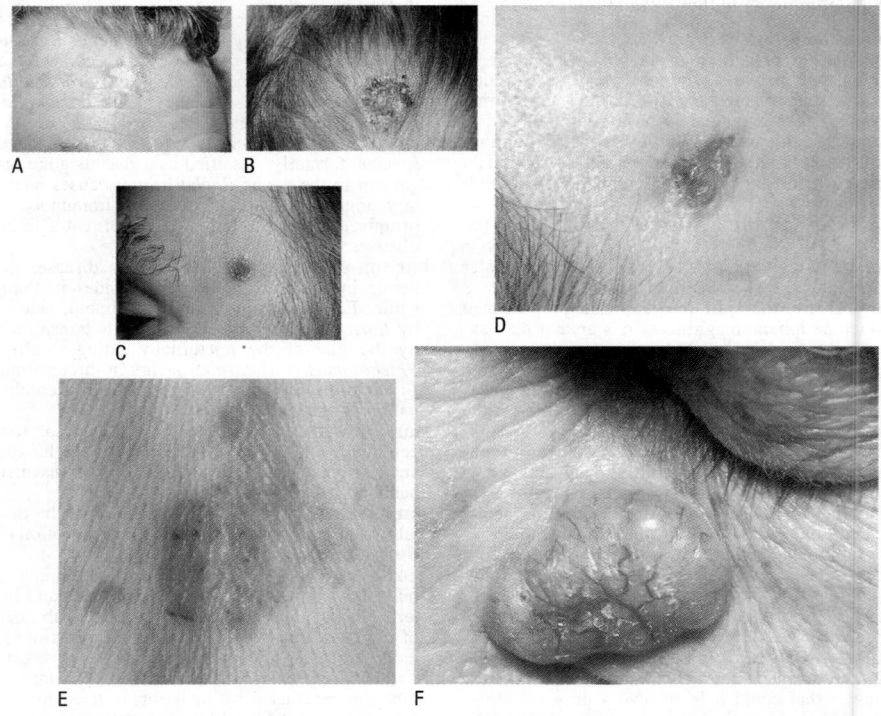

**basal cell carcinomas:** (A) morpheaform, (B), (D) ulcerated, (C), (F) nodular, (E) superficial

ent normally but is absent in pyramidal lesions. SYN finger-thumb reflex, Mayer reflex.

**ba·sal lam·i·na of cil·i·ary bod·y** the inner layer of the ciliary body, continuous with the basal layer of the choroid and supporting the pigment epithelium of the ciliary retina.

**ba·sal lam·i·na of neu·ral tube** the ventral division of the lateral walls of the neural tube in the embryo; it contains neuroblasts giving rise to somatic and visceral motor neurons. SYN basal plate of neural tube.

**ba·sal lam·i·nar dru·sen** small, round, translucent lesions measuring 25–75 μm in diameter, which represent nodular thickening of the basement membrane of the retinal pigment eplithelium, often with an overlying focal detachment of the retinal pigment epithelium from Bruch membrane. SYN cuticular drusen.

**ba·sal lay·er** SYN stratum basale (1).

**ba·sal lay·er of cho·roid** SYN lamina basalis choroideae.

**ba·sal lin·e·ar dru·sen** deposits of long-spaced collagen located between the plasma membrane and basement membrane of the retinal pigment epithelium.

**ba·sal plate of neu·ral tube** SYN basal lamina of neural tube.

**ba·sal rod** SYN costa (2).

**ba·sal sub·stan·tia** basal structures associated with the amygdaloid complex and its connections; includes the basal nucleus (nucleus basalis [TA]) also called the nucleus of Gansser, the sublenticular extended nucleus (pars sublenticularis amygdalae [TA]), and bed nucleus of the stria terminalis (nucleus stria terminalis [TA]). SYN substantia basalis [TA].

**ba·sal ten·to·ri·al branch of in·ter·nal ca·rot·id ar·tery** a small branch from the cavernous part of the internal carotid artery to the base of the tentorium.

**ba·sal vein of Ro·sen·thal** (rō′zen-tahl) a large vein passing caudally and dorsally along the medial surface of the temporal lobe from which it receives tributaries; it empties into the great cerebral vein (of Galen) from the lateral side.

**base** (bās) **1.** the lower part or bottom; the part of a pyramidal or cone-shaped structure opposite the apex; the foundation. SYN basis [TA]. **2.** in pharmacy, the chief ingredient of a mixture. **3.** in chemistry, an electropositive element (cation) that unites with an anion to form a salt; a compound ionizing to yield hydroxyl ion. SYN alkali (2). SEE ALSO Brønsted base, Lewis base. **4.** nitrogen-containing organic compounds (e.g., purines, pyrimidines, amines, alkaloids, ptomaines) that act as Brønsted bases. **5.** cations, or substances forming cations. [L. and G. *basis*]

**base·ball fin·ger** an avulsion, partial or complete, of the long finger extensor from the base of the distal phalanx. SYN mallet finger (2).

**base def·i·cit** a decrease in the total concentration of blood buffer base, indicative of metabolic acidosis or compensated respiratory alkalosis.

**base ex·cess** a measure of metabolic alkalosis; the amount of strong acid that would have to be added per unit volume of whole blood to titrate it to pH 7.4 while at 37°C and at a carbon dioxide pressure of 40 mmHg.

**base of heart** that part of the heart that lies opposite the apex, formed mainly by the left atrium but to a small extent by the posterior part of the

right atrium; it is directed backward and to the right and is separated from the vertebral column by the esophagus and aorta. SYN basis cordis [TA].

**base in·crease at low le·vels** a hearing aid signal-processing strategy to increase gradually the amplification of low frequencies at low-intensity levels.

**base line** a line approximating the base of the skull, passing from the infraorbital ridge to the midline of the occiput, intersecting the superior margin of the external auditory meatus; the skull is in the anatomic position when the base line lies in the horizontal plane. SYN orbitomeatal line.

**base of lung** the lower concave part of the lung that rests upon the convexity of the diaphragm. SYN basis pulmonis [TA].

**base·ment mem·brane** an amorphous extracellular layer closely applied to the basal surface of epithelium and also investing muscle cells, fat cells, and Schwann cells; thought to be a selective filter and to serve both structural and morphogenetic functions. It is composed of three successive layers (lamina lucida, lamina densa, and lamina fibroreticularis), a matrix of collagen, and several glycoproteins. SYN basilemma.

**base of mo·di·o·lus of co·chlea** the part of the modiolus enclosed by the basal turn of the cochlea; it faces the lateral end of the internal acoustic meatus. SEE cochlear area.

**base pair** the complex of two heterocyclic nucleic acid bases, one a pyrimidine and the other a purine, brought about by hydrogen bonding between the purine and the pyrimidine; base pairing is the essential element in the structure of DNA. Usually guanine is paired with cytosine (G·C), and adenine with thymine (A·T) or uracil (A·U). The sequence of the complementary bases in either strand of a two-stranded DNA molecule codes for amino acids used in the manufacture of proteins. Trios of bases (codons) specify each of 20 amino acids. During protein synthesis (translation), messenger RNA and ribosomes read the order of amino acids from strings of DNA to create protein chains, which are then released into the cell.

**base of pha·lanx of foot** proximal, concave, articulating end of the bones of the toes. SYN basis phalangis pedis [TA].

**base of pha·lanx of hand** proximal, concave, articulating end of the bones of the fingers. SYN basis phalangis manus [TA].

**base·plate** (bās′plāt) a temporary form representing the base of a denture; used for making maxillomandibular (jaw) relation records and for the arrangement of teeth.

**base of skull** the sloping floor of the cranial cavity. It comprises both the external base of skull (external view) and the internal base of skull (internal view). SYN basis cranii [TA].

**base of sta·pes** the flat portion of the stapes that fits in the oval window. SYN basis stapedis [TA], footplate (1), foot-plate.

**base sta·tion** general term used for the EMS radio console in a hospital emergency department. Also used to refer to a hospital that provides direct medical control to prehospital providers.

**base u·nits** the fundamental units of length, mass, time, electric current, thermodynamic temperature, amount of substance, and luminous intensity in the International System of Units (SI); the names and symbols of the units for these quantities are meter (m), kilogram (kg), second (s), ampere (A), kelvin (K), mole (mol), and candela (cd). SEE ALSO International System of Units.

⌂**ba•si-, ba•so-, ba•sio-** base; basis. [G. and L. *basis*]

**ba•si•breg•mat•ic ax•is** a line extending from the basion to the bregma.

**ba•sic** (bā′sik) relating to a base.

**ba•sic dyes** dyes which ionize in solution to give positively charged ions or cations; the auxochrome group is an amine which can form a salt with an acid; solutions are usually slightly acidic.

**ba•sic fuch•sin** [CI 42500] a triphenylmethane dye whose dominant component is pararosanilin; an important stain in histology, histochemistry, and bacteriology.

**ba•sic fuch•sin-meth•y•lene blue stain** a stain for intact epoxy sections; semithick sections of plastic-embedded tissues have nuclei stained purple; collagen, elastic lamina, and connective tissue are stained blue; mitochondria, myelin, and lipid droplets are stained red; cytoplasm, smooth muscle cells, axoplasm, and chondroblast are stained pink.

**ba•sic•i•ty** (bā-sis′i-tē) **1.** the valence or combining power of an acid, or the number of replaceable atoms of hydrogen in its molecule. **2.** the characteristic(s) of being a chemical base.

**ba•sic life sup•port** emergency cardiopulmonary resuscitation, control of bleeding, treatment of shock, acidosis, and poisoning, stabilization of injuries and wounds, and basic first aid.

**ba•sic per•son•al•i•ty type 1.** an individual's unique, covert, or underlying personality propensities, whether or not they are behaviorally manifest or overt; **2.** personality characteristics of an individual which are also shared by a majority of the members of a social group.

**ba•si•cra•ni•al ax•is** a line drawn from the basion to the midpoint of the sphenoethmoidal suture.

**ba•si•cra•ni•al flex•ure** SYN pontine flexure.

**ba•sic stain** a dye in which the cation is the colored component of the dye molecule that binds to anionic groups of nucleic acids ($PO_4\equiv$) or acidic mucopolysaccharides.

*Ba•sid•i•ob•o•lus* (ba-sid′ē-ob-ō-lŭs) a genus of fungi. *Basidiobolus haptosporus* has been isolated from cases of zygomycosis (entomophthoramycosis basidiobolae). [Mod. L. *basidium*, dim. of G. *basis*, base, + L. *bolus*, fr. G. *bolos*, lump or clod]

**Ba•sid•i•o•my•co•ta** (ba-sid′ē-ō-mī-kō-tă) a phylum of fungi characterized by a spore-bearing organ, the basidium, that is usually a clavate cell that bears basidiospores after karyogamy and meiosis.

**ba•sid•i•um**, pl. **ba•sid•ia** (ba-sid′ē-ŭm, ba-sid′ē-ă) a cell or spore-bearing organ, usually club-shaped, that is characteristic of the Basidiomycota. It bears basidiospores externally after karyogamy and meiosis. It is composed of a swollen terminal cell situated on a slender stalk, and gives rise to slender filaments (sterigmata), usually four in number, from the ends of which the basidiospores are developed. [L., fr G. *basis*, base]

**ba•si•fa•cial** (bā′si-fā′shăl) relating to the lower portion of the face.

**ba•si•fa•cial ax•is** a line drawn from the subnasal point to the midpoint of the sphenoethmoidal suture. SYN facial axis.

**bas•i•lar, bas•i•la•ris** (bas′i-lăr, bas-i-lā′ris) relating to the base of a pyramidal or broad structure.

**bas•i•lar ar•tery** formed by union of the intracranial portions of the two vertebral arteries; runs along the clivus in the pontine cistern of the subarachnoid space from the lower to the upper border of the pons, where it bifurcates into the two posterior cerebral arteries; *branches*, anterior, inferior, cerebellar, labyrinthine, pontine, mesencephalic, and superior cerebellar. SYN arteria basilaris [TA].

**bas•i•lar lam•i•na** SYN basilar membrane.

**bas•i•lar mem•brane** the membrane extending from the bony spiral membrane to the basilar crest of the cochlea; it forms the greater part of the floor of the cochlear duct separating the latter from the scala tympani and it supports the spiral organ. SYN basilar lamina.

**bas•i•lar men•in•gi•tis** meningitis at the base of the brain, due usually to tuberculosis, syphilis, or any low-grade chronic granulomatous process; may result in an internal hydrocephalus.

**bas•i•lar pa•pil•la** the auditory sense organ of birds, amphibians, and reptiles; homologous to the spiral organ in mammals.

**bas•i•lar ver•te•bra** the lowest lumbar vertebra.

**ba•si•lat•er•al** (bā′si-lat′er-ăl) relating to the base and one or more sides of any part.

**ba•si•lem•ma** (bā-si-lem′ă) SYN basement membrane. [basi- + G. *lemma*, rind]

**ba•sil•ic vein** arises from the ulnar side of the dorsal venous network of the hand; it curves around the medial side of the forearm, communicates with the cephalic vein via the median cubital vein, and passes up the medial side of the arm to join the axillary vein.

**ba•si•on** (bā′sē-on) the middle point on the anterior margin of the foramen magnum, opposite the opisthion. [G. *basis*, a base]

**ba•sip•e•tal** (bā-sip′ĕ-tăl) **1.** in a direction toward the base. **2.** pertaining to asexual conidial production in fungi, in which successive budding of the basal conidium forms in unbranched chain with the youngest at the base. [basi- + L. *peto*, to seek]

**bas•i•pho•bia** (bās-i-fō′bē-ă) morbid fear of walking. [G. *basis*, a stepping, + *phobos*, fear]

**ba•sis** (bā′sis) [TA] SYN base (1). [L. and G.]

**ba•sis cor•dis** [TA] SYN base of heart.

**ba•sis cra•nii** [TA] SYN base of skull.

**ba•sis pha•lan•gis ma•nus** [TA] SYN base of phalanx of hand.

**ba•sis pha•lan•gis pe•dis** [TA] SYN base of phalanx of foot.

**ba•si•sphe•noid** (bā′si-sfē′noyd) relating to the base or body of the sphenoid bone.

**ba•sis pul•mo•nis** [TA] SYN base of lung.

**ba•sis sta•pe•dis** [TA] SYN base of stapes.

**bas•ket cell 1.** a neuron enmeshing the cell body of another neuron with its terminal axon ramifications; **2.** SYN smudge cells. **3.** a myoepithelial cell with branching processes that occurs basal to the secretory cells of certain salivary gland and lacrimal gland alveoli.

**bas•ket nu•cle•us** nuclear structure that may be seen in *Iodamoeba bütschlii* cysts and occasionally in trophozoites; in stained preparations, fibrils may be seen running between the karyosome and the chromatin granules.

**ba·so·e·ryth·ro·cyte** (bā′sō-e-rith′rō-sīt) a red blood cell that manifests changes of basophilic degeneration, such as basophilic stippling, punctate basophilia, or basophilic granules.

**ba·so·e·ryth·ro·cy·to·sis** (bā′sō-ĕ-rith′rō-sī-tō′sis) an increase of red blood cells with basophilic degenerative changes, frequently observed in hypochromic anemia.

**ba·so·lat·er·al** (bā-sō-lat′er-ăl) basal and lateral; specifically used to refer to one of the two major cytological divisions of the amygdaloid complex.

**ba·so·phil, ba·so·phile** (bā′sō-fil, bā-sō-fīl) **1.** a cell with granules that stain specifically with basic dyes. **2.** SYN basophilic. **3.** a phagocytic leukocyte of the blood characterized by basophilic granules containing heparin and histamine; except for its segmented nucleus, it is morphologically and physiologically similar to the mast cell though they originate from different stem cells in the bone marrow. See page B1. [baso- + G. *philēo*, to love]

**ba·so·phil ad·e·no·ma** a tumor of the adenohypophysis in which the cell cytoplasm stains with basic dyes, often ACTH-producing.

**ba·so·phil·ia** (bā-sō-fil′ē-ă) **1.** a condition in which there are more than the usual number of basophilic leukocytes in the circulating blood (basophilic leukocytosis) or an increase in the proportion of parenchymatous basophilic cells in an organ (in the bone marrow, basophilic hyperplasia). **2.** a condition in which basophilic erythrocytes are found in circulating blood, as in certain instances of leukemia, advanced anemia, malaria, and plumbism. **3.** the reaction of immature erythrocytes to basic dyes whereby the cells appear blue or contain bluish granules. SYN basophilism.

**ba·so·phil·ic** (bā′sō-fil′ik) denoting tissue components having an affinity for basic dyes. SYN basophil (2), basophile.

**ba·so·phil·ic leu·ke·mia, ba·so·phil·o·cyt·ic leu·ke·mi·a** a form of granulocytic leukemia in which there are unusually great numbers of basophilic granulocytes in the tissues and circulating blood. SYN mast cell leukemia.

**ba·so·phil·ic leu·ko·cyte** a polymorphonuclear leukocyte characterized by many large, coarse, metachromatic granules (dark purple or blueblack with Wright stain) that usually fill the cytoplasm and may almost mask the nucleus; they usually do not occur in increased numbers as the result of acute infectious disease; the granules, which contain heparin and histamine, may degranulate in response to hypersensitivity reactions and can be of significance in general inflammation. SYN mast leukocyte.

**ba·so·phil·ic leu·ko·pe·nia** a decrease in the number of basophilic granulocytes in the circulating blood.

**ba·soph·i·lism** (bā-sof′i-lizm) SYN basophilia.

**ba·so·squa·mous car·ci·no·ma, ba·si·squa·-mous car·ci·no·ma** a carcinoma of the skin which in structure and behavior is considered transitional between basal cell and squamous cell carcinoma.

**Bas·si·ni her·ni·orr·ha·phy** (ba-sē′nē) an operation for indirect inguinal hernia repair; after reduction of the hernia, the sac is twisted, ligated, and cut off, then a new inguinal floor is made by

uniting the edge of the internal oblique muscle to the inguinal ligament, placing on this the cord, and covering the latter by the external oblique muscle.

**bas·to·ki·nin** SYN uteroglobin.

**batch an·a·ly·zer** a discrete automated chemical analyzer in which the instrument system sequentially performs a single test on each of a group of samples.

**bath 1.** immersion of the body or any of its parts in water or any other yielding or fluid medium, or application of such medium in any form to the body or any of its parts. **2.** apparatus used in giving a bath of any form. **3.** fluid used for maintenance of metabolic activities or growth of living organisms, e.g., cells derived from body tissue. [A.S. *baeth*]

**bath·ing trunk ne·vus** a large hairy congenital pigmented nevus with a predilection for the entire lower trunk; malignant melanoma may develop in childhood.

**bath itch** SYN bath pruritus.

**bath·mo·tro·pic** (bath-mō-trō′pik) influencing nervous and muscular irritability in response to stimuli. [G. *bathmos*, threshold, + *tropē*, a turning]

⊿**ba·tho-** depth. SEE ALSO bathy-. [G. *bathos*, depth]

**bath·o·pho·bia** (bath-ō-fō′bē-ă) morbid fear of deep places or of looking into them. [G. *bathos*, depth, + *phobos*, fear]

**bath pru·ri·tus** itching produced by inadequate rinsing off of soap or by overdrying of skin from excessive bathing. SYN bath itch.

⊿**ba·thy-** depth. SEE ALSO batho-. [G. *bathys*, deep]

**bath·y·an·es·the·sia** (bath′ē-an-es-thē′zē-ă) loss of deep sensibility, i.e., from muscles, ligaments, tendons, bones, and joints. [G. *bathys*, deep, + *an-* priv. + *aisthēsis*, sensation]

**bath·y·es·the·sia** (bath′ē-es-thē′zē-ă) general term for all sensation from the tissues beneath the skin, i.e., muscles, ligaments, tendons, bones and joints. SEE ALSO myesthesia. [G. *bathys*, deep, + *aisthēsis*, sensation]

**bath·y·hy·per·es·the·sia** (bath-ē-hī′per-es-thē′zē-ă) exaggerated sensitiveness of deep structures, e.g., muscular tissue. [G. *bathys*, deep, + *hyper*, above, + *aisthēsis*, sensation]

**bath·y·hyp·es·the·sia** (bath-ē-hip′es-thē′zē-ă) impairment of sensation in the structures beneath the skin, e.g., muscle tissue. [G. *bathys*, deep, + *hypo*, under, + *aisthēsis*, sensation]

**Ba·tis·ta pro·ce·dure** (bah-tēs′tah) surgical reduction of one or both ventricles when they are excessively dilated. SYN ventricular reduction surgery.

**bat·tery** (bat′er-ē) a group or series of tests administered for analytic or diagnostic purposes. [M.E. *batri*, beaten metal, fr. O.Fr. *batre*, to beat]

**Ba·tis·ta op·er·a·tion** SYN left ventricular volume reduction surgery.

**bat·tle·dore pla·cen·ta** a placenta in which the umbilical cord is attached at the border; so-called because of the fancied resemblance to the racquet used in battledore, a precursor to badminton.

**bat·tle fa·tigue** a term used to denote psychiatric illness consequent to the stresses of battle. SEE ALSO war neurosis. SYN shell shock.

**bat·tle neu·ro·sis** SYN war neurosis.

**Bat·tle sign** (bat′ĕl) postauricular ecchymosis in cases of fracture of the base of the skull.

**Bau·de·loc·que op·er·a·tion** (bō-dĕ-lōk′) an incision through the posterior cul-de-sac of the vagina for the removal of the ovum, in extrauterine pregnancy.

**Bau·er chro·mic ac·id leu·co·fuch·sin stain** (bow-er) a stain for glycogen and fungi utilizing chromic acid as an oxidizing agent of polysaccharides, followed by Schiff reagent; glycogen and fungi cell walls appear deep red.

**Bau·er-Kir·by test** (bow-er ker-bē) a standardized test for microbiologic susceptibility performed by transferring a standardized pure culture of the organism of interest onto a sensitivity plate (Petri dish with Mueller-Hinton agar) and observing growth in the presence of disks containing antibiotics.

**Bau·er syn·drome** (bow-er) aortitis and aortic endocarditis as a little-recognized manifestation of rheumatoid arthritis.

**Baum·gar·ten glands** (bawm′gar-ten) SYN Henle glands.

**Baum·gar·ten veins** (bawm′gar-ten) nonobliterated remnants of the vena umbilicalis.

**Bayle dis·ease** (bāl) SYN paresis (2).

**bay·o·net ap·po·si·tion** relationship of two fracture fragments that lie next to each other rather than in end-to-end contact.

**ba·y·o·net for·ceps** forceps with offset blades, such as those for use through an otoscope.

**bay·o·net hair** a spindle-shaped developmental defect occurring at the tapered end of the hair.

**Bay·ou vi·rus** (bī-yu′) a species of Hantavirus in the U.S. causing hantavirus pulmonary syndrome; transmitted by the rice rat.

**Ba·zett for·mu·la** (baz′et) a formula for correcting the observed QT interval in the electrocardiogram for cardiac rate (R-R interval): corrected QT = Q-T sec/$\sqrt{RR}$ sec.

**Ba·zin dis·ease** (bah-zā′) SYN erythema induratum.

**BBB** blood-brain barrier.

**BBOT** 2,5-bis(5-$t$-butylbenzoxazol-2-yl)thiophene, a liquid scintillator.

**B cell co·re·cep·tor** a complex of three proteins associated with the B-cell receptor (CR2, CD19, and TAPA-1).

**B cell dif·fer·en·ti·at·ing fac·tor** SYN interleukin-4.

**B cell re·cep·tors** a complex comprising a membrane-bound immunoglobulin molecule and two associated signal-transducing α and β chains.

**B cells** SYN beta cells (1).

**B cell stim·u·la·tory fac·tor 2** SYN interleukin-6.

**B chain** a polypeptide component of insulin containing 30 amino acyl residues; insulin is formed by the linkage of a B chain to an A chain.

**BCL-2** an oncogene that inhibits apoptosis.

**BCR/ABL gene** a fusion gene produced when a segment of the Abelson protooncogene, ABL, from chromosome 9, translocates to the major breakpoint cluster region (M-BCR) on chromosome 22. The fusion gene produces a specific protein, P210. This fusion gene is found in chronic myelocytic leukemia (CML).

**Bdel·lo·vib·rio bac·ter·i·o·vo·rus** an unusual species of obligatory aerobic, Gram-negative, comma-shaped bacteria that penetrates the cell walls and infects other Gram-negative species of bacteria. It is used extensively for research pur-

poses, primarily in genetic recombinant studies; not known to be a human pathogen.

**BE** barium enema.

**bead·ed** (bēd′ed) **1.** marked by numerous small rounded projections, often arranged in a row like a string of beads. **2.** applied to a series of non-continuous bacterial colonies along the line of inoculation in a stab culture. **3.** denoting stained bacteria in which more deeply stained granules occur at regular intervals in the organism.

**bead·ed hair** SYN monilethrix.

**beak·ed pel·vis** SYN osteomalacic pelvis.

**beak·er cell** SYN goblet cell.

**beam** (bēm) **1.** any bar whose curvature changes under load. DENTISTRY frequently used instead of "bar." **2.** a collimated emission of light or other radiation, such as an x-ray beam. [O.H.G. *Boum*]

**B-E am·pu·ta·tion** *below*-the-*el*bow amputation.

**bear·ing down** expulsive effort of a parturient woman in the second stage of labor.

**bear·ing-down pain** a uterine contraction accompanied by straining and tenesmus; usually appearing in the second stage of labor.

**beat** (bēt) **1.** to strike; to throb or pulsate. **2.** a stroke, impulse, or pulsation, as of the heart or pulse. **3.** mechanical activity of a cardiac chamber produced by catching a stimulus generated elsewhere in the heart. [A.S. *beatan*]

**Beau lines** (bō) transverse grooves on the fingernails following fever, malnutrition, trauma, myocardial infarction or other severe or systemic illness.

**Bech·te·rew dis·ease** (bek-ter′yev) SYN spondylitis deformans.

**Bech·te·rew-Men·del re·flex** (bek-ter′yev-men′ dĕl) percussion of the dorsum of the foot causes flexion of the toes; present in a pyramidal lesion. SYN Mendel-Bechterew reflex.

**Bech·te·rew sign** (bek-ter′yev) paralysis of automatic facial movements, the power of voluntary movement being retained.

**Beck·er dis·ease** (bek′er) an obscure South African cardiomyopathy leading to rapidly fatal congestive heart failure and idiopathic mural endomyocardial disease.

**Beck·er mus·cu·lar dys·tro·phy** (bek′er) a hereditary muscle disorder of late onset, usually in the second or third decade, affecting the proximal muscles with characteristic pseudohypertrophy of the calves; clinical features similar to Duchenne muscular dystrophy but much milder and not a genetic lethal; X-linked recessive inheritance, with both Becker and Duchenne dystrophies caused by mutation in the dystrophin gene on Xp. Cf. Duchenne dystrophy.

**Beck·er ne·vus** (bek′er) a nevus first seen as an irregular pigmentation of the shoulders, upper chest, or scapular area, gradually enlarging irregularly and becoming thickened and hairy.

**Beck·er stain for spi·ro·chetes** a stain applied to thin films fixed in formaldehyde-acetic acid; preparations are treated successively with tannin, carbolic acid, and carbol fuchsin.

**Beck·mann ap·pa·ra·tus** (bek′mahn) apparatus for the accurate measurement of melting points and boiling points in connection with molecular weight determinations.

**Beck meth·od** (bek) a permanent opening into the stomach made from its greater curvature.

**Beck tri·ad** (bek) SYN acute compression triad.

**Beck·with-Wie·de·mann syn·drome** (bek′

with-vē′de-mahn) exomphalos, macroglossia, and gigantism, often with neonatal hypoglycemia; autosomal recessive inheritance.

**Béclard her•nia** (bā-klahr′) a hernia through the opening for the saphenous vein.

**Bec•que•rel,** Antoine H., French physicist and Nobel laureate, 1852–1908. SEE becquerel.

**bec•que•rel** (bek-ă-rel′) the SI unit of measurement of radioactivity, equal to 1 disintegration per second; 1 Bq = $0.027 \times 10^{-9}$ Ci. SEE ALSO absorption. [A.H. *Becquerel*]

**bed** (bed) **1.** in anatomy, a base or structure that supports another structure. **2.** a piece of furniture used for rest, recuperation, or treatment.

**bed•bug** SYN *Cimex.*

**Bed•nar aph•thae** (bed′nahr) traumatic ulcers located bilaterally on either side of the midpalatal raphe in infants.

**bed rest** maintenance of the recumbent position, in bed, to minimize activity and help recovery from disease; formerly used extensively in treatment of tuberculosis, myocardial infarction, and other diseases.

**bed•side test•ing** SYN point of care testing.

**bed•sore, bed sore** (bed′sōr) SYN decubitus ulcer.

**bed•wet•ting** SYN nocturnal enuresis.

**Beer law** (bār) the intensity of a color or of a light ray is inversely proportional to the depth of liquid through which it is transmitted; it is concluded that the absorption is dependent upon the number of molecules in the path of the ray.

**Bee•vor sign** (bē′vŏr) with paralysis of the lower portions of the recti abdominis muscles the umbilicus moves upward.

**be•hav•ior** (bē-hāv′yer) **1.** any response emitted by or elicited from an organism. **2.** any mental or motor act or activity. **3.** specifically, parts of a total response pattern. [M.E., fr. O. Fr. *avoir,* to have]

**be•hav•ior•al** (bē-hāv′yer-ăl) pertaining to behavior.

**be•hav•ior•al ep•i•dem•ic** an epidemic originating in behavioral patterns (in contrast to invading microorganisms); examples include medieval dancing mania, episodes of crowd panic.

**be•hav•ior•al ge•net•ics** the study of heritable factors in behavioral patterns, as by pedigree analysis, biochemical abnormality, or karyotypic analysis.

**be•hav•ior•al im•mu•no•gen** not smoking, regular exercise, and related health-enhancing personal habits and lifestyle of an individual which are associated with a decreased risk of physical illness and dysfunction, and with greater longevity.

**be•hav•ior•al ob•ser•va•tion au•di•o•me•try** a method of observing the motor responses of young children to test sound intensities to determine the hearing threshold.

**be•hav•ior•al path•o•gen** the personal habits and lifestyle behaviors of an individual that are associated with an increased risk of physical illness and dysfunction. Cf. behavioral immunogen.

**be•hav•ior•al psy•chol•o•gy** SYN behaviorism.

**be•hav•ior•al sci•enc•es** a collective term for those disciplines or branches of science, such as psychology, sociology, and anthropology, that derive their theories and methods from the study of the behavior of living organisms.

**be•hav•ior dis•or•der** general term used to de-

note mental illness or psychological dysfunction, specifically those mental, emotional, or behavioral subclasses for which organic correlates do not exist. SEE ALSO antisocial personality disorder.

**be•hav•ior•ism** (bē-hāv′yer-izm) a branch of psychology that formulates, through systematic observation and experimentation, the laws and principles which underlie the behavior of man and animals; its major contributions have been made in the areas of conditioning and learning. SYN behavioral psychology.

**be•hav•ior mod•i•fi•ca•tion** the systematic use of principles of conditioning and learning, especially operant or instrumental conditioning, to teach certain skills or to extinguish undesirable behaviors, attitudes, or phobias.

**be•hav•ior ther•a•py** an offshoot of psychotherapy involving the use of procedures and techniques associated with conditioning and learning for the treatment of a variety of psychological conditions.

**be•hav•iour•ism [Br.]** SEE behaviorism.

**Beh•çet syn•drome, Beh•çet dis•ease** (beh-chet′) a syndrome characterized by simultaneously or successively occurring recurrent attacks of genital and oral ulcerations (aphthae) and uveitis or iridocyclitis with hypopyon, often with arthritis; a phase of a generalized disorder, occurring more often in men than in women, with variable manifestations, including dermatitis, erythema nodosum, thrombophlebitis, and cerebral involvement. SYN uveoencephalitic syndrome.

**be•hind-the-ear hear•ing aid** hearing aid that rests on the medial aspect of the pinna.

**Beh•ring law** (bā′ring) parenteral administration of serum from an immunized person provides a relative, passive immunity to that disease (i.e., prevents it, or favorably modifies its course) in a previously susceptible person.

**Behr syn•drome** (bār) characterized by bilateral optic atrophy with temporal field defects, nystagmus, ataxia, spasticity, and mental retardation; probably autosomal recessive inheritance.

**bel** unit expressing the relative intensity of a sound. The intensity in bels is the logarithm (to the base 10) of the ratio of the power of the sound to that of a reference sound. Ordinarily, the reference sound is assumed to be one with a power of $10^{-16}$ watts per sq cm, approximately the threshold of a normal human ear at 1000 Hz. [A.G. *Bell,* Scottish-U.S. scientist, 1847–1922]

**belch•ing** SYN eructation. [A.S. *baelcian*]

**belle in•dif•fér•ence** SEE la belle indifférence.

**Bel•li•ni ducts** (be-lē′nē) SYN papillary ducts.

**Bell law** (bel) the ventral spinal roots are motor, the dorsal are sensory. SYN Magendie law.

**Bell pal•sy** paresis or paralysis, usually unilateral, of the facial muscles, caused by dysfunction of the 7th cranial nerve; probably due to a viral infection; usually demyelinating in type. SYN peripheral facial paralysis.

**Bell phe•nom•e•non** (bel) reflex upper deviation of the eye on attempted eye closure; seen with several disorders, including facial mononeuropathies, Guillain-Barré syndrome, and myasthenia gravis.

**bell-shap•ed curve** SYN gaussian distribution.

**Bell spasm** (bel) SYN facial tic.

**bel•ly** (bel′ē) **1.** the abdomen. **2.** the wide swelling part of a muscle. SYN venter (2). **3.** popularly, the stomach or womb. [O.E. *belig,* bag]

**bel·o·ne·pho·bia** (bel'ō-nē-fō'bē-ă) morbid fear of needles, pins, and other sharp-pointed objects. [G. *belonē,* needle, + *phobos,* fear]

**Bel·sey fun·do·pli·ca·tion** (bel'sē) partial (270°) fundoplication performed via thoracotomy.

**Bence Jones pro·tein·u·ria** (bens jōnz) presence of Bence Jones protein in the urine, indicative of multiple myeloma, amyloidosis, or Waldenström macroglobulinemia.

**Bence Jones re·ac·tion** (bens jōnz) the classic means of identifying Bence Jones protein, which precipitates when urine containing it is gradually warmed to 45° to 70°C, and redissolves as the urine is heated to near boiling.

**bench·mark·ing** use of the qualities or performance of an organization as a standard of comparison for one's own organization.

**Bend·er ge·stalt test** (ben'der) a psychological test used by neurologists and clinical psychologists to measure a person's ability to visually copy a set of geometric designs; useful for measuring visuospatial and visuomotor coordination to detect brain damage.

**bend·ing frac·ture** an injury in which a long bone or bones, usually the radius and ulna, are bent due to multiple microfractures, none of which can be seen by x-ray imaging.

**bends** (bendz) colloquialism for Caisson sickness; decompression sickness. [fr. convulsive posture of those so afflicted]

**Be·ne·dek re·flex** (ben'ĕ-dek) plantar flexion of the foot caused by tapping the anterior margin of the lower part of the fibula, while the foot is slightly dorsiflexed.

**Ben·e·dict test** a copper-reduction test for glucose in urine.

**Ben·e·dikt syn·drome** (ben'ĕ-dikt) hemiplegia with clonic spasm or tremor and oculomotor paralysis on the opposite side.

**be·nign** (bē-nīn') denoting the mild character of an illness or the nonmalignant character of a neoplasm. [thru O. Fr., fr. L. *benignus,* kind]

**be·nign co·i·tal ceph·al·al·gia** SYN coital headache.

**be·nign ex·er·tion·al head·ache** headache occurring with exertion or straining in the absence of any intracranial disease.

**be·nign hy·per·ten·sion** hypertension that runs a relatively long and symptomless course.

**be·nign in·fan·tile my·oc·lo·nus** a seizure disorder of infancy in which myoclonic movements occur in the neck, trunk, and extremities; the EEG is normal, and seizures do not persist beyond 2 years of age.

**be·nign in·oc·u·la·tion lym·pho·re·tic·u·lo·sis, be·nign in·oc·u·la·tion re·tic·u·lo·sis** SYN catscratch disease.

**be·nign lym·pho·cy·to·ma cu·tis** a soft red to violaceous skin nodule caused by dense infiltration of the dermis by lymphocytes and histiocytes. SYN cutaneous pseudolymphoma.

**be·nign mon·o·clo·nal gam·mop·a·thy** SYN monoclonal gammopathy of undetermined significance.

**be·nign par·ox·ys·mal po·si·tion·al ver·ti·go** a recurrent, brief form of positional vertigo oc-

curring in clusters; believed to result from displaced remnants of utricular otoconia.

**be·nign po·si·tion·al ver·ti·go** brief attacks of paroxysmal vertigo and nystagmus that occur solely with certain head movements or positions, e.g., with neck extension; due to labyrinthine dysfunction. SYN postural vertigo (1).

**be·nign pros·tatic hy·per·pla·sia (BPH)** progressive enlargement of the prostate due to hyperplasia of both glandular and stromal components, typically beginning in the fifth decade and sometimes causing obstructive or irritative symptoms or both; does not evolve into cancer.

**be·nign ter·tian fe·ver** SYN vivax malaria.

**be·nign tet·a·nus** a disorder marked by intermittent tonic muscular contractions of the extremities, especially the hands and feet (carpopedal spasm), accompanied by paresthesias and, when severe, by crowing respirations due to laryngospasm and seizures; results from hypocalcemia, caused by various disorders, including gastrointestinal abnormalities. SYN intermittent cramp (2).

**be·nign tu·mor** a tumor that does not form metastases and does not invade and destroy adjacent normal tissue. See page B7.

**Ben·nett frac·ture** (ben'ĕt) fracture dislocation of the first metacarpal bone at the carpal-metacarpal joint.

**Ben·nett move·ment** (ben'ĕt) a lateral, bodily shift of the condyles of the lower jaw during lateral excursions.

**Benn·hold Con·go red stain** an amyloid stain useful for amyloid detection in pathologic tissue; gives red staining of amyloid; also induces green birefringence to amyloid under polarized light.

**ben·tir·o·mide test** a test of pancreatic exocrine function that does not require duodenal intubation: orally administered bentiromide is cleaved by chymotrypsin within the lumen of the small intestine, releasing *p*-aminobenzoic acid which is absorbed and excreted in the urine; diminished urinary excretion of *p*-aminobenzoic acid suggests pancreatic insufficiency.

**ben·ton·ite floc·cu·la·tion test** a flocculation test for rheumatoid arthritis in which sensitized bentonite particles are added to inactivated serum; the test is positive if half of the particles are clumped while the other half remain in suspension.

**benz-** combining form denoting benzene.

**ben·zene ring** the closed-chain arrangement of the carbon and hydrogen atoms in the benzene molecule. SEE ALSO cyclic compound.

**ben·zo·yl** (ben'zō-yl) the benzoic acid radical, $C_6H_5CO—$, forming benzoyl compounds.

**ben·zyl·i·dene** (ben-zil'i-dēn) the hydrocarbon radical, $C_6H_5CH=$.

**ben·zyl·ox·y·car·bon·yl (Z)** (ben'zil-ok-sē-kar'bon-il) amino-protecting radical used (as the chloride) in peptide synthesis, yielding $PhCH_2OCO—NHR.$ SYN carbobenzoxy-.

**Bé·rard an·eu·rysm** (bā-rahr') an arteriovenous aneurysm in the tissues outside the injured vein.

**Ber·ar·di·nel·li syn·drome** (bĕr-ahr'dĭ-nel'ē) SYN congenital total lipodystrophy.

**be·reave·ment** (bĕ-rēv-ment) an acute state of intense psychological sadness and suffering experienced after the tragic loss of a loved one or some priceless possession. [M.E., *bireven,* to deprive, + -ment]

**Ber·ger dis·ease, Ber·ger fo·cal glo·mer·u·**

b
e

**lo•ne•phri•tis** (ber′gĕr) SYN focal glomerulonephritis.

**Ber•ger space** (ber′gĕr) the space between the patellar fossa of the vitreous and the lens.

**Berg•man sign** (bĕrg′mĕn) a radiographic finding in which 1) the ureter is dilated distal to a ureteral obstruction and 2) a catheter, passed retrograde, coils in the dilated ureter. SYN catheter coiling sign.

**Berg stain** (berg) a method for staining spermatozoa, utilizing a carbol-fuchsin solution followed by dilute acetic acid and methylene blue; spermatozoa are stained a brilliant red and most other structures appear blue to purple.

**ber•i•beri, ber•i ber•i** (ber′ē-ber′ē) a nutritional deficiency syndrome occurring in endemic form in eastern and southern Asia, sporadically in other parts of the world, and sometimes in alcoholics, resulting mainly from a dietary deficiency of thiamine; characterized by painful polyneuritis, and edema resulting from a high-output form of heart failure. SYN endemic neuritis. [Singhalese, extreme weakness]

**berke•li•um (Bk)** (berk′lē-um) an artificial transuranium radioactive element; atomic no. 97, atomic wt. 247.07. [*Berkeley,* Calif., city where first prepared]

**Ber•lin blue** (ber-lin′ bloo) [CI 77510] ferric ferrocyanide; a dye used to color injection masses for blood vessels and lymphatics, and in staining of siderocytes. SYN Prussian blue.

**Ber•lin e•de•ma** (bĕr-lin′) retinal edema after blunt trauma to the globe.

**ber•loque der•ma•ti•tis, ber•lock der•ma•ti•tis** a type of photosensitization resulting in deep brown pigmentation on exposure to sunlight after application of bergamot oil and other essential oils in perfume.

**Ber•nard-Can•non ho•me•o•sta•sis** (bār-nahr′ ka′nŏn) the set of mechanisms responsible for the cybernetic adjustment of physiological and biochemical states in postnatal life. SYN physiologic homeostasis.

**Ber•nays sponge** (bĕr-nāz′) a compressed disk of aseptic cotton that swells when moistened; used in packing cavities.

**Bern•hardt dis•ease** (bern′hahrt) SYN meralgia paraesthetica.

**Bern•heim syn•drome** (bārn′hīm) systemic congestion resembling the consequences of right heart failure (enlarged liver, distended neck veins, and edema) without pulmonary congestion in subjects with left ventricular enlargement from any cause; reduction in the size of the right ventricular cavity is found by contrast imaging or echocardiography or at postmortem due to encroachment by the hypertrophied or aneurysmal ventricular septum.

**Ber•noul•li law** (bĕr-noo′lē, bār-noo-ē′) when friction is negligible, the velocity of flow of a gas or fluid through a tube is inversely related to its pressure against the side of the tube; i.e., velocity is greatest and pressure lowest at a point of constriction.

**Bern•stein test** (bern′stēn) a test to establish that substernal pain is due to reflux esophagitis, performed by instillation of a weak hydrochloric acid solution directly into the lower esophagus. SYN acid perfusion test.

**ber•ry an•eu•rysm** a small saccular aneurysm of a cerebral artery that resembles a berry. Such aneurysms frequently rupture causing subarachnoid hemorrhage.

**Ber•thol•let law** (bār-tho-lā′) salts in solution always react with each other so as to form a less soluble salt, if possible.

*Ber•ti•el•la stu•der•i* (ber-tē-el′ă stood-er′ē) common tapeworm found in primates; incidental zoonotic infections in humans in the tropics have been reported.

**Ber•tin col•umns** (bār-ta′) SYN renal columns.

**be•ryl•li•o•sis** (be-ril-ē-ō′sis) beryllium poisoning characterized by granulomatous fibrosis of the lungs from chronic inhalation of beryllium.

**be•ryl•li•um** (be-ril′ē-ŭm) a white metal element belonging to the alkaline earths; atomic no. 4., atomic wt. 9.012182. [G. *beryllos,* beryl]

**Bes•nier-Boeck-Schau•mann dis•ease** (bā-nyä′ bek shaw′mahn) SYN sarcoidosis.

**Bes•nier pru•ri•go** (bā-nyä′) European term for prurigo, possibly atopic.

**Best car•mine stain** (best) a method for the demonstration of glycogen in tissues.

**Best dis•ease** (best) autosomal dominant macular degeneration beginning during the first years of life. SYN vitelliform retinal dystrophy.

**best fre•quen•cy** SYN characteristic frequency.

**bes•ti•al•i•ty** (bes-chē-al′i-tē) sexual relations between a human and an animal. SYN zooerastia. [L. *bestia,* beast]

**be•ta** (β) (bā′ta) **1.** second letter of the Greek alphabet. **2.** CHEMISTRY denotes the second in a series, the second carbon from a functional (e.g., carboxylic) group, or the direction of a chemical bond toward the viewer. For terms with the prefix β, see the specific term.

**be•ta-block•er** (bā′tă-blok′er) SYN β-adrenergic blocking agent.

**be•ta cells 1.** basophil cells of the anterior lobe of the hypophysis that contain basophil granules and are believed to produce gonadotropic hormones; SYN B cells. **2.** the predominant cells of the islets of Langerhans, which produce insulin.

**be•ta•cism** (bā′tă-sizm) a defect in speech in which the sound of *b* is given to other consonants. [G. *bēta,* the second letter of the alphabet]

**be•ta fi•bers** nerve fibers having conduction velocities of about 40 m/sec.

**be•ta gran•ule** a granule of a beta cell.

**Be•ta•her•pes•vir•i•nae** (bā′ta-her′pez-vir′ĭ-nē) a subfamily of Herpesviridae containing Cytomegalovirus and Roseolovirus.

**be•ta•ine** (bē′tă-ēn) **1.** an oxidation product of choline and a transmethylating intermediate in metabolism. **2.** a class of compounds related to betaine(1) (i.e., $R_3 N^=-CHR'-COO^-$).

**be•ta par•ti•cle** an electron, either positively (positron, $\beta^+$) or negatively (negatron, $\beta^-$) charged, emitted during beta decay of a radionuclide. SYN beta ray.

**be•ta ray** SYN beta particle.

**be•ta rhy•thm** a wave pattern in the electroencephalogram in the frequency band of 18 to 30 Hz. SYN beta wave.

**be•ta-thal•as•sae•mia [Br.]**

**be•ta•tron** (bā′tă-tron) a circular electron accelerator that is a source of either high energy electrons or x-rays.

**be•ta wave** SYN beta rhythm.

**Be•thes•da sys•tem, Be•thes•da class•i•fi•ca•tion** (bĕ-thes′da) a comprehensive system for reporting findings on cervical Papanicolaou smears; includes observations on the adequacy of the specimen, benign cellular changes (inflammation, infection), changes in squamous or glandular epithelial cells reflecting atypia or malignancy, and hormonal status. [*Bethesda*, Maryland, site of NIH]

**Be•thes•da u•nit** a measure of inhibitor activity: the amount of inhibitor that will inactivate 50% or 0.5 unit of a coagulation factor during the incubation period. [*Bethesda*, MD]

**Bet•ke-Klei•hau•er test** (bet′kĕ-klī′haw-er) a slide test for the presence of fetal red blood cells among those of the mother.

**Betz cells** (betz) large pyramidal cells in the motor area of the precentral gyrus of the cerebral cortex.

**Beu•ren syn•drome** supravalvular aortic stenosis with multiple areas of peripheral pulmonary arterial stenosis, mental retardation, and dental anomalies.

**be•zoar** (bē′zōr) a concretion formed in the alimentary canal of animals, and occasionally humans; formerly considered to be a useful medicine with magical properties and apparently still used for this purpose in some places; according to the substance forming the ball, may be termed trichobezoar (hairball), trichophytobezoar (hair and vegetable fiber mixed), or phytobezoar (foodball). [Pers. *padzahr*, antidote]

**B fi•bers** myelinated fibers autonomic nerves, with a diameter of 2 μm or less, conducting at a rate of 3 to 15 m/sec.

**Bi** bismuth.

△**bi- 1.** prefix meaning twice or double, referring to double structures, dual actions, etc. **2.** in chemistry, used to denote a partially neutralized acid (an acid salt); e.g., bisulfate. Cf. bis-, di-. [L.]

**Bi an•ti•gen** SYN Bile antigen. SEE blood group.

**bi•ar•tic•u•lar** (bī′ar-tik′yu-lăr) SYN diarthric.

**bi•as** (bī′as) **1.** systematic discrepancy between a measurement and the true value; may be constant or proportionate and may adversely affect test results. **2.** any trend in the collection, analysis, interpretation, publication, or review of data that can lead to conclusions that differ systematically from the truth; deviation of results or inferences from the truth, or processes leading to deviation. [Fr. *biais*, obliquity, perh. fr. L. *bifax*, two-faced]

**bi•au•ric•u•lar ax•is** a straight line joining the two auricles.

**bi•ax•i•al joint** one in which there are two principal axes of movement situated at right angles to each other; e.g., saddle joints.

**bi bi re•ac•tion, bi-bi re•ac•tion** a reaction catalyzed by a single enzyme in which two substrates and two products are involved; the ping-pong mechanism may be involved in such a reaction. Cf. mechanism.

**bi•cam•er•al** (bī-kam′er-ăl) having two chambers; denoting especially an abscess divided by a more or less complete septum. [bi- + L. *camera*, chamber]

**BICAP cau•tery** a form of bipolar electrocoagulation frequently used to arrest gastrointestinal bleeding.

**bi•cap•su•lar** (bī-kap′soo-lăr) having a double capsule.

**bi•car•bon•ate** (bī-kar′bon-āt) the ion remaining after the first dissociation of carbonic acid; a central buffering agent in blood.

**bi•car•di•o•gram** (bī-kar′dē-ō-gram) the com-

posite curve of an electrocardiogram representing the combined effects of the right and left ventricles.

**bi•cel•lu•lar** (bī-sel′yu-lăr) having two cells or subdivisions.

**bi•ceps** (bī′seps) a muscle with two origins or heads. Commonly used to refer to the biceps brachii muscle. [bi- + L. *caput*, head]

**bi•ceps bra•chii mus•cle** *origin*, long head from supraglenoidal tuberosity of scapula, short head from coracoid process; *insertion*, tuberosity of radius; *action*, flexes and supinates forearm (it is the primary supinator of the forearm); *nerve supply*, musculocutaneous. SYN musculus biceps brachii [TA].

**bi•ceps fe•mo•ris mus•cle** *origin*, long head (caput longum) from tuberosity of ischium, short head (caput breve) from lower half of lateral lip of linea aspera; *insertion*, head of fibula; *action*, flexes knee and rotates leg laterally; *nerve supply*, long head, tibial, short head, peroneal. SYN musculus biceps femoris [TA].

**bi•ceps re•flex** contraction of the biceps brachii muscle when its tendon of insertion is struck.

**Bi•chat fis•sure** (bē-shah′) the nearly circular fissure corresponding to the medial margin of the cerebral (pallial) mantle, marking the hilus of the cerebral hemisphere, consisting of the callosomarginal fissure and choroidal fissure along the hippocampus, both of which are continuous with the stem of the fissure of Sylvius at the anterior extremity of the temporal lobe.

**Bi•chat mem•brane** (bē-shah′) the inner elastic membrane of arteries.

**bi•cip•i•tal** (bī-sip′i-tăl) **1.** two-headed. **2.** relating to a biceps muscle. [bi- + L. *caput*, head]

**bi•cip•i•tal rib** fusion of first thoracic rib with cervical vertebra.

**bi•clo•nal** (bī-klō′năl) pertaining to or characterized by biclonality.

**bi•clon•al•i•ty** (bī-klōn-al′i-tē) a condition in which some cells have markers of one cell line and other cells have markers of another cell line, as in biclonal leukemias.

**bi•con•cave** (bī-kon′kāv) concave on two sides; denoting especially a form of lens. SYN concavoconcave.

**bi•con•cave lens** a lens that is concave on two opposing surfaces. SYN concavoconcave lens.

**bi•con•dy•lar joint** a synovial joint in which two distinct rounded surfaces of one bone articulate with shallow depressions on another bone.

**bi•con•vex** (bī-kon′veks) convex on two sides; denoting especially a form of lens. SYN convexoconvex.

**bi•con•vex lens** a lens with both surfaces convex. SYN convexoconvex lens.

**bi•cor•nate uter•us** a uterus that is more or less completely divided into two lateral horns as a result of imperfect fusion of the paramesonephric ducts during embryonic development; it differs from septate uterus, in which there is no external mark of separation; in uterus bicornis, the cervix may be single (uterus bicornis unicollis) or double (uterus bicornis bicollis).

**bi•cor•nous, bi•cor•nu•ate, bi•cor•nate** (bī-kōr′nŭs, bī-kōr-′nyu-āt, bī-kōr′nāt) two-horned; having two processes or projections. [bi- + L. *cornu*, horn]

△**bicro-** SYN pico- (2).

**bi•cron** (bī′kron) SYN picometer.

**bi·cus·pid** (bī-kŭs′pid) **1.** having two points, prongs, or cusps. **2.** SYN premolar. [bi- + L. *cuspis,* point]

**bi·cus·pid mur·mur** SYN Flint murmur.

**bi·cus·pid tooth** SYN premolar tooth.

**bi·cus·pid valve** SYN mitral valve.

**bi·dac·ty·ly** (bī-dak′ti-lē) abnormality in which the medial digits are lacking, with only the first and fifth represented. SEE ALSO ectrodactyly. [bi- + G. *daktylos,* finger]

**bi·di·rec·tion·al ven·tric·u·lar tach·y·car·dia** ventricular tachycardia in which the QRS complexes in the electrocardiogram are alternately mainly positive and mainly negative; many such cases may represent ventricular tachycardia with alternating forms of aberrant ventricular conduction.

**bi·dis·coi·dal pla·cen·ta** a placenta with two separate disk-shaped portions attached to opposite walls of the uterus, normal for certain monkeys and shrews, and occasionally found in humans.

**BIDS** *b*rittle hair, *i*mpaired intelligence, *d*ecreased fertility, and *s*hort stature; usually manifested as an inherited deficiency of a high-sulfur protein.

**Biel·schow·sky dis·ease** (byels-chov′skē) early childhood type of lipofuscinosis.

**Biel·schow·sky sign** (byels-chov′skē) in paralysis of a superior oblique muscle, tilting the head to the side of the involved eye causes that eye to rotate upward.

**Biel·schow·sky stain** (byels-chov′skē) a method of treating tissues with silver nitrate to demonstrate reticular fibers, neurofibrils, axons, and dendrites.

**Bier am·pu·ta·tion** (bēr) osteoplastic amputation of tibia and fibula.

**Bier hy·per·e·mia** (bēr) obsolete term for hyperemia produced by Bier method (2).

**Bier meth·od** (bēr) **1.** SYN intravenous regional anesthesia. **2.** treatment of various surgical conditions by reactive hyperemia.

**Bier·nac·ki sign** (byer-naht′skē) analgesia to percussion of the ulnar nerve in tabes dorsalis and dementia paralytica.

**bi·fid** (bī′fid) split or cleft; separated into two parts. [L. *bifidus,* cleft in two parts]

**bi·fid ep·i·glot·tis** congenital malformation in which the right and left sides of the epiglottis are not joined; associated with stridor and aspiration in the newborn due to the rotation of the two sides of the epiglottis into the glottis.

*Bi·fi·do·bac·te·ri·um* (bī′fī-dō-bak-tēr′ē-ŭm) a genus of anaerobic bacteria (family Actinomycetaceae) containing Gram-positive rods of highly variable appearance; freshly isolated strains characteristically show true and false branching, with bifurcated V and Y forms uniform or branched, and club or spatulate forms. They frequently stain irregularly; two or more granules may stain with methylene blue, while the remainder of the cell is unstained. They are not acid fast, are nonmotile, and do not produce spores; acetic and lactic acids are produced from glucose. Pathogenicity for humans is rare, although they have been found in the feces and alimentary tract of infants, older people, and animals. The type species is *Bifidobacterium bifidum.* [L. *bifidus,* cleft in two parts, + bacterium]

*Bi·fid·o·bac·ter·i·um den·ti·um* a bacterial species recovered in association with dental caries

and periodontal disease. It is also an opportunistic pathogen, recovered in mixed infections associated with abscess formation.

**bi·fid ton·gue** a structural defect of the tongue in which the extremity is divided longitudinally for a greater or lesser distance. SEE ALSO diglossia. SYN cleft tongue.

**bi·fo·cal** (bī-fō′kăl) having two foci.

**bi·fo·cal lens** a lens used in cases of presbyopia, in which one portion is suited for distant vision, the other for reading and close work in general.

**bi·fo·rate** (bī-fō′rāt) having two openings. [bi- + L. *foro,* pp. *-atus,* to bore, pierce]

**bi·fur·cate, bi·fur·cat·ed** (bī-fer′kāt, bī-fer-′kā-ted) forked; two-pronged; having two branches. [bi- + L. *furca,* fork]

**bi·fur·ca·tion** (bī-fer-kā′shŭn) a forking; a division into two branches.

**big ACTH** a form of ACTH, produced by certain tumors, not immunochemically distinguishable from little ACTH but not exerting any of the biological effects characteristic of ACTH.

**bi·gem·i·nal pulse** a pulse in which the beats occur in pairs. SYN coupled pulse, pulsus bigeminus.

**bi·gem·i·nal rhy·thm** cardiac rhythm in which each beat of the dominant rhythm (sinus or other) is followed by a premature beat, with the result that the heartbeats occur in pairs (bigeminy). SYN coupled rhythm.

**bi·gem·i·ny** (bī-jem′i-nē) pairing; especially, the occurrence of heartbeats in pairs. [bi- + L. *geminus,* twin]

**bi·lat·er·al** (bī-lat′er-ăl) relating to, or having, two sides. [bi- + L. *latus,* side]

**bi·lat·er·al co·or·din·a·tion** the ability to coordinate the two sides of the body.

**bi·lat·er·al her·maph·ro·dit·ism** true hermaphroditism with an ovotestis on each side.

**bile** (bīl) the yellowish brown or green fluid secreted by the liver and discharged into the duodenum, where it aids in the emulsification of fats, increases peristalsis, and retards putrefaction; contains sodium glycocholate and sodium taurocholate, cholesterol, biliverdin and bilirubin, mucus, fat, lecithin, cells, and cellular debris. [L. *bilis*]

**bile ac·ids** steroid acids found in bile; e.g., taurocholic and glycocholic acids, used therapeutically when biliary secretion is inadequate and for biliary colic. Their physiological roles include fat emulsification.

**Bile an·ti·gen** SYN Bi antigen.

**bile duct** any of the ducts conveying bile between the liver and the intestine, including hepatic, cystic, and common bile duct. SYN biliary duct.

**bile pig·ments** coloring matter in the bile derived from porphyrins by rupture of a methane bridge; e.g., bilirubin, biliverdin.

**bi·le·vel pos·i·tive air·way pres·sure (BiPAP)** a mode of mechanical ventilatory support in which two levels of continuous positive airway pressure (CPAP) are delivered to the patient: (1) inspiratory positive airway pressure (IPAP); (2) expiratory positive airway pressure (EPAP).

**bil·har·zi·al dys·en·tery** dysentery due to infection with *Schistosoma mansoni, S. haematobium,* or *S. japonicum.*

△**bili-** bile. [L. *bilis,* bile]

**bil·i·ary** (bil′ē-ār-ē) relating to bile or the biliary tract. SYN bilious (1).

**bil·i·ary a·tre·sia** atresia of the major bile ducts, causing cholestasis and jaundice, which does not become apparent until several days after birth; periportal fibrosis develops and leads to cirrhosis, with proliferation of small bile ducts and giant cell transformation of hepatic cells. Cf. neonatal hepatitis.

**bil·i·ary can·a·lic·u·lus** one of the intercellular channels, 1 μm or less in diameter, that occur between liver cells forming the first portion of the bile system.

**bil·i·ary cir·rho·sis** cirrhosis due to biliary obstruction, which may be a primary intrahepatic disease or secondary to obstruction of extrahepatic bile ducts; the latter may lead to cholestasis and proliferation in small bile ducts with fibrosis, but marked disturbance of the lobular pattern is infrequent.

**bil·i·ary duct** SYN bile duct.

**bil·i·ary duc·tules** the excretory ducts of the liver that connect the interlobular ductules to the right (or left) hepatic duct. SYN ductuli biliferi.

**bil·i·gen·e·sis** (bil-i-jen′ĕ-sis) bile production. [bili- + G. *genesis*, production]

**bil·i·gen·ic** (bil-i-jen′ik) bile-producing.

**bil·ious** (bil′yŭs) **1.** SYN biliary. **2.** relating to or characteristic of biliousness. **3.** formerly, denoting a temperament characterized by a quick, irritable temper. SYN choleric.

**bil·i·ra·chia** (bil-i-rā′kē-ă) occurrence of bile pigments in the spinal fluid. [bili- + G. *rhachis*, spine]

**bil·i·ru·bin** (bil-i-roo′bin) a yellow bile pigment found as sodium bilirubinate (soluble), or as an insoluble calcium salt in gallstones, formed from hemoglobin during normal and abnormal destruction of erythrocytes by the reticuloendothelial system. Excess bilirubin is associated with jaundice. [bili- + L. *ruber*, red]

**bil·i·ru·bi·ne·mia** (bil′i-roo-bin-ē′mē-ă) the presence of bilirubin in the blood, where it is normally present in relatively small amounts; the term is usually used in relation to increased concentrations observed in various pathologic conditions where there is excessive destruction of erythrocytes or interference with the mechanism of excretion in the bile. Determination of the quantity of bilirubin in the blood serum reveals two fractions, namely direct reacting (conjugated) and indirect reacting (nonconjugated) bilirubin; determination of conjugated and total bilirubin in serum is an important and frequently used clinical laboratory test. [bilirubin + G. *haima*, blood]

**bil·i·ru·bin en·ceph·a·lop·a·thy** SYN kernicterus.

**bil·i·ru·bin·oids** (bil-i-roo′bin-oydz) generic term denoting intermediates in the conversion of bilirubin to stercobilin by reductive enzymes in intestinal bacteria; most are found in normal urine and feces.

**bil·i·ru·bi·nu·ria** (bil′i-roo-bi-nyu′rē-ă) the presence of bilirubin in the urine. [bilirubin + G. *ouron*, urine]

**bil·i·u·ria** (bil-ē-yu′rē-ă) the presence of various bile salts, or bile, in the urine. SYN choleuria, choluria. [bili- + G. *ouron*, urine]

**Bil·lings meth·od** (bil′ingz) a contraceptive method that involves periods of abstinence determined by changes in cervical mucus.

**Bill ma·neu·ver** (bil) forceps rotation of the fetal head at mid-pelvis before extraction of the head.

**Bill·roth op·er·a·tion I** (bil′rōt) excision of the pylorus and antrum and partial closure of the gastric end with end-to-end anastomosis of stomach and duodenum.

**Bill·roth op·er·a·tion II** (bil′rōt) excision of the pylorus and antrum with closure of the cut ends of the duodenum and stomach, followed by a gastrojejunostomy.

**bi·lo·bate, bi·lobed** (bī-lō′bāt, bī′lōbd) having two lobes.

**bi·lob·u·lar** (bī-lob′yu-lăr) having two lobules.

**bi·loc·u·lar, bi·loc·u·late** (bī-lok′yu-lăr, bī-lok′yu-lāt) having two compartments or spaces. [bi- + L. *loculus*, dim. of *locus*, a place]

**bi·loc·u·lar joint** one in which the intra-articular disk is complete, dividing the joint into two distinct cavities.

**bi·mal·le·o·lar frac·ture** (bī-mă-lē′ō-lar frak′cher) fracture of both medial and lateral malleoli. SEE ALSO malleolus.

**bi·man·u·al** (bī-man′yu-ăl) relating to, or performed by, both hands. [bi- + L. *manus*, hand]

**bi·man·u·al ver·sion** turning of the baby *in utero*, performed by the hands acting upon both extremities of the fetus; it may be external version or combined version.

**bi·mas·toid** (bī-mas′toyd) relating to both mastoid processes.

**bi·max·il·lary** (bī-mak′si-lār-e) relating to both the right and left maxillae; sometimes used when describing something affecting both halves of the upper jaw.

**bi·na·ry** (bī′nār-ē) **1.** comprising two components, elements, molecules, etc. **2.** denoting a choice of two mutually exclusive outcomes for one event (e.g., male or female; heads or tails; affected or unaffected). [L. *binarius*, consisting of two, fr. *bini*, two at a time]

**bi·na·ry dig·it 1.** the smallest unit of digital information expressed in the binary system of notation (either 0 or 1). **2.** the signal in computing.

**bi·na·ry fis·sion** simple fission in which the two new cells are approximately equal in size.

**bin·au·ral** (bin-aw′răl) relating to both ears. SYN binotic. [L. *bini*, a pair, + *auris*, ear]

**bi·nau·ral dip·la·cu·sis** a diplacusis in which the same sound is heard differently by the two ears.

**bind·er** (bīnd′er) **1.** a broad bandage, especially one encircling the abdomen. **2.** anything that binds.

**Bi·net scale, Bi·net test** (bē-nā′) SYN Stanford-Binet intelligence scale.

**Bing re·flex** (bing) when the foot is passively dorsiflexed, plantar flexion occurs if any point on the ankle between the two malleoli is tapped.

**bin·oc·u·lar** (bin-ok′yu-lăr) adapted to the use of both eyes; said of an optical instrument. [L. *bini*, paired, + *oculus*, eye]

**bin·oc·u·lar mi·cro·scope** a microscope having two eyepieces; it may be a compound microscope or a stereoscopic microscope.

**bin·oc·u·lar vi·sion** vision with a single image, by both eyes simultaneously.

**bi·no·mi·al** (bī-nō′mē-ăl) a set of two terms or names; in the probabilistic or statistical sense it corresponds to a Bernoulli trial. [bi- + G. *nomos*, name]

**bin·ot·ic** (bin-ot'ik) SYN binaural. [L. *bini,* a pair, + G. *ous* (*ōt-*), ear]

**Bins·wan·ger dis·ease** (bin-swăng-ĕr) one of the causes of multi-infarct dementia, in which there are many infarcts and lacunae in the white matter, with relative sparing of the cortex and basal ganglia.

**bi·nu·cle·ar, bi·nu·cle·ate** (bī-noo'klē-ăr, bī-noo-'klē-āt) having two nuclei.

**bi·nu·cle·o·late** (bī-noo'klē-ō-lāt) having two nucleoli.

⚠**bio-** combining form denoting life. [G. *bios,* life]

**bi·o·a·cous·tics** (bī'ō-ă-koos'tiks) the science dealing with the effects of sound or vibration on living organisms.

**bi·o·ac·tive non·nu·tri·ent** SYN phytochemical.

**bi·o·as·say** (bī-ō-as'ā) determination of the potency or concentration of a compound by its effect upon animals, isolated tissues, or microorganisms, as contrasted with analysis of its chemical or physical properties.

**bi·o·a·vail·a·bil·i·ty** (bī'ō-ă-vāl'ă-bil'i-tē) the physiological availability of a given amount of a drug, as distinct from its chemical potency; proportion of the administered dose which is absorbed into the bloodstream.

**bi·o·bur·den** (bī'ō-ber'den) degree of microbial contamination or microbial load; the number of microorganisms contaminating an object.

**bi·o·chem·i·cal** (bī-ō-kem'i-kăl) relating to biochemistry.

**bi·o·chem·i·cal mod·u·la·tion** term describing the modulation (either enhancement of activity or reduction of toxicity) of a chemotherapeutic agent by another agent, which may or may not have antineoplastic activity of its own.

**bi·o·chem·i·cal pro·file** a combination of biochemical tests usually performed with automated instrumentation.

**bi·o·chem·is·try** (bī-ō-kem'is-trē) the chemistry of living organisms and of the chemical, molecular, and physical changes occurring therein. SYN biologic chemistry, physiologic chemistry.

**bi·o·cid·al** (bī-ō-sī'dăl) destructive of life; particularly pertaining to microorganisms. [bio- + L. *caedo,* to kill]

**biocompatibility** (bī'ō-kom-pat-i-bil'i-tē) the relative ability of a material to interact favorably with a biological system. [bio- + compatibility]

**bi·o·cy·ber·net·ics** (bī'ō-sī-ber-net'iks) the science of communication and control within a living organism, particularly on a molecular basis.

**bi·o·de·grad·a·ble** (bī'ō-dē-grād'ă-bl) denoting a substance that can be chemically degraded or decomposed by natural effectors (e.g., weather, soil bacteria, plants, animals).

**bi·o·de·gra·da·tion** SYN biotransformation.

**bi·o·e·lec·tri·cal im·pe·dance a·nal·y·sis** method of determining body fat, fat-free body mass, and total body water by measuring resistance to the flow of a small electrical current passed through the body.

**bi·o·en·er·get·ics** study of diverse means for energy transfer for biologic work within living organisms.

**bi·o·feed·back** (bī-ō-fēd'bak) a training technique that enables an individual to gain some element of voluntary control over autonomic body functions; based on the learning principle that a desired response is learned when received information such as a recorded increase in skin temperature (feedback) indicates that a specific thought complex or action has produced the desired physiological response.

**bi·o·gen·e·sis** (bī-ō-jen'ĕ-sis) **1.** term given by Huxley to the principle that life originates from preexisting life only and never from nonliving material. SEE spontaneous generation, recapitulation theory. **2.** SYN biosynthesis. [bio- + G. *genesis,* origin]

**bi·o·ge·net·ic** (bī'ō-jĕ-net'ik) relating to biogenesis.

**bi·o·in·for·mat·ics** a scientific discipline encompassing all aspects of biologic information acquisition, processing, storage, distribution, analysis, and interpretation that combines the tools and techniques of mathematics, computer science, and biology with the aim of understanding the biologic significance of a variety of data.

**bi·o·in·stru·ment** (bī'ō-in'str-oo-ment) a sensor or device attached to or embedded in the body to record and transmit physiologic data to a receiving station.

**bi·o·ki·net·ics** (bī'ō-ki-net'iks) the study of the growth changes and movements that developing organisms undergo. [bio- + G. *kinēsis,* motion]

**bi·o·log·ic, bi·o·log·i·cal** (bī'ō-loj'ik, bī'ō-loj'i-kăl) relating to biology.

**bi·o·log·i·cal sam·pling** denotes sampling that can be taken without jeopardy to the whole organism (e.g., for hematological or biochemical study).

**bi·o·log·i·cal vec·tor** a vector, such as the *Anopheles* mosquito for malarial agents or the tsetse fly for agents of African sleeping sickness, in which the agent multiplies prior to being transmitted to another host.

**bi·o·log·ic as·say** SYN biotest.

**bi·o·log·i·c chem·is·try** SYN biochemistry.

**bi·o·log·i·c con·trol** control of living organisms, including vectors and reservoirs of disease, by using their natural enemies (predators, parasites, competitors).

**bi·o·log·ic ev·o·lu·tion** the doctrine that all forms of animal or plant life have been derived by gradual changes from simpler forms and ultimately unicellular organisms. SYN organic evolution.

**bi·o·log·ic half-life** the time required for one-half of an amount of a substance to be lost through biologic processes.

**bi·o·log·ic im·mu·no·ther·a·py** SYN immunotherapy.

**bi·o·log·ic in·di·ca·tor** a preparation of nonpathogenic microorganisms, usually bacterial spores, carried by an ampule or specially impregnated paper enclosed within a package during sterilization and subsequently incubated to verify that the spores were killed by the sterilization process.

**bi·o·log·ic psy·chi·a·try** a branch of psychiatry that emphasizes molecular, genetic, and pharmacologic methods in the diagnosis and treatment of mental disorders.

**bi·o·log·ic re·sponse mod·i·fi·er** agent that modifies host responses to neoplasms by enhancing immune systems or reconstituting impaired immune mechanisms.

**bi·o·log·ic vec·tor** a vector, such as the *Anopheles* mosquito for malarial agents or the tsetse fly for agents of African sleeping sickness, in which the agent multiplies prior to being transmitted to another host.

**bi·ol·o·gist** (bī-ol′ō-jist) a specialist or expert in biology.

**bi·ol·o·gy** (bī-ol′ō-jē) the science concerned with the phenomena of life and living organisms. [bio- + G. *logos,* study]

**bi·o·mass** (bī′ō-mas) the total weight of all living things in a given area, biotic community, species population, or habitat; a measure of total biotic productivity.

**bi·o·ma·te·ri·al** (bī′ō-ma-tē′rē-al) a synthetic or semisynthetic material used in a biological system to construct an implantable prosthesis and chosen for its biocompatibility. [bio- + material]

**bi·ome** (bī′ōm) the total complex of biotic communities occupying and characterizing a particular geographic area or zone. [bio- + -ome]

**bi·o·me·chan·i·cal a·nal·y·sis** SYN activity analysis.

**bi·o·me·chan·i·cal frame of ref·er·ence 1.** an intervention approach used when a person cannot maintain posture through appropriate involuntary muscle activity because of neuromuscular or musculoskeletal dysfunction; artificial supports are provided, temporarily or permanently; **2.** a therapeutic technique in which strength, endurance, and range of motion are increased in patients who have dysfunction in the peripheral nervous system or the musculoskeletal, integumentary, or cardiopulmonary systems.

**bi·o·me·chan·ics** (bī-ō-me-kan′iks) the science concerned with the action of forces, internal or external, on the living body.

**bi·o·med·i·cal** (bī-ō-med′i-kăl) **1.** pertaining to aspects of the biologic sciences that relate to or underlie medicine. **2.** biological and medical, i.e., encompassing both the science(s) and the art of medicine.

**bi·o·med·i·cal mod·el** a conceptual model of illness that excludes psychological and social factors.

**bi·o·mem·brane** (bī-ō-mem′brān) a structure bounding a cell or cell organelle; it contains lipids, proteins, glycolipids, steroids, etc. SYN membrana [TA], membrane (2).

**bi·o·me·tri·cian** (bī-o-me-tri′shăn) one who specializes in the science of biometry.

**bi·om·e·try** (bī-om′ě-trē) the application of statistical methods to the study of numerical data based on biological observations and phenomena. [bio- + G. *metron,* measure]

**bi·o·mi·cro·scope** (bī-ō-mī′krō-skōp) SYN slit-lamp.

**bi·o·mi·cros·co·py** (bī′ō-mī-kros′kŏ-pē) **1.** microscopic examination of living tissue in the body. **2.** examination of the cornea, aqueous humor, lens, vitreous humor, and retina by use of a slitlamp combined with a binocular microscope.

**bi·o·ne·cro·sis** (bī-ō-ne-krō′sis) SYN necrobiosis.

**bi·on·ic** (bī-on′ik) relating to or developed from bionics.

**bi·on·ics** (bī-on′iks) **1.** the science of biologic functions and mechanisms as applied to electronic technology. **2.** the science of applying the knowledge gained by studying the characteristics of living organisms to the formulation of nonorganic devices and techniques. [bio- + electronics]

**bi·o·phar·ma·ceu·tics** (bī′ō-far-mă-soo′tiks) the study of the physical and chemical properties of

a drug, and its dosage form, as related to the onset, duration, and intensity of drug action.

**bi·o·phys·ics** (bī-ō-phyz′iks) **1.** the study of biological processes and materials by means of the theories and tools of physics. **2.** the study of physical processes (e.g., electricity, luminescence) occurring in organisms.

**▯ bi·op·sy** (bī′op-sē) **1.** process of removing tissue from living patients for diagnostic examination. **2.** a specimen obtained by biopsy. See page 117. [bio- + G. *opsis,* vision]

**bi·o·psy·cho·so·cial mod·el** a conceptual model that assumes that psychological and social factors must also be included along with the biological in understanding a person's medical illness or disorder.

**bi·op·tome** (bī-op′tōm) a biopsy instrument passed through a catheter into the heart to obtain tissue for diagnosis. [*biop*sy + G. *tomē,* a cutting]

**bi·o·rhythm** (bī′ō-ridh-m) a biologically inherent cyclic variation or recurrence of an event or state, such as the sleep cycle, circadian rhythms, or periodic diseases. [bio- + G. *rhythmos,* rhythm]

**bi·o·safe·ty** (b-ī′ō-saf′tē) safety measures applied to the handling of biological materials or organisms with a known potential to cause disease in humans.

**bi·o·so·cial** (bī-ō-sō′shŭl) involving the interplay of biological and social influences.

**bi·o·spec·trom·e·try** (bī′ō-spek-trom′ě-trē) spectroscopic determination of the types and amounts of various substances in living tissue or fluid from a living body. [bio- + L. *spectrum,* an image, + G. *metron,* measure]

**bi·o·spec·tros·co·py** (bī′ō-spek-tros′kŏ-pē) spectroscopic examination of specimens of living tissue, including fluids removed therefrom. [bio- + L. *spectrum,* image, + G. *skopeō,* to examine]

**bi·o·sphere** (bī′ō-sfēr) all the regions in the world where living organisms are found. [bio- + G. *sphaira,* sphere]

**bi·o·sta·tis·tics** (bī′ō-stă-tis′tiks) the science of statistics applied to biological or medical data.

**bi·o·syn·the·sis** (bī-ō-sin′thě-sis) formation of a chemical compound by enzymes, either in the organism (*in vivo*) or by fragments or extracts of cells (*in vitro*). SYN biogenesis (2).

**bi·o·syn·thet·ic** (bī′ō-sin-thet′ik) relating to or produced by biosynthesis.

**bi·o·sys·tem** (bī′ō-sis-tem) a living organism or any complete system of living things that can, directly or indirectly, interact with others.

**bi·o·ta** (bī-ō′tă) the collective flora and fauna of a region. [Mod. L., fr. G. *bios,* life]

**Bi·ot breath·ing sign** (bē-ō′) irregular periods of apnea alternating with four or five deep breaths; seen with increased intracranial pressure.

**bi·o·te·lem·e·try** (bī-ō-tel-em′ě-trē) the technique of monitoring vital processes and transmitting data without wires to a point remote from the subject.

**bi·o·test** a method for assessing the effect of a compound, technique, or procedure on an organism. SYN biologic assay.

**bi·ot·ic** (bī-ot′ik) pertaining to life.

**bi·o·tin** (bī′ō-tin) *cis*-Hexahydro-2-oxo-1*H*-thieno[ 3,4-*d*]imidazoline-4-valeric acid; the D-isomer component of the vitamin $B_2$ complex occurring in or required by most organisms and inactivated by avidin; participates in biological carboxylations.

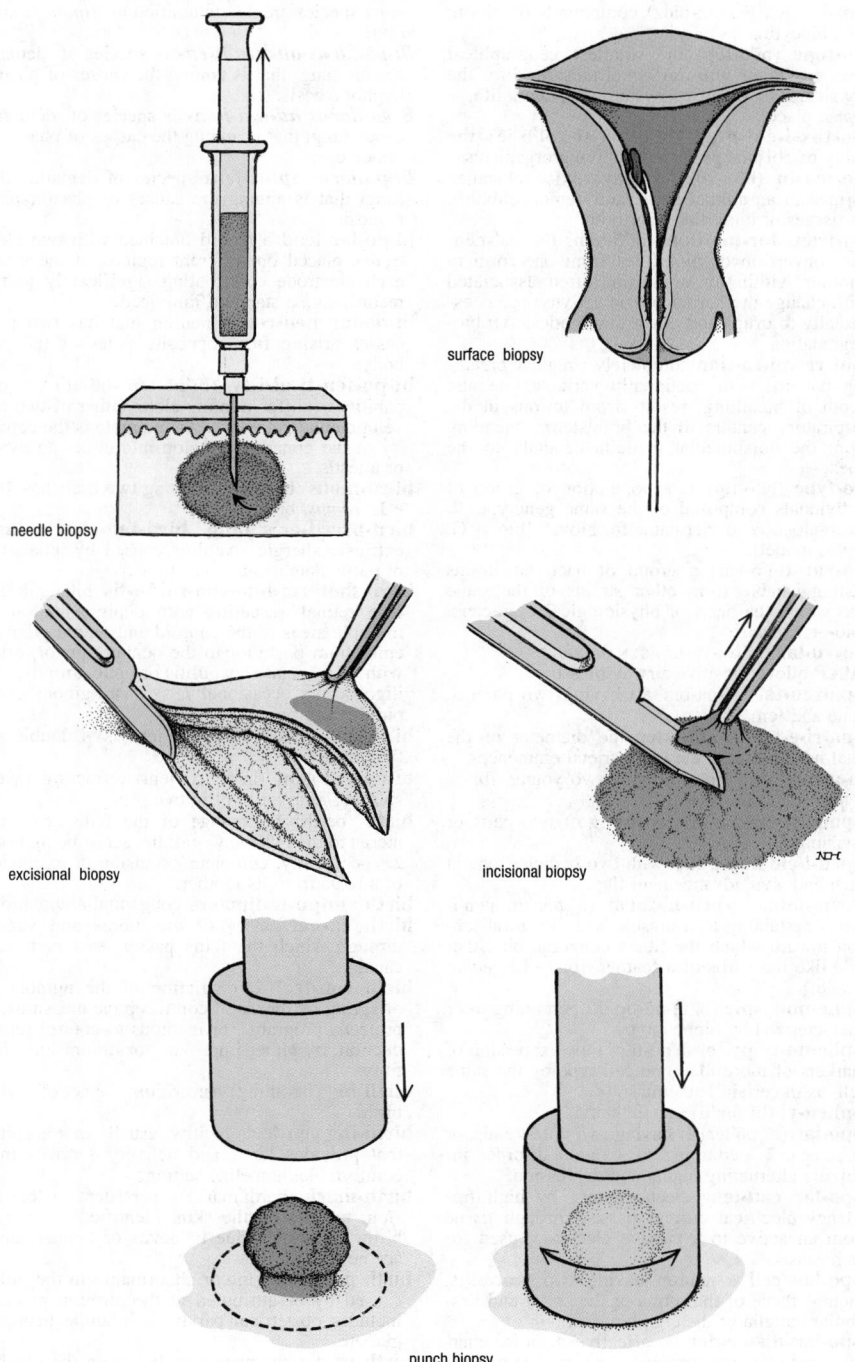

needle biopsy

surface biopsy

excisional biopsy

incisional biopsy

punch biopsy

**biopsy**

**bi·ot·i·nides** (bī-ot'i-nīdz) compounds of biotin; e.g., biocytin.

**bi·o·tope** (bī'ō-tōp) the smallest geographical area providing uniform conditions for life; the physical part of an ecosystem. [G. *bios,* life, + *topos,* place]

**bi·o·tox·i·col·o·gy** (bī'ō-tok-si-kol'ō-jē) the study of poisons produced by living organisms.

**bi·o·tox·in** (bī-ō-tok'sin) any toxic substance formed in an animal body, and demonstrable in its tissues or body fluids, or both.

**bi·o·trans·for·ma·tion** (bī'ō-trans-fōr-mā'shŭn) the conversion of molecules from one form to another within an organism, often associated with change in pharmacologic activity; refers especially to drugs and other xenobiotics. SYN biodegradation.

**Bi·ot res·pi·ra·tion** completely irregular breathing pattern, with continually variable rate and depth of breathing; results from lesions in the respiratory centers in the brainstem, extending from the dorsomedial medulla caudally to the obex.

**bi·o·type** (bī'ō-tīp) **1.** a population or group of individuals composed of the same genotype. **2.** BACTERIOLOGY former name for biovar. [bio- + G. *typos,* model]

**bi·o·var** (bī'ō-var) a group of bacterial strains distinguishable from other strains of the same species on the basis of physiological characters. [bio- + *variant*]

**bi·o·vu·lar** (bī'ov-yu-lar) SYN diovular.

**BiPAP** bilevel positive airway pressure.

**bi·pa·ren·tal** (bī-pa-ren'tăl) having two parents, male and female.

**bi·pa·ri·e·tal di·am·e·ter** the diameter of the fetal head between the two parietal eminences.

**bip·a·rous** (bip'ă-rŭs) bearing two young. [bi- + L. *pario,* to give birth]

**bi·par·tite** (bī-par'tīt) consisting of two parts or divisions.

**bi·ped·i·cle flap** a flap with two pedicles, one at each end. SYN advancement flap.

**bi·pen·nate, bi·pen·ni·form** (bī-pen'āt, pen'i-fōrm) pertaining to a muscle with a central tendon toward which the fibers converge on either side like the barbs of a feather. [bi- + L. *penna,* feather]

**bi·phe·no·ty·pic** (bī'fē-nō-tip'ik) pertaining to or characterized by biphenotypy.

**bi·phe·no·ty·py** (bī-fē'nō-tī'pē) the expression of markers of more than one cell type by the same cell, as in certain leukemias.

**bi·phen·yl** (bī-fen'il) SYN diphenyl.

**bi·po·lar** (bī-pō'ler) **1.** having two poles, ends, or extremes. **2.** pertaining to a mood disorder involving alternating mania and depression.

**bi·po·lar cau·tery** electrocautery by high frequency electrical current passed through tissue from an active to a passive electrode; used for hemostasis.

**bi·po·lar cell** a neuron having two processes, such as those of the retina or the spiral and vestibular ganglia of the eighth nerve.

**bi·po·lar dis·or·der** an affective disorder characterized by the occurrence of alternating periods of euphoria (mania) and depression. SYN manic-depressive psychosis.

**Bi·po·lar·is** (bī-pō-la'ris) genus of dematiaceous fungi that are among the causes of phaeohyphomycosis; some *Drechslera* and *Helminthospo-*

*rium* species are now classified as *Bipolaris* species.

**Bi·po·lar·is au·stra·li·en·sis** species of dematiaceous fungi that is among the causes of phaeohyphomycosis.

**Bi·po·lar·is ha·wai·i·en·sis** species of dematiaceous fungi that is among the causes of phaeohyphomycosis.

**Bi·po·lar·is spi·ci·fera** species of dematiaceous fungi that is among the causes of phaeohyphomycosis.

**bi·po·lar lead** a record obtained with two electrodes placed on different regions of the body, each electrode contributing significantly to the record; e.g., a standard limb lead.

**bi·po·lar neu·ron** a neuron that has two processes arising from opposite poles of the cell body.

**bi·po·ten·ti·al·i·ty** (bī'pō-ten-shē-al'i-tē) capability of differentiating along either of two developmental pathways. An example is the capacity of the gonad to develop into either an ovary or a testis.

**bi·ra·mous** (bī-rā'mŭs) having two branches. [bi- + L. *ramus,* branch]

**bird-breed·er's lung, bird-fan·ci·er's lung** extrinsic allergic alveolitis caused by inhalation of particulate avian emanations.

**bird shot ret·i·no·cho·roid·i·tis** bilateral diffuse retinal vasculitis with depigmentation of multiple areas of the choroid and retinal pigment epithelium posterior to the ocular equator, often with an associated papillitis or optic atrophy; vitiligo occurs occasionally. SYN vitiliginous choroiditis.

**bi·re·frin·gence** (bī-rē-frin'jens) SYN double refraction.

**bi·re·frin·gent** (bī-rē-frin'jent) refracting twice; splitting a ray of light in two.

**birth** (berth) **1.** passage of the fetus from the uterus to the outside world; the act of being born. **2.** specifically, complete expulsion or extraction of a fetus from its mother.

**birth am·pu·ta·tion** SYN congenital amputation.

**birth ca·nal** cavity of the uterus and vagina through which the fetus passes. SYN parturient canal.

**birth con·trol 1.** restriction of the number of offspring by means of contraceptive measures; **2.** projects, programs, or methods to control reproduction, by either improving or diminishing fertility.

**birth·ing** (ber'thing) parturition; the act of giving birth.

**birth·ing cen·ter** a facility, usually in a hospital, that provides labor and delivery services in a comfortable, homelike setting.

**birth·mark** (berth'mark) a persistent visible lesion, usually on the skin, identified at or near birth; commonly due to nevus or hemangioma. SEE nevus (1).

**birth pal·sy** any motor abnormality in the infant caused by or attributed to the birthing process; includes obstetrical paralysis, infantile hemiplegia, etc.

**birth rate** a summary rate based on the number of live births in a population over a given period, usually one year; the numerator is the number of live births, the denominator is the midyear population.

**birth trau·ma 1.** physical injury to an infant

during its delivery; **2.** the supposed emotional injury, inflicted by events incident to birth, upon an infant which allegedly appears in symbolic form in patients with mental illness.

**birth weight** in humans, the first weight of an infant obtained within less than the first 60 completed minutes after birth; a full-size infant is one weighing 2500 g or more; a low birth weight is less than 2500 g.

△**bis-** **1.** prefix signifying two or twice. **2.** CHEMISTRY used to denote the presence of two identical but separated complex groups in one molecule. Cf. bi-, di-. [L.]

**2,5-bis(5-***t***-bu•tyl•ben•zox•a•zol-2-yl)thi•o•phene (BBOT)** a scintillator used in radioactivity measurements by scintillation counting.

**Bisch•of my•e•lot•o•my** (bish'of) longitudinal incision of the spinal cord through the lateral column for treatment of spasticity of the lower extremities.

**bis in die** (bis in dē'ā) twice a day. [L.]

**bi•sex•u•al** (bī-seks'yu-ăl) **1.** having gonads of both sexes. SEE ALSO hermaphroditism. **2.** denoting an individual who engages in both heterosexual and homosexual relations.

**bis•fer•i•ous** (bis-fēr'ē-ŭs) striking twice; said of the pulse. [L. *bis,* twice, + *ferio,* to strike]

**bis•fer•i•ous pulse** (bis-fer'ē-ŭs) an arterial pulse with peaks that may be palpable. SYN pulsus bisferiens.

**Bish•op score** (bish'op) system to determine the inducibility of the cervix in a pregnant patient, based on dilation, effacement, station, and cervical consistency and position.

**Bish•op sphyg•mo•scope** (bish'op) an instrument for measuring the blood pressure, with special reference to diastolic pressure; the tube is filled with a solution of cadmium borotungstate, and the scale is the reverse of that of a mercurial manometer, the pressure being made directly by the weight of the liquid and not by compressed air.

**bis•il•i•ac** (bis-il'ē-ak) relating to any two corresponding iliac parts or structures, as the iliac bones or iliac fossae.

**bis•muth (Bi)** (biz'mŭth) a trivalent metallic element; atomic no. 83, atomic wt. 20.98037. Several of its salts are used in medicine. [Ger. *Wismut, weisse Masse,* white mass]

**bis•muth line** a black zone on the free marginal gingiva, often the first sign of poisoning from prolonged parenteral administration of bismuth.

**bis•mu•tho•sis** (biz-mŭ-thō'sis) chronic bismuth poisoning.

**bis•muth•yl** (biz'mŭ-thil) the group, BiO⁺, that behaves chemically as the ion of a univalent metal; its salts are subsalts of bismuth.

**1,3-bis•phos•pho•glyc•er•ate** (won-thrē bis-fos'fō-glis'er-āt) an intermediate in glycolysis which enzymatically reacts with ADP to generate ATP and 3-phosphoglycerate.

**2,3-bis•phos•pho•glyc•er•ate** an intermediate in the Rapoport-Luebering shunt, formed between 1,3-bisphosphoglycerate and 3-phosphoglycerate; an important regulator of the affinity of hemoglobin for oxygen; an intermediate of phosphoglycerate mutase.

**bis•tou•ry** (bis'too-rē) a long, narrow-bladed knife, with a straight or curved edge and sharp or blunt point (probe-point); used for opening or slitting cavities or hollow structures. [Fr. *bistouri,* fr. It. dialect *bistori,* perh. fr. *Pistoia,* Italy]

**bi•sul•fate** (bī-sŭl'fāt) a salt containing $HSO_4^-$. SYN acid sulfate.

**bi•sul•fide** (bī-sŭl'fīd) a compound of the anion HS⁻; an acid sulfide.

**bi•sul•fite** (bī-sŭl'fīt) a salt or ion of $HSO_3^-$.

**bite** (bīt) **1.** to incise or seize with the teeth. **2.** the act of incision or seizure with the teeth. **3.** a morsel of food held between the teeth. **4.** term used to denote the amount of pressure developed in closing the jaws. **5.** undesirable jargon for terms such as interocclusal record, maxillomandibular registration, denture space, and interarch distance. **6.** a wound or puncture of the skin made by animal or insect. SEE bites. [A.S. *bītan*]

**bite a•nal•y•sis** SYN occlusal analysis.

**bite•plate, bite•plane** (bīt'plāt, bīt'plān) a removable appliance that incorporates a plane of acrylic designed to occlude with the opposing teeth.

**bites** (bīts) penetration of the skin (puncture or laceration) causing reactions that result from 1) mechanical injury; 2) injection of toxic material such as snake or scorpion venom; 3) injection of antigenic substance, especially by insect or arthropod bites, capable of inducing and eliciting allergic sensitization; 4) introduction of otherwise saprophytic flora such as *Staphylococcus pyogenes* in the instance of human bites; 5) invasion of the tissue as in myiasis; 6) transmission of disease such as typhus and rabies. [see bite]

**bite•wing film** a special packaging of radiographic film that allows appendage of the film package to be held between the occlusal surfaces of the teeth. See page 364.

**bite•wing ra•di•o•graph, bite•wing** (bīt'wing) intraoral film adapted to show the coronal portion and cervical third of the root of the teeth in near occlusion; especially useful in detecting interproximal caries and determining alveolar septal height.

**bi•ther•mal ca•lor•ic test** a test of vestibular function in which each ear canal is alternately or simultaneously irrigated with water at 7°C above or below body temperature; the nystagmus produced may be monitored for direction, amplitude, speed of the slow component, and duration. SEE ALSO Bárány sign.

**Bi•tot spots** (bē-tō') any of numerous small, circumscribed, lusterless, grayish white, foamy, greasy, triangular deposits on the bulbar conjunctiva adjacent to the cornea in the area of the palpebral fissure in both eyes; occurs in vitamin A deficiency.

**bi•tro•chan•ter•ic** (bī-trō-kan-ter'ik) relating to two trochanters, either to the two trochanters of one femur or to both greater trochanters.

**Bit•torf re•ac•tion** (bit'orf) in cases of renal colic, pain radiating to the kidney upon squeezing the testicle or pressing the ovary.

**bi•u•ret** (bī-yu-ret') obtained by eliminating one $NH_3$ between two urea molecules. Used in protein determinations. SYN carbamoylurea.

**bi•u•ret re•ac•tion, bi•u•ret test** the formation of biuret, which gives a violet color due to the reaction of a polypeptide of more than three amino acids with $CuSO_4$ in strongly alkaline solution; used for the detection and quantitation of polypeptides or protein in biological fluids.

**bi•va•lence, bi•va•len•cy** (bī-vā'lens, bī-vā'len-sē) a combining power (valence) of 2. SYN divalence, divalency.

**bi·va·lent** (bī-vā′lent) **1.** having a combining power (valence) of two. SYN divalent. **2.** CYTOLOGY a structure consisting of two paired homologous chromosomes, each split into two sister chromatids, as seen during the pachytene stage of prophase in meiosis.

**bi·va·lent chro·mo·some** a pair of chromosomes temporarily united.

**bi·ven·tral** (bī-ven′tral) SYN digastric (1).

**Biz·zo·ze·ro red cells** nucleated red blood cells in human blood.

**Bjer·rum sco·to·ma** (byer′oom) a comet-shaped scotoma, occurring in glaucoma, attached at the temporal end to the blind spot or separated from it by a narrow gap; the defect widens as it extends above and nasally curves around the fixation spot, and then extends downward to end exactly at the nasal horizontal meridian.

**Björn·stad syn·drome** (byōrn′stahd) pili torti associated with sensorineural hearing loss, the severity of distortion and brittleness of the hair correlated with the degree of hearing impairment; autosomal dominant inheritance.

**Bk** berkelium.

**B-K am·pu·ta·tion** *b*elow-the-*k*nee amputation.

**black cat·a·ract** a cataract in which the lens is hardened and of a dark brown color.

**Black clas·si·fi·ca·tion** (blak) a classification of cavities of the teeth based upon the tooth surface(s) involved.

**Black Creek Ca·nal vi·rus** (blak crēk) a species of Hantavirus in the U.S. causing hantavirus pulmonary syndrome; transmitted by the cotton rat. [Black Creek Canal in Florida where the cotton rats were captured from which the virus was first isolated]

**black death** term applied to the worldwide epidemic of the 14th century, of which some 60 million persons are said to have died; the descriptions indicate that it was pneumonic plague.

**black eye** ecchymosis of the lids and their surroundings.

**black globe ther·mom·e·ter** ambient air thermometer, whose bulb is enclosed in a black metal sphere that absorbs radiant energy from the surroundings so as to measure heat gained from this source.

**black·head** (blak′hed) **1.** SYN open comedo. **2.** SYN histomoniasis.

**black im·por·ted fire ant** SYN *Solenopsis richteri.*

**black lung** a form of pneumoconiosis, common in coal miners, characterized by deposit of carbon particles in the lung. SYN miner's lung (2).

**black·out** (blak′owt) **1.** temporary loss of consciousness due to decreased blood flow to the brain. **2.** momentary loss of consciousness as in an absence. **3.** temporary loss of vision, without alteration of consciousness, due to positive (> normal) g (gravity) forces; caused by temporary decreased blood flow in the central retinal artery, and seen mostly in aviators. **4.** a transient episode that occurs during a state of intense intoxication (alcoholic blackout) for which the person has no recall, although not unconscious (as observed by others).

**black tongue** black to yellowish-brown discoloration of the dorsum of the tongue due to staining by exogenous material such as the components of tobacco; usually superimposed on hairy tongue. SYN lingua nigra, melanoglossia.

**black·wa·ter fe·ver** hemoglobinuria resulting from severe hemolysis occurring in falciparum malaria.

**blad·der** (blad′er) **1.** a distensible musculomembranous organ serving as a receptacle for fluid, as the gallbladder or urinary bladder. SEE detrusor. **2.** SYN urinary bladder. SYN vesica (1). [A.S. *blaedre*]

**blad·der ear** protrusion of a portion of the bladder into proximal inguinal canal; often seen in pediatric voiding cystourethrogram and rarely of clinical significance.

**Blag·den law** (blag′den) the depression of the freezing point of dilute solutions is proportional to the amount of the dissolved substance.

**Blain·ville ears** (blān′vil) asymmetry in size or shape of the auricles.

**Blair-Brown graft** (blār-brŏwn) a split-thickness graft of intermediate thickness.

**Bla·lock-Taus·sig op·er·a·tion** (blā′lok taw′sig) an operation for congenital malformations of the heart, in which an abnormally small volume of blood passes through the pulmonary circuit; blood from the systemic circulation is directed to the lungs by anastomosing the right or left subclavian artery to the right or left pulmonary artery.

**Bla·lock-Taus·sig shunt** (blā′lok taw′sig) a palliative subclavian artery to pulmonary artery anastomosis.

**blanch** (blantsh) **1.** to become white or pale, as skin or mucous membrane affected by vasoconstriction. **2.** to whiten or bleach a surface or substance. [O.Fr. *blanchir*, fr. *blanc*, white]

**bland di·et** a regular diet omitting foods that mechanically or chemically irritate the gastrointestinal tract.

**blank** a solution consisting of all of the analytical components except the compound to be measured; this is used to establish a baseline of measurement intensity against which the compound of interest is compared. [M.E. white, fr. O.Fr. *blanc*, fr. Germanic]

**blan·ket** a covering.

**blan·ket su·ture** a continuous lock-stitch used to approximate the skin of a wound.

**blast** (blăst) general term for immature or precursor cell. [G. *blastos*, germ]

△**-blast** an immature precursor cell of the type indicated by the preceding word. [G. *blastos*, germ]

**blast cell** an immature precursor cell; e.g., erythroblast, lymphoblast, neuroblast. SEE ALSO -blast.

**blas·te·ma** (blas-tē′mǎ) **1.** the primordial cellular mass (precursor) from which an organ or part is formed. **2.** a cluster of cells competent to initiate the regeneration of a damaged or ablated structure. [G. a sprout]

**blas·tem·ic** (blas-tēm′ik) relating to the blastema.

**blast in·ju·ry** tearing of lung tissue or rupture of abdominal viscera without external injury, as by the force of an explosion.

△**blasto-** pertaining to the process of budding by cells or tissue. [G. *blastos*, germ]

**blas·to·cele** (blas′tō-sēl) the cavity in the blastula of a developing embryo. SYN cleavage cavity, segmentation cavity. [blasto- + G. *koilos*, hollow]

**blas·to·cel·ic** (blas-tō-sē′lik) relating to the blastocele.

**Blas·to·co·nid·i·um** (blas'tō-kǒ-nid'ē-ŭm) a holoblastic conidium that is produced singly or in chains, and detached at maturity leaving a bud scar, as in the budding of a yeast cell. [blasto- + conidium]

**blas·to·cyst** (blas'tō-sist) the modified blastula stage of mammalian embryos, consisting of the inner cell mass and a thin trophoblast layer enclosing the blastocyst cavity. SYN blastodermic vesicle. [blasto- + G. *kystis,* bladder]

**blas·to·cyte** (blas'tō-sīt) an undifferentiated blastomere of the morula, blastula, or blastocyst stage of an embryo. [blasto- + G. *kytos,* cell]

**blas·to·cy·to·ma** (blas'tō-sī-tō'mǎ) SYN blastoma.

**blas·to·derm, blas·to·der·ma** (blas'tō-derm, blas-tō-der'ma) the thin, disk-shaped cell mass of a young embryo and its extraembryonic extensions over the surface of the yolk; when fully formed, all three primary germ layers (ectoderm, endoderm, and mesoderm) are present. SYN germ membrane, germinal membrane. [blasto- + G. *derma,* skin]

**blas·to·der·mal, blas·to·der·mic** (blas-tō-der'mǎl, blas-tō-der'mik) relating to the blastoderm.

**blas·to·der·mic ves·i·cle** SYN blastocyst.

**blas·to·disk** (blas'tō-disk) **1.** the disk of active cytoplasm at the animal pole of a telolecithal egg. **2.** the blastoderm, especially in very young stages when its extent is small.

**blas·to·gen·e·sis** (blas-tō-jen'ě-sis) **1.** reproduction of unicellular organisms by budding. **2.** development of an embryo during cleavage and germ layer formation. **3.** transformation of small lymphocytes of human peripheral blood in tissue culture into large, morphologically primitive blast-like cells capable of undergoing mitosis. [blasto- + G. *genesis,* origin]

**blas·to·ge·net·ic, blas·to·gen·ic** (blas'tō-je-net'ik, blas-tō-jen'ik) relating to blastogenesis.

**blas·to·ma** (blas-tō'mǎ) a neoplasm composed chiefly or entirely of immature undifferentiated cells (i.e., blast forms), with little or virtually no stroma. SYN blastocytoma. [blasto- + G. *-oma,* tumor]

**blas·to·mere** (blas'tō-mēr) one of the cells resulting from cleavage of a fertilized oocyte. [blasto- + G. *meros,* part]

*Blas·to·my·ces der·ma·tit·i·dis* (blas-tō-mī'sēz der-mǎ-tit'i-dis) a dimorphic soil fungus that causes blastomycosis. It grows in mammalian tissues as budding cells and in culture as a white to buff-colored filamentous fungus bearing spherical or ovoid conidia. [blasto- + G. *mykēs,* fungus]

**blas·to·my·co·sis** (blas'tō-mī-kō'sis) a chronic granulomatous and suppurative disease caused by *Blastomyces dermatitidis;* originates as a respiratory infection and disseminates, usually with pulmonary, osseous, and/or cutaneous involvement predominating. Formerly called North American blastomycosis, the disease now has been found in African states as well as in Canada and the U.S. SYN Gilchrist disease.

**blas·to·pore** (blas'tō-pōr) the opening into the archenteron formed by invagination of the blastula to form a gastrula. [blasto- + G. *poros,* opening]

*Blas·to·schiz·o·my·ces* (blas'tō-skiz-ō-mī'sēz) a genus of yeastlike fungi.

*Blas·to·schiz·o·my·ces cap·i·ta·tus* fungal species that causes severe disseminated infection in immunosuppressed patients; formerly classified as a species of *Geotrichum.*

**blas·tu·la** (blas'tyu-lǎ) an early stage of an embryo formed by the rearrangement of the blastomeres of the morula to form a hollow sphere. [G. *blastos,* germ]

**blas·tu·lar** (blas'tyu-lar) pertaining to the blastula.

**blas·tu·la·tion** (blas-tyu-lā'shǔn) formation of the blastula or blastocyst from the morula.

**Bla·tin syn·drome** (blah-tā') SYN hydatid thrill.

**bleb** (blěb) **1.** a large flaccid vesicle. **2.** an acquired lung cyst, usually less than 1 cm in diameter, similar to but smaller than a bulla, which is thought to be the most common cause of spontaneous pneumothorax. Blebs occur mainly in the apex of the lung.

**bleed** (blēd) to lose blood as a result of rupture or severance of blood vessels.

**bleed·ing time** the time interval between the appearance of the first drop of blood and the removal of the last drop following puncture of the ear lobe or the finger, usually 1 to 3 minutes; it is prolonged in cases of thrombocytopenia, diminished prothrombin, phosphorus poisoning, or chloroform poisoning, and in some liver diseases; it is normal in hemophilia.

**blem·ish** (blě'mish) **1.** a small circumscribed alteration of the skin considered to be unesthetic but insignificant. **2.** to alter the skin, rendering an unesthetic appearance.

△**blen·no-, blenn-** mucus. [G. *blenna, blennos*]

**blen·noid** (blen'oyd) SYN muciform. [blenno- + G. *eidos,* resemblance]

**bleph·ar·ad·e·ni·tis, bleph·a·ro·ad·e·ni·tis** (blef'ar-ad-ě-nī'tis, blef'ǎ-rō-ad-ě-nī'tis) inflammation of the meibomian glands or the marginal glands of Moll or Zeis. [blephar- + G. *adēn,* gland, + *-itis,* inflammation]

**bleph·a·rec·to·my** (blef'a-rek'tō-mē) excision of all or part of an eyelid. [blepharo- + G. *ektomē,* excision]

**bleph·ar·e·de·ma** (blef'ar-ě-dē'mǎ) edema of the eyelids, causing swelling and often a baggy appearance.

**bleph·a·ri·tis** (blef'ǎ-rī'tis) inflammation of the eyelids. [blepharo- + G. *-itis,* inflammation]

△**ble·pha·ro-, ble·phar-** eyelid. [G. *blepharon,* an eyelid]

**bleph·a·ro·ad·e·no·ma** (blef'ǎ-rō-ad-ě-nō'mǎ) a tumor or adenoma of a gland of the eyelid. [blepharo- + G. *adēn,* gland, + *-oma,* tumor]

**bleph·a·ro·chal·a·sis** (blef'ǎ-rō-kal'ǎ-sis) redundancy of the skin of the upper eyelids so that a fold of skin hangs down, often concealing the tarsal margin when the eye is open. [blepharo- + G. *chalasis,* a slackening]

**bleph·a·ro·col·o·bo·ma** (blef'ǎ-rō-kol-ō-bō'mǎ) a defect of the eyelid; may be congenital or acquired. [blepharo- + coloboma]

**bleph·a·ro·con·junc·ti·vi·tis** (blef'ǎ-rō-kon-jŭnk-ti-vī'tis) inflammation of the palpebral conjunctiva.

**bleph·a·ro·ker·a·to·con·junc·ti·vi·tis** (blef'ǎ-rō-ker'ǎ-tō-kon-jŭnk-ti-vī'tis) an inflammation involving the eyelids, cornea, and conjunctiva.

**bleph·a·ron** SYN eyelid.

**bleph·a·ro·phi·mo·sis** (blef'ǎ-rō-fi-mō'sis) decrease in the size of the palpebral aperture without fusion of lid margins. SYN blepharostenosis. [blepharo- + G. *phimōsis,* an obstruction]

**bleph·a·ro·plas·tic** (blef′ă-rō-plas′tik) relating to blepharoplasty.

**bleph·a·ro·plas·ty** (blef′ă-ro-plast-tē) any operation for the correction of a defect in the eyelids. [blepharo- + G. *plassō*, to form]

**bleph·a·ro·ple·gia** (blef′ă-rō-plē′jē-ă) paralysis of an eyelid. [blepharo- + G. *plēgē*, stroke]

**bleph·a·rop·to·sis, bleph·ar·op·to·sia** (blef′ă-rop′tō-sis, blef′ă-rop-tō′sē-ă) drooping of the upper eyelid. SYN ptosis (2). [blepharo- + G. *ptōsis, a falling*]

**bleph·a·rop·to·sis a·di·po·sa** blepharoptosis causing skin to hang over the free border of the eyelid.

**bleph·a·ro·spasm, bleph·a·ro·spas·mus** (blef′ă-rō-spazm, blef′ă-rō-spaz′mŭs) involuntary spasmodic contraction of the orbicularis oculi muscle.

**bleph·a·ro·stat** (blef′ă-rō-stat) SYN eye speculum. [blepharo- + G. *statos*, fixed]

**bleph·a·ro·ste·no·sis** (blef′ă-rō-ste-nō′sis) SYN blepharophimosis. [blepharo- + G. *stenōsis*, a narrowing]

**bleph·a·ro·syn·ech·ia** (blef′ă-rō-sin-ek′ē-ă) adhesion of the eyelids to each other or to the eyeball. [blepharo- + G. *synecheia*, continuity, fr. *syn-echō*, to hold together]

**bleph·a·rot·o·my** (blef-ă-rot′ō-mē) a cutting operation on an eyelid. [blepharo- + G. *tomē*, incision]

**blind** (blīnd) unable to see; without useful sight. SEE blindness.

**blind fis·tu·la** a fistula that ends in a cul-de-sac, being open at one extremity only. SYN incomplete fistula.

**blind loop syn·drome** a group of symptoms that result from the overgrowth of bacteria (primarily anaerobic) in a surgically bypassed or disconnected segment of intestine: local or systemic infection, fat malabsorption, and vitamin $B_{12}$ and folate deficiencies.

**blind·ness** (blīnd′nes) 1. loss of the sense of sight; absolute blindness connotes no light perception. SEE ALSO amblyopia, amaurosis. 2. loss of visual appreciation of objects although visual acuity is normal. 3. absence of the appreciation of sensation, e.g., taste blindness. SYN typhlosis.

**blind spot 1.** SYN physiologic scotoma. **2.** SYN mental scotoma. **3.** SYN optic disk.

**blink** (blink) to close and open the eyes rapidly; an involuntary act by which the tears are spread over the conjunctiva, keeping it moist.

**blink re·sponse, blink re·flex** a response elicited during nerve conduction studies, consisting of muscle action potentials evoked from orbicularis oculi muscles after brief electric or mechanical stimuli to the cutaneous area supplied by the ophthalmic branch of the trigeminal nerve. Characteristically, there is an early response (approximately 10 ms after stimulus) ipsilateral to the stimulation site (labeled R1) and bilateral late responses (approximately 30 ms after stimulus; labeled R2); the latter are responsible for the visible twitch of the orbicularis oculi muscles.

**blis·ter 1.** a fluid-filled thin-walled structure under the epidermis or within the epidermis (subepidermal or intradermal). **2.** to form a blister with heat or some other vesiculating agent.

**blis·ter·ing** SYN vesiculation (1).

**blis·ter·ing dis·tal dac·ty·li·tis** infection of the

volar fat pad of the distal phalanx of the finger by group A β-hemolytic streptococci.

**bloat, bloat·ing** (blōt, blōt′ing) abdominal distention from swallowed air or intestinal gas.

**block** (blok) **1.** to obstruct; to arrest passage through. **2.** a condition in which the passage of an electrical impulse is arrested, wholly or in part, temporarily or permanently. **3.** SYN atrioventricular block. [Fr. *bloquer*]

**block·ade** (blok′ād) **1.** intravenous injection of colloidal dyes or other substances whereby the reaction of the reticuloendothelial cells to other influences (e.g., by phagocytosis) is temporarily prevented. **2.** arrest of peripheral nerve conduction or transmission at autonomic synaptic junctions, autonomic receptor sites, or myoneural junctions by a drug.

**block an·es·the·sia** SYN conduction anesthesia.

**block·er** (blok′er) **1.** an instrument used to obstruct a passage. **2.** SEE blocking agent.

**block·ing ac·tiv·i·ty** repression or elimination of electrical activity in the brain by the arrival of a sensory stimulus.

**block·ing agent** a class of drugs that inhibit (block) a biologic activity or process; frequently called "blockers."

**block·ing an·ti·bod·y 1.** antibody which, in certain concentrations, does not cause precipitation after combining with specific antigen, and which, in this combined state, "blocks" activity of additional antibody added to increase the concentration to a level at which precipitation would ordinarily occur; **2.** the IgG class of immunoglobulin which combines specifically with an atopic allergen but does not elicit a type I allergic reaction, the combined IgG antibody "blocking" available IgE class (reaginic) antibody activity.

**Blocq dis·ease** (blok) SYN astasia-abasia.

**Blom-Singer valve** (blom-sing′er) a prosthesis for maintaining the patency of a tracheoesophageal puncture for vocal rehabilitation after laryngectomy.

**blood** (blŭd) the fluid and its suspended formed elements that are circulated through the heart, arteries, capillaries, and veins; blood is the means by which 1) oxygen and nutritive materials are transported to the tissues, and 2) carbon dioxide and various metabolic products are removed for excretion. The blood consists of a pale yellow or gray-yellow fluid, plasma, in which are suspended red blood cells (erythrocytes), white blood cells (leukocytes), and platelets. SEE ALSO arterial blood, venous blood. See page B1. [A.S. *blōd*]

**blood-air bar·ri·er** the material intervening between alveolar air and the blood; it consists of a nonstructural film or surfactant, alveolar epithelium, basement lamina, and endothelium.

**blood al·bu·min** SYN serum albumin.

**blood-a·que·ous bar·ri·er** a selectively permeable barrier between the capillary bed in the ciliary body and the aqueous humor.

**blood bank** a place, usually a separate part or division of a hospital laboratory or a separate free-standing facility, in which blood is collected from donors, typed, separated into several components, stored, and/or prepared for transfusion to recipients.

**blood blis·ter** a blister containing blood; resulting from a pinch or crushing injury.

**blood boost·ing** SYN blood doping.

**blood-brain bar•ri•er (BBB)** a selective mechanism opposing the passage of most ions and large-molecular weight compounds from the blood to brain tissue.

**blood cap•il•lary** (blŭd kap'i-lār-ē) (symbol c, as a subscript) a vessel whose wall consists of endothelium and its basement membrane; its diameter, when the capillary is open, is about 8 µm; with the electron microscope, fenestrated capillaries and continuous capillaries are distinguished.

**blood-ce•re•bro•spi•nal flu•id bar•ri•er, blood-CSF bar•ri•er** a barrier located at the tight junctions which surround and connect the cuboidal epithelial cells on the surface of the choroid plexus; capillaries and connective tissue stroma of the choroid do not represent a barrier to protein tracers or dyes.

**blood count** calculation of the number of red (RBC) or white (WBC) blood cells in a cubic millimeter of blood, by counting the cells in an accurate volume of diluted blood.

**blood cyst** SYN hemorrhagic cyst.

**blood disk** SYN platelet.

**blood dop•ing** infusion of red blood cells, usually freeze-preserved autologous blood, to increase hematocrit and hemoglobin levels; used by endurance athletes to increase blood's oxygen-carrying capacity and thus enhance endurance performance. SYN blood boosting, induced erythrocythemia.

**blood dys•cra•sia** a diseased state of the blood; usually refers to abnormal cellular elements of a permanent character.

**blood gas a•nal•y•sis** the direct electrode measurement of the partial pressure of oxygen and carbon dioxide in the blood.

**blood gas•es** a clinical expression for the determination of the partial pressures of oxygen and carbon dioxide in blood.

**blood group** a system of genetically determined antigens or agglutinogens located on the surface of the erythrocyte. Because of the antigen differences existing between individuals, blood groups are significant in blood transfusions, maternal-fetal incompatibilities (erythroblastosis fetalis), tissue and organ transplantation, disputed paternity cases, and in genetic and anthropologic studies; certain blood groups have been supposed to be related to susceptibility or resistance to certain diseases. Often used as synonymous with blood type.

**blood group an•ti•gen** generic term for any inherited antigen found on the surface of erythrocytes that determines a blood grouping reaction with specific antiserum; antigens of the ABO and Lewis blood groups may be found also in saliva and other body fluids.

**blood group•ing** the classification of blood samples by means of laboratory tests of their agglutination reactions with respect to one or more blood groups.

**blood group-spe•cif•ic sub•stanc•es A and B** solution of complexes of polysaccharides and amino acids that reduces the titer of anti-A and anti-B isoagglutinins in serum from group O persons; used to render group O blood reasonably safe for transfusion into persons of group A, B, or AB, but does not affect any incompatibility that results from various other factors, such as Rh.

**blood•less op•er•a•tion** an operation performed with negligible loss of blood.

**blood•let•ting** (blŭd'let-ing) removing blood, usually from a vein; used in congestive heart failure and polycythemia.

**blood plas•ma** SYN plasma (1).

**blood plas•ma frac•tions** portions of the blood plasma as separated by electrophoresis or other technique.

**blood poi•son•ing** SEE septicemia, pyemia.

**blood pool imag•ing** nuclear medicine study using a radionuclide that is confined to the vascular compartment.

**blood pres•sure** the pressure or tension of the blood within the systemic arteries, maintained by the contraction of the left ventricle, the resistance of the arterioles and capillaries, the elasticity of the arterial walls, as well as the viscosity and volume of the blood; expressed as relative to the ambient atmospheric pressure.

**blood re•la•tion•ship** SYN consanguinity.

**blood•shot** (blŭd'shot) denoting locally congested smaller blood vessels of a part (e.g., the conjunctiva) which are dilated and visible.

**blood•stream** (blŭd'strēm) the flowing blood as it is encountered in the circulatory system as distinguished from blood that has been removed from the circulatory system or sequestered in a part.

**blood sug•ar** SEE glucose.

**blood-thy•mus barrier** a sheath of pericytes and epithelial reticular cells around thymic capillaries that prevents the developing T lymphocytes of the thymus from being exposed to circulating antigens.

**blood type** the specific reaction pattern of erythrocytes of an individual to the antisera of one blood group; e.g., the ABO blood group consists of four major blood types: O, A, B, and AB. This classification depends on the presence or absence of two major antigens: A or B. Type O occurs when neither is present and type AB when both are present. See Blood Groups appendix.

**blood u•rea ni•tro•gen (BUN)** nitrogen, in the form of urea, in the blood; the most prevalent of nonprotein nitrogenous compounds in blood; blood normally contains 10 to 15 mg of urea/100 ml. SEE ALSO urea nitrogen.

**blood ves•sel** any vessel conveying blood: arteries, arterioles, capillaries, venules, veins. conveying blood.

**Bloom syn•drome** (bloom) congenital telangiectatic erythema, primarily in butterfly distribution, of the face and occasionally of the hands and forearms, with sun sensitivity of skin lesions and dwarfism with normal body proportions except for a narrow face and dolichocephalic skull; chromosomes are excessively unstable and there is a predisposition to malignancy; autosomal recessive inheritance, caused by mutation in the Bloom syndrome gene (BLM) on chromosome 15q.

**blot** SEE Northern blot analysis, Southern blot analysis, Western blot analysis, zoo blot analysis.

**Blount dis•ease** (blunt) tibia vara; nonrachitic bowlegs in children.

**blow-bot•tles** a device used to prevent atelectasis and maintain lung expansion in postsurgical patients. It consists of two 1-L bottles connected by a tube; with a series of slow exhalations, each preceded by a deep inhalation, the patient forces water from one bottle to the other. This device has largely been replaced by other adjuncts to lung expansion and airway clearance therapy. SEE ALSO incentive spirometer.

**blow-out frac•ture** a fracture of the floor of the orbit, without a fracture of the rim, produced by a blow on the globe with the force being transmitted via the globe to the orbital floor.

**blue ba•by** a child born cyanotic because of a congenital cardiac or pulmonary defect causing incomplete oxygenation of the blood.

**blue•ber•ry muf•fin ba•by** jaundice and purpura, especially of the face in the newborn, which may result from intrauterine viral infection.

**blue cat•a•ract** coronary cataract of bluish color.

**blue dome cyst 1.** one of a number of small dark blue nodules or cysts in the vaginal fornix due to retained menstrual blood in endometriosis affecting this region; **2.** a benign retention cyst of the mammary gland in fibrocystic disease, containing a pale slightly yellow fluid which gives a blue color to the cyst when seen through the surrounding fibrous tissue.

**blue-green bac•te•ria** SEE Cyanobacteria.

**blue line** a bluish line along the free border of the gingiva, occurring in chronic heavy metal poisoning.

**blue ne•vus** a dark blue or blue-black nevus covered by smooth skin and formed by heavily pigmented spindle-shaped or dendritic melanocytes in the reticular dermis.

**blue pus** pus tinged with pyocyanin, a product of *Pseudomonas aeruginosa*.

**blue rub•ber-bleb nevi** a syndrome characterized by erectile, easily compressible, thin-walled hemangiomatous nodules, widely distributed in the skin and in the alimentary canal; lesions in the gut may perforate or cause hemorrhage.

**blues** (blooz) state of depression or sadness. [slang, fr. *blue devils*]

**blue spot 1.** SYN macula cerulea. **2.** SYN mongolian spot.

**Blum•berg sign** (blum′bĕrg) pain felt upon sudden release of steadily applied pressure on a suspected area of the abdomen, indicative of peritonitis. SYN rebound tenderness.

**blunt•ed af•fect** a disturbance in mood manifested by a severe reduction in the expression of feeling.

**blunt-end•ed DNA, blunt-end** double-stranded DNA in which at least one of the ends has no unpaired bases.

**blush** (blŭsh) **1.** a sudden and brief redness of the face and neck due to emotion. **2.** in angiography, used metaphorically to describe neovascularity or, in some cases, extravasation. [M.E., fr. O.E. *blyscan*,]

**B lym•pho•cyte** a lymphocyte that resembles the bursa-derived lymphocyte of birds in that it is responsible for the production of immunoglobulins, i.e., it is the precursor of the plasma cell and expresses immunoglobulins on its surface but does not release them. It does not play a direct role in cell-mediated immunity. SEE ALSO T lymphocyte.

**BMI** body mass index.

**B-mode** a two-dimensional diagnostic ultrasound presentation of echo-producing interfaces in a single plane; the intensity of the echo is represented by modulation of the brightness (B) of the

spot, and the position of the echo is determined from the position of the transducer and the transit time of the acoustical pulse.

**Boch•da•lek her•nia** (bok′dĕl-ĕk) SYN congenital diaphragmatic hernia.

**Bo•dan•sky u•nit** (bō-dan′skē) that amount of phosphatase that liberates 1 mg of phosphorus as inorganic phosphate during the first hour of incubation with a buffered substrate containing sodium β-glycerophosphate.

**body** (bod′ē) **1.** the head, neck, trunk, and extremities. The human body, consisting of head (caput), neck (collum), trunk (truncus), and limbs (membra). **2.** the material part of a human, as distinguished from the mind and spirit. **3.** the principal mass of any structure. **4.** a thing; a substance. SEE ALSO corpus, soma. SYN corpus (1) [TA]. [A.S. *bodig*]

**body cav•i•ty** the collective visceral cavity of the trunk (thoracic cavity plus abdominopelvic cavity), bounded by the superior thoracic aperture above, the pelvic floor below, and the body walls (parietes) in between. SYN celom (2), celoma.

**body of hy•oid bone** the body of the hyoid bone, from which the greater and lesser horns extend.

**body im•age 1.** the cerebral representation of all body sensation organized in the parietal cortex; **2.** personal conception of one's own body as distinct from one's actual body or the conception other persons have of it.

■ **body mass in•dex (BMI)** a rough method of assessing nutritional status; correlates with risk of disease and death due to causes associated with obesity; because it does not distinguish excess adiposity from excess lean body mass, it is not useful in competitive athletes, body builders, pregnant women, or children. See page APP 128.

**body me•chan•ics** the application of physical principles to achieve maximum efficiency and to limit risk of physical stress or injury to the practitioner of physical therapy, massage therapy, chiropractic or osteopathic manipulation. SEE ALSO ergonomics.

**body scheme** a kinesthetic awareness of body parts and the relationship of those parts to one another and to objects in the environment. SYN kinesthetic awareness.

**body of stom•ach** the part of the stomach that lies between the fundus above and the pyloric antrum below; its boundaries are poorly defined.

**body sub•stance iso•la•tion** precautions taken by health care providers and others to avoid contact with blood and other body fluids.

**body sur•face a•re•a (BSA)** the area of the external surface of the body, expressed in square meters (m²); used to calculate metabolic, electrolyte, nutritional requirements, drug dosage, and expected pulmonary function measurements.

**body•work** any technique involving touch, massage, manipulation and/or energetic principles for the improvement or restoration of health. SEE ALSO massage therapy.

**Boeck dis•ease** (berk) SYN sarcoidosis.

**Boeck and Drbohlav Locke-egg-se•rum me•di•um** (berk and drb-ohl-ahf-lok) medium of whole eggs, human serum, and rice powder used to detect the presence of intestinal amebae, primarily *Entamoeba histolytica*.

**Boeh•mer he•ma•tox•y•lin** (ber-mer) an alum type of hematoxylin in which natural ripening occurs in about 8 to 10 days, and the solution is good for many months.

**Boer·haa·ve syn·drome** (boor′hah-vē) spontaneous rupture of the lower esophagus, a variant of Mallory-Weiss syndrome.

**Bohn no·dule** (bon) tiny buccal and palatal cysts in newborns derived from epithelial remnants of mucous gland tissue.

**Bohr at·om** (bor) a concept or model of the atom in which the negatively charged electrons move in circular or elliptical orbits around the positively charged nucleus, energy being emitted or absorbed when electrons change from one orbit to another.

**Bohr ef·fect** (bor) the effect of $H^+$ concentration on the affinity of hemoglobin for oxygen. As the $H^+$ concentration increases, the oxygen affinity decreases, causing a release of more oxygen to the tissue. One of the most important buffer systems in the body.

**Bohr e·qua·tion** (bor) an equation to calculate the respiratory dead space from the fact that gas expired from the lungs is a mixture of gas from the dead space and gas from the alveoli, i.e., the dead space volume divided by the tidal volume equals the difference between alveolar and mixed expired gas composition, divided by the difference between alveolar and inspired gas composition; gas composition can be expressed in any consistent units of concentration or partial pressure of oxygen or carbon dioxide.

**Bohr the·o·ry** (bor) theory that spectrum lines are produced by the quantized emission of radiant energy when electrons drop from an orbit of a higher to one of a lower energy level, or 2) by absorption of radiation when an electron rises from a lower to a higher energy level.

**boil** (boyl) SYN furuncle. [A.S. *byl*, a swelling]

**boil·er·mak·er's hear·ing loss** SYN noise-induced hearing loss.

**Bo·ley gauge** (bō′lē) a vernier, metric caliper used in dentistry to measure tooth, arch, and facial dimensions.

**bo·lus** (bō′lŭs) **1.** a single, relatively large quantity of a substance, usually one intended for therapeutic use, such as a bolus dose of a drug. **2.** a masticated morsel of food or another substance ready to be swallowed, such as a bolus of barium for x-ray studies. **3.** in high-energy radiation therapy, a quantity of tissue-equivalent material placed next to the irradiated region to increase the dose of secondary radiation to the superficial tissues. [L. fr. G. *bōlos,* lump, clod]

**Bom·bay blood type** blood type of individuals who possess the genes for A and B antigens but are unable to express the genes because they lack the gene for H antigen, a required precursor of A and B. Individuals with this blood type frequently have anti-H in their blood.

**bomb cal·o·rim·e·ter** an instrument for determining the potential energy of organic substances, including those in foods. In consists of a hollow steel container, lined with platinum and filled with pure oxygen, into which a weighed quantity of substance is placed and ignited with an electric fuse; the heat produced is absorbed by water surrounding the bomb and, from the rise in temperature, the calories liberated are calculated. See this page.

**bond** in chemistry, the force holding two neighboring atoms in place and resisting their separa-

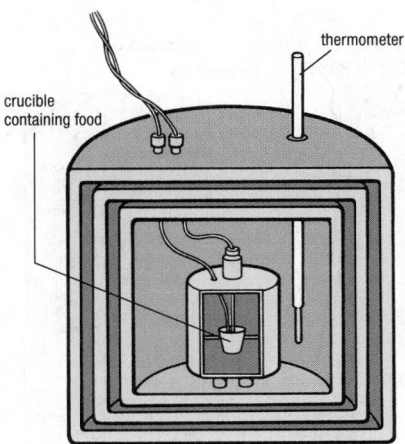

**bomb calorimeter:** measures heat produced by complete combustion of food sample

tion; a bond is electrovalent if it consists of the attraction between oppositely charged groups, or covalent if it results from the sharing of one, two, or three pairs of electrons by the bonded atoms.

**bonding** (bon′ding) formation of a close and enduring emotional attachment, such as between parent and child, lovers, or husband and wife.

**bone** (bōn) **1.** a hard connective tissue consisting of cells embedded in a matrix of mineralized ground substance and collagen fibers. The fibers are impregnated with a form of calcium phosphate similar to hydroxyapatite as well as with substantial quantities of carbonate, citrate sodium, and magnesium; by weight, bone is composed of 75% inorganic material and 25% organic material; a portion of osseous tissue of definite shape and size, forming a part of the animal skeleton; in man there are 200 distinct ossa in the skeleton, not including the ossicula auditus of the tympanic cavity or the ossa sesamoidea other than the two patellae. Bone consists of a dense outer layer of compact substance or cortical substance covered by the periosteum, and an inner loose, spongy substance; the central portion of a long bone is filled with marrow. **2.** a mass of this tissue of definite shape and size, forming a part of the animal skeleton. A bone consists of a dense outer layer of compact substance or cortex covered by the periosteum and an inner loose, spongy substance; the central portion of a long bone is filled with marrow. For definitions of bones as part of the animal skeleton, see os. See page 126. SYN os [TA]. [A.S. *bān*]

**bone block** a surgical procedure in which the bone adjacent to the joint is modified to limit the motion of the joint mechanically.

**bone block fu·sion** a method of fusing two bones in which a block of bone graft is placed between the two surfaces to obtain fusion and correct preexisting deformity.

**bone can·a·lic·u·lus** canaliculus connecting bone lacunae with one another or with a haver-

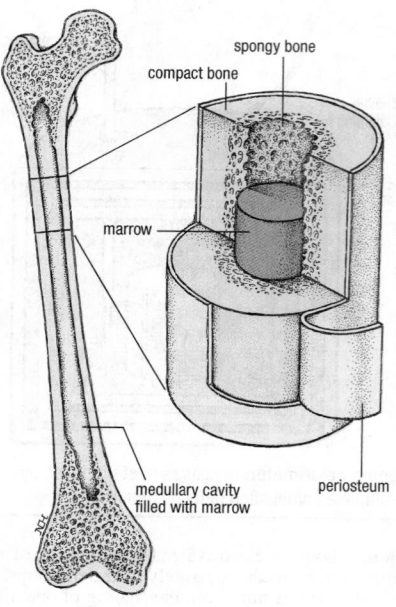

spongy bone
compact bone
marrow
medullary cavity filled with marrow
periosteum

**bone**

sian canal; contains the interconnecting cytoplasmic processes of osteocytes.

**bone con·duc·tion** in relation to hearing, the transmission of sound to the inner ear through vibrations applied to the bones of the skull.

**bone den·si·ty** quantitative measurement of the mineral content of bone, used as an indicator of the structural strength of the bone and as a screen for osteoporosis

**bone flap** portion of cranium removed but left attached to overlying muscle-fascial blood supply; term is often used incorrectly for a completely detached cranial section, i.e., a bone graft.

**bone for·ceps** a strong forceps used for seizing or removing fragments of bone.

**bone·let** (bōn′let) SYN ossicle.

**bone mar·row** the tissue filling the cavities of bones, having a stroma of reticular fibers and cells.

**bone mar·row trans·plan·ta·tion** grafting of bone marrow tissue; of value in aplastic anemia, primary immunodeficiency, and acute leukemia (following total body irradiation).

**bone ma·trix** the intercellular substance of bone tissue consisting of collagen fibers, ground substance, and inorganic bone salts.

**bone scan** x-ray examination of bone after injection of radioactive material, to identify areas of injury, disease, or regeneration. See page B12.

**bones of dig·its** the phalanges and sesamoid bones of the fingers and toes.

**bone spur** SYN heel spur.

**bones of skull, bones of cra·ni·um** the paired inferior nasal concha, lacrimal, maxilla, nasal, palatine, parietal, temporal, and zygomatic; and the unpaired ethmoid, frontal, occipital, sphenoid, and vomer. SYN ossa cranii [TA], cranial bones.

**bone tis·sue** SYN osseous tissue.

**Bon·hoef·fer sign** (bon′hĕrf-ĕr) loss of normal muscle tone in chorea.

**bonk·ing** SYN hitting the wall.

**Bon·net cap·sule** (bō-nā′) the anterior part of the vagina bulbi.

**Bon·nier syn·drome** (bon-yā′) a syndrome due to a lesion of Deiters nucleus and its connection; the symptoms include ocular disturbances (e.g., paralysis of accommodation, nystagmus, diplopia), as well as deafness, nausea, thirst, anorexia, and symptoms referable to the involvement of the vagus centers.

**bon·y am·pul·lae of sem·i·cir·cu·lar ca·nals** a circumscribed dilation of one extremity of each of the three bony semicircular canals, anterior, posterior, and lateral; each contains a membranous ampulla of the semicircular ducts.

**bon·y an·ky·lo·sis** SYN synostosis.

**bon·y lab·y·rinth** a series of cavities (cochlea, vestibule, and semicircular canals) contained within the otic capsule of the petrous portion of the temporal bone; the bony labyrinth is filled with perilymph, in which the delicate, endolymph-filled membranous labyrinth is suspended.

**bon·y pal·ate** a concave elliptical bony plate, constituting the roof of the oral cavity, formed of the palatine process of the maxilla and the horizontal plate of the palatine bone on either side.

**bon·y sem·i·cir·cu·lar ca·nals** the three bony tubes in the labyrinth of the ear within which the membranous semicircular ducts are located; they lie in planes at right angles to each other and are known as anterior semicircular canal, posterior semicircular canal, and lateral semicircular canal.

**BOOP** bronchiolitis obliterans with organizing pneumonia, an idiopathic form of bronchiolitis obliterans.

**boost·er, boost·er dose** a dose given at some time after an initial dose to enhance the effect, said usually of antigens for the production of antibodies.

**boot** (boot) a boot-shaped appliance. [M.E. *bote*, fr. O.Fr.]

**bor·bo·ryg·mus**, pl. **bor·bo·ryg·mi** (bōr-bō-rig′mŭs, bōr-bō-rig′mī) rumbling or gurgling noises produced by movement of gas, fluid, or both in the alimentary canal, and audible at a distance. [G. *borborygmos*, rumbling in the bowels]

**bor·der** (bōr′der) the part of a surface that forms its outer boundary. SEE ALSO margin. SYN margo [TA].

**bor·der·line ovar·i·an tu·mor** an ovarian surface epithelial tumor in which the growth pattern is intermediate between benign and malignant; includes mucinous, serous, endometrioid, and Brenner tumors of the ovary; highly curable but may recur after surgical removal.

**bor·der·line per·son·al·i·ty dis·or·der** a mental disorder in which the symptoms are not continually psychotic yet are not strictly neurotic: may include impulsivity and unpredictability, unstable interpersonal relationships, inappropriate or uncontrolled anger, identity disturbances, rapid shifts of mood, suicidal acts, self-mutilations, job and marital instability, chronic feelings of emptiness or boredom, and intolerance of being alone.

**bor·der move·ment** the limit of movement of the lower jaw as recorded in the sagittal and horizontal planes. Often referred to as the envelope of motion.

**Bor·de·tel·la** (bōr-dĕ-tel′ă) a genus of strictly aerobic bacteria (family Brucellaceae) containing minute Gram-negative coccobacilli. Motile and nonmotile species occur; motile cells are peritrichous. The metabolism of these organisms is respiratory. They require nicotinic acid, cysteine, and methionine; hemin (X factor) and coenzyme I (V factor) are not required. They are parasites and pathogens of the mammalian respiratory tract. The type species is *Bordetella pertussis*. [J. Bordet]

**Bor·de·tel·la bron·chi·sep·ti·ca** a bacterial species found in a broad range of animal species, causing atrophic rhinitis of swine, bronchopneumonia in rodents, and a highly contagious bronchopneumonia in dogs. It is a rare cause of opportunistic respiratory tract infection in immunocompromised patients.

**Bor·de·tel·la hin·zi·i** a newly described bacterial species isolated from a few human blood cultures and respiratory secretions, as well as from poultry respiratory secretions.

**Bor·de·tel·la hol·mi·e·si·i** a newly described bacterial species isolated from human blood cultures, primarily from immunocompromised patients.

**Bor·de·tel·la per·tus·sis** a species that causes whooping cough; it produces cell-destroying toxins and causes thick mucus to collect in the airway. The type species of the genus *Bordetella*.

**Borg scale** SYN rating of perceived exertion.

**Born·holm dis·ease** SYN epidemic pleurodynia. [*Bornholm,* Danish island in the Baltic where the d. was first described]

**Born·holm dis·ease vi·rus** SYN epidemic pleurodynia virus.

**bo·ron (B)** (bōr′on) a nonmetallic trivalent element, atomic no. 5, atomic wt. 10.811; occurs as a hard crystalline mass or as a brown powder, and forms borates and boric acid. A nutritional need has been reported in pregnant women. [Pers. *Burah*]

**Bor·rel blue stain** (bō-rel′) a stain for demonstrating spirochetes, treponemes, and Borrelia organisms, using silver oxide (prepared by means of mixing solutions of silver nitrate and sodium bicarbonate) and methylene blue.

**Bor·rel·ia** (bō-rē′lē-ă) a genus of bacteria (family Treponemataceae) containing cells 8–16 μm in length, with coarse, shallow, irregular spirals and tapered, finely filamented ends. These organisms are parasitic on many forms of animal life, are generally hematophytic, or are found on mucous membranes; most are transmitted to animals or humans by the bites of arthropods. The type species is *Borrelia anserina*. [A. *Borrell*]

**Bor·rel·ia af·ze·li·i** a bacterial genospecies of *Borrelia burgdorferi sensu lato* causing Lyme disease in Europe and Asia; transmitted by the tick *Ixodes ricinus* in central and western Europe and by the tick *Ixodes persulcatus* in Eurasia from the Baltic Sea to the Pacific Ocean. SEE ALSO *Borrelia burgdorferi sensu stricto.*

**Bor·rel·ia burg·dor·fer·i** a species causing Lyme disease. The vector transmitting this spirochete to humans is the tick, *Ixodes scapularis.*

**Bor·rel·ia burg·dor·fer·i sen·su lat·o** a bacterial complex causing Lyme disease that is composed of several genospecies including *Borrelia*

*burgdorferi sensu stricto, Borrelia garinii* and *Borrelia afzelii.*

**Bor·rel·ia burg·dor·fer·i sen·su strict·o** a bacterial genospecies of *Borrelia burgdorferi sensu lato* causing Lyme disease in North America and Europe; transmitted by the tick *Ixodes scapularis* in the eastern and central United States, by the tick *Ixodes pacificus* in the western United States, and by the tick *Ixodes ricinus* in Europe. SEE ALSO *Borrelia garinii.*

**Bor·rel·ia gar·i·ni·i** a bacterial genospecies of *Borrelia burgdorferi sensu lato* causing Lyme disease in Europe and Asia; transmitted by the tick *Ixodes ricinus* in central and western Europe and by the tick *Ixodes persulcatus* in Eurasia from the Baltic Sea to the Pacific Ocean. SEE ALSO *Borrelia burgdorferi sensu stricto.*

**bor·re·li·o·sis** (bō-rē-lē-ō′sis) disease caused by bacteria of the genus *Borrelia.*

**Bo·sin dis·ease** (bō′sin) SYN subacute sclerosing panencephalitis.

**boss** (baws) **1.** a protuberance; a circumscribed rounded swelling. **2.** the prominence of a kyphosis. [M. E. *boce,* fr. O. Fr.]

**bos·se·lat·ed** (baws′ĕ-lā-ted) marked by numerous bosses or rounded protuberances. [Fr. *bosseler,* to emboss]

**Bo·tal·lo duct** (bō-tah′lō) SYN ductus arteriosus.

**Bo·tal·lo fo·ra·men** (bō-tah′lō) the orifice of communication between the two atria of the fetal heart. SEE ALSO foramen ovale.

**bot·ry·oid** (bot′rē-oyd) having numerous rounded protuberances resembling a bunch of grapes. SYN staphyline, uviform. [G. *botryoidēs,* like a bunch of grapes (*botrys*)]

**bot·ry·oid sar·co·ma** a polypoid form of embryonal rhabdomyosarcoma which occurs in children, most frequently in the urogenital tract, characterized by the formation of grossly apparent grapelike clusters of neoplastic tissue; neoplasms of this type grow relatively rapidly and are highly malignant.

**Böt·tcher cells** (bĕrt′shĕr) cells of the basilar membrane of the cochlea.

**Böt·tcher crys·tals** (bĕrt′shĕr) small crystals observed microscopically in prostatic fluid that is treated with a drop or two of 1% solution of ammonium phosphate.

**Böt·tcher space** (bĕrt′shĕr) SYN endolymphatic sac.

**bot·tle** (bot′tl) a container for liquids.

**bot·u·li·nus tox·in** a potent neurotoxin from *Clostridium botulinum.*

**bot·u·lism** (bot′yu-lizm) food poisoning caused by the ingestion of the neurotoxin produced by *Clostridium botulinum,* usually in improperly canned or preserved food; causes paralysis and can be fatal. SEE ALSO *Clostridium botulinum.* [L. *botulus,* sausage]

**bou·bas** (boo′bahs) SYN yaws. [native Brazilian]

**Bou·chard dis·ease** (boo-shahr′) myopathic dilation of the stomach.

**Bou·chut tube** (boo-shoo′) a short cylindrical tube used in intubation of the larynx.

**bou·gie** (boo′zhē) a cylindrical instrument, usually somewhat flexible and yielding, used for calibrating or dilating constricted areas in tubular organs, such as the urethra or esophagus; sometimes containing a medication for local application. [Fr. candle]

**bou·gie·nage** (boo-zhē-nahzh′) examination or

treatment of the interior of any canal by the passage of a bougie or cannula.

**Bou·in fix·a·tive** (boo-ã′) a solution of glacial acetic acid, formalin, and picric acid, useful for soft and delicate tissues (as those of embryos) and small pieces of tissues; it preserves glycogen and nuclei and permits brilliant staining, but penetrates slowly, distorts kidney tissue and mitochondria, and does not permit Feulgen stain for DNA.

**boundaries** (bown′dar-′es) limits of one's personal space, including physical, psychosocial, or interpersonal domains.

**bou·quet** (boo-ka′) a cluster or bunch of structures, especially of blood vessels, suggesting a bouquet. [Fr.]

**Bour·don gauge** a type of flow-regulating device used in the delivery of medical gas.

**bou·ton** (boo-ton′) a button, pustule, or knob-like swelling. [Fr. button]

**bou·ton de Bagh·dad** the lesion occurring in cutaneous leishmaniasis.

**bou·ton·neuse fe·ver** tick-borne infection with *Rickettsia conorii* seen in Africa, Europe, the Middle East, and India. SYN tick typhus.

**bou·ton·nière de·form·it·y** (boo-tawn-yar′ dē-fōr′mi-tē) rupture of the central slip of a digital extensor tendon at the middle phalanx, marked by extension of the metacarpopophalangeal and distal interphalangeal joints and flexion of the proximal interphalangeal joint. [Fr., buttonhole]

**Bo·vie** an instrument used for electrosurgical dissection and hemostasis. Frequently used as a verb, i.e., to Bovie something is to dissect or cauterize it with the Bovie instrument.

**bo·vine** (bō′vīn) relating to cattle. [L. *bos* (*bov-*), ox]

**bo·vine ba·be·si·o·sis** an infectious disease of cattle caused by *Babesia* species and transmitted by ticks. SYN tick fever (3).

**bo·vine se·rum al·bu·min (BSA)** a source of albumin commonly used in *in vitro* biological studies.

**bo·vine spon·gi·form en·ceph·a·lop·a·thy** a disease of cattle first reported in 1986 in Great Britain; characterized clinically by apprehensive behavior, hyperesthesia, and ataxia, and histologically by spongiform changes in the gray matter of the brainstem; caused by a prion, like spongiform encephalopathies of other animals (e.g., scrapie) and human beings (Creutzfeldt-Jakob disease). SEE Creutzfeldt-Jakob disease.

**bow** (bō) any device bent in a simple curve or semicircle and possessing flexibility. [A.S. boga]

**Bow·ditch law** (bō′dich) consistently total response to any effective stimulus. SYN all or none law.

**bow·el** SYN intestinum. [through the Fr. from L. *botulus,* sausage]

**bow·el by·pass** SYN jejunoileal bypass.

**bow·el sounds** relatively high-pitched abdominal sounds caused by propulsion of intestinal contents through the lower alimentary tract.

**ⅈ Bow·en dis·ease** (bō′wen) a form of intraepidermal carcinoma characterized by the development of slowly enlarging pinkish or brownish papules or eroded plaques covered with a thickened horny layer; microscopically, there is dyskeratosis with large round epidermal cells with large nuclei and pale-staining cytoplasm which are

scattered through all levels of the epidermis. See page B7.

**Bow·ie stain** (bō′wē) a stain for juxtaglomerular granules in which the kidney sections are stained in a mixture of Biebrich scarlet red and ethyl violet; juxtaglomerular granules and elastic fibers are stained a deep purple, erythrocytes are amber, and background tissue appears in shades of red.

**bow·leg, bow-leg** (bō′leg) SYN genu varum.

**bowl·er's thumb** compression of the digital nerve on the medial aspect of the thumb, leading to paresthesia in the thumb.

**Bow·man cap·sule** (bō′măn) SYN glomerular capsule.

**Bow·man mem·brane, Bow·man lay·er** (bō′măn) SYN anterior elastic lamina of cornea.

**Bow·man probe** (bō′măn) a double-ended probe for the lacrimal duct.

**box** (boks) container; receptacle. [L.L. *buxis,* fr. G. *puxis,* box tree]

**box·er's frac·ture** fracture of the neck of a metacarpal bone (most often the fifth) with volar displacement of the head of the bone. SYN fracture of fifth metacarpal.

**box jel·ly** SYN Chiropsalmus quadrumanus.

**Boyd com·mu·ni·cat·ing per·fo·ra·tion vein** a vein connecting the superficial and deep venous systems in the anteromedial calf.

**Boy·den meal** (boy′den) a meal consisting of three or four egg yolks, beaten up in milk, used to test the evacuation time of the gallbladder; two-thirds to three-quarters of the contents will normally be evacuated within 40 minutes.

**Boy·er cyst** (bwah-yā) a subhyoid cyst.

**Boyle law** (boyl) at constant temperature, the volume of a given quantity of gas varies inversely with its absolute pressure. SYN Mariotte law.

**Boze·man-Fritsch cath·e·ter** (bōz′măn fritch) a slightly curved double-channel uterine catheter with several openings at the tip.

**Boze·man op·er·a·tion** (bōz′măn) an operation for uterovaginal fistula, the cervix uteri being attached to the bladder and opening into its cavity.

**Boze·man po·si·tion** (bōz′măn) knee-elbow position, the patient being strapped to supports.

**Boz·zo·lo sign** (bōt-sō′lō) pulsating vessels in the nasal mucous membrane, noted occasionally in thoracic aneurysm.

**BP** blood pressure.

**BPF** bronchopleural fistula.

**BP fis·tu·la** SYN bronchopleural fistula.

**BPH** benign prostatic hyperplasia.

**Br** bromine.

**brace** (brās) an orthosis or orthopedic appliance that supports or holds in correct position any movable part of the body and that allows motion of the part, in contrast to a splint, which prevents motion of the part. [M. E., fr. O. Fr., fr. L. *bracchium,* arm, fr. G. *brachion*]

**brac·es** (brā′sez) colloquialism for orthodontic appliances.

**bra·chia** (brā′kē-ă) plural of brachium.

**brach·i·al** (brā′kē-ăl) relating to the arm.

**brach·i·al ar·tery** *origin,* is a continuation of the axillary beginning at the inferior border of the teres major muscle; *branches,* deep brachial, superior ulnar collateral, inferior ulnar collateral, muscular, and nutrient; terminates in the cubital fossa by bifurcating into radial and ulnar arteries. SYN arteria brachialis [TA].

**bra·chi·al·gia** (brā-kē-al′jē-ă) pain in the arm. [L. *brachium*, arm, + *algos*, pain]

**bra·chi·a·lis mus·cle** *origin*, lower two-thirds of anterior surface of humerus; *insertion*, coronoid process of ulna; *action*, flexes elbow; *nerve supply*, musculocutaneous, usually with a minor contribution from the radial. SYN musculus brachialis [TA].

**bra·chi·al plex·us** a complex web of spinal nerves arising from the cervical spine which innervate the upper extremities.

**bra·chi·al plex·us in·ju·ry** damage to the brachial plexus related to delivery; associated with excessive lateral stretching of the head, typically in cases of shoulder dystocia or breech deliveries.

**bra·chi·al veins** venae comitantes of the brachial artery which empty into the axillary vein.

△**bra·chio-** **1.** SYN arm (1). **2.** SYN radial. [L. *brachium*]

**bra·chi·o·ce·phal·ic** (brā′kē-ō-se-fal′ik) relating to both arm and head.

**bra·chi·o·ce·phal·ic ar·te·ri·tis** giant-cell arteritis seen in older adults; characterized by inflammatory lesions in medium sized arteries, most commonly in the head, neck and/or shoulder girdle area. Erythrocyte sedimentation rate is elevated. Visual loss can occur.

**bra·chi·o·ce·phal·ic trunk** *origin*, arch of aorta; *branches*, right subclavian and right common carotid; occasionally it gives off the thyroidea ima. SYN truncus brachiocephalicus [TA].

**bra·chi·o·ce·phal·ic veins** formed by the union of the internal jugular and subclavian veins; other tributaries of the right brachiocephalic vein are the right vertebral and internal thoracic veins, and the right lymphatic duct; other tributaries of the left brachiocephalic vein are the left vertebral, internal thoracic, superior intercostal, thyroidea ima, and various anterior pericardial, bronchial, mediastinal veins, and the thoracic duct. SYN venae rachiocephalicae [TA], innominate veins.

**bra·chi·o·cru·ral** (brā′kē-ō-kroo′răl) relating to both arm and thigh.

**bra·chi·o·cu·bi·tal** (brā′kē-ō-kyu′bi-tăl) relating to both arm and elbow or to both arm and forearm.

**bra·chi·o·ra·di·a·lis mus·cle** *origin*, lateral supracondylar ridge of humerus; *insertion*, front of base of styloid process of radius; *action*, flexes elbow and assists slightly in supination; *nerve supply*, (common) radial. SYN musculus brachioradialis [TA].

**bra·chi·um**, pl. **bra·chia** (brak′ē-ŭm, brā′kē-ă) **1.** SYN arm (1). **2.** an anatomic structure resembling an arm. [L. arm, prob. akin to G. *brachiōn*]

**bra·chi·um of in·fe·ri·or col·lic·u·lus** a fiber bundle passing from the inferior colliculus on either side of the brainstem along the lateral border of the superior colliculus to the posterior part of the thalamus where it enters the medial geniculate body. It forms part of the major ascending auditory pathway.

**bra·chi·um of su·pe·ri·or col·lic·u·lus** a band of fibers of the optic tract bypassing the lateral geniculate body to terminate in the superior colliculus and pretectal region.

**Bracht ma·neu·ver** (brokt) delivery of a fetus in breech position by extension of the legs and trunk of the fetus over the symphysis pubis and abdomen of the mother; the fetal head is born spontaneously as the legs and trunk are lifted above the maternal pelvis, and as the body of the infant is extended by the operator.

△**brachy-** short. [G. *brachys*, short]

**brach·y·ba·sia** (brak-ē-bā′sē-ă) the shuffling gait of pyramidal tract disease. [brachy- + G. *basis*, a stepping]

**brach·y·ba·so·camp·to·dac·ty·ly** (brak-ē-bā′sō-kamp-tō-dak′ti-lē) disproportionate shortness and crookedness of the fingers. [brachy- + G. *basis*, base, + *campylos*, curved, + *daktylos*, finger]

**brach·y·ba·so·pha·lan·gia** (brak-ē-bā′sō-fă-lan′jē-ă) abnormal shortness of the proximal phalanges. [brachy- + G. *basis*, base, + phalanx]

**brach·y·car·dia** (brak-ē-kar′dē-ă) SYN bradycardia.

**brach·y·chei·lia, brach·y·chi·lia** (brak′ē-kī′lē-ă) abnormal shortness of the lips. [brachy- + G. *cheilos*, lip]

**brach·y·dac·ty·ly** (brak-ē-dak′ti-lē) abnormal shortness of the fingers. [brachy- + G. *daktylos*, finger]

**bra·ch·yg·na·thia** (brak-ig-nā′thē-ă) abnormal shortness or recession of the mandible. SEE ALSO micrognathia. [brachy- + G. *gnathos*, jaw]

**brach·y·me·lia** (brak-ē-mē′lē-ă) disproportionate shortness of the limbs. [brachy- + G. *melos*, limb]

**brach·y·me·so·pha·lan·gia** (brak-ē-mes′ō-fă-lan′jē-ă) abnormal shortness of the middle phalanges. [brachy- + G. *mesos*, middle, + phalanx]

**brach·y·met·a·car·pia** (brak′ē-met-ă-car′pē-ă) abnormal shortness of the metacarpals, especially the fourth and fifth.

**brach·y·met·a·tar·sia** (brak′ē-met-ă-tar′sē-ă) abnormal shortness of the metatarsals.

**brach·y·o·dont** (brak′ē-ō-dont) a tooth in which the root length exceeds that of the crown. [brachy- + G. *odous*, tooth]

**brach·y·o·nych·ia** (brak′ē-ō-nik′ē-ă) short nails, in which the width of the nail plate and nail bed is greater than the length. [G. *brachys*, short + *onyx, onychos*, nail, + suffix -*ia*, condition]

**brach·y·pel·lic pel·vis** a pelvis in which the transverse diameter is more than 1 cm longer but less than 3 cm longer than the anteroposterior diameter.

**brach·y·pha·lan·gia** (brak′ē-fă-lan′jē-ă) abnormal shortness of the phalanges. [brachy- + phalanx]

**brach·y·syn·dac·ty·ly** (brak′ē-sin-dak′ti-lē) abnormal shortness of fingers or toes combined with a webbing between the adjacent digits. [brachy- + syndactyly]

**brach·y·te·le·pha·lan·gia** (brak-ē-tel′ĕ-fă-lan′jē-ă) abnormal shortness of the distal phalanges. [brachy- + G. *telos*, end, + phalanx]

**brach·y·ther·a·py** (brak-ē-thār′ă-pē) radiotherapy in which the source of irradiation is placed close to the surface of the body or within a body cavity; e.g., application of radium to the cervix.

**Brad·bu·ry-Eg·gle·ston syn·drome** (brad′bĕ-rē eg′ĕl-stĕn) SYN pure autonomic failure.

**Brad·ford frame** (brad′ford) an oblong rectangular frame made of pipe, over which are stretched transversely two strips of canvas; permits trunk and lower extremities of a bed-ridden patient to move as a unit.

△**bra·dy-** slow. [G. *bradys*, slow]

**bra·dy·ar·rhyth·mia** (brad′ē-ă-rith′mē-ă) any

disturbance of the heart's rhythm resulting in a rate under 60 beats per minute. [brady- + G. *a-priv.* + *rhythmos,* rhythm]

**bra·dy·arth·ria** (brad-ē-arth′rē-ă) a form of dysarthria characterized by an abnormal slowness or deliberateness of speech. SYN bradyglossia (2), bradylalia, bradylogia. [brady- + G. *arthroō,* to utter distinctly, fr. *arthron,* a joint]

**bra·dy·car·dia** (brad-ē-kar′dē-ă) slowness of the heartbeat, usually a rate under 60 beats per minute. SYN brachycardia. [brady- + G. *kardia,* heart]

**brad·y·car·di·ac, bra·dy·car·dic** (brad-ē-kar′dē-ak, brad-ē-kar′dik) relating to or characterized by bradycardia.

**bra·dy·di·as·to·le** (brad-ē-dī-as′tō-lē) prolongation of the diastole of the heart.

**bra·dy·es·the·sia** (brad-ē-es-thē′zē-ă) slow sensory perception. [brady- + G. *aisthēsis,* sensation]

**bra·dy·glos·sia** (brad-ē-glos′ē-ă) **1.** slow or difficult tongue movement. **2.** SYN bradyarthria. [brady- + G. *glōssa,* tongue]

**bra·dy·ki·ne·sia** (brad-ē-kin-ē′zē-ă) a decrease in spontaneity and movement. One of the features of extrapyramidal disorders, such as Parkinson disease. [brady- + G. *kinēsis,* movement]

**bra·dy·ki·net·ic** (brad-ē-ki-net′ik) characterized by or pertaining to slow movement.

**bra·dy·ki·nin** (brad-ē-kī′nin) the nonapeptide Arg-Pro-Pro-Gly-Phe-Ser-Pro-Phe-Arg, normally present in blood in an inactive form; one of the plasma kinins, a potent vasodilator and mediator of anaphylaxis. [brady- + G. *kineō,* to move]

**bra·dy·la·lia** (brad-ē-lā′lē-ă) SYN bradyarthria. [brady- + G. *lalia,* speech]

**bra·dy·lex·ia** (brad-ē-lek′sē-ă) abnormal slowness in reading. [brady- + G. *lexis,* word]

**bra·dy·lo·gia** (brad-ē-lō′jē-ă) SYN bradyarthria. [brady- + G. *logos,* word]

**bra·dyp·nea** (brad-ip-nē′ă) abnormal slowness of respiration, specifically a low respiratory frequency. [brady- + G. *pnoē,* breathing]

**bra·dy·sper·ma·tism** (brad-ē-sper′mă-tizm) absence of ejaculatory force, so that the semen trickles away slowly. [brady, + G. *sperma* (*spermat-*), seed, + ism]

**bra·dy·sphyg·mia** (brad-ē-sfig′mē-ă) slowness of the pulse; can occur without bradycardia, as in ventricular bigeminy when every other beat may fail to produce a peripheral pulse. [brady- + G. *sphygmos,* pulse]

**bra·dy·stal·sis** (brad-ē-stahl′sis) slow bowel motion. [G. *bradys,* slow, + (*peri*) *stalsis,* contracting around]

**bra·dy·to·cia** (brad-ē-tō′sē-ă) tedious labor; slow delivery. [brady- + G. *tokos,* childbirth]

**bra·dy·u·ria** (brad-ē-yu′rē-ă) slow micturition. [brady- + G. *ouron,* urine]

**Brain,** W. Russell, Lord, English physician, 1895–1966. SEE Brain reflex.

**brain** (brān) that part of the central nervous system contained within the cranium. SEE ALSO encephalon. Cf. cerebrum, cerebellum. See this page. [A.S. *braegen*]

**brain at·tack** SYN stroke (1).

**brain·case** (brān′kās) SYN neurocranium.

**brain con·cus·sion** a clinical syndrome due to mechanical, usually traumatic, forces; characterized by immediate and transient impairment of

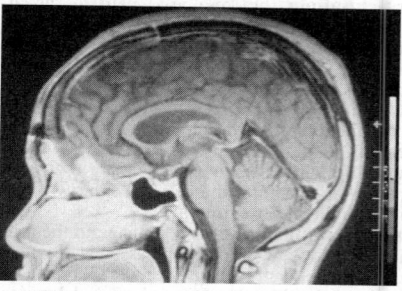

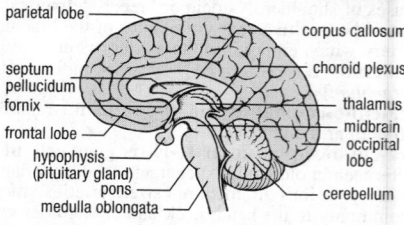

parietal lobe — corpus callosum
septum pellucidum — choroid plexus
fornix — thalamus
frontal lobe — midbrain
hypophysis (pituitary gland) — occipital lobe
pons — cerebellum
medulla oblongata —

**brain:** (above) magnetic resonance image (MRI) of a normal brain; (below) illustration of the same midsagittal view

neural function, such as alteration of consciousness, disturbance of vision and equilibrium, etc.

**Brain re·flex** (brān) SYN quadripedal extensor reflex.

**brain·stem, brain stem** (brān′stem) originally, the entire unpaired subdivision of the brain, composed of the rhombencephalon, mesencephalon, and diencephalon as distinguished from the brain's only paired subdivision, the telencephalon. More recently, the connotation of the term has undergone several arbitrary modifications: some use it to denote no more than rhombencephalon plus mesencephalon, distinguishing that complex from the prosencephalon (diencephalon plus telencephalon); others restrict it even further to refer exclusively to the rhombencephalon. From both developmental and architectural viewpoints, the original interpretation seems preferable.

**brain·stem au·di·tory e·voked po·ten·tial** responses triggered by click stimuli, which are generated in the acoustic nerve and brainstem auditory pathways; recorded over the scalp.

**brain·stem evoked re·sponse (BSER)** SYN auditory brainstem response.

**brain·stem e·voked re·sponse au·di·om·e·try, BSER au·di·om·e·try** SYN auditory brainstem response audiometry.

**brain sug·ar** D-galactose. SEE galactose.

**brain swell·ing** a pathologic entity, localized or generalized, characterized by an increase in bulk of brain tissue, due to expansion of the intravascular (congestion) or extravascular (edema) compartments that may coexist or may occur separately and be clinically indistinguishable; clinical manifestations depend on disturbed neuronal function due to local swelling, shifting of intracranial structures, and the effects of intracranial hypertension or circulatory disturbance.

**brain·wash·ing** (brān′wash′ing) inducing a person to modify his attitudes and behavior in certain directions through various forms of psychological pressure or torture.

**brain wave** colloquialism for electroencephalogram.

**brak·ing ra·di·a·tion** SYN Bremsstrahlung radiation.

**branch** an offshoot; in anatomy, one of the primary divisions of a nerve or blood vessel. A branch. SEE ramus, artery, nerve, vein. SYN ramus (1). [Fr. *branche,* related to L. *branchium,* arm]

**branch·er gly·co·gen stor·age dis·ease** type of glycogen storage disease, due to deficiency of amylo-1,4-1,6-transglucosidase (brancher enzyme).

**bran·chi·al arch** SYN pharyngeal arch.

**bran·chi·al cleft** the branchial ectodermal grooves of mammalian embryos, which are imperforate, rudimentary homologues of gill clefts in fishes. SEE pharyngeal cleft.

**branch·ing** dividing into parts; sending out offshoots; bifurcating.

**bran·chi·o·mo·tor nu·clei** collective term for those motoneuronal nuclei of the brainstem that develop from the branchiomotor column of the embryo and innervate striated muscle fibers.

**bran·chi·o·o·to·re·nal syn·drome** an autosomal dominant disorder characterized by anomalies of the pharyngeal arch (branchial arch) derivatives, sensory hearing impairment, and renal abnormalities.

**Brandt-An·drews ma·neu·ver** (brahnt an′ droos) the expression of the placenta by grasping the umbilical cord with one hand and placing the other hand on the abdomen, with the fingers over the anterior surface of the uterus at the junction of the lower uterine segment and the corpus uteri.

*Bran·ha·mel·la* (bran-hă-mel′ă) a subgenus of aerobic, nonmotile, non–spore-forming bacteria containing Gram-negative cocci that occur in pairs with adjacent sides flattened. They are found in the mucous membranes of the upper respiratory tract and occasionally cause respiratory infections and otitis media. [Sara *Branham*]

**Bran·ham sign** (bran′hĕm) bradycardia following compression or excision of an arteriovenous fistula.

**bran·ny** (bran′ē) denoting desquamation of small husk-like scales. [M.E. *bran,* broken coat of cereal grain]

**Bras·dor meth·od** (bras′dōr) treatment of aneurysm by ligation of the artery immediately below (on the distal side of) the tumor.

**brass found·er's fe·ver** an occupational disease, characterized by malaria-like symptoms, due to inhalation of particles and fumes of metallic oxides.

**Braun a·nas·to·mo·sis** (brown) after a loop gastroenterostomy, anastomosis between afferent and efferent loops of jejunum.

**brawny** (brahw′nē) thickened (lichenified) and dusky (a darkened hue), as of a swelling. [M.E. fleshy]

**brawn·y e·de·ma** SYN nonpitting edema.

**Brax·ton Hicks sign** (braks′tŏn-hix) irregular uterine contractions occurring after the third month of pregnancy.

**Bra·zel·ton Ne·o·na·tal Be·hav·i·or·al As·sess·ment Scale** a scale used by obstetricians, pediatricians, and pediatric psychologists to assess the sensory, motor, emotional and physical development of the neonate, usually beginning at birth or in the first month of life.

**BRCA1 gene** a tumor suppressor gene on chromosome 17 at locus 17q21, isolated in 1994; encodes p53 protein, which prevents cells with damaged DNA from dividing; carriers of germline mutations in BRCA1 are predisposed to develop both breast and ovarian cancer. SEE ALSO BRCA2 gene, carcinoma of the breast.

**BRCA2 gene** a tumor suppressor gene identified in 1995 on chromosome 13 at locus 13q12–q13; a large gene consisting of 27 exons distributed over 70kb, encoding a protein of 3418 amino acids; carriers of germline mutations in BRCA2 have an increased risk, similar to that of those with BRCA1 mutations, of developing breast cancer and a moderately increased risk of ovarian cancer; BRCA2 families also exhibit an increased incidence of male breast, pancreatic, prostate, laryngeal, and ocular cancers. SEE ALSO BRCA1 gene, carcinoma of the breast.

**break-even point** the point in sales volume at which total revenues equal total costs. Sales volume below the break-even point will cause a negative cash flow (loss); sales volume above the break-even point will result in a profit. This point is calculated to help determine whether a new test or procedure should be offered by a health care provider based on projected sales volume.

**break·point** (brāk′poynt) in helminth epidemiology, the critical mean wormload in a community, below which the helminth mating frequency is too low to maintain reproduction. Below this level, helminth infection in the community will progressively decline, ultimately to zero.

**breast** (brest) **1.** the pectoral surface of the thorax. **2.** the organ of milk secretion; one of two hemispheric projections situated in the subcutaneous layer over the pectoralis major muscle on either side of the chest of the mature female; it is rudimentary in the male. SYN mamma [TA], teat (2). [A.S. *breōst*]

**breast bone** SYN sternum.

**breast pump** a suction instrument for withdrawing milk from the breast.

**breath** (breth) **1.** the respired air. **2.** an inspiration. **3.** a single cycle of inhalation followed by exhalation. [A.S. *braeth*]

**breath-hold·ing test** a rough index of cardiopulmonary reserve measured by the length of time that a subject can voluntarily stop breathing; normal duration is 30 seconds or more; diminished cardiac or pulmonary reserve is indicated by a duration of 20 seconds or less.

**breath·ing** (brēdh′ing) inhalation and exhalation of air or gaseous mixtures. [A.S. *braeth*]

**breath·ing bag** a collapsible reservoir from which gases are inhaled and into which gases may be exhaled during general anesthesia or artificial ventilation. SYN reservoir bag.

**breath·ing re·serve** the difference between the pulmonary ventilation (i.e., the volume of air breathed under ordinary resting conditions) and the maximum breathing capacity.

**breath sounds** a murmur, bruit, fremitus, rhonchus, or rale heard on auscultation over the lungs or any part of the respiratory tract. SYN respiratory sounds.

**breath test** any diagnostic test in which endogenous or exogenous materials are measured in samples of breath as a means of identifying pathologic processes; examples include hydrogen breath testing for lactose intolerance or urea breath testing to detect gastric colonization with *Helicobacter pylori.*

**Bre·da dis·ease** (brā-dah) SYN espundia.

**breech** (brēch) SYN buttocks. [A.S. *brēc*]

**breech pre·sen·ta·tion** presentation of any part of the pelvic extremity of the fetus, the nates, knees, or feet; more properly only of the nates; frank breech presentation occurs when the fetus presents by the pelvic extremity; the thighs may be flexed and the legs extended over the anterior surfaces of the body; in **full breech presentation**, the thighs may be flexed on the abdomen and the legs upon the thighs, in **footling presentation**, **foot presentation** the feet may be the lowest part; in **incomplete foot presentation**, **incomplete knee presentation**, one leg may retain the position which is typical of one of the above-mentioned presentations, while the other foot or knee may present.

**breg·ma** (breg′mă) the point on the skull corresponding to the junction of the coronal and sagittal sutures. [G. the forepart of the head]

**breg·mat·ic** (breg-mat′ik) relating to the bregma.

**Brems·strah·lung ra·di·a·tion** (brĕmz′strah-lŭng rā-dē-ā′shŭn) when a high-speed electron from the cathode stream is slowed down and pulled off course by the positive pull of the target, this represents a loss of energy which is given up as heat and an x-ray photon. Most x-rays in medicine and dentistry are of Bremsstrahlung origin. SYN braking radiation. [Ger. *Bremse,* brake, + *Strahlung,* radiation]

**Bren·ner tu·mor** (bre′ner) a benign neoplasm of the ovary, consisting chiefly of fibrous tissue that contains nests of cells resembling transitional type epithelium, as well as glandlike structures that contain mucin; origin is controversial, but it may arise from Walthard cell rest; ordinarily found incidentally in ovaries removed for other reasons, especially in postmenopausal women.

**Bres·low thick·ness** (brez′lō) maximal thickness of a primary cutaneous melanoma measured in tissue sections from the top of the epidermal granular layer, or from the ulcer base (if the tumor is ulcerated), to the bottom of the tumor; metastatic rates correlate closely with tumor thickness.

**Breus mole** (brois) an aborted ovum in which the fetal surface of the placenta presents numerous hematomata with an absence of blood vessels in the chorion and an ovum much smaller in size than normal in relation to the duration of the pregnancy.

**bre·ve·tox·in** (brev′e-tok′sin) structurally unique neurotoxins produced by the "red tide" dinoflagellate *Ptychodiscus brevis Davis* (*Gymnodinium breve Davis*) a species of algae responsible for large fish kills and mollusk and human food poisoning in the Gulf of Mexico and along the Florida coast. Unlike previously isolated dinoflagellate toxins, such as saxitoxin, which are water-soluble sodium channel blockers, the brevotoxins are lipid-soluble sodium channel activators. Used as tools in neurobiologic research.

***Brev·i·bac·ter·ium*** (brev-ĕ-bak-tēr′ē-ŭm) a bacterial genus of nonmotile, nonsporeforming, Gram-positive rods found as normal human skin flora and in raw milk and on the surface of cheeses; some species, recovered from patients with septicemia and from the peritoneum of patients undergoing peritoneal dialysis, appear to be opportunistic human pathogens.

**brev·i·col·lis** (brev-ē-kol′is) abnormal shortness of the neck. [L. *brevis,* short, + *collum,* neck]

**bre·vis** (brev′is) brief, short. [L. short]

**Brew·er infarct** (broo′ĕr) a dark-red, wedge-shaped area resembling an infarct, seen on section of a kidney in pyelonephritis.

**Brick·er op·er·a·tion** (brik′ĕr) an operation utilizing an isolated segment of ileum to collect urine from the ureters and conduct it to the skin surface.

**bridge** (brij) **1.** the upper part of the ridge of the nose formed by the nasal bones. **2.** one of the threads of protoplasm that appear to pass from one cell to another. **3.** SYN fixed partial denture.

**bridge·work** (brij′werk) SYN partial denture.

**bri·dle su·ture** a suture passed through the superior rectus muscle to rotate the globe downward in eye surgery.

**Brigg test** a test using the reduction of molybdate to follow the excretion of homogentisic acid.

**Brill dis·ease** (bril) SYN Brill-Zinsser disease.

**Brill-Zins·ser dis·ease** (bril-zin′sĕr) an endogenous reinfection in persons who previously had epidemic typhus fever; it is mild and may be mistaken for endemic (murine) typhus. SYN Brill disease, recrudescent typhus.

**brim** the upper edge or rim of a hollow structure.

**Bri·quet a·tax·ia** (brē-kā′) weakening of the muscle sense and increased sensibility of the skin, in hysteria.

**Bri·quet dis·ease** hysterical neurosis, conversion type.

**Bri·quet syn·drome** (brē-kā′) a chronic but fluctuating mental disorder, usually of young women, characterized by frequent complaints of physical illness involving multiple organ systems simultaneously.

**brise·ment forcé** (briz-mon′fōr-sā′) procedure infrequently used to treat frozen shoulder in which a forceful manipulation is performed to restore range of motion that usually results in torn adhesions and adjacent joint capsule. [Fr. forcible breaking]

**Bris·saud dis·ease** (brē-sō′) SYN tic.

**Bris·saud re·flex** tickling the sole causes a contraction of the tensor fasciae latae muscle, even when there is no responsive movement of the toes.

**Brit·ish ther·mal u·nit (BTU)** the quantity of heat required to raise one pound of water from 3.9°C to 4.4°C; equal to 251.996 calories or to 1055.056 joules.

**brit·tle bones** SYN osteogenesis imperfecta.

**brit·tle di·a·be·tes** diabetes mellitus in which there are marked fluctuations in blood glucose concentrations that are difficult to control.

**broach** (brōch) a dental instrument for removing the pulp of a tooth or exploring the canal.

**Broad·bent law** (brod′bent) lesions of the upper segment of the motor tract cause less marked paralysis of muscles that habitually produce bilateral movements than of those that commonly act independently of the opposite side.

**Broad·bent sign** (brod′bent) a retraction of the thoracic wall, synchronous with cardiac systole, visible anywhere, but particularly in the left posterior axillary line; a sign of adherent pericardium.

**broad lig·a·ment of the uter·us** the peritoneal fold passing from the lateral margin of the uterus to the wall of the pelvis on either side and ensheathing the ovaries and uterine tubes. SYN ligamentum latum uteri [TA].

**broad spec·trum** a term indicating activity of an antibiotic against a wide variety of microorganisms.

**broad-spec·trum an·ti·bi·ot·ic** an antibiotic having a wide range of activity against both Gram-positive and Gram-negative organisms.

**Bro·ca a·pha·sia** (brō′kah) SYN motor aphasia.

**Bro·ca cen·ter** (brō′kah) the posterior part of the inferior frontal gyrus of the left or dominant hemisphere, corresponding approximately to Brodmann area 44; Broca identified this region as an essential component of the motor mechanisms governing articulated speech. SYN motor speech center.

**Bro·ca vi·su·al plane** (brō′kah) a plane drawn through the visual axes of each eye.

**Bro·die ab·scess** (brō′dē) a chronic abscess of bone surrounded by dense fibrous tissue and sclerotic bone.

**Bro·die dis·ease** (brō′dē) **1.** SYN Brodie knee. **2.** hysterical spinal neuralgia, simulating Pott disease, following a trauma.

**Bro·die knee** (brō′dē) chronic hypertrophic synovitis of the knee. SYN Brodie disease (1).

⚠**brom-, bromo-** prefixes that indicate bromine or a foul odor. [G. *brōmos,* a stench]

**bro·mate** (brō′māt) salt or anion of bromic acid.

**bro·mat·ed** (brō′māt-ĕd) combined or saturated with bromine or any of its compounds. SYN brominated.

**bro·mide** (brō′mīd) the anion Br⁻; salt of hydrogen bromide (HBr); several salts formerly used as sedatives, hypnotics, and anticonvulsants.

**bro·mi·dro·sis, brom·hi·dro·sis** (brom-ĭ-drō′sis) fetid or foul-smelling perspiration. SYN osmidrosis. [G. *brōmos,* a stench, + *hidrōs,* perspiration]

**bro·min·at·ed** (brō′min-āt-ĕd) SYN bromated.

**bro·mine (Br)** (brō′mēn, brō-min) a nonmetallic, reddish, volatile, liquid element; atomic no. 35, atomic wt. 79.904; valences 1 to 7, inclusive; it unites with hydrogen to form hydrobromic acid, and this reacts with many metals to form bromides, some of which are used in medicine. [Fr. *brome,* bromine, fr. G. *bromos,* stench]

**bro·mism, bro·min·ism** (brō′mizm, brō′min-izm) chronic bromide intoxication, characterized by headache, drowsiness, confusion and occasionally violent delirium, muscular weakness, cardiac depression, an acneform eruption, foul breath, anorexia, and gastric distress.

**bro·mo·der·ma** (brō-mō-der′mă) an acneform or granulomatous eruption due to hypersensitivity to bromide. [bromide + G. *derma,* skin]

**bro·mo·sul·fo·phthal·e·in** SYN sulfobromophthalein sodium.

**brom·phe·nol test** a colorimetric test for measurement of protein, albumin, and globulin in the urine by use of reagent strips.

**Bromp·ton cock·tail** (bromp′tŏn) a cocktail of morphine and cocaine usually used for analgesia in terminal cancer patients; the formulations vary, but typically it contains 15 mg of morphine hydrochoride and 10 mg of cocaine hydrochloride per 10 ml of the cocktail. [*Brompton* Chest Hospital, London, England, where developed]

**brom·sul·fo·phthal·e·in** SYN sulfobromophthalein sodium.

**bron·chi** (brong′kī) plural of bronchus.

**bron·chia** (brong′kē-ă) the smaller divisions of the bronchi. SEE ALSO bronchus, bronchiole. [G. pl. of *bronchion,* dim. of *bronchos,* trachea]

**bron·chi·al** (brong′kē-ăl) relating to the bronchi.

**bron·chi·al ad·e·no·ma** a benign or malignant polypoid epithelial tumor of bronchial mucosa, arising deep to the surface epithelium, possibly from mucous glands or their ducts.

**bron·chi·al ar·te·ri·og·ra·phy** radiography of bronchial arteries by selective injection of the intercostal arteries from which they arise.

**bron·chi·al asth·ma** a condition of the lungs in which there is widespread narrowing of airways, varying over short periods of time either spontaneously or as a result of treatment, due in varying degrees to contraction (spasm) of smooth muscle, edema of the mucosa, chronic or recurrent local inflammation of the submucosa with eventual fibrosis, and excessive mucus in the lumen of the bronchi and bronchioles; these changes are caused by the local release of spasmogens and vasoactive substances (e.g., histamine, or certain leukotrienes or prostaglandins) in the course of an allergic process.

**bron·chi·al branch·es of tho·rac·ic aor·ta** the bronchial branches or arteries, vessels, or nerves distributed to the bronchi; the following have branches so named: 1) thoracic aorta; 2) internal thoracic artery; 3) vagus nerves.

**bron·chi·al glands 1.** SYN bronchopulmonary lymph nodes. **2.** mucous and seromucous glands whose secretory units lie outside the muscle of the bronchi.

**bron·chi·al hy·giene** those activities contributing to the removal of bronchial secretions and the maintenance of clear airways.

**bron·chi·al mu·cous gland ad·e·no·ma** a rare benign tumor arising from the mucous glands of bronchial mucosa.

**bron·chi·al pneu·mo·nia** SYN bronchopneumonia.

**bron·chi·al prov·o·ca·tion** a procedure for identifying and characterizing hyperresponsive airways by having the subject inhale an agent known to cause (or suspected of causing) a decrease in pulmonary function.

**bron·chi·al ste·no·sis** narrowing of the lumen of a bronchial tube.

**bron·chi·al veins** many veins running in front of and behind the bronchi and uniting into two main trunks which empty on the right side into the azygos vein, on the left into the accessory hemiazygos or the left superior intercostal vein.

**bron·chic cells** SYN pulmonary alveolus.

**bron·chi·ec·ta·sis** (brong-kē-ek′tă-sis) chronic dilation of bronchi or bronchioles as a sequel of inflammatory disease or obstruction. [bronchi- + G. *ektasis,* a stretching]

**bron·chi·ec·tat·ic** (brong-kē-ek-tat′ik) relating to bronchiectasis.

**bron·chi in·tra·seg·men·ta·les** SYN intrasegmental bronchi.

**bron·chil·o·quy** (brong-kil′ō-kwē) rarely used term for bronchophony [bronchi- + L. *loquor,* to speak]

**bron·chi·o·gen·ic** (brong-kē-ō-jen′ik) SYN bronchogenic.

**bron·chi·o·lar aden·o·car·cin·o·ma** SYN alveolar cell carcinoma.

**bron·chi·o·lar car·ci·no·ma** a carcinoma, thought to be derived from epithelium of terminal bronchioles, in which the neoplastic tissue extends along the alveolar walls and grows in small masses within the alveoli; may be diffuse, nodular, or lobular; the neoplastic cells are cuboidal or columnar and form papillary structures; metastases are infrequent. SYN alveolar cell carcinoma, bronchiolo-alveolar carcinoma.

**bron·chi·ole** (brong'kē-ōl) one of approximately six generations of increasingly finer subdivisions of the bronchi, each less than 1 mm in diameter, and having no cartilage in its wall, but relatively abundant smooth muscle and elastic fibers. SYN bronchiolus [TA].

**bron·chi·o·lec·ta·sis** (brong'kē-ō-lek'tă-sis) bronchiectasis involving the bronchioles. [bronchiole + G. *ektasis*, a stretching]

**bron·chi·o·li** (brong-kē'ō-lī) plural of bronchiolus.

**bron·chi·ol·i·tis** (brong-kē-ō-lī'tis) inflammation of the bronchioles, often associated with bronchopneumonia. [bronchiole + -*itis*, inflammation]

**bron·chi·ol·i·tis fi·bro·sa ob·li·te·rans, bron·chi·ol·i·tis ob·lit·e·rans** obstruction of bronchioles and alveolar ducts by fibrous granulation tissue induced by mucosal ulceration; the condition may follow inhalation of irritant gases (see silo-filler's lung) or may complicate pneumonia (see BOOP); associated with obstructive findings (see unilateral hyperlucent lung, Swyer-James syndrome).

**bron·chi·ol·i·tis ob·li·te·rans with or·ga·niz·ing pneu·mo·ni·a (BOOP)** bronchiolitis fibrosa obliterans complicated by pneumonia with organization.

⚠**bron·chi·o·lo-** bronchiole. [L. *bronchiolus*]

**bron·chi·o·lo-al·ve·o·lar car·ci·no·ma** SYN bronchiolar carcinoma.

**bron·chi·o·lus,** pl. **bron·chi·o·li** (brong-kē'ō-lŭs, brong-kē'ō-lī) [TA] SYN bronchiole. [Mod. L. dim. of *bronchus*]

**bron·chi·o·ste·no·sis** (brong'kē-ō-sten-ō'sis) narrowing of the lumen of a bronchial tube.

**bron·chit·ic** (brong-kit'ik) relating to bronchitis.

**bron·chi·tis** (brong-kī'tis) inflammation of the mucous membrane of the bronchial tubes.

⚠**bron·cho-, bronch-, bron·chi-** bronchus. [G. *bronchos*, windpipe]

**bron·cho·al·ve·o·lar** (brong'kō-al-vē'ō-lăr) SYN bronchovesicular.

**bron·cho·al·ve·o·lar car·ci·no·ma** SYN alveolar cell carcinoma.

**bron·cho·al·ve·o·lar flu·id** a fluid containing several lytic enzymes that serves to remove inspired particulates from the pulmonary airways.

**bron·cho·al·ve·o·lar la·vage** a procedure performed via fiberoptic bronchoscopy, during which a distal airway is occluded and liquid is then introduced into the airway and recovered for examination of cell types and microorganisms.

**bron·cho·cav·ern·ous** (brong-kō-kav'er-nŭs) relating to a bronchus or bronchial tube and a pathologic pulmonary cavity.

**bron·cho·cele** (brong'kō-sēl) a circumscribed dilation of a bronchus. [broncho- + G. *kēlē*, hernia]

**bron·cho·cen·tric gran·u·lo·ma·to·sis** a severe form of allergic bronchopulmonary aspergillosis.

**bron·cho·con·stric·tor** (brong-kō-kon-strik'ter)

1. causing a reduction in caliber of a bronchus or bronchial tube. 2. an agent that possesses this action (e.g., histamine).

**bron·cho·di·la·tion** (brong'kō-dil-ă-shŭn) increase in caliber of the bronchi and bronchioles in response to pharmacologically active substances or autonomic nervous activity.

**bron·cho·di·la·tor** (brong-kō-dī'lă-ter) 1. causing an increase in caliber of a bronchus. 2. an agent that possesses this power (e.g., epinephrine).

**bron·cho·e·soph·a·gol·o·gy** (brong'kō-ē-sof-ă-gol'ō-jē) the specialty concerned with the diagnosis and treatment of diseases of the tracheobronchial tree and esophagus by endoscope and other means. [broncho- + G. *oisophagos*, esophagus, + *logos*, study]

**bron·cho·e·soph·a·gos·co·py** (brong'kō-ē-sof-ă-gos'kŏ-pē) examination of the tracheobronchial tree and esophagus with appropriate endoscopes.

**bron·cho·fi·ber·scope** (brong-kō-fī'ber-skōp) a fiberoptic endoscope adapted for visualization of the trachea and bronchi.

**bron·cho·gen·ic** (brong-kō-jen'ik) of bronchial origin; emanating from the bronchi. SYN bronchiogenic.

🔲**bron·cho·gen·ic car·ci·no·ma** squamous cell or oat cell carcinoma that arises in the mucosa of the large bronchi; local growth causes bronchial obstruction and is observed radiologically as an enlarging lung mass; malignant tumor cells can be detected in the sputum, and they metastasize early to the thoracic lymph nodes and to the brain, adrenal glands, and other organs via the bloodstream. See this page.

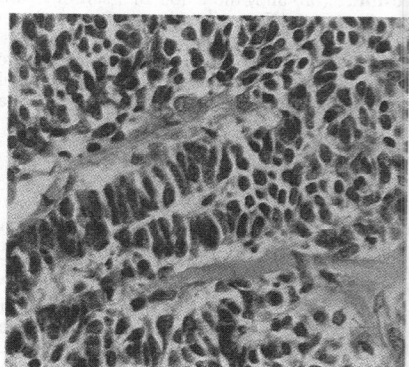

**bronchogenic carcinoma:** small cell

**bron·cho·gen·ic cyst** a cyst lined by ciliated columnar epithelium believed to represent bronchial differentiation; smooth muscle and mucous glands may be present.

**bron·cho·gram** (brong'kō-gram) a radiograph obtained by bronchography; radiographic visualization of a bronchus. [broncho- + G. *gramma*, a writing]

**bron·cho·lith** (brong'kō-lith) a hard concretion in a bronchus or bronchial tube. [broncho- + G. *lithos*, stone]

**bron·cho·li·thi·a·sis** (brong'kō-li-thī'ă-sis) bronchial inflammation or obstruction caused by broncholiths.

**bron·cho·ma·la·cia** (brong'kō-mă-lā'shē-ă) degeneration of elastic and connective tissue of bronchi and trachea. [broncho- + G. *malakia,* a softening]

**bron·cho·my·co·sis** (brong'kō-mī-kō'sis) any fungus disease of the bronchial tubes or bronchi. [broncho- + G. *mykēs,* fungus]

**bron·choph·o·ny** (brong-kof'ō-nē) increased intensity and clarity of voice sounds heard over a bronchus surrounded by consolidated lung tissue. SEE ALSO tracheophony. [broncho- + G. *phōnē,* voice]

**bron·cho·plas·ty** (brong'kō-plas-tē) surgical alteration of the configuration of a bronchus. [broncho- + G. *plastos,* formed]

**bron·cho·pleu·ral fis·tu·la (BPF)** communication between a bronchus and the pleural cavity; usually caused by necrotizing pneumonia or empyema; also may follow pulmonary surgery or irradiation. SYN BP fistula.

**bron·cho·pneu·mo·nia** (brong'ko-noo-mō'nē-ă) acute inflammation of the walls of the smaller bronchial tubes, with varying amounts of pulmonary consolidation due to spread of the inflammation into peribronchiolar alveoli and the alveolar ducts; may become confluent or may be hemorrhagic. SYN bronchial pneumonia.

**bron·cho·pul·mo·nary** (brong-kō-pul'mō-nār-ē) relating to the bronchi and the lungs.

**bron·cho·pul·mo·nary dys·pla·sia** chronic pulmonary insufficiency arising from long-term artificial pulmonary ventilation; seen more frequently in premature infants than in mature infants.

**bron·cho·pul·mo·nary lymph nodes** lymph nodes in the hilum of the lung that receive lymph from the pulmonary nodes, and drain to the tracheobronchial nodes. SYN bronchial glands (1).

**bron·cho·pul·mo·nary seg·ment** the largest subdivision of a lobe of the lung; it is supplied by a direct tertiary (lobular) bronchus and a tertiary branch of the pulmonary artery; it is separated from adjacent segments by connective tissue septa.

**bron·cho·pul·mo·nary se·ques·tra·tion** a congenital anomaly in which a mass of lung tissue becomes isolated, during development, from the rest of the lung; the bronchi in the mass are usually dilated or cystic and are not connected with the bronchial tree; it is supplied by a branch of the aorta.

**bron·chor·rha·phy** (brong-kōr'ă-fē) suture of a wound of the bronchus. [broncho- + G. *rhaphē,* a seam]

**bron·chor·rhea** (brong'kō-rē'ă) excessive secretion of mucus from the bronchial mucous membrane. [broncho- + G. *rhoia,* a flow]

**bron·chor·rhoea [Br.]** SEE bronchorrhea.

**bron·cho·scope** (brong'kō-skōp) an endoscope for inspecting the interior of the tracheobronchial tree. [broncho- + G. *skopeō,* to view]

**bron·chos·co·py** (brong-kos'kŏ-pē) inspection of the interior of the tracheobronchial tree through a bronchoscope. See this page and B8.

**bron·cho·spasm** (brong'kō-spazm) contraction of smooth muscle in the walls of the bronchi and bronchioles, causing narrowing of the lumen.

**bron·cho·spi·rog·ra·phy** (brong'kō-spī-rog'ră-fē) use of a single-lumen endobronchial tube for measurement of ventilatory function of one lung.

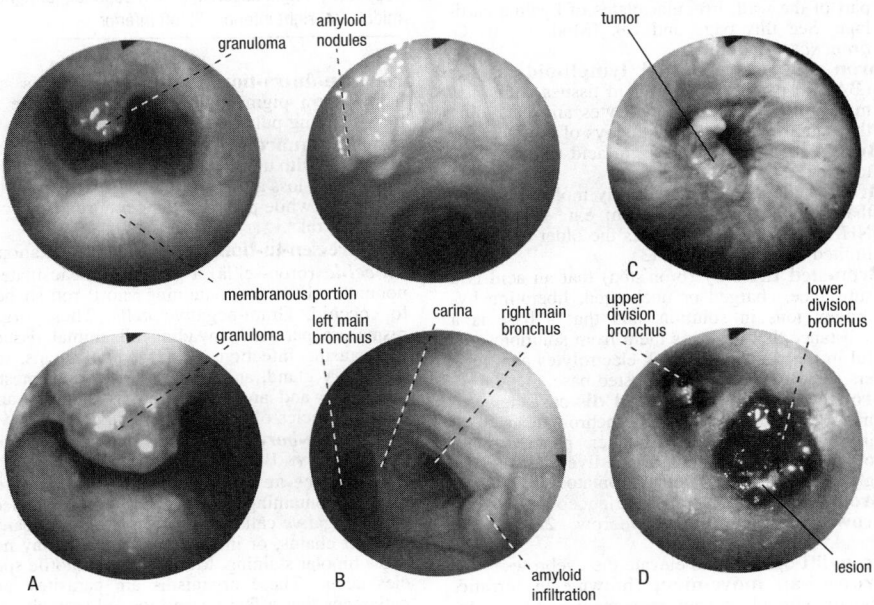

**bronchoscopic views:** (A) tuberculosis of the trachea in a 62-year-old female, (B) amyloidosis of trachea and bronchi in a 68-year-old male, (C) small-cell carcinoma in a 79-year-old male, (D) metastasis of melanoma in a 65-year-old female

[broncho- + L. *spiro,* to breathe, + G. *graphō,* to write]

**bron·cho·spi·rom·e·ter** (brong′kō-spī-rom′ĕ-ter) a device for measurement of rates and volumes of airflow into each lung separately, using a double-lumen endobronchial tube. [broncho- + L. *spiro,* to breathe, + G. *metron,* measure]

**bron·cho·spi·rom·e·try** (brong′kō-spī-rom′ĕ-trē) use of a bronchospirometer to measure ventilatory function of each lung separately.

**bron·cho·stax·is** (brong′kō-stak′sis) hemorrhage from the bronchi. [broncho- + G. *staxis,* a dripping]

**bron·cho·ste·no·sis** (brong-kō-sten-ō′sis) chronic narrowing of a bronchus.

**bron·chos·to·my** (brong-kos′tō-mē) surgical formation of a new opening into a bronchus. [broncho- + G. *stoma,* mouth]

**bron·chot·o·my** (brong-kot′ō-mē) incision of a bronchus.

**bron·cho·tra·che·al** (brong-kō-trā′kē-ăl) relating to the trachea and bronchi.

**bron·cho·ve·sic·u·lar** (brong′kō-vĕ-sik′yu-lăr) relating to the bronchioles and alveoli in the lungs. SYN bronchoalveolar.

**bron·chus,** pl. **bron·chi** (brong′kŭs, brong′kī) one of the two subdivisions of the trachea serving to convey air to and from the lungs. The trachea divides into right and left main bronchi, which in turn form lobar, segmental, and subsegmental bronchi. The intrapulmonary bronchi have a lining of pseudostratified ciliated columnar epithelium and a lamina propria with abundant longitudinal networks of elastic fibers; there are spirally arranged bundles of smooth muscle, abundant mucoserous glands, and, in the outer part of the wall, irregular plates of hyaline cartilage. See this page and B8. [Mod. L., fr. G. *bronchos,* windpipe]

**bron·chus-as·so·ci·at·ed lymph·oid tis·sue (BALT)** patches of lymphoid tissues composed mainly of B and T lymphocytes and extending throughout the bronchial airways of the lung.

**Brøn·sted ac·id** (brø′stĕd) an acid that is a proton donor.

**Brøn·sted base** (brøn′stĕd) any molecule or ion that combines with a proton; e.g., OH⁻, CN⁻, NH₃; this definition replaces the older and more limited concepts of base (3).

**Brøn·sted the·o·ry** (brøn′stĕd) that an acid is a substance, charged or uncharged, liberating hydrogen ions in solution, and that a base is a substance that removes them from solution; useful in the concept of weak electrolytes and buffers. Cf. Brønsted acid, Brønsted base.

**bronze di·a·be·tes, bronzed dis·ease** diabetes mellitus associated with hemochromatosis, with iron deposits in the skin, liver, pancreas, and other viscera, often with severe liver damage and glycosuria. SEE ALSO hemochromatosis.

**Brooke tu·mor** (brook) SYN trichoepithelioma.

**brow 1.** the eyebrow. SEE eyebrow. **2.** SYN forehead. [A.S. *brū*]

**brow·lift** operation to elevate the eyebrows.

**brown·i·an move·ment** (brown′ē-ăn) erratic, nondirectional, zigzag movement observed by microscope in suspensions of particles in fluid, resulting from the jostling or bumping of the larger particles by the molecules in the suspending medium. SYN molecular movement, pedesis.

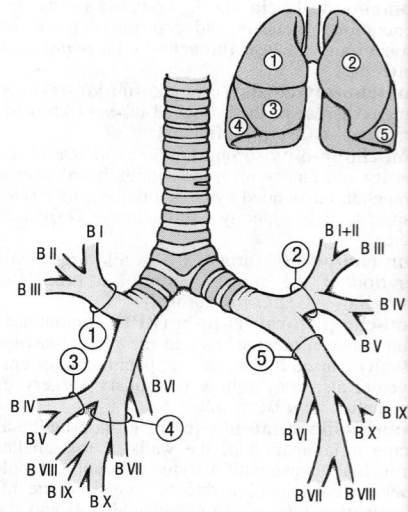

**segmental bronchi:** right lung: (B I) apical, (B II) posterior, (B III) anterior, (B IV) lateral, (B V) medial, (B VI) apical, (B VII) medial basal, (B VIII) anterior basal, (B IX) lateral basal, (B X) posterior basal; left lung: (B I+II) apicoposterior, (B III) anterior, (B IV) superior lingular, (B V) inferior lingular, (B VI) apical, (B VII) medial basal, (B VIII) anterior basal, (B IX) lateral basal, (B X) posterior basal; lobes of lungs supplied: (1) right superior, (2) left superior, (3) right middle, (4) right inferior, (5) left inferior

**brown in·du·ra·tion of the lung** fibrosis and hemosiderin pigmentation of the lungs due to long-standing pulmonary congestion.

**Brown-Sé·quard syn·drome** (broon-sā-kahr′) syndrome with unilateral spinal cord lesions, proprioception loss and weakness occur ipsilateral to the lesion, while pain and temperature loss occur contralateral.

**brow pre·sen·ta·tion** SEE cephalic presentation.

*Bru·cel·la* (broo-sel′lă) a genus of encapsulated, nonmotile bacteria containing short, rod-shaped to coccoid, Gram-negative cells. These organisms are parasitic, invading all animal tissues and causing infection of the genital organs, the mammary gland, and the respiratory and intestinal tracts, and are pathogenic for humans and various species of domestic animals.

*Bru·cel·la a·bor·tus* a species that causes undulant fever. SYN Bang bacillus.

*Bru·cel·la·ce·ae* (broo-sel-ā′sē-ē) a family of bacteria containing small, coccoid to rod-shaped, Gram-negative cells which occur singly, in pairs, in short chains, or in groups. The cells may not show bipolar staining. Motile and nonmotile species occur. These organisms are parasites and pathogens that affect warm-blooded animals, including humans. The type genus is *Brucella.*

*Bru·cel·la mel·i·ten·sis* a species that causes brucellosis in humans; it is the type species of the genus *Brucella.*

*Bru·cel·la su·is* a species causing brucellosis in

humans; may also infect horses, dogs, cows, monkeys, goats, and laboratory animals.

**bru·cel·lo·sis** (broo-sel-ō′sis) an infectious disease caused by *Brucella*, characterized by fever, sweating, weakness, and aching, and transmitted to humans by direct contact with diseased animals or through ingestion of infected meat or milk. SYN undulant fever.

**Bruce pro·to·col** (broos) a standardized protocol for electrocardiogram-monitored exercise using increasing speeds and elevations of the treadmill; a test for ischemia usually due to coronary artery disease. SEE ALSO stress test.

**Bruch mem·brane** SYN lamina basalis choroideae.

**Bruck dis·ease** (brook) a disease marked by osteogenesis imperfecta, ankylosis of the joints, and muscular atrophy.

**Brud·zin·ski sign** (broo-jin′skē) **1.** in meningitis, on passive flexion of the leg on one side, a similar movement occurs in the opposite leg. **2.** in meningitis, involuntary flexion of the knees and hips following flexion of the neck while supine.

**Brug fil·a·ri·a·sis** infection with filarial organism *Brugia malayi*, which causes adenitis, fever, lymphangitis, and sometimes elephantiasis; occurs primarily in southeast Asia, India, Indonesia, China, Japan, Korea, and the Philippines.

**bruise** (brooz) an injury producing a hematoma or diffuse extravasation of blood without rupture of the skin. [M.E. *bruisen*, fr. O.Fr., fr. Germanic]

**bru·it** (broo-ē′) a harsh or musical intermittent auscultatory sound, especially an abnormal one. [Fr.]

**bru·it de tam·bour** (broo-ē′ dĕ tăm-boor′) reverberating, musical tone heard as the second heart sound over the aortic area, associated with syphilitic aortic valvular disease. [Fr. sound of drum]

**Brun·ner glands** (broon′ĕr) SYN duodenal glands.

**Brunn mem·brane** (broon) the epithelium of the olfactory region of the nose.

**Bruns nys·tag·mus** (broonz) a fine, jerking (vestibular) nystagmus on horizontal gaze in one direction, together with a slower, larger amplitude (gaze, paretic) nystagmus on looking in the opposite direction; due to lateral brainstem compression, usually by a cerebellar-pontine angle mass such as an acoustic neuroma.

**brush** (brŭsh) an instrument consisting of flexible bristles attached to a handle or to the tip of a catheter. [A.S. *byrst,* bristle]

**brush bi·op·sy** obtained by abrading the surface of a lesion with a brush to obtain cells and tissue for microscopic examination.

**brush bor·der** an epithelial surface bearing closely packed microvilli about 2 μm long, such as occurs in the proximal tubule of the nephron.

**brush cath·e·ter** a ureteral catheter with a finely bristled brush tip that is endoscopically passed into the ureter or renal pelvis and by gentle to-and-fro movement brushes cells from the surface of suspected tumors.

**Brush·field spots** (brush′fēld) light-colored condensations of the surface of the mid-iris; seen in Down syndrome.

**Bru·ton a·gam·ma·glob·u·li·ne·mia** (broo′tŏn) an X-linked condition, with hypo- or agammaglobulinemia; the immune deficiency becomes apparent as maternally transmitted immunoglobulin levels decline in early infancy.

**brux·ism** (brŭk′sizm) a clenching of the teeth, associated with forceful lateral or protrusive jaw movements, resulting in rubbing, gritting, or grinding together of the teeth, usually during sleep; sometimes a pathologic condition. SEE ALSO parafunction. [G. *bruchō,* to grind the teeth]

**Bry·ant trac·tion** (brī′ănt) traction upon the lower limb placed vertically, employed especially in fractures of the femur in children.

**Bry·ant tri·an·gle** (brī′ănt) in fracture of the neck of the femur, to determine upward displacement of the trochanter, lines are drawn on the body to form a triangle: line *a* is drawn around the body at the level of the anterior superior iliac spines; line *b*, perpendicular to line *a*, is drawn to the greater trochanter of the femur; line *c* is drawn from the trochanter to the iliac spine; upward displacement is measured along line *b*. SYN iliofemoral triangle.

**BSA** bovine serum albumin; body surface area.

**BSER** brainstem evoked response. SEE brainstem evoked response audiometry.

**BTPS** symbol indicating that a gas volume has been expressed as if it were *s*aturated with water vapor at *b*ody *t*emperature (37°C) and at the ambient barometric *p*ressure; used for measurements of lung volumes.

**BTU** British thermal unit.

**bu·ba mad·re** (boo′bă mah′dre) SYN mother yaw.

**bu·bas** (boo′bahs) SYN yaws.

**bub·ble gum der·ma·ti·tis** allergic contact dermatitis developing about the lips in children who chew bubble gum; caused by plastics in the gum.

**bubble-through hu·mid·i·fi·er** a device that humidifies therapeutic gas (e.g., oxygen) by bubbling the gas through water.

**bu·bo** (boo′bō) inflammatory swelling of one or more lymph nodes, usually in the groin. [G. *boubōn,* the groin, a swelling in the groin]

**bu·bon·al·gia** (boo′bon-al′jē-ă) rarely used term for pain in the groin. [G. *boubōn,* groin, + *algos,* pain]

**bu·bon·ic** (boo-bon′ik) relating in any way to a bubo.

**bu·bon·ic plague** the usual form of plague marked by inflammatory enlargement of the lymphatic glands in the groins, axillae, or other parts.

**buc·ca,** gen. and pl. **buc·cae** (bŭk′ă, bŭk′sē) SYN cheek. [L.]

**buc·cal** (bŭk′ăl) pertaining to, adjacent to, or in the direction of the cheek.

**buc·cal ar·tery, buc·ci·na·tor ar·ter·y** *origin,* maxillary; *distribution,* buccinator muscle, skin, and mucous membrane of cheek; *anastomoses,* buccal branch of facial. SYN arteria buccalis [TA].

**buc·cal glands** numerous racemose, mucous, or serous glands in the submucous tissue of the cheeks. SYN genal glands.

**buc·cal nerve** a sensory branch of the mandibular division of the trigeminal nerve; it passes downward emerging from beneath the ramus of the mandible to run forward on the buccinator muscle, piercing (but not supplying) it to innervate buccal mucous membrane and skin of the cheek near the angle of the mouth. SYN nervus buccalis [TA].

**buc·ci·na·tor mus·cle** *origin,* posterior portion of alveolar portion of maxilla and mandible and pterygomandibular raphe; *insertion,* orbicularis oris at angle of mouth; *action*, flattens cheek, retracts angle of mouth; *nerve supply*, facial. Plays an important role in mastication, working with tongue to keep food between teeth; when it is paralyzed, food accumulates in the oral vestibule. SYN musculus buccinator [TA].

**buc·co-** cheek. [L. *bucca*]

**buc·co·gin·gi·val** (bŭk-ō-jin′ji-văl) relating to the cheek and the gum.

**buc·co·la·bi·al** (bŭk-ō-lā′bē-ăl) **1.** relating to both cheek and lip. **2.** DENTISTRY referring to that aspect of the dental arch or those surfaces of the teeth in contact with the mucosa of lip and cheek.

**buc·co·lin·gual** (bŭk-ō-ling′wăl) **1.** pertaining to the cheek and the tongue. **2.** DENTISTRY referring to that aspect of the dental arch or those surfaces of the teeth in contact with the mucosa of the lip or cheek and the tongue.

**buc·co·pha·ryn·ge·al** (bŭk′ō-fă-rin′jē-ăl) relating to both cheek or mouth and pharynx.

**buc·co·ver·sion** (bŭk′ō-ver-zhŭn) malposition of a posterior tooth from the normal line of occlusion toward the cheek.

**Buch·wald at·ro·phy** (book′wahld) a progressive form of cutaneous atrophy.

**buck·et-han·dle tear 1.** a tear in the central part of a semilunar cartilage. **2.** a tear in one of the menisci of a knee joint, near the rim and following its curvature, which can allow a flap of cartilage to impede movement of the joint.

**Buck ex·ten·sion** (buk) apparatus for applying longitudinal skin traction on the leg through contact between the skin and adhesive tape.

**buck·led in·nom·i·nate ar·tery** elongation of the innominate artery manifest as a pulsating mass in the right supraclavicular space and as a radiographic appearance mimicking an aneurysm or tumor of the apex of the right lung or superior mediastinum.

**buck tooth** an anterior tooth in labioversion.

**Buck·y di·a·phragm** (buk′ē) in radiography, a diaphragm with a moving grid that avoids grid shadows. SYN Potter-Bucky diaphragm.

**bud** (bŭd) **1.** an outgrowth that resembles the bud of a plant, usually pluripotential, and capable of differentiating and growing into a definitive structure. **2.** to give rise to such an outgrowth. SEE ALSO gemmation. **3.** a small outgrowth from a parent cell; a form of asexual reproduction.

**bud·ding** (bŭd′ing) SYN gemmation.

**Budd syn·drome** (bud) SYN Chiari syndrome.

**Buer·ger dis·ease** (bĕr′gĕr) SYN thromboangiitis obliterans.

**buf·fa·lo neck** combination of moderate kyphosis with thick heavy fat pad on the neck, seen especially in persons with Cushing disease or syndrome.

**buff·er** (bŭf′er) **1.** a mixture of an acid and its conjugate base (salt), such as $H_2CO_3/HCO_3^-$; $H_2PO_4^-/HPO_4^{2-}$, which, when present in a solution, resists changes in pH that would otherwise occur in the solution when acid or alkali is added to it. SEE ALSO conjugate acid-base pair. **2.** to add a buffer to a solution and thus give it the property of resisting a change in pH.

**buff·er val·ue** the power of a substance in solution to absorb acid or alkali without change in pH; this is highest at a pH value equal to the $pK_a$ value of the acid of the buffer pair.

**buf·fy coat** the light-colored layer of blood that is seen when anticoagulated blood is centrifuged or

allowed to stand. It appears as a layer between the plasma and red cells and is composed of leukocytes and platelets.

**buf·fy coat con·cen·tra·tion** centrifugation of whole blood containing anticoagulant to obtain a buffy coat layer containing white blood cells; blood films for staining can be prepared from this layer of cells and examined for the presence of parasites (trypanosomes and intracellular leishmaniae).

**bulb** (bŭlb) **1.** any globular or fusiform structure. SYN bulbus [TA]. **2.** a short, vertical underground stem of plants, as of onion and garlic. [L. *bulbus*, a bulbous root]

**bul·bar** (bŭl′bar) **1.** relating to a bulb. **2.** relating to the rhombencephalon (hindbrain). **3.** bulbshaped; resembling a bulb.

**bul·bar my·e·li·tis** inflammation of the medulla oblongata.

**bul·bar pal·sy** flaccid paralysis of the motor units of any or all cranial nerves. Bulbar palsies may also be identifed by the specific nerve affected, such as facial palsy or hypoglossal palsy. SEE ALSO cranial nerves.

**bul·bar pa·ral·y·sis** SYN progressive bulbar paralysis.

**bulb of cor·pus spon·gi·o·sum** SYN bulb of penis.

**bulb of eye** SYN eyeball.

**bulb of hair** hair bulb, the lower expanded extremity of the hair follicle that fits like a cap over the papilla pili.

**bul·bi** (bŭl′bī) plural of bulbus.

**bul·bi·tis** (bŭl-bī′tis) inflammation of the bulbous portion of the urethra.

**bul·bo-** bulb; bulbus [L. *bulbus*]

**bul·boid** (bŭl′boyd) bulb-shaped. [bulbo- + G. *eidos*, resemblance]

**bul·bo·spi·nal** (bŭl-bō-spī′năl) relating to the medulla oblongata and spinal cord, particularly to nerve fibers interconnecting the two. SYN spinobulbar.

**bul·bo·u·re·thral** (bŭl′bō-yu-rē′thrăl) relating to the bulbus penis and the urethra. SYN urethrobulbar.

**bul·bo·u·re·thral gland** one of two small compound racemose glands, that produce a mucoid secretion, lying side by side along the membranous urethra just above the bulb of the corpus spongiosum; they discharge through a small duct into the spongy portion of the urethra. SYN Cowper gland.

**bul·bous bou·gie** a bougie with a bulb-shaped tip, some of which are shaped like an acorn or an olive.

**bulb of pe·nis** the expanded posterior part of the corpus spongiosum of the penis lying in the interval between the crura of the penis. SYN bulbus penis [TA], bulb of corpus spongiosum, bulb of urethra.

**bulb ther·mom·e·ter** standard thermometer used to record ambient air temperature.

**bulb of u·re·thra** SYN bulb of penis.

**bul·bus**, gen. and pl. **bul·bi** (bŭl′bŭs, bŭl′bī) [TA] SYN bulb (1). [L. a plant bulb]

**bul·bus a·or·tae** [TA] SYN aortic bulb.

**bul·bus oc·u·li** [TA] SYN eyeball.

**bul·bus ol·fac·to·ri·us** [TA] SYN olfactory bulb.

**bul·bus pe·nis** [TA] SYN bulb of penis.

**bulb of ves·ti·bule** a mass of erectile tissue on

either side of the vagina united anterior to the urethra by the commissura bulborum.

**bu·lim·ia** (boo-lim'ē-ă) SYN bulimia nervosa. [G. *bous,* ox, + *limos,* hunger]

**bu·lim·ia ner·vo·sa** a chronic morbid disorder involving repeated and secretive episodic bouts of eating characterized by uncontrolled rapid ingestion of large quantities of food over a short period of time (binge eating), followed by self-induced vomiting, use of laxatives or diuretics, fasting, or vigorous exercise in order to prevent weight gain; often accompanied by feelings of guilt, depression, or self-disgust. SYN bulimia.

**bu·lim·ic** (boo-lim'ik) relating to, or suffering from, bulimia nervosa.

🛈 **bul·la,** gen. and pl. **bul·lae** (bul'ă, bul-'ē) **1.** a large blister appearing as a circumscribed area of separation of the epidermis from subepidermal structures or as a circumscribed area of separation of epidermal cells caused by the presence of serum, or an injected substance. **2.** a bubblelike structure. See page B4. [L. bubble]

**bull·dog for·ceps** a forceps for occluding a blood vessel.

**bul·lec·to·my** (bul-ek'tō-mē) resection of a bulla; helpful in treating some forms of bullous emphysema, in which giant bullae compress functioning lung tissue.

**bul·let for·ceps** a forceps with thin curved blades with serrated grasping surfaces, for extracting a bullet from tissues.

**bull neck** a heavy thick neck caused by hypertrophied muscles or enlarged cervical lymph nodes.

**bul·lous** (bul'ŭs) relating to, of the nature of, or marked by, bullae.

**bul·lous con·gen·i·tal ich·thy·o·si·form eryth·ro·der·ma** (bul'ŭs kon-jen'i-tal ik-thē-ō'si-fōrm ĕr-ē-thrō-der-mă) diffusely red, eroded skin at birth, with subsequent scaling, tending to improve in later life, characterized by generalized epidermolytic hyperkeratosis.

**bul·lous em·phy·se·ma** emphysema in which the enlarged airspaces are one to several cm in diameter, often visible on chest radiographs. Thin-walled air sacs under tension compress pulmonary tissue, either single or multiple.

**bul·lous im·pe·ti·go of new·born** disseminated bullous lesions appearing soon after birth, caused by infection with *Staphylococcus aureus.* SYN impetigo neonatorum (2), pemphigus gangrenosus (2).

**bul·lous ker·a·top·a·thy** edema of the corneal stroma and epithelium; occurs in Fuchs epithelial dystrophy, advanced glaucoma and iridocyclitis, and sometimes after intraocular lens implantation.

**bul·lous pem·phi·goid** a chronic, generally benign disease, most commonly of old age, characterized by tense nonacantholytic bullae in which serum antibodies are localized to the epidermal basement membrane, causing detachment of the entire thickness of the epidermis.

**Bum·ke pu·pil** (boom'ke) dilation of the pupil in response to anxiety or other psychic stimuli.

**BUN** blood urea nitrogen.

**bun·dle** (bŭn'dl) a structure composed of a group of fibers, muscular or nervous; a fasciculus.

**bun·dle-branch block** intraventricular block due to interruption of conduction in one of the two main branches of the bundle of His and

manifested in the electrocardiogram by marked prolongation of the QRS complex.

**bun·ion** (bŭn'yŭn) a localized swelling at either the medial or dorsal aspect of the first metatarsophalangeal joint, caused by bursal inflammation and fibrosis; a medial bunion is usually associated with hallux valgus. [O.F. *buigne,* bump on the head]

**bun·ion·ec·to·my** (bŭn-yŭn-ek'tō-mē) excision of a bunion.

**Bun·nell su·ture** (bĕ-nel') a method of tenorrhaphy using a pull-out wire affixed to buttons.

**bunodont** (boo'nō-dont) a tooth having low, rounded cusps. [G. *bounos,* mound, + *odous* (*odont-* ), tooth]

**Bun·sen burn·er** (bun'sĕn) a gas lamp supplied with openings admitting sufficient air that carbon is completely burned, giving a hot but only slightly luminous flame. [R.W. Bunsen]

**Bunsen sol·u·bil·i·ty co·ef·fi·cient (al·pha)** (bun'sĕn) the milliliters of gas STPD dissolved per milliliter of liquid and per atmosphere (760 mmHg) partial pressure of the gas at any given temperature.

**bun·ya·vi·rus en·ceph·a·li·tis** encephalitis of abrupt onset, with severe frontal headache and low-grade to moderate fever, caused by members of the genus *Bunyavirus.*

**buph·thal·mia, buph·thal·mus, buph·thal·mos** (boof-thal'mē-ă, boof-thal'mŭs, boof-thal' mos) an affection of infancy, marked by an increase of intraocular pressure with enlargement of the eyeball. SYN congenital glaucoma. [G. *bous,* ox, + *ophthalmos,* eye]

**bur** (ber) a rotary cutting instrument, used in dentistry, consisting of a small metal shaft and a head designed in various shapes; used at various rotational velocities for excavating decay, shaping cavity forms, and for reduction of tooth structure. SEE ALSO burr.

**bu·ret, bu·rette** (boo-ret') a graduated glass tube with a tap as its lower end; used for measuring liquids in volumetric chemical analyses. [Fr.]

**Bur·ger tri·an·gle** (bĕr'gĕr) a scalene triangle representing the frontal plane electrocardiographic leads comparable to, but more accurate than, the Einthoven triangle. SEE Einthoven triangle.

**bur·ied flap** a flap denuded of both surface epithelium and superficial dermis and transferred into the subcutaneous tissues.

**bur·ied su·ture** any suture placed entirely below the surface of the skin.

***Burk·hol·deria*** (berk-hol-der'ē-ă) a genus of motile, non–spore-forming Gram-negative rods, containing significant species of human pathogens formerly classified as members of the genus *Pseudomonas.*

***Burk·hol·der·ia cep·a·ci·a*** a bacterial species found in rotted onions and in clinical specimens; commonly found in respiratory secretions in patients with cystic fibrosis, it is frequently resistant to many antibiotics.

***Burk·hol·der·ia mal·le·i*** a bacterial species infectious to horses and donkeys, causing glanders and farcy. SYN *Pseudomonas mallei.*

***Burk·hol·der·ia pseu·do·mal·le·i*** a species found in cases of melioidosis in humans and other animals and in soil and water in tropical regions.

**Bur·kitt lym·pho·ma** (bĕr'kit) a form of malig-

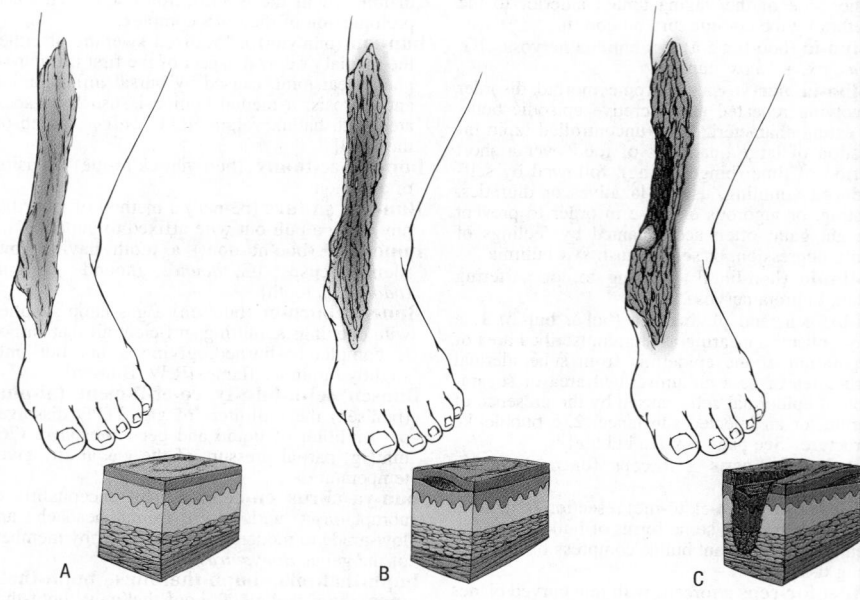

**burns:** (A) superficial burn; (B) partial-thickness burn; (C) full-thickness burn

nant lymphoma reported in African children, frequently involving the jaw and abdominal lymph nodes. Geographic distribution of Burkitt lymphoma suggests that it is found in areas with endemic malaria. It is primarily a B-cell neoplasm and is believed to be caused by Epstein-Barr virus, a member of the family Herpesviridae, which can be isolated from tumor cells in culture; occasional cases of lymphoma with similar features have been reported in the United States.

**burn** (bern) **1.** to cause a lesion by heat or a similar lesion by some other agent. **2.** a sensation of pain caused by excessive heat, or similar pain from any cause. **3.** a lesion caused by heat or any cauterizing agent, including friction, caustic agents, electricity, or electromagnetic energy; types of burns resulting from different agents are relatively specific and diagnostic. The division of burns into three degrees (first degree, second degree, and third degree) reflects the severity of skin damage (erythema, blisters, charring, respectively). See this page. [A.S. *baernan*]

**Bur·nett syn·drome** (běr-net′) SYN milk-alkali syndrome.

**burn·ing mouth syn·drome** a clinical condition in which the patient complains of a burning sensation in the oral cavity, although the appearance of the oral mucosa is normal; the cause has not been determined.

**burn·ing ton·gue** SYN glossodynia.

**burn·ing ton·gue syn·drome** a syndrome of pain in the tongue without apparent lesions, often associated with ageusia; more common in elderly women.

**bur·nish·er** (ber′nish-er) an instrument for smoothing and polishing the surface or edge of a dental restoration. [O. F. *burnir*, to polish]

**burn·out** SYN overtraining syndrome.

**Bu·row so·lu·tion** (boor′ov) a preparation of aluminium subacetate and glacial acetic acid, used for its antiseptic and astringent action on the skin.

**Bu·row tri·an·gle** (boor′ov) a triangle of skin and subcutaneous fat excised so that a flap can be advanced without buckling the adjacent tissue.

**burr** (ber) a drilling tool for enlarging a trephine hole in the cranium. SEE ALSO bur.

**bur·sa,** pl. **bur·sae** (ber′să, ber′sē) [TA] a closed sac or envelope lined with synovial membrane and containing fluid, usually found or formed in areas subject to friction; e.g., over an exposed or prominent part or where a tendon passes over a bone. [Mediev. L., a purse]

**bur·sae** (ber′sē)

**bur·sal** (ber′săl) relating to a bursa.

**bur·sal syn·o·vi·tis** SYN bursitis.

**bur·sa of pi·ri·for·mis** a small bursa located between the tendons of the piriformis and superior gemellus and the femur.

**bur·sa of ten·do cal·ca·ne·us** bursa between the tendo calcaneus and the upper part of the posterior surface of the calcaneum. SYN retrocalcaneal bursa.

**bur·sec·to·my** (ber-sek′tŏ-mē) surgical removal of a bursa. [bursa + G. *ektomē*, excision]

**bur·si·tis** (ber-sī′tis) inflammation of a bursa. SYN bursal synovitis.

**bur·so·lith** (ber′sō-lith) a calculus formed in a bursa. [bursa + G. *lithos*, stone]

**bur·sop·a·thy** (ber-sop′ă-thē) any disease of a bursa.

**bur·sot·o·my** (ber-sot′ō-mē) incision through the wall of a bursa. [bursa + G. *tomē*, a cutting]

**Bur·ton line** (ber′ton) a bluish line on the free

border of the gingiva, occurring in lead poisoning.

**Bu·sac·ca nod·ules** (boo-sah'kah) inflammatory, granulomatous nodules located away from the pupillary margin of the iris.

**Busch·ke dis·ease** (boosh'kĕ) SYN scleredema adultorum.

**Bus·quet dis·ease** (boos-kā') an osteoperiostitis of the metatarsal bones, leading to exostoses on the dorsum of the foot.

**Bus·se-Busch·ke dis·ease** (bow'sĕ boosh'kĕ) SYN cryptococcosis.

**bu·tane** (byu'tān) a gaseous hydrocarbon present in natural gas.

**bu·tan·o·yl** (byu'tan-ō-il) the radical of butanoic acid. SYN butyryl.

**buthionine sulfoximine** (boo-thī-ō-nēn sul-fox'ĭ-mēn) a compound that decreases intracellular glutathione by inhibition of its synthesis.

**but·ter** (bŭt'er) **1.** a coherent mass of milk fat, obtained by churning or shaking cream until the separate fat globules run together, leaving a liquid residue, buttermilk. **2.** a soft solid having the consistency of butter. [L. *butyrum*, G. *boutyros*, prob. fr. *bous*, cow, + *tyros*, cheese]

**but·ter·fly** (bŭt'er-flī) **1.** any structure or apparatus resembling in shape a butterfly with outstretched wings. **2.** a scaling erythematous lesion on each cheek, joined by a narrow band across the nose; seen in lupus erythematosus and seborrheic dermatitis.

**but·ter·fly pat·tern** bilateral, symmetric, pulmonary alveolar opacities sparing the periphery, on chest radiographs; usually caused by pulmonary edema.

**but·tocks** (bŭt'oks) the two gluteal prominences. SYN nates [TA], breech, clunes.

**but·ton** (bŭt'ŏn) a structure, lesion, or device of knob shape. [M.E., fr. O.Fr. *bouton*, fr. *bouter*, to thrust, fr. Germanic]

**but·ton·hole** (bŭt'ŏn-hōl) **1.** a short straight cut made through the wall of a cavity or canal. **2.** the contraction of an orifice down to a narrow slit; i.e., the so-called mitral buttonhole in extreme mitral stenosis.

**but·ton su·ture** a suture in which the threads are passed through the holes of a button and then tied; used to reduce the danger of the threads cutting through the flesh.

**but·tress plate** a metal plate used to support the internal fixation of a fracture.

**bu·tyl** (byu'til) a radical of *n*-butane.

**bu·ty·ra·ce·ous** (byu-tir-ā'shĭ-us) buttery in consistency.

**bu·ty·rate** (byu'ti-rāt) a salt or ester of butyric acid.

**bu·tyr·ic ac·id** (byu-tir'ik as'id) an acid of unpleasant odor occurring in butter, cod liver oil, sweat, and many other substances.

**bu·ty·roid** (byu'ti-royd) **1.** buttery. **2.** resembling butter.

**bu·tyr·ous** (byu'ti-rŭs) denoting a tissue or bacterial growth of butter-like consistency.

**bu·tyr·yl** (byu'ti-ril) SYN butanoyl.

**Buz·zard ma·neu·ver** (buz'ărd) testing the patellar reflex while the sitting patient makes firm pressure on the floor with the toes.

**B19 vi·rus** a human parvovirus associated with arthritis and arthralgia and a number of specific clinical entities, including erythema infectiosum and aplastic crisis in the presence of hemolytic anemia.

**BVM** bag-valve-mask device.

**By·ars flap** (bī'arz) skin flap made of dorsal prepuce to resurface the ventral penis in patients with chordee and/or hypospadias.

**by·pass** (bī'pas) **1.** a shunt or auxiliary flow. **2.** to create new flow from one structure to another through a diversionary channel. SEE ALSO shunt.

**bys·si·no·sis** (bis-i-nō'sis) obstructive airway disease in people who work with unprocessed cotton, flax, or hemp; caused by reaction to material in the dust. [G. *byssos*, flax, + *-osis*, condition]

**by·stand·er ly·sis** complement-mediated lysis of nearby cells in the vicinity of a complement activation site.

# C

**C 1.** large calorie; carbon; cathodal; cathode; Celsius; cervical vertebra (C1 to C7); closure (of an electrical circuit); congius (gallon); contraction; coulomb; curie; cylinder; cylindrical lens; cytidine; cysteine; cytosine; component of complement (C1 1/N C9); third substrate in a multisubstrate enzyme-catalyzed reaction. **2.** when followed by subscript letters, e.g., $C_{In}$, indicates renal clearance of a substance (e.g., inulin). When followed by subscript numbers, e.g., $C_{19}$, indicates the number of carbon atoms in a molecule.

**c 1.** centi-; small calorie; centum; concentration; speed of light in a vacuum; circumference; curie. **2.** as a subscript, refers to blood capillary.

**CA** carcinoma; cardiac arrest; cancer; chronologic age; cytosine arabinoside.

**CA-125** cancer antigen 125 test.

**$^{47}$Ca** calcium-47.

**CA-125 an·ti·gen** tumor marker elevated in 85% of women with advanced ovarian cancer. SEE ALSO cancer antigen 125 test.

**CA-15-3 an·ti·gen** antigen present in some patients with breast cancer.

**CA-19-9 an·ti·gen** tumor antigen present in cholangiocarcinomas and pancreatic carcinomas.

**ca·ble graft** a multiple strand nerve graft arranged as a pathway for regeneration of axons.

**Cab·ot ring bod·ies** (kab'ĕt) ring-shaped or figure-of-eight structures that stain red with Wright stain, found in red blood cells in severe anemias, possibly a remnant of the nuclear membrane; a form of basophilic degenerative process.

**ca·chec·tic** (kă-kek'tik) relating to or suffering from cachexia.

**cac·hec·tin** (kăk-ek'tin) a polypeptide hormone, produced by endotoxin-activated macrophages, which has the ability to modulate adipocyte metabolism, lyse tumor cells *in vitro*, and induce hemorrhagic necrosis of certain transplantable tumors *in vivo*. SYN tumor necrosis factor. [G. *kakos*, bad, + *hexis*, condition of body]

**ca·chex·ia** (kă-kek'sē-ă) a general weight loss and wasting occurring in the course of a chronic disease or emotional disturbance. [G. *kakos*, bad, + *hexis*, condition of body]

**ca·chex·ia hy·po·phys·e·o·pri·va** a condition following total removal of the hypophysis cerebri resulting in panhypopituitarism marked by a fall of body temperature, electrolyte imbalance, and hypoglycemia, followed by coma and death.

**ca·chex·ia stru·mi·pri·va** SYN cachexia thyropriva.

**ca·chex·ia thy·ro·pri·va** signs and symptoms of hypothyroidism (with or without myxedema) resulting from the loss of thyroid tissue, either from surgery, radiotherapy, or disease. SYN cachexia strumipriva.

**cach·in·na·tion** (kak-i-nā'shŭn) laughter without apparent cause, often observed in schizophrenia. [L. *cachinno*, to laugh immoderately and loudly]

⚠ **ca·co-, cac-, ca·ci-** bad; ill. Cf. mal-. [G. *kakos*]

**cac·o·geu·sia** (kak-ō-goo'sē-ă) a bad taste. [caco- + G. *geusis*, taste]

**cac·o·me·lia** (kak-ō-mē'lē-ă) congenital deformity of one or more limbs. [caco- + G. *melos*, limb]

**ca·cos·mia** (kă-koz'mē-ă) a subjective perception of nonexistent disagreeable odors. [G. *kakosmia*,

a bad smell, fr. *kakos*, bad, + *osmē*, the sense of smell]

**cac·u·men**, pl. **cac·u·mi·na** (kak-yu'men, kak-yu'mi-nă) the top or apex of a plant or an anatomic structure. [L. summit]

**ca·dav·er** (kă-dav'er) a dead body. SYN corpse. [L. fr. *cado*, to fall]

**ca·dav·er·ic** (kă-dav'er-ik) relating to a dead body.

**ca·dav·er·ine** (kă-dav'er-in) a foul-smelling diamine formed by bacterial decarboxylation of lysine; poisonous and irritating to the skin.

**ca·dav·er·ous** (kă-dav'er-ŭs) having the pallor and appearance of a corpse.

**cad·her·in** (kad-hēr'in) one of a class of integral-membrane glycoproteins that has a role in cell-cell adhesion and is important in morphogenesis and differentiation; E-cadherin is also known as uvomorulin and is concentrated in the belt desmosome in epithelial cells; N-cadherin is found in nerve, muscle, and lens cells and helps to maintain the integrity of neuronal aggregates; P-cadherin is expressed in placental and epidermal cells. [cell + adhere + -in]

**cad·mi·um (Cd)** (kad'mē-ŭm) a metallic element, atomic no. 48, atomic wt. 112.411; its salts are poisonous and little used in medicine. Various compounds of cadmium are used commercially in metallurgy, photography, electrochemistry, etc.; a few have been used as ascaricides, antiseptics, and fungicides. [L. *cadmia*, fr. G. *kadmeia* or *kadmia*, an ore of zinc, calamine]

**ca·du·ce·us** (kă-doo'sē-ŭs) a staff with two oppositely twined serpents and surmounted by two wings; emblem of the U.S. Army Medical Corps. SEE ALSO staff of Aesculapius. [L. the staff of Mercury; G. *kēryx* herald, the staff of Hermes]

⚠ **cae-** for words so beginning, see under ce-.

**cae·cum [Br.]** SEE cecum.

**caf·feine** (kaf'ēn) an alkaloid obtained from the dried leaves of *Thea sinensis*, tea, or the dried seeds of *Coffea arabica*, coffee; used as a central nervous system stimulant, diuretic, circulatory and respiratory stimulant, and as an adjunct in the treatment of headaches.

**caf·fein·ism** (kaf'ēn-izm) caffeine intoxication characterized by restlessness, tremulousness, excitement, insomnia, flushed face, diuresis, and gastrointestinal complaints, brought on by the ingestion of substances containing caffeine.

**cage** (kāj) **1.** an enclosure made partly or completely of open work and commonly used to house animals. **2.** a structure resembling such an enclosure. SYN cavea. [M.E., fr. O.Fr., fr. L. *cavea*, hollow, stall]

**Cagot ear** (kă-gō' ēr) an auricle having no lobulus. [a people in the Pyrenees among whom physical stigmata are common]

**Cain com·plex** extreme envy or jealousy of a brother, leading to hatred. [*Cain*, biblical personage]

**cais·son dis·ease** (kā'son dis'ēz) SYN decompression sickness. [Fr. *caisson* (fr. *caisse*, a chest) a water-tight box or cylinder containing air under high pressure used in sinking structural pilings underwater]

**Ca·jal as·tro·cyte stain** (kah-hahl') a method for demonstrating astrocytes by impregnation in a solution containing gold chloride and mercuric chloride.

**cake kid•ney** a solid, irregularly lobed organ of bizarre shape, usually situated in the pelvis toward the midline, produced by fusion of the renal anlagen (primordia of the kidneys).

**cal** small calorie.

**cal•a•mus** (kal′ă-mŭs) a reed-shaped structure. [L. reed, a pen]

**cal•a•mus scrip•to•ri•us** inferior part of the rhomboid fossa; the narrow lower end of the fourth ventricle between the two clavae. [L. writing pen]

**cal•cae•mia [Br.]** SYN hypercalcemia.

**cal•ca•ne•al, cal•ca•ne•an** (kal-kā′nē-al, kal-kā′ nē-an) relating to the calcaneus or heel bone.

**cal•ca•ne•al a•poph•y•si•tis** SYN Sever disease.

**cal•ca•ne•al pe•te•chi•ae** traumatic hemorrhage into the stratum corneum of the heel which may persist for several weeks as centrally confluent black dots.

**cal•ca•ne•al spur** SYN heel spur.

⚠️ **cal•ca•neo-** the calcaneus. [L. *calcaneum*, heel]

**cal•ca•ne•o•a•poph•y•si•tis** (kal-kā′nē-ō-ă-pof-i-sī′tis) inflammation at the posterior part of the os calcis, at the insertion of the Achilles tendon.

**cal•ca•ne•o•as•trag•a•loid** (kal-kā′nē-ō-as-trag′ ă-loyd) relating to the calcaneus, or os calcis, and the talus, or astragalus.

**cal•ca•ne•o•cu•boid** (kal-kā′nē-ō-kyu′boyd) relating to the calcaneus and the cuboid bone.

**cal•can•e•o•dyn•ia** (kal-kā′nē-ō-din′ē-ă) SYN painful heel. [calcaneo- + G. *odynē*, pain]

**cal•ca•ne•o•na•vic•u•lar** (kal-kā′nē-ō-na-vik′yu-lăr) relating to the calcaneus and the navicular bone.

**cal•ca•ne•o•tib•i•al** (kal-kā′nē-ō-tib′ē-ăl) relating to the calcaneus and the tibia.

**cal•ca•ne•um** (kal-kā′nē-ŭm) SYN calcaneus (1). [L. the heel]

**cal•ca•ne•us**, gen. and pl. **cal•ca•nei** (kal-kā′nē-ŭs, kal-kā′nē-ī) **1.** [TA] the largest of the tarsal bones; it forms the heel and articulates with the cuboid anteriorly and the talus above. SYN calcaneum, heel bone. **2.** SYN talipes calcaneus. [L. the heel (another form of *calcaneum*)]

**cal•car** (kal′kar) **1.** a small projection from any structure; internal spurs (septa) at the level of division of arteries and confluence of veins when branches or roots form an acute angle. **2.** a spine or projection from a bone. SYN spur. [L. spur, cock's spur]

**cal•car•e•ous** (kal-kā′rē-ŭs) chalky; relating to or containing lime or calcium, or calcific material. [L. *calcarius,* pertaining to lime, fr. *calx,* lime]

**cal•car•e•ous cor•pus•cles** rounded masses composed of concentric layers of calcium carbonate, characteristic of tapeworm tissue.

**cal•car•e•ous de•gen•er•a•tion** in a precise sense, not a degenerative process *per se,* but the deposition of insoluble calcium salts in tissue that has degenerated and become necrotic, as in dystrophic calcification.

**cal•car•e•ous in•fil•tra•tion** SYN calcification.

**cal•ca•rine** (kal′kă-rēn) **1.** relating to a calcar. **2.** spur-shaped.

**cal•ca•rine sul•cus** a deep fissure on the medial aspect of the cerebral cortex, extending on an arched line from the isthmus of the fornicate gyrus back to the occipital pole, marking the border between the lingual gyrus below and the cuneus above it. The cortex in the depth of the sulcus corresponds to the horizontal meridian of the contralateral half of the visual field.

**cal•car•i•u•ria** (kal-kar-ē-yu′rē-ă) excretion of calcium (lime) salts in the urine. [L. *calcarius,* of lime, + G. *ouron,* urine]

**cal•ce•mia** (kal-sē′mē-ă) SYN hypercalcemia.

**cal•ces** (kal′sēz) plural of calx.

**cal•ci•co•sis** (kal-si-kō′sis) pneumoconiosis from the inhalation of limestone dust.

**cal•ci•di•ol** (kal-sĭ-dī′ol) 25-hydroxycholecalciferol (a 3,25-diol); the first step in the biological conversion of vitamin $D_3$ to the more active form, calcitriol; it is more potent than vitamin $D_3$.

**cal•cif•er•ol** (kal-sif′er-ol) SYN ergocalciferol.

**cal•ci•fi•ca•tion** (kal′si-fi-kā′shŭn) **1.** deposition of lime or other insoluble calcium salts. **2.** a process in which tissue or noncellular material in the body becomes hardened as the result of precipitates or larger deposits of insoluble salts of calcium (and also magnesium), especially calcium carbonate and phosphate (hydroxyapatite) normally occurring only in the formation of bone and teeth. SYN calcareous infiltration. [L. *calx,* lime, + *facio,* to make]

**cal•cif•ic bur•si•tis** inflammation of a bursa that results in the deposition of calcium salts; most commonly associated with subdeltoid bursitis.

**cal•cif•ic ten•don•i•tis** chronic tendonitis with formation of mineral deposits in and around the tendon.

**cal•ci•fy** (kal′si-fī) to deposit or lay down calcium salts, as in the formation of bone.

**cal•ci•fy•ing o•don•to•gen•ic cyst, cal•ci•fy•ing and ker•a•tin•iz•ing o•don•to•gen•ic cyst** a mixed radiolucent-radiopaque lesion of the jaws with features of both a cyst and a solid neoplasm; characterized by ghost cell keratinization, dentinoid, and calcification.

**cal•ci•neu•rin** (kal-sē-noor′in) a calcium-dependent serine-threonine phosphatase involved in T-cell signaling transcription; the reaction cascade in which it resides is referred to as the calcineurin pathway. [calcium + G. *neuron,* nerve, + -in]

**cal•ci•no•sis** (kal-si-nō′sis) a condition characterized by the deposition of calcium salts in nodular foci in various tissues. [calcium + -osis, condition]

**cal•ci•no•sis cir•cum•scrip•ta** localized deposits of calcium salts in the skin and subcutaneous tissues, usually surrounded by a zone of granulomatous inflammation; clinically, the lesions resemble the tophi of gout.

**cal•ci•no•sis u•ni•ver•sa•lis** diffuse deposits of calcium salts in the skin and subcutaneous tissues, connective tissue, and other sites; may be associated with dermatomyositis, occurs more frequently in young persons, and is often fatal; serum levels of calcium and phosphorus are generally within normal limits.

**cal•ci•phil•ia** (kal-si-fil′ē-ă) a condition in which the tissues manifest an unusual affinity for calcium salts. [calcium + G. *phileō,* to love]

**cal•ci•phy•lax•is** (kal′si-fī-lak′sis) a condition of induced systemic hypersensitivity in which tissues respond to appropriate challenging agents with a sudden, but sometimes evanescent, local calcification.

**cal•ci•priv•ic** (kal-si-priv′ik) deprived of calcium.

**cal·ci·to·nin** (kal-si-tō'nin) a peptide hormone, of which eight forms are known; produced by the parathyroid, thyroid, and thymus glands; its action is opposite to that of parathyroid hormone in that calcitonin increases deposition of calcium and phosphate in bone and lowers the level of calcium in the blood. [calci- + G. *tonos*, stretching, + -in]

**cal·ci·to·nin gene-re·lat·ed pep·tide** a second product transcribed from the calcitonin gene. CGRP is found in a number of tissues including nervous tissue. It is a vasodilator that may participate in the cutaneous tingle response.

**cal·ci·um**, gen. **cal·cii** (kal'sē-ŭm, kal-sē-ī) a metallic bivalent element; atomic no. 20, atomic wt. 40.078, density 1.55, melting point 842°C. Many calcium salts have crucial uses in metabolism and in medicine. Calcium salts are responsible for the radiopacity of bone, calcified cartilage, and arteriosclerotic plaques in arteries. [Mod. L. fr. L. *calx*, lime]

**cal·ci·um-47** (⁴⁷Ca) a radioisotope of calcium with a half-life of 4.54 days, used in the diagnosis of disorders of calcium metabolism.

**cal·ci·um chan·nel block·er** a class of drugs with the capacity to prevent calcium ions from passing through biologic membranes. These agents are used to treat hypertension, angina pectoris, and cardiac arrhythmias; examples include nifedipine, diltiazem, and verapamil.

**cal·ci·um chan·nel-block·ing a·gent** a class of drugs that have the ability to inhibit movement of calcium ions across the cell membrane; of value in the treatment of cardiovascular disorders. SYN slow channel-blocking agent.

**cal·ci·um group** the metals of the alkaline earths: beryllium, magnesium, calcium, strontium, barium, and radium.

**cal·ci·um pump** a membranal protein that can transport calcium ions across the membrane using energy from ATP.

**cal·ci·u·ria** (kal-sē-yu'rē-ă) the urinary excretion of calcium; sometimes used as a synonym for hypercalciuria.

**cal·co·dyn·ia** (kal-kō-din'ē-ă) SYN painful heel. [L. *calx*, heel, + G. *odynē*, pain]

**cal·co·sphe·rite** (kal-kō-sfēr'īt) a tiny, spheroidal, concentrically laminated body containing deposits of calcium salts; found in papillary carcinoma of the thyroid and ovary and in meningioma. SYN psammoma bodies (3). [L. *calx*, lime, + G. *sphaira*, sphere]

**cal·cu·li** (kal'kyu-lī) plural of calculus.

**cal·cu·lo·sis** (kal-kyu-lō'sis) the tendency or disposition to form calculi or stones. [L. *calculus*, small stone, + G. *-osis*, condition]

**cal·cu·lus**, gen. and pl. **cal·cu·li** (kal'kyu-lŭs, kal'kyu-lī) a concretion formed in any part of the body, most commonly in the passages of the biliary and urinary tracts; usually composed of salts of inorganic or organic acids, or of other material such as cholesterol. SYN stone (1). [L. a pebble, a calculus]

**Cald·well-Luc op·er·a·tion** (kahld'well-loo-k) an intraoral procedure for opening into the maxillary antrum through the supradental (canine) fossa above the maxillary premolar teeth. SYN Luc operation.

**Cald·well-Mo·loy clas·si·fi·ca·tion** (kahld'well mě-loi') a classification of the variations in the female pelvis; namely gynecoid, android, anthropoid, and platypelloid pelvis, based on the type of the posterior and anterior segments of the inlet.

**cal·e·fa·cient** (kal-ĕ-fā'shent) 1. making warm or hot. 2. an agent causing a sense of warmth in the part to which it is applied. [L. *calefacio*, fr. *caleo*, to be warm, + *facio*, to make]

**calf**, pl. **calves** (kaf, kavz) SYN sural region. [Gael. *kalpa*]

**calf bone** SYN fibula. [O.N. *kalfi*, fibula]

**cal·i·ber** (kal'i-ber) the diameter of a hollow tubular structure. [Fr. *calibre*, of uncert. etym.]

**cal·i·brate** (kal'i-brāt) 1. to graduate or standardize any measuring instrument. 2. to measure the diameter of a tubular structure.

**cal·i·bra·tion curve** the graphic or mathematic relationship between the readings obtained in an analytic process and the quantity of analyte in a calibration. The relationship is often a straight line rather than a curve.

**cal·i·bra·tion in·ter·val** the period of time or series of measurements during which calibration can be expected to remain stable within specified and documented limits.

**cal·i·bra·tor** (kal'ĭ-brā-ter) a standard or reference material or substance used to standardize or calibrate an instrument or laboratory procedure.

**cal·i·ce·al** (kal'i-seāl) relating to the calyx.

**cal·i·ce·al di·ver·tic·u·lum** a congenital or acquired distention of a kidney calix that renders it susceptible to calculus formation.

**Cal·i·ci·vi·ri·dae** (kal'i-sē-ver'ĭ-dē) a family of RNA viruses associated with epidemic viral gastroenteritis and certain forms of hepatitis.

**cal·i·cot·o·my, cal·i·cec·to·my** (kal-ĭ-sot'ō-mē, kal-i-sek'tō-mē) incision into a calix, usually for removal of a calculus. [calix, + G. *tomē*, a cutting]

**ca·lic·u·lus**, pl. **ca·lic·u·li** (kă-lik'yu-lŭs, kă-lik' yulī) a bud-shaped or cup-shaped structure, resembling the closed calyx of a flower. [L. dim. from G. *kalyx*, the cup of a flower]

**ca·li·ec·ta·sis** (kā-lē-ek'tă-sis) dilation of the calices, usually due to obstruction or infection.

**Cal·i·for·nia vi·rus** a serologic group of the genus *Bunyavirus*, comprising over 14 strains including La Crosse and Tahyna virus, and the type strain, California virus, which causes encephalitis, chiefly in the age group 4 to 14 years.

**cal·i·for·ni·um (Cf)** (kal-i-fōr'nē-ŭm) an artificial transuranium element, symbol Cf, atomic no. 98, atomic wt. 251.08. [*California*, state and university where first prepared]

**ca·li·o·plas·ty** (kā'lē-ō-plas-tē) surgical reconstruction of a calix, usually designed to increase its lumen at the infundibulum.

**ca·li·or·rha·phy** (kā'lē-ōr-a-fē) 1. suturing of a calix. 2. plastic surgery of a dilated or obstructed calix to improve urinary drainage, often requiring combination of two or more calices or the massive movement of renal pelvic mucosa to rebuild the caliceal drainage system. [calix, + G. *rhaphē*, suture, seam]

**cal·i·pers** (kal'i-perz) an instrument used for measuring diameters. [a corruption of *caliber*]

**cal·is·then·ics** (kal-is-then'iks) systematic practice of various exercises with the object of preserving health and increasing physical strength. [G. *kalos*, beautiful, + *sthenos*, strength]

**ca·lix** (kā'liks) SYN calyx. [L. fr. G. *kalyx*, the cup of a flower]

**Cal·kins sign** (kǎl′kinz) the change of shape of the uterus from discoid to ovoid, indicating placental separation from the uterine wall.

**Cal·la·han meth·od** (kal′a-han) SYN chloropercha method.

**Cal·lan·der am·pu·ta·tion** (kal′ǎn-der) tenontoplastic amputation through the femur at the knee. SYN knee disarticulation amputation.

**Call-Ex·ner bod·ies** (kǎl-eks′ner) small fluid-filled spaces between granulosal cells in ovarian follicles and in ovarian tumors of granulosal origin; they may form a rosette-like structure.

**cal·lo·sal** (ka-lō′sǎl) relating to the corpus callosum.

**cal·los·i·ty** (ka-los′i-tē) a circumscribed thickening of the keratin layer of the epidermis as a result of repeated friction or intermittent pressure. SYN callus (1), keratoma (1), poroma (1), tyloma. [L. fr. *callosus,* thick-skinned]

**cal·lous** (kal′ŭs) relating to a callus or callosity.

**cal·lus** (kal′ŭs) 1. SYN callosity. 2. a composite mass of tissue that forms at a fracture site to establish continuity between the bone ends; it is composed initially of uncallused fibrous tissue and cartilage, and ultimately of bone. [L. hard skin]

**cal·mod·u·lin** (kal-mod′yu-lin) a protein that binds calcium ions, thereby becoming the agent for many of the cellular effects long ascribed to calcium ions. [*calc*ium + *modul*ate]

*Ca·lo·di·um* (ka-lō′dē-ŭm) one of three trichurid nematode genera, commonly referred to as *Capillaria.*

**ca·lor** (kā′lōr) heat, as one of the four signs of inflammation (c., rubor, tumor, dolor) enunciated by Celsus. [L.]

**Ca·lo·ri bur·sa** (kah-lō′rē) a bursa between the arch of the aorta and the trachea.

**ca·lor·ic** (kǎ-lōr′ik) 1. relating to a calorie. 2. relating to heat. [L. *calor,* heat]

**ca·lor·ic nys·tag·mus** jerky nystagmus induced by labyrinthine stimulation with hot or cold water in the ear.

**ca·lor·ic stim·u·la·tion** in treatment of swallowing disorders, the use of hot or (usually) cold temperature to increase awareness of the bolus in the mouth and pharynx; for example, the use of ice slush rather than a room temperature food of similar consistency.

**ca·lor·ic test** SYN Bárány caloric test.

**cal·o·rie** (kal′ō-rē) a unit of heat content or energy. The amount of heat necessary to raise 1 g of water from 14.5°C to 15.5°C (small calorie). Calorie is being replaced by joule, the SI unit equal to 0.239 calorie. SEE ALSO British thermal unit. [L. *calor,* heat]

**ca·lor·i·gen·ic** (kǎ-lōr-i-jen′ik) 1. capable of generating heat. 2. stimulating metabolic production of heat. SYN thermogenetic (2), thermogenic. [L. *calor,* heat, + G. *genesis,* production]

**cal·o·rim·e·ter** (kal-ō-rim′ě-ter) an apparatus for measuring the amount of heat liberated in a chemical reaction. [L. *calor,* heat, + G. *metron,* measure]

**cal·o·ri·met·ric** (kǎ′lōr-i-met′rik) relating to calorimetry.

**cal·o·rim·e·try** (kal-ō-rim′ě-trē) measurement of the amount of heat given off by a reaction or group of reactions (as by an organism).

**cal·var·ia,** pl. **cal·var·i·ae** (kal-vā′rē-ă, kal-vā′ rē-ē) [TA] the upper domelike portion of the skull. SYN skullcap. [L. a skull]

**cal·var·i·um** (kal-vār′ē-ŭm) USAGE NOTE: incorrectly used for calvaria.

**calx,** gen. **cal·cis,** pl. **cal·ces** (kalks, kal′sis, kal′ sēz) 1. SYN lime (1). [L. limestone] 2. the posterior rounded extremity of the foot. SYN heel (1). [L. heel]

*Ca·lym·ma·to·bac·te·ri·um* (kǎ-lim′mǎ-tō-bak-tēr′ē-ŭm) a genus of nonmotile bacteria containing Gram-negative, pleomorphic rods with single or bipolar condensations of chromatin; cells occur singly and in clusters. The organisms are pathogenic only for man. The type species is *Calymmatobacterium granulomatis;* this species causes granuloma inguinale. [G. *kalymma,* hood, veil, + *baktērion,* rod]

**ca·lyx,** pl. **ca·li·ces** (kā′liks, kal′i-sēz) a flower-shaped or funnel-shaped structure; specifically one of the branches or recesses of the pelvis of the kidney into which the orifices of the malpighian renal pyramids project. SYN calix. [G. cup of a flower]

**CAM** cell adhesion molecule.

**cam·era,** pl. **cam·er·ae, cam·er·as** (kam′er-ă, kam′er-ē) 1. a closed box; especially one containing a lens, shutter, and light-sensitive film or plates for photography. 2. in anatomy, any chamber or cavity, such as one of the chambers of the heart, or eye. [L. a vault]

**cam·er·a an·te·ri·or bul·bi oc·u·li** [TA] SYN anterior chamber of eyeball.

**cam·er·ae bul·bi** [TA] SYN chambers of eyeball.

**cam·er·a oc·u·li** SEE anterior chamber of eyeball, posterior chamber of eyeball.

**cam·er·a pos·tre·ma** SYN postremal chamber of eyeball.

**cam·er·as**

**cam·er·a vit·rea** SYN postremal chamber of eyeball.

**cAMP** adenosine 3′,5′-cyclic monophosphate (cyclic AMP).

**camp fe·ver** 1. SYN typhus. 2. any epidemic febrile illness affecting troops in an encampment.

**cam·pim·e·ter** (kam-pim′ě-ter) a small tangent screen used to measure central visual field. [L. *campus,* field, + G. *metron,* measure]

**cAMP re·cep·tor pro·tein (CRP)** SYN catabolite (gene) activator protein.

**camp·to·cor·mia** (kamp-tō-kōr′mē-ă) static, often marked forward flexion of the trunk; usually manifestation of conversion reaction. SYN camptospasm. [G. *kamptos,* bent, + *kormos,* trunk of a tree]

**camp·to·dac·ty·ly, camp·to·dac·tyl·ia** (kamp-tō-dak′ti-lē, kamp-tō-dak-til′ē-ă) permanent flexion of one or both interphalangeal joints of one or more fingers, usually the little finger; often congenital in origin. [G. *kamptos,* bent, + *daktylos,* finger]

**camp·to·me·lia** (kamp-tō-mē′lē-ă) a skeletal dysplasia characterized by a bending of the long bones of the limbs, resulting in a permanent bowing or curvature of the affected part. [G. *kamptos,* bent, + *melos,* limb]

**camp·to·mel·ic** (kamp-tō-mel′ik) denoting or characteristic of camptomelia.

**camp·to·mel·ic dwarf·ism** dwarfism with shortening of the lower limbs due to anterior bending of the femur and tibia.

**camp•to•spasm** (kamp′tō-spazm) SYN campto-cormia.

**camp•to•thec•in** (kamp-tō-thek′in) plant alka-loids consisting of a pentacyclic structure with a lactone ring; inhibitors of topoisomerase I, i.e., topotecan and irinotecan (CPT-11). [Camptotheca, genus name of botanic source]

*Cam•py•lo•bac•ter* (kam′pi-lō-bak′ter) a genus of bacteria containing Gram-negative, non-spore-forming, spirally curved rods with a single polar flagellum at one or both ends of the cell; they are motile with a characteristic corkscrew-like mo-tion. The type species, *Campylobacter fetus*, con-tains various subspecies, particularly *Campylo-bacter jejuni*, that can cause acute bacterial gas-troenteritis. [G. *campylos,* curved, + *baktron,* staff or rod]

*Cam•py•lo•bac•ter co•li* a thermophilic bacterial species that causes first watery, then inflamma-tory, diarrheal disease in humans and in piglets.

*Cam•py•lo•bac•ter con•cis•us* a catalase-nega-tive bacterial species isolated from normal hu-man fecal flora, gingival crevices in periodontal disease, and occasionally blood.

*Cam•py•lo•bac•ter fe•tus* a species that contains various subspecies which can cause human infec-tions as well as abortion in sheep and cattle; it is the type species of the genus *Campylobacter.*

*Cam•py•lo•bac•ter hy•o•in•tes•ti•na•lis* a bacte-rial species that causes an enteropathy in pigs; has been recovered from fecal specimens in hu-mans with diarrhea and with proctitis, but its pathogenic role has not been defined.

**cam•py•lo•bac•ter•i•o•sis** (kam′pi-lō-bak′ter-ē-ō′sis) infection caused by microaerophilic bacte-ria of the genus *Campylobacter.*

*Cam•py•lo•bac•ter je•ju•ni* a species that causes an acute gastroenteritis of sudden onset with con-stitutional symptoms (malaise, myalgia, arthral-gia, and headache) and cramping abdominal pain; potential sources of human infection in-clude poultry, cattle, sheep, pigs, and dogs.

*Cam•py•lo•bac•ter la•ri* a bacterial species pri-marily carried in birds, but associated with wa-ter-borne enteritis and occasionally septicemia in humans.

**ca•nal** (kă-nal′) a duct or channel; a tubular struc-ture. SYN canalis [TA]. [L. *canalis*]

**ca•na•les** (kă-nā′lēz) plural of canalis.

**can•a•lic•u•lar** (kan-ă-lik′yu-lăr) relating to a canaliculus. [L. *canaliculus,* small channel, dim. fr. *canalis,* canal + suffix *-ar,* pertaining to]

**can•a•lic•u•li** (kan-ă-lik′yu-lī) plural of canalicu-lus.

**can•a•lic•u•li den•ta•les** [TA] minute, wavy, branching tubes or canals in the dentin; they con-tain the long cytoplasmic processes of odonto-blasts and extend radially from the pulp to the dentoenamel junction. SYN dentinal canals, denti-nal tubules.

**can•a•lic•u•li•tis** (kan′ă-lik-yu-lī′tis) inflamma-tion of the lacrimal canaliculus. [canaliculus + G. *-itis,* inflammation]

**can•a•lic•u•li•za•tion** (kan-ă-lik′yu-lī-zā′shŭn) the formation of canaliculi, or small canals, in any tissue.

**can•a•lic•u•lus,** pl. **can•a•lic•u•li** (kan-ă-lik′yu-lŭs) [TA] a small canal or channel. SEE ALSO iter. [L. dim. fr. *canalis,* canal]

**ca•na•lis,** pl. **ca•na•les** (ka-nā′lis, kă-nā′lēz) [TA] SYN canal. [L.]

**ca•na•lis ad•duc•to•ri•us** [TA] SYN adductor ca-nal.

**ca•na•lis an•a•lis** [TA] SYN anal canal.

**ca•na•lis ca•ro•ti•cus** [TA] SYN carotid canal.

**ca•na•lis car•pi** [TA] SYN carpal tunnel.

**ca•na•lis cer•vi•cis uter•i** [TA] SYN cervical ca-nal.

**ca•na•lis fe•mo•ra•lis** [TA] SYN femoral canal.

**ca•na•lis hy•po•glos•sa•lis** [TA] SYN hypoglossal canal.

**ca•na•lis in•ci•si•vus** [TA] SYN incisive canal.

**ca•na•lis in•fra•or•bi•ta•lis** [TA] SYN infraor-bital canal.

**ca•na•lis in•gui•na•lis** [TA] SYN inguinal canal.

**ca•na•lis mus•cu•lo•tu•ba•ri•us** [TA] SYN mus-culotubal canal.

**ca•na•lis na•so•lac•ri•ma•lis** [TA] SYN nasolac-rimal canal.

**ca•na•lis nu•tri•ci•us** [TA] SYN nutrient canal.

**ca•na•lis ob•tu•ra•to•ri•us** [TA] SYN obturator canal.

**ca•na•lis op•ti•cus** [TA] SYN optic canal.

**ca•na•lis pte•ry•goi•de•us** [TA] SYN pterygoid canal.

**ca•na•lis pu•den•da•lis** [TA] SYN pudendal ca-nal.

**ca•na•lis py•lo•ri•cus** [TA] SYN pyloric canal.

**ca•na•lis ra•di•cis den•tis** [TA] SYN root canal of tooth.

**ca•na•lis sa•cra•lis** [TA] SYN sacral canal.

**ca•na•lis spi•ra•lis co•chle•ae** [TA] SYN co-chlear canal.

**ca•na•lis spi•ra•lis mo•di•o•li** [TA] SYN spiral canal of modiolus.

**ca•na•lis ver•te•bra•lis** [TA] SYN vertebral canal.

**can•a•li•za•tion** (kan-ăl-ī-zā′shŭn) the formation of canals or channels in a tissue.

**ca•nal for phar•yn•go•tym•pan•ic tube** the in-ferior division of the musculotubular canal that forms the bony part of the pharyngotympanic (auditory) tube. SYN semicanalis tubae auditoriae.

**ca•nals for less•er pal•a•tine nerves** canals lo-cated in the posterior part of the palatine bone.

**Can•a•van dis•ease** (kan′ă-van) progressive de-generative disease of infancy; mostly affecting Ashkenazi Jewish babies; onset typically within the first 3–4 months of birth; characterized by megalencephaly, optic atrophy, blindness, psy-chomotor regression, hypotonia, and spasticity; there is increased urinary excretion of *N*-acety-laspartic acid. MRI shows enlarged brain, de-creased attenuation of cerebral and cerebellar white matter, and normal ventricles; pathologi-cally, there is increased brain volume and weight and spongy degeneration in the subcortical white matter. Autosomal recessive inheritance, caused by mutation in the aspartoacyclase A gene (ASPA) on chromosome 17p in Jewish and non-Jewish affected individuals. SEE ALSO leukodys-trophy.

**can•cel•lat•ed** (kan′sĕ-lā-ted) SYN cancellous. [L. *cancello,* to make a lattice work]

**can•cel•lous** (kan′sĕ-lŭs) denoting bone that has a lattice-like or spongy structure. SYN cancellated.

**can•cel•lous bone** SYN substantia spongiosa.

**can•cel•lous tis•sue** latticelike or spongy osseous tissue.

**can•cel•lus,** pl. **can•cel•li** (kan-sel′ŭs, kan′se-lī) a lattice-like structure, as in spongy bone. [L. a grating, lattice]

**can•cer (CA)** (kan′ser) general term for malignant neoplasms; carcinoma or sarcoma, especially the former. [L. a crab, a cancer]

**can·cer an·ti·gen 125 test** test for cell-surface antigen found on derivatives of coelomic epithelium. Elevated levels of this antigen are associated with ovarian malignancy and benign pelvic disease such as endometriosis.

**can·cer fam·i·ly** a group of blood relatives of whom several have had cancer.

**can·cer·o·pho·bia** (kan'ser-ō-fō'bē-ă) a morbid fear of acquiring a malignant growth. SYN carcinophobia. [cancer + G. *phobos*, fear]

**can·cer·ous** (kan'ser-ŭs) relating to or pertaining to a malignant neoplasm, or being afflicted with such a process.

**can·cra** (kang'kră) plural of cancrum.

**can·cri·form** (kang'kri-fōrm) resembling cancer.

**can·crum**, pl. **can·cra** (kang'krŭm, kang'kră) a gangrenous, ulcerative, inflammatory lesion. [Mod. L., fr. L. *cancer*, crab]

**can·de·la** (kan'de-lă) the SI unit of luminous intensity, 1 lumen per m²; the luminous intensity, in a given direction, of a source that emits monochromatic radiation of frequency $540 \times 10^{12}$ hertz and that has a radiant intensity in that direction of 1/683 watt per steradian (solid angle). [L.]

*Can·di·da* (kan'did-ă) a genus of yeastlike fungi found in nature; a few species are isolated from the skin, feces, and vaginal and pharyngeal tissue, but the gastrointestinal tract is the source of the single most important species, *Candida albicans*. [L. *candidus*, dazzling white]

*Can·di·da gla·brat·a* a fungal species that is a cause of human candidiasis; formerly classified as *Torulopsis glabrata*.

*Can·di·da par·a·psi·lo·sis* a species of limited pathogenicity that may cause endocarditis, paronychia, and otitis externa.

*Can·di·da tro·pi·ca·lis* a species occasionally associated with candidiasis.

**can·di·de·mia** (kan-di-dē'mē-ă) presence of cells of *Candida* species in the peripheral blood. [*Candida* + G. *haima*, blood]

**can·di·di·a·sis** (kan-di-dī'ă-sis) infection with, or disease caused by, *Candida*, especially *C. albicans*. This disease usually results from debilitation (as in immunosuppression and especially AIDS), physiologic change, prolonged administration of antibiotics, and barrier breakage. See this page. SYN candidosis, moniliasis.

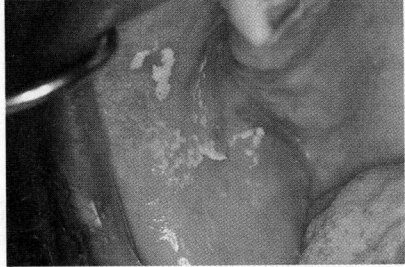

**candidiasis** of buccal mucosa

**can·di·do·sis** (kan-di-dō'sis) SYN candidiasis.
**can·dle-me·ter** (kan'dl-mē'ter) SYN lux.
**ca·nine** (kā'nīn) **1.** relating to a dog. **2.** relating to

the canine teeth. **3.** SYN canine tooth. **4.** referring to the cuspid tooth. [L. *caninus*]

**ca·nine tooth** a tooth having a crown of thick conical shape and a long, slightly flattened conical root; there are two canine teeth in each jaw, one on either side adjacent to the distal surface of the lateral incisors, in both the deciduous and the permanent dentition. SYN dens caninus [TA], canine (3), cuspid (2), eye tooth.

**ca·ni·ti·es** (kă-nish'ē-ēz) graying of hair. [L., fr. *canus*, hoary, gray]

**can·ker** (kang'ker) **1.** in cats and dogs, acute inflammation of the external ear and auditory canal. SEE aphtha. **2.** an outmoded term for aphthae. [L. *cancer*, crab, malignant growth]

**can·ker sores** SYN aphtha (2).

**can·nab·i·noids** (ka-nab'i-noydz) organic substances present in *Cannabis sativa*, having a variety of pharmacologic properties.

**can·na·bis** (kan'ă-bis) the dried flowering tops of the pistillate plants of *Cannabis sativa* (family Moraceae) containing isomeric tetrahydrocannabinols, cannabinol, and cannabidiol. Preparations of cannabis are smoked or ingested to induce psychotomimetic effects such as euphoria, hallucinations, drowsiness, and other mental changes. Cannabis was formerly used as a sedative and analgesic; now available for restricted use in management of iatrogenic anorexia, especially that associated with oncologic chemotherapy and radiation therapy. Known by many colloquial or slang terms such as marijuana; marihuana; pot; grass; bhang; charas; ganja; hashish. [L., fr. G. *kannabis*, hemp]

**can·na·bism** (kan'ă-bizm) poisoning by preparations of cannabis.

**Can·niz·za·ro re·ac·tion** (kahn'ē-tsah'rō) formation of an acid and an alcohol by the simultaneous oxidation of one aldehyde molecule and reduction of another; a dismutation: $2RCHO \rightarrow RCOOH + RCH_2OH$; when the aldehydes are not identical, this is referred to as a crossed Cannizzaro reaction.

**can·non·ball pulse** SYN water-hammer pulse.

**Can·non point** the location in the mid-transverse colon at which innervation by superior and inferior mesenteric plexuses overlap at the junction of the primitive midgut and hindgut, frequently resulting in narrowing evident on barium enema. SYN Cannon ring.

**Can·non ring** (kan'ŏn) SYN Cannon point.

**can·nu·la** (kan'yu-lă) a tube which can be inserted into a cavity, usually by means of a trocar filling its lumen; after insertion of the cannula, the trocar is withdrawn and the cannula remains as a channel for the transport of fluid. [L. dim. of *canna*, reed]

**can·nu·la·tion, can·nu·li·za·tion** (kan-yu-lā' shŭn, kan-yu-lī-zā'shŭn) insertion of a cannula.

**CANS** central auditory nervous system.

**Can·tel·li sign** (kahn-tĕ'lē) SEE doll's eye sign.

**can·ter·ing rhy·thm** SYN gallop.

**can·thal** (kan'thăl) relating to a canthus.

**can·thec·to·my** (kan-thek'tō-mē) excision of a palpebral canthus. [G. *kanthos*, canthus, + *ektomē*, excision]

**can·thi** (kan'thī) plural of canthus.

**can·thi·tis** (kan-thī'tis) inflammation of a canthus.

**can·thol·y·sis** (kan-thol'i-sis) SYN cantholysis (1). [G. *kanthos*, canthus, + *lysis*, loosening]

**can·tho·me·a·tal plane** plane passing through the two lateral angles of the eye and the center of the external acoustic meatus; this plane lies approximately midway between the Frankfort and the supraorbitomeatal planes.

**can·tho·plas·ty** (kan'thō-plas-tē) **1.** an operation for lengthening the palpebral fissure by incision through the lateral canthus. SYN cantholysis. **2.** an operation for restoration of the canthus. [G. *kanthos*, canthus, + *plassō*, to form]

**can·thor·rha·phy** (kan-thōr'ă-fē) suture of the eyelids at either canthus. [G. *kanthos*, canthus, + *rhaphē*, suture]

**can·thot·o·my** (kan-thot'ō-mē) slitting of the canthus. [G. *kanthos*, canthus, + *tomē*, incision]

**can·thus**, pl. **can·thi** (kan'thŭs, kan'thī) the angle of the eye. [G. *kanthos*, corner of the eye]

**can·ti·le·ver bridge** a fixed partial bridge denture in which the pontic is retained only on one side by an abutment tooth.

**CAP** catabolite (gene) activator protein.

**cap** (kap) **1.** any anatomic structure that resembles a cap or cover. **2.** a protective covering for an incomplete tooth. **3.** colloquialism for restoration of the coronal part of a natural tooth by means of an artificial crown. **4.** the nucleotide structure found at the 5′ terminus of many eukaryotic messenger RNAs.

**ca·pac·i·ta·tion** (kă-pas'i-tā'shŭn) a process whereby the glycoprotein coat and seminal proteins are removed from the acrosome of a sperm. Once capacitation has occurred, perforation of the acrosome can occur. [L. *capacitas*, fr. *capax*, capable of]

**ca·pac·i·tor** (kă-pas'i-ter) a device for holding a charge of electricity. SYN condenser (4).

**ca·pac·i·ty** (kă-pas'i-tē) **1.** the potential cubic contents of a cavity or receptacle. **2.** power to do. SEE ALSO volume. [L. *capax*, able to contain; fr. *capio*, to take]

**cap·ac·tins** (kap-ak'tinz) a class of proteins capping the ends of actin filaments.

**CAPD** continuous ambulatory peritoneal dialysis.

**cap·e·line ban·dage** a bandage covering the head or an amputation stump like a cap. [L. *capella*, a cap]

**Cap·gras syn·drome** (kahp'grah) the delusional belief that a person (or persons) close to the schizophrenic patient has been substituted for by one or more impostors; may have an organic etiology.

**Cap·il·la·ria gran·u·lo·ma** granulomatous lesions found in the liver and lung are a tissue response at the site of eggs or worms.

**cap·il·lar·i·o·mo·tor** (kap-i-lār'ē-ō-mō'tŏr) vasomotor, with special reference to the capillaries.

**cap·il·lar·i·tis** (kap'i-lar-ī'tis) inflammation of a capillary or capillaries.

**cap·il·lar·i·ty** (kap-i-lār'i-tē) the rise of liquids in narrow tubes or through the pores of a loose material, as a result of capillary action.

**cap·il·la·rop·a·thy** (kap'i-lă-rop'ă-thē) any disease of the capillaries, often applied to vascular changes in diabetes mellitus. SYN microangiopathy. [capillary + G. *pathos*, disease]

**cap·il·lary** (kap'i-lār-ē) **1.** resembling a hair; fine; minute. **2.** a capillary vessel; e.g., blood capillary, lymph capillary. **3.** relating to a blood or lymphatic capillary vessel. See this page. [L. *capillaris*, relating to hair]

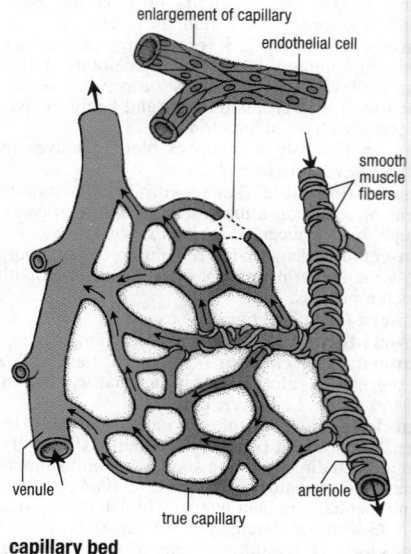

enlargement of capillary
endothelial cell
smooth muscle fibers
venule
arteriole
true capillary

**capillary bed**

**cap·il·lary ar·te·ri·ole** a minute artery that terminates in a capillary.

**cap·il·lary at·trac·tion** the force that causes fluids to rise up very fine tubes or pass through the pores of a loose material.

**cap·il·lary bed** the capillaries considered collectively and their volume capacity for blood.

**cap·il·lary drain·age** drainage by means of a wick of gauze or other material.

**cap·il·lary fil·ling** the return of a normal pink color to an area of skin, or a nail bed, after cutaneous capillaries have been emptied of blood by firm digital pressure; the promptness of return is a rough measure of general and vascular competence.

**cap·il·lary frac·ture** SYN hairline fracture.

**cap·il·lary fra·gil·i·ty** the susceptibility of capillaries to breakage and extravasation of red cells under conditions of increased stress.

**cap·il·lary he·man·gi·o·ma** an overgrowth of capillary blood vessels, seen most commonly in the skin, at or soon after birth, as a soft bright red to purple nodule or plaque that usually disappears by the fifth year. The most common type of hemangioma. SYN nevus vascularis, nevus vasculosus.

**cap·il·lary lake** the total mass of blood contained in capillary vessels.

**cap·il·lary vein** SYN venule.

**ca·pi·ta** (kap'i-tă) plural of caput.

**cap·i·tate** (kap'i-tāt) **1.** the largest of the carpal bones; located in the distal row. SYN capitate bone. **2.** head-shaped; having a rounded extremity. [L. *caput* (*capit*-), head]

**cap·i·tate bone** SYN capitate (1).

**cap·i·ta·tion** (kap'i-tā'shŭn) a system of medical reimbursement wherein the provider is paid an annual fee per covered patient by an insurer or other financial source, which aggregate fees are intended to reimburse all provided services. SEE

ALSO managed care. [L.L. *capitatio*, fr. *caput*, head]]

**cap·i·tel·lum** (kap-i-tel'ŭm) **1.** SYN capitulum (1). **2.** SYN capitulum of humerus. [L. dim. of *caput*, head]

**ca·pit·u·la** (kă-pit'yu-lă) plural of capitulum.

**ca·pit·u·lar** (kă-pit'yu-lăr) relating to a capitulum.

**ca·pit·u·lum**, pl. **ca·pit·u·la** (kă-pit'yu-lŭm, kă-pit'yu-lă) **1.** a small head or rounded articular extremity of a bone. SYN capitellum (1). SEE ALSO caput. **2.** the bloodsucking, probing, sensing, and holdfast mouthparts of a tick, including the basal supporting structure; relative size and shape of mouthparts forming the capitulum are characteristic for the genera of hard ticks. [L. dim. of *caput*, head]

**ca·pit·u·lum of hu·mer·us** the small rounded eminence on the lateral half of the distal end of the humerus for articulation with the radius. SYN capitellum (2).

**Cap·lan syn·drome** (kap'lăn) intrapulmonary nodules, histologically similar to subcutaneous rheumatoid nodules, associated with rheumatoid arthritis and pneumoconiosis in coal workers.

*Cap·no·cy·to·pha·ga* (kap'nō-sī-tŏf'a-ga) a genus of Gram-negative, fusiform-shaped bacteria associated with human periodontal disease.

**cap·no·gram** (kap'nō-gram) a continuous record of the carbon dioxide content of expired air. [G. *kapnos*, smoke, + *gramma*, something written]

**cap·no·graph** (kap'nō-graf) instrument by which a continuous graph of the carbon dioxide content of expired air is obtained.

**cap·no·met·er** (kap-nom'ĕ-ter) an instrument which measures the carbon dioxide concentration of exhaled air. SYN $CO_2$ analyzer. [G. *kapnos*, smoke, + *metron*, a measure]

**cap·no·met·ry** (kap-nom'ĕ-trē) the process of measuring and recording the carbon dioxide concentration of exhaled air at the patient's airway using a capnometer.

**cap·rate** (kap'rāt) a salt or ester of capric acid.

*n*-**cap·ric ac·id** (en-kap'rik as'id) a fatty acid found among the hydrolysis products of fat in goat's milk, cow's milk, and other substances. Cf. *n*-caproic acid, caprylic acid.

*n*-**ca·pro·ic ac·id** (en-kap-rō'ik as'id) a fatty acid found among the hydrolysis products of fat in butter, coconut oil, and some other substances.

**cap·ro·yl** (kap'rō-il) the acyl radical of caproic acid.

**cap·ro·y·late** (kap'rō-i-lāt) a salt or ester of caproic acid.

**cap·ry·late** (kap'ri-lāt) a salt or ester of caprylic acid.

**ca·pryl·ic ac·id** (kap-ril'ik as'id) a fatty acid found among the hydrolysis products of fat in butter, coconut oil, and other substances.

**cap·sid** (kap'sid) SEE virion.

**cap·su·la**, gen. and pl. **cap·su·lae** (kap'soo-lă, kap'soo-lē) [TA] **1.** a membranous structure, usually dense collagenous connective tissue, that envelops an organ, a joint, or any other part. **2.** an anatomic structure resembling a capsule or envelope. SYN capsule (1). [L. dim. of *capsa*, a chest or box]

**cap·su·la ar·ti·cu·la·ris** [TA] SYN articular capsule.

**cap·su·la ex·ter·na** [TA] SYN external capsule.

**cap·su·la fi·bro·sa pe·ri·vas·cu·la·ris he·pa·tis** [TA] SYN fibrous capsule of liver.

**cap·su·la in·ter·na** [TA] SYN internal capsule.

**cap·su·lar** (kap'soo-lăr) relating to any capsule.

**cap·su·lar an·ti·gen** that found only in the capsules of certain microorganisms; e.g., the specific polysaccharides of various types of pneumococci.

**cap·su·lar cat·a·ract** a cataract in which the opacity affects the capsule only.

**cap·su·lar lig·a·ment** thickened portions of the fibrous membrane of an articular capsule.

**cap·su·lar pat·tern** the pattern of limitation in range of motion exhibited by specific joints when inflamed; for example, the glenohumeral joint shows more limitation in external rotation than in internal rotation whereas the knee joint shows more limitation in flexion than in extension.

**cap·su·lar space** the slitlike space between the visceral and parietal layers of the capsule of the renal corpuscle; it opens into the proximal tubule of the nephron at the neck of the tubule.

**cap·sule** (kap'sool) **1.** SYN capsula. **2.** a fibrous tissue layer enveloping an organ or a neoplasm. **3.** a solid dosage form in which the drug is enclosed in either a hard or soft shell of soluble material. **4.** a hyaline glycosaminoglycan sheath on the wall of a fungus cell, blastoconidium, or spore. [L. *capsula*, dim. of *capsa*, box]

**cap·sule for·ceps** forceps used for removing the capsule of the lens in extracapsular extraction of a cataract.

**cap·sule of lens** the capsule enclosing the lens of the eye.

**cap·su·li·tis** (kap'soo-lī'tis) inflammation of the capsule of an organ or part, as of the liver or the lens of the eye.

**cap·su·lo·len·tic·u·lar** (kap'soo-lō-len-tik'yu-lăr) referring to the lens of the eye and its capsule.

**cap·su·lo·len·tic·u·lar cat·a·ract** a cataract in which both the lens and its capsule are involved. SEE ALSO membranous cataract.

**cap·su·lo·plas·ty** (kap'soo-lō-plas-tē) plastic surgery of a capsule; more specifically, the capsule of a joint. [L. *capsula*, capsule, + G. *plastos*, formed]

**cap·su·lor·rha·phy** (kap-soo-lōr'ă-fē) suture of a tear in any capsule; specifically, suture of a joint capsule to prevent recurring dislocation of the articulation. [L. *capsula*, capsule, + *rhaphē*, suture]

**cap·su·lor·rhex·is** (kap-soo-lō-reks'sis) technique used in cataract surgery by which a continuous circular tear is made in the anterior lens capsule. [L. *capsula*, capsule, + G. *rhēxis*, rupture]

**cap·su·lot·o·my** (kap-soo-lot'ō-mē) **1.** division of a capsule as around a breast implant. **2.** creation of an opening through a capsule; e.g., of a scar around a foreign body. **3.** incision of the capsule of the lens in the extracapsular cataract operation. [L. *capsula*, capsule, + G. *tomē*, a cutting]

**cap·ture** (kap'cher) catching and holding a particle or an electrical impulse originating elsewhere. [L. *capio*, pp. -*tus*, to take, seize]

**ca·put**, gen. **ca·pi·tis**, pl. **ca·pi·ta** (kap'ut, kap'i-tis, kap'i-tă) **1.** the upper or anterior extremity of the animal body, containing the brain and the organs of sight, hearing, taste, and smell. **2.** the upper, anterior, or larger extremity, expanded or rounded, of any body, organ, or other anatomic structure. **3.** the rounded extremity of a bone. **4.** that end of a muscle which is attached to the less movable part of the skeleton. [L.]

**ca·put me·du·sae 1.** varicose veins radiating from the umbilicus, seen in the Cruveilhier-Baumgarten syndrome; **2.** dilated ciliary arteries girdling the corneoscleral limbus in rubeosis iridis. SYN Medusa head. [*Medusa*, G. myth. char.]

**ca·put suc·ce·da·ne·um** an edematous swelling formed on the presenting portion of the scalp of an infant during birth.

**Ca·ra·bel·li cusp** (kah-rĕ-bel'ē) a cusp found on the lingual surface of the mesiolingual cusp of upper molars, ranging in size from a pit to a large cusp.

△**carb-, car·bo-** prefixes indicating carbon, especially the attachment of a group containing a carbon atom. [L. *carbo*, charcoal]

**car·ba·mate** (kar'bă-māt) **1.** a salt or ester of carbamic acid forming the basis of urethane hypnotics. **2.** a group of cholinesterase-inhibiting insecticides resembling organophosphates. SYN carbamoate.

**car·bam·ic ac·id** (kar-bam'ik as'id) a hypothetical acid, $NH_2$-COOH, forming carbamates; the acyl radical is carbamoyl.

**car·bam·i·no com·pound** any carbamic acid derivative formed by the combination of carbon dioxide with a free amino group to form an *N*-carboxyl group.

**carb·a·mi·no·he·mo·glo·bin** (kar-bam'i-nō-hē-mō-glō'bin) carbon dioxide bound to hemoglobin by means of a reactive amino group on the latter; approximately 20% of the total carbon dioxide in blood is combined with hemoglobin in this manner.

**car·ba·moate** (kar'ba-mōt) SYN carbamate.

**car·bam·o·yl** (kar'bă-mō-il) the acyl radical, $NH_2$-CO-, the transfer of which plays an important role in certain biochemical reactions. SYN carbamyl.

*N*-**car·bam·o·yl·as·par·tic acid** (kar'bă-mō-il-as-par'tik as'id) SYN ureidosuccinic acid.

**car·bam·o·yl·trans·fer·as·es** (kar'bă-mō-il-trans'fer-ās-ĕz) [EC group 2.1.3] enzymes transferring carbamoyl groups from one compound to another. SYN transcarbamoylases.

**car·bam·o·yl·u·rea** (kar'bă-mō-il-yu-rē'ă) SYN biuret.

**car·ba·myl** (kar'bă-mil) SYN carbamoyl.

**car·bo·ben·zoxy-** (kar'bō-ben-zok'sē) SYN benzyloxycarbonyl.

**car·bo·gen** (kar'bō-jen) a mixture of 10% carbon dioxide and 90% oxygen used for inhalation therapy to produce vasodilation. [*carbo*n dioxide + oxy*gen*]

**car·bo·hy·drate load·ing** combination of diet and exercise to significantly increase muscle and liver glycogen content. Frequently used by endurance athletes to enhance performance. SYN glycogen loading, glycogen supercompensation.

**car·bo·hy·drates** (kar-bō-hī'drāts) class name for the aldehydic or ketonic derivatives of polyhydric alcohols. Most such compounds have formulas that may be written $C_n(H_2O)_n$, although they are not true hydrates. The group includes simple sugars (monosaccharides, disaccharides, etc.), as well as macromolecular (polymeric) substances such as starch, glycogen, and cellulose polysaccharides. SEE ALSO saccharides.

**car·bo·hy·drat·u·ria** (kar'bō-hī-dră-tyu'rē-ă) excretion of one or more carbohydrates in the urine.

**car·bo·lu·ria** (kar-bō-lyu'rē-ă) the presence of phenol (carbolic acid) in the urine. [carbolic acid + G. *ouron*, urine]

**car·bon (C)** (kar'bŏn) a nonmetallic tetravalent element, atomic no. 6, atomic wt. 12.011; the major bioelement. It has two natural isotopes, $^{12}C$ and $^{13}C$ (the former, set at 12.00000, being the standard for all molecular weights), and two artificial, radioactive isotopes of interest, $^{11}C$ and $^{14}C$. The element occurs in diamond, graphite, charcoal, coke, and soot, and in the atmosphere as $CO_2$. Its compounds are found in all living tissues, and the study of its vast number of compounds constitutes most of organic chemistry. [L. *carbo*, coal]

**car·bon·ate** (kar'bŏn-āt) **1.** a salt of carbonic acid. **2.** the ion $CO_3^=$.

**car·bon di·ox·ide** the product of the combustion of carbon with an excess of air; in concentrations not less than 99.0% by volume of $CO_2$, used as a respiratory stimulant.

**car·bon di·ox·ide com·bin·ing pow·er** a measurement of the total $CO_2$ that can be bound as $HCO_2$ at a $P_{CO_2}$ of 40 mmHg at 25 C by serum, plasma, or whole blood.

**car·bon di·ox·ide cy·cle, car·bon cy·cle** the circulation of carbon as $CO_2$ from the expired air of animals and decaying organic matter to plant life where it is synthesized (through photosynthesis) to carbohydrate material, from which, as a result of catabolic processes in all life, it is again ultimately released to the atmosphere as $CO_2$.

**car·bon di·ox·ide pro·duc·tion ($\dot{V}CO_2$)** the volume of carbon dioxide produced by the body in one minute; it is reported in liters or ml per minute at STPD.

**car·bon mon·ox·ide (CO)** a colorless, practically odorless, and poisonous gas formed by the incomplete combustion of carbon; its toxic action is due to its strong affinity for hemoglobin, myoglobin, and the cytochromes, reducing oxygen transport and blocking oxygen utilization.

**car·bon mon·ox·ide he·mo·glo·bin** SYN carboxyhemoglobin.

**car·bon mon·ox·ide poi·son·ing** a potentially fatal acute or chronic intoxication caused by inhalation of carbon monoxide gas which competes favorably with oxygen for binding with hemoglobin (carboxyhemoglobinemia) and thus interferes with the transportation of oxygen and carbon dioxide by the blood.

**car·bon·yl** (kar'bŏn-il) the characteristic group, —CO—, of the ketones, aldehydes, and organic acids.

△**car·boxy-** combining form indicating addition of CO or $CO_2$.

**car·box·y·he·mo·glo·bin** (kar-bok'sē-hē-mō-glō'bin) a stable union of carbon monoxide with hemoglobin. The formation of carboxyhemoglobin prevents the normal transfer of carbon dioxide and oxygen during the circulation of blood; thus, increasing levels of carboxyhemoglobin result in various degrees of asphyxiation, including death. SYN carbon monoxide hemoglobin.

**car·box·y·he·mo·glo·bi·ne·mia** (kar-bok'sē-hē'mō-glō-bi-nē'mē-ă) presence of carboxyhemoglobin in the blood, as in carbon monoxide poisoning.

**car·box·yl** (kar-bok′sil) the characterizing group (—COOH) of organic acids.

**car·box·yl·ase** (kar-bok′sil-ās) one of several carboxy-lyases catalyzing the addition of $CO_2$ to another molecule to create an additional —COOH group.

**car·box·yl·a·tion** (kar-bok-si-lā′shŭn) addition of $CO_2$ to an organic acceptor to yield a —COOH group; catalyzed by carboxylases.

**car·box·yl·trans·fer·as·es** (kar-bok-sil-trans′fer-ās-ez) [EC group 2.1.3] enzymes transferring carboxyl groups from one compound to another. SYN transcarboxylases.

**car·box·y·pep·ti·dase** (kar-bok-sē-pep′ti-dās) a hydrolase that removes the amino acid at the free carboxyl end of a polypeptide chain; an exopeptidase.

**car·bun·cle** (kar′bŭng-kl) **1.** deep-seated pyogenic infection of the skin and subcutaneous tissues, usually arising in several contiguous hair follicles, with formation of connecting sinuses. **2.** SYN anthrax. [L. *carbunculus,* dim. of *carbo,* a live coal, a carbuncle]

**car·bun·cu·lar** (kar-bŭng′kyu-lăr) relating to a carbuncle.

**car·bun·cu·lo·sis** (kar-bŭng-kyu-lō′sis) a condition marked by the occurrence of several carbuncles simultaneously or within a short period of time.

**car·cin·ae·mia [Br.]** SEE carcinemia.

**car·ci·ne·mia** (kar-sĭ-nē′mē-ă) the presence of malignant cells in the blood. [carcin- + G. *haima,* blood]

△**car·ci·no-, car·cin-** cancer; crab. [G. *karkinos,* crab, cancer]

**car·ci·no·em·bry·on·ic** (kar′si-nō-em-brē-on′ik) pertaining to a substance found in embryonic tissue but absent from adult tissue except in certain carcinomas of the lung, digestive tract, and pancreas.

**car·ci·no·em·bry·on·ic an·ti·gen (CEA)** a glycoprotein constituent of the glycocalyx of embryonic endodermal epithelium, generally absent from adult cells with the exception of some carcinomas. It may also be detected in the serum of patients with colon cancer.

**car·cin·o·gen** (kar-sin′ō-jen, kar′si-nō-jen) any cancer-producing substance or organism, such as polycyclic aromatic hydrocarbons, or agents such as certain types of irradiation. [carcino- + G, *-gen,* producing]

**car·ci·no·gen·e·sis** (kar′si-nō-jen′ĕ-sis) the origin, production, or development of cancer, including carcinomas and other malignant neoplasms. [carcino- + G. *genesis,* generation]

**car·ci·no·gen·ic** (kar′si-nō-jen′ik) causing cancer.

**car·ci·noid syn·drome** a combination of symptoms and lesions usually produced by the release of serotonin from carcinoid tumors of the gastrointestinal tract that have metastasized to the liver; consists of irregular mottled blushing, flat angiomas of the skin, acquired tricuspid and pulmonary stenosis often with regurgitation, diarrhea, bronchial spasm, mental aberration, and excretion of large quantities of 5-hydroxyindoleacetic acid.

**car·ci·noid tu·mor** a neoplasm composed of cells of medium size, with moderately small vesicular nuclei; neoplastic cells are frequently palisaded at the periphery of small groups. Such neoplasms occur in the gastrointestinal tract, the lungs, and other sites, with approximately 90% in the appendix. SEE ALSO carcinoid syndrome. SYN argentaffinoma.

**car·ci·no·lyt·ic** (kar′si-nō-lit′ik) destructive to the cells of carcinoma. [carcino- + G. *lytikos,* causing a solution]

⊞**car·ci·no·ma (CA),** pl. **car·ci·no·mas, car·cin·o·ma·ta** (kar-si-nō′mă, kar-si-nō′măz, kar-si-nō′mă-tă) any of the various types of malignant neoplasm derived from epithelial tissue, occurring more frequently in the skin and large intestine in both sexes, the lung and prostate gland in men, and the lung and breast in women. Carcinomas are identified histologically on the basis of invasiveness and the changes that indicate anaplasia, i.e., loss of polarity of nuclei, loss of orderly maturation of cells (especially in squamous cell type), variation in the size and shape of cells, hyperchromatism of nuclei (with clumping of chromatin), and increase in the nuclear-cytoplasmic ratio. Carcinomas may be undifferentiated, or the neoplastic tissue may resemble (to varying degree) one of the types of normal epithelium. See page B8. [G. *karkinōma,* fr. *karkinos,* cancer, + *-oma,* tumor]

**car·ci·no·ma of the breast** a malignant tumor arising from epithelial cells of the female (and occasionally the male) breast, usually adenocarcinoma arising from ductal epithelium.

**car·ci·no·ma of the pro·state** a malignant neoplasm arising from glandular epithelial cells of the prostate gland.

**car·ci·no·ma in si·tu (CIS)** a lesion characterized by cytologic changes of the type associated with invasive carcinoma, but with the pathologic process limited to the lining epithelium and without histologic evidence of extension to adjacent structures. The lesion is presumed to be the precursor of invasive carcinoma, i.e., a localized and curable phase of carcinoma.

**car·ci·no·ma·ta** (kar-si-nō′mă-tă) alternative plural of carcinoma.

**car·ci·no·ma·to·sis** (kar′si-nō-mă-tō′sis) widespread dissemination of carcinoma in various organs or tissues of the body. SYN carcinosis.

**car·ci·nom·a·tous** (kar-si-nom′ă-tŭs) pertaining to or manifesting the properties of carcinoma.

**car·ci·no·pho·bia** (kar′sin-ō-fō′bē-ă) SYN cancerophobia.

**car·ci·no·sar·co·ma** (kar′si-nō-sar-kō′mă) a malignant neoplasm that contains elements of carcinoma and sarcoma so extensively intermixed as to indicate neoplasia of epithelial and mesenchymal tissue.

**car·ci·no·sis** (kar-si-nō′sis) SYN carcinomatosis.

**Car·den am·pu·ta·tion** (kahr′den) transcondylar amputation of the leg; the femur is sawed through the condyles just above the articular surface.

**car·di·ac ar·rest (CA)** complete cessation of cardiac activity either electric, mechanical, or both; may be purposely induced for therapeutic reasons.

**car·di·ac ar·rhyth·mia** SEE cardiac dysrhythmia.

**car·di·ac asth·ma** an asthmatic attack due to the pulmonary congestion and edema caused by left ventricular failure.

**car·di·ac care tech·ni·cian** SYN emergency medical technician–intermediate.

**car·di·ac cath·e·ter** SYN intracardiac catheter.

**car·di·ac cir·rho·sis** an extensive fibrotic reaction within the liver as a result of chronic constrictive pericarditis or prolonged congestive heart failure; true cirrhosis with fibrous bridging of lobules is unusual.

**car·di·ac cy·cle** the complete round of cardiac systole and diastole with the intervals between, commencing with any event in the heart's action and ending when same event is repeated.

**car·di·ac de·com·pres·sion** incision into the pericardium or aspiration of fluid from pericardium to relieve pressure due to blood or other fluid in the pericardial sac. SYN pericardial decompression.

**car·di·ac dys·rhyth·mia** any abnormality in the rate, regularity, or sequence of cardiac activation.

**car·di·ac e·de·ma** edema resulting from congestive heart failure.

**car·di·ac gan·glia** parasympathetic ganglia of the cardiac plexus lying between the arch of the aorta and the bifurcation of the pulmonary artery.

**car·di·ac gat·ing** using an electronic signal from the cardiac cycle to trigger an event, such as in imaging separate phases of cardiac contraction.

**car·di·ac gland** a coiled tubular gland located in the cardiac region of the stomach; secretes primarily mucus.

**car·di·ac his·ti·o·cyte** a large mononuclear cell found in connective tissue of the heart wall in inflammatory conditions, especially in the Aschoff body. SYN Anitschkow cell, Anitschkow myocyte.

**car·di·ac in·dex** the amount of blood ejected by the heart in a unit of time divided by the body surface area; usually expressed in liters per minute per square meter.

**car·di·ac in·suf·fi·cien·cy** SYN heart failure (1).

**car·di·ac jel·ly** the gelatinous, noncellular material between the endothelial lining and the myocardial layer of the heart in very young embryos; later in development it serves as a substratum for cardiac mesenchyme.

**car·di·ac mur·mur** a murmur produced within the heart, at one of its valvular orifices or across ventricular septal defects.

**car·di·ac mus·cle** the muscle forming the myocardium, consisting of anastomosing transversely striated muscle fibers formed of cells united at intercalated disks. SYN muscle of heart.

**car·di·ac neu·ro·sis** anxiety concerning the state of the heart, as a result of palpitation, chest pain, or other symptoms not due to heart disease; a form of hypochondriasis. SYN cardioneurosis.

**car·di·ac notch** a deep notch between the esophagus and fundus of the stomach.

**car·di·ac or·i·fice** the trumpet-shaped opening of the esophagus into the stomach.

**car·di·ac plex·us** a wide-meshed network of cardiopulmonary and splanchnic nerves arising from the afferent and autonomic nerve fibers (sympathetic) and vagus (parasympathetic) nerves, surrounding the arch of the aorta, the pulmonary artery, and continuing to the atria, ventricles, and coronary vessels.

**car·di·ac re·ha·bil·i·ta·tion** a systematic program of exercise and nutritional, behavioral, and vocational counseling to optimize the recovery and physiologic capacity of the patient with car-

diovascular disease, particularly during recovery after myocardial infarction.

**car·di·ac res·cue tech·ni·cian** SYN emergency medical technician–intermediate.

**car·di·ac re·serve** the work which the heart is able to perform beyond that required under the ordinary circumstances of daily life, depending upon the state of the myocardium and the degree to which, within physiologic limits, the cardiac muscle fibers can be stretched by the volume of blood reaching the heart during diastole.

**car·di·ac souf·fle** a soft, puffing heart murmur.

**car·di·ac sphinc·ter** a physiologic sphincter at the esophagogastric junction.

**car·di·ac tam·pon·ade** compression of the heart due to critically increased volume of fluid in the pericardium.

**car·di·ac val·vu·lar in·com·pe·tence** failure of a valve to close its aperture completely and prevent regurgitation of blood.

**car·di·ec·ta·sia** (kar'dē-ek-tā'zē-ă) SYN ectasia cordis. [cardi- + G. *ektasis*, a stretching]

**car·di·nal lig·a·ment** a fibrous band attached to the uterine cervix and the vault of the lateral fornix of the vagina; continuous with the tissue ensheathing the pelvic vessels.

**car·di·nal points 1.** the four points in the pelvic inlet toward one of which the occiput of the baby is usually directed in case of head presentation: two sacroiliac articulations and the two iliopectineal eminences corresponding to the acetabula; **2.** six points of a compound optical system: the anterior focal point, the posterior focal point, the two principal points, and the two nodal points.

**car·di·nal symp·tom** the primary or major symptom of diagnostic importance.

**car·di·nal veins** the major systemic venous channels in adult primitive vertebrates and in the embryos of higher vertebrates; the **anterior cardinal veins** are the major drainage channels from the cephalic part of the body, and the **posterior cardinal veins**, from the caudal part; the **common cardinal veins**, formed by the anastomosis of the anterior and posterior cardinal veins, are the main systemic return channels to the heart.

△**cardio-, cardi-** the heart. [G. *kardia*, heart]

**car·di·o·ac·cel·er·a·tor** (kar'dē-ō-ak-sel'er-ā-ter) accelerator of the heart beat.

**car·di·o·ac·tive** (kar'dē-ō-ak'tiv) influencing the heart.

**car·di·o·a·or·tic** (kar'dē-ō-ā-ōr'tik) relating to the heart and the aorta.

**car·di·o·ar·te·ri·al** (kar'dē-ō-ar-tēr'ē-ăl) relating to the heart and the arteries.

***Car·di·o·bac·te·ri·um*** (kar'dē-ō-bak-tē'rē-ŭm) a genus of nonmotile, pleomorphic, Gram-negative, facultatively anaerobic, rod-shaped bacteria found in the nasal flora and associated with endocarditis in humans. The type species is *Cardiobacterium hominis*.

***Car·di·o·bac·te·ri·um hom·i·nis*** a species that causes endocarditis in humans. The type species of *Cardiobacterium*. SEE HACEK group.

***Car·di·o·bac·te·ri·um vi·o·la·ce·um*** a motile, Gram-negative, non–spore-bearing rod, found in soil in tropical and subtropical environments; a cause of human infections including septicemia, pneumonia, wound infections, and abscesses; infection can be rapidly fatal, and may relapse after cessation of antibiotic therapy.

**car·di·o·cele** (kar'dē-ō-sēl) a herniation or protrusion of the heart through an opening in the diaphragm, or through a wound. [cardio- + G. *kēlē,* hernia]

**car·di·o·cha·la·sia** (kar'dē-ō-kă-lā'zē-ă) achalasia of the cardia.

**car·di·o·dy·nam·ics** (kar'dē-ō-dī-nam'iks) the mechanics of the heart's action, including its movement and the forces generated thereby.

**car·di·o·dyn·ia** (kar'dē-ō-din'ē-ă) pain in the heart. [cardio- + G. *odynē,* pain]

**car·di·o·e·soph·a·ge·al** (kar'dē-ō-ē-sof-ă-jē'ăl) denoting the junction of the esophagus and cardiac part of the stomach.

**car·di·o·e·soph·a·ge·al junc·tion** the abrupt transition from esophageal mucosa to that of the cardiac portion of stomach, demarcated internally in the living by the z-line, and approximated externally by the cardiac notch.

**car·di·o·gen·ic** (kar'dē-ō-jen'ik) of cardiac origin.

**car·di·o·gen·ic shock** shock resulting from decline in cardiac output secondary to serious heart disease, usually myocardial infarction.

**car·di·o·gram** (kar'dē-ō-gram) **1.** the graphic tracing made by the stylet of a cardiograph. **2.** any recording derived from the heart, with such prefixes as apex-, echo-, electro-, phono-, or vector- being understood. [cardio- + G. *gramma,* a diagram]

**car·di·o·graph** (kar'dē-ō-graf) an instrument for recording graphically the movements of the heart, constructed on the principle of the sphygmograph. [cardio- + G. *graphō,* to write]

**car·di·og·ra·phy** (kar-dē-og'ră-fē) the use of the cardiograph.

**car·di·o·he·pat·ic** (kar'dē-ō-hĕ-pat'ik) relating to the heart and the liver.

**car·di·o·ky·mo·gram** (kar'dē-ō-kī'mō-gram) record made by a cardiokymograph.

**car·di·o·ky·mo·graph** (kar'dē-ō-kī'mō-graf) device placed on the chest to record anterior left ventricle segmental wall motion; consists of a plate transducer with recording probe; changes in wall motion affect the magnetic field and thus the oscillatory frequency, which is recorded on a waveform polygraph.

**car·di·o·ky·mog·ra·phy** (kar'dē-ō-kī-mog'ră-fē) use of a cardiokymograph.

**car·di·o·lip·in** (kar'dē-ō-lip'in) a 1,3-bis-(phosphatidyl)glycerol found in many biomembranes with immunological properties; used in serological diagnosis of syphilis.

**car·di·ol·o·gist** (kar-dē-ol'ō-jist) physician specializing in cardiology.

**car·di·ol·o·gy** (kar-dē-ol'ō-jē) the medical specialty concerned with the diagnosis and treatment of heart disease. [cardio- + G. *logos,* study]

**car·di·o·ma·la·cia** (kar'dē-ō-mă-lā'shē-ă) softening of the walls of the heart. [cardio- + G. *malakia,* softness]

**car·di·o·meg·a·ly** (kar-dē-ō-meg'ă-lē) enlargement of the heart. SYN macrocardia, megalocardia. [cardio- + G. *megas,* large]

**car·di·o·mo·til·i·ty** (kar'dē-ō-mō-til'ĭ-tē) movements of the heart.

**car·di·o·mus·cu·lar** (kar'dē-ō-mŭs'kyu-lăr) pertaining to the cardiac musculature.

**car·di·o·my·o·li·po·sis** (kar'dē-ō-mī'ō-li-pō'sis) fatty degeneration of the myocardium. [cardio- + G. *mys,* muscle, + *lipos,* fat, + *-osis,* condition]

**car·di·o·my·op·a·thy** (kar'dē-ō-mī-op'ă-thē)

disease of the myocardium; a primary disease of heart muscle in the absence of a known underlying etiology. SYN myocardiopathy. [cardio- + G. *mys,* muscle, + *pathos,* disease]

**car·di·o·my·o·plas·ty** (kar'dē-ō-mī'ō-plas-tē) an operation that uses latissimus dorsi muscle to assist cardiac function. The muscle is moved into the thorax through the bed of the resected second or third rib, wrapped around the left and right ventricles, and stimulated to contract during cardiac systole by means of an implanted burst-stimulator.

**car·di·o·neph·ric** (kar'dē-ō-nef'rik) SYN cardiorenal.

**car·di·o·neu·ral** (kar'dē-ō-noor'ăl) relating to the nervous control of the heart. [cardio- + G. *neuron,* nerve]

**car·di·o·neu·ro·sis** (kar'dē-ō-noo-rō'sis) SYN cardiac neurosis.

**car·di·o·o·men·to·pexy** (kar'dē-ō-ō-men'tō-pek-sē) operation for the attachment of omentum to the heart with the object of improving its blood supply. [cardio- + omentum, + G. *pēxis,* fixation]

**car·di·op·a·thy** (kar-dē-op'ă-thē) any disease of the heart. [cardio- + G. *pathos,* disease]

**car·di·o·per·i·car·di·o·pexy** (kar'dē-ō-pār-i-kar'dē-ō-pek-sē) an operation to increase the blood supply to the myocardium; magnesium silicate is spread within the pericardial sac, or the sac is mechanically abraded, to cause an adhesive pericarditis and an increase in blood supply to develop. [cardio- + pericardium, + G. *pēxis,* fixation]

**car·di·o·pho·bia** (kar'dē-ō-fō'bē-ă) morbid fear of heart disease.

**car·di·o·phren·ic an·gle** the angle between the heart and the diaphragm at either side of the cardiac projection, usually as seen in a postero-anterior chest x-ray.

**car·di·o·plas·ty** (kar'dē-ō-plas-tē) an operation on the cardia of the stomach. SYN esophagogastroplasty, oesophagogastroplasty. [cardio- (2) + G. *plastos,* formed]

**car·di·o·ple·gia** (kar'dē-ō-plē'jē-ă) **1.** paralysis of the heart. **2.** an elective stopping of cardiac activity temporarily by injection of chemicals, selective hypothermia, or electrical stimuli. [cardio- + G. *plēgē,* stroke]

**car·di·o·ple·gic** (kar-dē-ō-plē'jik) relating to cardioplegia.

**car·di·o·ple·gic ar·rest** stoppage of electrical and mechanical cardiac activity, used by surgeons when operating upon the heart.

**car·di·op·to·sia, car·di·op·to·sis** (kar'dē-op-tō'sē-ă, kar'dē-op-tō'sis; kar'dē-op'tŏ-sis) a condition in which the heart is unduly movable and displaced downward, as distinguished from bathycardia. [cardio- + G. *ptōsis,* a falling]

**car·di·o·pul·mo·nary** (kar'dē-ō-pŭl'mŏ-ner-ē) relating to the heart and lungs. SYN pneumocardial.

**car·di·o·pul·mo·nary by·pass** diversion of the blood flow returning to the heart through a pump oxygenator (heart-lung machine) and then returning it to the arterial side of the circulation; used in operations upon the heart to maintain extracorporeal circulation.

**car·di·o·pul·mo·nary mur·mur** an innocent extracardiac murmur, synchronous with the heart's beat but disappearing when the breath is held, believed due to movement of air in a seg-

c
a

ment of lung compressed by the contracting heart.

**car·di·o·pul·mo·nary re·sus·ci·ta·tion (CPR)** restoration of cardiac output and pulmonary ventilation following cardiac arrest and apnea, using artificial respiration and manual closed chest compression or open chest cardiac massage.

**car·di·o·py·lo·ric** (kar'dē-ō-pi-lōr'ik) relating to the cardiac and pyloric extremities of the stomach.

**car·di·o·re·nal** (kar'dē-ō-rē'năl) relating to the heart and the kidney. SYN cardionephric, nephrocardiac.

**car·di·or·rha·phy** (kar-dē-ōr'ă-fē) suture of the heart wall. [cardio- + G. *rhaphē,* suture]

**car·di·or·rhex·is** (kar-dē-ō-rek'sis) rupture of the heart wall. [cardio- + G. *rhēxis,* rupture]

**car·di·o·se·lec·tive** (kar'dē-ō-sĕ-lek'tiv) denoting or having the properties of cardioselectivity.

**car·di·o·se·lec·tiv·i·ty** (kar'dē-ō-sĕ-lek-tiv'i-tē) the relatively predominant cardiovascular pharmacologic effect of a drug with multipharmacologic effects; used especially when describing beta-blocking agents.

**car·di·o·spasm** (kar'dē-ō-spazm) SYN esophageal achalasia.

**car·di·o·sphyg·mo·graph** (kar'dē-ō-sfig'mō-graf) an instrument for recording graphically the movements of the heart and the radial pulse. [cardio- + G. *sphygmos,* pulse, + *graphō,* to write]

**car·di·o·ta·chom·e·ter** (kar'dē-ō-tă-kom'ĕ-ter) an instrument for measuring heart rate. [cardio- + G. *tachos,* rapidity, + *metron,* measure]

**car·di·o·tho·rac·ic ra·tio** the ratio of the horizontal diameter of the heart to the inner diameter of the rib cage at its widest point as determined on a chest roentgenogram.

**car·di·ot·o·my** (kar-dē-ot'ŏ-mē) **1.** incision of a heart wall. **2.** incision of the cardiac part of the stomach. [cardio- + G. *tomē,* incision]

**car·di·o·ton·ic** (kar'dē-ō-ton'ik) exerting a favorable, so-called tonic effect upon the action of the heart; usually intended to indicate increased force of contraction. [cardio- + G. *tonos,* tension]

**car·di·o·tox·ic** (kar'dē-ō-tok'sik) having a deleterious effect upon the action of the heart, due to poisoning of the cardiac muscle or of its conducting system. [cardio- + G. *toxikon,* poison]

**car·di·o·val·vu·li·tis** (kar'dē-ō-val-vyu-lī'tis) inflammation of the heart valves.

**car·di·o·vas·cu·lar** (kar'dē-ō-vas'kyu-lăr) relating to the heart and the blood vessels or the circulation. SYN cardiovasculare. [cardio- + L. *vasculum,* vessel]

**car·di·o·vas·cu·lar drift** the gradual time-dependent downward "drift" in several cardiovascular responses, most notably stroke volume (with concomitant heart rate increase), during prolonged steady-rate exercise. The progressive increase in heart rate with cardiovascular drift during exercise decreases end-diastolic volume and hence stroke volume.

**cardiovasculare** SYN cardiovascular.

**car·di·o·ver·sion** (kar'dē-ō-ver'zhŭn) restoration of the heart's rhythm to normal by electrical countershock. [cardio- + con*version*]

**car·di·o·ver·ter** (kar'dē-ō-ver'ter) a machine used to perform cardioversion.

**car·di·tis** (kar-dī'tis) inflammation of the heart.

**care** (kār) in medicine and public health, a general term for the application of knowledge to the benefit of a community or individual.

**care·giver 1.** general term for a physician, nurse, or other healthcare practitioner who cares for patients. **2.** any person, including a family member, who provides care or assistance to one who is ill.

**care·plan** a written, well thought out, and prepared plan of nursing care outlining all the patient's needs and ways of meeting them. A dynamic, not static, document, more like a worksheet that is usually initiated by the admitting nurse and then is subject to ongoing reassessment and change by all nursing staff caring for the patient. The careplan ensures some consistency of care and team work. SYN plan of care.

**Car·ey Coombs mur·mur** (ka'rē koomz) a blubbering apical middiastolic murmur occurring in the acute stage of rheumatic mitral valvulitis and disappearing as the valvulitis subsides.

**Car·hart notch** (kahr'hart) isolated depression around 200 Hz in the bone-conduction audiogram of patients with otosclerosis. SEE air-bone gap. SEE ALSO otosclerosis.

**car·ies,** pl. **car·ies** (kār'ēz, kār'ēz) microbial destruction or necrosis of teeth. See this page. [L. dry rot]

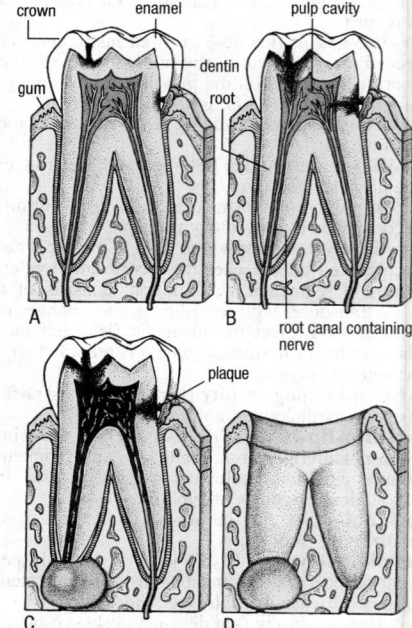

**caries:** (zones of dental caries shown in black); (A) acid, enzymes, or both produced by oral bacteria break down to form cavities; (B) bacteria penetrate dentin to invade pulp cavity; (C) infection destroys pulp and extends through left root canal to cause periapical disease; (D) tooth has been lost, leaving periapical cyst on the left

**ca·ri·na,** pl. **ca·ri·nae** (kă-rī'nă, kă-rī'nē) a term applied to anatomic structures forming a projecting central ridge. See page B8. [L. the keel of a boat]

**car·i·nate** (kar'i-nāt) shaped like a keel; relating to or resembling a carina.

**car·i·nate ab·do·men** a sloping of the sides with prominence of the central line of the abdomen.

△**cario-** caries. [L. *caries*]

**car·i·o·gen·e·sis** (kā'rē-ō-jen'ĕ-sis) the process of producing caries; the mechanism of caries production.

**car·i·o·gen·ic** (kā'rē-ō-jen'ik) producing caries; usually said of diets.

**car·i·o·ge·nic·i·ty** (kā'rē-ō-jĕ-nis'i-tē) potential for caries production.

**car·i·ol·o·gy** (kā-rē-ol'ō-jē) the study of dental caries and cariogenesis.

**car·i·ous** (kār'ē-ŭs) relating to or affected with caries.

**Car·len tube** (kahr'len) a double-lumen, flexible endobronchial tube used for bronchospirometry, for isolation of one lung to prevent contamination or secretions from the contralateral lung, or for ventilation of one lung.

**Car·man sign** (cahr'măn) in gastric radiology, the appearance of a contrast-filled malignant ulcer, which does not extend beyond the line of the gastric wall as a benign ulcer would; also has a thick overhanging rim of tumor tissue.

**car·min·a·tive** (kar-min'ă-tiv) an agent such as peppermint oil that is taken after a meal to facilitate belching through relaxation of the lower esophageal sphincter, thereby averting passage of swallowed air into the intestine as flatus. [L. *carmino*, pp. -*atus*, to card wool; special Mod. L. usage, to expel wind]

**car·mine** (kar'mēn) [CI 75470] red coloring matter used as a histology stain produced from coccinellin derived from cochineal; treatment of coccinellin with alum forms an aluminum lake of carminic acid, the essential constituent of carmine. [Mediev. L. *carminus*, contr. fr. *carmisinus*, fr. Ar. *qirmizē*, the cochineal insect]

**car·min·o·phil, car·min·o·phile, car·mi·noph·i·lous** (kar-min'ō-fil, kar-min'ō-fīl, kar-mi-nof'i-lŭs) staining readily with carmine dyes. [G. *phileō*, to love]

**car·nas·si·al tooth** a long-bladed premolar or molar of the Carnivora that has a cutting or shearing action, as in dogs or cats. SYN sectorial tooth.

**Car·nett sign** (kahr-net') disappearance of abdominal tenderness to palpation when the anterior abdominal muscles are contracted, indicating pain of intra-abdominal origin; persistence of tenderness suggests a source in the abdominal wall, which is also indicated when tenderness is caused by gently pinching a fold of skin and fat between the thumb and forefinger.

**car·ni·tine** (kar'ni-tēn) the L-isomer is a thyroid inhibitor found in muscle, liver, and meat extracts; L-carnitine is an acyl carrier with respect to the mitochondrial membrane; it thus stimulates fatty acid oxidation. [L. *caro, carn-*, flesh, + ine]

**Car·noy fix·a·tive** (kahr'noy) ethanol, chloroform, and acetic acid (6:3:1) or ethanol and acetic acid (3:1), an extremely rapid fixative used for glycogen preservation and as a nuclear fixative.

**Ca·ro·li dis·ease, Ca·ro·li syn·drome** (kah-rō-lē') congenital cystic dilation of the intrahepatic bile ducts, sometimes associated with intrahepatic stones and biliary obstruction.

**car·o·tene** (kar'ŏ-tēn) yellow-red pigments (lipochromes) widely distributed in plants and animals, notably in carrots, and closely related in structure to the xanthophylls and lycopenes and to the open-chain squalene; they include precursors of the vitamins A (provitamin A carotenoids).

**β-car·o·tene-cleav·age en·zyme** SYN β-carotene 15,15'-dioxygenase.

**β-car·o·tene 15,15'-di·ox·y·gen·ase** (bā'ta-kar'ŏ-tēn- dī-oks'ē-jen-āz) an enzyme catalyzing the reaction of β-carotene plus $O_2$ producing two retinals. SYN β-carotene-cleavage enzyme.

**car·o·ten·e·mia** (kar'ŏ-te-nē'mē-ă) carotene in the blood, especially pertaining to increased quantities, which sometimes cause a pale yellow-red pigmentation of the skin that may resemble icterus. SYN xanthemia.

**car·o·ten·o·der·ma** (ka-rŏt'en-ō-der-mă) SYN carotenosis cutis. [carotene + G. *derma*, skin]

**ca·rot·e·noid** (ka-rŏt'e-noyd) 1. resembling carotene; having a yellow color. 2. one of the carotenoids.

**ca·rot·e·noids** (ka-rŏt'e-noydz) generic term for a class of carotenes and their oxygenated derivatives (xanthophylls). Many carotenoids have anticancer activities.

**car·o·te·no·sis cu·tis** (kar-ŏ-te-nō'sis kyu'tis) a harmless reversible yellow coloration of the skin caused by an increase in carotene content. SYN carotenoderma.

**ca·rot·i·co·cav·er·nous fis·tu·la** SYN carotid-cavernous fistula.

**ca·rot·i·co·tym·pan·ic** (ka-rŏt'i-kō-tim-pan'ik) relating to the carotid canal and the tympanum.

**ca·rot·i·co·tym·pan·ic ar·ter·ies (of internal carotid artery)** small branches from the petrous part of the internal carotid artery supplying the tympanic cavity; anastomose with the anterior tympanic and maxillary arteries.

**ca·rot·id** (ka-rŏt'id) pertaining to any carotid structure. [G. *karōtides*, the carotid arteries, fr. *karoō*, to put to sleep (because compression of the c. artery results in unconsciousness)]

**ca·rot·id bod·y** a small epithelioid structure located just above the bifurcation of the common carotid artery on each side. It serves as a chemoreceptor organ responsive to oxygen lack, carbon dioxide excess, and increased hydrogen ion concentration. SYN intercarotid body.

**ca·rot·id bru·it** a systolic murmur heard in the neck but not at the aortic area; any bruit produced by blood flow in a carotid artery.

**ca·rot·id ca·nal** a passage through the petrous part of the temporal bone from its inferior surface upward, medially, and forward to the apex where it opens into the foramen lacerum. It transmits the internal carotid artery and plexuses of veins and autonomic nerves. SYN canalis caroticus [TA].

**ca·rot·id-cav·ern·ous fis·tu·la** a fistulous communication between the cavernous sinus and the traversing internal carotid artery, of spontaneous or traumatic origin; common manifestations are a pulsating unilateral exophthalmos and a detectable cranial bruit. SYN caroticocavernous fistula.

**ca·rot·id gan·gli·on** a small ganglionic swelling on filaments from the internal carotid plexus, lying on the undersurface of the carotid artery in the cavernous sinus.

**ca·rot·id sheath** the dense fibrous investment of the carotid artery, internal jugular vein, and vagus nerve on each side of the neck, deep to the sternocleidomastoid muscle; the layers of cervical fascia blend with it. SYN vagina carotica [TA].

**ca·rot·id si·nus** a slight dilation of the common carotid artery at its bifurcation into external and internal carotids; it contains baroreceptors which, when stimulated, cause slowing of the heart, vasodilation, and a fall in blood pressure and is innervated primarily by the glossopharyngeal nerve.

**ca·rot·id si·nus re·flex** a normal reflex relating to the carotid sinus syndrome, which results from hypersensitivity or hyperactivation of the carotid sinus.

**ca·rot·id si·nus syn·co·pe** syncope resulting from overactivity of the carotid sinus; attacks may be spontaneous or produced by pressure on a sensitive carotid sinus.

**ca·rot·id si·nus syn·drome** stimulation of a hyperactive carotid sinus, causing a marked fall in blood pressure due to vasodilation, cardiac slowing, or both; syncope with or without convulsions or A-V block may occur.

**ca·rot·id tri·an·gle** a space bounded by the superior belly of the omohyoid muscle, anterior border of the sternocleidomastoid, and posterior belly of the digastric; it contains the bifurcation of the common carotid artery.

**ca·rot·o·dyn·ia** (ka-rot′ō-din′ē-ă) pain caused by pressure on the carotid artery. [G. *odynē*, pain]

**car·pal** (kar′păl) relating to the carpus.

**car·pal bones** eight bones arranged in two rows that articulate proximally with the radius and indirectly with the ulna, and distally with the five metacarpal bones. SYN carpus (2) [TA].

**car·pal joints 1.** SYN intercarpal joints. **2.** SYN wrist joint.

**car·pal tun·nel** the passageway deep to the transverse carpal ligament between tubercles of the scaphoid and trapezoid bones on the radial side and the pisiform and hook of the hamate on the ulnar side, through which the median nerve and the flexor tendons of the fingers and thumb pass. SYN canalis carpi [TA].

**ⓘ car·pal tun·nel syn·drome** the most common nerve entrapment syndrome, characterized by nocturnal hand paresthesia and pain, and sometimes sensory loss and wasting in the median hand distribution; caused by entrapment of the median nerve at the wrist, within the carpal tunnel. See this page.

**car·pec·to·my** (kar-pek′tō-mē) excision of a portion or all of the carpus. [G. *karpos*, wrist, + *ektomē*, excision]

**Car·pen·ter syn·drome** (kahr′pĕn-tĕr) the association of primary hypothyroidism, primary adrenocortical insufficiency, and diabetes mellitus. [C.C.J. Carpenter]

**carp mouth** a mouth like that of the carp, with downturning of the corners; observed in Cornelia de Lange syndrome and Silver-Russell dwarfism.

*Car·po·gly·phus* (kar-pō-glif′us) a genus of mites including *Carpoglyptus passularum*, the fruit mite, which causes a dermatitis among handlers of dried fruit. [G. *karpos*, fruit, + *glyphō*, to carve]

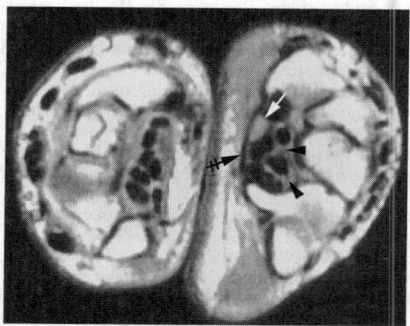

**carpal tunnel syndrome:** MRI of both wrists; swelling of left median nerve (white arrow), increased fluid between flexor tendons within tunnel (black arrowheads) and slight bowing of the flexor retinaculum (crossed arrow)

**car·po·met·a·car·pal** (kar′pō-met-ă-kar′păl) relating to both carpus and metacarpus.

**car·po·met·a·car·pal joints** the synovial joints between the carpal and metacarpal bones; these are all plane joints except that of the thumb, which is saddle-shaped.

**car·po·ped·al** (kar′pō-ped′ăl) relating to the wrist and the foot, or the hands and feet; denoting especially carpopedal spasm. [G. *karpos*, wrist, + L. *pes* (*ped-*), foot]

**car·po·ped·al con·trac·tion** SYN carpopedal spasm.

**car·po·ped·al spasm** spasm of the feet and hands observed in hyperventilation, calcium deprivation, and tetany: flexion of the hands at the wrists and of the fingers at the metacarpophalangeal joints and extension of the fingers at the phalangeal joints; the feet are dorsiflexed at the ankles and the toes plantar flexed. SYN carpopedal contraction.

**car·pus**, gen. and pl. **car·pi** (kar′pŭs, kar′pī) [TA] **1.** SYN wrist. **2.** SYN carpal bones. [Mod. L. fr. Gr. *karpos*]

**Car·rel treat·ment** (kah-rel′) treatment of wound surfaces by intermittent flushing with Dakin solution.

**car·ri·er** (kā′rē-er) **1.** a person or animal that harbors a specific infectious agent in the absence of discernible clinical disease and serves as a potential source of infection. **2.** any chemical capable of accepting an atom, radical, or subatomic particle from one compound, then passing it to another. **3.** a substance which, by having chemical properties closely related to or indistinguishable from those of a radioactive tracer, is able to carry the tracer through a precipitation or similar chemical procedure. SEE ALSO label, tracer. **4.** a large immunogen which when coupled to a hapten will facilitate an immune response to the hapten.

**car·ri·er screen·ing** indiscriminate examination of members of a population to detect heterozygotes for serious disorders and counsel about the risks of marriages with other carriers, and by antenatal diagnosis where a married couple are both carriers.

**Car·ri·ón dis·ease** (kah-rē-ōn′) SYN Oroya fever.

**car·ry·ing an·gle** the angle between the humerus and ulna when the arm is in anatomic position.

**car·ry·ing ca·pac·i·ty** an estimate of the number of people that a region, a nation, or the planet can sustain.

**carry-over** (kăr′ē-ō′ver) the phenomenon by which part of the analyte present in a sample appears to be present in the next or following samples in the same analytic process. This is most noticeable when a sample of low analyte concentration follows one of very high concentration.

**car sick·ness** a form of motion sickness caused by riding on a train or in an automobile or bus.

**car·ti·lage** (kăr′ti-lij) a connective tissue characterized by its nonvascularity and firm consistency; consists of cells (chondrocytes), an interstitial matrix of fibers (collagen), and a ground substance (proteoglycans); found primarily in joints, the walls of the thorax, and tubular structures such as the larynx, air passages, and ears; comprises most of the skeleton in early fetal life, but is slowly replaced by bone. There are three kinds of cartilage: hyaline cartilage, elastic cartilage, and fibrocartilage. SYN cartilago [TA], gristle. [L. *cartilago* (*cartilagin-*), gristle]

**car·ti·lage bone** SYN endochondral bone.

**car·ti·lage cap·sule** the more intensely basophilic matrix in hyaline cartilage surrounding the lacunae in which the cartilage cells lie. SYN territorial matrix.

**cartilage-hair hypoplasia** a skeletal dysplasia prevalent among the Amish, characterized by short-limb dwarfism, sparse, light-colored hair, T-cell immunologic defect rendering them susceptible to infections, and radiographic findings of metaphyseal dysplasia. Autosomal recessive inheritance, the gene maps to 9p. SYN McKusick metaphyseal dysplasia.

**car·ti·lage la·cu·na** a cavity within the matrix of cartilage, occupied by a chondrocyte. SYN cartilage space.

**car·ti·lage ma·trix** the intercellular substance of cartilage consisting of fibers and ground substance.

**car·ti·lage space** SYN cartilage lacuna.

**car·ti·la·gi·nes** (kar-ti-laj′i-nĕz) plural of cartilago.

**car·ti·la·gi·nes tra·che·a·les** [TA] SYN tracheal cartilages.

**car·ti·lag·i·noid** (kar-ti-laj′i-noyd) SYN chondroid (1).

**car·ti·lag·i·nous** (kar-ti-laj′i-nŭs) relating to or consisting of cartilage. SYN chondral.

**car·ti·lag·i·nous joint** a joint in which the apposed bony surfaces are united by cartilage. SYN synarthrodial joint (2).

**car·ti·la·go**, pl. **car·ti·la·gi·nes** (kar-ti-lă′gō, kar-ti-laj′i-nĕz) [TA] SYN cartilage. [L. gristle]

**car·ti·la·go ar·y·te·noi·dea** [TA] SYN arytenoid cartilage.

**car·ti·la·go au·ric·u·lae** [TA] SYN auricular cartilage.

**car·ti·la·go cor·ni·cu·la·ta** [TA] SYN corniculate cartilage.

**car·ti·la·go cos·ta·lis** [TA] SYN costal cartilage.

**car·ti·la·go cri·coi·dea** [TA] SYN cricoid cartilage.

**car·ti·la·go cu·ne·i·for·mis** [TA] SYN cuneiform cartilage.

**car·ti·la·go ep·i·glot·ti·ca** [TA] SYN epiglottic cartilage.

**cartilago epiphysialis** [TA] SYN epiphysial plate.

**car·ti·la·go na·si la·te·ra·lis** [TA] SYN lateral cartilage of nose.

**car·ti·la·go thy·roi·dea** [TA] SYN thyroid cartilage.

**car·ti·la·go vo·me·ro·na·sa·lis** [TA] SYN vomeronasal cartilage.

**ca·run·cle** (kar′ŭng-kl) a small, fleshy protuberance, or any structure suggesting such a shape.

**ca·run·cu·la**, pl. **ca·run·cu·lae** (kă-rŭng′kyu-lă, kă-rŭng′kyu-lē) a small, fleshy protuberance. [L. a small fleshy mass, fr. *caro*, flesh]

**Ca·rus curve, Ca·rus cir·cle** (kah′rĕs) an imaginary curved line obtained from a mathematical formula, supposed to indicate the outlet of the pelvic canal.

**Car·val·lo sign** (kahr-vah′yō) an increase in the intensity of the pansystolic murmur of tricuspid regurgitation during or at the end of inspiration, which distinguishes tricuspid from mitral involvement.

△**ca·ryo-** nucleus. SEE karyo-. [G. *karyon*, nut, kernel]

**Ca·sal neck·lace** (kah-sahl′) a dermatitis partly or completely encircling the lower part of the neck in pellagra.

**cas·cade** (kas-kād′) **1.** a series of sequential interactions, as of a physiological process, which once initiated continues to the final one; each interaction is activated by the preceding one, sometimes with cumulative effect. **2.** to spill over, especially rapidly. [Fr., fr. It. *cascare*, to fall]

**cas·cade stom·ach** a radiographic description: when contrast material is swallowed while the patient is in the upright position, the gastric fundus acts as a reservoir until contrast overflows (cascades) into the antrum; a normal variant in a horizontal stomach.

**case** (kās) **1.** an instance of disease with its attendant circumstances. Cf. patient. **2.** a box or container. [L. *casus*, an occurrence]

**ca·se·a·tion** (kā-sē-ā′shŭn) a form of coagulation necrosis in which the necrotic tissue resembles cheese and contains a mixture of protein and fat that is absorbed very slowly; occurs particularly in tuberculosis. SEE ALSO caseous necrosis. [L. *caseus*, cheese]

**case fa·tal·i·ty rate** the proportion of individuals contracting a disease that die of that disease.

**ca·sein** (kā′sē-in, kā′sēn) the principal protein of cow's milk and the chief constituent of cheese.

**case man·age·ment** a process whereby covered persons with specific health care needs are identified and an efficient treatment plan is formulated and implemented to produce the most cost-effective outcomes.

**case mix** the relative numbers of various types of patients being treated as categorized by DRG, severity of illness, and other indicators; used as a tool for managing and planning health care services.

**ca·se·ous** (kā′sē-ŭs) pertaining to or manifesting the features of tissue affected by caseation.

**ca·se·ous de·gen·er·a·tion** SYN caseous necrosis.

**ca·se·ous ne·cro·sis, ca·se·a·tion ne·cro·sis** necrosis characteristic of certain inflammations (e.g., tuberculosis, histoplasmosis); affected tissue manifests the friable, crumbly consistency and dull, opaque quality observed in cheese. SYN caseous degeneration.

**ca·se·ous os·te·i·tis** tuberculous caries in bone.

**Ca·so·ni an·ti·gen** (kah-sō′nē) skin-test antigen composed of sterile hydatid fluid; used in test for hydatid disease.

**cas·sette** (kă-set′) **1.** a plate, film, or tape holder for use in photography or radiography. A radiographic cassette contains two intensifying screens and a sheet of x-ray film. **2.** a perforated holder in which tissue blocks are placed for paraffin embedding. [Fr., dim. of *casse*, box]

**cast** (kast) **1.** an object formed by the solidification of a liquid poured into a mold. **2.** rigid encasement of a part, as with plaster, fiberglass, or a plastic, for purposes of immobilization. **3.** an elongated or cylindrical mold formed in a tubular structure (e.g., renal tubule, bronchiole) that may be observed in histologic sections or in material such as urine or sputum; results from inspissation of fluid material secreted or excreted in the tubular structures. **4.** restraint of a large animal, usually a horse, with ropes and harnesses in a recumbent position. **5.** in dentistry, a positive reproduction of the form of the tissues of the upper or lower jaw, which is made by the solidification of plaster, metal, etc., poured into an impression, and over which denture bases or other dental restorations may be fabricated. [M.E. *kasten,* fr. O.Norse *kasta*]

**cast brace** (kast brās) a specially designed plaster or plastic cast incorporating hinges and other brace components; used in the treatment of fractures to promote early activity and early joint motion.

**cas·trate** (kas′trāt) to remove the testicles or the ovaries. [L. *castro,* pp. *-atus,* to deprive of generative power (male or female)]

**cas·tra·tion** (kas-trā′shŭn) **1.** removal of the testicles or ovaries. **2.** SEE castration complex. [see castrate]

**cas·tra·tion cells** altered basophilic cells of the anterior lobe of the pituitary that develop following castration; the body of the cell is occupied by a large vacuole that displaces the nucleus to the periphery, giving the cell a resemblance to a signet ring. SYN signet ring cells.

**cas·tra·tion com·plex 1.** a child's fear of injury to the genitals by the parent of the same sex as punishment for unconscious guilt over oedipal feelings; **2.** fantasied loss of the penis by a female or fear of its actual loss by a male; **3.** unconscious fear of injury from those in authority.

**CAT** computerized axial tomography; chloramphenicol acetyl transferase.

△**cata-** down; opposite of ana-. SEE ALSO kata-. Cf. de-. [G. *kata,* down]

**cat·a·bi·ot·ic** (kat′ă-bī-ot′ik) used up in the carrying on of the vital processes other than growth, or in the performance of function, referring to the energy derived from food. [cata- + G. *biōtikos,* relating to life]

**cat·a·bol·ic** (kat-ă-bol′ik) relating to or promoting catabolism.

**ca·tab·o·lism** (kă-tab′ō-lizm) **1.** the breaking down in the body of complex chemical compounds into simpler ones, often accompanied by the liberation of energy. **2.** the sum of all degradative processes. Cf. anabolism, metabolism. [G. *katabolē,* a casting down]

**ca·tab·o·lite** (kă-tab′ō-līt) any product of catabolism.

**ca·tab·o·lite (gene) ac·ti·va·tor pro·tein (CAP)** a protein that can be activated by cAMP, whereupon it affects the action of RNA polymerase by binding it with it or near it on the DNA to be transcribed. SYN cAMP receptor protein.

**cat·a·chron·o·bi·ol·o·gy** (kat′ă-kron′ō-bī-ol′ō-jē) the study of the deleterious effects of time on a living system. [cata- + G. *chronos,* time, + biology]

**ca·ta·crot·ic** (kat-ă-krot′ik) relating to or characterized by catacrotism.

**ca·tac·ro·tism** (kă-tak′rō-tizm) a condition of the pulse in which there are one or more secondary expansions of the artery following the main beat, producing secondary upward waves on the downstroke of the pulse tracing. [cata- + G. *krotos,* beat]

**cat·a·di·crot·ic** (kat′ă-dī-krot′ik) relating to or characterized by catadicrotism.

**cat·a·di·cro·tism** (kat-ă-dī′krō-tizm) a condition of the pulse marked by two minor expansions of the artery following the main beat, producing two secondary upward waves on the downstroke of the pulse tracing. [cata + G. *di-,* two, + *krotos,* beat]

**cat·a·dro·mous** (kat-ă-drō′mus) migrating from fresh water to the ocean to spawn. SEE ALSO anadromous.

**cat·a·gen** (kat′ă-jen) a regressing phase of the hair growth cycle during which cell proliferation ceases, the hair follicle shortens, and an anchored club hair is produced.

**cat·a·gen·e·sis** (kat-ă-jen′ĕ-sis) SYN involution. [cata- + G. *genesis,* origin]

**cat·a·lase** (kat′ă-lās) a hemoprotein catalyzing the decomposition of hydrogen peroxide to water and oxygen ($2H_2O_2 \rightarrow O_2 + 2H_2O$).

**cat·a·lep·sy** (kat′ă-lep-sē) a morbid condition characterized by waxy rigidity of the limbs, lack of response to stimuli, mutism and inactivity; occurs with some psychoses, especially catatonic schizophrenia. [G. *katalēpsis,* a seizing, catalepsy, fr. *kata,* down, + *lēpsis,* a seizure]

**cat·a·lep·tic** (kat-ă-lep′tik) relating to, or suffering from, catalepsy.

**cat·a·lep·toid** (kat-ă-lep′toyd) simulating or resembling catalepsy.

**ca·tal·y·sis** (kă-tal′i-sis) the effect that a catalyst exerts upon a chemical reaction. [G. *katalysis,* dissolution]

**cat·a·lyst** (kat′ă-list) a substance that accelerates a chemical reaction but is not consumed or changed permanently thereby.

**cat·a·lyt·ic** (kat-ă-lit′ik) relating to or effecting catalysis.

**cat·a·lyze** (kat′ă-līz) to act as a catalyst.

**cat·a·me·ni·al pneu·mo·tho·rax** pneumothorax occurring in young women during menstruation, usually on the right side.

**cat·am·ne·sis** (kat-am-nē′sis) the medical history of a patient after an illness; the follow-up history. [cata- + G *mnēmē,* memory]

**cat·am·nes·tic** (kat-am-nes′tik) related to catamnesis.

**cat·a·pha·sia** (kat-ă-fā′zē-ă) SYN verbigeration. [cata- + G. *phasis,* a saying]

**ca·taph·o·ra** (kă-taf′ō-ră) semicoma or somnolence interrupted by intervals of partial consciousness. [G. a falling down]

**cat·a·pla·sia, cat·a·pla·sis** (kat-ă-plā′sē-ă, kat-ă-plā′sis) a degenerative change in cells or tissues that is the reverse of constructive or developmental change; a return to an earlier or embryonic stage. SYN retrogression. [cata- + G. *plasis,* a molding]

**cat·a·plec·tic** (kat-ă-plek′tik) **1.** developing suddenly. **2.** pertaining to cataplexy.

**cat·a·plexy** (kat′ă-plek-sē) a transient attack of extreme generalized muscular weakness, often precipitated by an emotional state such as laughing, surprise, fear, or anger. [cata- + G. *plēxis,* a blow, stroke]

**cat·a·ract** (kat′ă-rakt) complete or partial opacity of the ocular lens. See this page. [L. *cataracta,* fr. G. *katarrhaktēs,* a downrushing, a waterfall, fr. *kata- rrhēgnymi,* to break down, rush down]

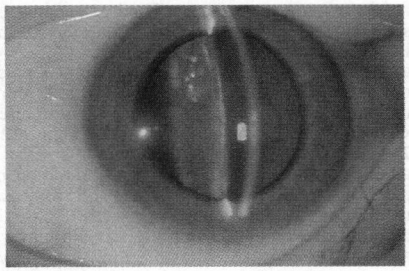

**cataract**

**cat·a·rac·to·gen·ic** (kat′ă-rak-tō-jen′ik) cataract-producing.

**cat·a·rac·tous** (kat-ă-rak′tŭs) relating to a cataract.

**ca·tarrh** (kă-tahr′) inflammation of a mucous membrane with increased flow of mucus or exudate. [G. *katarrheō,* to flow down]

**ca·tarrh·al** (kă-tah′răl) relating to or affected with catarrh.

**ca·tarrh·al gas·tri·tis** gastritis with excessive secretion of mucus.

**ca·tarrh·al in·flam·ma·tion** an inflammatory process that may occur in any mucous membrane, and is characterized by hyperemia of the mucosal vessels, edema of the interstitial tissue, enlargement of the secretory epithelial cells, and an irregular layer of viscous, mucinous material on the surface.

**cat·a·stal·sis** (kat-ă-stahl′sis) a contraction wave resembling ordinary peristalsis but not preceded by a zone of inhibition. [G. *kata-stellō,* to put in order, check]

**cat·a·stal·tic** (kat-ă-stahl′tik) **1.** inhibitory, restricting, or restraining. **2.** an inhibitory or checking agent, such as an astringent or antispasmodic. [cata- + G. *staltos,* contracted, fr. *stellō,* to contract]

**cat·a·stroph·ic re·ac·tion** the disorganized behavior that is the response to a severe shock or threatening situation with which the person cannot cope.

**cat·a·to·nia** (kat-ă-tō′nē-ă) a syndrome of psychomotor disturbances characterized by periods of physical rigidity, negativism, or stupor; may occur in schizophrenia, mood disorders, or or-ganic mental disorders. [G. *katatonos,* stretching down, depressed, fr. *kata,* down, + *tonos,* tone]

**cat·a·ton·ic, cat·a·to·ni·ac** (kat-ă-ton′ik, kat-ă-tō′nē-ak) relating to, or characterized by, catatonia.

**cat·a·ton·ic ri·gid·i·ty** rigidity associated with catatonic psychotic states in which all muscles exhibit flexibilitas cerea.

**cat·a·ton·ic schiz·o·phre·nia** schizophrenia characterized by marked disturbance, which may involve stupor, negativism, rigidity, excitement, or posturing; sometimes there is rapid alteration between the extremes of excitement and stupor. Associated features include stereotypic behavior, mannerisms, and waxy flexibility; mutism is particularly common.

**cat·a·tri·crot·ic** (kat′ă-trī-krot′ik) relating to or characterized by catatricrotism.

**cat·a·tri·cro·tism** (kat-ă-trī′krō-tizm) a condition of the pulse marked by three minor expansions of the artery following the main beat, producing three secondary upward waves on the downstroke of the pulse tracing. [cata- + G. *tri-,* three, + *krotos,* beat]

**cat·e·chol·a·mines** (kat-ĕ-kol′ă-mēnz) pyrocatechols with an alkylamine side chain; examples of biochemical interest are epinephrine, norepinephrine, and L-dopa. Catecholamines are major elements in responses to stress.

**cat·e·chol ox·i·dase (di·mer·iz·ing)** an enzyme oxidizing a catechol, with $O_2$, to a diphenylenedioxide quinone (e.g., 4 catechol + $3O_2$ → 2 dibenzo[1,4]-2,3-dione + $6H_2O$).

**cat·e·gor·i·cal trait** GENETICS a feature that can conveniently and effectively be analyzed by sorting into classes either because there is no satisfactory way of measuring it or because it falls into natural classes so that the variation among classes far exceeds that within classes; existence of categories suggests but does not prove the operation of a major, simple, underlying cause.

**cat·e·gor·i·za·tion** a process by which a hospital self-designates providing a specialized service. Criteria for categorization may be internal or based on national standards. Differs from designation, which is a legal process with external review.

**cat·en·ate** (kat′e-nāt) to connect in a series of links like a chain. [L. *catenatus,* chained together, fr. *catena,* chain]

**cat·en·in** (ka-tēn′in) cytoplasmic molecule that serves as a link between cadherins and the cytoskeleton of cells, allowing the formation of adherent junctions. There are two types: β-catenin, which is linked to the cadherin itself and α-catenin, which associates with actin microfilaments. [L. *catena,* chain, + -in]

**cat·er·pil·lar** (kat′er-pil′er) the wormlike larval stage of a butterfly or a moth. [M.E. *catirpeller,* fr. O.Fr. *cate,* cat, + *pelose,* hairy]

**cat·er·pil·lar flap** a tubed flap transferred end-over-end (in stages) from the donor area to a distant recipient area. SYN waltzed flap.

**cat·gut** (kat′gŭt) an absorbable surgical suture material made from the collagenous fibers of the submucosa of certain animals, usually sheep or cows. [probably from *kit,* a small violin, through confusion with *kit,* a small cat]

**ca·thar·sis** (kă-thar′sis) **1.** SYN purgation. **2.** the release or discharge of emotional tension or anxiety by psychoanalytically guided emotional reliving of past, especially repressed, events. [G. *katharsis,* purification, fr. *katharos,* pure]

**ca·thar·tic** (kă-thar′tik) **1.** relating to catharsis. **2.** an agent having purgative action.

**ca·thec·tic** (kă-thek′tik) pertaining to cathexis.

**cath·e·ter** (kath′ĕ-ter) **1.** a flexible tubular instrument to allow passage of fluid from or into a body cavity or blood vessel. SEE ALSO line (3). **2.** especially a catheter designed to be passed through the urethra into the bladder to drain it of urine. [G. *kathetēr,* fr. *kathiĕmi,* to send down]

**cath·e·ter coil·ing sign** SYN Bergman sign.

**cath·e·ter em·bo·lus** coiled worm-shaped platelet and fibrin aggregates produced during vascular catheterization, originating on the catheter or its guide wire; embolization of the catheter itself.

**cath·e·ter·i·sa·tion [Br.]** SEE catheterization.

**cath·e·ter·i·za·tion** (kath′ĕ-ter-ĭ-zā′shŭn) passage of a catheter.

**ca·thex·is** (kă-thek′sis) a conscious or unconscious attachment of psychic energy to an idea, object, or person. [G. *kathexis,* a holding in, retention]

**cath·o·dal (C)** (kath′ō-dăl) of, pertaining to, or emanating from a cathode.

**cath·ode (C)** (kath′ōd) **1.** the negative pole of a galvanic battery or the electrode connected with it; the electrode to which positively charged ions (cations) migrate. Cf. anode. **2.** negatively charged part of the x-ray tube head; it contains the tungsten filament. SYN negative electrode. [G. *kathodos,* a way down, fr. *kata,* down, + *hodos,* a way]

**cat·i·on** (kat′ī-on) an ion carrying a charge of positive electricity, therefore going to the negatively charged cathode. [G. *kation,* going down]

**cat·i·on ex·change** the process by which a cation in a liquid phase exchanges with another cation present as the counter-ion of a negatively charged solid polymer (cation exchanger). Cation exchange may be used chromatographically, to separate cations, and medicinally, to remove a cation. SEE ALSO anion exchange.

**cat·i·on-ex·change res·in** SEE cation exchange.

**cat·scratch dis·ease (CSD), cat·scratch fe·ver** an infection that causes chronic benign adenopathy in most cases, especially in children and young adults, usually associated with a cat scratch or bite. In most cases it is caused by the bacterium *Bartonella henselae.* The lymphadenopathy usually resolves spontaneously within a period of several months. The infection may cause other clinical symptoms such as fever of unknown origin, encephalitis, microabscess in the liver and spleen, and osteomyelitis. SYN benign inoculation lymphoreticulosis, benign inoculation reticulosis, regional granulomatous lymphadenitis.

**cau·da,** pl. **cau·dae** (kaw′dă, kaw′dē) [TA] SYN tail. [L. a tail]

**cau·dad** (kaw′dad) **1.** in a direction toward the tail. **2.** situated nearer the tail in relation to a specific reference point; opposite of craniad. SEE ALSO inferior. See page APP 89.

**cau·da e·qui·na** [TA] the bundle of spinal nerve roots arising from the lumbosacral enlargement and medullary cone and running through the lumbar cistern (subarachnoid space) within the vertebral canal below the first lumbar vertebra; it comprises the roots of all the spinal nerves below the first lumbar. [L. horse tail]

**cau·dal** (kaw′dăl) **1.** pertaining to the tail. **2.** VETERINARY ANATOMY denoting a position nearer to the tail. See page APP 89. [Mod. L. *caudalis*]

**cau·dal an·es·the·sia** regional anesthesia by injection of local anesthetic solution into the epidural space via the sacral hiatus.

**cau·dal flex·ure** the bend in the lumbosacral region of the embryo. SYN sacral flexure.

**cau·dal trans·verse fis·sure** SYN porta hepatis.

**cau·date lobe** SYN lobus caudatus.

**cau·date nu·cle·us** an elongated curved mass of gray matter, consisting of an anterior thick portion, the caput, or head, which protrudes into the anterior horn of the lateral ventricle, a portion extending along the floor of the body of the lateral ventricle, known as the corpus or body, and an elongated curved thin portion, the cauda or tail, which curves downward, backward, and forward in the temporal lobe in the wall of the lateral ventricle.

**cau·date pro·cess** a narrow band of hepatic tissue connecting the caudate and right lobes of the liver posterior to the porta hepatis.

**caul, cowl** (kawl) **1.** the amnion, either as a piece of membrane capping the baby's head at birth or the whole membrane when delivered unruptured with the baby. SYN galea (4), veil (2), velum (2). **2.** SYN greater omentum. [Gaelic, *call,* a veil]

**cau·li·flow·er ear** thickening and induration of the ear with distortion of contours following extravasation of blood within its tissues; a chronic deformity following (usually) repeated trauma.

**cau·mes·the·sia** (kaw-mes-thē′zē-ă) subjective heat sensation of uncomfortably high temperature; a type of thermal dysesthesia. [G. *kauma,* heat, + *aisthēsis,* sensation]

**cau·sal·gia** (kaw-zal′jē-ă) persistent severe burning sensation, usually following partial injury of a peripheral nerve, accompanied by trophic changes (thinning of skin, loss of sweat glands and hair follicles). [G. *kausis,* burning, + *algos,* pain]

**caus·tic** (kaws′tik) **1.** exerting an effect resembling a burn. **2.** an agent producing this effect. **3.** denoting a solution of a strong alkali; e.g., caustic soda, NaOH. [G. *kaustikos,* fr. *kaiō,* to burn]

**cau·ter·i·sa·tion [Br.]** SEE cauterization.

**cau·ter·ise [Br.]** SEE cauterize.

**cau·ter·i·za·tion** (kaw-ter-ĭ-zā′shŭn) the act of cauterizing. SEE ALSO cautery.

**cau·ter·ize** (kaw′ter-īz) to apply a cautery; to burn with a cautery.

**cau·tery** (kaw′ter-ē) **1.** an agent or device used for scarring, burning, or cutting the skin or other tissues by means of heat, cold, electric current, or caustic chemicals. **2.** use of a cautery. [G. *kautēr-ion,* a branding iron]

**ca·va** (kā′vă) SEE inferior vena cava, superior vena cava.

**ca·va·gram** (kā′vă-gram) SYN cavogram.

**ca·val** (kā′văl) relating to a vena cava.

**cave** (kāv) a hollow or enclosed space or cavity. SEE ALSO cavern, cavity.

**cavea** SYN cage.

**cav·ea tho·ra·cis** [TA] SYN thoracic cage.

**cav·e·o·la,** pl. **cav·e·o·lae** (kāv-ē-ō′lă, kāv-ē-ō′lē) a small pocket, vesicle, cave, or recess communicating with the outside of a cell and extending inward, indenting the cytoplasm and the cell membrane. Caveolae are considered to be sites of uptake of materials into the cell, expulsion of materials from the cell, or addition or removal of cell (unit) membrane to or from the cell surface. [L.]

**cav·ern** (kav′ern) an anatomic cavity with many interconnecting chambers. SEE ALSO cave, cavity.

**cav·er·nil·o·quy** (kav-er-nil′ŏ-kwē) low-pitched resonant pectoriloquy heard over a lung cavity. [L. *caverna,* cavern, + *loquor,* to talk]

**cav·er·ni·tis, cav·er·no·si·tis** (kav-er-nī′tis, kav′-er-nō-sī′tis) inflammation of the corpus cavernosum penis.

**cav·ern·ous** (kav′er-nŭs) relating to a cavern or a cavity; containing many cavities.

**cav·ern·ous an·gi·o·ma** vascular malformation composed of sinusoidal vessels without a large feeding artery.

**cavernous body** SEE corpus cavernosum clitoridis, corpus cavernosum penis.

**cav·ern·ous he·man·gi·o·ma** a vascular malformation containing large blood-filled spaces, due apparently to dilation and thickening of the walls of the capillary loops; in the skin, extends more deeply than a capillary hemangioma and is less likely to regress spontaneously. See page B5.

**cav·ern·ous nerves of clit·o·ris** nerves corresponding to the cavernous nerves of penis in the male, arising from the vesicular portion of the pelvic plexus. SYN nervi cavernosi clitoridis [TA].

**cav·ern·ous nerves of pe·nis** two nerves, major and minor, derived from the prostatic portion of the pelvic plexus supplying sympathetic and parasympathetic fibers to the helicine arteries and arteriovenous anastomoses of the corpus cavernosum stimulating erection. SYN nervi cavernosi penis [TA].

**cav·ern·ous plex·us of con·chae** erectile tissue in the mucous membrane covering the conchae of the nasal cavity.

**cav·ern·ous rale** a resonating, bubbling sound caused by air entering a cavity partly filled with fluid.

**cav·ern·ous si·nus** a paired dural venous sinus on either side of the sella turcica, the two being connected by anastomoses, the anterior and posterior intercavernous sinus, in front of and behind the hypophysis, respectively, making thus the circular sinus; the cavernous sinus is unique among dural venous sinuses in being trabeculated; coursing within the sinus are the internal carotid artery and the abducent nerve. SYN sinus cavernosus [TA].

**cav·ern·ous si·nus branch of in·ter·nal ca·rot·id ar·tery** a number of small branches of the cavernous part of the internal carotid artery. SEE ganglionic branch of internal carotid artery, basal tentorial branch of internal carotid artery, marginal tentorial branch of internal carotid artery.

**cav·ern·ous space** an anatomic cavity with many interconnecting chambers.

**cav·ern·ous trans·for·ma·tion of por·tal vein** replacement of the portal vein by a number of collateral channels, a consequence of thrombosis.

**cav·ern·ous veins of pe·nis** the cavernous venous spaces in the erectile tissue of the penis.

**cav·i·tary** (kav′i-tā-rē) relating to a cavity or having a cavity or cavities.

**cav·i·tas,** pl. **cav·i·ta·tes** (kav′i-tas, kav-i-tā′tēs) SYN cavity. [Mod. L.]

**cav·i·ta·tion** (kav-i-tā′shŭn) **1.** formation of a cavity, as in the lung in tuberculosis. **2.** the pro-

duction of small vapor-containing bubbles or cavities in a liquid by ultrasound.

**ca·vi·tis** (kā-vī′tis) SYN celophlebitis.

**cav·i·ty** (kav′i-tē) **1.** a hollow space; hole. SEE cave, cavitas, cavernous space. **2.** lay term for the loss of tooth structure due to dental caries. SYN cavitas, cavum. [L. *cavus,* hollow]

**cav·i·ty of sep·tum pel·lu·ci·dum** a slitlike, fluid-filled space of variable width between the left and right transparent septum, which occurs in fewer than 10% of human brains and may communicate with the third ventricle.

**ca·vo·gram** (kā′vō-gram) an angiogram of a vena cava. SYN cavagram. [(vena) cava + G. *gramma,* a writing]

**ca·vog·ra·phy** (kā-vog′ră-fē) SYN venacavography.

**ca·vo·pul·mo·nary a·nas·to·mo·sis** a means of palliating cyanotic heart disease by anastomosing the right pulmonary artery to the superior vena cava.

**ca·vo·sur·face** (kā-vō-ser′făs) relating to a cavity and the surface of a tooth.

**ca·vo·sur·face an·gle** the angle formed by the junction of a cavity wall and the surface of the tooth.

**ca·vum,** pl. **ca·va** (kā′vŭm, kā′vă) SYN cavity. [L. ntr. of adj. *cavus,* hollow]

**C-band·ing stain** a selective chromosome banding stain used in human cytogenetics, employing Giemsa stain after most of the DNA is denatured or extracted by treatment with alkali, acid, salt, or heat; only heterochromatic regions close to the centromeres and rich in satellite DNA stain, with the exception of the Y chromosome, whose long arm usually stains throughout.

**CBC** complete blood count.

**CBG** corticosteroid-binding globulin.

**CC** chief complaint.

**cc, c.c., c.c.** cubic centimeter.

**CCK** cholecystokinin.

**CCU** coronary care unit; critical care unit.

**CD** curative dose; circular dichroism; cluster of differentiation.

**Cd** cadmium.

**CDC** Centers for Disease Control and Prevention; previously known as the Communicable Disease Center.

**CD4/CD8 count** the ratio of the number of helper-inducer T lymphocytes to cytotoxic-suppressor T lymphocytes, as measured by monoclonal antibodies to the CD4 surface antigen found on helper-inducer T cells, and the CD8 surface antigen found on cytotoxic-suppressor T cells. In healthy individuals, the H/S ratio ranges between 1.6 and 2.2. The CD4/CD8 count is used to monitor for signs of organ rejection after transplants, and to assess the degree of immune compromise in HIV patients.

**cDNA** complementary DNA.

**CDP** cytidine 5′-diphosphate.

**Ce** cerium.

**CEA** carcinoembryonic antigen.

**ce·ca** (sē′kă) plural of cecum.

**ce·cal** (sē′kăl) **1.** relating to the cecum. **2.** ending blindly or in a cul-de-sac.

**ce·cec·to·my** (sē-sek′tō-mē) excision of the cecum. SYN typhlectomy. [ceco- + G. *ektomē,* excision]

**ce·ci·tis** (sē-sī′tis) inflammation of the cecum. SYN typhlenteritis, typhlitis, typhloenteritis.

△**ce•co-, cec-** the cecum. SEE ALSO typhlo- (1). Cf. typhlo-. [L. *caecum,* cecum, blind]

**ce•co•cen•tral sco•to•ma** a scotoma involving the optic disk area (blind spot) and the papillomacular fibers; there are three forms: 1) the cecocentral defect which extends from the blind spot toward or into the fixation area; 2) angioscotoma; 3) glaucomatous nerve-fiber bundle scotoma, due to involvement of nerve-fiber bundles at the edge of the optic disk.

**ce•co•co•los•to•my** (sē′kō-kō-los′tō-mē) formation of an anastomosis between cecum and colon.

**ce•co•il•e•os•to•my** (sē′kō-il-ē-os′tō-mē) SYN ileocecostomy.

**ce•co•pexy** (sē′kō-pek-sē) operative anchoring of a movable cecum. SYN typhlopexy, typhlopexia. [ceco- + G. *pexis,* fixation]

**ce•co•pli•ca•tion** (sē′kō-plĭ-kā′shŭn) operative reduction in size of a dilated cecum by the formation of folds or tucks in its wall. [ceco- + L. *plico,* pp. *-atus,* to fold]

**ce•cor•rha•phy** (sē-kōr′ă-fē) suture of the cecum. SYN typhlorrhaphy. [ceco- + G. *rhaphē,* suture]

**ce•co•sig•moid•os•to•my** (sē′kō-sig-moy-dos′tō-mē) formation of a communication between the cecum and the sigmoid colon.

**ce•cos•to•my** (sē-kos′tō-mē) operative formation of a cecal fistula. SYN typhlostomy. [ceco- + G. *stoma,* mouth]

**ce•cot•o•my** (sē-kot′ō-mē) incision into the cecum. SYN typhlotomy. [ceco- + G. *tome,* incision]

**ce•co•u•re•ter•o•cele** (sē′cō-yu-rē′ter-ō-sēl) a ureterocele that extends far along the urethra, sometimes even through the urethral meatus.

**ce•cro•pins** (sē-krō-pinz) antibacterial peptides consisting of two amphipathic α-helix components.

**ce•cum,** pl. **ce•ca** (sē′kŭm, sē′kă) **1.** the cul-de-sac, about 6 cm in depth, lying below the terminal ileum forming the first part of the large intestine. **2.** any similar structure ending in a cul-de-sac. [L. ntr. of *caecus,* blind]

***Ced•e•cea*** (sed-e′sē-ă) a genus in the Enterobacteriaceae group that includes the species *Cedecea davisae* (the type strain), *Cedecea lapagei,* and *Cedecea neteri;* they have been recovered from the human respiratory tract, but their role in disease has not yet been delineated.

**CEJ** SEE cementoenamel junction.

△**-cele** swelling; hernia. [G. *kēlē,* tumor]

**ce•li•ac** (sē′lē-ak) relating to the abdominal cavity. [G. *koilia,* belly]

**ce•li•ac ar•tery** SYN celiac trunk.

**ce•li•ac dis•ease** a disease occurring in children and adults characterized by sensitivity to gluten, with chronic inflammation and atrophy of the mucosa of the upper small intestine; manifestations include diarrhea, malabsorption, steatorrhea, and nutritional and vitamin deficiencies. SYN gluten enteropathy.

**ce•li•ac gan•glia** the largest and highest group of prevertebral sympathetic ganglia, located on the superior part of the abdominal aorta, on either side of the origin of the celiac artery; contains sympathetic neurons whose unmyelinated postganglionic axons innervate the stomach, liver, gallbladder, spleen, kidney, small intestine, and ascending and transverse colon.

**ce•li•ac lymph nodes** nodes located along the celiac trunk which drain lymph from the stomach, duodenum, pancreas, spleen, and biliary tract and drain to the cisterna chyli via the right and left intestinal lymphatic trunks.

**ce•li•ac plex•us** the most substantial, superior portion of the abdominal aortic plexus lying anterior to the aorta at the level of origin of the celiac trunk (vertebral level T-12); the celiac ganglia lie within the plexus; it is formed by contributions from the greater splanchnic and vagus (especially the posterior or right vagus) nerves and communicating branches to and from the superior mesenteric and renal plexuses and ganglia; most sympathetic, parasympathetic and visceral afferent fibers serving the abdominal viscera pass through this plexus. SYN plexus celiacus [TA].

**ce•li•ac plex•us re•flex** arterial hypotension coincident with surgical manipulations in the upper abdomen during general anesthesia.

**ce•li•ac trunk** *origin,* abdominal aorta just below diaphragm; *branches,* left gastric, common hepatic, splenic. SYN truncus celiacus [TA], arteria celiaca, celiac artery.

△**celio-** the abdomen. SEE ALSO celo- (3). [G. *koilia,* belly]

**ce•li•o•cen•te•sis** (sē′lē-ō-sen-tē′sis) rarely used term for paracentesis of the abdomen. [celio- + G. *kentēsis,* puncture]

**ce•li•or•rha•phy** (sē-lē-ōr′ă-fē) suture of a wound in the abdominal wall. SYN laparorrhaphy. [celio- + G. *rhaphē,* seam]

**ce•li•os•co•py** (sē-lē-os′kŏ-pē) SYN peritoneoscopy. [celio- + G. *skopeō,* to view]

**ce•li•ot•o•my** (sē-lē-ot′ō-mē) transabdominal incision into the peritoneal cavity. SYN abdominal section, laparotomy (2), ventrotomy. [celio- + G. *tome,* incision]

**ce•li•tis** (sē-lī′tis) any inflammation of the abdomen. [G. *koilia,* belly, + *-itis,* inflammation]

**cell** (sel) **1.** the smallest unit of living structure capable of independent existence, composed of a membrane-enclosed mass of protoplasm and containing a nucleus or nucleoid. Cells are highly variable and specialized in both structure and function, though all must at some stage replicate proteins and nucleic acids, utilize energy, and reproduce themselves. **2.** a small closed or partly closed cavity; a compartment or hollow receptacle. **3.** a container of glass, ceramic, or other solid material within which chemical reactions generating electricity take place. [L. *cella,* a storeroom, a chamber]

**cell ad•he•sion mol•e•cule (CAM)** proteins that hold cells together, e.g., uvomorulin, and hold them to their substrates, e.g., laminin.

**cell bod•y** the part of the cell containing the nucleus.

**cell bridg•es** SYN intercellular bridges.

**cell cul•ture** the maintenance or growth of dispersed cells after removal from the body, commonly on a glass surface immersed in nutrient fluid.

**cell cy•cle** the periodic biochemical and structural events occurring during proliferation of cells such as in tissue culture.

**cell fu•sion** the merging of the contents of two cells by artificial means without the destruction of either, resulting in a heterokaryon that, for at least a few generations, will reproduce its kind; an important method in assignment of loci to chromosomes.

**cell in•clu•sions 1.** the residual elements of the

cytoplasm that are metabolic products of the cell, e.g., pigment granules or crystals; SYN metaplasm. **2.** storage materials such as glycogen or fat; **3.** engulfed material such as carbon or other foreign substances. SEE ALSO inclusion bodies.

**cell line 1.** in tissue culture, the cells growing in the first or later subculture from a primary culture. **2.** a clone of cultured cells derived from an identified parental cell type.

**cell-me·di·at·ed im·mu·ni·ty (CMI), cel·lu·lar im·mu·ni·ty** immune responses which are initiated by T lymphocytes and mediated by T lymphocytes, macrophages, or both (e.g., graft rejection, delayed-type hypersensitivity).

**cell-me·di·at·ed re·ac·tion** immunological reaction of the delayed type, involving chiefly T lymphocytes, important in host defense against infection, in autoimmune diseases, and in transplant rejection. SEE ALSO skin test.

**cell mem·brane** the protoplasmic boundary of all cells that controls permeability and may serve other functions through surface specializations; e.g., active ion transport, absorption by formation of pinocytotic vesicles, and antigen recognition; its fine structure is trilaminar and consists of the electron-dense lamina externa and lamina interna with an electron-lucent lamina intermedia. SYN plasma membrane, plasmalemma, Wachendorf membrane (2).

**cell nest** a small focus or accumulation of one type of cell that is different from the other cells in the tissue.

**cel·lu·la,** gen. and pl. **cel·lu·lae** (sel′yu-lă, sel′yu-lē) **1.** in gross anatomy, a small but macroscopic compartment. SYN cellule. **2.** in histology, a cell. [L. a small chamber, dim. of *cella*]

**cel·lu·lar** (sel′yu-lăr) **1.** relating to, derived from, or composed of cells. **2.** having numerous compartments or interstices. [L. *cellula*, dim. of *cella*, storeroom]

**cel·lu·lar bi·ol·o·gy** SYN cytology.

**cel·lu·lar im·mu·no·de·fi·cien·cy with ab·nor·mal im·mu·no·glob·u·lin syn·the·sis** a group of disorders of unknown cause, associated with recurrent bacterial, fungal, protozoal, and viral infections; there is thymic hypoplasia with depressed cellular (T-lymphocyte) immunity combined with defective humoral (B-lymphocyte) immunity.

**cel·lu·lar in·fil·tra·tion** migration of cells from their sources of origin, or direct extension of cells as a result of unusual growth and multiplication; used especially with reference to such changes associated with inflammations and certain types of malignant neoplasms.

**cel·lu·lar·i·ty** (sel-yu-lar′i-tē) the degree, quality, or condition of cells that are present.

**cel·lu·lar pa·thol·o·gy 1.** the interpretation of diseases in terms of cellular alterations; **2.** sometimes used as a synonym for cytopathology (1).

**cel·lu·lase** (sel′yu-lās) endo-1,4-β-glucase; an enzyme catalyzing the hydrolysis of 1,4-β-glucoside links in cellulose. Used to produce digestive tablets and in the removal of cellulose from foods for special diets.

**cel·lule** (sel′yul) SYN cellula (1).

**cel·lu·li·ci·dal** (sel′yu-li-sī′dăl) destructive to cells. [cellula + L. *caedo*, to kill]

**cel·lu·lif·u·gal** (sel-yu-lif′yu-găl) moving from, or extending in a direction away from a cell or cell body. [cellula + L. *fugio*, to flee]

**cel·lu·lip·e·tal** (sel-yu-lip′ĕ-tăl) moving toward, or extending in a direction toward, a cell or cell body. [cellula + L. *peto*, to seek]

**cel·lu·lite** (sel′yu-līt) **1.** colloquial term for deposits of fat and fibrous tissue causing dimpling of the overlying skin. **2.** SYN lipoedema.

**cel·lu·li·tis** (sel-yu-lī′tis) inflammation of subcutaneous, loose connective tissue (formerly called cellular tissue).

**cell wall** the outer layer or membrane of some animal and plant cells; in the latter, it is mainly cellulose.

**cell wall–defective bacteria** bacteria with absent or damaged cell walls; morphologically, they may become spheroplasts, round structures with little or no cell wall, or they may develop filamentous forms, with or without bulbous, extruded portions.

△**ce·lo- 1.** the celom. [G. *koilōma*, hollow (celom)] **2.** hernia. [G. *kēlē*, hernia] **3.** the abdomen. SEE ALSO celio-. [G. *koilia*, belly]

**ce·lom, ce·lo·ma** (sē′lom, sē-lō′mă) **1.** the cavity between the splanchnic and somatic mesoderm in the embryo. **2.** SYN body cavity. [G. *koilōma*, a hollow]

**ce·lom·ic** (sē-lom′ik) relating to the body cavity.

**ce·lo·phle·bi·tis** (sē-lō-flĕ-bī′tis) inflammation of a vena cava. SYN cavitis. [G. *koilos*, hollow, + phlebitis]

**CELO vi·rus** a virus with characteristics of adenovirus, and similar to quail bronchitis virus.

**Cel·si·us (C)** SEE Celsius scale.

**Cel·si·us scale** (sel′sē-ŭs) a temperature scale that is based upon the triple point of water (defined to be 273.16 K) and assigned the value of 0.01°C; this has replaced the centigrade scale because the triple point of water can be more accurately measured than the ice point; for most practical purposes, the two scales are equivalent.

**ce·ment** (se-ment′) **1.** SYN cementum. **2.** in dentistry, a nonmetallic material used for luting, filling, or permanent or temporary restorative purposes, made by mixing components into a plastic mass that sets, or as an adherent sealer in attaching various dental restorations in or on the tooth. [see cementum]

**ce·ment di·sease** the osteolysis that frequently occurs in association with loosening of cemented total hip replacements; the microscopic particles of polymethylmethacrylate cement induce a biologic reaction by osteoclasts leading to bone resorption and progressive bone loss.

**ce·ment·i·cle** (se-men′ti-kl) a calcified spherical body, composed of cementum lying free within the periodontal membrane, attached to the cementum or imbedded within it.

**ce·ment line** the refractile boundary of an osteon or interstitial lamellar system in compact bone.

**ce·ment·o·blast** (se-men′tō-blast) one of the cells concerned with the formation of the layer of cementum on the roots of teeth. [L. *cementum*, cement, + G. *blastos*, germ]

**ce·ment·o·blas·to·ma** (se-men′tō-blas-tō′mă) a benign odontogenic tumor of functional cementoblasts; it appears as a mixed radiolucent-radiopaque lesion attached to a tooth root.

**ce·ment·o·cla·sia** (se-men-tō-klā′zē-ă) destruction of cementum by cementoclasts. [L. *cementum*, cement, + G. *klasis*, fracture]

**ce·ment·o·clast** (se-men′tō-klast) one of the multinucleated giant cells, identical with osteoclasts, that are associated with the resorption of cementum. [L. *cementum,* cement, + G. *klastos,* broken]

**ce•ment•o•cyte** (se-men'tō-sīt) an osteocyte-like cell with numerous processes, trapped in a lacuna in the cementum of the tooth. [L. *cementum,* cement, + G. *kytos,* cell]

**ce•ment•o•den•tin•al junc•tion** the surface at which the cementum and dentin of the root of a tooth are joined.

**ce•men•to•e•nam•el junc•tion** the surface at which the enamel of the crown and the cementum of the root of a tooth are joined. SEE ALSO cervical line.

**ce•men•to•ma** (se-men-tō'mă) any benign cementum-producing tumor; four types are recognized: 1) periapical cemental dysplasia, 2) central ossifying fibroma, 3) cementoblastoma, 4) sclerotic cemental mass. When the type is not specified, cementoma usually refers to periapical cemental dysplasia. [L. *cementum,* cement, + G. *-ōma,* tumor]

**ce•men•to•os•si•fy•ing fi•bro•ma** a form of fibroma with cementicles and bone rimmed with osteoblasts in moderately cellular stroma.

**ce•men•tum** (se-men'tŭm) a layer of bone-like mineralized tissue covering the dentin of the root and neck of a tooth that blends with the fibers of the periodontal ligament. SYN cement (1). [L. *caementum,* rough quarry stone, fr. *caedo,* to cut]

**ce•nes•the•sia** (sē-nes-thē'zē-ă) the general sense of bodily existence; the sensation caused by the functioning of the internal organs. [G. *koinos,* common, + *aisthēsis,* sensation]

**ce•nes•the•sic, ce•nes•thet•ic** (sē-nes-thet'ik, sē-nes-thet'ik) relating to cenesthesia.

△**ce•no-** 1. shared in common. [G. *koinos,* common] 2. new, fresh. [G. *kainos,* new] 3. emptiness (rare). SEE ALSO coeno-. [G. *kenos,* empty]

**cenocyte** (sē'nō-sīt) a multinucleate cell or hyphae without cross walls, characteristic of the hyphae of zygomycetes. [G. *koinos,* common, + *kytos,* cell]

**cen•o•site** (sē'nō-sīt) a facultative commensal organism that can sustain itself apart from its usual host. SYN coinosite. [G. *koinos,* common, + *sitos,* food]

**cen•sor** (sen'sŏr) PSYCHOANALYTIC THEORY the psychic barrier that prevents certain unconscious thoughts and wishes from coming to consciousness. [L. a judge, critic, fr. *censeo,* to value, judge]

**censoring** (sen'sŏr-ing) in epidemiology, (1) loss of subjects from a follow-up study for unknown reasons. (2) observations with unknown values from one end of a frequency distribution, beyond a measurement threshold.

**cen•sus** (sen'sus) an enumeration of a population, originally for taxation and military purposes, now with many other purposes; basic facts about all persons—age, sex, occupation, nature of residence, etc.— are recorded in the census, which often also includes some information about health status. [L., fr. *censeo,* to count]

**cen•ter** (sen'ter) 1. the middle point of a body; loosely, the interior of a body. A center of any kind, especially an anatomic center. 2. a group of nerve cells governing a specific function. 3. a facility performing a particular function or service for persons in the surrounding area. SYN centrum [TA]. [L. *centrum;* G. *kentron*]

**cen•ter of gra•vi•ty (COG)** the point on a body or system where, if pressure equal to the weight of the object is applied, forces acting on the object will be in equilibrium; the location of the COG in a human being in the anatomical position is just anterior to the second sacral vertebra.

**cen•ter of os•si•fi•ca•tion** a site of bone formation through accumulation of osteoblasts within connective tissue (membranous ossification), or of destruction of cartilage before onset of ossification (endochondral ossification). SYN centrum ossificationis [TA], ossific center, point of ossification.

**Cen•ters for Dis•ease Con•trol and Pre•ven•tion (CDC)** the federal facility for disease eradication, epidemiology, and education headquartered in Atlanta, Georgia, which encompasses the Center for Infectious Diseases, Center for Environmental Health, Center for Health Promotion and Education, Center for Prevention Services, Center for Professional Development and Training, and Center for Occupational Safety and Health. Formerly named Center for Disease Control (1970), Communicable Disease Center (1946).

**cen•te•sis** (sen-tē'sis) puncture, especially when used as a suffix, as in paracentesis. [G. *kentēsis,* puncture, fr. *kenteō,* to prick, pierce]

△**cen•ti-** (c) prefix used in the SI and metric systems to signify one hundredth ($10^{-2}$). [L. *centum,* one hundred]

**cen•ti•grade** (C) (sen'ti-grād) 1. basis of the former temperature scale in which 100 degrees separated the melting and boiling points of water. SEE Celsius scale. 2. one hundredth of a circle, equal to 3.6° of the astronomical circle. [L. *centum,* one hundred, + *gradus,* step, degree]

**cen•ti•gram** (sen'ti-gram) one hundredth of a gram.

**cen•tile** (sen'tīl) one-hundredth. [L. *centum,* one hundred, + *-ilis,* adj. suffix]

**cen•ti•li•ter** (sen'ti-lē-ter) 10 milliliters; one hundredth of a liter; 162.3073 minims (U.S.).

**cen•ti•me•ter (cm)** (sen'ti-mē-ter) one hundredth of a meter; 0.3937008 inch.

**cen•ti•me•ter-gram-sec•ond sys•tem (CGS, cgs)** the scientific system of expressing the fundamental physical units of length, mass, and time, and those derived from them, in centimeters, grams, and seconds; currently being replaced by the International System of Units based on the meter, kilogram, and second.

**cen•ti•me•ter-gram-sec•ond u•nit (CGS, cgs), cgs u•nit** an absolute unit of the centimeter-gram-second system.

**cen•ti•mor•gan (cM)** (sen'ti-mōr-găn) SEE morgan.

**cen•ti•nor•mal** (sen-ti-nōr'măl) one-hundredth normal; denoting the concentration of a solution.

**cen•ti•poise** (sen'ti-poyz) one hundredth of a poise.

**cen•tra** (sen'tră) plural of centrum.

**cen•trad** (sen'trad) 1. toward the center. 2. a unit of measurement of the refracting strength of a prism; it corresponds to the deviation of a ray of light, the arc of which is $^1/_{100}$ of the radius of the circle, or 0.57°.

**cen•tral am•pu•ta•tion** amputation in which the flaps are so united that the cicatrix runs across the end of the stump.

**cen•tral ap•nea** apnea as the result of medullary depression which inhibits respiratory movement.

**cen·tral a·re·o·lar cho·roi·dal dys·tro·phy** an autosomal dominant progressive disorder of vision loss with well-demarcated areas of atrophy of the pigmented layer of retina and choriocapillaris.

**cen·tral ar·tery of ret·i·na** a branch of the ophthalmic artery that penetrates the optic nerve 1 cm behind the eye to enter the eye at the optic papilla in the retina; it divides into superior and inferior temporal and nasal branches.

**cen·tral au·di·tory ner·vous sys·tem (CANS)** auditory neural pathway from the cochleas to the auditory cortex. SEE vestibulocochlear nerve [CN VIII].

**cen·tral ca·nal** the ependyma-lined lumen (cavity) of the neural tube, the cerebral part of which remains patent to form the ventricles of the brain, while the spinal part in the adult often is reduced to a solid strand of modified ependyma. SYN syringocele (1).

**central cloudy corneal dystrophy of François** (frahn-swah') an autosomal dominant opacification of the central corneal stroma consisting of cloudy polygonal areas.

**cen·tral cord syn·drome** quadriparesis most severely involving the distal upper extremities, with or without sensory loss and bladder dysfunction, usually due to ischemia from osteophytic or traumatic compression of the central part of the cervical spinal cord and/or artery.

**cen·tral cry·stal·line cor·ne·al dys·tro·phy of Sny·der** (sni'der) an autosomal dominant opacification of the central corneal stroma by needle-shaped polychromatic crystals.

**cen·tral deaf·ness** deafness due to disorder of the auditory system of the brainstem or cerebral cortex.

**cen·tral gan·glio·neu·ro·ma** SYN gangliocytoma.

**cen·tral gy·ri** the precentral and postcentral gyri.

**cen·tra·li·za·tion phe·nom·e·non** the relatively rapid change in the perceived location of pain, from more peripheral, or distal, to a more proximal, or central, location; commonly occurs during initial evaluation of patients with low back and radiating limb pain; helpful in determining the type and prognosis of physical therapy.

**cen·tral ne·cro·sis** necrosis involving the deeper or inner portions of a tissue, or an organ or its units.

**cen·tral ner·vous sys·tem (CNS)** the brain and the spinal cord.

**cen·tral os·si·fy·ing fi·bro·ma** a painless, slow-growing, expansile, sharply circumscribed benign fibro-osseous tumor of the jaws that is derived from cells of the periodontal ligament; presents initially as a radiolucency that becomes progressively more opaque as it matures.

**cen·tral os·te·i·tis 1.** SYN osteomyelitis. **2.** SYN endosteitis.

**cen·tral pal·mar space** the more medial of the central palmar spaces, bounded medially by the hypothenar compartment; related distally to the synovial tendon sheaths of digits 3 and 4 and proximally to the common flexor sheath.

**cen·tral pa·ral·y·sis** paralysis due to a lesion in the brain or spinal cord.

**cen·tral ret·i·nal ar·tery** a branch of the ophthalmic artery that penetrates the optic nerve 1 cm behind the eye (extraocular part) to enter the eye (intraocular part) at the optic papilla in the retina; it divides into superior and inferior tempo-

ral and nasal branches. SYN arteria centralis retinae [TA].

**cen·tral ret·i·nal fo·vea** a depression in the center of the macula retinae containing only cones and lacking blood vessels. SYN fovea centralis maculae luteae [TA].

**cen·tral sco·to·ma** a scotoma involving the fixation point.

**cen·tral spin·dle** in mitosis, a central group of microtubules (continuous fibers) that course uninterrupted, between the asters, in contrast to the microtubules attached to the individual chromosomes (spindle fibers).

**cen·tral sul·cus** a double-S-shaped fissure extending obliquely upward and backward on the lateral surface of each cerebral hemisphere at the boundary between frontal and parietal lobes.

**cen·tral vein of ret·i·na** formed by union of the retinal veins and accompanies the artery of the same name in the optic nerve. SYN vena centralis retinae [TA].

**cen·tral veins of liv·er** initial vein of the hepatic venous system, located in the center of the conceptual hepatic lobule, receiving blood from sinuses and draining into collecting veins that become hepatic veins. SYN Krukenberg veins.

**cen·tral vein of su·pra·re·nal gland** the single draining vein of the gland; it receives a number of medullary veins; on the right side it empties directly into the inferior vena cava and on the left into the left renal vein. SYN vena centralis glandulae suprarenalis [TA].

**cen·tral ve·nous cath·e·ter** a catheter passed through a peripheral or central vein, ending in the thoracic vena cava or right atrium, for measurement of venous pressure or for infusion of concentrated solutions; the peripheral end may connect to a subcutaneous chamber for percutaneous injections given over periods of months or may exit through the skin at a distance from the vein.

**cen·tral ve·nous pres·sure (CVP)** the pressure of the blood within the venous system in the superior and inferior vena cava, normally between 4 and 10 cm of water (1–3 mmHg); it is depressed in circulatory shock and deficiencies of circulating blood volume, and increased with cardiac failure and congestion of the venous circulation.

**cen·tral vi·sion** vision stimulated by an object imaged on the fovea centralis. SYN direct vision.

**cen·tren·ce·phal·ic** (sen'tren-se-fal'ik) relating to the center of the encephalon.

**cen·tri·ac·i·nar em·phy·se·ma** SYN centrilobular emphysema.

△**cen·tric** (sen'trik) **1.** having a center (of a specific kind or number) or having a specific thing as its center (of interest, focus, etc.). **2.** DENISSTRY pertaining to ideally centered occlusion, with optimum contact and intercuspation. [G. *kentron*, center]

**cen·tric fu·sion** SYN robertsonian translocation.

**cen·tric·i·put** (sen-tris'i-put) the central portion of the upper surface of the skull, between the occiput and the sinciput. [L. *centrum*, center, + *caput*, head]

**cen·tric oc·clu·sion 1.** the relation of opposing occlusal surfaces which provides the maximum contact and/or intercuspation; **2.** the occlusion of the teeth when the mandible is in centric relation to the maxillae. SYN acquired centric, habitual centric, intercuspal position.

**cen·tric re·la·tion** the relation of the lower to the upper jaw when the condyles are in their most posterior and superior position in the mandibular (glenoid) fossae. SYN terminal hinge position.

**cen·trif·u·gal** (sen-trif′yu-găl) **1.** denoting the direction of the force pulling an object outward (away) from an axis of rotation. **2.** sometimes, by analogy, extended to describe any movement away from a center. Cf. eccentric (2). [L. *centrum,* center, + *fugio,* to flee]

**cen·trif·u·gal nerve** SYN efferent nerve.

**cen·trif·u·ga·tion** (sen-trif-yu-gā′shŭn) sedimentation, by means of a centrifuge, of solids suspended in a fluid.

**cen·tri·fuge** (sen′tri-fyuj) **1.** an apparatus by means of which particles in suspension in a fluid are separated by spinning the fluid, the centrifugal force throwing the particles to the periphery of the rotated vessel. **2.** to submit to rapid rotary action, as in a centrifuge.

**cen·tri·lob·u·lar** (sen-tri-lob′yu-lăr) at or near the center of a lobule, e.g., of the liver.

**cen·tri·lob·u·lar em·phy·se·ma** emphysema affecting the lobules around their central bronchioles, causally related to bronchiolitis, and seen in coal-miner's pneumoconiosis. SYN centriacinar emphysema.

**cen·tri·ole** (sen′trē-ōl) tubular structures usually seen as paired organelles lying in the cytocentrum; centrioles may be multiple and numerous in some cells, such as the giant cells of bone marrow. [G. *kentron,* a point, center]

**cen·trip·e·tal** (sen-trip′ĕ-tăl) **1.** SYN afferent. **2.** denoting the direction of the force pulling an object toward an axis of rotation. SYN axipetal. [L. *centrum,* center, + *peto,* to seek]

**cen·trip·e·tal nerve** SYN afferent nerve.

⚠**cen·tro-** combining form denoting center. [G. *kentron*]

**cen·tro·ac·i·nar cell** a cell of the pancreatic ductule that occupies the lumen of an acinus; it secretes bicarbonate and water, providing an alkaline pH necessary for enzyme activity in the intestine.

**cen·tro·ki·ne·sia** (sen′trō-ki-nē′sē-ă) movement excited by a stimulus of central origin. [centro- + G. *kinēsis,* movement]

**cen·tro·ki·net·ic** (sen′trō-ki-net′ik) **1.** relating to centrokinesia. **2.** SYN excitomotor.

**cen·tro·me·di·an nu·cle·us** a large, lentil-shaped cell group, the largest and most caudal of the intralaminar nuclei, located within the lamina medullaris interna of the thalamus between the mediodorsal nucleus and ventrobasal nucleus; so called by Luys because of its prominent appearance on frontal sections midway between the anterior and posterior pole of the human thalamus. The nucleus receives numerous fibers from the internal segment of the globus pallidus by way of the thalamic fasciculus, ansa lenticularis, and lenticular fasciculus as well as projections from area 4 of the motor cortex; its major efferent connection is with the putamen although collaterals reach broad areas of the cerebral cortex.

**cen·tro·mere** (sen′trō-mēr) the nonstaining primary constriction of a chromosome; the centromere divides the chromosome into two arms, and its position is constant for a specific chromosome: near one end (acrocentric), near the center (metacentric), or between (submetacentric). [centro- + G. *meros,* part]

**cen·tro·some** (sen′trō-sōm) SYN cytocentrum. [centro- + G. *sōma,* body]

**cen·tro·sphere** (sen′trō-sfēr) the specialized cytoplasm of the cytocentrum. Contains the centrioles from which the astral fibers (microtubules) extend during mitosis. [centro- + G. *sphaira,* a ball, sphere]

**cen·tro·stal·tic** (sen-trō-stal′tik) relating to the center of motion. [centro- + G. *stallein,* set forth, fetch]

**cen·trum,** pl. **cen·tra** (sen′trŭm, sen′tră) [TA] SYN center. [L. fr. G. *kentron*]

**centrum ossificationis** [TA] SYN center of ossification.

**cen·tum (c)** (sĕn′tŭm) l. hundred [L. one hundred]

▣**ceph·a·lad** (sef′ă-lad) in a direction toward the head. SEE ALSO cranial (1). See page APP 89.

**ceph·a·lal·gia** (sef′al-al′jē-ă) SYN headache. [cephal- + G. *algos,* pain]

**ceph·al·e·de·ma** (sef′al-ĕ-dē′mă) edema of the head.

**ceph·al·hae·ma·to·ma [Br.]** SEE cephalhematoma.

**ceph·al·he·ma·to·cele, ceph·a·lo·he·ma·to·cele** (sef′ăl-hē-mat′ō-sēl, sef′ă-lō-hē-mat′ō-sēl) a cephalhematoma under the periosteum of the skull communicating with the dural sinuses. [cephal- + G. *haima,* blood, + *kēlē,* tumor]

**ceph·al·he·ma·to·ma, ceph·a·lo·he·ma·to·ma** (sef′ăl-hē-mă-tō′mă, sef′ă-lō-hē-mă-tō′mă) an effusion of blood beneath the periosteum of a cranial bone, seen frequently in a newborn as a result of birth trauma; contrasted with caput succedaneum, in which the effusion overlies the periosteum and consists of serum. SYN cephalohaematoma. [cephal- + G. *haima,* blood, + -*ōma,* tumor]

**ceph·al·hy·dro·cele** (sef-ăl-hī′drō-sēl) an accumulation of serous or watery fluid under the pericranium. [cephal- + G. *hydōr,* water, + *kēlē,* tumor]

▣**ce·phal·ic** (se-fa′lik) SYN cranial (1). See page APP 89.

**ceph·a·lic curve** curve conforming to that of the fetal head, used in reference to the shape of obstetrical forceps.

**ce·phal·ic flex·ure** the sharp, ventrally concave bend in the developing midbrain of the embryo. SYN cranial flexure, mesencephalic flexure.

**ce·phal·ic pole** the head end of the fetus.

**ce·phal·ic pre·sen·ta·tion** presentation of any part of the fetal head, usually the upper and back part as a result of flexion such that the chin is in contact with the thorax in vertex presentation; there may be degrees of flexion so that the presenting part is the large fontanel in sincipital presentation, the brow in brow presentation, or the face in face presentation.

**ceph·a·lic re·place·ment** in cases of shoulder dystocia when vaginal delivery cannot be effected, the fetal head is flexed and reinserted into the vagina to re-establish umbilical cord blood flow and delivery performed through cesarean section. SYN Zavanelli maneuver.

**ce·phal·ic tet·a·nus** a type of local tetanus that follows wounds to the face and head; after a brief incubation (1–2 days) the facial and ocular muscles become paretic yet undergo repeated tetanic spasms. The throat and tongue muscles may also be affected.

**ce·phal·ic vein** arises at the radial border of the dorsal venous rete of the hand, passes upward in front of the elbow and along the lateral side of the arm; it empties into the upper part of the axillary vein.

**ce·phal·ic ver·sion** version in which the fetus is turned so that the head presents; can be external cephalic version or internal cephalic version. SEE ALSO external cephalic version, internal cephalic version.

**ceph·a·li·tis** (sef-ă-lī′tis) SYN encephalitis.

△**ce·pha·lo-, cephal-** the head. [G. *kephalē*]

**ceph·a·lo·cau·dal ax·is** long axis of the body; the imaginary straight line in the median plane which runs from the apex of the skull through the center of the perineum and continuing between the lower limbs.

**ceph·a·lo·cele** (sef′ă-lō-sēl) protrusion of part of the cranial contents, e.g., meningocele, encephalocele. SEE ALSO encephalocele.

**ceph·a·lo·cen·te·sis** (sef′ă-lō-sen-tē′sis) passage of a hollow needle or trocar into the brain to drain or aspirate an abscess or the fluid of a hydrocephalus. [cephalo- + G. *kentēsis,* puncture]

**ceph·a·lo·dyn·ia** (sef′ă-lō-din′ē-ă) headache. [cephalo- + G. *odynē,* pain]

**ceph·a·lo·gy·ric** (sef′ă-lō-jī′rik) relating to rotation of the head. [cephalo- + G. *gyros,* a circle]

**ceph·a·lo·hae·ma·to·ma [Br.]** SYN cephalhematoma.

**ceph·a·lo·meg·a·ly** (sef′ă-lō-meg′ă-lē) enlargement of the head. [cephalo- + G. *megas,* great]

**ceph·a·lom·e·ter** (sef-ă-lom′ĕ-ter) an instrument used to position the head to produce oriented, reproducible lateral and posterior-anterior head films. SYN cephalostat. [cephalo- + G. *metron,* measure]

**ceph·a·lo·met·rics** (sef-ă-lō-met′riks) **1.** ORAL SURGERY, ORTHODONTICS the scientific measurement of the bones of the cranium and face, using a fixed, reproducible position for lateral radiographic exposure of skull and facial bones. **2.** a scientific study of the measurements of the head with relation to specific reference points; used for evaluation of facial growth and development, including soft tissue profile. [cephalo- + G. *metron,* measure]

**ceph·a·lom·e·try** (sef-ă-lom′ĕ-trē) measurements on the living head, or head without removal of the soft parts. SEE ALSO cephalometrics. [cephalo- + G. *metron,* measure]

**ceph·a·lo·mo·tor** (sef′ă-lō-mō′ter) relating to movements of the head.

**ceph·a·lop·a·thy** (sef-ă-lop′ă-thē) SYN encephalopathy. [cephalo- + G. *pathos,* suffering]

**ceph·a·lo·pel·vic** (sef′ă-lō-pel′vik) pertaining to the size of the fetal head in relation to the maternal pelvis.

**ceph·a·lo·pel·vic dis·pro·por·tion** a condition in which the fetal head is too large to traverse the maternal pelvis.

**ceph·a·lo·pel·vim·e·try** (sef′ă-lō-pel-vim′ĕ-trē) roentgenographic measurement of the dimensions of the pelvis and the fetal head. [cephalo- + pelvimetry]

**ceph·a·lo·stat** (sef′ă-lō-stat) SYN cephalometer. [cephalo- + G. *statos,* stationary]

**ce·phal·o·tho·rac·ic** (sef′ă-lō-thō-ras′ik) relating to the head and the chest.

△**-cep·tor** combining form denoting taker, receiver. [L. *capio,* pp. *captus,* to take]

**cer·am·i·dase** (ser-am′i-dās) an enzyme that hydrolyzes ceramides into sphingosine and a fatty acid. A deficiency of this enzyme is associated with Farber disease.

**cer·a·mide** (ser′ă-mīd) generic term for a class of sphingolipid, *N*-acyl (fatty acid) derivatives of a long chain base or sphingoid such as sphingenine or sphingosine. Ceramides accumulate in individuals with Farber disease.

△**cer·at-** SEE kerat-.

△**cer·a·to-** SEE kerato-.

**cer·a·to·cri·coid mus·cle** a fasciculus from the posterior cricoarytenoid muscle inserted into the inferior horn of the thyroid cartilage. SYN musculus ceratocricoideus [TA].

**cer·a·to·glos·sus** main, posterior part of hyoglossus muscle (vs. chondroglossus) arising from the greater horn of the hyoid bone.

**cer·car·ia,** pl. **cer·car·i·ae** (ser-kā′rē-ă, ser-kā′rē-ē) the free-swimming trematode larva that emerges from its host snail; it may penetrate the skin of a final host, encyst on vegetation, in or on fish, or penetrate and encyst in various arthropod hosts. Body and tail are greatly varied in form, and specialized function is adapted to the particular life cycle demands of each species. SEE ALSO sporocyst (1). [G. *kerkos,* tail]

**cer·ci** (ser′sī) plural of cercus.

**cer·clage** (ser-klahzh′) **1.** bringing into close opposition and binding together the ends of an obliquely fractured bone or the fragments of a broken patella by a ring or by an encircling, tightly drawn wire loop. **2.** operation for retinal detachment in which the choroid and retinal pigment epithelium are brought in contact with the detached sensory retina by a band encircling the sclera posterior. **3.** the placing of a nonabsorbable suture around an incompetent cervical os. SYN tiring. [Fr. an encircling, hooping, banding]

**cer·co·cys·tis** (ser-kō-sis′tis) a form of tapeworm larva that develops within the vertebrate host villus rather than in an invertebrate host. SEE ALSO cysticercus. [G. *kerkos,* tail, + *kystis,* bladder]

**cer·co·pith·e·crine her·pes·vi·rus** an herpesvirus, in the family Herpesviridae, affecting Old World monkeys, that is very similar morphologically to herpes simplex virus; fatal infection may occur in humans following the bite of an infected monkey, although other modes of transmission have also been documented.

**cer·cus,** gen. and pl. **cer·ci** (ser′kŭs, ser′sī) a stiff hairlike structure. [Mod. L., fr. G. *kerkos,* tail]

**ce·rea flex·i·bil·i·tas** (sē′rē-ă flek-si-bil′i-tas) "waxy flexibility," in which the limb remains where placed; often seen in catatonia. [L.]

**cer·e·bel·lar** (ser-e-bel′ar) relating to the cerebellum.

**cer·e·bel·lar cor·tex** the thin gray surface layer of the cerebellum, consisting of an outer molecular layer or stratum moleculare, a single layer of Purkinje cells (the ganglionic layer), and an inner granular layer or stratum granulosum.

**cer·e·bel·lar fissure** the deep furrows which divide the lobules of the cerebellum. SYN fissurae cerebelli [TA].

**cer·e·bel·lar gait** wide-based gait with lateral veering, unsteadiness, and irregularity of steps; often with a tendency to fall to one side, forward, or backward. SYN ataxic gait.

**cer·e·bel·lar hem·i·sphere** the large part of the cerebellum lateral to the vermis cerebelli.

**cer·e·bel·lar pe·dun·cle** pedunculus cerebellaris inferior, medius, and superior.

**cer·e·bel·li·tis** (ser-ĕ-bel-ī′tis) inflammation of the cerebellum.

△**cer·e·bel·lo-** the cerebellum. [L. *cerebrum*, brain, + *-ellum*, dim. suff.]

**cer·e·bel·lo·pon·tine ang·le** the recess at the junction of the cerebellum, pons, and medulla. SYN angulus pontocerebellaris [TA].

**cer·e·bel·lum**, pl. **ce·re·bel·la** (ser-e-bel′ŭm, ser-e-bel′ă) [TA] the large posterior brain mass lying dorsal to the pons and medulla and ventral to the posterior portion of the cerebrum; it consists of two lateral hemispheres united by a narrow middle portion, the vermis. [L. dim. of *cerebrum*, brain]

**ce·re·bra** (sĕ-rē′bră) plural of cerebrum.

**ce·re·bral** (ser′ĕ-brăl, sĕ-rē′brăl) relating to the cerebrum.

**ce·re·bral am·y·loid an·gi·op·a·thy** a pathological condition of small cerebral vessels characterized by deposits of amyloid in the vessel walls, which may lead to infarcts or hemorrhage; may also occur in Alzheimer disease. SEE ALSO congophilic angiopathy.

**ce·re·bral aq·ue·duct** an ependyma-lined canal in the mesencephalon about 20 mm long, connecting the third to the fourth ventricle.

**ce·re·bral cor·tex** the gray cellular mantle (1–4 mm thick) covering the entire surface of the cerebral hemisphere of mammals; characterized by a laminar organization of cellular and fibrous components such that its nerve cells are stacked in defined layers varying in number from one, as in the archicortex of the hippocampus, to five or six in the larger neocortex; the outermost (molecular or plexiform) layer contains very few cell bodies and is composed largely of the distal ramifications of the long apical dendrites issued perpendicularly to the surface by pyramidal and fusiform cells in deeper layers. From the surface inward, the layers as classified in K. Brodmann's parcellation are: 1) molecular or plexiform layer; 2) outer granular layer; 3) pyramidal cell layer; 4) inner granular layer; 5) inner pyramidal layer (ganglionic layer); and 6) multiform cell layer, many of which are fusiform. This multilaminate organization is typical of the neocortex (homotypic cortex; isocortex in O. Vogt's terminology), which in humans covers the largest part by far of the cerebral hemisphere. The more primordial heterotypic cortex or allocortex (Vogt) has fewer cell layers. A form of cortex intermediate between isocortex and allocortex, called juxtallocortex (Vogt) covers the ventral part of the cingulate gyrus and the entorhinal area of the parahippocampal gyrus.

On the basis of local differences in the arrangement of nerve cells (cytoarchitecture), Brodmann outlined 47 areas in the cerebral cortex which, in functional terms, can be classified into three categories: motor cortex (areas 4 and 6), characterized by a poorly developed inner granular layer (agranular cortex) and prominent pyramidal cell layers; sensory cortex, characterized by a prominent inner granular layer (granular cortex or koniocortex) and comprising the somatic sensory cortex (areas 1 to 3), the auditory cortex (areas 41 and 42), and the visual cortex (areas 17 to 19);

and association cortex, the vast remaining expanses of the cerebral cortex. See this page.

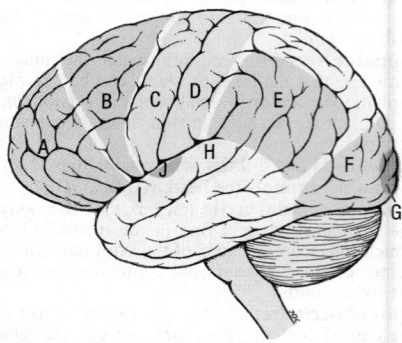

**cerebral cortex:** major functional areas: (A) biological intelligence, (B) premotor, (C) somatomotor, (D) somatosensory, (E) bodily awareness, (F) visual psychic, (G) visual sensory, (H) speech understanding, (I) auditory psychic, (J) auditory sensory

**ce·re·bral death** a clinical syndrome characterized by the permanent loss of cerebral and brain stem function, manifested by absence of responsiveness to external stimuli, absence of cephalic reflexes, and apnea. An isoelectric electroencephalogram for at least 30 minutes in the absence of hypothermia and poisoning by central nervous system depressants supports the diagnosis.

**ce·re·bral de·com·pres·sion** removal of a piece of the cranium, usually in the subtemporal region, with incision of the dura, to relieve intracranial pressure.

**ce·re·bral dom·i·nance** the fact that one hemisphere is dominant over the other and exercises greater influence over certain functions; the left cerebral hemisphere is usually dominant in the control of speech, language and analytical processing, and mathematics, while the right hemisphere (usually nondominant) processes spatial concepts and language as related to certain types of visual images; handedness (right-handed persons have left cerebral dominance) is considered a general example of cerebral dominance.

**ce·re·bral dys·pla·sia** abnormal development of the telencephalon.

**ce·re·bral e·de·ma** brain swelling due to increased volume of the extravascular compartment from the uptake of water in the neuropile and white matter. SEE ALSO brain swelling.

**ce·re·bral gi·gan·tism** a syndrome characterized by increased birth weight and length (above 90th percentile), accelerated growth rate for the first four or five years without elevation of serum growth hormone levels, and then reversion to normal growth rate; characteristic facies include prognathism, hypertelorism, antimongoloid slant, and dolichocephalic skull; moderate mental retardation and impaired coordination are also associated.

**ce·re·bral hem·i·sphere 1.** SYN hemisphere. **2.** the large mass of the telencephalon, on either side of the midline, consisting of the cerebral cortex and its associated fiber systems, together with the deeper-lying subcortical telencephalic nuclei (i.e., basal ganglia [nuclei]). SYN hemispherium (1).

▣ ce·re·bral hem·or·rhage hemorrhage into the substance of the cerebrum, usually in the region of the internal capsule by the rupture of the lenticulostriate artery. See this page. SYN hematencephalon.

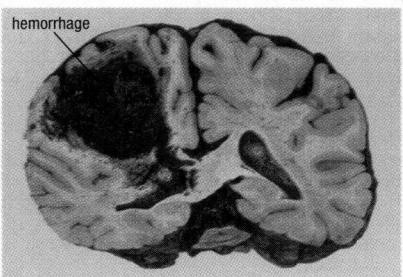

**hemorrhage:** autopsy specimen showing massive hemorrhage in the right cerebral hemisphere

ce·re·bral her·nia protrusion of brain substance through a defect in the skull.

ce·re·bral lo·cal·i·za·tion the mapping of the cerebral cortex into areas and the correlation of the various areas with cerebral function, or determining the site of a brain lesion, based on the signs and symptoms manifested by the patient or by neuroimaging.

ce·re·bral pal·sy defect of motor power and coordination related to damage of the brain.

ce·re·bral pe·dun·cle large bundles of corticofugal fibers forming the crus cerebri, plus the midbrain tegmentum; the substantia nigra, while a part of the base of the peduncle (basis pedunculi), is considered a structure separating the midbrain tegmentum from the crus cerebri. SEE ALSO crus cerebri.

ce·re·bral ves·i·cle each of the three divisions of the early embryonic brain (prosencephalon, mesencephalon, and rhombencephalon). SYN primary brain vesicle.

cer·e·bra·tion (ser-ĕ-brā'shŭn) activity of the mental processes; thinking. SEE ALSO cognition.

cer·e·bri·form (se-rē'bri-fōrm) resembling the external fissures and convolutions of the brain. [cerebri- + L. forma, shape, appearance, nature]

cer·e·bri·tis (ser-ĕ-brī'tis) focal inflammatory infiltrates in the brain parenchyma.

△cer·e·bro-, cer·e·br-, cer·e·bri- the cerebrum. SEE ALSO encephalo-. [L. cerebrum, brain]

cer·e·bro·ma SYN encephaloma.

cer·e·bro·ma·la·cia (ser'ĕ-brō-mă-lā'shē-ă) SYN encephalomalacia.

cer·e·bro·men·in·gi·tis (ser'ĕ-brō-men-in-jī'tis) SYN meningoencephalitis.

cer·e·brop·a·thy (ser-ĕ-brop'ă-thē) SYN encephalopathy.

cer·e·bro·scle·ro·sis (ser'ĕ-brō-sklēr-ō'sis) encephalosclerosis, hardening of the cerebral hemispheres. [cerebro- + G. sklērōsis, hardening]

cer·e·bro·side (ser'ĕ-brŏ-sīd) a class of glycosphingolipid; cerebrosides are found in the myelin sheath of nerve tissue.

cer·e·bro·spi·nal (sĕ-rē'brō-spī-năl) relating to the brain and the spinal cord.

cer·e·bro·spi·nal ax·is the central nervous system; the brain and spinal cord.

cer·e·bro·spi·nal flu·id (CSF) a fluid largely secreted by the choroid plexuses of the ventricles of the brain, filling the ventricles and the subarachnoid cavities of the brain and spinal cord.

cer·e·bro·spi·nal flu·id rhi·nor·rhea a discharge of cerebrospinal fluid from the nose.

cer·e·bro·spi·nal men·in·gi·tis SYN meningitis.

cer·e·bro·spi·nal pres·sure the pressure of the cerebrospinal fluid, normally 100 to 150 mm of water, relative to the ambient atmospheric pressure.

cer·e·brot·o·my (ser-ĕ-brot'ō-mē) incision of the brain. [cerebro- + G. tomē, incision]

cer·e·bro·vas·cu·lar (ser'ĕ-brō-vas'kyu-lăr) relating to the blood supply to the brain, particularly with reference to pathologic changes.

cer·e·bro·vas·cu·lar ac·ci·dent (CVA) an imprecise term for cerebral stroke.

cer·e·brum, pl. ce·re·bra, cer·e·brums (ser'ĕ-brŭm, sĕ-rē'brŭm; sĕ-rē'bră; ser'ĕ-brŭmz) [TA] originally referred to the largest portion of the brain; it now usually refers only to the parts derived from the telencephalon and includes mainly the cerebral hemispheres (cerebral cortex and basal ganglia). [L., brain]

ce·ri·um (Ce) (sēr'ē-ŭm) a metallic element, atomic no. 58, atomic wt. 140.115. [fr. Ceres, the planetoid]

cer·ti·fi·a·ble (ser-ti-fī'ă-bl) denoting a person showing disordered behavior of sufficient gravity to justify involuntary mental hospitalization.

cer·ti·fi·ca·tion (ser'ti-fi-kā'shŭn) 1. the attainment of board certification in a specialty. 2. the court procedure by which a patient is committed to a mental institution. 3. involuntary mental hospitalization.

cer·ti·fied milk cow's milk that does not have more than the maximal permissible limit of 10,000 bacteria per ml at any time prior to delivery to the consumer, and that must be cooled to 10°C or less and maintained at that temperature until delivery.

cer·ti·fied nurse-mid·wife a registered nurse with at least a master's degree in nursing and advanced education in the management of maternity. Certification is achieved through an organized program of study and national testing by the American College of Nurse-Midwives.

cer·ti·fied pas·teur·ized milk cow's milk in which the maximum permissible limit is 10,000 bacteria per ml before pasteurization and 500 bacteria per ml after pasteurization; it must be cooled to 7.2°C or less and maintained at that temperature until delivery.

cer·ti·fied ref·er·ence ma·ter·i·al (CRM) a reference material documented by or traceable to a certificate or publication from a reputable source and that states the values of the properties concerned.

ce·ru·lein (se-roo'lē-in) a decapeptide with hypotensive activity; stimulates smooth muscle and increases digestive secretions; it is similar in structure to cholecystokinin and the gastrins, but much more potent as a stimulant to gallbladder contraction; also stimulates release of insulin. [Fr. Hyla caerulea, from which isolated]

ce·ru·lo·plas·min (sĕ-roo'lō-plaz-min) a blue

copper-containing α-globulin of blood plasma; involved in copper transport and regulation, and can reduce $O_2$ directly without known intermediates. Ceruloplasmin is absent in congenital Wilson disease. [L. *caeruleus,* dark blue]

ce•ru•men (sĕ-roo'men) the soft, brownish yellow, waxy secretion (a modified sebum) of the ceruminous glands of the external auditory meatus. [L. *cera,* wax]

ce•ru•mi•nal (sĕ-roo'mi-năl) relating to cerumen.

ce•ru•mi•no•lyt•ic (sĕ-roo'mi-nō-lit'ik) any substance instilled into the external auditory canal to soften wax. [cerumen, + G. *lysis,* a loosening]

ce•ru•mi•no•sis (sĕ-roo-mi-nō'sis) excessive formation of cerumen.

ce•ru•mi•nous (sĕ-roo'mi-nŭs) relating to cerumen.

ce•ru•mi•nous glands apocrine sudoriferous glands in the external acoustic meatus. SYN glandulae ceruminosae (1) [TA].

cer•vi•cal (ser'vĭ-kal) relating to a neck, or cervix, in any sense. [L. *cervix (cervic-),* neck]

cer•vi•cal ca•nal a fusiform canal extending from the isthmus of the uterus to the opening of the uterus into the vagina. SYN canalis cervicis uteri [TA].

cer•vi•cal disk syn•drome pain, paresthesias, and sometimes weakness in the area of the distribution of one or more cervical roots, due to pressure of a protruded cervical intervertebral disk.

cer•vi•cal flex•ure the ventrally concave bend at the juncture of the brainstem and spinal cord in the embryo.

cer•vi•cal glands branched mucus-secreting glands in the mucosa of the cervix.

cer•vi•cal in•tra•ep•i•the•li•al ne•o•pla•si•a (CIN) dysplastic changes beginning at the squamocolumnar junction in the uterine cervix which may be precursors of squamous cell carcinoma: grade 1, mild dysplasia involving the lower one-third or less of the epithelial thickness; grade 2, moderate dysplasia with one-third to two-thirds involvement; grade 3, severe dysplasia or carcinoma in situ, with two-thirds to full-thickness involvement.

cer•vi•cal line a continuous anatomical irregular curved line marking the junction of the crown and the root of a tooth.

cer•vi•cal loop SYN ansa cervicalis.

cervical lordosis the normal, anteriorly convex curvature of the cervical segment of the vertebral column; a secondary curvature, acquired postnatally as the infant lifts its head. SYN lordosis cervicis [TA], lordosis colli.

cer•vi•cal or•tho•sis an orthosis designed to limit cervical spine motion to varying degrees, e.g., a soft cervical collar.

cer•vi•cal plex•us formed by loops joining the adjacent ventral primary rami of the first four cervical nerves and receiving gray communicating rami from the superior cervical ganglion; it lies deep to the sternocleidomastoid muscle, and sends out numerous cutaneous, muscular, and communicating rami.

cer•vi•cal preg•nan•cy the implantation and development of the impregnated ovum in the cervical canal.

cer•vi•cal rib a supernumerary rib articulating with a cervical vertebra, usually the seventh, but not reaching the sternum anteriorly. SEE ALSO cervical rib syndrome. SYN costa cervicalis [TA].

cer•vi•cal rib syn•drome 1) arterial thoracic outlet syndrome, in which the subclavian artery is compromised by a fully formed cervical rib, and 2) true neurogenic thoracic outlet syndrome, in which the proximal lower trunk of the brachial plexus is compromised by a radiolucent band extending from a rudimentary cervical rib to the first rib.

cer•vi•cal ver•te•brae [C1–C7] the seven segments of the vertebral column located in the neck. SYN vertebrae cervicales [C1–C7] [TA].

cer•vi•cec•to•my (ser-vi-sek'tō-mē) excision of the cervix uteri. SYN trachelectomy. [cervix + G. *ektomē,* excision]

cer•vi•ces (ser'vi-sēz) plural of cervix.

cer•vi•cis (ser'vi-sis) genitive of cervix.

cer•vi•ci•tis (ser-vi-sī'tis) inflammation of the mucous membrane, frequently involving also the deeper structures, of the cervix uteri. SYN trachelitis.

△cer•vi•co- a cervix, or neck, in any sense. [L. *cervix,* neck]

cer•vi•co•brach•i•al (ser'vi-kō-brā'kē-ăl) relating to the neck and the arm.

cer•vi•co•dyn•ia (ser'vi-kō-din'ē-ă) neck pain. SYN trachelodynia. [cervico- + G. *odynē,* pain]

cer•vi•co•fa•cial (ser'vi-kō-fā'shăl) relating to the neck and the face.

cer•vi•cog•ra•phy (ser-vi-kog'ră-fē) technique, equivalent to colposcopy, for photographing part or all of the uterine cervix. [cervix + G. *graphō,* to write]

cer•vi•co•oc•cip•i•tal (ser'vi-kō-ok-sip'i-tăl) relating to the neck and the occiput.

cer•vi•co•oc•u•lo•a•cous•tic syn•drome a disorder characterized by a congenitally short neck with fused cervical vertebrae (Klippel-Feil anomaly), sixth cranial nerve paralysis with retraction of the eye globe and narrowing of the palpebral fissure on adduction (Duane palsy), and sensorineural deafness; inheritance is thought to be multifactorial with limitation to females.

cer•vi•co•plas•ty (ser'vi-kō-plas-tē) plastic surgery on the cervix uteri or on the neck.

cer•vi•co•sco•py SYN acetowhitening.

cer•vi•co•tho•rac•ic (ser'vi-kō-thōr-as'ik) relating to: 1. the neck and thorax; 2. the transition between the neck and thorax; 3. the fusion of the cervical and thoracic vertebrae.

cer•vi•co•tho•rac•ic gan•gli•on a sympathetic trunk ganglion lying behind the subclavian artery near the origin of the vertebral artery, it is formed by the fusion of the inferior cervical ganglion, at the level of the seventh cervical vertebra, with the first thoracic ganglion. SYN ganglion cervicothoracicum [TA].

cervicothoracic orthosis a device designed to limit cervical spine motion by extending to cover more of the upper torso than a standard cervical orthosis.

cer•vi•cot•o•my (ser-vi-kot'ō-mē) incision into the cervix uteri. SYN trachelotomy. [cervico- + G. *tomē,* incision]

cer•vi•co•ves•i•cal (ser'vi-kō-ves'i-kăl) relating to the cervix of the uterus and the bladder.

cer•vix, gen. cer•vi•cis, pl. cer•vi•ces (ser'viks, ser'vi-sis, ser'vi-sēz) 1. SYN neck. 2. any neck-like structure. 3. SYN cervix of uterus. [L. neck]

cer•vix of uter•us the lower part of the uterus extending from the isthmus of the uterus into the vagina. It is divided into supravaginal and vagi-

**cer·vix of uter·us** the lower part of the uterus extending from the isthmus of the uterus into the vagina. It is divided into supravaginal and vaginal parts by its passage through the vaginal wall. SYN cervix (3).

**ce·sar·e·an hys·ter·ec·to·my** cesarean section followed by hysterectomy.

**ce·sar·e·an sec·tion** (sĕ-zar′ē-ăn) incision through the abdominal wall and the uterus (abdominal hysterotomy) for extraction of the fetus.

**ce·si·um (Cs)** (sē′zē-ŭm) a metallic element, atomic no. 55, atomic wt. 132.90543; a member of the alkali metal group. $^{137}$Cs (half-life equal to 30.1 years) is used in treatment of certain malignancies. [L. *caesius*, bluish gray]

**Ces·tan-Che·nais syn·drome** (sĕs-tahn shĕ-nā′) contralateral hemiplegia, hemianesthesia, and loss of pain and temperature sensibility, with ipsilateral hemiasynergia and lateropulsion, paralysis of the larynx and soft palate, enophthalmia, miosis, and ptosis, due to lesions of the brainstem.

**Ces·to·da** (ses-tō′dă) a subclass of tapeworms including the segmented tapeworms that parasitize humans and domestic animals. [G. *kestos*, girdle]

**ces·tode, ces·toid** (ses′tōd, ses′toyd) common name for tapeworms of the class Cestoidea or its subclasses, Cestoda and Cestodaria.

**Ces·toi·dea** (ses-toy′dē-ă) the tapeworms, a class of platyhelminth flatworms characterized by lack of an alimentary canal and a segmented body with a scolex or holdfast organ at one end; adult worms are vertebrate parasites, usually found in the small intestine. [G. *kestos*, girdle, + *eidos*, form]

**ce·tyl** (sē′til) the univalent radical $C_{16}H_{33}$– of cetyl alcohol.

**CF** citrovorum factor; coupling factor.

**Cf** californium.

**C fi·bers** unmyelinated fibers, 0.4 to 1.2 μm in diameter, conducting nerve impulses at a velocity of 0.7 to 2.3 m/sec.

**CFIDS** chronic fatigue and immune dysfunction syndrome.

**CFU** colony-forming unit.

**CGS, cgs** centimeter-gram-second. SEE centimeter-gram-second system.

**Chad·dock sign, Chad·dock re·flex** (chad′ĕk) when the external malleolar skin area is irritated, extension of the great toe occurs in cases of organic disease of the corticospinal reflex paths.

**Chad·wick sign** (chad′wik) a bluish discoloration of the cervix and vagina, a sign of pregnancy.

**chafe** (chāf) to cause irritation of the skin by friction. [Fr. *chauffer*, to heat, fr. L. *calefacio*, to make warm]

**Cha·gas dis·ease, Cha·gas-Cruz dis·ease** (shah′găs, shah′găs-krooz) SYN South American trypanosomiasis.

**cha·go·ma** (shă-gō′mă) the skin lesion in acute Chagas disease.

**chain** (chān) **1.** in chemistry, a series of atoms held together by one or more covalent bonds. **2.** in bacteriology, a linear arrangement of living cells that have divided in one plane and remain attached to each other. [L. *catena*]

**chain re·ac·tion** a self-perpetuating reaction in which a product of one step in the reaction itself serves to bring about the next step in the reaction, and so on. Cf. autocatalysis.

**chain re·flex** a series of reflexes, each serving as a stimulus for the next.

**chain of sur·vi·val** the American Heart Association's term for four major interventions designed to reduce sudden cardiac death—early access, early cardiopulmonary resuscitation (CPR), early defibrillation, and early advanced life support (ALS).

**chak·ra** an ancient Indian tradition of understanding human energy in a system of seven major vortices that activate and energize surrounding areas. Chakras are said to be accessed through the practice of polarity therapy, Reiki, and yoga. SEE ALSO polarity therapy.

**cha·la·sia, cha·la·sis** (kă-lā′zē-ă, kă-lā′sis) inhibition and relaxation of any previously sustained contraction of muscle, usually of a synergic group of muscles. [G. *chalaō*, to loosen]

**cha·la·zi·on**, pl. **cha·la·zia** (kă-lā′zē-on, kă-lā′zē-ă) a chronic inflammatory granuloma of a meibomian gland. SYN meibomian cyst, tarsal cyst. [G. dim. of *chalaza*, a sty]

**chal·i·co·sis** (kal-i-kō′sis) pneumoconiosis caused by the inhalation of dust incident to the occupation of stone cutting. [G. *chalix*, gravel]

**chal·lenge di·et** a diet in which one or more specific substances are included for the purpose of determining whether an abnormal reaction occurs.

**cha·lone** (kā′lōn) any of a number of mitotic inhibitors elaborated by a tissue and active only on that type of tissue, regardless of species; a reversible tissue-specific mitotic inhibitor. [G. + *chalaō*, to relax, + -one]

**cham·ber** (chām′ber) a compartment or enclosed space. SEE ALSO camera. [L. *camera*]

**chambers of eyeball** the cavities within the eyeball: anterior and posterior chambers, filled with aqueous, and the postremal (vitreous) chamber, occupied by the vitreous. SEE ALSO anterior chamber of eyeball, posterior chamber of eyeball, postremal chamber of eyeball. SYN camerae bulbi [TA].

**CHAMPUS** Civilian Health and Medical Program of the Uniformed Services.

**CHAMPVA** Civilian Health and Medical Program of the Veterans' Administration.

**Cham·py fix·a·tive** (chahm-pē′) a mixture of potassium bichromate, chromic acid, and osmic acid, considered an excellent cytologic fixative with advantages and disadvantages similar to those of Flemming fixative; it differs from Flemming fixative in substituting bichromate for acetic acid.

**chan·cre** (shang′ker) the primary lesion of syphilis, which begins at the site of infection after an interval of 10 to 30 days as a papule or area of infiltration, of dull red color, hard, and insensitive; the center usually becomes eroded or breaks down into an ulcer that heals slowly after 4 to 6 weeks. SYN hard chancre, hard ulcer. [Fr. indirectly from L. *cancer*]

**chan·cri·form** (shang′kri-fōrm) resembling chancre.

**chan·croid** (shang′kroyd) an infectious, painful, ragged venereal ulcer at the site of infection by *Haemophilus ducreyi*, beginning after an incubation period of 3 to 5 days; seen more commonly in men. SYN soft chancre, soft ulcer, venereal ulcer. [chancre + G. *eidos*, resemblance]

**Chand·ler syn·drome** (chand'ler) iris atrophy with corneal edema.

**change** (chānj) an alteration; in pathology, structural alteration of which the cause and significance is uncertain. SYN shift.

**change blind·ness** failure to observe large changes in the vision field that occur simultaneously with brief disturbances.

**chan·nel·op·a·thies** (chan-el-op'ath-ēz) SYN ion channel disorders. [channel + G. *pathos*, disease]

**cha·ot·ic rhy·thm** completely irregular cardiac rhythm at varying rates. SEE ALSO arrhythmia.

**chapped** (chapt) having or pertaining to skin, especially of the hands, that is dry, scaly, and fissured, owing to the action of cold or to the excess rate of evaporation of moisture from the skin surface. [M.E. *chap*, to chop, split]

**char·ac·ter** (kar'ak-ter) an attribute in individuals that is amenable to formal and logical analysis and may be used as the basis of generalizations about classes and other statements that transcend individuality. SYN characteristic (1). [G. *charakter*, stamp, mark, fr. *charassō*, to engrave]

**char·ac·ter dis·or·der** a term referring to a group of behavioral disorders, now replaced by a more general term, personality disorder, of which character disorders are now a subclass.

**char·ac·ter·is·tic** (kar'ak-ter-is'tik) **1.** SYN character. **2.** typical or distinctive of a particular disorder.

**char·ac·ter·is·tic fre·quen·cy** frequency at which a given neuron responds to the least sound intensity. SYN best frequency.

**char·ac·ter·is·tic ra·di·a·tion** when an incoming electron from the cathode stream that has enough energy to overcome the binding energy of electrons in the inner shells of the target material knocks the electron out of its shell, the outer electrons fall into the inner shell, giving up energy in the form of x-radiation. Produced at levels of greater than 69.5 kilovolts.

**char·ac·ter·iz·ing group** a group of atoms in a molecule that distinguishes the class of substances in which it occurs from all other classes; thus carbonyl (CO) is the characterizing group of ketones; COOH, of organic acids, etc.

**char·ac·ter neu·ro·sis** a subclass of personality disorders.

**char·coal** (char'kōl) carbon obtained by heating or burning wood with restricted access of air.

**Char·cot dis·ease** (shahr-kō') SYN amyotrophic lateral sclerosis.

**Char·cot gait** (shahr-kō') the gait of hereditary ataxia.

**Char·cot in·ter·mit·tent fe·ver** (shahr-kō') fever, chills, right upper quadrant pain, and jaundice associated with intermittently obstructing common duct stones.

**Char·cot joint** (shahr-kō') SYN neuropathic joint.

**Char·cot-Ley·den crys·tals** (shahr-kō' lī'den) crystals in the shape of elongated double pyramids, formed from eosinophils, found in the sputum in bronchial asthma.

**Char·cot-Ma·rie-Tooth dis·ease** (shahr-kō' mah-rē' tooth) SYN peroneal muscular atrophy.

**Char·cot syn·drome** (shahr-kō') SYN intermittent claudication.

**Char·cot tri·ad** (shahr-kō') **1.** in multiple (disseminated) sclerosis, the three symptoms: nystagmus, tremor, and scanning speech; **2.** combi-

nation of jaundice, fever, and upper abdominal pain that occurs as a result of cholangitis.

**Char·cot ver·ti·go** (shahr-kō') SYN tussive syncope.

**Char·gaff rule** (char'găf) in DNA the number of adenine units equals the number of thymine units; likewise, the number of guanine units equals the number of cytosine units.

**char·la·tan** (shar'lă-tăn) a medical fraud claiming to cure disease by useless procedures, secret remedies, and worthless diagnostic and therapeutic machines. SYN quack. [Fr., fr. It. *ciarlare*, to prattle]

**char·la·tan·ism** (shar'lă-tăn-izm) a fraudulent claim to medical knowledge; treating the sick without knowledge of medicine or authority to practice medicine.

**Charles law** (sharhlz) all gases expand equally on heating, namely, $\frac{1}{273.16}$ of their volume at 0°C for every degree Celsius. SYN Gay-Lussac law.

**char·ley horse** (char'lē hōrs) localized pain or muscle stiffness following a strain or contusion of a muscle. [slang]

**chart 1.** a recording of clinical data relating to a patient's case. **2.** SYN curve (2). **3.** in optics, symbols of graduated size for measuring visual acuity, or test types for determining far or near vision. SEE Snellen test type. [L. *charta*, sheet of papyrus]

**Char·ters meth·od** (chahr'terz) a method of toothbrushing using a restricted circular motion with the bristles inclined coronally at a 45 degree angle.

**Chaus·si·er sign** (shō-syā') severe pain in the epigastrium, a prodrome of eclampsia; may be of central origin or caused by distention of the capsule of liver by hemorrhage.

**Chayes meth·od** (chāyz) a method of replacing lost teeth using a mechanical device for the fixation and stabilization of the dental prosthesis which allows "movement in function" of the abutment teeth.

**Ché·di·ak-Hi·ga·shi syn·drome** (cha'de-ahk-hē-gah'shē) a genetic disorder associated with abnormalities of granulation and nuclear structure of all types of leukocytes and with the presence of peroxidase-positive granules, cytoplasmic inclusions, and Dohle bodies; characterized by hepatosplenomegaly, lymphadenopathy, anemia, neutropenia, partial albinism, nystagmus, photophobia, and susceptibilities to infection and lymphoma; death usually occurs in childhood; occurs in mink, cattle, mice, killer whales, and humans; autosomal recessive inheritance, caused by mutation in the Chediak-Higashi gene (CHS) on chromosome 1q.

**cheek** (chēk) the side of the face forming the lateral wall of the mouth. SYN bucca, gena, mala (1). [A. S. *ceáce*]

**cheek tooth** a posterior tooth; a premolar or molar.

**cheese work·er's lung** extrinsic allergic alveolitis caused by inhalation of spores of *Penicillium casei* from moldy cheese.

**chei·lec·to·my, chi·lec·to·my** (kī-lek'tō-mē) **1.** excision of a portion of the lip. **2.** chiseling away bony irregularities at osteochondral margin of a joint cavity that interfere with movements of the joint. [cheil- + G. *ektomē*, excision]

**cheil·ec·tro·pi·on, chil·ec·tro·pi·on** (kī-lek-trō'

pē-on) eversion of the lips or a lip. [cheil- + G. *ektropos,* a turning out]

**chei·li·tis, chi·li·tis** (kī-lī'tis) inflammation of the lips or of a lip. SEE ALSO cheilosis. [cheil- + G. *-itis,* inflammation]

**chei·li·tis gland·u·lar·is** an acquired disorder, of unknown etiology, of the lower lip characterized by swelling, ulceration, crusting, mucous gland hyperplasia, abscesses, and sinus tracts. SYN Volkmann cheilitis.

**chei·li·tis gran·u·lo·ma·to·sa** chronic, diffuse, soft swelling of the lips, of unknown etiology, microscopically characterized by noncaseating granulomatous inflammation. SYN Meischer syndrome.

⌂**cheilo-, cheil-** lips. SEE ALSO chilo-, labio-. [G. *cheilos,* lip]

**chei·lo·plas·ty, chi·lo·plas·ty** (kī'lō-plas-tē) plastic surgery of the lips. [cheilo- + G. *plastos,* formed]

**chei·lor·rha·phy, chi·lor·rha·phy** (kī-lōr'ă-fē) suturing of the lip. [cheilo- + G. *rhaphē,* suture]

**chei·lo·sis, chi·lo·sis** (kī-lō'sis) a condition characterized by dry scaling and fissuring of the lips. SEE ALSO cheilitis. [cheil- + G. *-osis,* condition]

**chei·lot·o·my, chi·lot·o·my** (kī-lot'ō-mē) incision into the lip. [cheilo- + G. *tomē,* incision]

**cheiralgia** (kīr-al'jē-ă) pain and paresthesia in the hand.

**cheiralgia paresthetica** compression neuropathy of the superficial branch of the radial nerve, marked by pain and paresthesia over the course of the nerve.

⌂**chei·ro-, cheir-** hand. SEE ALSO chiro-. [G. *cheir,* a hand]

**chei·rog·nos·tic, chi·rog·nos·tic** (kī'rog-nos'tik) able to distinguish between right and left, as of the hands or of which side of the body is touched. [cheiro- + G. *gnostikos,* perceptive]

**chei·ro·kin·es·the·sia** (kī'rō-kin-es-thē'zē-ă) the subjective sensation of movement of the hands. [cheiro- + G. *kinēsis,* movement, + *aisthēsis,* sensation]

**chei·ro·kin·es·thet·ic** (kī'rō-kin-es-thet'ik) relating to cheirokinesthesia.

**chei·ro·plas·ty, chi·ro·plas·ty** (kī'rō-plas-tē) rarely used term for plastic surgery of the hand. [cheiro- + G. *plastos,* formed]

**chei·ro·po·dal·gia, chi·ro·po·dal·gi·a** (kī'rō-pō-dal'jē-ă) pain in the hands and in the feet. [cheiro- + G. *pous,* foot, + *algos,* pain]

**chei·ro·pom·pho·lyx, chi·ro·pom·pho·lyx** (kī-rō-pom'fō-liks) SYN dyshidrosis. [cheiro- + G. *pompholyx,* a bubble, fr. *pomphos,* a blister]

**chei·ro·spasm, chi·ro·spasm** (kī'rō-spazm) spasm of the muscles of the hand, as in writer's cramp. [cheiro- + G. *spasmos,* spasm]

**che·late** (kē'lāt) **1.** to effect chelation. **2.** pertaining to chelation. **3.** a complex formed through chelation.

**che·la·tion** (kē-lā'shŭn) complex formation involving a metal ion and two or more polar groupings of a single molecule; can be used to remove an ion from participation in biological reactions, as in the chelation of $Ca^{2+}$ of blood by EDTA, which thus acts as an anticoagulant *in vitro.* [G. *chēlē,* claw]

**chem·ex·fo·li·a·tion** (kem'eks-fō-lē-ā'shŭn) a chemosurgical technique to remove acne scars or treat chronic skin changes caused by sunlight.

**chem·i·cal** (kem'i-kăl) relating to chemistry.

**chem·i·cal an·ti·dote** a substance that unites with a poison to form an innocuous chemical compound.

**chem·i·cal at·trac·tion** the force impelling atoms of different elements or molecules to unite to form new substances or compounds.

**chem·i·cal der·ma·ti·tis** allergic contact dermatitis or primary irritation dermatitis due to application of chemicals; usually characterized by erythema, edema, and vesiculation.

**chem·i·cal di·a·be·tes** SYN latent diabetes.

**chem·i·cal en·er·gy** energy liberated or absorbed by a chemical reaction, e.g., oxidation of carbon, or absorbed in the formation of a chemical compound.

**chem·i·cal per·i·to·ni·tis** peritonitis due to the escape of bile, contents of the gastrointestinal tract, or pancreatic juice into the peritoneal cavity; the contents of the fluid causes chemical injury, shock, and peritoneal exudation.

**chem·i·cal po·ten·tial** (μ) a measure of how the Gibbs free energy of a phase depends on any change in the composition of that phase.

**chem·i·cal preg·nan·cy** slight, unsustained rise in HCG levels.

**chem·i·cal re·pair** conversion of a free radical to a stable molecule.

**chem·i·cal sen·ses** the senses of smell and taste.

**chem·i·lu·mi·nes·cence** (kem'ō-loom-in-ess'ens) light produced by chemical action usually at, or below, room temperature.

**chem·i·lu·mi·nes·cence im·mun·o·as·say** an immunoassay technique in which the antigen or antibody is labeled with a molecule capable of emitting light during a chemical reaction; this light is used to measure the formation of the antigen-antibody complex.

**chem·ist** (kem'ist) **1.** a specialist or expert in chemistry. **2.** pharmacist (British).

**chem·is·try** (kem'is-trē) **1.** the science concerned with the atomic composition of substances, the elements and their interreactions, and the formation, decomposition, and properties of molecules. **2.** the chemical properties of a substance. **3.** chemical processes. [G. *chēmeia,* alchemy]

⌂**che·mo-, chem-** chemistry. [G. *chēmeia,* alchemy]

**che·mo·at·tract·ant** (kem'ō-ă-trak'tant) a chemical substance that influences the migration of cells. [chem- + attract + -i]

**che·mo·au·to·troph** (kem'ō-aw'tō-trōf, kē'mō-aw'tō-trōf) an organism that depends on inorganic chemicals for its energy and principally on carbon dioxide for its carbon. SYN chemolithotroph. [chemo- + G. *autos,* self, + *trophikos,* nourishing]

**che·mo·au·to·tro·phic** (kem'ō-aw-tō-trōf'ik) pertaining to a chemoautotroph. SYN chemolithotrophic.

**che·mo·cau·tery** (kem'ō-kaw-ter-ē, kē'mō-kaw-ter-ē) destruction of tissue by application of a chemical substance.

**che·mo·dec·to·ma** (kem'ō-dek-tō'mă, kē'mō-dek-tō'mă) a relatively rare, usually benign neoplasm originating in the chemoreceptor tissue of the carotid body, glomus jugulare, and aortic bodies. Cf. paraganglioma. SYN glomus jugulare tumor. [chemo- + G. *dektēs,* receiver, fr. *dechomai,* to receive, + *-oma,* tumor]

**che·mo·dec·to·ma·to·sis** (kem'ō-dek-tō-mă-to'sis, kē'mō-dek-tō-mă-to'sis) multiple tumors of perivascular tissue of chemoreceptor type, which have been reported in the lungs as minute neoplasms.

**che•mo•kines** several groups composed of usually 8–10 kD polypepide cytokines that are chemokinetic and chemotactic stimulating leukocyte movement and attraction. SYN intercrines.

**che•mo•ki•ne•sis** (kem'ō-ki-nē'sis, kē'mō-ki-nē' sis) stimulation of an organism by a chemical. [chemo- + G. *kinēsis*, movement]

**che•mo•ki•net•ic** (kem'ō-ki-net'ik) referring to chemokinesis.

**che•mo•lith•o•troph** (kem'ō-lith'ō-trōf, kē'mō-lith'ō-trōf) SYN chemoautotroph.

**che•mo•lith•o•tro•phic** (kem'ō-lith-ō-trōf'ik) SYN chemoautotrophic.

**che•mo•nu•cle•ol•y•sis** (kem'ō-noo-klē-ol'i-sis) injection of chymopapain into the herniated nucleus pulposus of an intervertebral disc.

**che•mo•or•ga•no•troph** (kem'ō-ōr'gă-nō-trōf, kē'mō-or'gă-nō-trōf) an organism that depends on organic chemicals for its energy and carbon. [chemo- + G. *organon*, organ, + *trophē*, nourishment]

**che•mo•or•ga•no•tro•phic** (kem'ō-ōr-gă-nō-trōf' ik) pertaining to a chemoorganotroph.

**che•mo•pro•phy•lax•is** (kem'ō-pro'fi-lak'sis, kē' mō-pro'fi-lak'sis) prevention of disease by the use of chemicals or drugs.

**che•mo•re•cep•tion** (kem-ō-ri-sep'shŭn) the ability to perceive chemicals in the environment that are odorants or tastants. SYN chemosensation.

**che•mo•re•cep•tive** (ke-mō-ri-sep'tiv) relating to chemoreception.

**che•mo•re•cep•tor** (kem'ō-ri-sep'tŏr) any cell that responds to a change in its chemical milieu with a nerve impulse. Such cells can be either 1) "transducer" cells innervated by sensory nerve fibers (e.g., the gustatory cells of the taste buds); or 2) nerve cells proper, such as the olfactory receptor cells of the olfactory mucosa.

**che•mo•re•sponse** (kē-mō-ri-sponz') a reaction to chemical stimulation.

**che•mo•sen•sa•tion** (ke-mō-sen-sā'shŭn) SYN chemoreception.

**che•mo•sen•si•tive** (kem-ō-sen'si-tiv, kē-mō-sen' si-tiv) capable of perceiving changes in the chemical composition of the environment.

**che•mo•sis** (kē-mō'sis) edema of the bulbar conjunctiva, forming a swelling around the cornea. [G. *chēmē*, a yawning, the cockle (from its gaping shell)]

**che•mo•sur•gery** (kem'ō-ser-jer-ē) excision of diseased tissue after it has been fixed *in situ* by chemical means.

**che•mo•tac•tic** (kem-ō-tak'tik, kē-mō-tak'tik) relating to chemotaxis.

**che•mo•tax•is** (kem-ō-tak'sis, kē-mo-tak'sis) movement of cells or organisms in response to chemicals. SYN chemotropism. [chemo- + G. *taxis*, orderly arrangement]

**che•mo•ther•a•peu•tic** (kem'ō-thār-ă-pyu'tik) relating to chemotherapy.

**che•mo•ther•a•py** (kem'ō-thār-ă-pē, kē'mō-thār-ă-pē) treatment of disease by means of chemical substances or drugs; usually used in reference to neoplastic disease. SEE ALSO pharmacotherapy.

**che•mot•ic** (ke-mot'ik) relating to chemosis.

**che•mot•ro•pism** (kĕ-mot'rōp'izm) SYN chemotaxis. [chemo- + G. *tropos*, direction, turn]

**CHEMTREC** Chemical Transportation Emergency Center, a service of the Chemical Manufacturers Association that provides round-the-clock advice on handling emergencies related to transport of hazardous material.

🔲 **cher•ry an•gi•o•ma** SYN senile hemangioma. See page B5.

**cher•ry-red spot** the ophthalmoscopic appearance of the normal choroid beneath the fovea centralis, appearing as a red spot surrounded by white retinal edema in central artery closure or lipid infiltration in sphingolipidosis. SYN Tay cherry-red spot.

**cher•ry-red spot my•oc•lo•nus syn•drome** a neuronal storage disorder in children characterized by a cherry red spot at the macula, progressive myoclonus, and easily controlled seizures; the result of sialidase deficiency. SYN sialidosis.

**che•rub•ism** (chār'ŭb-izm) progressive symmetric, painless swelling of the jaws beginning in early childhood and due to hereditary giant cell lesions manifested radiographically as multilocular radiolucencies. [Hebr. *kerubh*, cherub]

**chest** the anterior wall of the thorax; the breast. SEE ALSO thorax. SYN pectus [TA]. [A.S. *cest*, a box]

**chest leads** a unipolar electrocardiographic lead whose exploring electrode is on the chest overlying the heart or its vicinity; there are six standard chest leads, designated as $V_1$–$V_6$. SYN precordial leads.

**chest tube** a tube introduced into the intrapleural space to evacuate air or pleural fluid.

**chest wall** in respiratory physiology, the total system of structures outside the lungs that move as a part of breathing; it includes the rib cage, diaphragm, abdominal wall, and abdominal contents. SYN thoracic wall.

**chest wall com•pli•ance** the change in chest wall volume per unit change in transmural pressure; may be static or dynamic.

**Cheyne-Stokes res•pi•ra•tion** (chān-stōks) the pattern of breathing with gradual increase in depth and sometimes in rate to a maximum, followed by a decrease resulting in apnea; the cycles ordinarily are 30 seconds to 2 minutes in duration, with 5 to 30 seconds of apnea; seen with bilateral deep febrile hemisphere lesions, with metabolic encephalopathy and, characteristically, in coma from affection of the nervous centers of respiration.

**chi** (kī) **1.** the 22nd letter of the Greek alphabet, χ. **2.** in chemistry, denotes the 22nd in a series. **3.** symbol for the dihedral angle between the α-carbon and the side-chains of amino acids in peptides and proteins. **4.** in Oriental medical traditions, the force of energy existing in all life forms. Chi manifests as five different elements; these are labeled according to either the Oriental or Ayurvedic tradition. SEE ALSO five element theory.

**Chi•a•ri net** (kē-ah'rē) abnormal fibrous or lace-like strands in the right atrium, extending from the margins of the coronary or caval valves and attaching to the atrial wall along the line of the crista terminalis; results when resorption of the septum spurium is markedly less than normal.

**Chi•a•ri syn•drome** (kē-ah'rē) thrombosis of the hepatic vein with great enlargement of the liver and extensive development of collateral vessels, intractable ascites, and severe portal hypertension. SYN Budd syndrome.

**chi·asm** (kī′azm) **1.** an intersection or crossing of two lines. **2.** in anatomy, a decussation or crossing of two fibrous bundles, such as tendins, nerves, or tracts. **3.** in cytogenetics, the site at which two homologous chromosomes make contact (thus appearing to be crossed), enabling the exchange of genetic material during the prophase stage of meiosis. [G. *chiasma*]

**chi·as·ma**, pl. **chi·as·ma·ta** (kī-az′mă, kī-az′mă-tă) **1.** a decussation or crossing of two tracts, such as tendons or nerves; **2.** a site at which two homologous chromosomes appear to have exchanged material during meiosis. [G. *chiasma*, two crossing lines, fr. the letter *chi*, 3]

**chick·en breast** SYN pectus carinatum.

**chick·en fat clot** clot formed *in vitro* or postmortem from leukocytes and plasma of sedimented blood.

**chick·en·pox** (chik′en-poks) SYN varicella.

**chick·en·pox vi·rus** SYN varicella-zoster virus.

**chief ag·glu·ti·nin** SYN major agglutinin.

**chief cell** the predominant cell type of a gland.

**chief com·plaint (CC)** the primary symptom that a patient states as the reason for seeking medical care.

**chig·ger** (chig′er) the six-legged larva of *Trombicula* species; a bloodsucking stage of mites that includes the vectors of scrub typhus.

**chig·oe** (chig′ō) common name for *Tunga penetrans.*

**Chi·lai·di·ti syn·drome** (kē-lah-thē′tē) interposition of the colon between the liver and the diaphragm.

**chil·blain** (chil′blān) erythema, itching, and burning, especially of the dorsa of the fingers and toes, and of the heels, nose, and ears caused by vascular constriction on exposure to extreme cold (usually associated with high humidity); lesions can be single or multiple, and can become blistered and ulcerated. SYN erythema pernio. [chill + A.S. *blegen*, a blain]

**child a·buse** the psychological, emotional, and sexual abuse of a child, typically by a parent, stepparent, or parent surrogate. SEE domestic violence.

**child·bear·ing** (chīld′bār-ing) pregnancy and parturition.

**child·bed fe·ver** SYN puerperal fever.

**child·birth** (chīld′berth) the process of labor and delivery in the birth of a child. SEE ALSO birth. SYN parturition.

**child·hood** (chīld′hood) the period of life between infancy and puberty.

**child·hood ab·sence ep·i·lep·sy** a generalized epilepsy syndrome characterized by the onset of absence seizures in childhood, typically at age six or seven years. There is a strong genetic predisposition and girls are affected more often than boys. EEG reveals generalized 3 Hz spike-wave activity on a normal background. Prognosis for remission is good if the patient does not also have generalized tonic-clonic seizures. SEE ALSO absence.

**child·hood a·prax·ia** SYN developmental apraxia of speech.

**child psy·chi·a·try** the branch of psychiatry that deals with the emotional and mental disorders of children.

**chill 1.** a sensation of cold. **2.** a feeling of cold with shivering and pallor, accompanied by an elevation of temperature in the interior of the body; usually a prodromal symptom of an infectious disease due to the presence in the blood of foreign protein or toxins. SYN rigor (2). [A.S. *cele*, cold]

△**chi·lo-, chil-** lips. SEE ALSO cheilo-. [G. *cheilos*, lip]

**chi·me·ra** (ki-mēr′ă) **1.** the individual produced by grafting an embryonic part of one animal on to the embryo of another, either of the same or of another species. **2.** an organism that has received a transplant of genetically and immunologically different tissue, such as bone marrow. **3.** dizygotic twins that have immunologically distinct types of erythrocytes. **4.** sometimes used as a synonym for mosaic. Chimeric antibodies may have the Fab fragment from one species fused with the Fc fragment from another. **5.** a protein fusion in which two different proteins, usually from different species, are linked via peptide bonds; usually genetically engineered. **6.** any macromolecule fusion formed by two or more macromolecules from different species or from different genes. [L. *Chimaera*, G. *Chimaira*, mythic monster, (lit. a she-goat)]

**chi·mer·ic** (kī-mēr′ik) **1.** relating to a chimera. Cf. chimera (5). **2.** composed of parts that are of different origin and are seemingly incompatible.

**chin** the prominence formed by the anterior projection of the mandible, or lower jaw. SYN mentum. [A.S. *cin*]

**Chi·nese res·tau·rant syn·drome** development of chest pain, feelings of facial pressure, and sensation of burning over variable portions of the body surface after ingestion of food containing monosodium L-glutamate (MSG) by persons sensitive to this food additive.

**chip graft** a graft consisting of small pieces of cartilage or bone which are packed into a bone defect.

**chip sy·ringe** a tapered metal tube through which air is forced from a rubber bulb or pressure tank to blow debris from, or to dry, a cavity in preparing teeth for restoration.

**chi·ral·i·ty** (kī-ral′i-tē) the property of nonidentity of an object with its mirror image; used in chemistry with respect to stereochemical isomers. [G. *cheir*, hand]

△**chi·ro-, chir-** the hand. SEE ALSO cheiro-. [G. *cheir*, hand]

**chi·rop·o·dist** (kī-rop′ō-dist) SYN podiatrist. [chiro- + G. *pous*, foot]

**chi·rop·o·dy** (kī-rop′ō-dē) SYN podiatry.

**chi·ro·prac·tic** (kī-rō-prak′tik) the system that in theory uses the recuperative powers of the body and the relationship between the musculoskeletal structures and functions of the body, particularly of the spinal column and the nervous system, in the restoration and maintenance of health. [chiro- + G. *praktikos*, efficient]

**chi·ro·prac·tor** (kī-rō-prak′tŏr) one who is licensed and certified to practice chiropractic.

***Chi·ro·psal·mus*** a genus of the invertebrate phylum Cnidaria that includes the sea wasp.

***Chi·ro·psal·mus qua·dru·ma·nus*** the sea wasp, the most venomous jellyfish inhabiting the waters surrounding the United States. SEE ALSO jellyfish. SYN box jelly, sea wasp.

**chi-square test** (kī-skwār test) a statistical method of assessing the significance of a difference, as when the data from two or more samples are represented by a discrete number such as the numbers of females and males attending each of two colleges.

**chi·tin** (kī'tin) a polymer of *N*-acetyl-D-glucosamine similar in structure to cellulose and the second most abundant polysaccharide in nature, comprising the horny substance in the exoskeleton of beetles, crabs, certain microorganisms, etc.

**chi·tin·ous** (kī'tin-ŭs) of or relating to chitin.

**CHL** crown-heel length.

**Chla·myd·ia** (kla-mid'ē-ă) the single genus of the family Chlamydiaceae, including all the agents of the psittacosis-lymphogranuloma-trachoma disease groups. [G. *chlamys*, cloak]

**chla·myd·ia** (kla-mid'ē-ă, pl. **chla·myd·i·ae** (kla-mid'ē-ă, kla-mid'ē-ē) a vernacular term used to refer to any member of the genus *Chlamydia*.

**Chlam·y·di·a·ce·ae** (kla-mid'ē-ā'sē-ē) a family of the order Chlamydiales (formerly included in the order Rickettsiales) that includes the agents of the psittacosis-lymphogranuloma-trachoma group. The family contains small, coccoid, Gram-negative bacteria that resemble rickettsiae but differ from them by possessing a unique, obligately intracellular developmental cycle; intracytoplasmic microcolonies give rise to infectious forms by division.

**chla·myd·i·al** (kla-mid'ē-ăl) relating to or caused by any bacterium of the genus *Chlamydia*.

**Chla·myd·ia pneu·mo·ni·ae** a species that causes pneumonia and upper and lower respiratory disease. SYN TWAR.

**Chla·myd·ia psit·ta·ci** organisms that resemble *Chlamydia trachomatis*, but which do not produce glycogen and are not susceptible to sulfadiazine. Various strains of this species cause psittacosis in humans and ornithosis in birds.

**Chla·myd·ia tra·cho·ma·tis** spherical nonmotile organisms that accumulate glycogen and are susceptible to sulfadiazine and tetracycline; various strains of this species cause trachoma, inclusion and neonatal conjunctivitis, lymphogranuloma venereum, nonspecific urethritis, epididymitis, cervicitis, salpingitis, proctitis, and pneumonia; chief agent of bacterial sexually transmitted diseases in the U.S.; the type species of the genus *Chlamydia*.

**chla·myd·i·o·sis** (kla-mid-ē-ō'sis) general term for diseases caused by *Chlamydia* species. SEE ALSO ornithosis, psittacosis.

**chlo·as·ma** (klō-az'mă) melanoderma or melasma characterized by brown patches of irregular shape and size on the face and elsewhere; if confluent, facial patches are called the mask of pregnancy, and are associated most commonly with pregnancy and use of oral contraceptives. [G. *chloazō*, to become green]

△**chlor-, chlor·o-** 1. green. 2. chlorine. [G. *chloros*, green]

**chlor·ac·ne, chlo·rine ac·ne** (klōr-ak'nē) an occupational acne-like eruption due to prolonged contact with certain chlorinated compounds.

**chlor·am·phen·i·col** (klōr-am-fen'i-kol) D-(-)-*threo*-2,2-Dichloro-*N*-[β-hydroxy-α-(hydroxymethyl)-*p*-nitrophenethyl]acetamide; an antibiotic originally obtained from *Streptomyces venezuelae*. It is effective against a number of pathogenic microorganisms including *Staphylococcus aureus*, *Brucella abortus*, Friedländer bacillus, and the organisms of typhoid, typhus, and Rocky Mountain spotted fever; active by mouth. A serious reaction resulting in marrow damage

with agranulocytosis or aplastic anemia may occur.

**chlor·am·phen·i·col a·ce·tyl trans·fer·ase (CAT)** a bacterial enzyme often used as a marker for examining the control of eucaryotic gene expression.

**chlo·rate** (klōr'āt) a salt of chloric acid.

**chlor·hy·dria** (klōr-hī'drē-ă) SYN hyperchlorhydria.

**chlo·ride** (klōr'īd) a compound containing chlorine, at a valence of −1, as in the salts of hydrochloric acid.

**chlo·ride shift** when $CO_2$ enters the blood from the tissues, it passes into the red blood cell and is converted by carbonate dehydratase to bicarbonate ($HCO_3^-$); $HCO_3^-$ ion passes out into the plasma while $Cl^-$ migrates into the red blood cell. Reverse changes occur in the lungs when $CO_2$ is eliminated from the blood. SYN Hamburger phenomenon.

**chlor·i·du·ria** (klōr-i-dyu'rē-ă) SYN chloruresis.

**chlo·ri·nat·ed** (klōr'in-āt-ĕd) having been treated with chlorine.

**chlo·rine (Cl)** (klōr'ēn) 1. a greenish, toxic, gaseous element; atomic no. 17, atomic wt. 35.4527; a halogen used as a disinfectant and bleaching agent in the form of hypochlorite or of chlorine water, because of its oxidizing power. One of the bioelements. 2. the molecular form of chlorine (1), $Cl_2$. [G. *chloros*, greenish yellow]

**chlo·rine group** the halogens.

**chlo·rite** (klōr'īt) a salt of chlorous acid; the radical $ClO_2^-$.

**chlo·ro·form·ism** (klōr'ō-fōrm-izm) habitual chloroform inhalation, or the symptoms caused thereby.

**chlo·ro·ma, chlo·ro·leu·ke·mia** (klō-rō'mă, klōr'ō-loo-kē'mē-ă) a condition characterized by green masses of abnormal cells (in most instances, myeloblasts), especially in relation to the periosteum of the skull, spine, and ribs; the clinical course is similar to that of acute myeloid leukemia. SEE ALSO granulocytic sarcoma. SYN chloromyeloma. [chloro- + G. *-ōma*, tumor]

**chlo·ro·my·e·lo·ma** (klōr'ō-mī-ĕ-lō'mă) SYN chloroma. [chloro- + G. *myelos*, marrow, + *-ōma*, tumor]

**chlo·ro·per·cha meth·od** a method of filling the root canals of teeth by dissolving gutta-percha cones in a chloroform-rosin medium within the root canal. SYN Callahan method, Johnson method.

**chlo·ro·phyll** (klōr'ō-fil) a complex of light-absorbing green pigments that, in living plants, convert light energy into oxidizing and reducing power, thus fixing $CO_2$ and evolving $O_2$; the naturally occurring forms are chlorophyll *a*, *b*, *c*, and *d*.

**chlo·rop·sia** (klo-rop'sē-ă) a condition in which objects appear to be colored green, as may occur in digitalis intoxication. [chloro- + G. *opsis*, eyesight]

**chlo·rot·ic** (klō-rot'ik) pertaining to or having the characteristic features of chlorosis.

**chlor·u·re·sis, chlor·u·ria** (klōr-yu-rē'sis, klōr-yu'rē-ă) the excretion of chloride in the urine. SYN chloriduria.

**chlor·u·ret·ic** (klōr-yu-ret'ik) increasing the excretion of chloride in the urine.

**cho·a·na,** pl. **cho·a·nae** (kō-an-ă, kō'an-ē) the opening into the nasopharynx of the nasal cavity

**c**
**h**

on either side. USAGE NOTE: Often incorrectly called posterior choana(e). [Mod. L. fr. G. *choanē*, a funnel]

**choc•o•late cyst** cyst of the ovary with intracavitary hemorrhage and formation of a hematoma containing old brown blood; often seen with endometriosis of the ovary but occasionally with other types of cysts.

**Cho•dzko re•flex** (hahj′kă) contractions of several muscles of the shoulder girdle and arm when the manubrium sterni is percussed.

**choke** (chōk) to prevent respiration by compression or obstruction of the larynx or trachea. [M.E. *choken*, fr. O.E. *āceōcian*]

**choked disk** SYN papilledema.

**chokes** (chōks) a manifestation of decompression sickness or altitude sickness characterized by dyspnea, coughing, and choking.

**cho•la•gog•ic** (kō-lă-goj′ik) SYN cholagogue (2).

**cho•la•gogue** (kō′lă-gog) **1.** an agent that promotes the flow of bile into the intestine, especially as a result of contraction of the gallbladder. **2.** relating to such an agent or effect. SYN cholagogic. [chol- + G. *agōgos*, drawing forth]

**chol•an•gi•ec•ta•sis** (kō-lan-jē-ek′tă-sis) dilation of the bile ducts, usually as a sequel to obstruction. [chol- + G. *angeion*, vessel, + *ektasis*, a stretching]

**chol•an•gi•o•car•ci•no•ma** (kō-lan′jē-ō-kar-si-nō′mă) an adenocarcinoma, primarily in intrahepatic bile ducts, composed of ducts lined by cuboidal or columnar cells that do not contain bile, with abundant fibrous stroma.

**chol•an•gi•o•en•ter•os•to•my** (kō-lan′jē-ō-en-ter-os′tō-mē) surgical anastomosis of bile duct to intestine.

**chol•an•gi•o•fi•bro•sis** (kō-lan′jē-ō-fī-brō′sis) fibrosis of the bile ducts. [chol- + G. *angeion*, vessel, + fibrosis]

**chol•an•gi•o•gas•tros•to•my** (kō-lan′jē-ō-gastros′tō-mē) formation of a communication between a bile duct and the stomach. [chol- + G. *angeion*, vessel, + *gastēr*, belly, + *stoma*, mouth]

**chol•an•gi•o•gram** (kō-lan′jē-ō-gram) the radiographic record of the bile ducts obtained by cholangiography.

**chol•an•gi•og•ra•phy** (kō-lan-jē-og′ră-fē) radiographic examination of the bile ducts. [chol- + G. *angeion*, vessel, + *graphō*, to write]

**chol•an•gi•ole** (kō-lan′jē-ōl) a ductule occurring between a bile canaliculus and an interlobular bile duct. [chol- + G. *angeion*, vessel, + *-ole*, small]

**chol•an•gi•o•lit•ic cir•rho•sis** a form of cirrhosis in which there is diffuse inflammation of the cholangioles, with inflammation, fibrosis, and regeneration; characterized by chronicity, relapses, and febrile episodes.

**chol•an•gi•o•lit•ic hep•a•ti•tis** hepatitis with inflammatory changes around small bile ducts, producing mainly obstructive jaundice; may be due to viral infection or bacterial infection ascending biliary tree because of obstruction.

**chol•an•gi•o•li•tis** (kō-lan′jē-ō-lī′tis) inflammation of the small bile radicles or cholangioles.

**chol•an•gi•o•ma** (kō-lan′jē-ō′mă) a neoplasm of bile duct origin, especially within the liver; may be either benign or malignant (cholangiocarcinoma). [chol- + G. *angeion*, vessel, + *-oma*, tumor]

**chol•an•gi•o•pan•cre•a•tog•ra•phy** (kō-lan′jē-ō-pan-krē-ă-tog′ră-fē) radiographic examination of the bile ducts and pancreas.

**chol•an•gi•os•co•py** (kō-lan-jē-os′kŏ-pē) visual examination of bile ducts utilizing a fiberoptic endoscope. [chol- + G. *angeion*, vessel, + *skopeō*, to examine]

**chol•an•gi•os•to•my** (kō-lan-jē-os′tō-mē) formation of a fistula into a bile duct. [chol- + G. *angeion*, vessel, + *stoma*, mouth]

**chol•an•gi•ot•o•my** (kō-lan-jē-ot′ō-mē) incision into a bile duct. [chol- + G. *angeion*, vessel, + *tomē*, incision]

**chol•an•gi•tis, cho•lan•ge•i•tis** (kō-lan-jī′tis, kō′lan-jē-ī′tis) inflammation of a bile duct or the entire biliary tree. [chol- + G. *angeion*, vessel, + *-itis*, inflammation]

**cho•lan•o•poi•e•sis** (kō′lan-ō-poy-ē′sis) synthesis by the liver of cholic acid or its conjugates, or of natural bile salts. [chol- + G. *anō*, upward, + *poiēsis*, making]

**cho•lan•o•poi•et•ic** (kō′lan-ō-poy-et′ik) pertaining to or promoting cholanopoiesis.

**cho•late** (kō′lāt) a salt or ester of a cholic acid.

△**cho•le-, chol-, cho•lo-** bile. Cf. bili-. [G. *cholē*]

**cho•le•cal•cif•er•ol** (kō′lē-kal-sif′er-ol) probably the vitamin D of animal origin found in the skin, fur, and feathers of animals and birds exposed to sunlight, and also in butter, brain, fish oils, and egg yolk. SYN vitamin D₃.

**cho•le•cyst** (kō′le-sist) SYN gallbladder.

**cho•le•cys•ta•gog•ic** (kō′lē-sis-tă-goj′ik) stimulating activity of the gallbladder.

**cho•le•cys•ta•gogue** (kō-lē-sis′tă-gog) a substance that stimulates activity of the gallbladder. [chole- + G. *kystis*, bladder, + *agōgos*, leader]

**cho•le•cys•tec•ta•sia** (kō′lē-sis-tek-tā′zē-ă) rarely used term for dilation of the gallbladder. [chole- + G. *kystis*, bladder, + *ektasis*, extension]

**cho•le•cys•tec•to•my** (kō′lē-sis-tek′tō-mē) surgical removal of the gallbladder. [chole- + G. *kystis*, bladder, + *ektomē*, excision]

**cho•le•cyst•en•ter•os•to•my** (kō′lē-sist-en-ter-os′tō-mē) formation of a direct communication between the gallbladder and the intestine. [chole- + G. *kystis*, bladder, + *enteron*, intestine, + *stoma*, mouth]

**cho•le•cys•tic** (kō-lē-sis′tik) relating to the cholecyst, or gallbladder.

**cho•le•cys•tis** (kō-lē-sis′tis) SYN gallbladder. [chole- + G. *kystis*, bladder]

**cho•le•cys•ti•tis** (kō′lē-sis-tī′tis) inflammation of the gallbladder. [chole- + G. *kystis*, bladder, + *-itis*, inflammation]

**cho•le•cys•to•co•los•to•my** (kō′lē-sis′tō-kō-los′tō-mē) establishment of a communication between the gallbladder and the colon. SYN colocholecystostomy. [chole- + G. *kystis*, bladder, + *kōlon*, colon, + *stoma*, mouth]

**cho•le•cys•to•du•o•de•nos•to•my** (kō-lē-sis′tō-doo-ō-dē-nos′tō-mē) establishment of a direct communication between the gallbladder and the duodenum. SYN duodenocholecystostomy, duodenocystostomy (1). [chole- + G. *kystis*, bladder, + L. *duodenum* + G. *stoma*, mouth]

**cho•le•cys•to•gas•tros•to•my** (kō-lē-sis′tō-gastros′tō-mē) establishment of a communication between the gallbladder and the stomach. [chole- + G. *kystis*, bladder, + *gastēr*, stomach, + *stoma*, mouth]

**cho•le•cys•to•gram** (kō-lē-sis′tō-gram) the radiographic record of the gallbladder obtained by cholecystography.

**cho·le·cys·tog·ra·phy** (kō-lē-sis-tog'ră-fē) radiographic study of the gallbladder after oral administration of a cholecystopaque; or scintigraphic imaging of the gallbladder and central bile ducts after administration of a radiopharmaceutical secreted by the liver. [chole- + G. *kystis*, bladder, + *grapho*, to write]

**cho·le·cys·to·il·e·os·to·my** (kō-lē-sis'tō-il-ē-os'tō-mē) establishment of a communication between the gallbladder and the ileum. [chole- + G. *kystis*, bladder, + ileum + G. *stoma*, mouth]

**cho·le·cys·to·je·ju·nos·to·my** (kō-lē-sis'tō-jē-joo-nos'tō-mē) establishment of a communication between the gallbladder and the jejunum. [chole- + G. *kystis*, bladder, + jejunum, + G. *stoma*, mouth]

**cho·le·cys·to·ki·net·ic** (kō'lē-sis'tō-ki-net'ik) promoting emptying of the gallbladder.

**cho·le·cys·to·ki·nin (CCK)** (kō'lē-sis-tō-kī'nin) a polypeptide hormone liberated by the upper intestinal mucosa on contact with gastric contents; stimulates contraction of the gallbladder and secretion of pancreatic juice.

**cho·le·cys·to·li·thi·a·sis** (kō-lē-sis'tō-li-thī'ă-sis) presence of one or more gallstones in the gallbladder. [chole- + G. *kystis*, bladder, + *lithos*, stone]

**cho·le·cys·top·a·thy** (kō'lē-sis-top'ă-thē) disease of the gallbladder.

**cho·le·cys·to·pexy** (kō-lē-sis'tō-pek-sē) suture of the gallbladder to the abdominal wall. [chole- + G. *kystis*, bladder, + *pēxis*, fixation]

**cho·le·cys·tor·rha·phy** (kō'lē-sis-tōr'ă-fē) suture of an incised or ruptured gallbladder. [chole- + G. *kystis*, bladder, + *rhaphē*, sewing]

**cho·le·cys·to·so·nog·ra·phy** (kō-lē-sis'tō-sō-nog'ră-fē) ultrasonic examination of the gallbladder. [cholecysto- + sonography]

**cho·le·cys·tos·to·my** (kō'lē-sis-tos'tō-mē) establishment of a fistula into the gallbladder. [chole- + G. *kystis*, bladder, + *stoma*, mouth]

**cho·le·cys·tot·o·my** (kō'lē-sis-tot'ō-mē) incision into the gallbladder. [chole- + G. *kystis*, bladder, + *tomē*, incision]

**cho·le·doch·al** (kō-led'ō-kal) relating to the common bile duct.

**cho·le·doch·al cyst** cyst originating from common bile duct; usually becomes apparent early in life as a right upper abdominal mass in association with jaundice.

**cho·led·o·chec·to·my** (kō-led-ō-kek'tō-mē) surgical removal of a portion of the common bile duct. [choledoch- + G. *ektomē*, excision]

**cho·led·o·chi·tis** (kō-led-ō-kī'tis) inflammation of the common bile duct. [choledoch- + G. *-itis*, inflammation]

△**cho·led·o·cho-, cho·le·doch-** the ductus choledochus (the common bile duct). [G. *cholēdochos*, containing bile, fr. *cholē*, bile, + *dechomai*, to receive]

**cho·led·o·cho·du·o·de·nos·to·my** (kō-led'ō-kō-doo'ō-dē-nos'tō-mē) formation of a communication, other than the natural one, between the common bile duct and the duodenum. [choledocho- + duodenum + G. *stoma*, mouth]

**cho·led·o·cho·en·ter·os·tomy** (kō-led'ō-kō-en-ter-os'tō-mē) establishment of a communication, other than the natural one, between the common bile duct and any part of the intestine.

[choledocho- + G. *enteron*, intestine, + *stoma*, mouth]

**cho·led·o·cho·je·ju·nos·to·my** (kō-led'ō-kō-jē-joo-nos'tō-mē) anastomosis between the common bile duct and the jejunum. [choledocho- + jejuno- + G. *stoma*, mouth]

**cho·led·o·cho·li·thi·a·sis** (kō-led'ō-kō-lith-ī'ă-sis) presence of a gallstone in the common bile duct.

**cho·led·o·cho·li·thot·o·my** (kō-led'ō-kō-li-thot'ō-mē) incision of the common bile duct for the extraction of an impacted gallstone. [choledocho- + G. *lithos*, stone, + *tomē*, incision]

**cho·led·o·cho·plas·ty** (kō-led'ō-kō-plas-tē) plastic surgery of the common bile duct. [choledocho- + G. *plastos*, formed]

**cho·led·o·chor·rha·phy** (kō-led-ō-kōr'ă-fē) suturing together the divided ends of the common bile duct. [choledocho- + G. *rhaphē*, suture]

**cho·led·o·chos·to·my** (kō-led-ō-kos'tō-mē) establishment of a fistula into the common bile duct. [choledocho- + G. *stoma*, mouth]

**cho·led·o·chot·o·my** (kō-led-ō-kot'ō-mē) incision into the common bile duct. [choledocho- + G. *tomē*, incision]

**cho·led·o·chous** (kō-led'ō-kŭs) containing or conveying bile.

**cho·le·ic** (kō-lē'ik) SYN cholic.

**cho·le·ic ac·ids** compounds of bile acids and sterols.

**cho·le·lith** (kō'lē-lith) SYN gallstone. [chole- + G. *lithos*, stone]

▣ **cho·le·li·thi·a·sis** (kō'lē-li-thī'ă-sis) presence of concretions in the gallbladder or bile ducts. See this page.

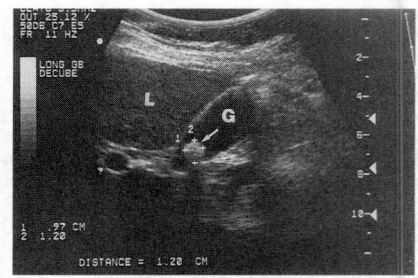

**cholelithiasis:** ultrasound shows single stone (arrow) measuring 1.2 X 0.97 cm in the dependent portion of the gallbladder; (L) liver, (G) gallbladder

**cho·le·li·thot·o·my** (kō'lē-li-thot'ō-mē) operative removal of a gallstone. [chole- + G. *lithos*, stone, + *tomē*, incision]

**cho·le·lith·o·trip·sy** (kō-lē-lith'ō-trip-sē) the crushing of a gallstone. [chole- + G. *lithos*, stone, + *tripsis*, a rubbing]

**cho·lem·e·sis** (kō-lem'ě-sis) vomiting of bile. [chole- + G. *emesis*, vomiting]

**cho·le·mia** (kō-lē'mē-ă) the presence of bile salts in the circulating blood. [chole- + G. *haima*, blood]

**cho·lem·ic** (kō-lē'mik) relating to cholemia.

**cho·le·per·i·to·ne·um** (kō'lē-per-i-tō-nē'ŭm) bile in the peritoneum, which may lead to bile peritonitis.

**cho•le•poi•e•sis** (kō'lē-poy-ē'sis) formation of bile. [chole- + G. *poiēsis,* making]

**cho•le•poi•et•ic** (kō'lē-poy-et'ik) relating to the formation of bile.

**chol•era** (kol'er-ă) an acute epidemic infectious disease caused by the bacterium *Vibrio cholerae,* occurring primarily in Asia. A toxin elaborated by the bacterium activates the adenylate cyclase of the mucosa, causing active secretion of an isotonic fluid resulting in watery diarrhea, loss of fluid and electrolytes, and dehydration and collapse, but no gross morphologic change in the intestinal mucosa. [L. a bilious disease, fr. G. *cholē,* bile]

**chol•er•a•ic** (kol'er-ā'ik) relating to cholera.

**chol•er•a•ic di•ar•rhea** SYN summer diarrhea.

**cho•le•re•sis** (kō-ler-ē'sis) the secretion of bile, as opposed to the expulsion of bile, by the gallbladder. [chole- + G. *hairesis,* a taking]

**cho•le•ret•ic** (kol-er-et'ik) **1.** relating to choleresis. **2.** an agent, usually a drug, that stimulates the liver to increase bile output.

**chol•er•ic** (kol'er-ik) SYN bilious (3).

**chol•er•i•form** (kol'er-i-fōrm) resembling cholera. SYN choleroid.

**chol•er•ine** (kol'er-ēn) a mild form of diarrhea seen during epidemics of Asiatic cholera.

**chol•er•oid** (kol'er-oyd) SYN choleriform.

**cho•ler•rha•gic** (kō-lē-raj'ik) referring to the flow of bile.

**cho•le•sta•sia, cho•le•sta•sis** (kō-les-tā'sē-ă, kō-les'tā-sis) an arrest in the flow of bile. [chole- + G. *stasis,* a standing still]

**cho•le•sta•sis of preg•nan•cy** SYN intrahepatic cholestasis of pregnancy.

**cho•le•stat•ic** (kō-les-tat'ik) tending to diminish or stop the flow of bile.

**cho•le•stat•ic jaun•dice** jaundice produced by inspissated bile or bile plugs in small biliary passages in the liver.

🔲 **cho•les•te•a•to•ma** (kō-les-tē-ă-tō'mă) **1.** a mass of keratinizing squamous epithelium and cholesterol in the middle ear, usually resulting from chronic otitis media, with squamous metaplasia or extension of squamous epithelium inward to line an expanding cystic cavity that may involve the mastoid and erode surrounding bone. **2.** an epidermoid cyst arising in the central nervous system in man or animals. See page B16. [cholesterol + G. *stear (steat-),* tallow, + *-ōma,* tumor]

**cho•les•ter•e•mia, cho•les•ter•ol•e•mia** (kō-lester-ē'mē-ă, kō-les'ter-ol-ē'mē-ă) the presence of excessive cholesterol in the blood. SYN cholesterolaemia. [cholesterol + G. *haima,* blood]

**cho•les•ter•in•ized an•ti•gen** cardiolipin to which cholesterol has been added.

**cho•les•ter•ol** (kō-les'ter-ol) 5-cholesten-3β-ol; the most abundant steroid in animal tissues; circulates in the plasma complexed to proteins of various densities and plays an important role in the pathogenesis of atheroma formation in arteries.

**cho•les•ter•ol•ae•mia [Br.]** SYN cholesteremia.

**cho•les•ter•ol em•bo•lism** embolism of lipid debris from an ulcerated atheromatous deposit, generally from a large artery to small arterial branches; it is usually small and rarely causes infarction. SYN atheromatous embolism.

**cho•les•ter•ol es•ter sto•rage dis•ease** a lipidosis caused by a deficiency of lysosomal acid li-

pase activity resulting in widespread accumulation of cholesterol esters and triglycerides in viscera with xanthomatosis, adrenal calcification, hepatosplenomegaly, foam cells in bone marrow and other tissues, and vacuolated lymphocytes in peripheral blood; autosomal recessive inheritance, caused by mutation in the lysosomal and lipase gene (LIPA) on chromosome 10q. SYN Wolman disease, Wolman xanthomatosis.

**cho•les•ter•ol gran•u•lo•ma** granuloma with prominent clefts of cholesterol surrounded by foreign-body giant cells found in chronic otitis media and sinusitis.

**cho•les•ter•ol•o•sis, cho•les•ter•o•sis** (kō-les'ter-ol-ō'sis, kō'les-ter-ō'sis) **1.** a condition resulting from a disturbance in metabolism of lipids, characterized by deposits of cholesterol in tissue. **2.** cholesterol crystals in the anterior chamber of the eye, as in aphakia with associated retinal separation.

**cho•les•ter•ol•u•ria** (kō-les'ter-ol-yu're-ă) the excretion of cholesterol in the urine.

**cho•le•u•ria** (kō-lē-yu'rē-ă) SYN biliuria.

**cho•lic** (kō'lik) relating to the bile. SYN choleic.

**cho•lic ac•id** a family of steroids comprising the bile acids (or salts), generally in conjugated form (e.g., glycocholic and taurocholic acids); cholic acids are derived from cholesterol.

**cho•line** (kō'lēn) found in most animal tissues. It is included in the vitamin B complex; as acetylcholine it is essential for synaptic transmission. Several salts of choline are used in medicine.

**cho•line a•ce•tyl•trans•fer•ase** an enzyme catalyzing the condensation of choline and acetylcoenzyme A, forming *O*-acetylcholine and coenzyme A.

**cho•line ki•nase** an enzyme that catalyzes the formation of *O*-phosphocholine and ADP from choline and ATP.

**cho•lin•er•gic** (kōl-in-ĕr'jik) relating to nerve cells or fibers that employ acetylcholine as their neurotransmitter. Cf. adrenergic. [choline + G. *ergon,* work]

**cho•lin•er•gic block•ade 1.** inhibition by a drug of nerve impulse transmission at autonomic ganglionic synapses (ganglionic blockade), at postganglionic parasympathetic effector cells (e.g., by atropine), and at myoneural junctions (myoneural blockade); **2.** the inhibition of a cholinergic agent.

**cho•lin•er•gic fi•bers** nerve fibers that transmit impulses to other nerve cells, muscle fibers, or gland cells by the medium of the transmitter substance acetylcholine.

**cho•lin•er•gic re•cep•tors** chemical sites in effector cells or at synapses through which acetylcholine exerts its action.

**cho•lin•er•gic ur•ti•car•ia** a form of physical or nonallergic urticaria initiated by heat (e.g., hot baths, physical exercise, pyrexia, exposure to sun or to a warm room) or by excitement; the rather distinctive lesions consist of pruritic areas 1 to 2 mm in diameter surrounded by bright red macules. SYN heat urticaria.

**cho•lin•es•ter•ase** (kō-lin-es'ter-ās) one of a family of enzymes capable of catalyzing the hydrolysis of acylcholines and a few other compounds. Found in cobra venom.

**cho•lin•es•ter•ase in•hib•i•tor** a drug, such as neostigmine, which, by inhibiting biodegradation of acetylcholine, restores myoneural function in myasthenia gravis or after nondepolarizing neuromuscular relaxants have been administered.

**cho·lin·o·cep·tive** (kō'lin-ō-sep'tiv) referring to chemical sites in effector cells with which acetylcholine unites to exert its actions. Cf. adrenoceptive. [acetylcholine + L. *capio*, to take]

**cho·li·no·lyt·ic** (kō'lin-ō-lit'ik) preventing the action of acetylcholine. [acetylcholine + G. *lysis*, loosening]

**chol·i·no·mi·met·ic** (kōl'i-nō-mi-met'ik) having an action similar to that of acetylcholine; term proposed to replace the less accurate term, parasympathomimetic. Cf. adrenomimetic. [acetylcholine + G. *mimētikos*, imitating]

**cho·lin·o·re·ac·tive** (kō'lin-ō-rē-ak'tiv) responding to acetylcholine and related compounds.

**chol·i·no·re·cep·tors** (kōl'i-nō-rē-sep'terz) SEE cholinergic receptors.

**cho·lo·yl** (kō'lō-il) the radical of cholic acid or cholate.

**chol·ur·ia** (kōl-yu'rē-ă) SYN biliuria. [G. *cholē*, bile, + *ouron*, urine]

**chon·dral** (kon'drăl) SYN cartilaginous. [G. *chondros*, cartilage]

**chon·dral frac·ture** fracture involving the articular cartilage of a joint. SEE ALSO articular cartilage.

**chon·dral·gia** (kon-dral'jē-ă) SYN chondrodynia. [G. *chondros*, cartilage, + *algos*, pain]

**chon·drec·to·my** (kon-drek'tō-mē) excision of cartilage. [G. *chondros*, cartilage, + *ektomē*, excision]

**chon·dri·fi·ca·tion** (kon'dri-fi-kā'shŭn) conversion into cartilage. [G. *chondros*, cartilage, + L. *facio*, to make]

**chon·dri·fi·ca·tion cen·ter** site of primitive cartilage formation in the fetus.

**chon·dri·tis** (kon-drī'tis) inflammation of cartilage. [G. *chondros*, cartilage, + *-itis*, inflammation]

△**chon·dro-, chon·dri·o-** 1. cartilage or cartilaginous. 2. granular or gritty substance. [G. *chondrion*, dim. of *chondros*, groats (coarsely ground grain), grit, gristle, cartilage]

**chon·dro·blast** (kon'drō-blast) a dividing cell of growing cartilage tissue. SYN chondroplast. [chondro- + G. *blastos*, germ]

**chon·dro·blas·to·ma** (kon'drō-blas-tō'mă) a benign tumor arising in the epiphyses of long bones, consisting of highly cellular tissue resembling fetal cartilage.

**chon·dro·cal·ci·no·sis** (kon'drō-kal-si-nō'sis) calcification of cartilage. [chondro- + calcium + G. *-osis*, condition]

**chon·dro·clast** (kon'drō-klast) a multinucleated giant cell involved in the resorption of calcified cartilage; morphologically identical to osteoblasts. [chondro- + G. *klastos*, broken in pieces]

**chon·dro·cos·tal** (kon-drō-kos'tăl) SYN costochondral. [chondro- + L. *costa*, rib]

**chon·dro·cra·ni·um** (kon-drō-krā'nē-ŭm) a cartilaginous skull; the cartilaginous parts of the developing skull. [chondro- + G. *kranion*, skull]

**chon·dro·cyte** (kon'drō-sīt) a nondividing cartilage cell; occupies a lacuna within the cartilage matrix. [chondro- + G. *kytos*, a hollow (cell)]

**chon·dro·dyn·ia** (kon-drō-din'ē-ă) pain in cartilage. SYN chondralgia. [chondro- + G. *odynē*, pain]

**chon·dro·dys·pla·sia** (kon'drō-dis-plā'zē-ă) SYN chondrodystrophy. [chondro- + G. *dys*, bad, + *plasis*, a molding]

**chon·dro·dys·pla·sia cal·cif·i·cans con·gen·i·ta** a form of hereditary chondrodysplasia characterized by asymmetric calcifications and dysplastic skeletal changes and relatively good prognosis. SYN Conradi disease.

**chon·dro·dys·tro·phic dwarf·ism** SEE chondrodystrophy.

**chon·dro·dys·tro·phy, chon·dro·dys·tro·phia** (kon-drō-dis'trō-fē, kon'drō-dis-trō'fē-ă) a disturbance in the development of the cartilage of the long bones, especially of the epiphysial plates, resulting in arrested growth and dwarfism in which the limbs are abnormally short, but the head and trunk are essentially normal. SYN chondrodysplasia. [chondro- + G. *dys*, bad, + *trophē* nourishment]

**chon·dro·dys·tro·phy with sen·sor·i·neu·ral deaf·ness** a skeletal dysplasia characterized by dwarfism, flat nasal bridge, cleft palate, sensorineural deafness, large epiphyses, and flattening of the vertebral bodies; autosomal recessive inheritance, caused by mutation in the type XI collagen gene (COL11A2) on chromosome 6p; dominant forms exist. SYN Nance-Insley syndrome, Nance-Sweeney chondrodysplasia, otospondylomegaepiphyseal dysplasia.

**chon·dro·ec·to·der·mal dys·pla·sia** triad of chondrodysplasia, ectodermal dysplasia, and polydactyly, with congenital heart defects in over half of patients; autosomal recessive inheritance.

**chon·dro·fi·bro·ma** (kon'drō-fī-brō'mă) SYN chondromyxoid fibroma.

**chon·dro·gen·e·sis** (kon-drō-jen'ĕ-sis) formation of cartilage. SYN chondrosis. [chondro- + G. *genesis*, origin]

**chon·droid** (kon'droyd) 1. resembling cartilage. SYN cartilaginoid. 2. maldeveloped cartilage, primarily cellular with a basophilic matrix and thin or nonexistent capsules. [chondro- + G. *eidos*, resemblance]

**chon·droid tis·sue** 1. in an adult, tissue resembling cartilage; SYN pseudocartilage. 2. in an embryo, an early stage in cartilage formation.

**chon·drol·y·sis** (kon-drol'i-sis) disappearance of articular cartilage as the result of disintegration or dissolution of the cartilage matrix and cells.

**chon·dro·ma** (kon-drō'mă) a benign neoplasm derived from mesodermal cells that form cartilage. [chondro- + G. *-ōma*, tumor]

**chon·dro·ma·la·cia** (kon'drō-mă-lā'shē-ă) softening of any cartilage. [chondro- + G. *malakia*, softness]

**chon·dro·ma·la·cia pa·tel·lae** degenerative condition in the articular cartilage of the patella caused by abnormal compression or shearing forces at the knee joint; may cause patellalgia.

**chon·dro·ma·to·sis** (kon'drō-mă-tō'sis) presence of multiple tumorlike foci of cartilage.

**chon·dro·ma·tous** (kon-drō'mă-tŭs) pertaining to or manifesting the features of a chondroma.

**chon·dro·mere** (kon'drō-mēr) a cartilage unit of the fetal axial skeleton; a primordial cartilaginous vertebra together with its costal component. [chondro- + G. *meros*, part]

**chon·dro·myx·oid fi·bro·ma, chon·dro·myx·o·ma** (kon'drō-mik-sō'mă) an uncommon benign bone tumor, occurring most frequently in the tibia of adolescents and young adults, composed of lobulated myxoid tissue with scanty chondroid foci. SYN chondrofibroma.

**chon·dro·nec·tin** (kon-drō-nek'tin) a glycoprotein of cartilage matrix that mediates the adhesion of chondrocytes to type II collagen. [chondro- + L. *necto*, to bind, + -in]

**chon·dro·os·se·ous** (kon-drō-os'ē-ŭs) relating to cartilage and bone.

**chon·dro·os·te·o·dys·tro·phy** (kon'drō-os'tē-ō-dis'trō-fē) term used for a group of disorders of bone and cartilage which includes Morquio syndrome and similar conditions. SYN osteochondrodystrophy.

**chon·drop·a·thy** (kon-drop'ă-thē) any disease of cartilage. [chondro- + G. *pathos*, suffering]

**chon·dro·phyte** (kon'drō-fīt) an abnormal cartilaginous mass that develops at the articular surface of a bone. [chondro- + G. *phytos*, a growth]

**chon·dro·plast** (kon'drō-plast) SYN chondroblast. [chondro- + G. *plastos*, formed]

**chon·dro·plas·ty** (kon'drō-plas-tē) reparative or plastic surgery of cartilage. [chondro- + G. *plastos*, formed]

**chon·dro·po·ro·sis** (kon'drō-pōr-ō'sis) condition of cartilage in which spaces appear, either normal (in the process of ossification) or pathologic. [chondro- + L. *porosus*, porous]

**chon·dro·sar·co·ma** (kon'drō-sar-kō'mă) a malignant neoplasm derived from cartilage cells.

**chon·dro·sis** (kon-drō'sis) SYN chondrogenesis.

**chon·dro·ster·nal** (kon-drō-ster'năl) **1.** relating to a sternal cartilage. **2.** relating to the costal cartilages and the sternum.

**chon·dro·ster·no·plas·ty** (kon-drō-ster'nō-plas-tē) surgical correction of malformations of the sternum.

**chon·drot·o·my** (kon-drot'ō-mē) division of cartilage. [chondro- + G. *tomē*, a cutting]

**chon·dro·xi·phoid** (kon-drō-zif'oyd) relating to the xiphoid or ensiform cartilage. [chondro- + G. *xiphos*, sword, + *eidos*, appearance]

**Cho·part am·pu·ta·tion** (shō-pahr') amputation through the midtarsal joint; i.e., between the tarsal navicular and the calcaneocuboid joints. SYN mediotarsal amputation.

△**chord-** cord. SEE ALSO cord-. [G. *chordē*]

**chor·da**, pl. **chor·dae** (kōr'dă, kōr'dē) [TA] a tendinous or a cord-like structure. SEE ALSO cord. [L., cord]

**chor·dae ten·di·ne·ae cor·dis** [TA] SYN chordae tendineae of heart.

**chordae tendineae falsae** [TA] SYN false chordae tendineae.

**chor·dae ten·din·e·ae of heart** the tendinous strands running from the papillary muscles to the leaflets of the atrioventricular (mitral and tricuspid) valves. Based on their shape, position, or specific area of attachment to the leaflets, several varieties have been described: fan-shaped chordae, rough zone chordae, free-edge chordae, deep chordae, and basal chordae. SYN chordae tendineae cordis [TA], tendinous cords.

**chor·dae ten·din·e·ae spur·i·ae** SYN false chordae tendineae.

**chord·al** (kōr'dăl) relating to any chorda or cord, especially the notochord.

**Chor·da·ta** (kor-dā'tă) the phylum that includes the vertebrates, defined by possession of: 1) a single dorsal nerve cord (the brain and spinal cord of mammals); 2) a cartilaginous rod, the notochord, which forms dorsal to the primitive

gut in the early embryo, and is surrounded and replaced by the vertebral column in the subphylum vertebrata; 3) by presence at some stage in development of gill slits in the pharynx or throat. [L. *chorda*, fr. G. *chordē*, a string]

**chor·date** (kōr'dāt) an animal of the phylum *Chordata*.

**chor·da tym·pa·ni** [TA] a nerve given off from the facial nerve in the facial canal that passes through the posterior canaliculus of the chorda tympani into the tympanic cavity, crosses over the tympanic membrane and handle of the malleus, and passes out through the anterior canaliculus of the chorda tympani in the petrotympanic fissure to join the lingual branch of the mandibular nerve in the infratemporal fossa; it conveys taste sensation from the anterior two-thirds of the tongue and carries parasympathetic preganglionic fibers to the submandibular ganglion, for innervation of the submandibular and sublingual salivary glands.

**chor·dee** (kōr-dē') **1.** painful erection of the penis in gonorrhea or Peyronie disease, with curvature resulting from lack of distensibility of the corpus cavernosum urethrae. **2.** ventral curvature of the penis, most apparent on erection, as seen in hypospadias due to congenital shortness of the ventral skin and, on rare occasions, in patients with a normally situated meatus. [Fr. corded]

**chor·di·tis** (kōr-dī'tis) inflammation of a cord; usually a vocal cord. [G. *chordē*, cord, + -*itis*, inflammation]

**chor·do·ma** (kōr-dō'mă) a rare neoplasm of skeletal tissue in adults, derived from persistent portions of the notochord. [(noto)chord + G. -*oma*, tumor]

**chor·do·skel·e·ton** (kōr-dō-skel'ĕ-tŏn) the part of the embryonic skeleton that develops in conjunction with the notochord.

**chor·dot·o·my** (kōr-dot'ō-mē) SYN cordotomy.

**cho·rea** (kōr-ē'ă) irregular, spasmodic, involuntary movements of the limbs or facial muscles, often accompanied by hypotonia. The location of the responsible cerebral lesion is not known. [L. fr. G. *choreia*, a choral dance, fr. *choros*, a dance]

**cho·re·al** (kōr-ē'ăl) relating to chorea.

**cho·re·ic** (kōr-ē'ik) relating to or of the nature of chorea.

**cho·re·ic a·ba·sia** abasia related to choreiform movements of the legs.

**cho·re·ic move·ment** an involuntary spasmodic twitching or jerking in groups of muscles not associated in the production of definite purposeful movements.

**cho·re·i·form** (kōr-ē'i-fōrm) SYN choreoid.

△**cho·re·o-** chorea.

**cho·re·o·ath·e·toid** (kōr'ē-ō-ath'ĕ-toyd) pertaining to or characterized by choreoathetosis.

**cho·re·o·ath·e·to·sis** (kōr'ē-ō-ath-ĕ-tō'sis) abnormal movements of body of combined choreic and athetoid pattern. [choreo- + G. *athētos*, unfixed, + -*ōsis*, condition]

**cho·re·oid** (kōr'ē-oyd) resembling chorea. SYN choreiform.

**cho·re·o·phra·sia** (kōr'ē-ō-frā'zē-ă) continual repetition of meaningless phrases. [choreo- + G. *phrasis*, speaking]

△**cho·ri·o-** any membrane, especially that enclosing the fetus. [G. *chorion*, membrane]

**cho·ri·o·ad·e·no·ma** (kō'rē-ō-ad-ĕ-nō'mă) a benign neoplasm of chorion, especially with hydatidiform mole formation.

**cho•ri•o•al•lan•to•ic** (kō'rē-ō-al-an-tō'ik) pertaining to the chorioallantois.

**cho•ri•o•al•lan•to•is** (kō'rē-ō-ă-lan'tō-is) extraembryonic membrane formed by the fusion of the allantois with the serosa or false chorion. In mammals it forms the fetal portion of the placenta; in avian embryos it is fused with the shell.

**cho•ri•o•am•ni•o•ni•tis** (kō'rē-ō-am'nē-ō-nī'tis) infection involving the chorion, amnion, and amniotic fluid; usually the placental villi and decidua are also involved.

**cho•ri•o•an•gi•o•ma** (kō'rē-ō-an-jē-ō'mă) benign tumor of placental blood vessels, usually of no clinical significance. SEE ALSO chorioangiosis. [chorion + angioma]

**cho•ri•o•an•gi•o•sis** (kō'rē-ō-an-jē-ō'sis) an abnormal increase in the number of vascular channels in placental villi; severe chorioangiosis is associated with a high incidence of neonatal death and major congenital malformations. [chorio- + G. *angeion,* vessel, + -*osis,* condition]

**cho•ri•o•cap•il•la•ris** (kō'rē-ō-kap-i-lā'ris) SYN choriocapillary layer.

**cho•ri•o•cap•il•la•ry lay•er** the internal layer of the choroidea of the eye, composed of a very close capillary network. SYN lamina choroidocapillaris [TA], choriocapillaris, entochoroidea, Ruysch membrane.

**cho•ri•o•car•ci•no•ma** (kō'rē-ō-kar-si-nō'mă) a highly malignant neoplasm derived from placental syncytial trophoblasts and cytotrophoblasts; villi are not formed; neoplastic cells invade blood vessels. Hemorrhagic metastases are found in the lungs, liver, brain, and vagina; choriocarcinoma may follow any type of pregnancy, especially hydatidiform mole, and occasionally originates in teratoid neoplasms of the ovaries or testes. SYN chorioepithelioma.

**cho•ri•o•cele** (kō'rē-ō-sēl) a hernia of the choroid coat of the eye through a defect in the sclera. [chorio- + G. *kēlē,* hernia]

**cho•ri•o•ep•i•the•li•o•ma** (kō'rē-ō-ep-i-thē-lē-ō'mă) SYN choriocarcinoma.

⚠**cho•ri•oid-, cho•ri•oid•o-** for words beginning thus and not found here, see choroid-, choroido-.

**cho•ri•o•men•in•gi•tis** (kō-rē-ō-men-in-jī'tis) a cerebral meningitis in which there is a more or less marked cellular infiltration of the meninges, often with a lymphocytic infiltration of the choroid plexuses.

**cho•ri•on** (kō'rē-on) the multilayered, outermost fetal membrane consisting of extraembryonic somatic mesoderm, trophoblast, and, on the maternal surface, villi bathed by maternal blood; as pregnancy progresses, part of the chorion becomes the definitive fetal placenta. SYN membrana serosa (1). [G. *chorion,* membrane enclosing the fetus]

**cho•ri•on•ic** (kō-rē-on'ik) relating to the chorion.

**cho•ri•on•ic ep•i•the•li•o•ma** obsolete term for choriocarcinoma.

**cho•ri•on•ic go•nad•o•tro•pic hor•mone, cho•ri•on•ic go•nad•o•tro•phic hor•mone** SYN chorionic gonadotropin.

**cho•ri•on•ic go•nad•o•tro•pin** a glycoprotein with a carbohydrate fraction composed of D-galactose and hexosamine, produced by the placental trophoblastic cells; its most important role appears to be stimulation, during the first trimes-

ter, of ovarian secretion of the estrogen and progesterone required for the integrity of the conceptus; it appears to play no significant role in the last two trimesters of pregnancy, as the estrogen and progesterone are then formed by the placenta. Testing for the beta fraction of human chorionic gonadotropin is the basis for most serum and urine pregnancy tests. SYN anterior pituitary-like hormone, chorionic gonadotropic hormone, chorionic gonadotrophic hormone.

**cho•ri•on•ic growth hor•mone-pro•lac•tin** SYN human placental lactogen.

**cho•ri•on•ic vil•li** vascular processes of the chorion of the embryo entering into the formation of the placenta.

**cho•ri•on•ic vil•lus bi•op•sy** transcervical or transabdominal sampling of the chorionic villi for genetic analysis.

**cho•ri•o•ret•i•nal** (kō-rē-ō-ret'i-năl) relating to the choroid coat of the eye and the retina. SYN retinochoroid.

**cho•ri•o•ret•i•ni•tis** (kō'rē-ō-ret-i-nī'tis) SYN retinochoroiditis.

**cho•ri•o•ret•i•nop•a•thy** (kō'rē-ō-ret-i-nop'ă-thē) a primary abnormality of the choroid with extension to the retina. SEE ALSO choroidopathy.

**cho•ris•ta** (kō-ris'tă) a focus of tissue that is histologically normal per se, but is not normally found in the organ or structure in which it is located. Cf. choristoma. [G. *chōristos,* separated]

**cho•ris•to•ma** (kō-ris-tō'mă) a mass formed by maldevelopment of tissue of a type not normally found at that site. [G. *chōristos,* separated, + -*ōma*]

**cho•roid** (kō'royd) the middle vascular tunic of the eye lying between the retina and the sclera. SYN choroidea [TA]. [G. *choroeidēs,* a false reading for *chorioeidēs,* like a membrane]

**cho•roi•dal** (kō-roy'dăl) relating to the choroid (choroidea).

**cho•roi•dal ne•o•vas•cu•lar•i•za•tion** ingrowth of new vessels from the choriocapillaris into the subretinal pigment epithelium and the retina; space associated with damage to the outer retina.

**cho•roi•dal ne•o•vas•cu•lar•i•za•tion type 1** ingrowth of new vessels from the choriocapillaris into the subretinal pigment epithelial space; associated with damage to the outer retina.

**cho•roi•dal ne•o•vas•cu•lar•i•za•tion type 2** ingrowth of new vessels from the choriocapillaris into the subretinal space; associated with damage to the outer retina.

**cho•roid cap•il•lary lay•er** SEE choriocapillary layer.

**cho•roi•dea** (kō-royd'ē-ă) [TA] SYN choroid. [SEE *choroid*]

**cho•roid•er•ae•mia [Br.]** SEE choroideremia.

**cho•roid•er•e•mia** (kō-roy-der-ē'mē-ă) progressive degeneration of the choroid in males, occasionally in females, beginning with peripheral pigmentary retinopathy, followed by atrophy of the retinal pigment epithelium and of the choriocapillaris, night blindness, progressive constriction of visual fields, and finally complete blindness; X-linked inheritance; heterozygous females show a pigmentary retinopathy but without visual defect or peripheral progression SYN progressive choroidal atrophy, progressive tapetochoroidal dystrophy. [choroid + G. *erēmia,* absence]

**cho•roid glo•mus** a marked enlargement of the

choroid plexus of the lateral ventricle at the junction of the central part with the inferior horn.

**cho·roid·i·tis** (kō-roy-dī′tis) inflammation of the choroid. Cf. choroidopathy, chorioretinopathy.

△**cho·roid·o-** the choroid.

**cho·roid·o·cy·cli·tis** (kō-roy′dō-sī-klī′tis) inflammation of the choroid coat and the ciliary body. [choroido- + G. *kyklos,* circle]

**cho·roid·op·a·thy** (kō-roy-dop′ă-thē) noninflammatory degeneration of the choroid.

**cho·roid·o·ret·i·ni·tis** (kō-roy′dō-ret-i-nī′tis) SYN retinochoroiditis.

**cho·roid plex·us** a vascular proliferation or fringe of the tela choroidea in the third, fourth and lateral cerebral ventricles; it secretes cerebrospinal fluid thereby regulating to some degree the intraventricular pressure.

**cho·roid te·la of third ven·tri·cle** a double fold of pia mater, enclosing subarachnoid trabeculae, between the fornix above and the epithelial roof of the third ventricle and the thalami below; at each lateral margin is a vascular fringe projecting into the choroidal fissure of the lateral ventricle; on its undersurface are several small vascular projections filling the folds of the ependymal roof of the third ventricle. SYN tela choroidea ventriculi tertii [TA].

**cho·ro·pleth·ic map** a method of mapping to display quantitative information such as death rates in defined jurisdictions (states, counties, etc.) by color coding or shading. [G. *chōros,* district, + *plēthos,* multitude, + -ic]

**Chris·tian dis·ease, Chris·tian syn·drome** (kris′chĕn, kris′chĕn) **1.** SYN Hand-Schüller-Christian disease. **2.** SYN relapsing febrile nodular nonsuppurative panniculitis.

**Christ·mas dis·ease** SYN hemophilia B.

**Christ·mas fac·tor** SYN factor IX.

△**chrom-, chro·mat-, chro·mat·o-, chro·mo-** color. [G. *chrōma*]

**chro·maf·fin** (krō′maf-in) giving a brownish yellow reaction with chromic salts; denoting certain cells in the medulla of the adrenal glands and in paraganglia. SYN chromatophil (3), chromophil (3), chromophile, pheochrome (1). [chrom- + L. *affinis,* affinity]

**chro·maf·fin bod·y** SYN paraganglion.

**chro·maf·fin cell** a cell that stains with chromic salts, in adrenal medulla and paraganglia of the sympathetic nervous system.

**chro·maf·fin·o·ma** (krō-maf-in-ō′mă) a neoplasm composed of chromaffin cells occurring in the adrenal medullae, the organs of Zuckerkandl, or the paraganglia of the thoracolumbar sympathetic chain; some chromaffinomas secrete catecholamines. SEE ALSO pheochromocytoma. SYN chromaffin tumor.

**chro·maf·fin·op·a·thy** (krō′maf-in-op′ă-thē) any pathologic condition of chromaffin tissue, as in the adrenal medullae or the organs of Zuckerkandl. [chromaffin + G. *pathos,* suffering]

**chro·maf·fin tis·sue** a cellular tissue, vascular and well supplied with nerves, made up chiefly of chromaffin cells; it is found in the medulla of the suprarenal glands and, in smaller collections, in the paraganglia.

**chro·maf·fin tu·mor** SYN chromaffinoma.

**chro·mat·ic** (krō-mat′ik) of or pertaining to color or colors; produced by, or made in, a color or colors.

**chro·mat·ic ab·er·ra·tion** the difference in focus or magnification of an image arising because of a difference in the refraction of different wavelengths composing white light. SYN chromatism (2).

**chro·ma·tic chart** SYN color chart.

**chromatic vi·sion** SYN chromatopsia.

**chro·ma·tid** (krō′mă-tid) each of the two strands formed by longitudinal duplication of a chromosome that becomes visible during prophase of mitosis or meiosis; the two chromatids are joined by the still undivided centromere; after the centromere has divided at metaphase and the two chromatids have separated, each chromatid becomes a chromosome. [G. *chrōma,* color, + -id (2),]

**chro·ma·tin** (krō′ma-tin) the genetic material of the nucleus, consisting of deoxyribonucleoprotein. During mitotic division the chromatin condenses into chromosomes. [G. *chrōma,* color]

**chro·ma·tin bod·y** the genetic apparatus of bacteria. SEE nucleus (2).

**chro·ma·tism** (krō′mă-tizm) **1.** abnormal pigmentation. **2.** SYN chromatic aberration. [G. *chrōma,* color]

**chro·ma·tog·e·nous** (krō-mă-toj′ĕ-nŭs) producing color; causing pigmentation. [chromato- + -gen, producing]

**chro·mat·o·gram** (krō-mat′ō-gram) the graphic record produced by chromatography.

**chro·mat·o·graph·ic** (krō′mat-ō-graf′ik) pertaining to chromatography.

**chro·mat·og·ra·phy** (krō-mă-tog′ră-fē) the separation of chemical substances and particles by differential movement through a two-phase system. SYN absorption chromatography. [chromato- + G. *graphō,* to write]

**chro·ma·tol·y·sis** (krō-mă-tol′i-sis) the disintegration of the granules of chromophil substance (Nissl bodies) in a nerve cell body which may occur after exhaustion of the cell or damage to its peripheral process. SYN chromolysis. [chromato- + G. *lysis,* dissolution]

**chro·mat·o·lyt·ic** (krō-mă-tō-lit′ik) relating to chromatolysis.

**chro·mat·o·phil** (krō-mat′ō-fil) **1.** SYN chromophilic. **2.** SYN chromophil (2). **3.** SYN chromaffin.

**chro·mat·o·phil·ia** (krō′mă-tō-fil′ē-ă) SYN chromophilia.

**chro·mat·o·phil·ic, chro·ma·toph·i·lous** (krō-mă-tō-fil′ik, krō′mă-tof′i-lŭs) SYN chromophilic.

**chro·mat·o·pho·bia** (krō′mă-tō-fō′bē-ă) SYN chromophobia.

**chro·mat·o·phore** (krō-mat′ō-fōr) **1.** a colored plastid, due to the presence of chlorophyll or other pigments, found in certain forms of protozoa. **2.** melanophage; a pigment-bearing phagocyte found chiefly in the skin, mucous membrane, and choroid coat of the eye, and also in melanomas. **3.** SYN chromophore. **4.** a colored plastid in plants; e.g., chloroplasts, leukoplasts, etc. [chromato- + G. *phoros,* bearing]

**chro·ma·top·sia** (krō-mă-top′sē-ă) a condition in which objects appear to be abnormally colored or tinged with color. SYN chromatic vision, colored vision. Cf. dyschromatopsia. [chromato- + G. *opsis,* vision]

**chro·ma·tu·ria** (krō-mă-tyu′rē-ă) abnormal coloration of the urine. [chromato- + G. *ouron,* urine]

**chrome** (krōm) chromium, especially as a source of pigment. [G. *chrŏma* color]

△-**chrome** a word termination indicating relationship to color. [G. *chrŏma* color]

**chro·mes·the·sia** (krō-mes-thē'zē-ă) **1.** the color sense. **2.** a condition in which non-visual stimuli, such as taste or smell, cause the perception of color. [G. *chrōma,* color, + *aisthēsis,* sensation]

**chrom·hi·dro·sis** (krōm-ĭ-drō'sis) a rare condition characterized by the excretion of sweat containing pigment. [chrom- + G. *hidros,* sweat]

**chro·mic phos·phate** <sup>32</sup>P col·loi·dal sus·pen·sion a pure β-emitting colloidal, nonabsorbable radiopharmaceutical administered into body cavities such as the pleural or peritoneal spaces to control malignant effusions. SEE ALSO sodium phosphate <sup>32</sup>P.

**chro·mi·um (Cr)** (krō'mē-ŭm) a metallic element, atomic no. 24, atomic wt. 51.9961. A dietary essential bioelement. <sup>51</sup>Cr (half-life of 27.70 days) is used as a diagnostic aid in many disorders (e.g., gastrointestinal protein loss). [G. *chroma,* color]

**chro·mi·um pic·o·lin·ate** a chromium salt taken by many athletes with the unsubstantiated belief that additional chromium promotes muscle growth, curbs appetite, and fosters body fat loss.

**chro·mo·blast** (krō'mō-blast) an embryonic cell with the potential of developing into a pigment cell. [chromo- + G. *blastos,* germ]

**chro·mo·blas·to·my·co·sis** (krō'mō-blas'tō-mī-kō'sis) a localized chronic mycosis of the skin and subcutaneous tissues characterized by skin lesions so rough and irregular as to present a cauliflower-like appearance; caused by dematiaceous fungi such as *Phialophora verrucosa, P. dermatitidis, Fonsecaea pedrosoi, F. compacta,* and *Cladosporium carrionii;* fungal cells resembling copper pennies form rounded sclerotic bodies in tissue, with epidermal hyperplasia and intraepidermal microabscesses. SYN chromomycosis. [chromo- + G. *blastos,* germ, + *mykē,* fungus, + *-osis,* condition]

**chro·mo·cys·tos·co·py** (krō'mō-sis-tos'kŏ-pē) SYN cystochromoscopy. [chromo- + G. *kystis,* bladder, + *skopeō,* to view]

**chro·mo·cyte** (krō'mō-sīt) any pigmented cell, such as a red blood corpuscle. [chromo- + G. *kytos,* cell]

**chro·mo·gen** (krō'mō-jen) **1.** a substance, itself without definite color, that may be transformed into a pigment. **2.** a microorganism that produces pigment.

**chro·mo·gen·e·sis** (krō-mō-jen'ĕ-sis) production of coloring matter or pigment. [chromo- + G. *genesis,* production]

**chro·mo·gen·ic** (krō-mō-jen'ik) **1.** denoting a chromogen. **2.** relating to chromogenesis.

**chro·mol·y·sis** (krō-mol'ĭ-sis) SYN chromatolysis.

**chro·mo·mere** (krō'mō-mēr) **1.** a condensed segment of a chromonema; densely staining bands visible in chromosomes under certain conditions. **2.** SYN granulomere. [chromo- + G. *meros,* a part]

**chro·mo·my·co·sis** (krō'mō-mī-kō'sis) SYN chromoblastomycosis. [chromo- + G. *mykēs,* fungus, + *-osis,* condition]

**chro·mo·ne·ma,** pl. **chro·mo·ne·ma·ta** (krō-mō-nē'mă, krō-mō-nē'ma-tă) the coiled filament in which the genes are located, which extends the entire length of a chromosome. [chromo- + G. *nēma,* thread]

**chro·mo·phil, chro·mo·phile** (krō'mō-fil, krō'mō-fīl) **1.** SYN chromophilic. **2.** a cell or any histologic element that stains readily. SYN chromatophil (2). **3.** SYN chromaffin. [chromo- + G. *phileō,* to love]

**chro·mo·phil ad·e·no·ma** any adenoma composed of cells that stain readily.

**chro·mo·phil·ia** (krō-mō-fil'ē-ă) the property possessed by most cells of staining readily with appropriate dyes. SYN chromatophilia. [chromo- + G. *phileō,* to love]

**chro·mo·phil·ic, chro·moph·i·lous** (krō-mō-fil'ik, krō-mof'i-lŭs) staining readily; denoting certain cells and histologic structures. SYN chromatophil (1), chromatophilic, chromatophilous, chromophil (1), chromophile.

**chro·mo·phobe** (krō'mō-fōb) resistant to stains, staining with difficulty or not at all; denoting certain degranulated cells in the anterior lobe of the pituitary gland. SYN chromophobic. [chromo- + G. *phobos,* fear]

**chro·mo·phobe ad·e·no·ma, chro·mo·pho·bic ad·e·no·ma** a tumor of the adenohypophysis whose cells do not stain with either acid or basic dyes.

**chro·mo·phobe cell** cells in the adenohypophysis without stainable cytoplasmic granules.

**chro·mo·pho·bia** (krō-mō-fō'bē-ă) **1.** resistance to stains on the part of cells and tissues. **2.** a morbid dislike of colors. SYN chromatophobia. [chromo- + G. *phobos,* fear]

**chro·mo·pho·bic** (krō-mō-fō'bik) SYN chromophobe. [chromo- + *phobos,* fear]

**chro·mo·phore** (krō'mō-fōr) the atomic grouping upon which the color of a substance depends. SYN chromatophore (3). [chromo- + G. *phoros,* bearing]

**chro·mo·phor·ic, chro·moph·o·rous** (krō-mō-fōr'ik, krō-mof'ŏr-ŭs) **1.** relating to a chromophore. **2.** producing or carrying color; denoting certain microorganisms.

**chro·mo·som·al** (krō'mō-sō'măl) pertaining to chromosomes.

**chro·mo·som·al de·le·tion** a microscopically evident loss of part of a chromosome. SEE ALSO monosomy.

**chro·mo·som·al in·sta·bil·i·ty syn·dromes, chro·mo·som·al break·age syn·dromes** a group of mendelian conditions associated with chromosomal instability and breakage *in vitro,* they often manifest an increased tendency to certain types of malignancies. SEE fragile X chromosome, xeroderma pigmentosum.

**chro·mo·som·al map** a formal, stylized representation of the karyotype and of the positioning and ordering on it of those loci that have been localized by any of several mapping methods.

**chro·mo·som·al re·gion** that part of a chromosome defined either by anatomical details, notably banding, or by its linkages (linkage group).

**chro·mo·som·al syn·drome** general designation for syndromes due to chromosomal aberrations; typically associated with mental retardation and multiple congenital anomalies.

**chro·mo·som·al trait** a trait dependent on a recurrent chromosomal aberration.

**chro·mo·some** (krō'mō-sōm) one of the bodies (normally 46 in humans) in the cell nucleus that is the bearer of genes, has the form of a delicate chromatin filament during interphase, contracts to form a compact cylinder segmented into two arms by the centromere during metaphase and anaphase stages of cell divison, and is capable of reproducing its physical and chemical structure through successive cell divisons. [chromo- + G. *sōma*, body]

**chro•mo•some ab•er•ra•tion** any deviation from the normal number or morphology of chromosomes; also the phenotypic consequences thereof.

**chro•mo•some band** a region of darker or contrasting staining across the width of a chromosome; the pattern of bands is characteristic for most chromosomes. SEE banding.

**chro•mo•some map•ping** the process of determining the position of loci on specific chromosomes and constructing a diagram of each chromosome showing the relative positions of loci; techniques include family studies with linkage analysis, somatic cell hybridization, and chromosome deletion mapping.

**chro•mo•some sat•el•lite** a small chromosomal segment separated from the main body of the chromosome by a secondary constriction; in humans it is usually associated with the short arm of an acrocentric chromosome.

**chro•mo•some walk•ing** a process of extending a genetic map by successive hybridization steps.

**chro•nax•ie** (krō′nak-sē) a measurement of excitability of nervous or muscular tissue; the shortest duration of an effective electrical stimulus having a strength equal to twice the minimum strength required for excitation. [G. *chronos*, time, + *axia*, value]

**chron•ic** (kron′ik) **1.** referring to a health-related state, lasting a long time. **2.** referring to exposure, prolonged or long-term, sometimes meaning also low-intensity. **3.** the U.S. National Center for Health Statistics defines a chronic condition as one of three months' duration or longer. [G. *chronos*, time]

**chron•ic a•dre•no•cor•ti•cal in•suf•fi•cien•cy** adrenocortical insufficiency usually as the result of idiopathic atrophy or destruction of both adrenal glands by tuberculosis, an autoimmune process, or other diseases. SYN Addison disease.

**chron•ic a•troph•ic thy•roid•i•tis** replacement of the thyroid gland by fibrous tissue, the commonest cause of myxedema in older persons.

**chron•ic bron•chi•tis** a condition of the bronchial tree characterized by cough, hypersecretion of mucus, and expectoration of sputum over a long period of time, associated with frequent bronchial infections; usually due to smoking.

**chron•ic des•qua•ma•tive gin•gi•vi•tis** a gingival condition of unknown etiology in middle-aged and older women, characterized by erythema, mucosal atrophy, and desquamation, and usually accompanied by a burning sensation and pain; diagnosis is usually made by biopsy and direct immunofluorescence. SYN gingivosis.

**chron•ic er•y•thre•mic my•e•lo•sis** SYN myelodysplastic syndrome.

**chron•ic fa•tigue and im•mune dys•func•tion syn•drome (CFIDS)** SYN chronic fatigue syndrome.

**chron•ic fa•tigue syn•drome** clinically evaluated new onset debilitating fatigue not substantially relieved by rest and concurrent four of eight symptoms persisting or occurring during six or more consecutive months and not predating the fatigue: substantial short-term memory impairment or concentration; sore throat; tender lymph nodes; muscle and multi-joint pain; unusual headache; unrefreshing sleep; postexertional malaise lasting more than 24 hours; of unknown etiology. SYN chronic fatigue and immune dysfunction syndrome, myalgic encephalomyelitis.

**chron•ic fi•bros•ing pan•cre•a•ti•tis** inflammation of the pancreas consisting of fibrosis, acinar atrophy, and calcification. Clinically, it follows a protracted course with relapses and remissions, and is usually due to alcohol abuse or malnutrition.

**chron•ic gran•u•lo•cyt•ic leu•ke•mia** SYN chronic myelocytic leukemia.

**chron•ic gran•u•lom•a•tous dis•ease** a congenital defect in the killing of phagocytosed bacteria by polymorphonuclear leukocytes. As a result there is an increased susceptibility to severe infection.

**chron•ic in•flam•ma•tion** an inflammation that may begin with a relatively rapid onset or in a slow, insidious, and even unnoticed manner, tends to persist for several weeks, months, or years and has a vague and indefinite termination; characterized histopathologically by infiltrates of small, round cells (lymphocytes), fibrosis, and granuloma formation.

**chron•ic in•ter•sti•tial sal•pin•gi•tis** salpingitis in which fibrosis or mononuclear cell infiltration involves all layers of the uterine or auditory tube. SYN pachysalpingitis.

**chron•ic ma•lar•ia** malaria that develops after frequently repeated attacks of one of the acute forms, usually falciparum malaria; it is characterized by profound anemia, enlargement of the spleen, emaciation, mental depression, sallow complexion, edema of ankles, feeble digestion, and muscular weakness.

**chron•ic moun•tain sick•ness** loss of high altitude tolerance after prolonged exposure (e.g., by residence), characterized by extreme polycythemia, exaggerated hypoxemia, and reduced mental and physical capacity; relieved by descent. SYN Monge disease.

**chron•ic mye•lo•cy•tic leu•ke•mia** a heterogeneous group of myeloproliferative disorders that may evolve into acute leukemia in late stages (i.e., blast crisis.) SYN chronic granulocytic leukemia, chronic myelogenous leukemia, chronic myeloid leukemia.

**chron•ic my•e•log•e•nous leu•ke•mia** SYN chronic myelocytic leukemia.

**chron•ic my•e•loid leu•ke•mia** SYN chronic myelocytic leukemia.

**chron•ic ob•struc•tive pul•mo•nary dis•ease (COPD)** general term used for those diseases with permanent or temporary narrowing of small bronchi, in which forced expiratory flow is slowed, especially when no etiologic or other more specific term can be applied.

**chron•ic pos•ter•i•or lar•yn•gi•tis** a form of laryngitis involving principally the interarytenoid area; thought to be caused by regurgitation of gastric contents.

**chron•ic pro•gress•ive ex•ter•nal oph•thal•-mo•ple•gia** a specific type of slowly worsening weakness of the ocular muscles, usually associated with a pigmentary retinopathy. SEE Kearns-Sayre syndrome, oculopharyngeal dystrophy.

**chron·ic re·laps·ing pan·cre·a·ti·tis** repeated exacerbations of pancreatitis in patient with chronic inflammation of that organ.

**chron·ic shock** the state of peripheral circulatory insufficiency developing in elderly patients with a debilitating disease, e.g., carcinoma; a subnormal blood volume makes the patient susceptible to hemorrhagic shock as a result of even a moderate blood loss such as may occur during an operation.

**chron·ic try·pan·o·so·mi·a·sis** SYN Gambian trypanosomiasis.

**chron·ic ul·cer** a longstanding ulcer with fibrous scar tissue in the floor of the ulcer.

△**chro·no-** time. [G. *chronos*]

**chro·no·bi·ol·o·gy** (kron'ō-bī-ol'ō-jē) that aspect of biology concerned with the timing of biological events, especially repetitive or cyclic phenomena. [chrono- + G. *bios*, life, + *logos*, study]

**chro·no·log·ic age (CA)** age expressed in years and months; used as a measurement against which to evaluate a child's mental age in computing the Stanford-Binet intelligence quotient.

**chron·o·on·col·o·gy** (kron'ō-on-kol'ō-jē) the study of the influence of biological rhythms on neoplastic growth. [G. *chronos*, time, + oncology]

**chro·no·tro·pic** (kron'ō-trop'ik) affecting the rate of rhythmic movements such as the heartbeat.

**chro·not·ro·pism** (kron-ot'rō-pizm) modification of the rate of a periodic movement, e.g., the heartbeat, through some external influence. [chrono- + G. *tropē*, turn, change]

△**chrys-, chrys·o-** gold; corresponds to L. *auro-*. [G. *chrysos*]

**Chrys·a·or·a** (kris'ă-ōr-a) a genus of the invertebrate phylum Cnidaria that includes the sea nettle.

**Chrys·a·or·a quin·que·cir·rha** the sea nettle, a jellyfish that can inflict moderate to severe stings. SEE ALSO jellyfish. SYN sea nettle.

**chry·si·a·sis** (kri-sī'ă-sis) a permanent slate-gray discoloration of the skin and sclera resulting from deposition of gold in the connective tissue of the skin and eye together with increased melanin formation after administration of gold. SYN chrysoderma. [G. *chrysos*, gold]

**chrys·o·der·ma** (kris-ō-der'mă) SYN chrysiasis. [G. *chrysos*, gold, + *derma*, skin]

**Chrys·ops** (kris'ops) the deerfly, a genus of biting flies with about 80 North American species; *Chrysops discalis* is a vector of *Francisella tularensis* in the U.S.; *Chrysops dimidiatus* and *Chrysops silaceus* are the principal vectors of *Loa loa* in west Africa. [G. *chrysos*, gold, + *ōps*, eye]

**chrys·o·ther·a·py** (kris-ō-thār'ă-pē) treatment of disease by the administration of gold salts. [G. *chrysos*, gold]

**Chvos·tek sign** (kvos'tĕk) facial irritability in tetany, unilateral spasm of the orbicularis oculi or orbicularis oris muscle being excited by a slight tap over the facial nerve just anterior to the external auditory meatus. SYN Weiss sign.

△**chyl-** SEE chylo-, chyle. [G. *chylos*, juice, chyle]

△**-chyl** SEE chyl-.

**chy·lan·gi·o·ma** (kī-lan-jē-ō'mă) a mass of prominent, dilated lacteals and larger intestinal lymphatic vessels. [chyl- + G. *angeion*, vessel, + *-ōma*, tumor]

**chyle** (kīl) a turbid white or pale yellow fluid taken up by the lacteals from the intestine during digestion and carried by the lymphatic system via the thoracic duct into the circulation. [G. *chylos*, juice]

**chyle fis·tu·la** a leak of chyle from a lymph vessel to the skin surface; a complication of radical neck dissection when the thoracic duct is injured.

**chy·le·mia** (kī-lē'mē-ă) the presence of chyle in the circulating blood. [chyl- + G. *haima*, blood]

**chyle ves·sel** SYN lacteal (2).

△**chy·li-** SEE chyl-.

**chy·li·fac·tion** (kī-li-fak'shŭn) SYN chylopoiesis. [chyl- + L. *facio*, to make]

**chy·li·fac·tive** (kī-li-fak'tiv) SYN chylopoietic.

**chy·lif·er·ous** (kī-lif'er-ŭs) conveying chyle. SYN chylophoric. [chyl- + L. *fero*, to carry]

**chy·li·fi·ca·tion** (kī'li-fi-kā'shŭn) SYN chylopoiesis.

**chy·li·form** (kī'li-fōrm) resembling chyle.

△**chy·lo-** chyle. [G. *chylos*, juice.]

**chy·lo·cele** (kī'lō-sēl) a cystlike lesion resulting from the effusion of chyle into the tunica vaginalis propria and cavity of the tunica vaginalis testis. [chylo- + G. *kēlē*, tumor]

**chy·lo·der·ma** (kī-lō-der'mă) SYN elephantiasis scroti. [chylo- + G. *derma*, skin]

**chy·lo·me·di·as·ti·num** (kī'lō-mē-dē-as-tī'nŭm) abnormal presence of chyle in the mediastinum.

**chy·lo·mi·cron**, pl. **chy·lo·mi·cra, chy·lo·mi·crons** (kī-lō-mī'kron, kī-lō-mī'kră, kī-lō-mī' kronz) a droplet of reprocessed lipid synthesized in epithelial cells of the small intestine; the least dense of the plasma lipoproteins. [chylo- + G. *micros*, small]

**chy·lo·mi·cro·ne·mia** (kī'lō-mī-krō-nē'mē-ă) the presence of chylomicrons, especially an increased number, in the circulating blood, as in type I familial hyperlipoproteinemia.

**chy·lo·per·i·car·di·um** (kī'lō-pār-i-kar'dē-ŭm) a milky pericardial effusion resulting from obstruction of the thoracic duct, from trauma, or of idiopathic origin.

**chy·lo·per·i·to·ne·um** (kī'lō-per-i-tō-nē'ŭm) SYN chylous ascites.

**chy·lo·phor·ic** (kī-lō-fōr'ik) SYN chyliferous. [chylo- + G. *phoros*, bearing]

**chy·lo·pneu·mo·tho·rax** (kī'lō-noo-mō-thōr' aks) free chyle and air in the pleural space.

**chy·lo·poi·e·sis** (kī'lō-poy-ē'sis) formation of chyle in the intestine. SYN chylifaction, chylification. [chylo- + G. *poiesis*, a making]

**chy·lo·poi·et·ic** (kī'lō-poy-et'ik) relating to chylopoiesis. SYN chylifactive.

**chy·lo·sis** (kī-lō'sis) the formation of chyle from the food in the intestine, its digestion and absorption by the intestinal mucosa, and its mixture with the blood and conveyance to the tissues.

**chy·lo·tho·rax** (kī-lō-thōr'aks) an accumulation of milky chylous fluid in the pleural space, usually on the left.

**chy·lous** (kī'lŭs) relating to chyle.

**chy·lous as·ci·tes, as·ci·tes chy·lo·sus** presence in the peritoneal cavity of a milky fluid containing suspended fat, ordinarily caused by an obstruction or injury of the thoracic duct or cisterna. SYN chyloperitoneum.

**chy·lu·ria** (kī-lyu'rē-ă) the passage of chyle in

the urine; a form of albiduria. [chyl- + G. *ouron,* urine]

**chyme** (kīm) the semifluid mass of partly digested food passed from the stomach into the duodenum. SYN pulp (3). [G. *chymos,* juice]

**chy·mi·fi·ca·tion** (kī-mi-fi-kā′shŭn) SYN chymopoiesis. [G. *chymos,* juice, + L. *facio,* to make]

**chy·mo·poi·e·sis** (kī′mō-poy-ē′sis) the production of chyme; the physical state of food (semifluid) brought about by digestion in the stomach. SYN chymification. [G. *chymos,* juice, chyme, + *poiesis,* a making]

**chy·mo·sin** (kī′mō-sin) a proteinase structurally homologous with pepsin; the milk-curdling enzyme obtained from the stomach of the calf. SYN rennin.

**chy·mo·tryp·sin** (kī-mō-trip′sin) a serine proteinase of the gastrointestinal tract, synthesized in the pancreas as chymotrypsinogen; used in the treatment of inflammation and edema associated with trauma and to facilitate intracapsular cataract extraction.

**chy·mo·tryp·sin·o·gen** (kī′mō-trip-sin′ō-jen) the precursor of chymotrypsin. Converted to π-chymotrypsin by the action of trypsin.

**CI** Colour Index.

**Ci** curie.

**Ci·ac·cio stain** (chah′chō) a method for demonstrating complex insoluble intra-cellular lipids using fixation in a formalin-dichromate solution, embedding in paraffin, staining with Sudan III or IV, and examination in aqueous mountant.

**Cian·ca syn·drome** (chē-ahn-kah) a severe form of infantile esotropia characterized by cross-fixation and tight medial rectus muscles.

**CIC** completely in the canal hearing aid.

**cic·a·trec·to·my** (sik-ă-trek′tō-mē) excision of a scar. [L. *cicatrix,* scar, + G. *ektomē,* excision]

**cic·a·tri·ces** (sik-ă-trī′sēz) plural of cicatrix.

**cic·a·tri·cial** (sik-ă-trish′ăl) relating to a scar.

**cic·a·tri·cial al·o·pe·cia** SYN scarring alopecia. [L. *cicatrix, cicatricis,* scar + suffix *-al,* characterized by]

**cic·a·tri·cial pem·phi·goid** a chronic disease that produces adhesions and progressive cicatrization and shrinkage of the conjunctival, oral, and vaginal mucous membranes.

**cic·a·trix,** pl. **cic·a·tri·ces** (sik′ă-triks, si-kā′triks; sik-ă-trī′sēz) a scar. [L.]

**cic·a·tri·za·tion** (sik′ă-tri-zā′shŭn) **1.** the process of scar formation. **2.** the healing of a wound otherwise than by first intention.

**ci·clo·pir·ox·ol·a·mine** (sī-klō-pir′oks-ōl′ă-mēn) a broad-spectrum antifungal agent used to treat a variety of fungus and yeast skin infections.

♻ **-ci·dal** SEE -cide.

♻ **-cide** a word ending denoting an agent that kills (e.g., insecticide), or the act of killing (e.g., suicide). [L. *-cida, -cidium,* fr. *caedo,* to kill]

**cig·a·rette drain** a wick of gauze wrapped in rubber tissue, providing capillary drainage.

**cil·ia** (sil′ē-ă) plural of cilium.

**cil·i·ary** (sil′ē-ar-ē) **1.** relating to any cilia or hairlike processes, specifically, the eyelashes. **2.** relating to certain of the structures of the eyeball. [Mod. L. *ciliaris,* relating to or resembling an eyelid, or eyelash, fr. L. *cilium,* eyelid]

**cil·i·ary bod·y** a thickened portion of the vascular tunic of the eye between the choroid and the iris; it consists of three parts or zones: orbiculus ciliaris, corona ciliaris, and ciliary muscle. SYN corpus ciliare [TA].

**cil·i·ary disk** SYN orbiculus ciliaris.

**ciliary dyskinesis 1.** absent or impaired motion of the cilia, occurring as a primary or secondary disorder; SEE ALSO Kartagener syndrome. **2.** associated with recurrent infections in the respiratory tract.

**cil·i·ary gan·gli·on** a small parasympathetic ganglion lying in the orbit between the optic nerve and the lateral rectus muscle; it receives preganglionic innervation from the Edinger-Westphal nucleus by way of the oculomotor nerve, and in turn gives rise to postganglionic fibers that innervate the ciliary muscle and the sphincter of the iris (sphincter pupillae muscle).

**cil·i·ary glands** a number of modified apocrine sudoriferous glands in the eyelids, with ducts that usually open into the follicles of the eyelashes. SYN Moll glands.

**cil·i·ary move·ment** the rhythmic, sweeping movement of epithelial cell cilia, of ciliate protozoans, or the sculling movement of flagella, effected possibly by the alternate contraction and relaxation of contractile threads (myoids) on one side of the cilium or flagellum.

**cil·i·ary mus·cle** the smooth muscle of the ciliary body; it consists of circular fibers (Müller muscle) and radiating fibers (meridional fibers, or Brücke muscle); *action,* in contracting, its diameter is reduced (like a sphincter), reducing tensile (stretching) forces on lens, allowing it to thicken for near vision (accommodation). SYN musculus ciliaris [TA].

**cil·i·ary pro·cess** one of the radiating pigmented ridges, usually seventy in number, on the inner surface of the ciliary body, increasing in thickness as they advance from the orbiculus ciliaris to the external border of the iris; these, together with the folds (plicae) in the furrows between them, constitute the corona ciliaris.

**cil·i·ary ring** SYN orbiculus ciliaris.

**cil·i·ary veins** several small veins, anterior and posterior, coming from the ciliary body and emptying into the superior and inferior ophthalmic veins.

**cil·i·ary zone** the outer, wider zone of the anterior surface of the iris, separated from the pupillary zone by the collarette.

**cil·i·ary zon·ule** a series of delicate meridional fibers arising from the inner surface of the orbiculus ciliaris that run in bundles between, and in a very thin layer over, the ciliary processes; at the inner border of the corona, the fibers diverge into two groups that are attached to the capsule on the anterior and posterior surfaces of the lens close to the equator; the spaces between these two layers of fibers are filled with aqueous humor. SYN zonula ciliaris [TA], suspensory ligament of lens, Zinn zonule.

**Ci·li·a·ta** (sil-ē-ā′tă) a class within the phylum Ciliophora. Typical members, such as *Paramecium* or *Balantidium coli* (a parasite of man) possess two distinctive nuclei, a macronucleus and a micronucleus; only the latter bears the hereditary material exchanged in conjugation, a form of sexual reproduction found only in the Ciliata. [L. *cilium,* eyelid]

**cil·i·at·ed** (sil′ē-ā-ted) having cilia.

**cil·i·at·ed ep·i·the·li·um** any epithelium having motile cilia on the free surface.

**cil·i·ates** (sil'ē-āts) common name for members of the Ciliata.

**cil·i·ec·to·my** (sil-ē-ek'tō-mē) SYN cyclectomy.

△**cil·i·o-, cil·i-** cilia or ciliary, in any sense; eyelashes. [L. *cilium,* eyelid (eyelash)]

**cil·i·o·cy·toph·thor·ia** (sil'ē-ō-sī-tof-thōr-ē-ă) a detached ciliary tuft (a remnant of ciliated epithelium), that can be seen in a variety of body fluids, especially peritoneal, amnionic, and respiratory specimens; they are motile and can be confused with ciliated or flagellated protozoa. [fr. Cilio- + cyto- + G. *phthora* corruption, decay, + *-ium,* noun suffix]

**cil·i·o·ret·i·nal** (sil'ē-ō-ret'i-năl) pertaining to the ciliary body and the retina.

**cil·i·o·scle·ral** (sil'ē-ō-sklē'răl) relating to the ciliary body and the sclera.

**cil·i·o·spi·nal** (sil'ē-ō-spī'nal) relating to the ciliary body and the spinal cord; denoting in particular the ciliospinal center.

**cil·i·o·spi·nal cen·ter** the preganglionic motor neurons in the first thoracic segment of the spinal cord which give rise to the sympathetic innervation of the dilator muscle of the pupil.

**cil·i·o·spi·nal re·flex** SYN pupillary-skin reflex.

**cil·i·um,** pl. **cil·ia** (sil'ē-ŭm, sil'ē-ă) **1.** SYN eyelash. **2.** a motile extension of a cell surface, e.g., of certain epithelial cells, containing nine longitudinal double microtubules arranged in a peripheral ring, together with a central pair. [L. an eyelid]

***Ci·mex*** (sī'meks) a genus of bedbugs of the family Cimicidae in the order Hemiptera, with flat, reddish-brown, wingless bodies, prominent lateral eyes, a three-jointed beak, and a characteristic odor from thoracic stink glands; an abundant pest in human abodes. Although its bite produces characteristic linear groups of pruritic wheals with a central hemorrhagic punctum, the bedbug is not a proven vector of human disease, with the possible exception of hepatitis B. SYN bedbug. [L. *cimex,* bug, L. *lectulus,* a bed]

**CIN** cervical intraepithelial neoplasia.

△**cine-, cin-** movement, usually relating to motion pictures. [G. *kineō,* to move]

**cin·e·an·gi·o·car·di·og·ra·phy** (sin'ē-an'jē-ō-kar-dē-og'ră-fē) motion pictures of the passage of a contrast medium through chambers of the heart and great vessels.

**cin·e·flu·o·rog·ra·phy** (sin'ē-floor-og'ră-fē) SYN cineradiography.

**cin·e·plas·tic am·pu·ta·tion, cin·e·plas·tics** (sin-ē-plas'tiks) a method of amputation of an extremity whereby the muscles and tendons are so arranged in the stump that they are able to execute independent movements and to communicate motion to a specially constructed prosthetic apparatus. SYN kineplastics.

**cin·e·ra·di·og·ra·phy** (sin'ē-rā-dē-og'ră-fē) radiography of an organ in motion, e.g., the heart, the gastrointestinal tract. SYN cinefluorography.

**ci·ne·rea** (si-nē'rē-ă) the gray substance of the brain and other parts of the nervous system. [L. fem. of *cinereus,* ashy, fr. *cinis,* ashes]

**ci·ne·re·al** (si-nē'rē-ăl) relating to the gray matter of the nervous system.

**cin·gu·late** (sin'gyu-lāt) relating to a cingulum.

**cin·gu·late gy·rus** a long, curved convolution of the medial surface of the cortical hemisphere, arched over the corpus callosum from which it is separated by the deep sulcus of corpus callosum; together with the parahippocampal gyrus, with which it is continuous behind the corpus callosum, it forms the fornicate gyrus.

**cin·gu·late sul·cus** a fissure on the mesial surface of the cerebral hemisphere, bounding the upper surface of the cingulate gyrus (callosal convolution); the anterior portion is called the pars subfrontalis; the posterior portion which curves up to the superomedial margin of the hemisphere and borders the paracentral lobule posteriorly, the pars marginalis.

**cin·gu·lot·o·my, cin·gu·lec·to·my** (sin-gyu-lot'ō-mē, sin-gyu-lek'tō-mē) electrolytic destruction of the anterior cingulate gyrus and callosum. [cingulum + G. *tomē,* a cutting]

**cin·gu·lum,** gen. **cin·gu·li,** pl. **cin·gu·la** (sin'gyu-lŭm, sin'gyu-lē, sin'gyu-lă) [TA] **1.** SYN girdle. **2.** a well-marked fiber bundle passing longitudinally in the white matter of the cingulate gyrus; the bundle extends from the region of the anterior perforated substance back over the dorsal surface of the corpus callosum; behind the splenium of the latter it curves down and then forward in the white matter of the parahippocampal gyrus; composed largely of fibers from the anterior thalamic nucleus to the cingulate and parahippocampal gyri, it also contains association fibers connecting these gyri with the frontal cortex, and their various subdivisions with each other. **3.** the lingual portion of an incisor or canine tooth, which forms a convexity on the cervical third of the crown. **4.** the cervical third of the crown of a molar, which is the source of the developing cusps. [L. girdle, fr. *cingo,* to surround]

**cir·ca·di·an** (ser-kā'dē-ăn) relating to biologic variations or rhythms with a cycle of about 24 hours. Cf. infradian, ultradian. [L. *circa,* about, + *dies,* day]

**cir·ci·nate** (ser'si-nāt) circular; ring-shaped. [L. *circinatus,* made round, pp. of *circino,* to make round, fr. *circinus,* a pair of compasses]

**cir·cle** (ser'kl) **1.** a ring-shaped structure or group of structures. **2.** a line or process with every point equidistant from the center. SYN circulus [TA]. [L. *circulus*]

**cir·cle ab·sorp·tion an·es·the·sia** inhalation anesthesia in which a circuit with carbon dioxide absorbent is used for complete (closed) or partial (semiclosed) rebreathing of exhaled gases.

**cir·cuit** (ser'kĭt) the path or course of flow of cases or electric or other currents. [L. *circuitus,* a going round, fr. *circum,* around, + *eo,* pp. *itus,* to go]

**cir·cuit re·sis·tance train·ing (CRT)** modification of standard strength training emphasizing relatively light load (40–60% of maximum strength) and continuous exercise to provide a more general conditioning to improve body composition, muscular strength and endurance, and cardiovascular fitness. SYN circuit training, circuit weight training.

**cir·cuit train·ing, cir·cuit weight train·ing** SYN circuit resistance training.

**cir·cu·lar am·pu·ta·tion** amputation performed by a circular incision through the skin, the muscles being similarly divided higher up, and the bone higher still.

**cir·cu·lar di·chro·ism (CD)** the change from circular polarization to elliptical polarization of monochromatic, circularly polarized light in the immediate vicinity of the absorption band of the substance through which the light passes.

**cir·cu·lar folds of small intestine** the numerous folds of the mucous membrane of the small intestine, running transversely for about two-thirds of the circumference of the gut. SYN plicae circulares intestini tenuis [TA], Kerckring folds, Kerckring valves.

**cir·cu·lar si·nus** 1. dural venous formation which surrounds the hypophysis, composed of right and left cavernous sinuses and the intercavernous sinuses; 2. a venous sinus at the periphery of the placenta; 3. SYN sinus venosus sclerae.

**cir·cu·la·tion** (ser-kyu-lā′shŭn) movements in a circle, or through a circular course, or through a course which leads back to the same point; usually referring to blood circulation unless otherwise specified. [L. *circulatio*]

**cir·cu·la·to·ry** (ser′kyu-lă-tō-rē) 1. relating to the circulation. 2. SYN sanguiferous.

**cir·cu·lus**, gen. and pl. **cir·cu·li** (ser′kyu-lŭs, ser′kyu-lī) [TA] SYN circle. 2. a circle formed by connecting arteries, veins, or nerves. [L. dim. of *circus*, circle]

⚠**cir·cum-** a circular movement, or a position surrounding the part indicated by the word to which it is joined. SEE ALSO peri-. [L. around]

**cir·cum·a·nal glands** large apocrine sweat glands surrounding the anus.

**cir·cum·ar·tic·u·lar** (ser′kŭm-ar-tik′yu-lăr) surrounding a joint. [circum- + L. *articulus*, joint]

**cir·cum·ax·il·lary** (ser-kŭm-ak′si-lār-ē) around the axilla.

**cir·cum·cise** (ser′kŭm-sīz) to perform circumcision, especially of the prepuce.

**cir·cum·ci·sion** (ser-kŭm-sizh′ŭn) 1. operation to remove part or all of the prepuce. SYN peritomy (2). 2. cutting around an anatomical part (e.g., the areola of the breast). SYN peritectomy (2). [L. *circumcido*, to cut around, fr. *circum*, around, + *caedo*, to cut]

**cir·cum·duc·tio** [TA] SYN circumduction.

**cir·cum·duc·tion** (ser-kŭm-dŭk′shŭn) 1. movement of a part, e.g., an extremity, in a circular direction. 2. SYN cycloduction. SYN circumductio [TA]. [circum- + L. *duco*, pp. *ductus*, to draw]

**cir·cum·fer·ence (c)** (ser-kŭm′fer-ens) the outer boundary, especially of a circular area. SYN circumferentia [TA]. [L. *circumferentia, a bearing around*]

**cir·cum·fer·en·tia** (ser-kŭm-fer-en′shē-ă) [TA] SYN circumference. [L. a bearing around]

**cir·cum·fer·en·tial fi·bro·car·ti·lage** a ring of fibrocartilage around the articular end of a bone, serving to deepen the joint cavity.

**cir·cum·fer·en·tial la·mel·la** a bony lamella that encircles the outer or inner surface of a bone.

**cir·cum·flex** (ser′kŭm-fleks) describing an arc of a circle or that which winds around something; denotes several anatomic structures: arteries, veins, nerves, and muscles. [circum- + L. *flexus*, to bend]

**cir·cum·flex scap·u·lar ar·tery** *origin*, subscapular; *distribution*, muscles of shoulder and scapular region; *anastomoses*, branches of suprascapular and transverse cervical.

**cir·cum·or·bit·al** (ser-kŭm-ōr′bi-tăl) around the orbit. SYN periorbital (2).

**cir·cum·scribed** (ser′kŭm-skrībd) bounded by a line; limited or confined. [circum- + L. *scribo*, to write]

**cir·cum·scribed myx·e·de·ma** nodules and plaques of mucoid edema of the skin, usually in the pretibial region, occurring in some patients with hyperthyroidism. SYN pretibial myxedema.

**cir·cum·scribed pos·ter·i·or ker·a·to·co·nus** congenital corneal defect characterized by a craterlike defect on the posterior corneal surface.

**cir·cum·spor·o·zo·ite pro·tein** one of two proteins (the other is thrombospondin-related adhesive protein) involved in sporozoite recognition of host cells in malaria.

**cir·cum·stan·ti·al·i·ty** (ser′kŭm-stan-shē-al′i-tē) a disturbance in the thought process in which one gives an excessive amount of detail that is often tangential, elaborate, and irrelevant, to avoid making a direct statement or answer to a question; observed in schizophrenia and in obsessional disorders. Cf. tangentiality. [L. *circumsto*, pr. p. *-stans*, to stand around]

**cir·cum·val·late** (ser-kŭm-val′āt) denoting a structure surrounded by a wall, as the circumvallate (vallate) papillae of the tongue. [circum- + L. *vallum*, wall]

**cir·cum·val·late pa·pil·lae** SYN vallate papilla.

**cir·cum·ven·tric·u·lar or·gans** four small areas at the base of the brain that are outside the blood-brain barrier. They are neurohypophysis, area postrema, organum vasculosum of the lamina terminalis, and subfornical organ (SFO).

**cir·cum·vo·lute** (ser-kŭm-vol′yut) twisted around; rolled about. [L. *circum-volvo*, pp. *-volutus*, to roll around]

**cir·cum·zy·go·mat·ic wir·ing** a means of fixation for mandibular fractures in which the mandible is fastened to the zygomatic arches with wire.

**cir·rho·sis** (sir-rō′sis) endstage liver disease characterized by diffuse damage to hepatic parenchymal cells, with nodular regeneration, fibrosis, and disturbance of normal architecture; associated with failure in the function of hepatic cells and interference with blood flow in the liver, frequently resulting in jaundice, portal hypertension, ascites, and ultimately biochemical and functional signs of hepatic failure. [G. *kirrhos*, yellow (liver), + *-osis*, condition]

**cir·rhot·ic** (sir-rot′ik) relating to or affected with cirrhosis or advanced fibrosis.

**cir·soid an·eu·rysm** dilation of a group of blood vessels owing to congenital malformation with arteriovenous shunting. SYN racemose aneurysm.

**CIS** carcinoma in situ.

⚠**cis-** 1. prefix meaning on this side, on the near side; opposite of trans-. 2. GENETICS a prefix denoting the location of two or more genes on the same chromosome of a homologous pair, in coupling. 3. ORGANIC CHEMISTRY a form of geometric isomerism in which similar functional groups are attached on the same side of the plane that includes two adjacent, fixed carbon atoms in a ring structure. 4. ORGANIC CHEMISTRY a form of geometric isomerism with regard to carbon-carbon double bonds. Identical functional groups on the same side of the double bond are cis-. When the four moieties attached to the carbons of the double bond are all different, then the E/Z nomenclature has to be followed. [L.]

**cis·tern** (sis′tern) 1. any cavity or enclosed space serving as a reservoir, especially for chyle, lymph, or cerebrospinal fluid. 2. an ultramicroscopic space occurring between the membranes of the flattened sacs of the endoplasmic reticulum, the Golgi complex, or the two membranes of the nuclear envelope. SYN cisterna [TA]. [L. *cisterna*]

cis•ter•na, gen. and pl. cis•ter•nae (sis-ter'nă, sis-ter'nē) [TA] SYN cistern. [L. an underground cistern for water, fr. *cista,* a box]

cis•ter•nal (sis-ter'năl) relating to a cisterna.

cis•ter•nal punc•ture passage of a hollow needle through the posterior atlantooccipital membrane into the cisterna cerebellomedullaris.

cis•tern•og•ra•phy (sis'tern-og'ră-fē) the radiographic study of the basal cisterns of the brain after the subarachnoid introduction of contrast medium, or a radiopharmaceutical with a suitable detector. [cisterna + G. *graphō,* to write]

cis•tron (sis'tron) 1. the smallest functional unit of heritability; a length of chromosomal DNA associated with a single biochemical function. In modern molecular biology, the cistron is essentially equivalent to the structural gene. 2. the genetic unit defined by the *cis/trans* test. [*cis tr*-ans + -on]

cit•rate (sit'rāt, sī'trāt) a salt or ester of citric acid; used as anticoagulants because they bind calcium ions.

cit•ric ac•id (sit'rik as'id) the acid of citrus fruits, widely distributed in nature and a key intermediate in intermediary metabolism.

cit•ric ac•id cy•cle SYN tricarboxylic acid cycle.

ci•trov•o•rum fac•tor (CF) SYN folinic acid.

ci•trul•line (sit'rul-ēn) an amino acid formed from L-ornithine in the course of the urea cycle as well as a product in nitric oxide biosynthesis; also found in watermelon (*Citrullus vulgaris*) and in casein. Elevated in individuals with a deficiency of argininosuccinate synthetase or argininosuccinate lyase.

cit•rul•li•nu•ria (sit'rŭl-i-nyu'rē-ă) enhanced urinary excretion of citrulline; a manifestation of citrullinemia.

Ci•vil•ian Health and Med•i•cal Pro•gram of the U•ni•formed Ser•vic•es (CHAMPUS) provides medical care and hospitalization in civilian hospitals by civilian physicians for military personnel, active or retired, and their dependents or survivors when governmental medical facilities are not available.

Ci•vil•ian Health and Med•i•cal Pro•gram of the Vet•er•ans' Ad•min•is•tra•tion (CHAMPVA) provides medical care and hospitalization in civilian hospitals by civilian physicians for dependents or survivors of veterans with service-related disabilities when governmental medical facilities are not available.

CJD Creutzfeldt-Jakob disease.

Cl chlorine.

Cla•do point (klah-dō') a point at the junction of the interspinous and right semilunar lines, at the lateral border of the rectus abdominis muscle, where marked tenderness on pressure is felt in some cases of appendicitis.

clad•o•spo•ri•o•sis (klad'ō-spō-rē-ō'sis) infection with a fungus of the genus *Cladosporium.*

*Clad•o•spo•ri•um* (klad-ō-spōr'i-ŭm) a genus of fungi having dematiaceous or dark-colored conidiophores with oval or round spores, commonly isolated in soil or plant residues. [G. *klados,* a branch, + *sporos,* seed]

*Clad•o•spo•ri•um* (*Xylohypha*) *ban•ti•a•num* a species of fungi that causes cerebral cladosporio-

sis; probably synonymous with *Cladosporium trichoides.*

clair•voy•ance (klār-voy'ans) perception of objective events (past, present, or future) not ordinarily discernible by the senses; a type of extrasensory perception. [Fr.]

clamp (klamp) an instrument for compression of a structure. Cf. forceps. [M.E., fr. Middle Dutch *klampe*]

clamp for•ceps a forceps with pronged jaws designed to engage the jaws of a rubber dam clamp so that they may be separated to pass over the widest buccolingual contour of a tooth. SYN rubber dam clamp forceps.

clam•shell in•ci•sion, clam•shell thor•a•cot•o•my incision made up of bilateral submammary anterior thoracotomies connected by a transverse sternotomy and providing access similar to that of a standard sternotomy. SEE ALSO transverse thoracosternotomy.

clang as•so•ci•a•tion psychic associations resulting from sounds; often encountered in the manic phase of manic-depressive psychosis.

Clap•ton line (klap'tŏn) a greenish discoloration of the marginal gingiva in cases of chronic copper poisoning.

cla•rif•i•cant (kla-rif'i-kant) an agent that makes a turbid liquid clear. [L. *clarus,* clear, + *facio,* to make]

Clark lev•el (klark) the level of invasion of primary malignant melanoma of the skin; limited to the epidermis, I; into the underlying papillary dermis, II; to the junction of the papillary and reticular dermis, III; into the reticular dermis, IV; into the subcutaneous fat, V. The prognosis is worse with each successive deeper level of invasion.

clasp 1. a part of a removable partial denture that acts as a direct retainer and/or stabilizer for the denture by partially surrounding or contacting an abutment tooth. 2. a direct retainer of a removable partial denture, usually consisting of two arms joined by a body which connects with an occlusal rest; at least one arm of a clasp usually terminates in the infrabulge (gingival convergence) area of the tooth enclosed.

clasp-knife spas•tic•i•ty, clasp-knife ri•gid•i•ty initial increased resistance to stretch of the extensor muscles of a joint that give way rather suddenly allowing the joint then to be easily flexed; the rigidity is due to an exaggeration of the stretch reflex.

class (klas) in biologic classification, the next division below the phylum (or subphylum) and above the order. [L. *classis,* a class, division]

class I an•ti•gens cell-membrane–bound glycoproteins that are coded by genes of the major histocompatibility complex.

class I mol•e•cule a major histocompatibility complex antigen made up of two noncovalently bonded polypeptide chains, one glycosylated, heavy, and variable with antigen specificity; the other chain is $\beta_2$-microglobulin.

class II an•ti•gens a cell-membrane glycoprotein encoded by genes of the major histocompatibility complex. These antigens are distributed on antigen-presenting cells such as macrophages, B cells, and dendritic cells.

class II mol•e•cule a major histocompatibility complex membrane-piercing antigen made up of two noncovalently bonded polypeptide chains designated α and β.

**class III an•ti•gens** non–cell-membrane molecules that are encoded by the S region of the major histocompatibility complex. These antigens are not involved in determining histocompatibility and include the complement proteins.

**clas•sic cho•roi•dal neo•vas•cu•lar•i•za•tion** well-demarcated areas of hyperfluorescence observed in the early phases of a retinal angiogram.

**clas•si•c he•mo•phil•ia** SYN hemophilia A.

**clas•sic mi•graine** a form of hemicrania migraine preceded by a scintillating scotoma (teichopsia).

**clas•si•fi•ca•tion** (klas'i-fi-kā'shŭn) a systematic arrangement into classes or groups based on perceived common characteristics; a means of giving order to a group of disconnected facts.

**clas•tic** (klas'tik) breaking up into pieces, or exhibiting a tendency so to break or divide. [G. *klastos,* broken]

**clas•to•gen•ic** (klas-tō-jen'ik) relating to the action of a clastogen.

**clas•to•thrix** (klas'tō-thriks) SYN trichorrhexis nodosa. [G. *klastos,* broken, + *thrix,* hair]

**clath•rate** (klath'rāt) a type of inclusion compound in which small molecules are trapped in the cage-like lattice of macromolecules. [L. *clathrare,* pp. *-atus,* to furnish with a lattice]

**Claude syn•drome** (klōd) midbrain syndrome with oculomotor palsy on the side of the lesion and incoordination on the opposite side.

**clau•di•ca•tion** (klaw-di-kā'shŭn) limping, usually referring to intermittent claudication. [L. *claudicatio,* fr. *claudico,* to limp]

**clau•di•ca•tory** (klaw'di-kă-tōr-ē) relating to claudication, especially intermittent claudication.

**Clau•di•us cells** (klaw'dē-ŭs) columnar cells on the floor of the ductus cochlearis external to the organ of Corti.

**claus•tral** (klaws'trăl) relating to the claustrum.

**claus•tro•pho•bia** (klaw-strō-fō'bē-ă) a morbid fear of being in a confined place. [L. *claustrum,* an enclosed space, + G. *phobos,* fear]

**claus•tro•pho•bic** (klaw-strō-fō'bik) relating to or suffering from claustrophobia.

**claus•trum,** pl. **claus•tra** (klaws'trŭm, klaws'tră) **1.** one of several anatomic structures bearing a resemblance to a barrier. **2.** [TA] a thin, vertically placed lamina of gray matter lying close to the putamen, from which it is separated by the external capsule. Cells of the claustrum have reciprocal connections with sensory areas of the cerebral cortex. [L. barrier]

**cla•vi** (klā'vī) plural of clavus.

**clav•i•cle** (klav'i-kl) a doubly curved long bone that forms part of the shoulder girdle. Its medial end articulates with the manubrium sterni at the sternoclavicular joint, its lateral end with the acromion of the scapula at the acromioclavicular joint. SYN clavicula [TA], collar bone.

**cla•vic•u•la,** pl. **cla•vic•u•lae** (klă-vik'yu-lă) [TA] SYN clavicle. [L. *clavicula,* a small key, fr. *clavis,* key]

**cla•vic•u•lar** (kla-vik'yu-lăr) relating to the clavicle.

**cla•vus,** pl. **cla•vi** (klā'vŭs, klā'vī) a small conical callosity caused by pressure over a bony prominence, usually on a toe. SYN corn, heloma. [L. a nail, wart, corn]

**claw•foot, claw foot** (klaw'fut) a fixed contracture of the foot characterized by hyperextension

at the metatarsophalangeal joint and flexion at the interphalangeal joints.

**claw•hand, claw hand** (klaw'hand) atrophy of the interosseous muscles of the hand with hyperextension of the metacarpophalangeal joints and flexion of the interphalangeal joints.

**CLB** cyanobacterialike, coccidialike or *Cryptosporidium*-like organisms that have now been identified as coccidia in the genus *Cyclospora* (*C. cayetanensis*).

**clean in•ter•mit•tent blad•der cath•e•ter•i•za•tion** a common way for patients with neurogenic bladders that do not empty normally to empty their bladders on a routine schedule.

**clear•ance** (klēr'ans) **1.** (*C* with a subscript indicating the substance removed). Removal of a substance from the blood, e.g., by renal excretion, expressed in terms of the volume flow of arterial blood or plasma that would contain the amount of substance removed per unit time; measured in ml/min. **2.** a condition in which bodies may pass each other without hindrance, or the distance between bodies. **3.** removal of something from some place; e.g., "esophageal acid clearance" refers to removal from the esophagus of some acid that has refluxed into it from the stomach, evaluated by the time taken for restoration of a normal pH in the esophagus.

**clear cell 1.** a cell in which the cytoplasm appears empty with the light microscope, as occurs in certain secretory cells of eccrine sweat glands and in the parathyroid glands when the glycogen is unstained; **2.** any cell, particularly a neoplastic one, containing abundant glycogen or other material that is not stained by hematoxylin or eosin, so that the cell cytoplasm is very pale in routinely stained sections.

**clear cell car•cin•o•ma** SYN mesonephroma.

**clear cell car•cin•o•ma of sal•i•vary glands** a malignant tumor, comprising several subtypes such as clear cell oncocytoma, hyalinizing clear cell carcinoma, epithelial-myoepithelial (intercalated duct) carcinoma.

**clear•ing fac•tors** lipoprotein lipases that appear in plasma during lipemia and catalyze hydrolysis of triglycerides only when the latter are bound to protein and when an acceptor (e.g., serum albumin) is present, thus "clearing" the plasma.

**clear lay•er of ep•i•der•mis** SYN stratum lucidum.

**cleav•age** (klēv'ij) **1.** series of mitotic cell divisions occurring in the oocyte immediately after fertilization. SEE ALSO cleavage division. **2.** splitting of a complex molecule into two or more simpler molecules. SYN scission (2). **3.** linear clefts in the skin indicating the direction of the fibers in the dermis. SEE ALSO cleavage lines.

**cleav•age cav•i•ty** SYN blastocele.

**cleav•age di•vi•sion** the rapid mitotic division of the zygote with decrease in size of individual cells or blastomeres and the formation of a morula. SEE ALSO cleavage (1).

**cleav•age lines** lines which can be extrapolated by connecting linear openings made when a round pin is driven into the skin of a cadaver, resulting from the principal axis of orientation of the subcutaneous connective tissue (collagen) fibers of the dermis; they vary in direction with the region of the body surface.

**cleav•age pro•duct** a substance resulting from

the splitting of a molecule into two or more simpler molecules.

**cleav•age site** SYN restriction site.

**cleav•age spin•dle** the spindle formed during the cleavage of a zygote or its blastomeres.

**cleft** (kleft) a fissure.

**cleft hand** a congenital deformity in which the division between the fingers, especially between the third and fourth, extends into the metacarpal region. SYN split hand.

**cleft lip** a congenital facial deformity of the lip (usually the upper lip) due to failure of fusion of the medial and lateral nasal prominences and maxillary process; frequently associated with cleft alveolus and cleft palate. SYN harelip.

**cleft pal•ate** a congenital fissure in the median line of the palate, often associated with cleft lip. Often occurs as a feature of a syndrome or generalized condition, e.g., diastrophic dwarfism or spondyloepiphyseal dysplasia congenita; its general genetic behavior resembles that of cleft lip. SYN palatoschisis.

**cleft spine** SEE spina bifida.

**cleft ton•gue** SYN bifid tongue.

**clei•dal** (klī′dăl) relating to the clavicle. SYN clidal.

**clei•do-, cleid-** the clavicle; also spelled clido-, clid-. [G. *kleis*, bar, bolt]

**clei•do•cos•tal** (klī-dō-kos′tăl) relating to the clavicle and a rib. SYN clidocostal. [cleido- + L. *costa*, rib]

**clei•do•cra•ni•al** (klī′dō-krā′nē-ăl) relating to the clavicle and the cranium. SYN clidocranial. [G. *kleis*, clavicle, + *kranion*, cranium]

**clei•dot•o•my** (klī-dot′ō-mē) cutting the clavicle of a dead fetus to effect a vaginal delivery. [cleido- + -tomy]

**-clei•sis** closure. [G. *kleisis*, a closing]

**clenched fist sign** in angina pectoris, pressing of the clenched fist against the chest to indicate the constricting, pressing quality of the pain.

**CLIA** Clinical Laboratory Improvement Amendments.

**CLIA '67** Clinical Laboratory Improvement Act of 1967.

**CLIA '88** Clinical Laboratory Improvement Amendments of 1988.

**click** (klik) a slight, sharp sound.

**cli•dal** (klī′dăl) SYN cleidal.

**cli•do-, clid-** the clavicle. SEE ALSO cleido-. [G. *kleis*, bar, bolt]

**cli•do•cos•tal** (klī-dō-kos′tăl) SYN cleidocostal.

**cli•do•cra•ni•al** (klī-dō-krā′nē-ăl) SYN cleidocranial.

**client** (klī′ent) a patron or customer; one who receives a professional service from another; one who seeks or receives advise or therapy from a paramedical professional. [L. *cliens*, protégé, dependent]

**cli•ent-cen•tered ther•a•py** a system of nondirective psychotherapy based on the assumption that the client (patient) both has the internal resources to improve and is in the best position to resolve personality dysfunction.

**cli•mac•ter•ic** (klī-mak′ter-ik, klī-mak-ter′ik) **1.** the period of endocrinal, somatic, and transitory psychologic changes occurring in the menopause. **2.** a critical period of life. [G. *klimaktēr*, the rung of a ladder]

**cli•max** (klī′maks) **1.** the height or acme of a

disease; its stage of greatest severity. **2.** SYN orgasm. [G. *klimax*, staircase]

**clin•i•cal** (klin′i-kl) **1.** relating to the bedside of a patient. **2.** denoting the symptoms and course of a disease, as distinguished from the laboratory findings of anatomical changes. **3.** relating to a clinic.

**clin•i•cal a•nat•o•my** the practical application of anatomic knowledge to diagnosis and treatment.

**clin•i•cal crown** that portion of the anatomic crown of a tooth that is present in the oral cavity.

**clin•i•cal di•ag•no•sis** a diagnosis made from a study of the signs and symptoms of a disease.

**clin•i•cal end point** traditional medical measures of a diagnostic or therapeutic impact that may or may not be perceived by the patient.

**clin•i•cal fit•ness** absence of frank disease or of subclinical precursors.

**clin•i•cal ge•net•ics** genetics applied to the diagnosis, prognosis, management, and prevention of genetic diseases. Cf. medical genetics.

**clin•i•cal in•di•ca•tor** a measure, process, or outcome used to judge a particular clinical situation and indicate whether the care delivered was appropriate.

**Clin•i•cal Lab•o•ra•to•ry Im•prove•ment A•mend•ments (CLIA)** federal legislation, and the personnel and procedures established by it under the aegis of the Health Care Financing Administration (HCFA), for the surveillance and regulation of all clinical laboratory procedures in the U.S.

**Clin•i•cal Lab•o•ra•to•ry Im•prove•ment Act of 1967 (CLIA '67)** federal law (Public Law 90-174) regulating medical laboratories that process more than 100 specimens per year in interstate commerce. Usually affects only large, independent laboratories. SEE ALSO Clinical Laboratory Improvement Amendments of 1988.

**Clin•i•cal Lab•o•ra•to•ry Im•prove•ment A•mend•ments of 1988 (CLIA '88)** amendments enacted by U.S. Congress in 1988 (Public Law 100-578) to revise and expand the Clinical Laboratory Improvement Act of 1967 and Medicare and Medicaid provisions. The amendments classify and regulate laboratories based on the complexity of procedures being performed and establish personnel qualifications. These rules apply to all testing sites, but several procedures and tests have waivers from these regulations. SEE ALSO Clinical Laboratory Improvement Act of 1967.

**clin•i•cal le•thal** a disorder that culminates in premature death.

**clin•i•cal med•i•cine** the study and practice of medicine in relation to the care of patients; the art of medicine as distinguished from laboratory science.

**clin•i•cal nurse spe•cial•ist** a registered nurse with at least a master's degree who has advanced education in a particular area of clinical practice such as oncology or psychiatry.

**clin•i•cal path** a map that outlines the entire track or path a patient is expected to follow throughout the course of treatment and beyond.

**clin•i•cal pa•thol•o•gy 1.** any part of the medical practice of pathology as it pertains to the care of patients; **2.** the subspecialty in pathology concerned with the theoretical and technical aspects of chemistry, immunohematology, microbiology, parasitology, immunology, hematology, and other fields as they pertain to the diagnosis of disease.

**clin·i·cal prac·tice guide·lines** a formal statement about a defined task or function in clinical practice, such as desirable diagnostic tests or the optimal treatment regimen for a specific diagnosis; generally based on the best available evidence, e.g., randomized controlled trials that have been assessed by a Cochrane collaborating group. SEE ALSO Cochrane collaboration.

**clin·i·cal psy·chol·o·gy** a branch of psychology that specializes in both discovering new knowledge and in applying the art and science of psychology to persons with emotional or behavioral disorders; subspecialities include clinical child psychology and pediatric psychology.

**clin·i·cal root of tooth** that portion of a tooth embedded in the investing structures; the portion of a tooth not visible in the oral cavity. SYN radix clinica dentis [TA].

**clin·i·cal ther·mom·e·ter** a small, self-registering thermometer, consisting of a simple scaled glass tube containing mercury, used for taking the temperature of the body.

**cli·ni·cian** (klin-ish′ŭn) a health professional engaged in the care of patients, as distinguished from one working in other areas.

**clin·i·co·path·o·log·ic** (klin′i-kō-path-ō-loj′ik) pertaining to the signs and symptoms manifested by a patient, and also the results of laboratory studies, as they relate to the findings in the gross and histologic examination of tissue by means of biopsy or autopsy, or both.

♻**cli·no-** a slope (inclination or declination) or bend. [G. klinō, to slope, incline, or bend]

**cli·no·ceph·a·ly** (klī′nō-sef′ă-lē) craniosynostosis in which the upper surface of the skull is concave, presenting a saddle-shaped appearance in profile. SYN saddle head. [clino- + G. kephalē, head]

**cli·no·dac·ty·ly** (klī′nō-dak′ti-lē) permanent deflection of one or more fingers. [clino- + G. daktylos, finger]

**cli·noid pro·cess** one of three pairs of bony projections from the sphenoid bone: anterior clinoid process, the recurved posterior angle of the lesser wing; middle clinoid process, a little spur of bone on the body of the sphenoid, posterolateral to the tuberculum sellae; posterior clinoid process, a spur of bone at each superior angle of the dorsum sellae.

**CLIP** corticotropin-like intermediate-lobe peptide.

**clip** (klip′) a fastener used to hold a part or thing together with another.

**clip for·ceps** a small forceps with spring catch to hold a bleeding vessel.

**clith·ro·pho·bia** (klīth-rō-fō′bē-ă) morbid fear of being locked in. [G. kleithron, a bolt, + phobos, fear]

**clit·o·ri·dec·to·my** (klit′ŏ-ri-dek′tō-mē) removal of the clitoris. [clitoris + G. ektomē, excision]

**clit·o·ri·di·tis** (klit′ŏ-rĭ-dī′tis) inflammation of the clitoris. SYN clitoritis. [clitoris + G. -itis, inflammation]

**clit·o·ris**, pl. **cli·to·ri·des** (klit′ŏ-ris, klītō-r′ĭ-dēz) [TA] a cylindric, erectile body, rarely exceeding 2 cm in length, situated at the most anterior portion of the vulva and projecting between the branched limbs or laminae of the labia minora,

which form its prepuce and frenulum. It consists of a glans, a corpus, and two crura. [G. kleitoris]

**clit·o·rism** (klit′ŏ-rizm) prolonged and usually painful erection of the clitoris; the analogue of priapism.

**clit·o·ri·tis** (klit′ŏ-rī′tis) SYN clitoriditis.

**clit·or·o·meg·a·ly** (klit′ŏr-ō-meg′ă-lē) an enlarged clitoris. [clitoris + G. megas, great]

**cli·vus**, pl. **cli·vi** (klī′vŭs, klī′vī) [TA] 1. a downward sloping surface. 2. the sloping surface from the dorsum sellae to the foramen magnum composed of part of the body of the sphenoid and part of the basal part of the occipital bone. [L. slope]

**clo·a·ca** (klō-ā′kă) 1. in early embryos, the endodermally lined chamber into which the hindgut and allantois empty. 2. in birds and monotremes, the common chamber into which the hindgut, bladder, and genital ducts empty. [L. sewer]

**clo·a·cal** (klō-ā′kăl) pertaining to the cloaca.

**clo·a·cal mem·brane** a transitory membrane in the caudal area of the ventral wall of the embryo, separating the endodermal from the ectodermal cloaca; it is divided into anal and genitourinary membranes that break down during the eighth to ninth week to establish the external opening for the alimentary and genitourinary tracts.

**clo·a·co·gen·ic car·ci·no·ma** 1. a type of squamous cell carcinoma of the anus originating in tissues arising from, or in remnants of, the cloaca. 2. in oncology, anal cancer arising proximal to the pectinate line. SYN cuboidal carcinoma. [cloaca + -genic]

**clo·nal** (klō′năl) pertaining to a clone.

**clo·nal se·lec·tion the·o·ry** a theory which states that each lymphocyte has membrane-bound immunoglobulin receptors specific for a particular antigen and once the receptor is engaged, proliferation of the cell occurs such that a clone of antibody producing cells (plasma cell) is produced.

**clone** (klōn) 1. a colony of organisms or cells derived from a single organism or cell by asexual reproduction, all having identical genetic constitutions. 2. to produce such a colony or individual. 3. a short section of DNA which has been copied by means of gene cloning. SEE cloning. [G. klōn, slip, cutting used for propagation]

**clo·nic** (klon′ik) relating to or characterized by clonus.

**clo·nic con·vul·sion** a convulsion in which the contractions are intermittent, the muscles alternately contracting and relaxing.

**clon·ic·i·ty** (klon-is′i-tē) the state of being clonic.

**clon·i·co·ton·ic** (klon′i-kō-ton′ik) both clonic and tonic; said of certain forms of muscular spasm.

**clo·nic spasm** alternate involuntary contraction and relaxation of a muscle.

**clo·nic state** movement marked by repetitive muscle contractions and relaxations in rapid succession.

**clon·ing** (klōn′ing) 1. growing a colony of genetically identical cells or organisms in vitro. 2. transplantation of a nucleus from a somatic cell to an ovum, which then develops into an embryo; many identical embryos can thus be generated by asexual reproduction. 3. with blastocysts, dividing a cluster of cells through microsurgery and transferring one-half of the cells to a zona pellucida that has been emptied of its contents. The resulting embryos, genetically identical, may be implanted in an animal for gestation. **4.** a recombinant DNA technique used to produce millions of copies of a DNA fragment. The fragment is spliced into a cloning vehicle (i.e., plasmid, bacteriophage, or animal virus). The cloning vehicle penetrates a bacterial cell or yeast (the host), which is then grown in vitro or in an animal host. In some cases, as in the production of genetically engineered drugs, the inserted DNA becomes activated and alters the chemical functioning of the host cell.

**clon·ing vec·tor** an autonomously replicating plasmid or phage with regions that are not essential for its propagation in bacteria and into which foreign DNA can be inserted; this foreign DNA is replicated and propagated as if it were a normal component of the vector.

**clo·nism** (klon′izm) a long continued state of clonic spasms.

**clo·no·gen·ic** (klō-nō-jen′ik) arising from or consisting of a clone.

**clo·nor·chi·a·sis** (klō-nōr-kī′ă-sis) a disease caused by the fluke *Clonorchis sinensis*, affecting the distal bile ducts after ingestion of raw, smoked, or undercooked fish or raw crayfish; repeated or chronic infection induces an intense proliferative and granulomatous condition.

*Clo·nor·chis si·nen·sis* (klō-nōr′kis sī-nen′sis) the Chinese liver fluke, a species of trematodes that in the Far East infects the bile passages; fish serve as second intermediate hosts and snails as the first intermediate hosts.

**clon·o·spasm** (klon′ō-spazm) SYN clonus.

**clo·nus** (klō′nŭs) a form of movement marked by contractions and relaxations of a muscle, occurring in rapid succession seen with, among other conditions, spasticity and some seizure disorders. SEE ALSO contraction. SYN clonospasm. [G. *klonos*, a tumult]

**Clo·quet her·nia** (klō-kā′) a femoral hernia perforating the aponeurosis of the pectineus and insinuating itself between this aponeurosis and the muscle, lying therefore behind the femoral vessels.

**closed an·es·the·sia** inhalation anesthesia in which there is total rebreathing of all exhaled gases, except carbon dioxide which is absorbed; gas flow into the anesthetic circuit consists only of oxygen, in amounts equal to the patient's metabolic consumption, plus small amounts of other gases (e.g., nitrous oxide) which undergo continued uptake by and distribution in the patient.

**closed chain com·pound** SYN cyclic compound.

**▣ closed chest mas·sage** rhythmic compression of the heart between sternum and spine by depressing the lower sternum with the heels of the hands, the patient lying supine. See this page.

**closed-cir·cuit he·li·um di·lu·tion** a gas dilution technique for measuring the functional residual capacity (FRC); the subject rebreathes helium from a spirometer while oxygen is added and carbon dioxide is removed to maintain a constant system volume.

**closed cir·cuit meth·od** a method for measuring oxygen consumption in which the subject rebreathes an initial quantity of oxygen through a carbon dioxide absorber and the decrease in the volume of oxygen being rebreathed is noted.

**closed cir·cuit spi·rom·e·try** measurement of

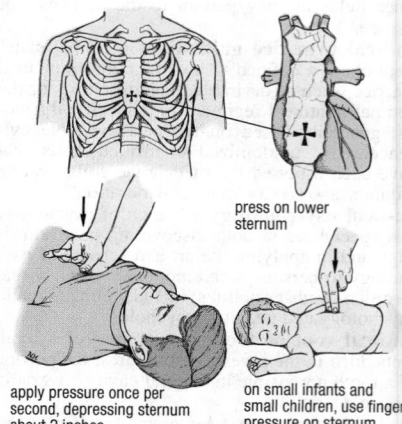

press on lower sternum

apply pressure once per second, depressing sternum about 2 inches

on small infants and small children, use finger pressure on sternum

**external cardiac compression**

$CO_2$ and $O_2$ in inspired and expired air by means of a device that, along with the subject's respiratory tract, forms a closed circuit.

**closed com·e·do** a comedo with a narrow or obstructed opening on the skin surface; closed comedos may rupture, producing a low-grade dermal inflammatory reaction. SYN whitehead (2).

**closed dis·lo·ca·tion** a dislocation not complicated by an external wound. SYN simple dislocation.

**closed drain·age** drainage of a body cavity via a water- or air-tight system.

**closed frac·ture** a fracture in which skin is intact at site of fracture. SYN simple fracture.

**closed head in·ju·ry** a head injury in which continuity of the scalp and mucous membranes is maintained.

**closed hos·pi·tal** a hospital that restricts membership on its attending or consulting staff, and thereby limits who may admit and treat patients.

**closed loop ob·struc·tion** obstruction of a segment of intestine either rotated on a fixed point (volvulus) or herniated through a fibrous opening (as under an adhesion or into a hernia); frequently associated with impaired perfusion ultimately resulting in gangrene.

**closed re·duc·tion of frac·tures** reduction by manipulation of bone, without incision in the skin.

**closed sur·gery** surgery without incision into skin, e.g., reduction of a fracture or dislocation.

**close-packed po·si·tion** joint position in which contact between the articulation structures is maximal. SYN joint extension.

**clos·ing snap** the accentuated first heart sound of mitral stenosis, related to closure of the abnormal valve.

**clos·ing vol·ume** the lung volume at which the flow from the lower parts of the lungs becomes severely reduced or stops during expiration, presumably because of airway closure; measured by the sharp rise in expiratory concentration of a tracer gas that had been inspired at the beginning of a breath that started from residual volume.

**clos·trid·i·al** (klos-trid′ē-ăl) relating to any bacterium of the genus *Clostridium.*

***Clos·trid·i·um*** (klos-trid′ē-ŭm) a genus of anaerobic (or anaerobic, aerotolerant), sporeforming, motile (occasionally nonmotile) bacteria containing Gram-positive rods. Exotoxins are sometimes produced by these organisms. They may cause disease in man and other animals. They are generally found in soil and in the intestinal tract of man and other animals. The type species is *Clostridium butyricum.* [G. *klōstēr*, a spindle]

**clos·trid·i·um,** pl. **clos·trid·ia** (klos-trid′ē-ŭm, klos-trid′ē-ă) a vernacular term used to refer to any member of the genus *Clostridium.*

***Clos·trid·i·um bi·fer·men·tans*** a species found in putrid meat and gaseous gangrene; also commonly in soil, feces, and sewage. Its pathogenicity varies from strain to strain.

***Clos·trid·i·um bot·u·li·num*** a species that occurs widely in nature and is a frequent cause of food poisoning (botulism) from preserved meats, fruits, or vegetables that have not been properly sterilized before canning.

***Clos·trid·i·um his·to·lyt·i·cum*** a species found in war wounds, where it induces necrosis of tissue; it produces a cytolytic exotoxin that causes local necrosis and sloughing on injection; it is not toxic on feeding; it is pathogenic for small laboratory animals.

***Clos·trid·i·um nov·y·i*** a species causing gaseous gangrene and necrotic hepatitis.

***Clos·trid·i·um par·a·bot·u·lin·um*** a species that produces a powerful exotoxin and is pathogenic for man and other animals.

***Clos·trid·i·um per·frin·gens*** a species that is the chief causative agent of gas gangrene; it may also be involved in causing enteritis, appendicitis, and puerperal fever; it is one of the most common causes of food poisoning in the U.S. SYN *Clostridium welchii, gas bacillus, Welch bacillus.*

***Clos·trid·i·um per·frin·gens* al·pha tox·in** a phospholipase produced by *Clostridium perfringens* that increases vascular permeability and produces necrosis.

***Clos·trid·i·um per·frin·gens* be·ta tox·in** a substance produced by *Clostridium perfringens* that causes necrosis and induces hypertension by causing release of catecholamine.

***Clos·trid·i·um per·frin·gens* en·ter·o·tox·in** a toxin produced by *Clostridium perfringens* that alters membrane permeability.

***Clos·trid·i·um per·frin·gens* ep·si·lon tox·in** a toxin produced by *Clostridium perfringens* that increases the permeability of the gastrointestinal wall.

***Clos·trid·i·um per·frin·gens* i·o·ta tox·in** a binary toxin produced by *Clostridium perfringens* responsible for necrosis and increased vascular permeability.

***Clos·tri·di·um sor·del·li·i*** a bacterial strain that produces multiple toxins including a lecithinase, hemolysin, and a fibrinolysin, which result in edema and potentially fatal hypotension, and necrotic infections in humans. It is especially associated with abdominal and gynecologic posttraumatic and postoperative wound infection; also causes big head in rams.

***Clos·trid·i·um te·ta·ni*** a species that causes tetanus; it produces a potent exotoxin (neurotoxin) that is intensely toxic for humans and other animals when formed in tissues or injected, but not when ingested.

***Clos·trid·i·um welch·i·i*** SYN *Clostridium perfringens.*

**clo·sure** (klō′zhŭr) **1.** the completion of a reflex pathway. **2.** the place of coupling between stimuli in the establishment of conditioned learning. **3.** to achieve or experience a sense of completion in a mental task. **4.** definitive repair of an open wound, traumatic or surgical.

**clo·sure prin·ci·ple** PSYCHOLOGY the principle that when one views fragmentary stimuli forming a nearly complete figure (e.g., an incomplete rectangle) one tends to ignore the missing parts and perceive the figure as whole. SEE gestalt.

**clot** (klot) **1.** to coagulate, said especially of blood. **2.** a soft, nonrigid, insoluble mass formed when a liquid (e.g., blood or lymph) gels. [O.E. *klott*, lump]

**clot·ting fac·tor** any of the various plasma components involved in the clotting process.

**cloud·y swell·ing** swelling of cells due to injury to the membranes affecting ionic transfer; causes an accumulation of intracellular water. SYN hydropic degeneration, parenchymatous degeneration.

**clubbed dig·it** SEE clubbing.

**clubbed fin·gers** SEE clubbing.

**club·bing** (klŭb′ing) a condition affecting the fingers and toes in which proliferation of distal tissues, especially the nail beds, results in thickening and widening of the extremities of the digits; the nails are abnormally curved and shiny. See page 196.

**club·foot, club foot** (klŭb′fut) SYN talipes equinovarus.

**club hair** a hair in resting state, prior to shedding, in which the bulb has become a club-shaped mass.

**club·hand, club hand** (klŭb′hand) congenital or acquired angulation deformity of the hand associated with partial or complete absence of radius or ulna; usually with intrinsic deformities in the hand in congenital variants.

**clue cell** a type of vaginal epithelial cell that appears granular and is coated with coccobacillary organisms; seen in bacterial vaginosis.

**clump·ing** (klŭmp-ing) the massing together of bacteria or other cells or particles suspended in a fluid.

**clu·ne·al** (kloo′nē-ăl) pertaining to the clunes.

**clu·nes** (kloo′nēz) SYN buttocks. [pl. of L. *clunis,* buttock]

**cluster of differentiation (CD)** cell membrane molecules that are used to classify leukocytes into subsets. CD molecules are classified by monoclonal antibodies. There are four general types: type I transmembrane proteins have their COOH-termini in the cytoplasm and their $NH_2$-termini outside the cell; type II transmembrane proteins have their $NH_2$-termini in the cytoplasm and their COOH-termini outside the cell; type III transmembrane proteins cross the plasma membrane more than once and hence may form transmembrane channels; and glycosylphosphatidylinositol-anchored proteins (type IV), which are tethered to the lipid bilayer via a glycosylphosphatidylinositol anchor.

**clus·ter of dif·fer·en·ti·a·tion 2** a glycoprotein that is expressed on all peripheral T cells, large granular lymphocytes and most, but not all, thy-

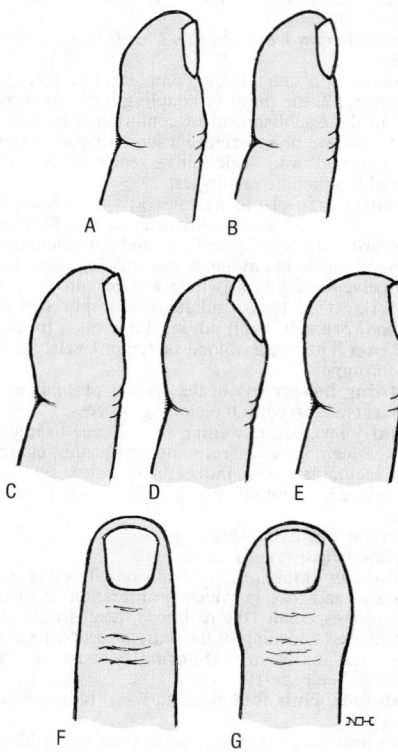

**varieties of digital clubbing:** (A) normal, (B) increased curvature on nail, (C) mild clubbing, (D) parrot's beak type, (E) watch glass type, (F) normal, (G) drumstick type

mocytes. CD2 is involved in signal transduction and cell adhesion.

**clus·ter of dif·fer·en·ti·a·tion 3** a complex of 5 polypeptides associated with the T cell receptor and is involved in signal transduction.

**clus·ter of dif·fer·en·ti·a·tion 4** a glycoprotein found on various subsets of T cells, i.e., usually on helper and some T cytotoxic cells.

**clus·ter of dif·fer·en·ti·a·tion 8** membrane glycoprotein found on subsets of T lymphocytes. CD8 is expressed on T cytotoxic cells and T suppressor cells.

**cluster of differentiation (CD) antigen** an antigen (marker) on the surface of a cell, usually a lymphocyte.

**clus·ter head·ache** possibly due to a hypersensitivity to histamine; characterized by recurrent, severe, unilateral orbitotemporal headaches associated with ipsilateral photophobia, lacrimation, and nasal congestion. SYN histaminic headache, Horton headache.

**cluttering** (klut'er-ing) speech disorder characterized by rapid, jerky utterances with many omissions and transpositions of speech sounds; sometimes confused with stuttering. SEE stuttering.

**cly·sis** (klī'sis) **1.** an infusion of fluid, usually subcutaneously, for therapeutic purposes. **2.** formerly, a fluid enema; later, the washing out of material from any body space or cavity by fluids. [G. *klysis,* a drenching by a clyster]

**Cm** curium.

**cM** centimorgan.

**cm** centimeter; cm² for square centimeter; cm³ for cubic centimeter.

**CMA** Certified Medical Assistant.

**cmc** critical micelle concentration.

**CMI** cell-mediated immunity.

**CML** cell-mediated lymphocytotoxicity.

**CMP** cytidine 5′-monophosphate (secondarily, any cytidine monophosphate).

**CMT** Certified Medical Transcriptionist. SEE medical transcriptionist.

**CMV 1.** cytomegalovirus. **2.** a cancer drug combination treatment consisting of cisplatin, methotrexate, and vinblastine, used in the treatment of bladder and other malignancies.

**CNS 1.** central nervous system. **2.** symbol for the thiocyanate radical, CNS⁻ or —CNS.

**CO** carbon monoxide.

**Co** cobalt; coccygeal.

△**co-** SEE con-.

**CoA** coenzyme A.

**co·ad·ap·ta·tion** (kō′ad-ap-tā′shŭn) GENETICS the operation of selection jointly on two or more loci.

**co·ag·glu·ti·nin** (kō-ă-gloo′ti-nin) a substance that does not agglutinate an antigen, but does result in agglutination of antigen that is coated with univalent antibody. SEE ALSO conglutination.

**co·ag·u·la** (kō-ag′yu-lă) plural of coagulum.

**co·ag·u·la·ble** (kō-ag′yu-lă-bl) capable of being coagulated or clotted.

**co·ag·u·lant** (kō-ag′yu-lant) **1.** an agent that causes, stimulates, or accelerates coagulation, especially with reference to blood. **2.** SYN coagulative.

**co·ag·u·late** (kō-ag′yu-lāt) **1.** to convert a fluid or a substance in solution into a solid or gel. **2.** to clot; to curdle; to change from a liquid to a solid or gel. [L. *coagulo,* pp. *-atus,* to curdle]

**co·ag·u·la·tion** (kō-ag-yu-lā′shŭn) **1.** clotting; the process of changing from a liquid to a solid, said especially of blood. **2.** a clot or coagulum. **3.** transformation of a sol into a gel or semisolid mass.

**co·ag·u·la·tion ne·cro·sis** a type of necrosis in which the affected cells or tissue are converted into a dry, dull, homogeneous eosinophilic mass without nuclei, as a result of the coagulation of protein as occurs in an infarct.

**co·ag·u·la·tion time** the time required for blood to coagulate; prolonged in hemophilia and in the presence of obstructive jaundice, some anemias and leukemias, and some of the infectious diseases.

**co·ag·u·la·tive** (kō-ag′yu-lă-tiv) causing coagulation. SYN coagulant (2).

**co·ag·u·lop·a·thy** (kō-ag-yu-lop′ă-thē) a disease affecting the coagulability of the blood.

**co·ag·u·lum**, pl. **co·ag·u·la** (kō-ag′yu-lŭm, kō-ag′yu-lă) a clot or a curd; a soft, nonrigid, insoluble mass formed when a sol undergoes coagulation. [L. a means of coagulating, rennet]

**co·al·co·hol·ic** (kō-al-kō-hol′ik) **1.** the person(s) who enables an alcoholic by assuming responsibilities on the alcoholic's behalf, minimizing or denying the problem drinking, or making amends for the alcoholic's behavior. **2.** pertaining to the co-alcoholic or to co-alcoholism.

**co•al•co•hol•ism** (kō-al′kō-hol-izm) the constellation of attitudes, attributes, and behaviors of the person who enables the alcoholic, which are necessary for the attainment of a symbiotic balance between alcoholic and co-alcoholic. SEE ALSO symbiosis.

**co•a•les•cence** (kō-ă-les′ens) fusion of originally separate parts. SYN concrescence (1).

**coal wor•ker's pneu•mo•co•ni•o•sis** SYN anthracosilicosis.

**CO₂ analyzer** SYN capnometer.

**co•ap•ta•tion** (kō-ap-tā′shŭn) joining or fitting together of two surfaces; e.g., the lips of a wound or the ends of a broken bone. [L. *co-apto*, pp. *-aptatus*, to fit together]

**co•ap•ta•tion splint** a short splint designed to prevent overriding of the ends of a fractured bone, usually supplemented by a longer splint to fix the entire limb.

**co•ap•ta•tion su•ture** SYN apposition suture.

**co•arct** (kō-arkt′) to restrict or press together. SYN coarctate (1). [L. *co-arcto*, pp. *-arctatus*, to press together]

**co•arc•tate** (kō-ark′tāt) **1.** SYN coarct. **2.** pressed together.

**co•arc•ta•tion** (kō-ark-tā′shŭn) a constriction, stricture, or stenosis, usually of the aorta.

**CoAS–, CoASH** symbols for the coenzyme A radical and reduced coenzyme A, respectively.

**coat** (kōt) **1.** the outer covering or envelope of an organ or part. **2.** one of the layers of membranous or other tissues forming the wall of a canal or hollow organ. SEE tunic.

**coat•ed tongue** a tongue with a whitish layer on its upper surface, composed of epithelial debris, food particles, and bacteria; often an indication of indigestion or of fever.

**Coats dis•ease** (kōts) SYN exudative retinitis.

**COB** Coordination of Benefits.

**co•bal•a•min** (kō-bal′ă-min) general term for compounds containing the dimethylbenzimidazolylcobamide nucleus of vitamin B₁₂.

**co•balt (Co)** (kō′bawlt) a steel-gray metallic element, atomic no. 27, atomic wt. 58.93320; a bioelement and a constituent of vitamin B₁₂; certain of its compounds are pigments, e.g., cobalt blue. [Ger. *kobalt*, goblin or evil spirit]

**cob•bler's su•ture** SYN doubly armed suture.

**Cobb meth•od** (kob) a technique used in scoliosis to determine the degree of curvature of the spine; the measurement is made by drawing a perpendicular to a line drawn across the superior endplate of the upper-end (most tilted) vertebra and the inferior endplate of the lower-end vertebra; the angle formed by the intersection of the two perpendicular lines is the Cobb angle, which is the measure of the magnitude of the curve.

**Cobb syn•drome** (kob) cutaneous angiomas, usually in a dermatomal distribution on the trunk, associated with vascular abnormality of the spinal cord and resulting neurologic symptoms.

**co•caine** (kō-kān′) a crystalline alkaloid obtained from the leaves of *Erythroxylon coca* (family Erythroxylaceae) and other species of *Erythroxylon*, or by synthesis from ecgonine or its derivatives; a potent central nervous system stimulant, vasoconstrictor, and topical anesthetic, widely abused as a euphoriant and associated with the risk of severe adverse physical and mental effects.

**co•caine hy•dro•chlor•ide** a water-soluble salt used for local anesthesia of the eye or mucous membranes.

**co•car•cin•o•gen** (kō-kar′si-nō-jen) a substance that works symbiotically with a carcinogen in the production of cancer.

**coc•cal** (kok′ăl) relating to cocci.

**coc•ci** (kok′sī) plural of coccus.

**Coc•cid•ia** (kok-sid′ē-ă) a subclass of protozoa in which mature trophozoites are small and typically intracellular. [Mod. L., fr. G. *kokkos*, berry]

**coc•cid•i•al** (kok-sid′ē-ăl) relating to coccidia.

**coc•cid•i•oi•dal** (kok-sid-ē-oy′dăl) referring to the disease or to the infecting organism of coccidioidomycosis.

**Coc•cid•i•oi•des** (kok-sid-ē-oy′dēz) a genus of fungi found in the soil of the semi-arid areas of the Southwestern U.S. and smaller areas throughout Central and South America. The only pathogenic species, *Coccidioides immitis*, causes coccidioidomycosis. [coccidium + G. *eidos*, resemblance]

**coc•cid•i•oi•do•ma** (kok-sid′ē-oy-dō′mă) a benign localized residual granulomatous lesion or scar in a lung following primary coccidioidomycosis.

**coc•cid•i•oi•do•my•co•sis** (kok-sid-ē-oy′dō-mī-kō′sis) a variable, benign, severe, or sometimes fatal systemic mycosis due to inhalation of arthroconidia of *Coccidioides immitis*. In benign forms of the infection, the lesions are limited to the upper respiratory tract, lungs, and near lymph nodes; in a low percentage of cases, the disease disseminates to other organs, meninges, bones, joints, and skin and subcutaneous tissues. [coccidioides + G. *mykēs*, fungus, + *-osis*, condition]

**coc•cid•i•o•sis** (kok-sid-ē-ō′sis) group name for diseases due to any species of coccidia; a common disease of many species of domestic animals and birds; both intestinal and pulmonary coccidiosis have been reported in human individuals with AIDS.

**coc•cid•i•um**, pl. **coc•cid•ia** (kok-sid′ē-ŭm, kok-sid′ē-ă) common name given to protozoan parasites in which schizogony occurs within epithelial cells, generally in the intestine. Coccidia are parasitic in domestic and wild birds and mammals, occasionally in humans; the majority are nonpathogenic. SEE *Isospora*. [Mod. L. dim. of G. *kokkos*, berry]

**coc•co•bac•il•lary** (kok′ō-bas′i-lār-ē) relating to a coccobacillus.

**coc•co•ba•cil•lus** (kok′ō-bă-sil′ŭs) a short, thick bacterial rod of the shape of an oval or slightly elongated coccus. [G. *kokkos*, berry]

**coc•coid** (kok′oyd) resembling a coccus. [G. *kokkos*, berry, + *eidos*, resemblance]

**coc•cus**, pl. **coc•ci** (kok′ŭs, kok′sī) **1.** a bacterium of round, spheroidal, or ovoid form. **2.** SYN cochineal. [G. *kokkos*, berry]

**coc•cy•al•gia** (kok-sē-al′jē-ă) SYN coccygodynia. [coccyx + G. *algos*, pain]

**coc•cy•dyn•ia** (kok-sē-din′ē-ă) SYN coccygodynia. [coccyx + G. *ōdyne, pain*]

**coc•cyg•eal (Co)** (kok-sij′ē-ăl) relating to the coccyx.

**coc•cyg•eal bod•y** an arteriovenous (arteriolovenular) anastomosis supplied by the middle sacral artery and located on the pelvic surface of the coccyx.

**coc•cyg•eal gan•gli•on** SYN ganglion impar.

**coc•cyg•eal nerve [Co]** a small nerve, the lowest of the spinal nerves, entering into the formation of the coccygeal plexus. SYN nervus coccygeus [TA].

**coc•cyg•eal plex•us** a small plexus formed by the fifth sacral and the coccygeal nerves; it gives origin to the anococcygeal nerves.

**coc•cyg•eal si•nus** a fistula opening in the region of the coccyx, being the result of incomplete closure of the caudal end of the neurenteric canal. SEE ALSO pilonidal sinus.

**coc•cy•ge•al ver•te•brae Co1–Co4** the four terminal segments of the vertebral column, usually fused to form the coccyx. SYN vertebrae coccygeae [Co1–Co4] [TA].

**coc•cy•gec•to•my** (kok-sē-jek'tō-mē) removal of the coccyx. [coccyx + G. *ektomē,* excision]

**coc•cyg•e•us mus•cle** *origin,* spine of ischium and sacrospinous ligament; *insertion,* sides of lower part of sacrum and upper part of coccyx; *action,* assists in support of pelvic floor, especially when intra-abdominal pressures increase; *nerve supply,* third and fourth sacral. SYN musculus coccygeus [TA].

**coc•cy•go•dyn•ia** (kok'si-gō-din'ē-ă) pain in the coccygeal region. SYN coccyalgia, coccydynia, coccyodynia. [coccyx + G. *odynē,* pain]

**coc•cy•got•o•my** (kok-sē-got'ō-mē) operation for freeing the coccyx from its attachments. [coccyx + G. *tomē,* a cutting]

**coc•cy•o•dyn•ia** (kok'sē-ō-din'ē-ă) SYN coccygodynia.

**coc•cyx,** gen. **coc•cy•gis,** pl. **coc•cy•ges** (kok' siks, kok'si-jis, kok'si-jēs) [TA] the small bone at the end of the vertebral column in man, formed by the fusion of four rudimentary vertebrae; it articulates above with the sacrum. [G. *kokkyx,* a cuckoo, the coccyx]

**coch•i•neal** (kotch'i-nēl) [CI 75470] the dried female insects, *Coccus cacti,* enclosing the young larvae, or the dried female insect, *Dactylopius coccus,* containing eggs and larvae, from which coccinellin is obtained; used as a red coloring agent and a stain. SEE carmine. SYN coccus (2). [O.Sp. *cochinilla,* wood louse, fr. G. *kokkinos,* berry]

**▣ co•chlea,** pl. **co•chle•ae** (kok'lē-ă, kok'lē-ē) [TA] a cone-shaped cavity in the petrous portion of the temporal bone, forming one of the divisions of the labyrinth or internal ear. It consists of a spiral canal making two and a half turns around a central core of spongy bone, the modiolus; this spiral canal of the cochlea contains the membranous cochlea, or cochlear duct, in which is the spiral organ (Corti organ). See this page. [L. snail shell]

**co•chle•ar** (kok'lē-ăr) relating to the cochlea.

**coch•le•ar ar•ea** the area inferior to the transverse crest of the fundus of the internal acoustic meatus through which the filaments of the cochlear nerve pass to enter the cochlea; forms the base of the conical modiolus about which the cochlear canal spirals. SEE base of modiolus of cochlea. SYN area cochlea [TA].

**co•chle•ar ca•nal** the winding tube of the bony labyrinth which makes two and a half turns about the modiolus of the cochlea; it is divided incompletely into two compartments by a winding shelf

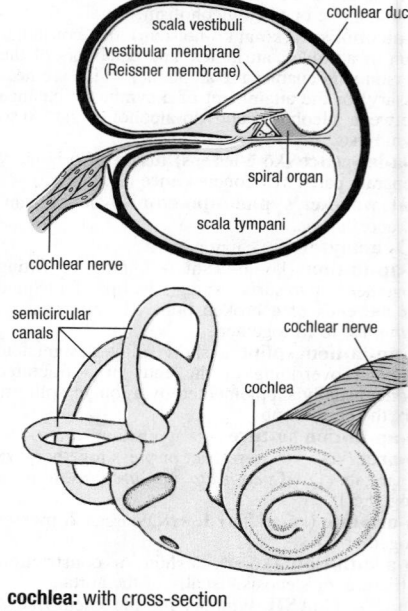

**cochlea:** with cross-section

---

of bone, the bony spiral lamina. SYN canalis spiralis cochleae [TA].

**co•chle•ar can•a•lic•u•lus** a minute canal in the temporal bone that passes from the cochlea inferiorly to open in front of the medial side of the jugular fossa. It contains the perilymphatic duct.

**coch•le•ar drill-out** implantation of electrodes in a cochlea in which the lumen of the scala tympani has been obliterated by the deposition of new bone due to the inflammatory process in labyrinthitis; the cochlear wall and new bone are drilled away so that the electrodes can be placed close to the remaining neurons of the auditory division of the eighth cranial nerve.

**co•chle•ar duct** a spirally arranged membranous tube suspended within the cochlea, occupying the lower portion of the scala vestibuli; it begins by a blind extremity, the vestibular cecum, in the cochlear recess of the vestibule; and ends in another blind extremity, the cecum cupulare or lagena, at the cupola of the cochlea; it contains endolymph and communicates with the sacculus by the ductus reuniens; the spiral organ (organ of Corti), the neuroepithelial receptor organ for hearing, occupies the floor of the duct. SYN scala media [TA].

**coch•le•ar dys•pla•sia** failure of the bony cochlea to develop completely.

**coch•le•ar hair cells** sensory cells in the organ of Corti in synaptic contact with sensory as well as efferent fibers of the cochlear auditory nerve; from the apical end of each cell about 100 stereocilia extend from the surface and make contact with the tectorial membrane. SYN Corti cells.

**coch•le•ar im•plant** amplification device surgically implanted with its stimulating electrodes inserted directly into the nonfunctioning cochlea. SEE hearing aid. SEE ALSO amplification.

**co•chle•ar joint** a hinge joint in which the elevation and depression, respectively, on the opposing articular surfaces form part of a spiral, flexion being accompanied by a certain amount of lateral deviation. SYN spiral joint.

**coch·lear mic·ro·phon·ic** (kok′lē-ar mī-krō-fon′ik) bioelectric potentials produced by the hair cells of the spiral organ (organ of Corti) in response to sound that faithfully represent the frequency and intensity of the acoustic stimulation.

**co·chle·ar nerve** the part of the vestibulocochlear nerve peripheral to the cochlear root; it is composed of fibers whose central nerve processes arise from the bipolar neurons of the spiral ganglion and which have their peripheral processes on the four rows of neuroepithelial cells (hair cells) of the spiral organ. SYN auditory nerve.

**coch·le·i·tis** (ko-klē-ī′tis) inflammation of the cochlea. [cochlea + G. -itis, inflammatio]

**co·chle·o·pal·pe·bral re·flex** a form of the wink reflex in which there is a contraction, sometimes very slight, of the orbicularis palpebrarum muscle when a sudden noise is made close to the ear; it is absent in labyrinthine disease with total deafness. SYN startle reflex (2).

**coch·le·o·topic** (ko-klē-ō-top′ik) referring to the frequency-responsive organization of the central auditory pathways in the brain. [cochlea + G. topos, place, + -ic]

**co·chle·o·ves·tib·u·lar** (kok′lē-ō-ves-tib′yu-lăr) relating to the cochlea and the vestibule of the ear.

**Coch·rane col·lab·o·ra·tion** (kok′răn) a worldwide network of clinical epidemiologists who review and publish results of randomized controlled trials. The aim is to provide improved data for use in evidence-based medicine and for setting clinical practice guidelines. SEE ALSO evidence-based medicine, clinical practice guidelines.

**Cock·ayne syn·drome** (kok-ān′) dwarfism, precociously senile appearance, pigmentary degeneration of the retina, optic atrophy, deafness, sensitivity to sunlight, microcephaly, and mental retardation; autosomal recessive inheritance associated with defective excision repair of DNA. There are various complementation groups.

**cock·tail** (kok′tāl) a mixture that includes several ingredients or drugs.

**co·con·trac·tion** OCCUPATIONAL THERAPY simultaneous contraction of both the agonist and the antagonist around a joint to hold a stable position.

**code** (kōd) **1.** a set of rules, principles, or ethics. **2.** any system devised to convey information or facilitate communication. **3.** term used in hospitals to describe an emergency situation requiring trained members of the staff, such as a cardiopulmonary resuscitation team, or the signal to summon such a team. **4.** a numerical system for ordering and classifying information, e.g., about diagnostic categories. [L. codex, book]

**coding** (kō′ding) assigning a number to a disease process, surgical procedure, or other type of health care service for the purpose of reimbursement, health care planning, and research.

**cod·ing se·quence** the portion of DNA that codes for transcription of messenger RNA. SEE exon.

**Codman tri·an·gle** (kod′măn) RADIOLOGY the interface between growing bone tumor and normal

bone, presenting as an incomplete triangle formed by periosteum.

**Cod·man tu·mor** (kod′măn) chondroblastoma of the proximal humerus.

**co·do·cyte** SYN target cell.

**co·dom·i·nant** (kō-dom′i-nant) in genetics, denoting an equal degree of dominance of two genes, both being expressed in the phenotype of the individual; e.g., genes A and B of the ABO blood group are codominant; individuals with both are type AB.

**co·dom·i·nant in·her·i·tance** inheritance in which two alleles are individually expressed in the presence of each other.

**co·dom·i·nant trait** SEE codominant.

**co·don** (kō′don) a set of three consecutive nucleotides in a strand of DNA or RNA that provides the genetic information to code for a specific amino acid which will be incorporated into a protein chain or serve as a termination signal. SYN triplet (3). [code + -on]

△**coe-** for words so beginning, and not found here, see ce-.

**co·ef·fi·cient** (kō-ĕ-fish′ĕnt) **1.** the expression of the amount or degree of any quality possessed by a substance, or of the degree of physical or chemical change normally occurring in that substance under stated conditions. **2.** the ratio or factor that relates a quantity observed under one set of conditions to that observed under standard conditions, usually when all variables are either 1 or a simple power of 10. [L. co- + efficio (exfacio), to accomplish]

**coefficient of variation (CV)** a unitless number used to describe dispersion of data. It allows comparison of standard deviations of test results expressed in different units. It is calculated from the standard deviation (s) and mean (x). CV = 100s ÷ x.

**Coe·len·ter·a·ta** (sē-len-tĕ-rā′tă) one of the major phyla of invertebrates, to which such forms as jellyfish belong.

**coe·len·ter·ate** (sē-len′ter-at) common name for members of the Coelenterata.

**coelom, pl. coeloma [Br.]** SEE celom.

△**coeno-** shared in common. SEE ALSO ceno-. [G. koinos, common]

**coe·no·cyte [Br.]** SEE cenocyte.

**co·en·zyme** (kō-en′zīm) a substance (excluding solo metal ions) that enhances or is necessary for the action of enzymes; coenzymes are of smaller molecular size than the enzymes themselves; several vitamins are coenzyme precursors. SYN cofactor (1).

**co·en·zyme A (CoA)** a coenzyme containing pantothenic acid, adenosine 3′-phosphate 5′-pyrophosphate, and cysteamine; involved in the transfer of acyl groups, notably in transacetylations.

**co·en·zyme Q (Q)** quinones with isoprenoid side chains (specifically, ubiquinones) that mediate electron transfer between cytochrome b and cytochrome c.

**coeur** (koor) SYN heart. [Fr.]

**coeur en sa·bot** (koor awn sah-bō′) the radiographic configuration of the heart in the tetralogy of Fallot; the elevated apex gives a silhouette like that of a wooden shoe.

**Coe vi·rus** (kō) a virus serologically identical with the A-21 strain of coxsackievirus; the cause of a common-cold-like disease in military recruits.

**co•fac•tor** (kō′fak′ter) **1.** SYN coenzyme. **2.** an atom or molecule essential for the action of a large molecule; e.g., heme in hemoglobin, magnesium in chlorophyll.

**COG** center of gravity.

**Co•gan-Reese syn•drome** (kō′gan-rēs) SYN iridocorneal endothelial syndrome.

**cog•ni•tion** (kog-ni′shŭn) **1.** the mental activities associated with thinking, learning, and memory. **2.** any process whereby one acquires knowledge. [L. *cognitio*]

**cog•ni•tive** (kog′ni-tiv) pertaining to cognition.

**cog•ni•tive dis•so•nance** a motivational state which exists when a person's attitudes, perceptions, and related cognitive state are inconsistent with each other, e.g., hating African Americans as a group but admiring Martin Luther King, Jr.

**cog•ni•tive lat•er•al•i•ty quo•tient** test for difference in cognitive performance of left and right sides of the brain.

**cog•ni•tive ther•a•py** any of a variety of techniques in psychotherapy that utilizes guided self-discovery, imaging, self-instruction, symbolic modeling, and related forms of explicitly elicited cognitions as the principal mode of treatment.

**cog•wheel res•pi•ra•tion** the inspiratory sound being broken into two or three by silent intervals.

**cog•wheel ri•gid•i•ty** a type of rigidity seen in parkinsonism in which the muscles respond with cogwheel-like jerks to the use of constant force in bending the limb.

**co•he•sion** (kō-hē′zhŭn) the attraction between molecules or masses that holds them together. [L. *co-haereo*, pp. *-haesus*, to stick together]

**co•hort** (kō′hōrt) **1.** component of the population born during a particular period and identified by period of birth so that its characteristics can be ascertained as it enters successive time and age periods. **2.** any designated group followed or traced over a period, as in an epidemiological cohort study. [L. *cohors*, retinue, military unit]

**coil** (kōil) **1.** a spiral or series of loops. **2.** an object made of wire wound in a spiral configuration, used in electronic applications, or a loop of wire used as an antenna.

**coin•o•site** (koyn′ō-sīt) SYN cenosite.

**co•i•tal** (kō′i-tăl) pertaining to coitus.

**co•i•tal head•ache** a form of benign exertional headache occurring during sexual activity. SYN benign coital cephalalgia.

**co•i•tion** (kō-ish′ŭn) SYN coitus. [L. *co-eo*, pp. *-itus*, to come together]

**co•i•tus** (kō′i-tŭs) sexual union between male and female. SYN coition, copulation (1), pareunia, sexual intercourse. [L.]

**co•i•tus in•ter•rup•tus** sexual intercourse that is interrupted before the male ejaculates.

**co•i•tus re•ser•va•tus** coitus in which ejaculation is postponed or suppressed.

*Co•ker•o•my•ces* (kō′ker-ō-mī′sēz) a fungal genus in the order Mucorales; a rare cause of disease in humans.

**col** (kol) a crater-like area of the interproximal oral mucosa joining the lingual and buccal interdental papillae.

**cold** (kōld) **1.** a low temperature; the sensation produced by a temperature notably below an accustomed norm or a comfortable level. **2.** popular term for a virus infection involving the upper respiratory tract and characterized by congestion of the mucosa, watery nasal discharge, and general malaise, with a duration of 3 to 5 days. SEE ALSO rhinitis. SYN frigid (1).

**cold ab•scess 1.** an abscess without heat or other usual signs of inflammation; **2.** SYN tuberculous abscess.

**cold ag•glu•ti•na•tion** agglutination of red blood cells by their own serum (see autoagglutination), or by any other serum when the blood is cooled below body temperature; seen occasionally in the blood of normal persons or as a pathologic finding in mycoplasmal pneumonia, infectious mononucleosis, certain protozoan infections, or lymphoproliferative neoplasms. SEE autoagglutination.

**cold ag•glu•ti•nin** an antibody which reacts more efficiently at temperatures below 37°C.

**cold cure res•in, cold-cur•ing res•in** SYN autopolymer resin.

**cold di•u•re•sis** increased excretion of urine in a cold environment.

**cold knife con•i•za•tion** obtaining a cone of endocervical tissue with a cold knife blade so as to preserve histological characteristics and avoid desiccating tissue.

**cold nod•ule** a thyroid nodule with a much lower uptake of radioactive iodine than the surrounding parenchyma; about one in four prove to be malignant.

**cold-sen•si•tive en•zyme** an enzyme that loses its stability as the temperature is lowered.

**cold sore** colloquialism for herpes simplex.

**cold stage** the stage of chill in a malarial paroxysm.

**cold ther•a•py** SYN cryokinetics.

**cold ul•cer** a small, gangrenous ulcer on the extremities; due to defective circulation.

**cold ur•ti•ca•ria** hypersensitivity to cold leading to superficial vascular reaction manifested by transient itching, erythema, and hives. SEE ALSO hypothermia.

**col•ec•to•my** (kō-lek′tō-mē) excision of a segment or all of the colon. [G. *kolon*, colon, + *ektomē*, excision]

**co•li•bac•il•lo•sis** (kō′li-bas-i-lō′sis) diarrheal disease caused by the bacterium *Escherichia coli*. Often called enteric colibacillosis.

**col•ic** (kol′ik) **1.** relating to the colon. **2.** spasmodic pains in the abdomen. **3.** in young infants, paroxysms of gastrointestinal pain, with crying and irritability, due to a variety of causes, such as swallowing of air, emotional upset, or overfeeding. [G. *kōlikos*, relating to the colon]

**col•i•cin** (kol′i-sin) bacteriocin produced by strains of *Escherichia coli* and other enterobacteria. [*(Escherichia) coli* + bacteriocin]

**col•icky** (kol′i-kē) denoting or resembling the pain of colic.

**col•i•form ba•cil•li** (kō′li-fōrm bă-sil′ī) common name for *Escherichia coli* that is used as an indicator of fecal contamination of water, measured in terms of coliform count. Occasionally used to refer to all lactose-fermenting enteric bacteria.

**col•in•e•ar•i•ty** (kol′in-ē-ar′i-tē) **1.** lying in a straight line. **2.** the phenomonon that the orderings of the corresponding elements of DNA, the RNA transcribed from it, and the amino acid sequence translated from the RNA are identical. [L. *collineo*, to direct in a straight line]

**co•li•pase** (kō′lip-ās) a small protein in pancreatic

juice that is essential for the efficient action of pancreatic lipase. [co- + lipase]

**co·li·phage** (kol'i-fāj) a bacteriophage with an affinity for one or another strain of *Escherichia coli*. [*(Escherichia) coli* + bacteriophage]

**co·li·tis** (kō-lī'tis) inflammation of the colon. [G. *kōlon,* colon, + *-itis,* inflammation]

**col·la** (kol'ă) plural of collum.

**col·la·gen** (kol'lă-jen) the major protein of the white fibers of connective tissue, cartilage, and bone; insoluble in water but can be altered to easily digestible, soluble gelatins by boiling in water, dilute acids, or alkalies. SEE ALSO collagen fiber. SYN ossein, osseine, ostein, osteine. [G. *koila,* glue, + *-gen,* producing]

**col·la·gen·ase** (kol-ă'jĕ-nās) a proteolytic enzyme that acts on one or more of the collagens.

**col·la·gen dis·ease, col·la·gen-vas·cu·lar dis··ease** a group of generalized diseases affecting connective tissue and frequently characterized by fibrinoid necrosis or vasculitis; in some collagen diseases, auto-immunization, particularly antinuclear antibodies, has been shown and circulating immune complexes are found. The term is not entirely acceptable because there is no evidence that collagen is primarily involved; "collagen" was once synonymous with "connective tissue" rather than describing a specific fibrinous protein in that tissue. SEE ALSO connective-tissue disease.

**col·la·gen fi·ber, col·lag·e·nous fi·ber** an individual fiber that varies in diameter from less than 1 μm to about 12 μm and is composed of fibrils; the fibers, which are usually arranged in bundles, undergo some branching and are of indefinite length; chemically the fiber is a glycoprotein, collagen, which yields gelatin upon boiling; they make up the principal element of irregular connective tissue, tendons, aponeuroses, and most ligaments, and occur in the matrix of cartilage and osseous tissue. SYN white fiber (2).

**col·la·gen·ic** (kol-ă-jen'ik) SYN collagenous.

**col·la·gen im·plan·ta·tion** SYN collagen injection.

**col·la·gen in·jec·tion** correction of superficial soft tissue deformities, acne scars, or age-related skin changes by injection (implantation) of collagen; bovine collagen preparations are commonly used. Prior intradermal testing is necessary to exclude hypersensitivity. SYN collagen implantation.

**col·lag·e·ni·za·tion** (ko-laj'ĕ-ni-zā'shŭn) **1.** replacement of tissues or fibrin by collagen. **2.** synthesis of collagen by fibroblasts.

**col·lag·e·no·lyt·ic** (ko-laj'ĕ-nō-lit'ik) causing the lysis of collagen, gelatin, and other proteins containing proline. [collagen + G. *lysis,* dissolving]

**col·lag·e·nous** (ko-laj'ĕ-nŭs) producing or containing collagen. SYN collagenic.

**col·lag·e·nous co·li·tis** colitis occurring mostly in middle-aged women and characterized by persistent watery diarrhea and a deposit of a band of collagen beneath the basement membrane of colon surface epithelium.

**col·lapse** (kō-laps') **1.** a condition of extreme prostration. **2.** a state of profound physical depression. **3.** a falling together of the walls of a structure or the failure of a physiological system. [L. *col-labor,* pp. *-lapsus,* to fall together]

**col·lar bone** SYN clavicle.

**col·lar-but·ton ab·scess** an abscess consisting of two cavities connected by a narrow channel,

usually formed by rupture of an abscess through an overlying fascia. SYN shirt-stud abscess.

**col·lat·er·al** (ko-lat'er-ăl) **1.** indirect, subsidiary, or accessory to the main thing; side by side. **2.** a side branch of a nerve axon or blood vessel.

**col·lat·er·al ar·tery 1.** one that runs parallel with a nerve or other structure; **2.** one through which a collateral circulation is established.

**col·lat·er·al cir·cu·la·tion** circulation maintained in small anastomosing vessels when the main vessel is obstructed.

**col·lat·er·al hy·per·e·mia** increased blood flow through abundant collateral channels when the circulation through the main artery to a part is arrested.

**col·lat·er·al in·her·i·tance** the appearance of characters in collateral members of a family group, as when an uncle and a niece show the same character inherited from a common ancestor.

**col·lat·er·al sul·cus** a long, deep sagittal fissure on the undersurface of the temporal lobe, marking the border between the fusiform gyrus laterally and the hippocampal and lingual gyri medially; the great depth of the collateral sulcus results in a bulging of the floor of the occipital and temporal horn of the lateral ventricle, the collateral eminence.

**col·lat·er·al ves·sel 1.** a branch of an artery running parallel with the parent trunk; **2.** a vessel that runs in parallel with another vessel, nerve, or other long structure.

**col·lec·tive un·con·scious** JUNGIAN PSYCHOLOGY the combined engrams or memory potentials inherited from an individual's phylogenetic past.

**Col·les frac·ture** (kol'ēz) a fracture of the distal radius with displacement and/or angulation of the distal fragment dorsally.

**col·lic·u·lar ar·te·ry** *origin:* precommunicating part (P1 segment) of posterior cerebral artery; *distribution:* to superior and inferior colliculi (corpora quadrigemina) of tectum of midbrain. SYN arteria quadrigeminalis.

**col·lic·u·lec·to·my** (ko-lik-yu-lek'tō-mē) excision of the colliculus seminalis.

**col·lic·u·li·tis** (ko-lik-yu-lī'tis) inflammation of the urethra in the region of the colliculus seminalis.

**col·lic·u·lus,** pl. **col·lic·u·li** (ko-lik'yu-lŭs, ko-lik-yu-lī) a small elevation above the surrounding parts. [L. mound, dim. of *collis,* hill]

**Col·lier sign** (kol'yer) unilateral or bilateral lid retraction due to midbrain lesion; occurring at any age. SEE setting sun sign, Epstein sign.

**col·lier's lung** SYN anthracosis.

**col·li·ma·tion** (kol-i-mā'shŭn) the process, in x-ray, of restricting and confining the x-ray beam to a given area and, in nuclear medicine, of restricting the detection of emitted radiations from a given area of interest. [L. *collineo,* to direct in a straight line]

**col·li·qua·tion** (kol-i-kwā'shŭn) **1.** excessive discharge of fluid. **2.** liquefaction in the process of necrosis. [L. *col-,* together, + *liquo,* pp. *liquatus,* to cause to melt]

**col·liq·ua·tive** (ko-lik'wă-tiv) denoting or characteristic of colliquation.

**Col·lis-Bel·sey fun·do·pli·ca·tion** (kol'is-bel' sē) SYN Collis-Nissen fundoplication.

**Col·lis-Nis·sen fun·do·pli·ca·tion** (kol'is-nis' en) operation for fundoplication in the presence of a shortened esophagus; the esophagus is lengthened by tubular stapling of the gastric cardia, and the fundoplication is then performed around this neo-esophagus. SYN Collis-Belsey fundoplication.

**col•loid** (kol′oyd) **1.** aggregates of atoms or molecules in a finely divided state (submicroscopic), dispersed in a gaseous, liquid, or solid medium, and resisting sedimentation, diffusion, and filtration, thus differing from precipitates. SEE ALSO hydrocolloid. **2.** gluelike. **3.** a translucent, yellowish, homogeneous material of the consistency of glue, less fluid than mucoid or mucinoid, found in the cells and tissues in a state of colloid degeneration. SYN colloidin. **4.** the stored secretion within follicles of the thyroid gland. [G. *kolla,* glue, + *eidos,* appearance]

**col•loid ac•ne** SYN colloid milium.

**col•loi•dal** (ko-loyd′ăl) denoting or characteristic of a colloid.

**col•loi•dal gel** a colloid that has developed resistance to flow because of chemical or thermal change.

**col•loi•dal so•lu•tion** a dispersoid, emulsoid, or suspensoid.

**col•loid bath** a bath prepared by adding soothing agents such as sodium bicarbonate or oatmeal to the bath water to relieve skin irritation and pruritus.

**col•loid car•ci•no•ma** SYN mucinous carcinoma.

**col•loid de•gen•er•a•tion** a degeneration similar to mucoid degeneration, in which the material is inspissated.

**col•loid goi•ter** a form of goiter in which the contents of the follicles increase greatly, causing pressure atrophy of the epithelium so that the gelatinous matter predominates in the tumor.

**col•loi•din** (ko-loy′din) SYN colloid (3).

**col•loid milium** (kol′loyd mil′ē-ŭm) yellow papules developing in sun-damaged skin of the head and backs of the hands, composed of colloid material in the dermis resembling amyloid but with a different ultrastructure. SYN colloid acne, colloid pseudomilium. [L. *milium,* millet]

**col•loid pseu•do•mil•i•um** SYN colloid milium.

**col•lum,** pl. **col•la** (kol′ŭm, kol′ă) SYN neck. [L.]

**col•lum pan•cre•at•i•cus** [TA] SYN neck of pancreas.

**col•lyr•i•um** (ko-lir′ē-ŭm) originally, any preparation for the eye; now, an eyewash. [G. *kollyrion,* poultice, eye salve]

△**col•o-** the colon. [G. *kolon*]

▤**col•o•bo•ma** (kol-ō-bō′mă) any defect, congenital, pathologic, or artificial, especially of the eye due to incomplete closure of the optic fissure. See page B15. [G. *kolobōma,* lit., the part taken away in mutilation, fr. *koloboō,* to dock, mutilate]

**col•o•bo•mat•ous mi•croph•thal•mia** a congenital defect occurring along an embryonic fissure in a small eye, sometimes associated with cysts.

**co•lo•cen•te•sis** (kō′lō-sen-tē′sis) puncture of the colon with a trochar or scalpel to relieve distention. SYN colopuncture. [colo- + G. *kentēsis,* a puncture]

**co•lo•cho•le•cys•tos•to•my** (kō′lō-kō-lē-sis-tos′tō-mē) SYN cholecystocolostomy.

**co•lo•co•los•to•my** (kō′lō-kō-los′tō-mē) establishment of a communication between two non-

continuous segments of the colon. [colo- + colo- + G. *stoma,* mouth]

**co•lo•en•ter•i•tis** (kō′lō-en-ter-ī′tis) SYN enterocolitis.

**co•lon** (kō′lon) the division of the large intestine extending from the cecum to the rectum. [G. *kolon*]

**co•lon•ic** (ko-lon′ik) relating to the colon.

**co•lon•op•a•thy, co•lop•a•thy** (kō-lŏ-nop′ă-thē, kō-lop′ă-thē) rarely used term for any disordered condition of the colon.

▤**co•lon•o•scope** (kō-lon′ō-skōp) an elongated endoscope, usually fiberoptic. See this page and B9.

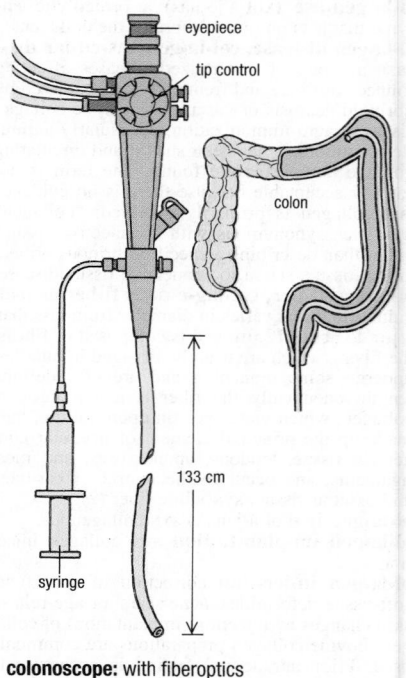

**colonoscope:** with fiberoptics

▤**co•lon•os•co•py, co•los•co•py** (kō-lon-os′kŏ-pē, kō-los′kŏ-pē) visual examination of the inner surface of the colon by means of a colonoscope. See this page and B9. [colon + G. *skopeō,* to view]

**co•lon sig•moid•e•um** [TA] SYN sigmoid colon.

**col•o•ny** (kol′ŏ-nē) **1.** a group of cells growing on a solid nutrient surface, each arising from the multiplication of an individual cell; a clone. **2.** a group of people with similar interests, living in a particular location or area. [L. *colonia,* a colony]

**col•o•ny-form•ing u•nit (CFU)** a stem cell in culture capable of proliferating and differentiating into more mature cells. If the CFU is committed to a specific cell line it is designated by an additional letter to indicate its commitment; e.g., CFU-E is committed to erythroid maturation; CFU-GM is committed to granulocyte/monocyte maturation.

**col•o•ny-stim•u•lat•ing fac•tors (CSF)** a group

of glycoprotein growth factors regulating differentiation in myeloid cell lines.

**col•o•pexy** (kol′ō-pek-sē) attachment of a portion of the colon to the abdominal wall. [colo- + G. *pēxis,* fixation]

**co•lo•pli•ca•tion** (kō′lō-pli-kā′shŭn) reduction of the lumen of a dilated colon by making folds or tucks in its walls. [colo- + Mod. L. *plica,* fold]

**co•lo•proc•ti•tis** (kō′lō-prok-tī′tis) inflammation of both colon and rectum. SYN colorectitis. [colo- + G. *prōktos,* anus (rectum), + *-itis,* inflammation]

**co•lo•proc•tos•to•my** (kō′lō-prok-tos′tō-mē) establishment of a communication between the rectum and a discontinuous segment of the colon. SYN colorectostomy. [colo- + G. *prōktos,* anus (rectum), + *stoma,* mouth]

**co•lop•to•sis, co•lop•to•sia** (kō-lop-tō′sis, kō-lop-tō′sē-ă) downward displacement, or prolapse, of the colon, especially of the transverse portion. [colo- + G. *ptōsis,* a falling]

**co•lo•punc•ture** (kō-lō-pŭnk′cher) SYN colocentesis.

**col•or** (kŭl′ŏr) **1.** that aspect of the appearance of objects and light sources that may be specified as to hue, lightness (brightness), and saturation. **2.** that portion of the visible (370-760 nm) electromagnetic spectrum specified as to wavelength, luminosity, and purity. [L.]

**Col•o•ra•do tick fe•ver** an infection caused by Colorado tick fever virus and transmitted to humans by *Dermacentor andersoni;* the symptoms are mild, there is no rash, fever is not excessive, and the disease is rarely fatal. SYN tick fever (5).

**Col•o•ra•do tick fe•ver vi•rus** a virus of the genus *Orbivirus,* found in the Rocky Mountain region of the United States and transmitted by the tick, *Dermacentor andersoni;* it causes Colorado tick fever.

**col•or ag•no•sia** inability to name or identify colors; caused by lesions of the dominant occipital and temporal lobes.

**col•or blind•ness** misleading term for anomalous or deficient color vision; complete color blindness is the absence of one of the primary cone pigments of the retina. SEE protanopia, deuteranopia, tritanopia.

**col•or chart** an assembly of chromatic samples used in checking color vision. SYN chromatic chart.

**co•lo•rec•tal** (kol′ō-rek′tăl) relating to the colon and rectum, or to the entire large bowel.

**co•lo•rec•ti•tis** (kō′lō-rek-tī′tis) SYN coloproctitis.

**co•lo•rec•tos•to•my** (kō′lō-rek-tos′tō-mē) SYN coloproctostomy.

**col•ored vi•sion (VC)** SYN chromatopsia.

**col•or hear•ing** a subjective perception of color produced by certain sounds. SYN pseudochromesthesia (2).

**col•or•im•e•ter** (kŏl-er-im′ĕ-ter) an optic device for determining the color and/or intensity of the color of a liquid.

**col•or•i•met•ric** (kŭl′ŏr-i-met′rik) relating to colorimetry.

**col•or•im•e•try** (kŭl′ŏr-im′ĕ-trē) a procedure for quantitative chemical analysis, based on comparison of the color developed in a solution of the test material with that in a standard solution; the two solutions are observed simultaneously in a colorimeter, and quantitated on the basis of the absorption of light.

**co•lor•rha•gia** (kō-lō-rā′jē-ă) an abnormal discharge from the colon. [colo- + G. *rhēgnymi,* to burst forth]

**co•lor•rha•phy** (kō-lōr′ă-fē) suture of the colon. [colo- + G. *rhaphē,* suture]

**col•or sco•to•ma** an area of depressed color vision in the visual field.

**col•or taste** a form of synesthesia in which the color sense and taste are associated, with stimulation of either sense inducing a subjective sensation in the associated sense. SYN pseudogeusesthesia.

**co•lo•sig•moi•dos•to•my** (kō′lō-sig-moy-dos′tō-mē) establishment of an anastomosis between any other part of the colon and the sigmoid colon.

**co•los•to•my** (kō-los′tō-mē) establishment of an artificial cutaneous opening into the colon. See this page. [colo- + G. *stoma,* mouth]

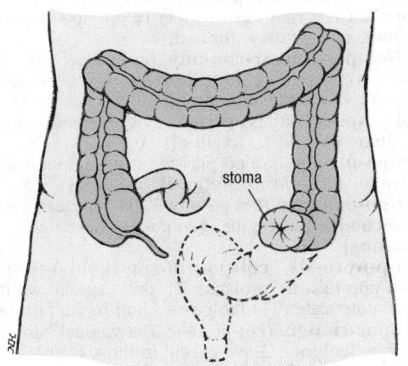

**colostomy:** stoma opens on anterior abdominal wall

**co•los•to•my bag** a bag worn over an artificial anus to collect feces.

**co•los•tric** (kō-los′trik) relating to the colostrum.

**co•los•tror•rhea** (kō-los-trōr-rē′ă) abnormally profuse secretion of colostrum. [colostrum, + G. *rhoia,* flow]

**co•los•trum** (kō-los′trŭm) a thin white opalescent fluid, the first milk secreted at the termination of pregnancy; it differs from the milk secreted later by containing more lactalbumin and lactoprotein; colostrum is also rich in antibodies which confer passive immunity to the newborn. SYN foremilk. [L.]

**co•lot•o•my** (kō-lot′ō-mē) incision into the colon. [colo- + G. *tomē,* incision]

**col•our•im•e•ter [Br.]** SEE colorimeter.

**col•our•im•e•try [Br.]** SEE colorimetry.

**Col•our In•dex (CI)** a publication concerned with the chemistry of dyes, with each listed dye identified by a five-digit Colour Index number, e.g., methylene blue is Colour Index 52015.

**col•pa•tre•sia** (kol-pa-trē′zē-ă) SYN vaginal atresia. [colp- + G. *atrētos,* imperforate]

**col•pec•ta•sis, col•pec•ta•sia** (kol-pek′tă-sis, kol-pek-tā′si-ă) distention of the vagina. [colp- + G. *aktasis,* stretching]

**col•pec•to•my** (kol-pek′tō-mē) SYN vaginectomy. [colp- + G. *ektomē,* excision]

△**colpo-, colp-** the vagina. SEE ALSO vagino-. [G. *kolpos*, fold or hollow]

**col·po·cele** (kol'pō-sēl) **1.** a hernia projecting into the vagina. SYN vaginocele. **2.** SYN colpoptosis. [colpo- + G. *kēlē,* hernia]

**col·po·clei·sis** (kol-pō-klī'sis) operation for obliterating the lumen of the vagina. [colpo- + G. *kleisis,* closure]

**col·po·cys·to·cele** (kol-pō-sis'tō-sēl) SYN cystocele. [colpo- + G. *kystis,* bladder, + *kēlē,* hernia]

**col·po·cys·to·plas·ty** (kol-pō-sis'tō-plas-tē) plastic surgery to repair the vesicovaginal wall. [colpo- + G. *kystis,* bladder, + *plastos,* formed]

**col·po·dyn·ia** (kol-pō-din'ē-ă) SYN vaginodynia. [colpo- + G. *odynē,* pain]

**col·po·mi·cros·co·py** (kol'pō-mī-kros'kŏ-pē) direct observation and study of cells in the vagina and cervix magnified *in vivo,* in the undisturbed tissue, by means of a colpomicroscope.

**col·po·per·i·ne·o·plas·ty** (kol'pō-pār-i-nē'ō-plas-tē) SYN vaginoperineoplasty. [colpo- + perineum, + G. *plastos,* formed]

**col·po·per·i·ne·or·rha·phy** (kol'pō-per-i-nē-ōr'ă-fē) SYN vaginoperineorrhaphy. [colpo- + perineum, + G. *rhaphē,* sewing]

**col·po·pexy** (kol'pō-pek-sē) SYN vaginofixation. [colpo- + G. *pēxis,* fixation]

**col·po·plas·ty** (kol'pō-plas-tē) SYN vaginoplasty. [colpo- + G. *plastos,* formed]

**col·po·poi·e·sis** (kol'pō-poy-ē'sis) surgical construction of a vagina. [colpo- + G. *poiēsis,* a making]

**col·po·pto·sis, col·po·pto·sia** (kol-pō-tō'sis, kol-pōp-tō'si-ă) prolapse of the vaginal walls. SYN colpocele (2). [colpo- + G. *ptōsis,* a falling]

**col·por·rha·gia** (kol-pō-rā'jē-ă) a vaginal hemorrhage. [colpo-+ G. *rhēgnymi,* to burst forth]

**col·por·rha·phy** (kol-pōr'ă-fē) repair of a rupture of the vagina by excision and suturing of the edges of the tear. [colpo- + G. *rhaphē,* suture]

**col·por·rhex·is** (kol-pō-rek'sis) tearing of the vaginal wall. [colpo- + G. *rhēxis,* rupture]

**col·po·scope** (kol'pō-skōp) endoscopic instrument that magnifies cells of the vagina and cervix *in vivo* to allow direct observation and study of these tissues.

**col·pos·co·py** (kol-pos'kŏ-pē) examination of vagina and cervix by means of an endoscope. [colpo- + G. *skopeō,* to view]

**col·po·spasm** (kol'pō-spazm) spasmodic contraction of the vagina.

**col·po·ste·no·sis** (kol'pō-sten-ō'sis) narrowing of the lumen of the vagina. [colpo- + G. *stenōsis,* narrowing]

**col·po·ste·not·o·my** (kol'pō-sten-ot'ō-mē) surgical correction of a colpostenosis. [colpo- + G. *stenōsis,* narrowing, + *tomē,* incision]

**col·po·sus·pen·sion** (kol'pō-sus-pen'shŭn) suture fixation of the lateral vaginal fornix to Cooper ligament on each side, as a modification and enhancement of the standard Marshall-Marchetti-Kranz urethrovesical suspension for stress urinary incontinence due to cystocele. [colpo- + suspension]

**col·pot·o·my** (kol-pot'ō-mē) SYN vaginotomy. [colpo- + G. *tomē,* incision]

**col·po·xe·ro·sis** (kol-pō-zē-rō'sis) abnormal dryness of the vaginal mucous membrane. [colpo- + G. *xērōsis,* dryness]

**Col·ti·vi·rus** (kol'tē-vī-rus) a genus in the family Reoviridae that causes Colorado tick fever. [*Colorado tick* fever + virus]

**col·u·mel·la,** pl. **col·u·mel·lae** (kol-oo-mel'ă, kol-oo-mel'ē) **1.** a small column. SYN columnella. **2.** in fungi, a sterile invagination of a sporangium, as in Zygomycetes. [L. dim. of *columna,* column]

**col·umn** (kol'ŭm) **1.** an anatomic part or structure in the form of a pillar or cylindric funiculus. SEE ALSO fascicle. **2.** a vertical object (usually cylindrical), mass, or formation. SYN columna [TA]. [L. *columna*]

**co·lum·na,** gen. and pl. **co·lum·nae** (ko-lŭm'nă, ko-lŭm'nē) [TA] SYN column. [L.]

**co·lum·nae an·a·les** [TA] SYN anal columns.

**co·lum·nae gri·se·ae** [TA] SYN gray columns.

**co·lum·nae re·na·les** [TA] SYN renal columns.

**co·lum·nar ep·i·the·li·um** epithelium formed of a single layer of prismatic cells taller than they are wide.

**co·lum·na ver·te·bra·lis** [TA] SYN vertebral column.

**col·umn chro·ma·tog·ra·phy** a form of partition, adsorption, ion exchange, or affinity chromatography in which one phase is liquid (aqueous) flowing down a column packed with the second phase, a solid.

**co·lum·nel·la,** pl. **col·um·nel·lae** (ko-lŭm-nel'ă, ko-lŭm'nel'ē) SYN columella (1). [L. dim. of *columna,* a column; another form of *columella*]

**col·umn of for·nix** that part of the fornix that curves down in front of the thalamus and the interventricular foramen of Monro, then continues through the hypothalamus to the mammillary body; consisting primarily of fibers originating in the hippocampus and subiculum, the column of fornix is the direct continuation of the body of the fornix.

△**com-** SEE con-.

**co·ma** (kō'mă) **1.** a state of profound unconsciousness from which one cannot be roused; may be due to the action of an ingested toxic substance or of one formed in the body, to trauma, or to disease. [G. *kōma,* deep sleep, trance] **2.** an aberration of spherical lenses; occurring in cases of oblique incidence (e.g., the image of a point becomes comet-shaped). [G. *kome,* hair] **3.** SYN coma aberration.

**co·ma ab·er·ra·tion** the distortion of image formation created when a bundle of light rays enters an optical system not parallel to the optic axis. SYN coma (3). [G. *kome,* hair, foliage]

**co·ma scale** a clinical scale to assess impaired consciousness; assessment may include motor responsiveness, verbal performance, and eye opening, as in the Glasgow (Scotland) coma scale, or the same three items and dysfunction of cranial nerves, as in the Maryland (U.S.) coma scale.

**co·ma·tose** (kō'mă-tōs) in a state of coma.

**com·bined glau·co·ma** glaucoma with angle-closure and open-angle mechanisms in the same eye.

**com·bined im·mu·no·de·fi·cien·cy** immunodeficiency of both the B-lymphocytes and T-lymphocytes.

**com·bined meth·ods** varying combinations of the oral auditory method and the manual visual method of education of deaf children. SEE ALSO oral auditory method, manual visual method, total communication.

**com·bined preg·nan·cy** coexisting uterine and ectopic pregnancy.

**com·bined ver·sion** bipolar version by means of one hand in the vagina, the other on the abdominal wall.

**com·bus·ti·ble** (kom-bus'ti-bl) capable of combustion.

**com·bus·tion** (kom-bŭs'chŭn) burning, the rapid oxidation of any substance accompanied by the production of heat and light. [L. *comburo*, pp. *-bustus*, to burn up]

**Com·by sign** (kom'bē) an early sign of measles, consisting of thin, whitish patches on the gums and buccal mucous membrane, formed of desquamating epithelial cells.

**com·e·do**, pl. **com·e·dos**, **com·e·do·nes** (kom'ē-dō, kom'ē-dōz, kom-ē-dō'nēz) a dilated hair follicle infundibulum filled with keratin squamae, bacteria, particularly *Propionibacterium acnes*, and sebum; the primary lesion of acne vulgaris. [L. a glutton, fr. *com-edo*, to eat up]

**com·e·do·car·ci·no·ma** (ko-m'ē-dō-kar-si-nō'mă) form of carcinoma of the breast or other organ in which plugs of necrotic malignant cells may be expressed from the ducts.

**com·e·do·gen·ic** (kom'ē-dō-jen'ik) tending to promote the formation of comedones. [comedo + G. *genesis*, production]

**co·mes**, pl. **com·i·tes** (kō'mēz, kom'i-tēz) a blood vessel accompanying another vessel or a nerve; the veins accompanying an artery, often two in number, are called venae comitantes or venae comites. [L. a companion, fr. *com-*, together, + *eo*, pp. *itus*, to go]

**com·fort zone** the temperature range between 28°C and 30°C at which the naked body is able to maintain the heat balance without either shivering or sweating; in the clothed body the range is from 13°C to 21°C.

**com·i·tant ar·te·ry of me·di·an nerve** SYN median artery.

**com·i·tant stra·bis·mus** a condition in which the degree of strabismus is the same in all directions of gaze.

**com·ma ba·cil·lus** SYN *Vibrio cholerae.*

**com·mand hal·lu·ci·na·tion** a symptom, usually auditory but sometimes visual, consisting of a message, from no external source, to do something.

**com·man·do pro·ce·dure** an operation for malignant tumors of the floor of the oral cavity, involving resection of portions of the mandible in continuity with the oral lesion and radical neck dissection.

**com·men·sal** (kŏ-men'săl) **1.** pertaining to or characterized by commensalism. **2.** an organism participating in commensalism.

**com·men·sal·ism** (kŏ-men'săl-izm) a symbiotic relationship in which one species derives benefit and the other is unharmed. Cf. metabiosis, mutualism, parasitism. [L. *con-*, with, together, + *mensa*, table]

**com·mi·nut·ed** (kom'i-noo-ted) broken into several pieces; denoting especially a fractured bone. [L. *com-minuo*, pp. *-minutus*, to make smaller, break into pieces, fr. *minor*, less]

**com·mi·nut·ed frac·ture** a fracture in which the bone is broken into pieces.

**com·mi·nu·tion** (kom-i-noo'shŭn) a breaking into several pieces.

**com·mis·su·ra**, gen. and pl. **com·mis·su·rae**

(kom-i-syur'ă, kom-is-yur'ē) [TA] SYN commissure. [L. a joining together, seam, fr. *com- mitto*, to send together, combine]

**com·mis·su·rae su·pra·op·ti·cae** [TA] the commissural fibers that lie above and behind the optic chiasm. SYN supraoptic commissures.

**com·mis·sur·al** (kom-i-syur'ăl) relating to a commissure.

**com·mis·sur·al fi·bers** nerve fibers crossing the midline and connecting two corresponding parts or regions of the nervous system.

**com·mis·sur·a pos·te·ri·or ce·re·bri** [TA] SYN posterior cerebral commissure.

**com·mis·sure** (kom'i-syur) **1.** angle or corner of the eye, lips, or labia. **2.** a bundle of nerve fibers passing from one side to the other in the brain or spinal cord. SYN commissura [TA].

**com·mis·sur·ot·o·my** (kom'i-syur-ot'ō-mē) **1.** surgical division of any commissure, fibrous band, or ring via surgery or a balloon catheter technique. **2.** SYN midline myelotomy.

**com·mon an·ti·gen** cross-reacting antigen (epitope), a common antigen that occurs in two or more different molecules or organisms. SYN heterogenic enterobacterial antigen.

**com·mon ba·sal vein** the tributary to the inferior pulmonary vein (right and left) that receives blood from the superior and inferior basal veins.

**com·mon bile duct** a duct formed by the union of the hepatic and cystic ducts; it discharges at the duodenal papilla.

**com·mon coch·le·ar ar·te·ry** *origin:* as a terminal branch, with the anterior vestibular artery, of the labyrinthine artery; *distribution:* runs in the cochlear axis of modiolus serving the spiral ganglia; sends the proper cochlear artery to the cochlear duct and supplies the apical two turns of the spiral modiolar artery. SYN arteria cochlearis communis [TA].

**com·mon fa·cial vein** a short vessel formed by the union of the facial vein and the retromandibular vein, emptying into the jugular vein; considered to be a continuation of the facial vein in the NA.

**com·mon he·pa·tic duct** the part of the biliary duct system that is formed by the confluence of right and left hepatic ducts. At the porta hepatis it is joined by the cystic duct to become the bile duct (common bile duct).

**com·mon mi·graine** a form of migraine headache without the visual prodrome, that is not limited on one side of the head but nevertheless is recognizable as migraine because of the stereotyped course; the tendency to nausea, photophobia, and phonophobia; and the relief produced by sleep.

**com·mon path·way of co·ag·u·la·tion** a part of the coagulation system where the intrinsic and extrinsic pathways converge to activate factor X. Coagulation factors X, V, II, and fibrinogen are part of this pathway. Both the APTT and PT test the integrity of this system.

**com·mon ten·di·nous ring of extraocular muscles** a fibrous ring that surrounds the optic canal and the medial part of the superior orbital fissure; it gives origin to the four rectus muscles of the eye and is partially fused with the sheath of the optic nerve. SYN anulus of Zinn.

**com·mu·ni·ca·ble** (kŏ-myun'i-kă-bl) capable of being communicated or transmitted; said especially of disease.

C
O

**com·mu·ni·ca·ble dis·ease** any disease that is transmissible by infection or contagion directly or through the agency of a vector.

**com·mu·ni·cat·ing ar·tery** an artery that connects two larger arteries.

**com·mu·ni·cat·ing branch** a bundle of nerve fibers passing from one named nerve to join another.

**com·mu·ni·ca·ting branch of fib·u·lar ar·te·ry** the communicating branch of the fibular (peroneal) artery.

**com·mu·ni·cat·ing branch of in·ter·nal lar·yn·ge·al nerve with re·cur·rent lar·yn·ge·al nerve** branch of internal branch of superior laryngeal nerve communicating with the recurrent laryngeal nerve in the wall of the laryngopharynx supplying sensory fibers to the latter.

**com·mu·ni·cat·ing hy·dro·ceph·a·lus** type of hydrocephalus in which there is an abnormality in cerebrospinal fluid absorption; there is no obstruction to cerebrospinal fluid flow in the ventricular system or where the cerebrospinal fluid passes into the spinal canal.

**com·mu·ni·ca·tion** (kŏ-myu-ni-kā′shŭn) **1.** an opening or connecting passage between two structures. **2.** ANATOMY a joining or connecting; said of fibrous, solid structures, e.g., tendons and nerves. **3.** the exchange of information between individuals using symbol systems such as spoken language or writing but also including elements such as icons, gestures, tone of voice, and facial expression. [L. *communicatio*]

**com·mu·ni·ca·tion board** any arrangement of letters, words, symbols, or pictures designed to aid an individual whose expressive language ability is inadequate. SEE augmentative and alternative communication. SYN conversation board, language board.

**com·mu·ni·ca·tion dis·or·der** any impairment of hearing, language, or speech that interferes with the ability to transmit or receive linguistic information. SYN communicative disorder.

**com·mu·ni·ca·tive dis·or·der** SYN communication disorder.

**com·mu·ni·ty** (kŏ-myu′ni-tē) a group of persons united by some common feature or shared interest; the social context in which professional services are provided. A community may be united by physical or geographic factors, on one or more common characteristics such as age, gender, developmental level, culture, or health/disability status, or on a shared perspective. SEE ALSO community-based practice. [L. *communitas,* fellowship, fr. *communis,* common]

**com·mu·ni·ty-based prac·tice** delivery of skilled services by a health practitioner with emphasis on the perspectives and methods of a specific profession. Typically this type of practice is initiated by the medical profession and relies on referrals from other professionals.

**com·mu·ni·ty-built prac·tice** delivery of skilled services by a health practitioner with emphasis on wellness and on the strengths and capacities of the client. Typically such a practice provides expert knowledge that is not otherwise available to the client and ends when the needs calling it into existence have been met.

**com·mu·ni·ty men·tal health cen·ter** a mental health treatment center located in a neighborhood catchment area close to the homes of patients, introduced in the 1960s via new federal legisla-

tion designed to replace the large state hospitals, which usually were located in remote rural areas; features include offering a series of comprehensive services by one or more members of the four mental health professions, provision of continuity of care, participation of consumers in the centers, community location to provide accessibility, a combination of indirect or preventive and direct services, the use of program-centered as well as case-centered consultation, a requirement for program evaluation, and various linkages to a variety of health and human services.

**Com·mu·ni·ty Pe·ri·o·don·tal In·dex of Treat·ment Needs (CPITN)** an assessment of periodontal treatment needs that divides the mouth into sextants and uses a standard probe for the examinations.

**com·mu·ni·ty psy·chi·a·try** psychiatry focusing on the detection, prevention, early treatment, and rehabilitation of individuals with emotional disorders and social deviance as they develop in the community.

**com·mu·ni·ty psy·chol·o·gy** the application of psychology to community programs, e.g., in the schools, correctional and welfare systems, and community mental health centers.

**Co·mol·li sign** (kom-ōl′ē) in cases of fracture of the scapula, a typical triangular cushion-like swelling appears, corresponding to the outline of the scapula.

**co·mor·bid·i·ty** (kō-mōr-bid′i-tē) a concomitant but unrelated pathologic or disease process; usually used in epidemiology to indicate the coexistence of two or more disease processes. [co- + L. *morbidus,* diseased]

**com·pact bone** the compact, noncancellous portion of bone that consists largely of concentric lamellar osteons and interstitial lamellae. SYN substantia compacta [TA], compact substance.

**com·pact sub·stance** SYN compact bone.

**com·par·a·tive a·nat·o·my** the comparative study of animal structure with regard to homologous organs or parts.

**com·par·a·tive pa·thol·o·gy** the pathology of diseases of animals, especially in relation to human pathology.

**com·par·ti·men·tum** [TA] SYN compartment.

**com·part·ment 1.** partitioned off portion of a larger bound space; a separate section or chamber; the compartments of the limbs are bound deeply by bones and intermuscular septa and superficially by deep fascia and generally are not in communication with the other compartments, and thus infection or increased pathologic pressure may be limited to a compartment; muscles contained within the compartments of the limbs share similar functions and innervation. **2.** a separate division; specifically, a structural or biochemical portion of a cell that is separated from the rest of the cell. SYN compartimentum [TA].

**com·part·ment syn·drome** condition in which increased intramuscular pressure in a confined anatomical space brought on by overactivity or trauma impedes blood flow and function of tissues within that space. SYN compression syndrome (2).

**com·pen·sat·ed ac·i·do·sis** an acidosis in which the pH of body fluids is normal; compensation is achieved by respiratory or renal mechanisms.

**com·pen·sat·ed al·ka·lo·sis** alkalosis in which there is a change in bicarbonate but the pH of body fluids approaches normal; respiratory alkalosis may be compensated by increased production of metabolic acids or increased renal excretion of bicarbonate; metabolic alkalosis is rarely compensated by hypoventilation.

**com·pen·sat·ing curve** the curve of Spee applied to dentures. SEE ALSO curve of Spee.

**com·pen·sa·tion** (kom-pen-sā′shŭn) **1.** a process in which a tendency for a change in a given direction is counteracted by another change so that the original change is not evident. **2.** an unconscious mechanism by which one tries to make up for fancied or real deficiencies. [L. *com-penso,* pp. *-atus,* to weigh together, counterbalance]

**com·pen·sa·tion neu·ro·sis** the development of symptoms of neurosis believed to be motivated by the desire for, and hope of, monetary or interpersonal gain.

**com·pen·sa·to·ry** (kom-pen′să-tōr-ē) providing compensation; making up for a deficiency or loss.

**com·pen·sa·to·ry cir·cu·la·tion** circulation established in dilated collateral vessels when the main vessel of the part is obstructed.

**com·pen·sa·to·ry hy·per·tro·phy** increase in size of an organ or part of an organ or tissue, when called upon to do additional work or perform the work of destroyed tissue or of a paired organ.

**com·pen·sa·to·ry move·ment** movement used habitually to achieve functional motor skills when a normal movement pattern has not been established or is unavailable, e.g., hyperextension of the neck. It is influenced by abnormal postural tone, reflexes, or movement.

**com·pen·sa·to·ry pause** the pause following an extrasystole, when the pause is long enough to compensate for the prematurity of the extrasystole; the short cycle ending with the extrasystole plus the pause following the extrasystole together equal two of the regular cycles.

**com·pen·sa·to·ry pol·y·cy·the·mia** a secondary polycythemia resulting from anoxia, e.g., in congenital heart disease, pulmonary emphysema, or prolonged residence at a high altitude.

**com·pe·tence** (kom′pĕ-tens) **1.** the quality of being competent or capable of performing an allotted function. **2.** the normal tight closure of a cardiac valve. **3.** the ability of a group of embryonic cells to respond to an inducer. **4.** the ability of a (bacterial) cell to take up free DNA, which may lead to transformation. **5.** in psychiatry, the mental ability to distinguish right from wrong and to manage one's own affairs, or to assist one's counsel in a legal proceeding. **6.** the state of reactivity of a cell, tissue, or organism that allows it to respond to certain stimuli. [Fr. *competence,* fr. L.L. *competentia,* congruity]

**com·pe·tence test·ing** SYN skills validation.

**com·pet·i·tive bind·ing as·say** an assay in which a binder competes for labeled versus unlabeled ligand; following separation of free and bound ligand, the ligand is quantitated by relating bound and unbound ratios to known standards. SEE ALSO enzyme-linked immunosorbent assay, immunoassay, enzyme-multiplied immunoassay technique, radioimmunoassay.

**com·pet·i·tive in·hi·bi·tion** blocking of the action of an enzyme by a compound that binds to the free enzyme, preventing the substrate from

binding and thus prevents the enzyme from acting on that substrate. SYN selective inhibition.

**com·plaint** (kom-plānt′) a disorder, disease, or symptom, or the description of it. [O. Fr. *complainte,* fr. L. *complango,* to lament]

**com·ple·ment** (kom′plĕ-ment) Ehrlich's term for the thermolabile substance, normally present in serum, that is destructive to certain bacteria and other cells sensitized by a specific complement-fixing antibody. Complement is a group of at least 20 distinct serum proteins, the activity of which is affected by a series of interactions resulting in enzymatic cleavages and which can follow one or the other of at least two pathways. In the case of immune hemolysis (classical pathway), the complex comprises nine components (designated C1 through C9) that react in a definite sequence and the activation of which is usually effected by the antigen-antibody complex; only the first seven components are involved in chemotaxis, and only the first four are involved in immune adherence or phagocytosis or are fixed by conglutinins. An alternative pathway (see properdin system) may be activated by factors other than antigen-antibody complexes and involves components other than C1, C4, and C2 in the activation of C3. SEE ALSO component of complement. [L. *complementum,* that which completes, fr. *com-pleo,* to fill up]

**com·ple·men·tal air** SYN inspiratory reserve volume.

**com·ple·men·tar·i·ty** (kom-plĕ-men-tār′i-tē) **1.** the degree of base-pairing between two sequences of DNA and/or RNA molecules. **2.** the degree of affinity, or fit, of antigen and antibody combining sites.

**com·ple·men·ta·ry air** SYN inspiratory capacity.

**com·ple·men·ta·ry DNA (cDNA) 1.** single-stranded DNA that is complementary to messenger RNA; **2.** DNA that has been synthesized from mRNA by the action of reverse transcriptase.

**com·ple·men·ta·ry hy·per·tro·phy** increase in size or expansion of part of an organ or tissue to fill the space left by the destruction of another portion of the same organ or tissue.

**com·ple·men·ta·ry med·i·cine** SYN alternative medicine.

**com·ple·men·ta·tion** (kom′plĕ-men-tā′shŭn) **1.** interaction between two defective viruses permitting replication under conditions inhibitory to the single virus. **2.** interaction between two genetic units, one or both of which are defective, permitting the organism containing these units to function normally, whereas it could not do so if either unit were absent.

**com·ple·ment bind·ing as·say** a test for the detection of immune complexes.

**com·ple·ment che·mo·tac·tic fac·tor** the activated complex of the fifth, sixth, and seventh components of complement (C567) which induces chemotaxis of polymorphonuclear leukocytes.

**com·ple·ment fix·a·tion** fixation of complement in a serum by an antigen-antibody combination whereby it is rendered unavailable to complete a reaction in a second antigen-antibody combination for which complement is necessary; the second system usually serves as an indicator (red blood cells plus specific hemolysin); if complement is fixed with the first antigen-antibody un-

C
0

ion, hemolysis does not occur, but, if complement is not so removed, it causes hemolysis in the second system.

**com·ple·ment-fix·a·tion test** an immunological test for determining the presence of a particular antigen or antibody when one of the two is known to be present, based on the fact that complement is "fixed" in the presence of antigen and its specific antibody.

**com·ple·ment-fix·ing an·ti·bod·y** antibody that combines with and sensitizes antigen leading to the activation of complement, which may result in cell lysis.

**com·ple·ment path·ways 1.** the classical complement pathway (initiated usually by binding of C1 to IgG or IgM antibody to C1)is a complex of three subunits: C1q, C1r, and C1s. After C1q is bound, C1r (an overbar indicates enzymatic activity) cleaves C1s to C1s. C1s cleaves both C4 into C4a and C4b as well as C2 into C2a and C2b. C2b combines with C4b to form C4b2b, which is a C3 convertase. C3 convertase cleaves C3 into C3a and C3b. C3b joins C4bC2b to form a C5 convertase (also known as C4b2b3b), which cleaves C5 into C5a and C5b. Once C5b is bound to the cell surface the remainder of the complement components (C6–C9) as well as C5b form the membrane attack complex (MAC). MAC causes a hole in the cell membrane. **2.** in the alternative complement pathway, surface-bound C3b binds Factor B, which is cleaved by Factor D into Ba and Bb. C3bBb is an unstable C3 convertase unless properdin (P) binds to it to form C3bBbP. The stable C3 convertase generates more C3b. When a complex of C3bBbC3b is formed, this is the alternative pathway C5 convertase. From C5b through C9, the classical and alternative pathways are the same. **3.** in the lectin-binding pathway, mannose-binding protein (MBP) initiates the pathway, which then uses components of the classical complement pathway. Some of the "a" components of both pathways have various biologic activities, i.e., C3a is an anaphylatoxin.

**com·ple·ment u·nit** the smallest amount (highest dilution) of complement that will cause hemolysis of a unit of red blood cells in the presence of a hemolysin unit.

**com·plete an·dro·gen in·sen·si·tiv·i·ty syn·drome** SYN testicular feminization syndrome.

**com·plete an·ti·bod·y** SYN saline agglutinin.

**com·plete an·ti·gen** any antigen capable of stimulating the formation of antibody with which it reacts *in vivo* or *in vitro*, as distinguished from incomplete antigen (hapten).

**com·plete A-V block, com·plete AV block** SEE atrioventricular block.

**com·plete blood count (CBC)** a combination of the following determinations: red blood cell count, white blood cell count, erythrocyte indices, hematocrit, and differential blood count.

**com·plete car·cin·o·gen** a chemical carcinogen that is able to induce cancer without provocation by a tumor-promoting agent introduced during therapy.

**com·plete den·ture** a dental prosthesis which is a substitute for the lost natural dentition and associated structures of the maxillae or mandible.

**com·plete fis·tu·la** a fistula that is open at both ends.

**com·plete her·nia** an indirect inguinal hernia in which the contents extend into the tunica vaginalis.

**com·plete·ly in the ca·nal hear·ing aid (CIC)** a hearing aid that fits entirely in the external auditory canal and is not visible at the surface of the body.

**com·plete mas·toi·dec·to·my** an operation to exenterate the air cell system from the mastoid process of the temporal bone for the drainage of the suppuration in acute mastoiditis.

**com·plete pos·ter·i·or la·ryn·ge·al cleft** SEE laryngotracheoesophageal cleft.

**com·plete trans·duc·tion** transduction in which the transferred genetic fragment is fully integrated in the genome of the recipient bacterium.

**com·plex** (kom'pleks) **1.** PSYCHIATRY an organized constellation of feelings, thoughts, perceptions, and memories that may be in part unconscious and may strongly influence associations and attitudes. **2.** CHEMISTRY the relatively stable combination of two or more compounds into a larger molecule without covalent binding. **3.** a composite of chemical or immunologic structures. **4.** an anatomic structure made up of three or more interrelated parts. **5.** an informal term used to denote a group of individual structures known or believed to be anatomically, embryologically, or physiologically related. [L. *complexus*, woven together]

**com·plex en·do·me·tri·al hy·per·pla·sia** closely packed endometrial glands, with a single layer of cells with slightly enlarged nuclei that are generally basally located. SYN adenomatous hyperplasia.

**com·plex frac·ture** a fracture with significant soft tissue injury.

**com·plex·ion** (kom-plek'shŭn) the color, texture, and general appearance of the skin of the face. [L. *complexio*, a combination, (later) physical condition]

**com·plex learn·ing pro·cess·es** those processes that require the use of symbolic manipulations, as in reasoning.

**com·plex mo·tor sei·zure** seizure characterized by muscles of each limb contracting asynchronously and sequentially to produce a movement that may resemble voluntary activity.

**com·plex o·don·to·ma** an odontoma in which the various odontogenic tissues are organized in a haphazard arrangement with no resemblance to teeth.

**com·plex par·tial sei·zure** a partial seizure with impairment of consciousness without features of a generalized seizure. Complex partial seizures are commonly associated with automatisms.

**com·plex pleu·ral ef·fu·sion** a pleural effusion without actual infection but with signs of a high degree of inflammation (e.g., low pH, low glucose, high lactate dehydrogenase, many white cells).

**com·plex pre·cip·i·tat·ed ep·i·lep·sy** a form of reflex epilepsy initiated by specialized sensory stimuli, e.g., certain visual patterns.

**com·plex sound** a sound composed of a number of sounds of different frequencies.

**com·plex·us** (kom-plek'sŭs) obsolete term for semispinalis capitis muscle. [L. an embracing, encircling]

**com·plex·us stim·u·lans cor·dis** [TA] SYN conducting system of heart.

**com·pli·ance** (kom-plī'ans) **1.** a measure of the

distensibility of a chamber expressed as a change in volume per unit change in pressure. **2.** the consistency and accuracy with which a patient follows the regimen prescribed by a physician or other health professional. Cf. adherence (2), maintenance. **3.** PHYSIOLOGY a measure of the ease with which a hollow viscus (e.g., lung, urinary bladder, gallbladder) may be distended, *i.e.*, the volume change resulting from the application of a unit pressure differential between the inside and outside of the viscus; the reciprocal of elastance. **4.** observance of rules or guidelines, as those governing provision of medical services and billing for them; fulfillment of a requirement. [M.E. fr. O. Fr., fr. L. *compleo*, to fulfill]

**com·pli·ca·tion** (kom-pli-kā′shŭn) a morbid process or event occurring during a disease that is not an essential part of the disease, although it may result from it or from independent causes.

**com·po·nent** (kom-pō′nent) an element forming a part of the whole. [L. *com-pono*, pp. *-positus*, to place together]

**com·po·nent of com·ple·ment (C)** any one of the nine distinct protein units (designated C1 through C9) that effect the immunological activities associated with complement.

**com·po·nent man·age·ment** the approach to health care cost containment that involves trying to control individual components such as drug, hospitalization, or laboratory testing costs. SEE ALSO managed care.

**com·pos·ite flap, com·pound flap** a flap of two or more elements incorporating underlying muscle, bone, or cartilage.

**com·pos·ite graft** a graft composed of several structures, such as skin and cartilage or a full-thickness segment of the ear.

**com·pos men·tis** (kom′pos men′tis) of sound mind; usually used in its opposite form, *non compos mentis*. [L. possessed of one's mind; *compos*, having control, + *mens* (*ment-*), mind]

**com·pound** (kom′pownd) **1.** in chemistry, a substance formed by the covalent or electrostatic union of two or more elements, generally differing entirely in physical characteristics from any of its components. **2.** in pharmacy, denoting a preparation containing several ingredients. [through O.Fr., fr. L. *compono*]

**com·pound ac·tion po·ten·tial** the combined potentials resulting from activation of the auditory division of the eighth cranial nerve.

**com·pound an·eu·rysm** an aneurysm in which some of the coats of the artery are ruptured, others intact.

**com·pound dis·lo·ca·tion** SYN open dislocation.

**com·pound frac·ture** SYN open fracture.

**com·pound gland** a gland whose larger excretory ducts branch repeatedly into smaller ducts, which ultimately drain secretory units.

**com·pound het·er·o·zy·gote** MEDICAL GENETICS the presence of two different mutant alleles at the same loci.

**com·pound hy·per·o·pic a·stig·ma·tism** astigmatism in which all meridians are hyperopic but to different degrees.

**com·pound joint** a joint composed of three or more skeletal elements, or in which two anatomically separate joints function as a unit.

**com·pound mi·cro·scope** a microscope having two or more magnifying lenses.

**com·pound my·o·pic a·stig·ma·tism** astigma-

tism in which all meridians are myopic but to different degrees.

**com·pound o·don·to·ma** an odontoma in which the odontogenic tissues are organized and resemble anomalous teeth.

**com·pound pre·sen·ta·tion** prolapse of an extremity, usually a hand, along with the presenting part during the second stage of labor, with both in the pelvis simultaneously.

**com·pre·hen·sion** (kom-prē-hen′shŭn) knowledge or understanding of an object, situation, event, or verbal statement.

**com·press** (kom′pres) a pad of gauze or other material applied for local pressure. [L. *com-primo*, pp. *-pressus*, to press together]

**com·pres·si·ble vol·ume** the volume of gas compressed (and therefore lost) in the mechanical ventilator circuit per delivered pressure; most systems have compressible volume loss factors of 3 to 5 ml/cm $H_2O$; some newer mechanical ventilators calculate the loss factor and monitor gas delivery so that the set volume is the volume that actually enters the patient's airway.

**com·pres·sion** (kom-presh′ŭn) a squeezing together; the exertion of pressure on a body so as to tend to increase its density; the decrease in a dimension of a body under the action of two external forces directed toward one another.

**com·pres·sion cy·a·no·sis** cyanosis accompanied by edema and petechial hemorrhages over the head, neck, and upper part of the chest, as a venous reflex resulting from severe compression of the thorax or abdomen; the conjunctiva and retinas are similarly affected.

**com·pres·sion frac·ture** a fracture causing loss of height of the vertebral body either by trauma or by pathology; it occurs most commonly in thoracic and lumbar spines. A common sequela of osteoporosis.

**com·pres·sion lim·it·ing** a hearing aid circuit in which amplification is reduced at high input levels.

**com·pres·sion neu·rop·a·thy** a focal nerve lesion produced when sustained pressure is applied to a localized portion of the nerve, either from an external or internal source.

**com·pres·sion pa·ral·y·sis** paralysis due to external pressure on a nerve.

**com·pres·sion plate** a plate for internal fracture fixation with screw holes so designed that insertion of screws draws bone fragments more firmly together.

**com·pres·sion syn·drome 1.** SYN crush syndrome. **2.** SYN compartment syndrome.

**com·pres·sion ther·a·py** use of circumferential elastic tubing, bandages, or a custom garment to apply pressure in such conditions as burns, lymphedema, edema, and venous stasis.

**com·pres·sor** (kom-pres′er) **1.** a muscle, contraction of which causes compression of any structure. **2.** an instrument for making pressure on a part, especially on an artery to prevent loss of blood.

**com·pul·sion** (kom-pŭl′shŭn) uncontrollable impulses to perform an act, often repetitively, as an unconscious mechanism to avoid unacceptable ideas and desires which, by themselves, arouse anxiety; the anxiety becomes fully manifest if performance of the compulsive act is prevented; may be associated with obsessive thoughts. [L. *com-pello* pp. *-pulsus*, to drive together, compel]

**com•pul•sive** (kom-pŭl′siv) influenced by compulsion; of a compelling and irresistible nature.

**com•pul•sive i•dea** a fixed and repetitively recurring idea.

**com•pul•sive per•son•al•i•ty** a personality characterized by rigidity, extreme inhibition, perfectionism, and excessive concern with conformity and adherence to standards of conscience either for the individual or for others.

◨**com•put•ed to•mog•ra•phy (CT)** imaging anatomical information from a cross-sectional plane of the body, each image generated by a computer synthesis of x-ray transmission data obtained in many different directions in a given plane. See page B14. SYN computerized axial tomography.

**com•pu•ter-based pa•tient re•cord (CPR)** electronic health record that integrates all of a patient's health care information into a database for accessibility; the CPR supports patient care decision making and research.

**com•put•er•ized ax•i•al to•mog•ra•phy (CAT)** SYN computed tomography.

△**con-** with, together, in association; appears as com- before p, b, or m, as col- before l, and as co- before a vowel; corresponds to G. *syn-*. [L. *cum,* with, together]

**conA, con A** concanavalin A.

**co•nar•i•um** (kō-nā′rē-ŭm) SYN pineal body. [G. *kōnarion* (dim. of *kōnos,* cone), the pineal body]

**co•na•tion** (kō-nā′shŭn) the conscious tendency to act, usually an aspect of mental process; historically aligned with cognition and affection, but more recently used in the wider sense of impulse, desire, purposeful striving. [L. *conātio,* an undertaking, effort]

**co•na•tive** (kon′ă-tiv) pertaining to, or characterized by, conation.

**con•ca•nav•a•lin A (conA, con A)** (kon-kă-nav′ ă-lin ā) a phytomitogen, extracted from the jack bean (*Canavalia ensiformis*) that agglutinates the blood of mammals and reacts with glucosans; like other phytohemagglutinins, con A stimulates T lymphocytes more vigorously than it does B lymphocytes.

**Con•ca•to dis•ease** (kon-kah′tō) SYN polyserositis.

**con•cave** (kon′kāv) having a depressed or hollowed surface. [L. *concavus,* arched or vaulted]

**con•cave lens** a diverging minus power lens.

**con•cav•i•ty** (kon-kav′i-tē) a hollow or depression, with more or less evenly curved sides, on any surface.

**con•ca•vo•con•cave** (kon-kā′vō-kon′kāv) SYN biconcave.

**con•ca•vo•con•cave lens** SYN biconcave lens.

**con•ca•vo•con•vex** (kon-kā′vō-kon′veks) concave on one surface and convex on the opposite surface.

**con•ca•vo•con•vex lens** a converging meniscus lens that is concave on one surface and convex on the opposite surface.

**con•cealed hem•or•rhage** SYN internal hemorrhage.

**con•cen•tra•tion (c)** (kon-sen-trā′shŭn) **1.** a preparation made by extracting a crude drug, precipitating from the solution, and drying. **2.** increasing the amount of solute in a given volume of solution by evaporation of the solvent. **3.** the quantity of a substance per unit volume or weight. In renal physiology, symbol U for urinary concentration, P for plasma concentration;

in respiratory physiology, symbol C for amount per unit volume in blood, F for fractional concentration (mole fraction or volume per volume) in dried gas; subscripts indicate location and chemical species. [L. *con-,* together, + *centrum,* center]

**concentrator** (kon′sen-trā′ter) a device for making a substance stronger or purer.

**con•cen•tric** (kon-sen′trik) having a common center; said of two or more circles or spheres having a common center.

**con•cen•tric con•trac•tion** a shortening contraction in which a muscle's attachments are drawn toward one another as the muscle contracts and overcomes an external resistance.

**con•cen•tric hy•per•tro•phy** thickening of the walls of the heart or any cavity with apparent diminution of the capacity of the cavity.

**con•cen•tric la•mel•la** one of the concentric tubular layers of bone surrounding the central canal in an osteon. SYN haversian lamella.

**con•cept** (kon′sept) **1.** an abstract idea or notion. **2.** an explanatory variable or principle in a scientific system. SYN conception (1). [L. *conceptum,* something understood, pp. ntr. of *concipio,* to receive, apprehend]

**con•cept for•ma•tion** PSYCHOLOGY the learning to conceive and respond in terms of abstract ideas based upon an action or object.

**con•cep•tion** (kon-sep′shŭn) **1.** SYN concept. **2.** act of forming a general idea or notion. **3.** act of conceiving, or becoming pregnant; fertilization of the oocyte (ovum) by a sperm (spermatozoon) to form a viable zygote. [L. *conceptio;* see concept]

**con•cep•tu•al** (kon-sep′chŭ-ăl) relating to the formation of ideas, usually higher order abstractions, to mental conceptions.

**con•cep•tus,** pl. **conceptus** (kon-sep′tŭs) the products of conception, i.e., embryo and membranes.

**con•cha,** pl. **con•chae** (kon′kă, kon′kē) in anatomy, a structure comparable to a shell in shape, as the auricle or pinna of the ear or a turbinated bone in the nose. [L. a shell]

**con•cha of ear** the large hollow, or floor of the auricle, between the anterior portion of the helix and the antihelix; it is divided by the crus of the helix into the cymba above and the cavum below.

**con•cha san•to•ri•ni** SYN supreme nasal concha.

**con•com•i•tant symp•tom** SYN accessory symptom.

**con•cor•dance** (kon-kōr′dans) agreement in the types of data that occur in natural pairs. [L. *concordia,* agreeing, harmony]

**con•cor•dance rate** the rate of occurrence of a trait, behavior, or action in members of a specified group that are concordant for a trait of interest. Broadly, it is taken as evidence of causal connection.

**con•cor•dant** (kon-kōr′dant) denoting or exhibiting concordance.

**con•cor•dant al•ter•nans** simultaneous occurrence of right ventricular and pulmonary artery alternans with left ventricular and peripheral pulsus alternans.

**con•cor•dant al•ter•na•tion** alternation in either the mechanical or electrical activity of the heart, occurring in both systemic and pulmonary circulations.

**con•cor•dant chan•ges e•lec•tro•car•di•o•-**

**gram** the presence of more than one waveform change, each in the same direction (polarity).

**con·cres·cence** (kon-krĕs′ens) **1.** SYN coalescence. **2.** DENTISTRY the union of the roots of two adjacent teeth by cementum.

**con·crete think·ing** thinking of objects or ideas as specific items rather than as an abstract representation of a more general concept, as contrasted with abstract thinking (e.g., perceiving a chair and a table as individual useful items and not as members of the general class, furniture).

**con·cre·tio cor·dis** (kon-krē′shē-ō kōr′dis) extensive adhesion between parietal and visceral layers of the pericardium with partial or complete obliteration of the pericardial cavity. SYN internal adhesive pericarditis.

**con·cre·tion** (kon-krē′shŭn) formation of solid material by the aggregation of discrete units or particles. [L. *cum*, together, + *crescere*, to grow]

**con·cur·rent dis·in·fec·tion** application of disinfective measures as soon as possible after discharge of infectious material from the body of an infected person, or after soiling of articles with such infectious discharges.

**con·cus·sion** (kon-kŭsh′ŭn) **1.** a violent shaking or jarring. **2.** an injury of a soft structure, as the brain, resulting from a blow or violent shaking. [L. *concussio*, fr. *con- cutio*, pp. *-cussus*, to shake violently]

**con·den·sa·tion** (kon-den-sā′shŭn) **1.** making more solid or dense. **2.** the change of a gas to a liquid, or of a liquid to a solid. **3.** PSYCHOANALYSIS an unconscious mental process in which one symbol stands for a number of others. **4.** DENTISTRY the process of packing a filling material into a cavity, using such force and direction that no voids result. [L. *con- denso*, pp. *-atus*, to make thick, condense]

**con·dens·er** (kon-den′ser) **1.** an apparatus for cooling a gas to a liquid, or a liquid to a solid. **2.** in dentistry, a manual or powered instrument used for packing a plastic or unset material into a cavity of a tooth; variation in sizes and shapes allows conformation of the mass to the cavity outline. **3.** the simple or compound lens on a microscope that is used to supply the illumination necessary for visibility of the specimen under observation. **4.** SYN capacitor.

**con·di·tion** (kon-dish′ŭn) **1.** to train; to undergo conditioning. **2.** BEHAVIORAL PSYCHOLOGY a certain response elicited by a specifiable stimulus or emitted in the presence of certain stimuli with reward of the response during prior occurrence. **3.** referring to several classes of learning in the behavioristic branch of psychology. [L. *conditio*, fr. *condico*, to agree]

**con·di·tioned re·flex (Cr)** a reflex that is gradually developed by training and association through the frequent repetition of a definite stimulus. SEE conditioning.

**con·di·tioned re·sponse** a response already in an individual's repertoire but which, through repeated pairings with its natural stimulus, has been acquired or conditioned anew to a previously neutral or conditioned stimulus. SEE conditioning. Cf. unconditioned response.

**con·di·tioned stim·u·lus 1.** a stimulus applied to one of the sense organs which are an essential and integral part of the neural mechanism underlying a conditioned reflex; **2.** a neutral stimulus, when paired with the unconditioned stimulus in simultaneous presentation to an organism, capable of eliciting a given response.

**con·di·tion·ing** (kon-dish′ŭn-ing) the process of acquiring, developing, educating, establishing, learning, or training new responses in an individual; a change in the frequency or form of behavior as a result of the influence of the environment.

**con·dom** (kon′dom) sheath or cover for the penis or vagina, for use in the prevention of conception or infection during coitus.

**con·duc·tance** (kon-dŭk′tans) **1.** a measure of conductivity; the ratio of the current flowing through a conductor to the difference in potential between the ends of the conductor; the conductance of a circuit is the reciprocal of its resistance. **2.** the ease with which a fluid or gas enters and flows through a conduit, air passage, or respiratory tract; the flow per unit pressure difference.

**con·duct dis·or·der** a mental disorder of childhood or adolescence characterized by a persistent pattern of violating societal norms and the rights of others; children with the disorder may exhibit physical aggression, cruelty to animals, vandalism and robbery, along with truancy, cheating, and lying. SEE borderline personality disorder.

**con·duct·ing sys·tem of heart** the system of atypical cardiac muscle fibers comprising the sinoatrial node, internodal tracts, atrioventricular node and bundle, the bundle branches, and their terminal ramifications into the Purkinje network; sometimes also called cardionector. SYN complexus stimulans cordis [TA].

**con·duc·tion** (kon-dŭk′shŭn) **1.** the act of transmitting or conveying certain forms of energy, such as heat, sound, or electricity, from one point to another, without evident movement in the conducting body. **2.** the transmission of stimuli of various sorts by living protoplasm. [L. *con- duco*, pp. *ductus*, to lead, conduct]

**con·duc·tion an·al·ge·sia** SYN regional anesthesia.

**con·duc·tion an·es·the·sia** regional anesthesia in which local anesthetic solution is injected about nerves to inhibit nerve transmission; includes spinal, epidural, nerve block, and field block anesthesia, but not local or topical anesthesia. SYN block anesthesia.

**con·duc·tion a·pha·sia** a form of aphasia in which the patient understands spoken and written words, is aware of his deficit, and can speak and write, but skips or repeats words, or substitutes one word for another (paraphasia); word repetition is severely impaired. The responsible lesion is in the associate tracts connecting the various language centers. SYN associative aphasia.

**con·duc·tive deaf·ness** hearing impairment caused by interference with sound or transmission through the external canal, middle ear, or ossicles.

**con·duc·tive hear·ing im·pair·ment** a form of hearing impairment due to a lesion in the external auditory canal or middle ear.

**con·duc·tive hear·ing loss** hearing loss caused by an obstruction or lesion in the outer ear, middle ear, or both. SEE ALSO air-bone gap.

**con·duc·tive heat** heat transmitted by direct contact, as by an electric pad or hot-water bottle.

**con·duc·tiv·i·ty** (kon-dŭk-tiv′i-tē) **1.** the power of transmission or conveyance of certain forms of energy, as heat, sound, and electricity, without perceptible motion in the conducting body. **2.** the property, inherent in living protoplasm, of transmitting a state of excitation; e.g., in muscle or nerve.

**con·duc·tor** (kon-dŭk′ter) **1.** a probe or sound with a groove along which a knife is passed in slitting open a sinus or fistula; a grooved director. **2.** any substance possessing conductivity.

**con·duit** (kon′doo-it) a channel.

**con·du·pli·cate** (kon-doo′pli-kāt) folded upon itself lengthwise. [L. *con-*, with, + *duplico,* pp. *-atus*]

**con·dy·lar** (kon′di-lăr) relating to a condyle.

**con·dy·lar ca·nal** the inconstant opening through the occipital bone posterior to the condyle on each side that transmits the occipital emissary vein.

**con·dy·lar fos·sa** a depression behind the condyle of the occipital bone in which the posterior margin of the superior facet of the atlas lies in extension.

**con·dy·lar joint** SYN ellipsoidal joint.

**con·dy·lar·thro·sis** (kon′di-lar-thrō′sis) a joint, like that of the knee, formed by condylar surfaces. [G. *kondylos,* condyle, + *arthrōsis,* a jointing]

**con·dyle** (kon′dīl) a rounded articular surface at the extremity of a bone. SYN condylus.

**con·dy·lec·to·my** (kon-di-lek′tō-mē) excision of a condyle. [G. *kondylos,* condyle, + *ektomē,* excision]

**con·dy·loid** (kon′di-loyd) relating to or resembling a condyle. [G. *kondylōdēs,* like a knuckle, fr. *kondylos,* condyle, + *eidos,* resemblance]

**con·dy·lo·ma,** pl. **con·dy·lo·ma·ta** (kon-di-lō′mă, kon-di-lō-mah′tă) a wartlike excrescence on the skin of the genitals, perineum, or anus. [G. *kondylōma,* a knob]

🔲**con·dy·lo·ma a·cu·mi·na·tum** a warty growth on the external genitals or at the anus, consisting of fibrous overgrowths covered by thickened epithelium showing koilocytosis, due to sexually transmitted infection with human papilloma virus; malignant change is associated with particular types of the virus. See page B3. SYN genital wart, venereal wart.

**con·dy·lo·ma la·tum** a secondary syphilitic eruption of flat-topped papules, found at the anus and wherever contiguous folds of skin produce heat and moisture. SYN flat condyloma (1).

**con·dy·lom·a·tous** (kon-di-lō′mă-tŭs) relating to a condyloma.

**con·dy·lot·o·my** (kon-di-lot′ō-mē) division, without removal, of a condyle. [G. *kondylos,* condyle, + *tomē,* incision]

**con·dy·lus** (kon′di-lŭs) SYN condyle. [L. fr. G. *kondylos,* knuckle, the knuckle of any joint]

**cone** (kōn) **1.** a surface joining a circle to a point above the plane (containing the circle). **2.** the photosensitive, outward-directed, conical process of a cone cell essential for sharp vision and color vision; cones are the only photoreceptor in the fovea centralis and become interspersed with increasing numbers of rods toward the periphery of the retina. **3.** metallic cylinder or truncated cone, either circular or square in cross-section, used to confine a beam of x-rays. SYN conus (1). [G. *kōnos,* cone]

△**-cone** the cusp of a tooth in the upper jaw.

**cone cell** one of the two types of visual receptor cells of the retina, essential for visual acuity and color vision; the second type is the rod cell.

**cone down 1.** to narrow a beam of x-rays to a region of interest using a collimator or cone (3). **2.** colloq., to delimit one's attention or activities.

**cone gran·ule** nucleus of a retinal cell connecting with one of the cones.

**cone of light** SYN pyramid of light.

**cone-rod re·ti·nal dys·tro·phy** a disorder affecting the retinal cones more than the rods, characterized by diminished central vision and color vision.

**con·fab·u·la·tion** (kon′fab-yu-lā′shŭn) the making of bizarre and incorrect responses, and a readiness to give a fluent but tangential answer, with no regard whatever to facts, to any question put; seen in amnesia, presbyophrenia, and Wernicke-Korsakoff syndrome. [L. *con-fabulor,* pp. *-fabulatus,* to talk together, fr. *fabula,* narrative]

**con·fec·tion** (kon-fek′shŭn) a pharmaceutical preparation consisting of a drug mixed with honey or syrup; a soft solid, sometimes used as an excipient for pill masses. [L. *confectio*]

**con·fi·den·ti·al·i·ty** (kon′fi-den-shē-al′i-tē) the statutorily protected right and duty of health professionals not to disclose information acquired during consultation with a patient. [L. *con-fido,* to trust, be assured]

**con·fig·u·ra·tion** (kon-fig-yu-rā′shŭn) **1.** the general form of a body and its parts. **2.** CHEMISTRY the spatial arrangement of atoms in a molecule. The configuration of a compound (e.g., a sugar) is the unique spatial arrangement of its atoms, on which no other arrangement of these atoms can be superimposed with complete correspondence. Cf. conformation.

**con·fine·ment** (kon-fīn′ment) lying-in; giving birth to a child. [L. *confine* (ntr.), a boundary, confine, fr. *con-* + *finis,* boundary]

**con·flict** (kon′flikt) tension or stress experienced by an organism when satisfaction of a need, drive, motive, or wish is thwarted by the presence of other attractive or unattractive needs, drives, or motives.

**con·flict of in·ter·est** a conflict between the personal interests and professional responsibilities of a health provider toward a patient or other consumer.

**con·flu·ence** (kon′floo-ĕns) a flowing together; a joining of two or more streams. [L. *confluens*]

**con·flu·ent** (kon′floo-ent) **1.** joining; running together; denoting certain skin lesions which become merged, forming a patch; denoting a disease characterized by lesions which are not discrete, or distinct one from the other. **2.** denoting a bone formed by the blending together of two originally distinct bones. [L. *con-fluo,* to flow together]

**con·fo·cal mi·cro·scope** a microscope that allows the observer to visualize objects in a single plane of focus, thereby creating a sharper image (usually the objects are fluorescent molecules); a refinement of this microscope uses optical sectioning and a computer to record serial sections. This permits three-dimensional reconstruction.

**con·for·ma·tion** (kon-fōr-mā′shŭn) the spatial arrangement of a molecule achieved by rotation of groups about single covalent bonds, without breaking any covalent bonds. Cf. configuration.

**con·found·ing** (kon-fown′ding) **1.** a situation in

which the effects of two or more processes are not separated; the distortion of the apparent effect of an exposure on risk, brought about by the association with other factors that can influence the outcome. **2.** a relationship between the effects of two or more causal factors observed in a set of data, such that it is not logically possible to separate the contribution of any single causal factor to the observed effects.

**con•fu•sion** (kon-fyu´zhŭn) a mental state in which reactions to environmental stimuli are inappropriate because the subject is bewildered, perplexed, or disoriented. [L. *confusio,* a confounding]

**con•ge•ner** (kon´jē-ner) **1.** one of two or more things of the same kind, as of animal or plant with respect to classification. **2.** one of two or more muscles with the same function. [L. *con-,* with, + *genus,* race]

**con•gen•i•tal** (kon-jen´i-tăl) existing at birth, referring to mental or physical traits, anomalies, malformations, or diseases, which may be either hereditary or due to an influence occurring during gestation up to the moment of birth. USAGE NOTE Often misused as a synonym of hereditary. [L. *congenitus,* born with]

**con•gen•i•tal a•fi•brin•o•gen•e•mia** a rare disorder of blood coagulation in which little or no fibrinogen can be found in plasma.

**con•gen•i•tal am•pu•ta•tion** amputation produced *in utero;* attributed to the pressure of constricting bands (amniotic). SYN amnionic amputation, amputation (1), birth amputation, intrauterine amputation, spontaneous amputation (1).

**con•gen•i•tal a•ne•mia** SYN erythroblastosis fetalis.

**con•gen•i•tal di•a•phrag•mat•ic her•nia** absence of the pleuroperitoneal membrane (usually on the left) or an enlarged Morgagni foramen which allows protrusion of abdominal viscera into the chest. SYN Bochdalek hernia.

**con•gen•i•tal ec•to•der•mal de•fect, con•gen•i•tal ec•to•der•mal dys•pla•si•a** incomplete development of the epidermis and skin appendages; the skin is smooth and hairless, the facies abnormal, and the teeth and nails may be affected; sweating may be deficient.

**con•gen•i•tal e•ryth•ro•poi•et•ic por•phyr•ia** enhanced porphyrin formation by erythroid cells in bone marrow, leading to severe porphyrinuria, often with hemolytic anemia and persistent cutaneous photosensitivity; caused by a deficiency of uroporphyrinogen III cosynthetase.

**con•gen•i•tal glau•co•ma** SYN buphthalmia.

**con•gen•i•tal Heinz bod•y he•mo•ly•tic a•ne•mia** a group of congenital hemolytic anemias caused by inheritance of an unstable hemoglobin variant. An amino acid substitution in one of the hemoglobin chains prevents the hemoglobin from folding into its normal conformation, alters the alpha-helix structure or subunit interaction sites, or affects the binding of heme to globin. The hemoglobin denatures into Heinz bodies, which attach to the cell membrane and cause membrane injury and premature destruction of the cell.

**con•gen•i•tal he•mo•lyt•ic a•ne•mia** accelerated destruction of red blood cells due to an inherited defect, such as in the membrane in hereditary spherocytosis.

**con•gen•i•tal he•red•i•tary en•do•the•li•al**

**dys•tro•phy** a dominantly or recessively inherited condition characterized by a cloudy, thickened cornea at birth or in the neonatal period.

**con•gen•i•tal hip dys•pla•sia** a developmental abnormality in which a neonate's hips easily become dislocated; etiology is complex, with mechanical, familial, hormonal, and obstetric factors all contributing; female predominance is 9:1. SYN developmental hip dysplasia.

**con•gen•i•tal hy•po•plas•tic a•ne•mia** congenital nonregenerative, familial hypoplastic, or pure red cell anemia; erythrogenesis imperfecta; Diamond-Blackfan syndrome; anemia resulting from congenital hypoplasia of the bone marrow, which is grossly deficient in erythroid precursors while other elements are normal; anemia is progressive and severe, but leukocyte and platelet counts are normal or slightly reduced; survival of transfused erythrocytes is normal.

**con•gen•i•tal hy•po•thy•roid•ism** lack of thyroid secretion. SEE infantile hypothyroidism.

**con•gen•i•tal ich•thy•o•si•form e•ryth•ro•der•ma** a genodermatosis characterized by diffuse chronic erythema and scale formation, which occurs in bullous and nonbullous forms. SYN ichthyosiform erythroderma.

**con•gen•i•tal meg•a•co•lon, meg•a•co•lon con•ge•ni•tum** congenital dilation and hypertrophy of the colon due to absence (aganglionosis) or marked reduction (hypoganglionosis) in the number of ganglion cells of the myenteric plexus of the rectum and a varying but continuous length of gut above the rectum. SYN Hirschsprung disease.

**con•gen•i•tal ne•vus** a melanocytic nevus that is visible at birth, is often larger than an acquired nevus, and more frequently involves deeper structures.

**con•gen•i•tal nys•tag•mus 1.** nystagmus present at birth or caused by lesions sustained *in utero* or at the time of birth; **2.** inherited nystagmus, usually X-linked, without associated neurologic lesions and nonprogressive. **3.** the nystagmus associated with albinism, achromatopsia, and hypoplasia of the macula.

**con•gen•i•tal par•a•my•o•to•nia, pa•ra•my•o•to•nia con•gen•i•ta** a nonprogressive myotonia induced by exposure of muscles to cold; there are episodes of intermittent flaccid paralysis, but no atrophy or hypertrophy of muscles; autosomal dominant inheritance. There is a variant autosomal dominant form in which cold is not a provoking factor. SYN Eulenburg disease.

**con•gen•i•tal py•lor•ic ste•no•sis** SYN hypertrophic pyloric stenosis.

**con•gen•i•tal stri•dor** crowing inspiration occurring at birth or within the first few months of life; sometimes without apparent cause and sometimes due to abnormal flaccidity of epiglottis or arytenoids.

**con•gen•i•tal syph•i•lis** syphilis acquired by the fetus *in utero,* thus present at birth.

**con•gen•i•tal to•tal li•po•dys•tro•phy** characterized by almost complete lack of subcutaneous fat, accelerated rate of growth and skeletal development during the first 3–4 years of life, muscular hypertrophy, cardiac enlargement, hepatosplenomegaly, acanthosis nigricans, hypertrichosis, renal enlargement, hypertriglyceridemia, and hypermetabolism; autosomal recessive inheri-

**con·gen·i·tal tox·o·plas·mo·sis** transmitted *in utero* to the fetus, observed as three syndromes: 1) acute: most of the organs contain foci of necrosis in association with fever, jaundice, hydrocephaly, encephalomyelitis, pneumonitis, cutaneous rash, ophthalmic lesions, hepatomegaly, and splenomegaly; 2) subacute: most of the lesions are partly healed or calcified, but those in the brain and eye seem to remain active, inasmuch as chorioretinitis is observed in more than 80% of diseased infants; 3) chronic: usually not recognized during the newborn period, but chorioretinitis and cerebral lesions may be detected weeks to years later.

**con·gen·i·tal valve** an abnormal lining fold obstructing a passage.

**con·gen·i·tal vir·i·liz·ing ad·re·nal hy·per··pla·sia** any inborn error of metabolism causing hyperplasia of the adrenal cortex and overproduction of virilizing hormones. Most forms are due to partial or complete 21-hydroxylase deficiency, leading to increased ACTH production by the pituitary, stimulating adrenal growth and function. Clinical features include ambiguous genitalia, virilization, and salt-wasting.

**con·gest·ed** (kon-jes'ted) containing an abnormal amount of blood; in a state of congestion.

**con·ges·tion** (kon-jes'chŭn) presence of an abnormal amount of fluid in the vessels or passages of a part or organ; especially, of blood due either to increased influx or to an obstruction to the return flow. SEE ALSO hyperemia. [L. *congestio,* a bringing together, a heap, fr. *con-gero,* pp. *-gestus,* to bring together]

**con·ges·tive** (kon-jes'tiv) relating to congestion.

**con·ges·tive heart fail·ure** SYN heart failure (1).

**con·ges·tive sple·no·meg·a·ly** enlargement of the spleen due to passive congestion; sometimes used as a synonym for Banti syndrome.

**con·glo·bate** (kon-glō'bāt) formed in a single rounded mass. [L. *con-globo,* pp. *-atus,* to gather into a *globus,* ball]

**con·glom·er·ate** (kon-glom'ĕ-răt) composed of several parts aggregated into one mass. [L. *con-glomero,* pp. *-atus,* to roll together, fr. *glomus,* a ball]

**con·glu·ti·nant** (kon-gloo'ti-nant) adhesive, promoting the union of a wound. [L. *con-glutino,* pp. *-atus,* to glue together, fr. *gluten,* glue]

**con·glu·ti·na·tion** (kon-gloo-ti-nā'shŭn) **1.** SYN adhesion (1). **2.** agglutination of antigen-(erythrocyte)-antibody-complement complex by normal bovine serum (and certain other colloidal materials); the procedure provides a means of detecting the presence of nonagglutinating antibody.

**con·go·phil·ic** (kon-gō-fil'ik) denoting any substance that takes a Congo red stain.

**con·go·phil·ic an·gi·op·a·thy** a condition of blood vessels characterized by deposits in the vessel walls of a substance, usually amyloid, that takes a Congo red stain. SEE ALSO cerebral amyloid angiopathy.

**Con·go red** (kong'gō) [CI 22120] an acid direct cotton dye, used as an indicator (pH 3.0, blue-violet, to pH 5.0, red) in testing for free hydrochloric acid in gastric contents; the dye is absorbed by amyloid and induces green fluorescence to amyloid in polarized light; used as a laboratory aid in the diagnosis of amyloidosis and as a histologic stain.

**co·ni** (kō'nī) plural of conus.

**con·i·cal cor·nea** SYN keratoconus.

**con·i·cal pa·pil·lae** numerous projections on the dorsum of the tongue, scattered among the filiform papillae and similar to them, but shorter.

△ **-co·nid** the cusp of a tooth in the lower jaw.

*Co·nid·i·o·bo·lus* a fungal genus in the family Entomophthoraceae, widely distributed in soil and among plants, insects, and amphibians. *C. coronatus* causes conidiobolomycosis, a chronic granulomatous disease of submucosal and subcutaneous tissues.

**co·ni·o·fi·bro·sis** (kō'nē-ō-fī-brō'sis) fibrosis produced by dust, especially of the lungs by inhaled dust. [G. *konis,* dust, + fibrosis]

**co·ni·o·phage** (kō'nē-ō-fāj) SYN alveolar macrophage. [G. *konis,* dust, + *phagō,* to eat]

**co·ni·o·sis** (kō-nē-ō'sis) any disease or morbid condition caused by dust. [G. *konis,* dust]

**con·i·za·tion** (kō-nī-zā'shŭn) excision of a cone of tissue, e.g., mucosa of the cervix uteri.

**con·joined a·nas·to·mo·sis** the joining together of two small blood vessels by side-to-side elliptical anastomosis to create a single larger stoma for subsequent end-to-end anastomosis.

**con·joined twins** monozygotic twins with varying extent of union and different degrees of residual duplication. The various types of union are named by the use of a prefix designating the region that is united and adding the suffix *-pagus,* meaning fused (e.g., craniopagus, thoracopagus); the various types of residual duplication are named by designating the parts duplicated and adding the suffix *-didymus,* or *-dymus,* meaning twin (e.g., cephalodidymus, cephalodidymus).

**con·ju·gant** (kon'jŭ-gant) a member of a mating pair of organisms or gametes undergoing conjugation. [L. *con-jugo,* to join]

**con·ju·ga·ta** (kon-jŭ-gā'tă) any conjugate diameter of the pelvis. SEE conjugate. [L. fem. of *conjugatus,* pp. of *con-jugo,* to join together]

**con·ju·gate** (kon'jŭ-gāt) **1.** joined or paired. SYN conjugated. **2.** a conjugate diameter of the pelvis. The distance between any two specified points on the periphery of the pelvic canal. [L. *conjugatus,* joined together. See conjugata]

**con·ju·gate ac·id-base pair** in prototonic solvents, acetic acid), two molecular species differing only in the presence or absence of a hydrogen ion; the basis of buffer action.

**con·ju·gat·ed** (kon'jŭ-gāt-ed) SYN conjugate (1).

**con·ju·gat·ed an·ti·gen** SYN conjugated hapten.

**con·ju·gat·ed dou·ble bonds** two or more double bonds separated by each single bond.

**con·ju·gate de·vi·a·tion of the eyes 1.** rotation of the eyes equally and simultaneously in the same direction, as occurs normally; **2.** a condition in which both eyes are turned to the same side as a result of either paralysis or muscular spasm.

**con·ju·gat·ed hap·ten** a hapten that may cause the production of antibodies when it has been covalently linked to protein. SYN conjugated antigen.

**con·ju·gat·ed pro·tein** protein attached to some other molecule or molecules (not amino acid in nature) otherwise than as a salt. SEE ALSO prosthetic group. Cf. simple protein.

**con·ju·gate fo·ra·men** a foramen formed by the notches of two bones in apposition.

**con·ju·gate fo·ra·men** a foramen formed by the notches of two bones in apposition.

**con·ju·gate nys·tag·mus** a nystagmus in which the two eyes move simultaneously in the same direction.

**con·ju·gate of pel·vic in·let** distance from the promontory of the sacrum to the upper posterior edge of the pubic symphysis.

**con·ju·gate point** a point so related to another that an object at one is imaged at the other.

**con·ju·ga·tion** (kon-jŭ-gā′shŭn) **1.** the union of two unicellular organisms or of the male and female gametes of multicellular forms followed by partition of the chromatin and the production of two new cells. **2.** bacterial conjugation, effected by simple contact, through which transfer genes and other genes of the plasmid are transferred to recipient bacteria through pili. **3.** sexual reproduction among protozoan ciliates, during which two individuals of appropriate mating types fuse along part of their lengths; their macronuclei degenerate and the micronuclei in each macronucleus divide several times (including a meiotic division); one of the resulting haploid pronuclei passes from each conjugant into the other and fuses with the remaining haploid nucleus in each conjugant; the organisms then separate (becoming exconjugants), undergo nuclear reorganization, and subsequently divide by asexual mitosis. **4.** the combination, especially in the liver, of certain toxic substances formed in the intestine, drugs, or steroid hormones with glucuronic or sulfuric acid; a means by which the biological activity of certain chemical substances is terminated and the substances made ready for excretion. **5.** the formation of glycyl or tauryl derivatives of the bile acids. [L. *con-jugo,* pp. *-jugatus,* to join together]

**con·ju·ga·tive plas·mid** a plasmid that can effect its own intercellular transfer by means of conjugation; this transfer is accomplished by a bacterium being rendered a donor, usually with specialized pili.

**con·junc·ti·va,** pl. **con·junc·ti·vae** (kon-jŭnk-tī′vă, kon-jŭnk-tī′vē) the mucous membrane investing the anterior surface of the eyeball and the posterior surface of the lids. [L. fem. of *conjunctivus,* from *conjungo,* pp. *-junctus,* to bind together]

**con·junc·ti·val** (kon-jŭnk-tī′văl) relating to the conjunctiva.

**con·junc·ti·val re·flex** closure of the eyes in response to irritation of the conjunctiva.

**con·junc·ti·val ring** a narrow ring at the junction of the periphery of the cornea with the conjunctiva.

**con·junc·ti·val sac** the space bound by the conjunctival membrane between the palpebral and bulbar conjunctiva, into which the lacrimal fluid is secreted; it opens anteriorly between the eyelids. SYN saccus conjunctivalis [TA].

**con·junc·ti·val var·ix** SYN varicula.

**con·junc·ti·val veins** the veins of the conjunctiva which drain primarily to the ophthalmic veins.

**con·junc·ti·vi·tis** (kon-jŭnk-ti-vī′tis) inflammation of the conjunctiva.

**con·junc·ti·vo·chal·a·sis** (kon-junk′ti-vō-kal′ă-sis) condition in which redundant bulbar conjunctiva billows over the eyelid margin or covers the lower punctum. [conjunctiva + G. *chalasis,* a loosening]

**con·junc·ti·vo·plas·ty** (kon-jŭngk′ti-vō-plas-tē) plastic surgery on the conjunctiva.

**con·nect·ing car·ti·lage** the cartilage in a cartilaginous joint such as the symphysis pubis. SYN interosseous cartilage.

**con·nec·tion** (kŏ-nek′shŭn) a union of elements or things; a connecting structure. SYN connexus.

**con·nec·tive tis·sue** the supporting or framework tissue of the animal body, formed of fibrous and ground substance with more or less numerous cells of various kinds; it is derived from the mesenchyme, and this in turn from the mesoderm. The varieties of connective tissue are: areolar or loose; adipose; dense, regular or irregular, white fibrous; elastic; mucous; and lymphoid tissue; cartilage; and bone. Blood and lymph may be regarded as connective tissues, the ground substance of which is a liquid. SYN interstitial tissue.

**con·nec·tive-tis·sue dis·ease** a group of generalized diseases affecting connective tissue, especially those not inherited as mendelian characteristics; rheumatic fever and rheumatoid arthritis were first proposed as such diseases, and other so-called collagen diseases have been added. SEE ALSO collagen disease.

**con·nec·tive tu·mor** any tumor of the connective tissue group, such as osteoma, fibroma, sarcoma.

**con·nec·tor** (kŏn-nec′-tōr) in dentistry, a part of a partial denture which unites its components.

**Con·nell su·ture** (kon′ĕl) a continuous suture used for inverting the gastric or intestinal walls in performing an anastomosis.

**con·nex·in 26** (kon-eks′in) the gap junction protein, the gene for which (Cx26) when mutated, accounts for a major portion of recessive nonsyndromic hearing impairment.

**con·nex·us** (ko-nek′sŭs) SYN connection. [L.]

**Conn syn·drome** (kon) SYN primary aldosteronism.

**co·noid** (kō′noyd) **1.** a cone-shaped structure. **2.** part of the apical complex characteristic of the protozoan subphylum, Apicomplexa; seen in sporozoites, merozoites, or other developmental stages of sporozoans, less well developed in the piroplasms (families Babesiidae and Theileriidae). The function of the conoid is unknown, but it is thought to be an organelle of penetration into the host cell, possibly aided by a protrusible form of the conoid. [G. *kōnoeidēs,* cone-shaped]

**co·noid tu·ber·cle** the prominence near the lateral end of the inferior surface of the clavicle that gives attachment to the conoid ligament.

**Con·ra·di dis·ease** (kon-rah′dē) SYN chondrodysplasia calcificans congenita.

**Con·ra·di-Hü·ner·mann syn·drome** (kon-rah′dē hyu′nĕr-mahn) one of the syndromes of chondrodysplasia punctata, autosomal dominant, with variable skin keratinization disorders and facial, cardiac, optic, and central nervous system abnormalities; epiphyseal stippling is also present.

**Con·ra·di line** (kon-rah′dē) a line extending from the base of the ensiform cartilage to the apex beat of the heart, corresponding approximately to the lower edge of the cardiac area.

**con·san·guin·e·ous** (kon-sang-gwin′ē-ŭs) denoting consanguinity. [L. *cum,* with, + *sanguis,* blood: *consanguineus*]

**con·san·guin·i·ty** (kon-sang-gwin′i-tē) kinship

because of common ancestry. SYN blood relationship. [L. *consanguinitas,* blood relationship]

**con·scious** (kon'shŭs) **1.** aware; having present knowledge or perception of oneself, one's acts and surroundings. **2.** denoting something occurring with the perceptive attention of the individual, as a conscious act or idea, distinguished from automatic or instinctive. [L. *conscius,* knowing]

**con·scious·ness** (kon'shŭs-nes) the state of being aware, or perceiving physical facts or mental concepts; a state of general wakefulness and responsiveness to environment; a functioning sensorium. [L. *con-scio,* to know, to be aware of]

**con·sec·u·tive am·pu·ta·tion** a revision or secondary amputation of a limb.

**con·sen·su·al** (kon-sen'shoo-ăl) denoting what something is by the fact of agreement between the perceiving of several persons. SYN reflex (3). [L. *con-,* with, + *sensus,* sensation]

**con·ser·va·tive** (kon-ser'vă-tiv) denoting treatment by gradual, limited, or well-established procedures, as opposed to radical.

**con·sis·ten·cy prin·ci·ple** PSYCHOLOGY the desire of human beings to be consistent, especially in their attitudes and beliefs; theories of attitude formation and change based on the consistency principle include balance theory, which suggests that individuals seek to avoid incongruity in their various attitudes.

**con·sol·i·da·tion** (kon-sol-i-dā'shŭn) solidification into a firm dense mass; applied especially to inflammatory induration of a normally aerated lung due to the presence of cellular exudate in the pulmonary alveoli. [L. *consolido,* to make thick, condense, fr. *solidus,* solid]

**con·spi·cu·i·ty** (kon-spi-kyu'i-tē) the visibility of a structure of interest on a radiograph, a function of the inherent contrast of the structure and the complexity (noise) of the surrounding image.

**con·stan·cy** (kon'stan-sē) the quality of being constant. [L. *constantia,* fr. *consto,* to stand still]

**con·stant** (kon'stănt) a quantity that, under stated conditions, does not vary with changes in the environment.

**con·sti·pate** (kon'sti-pāt) to cause constipation.

**con·sti·pat·ed** (kon'sti-pāt-ed) suffering from constipation.

**con·sti·pa·tion** (kon-sti-pā'shŭn) a condition in which bowel movements are infrequent or incomplete. [L. *con-stipo,* pp. *-atus,* to press together]

**con·sti·tu·tion** (kon-sti-too'shŭn) **1.** the physical makeup of a body, including the mode of performance of its functions, the activity of its metabolic processes, the manner and degree of its reactions to stimuli, and its power of resistance to the attack of pathogenic organisms. **2.** CHEMISTRY the number and kind of atoms in the molecule and the relation they bear to each other. [L. *constitutio,* constitution, disposition, fr. *constituo,* pp. *-stitutus,* to establish, fr. *statuo,* to set up]

**con·sti·tu·tion·al** (kon-sti-too'shŭn-ăl) **1.** relating to a body's constitution. **2.** general; relating to the system as a whole; not local.

**con·sti·tu·tion·al re·ac·tion** a generalized reaction in contrast to a focal or local reaction; in allergy the immediate or delayed response, following the introduction of an allergen, occurring at sites remote from that of injection.

**con·sti·tu·tion·al symp·tom** a symptom indicating a systemic effect of a disease; e.g., weight loss.

**con·stric·tio** [TA] SYN constriction (1).

**con·stric·tion** (kon-strik'shŭn) **1.** a normally or pathologically constricted or narrowed portion of a luminal structure. SYN constrictio [TA]. SEE ALSO stricture, stenosis. **2.** the act or process of binding or contracting, becoming narrowed; the condition of being constricted or squeezed. **3.** a subjective sensation of pressure or tightness, as if the body or any part were tightly bound or squeezed. [L. *con-stringo,* pp. *-strictus,* to draw together]

**con·stric·tion ring 1.** spastic stricture of the uterine cavity resulting when a zone of muscle goes into local tetanic contraction and forms a tight constriction about some part of the fetus; **2.** SYN amnionic band.

**con·stric·tive bron·chi·ol·i·tis** obliteration of bronchioles by scarring following bronchiolitis obliterans.

**con·stric·tive per·i·car·di·tis** postinflammatory thickening and scarring of the membrane producing constriction of the cardiac chambers; may be acute, subacute, or chronic. Formerly called chronic constrictive pericarditis.

**con·stric·tor** (kon-strik'ter) **1.** anything that binds or squeezes a part. **2.** a muscle, the action of which is to narrow a canal; a sphincter. [L. fr. *constringo,* to draw together]

**con·sul·tant** (kon-sŭl'tant) **1.** a physician or surgeon who does not take full responsibility for a patient, but acts in an advisory capacity, deliberating with and counseling the attending physician or surgeon. **2.** a member of a hospital staff who has no active service but stands ready to advise in any case, at the request of the attending physician or surgeon. [L. *consulto,* pp. *-atus,* to deliberate, ask advice]

**con·sul·ta·tion** (kon-sŭl-tā'shŭn) meeting of two or more physicians or surgeons to evaluate the nature and progress of disease in a particular patient and to establish diagnosis, prognosis, and/or therapy.

**con·sult·ing staff** specialists affiliated with a hospital who serve in an advisory capacity to the attending staff.

**con·sump·tion** (kon-sŭmp'shŭn) the using up of something, especially the rate at which it is used. [L. *con-sumo,* pp. *-sumptus,* to take up wholly, use up, waste]

**con·sump·tion co·ag·u·lop·a·thy** a disorder in which marked reductions develop in blood concentrations of platelets with exhaustion of the coagulation factors in the peripheral blood as a result of disseminated intravascular coagulation.

**con·tact** (kon'takt) **1.** the touching or apposition of two bodies. **2.** a person who has been exposed to a contagious disease. [L. *con- tingo,* pp. *-tactus,* to touch, seize, fr. *tango,* to touch]

**con·tact al·ler·gy** SYN allergic contact dermatitis.

**con·tac·tant** (kon-tak'tănt) any allergen that elicits manifestations of hypersensitivity by direct contact with skin or mucosa.

**con·tact chei·li·tis** inflammation of the lips resulting from contact with a primary irritant or specific allergen, including ingredients of lipsticks.

**con·tact der·ma·ti·tis** dermatitis resulting from cutaneous contact with a specific allergen (allergic contact dermatitis) or irritant (irritant contact dermatitis).

**con·tact hy·ster·o·scope** hysteroscope with a graded refractive index rod lens; it does not require distension for visualization and affords very short focal length views; suitable for localizing hemorrhages.

**con·tact in·hi·bi·tion** cessation of replication of dividing cells that come into contact, as in the center of a healing wound.

**con·tact lens** a lens that fits over the cornea and sclera or cornea only; used to correct refractive errors.

**con·tact splint** a slotted plate, held by screws, used in the treatment of fracture of long bones.

**con·tact-type der·ma·ti·tis** dermatitis resembling contact dermatitis or eczema, but caused by an ingested or injected allergen, usually a drug, and with a widespread or generalized distribution.

**con·tact ul·cer** ulceration of the vocal folds along their posterior borders, overlying the vocal processes of the arytenoid cartilages. Usually caused by vocal abuse; results in hoarse voice.

**con·tact with re·al·i·ty** correctly interpreting external phenomena in relation to the norms of one's social or cultural milieu.

**con·ta·gion** (kon-tā′jŭn) **1.** SYN contagium. **2.** transmission of infection by direct contact, droplet spread, or contaminated fomites. **3.** production via suggestion or imitation of a neurosis or psychosis in several or more members of a group. [L. *contagio;* fr. *contingo,* to touch closely]

**con·ta·gious** (kon-tā′jŭs) relating to contagion; communicable or transmissible by contact with the sick or their fresh secretions or excretions.

**con·ta·gious dis·ease** an infectious disease transmissible by direct or indirect contact; now used synonymously with communicable disease.

**con·ta·gious·ness** (kon-tā′jŭs-nes) the quality of being contagious.

**con·ta·gium** (kon-tā′jē-ŭm) the agent of an infectious disease. SYN contagion (1). [L. a touching]

**con·tained disk her·ni·a·tion** herniated disk material that remains covered by a thin layer of posterior annulus fibrosus or posterior longitudinal ligament; a disk protrusion is an example of a contained disk herniation.

**con·tam·i·nant** (kon-tam′i-nant) an impurity; any extraneous material associated with a chemical, a pharmaceutical preparation, a physiologic principle, or an infectious agent.

**con·tam·i·nate** (kon-tam′i-nāt) to cause or result in contamination. [L. *con-tamino,* to mingle, corrupt]

**con·tam·i·na·tion** (kon-tam-i-nā′shŭn) **1.** the presence of an infectious agent on a body surface; also on or in clothes, bedding, toys, surgical instruments or dressings, or other inanimate articles or substances including water, milk and food or that infectious agent itself. **2.** EPIDEMIOLOGY the situation that exists when a population being studied for one condition or factor also possesses other conditions or factors that modify results of the study. **3.** freudian term for a fusion and condensation of words. [L. *contamino,* pp. *-atus,* to stain, defile]

**con·tent** (kon′tent) **1.** that which is contained within something else, usually in this sense in the plural form, contents. **2.** in psychology, the form

of a dream as presented to consciousness. **3.** ambiguous usage for concentration (3); e.g., blood hemoglobin content could mean either its concentration or the product of its concentration and the blood volume. [L. *contentus,* fr. *con-tineo,* pp. *-tentus,* to hold together, contain]

**con·tent a·nal·y·sis** any of a variety of techniques for classification and study of the verbal products of normal or of psychologically impaired individuals.

**con·tig map** a physical map of a chromosome or stretch of DNA constructed from sets of overlapping and order clones (contig).

**con·ti·gu·i·ty** (kon-ti-gyu′i-tē) **1.** contact without structural continuity, e.g., the contact of the bones entering into the formation of a cranial suture. Cf. continuity. **2.** occurrence of two or more objects, events, or mental impressions together in space or time. [L. *contiguus,* touching, fr. *contingo,* to touch]

**con·tig·u·ous** (kon-tig′yu-ŭs) adjacent or in actual contact.

**con·ti·nence** (kon′ti-nens) **1.** moderation, temperance, or self-restraint in respect to the appetites, especially to sexual intercourse. **2.** the ability to retain urine and/or feces until a proper time for their discharge. [L. *continentia,* fr. *con- tineo,* to hold back]

**con·ti·nu·i·ty** (kon-ti-nu′i-tē) absence of interruption, a succession of parts intimately united, e.g., the unbroken conjunction of cells and structures that make up a single bone of the skull. Cf. contiguity. [L. *continuus,* continued]

**con·tin·u·ous am·bu·la·to·ry per·i·to·ne·al di·al·y·sis (CAPD)** method of peritoneal dialysis performed in ambulatory patients with influx and efflux of dialysate during normal activities.

**con·tin·u·ous bar re·tain·er** a metal bar, usually resting on lingual surfaces of teeth, to aid in their stabilization and to act as indirect retainers.

**con·tin·u·ous cap·il·lary** a capillary in which small vesicles (caveolae) are numerous and pores are absent.

**con·tin·u·ous flow an·a·lyz·er** an automated chemical analyzer in which the samples and reagents are pumped continuously through a system of modules interconnected by tubing.

**con·tin·u·ous in·ter·leaved sam·pling** a strategy in speech processing for cochlear implants in which brief pulses are presented to each electrode in a nonoverlapping sequence.

**con·tin·u·ous mur·mur** a murmur that is heard without interruption throughout systole and into diastole.

**con·tin·u·ous o·to·a·cou·stic e·mis·sion** a form of evoked otoacoustic emission in which the emission is of the same frequency as the stimulus and persists as long as the stimulus.

**con·tin·u·ous pos·i·tive air·way pres·sure (CPAP)** a technique of respiratory therapy, in either spontaneously breathing or mechanically ventilated patients, in which airway pressure is maintained above atmospheric pressure throughout the respiratory cycle by pressurization of the ventilatory circuit.

**con·tin·u·ous pos·i·tive pres·sure breath·ing (CPPB), con·tin·u·ous pos·i·tive pres·sure ven·ti·la·tion** SYN controlled mechanical ventilation.

**con·tin·u·ous su·ture** an uninterrupted series of

stitches using one suture; the stitching is fastened at each end by a knot. SYN uninterrupted suture.

**con·tin·u·ous train·ing** use of steady-state exercise to overload the aerobic system of energy transfer. Because of its submaximal nature, exercise continues for considerable time in relative comfort; ideal exercise for weight loss and improved health. SYN long slow distance training, LSD training.

**con·tin·u·ous wave la·ser** a laser in which energy output is constant.

**con·tour** (kon′toor) **1.** the outline of a part; the surface configuration. **2.** DENTISTRY to restore the normal outlines of a broken or otherwise misshapen tooth, or to create the external shape or form of a prosthesis. [L. *con-* (intens.), + *torno,* to turn (in a lathe), fr. *tornus,* a lathe]

△**con·tra-** opposed, against. SEE ALSO counter-. Cf. anti-. [L.]

**con·tra·an·gle** (kon′tră-ang′gl) **1.** one of the double or triple angles in the shank of an instrument by means of which the cutting edge or point is brought into the axis of the handle. **2.** an extension piece added to the end of a dental handpiece which, through a set of bevel gears, changes the angle of the axis of rotation of the bur in relation to the axis of the handpiece.

**con·tra·ap·er·ture** (kon′tră-ap′er-choor) SYN counteropening.

**con·tra·cep·tion** (kon-tră-sep′shŭn) prevention of conception or impregnation.

**con·tra·cep·tive** (kon-tră-sep′tiv) **1.** an agent for the prevention of conception. **2.** relating to any measure or agent designed to prevent conception. [L. *contra,* against, + conceptive]

**con·tra·cep·tive de·vice** a device used to prevent pregnancy; e.g., occlusive diaphragm, condom, intrauterine device.

**con·tra·cep·tive sponge** a resilient, hydrophilic sponge of polyurethane foam impregnated with a spermicide; contraception is achieved by action of the spermicide.

**con·tract** (kon-trakt′) **1.** to shorten; to become reduced in size; in the case of muscle, either to shorten or to undergo an increase in tension. **2.** to acquire by contagion or infection. **3.** (kon′trakt) an explicit bilateral commitment by psychotherapist and patient to a defined course of action to attain the goal of the psychotherapy. [L. *con-traho,* pp. *-tractus,* to draw together]

**con·tract·ed kid·ney** a diffusely scarred kidney in which fibrous tissue and ischemic atrophy lead to reduction in the size of the organ.

**con·tract·ed pel·vis** a pelvis with less than normal measurements in any diameter.

**con·trac·tile** (kon-trak′tīl) having the property of contracting.

**con·trac·til·i·ty** (kon-trak-til′i-tē) the ability or property of a substance, especially of muscle, of shortening, or becoming reduced in size, or developing increased tension.

**con·trac·tion** (C) (kon-trak′shŭn) **1.** a shortening or increase in tension; denoting the normal function of muscle. **2.** a shrinkage or reduction in size. **3.** heart beat, as in premature contraction. [L. *contractus,* drawn together]

**contraction stress test** SYN oxytocin challenge test.

**con·trac·tu·al psy·chi·a·try** psychiatric intervention voluntarily assumed by the patient, who is prompted by his personal difficulties or suffer-

ing and who retains control over his participation with the psychiatrist.

**con·trac·ture** (kon-trak′choor) static muscle shortening due to tonic spasm or fibrosis, to loss of muscular balance, the antagonists being paralyzed or to a loss of motion of the adjacent joint. [L. *contractura,* fr. *con-traho,* to draw together]

**con·tra·fis·sura** (kon′tră-fi-shyur′ă) fracture of a bone, as in the skull, at a point opposite that where the blow was received. [L. *contra,* against, counter, + *fissura,* fissure]

**con·tra·in·di·ca·tion** (kon-tră-in-di-kā′shŭn) any special symptom or circumstance that renders the use of a remedy or the carrying out of a procedure inadvisable, usually because of risk.

**con·tra·lat·er·al** (kon-tră-lat′er-ăl) relating to the opposite side, as when pain is felt or paralysis occurs on the side opposite to that of the lesion. SYN heterolateral. [L. *contra,* opposite, + *latus,* side]

**con·tra·lat·er·al hem·i·ple·gia** paralysis occurring on the side opposite to the causal central lesion.

**con·tra·lat·er·al rout·ing of sig·nals** a hearing aid configuration for greater hearing loss in one ear than the other in which sound is picked up by the microphone at the worse hearing ear and delivered to the better hearing ear.

**con·trast** (kon′trast) **1.** a comparison in which differences are demonstrated or enhanced. **2.** RADIOLOGY the difference between the image densities of two areas. [L. *contra,* against, + *sto,* pp. *status,* to stand]

**con·trast bath** a bath in which a part is immersed in hot water for a period of a few minutes and then in cold, the hot and cold periods alternated regularly at intervals, usually half-hours; used to increase the blood flow to the part.

**con·trast me·di·um** any internally administered substance that has a different opacity from soft tissue on radiography or computed tomography; used to opacify parts of the gastrointestinal tract, blood vessels, or the genitourinary tract.

**con·trast sen·si·tiv·i·ty test·ing** examination of the visual recognition of the variation in brightness of an object.

**con·trast stain** a dye used to color one portion of a tissue or cell which remained unaffected when the other part was stained by a dye of different color.

**con·tre·coup** (kawn-tr-koo′) denoting the manner of a contrafissura, as in the skull, at a point opposite that at which the blow was received. SEE ALSO contrecoup injury. [Fr. counter-blow]

**con·tre·coup in·ju·ry, con·tre·coup in·ju·ry of brain** injury occurring at a site other than that at which a blow is received, due to indirect transmission of force.

**con·trol** (kon-trōl′) **1.** (v.) to regulate, restrain, correct, restore to normal. **2.** (n.) ongoing operations or programs aimed at reducing a disease. **3.** (n.) members of a comparison group who differ in disease experience or allocation to a regimen from the subjects of a study. **4.** (v.) in statistics, to adjust or take into account extraneous influences. [Mediev. L. *contrarotulum,* a counterroll for checking accounts, fr. L. *rotula,* dim. of *rota,* a wheel]

**Con·trol of Com·mun·i·ca·ble Dis·eas·es Man·u·al** the internationally recognized authoritative manual (17th edition in the year 2000), published by the American Public Health Association.

**con·trol ex·per·i·ment** an experiment used to check another, to verify the result, or to demonstrate what would have occurred had the factor under study been omitted. SEE ALSO control.

**con·trol group** a group of subjects participating in the same experiment as another group of subjects, but which is not exposed to the variable under investigation. SEE ALSO experimental group.

**con·trolled me·chan·i·cal ven·ti·la·tion** artificial ventilation in which all inspirations are provided by positive pressure applied to the airway. SYN continuous positive pressure breathing, continuous positive pressure ventilation, intermittent positive pressure breathing, intermittent positive pressure ventilation.

**con·trolled sub·stance** a substance subject to the Controlled Substances Act (1970), which regulates the prescribing and dispensing, as well as the manufacturing, storage, sale, or distribution of substances assigned to five schedules according to their 1) potential for or evidence of abuse, 2) potential for psychic or physiologic dependence, 3) contributing a public health risk, 4) harmful pharmacologic effect, or 5) role as a precursor of other controlled substances.

**con·trol sy·ringe** a type of Luer-Lok syringe with thumb and finger rings attached to the proximal end of the barrel and to the tip of the plunger, allowing operation of the syringe with one hand. SYN ring syringe.

**con·tu·sion** (kon-too′shŭn) any mechanical injury (usually caused by a blow) resulting in hemorrhage beneath unbroken skin. SEE ALSO bruise. [L. *contusio,* a bruising]

***Co·nus*** (kō′nŭs) a genus of shellfish that inhabits the shores of some South Pacific islands. Several species are poisonous, their sting or spine causing acute pain, edema, numbness, spreading paralysis, and sometimes coma and death.

**co·nus**, pl. **co·ni** (kō′nŭs, kō′nī) **1.** SYN cone. **2.** posterior staphyloma in myopic choroidopathy. [L. fr. G. *kōnos,* cone]

**co·nus ar·te·ri·o·sus** [TA] SYN arterial cone.

**co·nus me·dul·la·ris** [TA] SYN medullary cone.

**con·va·les·cence** (kon-vă-les′ens) a period between the end of a disease and the patient's restoration to complete health. [L. *con-valesco,* to grow strong, fr. *valeo,* to be strong]

**con·va·les·cent** (kon-vă-les′ent) **1.** getting well or one who is getting well. **2.** denoting the period of convalescence.

**con·vec·tion** (kon-vek′shŭn) conveyance of heat in liquids or gases by movement of the heated particles, as when the layer of water at the bottom of a heated pot rises or the warm air of a room ascends to the ceiling. [L. *con-veho,* pp. *-vectus,* to carry or bring together]

**con·vec·tive heat** heat conveyed by a warm medium, such as air or water, in motion from its source.

**con·ven·tion·al signs** signs that acquire their function through social (linguistic) custom; e.g., words, mathematical symbols.

**con·ven·tion·al tho·ra·co·plas·ty** resection of ribs to allow inward retraction of the chest wall to reduce size of the pleural space; may be used in the treatment of empyema.

**con·ver·gence** (kon-ver′jens) **1.** the tending of

two or more objects toward a common point. **2.** the direction of the visual lines to a near point. [L. *con-vergere,* to incline together]

**con·ver·gence ex·cess** that condition in which an esophoria or esotropia is greater for near vision than for far vision.

**con·ver·gence in·suf·fi·cien·cy** that condition in which an esophoria or esotropia is more marked for far vision than for near vision.

**con·ver·gent** (kon-ver′jent) tending toward a common point.

**con·ver·gent ev·o·lu·tion** the evolutionary development of similar structures in two or more species, often widely separated phylogenetically, in response to similarities of environment; for example, the wings in insects, birds, and flying mammals.

**con·ver·gent stra·bis·mus** SYN esotropia.

**con·ver·sa·tion board** SYN communication board.

**con·ver·sion** (kon-ver′zhŭn) **1.** SYN transmutation. **2.** an unconscious defense mechanism by which the anxiety which stems from an unconscious conflict is converted and expressed symbolically as a physical symptom; transformation of an emotion into a physical manifestation, as in conversion hysteria. SEE conversion hysteria. **3.** VIROLOGY the acquisition by bacteria of a new property associated with presence of a prophage. SEE ALSO lysogeny. [L. *con-verto,* pp. *-versus,* to turn around, to change]

**con·ver·sion dis·or·der** a mental disorder in which an unconscious emotional conflict is expressed as an alteration or loss of physical functioning, usually controlled by the voluntary nervous system.

**con·ver·sion hys·te·ria** hysteria characterized by the substitution of physical signs or symptoms such as blindness, deafness, and paralysis for anxiety. SYN conversion hysteria neurosis, conversion reaction.

**con·ver·sion hys·te·ria neu·ro·sis** SYN conversion hysteria.

**con·ver·sion re·ac·tion** SYN conversion hysteria.

**con·ver·sive heat** heat produced in a body by the absorption of waves that are not in themselves hot, such as the sun's rays or infrared radiation.

**con·ver·tase** (kon′ver-tās) proteases of complement that convert one component into another. SEE component of complement.

**con·ver·tin** (kon-ver′tin) active form of factor VII designated VIIa.

**con·vex** (kon′veks, kŏn-veks′) applied to a surface that is evenly curved outward, as the segment of a sphere. [L. *convexus,* vaulted, arched, convex, fr. *con-veho,* to bring together]

**con·vex lens** a converging lens.

**con·vex·o·con·cave** (kon-vek′sō-kon′kāv) convex on one surface and concave on the opposite surface.

**con·vex·o·con·cave lens** a minus power lens having one surface convex and the opposite surface concave, with the latter having the greater curvature.

**con·vex·o·con·vex** (kon-vek′sō-kon′veks) SYN biconvex.

**con·vex·o·con·vex lens** SYN biconvex lens.

**con·vo·lut·ed part of kid·ney lob·ule** proximal and distal convoluted tubules and the associated renal corpuscles supplied by branches of the interlobular arteries. SYN renal labyrinth.

**con·vo·lu·ted sem·i·nif·er·ous tu·bule** SYN seminiferous tubule.

**con·vo·lu·ted tu·bule** either of two coiled segments of the renal tubule; the proximal convoluted tubule leads from the capsule of the kidney to the straight portion of the proximal tubule; the distal convoluted tubule is formed from the ascending limb of Henle loop and ends in a collecting tubule. SYN tubuli contorti (1).

**con·vo·lu·tion** (kon-vō-loo′shŭn) **1.** a coiling or rolling of an organ. **2.** specifically, a gyrus of the cerebral or cerebellar cortex. [L. *convolutio*]

**con·vul·sion** (kon-vŭl′shŭn) **1.** a violent spasm or series of jerkings of the face, trunk, or extremities. **2.** SYN seizure (2). [L. *convulsio*, fr. *con-vello*, pp. -*vulsus*, to tear up]

**con·vul·sive** (kon-vŭl′siv) relating to convulsions; marked by or producing convulsions.

**Cooke spec·u·lum** (kuk) a three-pronged speculum for rectal examinations and operations.

**Coo·ley a·ne·mia** (koo′lē) SYN thalassemia major.

**Coombs se·rum** (koomz) SYN antihuman globulin.

**Coombs test** (koomz) a test for antibodies, the so-called anti–human globulin test using either the direct or indirect Coombs tests.

**Coo·per her·nia** (koo′pĕr) a femoral hernia with two sacs, the first being in the femoral canal, and the second passing through a defect in the superficial fascia and appearing immediately beneath the skin. SYN Hey hernia.

**Coo·per her·ni·o·tome** (koo′pĕr) a slender bistoury with short cutting edge for dividing the constricting tissues at the neck of a hernial sac.

**Cooper-Rand art·i·fi·cial lar·ynx** (koo′pĕr-rand) an electronic device for vocal rehabilitation after laryngectomy that produces an intraoral sound articulated into speech with the pharynx, palate, tongue, lips, and teeth.

**co·or·di·na·tion** (kō-ōr′di-nā′shun) the harmonious working together of interrelated structures, especially of several muscles or muscle groups in the execution of complicated movements. [L. *co-*, together, + *ordino*, pp. -*atus*, to arrange, fr. *ordo* (*ordin-*), arrangement, order]

**Co·or·di·na·tion of Ben·e·fits (COB)** a clause in insurance policies for patients with more than one carrier to provide a maximum of 100% benefits. One carrier is designated as primary carrier; a second carrier covers any remaining costs not covered by the primary carrier.

**co-oximeter** (kō′oks-im′ĭ-ter) SYN oximeter.

**COPD** chronic obstructive pulmonary disease.

**cope** (kōp) **1.** the upper half of a flask in the casting art; hence applicable to the upper or cavity side of a denture flask. **2.** an act that enables one to adjust to the environmental circumstances.

**Cope clamp** (kōp) a clamp used in excision of colon and rectum.

**co·pol·y·mer** (kŏ′pol-i-mer) a polymer in which two or more monomers or base units are combined.

**co·pol·y·mer-1** acetate salt of a mixture of synthetic polypeptides composed of four amino acids; used to reduce the relapse rate with relapsing-remitting multiple sclerosis.

**cop·per (Cu)** (kop′er) a metallic element, atomic no. 29, atomic wt. 63.546; several of its salts are used in medicine. A bioelement found in a number of proteins. [L. *cuprum*, orig. *Cyprium*, fr. Cyprus, where it was mined]

**Cop·pet law** (kop-eh′) solutions having the same freezing point have equal concentrations of dissolved substances.

**cop·rem·e·sis** (kop-rem′ĕ-sis) SYN fecal vomiting. [G. *kopros*, dung, + emesis]

△**co·pro-** filth, dung, usually used in referring to feces. SEE ALSO scato-, sterco-. [G. *kopros*, dung]

**cop·ro·an·ti·bod·ies** (kop′rō-an′ti-bod-ēz) antibodies found in the intestine and in feces; they probably are formed by plasma cells in the intestinal mucosa and consist chiefly of the IgA class.

**cop·ro·lag·nia** (kop-rō-lag′nē-ă) a form of sexual perversion in which the thought or sight of excrement causes pleasurable sensation. [copro- + G. *lagneia*, lust]

**cop·ro·la·lia** (kop-rō-lā′lē-ă) involuntary utterances of vulgar or obscene words; seen in Gilles de la Tourette syndrome. [copro- + G. *lalia*, talk]

**cop·ro·lith** (kop′rō-lith) a hard mass consisting of inspissated feces. SYN fecalith, stercolith. [copro- + G. *lithos*, stone]

**co·prol·o·gy** (kop-rol′ō-jē) SYN scatology (1). [copro- + G. *logos*, study]

**cop·ro·ma** (kop-rō′mă) an accumulation of inspissated feces in the colon or rectum giving the appearance of an abdominal tumor. SYN fecaloma, stercoroma. [copro- + G. -*ōma*, tumor]

**cop·ro·pha·gia** (kop′rō-fā′jya) the eating of excrement.

**cop·ro·phil, cop·ro·phil·ic** (kop′rō-fil, kop-rō-fil′ik) **1.** denoting microorganisms occurring in fecal matter. **2.** relating to coprophilia. [see coprophilia]

**cop·ro·phil·ia** (kop-rō-fil′ē-ă) **1.** attraction of microorganisms to fecal matter. **2.** PSYCHIATRY a morbid attraction to, and interest in (with a sexual element), fecal matter. [copro- + G. *philos*, fond]

**cop·ro·pho·bia** (kop-rō-fō′bē-ă) morbid fear of defecation and feces. [copro- + G. *phobos*, fear]

**cop·ro·por·phyr·ia** (kop′rō-pōr-fir′ē-ă) presence of coproporphyrins in the urine, as in variegate porphyria.

**cop·ro·por·phy·rin** (kop-rō-pōr′fi-rin) one of two porphyrin compounds found normally in feces as a decomposition product of bilirubin (hence, from hemoglobin); certain corproporphyrins are elevated in certain porphyrias. SEE ALSO porphyrinogens.

**cop·ro·stas·is** (cop-rō-stā′sis) impaction of feces in the colon and sometimes the small intestine. [copro- + G. *stasis*, a standing]

**cop·u·la** (kop′yu-lă) **1.** ANATOMY a narrow part connecting two structures, e.g., the body of the hyoid bone. **2.** a swelling that is formed during the early development of the tongue by the medial portion of the second pharyngeal arch (branchial arch in fish); it is overgrown by the hypobranchial eminence and is not present in the adult tongue. [L. a bond, tie]

**cop·u·la·tion** (kop-yu-lā′shŭn) **1.** SYN coitus. **2.** in protozoology, conjugation between two cells that do not fuse but separate after mutual fertilization; observed in the ciliophora, as in *Paramecium*. [L. *copulatio*, a joining]

**cop·u·line** any of several pheromones that occur in vaginal secretions; men who were exposed to copulines rated women as more attractive, especially those women considered less attractive by controls tested with water. Copulines from ovulatory (but not menstrual or premenstrual) women caused a rise in salivary testosterone in men.

**cor**, gen. **cor·dis** (kōr, kōr'dis) [TA] SYN heart. [L.]

**cor·a·co·a·cro·mi·al** (kōr'ă-kō-ă-krō'mē-ăl) relating to the coracoid and acromial processes. SYN acromiocoracoid.

**cor·a·co·a·cro·mi·al lig·a·ment** the heavy arched fibrous band that passes between the coracoid process and the acromion above the shoulder joint; the osseofibrous arch thus formed prevents upward dislocation of the shoulder (glenohumeral) joint. SYN ligamentum coracoacromiale [TA].

**cor·a·co·bra·chi·a·lis mus·cle** origin, coracoid process of scapula; insertion, middle of medial border of humerus; action, adducts and flexes the arm; resists downward dislocation of shoulder joint; nerve supply, musculocutaneous. SYN musculus coracobrachialis [TA].

**cor·a·co·cla·vic·u·lar** (kōr'ă-kō-kla-vik'yu-lăr) relating to the coracoid process and the clavicle. SYN scapuloclavicular (2).

**cor·a·co·cla·vic·u·lar lig·a·ment** the strong ligament that unites the clavicle to the coracoid process; it is subdivided into the conoid ligament and the trapezoid ligament. The free upper limb is passively suspended from the clavicular "strut" by the coracoclavicular ligament; the ligament also plays an important role in preventing dislocation of the acromioclavicular joint. SYN ligamentum coracoclaviculare [TA].

**cor·a·co·hu·mer·al** (kōr'ă-kō-hyu'mer-ăl) relating to the coracoid process and the humerus.

**cor·a·coid** (kōr'ă-koyd) shaped like a crow's beak; denoting a process of the scapula. [G. korakōdēs, like a crow's beak, fr. korax, raven, + eidos, appearance]

**cor·a·coid pro·cess** a long curved projection from the neck of the scapula overhanging the glenoid cavity; it gives attachment to the short head of the biceps, the coracobrachialis, and the pectoralis minor muscles, and the conoid and coracoacromial ligaments.

**cor a·di·po·sum** SYN fatty heart (2).

**cor bi·loc·u·la·re** a heart in which the interatrial and interventricular septa are absent or incomplete.

**cor bovinum** SYN ox heart.

**cord** (kōrd) **1.** in anatomy, any long ropelike structure. A small, cordlike structure composed of several to many longitudinally oriented fibers, vessels, ducts, or combinations thereof. SEE ALSO chorda. **2.** in histopathology, a line of tumor cells only one cell in width. SYN funiculus [TA], funicle. [L. chorda, a string]

△**cord-** SEE chord-.

**cor·date** (kōr'dāt) heart-shaped.

**cor·date pel·vis, cor·di·form pel·vis** a pelvis with sacrum projecting forward between the ilia, giving to the brim a heart shape.

**cord blood** blood present in the umbilical vessels at the time of delivery.

**cor·dec·to·my** (kōr-dek'tō-mē) excision of a part or whole of a cord. [G. chordē, cord, + ektomē, excision]

**cor·di·form** (kōr'di-fōrm) heart-shaped. [L. cor (cord-), heart, + forma, shape]

**cor·di·form uter·us** an incomplete uterus bicor-

nis with a wedge-shaped depression at the fundus.

**cor·do·cen·te·sis** (cor-dō-cen-tē'sis) transabdominal blood sampling of the fetal umbilical cord, performed under ultrasound guidance. SYN funipuncture. [cord + G. kentēsis, puncture]

**cor·do·pexy** (kōr'dō-pek-sē) **1.** operative fixation of any displaced anatomical cord. **2.** lateral fixation of one or both vocal cords to correct glottic stenosis. [G. chordē, cord, + pēxis, fixation]

**cor·dot·o·my** (kōr-dot'ō-mē) **1.** any operation on the spinal cord. **2.** division of tracts of the spinal cord, which may be performed percutaneously (stereotactic cordotomy) or after laminectomy (open cordotomy) by various techniques such as incision or radio frequency coagulation. **3.** incision through the membranous vocal fold to widen the posterior glottis in bilateral vocal paralysis. SYN chordotomy. [G. chordē, cord, + tomē, a cutting]

△**core-, cor·e·o-, cor·o-** the pupil (of the eye). [G. korē, pupil]

**co·re·cep·tor** a cell surface protein that increases the sensitivity of the antigen receptor to antigen by binding to other ligands.

**cor·ec·to·pia** (kōr-ek-tō'pē-ă) eccentric location of the pupil so that it is not in the center of the iris. [G. korē, pupil, + ektopos, out of place]

**co·rel·y·sis** (kō-rĕl-ĭ-sis) a rarely used term for freeing of adhesions between lens capsule and the iris. [G. korē, pupil, + lysis, a loosening]

**cor·e·o·plas·ty** (kōr'ē-ō-plas-tē) the procedure to correct a misshapen, miotic, or occluded pupil. [G. korē, pupil, + plassō, to form]

**cor·e·pexy** (kōr'ĕ-peks-ē) a suturing of the iris to modify the shape or size of the pupil.

**cor·e·praxy** (kōr-e-prak'sē) a procedure designed to widen a small pupil. [G. korē, pupil, + praxis, action]

**co·re·pres·sor** (kō-rē-pres'ŏr) a molecule, usually a product of a specific metabolic pathway, that combines with and activates a repressor produced by a regulator gene. The repressor then attaches to an operator gene site and inhibits activity of the structural genes. This homeostatic mechanism regulates enzyme production in repressible enzyme systems.

**core tem·per·a·ture** the temperature of the interior of the body.

**Co·ri cy·cle** (kō'rē) the phases in the metabolism of carbohydrate: 1) glycogenolysis in the liver; 2) passage of glucose into the circulation; 3) deposition of glucose in the muscles as glycogen; 4) glycogenolysis during muscular activity and conversion to lactate, which is converted to glycogen in the liver.

**Co·ri dis·ease** (kō'rē) SYN type 3 glycogenosis.

**co·ri·um**, pl. **co·ria** (kō'rē-ŭm, kō'rē-ă) SYN dermis. [L. skin, hide, leather]

**cork·screw ves·sels** SYN hairpin vessels.

**corn** (kōrn) SYN clavus. [L. cornu, horn, hoof]

**cor·nea** (kōr'nē-ă) [TA] the transparent tissue constituting the anterior sixth of the outer wall of the eye, with a 7.7 mm radius of curvature as contrasted with the 13.5 mm of the sclera; it consists of stratified squamous epithelium continuous with that of the conjunctiva, a substantia propria, regularly arranged collagen imbedded in mucopolysaccharide, and an inner layer of endothelium. It is the chief refractory structure of the eye. [L. fem. of corneus, horny]

**cor·ne·al** (kōr′nē-ăl) relating to the cornea.

**cor·ne·al a·stig·ma·tism** astigmatism due to a defect in the curvature of the corneal surface.

**cor·ne·al cor·pus·cles** connective tissue cells found between the laminae of fibrous tissue in the cornea.

**cor·ne·al graft** SYN keratoplasty.

**cor·ne·al lay·er** SYN stratum corneum epidermidis.

**cor·ne·al pan·nus** fibrovascular connective tissue that proliferates in the anterior layers of the peripheral cornea in inflammatory corneal disease, particularly trachoma in which the pannus involves the superior cornea.

**cor·ne·al re·flex 1.** a contraction of the eyelids when the cornea is lightly touched with a camel-hair pencil; **2.** reflection of light from the surface of the cornea.

**cor·ne·al space** one of the stellate spaces between the lamellae of the cornea, each of which contains a cell or corneal corpuscle. SYN lacuna (4).

**cor·ne·al staph·y·lo·ma** SYN anterior staphyloma.

**cor·nea pla·na** a congenital disorder in which the arc curvature of the cornea is flatter than normal, leaving the eye hyperopic.

**cor·ne·o·cyte en·ve·lope** an electron-dense layer of highly cross-linked protein on the cytoplasmic surface of the cell membrane of epidermal corneocytes.

**cor·ne·o·sclera** (kōr′nē-ō-sklēr′ă) the combined cornea and sclera when considered as forming the external coat of the eyeball.

**cor·ne·o·scler·al** (kōr′nē-ō-sklēr′ăl) pertaining to the cornea and sclera.

**cor·ne·ous** (kōr′nē-ŭs) SYN horny. [L. corneus, fr. cornu, horn]

**Cor·ner tam·pon** (kor′nĕr) a plug of omentum stuffed into a wound of the stomach or intestine as a temporary tampon.

**cor·nic·u·late** (kōr-nik′yu-lāt) **1.** resembling a horn. **2.** having horns or horn-shaped appendages. [L. corniculatus, horned]

**cor·nic·u·late car·ti·lage** a conical nodule of elastic cartilage surmounting the apex of each arytenoid cartilage. SYN cartilago corniculata [TA].

**cor·nic·u·lum** (kōr-nik′yu-lŭm) a cornu of small size. [L. dim. of cornu, horn]

**cor·ni·fi·ca·tion** (kōr-ni-fi-kā′shŭn) SYN keratinization. [L. cornu, horn, + facio, to make]

**cor·nu,** gen. **cor·nus,** pl. **cor·nua** (kōr′noo, kōr′ nŭs, kōr′noo-ă) **1.** SYN horn. **2.** any structure composed of horny substance. **3.** one of the coronal extensions of the dental pulp underlying a cusp or lobe. **4.** the major subdivisions of the lateral ventricle in the cerebral hemisphere (the frontal horn, occipital horn, and temporal horn). SEE ALSO lateral ventricle. **5.** the major divisions of the gray columns of the spinal cord (anterior horn, lateral horn, posterior horn). [L. horn]

**cor·nu·al** (kōr′noo-ăl) relating to a cornu.

**cor·nu·al preg·nan·cy** the implantation and development of the impregnated ovum in one of the cornua of the uterus.

**cor·nu am·mo·nis** (am-mon′is) [TA] SYN Ammon horn.

**cor·nu an·te·ri·us** [TA] SYN anterior horn.

**cor·nu pos·te·ri·us** SYN posterior horn.

**co·ro·na,** pl. **co·ro·nae** (kō-rō′nă, kōr′ŏ-nē) [TA] SYN crown. [L. garland, crown, fr. G. korōnē]

**cor·o·nad** (kōr′ŏ-nad) in a direction toward any corona.

**co·ro·na of glans pe·nis** the prominent posterior border of the glans penis.

**cor·o·nal** (kōr′ŏ-năl) relating to a corona or the coronal plane.

🔒**cor·o·nal plane** a vertical plane at right angles to a sagittal plane, dividing the body into anterior and posterior portions. See page APP 88. SYN frontal plane.

**cor·o·nal su·ture** the line of junction of the frontal with the two parietal bones of the skull.

**co·ro·na ra·di·a·ta** [TA] **1.** a fan-shaped fiber mass on the white matter of the cerebral cortex, composed of the widely radiating fibers of the internal capsule; **2.** a single layer of columnar cells derived from the cumulus oophorus, which anchor on the pellucid zone of the oocyte in a secondary follicle. SYN radiate crown.

**cor·o·na·ri·tis** (kōr′ō-nă-rī′tis) inflammation of coronary artery or arteries.

**cor·o·nary** (kōr′o-nār-ē) **1.** relating to or resembling a crown. **2.** encircling; denoting various anatomic structures, e.g., nerves, blood vessels, ligaments. **3.** specifically, denoting the coronary blood vessels of the heart; colloquially, myocardial infarction or coronary thrombosis. [L. coronarius; fr. corona, a crown]

**cor·o·nary an·gi·og·ra·phy** imaging of the circulation of the myocardium by injection of contrast medium, usually by selective catheterization of each coronary artery, formerly by injection at the root of the aorta.

🔒**cor·o·nary ar·ter·ies 1.** right coronary artery: origin, right aortic sinus; distribution, it passes around the right side of the heart in the coronary sulcus, giving branches to the right atrium and ventricle, including the atrioventricular branches and the posterior interventricular branch. **2.** left coronary artery: origin, left aortic sinus; distribution, divides into two major branches, anterior interventricular which descends in anterior interventricular sulcus, and circumflex branch which passes to the diaphragmatic surface of left ventricle; it gives atrial, ventricular, and atrioventricular branches. See page 223.

**cor·o·nary ar·tery by·pass** conduit, usually a vein graft or internal mammary artery, surgically interposed between the aorta and a coronary artery branch to coronary shunt blood beyond an obstruction.

**cor·o·nary by·pass** vein grafts or other conduits shunting blood from the aorta to branches of the coronary arteries, to increase the flow beyond the local obstruction.

**cor·o·nary care u·nit (CCU)** a group of beds within a hospital set aside for the care of patients having or suspected of having myocardial infarction.

**cor·o·nary cat·a·ract** peripheral cortical developmental cataract occurring just after puberty; transmitted as a hereditary dominant characteristic.

**cor·o·nary fail·ure** acute coronary insufficiency.

**cor·o·nary groove** a groove on the outer surface of the heart marking the division between the atria and the ventricles.

**cor·o·nary in·suf·fi·cien·cy** inadequate coronary circulation leading to anginal pain.

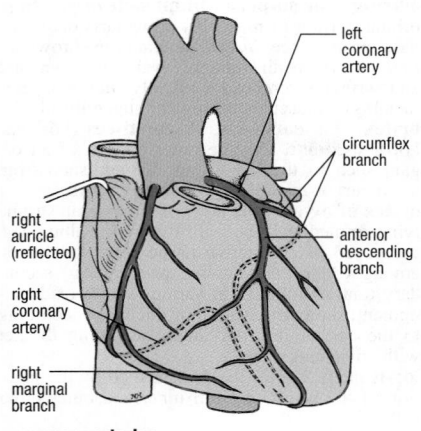

right
auricle
(reflected)

right
coronary
artery

right
marginal
branch

left
coronary
artery

circumflex
branch

anterior
descending
branch

**coronary arteries**

**cor•o•nary oc•clu•sion** blockage of a coronary vessel, usually by thrombosis or atheroma, often leading to myocardial infarction.

**cor•o•nary si•nus** a short trunk receiving most of the cardiac veins, beginning at the junction of the great cardiac vein and the oblique vein of the left atrium, running in the posterior part of the coronary sulcus and emptying into the right atrium between the inferior vena cava and the atrioventricular orifice.

**cor•o•nary throm•bo•sis** coronary occlusion by thrombus formation, usually the result of atheromatous changes in the arterial wall and usually leading to myocardial infarction.

**Co•ro•na•vir•i•dae** (kō-rō'nă-vir'i-dē) a family of single-stranded RNA-containing viruses, some of which cause upper respiratory tract infections in man similar to the "common cold." [L. *corona,* garland, crown]

**Co•ro•na•vi•rus** (kō-rō'nă-vī'rŭs) a genus in the family Coronaviridae that is associated with upper respiratory tract infections and possibly gastroenteritis in man.

**co•ro•na•vi•rus** (kō-rō'nă-vī'rŭs) any virus of the family Coronaviridae.

**cor•o•ner** (kōr'on-er) an official whose duty it is to investigate sudden, suspicious, or violent death to determine the cause; in some communities, the office has been replaced by that of medical examiner. [L. *corona,* a crown]

**cor•o•noi•dec•to•my** (kōr'ŏ-noy-dek'tō-mē) surgical removal of the coronoid process of the mandible. [coronoid + G. *ektomē,* excision]

**cor•o•noid pro•cess** a sharp triangular projection from a bone; coronoid process of the mandible, the triangular anterior process of the mandibular ramus, giving attachment to the temporal muscle; coronoid process of the ulna, a bracketlike projection from the anterior portion of the proximal extremity of the ulna; its anterior surface gives attachment to the brachialis, its proximal surface enters into the formation of the trochlear notch.

**cor•po•ra** (kōr'pōr-ă) plural of corpus.

**cor•po•ra ar•e•na•cea** small calcareous concretions in the stroma of the pineal and other central nervous system tissues. SYN psammoma bodies (2).

**cor•po•ra par•a•a•or•ti•ca** [TA] SYN paraaortic bodies.

**cor•po•re•al** (kōr-pō'rē-ăl) pertaining to the body, or to a corpus.

**corpse** (kōrps) SYN cadaver. [L. *corpus,* body]

**cor•pu•lence, cor•pu•len•cy** (kōr'pyu-lens, kōr'pyu-len-sē) SYN obesity. [L. *corpulentia,* magnification of *corpus,* body]

**cor•pu•lent** (kōr'pyu-lent) SYN obese.

**cor pul•mo•na•le** chronic cor pulmonale is characterized by hypertrophy of the right ventricle resulting from disease of the lungs; acute cor pulmonale is characterized by dilation and failure of the right side of the heart due to pulmonary embolism. In both types, characteristic electrocardiogram changes occur, and in later stages there is usually right-sided cardiac failure.

**cor•pus,** gen. **cor•po•ris,** pl. **cor•po•ra** (kōr'pŭs, kōr-pōr-is, kōr'pōr-ă) [TA] **1.** SYN body. **2.** any body or mass. **3.** the main part of an organ or other anatomic structure, as distinguished from the head or tail. SEE ALSO body, shaft, soma. [L. body]

**cor•pus al•bi•cans** [TA] a retrogressed corpus luteum, characterized by a shrinking cicatricial core surrounded by an amorphous, convoluted, completely hyalinized lutein zone. SYN albicans (2).

**cor•pus am•y•la•ce•um,** pl. **cor•po•ra am•y•la•ce•a** one of a number of small ovoid or rounded, sometimes laminated, bodies resembling a grain of starch and found in nervous tissue, in the prostate, and in pulmonary alveoli. SYN amnionic corpuscle.

**cor•pus cal•lo•sum** [TA] the great commissural plate of nerve fibers interconnecting the cortical hemispheres (with the exception of most of the temporal lobes which are interconnected by the anterior commissure). Lying at the floor of the longitudinal fissure, and covered on each side by the cingulate gyrus, it is arched from behind forward and is thick at each extremity (splenium and genu) but thinner in its long central portion (truncus); it curves back underneath itself at the genu to form the rostrum of the corpus callosum.

**cor•pus ca•ver•no•sum cli•to•ri•dis** [TA] one of the two parallel columns of erectile tissue forming the body of the clitoris; they diverge at the root to form the crura of the clitoris.

**cor•pus ca•ver•no•sum pe•nis** [TA] one of two parallel columns of erectile tissue forming the dorsal part of the body of the penis; they are separated posteriorly, forming the crura of the penis.

**cor•pus ci•li•a•re** [TA] SYN ciliary body.

**cor•pus•cle** (kōr'pŭs-l) **1.** a small mass or body. **2.** a blood cell. SYN corpusculum. [L. *corpusculum,* dim. of *corpus,* body]

**cor•pus•cu•la ar•tic•u•la•ria** [TA] SYN articular corpuscles.

**cor•pus•cu•la gen•i•ta•lia** [TA] SYN genital corpuscles.

**cor•pus•cu•la la•mel•lo•sa** [TA] SYN lamellated corpuscles.

**cor•pus•cu•lar** (kōr-pŭs'kyu-lăr) relating to a corpuscle.

**cor•pus•cu•lar ra•di•a•tion** radiation consisting of streams of subatomic particles such as protons, electrons, neutrons, etc.

**cor•pus•cu•lum,** pl. **cor•pus•cu•la** (kōr-pŭs'kyu-lŭm, kōr'pŭs-kyu-lă) SYN corpuscle.

**cor·pus·cu·lum re·nis,** pl. **cor·pus·cu·la re·nis** SYN renal corpuscle.

**cor·pus fim·bri·a·tum 1.** SYN fimbria hippocampi. **2.** the outer, ovarian extremity of the oviduct.

**cor·pus ge·ni·cu·la·tum la·te·ra·le** [TA] SYN lateral geniculate body.

**cor·pus he·mor·rha·gi·cum** a hematoma with a lining formed by the thinned-out bright yellow lutein zone; gradual resorption of the blood elements leaves a cavity filled with a clear fluid, i.e., a corpus luteum cyst.

**cor·pus lu·te·um** [TA] the yellow endocrine body formed in the ovary at the site of a ruptured ovarian follicle; a stage of proliferation and vascularization precedes full maturity; later, a bright yellow lutein zone is traversed by trabeculae of theca interna containing numerous blood vessels; the corpus luteum secretes estrogen, as did the follicle, and also secretes progesterone. If pregnancy does not occur, it is called a corpus luteum spurium, which undergoes progressive retrogression to a corpus albicans. If pregnancy does occur, it is called a corpus luteum verum, which increases in size, persisting to the fifth or sixth month of pregnancy before retrogression.

**cor·pus lu·te·um cyst** persistent corpus luteum with cyst formation.

**cor·pus lu·te·um hor·mone** SYN progesterone.

**cor·pus mam·mil·la·re** [TA] SYN mammillary body.

**cor·pus o·li·va·re** [TA] SYN oliva.

**cor·pus pi·nea·le** [TA] SYN pineal body.

**cor·pus spon·gi·o·sum pe·nis** [TA] the median column of erectile tissue located between and ventral to the two corpora cavernosa penis; posteriorly it expands into the bulbus penis and anteriorly it terminates as the enlarged glans penis; it is traversed by the urethra.

**cor·pus spon·gi·o·sum u·re·thrae mu·li·e·bris** the submucous coat of the female urethra, containing a venous network that insinuates itself between the muscular layers, giving to them an erectile nature.

**cor·pus stri·a·tum** [TA] SYN striate body.

**cor·pus vit·re·um** [TA] SYN vitreous body. SEE ALSO vitreous.

**cor·rec·tive** (kō-rek'tiv) **1.** counteracting, modifying, or changing what is injurious. **2.** a drug that modifies or corrects an undesirable or injurious effect of another drug. [L. *cor-rigo* (*conr-*), pp. *-rectus,* to set right, fr. *rego,* to keep straight]

**cor·re·spon·dence** (kŏr-ĕ-spon'dens) in optics, those points on each retina that have the same visual direction.

**Cor·ri·gan dis·ease** (kōr'i-găn) SYN aortic regurgitation.

**Cor·ri·gan sign** (kōr'i-găn) a full, hard pulse followed by a sudden collapse easily palpated and occurring in aortic regurgitation.

**cor·rin** (kōr'in) the cyclic system of four pyrrole rings forming corrinoids, which are the central structure of the vitamins $B_{12}$ and related compounds. [fr. *core* (of vitamin $B_{12}$ molecule)]

**cor·ro·sive** (kŏ-rō'siv) **1.** causing corrosion. **2.** an agent that produces corrosion; e.g., a strong acid or alkali.

**cor·ru·ga·tor** (kōr'ŭ-gā-ter) a muscle that draws together the skin, causing it to wrinkle. [L. *cor-rugo* (*conr-*), pp. *-atus,* to wrinkle, fr. *ruga,* a wrinkle]

**cor·ru·ga·tor su·per·ci·lii mus·cle** *origin,* from orbital portion of musculus orbicularis oculi and nasal prominence; *insertion,* skin of eyebrow; *action,* draws medial end of eyebrow downward and wrinkles forehead vertically; *nerve supply,* facial. SYN musculus corrugator supercilii [TA].

**cor·tex,** gen. **cor·ti·cis,** pl. **cor·ti·ces** (kōr'teks, kōr-ti-sis, kōr'ti-sēz) the outer portion of an organ, such as the kidney, as distinguished from the inner, or medullary, portion. [L. bark]

**cor·tex of o·va·ry** the layer of the ovarian stroma lying immediately beneath the tunica albuginea, composed of connective tissue cells and fibers, among which are scattered primary and secondary (antral) follicles in various stages of development; the cortex varies in thickness according to the age of the individual, becoming thinner with advancing years.

**Cor·ti arch** (kōr'tē) the arch formed by the junction of the heads of Corti inner and outer pillar cells.

**cor·ti·cal** (kōr'ti-kăl) relating to a cortex.

**cor·ti·cal ar·ter·ies** branches of the anterior, middle, and posterior cerebral arteriesy that supply the cerebral cortex.

**cor·ti·cal au·di·om·e·try** measurement of the potentials that arise in the auditory system above the level of the brainstem.

**cor·ti·cal blind·ness** loss of sight due to an organic lesion in the visual cortex.

**cor·ti·cal bone** the superficial thin layer of compact bone. SYN substantia corticalis [TA], cortical substance.

**cor·ti·cal cat·a·ract** a cataract in which the opacity affects the cortex of the lens.

**cor·ti·cal deaf·ness** deafness resulting from bilateral lesions of the primary receptive area of the temporal lobe.

**cor·ti·cal hor·mones** steroid hormones produced by the adrenal cortex.

**cor·ti·cal lob·ules of kid·ney** one of the subdivisions of the kidney, consisting of a medullary ray and that portion of the convoluted port (renal corpuscles and convoluted tubules) associated with its collecting duct.

**cor·ti·cal ra·di·ate ar·te·ries** the branches of the arcuate arteries of the kidney radiating outward through the renal columns and cortex and supplying the glomeruli.

**cor·ti·cal sub·stance** SYN cortical bone.

**Cor·ti ca·nal** (kōr'tē) SYN Corti tunnel.

**Cor·ti cells** (kōr'tē) SYN cochlear hair cells.

**cor·ti·ces** (kōr'ti-sēz) plural of cortex.

**cor·ti·cif·u·gal, cor·ti·cof·u·gal** (kōr-ti-sif'yu-găl, kōr'ti-kō-fyu'găl) passing in a direction away from the outer surface; denoting especially nerve fibers conveying impulses away from the cerebral cortex. [L. *cortex,* rind, bark, + *fugio,* to flee]

**cor·ti·cip·e·tal** (kōr-ti-sip'e-tăl) passing in a direction toward the outer surface; denoting nerve fibers conveying impulses toward the cerebral cortex. [L. *cortex,* rind, bark, + *peto,* to seek]

**cor·ti·co·ba·sal de·gen·er·a·tion** a rare, progressive disease involving both cerebral cortex and extrapyramidal structures; clinically manifested as disturbances of voluntary movements and rigidity; pathologic characteristics include degeneration of the cerebral cortex with balloon neurons and degeneration of the substantia nigra.

**cor·ti·co·bul·bar** (kōr'ti-kō-bŭl'bar) pertaining to corticofugal fibers projecting to the rhombencephalon that terminate 1) directly on some motor cranial nerve nuclei, 2) in the reticular formation, or 3) on sensory relay nuclei, such as the cuneate, gracile, and spinal trigeminal nucleus.

**cor·ti·coid** (kōr′ti-koyd) **1.** having an action similar to that of a hormone of the adrenal cortex. **2.** any substance exhibiting this action. **3.** SYN corticosteroid.

**cor·ti·co·lib·er·in** (kōr′ti-kō-lib′er-in) SYN corticotropin-releasing hormone. [corticosteroid + L. *libero,* to free, + -in]

**cor·ti·co·ste·roid** (kōr′ti-kō-stēr′oyd) a steroid produced by the adrenal cortex (i.e., adrenal corticoid); a corticoid containing a steroid. SYN corticoid (3).

**cor·ti·co·ste·roid-bind·ing glob·u·lin (CBG)** SYN transcortin.

**cor·ti·co·troph** (kōr′ti-kō-trof) a cell of the adenohypophysis that produces adrenocorticotropic hormone (ACTH).

**cor·ti·co·tro·pin** (kōr′ti-kō-trō′pin) **1.** SYN adrenocorticotropic hormone. **2.** SYN β-corticotropin. [G. *tropē,* a turning]

β-**cor·ti·co·tro·pin** acid- or pepsin-degraded β-corticotropin. SYN corticotropin (2).

**cor·ti·co·trop·in-like in·ter·me·di·ate-lobe pep·tide (CLIP)** product of propiomelanocortin with unknown function.

**cor·ti·co·tro·pin-re·leas·ing fac·tor (CRF)** SYN corticotropin-releasing hormone.

**cor·ti·co·tro·pin-re·leas·ing hor·mone (CRH)** a factor secreted by the hypothalamus that stimulates the pituitary to release adrenocorticotropic hormone. SYN corticoliberin, corticotropin-releasing factor.

**Cor·ti·co·vi·rus** only genus in family of Corticoviridae.

**cor·ti·lymph** (kōr′tē-limf) the fluid in Corti tunnel.

**Cor·ti mem·brane** (kōr′tē) SYN tectorial membrane of cochlear duct.

**Cor·ti or·gan** (kōr′tē) SYN spiral organ.

**cor·ti·sol** (kōr′ti-sol) SYN hydrocortisone.

**cor·ti·sone** (kōr′ti-sōn) a glucocorticoid not normally secreted in significant quantities by the human adrenal cortex. It exhibits no biological activity until converted to hydrocortisone (cortisol); it acts upon carbohydrate metabolism and influences the nutrition and growth of connective (collagenous) tissues.

**Cor·ti tun·nel** (kōr′tē) the spiral canal in the organ of Corti, formed by the outer and inner pillar cells or rods of Corti; it is filled with fluid and occasionally crossed by nonmedullated nerve fibers. SYN Corti canal.

**cor tri·at·ri·a·tum** a heart with three atrial chambers, the left atrium being subdivided by a transverse septum with a single small opening which separates the openings of the pulmonary veins from the mitral valve.

**cor tri·lo·cu·la·re** three-chambered heart due to absence of the interatrial or the interventricular septum.

**Cor·vi·sart fa·ci·es** (kor′vē-sahr′) the characteristic facies seen in cardiac insufficiency or aortic regurgitation; a swollen, purplish, cyanotic face with shiny eyes and puffy eyelids; nonspecific.

**co·rym·bi·form** (kŏ-rim′bi-fōrm) denoting the flower-like clustering configuration of skin lesions in granulomatous diseases (e.g., syphilis, tuberculosis). [L. *corymbus,* cluster, garland]

**Cor·y·ne·bac·te·ri·um** (kŏ-rī′nē-bak-tēr′ē-ŭm) a genus of nonmotile (except for some plant pathogens), aerobic to anaerobic bacteria (family Corynebacteriaceae) containing irregularly staining, Gram-positive, straight to slightly curved, often club-shaped rods which, as a result of snapping division, show a picket fence arrangement. These organisms are widely distributed in nature. The best known species are parasites and pathogens of humans and domestic animals. The type species is *Corynebacterium diphtheriae.* [G. *coryne,* a club, + *bacterium,* a small rod]

**cor·y·ne·bac·te·ri·um,** pl. **cor·y·ne·bac·te·ria** (kŏ-rī′nē-bak-tēr′ē-ŭm, kŏ-rī′nē-bak-tēr′ē-ă) a vernacular term used to refer to any member of the genus *Corynebacterium.*

**Cor·y·ne·bac·te·ri·um am·y·co·la·tum** a species found as normal skin flora, it causes septicemia, frequently associated with venous access devices, and has also been recovered from urinary tract infections and mixed flora abscesses.

**Cor·y·ne·bac·te·ri·um diph·the·ri·ae** type species of the genus *Corynebacterium,* the cause of diphtheria. It induces a severe membranous pharyngitis and produces an exotoxin that damages myocardium and other tissues; may also infect superficial wounds; an asymptomatic carrier state is common. SYN Loeffler bacillus.

**Cor·y·ne·bac·te·ri·um glu·cu·ron·o·ly·ti·cum** a species isolated from patients with urinary tract infections.

**Cor·y·ne·bac·te·ri·um jei·kei·um** species associated with septicemia and skin lesions in immunocompromised patients, especially associated with venous access devices.

**Cor·y·ne·bac·te·ri·um ma·tru·cho·ti·i** a species recovered in mixed infections from human eye specimens.

**co·ry·za** (kŏ-rī′ză) SYN acute rhinitis. [G.]

**Co·ry·za·vi·rus** (kŏ-rī′ză-vī′rŭs) former name for *Rhinovirus.*

**cos·me·sis** (koz-mē′sis) a concern in therapeutics, especially in surgical operations, for the appearance of the patient. [G. *kosmēsis,* an adorning, fr. *kosmeō,* to order, arrange, adorn, fr. *kosmos,* order]

**cos·met·ic** (koz-met′ik) **1.** relating to cosmesis. **2.** relating to the use of cosmetics.

**cos·met·ics** (koz-met′iks) composite term for a variety of adornments and camouflages applied to the skin, lips, hair, and nails in accordance with cultural dictates.

**cos·met·ic sur·gery** surgery in which the principal purpose is to improve the appearance, usually with the connotation that the improvement sought is beyond the normal appearance, and its acceptable variations, for the age and the ethnic origin of the patient.

**cos·mo·pol·i·tan** (koz-mō-pol′i-tan) BIOLOGICAL SCIENCES a term denoting worldwide distribution. [G. *kosmos,* universe, + *polis,* city-state]

**cos·ta,** gen. and pl. **cos·tae** (kos′tă, kos′tē) [TA] **1.** SYN rib. **2.** a rodlike internal supporting organelle that runs along the base of the undulating membrane of certain flagellate parasites such as *Trichomonas.* SYN basal rod. [L.]

**cos·ta cer·vi·ca·lis** [TA] SYN cervical rib.

**cos·tae fluc·tu·an·tes [XI–XII]** [TA] SYN floating ribs [XI–XII].

**cos·tae spu·ri·ae** [TA] SYN false ribs.

**cos·tae ve·rae** [TA] SYN true ribs [I–VII].

**cos·tal** (kos′tăl) relating to a rib.

**cos·tal an·gle** the rather abrupt change in curvature of the body of a rib posteriorly, such that the neck and head of the rib are directed upward. SYN angulus costae [TA].

**cos·tal arch** that portion of the inferior aperture of the thorax formed by the articulated cartilages of the seventh to tenth (false) ribs.

**cos·tal car·ti·lage** the cartilage forming the anterior continuation of a rib, providing the means by which it reaches and articulates with the sternum. SYN cartilago costalis [TA].

**cos·tal·gia** (kos-tal′jē-ă) SYN pleurodynia. [L. *costa,* rib, + G. *algos,* pain]

**cos·tec·to·my** (kos-tek′tō-mē) excision of a rib. [L. *costa,* rib, + G. *ektomē,* excision]

**co·stim·u·la·tory mol·e·cule** membrane-bound or secreted product of accessory cells that is required for signal transduction.

△**cos·to-** the ribs. [L. *costa,* rib]

**cos·to·ax·il·lary vein** one of a number of anastomotic veins connecting the intercostal veins of the first to seventh intercostal spaces with the lateral thoracic or the thoracoepigastric vein.

**cos·to·cer·vi·cal trunk, cos·to·cer·vi·cal ar·ter·y** a short artery that arises from the subclavian artery on each side and divides into deep cervical and superior intercostal branches, the latter dividing usually to form the first and second posterior intercostal arteries. SYN truncus costocervicalis [TA].

**cos·to·chon·dral** (kos-tō-kon′drăl) relating to the costal cartilages. SYN chondrocostal.

**cos·to·chon·dri·tis** (kos′tō-kon-drī′tis) inflammation of one or more costal cartilages, characterized by local tenderness and pain of the anterior chest wall that may radiate, but without the local swelling typical of Tietze syndrome. [costo- + G. *chondros,* cartilage, + *-itis,* inflammation]

**cos·to·cla·vic·u·lar** (kos-tō-klă-vik′yu-lăr) relating to the ribs and the clavicle.

**cos·to·cla·vic·u·lar lig·a·ment** the ligament that connects the first rib and the clavicle near its sternal end; limits elevation of shoulder (at sternoclavicular joint). SYN ligamentum costoclaviculare [TA], rhomboid ligament.

**cos·to·cor·a·coid** (kos-tō-kōr′ă-koyd) relating to the ribs and the coracoid process of the scapula.

**cos·to·gen·ic** (kos-tō-jen′ik) arising from a rib.

**cos·to·phren·ic an·gle** the angle between the costal and diaphragmatic parietal pleura as they meet at the costodiaphragmatic line of pleura reflection. Used as a synonym in radiology to identify the costodiaphragmatic recess.

**cos·to·scap·u·lar** (kos-tō-skap′yū-lăr) relating to the ribs and the scapula.

**cos·to·ster·nal** (kos-tō-ster′năl) pertaining to the ribs and the sternum.

**cos·to·ster·no·plas·ty** (kos-tō-ster′nō-plas-tē) operation to correct a malformation of the anterior chest wall. [costo- + G. *sternon,* chest, + *plastos,* formed]

**cos·tot·o·my** (kos-tot′ō-mē) division of a rib. [costo- + G. *tomē,* a cutting]

**cos·to·trans·verse** (kos-tō-trans-vers′) relating to the ribs and the transverse processes of the vertebrae articulating with them.

**cos·to·trans·ver·sec·to·my** (kos′tō-tranz-ver-sek′tō-mē) excision of a proximal portion of a rib and the articulating transverse process.

**cos·to·trans·verse lig·a·ment** the ligament that connects the dorsal aspect of the neck of a rib to the ventral aspect of the corresponding transverse process. SYN ligamentum costotransversarium [TA].

**cos·to·ver·te·bral** (kos-tō-ver′tĕ-brăl) relating to the ribs and the bodies of the thoracic vertebrae with which they articulate. SYN vertebrocostal (1).

**cos·to·ver·te·bral an·gle** the acute angle formed between either twelfth rib and the vertebral column.

**cos·to·xi·phoid** (kos-tō-zī′foyd) relating to the ribs and the xiphoid cartilage of the sternum.

**Co·tard syn·drome** (kō-tahr′) psychotic depression involving delusion of the existence of one's body, along with ideas of negation and suicidal impulses.

**Côte-d'Ivoire virus** (kōt dē-vwah) a variant of Ebola virus. SYN Ebola virus Côte-d'Ivoire.

**co·throm·bo·plas·tin** (ko-throm-bo-plas-tin) SYN factor VII.

**co·trans·port** (kō-trans′pōrt) the transport of one substance across a membrane, coupled with the simultaneous transport of another substance across the same membrane in the same direction.

**Cot·te op·er·a·tion** (kot) SYN presacral neurectomy.

**cot·ton-fi·ber em·bo·lism** embolism by cotton fibers from sterile gauze used in intravenous medication or transfusion; may form as foreign body granulomas in small pulmonary arteries.

**cot·ton-wool patch·es** white, fuzzy areas on the surface of the retina (accumulations of cellular organelles) caused by damage (usually infarction) of the retinal fiber layer.

**cot·y·le·don** (kot-i-lē′don) **1.** in plants, a seed leaf, the first leaf to grow from a seed. **2.** a placental unit. [G. *kotylēdon,* any cup-shaped hollow]

**cot·y·loid** (kot′i-loyd) **1.** cup-shaped; cuplike. **2.** relating to the cotyloid cavity or acetabulum. [G. *kotylē,* a small cup, + *eidos,* appearance]

**cot·y·loid cav·i·ty** SYN acetabulum.

**cot·y·loid joint** SYN ball-and-socket joint.

**cough** (kawf) **1.** a sudden expulsion of air through the glottis, occurring immediately on opening the previously closed glottis, and excited by mechanical or chemical irritation of the trachea or bronchi, or by pressure from adjacent structures. **2.** to force air through the glottis by a series of expiratory efforts. [echoic]

**cough re·flex** the reflex which mediates coughing in response to irritation of the larynx or tracheobronchial tree.

**cou·lomb (C, Q)** (koo-lom′) the unit of electrical charge, equal to $3 \times 10^9$ electrostatic units; the quantity of electricity delivered by a current of 1 ampere in 1 second; equal to 1/96,485 faraday. [C. A. de *Coulomb,* Fr. physicist, 1736–1806]

**cou·lom·e·try** (koo-lŏm′ĕt-rē) a titration technique in which the titrant is electrochemically generated. The $Ag^+$ titrant in the chloridometer is commonly used to determine the concentration of chloride in the sample. [coulomb + -metry]

**Cou·mel tach·y·car·dia** (koo-mā′) a persistent junctional reciprocating tachycardia that usually uses a slowly conducting posteroseptal pathway for the retrograde journey.

**coun·sel·ing** (kown-sel-ing) a professional relationship and activity in which one person endeavors to help another to understand and to solve his or her adjustment problems; the giving of advice, opinion, and instruction to direct the judgment or conduct of another. SEE psychotherapy. [L. *consilium,* deliberation]

**coun·sel·ling [Br.]** SEE counseling.

**count** (kownt) **1.** a tally of instruments and materials performed at the beginning of a surgical operation and again before the incision is closed, to ensure that no foreign object remains in the patient. **2.** to enumerate or score.

**count·er** (kown′ter) a device that counts.

△**count·er-** opposite, opposed, against. SEE ALSO contra-. [L. *contra,* against]

**count·er·con·di·tion·ing** (kown′ter-kon-dish′ŭn-ing) any behavior therapy in which a second conditioned response (e.g., approaching or even touching a snake) is introduced for the purpose of counteracting or nullifying a previously conditioned or learned response (e.g., fear and avoidance of snakes).

**count·er·cur·rent mech·a·nism** a system in the renal medulla that facilitates concentration of the urine as it passes through the renal tubules.

**count·er·ex·ten·sion** (kown′ter-eks-ten′shŭn) SYN countertraction.

**count·er·im·mu·no·e·lec·tro·pho·re·sis** (kown′ter-im′yu-nō-ē-lek′trō-fōr-ē′sis) immunoelectrophoresis in which antigen is placed in wells cut in the sheet of agar gel toward the cathode, and antiserum is placed in wells toward the anode; antigen and antibody, moving in opposite directions, form precipitates in the area between the cells where they meet in concentrations of optimal proportions.

**count·er·in·ci·sion** (kown′ter-in-sizh′ŭn) a second incision adjacent to a primary incision.

**count·er·ir·ri·tant** (kown-ter-ir′i-tant) **1.** an agent that causes irritation or a mild inflammation of the skin in order to relieve symptoms of a deep-seated inflammatory process. **2.** relating to or producing counterirritation.

**count·er·ir·ri·ta·tion** (kown′ter-ir-i-tā′shŭn) irritation or mild inflammation (redness, vesication, or pustulation) of the skin excited for the purpose of relieving symptoms of an inflammation of the deeper structures. SYN revulsion (1).

**count·er·o·pen·ing** (kown′ter-ō-pen-ing) a second opening made at the dependent part of an abscess or other cavity containing fluid, which is not draining satisfactorily through an opening previously made. SYN contraaperture, counterpuncture.

**count·er·pul·sa·tion** (kown′ter-pŭl-sā′shŭn) a means of assisting the failing heart by automatically removing arterial blood just before and during ventricular ejection and returning it to the circulation during diastole; a balloon catheter is inserted into the aorta and activated by an automatic mechanism triggered by the ECG.

**count·er·punc·ture** (kown′ter-pŭnk-cher) SYN counteropening.

**count·er·shock** (kown′ter-shok) an electric shock applied to the heart to terminate a disturbance of its rhythm.

**count·er·stain** (kown′ter-stān) a second stain of a different color, having affinity for tissues, cells, or parts of cells other than those taking the primary stain, used to render more distinct the parts taking the first stain.

**count·er·trac·tion** (kown-ter-trak′shŭn) the resistance, or back-pull, made to traction or pulling on a limb; e.g., in the case of traction made on the leg, countertraction may be effected by raising the foot of the bed so that the weight of the body pulls against the weight attached to the limb. SYN counterextension.

**count·er·trans·fer·ence** (kown′ter-trans-fer′ens) PSYCHOANALYSIS the analyst's transference (often unconscious) toward the patient of his or her emotional needs and feelings, with personal involvement to the detriment of the desired objective analyst-patient relationship.

**count·er·trans·port** (kown-ter-tranz′pōrt) the transport of one substance across a membrane, coupled with the simultaneous transport of another substance across the same membrane in the opposite direction.

**count·ing cham·ber** a standardized ruled-glass slide used for counting cells (especially erythrocytes and leukocytes) and other particulate material in a measured volume of fluid; such slides are frequently known as hemocytometers.

**coup de glotte** SYN glottal attack.

**coup in·ju·ry of brain** an injury occurring directly beneath the skull at the area of impact.

**cou·ple** (kŭ′pl) to copulate; to perform coitus; said especially of the lower animals.

**cou·pled pulse** SYN bigeminal pulse.

**cou·pled rhy·thm** SYN bigeminal rhythm.

**cou·pling** (kŭp′ling) **1.** the repeated pairing of a normal sinus beat with a ventricular extrasystole. **2.** a condition in which one or more products of a reaction are the subsequent reactants (or substrates) of a second reaction.

**cou·pling fac·tors** proteins that restore phosphorylating ability to mitochondria that have lost it.

**Cour·nand dip** (koor-nahn′) in constrictive pericarditis, rapid early diastolic fall and reascent of the ventricular pressure curve to an elevated plateau (square root configuration).

**Cour·voi·sier gall·blad·der** (koor-vwah′zē-ā′) an enlarged, often palpable gallbladder in a patient with carcinoma of the head of the pancreas. It is associated with jaundice due to obstruction of the common bile duct. SEE Courvoisier law.

**Cour·voi·sier law** (koor-vwah′zē-ā′) painless enlargement of the gallbladder with jaundice is likely to result from carcinoma of the head of the pancreas and not from a stone in the common duct, because in the latter the gallbladder is usually scarred from infection and does not distend.

**cou·vade** (koo-vahd′) a primitive custom in certain cultures in which a man develops labor pains while his wife is in labor and then submits to the same postpartum purification rites and taboos. [Fr. *couver,* to hatch]

**Cou·ve·laire uter·us** (koo-vĕ-lār′) extravasation of blood into the uterine musculature and beneath the uterine peritoneum in association with severe forms of abruptio placentae.

**co·va·lent** (kō-vāl′ent) denoting an interatomic bond characterized by the sharing of 2, 4, or 6 electrons.

**cov·er·age** (kov′er-ej) a measure of the extent to which the services rendered cover the potential need for these services in a community; applied specifically to such services as immunization in developing countries.

**cov·ert sen·si·ti·za·tion** aversive conditioning or training to abolish an unwanted behavior, during which the patient is taught to imagine unpleasant and related aversive consequences while engaging in the unwanted habit.

**cov•er-un•cov•er test** a test to detect strabismus; the patient's attention is directed to a small fixation object, one eye is covered and after a few seconds, uncovered; if the uncovered eye moves to see the picture, strabismus is present.

**Cow•den dis•ease** (kow'dĕn) hypertrichosis and gingival fibromatosis from infancy, accompanied by postpubertal fibroadenomatous breast enlargement; papules of the face are characteristic of multiple trichilemmomas.

**Cow•dry type A in•clu•sion bod•ies** (kow'drē) dropletlike masses of acidophilic material surrounded by clear halos within nuclei, with margination of chromatin on the nuclear membrane as seen in human herpesvirus–infected cells.

**Cow•dry type B in•clu•sion bod•ies** (kow'drē) obsolete term for dropletlike masses of acidophilic material surrounded by clear halos within nuclei, without other nuclear changes during early stages of development of the inclusion as seen in poliomyelitis.

**Cow•per cyst** (kow'per) a retention cyst of a bulbourethral gland.

**Cow•per gland** (kow'per) SYN bulbourethral gland.

**cow•per•i•an** (kow-pēr'ē-an) relating to or described by Cowper.

**cow•per•i•tis** (kow-per-ī'tis) inflammation of Cowper gland.

**coxa**, gen. and pl. **cox•ae** (kok'să, kok'sē) **1.** SYN hip bone. **2.** SYN hip joint. [L]

**cox•al•gia** (koks-al'jē-ă) SYN coxodynia. [L. *coxa,* hip, + G. *algos,* pain]

**cox•a mag•na** enlargement, and often deformation of the femoral head; usually refers to a sequela of Legg-Calvé-Perthes disease or osteoarthritis.

**cox•a val•ga** alteration of the angle made by the axis of the femoral neck to the axis of the femoral shaft, so that the angle exceeds 135°; the femoral neck is in more of a straight-line relationship to the shaft of the femur.

**cox•a va•ra** alteration of the angle made by the axis of the femoral neck to the axis of the femoral shaft so that the angle is less than 135°; the femoral neck becomes more horizontal.

**Cox•i•el•la** (kok-sē-el'ă) a genus of filterable bacteria (order Rickettsiales) containing small, pleomorphic, rod-shaped or coccoid, Gram-negative cells which occur intracellularly in the cytoplasm of infected cells and possibly extracellularly in infected ticks. These organisms have not been cultivated in cell-free media; they are parasitic on man and other animals. The type species is *Coxiella burnetii.* [H. R. Cox, U.S. bacteriologist, *1907]

**Cox•i•el•la bur•ne•ti•i** a species that causes Q fever in man; it is more resistant than other rickettsiae and may be passed via aerosols as well as living vectors. Acute pneumonia and chronic endocarditis are also associated with this species. The type species of the genus *Coxiella.*

**cox•o•dyn•ia** (koks-ō-din'ē-ă) pain in the hip joint. SYN coxalgia. [L. *coxa,* hip, + G. *odynē,* pain]

**cox•o•fem•o•ral** (kok-sō-fem'ŏ-răl) relating to the hip bone and the femur.

**cox•o•tu•ber•cu•lo•sis** (koks'ō-too-ber-kyu-lō' sis) tuberculous hip-joint disease.

**Cox•sack•ie en•ceph•a•li•tis** a viral encephalitis, seen mainly in infants and involving principally the gray matter of the medulla and cord, caused by *Enterovirus* Coxsackie B.

**Cox•sack•ie•vi•rus, Cox•sack•ie vi•rus** (kok-sak'ē-vī'rŭs) a group of picornaviruses causing myositis, paralysis, and death in young mice, and responsible for a variety of diseases in man, although inapparent infections are common. They are divided antigenically into two groups, A and B, each of which includes a number of serological types. Type A viruses cause herpangina and hand-foot-and-mouth disease; type B viruses cause epidemic pleurodynia; both type viruses may cause aseptic meningitis, myocarditis and pericarditis, and acute onset juvenile diabetes. [*Coxsackie,* N.Y., where first isolated]

**CPAP** continuous positive airway pressure.

**CPITN** Community Periodontal Index of Treatment Needs.

**CPPB** continuous positive pressure breathing.

**CPR** cardiopulmonary resuscitation; computer-based patient record.

**cps** cycles per second.

**CPT** Current Procedural Terminology.

**Cr** conditioned reflex; crown-rump length.

**Cr 1.** chromium. **2.** creatinine.

**crack** (krăk) **1.** a fissure. **2.** SEE crack cocaine. [slang]

**crack co•caine** a derivative of cocaine, usually smoked, producing brief, intense euphoria. Crack cocaine is relatively inexpensive and extremely addictive; dependency can develop in less than 2 weeks. Like snorted or injected cocaine, it has both acute and chronic adverse effects, including heart and nasopharyngeal damage, seizures, sudden death, and psychosis. SEE ALSO street drug.

**cracked heel** SYN keratoderma plantare sulcatum.

**crac•kle** (krak'l) short, sharp, or rough sounds heard with a stethoscope over the chest. Most often heard in pleurisy with fibrinous exudate. [echoic]

**cra•dle** (krā'dl) a frame used to keep bedclothes from coming in contact with a patient. [M.E. *cradel*]

**cra•dle cap** colloquialism for seborrheic dermatitis of the scalp of the newborn.

**cramp** (kramp) **1.** a painful muscle spasm caused by prolonged tetanic contraction. **2.** a localized muscle spasm related to occupational use, qualified according to the occupation of the sufferer; e.g., writer's cramp. [M.E. *crampe,* fr. O. Fr., fr. Germanic]

**Cramp•ton test** (kramp'tŏn) a test for physical condition and resistance; a record is made of the pulse and the blood pressure in the recumbent and in the standing position, and the difference is graded from the theoretical perfection of 100 (seldom attained) downward (a reading of 75 is considered excellent, 65 poor).

**Cran•dall syn•drome** (kran'dăl) characterized by pili torti, sensorineural deafness, and hypogonadism; a familial trait in which there is a deficiency of luteinizing and growth hormones. SEE ALSO Björnstad syndrome.

**cra•nia** (krā'nē-ă) plural of cranium.

**cra•ni•ad** (krā'nē-ad) situated nearer the head in relation to a specific reference point; opposite of caudad. SEE ALSO superior.

**cra•ni•al** (krā'nē-ăl) **1.** relating to the cranium or

head. SYN cephalic. SEE ALSO cephalad. **2.** SYN superior (2).

**cra·ni·al a·rach·noid ma·ter** that portion of the arachnoid that lies within the cranial cavity and surrounds the brain and the cranial portion of the subarachnoid space. In several sites it is relatively widely separated from the pia mater, creating the cranial subarachnoid cisterns. SYN arachnoidea mater cranialis [TA], arachnoid of brain, arachnoidea mater encephali.

**cra·ni·al ar·te·ri·tis** SYN temporal arteritis.

**cra·ni·al bones** SYN bones of skull.

**cra·ni·al cav·i·ty** the space within the skull occupied by the brain, its coverings, and cerebrospinal fluid. SYN intracranial cavity.

**cra·ni·al flex·ure** SYN cephalic flexure.

**cra·ni·al nerves** those nerves that emerge from, or enter, the cranium or skull, in contrast to the spinal nerves, which emerge from the spine or vertebral column. The twelve paired cranial nerves are the olfactory, optic, oculomotor, trochlear, trigeminal, abducent, facial, vestibulocochlear, glossopharyngeal, vagal, accessory, and hypoglossal nerves. See this page. SYN nervi craniales [TA].

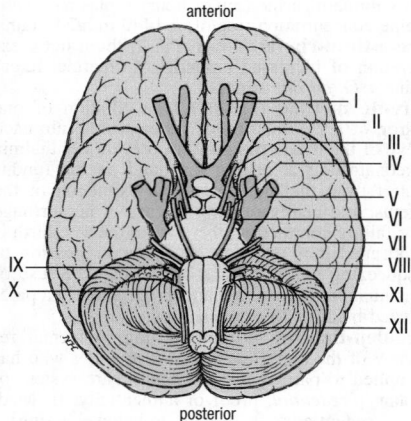

anterior

posterior

**cranial nerves:** (inferior view): (I) olfactory, (II) optic, (III) oculomotor, (IV) trochlear, (V) trigeminal, (VI) abducens, (VII) facial, (VIII) vestibulocochlear, (IX) glossopharyngeal, (X) vagus, (XI) accessory, (XII) hypoglossal

**cra·ni·al pia ma·ter** the pia mater found specifically around the brain; contiguous with the arachnoid mater via the arachnoid trabeculae. SEE ALSO pia mater. SYN pia mater encephali [TA].

**cra·ni·al root of ac·ces·so·ry nerve** the roots of the accessory nerve which arise from the medulla; the nerve fibers of the cranial root join the intracranial portion of the vagus nerve and are distributed to the pharyngeal plexus, providing the motor innervation of the soft palate (except the tensor veli palati) and the pharynx.

**cra·ni·al su·tures** the sutures between the bones of the skull.

**cra·ni·al ver·te·bra** a segment of the skull regarded as homologous with a segment of the vertebral column.

**cra·ni·ec·to·my** (krā′nē-ek′tō-mē) excision of a portion of the skull. [G. *kranion*, skull, + *ektomē*, excision]

**cra·ni·o-, cra·ni-** the cranium. Cf. cerebro-. [G. *kranion*, skull]

**cra·ni·o·cele** (krā′nē-ō-sēl) SYN encephalocele. [cranio- + G. *kēlē*, hernia]

**cra·ni·o·ce·re·bral** (krā′nē-ō-ser′ē-brăl) relating to the skull and the brain.

**cra·ni·o·fa·cial** (krā′nē-ō-fā′shăl) relating to both the face and the cranium.

**cra·ni·o·fa·cial dys·junc·tion frac·ture** a complex fracture in which the facial bones are separated from the cranial bones.

**cra·ni·o·fe·nes·tria** (krā′nē-ō-fe-nes′trē-ă) SYN craniolacunia. [cranio- + L. *fenestra*, window]

**cra·ni·o·la·cu·nia** (krā′nē-ō-lă-koo′nē-ă) incomplete formation of the bones of the vault of the fetal skull so that there are nonossified areas in the calvaria. SYN craniofenestria. [cranio- + L. *lacuna*, cleft]

**cra·ni·o·ma·la·cia** (krā′nē-ō-mă-lā′shē-ă) softening of the bones of the skull. [cranio- + G. *malakia*, softness]

**cra·ni·o·met·ric points** fixed points on the skull used as landmarks in craniometry.

**cra·ni·op·a·thy** (krā-nē-op′ă-thē) any pathological condition of the cranial bones. [cranio- + G. *pathos*, suffering]

**cra·ni·o·pha·ryn·ge·al** (krā′nē-ō-fă-rin′jē-ăl) relating to the skull and to the pharynx.

**cra·ni·o·pha·ryn·gi·o·ma** (krā′nē-ō-fă-rin-jē-ō′mă) a suprasellar neoplasm that develops from Rathke pouch; the histologic pattern consists of nesting of squamous epithelium bordered by radially arranged cells. SYN Rathke pouch tumor. [cranio- + pharyngio- + -oma]

**cra·ni·o·plas·ty** (krā′nē-ō-plas-tē) plastic surgery of the skull; a surgical correction of a skull defect. [cranio- + G. *plastos*, formed]

**cra·ni·o·punc·ture** (krā′nē-ō-pŭnk′choor) puncture of the brain for exploratory purposes.

**cra·ni·or·rha·chis·chi·sis** (krā′nē-ō-ră-kis′ki-sis) severe congenital malformation in which there is incomplete closure of the skull and vertebral column. [cranio- + G. *rhachis*, spine, + *schisis*, a cleaving]

**cra·ni·o·sa·cral** (krā′nē-ō-sā′krăl) denoting the cranial and sacral origins of the parasympathetic division of the autonomic nervous system.

**cra·ni·o·sac·ral ther·a·py** a bodywork modality that focuses on identifying and resolving restrictions in the dural sheath which are said to cause restrictions in fascia throughout the body. Practitioners perform therapy by means of palpation of the theoretical but unproven and unmeasurable rhythmic movements of cerebrospinal fluid.

**cra·ni·os·chi·sis** (krā-nē-os′ki-sis) congenital malformation in which there is incomplete closure of the skull. Usually accompanied by grossly defective development of the brain. [cranio- + G. *schisis*, a cleavage]

**cra·ni·o·scle·ro·sis** (krā′nē-ō-skler-ō′sis) thickening of the skull. [cranio- + G. *sklēros*, hard, + *-osis*, condition]

**cra·ni·o·spi·nal** (krā′nē-ō-spī′năl) relating to the cranium and spinal column.

**cra·ni·o·spi·nal sensory gan·glia** a term collectively designating the sensory ganglia on the dorsal (posterior) roots of spinal nerves and on those cranial nerves that contain general sensory and taste fibers; also called encephalospinal ganglia.

**cra·ni·o·ste·no·sis** (krā′nē-ō-sten-ō′sis) premature closure of cranial sutures resulting in malformation of the skull. [cranio- + G. *stenōsis,* a narrowing]

**cra·ni·o·syn·os·to·sis** (krā′nē-ō-sin′os-tō′sis) premature ossification of the skull and obliteration of the sutures.

**cra·ni·o·tabes** (krā′nē-ō-tā′bēz) a disease marked by areas of thinning and softening in the bones of the skull and widening of the sutures and fontanelles. Usually of syphilitic or rachitic origin. [cranio- + L. *tabes,* a wasting]

**cra·ni·ot·o·my** (krā-nē-ot′ō-mē) opening into the skull, either by attached or detached craniotomy or by trephination. [cranio- + G. *tomē,* incision]

**cra·ni·o·tym·pan·ic** (krā′nē-ō-tim-pan′ik) relating to the skull and the middle ear.

**cra·ni·um,** pl. **cra·nia** (krā′nē-ŭm, krā′nē-ă) SYN skull. [Mediev. L. fr. G. *kranion*]

**crank test** SYN anterior apprehension test.

**crash cart** a movable collection of emergency equipment and supplies meant to be readily available for resuscitative effort. It includes medication as well as the equipment for defibrillation, intubation, intravenous medication, and passage of central lines.

**cra·vat ban·dage** a bandage made by bringing the point of a triangular bandage to the middle of the base and then folding lengthwise to the desired width.

**C-re·ac·tive pro·tein (CRP)** a β-globulin found in the serum of various persons with certain inflammatory, degenerative, and neoplastic diseases; although the protein is not a specific antibody, it precipitates *in vitro* the C polysaccharide present in all types of pneumococci.

**cream** (krēm) **1.** the upper fatty layer which forms in milk on standing or which is separated from it by centrifugation; it contains about the same amount of sugar and protein as milk, but from 12 to 40% more fat. **2.** any whitish viscid fluid resembling cream. **3.** a semisolid emulsion of either the oil-in-water or the water-in-oil type, ordinarily intended for topical use. [L. *cremor,* thick juice, broth]

**crease** (krēs) a line or linear depression as produced by a fold. SEE ALSO fold, groove, line.

**cre·a·ti·nase** (krē′ă-tǐ-nās) an enzyme catalyzing the hydrolysis of creatine to sarcosine and urea.

**cre·a·tine** (krē′ă-tēn, krē′ă-tin) occurs in urine, sometimes as such, but generally as creatinine, and in muscle, generally as phosphocreatine. Elevated in urine in muscular dystrophy.

**cre·a·tine ki·nase** an enzyme catalyzing the reversible transfer of phosphate from phosphocreatine to ADP, forming creatine and ATP; of importance in muscle contraction. Certain isozymes are elevated in plasma following myocardial infarctions.

**cre·a·tine ki·nase iso·en·zymes** the isoenzymes of creatine kinase: CK-MM, the predominant form, found primarily in skeletal muscle; CK-MB, found in cardiac muscle, tongue, diaphragm, and in small amounts in skeletal muscle; and CK-BB found in the brain, smooth muscle, thyroid, lungs, and prostate. Elevations can help in the differential diagnosis of a variety of states, with CK-MB elevations as an important marker following myocardial infarctions, elevations in

CK-MM an indicator of muscle disease, and elevations in CK-BB an occasional finding following brain infarcts, bowel infarcts, or in the presence of certain malignancies.

**cre·a·ti·ne·mia** (krē′ă-ti-nē′mē-ă) the presence of abnormal concentrations of creatine in peripheral blood. [creatine + G. *haima,* blood]

**cre·a·tine phos·phate** SYN phosphocreatine.

**cre·at·i·nin·ase** (krē-at′i-nin-ās) an amidohydrolase catalyzing the conversion of creatine to creatinine.

**cre·at·i·nine (Cr)** (krē-at′i-nēn, krē-at′i-nin) a component of urine and the final product of creatine catabolism; formed by the nonenzymatic dephosphorylative cyclization of phosphocreatine to form the internal anhydride of creatine. Documented ergogenic benefits of creatine administration include enhanced performance in all-out exercise of up to 30-seconds' duration and facilitated recovery from repeated bouts of intense exercise.

**cre·at·i·nine clear·ance** a mathematical calculation of the total amount of creatinine excreted in the urine over a period of time. It tests renal function. The calculation is: creatinine clearance (ml/min) = urine creatinine concentration (mg/dl) × volume of urine (ml/24 hour) ÷ plasma creatinine concentration (mg/dl) x 1440 min/24 hour.

**cre·a·tin·u·ria** (krē′ă-ti-nyu′rē-ă) the urinary excretion of increased amounts of creatine. [creatine + G. *ouron,* urine]

**Cre·dé method** (krě-dā′) **1.** instillation of one drop of a 2% solution of silver nitrate into each eye of the newborn infant, to prevent ophthalmia neonatorum; **2.** resting the hand on the fundus uteri from the moment of the expulsion of the fetus, and gently rubbing in case of hemorrhage or failing contraction; then, when the afterbirth is loosened it is expelled by firm compression or squeezing of the fundus by the hand; **3.** use of manual pressure on a bladder, particularly a paralyzed bladder, to express urine.

**cre·den·tial·ing** (krĭ-den′shal-ing) a formal review of the qualifications of a provider who has applied to participate in a health care system or plan. [*credential,* proof of authenticity, fr. Med. L. *credentialis,* fr. *credo,* to believe, + -ing]

**cre·mas·ter** (krē-mas′ter) SEE cremaster muscle. [G. *kremastēr,* a suspender, fr. *kremannymi,* to hang]

**crem·as·ter·ic** (krē-mas-ter′ik) relating to the cremaster.

**crem·as·ter·ic ar·tery** *origin,* inferior epigastric; *distribution,* coverings of spermatic cord; *anastomoses,* external pudendal, spermatic, and perineal arteries. SYN arteria cremasterica [TA].

**crem·as·ter·ic re·flex** a drawing up of the scrotum and testicle of the same side when the skin over Scarpa triangle or on the inner side of the thigh is scratched.

**cre·mas·ter mus·cle** *origin,* from internal oblique muscle and inguinal ligament; *insertion,* cremasteric fascia (spermatic cord); *action,* raises testicle; *nerve supply,* genital branch of genitofemoral; in the male the muscle envelops the spermatic cord and testis; in the female, the round ligament of the uterus. SYN musculus cremaster [TA].

**crem·no·cele** (krem′nō-sēl) a protrusion of intestine into the labium majus. [G. *krēmnos,* overhanging cliff, labium pudendi, + *kēlē,* hernia]

**cre•na**, pl. **cre•nae** (krē′nă, krē′nē) a V-shaped cut or the space created by such a cut; one of the notches into which the opposing projections fit in the cranial sutures. [L. a notch]

**cre•nate, cre•nat•ed** (krē′nāt, krē′nā-ted) indented; denoting the outline of a shriveled red blood cell, as observed in a hypertonic solution. [L. *crena*, a notch]

**creno•cyte** (krē′nō-sīt) a red blood cell with serrated, notched edges. [L. *crena*, a notch, + G. *kytos,* a hollow (cell)]

**crep•i•tant** (krep′i-tant) **1.** relating to or characterized by crepitation. **2.** denoting a fine bubbling noise (rale) produced by air entering fluid in lung tissue; heard in pneumonia and in certain other conditions. **3.** the sensation imparted to the palpating finger by gas or air in the subcutaneous tissues.

**crep•i•tant rale** a fine bubbling or crackling sound produced by air mixing with very thin secretions in the smaller bronchial tubes.

**crep•i•ta•tion** (krep-i-tā′shŭn) **1.** crackling; the quality of a fine bubbling sound (rale) that resembles noise heard on rubbing hair between the fingers. **2.** the sensation felt on placing the hand over the seat of a fracture when the broken ends of the bone are moved, or over tissue, in which gas gangrene is present. **3.** noise or vibration produced by rubbing bone or irregular cartilage surfaces together as by movement of patella against femoral condyles in arthritis and other conditions. SYN crepitus (1). [see crepitus]

**crep•i•tus** (krep′i-tŭs) **1.** SYN crepitation. **2.** a noisy discharge of gas from the intestine. [L. fr. *crepo,* to rattle]

**cre•scen•do an•gi•na** angina pectoris that occurs with increasing frequency, intensity, or duration.

**cre•scen•do mur•mur** a murmur that increases in intensity and suddenly ceases; the presystolic murmur of mitral stenosis is a common example.

**cres•cent** (kres′ent) **1.** any figure of the shape of the moon in its first quarter. **2.** the figure made by the gray columns or cornua on cross-section of the spinal cord. **3.** SYN malarial crescent. [L. *cresco,* pp. *cretus,* to grow]

**cres•cent cell a•ne•mia** SYN sickle cell anemia.

**cres•cen•tic** (kres-sen′tik) shaped like a crescent.

**cres•cent sign 1.** in radiography of the lung, a crescent of gas near the top of a mass lesion, signifying cavitation with a space above the debris; seen in aspergilloma, hydatidoma; **2.** in computed tomography, a high attenuating layer of new blood in an aneurysm; indicates a ruptured abdominal aortic aneurysm; **3.** in diagnostic ultrasound, a sonolucent crescentic layer in a tumor mass, typically necrosis in stromal tumors of the small bowel; **4.** in diagnostic ultrasound, a hyperechoic crescent, representing the entering limb of an intussusception; also known as crescent-in-a-doughnut; **5.** in osteoradiology, a subcortical lucent crescent in the femoral head, signifying osteonecrosis. SYN meniscus sign.

**cre•sol red** (krē′sol) an acid-base indicator with a pK value of 8.3; yellow at pH values below 7.4, red above 9.0.

**CREST** calcinosis, *R*aynaud phenomenon, *e*sophageal motility disorders, *s*clerodactyly, and *t*elangiectasia.

**crest** (krest) **1.** a ridge, especially a bony ridge. **2.** the ridge of the neck of a male animal, especially of a stallion or bull. **3.** feathers on the top of a bird's head, or fin rays on the top of a fish's head. SYN crista [TA]. [L. *crista*]

**crest of head of rib** the ridge that separates the superior and inferior articular surfaces of the head of a rib.

**crest of pal•a•tine bone, pal•a•tine crest** a transverse ridge near the posterior border of the bony palate, located on the inferior surface of the horizontal plate of the palatine bone.

**crests of nail matrix** the numerous longitudinal ridges of the nail bed distal to the lunula.

**CREST syn•drome** a variant of scleroderma characterized by *c*alcinosis, *R*aynaud phenomenon, *e*sophageal motility disorders, *s*clerodactyly, and *t*elangiectasia.

**Cres•y•lecht vi•o•let stain** a stain used for identification of *Pneumocystis carinii.*

**cre•tin** (krē′tin) an individual exhibiting cretinism. [Fr. *crétin*]

**cre•tin•ism** (krē′tin-izm) obsolete term for congenital hypothyroidism. SEE infantile hypothyroidism.

**cre•tin•oid** (krē′tin-oyd) resembling a cretin; presenting symptoms similar to those of cretinism.

**cre•tin•ous** (krē′tin-ŭs) relating to cretinism or a cretin; affected with cretinism.

**Creutzfeldt-Jakob disease (CJD)** a progressive neurologic disorder, one of the subacute spongiform encephalopathies caused by prions. Clinical features of CJD include a progressive cerebellar syndrome, including ataxia, abnormalities of gait and speech, and dementia. In most patients, these symptoms are followed by involuntary movements (myoclonus) and the appearance of a typical diagnostic electroencephalogram tracing (burst suppression, consisting of intermittent sharp and slow wave complexes on a flat background). The average survival is less than 1 year after onset of symptoms. Changes in the CSF are absent or nonspecific. Mild cortical atrophy and ventricular dilation may be grossly evident. On microscopic examination the distinctive finding is spongiform encephalopathy in gray matter throughout the brain and spinal cord. Severe neuronal loss and gliosis are also present and mild demyelination may occur. Ultrastructural changes include formation of intracytoplasmic vacuoles, the basis for the spongy appearance. CJD occurs worldwide at a rate of about 1–2 cases per million population per year; most cases are sporadic, but 10–12% are inherited. The peak incidence is between 55 and 65 years of age; the disease is rare before age 30. Cases of iatrogenic Creutzfeldt-Jakob disease have been associated with corneal transplants, electrode implants, dura mater grafts, and administration of human growth hormone. CJD is caused by a prion protein (an abnormal isoform of amyloid protein) that serves as a nucleating factor, inducing abnormalities in other proteins. This protein is detectable by Western blot early in the course of clinical disease. Prion diseases besides CJD include Gerstmann-Sträussler-Scheinker syndrome, fatal familial insomnia, and kuru in humans; scrapie in sheep and goats; bovine spongiform encephalopathy (mad cow disease) in cattle; and similar encephalopathies and wasting syndromes in other species. All these diseases have been shown to be transmissible in laboratory animals. SEE ALSO bovine spongiform encephalopathy.

**crev·ice** (krev'is) a crack or small fissure, especially in a solid substance. [Fr. *crevasse*]

**cre·vic·u·lar** (krĕ-vik'yu-lăr) **1.** relating to any crevice. **2.** DENTISTRY relating especially to the gingival crevice or sulcus.

**CRF** corticotropin-releasing factor.

**CRH** corticotropin-releasing hormone.

**crib-bit·ing** (krib-bīt'ing) a behavior disorder of horses in which the animal grasps the edge of a convenient fixture and presses down, raising the floor of its mouth, forcing the soft palate open, and sometimes swallowing air. SEE aerophagia.

**crib death** SYN sudden infant death syndrome.

**cri·bra** (krī'bră) plural of cribrum.

**crib·rate** (krib'rāt) SYN cribriform.

**cri·bra·tion** (kri-brā'shŭn) **1.** sifting; passing through a sieve. **2.** the condition of being cribrate or numerously pitted or punctured.

**crib·ri·form** (krib'ri-fōrm) sievelike; containing many perforations. SYN cribrate, polyporous. [L. *cribrum,* a sieve, + *forma,* form]

**crib·ri·form plate of eth·moid bone** a horizontal lamina from which are suspended the labyrinth, on either side, and the lamina perpendicularis in the center; it fits into the ethmoidal notch of the frontal bone and supports the olfactory lobes of the cerebrum, being pierced with numerous openings for the passage of the olfactory nerves. SYN lamina cribrosa ossis ethmoidalis [TA], cribrum.

**cri·brum,** pl. **cri·bra** (krī'brŭm, krib'rŭm; krī'bră) SYN cribriform plate of ethmoid bone. [L. a sieve]

**cri·co·ar·y·te·noid** (krī'kō-ar-i-tē'noyd) relating to the cricoid and arytenoid cartilages.

**cri·coid** (krī'koyd) ring-shaped; denoting the cricoid cartilage. [L. *cricoideus,* fr. G. *krikos,* a ring, + *eidos,* form]

**cri·coid car·ti·lage** the lowermost of the laryngeal cartilages; it is shaped like a signet ring, being expanded into a nearly quadrilateral plate (lamina) posteriorly; the anterior portion is called the arch (arcus). SYN cartilago cricoidea [TA].

**cri·coid split op·er·a·tion** an operation to repair subglottic stenosis by transecting the anterior and posterior aspects of the ring of the cricoid cartilage, with or without the insertion of grafts to reconstruct the subglottic lumen.

**cri·co·pha·ryn·ge·al** (krī'kō-fă-rin'jē-ăl) relating to the cricoid cartilage and the pharynx; a part of the inferior constrictor muscle of the pharynx. SEE inferior constrictor muscle of pharynx.

**cri·co·pha·ryn·ge·al ach·a·la·sia** functional obstruction at the level of the upper esophageal sphincter due to failure of relaxation of the cricopharyngeal muscles; often associated with a pharyngoesophageal diverticulum. SYN achalasia of the upper sphincter, hypertensive upper esophageal sphincter.

**cri·co·thy·roid** (krī-kō-thī'royd) relating to the cricoid and thyroid cartilages.

**cri·co·thy·roid mus·cle** *origin,* anterior surface of arch of cricoid; *insertion,* the anterior or straight part passes upward to ala of thyroid; the posterior or oblique part passes more outward to inferior horn of thyroid; *action,* makes vocal folds tense, increasing the pitch of voice tone; *nerve supply,* external laryngeal branch of superior laryngeal nerve (from vagus). SYN musculus cricothyroideus [TA].

**cri·co·thy·rot·o·my** (krī'kō-thī-rot'ō-mē) inci-

sion through the skin and cricothyroid membrane for relief of respiratory obstruction; used prior to or in place of tracheotomy in certain emergency respiratory obstructions. SYN intercricothyrotomy. [cricoid + thyroid + G. *tomē,* incision]

**cri·cot·o·my** (krī-kot'ō-mē) division of the cricoid cartilage, as in cricoid split, to enlarge the subglottic airway. [cricoid + G. *tomē,* incision]

**cri-du-chat syn·drome, cat-cry syn·drome** a disorder due to deletion of the short arm of chromosome 5, characterized by microcephaly, hypertelorism, antimongoloid palpebral fissures, epicanthal folds, micrognathia, strabismus, mental and physical retardation, and a characteristic high-pitched catlike whine.

**Crig·ler-Naj·jar syn·drome** (krig'ler nah'jahr) a defect in ability to form bilirubin glucuronide due to deficiency of bilirubin-glucuronide glucuronosyltransferase; characterized by familial nonhemolytic jaundice and, in its severe form, by irreversible brain damage in infancy that resembles kernicterus and may be fatal.

**Crile clamp** (krīl) a clamp for temporary stoppage of blood flow.

**crim·i·nal a·bor·tion** termination of pregnancy without legal justification.

**crim·i·nal psy·chol·o·gy** the study of the mind and its workings in relation to crime. SEE forensic psychology.

**crin·o·gen·ic** (krin-ō-jen'ik) causing secretion; stimulating a gland to increased function. [G. *krinō,* to separate, + *-gen,* to produce]

**crin·oph·a·gy** (krin-of'ă-jē) disposal of excess secretory granules by lysosomes.

**cri·sis,** pl. **cri·ses** (krī'sis, krī'sēz) **1.** a sudden change, usually for the better, in the course of an acute disease, in contrast to gradual improvement by lysis. **2.** a paroxysmal pain in an organ or circumscribed region of the body occurring in the course of tabetic neurosyphilis. **3.** a convulsive attack. [G. *krisis,* a separation, crisis]

**cris·ta,** pl. **cris·tae** (kris'tă, kris'tē) [TA] SYN crest. [L. crest]

**cris·ta gal·li** [TA] the triangular midline process of the ethmoid bone extending superiorly from the cribriform plate; it gives anterior attachment to the falx cerebri.

**cri·te·ri·on,** pl. **cri·te·ria** (krī-tēr'ē-on, crī-tēr-ē-ă) **1.** a standard or rule for judging; usually plural (criteria) denoting a set of standards or rules. **2.** in psychology, a standard such as school grades against which test scores on intelligence tests or other measured behaviors are validated. **3.** a list of manifestations of a disease or disorder, a certain number of which must be present to warrant diagnosis in a given patient. [G. *kritērion,* a standard]

**crit·i·cal ap·prai·sal** the process used to systematically locate and evaluate evidence for its validity and usefulness. It is an integral part of evidence-based practice. SEE ALSO evidence-based practice.

**crit·i·cal care u·nit (CCU)** SYN intensive care unit.

**crit·i·cal in·ci·dent stress man·age·ment** a process of providing mental health management and support to providers who have experienced a critical stress incident.

**crit·i·cal lim·it** the upper or lower boundary of a laboratory test result that indicates a life-threatening value.

**crit·i·cal mi·celle con·cen·tra·tion (cmc)** the concentration at which an amphipathic molecule (e.g., a phospholipid) will form a micelle.

**crit·i·cal or·gan** the organ or physiologic system that for a given source of radiation would first reach its legally defined maximum permissible radiation exposure as the dose of radiopharmaceutical is increased.

**crit·i·cal path·way** a schedule of medical and nursing procedures, including diagnostic tests, medications, and consultations, designed to provide practice guidelines for the efficient, coordinated treatment of a specific condition.

**crit·i·cal tem·per·a·ture** the temperature of a gas above which it is no longer possible by use of any pressure, however great, to convert it into a liquid.

**CRL** crown-rump length.

**CRM** certified reference material.

**cRNA** complementary ribonucleic acid.

**croc·o·dile tears syn·drome** a flow of tears, usually unilateral, upon eating or the anticipation of eating; this happens when nerve fibers originally destined for a salivary gland are damaged and regrow, aberrantly, into the lacrimal gland.

**Crocq dis·ease** (krŏk) SYN acrocyanosis.

**Crohn dis·ease** (krōn) SYN regional enteritis.

**Crooke gran·ules** (kruk) lumpy masses of basophilic material in the basophil cells of the anterior lobe of the pituitary, associated with Cushing disease, or following the administration of ACTH.

**Crooke hy·a·line change** (kruk) replacement of cytoplasmic granules of basophil cells of the anterior pituitary by homogeneous hyaline material; a characteristic finding in Cushing syndrome, but usually not present in the cells of a basophil adenoma.

**Crookes glass** (kruks) a spectacle lens combined with metallic oxides to absorb ultraviolet or infrared rays.

**cross** (kros) **1.** any figure in the shape of a cross formed by two intersecting lines. SYN crux. **2.** a method of hybridization or the hybrid so produced. [F. *croix,* L. *crux*]

**cross·bite** (kros′bīt) an abnormal relation of one or more teeth of one arch to the opposing tooth or teeth of the other arch due to labial, buccal, or lingual deviation of tooth position, or to abnormal jaw position.

**cross·bite tooth** a posterior tooth designed to permit the modified cusp of the upper tooth to be positioned in the fossae of the lower tooth.

**cross-dress·ing** (kros′ dres′ing) clothing oneself in attire generally associated with the opposite sex. SEE transvestism.

**crossed di·plo·pia** diplopia in which the image seen by the right eye is to the left of the image seen by the left eye.

**crossed em·bo·lism 1.** obstruction of a systemic artery by an embolus originating in the venous system which passes through a septal defect, patent foramen ovale, or other shunt to the arterial system; **2.** obstruction by a minute embolism that passes through the pulmonary capillaries from the venous to the arterial system.

**crossed ex·ten·sion re·flex** reflex extension of the joints of an extremity accompanying a flexion reflex in the contralateral extremity, induced by application to the contralateral extremity of a painful stimulus distally.

**crossed eyes, cross-eye** (kros′ī) SYN strabismus.

**crossed re·flex** a reflex movement on one side of the body in response to a stimulus applied to the opposite side.

**crossed re·nal ec·to·pia** ectopic kidney located on opposite (contralateral) side of midline from its ureteral insertion into bladder. In most instances, the two renal moieties are fused (crossed fused ectopia).

**cross flap** a skin flap transferred from one part of the body to a corresponding part, as from one arm to the other.

**cross-hy·brid·i·sa·tion [Br.]** SEE cross hybridization.

**cross hybridization** (kros hī-brĭd-ĭ-zā-shun) annealing of a DNA probe to an imperfectly matching DNA molecule.

**cross in·fec·tion** infection spread from one source to another, person to person, animal to person, person to animal, animal to animal.

**cross·ing-over, cross·o·ver** (kros-ing-ō′ver, kros′ō-ver) **1.** reciprocal exchange of material between two paired chromosomes during meiosis, resulting in the transfer of a block of genes from each chromosome to its homologue. **2.** refers to the phenomenon of sound presented to one ear may be perceived in the other ear by passing around the head by air conduction or through the head by bone conduction.

**cross-le·vel bi·as** a bias due to aggregation at the population level of causes and/or effects that are unlike at the individual level; can occur in ecologic studies.

**cross-match·ing** (kros′match-ing) **1.** a test for incompatibility between donor and recipient blood, carried out before transfusion to avoid hemolytic reactions between the donor's red blood cells and antibodies in the recipient's plasma, or the reverse; performed by mixing a sample of red blood cells of the donor with plasma of the recipient (*major crossmatch*) and the red blood cells of the recipient with the plasma of the donor (*minor crossmatch*). Incompatibility is indicated by clumping of red blood cells and contraindicates use of the donor's blood. **2.** in allotransplantation of solid organs (e.g., kidney), a test for identification of antibody in the serum of potential allograft recipients which reacts directly with the lymphocytes or other cells of a potential allograft donor; presence of these antibodies usually, if not always, contraindicates the performance of the transplantation because virtually all such grafts will be subject to a hyperacute type of rejection.

**cross-over stud·y** a study in which the subject is switched from the experimental to the control procedure (or vice versa).

**cross-re·act·ing ag·glu·ti·nin** SYN group agglutinin.

**cross-re·act·ing an·ti·bod·y 1.** antibody specific for group antigens, i.e., those with identical functional groups; **2.** antibody for antigens that have functional groups of closely similar, but not identical, chemical structure.

**cross-re·ac·tion** a specific reaction between an antiserum and an antigen complex other than the antigen complex that evoked the various specific antibodies of the antiserum. It is due to at least one antigenic determinant that is included among the determinants of the other complex.

**cross sec·tion 1.** a planar or two-dimensional

view, diagram, or image of the internal structure of the body, part of the body, or any anatomic structure afforded by slicing, actually or through imaging (radiographic, magnetic, or microscopic) techniques, the body or structure along a particular plane; **2.** the slice or section of a given thickness created by actual serial parallel cuts through a structure or by the application of imaging technique.

**cross-sec•tion•al stud•y** a study in which groups of individuals of different types are composed into one large sample and studied at only a single point in time (e.g., a survey in which all voters, regardless of age, religion, gender, or geographic location, are sampled in one day). SYN synchronic study.

**cross-ta•ble lat•er•al pro•jec•tion** lateral projection radiography of a supine subject using a horizontal x-ray beam.

**cross-ta•per** (kros tā′per) a practice in pharmacotherapy of lowering the dosage of one medication while simultaneously increasing the dosage of another medication.

**cross tol•er•ance** the resistance to one or several effects of a compound as a result of tolerance developed to a pharmacologically similar compound.

**croup** (kroop) **1.** laryngotracheobronchitis in infants and young children caused by parainfluenza viruses 1 and 2. **2.** any affection of the larynx in children, characterized by difficult and noisy respiration and a hoarse cough. [Scots, probably from A.S. *kropan,* to cry aloud]

**croup-as•so•ci•at•ed vi•rus** parainfluenza virus type 2. SEE parainfluenza viruses.

**croup•ous** (kroo′pŭs) relating to croup; marked by a fibrinous exudation.

**croup•ous mem•brane** SYN false membrane.

**Crou•zon syn•drome** (kroo′zon) craniosynostosis with broad forehead, ocular hypertelorism, exophthalmos, beaked nose, and hypoplasia of the maxilla.

**crowd•ing** (krowd′ing) a condition in which the teeth are crowded, assuming altered positions such as bunching, overlapping, displacement in various directions, torsiversion, etc.

**crowd•ing phe•nom•e•non** a characteristic of amblyopic vision in which vision is better for single optotype presentation than multiple, simultaneous optotype presentation.

**Crowe-Da•vis mouth gag** (krō-dā′vis) instrument used for opening the mouth, depressing the tongue, maintaining the airway, and transmitting volatile anesthetics during tonsillectomy or other oropharyngeal surgery.

**crown** (krown) **1.** any structure, normal or pathologic, resembling or suggesting a crown or a wreath. **2.** DENTISTRY that part of a tooth that is covered with enamel, or an artificial substitute for that part. SYN corona [TA]. [L. *corona*]

**crown-heel length (CHL)** length of an outstretched embryo or fetus from skull vertex to heel.

**crown•ing** (krown′ing) **1.** preparation of the natural crown of a tooth and covering the prepared crown with a veneer of suitable dental material (gold or non-precious metal casting, porcelain, plastic, or combinations). **2.** that stage of childbirth when the fetal head has negotiated the pelvic outlet and the largest diameter of the head is encircled by the vulvar ring.

**crown-rump length (Cr, CRL)** a measurement from the skull vertex to the midpoint between the apices of the buttocks of an embryo or fetus, which permits approximation of embryonic or fetal age.

**CRP** cAMP receptor protein; C-reactive protein.

**CRT** circuit resistance training.

**cru•ces** (kroo′sēz) plural of crux.

**cru•ces pi•lo•rum** crosslike figures formed by hairs growing from two directions that meet and then separate in a direction perpendicular to the original orientation.

**cru•ci•ate** (kroo′shē-āt) shaped like, or resembling, a cross. [L. *cruciatus*]

**cru•ci•ate a•nas•to•mo•sis, cru•cial a•nas•to•mo•sis** a four-way anastomosis between branches of the first perforating branch of the deep femoral, inferior gluteal and medial and lateral circumflex femoral arteries, located posterior to the upper part of the femur.

**cru•ci•ate lig•a•ments** major ligaments that crisscross the knee in the anteroposterior direction, providing stability in that plane. SEE ALSO Lachman test.

**cru•ci•ate mus•cle** a general type of muscle in which the muscles or bundles of muscle fibers cross in an X-shaped configuration; e.g., the oblique arytenoid muscles.

**cru•ra** (kroo′rā) plural of crus.

**cru•ra of the di•a•phragm** the muscular origins of the diaphragm from the bodies of the upper lumbar vertebrae that pass the aorta upward to the central tendon. SYN crura diaphragmatis [TA].

**cru•ra di•a•phrag•ma•tis** [TA] SYN crura of the diaphragm.

**cru•ral** (kroo′răl) relating to the leg or thigh, or to any crus.

**cru•ral her•nia** SYN femoral hernia.

**cru•ral in•ter•os•se•ous nerve** a nerve given off from one of the muscular branches of the tibial nerve which passes down over the posterior surface of the interosseous membrane supplying it and the two bones of the leg. SYN nervus interosseus cruris [TA].

**cru•ral sheath** SYN femoral sheath.

**cru•ris** (kroo′ris)

**crus**, gen. **cru•ris**, pl. **cru•ra** (kroos, kroo′ris, kroo′rā) [TA] **1.** SYN leg. **2.** any anatomic structure resembling a leg; usually (in the plural) a pair of diverging bands or elongated masses. SEE ALSO limb. [L.]

**crus ce•re•bri** [TA] specifically, the massive bundle of corticofugal nerve fibers passing longitudinally on the ventral surface of the midbrain on each side of the midline; it consists of fibers descending from the cortex to the tegmentum of the brainstem, pontine gray matter, and spinal cord. SEE ALSO cerebral peduncle.

**crus cli•to•ris** [TA] SYN crus of clitoris.

**crus of clit•o•ris** the continuation on each side of the corpus cavernosum of the clitoris which diverges from the body posteriorly and is attached to the pubic arch. SYN crus clitoris [TA].

**crus for•ni•cis** [TA] that part of the fornix that rises in a forward curve behind the thalamus to continue forward as the body for fornix ventral to the corpus callosum.

**crush syn•drome** the shocklike state that follows release of a limb or limbs or the trunk and pelvis after a prolonged period of compression, as by a heavy weight; characterized by suppression of urine, probably the result of damage to the renal tubules by myoglobin from the damaged muscles. SYN compression syndrome (1).

**crus pe·nis** [TA] SYN crus of penis.

**crus of pe·nis** the posterior, tapering portion of the corpus cavernosum penis which diverges from its contralateral partner to be attached to the ischiopubic ramus. SYN crus penis [TA].

■**crust** (krŭst) **1.** a hard outer layer or covering; cutaneous crusts are often formed by dried serum or pus on the surface of a ruptured blister or pustule. **2.** a scab. See page B5. SYN crusta. [L. *crusta*]

**crus·ta**, pl. **crus·tae** (krŭs'tă, krŭs'tē) SYN crust. [L.]

**crus·ta lac·tea** seborrhea of the scalp in an infant. SYN milk crust.

**crutch** (krŭtch) a device used singly or in pairs to assist in walking when the act is impaired by a lower extremity (or trunk) disability; it transfers all or part of weight-bearing to the upper extremity. [A. S. *cryce*]

**Cru·veil·hier-Baum·gar·ten sign, Cru·veil·-hier-Baum·gar·ten mur·mur** (kroo-vāl-yā' bawm'gahr-tĕn, kroo-vāl-yā' bawm'gahr-tĕn) a murmur over the umbilicus often in the presence of caput medusae, resulting from portal hypertension, usually with hepatic cirrhosis; recanalization of the umbilical vein with reverse blood flow from the liver into the abdominal wall veins creates the murmur.

**Cru·veil·hier dis·ease** (kroo-vāl-yā') SYN amyotrophic lateral sclerosis.

**crux**, pl. **cru·ces** (krŭks, kroo'sēz) a junction or crossing. SYN cross (1). [L.]

**Cruz try·pan·o·so·mi·a·sis** (krooz) SYN South American trypanosomiasis.

**cry·al·ge·sia** (krī-al-jē'zē-ă) pain caused by cold. SYN crymodynia. [G. *kryos*, cold, + *algos*, pain]

**cry·an·es·the·sia** (krī'an-es-thē'zē-ă) inability to perceive cold. [G. *kryos*, cold, + *an-* priv. + *aisthēsis*, sensation]

**cry·es·the·sia** (krī-es-thē'zē-ă) **1.** a subjective sensation of cold. **2.** sensitiveness to cold. [G. *kryos*, cold, + *aisthēsis*, sensation]

**cry for help** telephone calls, notes left in conspicuous places, and other behaviors that communicate extreme distress and possible consideration of suicide.

△**crymo-** cold. SEE ALSO cryo-, psychro-. [G. *krymos*,]

**cry·mo·dyn·ia** (krī-mō-din'ē-ă) SYN cryalgesia. [crymo- + G. *odynē*, pain]

**cry·mo·phil·ic** (krī-mō-fil'ik) preferring cold; denoting microorganisms which thrive best at low temperatures. SYN cryophilic. [crymo- + G. *philos*, fond]

**cry·mo·phy·lac·tic** (krī'mō-fi-lak'tik) resistant to cold, said of certain microorganisms that are not destroyed even by freezing temperatures. SYN cryophylactic. [crymo- + G. *phylaxis*, a guarding against]

△**cry·o-, cry-** cold. SEE ALSO crymo-, psychro-. [G. *kryos*,]

**cry·o·an·es·the·sia** (krī-ō-an-es-thē'zē-ă) localized application of cold as a means of producing regional anesthesia. SYN refrigeration anesthesia.

**cry·o·cau·tery** (krī'ō-kaw'ter-ē) any substance, such as liquid air or carbon dioxide snow, or a low temperature instrument, the application of which causes destruction of tissue by freezing.

**cry·o·ex·trac·tion** (krī'ō-ek-strak'shŭn) removal of cataracts by the adhesion of a freezing probe to the lens; now rarely done.

**cry·o·fi·brin·o·gen** (krī'ō-fī-brin'ō-jen) an abnormal type of fibrinogen very rarely found in human plasma; it is precipitated upon cooling, but redissolves when warmed to room temperature.

**cry·o·fi·brin·o·gen·e·mia** (krī'ō-fī-brin'ō-je-nē' mē-ă) the presence in the blood of cryofibrinogens.

**cry·o·frac·ture** (krī-ō-frak'cher) SYN freeze fracture. [cryo- + fracture]

**cry·o·gen·ic** (krī-ō-jen'ik) **1.** denoting or characteristic of a cryogen. **2.** relating to cryogenics.

**cry·o·glob·u·lin·e·mia** (krī'ō-glob'yu-li-nē'mē-ă) the presence of abnormal quantities of cryoglobulin in the blood plasma.

**cry·o·glob·u·lins** (krī-ō-glob'yu-linz) abnormal plasma proteins characterized by precipitating, gelling, or crystallizing when serum or solutions of them are cooled; they may appear in patients with multiple myeloma.

**cryokinetics** (krī-ō-kǐ-nět'iks) the combination of cryotherapy with exercise. SEE ALSO cryotherapy. SYN cold therapy. [cryo- + kinetics]

**cry·ol·y·sis** (krī-ol'i-sis) destruction by cold. [cryo- + G. *lysis*, dissolution]

**cry·op·a·thy** (krī-op'ă-thē) a morbid condition in which exposure to cold is an important factor. [cryo- + G. *pathos*, suffering]

**cry·o·pexy** (krī'ō-pek-sē) in retinal detachment surgery, sealing the sensory retina to the pigment epithelium and choroid by a freezing probe applied to the sclera. [cryo- + G. *pēxis*, a fixing in place]

**cry·o·phil·ic** (krī-ō-fil'ik) SYN crymophilic. [cryo- + G. *philos*, fond]

**cry·o·phy·lac·tic** (krī'ō-fī-lak'tik) SYN crymophylactic.

**cry·o·pre·cip·i·tate** (krī'ō-prē-sip'i-tāt) precipitate that forms when soluble material is cooled, especially with reference to the precipitate that forms in normal blood plasma which has been subjected to cold precipitation and which is rich in factor VIII.

**cry·o·pres·er·va·tion** (krī'ō-pres-er-vā'shŭn) maintenance of the viability of excised tissues or organs at extremely low temperatures.

**cry·o·probe** (krī'ō-prōb) an instrument used in cryosurgery to apply extreme cold to a selected area. [cryo- + L. *probo*, to test]

**cry·o·pro·tein** (krī-ō-prō'tēn) a protein that precipitates from solution when cooled and redissolves upon warming.

**cry·os·co·py** (krī-os'kǒ-pē) the determination of the freezing point of a fluid, usually blood or urine, compared with that of distilled water. [cryo- + G. *skopeō*, to examine]

**cry·o·sur·gery** (krī-ō-ser'jer-ē) an operation using freezing temperature (achieved by liquid nitrogen or carbon dioxide) to destroy tissue.

**cry·o·ther·a·py** (krī-ō-thār'ă-pē) the use of cold in the treatment of disease or injury.

**cry·o·tol·er·ant** (krī-ō-tol'er-ant) tolerant of very low temperatures.

**crypt** (kript) a pitlike depression or tubular recess.

**crypt ab·scess·es** abscesses in crypts of Lieberkühn, a characteristic feature of ulcerative colitis.

**cryp·tec·to·my** (krip-tek'tō-mē) excision of a

tonsillar or other crypt. [crypt + G. *ektomē*, excision]

**cryp·tic** (krip'tik) hidden; occult; larvate. [G. *kryptikos*]

**cryp·ti·tis** (krip-tī'tis) inflammation of a follicle or glandular tubule, particularly in the rectum.

△**cryp·to-, crypt-** hidden, obscure; without apparent cause. [G. *kryptos*, hidden, concealed]

**cryp·to·chrome** (krip'tō-krōm) flavoprotein ultraviolet-A receptor involved in circadian rhythm entrainment in plants, insects, and mammals.

**cryp·to·coc·co·sis** (krip'tō-kok-ō'sis) infection by *Cryptococcus neoformans*, causing a pulmonary, disseminated, or meningeal mycosis. The most familiar and readily recognized form involves the central nervous system, with subacute or chronic meningitis. SYN Busse-Buschke disease.

**Cryp·to·coc·cus** (krip-tō-kok'ŭs) a genus of yeastlike fungi that reproduce by budding. [crypto- + G. *kokkos*, berry]

**cryp·to·gen·ic** (krip-tō-jen'ik) of obscure, indeterminate etiology or origin, in contrast to phanerogenic. [crypto- + G. *genesis*, origin]

**cryp·to·gen·ic fi·bros·ing al·ve·o·li·tis** SYN idiopathic pulmonary fibrosis.

**cryp·to·gen·ic sep·ti·ce·mia** a form of septicemia in which no primary focus of infection can be found.

**cryp·to·lith** (krip'tō-lith) a concretion in a gland follicle. [crypto- + G. *lithos*, stone]

**cryp·to·men·or·rhea** (krip'tō-men-ō-rē'ă) occurrence each month of the general symptoms of the menses without any flow of blood, as in cases of imperforate hymen. [crypto- + G. *mēn*, month, + *rhoia*, flow]

**cryp·to·po·dia** (krip-tō-pō'dē-ă) a swelling of the lower part of the leg and the foot, in such a manner that there is great distortion and the sole seems to be a flattened pad. [crypto- + G. *pous*, foot]

**cryp·tor·chi·dism** (krip-tōr'ki-dizm) SYN cryptorchism.

**cryp·tor·chi·do·pexy** (krip-tōr'ki-dō-pek'sē) SYN orchiopexy. [crypto- + G. *orchis*, testis, + *pēxis*, fixation]

**cryp·tor·chism** (krip-tōr'kizm) failure of one or both of the testes to descend. SYN cryptorchidism.

**cryp·to·spo·rid·i·o·sis** (krip'tō-spō-rid-ē-ō'sis) an enteric disease caused by waterborne protozoan parasites of the genus *Cryptosporidium*; disease in immunocompetent persons is manifest as a self-limiting diarrhea, whereas in immuno-compromised persons it is manifest as a prolonged severe diarrhea that can be fatal.

**Cryp·to·spo·rid·i·um** (krip'tō-spō-rid'ē-ŭm) a genus of coccidian sporozoans (family Cryptosporidiidae, suborder Eimeriina) that are important pathogens of calves and other domestic animals, and common opportunistic parasites of humans that flourish under conditions of compromised immune function; can cause self-limiting diarrhea in immunocompetent persons.

**Cryp·to·spo·rid·i·um par·vum** sporozoan species that is an important cause of neonatal diarrhea in calves and lambs; causes mild, self-limiting to severe, chronic diarrhea in humans.

**cryp·to·zy·gous** (krip-tō-zī'gŭs) having a narrow face as compared with the width of the cranium, so that, when the skull is viewed from above, the zygomatic arches are not visible. [crypto- + G. *zygon*, yoke]

**crypts of Lie·ber·kühn** (lē'ber-kēn) SYN intestinal glands.

**crys·tal** (kris'tăl) a solid of regular shape and, for a given compound, characteristic angles, formed when an element or compound solidifies slowly enough, as a result either of freezing from the liquid form or of precipitating out of solution, to allow the individual molecules to take up regular positions with respect to one another. [G. *krystallos*, clear ice, crystal]

**crys·tal·lin** (kris'tă-lin) a type of protein found in the lens of the eye.

**crys·tal·line** (kris'tă-lēn) **1.** clear; transparent. **2.** relating to a crystal or crystals.

**crys·tal·li·za·tion** (kris'tăl-i-zā'shŭn) assumption of a crystalline form when a vapor or liquid becomes solidified, or a solute precipitates from solution.

**crys·tal·loid** (kris'tăl-oyd) **1.** resembling a crystal, or being such. **2.** a body that in solution can pass through a semipermeable membrane, as distinguished from a colloid, which cannot do so.

**crys·tal·lu·ria** (kris-tă-lyu'rē-ă) the excretion of crystalline materials in the urine.

**Cs** cesium.

**CSD** catscratch disease.

**C-sec·tion** SEE cesarean section.

**CSF** cerebrospinal fluid; colony-stimulating factors.

**CT** computed tomography. See page B14.

**CTD** cumulative trauma disorders.

**Cte·no·ce·phal·i·des** (tē-nō-se-fal'i-dēz) a genus of fleas. *Ctenocephalides canis* (dog flea) and *Ctenocephalides felis* (cat flea) are nearly universal ectoparasites of household pets; will attack humans when starving owing to absence of pets. [G. *ktenōdēs*, like a cockle, + *kephalē*, head]

**C ter·mi·nus** the end of a peptide or protein having a free carboxyl (–COOH) group.

**CTP** cytidine 5′-triphosphate.

**CT pel·vim·e·try** procedure for measurement of the bony pelvis and fetal head through use of CT images; currently the more accurate imaging technique.

**Cu** copper.

**cu·bic cen·ti·me·ter** (cc, c.c., c.c.) one thousandth of a liter; 1 milliliter.

**cu·bi·tal** (kyu'bi-tăl) relating to the elbow or to the ulna.

**cu·bi·tal joint** SYN elbow joint.

**cu·bi·tal nerve** SYN ulnar nerve.

**cu·bi·tal tun·nel syn·drome** a group of symptoms that develop from compression of the ulnar nerve within the cubital tunnel at the elbow; can include paresthesia into the 4th and 5th digits and weakness of the intrinsic muscles of the hand.

**cu·bi·tus,** gen. and pl. **cu·bi·ti** (kyu'bi-tŭs, kyu'bi-tī) [Ta] **1.** SYN elbow (2). **2.** SYN ulna. [L. elbow]

**cu·bi·tus val·gus** deviation of the extended forearm to the outer (radial) side of the axis of the limb.

**cu·bi·tus var·us** deviation of the extended forearm to the inward (ulnar) side of the axis of the limb.

**cu·boid, cu·boi·dal** (kyu'boyd, kyu-boy'dăl) **1.** resembling a cube in shape. **2.** relating to the os cuboideum. [G. *kybos*, cube, + *eidos*, resemblance]

**cu·boi·dal car·ci·no·ma** SYN cloacogenic carcinoma.

**cu·boi·dal ep·i·the·li·um** simple epithelium with cells appearing as cubes in a vertical section but as polyhedra in surface view.

**cu·boid bone** the lateral bone of the distal row of the tarsus, articulating with the calcaneus, lateral cuneiform, navicular (occasionally), and fourth and fifth metatarsal bones.

**cued speech** a system of communication in which a person with profound hearing impairment in which handshapes are used to cue sounds to supplement spoken language.

**cuff** (kŭf) any structure shaped like a cuff.

**cul-de-sac,** pl. **culs-de-sac** (kŭl-de-sak′) **1.** a blind pouch or tubular cavity closed at one end; e.g., diverticulum; cecum. **2.** SYN rectouterine pouch. [Fr. bottom of a sack]

**cul·do·cen·te·sis** (kŭl′dō-sen-tē′sis) aspiration of fluid from the cul-de-sac by puncture of the vaginal vault near the midline between the uterosacral ligaments. [cul-de-sac + G. *kentēsis,* puncture]

**cul·do·plas·ty** (kŭl′dō-plas-tē) plastic surgery to remedy relaxation of the posterior fornix of the vagina. [cul-de-sac + G. *plastos,* formed]

**cul·do·scope** (kŭl′dō-skōp) endoscopic instrument used in culdoscopy.

**cul·dos·co·py** (kŭl-dos′kŏ-pē) introduction of an endoscope through the posterior vaginal wall for viewing the rectovaginal pouch and pelvic viscera. [cul-de-sac + G. *skopeō,* to view]

**Cu·lex** (kyu′leks) a genus of mosquitoes including over 2,000 species. Largely tropical but worldwide in distribution; they are vectors for a number of diseases of man and of domestic and wild animals and birds. [L. gnat]

**Cu·lex ni·gri·pal·pus** mosquito species that is a vector of St. Louis encephalitis within the United States.

**Cu·lex res·tu·ans** mosquito species that is a secondary or suspected vector of Eastern equine encephalitis and Western equine encephalitis within the United States.

**Cu·lex sa·li·na·ri·us** mosquito species that is a secondary or suspected vector of Eastern equine encephalitis within the United States.

**cu·li·ci·dal** (kyu-li-sī′dăl) destructive to mosquitoes. [L. *culex,* gnat, + *caedo,* to kill]

**cu·li·cide** (kyu′li-sīd) an agent that destroys mosquitoes.

**Cu·li·coi·des** (kyu-li-koy′dēz) a genus of minute biting gnats or midges, vectors of several nonpathogenic human filariae (*Mansonella, Dipetalonema*). [L. *culex,* gnat]

**Cu·li·se·ta** (kū-lis′ē-ta) a genus of mosquitoes (family Culicidae). They are vectors for a number of diseases of humans and of domestic and wild animals and birds.

**Cu·lis·e·ta in·or·na·ta** mosquito species that is a secondary or suspected vector of Western equine encephalitis and California group encephalitis within the United States.

**Cul·len sign** (kŭl′len) periumbilical darkening of the skin from blood, a sign of intraperitoneal hemorrhage, especially in ruptured ectopic pregnancy.

**cul·ti·va·tion** (kŭl-ti-vā′shŭn) SYN culture. [Mediev. L. *cultivo,* pp. *-atus,* fr. L. *colo,* pp. *cultus,* to till]

**cul·tur·al di·ver·si·ty** (kul′choo-ral dĭ-ver′sĭ-tē)

the inevitable variety in customs, attitudes, practices, and behavior that exists among groups of individuals from different ethnic, racial, or national backgrounds who come into contact.

**cul·tur·al shock** a form of stress associated with the beginning of an individual's assimilation into a new and vastly different culture.

**cul·ture** (kŭl′chŭr) **1.** the propagation of microorganisms on or in media of various kinds. **2.** a mass of microorganisms on or in a medium. **3.** the propagation of mammalian cells, i.e., cell culture. SEE cell culture. **4.** set of beliefs, values, artistic, historical, religious characteristics, customs, etc. common to a community or nation. SYN cultivation. [L. *cultura,* tillage, fr. *colo,* pp. *cultus,* to till]

**cul·ture me·di·um** a substance, either solid or liquid, used for the cultivation, isolation, identification, or storage of microorganisms. SYN medium (3).

**Cum·mer clas·si·fi·ca·tion** (kum′ĕr) a listing of several types of removable partial dentures in accordance with the distribution of direct retainers.

**cu·mu·la·tive** (kyu′myu-lă-tiv) tending to accumulate or pile up, as with certain drugs that may have a cumulative effect.

**cu·mu·la·tive ac·tion** SYN cumulative effect.

**cu·mu·la·tive ef·fect** the condition in which repeated administration of a drug may produce effects that are more pronounced than those produced by the first dose. SYN cumulative action.

**cu·mu·la·tive trau·ma dis·or·ders (CTD)** chronic disorders involving tendon, muscle, joint, and nerve damage, often resulting from work-related physical activities. CTDs, including repetitive motion disorders and carpal tunnel syndrome, result when the body is subjected to direct pressure, vibration, or repetitive movements for prolonged periods. SYN repetitive strain disorders.

**cu·ne·ate** (kyu′nē-āt) wedge-shaped. [L. *cuneus,* wedge]

**cu·ne·ate fas·cic·u·lus, cu·ne·ate fu·nic·u·lus** the larger lateral subdivision of the posterior funiculus.

**cu·ne·ate nu·cle·us** the larger Burdach nucleus; one of the three nuclei of the posterior column of the spinal cord; located near the dorsal surface of the medulla oblongata at and below the level of the obex, the nucleus receives posterior root fibers corresponding to the sensory innervation of the arm and hand of the same side; together with its medial companion, the gracile nucleus, it is the major source of origin of the medial lemniscus.

**cu·ne·i·form bone** SEE triquetral bone.

**cu·ne·i·form car·ti·lage** a small nonarticulating rod of elastic cartilage in the aryepiglottic fold anterolateral and somewhat superior to the corniculate cartilage. SYN cartilago cuneiformis [TA].

**cu·ne·o·cu·boid** (kyu′nē-ō-kyu′boyd) relating to the lateral cuneiform and the cuboid bones.

**cu·ne·o·na·vic·u·lar** (kyu-nē-ō-na-vik′yu-lăr) relating to the cuneiform and the navicular bones.

**cu·ne·us,** pl. **cu·nei** (kyu′nē-ŭs, kyu′nē-ī; kyu′nē-ī) that region of the medial aspect of the occipital lobe of each cerebral hemisphere bounded by the parietooccipital fissure and the calcarine fissure. [L. *wedge*]

**cu·nic·u·lus**, pl. **cu·nic·u·li** (kyu-nik′yu-lŭs -lī) the burrow of the scabies mite in the epidermis. [L. a rabbit; an underground passage]

**cun·ni·lin·gus** (kŭn-i-ling′gŭs) oral stimulation of the vulva or clitoris; contrasted with fellatio, which is the oral stimulation of the penis. [L. *cunnus,* pudendum, + *lingo,* to lick]

**cup** (kŭp) **1.** an excavated or cup-shaped structure, either anatomic or pathologic. **2.** SYN cupping glass. [A.S. *cuppe*]

**cup bi·op·sy for·ceps** a slender flexible forceps with movable cup-shaped jaws, used to obtain biopsy specimens through an endoscope.

**cup:disc ratio** the ratio between the diameter of the cupped or depressed central zone of the optic disc and the diameter of the entire disc; normally less than 1:3, it is increased in glaucoma.

**Cu·pid's bow** (kyu′pidz) the contour of the superior margin of the upper lip.

**cu·po·la** (koo′pŏ-lă) SYN cupula.

**cup·ping** (kŭp′ing) **1.** formation of a hollow, or cup-shaped excavation. **2.** application of a cupping glass. SEE ALSO cup.

**cup·ping glass** a glass vessel, from which the air has been exhausted by heat or a special suction apparatus, formerly applied to the skin in order to draw blood to the surface. SEE ALSO cupping, cup. SYN cup (2).

**cu·pu·la**, pl. **cu·pu·lae** (koo′poo-lă, kyu′pyu-lă; koo′poo-lē, kyu′pyu-lē) [TA] a cup-shaped or domelike structure. SYN cupola. [L. dim. of *cupa,* a tub]

**cu·pu·lar ce·cum of the co·chle·ar duct** the upper blind extremity of the cochlear duct. SYN lagena (1).

**cu·pu·li·form cat·a·ract** a common form of senile cataract often confined to a region just within the posterior capsule.

**cu·pu·lo·gram** (koo′poo-lō-gram) a graphic representation of vestibular function relative to normal performance.

**cur·a·tive** (kyur′ă-tiv) **1.** that which heals or cures. **2.** tending to heal or cure.

**cur·a·tive dose (CD) 1.** the quantity of any substance required to effect the cure of a disease or that will correct the manifestations of a deficiency of a particular factor in the diet; **2.** effective dose used with therapeutically applied compounds.

**cure** (kyur) **1.** to heal; to make well. **2.** a restoration to health. **3.** a special method or course of treatment. **4.** hardening of certain materials with time or by the application of heat, light, or chemical agents, e.g., polymerization of acrylic denture-based material. [L. *curo,* to care for]

**cu·ret·ment** (kyu-ret′ment) SYN curettage.

**cu·ret·tage** (kyu-rĕ-tahzh′) a scraping, usually of the interior of a cavity or tract, for the removal of new growths or other abnormal tissues, or to obtain material for tissue diagnosis. SYN curetment, curettement.

**cu·rette, cu·ret** (kyu-ret′) instrument in the form of a loop, ring, or scoop with sharpened edges attached to a rod-shaped handle, used for curettage. [Fr.]

**cu·rette·ment** (kyu-ret′ment) SYN curettage.

**cu·rie (c, C, Ci)** (kyu′rē) a unit of measurement of radioactivity, $3.70 \times 10^{10}$ disintegrations per second; superseded by the S.I. unit, the becquerel

(1 disintegration per second). [Marie (1867–1934) and Pierre (1859–1906) *Curie,* French chemists and physicists and Nobel laureates]

**cu·ri·um (cm)** (kyu′rē-ŭm) an element, atomic no. 96, atomic wt. 247.07, not occurring naturally on earth, but first formed artificially in 1944 by bombarding $^{239}$Pu with alpha particles; the most stable of the curium isotopes is $^{247}$Cm, with a half-life of 15.6 million years. [see curie]

**Curling ul·cer** SYN stress ulcer.

**cur·rant jel·ly clot** a jelly-like mass of red blood cells and fibrin formed by the *in vitro* or postmortem clotting of whole or sedimented blood.

**cur·rent** (ker′rĕnt) a stream or flow of fluid, air, or electricity. [L. *currens,* pres. p. of *curro,* to run]

**Cur·rent Pro·ce·du·ral Ter·min·o·lo·gy (CPT)** a coding system for all medical procedures and services, published by the American Medical Association (as *Physicians' Current Procedural Terminology*) and revised annually.

**Cursch·mann spi·ral** (koorsh′mahn) a spirally twisted mass of mucus occurring in the sputum in bronchial asthma.

**curse** (kers) an affliction thought to be invoked by a malevolent spirit.

**cur·va·tu·ra**, pl. **cur·va·tu·rae** (ker′vă-too′ră, ker′vă-too′rē) SYN curvature. [L.]

**cur·va·ture** (ker′vă-choor) a bending or flexure. SEE angulation. SYN curvatura. [L. *curvatura,* fr. *curvo,* pp. -*atus,* to bend, curve]

**cur·va·ture ab·er·ra·tion** lack of spatial correspondence causing the image of a straight extended object to appear curved.

**cur·va·ture hy·per·o·pia** hyperopia due to decreased refraction of the anterior ocular segment.

**cur·va·ture my·o·pia** myopia due to refractive errors resulting from excessive corneal curvature.

**curve** (kerv) **1.** a nonangular continuous bend or line. **2.** a chart or graphic representation, by means of a continuous line connecting individual observations, of the course of a physiologic activity, of the number of cases of a disease in a given period, or of any entity that might be otherwise presented by a table of figures. SYN chart (2). [L. *curvo,* to bend]

**curve of oc·clu·sion 1.** a curved surface which makes simultaneous contact with the major portion of the incisal and occlusal prominences of the existing teeth; **2.** the curve of a dentition on which the occlusal surfaces lie.

**curve of Spee** (shpā) an anatomic curvature determined by the occlusal surfaces of the teeth following the anterior mandibular cusp tips to the buccal cusp tips of the mandibular posterior teeth. SYN von Spee curve.

**curve of Wil·son** (wil′son) the curvature in a frontal plane through the cusp tips of both the right and left molars.

**Cush·ing ba·soph·i·lism** (kush′ing) SYN Cushing syndrome.

**Cush·ing dis·ease** (kush′ing) adrenal hyperplasia (Cushing syndrome) caused by an ACTH-secreting basophil adenoma of the pituitary.

**Cush·ing dis·ease of the o·men·tum** (kush′ing) central obesity in association with glucocorticoid excess, in which adipose stromal cells of the omental fat, but not subcutaneous tissue, can generate active cortisol from inactive cortisone. Patients have increased cortisol production and urinary cortisol excretion but no abnormality in the hypothalamico-pituitary-adrenal axis.

**cush·ing·oid** (kush'ing-oyd) resembling the signs and symptoms of Cushing disease or syndrome: buffalo hump obesity, striations, adiposity, hypertension, diabetes, and osteoporosis, usually due to exogenous corticosteroids.

**Cush·ing su·ture** (kush'ing) a running horizontal mattress suture used to approximate two adjacent surfaces.

**Cush·ing syn·drome** (kush'ing) a disorder resulting from increased adrenocortical secretion of cortisol (giving clinical picture of Cushing disease), due to any one of several sources: ACTH-dependent adrenocortical hyperplasia or tumor, ectopic ACTH-secreting tumor, or excessive administration of steroids; characterized by truncal obesity, moon face, acne, abdominal striae, hypertension, decreased carbohydrate tolerance, protein catabolism, psychiatric disturbances, and osteoporosis, amenorrhea, and hirsutism in females; when associated with an ACTH-producing adenoma, called Cushing disease. SYN Cushing basophilism.

**cush·ion** (kush'ŭn) ANATOMY any structure resembling a pad or cushion.

**cusp** (kŭsp) **1.** DENTISTRY a conical elevation arising on the surface of a tooth from an independent calcification center. **2.** a leaflet of a cardiac valve. SYN cuspis [TA]. [L. *cuspis,* point]

**cus·pal** (kŭs'păl) pertaining to a cusp.

**cusp and groove pat·tern** the arrangement of the cusps and grooves on molars; in the lower molars there are four principal ones, Y-5, Y-4, +5 and +4

**cusp height 1.** the shortest distance between the tip of a cusp and its base plane; **2.** the shortest distance between the deepest part of the central fossa of a posterior tooth and a line connecting the points of the cusps of the tooth.

**cus·pid** (kŭs'pid) **1.** having but one cusp. **2.** SYN canine tooth. [L. *cuspis,* point]

**cus·pi·date** (kŭs'pi-dāt) having a cusp or cusps.

**cus·pis,** pl. **cus·pi·des** (kŭs'pis, kŭs'pi-dēz) [TA] SYN cusp. [L. a point]

**cusp ridge** an elevation extending both mesially and distally from the cusp tip of molars and premolars, thus forming the lingual and buccal boundaries of the occlusal surface.

**cu·ta·ne·ous** (kyu-tā'nē-ŭs) relating to the skin. [L. *cutis,* skin]

**cu·ta·ne·ous an·cy·lo·sto·mi·a·sis** cutaneous larva migrans caused by larvae of hookworms. SYN swimmer's itch (1), water itch (1).

**cu·ta·ne·ous branch of an·te·ri·or branch of ob·tu·ra·tor nerve** branch of the anterior branch of obturator nerve supplying skin of medial thigh above knee.

**cu·ta·ne·ous branch of mixed nerve** branch of a mixed spinal nerve (or its derivatives) innervating skin; such branches would convey mostly somatic sensory but also visceral motor fibers (postsynaptic sympathetic fibers for vasomotion and pilomotion).

**cu·ta·ne·ous horn** a protruding keratotic growth of the skin; the base may show changes of actinic keratosis or carcinoma.

**cu·ta·ne·ous lar·va mi·grans** an advancing serpiginous or netlike tunneling in the skin, with marked pruritus, caused by wandering hookworm larvae not adapted to intestinal maturation

in man; especially common in the eastern and southern coastal U.S. and other tropical and subtropical coastal areas; various hookworms of dogs and cats have been implicated, chiefly *Ancylostoma braziliense* in the U.S., but also *Ancylostoma caninum* of dogs, *Uncinaria stenocephalia,* the European dog hookworm, and *Bunostomum phlebotomum,* the cattle hookworm; *Strongyloides* species of animal origin may also contribute to human cutaneous larva migrans.

**cu·ta·ne·ous leish·man·i·a·sis** infection with promastigotes (leptomonads) of *Leishmania tropica* and of *L. major* inoculated into the skin by the bite of an infected sandfly, *Phlebotomus* (commonly *P. papatasi*); it is endemic in parts of Asia Minor, northern Africa, and India. The ulcer begins as a papule that enlarges to a nodule and then breaks down into an ulcer. Two distinctive clinical and epidemiological diseases are recognized, the more common and widespread zoonotic rural disease with a moist acute form, caused by *L. major,* with reservoir rodent hosts; and an urban, anthroponotic, dry, chronic form of leishmaniasis caused by *L. tropica,* without a reservoir host, and now largely controlled. SEE zoonotic cutaneous leishmaniasis. SYN Old World leishmaniasis, tropical sore.

**cu·ta·ne·ous leish·man·i·a·sis gran·u·lo·ma** lymphocytic granuloma with a necrotic center found during the healing process.

**cu·ta·ne·ous mus·cle** a muscle that lies in the subcutaneous tissue and attaches to the skin; it may or may not have a bony attachment. The muscles of expression are the chief examples of cutaneous muscles in the human.

**cu·ta·ne·ous nerve** a mixed nerve supplying a region of the skin, including its sensory endings, blood vessels, smooth muscle and glands.

**cu·ta·ne·ous pseu·do·lym·pho·ma** SYN benign lymphocytoma cutis.

**cu·ta·ne·ous tu·ber·cu·lo·sis** pathologic lesions of the skin caused by *Mycobacterium tuberculosis.*

**cu·ta·ne·ous vas·cu·li·tis** an acute form of vasculitis which may affect the skin only, but also may involve other organs, with a polymorphonuclear infiltrate in the walls of and surrounding small (dermal) vessels. Nuclear fragments are formed by karyorrhexis of the neutrophils. SEE ALSO leukocytoclastic vasculitis.

**cut·down** (kŭt'down) dissection of a vein for insertion of a cannula or needle for the administration of intravenous fluids or medication. SYN venostomy.

**cu·ti·cle** (kyu'ti-kl) **1.** an outer thin layer, usually horny in nature. SYN cuticula (1). **2.** the layer, chitinous in some invertebrates, which occurs on the surface of epithelial cells. **3.** SYN epidermis. [L. *cuticula,* dim. of *cutis,* skin]

**cu·tic·u·la,** pl. **cu·tic·u·lae** (kyu-tik'yu-lă, kyu-tik'yu-lē) **1.** SYN cuticle (1). **2.** SYN epidermis. [L. cuticle]

**cu·tic·u·lar dru·sen** SYN basal laminar drusen.

**cu·ti·re·ac·tion** (kyu'ti-rē-ak'shŭn) the inflammatory reaction to a skin test in a sensitive (allergic) subject. [L. *cutis,* skin, + reaction]

**cu·tis** (kyu'tis) [TA] SYN skin. [L.]

**cu·tis an·se·ri·na** contraction of the arrectores pilorum produced by cold, fear, or other stimulus, causing the follicular orifices to become prominent.

**cu·tis lax·a** [TA] a congenital or acquired condition characterized by deficient elastic fibers of the skin, which may hang in folds; vascular anomalies may be present. SYN pachydermatocele.

**cu·tis mar·mo·ra·ta** a normal, physiologic, pink, marble-like mottling of the skin in infants, persisting abnormally in some children on exposure to cold.

**cu·tis mar·mo·ra·ta tel·an·gi·ec·tat·i·ca con··gen·i·ta** capillary-venous cutaneous malformation with "marbled" appearance. SYN Van Lohuizen syndrome.

**cu·tis plate** SYN dermatome (2).

**cu·tis rhom·boi·da·lis nu·chae** geometric furrowed configurations of the skin of the back of the neck as a result of prolonged exposure to sunlight with solar elastosis.

**cu·tis ve·ra** SYN dermis.

**cutpoint** (kut'poynt) arbitrary value on an ordinal scale such as blood pressure, beyond which values are regarded as clinically abnormal.

**Cu·vier ducts** (kū-vē-ā') obsolete term for the common cardinal veins.

**Cu·vier veins** (kū-vē-ā') the common cardinal veins of the embryo. SEE cardinal veins.

**CV** coefficient of variation.

**CVA** cerebrovascular accident.

**CVP** central venous pressure.

**cy·a·nide** (sī'an-īd) 1. the radical –CN or ion (CN)⁻. The ion is extremely poisonous, forming hydrocyanic acid in water; inhibits respiratory enzymes. 2. a salt of HCN or a cyano-containing molecule.

**cy·an·met·he·mo·glo·bin** (sī'an-met-hē'mō-glō-bin) a relatively nontoxic compound of cyanide with methemoglobin, which is formed when methylene blue is administered in cases of cyanide poisoning.

△**cy·an·o-, cy·an-** 1. blue. 2. chemical prefix frequently used in naming compounds that contain the cyanide group, CN. [G. *kyanos,* a dark blue substance]

**Cy·a·no·bac·te·ria** (sī'ă-nō-bak-tēr'ē-ă) a division of the kingdom Prokaryotae consisting of unicellular or filamentous bacteria that are either nonmotile or possess a gliding motility, reproduce by binary fission, and perform photosynthesis with the production of oxygen. SYN Cyanophyceae.

**cy·an·o·bac·te·ri·um·like bod·ies** SYN *Cyclospora.*

**cy·a·no·co·bal·a·min** (sī'an-ō-kō-bal'ă-min) a complex of cyanide and cobalamin, as in vitamin $B_{12}$.

**cy·an·o·phil, cy·an·o·phile** (sī'an-ō-fil, sī'an-ō-fīl) a cell or element that is differentially colored blue by a staining procedure. [cyano- + G. *philos,* fond]

**cy·a·noph·i·lous** (sī-ă-nof'i-lŭs) readily stainable with a blue dye.

**Cy·a·no·phy·ce·ae** (sī'ă-nō-fī'sē-ē) SYN Cyanobacteria. [cyano- + G. *phykos,* seaweed]

**cy·a·nop·sia** (sī-ă-nop'sē-ă) a condition in which all objects appear blue; may temporarily follow cataract extraction. [cyano- + G. *opsis,* vision]

**cy·a·nosed** (sī'ă-nōst) SYN cyanotic.

**cy·a·nose tar·dive** (sē-ă-nōs' tar-dēv') cyanosis developing in congenital heart disease only after the heart begins to fail. SYN tardive cyanosis. [F. delayed cyanosis]

**cy·a·no·sis** (sī-ă-nō'sis) a dark bluish or purplish coloration of the skin, nail beds, lips, or mucous membranes due to deficient oxygenation of the blood, evident when reduced hemoglobin in the blood exceeds 5 g per 100 ml. [G. dark blue color, fr. *kyanos,* blue substance]

**cy·a·not·ic** (sī-ă-not'ik) relating to or marked by cyanosis. SYN cyanosed.

**cy·a·not·ic in·du·ra·tion** induration related to persistent, chronic venous congestion in an organ or tissue, frequently resulting in fibrous thickening of the walls of the veins and eventual fibrosis of adjacent tissue.

**cy·ber·net·ics** (sī-ber-net'iks) 1. the comparative study of electronic calculators and the human nervous system, with intent to explain the functioning of the brain. 2. the science of control and communication in both living and nonliving systems; characteristically, control is governed by feedback, that is, by communication within the system concerning the difference between the actual and the desired result, action then being modified so as to minimize this difference. SEE ALSO feedback. [G. *kybernētica,* things pertaining to control or piloting]

**cy·clar·thro·di·al** (sī-klar-thrō'dē-ăl) relating to a cyclarthrosis.

**cy·clar·thro·sis** (sī-klar-thrō'sis) a joint capable of rotation. [cyclo- + G. *arthrōsis,* articulation]

**cy·clase** (sī'klās) descriptive name applied to an enzyme that forms a cyclic compound; e.g., adenylate cyclase.

**cy·cle** (sī'kl) 1. a recurrent series of events. 2. a recurring period of time. 3. one successive compression and rarefaction of a wave, as of a sound wave. [G. *kyklos,* circle]

**cy·clec·to·my** (sī-klek'tō-mē, sik-lek'tō-mē) excision of a portion of the ciliary body. SYN ciliectomy. [cyclo- + G. *ektomē,* excision]

**cycle length al·ter·nans** a succession of alternately long and short diastolic intervals.

**cy·clen·ceph·a·ly, cy·clen·ce·pha·lia** (sī-klen-sef'ă-lē, sī-klen-se-fā'lē-ă) condition in a malformed fetus characterized by poor development and a varying degree of fusion of the two cerebral hemispheres. SYN cyclocephaly, cyclocephalia. [cyclo- + G. *enkephalos,* brain]

**cy·cles per sec·ond (cps)** the number of successive compressions and rarefactions per second of a sound wave. The preferred designation for this unit of frequency is hertz.

**cy·clic** (sī'klik, sik'lik) 1. pertaining to, or characteristic of, a cycle; occurring periodically, denoting the course of the symptoms in certain diseases or disorders. 2. CHEMISTRY pertaining to a molecule containing a ring of atoms; denoting a cyclic compound.

**cy·clic AMP** SYN adenosine 3',5'-cyclic monophosphate.

**3',5'-cy·clic AMP syn·the·tase** SYN adenylate cyclase.

**cy·clic com·pound** any compound in which the constituent atoms, or any part of them, form a ring. Used mainly in organic chemistry. SYN closed chain compound.

**cy·clin D** protein involved in progression to cell division.

**cy·clist's nip·ples** nipple irritation due to the combined effects of perspiration and wind-chill producing cold, painful nipples.

**cy·clist's pal·sy** paresthesia of the ulnar nerve in

cyclists resulting from leaning on the handlebars for an extended period. SYN ulnar nerve compression syndrome.

**cy·cli·tis** (sī-klī'tis) inflammation of the ciliary body. [G. *kyklos,* circle (ciliary body), + *-itis,* inflammation]

⚠**cy·clo-, cycl-** 1. a circle or cycle; the ciliary body. 2. CHEMISTRY a molecule consisting of atoms in a ring. [G. *kyklos,* circle]

**cy·clo·ceph·a·ly, cy·clo·ce·pha·lia** (sī-klō-sef'ă-lē, sī-klō-sĕ-fā'lē-ă) SYN cyclencephaly. [cyclo- + G. *kephalē,* head]

**cy·clo·cho·roid·i·tis** (sī'klō-kō-roy-dī'tis) inflammation of the ciliary body and the choroid.

**cy·clo·cry·o·ther·a·py** (sī'klō-krī'ō-thār'ă-pē) transscleral freezing of the ciliary body in the treatment of glaucoma.

**cy·clo·di·al·y·sis** (sī'klō-dī-al'i-sis) establishment of a communication between the anterior chamber and the suprachoroidal space in order to reduce intraocular pressure in glaucoma. [cyclo- + G. *dialysis,* separation]

**cy·clo·di·a·ther·my** (sī'klō-dī-ă-ther'mē) diathermy applied to the sclera adjacent to the ciliary body in the treatment of glaucoma.

**cy·clo·duc·tion** (sī-klō-dŭk'shŭn) rotation of the eye around its visual axis. SYN circumduction (2). [cyclo- + L. *duco,* pp. *ductus,* to draw]

**cy·clo·pep·tide** (sī-klō-pep'tīd) a polypeptide lacking terminal —$NH_2$ and —COOH groups by virtue of their combination to form another peptide link, forming a ring.

**cy·clo·pho·ras·es** (sī-klō-fōr'ās-ez) the group of enzymes in mitochondria that catalyze the complete oxidation of pyruvic acid to carbon dioxide and water; essentially, those enzymes and coenzymes involved in the tricarboxylic acid cycle.

**cy·clo·pho·ria** (sī-klō-fō'rē-ă) abnormal tendency for each eye to rotate around its anteroposterior axis, the rotation being prevented by visual fusional impulses. [cyclo- + G. *phora,* movement]

**cy·clo·pho·to·co·ag·u·la·tion** (sī'klō-fō'tō-kō-ag-yu-lā'shŭn) photocoagulation of the ciliary processes to reduce the secretion of aqueous humor in glaucoma. [cyclo- + photocoagulation]

**cy·clo·pia** (sī-klō'pē-ă) a congenital defect in which the two orbits merge to form a single cavity containing one eye, its origin evidenced by fusion of the right and left optic primordia, and in which the nose is absent; usually combined with cyclencephaly. SYN synophthalmia. [G. *Kyklōps,* mythic one-eyed giant, fr. *kyklos,* circle, + *ōps,* eye]

**cy·clo·pi·an** (sī-klō'pē-an) denoting or relating to cyclopia.

**cy·clo·ple·gia** (sī-klō-plē'jē-ă) loss of power in the ciliary muscle of the eye; may be by denervation or by pharmacologic action. [cyclo- + G. *plēgē,* stroke]

**cy·clo·ple·gic** (sī-klō-plē'jik) 1. relating to cycloplegia. 2. a drug that paralyzes the ciliary muscle and thus the power of accommodation.

**Cy·clo·spo·ra** (sī-klō-spōr'ă) a *Cryptosporidium*-like genus of coccidian parasites reported from millipedes, reptiles, insectivores, and a rodent species. Cyclospora is characterized by acid-fast oocysts with two sporocysts, each with two sporozoites. Cyclospora is implicated as the cause of a widespread, prolonged but self-limited human diarrhea in patients in the Americas, Caribbean

countries, Southeast Asia, and eastern Europe previously reported as caused by cyanobacteriumlike bodies. SYN cyanobacteriumlike bodies.

*Cy·clo·spor·a caye·tan·en·sis* a species causing enteritis with persistent diarrhea; usually acquired by ingestion of contaminated water or food.

**cy·clo·thy·mia** (sī-klō-thī'mē-ă) a mental disorder characterized by marked swings of mood from depression to hypomania but not to the degree that occurs in bipolar disorder. [cyclo- + G. *thymos,* rage]

**cy·clo·thy·mic dis·or·der** an affective disorder characterized by mood swings including periods of hypomania and depression; a form of depressive disorder.

**cy·clo·thy·mic per·son·al·i·ty** a personality disorder in which a person experiences regularly alternating periods of elation and depression, usually not related to external circumstances.

**cy·clot·o·my** (sī-klot'ō-mē) operation of cutting the ciliary muscle. [cyclo- + G. *tomē,* incision]

**cy·clo·tro·pia** (sī-klō-trō'pē-ă) a disparity of ocular position in which one eye is rotated around its visual axis, with respect to the other eye. [cyclo- + G. *tropē,* a turn, turning]

**Cyd** cytidine.

**cyl·in·der (C)** (sil'in-der) 1. a cylindrical lens. 2. a cylindrical or rodlike renal cast. 3. a cylindrical metal container for gases stored under high pressure. [G. *kylindros,* a roll]

**cyl·in·dri·cal lens (C)** a lens in which one of the surfaces is curved in one meridian and less curved in the opposite meridian; commonly used to correct the visual distortion resulting from astigmatism. SYN astigmatic lens.

**cyl·in·dro·ad·e·no·ma** (sil'in-drō-ad-ĕ-nō'mă) SYN cylindroma.

**cyl·in·dro·ma** (sil-in-drō'mă) a histologic type of epithelial neoplasm, frequently malignant, characterized by islands of neoplastic cells embedded in a hyalinized stroma; may form from ducts of glands, especially in salivary glands, skin, and bronchi. SYN cylindroadenoma. [G. *kylindros,* cylinder, *-oma,* tumor]

**cyl·in·drom·a·tous car·ci·no·ma** SYN adenoid cystic carcinoma.

**cyl·in·dru·ria** (sil-in-dr-yu'rē-ă) the presence of renal cylinders or casts in the urine.

**cym·bo·ce·phal·ic, cym·bo·ceph·a·lous** (sim-bō-se-fal'ik, sim-bō-sef'ă-lŭs) relating to cymbocephaly.

**cym·bo·ceph·a·ly** SYN scaphocephaly. [G. *kymbē,* the hollow of a vessel, a boat-shaped structure, *kephalē,* head]

**cyn·ic spasm** SYN risus caninus.

**cy·no·ceph·a·ly** (sī-nō-sef'ă-lē) craniostenosis in which the skull slopes back from the orbits, producing a resemblance to the head of a dog. [G. *kyōn,* dog, + *kephalē,* head]

**cy·no·pho·bia** (sī-nō-fō'bē-ă) morbid fear of dogs. [G. *kyōn,* dog, + *phobos,* fear]

**CYP** abbreviation for cytochrome P450 enzymes; usually followed by an arabic numeral, a letter, and another arabic numeral (e.g., CYP 2D6). These enzymes are found in and on the smooth endoplasmic reticulum of liver and other cells and are responsible for a large number of drug biotransformation reactions.

**CYP 1A2** microsomal enzyme, the substrates of which include theophylline, antidepressants, and tacrine. It is inhibited by grapefruit juice and quinolones, and induced by smoking, phenobarbital, phenytoin, rifampin, and omeprazole.

**CYP 3A** a cytochrome P450 isoform found in the gastrointestinal tract as well as hepatic and other cells; substrates include benzodiazepines, calcium channel blockers, antihistamines, steroid hormones, and protease inhibitors. Inhibited by antidepressants, azole antifungals, cimetidine, and erythromycin. Induced by phenobarbital, phenytoin, rifampin, and carbamazepine.

**CYP 2C9** microsomal enzyme responsible for the oxidation of S-warfarin, phenytoin, and numerous NSAIDs. Inhibitors include azole antifungals (e.g., ketoconazole, itraconazole, metronidazole); induced by rifampin.

**CYP 2C19** microsomal enzyme partially responsible for the oxidation of clomipramine, diazepam, propranolol, imipramine, and omeprazole. Inhibited by fluoxetine, sertraline, omeprazole, and ritonavir.

**CYP 2D6** an isoenzyme that metabolizes many antidepressants, antipsychotic agents, beta adrenergic blockers, and codeine. It is inhibited by cimetidine and several antidepressants and antipsychotics.

**CYP 2E1** microsomal enzyme that participates in the oxidation of ethanol and acetaminophen. Inhibited by disulfiram and induced by ethanol and isoniazid (INH). Believed to be responsible for the hepatotoxic metabolite of acetaminophen.

**Cys** cysteine (half-cystine) or its mono- or diradical.

🔲 **cyst** (sist) 1. a bladder. 2. an abnormal sac containing gas, fluid, or a semisolid material, with a membranous lining. SEE ALSO pseudocyst. See page B4. [G. *kystis*, bladder]

**cyst•ad•e•no•car•ci•no•ma** (sist-ad′en-ō-kar-si-nō′mă) a malignant neoplasm derived from glandular epithelium, in which cystic accumulations of retained secretions are formed; the neoplastic cells manifest varying degrees of anaplasia and invasiveness, and local extension and metastases occur; cystadenocarcinomas develop frequently in the ovaries, where pseudomucinous and serous types are recognized.

**cyst•ad•e•no•ma** (sist′ad-ĕ-nō′mă) a histologically benign neoplasm derived from glandular epithelium, in which cystic accumulations of retained secretions are formed. SYN cystoadenoma.

**cyst•al•gia** (sist-al′jē-ă) pain in a bladder, especially the urinary bladder. [cyst- + G. *algos*, pain]

**cys•ta•thi•o•nase** (sis-tă-thī′ō-nās) SYN cystathionine γ-lyase.

**cys•ta•thi•o•nine** (sis-tă-thī′ō-nēn) an intermediate in the conversion of L-methionine to L-cysteine; cleaved by cystathionases.

**cys•ta•thi•o•nine γ-ly•ase** a liver enzyme that catalyzes the hydrolysis of L-cystathionine to L-cysteine and 2-ketobutyrate. A deficiency of this enzyme results in cystathioninuria. A step in methionine catabolism and in cysteine biosynthesis. SYN cystathionase.

**cys•tec•ta•sia, cys•tec•ta•sy** (sis-tek-tā′zē-ă, sis-tek′tă-sē) dilation of the bladder. [cyst- + G. *ektasis*, a stretching]

**cys•tec•to•my** (sis-tek′tō-mē) 1. excision of the the urinary bladder. 2. excision of the gallbladder (cholecystectomy). 3. removal of a cyst. [cyst- + G. *ektomē*, excision]

**cys•te•ic ac•id** (sis-tā′ik as′id) an oxidation pro-

duct of cysteine, and a precursor of taurine and isethionic acid.

**cys•te•ine (C, Cys)** (sis′ta-ēn) an amino acid found in most proteins; especially abundant in keratin.

**cys•tic** (sis′tik) 1. relating to the urinary bladder or gallbladder. 2. relating to a cyst. 3. containing cysts.

**cys•tic ac•ne** severe acne in which the predominant lesions are follicular cysts which rupture and scar.

**cys•tic ar•tery** *origin*, right branch of hepatic; *distribution*, gall bladder and visceral surface of the liver. SYN arteria cystica [TA].

**cys•tic dis•ease of the breast** fibrocystic condition of the breasts.

**cys•tic duct, cys•tic gall duct** the ductus leading from the gallbladder; it joins the hepatic duct to form the common bile duct.

**cys•ti•cer•co•sis** (sis′ti-ser-kō′sis) 1. disease caused by encystment of cysticercus larvae (e.g., *Taenia solium* or *T. saginata*) in subcutaneous, muscle, or central nervous system tissues; cysticercosis is typically developed in swine and cattle, producing measly pork and beef. In humans, it results from the hatching of the eggs of *Taenia solium* in the intestines or by accidental ingestion of eggs from human feces; encystment in the brain may cause serious nervous damage, and encystment in the eye (usually the rear chamber) may cause ophthalmic damage. 2. larval infections in animals with other taeniid tapeworm larvae.

*Cys•ti•cer•cus* (sis-ti-ser′kŭs) the encysted larva of taenioid tapeworms. SEE cysticercus. [G. *kystis*, bladder, + *kerkos*, tail]

**cys•ti•cer•cus**, pl. **cys•ti•cer•ci** (sis-ti-ser′kŭs, sis′ti-ser′sī) the larval form of certain *Taenia* species, typically found in muscles of mammalian intermediate hosts; it consists of a fluid-filled bladder in which the invaginated cestode scolex develops. SEE ALSO *Taenia saginata, Taenia solium*. [G. *kystis*, bladder, + *kerkos*, tail]

**cys•tic fi•bro•sis, cys•tic fi•bro•sis of the pan•cre•as** a congenital metabolic disorder, inherited as an autosomal trait, in which secretions of exocrine glands are abnormal; excessively viscid mucus causes obstruction of passageways (including pancreatic and bile ducts, intestines, and bronchi), and the sodium and chloride content of sweat are increased throughout the patient's life; symptoms usually appear in childhood and include meconium ileus, poor growth despite good appetite, malabsorption and foul bulky stools, chronic bronchitis with cough, recurrent pneumonia, bronchiectasis, emphysema, clubbing of the fingers, and salt depletion in hot weather. Detailed genetic mapping and molecular biology have been accomplished by the methods of reverse genetics.

**cys•tic goi•ter** an enlargement in the thyroid region due to the presence of one or more cysts within the gland.

**cys•tic lymph node** a lymph node at the neck of the gallbladder draining lymph into the hepatic nodes.

**cys•tic veins** veins, usually anterior and posterior, which drain the neck of the gallbladder and cystic duct, along which they pass to enter the right branch of the portal vein; they communicate extensively with surrounding veins of the stomach, duodenum and pancreas.

**cys·ti·form** (sis′ti-fōrm) SYN cystoid (1).

**cys·tine** (sis′tīn) the disulfide product of two cysteines in which two –SH groups become one –S–S– group; sometimes occurs as a deposit in the urine, or forming a vesical calculus.

**cys·tine cal·cu·lus** a calculus composed of cystine, soft and faintly radiopaque.

**cys·ti·ne·mia** (sis-ti-nē′mē-ă) the presence of cystine in the blood. [cystine + G. *haima*, blood]

**cys·ti·nu·ria** (sis-ti-nyu′rē-ă) excessive urinary excretion of cystine, along with lysine, arginine, and ornithine, arising from defective transport systems for these acids in the kidney and intestine; renal function is sometimes compromised by cystine crystalluria and nephrolithiasis; occurs in certain heritable diseases, such as Fanconi syndrome (cystinosis) and hepatolenticular degeneration. [cystine + G. *ouron*, urine]

**cys·ti·tis** (sis-tī′tis) inflammation of the urinary bladder. [cyst- + G. *-itis*, inflammation]

**cys·ti·tis cys·ti·ca** cystitis glandularis with the formation of cysts.

**cys·ti·tis glan·du·la·ris** chronic cystitis with glandlike metaplasia of transitional epithelium.

**cys·to-, cys·ti-, cyst-** combining forms relating to: **1.** the bladder. **2.** the cystic duct. **3.** a cyst. Cf. vesico-. [G. *kystis*, bladder, pouch]

**cys·to·ad·e·no·ma** (sis′tō-ad-ĕ-nō′mă) SYN cystadenoma.

**cys·to·car·ci·no·ma** (sis′tō-kar-si-nō′mă) a carcinoma in which cystic degeneration has occurred; sometimes used incorrectly as a term for cystadenocarcinoma. SYN cystoepithelioma.

**cys·to·cele** (sis′tō-sēl) hernia of the bladder usually into the vagina and introitus. SYN colpocystocele, vesicocele. [cysto- + G. *kēlē*, hernia]

**cys·to·chro·mos·co·py** (sis′tō-krō-mos′kŏ-pē) examination of the interior of the bladder after administration of a dye to aid in the identification or study of the function of the ureteral orifices. SYN chromocystoscopy. [cysto- + G. *chrōma*, color + *skopeō*, to view]

**cys·to·du·o·de·nal lig·a·ment** a peritoneal fold that sometimes passes from the gallbladder to the first part of the duodenum.

**cys·to·du·o·de·nos·to·my** (sis′tō-doo′ō-dē-nos′tō-mē) drainage of a cyst, usually pancreatic pseudocyst, into duodenum. SYN duodenocystostomy (2). [cysto- + duodenum, + G. *stoma*, mouth]

**cys·to·ep·i·the·li·o·ma** (sis′tō-ep-i-thē-lē-ō′mă) SYN cystocarcinoma.

**cys·to·fi·bro·ma** (sis′tō-fī-brō′mă) a fibroma in which cysts or cystlike foci have formed.

**cys·to·gram** (sis′tō-gram) radiographic demonstration of the bladder filled with contrast medium.

**cys·tog·ra·phy** (sis-tog′ră-fē) radiography of the bladder following injection of a radiopaque substance. [cysto- + G. *graphō*, to write]

**cys·toid** (sis′toyd) **1.** bladder-like, resembling a cyst. SYN cystiform, cystomorphous. **2.** a tumor resembling a cyst, with fluid, granular, or pulpy contents, but without a capsule. [cysto- + G. *eidos*, appearance]

**cys·toid mac·u·lop·a·thy** cystic degeneration of the central retina that may occur after cataract extraction, in senile macular degeneration, and in other retinal abnormalities.

**cys·to·li·thi·a·sis** (sis′tō-li-thī′ă-sis) the presence of a vesical calculus. [cysto- + G. *lithos*, stone, + *-iasis*, condition]

**cys·to·lith·ic** (sis-tō-lith′ik) relating to a vesical calculus.

**cy·sto·lith·o·la·paxy** (sis′tō-lith-ō-lă-paks-ē) removal of bladder calculi by intravesical crushing and then irrigating to remove fragments. [cysto- + G. *lithos*, stone, + *lapaxis*, an emptying out]

**cys·to·li·thot·o·my** (sis′tō-li-thot′ō-mē) removal of a stone from the bladder through an incision in its wall. [cysto- + G. *lithos*, stone, + *tomē*, incision]

**cys·to·ma** (sis-tō′mă) a cystic tumor; a new growth containing cysts. [cyst- + G. *-oma*, tumor]

**cys·tom·e·ter** (sis-tom′ĕ-ter) a device for studying bladder function by measuring capacity, sensation, intravesical pressure, and residual urine. [cysto- + G. *metron*, measure]

**cys·to·met·ro·gram** (sis-tō-met′rō-gram) a graphic recording of urinary bladder pressure at various volumes. [cysto- + G. *metron*, measure, + *gramma*, a writing]

**cys·tom·e·try, cys·to·me·trog·ra·phy** (sis-tom′ĕ-trē, sis′tō-mĕ-trog′ră-fē) a method for measurement of the pressure/volume relationship of the bladder. SEE cystometer.

**cys·to·mor·phous** (sis-tō-mōr′fŭs) SYN cystoid (1). [cysto- + G. *morphē*, form]

**cys·to·pan·en·dos·co·py** (sis′tō-pan-en-dos′kŏ-pē) inspection of the interior of the bladder and urethra by means of specially designed endoscopes introduced in retrograde fashion through the urethra and into the bladder. [cysto- + panendoscope]

**cys·to·pa·ral·y·sis** (sis-tō-pă-ral′i-sis) SYN cystoplegia.

**cys·to·pexy** (sis′tō-pek-sē) surgical attachment of the gallbladder or of the urinary bladder to the abdominal wall or to other supporting structures. [cysto- + G. *pēxis*, fixation]

**cys·to·plas·ty** (sis′tō-plas-tē) any reconstructive operation on the urinary bladder. Cf. ileocystoplasty. [cysto- + G. *plastos*, formed]

**cys·to·ple·gia** (sis-tō-plē′jē-ă) paralysis of the bladder. SYN cystoparalysis. [cysto- + G. *plēgē*, a stroke]

**cystoptosis, cys·to·pto·si·a** (sis-top-tō′sis) prolapse of the vesical mucous membrane into the urethra. [cysto- + G. *ptosis*, a falling]

**cys·to·py·e·li·tis** (sis′tō-pī-el-ī′tis) inflammation of both the bladder and the pelvis of the kidney. [cysto- + G. *pyelos*, trough (pelvis), + *-itis*, inflammation]

**cys·to·py·e·lo·ne·phri·tis** (sis-tō-pī′el-ō-nef-rī′tis) inflammation of the bladder, the pelvis of the kidney, and the kidney parenchyma. [cysto- + G. *pyelos*, trough (pelvis), + *nephros*, kidney, + *-itis*, inflammation]

**cys·to·rec·tos·to·my** (sis-tō-rek-tos′tō-mē) SYN vesicorectostomy. [cysto + rectum + G. *stoma*, mouth]

**cys·tor·rha·phy** (sis-tōr′ă-fē) suture of a wound or defect in the urinary bladder. [cysto- + G. *rhaphē*, a sewing]

**cys·tor·rhea** (sis′tō-rē-ă) a mucous discharge from the bladder. [cysto- + G. *rhoia*, a flow]

**cys·to·sar·co·ma** (sis′tō-sar-kō′mă) a sarcoma in which the formation of cysts or cystlike foci has occurred.

**cys·to·scope** (sis'tō-skōp) a lighted tubular endoscope for examining the interior of the bladder. [cysto- + G. *skopeō*, to examine]

**cys·to·scop·ic u·rog·ra·phy** SYN retrograde urography.

**cys·tos·co·py** (sis-tos'kŏ-pē) the inspection of the interior of the bladder by means of a cystoscope.

**cys·tos·to·my** (sis-tos'tō-mē) creation of an opening into the urinary bladder. SYN vesicostomy. [cysto- + G. *stoma*, mouth]

**cys·to·tome** (sis'tō-tōm) **1.** an instrument for incising the urinary bladder or gallbladder. **2.** a surgical instrument used for incising the capsule of a lens.

**cys·tot·o·my** (sis-tot'ō-mē) incision into urinary bladder or gallbladder. SYN vesicotomy. [cysto- + G. *tomē*, incision]

**cys·to·u·re·ter·i·tis** (sis'tō-yū-rē-ter-ī'tis) inflammation of the bladder and of one or both ureters.

**cys·to·u·re·ter·o·gram** (sis'tō-yū-rē'ter-ō-gram) radiographic demonstration of the bladder and ureters.

**cys·to·u·re·ter·og·ra·phy** (sis'tō-yu-rē'ter-og'rǎ-fē) radiography of the bladder and ureters.

**cys·to·u·re·thri·tis** (sis'tō-yu-rē-thrī'tis) inflammation of the bladder and of the urethra.

**cys·to·u·re·thro·gram** (sis-tō-yu-rēth'rō-gram) an x-ray image made during voiding and with the bladder and urethra filled with contrast medium to demonstrate the urethra. SYN voiding cystogram.

**cys·to·u·re·throg·ra·phy** (sis'tō-yu'rē-throg'rǎ-fē) radiography of the bladder and urethra during voiding, following filling of the bladder with a radiopaque contrast medium either by intravenous injection or retrograde catheterization.

**cys·to·u·re·thro·scope** (sis-tō-yu-rē'thrō-skōp) an instrument combining the uses of a cystoscope and a urethroscope, whereby both the bladder and urethra can be visually inspected.

**Cyt** cytosine.

**cy·ta·pher·e·sis** (sī'tǎ-fĕ-rē'sis) a procedure in which various cells can be separated from the withdrawn blood and retained, with the plasma and other formed elements retransfused into the donor. [cyt- + G. *aphairesis*, a withdrawal]

△**-cyte** cell. [G. *kyton*, a hollow (cell)]

**cyt·i·dine** (**C, Cyd**) (sī'ti-dēn) a major component of ribonucleic acids. SYN cytosine ribonucleoside.

**cyt·i·dine 5'-di·phos·phate** (**CDP**) an ester, at the 5' position, between cytidine and diphosphoric acid.

**cyt·i·dine 5'-tri·phos·phate** (**CTP**) an ester, at the 5' position, between cytidine and triphosphoric acid.

**cyt·i·dyl·ic ac·id** (sī-ti-dil'ik as'id) cytidine monophosphate (five are possible, depending on the site of attachment of the phosphate to the ribosyl OHs); a constituent of ribonucleic acids.

△**cy·to-, cyt-** a cell. [G. *kytos*, a hollow (cell)]

**cy·to·ar·chi·tec·ture** (sī'tō-ar'ki-tek-cher) the arrangement of cells in a tissue; the term commonly refers to the arrangement of nerve-cell bodies in the brain, especially the cerebral cortex.

**cy·to·cen·trum** (sī-tō-sen'trŭm) a zone of cytoplasm containing one or two centrioles but devoid of other organelles; usually located near the nucleus of a cell. SYN centrosome, microcentrum. [cyto- + G. *kentron*, center]

**cy·to·chem·is·try** (sī'tō-kem'is-trē) the study of intracellular distribution of chemicals, reaction sites, enzymes, etc., often by means of staining reactions, radioactive isotope uptake, selective metal distribution in electron microscopy, or other methods. SYN histochemistry.

**cy·to·chrome** (sī'tō-krōm) a class of hemoprotein whose principal biological function is electron and/or hydrogen transport by virtue of a reversible valency change of the heme iron. Many variants exist, particularly among bacteria and in green plants and algae, one being a variant of the *c* type cytochrome called cytochrome *f*. The mitochondrial system of cytochromes provides electron transport through cytochrome *c* oxidase to molecular oxygen as the terminal electron acceptor (respiration). [cyto- + G. *chrōma*, color]

**cy·to·chrome P-450 sys·tem** a heterogeneous group of enzymes that catalyze various oxidative reactions in the human liver, intestine, kidney, lung, and central nervous system; these enzymes are involved in the metabolism of many endogenous and exogenous substrates, including drugs, toxins, hormones, and natural plant products. Cytochrome P-450 enzymes are classified on the basis of chemical structure (amino acid sequencing). The designation of each enzyme is CYP followed by a numeral for the family to which it has been assigned, a letter for its subfamily, and sometimes a second numeral for the individual enzyme.

**cy·toc·i·dal** (sī-tō-sī'dǎl) causing the death of cells. [cyto- + L. *caedo*, to kill]

**cy·to·cide** (sī'tō-sīd) an agent that is destructive to cells. [cyto- + L. *caedo*, to kill]

**cy·toc·la·sis** (sī-tok'lǎ-sis) fragmentation of cells. [cyto- + G. *klasis*, a breaking]

**cy·to·clas·tic** (sī-tō-klas'tik) relating to cytoclasis.

**cy·to·di·ag·no·sis** (sī'tō-dī-ag-nō'sis) diagnosis of a pathologic process by means of microscopic study of cells.

**cy·to·gen·e·sis** (sī-tō-jen'ĕ-sis) the origin and development of cells. [cyto- + G. *genesis*, origin]

**cy·to·ge·net·i·cist** (sī'tō-jĕ-net'i-sist) a specialist in cytogenetics.

**cy·to·ge·net·ics** (sī'tō-jĕ-net'iks) the branch of genetics concerned with the structure and function of the cell, especially the chromosomes. Modern molecular cytogenetics involves the microscopic study of chromosomes that have been arranged as karyotypes. Individuals can be classified according to characteristic banding patterns that appear when the karyotypes are exposed to certain dyes. In addition, DNA probes may be applied to locate specific gene sequences. Cytogenetic techniques are used to test for inherent errors of metabolism, for disorders such as Down syndrome, and to determine sex in cases where anatomy is inconclusive.

**cy·to·gen·ic** (sī-tō-jen'ik) relating to cytogenesis.

**cy·to·gen·ic re·pro·duc·tion** reproduction by means of unicellular germ cells; includes both sexual reproduction and asexual reproduction by means of spores.

**cy·tog·e·nous** (sī-toj'ĕ-nŭs) cell-forming.

**cy·to·glu·co·pe·nia** (sī'tō-gloo-kō-pē'nē-ă) an intracellular deficiency of glucose. [cyto- + glucose + G. *penia*, poverty]

**cy·toid** (sī'toyd) resembling a cell. [cyto- + G. *eidos*, resemblance]

**cy·to·ker·a·tin** (sī-tō-ker-a-tinz) SYN keratin.

**cy·to·kine** (sī′tō-kīn) hormone-like proteins, secreted by many cell types, which regulate the intensity and duration of immune responses and are involved in cell-to-cell communication. SEE ALSO interferon, interleukin, lymphokine. [cyto- + G. *kinēsis,* movement]

**cy·to·ki·ne·sis** (sī′tō-ki-nē′sis) changes occurring in the protoplasm of the cell outside the nucleus during cell division. [cyto- + G. *kinēsis,* movement]

**cy·to·log·ic** (sī-tō-loj′ik) relating to cytology.

**cy·to·log·ic smear** a type of cytologic specimen made by smearing a sample (obtained by a variety of methods from a number of sites), then fixing it and staining it, usually with 95% ethyl alcohol and Papanicolaou stain.

**cy·tol·o·gist** (sī-tol′ō-jist) one who specializes in cytology.

**cy·tol·o·gy** (sī-tol′ō-jē) the study of the anatomy, physiology, pathology, and chemistry of the cell. SYN cellular biology. [cyto- + G. *logos,* study]

**cy·tol·y·sin** (sī-tol′i-sin) a substance i.e., an antibody that effects partial or complete destruction of an animal cell; may require complement. SEE ALSO perforin.

**cy·tol·y·sis** (sī-tol′i-sis) the dissolution of a cell. [cyto- + G. *lysis,* loosening]

**cy·to·ly·so·some** (sī-tō-lī′sō-sōm) a variety of secondary lysosome that contains the remnants of mitochondria, ribosomes, or other organelles.

**cy·to·lyt·ic** (sī-tō-lit′ik) pertaining to cytolysis; possessing a solvent or destructive action on cells.

**cy·to·me·ga·lic in·clu·sion dis·ease** the presence of inclusion bodies within the cytoplasm and nuclei of enlarged cells of various organs of newborn infants dying with jaundice, hepatomegaly, splenomegaly, purpura, thrombocytopenia, and fever; the condition also occurs, at all ages, as a complication of other diseases in which immune mechanisms are severely depressed, and has been found incidentally in salivary gland epithelium, apparently as a localized or mild infection (salivary gland virus disease). SYN cytomegalovirus disease, inclusion body disease.

**cy·to·meg·a·lo·vi·rus (CMV)** (sī-tō-meg′ă-lō-vī′rŭs) a group of herpesviruses infecting humans and other animals, many having special affinity for salivary glands, and causing development of characteristic inclusions in the cytoplasm or nucleus. Most infections are asymptomatic, but if symptoms are present, they manifest as mononucleosis-like illness. Congenital infection may cause malformation or fetal death; infection in immunocompromised persons may be life-threatening. SYN human herpesvirus 5. [cyto- + G. *megas,* big]

**cy·to·meg·a·lo·vi·rus dis·ease** SYN cytomegalic inclusion disease.

**cy·to·met·a·pla·sia** (sī′tō-met-ă-plā′zē-ă) change of form or function of a cell, other than that related to neoplasia. [cyto- + G. *metaplasis,* transformation]

**cy·tom·e·ter** (sī-tom′ĕ-ter) a device used to count and measure cells, especially blood cells, either visually (with a microscope) or automatically (as in flow cytometry). [cyto- + G. *metron,* measure]

**cy·tom·e·try** (sī-tom′ĕ-trē) the counting of cells, especially blood cells, using a cytometer or hemocytometer.

**cy·to·mor·phol·o·gy** (sī′tō-mōr-fol′ō-jē) the study of the structure of cells.

**cy·to·mor·pho·sis** (sī′tō-mōr-fō′sis) changes that the cell undergoes during the various stages of its existence. SEE ALSO prosoplasia. [cyto- + G. *morphōsis,* a shaping]

**cy·to·path·ic** (sī-tō-path′ik) pertaining to or exhibiting cytopathy.

**cy·to·path·o·gen·ic** (sī′tō-path-ō-jen′ik) pertaining to an agent or substance that causes a diseased condition in cells, in contrast to histologic changes; used especially with reference to effects observed in cells in tissue cultures.

**cy·to·path·o·gen·ic vi·rus** a virus whose multiplication leads to degenerative changes in the host cell.

**cy·to·path·o·log·ic, cy·to·path·o·log·i·cal** (sī′tō-pa-thō-loj′ik, sī′tō-pa-thō-loj′i-kăl) **1.** denoting cellular changes in disease. **2.** relating to cytopathology.

**cy·to·pa·thol·o·gist** (sī′tō-pa-thol′ō-jist) a physician specially trained and experienced in cytopathology.

**cy·to·pa·thol·o·gy** (sī′tō-pa-thol′ō-jē) **1.** the study of disease changes within individual cells or cell types. **2.** SYN exfoliative cytology.

**cy·top·a·thy** (sī-top′ă-thē) any disorder of a cell or anomaly of any of its constituents. [cyto- + G. *pathos,* disease]

**cy·to·pe·nia** (sī-tō-pē′nē-ă) a reduction, i.e., hypocytosis, or a lack of cellular elements in the circulating blood. [cyto- + G. *penia,* poverty]

**cy·toph·a·gous** (sī-tof′ă-gŭs) devouring, or destructive to, cells.

**cy·toph·a·gy** (sī-tof′ă-jē) devouring of other cells by phagocytes. [cyto- + G. *phagō,* to devour]

**cy·to·phil·ic** (sī-tō-fil′ik) SYN cytotropic. [cyto- + G. *philos,* fond]

**cy·to·phil·ic an·ti·bod·y** SYN cytotropic antibody.

**cy·to·pho·tom·e·try** (sī′tō-fō-tom′ĕ-trē) a method of measuring the absorption of monochromatic light by stained microscopic structures (e.g., chromosomes, nuclei, whole cells) with the aid of a photoelectric cell; also used to measure emitted light from such objects by fluorescence in combination with selected fluorochrome dyes. [cyto- + G. *phōs,* light + *metron,* measure]

**cy·to·phy·lac·tic** (sī′tō-fī-lak′tik) relating to cytophylaxis.

**cy·to·phy·lax·is** (sī′tō-fī-lak′sis) protection of cells against lytic agents. [cyto- + G. *phylaxis,* a guarding]

**cy·to·plasm** (sī′tō-plazm) the substance of a cell, exclusive of the nucleus, that contains various organelles and inclusions within a colloidal protoplasm. SEE ALSO protoplasm, hyaloplasm, cytosol. [cyto- + G. *plasma,* thing formed]

**cy·to·plas·mic** (sī-tō-plaz′mik) relating to the cytoplasm.

**cy·to·plas·mic bridg·es** SYN intercellular bridges.

**cy·to·plas·mic in·clu·sion bod·ies** SEE inclusion bodies.

**cy·to·plas·mic in·her·i·tance** transmission of characters dependent on self-perpetuating elements not nuclear in origin (e.g., mitochondrial DNA).

**cy·to·plast** (sī′tō-plast) the living intact cytoplasm that remains following cell enucleation. [cyto- + G. *plastos,* formed]

c
y

**cy•to•re•duc•tive ther•a•py** therapy with the intention of reducing the number of cells in a lesion, usually a malignancy.

**cy•to•screen•er** (sī'tō-skrēn'er) SYN cytotechnologist.

**cy•to•sine (Cyt)** (sī'tō-sēn) a pyrimidine found in nucleic acids.

**cy•to•sine ar•a•bi•no•side (CA) 1.** a synthetic nucleoside used as an antimetabolite in the treatment of neoplasms. **2.** incorrect term for arabinosylcytosine.

**cy•to•sine ri•bo•nu•cle•o•side** SYN cytidine.

**cy•to•sis** (sī-tō'sis) **1.** a condition in which there is more than the usual number of cells, as in the spinal fluid in meningitis. **2.** frequently used with a prefixed combining form as a means of describing certain features pertaining to cells; e.g., isocytosis, equality in size; polycytosis, abnormal increase in number. [cyto- + G. -osis, condition]

**cy•to•skel•e•ton** (sī-tō-skel'ĕ-ton) the tonofilaments, keratin, desmin, neurofilaments, or other intermediate filaments serving as supportive cytoplasmic elements to stiffen cells or to organize intracellular organelles.

**cy•to•sol** (sī'tō-sol) cytoplasm exclusive of the mitochondria, endoplasmic reticulum, and other membranous components. [cyto- + "sol," abbrev. of soluble]

**cy•to•sol•ic** (sī-tō-sol'ik) relating to or contained in the cytosol.

**cy•to•some** (sī'tō-sōm) **1.** the cell body exclusive of the nucleus. **2.** one of the osmiophilic bodies that are 1 μm or less in diameter, have concentric lamellae, and occur in the great alveolar cells of the lung. SYN multilamellar body. [cyto- + G. sōma, body]

**cy•tos•ta•sis** (sī-tos'tă-sis) the slowing of movement and accumulation of blood cells, especially polymorphonuclear leukocytes, in the capillaries, as in a region of inflammation; obstruction of a capillary as the result of accumulated leukocytes. [cyto- + G. stasis, standing]

**cy•to•stat•ic** (sī-tō-stat'ik) characterized by cytostasis.

**cy•to•tac•tic** (sī-tō-tak'tik) relating to cytotaxis.

**cy•to•tax•is, cy•to•tax•ia** (sī-tō-tak'sis, sī-tō-tak' sē-ă) the attraction (**positive cytotaxis**) or repulsion (**negative cytotaxis**) of cells for one another. [cyto- + G. taxis, arrangement]

**cy•to•tech•nol•o•gist** (sī'tō-tek-nol'ŏ-jist) a person with special training in cytopathology who is responsible for screening Pap smears and determining which are negative and which require further review by a pathologist. SEE ALSO Pap smear, Pap test. SYN cytoscreener.

**cy•toth•e•sis** (sī-toth'ĕ-sis) the repair of injury in a cell; the restoration of cells. [cyto- + G. thesis, a placing]

**cy•to•tox•ic** (sī-tō-tok'sik) detrimental or destructive to cells; pertaining to the effect of noncytophilic antibody on specific antigen, frequently, but not always, mediating the action of complement.

**cy•to•tox•ic•i•ty** (sī-tō-tok-sis'i-tē) the quality or state of being cytotoxic.

**cy•to•tox•ic re•ac•tion** an immunologic (allergic) reaction in which noncytotropic IgG or IgM antibody combines with specific antigen on cell surfaces; the resulting complex initiates the activation of complement which causes cell lysis or other damage, or, in the absence of complement, may lead to phagocytosis or may enhance T lymphocyte involvement.

**cy•to•tox•in** (sī'tō-tok'sin) a specific substance, which may or may not be antibody, that inhibits or prevents the functions of cells, causes destruction of cells, or both. [cyto- + G. toxikon, poison]

**cy•to•tro•pho•blast** (sī-tō-trof'ō-blast) the inner cellular layer of the trophoblast.

**cy•to•tro•pho•blas•tic cells** stem cells that fuse to form the overlying syncytiotrophoblast of placental villi. SYN Langhans cells (2).

**cy•to•tro•pic** (sī-tō-trop'ik) having an affinity for cells. SYN cytophilic.

**cy•to•tro•pic an•ti•bod•y** antibody that has an affinity for certain kinds of cells, in addition to and unrelated to its specific affinity for the antigen that induced it, because of the properties of the Fc portion of the heavy chain. SEE ALSO heterocytotropic antibody, homocytotropic antibody. SYN anaphylactic antibody, cytophilic antibody.

**cy•tot•ro•pism** (sī-tot'rō-pizm) **1.** affinity for cells. **2.** affinity for specific cells, especially the ability of viruses to localize in and damage specific cells. [cyto- + G. tropos, a turning]

**cy•tu•ria** (sī-tyu'rē-ă) the passage of cells in unusual numbers in the urine. [G. kytos, cell, + ouron, urine]

**Cza•pek so•lu•tion a•gar** (chah'pek) a culture medium used for the cultivation of fungus species and for identification of Aspergillus and Penicillium species.

**Czer•ny-Lem•bert su•ture** (cher'nē-lem'bert) an intestinal suture in two rows combining the Czerny suture (first) and the Lembert suture (second).

**Czer•ny su•ture** (cher'nē) the first row of the Czerny-Lembert intestinal suture; the needle enters the serosa and passes out through the submucosa or muscularis, and then enters the submucosa or muscularis of the opposite side and emerges from the serosa.

# D

$\Delta$, $\delta$ delta. SEE delta.

**d** deci-; *dexter* [L], right; diameter; day.

⚠**d-** prefix indicating a chemical compound to be dextrorotatory; should be avoided when (+) or (−) could be used. Cf. L-.

⚠**D-** prefix indicating that a chemical compound is sterically related to D-glyceraldehyde, the basis of stereochemical nomenclature. Cf. lambda.

⚠**-d** suffix indicating the presence of deuterium in a compound in concentrations above normal, thus labelling the compound; subscripts ($d_2$, $d_3$, etc.) indicate the number of such atoms so fortified.

**DA** developmental age.

**Da** dalton.

**dA, dAdo** deoxyadenosine.

**da** deca-.

**Da·ae dis·ease** (dah'ĕ) SYN epidemic pleurodynia.

⚠**da·cry·o-, da·cry-** tears; lacrimal sac or duct. [G. *dakryon*, tear]

**dac·ry·o·ad·e·ni·tis** (dak-rē-ō-ad-ĕ-nī'tis) inflammation of the lacrimal gland. [dacryo- + G. *adēn*, gland, + -*itis*, inflammation]

**dac·ry·o·blen·nor·rhea** (dak-rē-ō-blen-ō-rē'ă) a chronic discharge of mucus from a lacrimal sac. [dacryo- + G. *blenna*, mucus, + *rhoia*, flow]

**dac·ry·o·cele** (dak'rē-ō-sēl) SYN dacryocystocele.

**dac·ry·o·cyst** (dak'rē-ō-sist) SYN lacrimal sac. [dacryo- + G. *kystis*, sac]

**dac·ry·o·cys·tal·gia** (dak'rē-ō-sis-tal'jē-ă) pain in the lacrimal sac. [dacryocyst + G. *algos*, pain]

**dac·ry·o·cys·tec·to·my** (dak'rē-ō-sis-tek'tō-mē) surgical removal of the lacrimal sac. [dacryocyst + G. *ektomē*, excision]

**dac·ry·o·cys·to·cele** (dak'rē-ō-sis'tō-sēl) enlargement of the lacrimal sac with fluid. SYN dacryocele. [dacryocyst + G. *kēlē*, hernia]

**dac·ry·o·cys·tog·ra·phy (DCG)** (dak'rē-ō-sis-tog'ra-fē) radiography of the lacrimal drainage system by introduction of a contrast agent. [dacryocyst + -o- + G. *graphō*, to scratch, to write]

**dac·ry·o·cys·to·rhi·nos·to·my** (dak'rē-ō-sis'tō-rī-nos'tō-mē) an operation providing an anastomosis between the lacrimal sac and the nasal mucosa through an opening in the lacrimal bone. [dacryocyst + G. *rhis* (*rhin-*), nose, + *stoma*, mouth]

**dac·ry·o·cys·tot·o·my** (dak'rē-ō-sis-tot'ō-mē) incision of the lacrimal sac. [dacryocyst + G. *tomē*, incision]

**dac·ry·o·cyte** (dăk'rē-ō-sīt) an abnormally shaped red cell with a single point or elongation; also called a teardrop. This form of poikilocyte is associated with myelofibrosis with myeloid metaplasia. SYN teardrop cell. [dacryo- + -cyte]

**dac·ry·o·hem·or·rhea** (dak'rē-ō-hem-ō-rē'ă) bloody tears. [dacryo- + G. *haima*, blood, + *rhoia*, flow]

**dac·ry·o·lith** (dak'rē-ō-lith) a concretion in the lacrimal apparatus. SYN ophthalmolith, tear stone. [dacryo- + G. *lithos*, stone]

**dac·ry·o·li·thi·a·sis** (dak'rē-ō-li-thī'ă-sis) the formation and presence of dacryoliths.

**dac·ry·ops** (dak'rē-ops) 1. excess of tears in the eye. 2. a cyst of a duct of the lacrimal gland. [dacryo- + G. *ōps*, eye]

**dac·ry·o·py·or·rhea** (dak'rē-ō-pī-ō-rē'ă) the discharge of tears containing leukocytes. [dacryo- + G. *pyon*, pus, + *rhoia*, flow]

**dac·ry·or·rhea** (dak'rē-ō-rē'ă) an excessive secretion of tears. [dacryo- + G. *rhoia*, flow]

**dac·ry·or·rhoea [Br.]** SEE dacryorrhea.

**dac·ry·o·ste·no·sis** (dak'rē-ō-ste-nō'sis) stricture of a lacrimal or nasal duct. [dacryo- + G. *stenōsis*, narrowing]

**dac·tyl** (dak'til) SYN digit. [G. *daktylos*]

**dac·ty·li·tis** (dak-ti-lī'tis) inflammation of one or more fingers.

⚠**dac·ty·lo-, dac·tyl-** the fingers, and (less often) toes. See entries under digit. [G. *daktylos*, finger]

**dac·ty·lo·camp·sis** (dak'ti-lō-kamp'sis) permanent flexion of the fingers. [dactylo- + G. *kampsis*, bending]

**dac·ty·lo·gry·po·sis** (dak'ti-lō-gri-pō'sis) permanent curvature or deformity of the fingers. [dactylo- + G. *grypōsis*, a crooking]

**dac·tyl·o·meg·a·ly** (dak'til-ō-meg'ă-lē) SYN megadactyly. [dactylo- + G. *megas*, large]

**dac·ty·lus**, pl. **dac·ty·li** (dak'ti-lŭs, dak'ti-lī) SYN digit. [G. *daktylos*]

**Da Fa·no stain** (dah fah'nō) a silver stain that produces a blackening of Golgi elements after tissues are fixed in a mixture of nitrate and formalin.

**Dal·rym·ple sign** (dal'rim-pĕl) retraction of the upper eyelid in Graves disease, causing abnormal wideness of the palpebral fissure.

**Dal·ton,** John, English chemist, mathematician, and natural philosopher, 1766–1844. SEE Dalton law.

**dal·ton (Da)** (dawl'tŏn) term unofficially used to indicate a unit of mass equal to $1/_{12}$ the mass of a carbon-12 atom, 1.0000 in the atomic mass scale; numerically, but not dimensionally, equal to molecular or particle weight (atomic mass units). [J. *Dalton*]

**Dal·ton law** (dawl'ton) each gas in a mixture of gases exerts a pressure proportionate to the percentage of the gas and independent of the presence of the other gases present. SYN law of partial pressures.

**DALYs** disability-adjusted life years.

**dam 1.** any barrier to the flow of fluid. **2.** SURGERY, DENTISTRY a sheet of thin rubber arranged so as to shut off the part operated upon from the access of fluid. [A.S. *fordemman*, to stop up]

**dAMP** deoxyadenylic acid.

**damp 1.** humid; moist. **2.** atmospheric moisture. **3.** foul air in a mine; air charged with carbon oxides (black or choke damp) or with various explosive hydrocarbon vapors (firedamp).

**Da·na op·er·a·tion** (dā'nă) SYN posterior rhizotomy.

**dance** (dans) involuntary movements related to brain damage.

**Dance sign** (dans) a slight retraction in the neighborhood of the right iliac fossa in some cases of intussusception.

**dan·der 1.** a fine scaling of the skin and scalp. SEE ALSO dandruff. **2.** a normal effluvium of animal hair or coat capable of causing allergic responses in atopic persons.

**dan·druff** (dan'drŭf) the presence, in varying amounts, of white or gray scales in the hair of the scalp, due to exfoliation of the epidermis. SEE ALSO seborrheic dermatitis. SYN scurf, seborrhea sicca (2).

**Dan•dy op•er•a•tion** (dan'dē) SEE third ventriculostomy, trigeminal rhizotomy.

**Dan•dy-Walk•er syn•drome** (dan'dē-wŏk'er) developmental anomaly of the fourth ventricle associated with atresia of the foramina of Luschka and Magendie that results in cerebellar hypoplasia, hydrocephalus, and posterior fossa cyst formation.

**Dane par•ti•cles** (dān) the larger spherical forms of hepatitis-associated antigens; they comprise the virion of hepatitis B virus.

**Dane stain** (dān) a stain for prekeratin, keratin, and mucin that employs hemalum, phloxine, Alcian blue, and orange G; nuclei appear orange to brown, acid mucopolysaccharides pale blue, and keratins orange to red-orange.

**Dan•forth sign** (dan'fōrth) shoulder pain on inspiration, due to irritation of the diaphragm by a hemoperitoneum in ruptured ectopic pregnancy.

**Dan•iels•sen dis•ease** (dan-yel'sen) SYN anesthetic leprosy.

**DANS** 1-dimethylaminonaphthalene-5-sulfonic acid; a green fluorescing compound used in immunohistochemistry to detect antigens.

**dan•syl (Dns, DNS)** (dan'sil) The 5-dimethylaminonaphthalene-1-sulfonyl radical; a blocking agent for $NH_2$ groups, used in peptide synthesis.

**d'Ar•cet met•al** (dahr-sā') an alloy of lead, bismuth, and tin; used in dentistry.

**Da•ri•er dis•ease** (dah-rē-ā') SYN keratosis follicularis.

**Da•ri•er sign** (dah-rē-ā') urtication on stroking of cutaneous lesions of urticaria pigmentosa (mastocytosis).

**dark ad•ap•ta•tion** the visual adjustment occurring under reduced illumination in which the retinal sensitivity to light is increased. SEE ALSO dark-adapted eye. SYN scotopic adaptation.

**dark-a•dapt•ed eye** an eye that has been in darkness or semidarkness and has undergone regeneration of rhodopsin (visual purple), which renders it more sensitive to reduced illumination. SYN scotopic eye.

**dark-field mi•cro•scope** a microscope that has a special condenser and objective with a diaphragm or stop that scatters light from the object observed, with the result that the object appears bright on a dark background.

**Dar•row red** a basic oxazin dye, $C_{18}H_{14}N_3O_2Cl$, used as a substitute for cresyl violet acetate in the staining of Nissl substance. [Mary A. *Darrow*, U.S. stain technologist, 1894–1973]

**dar•win•i•an** (dar-win'ē-an) relating to or ascribed to Darwin.

**dar•win•i•an ev•o•lu•tion** the proposition that the phylogeny of all species is wholly ascribable to random variation (mutation) in genotypes and the operation of preferential survival of those resulting phenotypes most suited to survive in the contemporary environment.

**dar•win•i•an re•flex** (dar-win'ē-ăn) the tendency of young infants to grasp a bar and hang suspended. Cf. grasping reflex.

**dar•win•i•an tu•ber•cle** (dar-win'ē-ăn) SYN auricular tubercle.

**DAS** developmental apraxia of speech.

**da•ta** facts (usually established by observation, measurement, or experiment) used as a basis for inference, testing, models, etc. The word is plural and takes a plural verb.

**data dic•tion•a•ry** standardized set of definitions of all data elements collected in a given health care facility.

**date boil, Del•hi boil, Jer•i•cho boil** the lesion occurring in cutaneous leishmaniasis.

**da•tum** (dā'tŭm) an individual piece of information used in a scholarly field. [L., *given*, fr. *do*, pp. *datum*, to give]

**da•tum plane** an arbitrary plane used as a base from which to make craniometric measurements.

**daugh•ter** (daw'ter) in nuclear medicine, an isotope that is the disintegration product of a radionuclide. SEE daughter isotope, radionuclide generator. [O.E. *dohtor*]

**daugh•ter cell** one of the two or more cells formed in the division of a parent cell.

**daugh•ter cyst** a secondary cyst, usually multiple, derived from a mother cyst.

**daugh•ter iso•tope** an element produced by radioactive decay of another. SEE ALSO radionuclide generator.

**daugh•ter star** one of the figures forming the diaster. SYN polar star.

**dau•no•ru•bi•cin** (daw'nō-roo'bĭ-sin) SYN rubidomycin.

**Da•vi•el op•er•a•tion** (dah-vē-el') extracapsular cataract extraction.

**Da•vi•el spoon** (dah-vē-el') a small ovoid instrument for removing the remains of a cataract after discission.

**Davis battery model of transduction** (dā'vis) a concept in which the positive endocochlear potential and the negative intracellular potential of the hair cells provide the electromotive force to pass current through the reticular lamina of the organ of Corti.

**Da•vis graft** (dā'vis) "pinch grafts," i.e., small pieces (2–3 mm) of full-thickness skin grafts.

**dawn phe•nom•e•non** abrupt increases in fasting levels of plasma glucose concentrations between 5 and 9 AM in the absence of antecedent hypoglycemia; occurs in diabetic patients receiving insulin therapy.

**Daw•son en•ceph•a•li•tis** (daw'sŏn) SYN subacute sclerosing panencephalitis.

**day blind•ness** SYN hemeralopia.

**DB, db** decibel.

**DC** direct current.

**D & C** dilation and curettage.

**DCG** dacryocystography.

**dCMP** deoxycytidylic acid.

**d-dimer** (dī'mer) a covalently cross-linked degradation product released from the cross-linked fibrin polymer during plasmin-mediated fibrinolysis; laboratory measurements of this product made using latex bead or ELISA assays can be used to identify the presence of fibrinolysis.

**D & E** dilation and evacuation.

△**de- 1.** away from, cessation, without; sometimes has an intensive force. **2.** for names with this prefix not found here, see under the principal part of the name. [L. *de*, from, away]

**de•ac•yl•ase** (dē-as'il-ās) **1.** a member of the subclass of hydrolases (EC class 3), especially of that subclass of esterases, lipases, lactonases, and hydrolases (EC subclass 3.1). **2.** any enzyme catalyzing the hydrolytic cleavage of an acyl group (R-CO-) in an ester linkage; also includes enzymes cleaving amide linkages (EC subclass 3.5) and similar acyl compounds.

**dead arm syndrome** sensory diminution or loss

in the arm after anterior shoulder dislocation or subluxation.

**dead-end host** a host from which infectious agents are not transmitted to other susceptible hosts.

**dead-in-bed syndrome** the finding of young, insulin-dependent diabetics without previous illness or abnormal glucose control dead in bed in the morning. Assumed to be due to hypoglycemia but it has been difficult to establish that fact postmortem. Usually occurs in diabetics taking three daily doses of insulin, suggesting inadvertent administration of erroneous dose, with lack of awareness of hypoglycemia during sleep.

**dead pulp** SYN necrotic pulp.

**dead space 1.** a cavity, potential or real, remaining after the closure of a wound which is not obliterated by the operative technique; **2.** SEE anatomic dead space, physiologic dead space.

**deaf** (def) unable to hear; hearing indistinctly; hard of hearing. [A.S. *deáf*]

**de·af·fer·en·ta·tion** (dē-af′er-en-tā′shŭn) a loss of the sensory input from a portion of the body, usually caused by interruption of the peripheral sensory fibers. [L. *de,* from, + afferent]

**deaf·mut·ism** (def-myu′tizm) inability to speak, due to congenital or early acquired profound deafness.

**deaf·ness** (def′nes) general term for loss of the ability to hear, without designation of the degree or cause of the loss.

**de·al·co·hol·i·za·tion** (dē-al′kō-hol-i-zā′shŭn) the removal of alcohol from a fluid; in histologic technique, the removal of alcohol from a specimen that has been previously immersed in this fluid.

**de·am·i·dase** (dē-am′i-dā-sez) SYN amidohydrolase.

**de·am·i·da·tion, de·am·i·di·za·tion** (dē-am-i-dā′shŭn, dē-am′i-di-zā′shŭn) the hydrolytic removal of an amide group.

**de·am·i·diz·ing en·zyme** SYN amidohydrolase.

**de·am·i·nas·es** (dē-am′i-nā-sez) [EC group 3.5.4] enzymes catalyzing simple hydrolysis of C—NH$_2$ bonds of purines, pyrimidines, and pterins. SYN deaminating enzymes.

**de·am·i·nat·ing en·zymes** SYN deaminases.

**de·am·i·na·tion, de·am·i·ni·za·tion** (dē-am-i-nā′shŭn, dē-am′i-ni-zā′shŭn) removal, usually by hydrolysis, of the NH$_2$ group from an amino compound.

**Dean flu·o·ro·sis in·dex** (dēn) an index that measures the degree of mottled enamel (fluorosis) in teeth; used most often in epidemiological field studies.

**de·ar·te·ri·al·i·za·tion** (dē-ar-tēr′ē-ăl-i-zā′shŭn) changing the character of arterial blood to that of venous blood; i.e., deoxygenation of blood.

**death** (dĕth) the cessation of life. In lower multicellular organisms, death is a gradual process at the cellular level, because tissues vary in their ability to withstand deprivation of oxygen; in higher organisms, a cessation of integrated tissue and organ functions; in humans, manifested by the loss of heartbeat, by the absence of spontaneous breathing, and by cerebral death. SYN mors. [A.S. *dēath*]

**death in·stinct** the instinct of all living creatures toward self-destruction, death, or a return to the inorganic lifelessness from which they arose.

**death rate** an estimate of the proportion of the population that dies during a specified period, usually a year; the numerator is the number of people dying, the denominator is the number in the population, usually an estimate of the number at the midperiod. SYN mortality rate, mortality (2).

**Dea·ver in·ci·sion** (dē′ver) an incision in the right lower abdominal quadrant, with medial displacement of the rectus muscle.

**Dea·ver meth·od** (dē′ver), a method of motor reeducation.

**De·Bak·ey clas·si·fi·ca·tion of a·or·tic dis·-sec·tion** (dĕ-bā′kē) consists of three types: Type I extends into the transverse arch and distal aorta and type II is confined to the ascending aorta; type III dissections begin in the descending aorta, with type IIIA extending toward the diaphragm and type IIIB extending below it.

**de·band·ing** (dē-band′ing) the removal of fixed orthodontic appliances.

**de·bil·i·tat·ing** (dĕ-bil′i-tāt-ing) denoting or characteristic of a morbid process that causes weakness.

**de·bond** (dē-bond′) to separate a dental appliance such as an orthodontic band from the tooth to which it has been attached or bonded by a resin cement. [de- + bond]

**de·branch·ing en·zymes** enzymes that bring about destruction of branches in glycogen; a mixture of transferases and hydrolases.

**de·bris** (de-brē) a useless accumulation of miscellaneous particles; waste in the form of fragments. [Fr. *débris,* fr. O.Fr. *desbrisier,* to break apart, (fr. *des-* down, away + *brisier* to break) rubble, rubbish]

**debt** (det) a deficit; a liability. [L. *debitum,* debt]

**de·bulk·ing op·er·a·tion** excision of a major part of a malignant tumor which cannot be completely removed, so as to enhance the effectiveness of subsequent radio- or chemotherapy.

△**de·ca-** (da) prefix used in the SI and metric systems to signify 10. Also spelled deka-. [G. *deka,* ten]

**de·cal·ci·fi·ca·tion** (dē′kal-si-fi-kā′shŭn) **1.** removal of calcium salts from bones and teeth, either *in vitro* or as a result of a pathologic process. **2.** precipitation of calcium from blood as by oxalate or fluoride, or the conversion of blood calcium to an un-ionized form as by citrate, thus preventing or delaying coagulation. [L. *de-,* away, + *calx* (*calc*-), lime, + *facio,* to make]

**de·cal·ci·fy·ing** (dē-kal′si-fī-ing) denoting an agent, measure, or process that causes decalcification.

**de·can·nul·a·tion** (dē-kan-yu-lā′shŭn) planned or accidental removal of a tracheostomy tube.

**de·ca·pac·i·ta·tion** (dē′kă-pas-i-tā′shŭn) prevention of spermatozoa from undergoing capacitation and thus from becoming able to fertilize oocytes (ova).

**de·cap·i·ta·tion** (dē-kap-i-tā′shŭn) removal of a head.

**de·cap·su·la·tion** (dē-kap-soo-lā′shŭn) incision and removal of a capsule or enveloping membrane.

**de·car·box·yl·ase** (dē-kar-boks′ē-lās) any enzyme (EC subclass 4.1.1) that removes a molecule of carbon dioxide from a carboxylic group.

**de·car·box·yl·a·tion** (dē′kar-boks-ē-lā′shŭn) a reaction involving the removal of a molecule of carbon dioxide from a carboxylic acid.

**d**
**e**

**de·cay** (dē-kā′) **1.** destruction of an organic substance by slow combustion or gradual oxidation. **2.** SYN putrefaction. **3.** to deteriorate; to undergo slow combustion or putrefaction. **4.** DENTISTRY caries. **5.** PSYCHOLOGY loss of information registered by the senses and processed into short-term memory. SEE ALSO memory. **6.** loss of radioactivity over time; spontaneous emission of radiation or charged particles or both from an unstable nucleus. [L. *de,* down, + *cado,* to fall]

**de·cay con·stant** the fractional change in the number of atoms of a radionuclide which occurs in unit time; the constant l in the equation for the fraction (DN/N) of the number of atoms (N) of a radionuclide disintegrating in time *Dt, DN/N = − lDt.* SYN radioactive constant.

**de·cay the·o·ry** a theory of forgetting based on the premise that an engram or memory trace dissipates progressively with time during the interval when it is not activated.

**de·cer·e·brate** (dē-ser′ĕ-brāt) **1.** to cause decerebration. **2.** denoting an animal so prepared, or a patient whose brain has suffered an injury causing neurologic impairment comparable to that of a decerebrate animal.

**de·cer·e·brate ri·gid·i·ty** a postural change that occurs in some comatose patients, consisting of episodes of opisthotonos, rigid extension of the limbs, internal rotation of the upper extremities, and marked plantar flexion of the feet; produced by a variety of metabolic and structural brain disorders. SEE ALSO decorticate rigidity.

**de·cer·e·bra·tion** (dē-ser′ĕ-brā′shŭn) removal of the brain above the lower border of the corpora quadrigemina, or a complete section of the brain at this level or somewhat below.

**de·cho·les·ter·ol·i·za·tion** (dē′kō-les′ter-ol-i-zā′shŭn) therapeutic reduction of the cholesterol concentration of the blood.

△**de·ci-** **(d)** prefix used in the SI and metric system to signify one-tenth (10⁻). [L. *decimus,* tenth]

**dec·i·bel (DB, db)** (des′i-bel) one-tenth of a bel; unit for expressing the relative loudness of sound on a logarithmic scale. [L. *decimus,* tenth, + bel]

**de·cid·ua** (dē-sid′yu-ă) SYN deciduous membrane. [L. *deciduus,* falling off (qualifying *membrana,* membrane, understood)]

**de·cid·u·a ba·sa·lis** [TA] the area of endometrium between the implanted chorionic sac and the myometrium, which develops into the maternal part of the placenta. SYN decidua serotina.

**de·cid·u·a cap·su·lar·is** [TA] the layer of endometrium overlying the implanted chorionic sac; it becomes progressively attenuated as the chorionic sac enlarges and, by the fourth month, is squeezed against the decidua parietalis and thereafter undergoes rapid regression. SYN decidua reflexa, membrana adventitia.

**de·cid·u·al** (dē-sid′yu-ăl) relating to the decidua.

**de·cid·u·al cell** an enlarged, ovoid connective tissue cell appearing in the endometrium of pregnancy.

**de·cid·u·a men·stru·a·lis** the succulent mucous membrane of the nonpregnant uterus at the menstrual period.

**de·cid·u·a pa·ri·e·tal·is** the altered endometrium lining the main cavity of the pregnant uterus other than at the site of attachment of the chorionic sac. SYN decidua vera.

**de·cid·u·a po·ly·po·sa** decidua parietalis showing polypoid projections of the endometrial surface.

**de·cid·u·a re·flex·a** SYN decidua capsularis.

**de·cid·u·a ser·o·ti·na** SYN decidua basalis.

**de·cid·u·a spon·gi·o·sa** the portion of the decidua basalis attached to the myometrium.

**de·cid·u·a·tion** (dē-sid-yu-ā′shŭn) shedding of endometrial tissue during menstruation. [L. *deciduus,* falling off]

**de·cid·u·a ve·ra** SYN decidua parietalis.

**de·cid·u·i·tis** (dē-sid-yu-ī′tis) inflammation of the decidua.

**de·cid·u·o·ma** (dē-sid-yu-ō′mă) an intrauterine mass of decidual tissue, probably the result of hyperplasia of decidual cells retained in the uterus. SYN placentoma.

**de·cid·u·ous** (dē-sid′yu-ŭs) **1.** not permanent; denoting that which eventually falls off. **2.** DENTISTRY referring to the first or primary dentition. SEE deciduous tooth. [L. *deciduus,* falling off]

**de·cid·u·ous den·ti·tion** SYN deciduous tooth. See this page.

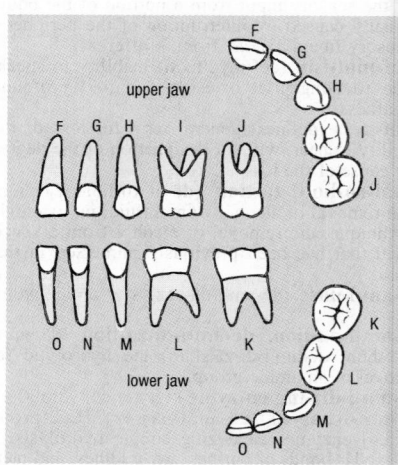

**deciduous dentition, half view, left side**
(lettering code, universal system of deciduous teeth): central incisor F, O; lateral incisor G, N; canine H, M; first molar I, L; second molar J, K

**de·cid·u·ous mem·brane** the mucous membrane of the pregnant uterus that has undergone changes, under the influence of the ovulation cycle, to fit it for the implantation and nutrition of the oocyte; so-called because the membrane is cast off after labor. SYN decidua, membrana decidua.

**de·cid·u·ous tooth** one of the first set of teeth, comprising 20 in all, that erupts between the mean ages of 6 and 28 months of life. SYN dens deciduus [TA], baby tooth, deciduous dentition, milk dentition, milk tooth, primary dentition, primary tooth, temporary tooth.

**dec·i·me·ter** (des′i-mē-ter) one-tenth of a meter.

**de·ci·me·tre [Br.]** SEE decimeter.

**de·clamp·ing phe·nom·e·non** shock or hypotension following abrupt release of clamps from a large portion of the vascular bed, as from the aorta; apparently caused by transient pooling of blood in a previously ischemic area. SYN declamping shock.

**de·clamp·ing shock** SYN declamping phenomenon.

**dec·li·na·tion** (dek-li-nā'shŭn) a bending, sloping, or other deviation from a normal vertical position. [L. *declinatio*, a bending aside]

**de·clive** (dē-klīv'ē) [TA] the posterior sloping portion of the monticulus of the vermis of the cerebellum; vermal lobule caudal to the primary fissure. SYN declivis. [L. *declivis*, sloping downward, fr. *clivus*, a slope]

**de·cli·vis** (dē-klī'vis) SYN declive.

**de·com·pen·sa·tion** (de'kom-pen-sā'shŭn) **1.** a failure of compensation in heart disease. **2.** the appearance or exacerbation of a mental disorder due to failure of defense mechanisms.

**de·com·po·si·tion** (dē'kom-pō-zish'ŭn) SYN putrefaction.

**de·com·pres·sion** (dē'kom-presh-ŭn) removal of pressure. [L. *de-*, from, down, + *com-primo*, pp. *-pressus*, to press together]

**de·com·pres·sion sick·ness** a symptom complex caused by the escape from solution in the body fluids of nitrogen bubbles absorbed originally at high atmospheric pressure, as a result of abrupt reduction in atmospheric pressure (either rapid ascent to high altitude or return from a compressed-air environment); it is characterized by headache, pain in the arms, legs, joints, and epigastrium, itching of the skin, vertigo, dyspnea, coughing, choking, vomiting, weakness and sometimes paralysis, and severe peripheral circulatory collapse. SYN caisson disease.

**de·con·ges·tant** (dē-kon-jes'tant) **1.** having the property of reducing congestion. **2.** an agent that possesses this action.

**de·con·tam·i·na·tion** (dē'kon-tam-i-nā'shŭn) removal or neutralization of poisonous gas or other injurious agents from the environment.

**de·cor·ti·cate ri·gid·i·ty** a unilateral or bilateral postural change, in which the upper extremities are flexed and adducted and the lower extremities are held in rigid extension; due to structural lesions of the thalamus, internal capsule, or cerebral white matter.

**de·cor·ti·ca·tion** (dē-kōr-ti-kā'shŭn) **1.** removal of the cortex, or external layer, beneath the capsule from any organ or structure. **2.** an operation for removal of the clot and scar tissue that form after a hemothorax or neglected empyema. [L. *decortico*, pp. *-atus*, to deprive of bark, fr. *de*, from, + *cortex*, rind, bark]

**de·coy cell** benign exfoliated epithelial cell with pyknotic nucleus seen in urinary infections; may be mistaken for malignant cell.

**de·cru·des·cence** (dē-kroo-des'ens) abatement of the symptoms of disease. [L. *de*, from, + *crudesco*, to become worse, fr. *crudus*, crude]

**de·cu·bi·tal** (dē-kyu'bi-tăl) relating to a decubitus ulcer.

**de·cu·bi·tus** (dē-kyu'bi-tŭs) **1.** the position of the patient in bed; e.g., dorsal decubitus, lateral decubitus. SEE ALSO decubitus film. **2.** sometimes used in referring to a decubitus ulcer. [L. *decumbo*, to lie down]

**de·cu·bi·tus film** a radiograph exposed with the subject in the decubitus position; named for the side that is dependent.

**⬛ de·cu·bi·tus pro·jec·tion** RADIOLOGY procedure in which a patient to be x-rayed is placed in a decubitus position, with the x-ray beam directed horizontally. See page APP 95.

**⬛ de·cu·bi·tus ul·cer** focal ischemic necrosis of skin and underlying tissues at sites of constant pressure or recurring friction in persons confined to bed or immobilized by illness; malnutrition worsens the prognosis. SEE decubitus. See this page. SYN bedsore, bed sore, pressure sore, pressure ulcer.

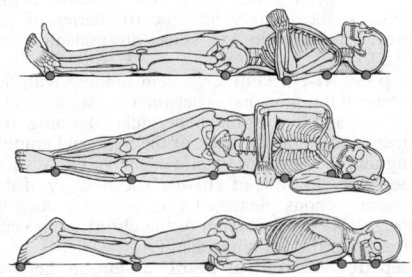

**decubitus ulcer:** most common sites due to proximity of bone to skin

**de·cus·sate** (dē'kŭ-sāt, dē-kŭs'āt) **1.** to cross. **2.** crossed like the arms of an X. [L. *decusso*, pp. *-atus*, to make in the form of an X, fr. *decussis*, a large, bronze Roman coin marked with an X to indicate its denomination]

**de·cus·sa·tio**, pl. **de·cus·sa·ti·o·nes** (dē-kŭ-sā'shē-ō, dē-kŭ-sā'shē-ō'nēz) **1.** in general, any crossing over or intersection of parts. **2.** the intercrossing of two homonymous fiber bundles as each crosses over to the opposite side of the brain in the course of its ascent or descent through the brainstem or spinal cord. SYN decussation. [L. (see decussate)]

**de·cus·sa·tio lem·ni·sco·rum** SYN decussation of medial lemniscus.

**de·cus·sa·tion** (dē-kŭ-sā'shŭn) SYN decussatio. [L. *decussatio*]

**de·cus·sa·ti·o·nes teg·men·ti** SYN tegmental decussations.

**de·cus·sa·tion of me·di·al lem·nis·cus** the intercrossing of the fibers of the left and right medial lemniscus ascending from the gracile and cuneate nuclei, immediately rostral to the level of the decussation of the pyramidal tracts in the medulla oblongata. SYN decussatio lemniscorum.

**de·cus·sa·tion of su·pe·ri·or cer·e·bel·lar pe·dun·cles** the decussation of the left and right superior cerebellar peduncles in the tegmentum of the caudal mesencephalon.

**de·cus·sa·tio py·ra·mi·dum** [TA] SYN pyramidal decussation.

**de·dif·fer·en·ti·a·tion** (dē-dif'er-en-shē-ā'shŭn) **1.** the return of parts to a more homogeneous state. **2.** SYN anaplasia.

**de·duc·tion** (dē-duk'shŭn) the logical derivation of a conclusion from certain premises. The conclusion will be true if the premises are true and the deductive argument is valid. Cf. induction (9).

**deep ar·tery of arm** SYN profunda brachii artery.

**deep ar·tery of clit·o·ris** the deep terminal branch of the internal pudendal artery in the female; it supplies the crus of the clitoris. SYN arteria profunda clitoridis [TA].

**deep ar•tery of pe•nis** *origin*, terminal branch (with dorsal artery of penis) of the internal pudendal artery; *distribution*, corpus cavernosum of the penis via capillary beds and via helicine arteries and arteriovenous anastomoses to produce erection. SYN arteria profunda penis [TA].

**deep ce•re•bral veins** the numerous veins draining the deep structures of the cerebral hemispheres; they empty into the tributaries of the great cerebral vein. SYN venae profundae cerebri [TA].

**deep cer•vi•cal vein** large vein running with the artery of the same name between the semispinalis capitis and semispinalis cervicis, draining the deep muscles at the back of the neck and emptying into the brachiocephalic or the vertebral vein.

**deep dor•sal vein of clit•o•ris** a tributary of the vesical venous plexus; it runs a course deep to the fascia on the dorsum of the clitoris. SYN vena dorsalis profunda clitoridis [TA].

**deep dor•sal vein of pe•nis** a vein on the dorsum of the penis deep to the fascia of the penis; it is a tributary to the prostatic venous plexus. SYN vepna dorsalis profunda penis [TA].

**deep fa•cial vein** the communicating vein that passes from the pterygoid venous plexus of the infratemporal fossa to the facial vein; it is devoid of valves.

**deep fas•cia** a thin fibrous membrane, devoid of fat, that invests the muscles, separating the several groups and the individual muscles, forms sheaths for the nerves and vessels, becomes specialized around the joints to form or strengthen ligaments, envelops various organs and glands, and binds all the structures together into a firm compact mass.

**deep fas•cia of thigh** the strong deep fascia of the thigh, enveloping the muscles of the thigh and thickened laterally as the iliotibial tract.

**deep fem•o•ral vein** accompanies the deep femoral artery, receiving perforating veins from the lateral and posterior aspects of the thigh. It joins the femoral vein in the femoral triangle, usually in common with the medial and lateral circumflex femoral veins.

**deep in•gui•nal ring** the opening in the transversalis fascia through which the ductus deferens (or round ligament in the female) and gonadal vessels enter the inguinal canal. Located midway between anterior superior iliac spine and pubic tubercle, it is bounded medially by the lateral umbilical ligament (inferior epigastric vessels) and inferiorly by the inguinal ligament. Indirect inguinal hernias exit the abdominal cavity via the deep inguinal ring

**deep lin•gual ar•tery** termination of lingual artery, *distribution*, muscles and mucous membrane of under surface of tongue.

**deep lin•gual vein** the principal vein of the tongue that accompanies the deep lingual artery and joins the lingual vein. It drains the body and apex of the tongue, running posteriorly near the median plane; often visible through the mucosa on the underside of the tongue, to each side of the frenulum.

**deep plantar (arterial) arch 1.** the arterial arch formed by the lateral plantar artery running across the bases of the metatarsal bones and anastomosing with the dorsalis pedis artery via

the deep plantar artery; **2.** either of two bony arches of the foot, longitudinal arch or transverse arch.

**deep plan•tar ar•tery** deep plantar branch of arcuate artery or its first metatarsal artery branch that penetrates the foot between first and second metatarsal bones to anastomose with the termination of the plantar arterial arch. SYN arteria plantaris profunda [TA].

**deep re•flex** an involuntary muscular contraction following percussion of a tendon or bone. SYN jerk (2).

**deep tem•po•ral nerves** two branches, anterior and posterior, from the mandibular nerve, supplying the temporalis muscle and periosteum of the temporal fossa. SYN nervi temporales profundi [TA].

**deep ten•don re•flex** SYN myotatic reflex.

**deep tis•sue mas•sage** a group of massage techniques designed to access deep layers of muscle and fascia in order to improve alignment, reduce levels of resting tension, and create more efficient postural and movement patterns. Includes rolfing, myofascial release, structural integration.

**deep trans•verse per•i•ne•al mus•cle** *origin*, ramus of ischium; *insertion*, with its fellow in a median raphe; *action*, assists sphincter urethrae with some sphincteric action on vagina in female; *nerve supply*, pudendal (dorsal nerve of penis/clitoris). SYN musculus transversus perinei profundus [TA].

**deep vein of pe•nis** the vein deep to the deep fascia on the dorsum of the penis; it enters the prostatic plexus by passing through a gap between the arcuate pubic ligament and the transverse perineal ligament.

**deep veins of clit•o•ris** the veins that pass from the dorsum of the clitoris to join the vesical plexus.

**deep ve•nous throm•bo•sis** formation of one or more thrombi in the deep veins, usually of the lower extremity or in the pelvis. Carries a high risk of pulmonary embolism. SEE ALSO thrombophlebitis.

**def, DEF** decayed, extracted, or filled tooth.

**de•fae•ca•tion [Br.]** SEE defecation.

**def caries index** an index of past caries experience that includes decayed, extracted, and filled deciduous teeth; sometimes the extracted portion (e) is not included.

**def•e•cate** (def′ĕ-kāt) to perform defecation.

**def•e•ca•tion** (def-ĕ-kā′shŭn) the discharge of feces from the rectum. SYN movement (3). [L. *defaeco*, pp. *-atus*, to remove the dregs, purify]

**de•fec•og•ra•phy** (de-fĕ-kog′ră-fē) radiographic examination of the act of defecation of a radiopaque stool. [defecation + G. *graphō*, to write]

**de•fect** (dē′fekt) an imperfection, malformation, dysfunction, or absence; a qualitative departure from what is expected. USAGE NOTE Often confused with deficiency, which is a quantitative shortcoming. [L. *deficio*, pp. *-fectus*, to fail, to lack]

**de•fec•tive** (dē-fek′tiv) denoting or exhibiting a defect; imperfect; a failure of quality.

**de•fec•tive bac•te•ri•o•phage** a temperate bacteriophage mutant whose genome does not contain all of the normal components and cannot become a fully infectious virus, yet can replicate indefinitely in the bacterial genome as defective probacteriophage; many defective bacteriophages are mediators of transduction.

**de·fec·tive vi·rus** a virus particle that contains insufficient nucleic acid to provide for production of all essential viral components.

**de·fense** (dē-fens′) the psychological mechanisms used to control anxiety, e.g., rationalization, projection. [L. *defendo*, to ward off]

**de·fense mech·a·nism 1.** a psychological means of coping with conflict or anxiety, e.g., conversion, denial, dissociation, rationalization, repression, sublimation; **2.** the psychic structure underlying a coping strategy; **3.** immunological mechanism vs. nonspecific defense mechanism.

**de·fen·sins** (dē-fen′sinz) a class of basic antibiotic peptides, found in neutrophils, that apparently kill bacteria by causing membrane damage. [L. *de-fendo*, pp. *de-fensum*, to repel, avert, + -in]

**de·fen·sive med·i·cine** diagnostic or therapeutic measures conducted primarily as a safeguard against possible subsequent malpractice liability.

**de·fen·sive·ness** (dē-fen′siv-nes) excessive reaction to sensory stimuli.

**def·er·ent** (def′er-ent) carrying away. [L. *deferens*, pres. p. of *defero*, to carry away]

**def·er·ent duct** SYN ductus deferens.

**def·er·en·tec·to·my** (def′er-en-tek′tō-mē) SYN vasectomy. [(ductus) deferens, + G. *ektomē*, excision]

**def·er·en·tial** (def-er-en′shăl) relating to the ductus deferens.

**def·er·en·ti·tis** (def′er-en-tī′tis) inflammation of the ductus deferens. SYN vasitis.

**de·fer·ves·cence** (def-er-ves′ens) falling of an elevated temperature; abatement of fever. [L. *defervesco*, to cease boiling, fr. *de-* neg. + *fervesco*, to begin to boil]

**de·fi·bril·la·tion** (dē-fib-ri-lā′shŭn) the arrest of fibrillation of the cardiac muscle (atrial or ventricular) with restoration of the normal rhythm.

**de·fi·bril·la·tor** (dē-fib′ri-lā-ter) **1.** any agent or measure, e.g., an electric shock, that arrests fibrillation of the atria or ventricles and restores the normal rhythm. **2.** the machine designed to administer a defibrillating electric shock.

**de·fi·bri·na·tion** (dē-fī-bri-nā′shŭn) removal of fibrin from the blood, usually by means of constant agitation while the blood is collected in a container with glass beads or chips.

**de·fi·cien·cy** (dē-fish′en-sē) an insufficient quantity of some substance (as in dietary deficiency, hemoglobin deficiency as in marrow aplasia), organization (as in mental deficiency), activity (as in enzyme deficiency or reduced oxygen-carrying capacity of the blood), etc., of which the amount present is of normal quality. SEE ALSO deficiency disease. [L. *deficio*, to fail, fr. *facio*, to do]

**de·fi·cien·cy dis·ease** any disease resulting from undernutrition or an inadequacy of calories, proteins, essential amino acids, fatty acids, vitamins, or trace minerals.

**de·fi·cien·cy symp·tom** manifestation of a lack, in varying degrees, of some substance (e.g., hormone, enzyme, vitamin) necessary for normal structure and/or function of an organism.

**def·i·cit** (def′i-sit) the result of consuming or losing something faster than it is being replenished or replaced. [L. *deficio*, to fail]

**de·fin·i·tive host** one in which a parasite reaches the adult or sexually mature stage.

**de·flec·tion** (dē-flek′shŭn) **1.** a moving to one side. **2.** in the electrocardiogram, a deviation of the curve from the isoelectric base line; any wave or complex of the electrocardiogram. [L. *deflecto*, pp. *-flexus*, to bend aside]

**de·flex·ion** (dē′fleks-shŭn) term used to describe the position of the fetal head in relation to the maternal pelvis in which the head is descending in a nonflexed or extended attitude. [de- + L. *flexio*, a bending, fr. *flecto*, pp. *flexum*, to bend]

**de·flu·vi·um** (dē-floo′vē-ŭm) SYN defluxion. [L., fr. *de-fluo*, pp. *-fluxus*, to flow down]

**de·flux·ion** (dē-flŭk′shŭn) **1.** a falling down or out, as of the hair. SEE ALSO effluvium. **2.** a flowing down or discharge of fluid. SYN defluvium. [L. *defluxio*, *de-fluo*, pp. *-fluxus*, to flow down]

**de·for·ma·tion** (dē-fōr-mā′shŭn) **1.** deviation of form from the normal; specifically, an alteration in shape and/or structure of a previously normally formed part. It occurs after organogenesis and often involves the musculoskeletal system (e.g., clubfoot). **2.** SYN deformity. **3.** RHEOLOGY the change in the physical shape of a mass by applied stress. [L. *de-formo*, pp. *-atus*, to deform, fr. *forma*, form]

**de·for·mi·ty** (dē-fōr′mi-tē) a permanent structural deviation from the normal shape or size, resulting in disfigurement; may be congenital or acquired. SYN deformation (2).

**defs, DMFS** decayed, filled, or missing tooth surfaces.

**deft, DMFT** decayed, missing, or filled teeth.

**de·gen·er·ate 1.** (dē-jen′er-āt) to pass to a lower level of mental, physical, or moral state; to fall below the normal or acceptable type or state. **2.** (dē-jen′ĕ-răt) below the normal or acceptable; that which has passed to a lower level.

**de·gen·er·a·tion** (dē-jen-er-ā′shŭn) **1.** deterioration; passing from a higher to a lower level or type. **2.** a worsening of mental, physical, or moral qualities. **3.** a retrogressive pathologic change in cells or tissues, in consequence of which their functions are often impaired or destroyed; sometimes reversible; in the early stages, necrosis results. [L. *degeneratio*]

**de·gen·er·a·tive** (dē-jen′er-ă-tiv) relating to degeneration.

**de·gen·er·a·tive joint dis·ease** SYN osteoarthritis.

**de·glov·ing** (dē-glov′ing) **1.** intraoral surgical exposure of the anterior mandible used in various orthognathic surgical operations such as genioplasty or mandibular alveolar surgery. **2.** SEE degloving injury.

**de·glov·ing in·ju·ry** avulsion of the skin of the hand (or foot) in which the part is skeletonized by removal of most or all of the skin and subcutaneous tissue.

**de·glu·ti·tion** (dē-gloo-tish′ŭn) the act of swallowing. [L. *de-glutio*, to swallow]

**de·glu·ti·tion syn·co·pe** faintness or unconsciousness upon swallowing. This is nearly always due to excessive vagal effect on a heart that may already have bradycardia or atrioventricular block.

**deg·ra·da·tion** (deg-ră-dā′shŭn) the change of a chemical compound into a less complex compound. [L. *degradatus*, degrade]

**de·gree** (dĕ-grē′) **1.** one of the divisions on the scale of a measuring instrument such as a thermometer, barometer, etc. See Comparative Temperature Scales appendix. SEE scale. **2.** the 360th part of the circumference of a circle. **3.** a position or rank within a graded series. **4.** a measure of damage to tissue. [Fr. *degré;* L. *gradus,* a step]

**de•gus•ta•tion** (dē-gŭs-tā′shŭn) **1.** the act of tasting. **2.** the sense of taste. [L. *degustatio,* fr. *de-gusto,* pp. *-atus,* to taste]

**De•hio test** (de-hē-o) if an injection of atropine relieves bradycardia, the condition is due to action of the vagus; if it does not, the condition may be due to an affection of the heart itself.

**de•his•cence** (dē-his′ens) a bursting open, splitting, or gaping along natural or sutured lines. [L. *dehisco,* to split apart or open]

**de•hy•drase** (dē-hī′drās) former name for dehydratase.

**de•hy•dra•tase** (dē-hī′drā-tās) a subclass (EC 4.2.1) of lyases (hydro-lyases) that remove H and OH as $H_2O$ from a substrate, leaving a double bond, or add a group to a double bond by the elimination of water from two substances to form a third.

**de•hy•dra•tion** (dē-hī-drā′shŭn) **1.** deprivation of water. SYN anhydration. **2.** process of losing body water, progressing either from the hyperhydrated state to euhydration or from euhydration downward to hypohydration. **3.** SYN exsiccation (2). **4.** SYN desiccation.

△**dehydro-** prefix used in the names of chemical compounds that differ from more familiar compounds in the absence of two hydrogen atoms; e.g., dehydroascorbic acid, which resembles ascorbic acid in all structural features except for its lack of two hydrogen atoms that are present in the ascorbic acid molecule. In systematic nomenclature, didehydro- is preferred as being more exact.

**11-de•hy•dro•cor•ti•co•ster•one** (el-ev′en-dē-hī′drō-kōr-ti-kos′ter-ōn) a metabolite of corticosterone, found in the adrenal cortex.

**de•hy•dro•epi•and•ros•ter•one (DHEA)** steroid agent related to male hormones that have been advocated as able to prevent physiologic consequences of aging, without studies that show benefit or safety.

**de•hy•dro•gen•ase** (dē-hī′drō-jen-ās) class name for those enzymes that oxidize substrates by catalyzing removal of hydrogen from metabolites (hydrogen donors) and transferring it to other substances (hydrogen acceptors).

**de•hy•dro•gen•a•tion** (dē-hī′drō-jen-ā′shŭn) removal of a pair of hydrogen atoms from a compound by the action of enzymes (dehydrogenases) or other catalysts.

**de•in•sti•tu•tion•al•i•za•tion** (dē′in-sti-too′shŭn-ăl-i-zā-shŭn) the discharge of institutionalized patients from a mental hospital into treatment programs in half-way houses and other community-based programs.

**DEJ** dentinoenamel junction.

**de•jec•tion** (dē-jek′shŭn) **1.** SYN depression (4). **2.** the discharge of excrementitious matter. **3.** the matter so discharged. [L. *dejectio,* fr. *de- jicio,* pp. *-jectus,* to cast down]

**De•je•rine dis•ease** (dĕ-zhĕ-rēn′) SYN Dejerine-Sottas disease.

**De•je•rine hand phe•nom•e•non** (dĕ-zhĕ-rēn′) clonic contractions of the flexors of the hand (wrist) on tapping the dorsum of the hand or the volar side of the forearm near the wrist; occurs in normal persons but is exaggerated in pyramidal tract lesions.

**De•je•rine sign** (dĕ-zhĕ-rēn′) aggravation of symptoms of root irritation by the acts of coughing, sneezing, or straining to defecate.

**De•je•rine-Sot•tas dis•ease** (dĕ-zhĕ-rēn′ sō′tăs) a familial type of demyelinating sensorimotor polyneuropathy that begins in early childhood and is slowly progressive; clinically characterized by foot pain and paresthesias, followed by symmetrical weakness and wasting of the distal limbs; one of the causes of stork legs; patients are wheelchair-bound at an early age; peripheral nerves are palpably enlarged and non-tender; pathologically, onion bulb formation is seen in the nerves: whorls of overlapping, intertwined Schwann cell processes that encircle bare axons; usually autosomal recessive inheritance. SYN Dejerine disease, progressive hypertrophic polyneuropathy.

△**de•ka-** SEE deca-.

**Del•a•field he•ma•tox•y•lin** (del′ă-fēld) an alum type of hematoxylin used in histology; natural ripening takes about 2 months and the solution is good for years.

**de•lam•i•na•tion** (dē-lam-i-nā′shŭn) division into separate layers. [L. *de,* from, + *lamina,* a thin plate]

**de•layed al•ler•gy** a type IV allergic reaction; so called because in a sensitized subject the reaction becomes evident hours after contact with the allergen (antigen), reaches its peak after 36 to 48 hours, then recedes slowly. Associated with cell-mediated responses. SEE ALSO delayed reaction. Cf. immediate allergy.

**de•layed den•ti•tion** delayed eruption of the teeth.

**de•layed flap** a flap raised in its donor area in two or more stages to increase its chances of survival after transfer.

**de•layed graft** application of a skin graft after waiting several days for healthy granulations to form.

**de•layed on•set musc•le sore•ness (DOMS)** residual muscle soreness that appears within 24 hours and may last for several days after unaccustomed heavy muscular activity, particularly with eccentric muscle actions; related to actual muscle cell damage.

**de•layed pu•ber•ty** lack of any signs of puberty by age 14 years in either sex.

**de•layed re•ac•tion** a local or generalized immune response that begins 24 to 48 hours after exposure to an antigen. SEE cell-mediated reaction.

**Del•bet sign** (del′bā) in aneurysm of a main artery, maintenance of nutrition in distal tissues indicates efficient collateral circulation even when the pulse has disappeared.

**de•lead** (dē-led′) to cause the mobilization and excretion of lead deposited in the bones and other tissues, as by the administration of a chelating agent.

**del•e•te•ri•ous** (del-ĕ-tēr′ē-ŭs) injurious; noxious; harmful. [G. *dēlētērios,* fr. *dēleomai,* to injure]

**de•le•tion** (dĕ-lē′shŭn) in genetics, any spontaneous elimination of part of the normal genetic complement, whether cytogenetically visible (chromosomal deletion) or inferred from phenotypic evidence (point deletion). [L. *deletio,* destruction]

**del·i·ques·cence** (del-i-kwes′ens) becoming damp or liquid by absorption of water from the atmosphere; a property of certain salts, such as CaCl₂. [L. *de-liquesco,* to melt or become liquid]

**de·lir·i·ous** (dē-lir′ē-ŭs) in a state of delirium.

**de·lir·i·um,** pl. **de·li·ria** (dē-lir′ē-ŭm, dē-lir′ē-ă) an altered state of consciousness, consisting of confusion, distractibility, disorientation, disordered thinking and memory, defective perception (illusions and hallucinations), prominent hyperactivity, agitation and autonomic nervous system overactivity; caused by a number of toxic structural and metabolic disorders. [L. fr. *deliro,* to be crazy, fr. *de-* + *lira,* a furrow (*i.e.,* go out of the furrow)]

**de·lir·i·um tre·mens (DT)** a severe, sometimes fatal, form of delirium due to alcoholic withdrawal following a period of sustained intoxication. SYN oenomania. [L. pres. p. of *tremo,* to tremble]

**de·liv·er** (dē-liv′er) **1.** to assist a woman in childbirth. **2.** to extract from an enclosed place, as the fetus from the womb, an object or foreign body, e.g., a tumor from its capsule or surroundings, or the lens of the eye in cases of cataract. [fr. O. Fr. fr. L. *de-* + *liber,* free]

**de·liv·ery** (dē-liv′er-ē) passage of the fetus and the placenta from the genital canal into the external world.

**del·le** (del′eh) the central lighter-colored portion of the erythrocyte, as observed in a stained film of blood. [Ger. *Delle,* low ground, pit]

**del·len** (del′en) shallow, saucer-like, clearly defined excavations at the margin of the cornea, about 1.5 by 2 mm, due to localized dehydration; also called Fuchs dellen. [Ger. pl. of *Delle,* low ground, pit]

**del·phi·an node** a midline prelaryngeal lymph node, adjacent to the thyroid gland, enlargement of which is indicative of thyroid disease or early metastasis from the subglottic larynx.

**del·ta** (Δ, δ) (del′tă) **1.** fourth letter of the Greek alphabet. **2.** CHEMISTRY a double bond, usually with a superscript to indicate position in a chain (Δ⁵); application of heat in a reaction (A $\overset{\Delta}{\to}$ B); absence of heat treatment ($\cancel{\Delta}$); distance between two atoms in a molecule, or position of a substituent located on the fourth atom from the carboxyl or other primary functional group (δ); change (Δ); thickness (δ); chemical shift in NMR (δ). **3.** ANATOMY a triangular surface.

**del·ta a·gent** SYN hepatitis D virus.

**del·ta bil·i·ru·bin** the fraction of bilirubin covalently bound to albumin.

**del·ta cell 1.** a variety of cell in the anterior lobe of the hypophysis that has basophilic granules; **2.** a cell of the islets of Langerhans, with fine granules that stain with aniline blue; secretes somatostatin.

**del·ta check** a comparison of consecutive values for a given test in a patient's laboratory file used to detect abrupt changes, usually generated as a part of computer-based quality control programs.

**del·ta fibers** nerve fibers with conduction velocities in the range of 8–30 m/sec.

**del·ta gran·ule** a granule of a delta cell.

**del·ta hep·a·ti·tis** SYN viral hepatitis type D.

**del·ta rhythm** a wave pattern in the electroencephalogram in the frequency band of 1.5 to 4.0 Hz. SYN delta wave (2).

**del·ta wave 1.** a premature upstroke of the QRS

complex due to an atrioventricular bypass tract as in WPW syndrome; **2.** SYN delta rhythm.

**del·toid** (del′toyd) **1.** resembling the Greek letter delta (Δ); triangular. **2.** SYN deltoid muscle. [G. *deltoeidēs,* shaped like the letter *delta*]

**del·toid lig·a·ment** compound ligament consisting of four component ligaments which pass downward from the medial malleolus of the tibia to the tarsal bones: 1) tibionavicular ligament (pars tibionavicularis [TA]), 2) tibiocalcaneal ligament (pars tibiocalcanea [TA]), 3) anterior tibiotalar ligament (pars tibiotalaris anterior, and 4) posterior tibiotalar ligament (pars tibiotalaris posterior). SYN ligamentum deltoideum.

**del·toid mus·cle** *origin,* lateral third of clavicle, lateral border of acromion process, lower border of spine of scapula; *insertion,* lateral side of shaft of humerus a little above its middle (deltoid tuberosity); *action,* abduction, flexion, extension, and rotation of arm; *nerve supply,* axillary from fifth and sixth cervical spinal cord segments through brachial plexus. SYN musculus deltoideus [TA], deltoid (2).

**de·lu·sion** (dē-loo′zhŭn) a false belief or wrong judgment held with conviction despite incontrovertible evidence to the contrary. [L. *de-ludo,* pp. *-lusus,* to play false, deceive, fr. *ludo,* to play]

**de·lu·sion·al** (dē-loo′zhŭn-ăl) relating to a delusion.

**de·lu·sion of gran·deur** a delusion in which one believes oneself possessed of great wealth, intellect, importance, power, etc.

**de·lu·sion of ne·ga·tion** a delusion in which one imagines that the world and all that relates to it have ceased to exist.

**de·lu·sion of per·se·cu·tion, per·se·cu·to·ry de·lu·sion** a false notion that one is being persecuted; characteristic symptom of paranoid schizophrenia.

**de·mand ox·y·gen de·li·very de·vice** an electronic device that conserves oxygen by sensing the initiation of an inspiratory effort and then delivering oxygen only during the inspiratory phase.

**de·mand pace·mak·er** a form of artificial pacemaker usually implanted into cardiac tissue because its output of electrical stimuli can be inhibited by endogenous cardiac electrical activity.

**de·mat·i·a·ceous** (dē-mat-ē-ā′shŭs) denoting dark conidia and/or hyphae, usually brown or black; used frequently to denote dark-colored fungi.

**de·mat·i·a·ceous fun·gi** (de-măt′ē-ā-cē-ous) dark fungi that form melanin. [Mod. L. *Dematium* (genus name), fr. g. *demation,* fine strand, fr. *dema,* band, fr. *deō,* to bind + suffix *-aceous,* characterized by]

**de·men·tia** (dē-men′shē-ă) the loss, usually progressive, of cognitive and intellectual functions, without impairment of perception or consciousness; caused by a variety of disorders including severe infections and toxins, but most commonly associated with structural brain disease. Characterized by disorientation, impaired memory, judgment, and intellect, and a shallow labile affect. SYN amentia. [L. fr. *de-* priv. + *mens,* mind]

△**dem·i-** half, lesser. SEE ALSO hemi-, semi-. [Fr. fr. L. *dimidius,* half]

**dem·i·gaunt·let ban·dage** a gauntlet bandage that covers only the hand, leaving the fingers exposed.

**dem·i·lune** (dem'ē-loon) **1.** a small body with a form similar to that of a half-moon or a crescent. **2.** term frequently used for the gametocyte of *Plasmodium falciparum*. [Fr. half-moon]

**de·min·er·al·i·za·tion** (dē-min'er-ăl-ī-zā'shŭn) a loss or decrease of the mineral constituents of the body or individual tissues, especially of bone.

***Dem·o·dex*** (dem'ō-deks) a genus of minute mites that inhabit the skin and are usually found in the sebaceous glands and hair follicles. [G. *dēmos*, tallow, + *dēx*, a woodworm]

**dem·o·di·co·sis** (dem-ō-di-cō'sis) infestation by mites of the species *Demodex*, chiefly involving hair follicles and characterized by varying degrees of local inflammation and immune response.

**de·mog·ra·phy** (dĕ-mog'ră-fē) the study of populations, especially with reference to size, density, fertility, mortality, growth rate, age distribution, migration, and vital statistics. [G. *demos*, people, + *graphō*, to write]

**De Mor·gan spot** (dĕ mōr'găn) SYN senile hemangioma.

**de·mul·cent** (de-mŭl'sent) **1.** soothing; relieving irritation. **2.** an agent, such as a mucilage or oil, that soothes and relieves irritation, especially of the mucous surfaces. [L. *de-mulceo*, pp. *-mulctus*, to stroke lightly, to soften]

**de Mus·set sign** (dĕ moo-sā') SYN Musset sign.

**de·my·e·li·nat·ing dis·ease** generic term for a group of diseases, of unknown cause, in which there is extensive loss of the myelin in the central nervous system, as in multiple sclerosis.

**de·my·e·li·na·tion, de·my·e·lin·i·za·tion** (dē-mī'ĕ-li-nā'shŭn, dē-mī'ĕ-lin-i-za'shŭn) loss of myelin with preservation of the axons or fiber tracts. Central demyelination occurs within the central nervous system (e.g., the demyelination seen with multiple sclerosis); peripheral demyelination affects the peripheral nervous system (e.g., the demyelination seen with Guillain-Barré syndrome).

**de·my·e·lin·i·sa·tion [Br.]** SEE demyelinization.

**de·na·tur·a·tion** (dē-na-tyu-rā'shŭn) the process of becoming denatured.

**de·na·tured** (dē-nāt'yu-rd) **1.** made unnatural or changed from the normal; often applied to proteins or nucleic acids heated or otherwise treated to the point where tertiary structural characteristics are altered. **2.** adulterated, as by addition of methanol to ethanol.

**den·dri·form** (den'dri-fōrm) tree-shaped, or branching. SYN arborescent, dendritic (1), dendroid. [G. *dendron*, tree, + L. *forma*, form]

**den·dri·form ker·a·ti·tis, den·drit·ic ker·a·ti·tis** a form of herpetic keratitis.

**den·drite** (den'drīt) **1.** one of the two types of branching protoplasmic processes of the nerve cell (the other being the axon). SYN dendritic process, dendron, neurodendrite. **2.** a crystalline treelike structure formed during the freezing of an alloy. [G. *dendritēs*, relating to a tree]

**den·drit·ic** (den-drit'ik) **1.** SYN dendriform. **2.** relating to the dendrites of nerve cells.

**den·drit·ic cell** cell of neural crest origin with extensive processes; they develop melanin early.

**den·drit·ic cor·ne·al ul·cer** keratitis caused by herpes simplex virus.

**den·drit·ic pro·cess** SYN dendrite (1).

**den·drit·ic spines** variably long excrescences of nerve cell dendrites, varying in shape from small knobs to thornlike or filamentous processes, usually more numerous on distal dendrite arborizations than on the proximal part of dendritic trunks; they are a preferential site of synaptic axodendritic contact; sparse or absent in some types of nerve cells (motor neurons, the large cells of the globus pallidus, stellate cells of the cerebral cortex), exceedingly numerous in others such as the pyramidal cells of the cerebral cortex and the Purkinje cells of the cerebellar cortex. SYN gemmule (2).

**den·droid** (den'droyd) SYN dendriform. [G. *dendron*, tree, + *eidos*, appearance]

**den·dron** SYN dendrite (1). [G. a tree]

**de·ner·vate** (dē-ner'vāt) to cause denervation.

**de·ner·va·tion** (dē-ner-vā'shŭn) loss of nerve supply.

**den·gue, den·gue hem·or·rhag·ic fe·ver, den·gue fe·ver** (den'gā) a disease of tropical and subtropical regions, caused by dengue virus and transmitted by a mosquito of the genus *Aedes*. Four grades of severity are recognized: grade I, fever and constitutional symptoms; grade II, spontaneous bleeding (of skin, gums, or gastrointestinal tract); grade III, agitation and circulatory failure; grade IV, profound shock. [Sp. corruption of "dandy" fever]

**den·gue vi·rus** a virus of the genus *Flavivirus;* the etiologic agent of dengue in humans and also occurring in monkeys and chimpanzees, usually as inapparent infection; four serotypes are recognized; transmission is effected by mosquitoes of the genus *Aedes*.

**de·ni·al** (dē-nī'ăl) an unconscious defense mechanism used to allay anxiety by denying the existence of important conflicts or troublesome impulses. SYN negation. [M.E., fr, O. Fr., fr. L. *denegare*, to say no]

**den·i·da·tion** (den-i-dā'shŭn) exfoliation of the superficial portion of the mucous membrane of the uterus; stripping off of the menstrual decidua. [L. *de*, from, + *nidus*, nest]

**Den·is Browne pouch** (de'nis brown) a pocket formed between Scarpa and external oblique fascia adjacent to external inguinal ring; a common lodging site for an undescended testis (as in cryptorchism).

**Den·is Browne splint** (de'nis brown) a light aluminum splint applied to the lateral aspect of the leg and foot; used for clubfoot.

**Den·nie-Mor·gan fold, Den·nie line** (den'ē mōr'găn, den'ē) a fold or line below each lower eyelid caused by edema in atopic dermatitis.

**dens**, pl. **den·tes** (denz, den'tēz) [TA] **1.** SYN tooth. **2.** a strong toothlike process projecting upward from the body of the axis, or epistropheus, around which the atlas rotates. SYN odontoid process of epistropheus. [L.]

**dens ca·ni·nus**, pl. **den·tes ca·ni·ni** [TA] SYN canine tooth.

**dens de·ci·du·us**, pl. **den·tes de·ci·du·i** [TA] SYN deciduous tooth.

**dens in den·te** a developmental disturbance in tooth formation resulting from invagination of the epithelium associated with crown development into the area destined to become pulp space; after calcification there is an invagination of enamel and dentin into the pulp space, giving the radiographic appearance of a "tooth within a tooth."

**dense bo·dies 1.** granules in the central granulomere of blood platelets that take up and store serotonin from plasma; **2.** electron-dense bodies containing α-actinin in the cytoplasm of smooth muscle cells, believed to be homologous to the Z-lines of striated muscle.

**den·sim·e·ter** (den-sim′ĕ-ter) SYN densitometer (1). [L. *densitas,* density, + G. *metron,* measure]

**dens in·ci·si·vus,** pl. **den·tes in·ci·si·vi** [TA] SYN incisor tooth.

**den·si·tom·e·ter** (den-si-tom′ĕ-ter) **1.** an instrument for measuring the density of a fluid. SYN densimeter. **2.** an instrument for measuring, by virtue of relative turbidity, the growth of bacteria in broth; useful in microbiologic assay of nutrients and antibiotics, phage studies, etc. **3.** an instrument for measuring the density of components (e.g., protein fractions) separated by electrophoresis or chromatography, utilizing light absorption or reflection. **4.** an electronic instrument for measuring the blackening of radiographic film by x-ray exposure; used for film sensitometry, bone densitometry, measurement of line spread function (microdensitometer). [L. *densitas,* density, + G. *metron,* measure]

**den·si·tom·e·try** (den-si-tom′ĕ-trē) SYN underwater weighing.

**den·si·ty** (den′si-tē) **1.** the compactness of a substance; the ratio of mass to unit volume, usually expressed as g/cm$^3$ (kg/m$^3$ in the SI system). **2.** the quantity of electricity on a given surface or in a given time per unit of volume. **3.** in radiological physics, the opacity to light of an exposed radiographic or photographic film; the darker the film, the greater the measured density. **4.** in clinical radiology, a less-exposed area on a film, corresponding to a region of greater x-ray attenuation (radiopacity) in the subject; the more light transmitted by the film, the greater the density of the subject; this is not actually the opposite of the prior definition, since one concerns film density and the other subject density. [L. *densus,* thick]

**dens mo·la·ris,** pl. **den·tes mo·la·res** [TA] SYN molar tooth. SEE ALSO molar.

**dens per·ma·nens,** pl. **den·tes per·ma·nen·tes** [TA] SYN permanent tooth.

**dens pre·mo·la·ris,** pl. **den·tes pre·mo·la·res** [TA] SYN premolar tooth.

**dens se·ro·ti·nus** [TA] SYN third molar.

◁**dent-, den·ti-, den·to-** teeth; dental. SEE ALSO odonto-. [L. *dens,* tooth]

**den·tal** (den′tăl) relating to the teeth. [L. *dens,* tooth]

**den·tal ab·scess, den·to·al·ve·o·lar ab·scess** SYN alveolar abscess.

**den·tal ac·qui·red pel·li·cle** a thin membranous layer, amorphous, acellular, and organic, that forms on exposed tooth surfaces, dental restorations, and dental calculus deposits.

**den·tal anat·o·my** that branch of gross anatomy concerned with the morphology of teeth, their location, position, and relationships.

**den·tal an·ky·lo·sis** rigid fixation of a tooth to the surrounding alveolus as a result of ossification of the ligament; prevents eruption and orthodontic movement.

**den·tal an·thro·po·lo·gy** a branch of physical anthropology concerned with the origin, evolution, and development of the dentitions of primates, especially humans, and the relationship to their physical, social, and cultural relationships.

**den·tal arch** the curved structure formed by the natural dentition or the residual ridge, which remains after the loss of the natural teeth.

**den·tal as·sis·tant** a person trained to provide support to a dentist with general tasks ranging from clerical work and assistance at chairside to laboratory, infection control, and radiographic work.

**den·tal bulb** the papilla, derived from mesoderm, that forms the part of the primordium of a tooth that is situated within the cup-shaped enamel organ.

**den·tal cal·cu·lus 1.** calcified deposits formed around the teeth; may appear as subgingival or supragingival calculus; **2.** SYN tartar (2).

**den·tal crypt** the space filled by the dental follicle.

**den·tal fol·li·cle** the dental sac with its enclosed odontogenic organ and developing tooth.

**den·tal for·ceps** forceps used to luxate teeth and remove them from the alveolus. SYN extracting forceps.

**den·tal for·mu·la** a statement in tabular form of the number of each kind of teeth in the jaw.

**den·tal ger·i·at·rics** treatment of dental problems peculiar to advanced age. SYN gerodontics, gerodontology.

**den·tal·gia** (den-tal′jē-ă) SYN toothache. [L. *dens,* tooth, + G. *algos,* pain]

**den·tal gran·u·lo·ma** SYN periapical granuloma.

**den·tal hy·gien·ist** a licensed, professional auxiliary in dentistry who is both an oral health educator and clinician, and who uses preventive, therapeutic, and educational methods for the control of oral diseases.

▣**den·tal im·plants** crowns, bridges, or dentures attached permanently to the jaw by means of various types of metal anchors. See page 258.

**den·tal or·gan** SYN enamel organ.

**den·tal pa·pil·la** a projection of the mesenchymal tissue of the developing jaw into the cup of the enamel organ; its outer layer becomes a layer of specialized columnar cells, the odontoblasts, which form the dentin of the tooth.

**den·tal plaque 1.** the noncalcified accumulation mainly of oral microorganisms and their products, that adheres tenaciously to the teeth and is not readily dislodged; **2.** SYN bacterial plaque.

**den·tal pub·lic health** the science and art of preventing and controlling dental diseases and promoting dental health through organized community efforts. One of the dental specialties.

**den·tal pulp, den·ti·nal pulp** the soft tissue within the pulp cavity, consisting of connective tissue containing blood vessels, nerves and lymphatics, and at the periphery a layer of odontoblasts capable of internal repair of the dentin. SYN pulp (2), tooth pulp.

**den·tal ridge** the prominent border of a cusp or margin of a tooth.

**den·tal sac** the outer connective tissue envelope surrounding a developing tooth; also applied to the mesenchymal concentration that is the primordium of the sac. SEE ALSO dental follicle.

**den·tal sur·geon** a general practitioner of dentistry. SYN oral surgeon.

**den·tal sy·ringe** a breech-loading metal cartridge syringe into which fits a hermetically sealed glass cartridge containing anesthetic solution.

**den·tate** (den′tāt) notched; toothed; cogged. [L. *dentatus,* toothed]

d
e

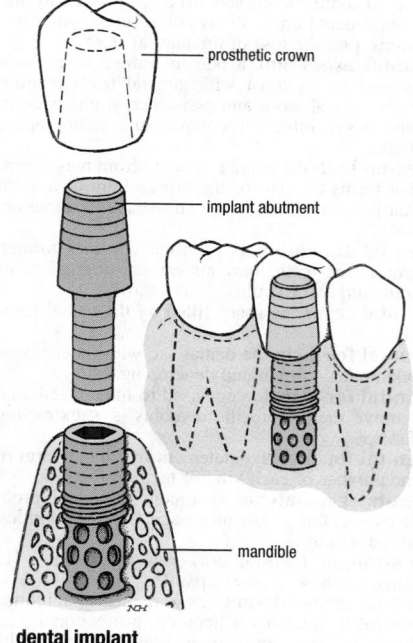

prosthetic crown

implant abutment

mandible

**dental implant**

**den·tate gy·rus** one of the two interlocking gyri composing the hippocampus, the other one being the Ammon horn.

**den·tate nu·cle·us of cer·e·bel·lum** the most lateral and largest of the cerebellar nuclei; it receives the axons of the Purkinje cells of the neocerebellum (lateral areas of cerebellar cortex); together with the more medially located globosus and emboliform nuclei it is the major source of fibers composing the massive superior cerebellar peduncle or brachium conjunctivum. SYN nucleus dentatus [TA].

**den·tate su·ture** SYN serrate suture.

**den·tes** (den'tēz) plural of dens. [L.]

**den·ti·cle** (den'ti-kl) **1.** SYN endolith. **2.** a tooth-like projection from a hard surface. [L. *denticulus*, a small tooth]

**den·ti·frice** (den'ti-fris) any preparation used in the cleansing of the teeth, e.g., a tooth powder, toothpaste, or tooth wash. [L. *dentifricium*, fr. *dens*, tooth, + *frico*, pp. *frictus*, to rub]

**den·tig·er·ous** (den-tij'er-ŭs) arising from or associated with teeth, as a dentigerous cyst. [denti- + L. *gero*, to bear]

**den·tig·er·ous cyst** an odontogenic cyst derived from the reduced enamel epithelium surrounding the crown of an impacted, unerupted, or embedded tooth. SYN follicular cyst (2).

**den·ti·la·bi·al** (den'ti-lā'bē-ăl) relating to the teeth and lips. [denti- + L. *labium*, lip]

**den·ti·lin·gual** (den-ti-ling'gwăl) relating to the teeth and tongue. [denti- + L. *lingua*, tongue]

**den·tin** (den'tin) the ivory forming the mass of the tooth. Calcified tissue that is not as hard as enamel but harder than cementum. About 20% is organic matrix, mostly a fibrous protein collagen, with some elastin and a small amount of muco-

polysaccharide; the inorganic fraction (70%) is mainly hydroxyapatite, with some carbonate, magnesium, and fluoride. The dentin is traversed by closely packed tubules running from the pulp cavity outward; within the tubules are processes from the odontoblasts. SYN dentinum. [L. *dens*, tooth]

**den·ti·nal** (den'ti-năl) relating to dentin.

**den·ti·nal ca·nals** SYN canaliculi dentales.

**den·ti·nal·gia** (den-ti-nal'jē-ă) dentinal sensitivity or pain. [dentin + G. *algos*, pain]

**den·ti·nal la·mi·na cyst** a small keratin-filled cyst, usually multiple, on the alveolar ridge of new-born infants; it is derived from remnants of the dental lamina.

**den·ti·nal sheath** a layer of tissue relatively resistant to the action of acids, which forms the walls of the dentinal tubules.

**den·ti·nal tu·bules** SYN canaliculi dentales.

**den·tin bridge** a deposit of reparative dentin or other calcific substances which forms across and reseals exposed tooth pulp tissue.

**den·tin dys·pla·sia** a hereditary disorder of the teeth, involving both primary and permanent dentition, in which the clinical morphology and color of the teeth are normal, but the teeth radiographically exhibit short roots, obliteration of the pulp chambers and canals, and mobility and premature exfoliation.

**den·tin·o·ce·men·tal** (den'ti-nō-se-men'tăl) relating to the dentin and cementum of teeth.

**den·tin·o·e·nam·el** (den'ti-nō-ē-nam'ĕl) relating to the dentin and enamel of teeth. SYN amelodentinal.

**den·tin·o·e·nam·el junc·tion (DEJ)** the surface at which the enamel and the dentin of the crown of a tooth are joined.

**den·tin·o·gen·e·sis** (den'ti-nō-jen'ĕ-sis) the process of dentin formation in the development of teeth. [dentin + G. *genesis*, production]

**den·tin·o·gen·e·sis im·per·fec·ta** a hereditary disorder of the teeth characterized by translucent gray to yellow-brown teeth involving both primary and permanent dentition; the enamel fractures easily, leaving exposed dentin which undergoes rapid attrition; radiographically, the pulp chambers and canals appear obliterated and the roots are short and blunted; sometimes occurs in association with osteogenesis imperfecta.

**den·ti·noid** (den'ti-noyd) **1.** resembling dentin. **2.** SYN dentinoma. [dentin + G. *eidos*, resembling]

**den·ti·no·ma** (den'ti-nō'mă) a rare benign odontogenic tumor consisting microscopically of dysplastic dentin and strands of epithelium within a fibrous stroma. SYN dentinoid (2). [dentin + G. *-oma*, tumor]

**den·ti·num** (den'ti-nŭm) SYN dentin. [L. *dens*, tooth]

**den·tip·a·rous** (den-tip'ă-rŭs) tooth-bearing. [denti- + L. *pario*, to bear]

**den·tist** a legally qualified practitioner of dentistry.

**den·tis·try** (den'tis-trē) the healing science and art concerned with the embryology, anatomy, physiology, and pathology of the oral-facial complex, and with the prevention, diagnosis, and treatment of deformities, pathoses, and traumatic injuries thereof.

**den·ti·tion** (den-tish'ŭn) the natural teeth, as considered collectively, in the dental arch; may be deciduous, permanent, or mixed. [L. *dentitio,* teething]

**den·to·al·ve·o·lar** (den'to-al-vē'ō-lăr) usually, denoting that portion of the alveolar bone immediately about the teeth; used also to denote the functional unity of teeth and alveolar bone.

**den·tu·lous** (den'tyu-lŭs) having natural teeth present in the mouth.

**den·ture** (den'tyur) **1.** an artificial substitute for missing natural teeth and adjacent tissues. **2.** sometimes used to denote the dentition of animals.

**den·ture base 1.** that part of a denture which rests on the oral mucosa and to which teeth are attached; **2.** that part of a complete or partial denture which rests upon the basal seat and to which teeth are attached. SYN saddle (2).

**den·ture bor·der 1.** the limit or boundary or circumferential margin of a denture base; **2.** the margin of the denture base at the junction of the polished surface with the impression (tissue) surface; **3.** the extreme edges of a denture base at the buccolabial, lingual, and posterior limits. SYN periphery (2).

**den·ture foun·da·tion** that portion of the oral structures which is available to support a denture.

**den·ture sta·bil·i·ty** the quality of a denture to be firm, steady, constant, and resist change of position when functional forces are applied. SYN stabilization (2).

**de·nu·cle·at·ed** (dē-noo'klē-ā-ted) deprived of a nucleus.

**de·nu·da·tion** (den-yu-dā'shŭn) depriving of a covering or protecting layer; the act of laying bare, as in the removal of the epithelium from an underlying surface. [L. *de-nudo,* to lay bare, fr. *de,* from, + *nudus,* naked]

**de·nude** (dē'nyud) to perform denudation.

**Denver De·vel·op·men·tal Screen·ing Test** a scale used by psychologists and pediatricians to assess the developmental, intellectual, motor, and social maturity of children at any age level from birth to adolescence.

**de·o·dor·ant** (dē-ō'der-ant) **1.** eliminating or masking a smell, especially an unpleasant one. **2.** an agent having such an action; especially a cosmetic combined with an antiperspirant. SYN deodorizer. [L. *de-* priv. + *odoro,* pp. *-atus,* to give an odor to, fr. *odor,* a smell]

**de·o·dor·iz·er** (dē-ō'der-īz-er) SYN deodorant (2).

**de·os·si·fi·ca·tion** (dē-os'i-fi-kā'shŭn) removal of the mineral constituents of bone. [L. *de,* from, + *os,* bone, + *facio,* to make]

**de·ox·y·a·den·o·sine (dA, dAdo)** (dē-oks'ē-ă-den'ō-sēn) 2'-deoxyribosyladenine, one of the four major nucleosides of DNA (the others being deoxycytidine, deoxyguanosine, and thymidine). The 5' derivative is also an important component of one form of vitamin B₁₂. Deoxyadenosine accumulates in individuals with severe combined immunodeficiency disease.

**de·ox·y·ad·e·nyl·ic ac·id (dAMP)** (dē-oks'ē-ad-en-il'ik as'id) deoxyadenosine monophosphate, a hydrolysis product of DNA, differing from adenylic acid in containing deoxyribose in place of ribose. SYN adenine deoxyribonucleotide.

**de·ox·y·cho·late** (dē-oks-ē-kō'lāt) a salt or ester of deoxycholic acid.

**de·ox·y·cho·lic ac·id** (dē-oks-ē-kō'lik as'id) a

bile acid and choleretic; used in biochemical preparations as a detergent.

**de·ox·y·cor·ti·cos·ter·one** (dē-oks'ē-kōr-ti-kos'ter-ōn) an adrenocortical steroid, principally a biosynthetic precursor of corticosterone and possibly aldosterone, that rarely appears in adrenocortical secretions; a potent mineralocorticoid with no appreciable glucocorticoid activity. SYN 21-hydroxyprogesterone.

**de·ox·y·cyt·i·dine** (dē-oks-ē-sī'ti-dēn) 2'-deoxyribosylcytosine, one of the four major nucleosides of DNA (the others being deoxyadenosine, deoxyguanosine, and thymidine).

**de·ox·y·cyt·i·dyl·ic ac·id (dCMP)** (dē-oks'ē-sī-ti-dil'ik as'id) deoxycytidine monophosphate, a hydrolysis product of DNA.

**de·ox·y·gua·no·sine** (dē-oks-ē-gwan'ō-sēn) one of the four major nucleosides of DNA (the others being deoxyadenosine, deoxycytidine, and thymidine). Found to accumulate in individuals with purine nucleoside phosphorylase deficiency.

**de·ox·y·gua·nyl·ic ac·id (dGMP)** (dē-oks-ē-gwan-il'ik as'id) deoxyguanosine monophosphate, a hydrolysis product of DNA. SYN guanine deoxyribonucleotide.

**de·ox·y·haem·o·glo·bin [Br.]** SEE deoxyhemoglobin.

**de·ox·y·hem·o·glo·bin** (dē-oks-ē-hē'mō-glō-bin) the reduced form of hemoglobin, resulting when oxyhemoglobin loses its oxygen. [de- + oxy- + hemoglobin]

**de·ox·y·ri·bo·nu·cle·ase (DNase, DNAase)** (dē-oks'ē-rī-bō-noo'klē-ās) any enzyme (phosphodiesterase) hydrolyzing phosphodiester bonds in DNA. SEE ALSO endonuclease, nuclease.

**de·ox·y·ri·bo·nu·cle·ic ac·id (DNA)** (dē-oks'ē-rī'bō-noo-klē'ik as'id) the type of nucleic acid containing deoxyribose as the sugar component and found principally in the nuclei (chromatin, chromosomes) and mitochondria of animal and plant cells, usually loosely bound to protein (hence the term deoxyribonucleoprotein); considered to be the autoreproducing component of chromosomes and of many viruses, and the repository of hereditary characteristics. Its linear macromolecular chain consists of deoxyribose molecules esterified with phosphate groups between the 3'- and 5'-hydroxyl groups; linked to this structure are the purines adenine (A) and guanine (G) and the pyrimidines cytosine (C) and thymine (T). DNA may be open-ended or circular, single- or double-stranded, and many forms are known, the most commonly described of which is double-stranded, wherein the pyrimidines and purines cross-link through hydrogen bonding in the schema A-T and C-G, bringing two antiparallel strands into a double helix. Chromosomes are composed of double-stranded DNA; mitochondrial DNA is circular.

**de·ox·y·ri·bo·nu·cle·o·pro·tein** (dē-oks'ē-rī-bō-noo'klē-ō-prō'tēn) the complex of DNA and protein in which DNA is usually found upon cell disruption and isolation.

**de·ox·y·ri·bo·nu·cle·o·side** (dē-oks'ē-rī-bō-noo'klē-ō-tīd) a nucleoside component of DNA containing 2-deoxy-D-ribose; the condensation product of deoxy-D-ribose with purines or pyrimidines.

**de·ox·y·ri·bo·nu·cle·o·tide** (dē-oks'ē-rī-bō-nū'klē-ō-tīd) a nucleotide component of DNA containing 2-deoxy-D-ribose; the phosphoric ester of deoxyribonucleoside; formed in nucleotide biosynthesis.

**de·ox·y·ri·bose** (dē-oks-ē-rī′bōs) a deoxypentose, 2-deoxy-D-ribose being the most common example, occurring in DNA and responsible for its name.

**de·ox·y·ribo·vi·rus** (dē-ok′sē-vī′rŭs) SYN DNA virus.

**de·ox·y sug·ar** a sugar containing fewer oxygen atoms than carbon atoms and in which, consequently, one or more carbons in the molecule lack an attached hydroxyl group.

**de·ox·y·thy·mi·dine (dT)** (dē-oks′ē-thī′mi-dēn) SYN thymidine.

**de·ox·y·thy·mi·dyl·ic ac·id (dTMP)** (dē-oks′ē-thī-mi-dil′ik as′id) a component of DNA; originally and properly called thymidylic acid, but use of deoxy- is less ambiguous, as ribothymidylic acid is now known to exist.

**de·pen·dence** (dē-pen′dens) the quality or condition of relying upon, being influenced by, or being subservient to a person or object reflecting a particular need. [L. *dependeo*, to hang from]

**de·pen·dent drain·age** drainage from the lowest part and into a receptacle at a level lower than the structure being drained.

**de·pen·dent e·de·ma** a clinically detectable increase in extracellular fluid volume localized in a dependent area, as of a limb, characterized by swelling or pitting.

**de·pen·dent per·son·al·i·ty** a personality disorder in which a person passively allows others to assume responsibility for making decisions.

**de·per·son·al·i·sa·tion [Br.]** SEE depersonalization.

**de·per·son·al·i·za·tion** (dē-per′sŏn-ăl-i-zā′shŭn) a state in which a person loses the feeling of his own identity in relation to others in his family or peer group, or loses the feeling of his own reality.

**de·phas·ing** (dē-fāz′ing) MAGNETIC RESONANCE the gradual loss of orientation of the magnetic atomic nuclei due to random molecular energy transfer or relaxation following alignment by a radiofrequency pulse.

**de·pig·men·ta·tion** (dē-pig-men-tā′shŭn) loss of pigment which may be partial or complete. SEE ALSO achromia (1).

**dep·i·late** (dep′i-lāt) to remove hair by any means. Cf. epilate. [L. *de-pilo*, pp. *-atus*, to deprive of hair, fr. *de-* neg. + *pilo*, to grow hair]

**dep·i·la·tion** (dep-i-lā′shŭn) SYN epilation.

**de·pil·a·to·ry** (dē-pil′ă-tō-rē) pertaining to removal of hair at the surface of the skin, as through shaving or the application of alkaline chemical hair removal products. 2. an agent having this action. Cf. epilatory.

**de·po·lar·i·za·tion** (dē-pō′lăr-i-zā′shŭn) the destruction, neutralization, or change in direction of polarity.

**de·po·lar·iz·ing block** skeletal muscle paralysis associated with loss of polarity of the motor end-plate, as occurs following administration of succinylcholine.

**de·pol·y·mer·ase** (dē-pol′i-mer-ās) an enzyme catalyzing the hydrolysis of a macromolecule to simpler components. SEE nuclease.

**de·pol·y·mer·i·sa·tion [Br.]** SEE depolymerization.

**de·po·lym·er·i·za·tion** (dē-po-lim′er-ĭ-zā′shŭn)

the dismantling of a polymer into individual monomers.

**de·pres·sant** (dē-pres′ănt) 1. diminishing functional tone or activity. 2. an agent that reduces nervous or functional activity, such as a sedative or anesthetic. [L. *de-primo*, pp. *-pressus*, to press down]

**de·pressed** (dē-prest′) 1. flattened from above downward. 2. below the normal level or the level of the surrounding parts. 3. below the normal functional level. 4. dejected; low in spirits.

**de·pressed skull frac·ture** a fracture with inward displacement of a part of the calvarium; may or may not be associated with disruption of the underlying dura or cerebral cortex.

**de·pres·sion** (dē-presh′ŭn) 1. reduction of the level of functioning. 2. a hollow or sunken area. 3. displacement of a part downward or inward. 4. a temporary mental state or chronic mental disorder characterized by feelings of sadness, loneliness, despair, low self-esteem, and self-reproach; accompanying signs include psychomotor retardation or less frequently agitation, withdrawal from social contact, and vegetative states such as loss of appetite and insomnia. SYN dejection (1). [L. *depressio*, fr. *deprimo*, to press down]

**de·pres·sor** (dē-pres′ŏr) 1. a muscle that flattens or lowers a part. 2. anything that depresses or retards functional activity. 3. an instrument or device used to push certain structures out of the way during an operation or examination. 4. an agent that decreases blood pressure. [L. *de-primo*, pp. *-pressus*, to press down]

**de·pres·sor an·gu·li o·ris mus·cle** *origin*, lower border of mandible anteriorly; *insertion*, blends with other muscles in lower lip near angle of mouth; *action*, pulls down corners of mouth; *nerve supply*, facial. SYN musculus depressor anguli oris [TA], triangular muscle (2).

**de·pres·sor fi·bers** sensory nerve fibers having pressure-sensitive endings; situated in the walls of certain arteries; capable of activating blood-pressure-lowering brainstem mechanisms when stimulated by an increase in intraarterial pressure.

**de·pres·sor la·bii in·fe·ri·o·ris mus·cle** *origin*, anterior portion of lower border of mandible; *insertion*, orbicularis oris musculus and skin of lower lip; *action*, depresses lower lip; *nerve supply*, facial. SYN musculus depressor labii inferioris [TA].

**de·pres·sor sep·ti mus·cle** a vertical fasciculus from the orbicularis oris musculus passing upward along the median line of the upper lip, and inserted into the cartilaginous septum of the nose; *action*, depresses septum; *nerve supply*, facial. SYN musculus depressor septi [TA].

**de·pres·sor su·per·ci·lii mus·cle** fibers of the orbital part of the orbicularis oculi musculus insert in the eyebrow; *action*, depresses eyebrow; *nerve supply*, facial. SYN musculus depressor supercilii [TA].

**dep·ri·va·tion** (dep′ri-vā′shŭn) absence, loss, or withholding of something needed.

**depth** distance from the surface downward.

**depth per·cep·tion** the visual ability to judge depth or distance.

**de Quer·vain dis·ease** (dĕ kār-vā′) fibrosis of the sheath of a tendon of the thumb.

**de Quer·vain tenosynovitis** (dĕ kār-vā′) inflammation of the tendons of the first dorsal compartment of the wrist, which includes the abductor pollicis longus and extensor pollicis brevis; diagnosed by a specific provocative test (Finkelstein test).

**de Quer·vain thy·roid·i·tis** (dĕ kār-vā′) SYN subacute granulomatous thyroiditis.

**de·range·ment** (dē-rānj′ment) **1.** a disturbance of the regular order or arrangement. **2.** rarely used term for a mental disturbance or disorder. [Fr.]

**de·re·al·i·za·tion** (dē-rē′ă-li-zā′shŭn) an alteration in one's perception of the environment such that things that are ordinarily familiar seem strange, unreal, or two-dimensional.

**de·re·ism** (dē′rē-izm) mental activity in fantasy in contrast to reality. [L. *de*, away, + *res*, thing]

**de·re·is·tic** (dē-rē-is′tik) living in imagination or fantasy with thoughts that are incongruent with logic or experience.

**der·en·ceph·a·ly** (dār-en-sef′ă-lē) cervical rachischisis and anencephaly, a malformation involving an open neurocranium with a rudimentary brain usually crowded back toward bifid cervical vertebrae. [G. *derē*, neck, + *enkephalos*, brain]

**de·re·pres·sion** (dē-rē-presh′ŭn) a homeostatic mechanism for regulating enzyme production in an inducible enzyme system: an inducer, usually a substrate of a specific enzyme pathway, by combining with an active repressor (produced by a regulator gene) deactivates it.

**der·i·va·tion** (dār-i-vā′shŭn) the source, origin, or evolutionary course of a structure or process. SYN revulsion (2). [L. *derivatio*, fr. *derivo*, pp. *-atus*, to draw off, fr. *rivus*, a stream]

**de·riv·a·tive** (dĕ-riv′ă-tiv) **1.** relating to or producing derivation. **2.** something produced by modification of something preexisting. **3.** specifically, a chemical compound produced from another compound in one or more steps, as in replacement of H by an alkyl, acyl, or amino group.

⟁**derm-, der·ma-** the skin; corresponds to the L. *cut-*. See entries under cut. [G. *derma*]

**der·ma·brad·er** (derm′ă-brād-er) a motor-driven device used in dermabrasion.

**der·ma·bra·sion** (der-mă-brā′zhŭn) operative procedure used to remove acne scars or pits performed with sandpaper, rotating wire brushes, or other abrasive materials. SYN planing.

**Der·ma·cen·tor** (der-mă-sen′ter) an ornate, characteristically marked genus of hard ticks (family Ixodidae) that possess eyes and 11 festoons; it consists of some 20 species whose members commonly attack dogs, humans, and other mammals. [derm- + G. *kentōr*, a goader]

**Der·ma·cen·tor an·der·so·ni** the wood tick; vector of Rocky Mountain spotted fever; also transmits tularemia and causes tick paralysis.

**Der·ma·cen·tor mar·gin·a·tus** a tick species found across Europe and the vector of a human rickettsiosis caused by *Rickettsia slovaca*.

**Der·ma·cen·tor va·ri·a·bi·lis** the American dog tick, a common pest of dogs along the eastern seaboard of the U.S., a vector of tularemia, and a principal vector of *Rickettsia rickettsii* which causes Rocky Mountain spotted fever in the central and eastern U.S.; may also cause tick paralysis.

**Der·ma·coc·cus** (der-ma-kok′us) a genus of Gram-positive, aerobic cocci found on human skin.

**der·mal** (der′măl) relating to the skin. SYN dermatic, dermatoid (2), dermic.

**der·mal graft** a graft of dermis, made from skin by cutting away a thin split-thickness graft.

**der·mal pa·pil·lae** SYN papilla of dermis.

**der·mal si·nus** a sinus lined with epidermis and skin appendages extending from the skin to some deeper-lying structure, most frequently the spinal cord.

⟁**dermat-** the skin. SEE ALSO derm-, dermato-, dermo-. [G. *derma*]

**der·mat·ic** (der-mat′ik) SYN dermal.

**der·ma·ti·tis**, pl. **der·ma·tit·i·des** (der-mă-tī′tis, der-mă-tit′i-dēz) inflammation of the skin. [derm- + G. *-itis*, inflammation]

**dermatitis-causing caterpillar** one of several species whose hairs can cause an allergic dermatitis; the saddleback caterpillar (*Sibine stimulea*) and the brown-tail moth (*Euproctis chrysorrhoea*) are common examples.

**der·ma·ti·tis ex·fo·li·a·ti·va in·fan·tum, der·ma·ti·tis ex·fo·li·a·ti·va ne·o·na·to·rum** a generalized pyoderma accompanied by exfoliative dermatitis, with constitutional symptoms, affecting young infants, which may result from atopic dermatitis, Leiner disease, or staphylococcal scalded skin syndrome. SYN impetigo neonatorum (1).

**der·ma·ti·tis gan·gre·no·sa in·fan·tum** a bullous or pustular eruption, of uncertain origin, followed by necrotic ulcers or extensive gangrene in children under 2 years of age; if untreated, death may result from hematogenous infection, such as liver abscess. SYN pemphigus gangrenosus (1).

⊞**der·ma·ti·tis her·pet·i·for·mis** a chronic disease of the skin marked by a symmetric itching eruption of vesicles and papules that occur in groups; relapses are common; associated with gluten-sensitive enteropathy and IgA immune complexes beneath the epidermis of lesioned and normal-appearing skin. See page B6. SYN Duhring disease.

**der·ma·ti·tis me·di·ca·men·to·sa** SYN drug eruption.

**der·ma·ti·tis pa·pil·la·ris ca·pil·li·tii** SYN acne keloid.

**der·ma·ti·tis re·pens** SYN pustulosis palmaris et plantaris. [L. creeping]

⟁**dermato-** SEE derm-. [G. *derma*, skin]

**der·mat·o·cha·la·sis** (der′mă-tō-kă-lā′sis) a congenital or acquired condition characterized by elastic fibers of the skin, which may hang in folds; vascular anomalies may be present; inheritance is either autosomal dominant or recessive, the latter sometimes in association with pulmonary emphysema and diverticula of the alimentary tract or bladder. The dominant form is caused by mutation in the elastin gene (ELN) on 7q. There is also an X-linked form that is due to mutation in the Menkes gene (MNK), encoding copper-transporting ATPase on Xq. [dermato- + G. *chalasis*, a loosening]

**der·mat·o·fi·bro·ma** (der′mă-tō-fī-brō′mă) a slowly growing benign skin nodule consisting of poorly demarcated cellular fibrous tissue enclosing collapsed capillaries, with scattered hemosiderin-pigmented and lipid macrophages. The following terms are considered by some to be synonymous with, and by others to be varieties of, dermatofibroma: sclerosing hemangioma, fibrous histiocytoma, nodular subepidermal fibrosis.

d
e

**der·mat·o·glyph·ics** (der′mă-tō-glif′iks) **1.** the configurations of the characteristic ridge patterns of the volar surfaces of the skin; in the human hand, the distal segment of each digit has three types of configurations: whorl, loop, and arch. SEE ALSO fingerprint. **2.** the science or study of these configurations or patterns. [dermato- + *glyphē,* carved work]

**der·ma·tog·ra·phism** (der-mă-tog′ră-fizm) a form of urticaria in which whealing occurs in the site and in the configuration of application of stroking (pressure, friction) of the skin. SYN dermography, dermographism, dermography. [dermato- + G. *graphō,* to write]

**der·ma·toid** (der′mă-toyd) **1.** resembling skin. SYN dermoid (1). **2.** SYN dermal.

**der·ma·tol·o·gist** (der-mă-tol′ō-jist) a physician who specializes in the diagnosis and treatment of cutaneous diseases and related systemic diseases.

**der·ma·tol·o·gy** (der-mă-tol′ō-jē) the branch of medicine concerned with the study of the skin, diseases of the skin, and the relationship of cutaneous lesions to systemic disease. [dermato- + G. *logos,* study]

**der·ma·tol·y·sis** (der-mă-tol′i-sis) loosening of the skin or atrophy of the skin by disease; erroneously used as a synonym for cutis laxa. [dermato- + G. *lysis,* a loosening]

**der·ma·to·ma** (der-mă-tō′mă) a circumscribed thickening or hypertrophy of the skin. [dermato- + G. *-oma,* tumor]

**🔲 der·ma·tome** (der′mă-tōm) **1.** an instrument for cutting thin slices of skin for grafting, or excising small lesions. **2.** the dorsolateral part of an embryonic somite. SYN cutis plate. **3.** the area of skin supplied by cutaneous branches from a single spinal nerve; neighboring dermatome may overlap. See this page. [dermato- + G. *tomē,* a cutting]

**der·mat·o·meg·a·ly** (der′mă-tō-meg′ă-lē) congenital or acquired defect in which the skin hangs in folds. [dermato- + G. *megas,* large]

**der·mat·o·mere** (der′mă-tō-mēr) a metameric area of the embryonic integument. [dermato- + G. *meros,* part]

**der·mat·o·my·co·sis** (der′mă-tō-mī-kō′sis) fungus infection of the skin caused by dermatophytes, yeasts, and other fungi. Cf. dermatophytosis.

**der·mat·o·my·o·ma** (der′mă-tō-mī-ō′mă) SYN leiomyoma cutis. [dermato- + G. *mys,* muscle, + *-oma,* tumor]

**🔲 der·mat·o·my·o·si·tis** (der′mă-tō-mī-ō-sī′tis) a progressive condition characterized by symmetric proximal muscular weakness with elevated muscle enzyme levels and a skin rash, typically a purplish-red or heliotrope erythema on the face, and edema of the eyelids and periorbital tissue; affected muscle tissue shows degeneration of fibers with a chronic inflammatory reaction; occurs in children and adults, and in the latter may be associated with visceral cancer. See page B4. [dermato- + G. *mys,* muscle, + *-itis,* inflammation]

**der·mat·o·neu·ro·sis** (der′mă-tō-noo-ro′sis) any cutaneous eruption due to emotional stimuli.

**der·mat·o·pa·thol·o·gy** (der′mă-tō-pa-thol′ō-jē) histopathology of the skin and subcutis, and study of the causes of skin disease.

**der·ma·top·a·thy** (der′mă-top′ă-thē) any disease

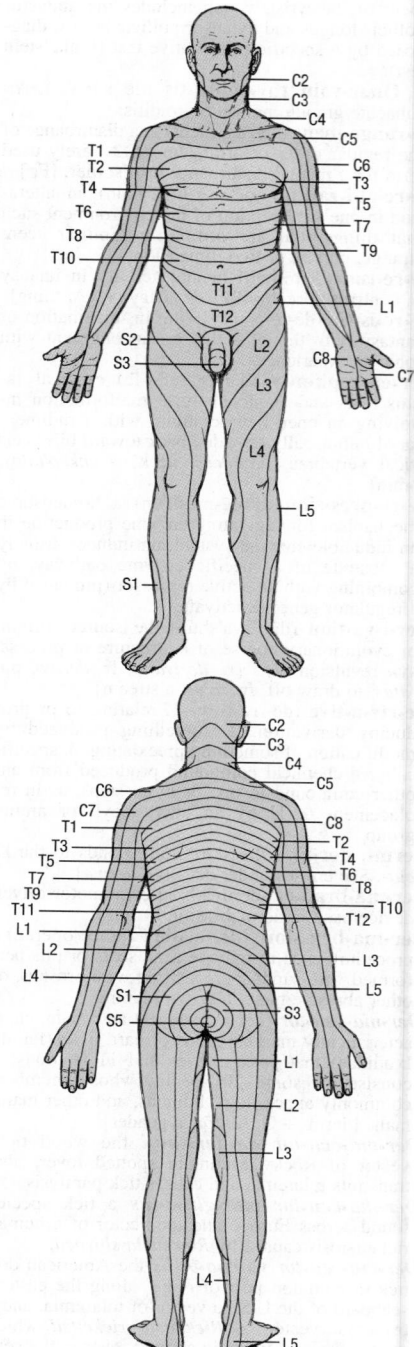

**dermatomes:** areas of skin supplied by cutaneous branches of spinal nerves

of the skin. SYN dermopathy. [dermato- + G. *pathos*, suffering]

**Der·ma·toph·a·goi·des pter·o·nys·si·nus** (der-mă-tof-ă-goy′dēz ter-ō-ni-sī′nŭs) a species of mites found in house dust and a common cause of atopic asthma. [dermato- + G. *phagō*, to eat; ptero- + G. *nyssō*, to prick, stab]

**der·mat·o·phy·lax·is** (der′mă-tō-fī-lak′sis) protection of the skin against potentially harmful agents; e.g., infection, excessive sunlight, noxious agents. [dermato- + G. *phylaxis*, protection]

**der·mat·o·phyte** (der′mă-tō-fīt) a fungus that causes superficial infections of the skin, hair, and/or nails, i.e., keratinized tissues. Species of *Epidermophyton*, *Microsporum*, and *Trichophyton* are regarded as dermatophytes, but causative agents of tinea versicolor, tinea nigra, and cutaneous candidiasis are not so classified. [dermato- + G. *phyton*, plant]

**der·mat·o·phy·tid** (der-mă-tof′i-tid) an allergic manifestation of dermatophytosis at a site distant from that of the primary fungous infection. The lesions, usually small vesicles on the hands and/or arms, are devoid of the fungus and may become extensive, covering wide areas of the body and causing extreme discomfort to the patient. SEE ALSO -id (1), id reaction.

**der·mat·o·phy·to·sis** (der′mă-tō-fī-tō′sis) an infection of the hair, skin, or nails caused by any one of the dermatophytes. The lesions are characterized by erythema, small papular vesicles, fissures, and scaling. Common sites of infection are the feet (tinea pedis), nails (onychomycosis), and scalp (tinea capitis). Cf. dermatomycosis.

**der·mat·o·plas·ty** (der′ma-tō-plas-tē) plastic surgery of the skin, as by skin grafting. SYN dermoplasty. [dermato- + G. *plastos*, formed]

**der·mat·o·pol·y·neu·ri·tis** (der′mă-tō-pol′ē-noo-rī′tis) SYN acrodynia (2).

**der·mat·o·scle·ro·sis** (der′mă-tō-skler-ō′sis) SYN scleroderma. [dermato- + G. *sklēroō*, to harden]

**der·ma·to·sis**, pl. **der·ma·to·ses** (der-mă-tō′sis, der-mă-tō′-sēz) nonspecific term used to denote any cutaneous abnormality or eruption. [dermato- + G. *-osis*, condition]

**der·ma·to·sis me·di·ca·men·to·sa** SYN drug eruption.

**der·mat·o·ther·a·py** (der′mă-tō-thār′ă-pē) treatment of skin diseases.

**der·mat·o·tro·pic** (der′mă-tō-trop′ik) having an affinity for the skin. SYN dermotropic. [dermato- + G. *trōpe*, a turning]

**der·mic** (der′mik) SYN dermal.

**der·mis** (der′mis) a layer of skin composed of a superficial thin layer that interdigitates with the epidermis, the stratum papillare, and the stratum reticulare; it contains blood and lymphatic vessels, nerves and nerve endings, glands, and, except for glabrous skin, hair follicles. SYN corium, cutis vera. [G. *derma*, skin]

**der·mo-** SEE derm-. [G. *derma*, skin]

**Der·mo·bac·ter** (der-mō-bak′ter) a bacterial genus of nonmotile, non–spore-bearing Gram-positive rods, recovered from human skin. *Dermobacter hominis* has been found in blood cultures.

**der·mo·blast** (der′mō-blast) one of the mesodermal cells from which the corium is developed. [dermo- + G. *blastos*, germ]

**der·mo·graph·ia, der·mog·ra·phism, der·-**

**mog·ra·phy** (der-mō-graf′ē-ă, der-mog′ră-fizm, der-mog′ră-fē) SYN dermatographism.

**der·mo·haem·al [Br.]** possessing both dermal and haemal structures, as in certain fishes.

**der·moid** (der′moyd) **1.** SYN dermatoid (1). **2.** SYN dermoid cyst. [dermo- + G. *eidos*, resemblance]

**der·moid cyst** a tumor consisting of displaced ectodermal structures along lines of embryonic fusion, the wall being formed of epithelium-lined connective tissue, including skin appendages and containing keratin, sebum, and hair. SYN dermoid tumor, dermoid (2).

**der·moid tu·mor** SYN dermoid cyst.

**der·mop·a·thy** (der-mop′ă-thē) SYN dermatopathy.

**der·mo·plas·ty** (der′mō-plas-tē) SYN dermatoplasty.

**der·mo·tro·p·ic** (der-mō-trop′ik) SYN dermatotropic.

**der·mo·vas·cu·lar** (der-mō-vas′kyu-lăr) pertaining to the blood vessels of the skin. [dermo- + L. *vasculum*, small vessel]

**de·ro·ta·tion** (dē-rō-tā′shŭn) **1.** a turning back. **2.** ORTHOPEDICS the correction of a rotation deformity by turning or rotating the deformed structure toward a normal position. [L. *de*, away, + *rotatio*, turning]

**DES** diethylstilbestrol.

**des-** CHEMISTRY a prefix indicating absence of some component of the principal part of the name; largely replaced by de- (e.g., deoxyribonucleic acid, dehydro-).

**de·sat·u·ra·tion** (dē′sat-yu-rā′shŭn) the act, or the result of the act, of making something less completely saturated; more specifically, the percentage of total binding sites remaining unfilled, e.g., when hemoglobin is 70% saturated with oxygen and nothing else, its desaturation is 30%. Cf. saturation (5).

**De·sault ban·dage** (dĕ-sō′) a bandage for fracture of the clavicle; the elbow is bound to the side, with a pad placed in the axilla.

**Des·cartes law** (dā-kahrt′) SYN law of refraction.

**des·ce·me·ti·tis** (des′ĕ-mĕ-tī′tis) inflammation of Descemet membrane.

**Des·ce·met mem·brane** (des-ĕ-mā) SYN posterior elastic lamina of cornea.

**des·ce·met·o·cele** (des-ĕ-met′ō-sēl) a bulging forward of Descemet membrane caused by the destruction of the substance of the cornea by infection.

**des·cend·ing co·lon** the part of the colon extending from the left colic flexure to the pelvic brim.

**des·cend·ing de·gen·er·a·tion 1.** orthograde (wallerian) degeneration of an injured nerve fiber; i.e., distal to the lesion; **2.** degeneration caudal to the level of a spinal cord lesion.

**des·cend·ing ge·nic·u·lar ar·tery** *origin*, femoral, in adductor canal; *distribution*, penetrates vasoadductor fascia to supply knee joint and adjacent parts; *anastomoses*, medial superior genicular, medial inferior genicular, lateral superior genicular, lateral inferior genicular and anterior tibial recurrent arteries, i.e., articular network of knee. SYN arteria descendens genus [TA].

**de·scen·sus** (dē-sen′sŭs) descent of the testis from the abdomen into the scrotum during the seventh and eighth months of intrauterine life. SEE ALSO ptosis, procidentia. SYN descent (1). [L.]

**de·scen·sus tes·tis** [TA] descent of the testis from the abdomen into the scrotum during the seventh and eighth months of intrauterine life.

**de·scent** (dē-sent′) **1.** SYN descensus. **2.** OBSTETRICS the passage of the presenting part of the fetus into and through the birth canal. [L. descensus]

**DES daughter** the daughter of a woman who received diethylstilbestrol during pregnancy; DES daughters are at risk of deformity, adenosis, and other epithelial changes of the vagina and cervix, including clear cell adenocarcinoma.

**de·sen·si·ti·sa·tion [Br.]** SEE desensitization.

**de·sen·si·tiz·a·tion** (dē-sen′si-ti-zā′shŭn) **1.** the reduction or abolition of allergic sensitivity or reactions to the specific antigen (allergen). SYN antianaphylaxis. **2.** the act of removing an emotional complex.

**de·sen·si·tize** (dē-sen′si-tīz) **1.** to reduce or remove any form of sensitivity. **2.** to effect desensitization (1). **3.** DENTISTRY to eliminate or subdue the painful response of exposed, vital dentin to irritative agents or thermal changes.

**des·e·tope** (dē′se-tōp) that part of the Class II major histocompatibility molecule that interacts with the antigen. [*de*terminant *se*lection + -tope]

**des·flu·rane** (des′floor′ān) an inhalation anesthetic with physical characteristics that provide rapid induction of and recovery from anesthesia.

**des·ic·cant** (des′i-kant) **1.** drying; causing or promoting dryness. SYN desiccative. **2.** an agent that absorbs moisture; a drying agent. SYN exsiccant. [L. *de-sicco,* pp. *-siccatus,* to dry up]

**des·ic·cate** (des′i-kāt) to dry thoroughly; to render free from moisture. SYN exsiccate.

**des·ic·ca·tion** (des-i-kā′shŭn) the process of being desiccated. SYN dehydration (4), exsiccation (1).

**des·ic·ca·tive** (des-i-kā′tiv) SYN desiccant (1).

**de·sig·na·tion** a legal process by which a hospital is formally designated to provide a specialized service. Usually requires meeting set standards and an external review, e.g., trauma center.

**Des·mar·res re·trac·tor** (dah-măr′ah) an instrument used to withdraw an eyelid.

**des·min** (dez′minz) any of various proteins found in intermediate filaments that copolymerize with vimentin to form constituents of connective tissue, cell walls, and filaments. Found in Z disk of skeletal and cardiac muscle cells.

**des·mi·tis** (dez-mī′tis) inflammation of a ligament. [desm- + G. *-itis,* inflammation]

⚠ **des·mo-, desm-** fibrous connection; ligament. [G. *desmos,* a band]

**des·mo·cra·ni·um** (dez-mō-krā′nē-ŭm) the mesenchymal primordium of the cranium.

**des·mo·den·ti·um, des·mo·don·ti·um** the collagen fibers, running from the cementum to the alveolar bone, that suspend a tooth in its socket; they include apical, oblique, horizontal, and alveolar crest fibers, indicating that the orientation of the fibers varies at different levels.

**des·mog·e·nous** (dez-moj′ĕ-nŭs) of connective tissue or ligamentous origin or causation; e.g., denoting a deformity due to contraction of ligaments, fascia, or a scar. [desmo- + G. *-gen,* producing]

**des·moid** (dez′moyd) **1.** fibrous or ligamentous. **2.** a nodule or mass of firm scarlike connective tissue resulting from active proliferation of fibroblasts, occurring most frequently in the abdominal muscles of women who have borne children. SYN desmoid tumor. [desmo- + G. *eidos,* appearance, form]

**des·moid tu·mor** SYN desmoid (2).

**des·mo·las·es** (dez′mō-lā′sez) enzymes catalyzing reactions other than those involving hydrolysis; e.g., those involving oxidation and reduction, isomerization, the breaking of carbon-carbon bonds.

**des·mop·a·thy** (dez-mop′ă-thē) any disease of the ligaments. [desmo- + G. *pathos,* suffering]

**des·mo·pla·sia** (dez-mō-plā′zē-ă) hyperplasia of fibroblasts and disproportionate formation of fibrous connective tissue, especially in the stroma of a carcinoma. [desmo- + G. *plasis,* a molding]

**des·mo·plas·tic** (des-mō-plas′tik) **1.** causing or forming adhesions. **2.** causing fibrosis in the vascular stroma of a neoplasm.

**des·mo·plas·tic fi·bro·ma** a benign fibrous tumor of bone affecting children and young adults; cortical destruction may result.

**des·mo·plas·tic small cell tu·mor** a high-grade malignant tumor found most often in the abdomen of adolescent males; typically tumor cells contain both desmin and keratin, i.e., show hybrid features like fetal mesothelial cells; the exact nature of these cells remains unknown.

**des·mo·plas·tic trich·o·ep·i·the·li·o·ma** a solitary, hard, annular, centrally depressed papule, occurring usually in women on the face, consisting of dermal strands of basaloid cells and small keratinous cysts within sclerotic desmoplastic stroma.

**des·mo·pres·sin** (des-mō-pres′in) an analog of vasopressin (antidiuretic hormone, ADH) possessing powerful antidiuretic activity.

**des·mo·some** (dez′mō-sōm) a site of adhesion between two epithelial cells, consisting of a dense attachment plaque separated from a similar structure in the other cell by a thin layer of extracellular material. SYN macula adherens. [desmo- + G. *sōma,* body]

**de·spe·ci·a·tion** (dē-spē′shē-ā′shŭn) **1.** alteration or loss of species characteristics. **2.** removal of species-specific antigenic properties from a foreign protein.

**des·qua·ma·tion** (des-kwă-mā′shŭn) the shedding of the cuticle in scales or of the outer layer of any surface.

**des·qua·ma·tive** (des-kwam′ă-tiv) relating to or marked by desquamation.

**de·sulf·hy·dras·es** (dē′sulf-hī′drā-sez) enzymes or groups of enzymes catalyzing the removal of a molecule of $H_2S$ or substituted $H_2S$ from a compound, as in the conversion of cysteine to pyruvic acid by cysteine desulfhydrase (cystathionine γ-lyase).

**de·sul·phur·i·sa·tion [Br.]** SEE desulphurization.

**de·sul·phur·i·za·tion** (dē-sul′fer-ĭ-zā-shŭn) the process of removing sulphur from a molecule.

**de·tach·ment** (dē-tach′ment) **1.** a voluntary or involuntary feeling or emotion that accompanies a sense of separation from normal associations or environment. **2.** separation of a structure from its support.

**de·tailed phy·si·cal ex·am·i·na·tion** a head-to-toe patient assessment that follows the focused history and physical exam and is more thorough than the rapid trauma assessment or rapid medical assessment.

**de·tec·tor** (dē-tek′ter) the component of a laboratory instrument which detects the chemical or physical signal indicating the presence or quantity of the substance of interest.

**de·tec·tor coil** a coil used in magnetic resonance imaging as an antenna to record radiofrequency emissions of stimulated nuclei, e.g., body coil, head coil.

**de·ter·gent** (dē-ter′jent) **1.** cleansing. **2.** a cleansing or purging agent, usually salts of long-chain aliphatic bases or acids which, through a surface action that depends on their possessing both hydrophilic and hydrophobic properties, exert cleansing (oil-dissolving) and antibacterial effects. [L. *de-tergeo,* pp. *-tersus,* to wipe off]

**de·te·ri·o·ra·tion** (dē-tēr′i-ō-rā′shŭn) the process or condition of becoming worse. [L. *deterior,* worse]

**de·ter·mi·nant** (dē-ter′mi-nănt) the factor that contributes to the generation of a trait. [L. *determans,* determining, limiting]

**de·ter·mi·na·tion** (dē-ter-mi-nā′shŭn) **1.** a change, for the better or for the worse, in the course of a disease. **2.** a general move toward a given point. **3.** the measurement or estimation of any quantity or quality in scientific or laboratory investigation. **4.** discernment of a state or category (e.g., in diagnosis). **5.** a process, both necessary and sufficient, whereby an effect is caused. [L. *de-termino,* pp. *-atus,* to limit, determine, fr. *terminus,* a boundary]

**de·ter·mi·nism** (dē-ter′mi-nizm) the proposition that all behavior is caused exclusively by genetic and environmental influences with no random components, and independent of free will. [L. *determino,* to limit, fr. *terminus,* boundary + -ism]

**de·tox·i·cate, de·tox·i·fy** (dē-tok′si-kāt, dē-tok′si-fī) to diminish or remove the poisonous quality of any substance; to lessen the virulence of any pathogenic organism. [L. *de,* from, + *toxicum,* poison]

**de·tox·i·ca·tion** (dē-tok-si-kā′shŭn) **1.** recovery from the toxic effects of a drug. **2.** removal of the toxic properties from a poison. **3.** metabolic conversion of pharmacologically active principles to pharmacologically less active principles. SYN detoxification.

**de·tox·i·fi·ca·tion** (dē-tok′si-fi-kā′shŭn) SYN detoxication.

**de·train·ing** SYN reversal.

**de·tri·tion** (dē-trish′ŭn) a wearing away by use or friction. [L. *de-tero,* pp. *-tritus,* to rub off]

**de·tri·tus** (dē-trī′tŭs) any broken-down material, carious or gangrenous matter, gravel, etc. [L. (see detrition)]

**de·tru·sor** (dē-troo′ser) a muscle that has the action of expelling a substance. [L. *detrudo,* to drive away]

**de·tru·sor·rha·phy** (dē-troo′-sor-a-fē) a procedure in which bladder muscle (detrusor) is reconstructed around the ureterovesical junction to form a competent one-way valve. SEE ALSO ureteroneocystostomy. SYN extravesical reimplantation. [detrusor + G. *rhaphē,* a seam]

**de·tu·mes·cence** (dē-too-mes′ens) subsidence of a swelling. [L. *de,* from, + *tumesco,* to swell up, fr. *tumeo,* to swell]

**deu·ter·an·o·pia** (doo′ter-ă-nō′pē-ă) a congenital abnormality of the retina in which there are two rather than three retinal cone pigments (dichromatism) and complete insensitivity to middle wavelengths (green). [G. *deuteros,* second, + anopia]

⚠**deu·ter·io-** prefix indicating "containing deuterium."

**deu·te·ri·um** (doo-tēr′ē-ŭm) SYN hydrogen-2. [G. *deuteros,* second]

⚠**deu·tero-, deut-, deu·to-** two, or second (in a series); secondary. [G. *deuteros,* second]

**deu·ter·o·my·ce·tes** (doo′ter-ō-mī-sē′tēz) members of the class Deuteromycetes or the phylum Deuteromycota.

**deu·ter·o·path·ic** (doo′ter-ō-path′ik) relating to a deuteropathy.

**deu·ter·op·a·thy** (doo-ter-op′ă-thē) a secondary disease or symptom. [deutero- + G. *pathos,* suffering]

**deu·ter·o·plasm** (doo′ter-ō-plazm) SYN deutoplasm. [deutero- + G. *plasma,* thing formed]

**deu·to·nymph** (doo′to-nimf) the third stage of a mite.

**deu·to·plasm** (doo′tō-plazm) the yolk of a meroblastic egg; the nonliving material in the cytoplasm, especially that stored in the oocyte as food for the developing embryo, the commonest types being lipoid droplets and yolk granules. SYN deuteroplasm. [deuto- + G. *plasma,* thing formed]

**de·vas·cu·lar·i·za·tion** (dē-vas′kyu-lăr-i-zā′shŭn) occlusion of all or most of the blood vessels to any part or organ. [L. *de,* away, + *vasculum,* small vessel, + G. *izo,* to cause]

**de·vel·op·er** (dē-vel′ŏp-er) **1.** an individual or procedure that develops. **2.** SYN eluent. **3.** the chemicals used to develop film by reducing the light-activated silver halide molecules to atomic silver.

**de·vel·op·ment** (dē-vel′ŏp-ment) **1.** the act or process of natural progression in physical and psychological maturation from a previous, lower, or embryonic stage to a later, more complex, or adult stage. **2.** the process of chromatography.

**de·vel·op·men·tal age (DA) 1.** age estimated by anatomic development since fertilization; **2.** age of an individual estimated from the degree of anatomic, physiologic, mental, and emotional maturation.

**de·vel·op·men·tal a·nat·o·my** anatomy of the structural changes of an individual from fertilization to adulthood; includes embryology, fetology, and postnatal development.

**de·vel·op·men·tal a·nom·a·ly** an anomaly established during intrauterine life; a congenital anomaly.

**de·vel·op·men·tal a·prax·ia of speech (DAS)** severe articulatory disturbance in childhood characterized by multiple and inconsistent errors in production of voluntary sequences of phonemes, but not due to weakness or spasticity of speech musculature (i.e., not dysarthria). SYN childhood apraxia, developmental dyspraxia of speech.

**de·vel·op·men·tal dis·a·bil·i·ty** loss of function brought on by prenatal and postnatal events in which the predominant disturbance is in the acquisition of cognitive, language, motor, or social skills; e.g., mental retardation, autistic disorder, learning disorder, and attention-deficit hyperactivity disorder.

**de·vel·op·men·tal dys·prax·ia of speech** SYN developmental apraxia of speech.

**de·vel·op·men·tal grooves** fine lines found in

the enamel of a tooth that mark the junction of the lobes of the crown in its development. SYN developmental lines.

**de·vel·op·men·tal hip dys·pla·sia** SYN congenital hip dysplasia.

**de·vel·op·men·tal lines** SYN developmental grooves.

🔲 **de·vel·op·men·tal mile·stones** a stage in the neuromuscular, mental, or social maturation of an infant or young child, generally marked by the attainment of a capacity or skill, such as rolling over, sitting with good head control, smiling spontaneously, laughing, and following moving objects with the eyes; all of these occur by the age of 2–4 months in the normal infant. See this page.

**de·vel·op·men·tal psy·chol·o·gy** the study of the psychological, physiological, and behavioral changes in an organism that occur from birth to old age.

**De·ven·ter pel·vis** (dā′věn-těr) a pelvis with shortened anteroposterior diameter.

**de·vi·ance** (dē′vē-ans) SYN deviation (3).

**de·vi·ant** (dē′vē-ant) **1.** denoting or indicative of deviation. **2.** an individual exhibiting deviation, especially sexual.

**de·vi·a·tion** (dē-vē-ā′shŭn) **1.** a turning away or aside from the normal point or course. **2.** an abnormality. **3.** PSYCHIATRY, BEHAVIORAL SCIENCES a departure from an accepted norm, role, or rule. SYN deviance. **4.** a statistical measure representing the difference between an individual value in a set of values and the mean value in that set. [L. *devio*, to turn from the straight path, fr. *de*, from, + *via*, way]

**De·vic dis·ease** (dě-vēk′) SYN neuromyelitis optica.

**de·vice** (dē-vīs′) an appliance, usually mechanical, designed to perform a specific function, such as prosthesis or orthesis. [M.E., fr. O. Fr. *devis*, fr. L. *divisum*, divided]

**dev·il's grip** SYN epidemic pleurodynia.

**de·vi·om·e·ter** (dē-vē-om′ě-ter) a form of strabismometer.

**de·vi·tal·ized** (dē-vī′tăl-īzd) devoid of life; dead.

**de Weck·er scis·sors** (dě wek-ěr) a small scissors with sharp points for intraocular cutting of the iris and lens capsule.

**dex·ter** (deks′ter) located on or relating to the right side. [L. fr. *dextra*, neut. *dextrum*]

**dex·trad** (deks′trad) toward the right side. [L. *dexter*, right, + *ad*, to]

**dex·tral** (deks′trăl) SYN right-handed.

**dex·tral·i·ty** (deks-tral′i-tē) right-handedness; preference for the right hand in performing manual tasks.

**dex·tran·ase** (deks′tran-ās) an enzyme hydrolyzing 1,6-α-D-glucosidic linkages in dextran; used in the prevention of caries.

**dex·trase** (deks′trās) nonspecific term for the complex of enzymes that converts dextrose (D-glucose) into lactic acid.

**dex·tri·nase** (deks′tri-nās) any of the enzymes catalyzing the hydrolysis of dextrins; e.g., amylo-1,6-glucosidase, dextrin dextranase.

**dex·trin dex·tran·ase** (deks′trin deks′tran-āz) a glucosyltransferase transferring 1,4-α-D-glucosyl residues, thus catalyzing the synthesis of dextrans from dextrins by glucose transfer.

**α-dex·trin en·do-1,6-α-glu·co·si·dase** an enzyme with action similar to that of isoamylase; it

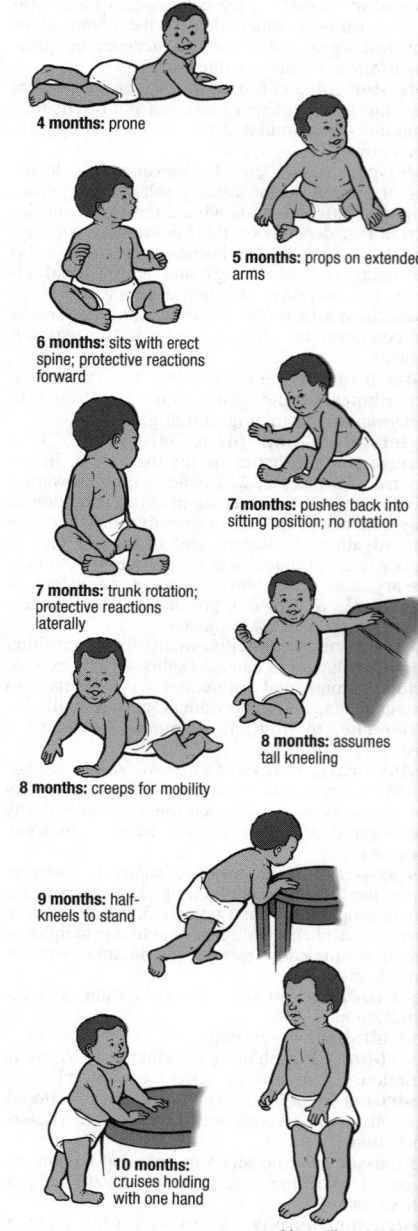

**4 months:** prone

**5 months:** props on extended arms

**6 months:** sits with erect spine; protective reactions forward

**7 months:** pushes back into sitting position; no rotation

**7 months:** trunk rotation; protective reactions laterally

**8 months:** assumes tall kneeling

**8 months:** creeps for mobility

**9 months:** half-kneels to stand

**10 months:** cruises holding with one hand

**11 months:** stands

**developmental milestones**

cleaves 1,6-α-glucosidic linkages in pullalan, amylopectin, and glycogen, and in α- and β-amylase limit-dextrins of amylopectin and glycogen. Cf. isoamylase.

**dex·tri·no·sis** (deks-trin-ō′sis) SYN glycogenosis.

**dex·tri·nu·ria** (deks-tri-nyu′rē-ă) the passage of dextrin in the urine.

**dextro-, dextr-** **1.** right, toward, or on the right side. **2.** dextrorotatory. [L. *dexter*, on the right-hand side]

**dex·tro·am·phet·a·mine sul·fate** (deks'trō-am-fet'ă-mēn sul'fāt) (+)-α-methylphenethylamine sulfate; similar in action to racemic amphetamine sulfate, but more stimulating to the central nervous system; sympathomimetic and appetite depressant.

**dex·tro·car·dia** (deks'trō-kar'dē-ă) displacement of the heart to the right, either as dextroposition, with simple displacement to the right, or as cardiac heterotaxia, with complete transposition of the right and left chambers, resulting in a heart that is the mirror image of a normal heart. [dextro- + G. *kardia*, heart]

**dex·tro·car·dia with si·tus in·ver·sus** displacement of the heart to the right side of the thorax with mirror transposition of the cardiac chambers together with transposition of the abdominal viscera.

**dex·tro·gas·tria** (deks-trō-gas'trē-ă) condition in which the stomach is displaced to the right; may represent either simple displacement or situs inversus. Usually associated with dextrocardia. [dextro- + G. *gastēr*, stomach]

**dex·tro·gy·ra·tion** (deks'trō-jī-rā'shŭn) a twisting to the right. [dextro- + L. *gyro*, pp. *-atus*, to turn in a circle, fr. *gyrus*, circle]

**dex·tro·e·dal** (deks-trop'ĕ-dăl) denoting one who uses the right leg in preference to the left. SYN right-footed. [dextro- + L. *pes* (*ped*-), foot]

**dex·tro·po·si·tion** (deks'trō-pō-zi'shŭn) abnormal right-sided location or origin of a normally left-sided structure, e.g., origin of the aorta from the right ventricle.

**dex·tro·po·si·tion of the heart** SEE dextrocardia.

**dex·tro·ro·ta·to·ry** (deks-trō-rō'tă-tōr-ē) denoting dextrorotation, or certain crystals or solutions capable of such action; as a chemical prefix, usually abbreviated *d*-. Cf. levorotatory.

**dex·trose** (deks'trōs) SEE glucose.

**dex·tro·si·nis·tral** (deks'trō-si-nis'trăl) in a direction from right to left. [dextro- + L. *sinister*, left]

**dex·tro·tor·sion** (deks-trō-tōr'shŭn) **1.** a twisting to the right. **2.** OPHTHALMOLOGY a conjugate rotation of the upper pole of both corneas to the right. [dextro- + L. *torsio*, a twisting]

**dex·tro·tro·p·ic** (dek-trō-trop'ik) turning to the right. [dextro- + G. *tropos*, a turn]

**dex·tro·ver·sion** (deks'trō-ver'zhŭn) **1.** version toward the right. **2.** in ophthalmology, a conjugate rotation of both eyes to the right. [dextro- + L. *verto*, pp. *versus*, to turn]

**df, DF** decayed and/or filled teeth.

**dGMP** deoxyguanylic acid.

**DHEA** dehydroepiandrosterone.

**DHEAS** abbreviation for the sulfate salt of dehydroepiandrosterone.

**di-** **1.** two, twice. **2.** CHEMISTRY often used in place of bis- when not likely to be confusing; e.g., dichloro- compounds. Cf. bi-, bis-. [G. *dis*, two]

**di·a-** through, throughout, completely. [G. *dia*, through]

**di·a·be·tes** (dī-ă-bē'tēz) either diabetes insipidus or diabetes mellitus, diseases having in common the symptom polyuria; when used without qualification, refers to diabetes mellitus. [G. *diabētēs*, a compass, a siphon, diabetes]

**di·a·be·tes in·sip·i·dus** chronic excretion of very large amounts of pale urine of low specific gravity, causing dehydration and extreme thirst; ordinarily results from inadequate output of pituitary antidiuretic hormone. SEE ALSO nephrogenic diabetes insipidus.

**di·a·be·tes in·ter·mit·tens** diabetes mellitus in which there are periods of relatively normal carbohydrate metabolism followed by relapses to the previous diabetic state.

**di·a·be·tes mel·li·tus (DM)** a metabolic disease in which carbohydrate utilization is reduced and that of lipid and protein enhanced; it is caused by an absolute or relative deficiency of insulin and is characterized, in more severe cases, by chronic hyperglycemia, glycosuria, water and electrolyte loss, ketoacidosis, and coma; long-term complications include development of neuropathy, retinopathy, nephropathy, generalized degenerative changes in large and small blood vessels, and increased susceptibility to infection. SEE ALSO insulin-dependent diabetes mellitus, non-insulin-dependent diabetes mellitus. [L. sweetened with honey]

**di·a·bet·ic** (dī-ă-bet'ik) **1.** relating to or suffering from diabetes. **2.** one who suffers from diabetes.

**di·a·bet·ic ac·i·do·sis** decreased pH and bicarbonate concentration in the body fluids caused by accumulation of ketone bodies in diabetes mellitus.

**di·a·bet·ic a·my·ot·ro·phy** a type of diabetic neuropathy that primarily affects elderly patients with diabetes mellitus; clinically characterized by unilateral or bilateral anterior thigh pain, weakness, and atrophy; one type of diabetic polyradiculopathy. Sometimes referred to, erroneously, as diabetic femoral neuropathy.

**di·a·bet·ic co·ma** coma that develops in severe and inadequately treated diabetes mellitus and is commonly fatal, unless appropriate therapy is instituted promptly; results from reduced oxidative metabolism of the central nervous system that, in turn, stems from severe ketoacidosis and possibly also from the histotoxic action of the ketone bodies and disturbances in water and electrolyte balance.

**di·a·bet·ic der·mop·a·thy** small macules and papules of the extensor surfaces of the extremities, most commonly the shins of diabetics, which become atrophic, hyperpigmented, and occasionally undergo ulceration with scarring; may be a manifestation of microangiopathy.

**di·a·bet·ic di·et** a dietary adjustment for patients with diabetes mellitus intended to decrease the need for insulin or oral diabetic agents and control weight by adjusting caloric and carbohydrate intake.

**di·a·bet·ic glo·mer·u·lo·scle·ro·sis** rounded hyaline or laminated nodules in the periphery of the glomeruli with capillary basement membrane thickening and increased mesangial matrix occurring in long-standing diabetes, proteinuria, and ultimately renal failure. SYN intercapillary glomerulosclerosis.

**di·a·bet·ic neph·ro·pa·thy** a syndrome occurring in people with diabetes mellitus and characterized by albuminuria, hypertension, and progressive renal insufficiency.

**di·a·bet·ic neu·rop·a·thy** a generic term for any diabetes mellitus-related disorder of the peripheral nervous system, autonomic nervous system, and some cranial nerves. This most commonly occurring of the chronic complications of diabetes takes two forms, peripheral (with dulling of the sensations of pain, temperature, and pressure, especially in the lower legs and feet), and autonomic (with alternating bouts of diarrhea and constipation, impotence, and reduced cardiac function).

**🔲 di•a•bet•ic ret•i•nop•a•thy** retinal changes occurring in diabetes of long duration, marked by hemorrhages, microaneurysms, and sharply defined waxy deposits, or by proliferative retinopathy. See page B15.

**di•a•be•to•gen•ic** (dī′ă-bē-tō-jen′ik) causing diabetes.

**di•a•be•tog•en•ous** (dī′ă-bĕ-toj′en-ŭs) caused by diabetes.

**di•a•be•tol•o•gy** (dī′ă-be-tol′ō-jē) the field of medicine concerned with diabetes.

**di•a•ce•tic ac•id** (dī-ă-sē′tik as′id, dī-ă-set′ik as′ id) SYN acetoacetic acid.

**di•a•ce•tyl•mon•ox•ime** (dī-as′ĕ-til-mon-ok′sīm) a 2-oxo-oxime that can reactivate phosphorylated acetylcholinesterase *in vitro* and *in vivo;* it penetrates the blood-brain barrier.

**di•a•chron•ic** (dī-ă-kron′ik) systematically observed over time in the same subjects throughout as opposed to synchronic or cross-sectional. [dia- + G. *chronos*, time]

**di•a•chron•ic stu•dy** a study of the natural course of a life or disorder in which a cohort of subjects is serially observed over a period of time and no assumptions need be made about the stability of the system.

**di•a•crit•ic, di•a•crit•i•cal** (dī-ă-krit′ik, dī-ă-krit′ i-kăl) distinguishing; diagnostic; allowing of distinction. [G. *diakritikos*, able to distinguish]

**di•ad** (dī′ad) **1.** the transverse tubule and a cisterna in cardiac muscle fibers. **2.** SYN dyad (1).

**di•ad•o•cho•ki•ne•sia, di•ad•o•cho•ki•ne•sis** (dī-ad′ō-kō-ki-nē′zē-ă, dī-ad′ō-kō-ki-nē′sis) the normal power of alternately bringing a limb into opposite positions, as of flexion and extension or of pronation and supination. [G. *diadochos,* working in turn, + *kinēsis,* movement]

**di•ad•o•cho•ki•net•ic** (dī-ad′ō-kō-ki-net′ik) relating to diadochokinesia.

**di•ae•re•tic [Br.]** SEE dieretic.

**di•ag•nose** (dī-ag-nōs′) to make a diagnosis.

**di•ag•no•sis** (dī-ag-nō′sis) the determination of the nature of a disease. [G. *diagnōsis,* a deciding]

**di•ag•no•sis by ex•clu•sion** a diagnosis made by excluding those diseases to which only some of the patient's symptoms might belong, leaving one disease as the most likely diagnosis, although no definitive tests or findings establish that diagnosis.

**di•ag•no•sis-re•lat•ed group (DRG)** a classification of patients by diagnosis or surgical procedure (sometimes including age) into major diagnostic categories (each containing specific diseases, disorders, or procedures) for the purpose of determining payment of hospitalization charges, based on the premise that treatment of similar medical diagnoses generates similar costs.

**di•ag•nos•tic** (dī-ag-nos′tik) **1.** relating to or aiding in diagnosis. **2.** establishing or confirming a diagnosis.

**di•ag•nos•ti•cian** (dī′ag-nos-tish′ăn) one who is skilled in making diagnoses.

**di•ag•nos•tic ra•di•o•logy** SYN radiology (2).

**di•ag•nos•tic spec•i•fic•i•ty 1.** the probability (P) that, given the absence of disease (D), a normal test result (T) excludes disease; i.e., P(T/D). **2.** specificity (%) = number of individuals without the disease who test negative × 100 ÷ total number of individuals tested without the disease.

**Di•ag•nos•tic and Sta•tis•ti•cal Man•u•al (DSM)** an American Psychiatric Association publication that classifies mental illnesses. Currently in its fourth edition (DSM-IV), the manual provides health practitioners with a comprehensive system for diagnosing mental illnesses based on specific clinical and behavioral symptoms.

**di•ag•nos•tic ul•tra•sound** the use of ultrasound to obtain images for medical diagnostic purposes.

**di•ag•o•nal con•ju•gate** the anteroposterior dimension of the inlet; the clinical distance from the promontory of the sacrum to the lower margin of the symphysis pubica. SYN false conjugate (1).

**di•a•gram** a simple, graphic depiction of an idea or object.

**di•a•ki•ne•sis** (dī′ă-ki-nē′sis) final stage of prophase in meiosis I, in which the chromosomes continue to shorten and the nucleolus and nuclear membrane disappear. [G. *dia,* through, + *kinēsis,* movement]

**di•al•y•sance** (dī-al′i-sans) the number of milliliters of blood completely cleared of any substance by an artificial kidney or by peritoneal dialysis in a unit of time; conventional clearance formulas are expressed as mm/min. [fr. dialysis]

**di•al•y•sate** (dī-al′i-sāt) that part of a mixture that passes through a dialyzing membrane. SYN diffusate.

**di•al•y•sis** (dī-al′i-sis) a form of filtration to separate crystalloid from colloid substances (or smaller molecules from larger ones) in a solution by interposing a semipermeable membrane between the solution and water; the crystalloid (smaller) substances pass through the membrane into the water on the other side, the colloids do not. SYN diffusion (2). [G. a separation, fr. *dialyo,* to separate]

**di•al•y•sis en•ceph•a•lop•a•thy syn•drome, di•al•y•sis de•men•ti•a** a progressive, often fatal, diffuse encephalopathy occurring in patients on chronic hemodialysis.

**di•al•y•sis ret•i•nae** congenital or traumatic separation of the peripheral sensory retina from the retinal pigment epithelium at the ora serrata, often causing a retinal detachment.

**di•a•lyz•er** (dī′ă-lī-zer) the apparatus for performing dialysis; a membrane used in dialysis.

**di•a•me•lia** (dī-ă-mē′lē-ă) absence of two limbs.

**di•am•e•ter** (dī-am′ĕ-ter) **1.** a straight line connecting two opposite points on the surface of a more or less spherical or cylindrical body, or at the boundary of an opening or foramen, passing through the center of such body or opening. **2.** the distance measured along such a line. [G. *diametros,* fr. *dia,* through, + *metron,* measure]

**Dia•mond TYM med•i•um** (dī′mond) medium of trypticase, yeast extract, maltose, and serum used to detect the presence of *Trichomonas vaginalis.*

**Di•an•a com•plex** (dī-a′nă) ideas leading to the adoption of masculine traits and behavior in a female. [*Diana,* L. myth. char.]

**di•a•pause** (dī′ă-pawz) a period of biological quiescence or dormancy with decreased metabolism; an interval in which development is arrested or greatly slowed. [dia- + G. *pausis*, pause]

**di•a•pe•de•sis** (dī'ă-pĕ-dē'sis) the passage of blood, or any of its formed elements, through the intact walls of blood vessels. SYN migration (2). [G. *dia*, through, + *pēdēsis*, a leaping]

**di•a•per der•ma•ti•tis, di•a•per rash** colloquially referred to as diaper, ammonia, or napkin rash; dermatitis of thighs and buttocks resulting from exposure to urine and feces in infants' diapers. Formerly attributed to ammonia formation; moisture, bacterial growth, and alkalinity may all induce lesions.

**di•aph•a•nos•cope** (dī-af'ă-nō-skōp) an instrument for illuminating the interior of a cavity to determine the translucency of its walls. [G. *diaphanēs*, transparent, + *skopeō*, to examine]

**di•aph•a•nos•co•py** (dī-af-ă-nos'kŏ-pē) examination of a cavity with a diaphanoscope.

**di•a•phe•met•ric** (dī'ă-fĕ-met'rik) relating to the determination of the degree of tactile sensibility. [G. *dia*, through, + *haphē*, touch, + *metron*, measure]

**di•a•pho•re•sis** (dī'ă-fō-rē'sis) SYN perspiration (1). [G. *diaphorēsis*, fr. *dia*, through, + *phoreō*, to carry]

**di•a•pho•ret•ic** (dī-ă-fō-ret'ik) **1.** relating to, or causing, perspiration. **2.** an agent that increases perspiration.

**di•a•phragm** (dī'ă-fram) **1.** the musculomembranous partition between the abdominal and thoracic cavities. SYN diaphragma (2), midriff. **2.** a thin disk pierced with an opening, used in a microscope, camera, or other optical instrument in order to shut out the marginal rays of light, thus giving a more direct illumination. **3.** a flexible ring covered with a dome-shaped sheet of elastic material used in the vagina to prevent pregnancy. **4.** in radiography, a grid (2). [G. *diaphragma*]

**di•a•phrag•ma,** pl. **di•a•phrag•ma•ta** (dī-ă-frag'mă, dī-ă-frag'mă-tă) **1.** a thin partition separating adjacent regions. **2.** [TA] SYN diaphragm (1). [G. *diaphragma*, a partition wall, midriff]

**di•a•phrag•ma sel•lae** [TA] a fold of dura mater extending transversely across the sella turcica and roofing over the hypophyseal fossa; it is perforated in its center for the passage of the infundibulum. SYN diaphragm of sella turcica.

**di•a•phrag•mat•ic** (dī'ă-frag-mat'ik) relating to a diaphragm. SYN phrenic (1).

**di•a•phrag•mat•ic flut•ter** rapid rhythmical contractions (average, 150 per minute) of the diaphragm, simulating atrial flutter clinically and sometimes electrocardiographically.

**di•a•phrag•mat•ic her•nia** protrusion of abdominal contents into the chest through a weakness in the respiratory diaphragm; a common type is the hiatal hernia.

**di•a•phrag•mat•ic lig•a•ment of the mes•o••neph•ros** the segment of the urogenital ridge that extends from the mesonephros to the diaphragm; becomes the suspensory ligament of the ovary.

**di•a•phrag•mat•ic pleu•ri•sy** SYN epidemic pleurodynia.

**di•a•phragm of sel•la turcica** SYN diaphragma sellae.

**di•a•phy•sec•to•my** (dī'ă-fi-sek'tō-mē) partial or complete removal of the shaft of a long bone. [diaphysis + G. *ektomē*, excision]

**di•a•phys•i•al** (dī-ă-fiz'ē-ăl) relating to a diaphysis.

**di•aph•y•sis,** pl. **di•aph•y•ses** (dī-af'i-sis, dī-af'i-sēz) [TA] SYN shaft. [G. a growing between]

**di•a•pi•re•sis** (dī'ă-pī-rē'sis) passage of colloidal or other small particles of suspended matter through the unruptured walls of the blood vessels. SEE ALSO diapedesis. [G. *diapeirō*, to drive through, fr. *peirō*, to pierce]

**di•ar•rhea** (dī-ă-rē'ă) an abnormally frequent discharge of semisolid or fluid fecal matter from the bowel. [G. *diarrhoia*, fr. *dia*, through, + *rhoia*, a flow, a flux]

**di•ar•rhe•al, di•ar•rhe•ic** (dī-ă-rē'ăl, dī-ă-rē'ik) relating to diarrhea. SYN diarrhetic.

**di•ar•rhe•tic** SYN diarrheal.

**di•ar•rhoe•al [Br.]** SEE diarrheal.

**di•ar•thric** (dī-ar'thrik) relating to two joints. SYN biarticular, diarticular. [G. *di-*, two, + *arthron*, joint]

**di•ar•thro•di•al joint** SYN synovial joint.

**di•ar•thro•sis,** pl. **di•ar•thro•ses** (dī-ar-thrō'sis, dī-ar-thrō'sēz) SYN synovial joint. [G. articulation]

**di•ar•tic•u•lar** (dī-ar-tik'yu-lăr) SYN diarthric.

**di•as•chi•sis** (dī-as'ki-sis) a sudden inhibition of function produced by an acute focal disturbance in a portion of the brain at a distance from the original seat of injury, but anatomically connected with it through fiber tracts. [G. a splitting]

**di•a•scope** (dī'ă-skōp) a flat glass plate through which one can examine superficial skin lesions by means of pressure. [G. *dia*, through, + *skopeō*, to view]

**di•as•co•py** (dī-as'kŏ-pē) examination of superficial skin lesions with a diascope. [G. *dia*, through, + *skopeō*, to see]

**di•a•stal•sis** (dī-ă-stahl'sis) the type of peristalsis in which a region of inhibition precedes the wave of contraction, as seen in the intestinal tract. [G. an arrangement]

**di•a•stal•tic** (dī-ă-stahl'tik) pertaining to diastalsis.

**di•as•ta•sis** (dī-as'tă-sis) **1.** any simple separation of normally joined parts. SYN divarication. **2.** the mid-portion of diastole when the blood enters the ventricle slowly or ceases to enter prior to atrial systole. Diastasis duration is in inverse proportion to heart rate and is absent at very high heart rates. [G. a separation]

**di•as•tas•u•ria** (dī-as-tās-yu'rē-ă) SYN amylasuria.

**di•a•stat•ic** (dī-ă-stat'ik) relating to a diastasis.

**di•a•ste•ma,** pl. **di•a•ste•ma•ta** (dī'ă-stē'mă, dī-ă-stē'mă-tă) [TA] **1.** fissure or abnormal opening in any part, especially if congenital. **2.** space between two adjacent teeth in the same dental arch. **3.** a space between the upper central incisors in humans, or a space between two adjacent teeth in the same dental arch, especially that between the upper lateral incisor and the adjacent canine, into which the lower canine closes in the Carnivora such as dogs. [G. *diastēma*, an interval]

**di•a•ste•ma•to•cra•nia** (dī-ă-stē'mă-tō-krā'nē-ă) congenital sagittal fissure of the skull. [G. *diastēma*, an interval, + *kranion*, skull]

**di•a•ste•ma•to•my•e•lia** (dī-ă-stē'mă-tō-mī-e'lē-ă) complete or incomplete sagittal division of the spinal cord by an osseous or fibrocartilaginous septum. [G. *diastēma*, interval, + *myelon*, marrow]

**di·as·to·le** (dī-as'tō-lē) normal postsystolic dilation of the heart cavities, during which they fill with blood; diastole of the atria precedes that of the ventricles; diastole of either chamber alternates rhythmically with systole or contraction of that chamber. [G. *diastolē*, dilation]

**di·a·stol·ic** (dī-ă-stol'ik) relating to diastole.

**di·a·stol·ic mur·mur (DM)** a murmur heard during diastole.

**di·a·stol·ic pres·sure** the intracardiac pressure during or resulting from diastolic relaxation of a cardiac chamber; the lowest arterial blood pressure reached during any given ventricular cycle.

**di·a·stol·ic thrill** a thrill felt over the precordium or over a blood vessel during ventricular diastole.

**di·as·tro·phic dys·pla·sia** a skeletal dysplasia characterized by scoliosis, hitchhiker's thumb due to shortening of the first metacarpal bone, cleft palate, malformed ear with calcification, chondritis, shortening of the Achilles tendon, clubbed foot, and characteristic radiologic findings; autosomal recessive inheritance, caused by mutation in the diastrophic dysplasia sulfate transporter gene (DTDST) on chromosome 5q.

**di·a·tax·ia** (dī'ă-tak'sē-ă) ataxia affecting both sides of the body.

**di·a·ther·mal** (dī-ă-ther'mal) SYN diathermic. [G. *dia*, through, + *thermē*, heat]

**di·a·ther·ma·nous** (dī-ă-ther'man-ŭs) permeable by heat rays. SYN transcalent. [G. *dia-thermaino*, to heat through, fr. *thermos*, hot]

**di·a·ther·mic** (dī-ă-ther'mik) relating to, characterized by, or affected by diathermy. SYN diathermal.

**di·a·ther·my** (dī'ă-ther-mē) therapeutic use of short or ultrashort waves of electromagnetic energy to heat muscular tissue. [G. *dia*, through, + *thermē*, heat]

**di·ath·e·sis** (dī-ath'ĕ-sis) the constitutional or inborn state disposing to a disease, group of diseases, or metabolic or structural anomaly. [G. arrangement, condition]

**di·a·thet·ic** (dī-ă-thet'ik) relating to a diathesis.

**di·a·to·ma·ceous earth** a powder made of desiccated diatom material; used as a filtering agent, adsorbent, and abrasive in many chemical operations.

**di·a·tom·ic** (dī-ă-tom'ik) **1.** denoting a compound with a molecule made up of two atoms. **2.** denoting any ion or atomic grouping composed of two atoms only.

△**di·a·zo-** prefix denoting a compound containing the ≡C–N=N–X grouping, where X is not carbon (except for CN), or the grouping $N_2$ attached by one atom to carbon. Cf. azo-. [G. *di-*, two, + Fr. *azote*, nitrogen]

**di·ba·sic** (dī-bā'sik) having two replaceable hydrogen atoms, denoting an acid with two ionizable hydrogen atoms.

**di·bu·caine num·ber (DN)** (dī-byu'kān num'ber) a test for differentiation of one of several forms of atypical pseudocholinesterases that are unable to inactivate succinylcholine at normal rates; based upon percent inhibition of the enzymes by dibucaine. SEE ALSO fluoride number.

**DIC** disseminated intravascular coagulation.

**di·car·box·yl·ic ac·id cy·cle 1.** that portion of the tricarboxylic acid cycle involving the dicarboxylic acids (succinic, fumaric, malic, and oxaloacetic acids); **2.** a cyclic scheme in which certain steps of the tricarboxylic acid cycle are used

with the glyoxylate cycle; important in the utilization of glyoxylic acid in microorganisms.

**di·cen·tric** (dī-sen'trik) having two centromeres, an abnormal state.

**di·cho·ri·al, di·cho·ri·on·ic** (dī-kō'rē-ăl, dī-kō-rē-on'ik) showing evidence of two chorions. [G. *di-*, two, + chorion]

**di·cho·ri·on·ic di·am·ni·on·ic pla·cen·ta** SEE twin placenta.

**di·chro·ic** (dī-krō'ik) relating to dichroism.

**di·chro·ism** (dī'krō-izm) the property of seeming to be differently colored when viewed from emitted light and from transmitted light. [G. *di-*, two, + *chrōa*, color]

**di·chro·mate** (dī-krō'māt) a compound containing the radical $Cr_2O_7^=$.

**di·chro·mat·ic** (dī-krō-mat'ik) **1.** having or exhibiting two colors. **2.** relating to dichromatism (2).

**di·chro·ma·tism** (dī-krō'mă-tizm) **1.** the state of being dichromatic (1). **2.** the abnormality of color vision in which only two of the three retinal cone pigments are present, as in protanopia, deuteranopia, and tritanopia. SYN dichromatopsia. [G. *di-*, two, + *chrōma*, color]

**di·chro·ma·top·sia** (dī-krō-mă-top'sē-ă) SYN dichromatism (2). [G. *di-*, two, + *chrōma*, color, + *opsis*, vision]

**Dick·ens shunt** (dik'enz) SYN pentose phosphate pathway.

**Dick test** (dik) an intracutaneous test of susceptibility to the erythrogenic toxin of *Streptococcus pyogenes* responsible for the rash and other manifestations of scarlet fever.

**DICOM** Digital Imaging and Communications in Medicine, a joint standard of the American College of Radiology and National Equipment Manufacturers Association; specifies entities (or objects) and functions (or services) to allow communication between various image sources and other computer devices, such as archives or workstations.

**di·co·ria** (dī-kō'rē-ă) SYN diplocoria. [G. *di-*, two, + *korē*, pupil]

***Di·cro·coe·li·um*** (dī-krō-sē'lē-um) a genus of digenetic trematodes inhabiting the biliary tract of herbivores. The lancet fluke, *D. dentriticum*, is rarely found in humans but is an important parasite of sheep. [G. *dikroos*, forked, + *koilia*, belly]

**di·crot·ic** (dī-krot'ik) relating to dicrotism. [G. *dikrotos*, double-beating]

**di·crot·ic notch** (dī-krot'ik nawch) the acute drop in arterial pressure pulse curves following the systolic peak, corresponding to the incisura of the displacement pulse curve.

**di·crot·ic pulse** a pulse which is marked by a double beat, the second, due to a palpable dicrotic wave, being weaker than the first.

**di·cro·tism** (dī'krō-tizm) that form of the pulse in which a double beat can be appreciated at any arterial pulse for each beat of the heart; due to accentuation of the dicrotic wave. [G. *di-*, two, + *krotos*, a beat]

**dicta-** (dik'ta) two hundred. [G.]

**dic·ty·o·ma** (dik-tē-ō'mă) a benign tumor of the ciliary epithelium with a net-like structure resembling embryonic retina. [G. *dikyton*, net (retina), + *-oma*, tumor]

**di·dac·tic** (dī-dak'tik) instructive; denoting medical teaching by lectures or textbooks, as distinguished from clinical demonstrations with patients or laboratory exercises. [G. *didaktikos,* fr. *didaskō,* to teach]

**di·dac·ty·lism** (dī-dak′ti-lizm) congenital condition of having two fingers on a hand or two toes on a foot. [G. *di-,* two, + *daktylos,* finger or toe]

**di·del·phic** (dī-del′fik) having or relating to a double uterus. [G. *di-,* two, + *delphys,* womb]

⚠ **did·ym-, did·y·mo-** the didymus, testis. [G. *didymos,* twin]

**did·y·mus** (did′ē-mŭs) SYN testis. [G. *didymos,* a twin, pl. *didymoi,* testes]

⚠ **-did·y·mus** a conjoined twin, with the first element of the complete word designating fused parts. SEE ALSO -dymus, -pagus. [G. *didymos,* twin]

**di·e·cious** (dī-ē′shŭs) denoting animals or plants that are sexually distinct, the individuals being of one or the other sex. [G. *di-,* two, + *oikia,* house]

**di·en·ceph·a·lon,** pl. **di·en·ceph·a·la** (dī-en-sef′ă-lon, dī-en-sef′ă-lă) that part of the prosencephalon composed of the epithalamus, dorsal thalamus, subthalamus, and hypothalamus. [G. *dia,* through, + *enkephalos,* brain]

***Di·ent·a·moe·ba frag·i·lis*** (dī-ent-ă-mē′bă fraj′i-lis) a species of small ameba-like flagellates related to *Trichomonas,* parasitic in the large intestine of humans and certain monkeys; usually nonpathogenic, but sometimes causing low-grade inflammation with mucous diarrhea.

**di·ent·a·moe·bia·sis** (dī-ent-ă-mē-bī′ă-sis) infection with protozoa of the genus *Dientamoeba.*

**di·er·e·sis** (dī-er′ĕ-sis) SYN solution of continuity. [G. *diairesis,* a division]

**dieretic** (dī-er-et′ik) 1. Relating to dieresis. 2. Dividing; ulcerating; corroding.

**di·es·trous** (dī-es′trŭs) pertaining to diestrus.

**di·es·trus** (dī-es′trŭs) a period of sexual quiescence intervening between two periods of estrus. [G. *dia,* between, + *oistros,* desire]

**di·et** (dī′et) 1. food and drink in general. 2. a prescribed course of eating and drinking in which the amount and kind of food, as well as the times at which it is to be taken, are regulated for therapeutic purposes. 3. reduction of caloric intake so as to lose weight. 4. to follow any prescribed or specific diet. [G. *diaita,* a way of life; a diet]

**di·e·tary** (dī′ĕ-tār-ē) relating to the diet.

**di·e·tary a·men·or·rhea** loss of menstrual function due to severe weight loss or gain.

**di·e·tary fi·ber** the plant polysaccharides and lignin that are resistant to hydrolysis by the digestive enzymes in humans.

**Di·e·ta·ry Re·fer·ence In·take (DRI)** a set of values for the dietary nutrient intakes of healthy people in the United States and Canada, used for planning and assessing diets. Include the Recommended Dietary Allowance (RDA), the Adequate Intake (AI), the Tolerable Upper Limit (TUL), and the Estimated Average Intake (EAI). Will eventually replace the U.S. Recommended Daily Allowance and the Canadian Recommended Nutrient Intake (RNI). See appendix.

**Die·ter·le stain** (dē-ter-lĕ) stain used to demonstrate spirochetes and Leishman-Donovan bodies; employs silver nitrate and uranium nitrate.

**di·e·tet·ic** (dī′ĕ-tet′ik) 1. relating to the diet. 2. descriptive of food that, naturally or through processing, has a low caloric content.

**di·e·tet·ics** (dī-ĕ-tet′iks) the practical application of diet in the prophylaxis and treatment of disease.

**di·eth·yl·stil·bes·trol (DES)** (dī-eth′il-stil-bes′trol) a synthetic nonsteroidal estrogenic compound. Sometimes used as a postcoital antipregnancy agent to prevent implantation of the fertilized ovum. The first demonstrated transplacental carcinogen responsible for a delayed clear cell vaginal carcinoma in female offspring of mothers who took the drug during pregnancy when the drug was erroneously thought to prevent threatened abortion. SYN stilboestrol.

**di·e·ti·tian** (dī-ĕ-tish′ŭn) an expert in dietetics.

**Die·tl cri·sis** (dē′tĕl) intermittent pain, sometimes with nausea and emesis, caused by intermittent proximal obstruction of ureter.

**di·et qua·li·ty in·dex** a measure of the quality of the diet using a composite of eight recommendations regarding the consumption of foods and nutrients from the National Academy of Sciences (NAS). Meeting the standard is assigned a value of 0, within 30% of goal a value of 1, differing by more than 30% a 2. The resulting index can be a figure of between 0–16, the lower the better. The NAS recommendations include reducing total fat intake to 30% or less of total energy; reducing saturated fatty-acid intake to less than 10% of energy; reducing cholesterol intake to less than 300 mg daily; eating 5 or more servings daily of vegetables and fruits; increasing intake of starches and other complex carbohydrates by eating 6 or more servings daily of bread, cereal, and legumes; maintaining protein intake at moderate levels (levels lower than twice the RDA); limiting total daily intake of sodium to 2400 mg or less; and maintaining adequate calcium intake (approximately the RDA).

**Dieu·la·foy le·sion** (dyoo-lah-fwah) an abnormally large submucosal artery located in the proximal stomach, which may be the site of acute and recurrent episodes of massive hemorrhage.

**dif-** (L.) Prefix: separation, taking apart, in two, reversal, not, un-.

**dif·fer·ence** (dif′er-ens) the magnitude or degree by which one quality or quantity differs from another of the same kind.

**dif·fer·ence li·men** a barely noticeable change in the intensity or frequency of a stimulus.

**dif·fer·en·tial di·ag·no·sis** the determination of which of two or more diseases with similar symptoms is the one from which the patient is suffering, by a systematic comparison and contrasting of the clinical findings. SYN differentiation (2).

**dif·fe·ren·tial dis·play** the use of reverse transcriptase and polymerase chain reaction technologies to amplify mRNA from specific cells or tissues and then to compare them directly with amplified mRNA from another cell or tissue.

**dif·fer·en·tial u·re·ter·al cath·e·ter·i·za·tion test** a study performed to determine various functional parameters of one kidney compared to the other; ureteral catheters are inserted at cystoscopy into the ureter or renal pelvis bilaterally, and simultaneous measurements are made of urine flow rate, insulin, or PAH (if infused), endogenous creatinine, or various urinary solutes.

**dif·fer·en·ti·a·tion** (dif′er-en-shē-ā′shŭn) 1. the acquisition or possession of one or more characteristics or functions different from that of the original type. SYN specialization (2). 2. SYN differential diagnosis. 3. partial removal of a stain

d
i

from a histologic section to accentuate the staining differences of tissue components.

**dif•frac•tion** (di-frak′shŭn) deflection of the rays of light from a straight line in passing by the edge of an opaque body or in passing an obstacle of about the size of the wavelength of the light. [L. *dif- fringo,* pp. *-fractus,* to break in pieces]

**dif•fu•sate** (di-fyu′zāt) SYN dialysate. [L. *dif-fundo,* pp. *-fusus,* to pour in different directions]

**dif•fuse** (di-fyus) **1.** (di-fyūz′) to disseminate; to spread about. **2.** (di-fyūs′) disseminated; spread about; not restricted. [L. *dif-fundo,* pp. *-fusus,* to pour in different directions]

**dif•fuse ab•scess** a collection of pus not circumscribed by a well-defined capsule.

**dif•fuse cu•ta•ne•ous leish•man•i•a•sis** leishmaniasis caused by several New and Old World species and strains of *Leishmania.* The condition is associated with a suppressed cell-mediated immune response.

**dif•fuse cu•ta•ne•ous mas•to•cy•to•sis** a benign process consisting of focal cutaneous infiltrates composed of mast cells; lesions are flat or slightly elevated, form wheals and itch when stroked; bone lesions may occur.

**dif•fuse hy•per•ker•a•to•sis of palms and soles** an autosomal dominant disorder with onset in early infancy; characterized by hyperkeratotic, scaling plaques and often hyperhidrosis on the palms and soles.

**dif•fuse id•i•o•path•ic skel•e•tal hy•per•os•to•sis** a generalized spinal and extraspinal articular disorder characterized by calcification and ossification of ligaments, particularly of the anterior longitudinal ligament; distinct from ankylosing spondylitis or degenerative joint disease. SYN Forestier disease.

**dif•fuse in•ju•ries** injury over a large body area usually resulting from encounters with low velocity-high mass forces.

**dif•fuse Le•wy body di•sease** (lā-vē) a degenerative cerebral disorder of the elderly, characterized initially by progressive dementia or psychosis, and subsequently by parkinsonian findings, usually with severe rigidity; other manifestations include involuntary movements, myoclonus, dysphagia, and orthostatic hypotension. Pathologically, Lewy bodies are present diffusely in the nuclei of the hypothalamus, basal forebrain, and brainstem. SYN Lewy body dementia.

**dif•fuse ob•struc•tive em•phy•se•ma** the major component of chronic obstructive lung disease.

**dif•fuse un•i•la•ter•al sub•a•cute neu•ro•re•tin•i•tis (DUSN)** inflammation of the neurosensory retina caused by infiltration by a roundworm such as *Baylis ascaris* or *Ancylostoma* species.

**dif•fuse wax•y spleen** a condition of amyloid degeneration of the spleen, affecting chiefly the extrasinusoidal tissue spaces of the pulp.

**dif•fus•i•ble** (di-fyuz′i-bl) capable of diffusing.

**dif•fus•i•ble stim•u•lant** a stimulant that produces a rapid but temporary effect.

**dif•fus•ing ca•pac•i•ty** (di-fyuz′ing kă-pasĭ-tē) the amount of oxygen taken up by pulmonary capillary blood per minute per unit average oxygen pressure gradient between alveolar gas and pulmonary capillary blood; units are: ml/min/mmHg; also applied to other gases such as carbon monoxide.

**dif•fu•sion** (di-fyu′zhŭn) **1.** the random movement of molecules or ions or small particles in solution or suspension toward a uniform distribution throughout the available volume. **2.** SYN dialysis.

**dif•fu•sion an•ox•ia** diffusion hypoxia severe enough to result in the absence of oxygen in alveolar gas.

**dif•fu•sion co•ef•fi•cient** the mass of material diffusing across a unit area in unit time under a concentration gradient of unity.

**dif•fu•sion hy•pox•ia** decrease in alveolar oxygen tension when room air is inhaled at the conclusion of nitrous oxide anesthesia, because nitrous oxide diffusing out of the blood dilutes the alveolar oxygen.

**dif•fu•sion res•pi•ra•tion** maintenance of oxygenation during apnea by intratracheal insufflation of oxygen at high flow rates.

**di•gas•tric** (dī-gas′trik) **1.** having two bellies; denoting especially a muscle with two fleshy parts separated by an intervening tendinous part. SYN biventral. SEE digastric muscle. **2.** relating to the digastric muscle; denoting a fossa or groove with which it is in relation and a nerve supplying its posterior belly. [G. *di-,* two, + *gastēr,* belly]

**di•gas•tric fos•sa** a hollow on the posterior surface of the base of the mandible, on either side of the median plane, giving attachment to the anterior belly of the digastric muscle.

**di•gas•tric mus•cle 1.** one of the suprahyoid group of muscles consisting of two bellies united by a central tendon which is connected to the body of the hyoid bone; *origin,* by posterior belly from the digastric groove medial to the mastoid process; *insertion,* by anterior belly into lower border of mandible near midline; *action,* elevates the hyoid when mandible is fixed; depresses the mandible when hyoid is fixed; *nerve supply,* posterior belly from facial, anterior belly by nerve to the mylohyoid from the mandibular division of trigeminal; **2.** a muscle with two fleshy bellies separated by a fibrous insertion; SYN musculus digastricus [TA].

**di•gas•tric tri•an•gle** SYN submandibular triangle.

**di•gen•e•sis** (dī-jen′ĕ-sis) reproduction in distinctive patterns in alternate generations, as seen in the nonsexual (invertebrate) and the sexual (vertebrate) cycles of digenetic trematode parasites. [G. *di-,* two, + G. *genesis,* generation]

**di•ge•net•ic** (dī-jĕ-net′ik) **1.** pertaining to or characterized by digenesis. SYN heteroxenous. **2.** pertaining to the digenetic fluke.

**di•gest** (di-jest′ dī-jest) **1.** (di-jest′, dī-) to soften by moisture and heat. **2.** (di-jest′, dī-) to hydrolyze or break up into simpler chemical compounds by means of hydrolyzing enzymes or chemical action. **3.** (dī′jest) the materials resulting from digestion or hydrolysis. [L. *digero,* pp. *-gestus,* to force apart, divide, dissolve]

**di•ges•tant** (dī-jes′tănt) **1.** aiding digestion. **2.** an agent that favors or assists the process of digestion. SYN digestive (2).

**di•ges•tion** (dī-jes′chŭn) **1.** the process of making a digest. **2.** the mechanical, chemical, and enzymatic process whereby ingested food is converted into material suitable for assimilation for synthesis of tissues or liberation of energy. [L. *digestio.* See digest]

**di•ges•tive** (di-jes′tiv, dī-) **1.** relating to digestion. **2.** SYN digestant (2).

**di·ges·tive sys·tem** the digestive tract from the mouth to the anus with all its associated glands and organs. See page A23.

**di·ges·tive tract** the passage leading from the mouth to the anus through the pharynx, esophagus, stomach, and intestine. SYN alimentary canal, alimentary tract.

**dig·it** (dij'it) a finger or toe. SYN digitus [TA], dactyl, dactylus. [L. *digitus*]

**dig·i·tal** (dij'i-tăl) relating to or resembling a digit or digits or an impression made by them; based on numerical methodology.

**dig·i·tal crease** one of the grooves on the palmar surface of a finger, at the level of an interphalangeal joint.

**dig·i·tal hear·ing aid** programmable hearing aid that can be customized to the extent of the user's hearing loss.

**dig·i·tal·i·sa·tion [Br.]** SEE digitalization.

**dig·i·tal·i·za·tion** (dij'i-tal-i-zā'shŭn) administration of digitalis until sufficient amounts are present in the body to produce the desired therapeutic effects.

**dig·i·tal ra·di·og·ra·phy** computed radiography or computer processing of a digitized image from a conventional image-intensifier and video camera. SEE DSA.

**dig·i·tal re·flex** SYN Hoffmann sign (2).

**dig·i·tal sub·trac·tion an·gi·og·ra·phy (DSA)** computer-assisted roentgenographic angiography permitting visualization of vascular structures without superimposed bone and soft tissue density; images made before and after contrast injection allow subtraction (separation and removal) of opacities not enhanced by the contrast medium. Other image-processing can be performed. Contrast material may be injected intravenously or in lower-than-usual amount intra-arterially.

**dig·i·tate** (dij'i-tāt) marked by a number of finger-like processes or impressions. [L. *digitatus*, having fingers, fr. *digitus*, finger]

**dig·i·ta·tion** (dij-i-tā'shŭn) a process resembling a finger. [Mod. L. *digitatio*]

**dig·i·tus**, pl. **dig·i·ti** (dij'i-tŭs, dij'i-tī) [TA] SYN digit. [L.]

**di·glos·sia** (dī-glos'ē-ă) a developmental condition that results in a longitudinal split in the tongue. SEE ALSO bifid tongue. [G. *di-*, two, + *glōssa*, tongue]

**di·het·er·o·zy·gote** (dī-het'er-ō-zī'gōt) an individual heterozygous at two loci of interest, especially in genetic linkage analysis.

**di·hy·drate** (dī-hī'drāt) a compound with two molecules of water of crystallization.

**di·hy·dric al·co·hol** alcohol containing two OH groups in its molecule; e.g., ethylene glycol.

△**di·hy·dro-** prefix indicating the addition of two hydrogen atoms. [G. *di*, two + *hydōr*, water]

**7,8-di·hy·dro·fo·lic ac·id** (sev'en-āt-dī-hī-drō-fō'lik as'id) intermediate between folic acid and 5,6,7,8-tetrahydrofolic acid.

**di·hy·dro·gen** SYN hydrogen (2).

**di·hy·dro·lip·o·am·ide ace·tyl·trans·fer·ase** (dī-hī'drō-lip-ō-am'id ă-sē-til-trans'fer-ās) an enzyme transferring acetyl from $S^6$-acetyl-dihydrolipoamide to coenzyme A. A part of many enzyme complexes (e.g., pyruvate dehydrogenase complex). SYN lipoate acetyltransferase, thioltransacetylase A.

**di·hy·dro·or·o·tate** (dī-hī'drō-ōr-ō'tāt) L-5,6-dihydroorotate; an intermediate in the biosynthesis of pyrimidines.

**di·hy·dro·pte·ro·ic ac·id** (dī-hī'drō-te-rō'ik as'id) an intermediate in the formation of folic acid; a compound of 6-hydroxymethylpterin and *p*-aminobenzoic acid, the combining of which is inhibited by sulfonamides.

**di·hy·dro·ur·i·dine** (dī-hī-drō-yur'i-dēn) uridine in which the 5,6- double bond has been saturated by addition of two hydrogen atoms; a rare constituent of transfer ribonucleic acids.

△**di·hy·drox·y-** prefix denoting addition of two hydroxyl groups; as a suffix, becomes -diol.

**di·hy·drox·y·ac·e·tone** (dī'hī-drok-sē-as'e-tōn) the simplest ketose.

**2,8-di·hy·drox·y·a·de·nine li·thi·a·sis** formation of calculi of 2,8-dihydroxyadenine due to a deficiency or reduced activity of adenine phosphoribosyltransferase.

**di·i·o·dide** (dī-ī'ō-dīd) a compound containing two atoms of iodine per molecule.

△**di·i·o·do-** prefix indicating two atoms of iodine. [G. *di*, + *ioeidēs*, violet flower color]

**di·i·o·do·ty·ro·sine (DIT)** (di'ī-ō-dō-tī'rō-sēn) an intermediate in the biosynthesis of thyroid hormone.

**di·ke·tone** (dī-kē'tōn) a molecule containing two carbonyl groups; e.g., acetylacetone ($CH_3COCH_2COCH_3$).

**di·ke·to·pi·per·a·zines** (dī-kē'tō-pī-per'ă-zēnz) a class of organic compounds with a closed ring structure formed from two α-amino acids by the joining of the α-amino group of each to the carboxyl group of the other.

**di·lac·er·a·tion** (dī-las-er-ā'shŭn) displacement of some portion of a developing tooth, which is then further developed in its new relation, so that its root or crown is sharply angulated. [L. *di-lacero*, pp. *laceratus*, to tear in pieces, fr. *lacer*, mangled]

**di·late** (dī'lāt) to perform or undergo dilation.

**di·lat·ed pore** an enlarged follicular opening of the skin, with a keratinous plug and occasional lanugo or mature hair.

**di·la·tion, dil·a·ta·tion** (dī-lā'shŭn, dil-ă-tā'shŭn) **1.** physiologic or artificial enlargement of a hollow structure or opening. **2.** the act of stretching or enlarging an opening or the lumen of a hollow structure. [L. *dilato*, pp. *dilatatus*, to spread out, dilate]

**di·la·tion and cu·ret·tage (D & C)** dilation of the cervix and curettement of the endometrium.

**di·la·tion and e·vac·u·a·tion (D & E)** dilation of the cervix and removal of the products of conception.

**di·la·tion and ex·trac·tion** a form of abortion in which the cervix is dilated and the fetus extracted in pieces using surgical forceps; technique used to complete a second trimester spontaneous abortion or as a form of induced abortion.

**di·la·tion and suc·tion** SYN suction curettage.

**di·la·tor, dil·a·ta·tor** (dī-lā'tĕr, dil'ă-tā'tĕr) **1.** an instrument designed for enlarging a hollow structure or opening. **2.** a muscle that pulls open an orifice. **3.** a substance that causes dilation or enlargement of an opening or the lumen of a hollow structure.

**di·la·tor mus·cle** a muscle which opens an orifice or dilates the lumen of an organ; it is the dilating or opening component of a pylorus (the other component is the sphincter muscle).

d
i

**di·la·tor pu·pil·lae mus·cle** the radial muscular fibers extending from the sphincter pupillae to the ciliary margin; some anatomists regard them as elastic, not muscular, in humans. SYN musculus dilatator pupillae [TA].

**di·la·tor tu·bae mus·cle** that portion of the musculus tensor veli palatini that attaches to the mucous membrane of the auditory tube; formerly described as a separate muscle. SYN musculus dilatator tubae [TA].

**di·lep·tic sei·zure** seizure characterized by impaired awareness of, interaction with, or memory of ongoing events.

**dil·u·ent** (dil'y-ent) **1.** ingredient in a medicinal preparation which lacks pharmacological activity but is pharmaceutically necessary or desirable. May be a liquid for the dissolution of drugs to be injected, ingested, or inhaled. **2.** diluting; denoting that which dilutes. USAGE NOTE: Often misspelled dilutent, or erroneously so pronounced.

**di·lute** (dī-loot') **1.** to reduce the concentration, strength, quality, or purity of a solution or mixture. **2.** diluted; denoting a solution or mixture so altered. [L. *di-luo*, to wash away, dilute]

**di·lute Rus·sell's vi·per ven·om test (DRVVT)** a test used to confirm the presence of a lupus anticoagulant.

**di·lu·tion** (dī-loo'shŭn) **1.** the act of being diluted. **2.** a diluted solution or mixture. **3.** MICROBIOLOGY a method for counting the number of viable cells in a suspension; a sample is diluted to the point where an aliquot, when plated, yields a countable number of separate colonies.

**di·me·lia** (dī-mē'lē-ă) congenital duplication of the whole or a part of a limb. [G. *di-*, two, + *melos*, limb]

**di·men·sion** (di-men'shŭn) scope, size, magnitude; denoting, in the plural, linear measurements of length, width, and height.

**di·mer** (dī'mer) a compound or unit produced by the combination of two like molecules; in the strictest sense, without loss of atoms (thus nitrogen tetroxide, $N_2O_4$, is the dimer of nitrogen dioxide, $NO_2$), but usually by elimination of $H_2O$ or a similar small molecule between the two (e.g., a disaccharide), or by simple noncovalent association (as of two identical protein molecules); higher orders of complexity are called trimers, tetramers, oligomers, and polymers. [G. *di-*, two, + -mer]

**di·mer·ic** (dī'mer-ik) having the characteristics of a dimer.

**di·meth·yl sulf·ox·ide** (dī-meth'il) methyl sulfoxide; a penetrating solvent, enhancing absorption of therapeutic agents from the skin; used in the treatment of interstitial cystitis.

**di·mor·phic** (dī-mōr'fik) **1.** in fungi, a term referring to growth and reproduction in two forms: mold and yeast. SYN dimorphous (2). **2.** SYN dimorphous (1).

**di·mor·phism** (dī-mōr'fizm) existence in two shapes or forms; denoting a difference of crystalline form exhibited by the same substance, or a difference in form or outward appearance between individuals of the same species. [G. *di-*, two, + *morphē*, shape]

**di·mor·phous** (dī-mōr'fŭs) **1.** having the property of dimorphism. SYN dimorphic (2). **2.** SYN dimorphic (1).

**dim·ple** (dim'pl) **1.** a natural indentation, usually circular and of small area, in the chin, cheek, or sacral region. **2.** a depression of similar appearance to a dimple, resulting from trauma or the contraction of scar tissue. **3.** to cause dimples.

**dimp·ling** (dim'pling) **1.** causing dimples. **2.** a condition marked by the formation of dimples, natural or artificial.

**di·ni·tro·phen·yl·hy·dra·zine test** a screening test for maple syrup urine disease; the addition of 2,4-dinitrophenylhydrazine in HCl to urine gives a chalky white precipitate in the presence of ketoacids.

**din·ner pad** a pad of moderate thickness placed over the pit of the stomach before the application of a plaster jacket; after the plaster has set the pad is removed, leaving space for varying degrees of abdominal distention.

**Di·no·fla·gel·li·da** an order in the phylum Sarcomastigophora characterized by the presence of two flagella so placed as to cause the organism to have a whirling motility. Its outer surface is composed of cellulose-containing plates whose size and number vary with genus and species.

**⚠-di·ol** (dī'ol) **1.** suffix form of the prefix dihydroxy. **2.** a member of a class of compounds containing two hydroxyl groups.

**di·op·ter** (dī-op'ter) the unit of refracting power of lenses, denoting the reciprocal of the focal length expressed in meters. [G. *dioptra*, a leveling instrument]

**di·op·tric ab·er·ra·tion** SYN spherical aberration.

**di·op·trics** (dī-op'triks) the branch of optics concerned with the refraction of light.

**di·otic** (dī-ot'ik) simultaneous presentation of the same sound to each ear. [di- + otic]

**di·ov·u·lar** (dī'ov-yu-lar) relating to two oocytes (ova). SYN biovular. [di- + Mod. L. *ovulum*, dim. of L. *ovum*, egg]

**di·ov·u·la·to·ry** (dī-ō'vyu-lă-tō'rē) releasing two oocytes (ova) in one ovarian cycle.

**di·ox·ide** (dī-oks'īd) a molecule containing two atoms of oxygen; e.g., carbon dioxide, $CO_2$.

**di·ox·in** (dī-oks'in) **1.** a ring consisting of two oxygen atoms, four CH groups, and two double bonds; the positions of the oxygen atoms are specified by prefixes, as in 1,4-dioxin. **2.** abbreviation for dibenzo[*b*,*e*][1,4]dioxin. **3.** 2,3,7,8-tetrachlorodibenzo[*b*,*e*][1,4]dioxin; a contaminant in the herbicide, 2,4,5-T; its potential toxicity, carcinogenicity, and teratogenicity are controversial.

**di·ox·y·gen·ase** (dī-oks'ē-jen-ās) an oxidoreductase that incorporates two atoms of oxygen (from one molecule of $O_2$) into the (reduced) substrate.

**dip 1.** a downward inclination or slope. **2.** a preparation for coating a surface by submersion, as for the destruction of skin parasites. [M.E. *dippen*]

**di·pep·ti·dase** (dī-pep'ti-dās) [EC 3.4.13.11.] a hydrolase catalyzing the hydrolysis of a dipeptide to its constituent amino acids.

**di·pep·tide** (dī-pep'tīd) a combination of two amino acids by means of a peptide (–CO–NH–) link.

**di·pep·ti·dyl pep·ti·dase** (dī-pep-tī'dil pep'ti-dās) a hydrolase occurring in two forms: **dipeptidyl peptidase I**, dipeptidyl transferase, cleaving dipeptides from the amino end of polypeptides; **dipeptidyl peptidase II**, with properties similar to those of I, has a different specificity.

**di·pep·ti·dyl trans·fer·ase** (dī-pep-tī'dil trans'

fer-ās) cleaving dipeptides from the amino end of polypeptides. SEE dipeptidyl peptidase.

**di•phal•lus** (dī-fal′ŭs) congenital duplication, partial or complete, of the penis. May also be associated with exstrophy of the urinary bladder. [G. *di-*, two, + *phallos,* penis]

**di•pha•sic** (dī-fā′zik) occurring in or characterized by two phases or stages.

**di•phen•yl** (dī-fen′il) phenylbenzene; colorless liquid; used as heat transfer agent, frequently as polychlorinated biphenyls (PCBs); as fungistat for oranges and in organic syntheses. Produces convulsions and central nervous system depression. SYN biphenyl.

**2,5-di•phen•yl•ox•a•zole (PPO)** (too-fīv-dī′fen-il-oks′ă-zōl) a scintillator used in radioactivity measurements by scintillation counting.

**di•phos•pha•tase** (dī-fos′fa-tāz) SYN pyrophosphatase.

**1,3-di•phos•pho•glyc•er•ate** (won-thrē-dī-fos′fō-glis′er-āt) an intermediate in glycolysis which enzymatically reacts with ADP to generate ATP and 3-phosphoglycerate.

**2,3-di•phos•pho•glyc•er•ate** an intermediate in the Rapoport-Luebering shunt, formed between 1,3-P$_2$Gri and 3-phosphoglycerate; an important regulator of the affinity of hemoglobin for oxygen; an intermediate of phosphoglycerate mutase.

**di•phos•pho•py•ri•dine nu•cle•o•tide (DPN)** (dī′fos-fō-pir′i-dēn noo′klē-ō-tīd) SYN nicotinamide adenine dinucleotide.

**diph•the•ria** (dif-thēr′ē-ă) a specific infectious disease due to *Corynebacterium diphtheriae* and its highly potent toxin; marked by severe inflammation with formation of a thick membranous coating of the pharynx, the nose, and sometimes the tracheobronchial tree; the toxin produces degeneration in peripheral nerves, heart muscle, and other tissues. Had a high fatality rate, especially in children; now rare due to an effective toxoid. [G. *diphthera,* leather]

**diph•the•ri•al, diph•the•rit•ic** (dif-thēr′ē-ăl, dif-thĕ-rit′ik) relating to diphtheria, or the membranous exudate characteristic of this disease.

**diph•the•ria tox•oid, tet•a•nus tox•oid, and per•tus•sis vac•cine** a vaccine available in three forms: 1) diphtheria and tetanus toxoids plus pertussis vaccine (DTP); 2) tetanus and diphtheria toxoids, adult type (Td); and 3) tetanus toxoid (T); used for active immunization against diphtheria, tetanus, and whooping cough.

**diph•the•rit•ic mem•brane** the false membrane forming on the mucous surfaces in diphtheria.

**diph•the•roid** (dif′thĕ-royd) **1.** one of a group of local infections suggesting diphtheria, but caused by microorganisms other than *Corynebacterium diphtheriae.* SYN pseudodiphtheria. **2.** any microorganism resembling *Corynebacterium diphtheriae.* [diphtheria + G. *eidos,* resemblance]

**di•phyl•lo•both•ri•a•sis** (dī-fil′ō-both-rī′ă-sis) infection with the cestode *Diphyllobothrium latum;* human infection is caused by ingestion of raw or inadequately cooked fish infected with the plerocercoid larva. Leukocytosis and eosinophilia may occur; if the worm is high enough in the alimentary canal, it may preempt the supply of vitamin B$_{12}$ or alter its absorption, leading to hyperchromic macrocytic anemia.

*Di•phyl•lo•both•ri•um* (dī-fil-lō-both′rē-ŭm) a large genus of tapeworms (order Pseudophyl-

lidea) characterized by a spatulate scolex with dorsal and ventral sucking grooves or bothria. Several species are found in humans, although only one, *Diphyllobothrium latum,* is of widespread importance. [G. *di-,* two, + *phyllon,* leaf, + *bothrion,* little ditch]

**di•phy•o•dont** (dif′ē-ō-dont) developing two successive sets of teeth, as occurs in humans and most other mammals. [G. *di-,* two, + *phyō,* to produce, + *odous* (*odont-*), tooth]

**dip•la•cu•sis** (dip-lă-koo′sis) abnormal perception of sound, either in time or in pitch, so that one sound is heard as two. [G. *diplous,* double, + *akousis,* a hearing]

**di•ple•gia** (dī-plē′jē-ă) paralysis of corresponding parts on both sides of the body. [G. *di-,* two, + *plēgē,* a stroke]

△**dip•lo-** double, twofold. SEE haplo-. [G. *diploos,* double]

**dip•lo•ba•cil•lus** (dip′lō-bă-sil′ŭs) two rod-shaped bacterial cells linked end to end. [diplo- + bacillus]

**dip•lo•bac•te•ria** (dip′lō-bak-tēr′ē-ă) bacterial cells linked together in pairs.

**dip•lo•blas•tic** (dip-lō-blas′tik) formed of two germ layers. [diplo- + G. *blastos,* germ]

**dip•lo•car•dia** (dip-lō-kar′dē-ă) an anomaly in which the two lateral halves of the heart are separated to varying degrees by a central fissure. [diplo- + G. *kardia,* heart]

**dip•lo•coc•cus,** pl. **dip•lo•coc•ci** (dip′lō-kok′ŭs, dip′lō-kok′sī) spherical or ovoid bacterial cells joined together in pairs. [diplo- + G. *kokkos,* berry]

**dip•lo•co•ria** (dip-lō-kō′rē-ă) the occurrence of two pupils in the eye. SYN dicoria. [diplo- + G. *korē,* pupil]

**dip•lo•gen•e•sis** (dip-lō-jen′ĕ-sis) production of a double fetus or of one with some parts doubled. [diplo- + G. *genesis,* production]

**di•plo•ic vein** one of the veins in the diploë of the cranial bones, connected with the cerebral sinuses by emissary veins; the main diploic veins are the frontal, anterior temporal, posterior temporal, and occipital. SYN Dupuytren canal.

**dip•loid** (dip′loyd) denoting the state of a cell containing two haploid sets derived from the father and from the mother respectively; the normal chromosome complement of somatic cells (in humans, 46 chromosomes). [diplo- + G. *eidos* resemblance]

**dip•lo•my•e•lia** (dip-lō-mī-ē′lē-ă) complete or incomplete doubling of the spinal cord; may be accompanied by a bony septum of the vertebral canal. [diplo- + G. *myelon,* marrow]

**dip•lo•ne•ma** (dip-lō-nē′mă) the doubled form of the chromosome strand visible at the diplotene stage of meiosis. [diplo- + G. *nēma,* thread]

**dip•lop•a•gus** (dip-lop′ă-gŭs) general term for conjoined twins, each with fairly complete bodies, although one or more internal organs may be in common. SEE conjoined twins. [diplo- + G. *pagos,* something fixed]

**dip•lo•pho•nia** (dĭp-lō-fō′nē-ă) vibration of both the ventricular folds and the vocal folds, producing two simultaneous voice tones. [diplo- + -phonia]

**dip•lo•pia** (di-plō′pē-ă) the condition in which a single object is perceived as two objects. SYN double vision. [diplo- + G. *ōps,* eye]

**dip•lo•some** (dip′lō-sōm) paired allosomes; the

pair of centrioles of mammalian cells. [diplo- + G. *sōma*, body]

**dip•lo•so•mia** (dip-lō-sō′mē-ă) condition in which twins who seem functionally independent are joined at one or more points. SEE conjoined twins. [diplo- + G. *sōma*, body]

**dip•lo•tene** (dip′lō-tēn) the late stage of prophase in meiosis in which the paired homologous chromosomes begin to repel each other and move apart. [diplo- + G. *tainia*, band]

**di•po•lar i•ons** ions possessing both a negative charge and a positive charge, each localized at a different point in the molecule, which thus has both positive and negative "poles." SYN zwitterions.

**di•pole** a pair of separated electrical charges, one or more positive and one or more negative; or a pair of separated partial charges. SYN doublet (2).

**dip•se•sis** (dip-sē′sis) an abnormal or excessive thirst, or a craving for unusual forms of drink. SYN dipsosis. [G. *dipseō*, to thirst]

**dip•so•ma•nia** (dip-sō-mā′nē-ă) a recurring compulsion to drink alcoholic beverages to excess. SEE alcoholism. [G. *dipsa*, thirst, + *mania*, madness]

**dip•so•sis** (dip-sō′sis) SYN dipsesis. [G. *dipsa*, thirst, + -*osis*, condition]

**dip•so•ther•a•py** (dip′sō-thār′ă-pē) treatment of certain diseases by abstention, as far as possible, from liquids.

**dip•stick** a strip of plastic or paper bearing one or more dots or squares of reagent, used to perform qualitative or semiquantitative tests on urine; results of tests are read as color changes.

**Dip•tera** (dip′ter-ă) an important order of insects (the two-wing flies and gnats), including many significant disease vectors such as the mosquito, tsetse fly, sandfly, and biting midge. [G. *di-*, two, + *pteron*, wing]

**dip•ter•an** (dip′ter-an) denoting insects of the order Diptera.

**dip•ter•ous** (dip′ter-ŭs) relating to or characteristic of the order Diptera.

**dip•y•li•di•a•sis** (dip′i-li-dī′ă-sis) infection of carnivores and man with the cestode *Dipylidium caninum.*

**Dip•y•lid•i•um ca•ni•num** (dip-ĭ-lid′ē-ŭm kā-nī′nŭm) the commonest species of dog tapeworm, the double-pored tapeworm, the larvae of which are harbored by dog fleas or lice; the worm occasionally infects humans. [G. *dipylos*, with two entrances; L. ntr. of *caninus*, pertaining to *canis*, dog]

**dir-** SEE dif-.

**di•rect cal•o•rim•e•try** measurement of the heat produced by a reaction, as distinguished from measurement of something other than heat production.

**di•rect Coombs test** (koomz) a test for detecting sensitized erythrocytes in erythroblastosis fetalis and in cases of acquired immune hemolytic anemia: the patient's erythrocytes are washed with saline to remove serum and unattached antibody protein, then incubated with Coombs anti-human globulin (usually serum from a rabbit or goat previously immunized with human globulin); after incubation, the system is centrifuged and examined for agglutination, which indicates the presence of so-called incomplete or univalent antibodies on the surface of the erythrocytes.

**di•rect cur•rent (DC)** a current that flows only in one direction; e.g., that derived from a battery; sometimes referred to as galvanic current.

**di•rect flap** a flap raised completely and transferred at the same stage. SYN immediate flap.

**di•rect frac•ture** a fracture, especially of the skull, occurring at the point of injury.

**di•rect im•mu•no•fluor•es•cence** fluorescence microscopy of tissue from lesions after application of labeled antibody. SEE ALSO fluorescent antibody technique.

**di•rec•tion•al pre•pon•der•ance** a right or left predominance of nystagmus calculated from the responses to the binaural, bithermal caloric test.

**di•rec•tion•al weak•ness** a right or left decrement of nystagmus, calculated from the responses to the binaural, bithermal caloric test.

**di•rect lar•yn•gos•co•py** inspection of the larynx by means of either a rigid, hollow instrument or a fiberoptic cable.

**direct medical control** medical control provided directly to a prehospital provider by a physician or authorized health care provider; usually provided via the Emergency Medical Service radio system base station.

**di•rect nu•cle•ar di•vi•sion** SYN amitosis.

**di•rect oph•thal•mo•scope** an instrument designed to visualize the interior of the eye, with the instrument relatively close to the subject's eye and the observer viewing an upright magnified image.

**di•rec•tor** (dī-rek′ter) **1.** a smoothly grooved instrument used with a knife to limit the incision of tissues. SYN staff (2). **2.** the head of a service or specialty division. [L. *dirigo*, pp. -*rectus*, to arrange, set in order]

**di•rect re•act•ing bil•i•ru•bin** the fraction of serum bilirubin which has been conjugated with glucuronic acid in the liver cell to form bilirubin diglucuronide; so called because it reacts directly with the Ehrlich diazo reagent; increased levels are found in hepatobiliary diseases, especially of the obstructive variety.

**di•rect trans•fu•sion** transfusion of blood from the donor to the recipient, either through a tube connecting their blood or by suturing the vessels together. SYN immediate transfusion.

**di•rect vi•sion** SYN central vision.

**di•rect wet mount ex•am•i•na•tion** microscopic review at low (100×) and high dry (400×) total magnifications of saline and fresh fecal specimen to detect parasites, including motile protozoan trophozoites.

**dir. prop.** L. *direction propria*, with proper direction.

**dirt-eat•ing** SYN geophagia.

△**dis-** in two, apart; un-, not; very. Cf. dys-. [L. separation]

**dis•a•bil•i•ty** (dis-ă-bil′i-tē) **1.** any restriction or lack of ability to perform an activity in a manner or within the range considered normal for a human being. **2.** an impairment or defect of one or more organs or members.

**dis•a•bil•i•ty-ad•just•ed life years (DALYs)** a measure of the burden of disease on a defined population, based on adjustment of life expectancy to allow for long-term disability as estimated from official statistics. SEE ALSO global burden of disease.

**di•sac•cha•ride** (dī-sak′ă-rīd) a condensation product of two monosaccharides by elimination of water.

**dis·ag·gre·ga·tion** (dis'ag-grĕ-gā'shŭn) **1.** a breaking up into component parts. **2.** an inability to coordinate various sensations and failure to comprehend their mutual relations. [L. *dis-*, separating, + *ag- grego* (*adg-*), pp. *-gregatus*, to add to something]

**dis·ar·tic·u·la·tion** (dis-ar-tik-yu-lā'shŭn) amputation of a limb through a joint, without cutting of bone. SYN exarticulation. [L. *dis-*, apart, + *articulus*, joint]

**dis·as·so·ci·a·tion** (dis'ă-sō-sē-ā'shŭn) SYN dissociation (1).

**disc** (disk) SEE disk.

**dis·charge** (dis'charj) **1.** that which is emitted or evacuated, as an excretion or a secretion. **2.** the activation or firing of a neuron.

**dis·chro·na·tion** (dis-krō-nā'shŭn) a disturbance in the consciousness of time. [L. *dis-*, apart, + G. *chronos*, time]

**dis·ci** (dis'kī) plural of discus.

**dis·ci·form** (dis'ki-fōrm) disk-shaped.

**dis·ci·form de·gen·er·a·tion** subretinal neovascularization with retinal separation and hemorrhage leading finally to a circular mass of fibrous tissue with marked loss of visual acuity.

**dis·ci·form ker·a·ti·tis** large disk-shaped infiltration of the central or paracentral corneal stroma. This lesion is deep and nonsuppurative and is seen in virus infections, particularly herpetic.

**dis·cis·sion** (di-sish'ŭn) **1.** incision or cutting through a part. **2.** OPHTHALMOLOGY opening of the capsule and breaking up of the cortex of the lens with a needle knife or laser. [L. *di- scindo*, pp. *-scissus*, to tear asunder]

**dis·clos·ing a·gent** selective dye in solution, tablet, or lozenge form used to visualize and identify bacterial plaque on the surfaces of the teeth.

**dis·clos·ing so·lu·tion** a solution that selectively stains all soft debris, pellicle, and bacterial plaque on teeth; used as an aid in identifying bacterial plaque.

**dis·coid** (dis'koyd) **1.** resembling a disk. **2.** DENTISTRY an excavating or carving instrument having a circular blade with a cutting edge around the periphery. [disco- + G. *eidos*, appearance]

**dis·coid lu·pus er·y·the·ma·to·sus** a form of lupus erythematosus in which cutaneous lesions appear on the face and and elsewhere; these are atrophic plaques with erythema, hyperkeratosis, follicular plugging, and telangiectasia.

**dis·con·tin·u·a·tion test** a test to determine whether a certain drug is responsible for a reaction by observation of a remission of symptoms following cessation of its use.

**dis·co·pla·cen·ta** (dis-kō-pla-sen'tă) a placenta of discoid shape.

**dis·cor·dance** (dis-kōr'dans) dissociation of two characteristics in the members of a sample from a population; used as a measure of dependence. Cf. concordance.

**dis·cor·dant al·ter·nans** presence of right ventricular and pulmonary artery alternans with peripheral pulsus alternans, but with the strong beat of the right ventricle coinciding with the weak beat of the left and vice versa.

**dis·cor·dant al·ter·na·tion** alternation in cardiac activities of either the systemic or the pulmonary circulation, but not of both, or in both but oppositely directed in each.

**dis·cor·dant chan·ges e·lec·tro·car·di·o··gram** the presence of more than one waveform change, each in a different direction (polarity).

**dis·crete** (dis-krēt') separate; distinct; not joined to or incorporated with another; denoting especially certain lesions of the skin. [L. *dis- cerno*, pp. *-cretus*, to separate]

**dis·crete a·na·ly·zer** an automated chemical analyzer in which the instrument performs tests on samples that are kept in discrete containers in contrast to a continuous flow analyzer.

**dis·crim·i·nant stim·u·lus** a stimulus which can be differentiated from all other stimulus in the environment because it has been, and continues to serve as, an indicator of a potential reinforcer.

**dis·crim·i·na·tion** (dis'krim-i-nā'shŭn) the capacity or act of distinguishing between different things; the ability to perceive different things as different, or to repond to them differently. [L. *discrimino*, pp. *-atus*, to separate]

**dis·cri·mi·na·tion score** the percentage of words that a subject can repeat correctly from a list of phonetically balanced words presented at 25–40 dB above the speech reception threshold.

**dis·cus**, pl. **dis·ci** (dis'kŭs, dis'kī) [TA] SYN lamella (2). [L. fr. G. *diskos*, a quoit, disk]

**dis·cus ner·vi op·ti·ci** [TA] SYN optic disk.

**dis·ease** (di-zēz') **1.** an interruption, cessation, or disorder of body functions, systems, or organs. SYN illness, morbus, sickness. **2.** a morbid entity characterized usually by at least two of these criteria: recognized etiologic agent(s), identifiable group of signs and symptoms, or consistent anatomical alterations. SEE ALSO syndrome. **3.** literally, dis-ease, the opposite of ease. [Eng. *dis- priv.* + ease]

**dis·ease de·ter·mi·nants** any variables that directly or indirectly influence the frequency of occurrence and/or the distribution of any given disease; these include specific disease agents, host characteristics, and environmental factors.

**dis·ease-mod·i·fy·ing an·ti·rheu·ma·tic drugs (DMARD)** agents that apparently alter the course and progression of rheumatoid arthritis, as opposed to more rapidly acting substances that suppress inflammation and decrease pain, but do not prevent cartilage or bone erosion or progressive disability.

**dis·en·gage·ment** (dis-en-gāj'ment) **1.** the act of setting free or extricating; in childbirth, the emergence of the head from the vulva. **2.** ascent of the presenting part from the pelvis after the inlet has been negotiated. [Fr.]

**dis·e·qui·lib·ri·um** (dis-ē'kwi-lib'rē-ŭm) a disturbance or absence of equilibrium.

**dis·flu·en·cy** SYN dysfluency.

**dis·flu·ent** (dis-floo'ent) relating to disfluency.

**dis·ger·mi·no·ma** (dis-jer-mi-nō'mă) SYN dysgerminoma.

**dis·im·pac·tion** (dis'im-pak'shŭn) **1.** separation of impaction in a fractured bone. **2.** removal of impacted feces, usually manually.

**dis·in·fect** (dis-in-fekt') to destroy pathogenic microorganisms in or on any substance or to inhibit their growth and vital activity.

**dis·in·fec·tant** (dis-in-fek'tănt) **1.** capable of destroying pathogenic microorganisms or inhibiting their growth. **2.** an agent that possesses this property.

**dis·in·fec·tion** (dis-in-fek'shŭn) destruction of pathogenic microorganisms or their toxins or vectors by direct exposure to chemical or physical agents.

**dis·in·te·gra·tion** (dis-in-tĕ-grā'shŭn) **1.** loss or separation of the component parts of a substance, as in catabolism or decay. **2.** disorganization of psychic and behavioral processes. [dis- + L. *integer*, whole, intact]

**dis·junc·tion** (dis-jŭnk'shŭn) the normal separation of pairs of chromosomes at the anaphase stage of meiosis I or II. [dis- + L. *junctio*, a joining, fr. *jungo*, pp. *junctum*, to join]

**disk 1.** A round, flat plate; any approximately flat circular structure. **2.** SYN lamella (2). **3.** in dentistry, a circular piece of thin paper or other material, coated with an abrasive substance, used for cutting and polishing teeth and fillings. [L. *discus*; G. *diskos*, a quoit, disk]

**disk·ec·to·my** (dis-kek'tō-mē) excision, in part or whole, of an intervertebral disk. SYN diskotomy. [disco- + G. *ektomē*, excision]

**disk e·lec·tro·pho·re·sis** a modification of gel electrophoresis in which a discontinuity (pH, gel pore size) is introduced near the origin to produce a lamina (disk) of the materials being separated; the separating bands retain their discoid shape as they move through the gel.

**disk her·ni·a·tion** extension of disk material beyond the posterior anulus fibrosus and posterior longitudinal ligament and into the spinal canal.

**dis·ki·tis** (dis-kī'tis) nonbacterial inflammation of an intervertebral disk or disk space.

△**dis·ko-** a disk; disk-shaped. [G. *diskos*]

**dis·ko·gen·ic** (dis'kō-gen'ik) denoting a disorder originating in or from an intervertebral disk. [disco- + G. *genesis*, origin]

**dis·kop·a·thy** (dis-kop'ă-thē) disease of a disk, particularly of an invertebral disk. [disco- + G. *pathos*, disease]

**dis·kot·o·my** (dis-kot'ō-mē) SYN diskectomy. [disco- + G. *tomē*, incision]

**disk syn·drome** a constellation of symptoms and signs, including pain, paresthesias, sensory loss, weakness, and impaired reflexes, due to a compressive radiculopathy caused by intervertebral disk pressure.

**dis·lo·cate** (dis'lō-kāt) to luxate; to put out of joint.

▣**dis·lo·ca·tion** (dis-lō-kā'shŭn) displacement of an organ or any part; specifically a disturbance or disarrangement of the normal relation of the bones entering into the formation of a joint. See this page. SYN luxation (1). [L. *dislocatio*, fr. *dis-*, apart, + *locatio*, a placing]

**dis·lo·ca·tion frac·ture** a fracture of a bone near an articulation with its concomitant dislocation from that joint.

**dis·mem·ber** (dis-mem'ber) to amputate an arm or leg.

**dis·mu·tase** (dis'myu-tās) generic name for enzymes catalyzing the reaction of two identical molecules to produce two molecules in differing states of oxidation or phosphorylation.

**dis·or·der** (dis-ōr'der) a disturbance of function, structure, or both, resulting from a genetic or embryologic failure in development or from exogenous factors such as poison, trauma, or disease.

**dis·or·ga·ni·za·tion** (dis-ōr'gan-i-zā'shŭn) destruction of an organ or tissue with consequent loss of function.

**dis·or·ga·nized schiz·o·phre·nia** a severe form of schizophrenia characterized by the predominance of incoherence, blunted, inappropriate or silly affect, and the absence of systematized delusions. SYN hebephrenic schizophrenia.

**dis·o·ri·en·ta·tion** (dis'ōr-ē-en-tā'shŭn) loss of the sense of familiarity with one's surroundings (time, place, and person); loss of one's bearings.

**dis·pen·sa·ry** (dis-pen'ser-ē) **1.** a physician's office, especially the office of one who dispenses

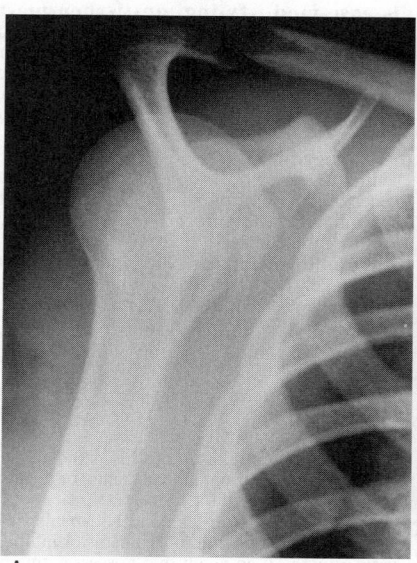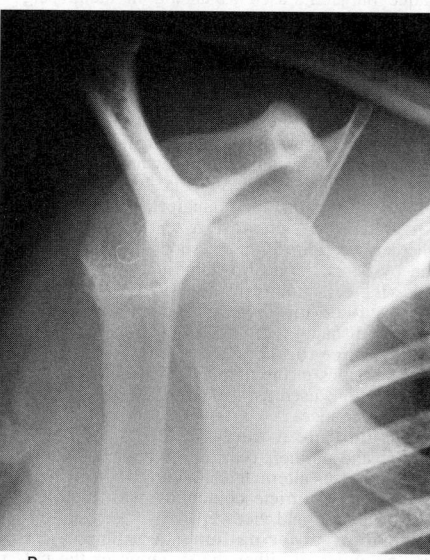

**dislocation:** (A) normal scapular view of shoulder; (B) anterior dislocation of shoulder

medicines. **2.** the office of a hospital pharmacist, where medicines are given out on physicians' orders. **3.** an outpatient department of a hospital. [L. *dis-penso,* pp. *-atus,* to distribute by weight, fr. *penso,* to weigh]

**Dis·pen·sa·to·ry** (dis-pen′să-tō-rē) a work originally intended as a commentary on the Pharmacopeia, but now more of a supplement to that work, which contains an account of the sources, mode of preparation, physiologic action, and therapeutic uses of most of the agents, official and nonofficial, used in the treatment of disease. [L. *dispensator,* a manager, steward; see dispensary]

**dis·pense** (dis-pens′) to give out medicine and other necessities to the sick; to fill a medical prescription.

**dis·perse** (dis-pers′) to dissipate, to cause disappearance of, to scatter, to dilute.

**dis·per·sion** (dis-per′zhŭn) **1.** the act of dispersing or of being dispersed. **2.** incorporation of the particles of one substance into the mass of another, including solutions, suspensions, and colloidal dispersions (solutions). **3.** specifically, what is usually called a colloidal solution. **4.** the extent or degree in which values of a statistical frequency distribution are scattered about a mean or median value. [L. *dispersio*]

**dis·per·sion me·di·um** SYN external phase.

**di·spi·reme** (dī-spī′rēm) the double chromatin skein in the telophase of mitosis. [G. *di-,* twice, + *speirēma,* coil, convolution]

**dis·placed frac·ture** a fracture in which the fragments are separated and are not in alignment.

**dis·place·ment** (dis-plās′ment) **1.** removal from the normal location or position. **2.** the adding to a fluid (particularly a gas) in an open vessel one of greater density whereby the first is expelled. **3.** CHEMISTRY a change in which one element, radical, or molecule is replaced by another, or in which one element exchanges electric charges with another by reduction or oxidation. **4.** PSYCHIATRY the transfer of impulses from one expression to another, as from fighting to talking.

**dis·po·si·tion** followup list detailed in the health care record, after initial episode of care, of services and treatments to be provided to the patient.

**dis·pro·por·tion** (dis-prō-pōr′shŭn) lack of proportion or symmetry.

**dis·sect** (di-sekt′) **1.** to cut apart or separate the tissues of the body for study. **2.** SURGERY to separate structures along natural lines or planes of cleavage. [L. *dis-seco,* pp. *-sectus,* to cut asunder]

**dis·sect·ing an·eu·rysm** splitting or dissection of an arterial wall by blood entering through an intimal tear or by interstitial hemorrhage; more common in the aorta.

**dis·sect·ing cel·lu·li·tis** a chronic dissecting folliculitis of the scalp.

**dis·sec·tion** (di-sek′shŭn) the act of dissecting. SYN anatomy (3), necrotomy (1).

**dis·sec·tion tu·ber·cle** SYN postmortem wart.

**dis·sec·tor** (dis-ek′ter) **1.** one who dissects. **2.** a written guide for dissection. **3.** instrument for dissecting.

**dis·sem·i·nat·ed** (di-sem′i-nā-ted) widely scattered throughout an organ, tissue, or the body. [L. *dis-semino,* pp. *-atus,* to scatter seed, fr. *semen* (*-min-*), seed]

**dis·sem·i·nated coc·cid·i·oi·do·my·co·sis** a se-

vere, chronic, and progressive form of coccidioidomycosis with spread from the lung to other organs. Patients with this disease are usually significantly immunocompromised.

**dis·sem·i·nat·ed in·tra·vas·cu·lar co·ag·u·la·tion (DIC)** a hemorrhagic syndrome that occurs following the uncontrolled activation of clotting factors and fibrinolytic enzymes throughout small blood vessels; fibrin is deposited, platelets and clotting factors are consumed, and fibrin degradation products inhibit fibrin polymerization, resulting in tissue necrosis and bleeding. SEE ALSO consumption coagulopathy.

**dis·sem·i·nat·ed lu·pus er·y·the·ma·to·sus** SYN systemic lupus erythematosus.

**dis·sem·i·nat·ed tu·ber·cu·lo·sis** SYN acute tuberculosis.

**dis·sim·u·la·tion** (di-sim-yu-lā′shŭn) concealment of the truth about a situation, especially about a state of health or during a mental status examination, as by a malingerer or someone with a factitious disorder. [L. *dissimulatio,* fr. *dissimulo,* to feign, fr. *dis,* apart, + *simillis,* same]

**dis·so·ci·at·ed an·es·the·sia** loss of some types of sensation with persistence of others; most often used in context of nerve blocks, wherein a loss of sensation for pain and temperature occurs without loss of tactile sense.

**dis·so·ci·at·ed hor·i·zon·tal de·vi·a·tion** a tendency often associated with repaired congenital esotropia in which an eye abducts when it is covered, in violation of Hering law.

**dis·so·ci·at·ed nys·tag·mus** a nystagmus in which the movements of the two eyes are dissimilar in direction, amplitude, and periodicity.

**dis·so·ci·at·ed ver·ti·cal de·vi·a·tion** a tendency often associated with congenital esotropia, in which an eye elevates, abducts, and extorts when covered, in violation of Hering law.

**dis·so·ci·a·tion** (di-sō-shē-ā′shŭn) **1.** separation, or a dissolution of relations. SYN disassociation. **2.** the change of a complex chemical compound into a simpler one by any lytic reaction, by ionization, by heterolysis, or by homolysis. **3.** an unconscious separation of a group of mental processes from the rest, resulting in an independent functioning of these processes and a loss of the usual associations; for example, a separation of affect from cognition. SEE multiple personality. **4.** a state used as an essential part of a technique for healing in psychology and psychotherapy, for instance in hypnotherapy or the neurolinguistic programming technique of time-line therapy. SEE ALSO Time-Line therapy. **5.** the translocation between a large chromosome and a small supernumerary one. **6.** separation of the nuclear components of a heterokaryotic dikaryon. [L. *dis-socio,* pp. *-atus,* to disjoin, separate, fr. *socius,* partner, ally]

**dis·so·ci·a·tion move·ment** ability to differentiate movements among the various parts of the body.

**dis·so·ci·a·tion sen·si·bil·i·ty** the loss of the pain and the thermal senses with preservation of tactile sensibility or vice versa.

**dis·so·ci·a·tive an·es·the·sia** a form of general anesthesia, but not necessarily complete unconsciousness, characterized by catalepsy, catatonia, and amnesia, especially that produced by phenylcyclohexylamine compounds, including ketamine.

d
i

**dis·so·ci·a·tive iden·ti·ty dis·or·der** a disorder in which two or more distinct conscious personalities alternately prevail in the same person, sometimes without any one personality being aware of the other(s).

**dis·so·ci·a·tive re·ac·tion** reaction characterized by such dissociative behavior as amnesia, fugues, sleepwalking, and dream states.

**dis·solve** (di-zolv′) to change or cause to change from a solid to a dispersed form by immersion in a fluid of suitable properties. [L. *dis-solvo,* pp. *-solutus,* to loose asunder, to dissolve]

**dis·so·nance** (dis′ō-năns) SOCIAL PSYCHOLOGY an aversive state which arises when an individual is minimally aware of internal inconsistency or conflict. [L. *dissonus,* discordant, confused]

**dis·tad** (dis′tad) toward the periphery; in a distal direction.

**dis·tal** (dis′tăl) **1.** situated away from the center of the body, or from the point of origin; specifically applied to the extremity or distant part of a limb or organ. **2.** DENTISTRY away from the median sagittal plane of the face, following the curvature of the dental arch. See page APP 89. SYN distalis. [L. *distalis*]

**dis·tal an·gle** the angle formed by the meeting of the distal with the labial (or buccal) or lingual surface of a tooth.

**dis·tal end** the posterior extremity of a dental appliance. SYN heel (2).

**dis·tal il·e·i·tis, re·gion·al il·e·i·tis, ter·mi·nal il·e·i·tis** SYN regional enteritis.

**dis·tal in·tes·ti·nal ob·struc·tive syn·drome** a syndrome seen in cystic fibrosis secondary to impaction with feces and inspissated mucus.

**dis·ta·lis** (dis-tā′lis) SYN distal.

**dis·tal oc·clu·sion 1.** a tooth occluding in a position distal to normal; SYN retrusive occlusion (2). **2.** SYN distocclusion.

**distal sple·no·re·nal shunt** anastomosis of the splenic vein to the left renal vein, usually end-to-side, for control of portal hypertension.

**dis·tance** (dis′tans) the measure of space between two objects. [L. *distantia,* fr. *di-sto,* to stand apart, be distant]

**dis·tant flap** a flap in which the donor site is distant from the recipient area.

**dis·ten·tion, dis·ten·sion** (dis-ten′shŭn) the act or state of being distended or stretched. SEE ALSO dilation. [L. *dis-tendo,* to stretch apart]

**dis·til·late** (dis′ti-lāt) the product of distillation.

**dis·til·la·tion** (dis-ti-lā′shŭn) volatilization of a liquid by heat and subsequent condensation of the vapor; a means of separating the volatile from the nonvolatile, or the more volatile from the less volatile, part of a liquid mixture. [L. *de-(di-)stillo,* pp. *-atus,* to drop down]

**dis·to·buc·cal** (dis-tō-bŭk′kăl) relating to the distal and buccal surfaces of a tooth; denoting the angle formed by their junction.

**dis·to·buc·co·oc·clu·sal** (dis′tō-bŭk′ŏ-ō-kloo′săl) relating to the distal, buccal, and occlusal surfaces of a premolar or molar tooth; denoting especially the angle formed by the junction of these surfaces.

**dis·to·buc·co·pul·pal** (dis′tō-bŭk′ō-pŭl′păl) relating to the point (trihedral) angle formed by the junction of a distal, buccal, and pulpal wall of a cavity.

**dis·to·cer·vi·cal** (dis-tō-ser′vi-kăl) relating to the line angle formed by the junction of the distal and cervical (gingival) walls of a class V cavity.

**dis·to·clu·sal** (dis-tō-kloo′săl) **1.** relating to or characterized by distoclusion. **2.** denoting a compound cavity or restoration involving the distal and occlusal surfaces of a tooth. **3.** denoting the line angle formed by the distal and occlusal walls of a class V cavity.

**dis·to·clu·sion** (dis-tō-kloo′zhŭn) a malocclusion in which the mandibular arch articulates with the maxillary arch in a position distal to normal; in Angle classification, a Class II malocclusion. SYN distal occlusion (2).

**dis·to·gin·gi·val** (dis-tō-jin′ji-văl) relating to the junction of the distal and gingival walls of a tooth cavity.

**dis·to·in·ci·sal** (dis′tō-in-sī′zăl) relating to the line (dihedral) angle formed by the junction of the distal and incisal walls of a class V cavity in an anterior tooth or formed by the distal and incisal surfaces of a tooth.

**dis·to·la·bi·al** (dis-tō-lā′bē-ăl) relating to the distal and labial surfaces of a tooth; denoting the angle formed by their junction.

**dis·to·la·bi·o·pul·pal** (dis′tō-lā′bē-ō-pŭl′păl) relating to the point (trihedral) angle formed by the junction of distal, labial, and pulpal walls of the incisal part of a class IV (mesioincisal) cavity.

**dis·to·lin·gual** (dis-tō-ling′gwăl) relating to the distal and lingual surfaces of a tooth; denoting the angle formed by their junction.

**dis·to·lin·guo·oc·clu·sal** (dis′tō-ling′gwō-ŏ-kloo′zăl) relating to the distal, lingual, and occlusal surfaces of a bicuspid or molar tooth; denoting especially the angle formed by the junction of these surfaces.

**dis·to·mo·lar** (dis-tō-mō′lăr) a supernumerary tooth located in the region posterior to the third molar tooth.

**dis·to·pul·pal** (dis-tō-pŭl′păl) relating to the line (dihedral) angle formed by the junction of the distal and pulpal walls of a cavity.

**dis·tor·tion** (dis-tōr′shŭn) **1.** in psychiatry, a defense mechanism that helps to repress or disguise unacceptable thoughts. **2.** in dental impressions, the permanent deformation of the impression material after the registration of an imprint. **3.** a twisting out of normal shape or form. **4.** in ophthalmology, unequal magnification over a field of view. [L. *distortio,* fr. *dis-torqueo,* to wrench apart]

**dis·tor·tion ab·er·ra·tion** the faulty formation of an image arising because the magnification of the peripheral part of an object is different from that of the central part when viewed through a lens.

**dis·tor·tion-prod·uct o·to·a·cous·tic e·mis·sion** a form of evoked otoacoustic emission in which a third frequency is produced when two pure tones are used as the stimulus.

**dis·to·ver·sion** (dis′tō-ver-zhŭn) malposition of a tooth distal to normal, in a posterior direction following the curvature of the dental arch.

**dis·trac·tion** (dis-trak′shŭn) **1.** difficulty or impossibility of concentration or fixation of the mind. **2.** manipulation or traction of a limb to separate bony fragments or joint surfaces. [L. *dis-traho,* pp. *-tractus,* to pull in different directions]

**dis·trac·tion os·te·o·ge·ne·sis** a technique of inducing new bone formation by dividing a bone and applying tension through an external fixation device to lengthen the bone.

**dis•tress** (dis-tres′) mental or physical suffering or anguish. [L. *distringo*, to draw asunder]

**dis•tri•bu•tion** (dis-tri-byu′shŭn) **1.** the passage of the branches of arteries or nerves to the tissues and organs. **2.** the area in which the branches of an artery or a nerve terminate, or the area supplied by such an artery or nerve. **3.** the relative numbers of individuals in each of various categories or populations, such as in different age, sex, or occupational samples. [L. *dis-tribuo*, pp. *-tributus*, to distribute, fr. *tribus*, a tribe]

**dis•trix** (dis′triks) splitting of the hairs at their ends. [G. *dis*, twice, + *thrix*, hair]

**dis•tro•pin** SYN dystrophin.

**di•sul•fate** (dī-sŭl′fāt) a molecule containing two sulfates.

**di•sul•fide** (dī-sŭl′fīd) **1.** a molecule containing two atoms of sulfur to one of the reference element, e.g., CS$_2$, carbon disulfide. **2.** a compound containing the —S—S— group, e.g., cystine.

**di•sul•fide bond** a single bond between two sulfurs; specifically, the —S—S— link binding two peptide chains (or different parts of one peptide chain).

**DIT** diiodotyrosine.

**di•ter•penes** (dī-ter′pēnz) hydrocarbons or their derivatives containing 4 isoprene units, hence containing 20 carbon atoms and 4 branched methyl groups; e.g., vitamin A, retinene, aconitine.

**Ditt•rich plug** (dit′rik) a minute, dirty-grayish, ill-smelling mass of bacteria and fatty acid crystals in the sputum in pulmonary gangrene and fetid bronchitis.

**di•u•re•sis** (dī-yu-rē′sis) excretion of urine; commonly denotes production of unusually large volumes of urine. [G. *dia*, throughout, completely, + *ourēsis*, urination]

**di•u•ret•ic** (dī-yu-ret′ik) **1.** promoting the excretion of urine. **2.** an agent that increases the amount of urine excreted.

**di•ur•nal** (dī-er′nǎl) **1.** pertaining to the daylight hours; opposite of nocturnal. **2.** repeating once each 24 hours, e.g., a diurnal variation or a diurnal rhythm. Cf. circadian. [L. *diurnus*, of the day]

**di•va•lence, di•va•len•cy** (dī-vā′lens, dī-vā′len-sē) SYN bivalence.

**di•va•lent** (dī-vā′lent) SYN bivalent (1).

**di•var•i•ca•tion** (dī′var-i-kā′shŭn) SYN diastasis (1). [L. *divaricare*, to spread asunder]

**di•ver•gence** (dī-ver′jens) **1.** a moving or spreading apart or in different directions. **2.** the spreading of branches of the neuron to form synapses with several other neurons. [L. *di-*, apart, + *vergo*, to incline]

**di•ver•gence in•suf•fi•cien•cy** that condition in which an exophoria or exotropia is more marked for near vision than for far vision.

**di•ver•gence pa•re•sis** an esodeviation of the eyes that is greater in the distance than near, which may be a sign of central nervous system disease or a mild bilateral sixth nerve palsy.

**di•ver•gent** (dī-ver′jent) moving in different directions; radiating.

**di•ver•gent stra•bis•mus** SYN exotropia.

**di•ver•sion** the process of rerouting an ambulance to another facility other than the closest appropriate facility.

**di•ver•tic•u•la** (dī-ver-tik′yu-lă) plural of diverticulum.

**di•ver•tic•u•la of co•lon** diverticula, which are herniations of mucosa and submucosa between fibers of the major muscle layer (muscularis propria) of the colon; can cause bleeding and episodes of severe inflammation.

**di•ver•tic•u•lar** (dī-ver-tik′yu-lăr) relating to a diverticulum.

**di•ver•tic•u•lec•to•my** (dī′ver-tik-yu-lek′tō-mē) excision of a diverticulum.

**di•ver•tic•u•li•tis** (dī′ver-tik-yu-lī′tis) inflammation of a diverticulum, especially of the small pockets in the wall of the colon which fill with stagnant fecal material and become inflamed; rarely, they may cause obstruction, perforation, or bleeding.

**di•ver•tic•u•lo•ma** (dī′ver-tik-yu-lō′mă) development of a granulomatous mass in the wall of the colon. [diverticulum + G. *-oma*, tumor]

**di•ver•tic•u•lo•sis** (dī′ver-tik-yu-lō′sis) presence of a number of diverticula of the intestine, common in middle age; the lesions are acquired pulsion diverticula. See page B9.

**di•ver•tic•u•lum**, pl. **di•ver•tic•u•la** (dī-ver-tik′yu-lŭm, dī-ver-tik′yu-lă) a pouch or sac opening from a tubular or saccular organ, such as the gut or bladder. [L. *deverticulum* (or *di-*), a by-road, fr. *de-verto*, to turn aside]

**div•ing goi•ter** a freely movable goiter that is sometimes above and sometimes below the sternal notch. SYN wandering goiter.

**div•ing re•flex** a reflex by which immersing the face or body in water, especially cold water, tends to cause bradycardia and peripheral vasoconstriction; relatively minor in most humans.

**di•vi•sio** SYN division.

**di•vi•sio au•to•nom•i•ca sys•tem•a•tis ner•vo•si per•i•pher•i•ci** [TA] SYN autonomic division of nervous system.

**di•vi•si•o la•ter•a•lis dex•tra he•pa•tis** [TA] SYN right lateral division of liver.

**di•vi•sio la•ter•a•lis si•nis•tra he•pa•tis** [TA] SYN left lateral division of liver.

**di•vi•sio me•di•a•lis dex•tra he•pa•tis** [TA] SYN right medial division of liver.

**di•vi•sio me•di•a•lis si•nis•tra he•pa•tis** [TA] SYN left medial division of liver.

**di•vi•sion** (di-vizh′ŭn) a separating into two or more parts. SYN divisio.

**di•vi•sion•al block** arrest of the impulse in one of the assumed two main divisions of the left branch of the bundle of His; i.e., in either the anterior (superior) division or the posterior (inferior) division.

**di•vul•sion** (di-vŭl′shŭn) **1.** removal of a part by tearing. **2.** forcible dilation of the walls of a cavity or canal.

**di•vul•sor** (di-vŭl′sĕr) an instrument for forcible dilation of the urethra or other canal or cavity.

**Dix-Hall•pike ma•neu•ver** (diks-hahl′pīk) test for eliciting paroxysmal vertigo and nystagmus in which the patient is brought from the sitting to the supine position with the head hanging over the examining table and turned to the right or left; vertigo and nystagmus are elicited when the head is rotated toward the affected ear.

**di•zy•got•ic, di•zy•gous** (dī′zī-got′ik, dī-zī′gŭs) relating to twins derived from two separate zygotes but sharing a common intrauterine environment. [G. *di-*, two, + *zygotos*, yoked together]

**di•zy•got•ic twins** twins derived from two zygotes. SYN fraternal twins, heterologous twins.

**diz•zi•ness** (diz′i-nes) imprecise term commonly used by patients in an attempt to describe various symptoms such as faintness, vertigo, disequilibrium, or unsteadiness. SEE ALSO vertigo. [A. S. *dyzig,* foolish]

**djen•kol poi•son•ing** poisoning believed to result from eating excessive amounts of a bean, *Pitecolobium lobatum;* symptoms are pain in the renal region, dysuria, and later anuria; the djenkol bean has a high vitamin B content and is used for food despite its toxic qualities.

⌂**DL-** prefix (in small capital letters) denoting a substance consisting of equal quantities of the two enantiomorphs, D and L; replaces the older *dl-* (in lower case italics) as a more exact definition of structure.

**DM** adamsite; diabetes mellitus; diastolic murmur; dopamine.

**DMARD** disease-modifying antirheumatic drugs.

**DMF caries index** an index of past caries experience that includes decayed, missing, and filled permanent teeth. DMFT is used when permanent teeth are referred to and DMFS is the index that includes the surfaces of permanent teeth.

**DN** dibucaine number.

🔳**DNA** deoxyribonucleic acid. See this page.

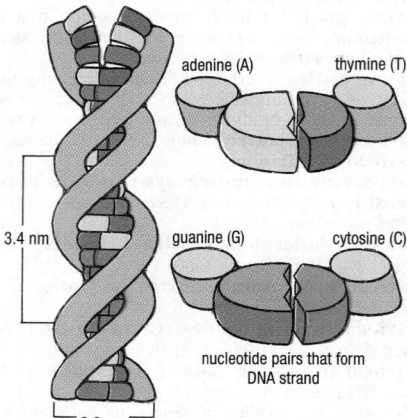

adenine (A) thymine (T)

3.4 nm guanine (G) cytosine (C)

nucleotide pairs that form DNA strand

2.0 nm

**DNA** (deoxyribonucleic acid)

**DNA fin•ger•print•ing** a technique used to compare individuals by molecular genotyping. DNA is isolated from a specific individual, digested, and fractionated according to size. A Southern hybridization with a radiolabeled repetitive DNA probe provides an autoradiographic pattern unique to the individual. DNA fingerprinting offers a statistical basis for evaluating the probability that samples of blood, hair, semen, or tissue have originated from a given individual.

**DNA he•lix** SYN Watson-Crick helix.

**DNA mar•kers** segments of chromosomal DNA known to be linked with heritable traits or diseases. Although the markers themselves do not produce the conditions, they exist in concert with the genes responsible and are passed on with them. Certain markers, restriction fragment length polymorphisms, consist of segments of

DNA that can be identified on autoradiographs (produced after digestion of the DNA by restriction enzymes and segregation of the resulting fragments through gel electrophoresis).

**DNA pol•y•mor•phism** a condition in which one of two different but normal nucleotide sequences can exist at a particular site in DNA.

**DNA-RNA hy•brid** double-stranded polynucleic acids in which one strand is DNA and the other strand is the complementary RNA; formed during transcription and during multiplication of oncogenic RNA viruses.

**DNase, DNAase** deoxyribonuclease.

**DNA vi•rus** a major group of animal viruses in which the core consists of deoxyribonucleic acid (DNA); it includes parvoviruses, papovaviruses, adenoviruses, herpesviruses, poxviruses, and other unclassified DNA viruses. SYN deoxyribovirus.

**DNR** do not resuscitate.

**Dns, DNS** dansyl.

**DOA** dead on arrival.

**doc•tor** (dok′ter) **1.** a title conferred by a university on one who has followed a prescribed course of study, or given as a title of distinction; as doctor of medicine, laws, philosophy, etc. **2.** a physician, especially one upon whom has been conferred the degree of M.D. by a university or medical school. [L. a teacher, fr. *doceo,* pp. *doctus,* to teach]

**Döderlein ba•cil•lus** (dĕr′der-līn) a large, Gram-positive bacterium occurring in normal vaginal secretions; thought by some to be identical with *Lactobacillus acidophilus.*

**dol** (dōl) a unit measure of pain. [L. *dolor,* pain]

⌂**dol•i•cho-** Long. [G. *dolichos*]

**dol•i•cho•ce•phal•ic, dol•i•cho•ceph•a•lous** (dol-i-kō-sĕ-fal′ik, dol-i-kō-sef′ă-lŭs) having a disproportionately long head; denoting a skull with a cephalic index below 75. [dolicho- + G. *kephalē,* head]

**dol•i•cho•fa•cial** (dol-i-kō-fā′shăl) SYN dolichoprosopic.

**dol•i•chol** (dol′i-kol) polyisoprenes in which the terminal member is saturated and oxidized to an alcohol, usually phosphorylated and often glycosylated; found in endoplasmic reticulum, but not in mitochondrial or plasma membranes; urinary levels are elevated in disorders exhibiting abnormal skin, rectal, or brain profiles in electron microscopy of biopsies.

**dol•i•cho•pel•ic, dol•i•cho•pel•vic** (dol-i-kō-pel′ik, dol-i-kō-pel′vik) having a disproportionately long pelvis; denoting a pelvis with a pelvic index above 95. [dolicho- + G. *pellis,* bowl (pelvis)]

**dol•i•cho•pel•ic pel•vis** a pelvis in which the anteroposterior diameter is longer than the transverse.

**dol•i•cho•pro•sop•ic, dol•i•cho•pro•so•pous** (dol-i-kō-pros-ō′pik, dol-i-kō-pros′ō-pŭs) having a disproportionately long face. SYN dolichofacial. [dolicho- + G. *prosōpikos,* facial]

**doll's eye sign** reflex movement of the eyes in the opposite direction to that in which the head is moved, e.g., the eyes being lowered as the head is raised, and the reverse (Cantelli sign); an indication of functional integrity of the brainstem tegmental pathways and cranial nerves involved in eye movement.

**do•lor** (dō′lōr) pain, as one of the four signs of

inflammation (d., calor, rubor, tumor) enunciated by Celsus. [L.]

**do·lo·rif·ic** (dō-lōr-if'ik) pain-producing.

**do·lo·rim·e·try** (dō-lō-rim'ĕ-trē) the measurement of pain. [L. *dolor,* pain, + G. *metron,* measure]

**do·main** (dō-mān') **1.** homologous unit of approximately 110–120 amino acids, groups of which make up the light and heavy chains of the immunoglobulin molecule; each serves a specific function. The light chain has two domains, one in the variable region and one in the constant region of the chain; the heavy chain has four to five domains, depending upon the class of immunoglobulin, one in the variable region and the remaining ones in the constant region. **2.** a region of a protein having some distinctive physical feature or role. **3.** an independently folded, globular structure composed of one section of a polypeptide chain. A domain may interact with another domain; it may be associated with a particular function. Domains can vary in size. [Fr. *domaine,* fr. L. *dominium,* property, dominion]

**do·mes·tic vi·o·lence** intentionally inflicted injury perpetrated by and on family member(s); varieties include spouse abuse, child abuse, and sexual abuse, including incest. Various kinds of abuse, such as sexual abuse, also happen outside of the family unit.

**dom·i·cil·i·at·ed** (dō-mi-sil'ē-āt-ed) a state of close association of an organism within human abodes or activities, such that partial domestication results, leading to the organism's dependence on continued association with the human environment; this frequently results in the domiciliated organism becoming a noxious pest, a vector, or an intermediate host of human disease. [L. *domicilium,* a dwelling]

**dom·i·nance** (dom'i-nans) the state of being dominant.

**dom·i·nance of traits** an expression of the apparent physiologic relationship existing between two or more genes that may occupy the same chromosomal locus (alleles). At a specific locus there are three possible combinations of two allelic genes, *A* and *a*: two homozygous (*AA* and *aa*) and one heterozygous (*Aa*). If a heterozygous individual presents only the hereditary characteristic determined by gene *A*, but not *a*, *A* is said to be dominant and *a* recessive; in this case, *AA* and *Aa*, although genotypically distinct, should be phenotypically indistinguishable. If *AA*, *Aa*, and *aa* are distinguishable, each from the others, *A* and *a* are codominant.

**dom·i·nant** (dom'i-nant) **1.** ruling or controlling. **2.** in genetics, denoting an allele possessed by one of the parents of a hybrid which is expressed in the latter to the exclusion of a contrasting allele (the recessive) from the other parent. [L. *dominans,* pres. p. of *dominor,* to rule, fr. *dominus,* lord, master, fr. *domus,* house]

**dom·i·nant char·ac·ter** an inherited character expressed in either the homozygous or heterozygous state. SEE phenotype.

**dom·i·nant eye** the eye that is customarily used for monocular tasks.

**dom·i·nant gene** SEE dominance of traits.

**dom·i·nant hem·i·sphere** that cerebral hemisphere containing the representation of speech and controlling the arm and leg used preferentially in skilled movements; usually the left hemisphere.

**dom·i·nant i·dea** an idea that governs all one's actions and thoughts.

**dom·i·nant in·her·i·tance** SEE dominance of traits.

**dom·i·nant op·tic at·ro·phy** an autosomal dominant bilateral optic neuropathy characterized by insidious preschool vision loss. SYN Kjer optic atrophy.

**dom·i·nant trait** an outstanding mental or physical characteristic; SEE dominance of traits.

**DOMS** delayed onset muscle soreness.

**Do·nath-Land·stein·er an·ti·bo·dy** (dō'nath-lahnd'shtī-nĕr) an IgG antibody associated with paroxysmal cold hemoglobinuria. The antibody is biphasic, reacting with erythrocytes at temperatures below 15° C, which fixes complement to the cell membrane. Upon warming to body temperature, the antibody detaches, but the terminal complement components are activated on the cell membrane, causing hemolysis. SEE ALSO hemoglobinuria.

**Do·nath-Land·stei·ner phe·nom·e·non** (dō'nath-lahnd'shtī-nĕr) the hemolysis which results in a sample of blood of a subject with paroxysmal hemoglobinuria when the sample is cooled to around 5°C and then warmed again.

**Don·ders law** (don'dĕrz) the rotation of the eyeball is determined by the distance of the object from the median plane and the line of the horizon.

**Don Juan** (don hwahn) PSYCHIATRY a term used to denote males with compulsive sexual or romantic overactivity, usually with a succession of female partners. [legendary Spanish nobleman]

**do·nor** (dō'ner) **1.** an individual from whom blood, tissue, or an organ is taken for transplantation. **2.** a compound that will transfer an atom or a radical to an acceptor. **3.** an atom that readily yields electrons to an acceptor. [L. *dono,* pp. *donatus,* to donate, to give]

**Don·o·van bod·ies** (don'ĕ-văn) clusters of blue or black staining, bipolar chromatin condensations in large mononuclear cells in granulation tissue infected with *Calymmatobacterium granulomatis.*

**don·o·va·no·sis** (don'ō-vă-nō'sis) SYN granuloma inguinale.

**Do·pa, DO·PA, Do·pa** (dō'pă) an intermediate in the catabolism of L-phenylalanine and L-tyrosine, and in the biosynthesis of norepinephrine, epinephrine, and melanin; the L form, levodopa, is biologically active.

**do·pa·mine (DM)** (dō'pă-mēn) 3,4-dihydroxyphenylethylamine; an intermediate in tyrosine metabolism and precursor of norepinephrine and epinephrine.

**doping** (dōp'ing) the administration of foreign substances to an individual; often used in reference to athletes who try to enhance physiologic function and exercise performance.

**Dopp·ler** (dop'ler), Christian J., Austrian mathematician and physicist in U.S., 1803–1853. SEE Doppler echocardiography, Doppler effect, Doppler shift, Doppler ultrasonography.

**Dopp·ler** (dop'ler) a diagnostic instrument that emits an ultrasonic beam into the body; the ultrasound reflected from moving structures changes its frequency (Doppler effect). Of diagnostic value in peripheral vascular and cardiac disease.

d
o

**Dopp·ler co·lor flow** (dop'ler) a computer-generated color image produced by Doppler ultrasonography in which different directions of flow are represented by different hues. SEE Doppler ultrasonography.

**Dopp·ler ech·o·car·di·og·ra·phy** (dop'ler) use of Doppler ultrasonography techniques to augment two-dimensional echocardiography by allowing velocities to be registered within the echocardiographic image. SEE ALSO duplex ultrasonography, Doppler ultrasonography.

**Dopp·ler ef·fect** (dop'ler) a change in frequency observed when the sound and observer are in relative motion away from or toward each other. SEE ALSO Doppler shift.

**Dopp·ler shift** (dop'ler) the magnitude of the frequency change in hertz when sound and observer are in relative motion away from or toward each other. SEE ALSO Doppler effect.

**[i] Dopp·ler ul·tra·so·nog·ra·phy** (dop'ler) application of the Doppler effect in ultrasound to detect movement of scatterers (usually red blood cells) by the analysis of the change in frequency of the returning echoes. See this page and B10.

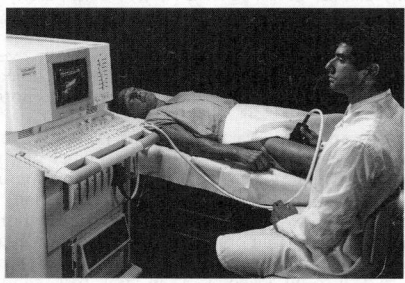

A

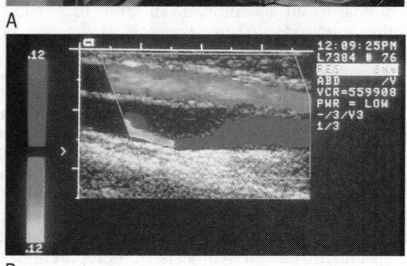

B

**Doppler ultrasonography:** (A) vascular imaging, (B) color flow Doppler showing femoral vein thrombus

**Do·rel·lo ca·nal** (dō-rel'ō) a bony canal sometimes found at the tip of the temporal bone enclosing the abducens nerve and inferior petrosal sinus as these two structures enter the cavernous sinus.

**Do·ren·dorf sign** (dōr'ĕn-dorf) fullness of one supraclavicular groove in aneurysm of the aortic arch.

**Dor fundoplication** (dōr) a partial (180°) and anterior fundoplication, popular in Europe and South America and most often used along with a myotomy for the treatment of achalasia.

**dor·sa** (dōr'să) plural of dorsum.

**dor·sad** (dor'sad) toward or in the direction of the back. [L. *dorsum,* back, + *ad,* to]

**dor·sal** (dōr'săl) **1.** pertaining to the back or any dorsum. **2.** SYN posterior (2). [Mediev. L. *dorsalis,* fr. *dorsum,* back]

**dor·sal ar·tery of clit·o·ris** one of the two terminal branches of the internal pudendal artery in the female, the other being the deep artery of the clitoris. SYN arteria dorsalis clitoridis [TA].

**dor·sal ar·tery of pe·nis** the dorsal terminal branch of the internal pudendal artery in the male. SYN arteria dorsalis penis [TA].

**dor·sal dig·i·tal ar·tery** one of the collateral digital branches of the dorsal metatarsal arteries in the foot, and/or of the dorsal metacarpal arteries in the hand.

**dor·sal dig·i·tal nerves of foot** nerves supplying the skin of the dorsal aspect of the proximal and middle phalanges of the toes. SYN nervi digitales dorsales pedis [TA].

**dor·sal dig·i·tal nerves of hand** terminal branches of the radial and ulnar nerves in the hand supplying the skin of the dorsal surface of the proximal and middle phalanges of the fingers. SYN nervi digitales dorsales manus [TA].

**dor·sal flex·ure** a flexure in the mid-dorsal region in the embryo.

**dor·sal·gia** (dōr-sal'jē-ă) pain in the upper back. [L. *dorsum,* back, + G. *algos,* pain]

**dor·sal hy·po·thal·a·mic ar·ea** a relatively small region of the hypothalamus located ventral to the hypothalamic sulcus; contains the following nuclei: portions of the dorsomedial nucleus (nucleus dorsomedialis [TA]), endopeduncular nucleus (nucleus endopeduncularis [TA]), and portions of the nucleus of the ansa lenticularis (nucleus ansae lenticularis [TA]).

**dor·sa·lis pe·dis ar·tery** continuation of anterior tibial artery after crossing ankle; *branches,* lateral tarsal, arcuate, dorsal metatarsal; *anastomosis,* lateral plantar, forms the plantar arch.

**dor·sal mid·brain syn·drome** SYN Parinaud syndrome.

**dor·sal na·sal ar·tery** *origin,* ophthalmic; external artery of the nose; *distribution,* skin of side of root of nose; *anastomoses,* angular artery. SYN external nasal artery.

**dor·sal nerve of clit·o·ris** the deep terminal branch of the pudendal, supplying especially the glans clitoridis after passing through the musculature of the urogenital diaphragm, to run along the dorsum of the clitoral shaft. SYN nervus dorsalis clitoridis [TA].

**dor·sal nerve of pe·nis** the deep terminal branch of the pudendal which runs through the urogenital diaphragm giving branches, then runs along the dorsum of the penis, supplying the skin of the penis, the prepuce, the corpora cavernosa, and the glans. SYN nervus dorsalis penis [TA].

**dor·sal nu·cle·us of thal·a·mus** one of the major subdivisions of the thalamus; the composite dorsal nucleus includes the nucleus lateralis anterior or dorsalis, nucleus lateralis intermedius, nucleus lateralis posterior, and pulvinar; together, these cell groups form most of the free dorsal surface of the posterior half of the thalamus and project to a very large region of parietal, occipitoparietal, and temporal cortex; its afferent connections are largely obscure, but the nucleus lateralis posterior and the pulvinar receive a projection from the superior colliculus.

**dor·sal nu·cle·us of va·gus nerve** the visceral motor nucleus located in the vagal trigone (ala cinerea) of the floor of the fourth ventricle. It gives rise to the parasympathetic fibers of the vagus nerve innervating the heart muscle and the smooth musculature and glands of the respiratory and intestinal tracts.

**dor·sal ra·di·o·car·pal lig·a·ment** the ligament that extends from the distal end of the radius posteriorly to the proximal row of carpal bones.

**dor·sal root** the sensory root of a spinal nerve, having a dorsal root ganglion containing the nerve cell bodies of the fibers conveyed by the root in its distal end.

**dor·sal scap·u·lar ar·tery** *origin*, subclavian or as the deep branch of the transverse cervical; *distribution*, passes deep to the rhomboid muscles, supplying them and other muscles and skin along the vertebral border of the scapula; *anastomoses*, suprascapular and scapular circumflex.

**dor·sal scap·u·lar nerve** arises from ventral primary rami of the fifth to seventh cervical nerves and passes downward to supply the levator scapulae and the rhomboideus major and minor muscles. SYN nervus dorsalis scapulae [TA].

**dor·sal scap·u·lar vein** the vena comitans of the descending scapular artery; it is a tributary to the subclavian or the external jugular vein.

**Dor·set cul·ture egg me·di·um** (dōr′set) a medium for cultivating *Mycobacterium tuberculosis;* it consists of the whites and yolks of four fresh eggs and a solution of sodium chloride.

**dor·si·flex·ion** (dōr-si-flek′shŭn) turning upward of the foot or toes or of the hand or fingers.

**dor·si·spi·nal** (dōr′si-spī′năl) relating to the vertebral column, especially to its dorsal aspect.

**dor·so·ceph·a·lad** (dōr′sō-sef′ă-lad) toward the occiput, or back of the head. [L. *dorsum*, back, + G. *kephalē*, head, + L. *ad*, to]

**dor·so·lat·er·al** (dōr-sō-lat′er-ăl) relating to the back and the side.

**dor·so·lat·er·al fas·cic·u·lus** a longitudinal bundle of thin, unmyelinated and poorly myelinated fibers capping the apex of the posterior horn of the spinal gray matter, composed of posterior root fibers and short association fibers that interconnect neighboring segments of the posterior horn.

**dor·so·lat·er·al sul·cus** SYN posterolateral sulcus.

**dor·so·lum·bar** (dōr-sō-lŭm′bar) referring to the back in the region of the lower thoracic and upper lumbar vertebrae.

**dor·so·ven·trad** (dōr-sō-ven′trad) in a direction from the dorsal to the ventral aspect.

**dor·sum**, gen. **dor·si**, pl. **dor·sa** (dōr′sŭm, dōr-sī, dōr′să) [TA] **1.** the back of the body. **2.** the upper or posterior surface, or the back, of any part. [L. back]

**dos·age** (dō′sij) **1.** the giving of medicine or other therapeutic agent in prescribed amounts. **2.** the size, frequency, and number of doses of medicine to be given. USAGE NOTE: Sometimes incorrectly used for dose. Cf. dose.

**dose** (dī′pōl) the quantity of a drug or other remedy to be taken or applied all at one time or in fractional amounts within a given period. USAGE NOTE: Sometimes incorrectly used for dosage. Cf. dosage (2). [G. *dosis*, a giving]

**dose e·qui·va·lent li·mits** radiation exposure limits for radiation workers. Will replace maximum permissible dose.

**dos·im·e·ter** (dō-sim′ĕ-ter) **1.** a device for measuring radiation, especially x-rays. **2.** in pulmonary function testing, a device, which can be triggered automatically by a sensor near the subject's mouth or manually by a technician, that allows for the delivery of a reproducible dose from a nebulizer. [G. *dosis,* dose, + *metron,* measure]

**do·sim·e·try** (dō-sim′ĕ-trē) measurement of radiation exposure, especially x-rays or gamma rays; calculation of radiation dose from internally administered radionuclides.

**dot** (dŏt) a small spot.

**dot·age** (dō′tij) the deterioration of previously intact mental powers, common in old age.

**dou·ble blind ex·per·i·ment** an experiment conducted with neither experimenter nor subjects knowing which experiment is the control; prevents bias in recording results. SEE ALSO double-masked experiment.

**dou·ble bond** a covalent bond resulting from the sharing of two pairs of electrons; e.g., $H_2C{=}CH_2$ (ethylene).

**dou·ble-chan·nel cath·e·ter** a catheter with two lumens, allowing irrigation and aspiration. SYN two-way catheter.

**dou·ble com·part·ment hy·dro·ceph·a·lus** independent supra- and infratentorial hydrocephalus usually due to a veil occlusion of the aqueduct of midbrain.

**dou·ble con·trast en·e·ma** SYN air contrast enema.

**double e·le·va·tor pal·sy** limited elevation of an eye in abduction and adduction, implying paresis of the superior rectus and inferior oblique muscles, although many cases are due to restriction of the inferior rectus muscle.

**dou·ble flap am·pu·ta·tion** amputation in which a flap is cut from the soft parts on either side of the limb.

**dou·ble he·lix** SYN Watson-Crick helix.

**dou·ble-masked ex·per·i·ment** a double-blind study conducted so that neither the subject nor the observer knows the identity of the control or variable.

**dou·ble pneu·mo·nia** lobar pneumonia involving both lungs.

**dou·ble pro·duct** the product of systolic blood pressure multiplied by the heart frequency; a measure of heart work load. SEE ALSO Robinson index.

**dou·ble re·frac·tion** the property of having more than one refractive index according to the direction of the transmitted light. SYN birefringence.

**double ring sign** two concentric rings around the optic nerve characteristic of optic nerve hypoplasia.

**dou·ble stain** a mixture of two dyes, each of which stains different portions of a tissue or cell.

**dou·blet** (dŭb′let) **1.** a combination of two lenses designed to correct the chromatic and spherical aberration. **2.** SYN dipole. **3.** any sequence of two nucleotides in a polynucleotide strand. **4.** a closely spaced pair of peaks or lines in a spectrum.

**dou·ble vi·sion** SYN diplopia.

**dou·bling time** the time it takes for the number of cells in a neoplasm to double, with shorter doubling times implying more rapid growth.

**dou·bly armed su·ture** a suture with a needle attached at both ends. SYN cobbler's suture.

**dou·bly het·er·o·zy·gous** denoting that genotype in which a parent is heterozygous at both loci, the state that on average contains the maximum information about the linkage.

**douche** (doosh) **1.** a current of water, gas, or vapor directed against a surface or projected into a cavity. **2.** an instrument for giving a douche. **3.** to apply a douche. [Fr. fr. *doucher*, to pour]

**douche bath** the local application of water in the form of a large jet or stream.

**Doug·las bag** (dŭg'lăs) a large bag in which expired gas is collected for several minutes to determine oxygen consumption in humans under conditions of actual work. [C.G. Douglas]

**dove·tail stress-bro·ken abut·ment** an abutment connected to a fixed partial denture by a nonrigid connector that is trapezoidal in cross-section.

**dow·a·ger's hump** postmenopausal cervical kyphosis of older women due to osteoporosis and compression fractures of vertebra.

**dowel graft** a circular bone graft harvested with special instruments, used in orthopedic surgery as a structural bone graft to obtain fusion between two adjacent vertebrae.

**Dow·ney cell** (down'ē) the atypical lymphocyte of infectious mononucleosis.

**down·growth** (doun-grōth) something that grows downward; the process of growing in a downward direction.

**Downs a·nal·y·sis** (downz) a series of cephalometric criteria used as an aid in orthodontic diagnosis.

**Down syn·drome** (down) a chromosomal dysgenesis syndrome consisting of a variable constellation of abnormalities caused by triplication or translocation of chromosome 21. The abnormalities include mental retardation, retarded growth, flat hypoplastic face with short nose, prominent epicanthic skin folds, small, low-set ears with prominent antihelix, fissured and thickened tongue, laxness of joint ligaments, pelvic dysplasia, broad hands and feet, stubby fingers, and transverse palmar crease. Lenticular opacities and heart disease are common. The incidence of leukemia is increased and Alzheimer disease is almost inevitable by age 40. SYN trisomy 21 syndrome.

**dox·a·cu·ri·um chlo·ride** (doks'a-koo'rē-um klō'rīd) a nondepolarizing neuromuscular blocking drug similar to pancuronium but without cardiovascular side effects.

**Doyère em·i·nence** (dwah-ēr') a slight elevation on the surface of a striated muscle corresponds to the site of the motor endplate.

**Doyle op·er·a·tion** (dōil) paracervical uterine denervation.

**DPN** diphosphopyridine nucleotide.

**DPN⁺** oxidized diphosphopyridine nucleotide.

**DPT** diphtheria-pertussis-tetanus (vaccine).

**DR** reaction of degeneration.

**dr** dram.

**dra·cun·cu·li·a·sis, dra·cun·cu·lo·sis** (dra-kŭng-kyu-lī'ă-sis, dra-kŭng-kyu-lō'sis) infection with *Dracunculus medinensis*.

***Dra·cun·cu·lus*** (dra-kŭng'kyu-lŭs) a genus of nematodes that have some resemblances to true filarial worms; however, adults are larger and the

intermediate host is a freshwater crustacean rather than an insect. [L. dim. of *draco*, serpent]

**draft 1.** a current of air in a confined space. **2.** a quantity of liquid medicine ordered as a single dose.

**drain** (drān) **1.** to remove fluid from a cavity as it forms, e.g., to drain an abscess. **2.** a device, usually in the shape of a tube or wick, for removing fluid as it collects in a cavity, especially a wound cavity. [A. S. *drehnian*, to draw off]

**drain·age** (drān'ij) continuous flow or withdrawal of fluids from a wound or other cavity.

**drain·age tube** a tube introduced into a wound or cavity to facilitate removal of a fluid.

**dram (dr)** a unit of weight: $^1/_8$ oz.; 60 gr, apothecaries' weight; $^1/_{16}$ oz., avoirdupois weight. Cf. fluidram. [see drachm]

**drape** (drāp) **1.** to cover parts of the body other than those to be examined or operated upon. **2.** the cloth or materials used for such cover. [M.E., fr. L.L. *drappus*, cloth]

**Dra·per law** (drā'per) a chemical change is produced in a photochemical substance only by those light rays that are absorbed by that substance.

**draw·er sign** in a knee examination, abnormal forward or backward sliding of the tibia with respect to the femur indicating laxity or tear of the anterior (forward slide) or posterior (backward slide) cruciate ligaments of the knee. SYN drawer test.

**draw·er test** SYN drawer sign.

**dream** (drēm) mental activity during sleep in which events, thought, emotions, and images are experienced as real.

**dream·y state** the semiconscious state associated with an epileptic attack.

**drep·a·no·cyte** (drep'ă-nō-sīt) SYN sickle cell. [G. *drepane*, sickle, + *kytos*, a hollow (cell)]

**drep·a·no·cyt·ic** (drep'ă-nō-sit'ik) relating to or resembling a sickle cell.

**drep·a·no·cyt·ic a·ne·mia** SYN sickle cell anemia.

**dress·ing** (dres'ing) the material applied, or the application itself of material, to a wound for protection, absorbance, drainage, etc.

**dress·ing for·ceps** a forceps for general use in dressing wounds, removing fragments of necrotic tissue, small foreign bodies, etc.

**Dress·ler beat** (dres'ler) fusion beat interrupting a ventricular tachycardia and producing a normally narrow QRS complex as a result of the fusion of two impulses, one impulse from the ventricular tachycardia and the other from a supraventricular focus; Dressler beats strongly support the diagnosis of ventricular tachycardia by interruption of it.

**Dress·ler syn·drome** (dres'ler) recurrent pericarditis following acute myocardial infarction.

**DRG** diagnosis-related group.

**DRI** Dietary Reference Intake.

**drift 1.** a gradual movement, as from an original position. **2.** a gradual change in the value of a random variable over time as a result of various factors, some random and some systematic effects of trend, manipulation, etc.

**drill-out** a drilling away; scooping out.

**Drin·ker res·pi·ra·tor** (dring'kĕr) a mechanical respirator in which the body except the head is encased within a metal tank, which is sealed at the neck with an airtight gasket; artificial respiration is induced by making the air pressure inside alternately negative and positive. SYN iron lung.

**drip 1.** to flow a drop at a time. **2.** a flowing in drops.

**drive 1.** a basic compelling urge. **2.** PSYCHOLOGY classified as either innate (e.g., hunger) or learned (e.g., hoarding) and appetitive (e.g., hunger, thirst, sex) or aversive (e.g., fear, pain, grief). SEE ALSO motive.

**driv•ing** (drīv'ing) the induction of a frequency in the electroencephalogram by sensory stimulation at this frequency.

**drom•o•graph** (drom'ō-graf) an instrument for recording the rapidity of the blood circulation. [G. *dromos,* a running, + *graphō,* to record]

**drom•o•ma•nia** (drom-ō-mā'nē-ă) an uncontrollable impulse to wander or travel. [G. *dromos,* a running, + *mania,* insanity]

**dro•mo•tro•pic** (drō-mō-trop'ik) influencing the velocity of conduction of excitation, as in nerve or cardiac muscle fibers. [G. *dromos,* a running, + *tropē,* a turn]

**drop 1.** to fall, or to be dispensed or poured in globules. **2.** a liquid globule. **3.** a volume of liquid regarded as a unit of dosage, equivalent in the case of water to about 1 minim. [A.S. *droppan*]

**drop at•tack** an episode of sudden falling that occurs during standing or walking, without warning and without loss of consciousness, vertigo, or postictal behavior. The patients are usually elderly and have normal electroencephalograms; of unknown cause.

**dropfoot, drop foot** SEE footdrop.

**drop hand** SYN wrist-drop.

**drop•let** (drop'let) a diminutive drop, such as a particle of moisture discharged from the mouth during coughing, sneezing, or speaking; these may transmit infections to others by their airborne passage. [drop + -*let,* dim. suffix]

**drop•let in•fec•tion** infection acquired through the inhalation of droplets or aerosols of saliva or sputum containing virus or other microorganisms expelled by another person during sneezing, coughing, laughing, or talking.

**drown•ing** death from suffocation induced by immersion in water or other fluid, with filling of pulmonary air spaces and passages with fluid to the detriment of gas exchange. [M.E. *drounen*]

**drows•i•ness** (drow'zē-nes) a state of impaired awareness associated with a desire or inclination to sleep.

**drug** (drŭg) **1.** therapeutic agent; any substance, other than food, used in the prevention, diagnosis, alleviation, treatment, or cure of disease. For types or classifications of drugs, see the specific name. SEE ALSO agent. **2.** to administer or take a drug, usually implying an overly large quantity or a narcotic. **3.** general term for any substance, stimulating or depressing, that can be habituating or addictive, especially a narcotic. [M.E. *drogge*]

**drug a•buse** habitual use of drugs not needed for therapeutic purposes, such as solely to alter one's mood, affect, or state of consciousness, or to affect a body function unnecessarily (as in laxative abuse); nonmedical use of drugs.

**drug e•rup•tion** any eruption caused by the ingestion, injection, or inhalation of a drug, most often the result of allergic sensitization; reactions to drugs applied to the cutaneous surface are not generally designated as drug eruption, but as contact-type dermatitis. SYN dermatitis medicamentosa, dermatosis medicamentosa, drug rash.

**drug-fast** pertaining to microorganisms that resist or become tolerant to an antibacterial agent.

**drug hol•i•day** intervals when a chronically medicated patient temporarily stops taking the medication; used to allow some recuperation of normal functions and/or to maintain sensitivity to the drug(s).

**drug in•ter•ac•tions** the pharmacological result, either desirable or undesirable, of drugs interacting with other drugs, with endogenous physiologic chemical agents (e.g., MAOI with epinephrine), with components of the diet, and with chemicals used in diagnostic tests or the results of such tests.

**drug psy•cho•sis** psychosis following or precipitated by ingestion of a drug.

**drug rash** SYN drug eruption.

**drug re•sis•tance** the capacity of disease-causing pathogens to withstand drugs previously toxic to them; achieved by spontaneous mutation or through selective pressure after exposure to the drug in question.

**drug tet•a•nus** tonic spasms caused by strychnine or other tetanic. SYN toxic tetanus.

**Drug Use Re•view** a program that reviews, analyzes, and interprets rates, costs, and appropriateness of drug usage within specific health care environments.

**drug u•ti•li•za•tion re•view, drug use e•val•u•a•tion** an authorized, structured, ongoing program that collects, analyzes, and interprets drug use patterns to improve the quality of drug use and patient outcomes.

**drum, drum•head** (drŭm, drŭm'hed) SYN tympanic membrane.

**drum mem•brane** SYN tympanic membrane.

**Drum•mond sign** (drŭm'ŏnd) in certain cases of aortic aneurysm, a puffing sound, synchronous with cardiac systole, heard from the nostrils, when the mouth is closed.

**drunk•en•ness** (drŭnk'en-nes) intoxication, usually alcoholic.

**dru•sen** (droo'sen) small bright structures seen in the retina and in the optic disc. [Ger. pl. of *Druse,* stony nodule, geode]

**DRVVT** dilute Russell's viper venom test.

**dry ab•scess** the remains of an abscess after the pus is absorbed.

**dry cough** a cough not accompanied by expectoration; a nonproductive cough.

**dry gan•grene** a form of gangrene in which the involved part is dry and shriveled. SYN mummification (1).

**dry joint** a joint affected with atrophic desiccating changes.

**Dry•o•pi•the•cus pat•tern 1.** The ancestral pattern of cusps and grooves in humans. **2.** A Y-5 cusp and groove pattern. SEE ALSO cusp and groove pattern.

**dry pleu•ri•sy** pleurisy with a fibrinous exudation, without an effusion of serum, resulting in adhesion between the opposing surfaces of the pleura. SYN adhesive pleurisy, fibrinous pleurisy, plastic pleurisy.

**dry rale** a harsh or musical breath sound produced by a constriction in a bronchial tube or the presence of a viscid secretion narrowing the lumen.

**dry syn·o·vi·tis** synovitis with little serous or purulent effusion. SYN synovitis sicca.

**dry vom·it·ing** SYN retching.

**DSA** digital subtraction angiography.

**DSM** Diagnostic and Statistical Manual.

**DT** delirium tremens; duration tetany.

**dT** deoxythymidine.

**DTaP** diphtheria, tetanus, and acellular pertussis vaccine.

**dTDP** thymidine 5′-diphosphate.

**dThd** thymidine.

**dTMP** deoxythymidylic acid.

**DTR** deep tendon reflex.

**du·al·ism** (doo′ăl-izm) **1.** CHEMISTRY theory that every compound, no matter how many elements enter into it, is composed of two parts, one electrically negative, the other positive; applicable to polar compounds but not to nonpolar compounds. **2.** HEMATOLOGY the concept that blood cells have two origins, i.e., lymphogenous and myelogenous. **3.** the theory that the mind and body are two distinct systems, independent and different in nature. [L. *dualis,* relating to two, fr. *duo,* two]

**Du·bois ab·scess·es** (doo-bwah′) small cysts of the thymus containing polymorphonuclear leukocytes but lined by squamous epithelium; reported in congenital syphilis but also found in the absence of syphilis.

**Du·Bois for·mu·la** (doo-bwah′) a formula for predicting a man's surface area from weight and height: $A = 71.84W^{0.425} H^{0.725}$, where $A$ = surface area in cm$^2$, $W$ = weight in kg, and $H$ = height in cm.

**Du·bo·witz score** (doo′bō-wits) a method of clinical assessment of gestational age in the newborn that includes neurological criteria for the infant's maturity and other physical criteria to determine the gestational age of the infant; useful from birth to 5 days of life.

**Du·chenne-A·ran dis·ease** (doo-shen′ ah-rah′) SYN amyotrophic lateral sclerosis.

**Du·chenne dis·ease** (doo-shen′) SYN Duchenne dystrophy.

**Du·chenne dys·tro·phy** (doo-shen′) the most common childhood muscular dystrophy, with onset usually before age 6. Characterized by symmetrical weakness and wasting of first the pelvic and crural muscles and then the pectoral and proximal upper extremity muscles; pseudohypertrophy of some muscles, especially the calf; heart involvement; sometimes mild mental retardation; progressive course and early death, usually in adolescence. X-linked inheritance (affects males and transmitted by females). SYN Duchenne disease.

**Du·chenne-Erb pa·ral·y·sis** (doo-shen′ ārb) SYN Erb palsy.

**Du·chenne sign** (doo-shen′) falling in of the epigastrium during inspiration in paralysis of the diaphragm.

**Duck·worth phe·nom·e·non** (duk′werth) respiratory arrest before cardiac arrest as a result of intracranial disease.

**Du·crey ba·cil·lus** (doo-krā′) SYN *Haemophilus ducreyi.*

**duct** (dŭkt) a tubular structure giving exit to the secretion of a gland, or conducting any fluid. SEE ALSO canal. SYN ductus [TA]. [L. *duco,* pp. *ductus,* to lead]

**duc·tal** (dŭk′tăl) relating to a duct.

**duc·tal an·eu·rysm** aneurysm of the patent ductus arteriosus, occurs either in infants or adults. SYN ductus diverticulum.

**duc·tile** (dŭk′tĭl) denoting the property of a material that allows it to be bent, drawn out (as a wire), or otherwise deformed without breaking. [L. *ductilis,* capable of being led or drawn]

**duct·less** (dŭkt′les) having no duct; denoting certain glands having only an internal secretion.

**duct·less glands** SYN endocrine glands.

**duc·tu·lar** (dŭkt′yu-lăr) relating to a ductule.

**duc·tule** (dŭkt′yul) a minute duct. SYN ductulus [TA].

**duc·tu·li bil·i·fe·ri** SYN biliary ductules.

**duc·tu·li ef·fe·ren·tes tes·tis** [TA] SYN efferent ductules of testis.

**duc·tu·li pros·ta·ti·ci** [TA] SYN prostatic ductules.

**duc·tu·lus,** pl. **duc·tu·li** (dŭkt′yu-lŭs, dŭk-tyu-lī) [TA] SYN ductule. [Mod. L. dim. of L. *ductus,* duct]

**duc·tu·lus al·ve·o·la·ris,** pl. **duc·tu·li al·ve·o·la·res** SYN alveolar duct.

**duc·tus,** gen. and pl. **duc·tus** (dŭk′tŭs) [TA] SYN duct. [L. a leading, fr. *duco,* pp. *ductus,* to lead]

**duc·tus ar·te·ri·o·sus** a fetal vessel connecting the left pulmonary artery with the descending aorta; in the first two months after birth, it normally changes into a fibrous cord, the ligamentum arteriosum; occasional postnatal failure to close causes a surgically correctable cardiovascular handicap. SYN arterial canal, arterial duct, Botallo duct.

**duc·tus def·er·ens** [TA] the secretory duct of the testicle, running from the epididymis, of which it is the continuation, to the prostatic urethra where it terminates as the ejaculatory duct. SYN arteriola glomerularis efferens [TA], deferent duct, spermatic duct, spermiduct (1), vas deferens.

**duc·tus di·ver·ti·cu·lum** SYN ductal aneurysm.

**duc·tus pan·cre·at·i·cus ac·ces·so·ri·us** [TA] SYN accessory pancreatic duct.

**duc·tus ve·no·sus** in the fetus, continuation of the left umbilical vein through the liver to the inferior vena cava; after birth, its lumen becomes obliterated, forming the ligamentum venosum.

**Dugas test** (doo-gah′) in the case of an injured shoulder, if the elbow cannot be made to touch the chest while the hand rests on the opposite shoulder, the injury is a dislocation and not a fracture of the humerus.

**Duh·ring dis·ease** (doo′ring) SYN dermatitis herpetiformis.

**Dührssen in·ci·sions** (dēr′sen) three surgical incisions of an incompletely dilated cervix, corresponding roughly to 2, 6, and 10 o'clock, used as a means of effecting immediate delivery of the fetus when there is an entrapped head during a breech delivery.

**Dukes clas·si·fi·ca·tion** (dooks) a classification of the extent of invasion of a resected adenocarcinoma of the colon or rectum commonly modified as follows: A (Dukes A), confined to the mucosa; $B_1$, into the muscularis mucosae; $B_2$, through the muscularis mucosae; $C_1$, limited to the bowel wall, with nodal metastases; $C_2$, through the bowel wall, with nodal metastases.

**Dukes dis·ease** (dooks) SYN exanthema subitum.

**dull** (dŭl) not sharp or acute, in any sense; qualifying a surgical instrument, the action of the mind, pain, a sound (especially the percussion note), etc. [M.E. *dul*]

**Du·mont·pal·li·er pes·sa·ry** (doo-mŏn-pal-yā′) an elastic ring pessary. SYN Mayer pessary.

**dump·ing syn·drome** a syndrome that occurs after eating, most often seen in patients with shunts of the upper alimentary canal; characterized by flushing, sweating, dizziness, weakness, and vasomotor collapse, occasionally with pain and headache; results from rapid passage of large amounts of food into the small intestine, with an osmotic effect removing fluid from plasma and causing hypovolemia. SYN early dumping syndrome, postgastrectomy syndrome.

**Dun·can dis·ease** (dŭn′kăn) SYN X-linked lymphoproliferative syndrome.

**Dun·can mech·a·nism** (dŭn′kăn) passage of the placenta from the uterus with the rough side foremost.

**Dun·can pla·cen·ta** (dŭn′kăn) a separated placenta that appears at the vulva with the chorionic surface outward.

**du·o·de·nal** (doo′ō-dē′năl) relating to the duodenum.

**du·o·de·nal am·pul·la** the dilated portion of the superior part of the duodenum; SEE ALSO duodenal cap.

**du·o·de·nal cap** the first portion of the duodenum, as seen in a roentgenogram or by fluoroscopy.

**du·o·de·nal glands** small, branched, coiled tubular glands that occur mostly in the submucosa of the first third of the duodenum; they secrete an alkaline mucoid substance that serves to neutralize gastric juice. SYN Brunner glands.

**du·o·de·nec·to·my** (doo-ō-dĕ-nek′tō-mē) excision of the duodenum. [duodenum + G. *ektomē,* excision]

**du·o·de·ni·tis** (doo-od-ĕ-nī′tis) inflammation of the duodenum.

△**du·o·de·no-** combining form relating to the duodenum. [L. *duodenum (digitorum),* breadth of 12 fingers]

**du·o·de·no·cho·lan·gi·tis** (doo-ō-dē′nō-kō-lan-jī′tis) inflammation of the duodenum and common bile duct. [duodeno- + G. *cholē,* bile, + *angeion,* vessel, + *-itis,* inflammation]

**du·o·de·no·cho·le·cys·tos·to·my** (doo-ō-dē′nō-kō-lē-sis-tos′tō-mē) SYN cholecystoduodenostomy. [duodeno- + G. *cholē,* bile, + *kystis,* bladder, + *stoma,* mouth]

**du·o·de·no·cho·led·o·chot·o·my** (doo-ō-dē′nō-kō-led-ō-kot′ō-mē) incision into the common bile duct and the adjacent portion of the duodenum. [duodeno- + G. *choledochus,* bile duct, + *tomē,* incision]

**du·o·de·no·cys·tos·to·my** (doo-ō-dē′nō-sis-tos′tō-mē) **1.** SYN cholecystoduodenostomy. **2.** SYN cystoduodenostomy. **3.** SYN pancreatic cystoduodenostomy.

**du·o·de·no·en·ter·os·to·my** (doo-ō-dē′nō-en-ter-os′tō-mē) establishment of communication between the duodenum and another part of the intestinal tract. [duodeno- + G. *enteron,* intestine, + *stoma,* mouth]

**du·o·de·no·je·ju·nal flex·ure** an abrupt bend in the small intestine at the junction of the duodenum and jejunum. SYN flexura duodenojejunalis [TA].

**du·o·de·no·je·ju·nos·to·my** (doo-ō-dē′nō-jĕ-joo-nos′tō-mē) operative formation of an artificial communication between the duodenum and the jejunum. [duodeno- + jejunum, + G. *stoma,* mouth]

**du·o·de·nol·y·sis** (doo-ō-dĕ-nol′i-sis) incision of adhesions to the duodenum. [duodeno- + G. *lysis,* a freeing]

**du·o·de·nor·rha·phy** (doo-ō-dĕ-nōr′ă-fē) suture of a tear or incision in the duodenum. [duodeno- + G. *rhaphē,* a seam]

**du·o·de·nos·co·py** (doo-ō-dĕ-nos′kŏ-pē) inspection of the interior of the duodenum through an endoscope. [duodeno- + G. *skopeō,* to examine]

**du·o·de·nos·to·my** (doo-ō-dĕ-nos′tō-mē) establishment of a fistula into the duodenum. [duodeno- + G. *stoma,* mouth]

**du·o·de·not·o·my** (doo-ō-dĕ-not′ō-mē) incision of the duodenum. [duodeno- + G. *tomē,* incision]

**du·o·de·num,** gen. **du·o·de·ni,** pl. **du·o·de·na** (doo-od′ĕ-nŭm, doo-od′ĕ-nī, doo-od′ĕ-nă) [TA] the first division of the small intestine, about 25 cm in length, extending from the pylorus to the junction with the jejunum at the level of the first or second lumbar vertebra on the left side. It is divided into the superior part, the first part of which is the duodenal cap, the descending part, into which the bile and pancreatic ducts open, the horizontal (inferior) part and the ascending part, terminating at the duodenojejunal junction. [Mediev. L. fr. L. *duodeni,* twelve]

**du·plex kid·ney** a kidney in which two pelviocaliceal systems are present.

**du·plex ul·tra·so·nog·ra·phy** the combination of real-time and Doppler ultrasonography.

**du·plex uter·us** any uterus with double lumen (uterus didelphys, uterus bicornis bicollis, or septate uterus).

**du·pli·ca·tion** (doo-pli-kā′shŭn) **1.** a doubling. SEE ALSO reduplication. **2.** inclusion of two copies of the same genetic material in a genome; an important step in diversification of genomes; as in the evolution of the (non-allelic) hemoglobin chains from a common ancestor. [L. *duplicatio,* a doubling, fr. *duplico,* to double]

**du·pli·ca·tion of chro·mo·somes** a chromosome aberration resulting from unequal crossing over or exchange of segments between two homologous chromosomes; one chromosome of the pair loses a small segment, while the other gains this segment; the chromosome gaining the segment has undergone duplication while its homologue has undergone deletion.

**Du·puy-Du·temps op·er·a·tion** (doo-pwē′ doo-tah′) a modified dacryocystorhinostomy for stenosis of the lacrimal duct.

**Du·puy·tren am·pu·ta·tion** (doo-pwē-trah′) amputation of the arm at the shoulder joint.

**Du·puy·tren ca·nal** (doo-pwē-trah′) SYN diploic vein.

**Du·puy·tren con·trac·ture** (doo-pwē-trah′) a disease of the palmar fascia resulting in thickening and shortening of fibrous bands on the palmar surface of the hand and fingers resulting in a characteristic flexion deformity of the fourth and fifth digits.

**Du·puy·tren dis·ease of the foot** (doo-pwē-trah′) SYN plantar fibromatosis.

**Du·puy·tren frac·ture** (doo-pwē-trah′) fracture of lower part of fibula, with dislocation of ankle.

**Du·puy·tren hy·dro·cele** (doo-pwē-trah′) bilocular hydrocele in which the sac fills the scrotum

d
u

and also extends into the abdominal cavity beneath the peritoneum.

**Du•puy•tren sign** (doo-pwē-trah') **1.** in congenital dislocation, free up and down movement of the head of the femur occurs upon intermittent traction; **2.** a crackling sensation on pressure over the bone in certain cases of sarcoma.

**Du•puy•tren su•ture** (doo-pwē-trah') a continuous Lembert suture.

**Du•puy•tren tour•ni•quet** (doo-pwē-trah') an instrument for compression on the abdominal aorta.

**du•ra** (doo'rǎ) SYN dura mater. [L. fem. of *durus,* hard]

**dur•able pow•er of at•tor•ney 1.** SYN advance directive. **2.** SYN living will.

**du•ral** (doo'rǎl) relating to the dura mater.

**dur•al ca•ver•nous si•nus fis•tu•la** a vascular shunt between the meningeal branches of the internal or external carotid arteries and the cavernous sinus.

**du•ral sheath** an extension of the dura mater that ensheathes the roots of spinal nerves or, more particularly, the vagina externa nervi optici.

**du•ral ve•nous si•nus•es** endothelium-lined venous channels in the dura mater. SYN venous sinuses.

**du•ra mat•er** (doo'rǎ mā'ter) [TA] pachymeninx (as distinguished from leptomeninx, the combined pia mater and arachnoid); a tough, fibrous membrane forming the outer covering of the central nervous system. SYN dura. [L. hard mother, mistransl. of Ar. *umm al-jāfīyah,* tough protector or covering]

**du•ra•tion** (doo-rā'shŭn) a continuous period of time.

**du•ra•tion tet•a•ny (DT)** a tonic spasm occurring in degenerated muscles upon application of a strong galvanic current.

**Dürck nodes** (dērk) perivascular chronic inflammatory infiltrates in the brain, occurring in human trypanosomiasis.

**Du•ret hem•or•rhage** (doo-rā') small brainstem hemorrhage resulting from brainstem distortion secondary to transtentorial herniation.

**Du•ret le•sion** (doo-rā') small hemorrhage(s) in the floor of the fourth ventricle or beneath the aqueduct of Sylvius.

**Dur•ham rule** (doo-răm) an American test of criminal responsibility (1954): "an accused is not criminally responsible if his unlawful act was the product of mental disease or mental defect."

**Dur•ham tube** (doo-răm) a jointed tracheotomy tube.

**Du•ro•zi•ez dis•ease** (doo-rō'zē-ā') congenital stenosis of the mitral valve.

**Du•ro•zi•ez mur•mur** (doo-rō'zē-ā') a two-phase murmur over peripheral arteries, especially the femoral artery, due to rapid ebb and flow of blood during aortic insufficiency.

**DUSN** diffuse unilateral subacute neuroretinitis.

**dust cell** SYN alveolar macrophage.

**Dut•ton dis•ease** (dŭt'ŏn) African tick-borne relapsing fever caused by *Borrelia duttonii* and spread by the soft tick, *Ornithodoros moubata.*

**duty cycle** ($t_i/t_{tot}$) the ratio of inspiratory ($t_i$) time to total-breathing-cycle time ($t_{tot}$).

**Du•ven•hage vi•rus** a species of Lyssavirus causing a rabieslike disease in humans in Africa; transmitted by the bite of insectivorous bats. [the virus was named after its first victim, a man infected near Pretoria, South Africa]

**DVT** deep venous thrombosis.

**dwarf** (dwôrf) an abnormally undersized person with disproportion among the bodily parts. SEE dwarfism. [A.S. *dweorh*]

**dwarf•ism** (dwôrf'izm) a condition in which the standing height of the subject is below the 3rd percentile.

**Dwy•er os•te•o•to•my** (dwī'er), a procedure for clubfoot.

**Dy** dysprosium.

**dy•ad** (dī'ad) **1.** a pair. SYN diad (2). **2.** CHEMISTRY a bivalent element. **3.** a pair of persons in an interactional situation, e.g., patient and therapist, husband and wife. **4.** the double chromosome resulting from the splitting of a tetrad during meiosis. [G. *dyas,* the number two, duality]

**dye** (dī) a stain or coloring matter; a compound consisting of chromophore and auxochrome groups attached to one or more benzene rings, its color being due to the chromophore and its dyeing affinities to the auxochrome. Dyes are used for intravital coloration of living cells, staining tissues and microorganisms, as antiseptics and germicides, and some as stimulants of epithelial growth. Commonly used for radiographic contrast medium. [A.S. *deah, deag*]

**dye dis•ap•pear•ance test** SYN fluorescein instillation test.

**△-dymus 1.** suffix to be combined with number roots; e.g., didymus, tridymus, tetradymus. **2.** occasionally used for -tridymus. [G. -*dymos,* fold]

**dy•nam•ic com•pli•ance** compliance measured during cyclic variations in the volume of a distensible vessel; the ratio of the change in volume to the change in distending pressure when the pressure change is measured between points in time at which the rate of volume change is zero.

**dy•nam•ic con•stant ex•ter•nal re•sis•tance train•ing** resistance training in which external resistance does not change; joint flexion and extension occurs with each repetition. Formerly (but incorrectly) referred to as isotonic exercise.

**dy•nam•ic e•qui•lib•ri•um** SYN equilibrium (2).

**dy•nam•ic il•e•us** intestinal obstruction due to spastic contraction of a segment of the bowel. SYN spastic ileus.

**dy•nam•ic move•ment** smooth, controlled, coordinated action based on a point of stability as its support.

**dy•nam•ic pos•tur•o•gra•phy** a measurement of postural stability under varying visual and proprioceptive inputs. SYN posturography.

**dy•nam•ic psy•chi•a•try** SYN psychoanalytic psychiatry.

**dy•nam•ic psy•chol•o•gy** a psychologic approach that concerns itself with the causes of behavior.

**dy•nam•ic re•frac•tion** refraction of the eye during accommodation.

**dy•nam•ics** (dī-nam'iks) **1.** the science of motion in response to forces. **2.** PSYCHIATRY the determination of how emotional and mental disorders develop. **3.** BEHAVIORAL SCIENCES any of the numerous intrapersonal and interpersonal influences or phenomena associated with personality development and interpersonal processes. [G. *dynamis,* force]

**dy•nam•ic splint** a splint utilizing springs or elastic bands that aids in movements initiated by the patient by controlling the plane and range of motion. SYN active splint, functional splint (1).

△**dynamo-** combining form, force, energy. [G. *dynamis*, power]

**dy·na·mo·gen·e·sis** (dī'nă-mō-jen'ĕ-sis) the production of force, especially of muscular or nervous energy. [dynamo- + G. *genesis*, production]

**dy·na·mo·gen·ic** (dī'nă-mō-jen'ik) producing power or force, especially nervous or muscular power or activity.

**dy·nam·o·graph** (dī-nam'ō-graf) an instrument for recording the degree of muscular power. [dynamo- + G. *graphō*, to write]

**dy·na·mom·e·ter** (dī-nă-mom'ĕ-ter) an instrument for measuring the degree of muscular power. SYN ergometer. [dynamo- + G. *metron*, measure]

**dyne** (dīn) the unit of force in the CGS system, replaced in the SI system by the newton (1 newton = $10^5$ dynes), that gives a body of 1 g mass an acceleration of 1 cm/sec$^2$; expressed as $F$ (dynes) = $m$ (grams) × $a$ (cm/sec$^2$). [G. *dynamis*, force]

**dyn·ein** (dīn'ēn) a protein associated with motile structures, exhibiting adenosine triphosphatase activity; it forms "arms" on the outer tubules of cilia and flagella. SEE ALSO tubulin. [dyne + protein]

△**dys-** bad, difficult, un-, mis-; opposite of eu-. Cf. dis-. [G.]

**dys·a·cu·sis, dys·a·cu·si·a, dys·a·cou·sia** (dis-ă-koo'sis, dis-ă-koo'sē-ă) **1.** any impairment of hearing involving difficulty in processing details of sound as opposed to any loss of sensitivity to sound. **2.** pain or discomfort in the ear from exposure to sound. [dys- + G. *akousis*, hearing]

**dys·a·phia** (dis-ā'fē-ă, dis-af'ē-ă) impairment of the sense of touch. [dys- + G. *haphē*, touch]

**dys·ar·te·ri·ot·o·ny** (dis-ar-tēr-ē-ot'ō-nē) abnormal blood pressure, either too high or too low. [dys- + G. *artēria*, artery, + *tonos*, tension]

**dys·ar·thria** (dis-ar'thrē-ă) a disturbance of speech and language due to emotional stress, to brain injury, or to paralysis, incoordination, or spasticity of the muscles used for speaking. SYN dysarthrosis (1). [dys- + G. *arthroō*, to articulate]

**dysarthria–clumsy hand syndrome** a disorder characterized by dysarthria and a clumsiness of one hand, caused by a lacunar stroke in the basis pontis.

**dys·ar·thric** (dis-ar'thrik) relating to dysarthria.

**dys·ar·thro·sis** (dis-ar-thrō'sis) **1.** SYN dysarthria. **2.** malformation of a joint. **3.** a false joint. [dys- + G. *arthrōsis*, joint]

**dys·au·to·no·mia** (dis'aw-tō-nō'mē-ă) abnormal functioning of the autonomic nervous system. [dys- + G. *autonomia*, self-government]

**dys·ba·rism** (dis'bar-izm) general term for the symptom complex resulting from exposure to decreased or changing barometric pressure, including all physiologic effects resulting from such changes with the exception of hypoxia, and including the effects of rapid decompression. [dys- + G. *baros*, weight]

**dys·ba·sia** (dis-bā'zē-ă) **1.** difficulty in walking. **2.** the difficult or distorted walking that occurs in persons with certain mental disorders. [dys- + G. *basis*, a step]

**dys·bu·lia** (dis-boo'lē-ă) weakness and uncertainty of volition. [dys- + G. *boulē*, will]

**dys·bu·lic** (dis-boo'lik) relating to, or characterized by, dysbulia.

**dys·cal·cu·lia** (dis-kal-kyu'lē-ă) difficulty in performing simple mathematical problems; commonly seen in parietal lobe lesions. [dys- + L. *calculo*, to compute, fr. *calculus*, pebble, counter]

**dys·ce·pha·lia** (dis-sĕ-fā'lē-ă) malformation of the head and face. [dys- + G. *kephalē*, head]

**dys·chei·ral, dys·chi·ral** (dis-kī'răl) relating to dyscheiria.

**dys·che·zia** (dis-kē'zē-ă) difficulty in defecation. [dys- + G. *chezō*, to defecate]

**dys·chon·dro·gen·e·sis** (dis-kon-drō-jen'ĕ-sis) abnormal development of cartilage. [dys- + G. *chondros*, cartilage, + *genesis*, production]

**dys·chon·dro·pla·sia** (dis-kon-drō-plā'zē-ă) SYN enchondromatosis. [dys- + G. *chondros*, cartilage, + *plasis*, a forming]

**dys·chro·ma·top·sia** (dis'krō-mă-top'sē-ă) a condition in which the ability to perceive colors is not fully normal. Cf. dichromatism, monochromatism, chromatopsia. [dys- + G. *chrōma*, color, + *opsis*, vision]

**dys·chro·mia** (dis-krō'mē-ă) any abnormality in the color of the skin.

**dys·co·ria** (dis-kō'rē-ă) abnormality in the shape of the pupil. [dys- + G. *korē*, pupil of eye]

**dys·cra·sia** (dis-krā'zē-ă) **1.** a morbid general state resulting from the presence of abnormal material in the blood, usually applied to diseases affecting blood cells or platelets. **2.** old term indicating disease. [G. bad temperament, fr. dys- + *krasis*, a mixing]

**dys·cra·sic, dys·crat·ic** (dis-krā'zik, krat'ik) pertaining to or affected with dyscrasia.

**dys·en·ter·ic** (dis-en-tār'ik) relating to or suffering from dysentery.

**dys·en·tery** (dis'en-tār-ē) a disease marked by frequent watery stools, often with blood and mucus, and characterized clinically by pain, tenesmus, fever, and dehydration. [G. *dysenteria*, fr. *dys-*, bad, + *entera*, bowels]

**dys·er·e·thism** (dis-er'ĕ-thizm) a condition of slow response to stimuli. [dys- + G. *erethismos*, irritation]

**dys·er·gia** (dis-er'jē-ă) lack of harmonious action between the muscles concerned in executing any definite voluntary movement. [dys- + G. *ergon*, work]

**dys·es·the·sia** (dis-es-thē'zē-ă) **1.** impairment of sensation short of anesthesia. **2.** a condition in which a disagreeable sensation is produced by ordinary stimuli; caused by lesions of the sensory pathways, peripheral or central. **3.** abnormal sensations experienced in the absence of stimulation. [G. *dysaisthēsia*, fr. *dys-*, hard, difficult, + *aisthēsis*, sensation]

**dys·fi·brin·o·ge·ne·mia** (dis'fī-brin'ō-jĕ-nē'mē-ă) an autosomal dominant disorder of qualitatively abnormal fibrinogens of various types, resulting in abnormalities of coagulation tests (bleeding time, clotting time, thrombin time); symptoms vary from none to abnormal bleeding and excessive clotting.

**dys·flu·en·cy** (dis-floo'ĕn-sē) speech interrupted in its forward flow by hesitations, repetitions, or prolongations of sounds. Although dysfluencies are the common manifestation of a stuttering disorder, they are also present in normal speech, particularly during speech development in young children. SEE stuttering. SYN disfluency, nonfluency.

**dys·func·tion** (dis-fŭnk'shŭn) difficult or abnormal function.

**dys·gam·ma·glob·u·lin·e·mia** (dis-gam'ă-glob'yu-li-nē'mē-ă) an immunoglobulin abnormality, especially a disturbance of the percentage distribution of γ-globulins.

**dys·gen·e·sis** (dis-jen'ĕ-sis) defective development. [dys- + G. *genesis*, generation]

**dys·gen·ic** (dis-jen'ik) applying to factors that have a detrimental effect upon hereditary qualities, physical or mental.

**dys·ger·mi·no·ma** (dis-jer-mi-nō'mă) a rare malignant neoplasm of the ovary composed of undifferentiated gonadal germinal cells and occurring more frequently in patients less than 20 years of age. The neoplasms contain foci of necrosis and hemorrhage, and tend to be encapsulated; characteristically, they spread by way of lymphatic vessels, but widespread metastases also occur. SYN disgerminoma. [dys- + L. *germen*, a bud or sprout, + G. *-ōma*, tumor]

**dys·geu·sia** (dis-goo'zē-ă) impairment or perversion of the gustatory sense. [dys- + G. *geusis*, taste]

**dys·gna·thia** (dis-nath'ē-ă) any abnormality that extends beyond the teeth and includes the maxilla or mandible, or both. [dys- + G. *gnathos*, jaw]

**dys·gnath·ic** (dis-nath'ik) pertaining to or characterized by abnormality of the maxilla and mandible.

**dys·gno·sia** (dis-nō'sē-ă) any cognitive disorder, i.e., any mental illness. [G. *dysgnōsia*, difficulty of knowing]

**dys·har·mo·ni·ous re·tin·al cor·re·spon··dence** a type of anomalous retinal correspondence in which the angle of the visual direction of the two retinas is different from the objective angle of the strabismus.

**dys·hem·a·to·poi·e·sis, dys·he·mo·poi·e·sis** (dis-hē'mă-tō-poy-ē'sis, dis-hē'mō-poy-ē'sis) defective formation of the blood. [dys- + G. *haima* (*haimat-*), blood, + *poiēsis*, making]

**dys·hem·a·to·poi·et·ic, dys·he·mo·poi·et·ic** (dis-hē'mă-tō-poy-et'ik, dis-hē'mō-poy-et'ik) pertaining to or characterized by dyshematopoiesis.

**dys·hi·dro·sis, dys·hi·dro·tic ec·ze·ma** (dis-ĭ-drō'sis) a vesicular or vesicopustular eruption of multiple causes that occurs primarily on the volar surfaces of the hands and feet; the lesions spread peripherally but have a tendency to central clearing. SYN cheiropompholyx, chiropompholyx. [dys- + G. *hidrōs*, sweat]

**dys·kar·y·o·sis** (dis-kar-ē-ō'sis) abnormal maturation seen in exfoliated cells that have normal cytoplasm but hyperchromatic nuclei, or irregular chromatin distribution; may be followed by the development of a malignant neoplasm. [dys- + G. *karyon*, nucleus, + *-ōsis*, condition]

**dys·kar·y·ot·ic** (dis-kar-ē-ot'ik) pertaining to or characterized by dyskaryosis.

**dys·ker·a·to·ma** (dis-ker-ă-tō'mă) a skin tumor exhibiting dyskeratosis. [dys- + G. *keras*, horn, + *-oma*, tumor]

**dys·ker·a·to·sis** (dis'ker-ă-tō'sis) **1.** premature keratinization in individual epithelial cells that have not reached the keratinizing surface layer; dyskeratotic cells generally become rounded, and they may break away from adjacent cells and fall

off. **2.** epidermalization of the conjunctival and corneal epithelium. **3.** a disorder of keratinization. [dys- + G. *keras*, horn, + *-osis*, condition]

**dys·ker·a·tot·ic** (dis'ker-a-tot'ik) relating to or characterized by dyskeratosis.

**dys·ki·ne·sia, dys·ki·ne·sis** (dis-ki-nē'zē-ă) difficulty in performing voluntary movements. Term usually used in relation to various extrapyramidal disorders. [dys- + G. *kinēsis*, movement]

**dys·ki·ne·sia al·ge·ra** a hysterical condition in which active movement causes pain.

**dys·ki·ne·sia in·ter·mit·tens** intermittent disability of the limbs due to impairment of circulation.

**dys·ki·ne·sia syn·drome** (dis-ki-nē'zē-ă sin' drōm) a genetic disorder in which the clearance of mucus is sluggish and bronchiectasis is prevalent and intractable. There is evidence that the defect lies in dynein, a protein in the cilia. The pattern of inheritance is apparently autosomal recessive.

**dys·ki·net·ic** (dis-ki-net'ik) denoting or characteristic of dyskinesia.

**dys·lex·ia** (dis-lek'sē-ă) impaired reading ability with a competence level below that expected on the basis of the individual's level of intelligence, and in the presence of normal vision and letter recognition and normal recognition of the meaning of pictures and objects. [dys- + G. *lexis*, word, phrase]

**dys·lex·ic** (dis-lek'sik) relating to, or characterized by, dyslexia.

**dys·lo·gia** (dis-lō'jē-ă) impairment of speech and reasoning as the result of a mental disorder. [dys- + G. *logos*, speaking, reason]

**dys·ma·ture** (dis'mă-tyur) **1.** denoting faulty development or ripening; often connoting structural and/or functional abnormalities. **2.** OBSTETRICS denoting an infant whose birth weight is inappropriately low for its gestational age. **3.** immature development of the placenta so that normal function does not occur.

**dys·ma·tu·ri·ty** (dis'mă-yur-i-tē) syndrome of an infant born with relative absence of subcutaneous fat, wrinkling of the skin, prominent finger and toe nails, and meconium staining of skin and placental membranes; often associated with postmaturity or placental insufficiency.

**dys·me·lia** (dis-mē'lē-ă) congenital abnormality characterized by missing or foreshortened limbs, sometimes with associated vertebral column abnormalities; caused by metabolic disturbance at the time of primordial limb development. SEE amelia, phocomelia. [dys- + G. *melos*, limb]

**dys·men·or·rhea** (dis-men-ōr-ē'ă) difficult and painful menstruation. SYN menorrhalgia. [dys- + G. *mēn*, month, + *rhoia*, a flow]

**dys·met·ria** (dis-met'rē-ă) an aspect of ataxia, in which the ability to control the distance, power, and speed of an act is impaired. Usually used to describe abnormalities of movement caused by cerebellar disorders. SEE ALSO hypermetria, hypometria. [dys- + G. *metron*, measure]

**dys·mor·phism** (dis-mōr'fizm) abnormality of shape. [G. *dysmorphia*, badness of form]

**dys·mor·pho·gen·e·sis** (dis'mōr-fō-jen'ĕ-sis) the process of abnormal tissue formation. [dys- + G. *morphē*, form, + *genesis*, production]

**dys·mor·phol·o·gy** (dis-mōr-fol'ō-jē) the study of developmental structural defects. A branch of clinical genetics. [dys- + G. *morphē,* form, + *logos,* study]

**dys·my·o·to·nia** (dis-mī-ō-tō′nē-ă) abnormal muscular tonicity (either hyper- or hypo-). SEE dystonia. [dys- + G. *mys,* muscle, + *tonos,* tension, tone]

**dys·nys·tax·is** (dis-nis-tak′sis) a condition of half sleep. SYN light sleep. [dys- + G. *nystaxis,* drowsiness]

**dys·o·don·ti·a·sis** (dis′ō-don-tī′ă-sis) **1.** difficulty or irregularity in the eruption of the teeth. **2.** an imperfect dentition. [dys- + G. *odous,* tooth, + *-iasis,* condition]

**dys·on·to·gen·e·sis** (dis′on-tō-jen′ĕ-sis) defective embryonic development. [dys- + G. *ōn,* being, + *genesis,* origin]

**dys·on·to·ge·net·ic** (dis′on-tō-jĕ-net′ik) characterized by dysontogenesis.

**dys·o·rex·ia** (dis-ō-rek′sē-ă) diminished or perverted appetite. [dys- + G. *orexis,* appetite]

**dys·os·mia** (dis-oz′mē-ă) altered sense of smell. [dys- + G. *osmē,* smell]

**dys·os·te·o·gen·e·sis, dys·os·to·sis** (dis′os-tē-ō-jen′ĕ-sis, dis-os-tō′sis) defective bone formation. [dys- + G. *osteon,* bone, + *genesis,* production]

**dys·pa·reu·nia** (dis-pa-roo′nē-ă) occurrence of pain during sexual intercourse. [dys- + G. *pareunos,* lying beside, fr. *para,* beside, + *eunē,* a bed]

**dys·pep·sia** (dis-pep′sē-ă) impaired gastric function or "upset stomach" due to some disorder of the stomach; characterized by epigastric pain, sometimes burning, nausea, and gaseous eructation. SYN gastric indigestion. [dys- + G. *pepsis,* digestion]

**dys·pep·tic** (dis-pep′tik) relating to or suffering from dyspepsia.

**dys·pha·gia, dys·pha·gy** (dis-fā′jē-ă, dis′fă-jē) difficulty in swallowing. SYN aglutition. [dys- + G. *phagō,* to eat]

**dys·pha·sia** (dis-fā′zē-ă) SYN aphasia. [dys- + G. *phasis,* speaking]

**dys·pha·sic** (dis-fā′zic) SYN aphasiac.

**dys·phe·mia** (dis-fē′mē-ă) disordered phonation, articulation, or hearing due to emotional or mental deficits. [dys- + G. *phēmē,* speech]

**dys·pho·nia** (dis-fō′nē-ă) any disorder of phonation affecting voice quality or ability to produce voice. SEE aphonia. [dys- + G. *phōnē,* voice]

**dys·pho·ria** (dis-fōr′ē-ă) a mood of general dissatisfaction, restlessness, depression, and anxiety; a feeling of unpleasantness or discomfort. [dys- + G. *phora,* a bearing]

**dys·phra·sia** (dis-frā′zē-ă) SYN aphasia. [dys- + G. *phrasis,* speaking]

**dys·pig·men·ta·tion** (dis′pig-men-tā′shŭn) any abnormality in the formation or distribution of pigment, especially in the skin; usually applied to an abnormal reduction in pigmentation (depigmentation).

**dys·pla·sia** (dis-plā′zē-ă) abnormal tissue development. SEE ALSO heteroplasia. [dys- + G. *plasis,* a molding]

**dys·pla·sia ep·i·phys·e·a·lis mul·ti·plex** SYN multiple epiphysial dysplasia.

**dys·plas·tic** (dis-plas′tik) pertaining to or marked by dysplasia.

**dys·plas·tic ne·vus syn·drome, dys·plas·tic ne·vus** clinically atypical nevi having variable pigmentation and ill defined borders, with an increased risk for development of cutaneous malig-

nant melanoma; biopsies show melanocytic dysplasia.

**dysp·nea** (disp-nē′ă) shortness of breath, a subjective difficulty or distress in breathing, usually associated with disease of the heart or lungs; occurs normally during intense physical exertion or at high altitude. [G. *dyspnoia,* fr. *dys-,* bad, + *pnoē,* breathing]

**dysp·ne·ic** (disp-nē′ik) out of breath; relating to or suffering from dyspnea.

**dys·prax·ia** (dis-prak′sē-ă) impaired or painful functioning in any organ. [dys- + G. *praxis,* a doing]

**dys·prax·ia of speech** SYN verbal apraxia.

**dys·pro·si·um (Dy)** (dis-prō′sē-ŭm) a metallic element of the lanthanide (rare earth) series, atomic no. 66, atomic wt. 162.50. [G. *dysprositos,* hard to get at]

**dys·pro·tein·e·mia** (dis-prō′tēn-ē′mē-ă) an abnormality in plasma proteins, usually in immunoglobulins.

**dys·pro·tein·e·mic** (dis-prō-tēn-ē′mik) relating to dysproteinemia.

**dys·ra·phism, dys·raph·ia** (dis′ră-fizm, dis-raf′ē-ă) defective fusion, especially of the neural folds, resulting in status dysraphicus. [dys- + G. *rhaphē,* suture]

**dysreflexia** (dis′rē-flek′sē-a) a condition of disordered or inappropriate responses to stimuli. [dys- + reflex + -ia]

**dys·rhyth·mia** (dis-rith′mē-ă) defective rhythm. See also entries under rhythm. Cf. arrhythmia. [dys- + G. *rhythmos,* rhythm]

**dys·se·ba·cia, dys·se·ba·cea** (dis-sĕ-bā′shē-ă, dis′sē-bă′shē-ă) SYN seborrheic dermatitis. [dys- + L. *sebum,* grease]

**dys·som·nia** (dis-som′nē-ă) disturbance of normal sleep or rhythm pattern.

**dys·sta·sia** (dis-stā′zē-ă) difficulty in standing. [dys- + G. *stasis,* standing]

**dys·stat·ic** (dis-stat′ik) marked by difficulty in standing.

**dys·syn·er·gia** (dis-in-er′jē-ă) an aspect of ataxia, in which an act is not performed smoothly or accurately because of lack of harmonious association of its various components; usually used to describe abnormalities of movement caused by cerebellar disorders. [dys- + G. *syn,* with, + *ergon,* work]

**dys·syn·er·gia cer·e·bel·lar·is my·o·clo·ni·ca** a familial disorder beginning in late childhood, characterized by progressive cerebellar ataxia, action myoclonus and preserved intellect. Probably due to multiple causes, mitochondrial abnormalities being one.

**dys·thy·mia** (dis-thī′mē-ă) a chronic mood disorder manifested as depression for most of the day, more days than not, accompanied by some of the following symptoms: poor appetite or overeating, insomnia or hypersomnia, low energy or fatigue, low self-esteem, poor concentration, difficulty making decisions, and feelings of hopelessness. SEE endogenous depression, exogenous depression. [dys- + G. *thymos,* mind, emotion]

**dys·thy·mic** (dis-thī′mik) relating to dysthymia.

**dys·thy·mic dis·or·der** a chronic disturbance of mood characterized by mild depression or loss of interest in usual activities. SEE depression.

**dys·thy·roid or·bit·o·pa·thy** inflammation of the orbit in Graves disease.

**dys·to·cia** (dis-tō′sē-ă) difficult childbirth. [G. *dystokia,* fr. *dys-,* difficult, + *tokos,* childbirth]

**dys·to·nia** (dis-tō′nē-ă) a state of abnormal (either hypo- or hyper-) tonicity in any of the tissues. SYN torsion spasm. [dys- + G. *tonos,* tension]

**dys·to·nia mus·cu·lo·rum de·for·mans** a genetic, environmental, or idiopathic disorder, usually beginning in childhood or adolescence, marked by muscular contractions that distort the spine, limbs, hips, and sometimes the cranial-innervated muscles. The abnormal movements are increased by excitement and, at least initially, abolished by sleep. The musculature is hypertonic when in action, hypotonic when at rest.

**dys·ton·ic** (dis-ton′ik) pertaining to dystonia.

**dys·ton·ic re·ac·tion** a state of abnormal tension or muscle tone, similar to dystonia, produced as a side effect of certain antipsychotic medication; a severe form, where the eyes appear to roll up into the head, is called oculogyric crisis.

**dys·to·pia** (dis-tō′pē-ă) faulty or abnormal position of a part or organ. SYN malposition. [dys- + G. *topos,* place]

**dys·top·ic** (dis-top′ik) pertaining to, or characterized by, dystopia. SEE ALSO ectopic.

**dys·tro·phia** (dis-trō′fē-ă) SYN dystrophy. [L. fr. G. *dys-,* bad, + *trophē,* nourishment]

**dys·tro·phia ad·i·po·so·ge·ni·ta·lis** a disorder characterized primarily by obesity and hypogonadotrophic hypogonadism in adolescent boys; dwarfism is rare, and when present is thought to reflect hypothyroidism. Visual loss, behavioral abnormalities, and diabetes insipidus may occur. The most common causes are pituitary and hypothalamic neoplasms. SYN adiposogenital dystrophy, Fröhlich syndrome, hypophysial syndrome.

**dys·tro·phia e·pi·the·li·al·is cor·neae** a corneal dystrophy causing stromal edema and epithelial bullae, erosions, and scarring. SYN Fuchs epithelial dystrophy.

**dys·tro·phia un·gui·um** dystrophy of the nails.

**dys·tro·phic** (dis-trof′ik) relating to dystrophy.

**dys·tro·phic cal·ci·fi·ca·tion** calcification occurring in degenerated or necrotic tissue, as in hyalinized scars, degenerated foci in leiomyomas, and caseous nodules.

**dys·tro·phin** (dis-trō′fin) a protein found in the sarcolemma of normal muscle; it is missing in individuals with pseudohypertrophic muscular dystrophy and in other forms of muscular dystrophy. SYN distropin, dystropin.

**dys·tro·phy** (dis′trō-fē) progressive changes that may result from defective nutrition of a tissue or organ. SYN dystrophia. [dys- + G. *trophē,* nourishment]

**dys·tro·pin** SYN dystrophin.

**dys·u·ria** (dis-yu′rē-ă) difficulty or pain in urination. [dys- + G. *ouron,* urine]

**dys·u·ric** (dis-yu′rik) relating to or suffering from dysuria.

**dys·ver·sion** (dis-ver′zhŭn) a turning in any direction, less than inversion; particularly dysversion of the optic nerve head (situs inversus of the optic disk). [dys- + L. *verto,* to turn]

# E

η eta.

ε **1.** epsilon. SEE epsilon.   **2.** molar absorption coefficient.

**E 1.** exa-; extraction ratio; glutamic acid; energy; electromotive force; glutamyl; internal energy. **2.** as a subscript, refers to expired gas.

*E* entgegen.

e elementary charge; base of natural logarithms (2.71828...).

**Ea·gle ba·sal me·di·um** (ē-gĕl) a solution of various salts containing 13 naturally occurring amino acids, several vitamins, two antibiotics, and phenol red; used as a tissue culture medium.

**Ea·gle min·i·mum es·sen·tial me·di·um** (ē-gĕl) a tissue culture medium similar to Eagle basal medium but with different amounts and a few exclusions (e.g., antibiotics and phenol red).

**Eales dis·ease** (ēlz) peripheral retinal periphlebitis causing recurrent retinal or intravitreous hemorrhages in young adults.

■**ear** (ēr) the organ of hearing: composed of the **external ear**, which includes the auricle and the external acoustic, or auditory, meatus; the **middle ear**, or the tympanic cavity with its ossicles; and the **internal ear** or **inner ear**, or labyrinth, which includes the semicircular canals, vestibule, and cochlea. SEE ALSO auricle.   See this page. SYN auris [TA].   [A.S. *eáre*]

**ear·ache** (ēr'āk) pain in the ear. SYN otalgia, otodynia.

**ear bones** SYN auditory ossicles.

**ear·drum** (ēr'drŭm) SYN tympanic membrane.

**Ear·le so·lu·tion** (erl) a tissue culture medium containing $CaCl_2$, $MgSO_4$, KCl, $NaHCO_3$, NaCl, $NaH_2PO_4 \cdot H_2O$, and glucose.

**ear lobe crease** a diagonal crease found on one or both earlobes with a possible connection to coronary heart disease in males.

**ear·ly dis·charge** discharge of a woman and the newborn from the hospital within 24 hours of a vaginal delivery.

**ear·ly dump·ing syn·drome** SYN dumping syndrome.

**ear·piece** (ēr-pēs) a part of a device inserted into the external auditory canal to deliver sound to the ear.

**ear·plug** (ēr'plug) generic term for occlusive devices for the external auditory canal for protection of hearing against noise-induced hearing loss or to prevent water from getting into the ear. SEE ALSO hearing protector.

**earth** (erth) **1.** soil; the soft material of the land, as opposed to rock and sand. **2.** an easily pulverized mineral. **3.** an insoluble oxide of aluminum or of certain other elements characterized by a high melting point. [A.S. *eorthe*]

**eat·ing ep·i·lep·sy** epileptic seizures provoked by eating; a type of reflex epilepsy.

■**eat·ing-right py·ra·mid** USDA guidelines for sound nutrition that emphasize grains, vegetables, and fruits and downplay food sources high in animal protein, lipids, and dairy products. Recommendation for regular physical activity (≥ 30 min) is included in guidelines. See page APP 145.

**Ea·ton a·gent** (ē-ton) SYN *Mycoplasma pneumoniae*.

**E·berth lines** (ā'bĕrt) lines appearing between the cells of the myocardium when stained with silver nitrate.

**E·bo·la vi·rus** (ē-bō'lah) a virus morphologically similar to but antigenically distinct from Mar-

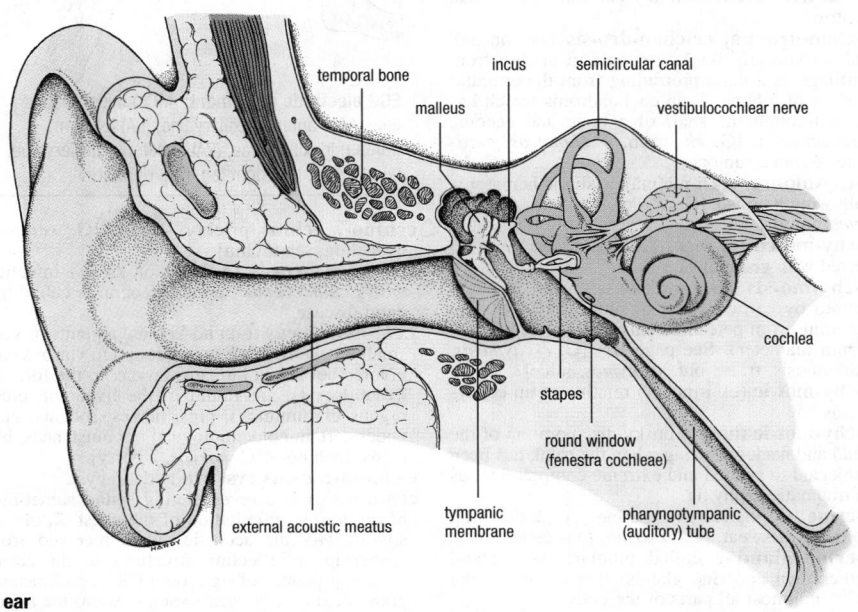

temporal bone

incus   semicircular canal

malleus   vestibulocochlear nerve

cochlea

stapes

round window (fenestra cochleae)

external acoustic meatus

tympanic membrane

pharyngotympanic (auditory) tube

ear

burg virus, in the family Filoviridae, which causes viral hemorrhagic fever.

**E·bo·la vi·rus Côte-d'Ivoire** (ē-bō′lah vī′ruŭs kōt dē vwah) SYN Côte-d'Ivoire virus.

**E·bo·la vi·rus Res·ton** (ē-bō′lah vī′ruŭs res′ton) SYN Reston virus.

**E·bo·la vi·rus Su·dan** (ē-bō′lah vī′ruŭs soo-dan′) SYN Sudan virus.

**E·bo·la vi·rus Za·ire** (ē-bō′lah vī′ruŭs zī-ēr′) SYN Zaire virus.

**Eb·stein a·nom·a·ly** (eb′shtīn) congenital downward displacement of the tricuspid valve into the right ventricle.

**Eb·stein sign** (eb′shtīn) in pericardial effusion, obtuseness of the cardiohepatic angle on percussion.

**EBT** electron beam tomography.

**eb·ur·na·tion** (ē-bŭr-nā′shŭn) a change in exposed subchondral bone in degenerative joint disease in which it is converted into a dense substance with a smooth surface like ivory. [L. *eburneus,* of ivory]

**ebur·ni·tis** (ē-bŭr-nī′tis) increased density and hardness of dentin, which may occur after the dentin is exposed. [L. *eburneus,* of ivory, + G. -itis, inflammation]

**EBV** Epstein-Barr virus.

**◁ec-** out of, away from. [G.]

**ec·cen·tric** (ek-sen′trik) **1.** abnormal or peculiar in ideas or behavior. **2.** situated away from a center or proceeding from a center. Cf. centrifugal (2). **3.** SYN peripheral. [G. *ek,* out, + *kentron,* center]

**ec·cen·tric con·trac·tion** a lengthening action in which a muscle's attachments are drawn away from one another by an external resistance, even though the muscle is activated.

**ec·cen·tric hy·per·tro·phy** thickening of the wall of the heart or other cavity, with dilation.

**ec·cen·tric oc·clu·sion** any occlusion other than centric.

**ec·chon·dro·ma, ec·chon·dro·sis** (ek-kon-drō′mă, ek-kon-drō′sis) **1.** a neoplasm arising from cartilage as a mass protruding from the articular surface of a bone. **2.** an enchondroma which has burst through the shaft of a bone and become pedunculated. [G. *ek,* from, + *chondros,* cartilage, + *-oma,* tumor]

**ec·chy·mo·ma** (ek-i-mō′mă) a slight hematoma following a bruise. [G. *ek,* out, + *chymos,* juice, + *-oma,* tumor]

**ec·chy·mosed** (ek′i-mōst) characterized by or affected with ecchymosis.

🔲 **ec·chy·mo·sis** (ek-i-mō′sis) a purplish patch caused by extravasation of blood into the skin, differing from petechiae only in size (larger than 3 mm diameter). See page B5. [G. *ekchymōsis,* ecchymosis, fr. *ek,* out, + *chymos,* juice]

**ec·chy·mot·ic** (ek-i-mot′ik) relating to an ecchymosis.

**ec·chy·mot·ic mask** a dusky discoloration of the head and neck occurring when the trunk has been subjected to sudden and extreme compression, as in traumatic asphyxia.

**ec·crine** (ek′rin) **1.** SYN exocrine (1). **2.** denoting the flow of sweat. [G. *ek-krino,* to secrete]

**ec·crine gland** a coiled tubular sweat gland (other than apocrine glands) that occurs in the skin on almost all parts of the body.

**ec·crine po·ro·ma** a poroma or acrospiroma of

the eccrine sweat glands, usually occurring on the sole of the foot.

**ec·cri·sis** (ek′ri-sis) **1.** the removal of waste products. **2.** any waste product; excrement. [G. separation]

**ec·cy·e·sis** (ek-sī-ē′sis) SYN ectopic pregnancy. [G. *ek,* out, + *kyēsis,* pregnancy]

**ec·dem·ic** (ek-dem′ik) denoting a disease brought into a region from without. [G. *ekdēmos,* foreign, from home, fr. *dēmos,* people]

**ECF** extracellular fluid.

**ECF-A** eosinophil chemotactic factor of anaphylaxis.

🔲 **ECG** electrocardiogram. See this page.

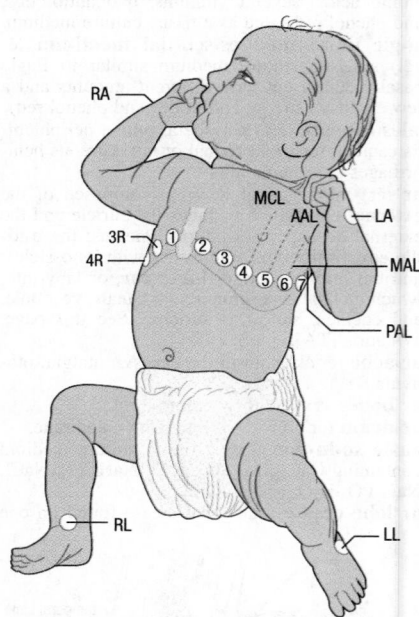

**ECG electrode placement:** (MCL) midclavicular line, (AAL) anterior axillary line, (LA) left arm, (MAL) midaxillary line, (PAL) posterior axillary line, (LL) left leg, (RL) right leg, (RA) right arm

**◁echino-, echin-** prickly, spiny. [G. *echinos,* hedgehog, sea urchin]

**echi·no·coc·co·sis** (ĕ-kī′nō-kok-kō′sis) infection with *Echinococcus;* larval infection is called hydatid disease.

**Echi·no·coc·cus** (ĕ-kī′nō-kok′ŭs) a genus of very small tapeworms; adults are found in various carnivores but not in humans; larvae, in the form of hydatid cysts, are found in the liver and other organs of ruminants, pigs, horses, rodents, and, under certain epidemiological circumstances, humans. [echino- + G. *kokkos,* a berry]

**e·chi·no·coc·cus cyst** SYN hydatid cyst.

**ech·o** (ek′ō) **1.** a reverberating sound sometimes heard during auscultation of the chest. **2.** ULTRASONOGRAPHY the acoustic signal received from scattering or reflecting structures or the corresponding pattern of light on a CRT or ultrasonogram. **3.** MAGNETIC RESONANCE IMAGING the signal detected following an inverting pulse. [G.]

**ech·o·a·cou·sia** (ek'ō-ă-koo'zē-ă) a subjective disturbance of hearing in which a sound appears to be repeated. [echo + G. *akouō*, to hear]

**ech·o·a·or·tog·ra·phy** (ek'ō-ā-ōr-tog'ră-fē) application of ultrasound techniques to the diagnosis and study of the aorta. [echo + aortography]

**ech·o·car·di·o·gram** (ek-ō-kar'dē-ō-gram) the ultrasonic record obtained by echocardiography. SEE ultrasonography. See page B10.

**ech·o·car·di·og·ra·phy** (ek'ō-kar-dē-og'ră-fē) the use of ultrasound in the investigation of the heart and great vessels and diagnosis of cardiovascular lesions. See this page. SYN ultrasound cardiography. [echo + cardiography]

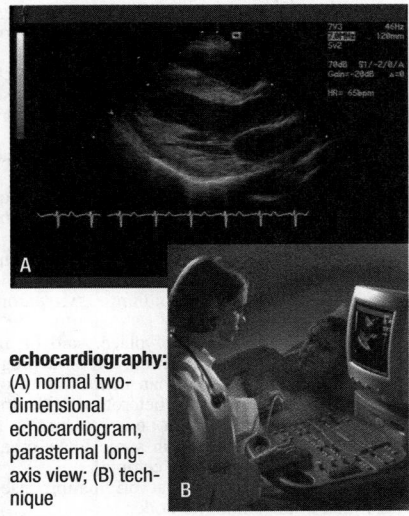

**echocardiography:** (A) normal two-dimensional echocardiogram, parasternal long-axis view; (B) technique

**ech·o·en·ceph·a·log·ra·phy** (ek'ō-en-sef-ă-log'ră-fē) the use of reflected ultrasound in the diagnosis of intracranial processes. [echo + encephalography]

**ech·o·gen·ic** (ek-ō-jen'ik) pertaining to a structure or medium (e.g., tissue) that is capable of producing echoes. Contrast with the terms hypoechoic, hyperechoic, and anechoic, which refer to the paucity, abundance, and absence of echoes displayed on the image.

**ech·o·gram** (ek'ō-gram) a record obtained using high frequency acoustic reflection techniques in any one of the various display modes, especially an echocardiogram. SEE ALSO ultrasonogram. [echo + G. *gramma*, a diagram]

**echog·ra·phy** (e-kog'ră-fē) SYN ultrasonography. [echo + G. *graphō*, to write]

**ech·o·la·lia** (ek-ō-lā'lē-ă) involuntary parrot-like repetition of a word or sentence just spoken by another person. Usually seen with schizophrenia. SYN echophrasia. [echo + G. *lalia*, a form of speech]

**ech·o·mim·ia** (ek-ō-mim'ē-ă) SYN echopathy. [echo + G. *mimēsis*, imitation]

**ech·o·mo·tism** (ek'ō-mō'tizm) SYN echopraxia. [echo + L. *motio*, motion]

**echop·a·thy** (ĕ-kop'ă-thē) a form of psychopathology, usually associated with schizophrenia, in which the words (echolalia) or actions (echo-

praxia) of another are imitated and repeated. SYN echomimia. [echo + G. *pathos*, suffering]

**ech·o·phra·sia** (ek-ō-frā'zē-ă) SYN echolalia. [echo + *phrasis*, speech]

**echo plan·ar** a method of magnetic resonance imaging that allows rapid image acquisition during free induction decay, using rapidly oscillating radiofrequency gradients.

**echo·prax·ia** (ek'ō-prak'sē-ă) involuntary imitation of movements made by another. SEE echopathy. SYN echomotism. [echo + G. *praxis*, action]

**ECHO vi·rus, echo·vi·rus** (ek'ō-vī-rŭs) an enterovirus isolated from humans; while there are many inapparent infections, certain of the several serotypes are associated with fever and aseptic meningitis, and some appear to cause mild respiratory disease.

**Eck fis·tu·la** (ek) transposition of the portal circulation to the systemic by making an anastomosis between the vena cava and portal vein and then ligating the latter close to the liver.

**ecla·bi·um** (ek-lā'bē-ŭm) eversion of a lip. [G. *ek*, out, + L. *labium*, lip]

**eclamp·sia** (ek-lamp'sē-ă) occurrence of one or more convulsions, not attributable to other cerebral conditions such as epilepsy or cerebral hemorrhage, in a patient with preeclampsia. [G. *eklampsis*, a shining forth]

**eclamp·tic** (ek-lamp'tik) relating to eclampsia.

**eclamp·to·gen·ic, eclamp·tog·e·nous** (ek-lamp-tō-jen'ik, ek-lamp-toj'ĕ-nŭs) causing eclampsia.

**eclipse pe·ri·od** the time between infection by (or induction of) a bacteriophage, or other virus, and the appearance of mature virus within the cell; an interval of time during which infective viral material cannot be recovered.

**ECMO** extracorporeal-membrane oxygenation.

**eco-** the environment. [G. *oikos*, house, household, habitation]

**eco·log·ic chem·is·try 1.** chemistry that concentrates on the effects of synthetic chemicals on the environment as well as the development of agents that are not harmful to the environment; **2.** the study of the molecular interactions between species and between species and the environment.

**eco·log·ic stu·dy** epidemiologic study in which the units of analysis are populations or groups of people rather than individuals.

**ecol·o·gy** (ē-kol'ō-jē) the branch of biology concerned with interrelationships among living organisms, encompassing the relations of organisms to each other, to the environment, and to energy balance within a given ecosystem. [eco- + G. *logos*, study]

**ecol·o·gy of hu·man per·for·mance** framework for understanding human performance as a transactional process through which the individual, the context, and performance of the task affect each other. Each transaction affects a person's future performance range and options.

**eco·sys·tem** (ē'kō-sis-tem) **1.** the fundamental unit in ecology, comprising the living organisms and the nonliving elements that interact in a defined region. **2.** a biocenosis (biotic community) and its biotope.

**eco·tax·is** (ē-kō-tak'sis) migration of lymphocytes from the thymus and bone marrow into tissues possessing an appropriate microenvironment. [eco- + G. *taxis*, order, arrangement]

e
c

**eco·tro·pic vi·rus** an oncornavirus that does not produce disease in its natural host but does replicate in tissue culture cells derived from the host species.

**ECP** eosinophil cationic protein.

**ec·phy·ma** (ek-fī'mă) a warty growth or protuberance. [G. a pimply eruption]

**ECS** electrocerebral silence.

**ECT** electroconvulsive therapy.

**ec·tad** (ek'tad) outward. [G. *ektos,* outside, + L. *ad,* to]

**ec·tal** (ek'tăl) outer; external. [G. *ektos,* outside]

**ec·ta·sia, ec·ta·sis** (ek-tā'zē-ă, ek'tă-sis) dilation of a tubular structure. [G. *ektasis,* a stretching]

△-**ectasia, -ectasis** dilation, expansion. [G. *ektasis,* a stretching]

**ec·ta·sia cor·dis** dilation of the heart. SYN cardiectasia.

**ec·tat·ic** (ek-tat'ik) relating to, or marked by, ectasis.

**ec·tat·ic em·phy·se·ma** obstructive airway disease with areas of dilatation of alveoli acini. Seen primarily in association with inherited deficiency of alpha₁ protease inhibitor. SEE panlobular emphysema.

**ec·ten·tal** (ek-ten'tăl) relating to both ectoderm and endoderm; denoting the line where these two layers join. [G. *ektos,* outside, + *entos,* within]

**ec·thy·ma** (ek-thī'mă) a pyogenic infection of the skin initiated by β-hemolytic streptococci and characterized by adherent crusts beneath which ulceration occurs; the ulcers heal with scar formation. [G. a pustule]

△**ec·to-, ect-** outer, on the outside. SEE ALSO exo-. [G. *ektos,* outside]

**ec·to·an·ti·gen** (ek-tō-an'ti-jen) any toxin or other excitor of antibody formation, separate or separable from its source. SYN exoantigen.

**ec·to·blast** (ek'tō-blast) **1.** SYN ectoderm. **2.** as used by some experimental embryologists, the original outer cell layer from which the primary germ layers are formed; in this sense, synonymous with protoderm. **3.** a cell wall. [ecto- + G. *blastos,* germ]

**ec·to·car·dia** (ek-tō-kar'dē-ă) congenital displacement of the heart. SYN exocardia. [ecto- + G. *kardia,* heart]

**ec·to·cer·vi·cal** (ek'tō-ser'vi-kăl) pertaining to the pars vaginalis of the cervix uteri that is lined with stratified squamous epithelium.

**ec·to·derm** (ek'tō-derm) the outer layer of cells in the embryo, after establishment of the three primary germ layers (ectoderm, mesoderm, endoderm). SYN ectoblast (1). [ecto- + G. *derma,* skin]

**ec·to·der·mal** (ek-tō-der'măl) relating to the ectoderm.

**ec·to·en·tad** (ek-tō-en'tad) from without inward.

**ec·to·en·zyme** (ek-tō-en'zīm) an enzyme that is excreted externally and that acts outside the organism.

**ec·tog·e·nous** (ek-toj'e-nŭs) SYN exogenous. [ecto- + G. *-gen,* producing]

**ec·to·glob·u·lar** (ek-tō-glob'yu-lăr) not within a globular body; specifically not within a red blood cell.

**ec·to·mere** (ek'tō-mēr) one of the blastomeres involved in formation of ectoderm. [ecto- + G. *meros,* part]

**ec·to·morph** (ek'tō-mōrf) a constitutional body type or build (biotype or somatotype) in which

tissues originating from the ectoderm predominate; from a morphological standpoint, the limbs predominate over the trunk. [ecto- + G. *morphē,* form]

**ec·to·mor·phic** (ek-tō-mōrf'ik) relating to, or having the characteristics of, an ectomorph.

△-**ec·to·my** removal of an anatomical structure. SEE ALSO -tomy. [G. *ektomē,* a cutting out]

**ec·top·a·gus** (ek-top'ă-gŭs) conjoined twins in which the bodies are joined laterally. SEE conjoined twins. [ecto- + G. *pagos,* something fixed]

**ec·to·par·a·site** (ek-tō-par'ă-sīt) a parasite that lives on the surface of the host body.

**ec·to·pia** (ek-tō'pē-ă) congenital displacement or malposition of any organ or part of the body. SYN ectopy, heterotopia (1). [G. *ektopos,* out of place, fr. *ektos,* outside, + *topos,* place]

**ec·to·pia cor·dis** congenital condition in which the heart is exposed on the thoracic wall because of maldevelopment of the sternum and pericardium.

**ec·to·pia len·tis** displacement of the lens of the eye.

**ec·to·pia len·tis et pu·pil·lae** disorder characterized by corectopia and a subluxed or dislocated lens.

**ec·to·pia pu·pil·lae con·gen·i·ta** displacement of the pupil present at birth.

**ec·to·pia tes·tis** SYN parorchidium. SYN parorchidium.

**ec·top·ic** (ek-top'ik) **1.** out of place; said of an organ not in its proper position, or of a pregnancy occurring elsewhere than in the cavity of the uterus. SYN aberrant (3), heterotopic (1), imperforate anus (2). **2.** CARDIOGRAPHY denoting a heartbeat that has its origin in some focus other than the sinoatrial node. [see ectopia]

**ec·top·ic beat** a cardiac beat originating elsewhere than at the sinoatrial node.

**ec·top·ic bone** proliferation of bone in an abnormal place.

**ec·top·ic preg·nan·cy** the development of an impregnated ovum outside the cavity of the uterus. SYN eccyesis.

**ec·top·ic schis·to·so·mi·a·sis** a clinical form of schistosomiasis that occurs outside of the normal site of parasitism (mesenteric vein or hepatic portals).

**ec·top·ic tach·y·car·dia** a tachycardia originating in a focus other than the sinus node, e.g., atrial, A-V junctional, or ventricular tachycardia.

**ec·top·ic tes·tis** a variant of undescended testis wherein testicular position is outside the usual pathway of descent. SEE ALSO ectopia testis.

**ec·top·ic u·re·ter·o·cele** a ureterocele extending distal to the bladder neck.

**ec·to·py** (ek'tō-pē) SYN ectopia.

**ec·tos·te·al** (ek-tos'tē-ăl) relating to the external surface of a bone. [ecto- + G. *osteon,* bone]

**ec·tos·to·sis** (ek-tos-tō'sis) ossification in cartilage beneath the perichondrium, or formation of bone beneath the periosteum. [ecto- + G. *osteon,* bone, + *-osis,* condition]

**ec·to·thrix** (ek'tō-thriks) a sheath of spores (conidia) on the outside of a hair. [ecto- + G. *thrix,* hair]

△**ec·tro-** congenital absence of a part. [G. *ektrōsis,* miscarriage]

**ec·tro·dac·ty·ly, ec·tro·dac·tyl·ia, ec·tro·dac·tyl·ism** (ek-trō-dak'ti-lē, ek-trō-dak-til'i-ă, ek-trō-dak′ti-lizm) congenital absence of all or part of one or more fingers or toes. Known also as split-hand/foot deformity, lobster claw. There are several varieties and the pattern of inheritance is usually irregular. [ectro- + G. *daktylos,* finger]

**ec·tro·dac·ty·ly–ec·to·der·mal dys·pla·sia–cleft·ing syn·drome** an autosomal recessive disorder resulting in defects of hands and feet; the ectodermal dysplasia causes anodontia and cleft palate.

**ec·tro·gen·ic** (ek-trō-jen′ik) relating to ectrogeny.

**ec·trog·e·ny** (ek-troj′ĕ-nē) congenital absence or defect of any bodily part. [ectro- + G. *-gen,* producing]

**ec·tro·me·lia** (ek-trō-mē′lē-ă) **1.** congenital hypoplasia or aplasia of one or more limbs. **2.** a disease of mice caused by the ectromelia virus; characterized by gangrenous loss of feet and necrotic areas in the internal organs; in laboratory mouse colonies, it usually results in high mortality rates. [ectro- + G. *melos,* limb]

**ec·tro·mel·ic** (ek-trō-mel′ik) pertaining to, or characterized by, ectromelia.

**ec·tro·pi·on, ec·tro·pi·um** (ek-trō′pē-on, ek-trō-pē-ŭm) a rolling outward of the margin of a part, e.g., of an eyelid. [G. *ek,* out, + *tropē,* a turning]

**ec·tro·pi·on u·ve·ae** eversion of the pigmented posterior epithelium of the iris at the pupillary margin.

**ec·trop·o·dy** (ek-trop′ō-dē) total or partial absence of a foot. [ectro- + G. *pous,* foot]

**ec·tro·syn·dac·ty·ly** (ek′trō-sin-dak′ti-lē) congenital anomaly marked by the absence of one or more digits and the fusion of others. [ectro- + G. *syn,* together, + *daktylos,* finger]

**ec·ze·ma** (ek′zĕ-mă) generic term for inflammatory conditions of the skin, particularly with vesiculation in the acute stage, typically erythematous, edematous, papular, and crusting; followed often by lichenification and scaling and occasionally by duskiness of the erythema and, infrequently, hyperpigmentation; often accompanied by sensations of itching and burning; the vesicles form by intraepidermal spongiosis. Sometimes referred to colloquially as tetter, dry tetter, scaly tetter. [G. fr. *ekzeō,* to boil over]

**ec·ze·ma her·pe·ti·cum** a febrile condition caused by cutaneous dissemination of herpesvirus type 1, occurring most commonly in children, consisting of a widespread eruption of vesicles rapidly becoming umbilicated pustules.

**ec·ze·ma mar·gi·na·tum** SYN tinea cruris.

**ec·ze·ma·toid** (ek-zem′ă-toyd) resembling eczema in appearance.

**ec·ze·ma·tous** (ek-zem′ă-tŭs) marked by or resembling eczema.

**ED** effective dose.

**ED$_{50}$** median effective dose.

**ede·ma** (e-dē′mă) an accumulation of an excessive amount of watery fluid in cells, tissues, or serous cavities. [G. *oidēma,* a swelling]

**edem·a·tous** (e-dem′ă-tŭs) marked by edema.

**eden·tate** (ē-den′tāt) SYN edentulous. [L. *edentatus*]

**eden·tu·lous** (ē-den′tyu-lŭs) toothless, having lost the natural teeth. SYN edentate. [L. *edentulus,* toothless]

**Ed·er-Pus·tow bou·gie** (ā′dĕr-poo′stō) a metal olive-shaped bougie with a flexible metal dilating system (for esophageal stricture).

**ed·e·tate** (ed′ĕ-tāt) USAN-approved contraction for ethylenediaminetetraacetate.

**Ed·i·son ef·fect** (ed′i-son) SYN thermionic emission.

**EDM** multiple epiphysial dysplasia.

**EDSS** expanded disability status scale.

**EEG** electroencephalogram; electroencephalography.

**eel** (ēl) any of a number of scaleless, snakelike fish. [M.E. *ele,* fr. O.E. *ael*]

**EENT** eye, ear, nose, and throat. See also ENT.

**ef·face·ment** (ē-fās′ment) the thinning out of the cervix just before or during labor.

**ef·fect** (e-fekt′) the result or consequence of an action. [L. *efficio,* pp. *effectus,* to accomplish, fr. *facio,* to do]

**ef·fec·tive con·ju·gate** the internal conjugate measured from the nearest lumbar vertebra to the symphysis, in spondylolisthesis. SYN false conjugate (2).

**ef·fec·tive dose (ED) 1.** the dose that produces the desired effect; when followed by a subscript (generally "ED$_{50}$"), it denotes the dose having such an effect on a certain percentage (e.g., 50%) of the test animals; ED$_{50}$ is the median effective dose; **2.** in radiation protection, the sum of the equivalent doses in all tissues and organs of the body weighted for tissue effects of radiation. The unit of effective dose is the sievert (Sv).

**ef·fec·tive·ness 1.** a measure of the accuracy or success of a diagnostic or therapeutic technique when carried out in an average clinical environment. **2.** the extent to which a treatment achieves its intended purpose.

**ef·fec·tive os·mot·ic pres·sure** that part of the total osmotic pressure of a solution that governs the tendency of its solvent to pass across a boundary, usually a semipermeable membrane.

**ef·fec·tive re·nal blood flow (ERBF)** the amount of blood flowing to the parts of the kidney that are involved with production of constituents of urine.

**ef·fec·tive re·nal plas·ma flow (ERPF)** the amount of plasma flowing to the parts of the kidney that have a function in the production of constituents of urine; the clearance of substances such as iodopyracet and *p*-aminohippuric acid, assuming that the extraction ratio in the peritubular capillaries is 100%.

**ef·fec·tive tem·per·a·ture** a comfort index or scale which takes into account the temperature of air, its moisture content, and movement.

**ef·fec·tor** (ē-fek′tŏr) **1.** a peripheral tissue that receives nerve impulses and reacts by contraction (muscle), secretion (gland), or a discharge of electricity (electric organ of certain bony fishes). **2.** a small metabolic molecule that by combining with a repressor gene depresses the activity of an operon. **3.** a small molecule that binds to a protein and, in so doing, alters the activity of that protein. **4.** a substance, technique, procedure, or individual that causes an effect. [L. producer]

**ef·fem·i·na·tion** (e-fem-i-nā′shŭn) acquisition of feminine characteristics, either physiologically as part of female maturation, or pathologically by individuals of either sex. [L. *ef-femino,* pp. *-atus,* to make feminine, fr. *ex,* out, + *femina,* woman]

**ef·fer·ent** (ef′er-ent) conducting outward from an organ or part; e.g., the efferent connections of a group of nerve cells, efferent blood vessels, or the excretory duct of an organ. [L. *efferens,* fr. *effero,* to bring out]

**ef•fer•ent duc•tules of tes•tis** one of 12 to 14 small seminal ducts leading from the testis to the head of the epididymis. SYN ductuli efferentes testis [TA].

**ef•fer•ent glo•mer•u•lar ar•te•ri•ole** the vessel that carries blood from the glomerular capillary network to the capillary bed of the proximal convoluted tubule. SYN vas efferens (2) [TA], efferent vessel.

**ef•fer•ent nerve** a nerve conveying impulses from the central nervous system to the periphery. SYN centrifugal nerve.

**ef•fer•ent ves•sel** SYN efferent glomerular arteriole.

**ef•fer•ves•cent salts** preparations made by adding sodium bicarbonate and tartaric and citric acids to the active salt; when thrown into water the acids break up the sodium bicarbonate, setting free the carbonic acid gas.

**ef•fi•cien•cy** (ĕ-fish'en-sē) **1.** the production of the desired effects or results with minimum waste of time, effort, or skill. **2.** a measure of effectiveness; specifically, the useful work output divided by the energy input.

**ef•fleu•rage** (e-fler-ahz') a form of massage consisting of long, unbroken strokes in which the hand conforms to the surface and follows the fiber direction of underlying structures. [Fr. *effleurer,* to touch lightly]

**ef•flo•resce** (e-flōr-es') to become powdery by losing the water of crystallization on exposure to a dry atmosphere. [L. *ef-floresco* (*exf-*), to blossom, fr. *flos* (*flor-*), flower]

**ef•flu•vi•um,** pl. **ef•flu•via** (e-floo'vē-ŭm, e-floo'v-ē-ă) shedding of hair. SEE ALSO defluxion (1). [L. a flowing out, fr. *ef-fluo,* to flow out]

**ef•fu•sion** (e-fyu'zhŭn) **1.** the escape of fluid from the blood vessels or lymphatics into the tissues or a cavity. **2.** a collection of the fluid effused. [L. *effusio,* a pouring out]

**EGD** esophagogastroduodenoscopy.

**eges•ta** (ē-jes'tă) unabsorbed food residues that are discharged from the digestive tract. [L. *e-gero,* pp. *-gestus,* to carry out, discharge]

**EGFR** epidermal growth factor receptor .

**egg** (eg) the female sexual cell or gamete. SEE ALSO oocyte. [A.S. *aeg*]

**egg al•bu•min** SYN ovalbumin.

**egg clus•ter** one of the clumps of cells resulting from the breaking up of the gonadal cords in the ovarian cortex; these clumps later develop into primary ovarian follicles.

**egg mem•brane** a primary egg membrane is produced from ovarian cytoplasm (e.g., a vitelline membrane); a secondary egg membrane is the product of the ovarian follicle (e.g., the zona pellucida); a tertiary egg membrane is secreted by the lining of the oviduct (e.g., a shell).

**egg•shell cal•ci•fi•ca•tion** a thin layer of calcification around an intrathoracic lymph node, usually in silicosis, seen on a chest radiograph.

**e•go** (ē'gō) PSYCHOANALYSIS one of the three components of the psychic apparatus in the freudian structural framework, the other two being the id and superego. The ego occupies a position between the primal instincts (pleasure principle) and the demands of the outer world (reality principle), and therefore mediates between the person and external reality by performing the important functions of perceiving the needs of the self, both physical and psychological, and the qualities and attitudes of the environment. It is also responsible for certain defensive functions to protect the person against the demands of the id and superego. [L. I]

**ego•bron•choph•o•ny** (ē'gō-brong-kof'ō-nē) egophony with bronchophony. [G. *aix* (*aig-*), goat, + *bronchos,* bronchus, + *phōnē,* voice]

**ego•cen•tric** (ē-gō-sen'trik) marked by extreme concentration of attention upon oneself, i.e., self-centered. SYN egotropic. [ego + G. *kentron,* center]

**ego•dys•ton•ic** (ē'gō-dis-ton'ik) repugnant to or at variance with the aims of the ego and related psychological needs of the individual (e.g., an obsessive thought or compulsive behavior); the opposite of ego-syntonic. [ego + G. *dys,* bad, + *tonos,* tension]

**e•go-dys•ton•ic ho•mo•sex•u•al•i•ty** a psychological or psychiatric disorder in which an individual experiences persistent distress associated with same-sex preference and a strong need to change the behavior or, at least, to alleviate the distress associated with the homosexuality.

**ego ide•al** the part of the personality that comprises the goals, aspirations, and aims of the self, usually growing out of the emulation of a significant person with whom one has identified.

**ego iden•ti•ty** the ego's sense of its own identity.

**ego•ma•nia** (ē-gō-mā'nē-ă) extreme self-centeredness, self-appreciation, or self-content. [ego + G. *mania,* frenzy]

**ego•phon•ic** (ē-gō-fon'ik) relating to egophony.

**egoph•o•ny** (ē-gof'ō-nē) a peculiar broken quality of the voice sounds, like the bleating of a goat, heard about the upper level of the fluid in cases of pleurisy with effusion. [G. *aix* (*aig-*), goat, + *phōnē,* voice]

**ego-syn•ton•ic** (ē'gō-sin-ton'ik) acceptable to the aims of the ego and the related psychological needs of the individual (e.g., a delusion); the opposite of ego-dystonic. [ego + G. *syn,* together, + *tonos,* tension]

**ego•tro•pic** (ē-gō-trop'ik) SYN egocentric. [ego + G. *tropē,* a turning]

**E•gyp•tian oph•thal•mia** (ē-jip'shŭn) SYN trachoma.

**e-health** health information on the Internet for patients, providers, and healthcare companies.

**EHEC** enterohemorrhagic *Escherichia coli.*

**Eh•ret phe•nom•e•non** (ār'et) a sudden throb felt by the finger on the brachial artery, as the pressure in the cuff falls during a blood pressure estimation; said to indicate fairly accurately the diastolic pressure.

**Ehr•lich ac•id he•ma•tox•y•lin stain** an alum type of hematoxylin stain used as a regressive staining method for nuclei, followed by differentiation to required staining intensity; the solution may be allowed to ripen naturally in sunlight or partially oxidized with sodium iodate.

**Ehr•lich a•ne•mia** (ār'lik) SYN aplastic anemia.

**Ehr•lich an•i•line crys•tal vi•o•let stain** (ār'lik) a stain for Gram-positive bacteria.

**Ehr•lich benz•al•de•hyde re•ac•tion** (ār'lik) a test for urobilinogen in the urine, by dissolving 2 g of dimethyl-*p*-aminobenzaldehyde in 100 mL of 5% hydrochloric acid and adding this reagent to urine; a red color in the cold indicates the presence of an excessive amount of urobilinogen.

**Ehr·lich·ia** (er-lik′ē-ă) a genus of small, often pleomorphic, coccoid to ellipsoidal, nonmotile, Gram-negative bacteria (order Rickettsiales) that occur either singly or in compact inclusions in circulating mammalian leukocytes; species are the etiologic agents of ehrlichiosis and are transmitted by ticks. The type species is *Ehrlichia canis*. [P. *Ehrlich*]

**Ehr·lich·ia chaf·feen·sis** a recently described species associated with human ehrlichiosis and carried by the tick vector, *Amblyomma americanum*, the Lone Star tick.

**Ehr·lich·ia e·qui** a bacterial species that causes human granulocytic ehrlichiosis; occurs in the Midatlantic, southern New England, and southern Midwest and is spread by ticks (*Ixodes*).

**Ehr·lich·ia pha·go·cy·to·phila** a bacterial species that causes human granulocytic ehrlichiosis; also causes tick-borne fever in cattle; occurs in the Midatlantic, southern New England, and southern Midwest and is spread by ticks (*Ixodes*).

**Ehr·lich in·ner body** (ār′lik) a round oxyphil body found in the red blood cell in hemolysis due to a specific blood poison. SYN Heinz-Ehrlich body.

**ehr·lich·i·o·sis** (er-lik-ē-ō′sis) a tickborn infection of human beings and dogs, caused by bacteria of the genus *Ehrlichia*, which produces manifestations similar to those of Rocky Mountain spotted fever.

**Ehr·lich phe·nom·e·non** (ār′lik) the difference between the amount of diphtheria toxin that will exactly neutralize one unit of antitoxin and that which, added to one unit of antitoxin, will leave one lethal dose free is greater than one lethal dose of toxin; i.e., it is necessary to add more than one lethal dose of toxin to a neutral mixture of toxin and antitoxin to make the mixture lethal (the basis of the L₊ dose).

**Ehr·lich pos·tu·late** (ār′lik) SYN side-chain theory.

**Ehr·lich the·o·ry** (ār′lik) SEE side-chain theory.

**Ehr·lich tri·ac·id stain** (ār′lik) a differential leukocytic stain comprised of saturated solutions of orange G, acid fuchsin, and methyl green.

**Ehr·lich tri·ple stain** (ār′lik) a mixture of indulin, eosin Y, and aurantia.

**EIA** enzyme immunoassay.

**Eich·horst cor·pus·cles** (īk′hōrst) the globular forms sometimes occurring in the poikilocytosis of pernicious anemia.

**Eich·horst neu·ri·tis** (īk′hōrst) SYN interstitial neuritis.

**Eick·en meth·od** (ī′kĕn) facilitation of hypopharyngoscopy by means of forward traction on the cricoid cartilage by a laryngeal probe.

**ei·co·sa·noids** (ī′kō-să-noydz) the physiologically active substances derived from arachidonic acid, i.e., the prostaglandins, leukotrienes, and thromboxanes; synthesized via a cascade pathway. [G. *eicosa-*, twenty, + *eidos*, form]

**EIEC** enteroinvasive *Escherichia coli*.

**eighth cra·ni·al nerve [CN VIII]** SYN vestibulocochlear nerve [CN VIII].

**Ei·ken·el·la cor·ro·dens** (ī-kĕ-nel′ă kōr-rō′denz) a species of nonmotile, rod-shaped, Gram-negative, facultatively anaerobic bacteria that is part of the normal flora of the adult human oral cavity but may be an opportunistic pathogen, especially in immunocompromised hosts. [M. *Eiken*, 1958]

**Ei·nar·son gal·lo·cy·a·nin-chrome al·um**

**stain** (īn′ăr-sŏn) a method for staining both RNA and DNA a deep blue; with proper controls, nucleic acid content of stained cells and nuclei may be estimated by cytophotometry; also useful for Nissl substance.

**ein·stein** (īn′stīn) a unit of energy equal to 1 mol quantum, hence to $6.0221367 \times 10^{23}$ quanta. The value of einstein, in kJ, is dependent upon the wavelength. [A. *Einstein*, German-born theoretical physicist and Nobel laureate in U.S., 1879–1955]

**ein·stein·i·um (Es)** (īn-stīn′ē-ŭm) an artificially prepared transuranium element, atomic no. 99, atomic wt. 252.0; it has many isotopes, all of which are radioactive ($^{252}$Es has the longest known half-life, 1.29 years).

**Ein·tho·ven law** (īn′tō-vĕn) in the electrocardiogram the potential of any wave or complex in lead II is equal to the sum of its potentials in leads I and III.

**Ein·tho·ven tri·an·gle** (īn′tō-vĕn) an imaginary equilateral triangle with the heart at its center, its equal sides representing the three standard limb leads of the electrocardiogram.

**Ei·sen·men·ger com·plex** (ī′sĕn-meng′ĕr) the combination of ventricular septal defect with pulmonary hypertension and consequent right-to-left shunt through the defect, with or without an associated overriding aorta.

**Ei·sen·men·ger syn·drome** (ī′sĕn-meng′ĕr) cardiac failure with significant right-to-left shunt producing cyanosis due to higher pressure on the right side of the shunt. Usually due to the Eisenmenger complex, a ventricular septal defect with right ventricular hypertrophy and dilatation, severe pulmonary hypertension, and frequent straddling of the defect by a misplaced aortic root.

**ejac·u·late** (ē-jak′yu-lāt) **1.** to expel suddenly, as of semen. **2.** semen expelled in ejaculation. [see ejaculation]

**ejac·u·la·tio** (ē-jak-yu-lā′shē-ō) SYN ejaculation.

**ejac·u·la·tion** (ē-jak-ū-lā′shŭn) the process that results in propulsion of semen from the genital ducts and urethra to the exterior; caused by the rhythmic contractions of the muscles surrounding the internal genital organs and the ischiocavernous and bulbocavernous muscles, resulting in an increase in pressure on the semen in the internal genital glands and the internal urethra. SYN ejaculatio. [L. *e-iaculo*, pp. *-atus*, to shoot out]

**ejac·u·la·to·ry** (ē-jak′yu-lă-tōr-ē) relating to an ejaculation.

**e·jac·u·la·to·ry duct** the duct formed by the union of the deferent duct and the excretory duct of the seminal vesicle, which opens into the prostatic urethra. SYN spermiduct (2).

**ejec·ta** (ē-jek′tă) SYN ejection (2). [L. ntr. pl. of *ejectus*, pp. of *ejicio*, to throw out]

**ejec·tion** (ē-jek′shŭn) **1.** the act of driving or throwing out by physical force from within. **2.** that which is ejected. SYN ejecta. [L. *ejectio*, from *ejicio*, to cast out]

**e·jec·tion mur·mur** a diamond-shaped systolic murmur produced by the ejection of blood into the aorta or pulmonary artery and ending by the time of the second heart sound component produced, respectively, by closing of the aortic or pulmonic valve.

**e·jec·tion pe·ri·od** SYN sphygmic interval.

△**eka-** prefix used to denote an undiscovered or just

discovered element in the periodic system before a proper and official name is assigned by authorities; e.g., eka-osmium, now plutonium. [Sanskrit *eka,* one]

**EKG** electrocardiogram.

**elab·o·ra·tion** (ē-lab′ōr-ā′shŭn) the process of working out in detail by labor and study. [L. *e-laborō,* pp. *-atus,* to labor, endeavor, fr. *labor,* toil, to work out]

**elas·tance** (ē-las′tans) **1.** a measure of the stiffness of a chamber expressed as a change in pressure per unit change in volume; the reciprocal of compliance. **2.** in medicine and physiology, usually a measure of the tendency of a hollow viscus (e.g., lung, urinary bladder, gallbladder) to recoil toward its original dimensions upon removal of a distending or compressing force.

**elas·tase** (ē-las′tās) a serine proteinase hydrolyzing elastin.

**elas·tic** (ē-las′tik) **1.** having the property of returning to the original shape after being compressed, bent, or otherwise distorted. **2.** a rubber or plastic band used in orthodontics as either a primary or adjunctive source of force to move teeth. The term is generally modified by an adjective to describe the direction of the force or the location of the terminal connecting points. [G. *elastreō,* epic form of *elaunō,* drive, push]

**elas·tic ban·dage** a bandage containing stretchable material; used to make local pressure.

**elas·tic car·ti·lage** a cartilage in which cells are surrounded by a territorial capsular matrix outside of which is an interterritorial matrix containing elastic fiber networks in addition to collagen fibers and ground substance. SYN yellow cartilage.

**elas·tic fi·bers** fibers that are 0.2 to 2 μm in diameter but may be larger in some ligaments; they branch and anastomose to form networks and fuse to form fenestrated membranes; the fibers and membranes consist of microfibrils about 10 nm wide and an amorphous substance containing elastin. SYN yellow fibers.

**elas·ti·cin** (ē-las′ti-sin) SYN elastin.

**elas·tic·i·ty** (ē-las-tis′i-tē) the quality or condition of being elastic.

**elas·tic la·mel·la** a thin sheet or membrane composed of elastic fibers.

**elas·tic lam·i·nae of ar·ter·ies** 1) external: the layer of elastic connective tissue lying immediately outside the smooth muscle of the tunica media; 2) internal: a fenestrated layer of elastic tissue of the tunica intima. SYN elastic layers of arteries.

**elas·tic lay·ers of ar·ter·ies** SYN elastic laminae of arteries.

**elas·tic mem·brane** a membrane formed of elastic connective tissue, present as fenestrated lamellae in the coats of the arteries and elsewhere.

**elas·tic tis·sue** a form of connective tissue in which the elastic fibers predominate; it constitutes the ligamenta flava of the vertebrae and the ligamentum nuchae, especially of quadrupeds; it occurs also in the walls of the arteries and of the bronchial tree, and connects the cartilages of the larynx.

**elas·tin** (ē-las′tin) a yellow elastic fibrous mucoprotein that is the major connective tissue protein of elastic structures (large blood vessels, tendons, and ligaments). SYN elasticin.

**elas·to·fi·bro·ma** (ē-las′tō-fī-brō′mă) a nonen-

capsulated slow-growing mass of poorly cellular, collagenous, fibrous tissue and elastic tissue; occurs usually in subscapular adipose tissue of old persons. [G. *elastos,* beaten, + L. *fibra, -oma* tumor]

**e·las·toid de·gen·er·a·tion 1.** SYN elastosis (2). **2.** hyaline degeneration of the elastic tissue of the arterial wall, seen during involution of the uterus.

**elas·to·ma** (ĕ-las-tō′mă) a tumor-like deposit of elastic tissue.

**elas·to·sis** (ĕ-las-tō′sis) **1.** degenerative change in elastic tissue. **2.** degeneration of collagen fibers, with altered staining properties resembling elastic tissue, or formation by fibroblast-activated ultraviolet or mast cell mediators of abnormal fibers. SYN elastoid degeneration (1), elastotic degeneration.

**e·las·tot·ic de·gen·er·a·tion** SYN elastosis (2).

**e·laun·in** (ē-law′nin) a component of elastic fibers formed from a deposition of elastin between oxytalan fibers; found in the connective tissue of the dermis, particularly in association with sweat glands. [G. *elaunō,* to drive]

**el·bow** (el′bō) **1.** the region of the upper limb between arm and forearm surrounding the elbow joint, especially posteriorly. **2.** the joint between the arm and the forearm. SYN cubitus (1). **3.** an angular body resembling a flexed elbow. [A.S. *elnboga*]

**el·bow bone** SYN olecranon.

**el·bowed bou·gie** a bougie with a sharply angulated bend near its tip.

**el·bow joint** a compound hinge synovial joint between the humerus and the bones of the forearm; it consists of the articulatio humeroradialis and the articulatio humeroulnaris. SYN cubital joint.

**el·der a·buse** the physical or emotional abuse, including financial exploitation, of an elderly person, by one or more of the individual's children, nursing home caregivers, or others.

**el·der·ly pri·mi·gra·vi·da** dated term referring to a woman older than 35 years who is pregnant for the first time.

**elec·tive a·bor·tion** an abortion without medical justification but done in a legal way, as in the United States.

**elec·tive mut·ism** mutism due to psychogenic causes.

**Elec·tra com·plex** (ē-lek′etră) unresolved conflicts during childhood toward the father which subsequently influence a woman's relationships with men. [*Electra,* daughter of Agamemnon]

**elec·tri·cal al·ter·nans** alternation in the amplitude of P waves, QRS complexes, or T wave as observed by electrocardiography.

**elec·tri·cal al·ter·na·tion of heart** a disorder in which the ventricular or atrial complexes or both are regular in time but of alternating pattern; detected by electrocardiography.

**elec·tri·cal ax·is** the net direction of the electromotive forces developed in the heart during its activation, usually represented in the frontal plane.

**elec·tri·cal di·as·to·le** period from end of T wave to beginning of next Q wave.

**elec·tri·cal fail·ure** failure in which the cardiac inadequacy is secondary to disturbance of the electrical impulse.

**elec·tri·cal sys·to·le** the duration of the QRS-T

complex (i.e., from the earliest Q wave to the end of the latest T wave on the ECG).

⌂**elec·tro-** electric, electricity. [G. *ēlektron,* amber (on which static electricity can be generated by friction)]

**elec·tro·a·cu·punc·ture** acupuncture in which needles are attached to a source of electric current.

**elec·tro·an·al·ge·sia** (ē-lek′trō-an-ăl-jē′zē-ă) analgesia induced by the passage of an electric current.

**elec·tro·an·es·the·sia** (ē-lek′trō-an-es-thē′zē-ă) anesthesia produced by an electric current.

**elec·tro·car·di·o·gram (ECG, EKG)** (ē-lek-trō-kar′dē-ō-gram) graphic record of cardiac action currents obtained with the electrocardiograph. [electro- + G. *kardia,* heart, + *gramma,* a drawing]

**elec·tro·car·di·o·graph** (ē-lek-trō-kar′dē-ō-graf) an instrument for recording the potential of the electrical currents that traverse the heart.

◨**elec·tro·car·di·og·ra·phy** (ē-lek′trō-kar-dē-og′ră-fē) **1.** a method of recording the electrical activity of the heart: impulse formation and conduction, depolarization and repolarization of atria and ventricles. **2.** the study and interpretation of electrocardiograms. See this page.

**elec·tro·cau·ter·i·za·tion** (ē-lek′trō-kaw′ter-i-zā′shŭn) cauterization by passage of high frequency current through tissue or by metal that has been electrically heated.

**elec·tro·cau·tery** (ē-lek′trō-kaw′ter-ē) **1.** an instrument for directing a high frequency current

through a local area of tissue. **2.** a metal cauterizing instrument heated by an electric current.

**elec·tro·ce·re·bral si·lence (ECS)** (ē-lek′trō-ser-ē′brăl sī′lens) flat or isoelectric encephalogram; an electroencephalogram with absence of cerebral activity from symmetrically placed electrode pairs; if such a record is present for 30 minutes in a clinically brain dead adult and if drug intoxication, hypothermia, and recent hypotension have been excluded, the diagnosis of cerebral death is supported. SYN flat electroencephalogram.

**elec·tro·chem·i·cal** (ē-lek′trō-kem′i-kăl) denoting chemical reactions involving electricity, and the mechanisms involved.

**elec·tro·co·ag·u·la·tion** (ē-lek′trō-kō-ag-yu-lā′shŭn) coagulation produced by an electrocautery.

**elec·tro·co·chle·o·gram** (ē-lek′trō-kok′lē-ō-gram) the record obtained by electrocochleography.

**elec·tro·co·chle·og·ra·phy** (ē-lek′trō-kok-lē-og′ră-fē) a measurement of the electrical potentials generated in the inner ear as a result of sound stimulation. [electro- + L. *cochlea,* snail shell, + G. *graphō,* to write]

**elec·tro·con·trac·til·i·ty** (ē-lek′trō-kon-trak-til′i-tē) the power of contraction of muscular tissue in response to an electrical stimulus.

**elec·tro·con·vul·sive** (ē-lek′trō-kon-vŭl′siv) denoting a convulsive response to an electrical stimulus. SEE electroshock therapy.

**elec·tro·con·vul·sive ther·a·py (ECT)** SYN electroshock therapy.

e
l

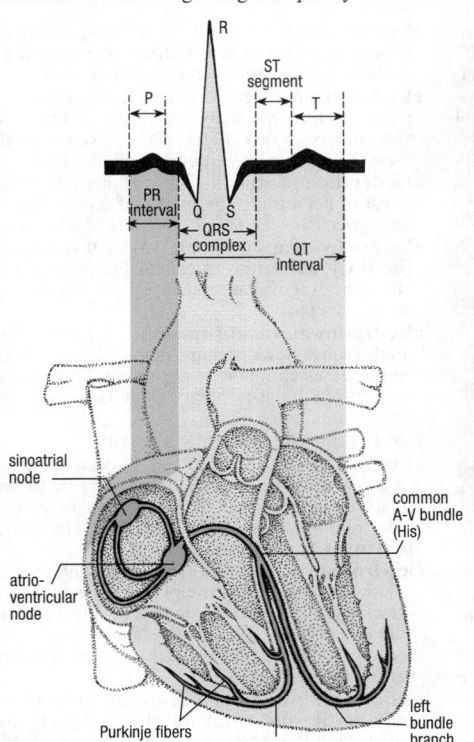

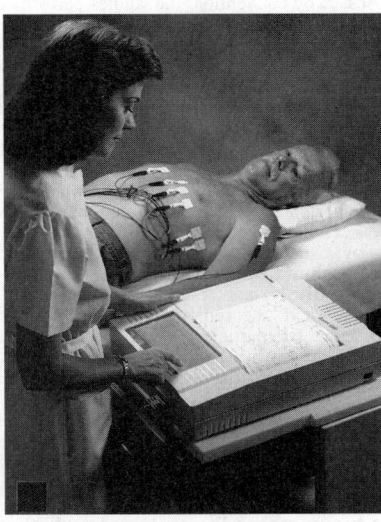

**electrocardiography (ECG):** (right) resting electrocardiogram; (left) an electrical picture of the heart is represented by positive and negative deflections on a graph labeled with the letters P,Q,R,S, and T, corresponding to the events of the cardiac cycle

**elec·tro·cor·ti·co·gram** (ē-lek-trō-kōr′ti-kō-gram) a record of electrical activity derived directly from the cerebral cortex.

**elec·tro·cor·ti·cog·ra·phy** (ē-lek′trō-kōr-ti-kog′ră-fē) the technique of recording the electrical activity of the cerebral cortex by means of electrodes placed directly on it.

**elec·trode** (ē-lek′trōd) **1.** device to record one of the two extremities of an electric circuit; one of the two poles of an electric battery or of the end of the conductors connected thereto. **2.** an electrical terminal specialized for a particular electrochemical reaction. [electro- + G. *hodos,* way]

**elec·trode cath·e·ter ab·la·tion** a method of ablating the site of origin of arrhythmias whereby high energy electric shocks are delivered by intravascular catheters.

**elec·tro·der·mal** (ē-lek′trō-der′măl) pertaining to electric properties of the skin, usually referring to altered resistance. [electro- + G. *derma,* skin]

**elec·tro·der·mal au·di·om·e·try** a form of electrophysiologic audiometry used to determine hearing thresholds by measuring changes in skin resistance as a conditioned response to noise stimuli.

**elec·tro·des·ic·ca·tion** (ē-lek′trō-des-i-kā′shŭn) destruction of lesions or sealing off of blood vessels (usually of the skin, but also of available surfaces of mucous membrane) by monopolar high-frequency electric current. [electro- + L. *desicco,* to dry up]

**elec·tro·di·ag·no·sis** (ē-lek′trō-dī-ag-nō′sis) **1.** the use of electronic devices for diagnostic purposes. **2.** by convention, the studies performed in the EMG laboratory, i.e., nerve conduction studies and needle electrode examination (EMG proper). SYN electroneurography. **3.** determination of the nature of a disease through observation of changes in electrical activity. SYN evoked electromyography.

**elec·tro·di·ag·nos·tic me·di·cine** the specific area of medical practice in which specially trained physicians use information from the clinical history and physical examination, along with the scientific method of recording and analyzing biologic electrical potentials, to diagnose and treat neuromuscular disorders.

**elec·tro·di·al·y·sis** (ē-lek′trō-dī-al′i-sis) in an electric field, the removal of ions from larger molecules and particles.

**elec·tro·en·ceph·a·lo·gram (EEG)** (ē-lek′trō-en-sef′ă-lō-gram) the record obtained by means of the electroencephalograph.

**elec·tro·en·ceph·a·lo·graph** (ē-lek′trō-en-sef′ă-lō-graf) a system for recording the electric potentials of the brain derived from electrodes attached to the scalp. [electro- + G. *encephalon,* brain, + *graphō,* to write]

**elec·tro·en·ceph·a·lo·graph·ic dys·rhyth·mia** a diffusely irregular brain wave tracing.

🔲 **elec·tro·en·ceph·a·log·ra·phy (EEG)** (ē-lek′trō-en-sef′ă-log′ră-fē) registration of the electrical potentials recorded by an electroencephalograph. See this page.

**elec·tro·en·dos·mo·sis** (ē-lek′trō-en-dos-mō′sis) endosmosis produced by means of an electric field.

**elec·tro·gas·tro·gram** (ē-lek′trō-gas′trō-gram) the record obtained with the electrogastrograph.

**elec·tro·gas·tro·graph** (ē-lek′trō-gas′trō-graf) an instrument used in electrogastrography.

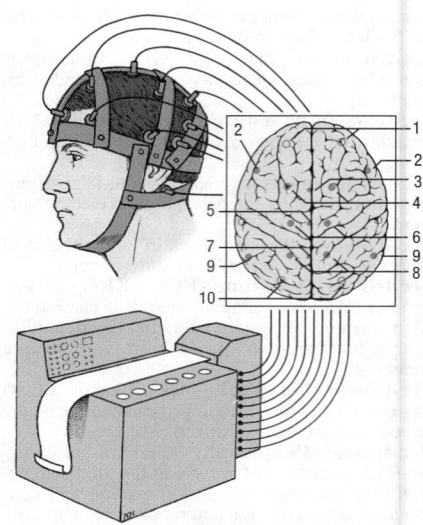

**electroencephalography:** insert shows leads used, (1) frontal, (2) temporal (front), (3) bregma, (4) precentral, (5) vertex, (6) central, (7) lambda, (8) parietal, (9) temporal (rear), (10) occipital

[electro- + G. *gastēr,* stomach, + *graphō,* to write]

**elec·tro·gas·trog·ra·phy** (ē-lek′trō-gas-trog′ră-fē) the recording of the electrical phenomena associated with gastric secretion and motility.

**elec·tro·gram** (ē-lek′trō-gram) **1.** any record on paper or film made by an electrical event. **2.** ELECTROPHYSIOLOGY a recording taken directly from the surface by unipolar or bipolar leads.

**elec·tro·he·mo·sta·sis** (ē-lek′trō-hē-mō-stā′sis) arrest of hemorrhage by means of an electrocautery. [electro- + G. *haima,* blood, + *stasis,* halt]

**elec·tro·hy·drau·lic shock wave lith·o·trip·sy (ESWL)** destruction of calculi (urinary tract or other) by fragmentation using shock waves sent transcutaneously.

**elec·tro·im·mu·no·dif·fu·sion** (ē-lek′trō-im′yu-nō-di-fyu′zhŭn) an immunochemical method that combines electrophoretic separation with immunodiffusion by incorporating antibody into the support medium.

**elec·tro·lar·ynx** SYN artificial larynx.

**elec·trol·y·sis** (ē-lek-trol′i-sis) **1.** decomposition of a salt or other chemical compound by means of an electric current. **2.** destruction of certain hair follicles by means of galvanic electricity. [electro- + G. *lysis,* dissolution]

**elec·tro·lyte** (ē-lek′trō-līt) any compound that, in solution, conducts electricity and is decomposed (electrolyzed) by it; an ionizable substance in solution. [electro- + G. *lytos,* soluble]

**elec·tro·lyt·ic** (ē-lek-trō-lit′ik) referring to or caused by electrolysis.

**elec·tro·mag·ne·tic ra·di·a·tion, elec·tro·mag·ne·tic spec·trum** wavelike energy propagated through matter or space. Varies widely in wavelength, frequency, photon energy, and properties. Is natural or artificial and includes radiowaves, microwaves, visible light, ultraviolet light, x-rays, gamma rays, and cosmic radiation.

**elec·tro·me·chan·i·cal dis·so·ci·a·tion** persistence of electrical activity in the heart without associated mechanical contraction; often a sign of cardiac rupture. SYN pulseless electrical activity.

**elec·tro·mech·an·i·cal sys·tole** the period from the beginning of the QRS complex to the first (aortic) vibration of the second heart sound. SYN QS₂ interval.

**elec·tro·mo·til·i·ty** (ē-lek′trō-mō-til′ĭ-tē) the motility of the auditory outer hair cells in response to electrical stimulation.

**elec·tro·mo·tive force (EMF)** the force (measured in volts) that causes the flow of electricity from one point to another.

**elec·tro·my·o·gram (EMG)** (ē-lek-trō-mī′ō-gram) a graphic representation of the electric currents associated with muscular action.

**elec·tro·my·o·graph** (ē-lek-trō-mī′ō-graf) an instrument for recording electrical currents generated in an active muscle.

**elec·tro·my·og·ra·phy** (ē-lek′trō-mī-og′ră-fē) **1.** the recording of electrical activity generated in muscle for diagnostic purposes; both surface and needle recording electrodes can be used, although characteristically the latter is employed, so that the procedure is also called needle electrode examination. **2.** umbrella term for the entire electrodiagnostic study performed in the EMG laboratory, including not only the needle electrode examination, but also the nerve conduction studies. [electro- + G. *mys*, muscle, + *graphō*, to write]

**elec·tron** (β−) (ē-lek′tron) one of the negatively charged subatomic particles that are distributed about the positive nucleus and with it constitute the atom; in mass they are estimated to be 1/1836.15 of a proton; when emitted from inside the nucleus of a radioactive substance, electrons are called beta particles. [electro- + -on]

**elec·tro·nar·co·sis** (ē-lek′trō-nar-kō′sis) production of insensibility to pain by the use of electrical current.

**elec·tron beam to·mog·raphy (EBT)** computed tomography in which the circular motion of the x-ray tube is replaced by rapid electronic positioning of the cathode ray around a circular anode, allowing full scans in tens of milliseconds.

**elec·tro·neg·a·tive** (ē-lek-trō-neg′ă-tiv) relating to or charged with negative electricity; referring to an element whose uncharged atoms have a tendency to ionize by adding electrons, thus becoming anions (e.g., oxygen, fluorine, chlorine).

**elec·tro·neu·rog·ra·phy** (ē-lek′trō-noo-rog′ră-fē) SYN electrodiagnosis (2).

**elec·tro·neu·ro·my·og·ra·phy** (ē-lek′trō-noor′ō-mī-og′ră-fē) a method of measuring changes in a peripheral nerve by combining electromyography of a muscle with electrical stimulation of the nerve trunk carrying fibers to and from the muscle.

**elec·tron·ic cell count·er** an automatic blood cell counter in which cells passing through an aperture alter resistance and are counted as voltage pulses, or in which cells passing through a flow cell deflect light; some types of counter are capable of multiple simultaneous measurements on each blood sample; e.g., leukocyte count, red

cell count, hemoglobin, hematocrit, and red cell indices.

**e·lec·tron mi·cro·scope** a visual and photographic microscope in which electron beams with wavelengths shorter than visible light are used instead of light, thereby allowing much greater resolution and magnification; in this technique, the electrons are transmitted through a very thin section of an embedded and dehydrated specimen maintained in a vacuum.

**elec·tron ra·di·og·ra·phy** radiographic imaging in which x-radiation is converted to a latent image and subsequently recovered by a printing process. SEE xeroradiography.

**elec·tron spin res·o·nance (ESR)** a spectrometric method, based on measurement of electron spins and magnetic moments, for detecting and estimating free radicals in reactions and in biological systems.

**elec·tron-volt (EV, ev)** the energy imparted to an electron by a potential of 1 volt; equal to $1.60218 \times 10^{-12}$ erg in the CGS system, or $1.60218 \times 10^{-19}$ joule in the SI system.

**elec·tro·nys·tag·mog·ra·phy (ENG)** (ē-lek′trō-nis′tag-mog′ră-fē) a method of nystagmography based on electro-oculography; skin electrodes are placed at outer canthi to register horizontal nystagmus or above and below each eye for vertical nystagmus. [electro- + nystagmus + G. *graphō*, to write]

**elec·tro·oc·u·lo·gram** (ē-lek′trō-ok′yu-lō-gram) a record of electric currents in electro-oculography.

**elec·tro·oc·u·log·ra·phy (EOG)** (ē-lek′trō-ok′yū-log′ră-fē) oculography in which electrodes placed on the skin adjacent to the eyes measure changes in standing potential between the front and back of the eyeball as the eyes move; a sensitive electrical test for detection of retinal pigment epithelium dysfunction.

**elec·tro·ol·fac·to·gram (EOG)** (ē-lek′trō-ol-fak′tō-gram) an electronegative wave of potential occurring on the surface of the olfactory epithelium in response to stimulation by an odor.

**elec·tro·pher·o·gram** (ē-lek-trō-fer′ō-gram) the densitometric or colorimetric pattern obtained from filter paper or similar porous strips on which substances have been separated by electrophoresis; may also refer to the strips themselves. SYN electrophoretogram.

**elec·tro·phil, elec·tro·phile** (ē-lek′trō-fil, ē-lek′trō-fīl) **1.** the electron-attracting atom or agent in an organic reaction. Cf. nucleophil. **2.** relating to an electrophil. SYN electrophilic. [electro- + G. *philos*, fond]

**elec·tro·phil·ic** (ē-lek-trō-fil′ik) SYN electrophil (2).

**elec·tro·pho·re·sis** (ē-lek-trō-fōr′ē-sis) the movement of particles in an electric field toward anode or cathode. SEE ALSO electropherogram. SYN ionophoresis, phoresis (1). [electro- + G. *phorēsis*, a carrying]

**elec·tro·pho·ret·ic** (ē-lek′trō-fōr-et′ik) relating to electrophoresis, as an electrophoretic separation. SYN ionophoretic.

**elec·tro·pho·ret·o·gram** (ē-lek′trō-fōr-et′ō-gram) SYN electropherogram.

**elec·tro·phren·ic res·pi·ra·tion** the rhythmical electrical stimulation of the phrenic nerve by an electrode applied to the skin at the motor points of the phrenic nerve; it is used in paralysis of the respiratory center resulting from acute bulbar poliomyelitis.

**elec·tro·ret·i·no·gram (ERG)** (ē-lek'trō-ret'i-nō-gram) a record of the retinal action currents produced in the retina by an adequate light stimulus. [electro- + retina + G. *gramma*, something written]

**elec·tro·ret·i·nog·ra·phy** (ē-lek'trō-ret'i-nog'ră-fē) the recording and study of the retinal action currents.

**elec·tro·scis·sion** (ē-lek'trō-si-shŭn) division of tissues by means of an electrocautery knife. [electro- + L. *scissio*, a splitting, fr. *scindo*, to split]

**elec·tro·shock** (ē-lek'trō-shok) SEE electroshock therapy.

**elec·tro·shock ther·a·py (EST)** a form of treatment of mental disorders in which convulsions are produced by the passage of an electric current through the brain. SYN electroconvulsive therapy.

**elec·tro·stat·ic bond** bond between atoms or groups carrying opposite charges (or, in some cases, partial charges).

**elec·tro·sur·gery** (ē-lek-trō-ser'jer-ē) division of tissues by high frequency current applied locally with a metal instrument or needle. SEE ALSO electrocautery.

**elec·tro·tax·is** (ē-lek-trō-tak'sis) reaction of plant or animal protoplasm to either an anode or a cathode. SEE ALSO tropism. SYN electrotropism. [electro- + G. *taxis*, orderly arrangement]

**elec·tro·ther·a·peu·tics, elec·tro·ther·a·py** (ē-lek'trō-thār-ă-pyu'tiks, ē-lek'trō-thār'ă-pē) use of electricity in the treatment of disease.

**elec·tro·ton·ic** (ē-lek-trō-ton'ik) relating to electrotonus.

**elec·trot·o·nus** (ē-lek-trot'ō-nŭs) changes in excitability and conductivity in a nerve or muscle cell caused by the passage of a constant electric current. [electro- + G. *tonos*, tension]

**elec·trot·ro·pism** (ē-lek-trot'rō-pizm, ē-lek-trō-trō'pizm) SYN electrotaxis. [electro- + G. *tropē*, a turning]

**ele·i·din** (ē-lē'ĭ-din) a refractile and weakly staining keratin present in the cells of the stratum lucidum of the palmar and plantar epidermis.

**el·e·ment** (el'ě-ment) **1.** a substance composed of atoms of only one kind, i.e., of identical atomic (proton) number, that therefore cannot be decomposed into two or more elements, and that can lose its chemical properties only by union with some other element or by a nuclear reaction changing the proton number. **2.** an indivisible structure or entity. **3.** a functional entity, frequently exogenous, within a bacterium, such as an extrachromosomal element. [L. *elementum*, a rudiment, beginning]

**el·e·men·ta·ry gran·ule** a particle of blood dust, or hemoconia.

**el·e·men·ta·ry par·ti·cle 1.** SYN platelet. **2.** one of the units occurring on the matrical surface of mitochondrial cristae; the particles may be concerned with the electron transport system.

△**el·eo-** oil. SEE ALSO oleo-. [G. *elaion*, olive oil]

**el·e·phan·ti·ac, el·e·phan·ti·as·ic** (el-ě-fan'tē-ak, el-ě-fan-tē-as'ik) relating to elephantiasis.

▮**el·e·phan·ti·a·sis** (el-ě-fan-tī'ă-sis) hypertrophy and fibrosis of the skin and subcutaneous tissue, especially of the lower extremities and genitalia, due to long-standing obstruction of lymphatic vessels, most commonly after years of infection by the filarial worms *Wuchereria bancrofti* or *Brugia malayi*. See this page. [G. fr. *elephas*, elephant]

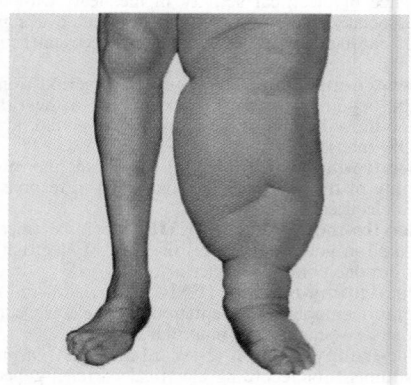

**elephantiasis:** lymphedema

**el·e·phan·ti·a·sis scro·ti** brawny swelling of the scrotum as a result of chronic lymphatic obstruction. SYN chyloderma.

**el·e·phan·toid fe·ver** lymphangitis and an elevation of temperature marking the beginning of endemic elephantiasis (filariasis).

**el·e·va·tion** (el-ě-vā'shŭn) SYN torus (2).

**el·e·va·tor** (el'ě-vā-tĕr) **1.** an instrument for prying up a sunken part, as the depressed fragment of bone in fracture of the skull, or for elevating tissues. **2.** a surgical instrument used to luxate and remove teeth and roots that cannot be engaged by the beaks of a forceps, or to loosen teeth and roots prior to forceps application. [L. fr. *e-levo*, pp. *-atus*, to lift up]

**el·e·va·tor mus·cle of scap·u·la** SYN levator scapulae muscle.

**el·e·va·tor mus·cle of soft pal·ate** SYN levator veli palatini muscle.

**el·e·va·tor mus·cle of up·per eye·lid** SYN levator palpebrae superioris muscle.

**elev·enth cra·ni·al nerve [CN XI]** SYN accessory nerve [CN XI].

**el·fin fa·cies syn·drome** SYN Williams syndrome.

**elim·i·na·tion** (ē-lim-i-nā'shŭn) expulsion; removal of waste material from the body; the getting rid of anything. [L. *elimino*, pp. *-atus*, to turn out of doors, fr. *limen*, threshold]

**e·lim·i·na·tion di·et** a diet designed to detect what component of the diet causes allergic manifestations in the patient; food items to which the patient may be sensitive are withdrawn separately and successively from the diet until that which causes the symptoms is discovered.

**ELISA** enzyme-linked immunosorbent assay.

**elix·ir** (ē-lik'ser) a clear, sweetened, hydroalcoholic liquid intended for oral use; elixirs contain flavoring substances and are used either as vehicles or for the therapeutic effect of the active medicinal agents. [Mediev. L., fr. Ar. *al-iksir*, the philosopher's stone]

**El·li·ot op·er·a·tion** (el'ē-ŏt) trephining of the eyeball at the corneoscleral margin to relieve tension in glaucoma.

**El·li·ot po·si·tion** (el′ē-ŏt) a supine position upon a double inclined plane or on a single inclined plane, with a cushion under the back at the level of the liver; used to facilitate abdominal section.

**El·li·ott law** (el′ē-ŏt) adrenaline acts upon those structures innervated by sympathetic nerve fibers.

**el·lip·soi·dal joint** a modified ball-and-socket synovial joint in which the joint surfaces are elongated or ellipsoidal; it is a biaxial joint, i.e., two axes of motion at right angles to each other. SYN condylar joint.

**el·lip·ti·cal am·pu·ta·tion** circular amputation in which the sweep of the knife is not exactly vertical to the axis of the limb, the outline of the cut surface being therefore elliptical.

**el·lip·to·cyte** (ē-lip′tō-sīt) an elliptical red blood corpuscle found normally in the lower vertebrates with the exception of Cyclostomata; in mammals it occurs normally only among the camels, hence cameloid cell. SYN ovalocyte. [G. *elleipsis,* a leaving out, an ellipse, + *kytos,* cell]

**el·lip·to·cy·to·sis** (ē-lip′tō-sī-tō′sis) a hereditary abnormality of hemopoiesis in which 50 to 90% of the red blood cells consist of rod forms and elliptocytes, often with an associated hemolytic anemia. SYN ovalocytosis.

**El·oes·ser flap** (el-es′ĕr) a surgically created open skin-lined tract for chronic drainage of an empyema, often following pneumonectomy.

**e·lon·ga·tion** RADIOLOGY radiographic distortion where the image appears longer than the actual image. Caused by insufficient vertical angulation.

**e·lon·ga·tion fac·tor** proteins that catalyze the elongation of peptide chains during protein biosynthesis. SYN transfer factor (3).

**El·schnig spots** (elsh′nig) isolated choroidal bright yellow or red spots with black pigment flecks at their borders, seen ophthalmoscopically in advanced hypertensive retinopathy.

**el·u·ant** (el′yu-ant) the material that has been eluted.

**el·u·ate** (el′yu-āt) the solution emerging from a column or paper in chromatography. [see elution]

**el·u·ent** (el′yu-ent) the mobile phase in chromatography. SYN developer (2). [see elution]

**elute** (ē-loot) to perform or accomplish an elution.

**elu·tion** (ē-loo′shŭn) **1.** the separation, by washing, of one solid from another. **2.** the removal, by means of a suitable solvent, of one material from another that is insoluble in that solvent, as in column chromatography. **3.** the removal of antibodies absorbed onto the erythrocyte surface. [L. *e-luo,* pp. *lutus,* to wash out]

△**el·y·tro-** the vagina. SEE ALSO colpo-, vagino-. [G. *elytron,* sheath (vagina)]

△**em-** SEE en-.

**EMA** epithelial membrane antigen.

**ema·ci·a·tion** (ē-mā-sē-ā′shŭn) abnormal thinness resulting from extreme loss of flesh. SYN wasting (1). [L. *e-macio,* pp. *-atus,* to make thin]

**em·a·na·tion** (em-ă-nā′shŭn) **1.** any substance that flows out or is emitted from a source or origin. **2.** the radiation from a radioactive element. [L. *e- mano,* pp. *-atus,* to flow out]

**emas·cu·la·tion** (ē-mas-kyu-lā′shŭn) castration of the male by removal of the testes and/or penis. [L. *emasculo,* pp. *-atus,* to castrate, fr. *e-* priv. + *masculus,* masculine]

**EMB** eosin-methylene blue. SEE eosin-methylene blue agar.

**em·balm** (em-bahlm′) to treat a dead body with chemicals to preserve it from decay. [L. *in,* in, + *balsamum,* balsam]

**Emb·den-Mey·er·hof path·way** (em′den-mī′ĕr-hof) the anaerobic glycolytic pathway by which D-glucose (most notably in muscle) is converted to lactic acid. Cf. glycolysis.

**em·bo·le** (em′bō-lē) **1.** reduction of a limb dislocation. **2.** formation of the gastrula by invagination. SYN emboly. [G. *embolē,* insertion]

**em·bo·lec·to·my** (em-bō-lek′tō-mē) removal of an embolus. [G. *embolos,* a plug (embolus), + *ektomē,* excision]

**em·bo·li** (em′bō-lī) plural of embolus.

**em·bol·ic** (em-bol′ik) relating to an embolus or to embolism.

**em·bol·i·form nu·cle·us** a small wedge-shaped nucleus in the central white substance of the cerebellum just internal to the hilus of the dentate nucleus; receives axons of Purkinje cells of the intermediate area of the cerebellar cortex; axons of these cells exit the cerebellum via the superior cerebellar peduncle. SYN embolus (2).

**em·bo·li·sa·tion [Br.]** SEE embolization.

**em·bo·lism** (em′bō-lizm) obstruction or occlusion of a vessel by an embolus. See this page. [G. *embolisma,* a piece or patch; lit. something thrust in]

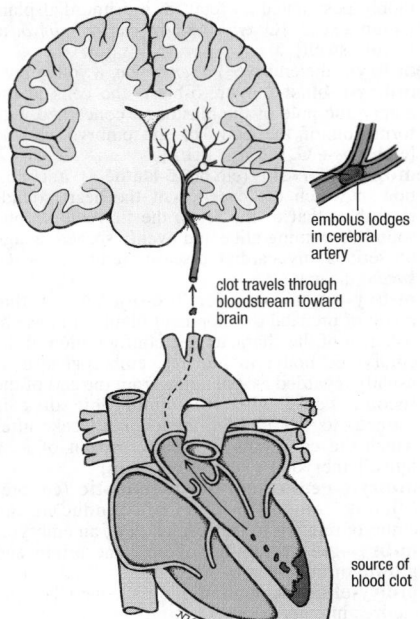

embolus lodges in cerebral artery

clot travels through bloodstream toward brain

source of blood clot

**embolism** (embolus arising from a mural thrombus of the left ventricle)

**em·bo·li·za·tion** (em′bol-i-zā′shŭn) **1.** the formation and release of an embolus into the circulation. **2.** therapeutic introduction of various substances into the circulation to occlude vessels, either to arrest or prevent hemorrhaging or to devitalize a structure or organ by occluding its blood supply.

**em•bo•lo•la•lia, em•bo•lo•phra•sia** (em′bō-lō-lā′lē-ă, em′bō-lō-frā′zē-ă) interjection of meaningless words into a sentence when speaking. [G. *embolos,* something thrown in, fr. *emballo,* to throw in, + *lalia,* speaking]

**em•bo•lo•ther•a•py** (em-bō-lō-thār′ă-pē) occlusion of arteries by insertion of blood clots, Gelfoam, coils, balloons, etc., with an angiographic catheter; used for control of inoperable hemorrhage or preoperative management of highly vascular neoplasms. [G. *embolos,* plug, + *therapeia,* medical treatment]

**em•bo•lus,** pl. **em•bo•li** (em′bō-lŭs, em′bō-lī) **1.** a plug, composed of a detached thrombus or vegetation, mass of bacteria, or other foreign body, occluding a vessel. **2.** SYN emboliform nucleus. [G. *embolos,* a plug, wedge or stopper]

**em•bo•ly** (em′bō-lē) SYN embole (2).

**em•bra•sure** (em-brā′sher) DENTISTRY an opening that widens outwardly or inwardly; specifically, that space adjacent to the interproximal contact area that spreads toward the facial, gingival, lingual, occlusal, or incisal aspect. [Fr. an opening in a wall for cannon]

**em•bryo** (em′brē-ō) **1.** an organism in the early stages of development. **2.** in humans, the developing organism from conception until approximately the end of the second month; developmental stages from this time to birth are commonly designated as fetal. **3.** a primordial plant within a seed. [G. *embryon,* fr. *en,* in, + *bryō,* to be full, swell]

△**em•bryo-** the embryo. [G. *embryon,* a young one]

**em•bry•o•blast** (em′brē-ō-blast) the cells at the embryonic pole of the blastocyst concerned with formation of the body of the embryo *per se.* [embryo- + G. *blastos,* germ]

**em•bry•o•car•dia** (em′brē-ō-kar′dē-ă) a condition in which the cadence of the heart sounds resembles that of the fetus, the first and second sounds becoming alike and evenly spaced; a sign of serious myocardial disease. [embryo- + G. *kardia,* heart]

**em•bry•o•gen•e•sis** (em′brē-ō-jen′ĕ-sis) that phase of prenatal development involved in establishment of the characteristic configuration of the embryonic body; in humans, embryogenesis is usually regarded as extending from the end of the second week, when the embryonic disk is formed, to the end of the eighth week, after which the conceptus is usually spoken of as a fetus. [embryo- + G. *genesis,* origin]

**em•bry•o•gen•ic, em•bry•o•ge•ne•tic** (em-brē-ō-jen′ik, em′brē-ō-jĕ-net′ik) producing an embryo; relating to the formation of an embryo.

**em•bry•og•e•ny** (em-brē-oj′ĕ-nē) the origin and growth of the embryo.

**em•bry•ol•o•gist** (em-brē-ol′ō-jist) one who specializes in embryology.

**em•bry•ol•o•gy** (em-brē-ol′ō-jē) science of the origin and development of the organism from fertilization of the oocyte to the end of the eighth week and, by extension, all subsequent states up to birth. [embryo- + G. *logos,* study]

**em•bry•o•ma** (em-brē-ō′mă) SYN embryonal tumor.

**em•bry•o•nal** (em′brē-ō′năl) relating to an embryo.

**em•bry•o•nal ar•ea, em•bry•on•ic ar•e•a** the

area of the blastoderm on either side of, and immediately cephalic to, the primitive streak where the component cell layers have become thickened.

**em•bry•o•nal car•ci•no•ma** a malignant neoplasm of the testis, composed of large anaplastic cells with indistinct cellular borders; embryonal carcinomas may be malignant teratomas without differentiated elements.

**em•bry•o•nal leu•ke•mia** SYN stem cell leukemia.

**em•bry•o•nal rhab•do•my•o•sar•co•ma** malignant neoplasm occurring in children, consisting of loose, spindle-celled tissue with rare cross-striations, and arising in many parts of the body in addition to skeletal muscles.

**em•bry•o•nal rhab•do•my•o•sar•co•mas** malignant neoplasms occurring in children, consisting of loose, spindle-celled tissue with rare cross-striations, and arising in many parts of the body in addition to skeletal muscles.

**em•bry•o•nal tu•mor, em•bry•on•ic tu•mor** a neoplasm, usually malignant, which arises during intrauterine or early postnatal development from an organ rudiment or immature tissue; it forms immature structures characteristic of the part from which it arises, and may form other tissues as well. The term includes neuroblastoma and Wilms tumor, and is also used to include certain neoplasms presenting in later life, this usage being based on the belief that such tumors arise from embryonic rests. SEE ALSO teratoma. SYN embryoma.

**em•bry•on•ic mem•brane** SYN fetal membrane.

**em•bry•on•ic shield** a thickened area of the embryonic blastoderm from which the embryo develops.

**em•bry•on•i•za•tion** (em′brē-on-i-zā′shŭn) reversion of a cell or tissue to an embryonic form.

**em•bry•o•noid** (em′brē-ō-noyd) resembling an embryo or a fetus. [embryo- + G. *eidos,* appearance]

**em•bry•o•ny** (em′brē-ō-nē) the forming of an embryo.

**em•bry•o•path•ic cat•a•ract** congenital cataract as a result of intrauterine infection, e.g., rubella.

**em•bry•op•a•thy** (em-brē-op′ă-thē) a morbid condition in the embryo or fetus. SYN fetopathy. [embryo- + G. *pathos,* disease]

**em•bry•o•plas•tic** (em-brē-ō-plas′tik) **1.** producing an embryo. **2.** relating to the formation of an embryo. [embryo- + G. *plassō,* to form]

**em•bry•ot•o•my** (em-brē-ot′ō-mē) any mutilating operation on the fetus to make possible its removal when delivery is impossible by natural means. [embryo- + G. *tomē,* cutting]

**em•bry•o•tox•ic•i•ty** (em′brē-ō-tok-sis′i-tē) injury to the embryo, which may result in death or in abnormal development of a part, owing to substances that enter the placental circulation.

**em•bry•o•tox•on** (em′brē-ō-tok′son) congenital opacity of the periphery of the cornea, a feature of osteogenesis imperfecta. [embryo- + G. *toxon,* bow]

**em•bry•o trans•fer** after artificial insemination in vitro, the fertilized oocyte (ovum) is transferred at the blastocyst stage to the recipient's uterus or oviduct.

**em•bry•o•troph** (em′brē-ō-trōf) **1.** nutritive material supplied to the embryo during development. Cf. hemotroph. **2.** in the implantation stages of deciduate placental mammals, fluid adjacent to the blastodermic vesicle; a mixture of the secretion of the uterine glands, cellular debris resulting from the trophoblastic invasion of the endometrium, and exuded plasma. [embryo- + G. *trophē,* nourishment]

**em·bry·o·tro·phic** (em'brē-ō-trof'ik) relating to any process or agency involved in the nourishment of the embryo.

**em·bry·ot·ro·phy** (em'brē-ot'rō-fē) the nutrition of the embryo. [embryo- + G. *trophē,* nourishment]

**E&M codes** Evaluation and Management codes.

**emed·ul·late** (ē-med'yu-lāt) to extract any marrow. [L. *e-,* from, + *medulla,* marrow]

**emei·o·cy·to·sis** (ē'mē-ō-sī-tō'sis) SYN exocytosis (2). [L. *emitto,* to send forth, + G. *kytos,* cell, + *-osis,* condition]

**emergence** (ē-mer'jens) a coming forth or becoming evident. [[L. *e-mergo,* arise, come forth]]

**emer·gen·cy hor·mo·nal con·tra·cep·tion** SYN morning after pill. SYN postcoital contraception.

**emer·gen·cy med·i·cal ser·vice** a firm or agency that provides emergency treatment for victims of sudden illness or trauma and transport to a treatment facility. SYN ambulance service.

**emer·gen·cy med·i·cal ser·vice sys·tem** a coordinated, community-based system for providing emergency care, including public access (911), prehospital responders (paramedics or emergency medical technicians), transport (ambulances, helicopters, etc.), receiving facilities, coordinated communications, and medical direction. SYN EMS system.

**emer·gen·cy med·i·cal tech·ni·cian** SYN prehospital provider.

**emer·gen·cy med·i·cal tech·ni·cian–ba·sic (EMT-B)** a certified prehospital provider who can perform basic life support (BLS); uses assessment-based approach to patient management. Minimum level of certification required to staff a BLS ambulance. SEE ALSO basic life support.

**emer·gen·cy med·i·cal tech·ni·cian–in·ter·me·di·ate (EMT-I)** a certified prehospital provider who can perform intermediate advanced life support (ALS); usually works under direct medical control. Minimum level of certification required to staff an ALS ambulance. SEE ALSO advanced life support. SYN cardiac care technician, cardiac rescue technician.

**emer·gen·cy med·i·cal tech·ni·cian–par·a·med·ic (EMT-P)** a licensed prehospital provider who can perform all aspects of advanced life support; usually works according to standing orders or protocols and uses a diagnostic approach to patient management. SEE ALSO prehospital provider.

**emer·gen·cy the·o·ry** a theory of the emotions, advanced by W.B. Cannon, that animal and human organisms respond to emergency situations by increased sympathetic nervous system activity including an increased catecholamine production with associated increases in blood pressure, heart and respiratory rates, and skeletal muscle blood flow.

**em·e·sis** (em'ě-sis) **1.** SYN vomiting. **2.** combining form, used in the suffix position, for vomiting. [G. fr. *emeō,* to vomit]

**emet·ic** (ě-met'ik) **1.** relating to or causing vomiting. **2.** an agent that causes vomiting. [G. *emetikos,* producing vomiting, fr. *emeō,* to vomit]

**em·e·to·ca·thar·tic** (em'ě-tō-kă-thar'tik) **1.** both emetic and cathartic. **2.** an agent that causes both vomiting and purging.

**EMF** electromotive force.

**EMG** electromyogram.

**EMG bi·o·feed·back** a form of biofeedback that uses an electromyographic measure of muscle tension as the physical symptom to be deconditioned, such as tension in the frontalis muscle in the head which can cause headaches.

△**-emia** blood. [G. *haima*]

**em·i·gra·tion** (em-i-grā'shŭn) the passage of white blood cells through the endothelium and wall of small blood vessels. [L. *e-migro,* pp. *-atus,* to emigrate]

**em·i·nence** (em'i-nens) a circumscribed area raised above the general level of the surrounding surface, particularly on a bone surface. SYN eminentia [TA]. [L. *eminentia*]

**em·i·nen·tia,** pl. **em·i·nen·ti·ae** (em-i-nen'shē-ă, em-i-nen'shē-ē) [TA] SYN eminence. [L. prominence, fr. *e-mineo,* to stand out, project]

**em·i·nen·tia py·ra·mi·da·lis** [TA] a conical projection posterior to the vestibular window in the middle ear; it is hollow and contains the stapedius muscle.

**em·i·o·cy·to·sis** (ē'mē-ō-sī-tō'sis) SYN exocytosis (2). [L. *emitto,* to send forth, + G. *kytos,* cell, + *-osis,* condition]

**em·is·sary** (em'i-sār-ē) **1.** relating to, or providing, an outlet or drain. **2.** SYN emissary vein. [see emissarium]

**em·is·sary vein** one of the channels of communication between the venous sinuses of the dura mater and the veins of the diploë and the scalp. SYN emissary (2).

**emis·sion** (ē-mish'ŭn) a discharge; referring usually to a discharge of the male internal genital organs into the internal urethra; the contents of the organs, including sperm cells, prostatic fluid, and seminal vesicle fluid, mix in the internal urethra with mucus from the bulbourethral glands to form semen. [L. *emissio,* fr. *e- mitto,* to send out]

**EMIT** enzyme-multiplied immunoassay technique.

**em·men·ia** (ě-men'ē-ă, ě-mē'nē-ă) SYN menses. [G. *emmēnos,* monthly]

**em·men·ic** (ě-men'ik) SYN menstrual.

**em·men·i·op·a·thy** (ě-men'ē-op'ă-thē) any disorder of menstruation. [G. *emmēnos,* monthly, + *pathos,* suffering]

**Em·met nee·dle** (em'ět) a strong needle with the eye in the point, having a wide curve, and set in a handle, used to pass a ligature around an undissected structure.

**Em·met op·er·a·tion** (em'ět) SYN trachelorrhaphy.

**em·me·tro·pia** (em-ě-trō'pē-ă) the state of refraction of the eye in which parallel rays, when the eye is at rest, are focused exactly on the retina. [G. *emmetros,* according to measure, + *ōps,* eye]

**em·me·tro·pic** (em-ě-trop'ik) pertaining to or characterized by emmetropia.

***Em·mon·sia par·va* var. *cres·cens*** the main fungal species causing adiaspiromycosis in animals and the only agent of human adiaspiromycosis; infection is acquired by inhaling conidia from the fungus growing in soil.

**Em•mon•sia par•va var. par•va** a fungal species causing adiaspiromycosis in animals.

**emol•lient** (ē-mol′ē-ent) **1.** soothing to the skin or mucous membrane. **2.** an agent that softens the skin or soothes irritation in the skin or mucous membrane. [L. *emolliens,* pres. p. of *e- mollio,* to soften]

**emo•tion** (ē-mō′shŭn) a strong feeling, aroused mental state, or intense state of drive or unrest directed toward a definite object and evidenced in both behavior and in psychologic changes, with accompanying autonomic nervous system manifestations. [L. *e-moveo,* pp. *-motus,* to move out, agitate]

**emo•tion•al** (ē-mō′shŭn-ăl) relating to or marked by an emotion.

**e•mo•tion•al dep•ri•va•tion** lack of adequate and appropriate interpersonal or environmental experiences, or both, usually in the early developmental years.

**e•mo•tion•al dis•or•der** SEE mental illness, behavior disorder.

**em•path•ic** (em-path′ik) relating to or marked by empathy.

**em•pa•thize** (em′pă-thīz) to feel empathy in relation to another person; to put oneself in another's place.

**em•pa•thy** (em′pă-thē) **1.** the ability to intellectually and emotionally sense the emotions, feelings, and reactions that another person is experiencing and to effectively communicate that understanding to the individual. Cf. sympathy (3). **2.** the anthropomorphization or humanizing of objects and the feeling of oneself as being in and part of them. [G. *en* (*em*), in, + *pathos,* feeling]

**em•phy•se•ma** (em-fi-sē′mă) **1.** presence of air in the interstices of the connective tissue of a part. **2.** a condition of the lung characterized by increase beyond the normal in the size of air spaces distal to the terminal bronchiole (those parts containing alveoli), with destructive changes in their walls and reduction in their number. Clinical manifestation is breathlessness on exertion, due to the combined effect (in varying degrees) of reduction of alveolar surface for gas exchange and collapse of smaller airways with trapping of alveolar gas in expiration; this causes the chest to be held in the position of inspiration ("barrel chest"), with prolonged expiration and increased residual volume. Symptoms of chronic bronchitis often, but not necessarily, coexist. Two structural varieties are panlobular (panacinar) emphysema and centrilobular (centriacinar) emphysema; paracicatricial, paraseptal, and bullous emphysema are also common. SYN pulmonary emphysema. [G. inflation of stomach, etc. fr. *en,* in, + *physēma,* a blowing, fr. *physa,* bellows]

**em•phy•sem•a•tous** (em-fi-sem′ă-tŭs) relating to or affected with emphysema.

**em•pir•ic** (em-pir′ik) **1.** SYN empirical. **2.** a member of a school of Graeco-Roman physicians who placed their confidence in and based their practice purely on experience, avoiding all speculation, theory, or abstract reasoning. **3.** modern: testing a hypothesis by careful observation, hence rationally based on experience. [see empirical]

**em•pir•i•cal** (em-pir′i-kăl) **1.** founded on practical experience, rather than on reasoning alone, but not proved scientifically, in contrast to rational (1). **2.** relating to an empiric (2). **3.** based on careful observational testing of a hypothesis; rational. SYN empiric (1). [G. *empeirikos;* fr. *empeiria,* experience, fr. *en,* in, + *peira,* a trial]

**em•pir•i•cal for•mu•la** CHEMISTRY a formula indicating the kind and number of atoms in the molecules of a substance, or its composition, but not the relation of the atoms to each other or the intimate structure of the molecule.

**em•pir•i•cal hor•op•ter** an experimentally determined ellipse passing through the optical centers of two eyes by which points adjacent to the point of fixation, both lying on the ellipse, are perceived to be stimulating corresponding retinal points.

**em•pir•ic risk** risk that is based on empirical evidence alone, without any appeal to formal theory or surmise.

**em•por•i•at•rics** (em-pōr-ē-at′riks) the specialty of travel medicine, dealing with diseases that travelers can acquire, especially in the tropics. [G. *emporion,* market, fr. *emporos,* traveler, merchant, + (*technē*) *iatrikē,* medical art]

**em•pros•thot•o•nos** (em′pros-thot′ō-nŭs) a tetanic contraction of the flexor muscles, curving the back with concavity forward. [G. *emprosthen,* forward, + *tonos,* tension]

**em•py•e•ma** (em-pi-ē′mă) pus in a body cavity; when used without qualification, refers specifically to pyothorax. [G. *empyēma,* suppuration, fr. *en,* in, + *pyon,* pus]

**em•py•e•mic** (em-pī-ē′mik) relating to empyema.

**em•py•e•sis** (em-pī-ē′sis) a pustular eruption. [G. suppuration]

**EMS** emergency medical service.

**EMSS** emergency medical service system.

**EMS sys•tem** SYN emergency medical service system.

**EMT-B** emergency medical technician–basic.

**EMT-I** emergency medical technician–intermediate.

**EMT-P** emergency medical technician–paramedic.

**emul•si•fi•er** (ē-mŭl′si-fī-er) an agent, such as gum arabic or egg yolk, used to make an emulsion of a fixed oil. Soaps, detergents, steroids, and proteins can act as emulsifiers.

**emul•sion** (ē-mŭl′shŭn) a system containing two immiscible liquids in which one is dispersed, in the form of very small globules (internal phase), throughout the other (external phase). [Mod. L. fr. *e-mulgeo,* pp. *-mulsus,* to milk or drain out]

**emul•soid** (ē-mŭl′soyd) a colloidal dispersion in which the dispersed particles are more or less liquid and exert a certain attraction on and absorb a certain quantity of the fluid in which they are suspended.

⌂**en-** in; appears as em- before b, p, or m. [G.]

**enam•el** (ē-nam′ĕl) the hard, acellular, inert substance covering the tooth. In its mature form, it is composed of an inorganic portion made up of 90% hydroxyapatite and 6-8% calcium carbonate, calcium fluoride, and magnesium carbonate, the remainder comprising an organic matrix of protein and glycoprotein; structurally, it is made up of oriented rods each of which consists of a stack of rodlets encased in an organic prism sheath. [M.E., fr. Fr. *enamailer,* to apply enamel, fr. *en,* on, + *amail,* enamel, fr. Germanic]

**enam•el cap** the enamel covering the crown of a tooth.

**enam·el crypt** the narrow, mesenchyme-filled space between the dental ledge and an enamel organ.

**enam·el germ** the enamel organ of a developing tooth; one of a series of knoblike projections from the dental lamina, later becoming bell-shaped and receiving in its hollow the dental papilla.

**enam·el hy·po·cal·ci·fi·ca·tion** a disturbance in the maturation of enamel due to improper calcification of the enamel matrix, resulting in the appearance of chalky, smooth surfaces on the crown. SEE ALSO enamel hypoplasia.

**enam·el hy·po·plas·ia** a disturbance in the developing ameloblasts during enamel matrix formation resulting in a pitted surface of the crown. SEE ALSO fluorosis.

**en·am·el·ins** a class of proteins that form the organic matrix of mature tooth enamel. [enamel + -in]

**enam·el lay·er** SYN ameloblastic layer.

**enam·el mem·brane** the internal layer of the enamel organ formed by the enamel cells.

**enam·el·o·gen·e·sis** (ē-nam'ĕl-ō-jen'ĕ-sis) SYN amelogenesis.

**enam·el·o·ma, enam·el pearl** (ē-nam-ĕl-ō'mă) a developmental anomaly in which there is a small nodule of enamel below the cementoenamel junction, usually at the bifurcation of molar teeth.

**enam·el or·gan** a circumscribed mass of ectodermal cells budded off from the dental lamina; it develops the ameloblast layer of cells, which produce the enamel cap of a developing tooth. SYN dental organ.

**en·an·them, en·an·the·ma** (en-an'them, en-an-thē'mă) a mucous membrane eruption, especially one occurring in connection with one of the exanthemas. [G. en, in, + anthēma, bloom, eruption, fr. antheō, to bloom]

**en·an·them·a·tous** (en-an-them'ă-tŭs) relating to an enanthem.

**en·an·the·sis** (en-an-thē'sis) the skin eruption of a general disease, such as scarlatina or typhoid fever. [G. en, in, + anthēsis, full bloom]

**en·ar·thro·di·al** (en-ar-thrō'dē-al) relating to an enarthrosis.

**en·ar·thro·di·al joint** SYN ball-and-socket joint.

**en·ar·thro·sis** (en-ar-thrō'sis) SYN ball-and-socket joint. [G. en-arthrōsis, a jointing where the ball is deep seat in the socket]

**en bloc** (ahn blok) in a lump; as a whole; used to refer to autopsy techniques in which visceral organs are removed in large blocks allowing the prosector to retain a continuity in organ architecture during the subsequent dissection. [Fr., in a lump]

**en·cap·su·la·tion** (en-kap-soo-lā'shŭn) enclosure in a capsule or sheath. [L. in + capsula, dim. of capsa, box]

**en·ceph·a·lal·gia** (en-sef-ă-lal'jē-ă) SYN headache. [encephalo- + G. algos, pain]

**en·ceph·a·la·tro·phic** (en-sef-ă-lă-trof'ik) relating to encephalatrophy.

**en·ceph·a·lat·ro·phy** (en-sef-ă-lat'rō-fē) atrophy of the brain. [encephalo- + G. a- priv. + trophē, nourishment]

**en·ce·phal·ic** (en'se-fal'ik) relating to the brain, or to the structures within the cranium.

**en·ceph·a·lit·ic** (en-sef-a-lit'ik) relating to encephalitis.

**en·ceph·a·li·tis**, pl. **en·ceph·a·lit·i·des** (en-sef-ă-lī'tis, en-sef-ă-lit'i-dēz) inflammation of the brain. SYN cephalitis. [G. enkephalos, brain, + -itis, inflammation]

**en·ceph·a·li·tis per·i·ax·i·a·lis dif·fu·sa** SYN Schilder disease.

*En·ceph·a·li·to·zo·on* (en-sef'ă-li-tō-zō'on) a genus of protozoan parasites, formerly considered part of the family Toxoplasmatidae, class Sporozoea, but now recognized as a member of the protozoan phylum Microspora, family Nosematidae. *Encephalitozoon cuniculi* is considered the primary microsporan parasite of mammals, commonly found in the brain and kidney tubules of rodents and carnivores and causing nosematosis in rabbits. [encephalitis + G. zōon, animal]

*En·ceph·a·li·to·zo·on hel·lem* a species of *Encephalitozoon* described from human ophthalmic infections causing punctate keratopathy and corneal ulceration in AIDS patients.

*En·ceph·a·li·to·zo·on in·tes·ti·na·le* a diarrheogenic microsporidian described in HIV-infected patients; disease may be localized to the gastrointestinal tract or may disseminate intravascularly.

⌒**en·ceph·a·lo-, en·ceph·al-** the brain. Cf. cerebro-. [G. enkephalos, brain]

**en·ceph·a·lo·cele** (en-sef'ă-lō-sēl) a congenital gap in the skull with herniation of brain substance. SYN craniocele. [encephalo- + G. kēlē, hernia]

**en·ceph·a·lo·gram** (en-sef'ă-lō-gram) the record obtained by encephalography. [encephalo- + G. gramma, a drawing]

**en·ceph·a·log·ra·phy** (en-sef-ă-log'ră-fē) radiographic representation of the brain. [encephalo- + G. graphō, to write]

**en·ceph·a·loid** (en-sef'ă-loyd) resembling brain substance; denoting a carcinoma of soft, brainlike consistency. [encephalo- + G. eidos, resemblance]

**en·ceph·a·lo·lith** (en-sef'ă-lō-lith) a concretion in the brain or one of its ventricles. [encephalo- + G. lithos, stone]

**en·ceph·a·lo·ma** (en-sef-ă-lō'mă) herniation of brain substance. SYN cerebroma.

**en·ceph·a·lo·ma·la·cia** (en-sef'ă-lō-mă-lā'shē-ă) abnormal softness of the cerebral parenchyma often due to ischemia or infarction. SYN cerebromalacia. [encephalo- + G. malakia, softness]

**en·ceph·a·lo·men·in·gi·tis** (en-sef'ă-lō-men-in-jī'tis) SYN meningoencephalitis. [encephalo- + G. mēninx, membrane, + -itis, inflammation]

**en·ceph·a·lo·me·nin·go·cele** (en-sef'ă-lō-me-ning'gō-sēl) SYN meningoencephalocele. [encephalo- + G. mēninx, membrane, + kēlē, hernia]

**en·ceph·a·lo·men·in·gop·a·thy** (en-sef'ă-lō-men-in-gop'ă-thē) SYN meningoencephalopathy.

**en·ceph·a·lo·mere** (en-sef'ă-lō-mēr) a neuromere. [encephalo- + G. meros, a part]

**en·ceph·a·lom·e·ter** (en-sef-ă-lom'ĕ-ter) an apparatus for indicating on the skull the location of the cortical centers. [encephalo- + G. metron, measure]

**en·ceph·a·lo·my·e·li·tis** (en-sef-ă-lō-mī'ĕ-lī'tis) inflammation of the brain and spinal cord. [encephalo- + G. myelon, marrow, + -itis, inflammation]

**en·ceph·a·lo·my·e·lo·cele** (en-sef'ă-lō-mī'ĕ-lō-sēl) congenital defect usually in the occipital region (foramen magnum) and cervical vertebrae, with herniation of the meninges, medulla, and spinal cord. [G. *enkephalos,* brain, + *myelon,* marrow, + *kēlē,* hernia]

**en·ceph·a·lo·my·e·lo·neu·rop·a·thy** (en-sef'ă-lō-mī'ĕ-lō-noo-rop'ă-thē) a disease involving the brain, spinal cord, and peripheral nerves.

**en·ceph·a·lo·my·e·lop·a·thy** (en-sef'ă-lō-mī-ĕ-lop'ă-thē) any disease of both brain and spinal cord. [G. *enkephalos,* brain, + *myelon,* marrow, + *pathos,* suffering]

**en·ceph·a·lo·my·e·lo·ra·dic·u·li·tis** (en-sef'ă-lō-mī'ĕ-lō-ră-dik'yu-lī-tis) SYN encephalomyelo-radiculopathy.

**en·ceph·a·lo·my·e·lo·ra·dic·u·lop·a·thy** (en-sef'ă-lō-mī'ĕ-lō-ră-dik'yu-lop-ă-thē) a disease process involving the brain, spinal cord, and spinal roots. SYN encephalomyeloradiculitis.

**en·ceph·a·lo·my·o·car·di·tis** (en-sef'ă-lō-mī'ō-kar-dī'tis) associated encephalitis and myocarditis; often caused by a viral infection such as in polio myelitis.

**en·ceph·a·lo·my·o·car·di·tis vi·rus** a picornavirus, probably of rodents; occasionally causes febrile illness with central nervous system involvement in humans.

**en·ceph·a·lon,** pl. **en·ceph·a·la** (en-sef'ă-lon, en-sef-ă-lă) [TA] that portion of the cerebrospinal axis contained within the cranium, composed of the prosencephalon, mesencephalon, and rhombencephalon. [G. *enkephalos,* brain, fr. *en,* in, + *kephalē,* head]

**en·ceph·a·lop·a·thy** (en-sef'ă-lop'ă-thē) any disorder of the brain. SYN cephalopathy, cerebropathy, encephalosis. [encephalo- + G. *pathos,* suffering]

**en·ceph·a·los·chi·sis** (en-sef-ă-los'ki-sis) developmental failure of closure of the rostral part of the neural tube. [encephalo- + G. *schisis,* fissure]

**en·ceph·a·lo·scle·ro·sis** (en-sef'ă-lō-sklēr-o'sis) a sclerosis, or hardening, of the brain. SEE ALSO cerebrosclerosis. [encephalo- + G. *sklērōsis,* hardening]

**en·ceph·a·lo·sis** SYN encephalopathy.

**en·ceph·a·lot·o·my** (en-sef-ă-lot'ō-mē) dissection or incision of the brain. [encephalo- + G. *tomē,* incision]

**en·chon·dro·ma** (en-kon-drō'mă) a benign cartilaginous growth starting within the medullary cavity of a bone originally formed from cartilage; enchondromas may distend the cortex, especially of small bones, and may be solitary or multiple (endochondromatosis). [Mod. L. fr. G. *en,* in, + *chondros,* cartilage, + *-oma,* tumor]

**en·chon·dro·ma·to·sis** (en-kon'drō-ma-tō'sis) a rarely familial, and probably hamartomatous proliferation of cartilage in the metaphyses of several bones, most commonly of the hands and feet, causing distorted growth in length or pathological fractures; chondrosarcoma frequently develops. When combined with hemangiomas in the cutaneous or visceral regions, called Maffucci syndrome. SYN dyschondroplasia.

**en·chon·drom·a·tous** (en-kon-drō'mă-tŭs) relating to or having the elements of enchondroma.

**en·clave** (en'klāv, ahn-klahv') an enclosure; a detached mass of tissue enclosed in tissue of another kind; seen especially in the case of isolated masses of gland tissue detached from the main gland. [Fr. fr. L. *clavis,* key]

**en·cod·ing** (en-kōd'ing) the first stage in the memory process, followed by storage and re-

trieval, involving processes associated with receiving or briefly registering stimuli through one or more of the senses and modifying that information.

**en·cop·re·sis** (en-kō-prē'sis) the repeated, generally involuntary passage of feces into inappropriate places (e.g., clothing); considered a mental disorder if it occurs in a child more than 4 years old. [G. *enkopros,* full of manure]

**en·coun·ter** a health care contact between the patient and the provider who is responsible for diagnosing and treating the patient.

**en·coun·ter group** a form of psychological sensitivity training that emphasizes the experiencing of individual relationships within the group and minimizes intellectual and didactic input; the group focuses on the present rather than concerning itself with the past or outside problems of its members.

**en·cyst·ed** (en-sis'ted) encapsulated by a membranous bag. [G. *kystis,* bladder]

**en·cyst·ed cal·cu·lus** a urinary calculus enclosed in a sac developed from the wall of the bladder. SYN pocketed calculus.

**end** an extremity, or the most remote point of an extremity.

**end·an·gi·i·tis, end·an·ge·i·tis** (end-an-jē-ī'tis) inflammation of the intima of a blood vessel. SYN endovasculitis. [endo- + G. *angeion,* vessel, + *-itis,* inflammation]

**end·a·or·ti·tis** (end'ā-ōr-tī'tis) inflammation of the intima of the aorta.

**end·ar·ter·ec·to·my** (end-ar-ter-ek'tō-mē) excision of diseased endothelial and media or most of the media of an artery, and also of occluding atheromatous deposits, so as to leave a smooth lining, mostly consisting of adventitia. [endo- + artery + G. *ektomē,* excision]

**end·ar·te·ri·tis** (end'ar-ter-ī'tis) inflammation of the intima of an artery. SYN endoarteritis.

**end·ar·te·ri·tis ob·li·te·rans, ob·lit·er·at·ing end·ar·te·ri·tis** an extreme degree of endarteritis proliferans closing the lumen of the artery. SYN arteritis obliterans, obliterating arteritis.

**end·ar·te·ri·tis pro·li·fe·rans, pro·lif·er·at·ing end·ar·te·ri·tis** chronic endarteritis accompanied by a marked increase of fibrous tissue in the intima.

**end ar·tery** an artery with insufficient anastomoses to maintain viability of the tissue supplied if occlusion of the artery occurs. SYN terminal artery.

**end·au·ral** (end-aw'răl) within the ear. [endo- + L. *auris,* ear]

**end·brain** SYN telencephalon.

**end bud** SYN tail bud.

**end bulb** one of the oval or rounded bodies in which the sensory nerve fibers terminate in mucous membrane.

**end-di·a·stol·ic vol·ume** the amount of blood in the ventricle immediately before a cardiac contraction begins; a measurement of cardiac filling between beats, related to diastolic function.

**en·dec·to·cide** a drug effective against both endoparasites and ectoparasites, e.g., the macrolide antibiotic avermectin. [*endo*parasite + *ecto*parasite + -cide]

**en·dem·ic** (en-dem'ik) present in a community or among a group of people; said of a disease prevailing continually in a region. Cf. epidemic, sporadic. [G. *endēmos*, native, fr. *en*, in, + *dē-mos*, the people]

**en·dem·ic dis·ease** continued prevalence of a disease in a specific population or area. SEE ALSO endemic.

**en·dem·ic he·ma·tu·ria** SYN schistosomiasis haematobium.

**en·dem·ic neu·ri·tis** SYN beriberi.

**en·dem·ic sta·bil·i·ty** a situation in which all factors influencing disease occurrence are relatively stable, resulting in little fluctuation in disease incidence over time; changes in one or more of these factors (e.g., reduction in proportion of individuals with immunity from exposure to infectious agent) can lead to an unstable situation in which major disease outbreaks occur. SYN enzootic stability.

**en·dem·ic ty·phus** SYN murine typhus.

**en·dem·o·ep·i·dem·ic** (en-dem′ō-ep-i-dem′ik) denoting a temporary large increase in the number of cases of an endemic disease.

**end·er·gon·ic** (en-der-gon′ik) referring to a chemical reaction that takes place with absorption of energy from its surroundings (i.e., a positive change in Gibbs free energy). Cf. exergonic. [endo- + G. *ergon*, work]

**end-feel** the texture of resistance felt when a joint reaches the end of its range of motion. Can be bony (bone-to-bone contact), springy (soft tissue approximation), abrupt (limited by protective muscle spasm), or empty (pain is felt well before the end of a normal range of motion, but no organic resistance is identified). Abnormal endfeel can indicate causes of joint dysfunction.

**end-feet** SYN axon terminals.

**end·ing 1.** a termination or conclusion. **2.** a nerve ending.

⚠**en·do-, end-** prefixes indicating within, inner, absorbing, or containing. SEE ALSO ento-. [G. *endon*, within]

**En·do a·gar** (en′dō) a medium containing peptone, lactose, dipotassium phosphate, agar, sodium sulfite, basic fuchsin, and distilled water; originally developed for the isolation of *Salmonella typhi*, this medium is now most useful in the bacteriological examination of water; coliform organisms ferment the lactose, and their colonies become red and color the surrounding medium; non-lactose-fermenting organisms produce clear, colorless colonies against the faint pink background of the medium. SYN Endo medium.

**en·do·an·eu·rys·mo·plas·ty** (en′dō-an-yu-riz′mō-plas-tē) SYN aneurysmoplasty.

**en·do·an·eu·rys·mor·rha·phy** (en′dō-an-yu-riz-mōr′ă-fē) SYN aneurysmoplasty. [endo- + G. *aneurysma*, aneurysm, + *rhaphē*, suture]

**en·do·ar·te·ri·tis** (en′dō-ar-ter-ī′tis) SYN endarteritis.

**en·do·blast** (en′dō-blast) entoderm. [endo- + G. *blastos*, germ]

**en·do·bron·chi·al tube** a single- or double-lumen tube with an inflatable cuff at the distal end that, after being passed through the larynx and trachea, is positioned so that ventilation is restricted to one lung; a single-lumen tube is placed in the mainstem bronchus of the lung; a double-lumen tube is positioned at the tracheal carina to permit ventilation of either or both lungs.

**en·do·car·dit·ic** (en′dō-kar-dit′ik) relating to endocarditis.

**en·do·car·di·tis** (en′dō-kar-dī′tis) inflammation of the endocardium.

**en·do·car·di·um**, pl. **en·do·car·dia** (en-dō-kar′dē-ŭm, en-dō-kar′d-ē-ă) the innermost tunic of the heart, which includes endothelium and subendothelial connective tissue; in the atrial wall, smooth muscle and numerous elastic fibers also occur. [endo- + G. *kardia*, heart]

**en·do·cer·vi·cal** (en′dō-ser′vi-kăl) **1.** within any cervix, specifically within the cervix uteri. **2.** relating to the endocervix.

**en·do·cer·vi·ci·tis** (en′dō-ser-vi-sī′tis) inflammation of the mucous membrane of the cervix uteri. SYN endotrachelitis.

**en·do·cer·vix** (en-dō-ser′viks) the mucous membrane of the cervical canal.

**en·do·chon·dral bone** a bone that develops in a cartilage environment after the latter is partially or entirely destroyed by calcification and subsequent resorption. SYN cartilage bone.

**en·do·chon·dral os·si·fi·ca·tion** formation of osseous tissue by the replacement of calcified cartilage; long bones grow in length by endochondral ossification at the epiphysial cartilage plate where osteoblasts form bone trabeculae on a framework of calcified cartilage.

**en·do·co·ag·u·la·tion** (en-dō-kō-ag-oo-lā′shŭn) SYN thermocoagulation.

**en·do·coch·le·ar po·ten·tial** the standing direct current potential in the endolymph relative to the perilymph, measuring positive 80 mV.

**en·do·co·li·tis** (en′dō-kō-lī′tis) simple catarrhal inflammation of the colon.

**en·do·cra·ni·al** (en-dō-krā′nē-ăl) **1.** within the cranium. **2.** relating to the endocranium.

**en·do·cra·ni·um** (en′dō-krā′nē-ŭm) the lining membrane of the cranium, or dura mater of the brain.

**en·do·crine** (en′dō-krin) **1.** secreting internally, most commonly into the systemic circulation; of or pertaining to such secretion. Cf. paracrine. **2.** the internal or hormonal secretion of a ductless gland. **3.** denoting a gland that furnishes an internal secretion. [endo- + G. *krinō*, to separate]

**en·do·crine glands** glands that have no ducts, their secretions being absorbed directly into the blood. SYN ductless glands.

**en·do·crine sys·tem** collective designation for those tissues capable of secreting hormones.

**en·do·cri·nol·o·gist** (en′dō-kri-nol′ō-jist) one who specializes in endocrinology.

**en·do·cri·nol·o·gy** (en′dō-kri-nol′ō-jē) the science and medical specialty concerned with the internal or hormonal secretions and their physiologic and pathologic relations. [endocrine + G. *logos*, study]

**en·do·cri·no·ma** (en′dō-kri-nō′mă) a tumor with endocrine tissue that retains the function of the parent organ, usually to an excessive degree.

**en·do·crin·o·path·ic** (en′dō-kri-nō-path′ik) relating to or suffering from an endocrinopathy.

**en·do·cri·nop·a·thy** (en′dō-kri-nop′ă-thē) a disorder in the function of an endocrine gland and the consequences thereof. [endocrine + G. *pathos*, disease]

**en·do·cys·ti·tis** (en′dō-sis-tī′tis) inflammation of the mucous membrane of the bladder. [endo- + G. *kystis*, bladder, + *-itis*, inflammation]

**en·do·cy·to·sis** (en′dō-sī-tō′sis) internalization of

substances from the extracellular environment through the formation of vesicles formed from the plasma membrane. SEE ALSO phagocytosis. Cf. exocytosis (2). [endo- + G. *kytos,* cell, + *-osis,* condition]

**en·do·derm** (en′dō-derm) the innermost of the three primary germ layers of the embryo (ectoderm, mesoderm, endoderm); from it are derived the epithelial lining of the primitive gut tract and the epithelial component of the glands and other structures (e.g., lower respiratory system) that develop as outgrowths from the gut tube. SYN entoderm, hypoblast. [endo- + G. *derma,* skin]

**en·do·der·mal cell** embryonic cells forming the yolk sac and giving rise to the epithelium of the alimentary and respiratory tracts and to the parenchyma of associated glands. SYN entodermal cell.

**en·do·der·mal cyst** cyst lined by columnar epithelium; presumed dermal in origin.

**en·do·don·tics, en·do·don·tia, en·do·don·tol·o·gy** (en-dō-don′tiks, en-dō-don′shē-ă, en′do-don-tol′ō-jē) a field of dentistry concerned with the diseases and injuries of the dental pulp and periapical tissues, and with the prevention, diagnosis, and treatment of diseases and injuries in these tissues. [endo- + G. *odous,* tooth]

**en·do·don·tist** (en-dō-don′tist) one who specializes in the practice of endodontics.

**en·do·en·ter·i·tis** (en′dō-en-ter-ī′tis) inflammation of the intestinal mucous membrane. [endo- + G. *enteron,* intestine, *-itis,* inflammation]

**end-of-life care** multidimensional and multidisciplinary physical, emotional, and spiritual care of the patient with terminal illness, including support of family and caregivers.

**en·dog·a·my** (en-dog′ă-mē) reproduction by conjugation between sister cells, the descendants of one original cell. [endo- + G. *gamos,* marriage]

**en·do·gen·ic tox·i·co·sis** SYN autointoxication.

**en·dog·e·nous** (en-doj′ĕ-nŭs) originating or produced within the organism or one of its parts. [endo- + G. *-gen,* production]

**en·dog·e·nous de·pres·sion** a descriptive syndrome for a cluster of symptoms and features occurring in the absence of external precipitants and believed to have a biologic origin; e.g., anhedonia, psychomotor agitation or retardation, diurnal mood variation with increased severity in the morning, early morning awakening and insomnia in the middle of the night, weight loss, self-reproach or guilt, and lack of reactivity to one's environment.

**en·dog·e·nous hy·per·glyc·er·i·de·mia** type IV familial hyperlipoproteinemia or, more commonly, a nonfamilial sporadic variety.

**en·dog·e·nous in·fec·tion** infection caused by an infectious agent already present in the body, the previous infection having been inapparent.

**en·dog·e·nous py·ro·gen (EP)** an endogenous protein that induces fever. Several (about 11) have been identified, including cytokines formed by components of the immune system, especially macrophages (e.g., interleukins 1 and 6, interferons and tumor necrosis factors).

**endo·glin** (en′dō-glin) a protein on the surface of endothelial cells that binds to transforming growth factor-β.

**en·do·in·tox·i·ca·tion** (en′dō-in-tok-si-kā′shŭn) poisoning by an endogenous toxin.

**en·do·lith** (en′dō-lith) a calcified body found in the pulp chamber of a tooth; may be composed of irregular dentin (true denticle) or due to ectopic calcification of pulp tissue (false denticle). SYN denticle (1), pulp stone. [endo- + G. *lithos,* stone]

**en·do·lymph** (en′dō-limf) the fluid contained within the membranous labyrinth of the inner ear.

**en·do·lym·phat·ic duct** a small membranous canal, connecting with both saccule and utricle of the membranous labyrinth, passing through the aqueduct of the vestibule, and terminating in a dilated blind extremity, the endolymphatic sac, on the posterior surface of the petrous portion of the temporal bone beneath the dura mater.

**en·do·lym·phat·ic sac** the dilated blind extremity of the endolymphatic duct. SYN saccus endolymphaticus [TA], Böttcher space.

**en·do·lym·phat·ic sac sur·gery** a generic term for several operations performed on the endolymphatic sac for the treatment of Ménière disease.

**en·do·lym·phat·ic shunt op·er·a·tion** an operation to establish a communication between the endolymphatic sac and the cerebrospinal fluid space for the treatment of Ménière disease.

**en·do·lym·phic** (en-dō-lim′fik) relating to the endolymph.

**En·do me·di·um** (en′dō) SYN Endo agar.

**en·do·me·tria** (en-dō-mē′trē-ă) plural of endometrium.

**en·do·me·tri·al** (en-dō-mē′trē-ăl) relating to or composed of endometrium.

**en·do·met·ri·al ab·la·tion** therapeutic selective endometrial destruction.

**en·do·met·ri·al hy·per·pla·sia** increase in the number of endometrial glands, usually secondary to hyperestrinism; classified as simple hyperplasia, complex hyperplasia, or complex hyperplasia with atypia; the latter may progress to adenocarcinoma.

**en·do·me·tri·al stro·mal sar·co·ma** a term sometimes used for a relatively rare sarcoma believed to be a form of endometriosis in which the lesions form multiple foci in the myometrium and in vascular spaces in other sites, and which consist of histologic and cytologic elements that resemble those of the endometrial stroma.

**en·do·me·tri·oid** (en-dō-mē′trē-oyd) microscopically resembling endometrial tissue.

**en·do·me·tri·oid car·ci·no·ma** adenocarcinoma of the ovary or prostate resembling endometrial adenocarcinoma, possibly arising from ovarian foci of endometriosis.

**en·do·me·tri·oid tu·mor** a tumor of the ovary containing epithelial or stromal elements resembling tumors of the endometrium.

**en·do·me·tri·o·ma** (en′dō-mē-trē-ō′mă) circumscribed mass of ectopic endometrial tissue in endometriosis. [endometrium + *-oma,* tumor]

**en·do·me·tri·o·sis** (en′dō-mē-trē-ō′sis) ectopic occurrence of endometrial tissue, frequently forming cysts containing altered blood. [endometrium + *-osis,* condition]

**en·do·me·tri·tis** (en′dō-mē-trī′tis) inflammation of the endometrium. [endometrium + *-itis,* inflammation]

**en·do·me·tri·um,** pl. **en·do·me·tria** (en′dō-mē′trē-ŭm, en-dō-mē′trē-ă) [TA] the mucous membrane forming the inner layer of the uterine wall; it consists of a simple columnar epithelium and a lamina propria that contains simple tubular uterine glands. The structure, thickness, and state of the endometrium undergo marked change with the menstrual cycle. [endo- + G. *mētra,* uterus]

**en·do·mi·to·sis** (en′dō-mī-tō′sis) SYN endopolyploidy.

**en·do·morph** (en′dō-mōrf) a constitutional body type or build (biotype or somatotype) in which tissues that originated in the endoderm prevail; from a morphological standpoint, the trunk predominates over the limbs. [endo- + G. *morphē,* form]

**en·do·mor·phic** (en′dō-mōr′fik) relating to, or having the characteristics of, an endomorph.

**En·do·my·ce·ta·les** (en′dō-mī-sē-tā′lēz) an order of Ascomycota that includes the yeasts.

**en·do·my·o·car·di·al** (en′dō-mī-ō-kar′dē-ăl) relating to the endocardium and the myocardium.

**en·do·my·o·car·di·al fi·bro·sis** thickening of the ventricular endocardium by fibrosis, involving the subendocardial myocardium, and sometimes the atrioventricular valves, with mural thrombosis, leading to progressive right and left ventricular failure with mitral and tricuspid insufficiency; occurs in adults and is endemic in parts of Africa.

**en·do·my·o·car·di·tis** (en-dō-mī′ō-kar-dī′tis) inflammation of both endocardium and myocardium.

**en·do·my·o·me·tri·tis** (en′dō-mī-ō-mē-trī′tis) sepsis involving the tissues of the uterus. [endo- + G. *mys,* muscle, + *mētra,* uterus, + *-itis,* inflammation]

**en·do·mys·i·um** (en′dō-miz′ē-ŭm, en′dō-mis′ē-ŭm) the fine connective tissue sheath surrounding a muscle fiber. [endo- + G. *mys,* muscle]

**en·do·neu·ri·um** (en-dō-noo′rē-ŭm) the innermost connective tissue supportive structure present in peripheral nerve trunks, found within the fascicles. With the perineurium and epineurium, the endoneurium composes the peripheral nerve stroma. SYN Henle sheath. [endo- + G. *neuron,* nerve]

**en·do·nu·cle·ase** (en-dō-noo′klē-ās) a nuclease (phosphodiesterase) that cleaves polynucleotides (nucleic acids) at interior bonds, thus producing poly- or oligonucleotide fragments of varying size. Cf. exonuclease.

**en·do·par·a·site** (en-dō-par′ă-sīt) a parasite living within the body of its host.

**en·do·pep·ti·dase** (en-dō-pep′ti-dās) an enzyme catalyzing the hydrolysis of a peptide chain at points well within the chain, not near termini; e.g., pepsin, trypsin. Cf. exopeptidase.

**en·do·per·i·car·di·tis** (en′dō-pār′i-kar-dī′tis) simultaneous inflammation of the endocardium and pericardium. [endo- + G. *peri,* around, + *kardia,* heart, + *-itis,* inflammation]

**en·do·per·i·my·o·car·di·tis** (en′dō-pār′i-mī′ō-kar-dī′tis) simultaneous inflammation of the heart muscle and of the endocardium and pericardium. [endo- + G. *peri,* around, + *mys,* muscle, + *kardia,* heart, + *-itis,* inflammation]

**en·do·per·i·to·ni·tis** (en-dō-per′i-tō-nī′tis) superficial inflammation of the peritoneum.

**en·do·phle·bi·tis** (en′dō-fle-bī′tis) inflammation of the intima of a vein. [endo- + G. *phleps (phleb-),* vein, + *-itis,* inflammation]

**en·doph·thal·mi·tis** (en-dof-thal-mī′tis) inflammation of the tissues within the eyeball. [endo- + G. *ophthalmos,* eye, + *-itis,* inflammation]

**en·do·plasm** (en′dō-plazm) the inner or medullary part of the cytoplasm, as opposed to the ectoplasm, containing the cell organelles.

**en·do·plas·mic re·tic·u·lum (ER)** the network of cytoplasmic tubules or flattened sacs (cisternae) with (rough ER) or without (smooth ER) ribosomes on the surface of their membranes in eukaryotes.

**en·do·pol·y·ploid** (en-dō-pol′ē-ployd) relating to endopolyploidy.

**en·do·pol·y·ploi·dy** (en-dō-pol′ē-ploy-dē) the process or state of duplication of the chromosomes without accompanying spindle formation or cytokinesis, resulting in a polyploid nucleus. SYN endomitosis. [endo- + polyploidy]

**en·do·rec·tal pull-through pro·ce·dure** removal of diseased rectal mucosa along with resection of the lower bowel, followed by anastomosis of the proximal stump to the anus, in order to spare rectal muscle function.

**en·do·re·du·pli·ca·tion** (en′dō-rē-doo′pli-kā′shŭn) a form of polyploidy or polysomy by redoubling of chromosomes, giving rise to four-stranded chromosomes at prophase and metaphase.

**end or·gan** the special structure containing the terminal of a nerve fiber in peripheral tissue such as muscle, tissue, skin, mucous membrane, or glands.

**en·dor·phin·er·gic** (en′dōr-fin-er′jik) relating to nerve cells or fibers that employ an endorphin as their neurotransmitter. [endorphin + G. *ergon,* work]

**en·do·sac** (en′dō-sak) a sac or bag used in laparoscopic surgery in which tissue is placed to facilitate removal or morcellation.

**en·do·sal·pin·gi·tis** (en′dō-sal-pin-jī′tis) inflammation of the lining membrane of the eustachian or the fallopian tube. [endo- + G. *salpinx (salping-),* tube, + *-itis,* inflammation]

**en·do·scope** (en′dō-skōp) an instrument for the examination of the interior of a tubular or hollow organ. [endo- + G. *skopeō,* to examine]

**en·do·scop·ic bi·op·sy** biopsy obtained by instruments passed through an endoscope or obtained by a needle introduced under endoscopic guidance.

**en·do·scop·ic ret·ro·grade chol·an·gi·o·pan·cre·a·tog·ra·phy (ERCP)** a method of cholangiopancreatography using an endoscope to inspect and cannulate the ampulla of Vater, with injection of contrast medium for radiographic examination of the pancreatic, hepatic, and common bile ducts.

**en·dos·co·pist** (en-dos′kŏ-pist) a specialist trained in the use of an endoscope.

**en·dos·co·py** (en-dos′kŏ-pē) examination of the interior of a canal or hollow viscus by means of a special instrument, such as an endoscope. [see endoscope]

**en·do·skel·e·ton** (en-dō-skel′ĕ-tŏn) the internal bony framework of the body; the skeleton in its usual context as distinguished from exoskeleton.

**en·do·so·nos·co·py** (en-dō-son′ŏ-skŏ-pē) a sonographic study carried out by transducers inserted into the body as miniature probes in the esophagus, urethra, bladder, vagina, or rectum.

**en·do·spore** (en′dō-spōr) **1.** a body formed within the vegetative cells of some bacteria, particularly those belonging to the genera *Bacillus* and *Clostridium.* **2.** a fungus spore borne within a cell or within the tubular end of a sporophore as in the spherule of *Coccidioides immitis*. [endo- + G. *sporos*, seed]

**en·dos·se·ous im·plant** SYN endosteal implant.

**en·dos·te·al** (en-dos'tē-ăl) relating to the endosteum.

**en·dos·te·al im·plant** an implant that is inserted into the alveolar and/or basal bone and protrudes through the mucoperiosteum. SYN endosseous implant.

**en·dos·te·i·tis, en·dos·ti·tis** (en'dos-tē-ī'tis, en' dos-tī'tis) inflammation of the endosteum or of the medullary cavity of a bone. SYN central osteitis (2), perimyelitis. [endo- + G. *osteon*, bone, + *-itis*, inflammation]

**en·dos·te·o·ma** (en-dos'tē-ō'mă) a benign neoplasm of bone tissue in the medullary cavity of a bone. SYN endostoma. [endo- + G. *osteon*, bone, + *-ōma*, tumor]

**en·dos·te·um** (en-dos'tē-ŭm) [TA] a layer of cells lining the inner surface of bone in the central medullary cavity. SYN medullary membrane. [endo- + G. *osteon*, bone]

**en·dos·to·ma** (en-dō-stō'mă) SYN endosteoma.

**en·do·ten·din·e·um** (en'dō-ten-din'ē-ŭm) the fine connective tissue surrounding secondary fascicles of a tendon. [endo- + L. *tendon*, tendon, + *-eus*, adj.; the whole, in its neuter form, used substantively]

**en·do·the·lia** (en-dō-thē'-lē-ă) plural of endothelium.

**en·do·the·li·al** (en-dō-thē'lē-ăl) relating to the endothelium.

**en·do·the·li·al dys·tro·phy of cor·nea** spontaneous loss of corneal endothelium leading to edema of the corneal stroma and epithelium.

**en·do·the·li·al leu·ko·cyte** old term for a monocyte, a type of leukocyte thought to be derived from reticuloendothelial tissue.

**en·do·the·li·al my·e·lo·ma** SYN Ewing tumor.

**en·do·the·li·oid** (en-dō-thē'lē-oyd) resembling endothelium.

**en·do·the·li·o·ma** (en'dō-thē-lē-ō'mă) generic term for a group of neoplasms, particularly benign tumors, derived from the endothelial tissue of blood vessels or lymphatic channels; endotheliomas may be benign or malignant. [endothelium + *-oma*, tumor]

**en·do·the·li·o·sis** (en'dō-thē-lē-ō'sis) proliferation of endothelium.

**en·do·the·li·um**, pl. **en·do·the·li·a** (en-dō-thē' lē-ŭm, en-dō-thē'-lē-ă) a layer of flat cells lining especially blood and lymphatic vessels and the heart. [endo- + G. *thēlē*, nipple]

**en·do·ther·mic** (en-dō-ther'mik) denoting a chemical reaction during which heat (enthalpy) is absorbed. Cf. exothermic (1). [endo- + G. *thermē*, heat]

**en·do·tho·rac·ic fas·cia** the extrapleural fascia that lines the wall of the thorax; it extends over the cupula of the pleura as the suprapleural membrane and also forms a thin layer between the diaphragm and pleura (phrenicopleura fascia).

**en·do·thrix** (en'dō-thriks) fungal spores (conidia) invading the interior of a hair shaft; there is no conspicuous external sheath of spores, as there is with ectothrix. [endo- + G. *thrix*, hair]

**en·do·tox·e·mia** (en'dō-tok-sē'mē-ă) presence in the blood of endotoxins, which, if derived from Gram-negative rod-shaped bacteria, may cause a

generalized Shwartzman phenomenon with shock.

**en·do·tox·ic** (en-dō-tok'sik) denoting an endotoxin.

**en·do·tox·i·co·sis** (en'dō-tok-si-kō'sis) poisoning by an endotoxin.

**en·do·tox·in** (en-dō-tok'sin) **1.** a bacterial toxin not freely liberated into the surrounding medium, in contrast to exotoxin. **2.** the complex phospho-lipid-polysaccharide macromolecules which form an integral part of the cell wall of strains of Gram-negative bacteria. The toxins may cause a state of shock accompanied by severe diarrhea, and, in smaller doses, fever and leukopenia followed by leukocytosis. SYN intracellular toxin.

**en·do·tra·che·al** (en'dō-trā'kē-ăl) within the trachea.

**en·do·tra·che·al an·es·the·sia** inhalation anesthesia technique in which anesthetic and respiratory gases pass through a tube placed in the trachea via the mouth or nose.

**en·do·tra·che·al in·tu·ba·tion** passage of a tube through the nose or mouth into the trachea for maintenance of the airway during anesthesia or for maintenance of an imperiled airway.

**en·do·tra·che·al tube** SYN tracheal tube.

**en·do·tra·che·li·tis** (en'dō-trak-el-ī'tis) SYN endocervicitis.

**en·do·vas·cu·li·tis** (en'dō-vas'kyu-lī'tis) SYN endangiitis.

**end-piece** the terminal part of the tail of a spermatozoon consisting of the axoneme and the flagellar membrane.

**end·plate, end-plate** (end'plāt) the ending of a motor nerve fiber in relation to a skeletal muscle fiber.

**end stage** the late, fully developed phase of a disease.

**end-sys·tol·ic vol·ume** the amount of blood in the ventricle at the end of the cardiac ejection period and immediately preceding the beginning of ventricular relaxation; a measurement of the adequacy of cardiac emptying, related to systolic function.

**end-tid·al** (end-tī'dăl) at the end of a normal expiration.

**end-to-end a·nas·to·mo·sis** anastomosis performed after cutting each structure to be joined in a plane perpendicular to the ultimate flow through the structures.

**en·dur·ance** sustaining of cardiac, pulmonary, and musculoskeletal exertion over time.

△**-ene** suffix applied to a chemical name indicating the presence of a carbon-carbon double bond; e.g., propene (unsaturated propane, $CH_3$—$CH$= $CH_2$). [G. *enos*, origin]

**en·e·ma** (en'ĕ-mă) a rectal injection to clear out the bowel or to administer drugs or food. [G.]

**en·ergy** (en'er-jē) the exertion of power; the capacity to do work, taking the forms of kinetic energy, potential energy, chemical energy, electrical energy, etc. [G. *energeia*, fr. *en*, in, + *ergon*, work]

**e·ner·gy bal·ance e·qua·tion** equation stating that body mass remains constant when caloric intake equals caloric expenditure. Any chronic imbalance on either side of the equation causes body mass to change.

**e·ner·gy sub·trac·tion** digital radiography using higher- and lower-energy exposures, either by double exposure at 2-kV levels or by interposing a copper filter that absorbs the lower-energy photons between two phosphor plates, with computer calculation of high-Z and low-Z images (bone and soft tissues, respectively); makes use of the fact that lower-energy x-rays are absorbed by more high-Z substances, such as calcium and copper, because of the photoelectric effect.

**en•er•va•tion** (en-er-vā'shŭn) failure of nerve force; weakening. [L. *enervo,* pp. *-atus,* to enervate, fr. *e-* priv. + *nervus,* nerve]

**ENG** electronystagmography.

**en•gage•ment** (en-gāj'ment) OBSTETRICS the mechanism by which the biparietal diameter of the fetal head enters the plane of the inlet.

**En•glish lock** articulation of the blades of obstetrical forceps consisting of a socket on the shank at the junction with the handle in a similar socket on the other shank; used in Simpson forceps.

**en•gorged** (en-gōrjd') absolutely filled; distended with fluid. SEE ALSO congested, hyperemic. [O. Fr. fr. Mediev. L. *gorgia,* throat, narrow passage, fr. L. *gurges,* a whirlpool]

**en•gram** (en'gram) in the mnemic hypothesis, a physical habit or memory trace made on the protoplasm of an organism by the repetition of stimuli. [G. *en,* in, + *gramma,* mark]

**en•graph•ia** (en-graf'ē-ă) the formation of engrams.

**en•hance•ment** (en-hans'ment) **1.** the act of augmenting. **2.** in immunology, the prolongation of a process or event by suppressing an opposing process.

**en•hanc•er** a genetic element that is important in the function of a specific promoter. [M.E. *enhauncen,* raise, increase, fr. O. Fr. *enhaucier,* fr. L.L. *inalto,* fr. *altus,* high, + *-er,* agent suffix]

**en•keph•a•lin•er•gic** (en-kef'ă-lin-er'jik) relating to nerve cells or fibers that employ an enkephalin as their neurotransmitter. [enkephalin + G. *ergon,* work]

**en•large•ment** (en-larj'ment) **1.** an increase in size; an anatomic swelling, enlargement, or prominence. **2.** an intumescence or swelling. SYN intumescence (1), intumescentia.

**en•large•ment of the ves•tib•u•lar a•que•duct** recessive hereditary hearing impairment associated with a large vestibular aqueduct.

△-**en•o•ic** suffix indicating an unsaturated acid. [-ene + -ic]

**enol** (ē'nol) a compound possessing a hydroxyl group (alcohol) attached to a doubly bonded (ethylenic) carbon atom (–CH=CH(OH)–). [-ene + -ol]

**eno•lase** (ē'nol-ās) an enzyme catalyzing the reversible dehydration of 2-phospho-D-glycerate to phospho*enol*pyruvate and water; a step in both glycolysis and gluconeogenesis; several isozymes exist; requires magnesium ion and is inhibited by F⁻.

**enology** (ē-nŏl'ō-jē) the study of wine. [G. *oinos,* wine + *logos,*study]

**en•oph•thal•mos** (en'of-thal'mos) recession of the eyeball within the orbit. [G. *en,* in, + *ophthalmos,* eye]

**en•os•to•sis** (en-os-tō'sis) a mass of proliferating bone tissue within a bone. [G. *en,* in, + *osteon,* bone, + *-osis,* condition]

**en•o•yl** (ēn'ō-il) the acyl radical of an unsaturated aliphatic acid. [-ene + -oyl]

**en•si•form** (en'si-fōrm) SYN xiphoid. [L. *ensis,* sword, + *forma,* appearance]

**en•si•form pro•cess** SYN xiphoid process.

**ENT** ears, nose, and throat. SEE otorhinolaryngology.

**en•tad** toward the interior. [G. *entos,* within, + L. *ad,* to]

**en•tal** (en'tăl) relating to the interior; inside. [G. *entos,* within]

**ent•am•e•bi•a•sis** (ent-ă-mē-bi'ă-sis) infection with *Entamoeba histolytica.* SEE amebiasis, amebic dysentery.

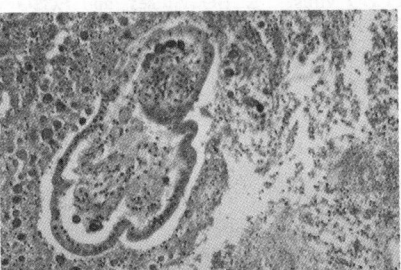*Ent•a•moe•ba* (ent-ă-mē'bă) a genus of ameba parasitic in the oral cavity, cecum, and large bowel of humans and other primates and in many domestic and wild mammals and birds; with the exception of *Entamoeba histolytica,* members of the genus appear to be relatively harmless inhabitants of the host. See this page. [G. *entos,* within + *amoibē,* change]

**Entamoeba histolytica:** many trophozoites are seen in an ulcerative colonic lesion; periodic acid–Schiff stain; X 80

*Ent•a•moe•ba dis•par* nonpathogenic species that occurs in the large intestine of humans; formerly considered *Entamoeba histolytica, Entamoeba dispar* is now considered a separate species; it is nonpathogenic and is not associated with symptomatic amebiasis in humans. Morphologically it resembles *Entamoeba histolytica;* however, the trophozoites are never found to contain ingested red blood cells.

*Ent•a•moe•ba po•lec•ki* a species of ameba commonly found in the intestines of pigs; also parasitizes monkeys, cattle, goats, sheep and dogs; also found in humans, where it does not produce symptoms; clinical importance lies in the possibility of confusing the organism with *Entamoeba histolytica.*

**en•ter•al** (en'ter-ăl) within, or by way of, the intestine or gastrointestinal tract, especially as distinguished from parenteral. A term used to describe tube feedings. [G. *enteron,* intestine]

**en•ter•al•gia** (en-ter-al'jē-ă) enterdynia; severe abdominal pain accompanying spasm of the bowel. SYN enterodynia. [entero- + G. *algos,* pain]

**en•ter•al hy•per•al•i•men•ta•tion** hyperalimentation by the administration of elemental nutrients via a catheter placed within the intestinal tract; usually used in patients with at least a portion of functional small intestine.

**en•ter•ec•ta•sis** (en-ter-ek'tă-sis) dilation of the bowel. [entero- + G. *ektasis,* a stretching]

**en•ter•ec•to•my** (en-ter-ek'tō-mē) resection of a

segment of the intestine. [entero- + G. *ektomē*, excision]

**en·ter·el·co·sis** (en-ter-el-kō'sis) ulceration of the bowel. [entero- + G. *helkos*, ulcer]

**en·ter·ic** (en-ter'ik) relating to the intestine. [G. *enterikos*, from *entera*, bowels]

**ent·er·ic coat·ed tab·let** a tablet coated with a substance that delays release of the medication until the tablet has passed through the stomach and into the intestine (enteron).

**en·ter·ic fe·ver** **1.** SYN typhoid fever. **2.** the group of typhoid and paratyphoid fevers.

**en·ter·i·coid fe·ver** a fever, neither paratyphoid nor typhoid, resembling the latter.

**en·ter·ic or·phan vi·rus·es** enteroviruses isolated from humans and other animals, "orphan" implying lack of known association with disease when isolated; many viruses of the group are now known to be pathogenic; they include ECBO viruses, ECHO viruses, and ECSO viruses.

**en·ter·ic tu·ber·cu·lo·sis** a complication of cavitary pulmonary tuberculosis usually resulting from expectoration and swallowing of bacilli that then infect areas of the digestive tract. SEE ALSO tuberculous enteritis.

**en·ter·ic vi·rus·es** viruses of the genus Enterovirus.

**en·ter·i·tis** (en-ter-ī'tis) inflammation of the intestine, especially of the small intestine. [entero- + G. -*itis*, inflammation]

**en·ter·i·tis ne·cro·ti·cans** enteritis with necrosis of the bowel wall caused by *Clostridium welchii*.

♻ **en·ter·o-, en·ter-** the intestines. [G. *enteron*, intestine]

**en·ter·o·a·nas·to·mo·sis** (en'ter-ō-an-as-tō-mō'sis) SYN enteroenterostomy.

*En·ter·o·bac·ter* (en'ter-ō-bak'ter) a genus of aerobic, facultatively anaerobic, non-spore-forming, motile bacteria (family Enterobacteriaceae) containing Gram-negative rods. The cells are peritrichous, and some strains have encapsulated cells. Glucose is fermented with the production of acid and gas. The Voges-Proskauer test is usually positive. Gelatin is slowly liquefied by the most commonly occurring forms (*Enterobacter cloacae*). These organisms occur in the feces of humans and other animals and in sewage, soil, water, and dairy products; recognized as an agent of common nosocomial infections of the urinary tract, lungs, or blood; somewhat resistant to antibiotics. This genus characteristically acquires resistance rapidly in part because of the presence of inducible β-lactamases; the type species is *Enterobacter cloacae*.

*En·ter·o·bac·ter sa·ka·za·ki·i* a bacterial species especially associated with nursery-acquired neonatal meningitis.

**en·ter·o·bi·a·sis** (en'ter-ō-bī'ă-sis) infection with *Enterobius vermicularis*, the human pinworm.

🔳 *En·te·ro·bi·us* (en-ter-ō'bī-ŭs) a genus of nematode worms which includes the pinworms (*Enterobius vermicularis*). See this page. [entero- + G. *bios*, life]

*En·te·ro·bi·us* **gran·u·lo·ma** lesions containing dead worms and eggs of the nematode are found in vagina, cervix, fallopian tubes, omentum, peritoneum, liver, kidneys, and lungs.

**en·ter·o·cele** (en'ter-o-sēl) **1.** a hernial protrusion through a defect in the rectovaginal or vesicovaginal pouch. [entero- + G. *kēlē*, hernia] **2.** SYN

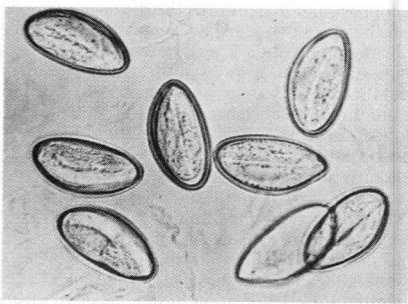

***Enterobius vermicularis*** (pinworm ova): transparent tape preparation

abdominal cavity. [entero- + G. *koilia*, a hollow] **3.** an intestinal hernia. [see 1]

**en·ter·o·cen·te·sis** (en'ter-ō-sen-tē'sis) puncture of the intestine with a hollow needle (trocar and cannula) to withdraw substances. [entero- + G. *kentēsis*, puncture]

**en·ter·o·ci·dal** (en-ter-ō-sī'dal) an agent that kills parasites residing in the gastrointestinal tract.

**en·ter·o·clei·sis** (en-ter-ō-klī'sis) occlusion of the lumen of the alimentary canal. [entero- + G. *kleisis*, a closing]

**en·ter·oc·ly·sis** (en-ter-ok'li-sis) **1.** SYN high enema. **2.** in radiography of the small intestine, filling by introduction of contrast medium through a catheter advanced into the duodenum or jejunum from above. [entero- + G. *klysis*, a washing out]

*En·ter·o·coc·cus* (en'ter-ō-kok'ŭs) genus of facultatively anaerobic, generally nonmotile, non–spore-forming, Gram-positive bacteria. Found in the intestinal tract of humans and animals, enterococci cause intraabdominal, wound and urinary tract infections. Type species is *E. faecalis*. *E. faecium* is also clinically significant.

**en·ter·o·coc·cus**, pl. **en·ter·o·coc·ci** (en'ter-ō-kok'ŭs, en-ter-o-kok'sī) a streptococcus that inhabits the intestinal tract. [entero- + G. *kokkos*, a berry]

*En·ter·o·coc·cus fae·cal·is* is a bacterial species found in human feces and in the intestines of many warm-blooded animals; occasionally found in urinary infections and in blood and heart lesions in subacute endocarditis; a major cause of nosocomial infection, especially in association with Gram-negative pathogens.

*En·ter·o·coc·cus fae·ci·um* the second most common species of this genus recovered in human infection; this species has low-level resistance to ampicillin, and in the U.S. and other countries where vancomycin is used frequently, resistant strains have been rapidly appearing as causes of nosocomial infections; in cases of septicemia in immunocompromised patients, fatality rates can be over 50%.

**en·ter·o·co·li·tis** (en'ter-ō-kō-lī'tis) inflammation of the mucous membrane of a greater or lesser extent of both small and large intestines. SYN coloenteritis. [entero- + G. *kolon*, colon, + -*itis*, inflammation]

**en·ter·o·co·los·to·my** (en'ter-ō-kō-los'tō-mē) establishment of an artificial opening between the small intestine and the colon. [entero- + G. *kōlon*, colon, + *stoma*, mouth]

**en·ter·o·cyst, en·ter·o·cys·to·ma** (en'ter-ō-sist, en'ter-ō-sis-tō'mă) a cyst of the wall of the intestine. [entero- + G. *kystis*, bladder]

**en·ter·o·cys·to·cele** (en'ter-ō-sis'tō-sēl) a hernia of both intestine and bladder wall. [entero- + G. *kystis*, bladder, + *kēlē*, hernia]

**en·ter·o·dyn·ia** (en'ter-ō-din'ē-ă) SYN enteralgia. [entero- + G. *odynē*, pain]

**en·ter·o·en·do·crine cells** a family of cells with argyrophilic granules occurring throughout the digestive tract and believed to produce at least 20 gastrointestinal hormones and neurotransmitters.

**en·ter·o·en·ter·os·to·my** (en'ter-ō-en-ter-os'tō-mē) establishment of a new communication between two segments of intestine. SYN enteroanastomosis, intestinal anastomosis.

**en·ter·o·gas·tric re·flex** peristaltic contraction of the small intestine induced by the entrance of food into the stomach. SEE ALSO gastrocolic reflex.

**en·ter·o·gas·tri·tis** (en'ter-ō-gas-trī'tis) SYN gastroenteritis. [entero- + G. *gastēr*, belly, + *-itis*, inflammation]

**en·ter·o·gas·trone** (en'ter-ō-gas'trōn) a hormone, obtained from intestinal mucosa, that inhibits gastric secretion and motility; secretion of enterogastrone is stimulated by exposure of duodenal mucosa to dietary lipids.

**en·ter·og·e·nous** (en-ter-oj'ĕ-nŭs) of intestinal origin. [entero- + G. *-gen*, producing]

**en·ter·og·e·nous cy·a·no·sis** apparent cyanosis caused by the absorption of nitrites or other toxic materials from the intestine with the formation of methemoglobin or sulfhemoglobin; the skin color change is due to the chocolate color of methemoglobin.

**en·ter·og·e·nous cyst** mediastinal cyst derived from cells sequestered from the primitive foregut; may be classified histologically as bronchogenic, esophageal, or gastric.

**en·ter·o·hem·or·rhag·ic Esch·e·rich·ia co·li (EHEC)** enterohemorrhagic strains of *Escherichia coli*, usually of the serotype 0157:H7; produces a toxin resembling that produced by *Shigella*; associated with damage to the epithelium, ischemia of the bowel, and necrosis of the colon. Apparently responsible for a hemorrhagic form of colitis without fever, which can be very severe, spread primarily by contaminated beef. May also cause microangiopathic hemolytic anemia, renal failure, and the hemolytic uremic syndrome.

**en·ter·o·he·pat·ic cir·cu·la·tion** circulation of substances such as bile salts which are absorbed from the intestine and carried to the liver, where they are secreted into the bile and again enter the intestine.

**en·ter·o·hep·a·ti·tis** (en'ter-ō-hep-ă-tī'tis) inflammation of both the intestine and the liver. [entero- + G. *hēpar* (*hēpat-*), liver, + *-itis*, inflammation]

**en·ter·o·hep·a·to·cele** (en'ter-ō-hep'ă-tō-sēl) congenital umbilical hernia containing intestine and liver. SEE omphalocele. [entero- + G. *hēpar* (*hēpat-*), liver, + *kēlē*, hernia]

**en·ter·o·in·va·sive Esch·e·rich·ia co·li (EIEC)** enteroinvasive strain of *Escherichia coli* that penetrates gut mucosa and multiplies in colon epithelial cells, resulting in shigellosis-like

changes of the mucosa. This strain produces a severe diarrheal illness that can resemble shigellosis except for the absence of vomiting and shorter duration of illness.

**en·ter·o·ki·ne·sis** (en'ter-ō-ki-nē'sis) muscular contraction of the alimentary canal. SEE ALSO peristalsis. [entero- + G. *kinēsis*, movement]

**en·ter·o·ki·net·ic** (en'ter-ō-ki-net'ik) relating to, or producing, enterokinesis.

**en·ter·o·lith** (en'ter-ō-lith) an intestinal calculus formed of layers of soaps and earthy phosphates surrounding a nucleus of some hard body such as a swallowed fruit stone or other indigestible substance. [entero- + G. *lithos*, stone]

**en·ter·o·li·thi·a·sis** (en'ter-ō-li-thī'ă-sis) presence of calculi in the intestine.

**en·ter·ol·o·gy** (en-ter-ol'ō-jē) the branch of medical science concerned especially with the intestinal tract. [entero- + G. *logos*, study]

**en·ter·ol·y·sis** (en-ter-ol'i-sis) division of intestinal adhesions. [entero- + G. *lysis*, dissolution]

**en·ter·o·meg·a·ly, en·ter·o·me·ga·lia** (en'ter-ō-meg'ă-lē, en-ter-ō-me-gā'lē-ă) SYN megaloenteron. [entero- + G. *megas*, great]

**en·ter·o·my·co·sis** (en'ter-ō-mī-kō'sis) an intestinal disease of fungal origin. [entero- + G. *mykēs*, fungus, + *-osis*, condition]

**en·ter·o·pa·re·sis** (en'ter-ō-pă-rē'sis, en'ter-ō-par'i-sis) rarely used term for a state of diminished or absent peristalsis with flaccidity of the muscles of the intestinal walls. [entero- + G. *paresis*, slackening, relaxation]

**en·ter·o·path·o·gen** (en'ter-ō-path'ō-jen) an organism capable of producing disease in the intestinal tract.

**en·ter·o·path·o·gen·ic** (en'ter-ō-path-ō-jen'ik) capable of producing disease in the intestinal tract.

**en·ter·o·path·o·gen·ic Esch·e·rich·ia co·li (EPEC)** enteropathogenic strain of *Escherichia coli;* organisms adhere to small bowel mucosa and produce characteristic changes in the microvilli. This strain produces symptomatic, sometimes serious, gastrointestinal illnesses, especially severe in neonates and young children; typically it produces toxins.

**en·ter·op·a·thy** (en-ter-op'ă-thē) an intestinal disease. [entero- + G. *pathos*, suffering]

**en·ter·o·pep·ti·dase** (en'ter-ō-pep'ti-dās) an intestinal proteolytic glycoenzyme from the duodenal mucosa that converts trypsinogen into trypsin (removes a hexapeptide from trypsinogen).

**en·ter·o·pex·y** (en'ter-ō-pek-sē) fixation of a segment of the intestine to the abdominal wall. [entero- + G. *pēxis*, fixation]

**en·ter·o·pto·sis, en·ter·o·pto·sia** (en'ter-ō-tō'sis, en'ter-ō-tō'sē-ă) abnormal descent of the intestines in the abdominal cavity, usually associated with falling of the other viscera. [entero- + G. *ptōsis*, a falling]

**en·ter·o·ptot·ic** (en'ter-ō-tot'ik) relating to or suffering from enteroptosis.

**en·ter·or·rha·gia** (en-ter-ō-rā'jē-ă) bleeding within the intestinal tract. [entero- + G. *rhēgnymi*, to burst forth]

**en·ter·or·rha·phy** (en-ter-ōr'ă-fē) suture of the intestine. [entero- + G. *rhaphē*, suture]

**en·ter·o·sep·sis** (en'ter-ō-sep'sis) sepsis occurring in or derived from the alimentary canal. [entero- + G. *sēpsis*, putrefaction]

**en·ter·o·spasm** (en'ter-ō-spazm) increased, irregular, and painful peristalsis. [entero- + G. *spasmos*, spasm]

**en·ter·o·sta·sis** (en-ter-os'tă-sis) intestinal stasis; a retardation or arrest of the passage of the intestinal contents. [entero- + G. *stasis*, a standing]

**en·ter·o·ste·no·sis** (en'ter-ō-sten-ō'sis) narrowing of the lumen of the intestine. [entero- + G. *stenōsis*, narrowing]

**⊞en·ter·os·to·my** (en-ter-os'tō-mē) an artificial anus or fistula into the intestine through the abdominal wall. See this page. [entero- + G. *stoma*, mouth]

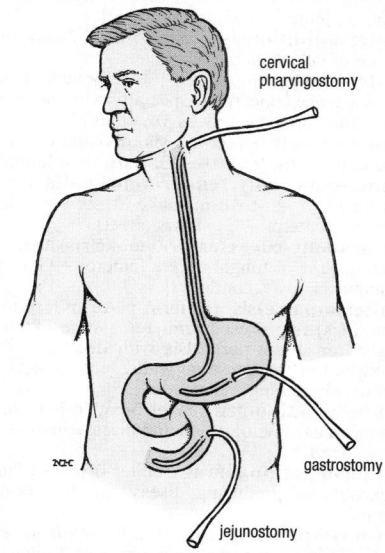

cervical
pharyngostomy

gastrostomy

jejunostomy

**enterostomy tubes:** flexible tubes passing through surgical openings into selected portions of the gastrointestinal tract, providing access for liquid food; a temporary alternative to enterostomy

**en·ter·ot·o·my** (en-ter-ot'ō-mē) incision into the intestine.

**en·ter·o·tox·ae·mia [Br.]** SEE enterotoxemia.

**en·ter·o·tox·e·mia** (en-ter-ō-tok-sē'mē-ă) the presence of an enterotoxin in the blood. [enterotoxin + G. *haima*, blood]

**en·ter·o·tox·i·gen·ic** (en'ter-ō-tok-si-jen'ik) denoting an organism containing or producing a toxin specific for cells of the intestinal mucosa.

**en·ter·o·tox·i·gen·ic** *Esch·e·rich·i·a co·li* **(ETEC)** enterotoxigenic strain of *Escherichia coli;* attaches to the duodenum or proximal small intestine mucosa, where it forms heat-stable and heat-labile toxins that activate adenylate cyclase, causing wasting diarrhea. Responsible for 40–70% of traveler's diarrhea; chiefly water-borne via human feces.

**en·ter·o·tox·in** (en'ter-ō-tok'sin) a cytotoxin specific for the cells of the intestinal mucosa.

**en·ter·o·tro·pic** (en'ter-ō-trop'ik) attracted by or affecting the intestine. [entero- + G. *tropikos*, turning]

*En·te·ro·vi·rus* (en'ter-ō-vī'rŭs) a large and diverse group of viruses that includes poliovirus

types 1 to 3, Coxsackievirus A and B, echoviruses, and the enteroviruses identified since 1969 and assigned type numbers.

**en·ter·o·zo·ic** (en'ter-ō-zō'ik) relating to an enterozoon.

**en·ter·o·zo·on** (en'ter-ō-zō'on) an animal parasite in the intestine. [entero- + G. *zōon*, animal]

**ent·ge·gen (*E*)** (ent-gā'gen) term used when the two higher ranking groups, attached to different carbon atoms in a carbon-carbon double bond, are on opposite sides of the double bond (hence, analogous to trans-). [Ger. opposite]

**en·thal·py (*H*)** (en'thal-pē) heat content, symbolized as *H;* a thermodynamic function, defined as $E + PV$, where $E$ is the internal energy of a system, $P$ the pressure, and $V$ the volume; the heat of a reaction, measured at constant pressure, is $\Delta H$. SYN heat (3). [G. *enthalpō*, to warm in]

**en·the·si·tis** (en-thĕ-sī'tis) traumatic disease occurring at the insertion of muscles where recurring concentration of stress provokes inflammation with a strong tendency toward fibrosis and calcification. [G. *enthetos*, implanted, + *-itis*, inflammation]

**en·the·so·path·ic** (en-thĕ-sō-path'ik) denoting or characteristic of enthesopathy.

**en·the·sop·a·thy** (en-thē-sop'ă-thē) a disease process occurring at the site of insertion of muscle tendons and ligaments into bones or joint capsules. [G. *en*, in, + *thesis*, a placing, + *pathos*, suffering]

△**en·to-, ent-** inner, or within. SEE ALSO endo-. [G. *entos*, within]

**en·to·blast** (en'tō-blast) **1.** pertaining to entoderm. **2.** cell nucleolus. [ento- + G. *blastos*, germ]

**en·to·cele** (en'tō-sēl) an internal hernia. [ento- + G. *kēlē*, hernia]

**en·to·cho·roi·dea** (en'tō-kō-roy'dē-ă) SYN choriocapillary layer. [ento- + G. *chorioeidēs*, choroid]

**en·to·co·nid** (en-tō-kō'nid) **1.** the distolingual cusp of human lower molars. **2.** one of the three cusps of the talonid. [ento- + G. *kōnos*, cone]

**en·to·derm** (en'tō-derm) SYN endoderm. [ento- + G. *derma*, skin]

**en·to·der·mal cell** SYN endodermal cell.

**en·to·ec·tad** (en-tō-ek'tad) from within outward. [G. *entos*, within, + *ektos*, without, + L. *ad*, to]

*En·to·lo·ma si·nu·a·tum* (en-tō-lō'mă sī-nyu-ā'tum) a species of mushroom capable of producing mycetismus gastrointestinalis.

**en·to·mi·on** (en-tō'mē-on) the tip of the mastoid angle of the parietal bone. [G. *entomē*, notch]

**en·to·mol·o·gy** (en-tō-mol'ō-jē) the science concerned with the study of insects. [G. *entomon*, insect, + *logos*, study]

*En·to·moph·thora* (en-tō-mof'thor-ă) a fungal genus reclassified as *Conidiobolus.*

*En·to·moph·thor·a co·ron·a·ta* a fungal genus reclassified as *Conidiobolus*, the cause of conidiobolomycosis.

*En·to·moph·thor·ales* (en-tō-mof'thor-al'ēz) an order of the fungal class Zygomycetes. The genera include conidiobolus, which causes a chronic granulomatous inflammation of a nasal and paranasal sinus mucosa (conidiobolomycosis) and Basidiobolus, which causes a chronic subcutaneous granuloma (basidiobolomycosis). When conidiobolomycosis and basidiobolomycosis are

en•to•moph•tho•ra•my•co•sis (en-tō-mof′thō-ră-mī-kō′sis) a disease caused by fungi of the genera *Basidiobolus* or *Conidiobolus;* tissues are invaded by broad nonseptate hyphae that become surrounded by eosinophilic material. A form of zygomycosis. SEE zygomycosis. [Entomophthorales (order name) + G. *mykēs,* fungus + -osis, condition]

En•to•mo•pox•vi•rus (en′tē-mō-poks-vī′rŭs) the genus of viruses (family Poxviridae) that comprises the poxviruses of insects; they seem not to multiply in vertebrates. [G. *entomon,* insect]

en•top•ic (ent-op′ik) placed within; occurring or situated in the normal place; opposed to ectopic. [G. *en,* within, + *topos,* place]

ent•op•tic (en-top′tik) within the eyeball. Often used to describe visual phenomena generated by mechanical or electrical stimulations of the retina. [ento- + G. *optikos,* relating to vision]

en•to•ret•i•na (en-tō-ret′i-nă) the layers of the retina from the outer plexiform to the nerve fiber layer inclusive.

en•to•zo•al (en-tō-zō′ăl) relating to entozoa.

en•to•zo•on, pl. en•to•zoa (en-tō-zō′on, en-tō-zō′ă) an animal parasite whose habitat is any of the internal organs or tissues. [ento- + G. *zōon,* animal]

en•train•ment mask a face mask designed to entrain atmospheric air in order to provide a constant fractional dilution of a pressurized gas, most commonly oxygen.

en•trap•ment neu•rop•a•thy a focal nerve lesion produced by constriction or mechanical distortion of the nerve, within a fibrous or fibroosseous tunnel, or by a fibrous band.

en•tro•pi•on, en•tro•pi•um (en-trō′pē-on, en-trō′pē-ŭm) **1.** inversion or turning inward of a part. **2.** the infolding of the margin of an eyelid. [G. *en,* in, + *tropē,* a turning]

en•tro•py (*S*) (en′trō-pē) that fraction of heat (energy) content not available for the performance of work, usually because (in a chemical reaction) it has been used to increase the random motion of the atoms or molecules in the system; thus, entropy is a measure of randomness or disorder. [G. *entropia,* a turning towards]

en•ty•py (en′ti-pē) a type of gastrulation seen in some early mammalian embryos in which the endoderm covers the embryonic and amniotic ectoderm; part of the preplacental trophoblast may also be covered. [G. *entypē,* pattern]

enu•cle•ate (ē-noo′klē-āt) to remove entirely; to shell like a nut, as in the removal of an eye from its capsule or a tumor from its enveloping capsule.

enu•cle•a•tion (ē-noo-klē-ā′shŭn) **1.** removal of an entire structure (such as an eyeball or tumor), without rupture, as one shells the kernel of a nut. **2.** removal or destruction of the nucleus of a cell. [L. *enucleo,* to remove the kernel, fr. *e,* out, + *nucleus,* nut, kernel]

en•u•re•sis (en-yu-rē′sis) urinary incontinence; may be intentional or involuntary but not due to a physical disorder. [G. *en-oureō,* to urinate in]

en•ve•lope (en′vĕ-lōp) in anatomy, a structure that encloses or covers.

en•ven•om•a•tion (en-ven-ō-mā′shŭn) the act of injecting a poisonous material (venom) by sting, spine, bite, or other venom apparatus.

en•vi•ron•ment (en-vī′ron-ment) the milieu; the aggregate of all of the external conditions and influences affecting the life and development of an organism. [Fr. *environ,* around]

en•vi•ron•men•tal psy•chol•o•gy the study and application by behavioral scientists and architects of how changes in physical space and related physical stimuli impact upon the behavior of individuals. SEE ALSO personal space.

en•zo•ot•ic (en-zō-ot′ik) denoting a temporal pattern of disease occurrence in an animal population in which the disease occurs with predictable regularity with only relatively minor fluctuations in its frequency over time. SEE epizootic, sporadic. Cf. epizootic, sporadic. [G. *en,* in, + *zōon,* animal]

en•zo•ot•ic sta•bil•i•ty SYN endemic stability.

en•zy•got•ic (en-zī-got′ik) derived from a single fertilized oocyte; denoting twins so derived. [G. *eis* (*en*), one, + zygote]

en•zy•got•ic twins SYN monozygotic twins.

en•zy•mat•ic (en-zī-mat′ik) relating to an enzyme.

en•zyme (en′zīm) a protein that acts as a catalyst to induce chemical changes in other substances, itself remaining apparently unchanged by the process. Enzymes, with the exception of those discovered long ago (e.g., pepsin, emulsin), are generally named by adding -ase to the name of the substrate on which the enzyme acts (e.g., glucosidase), the substance activated (e.g., hydrogenase), and/or the type of reaction (e.g., oxidoreductase, transferase, hydrolase, lyase, isomerase, ligase or synthetase—these being the six main groups in the Enzyme Nomenclature Recommendations of the International Union of Biochemistry). [G. + L. *en,* in + *zymē,* leaven]

en•zyme im•mu•no•as•say (EIA) assay using antibodies to detect the analyte of interest and an enzyme linked to the antigen-antibody complex. The enzyme reacts with a substrate to produce a product that is measured to quantitate the amount of antigen-antibody formed. SEE ALSO enzymelinked immunosorbent assay, enzyme-multiplied immunoassay technique.

en•zyme-linked im•mu•no•sor•bent as•say (ELISA) a sensitive method for serodiagnosis of specific infectious diseases; an *in vitro* competitive binding assay in which an enzyme and its substrate rather than a radioactive substance serve as the indicator system; in positive tests, the two yield a colored or other easily recognizable substance; the enzyme is linked to known immunoglobulin (or antigen) and in positive tests remains as part of the antigen-antibody complex available to react with its substrate when added.

en•zyme-mul•ti•plied im•mu•no•as•say tech•nique (EMIT) a type of immunoassay in which the ligand is labeled with an enzyme. SEE ALSO competitive binding assay, enzyme-linked immunosorbent assay.

en•zy•mol•o•gy (en-zī-mol′ō-jē) the branch of chemistry concerned with the properties and actions of enzymes. [enzyme + G. *logos,* study]

en•zy•mol•y•sis (en-zī-mol′i-sis) **1.** the splitting or cleavage of a substance into smaller parts by means of enzymatic action. **2.** lysis by the action of an enzyme. [enzyme + G. *lysis,* dissolution]

en•zy•mop•a•thy (en-zī-mop′ă-thē) any disturbance of enzyme function, including genetic de-

e
n

ficiency or defect in specific enzymes. [enzyme + G. *pathos,* disease]

**EOB** Explanation of Benefits.

**EOG** electro-oculography; electro-olfactogram.

**eo·sin** (ē'ō-sin) a fluorescent acid dye used for cytoplasmic stains and counterstains in histology and in Romanovsky-type blood stains. [G. *ēōs,* dawn]

**eo·sin B** the disodium salt of 4',5'-dibromo-2',7'-dinitrofluorescein. SYN eosin I bluish. [CI 45400]

**eo·sin I blu·ish** SYN eosin B.

**eo·sin-meth·yl·ene blue a·gar** agar composed of peptone, lactose, and sucrose and containing eosin and methylene blue, used to distinguish between lactose-fermenting and non-lactose-fermenting Gram-negative bacteria.

**eo·sin·o·pe·nia** (ē'ō-sin-ō-pē'nē-ă) an abnormally small number of eosinophils in the peripheral bloodstream. [eosino(phil) + G. *penia,* poverty]

🔲 **eo·sin·o·phil, eosin·o·phile** (ē-ō-sin'ō-fil, ē-ō-sin'ō-fīl) SYN eosinophilic leukocyte. See page B1. [eosin + G. *philos,* fond]

**eo·sin·o·phil ad·e·no·ma** SYN acidophil adenoma.

**eo·sin·o·phil ca·ti·on·ic pro·tein (ECP)** protein the level of which in serum of clotted blood reflects the rate of activation of circulating eosinophils.

**eo·sin·o·phil che·mo·tac·tic fac·tor of an·a·phy·lax·is** a peptide that is chemotactic for eosinophilic leukocytes and is released from disrupted mast cells.

**eo·sin·o·phil·ia** (ē-ō-sin'ō-fil-e-ă) SYN eosinophilic leukocytosis.

**eo·sin·o·phil·ia-my·al·gia syn·drome** a probable autoimmune disorder precipitated by contaminated L-tryptophan tablets, and characterized by fatigue, low-grade fever, myalgias, muscle tenderness and cramps, weakness, paresthesias of the extremities, and skin indurations; marked eosinophilia is noted on peripheral blood studies, serum aldolase increased and biopsies of peripheral nerve, muscle, skin, and fascia show microangiopathy and inflammation in connective tissue.

**eo·sin·o·phil·ic** (ē-ō-sin-ō-fil'ik) staining readily with eosin dyes; denoting such cell or tissue elements.

**eo·sin·o·phil·ic gran·u·lo·ma** a lesion observed more frequently in children and adolescents, occasionally in young adults, which occurs chiefly as a solitary focus in one bone, although multiple involvement is sometimes observed and similar foci may develop in the lung; characterized by numerous Langerhans cells and eosinophils, and occasional foci of necrosis; may be related to Hand-Schüller-Christian disease, possibly representing a benign form.

**eo·sin·o·phil·ic leu·ke·mia, eo·sin·o·phil·o·cyt·ic leu·ke·mi·a** a form of granulocytic leukemia in which there are conspicuous numbers of eosinophilic granulocytes in the tissues and circulating blood, or in which such cells are predominant.

**eo·sin·o·phil·ic leu·ko·cyte** a polymorphonuclear leukocyte characterized by prominent cytoplasmic granules that are bright yellow-red or orange when treated with Wright stain; the nuclei are usually larger than those of neutrophils and characteristically have two lobes; these leukocytes are motile phagocytes with distinctive anti-

parasitic functions. SYN eosinophil, eosinophile, oxyphil (2), oxyphile, oxyphilic leukocyte.

**eo·sin·o·phil·ic leu·ko·cy·to·sis** a form of relative leukocytosis in which the greatest proportionate increase is in the eosinophils. SYN eosinophilia.

**eo·sin·o·phil·ic leu·ko·pe·nia** a decrease in the number of eosinophilic granulocytes normally present in the circulating blood.

**eo·sin·o·phil·ic pneu·mo·nia** an immunologic disorder characterized by radiologic evidence of infiltrates accompanied by either peripheral blood eosinophilia or histopathologic evidence of eosinophilic infiltrates in lung tissue.

**eo·sin·o·phil·ic pus·tu·lar fol·lic·u·li·tis** a dermatosis characterized by sterile pruritic papules and pustules that coalesce to form plaques with papulovesicular borders; spontaneous exacerbations and remissions may be accompanied by peripheral leukocytosis, eosinophilia, or both, and may result in eventual destruction of hair follicles and formation of eosinophilic abscesses. The disease has been reported in AIDS, and a possibly separate form of eosinophilic pustular folliculitis occurs in infants. SYN Ofuji disease.

**eo·sin·o·phil·u·ria** (ē-ō-sin'ō-fil-yu'rē-ă) presence of eosinophils in the urine.

**eo·sin y, eo·sin Ys, eo·sin yel·low·ish** the disodium salt of 2',4',5',7'-tetrabromofluorescein. [C.I. 45380]

**EP** endogenous pyrogen.

**ep·ax·i·al** (ep-ak'sē-ăl) above or behind any axis, such as the spinal axis or the axis of a limb. [G. *epi,* upon, + L. *axis,* axis]

**EPEC** enteropathogenic *Escherichia coli.*

**ep·en·dy·ma** (ep-en'di-mă) [TA] the cellular membrane lining the central canal of the spinal cord and the brain ventricles. [G. *ependyma,* an upper garment]

**ep·en·dy·mal** (ep-en'di-măl) relating to the ependyma.

**ep·en·dy·mal cell** a cell lining the central canal of the spinal cord (those of pyramidal shape) or one of the brain ventricles (those of cuboidal shape).

**ep·en·dy·mi·tis** (ep-en-di-mī'tis) inflammation of the ependyma.

**ep·en·dy·mo·blast** (ep-en'di-mō-blast) an embryonic ependymal cell. [ependyma + G. *blastos,* germ]

**ep·en·dy·mo·cyte** (ep-en'di-mō-sīt) an ependymal cell. [ependyma + G. *kytos,* cell]

**ep·en·dy·mo·ma** (ep-en-di-mō'mă) a glioma derived from relatively undifferentiated ependymal cells; ependymomas may originate from the lining of any of the ventricles or, more commonly, from the central canal of the spinal cord.

**eph·apse** (ef'aps) a place where two or more nerve cell processes (axons, dendrites) touch without forming a typical synaptic contact; some form of neural transmission may occur at such nonsynaptic contact sites. [G. *ephapsis,* contact]

**eph·ap·tic** (e-fap'tik) relating to an ephapse.

**ephe·bic** (ĕ-fē'bik) rarely used term relating to the period of puberty or to a youth. [G. *ephēbikos,* relating to youth, fr. *hēbē,* youth]

**ephe·lis,** pl. **ephe·li·des** (ef-ē'lis, ef-ē'li-dēz) SYN freckle. [G.]

△**epi-** upon, following, or subsequent to. [G.]

**ep·i·an·dros·ter·one** (ep'i-an-dros'ter-ōn) inactive isomer of androsterone; found in urine and in testicular and ovarian tissue.

**ep·i·blast** (ep′i-blast) the component of the bilaminar embryonic disk that gives rise to ectoderm and mesoderm. The mesoderm then displaces the hypoblast cells and forms the entodermal cell layer on its inner surface. [epi- + G. *blastos*, germ]

**ep·i·blas·tic** (ep-i-blas′tik) relating to epiblast.

**ep·i·bleph·a·ron** (ep′i-blef′ă-ron) a congenital horizontal skin fold near the margin of the eyelid, caused by abnormal insertion of muscle fibers. In the upper lid, it simulates blepharochalasis; in the lower lid, it causes a turning inward of the lashes. [epi- + G. *blepharon*, eyelid]

**epib·o·ly, e·pib·o·le** (ē-pib′ō-lē) **1.** a process involved in gastrulation of telolecithal eggs in which, as a result of differential growth, some of the cells of the protoderm move over the surface toward the lips of the blastopore. **2.** growth of epithelium in an organ culture to surround the underlying mesenchymal tissue. [G. *epibolē*, a throwing or laying on]

**ep·i·bul·bar** (ep-i-bŭl′bar) upon a bulb of any kind; specifically, upon the eyeball.

**ep·i·can·thal fold** a fold of skin extending from the root of the nose to the medial termination of the eyebrow, overlapping the medial angle of the eye; its presence is normal in fetal life and in Asians.

**ep·i·car·dia** (ep-i-kar′dē-ă) the portion of the esophagus from where it passes through the diaphragm to the stomach. [epi- + G. *kardia*, heart]

**ep·i·car·di·al** (ep-i-kar′dē-ăl) **1.** relating to the epicardia. **2.** relating to the epicardium.

**ep·i·con·dy·lal·gia** (ep′i-kon-di-lal′jē-ă) pain in an epicondyle of the humerus or in the tendons or muscles originating therefrom. [epicondyle + G. *algos*, pain]

**ep·i·con·dyle** (ep-i-kon′dīl) a projection from a long bone near the articular extremity above or upon the condyle. SYN epicondylus [TA]. [epi- + G. *kondylos*, a knuckle]

**ep·i·con·dy·li·tis** (ep′i-kon-di-lī′tis) infection or inflammation of an epicondyle, or of associated tendons and other soft tissues, particularly the medial or lateral epicondyle of the humerus.

**ep·i·con·dy·lus**, pl. **ep·i·con·dy·li** (ep-i-kon′di-lŭs, ep-i-kon′di-lī) [TA] SYN epicondyle. [L.]

**ep·i·cra·ni·al ap·o·neu·ro·sis** the aponeurosis or intermediate tendon connecting the frontalis and occipitalis muscles to form the epicranius. SYN galea (2).

**ep·i·cra·ni·um** (ep-i-krā′nē-ŭm) the muscle, aponeurosis, and skin covering the cranium. [epi- + G. *kranion*, skull]

**ep·i·cra·ni·us** SEE epicranius muscle.

**ep·i·cra·ni·us mus·cle** composed of the epicranial aponeurosis and the muscles inserting into it, i.e., the occipitofrontalis musculus and temporoparietalis musculus. SYN musculus epicranius [TA].

**ep·i·cri·sis** (ep-i-krī′sis) a secondary crisis; a crisis terminating a recrudescence of morbid symptoms following a primary crisis.

**ep·i·crit·ic, ep·i·crit·ic sen·si·bil·i·ty** (ep-i-krit′ik) that aspect of somatic sensation which permits the discrimination and the topographic localization of the finer degrees of touch and temperature stimuli. Cf. protopathic. [G. *epikritikos*,

adjudicatory, fr. *epi*, on, + *krinō*, to separate, judge]

**ep·i·cys·ti·tis** (ep′i-sis-tī′tis) inflammation of the cellular tissue around the bladder. [epi- + G. *kystis*, bladder, + -*itis*, inflammation]

**ep·i·dem·ic** (ep-i-dem′ik) the occurrence in a community or region of cases of an illness, specific health-related behavior, or other health-related events clearly in excess of normal expectancy. Cf. endemic, sporadic. [epi- + G. *dēmos*, the people]

**ep·i·dem·ic dis·ease** marked increase in prevalence of a disease in a specific population or area, usually with an environmental cause, such as an infectious or toxic agent.

**ep·i·dem·ic gas·tro·en·ter·i·tis vi·rus** a RNA virus, about 27 nm in diameter, which has not been cultured *in vitro;* it is the cause of epidemic nonbacterial gastroenteritis; at least five antigenically distinct serotypes have been recognized, including the Norwalk agent. These viruses are classified with the Caliciviruses in the family Caliciviridae. SYN gastroenteritis virus type A.

**ep·i·dem·ic he·mo·glo·bi·nu·ria** the presence of hemoglobin in the urine of young infants, attended with cyanosis, jaundice, and other conditions; may be due to secondary methemoglobinemia; also called Winckel disease.

**ep·i·dem·ic hem·or·rhag·ic fe·ver** a condition characterized by acute onset of headache, chills and high fever, sweating, thirst, photophobia, coryza, cough, myalgia, arthralgia, and abdominal pain with nausea and vomiting; this phase lasts from three to six days and is followed by capillary and renal interstitial hemorrhages, edema, oliguria, azotemia, and shock; most varieties are caused by viruses and are are rodent-borne. SYN hemorrhagic fever with renal syndrome.

**ep·i·dem·ic·i·ty** (ep′i-dem-is′i-tē) the state of prevailing disease in epidemic form.

**ep·i·dem·ic ker·a·to·con·junc·ti·vi·tis** follicular conjunctivitis followed by subepithelial corneal infiltrates; often caused by adenovirus type 8, less commonly by other types. SYN virus keratoconjunctivitis.

**ep·i·dem·ic ker·a·to·con·junc·ti·vi·tis vi·rus** an adenovirus (type 8) causing epidemic keratoconjunctivitis, especially among shipyard workers, and also associated with outbreaks of swimming pool conjunctivitis. SYN shipyard eye.

**ep·i·dem·ic my·al·gia** SYN epidemic pleurodynia.

**ep·i·dem·ic my·o·si·tis, my·o·si·tis ep·i·dem·i·ca a·cu·ta** SYN epidemic pleurodynia.

**ep·i·dem·ic neu·ro·my·as·the·nia** an epidemic disease characterized by stiffness of the neck and back, headache, diarrhea, fever, and localized muscular weakness; probably viral in origin. SYN benign myalgic encephalomyelitis, Iceland disease.

**ep·i·dem·ic pa·rot·i·di·tis** an acute infectious and contagious disease caused by a *Paramyxovirus* and characterized by fever, inflammation and swelling of the parotid gland, sometimes of other salivary glands, and occasionally by inflammation of the testis, ovary, pancreas, or meninges. SYN mumps.

**ep·i·dem·ic par·o·ti·tis vi·rus** SYN mumps virus.

**ep·i·dem·ic pleu·ro·dyn·ia** an acute infectious disease usually occurring in epidemic form, characterized by paroxysms of pain, usually in the chest, and associated with strains of coxsackievirus type B. syn Bornholm disease, Daae disease, devil's grip, diaphragmatic pleurisy, epidemic myalgia, epidemic myositis, myositis epidemica acuta, Sylvest disease.

**ep·i·dem·ic pleu·ro·dyn·ia vi·rus** a Coxsackievirus, type B, that causes epidemic pleurodynia. syn Bornholm disease virus.

**ep·i·dem·ic pol·y·ar·thri·tis** a mild febrile illness of humans in Australia characterized by polyarthralgia and rash, caused by the Ross River virus and transmitted by mosquitoes.

**ep·i·dem·ic ro·se·o·la** syn rubella.

**ep·i·dem·ic ty·phus** typhus caused by *Rickettsia prowazekii* and spread by body lice; marked by high fever, mental and physical depression, and a macular and papular eruption; lasts for about two weeks and occurs when large crowds are brought together and personal hygiene is at a low ebb; recrudescences can occur.

**ep·i·de·mi·o·log·i·cal ge·net·ics** the study of genetics as a phenomenon of defined populations by the criteria, methods, and objectives of epidemiology rather than of population genetics.

**ep·i·de·mi·ol·o·gist** (ep-i-dē-mē-ol'ō-jist) an investigator who studies the occurrence of disease or other health-related conditions, states, or events in specified populations; one who practices epidemiology; the control of disease usually is also considered a task of the epidemiologist.

**ep·i·de·mi·ol·o·gy** (ep-i-dē-mē-ol'ō-jē) the study of the distribution and determinants of health-related states or events in specified populations, and the application of this study to control of health problems. [G. *epidēmios*, epidemic, + *logos*, study]

**ep·i·der·mal, ep·i·der·mat·ic** (ep-i-der'măl, ep-i-der-mat'ik) relating to the epidermis. syn epidermic.

**ep·i·der·mal cyst** a cyst formed of a mass of epidermal cells which, as a result of trauma, has been pushed beneath the epidermis; the cyst is lined with stratified squamous epithelium and contains concentric layers of keratin.

**epidermal growth factor receptor (EGFR)** receptor often upregulated in epithelial tumors.

**ep·i·der·mal·i·za·tion** (ep-i-der'mal-i-zā'shŭn) syn squamous metaplasia.

**e·pi·der·mal-mel·an·in unit** an association of one melanocyte with several surrounding epidermal keratinocytes, presumably one that favors the transfer of melanin granules from the melanocyte to the keratinocytes.

**ep·i·der·mal ridg·es** ridges of the epidermis of the palms and soles, where the sweat pores open. syn skin ridges.

**ep·i·der·mic** (ep-i-der'mik) syn epidermal.

**ep·i·der·mis**, pl. **ep·i·derm·i·des** (ep-i-derm'is, ep-i-derm'i-dēz) [TA] **1.** the superficial epithelial portion of the skin (cutis). The epidermis of the palms and soles has the following strata: stratum corneum (horny layer), stratum lucidum (clear layer), stratum granulosum (granular layer), stratum spinosum (prickle cell layer), and stratum basale (basal cell layer); in other parts of the body, the stratum lucidum may be absent. **2.** botany the outermost layer of cells in leaves and the young parts of plants. syn cuticle (3), cuticula (2). [G. *epidermis*, the outer skin, fr. *epi*, on, + *derma*, skin]

**ep·i·der·mi·tis** (ep-i-der-mī'tis) inflammation of the epidermis or superficial layers of the skin.

**ep·i·der·mo·dys·pla·sia** (ep-i-der'mō-dis-plā'zē-ă) faulty growth or development of the epidermis. [epidermis + G. *dys-*, bad, + *plasis*, a molding]

**ep·i·der·moid** (ep-i-der'moyd) **1.** resembling epidermis. **2.** a cholesteatoma or other cystic tumor arising from aberrant epidermal cells. [epidermis + G. *eidos*, appearance]

**ep·i·der·moid car·ci·no·ma** squamous cell carcinoma of the skin.

**ep·i·der·moid cyst** a spherical, unilocular cyst of the dermis, composed of encysted keratin and sebum; the cyst is lined by a keratinizing epithelium resembling the epidermis derived from the follicular infundibulum.

**ep·i·der·mol·y·sis** (ep'i-der-mol'i-sis) a condition in which the epidermis is loosely attached to the corium, readily exfoliating or forming blisters. [epidermis + G. *lysis*, loosening]

**ep·i·der·mol·y·sis bul·lo·sa** a group of inherited chronic noninflammatory skin diseases in which large bullae and erosions result from slight mechanical trauma; a form limited to the hands and feet is also called Weber-Cockayne syndrome.

*Ep·i·der·mo·phy·ton* (ep'i-der-mof'i-ton, ep'i-der'mō-fī'ton) a genus of fungi whose macroconidia are clavate and smooth-walled. The only species, *Epidermophyton floccosum*, is a common cause of tinea pedis and tinea cruris. [epidermis + G. *phyton*, plant]

**ep·i·der·mot·ro·pism** (ep-i-der-mot'rō-pizm) movement towards the epidermis, as in the migration of T lymphocytes into the epidermis in mycosis fungoides. [epidermis + G. *trope*, a turning]

**ep·i·did·y·mal** (ep-i-did'i-măl) relating to the epididymis.

**ep·i·did·y·mec·to·my** (ep'i-did-i-mek'tō-mē) operative removal of the epididymis. [epididymis + G. *ektome*, excision]

**ep·i·did·y·mis**, gen. **ep·i·did·y·mi·dis**, pl. **ep·i·did·y·mi·des** (ep-i-did'i-mis, ep-i-di-dim'i-dis, ep-i-di-dim'i-dēz) [TA] an elongated structure connected to the posterior surface of the testis, consisting of the head of the epididymis, body of epididymis, and tail of epididymis, which turns sharply upon itself to become the ductus deferens; the main component is the very convoluted duct of the epididymis, within the tail and the beginning of the ductus deferens. The epididymis stores and matures spermatozoa and transports them from testis to ductus deferens (vas deferens) [Mod. L. fr. G. *epididymis*, fr. *epi*, on, + *didymos*, twin, in pl. testes]

**ep·i·did·y·mi·tis** (ep-i-did-i-mī'tis) inflammation of the epididymis.

**ep·i·did·y·mo·or·chi·tis** (ep-i-did'i-mō-ōr-kī'tis) simultaneous inflammation of both epididymis and testis. [epididymis + G. *orchis*, testis]

**ep·i·did·y·mo·plas·ty** (ep-i-did'i-mō-plas-tē) surgical repair of the epididymis. [epididymis + G. *plastos*, formed]

**ep·i·did·y·mot·o·my** (ep'i-did-i-mot'ō-mē) incision into the epididymis, as in preparation for epididymovasostomy or for drainage of purulent material. [epididymis + G. *tome*, a cutting]

**ep·i·did·y·mo·vas·ec·to·my** (ep-i-did'i-mō-va-sek'tō-mē) surgical removal of the epididymis and vas deferens. [epididymis + vasectomy]

**ep·i·did·y·mo·va·sos·to·my** (ep-i-did'i-mō-va-sos'tō-mē) surgical anastomosis of the vas deferens to the epididymis. [epididymis + vasostomy]

**ep·i·du·ral** (ep-i-doo'răl) upon (or outside) the dura mater.

**ep·i·du·ral an·es·the·sia** regional anesthesia produced by injection of local anesthetic solution into the peridural space. SYN peridural anesthesia.

**ep·i·du·ral block** an obstruction in the epidural space; used inaccurately to refer to epidural anesthesia.

**ep·i·du·ral cav·i·ty** the space between the walls of the vertebral canal and the dura mater of the spinal cord.

🚹 **ep·i·du·ral he·ma·to·ma** SYN extradural hemorrhage. See this page.

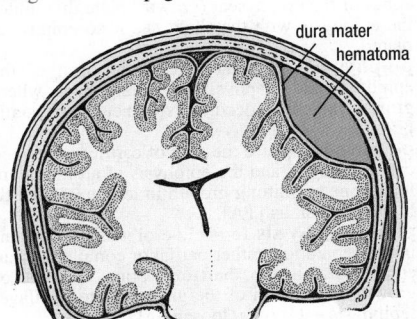

**epidural hematoma:** showing frontal section of brain

**ep·i·du·rog·ra·phy** (ep-i-doo-rog'ră-fē) radiographic visualization of the epidural space following the regional instillation of a radiopaque contrast medium.

**ep·i·es·tri·ol** (ep-i-es'trē-ol) SEE estriol.

**ep·i·gas·tral·gia** (ep'i-gas-tral'jē-ă) pain in the epigastric region. [epigastrium + G. *algos*, pain]

**ep·i·gas·tric** (ep-i-gas'trik) relating to the epigastrium.

**ep·i·gas·tric fos·sa** the slight depression in the midline just inferior to the xiphoid process of the sternum.

**ep·i·gas·tric her·nia** hernia through the linea alba above the navel.

**ep·i·gas·tric re·gion** the region of the abdomen located between the costal margins and the subcostal plane.

**ep·i·gen·e·sis** (ep-i-jen'ĕ-sis) 1. development of offspring from a zygote. 2. regulation of the expression of gene activity without alteration of genetic structure. [epi- + G. *genesis,* creation]

**ep·i·ge·net·ic** (ep'i-jĕ-net'ik) relating to epigenesis.

**ep·i·glot·tic, ep·i·glot·tid·e·an** (ep-i-glot'ik, ep-i-glo-tid'ē-an) relating to the epiglottis.

**ep·i·glot·tic car·ti·lage** a thin lamina of elastic cartilage forming the central portion of the epiglottis. SYN cartilago epiglottica [TA].

**ep·i·glot·ti·dec·to·my** (ep'i-glot-i-dek'tō-mē) excision of the epiglottis. [epiglottis + G. *ektomē,* excision]

**ep·i·glot·tis** (ep-i-glot'is) [TA] a leaf-shaped plate of elastic cartilage, covered with mucous membrane, at the root of the tongue, which serves as a diverter valve over the superior aperture of the larynx during the act of swallowing; it stands erect when liquids are being swallowed, but is passively bent over the aperture by solid foods being swallowed. [G. *epiglōttis,* fr. *epi* on, + *glōttis,* the mouth of the windpipe]

**ep·i·glot·ti·tis, ep·i·glot·ti·di·tis** (ep-i-glot-ī'tis, ep'i-glot-i-dī'tis) inflammation of the epiglottis, which may cause respiratory obstruction, especially in children; frequently due to infection by *Haemophilus influenzae* type b.

**ep·i·ker·a·to·phak·ia** (ep'i-ker'ă-tō-phak'ē-ă) modification of refractive error by application of a donor cornea to the anterior surface of the patient's cornea from which epithelium has been removed. [epi- + G. *keras,* horn, + *phakos,* lens]

**ep·i·late** (ep'i-lāt) to extract a hair; to remove the hair from a part by forcible extraction, electrolysis, or loosening at the root by chemical means. Cf. depilate. [L. *e,* out, + *pilus,* a hair]

**ep·i·la·tion** (ep-i-lā'shŭn) the act or result of removing hair. SYN depilation.

**epil·a·to·ry** (e-pil'ă-tō-rē) 1. pertaining to removal of hair by any method that also removes the entire hair shaft, as in plucking or the application of heated wax products that harden, allowing the patient to remove an entire mass of hair at the same time. 2. an agent having this action. Cf. depilatory.

**ep·i·lem·ma** (ep-i-lem'ă) the connective tissue sheath of nerve fibers near their termination. [epi- *lemma,* husk]

**ep·i·lep·sy** (ep'i-lep'sē) a chronic disorder characterized by paroxysmal brain dysfunction due to excessive neuronal discharge, and usually associated with some alteration of consciousness. The clinical manifestations of the attack may vary from complex abnormalities of behavior including generalized or focal convulsions to momentary spells of impaired consciousness. These clinical states have been subjected to a variety of classifications, none universally accepted to date and, accordingly, the terminologies used to describe the different types of attacks remain purely descriptive and nonstandardized; they are variously based on 1) the clinical manifestations of the seizure (motor, sensory, reflex, psychic or vegetative), 2) the pathologic substrate (hereditary, inflammatory, degenerative, neoplastic, traumatic, or cryptogenic), 3) the location of the epileptogenic lesion (rolandic, temporal, diencephalic regions), and 4) the time period at which the attacks occur (nocturnal, diurnal, menstrual). SYN fit (3), seizure disorder. [G. *epilēpsia,* seizure]

**ep·i·lep·tic** (ep-i-lep'tik) relating to, characterized by, or suffering from epilepsy.

**e·pi·lep·tic spasm** spasm characterized by a sudden flexion-extension, or mixed extension-flexion, predominantly proximal (including truncal muscles), which is usually more sustained than a myoclonic movement but not as sustained as a tonic seizure. Occurs frequently in clusters, with the individual events ranging in duration from myoclonic to tonic seizure components.

**ep·i·lep·ti·form** (ep-i-lep'ti-fōrm) SYN epileptoid.

**ep·i·lep·to·gen·ic, ep·i·lep·tog·e·nous** (ep-i-lep-tō-jen'ik, ep-i-lep-toj'ĕ-nŭs) causing epilepsy.

**ep·i·lep·to·gen·ic zone** a cortical region which on stimulation reproduces the patient's spontaneous seizure or aura.

e
p

**ep·i·lep·toid** (ep-i-lep'toyd) resembling epilepsy; denoting certain convulsions, especially of functional nature. SYN epileptiform. [G. *epilēpsia,* seizure, epilepsy, + *eidos,* resemblance]

**epi·lu·min·es·cence mi·cros·co·py** low-power microscopy (×50–×100), commonly a television microscope applied to a glass slide covering mineral oil on the surface of a skin lesion, e.g., to determine malignancy in pigmented lesions. SYN surface microscopy.

**ep·i·man·dib·u·lar** (ep-i-man-dib'yu-lăr) upon the lower jaw. [epi- + L. *mandibulum,* mandible]

**ep·i·men·or·rha·gia** (ep-i-men-ō-rā'jē-ă) prolonged and profuse menstruation occurring at any time, but most frequently at the beginning and end of menstrual life.

**ep·i·men·or·rhea** (ep-i-men-ō-rē'ă) too frequent menstruation, occurring at any time, but particularly at the beginning and end of menstrual life.

**ep·i·mer** (ep'i-mer) one of two molecules (having more than one chiral center) differing only in the spatial arrangement about a single chiral atom. SEE sugars. Cf. anomer. [epi- + G. *meros,* part]

**ep·i·mer·ase** (ep'i-mer-ās) [EC 5.1] a class of enzymes catalyzing epimeric changes.

**ep·i·mere** (ep'i-mēr) the dorsal part of the myotome. SEE myotome (3). [epi- + G. *meros,* part]

**ep·i·mor·pho·sis** (ep'i-mōr-fō'sis) regeneration of a part of an organism by growth at the cut surface. [epi- + G. *morphē,* shape]

**ep·i·mys·i·ot·o·my** (ep'i-mis-ē-ot'ō-mē) incision of the sheath of a muscle. [epimysium + G. *tomē,* a cutting]

**ep·i·mys·i·um** (ep-i-mis'ē-ŭm) [TA] the fibrous connective tissue envelope surrounding a skeletal muscle. [epi- + G. *mys,* muscle]

**ep·i·neph·rine** (ep'i-nef'rin) a catecholamine that is the chief neurohormone of the adrenal medulla. The L-isomer is the most potent stimulant (sympathomimetic) of adrenergic α- and β-receptors, resulting in increased heart rate and force of contraction, vasoconstriction or vasodilation, relaxation of bronchiolar and intestinal smooth muscle, glycogenolysis, lipolysis, and other metabolic effects; used in the treatment of bronchial asthma, acute allergic disorders, open-angle glaucoma, and heart block, and as a topical and local vasoconstrictor. SYN adrenaline. [epi- + G. *nephros,* kidney, + -ine]

**ep·i·neph·ros** (ep-i-nef'ros) SYN suprarenal gland. [epi- + G. *nephros,* kidney]

**ep·i·neu·ral** (ep-i-noo'răl) on a neural arch of a vertebra.

**ep·i·neu·ri·al** (ep-i-noo'rē-ăl) relating to the epineurium.

**ep·i·neu·ri·um** (ep-i-noo'rē-ŭm) [TA] the outermost supporting structure of peripheral nerve trunks, consisting of a condensation of areolar connective tissue; subdivided into those layers that surround the whole nerve trunk (epifascicular epineurium), and those layers which extend between the nerve fascicles (interfascicular epineurium). With the endoneurium and perineurium, the epineurium composes the peripheral nerve stroma. [epi- + G. *neuron,* nerve]

**ep·i·ot·ic cen·ter** the center of ossification of the petrous part of the temporal bone that appears posterior to the posterior semicircular canal.

**ep·i·phar·ynx** (ep'i-far'ingks) SYN nasopharynx. [G. *epi,* on, over, + pharynx]

**ep·i·phe·nom·e·non** (ep'i-fĕ-nom'ĕ-non) a symptom appearing during the course of a disease, not of usual occurrence, and not necessarily associated with the disease.

**epiph·o·ra** (ē-pif'ō-ră) an overflow of tears upon the cheek, due to imperfect drainage by the tear-conducting passages. SYN tearing. [G. a sudden flow, fr. *epi,* on, + *pherō,* to bear]

**ep·i·phys·e·al frac·ture** injury to the growth plate of a long bone in children and adolescents.

**ep·i·phys·i·al ar·rest** early and premature fusion between epiphysis and diaphysis.

**ep·i·phys·i·al car·ti·lage** paticular type of new cartilage produced by the epiphysis of a growing long bone; located on the epiphysial (distal) side of the zone of growth cartilage, it is a zone of relatively quiescent chondrocytes (the resting zone) of the epiphyseal (growth) plate that unites the epiphysis with the shaft. SEE ALSO epiphysial plate.

**ep·i·phys·i·al line** the line of junction of the epiphysis and diaphysis of a long bone where growth in length occurs. SYN linea epiphysialis [TA].

**ep·i·phys·i·al plate** the disk of cartilage between the metaphysis and the epiphysis of an immature long bone permitting growth in length. SYN cartilago epiphysialis [TA].

**epiph·y·si·ol·y·sis** (ep-i-fiz-ē-ol'i-sis) **1.** loosening or separation, either partial or complete, of an epiphysis from the shaft of a bone. **2.** arrest of growth by ablation of the growth plate cartilage. [epiphysis + G. *lysis,* loosening]

**epiph·y·sis,** pl. **epiph·y·ses** (e-pif'i-sis, e-pif'i-sēz) [TA] a part of a long bone developed from a center of ossification distinct from that of the shaft and separated at first from the latter by a layer of cartilage. [G. an excrescence, fr. *epi,* upon, + *physis,* growth]

**epiph·y·si·tis** (e-pif-i-sī'tis) inflammation of an epiphysis.

**ep·i·pi·al** (ep'i-pī'ăl) on the pia mater.

△**ep·i·plo-** omentum. SEE ALSO omento-. [G. *epiploon*]

**ep·i·plo·ic** (ep'i-plō'ik) SYN omental.

**ep·i·plo·ic fo·ra·men** the passage, below and behind the portal hepatis, connecting the two sacs of the peritoneum; it is bounded anteriorly by the hepatoduodenal ligament and posteriorly by a peritoneal fold over the inferior vena cava.

**ep·i·scle·ra** (ep'i-sklēr'ă) the connective tissue between the sclera and the conjunctiva. [epi- + sclera]

**ep·i·scle·ral** (ep-i-sklēr'ăl) **1.** upon the sclera. **2.** relating to the episclera.

**ep·i·scle·ral ar·tery** one of many small branches of the anterior ciliary arteries that arise as they perforate the sclera near the corneoscleral junction, and course on the sclera. SYN arteria episcleralis [TA].

**ep·i·scle·ral space** the space between the fascial sheath of the eyeball and the sclera.

**ep·i·scle·ral veins** a series of small venules in the sclera close to the corneal margin that empty into the anterior ciliary veins.

**ep·i·scle·ri·tis** (ep-i-skle-rī'tis) inflammation of the episcleral connective tissue. SEE ALSO scleritis.

△**ep·i·sio-** the vulva. SEE ALSO vulvo-. [G. *episeion,* pubic region]

**ep·i·si·o·per·i·ne·or·rha·phy** (e-piz'ē-ō-per'i-nē-ōr'ă-fē) repair of an incised or a ruptured perineum and lacerated vulva or repair of a surgical incision of the vulva and perineum. [episio- + G. *perinaion*, perineum, + *rhaphē*, a stitching]

**ep·i·si·o·plas·ty** (e-piz′ē-ō-plas-tē) plastic surgery of the vulva. [episio- + G. *plastos*, formed]

**ep·i·si·or·rha·phy** (e-piz-i-ōr′ră-fē) repair of a lacerated vulva or an episiotomy. [episio- + G. *rhaphē*, a stitching]

**ep·i·si·o·ste·no·sis** (e-piz′i-ō-stě-nō′sis) narrowing of the vulvar orifice. [episio- + G. *stenōsis*, narrowing]

**ep·i·si·ot·o·my** (e-piz-ē-ot′ō-mē) surgical incision of the vulva to prevent laceration at the time of delivery or to facilitate vaginal surgery. [episio- + G. *tomē*, incision]

**ep·i·so·de** (ep′i-sōd) an important event or series of events taking place in the course of continuous events, e.g., an episode of depression.

**epi·sode of care** all services provided to a patient with a medical problem within a specific period of time across a continuum of care in an integrated system.

**epi·so·dic hy·per·ten·sion** hypertension manifested intermittently, triggered by anxiety or emotional factors. SYN paroxysmal hypertension.

**ep·i·some** (ep′i-sōm) an extrachromosomal element (plasmid) that may either integrate into the bacterial chromosome of the host or replicate and function stably when physically separated from the chromosome. [epi- + G. *sōma*, body (chromosome)]

**ep·i·spa·di·as** (ep-i-spā′dē-ăs) a malformation in which the urethra opens on the dorsum of the penis; frequently associated with exstrophy of the bladder. [epi- + G. *spaō*, to tear or gouge]

**ep·i·sple·ni·tis** (ep-i-splē-nī′tis) inflammation of the capsule of the spleen.

**epis·ta·sis** (e-pis′tă-sis) 1. the formation of a pellicle or scum on the surface of a liquid, especially as on standing urine. 2. phenotypic interaction of non-allelic genes. 3. a form of gene interaction whereby one gene masks or interferes with the phenotypic expression of one or more genes at other loci; the gene whose phenotype is expressed is said to be "epistatic," while the phenotype altered or suppressed is then said to be "hypostatic". [G. scum; epi- + G. *stasis*, a standing]

**ep·i·stat·ic** (ep-is-tat′ik) relating to epistasis.

**ep·i·stax·is** (ep′i-stak′sis) profuse bleeding from the nose. SYN nosebleed. [G. fr. *epistazō*, to bleed at the nose, fr. *epi*, on, + *stazō*, to fall in drops]

**ep·i·sten·o·car·di·ac per·i·car·di·tis** pericarditis accompanying transmural myocardial infarction and limited to the area over the infarct.

**ep·i·ster·nal** (ep-i-ster′năl) 1. over or on the sternum. 2. relating to the episternum.

**ep·i·stro·phe·us** (ep-i-strō′fē-ŭs) SYN axis (5). [G. the pivot]

**ep·i·ten·din·e·um** (ep′i-ten-din′ē-ŭm) the white fibrous sheath surrounding a tendon. [L.]

**ep·i·thal·a·mus** (ep′i-thal′ă-mŭs) [TA] a small dorsomedial area of the thalamus corresponding to the habenula and its associated structures, the medullary stria, pineal body, and habenular commissure. [epi- + thalamus]

**ep·i·the·lia** (ep-i-thē′lē-ă) plural of epithelium.

**ep·i·the·li·al** (ep-i-thē′lē-ăl) relating to or consisting of epithelium.

**ep·i·the·li·al down·growth** the invasion of surface epithelium into the interior of the eye as a consequence of a penetrating ocular wound.

**ep·i·the·li·al dys·tro·phy** corneal dystrophy affecting primarily the epithelium and its basement membrane.

**ep·i·the·li·al·i·za·tion** (ep-i-thē′lē-ăl-i-zā′shŭn) formation of epithelium over a denuded surface. SYN epithelization.

**ep·i·the·li·al lam·i·na** the layer of modified ependymal cells that forms the inner layer of the tela choroidea, facing the ventricle.

**ep·i·the·li·al mem·brane an·ti·gen (EMA)** a heavily glycosylated, 70-kd protein complex, first isolated in human milk fat globulin; this antigen is present in a variety of glandular epithelia, especially in breast carcinoma cells, but may also be seen in cultured fibroblasts, lymphoid cells, and some stromal cells. Immunohistochemical staining may be used as a diagnostic aid in tissue diagnosis.

**ep·i·the·li·al pearl** SYN keratin pearl.

**ep·i·the·li·al plug** a mass of epithelial cells temporarily occluding an embryonic opening; the term is most commonly used with reference to the external nares.

**ep·i·the·li·oid** (ep-i-thē′lē-oyd) resembling or having some of the characteristics of epithelium. [epithelium + G. *eidos*, resemblance]

**ep·i·the·li·oid cell 1.** a nonepithelial cell having certain characteristics of epithelium; **2.** large mononuclear histiocytes having certain epithelial characteristics, particularly in tubercles where they are polygonal and have eosinophilic cytoplasm.

**ep·i·the·li·o·lyt·ic** (ep-i-thē′lē-ō-lit′ik) destructive to epithelium.

**ep·i·the·li·o·ma** (ep′i-thē-lē-ō′mă) **1.** an epithelial neoplasm or hamartoma of the skin, especially of skin appendage origin. **2.** a carcinoma of the skin derived from squamous, basal, or adnexal cells. [epithelium + G. *-ōma*, tumor]

**ep·i·the·li·om·a·tous** (ep-i-thē-lē-ō′mă-tŭs) pertaining to epithelioma.

**ep·i·the·li·op·a·thy** (ep′i-thē-lē-op′ă-thē) disease involving epithelium. [epithelium + G. *pathos*, suffering]

🔲 **ep·i·the·li·um**, pl. **ep·i·the·lia** (ep-i-thē′lē-ŭm, ep-i-thē′lē-ă) [TA] the purely cellular avascular layer covering all the free surfaces, cutaneous, mucous, and serous, including the glands and other structures derived therefrom. See page 328. [G. *epi*, upon, + *thēlē*, nipple, a term applied originally to the thin skin covering the nipples and the papillary layer of the border of the lips]

**ep·i·the·li·za·tion** (ep-i-thē-li-zā′shŭn) SYN epithelialization.

**ep·i·tope** (ep′i-tōp) the simplest form of an antigenic determinant, on a complex antigenic molecule, that can combine with antibody or T cell receptor. [epi- + -tope]

**ep·i·trich·i·um** (ep-i-trik′ē-ŭm) SYN periderm. [epi- + G. *trichion*, dim. of *thrix*, (*trich-*), hair]

**ep·i·tym·pan·ic** (ep-i-tim-pan′ik) above, or in the upper part of, the tympanic cavity or membrane.

**ep·i·tym·pan·ic re·cess** the upper portion of the tympanic cavity above the tympanic membrane; it contains the head of the malleus and the body of the incus.

**ep·i·zo·ic** (ep-i-zō′ik) living as a parasite on the skin surface.

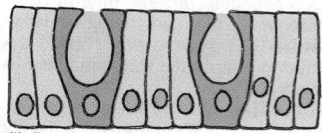

columnar epithelium
of intestines

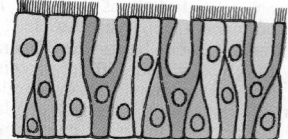

pseudostratified ciliated
columnar epithelium

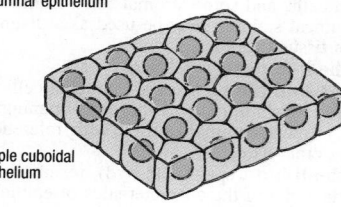

simple cuboidal
epithelium

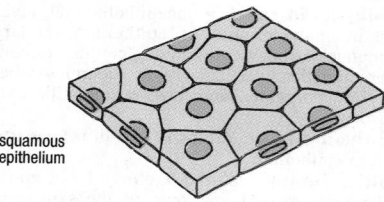

squamous
epithelium

**types of epithelium** (simplified schematic)

**ep·i·zo·ol·o·gy** (ep′i-zō-ol′ō-jē) SYN epizootiology. [epi- + G. *zōon,* animal, + *logos,* study]

**ep·i·zo·on,** pl. **ep·i·zoa** (ep-i-zō′on, ep-i-zō′ă) an animal parasite living on the body surface. [epi- + G. *zōon,* animal]

**ep·i·zo·ot·ic** (ep′i-zō-ot′ik) **1.** disease occurrence in an animal population with a frequency clearly in excess of the expected. **2.** an outbreak (epidemic) of disease in an animal population; often with the implication that it may also affect human populations. [epi- + G. *zōon,* animal]

**ep·i·zo·ot·i·ol·o·gy** (ep′i-zō-ot′ē-ol′ō-jē) epidemiology of disease in animal populations. SYN epizoology. [epi- + G. *zōon,* animal, + *logos,* study]

**EPO** exclusive provider organization.

**ep·o·nych·ia** (ep-ō-nik′ē-ă) infection involving the proximal nail fold.

**ep·o·nych·i·um** (ep-ō-nik′ē-ŭm) [TA] **1.** the thin, condensed, eleidin-rich layer of epidermis that precedes and initially covers the nail plate in the embryo. It normally degenerates by the eighth month except at the nail base, where it remains as the cuticle of the nail. **2.** the corneal layer of epidermis overlapping and in direct contact with the nail root proximally or the sides of the nail plate laterally, forming the undersurface of the nail wall or nail folds of the nail. SYN perionychium. **3.** the thin skin adherent to the nail at its

proximal portion. [G. *epi,* upon, + *onyx (onych-),* nail]

**ep·o·nym** (ep′ō-nim) the name of a disease, structure, operation, or procedure, usually derived from the name of the person who first discovered or described it. [G. *epōnymos,* named after]

**ep·o·nym·ic** (ep-ō-nim′ik) **1.** relating to an eponym. **2.** an eponym.

**ep·ox·y** (ē-pok′sē) chemical term describing an oxygen atom bound to two linked carbon atoms Generally, any cyclic ether, but commonly applied to a 3-membered ring. Epoxys are important chemical intermediates, and the basis of epoxy resins (polymers) formed from epoxy monomers.

**ep·si·lon** (ε) (ep′sil-on) **1.** fifth letter of the Greek alphabet. **2.** extinction coefficient. **3.** CHEMISTRY a position of a substituent located on the fifth atom from the carboxyl or other primary functional group. For terms with the prefix ε, see the specific term.

**ep·si·lon wave** late R wave (in lead $V_1$) of delayed right ventricular activation in arrhythmogenic RV dysplasia.

**Ep·stein-Barr vi·rus (EBV)** (ep′stīn băr) a herpesvirus that causes infectious mononucleosis and is also found in cell cultures of Burkitt lymphoma; associated with nasopharyngeal carcinoma. SYN human herpesvirus 4.

**Ep·stein pearls** (ep′stīn) multiple small, white, epithelial inclusion cysts found in the midline of the palate in newborn infants.

**Ep·stein sign** (ep′stīn) lid retraction in an infant giving it a frightened expression and a "wild glance." SEE setting sun sign, Collier sign.

**epu·lis** (ep-yu′lis) a nonspecific exophytic gingival mass. [G. *epoulis,* a gumboil]

**ep·u·loid** (ep′yu-loyd) a gingival mass that resembles an epulis.

**equa·tion** (ē-kwā′zhŭn) a statement expressing the equality of two things, usually with the use of mathematical or chemical symbols. [L. *aequare,* to make equal]

**equa·tion of mo·tion 1.** an expression of Newton's second law that relates forces, displacements, and their derivatives for a mechanical system. **2.** for the respiratory system, an equation that relates the forces involved in breathing to the displacements they produce. Typically, pressure differences are used to represent generalized forces and volume changes are used to represent generalized displacements. The simplest equation of motion written for the lungs states that the change in transpulmonary pressure is equal to the sum of an elastic term plus a flow resistive term: transpulmonary pressure change = elastance × tidal volume + resistance × change in flow.

**equa·to·ri·al plane** in metaphase of mitosis, the plane that touches all of the centromeres and their spindle attachments.

**equa·to·ri·al plate** the assembly of chromosomes in mitosis.

**equa·to·ri·al staph·y·lo·ma** a staphyloma occurring in the area of exit of the vortex veins. SYN scleral staphyloma.

**equi·ax·i·al** (ē′kwi-ak′sē-ăl) having axes of equal length.

**equil·i·bra·tion** (e-kwil-ĭ-brā′shŭn) **1.** the act of maintaining an equilibrium or balance. **2.** the act of exposing a liquid, e.g., blood or plasma, to a gas at a certain partial pressure until the partial pressures of the gas within and without the liquid are equal. **3.** DENTISTRY modification of occlusal forms of the teeth by grinding, with the intent of equalizing occlusal stress, producing simultaneous occlusal contacts, or harmonizing cuspal relations. **4.** CHROMATOGRAPHY the saturation of the stationary phase with the vapor of the elution solvent to be used.

**equi·lib·ri·um** (ē-kwi-lib'rē-ŭm) **1.** the condition of being evenly balanced; a state of repose between two or more antagonistic forces that exactly counteract each other. **2.** CHEMISTRY a state of apparent repose created by two reactions proceeding in opposite directions at equal speed; in chemical equations, sometimes indicated by two opposing arrows (↔) or (↔). SYN dynamic equilibrium. [L. *aequilibrium,* a horizontal position, fr. *aequus,* equal, + *libra,* a balance]

**equi·lib·ri·um di·al·y·sis** IMMUNOLOGY a method for determination of association constants for hapten-antibody reactions in a system in which the hapten (dialyzable) and antibody (nondialyzable) solutions are separated by semipermeable membranes.

**equine** (ē'kwīn) relating to, derived from, or resembling the horse, mule, ass, or other members of the genus *Equus.* [L. *equinus,* fr. *equus,* horse]

**equine in·fec·tious a·ne·mia** a worldwide infectious disease of horses and other equids, caused by equine infectious anemia virus and a member of the family Retroviridae, marked by general debility, remittent fever, staggering gait, progressive anemia, and loss of flesh; it is transmitted by bloodsucking insects and by contact, oral infection, or the use of unsterilized syringes and needles. SYN swamp fever (1).

**equine mor·bil·li·vi·rus** a species causing a fatal respiratory disease in horses and humans in Australia, with encephalitis also seen in some human cases. SYN Hendra virus.

**equi·no·val·gus** (ek'wi-nō-val'gŭs) SYN talipes equinovalgus.

**equi·no·var·us** (ek'wi-nō-vā'rŭs) SYN talipes equinovarus.

**equi·tox·ic** (ē-kwi-tok'sik) of equivalent toxicity.

**equiv·a·lence, equiv·a·len·cy** (ē-kwiv'ă-lens, ē-kwiv'ă-len-sē) the property of an element or radical of combining with or displacing, in definite and fixed proportion, another element or radical in a compound. [L. *aequus,* equal, + *valentia,* strength (valence)]

**equiv·a·lent** (ē-kwiv'ă-lent) **1.** equal in any respect. **2.** that which is equal in size, weight, force, or any other quality to something else. **3.** having the capability to counterbalance or neutralize each other. **4.** having equal valences. **5.** SYN gram equivalent. [see equivalence]

**ER** endoplasmic reticulum; emergency room.

**Er** erbium.

**Eran·ko flu·o·res·cence stain** exposure of frozen sections to formaldehyde, which produces a strong yellow-green fluorescence from cells containing norepinephrine.

**ERBF** effective renal blood flow.

**er·bi·um (Er)** (er'bē-ŭm) a rare earth (lanthanide) element, atomic no. 68, atomic wt. 167.26. [from Ytterby, a village in Sweden]

**Erb pal·sy, Erb pa·ral·y·sis** (erb) a type of brachial birth palsy in which there is paralysis of the muscles of the upper arm and shoulder girdle (deltoid, biceps, brachialis, and brachioradialis muscles) due to a lesion of the upper trunk of the brachial plexus or of the roots of the fifth and sixth cervical roots. SYN Duchenne-Erb paralysis.

**Erb-West·phal sign** (erb-vest'fahl) abolition of the patellar tendon reflex, in tabes and certain other diseases of the spinal cord, and occasionally also in brain disease. SYN Westphal sign.

**ERCP** endoscopic retrograde cholangiopancreatography.

**erec·tile** (ē-rek'tīl) capable of erection.

**e·rec·tile tis·sue** a tissue with numerous vascular spaces that may become engorged with blood.

**erec·tion** (ē-rek'shŭn) the condition of erectile tissue when filled with blood, which then becomes hard and unyielding; denoting especially this state of the penis. [L. *erectio,* fr. *erigo,* pp. *erectus,* to set up]

**erec·tor** (ērek'tŏr) **1.** one who or that which raises or makes erect. **2.** denoting specifically certain muscles having such action. SYN arrector. [Mod. L.]

**e·rec·tor mus·cles of hairs** SYN arrector muscle of hair.

**e·rec·tor spi·nae mus·cles, e·rec·tor mus·cle of spine** *origin,* from sacrum, ilium, and spines of lumbar vertebrae; it divides into three columns, iliocostalis musculus, longissimus musculus, and spinalis musculus, which insert into ribs and vertebrae with additional muscle slips joining the columns at successively higher levels; *action,* extends vertebral column; *nerve supply,* dorsal primary rami of spinal nerves. SYN musculus erector spinae [TA].

**er·e·thism** (er'ĕ-thizm) an abnormal state of excitement or irritation, either general or local. [G. *erethismos,* irritation]

**er·e·this·mic, er·e·this·tic, er·e·thit·ic** (er-ĕ-thiz'mik, er-ĕ-this'tik, er-ĕ-thit'ik) excited; marked by or causing erethism; irritable.

**ERG** electroretinogram.

**erg** the unit of work in the CGS system; the amount of work done by 1 dyne acting through 1 cm, 1 g cm$^2$ s$^{-2}$; in the SI system, 1 erg equals $10^{-7}$ joule. [G. *ergon,* work]

**er·ga·sia** (er-gā'zē-ă) **1.** any form of activity, especially mental. **2.** the total of functions and reactions of an individual. [G. work]

**er·gas·to·plasm** (er-gas'tō-plazm) SYN granular endoplasmic reticulum. [G. *ergastēr,* a workman, + *plasma,* something formed]

△**er·go-** work. [G. *ergon*]

**er·go·cal·cif·er·ol** (er'gō-kal-sif'er-ol) activated ergosterol, the vitamin D of plant origin; it arises from ultraviolet irradiation of ergosterol; used in prophylaxis and treatment of vitamin D deficiency. SYN calciferol, vitamin D$_2$.

**ergogenic aid** ergogenic aids have been classified as nutritional, pharmacologic, physiologic, or psychologic and range from use of accepted techniques such as carbohydrate loading to illegal and unsafe approaches such as anabolic-androgenic steroid use.

**er·go·graph** (er'gō-graf) an instrument for recording the amount of work done by muscular contractions, or the amplitude of contraction. [ergo- + G. *graphō,* to write]

**er·go·graph·ic** (er-gō-graf'ik) relating to the ergograph and the record made by it.

**ergolytic** (er-gō-lit'ik) pertaining to any substance

that impairs exercise performance. [ergo- + G. *lysis*, a loosening]

**er·gom·e·ter** (er-gom'ĕ-ter) SYN dynamometer. [ergo- + G. *metron*, measure]

**er·go·nom·ics** (er-gō-nom'iks) a branch of ecology concerned with human factors in the design and operation of machines and the physical environment. [ergo- + G. *nomos*, law]

**er·gos·ter·ol** (er-gos'ter-ol) the most important of the provitamins $D_2$; ultraviolet irradiation converts ergosterol to lumisterol, tachysterol, and ergocalciferol; main sterol in yeast.

**er·got** (er'got) the resistant, overwintering stage of the parasitic ascomycetous fungus *Claviceps purpurea*, a pathogen of cereal rye that transforms the seed of rye into a compact spurlike mass of fungal pseudotissue (the sclerotium) containing five or more optically isomeric pairs of alkaloids. The levorotary isomers induce uterine contractions, control bleeding, and alleviate certain localized vascular disorders (migraine headaches). [O. Fr. *argot*, cock's spur]

**er·got·ism** (er'got-izm) poisoning by a toxic substance contained in the sclerotia of the fungus, *Claviceps purpura*, growing on cereal rye; characterized by necrosis of the extremities (gangrene) due to contraction of the peripheral vascular bed. SYN Saint Anthony fire (1).

**erode** (ē-rōd') 1. to cause, or to be affected by, erosion. 2. to remove by ulceration. [L. *erodo*, to gnaw away]

**erog·e·nous** (ĕ-roj'ĕ-nŭs) capable of producing sexual excitement when stimulated. [G. *eros*, love, + *genos*, birth]

**erog·e·nous zone, ero·to·gen·ic zone** areas of the body, such as genitals and nipples, which elicit sexual arousal when stimulated.

**eros** (ē'ros, ār'os) PSYCHOANALYSIS the life principle representing all instinctual tendencies toward procreation and life. [G. love]

**E-ro·sette test** a test to identify T lymphocytes by mixing purified blood lymphocytes with serum and sheep erythrocytes; rosettes of erythrocytes form around human T lymphocytes on incubation.

**ero·sion** (ē-rō'zhŭn) 1. a wearing away or a state of being worn away, as by friction or pressure. 2. a shallow ulcer; in the stomach and intestine, an ulcer limited to the mucosa, with no penetration of the muscularis mucosae. 3. the wearing away of a tooth by nonbacterial chemical action; when the cause is unknown, it is referred to as idiopathic erosion. SYN odontolysis. See page B5. [L. *erosio*, fr. *erodo*, to gnaw away]

**ero·sive** (ē-rō'siv) 1. having the property of eroding or wearing away. 2. an eroding agent.

**erot·ic** (ĕ-rot'ik) lustful; relating to sexual passion; having the quality to produce sexual arousal. [G. *erōtikos*, relating to love, fr. *erōs*, love]

**ero·to·gen·ic** (er'ō-tō-jen'ik) capable of causing sexual excitement or arousal. [G. *erōs*, love, + *-gen*, production]

**ero·to·ma·nia** (er'ō-tō-mā'nē-ă) 1. excessive or morbid inclination to erotic thoughts and behavior. 2. the delusional belief that one is involved in a relationship with another, generally of higher socioeconomic status. [G. *erōs*, love, + *mania*, frenzy]

**ero·to·man·ic dis·or·der** the false belief that

one is loved by another such as a movie star or a casual acquaintance.

**ero·to·path·ic** (er'ō-tō-path'ik) relating to erotopathy.

**er·o·top·a·thy** (er-ō-top'ă-thē) any abnormality of the sexual impulse. [G. *erōs*, love, + *pathos*, suffering]

**ero·to·pho·bia** (er'ō-tō-fō'bē-ă) morbid aversion to the thought of sexual love and to its physical expression. [G. *erōs*, love, + *phobos*, fear]

**ERPF** effective renal plasma flow.

**er·ror** (er'ŏr) 1. a defect in structure or function. 2. BIOSTATISTICS 1) a mistaken decision, as in hypothesis testing or classification by a discriminant function; 2) the difference between the true value and the observed value of a variate, ascribed to randomness or misreading by an observer. 3. a false or mistaken belief; in biomedical and other sciences, there are many varieties of error, for example due to bias, inaccurate measurements, or faulty instruments.

**er·ror-prone po·ly·mer·ase chain re·ac·tion** use of PCR under conditions in which misincorporation of bases is favored, e.g., where random mutants are sought for a portion of amplified DNA.

**ERT** estrogen replacement therapy.

**eruc·ta·tion** (ē-rŭk-tā'shŭn) the voiding of gas or of a small quantity of acid fluid from the stomach through the mouth. SYN belching. [L. *eructo*, pp. *-atus*, to belch]

**erup·tion** (ē-rŭp'shŭn) 1. a breaking out, especially the appearance of lesions on the skin. 2. a rapidly developing dermatosis of the skin or mucous membranes, especially when appearing as a local manifestation of one of the exanthemata; an eruption is characterized, according to the nature of the lesion, as macular, papular, vesicular, pustular, bullous, nodular, erythematous, etc. 3. the passage of a tooth through the alveolar process and perforation of the gums until it reaches occlusion or contact with the opposing tooth. SEE ALSO emergence. [L. *e-rumpo*, pp. *-ruptus*, to break out]

**erup·tive** (ē-rŭp'tiv) characterized by eruption.

**e·rup·tive xan·tho·ma** the sudden appearance of groups of waxy, yellow or yellowish-brown papules with an erythematous halo, especially over extensors of the elbows and knees, and on the back and buttocks of patients with severe hyperlipemia, often familial or, more rarely, in severe diabetes.

**ERV** expiratory reserve volume.

**er·y·sip·e·las** (er-i-sip'ĕ-las) a specific, acute, cutaneous inflammatory disease caused by β-hemolytic streptococci and characterized by hot, red, edematous, brawny, and sharply defined eruptions; usually accompanied by severe constitutional symptoms. [G., fr. *erythros*, red + *pella*, skin]

**er·y·si·pel·a·tous** (er'i-si-pel'ă-tŭs) relating to erysipelas.

**er·y·sip·e·loid** (er-i-sip'ĕ-loyd) a specific, usually self-limiting, cellulitis of the hand caused by *Erysipelothrix rhusiopathiae;* appears as a dusky erythema with diamondlike configuration of the skin at the site of a wound sustained in handling fish or meat and may become generalized, with plaques of erythema and bullae, and occasionally, severe toxemia. [G. *erysipelas* + *eidos*, resemblance]

**Er•y•sip•e•lo•thrix** (ār-i-sip′ĕ-lō-thriks) a genus of bacteria containing nonmotile, Gram-positive, rod-shaped organisms which have a tendency to form long filaments. Members of this genus are parasitic on mammals, birds, and fish. The type species is *Erysipelothrix rhusiopathiae.* [erysipelas + G. *thrix,* hair]

**er•y•the•ma** (er-i-thē′mă) redness of the skin due to capillary dilatation. [G. *erythēma,* flush]

**er•y•the•ma ab ig•ne** SYN erythema caloricum.

**er•y•the•ma an•u•la•re** rounded or ringed lesions.

**er•y•the•ma an•u•la•re cen•tri•fu•gum** a chronic recurring erythematous eruption consisting of small and large annular lesions, with a scant marginal scale, usually of unknown cause.

**er•y•the•ma ar•thri•ti•cum ep•i•de•mi•cum** SYN Haverhill fever.

**er•y•the•ma ca•lo•ri•cum** a reticulated, pigmented, macular eruption that occurs, mostly on the shins, of bakers, stokers, and others exposed to radiant heat. SYN erythema ab igne.

**er•y•the•ma chro•ni•cum mi•grans** a raised erythematous ring with advancing indurated borders and central clearing, radiating from the site of a tick bite such as that by *Ixodes scapularis;* the characteristic skin lesion of Lyme disease, due to the spirochete *Borrelia burgdorferi.*

**er•y•the•ma dose** the minimum dose of x-rays or other form of radiation sufficient to produce erythema.

**er•y•the•ma in•du•ra•tum** recurrent hard subcutaneous nodules that frequently break down and form necrotic ulcers, usually on the calves and less frequently on the thighs or arms of middle-aged women; probably a form of nodular vasculitis. SYN Bazin disease.

**er•y•the•ma in•fec•ti•o•sum** a mild infectious exanthema of childhood characterized by an erythematous maculopapular eruption, resulting in a lacelike facial rash or "slapped cheek" appearance. Fever and arthritis may also accompany infection; caused by Parvovirus B 19. SYN fifth disease.

**er•y•the•ma i•ris** concentric rings of erythema varying in intensity, characteristic of erythema multiforme. SYN herpes iris (1).

**er•y•the•ma mar•gi•na•tum** a variant of erythema multiforme seen in rheumatic fever.

**er•y•the•ma mul•ti•for•me** an acute eruption of macules, papules, or subdermal vesicles presenting a multiform appearance, the characteristic lesion being the target or iris lesion over the dorsal aspect of the hands and forearms; its origin may be allergic, seasonal, or from drug sensitivity, and the eruption, although usually self-limited, may be recurrent or may run a severe course, sometimes with fatal termination (Stevens-Johnson syndrome). SYN herpes iris (2).

**er•y•the•ma no•do•sum** a panniculitis marked by the sudden formation of painful nodes on the extensor surfaces of the lower extremities, with lesions that are self-limiting but tend to recur; associated with arthralgia and fever; may be the result of drug sensitivity or associated with sarcoidosis and various infections. Deep biopsies show a septal panniculitis with infiltration by lymphocytes and scattered multinucleated giant cells.

**er•y•the•ma nu•chae** SYN Unna nevus.

**er•y•the•ma per•nio** SYN chilblain.

**er•y•them•a•tous** (er-i-them′ă-tŭs, er-i-thē′mă-tŭs) relating to or marked by erythema.

**er•y•the•ma•to•ve•sic•u•lar** (er-i-the′mă-tō-ve-sik′yu-lăr) denoting a condition characterized by erythema and vesiculation, as in allergic contact dermatitis.

**er•y•the•ma tox•i•cum** flushing of the skin due to allergic reaction to some toxic substance.

**er•y•the•ma tox•i•cum ne•o•na•to•rum** a common transient idiopathic eruption of erythema, small papules, and occasionally pustules filled with eosinophilic leukocytes overlying hair follicles of the newborn.

**er•y•thrae•mia [Br.]** SYN polycythemia vera.

**er•y•thral•gia** (ēr-i-thral′jē-ă) painful redness of the skin. SEE ALSO erythromelalgia. [erythro- + G. *algos,* pain]

**ery•thras•ma** (er-i-thraz′mă) an eruption of well-circumscribed reddish brown patches, in the axillae and groins especially, due to the presence of *Corynebacterium minutissimum* in the stratum corneum. [G. *erythrainō,* to redden]

**eryth•re•de•ma** (ĕ-rith-rē-dē′mă) SYN acrodynia (2). [erythro- + G. *oidēma,* swelling]

**er•y•thre•mia** (er-i-thrē′mē-ă) SYN polycythemia vera. [erythro- + G. *haima,* blood]

**er•y•threm•ic my•e•lo•sis** a neoplastic process of erythropoietic tissue, characterized by anemia, irregular fever, splenomegaly, hepatomegaly, hemorrhagic disorders, and numerous erythroblasts in blood. Acute and chronic forms are recognized, but in the latter there is less prominence of the immature cells; the former is also called Di Guglielmo disease and acute erythremia.

**er•y•thrism** (er′i-thrizm, ĕ-rith′rizm) redness of the hair with a ruddy, freckled complexion. [G. *erythros,* red]

**er•y•thris•tic** (er-i-thris′tik) relating to or marked by erythrism; having a ruddy complexion and reddish hair. SYN rufous.

△**eryth•ro-, erythr- 1.** combining form denoting red or red blood cell; corresponds to L. *rub-.* **2.** indicates the structure of erythrose in a larger sugar; used as such, it is italicized (e.g., 2-deoxy-D-*erythro*-pentose). [G. *erythros,* red]

**eryth•ro•blast** (ĕ-rith′rō-blast) the first generation of cells in the red blood cell series that can be distinguished from precursor endothelial cells. In normal maturation four stages of development can be recognized: 1) pronormoblast, 2) basophilic normoblast, 3) polychromatic normoblast, and 4) orthochromatic normoblast. [erythro- + G. *blastos,* germ]

**eryth•ro•blas•te•mia** (ĕ-rith′rō-blas-tē′mē-ă) the presence of nucleated red cells in the peripheral blood. [erythroblast + G. *haima,* blood]

**eryth•ro•blas•to•pe•nia** (ĕ-rith′rō-blas-tō-pē′nē-ă) a primary deficiency of erythroblasts in bone marrow, seen in aplastic anemia. [erythroblast + G. *penia,* poverty]

**eryth•ro•blas•to•sis** (ĕ-rith′rō-blas-tō′sis) the presence of erythroblasts in considerable number in the blood. [erythroblast + *-osis,* condition]

**e•ryth•ro•blas•to•sis fe•ta•lis** a grave hemolytic anemia that, in most instances, results from development in the mother of anti-Rh antibody in response to the Rh factor in the (Rh-positive) fetal blood; it is characterized by many erythroblasts in the circulation, and often generalized edema (hydrops fetalis) and enlargement of the liver and spleen; the disease is sometimes caused

e
r

by antibodies for antigens other than Rh. SYN congenital anemia, hemolytic disease of newborn, neonatal anemia, Rh antigen incompatibility.

**eryth·ro·blas·tot·ic** (ĕ-rith′rō-blas-tot′ik) pertaining to erythroblastosis, especially erythroblastosis fetalis.

**eryth·ro·cla·sis** (er-i-throk′lă-sis) fragmentation of the red blood cells. [erythro- + G. *klasis,* a breaking]

**eryth·ro·clas·tic** (ĕ-rith′rō-klas′tik) pertaining to erythroclasis; destructive to red blood cells.

**eryth·ro·cy·a·no·sis** (ĕ-rith′rō-sī-ă-nō′sis) a condition seen in girls and young women in which exposure of the limbs to cold causes them to become swollen and dusky red; it results from direct exposure to cold, but not freezing, temperatures. [erythro- + G. *kyanos,* blue, + *-osis,* condition]

**⊟ eryth·ro·cyte** (ĕ-rith′rō-sīt) a mature red blood cell. See this page. SYN haemacyte, hemacyte, red blood cell, red corpuscle. [erythro- + G. *kytos,* cell]

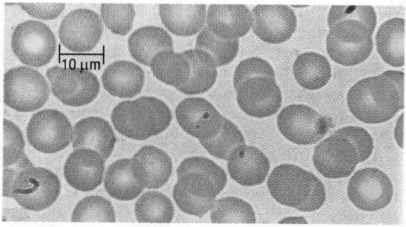

**erythrocytes:** in blood smear

**eryth·ro·cyte in·di·ces** calculations for determining the average size, hemoglobin content, and concentration of hemoglobin in red blood cells, specifically mean cell volume, mean cell hemoglobin, and mean cell hemoglobin concentration.

**eryth·ro·cyte sed·i·men·ta·tion rate (ESR)** the rate of settling of red blood cells in anticoagulated blood; increased rates are often associated with anemia or inflammatory states.

**eryth·ro·cy·thaem·ia [Br.]** SYN polycythemia.

**eryth·ro·cy·the·mia** (ĕ-rith′rō-sī-the′mē-ă) SYN polycythemia. [erythro- + G. *kytos,* cell, + *haima,* blood]

**eryth·ro·cyt·ic** (ĕ-rith-rō-sit′ik) pertaining to an erythrocyte.

**eryth·ro·cy·tic cycle** that pathogenic portion of the vertebrate phase of the life cycle of malarial organisms that takes place in the red blood cells.

**eryth·ro·cy·tic se·ries** the cells in the various stages of development in the red bone marrow leading to the formation of the erythrocyte, e.g., erythroblasts, normoblasts, erythrocytes.

**eryth·ro·cy·tol·y·sin** (ĕ-rith′rō-sī-tol′i-sin) SYN hemolysin (1).

**eryth·ro·cy·tol·y·sis** (ĕ-rith′rō-sī-tol′i-sis) SYN hemolysis. [erythrocyte + G. *lysis,* loosening]

**eryth·ro·cy·tor·rhex·is** (ĕ-rith′rō-sī-tō-rek′sis) a partial erythrocytolysis in which particles of protoplasm escape from the red blood cells, which then become crenated and deformed. SYN erythrorrhexis. [erythrocyte + G. *rhexis,* rupture]

**eryth·ro·cy·tos·chi·sis** (ĕ-rith′rō-sī-tos′ki-sis) a

breaking up of the red blood cells into small particles that morphologically resemble platelets. [erythrocyte + G. *schisis,* a splitting]

**eryth·ro·cy·to·sis** (ĕ-rith′rō-sī-tō′sis) polycythemia, especially that which occurs in response to some known stimulus.

**eryth·ro·de·gen·er·a·tive** (ĕ-rith′rō-de-jen′er-ă-tiv) pertaining to or characterized by degeneration of the red blood cells.

**eryth·ro·der·ma** (ĕ-rith-rō-der′mă) a nonspecific designation for intense and usually widespread reddening of the skin from dilatation of blood vessels, often preceding, or associated with exfoliation. SYN erythrodermatitis. [erythro- + G. *derma,* skin]

**e·ryth·ro·der·ma des·qua·ma·ti·vum** severe, extensive seborrheic dermatitis with exfoliative dermatitis, generalized lymphadenopathy, and diarrhea in the newborn; frequently occurs in undernourished, cachectic children. SYN Leiner disease.

**e·ryth·ro·der·ma pso·ri·a·ti·cum** extensive exfoliative dermatitis simulating psoriasis.

**eryth·ro·der·ma·ti·tis** (ĕ-rith′rō-der-mă-tī′tis) SYN erythroderma.

**eryth·ro·don·tia** (ĕ-rith-rō-don′shē-ă) reddish discoloration of the teeth, as may occur in porphyria. [erythro- + G. *odous,* tooth]

**er·y·thro·ed·e·ma [Br.]** SEE acrodynia.

**eryth·ro·gen·ic** (ĕ-rith-rō-jen′ik) **1.** producing red, as causing an eruption or a red color sensation. **2.** pertaining to the formation of red blood cells. [erythro- + *-gen,* producing]

**eryth·ro·gen·ic tox·in** SYN streptococcus erythrogenic toxin.

**er·y·throid** (er′i-throyd, ĕ-rith′royd) reddish in color.

**eryth·ro·ker·a·to·der·mia** (ĕ-rith′rō-ker-ă-tō-der′mē-ă) a neurocutaneous syndrome characterized by papulosquamous erythematous plaques with onset shortly after birth; ataxia, nystagmus, dysarthria, and decreased tendon reflexes appear later in life; symmetric progressive erythrokeratodermia is inherited as an autosomal dominant disorder and does not involve the palms and soles. [erythro- + G. *keras,* horn, + *derma,* skin, + *-ia,* condition]

**eryth·ro·ker·a·to·der·mia va·ri·a·bi·lis** a dermatosis characterized by hyperkeratotic plaques of bizarre, geographic configuration, associated with erythrodermic areas that may vary remarkably in size, shape, and position from day to day; hair, nails, and teeth are not affected; onset is usually in the first year of life; autosomal dominant or recessive inheritance, caused by mutation in the connexin gene encoding gap junction protein beta-3 (GJB3) on 1p.

**eryth·ro·ki·net·ics** (ĕ-rith′rō-ki-net′iks) the kinetics of erythrocytes from their generation to destruction. [erythro- + G. *kinēsis,* movement]

**eryth·ro·leu·ke·mia** (ĕ-rith′rō-loo-kē′mē-ă) simultaneous neoplastic proliferation of erythroblastic and leukoblastic tissues.

**eryth·ro·leu·ko·sis** (ĕ-rith′rō-loo-kō′sis) a condition resembling leukemia in which the erythropoietic tissue is affected in addition to the leukopoietic tissue.

**er·y·throl·y·sin** (er-i-throl′i-sin) SYN hemolysin (1).

**er·y·throl·y·sis** (er-i-throl′i-sis) SYN hemolysis.

**eryth·ro·mel·al·gia** (ĕ-rith′rō-mel-al′jē-ă) **1.** paroxysmal throbbing and burning pain in the skin often precipitated by exertion or heat, affecting the hands and feet, accompanied by a dusky mottled redness of the parts with increased skin temperature; may be associated with myeloproliferative disorders. **2.** a rare disorder of middle age, characterized by paroxysmal attacks of severe burning pain, reddening, hyperalgesia and sweating, involving one or more extremities, usually both feet; the attacks can be triggered by warmth, and are usually relieved by cold and limb elevation. SYN Mitchell disease, red neuralgia. [erythro- + G. *melos,* limb, + *algos,* pain]

**er•y•thron** (er′i-thron) the total mass of circulating red blood cells, and that part of the hematopoietic tissue from which they are derived.

**eryth•ro•ne•o•cy•to•sis** (ĕ-rith′rō-nē-ō-sī-tō′sis) the presence in the peripheral circulation of regenerative forms of red blood cells. [erythrocyte + G. *neos,* new, + *kytos,* cell, + *-osis,* condition]

**eryth•ro•pe•nia** (ĕ-rith-rō-pē′nē-ă) deficiency in the number of red blood cells. [erythrocyte + G. *penia,* poverty]

**eryth•ro•pha•gia** (ĕ-rith-rō-fā′jē-ă) phagocytic destruction of red blood cells. [erythrocyte + G. *phagō,* to eat, + -ia]

**eryth•ro•phag•o•cy•to•sis** (ĕ-rith′rō-fag′ō-sī-tō′sis) phagocytosis of erythrocytes.

**eryth•ro•phil** (ĕ-rith′rō-fil) **1.** staining readily with red dyes. SYN erythrophilic. **2.** a cell or tissue element that stains red. [erythro- + G. *philos,* fond]

**eryth•ro•phil•ic** (ĕ-rith-rō-fil′ik) SYN erythrophil (1).

**eryth•ro•pla•kia** (ĕ-rith-rō-plā′kē-ă) a red, velvety, plaquelike lesion of mucous membrane which often represents malignant change. [erythro- + G. *plax,* plate]

**eryth•ro•pla•sia** (ĕ-rith-rō-plā′zē-ă) erythema and dysplasia of the epithelium. [erythro- + G. *plassō,* to form]

**eryth•ro•pla•sia of Quey•rat** (kā-rah′) carcinoma *in situ* of the glans penis.

**eryth•ro•poi•e•sis** (ĕ-rith′rō-poy-ē′sis) the formation of red blood cells. [erythrocyte + G. *poiēsis,* a making]

**eryth•ro•poi•et•ic** (ĕ-rith′rō-poy-et′ik) pertaining to or characterized by erythropoiesis.

**eryth•ro•poi•et•ic por•phyr•ia** a classification of porphyria that includes congenital erythropoietic porphyria and erythropoietic protoporphyria.

**eryth•ro•poi•et•ic pro•to•por•phyr•ia** a benign disorder of porphyrin metabolism due to a deficiency of ferrochelatase and characterized by enhanced fecal excretion of protoporphyrin and increased protoporphyrin IX in red blood cells, plasma, and feces; solar urticaria or eczema develops on exposure to sunlight.

**eryth•ro•poi•e•tin** (ĕ-rith-rō-poy′ĕ-tin) a protein that enhances erythropoiesis by stimulating formation of proerythroblasts and release of reticulocytes from bone marrow; it is secreted by the kidney and possibly by other tissues.

**eryth•ro•pros•o•pal•gia** (ĕ-rith′rō-pros-ō-pal′jē-ă) a disorder similar to erythromelalgia, but with the pain and redness occurring in the face. [erythro- + G. *prosōpon,* face, + *algos,* pain]

**eryth•rop•sia** (ĕ-rith-rop′sē-ă) an abnormality of vision in which all objects appear to be tinged with red. [erythro- + G. *ōps,* eye]

**eryth•ror•rhex•is** (er′i-thrō-rek′sis, ĕ-rith-rō-rek′sis) SYN erythrocytorrhexis. [erythrocyte + G. *rhēxis,* rupture]

**er•y•thru•ria** (er-i-thr-yu′rē-ă) the passage of red urine. [erythro- + G. *ouron,* urine]

**Es** einsteinium.

**es•cape** (es-kāp′) CARDIOLOGY term used to describe the situation when a higher pacemaker defaults or A-V conduction fails and a lower pacemaker assumes the function of pacemaking for one or more beats.

**es•cape beat, es•caped beat** an automatic beat, usually arising from the A-V junction or ventricle, occurring after the next expected normal beat has defaulted; it is therefore always a late beat, terminating a longer cycle than the normal.

**es•cape rhythm** three or more consecutive impulses at a rate not exceeding the upper limit of the inherent pacemaker.

**es•char** (es′kar) a thick, coagulated crust or slough which develops following a thermal burn or chemical or physical cauterization of the skin. [G. *eschara,* a fireplace, a scab caused by burning]

**es•cha•rot•ic** (es-kă-rot′ik) caustic or corrosive. [G. *escharōtikos*]

**es•cha•rot•o•my** (es-kă-rot′ō-mē) surgical incision in an eschar to lessen constriction, as might be done following a burn. [eschar + G. *tomē,* incision]

**Esch•e•rich•ia** (esh-ĕ-rik′ē-ă) a genus of aerobic, facultatively anaerobic bacteria containing short, motile or nonmotile, Gram-negative rods. Motile cells are peritrichous. Glucose and lactose are fermented with the production of acid and gas. These organisms are found in feces; some are pathogenic to man, causing enteritis, peritonitis, cystitis, etc. It is the type genus of the family Enterobacteriaceae. The type species is *Escherichia coli.* [T. Escherich, German pediatrician and bacteriologist, 1857–1911]

**Esch•e•rich•ia co•li** a species that occurs normally in the intestines of man and other vertebrates, is widely distributed in nature, and is a frequent cause of infections of the urogenital tract and of diarrhea in infants; enteropathogenic strains (serovars) of *Escherichia coli* cause diarrhea due to enterotoxin, the production of which seems to be associated with a transferable episome; the type species of the genus.

**E se•lec•tin** cell surface receptor produced by endothelium.

**esoph•a•ge•al** (ē-sof′ă-jē′ăl, ē′sŏ-faj′ē-ăl) relating to the esophagus.

**esoph•a•ge•al a•cha•la•sia** an obstruction to the passage of food that develops in the terminal esophagus, caused by an autonomic nervous system abnormality. SYN achalasia of the cardia, cardiospasm.

**esoph•a•ge•al hi•a•tus** the opening in the right crus of the diaphragm, between the central tendon and the hiatus aorticus, through which pass the esophagus and the two vagus nerves.

**esoph•a•ge•al lead** an electrocardiographic lead passed down the throat into the esophagus to record the electrocardiogram at various levels of the esophagus; especially useful for certain types of arrhythmias. Similarly, a transducer for echocardiography can be passed into the esophagus.

**esoph•a•ge•al re•flux, gas•tro•e•soph•a•ge•al re•flux** SEE gastroesophageal reflux disease.

**esoph•a•ge•al speech** a technique for speaking

after total laryngectomy; phonation results from introducing air into the upper esophagus to allow vibration of the pharyngoesophageal (PE) segment.

**esoph·a·ge·al va·ri·ces** longitudinal venous varices at the lower end of the esophagus as a result of portal hypertension; they are superficial and liable to ulceration and massive bleeding. See page B8.

**esoph·a·ge·al veins** series of veins draining the submucous venous plexus of the esophagus; proceeding inferiorly from the cervical portion of the esophagus, they drain to the inferior thyroid vein, the superior intercostal veins, the azygos, accessory hemiazygos and hemiazygos veins, all of which are ultimately tributaries of the superior vena cava; the most inferior esophageal veins, from the cardiac portion of the esophagus, drain via the esophageal branches of the left gastric vein, a tributary of the portal vein. Thus, the submucosal veins of the inferior esophagus form a portocaval anastomoses, and are subject to the formation of varicosities in portal hypertension.

**esoph·a·gec·ta·sis, esoph·a·gec·ta·sia** (ē-sof-ă-jek'tă-sis, ē-sof-ă-jek-tā'zē-ă) dilation of the esophagus. [esophagus + G. *ektasis*, a stretching]

**esoph·a·gec·to·my** (ē-sof-ă-jek'tō-mē) excision of any part of the esophagus. [esophagus + G. *ektomē*, excision]

**esoph·a·gi** (ē-sof'ă-jī) plural of esophagus.

**esoph·a·gism** (ē-sof'ă-jizm) esophageal spasm causing dysphagia.

**esoph·a·gi·tis** (ē-sof-ă-jī'tis) inflammation of the esophagus.

**esoph·a·go·car·di·o·plas·ty** (ē-sof'ă-gō-kar'dē-ō-plas-tē) plastic surgery of the esophagus and cardiac end of the stomach.

**esoph·a·go·cele** (ē-sof'ă-gō-sēl) protrusion of the mucous membrane of the esophagus through a tear in the muscular coat. [esophagus + G. *kēlē*, hernia]

**esoph·a·go·du·o·den·os·to·my** (ē-sof'ă-gō-doo'ō-den-os'tō -mē) surgical formation of a direct communication between the esophagus and the duodenum, with or without removal of the stomach.

**esoph·a·go·en·ter·os·to·my** (ē-sof'ă-gō-en-ter-os'tō-mē) surgical formation of a direct communication between the esophagus and intestine. [esophagus + G. *enteron*, intestine, + *stoma*, mouth]

**esoph·a·go·gas·trec·to·my** (ē-sof'ă-gō-gas-trek'tō-mē) removal of a portion of the lower esophagus and proximal stomach for treatment of neoplasms or strictures of those organs, especially those lesions located at or near the cardioesophageal junction.

**e·soph·a·go·gas·tric junc·tion** terminal end of esophagus and beginning of stomach at the cardiac orifice; site of the physiologic inferior esophageal sphincter.

**esoph·a·go·gas·tro·a·nas·to·mo·sis** (ē-sof'ă-gō-gas'trō-ă-nas-tō-mō'sis) SYN esophagogastrostomy.

**esoph·a·go·gas·tro·du·o·de·nos·co·py (EGD)** (ĕ-sof'ă-gō-gas'trō-doo'ō-den-os-kŏ-pē) endoscopic examination of the esophagus, stomach and duodenum usually performed using a fiberoptic instrument. See page B8.

**esoph·a·go·gas·tro·plas·ty** (ē-sof'ă-gō-gas'trō-plas-tē) SYN cardioplasty.

**esoph·a·go·gas·tros·to·my** (ē-sof'ă-gō-gas-tros'tō-mē) anastomosis of esophagus to stomach, usually following esophagogastrectomy. SYN esophagogastroanastomosis, gastroesophagostomy. [esophagus + G. *gastēr*, stomach, + *stoma*, mouth]

**esoph·a·go·gram** (ē-sof'ă-gō-gram) a radiograph of the esophagus.

**esoph·a·gog·ra·phy** (ē-sof-ă-gog'ră-fē) radiography of the esophagus using swallowed or injected radiopaque contrast media; the technique of obtaining an esophagogram. [esophagus + G. *graphō*, to write]

**esoph·a·go·ma·la·cia** (ē-sof'ă-gō-mă-lā'shē-ă) softening of the walls of the esophagus. [esophagus + G. *malakia*, softness]

**esoph·a·go·my·ot·o·my** (ē-sof'ă-gō-mī-ot'ō-mē) treatment of esophageal achalasia by longitudinal division of the lowest part of the esophageal muscle down to the submucosal layer; some muscle fibers of the cardia may also be divided. [esophagus + G. *mys*, muscle, + *tomē*, incision]

**esoph·a·go·plas·ty** (ē-sof'ă-gō-plas-tē) plastic surgery of the wall of the esophagus. [esophagus + G. *plastos*, formed]

**esoph·a·go·pli·ca·tion** (ē-sof'ă-gō-pli-kā'shŭn) reduction in size of a dilated esophagus or of a pouch in it by making longitudinal folds or tucks in its wall. [esophagus + L. *plico*, to fold]

**esoph·a·go·pto·sis, esoph·a·go·pto·sia** (ē-sof'ă-gō-tō'sis, ē-sof'ă-gō-tō'sē-ă) relaxation and downward displacement of the walls of the esophagus. [esophagus + G. *ptōsis*, a falling]

**esoph·a·go·scope** (ē-sof'ă-gō-skōp) an endoscope for inspecting the interior of the esophagus. [esophagus + G. *skopeō*, to examine]

**esoph·a·gos·co·py** (ē-sof-ă-gos'kŏ-pē) inspection of the interior of the esophagus by means of an endoscope. [esophagus + G. *skopeō*, to examine]

**esoph·a·go·spasm** (ē-sof'ă-gō-spazm) spasm of the walls of the esophagus.

**esoph·a·go·ste·no·sis** (ē-sof'ă-gō-stĕ-nō'sis) stricture or a general narrowing of the esophagus. [esophagus + G. *stenōsis*, a narrowing]

**esoph·a·go·sto·mi·a·sis** (ē-sof'ă-gō'stō-mī'a-sĭs) intestinal parasitization by nematodes of the genus *Oesophagostomum*.

**esoph·a·gos·to·my** (ē-sof-ă-gos'tō-mē) surgical formation of an opening directly into the esophagus from without. [esophagus + G. *stoma*, mouth]

**esoph·a·got·o·my** (ē-sof-ă-got'ō-mē) an incision through the wall of the esophagus. [esophagus + G. *tomē*, an incision]

**esoph·a·gus**, pl. **esoph·a·gi** (ē-sof'ă-gŭs, ē-sof'ă-jī) the portion of the digestive canal between the pharynx and stomach. It is about 25 cm long and consists of three parts: the cervical part, from the cricoid cartilage to the thoracic inlet; the thoracic part, from the thoracic inlet to the diaphragm; and the abdominal part, below the diaphragm to the cardiac opening of the stomach. [G. *oisophagos*, gullet]

**es·o·pho·ria** (es-ō-fō'rē-ă) a tendency for the eyes to turn inward, prevented by binocular vision. [G. *esō*, inward, + *phora*, a carrying]

**es·o·phor·ic** (es-ō-fōr'ik) relating to or marked by esophoria.

**es·o·tro·pia** (es-ō-trō'pē-ă) the form of strabismus in which the visual axes converge; may be paralytic or concomitant, monocular or alternating, accommodative or nonaccommodative. SYN convergent strabismus. [G. *esō*, inward, + *tropē*, turn]

**es•o•tro•pic** (es-ō-trop′ik) relating to or marked by esotropia.

**ESP** extrasensory perception.

**es•pun•dia** (es-poon′dj-ah) a type of American leishmaniasis caused by *Leishmania braziliensis* that affects the mucous membranes, particularly in the nasal and oral region, resulting in grossly destructive changes; may develop metastatically from sores originally found elsewhere on the body. SYN Breda disease. [Sp., fr. L. *spongia,* sponge]

**ESR** erythrocyte sedimentation rate; electron spin resonance.

**es•sen•tial** (ĕ-sen′shăl) **1.** necessary, indispensable, (e.g., essential amino acids, essential fatty acids). **2.** characteristic of. **3.** determining. **4.** of unknown etiology. **5.** relating to an essence (e.g., essential oil). **6.** SYN intrinsic.

**es•sen•tial a•mi•no ac•ids** α-amino acids nutritionally required by an organism and which must be supplied in its diet (i.e., cannot be synthesized by the organism) either as free amino acid or in proteins.

**es•sen•tial dys•men•or•rhea** SYN primary dysmenorrhea.

**es•sen•tial hy•per•ten•sion** hypertension without known cause.

**es•sen•tial oil** plant product, usually somewhat volatile, giving the odors and tastes characteristic of the particular plant; usually, the steam distillates of plants or of oils obtained by pressing the rinds of plants. SEE ALSO volatile oil.

**es•sen•tial pru•ri•tus** itching that occurs independently of skin lesions.

**es•sen•tial tel•an•gi•ec•ta•sia 1.** localized capillary dilation of undetermined origin; **2.** SYN angioma serpiginosum.

**es•sen•tial throm•bo•cy•to•pe•nia** a primary form of thrombocytopenia, in contrast to secondary forms that are associated with metastatic neoplasms, tuberculosis, and leukemia involving the bone marrow, or with direct suppression of bone marrow by the use of chemical agents, or with other conditions.

**es•sen•tial trem•or** an action tremor of 4–8 Hz frequency that usually begins in early adult life and is limited to the upper limbs and head; called familial when it appears in several family members.

**Es•ser graft** (es′ĕr) SYN inlay graft.

**EST** electroshock therapy.

**es•ter** (es′ter) an organic compound containing the grouping, –X(O)–O–R (X = carbon, sulfur, phosphorus, etc.; R = radical of an alcohol), formed by the elimination of $H_2O$ between the –OH of an acid group and the –OH of an alcohol group.

**es•ter•ase** (es′ter-ās) a generic term for enzymes that catalyze the hydrolysis of esters.

**es•ter•i•fi•ca•tion** (es′ter′i-fi-kā′shŭn) the process of forming an ester, as in the reaction of ethanol and acetic acid to form ethyl acetate.

**es•the•sia** (es-thē′zē-ă) SYN perception. [G. *aisthēsis,* sensation]

△**es•the•si•o-** **1.** sensation, perception. [G. *aesthēsis,* sense perception]

**es•the•si•od•ic** (es-thē-zē-od′ik) conveying sensory impressions. SYN aesthesodic, esthesodic. [esthesio- + G. *hodos,* way]

**es•the•si•o•gen•e•sis** (es-thē′zē-ō-jen′ĕ-sis) the production of sensation, especially of nervous erethism. [esthesio- + G. *genesis,* origin]

**es•the•si•o•gen•ic** (es-thē-zē-ō-jen′ik) producing a sensation.

**es•the•si•om•e•ter** (es-thē-zē-om′ĕ-ter) an instrument for determining the state of tactile and other forms of sensibility. SYN tactometer. [esthesio- + G. *metron,* measure]

**es•the•si•om•e•try** (es-thē-zē-om′ĕ-trē) measurement of the degree of tactile or other sensibility.

**es•the•si•o•phys•i•ol•o•gy** (es-thē′zē-ō-fiz-ē-ol′ ō-jē) the physiology of sensation and the sense organs.

**es•the•sod•ic** (es′thē-zod′ik) SYN esthesiodic.

**es•thet•ic** (es-thet′ik) **1.** pertaining to the sensations. **2.** pertaining to esthetics (i.e., beauty). [G. *aisthēsis,* sensation]

**es•thet•ics** (es-thet′iks) the branch of philosophy concerned with art and beauty, especially with the components thereof.

**es•ti•mate** (es′tĭ-māt) **1.** a measurement or a statement about the value of some quantity that is known, believed, or suspected to incorporate some degree of error. **2.** the result of applying any estimator to a random sample of data. It is not a random variable but a realization of one, a fixed quantity, and it has no variance although commonly it also furnishes an estimate of what the variance of the estimator is. (Not to be confused with an estimator, which is a prescription for obtaining an estimate.) [L. *aestimo,* pp. *aestimatum,* to appraise]

**es•ti•val** (es′ti-văl) relating to or occurring in the summer. [L. *aestivus,* summer (adj.)]

**es•ti•va•tion** living through the summer in a quiescent, torpid state.

**es•ti•vo•au•tum•nal** (es′ti-vō-aw-tŭm′năl) relating to or occurring in summer and autumn. [L. *aestivus,* summer (adj.), + *autumnalis,* autumnal]

**Est•land•er op•er•a•tion** (est′lahnd-ĕr) use of an Estlander flap in plastic surgery of the lips.

**es•tra•di•ol** (es-tră-dī′ol) the most potent naturally occurring estrogen, formed by the ovary, placenta, testis, and possibly the adrenal cortex.

**es•tri•ol** (es′trē-ol) an estrogenic metabolite of estradiol, usually the predominant estrogenic metabolite found in urine (especially during pregnancy).

**es•tro•gen** (es′trō-jen) generic term for any substance, natural or synthetic, that exerts biological effects characteristic of estrogenic hormones. Estrogens are formed by the ovary, placenta, testes, and possibly the adrenal cortex, as well as by certain plants; stimulate secondary sexual characteristics, and exert systemic effects, such as growth and maturation of long bones; given after menopause or oophorectomy to lower the risk of heart attack and prevent osteoporosis; also used to prevent or stop lactation, suppress ovulation, and palliate carcinoma of the breast and prostate. [G. *oistrus,* estrus, + *-gen,* producing]

**es•tro•gen•ic** (es-trō-jen′ik) **1.** causing estrus in animals. **2.** having an action similar to that of an estrogen.

**es•tro•gen re•cep•tor** receptor for estrogens; its presence conveys a better prognosis for breast cancers.

**es•tro•gen re•place•ment ther•a•py (ERT)** administration of sex hormones to women after menopause or oophorectomy. SYN hormone replacement therapy.

**es·trone** (es'trōn) a metabolite of 17β-estradiol, commonly found in urine, ovaries, and placenta; with considerably less biological activity than the parent hormone.

**estrous** pertaining to estrus. SYN estrual, oestrual.

**es·trous cy·cle** the series of cyclic uterine, ovarian, and other changes that occur in higher animals.

**estrual** (es'troo-ăl) SYN estrous.

**es·tru·a·tion** (es-troo-ā'shŭn) SYN estrus.

**es·trus** (es'trŭs) that portion or phase of the sexual cycle of female animals characterized by willingness to permit coitus; readily detectable behavioral and other signs are exhibited by animals during this period. SYN estruation, heat (2). [G. *oistros*, mad desire]

**ESWL** electrohydraulic shock wave lithotripsy; extracorporeal shock wave lithotripsy

**Et** ethyl.

**eta (H, η)** (āt'a) the seventh letter of the Greek alphabet. **1.** CHEMISTRY denotes the position seven atoms from the carboxyl group or other primary functional group. **2.** viscosity.

**ETEC** enterotoxigenic *Escherichia coli.*

**eth·a·nol** (eth'an-ol) SYN alcohol (2).

**eth·en·yl** (eth'en-il) SYN vinyl.

**ether** (ē'ther) **1.** any organic compound in which two carbon atoms are independently linked to a common oxygen atom, thus containing the group –C–O–C–. SEE ALSO epoxy. **2.** loosely used to refer to diethyl ether. [G. *aithēr*, the pure upper air]

**ethe·re·al** (ē-thēr'ē-ăl) relating to or containing ether. [G. *aitherios*, etherial, fr. *aithēr*, the upper air]

**e·the·re·al oil** SYN volatile oil.

**eth·i·cal** (eth'i-kăl) relating to ethics; in conformity with the rules governing personal and professional conduct.

**eth·ics** (eth'iks) the branch of philosophy that deals with the distinction between right and wrong, with the moral consequences of human actions. [G. *ethikos*, arising from custom, fr. *ethos*, custom]

△**eth·mo-** **1.** ethmoid. **2.** the ethmoid bone. [G. *ēthmos*, sieve]

**eth·moid** (eth'moyd) **1.** resembling a sieve. **2.** relating to the ethmoid bone. SYN ethmoidal. [G. *ēthmos*, sieve, + *eidos*, resemblance]

**eth·moi·dal** (eth-moy'dăl) SYN ethmoid.

**eth·moi·dal crest** bony ridge which articulates with, or provides attachment for, any part of the ethmoid bone, especially the middle nasal concha.

**eth·moi·dal fo·ra·men** either of two foramina formed by grooves on either edge of the ethmoidal notch of the frontal bone, and completed by similar grooves on the ethmoid bone: anterior ethmoidal foramen, located in an anterior position; posterior ethmoidal foramen located in a posterior position.

**eth·moi·dal in·fun·dib·u·lum** a passage from the middle meatus of the nose communicating with the anterior ethmoidal cells and frontal sinus.

**eth·moi·dal lab·y·rinth** a mass of air cells with thin bony walls forming part of the lateral wall of the nasal cavity; the cells are arranged in three

groups, anterior, middle, and posterior, and are closed laterally by the orbital plate which forms part of the wall of the orbit.

**eth·moi·dal veins** accompany the anterior and posterior ethmoidal arteries and pass into the superior ophthalmic vein; they drain the ethmoidal sinuses.

**eth·moid bone** an irregularly shaped bone lying between the orbital plates of the frontal and anterior to the sphenoid bone; it consists of two lateral masses of thin plates enclosing air cells, attached above to a perforated horizontal lamina, the cribriform plate, from which descends a median vertical or perpendicular plate in the interval between the two lateral masses; the bone articulates with the sphenoid, frontal, maxillary, lacrimal, and palatine bones, the inferior nasal concha, and the vomer; it enters into the formation of the anterior cranial fossa, the orbits, and the nasal cavity.

**eth·moi·dec·to·my** (eth-moy-dek'tō-mē) removal of all or part of the mucosal lining and bony partitions between the ethmoid sinuses. [ethmo- + G. *ektomē*, excision]

**eth·moid·i·tis** (eth-moy-dī'tis) inflammation of the ethmoid sinuses.

**eth·mo·tur·bi·nals** (eth-mō-ter'bi-nalz) the conchae of the ethmoid bone; the superior and middle conchae; occasionally a third, the supreme concha, exists.

**eth·nic group** (eth'nik groop) a social group characterized by a distinctive social and cultural tradition maintained from generation to generation, a common history and origin and a sense of identification with the group.

**eth·no·cen·trism** (eth-nō-sen'trizm) the tendency to evaluate other groups according to the values and standards of one's own ethnic group, especially with the conviction that one's own ethnic group is superior to the other groups. [G. *ethnos*, race, tribe, + *kentron*, center of a circle]

**eth·o·phar·ma·col·o·gy** (eth'ō-far-mă-kol'ō-jē) the study of drug effects on behavior, relying on observation and description of species-specific elements (acts and postures during social encounters). [G. *ethos*, character, habit, + pharmacology]

**eth·oxy** (e-thok'sē) the monovalent radical, $CH_3CH_2O$–.

**eth·yl (Et)** (eth'il) the hydrocarbon radical, $CH_3CH_2$–.

**eth·yl al·co·hol** SYN alcohol (2).

**eth·yl·ate** (eth'i-lāt) a compound in which the hydrogen of the hydroxyl group of ethanol is replaced by a metallic atom, usually sodium or potassium; e.g., $C_2H_5ONa$, sodium ethylate.

**eth·yl·di·chlo·ro·ar·sine** (eth'il-dī-klōr-ō-ar'sēn) a blister agent used in World War I; irritating to the respiratory tract.

**eth·yl·i·dyne** (eth-il'i-dīn) the radical $CH_3C\equiv$.

**eti·o·la·tion** (ē-tē-ō-lā'shŭn) **1.** pallor resulting from absence of light, as in persons confined because of illness or imprisonment, or in plants bleached by being deprived of light. **2.** the process of blanching, bleaching, or making pale by withholding light. [Fr. *étioler*, to blanch]

**eti·o·log·ic** (ē'tē-ō-loj'ik) relating to etiology. SYN etiological.

**e·ti·o·lo·gi·cal** SYN etiologic.

**eti·ol·o·gy** (ē-tē-ol'ō-jē) **1.** the science and study of the causes of disease and their mode of operation. Cf. pathogenesis. **2.** the science of causes, causality; in common usage, cause. [G. *aitia,* cause, + *logos,* treatise, discourse]

**Eu** europium.

△**eu-** good, well; opposite of dys-, caco-. [G.]

**Eu·bac·te·ri·um** (yu′bak-tēr′ē-ŭm) a genus of anaerobic, nonsporeforming, nonmotile bacteria containing straight or curved Gram-positive rods which usually occur singly, in pairs, or in short chains. Usually these organisms attack carbohydrates. They may be pathogenic. Rarely associated with intraabdominal sepsis in humans. The type species is *Eubacterium limosum.*

**eu·chlor·hy·dria** (yu-klōr-hi′drē-ă) a condition in which free hydrochloric acid exists in normal amount in the gastric juice. [eu- + cholohydric (acid) + -ia]

**eu·cho·lia** (yu-kō′lē-ă) a normal state of the bile as regards quantity and quality. [eu- + G. *cholē,* bile]

**eu·chro·ma·tin** (yu-krō′mă-tin) the parts of chromosomes that, during interphase, are uncoiled dispersed threads and not stained by ordinary dyes; metabolically active, in contrast to the inert heterochromatin.

**Eu·co·le·us** (yu-kō′lē-us) one of three trichurid nematode genera, commonly referred to as *Capillaria.*

**eu·di·a·pho·re·sis** (yu-dī′ă-fō-rē′sis) normal free sweating. [eu- + G. *diaphorēsis,* perspiration]

**eu·gen·ic** (yu-jen′ik) relating to eugenics.

**eu·gen·ics** (yu-jen′iks) **1.** practices and policies, as of mate selection or of sterilization, that tend to better the innate qualities of progeny and human stock. **2.** practices and genetic counseling directed to anticipating genetic disability and disease. [G. *eugeneia,* nobility of birth, fr. *eu,* well, + *genesis,* production]

**eu·glob·u·lin** (yu-glob′yu-lin) that fraction of the serum globulin less soluble in $(NH_4)_2SO_4$ solution than the pseudoglobulin fraction.

**eu·gly·ce·mia** (yu-glī-sē′mē-ă) a normal blood glucose concentration. SYN normoglycaemia, normoglycemia. [eu- + G. *glykys,* sweet, + *haima,* blood]

**eu·gly·ce·mic** (yu-glī-sē′mik) denoting, characteristic of, or promoting euglycemia. SYN normoglycemic.

**eu·gna·thia** (yu-nā′thē-ă) an abnormality that is limited to the teeth and their immediate alveolar supports. [eu- + G. *gnathos,* jaw]

**eu·gon·ic** (yu-gon′ik) a term used to indicate that the growth of a bacterial culture is rapid and relatively luxuriant; used especially in reference to the growth of cultures of the human tubercle bacillus (*Mycobacterium tuberculosis*). [G. *eugonos,* productive, fr. *eu,* well, + *gonos,* seed, offspring]

**Eu·kar·y·o·tae, Eu·car·y·o·tae** (yu-kar-ē-ō′tē) a superkingdom of organisms characterized by eukaryotic cells; acellular members (kingdom Protoctista) are characterized by a single eukaryotic unit; more complex (multicellular) members have been assigned to the kingdoms Fungi, Plantae, and Animalia.

**eu·kar·y·ote** (yu-kar′ē-ōt) **1.** a cell containing a membrane-bound nucleus with chromosomes of DNA, RNA, and proteins, with cell division involving a form of mitosis in which mitotic spindles (or some microtubule arrangement) are involved; mitochondria are present, and, in photo-

synthetic species, plastids are found. Possession of a eukaryote type of cell characterizes the four kingdoms above the Monera or prokaryote level of complexity: Protoctista, Fungi, Plantae, and Animalia, combined into the superkingdom Eukaryotae. **2.** common name for members of the Eukaryotae. [eu- + G. *karyon,* kernel, nut]

**eu·kar·y·ot·ic** (yu′kar-ē-ot′ik) pertaining to or characteristic of a eukaryote.

**Eu·len·burg dis·ease** (oy′lĕn-bĕrg) SYN congenital paramyotonia.

**eu·me·tria** (yu-mē′trē-ă) graduation of the strength of nerve impulses to match the need. [G. moderation, goodness of meter]

**eu·my·ce·to·ma** (yu-mī-set-ō′ma) mycetoma caused by fungi. Cf. actinomycetoma.

**eu·nuch** (yu′nŭk) a male whose testes have been removed or have never developed. [G. *eunouchos,* chamberlain, fr. *eunē,* bed, + *echō,* to have]

**eu·nuch·oid** (yu′nŭ-koyd) resembling, or having the general characteristics of, a eunuch; usually indicating the physical habitus of a male in whom hypogonadism occurred before puberty. [G. *eunouchos,* eunuch, + *eidos,* resembling]

**eu·nuch·oid gi·gan·tism** gigantism with deficient development of sexual organs; may be of pituitary or gonadal origin; gigantism accompanied by body proportions typical of hypogonadism during adolescence.

**eu·nuch·oid·ism** (yu′nŭ-koyd-izm) a state in which testes are present but fail to function normally; may be of gonadal or pituitary origin.

**eu·pep·sia** (yu-pep′sē-ă) good digestion. [G., fr. *eu,* well, + *pepsis,* digestion]

**eu·pep·tic** (yu-pep′tik) digesting well; having a good digestion.

**eu·pep·tide** (yu-pep′tīd) a peptide containing normal peptide bonds (between α-carboxyl groups and α-amino groups). Cf. peptide. [G. *eu-,* normal, usual + peptide]

**eu·pho·ret·ic** (yu-fō-ret′ik) SYN euphoriant.

**eu·pho·ria** (yu-fōr′ē-ă) a feeling of well-being, commonly exaggerated and not necessarily well founded. [eu- + G. *pherō,* to bear]

**eu·pho·ri·ant** (yu-fōr′ē-ant) **1.** having the capability to produce a sense of well-being. **2.** an agent with such a capability. SYN euphoretic.

**eu·plas·tic lymph** lymph that contains relatively few leukocytes, but a comparatively high concentration of fibrinogen; such lymph clots fairly well and tends to become organized with fibrous tissue.

**eu·ploid** (yu′ployd) relating to euploidy.

**eu·ploidy** (yu′ploy-dē) the state of a cell containing whole haploid sets. [eu- + G. *-ploos,* -fold]

**eup·nea** (yu-p-nē′ă) easy, free respiration; the type observed in a normal individual under resting conditions. [G. *eupnoia,* fr. *eu,* well, + *pnoia,* breath]

**eu·prax·ia** (yu-prak′sē-ă) normal ability to perform coordinated movements. [eu- + G. *praxis,* a doing]

**eu·rhyth·mia** (yu-ridh′mē-ă) harmonious body relationships of the separate organs. [eu- + G. *rhythmos,* rhythm]

**Eu·ro·pe·an bat Lys·sa·vi·rus** two species (1 & 2) causing rabieslike diseases in humans in Europe; transmitted by bite of insectivorous bats.

**eu·ro·pi·um (Eu)** (yu-rō′pē-ŭm) an element of

e
u

the rare earth (lanthanide) group, atomic no. 63, atomic wt. 151.965. [L. *Europa*, Europe]

⌂**eu•ry-** broad, wide; opposite of steno-. [G. *eurys*, wide]

**eu•ry•bleph•a•ron** (yu-rē-blef′ă-ron) a congenital anomaly characterized by sagging of the lateral aspect of the lower eyelid away from the eye. [eury- + G. *blepharon*, eyelid]

**eu•ry•ce•phal•ic, eu•ry•ceph•a•lous** (yu′rē-se-fal′ik, yu′rē-sef′ă-lŭs) having an abnormally broad head; sometimes used in reference to a brachycephalic head. [eury- + G. *kephalē*, head]

**eu•ryg•nath•ic** (yu-rig-nath′ik) having a wide jaw.

**eu•ry•on** (yu′rē-on) the extremity, on either side, of the greatest transverse diameter of the head; a point used in craniometry. [G. *eurys*, broad]

**eu•sta•chi•an** (yu-stā′shŭn) described by or attributed to Bartolomeo Eustachio (1524–1574); usually referring to the auditory tube.

**eu•sta•chi•an tube** (yu-sta′shŭn, yu-stā′kĕ-un) SYN pharyngotympanic (auditory) tube.

**eu•stron•gyl•oi•des** (yu-stron-jil′oy-dēz) nematode found in fish, amphibians, and reptiles; human infections, manifested by gastrointestinal symptoms, are rare and related to consumption of raw fish; larvae are pinkish red.

**eu•sys•to•le** (yu-sis′tō-lē) a condition in which the cardiac systole is normal in force and time. [eu- + systole]

**eu•sys•tol•ic** (yu-sis-tol′ik) relating to eusystole.

**eu•tec•tic al•loy** an alloy, generally brittle and subject to tarnish and corrosion, with a fusion temperature lower than that of any of its components; used in dentistry mainly in solders.

**eu•tha•na•sia** (yu-thă-nā′zē-ă) 1. the intentional putting to death of a person with an incurable or painful disease, intended as an act of mercy. 2. a quiet, painless death. [eu- + G. *thanatos*, death]

**eu•then•ics** (yu-then′iks) the science concerned with establishing optimum living conditions for plants, animals, or humans, especially through proper provisioning and environment. [G. *eutheneō*, to thrive]

**eu•ther•mic** (yu-ther′mik) at an optimal temperature. [eu- + G. *thermos*, warm]

**eu•ton•ic** (yu-ton′ik) SYN normotonic (1). [eu- + G. *tonos*, tone]

**eu•tro•phia** (yu-trō′fē-ă) a state of normal nourishment and growth. [G. fr. *eu*, well, + *trophē*, nourishment]

**eu•tro•phic** (yu-trof′ik) relating to, characterized by, or promoting eutrophia.

**EV, ev** electron-volt.

**evac•u•ant** (ē-vak′yu-ant) 1. promoting an excretion, especially of the bowels. 2. an agent that increases excretion, especially a cathartic.

**evac•u•a•tion** (ē-vak-yu-ā′shŭn) 1. removal of material, especially wastes from the bowels by defecation. 2. SYN stool (2). 3. removal of air from a closed vessel; production of a vacuum.

**evac•u•a•tor** (ē-vak′yu-ā-tŏr) a mechanical evacuant; an instrument for the removal of fluid or small particles from a body cavity, or of impacted feces from the rectum.

**evag•i•na•tion** (ē-vaj-i-nā′shŭn) protrusion of some part or organ from its normal position. [L. *e*, out, + *vagina*, sheath]

**Eval•u•a•tion and Man•age•ment codes (E&M codes)** CPT codes that describe patient

encounters with healthcare professionals; used to evaluate and manage general health.

**ev•a•nes•cent** (ev-ă-nes′ent) of short duration. [L. *e*, out, + *vanesco*, to vanish]

**Ev•ans blue** (ev′ănz) [CI 23860] a diazo dye used for the determination of the blood volume on the basis of the dilution of a standard solution of the dye in the plasma after its intravenous injection; it binds to proteins and is also used as a vital stain for following diffusion through blood vessel walls.

**Ev•ans syn•drome** (ev′ănz) acquired hemolytic anemia and thrombocytopenia.

**evap•o•rate** (ē-vap′ōr-āt) to cause or undergo evaporation.

**evap•o•ra•tion** (ē-vap-ŏ-ra′shŭn) 1. a change from liquid to vapor form. 2. loss of volume of a liquid by conversion into vapor. SYN volatilization. [L. *e*, out, + *vaporo*, to emit vapor]

**event** an incident or occurrence; anything that happens.

**even•tra•tion** (ē′ven-trā′shŭn) 1. protrusion of omentum and/or intestine through an opening in the abdominal wall. SYN evisceration (3). 2. removal of the contents of the abdominal cavity. [L. *e*, out, + *venter*, belly]

**even•tra•tion of the di•a•phragm** extreme elevation of a half or part of the diaphragm, which is usually atrophic and abnormally thin.

🔳**ever•sion** (ē-ver′zhŭn) a turning outward, as of the eyelid or foot. See page APP 91. [L. *e-everto*, pp. *-versus*, to overturn]

**evert** (ē-vert′) to turn outward. [L. *e-verto*, to overturn]

**ev•i•dence-based me•di•cine** the process of applying relevant information derived from peer-reviewed medical literature to address a specific clinical problem; the application of simple rules of science and common sense to determine the validity of the information; and the application of the information to the clinical problem. SEE ALSO Cochrane collaboration, clinical practice guidelines.

**ev•i•dence-based prac•tice** the formulation of treatment decisions by using the best available research evidence and integrating this evidence with the practitioner's skill and experience.

**evis•cer•a•tion** (ē-vis-er-ā′shŭn) 1. SYN exenteration. 2. removal of the contents of the eyeball, leaving the sclera and sometimes the cornea. 3. SYN eventration (1). [L. *eviscero*, to disembowel]

**evo•ca•tion** (ev-ō-kā′shŭn, ē-vō-kā′shŭn) induction of a particular tissue produced by the action of an evocator during embryogenesis. [L. *evoco*, pp. *evocatus*, to call forth, evoke]

**evo•ca•tor** (ev′ō-kā-ter) a factor in the control of morphogenesis in the early embryo.

**evoked e•lec•tro•my•o•gra•phy** SYN electrodiagnosis.

**evoked o•to•a•cous•tic e•mis•sion** a form resulting from acoustic stimulation, as opposed to spontaneous otoacoustic emission.

**evoked re•sponse** an alteration in the electrical activity of a region of the nervous system through which an incoming sensory stimulus is passing.

**ev•o•lu•tion** (ev-ō-loo′shŭn) 1. a continuing process of change from one state, condition or form to another. 2. a progressive distancing between the genotype and the phenotype in a line of descent. [L. *e-volvo*, pp. *-volutus*, to roll out]

**ev·o·lu·tion·ary fit·ness** the probability that the line of descent from an individual with a specific trait will not eventually die out.

**evul·sion** (ē-vŭl'shŭn) a forcible pulling out or extraction. Cf. avulsion. [L. *evulsio*, fr. *e-vello*, pp. *-vulsus*, to pluck out]

**Ew·art pro·ce·dure** (yu'ărt) elevation of the larynx between the thumb and forefinger to elicit tracheal tugging.

**Ew·art sign** (yu'ărt) in large pericardial effusions, an area of dullness with bronchial breathing and bronchophony below the angle of the left scapula. SYN Pins sign.

**Ew·ing sar·co·ma** (yu'ing) SYN Ewing tumor.

**Ew·ing sign** (yu'ing) tenderness at the upper inner angle of the orbit at the point of attachment of the pulley of the superior oblique muscle, denoting closure of the outlet of the frontal sinus.

**Ew·ing tu·mor** (yu'ing) a malignant neoplasm which occurs usually before the age of 20 years, about twice as frequently in males, and in about 75% of patients involves bones of the extremities, including the shoulder girdle, with a predilection for the metaphysis; histologically, there are conspicuous foci of necrosis in association with irregular masses of small, regular, rounded, or ovoid cells (2–3 times the diameter of erythrocytes), with very scanty cytoplasm. SYN endothelial myeloma, Ewing sarcoma.

△**ex-** out of, from, away from. [L. and G. out of]

△**exa-** (**E**) prefix used in the SI and metric systems to signify one quintillion (10^{18}).

**ex·ac·er·ba·tion** (eg-zas-er-bā'shŭn) an increase in the severity of a disease or any of its signs or symptoms. [L. *ex- acerbo*, pp. *-atus*, to exasperate, increase, fr. *acerbus*, sour]

**ex·ae·re·sis [Br.]** SYN excision.

**ex·am·i·na·tion** (eg-zam-i-nā'shŭn) any investigation or inspection made for the purpose of diagnosis; usually qualified by the method used.

**ex·an·them** (eg-zan'them) SYN exanthema.

**ex·an·the·ma** (eg-zan-thē'mă) a skin eruption occurring as a symptom of an acute viral or coccal disease, as in scarlet fever or measles. SYN exanthem. [G. efflorescence, an eruption, fr. *anthos*, flower]

**ex·an·the·ma sub·i·tum** a disease due to herpes virus-6 of infants and young children, marked by sudden onset with fever lasting several days (sometimes with convulsions) and followed by a fine macular (sometimes maculopapular) rash that appears within a few hours to a day after the fever has subsided. SYN Dukes disease, roseola infantilis, roseola infantum, sixth disease.

**ex·an·them·a·tous** (eg-zan-them'ă-tŭs) relating to an exanthema.

**ex·ar·tic·u·la·tion** (eks-ar-tik-yu-lā'shŭn) SYN disarticulation. [L. *ex*, out, + *articulus*, joint]

**ex·cal·a·tion** (eks-kă-lā'shŭn) absence, suppression, or failure of development of one of a series of structures, as of a digit or vertebra. [G. *ex*, from, + *chalaō*, to abate, release]

**ex·ca·va·tio** (eks-kă-vā'shē-ō) [TA] SYN excavation (1). [L. fr. *ex-cavo*, pp. *-cavatus*, to hollow out, fr. *ex*, out, + *cavus*, hollow]

**ex·ca·va·tion** (eks-kă-vā'shŭn) **1.** a natural cavity, pouch, or recess. SYN excavatio [TA]. **2.** a cavity formed artificially or as the result of a pathologic process.

**ex·ca·va·tio rec·to·u·te·ri·na** [TA] SYN rectouterine pouch.

**ex·ca·va·tio rec·to·ve·si·ca·lis** [TA] SYN rectovesical pouch.

**ex·ca·va·tor** (eks'kă-vā-tŏr) **1.** an instrument like a large sharp spoon or scoop, used in scraping out pathologic tissue. **2.** DENTISTRY an instrument, generally a small spoon or curette, for cleaning out and shaping a carious cavity preparatory to filling.

**ex·ce·men·to·sis** (ek'sē-men-tō'sis) a nodular outgrowth of cementum on the root surface of a tooth.

**ex·cen·tric** (ek-sen'trik) alternative spelling for eccentric (2, 3).

**ex·cess** (ek'ses) that which is more than the usual or specified amount.

**ex·change** (eks-chānj') to substitute one thing for another, or the act of such substitution.

**ex·change trans·fu·sion** removal of most of a patient's blood followed by introduction of an equal amount from donors. SYN substitution transfusion, total transfusion.

**ex·ci·mer la·ser** laser used particularly for refractive procedures, consisting of photons in the ultraviolet spectrum emitted by unstable dimers of argon and fluoride. [*exc*ited d*imer*]

**ex·cip·i·ent** (ek-sip'ē-ent) a more or less inert substance added in a prescription as a diluent or vehicle or to give form or consistency when the remedy is given in pill form. [L. *excipiens;* pres. p. of *ex- cipio*, to take out]

**ex·cise** (ek-sīz') to cut out. SEE ALSO resect.

**ex·ci·sion** (ek-sizh'ŭn) **1.** the act of cutting out; the surgical removal of part or all of a structure or organ. SYN resection (3). SEE ALSO resection. **2.** MOLECULAR BIOLOGY a recombination event in which a genetic element is removed. SYN exaeresis, exeresis. [L. *excido*, to cut out]

**ex·ci·sion bi·op·sy** excision of tissue for gross and microscopic examination in such a manner that the entire lesion is removed. See page 117.

**ex·cit·a·bil·i·ty** (ek-sī'tă-bil'i-tē) having the capability of being excited.

**ex·cit·a·ble** (ek-sī'tă-bl) **1.** capable of quick response to a stimulus; having potentiality for emotional arousal. Cf. irritable. **2.** NEUROPHYSIOLOGY referring to a tissue, cell, or membrane capable of undergoing excitation in response to an adequate stimulus.

**ex·cit·a·ble ar·ea** SYN motor cortex.

**ex·ci·ta·tion** (ek-sī-tā'shŭn) **1.** the act of increasing the rapidity or intensity of physical or mental processes. **2.** NEUROPHYSIOLOGY the complete all-or-none response of a nerve or muscle to an adequate stimulus, ordinarily including propagation of excitation along the membranes of the cell or cells involved. SEE ALSO stimulation.

**ex·ci·ta·tion wave** a wave of altered electrical conditions that is propagated along a muscle fiber preparatory to its contraction.

**ex·cit·a·to·ry post·syn·ap·tic po·ten·tial** the change in potential which is produced in the membrane of the next neuron when an impulse which has an excitatory influence arrives at the synapse; it is a local change in the direction of depolarization; summation of these potentials can lead to discharge of an impulse by the neuron.

**ex·cit·ed state** the condition of an atom or molecule after absorbing energy, which may be the result of exposure to light, electricity, elevated temperature, or a chemical reaction; such activation may be a necessary prelude to a chemical reaction or to the emission of light.

**ex·cite·ment** (ek-sīt'ment) an emotional state sometimes characterized by its potential for impulsive or poorly controlled activity.

**ex·cit·ing eye** the injured eye in sympathetic ophthalmia.

**ex·ci·to·mo·tor** (ek-sī'tō-mō'ter) causing or increasing the rapidity of motion. SYN centrokinetic (2).

**ex·ci·to·re·flex nerve** a visceral nerve the special function of which is to cause reflex action.

**ex·ci·tor nerve** a nerve conducting impulses that stimulate to increase function.

**ex·clave** (eks-klāv') an outlying, detached portion of a gland or other part, such as the thyroid or pancreas; an accessory gland. [L. *ex,* out, + *-clave* (in enclave)]

**ex·clu·sion** (eks-kloo'zhŭn) a shutting out; disconnection from the main portion. [L. *ex- cludo,* pp. *-clusus,* to shut out]

**ex·clu·sive pro·vi·der or·gan·i·za·tion (EPO)** a managed care plan in which enrollees must receive their care from affiliated providers; treatment provided outside the approved network must be paid for by the patients. SEE ALSO managed care.

**ex·co·ri·ate** (eks-kō'rē-āt) to scratch or otherwise denude the skin by physical means.

▣ **ex·co·ri·a·tion** (eks-kō'rē-ā'shŭn) a scratch mark; a linear break in the skin surface, usually covered with blood or serous crusts. See page B5. [L. *excorio,* to skin, strip, fr. *corium,* skin, hide]

**ex·cre·ment** (eks'krĕ-ment) waste matter or any excretion cast out of the body; e.g., feces. [L. *excerno,* pp. *-cretus,* to separate]

**ex·cre·men·ti·tious** (eks'krĕ-men-tish'ŭs) relating to any excrement.

**ex·cres·cence** (eks-kres'ens) any outgrowth from a surface. [L. *ex- cresco,* pp. *-cretus,* to grow forth]

**ex·cre·ta** (eks-krē'tă) SYN excretion (2). [L. neut. pl. of *excretus,* pp. of *ex-cerno,* to separate]

**ex·crete** (eks-krēt') to separate from the blood and cast out; to perform excretion.

**ex·cre·tion** (eks-krē'shŭn) **1.** the process whereby the undigested residue of food and the waste products of metabolism are eliminated, material is removed to regulate the composition of body fluids and tissues, or substances are expelled to perform functions on an exterior surface. **2.** the product of a tissue or organ that is material to be passed out of the body. SYN excreta. Cf. secretion. [see excrement]

**ex·cre·to·ry** (eks'krĕ-tō-rē) relating to excretion.

**ex·cre·to·ry duct** a duct carrying the secretion from a gland or a fluid from any reservoir.

**ex·cre·to·ry ducts of lac·ri·mal gland** the 6–10 excretory ducts of the lacrimal gland that open into the superior fornix of the conjunctival sac.

**ex·cre·to·ry gland** a gland separating excrementitious or waste material from the blood.

**ex·cy·clo·pho·ria** (ek-sī-klō-fō'rē-ă) a cyclophoria in which the upper poles of each cornea tend to rotate laterally. [ex- + cyclo- + G. *phora,* a carrying]

**ex·cys·ta·tion** (ek-sis-tā'shŭn) the action of an encysted organism in escaping from its envelope.

**ex·e·mia** (ek-sē'mē-ă) a condition, as in shock, in which a considerable portion of the blood is re-

moved from the main circulation but remains within blood vessels in certain areas where it is stagnant. [G. *ex,* out of, + *haima,* blood]

**ex·en·ce·phal·ic** (eks'en-se-fal'ik) relating to exencephaly.

**ex·en·ceph·a·ly** (eks-en-sef'ă-lē) condition in which the neurocranium is defective with the brain exposed or extruding. [G. *ex,* out, + *enkephalos,* brain]

**ex·en·ter·a·tion** (eks-en-ter-ā'shŭn) removal of internal organs and tissues, usually radical removal of the contents of a body cavity. SYN evisceration (1). [G. *ex,* out, + *enteron,* bowel]

**ex·en·ter·i·tis** (eks-en-ter-ī'tis) inflammation of the peritoneal covering of the intestine. [G. *exō,* on the outside, + enteritis]

**ex·er·cise** (ek'ser-sīz) **1.** *active:* bodily exertion for the sake of restoring the organs and functions to a healthy state or keeping them healthy. **2.** *passive:* motion of limbs without effort by the patient.

**ex·er·cise econ·omy** energy required (usually measured as oxygen consumption) to maintain a constant velocity of movement. SYN movement economy.

**ex·er·cise-in·duced ane·mia** reduction in hemoglobin concentration to levels approaching clinical anemia, believed due to intense exercise training; generally occurs in the early phase of training and parallels the disproportionately large expansion in plasma volume in relation to total hemoglobin with training. SEE ALSO anemia. SYN sports anemia.

**ex·er·cise-in·duced asth·ma, ex·er·cise-in·duced bron·cho·spasm** bronchial spasm, edema, and mucus secretion brought about by exercise, particularly in cool, dry environment. Recovery usually occurs spontaneously within 90 minutes. A 10–15% reduction in pre-exercise values for FEV$_1$/FVC confirms diagnosis. SEE ALSO asthma.

**ex·er·cise-in·duced ur·ti·car·ia** a variant of cholinergic urticaria with larger lesions, induced by physical activity.

**exercise physiology** body of knowledge concerning physiologic, metabolic, and structural responses to acute and long-term physical activity.

**ex·er·cise pre·scrip·tion** formulation of individualized exercise program based on exercise frequency, intensity, and duration with consideration for the specificity of the training response. SEE ALSO prescription, specificity of training principle.

**ex·er·cise pres·sor re·flex** reflex afferent neural input to cardiovascular center in medulla from proprioceptors (mechanoreceptors and metaboreceptors) in active muscles during exercise.

**ex·er·cise ra·di·o·nu·clide an·gi·o·car·di·og·ra·phy** radionuclide angiocardiography while performing exercise, such as on a treadmill or bicycle.

**ex·er·cise stress test** SYN stress test.

**ex·er·e·sis** (ek-ser'ĕ-sis) SYN excision. [G. *exairesis,* a taking out, fr. *haireō,* to take, grasp]

**ex·er·gon·ic** (ek-ser-gon'ik) referring to a chemical reaction that takes place with release of Gibbs free energy to its surroundings. Cf. endergonic. [exo- + G. *ergon,* work]

**ex·fo·li·a·tion** (eks-fō-lē-ā'shŭn) **1.** detachment and shedding of superficial cells from any tissue surface. **2.** scaling or desquamation of the horny layer of epidermis. **3.** loss of deciduous teeth following physiological loss of root structure. [Mod. L. fr. L. *ex,* out, + *folium,* leaf]

**ex·fo·li·a·tive** (eks-fō′lē-ā-tiv) marked by exfoliation, desquamation, or profuse scaling. [Mod. L. *exfoliativus*]

**ex·fo·li·a·tive cy·tol·o·gy** the examination, for diagnostic purposes, of cells denuded from a neoplasm or an epithelial surface, recovered from exudate, secretions, or washings from tissue (e.g., sputum, vaginal secretion, gastric washings, urine). SYN cytopathology (2).

**ex·fo·li·a·tive der·ma·ti·tis** generalized exfoliation with scaling of the skin and usually with erythema (erythroderma); may be a drug reaction or associated with various benign dermatoses, lupus erythematosus, lymphomas, or of undetermined cause. SYN pityriasis rubra, Wilson disease (2).

**ex·fo·li·a·tive gas·tri·tis** gastritis with excessive shedding of mucosal epithelial cells.

**ex·fol·i·a·tive psor·i·a·sis** exfoliative dermatitis developing from chronic psoriasis, sometimes resulting from overtreatment of psoriasis.

**ex·ha·la·tion** (eks-hă-lā′shŭn) **1.** breathing out. SYN expiration (1). **2.** the giving forth of gas or vapor. **3.** any exhaled or emitted gas or vapor. [L. *ex-halo,* pp. *-halatus,* to breathe out]

**ex·hale** (eks-hāl′) **1.** to breathe out. SYN expire (1). **2.** to emit a gas, vapor, or odor.

**ex·haus·tion** (eg-zos′chŭn) **1.** extreme fatigue; inability to respond to stimuli. **2.** removal of contents; using up of a supply of anything. **3.** extraction of the active constituents of a drug by treating with water, alcohol, or other solvent. [L. *ex-haurio,* pp. *-haustus,* to draw out, empty]

**ex·hi·bi·tion·ism** (ek-si-bish′ŭn-izm) a morbid compulsion to expose a part of the body, especially the genitals, with the intent of provoking sexual interest in the viewer.

**ex·hi·bi·tion·ist** (ek-si-bish′ŭn-ist) one who engages in exhibitionism.

△**ex·o-** exterior, external, or outward. SEE ALSO ecto-. [G. *exō,* outside]

**ex·o·an·ti·gen** (ek-sō-an′ti-jen) SYN ectoantigen.

**ex·o·car·dia** (ek-sō-kar′dē-ă) SYN ectocardia.

**ex·o·crine** (ek′sō-krin) **1.** denoting glandular secretion delivered to an apical or luminal surface. SYN eccrine (1). **2.** denoting a gland that secretes outwardly through excretory ducts. [exo- + G. *krinō,* to separate]

**ex·o·crine gland** a gland from which secretions reach a free surface of the body by ducts.

**ex·o·cy·to·sis** (ek′sō-sī-to′sis) **1.** the appearance of migrating inflammatory cells in the epidermis. **2.** the process whereby secretory granules or droplets are released from a cell; the membrane around the granule fuses with the cell membrane, which ruptures, and the secretion is discharged. SYN emeiocytosis, emiocytosis. Cf. endocytosis. [exo- + G. *kytos,* cell, + *-osis,* condition]

**ex·o·de·vi·a·tion** (ek′sō-dē-vē-ā′shŭn) **1.** SYN exophoria. **2.** SYN exotropia.

**ex·o·don·tia** (ek-sō-don′shē-ă) the branch of dental practice concerned with the extraction of teeth. [exo- + G. *odous,* tooth]

**ex·o·don·tist** (ek-sō-don′tist) one who specializes in the extraction of teeth.

**ex·o·en·zyme** (ek-sō-en′zīm) SYN extracellular enzyme.

**ex·o·e·ryth·ro·cyt·ic stage** developmental stage of the malaria parasite (*Plasmodium*) in liver parenchyma cells of the vertebrate host before erythrocytes are invaded. The initial generation produces cryptozoites, the next generation metacryptozoites; reinfection of liver cells from blood cells apparently does not occur.

**ex·og·a·my** (ek-sog′ă-mē) sexual reproduction by means of conjugation of two gametes of different ancestry, as in certain protozoan species. [exo- + G. *gamos,* marriage]

**ex·o·gas·tru·la** (eks-ō-gas′troo-lă) an abnormal embryo in which the primordial gut has been everted.

**ex·og·e·nous** (eks-oj′ĕ-nŭs) originating or produced outside of the organism. SYN ectogenous. [exo- + G. *-gen,* production]

**ex·og·e·nous buf·fer** sodium bicarbonate or sodium citrate taken orally before competition by sprint-type athletes to raise extracellular pH; enhances performance in short-term, maximal exercise that generates high levels of muscle and blood lactate.

**ex·og·e·nous de·pres·sion** similar signs and symptoms as endogenous depression but the precipitating factors are social or environmental and outside the individual.

**ex·og·e·nous fi·bers** nerve fibers by which a given region of the central nervous system is connected with other regions; the term applies to both afferent and efferent fiber connections.

**ex·og·e·nous hy·per·glyc·er·i·de·mia** persistent hyperglyceridemia due to retarded rate of removal from plasma of chylomicrons of dietary origin.

**ex·og·e·nous py·ro·gens** drugs or substances that are formed by microorganisms and induce fever. Among the latter are lipopolysaccharides and lipoteichoic acid.

**ex·om·pha·los** (eks-om′fă-lŭs) **1.** protrusion of the umbilicus. SYN exumbilication (1). **2.** SYN umbilical hernia. **3.** SYN omphalocele. [G. *ex,* out, + *omphalos,* umbilicus]

**ex·on** (eks′on) a portion of a DNA that codes for a section of the mature messenger RNA from that DNA, and is therefore expressed ("translated" into protein) at the ribosome. [ex- + on]

**ex·o·nu·cle·ase** (eks-ō-noo′klē-ās) a nuclease that releases one nucleotide at a time, serially, beginning at one end of a polynucleotide (nucleic acid). Cf. endonuclease.

**ex·o·pep·ti·dase** (ek-s-ō-pep′ti-dās) an enzyme that catalyzes the hydrolysis of the terminal amino acid of a peptide chain; e.g., carboxypeptidase. Cf. endopeptidase.

*Ex·o·phi·a·la* (ek-sō-fī′ă-lă) a genus of pathogenic fungi having dematiaceous conidiophores. They cause mycetoma or phaeohyphomycosis; in cases of mycetoma, black granules develop in subcutaneous abscesses; in cases of phaeohyphomycosis, sclerotic bodies are found in tissues. [*exo* + G. *phialē,* a broad flat vessel]

*Ex·o·phi·a·la jean·selme·i* a species found in cases of mycetoma or phaeohyphomycosis.

*Ex·o·phi·a·la wer·nec·ki·i* a species that causes tinea nigra.

**ex·o·pho·ria** (eks′o-fō′rē-ă) tendency of the eyes to deviate outward when fusion is suspended. SYN exodeviation (1). [exo- + G. *phora,* a carrying]

**ex·o·phor·ic** (ek-s-ō-fōr′ik) relating to exophoria.

**ex·oph·thal·mic** (eks-of-thal′mik) relating to exophthalmos; marked by prominence of the eyeball.

**ex·oph·thal·mic goi·ter** any of the various forms of hyperthyroidism in which the thyroid gland is enlarged and exophthalmos is present.

**ex·oph·thal·mic oph·thal·mo·ple·gia** ophthalmoplegia with protrusion of the eyeballs due to increased water content of orbital tissues incidental to thyroid disorders, usually hyperthyroidism.

**ex·oph·thal·mom·e·ter** (eks-of-thal-mom′ĕ-ter) an instrument to measure the distance between the anterior pole of the eye and a fixed reference point, often the zygomatic bone. [exophthalmos + G. *metron,* measure]

**ex·oph·thal·mos, ex·oph·thal·mus** (eks-of-thal′mos) protrusion of one or both eyeballs; can be congenital and familial, or due to pathology, such as a retro-orbital tumor (usually unilateral) or thyroid disease (usually bilateral). SYN proptosis. [G. *ex,* out, + *ophthalmos,* eye]

**ex·o·phyte** (eks′ō-fīt) an exterior or external plant parasite. [exo- + G. *phyton,* plant]

**ex·o·phyt·ic** (eks-ō-fit′ik) **1.** pertaining to an exophyte. **2.** denoting a neoplasm or lesion that grows outward from an epithelial surface.

**ex·o·se·ro·sis** (eks′ō-se-rō′sis) serous exudation from the skin surface, as in eczema or abrasions.

**ex·o·skel·e·ton** (eks-ō-skel′ĕ-tŏn) **1.** all hard parts, such as hair, teeth, nails, feathers, dermal plates, and scales, developed from the ectoderm or somatic mesoderm in vertebrates. **2.** outer chitinous envelope of insects, certain Crustacea, and other invertebrates.

**ex·os·to·sis,** pl. **ex·os·to·ses** (eks-os-tō′sis, eks-os-tō′sēz) a cartilage-capped bony projection arising from any bone that develops from cartilage. SEE ALSO osteochondroma. See this page and B16. SYN hyperostosis (2), poroma (2). [exo- + G. *osteon,* bone, + *-osis,* condition]

**ex·o·ter·ic** (eks-ō-tēr′ik) of external origin; arising outside the organism. [G. *exōterikos,* outer]

**ex·o·ther·mic** (eks-ō-ther′mik) **1.** denoting a chemical reaction during which heat (i.e., enthalpy) is emitted. Cf. endothermic. **2.** relating to the external warmth of the body. [exo- + G. *thermē,* heat]

**ex·o·tox·ic** (eks-ō-tok′sik) **1.** relating to an exotoxin. **2.** relating to the introduction of an exogenous poison or toxin.

**ex·o·tox·in** (eks-ō-tok′sin) a specific, soluble, antigenic, usually heat labile, injurious substance elaborated by certain bacteria; it is formed within the cell, but is released into the environment where it is rapidly active in extremely small amounts; most exotoxins are protein in nature. SYN extracellular toxin.

**ex·o·tro·pia** (eks-ō-trō′pē-ă) that type of strabismus in which the visual axes diverge; may be paralytic or concomitant, monocular or alternating, constant or intermittent. SYN divergent strabismus, exodeviation (2), wall-eye (1). [exo- + G. *trope,* turn]

**ex·pand·a·ble stent** stent placed within the lumen of a structure, often percutaneously, that then shortens in its longitudinal dimension and increases its diameter, thereby increasing the inside dimension of the structure.

**ex·pan·ded dis·a·bil·i·ty sta·tus scale (EDSS)** a commonly used rating system for evaluating the degree of neurologic impairment in multiple

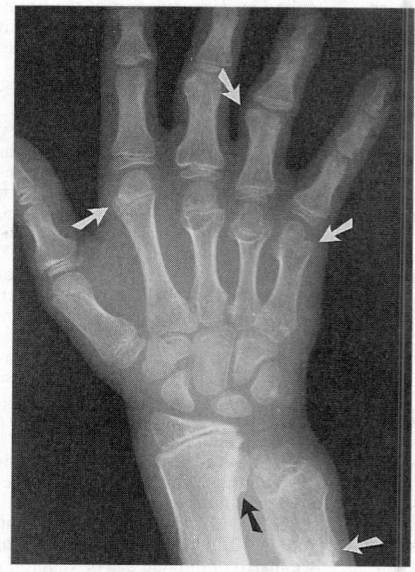

**exostosis:** several small osteochondromas (arrows)

sclerosis, based on neurologic findings, and not symptoms; there are 10 grades in all, in steps and half-steps (e.g., 4, 4.5, 5), with "1" being neurologically normal and "10" being death. SYN Kurtzke multiple sclerosis disability scale.

**ex·pan·sion** (eks-pan′shŭn) **1.** an increase in size as of chest or lungs. **2.** the spreading out of any structure, as a tendon. **3.** an expanse; a wide area. [L. *ex-pando,* pp. *-pansus,* to spread out]

**ex·pec·to·rant** (ek-spek′tō-rănt) **1.** promoting secretion from the mucous membrane of the air passages or facilitating its expulsion. **2.** an agent such as guaifenesin that thins respiratory tract mucus and promotes its removal from the tracheobronchial passages. [L. *ex,* out, + *pectus,* chest]

**ex·pec·to·rate** (ek-spek′tō-rāt) to spit; to eject saliva, mucus, or other fluid from the mouth.

**ex·pec·to·ra·tion** (ek-spek-tō-rā′shŭn) **1.** mucus and other fluids formed in the air passages and upper food passages (the mouth), and expelled by coughing. SEE ALSO sputum (1). **2.** the act of spitting; the expelling from the mouth of saliva, mucus, and other material from the air or upper food passages.

**ex·pen·di·ture** (eks-pen′dĭ-cher) the act of expending; an amount expended or used up. [L. *ex-pendo,* to weigh out, pay]

**ex·pe·ri·ence** (ek-spēr′ē-ens) the feeling of emotions and sensations, as opposed to thinking; involvement in what is happening rather than abstract reflection on an event or interpersonal encounter. [L. *experientia,* fr. *experior,* to try]

**ex·per·i·en·tial au·ra** epileptic aura characterized by altered perception of one's internal and/or external environment; may involve auditory, visual, olfactory, gustatory, somatosensory, or emotional altered perceptions. When one of the altered perceptions is clearly predominant, the specific aura classification should be used. SEE ALSO aura (1).

**ex·per·i·ment** (eks-per'i-ment) **1.** a study in which the investigator intentionally alters one or more factors under controlled conditions in order to study the effects of doing so. **2.** MAGNETIC RESONANCE the term applied to a pulse sequence. [L. *experimentum*, fr. *experior*, to test, try]

**ex·per·i·men·tal er·ror** the total error of measurement ascribed to the conduct of an empirical observation. It is commonly expressed as the standard deviation of replicated experiments. There may be many components, including those in the sampling procedure, the measurements, injudicious choice of a model, observer bias, etc.

**ex·per·i·men·tal group** a group of subjects exposed to the variable of an experiment, as opposed to the control group.

**ex·per·i·men·tal med·i·cine** the scientific investigation of medical problems by experimentation upon animals or by clinical research.

**ex·per·i·men·tal psy·chol·o·gy 1.** a subdiscipline within the science of psychology that is concerned with the study of conditioning, learning, perception, motivation, emotion, language, and thinking; **2.** also used in relation to subject-matter areas in which experimental, in contrast to correlational or socioexperiential, methods are emphasized.

**ex·per·i·ment·er ef·fects** the influence of the experimenter's behavior, personality traits, or expectancies on the results of that person's own research.

**ex·pi·ra·tion** (eks-pi-rā'shŭn) **1.** SYN exhalation (1). **2.** death. [L. *expiro* or *ex-spiro*, pp. -*atus*, to breathe out]

**ex·pi·ra·to·ry** (ek-spī'ră-tō-rē) relating to expiration.

**ex·pi·ra·to·ry re·serve vol·ume (ERV)** the maximal volume of air (about 1000 ml) that can be expelled from the lungs after a normal expiration. SYN reserve air, supplemental air.

**ex·pi·ra·to·ry stri·dor** a singing sound due to the semiapproximated vocal folds offering resistance to the escape of air.

**ex·pire** (ek-spīr') **1.** SYN exhale (1). **2.** to die.

**ex·pired gas 1.** any gas that has been expired from the lungs; **2.** often used synonymously with mixed expired gas.

**Ex·plan·a·tion of Ben·e·fits (EOB)** the report from an insurance carrier that explains benefits, deductibles, copayment responsibilities, and reasons for noncoverage of claims.

**ex·plant** (eks'plant) living tissue transferred from an organism to an artificial medium for culture.

**ex·plo·ra·tion** (eks-plōr-ā'shŭn) an active examination, usually involving endoscopy or a surgical procedure, to ascertain conditions present as an aid in diagnosis. [L. *ex-ploro*, pp. -*ploratus*, to explore]

**ex·plor·a·to·ry** (eks-plōr'ă-tōr-ē) relating to, or with a view to, exploration.

**ex·plor·er** (eks'plōr'er) a sharp pointed probe used to investigate natural or restored tooth surfaces in order to detect caries or other defects.

**ex·po·sure dose** the radiation dose, expressed in roentgens, delivered at a point in free air.

**ex·po·sure ker·a·ti·tis** inflammation of the cornea resulting from irritation caused by inability to close the eyelids.

**ex·press** (eks-pres') to press or squeeze out. [L. *ex-premo*, pp. -*pressus*, to press out]

**ex·pressed skull frac·ture** a fracture with outward displacement of a part of the cranium.

**ex·pres·sion** (eks-presh'ŭn) **1.** squeezing out; expelling by pressure. **2.** mobility of the features giving a particular emotional significance to the face. SYN facies (3) [TA]. **3.** any act by an individual. **4.** something that manifests something else.

**ex·pres·sion vec·tor** a vector (plasmid, yeast, or animal virus genome) used experimentally to introduce foreign genetic material into a propagatable host cell in order to replicate and amplify the foreign DNA sequences as a recombinant molecule (recombinant DNA cloning of sequences).

**ex·pres·sive a·pha·sia** a type of aphasia in which the greatest deficit is in speech production or language output; usually accompanied by a deficit in communicating by writing, signs, etc. The patient is aware of his impairment. The lesion typically includes the posterior frontal lobe. SYN anterior aphasia, motor aphasia, nonfluent aphasia.

**ex·pul·sive** (eks-pŭl'siv) tending to expel. [L. *ex-pello*, pp. -*pulsus*, to drive out]

**ex·pul·sive pains** effective labor pains, associated with contraction of the uterine muscle.

**ex·qui·site** (eks-kwiz'it) extremely intense, keen, sharp; said of pain or tenderness. [L. *exquiro*, pp. *exquisitus*, to search out]

**ex·san·gui·nate** (eks-ang'gwi-nāt) **1.** to remove or withdraw the circulating blood; to make bloodless. **2.** SYN exsanguine. [L. *ex*, out, + *sanguis* (-*guin*), blood]

**ex·san·gui·na·tion** (eks-ang'gwi-nā'shŭn) removal of blood; making exsanguine.

**ex·san·guine** (ek-sang'gwin) deprived of blood. SYN exsanguinate (2).

*Ex·se·ro·hi·lum* (eks'er-ō-hī'lum) a genus of fungi; a cause of human phaeohyphomycosis.

**ex·sic·cant** (eks-ik'ant) SYN desiccant.

**ex·sic·cate** (eks'i-kāt) SYN desiccate.

**ex·sic·ca·tion** (eks-i-kā'shŭn) **1.** SYN desiccation. **2.** the removal of water of crystallization. SYN dehydration (3). [L. *ex sicco*, pp. *siccatus*, to dry up]

**ex·sorp·tion** (eks-ōrp'shŭn) movement of substances from the blood into the lumen of the gut. [L. *ex*, out, + *sorbeo*, to suck]

**ex·stro·phy** (eks'trō-fē) congenital eversion of a hollow organ. [G. *ex*, out, + *strophē*, a turning]

**ex·stro·phy of the blad·der** a congenital gap in the anterior wall of the bladder and the adjacent abdominal wall, the interior and posterior wall of the bladder being exposed.

**ex·tend** (eks-tend') to straighten a limb, to diminish or extinguish the angle formed by flexion; to place the distal segment of a limb in such a position that its axis is continuous with that of the proximal segment. [L. *ex- tendo*, pp. -*tensus*, to stretch out]

**ex·ten·ded me·di·a·stin·o·scop·y** cervical mediastinoscopy in which, in addition to the standard pre- and paratracheal exploration, the mediastinoscope is passed anterior to the innominate artery and aortic arch to provide access to the subaortic (aortopulmonary window) and anterior mediastinal lymph nodes; an alternative to the Chamberlain procedure.

**ex·tend·ed rad·i·cal mas·tec·to·my** excision of the entire breast including the nipple, areola, and overlying skin, as well as the pectoral muscles and the lymphatic-bearing tissues of the axilla and chest wall and internal mammary chain of lymph nodes.

**ex·ten·ded thy·mec·to·my** thymectomy performed via combined sternotomy and a cervical incision to allow removal of all extraglandular thymic tissue. SYN maximal thymectomy.

**ex·ten·sion** (eks-ten'shŭn) **1.** the act of bringing the distal portion of a joint in continuity with the long axis of the proximal portion. **2.** a pulling or dragging force exerted on a limb in a distal direction. See page APP 90. [L. *extensio*, a stretching out]

**ex·ten·sor** (eks-ten'ser) a muscle the contraction of which causes movement at a joint with the consequence that the limb or body assumes a more straight line, or so that the distance between the parts proximal and distal to the joint is increased or extended; the antagonist of a flexor. SEE muscle. [L. one who stretches, fr. *ex-tendo*, to stretch out]

**ex·ten·sor car·pi ra·di·a·lis bre·vis mus·cle** *origin*, lateral epicondyle of humerus; *insertion*, base of third metacarpal bone; *action*, extends and abducts wrist radialward; *nerve supply*, radial. SYN musculus extensor carpi radialis brevis [TA], short radial extensor muscle of wrist.

**ex·ten·sor car·pi ra·di·a·lis lon·gus mus·cle** *origin*, lateral supracondylar ridge of humerus; *insertion*, back of base of second metacarpal bone; *action*, extends and deviates wrist radialward; *nerve supply*, radial. SYN musculus extensor carpi radialis longus [TA], long radial extensor muscle of wrist.

**ex·ten·sor car·pi ul·na·ris mus·cle** *origin*, lateral epicondyle of humerus (humeral head) and oblique line and posterior border of ulna (ulnar head); *insertion*, base of fifth metacarpal bone; *action*, extends and abducts wrist ulnarward; *nerve supply*, radial (posterior interosseous). SYN musculus extensor carpi ulnaris [TA], ulnar extensor muscle of wrist.

**ex·ten·sor di·gi·ti mi·ni·mi mus·cle** *origin*, lateral epicondyle of humerus; *insertion*, dorsum of proximal, middle, and distal phalanges of little finger; *action*, extends fingers; *nerve supply*, radial (posterior interosseous). SYN musculus extensor digiti minimi [TA], extensor muscle of little finger.

**ex·ten·sor di·gi·to·rum bre·vis mus·cle** *origin*, dorsal surface of calcaneus; *insertion*, by four tendons fusing with those of the extensor digitorum longus, and by a slip attached independently to the base of the proximal phalanx of the great toe; *action*, extends toes; *nerve supply*, deep peroneal. SYN musculus extensor digitorum brevis [TA], short extensor muscle of toes.

**ex·ten·sor di·gi·to·rum lon·gus mus·cle** *origin*, lateral condyle of tibia, upper two-thirds of anterior margin of fibula; *insertion*, by four tendons to the dorsal surfaces of the bases of the proximal, middle, and distal phalanges of the second to fifth toes; *action*, extends the four lateral toes; *nerve supply*, deep branch of peroneal. SYN musculus extensor digitorum longus [TA], long extensor muscle of toes.

**ex·ten·sor di·gi·to·rum mus·cle** *origin*, lateral epicondyle of humerus; *insertion*, by four ten-

dons into the base of the proximal and middle and base of the distal phalanges; *action*, extends fingers; *nerve supply*, radial (posterior interosseous). SYN musculus extensor digitorum [TA], extensor muscle of fingers.

**ex·ten·sor hal·lu·cis bre·vis mus·cle** the medial belly of extensor digitorum brevis, the tendon of which is inserted into the base of the proximal phalanx of the great toe. SYN musculus extensor hallucis brevis [TA], short extensor muscle of great toe.

**ex·ten·sor hal·lu·cis lon·gus mus·cle** *origin*, lateral surface of tibia and interosseous membrane; *insertion*, base of distal phalanx of great toe; *action*, extends the great toe; *nerve supply*, anterior tibial. SYN musculus extensor hallucis longus [TA].

**ex·ten·sor in·di·cis mus·cle** *origin*, dorsal surface of ulna; *insertion*, dorsal extensor aponeurosis of index finger; *action*, assists in extending the forefinger; *nerve supply*, radial. SYN musculus extensor indicis [TA], index extensor muscle.

**ex·ten·sor mus·cle of fin·gers** SYN extensor digitorum muscle.

**ex·ten·sor mus·cle of lit·tle fin·ger** SYN extensor digiti minimi muscle.

**ex·ten·sor ret·i·nac·u·lum** a strong fibrous band formed as a thickening of the antebrachial deep fascia, stretching obliquely across the back of the wrist, attaching deeply to ridges on the dorsal aspect of the radius, triquetral and pisiform bones, binding down the extensor tendons of the fingers and thumb.

**ex·te·ri·or·ize** (eks-tēr'ē-ōr-īz) **1.** to direct interests, thoughts, or feelings into a channel leading outside the self, to some definite aim or object. **2.** to expose an organ temporarily for observation, or permanently for purposes of physiologic experiment.

**ex·tern** (eks'tern) an advanced student or recent graduate who assists in the medical or surgical care of hospital patients. [F. *externe*, outside, a day scholar]

**ex·ter·nal** (eks-ter'năl) on the outside or farther from the center. USAGE NOTE: Often incorrectly used to mean lateral. [L. *externus*]

**ex·ter·nal base of skull** external aspect of the base of skull

**ex·ter·nal cap·sule** a thin lamina of white substance separating the claustrum from the putamen. It joins the internal capsule at either extremity of the putamen, forming a capsule of white matter external to the lenticular nucleus. SYN capsula externa [TA].

**ex·ter·nal ca·rot·id nerves** a number of sympathetic nerve fibers conveyed via the cephalic arterial ramus of the sympathetic trunk which extends from the superior cervical ganglion to the external carotid artery, forming the external carotid plexus. SYN nervi carotici externi [TA].

**ex·ter·nal ce·pha·lic ver·sion** version performed entirely by external manipulation. SEE ALSO cephalic version.

**ex·ter·nal con·ju·gate** the distance in a straight line between the depression under the last spinous process of the lumbar vertebrae and the upper edge of the pubic symphysis.

**ex·ter·nal ear** SEE ear.

**ex·ter·nal fis·tu·la** a fistula between a hollow viscus and the skin.

**ex•ter•nal fix•a•tion** fixation of fractured bones by splints, plastic dressings, or transfixion pins.

**ex•ter•nal gen•i•ta•lia** the vulva in the female, and the penis and scrotum in the male.

**ex•ter•nal nasal ar•tery** SYN dorsal nasal artery.

**ex•ter•nal na•sal veins** several vessels that drain the external nose, emptying into the angular or facial vein.

**ex•ter•nal nose** the visible portion of the nose which forms a prominent feature of the face; it consists of a root, dorsum and apex from above downward and is perforated inferiorly by two nostrils separated by a septum. SYN nasus (1).

**ex•ter•nal ob•lique mus•cle** origin, fifth to twelfth ribs; insertion, anterior half of lateral lip of iliac crest, inguinal ligament, and anterior layer of the rectus sheath; action, diminishes capacity of abdomen, draws thorax downward; nerve supply, thoracoabdominal nerves. SYN musculus obliquus externus abdominis [TA].

**ex•ter•nal ob•tu•ra•tor mus•cle** SYN obturator externus muscle.

**ex•ter•nal oc•cip•i•tal crest** a ridge extending from the external occipital protuberance to the border of the foramen magnum.

**ex•ter•nal oph•thal•mop•a•thy** any disease of the conjunctiva, cornea, or adnexa of the eye.

**ex•ter•nal oph•thal•mo•ple•gia** SYN ophthalmoplegia externa.

**ex•ter•nal os of uter•us** the vaginal opening of the uterus.

**ex•ter•nal phase** the medium or fluid in which a disperse is suspended. SYN dispersion medium.

**ex•ter•nal pu•den•dal ar•ter•ies** origin, femoral; distribution, skin over pubis, skin over penis and skin of scrotum or labium majus via anterior scrotal (labial) arteries; anastomoses, dorsal artery of penis or clitoris, posterior scrotal or labial arteries. SYN arteriae pudendae externae [TA].

**ex•ter•nal pu•den•dal veins** these correspond to the arteries of the same name; they empty into the great saphenous vein or directly into the femoral vein, and receive the superficial dorsal vein of the penis (or clitoris) and the anterior scrotal (or labial) veins.

**ex•ter•nal res•pi•ra•tion** the exchange of respiratory gases in the lungs as distinguished from internal or tissue respiration.

**ex•ter•nal trac•tion** a pulling force created by using fixed anchorage (e.g., a headcap or bed frame) outside the oral cavity; principally used in the management of midfacial fractures.

**ex•ter•nal u•re•thral or•i•fice 1.** the slitlike opening of the urethra in the glans penis; **2.** the external orifice of the urethra (in the female) in the vestibule, usually upon a slight elevation, the papilla urethrae.

**ex•ter•o•cep•tive** (eks′ter-ō-sep′tiv) relating to the exteroceptors; denoting the surface of the body containing the end organs adapted to receive impressions or stimuli from without. [L. exterus, outside, + capio, to take]

**ex•ter•o•cep•tor** (eks′ter-ō-sep′ter) one of the peripheral end organs of the afferent nerves in the skin or mucous membrane, which respond to stimulation by external agents. [L. exterus, external, + receptor, receiver]

**ex•ter•o•fec•tive** (eks′ter-ō-fek′tiv) pertaining to the response of the nervous system to external stimuli. [L. extero, from outside, + affectus, affected]

**ex•tinc•tion** (eks-tingk′shŭn) **1.** in behavior modification or classical or operant conditioning, a progressive decrease in the frequency of a response that is not positively reinforced. SEE conditioning. **2.** SYN absorbance. [L. extinguo, to quench]

**ex•tinc•tion co•ef•fi•cient (ep•sil•on)** SYN specific absorption coefficient.

**ex•tin•guish** (eks-ting′gwish) **1.** to abolish; to quench, as a flame; to cause loss of identity; to destroy. **2.** PSYCHOLOGY to abolish a conditioned response. SEE conditioning. [L. extinguo, to quench]

**ex•tir•pa•tion** (eks-tir-pā′shŭn) complete removal of an organ or diseased tissue. [L. extirpo, to root out, fr. stirps, a stalk, root]

**ex•tor•sion** (eks-tōr′shŭn) **1.** outward rotation of a limb or of an organ. **2.** conjugate rotation of the upper poles of each cornea outward. [L. extorsio, fr. ex- torqueo, to twist out]

△**ex•tra-** without, outside of. [L.]

**ex•tra•ax•i•al** (eks-tră-aks′ē-ăl) off the axis; applied to intracranial lesions that do not arise from the brain itself.

**ex•tra•cap•su•lar an•ky•lo•sis** stiffness of a joint due to induration or heterotopic ossification of the surrounding tissues. SYN spurious ankylosis.

**ex•tra•cap•su•lar lig•a•ments** ligaments associated with a synovial joint but separate from and external to its articular capsule.

**ex•tra•cel•lu•lar** (eks-tră-sel′yu-ler) outside the cells.

**ex•tra•cel•lu•lar en•zyme** an enzyme performing its functions outside a cell; e.g., the various digestive enzymes. SYN exoenzyme.

**ex•tra•cel•lu•lar flu•id (ECF) 1.** the interstitial fluid and the plasma, constituting about 20% of the weight of the body; **2.** sometimes used to mean all fluid outside of cells, usually excluding transcellular fluid.

**ex•tra•cel•lu•lar tox•in** SYN exotoxin.

**ex•tra•chro•mo•som•al el•e•ment, ex•tra•chro•mo•som•al ge•net•ic el•e•ment** SYN plasmid.

**ex•tra•chro•mo•som•al in•her•i•tance** transmission of characters dependent on some factor not connected with the chromosomes.

**ex•tra•cor•po•re•al** (eks′tră-kōr-pō′rē-ăl) outside of, or unrelated to, the body or any anatomic "corpus."

**ex•tra•cor•po•re•al cir•cu•la•tion** the circulation of blood outside of the body through a machine that temporarily assumes an organ's functions, e.g., through a heart-lung machine or artificial kidney.

**ex•tra•cor•po•re•al-mem•brane ox•y•gen•a•tion (ECMO)** a system to augment alveolar ventilation by gaseous diffusion across membranes outside the patient's body.

**ex•tra•cor•po•re•al shock wave lith•o•trip•sy (ESWL)** (eks′tră-kōr-pō′rē-ăl shŏk-wāv lith′ō-trip′sē) breaking up of renal or ureteral calculi by focused ultrasound energy.

**ex•tract 1.** (ek′strakt) a concentrated preparation of a drug obtained by removing the active constituents with suitable solvents, evaporating all or nearly all of the solvent, and adjusting the residual mass or powder to the prescribed standard. **2.** (ek-strakt′) to remove part of a mixture with a solvent. **3.** to perform extraction. [L. *ex-traho*, pp. *-tractus*, to draw out]

**ex·tract·ing for·ceps** SYN dental forceps.

**ex·trac·tion** (ek-strak′shŭn) **1.** luxation and removal of a tooth from its alveolus. **2.** partitioning of material (solute) into a solvent. **3.** the active portion of a drug; the making of an extract. **4.** surgical removal by pulling out. **5.** removal of the fetus from the uterus or vagina at or near the end of pregnancy, either manually or with instruments. **6.** removal by suction of the products of conception before a menstrual period has been missed. [L. *ex-traho*, pp. *-tractus*, to draw out]

**ex·trac·tion co·ef·fi·cient** the percentage of a substance removed from the blood or plasma in a single passage through a tissue.

**ex·trac·tion ra·ti·o (E)** the fraction of a substance removed from the blood flowing through the kidney.

**ex·trac·tives** (eks-trak′tivz) substances present in vegetable or animal tissue that can be separated by successive treatment with solvents and recovered by evaporation of the solution.

**ex·trac·tor** (eks-trak′ter) instrument for use in drawing or pulling out any natural part, as a tooth, or a foreign body.

**ex·tra·cys·tic** (eks-tră-sis′tik) outside of, or unrelated to, the gallbladder or urinary bladder or any cystic tumor.

**ex·tra·du·ral hem·or·rhage** an accumulation of blood between the skull and the dura mater. SYN epidural hematoma.

**ex·tra·em·bry·on·ic** (eks′tră-em-brē-on′ik) outside the embryonic body; referring, e.g., to structures providing protection and nutrition but discarded at birth without being incorporated in the body.

**ex·tra·mam·ma·ry Pa·get dis·ease** (pă′jĕt) an intraepidermal form of mucinous adenocarcinoma, most commonly in the anogenital region. SYN Paget disease (3).

**ex·tra·no·dal mar·gin·al zone lymph·o·ma** SYN MALToma.

**ex·tra·oc·u·lar mus·cles** the muscles within the orbit including the four rectus muscles (superior, inferior, medial and lateral); two oblique muscles (superior and inferior), and the levator of the superior eyelid (levator palpebrae superioris).

**ex·tra·per·i·to·ne·al fas·cia** the thin layer of fascia and adipose tissue between the peritoneum and fascia transversalis. SYN fascia subperitonealis [TA].

**ex·tra·phys·i·o·log·ic** (eks′tră-fiz-ē-ō-loj′ik) outside of the domain of physiology; more than physiologic, therefore pathologic.

**ex·tra·py·ram·i·dal dis·ease** a general term for a number of disorders caused by abnormalities of the basal ganglia or certain brain stem or thalamic nuclei; characterized by motor deficits, loss of postural reflexes, bradykinesia, tremor, rigidity, and various involuntary movements.

**ex·tra·py·ram·i·dal dys·ki·ne·si·a** abnormal involuntary movement attributed to pathological states of one or more parts of the striate body and characterized by insuppressible, stereotyped, automatic movements that cease only during sleep; e.g., Parkinson disease; chorea; athetosis; hemiballism.

**ex·tra·py·ram·i·dal mo·tor sys·tem** literally: all of the brain structures affecting bodily (somatic) movement, excluding the motor neurons,

the motor cortex, and the pyramidal (corticobulbar and corticospinal) tract. Despite its very wide literal connotation, the term is commonly used to denote in particular the striate body (basal ganglia), its associated structures (substantia nigra; subthalamic nucleus), and its descending connections with the midbrain.

**ex·tra·sac·cu·lar her·nia** SYN sliding hernia.

**ex·tra·sen·so·ry** (eks-tră-sen′sōr-ē) outside or beyond the ordinary senses; not limited to the senses, as in extrasensory perception.

**ex·tra·sen·so·ry per·cep·tion (ESP)** perception by means other than through the ordinary senses; e.g., telepathy, clairvoyance, precognition.

**ex·tra·sys·to·le** (eks′tră-sis′tō-lē) an ectopic beat from any source in the heart. SYN premature systole.

**ex·tra·thor·a·cic air·way ob·struc·tion** form of airway obstruction in which the site of airway narrowing is above the thoracic inlet. It can be variable (e.g., reduction in inspiratory but not expirator flows) or fixed (reduction in both inspiratory and expiratory flows).

**ex·trav·a·sate** (eks-trav′ă-sāt) **1.** to exude from or pass out of a vessel into the tissues, said of blood, lymph, or urine. **2.** the substance thus exuded. SYN suffusion (4). [L. *extra*, out of, + *vas*, vessel]

**ex·trav·a·sa·tion** (eks-trav′ă-sā′shŭn) the act of extravasating. [extra- + L. *vas*, vessel]

**ex·tra·vas·cu·lar flu·id** all fluid outside the blood vessels, i.e., intracellular, interstitial, and transcellular fluids; it constitutes about 48%–58% of the body weight.

**ex·tra·ver·sion** (eks-tră-ver′zhŭn) SYN extroversion.

**ex·tra·ves·i·cal re·im·plan·ta·tion** SYN detrusorrhaphy.

**ex·tre·mal quo·tient** the ratio of the rate in the jurisdiction with the highest rate of interventions such as surgical procedures to the rate in the jurisdiction with the lowest rate.

**in ex·tre·mis** (in eks-trē′mis) at the point of death. [L. *extremus*, last]

**ex·trem·i·tas** (eks-trem′i-tas) [TA] SYN extremity. SEE limb. [L. fr. *extremus*, last, outermost]

**ex·trem·i·ty** (eks-trem′i-tē) one of the ends of an elongated or pointed structure. Incorrectly used to mean limb. SYN extremitas [TA].

**ex·trin·sic** (eks-trin′sik) originating outside of the part where found or upon which it acts; denoting especially a muscle, such as extrinsic muscles of hand. [L. *extrinsecus*, from without]

**ex·trin·sic al·ler·gic al·ve·o·li·tis** pneumoconiosis resulting from hypersensitivity to organic dust, usually specified according to occupational exposure; in the acute form, respiratory symptoms and fever start several hours after exposure to the dust; in the chronic form, there is eventual diffuse pulmonary fibrosis after exposure over several years.

**ex·trin·sic co·a·gu·la·tion path·way** a part of the coagulation pathway that is activated by contact of factor VII in the blood with tissue factor (TF), an integral membrane protein of extravascular plasma membranes. The integrity of this pathway can be tested by the prothrombin time (PT).

**ex·trin·sic fac·tor** dietary vitamin $B_{12}$.

**ex·trin·sic in·cu·ba·tion pe·ri·od** (eks-trin′sik in-kyu-bā-shŭn pēr-ē-ŏd) time required for the development of a disease agent in a vector, from the time of uptake of the agent to the time when the vector is infective.

**ex·trin·sic sphinc·ter** a sphincter provided by circular muscular fibers extraneous to the organ.

**ex·tro·ver·sion** (eks′trō-ver′zhŭn) **1.** a turning outward. **2.** a trait involving social intercourse, as practiced by an extrovert. Cf. introversion. SYN extraversion. [incorrectly formed fr. L. *extra,* outside, + *verto,* pp. *versus,* to turn]

**ex·tro·vert, ex·tra·vert** (eks′trō-vert) a gregarious person whose chief interests lie outside the self, and who is socially self-confident and involved in the affairs of others. Cf. introvert.

**ex·trude** (eks-trood′) to thrust, force, or press out.

**ex·tru·sion** (eks-troo′zhŭn) **1.** a thrusting or forcing out of a normal position. **2.** the overeruption or migration of a tooth beyond its normal occlusal position.

**ex·tu·ba·tion** (eks′too-bā′shŭn) removal of a tube from an organ, structure, or orifice. [L. *ex,* out, + *tuba,* tube]

**ex·u·ber·ant** (ek-zoo′ber-ănt) denoting excessive proliferation or growth, as of granulation tissue. [L. *exubero,* to abound, be abundant]

**ex·u·date** (eks′oo-dāt) any fluid that has exuded out of a tissue or its capillaries because of injury or inflammation. Cf. transudate. SYN exudation (2). [L. *ex,* out, + *sudo,* to sweat]

**ex·u·da·tion** (eks-oo-dā′shŭn) **1.** the act or process of exuding. **2.** SYN exudate.

**ex·u·da·tion cyst** a cyst resulting from distention of a closed cavity, such as a bursa, by an excessive secretion of its normal fluid contents.

**ex·ud·a·tive** (eks-oo′dă-tiv) relating to the process of exudation or to an exudate.

**ex·u·da·tive dru·sen** accumulations of an amorphous and granular material, cytoplasmic processes, and bent fibers between the basement membrane of the retinal pigment epithelium and the inner collagenous zone of the lamina basalis choroidae; types of exudative drusen include hard drusen and soft drusen. SYN typical drusen.

**ex·ud·a·tive in·flam·ma·tion** inflammation in which the conspicuous or distinguishing feature is an exudate, which may be chiefly serous, serofibrinous, fibrinous, or mucous, or may be characterized by relatively large numbers of cells.

**ex·ud·a·tive ret·i·ni·tis, ret·i·ni·tis ex·u·da·ti·va** a chronic abnormality characterized by deposition of cholesterol and cholesterol esters in outer retinal layers and subretinal space. In adults, often preceded by uveitis; in children, often preceded by retinal vascular abnormalities. SYN Coats disease.

**ex·ude** (ek-zood′) in general, to ooze or pass gradually out of a body structure or tissue. [L. *ex,* out, + *sudo,* to sweat]

**ex·um·bil·i·ca·tion** (eks′ŭm-bil-i-kā′shŭn) **1.** SYN exomphalos (1). **2.** SYN umbilical hernia. **3.** SYN omphalocele. [L. *ex,* out, + *umbilicus,* navel]

**ex vi·vo** (ex vē′vō) referring to the use or positioning of a tissue or cell after removal from an organism while the tissue or cells remain viable. [L. from the living]

**eye** (ī) **1.** the organ of vision that consists of the eyeball and the optic nerve; SYN oculus [TA]. **2.** the area of the eye, including lids and other accessory organs of the eye; the contents of the orbit (common). See this page. [A.S. *eāge*]

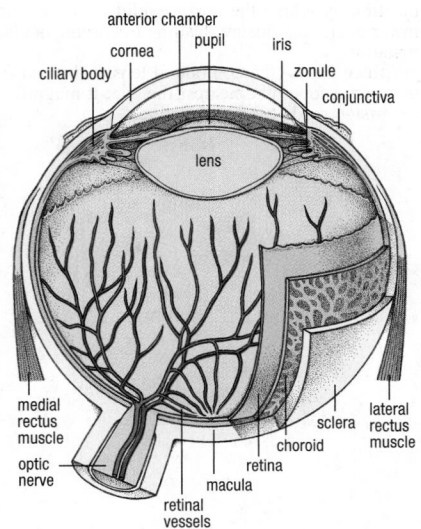

**eye** (cutaway superior view)

**eye·ball** (ī′bawl) the eye proper without the appendages. SYN bulbus oculi [TA], bulb of eye.

**eye bank** a place where corneas of eyes removed after death are preserved for subsequent keratoplasty.

**eye·brow** the crescentic line of hairs at the superior edge of the orbit. SYN supercilium (1) [TA].

**eye-clo·sure pu·pil re·ac·tion** a constriction of both pupils when an effort is made to close eyelids forcibly held apart. A variant of the pupil response to near vision. SYN Galassi pupillary phenomenon, Gifford reflex, Westphal pupillary reflex.

**eye cup** a small oval receptacle used to apply a liquid to the external eye.

**eye·glass·es** SYN spectacles.

**eye·grounds** (ī′growndz) the fundus of the eye as seen with the ophthalmoscope.

**eye·lash** one of the stiff hairs projecting from the margin of the eyelid. SYN cilium (1).

**eye·lash sign** in a case of apparent unconsciousness due to functional disease, such as conversion hysteria, stroking the eyelashes will occasion movement of the lids, but no such reflex will occur in case of severe organic brain lesion such as apoplexy, fracture of the skull, or other traumatism.

**eye·lid** one of the two movable folds covering the front of the eyeball when closed; formed of a fibrous core (tarsal plate) and the palpebral portions of the orbicularis oculi muscle covered with skin on the superficial, anterior surface and lined with conjunctiva on the deep, posterior surface; rapid contraction of the contained muscle fibers produces blinking; they each have fixed (orbital) and free margins, the latter separated centrally by the palpebral fissure, united at the lateral and medial palpebral commissures, and bearing eyelashes, the openings of tarsal and ciliary glands and (medially) the lacrimal puncta. SYN palpebra [TA], blepharon, lid.

**eye·lid im·bri·ca·tion** an abnormality of eyelid

position by which the upper eyelid overrides the lower eyelid on closure, leading to chronic ocular irritation.

**eye•piece** (ī′pēs) the compound lens at the end of the microscope tube nearest the eye; it magnifies the image made by the objective.

**eye spec•u•lum** an instrument for keeping the eyelids apart during inspection of or operation on the eye. SYN blepharostat.

**eye•strain** SYN asthenopia.

**eye tooth** SYN canine tooth.

# F

**F 1.** fractional concentration, followed by subscripts indicating location and chemical species; free energy; farad; faraday; Fahrenheit; visual field; fluorine; force; filial generation, followed by subscript numerals indicating indicating specified matings; phenylalanine. **2.** focus (1).

***F*** faraday, Faraday constant, force; free energy.

**f** femto-; respiratory frequency; fugacity; formyl.

**F0** fundamental frequency.

**F1.2** prothrombin fragment 1.2.

**Fab** SEE Fab fragment.

**FAB** SEE French-American-British classification system.

**FAB class·i·fi·ca·tion** French-American-British classification of acute leukemias based on the study of microscopic features and cytochemistry of blast cells; it subdivides acute myelogenous leukemias into eight groups ($M_0$–$M_7$) and acute lymphoblastic leukemias into 3 groups ($L_1$–$L_3$); widely used in clinical practice.

**fa·bel·la** (fa-bel'lă) a sesamoid bone in the tendon of the lateral head of the gastrocnemius muscle. [Mod. L. dim. of *faba,* bean]

**Fab frag·ment** the antigen-binding fragment of an immunoglobulin molecule, consisting of both a light chain and part of a heavy chain.

**Fa·bry dis·ease** (fah'brē) due to deficiency of α-galactosidase and characterized by abnormal accumulations of neutral glycolipids (e.g., globotriaosylceramide) in endothelial cells in blood vessel walls; clinical findings include angiokeratomas on the thighs, buttocks, and genitalia, hypohidrosis, paresthesia in extremities, cornea verticillata, and spokelike posterior subcapsular cataracts; death results from renal, cardiac, or cerebrovascular complications; X-linked recessive inheritance caused by mutation the α-galactosidase gene (GLA) on Xq.

**face** (fās) **1.** the front portion of the head; the visage including eyes, nose, mouth, forehead, cheeks, and chin; excludes ears. SYN facies (1) [TA]. **2.** SYN surface.

**face-bow** a caliperlike device used to record the relationship of the jaws to the temporomandibular joints; the record may then be used to orient a cast or model of the maxilla to the opening and closing axis of the articulator.

**face-lift** SEE rhytidectomy.

**face pre·sen·ta·tion** SEE cephalic presentation.

**fac·et, fa·cette** (fas'et, fă-set') **1.** a small smooth area on a bone or other firm structure. **2.** a worn spot on a tooth, produced by chewing or grinding. [Fr. *facette*]

**fac·e·tec·to·my** (fas-ĕ-tek'tō-mē) excision of a facet. [facet + G. *ektomē,* excision]

**fa·cial** (fā'shăl) relating to the face.

**fa·cial ar·tery** *origin,* external carotid; *branches,* ascending palatine, tonsillar and glandular branches, submental, inferior labial, superior labial, masseteric, buccal, lateral nasal branches, and angular. SYN arteria facialis [TA].

**fa·cial ax·is** SYN basifacial axis.

**fa·cial bones** the bones surrounding the mouth and nose and contributing to the orbits; they are the paired maxillae, zygomatic, nasal, lacrimal, palatine, and inferior nasal conchae; and the unpaired ethmoid, vomer, mandible, and hyoid.

**fa·cial ca·nal** the bony passage in the temporal bone through which the facial nerve passes; the facial canal commences at the internal auditory meatus with the horizontal part which passes at first anteriorly (medial crus of facial canal) then turns posteriorly at the geniculum of the facial canal to pass medial to the tympanic cavity (lateral crus of facial canal); finally, it turns downward (descending part of facial canal) to reach the stylomastoid foramen.

**fa·cial hem·i·ple·gia** paralysis of one side of the face, the muscles of the extremities being unaffected.

**fa·cial nerve [CN VII]** nerve with origin in the tegmentum of the lower portion of the pons; it emerges from the brain at the posterior border of the pons; it leaves the cranial cavity through the internal acoustic meatus where it is joined by the intermediate nerve, traverses the facial canal in the petrous portion of the temporal bone, and makes its exit through the stylomastoid foramen; after supplying the stapedius, occipitalis, auricular, stylohyoid, and posterior belly of the digastric muscles; its main trunk ramifies within the parotid gland forming the intraparotid plexus, the various branches of which pass to the muscles of facial expression. See this page. SYN nervus facialis [CN VII] [TA], seventh cranial nerve [CN VII].

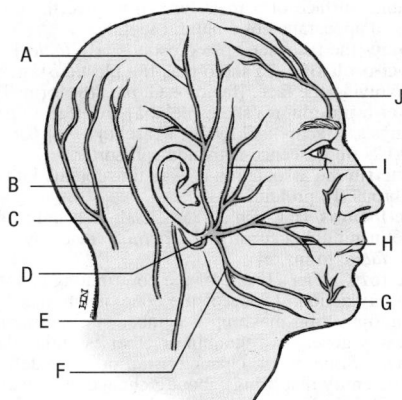

**facial and other nerves supplying the head and neck:** (A) auriculotemporal branch of facial nerve, (B) small occipital nerve, (C) greater occipital nerve, (D) facial nerve, (E) great auricular nerve, (F) mandibular branch of facial nerve, (G) mental nerve, (H) buccal branch of facial nerve, (I) temporal branch of facial nerve, (J) supraorbital nerve

**fa·cial pal·sy** SYN facial paralysis.

**fa·cial pa·ral·y·sis** paresis or paralysis of the facial muscles, usually unilateral, due to either a lesion involving the nucleus or the facial nerve or a supranuclear lesion in the cerebrum or upper brainstem. SYN facial palsy, facioplegia, prosopoplegia.

**fa·cial re·cess ap·proach** a surgical approach to

the middle ear from the mastoid through the recess lateral to the facial nerve canal.

**fa·cial spa·sm** SYN facial tic.

**fa·cial tic** involuntary twitching of the facial muscles, sometimes unilateral. SYN Bell spasm, facial spasm, palmus (1), prosopospasm.

**fa·cial vein** a continuation of the angular vein at the medial angle of the eye; it passes diagonally downward and outward, uniting with the retromandibular vein below the border of the lower jaw before emptying into the internal jugular vein.

△**-fac·ient** causing; one who or that which brings about. [L. *facio,* to make]

**fa·ci·es,** pl. **fa·ci·es** (fā'shē-ēz, fash'ē-ēz) [TA] **1.** SYN face (1). **2.** SYN surface. **3.** SYN expression (2). [L.]

**fa·cil·i·ta·ted com·mu·ni·ca·tion** method in which individuals who are unable to communicate effectively are aided by a "facilitator" who physically assists them to use augmentative communication systems such as a communication board or typewriter. SEE augmentative and alternative communication. SEE ALSO communication board.

**fa·cil·i·ta·tion** (fă-sil'i-tā'shŭn) enhancement or reinforcement of a reflex or other nervous activity by the arrival at the reflex center of other excitatory impulses. [L. *facilitas,* fr. *facilis,* easy]

**fac·ing** (fās'ing) a tooth-colored material (usually plastic or porcelain) used to hide the buccal or labial surface of a metal crown to give the outward appearance of a natural tooth.

△**fa·cio-** the face. SEE ALSO prosopo-. [L. *facies*]

**fa·ci·o·plas·ty** (fā'shē-ō-plas-tē) plastic surgery involving the face. [facio- + G. *plastos,* formed]

**fa·ci·o·ple·gia** (fā'shē-ō-plē'jē-ă) SYN facial paralysis. [facio- + G. *plēgē,* a stroke]

**FACS** fluorescence-activated cell sorter.

**F-ac·tin** the association of G-actin subunits into a fibrous (F) protein.

**fac·ti·tious** (fak-tish'ŭs) artificial; self-induced; not naturally occurring. [L. *factitius,* made by art, fr. *facio,* to make]

**fac·tor** (fak'ter) **1.** one of the contributing causes in any action. **2.** one of the components that by multiplication make up a number or expression. **3.** SYN gene. **4.** a vitamin or other essential element. **5.** an event, characteristic, or other definable entity that brings about a change in a health condition. **6.** a categorical independent variable, used to identify, by means of numerical codes, membership in a qualitatively identifiable group; for example, "overcrowding is a factor in disease transmission." [L. maker, causer, fr. *facio,* to make]

**fac·tor I** in the clotting of blood a factor that is converted to fibrin through the action of thrombin. SEE ALSO fibrinogen.

**fac·tor III** in the clotting of blood, tissue factor or thromboplastin; it initiates the extrinsic pathway by reacting with factor VII and calcium to form factor VIIa. SEE thromboplastin.

**fac·tor IV** in the clotting of blood, calcium ions.

**fac·tor V** a plasma factor in blood coagulation. Factor V does not have enzymatic action but participates in the common pathway of coagulation by binding factor Xa to platelet surfaces. Deficiency of this factor leads to a rare hemorrhagic tendency known as parahemophilia or hypoproaccelerinemia. SYN accelerator factor, plasma accelerator globulin, proaccelerin, prothrombin accelerator.

**fac·tor VII** a plasma factor in blood coagulation. Factor VII forms a complex with tissue thromboplastin and calcium to activate factor X. It accelerates the conversion of prothrombin to thrombin, in the presence of tissue thromboplastin, calcium, and factor V. SYN cothromboplastin, proconvertin, serum accelerator, serum prothrombin conversion accelerator.

**fac·tor VIII** a plasma factor in blood coagulation. Factor VIII participates in the clotting of the blood by forming a complex with factor IXa, platelets, and calcium and enzymatically catalyzing the activation of factor X. Deficiency of factor VIII is associated with classic hemophilia A. **Factor VIII:C** is the coagulant component of factor VIII, which circulates in the plasma complexed with **factor VIIIR** (von Willebrand factor), a glycoprotein that is synthesized by endothelial cells and megakaryocytes, and binds to arteries that have lost their endothelial cell linings, creating a surface to which platelets adhere. Disorders involving factor VIIIR form a heterogenous group of abnormalities called von Willebrand disease. SYN antihemophilic factor A, antihemophilic globulin A, proserum prothrombin conversion accelerator.

**fac·tor IX** in the clotting of blood, also known as: Christmas factor, plasma thromboplastin component, and antihemophilic globulin B, factor IX is required for the formation of intrinsic blood thromboplastin; deficiency causes hemophilia B. SYN antihemophilic globulin B, Christmas factor.

**fac·tor X** a plasma coagulation factor that assists in the conversion of prothrombin to thrombin. A deficiency of factor X will lead to impaired blood coagulation. SYN prothrombinase, Stuart factor, Stuart-Prower factor.

**fac·tor Xa** the active form of factor X; it is formed from factor X by limited proteolysis via factor VIIa and tissue factor (extrinsic pathway) or factor Ixa, VIIIa (intrinsic pathway). Factor Xa forms a complex with factor Va, phospholipid, and calcium to convert.

**fac·tor XI** a plasma coagulation factor; a component of the contact system which is absorbed from plasma and serum by glass and similar surfaces. Deficiency of factor XI results in a hemorrhagic tendency. SYN plasma thromboplastin antecedent.

**fac·tor XII** a plasma coagulation factor. When activated by glass or otherwise to its active form, factor XIIa (EC 3.4.21.38), a serine proteinase, it activates factors VII and XI and converts factor XI to its active form, factor XIa. Deficiency of factor XII results in great prolongation of the clotting time of venous blood, but only rarely in a hemorrhagic tendency. SYN Hageman factor.

**fac·tor XIII** a plasma coagulation factor catalyzed by thrombin into its active form, factor XIIIa, which cross-links subunits of the fibrin clot to form insoluble fibrin. SYN Laki-Lorand factor.

**fac·to·ri·al ex·per·i·ments** an experimental design in which two or more series of treatments are tried in all combinations.

**fac·ul·ta·tive** (fak-ŭl-tā'tiv) able to live under more than one specific set of environmental conditions; possessing an alternative pathway.

**fac·ul·ta·tive an·aer·obe** an anaerobe that

grows in the presence of air or under conditions of reduced oxygen tension.

**fac·ul·ta·tive hy·per·o·pia** SYN manifest hyperopia.

**fac·ul·ta·tive par·a·site** an organism that may either lead an independent existence or live as a parasite, in contrast to obligate parasite.

**fac·ul·ty** (fak'ŭl-tē) a natural or specialized power of a living organism.

**FAD** flavin adenine dinucleotide.

**Fa·den su·ture** a suture placed between an ocular rectus muscle and the posterior sclera to limit excessive action of the eyeball. [Ger. *Faden*, thread, twine]

**fae·cal [Br.]** SEE fecal.

**fae·ca·lith [Br.]** SEE fecalith.

**fae·ca·lu·ria [Br.]** SEE fecaluria.

**fae·ces [Br.]** SEE feces.

**fa·got cell** a neoplastic promyelocyte with bundles of Auer rods, found in hypergranular promyelocytic leukemia (M3).

**Fahr dis·ease** (fahr) progressive calcific deposition in the walls of blood vessels of the basal ganglia, in young to middle-aged persons; occasionally associated with mental retardation and extrapyramidal symptoms.

**Fahr·en·heit (F)** Gabriel D., German-Dutch physicist, 1686–1736. SEE Fahrenheit scale.

**Fahr·en·heit scale** (fār'ĕn-hīt) a thermometer scale in which the freezing point of water is 32°F and the boiling point of water 212°F; 0°F indicates the lowest temperature Fahrenheit could obtain by a mixture of ice and salt in 1724; °C = (5/9)(°F − 32).

**fail·ure** (fāl'yur) the state of insufficiency or non-performance.

**fail·ure to thrive** a condition in which an infant's weight gain and growth are far below usual levels for age.

**faint** (fānt) **1.** extremely weak; threatened with syncope. **2.** an episode of syncope. SEE ALSO syncope. [M.E., fr. O. Fr. *feindre*, to feign]

**fal·cate** (fal'kāt) SYN falciform.

**fal·ces** (fal'sēz) plural of falx.

**fal·ci·form** (fal'si-fōrm) having a crescentic or sickle shape. SYN falcate. [L. *falx*, sickle, + *forma*, form]

**fal·ci·form lig·a·ment** SYN falciform process.

**fal·ci·form lig·a·ment of liv·er** a crescentic fold of peritoneum extending to the surface of the liver from the diaphragm and anterior abdominal wall; the round ligament lies in its free inferior border; remnant of embryonic ventral mesogastrium. SYN ligamentum falciforme hepatis [TA].

**fal·ci·form pro·cess** a continuation of the inner border of the sacrotuberous ligament upward and forward on the inner aspect of the ramus of the ischium. SYN processus falciformis [TA], falciform ligament.

**fal·cip·a·rum ma·lar·ia** malaria caused by *Plasmodium falciparum* and characterized by malarial paroxysms of severe form that occur every 48 hours with acute cerebral, renal, or gastrointestinal manifestations in severe cases, chiefly caused by the large number of red blood cells affected and the tendency for infected red cells to become sticky and clump, thus blocking capillaries. SYN malignant tertian malaria.

**fal·cu·la** (fal'kyu-lă) SYN falx cerebelli. [L. dim. of *falx*]

**fal·cu·lar** (fal'kyu-lăr) **1.** resembling a sickle or falx. **2.** relating to the falx cerebelli or cerebri.

**fal·lo·pi·an** (fa-lō'pē-an) described by or attributed to Gabriele Fallopio (1523–1562); usually referring to the uterine tube.

**fal·lo·pi·an tube** (fă-lō'pē-ăn) SYN uterine tube.

**Fal·lot tet·rad** (fă-lō') SYN tetralogy of Fallot.

**Fal·lot tri·ad** (fă-lō') SYN trilogy of Fallot.

**false ane·mia** SYN pseudoanemia.

**false an·eu·rysm 1.** pulsating, encapsulated hematoma in communication with the lumen of a ruptured vessel; **2.** ventricular pseudoaneurysm, a cardiac rupture contained and loculated by pericardium, which forms its external wall. **3.** an aneurysm whose walls consist of adventitia and periarterial fibrous tissue and hematoma.

**false an·ky·lo·sis** SYN fibrous ankylosis.

**false bleph·a·rop·to·sis** SYN pseudoptosis.

**false cast** an elongated, ribbon-like mucous thread with poorly defined edges and pointed or split ends, often confused with a true urinary cast. SYN pseudocast.

**false chor·dae ten·din·eae** tendinous cords that, unlike the true chordae tendineae, do not attach to the leaflets of the atrioventricular valves. Instead they connect papillary muscles to each other or to the ventricular wall (including the interventricular septum), or merely pass between two points on the ventricular wall (including the septum). SYN chordae tendineae falsae [TA], chordae tendineae spuriae.

**False Claims Act (FCA)** Federal legislation that prohibits anyone from knowingly presenting a false or fraudulent claim to the federal government for payment. The act defines "knowingly" as either having actual knowledge that information is false or acting with reckless disregard of the truth or falsity of information.

**false con·ju·gate 1.** SYN diagonal conjugate. **2.** SYN effective conjugate.

**false di·ver·tic·u·lum** a diverticulum of the intestine that passes through a defect in the muscular wall of the gut and thus does not include a layer of muscle in its wall.

**false he·ma·tu·ria** SYN pseudohematuria.

**false her·maph·ro·dit·ism** SYN pseudohermaphroditism.

**false im·age** the image in the deviating eye in strabismus.

**false joint** SYN pseudarthrosis.

**false lu·men** in a dissecting aneurysm, the abnormal channel within the wall of the involved artery.

**false mem·brane** a thick, tough fibrinous exudate on the surface of a mucous membrane or the skin, as seen in diphtheria. SYN croupous membrane, neomembrane, plica (2), pseudomembrane.

**false mem·o·ry syn·drome** an apparent memory of an imagined event, usually traumatic and remote in time; generally used pejoratively to imply that the memory was engendered by the therapist facilitating its recovery; a controversial concept.

**false neg·a·tive** (fawls neg'ă-tiv) **1.** a test result which erroneously excludes an individual from a specific diagnostic or reference group. **2.** an individual excluded by erroneous test results from a particular diagnostic group. **3.** a false-negative result.

**false-neg·a·tive re·ac·tion** an erroneous or mistakenly negative response.

**false neu·ro·ma** SYN traumatic neuroma.

**false pel·vis** SYN greater pelvis.

**false pos·i·tive** (fawls pos'i-tiv) **1.** a test result which erroneously assigns an individual to a specific diagnostic or reference group. **2.** an individual included by erroneous test results in a particular diagnostic group. **3.** a false-positive result.

**false-pos·i·tive re·ac·tion** an erroneous or mistakenly positive response.

**false preg·nan·cy** a condition in which some signs and symptoms suggest pregnancy, although the woman is not pregnant. SYN pseudocyesis, pseudopregnancy (1).

**false ribs** five lower ribs on either side that do not articulate with the sternum directly. SYN costae spuriae [TA].

**false su·ture** one whose opposing margins are smooth or present only a few ill-defined projections.

**fal·set·to** (fahl-sĕt'ō) high-pitched voice produced by vibration of the anterior third of the vocal folds while the posterior folds are tightly adducted. SEE ALSO voice. [Ital., unnatural voice, fr. *falso,* false, + *-etto,* dim. suff.]

**false vo·cal cord** SYN vestibular fold.

**false wa·ters** a leakage of fluid prior to or in beginning labor, before the rupture of the amnion.

**fal·si·fi·ca·tion** (fawl'si-fi-kā'shŭn) the deliberate act of misrepresentation so as to deceive. [L. *falsus,* false, + *facio,* to make]

**falx**, pl. **fal·ces** (falks, fal'sēz) [TA] a sickle-shaped structure. [L. sickle]

**falx ce·re·bel·li** [TA] a short process of dura mater projecting forward from the internal occipital crest below the tentorium; it occupies the posterior cerebellar notch and the vallecula, and bifurcates below into two diverging limbs passing to either side of the foramen magnum. SYN falcula.

**falx ce·re·bri** [TA] the scythe-shaped fold of dura mater in the longitudinal fissure between the two cerebral hemispheres; it is attached anteriorly to the crista galli of the ethmoid bone and caudally to the upper surface of the tentorium.

**falx in·gui·na·lis** [TA] SYN inguinal falx.

**fa·mil·i·al** (fa-mil'ē-ăl) affecting more members of the same family than can be accounted for by chance, usually within a single sibship; commonly but incorrectly used to mean genetic. [L. *familia,* family]

**fa·mil·i·al ade·no·mat·ous pol·y·po·sis (FAP)** polyposis of the colon that usually begins in childhood; polyps increase in number, causing symptoms of chronic colitis; pigmented retinal lesions are frequently found; carcinoma of the colon almost invariably develops in untreated cases; autosomal dominant inheritance, caused by mutation in the adenomatous polyposis coli gene (APC) on 5q. In Gardner syndrome, which is allelic to FAP, there are extracolonic changes (desmoid tumors, osteomas, jaw cysts). SYN adenomatous polyposis coli, familial polyposis coli.

**fa·mil·i·al ag·gre·ga·tion** occurrence of a trait in more members of a family than can be readily accounted for by chance; presumptive but not cogent evidence of the operation of genetic factors.

**fa·mil·i·al a·min·o·gly·co·side o·to·tox·i·ci·ty** inherited susceptibility to sensory hearing loss upon administration of aminoglycoside antibiotics due to a mutation in the mitochondrial genome.

**fa·mil·i·al am·y·loid neu·rop·a·thy** a disorder in which various peripheral nerves are infiltrated with amyloid and their functions disturbed, an abnormal prealbumin is also formed and is present in the blood; characteristically, it begins during mid-life and is found largely in persons of Portuguese descent; autosomal dominant inheritance. Other rare clinical types occur.

**fa·mil·i·al dys·au·to·no·mia** a congenital syndrome with aberrations in autonomic nervous system function such as indifference to pain, diminished lacrimation, poor vasomotor homeostasis, motor incoordination, labile cardiovascular reactions, hyporeflexia, frequent attacks of bronchial pneumonia, hypersalivation with aspiration and difficulty in swallowing, hyperemesis, emotional instability, and an intolerance for anesthetics.

**fa·mil·i·al eryth·ro·pha·go·cy·tic lym·pho··his·ti·o·cy·tosis (FEL)** SYN familial hemophagocytic lymphohistiocytosis.

**fa·mil·i·al fat-in·duced hy·per·li·pe·mia** SYN type I familial hyperlipoproteinemia.

**fa·mil·i·al goi·ter** a group of heritable thyroid disorders in which goiter is commonly apparent first during childhood; often associated with skeletal and/or mental retardation, and with other signs of hypothyroidism that may develop with age.

**fa·mil·i·al he·mo·pha·go·cy·tic lymph·o·his··ti·o·cy·to·sis (FMLH)** an extremely rare, usually fatal disease of childhood characterized by multiorgan infiltration with activated macrophages and lymphocytes. The disease is often familial and appears to be inherited as an autosomal recessive trait. SYN familial erythrophagocytic lymphohistiocytosis.

**fa·mil·i·al hy·per·cho·les·ter·ol·e·mia** SYN type II familial hyperlipoproteinemia.

**fa·mil·i·al hy·per·cho·les·ter·ol·e·mia with hy·per·li·pe·mia** SYN type III familial hyperlipoproteinemia.

**fa·mil·i·al hy·per·chy·lo·mi·cro·ne·mia** SYN type I familial hyperlipoproteinemia.

**fa·mi·li·al hy·per·lip·o·pro·tein·e·mia** a group of diseases characterized by changes in concentration of β-lipoproteins and pre-β-lipoproteins and the lipids associated with them.

**fa·mil·i·al hy·per·tri·glyc·er·i·de·mia 1.** SYN type I familial hyperlipoproteinemia. **2.** SYN type IV familial hyperlipoproteinemia.

**fa·mil·i·al hy·per·tro·phic car·di·o·my·op·a··thy** familial form of hypertrophic cardiomyopathy.

**fa·mil·i·al jaun·dice** SYN hereditary spherocytosis.

**fa·mil·i·al non·he·mo·lyt·ic jaun·dice** mild jaundice due to increased amounts of unconjugated bilirubin in the plasma without evidence of liver damage, biliary obstruction, or hemolysis; thought to be due to an inborn error of metabolism in which the excretion of bilirubin by the liver is defective. SYN Gilbert disease.

**fa·mil·i·al par·ox·ys·mal pol·y·ser·o·si·tis** transient recurring attacks of abdominal pain, fever, pleurisy, arthritis, and rash; the condition is asymptomatic between attacks.

**fa·mil·i·al par·tial lip·o·dys·tro·phy** characterized by symmetric lipoatrophy of the trunk and limbs but the face is spared; with full rounded face, xanthomata, acanthosis nigricans, and insulin-resistant hyperglycemia; there is accumulation of fat around the neck and shoulders and genitalia. SYN Kobberling-Dunnigan syndrome.

**fa·mil·i·al pe·ri·od·ic pa·ral·y·sis** inherited muscle disorder manifested as recurrent episodes of marked generalized weakness. SEE hyperkalemic periodic paralysis, hypokalemic periodic paralysis, normokalemic periodic paralysis.

**fa·mil·i·al pol·yp·o·sis co·li** SYN familial adenomatous polyposis.

**fa·mil·i·al pseu·do·in·flam·ma·to·ry mac·u·lar de·gen·er·a·tion** macular degeneration that occurs during the fifth decade of life, with sudden development of a central scotoma in one eye followed rapidly by a similar lesion in the opposite eye. SYN Sorsby macular degeneration.

**fa·mil·i·al screen·ing** screening directed at close relatives of probands with diseases that may lie latent, as in age-dependent dominant traits, or that may involve risk to progeny, as X-linked traits.

**fam·i·ly** (fam′ĭ-lē) **1.** a group of two or more persons united by blood, adoptive, or marital ties, or the common law equivalent. **2.** in biologic classification, a taxonomic grouping at the level intermediate between the order and the tribe or genus. **3.** a group of substances closely related structurally. **4.** a group of proteins with characteristic sequence, pharmacologic, and/or signaling profiles. [L. *familia*]

**fam·i·ly med·i·cine** the medical specialty concerned with providing continuous, comprehensive care to all age groups, from first patient contact to terminal care, with special emphasis on care of the family as a unit.

**fam·i·ly prac·tice** a specialty of medicine in which the physician takes responsibility for the health and medical care of all members of a family group, regardless of age or gender, but usually does limited amounts of obstetrics and surgery.

**fam·i·ly ther·a·py** a type of group psychotherapy in which a family in conflict meets as a group with the therapist and explores its relationships and processes; focus is on the resolution of current issues between members rather than on individual members.

**Fan·co·ni a·ne·mia** (fahn-kō′nē) a type of idiopathic refractory anemia characterized by pancytopenia, hypoplasia of the bone marrow, and congenital anomalies, occurring in members of the same family (an autosomal recessive trait in at least five nonallelic types; the anemia is normocytic or slightly macrocytic, macrocytes and target cells may be found in the circulating blood, and the leukopenia usually is due to neutropenia. Congenital anomalies include short stature; microcephaly; hypogenitalism; strabismus; anomalies of the thumbs, radii, kidneys, and urinary tract; mental retardation; and microphthalmia. SYN Fanconi syndrome (1).

**Fan·co·ni syn·drome** (fahn-kō′nē) **1.** SYN Fanconi anemia. **2.** a group of conditions with characteristic disorders of renal tubular function, which may be classified as: 1) cystinosis, an autosomal recessive disease of early childhood; 2) adult Fanconi syndrome, a rare hereditary form,

probably due to a recessive gene different from that found in cystinosis, characterized by the tubular malfunction seen in cystinosis and by osteomalacia, but without cystine deposit in tissues; 3) acquired Fanconi syndrome, which may be associated with multiple myeloma or may result from chemical poisoning, injury, or persisting damage of proximal tubular epithelium due to various causes, leading to multiple defects of tubular function.

**fan·ta·sy** (fan′tă-sē) imagery that is more or less coherent, as in dreams and daydreams, yet unrestricted by reality. SYN phantasia. [G. *phantasia*, idea, image]

**FAP** familial adenomatous polyposis.

**Fa·ra·beuf am·pu·ta·tion** (fahr′ă-boof) **1.** amputation of the leg, the flap being large and on the outer side; **2.** amputation of the foot; disarticulation of the foot through the subtalar joint and the talo-navicular joint.

**Fa·ra·beuf tri·an·gle** (fahr′ă-boof) the triangle formed by the internal jugular and facial veins and the hypoglossal nerve.

**far·ad** (**F**) (fa′rad) a practical unit of electrical capacity; the capacity of a condenser having a charge of 1 coulomb under an electromotive force of 1 volt. [M. *Faraday*]

**Fa·ra·day** (far′ă-dā), Michael, English physicist and chemist, 1791–1867. SEE farad, faraday.

**far·a·day** (**F**, *F*) (fa′ră-dā) 96,485.309 coulombs per mole, the amount of electricity required to reduce one equivalent of a monovalent ion. [M. *Faraday*]

**Far·a·day con·stant** (*F*) (far′ă-dā) SEE faraday.

**Far·a·day laws** (far′ă-dā) **1.** the amount of an electrolyte decomposed by an electric current is proportional to the amount of the current; **2.** when the same current is passed through several electrolytes, the amounts of the different substances decomposed are proportional to their chemical equivalents.

**far-and-near su·ture** a suture consisting of alternate near and far stitches, used to approximate fascial edges.

**far·del** (far′del) the total measurable penalty that is incurred as a result of the occurrence of a genetic disease in one individual; one of two major quantitative considerations in the prognostic aspects of genetic counseling, the other being risk of occurrence. [M.E., fr. O. Fr., fr. Ar. *fardah*, bundle]

**farm·er's lung** a hypersensitivity pneumonitis characterized by fever and dyspnea, caused by inhalation of organic dust from moldy hay containing spores of actinomycetes and certain true fungi, which thrive in the elevated temperatures of hay lofts and silos.

**far point** that point in conjugate focus with the retina when the eye is not accommodating.

**Far·rant mount·ing flu·id** (far′ănt) an aqueous solution containing gum arabic, arsenic trioxide, glycerol, and water, used in mounting histologic sections directly from water; some modifications involve addition of potassium acetate to bring the pH up to neutrality and substitution of other preservatives like cresol or thymol for arsenic trioxide.

**Farr laws** (fahr) a set of mathematical formulae, axioms, and laws first enunciated in the annual reports submitted by William Farr to the Registrar General of England and Wales from 1839 to

1883. The laws deal with the relationship of incidence to prevalence, the natural history of epidemics, and mathematical features of common types of epidemic.

**far·sight·ed·ness** (far'sīt'ed-nes) SYN hyperopia.

**fart·lek train·ing** (fart'lek trān'ing) relatively unstructured interval-type training for aerobic fitness; consists of alternating intervals of fast and slow paced training over natural terrain (usually hilly countryside). SYN speed play. [Swed. *fart,* speed, + *lek,* play]

**Fas** a receptor present in cells that binds with Fas ligand to induce apoptosis. SEE ALSO Fas ligand.

**fas·cia,** pl. **fas·ci·ae, fas·ci·as** (fash'ē-ă, fash'ē-ē, fash'ē-ăs) [TA] a sheet of fibrous tissue that envelops the body beneath the skin; it also encloses muscles and groups of muscles, and separates their several layers or groups. [L. a band or fillet]

**fas·cia ad·he·rens** a broad intercellular junction in the intercalated disk of cardiac muscle that anchors actin filaments.

**fas·cia graft** a graft of fibrous tissue, usually the fascia lata.

**fas·cial** (fash'ē-ăl) relating to any fascia.

**fas·cial sheath of eye·ball** a condensation of connective tissue on the outer aspect of the sclera from which it is separated by a narrow cleftlike episcleral space; the sheath is attached to the sclera near the sclerocorneal junction and blends with the fascia of the extraocular muscles. SYN Tenon capsule.

**fas·cia mus·cu·li quad·ra·ti lum·bor·um** SYN anterior layer of thoracolumbar fascia.

**fas·cia pe·ri·nei su·per·fi·ci·a·lis** [TA] SYN superficial fascia of perineum.

**fas·ci·as** (fash'ē-ăs)

**fas·cia sub·per·i·to·ne·a·lis** [TA] SYN extraperitoneal fascia.

**fas·ci·cle** (fas'i-kl) a band or bundle of fibers, usually of muscle or nerve fibers; a nerve fiber tract. SYN fasciculus [TA].

**fas·cic·u·lar** (fa-sik'yu-lăr) relating to a fasciculus; arranged in the form of a bundle or collection of rods.

**fas·cic·u·lar de·gen·er·a·tion** muscular degeneration due to loss of motor neurons in the spinal cord or brainstem.

**fas·cic·u·lar graft** a nerve graft in which each bundle of fibers is approximated and sutured separately.

**fas·cic·u·la·tion** (fa-sik-yu-lā'shŭn) **1.** an arrangement in the form of fasciculi. **2.** involuntary contractions, or twitchings, of groups (fasciculi) of muscle fibers, a coarser form of muscular contraction than fibrillation.

**fas·cic·u·li** (fa-sik'yu-lī) plural of fasciculus.

**fas·cic·u·li pro·prii** [TA] Flechsig fasciculi or ground bundles (fasciculus anterior proprius and fasciculus lateralis proprius or lateral ground bundle); intersegmental fasciculi; ascending and descending association fiber systems of the spinal cord which lie deep in the anterior, lateral, and posterior funiculi adjacent to the gray matter. SYN ground bundles.

**fas·cic·u·lus,** gen. and pl. **fas·cic·u·li** (fă-sik'yu-lŭs, fa-sik'yu-lī) [TA] SYN fascicle. [L. dim. of *fascis,* bundle]

**fas·cic·u·lus lon·gi·tu·di·na·lis in·fe·ri·or** [TA] SYN inferior longitudinal fasciculus.

**fas·cic·u·lus lon·gi·tu·di·na·lis su·pe·ri·or** [TA] SYN superior longitudinal fasciculus.

**fas·ci·ec·to·my** (fash-ē-ek'tō-mē) excision of strips of fascia. [fascia + G. *ektomē,* excision]

**fas·ci·i·tis** (fash-ē-ī'tis) **1.** inflammation in fascia. **2.** reactive proliferation of fibroblasts in fascia.

△**fas·cio-** a fascia. [L. *fascia,* a band or fillet]

**fas·ci·od·e·sis** (fash-ē-od'ē-sis) surgical attachment of a fascia to another fascia or a tendon. [fascio- + G. *desis,* a binding together]

**fas·ci·o·la,** pl. **fas·ci·o·lae** (fa-sh-ē'ō-lă, fa-sh-ē' ō-lē) a small band or group of fibers. [L. dim. of *fascia,* band, fillet]

**fas·ci·o·lar** (fa-sh-ē'ō-lăr) relating to the gyrus fasciolaris.

**fas·ci·o·plas·ty** (fa-sh'ē-ō-plas-tē) plastic surgery of a fascia. [fascia + G. *plastos,* formed]

**fas·ci·or·rha·phy** (fa-sh-ē-ōr'ă-fē) suture of a fascia or aponeurosis. SYN aponeurorrhaphy. [fascio- + G. *rhaphē,* suture]

**fas·ci·ot·o·my** (fash-ē-ot'ō-mē) incision through a fascia; used in the treatment of certain vascular disorders and injuries when marked swelling is anticipated which could compromise blood flow; fasciotomy may be combined with embolectomy in the treatment of acute arterial embolism. [fascio- + G. *tomē,* incision]

**Fas li·gand** a molecule on the surface of cytotoxic T cells that binds to its receptor, Fas, on the surface of other cells, initiating apoptosis in the target cell. SEE ALSO Fas.

**Fas re·cep·tor** SEE Fas.

**fast 1.** durable; resistant to change; applied to stained microorganisms which cannot be decolorized. SEE ALSO acid-fast. **2.** not eating. [A.S. *foest,* firm, fixed]

**fast com·po·nent of ny·stag·mus** compensatory movement of the eyes in the vestibuloocular reflex.

**fas·tid·i·ous** (fas-tid'ē-ŭs) in bacteriology, having complex nutritional requirements.

**fas·tig·i·al nu·cle·us** the most medial of the cerebellar nuclei, lying medial to the interpositus nucleus, near the midline, in the white matter underneath the vermis of the cerebellar cortex. It receives the axons of Purkinje cells from all parts of the vermis. Its major projection is to the vestibular nuclei and medullary reticular formation.

**fas·tig·i·um** (fas-tij'ē-ŭm) **1.** [TA] apex of the roof of the fourth ventricle of the brain, an angle formed by the anterior and posterior medullary vela extending into the substance of the vermis. **2.** the acme or period of full development of a disease. [L. top, as of a gable; a pointed extremity]

**fast-neut·ron ra·di·a·tion ther·a·py** radiation therapy using high-energy neutrons from cyclotrons or proton accelerators.

**fast smear** a cytologic smear containing material from the vaginal pool and pancervical scrapings, mixed and prepared on one microscopic slide, smeared, and fixed immediately; used principally for routine screening of ovaries, endometrium, cervix, vagina, and hormonal states.

**fat 1.** SYN adipose tissue. **2.** common term for obese. **3.** a greasy, soft-solid material, found in animal tissues and many plants, composed of a mixture of glycerol esters; together with oils they make up the homolipids. **4.** a triacylglycerol or a mixture of triacylglycerols. [A.S. *faet*]

**fa·tal** (fā'tăl) pertaining to or causing death; denoting especially inevitability or inescapability of death. [L. *fatalis,* of or belonging to fate]

**fa·tal·i·ty rate** the death rate observed in a designated series of persons affected by a simultaneous event such as a disaster.

**fat cell** a connective tissue cell distended with one or more fat globules, the cytoplasm usually being compressed into a thin envelope, with the nucleus at one point in the periphery. SYN adipocyte, adipose cell.

**fat em·bo·lism** the occurrence of fat globules in the circulation following fractures of a long bone, in burns, in parturition, and in association with fatty degeneration of the liver; the emboli most commonly block pulmonary or cerebral vessels when symptoms referable to either or both of these regions appear.

**fat-free bo·dy mass (FFM)** body mass devoid of storage fat; a theoretical entity that contains the small percentage of non-sex-specific essential fat equivalent to approximately 3% of body mass (located chiefly within the central nervous system, bone marrow, and internal organs). SYN lean body mass.

**fat·i·ga·bil·i·ty** (fat′i-gă-bil′i-tē) a condition in which fatigue is easily induced.

**fa·tigue** (fă-tēg′) **1.** that state, following a period of mental or bodily activity, characterized by a lessened capacity for work and reduced efficiency of accomplishment, usually accompanied by a feeling of weariness, sleepiness, or irritability; may also supervene when, from any cause, energy expenditure outstrips restorative processes and may be confined to a single organ. **2.** sensation of boredom and lassitude due to absence of stimulation, monotony, or lack of interest in one's surroundings. [Fr., fr. L. *fatigo,* to tire]

**fat ne·cro·sis** the death of adipose tissue, characterized by the formation of small (1–4 mm), dull, chalky, gray or white foci. SYN steatonecrosis.

**fat-pad, fat pad** an accumulation of somewhat encapsulated adipose tissue.

**fat-sol·u·ble vi·ta·mins** those vitamins, soluble in fat solvents (nonpolar solvents) and relatively insoluble in water, marked in chemical structure by the presence of large hydrocarbon moieties in the molecule; e.g., vitamins A, D, E, K.

**fat-stor·ing cell** a multilocular fat-filled cell present in the perisinusoidal space in the liver. SYN lipocyte.

**fat tide** an increase in the fat content of blood and lymph following a meal.

**fat·ty** (fat′ē) oily or greasy; relating in any sense to fat.

**fat·ty ac·id** any acid derived from fats by hydrolysis (e.g., oleic, palmitic, or stearic acids); any long-chain monobasic organic acid; they accumulate in disorders associated with the peroxisomes.

**fat·ty ac·id–bind·ing pro·tein** SYN Z-protein.

**fat·ty ac·id ox·i·da·tion cy·cle** a series of reactions involving acyl-coenzyme A compounds; the major pathway of fatty acid catabolism in living tissue.

**ω-3 fat·ty ac·ids** a class of fatty acids that have a double bond three carbons from the methyl moiety; reportedly, they play a role in lowering cholesterol and LDL levels.

**fat·ty cir·rho·sis** early nutritional cirrhosis, especially in alcoholics, in which the liver is enlarged by fatty change, with mild fibrosis.

**fat·ty de·gen·er·a·tion** abnormal formation of microscopically visible droplets of fat in the cytoplasm of cells, as a result of injury. SYN adipose degeneration, steatosis (2).

**fat·ty heart 1.** fatty degeneration of the myocardium; **2.** accumulation of adipose tissue on the external surface of the heart with occasional infiltration of fat between the muscle bundles of the heart wall. SYN adiposis cardiaca, cor adiposum.

**fat·ty her·nia** SYN pannicular hernia.

**fat·ty in·fil·tra·tion** abnormal accumulation of fat droplets in the cytoplasm of cells, particularly of fat derived from outside the cells. SEE ALSO fatty degeneration.

**fat·ty kid·ney** a kidney in which there is fatty metamorphosis of the parenchymal cells, especially fatty degeneration.

**fat·ty liv·er** yellow discoloration of the liver due to fatty degeneration of liver parenchymal cells.

**fat·ty met·a·mor·pho·sis** the appearance of microscopically visible droplets of fat in the cytoplasm of cells. SEE ALSO fatty degeneration.

**fat·ty oil** an oil derived from both animals and plants; chemically, a glyceride of a fatty acid which, by substitution of the glycerine with an alkaline base, is converted into a soap; a fatty oil, in contrast to a volatile oil, is permanent and not capable of distillation.

**fau·ces,** gen. **fau·ci·um** (faw′sēz, faw′sē-ŭm) [TA] the space between the cavity of the mouth and the pharynx, bounded by the soft palate and the base of the tongue. [L. the throat]

**fau·cial** (faw′shăl) relating to the fauces.

**fau·cial ton·sil** SYN palatine tonsil.

**faul·ty un·ion** SYN fibrous union. SEE vicious union.

**fau·na** (faw′nă) the animal forms of a continent, district, locality, or habitat. [Mod. L. application of *Fauna,* sister of *Faunus,* a rural deity]

**fa·ve·o·late** (fā-vē′ō-lāt) pitted.

**fa·ve·o·lus,** pl. **fa·ve·o·li** (fā-vē′ō-lŭs, fā-vē′ō-lī) a small pit or depression. [Mod. L. dim. of *favus,* honeycomb]

**fa·vid** (fā′vid) an allergic reaction in the skin observed in patients who have favus.

**fa·vism** (fā′vizm) an acute condition seen following the ingestion of certain species of beans, e.g., *Vicia faba,* or inhalation of the pollen of its flower, in individuals with genetic erythrocytic deficiency of glucose 6-phosphate dehydrogenase; characterized by fever, headache, abdominal pain, severe anemia, prostration, and coma. [Ital. *favismo,* from *fava,* bean]

**Fav·re dys·tro·phy** (fahv′rĕ) SYN vitreotapetoretinal dystrophy.

**Fav·re-Ra·cou·chot dis·ease** (fahv′rĕ-ra-coo-shō) comedones developing on sun-damaged skin due to obstruction of pilosebaceous follicles by solar elastosis. SYN solar comedo.

**fa·vus** (fā′vŭs, fah′vŭs) a severe type of chronic ringworm of the scalp and nails; it occurs more frequently in the Mediterranean countries, southeastern Europe, southern Asia, and northern Africa. Differences in severity are related to hygiene. [L. honeycomb]

**Fa·zi·o-Londe dis·ease** (fahz′ē-ō-lōnd) a progressive bulbar palsy affecting the brainstem; due to motor neuron degeneration; a variant of spinal muscular atrophy.

**FCA** False Claims Act.

**Fc frag·ment, Fc** the crystallizable fragment of

an immunoglobulin molecule composed of part of the heavy chains and responsible for binding to antibody receptors on cells and the Clq component of complement.

**FDA** Food and Drug Administration of the United States Department of Health and Human Services.

**F.D.I. den·tal no·men·cla·ture** 1. A system of identifying teeth used worldwide that identifies each dental quadrant (1 through 4 for the permanent teeth and 5 through 8 for the deciduous teeth) and each tooth with a number indicating its location from the midline; e.g., 36 is the lower left first permanent molar and 62 is the upper left deciduous lateral incisor. 2. A system devised by the Fédération Dentaire Internationale.

**Fe** iron. [L. *ferrum,* iron]

**fear** (fēr) apprehension; dread; alarm; by having an identifiable stimulus, fear is differentiated from anxiety, which has no easily identifiable stimulus. [A.S. *faer*]

**feb·rile** (feb′ril, fē′brīl) denoting or relating to fever. SYN feverish (1), pyretic.

**feb·rile con·vul·sion** a brief seizure, lasting less than 15 minutes, seen in a neurologically normal infant or young child, associated with fever.

**fe·cal** (fē′kăl) relating to feces.

**fe·cal ab·scess** SYN stercoral abscess.

**fe·cal con·cen·tra·tion** preparation using centrifugation and either flotation or sedimentation methods to separate parasitic elements from fecal debris.

**fe·cal ex·am·i·na·tion** microscopic review of direct wet mounts, concentration methods, and permanent stained smears to recover and identify parasites from stool specimens.

**fe·cal fis·tu·la** SYN intestinal fistula.

**fe·cal·ith** (fē′kă-lith) SYN coprolith. [L. *faeces,* feces, + G. *lithos,* stone]

**fe·cal·oid** (fē′kă-loyd) resembling feces. [L. *faeces,* feces, + G. *eidos,* resemblance]

**fe·ca·lo·ma** (fē′kă-lō-mă) SYN coproma.

**fe·ca·lu·ria** (fē-kăl-yur′ē-ă) the commingling of feces with urine passed from the urethra in persons with a fistula connecting the intestinal tract and bladder. [L. *faeces,* feces, + G. *ouron,* urine]

**fe·cal vom·it·ing** vomitus with appearance and/or odor of feces suggestive of long-standing distal small bowel or colonic obstruction. SYN copremesis, stercoraceous vomiting.

**fe·ces** (fē′sēz) the matter discharged from the bowel during defecation, consisting of the undigested residue of the food, epithelium, the intestinal mucus, bacteria, and waste material from the food. SYN stercus. [L., pl. of *faex* (*faec-*), dregs]

**Fech·ner-Web·er law** (fek′ner-vā′ber) SYN Weber-Fechner law.

**fec·u·lent** (fek′yu-lent) foul. [L. *faeculentus,* full of excrement, fr. *faeces,* dregs, feces]

**fe·cund** (fē′kŭnd, fek′ŭnd) SYN fertile (1). [L. *fecundus,* fruitful]

**fe·cun·da·tion** (fē-kŭn-dā′shŭn) the act of rendering fertile. SEE ALSO fertilization.

**fe·cun·di·ty** (fē-kŭn′di-tē) the ability to produce live offspring.

**feed·back** (fēd′bak) **1.** in a given system, the return, as input, of some of the output, as a regulatory mechanism; e.g., regulation of a furnace by a thermostat. **2.** an explanation for the learning of motor skills: sensory stimuli set up by muscle contractions modulate the activity of the motor

system. **3.** the feeling evoked by another person's reaction to oneself. SEE biofeedback.

**feed·back in·hi·bi·tion** inhibition of activity by an end product of the pathway of which that activity is a part. SYN feedback mechanism.

**feed·back mech·an·ism** SYN feedback inhibition.

**feed·ing** (fēd′ing) giving food or nourishment.

**feed·ing tube** a flexible tube passed through the oral pharynx and into the esophagus and stomach, through which liquid food is fed.

**fee-for-ser·vice** payment made at the time of health care service; the amount varies according to the provider's estimate of the costs involved.

**fee-for-ser·vice in·sur·ance** insurance coverage that reimburses participants and providers following submission of a claim. Participants have few if any restrictions on which hospitals or doctors to use.

**Feer dis·ease** (fār) SYN acrodynia (2).

**FEES** fiberoptic endoscopic examination of swallowing.

**FEF** forced expiratory flow.

**FEL** familial erythrophagocytic lymphohistiocytosis.

**fe·line in·fec·tious a·ne·mi·a (FIA)** an acute or chronic anemia of domestic cats caused by the rickettsia *Haemobartonella felis.*

**fel·la·tio** (fē-lā′shē-ō) oral stimulation of the penis. [L.]

**fel·on** (fel′ŏn) a purulent infection or abscess involving the bulbous distal end of a finger. SYN whitlow. [M.E. *feloun,* malignant]

**felt·work 1.** a fibrous network. **2.** a close plexus of nerve fibrils. SEE neuropil.

**fe·male** (fē′māl) ZOOLOGY denoting the sex that bears the young or the ovum.

**fe·male ath·lete tri·ad** a combination of disordered eating, amenorrhea, and osteoporosis, commonly seen in adolescent and young adult female athletes.

**fe·male cath·e·ter** a short, nearly straight catheter for passage into the female bladder.

**fe·male cir·cum·ci·sion** a broad term referring to many forms of female genital cutting, ranging from removal of the clitoral prepuce to the removal of the clitoris, labia minora and parts of the labia majora, and infibulation; done for cultural, not medical, reasons.

**fe·male pat·tern al·o·pe·cia** diffuse partial hair loss in the centroparietal area of the scalp, with preservation of the frontal and temporal hair lines; the most frequent type of androgenic alopecia in women. See page 357.

**fe·male pseu·do·her·ma·phro·di·tism** pseudohermaphroditism with skeletal and genital anomalies but with female gonads and an XX karyotype. SYN androgyny (1).

**fem·i·nin·i·ty com·plex** PSYCHOANALYSIS the unconscious fear, in boys and men, of castration at the hands of the mother with resultant identification with the aggressor and envious desire for breasts and vagina.

**fem·i·ni·za·tion** (fem′i-ni-zā′shŭn) development of what are superficially external female characteristics by a male.

**fem·o·ral** (fem′ŏ-răl) relating to the femur or thigh.

**fem·o·ral ar·tery** *origin,* continuation of external iliac, beginning at inguinal ligament; *branches,* external pudendal, superficial epigastric, superficial circumflex iliac, profunda femoris, descending genicular, terminating as the popliteal artery as it passes through the adductor hiatus to enter the popliteal space. SYN arteria femoralis [TA].

**fem·o·ral ca·nal** the medial compartment of the femoral sheath. SYN canalis femoralis [TA].

**fem·o·ral her·nia** hernia through the femoral ring. SYN crural hernia, femorocele.

**fem·o·ral nerve** arises from the second, third, and fourth lumbar nerves in the substance of the psoas muscle and enters the thigh via the muscular lacuna beneath the inguinal ligament, lateral to the femoral vessels; it arborize within the femoral triangle into muscle branches to the sartorius, pectineus and quadriceps muscles and anterior femoral cutaneous nerves to the skin of the anterior and medial region of the thigh; its terminal branch is the saphenous nerve by which it supplies the skin of the medial leg and foot. SYN nervus femoralis [TA].

**fem·o·ral nut·ri·ent ar·tery** one of two arteries, superior and inferior, arising from the first and third perforating arteries, respectively (sometimes second and fourth).

**fem·o·ral sheath** the fascia enclosing the femoral vessels, formed by the transversalis fascia anteriorly and the iliac fascia posteriorly; two septa divide the sheath into three compartments, the lateral of which contains the femoral artery and the femoral branch of the genitofemoral nerve, the middle the femoral vein, and the medial is the femoral canal. SYN crural sheath.

**fem·o·ral tri·an·gle** a triangular space at the upper part of the thigh, bounded by the sartorius and adductor longus muscles and the inguinal ligament, with a floor formed laterally by the iliopsoas muscle and medially by the pectineus muscle; the branches of the femoral nerve are distributed within the femoral triangle; it is bisected by the femoral vessels, which enter the adductor canal at its apex. SYN trigonum femorale [TA], Scarpa triangle.

**fem·o·ral vein** a continuation of the popliteal vein; it accompanies the femoral artery through the adductor canal and into the femoral triangle where it lies within the femoral sheath; it becomes the external iliac vein as it passes deep to inguinal ligament. SYN vena femoralis [TA].

**fem·o·ro·cele** (fem′ŏ-rō-sēl) SYN femoral hernia. [L. *femur*, thigh, + G. *kēlē*, hernia]

**fem·o·ro·tib·i·al** (fem′ŏ-rō-tib′ē-ăl) relating to the femur and the tibia.

⚠**fem·to-** (f) SI and metric systems to signify one-quadrillionth ($10^{-15}$). [Danish and Norwegian *femten*, fifteen]

**fe·mur**, gen. **fe·mo·ris**, pl. **fem·o·ra** (fē′mŭr, fem′ŏ-ris, fem′ŏ-r-ă) [TA] **1.** the thigh. **2.** the long bone of the thigh, articulating with the hip bone proximally and the tibia and patella distally. SYN thigh bone. [L. thigh]

**fe·nes·tra**, pl. **fe·nes·trae** (fe-nes′tră, fe-nes′trē) **1.** an anatomic aperture, often closed by a membrane. **2.** an opening left in a cast or other form of fixed dressing in order to permit access to a wound or inspection of the part. **3.** the opening in one of the blades of an obstetrical forceps. **4.** a lateral opening in the sheath of an endoscopic instrument that allows lateral viewing or operative maneuvering through the sheath. **5.** openings in the wall of a tube, catheter, or trocar designed to promote better flow of air or fluids. SYN window. [L. window]

**fe·nes·tra co·chle·ae** [TA] an opening on the medial wall of the middle ear leading into the cochlea, closed in life by the secondary tympanic membrane. SYN round window.

**fen·es·trat·ed** (fen′es-trā′ted) having fenestrae or window-like openings.

**fen·es·trat·ed cap·il·lary** a capillary, found in renal glomeruli, intestinal villi, and some glands, in which ultramicroscopic pores of variable size occur.

**fen·es·trat·ed mem·brane** an elastic membrane, as in elastic laminae of arteries.

**fen·es·tra·tion** (fen-es-trā′shŭn) **1.** the presence of openings or fenestrae in a part. **2.** making openings in a dressing to allow inspection of the parts. **3.** DENTISTRY a surgical perforation of the mucoperiosteum and alveolar process to expose the root tip of a tooth to permit drainage of tissue exudate.

f
e

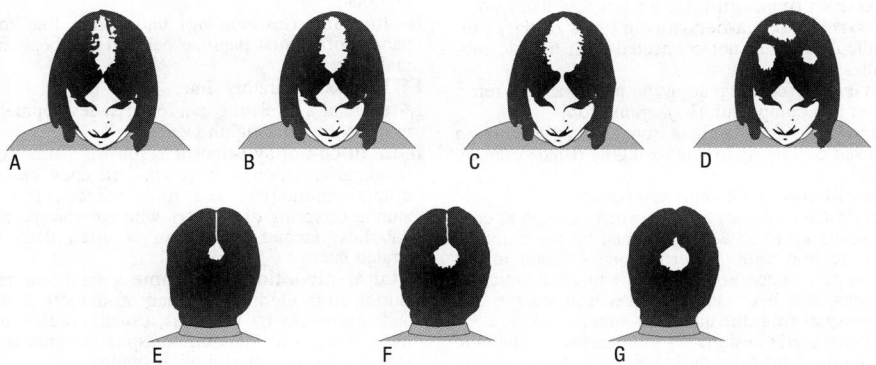

A          B                    C          D

E          F          G

**alopecia: female pattern alopecia,** (A) mild vertex hair loss, (B) moderate vertex hair loss, (C) more advanced vertex hair loss, (D) patchy hair loss; **male pattern alopecia,** (E) mild vertex hair loss, (F) moderate vertex hair loss, (G) more advanced vertex hair loss

**fe·nes·tra ves·tib·u·li** [TA] an oval opening on the medial wall of the tympanic cavity leading into the vestibule, closed by the foot of the stapes. SYN oval window.

**Fer·gu·son ref·lex** (fer′gŭ-sŏn) enhancement of uterine activity due to mechanical stretching of the lower uterine segment and cervix.

**Fer·gus·son in·ci·sion** (fer′gŭ-sŏn) an incision used in maxillectomy, along the junction of the nose and cheek, and bisecting the upper lip.

**fer·ment** (fer-ment′) to cause or to undergo fermentation. [L. *fermentum,* leaven]

**fer·men·ta·tion** (fer-men-tā′shŭn) **1.** a chemical change induced in a complex organic compound by the action of an enzyme, whereby the substance is split into simpler compounds. **2.** BACTERIOLOGY the anaerobic dissimilation of substrates with the production of energy and reduced compounds; the mechanism of fermentation does not involve a respiratory chain or cytochrome, hence oxygen is not the final electron acceptor as it is in oxidation. [L. *fermento,* pp. *-atus,* to ferment, from L. *fermentum,* yeast]

**fer·ment·a·tive** (fer-ment′ă-tiv) causing or having the ability to cause fermentation.

**fer·mi·um (Fm)** (fer′mē-ŭm) radioactive element, artificially prepared in 1955, atomic no. 100, atomic wt. 257.095; $^{257}$Fm has the longest known half-life (100.5 days). [E. *Fermi,* It.-U.S. physicist and Nobel laureate, 1901–1954]

**fern·ing** a term used to describe the pattern of arborization produced by a thin film of cervical mucus, secreted at midcycle, upon drying, which resembles somewhat a fern or a palm leaf.

**fern test 1.** a test for estrogenic activity; cervical mucus smears form a fern pattern at those times when estrogen secretion is elevated, as at the time of ovulation; **2.** a test to detect ruptured amniotic membranes.

**Fer·ra·ta cell** (fĕ-rah′tă) SYN hemohistioblast.

**fer·re·dox·ins** (fer-ĕ-dok′sinz) proteins containing iron and (labile) sulfur in equal amounts, displaying electron-carrier activity but no classical enzyme function. Ferredoxins are found in green plants, algae, and anaerobic bacteria, and are involved in several oxidation-reduction reactions in living organisms (e.g., nitrogen fixation).

**Fer·rein pyr·a·mid** (fer-ā′) SYN medullary ray.

**Fer·rein va·sa a·ber·ran·tia** (fer-ā′) biliary canaliculi that are not connected with hepatic lobules.

**△fer·ri-** prefix designating the presence of a ferric ion in a compound. [L. *ferrum,* iron]

**fer·ric** (fer′ik) relating to iron, especially denoting a salt containing iron in its higher (triad) valence, $Fe^{3+}$.

**fer·ri·heme** (fer′ē-hēm) SYN hematin.

**fer·ri·tin** (fer′ĭ-tin) an iron protein complex, containing up to 23% iron, formed by the union of ferric iron with apoferritin; it is found in the intestinal mucosa, spleen, bone marrow, reticulocytes, and liver, and regulates iron storage and transport from the intestinal lumen to plasma.

**△fer·ro-** prefix designating the presence of metallic iron or of the divalent ion $Fe^{2+}$. [L. *ferrum,* iron]

**fer·ro·ki·net·ics** (fār-ō-ki-net′iks) the study of iron metabolism using radioactive iron. [L. *ferrum,* iron, + G. *kinēsis,* movement]

**fer·ro·pro·teins** (fār-ō-prō′tēnz) proteins containing iron in a prosthetic group; e.g., heme, cytochrome.

**fer·rous** (fār′ŭs) relating to iron, especially denoting a salt containing iron in its lowest valence state, $Fe^{2+}$. [L. *ferreus,* made of iron]

**fer·ru·gi·na·tion** (fe-roo′ji-nā′shŭn) deposition of mineral including iron in the walls of small blood vessels and at the site of a dead neuron. [L. *ferrugo,* iron-rust]

**fer·ru·gi·nous** (fe-roo′ji-nŭs) **1.** iron-bearing; associated with or containing iron. **2.** of the color of iron rust. [L. *ferrugineus,* iron rust, rust-colored]

**Fer·ry line** (fer′ē) an iron line occurring in the corneal epithelium anterior to a filtering bleb.

**fer·tile** (fer′til) **1.** fruitful; capable of conceiving and bearing young. SYN fecund. **2.** impregnated; fertilized. [L. *fertilis,* fr. *fero,* to bear]

**fer·tile pe·ri·od** the period in a regularly menstruating woman's cycle, during which conception is most likely.

**fer·til·i·ty** (fer-til′i-tē) the capacity to beget or to conceive and bear offspring; refers to production of live offspring and hence does not include stillbirths.

**fer·til·i·za·tion** (fer′til-i-zā′shŭn) the process beginning with penetration of the secondary oocyte by the spermatozoon and completed by fusion of the male and female pronuclei.

**FESS** functional endoscopic sinus surgery.

**fes·ter 1.** to form pus or putrefy. **2.** to make inflamed. [L. *fistula*]

**fes·ti·nant** (fes′ti-nant) rapid; hastening; accelerating. [L. *festino,* to hasten]

**fes·ti·nat·ing gait, fes·ti·na·tion** (fes-ti-nā′shŭn) gait in which the trunk is flexed, legs are flexed at the knees and hips, but stiff, while the steps are short and progressively more rapid; characteristically seen with parkinsonism (1) and other neurologic diseases.

**fes·toon** (fes-toon′) **1.** a carving in the base material of a denture that simulates the contours of the natural tissue that is being replaced by the denture. **2.** a distinguishing characteristic of certain hard tick species, consisting of small rectangular areas separated by grooves along the posterior margin of the dorsum of both males and females. [thr. Fr. fr. L. *festum,* festival, hence festive decorations]

**fes·toon·ing** (fes-toon′ing) undulating, like the pattern of dermal papillae beneath a subepidermal blister.

**FET** forced expiratory time.

**fe·tal** (fē′tăl) **1.** relating to a fetus; **2.** development in utero after the eighth week.

**fe·tal al·co·hol syn·drome** a specific pattern of fetal malformation with growth deficiency, craniofacial anomalies, and limb defects, found among offspring of mothers who are chronic alcoholics; mental retardation is often demonstrated later.

**fe·tal as·pir·a·tion syn·drome** a syndrome resulting from uterine aspiration of amniotic fluid and meconium by the fetus, usually caused by hypoxia and often leading to aspiration pneumonia. SYN meconium aspiration syndrome.

**fe·tal death** death prior to the complete expulsion or extraction from the mother of a product of conception, irrespective of the duration of pregnancy. Fetal death is considered *early* if it takes place in the first 20 weeks of gestation; *middle* (intermediate) if it takes place from 21 to 28 weeks of gestation, and *late* if it takes place after 28 weeks.

**fe·tal dys·to·cia** (fē'tal) dystocia due to an abnormality of the fetus.

**fe·tal growth re·stric·tion** fetal weight ≤5th percentile for gestational age. SYN intrauterine growth retardation.

**fe·tal hy·drops, hy·drops fe·ta·lis** abnormal accumulation of serous fluid in the fetal tissues, as in erythroblastosis fetalis.

**fe·tal med·i·cine** study of the growth, development, care, and treatment of the fetus, and of environmental factors harmful to the fetus. SYN fetology.

**fe·tal mem·brane** a structure or tissue that develops from the fertilized oocyte but does not form part of the embryo proper. SYN embryonic membrane.

**fe·tal pla·cen·ta, pla·cen·ta fe·ta·lis** the chorionic portion of the placenta, containing the fetal blood vessels, from which the funis develops; specifically, in humans, it develops from the chorion frondosum or villous chorion.

**fe·tal scalp stim·u·la·tion** intrapartum test for fetal well-being; acceleration of the fetal heart rate in response to digital or forceps stimulation of scalp is associated with a normal scalp blood pH.

**fe·tal souf·fle** a blowing murmur, synchronous with the fetal heart beat, sometimes only systolic and sometimes continuous, heard on auscultation over the pregnant uterus.

**fe·tal was·tage** loss of an embryo or fetus through spontaneous abortion or stillbirth; usually expressed as a rate per 1000 pregnancies with respect to a particular cause, such as maternal infection or drug addiction.

**fe·ti·cide** (fē'ti-sīd) destruction of the embryo or fetus in the uterus. [L. *fetus* + *caedo*, to kill]

**fet·id** (fet'id, fē'tid) foul-smelling. [L. *foetidus*]

**fet·ish** (fet'ish) an inanimate object or nonsexual body part that is regarded as endowed with magic or erotic qualities. [Fr. *fétiche*, fr. L. *factitius*, made by art, artificial]

**fet·ish·ism** (fet'ish-izm) the act of worshiping or using for sexual arousal and gratification that which is regarded as a fetish.

**fe·to·glob·u·lin** (fē-tō-glob'yu-linz) one of a number of proteins found in fetal blood, of unknown function. α-fetoglobulin occurs in normal amounts in adults and in larger amounts in the fetus and pregnant mother, especially in the second trimester; elevated levels are also detected in patients with liver disease and neoplasms.

**fe·tol·o·gy** (fē-tol'ō-jē) SYN fetal medicine. [L. *fetus* + G. *logos*, study]

**fe·tom·e·try** (fē-tom'ĕ-trē) estimation of the size of the fetus, especially of its head, prior to delivery. [L. *fetus* + G. *metron*, measure]

**fe·top·a·thy** (fē-top'ă-thē) SYN embryopathy. [L. *fetus* + G. *pathos*, suffering, disease]

**fe·to·pla·cen·tal** (fē'tō-pla-sen'tăl) relating to the fetus and its placenta.

**fe·to·pro·tein, γ-fe·to·pro·tein, β-fe·to·pro·tein, α-fe·to·pro·tein (AFP)** (fē-tō-prō'tēn) fetal proteins found in small amounts in adults in the following forms: α-fetoprotein (AFP) increases in maternal blood during pregnancy; when detected by amniocentesis, is an important indicator of neural tube defects; used as a tumor

marker in adults with hepatocellular carcinoma; β-fetoprotein, although a fetal liver protein, has been detected in adult patients with liver disease; γ-fetoprotein occurs in various neoplasms. SEE ALSO fetoglobulin.

**fe·tor** (fē'tōr) a very offensive odor. [L. an offensive smell, fr. *feteo*, to stink]

**fe·tor he·pat·i·cus** a peculiar odor to the breath in persons with severe liver disease; caused by volatile aromatic substances that accumulate in the blood and urine due to defective hepatic metabolism.

**fe·to·scope** (fē'tō-skōp) 1. a fiberoptic endoscope used in fetology. 2. a stethoscope designed for listening to fetal heart sounds.

**fe·tos·co·py** (fē-tos'kŏ-pē) use of a fiberoptic endoscope to view the fetus and the fetal surface of the placenta transabdominally, and also for collection of fetal blood from the umbilical vein for antenatal diagnosis of fetal disorders.

**fe·to·tox·ic** (fē-tō-tok'sik) a substance that is poisonous to a fetus.

**fe·tu·in** (fē-too'in) a low molecular-weight globulin that constitutes nearly the total globulin in fetal blood. [fetus + -in]

**fe·tus**, pl. **fe·tus·es** (fē'tŭs, fē'tŭs-ez) 1. the unborn young of a viviparous animal after it has taken form in the uterus. 2. in humans, the product of conception from the end of the eighth week to the moment of birth. [L. offspring]

**fe·tus pap·y·ra·ceus** one of twin fetuses that has died and been pressed flat against the uterine wall by the growth of the living fetus.

**Feul·gen cy·to·met·ry** (foyl'gĕn) a form of cytometry using Feulgen-stained nuclei to characterize the chromatin pattern and nuclear distribution of DNA of cells.

**FEV** forced expiratory volume, with subscript indicating time interval in seconds.

**fe·ver** (fē'ver) a complex physiologic response to disease mediated by pyrogenic cytokines and characterized by a rise in core temperature, generation of acute phase reactants and activation of immunologic systems. SYN pyrexia. [A.S. *fefer*]

**fe·ver blis·ter** colloquialism for herpes simplex of the lips.

**fe·ver·ish** (fē'ver-ish) 1. SYN febrile. 2. having a fever.

**fe·ver of un·known or·i·gin (FUO)** a sustained elevation of temperature, lasting two weeks or longer, for which no explanation can be found despite vigorous diagnostic evaluation. SYN pyrexia of unknown origin.

**FF** filtration fraction.

**F fac·tor** SYN F plasmid.

**FFD** focal-film distance.

**FFM** fat-free body mass.

**FIA** feline infectious anemia.

**fi·ber** (fī'ber) a slender thread or filament. 1. a strand or filament; especially the extracellular filamentous structures peculiar to connective tissue. 2. the nerve cell axon with its glial envelope. 3. elongated, hence threadlike, cells such as muscle cells and the epithelial cells composing the major part of the eye lens. SYN fibra [TA]. [L. *fibra*]

**fi·ber·op·tic** (fī-ber-op'tik) pertaining to fiberoptics.

**fi·ber·op·tic en·dos·cop·ic ex·am·i·na·tion of swal·low·ing (FEES)** a diagnostic technique for evaluation of deviant swallowing patterns, using a transnasal fiberoptic endoscope to visualize the larynx and pharynx. SEE ALSO fiberoptics, endoscope.

**fi·ber·op·tics** (fī-ber-op'tiks) an optical system in which the image is conveyed by a compact bundle of small diameter, flexible, glass or plastic fibers.

**fi·ber·scope** (fī'ber-skōp) an optical instrument that transmits light and carries images back to the observer through a flexible bundle of small glass or plastic fibers. It is used to inspect interior portions of the body. SEE ALSO fiberoptics.

**fi·bra** (fī'bră) [TA] SYN fiber, fiber. [L.]

**fi·brae me·rid·i·o·na·les mus·cu·lar·is cil·i·ar·is** [TA] SYN meridional fibers of ciliary muscle.

**fi·bre [Br.]** SEE fiber.

**fi·bre-op·tic [Br.]** SEE fiberoptic.

**fi·bre-op·tics [Br.]** SEE fiberoptics.

**fi·bre·scope [Br.]** SEE fiberscope.

**fi·bril** (fī'bril) a minute fiber or component of a fiber. SYN fibrilla. [Mod. L. *fibrilla*]

**fi·bril·la**, pl. **fi·bril·lae** (fī-bril'ă, fī-bril'ē) SYN fibril. [Mod. L. dim. of L. *fibra*, a fiber]

**fi·bril·lar, fi·bril·lary** (fī'bri-lar, fi-bri-lar'ē) **1.** relating to a fibril. **2.** denoting the fine rapid contractions or twitchings of fibers or of small groups of fibers in skeletal or cardiac muscle. SYN filar (1).

**fi·bril·lary as·tro·cyte, fi·brous as·tro·cyte** a stellate astrocytic cell with long processes found mainly in the white matter of the brain and spinal cord and characterized by having bundles of glial filaments in its cytoplasm; origin of most astrocytomas.

**fi·bril·lary con·trac·tions** contractions occurring spontaneously in individual muscle fibers.

**fi·bril·late** (fī'bri-lāt) **1.** to make or to become fibrillar. **2.** SYN fibrillated. **3.** to be in a state of fibrillation (3).

**fi·bril·lat·ed** (fī'bri-lā-ted) composed of fibrils. SYN fibrillate (2).

**fi·bril·la·tion** (fī-bri-lā'shŭn) **1.** the condition of being fibrillated. **2.** the formation of fibrils. **3.** exceedingly rapid contractions or twitching of muscular fibrils, but not of the muscle as a whole. **4.** vermicular twitching, usually slow, of individual muscular fibers; commonly occurs in atria or ventricles of the heart as well as in recently denervated skeletal muscle fibers.

**fi·bril·lo·gen·e·sis** (fī'bril-ō-jen'ě-sis) the development of fine fibrils (as seen with the electron microscope) normally present in collagenous fibers of connective tissue.

**fi·brin** (fī'brin) an elastic filamentous protein derived from fibrinogen by the action of thrombin, which releases fibrinopeptides A and B from fibrinogen in coagulation of the blood; a component of thrombi, vegetations, and acute inflammatory exudates such as in diphtheria and lobar pneumonia. [L. *fibra*, fiber]

**fi·brin·ase** (fī'brin-ās) **1.** former term for factor XIII. **2.** SYN plasmin.

**fi·brin cal·cu·lus** a urinary calculus formed largely from fibrinogen in blood.

**fi·brin/fi·brin·o·gen deg·ra·da·tion pro·ducts** several poorly characterized small peptides that result from the action of plasmin on fibrinogen and fibrin in the fibrinolytic process.

△**fi·bri·no-** fibrin. [L. *fibra*, fiber]

**fi·bri·no·cel·lu·lar** (fī'bri-nō-sel'yu-lăr) com-

posed of fibrin and cells, as in certain types of exudates resulting from acute inflammation.

**fi·brin·o·gen** (fī-brin'ō-jen) a globulin of the blood plasma that is converted into fibrin by the action of thrombin in the presence of ionized calcium to produce coagulation of the blood; the only coagulable protein in the blood plasma of vertebrates; it is absent in afibrinogenemia and is defective in dysfibrinogenemia.

**fi·brin·o·ge·ne·mia** (fī-brin'ō-jě-nē'mē-ă) SYN hyperfibrinogenemia.

**fi·bri·no·gen·e·sis** (fī'bri-nō-jen'ě-sis) formation or production of fibrin.

**fi·bri·no·gen·ic, fi·bri·nog·e·nous** (fī'brin-ō-jen'ik, fī'bri-noj'ě-nŭs) **1.** pertaining to fibrinogen. **2.** producing fibrin.

**fi·brin·o·gen·ol·y·sis** (fī-brin'ō-jen-ol'i-sis) the inactivation or dissolution of fibrinogen in the blood. [fibrinogen + G. *lysis*, dissolution]

**fi·brin·o·gen·o·pe·nia** (fī-brin'ō-jen-ō-pē'nē-ă) a concentration of fibrinogen in the blood that is less than the normal. [fibrinogen + G. *penia*, poverty]

**fi·brin·oid** (fī'bri-noyd) **1.** resembling fibrin. **2.** a deeply or brilliantly acidophilic, homogeneous, refractile, proteinaceous material that: 1) is frequently formed in the walls of blood vessels and in connective tissue of patients with such diseases as disseminated lupus erythematosus, polyarteritis nodosa, scleroderma, dermatomyositis, and rheumatic fever; 2) is sometimes observed in healing wounds, chronic peptic ulcers, the placenta, necrotic arterioles of malignant hypertension, and other unrelated conditions. [fibrin + G. *eidos*, resemblance]

**fi·brin·oid de·gen·er·a·tion, fi·brin·ous de·gen·er·a·tion** a process resulting in acidophilic refractile deposits with staining reactions that resemble fibrin, occurring in connective tissue, blood vessel walls, and other sites.

**fi·bri·nol·y·sin** (fī-bri-nol-ŏ-lī'sīn) SYN plasmin.

**fi·bri·nol·y·sis** (fī-bri-nol'i-sis) hydrolysis of fibrin. [fibrino- + G. *lysis*, dissolution]

**fi·bri·no·lyt·ic** (fī-brin-ō-lit'ik) denoting, characterized by, or causing fibrinolysis.

**fi·bri·no·lyt·ic pur·pu·ra** purpura in which the bleeding is associated with rapid fibrinolysis of the clot.

**fi·bri·no·pep·tide** (fī'brin-ō-pep'tīd) one of two pairs of peptides (A and B) released from the amino-terminal ends of 2α- and 2β-chains of fibrinogen by the action of thrombin to form fibrin; they have a vasoconstrictive effect.

**fi·bri·no·pu·ru·lent** (fī'bri-nō-pyu'rŭ-lent) pertaining to pus or suppurative exudate that contains a relatively large amount of fibrin.

**fi·brin·ous** (fī'brin-ŭs) pertaining to or composed of fibrin.

**fi·brin·ous bron·chi·tis** inflammation of the bronchial mucous membrane, accompanied by a fibrinous exudation, with obstruction of air flow. SYN pseudomembranous bronchitis.

**fi·brin·ous in·flam·ma·tion** an exudative inflammation in which there is a disproportionately large amount of fibrin.

**fi·brin·ous per·i·car·di·tis** acute pericarditis with fibrinous exudate.

**fi·brin·ous pleu·ri·sy** SYN dry pleurisy.

**fi·brin·ous pol·yp** a misnomer for a mass of fibrin retained within the uterine cavity after childbirth.

## CONTENTS

## INDEX

### A

**Anatomy**

**Anatomical images provided by:**

# adam.com™

## A.D.A.M.
### Software, Inc.
1600 River Edge Parkway
Suite 800
Atlanta, GA 30328
(770) 980-0888
www.adam.com

Anatomy

Anatomy

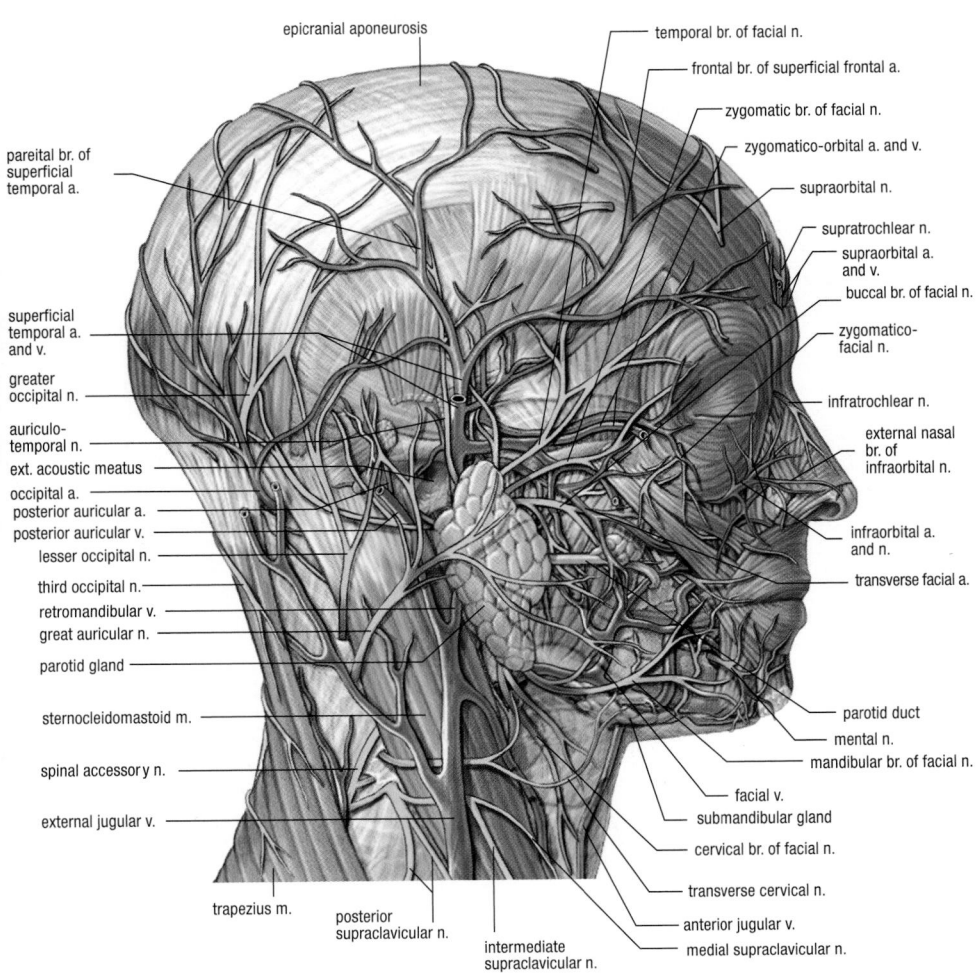

epicranial aponeurosis

temporal br. of facial n.

frontal br. of superficial frontal a.

zygomatic br. of facial n.

zygomatico-orbital a. and v.

pareital br. of superficial temporal a.

supraorbital n.

supratrochlear n.

supraorbital a. and v.

buccal br. of facial n.

superficial temporal a. and v.

zygomatico-facial n.

greater occipital n.

infratrochlear n.

auriculo-temporal n.

external nasal br. of infraorbital n.

ext. acoustic meatus

occipital a.

posterior auricular a.

posterior auricular v.

infraorbital a. and n.

lesser occipital n.

transverse facial a.

third occipital n.

retromandibular v.

great auricular n.

parotid gland

sternocleidomastoid m.

parotid duct

mental n.

mandibular br. of facial n.

spinal accessory n.

facial v.

submandibular gland

external jugular v.

cervical br. of facial n.

transverse cervical n.

trapezius m.

posterior supraclavicular n.

anterior jugular v.

medial supraclavicular n.

intermediate supraclavicular n.

Anatomy

Imagery © adam.com

A5

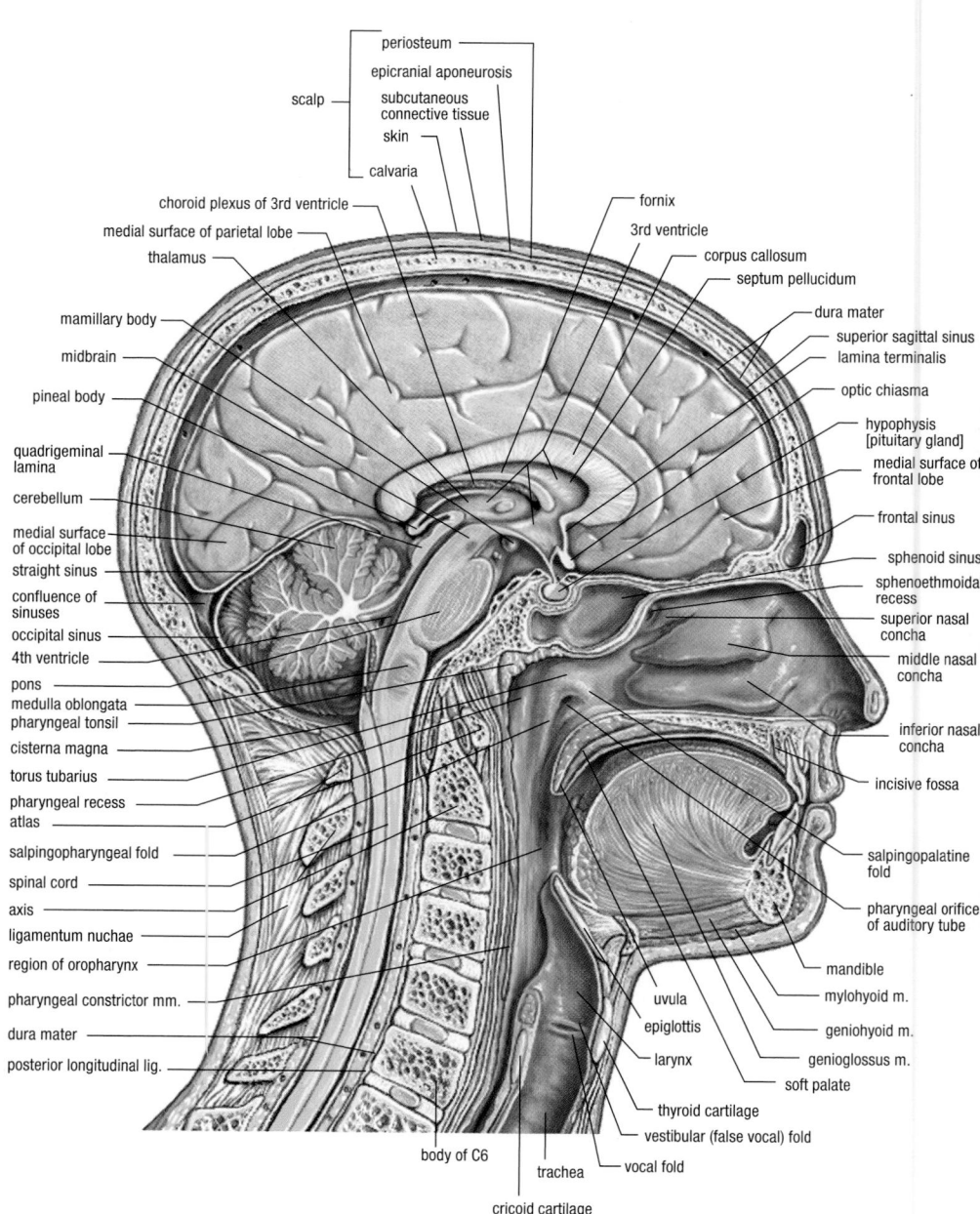

periosteum

epicranial aponeurosis

scalp

subcutaneous connective tissue

skin

calvaria

choroid plexus of 3rd ventricle

medial surface of parietal lobe

thalamus

mamillary body

midbrain

pineal body

quadrigeminal lamina

cerebellum

medial surface of occipital lobe

straight sinus

confluence of sinuses

occipital sinus

4th ventricle

pons

medulla oblongata

pharyngeal tonsil

cisterna magna

torus tubarius

pharyngeal recess

atlas

salpingopharyngeal fold

spinal cord

axis

ligamentum nuchae

region of oropharynx

pharyngeal constrictor mm.

dura mater

posterior longitudinal lig.

fornix

3rd ventricle

corpus callosum

septum pellucidum

dura mater

superior sagittal sinus

lamina terminalis

optic chiasma

hypophysis [pituitary gland]

medial surface of frontal lobe

frontal sinus

sphenoid sinus

sphenoethmoidal recess

superior nasal concha

middle nasal concha

inferior nasal concha

incisive fossa

salpingopalatine fold

pharyngeal orifice of auditory tube

mandible

mylohyoid m.

geniohyoid m.

genioglossus m.

soft palate

uvula

epiglottis

larynx

body of C6

trachea

cricoid cartilage

thyroid cartilage

vestibular (false vocal) fold

vocal fold

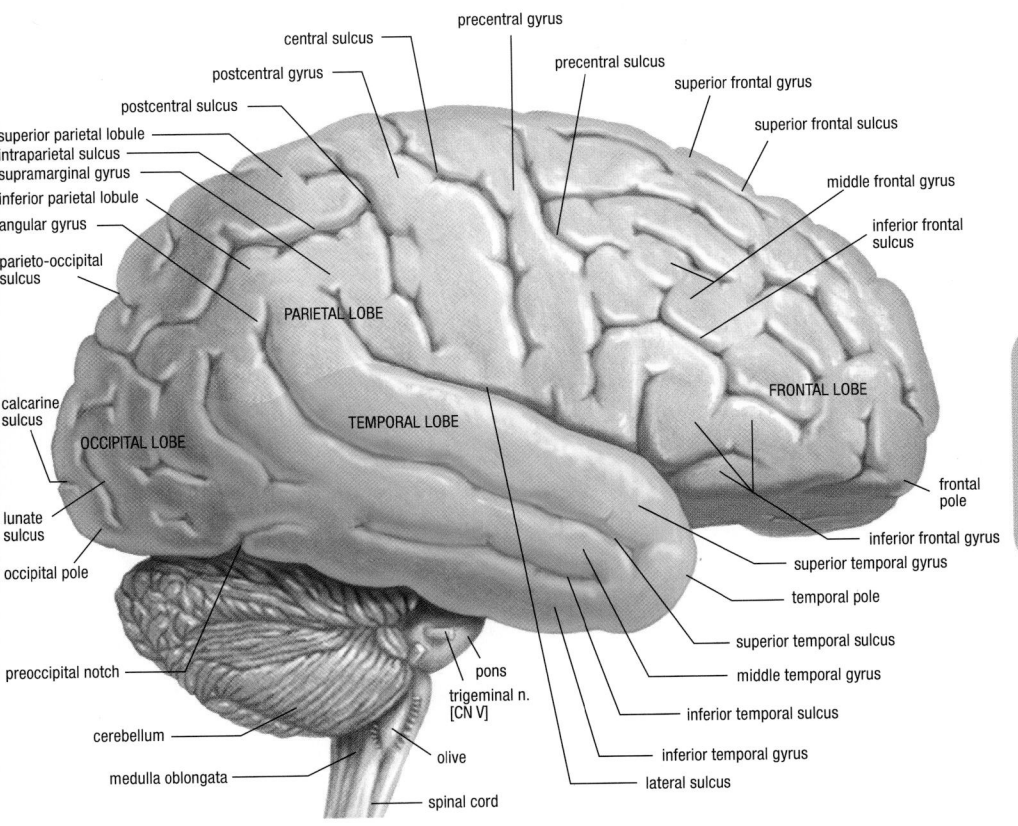

precentral gyrus

central sulcus

postcentral gyrus

postcentral sulcus

precentral sulcus

superior frontal gyrus

superior frontal sulcus

superior parietal lobule
intraparietal sulcus
supramarginal gyrus
inferior parietal lobule

middle frontal gyrus

angular gyrus

inferior frontal
sulcus

parieto-occipital
sulcus

PARIETAL LOBE

FRONTAL LOBE

calcarine
sulcus

OCCIPITAL LOBE

TEMPORAL LOBE

frontal
pole

lunate
sulcus

inferior frontal gyrus

superior temporal gyrus

occipital pole

temporal pole

superior temporal sulcus

preoccipital notch

pons

middle temporal gyrus

trigeminal n.
[CN V]

inferior temporal sulcus

cerebellum

olive

inferior temporal gyrus

medulla oblongata

lateral sulcus

spinal cord

Anatomy

Imagery © adam.com

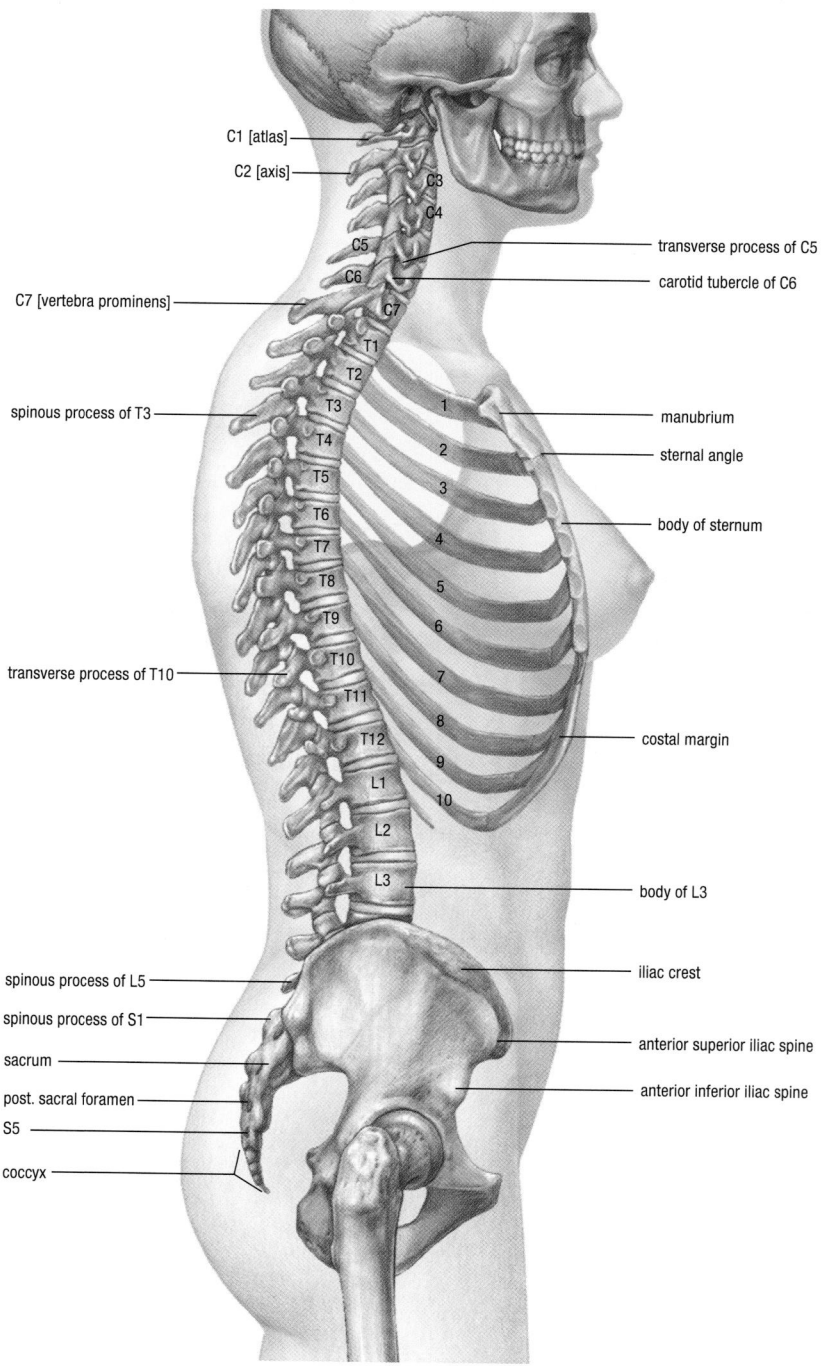

C1 [atlas]
C2 [axis]
C3
C4
C5
C6
transverse process of C5
carotid tubercle of C6
C7 [vertebra prominens]
C7
T1
T2
spinous process of T3
T3
1
manubrium
T4
2
sternal angle
T5
3
T6
4
body of sternum
T7
T8
5
T9
6
transverse process of T10
T10
7
T11
8
T12
costal margin
9
L1
10
L2
L3
body of L3
iliac crest
spinous process of L5
spinous process of S1
sacrum
anterior superior iliac spine
post. sacral foramen
anterior inferior iliac spine
S5
coccyx

Imagery © adam.com

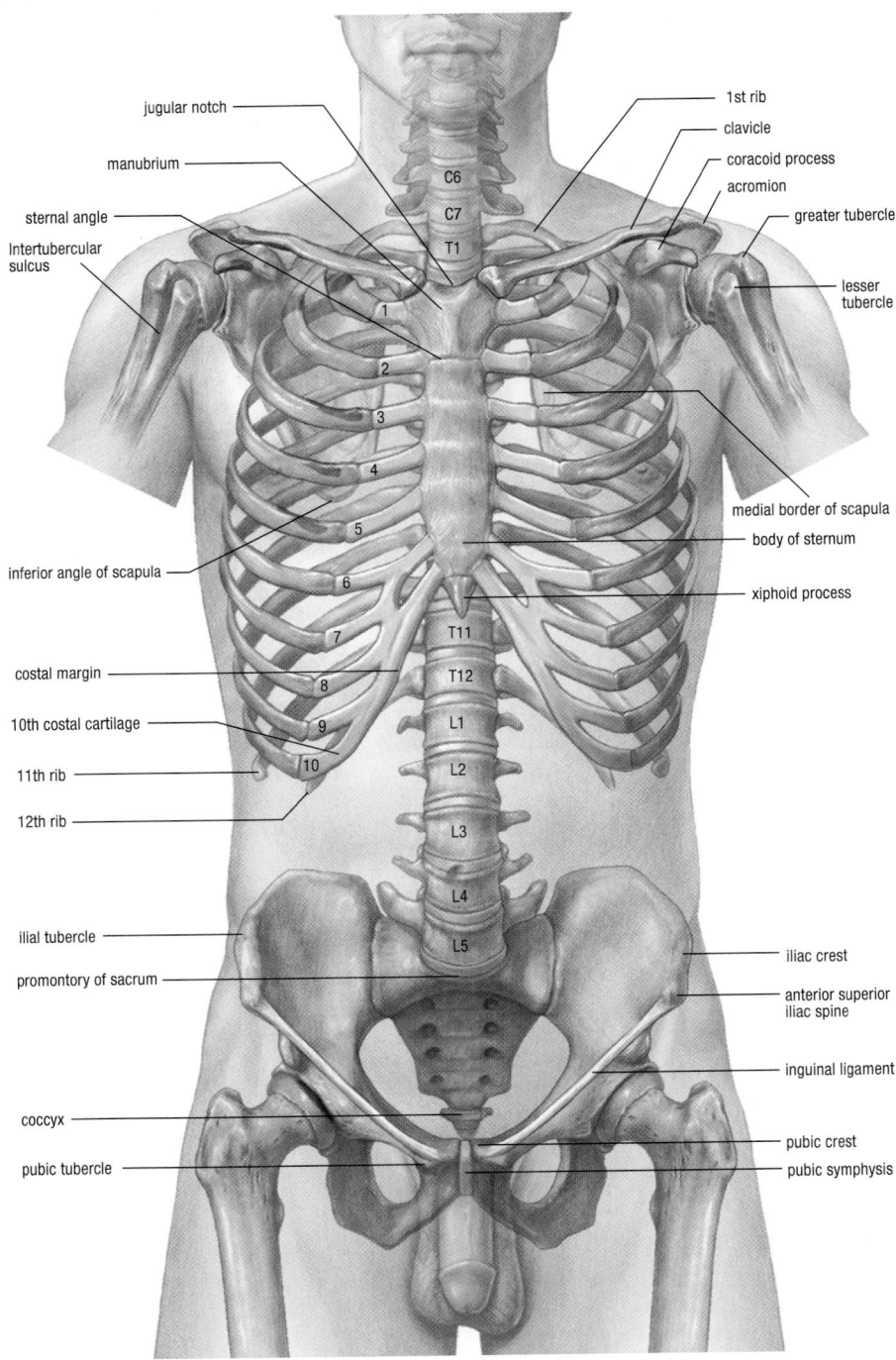

jugular notch

manubrium

sternal angle

Intertubercular
sulcus

inferior angle of scapula

costal margin

10th costal cartilage

11th rib

12th rib

ilial tubercle

promontory of sacrum

coccyx

pubic tubercle

1st rib

clavicle

coracoid process

acromion

greater tubercle

lesser
tubercle

medial border of scapula

body of sternum

xiphoid process

iliac crest

anterior superior
iliac spine

inguinal ligament

pubic crest

pubic symphysis

C6

C7

T1

T11

T12

L1

L2

L3

L4

L5

**Anatomy**

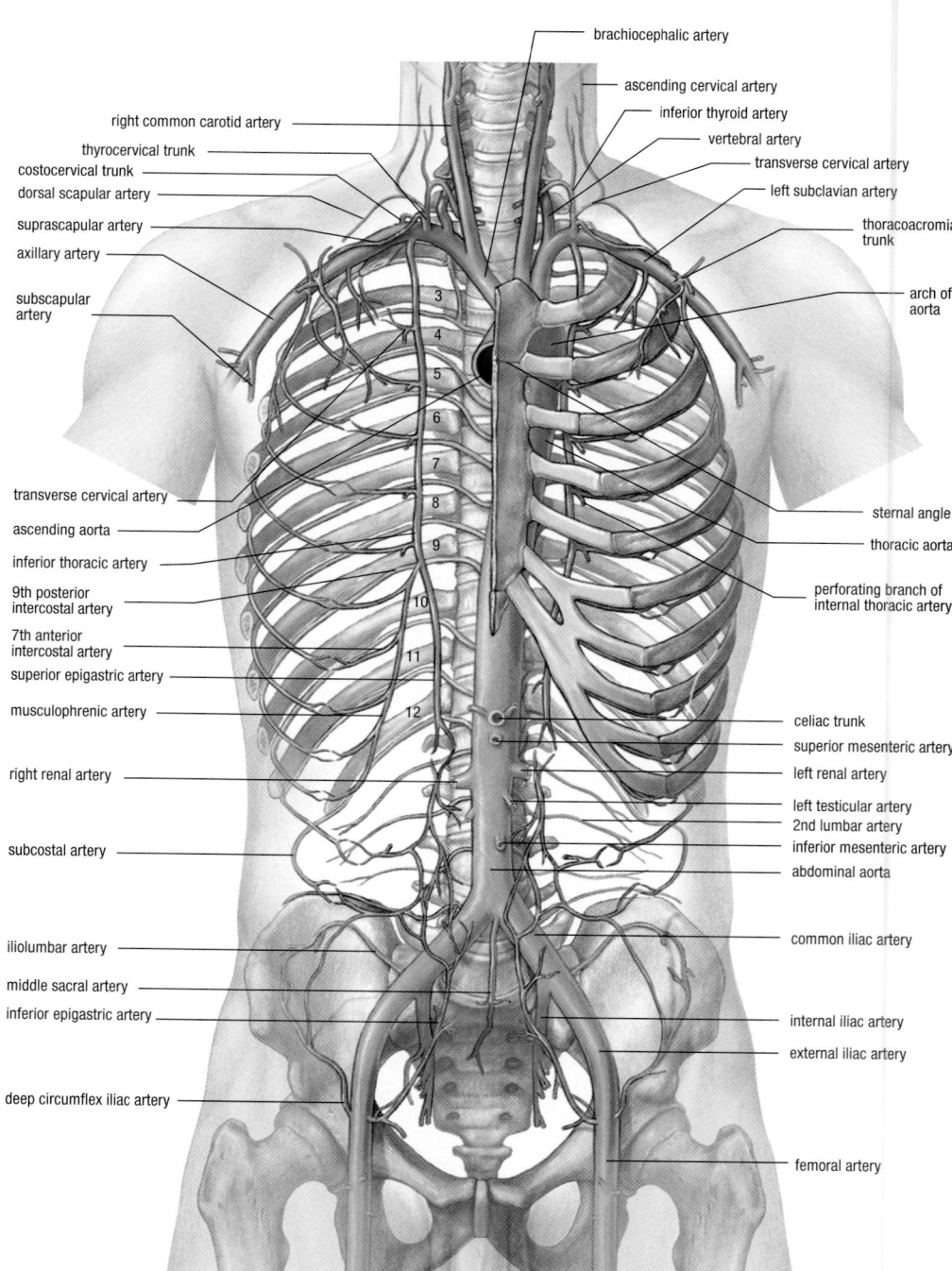

brachiocephalic artery

ascending cervical artery

right common carotid artery

inferior thyroid artery

thyrocervical trunk

vertebral artery

costocervical trunk

transverse cervical artery

dorsal scapular artery

left subclavian artery

suprascapular artery

thoracoacromial trunk

axillary artery

arch of aorta

subscapular artery

transverse cervical artery

sternal angle

ascending aorta

thoracic aorta

inferior thoracic artery

9th posterior intercostal artery

perforating branch of internal thoracic artery

7th anterior intercostal artery

superior epigastric artery

musculophrenic artery

celiac trunk

superior mesenteric artery

right renal artery

left renal artery

left testicular artery

2nd lumbar artery

subcostal artery

inferior mesenteric artery

abdominal aorta

iliolumbar artery

common iliac artery

middle sacral artery

inferior epigastric artery

internal iliac artery

external iliac artery

deep circumflex iliac artery

femoral artery

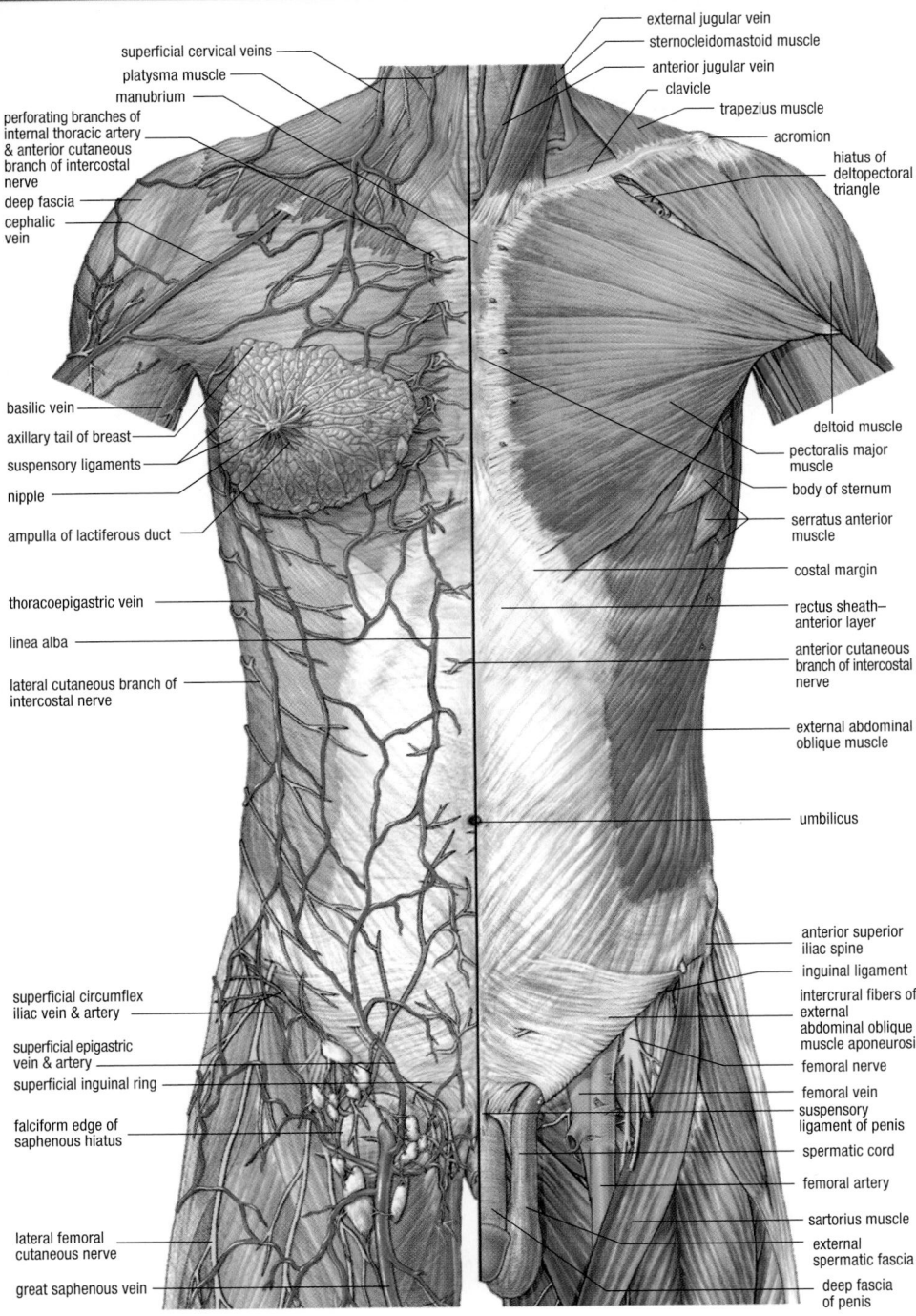

superficial cervical veins

platysma muscle

manubrium

perforating branches of internal thoracic artery & anterior cutaneous branch of intercostal nerve

deep fascia

cephalic vein

basilic vein

axillary tail of breast

suspensory ligaments

nipple

ampulla of lactiferous duct

thoracoepigastric vein

linea alba

lateral cutaneous branch of intercostal nerve

superficial circumflex iliac vein & artery

superficial epigastric vein & artery

superficial inguinal ring

falciform edge of saphenous hiatus

lateral femoral cutaneous nerve

great saphenous vein

external jugular vein

sternocleidomastoid muscle

anterior jugular vein

clavicle

trapezius muscle

acromion

hiatus of deltopectoral triangle

deltoid muscle

pectoralis major muscle

body of sternum

serratus anterior muscle

costal margin

rectus sheath–anterior layer

anterior cutaneous branch of intercostal nerve

external abdominal oblique muscle

umbilicus

anterior superior iliac spine

inguinal ligament

intercrural fibers of external abdominal oblique muscle aponeurosis

femoral nerve

femoral vein

suspensory ligament of penis

spermatic cord

femoral artery

sartorius muscle

external spermatic fascia

deep fascia of penis

**Anatomy**

Imagery © adam.com

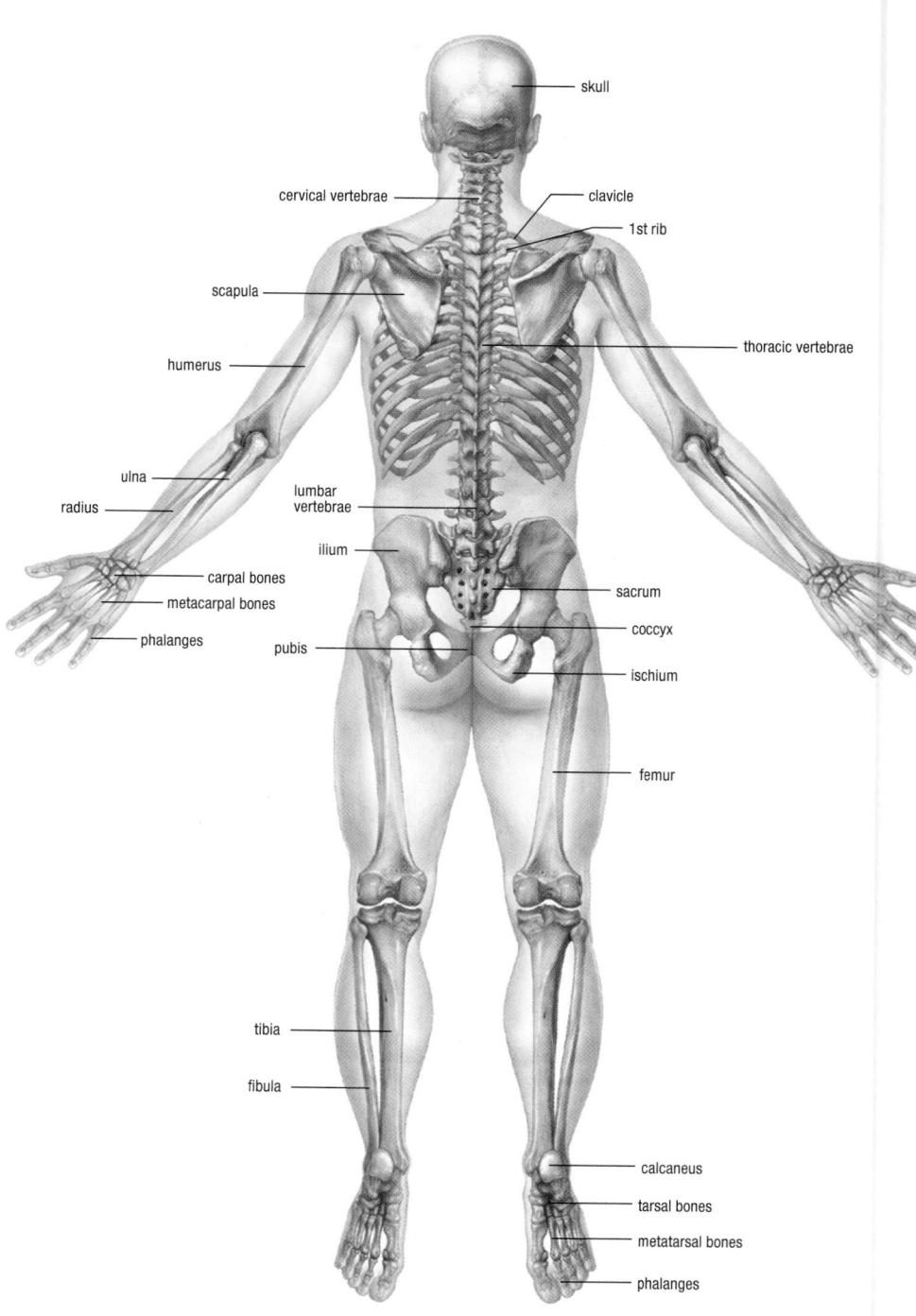

skull

cervical vertebrae

clavicle

1st rib

scapula

thoracic vertebrae

humerus

ulna

radius

lumbar vertebrae

ilium

carpal bones

metacarpal bones

phalanges

pubis

sacrum

coccyx

ischium

femur

tibia

fibula

calcaneus

tarsal bones

metatarsal bones

phalanges

Imagery © adam.com

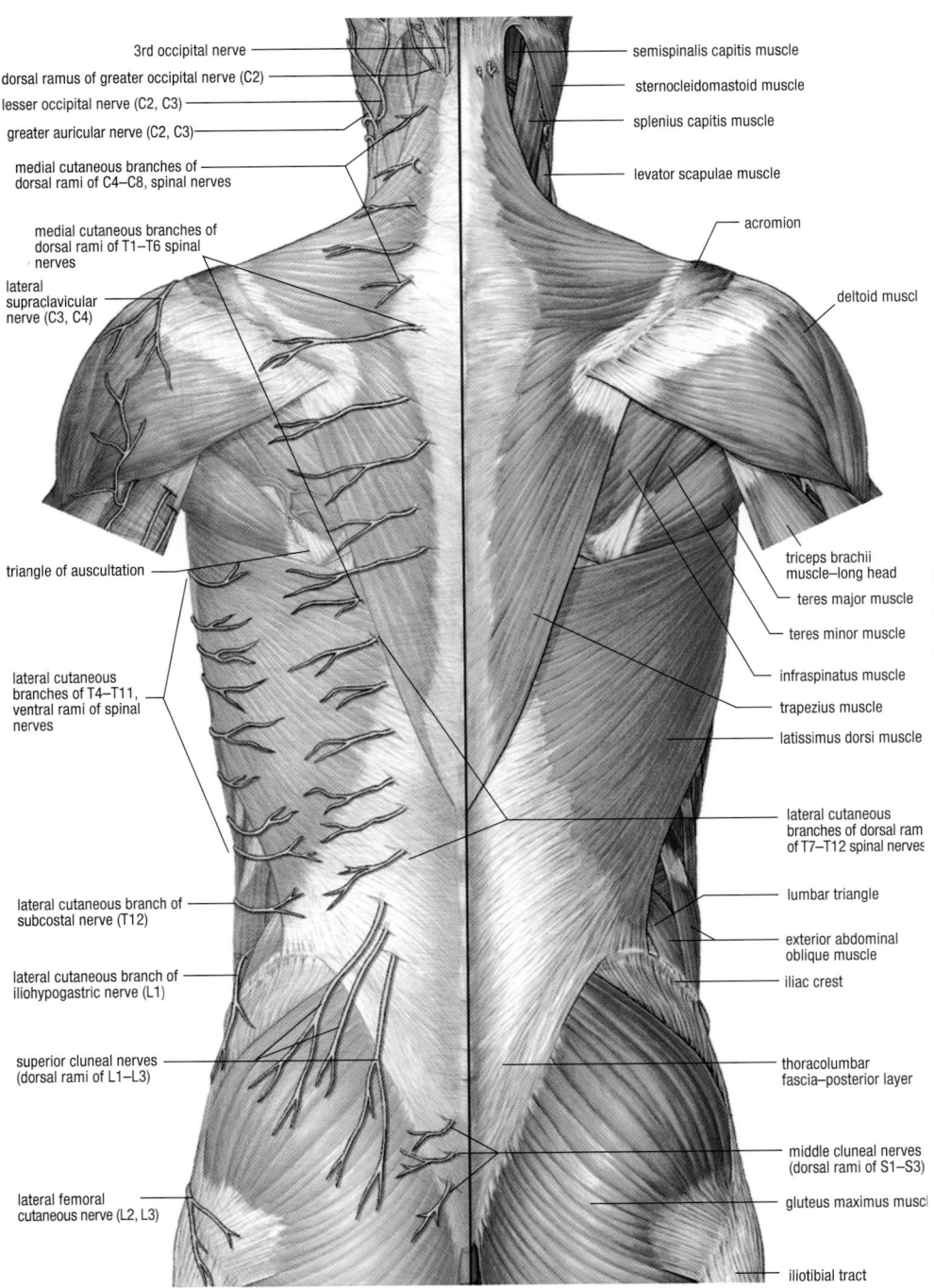

3rd occipital nerve

dorsal ramus of greater occipital nerve (C2)

lesser occipital nerve (C2, C3)

greater auricular nerve (C2, C3)

medial cutaneous branches of dorsal rami of C4–C8, spinal nerves

medial cutaneous branches of dorsal rami of T1–T6 spinal nerves

lateral supraclavicular nerve (C3, C4)

triangle of auscultation

lateral cutaneous branches of T4–T11, ventral rami of spinal nerves

lateral cutaneous branch of subcostal nerve (T12)

lateral cutaneous branch of iliohypogastric nerve (L1)

superior cluneal nerves (dorsal rami of L1–L3)

lateral femoral cutaneous nerve (L2, L3)

semispinalis capitis muscle

sternocleidomastoid muscle

splenius capitis muscle

levator scapulae muscle

acromion

deltoid muscl

triceps brachii muscle–long head

teres major muscle

teres minor muscle

infraspinatus muscle

trapezius muscle

latissimus dorsi muscle

lateral cutaneous branches of dorsal ram of T7–T12 spinal nerves

lumbar triangle

exterior abdominal oblique muscle

iliac crest

thoracolumbar fascia–posterior layer

middle cluneal nerves (dorsal rami of S1–S3)

gluteus maximus muscl

iliotibial tract

Anatomy

Imagery © adam.com

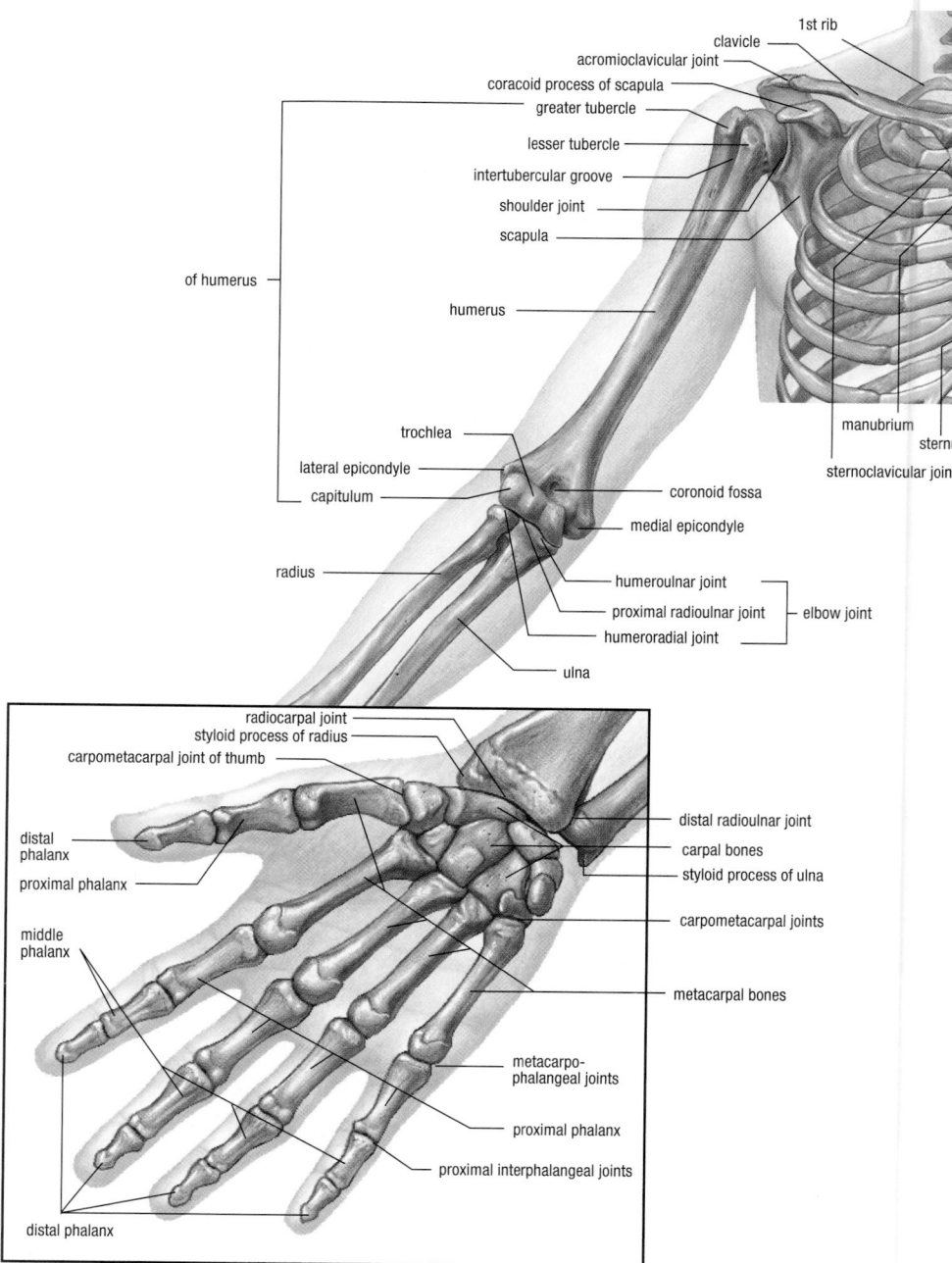

1st rib

clavicle

acromioclavicular joint

coracoid process of scapula

greater tubercle

lesser tubercle

intertubercular groove

shoulder joint

scapula

of humerus

humerus

manubrium

sternum

sternoclavicular joint

trochlea

lateral epicondyle

capitulum

coronoid fossa

medial epicondyle

radius

humeroulnar joint

proximal radioulnar joint — elbow joint

humeroradial joint

ulna

radiocarpal joint

styloid process of radius

carpometacarpal joint of thumb

distal phalanx

proximal phalanx

distal radioulnar joint

carpal bones

styloid process of ulna

carpometacarpal joints

metacarpal bones

middle phalanx

metacarpo-phalangeal joints

proximal phalanx

proximal interphalangeal joints

distal phalanx

Imagery © adam.com

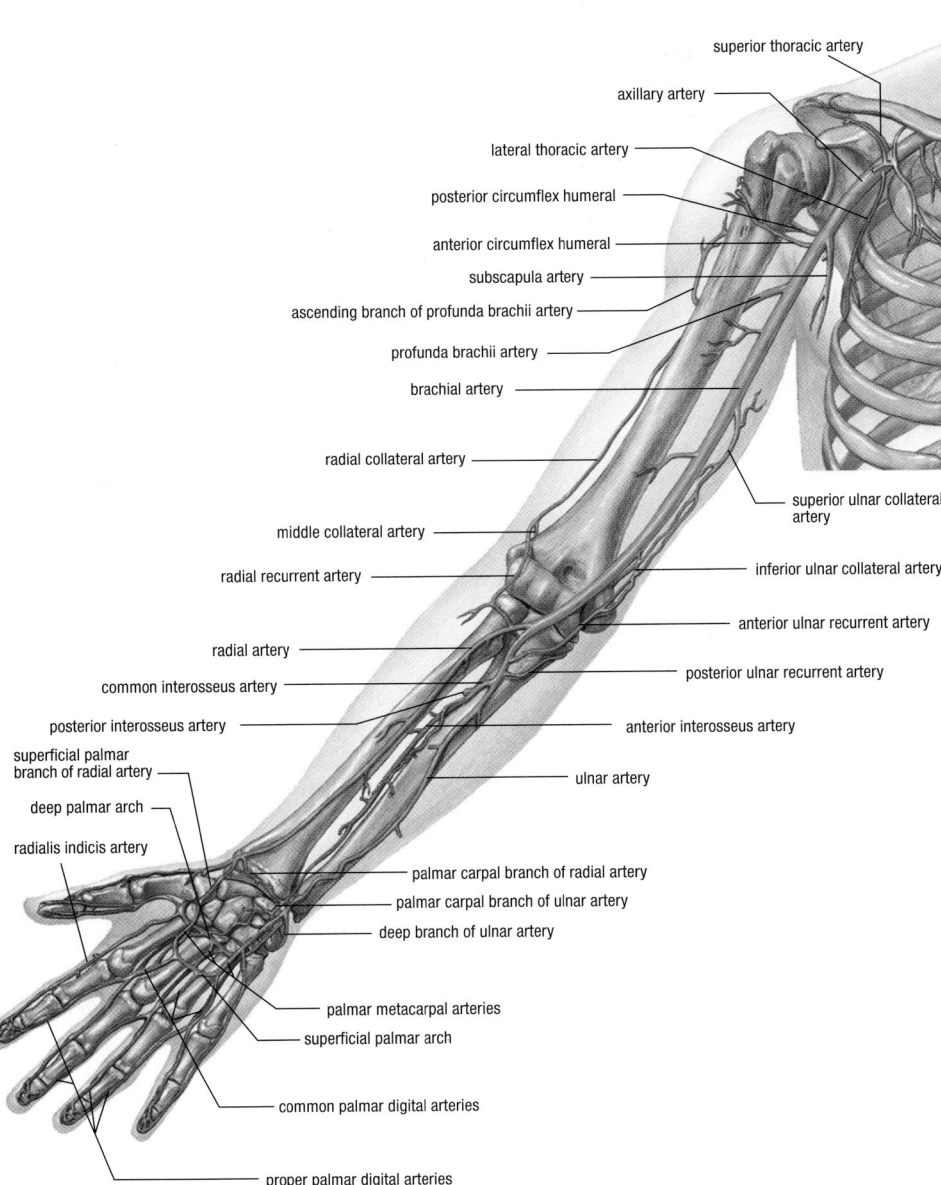

superior thoracic artery

axillary artery

lateral thoracic artery

posterior circumflex humeral

anterior circumflex humeral

subscapula artery

ascending branch of profunda brachii artery

profunda brachii artery

brachial artery

radial collateral artery

superior ulnar collateral artery

middle collateral artery

inferior ulnar collateral artery

radial recurrent artery

anterior ulnar recurrent artery

radial artery

posterior ulnar recurrent artery

common interosseus artery

posterior interosseus artery

anterior interosseus artery

superficial palmar branch of radial artery

ulnar artery

deep palmar arch

radialis indicis artery

palmar carpal branch of radial artery

palmar carpal branch of ulnar artery

deep branch of ulnar artery

palmar metacarpal arteries

superficial palmar arch

common palmar digital arteries

proper palmar digital arteries

Anatomy

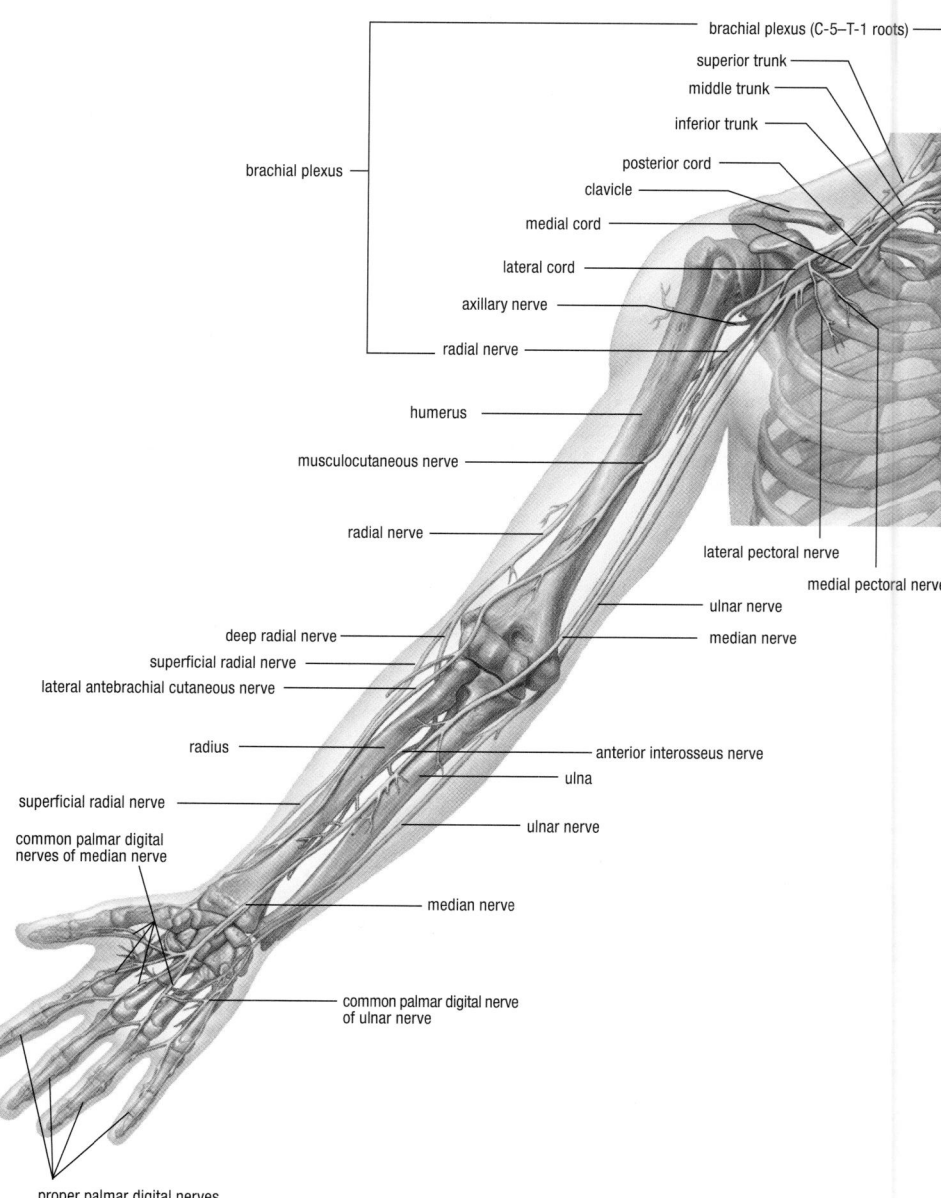

brachial plexus (C-5–T-1 roots)
superior trunk
middle trunk
inferior trunk
posterior cord
clavicle
medial cord
lateral cord
axillary nerve
radial nerve

brachial plexus

humerus

musculocutaneous nerve

radial nerve

lateral pectoral nerve
medial pectoral nerve

ulnar nerve
median nerve

deep radial nerve
superficial radial nerve
lateral antebrachial cutaneous nerve

radius
anterior interosseus nerve
ulna

superficial radial nerve
ulnar nerve

common palmar digital
nerves of median nerve

median nerve

common palmar digital nerve
of ulnar nerve

proper palmar digital nerves

Imagery © adam.com

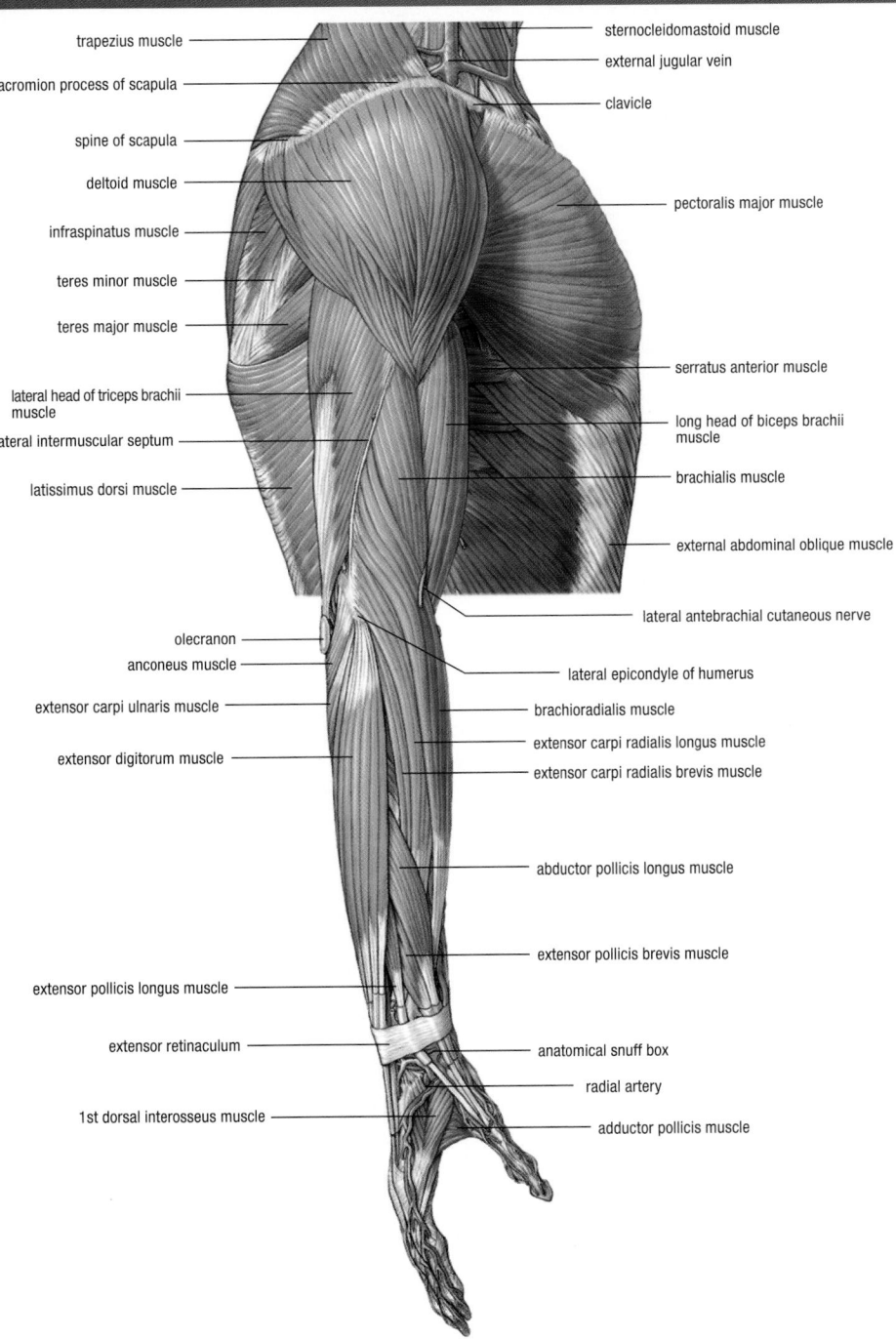

trapezius muscle

acromion process of scapula

spine of scapula

deltoid muscle

infraspinatus muscle

teres minor muscle

teres major muscle

lateral head of triceps brachii muscle

lateral intermuscular septum

latissimus dorsi muscle

olecranon

anconeus muscle

extensor carpi ulnaris muscle

extensor digitorum muscle

extensor pollicis longus muscle

extensor retinaculum

1st dorsal interosseus muscle

sternocleidomastoid muscle

external jugular vein

clavicle

pectoralis major muscle

serratus anterior muscle

long head of biceps brachii muscle

brachialis muscle

external abdominal oblique muscle

lateral antebrachial cutaneous nerve

lateral epicondyle of humerus

brachioradialis muscle

extensor carpi radialis longus muscle

extensor carpi radialis brevis muscle

abductor pollicis longus muscle

extensor pollicis brevis muscle

anatomical snuff box

radial artery

adductor pollicis muscle

Anatomy

Imagery © adam.com

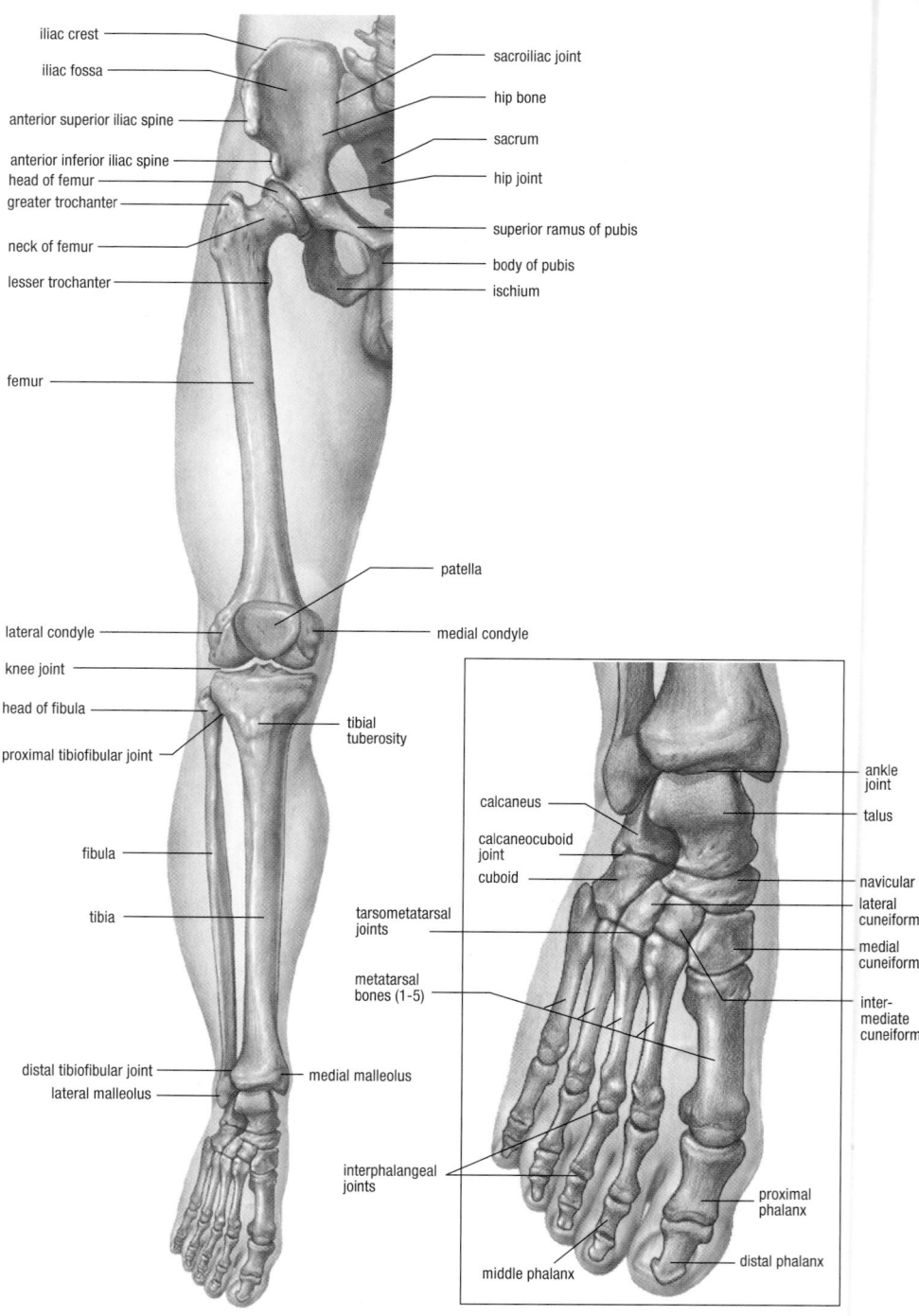

iliac crest

iliac fossa

anterior superior iliac spine

anterior inferior iliac spine

head of femur

greater trochanter

neck of femur

lesser trochanter

femur

sacroiliac joint

hip bone

sacrum

hip joint

superior ramus of pubis

body of pubis

ischium

patella

lateral condyle

medial condyle

knee joint

head of fibula

proximal tibiofibular joint

tibial tuberosity

fibula

tibia

distal tibiofibular joint

lateral malleolus

medial malleolus

tarsometatarsal joints

metatarsal bones (1-5)

interphalangeal joints

ankle joint

talus

calcaneus

calcaneocuboid joint

cuboid

navicular

lateral cuneiform

medial cuneiform

inter-mediate cuneiform

proximal phalanx

distal phalanx

middle phalanx

Imagery © adam.com

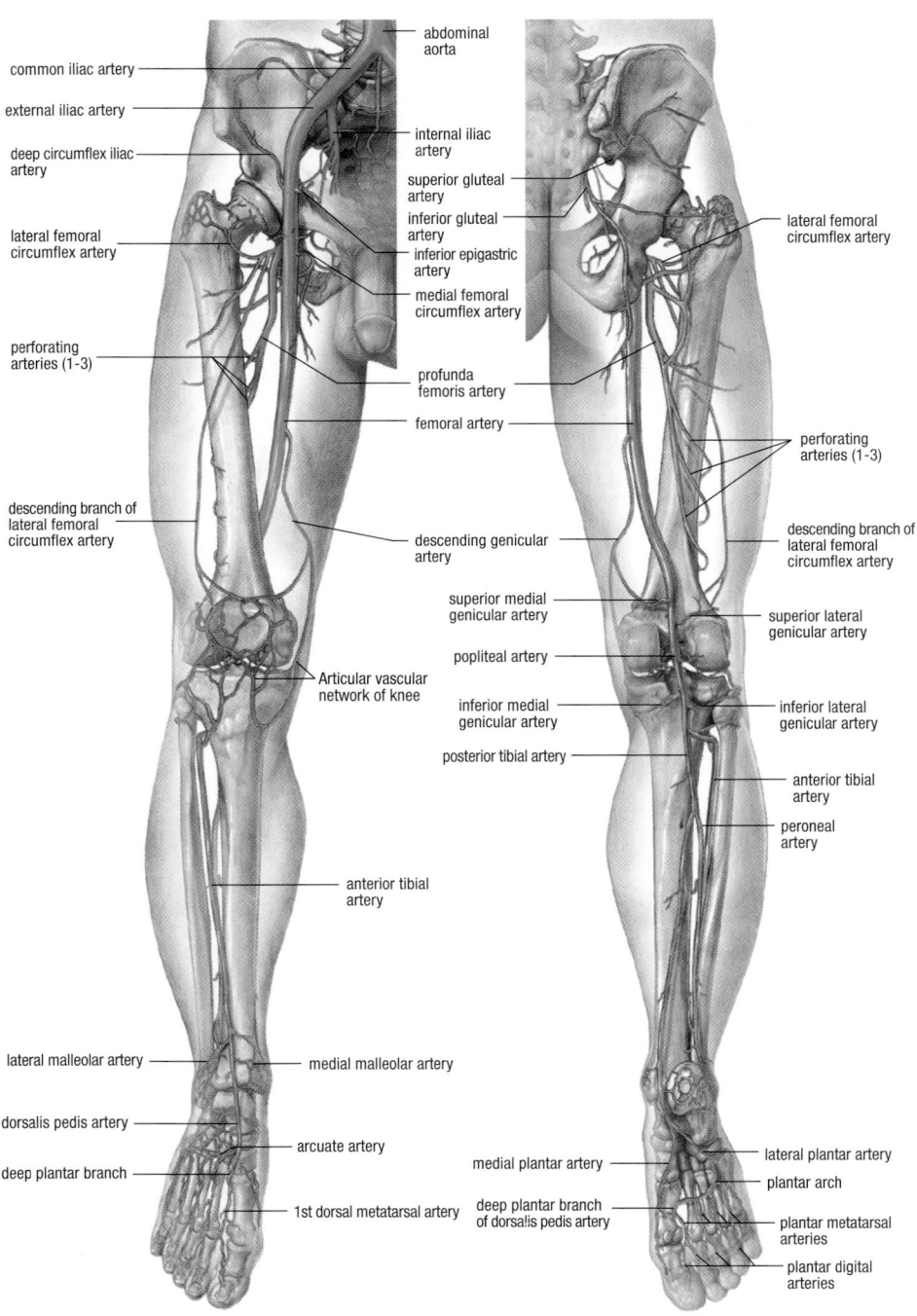

abdominal aorta

common iliac artery

external iliac artery

deep circumflex iliac artery

internal iliac artery

superior gluteal artery

inferior gluteal artery

lateral femoral circumflex artery

lateral femoral circumflex artery

inferior epigastric artery

medial femoral circumflex artery

perforating arteries (1-3)

profunda femoris artery

femoral artery

perforating arteries (1-3)

descending branch of lateral femoral circumflex artery

descending genicular artery

descending branch of lateral femoral circumflex artery

superior medial genicular artery

superior lateral genicular artery

popliteal artery

Articular vascular network of knee

inferior medial genicular artery

inferior lateral genicular artery

posterior tibial artery

anterior tibial artery

peroneal artery

anterior tibial artery

lateral malleolar artery

medial malleolar artery

dorsalis pedis artery

arcuate artery

deep plantar branch

medial plantar artery

lateral plantar artery

plantar arch

1st dorsal metatarsal artery

deep plantar branch of dorsalis pedis artery

plantar metatarsal arteries

plantar digital arteries

**Anatomy**

Imagery © adam.com

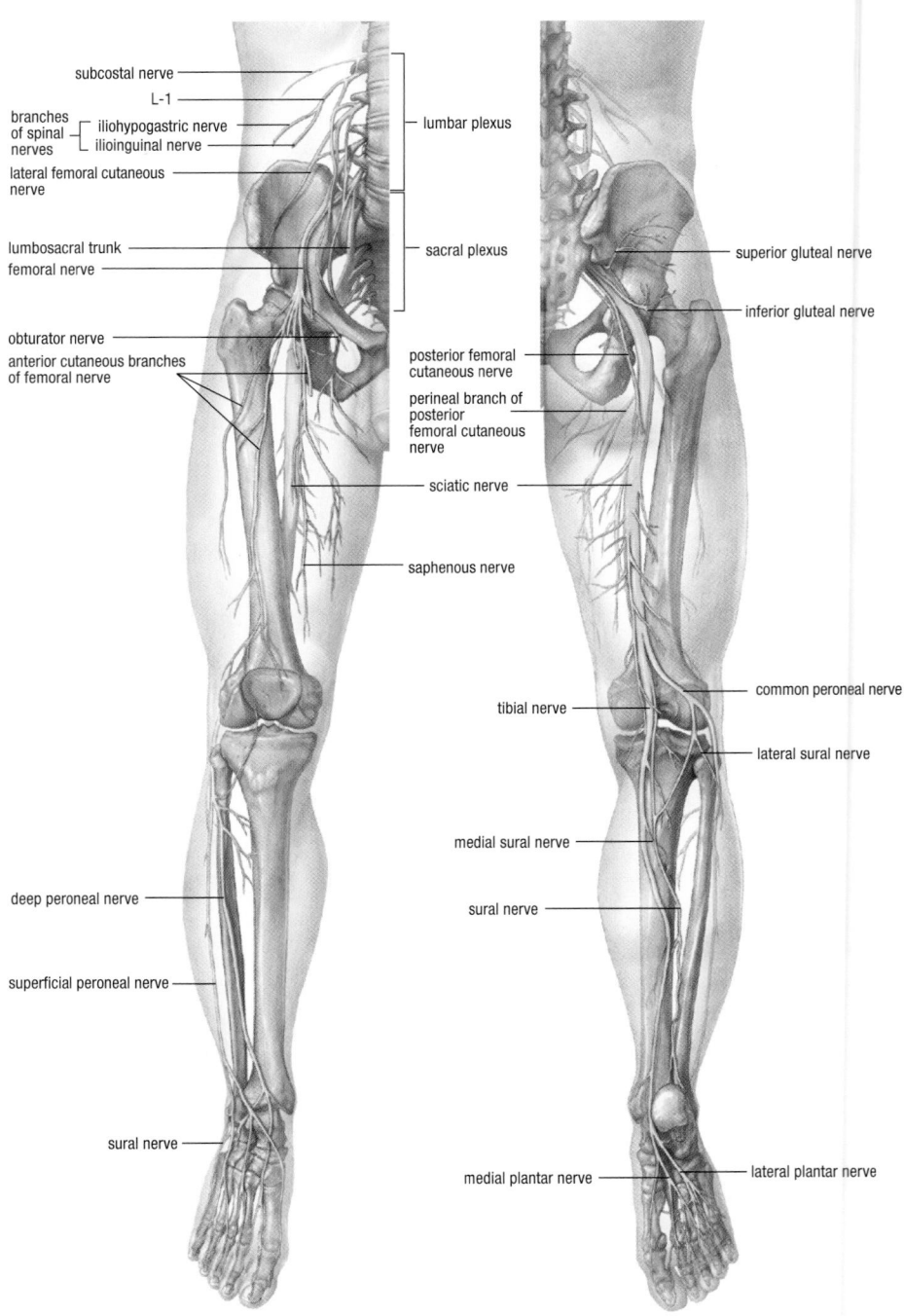

subcostal nerve

L-1

branches of spinal nerves — iliohypogastric nerve
— ilioinguinal nerve

lateral femoral cutaneous nerve

lumbosacral trunk

femoral nerve

obturator nerve

anterior cutaneous branches of femoral nerve

lumbar plexus

sacral plexus

superior gluteal nerve

inferior gluteal nerve

posterior femoral cutaneous nerve

perineal branch of posterior femoral cutaneous nerve

sciatic nerve

saphenous nerve

common peroneal nerve

tibial nerve

lateral sural nerve

medial sural nerve

deep peroneal nerve

sural nerve

superficial peroneal nerve

sural nerve

medial plantar nerve

lateral plantar nerve

Imagery © adam.com

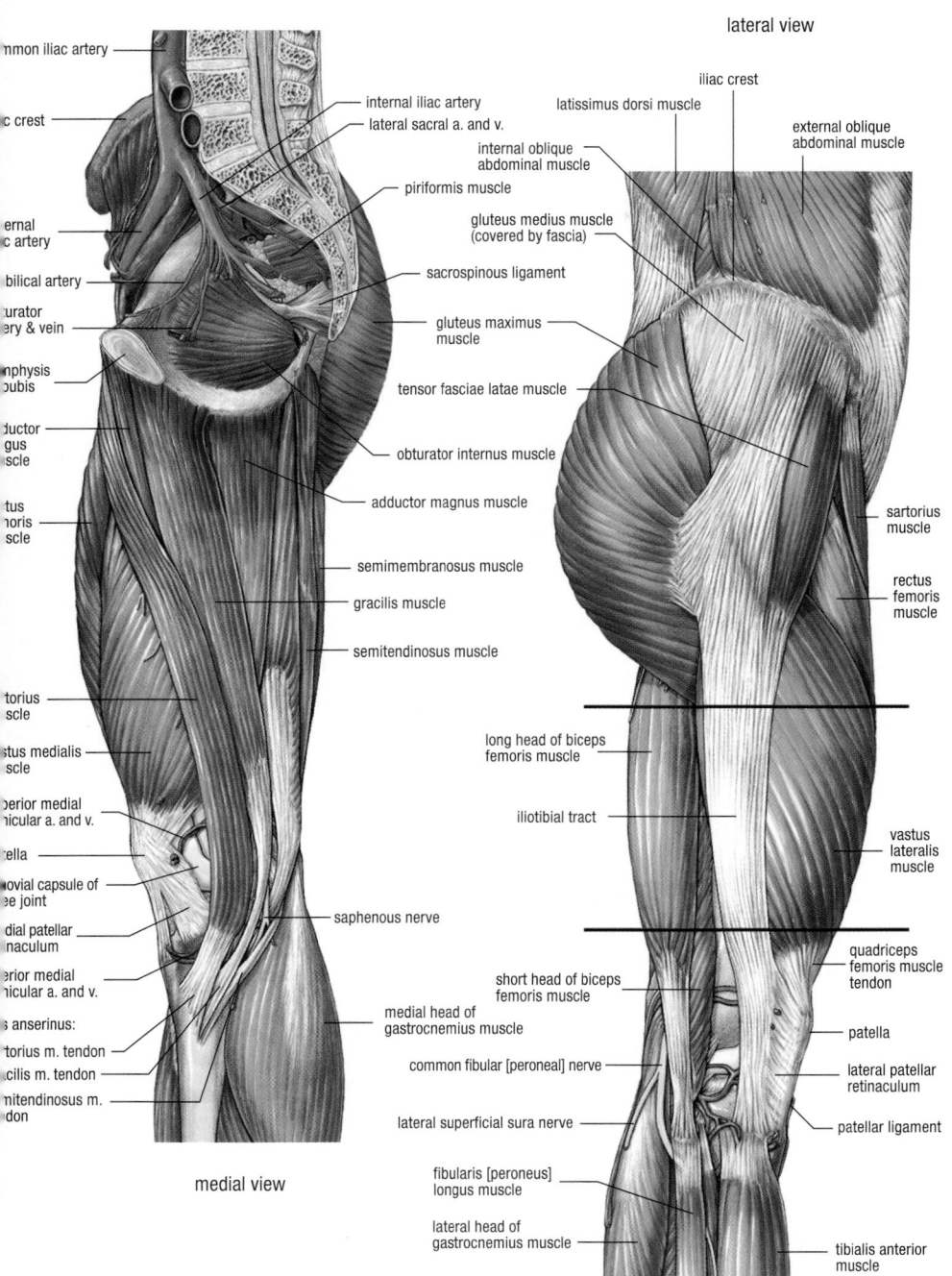

lateral view

mmon iliac artery

c crest

ernal c artery

bilical artery

turator ery & vein

nphysis ubis

ductor gus scle

tus noris scle

torius scle

stus medialis scle

perior medial nicular a. and v.

tella

ovial capsule of e joint

dial patellar naculum

erior medial nicular a. and v.

s anserinus:
torius m. tendon
cilis m. tendon
mitendinosus m. don

internal iliac artery
lateral sacral a. and v.
internal oblique abdominal muscle
piriformis muscle
gluteus medius muscle (covered by fascia)
sacrospinous ligament
gluteus maximus muscle
tensor fasciae latae muscle
obturator internus muscle
adductor magnus muscle
semimembranosus muscle
gracilis muscle
semitendinosus muscle

saphenous nerve

long head of biceps femoris muscle
iliotibial tract
short head of biceps femoris muscle
medial head of gastrocnemius muscle
common fibular [peroneal] nerve
lateral superficial sura nerve
fibularis [peroneus] longus muscle
lateral head of gastrocnemius muscle

latissimus dorsi muscle
iliac crest
external oblique abdominal muscle

sartorius muscle

rectus femoris muscle

vastus lateralis muscle

quadriceps femoris muscle tendon

patella

lateral patellar retinaculum

patellar ligament

tibialis anterior muscle

medial view

Anatomy

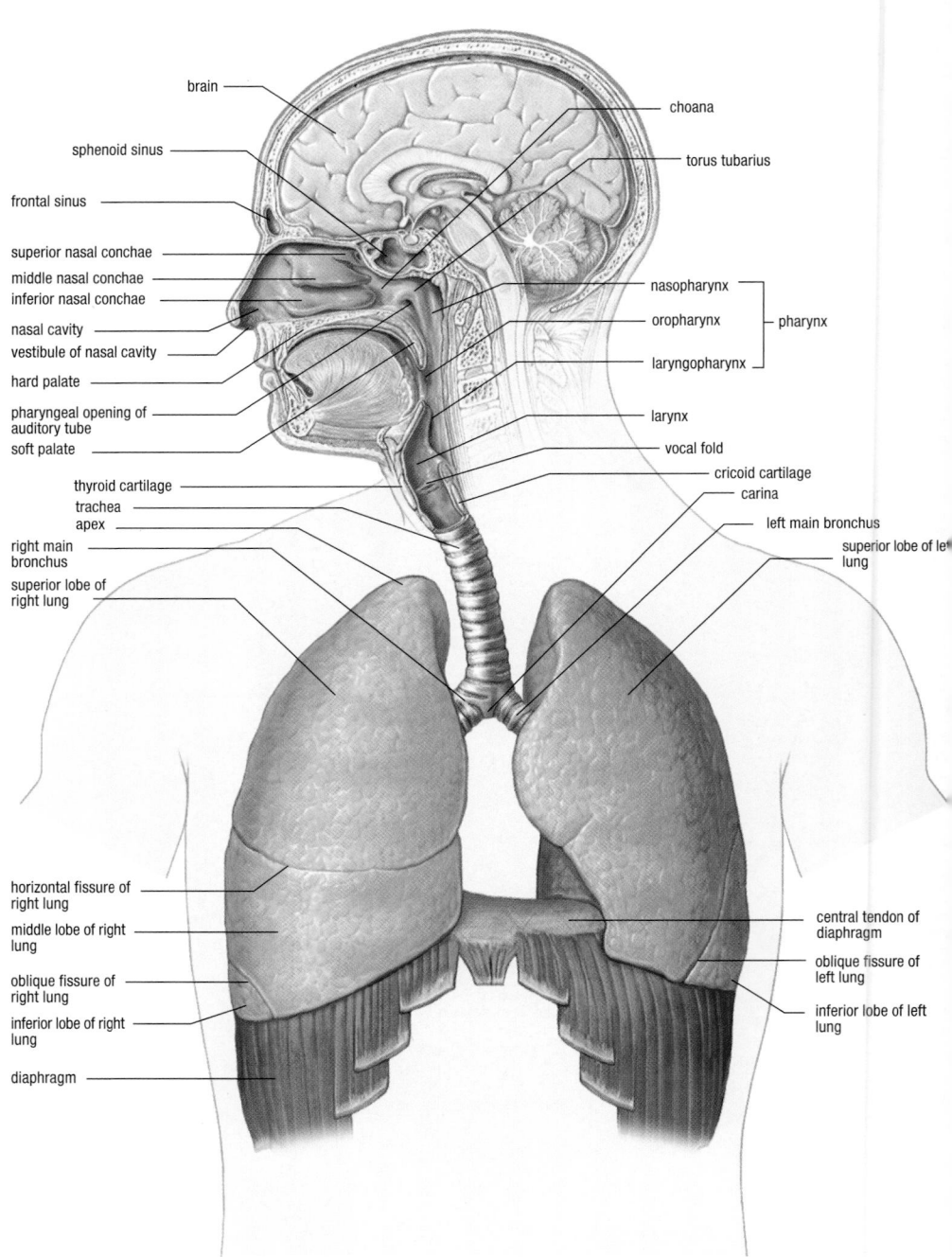

brain

choana

sphenoid sinus

torus tubarius

frontal sinus

superior nasal conchae

middle nasal conchae

inferior nasal conchae

nasopharynx

nasal cavity

oropharynx

pharynx

vestibule of nasal cavity

laryngopharynx

hard palate

pharyngeal opening of
auditory tube

larynx

soft palate

vocal fold

cricoid cartilage

thyroid cartilage

carina

trachea

apex

left main bronchus

right main
bronchus

superior lobe of le[ ]
lung

superior lobe of
right lung

horizontal fissure of
right lung

central tendon of
diaphragm

middle lobe of right
lung

oblique fissure of
left lung

oblique fissure of
right lung

inferior lobe of left
lung

inferior lobe of right
lung

diaphragm

Imagery © adam.com

A22

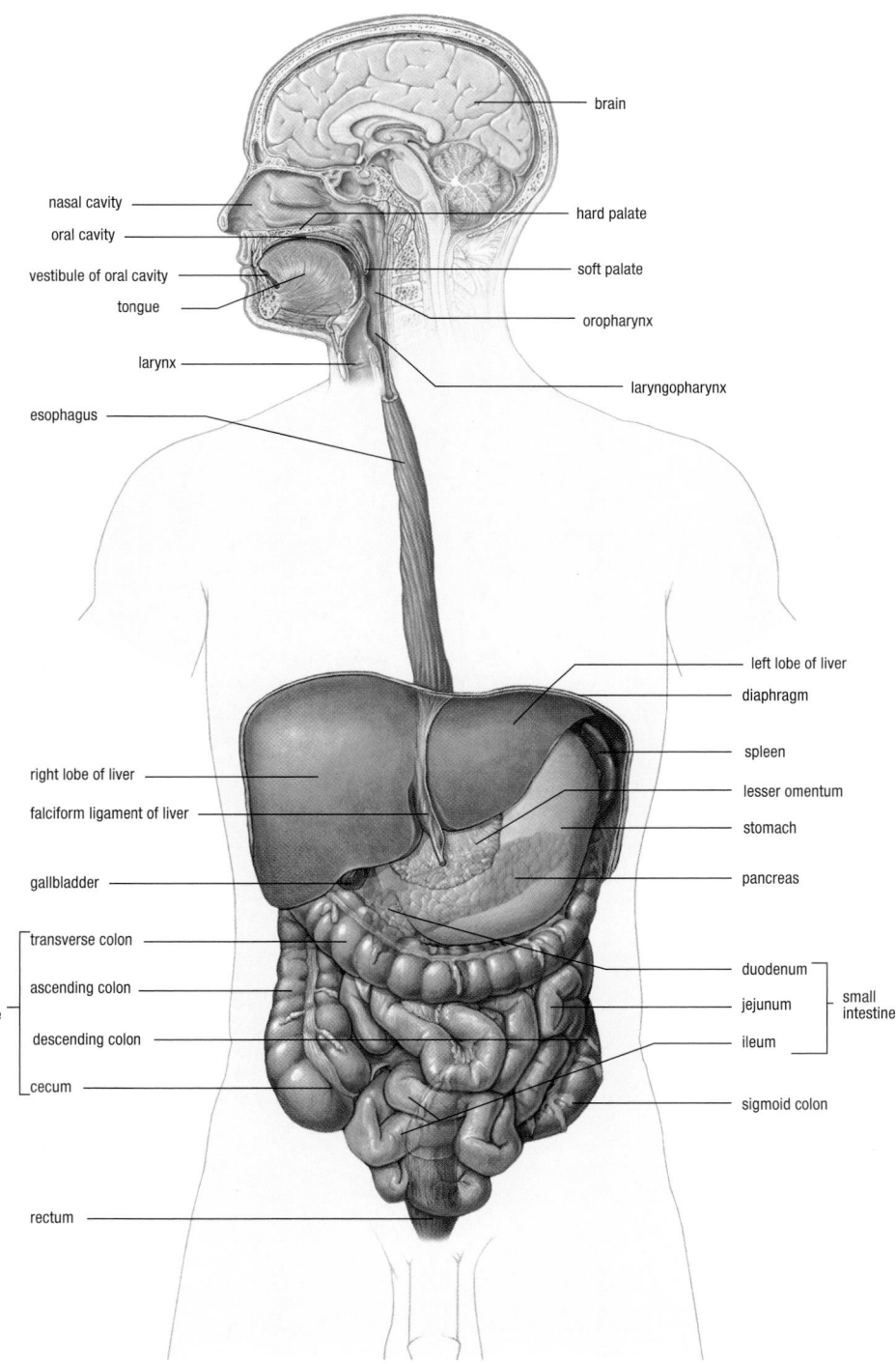

brain

nasal cavity

oral cavity

vestibule of oral cavity

tongue

larynx

esophagus

hard palate

soft palate

oropharynx

laryngopharynx

left lobe of liver

diaphragm

spleen

right lobe of liver

falciform ligament of liver

lesser omentum

stomach

gallbladder

pancreas

transverse colon

ascending colon

descending colon

cecum

large intestine

duodenum

jejunum

ileum

small intestine

sigmoid colon

rectum

Anatomy

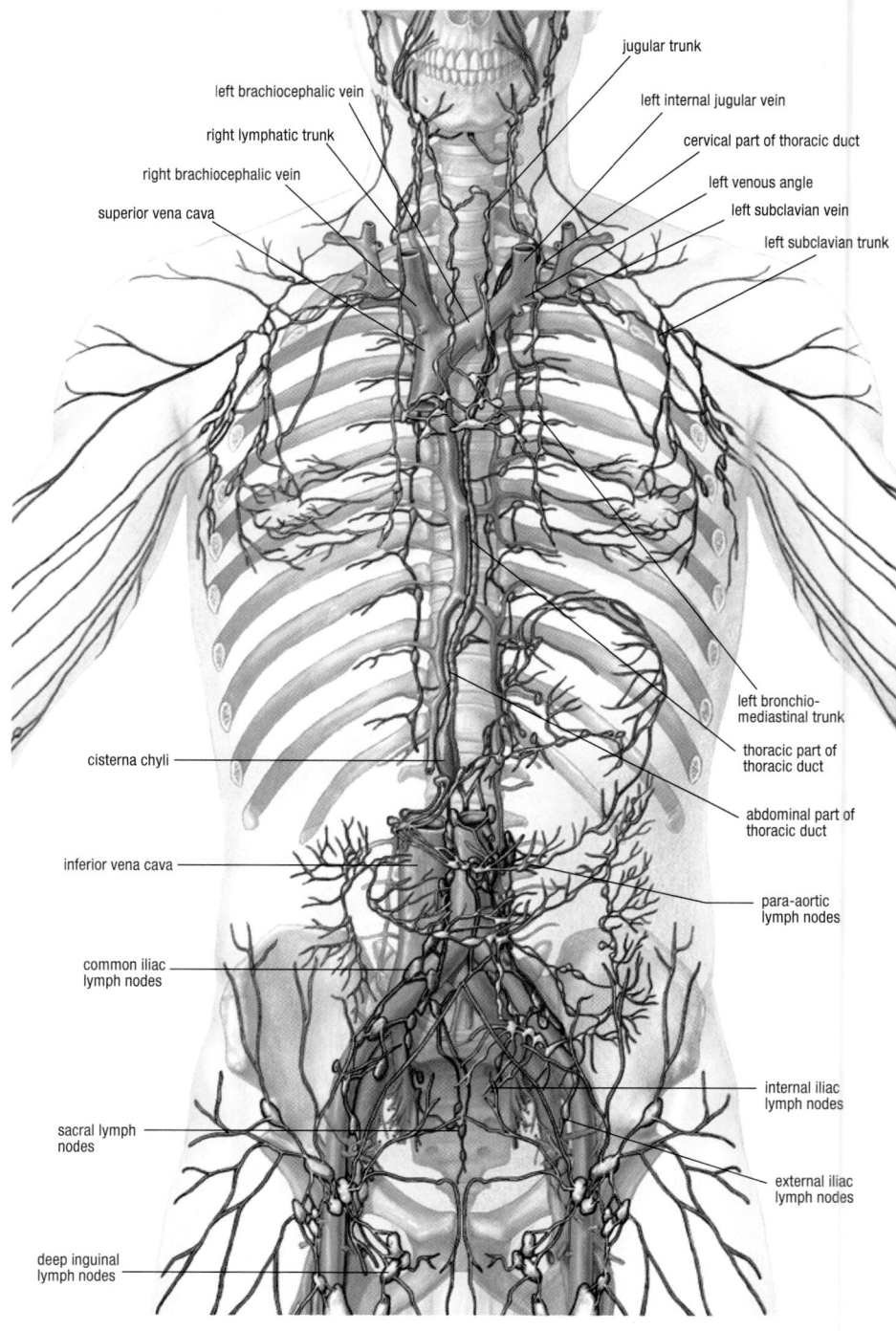

jugular trunk

left brachiocephalic vein

left internal jugular vein

right lymphatic trunk

cervical part of thoracic duct

right brachiocephalic vein

left venous angle

superior vena cava

left subclavian vein

left subclavian trunk

left bronchio-mediastinal trunk

thoracic part of thoracic duct

cisterna chyli

abdominal part of thoracic duct

inferior vena cava

para-aortic lymph nodes

common iliac lymph nodes

internal iliac lymph nodes

sacral lymph nodes

external iliac lymph nodes

deep inguinal lymph nodes

Imagery © adam.com

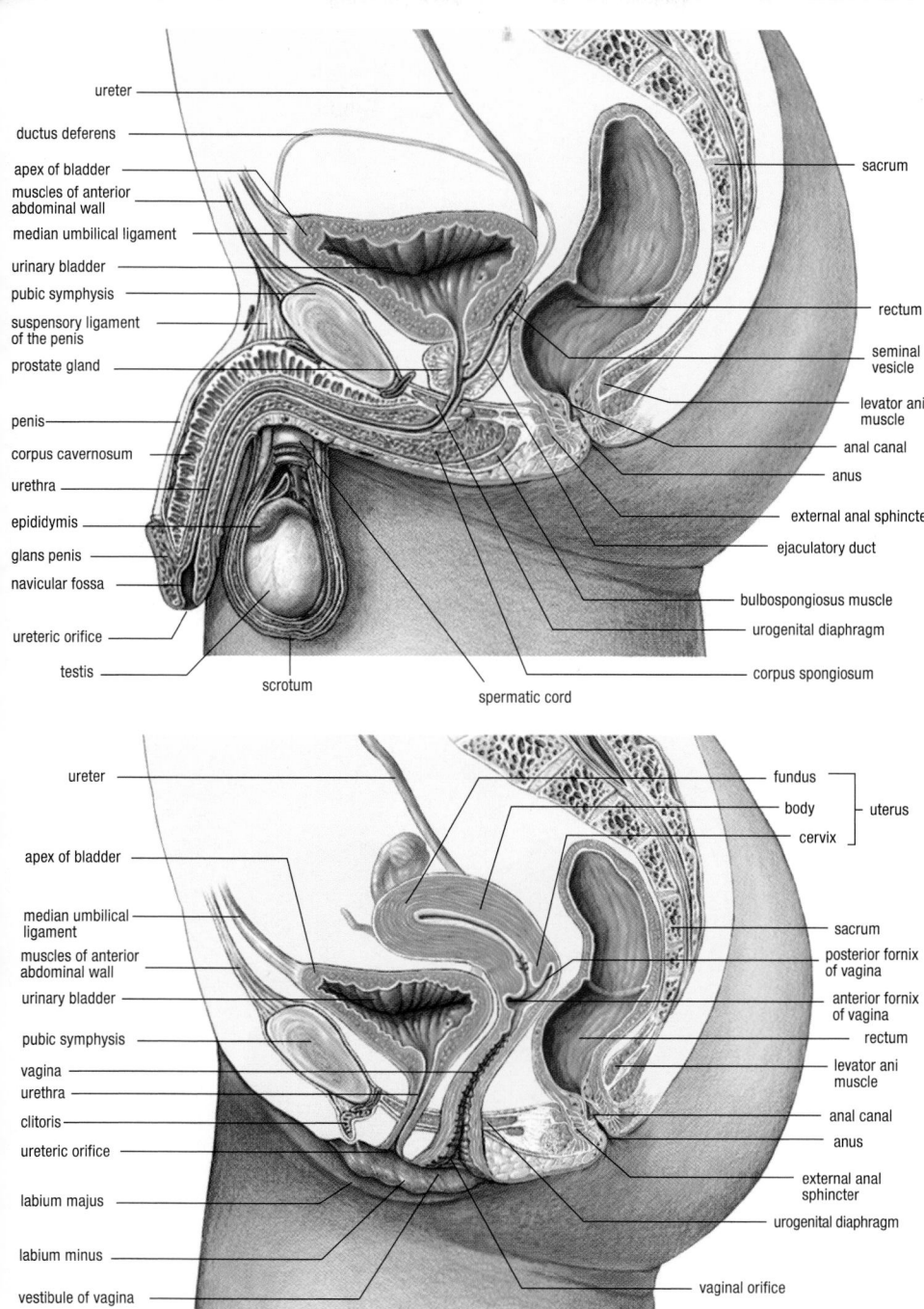

ureter
ductus deferens
apex of bladder
muscles of anterior abdominal wall
median umbilical ligament
urinary bladder
pubic symphysis
suspensory ligament of the penis
prostate gland
penis
corpus cavernosum
urethra
epididymis
glans penis
navicular fossa
ureteric orifice
testis
scrotum
spermatic cord

sacrum
rectum
seminal vesicle
levator ani muscle
anal canal
anus
external anal sphincter
ejaculatory duct
bulbospongiosus muscle
urogenital diaphragm
corpus spongiosum

ureter
apex of bladder
median umbilical ligament
muscles of anterior abdominal wall
urinary bladder
pubic symphysis
vagina
urethra
clitoris
ureteric orifice
labium majus
labium minus
vestibule of vagina

fundus
body — uterus
cervix
sacrum
posterior fornix of vagina
anterior fornix of vagina
rectum
levator ani muscle
anal canal
anus
external anal sphincter
urogenital diaphragm
vaginal orifice

**Anatomy**

Imagery © adam.com

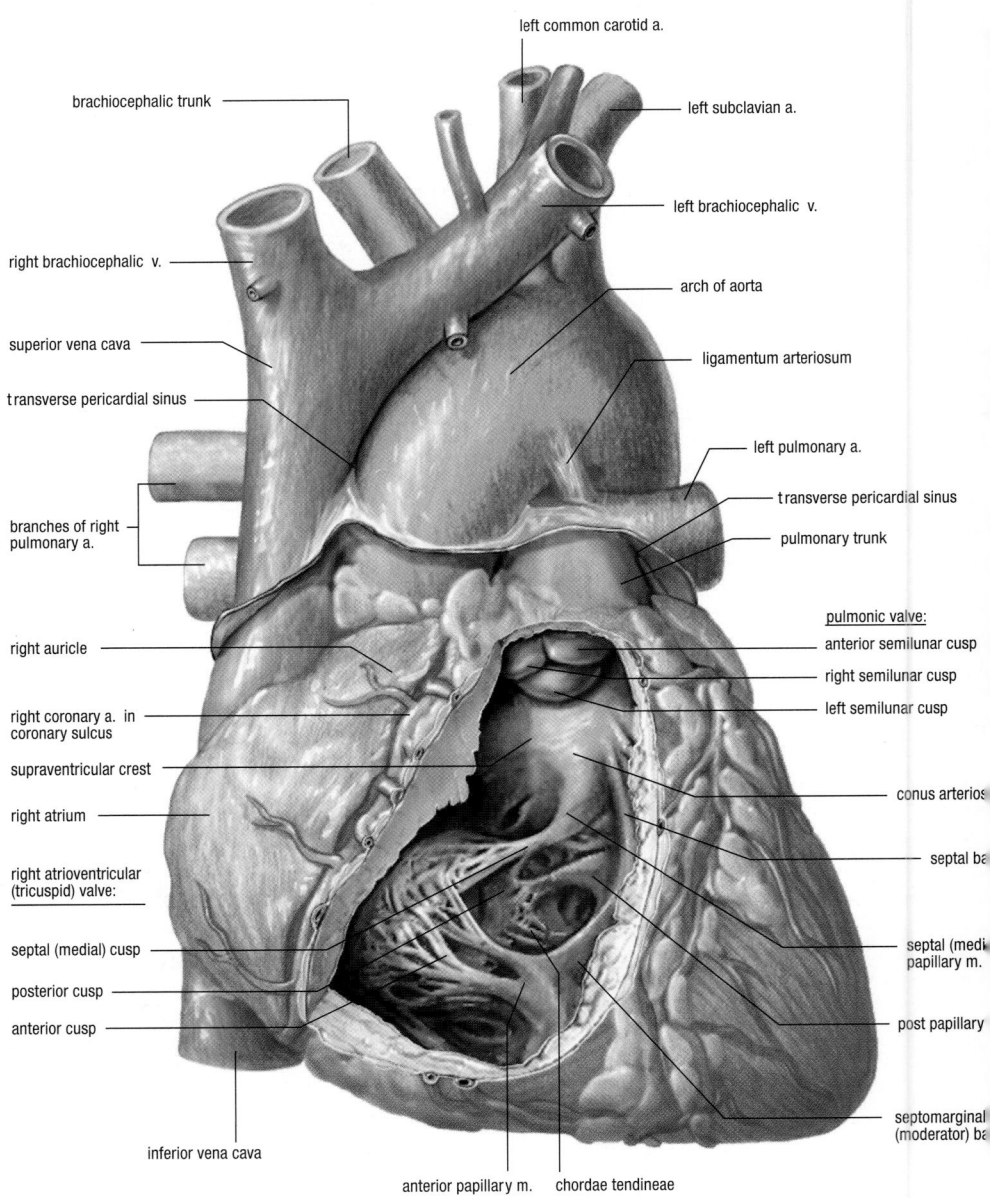

left common carotid a.

brachiocephalic trunk

left subclavian a.

left brachiocephalic v.

right brachiocephalic v.

arch of aorta

superior vena cava

ligamentum arteriosum

transverse pericardial sinus

left pulmonary a.

transverse pericardial sinus

branches of right pulmonary a.

pulmonary trunk

pulmonic valve:
anterior semilunar cusp

right auricle

right semilunar cusp

right coronary a. in coronary sulcus

left semilunar cusp

supraventricular crest

conus arterios

right atrium

septal ba

right atrioventricular (tricuspid) valve:

septal (medi) papillary m.

septal (medial) cusp

posterior cusp

anterior cusp

post papillary

inferior vena cava

septomarginal (moderator) ba

anterior papillary m.     chordae tendineae

Imagery © adam.com

**fi·bri·nu·ria** (fī-brin-yur′ē-ă) the passage of urine that contains fibrin. [fibrin + G. *ouron,* urine]

**fi·bro-, fibr-** fiber. [L. *fibra*]

**fi·bro·ad·e·no·ma** (fī′brō-ad-ĕ-nō′mă) a benign neoplasm derived from glandular epithelium, in which there is a conspicuous stroma of proliferating fibroblasts and connective tissue elements; commonly occurs in breast tissue. SYN fibroid adenoma, adenoma fibrosum.

**fi·bro·ad·i·pose** (fī-brō-ad′i-pōz) relating to or containing both fibrous and fatty structures.

**fi·bro·a·re·o·lar** (fī′brō-ă-rē′ō-lăr) denoting connective tissue that is both fibrous and areolar in character.

**fi·bro·blast** (fī′brō-blast) a stellate or spindle-shaped cell with cytoplasmic processes present in connective tissue, capable of forming collagen fibers; an inactive fibroblast is sometimes called a fibrocyte.

**fi·bro·blas·tic** (fī-brō-blas′tik) relating to fibroblasts.

**fi·bro·car·ci·no·ma** (fī′brō-kar-si-nō′mă) SYN scirrhous carcinoma.

**fi·bro·car·ti·lage** (fī-brō-kar′ti-lij) a variety of cartilage that contains visible type I collagen fibers; appears as a transition between tendons or ligaments or bones. SYN fibrocartilago.

**fi·bro·car·ti·lag·i·nous** (fī′brō-kar-ti-laj′i-nŭs) relating to or composed of fibrocartilage.

**fi·bro·car·ti·la·go** (fī′brō-kar-ti-lā′gō) SYN fibrocartilage.

**fi·bro·cel·lu·lar** (fī-brō-sel′yu-lăr) both fibrous and cellular.

**fi·bro·chon·dri·tis** (fī′brō-kon-drī′tis) inflammation of a fibrocartilage.

**fi·bro·chon·dro·ma** (fī′brō-kon-drō′mă) a benign neoplasm of cartilaginous tissue, in which there is a relatively unusual amount of fibrous stroma.

**fi·bro·cyst** (fī′brō-sist) any cystic lesion circumscribed by or situated within a conspicuous amount of fibrous connective tissue.

**fi·bro·cys·tic** (fī-brō-sis′tik) pertaining to or characterized by the presence of fibrocysts.

**fi·bro·cys·to·ma** (fī′brō-sis-tō′mă) a benign neoplasm, usually derived from glandular epithelium, characterized by cysts within a conspicuous fibrous stroma.

**fi·bro·e·las·tic** (fī′brō-ē-las′tik) composed of collagen and elastic fibers.

**fi·broid** (fī′broyd) **1.** resembling or composed of fibers or fibrous tissue. **2.** old term for certain types of leiomyoma, especially those occurring in the uterus. **3.** SYN fibroleiomyoma. [fibro- + G. *eidos,* resemblance]

**fi·broid ad·e·no·ma, ad·e·no·ma fi·bro·sum** SYN fibroadenoma.

**fi·broid cat·a·ract, fi·brin·ous cat·a·ract** a sclerotic hardening of the capsule of the lens, following exudative iridocyclitis.

**fi·broid·ec·to·my** (fī-broy-dek′tō-mē) removal of a fibroid tumor. [fibroid + G. *ektomē,* excision]

**fi·bro·la·mel·lar liv·er cell car·ci·no·ma** primary hepatic carcinoma in which malignant hepatocytes are intersected by fibrous lamellated bands. SYN oncocytic hepatocellular tumor.

**fi·bro·lei·o·my·o·ma** (fī′brō-lī′ō-mī-ō′mă) a leiomyoma containing non-neoplastic collagenous fibrous tissue, which may make the tumor hard; fibroleiomyoma usually arises in the myome-

trium, and the proportion of fibrous tissue increases with age. SYN fibroid (3), leiomyofibroma.

**fi·bro·li·po·ma** (fī′brō-li-pō′mă) a lipoma with an abundant stroma of fibrous tissue.

**fi·bro·ma** (fī-brō′mă) a benign neoplasm derived from fibrous connective tissue. [fibro- + G. *-oma,* tumor]

**fi·bro·ma·toid** (fī-brō′mă-toyd) a focus, nodule, or mass of proliferating fibroblasts that resembles a fibroma but is not regarded as neoplastic.

**fi·bro·ma·to·sis** (fī′brō-mă-tō′sis) **1.** a condition characterized by the occurrence of multiple fibromas, with a relatively large distribution. **2.** abnormal hyperplasia of fibrous tissue.

**fi·bro·ma·tous** (fī-brō′mă-tŭs) pertaining to, or of the nature of, a fibroma.

**fi·bro·mus·cu·lar** (fī′brō-mŭs′kyu-lăr) both fibrous and muscular; relating to both fibrous and muscular tissues.

**fi·bro·my·al·gia, fi·bro·my·al·gia syn·drome** a condition of chronic diffuse widespread aching and stiffness affecting muscles and soft tissues; diagnosis requires 11 of 18 specific tender points including the occiput, neck, shoulders, chest, elbows, gluteus, greater trochanter and knees; 4 kg touch pressure elicits painful response; tender points are found on both sides of the body and above and below the waist. There are primary and secondary forms.

**fi·bro·my·ec·to·my** (fī′brō-mī-ek′tō-mē) excision of a fibromyoma.

**fi·bro·my·o·ma** (fī′brō-mī-ō′mă) a leiomyoma that contains a relatively abundant amount of fibrous tissue.

**fi·bro·my·o·si·tis** (fī′brō-mī-ō-sī′tis) chronic inflammation of a muscle with an overgrowth, or hyperplasia, of the connective tissue. [fibro- + G. *mys,* muscle, + *-itis,* inflammation]

**fi·bro·myx·o·ma** (fī′brō-mik-sō′mă) a myxoma that contains a relatively abundant amount of mature fibroblasts and connective tissue. [fibro- + G. *myxa,* mucus, + *-ōma,* tumor]

**fi·bro·nec·tin** (fī-brō-nek′tin) glycoproteins found on cell membranes and in blood and other body fluids, which are thought to function as adhesive ligand-like molecules. Possible roles in other processes include transformation to malignancy. Deficiency of fibronectin is associated with Ehlers-Danlos syndrome. [L. *fibra,* fiber, + *nexus,* interconnection]

**fi·bro·neu·ro·ma** (fī′brō-noo-rō′mă) SYN neurofibroma.

**fi·bro·pap·il·lo·ma** (fī′brō-pap-i-lō′mă) a papilloma characterized by a conspicuous amount of fibrous connective tissue at the base and forming the cores upon which the neoplastic epithelial cells are massed.

**fi·bro·pla·sia** (fī-brō-plā′zē-ă) production of fibrous tissue, usually implying an abnormal increase of non-neoplastic fibrous tissue. [fibro- + G. *plasis,* a molding]

**fi·bro·plas·tic** (fī-brō-plas′tik) producing fibrous tissue. [fibro- + G. *plastos,* formed]

**fi·bro·re·tic·u·late** (fī′brō-re-tik′yu-lāt) relating to or consisting of a network of fibrous tissue.

**fi·bro·sar·co·ma** (fī′brō-sar-kō′mă) a malignant neoplasm derived from deep fibrous tissue, characterized by bundles of immature proliferating fibroblasts arranged in a distinctive herringbone pattern with variable collagen formation, which tends to invade locally and metastasize by the bloodstream.

**fi·bro·se·rous** (fī-brō-sē′rŭs) composed of fibrous tissue with a serous surface; denoting any serous membrane.

**fi·bros·ing co·lon·o·pa·thy** colonic fibrosis seen in cystic fibrosis patients, thought to be due to pancreatins.

**fi·bro·sis** (fī-brō′sis) formation of fibrous tissue as a reparative or reactive process, as opposed to formation of fibrous tissue as a normal constituent of an organ or tissue.

**fi·bro·sit·ic head·ache** headache centered in the occipital region due to fibrositis of the occipital muscles; tender areas are present and, commonly, tender nodules are found in the scalp in the lower occipital region.

**fi·bro·si·tis** (fī-brō-sī′tis) **1.** inflammation of fibrous tissue. **2.** obsolete term for fibromyalgia. [fibro- + G. -itis, inflammation]

**fi·brot·ic** (fī-brot′ik) pertaining to or characterized by fibrosis.

**fi·brous** (fī′brŭs) composed of or containing fibroblasts, and also the fibrils and fibers of connective tissue formed by such cells.

**fi·brous an·ky·lo·sis** stiffening of a joint due to the presence of fibrous bands between and about the bones forming the joint. SYN false ankylosis, pseudankylosis.

**fi·brous ar·tic·u·lar cap·sule** the outer fibrous part of the capsule of a synovial joint, which may in places be thickened to form capsular ligaments.

**fi·brous cap·sule** any fibrous envelope of a part; the fibrous capsule of an organ.

**fi·brous cap·sule of kid·ney** a fibrous membrane ensheathing the kidney.

**fi·brous cap·sule of liv·er** a layer of connective tissue ensheathing the hepatic artery, portal vein, and bile ducts as these ramify within the liver; SYN capsula fibrosa perivascularis hepatis [TA], Glisson capsule.

**fi·brous cor·ti·cal de·fect** a common 1 to 3 cm defect in the cortex of a bone, most commonly the lower femoral shaft of a child, filled with fibrous tissue. Nonosteogenic or nonossifying fibroma by convention refers to lesions greater than 3 cm in diameter. SYN nonosteogenic fibroma.

**fi·brous de·gen·er·a·tion** not a degeneration *per se*, but rather a reparative process; cells and foci of tissue previously affected with degenerative processes, and necrosis, are replaced by cellular fibrous tissue.

**fi·brous dys·pla·sia of bone** a disturbance in which bone undergoing physiologic lysis is replaced by abnormal fibrous tissue, resulting in asymmetric distortion and expansion of bone; may be confined to a single bone (monostotic fibrous dysplasia) or involve multiple bones (polyostotic fibrous dysplasia).

**fi·brous goi·ter** a firm hyperplasia of the thyroid and its capsule.

**fi·brous joint** a union of two bones by fibrous tissue such that there is no joint cavity and almost no motion possible; the types of fibrous joints are sutures, syndesmoses, and gomphoses. SYN immovable joint, synarthrodia, synarthrodial joint (1).

**fi·brous tis·sue** a tissue composed of bundles of collagenous white fibers between which are rows

of connective tissue cells; the tendons, ligaments, aponeuroses, and some of the membranes, such as the dura mater.

**fi·brous tu·ber·cle** a tubercle in which fibroblasts proliferate about the periphery (and into the cellular zones), eventually resulting in a rim or wall of cellular fibrous tissue or collagenous material around the tubercle.

**fi·brous un·ion** union of fracture by fibrous tissue. SEE nonunion, vicious union. SYN faulty union.

**fib·u·la** (fib′yu-lă) the lateral and smaller of the two bones of the leg; it is not-weight bearing and articulates with the tibia above and the tibia and talus below. SYN calf bone. [L. *fibula* (contr. fr. *figibula*), that which fastens, a clasp, buckle, fr. *figo*, to fix, fasten]

**fib·u·lar** (fib′yu-lăr) relating to the fibula. [L. *fibularis*]

**fib·u·lar ar·tery** SYN peroneal artery.

**fib·u·lar nut·ri·ent ar·tery** *origin*, fibular (peroneal); *distribution*, fibula.

**fib·u·lar tar·sal ten·din·ous sheaths** synovial tendon sheaths of flexor tendons enabling movement of tendons posterior to the lateral malleolus and across tarsal bones, passing deep to the fibular retinacula; includes (1) the common tendinous sheath of fibulares (peronei) muscles (vagina communis tendinum musculorum fibularium (peroneorum) [TA]; and (2) the plantar tendinous sheath of fibularis (peroneus) (vagina plantaris tendinis musculi fibularis (peronei) longi [TA]).

**fib·u·lar veins** SYN peroneal veins.

**fib·u·lo·cal·ca·ne·al** (fib′yu-lō-kal-kā′nē-ăl) relating to the fibula and the calcaneus.

**Fick laws of dif·fu·sion** (fik) **1.** the direction of movement of solutes by diffusion is always from a higher to a lower concentration and the diffusive flux $J_A$ of solute A across a plane at x is proportional to the concentration gradient of A at x; i.e., $J_A = -D(C_A/x)$; **2.** the increase of concentration of solute A with time, $C_A/t$, is directly proportional to the change in the concentration gradient, i.e., $C_A/t = D(fl^2/x^2)$.

**Fick meth·od** (fik) a method of calculating cardiac output or organ blood flow from measurements of oxygen consumption and of the difference in oxygen concentration between arterial and venous.

**Fi·coll-Hy·paque tech·nique** (fik′ol-hī-pāk) a density-gradient centrifugation technique for separating lymphocytes from other formed elements in the blood; the sample is layered onto a Ficoll-sodium metrizoate gradient of specific density; following centrifugation, lymphocytes are collected from the plasma-Ficoll interface.

**FID** free induction decay.

**Fied·ler my·o·car·di·tis** (fēd′ler) SYN acute isolated myocarditis.

**field** (fēld) a definite area of plane surface, considered in relation to some specific object. [A.S. *feld*]

**field block** regional anesthesia produced by infiltration of local anesthetic solution into tissues surrounding an operative field.

**Field rap·id stain** (fēld) a stain to permit rapid positive diagnosis of malaria in endemic areas by using thick films; it employs methylene blue and azure B in a phosphate buffer, with the preparation counterstained by eosin in a phosphate buffer.

**fifth cra·ni·al nerve [CN V]** SYN trigeminal nerve [CN V].

**fifth dis·ease** SYN erythema infectiosum. [after scarlatina, morbilli, rubella, and fourth d.]

**FIGLU** formiminoglutamic acid.

**fig·ure** (fig′yur) **1.** a form or shape. **2.** a person representing the essential aspects of a particular role. **3.** a form, shape, outline, or representation of an object or person. [L. *figura*, fr *fingo*, to shape, fashion]

**fig·ure and ground** that aspect of perception wherein the perceived is separated into at least two parts, each with different attributes but influencing one another. Figure is the most distinct; ground the least formed; e.g., a bird or tree (figure) seen against the sky (ground).

**fig·ure-ground per·cep·tion** differentiation between foreground and background forms and objects.

**fig·ure-of-8 ban·dage** a bandage applied alternately to two parts, usually two segments of a limb above and below the joint, in such a way that the turns describe the figure 8; used primarily for the treatment of fractures of the clavicle.

**fi·la** (fī′lă) plural of filum. [L.]

**fi·la·ceous** (fī-lā′shŭs) SYN filamentous. [L. *filum*, a thread]

**fil·a·ment** (fil′ă-ment) **1.** SYN filamentum. **2.** BACTERIOLOGY a fine threadlike form, unsegmented or segmented without constrictions. [L. *filamentum*, fr. *filum*, a thread]

**fil·a·men·tous** (fil-ă-men′tŭs) **1.** threadlike in structure. SYN filiform (1). **2.** composed of filaments or threadlike structures. SYN filaceous, filar (2).

**fil·a·men·tum**, pl. **fil·a·men·ta** (fil-ă-men′tŭm, fil-ă-men′tă) a fibril, fine fiber, or threadlike structure. SYN filament (1). [L.]

**fi·lar** (fī′lăr) **1.** SYN fibrillar. **2.** SYN filamentous. [L. *filum*, a thread]

**Fi·lar·ia** (fī-lar′ē-ă) nematodes classified in several genera of the family Onchocercidae; e.g., *Wuchereria bancrofti, Brugia malayi, Onchocerca volvulus, Mansonella perstans, M. streptocerca, M. ozzardi, Loa loa*, and *Dracunculus medinensis*. SEE ALSO filaria.

**fi·lar·ia**, pl. **fi·lar·i·ae** (fĭ-lar′ē-ă, fĭ-lar′ē-ē) common name for nematodes of the family Onchocercidae, which live as adults in the blood, tissue fluids, tissues, or body cavities of many vertebrates. The females lay partially embryonated eggs, the embryos uncoil and circulate in blood or tissue fluids as microfilariae; if ingested by an appropriate bloodsucking arthropod, larval stages develop; later, infective larvae may be deposited on another vertebrate host's skin when the arthropod seeks another blood meal. [L. *filum*, a thread]

**fi·lar·i·al** (fĭ-lā′rē-ăl) pertaining to a filaria (or filariae), including the microfilaria stage.

**fil·a·ri·a·sis** (fil-ă-rī′ă-sis) presence of filariae in the tissues of the body or in blood (microfilaremia) or tissue fluids (microfilariasis), occurring in tropical and subtropical regions; living worms cause minimal tissue reaction, which may be asymptomatic, but death of the adult worms leads to granulomatous inflammation and permanent fibrosis causing obstruction of the lymphatic

channels from dense hyalinized scars in the subcutaneous tissues; the most serious consequence is elephantiasis or pachyderma.

**fi·lar·i·ci·dal** (fĭ-lar-i-sī′dăl) fatal to filariae.

**fi·lar·i·cide** (fĭ-lar′i-sīd) an agent that kills filariae. [filaria + L. *caedo*, to kill]

**fi·lar·i·form** (fĭ-lar′i-fōrm) **1.** resembling filariae or other types of small nematode worms. **2.** thin or hairlike.

**Fi·la·tov flap** (fĭ-lah′tof) SYN tubed flap.

**Fi·la·tov-Gil·lies flap** (fĭ-lah′tof gil′ēz) SYN tubed flap.

**fil·i·al** (fil′ē-ăl) denoting the relationship of offspring to parents. SEE filial generation. [L. *filialis*, fr. *filius*, son, *filia*, daughter]

**fil·i·al gen·er·a·tion (F)** the offspring of a genetically specified mating: first filial generation (symbol $F_1$), the offspring of parents of contrasting genotypes; second filial generation ($F_2$), the offspring of two $F_1$ individuals; third filial generation ($F_3$), fourth filial generation ($F_4$), etc., the offspring in succeeding generations of continued inbreeding of $F_1$ descendents.

**fil·i·form** (fil′i-fōrm) **1.** SYN filamentous (1). **2.** BACTERIOLOGY denoting an even growth along the line of inoculation, either stroke or stab. [L. *filum*, thread]

**fil·i·form bou·gie** a very slender bougie usually used for gentle exploration of strictures or sinus tracts of small diameter where false passages can be encountered or created; the trailing end usually consists of a threaded cylinder into which the screw tip of a following bougie can be inserted.

**fil·i·form pa·pil·lae** numerous elongated conical keratinized projections on the dorsum of the tongue.

**fil·let** (fil′et) **1.** SYN lemniscus. **2.** a skein, loop of cord, or tape used for making traction on a part of the fetus. [Fr. *filet*, a band]

**fill·ing** (fil′ing) lay term for a dental restoration.

**fill·ing de·fect** displacement of contrast medium by a space-occupying lesion in a radiographic study of a contrast-filled hollow viscus, such as a polyp on a barium enema; also applied to defects in the otherwise uniform distribution of radionuclide in an organ, such as a metastasis in the liver on a $^{99m}$Tc-sulfur colloid scan.

**film 1.** a thin sheet of flexible material coated with a light-sensitive or x-ray-sensitive substance used in taking photographs or radiographs. **2.** a thin layer or coating. **3.** a radiograph (colloq.). See page 364.

**film badge** small packet of x-ray film and filters worn by radiation workers to monitor exposure to radiation on a monthly basis. SEE ALSO pocket dosimeter, thermoluminescent dosimeter.

**film·less ra·di·o·gra·phy** electronic acquisition and distribution of radiographic images, eliminating the handling and storage of film. SEE ALSO PACS.

**fi·lo·pres·sure** (fī-lō-presh′ŭr) temporary pressure on a blood vessel by a ligature, which is removed when the flow of blood has ceased. [L. *filum*, thread]

**fil·ter** (fil′ter) **1.** a porous substance through which a liquid or gas is passed in order to separate it from contained particulate matter or impurities. SYN filtrum. **2.** to use or to subject to the action of a filter. **3.** RADIOLOGY a device, used in both diagnostic and therapeutic radiology, that permits passage of useful x-rays and absorbs those that have a lower and less desirable energy. **4.** a device used in spectrophotometric analysis to isolate a segment of the spectrum. **5.** a mathematical algorithm applied to image data for the purpose of enhancing image quality, usually by suppression of high spatial frequency noise. [Mediev. L. *filtro,* pp. *-atus,* to strain through felt, fr. *filtrum,* felt]

**fil·ter·ing bleb** a blister of conjunctiva resulting from glaucoma surgery by which a flap of sclera is created in the eye wall, allowing aqueous humor to percolate out of the eye and underneath the conjunctiva, thus lowering intraocular pressure.

**fil·ter·ing op·er·a·tion** a surgical procedure for creation of a fistula between the anterior chamber of the eye and the subconjunctival space in treatment of glaucoma.

**fil·tra·ble, fil·ter·a·ble** (fil'tră-bl, fil'ter-ă-bl) capable of passing a filter; frequently applied to smaller viruses and some bacteria.

**fil·trate** (fil'trāt) that which has passed through a filter.

**fil·tra·tion** (fil-trā'shŭn) **1.** the process of passing a liquid or gas through a filter. **2.** RADIOLOGY the process of attenuating and hardening a beam of x-rays or gamma rays by interposing a filter (3) between the radiation source and the object being irradiated; inherent filtration is that which is caused by the apparatus itself, such as the glass of an x-ray tube, without addition of a filter. SYN percolation (1).

**fil·tra·tion an·gle** SYN iridocorneal angle.

**fil·tra·tion co·ef·fi·cient** a measure of a membrane's permeability to water; specifically, the volume of fluid filtered in unit time through a unit area of membrane per unit pressure difference, taking into account both hydraulic and osmotic pressures.

**fil·tra·tion frac·tion (FF)** the fraction of the plasma entering the kidney that filters into the lumen of the renal tubules, determined by dividing the glomerular filtration rate by the renal plasma flow; normally, it is around 0.17.

**fil·trum** (fil'trŭm) SYN filter (1). [Mediev. L.]

**fi·lum,** pl. **fi·la** (fī'lŭm, fī'lă) a structure of filamentous or threadlike appearance. [L. thread]

**fi·lum of spi·nal du·ra mat·er** the thread-like termination of the spinal dura mater, surrounding

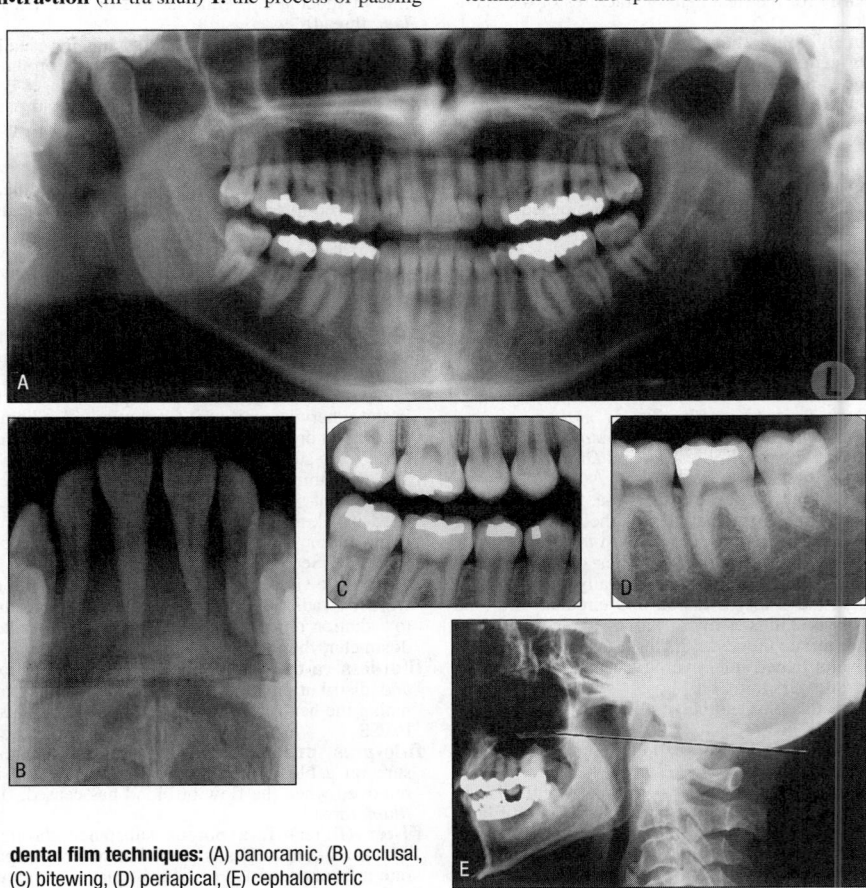

**dental film techniques:** (A) panoramic, (B) occlusal, (C) bitewing, (D) periapical, (E) cephalometric

and fused to the filum terminale of the cord, and attached to the deep dorsal sacrococcygeal ligament; extends from $S_{2-3}$ to $Co_2$ vertebral levels.

**fim•bria**, pl. **fim•bri•ae** (fim′brē-ă, fim′brē-ē) **1.** any fringelike structure. **2.** SYN pilus (2). [L. fringe]

**fim•bri•ae ova•ri•cae** [TA] SYN fimbriae of uterine tube.

**fim•bri•ae of uter•ine tube** the irregularly branched or fringed processes surrounding the ampulla at the abdominal opening of the uterine tube; most of the lining epithelial cells have cilia that beat toward the uterus. SYN fimbriae ovaricae [TA].

**fim•bria hip•po•cam•pi** [TA] a narrow sharp-edged crest of white fiber matter, continuous with the alveus hippocampi, attached to the medial border of the hippocampus; composed of efferent fibers of the hippocampus that form the fornix, fibers of the hippocampal commissure, and septohippocampal fibers. SYN corpus fimbriatum (1).

**fim•bri•ate, fim•bri•at•ed** (fim′brē-āt, fim′brē-ā-ted) having fimbriae.

**fim•bri•o•cele** (fim′brē-ō-sēl) hernia of the corpus fimbriatum of the oviduct. [L. *fimbria*, fringe, + G. *kēlē*, hernia]

**fine nee•dle bi•op•sy** removal of tissue or suspensions of cells through a small needle.

∎**fin•ger** (fing′ger) one of the digits of the hand. See this page. [A.S.]

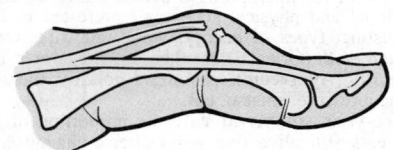

boutonnière deformity

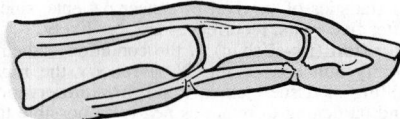

jersey finger (ruptured flexor digitorum profundus tendon)

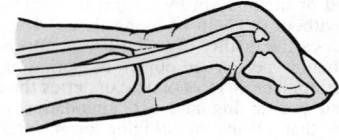

mallet finger

**finger: deformities and fractures**

---

**fin•ger ag•no•sia** inability to name or recognize individual fingers, of one's own or of other persons; most often caused by lesion of or near the angular gyrus of the dominant hemisphere.

**fin•ger-nose test** a test of voluntary eye-motor coordination of the upper limb(s); the subject is asked to slowly touch the tip of the nose with the extended index finger; assesses cerebellar function.

**fin•ger•print** (fing′ger-print′) **1.** an impression of the inked bulb of the distal phalanx of a finger,

showing the configuration of the surface ridges, used as a means of identification. SEE ALSO dermatoglyphics, Galton system of classification of fingerprints. **2.** term, sometimes used informally, referring to any analytic method capable of making fine distinctions between similar compounds or gel patterns; e.g., the pattern of an infrared absorption curve or of a two-dimensional paper chromatograph. **3.** in genetics, the analysis of DNA fragments to determine the identity of an individual or the paternity of a child.

**fin•ger•spel•ling** method of communication using specific finger and hand movements, representing letters of the alphabet, to spell words. SEE ALSO American Manual Alphabet.

**fin•ger-thumb re•flex** SYN basal joint reflex.

**fin•ger-to-fin•ger test** a test for coordination and position sense of the upper limbs; the subject is asked to approximate the ends of the index fingers; assesses cerebellar function.

**Fin•kel•stein test** (fing′kĕl-shtīn) test to detect de Quervain tenosynovitis in which the thumb is flexed into the palm and is covered by the remaining four digits; the wrist is then bent toward the ulna; positive result of test produces pain and crepitus along the path of the involved tendon.

**Fin•ney op•er•a•tion** (fin′ē) gastroduodenostomy that creates, by the technique of closure, a large opening to ensure free emptying from the stomach.

**fire ant** any of several species in the genus *Solenopsis* whose bite causes a fiery, burning sensation and sometimes severe allergic reactions.

**first aid** immediate assistance administered in the case of injury or sudden illness by a bystander or other lay person, before the arrival of trained medical personnel.

**first cra•ni•al nerve [CN I]** SYN olfactory nerves [CN I].

**first de•gree AV block** SEE atrioventricular block.

**first-de•gree burn** a burn involving only the epidermis and causing erythema and edema without vesiculation.

**first de•gree pro•lapse** SEE prolapse of the uterus.

**first heart sound ($S_1$)** occurs with ventricular systole and is mainly produced by closure of the atrioventricular valves.

**first mo•lar, first per•ma•nent mo•lar** sixth permanent tooth or fourth deciduous tooth in the maxilla and mandible on either side of the midsagittal plane of the head following the arch form.

**first-pass me•tab•o•lism, first-pass ef•fect** the intestinal and hepatic degradation or alteration of a drug or substance taken by mouth, after absorption, removing some of the active substance from the blood before it enters the general circulation.

**first re•spon•der 1.** the first person to arrive at the emergency scene (medical incident or trauma) to assist the patient or render immediate life-sustaining aid. **2.** the basic level of training and certification for prehospital medical responders, i.e., fire fighters and law enforcement personnel.

**first and se•cond pos•ter•i•or in•ter•cos•tal ar•ter•ies** terminal branches of the superior intercostal artery (from costocervical trunk) supplying upper two intercostal spaces.

**Fi•scher sign, Fi•scher symp•tom** (fish′ĕr) an

obsolete sign: in tuberculosis of the mediastinal or peribronchial glands, after bending the patient's head as far back as possible, auscultation over the manubrium sterni will sometimes reveal a continuous loud murmur caused by the pressure of the enlarged glands on the large mediastinal vessels.

**FISH** fluorescent in situ hybridization.

**Fish•berg con•cen•tra•tion test** (fish'bĕrg) a test of renal water conservation; after overnight fluid deprivation, morning urine samples are collected and specific gravity is measured.

**Fish•er ex•act test** the test for association in a two-by-two table that is based on the exact distribution of the frequencies within the table.

**Fish•er syn•drome** (fish'ĕr) a syndrome characterized by ophthalmoplegia, ataxia, and areflexia; a form of polyneuroradiculitis.

**fis•sion** (fish'ŭn) **1.** the act of splitting, e.g., amitotic division of a cell or its nucleus. **2.** splitting of the nucleus of an atom. [L. *fissio*, a cleaving, fr. *findo*, pp. *fissus*, to cleave]

**fis•sion pro•duct** an atomic species produced in the course of the fission of a larger atom such as $^{235}$U.

**fis•si•par•i•ty** (fis-i-par'i-tē) SYN schizogenesis. [L. *fissio*, cleaving, fr. *findo*, to cleave, + *pario*, to bring forth]

**fis•sip•a•rous** (fi-sip'ă-rŭs) reproducing or propagating by fission. [L. *findo*, pp. *fissus*, split, + *pario*, to produce]

**fis•su•la** (fiz'oo-la) diminutive of fissure; a small fissure or cleft.

**fis•su•la an•te fe•nes•tram** minute, slitlike passage in the labyrinthine wall of the tympanic cavity, extending obliquely from the region of the cochleaform process to the vestibule of the bony labyrinth, anterior to the oval window; it is considered to be an extension of the perilymphatic space, but is occupied by a small band of connective tissue that is continuous with the mucosa of the tympanic cavity.

**fis•su•ra,** pl. **fis•su•rae** (fi-soo'ră, fi-soo'rē) **1.** [TA] SYN fissure. **2.** NEUROANATOMY a particularly deep sulcus of the surface of the brain or spinal cord. [L. fr. *findo*, to cleave]

**fis•su•rae ce•re•bel•li** [TA] SYN cerebellar fissure.

**fis•su•ra li•ga•men•ti te•re•tis** [TA] SYN fissure of round ligament of liver.

**fis•su•ra li•ga•men•ti ve•no•si** [TA] SYN fissure of ligamentum venosum.

**fis•sure** (fish'ŭr) **1.** a deep furrow, cleft, or slit. SEE ALSO sulcus. **2.** in dentistry, a developmental break or fault in the tooth enamel. See page B5. SYN fissura (1). [L. *fissura*]

**fis•sured frac•ture** SYN linear fracture.

**fis•sured ton•gue** a painless condition of the tongue characterized by numerous grooves or furrows on the dorsal surface.

**fis•sure of lig•a•men•tum ve•no•sum** a deep cleft extending from the porta hepatis and the inferior vena cava between the left lobe and the caudate lobe; it lodges the ligamentum venosum and is thus a vestige of the fossa of the ductus venosus. SYN fissura ligamenti venosi [TA].

**fis•sure of round lig•a•ment of li•ver** a cleft on the inferior surface of the liver, running from the inferior border to the left extremity of the porta hepatis; it lodges the round ligament of the liver. SYN fissura ligamenti teretis [TA].

**fis•tu•la,** pl. **fis•tu•lae, fis•tu•las** (fis'tyu-lă, fis-tyu-lē, fis-tyu-lăs) an abnormal passage from one epithelialized surface to another; congenital, caused by disease or injury, or created surgically. [L. a pipe, a tube]

**fis•tu•la•tion, fis•tu•li•za•tion** (fis-tyu-lā'shŭn, fis-tyu-li-zā'shŭn) formation of a fistula in a part; becoming fistulous.

**fis•tu•lec•to•my** (fis-tyu-lek'tō-mē) excision of a fistula. SYN syringectomy. [fistula + G. *ektomē*, excision]

**fis•tu•lot•o•my** (fis-tyu-lot'ō-mē) incision or surgical enlargement of a fistula. SYN syringotomy. [fistula + G. *tomē*, incision]

**fis•tu•lous** (fis'tyu-lŭs) relating to or containing a fistula.

**fit 1.** an attack of an acute disease or the sudden appearance of some symptom, such as coughing. **2.** a convulsion. **3.** SYN epilepsy. **4.** DENTISTRY the adaptation of any dental restoration, e.g., of an inlay to the cavity preparation in a tooth, or of a denture to its basal seat. [A.S. *fitt*]

**FITC** fluorescein isothiocyanate.

**fit•ness** (fit'nes) **1.** well-being. **2.** suitability. **3.** POPULATION GENETICS a measure of the relative survival and reproductive success of a given individual or phenotype, or of a population subgroup. **4.** a set of attributes, primarily respiratory and cardiovascular, relating to ability to perform tasks requiring expenditure of energy.

**five el•e•ment theo•ry** an alternative medical system for interpreting a person's mental, emotional and physical states as manifested in five distinct types of energy: wood, air, fire, water and earth (Oriental) or ether, air, fire, water, and earth (Ayurvedic). SEE ALSO polarity therapy, acupressure, shiatsu, chi.

**five-year sur•viv•al rate** the proportion of patients still alive five years after a diagnosis or form of treatment is completed. Usually applied to statistics of survival of cancer patients, since, after five years, recurrences are less likely.

**fix•a•tion** (fik-sā'shŭn) **1.** the condition of being firmly attached or set. **2.** HISTOLOGY the rapid killing of tissue elements and their preservation and hardening to retain as nearly as possible the same relations they had in the living body. SYN fixing. **3.** CHEMISTRY the conversion of a gas into solid or liquid form by chemical reactions, with or without the help of living tissue. **4.** PSYCHOANALYSIS the quality of being firmly attached to a particular person or object or period in one's development. **5.** PHYSIOLOGICAL OPTICS the coordinated positioning and accommodation of both eyes that results in bringing or maintaining a sharp image of a stationary or moving object on the fovea of each eye. [L. *figo*, pp. *fixus*, to fix, fasten]

**fix•a•tion nys•tag•mus** nystagmus aggravated or induced by ocular fixation, arising as optokinetic nystagmus, or resulting from midbrain lesions.

**fix•a•tion sup•pres•sion** the reduction in induced or spontaneous nystagmus that occurs with visual fixation.

**fix•a•tive** (fik'să-tiv) **1.** serving to fix, bind, or make firm or stable. **2.** a substance used for the preservation of gross and histologic specimens of tissue, or individual cells, usually by denaturing and precipitating or cross-linking the protein constituents. SEE ALSO fluid, solution.

**fix•a•tor** (fik-sā'ter) a device providing rigid immobilization through external skeletal fixation by means of rods (fixators) attached to pins which are placed in or through the bone.

**fix·a·tor mus·cle** a muscle that acts as a stabilizer of one part of the body during movement of another part.

**fixed drug e·rup·tion** a type of drug eruption that recurs at a fixed site (or sites) following the administration of a particular drug.

**fixed end** for a given movement, the end of a bone that is held stationary (as a consequence of attachment or muscular fixation) while the other end of the bone (the mobile end) moves in response to muscle activity or gravity. SYN punctum fixa.

**fixed i·dea 1.** an exaggerated notion, belief, or delusion that persists, despite evidence to the contrary, and controls the mind; **2.** the obstinate conviction of a psychotic person regarding the correctness of a delusion.

**fixed mac·ro·phage** a relatively immotile macrophage found in connective tissue, lymph nodes, spleen, and bone marrow.

**fixed par·tial den·ture** a restoration of one or more missing teeth which cannot be readily removed by the patient or dentist; it is permanently attached to natural teeth or roots which furnish the primary support to the appliance. SYN bridge (3).

**fixed pu·pil** a stationary pupil unresponsive to all stimuli.

**fixed-rate pace·mak·er** an artificial pacemaker that emits electrical stimuli at a constant frequency.

**fixed vi·rus** rabies virus whose virulence for rabbits has been stabilized by numerous passages through this experimental host. SEE ALSO street virus.

**fix·er** in photography and radiography, a solution that removes both the unexposed and undeveloped silver halide crystals from the film emulsion and hardens the gelatin.

**fix·ing** (fik′sing) SYN fixation (2).

**flac·cid** (flak′sid, flas′id) relaxed, flabby, or without tone. [L. *flaccidus*]

**flac·cid dys·arth·ria** dysarthria associated with peripheral muscle weakness usually due to lower motor neuron disorders, causing hypernasality, imprecise consonants, breathy voice, and monotony of pitch. SEE hypernasality.

**flac·cid·i·ty** (flăk-sid′i-tē) the condition or state of being flaccid.

**fla·gel·la** (flă-jel′ă) plural of flagellum.

**fla·gel·lar** (fla-jel′ăr) relating to a flagellum or to the extremity of a protozoan.

**fla·gel·lar an·ti·gen** the heat-labile antigens associated with bacterial flagella, in contrast to somatic antigen. SEE ALSO H antigen.

**flag·el·late** (flaj′ĕ-lāt) **1.** possessing one or more flagella. **2.** a member of the class Mastigophora.

**flag·el·lat·ed** (flaj′ĕ-lā-ted) possessing one or more flagella.

**flag·el·la·tion** (flaj′ĕ-lā′shŭn) **1.** whipping either one's self or another as a means of arousing or heightening sexual feeling. **2.** the pattern of formation of flagella. [L. *flagellatus*, fr. *flagello*, to whip or scourge]

**flag·el·lo·sis** (flaj′ĕ-lō′sis) infection with flagellated protozoa in the intestinal or genital tract, e.g., trichomoniasis.

**fla·gel·lum**, pl. **fla·gel·la** (flă-jel′ŭm, flă-jel′ă) a whiplike locomotory organelle of constant structural arrangement consisting of nine double peripheral microtubules and two single central microtubules; it arises from a deeply staining basal granule, often connected to the nucleus by a fiber, the rhizoplast. [L. dim. of *flagrum*, a whip]

**flail chest** flapping chest wall; condition in which three or more consecutive ribs on the same side of the chest have been fractured in at least two places, with resulting instability of the chest wall, paradoxical respiratory movements of the injured segment, and loss of respiratory efficiency.

**flail joint** a joint with loss of function caused by loss of ability to stabilize the joint in any plane within its normal range of motion.

**flame cell** primitive, ciliated excretory cell in trematodes; the movement of the cilia on this cell within the miracidium larva within a schistosome egg indicates egg viability.

**flange** (flanj) that part of the denture base which extends from the cervical ends of the teeth to the border of the denture.

**flank** SYN latus.

**flank po·si·tion** a lateral recumbent position, but with the lower leg flexed, the upper leg extended, and convex extension of the upper side of the body; used for nephrectomy.

**flap 1.** mass or tongue of tissue for transplantation, vascularized by a pedicle or stem; specifically, a pedicle flap. SEE ALSO local flap, distant flap. **2.** an uncontrolled movement, as of the hands. SEE asterixis. [M.E. *flappe*]

**flap am·pu·ta·tion** an amputation in which flaps of the muscular and cutaneous tissues are made to cover the end of the bone. SYN flap operation (1).

**flap·less am·pu·ta·tion** an amputation without any tissue to cover the stump

**flap op·er·a·tion 1.** SYN flap amputation. **2.** DENTAL SURGERY an operation in which a portion of the mucoperiosteal tissues is surgically detached from the underlying bone or impacted tooth for better access and visibility in exploring the area covered by the tissue. SEE ALSO flap.

**flap·ping trem·or** SYN asterixis.

**flare** (flār) **1.** a gradual tapering or spreading outward. **2.** a diffuse redness of the skin extending beyond the local reaction to the application of an irritant; it is due to dilation of the arterioles and capillaries; depends upon an axon reflex set up by the liberation of a histamine-like substance in skin when injured. SEE ALSO triple response.

**flash 1.** a sudden and brief burst of light or heat. **2.** excess material extruded between the sections of a flask in the process of molding denture bases or other dental restorations.

**flash·back** an involuntary recurrence of some aspect of a hallucinatory experience or perceptual distortion occurring some time after ingestion of the hallucinogen that produced the original effect and without subsequent ingestion of the substance.

**flash blind·ness** a temporary loss of vision produced when retinal light-sensitive pigments are bleached by light more intense than that to which the retina is physiologically adapted at that moment.

**flash-lag ef·fect** the apparent lagging behind a moving object of a portion of it that flashes briefly.

**flash meth·od** sterilization of milk by raising it

rapidly to a temperature of 178°F, holding it there for a short time, and reducing it rapidly to 40°F.

**flask** a small receptacle, usually of glass, used for holding liquids, powder, or gases. [M.E. keg, fr. Fr. *flasque,* fr. Germanic]

**Fla·tau law** (flah'tow) a law concerning the excentric position of the long spinal tracts; the greater the distance the nerve fibers run lengthwise in the cord, the more they tend to be situated toward its periphery.

**flat bone** a type of bone characterized by its thin, flattened shape, such as the scapula or certain of the cranial bones.

**flat chest** a thorax in which the anteroposterior diameter is shorter than the average.

**flat con·dy·lo·ma 1.** SYN condyloma latum. **2.** a condyloma of the uterine cervix or other site caused by human papilloma virus infection and characterized histologically by koilocytosis without papillomatosis.

**flat e·lec·tro·en·ceph·a·lo·gram** SYN electrocerebral silence.

**flat flap** a flap in which during transfer the pedicle is left flat or open, i.e., untubed. SYN open flap.

**flat·foot** (flat'fŭt) SYN talipes planus.

**flat pel·vis** a pelvis in which the anteroposterior diameter is uniformly contracted, the sacrum being dislocated forward between the iliac bones.

**flat plate** JARGON an abdominal radiograph made with the subject supine and without contrast medium.

**flat·u·lence** (flat'yu-lens) presence of an excessive amount of gas in the stomach and intestines. [Mod. L. *flatulentus,* fr. L. *flatus,* a blowing, fr. *flo,* pp. *flatus,* to blow]

**flat·u·lent** (flat'yu-lent) relating to or suffering from flatulence.

**fla·tus** (flā'tŭs) gas or air in the gastrointestinal tract which may be expelled through the anus. [L. a blowing]

**flat wart** SYN verruca plana.

**flat·worm** (flat'werm) a member of the phylum Platyhelminthes, including the parasitic tapeworms and flukes.

**fla·vin, fla·vine** (flā'vin, flā-vēn, flav'in, flāv-ēn) a yellow acridine dye, preparations of which are used as antiseptics. [L. *flavus,* yellow]

**fla·vin ad·e·nine di·nu·cle·o·tide (FAD)** a condensation product of riboflavin and adenosine 5'-diphosphate; the coenzyme of various aerobic dehydrogenases, e.g., D-amino-acid oxidase and aldehyde dehydrogenase; strictly speaking, FAD is not a dinucleotide since it contains a sugar alcohol.

**fla·vin mon·o·nu·cle·o·tide (FMN)** riboflavin 5'-phosphate; the coenzyme of a number of oxidation-reduction enzymes; e.g., NADH dehydrogenase and L-amino acid oxidase. Strictly speaking, FMN is not a nucleotide since it contains a sugar alcohol instead of a sugar.

**Fla·vi·vi·rus** (flā'vi-vī-rŭs) a genus in the family Flaviviridae that includes yellow fever, dengue, and St. Louis encephalitis viruses. [L. *flavus,* yellow, + virus]

**Fla·vo·bac·te·ri·um** (flā-vō-bak-tēr'ē-ŭm) a genus of aerobic to facultatively anaerobic, nonsporeforming, motile and nonmotile bacteria containing Gram-negative rods. These organisms characteristically produce yellow, orange, red, or yellow-brown pigments. They are found in soil and fresh and salt water. Some species are pathogenic. [L. *flavus,* yellow]

**Fla·vo·bac·ter·i·um men·in·go·sep·ti·cum** among the normal flora of the human respiratory tract, this bacterial species is an occasional cause of nosocomial infection, including neonatal meningitis.

**fla·vo·en·zyme** (flā-vō-en'zīm) any enzyme that possesses a flavin nucleotide as coenzyme; e.g., xanthine oxidase, succinate dehydrogenase.

**fla·vo·pro·tein** (flā'vō-prō'tēn) a compound protein possessing a flavin as prosthetic group. Cf. flavoenzyme.

**flea** (flē) an insect of the order Siphonaptera, marked by lateral compression, sucking mouthparts, extraordinary jumping powers, and ectoparasitic adult life in the hair and feathers of warm-blooded animals.

**Flei·scher ring** (flīsh'er) an incomplete ring often present at the base of the keratoconus cone; it may be yellow or greenish from deposition of hemosiderin.

**Fleisch·ner lines** (flīsh'ner) coarse linear shadows on a chest radiograph, indicating bands of subsegmental atelectasis.

**Flem·ming fix·a·tive** (flem'ing) a mixture of chromic acid, osmic acid, and acetic acid that makes an excellent cytoplasmic and chromosomal fixative, especially when acetic acid is omitted; disadvantages are that it penetrates poorly, requires lengthy washing, and deteriorates rapidly.

**Flem·ming tri·ple stain** (flem'ing) a stain composed of safranin, methyl violet, and orange G.

**flesh 1.** living tissue, especially soft tissues as contrasted with bone; **2.** SYN muscular tissue. **3.** the meat of animals used for food. [A.S. *flaesc*]

**flesh fly** genera of flies including *Wohlfahrtia, Sarcophaga,* and *Parasarcophaga* that feed on feces and decaying meat or fish; can cause human disease.

**Flet·cher fac·tor** (flech'er) SYN prekallikrein.

**flex** (fleks) to bend; to move a joint in such a direction as to approximate the two parts which it connects. [L. *flecto,* pp. *flexus,* to bend]

**flex·i·bil·i·tas ce·rea** (flek-si-bil'i-tas sē'rē-ă) the rigidity of catalepsy which may be overcome by slight external force, but which returns at once, holding the limb firmly in the new position. [L. waxy flexibility]

**flex·i·bil·i·ty** range of motion about a joint dependent on the condition of surrounding structures. SEE range of motion.

**flex·i·ble en·do·scope** an optical instrument that transmits light and carries images back to the observer through a flexible bundle of small (about 10 μm) transparent fibers. It is used to inspect interior portions of the body. These instruments are generally equipped with mechanisms for steering and may have additional ports for allowing sampling and/or operative instruments along their axis to the internal site. SEE ALSO fiberoptics.

**flex·i·ble hy·ster·o·scope** steerable flexible hysteroscope of small diameter for operative or diagnostic procedures, that does not require an outer sheath, has fiberoptics for visualization, and must be used with a distending gas.

**flex·ion** (flek'shŭn) **1.** the act of flexing or bending, e.g., bending of a joint so as to approximate the parts it connects; bending of the spine so that the concavity of the curve looks forward. **2.** the condition of being flexed or bent. See page APP 90. SYN open-packed position (2). [L. *flecto,* pp. *flexus,* to bend]

**flex·ion-ex·ten·sion in·ju·ry** forceful application of a forward and backward movement of the unsupported head that may produce an injury to the cervical spine or the brain.

***Flex·ner ba·cil·lus*** (fleks′nĕr) SYN *Shigella flexneri.*

**flex·o·me·ter** SYN goniometer (3).

**flex·or** (flek′ser) a muscle the action of which is to flex a joint.

**flex·or car·pi ra·di·a·lis mus·cle** *origin,* common flexor origin of the medial condyle of humerus; *insertion,* anterior surface of the base of the second and most often sending a slip to that of the third metacarpal bone; *action,* flexes and abducts wrist radialward; *nerve supply,* median; its tendon travels in its own canal roofed by a layer of the transverse carpal ligament. SYN musculus flexor carpi radialis [TA], radial flexor muscle of wrist.

**flex·or car·pi ul·na·ris mus·cle** *origin,* humeral head from medial condyle of humerus, ulnar head from olecranon and upper three-fifths of posterior border of ulna; *insertion,* pisiform bone, but is continued to the fifth metacarpal bone via the pisometacarpal ligament; *action,* flexes and abducts wrist ulnarward; *nerve supply,* ulnar. SYN musculus flexor carpi ulnaris [TA], ulnar flexor muscle of wrist.

**flex·or di·gi·ti mi·ni·mi bre·vis mus·cle of foot** *origin,* base of metatarsal bone of the little toe and sheath of musculus peroneus longus; *insertion,* lateral surface of base of proximal phalanx of little toe; *action,* flexes the proximal phalanx of the little toe; *nerve supply,* lateral plantar. SYN musculus flexor digiti minimi brevis pedis [TA], short flexor muscle of little toe.

**flex·or di·gi·ti mi·ni·mi bre·vis mus·cle of hand** *origin,* hamulus of hamate bone; *insertion,* medial side of proximal phalanx of little finger; *action,* flexes proximal phalanx of little finger; *nerve supply,* ulnar. SYN musculus flexor digiti minimi brevis manus [TA], short flexor muscle of little finger.

**flex·or di·gi·to·rum bre·vis mus·cle** *origin,* medial tubercle of calcaneus and central portion of plantar fascia; *insertion,* middle phalanges of four lateral toes by tendons perforated by those of the flexor longus; *action,* flexes lateral four toes; *nerve supply,* medial plantar. SYN musculus flexor digitorum brevis [TA], short flexor muscle of toes.

**flex·or di·gi·to·rum lon·gus mus·cle** *origin,* middle third of posterior surface of tibia; *insertion,* by four tendons, perforating those of the flexor brevis, into bases of distal phalanges of four lateral toes; *action,* flexes second to fifth toes; *nerve supply,* tibial nerve. SYN musculus flexor digitorum longus [TA], long flexor muscle of toes.

**flex·or di·gi·to·rum pro·fun·dus mus·cle** *origin,* anterior surface of upper third of ulna; *insertion,* by four tendons, piercing those of the superficialis, into base of distal phalanx of each finger; *action,* flexes distal interphalangeal joint of fingers; *nerve supply,* ulnar and median (anterior in-

terosseous muscle). SYN musculus flexor digitorum profundus [TA].

**flex·or di·gi·to·rum su·per·fi·ci·a·lis mus·cle** *origin,* humeroulnar head from the medial epicondyle of the humerus, the medial border of the coronoid process, and a tendinous arch between these points, radial head from the oblique line and middle third of the lateral border of the radius; *insertion,* by four split tendons, passing to either side of the profundus tendons, into sides of middle phalanx of each finger; *action,* flexes proximal interphalangeal joint of the fingers; *nerve supply,* median. SYN musculus flexor digitorum superficialis [TA], superficial flexor muscle of fingers.

**flex·or hal·lu·cis bre·vis mus·cle** *origin,* medial surface of cuboid and middle and lateral cuneiform bones; *insertion,* by two tendons, embracing that of the flexor longus hallucis, into the sides of the base of the proximal phalanx of the great toe; *action,* flexes great toe; *nerve supply,* medial and lateral plantar. SYN short flexor muscle of great toe.

**flex·or hal·lu·cis lon·gus mus·cle** *origin,* lower two-thirds of posterior surface of fibula; *insertion,* base of distal phalanx of great toe; *action,* flexes great toe; *nerve supply,* medial plantar. SYN long flexor muscle of great toe.

**flex·or pol·li·cis bre·vis mus·cle** *origin,* superficial portion from flexor retinaculum of wrist, deep portion from ulnar side of first metacarpal bone; *insertion,* base of proximal phalanx of thumb; *action,* flexes proximal phalanx of thumb; *nerve supply,* median (superficial head) and deep branch of ulnar (deep head). Some authors consider the deep head to be the first in a series of four palmar interossei muscles of the hand. SYN short flexor muscle of thumb.

**flex·or pol·li·cis lon·gus mus·cle** *origin,* anterior surface of middle third of radius; *insertion,* distal phalanx of thumb; *action,* flexes distal phalanx of thumb; *nerve supply,* median palmar interosseous. SYN long flexor muscle of thumb.

**flex·or re·flex** flexion of ankle, knee, and hip when the foot is painfully stimulated; the crossed extension reflex occurs in association with it.

**flex·or ret·i·nac·u·lum of low·er limb** a wide band passing from the medial malleolus to the medial and upper border of the calcaneus and to the plantar surface as far as the navicular bone; it holds in place the tendons of the tibialis posterior, flexor digitorum longus, and flexor hallucis longus.

**flex·u·ra,** pl. **flex·u·rae** (flek-sh-yur′ă, flek-sh-yur′ē) [TA] SYN flexure. [L. a bending]

**flex·u·ra co·li dex·tra** [TA] SYN right colic flexure.

**flex·u·ra co·li si·nis·tra** [TA] SYN left colic flexure.

**flex·u·ra du·o·de·no·je·ju·na·lis** [TA] SYN duodenojejunal flexure.

**flex·ur·al** (flek′sh-yur-ăl) relating to a flexure.

**flex·ur·al psor·i·a·sis** psoriasis involving intertriginous folds, e.g., axillary and inguinal skin, which may resemble seborrheic dermatitis.

**flex·ure** (flek′sh-yur) a bend, as in an organ or structure. SYN flexura [TA]. [L. *flexura*]

**Flie·rin·ga ring** (flēr-ing-ah) a stainless steel ring sutured to the sclera to prevent collapse of the globe in difficult intraocular operations.

**flight or fight re·sponse** SEE emergency theory.

**flight of i·de·as** an uncontrollable symptom of the manic phase of a bipolar depressive disorder in which streams of unrelated words and ideas occur to the patient at a rate that is impossible to vocalize despite a marked increase in the individual's overall output of words. SEE ALSO mania.

**flight in·to dis·ease** gain through falling ill or assuming the sick role. SEE primary gain, secondary gain.

**flight in·to health** DYNAMIC PSYCHOTHERAPY the early but often only temporary disappearance of the symptoms that ostensibly brought the patient into therapy; a defense against the anxiety engendered by the prospect of further psychoanalytic exploration of the patient's conflicts.

**Flin·ders Is·land spot·ted fe·ver** (flin′dĕrz ī′lănd) a febrile disease caused by the bacterium *Rickettsia honei* in southeastern Australia and characterized by headache, myalgia, and maculopapular rash. [named after Flinders Island in Tasmania, Australia, from which the first cases of the disease were identified]

**Flint ar·cade** (flint) a series of vascular arches at the bases of the pyramids of the kidney.

**Flint mur·mur** (flint) a diastolic murmur, similar to that of mitral stenosis, heard best at the cardiac apex. SYN bicuspid murmur.

**flip an·gle** in a magnetic resonance imaging sequence, the rotation of the average axis of the protons induced by radiofrequency signals; low angles are used in rapid-imaging sequences and to show a signal from flowing blood.

**flit·ter** SYN impure flutter.

**float·er** (flōt′er) an object in the field of vision that originates in the vitreous body. SEE ALSO muscae volitantes.

**float·ing** (flōt′ing) **1.** free or unattached. **2.** unduly movable; out of the normal position; denoting an occasional abnormal condition of certain organs, such as the kidneys, liver, and spleen.

**float·ing car·ti·lage** a loose piece of cartilage within a joint cavity, detached from the articular cartilage or from a meniscus.

**float·ing kid·ney** the abnormally mobile kidney in nephroptosis. SYN wandering kidney.

**float·ing pa·tel·la** SYN ballottable patella.

**float·ing ribs [XI–XII]** the two lower ribs on either side that are not attached anteriorly. SYN costae fluctuantes [XI–XII] [TA], vertebral ribs.

**float·ing spleen** a spleen that is palpable because of excessive mobility from a relaxed or lengthened pedicle rather than because of enlargement. SYN lien mobilis, movable spleen.

**floc·cil·la·tion** (flok-si-lā′shŭn) an aimless plucking at the bedclothes, as if one were picking off threads or tufts of cotton. [Mod. L. *flocculus*]

**floc·cose** (flok′ōs) BACTERIOLOGY applied to a growth of short, curving filaments or chains closely but irregularly disposed. [L. *floccus*, a flock of wool]

**floc·cu·lar** (flok′yu-lăr) relating to a flocculus of any sort; specifically to the flocculus of the cerebellum.

**floc·cu·late** (flok′yu-lāt) to become flocculent.

**floc·cu·la·tion** (flok-yu-lā′shŭn) precipitation from solution in the form of fleecy masses; the process of becoming flocculent.

**floc·cu·lent** (flok′yu-lent) **1.** resembling tufts of cotton or wool; denoting a fluid, such as the urine, containing numerous shreds or fluffy particles of gray-white or white mucus or other mate-

rial. **2.** BACTERIOLOGY denoting a fluid culture in which there are numerous colonies either floating in the fluid medium or loosely deposited at the bottom.

**floc·cu·lus,** pl. **floc·cu·li** (flok′yu-lŭs, flok′yu-lī) **1.** a tuft or shred of cotton or wool or anything resembling it. **2.** [TA] a small lobe of the cerebellum at the posterior border of the middle cerebellar peduncle anterior to the biventer lobule; it is associated with the nodulus of the vermis; together, these two structures compose the vestibular part of the cerebellum. [Mod. L. dim. of L. *floccus*, a tuft of wool]

**flood** (flŭd) **1.** to bleed profusely from the uterus, as after childbirth or in cases of menorrhagia. **2.** colloquialism for a profuse menstrual discharge. [A.S. *flōd*]

**flood·ing** (flŭd′ing) **1.** bleeding profusely from the uterus, especially after childbirth or in severe cases of menorrhagia. **2.** a type of behavior therapy; a therapeutic strategy at the beginning of therapy, in which the patients imagine the most anxiety-producing scene and fully immerse (flood) themselves in it.

**floor plate** ventral midline thinning of the developing neural tube, a continuity between the basal laminae of either side; opposite of roof plate. SYN ventral plate.

**flo·ra** (flō′ră) **1.** plant life, usually of a certain locality or district. **2.** the population of microorganisms inhabiting the internal and external surfaces of healthy conventional animals. [L. *Flora*, goddess of flowers, fr. *flos* (*flor*-), a flower]

**flor·id** (flōr′id) **1.** of a bright red color; denoting certain cutaneous lesions. **2.** fully developed. [L. *floridus*, flowery]

**flo·ta·tion** (flō-tā′shŭn) a process for separating solids by their tendency to float upon or sink into a liquid.

**flo·ta·tion con·stant ($S_f$)** characteristic sedimentation behavior of a lipoprotein fraction of plasma in a centrifugal field in a medium of appropriate density, achieved by adding a salt or $D_2O$ to the plasma. SYN Svedberg of flotation.

**flo·ta·tion meth·od** flotation of helminth eggs on the surface of a liquid of high specific gravity when eggs are difficult to find in direct examination.

**flow** (flō) **1.** to bleed from the uterus less profusely than in flooding. **2.** the menstrual discharge. **3.** movement of a liquid or gas; specifically, the volume of liquid or gas passing a given point per unit of time. **4.** RHEOLOGY a permanent deformation of a body which proceeds with time. [A.S. *flōwan*]

**flow-con·trol·led ven·ti·la·tor** a ventilator designed to deliver mandatory breaths with a preset flow waveform.

**flow cy·tom·e·try** a method of measuring fluorescence from stained cells that are in suspension and flowing through a narrow orifice, usually with one or two lasers to activate the dyes; used to measure cell size, number, viability, and nucleic acid content.

**flow di·a·gram** a diagram composed of blocks connected by arrows representing steps in a process such as decision analysis.

**flow·ers** (flow′erz) a mineral substance in a powdery state after sublimation.

**flow·me·ter** (flō′mē-ter) **1.** a device for measuring the flow of liquid or gas. SEE ALSO pneumotachometer. **2.** a device for controlling the flow of medical gases as in the delivery of air or oxygen to a nebulizer.

**flow·vol·ume loop stu·dies** diagnostic methods in which inspiratory and expiratory flow-volume curves are used to determine the location of an obstruction in the tracheobronchial tree.

**flu** (floo) SYN influenza.

**fluc·tu·ate** (flŭk'tyu-āt) **1.** to move in waves. **2.** to vary, to change from time to time, as in referring to any quantity or quality (blood pressure, concentration of substance in urine or blood, secretory activity). [L. *fluctuo,* pp. *-atus,* to flow in waves]

**flu·ence** (floo'ens) a measure of the quantity of x-radiation in a beam in diagnostic radiology, either particle fluence, the number of photons entering a sphere of unit cross-sectional area, or energy fluence, the sum of the energies of the photons passing through a unit area. Cf. flux. [L. *fluentia,* a flowing, fr. *fluo,* to flow]

**flu·en·cy** (floo'en-sē) the smooth flow of speech sounds in connected discourse, without interruptions or repetitions. [L. *fluentia,*a flowing, fr. *fluo,* to flow]

**flu·ent a·pha·sia** SYN receptive aphasia.

**flu·id** (floo'id) **1.** a nonsolid substance, such as a liquid or gas, that tends to flow or conform to the shape of the container. **2.** consisting of particles or distinct entities that can readily change their relative positions; tending to move or capable of flowing. [L. *fluidus,* fr. *fluo,* to flow]

**flu·id·ex·tract** (floo-id-eks'trakt) pharmacopeial liquid preparation of vegetable drugs, made by percolation, containing alcohol as a solvent or as a preservative, or both, and so made that each milliliter contains the therapeutic constituents of 1 g of the standard drug that it represents.

**flu·id·ounce** (floo'id-owns') a measure of capacity: 8 fluidrams. The imperial fluidounce is a measure containing 1 avoirdupois ounce, 437.5 grains, of distilled water at 15.6°C, and equals 28.4 ml; the U.S. fluidounce is $^1/_{128}$ gallon, contains 454.6 grains of distilled water at 25°C, and equals 29.57 ml.

**flu·i·dram** (floo'i-dram') a measure of capacity: ⅛ of a fluidounce; a teaspoonful. The imperial fluidram contains 54.8 grains of distilled water, and equals 3.55 ml; the U.S. fluidram contains 57.1 grains of distilled water and equals 3.70 ml. Cf. dram.

**fluke** (flook) common name for members of the class Trematoda. All flukes of mammals (subclass Digenea) are internal parasites in the adult stage and are characterized by complex digenetic life cycles involving a snail initial host, in which larval multiplication occurs, and the release of swimming larvae (cercariae) which directly penetrate the skin of the final host (as in schistosomes), encyst on vegetation (as in *Fasciola*), or encyst in or on another intermediate host (as in *Clonorchis* and other fish-borne flukes). Blood flukes live in the mesenteric-portal bloodstream and associated vesical and pelvic venous plexuses; they include *Schistosoma haematobium* (the vesical blood fluke), *S. mansoni* (Manson intestinal blood fluke), and *S. japonicum* (the Oriental blood fluke). Other important flukes are *Paragonimus westermani* (bronchial or lung fluke), *Opisthorchis felineus* (cat liver fluke), *Clonorchis sinensis* (Chinese liver or Oriental fluke), *Heterophyes heterophyes* (Egyptian or small intestinal fluke), *Fasciolopsis buski* (large intestinal fluke), *Dicrocoelium dendriticum* (lancet fluke), *Fasciola hepatica* (liver or sheep liver fluke), and *Paramphistomum* (rumen fluke). [A.S. *flōc,* flatfish]

**flu·men,** pl. **flu·mi·na** (floo'men, floo'min-ă) a flowing, or stream. [L.]

△**fluor-, fluoro-** fluorine.

**fluorapatite** (floor-ap'ă-tīt) a form of hydroxyapatite in which fluoride ions have replaced some of the hydroxyl ions; as a component of teeth, fluorapatite resists acids from plaque-forming bacteria and high carbohydrate intake.

**flu·o·res·ce·in** (floor-es'ē-ĭn) [C.I. 45350] an orange-red crystalline powder that yields a bright green fluorescence in solution, and is reduced to fluorescin; a nontoxic, water-soluble indicator used diagnostically to trace water flow and to visualize corneal abrasions or ulcers.

**flu·o·res·ce·in in·stil·la·tion test** a test for patency of the lacrimal system; fluorescein instilled in the conjunctival sac can be recovered from the inferior nasal meatus. SYN dye disappearance test, Jones test.

**flu·o·res·ce·in iso·thi·o·cy·a·nate (FITC)** (floor-es'ē-ĭn ī'sō-thī-ō-sī'ă-nāt) a fluorochrome dye frequently coupled to antibodies which are used to locate and identify specific antigens.

**flu·o·res·cence** (floor-es'ens) emission of a longer wavelength radiation by a substance as a consequence of absorption of energy from a shorter wavelength radiation, continuing only as long as the stimulus is present; distinguished from phosphorescence in that, in the latter, emission persists for a perceptible period of time after the stimulus has been removed. [*fluor*spar + *-escence,* inchoative suffix]

**flu·o·res·cence-ac·ti·vat·ed cell sort·er (FACS)** (floor-es'ens ak-tĭ-vāt-ĕd sel sort-er) a machine that can separate and analyze cells, such as lymphocytes, which are labeled with fluorochrome-conjugated antibody, by their fluorescence and light scattering patterns.

**flu·o·res·cence mi·cros·co·py** a procedure based on the fact that fluorescent materials emit visible light when they are irradiated with ultraviolet or violet-blue visible rays; some materials manifest this property naturally, whereas others may be treated with fluorescent solutions (somewhat analogous to staining).

**flu·o·res·cent** (floor-es'ent) possessing the quality of fluorescence.

**flu·o·res·cent an·ti·body tech·nique** a procedure to test for antigen with a fluorescent antibody by one of two methods: *direct,* in which immunoglobulin (antibody) conjugated with a fluorescent dye is added to tissue and combines with specific antigen (microbe, or other), the resulting antigen-antibody complex being located by fluorescence microscopy; or *indirect,* in which unlabeled immunoglobulin (antibody) is added to tissue and combines with specific antigen, after which the antigen-antibody complex may be labeled with fluorescein-conjugated anti-immunoglobulin antibody, the resulting triple complex then being located by fluorescence microscopy.

**flu·o·res·cent screen** a screen coated with fluorescent crystals such as the calcium tungstate used in the fluoroscope.

f
l

**flu·or·es·cent in si·tu hy·brid·i·za·tion (FISH), flu·or·es·cence in si·tu hy·brid·i·za·tion** a method used to determine the chromosomal location or expression pattern of genomic DNA or cDNA fragments. The piece of DNA to be mapped (the "probe") is labeled with a fluorescent dye and hybridized to a chromosome preparation or to a tissue section. The probe anneals to complementary DNA or RNA sequences. Examination of the chromosomes or tissue section under a fluorescence microscope reveals the number, size, and location of the target sequences.

**flu·o·res·cent stain** a stain or staining procedure using a fluorescent dye or substance that will combine selectively with certain tissue components and that will then fluoresce upon irradiation with ultraviolet or violet-blue light.

**flu·o·res·cent trep·o·ne·mal an·ti·body-ab·sorp·tion test** a sensitive and specific serologic test for syphilis using a suspension of the Nichols strain of *Treponema pallidum* as antigen; the presence or absence of antibody in the patient's serum is indicated by an indirect fluorescent antibody technique.

**flu·o·ri·dat·ed tooth** a tooth exposed to fluorine salts during odontogenesis.

**flu·o·ri·da·tion** (floor'i-dā'shŭn) addition of fluorides to a community water supply, usually 1 ppm or less, to reduce incidence of dental decay.

**flu·o·ride** (floor'īd) a compound of fluorine with a metal, a nonmetal, or an organic radical; the anion of fluorine; inhibits enolase; found in bone and tooth apatite; fluoride has a cariostatic effect; high levels are toxic.

**flu·o·ride num·ber** the percent inhibition of pseudocholinesterase produced by fluorides; used to differentiate normal from atypical pseudocholinesterases. SEE ALSO dibucaine number.

**flu·o·ri·di·za·tion** (floor'i-di-zā'shŭn) therapeutic use of fluorides to reduce the incidence of dental decay; sometimes used to refer to the topical application of fluoride agents to the teeth.

**flu·o·rine (F)** (floor'ēn) a gaseous chemical element, atomic no. 9, atomic weight 18.9984032; $^{18}$F (half-life of 1.83 hours) is used as a diagnostic aid in various tissue scans. [L. *fluere*, flow]

**flu·o·ro·chrome** (floor'ō-krōm) any fluorescent dye used to label or stain.

**flu·o·rog·ra·phy** (floor-og'ră-fē) SYN photofluorography.

**flu·o·ro·im·mu·no·as·say** (floo-r'ō-im-yu-nō-as'ā) an immunoassay that has antigen or antibody labeled with a fluorophore.

**flu·o·rom·e·ter** (floor-om'ĕ-ter) a device employing an ultraviolet source, monochromators for selection of wavelength, and a detector of visible light; used in fluorometry.

**flu·o·rom·e·try** (floor-om'ĕ-trē) an analytic method for detecting fluorescent compounds, using a beam of ultraviolet light that excites the compounds and causes them to emit visible light. [fluoro- + G. *metron*, measure]

**flu·o·ro·pho·tom·e·try** (floor'ō-fō-tom'ĕ-trē) photomultiplier tube measurement of fluorescence emitted from the interior of the eye after intravenous administration of fluorescein; used to measure the rate of formation of aqueous humor or integrity of the retinal vasculature.

**flu·o·ro·scope** (floor'ō-skōp) an apparatus for rendering visible the patterns of x-rays which have passed through a body under examination, by interposing a glass plate coated with fluorescent materials, such as calcium tungstate; to examine a patient by fluoroscopy. [fluorescence + G. *skopeō*, to examine]

**flu·o·ro·scop·ic** (floor-ō-skop'ik) relating to or effected by means of fluoroscopy.

**flu·o·ros·co·py** (floor-os'kŏ-pē) examination of the tissues and deep structures of the body by x-ray, using the fluoroscope.

**flu·o·ro·sis** (floor-ō'sis) a condition caused by an excessive intake of fluorides, characterized mainly by mottling, staining, or hypoplasia of the enamel of the teeth.

**flush** (flŭsh) **1.** to wash out with a full stream of fluid. **2.** a transient erythema due to heat, exertion, stress, or disease. **3.** flat, or even with another surface, as a flush stoma.

**flut·ter** (flŭt'er) agitation; tremulousness. [A.S. *floterian*, to float about]

**flut·ter-fi·bril·la·tion** SYN impure flutter.

**flux** (flŭks) **1.** the discharge of a fluid material in large amount from a cavity or surface of the body. SEE ALSO diarrhea. **2.** material discharged from the bowels. **3.** a material used to remove oxides from the surface of molten metal and to protect it when casting; serves a similar purpose in soldering operations. Also, an ingredient in dental porcelain that by its lower melting temperature helps to bond the silica particles. **4.** (*J*) the moles of a substance crossing through a unit area of a boundary layer or membrane per unit of time. **5.** bidirectional movement of a substance at a membrane or surface. **6.** DIAGNOSTIC RADIOLOGY photon fluence per unit time. [L. *fluxus*, a flow]

**flux·ion·ary hy·per·e·mia** SYN active hyperemia.

**fly** (flī) a two-winged insect in the order Diptera. Important flies include *Simulium* (black fly), *Calliphora* (bluebottle fly), *Piophila casei* (cheese fly), *Chrysops* (deer fly), *Siphona irritans* (horn fly), *Fannia scolaris* (latrine fly), *Oestrus ovis* and *Gasterophilus hemorrhoidalis* (nose fly), *Cochliomyia hominivorax* (primary screw-worm fly) and *C. macellaria* (secondary screw-worm fly), *Stomoxys calcitrans* (stable fly), *Glossina* (tsetse fly), members of the insect order Trichoptera also have the common name fly. [A.S. *fleóge*]

**Fm** fermium.

**FMLH** familial hemophagocytic lymphohistiocytosis.

**FMN** flavin mononucleotide.

**FMR1** SYN fragile X syndrome.

**FNA** fine needle aspiration biopsy.

**foam cells** cells with abundant, pale-staining, finely vacuolated cytoplasm, usually histiocytes that have ingested or accumulated material that dissolves during tissue preparation, especially lipids. SEE ALSO lipophage.

**foam·y vi·rus·es** retroviruses found in primates and other mammals; so named because of lace-like changes produced in monkey kidney cells; syncytia are also produced.

**fo·cal** (fō'kăl) **1.** denoting a focus. **2.** relating to a localized area.

**fo·cal am·y·loi·do·sis** SYN nodular amyloidosis.

**fo·cal depth, depth of fo·cus** the greatest distance through which an object point can be moved while remaining in focus.

**fo·cal dis·tance** the distance from the center of a lens to its focus.

**fo·cal ep·i·lep·sy** epilepsy of various etiologies characterized by focal seizures or secondarily generalized tonic-clonic seizures. Ictal symptoms are often related to the brain region where the seizure begins focally. SYN localization-related epilepsy (2).

**fo·cal-film dis·tance (FFD)** the distance from the source of radiation (the focal spot of the x-ray tube) to the film or other image-receptor. SYN source-to-image distance.

**fo·cal glo·mer·u·lo·ne·phri·tis** glomerulonephritis affecting a small proportion of renal glomeruli which commonly presents with hematuria and may be associated with acute upper respiratory infection in young males, not usually due to streptococci; associated with IgA deposits in the glomerular mesangium and may also be associated with systemic disease, as in Henoch-Schönlein purpura. SYN Berger disease, Berger focal glomerulonephritis.

**fo·cal in·fec·tion** local infection that can serve as a source of disseminated or metastatic infection

**fo·cal in·ju·ry** injury to a small, concentrated area, usually caused by high velocity-low mass forces.

**fo·cal ne·cro·sis** occurrence of numerous small, well-circumscribed zones of tissue that manifest coagulative, caseous, or gummatous necrosis.

**fo·cal point** SEE anterior focal point, posterior focal point.

**fo·cal re·ac·tion** a reaction which occurs at the point of entrance of an infecting organism or of an injection, as in the Arthus phenomenon. SYN local reaction.

**fo·cal seg·men·tal glo·mer·u·lo·scle·ro·sis** segmental collapse of glomerular capillaries with thickened basement membranes and increased mesangial matrix; seen in some glomeruli of patients with nephrotic syndrome or mesangial proliferative glomerulonephritis.

**fo·cus**, pl. **fo·ci** (fō′kŭs, fō′sī) **1.** (F) the point at which the light rays meet after passing through a convex lens. **2.** the center, or the starting point, of a disease process. [L. a hearth]

**fo·cus·ed his·to·ry and phy·si·cal ex·am·i·na·tion** the second stage of patient assessment conducted by prehospital providers after the initial assessment of the stable responsive patient designed to identify additional injuries or conditions requiring emergency intervention.

**fo·cus·ed me·di·cal as·sess·ment** physical examination of a prehospital patient that focuses on body areas and systems as indicated by patient's chief complaint and initial assessment.

**fo·cus·ed trau·ma as·sess·ment** physical examination, focusing on a specific injury or suspected area of injury, of a prehospital patient before transport.

**foe·tal [Br.]** SEE fetal.

**foe·to·pla·cen·tal [Br.]** SEE fetoplacental.

**foe·to·tox·ic [Br.]** SEE fetotoxic.

**foe·tus [Br.]** SEE fetus.

**Fo·gar·ty cath·e·ter** (fō′gär-tē) a catheter commonly used to remove arterial emboli, thrombi from major veins or to remove stones from the biliary ducts. SYN balloon-tip catheter (3).

**Fo·gar·ty em·bo·lec·to·my cath·e·ter** (fō′gär-tē) a catheter with an inflatable balloon near its tip; used to remove emboli and thrombi from blood vessels or to remove stones from the biliary tract.

**fog·ging** (fog′ing) a method of refraction in which accommodation is relaxed by overcorrection with a convex spherical lens.

**fo·late** (fō′lāt) a salt or ester of folic acid.

**fold** (fōld) **1.** a ridge or margin apparently formed by the doubling back of a lamina. SEE ALSO plica. **2.** in the embryo, a transient elevation or reduplication of tissue in the form of a lamina.

**fold·a·ble in·tra·oc·u·lar lens** a lens often made of silicone or an acrylic polymer that may be doubled over for implantation into the eye following cataract removal.

**fold·ed-lung syn·drome** collapse of part of the lung caught between shrinking fibrous pleural scars, sometimes resulting from pleural asbestosis.

**Fo·ley cath·e·ter** (fō′lē) a urethral catheter with a retaining balloon. See this page.

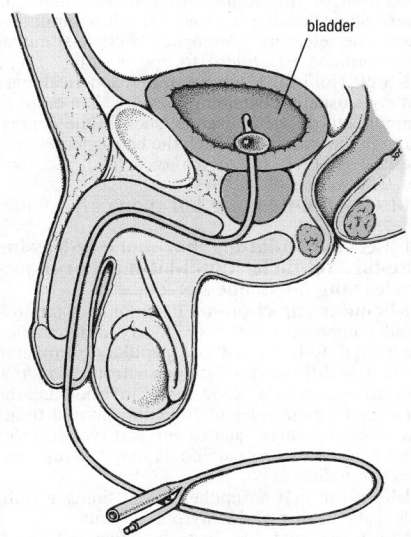

bladder

**Foley catheter**

**fo·lia** (fō′lē-ă) plural of folium.

**fo·li·ate pa·pil·lae** numerous projections arranged in several transverse folds upon the lateral margins of the tongue just in front of the palatoglossus muscle.

**fo·lic ac·id** (fō′lik as′id) **1.** collective term for pteroylglutamic acids and their oligoglutamic acid conjugates. **2.** pteroylmonoglutamic acid, a member of the vitamin B complex necessary for the production of red blood cells. It is present in liver, green vegetables, and yeast; used to treat folate deficiency and megaloblastic anemia.

**fo·lic ac·id an·ta·go·nist** modified pterins, such as aminopterin and amethopterin, that interfere with the action of folic acid and thus produce the symptoms of folic acid deficiency; have been used in cancer chemotherapy.

**fo·lie** (fō-lē′) old term for madness or insanity. [Fr. folly]

**fo·lie du doute** (fō-lē′-du-doot) an excessive doubting about all the affairs of life and a morbid scrupulousness concerning minutiae. [Fr. from doubt]

**fo·li·nate** (fō′li-nāt) a salt or ester of folinic acid.

**fo·lin·ic ac·id** (fō-lin′ik as′id) the active form of folic acid, which acts as a formyl group carrier in transformylation reactions; the calcium salt, leucovorin calcium, has therapeutic use. SYN citrovorum factor.

**Fo·lin re·ac·tion** (fō′lin) the reaction of amino acids in alkaline solution with 1,2-naphthoquinone-4-sulfonate (Folin reagent) to yield a red color; useful for quantitative assay.

**fo·li·um**, pl. **fo·lia** (fō′lē-ŭm, fō′lē-ă) a broad, thin, leaflike structure. [L. a leaf]

**folk med·i·cine** treatment of ailments by nonphysicians with remedies and simple measures based upon experience and knowledge handed on from generation to generation.

**fol·lib·er·in** (fol-lib′er-in) a decapeptide of hypothalamic origin capable of accelerating pituitary secretion of follitropin. SYN follicle-stimulating hormone-releasing factor, follicle-stimulating hormone-releasing hormone. [follicle-stimulating hormone + L. *libero*, to free, + -in]

**fol·li·cle** (fol′i-kl) **1.** a more or less spherical mass of cells usually containing a cavity. **2.** a crypt or minute cul-de-sac or lacuna, such as the depression in the skin from which the hair emerges. SYN folliculus [TA]. [L. *folliculus,* a small sac, dim. of *follis,* a pair of bellows]

**fol·li·cle-stim·u·lat·ing hor·mone** SYN follitropin.

**fol·li·cle-stim·u·lat·ing hor·mone-re·leas·ing fac·tor, fol·li·cle-stim·u·lat·ing hor·mone-re·leas·ing hor·mone** SYN folliberin.

**fol·lic·u·lar car·ci·no·ma** carcinoma of the thyroid composed of well or poorly differentiated epithelial follicles without papillary formation, which is difficult to distinguish from adenoma; the criteria include blood vessel invasion and the finding of metastases of follicular thyroid tissue in other structures such as cervical lymph nodes and bone; follicular carcinoma may take up radioactive iodine.

**fol·lic·u·lar cell** an epithelial cell lining a follicle, such as that of the thyroid or ovary.

**fol·lic·u·lar cyst 1.** a cystic graafian follicle; **2.** SYN dentigerous cyst.

**fol·lic·u·lar cys·ti·tis** chronic cystitis characterized by small mucosal nodules due to lymphocytic infiltration.

**fol·lic·u·lar goi·ter** SYN parenchymatous goiter.

**fol·lic·u·lar lym·pho·ma** SYN nodular lymphoma.

**fol·lic·u·lar stig·ma** the point where the graafian follicle is about to rupture on the surface of the ovary. SYN stigma (2).

**fol·lic·u·li** (fō-lik′yu-lī) plural of folliculus.

**fol·lic·u·li glan·du·lae thy·roi·de·ae** [TA] SYN thyroid follicles.

**fol·lic·u·li lin·gua·les** [TA] SYN lingual follicles.

**fol·lic·u·li lym·pha·ti·ci li·e·na·les** SYN splenic lymph follicles.

**fol·lic·u·li·tis** (fō-lik-yu-lī′tis) an inflammatory reaction in hair follicles; the lesions may be papules or pustules.

**fol·lic·u·li·tis bar·bae** SYN tinea barbae.

**fol·lic·u·li·tis de·cal·vans** a papular or pustular inflammation of the hair follicles of the scalp seen mostly in men, resulting in scarring and loss of hair in the affected area.

**fol·lic·u·li·tis ke·loi·da·lis** SYN acne keloid.

**fol·lic·u·li·tis u·ler·y·the·ma·to·sa re·ti·cu·la·ta** erythematous "ice-pick" or pitted scars on the cheeks; a scarring type of folliculitis, associated with keratosis pilaris.

**fol·lic·u·lo·ma** (fō-lik-yu-lō′mă) **1.** SYN granulosa cell tumor. **2.** cystic enlargement of a graafian follicle.

**fol·lic·u·lo·sis** (fō-lik-yu-lō′sis) presence of lymph follicles in abnormally great numbers.

**fol·lic·u·lus**, pl. **fol·lic·u·li** (fō-lik′yu-lŭs, fō-lik′yu-lī) SYN follicle. [L. a small sac, dim. of *follis,* bellows]

**fol·lic·u·lus lym·pha·ti·cus** SYN lymph follicle.

**fol·lic·u·lus pi·li** [TA] SYN hair follicle.

**Fol·ling dis·ease** (fahl′ing) SYN phenylketonuria.

**fol·li·stat·in** (fol-ĭ-stat′in) a peptide synthesized by granulosa cells in response to FSH, which suppresses FSH activity, probably by binding activins. [*follicle* + -stat + -in]

**fol·li·tro·pin** (fol-i-trō′pin) an acidic glycoprotein hormone of the anterior pituitary that stimulates the ovarian follicles and promotes follicular maturation and the secretion of estradiol; in the male, it stimulates the epithelium of the seminiferous tubules and is partially responsible for inducing spermatogenesis. SYN follicle-stimulating hormone. [*follicle* + G. *tropē,* a turning, + -in]

**fol·low·ing bou·gie** a flexible tapered bougie with a screw tip which is attached to the trailing end of a filiform bougie, to allow progressive dilation without danger of creating false passages.

**fo·mes**, pl. **fom·i·tes** (fō′mēz, fōm′i-tēz) objects such as clothing, towels, and utensils that harbor a disease agent and are capable of transmitting it; usually used in the plural. SYN fomite. [L. tinder, fr. *foveo,* to keep warm]

**fo·mite** (fō′mīt) SYN fomes.

**Fo·nio so·lu·tion** (fō′nē-ō) a diluent with magnesium sulfate, used for stained smears of blood platelets.

**fon·ta·nelle** (fon′tă-nel′) [TA] one of several membranous intervals at the margins of the cranial bones in the infant. SYN fonticulus [TA]. [Fr. dim. of *fontaine,* fountain, spring]

**fon·tic·u·lus**, pl. **fon·tic·u·li** (fon-tik′yu-lŭs, fon-tik′yu-lī) [TA] SYN fontanelle. [L. dim. of *fons* (*font-*), fountain, spring]

**food** (food) that which is eaten to supply necessary nutritive elements. [A.S. *fōda*]

**food ball** SYN phytobezoar.

**food poi·son·ing** poisoning in which the active agent is contained in ingested food.

**foot** (fŭt) **1.** the lower, pedal, podalic, extremity of the leg. SYN pes (1) [TA]. **2.** a unit of length, containing 12 inches, equal to 30.48 cm. [A.S. *fōt*]

**foot·can·dle** (fŭt′kan-dl) illumination or brightness equivalent to 1 lumen per square foot; replaced in the SI system by the candela.

**foot·drop** (fŭt′drop) partial or total inability to dorsiflex the foot, as a consequence of which the toes drag on the ground during walking unless a steppage gait is used; most often ultimately due to weakness of the dorsiflexor muscles of the foot (especially the tibialis anterior), but has many causes, including disorders of the central nervous system, motor unit, tendons, and bones.

**foot of hip·po·cam·pus** the anterior thickened extremity of the hippocampus.

**foot·ling** (fŭt′ling) a fetal foot, particularly one that descends into the birth canal in an incomplete breech presentation. [foot, fr. A. S. *fot*, + *-ling*, dim. suffix]

**foot·ling pre·sen·ta·tion, foot pre·sen·ta·tion** SEE breech presentation.

**foot·plate, foot-plate** (fŭt′plāt) 1. SYN base of stapes. 2. SYN pedicel.

**foot-pound** (fŭt′pownd) energy expended, or work done, in raising a mass of 1 pound a height of 1 foot vertically against gravitational force.

**foot-pound·al** (fŭt′pownd-ăl) energy exerted, or work done, when a force of 1 poundal displaces a body 1 foot in the direction of the force; equal to about 0.01 calorie.

**foot-pound-second sys·tem (FPS, fps)** a system of absolute units based on the foot, pound, and second.

**foot-pound-second u·nit (FPS, fps), FPS u··nit, fps unit** an absolute unit of the foot-pound-second system.

**foot pro·cess** SYN pedicel.

**Foot re·tic·u·lin im·preg·na·tion stain** (fut) a silver stain in which reticulin stains black and collagen stains golden brown; sections are floated on the surface of solutions to avoid contamination with silver debris.

**fo·ra·men**, pl. **fo·ram·i·na** (fō-rā′men, fō-ram′ĭ-nă) [TA] an aperture or perforation through a bone or a membranous structure. [L. an aperture, fr. *foro*, to pierce]

**fo·ra·men ce·cum me·dul·lae ob·lon·ga·tae** [TA] a small triangular depression at the lower boundary of the pons that marks the upper limit of the median fissure of the medulla oblongata.

**fo·ra·men mag·num** [TA] the large opening in the basal part of the occipital bone through which the spinal cord becomes continuous with the medulla oblongata. SYN great foramen.

**fo·ra·men man·di·bu·lae** [TA] SYN mandibular foramen.

**fo·ra·men ob·tu·ra·tum** [TA] SYN obturator foramen.

**fo·ra·men o·va·le, o·val fo·ra·men 1.** *foramen ovale cordis* [TA] in the fetal heart, the oval opening in the septum secundum; the persistent part of the septum primum acts as a valve for this interatrial communication during fetal life and normally postnatally becomes fused to the septum secundum to close it; **2.** *foramen ovale* [TA] a large oval opening in the base of the greater wing of the sphenoid bone, transmitting the mandibular nerve and a small meningeal artery;

**fo·ra·men ro·tun·dum** [TA] an opening in the base of the greater wing of the sphenoid bone, transmitting the maxillary nerve.

**fo·ra·men sphe·no·pa·la·ti·num** [TA] SYN sphenopalatine foramen.

**fo·ra·men spi·no·sum** [TA] an opening in the base of the greater wing of the sphenoid bone, anterior to the spine of the sphenoid, transmitting the middle meningeal artery.

**fo·ra·men su·pra·or·bi·ta·le** [TA] SYN supraorbital foramen.

**fo·ra·men zy·go·ma·ti·co·fa·ci·ale** [TA] SYN zygomaticofacial foramen.

**fo·ra·men zy·go·ma·ti·co·or·bi·ta·le** [TA] SYN zygomatico-orbital foramen.

**fo·ra·men zy·go·ma·ti·co·tem·po·ra·le** [TA] SYN zygomaticotemporal foramen.

**fo·ram·i·na** (fō-ram′i-nă) plural of foramen.

**fo·ram·i·na pa·la·ti·na mi·no·ra** [TA] SYN lesser palatine foramina.

**Forbes dis·ease** (fōrbz) SYN type 3 glycogenosis.

**force (F, F)** (fōrs) that which tends to produce motion in a body. [L. *fortis*, strong]

**forced beat 1.** an extrasystole supposedly precipitated in some way by the preceding normal beat to which it is coupled; **2.** an extrasystole caused by artificial stimulation of the heart.

**forced ex·pi·ra·to·ry flow (FEF)** expiratory flow during measurement of forced vital capacity; subscripts specify the exact parameter measured.

**forced ex·pi·ra·to·ry time (FET)** the time taken to expire a given volume or a given fraction of vital capacity during measurement of forced vital capacity; subscripts specify the exact parameters measured.

**forced ex·pi·ra·to·ry vol·ume (FEV)** the maximal volume that can be expired in a specific time interval when starting from maximal inspiration.

**forced feed·ing, forc·i·ble feed·ing 1.** giving liquid food through a nasal tube passed into the stomach; **2.** forcing a person to eat more food than desired.

**forced vi·tal ca·pac·i·ty (FVC)** vital capacity measured with the subject exhaling as rapidly as possible.

**force of mas·ti·ca·tion** the force created by the action of the muscles during mastication. SYN masticatory force.

**for·ceps** (fōr′seps) 1. an instrument for seizing a structure, and making compression or traction. Cf. clamp. 2. [TA] bands of white fibers in the brain, major forceps and minor forceps. [L. a pair of tongs]

**for·ceps de·liv·er·y** assisted birth of the child by an instrument designed to grasp the fetal head.

**for·ci·pres·sure** (fōr′si-presh-ŭr) a method of arresting hemorrhage by compressing a blood vessel with forceps.

**For·dyce an·gi·o·ker·a·to·ma** (fōr′dīs) an asymptomatic vascular papule appearing on the scrotum in adults.

**For·dyce spots, For·dyce gran·ules, For·dyce dis·ease** (fōr′dīs) a condition marked by the presence of numerous small, yellowish-white bodies or granules on the inner surface and vermilion border of the lips; histologically the lesions are ectopic sebaceous glands.

**fore·arm** (fōr′arm) the segment of the upper limb between the elbow and the wrist. SYN antebrachium [TA].

**fore·brain** (fōr′brān) SYN prosencephalon.

**fore·con·scious** (fōr′kon-shŭs) denoting memories, not at present in the consciousness, which can be evoked from time to time, or an unconscious mental process which becomes conscious only on the fulfillment of certain conditions. Cf. preconscious.

**fore·gut** (fōr′gŭt) the cephalic portion of the primordial digestive tube in the embryo. From its endoderm arises the epithelial lining of the pharynx, trachea, lungs, esophagus, and stomach, the first part and cranial half of the second part of the duodenum, and the parenchyma of the liver, gallbladder, and pancreas.

**fore·head** (fōr′ed, fōr′hed) the part of the face between the eyebrows and the hairy scalp. SYN brow (2), frons.

**for·eign body** anything in the tissues or cavities

of the body that has been introduced there from without, and that is not rapidly absorbable. See page B16.

**for·eign body gran·u·lo·ma** a granuloma caused by the presence of foreign particulate material in tissue, characterized by a histiocytic reaction with foreign body giant cells.

**Fo·rel de·cus·sa·tion** (fō-rel′) SEE tegmental decussations (2).

**fore·milk** (fōr′milk) SYN colostrum.

**fo·ren·sic** (fō-ren′sik) pertaining or applicable to personal injury, murder, and other legal proceedings. [L. *forensis,* of a forum]

**fo·ren·sic den·tis·try 1.** the relation and application of dental facts to legal problems, as in using the teeth for identifying the dead; **2.** the law in its bearing on the practice of dentistry.

**fo·ren·sic med·i·cine 1.** the relation and application of medical facts to legal matters; **2.** the law in its bearing on the practice of medicine. SYN legal medicine.

**fo·ren·sic psy·chi·a·try, le·gal psy·chi·a·try** the application of psychiatry in courts of law, e.g., in determinations for commitment, competency, fitness to stand trial, responsibility for crime.

**fo·ren·sic psy·chol·o·gy** the application of psychology to legal matters in a court of law.

**fore·play** (fōr′plā) stimulative sexual activity preceding sexual intercourse.

**fore·quar·ter am·pu·ta·tion** amputation of the arm with removal of the scapula and a portion of the clavicle.

**fore·shor·ten·ing** RADIOLOGY radiographic distortion occurring where the image appears shorter than the actual image. Caused by excessive vertical angulation.

**fore·skin** (fōr′skin) SYN prepuce.

**For·es·ti·er dis·ease** (fō′res-tē-ā′) SYN diffuse idiopathic skeletal hyperostosis.

**fore·wa·ters** (fōr′wah-terz) colloquialism for the bulging fluid-filled amniotic membrane presenting in front of the fetal head.

**fork 1.** a pronged instrument used for holding or lifting; **2.** an instrument resembling a fork in that it has tines or prongs.

**form** (fōrm) shape; mold. [L. *forma*]

△**-form** in the form, shape of; equivalent to -oid. SEE morpho-. [L. *-formis*]

**For·mad kid·ney** (fōr′mad) an enlarged and deformed kidney sometimes seen in chronic alcoholism.

**for·ma·lin-ether se·di·men·ta·tion con·cen·tra·tion** a sedimentation method to separate parasitic elements from fecal debris through centrifugation and the use of ether to trap debris in a separate layer from the parasites.

**for·ma·lin-ethyl a·ce·tate se·di·men·ta·tion con·cen·tra·tion** a sedimentation method to separate parasitic elements from fecal debris through centrifugation and the use of ethyl acetate (substitute for ether) to trap debris in a separate layer from the parasites.

**for·ma·lin pig·ment** a pigment formed when acid aqueous solutions of formaldehyde act on blood-rich tissues.

**for·mam·i·dase** (fōr-mam′i-dās) an enzyme catalyzing the hydrolysis of N-formyl-L-kynurenine to L-kynurenine and formate, a reaction of significance in L-tryptophan catabolism. SYN formylase.

**for·mant** (fōr′mant) tones and their overtones resulting from the production of vowel phonemes.

**for·mate** (fōr′māt) a salt or ester of formic acid; i.e., the monovalent radical HCOO– or the anion HCOO⁻.

**for·ma·tio,** pl. **for·ma·ti·o·nes** (fōr-mā′shē-ō, fōr′shē-ō′nēz) [TA] **1.** SYN formation. **2.** a structure of definite shape or cellular arrangement. [L. fr. *formo,* pp. *-atus,* to form]

**for·ma·tion** (fōr-mā′shŭn) **1.** shape, configuration, arrangement; the way in which anything is formed. **2.** that which is formed. **3.** the act of giving form and shape. SYN formatio (1) [TA].

**for·ma·tio re·tic·u·la·ris** [TA] SYN reticular formation.

**form con·stan·cy** recognition of forms and objects as the same although they appear in various environments, positions, and sizes.

**forme fruste,** pl. **for·mes frus·tes** (fōrm′ froost′ ) a partial, arrested, or inapparent form of disease. [Fr. unfinished form]

**for·mic ac·id** the smallest carboxylic acid; a strong caustic, used as an astringent and counterirritant.

**for·mi·ca·tion** (fōr-mi-kā′shŭn) a form of paresthesia or tactile hallucination; a sensation as if small insects were creeping under the skin. [L. *formica,* ant]

**for·mim·i·no·glu·tam·ic ac·id (FIGLU)** (fōr-mim′i-nō-gloo-tam′ik as′id) an intermediate metabolite in L-histidine catabolism in the conversion of L-histidine to L-glutamic acid, with the formimino group being transferred to tetrahydrofolic acid; it may appear in the urine of patients with folic acid or vitamin $B_{12}$ deficiency, or liver disease.

**for·min** (fōr′min) a family of proteins that participates in cell polarization, cytokinesis, and vertebrate limb formation. [L. *forma,* form, + -in]

**for·mol-gel test** a test to detect the greatly increased serum proteins in visceral leishmaniasis; one drop of full-strength formalin is added to 1 mL of serum, with rapid and complete coagulation indicating the positive reaction.

**for·mu·la,** pl. **for·mu·las, for·mu·lae** (fōr′myu-lă, fōr′myu-lăz, fōr′myu-lē) **1.** a recipe or prescription containing directions for the compounding of a medicinal preparation. **2.** CHEMISTRY a symbol or collection of symbols expressing the number of atoms of the element or elements forming one molecule of a substance, together with, on occasion, information concerning the arrangement of the atoms within the molecule, their electronic structure, their charge, the nature of the bonds within the molecule, etc. **3.** an expression by symbols and numbers of the normal order or arrangement of parts or structures. [L. dim. of *forma,* form]

**for·mu·lary** (fōr′myu-lā-rē) **1.** a collection of formulas for the compounding of medicinal preparations. SEE National Formulary, Pharmacopeia. **2.** an official list of drugs approved for prescribing or administration to patients of a hospital or HMO or to beneficiaries of a health insurance program.

**for·myl (f)** (fōr′mil) the radical, HCO–.

**for·my·lase** (fōr′mi-lās) SYN formamidase.

**N-for·myl·me·thi·o·nine** (en-fōr′mil-me-thī′ō-nēn) methionine acylated on the $NH_2$ group by a formyl (–CHO) group. This is the starting amino acid residue for virtually all bacterial polypeptides. It is also observed in mitochondria and chloroplasts of eukaryotes. SEE ALSO initiating codon.

**for·ni·cate** (fōr'ni-kāt) **1.** vaulted or arched; resembling a fornix. [L. *fornicatus,* arched, fr. *fornix,* vault, arch] **2.** to have sexual intercourse. [see fornication]

**for·ni·cate gy·rus** the horseshoe-shaped cortical convolution bordering the hilus of the cerebral hemisphere; its upper limb is formed by the cingulate gyrus, its lower by the parahippocampal gyrus; SYN gyrus fornicatus (1).

**for·ni·ca·tion** (fōr-ni-kā'shŭn) sexual intercourse, especially between unmarried partners. [L. *fornicatio,* an arched or vaulted basement (brothel)]

**for·nix,** gen. **for·ni·cis,** pl. **for·ni·ces** (fōr'niks, fōr'-ni-sis, fōr-ni-sēz) [TA] **1.** in general, an archshaped structure; often the arch-shaped roof (or roof portion) of an anatomic space. **2.** the compact, white fiber bundle by which the hippocampus of each cerebral hemisphere projects to the contralateral hippocampus and to the septum, anterior nucleus of the thalamus, and mammillary body. Arising from pyramidal cells of Ammon horn, the fibers of the fornix form the alveus hippocampi and the fimbria hippocampi, and in their further course compose, sequentially, the commissure of the fornix, also called the hippocampal commissure (commissura hippocampi [TA]), the crus of fornix (crus fornicis [TA]), the body of fornix (corpus fornicis [TA]), and the column of fornix (columna fornicis [TA]), which divides into a smaller portion of precommissural fibers that pass anterior to the anterior commissure to the septal area and a larger portion of postcommissural fibers that pass posterior to the anterior commissure to end mainly in the mammillary nuclei and to a lesser extent in the anterior thalamic nucleus. [L. arch, vault]

**for·nix of stom·ach** the domed or pocket-like portion of the stomach that lies superior to and to the left of the cardial orifice, in which, in the upright position, gas is often contained; formerly considered synonym with fundus of stomach; in Terminologia Anatomica, the fundus is the uppermost portion of the body of the stomach, whose mucosa includes the greatest density of fundic cells.

**For·si·us-Er·ik·sson al·bin·ism** (fōr'sē-ŭs-er'ik-sŏn) SYN ocular albinism 2.

**forsk·o·lin** (fōr'skŏ-lin) a phorbol ester that binds to and activates protein kinase C, thus mimicking the actions of diacylglycerol. [fr. *Coleus forskohlii,* taxonomic name of botanical source]

**För·ster uve·i·tis** (fēr'ster) syphilitic inflammation, with diffuse nodules involving the choroid and retinal vasculitis.

**Fort Bragg fe·ver** (fōrt brag) SYN pretibial fever.

**for·ti·fi·ca·tion spec·trum** the zigzag banding of light, resembling the walls of fortified medieval towns, that marks the margin of the scintillating scotoma of migraine.

**for·ward heart fail·ure** a concept that maintains that the phenomena of congestive heart failure result from the inadequate cardiac output, and especially from the consequent inadequacy of renal blood flow with resulting retention of sodium and water. Cf. backward heart failure.

**fos·sa,** gen. and pl. **fos·sae** (fos'ă, fos'ē) [TA] a depression usually more or less longitudinal in shape below the level of the surface of a part. [L. a trench or ditch]

**fos·sa ace·ta·bu·li** [TA] SYN acetabular fossa.

**fos·sa for gall·blad·der** a depression on the visceral surface of the liver anteriorly, between the quadrate and the right lobes, lodging the gallbladder.

**fos·sa o·va·lis 1.** [TA] an oval depression on the lower part of the septum of the right atrium; it is a vestige of the foramen ovale, and its floor corresponds to the septum primum of the fetal heart; **2.** SYN saphenous opening.

**fos·sa of ves·ti·bule of va·gi·na** the portion of the vestibule of the vagina between the frenulum of the labia minora and the posterior labial commissure of the vulva. SYN fossa vestibuli vaginae [TA].

**fos·sa ves·tib·u·li va·gi·nae** [TA] SYN fossa of vestibule of vagina.

**fos·sette** (fos-et') **1.** SYN fossula. **2.** a seldom-used term for corneal ulcer of small diameter. [Fr. dim. of *fosse,* a ditch]

**fos·su·la,** pl. **fos·su·lae** (fos'yu-lă, fos'yu-lē) [TA] **1.** a small fossa. **2.** a minor fissure or slight depression on the surface of the cerebrum. SYN fossette (1). [L. dim. of *fossa,* ditch]

**fos·su·la post fe·nes·tram** the small passage filled with connective tissue posterior to the oval window of the cochlea; a site of predilection for otosclerosis.

**Fos·ter frame** (fos'ter) a reversible bed similar to a Stryker frame.

**Fos·ter Ken·ne·dy syn·drome** (fos'ter ken'ĕ-dē) SYN Kennedy syndrome.

**Foth·er·gill dis·ease** (foth'ĕr-gil) **1.** SYN trigeminal neuralgia. **2.** SYN anginose scarlatina.

**Foth·er·gill neu·ral·gia** (foth'ĕr-gil) SYN trigeminal neuralgia.

**Foth·er·gill op·er·a·tion** (foth'ĕr-gil) SYN Manchester operation.

**Foth·er·gill sign** (foth'ĕr-gil) in rectus sheath hematoma, the hematoma produces a mass that does not cross the midline and remains palpable when the rectus muscle is tense.

**Fou·chet stain** (foo-shā') reagent employed to demonstrate bile pigments; paraffin sections are used for conjugated bile pigments, frozen sections for unconjugated ones.

**fou·lage** (foo-lahzh') kneading and pressure of the muscles, constituting a form of massage. [Fr. impression]

**foun·da·tion** (fown-dā'shŭn) a base; a supporting structure.

**found·er prin·ci·ple** the conditional probabilities of the frequencies of a set of genes at any future date depend on the initial composition of the founders of the population and have in general no tendency to revert to the composition of the population from which the founders were themselves derived.

**foun·tain de·cus·sa·tion** SEE tegmental decussation (1).

**foun·tain sy·ringe** an apparatus consisting of a reservoir for holding fluid, to the bottom of which is attached a tube with a suitable nozzle; used for vaginal or rectal injections, irrigating wounds, etc., the force of the flow being regulated by the height of the reservoir above the point of discharge.

**Four Cor·ners vi·rus** (fō kōr'nerz) SYN Sin Nombre virus. [from the section of the U.S.

where New Mexico, Colorado, Utah, and Arizona meet, site of a major occurrence]

**Fou·ri·er a·nal·y·sis** (foor-yā′) a mathematical approximation of a function as the sum of periodic functions (sine waves) of different frequencies; used in reconstruction of images in computed tomography and magnetic resonance imaging and in analysis of any kind of signal for its frequency content.

**Fou·ri·er trans·form** (foor-yā′) a mathematical technique of dividing a time-varying function or signal into components at different frequencies, giving the phase and amplitude of each; used in computed tomography and magnetic resonance image reconstruction transformation.

**fourth cra·ni·al nerve [CN IV]** SYN trochlear nerve [CN IV].

**fourth heart sound ($S_4$)** the sound produced in late diastole in association with ventricular filling due to atrial systole and related to reduced ventricular compliance. It may be normal at older ages but is nearly always abnormal at younger ages. It is common in ventricular hypertrophy, particularly with hypertension, and is almost invariable during acute myocardial infarction. Fourth heart sounds may arise from the right or left ventricle or both.

**fourth lum·bar nerve [L4]** the ventral branch of the nerve is forked to enter into the formation of both lumbar and sacral plexuses.

**fourth toe [IV]** fourth digit of foot.

**fourth ven·tri·cle** a cavity of irregular shape extending from the obex rostralward to its communication with the sylvian aqueduct, enclosed between the cerebellum dorsally and the rhombencephalic tegmentum ventrally, having a rhomboid-shaped floor (rhomboid fossa) and a tentlike roof which in its caudal part is formed by the tela choroidea and the posterior medullary velum, in its middle part by the white matter of the cerebellum, and in its narrowing rostral part (recessus superior) by the anterior medullary velum. The fourth ventricle reaches its greatest width at the pontomedullary transition, where it expands laterally behind the cerebellar peduncles into the spoutlike lateral recess, and its greatest height at the fastigial recess, which reaches up into the cerebellar white matter. Direct communication between the ventricular system and the subarachnoid space is established at the level of the fourth ventricle by a median opening in the tela choroidea, the medial aperture of the foramen of Magendie, which opens into the cerebellomedullary cistern, and on both sides by the lateral aperture or foramen of Luschka, which connects the lateral recess with the interpeduncular cistern.

**fo·vea**, pl. **fo·ve·ae** (fō′vē-ă, fō′vē-ē) [TA] any natural depression on the surface of the body, such as the axilla, or on the surface of a bone. Cf. dimple. [L. a pit]

**fo·vea cen·tra·lis maculae luteae** [TA] SYN central retinal fovea.

**fo·ve·ate, fo·ve·at·ed** (fō′vē-āt, fō′vē-ā-ted) pitted; having foveas or depressions on the surface.

**fo·ve·a·tion** (fō-vē-ā′shŭn) pitted scar formation, as in chickenpox. [L. *fovea,* a pit]

**fo·ve·o·la**, pl. **fo·ve·o·lae** (fō-vē′ō-lă, fō-vē′ō-lē) [TA] a minute fovea or pit. [Mod. L. dim. of L. *fovea,* pit]

**fo·ve·o·lar** (fō-vē′ō-lăr) pertaining to a foveola.

**fo·ve·o·late** (fō′vē-ō-lāt, fō-vē′ō-lāt) having minute pits (foveolae) or small depressions on the surface.

**Fo·vil·le syn·drome** (fō-vēl′) a form of alternating hemiplegia characterized by abducens paralysis on one side, paralysis of the extremities on the other.

**Fow·ler po·si·tion** (fowl′ĕr) a recumbent position in which the head of the bed is elevated 60–90 cm above the level.

**F plas·mid** the prototype conjugative plasmid associated with conjugation in the K-12 strain of *Escherichia coli.* SYN F factor.

**FPS, fps** foot-pound-second. SEE foot-pound-second system, foot-pound-second unit.

**Fr** 1. francium. 2. French scale.

**Frac·ca·ro** (frahc-cah′rō), M., Italian physician. SEE Parenti-Fraccaro syndrome.

**fractals** (frak′talz) mathematical patterns developed by Benoit Mandelbrot in 1977, in which small parts have the same shape as the whole. Blood vessels and the bronchial tree behave as fractals; some infections and neoplasms also behave as fractals. [Fr., fr. L. *fractus,* broken, pp. of *frango,* to break, + -al]

**frac·tion** (frak′shŭn) 1. the quotient of two quantities. 2. an aliquot portion or any portion.

**frac·tion·a·tion** (frak-shŭn-ā′shŭn) 1. separation of the components of a mixture. 2. the administration of a course of therapeutic radiation of a neoplasm in a planned series of fractions of the total dose, most often once a day for several weeks, in order to minimize radiation damage of contiguous normal tissues.

**frac·ture** (frak′cher) 1. to break. 2. a break, especially the breaking of a bone or cartilage. See page 379. [L. *fractura,* a break]

**frac·ture blis·ter** superficial epidermolysis that occurs in association, most commonly, with fractures of the leg and ankle and forearm and wrist; etiology represents a combination of excessive swelling and torsional injury to the overlying soft tissues.

**frac·ture by con·tre·coup** skull fracture at a point distant from the site of impact.

**frac·ture of fifth me·ta·car·pal** SYN boxer's fracture.

**frag·ile site** a nonstaining gap at a specific point on a chromosome, usually involving both chromatids, always at the same point on chromosomes of different cells from an individual or kindred.

**frag·ile X chro·mo·some** an X chromosome with a fragile site near the end of the long arm, resulting in the appearance of an almost detached fragment; frequently associated with X-linked mental retardation.

**frag·ile X syn·drome (FMR1)** an X-linked recessive syndrome consisting of mental retardation, a characteristic facies, and macroorchidism; DNA analysis shows abnormal trinucleotide repeats on the X chromosome near the end of its long arm, at Xq27.3; a constriction is demonstrable at this site on karyotyping after culture in folate-deficient medium. SYN FMR1, marker X syndrome, Martin-Bell syndrome.

**fra·gil·i·ty** (fră-jil′i-tē) brittleness; liability to break, burst, or disintegrate. [L. *fragilitas*]

**fra·gil·i·ty of the blood** SYN osmotic fragility.

**fra·gil·i·ty test** a test that measures the resistance of erythrocytes to hemolysis in hypotonic saline solutions; erythrocytes to be tested are added to

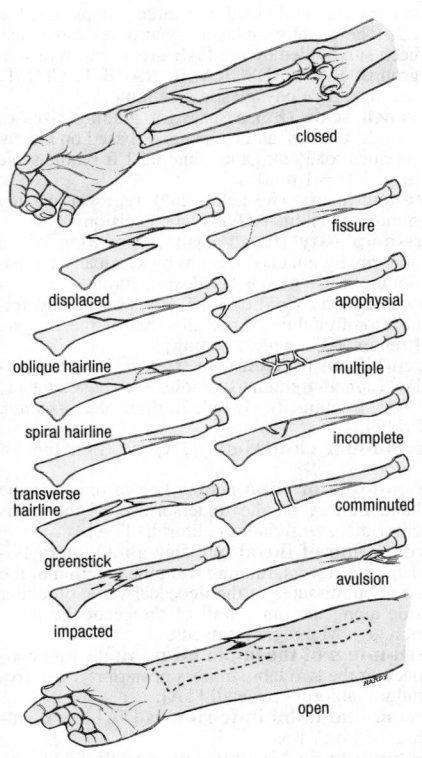

closed

fissure

displaced

apophysial

oblique hairline

multiple

spiral hairline

incomplete

transverse
hairline

comminuted

greenstick

avulsion

impacted

open

**types of fractures**

varying concentrations of saline and beginning and complete hemolysis are measured; in hereditary spherocytosis, the fragility of the erythrocytes is markedly increased, whereas in thalassemia and sickle cell anemia, the fragility of the erythrocytes is usually reduced.

**frag·ment** (frag′ment) a small part broken from a larger entity.

**frag·men·ta·tion** the breaking of an entity into smaller parts. SYN spallation (1).

**frambesia** (fram-bē′zē-ă) SYN yaws. [Fr. *framboise,* raspberry]

**fram·be·si·o·ma** (fram-bē-zē-ō′mă) SYN mother yaw. [frambesia + *-oma,* tumor]

**fram·bo·e·sia [Br.]** SYN yaws.

**frame** (frām) a supporting or integrating structure made of parts fitted together.

**frame·work re·gion** in immunology, a conserved sequence of amino acids on either side of the hypervariable regions in the variable domains of an immunoglobulin chain.

*Fran·ci·sel·la* (fran′si-sel′lă) a genus of nonmotile, nonsporeforming, aerobic bacteria that contain small, Gram-negative cocci and rods. Capsules are rarely produced and the cells may show bipolar staining. These organisms are highly pleomorphic; they do not grow on plain agar or in liquid media without special enrichment; they are pathogenic and cause tularemia in humans. The type species is *Francisella tularensis.*

*Fran·ci·sel·la tu·la·ren·sis* a species that causes

tularemia in man, transmitted to man from wild animals by bloodsucking insects or by contact with infected animals such as ticks; main sources of infection are rabbits and ticks; it can penetrate unbroken skin to cause infection; it is the type species of the genus *Francisella.*

**fran·ci·um (Fr)** (fran′sē-ŭm) radioactive element of the alkali metal series; atomic no. 87; half-life of most stable known isotope, $^{223}$Fr, is 21.8 minutes. [*France,* native country of Mlle. M. Perey, the discoverer]

**Francke nee·dle** (frahng-kĕ) a small lancet-shaped, spring-activated needle, used to evacuate a small effusion of blood.

**François** (frahn-swah′), Jules, contemporary Belgian ophthalmologist. SEE central cloudy corneal dystrophy of François.

**Frank** (frahngk), Otto, German physiologist, 1865–1944. SEE Frank-Starling curve.

**frank** unmistakable; manifest; clinically evident.

**frank breech pre·sen·ta·tion** SEE breech presentation.

**Frank·fort hor·i·zon·tal plane** (frahngk′fŏrt) a cephalometric plane that passes through the inferior borders of the bony orbits and the upper margins of the auditory meatus.

**Frank-Star·ling curve** (frahngk-stär′ling) SYN Starling curve.

**Fränt·zel mur·mur** (frahnt′zel) murmur of mitral stenosis when louder at its beginning and end than in its midportion.

**Fra·ser syn·drome** (frā′zer) an association of cryptophthalmus with multiple anomalies, including middle and outer ear malformations, cleft palate, laryngeal deformity, displacement of umbilicus and nipples, digital malformations, separation of symphysis pubis, maldevelopment of kidneys, and masculinization of genitalia in females; autosomal recessive inheritance.

**fra·ter·nal twins** SYN dizygotic twins.

**fraud** (frawd) an act of deliberate deception performed to acquire an unlawful benefit, such as the improper coding of health services in a claim for payment. [L. *fraus*]

**Fraun·ho·fer line** (frown′hōf-ĕr) any one of the more prominent absorption lines of the solar spectrum.

**Fra·zier nee·dle** (frā′zhĕr) a needle for draining lateral ventricles of brain.

**Fra·zier-Spil·ler op·er·a·tion** (frā′zher-spil′ĕr) SEE trigeminal rhizotomy.

**FRC** functional residual capacity.

**freck·le** (frek′l) yellowish or brownish macules developing on the exposed parts of the skin, especially in persons of light complexion; the lesions increase in number on exposure to the sun; the epidermis is microscopically normal except for increased melanin. SEE ALSO lentigo. SYN ephelis. [O. E. *freken*]

**Fre·det-Ram·stedt op·er·a·tion** (frĕ-dā′ rahm′shtet) SYN pyloromyotomy.

**Fred·rick·son clas·si·fi·ca·tion** (fred′rik-son) a classification system of hyperlipoproteinemia that uses plasma appearance, triglyceride values and total cholesterol values. There are five types: I, II, III, IV, V. SEE ALSO hyperlipoproteinemia.

**free as·so·ci·a·tion** an investigative psychoanalytic technique in which the patient verbalizes, without reservation or censor, the passing contents of his or her mind; the conflicts verbalized are the basis of the psychoanalyst's interpretations.

**free en·er·gy (F, F)** a thermodynamic function symbolized as $F$, or $G$ (Gibbs free energy), $=H - TS$, where $H$ is the enthalpy of a system, $T$ the absolute temperature, and $S$ the entropy; chemical reactions proceed spontaneously in the direction that involves a net decrease in the free energy of the system (i.e., $\Delta G < 0$).

**free flap** island flap in which the donor vessels are severed proximally, the flap is transported as a free object to the recipient area, and the flap is revascularized by anastomosing its supplying vessels to vessels there.

**free gin·gi·va** that portion of the gingiva that surrounds the tooth and is not directly attached to the tooth surface; the outer wall of the gingival sulcus.

**free graft** a graft transplanted without its normal attachments, or a pedicle, from one site to another.

**free in·duc·tion de·cay (FID)** in magnetic resonance imaging, the decay curve that is detected by the radiofrequency coil after the application of an excitation pulse, without additional pulses (free).

**free mac·ro·phage** an actively motile macrophage typically found in sites of inflammation.

**free nerve end·ings** a form of peripheral ending of sensory nerve fibers in which the terminal filaments end freely in the tissue.

**free rad·i·cal** a radical in its (usually transient) uncombined state; an atom or atom group carrying an unpaired electron and no charge. Free radicals may be involved as short-lived, highly active intermediates in various reactions in living tissue, notably in photosynthesis. The free radical nitric oxide, $NO\cdot$, plays an important role in vasodilation. SYN radical (4).

**free·way space** the space between the occluding surfaces of the maxillary and mandibular teeth when the mandible is in physiologic resting position. SYN interocclusal distance (2).

**freeze-dry·ing** (frēz'drī-ing) SYN lyophilization.

**freeze fracture** a procedure for preparing cells or other biological samples for electron microscopy in which the sample is frozen quickly and then broken with a sharp blow. SYN cryofracture.

**freez·ing** (frē'zing) congealing, stiffening, or hardening by exposure to cold.

**Freiberg dis·ease** (frī'bĕrg) osteonecrosis of second metatarsal head.

**Frej·ka pil·low splint** (frāj'kah) a pillow splint used for abduction and flexion of the femurs in treatment of congenital hip dysplasia or dislocation in infants.

**frem·i·tus** (frem'i-tŭs) a vibration imparted to the hand resting on the chest or other part of the body. SEE ALSO thrill. [L. a dull roaring sound, fr. *fremo*, pp. *-itus*, to roar, resound]

**frem·i·tus pec·to·ral·is** vibration on the chest wall produced by phonation.

**fre·na** (frē'nă) plural of frenum.

**fre·nal** (frē'năl) relating to any frenum.

**French-A·mer·i·can-Bri·tish clas·si·fi·ca·tion sys·tem (FAB)** a classification and nomenclature system for acute leukemias based on morphologic characteristics and cytochemical stain reactions. The acute myeloid leukemias are subdivided into eight FAB groups: M0, M1, M2, M3, M4, M5, M6, M7. The acute lymphoid leu-

kemias are subdivided into three groups: L1, L2, L3. The myelodysplastic syndromes have also been subdivided by the FAB group into five subgroups: RA, RARS, RAEB, RAEB-T, CMML. SEE ALSO myelodysplastic syndrome.

**French scale (Fr)** a scale for grading sizes of sounds, tubules, and catheters as based on a measurement of $\frac{1}{3}$ mm and equaling 1 fr on the scale (e.g., 3 fr = 1 mm).

**fre·nec·to·my** (frē-nek'tō-mē) removal of any frenum. [frenum + G. *ektomē*, excision]

**fre·no·plas·ty** (frē'nō-plas-tē) correction of an abnormally attached frenum by surgically repositioning it. [frenum + G. *plastos*, formed]

**fre·not·o·my** (frē-not'ō-mē) division of any frenum or frenulum, especially that of the tongue. [frenum + G. *tomē*, a cutting]

**fren·u·lum**, pl. **fren·u·la** (fren'yu-lŭm, fren'yu-lă) a small frenum or bridle. SYN habenula (1) [TA], frenum (3). [Mod. L. dim. of L. *frenum*, bridle]

**fren·u·lum cli·to·ri·dis** [TA] SYN frenulum of clitoris.

**fren·u·lum of clit·o·ris** the line of union of the labia minora on the undersurface of the glans clitoridis. SYN frenulum clitoridis [TA].

**fre·nu·lum of il·e·al or·i·fice** a fold, more evident in cadavers, running from the junction of the two commissures of the ileocecal valve on either side along the inner wall of the cecocolic junction. SYN Morgagni retinaculum.

**fren·u·lum of the la·bia mi·no·ra** the fold connecting the two labia minora posteriorly. SYN frenulum labiorum pudendi [TA].

**fre·nu·lum la·bii in·fe·ri·or·is** [TA] SYN frenulum of lower lip.

**fre·nu·lum la·bi·o·rum pu·den·di** [TA] SYN frenulum of the labia minora.

**fren·u·lum of low·er lip** the folds of mucous membrane extending from the gingiva to the midline of the lower (frenulum of the lower lip) and upper lips (frenulum of the upper lips), respectively. SYN frenulum labii inferioris [TA].

**fren·u·lum of pre·puce** a fold of mucous membrane passing from the undersurface of the glans penis to the deep surface of the prepuce. SYN frenulum preputii [TA].

**fre·nu·lum pre·pu·tii** [TA] SYN frenulum of prepuce.

**fre·num**, pl. **fre·na**, **fre·nums** (frē'nŭm, frē'nă, frē'-nŭmz) **1.** a narrow reflection or fold of mucous membrane passing from a more fixed to a movable part, serving to check undue movement of the part. **2.** an anatomic structure resembling such a fold. **3.** SYN frenulum. [L. a bridle, curb]

**fre·quen·cy (v)** (frē'kwen-sē) **1.** the number of regular recurrences in a given time, e.g., heartbeats, sound vibrations. **2.** ACOUSTICS the number of cycles of compression and rarefaction of a sound wave that occur in one second, expressed in hertz (Hz). **3.** the rate of vocal fold vibration (i.e., the number of times the glottis opens and closes in one second) during phonation; perceived as voice pitch. [L. *frequens*, repeated, often, constant]

**fret·ting** (fret'ing) abrasive polishing and wear of two metallic surfaces at their interface due to repetitive motion. [M.E., fr. O.E. *fretan*, to devour]

**freud·i·an** (froyd'ē-ăn) relating to or described by Sigmund Freud (1856-1939).

**freud·i·an psy·cho·a·nal·y·sis** (froyd'ē-ăn) the theory and practice of psychoanalysis and psychotherapy as developed by Sigmund Freud, based on: 1) his theory of personality, which postulates that psychic life is made up of instinctual and socially acquired forces, or the id, the ego, and a superego; 2) his discovery that the free-associated technique of verbalizing for the analyst all thoughts reveals the areas of conflict within a patient's personality; 3) that the vehicle for gaining this insight and readjusting one's personality is the learning a patient does, first developing a stormy emotional bond with the analyst (transference relationship) and next successfully learning to break this bond.

**freud·i·an slip** (froyd-ē-ăn) a mistake in speech or deed which presumably suggests some underlying motive, often sexual or aggressive in nature.

**Freud the·o·ry** (froyd) a comprehensive theory of how personality is formed and develops in normal and emotionally disturbed individuals; e.g., that an attack of conversion hysteria is due to a psychic trauma which was not adequately reacted to at the time it was received, and persists as an affect memory. SEE ALSO psychoanalysis.

**Freund ad·ju·vant** (froynd) SEE adjuvant.

**Freund a·nom·a·ly** (froynd) a narrowing of the upper aperture of the thorax by shortening of the first rib and its cartilage; formerly believed to predispose to tuberculosis because of defective expansion of the lung apex.

**Freund com·plete ad·ju·vant** (froynd) water-in-oil emulsion of antigen, to which killed mycobacteria or tuberculosis bacteria are added.

**Freund in·com·plete ad·ju·vant** (froynd) water-in-oil emulsion of antigen, without mycobacteria.

**Freund op·er·a·tion** (froynd) 1. total abdominal hysterectomy for uterine cancer; 2. chondrotomy to relieve Freund anomaly.

**Frey hairs** (frī) short hairs of varying degrees of stiffness, set at right angles into the end of a light wooden handle; used for assessing sensation.

**FRH** follitropin-releasing hormone.

**fri·a·ble** (frī'ă-bl) 1. said of tissue that readily tears, fragments, or bleeds when gently palpated or manipulated. 2. easily reduced to powder. 3. BACTERIOLOGY denoting a dry and brittle culture falling into powder when touched or shaken. [L. *friabilis,* fr. *frio,* to crumble]

**fric·tion** (frik'shŭn) 1. the act of rubbing the surface of an object against that of another; especially rubbing the limbs of the body to aid the circulation. 2. the force required for relative motion of two bodies that are in contact. 3. a group of movements in massage intended to move superficial layers over deeper structures, to reach deeper tissues, or to create heat. Includes static, cross-fiber, with-fiber, and circular frictions. [L. *frictio,* fr. *frico,* to rub]

**fric·tion rub** SYN friction sound.

**fric·tion sound** the sound, heard on auscultation, made by the rubbing of two opposed serous surfaces roughened by an inflammatory exudate, or, if chronic, by nonadhesive fibrosis. SYN friction rub.

**Fried·länd·er ba·cil·lus** (frēd'len-der) SYN *Klebsiella pneumoniae.*

**Fried·länd·er pneu·mo·nia** (frēd'len-der) a form of pneumonia caused by infection with *Klebsiella pneumoniae* (Friedländer bacillus), characteristically severe and lobar in distribution.

**Fried·man curve** (frēd'măn) SYN partogram.

**Fried·reich a·tax·ia** (frēd'rīk) a neurologic disorder characterized by ataxia, dysarthria, scoliosis, high-arched foot or pes cavus and paralysis of the muscles, especially of the lower extremities; onset usually in childhood or youth with sclerosis of the posterior and lateral columns of the spinal cord; autosomal recessive inheritance, caused by mutation involving trinucleotide repeat expansion in Friedreich ataxia gene (FRDA) on chromosome 9q.

**Fried·reich sign** (frēd'rīk) in adherent pericardium, sudden collapse of the previously distended veins of the neck at each diastole of the heart.

**frig·id** (frij'id) 1. SYN cold. 2. temperamentally, especially sexually, unresponsive. [L. *frigidus,* cold]

**fri·gid·i·ty** (fri-jid'i-tē) 1. inability in the female to achieve orgasm or any other satisfactory level of sexual response. 2. the state of being frigid (2).

**frog leg po·si·tion** supine with soles of feet together and knees apart to expose the perineum.

**Fröh·lich dwarf·ism** (frer'lik) dwarfism with Fröhlich syndrome.

**Fröh·lich syn·drome** (frer'lik) SYN dystrophia adiposogenitalis.

**Froin syn·drome** (frwahn) an alteration in the cerebrospinal fluid, which is yellowish and coagulates spontaneously in a few seconds after withdrawal, owing to its greatly increased protein (albumin and globulin) content; noted in loculated portions of the subarachnoid space isolated from spinal fluid circulation by an inflammatory or neoplastic obstruction.

**Fro·ment sign** (frō-maw') flexion of the distal phalanx of the thumb when a sheet of paper is held between the thumb and index finger in ulnar nerve palsy.

**frons,** gen. **fron·tis** (fronz, frŭn'tis) SYN forehead. [L.]

**front·ad** (frŭn'tad) toward the front.

**fron·tal** (frŭn'tăl) 1. in front; relating to the anterior part of a body. 2. referring to the frontal (coronal) plane or to the frontal bone or forehead. SYN frontalis.

**fron·tal ar·ea** SYN frontal cortex.

**fron·tal ar·tery** SYN supratrochlear artery.

**fron·tal bone** the large single bone forming the forehead and the upper margin and roof of the orbit on either side; it articulates with the parietal, nasal, ethmoid, maxillary, and zygomatic bones, and with the lesser wings of the sphenoid.

**fron·tal cor·tex** cortex of the frontal lobe of the cerebral hemisphere. SYN frontal area.

**fron·tal crest** a ridge arising at the termination of the sagittal sulcus on the cerebral surface of the frontal bone and ending at the foramen cecum.

**fron·ta·lis** (frŭn-tā'lis) SYN frontal. [L.]

**fron·tal lobe of cer·e·brum** the portion of each cerebral hemisphere anterior to the central sulcus.

**fron·tal lobe ep·i·lep·sy** epilepsy with seizures originating in the frontal lobe. Frontal lobe epilepsies have been divided into several specific syndromes including the syndrome of supplementary motor seizures, cingulate seizures, anterior frontal polar region seizures, orbital frontal seizures, dorsolateral seizures, opercular seizures, and seizures of the motor cortex.

**fron•tal nerve** a branch of the ophthalmic nerve which divides within the orbit into the supratrochlear and the supraorbital nerves. SYN nervus frontalis [TA].

**fron•tal plane** SYN coronal plane.

**fron•tal pole of cer•e•brum** the most anterior promontory of each cerebral hemisphere.

**fron•tal si•nus** a hollow paranasal sinus formed on either side in the lower part of the squama of the frontal bone; it communicates by the ethmoidal infundibulum with the middle meatus of the nasal cavity of the same side.

**fron•tal su•ture** the suture between the two halves of the frontal bone, usually obliterated by about the 6th year; if persistent it is called a metopic suture.

**fron•to•an•te•ri•or po•si•tion** a cephalic presentation of the fetus with its forehead directed toward the right (**right frontoanterior**, RFA) or to the left (**left frontoanterior**, LFA) of the acetabulum of the mother.

**fron•to•ma•lar** (frŭn'tō-mā'lăr) SYN frontozygomatic.

**fron•to•max•il•lary** (frŭn'tō-mak'si-lā-rē) relating to the frontal and the maxillary bones.

**fron•to•na•sal** (frŭn'tō-nā'zăl) relating to the frontal and the nasal bones.

**fron•to•oc•cip•i•tal** (frŭn'tō-ok-sip'i-tăl) relating to the frontal and the occipital bones, or to the forehead and the occiput.

**fron•to•pa•ri•e•tal** (frŭn'tō-pa-rī'ĕ-tăl) relating to the frontal and the parietal bones.

**fron•to•pos•te•ri•or po•si•tion** a cephalic presentation of the fetus with its forehead directed toward the right (**right frontoposterior**, RFP) or to the left (**left frontoposterior**, LFP) sacroiliac articulation of the mother.

**fron•to•tem•po•ral** (frŭn-tō-tem'pŏ-răl) relating to the frontal and the temporal bones.

**fron•to•trans•verse po•si•tion** a cephalic presentation of the fetus with its forehead directed toward the right (**right frontotransverse**, RFT) or to the left (**left frontotransverse**, LFT) iliac fossa of the mother.

**fron•to•zy•go•mat•ic** (frŭn'tō-zī'gō-mat'ik) relating to the frontal and zygomatic bones. SYN frontomalar.

**Frost** (frost), William A., English ophthalmologist, 1853–1935.

**Frost** (frost), Albert D., U.S. ophthalmologist, 1889–1945. SEE Frost suture.

**frost** a deposit resembling that of frozen vapor or dew.

**frost•bite** (frost'bīt) local tissue destruction resulting from exposure to extreme cold; in mild cases, it results in superficial, reversible freezing followed by erythema and slight pain; in severe cases, it can be painless or paresthetic and result in blistering, persistent edema, and gangrene.

**fros•ted branch an•gi•i•tis** angiitis characterized by inflammation of blood vessels with sheathing giving the appearance of branches on a tree.

**frost•ed liv•er** hyaloserositis of the liver.

**Frost su•ture** (frost) intermarginal suture between the eyelids to protect the cornea.

**frot•tage** (frō-tahzh') **1.** the rubbing movement in massage. **2.** production of sexual excitement by rubbing against someone. [F. a rubbing]

**fro•zen pel•vis** a condition in which the true pelvis is indurated throughout, especially by carcinoma.

**fro•zen sec•tion** a thin slice of tissue cut from a frozen specimen, often used for rapid microscopic diagnosis.

⌂**fruc•to-** chemical prefix denoting the fructose configuration. [L. *fructus*, fruit]

**fruc•to•fu•ra•nose** (frŭk-tō-foor'ă-nōs) fructose in furanose form.

**β-fruc•to•fu•ran•o•sid•ase** (frŭk'tō-foor-ă-nō-sīd'ās, fruk-) β-*h*-fructosidase; an enzyme hydrolyzing β-D-fructofuranosides and releasing free D-fructose; if the substrate is sucrose, the product is D-glucose plus D-fructose (invert sugar); invert sugar is more easily digestible than sucrose.

**fruc•to•ki•nase** (frŭk-tō-kī'nās) a liver enzyme that catalyzes the reaction of ATP and D-fructose to form fructose 6-phosphate and ADP; deficient in individuals with essential fructosuria (hepatic fructokinase deficiency).

**fruc•tose** (frŭk'tōs) D-*arabino*-2-hexulose; the D-isomer (also referred to as fruit sugar, levoglucose, levulose, and D-*arabino*-2-hexulose) is a 2-ketohexose that in D form is physiologically the most important of the ketohexoses and one of the two products of sucrose hydrolysis, and is metabolized or converted to glycogen in the absence of insulin. [L. *fructus*, fruit, + -ose]

**fruc•to•se•mia** (frook-tō-sē'mē-ă) presence of fructose in the circulating blood.

**fruc•to•side** (frook'tō-sīd) fructose in -C-O- linkage where the -C-O- group is the original 2 group of the fructose.

**fruc•to•su•ria** (frook-tōs-yur'ē-ă) excretion of fructose in the urine. [fructose + G. *ouron*, urine]

⌂**fruc•to•syl-** chemical prefix indicating fructose in -C-R- (not -C-O-R-) linkage through its carbon-2 (R usually C).

**fruit sug•ar** D-fructose. SEE fructose.

**frus•tra•tion** (frŭs'trā'shŭn) the thwarting of or inability to gratify a desire or to satisfy an urge or need. [L. *frustro*, pp. -*atus*, to deceive, disappoint, fr. *frustra* (adv.), in vain]

**FTA-ABS** fluorescent treponemal antibody absorption. SEE fluorescent treponemal antibody-absorption test.

**Fuchs ad•e•no•ma** (fyooks) a benign epithelial tumor of the nonpigmented epithelium of the ciliary body, rarely exceeding 1 mm in diameter.

**Fuchs black spot** (fyooks) an area of pigment proliferation in the macular region in degenerative myopia.

**Fuchs col•o•bo•ma** (fyooks) a congenital inferior crescent on the choroid at the edge of the optic disk; not associated with myopia.

**Fuchs en•do•the•li•al dys•tro•phy** (fyooks) common corneal dystrophy with autosomal dominant inheritance, characterized by keratopathia guttata with loss of endothelium and progressive corneal edema.

**Fuchs e•pi•thel•i•al dys•tro•phy** (fyooks) SYN dystrophia epithelialis corneae.

**Fuchs het•er•o•chro•mic cy•cli•tis** (fyooks) SYN Fuchs syndrome.

**fuch•sin** (fyook'sin) a nonspecific term referring to any of several red rosanilin dyes used as stains in histology and bacteriology. [Leonhard *Fuchs*, German botanist, 1501–1506]

**fuch•sin•o•phil** (fyook'si-nō-fil) **1.** staining readily with fuchsin dyes. SYN fuchsinophilic. **2.**

a cell or histologic element that stains readily with fuchsin. [fuchsin + G. *philos,* fond]

**fuch·sin·o·phil gran·ule** a granule that has an affinity for fuchsin.

**fuch·sin·o·phil·ic** (fyook′si-nō-fil′ik) SYN fuchsinophil (1).

**Fuchs spur** (fyooks) epithelial outgrowth of the dilator muscle of the pupil about midway in the breadth of the sphincter; part of the insertion of the dilator muscle onto the iris sphincter.

**Fuchs syn·drome** (fyooks) a syndrome characterized by corneal degeneration, heterochromia of the iris, iridocyclitis, keratic precipitates, and cataract; probably autosomal dominant inheritance. SYN Fuchs heterochromic cyclitis.

**Fuchs u·ve·itis** (fyooks) SYN heterochromic uveitis.

**fu·cose** (fyoo′kōs) 6-Deoxygalactose; a methylpentose, the L-configuration of which occurs in the mucopolysaccharides of the blood group substances, in human milk (as a polysaccharide), and elsewhere in nature. The D-configuration has been found in certain antibiotics.

**fu·gac·i·ty (f)** (fyoo-gas′i-tē) the tendency of the molecules in a fluid, as a result of all forces acting on them, to leave a given site in the body; the escaping tendency of a fluid, as in diffusion, evaporation, etc. [L. *fuga,* flight]

△**-fugal** movement away from the part indicated by the main portion of the word. [L. *fugio,* to flee]

△**-fuge** flight, denoting the place from which flight takes place or that which is put to flight. [L. *fuga* a running away]

**fugue** (fyoog) a condition in which an individual suddenly abandons a present activity or lifestyle and starts a new and different one, often in a different city; afterward, the individual alleges amnesia for events occurring during the fugue period, although earlier events are remembered and habits and skills are usually unaffected. [Fr. fr. L. *fuga,* flight]

**ful·crum,** pl. **ful·cra, ful·crums** (ful′krŭm, ful′krӑ, ful′krŭmz) a support or the point thereon on which a lever turns. [L. a bedpost, fr. *fulcio,* to prop up]

**ful·gu·rant** (ful′gyŭ-rănt) sharp and piercing. Cf. fulminant. SYN fulgurating (1). [L. *fulgur,* flashing lightning]

**ful·gu·rat·ing** (ful′gyŭ-rā-ting) 1. SYN fulgurant. 2. relating to fulguration.

**ful·gu·ra·tion** (ful-gyŭ-rā′shŭn) destruction of tissue by means of a high-frequency electric current: **direct fulguration** utilizes an insulated electrode with a metal point, which is connected to the uniterminal of the high-frequency apparatus, from which a spark of electricity is allowed to impinge on the area to be treated; **indirect fulguration** involves directly connecting the patient by a metal contact to the uniterminal and utilizing an active electrode to complete an arc from the patient. [L. *fulgur,* lightning stroke]

**ful·ler's earth 1.** an amorphous variety of kaolin of varying composition, containing an aluminum magnesium silicate. **2.** a refined clay sometimes used as a dusting powder or applied moistened with water as a form of poultice. Used as decolorizer for oils and other liquids, filtering medium, filler for rubber, and in agricultural formulations. [fr. *fulling,* an old process of cleaning wool with earth or clay]

**full-thick·ness graft** a graft of the full thickness

of mucosa and submucosa or of skin and subcutaneous tissue.

**ful·mi·nant** (ful′mi-nănt) occurring suddenly, with lightning-like rapidity, and with great intensity or severity. Cf. fulgurant. [L. *fulmino,* pp. *-atus,* to hurl lightning, fr. *fulmen,* lightning]

**ful·mi·nat·ing** (ful′mi-nā′ting) running a speedy course, with rapid worsening.

**fu·ma·rate hy·dra·tase** (fyu′mă-rāt hī′dră-tās) an enzyme catalyzing the reversible interconversion of fumaric acid and water to malic acid, a reaction of importance in the tricarboxylic acid cycle. Deficiency leads to mental retardation.

**fu·mar·ic ac·id** (fyu-mar′ik as′id) *trans*-butanedioic acid; an unsaturated dicarboxylic acid occurring as an intermediate in the tricarboxylic acid cycle.

**fu·mi·gant** (fyu′mi-gănt) a substance used in fumigation.

**fu·mi·gate** (fyu′mi-gāt) to expose to the action of smoke or of fumes of any kind as a means of disinfection or eradication. [L. *fumigo* pp. *-atus,* to fumigate, fr. *fumus,* smoke, + *ago,* to drive]

**fu·mi·ga·tion** (fyu-mi-gā′shŭn) the act of fumigating; the use of a fumigant.

**fum·ing** (fyum′ing) giving forth a visible vapor, a property of concentrated nitric, sulfuric, and hydrochloric acids, and certain other substances. [L. *fumus,* smoke]

**func·tio lae·sa** (fŭngk′shē-ō lē′să) impaired function; a fifth sign of inflammation added by Galen to those enunciated by Celsus (rubor, tumor, calor, and dolor). [L.]

**func·tion** (fŭngk′shŭn) 1. the special action or physiologic property of an organ or other part of the body. 2. to perform its special work or office, said of an organ or other part of the body. 3. the general properties of any substance, depending on its chemical character and relation to other substances, according to which it may be grouped among acids, bases, alcohols, esters, etc. 4. a particular reactive grouping in a molecule; e.g., a functional group, such as the –OH group of an alcohol. 5. a quality, trait, or fact that is so related to another as to be dependent upon and to vary with this other. [L. *functio,* fr. *fungor,* pp. *functus,* to perform]

**func·tion·al** (fŭnk′shŭn-ăl) 1. relating to a function. 2. not organic in origin; denoting a disorder with no known or detectable organic basis to explain the symptoms. SEE neurosis.

**func·tion·al ac·ti·vi·ty** 1. an activity that enhances performance, improves physiologic capacity, or prevents dysfunction; 2. an activity that allows one to meet the demands of the environment and daily life.

**func·tion·al a·nat·o·my** anatomy studied in its relation to function.

**func·tion·al blind·ness** apparent loss of vision related to suggestibility.

**func·tion·al con·ges·tion** hyperemia occurring during functional activity of an organ. SYN physiologic congestion.

**func·tion·al deaf·ness** SYN psychogenic deafness.

**func·tion·al dis·or·der, func·tion·al dis·ease** a physical disorder with no known or detectable organic basis to explain the symptoms. SEE behavior disorder, neurosis.

**func·tion·al dys·men·or·rhea** SYN primary dysmenorrhea.

f
u

**func·tion·al en·dos·cop·ic si·nus sur·ger·y (FESS)** a group of operations performed on the paranasal sinuses, with illumination and magnification through an endoscope.

**func·tion·al food** any food demonstrated to confer physiologic benefits or to reduce the risk of chronic disease besides serving as a nutrient.

**func·tion·al ge·nom·ics** the study of expressed genes in organisms, including the identity of the genes and the factors that control differential expression.

**func·tion·al hear·ing im·pair·ment** SYN psychogenic hearing impairment.

**func·tion·al mur·mur** a cardiac murmur not associated with a significant heart lesion. SYN innocent murmur.

**func·tion·al neck dis·sec·tion** operation to remove metastases to the lymph nodes of the neck; differs from a radical neck dissection by preserving any of the following structures: the sterno-cleidomastoid muscle, the spinal accessory nerve, and the internal jugular vein. SYN limited neck dissection.

**func·tion·al neu·ro·sur·gery** destruction or chronic excitation of a part of the brain to treat disordered behavior or function.

**func·tion·al oc·clu·sion 1.** any tooth contacts made within the functional range of the opposing teeth surfaces; **2.** occlusion which occurs during function.

**func·tion·al re·sid·u·al air** SYN functional residual capacity.

**func·tion·al re·sid·u·al ca·pac·i·ty (FRC)** the volume of gas remaining in the lungs at the end of a normal expiration; it is the sum of expiratory reserve volume and residual volume. SYN functional residual air.

**func·tion·al splint 1.** SYN dynamic splint. **2.** the joining of two or more teeth into a rigid unit by means of fixed restorations that cover all or part of the abutment teeth.

**func·tion·al test** assessment of an individual's ability to move a body part actively, against resistance, and in a specific movement pattern.

**fun·da·men·tal fre·quen·cy (F0) 1.** ACOUSTICS the basic frequency of a vibrating object or sound as opposed to its harmonics, or the principal component of a complex sound wave; **2.** the frequency of vocal fold vibration at the glottis, unaffected by resonance. SEE ALSO optimal pitch.

**fun·dec·to·my** (fŭn-dek'tō-mē) SYN fundusectomy. [fundus + G. ektomē, excision]

**fun·dic** (fŭn'dik) relating to a fundus.

**fun·di·form** (fŭn'di-fōrm) looped; sling-shaped. [L. funda, a sling, + forma, shape]

**fun·do·pli·ca·tion** (fŭn'dō-pli-kā'shŭn) suture of the fundus of the stomach around the esophagus to prevent reflux in repair of hiatal hernia. [fundus + L. plico, to fold]

**fun·dus,** pl. **fun·di** (fŭn'dŭs, fŭn-dī) the bottom or lowest part of a sac or hollow organ; that part farthest removed from the opening or exit; occasionally a broad cul-de-sac. [L. bottom]

**fun·du·sec·to·my** (fŭn-dŭ-sek'tō-mē) excision of the fundus of an organ. SYN fundectomy. [L. fundus, + G. ektomē, excision]

**fun·dus of eye** the portion of the interior of the eyeball around the posterior pole, visible through the ophthalmoscope. See page B15. SYN fundus oculi.

**fun·dus of gall·blad·der** the wide closed end of the gallbladder situated at the inferior border of the liver.

**fun·dus oc·u·li** SYN fundus of eye. SEE eye-grounds.

**fun·dus of stom·ach** the portion of the stomach that lies above the cardiac notch. SYN fundus ventriculi.

**fun·dus of u·ri·nary blad·der** the fundus is formed by the posterior wall which is somewhat convex. SYN fundus vesicae urinariae.

**fun·dus of uter·us** the upper rounded extremity of the uterus above the openings of the uterine (fallopian) tubes.

**fun·dus ven·tric·u·li** SYN fundus of stomach.

**fun·dus ve·si·cae u·ri·na·ri·ae** SYN fundus of urinary bladder.

**fun·gae·mia [Br.]** SEE fungemia.

**fun·gal** (fŭng'găl) SYN fungous.

**fun·gate** (fŭng'gāt) to grow exuberantly like a fungus.

**fun·ge·mia** (fŭn-jē'mē-ă) fungal infection disseminated by way of the bloodstream.

**Fun·gi** (fŭn'jī) a division of eukaryotic organisms that grow in irregular masses, without roots, stems, or leaves, and are devoid of chlorophyll or other pigments capable of photosynthesis. Each organism (thallus) is unicellular to filamentous, and possesses branched somatic structures (hyphae) surrounded by cell walls containing cellulose or chitin or both, and containing true nuclei. They reproduce sexually or asexually (spore formation), and may obtain nutrition from other living organisms as parasites or from dead organic matter as saprobes (saprophytes). [L. fungus, a mushroom]

**fun·gi** (fŭn'jī) plural of fungus.

**fun·gi·ci·dal** (fŭn-ji-sī'dăl) having a killing action on fungi. [fungus + L. caedo, to kill]

**fun·gi·cide** (fŭn'ji-sīd) any substance that has a destructive killing action upon fungi.

**fun·gi·form** (fŭn'ji-fōrm) shaped like a fungus or mushroom; applied to any structure with a broad, often branched, free portion and a narrower base.

**fun·gi·form pa·pil·lae** numerous minute elevations on the dorsum of the tongue, of a fancied mushroom shape, the tip being broader than the base; the epithelium of many of these papillae has taste buds.

**Fun·gi Im·per·fec·ti** (fŭn'jī im-per-fek'tī) a phylum of fungi in which sexual reproduction is not known or in which one of the mating types has not yet been discovered.

**fun·gi·stat·ic** (fŭn-ji-stat'ik) having an inhibiting action upon the growth of fungi. [fungus + G. statos, standing]

**fun·gi·tox·ic** (fŭn-ji-tok'sik) poisonous or in any way deleterious to the growth of fungi.

**fun·goid** (fŭng'goyd) resembling a fungus; denoting an exuberant morbid growth on the surface of the body.

**fun·gos·i·ty** (fŭng-gos'i-tē) a fungoid growth.

**fun·gous** (fŭng'gŭs) relating to a fungus. SYN fungal.

**fun·gus,** pl. **fun·gi** (fŭng'gŭs, fŭn'jī) a general term used to encompass the diverse morphological forms of yeasts and molds. Originally classified as primitive plants without chlorophyll, the fungi are placed in the kingdom Fungi and some in the kingdom Protista, along with algae, protozoa, and slime molds. Fungi share with bacteria the ability to break down complex organic substances and are essential to the recycling of carbon and other elements. Fungi are important as foods and to the fermentation process in the development of substances of industrial and medical importance, including alcohol, the antibiotics, other drugs, and antitoxins. Relatively few fungi are pathogenic for humans, whereas most plant diseases are caused by fungi. [L. *fungus,* a mushroom]

**fun·gus ball** a compact mass of fungal mycelium and cellular debris, 1 to 5 cm in diameter, residing within a lung cavity; usually produced by *Aspergillus fumigatus.* SEE ALSO aspergilloma (2).

**fu·nic** (fyu′nik) relating to the funis, or umbilical cord. SYN funicular (2).

**fu·ni·cle** (fyu′ni-kl) SYN cord.

**fu·nic·u·lar** (fyu-nik′yu-lăr) **1.** relating to a funiculus. **2.** SYN funic.

**fu·nic·u·lar graft** a nerve graft in which each funiculus (composed of two or more fasciculi) is approximated and sutured separately.

**fu·nic·u·lar pro·cess** the tunica vaginalis surrounding the spermatic cord.

**fu·nic·u·li·tis** (fyu-nik′yu-lī′tis) **1.** inflammation of a funiculus, especially of the spermatic cord. **2.** inflammation of the umbilical cord usually associated with chorioamnionitis. [funiculus + G. *-itis,* inflammation]

**fu·nic·u·lo·pexy** (fyu-nik′yu-lō-pek-sē) suturing of the spermatic cord to the surrounding tissue in the correction of an undescended testicle. [funiculus + G. *pēxis,* a fixing]

**fu·nic·u·lus,** pl. **fu·nic·u·li** (fyu-nik′yu-lŭs, fyu-nik′yu-lī) [TA] SYN cord. [L. dim. of *funis,* cord]

**fu·nic·u·lus sper·ma·ti·cus** [TA] SYN spermatic cord.

**fu·nic·u·lus um·bi·li·ca·lis** [TA] SYN umbilical cord.

**fu·ni·form** (fyu′ni-fōrm) ropelike. [L. *funis,* cord, + *forma,* shape]

**fu·ni·punc·ture** (fyu′nē-pŭnk′cher) SYN cordocentesis. [L. *funis,* cord, + puncture]

**fu·nis** (fyu′nis) **1.** SYN umbilical cord. **2.** a cordlike structure. [L. a rope, cord]

**funisitis** (fyu-ni-sī-tis) inflammation of the umbilical cord. [funis + -itis]

**fun·nel** (fŭn′ĕl) **1.** a hollow conical vessel with a tube of variable length proceeding from its apex, used in pouring fluids from one container to another, in filtering, etc. **2.** in anatomy, an infundibulum.

**fun·nel breast, fun·nel chest** SYN pectus excavatum.

**fun·nel plot** a graphic method of detecting publication bias. The estimate of risk derived from a set of epidemiologic studies used in a metaanalysis is plotted against sample size. If there is no publication bias, the plot is funnel-shaped; if studies giving significant results are more likely to be published than negative studies, the plot is asymmetric. SEE ALSO meta-analysis.

**fun·nel-shaped pel·vis** a pelvis in which the pelvic inlet dimensions are normal, but the outlet is contracted in the transverse or in both transverse and anteroposterior diameters.

**FUO** fever of unknown origin.

**fu·ra-2** a fluorescent indicator which binds calcium; it is excited at longer wavelengths when free of calcium than when calcium is bound; the ratio of fluorescence intensity at two excitation wavelengths provides a measure of free calcium

ion concentration; may be injected into cells to monitor moment-to-moment changes in intracellular free calcium ion concentration. SEE ALSO aequorin.

**fu·ra·nose** (fyur′ă-nōs) a saccharide unit or molecule containing the furan grouping. [furan + -ose(1)]

**fur·cal** (fer′kăl) forked.

**fur·ca·tion** (fer-kā′shŭn) **1.** a forking, or a forklike part or branch. **2.** DENTISTRY the region of a multirooted tooth at which the roots divide. [L. *furca,* fork]

**fur·fu·ra·ceous** (fer-fŭ-rā′shŭs) branny, or composed of small scales; denoting a form of desquamation. SYN pityroid. [L. *furfuraceus,* fr. *furfur,* bran]

**fu·ror ep·i·lep·ti·cus** (fu′rōr ep-i-lep′ti-kŭs) attacks of anger to which epileptic individuals are occasionally subject, occurring without apparent provocation and without disturbance of consciousness.

**fur·row** (fer′rō) a groove or sulcus. [A.S. *furh*]

**fu·run·cle** (fyu′rŭng-kl) a localized pyogenic infection, most frequently by *Staphylococcus aureus,* originating deep in a hair follicle. SYN boil, furunculus. [L. *furunculus,* a petty thief]

**fu·run·cu·lar** (fyu-rŭng′kyu-lăr) relating to a furuncle. SYN furunculous.

**fu·run·cu·loid** (fyu-rŭng′kyu-loyd) resembling a furuncle. [furunculus + G. *eidos,* resemblance]

**fu·run·cu·lo·sis** (fyu-rŭng-kyu-lō′sis) a condition marked by the presence of furuncles, often chronic and recurrent.

**fu·run·cu·lous** (fyu-rŭng′kyu-lŭs) SYN furuncular.

**fu·run·cu·lus,** pl. **fu·run·cu·li** (fyu-rŭng′kyu-lŭs, fyu-rŭng′kyu-lī) SYN furuncle. [L. a petty thief, a boil, dim. of *fur,* a thief]

*Fu·sar·i·um* (fyu-zā′rē-ŭm) a genus of rapidly growing fungi producing characteristic sickle-shaped, multiseptate macroconidia which can be mistaken for those produced by some dermatophytes. A few species can produce corneal ulcers; some are common colonizers of burned skin and some may cause disseminated hyalohyphomycosis. [L. *fusus,* spindle]

**fused kid·ney** a single, anomalous organ produced by fusion of the two renal anlagen (primordia of the kidneys).

**fu·si·form** (fyu′zi-fōrm) spindle-shaped; tapering at both ends. [L. *fusus,* a spindle, + *forma,* form]

**fu·si·form an·eu·rysm** an elongated spindle-shaped dilation of an artery.

**fu·si·form gy·rus** an extremely long convolution extending lengthwise over the inferior aspect of the temporal and occipital lobes, demarcated medially by the collateral sulcus from the lingual gyrus and the anterior part of the parahippocampal gyrus, laterally by the inferior temporal sulcus from the inferior temporal gyrus.

**fu·si·mo·tor** (fyu′zē-mō′ter) pertaining to the efferent innervation of intrafusal muscle fibers by gamma motor neurons. SEE ALSO neuromuscular spindle. [L. *fusus,* spindle, + *moveo,* to move]

**fu·sin** (fyoo′zin) a G protein–linked receptor present on certain human cells that is thought to be required for HIV fusion with a target cell. [fuse, fr. L. *fundo,* pp. *fusum,* to melt, + -in]

**fu·sion** (fyoo′zhŭn) **1.** liquefaction, as by melting by heat. **2.** union, as by joining together. **3.** the blending of slightly different images from each

*f u*

eye into a single perception. **4.** the joining of two or more adjacent teeth during their development by a dentinal union. SEE ALSO concrescence. **5.** joining of two genes, often neighboring genes. [L. *fusio,* a pouring, fr. *fundo,* pp. *fusus,* to pour]

**fu•sion beat** a beat triggered by more than a single electrical impulse, when the wave fronts coincide to act together on a single final pathway of activity; in the electrocardiogram, the atrial or ventricular complex when either atria or ventricles are activated jointly by two simultaneous or nearly simultaneous invading impulses.

*Fu•so•bac•te•ri•um* (fyoo′zō-bak-tēr′ē-ŭm) a genus of bacteria containing Gram-negative, non–spore-forming, obligately anaerobic rods which produce butyric acid as a major metabolic product. These organisms are found in cavities of humans and other animals; some species are pathogenic. [L. *fusus,* a spindle, + bacterium]

**fu•so•cel•lu•lar** (fyoo′zō-sel′yu-lăr) spindle-celled.

**fu•so•spi•ro•chae•tal [Br.]** SEE fusospirochetal.

**fu•so•spi•ro•chet•al** (fyoo-zō-spī-rō-kē′tăl) referring to the associated fusiform and spirochetal organisms found in the lesions of Vincent angina.

**fu•so•spi•ro•chet•al gin•gi•vi•tis** SYN necrotizing ulcerative gingivitis.

**Fut•cher line** (fooch′er) a dorsoventral line of pigmentation occurring symmetrically and bilaterally for about 10 cm along the lateral edge of the biceps muscle; it is seen in some African Americans.

**FVC** forced vital capacity.

**f wave, ff waves** atrial fibrillation wave.

**F waves** the waves of atrial flutter usually best seen in ECG leads 2, 3, and AVF. (A small f indicates atrial fibrillation).

# G

γ **1.** gamma. SEE gamma. **2.** activity coefficient; surface tension.

**G** newtonian constant of gravitation, gap (3); gauss; giga-; D-glucose, as in UDPG; guanosine, as in GDP; glycine; guanine.

**G** $G_{act}$ or $G^+$.

**g** gram.

**g** unit of acceleration based on the acceleration produced by the earth's gravitational attraction, where 1 $g$ = 980.621 cm/sec$^2$ (about 32.1725 ft/sec$^2$) at sea level and 45° latitude. At 30° latitude, $g$ equals 979.329 cm/sec$^2$.

**Ga** gallium.

**GABA** γ-aminobutyric acid.

**G-ac·tin** the globular (G) subunits of the actin molecule, having a molecular weight of 57,000 and containing one molecule of ATP.

**gad·o·lin·i·um (Gd)** (gad-ō-lin′ē-ŭm) an element of the lanthanide group, atomic no. 64, atomic wt. 157.25. The magnetic properties of this element are used in contrast media for magnetic resonance imaging. [mineral, gadolinite, from Johan *Gadolin*, Finnish chemist, 1760–1852]

**Gaens·len sign** (genz′len) pain on hyperextension of the hip with pelvis fixed by flexion of opposite hip; causes a torsion stress at the sacroiliac and lumbosacral joints.

**gag 1.** to retch; to cause to retch or heave. **2.** to prevent from talking. **3.** an instrument adjusted between the teeth to keep the mouth from closing during operations in the mouth or throat.

**gag re·flex** contact of a foreign body with the mucous membrane of the fauces causes retching or gagging.

**gain** (gān) **1.** profit; advantage. **2.** the ratio of output to input of an amplifying system, generally expressed in decibels. [M.E. *gayne*, booty, fr. O.Fr., fr. Germanic]

**Gaird·ner dis·ease** (gārd′ner) attacks of cardiac distress accompanied by apprehension.

**Gais·böck syn·drome** (gīs′bĕrk) SYN polycythemia hypertonica.

**gait** (gāt) manner of walking.

**Gal** galactose.

**ga·lac·ta·cra·sia** (gă-lak′tă-krā′zē-ă) abnormal composition of mother's milk. [galact- + G. *akrasia*, bad mixture, fr. *a*- priv. + *krasis*, a mixing]

**ga·lac·ta·gogue** (gă-lak′tă-gog) an agent that promotes the secretion and flow of milk. [galact- + G. *agōgos*, leading]

**ga·lac·tic** (gă-lak′tik) pertaining to milk; promoting the flow of milk.

△**ga·lac·to-, ga·lact-** milk. Cf. lact-. [G. *gala*]

**ga·lac·to·cele** (gă-lak′tō-sēl) retention cyst caused by occlusion of a lactiferous duct. SYN lactocele. [galacto- + G. *kēlē*, tumor]

**ga·lac·to·ki·nase** (gă-lak-tō-kī′nās) an enzyme (phosphotransferase) that, in the presence of ATP, catalyzes the phosphorylation of D-galactose to D-galactose 1-phosphate, the first step in the metabolism of D-galactose; galactokinase is deficient in one form of galactosemia.

**ga·lac·to·phore** (gă-lak′tō-fōr) SYN lactiferous ducts. [galacto- + G. *phoros*, bearing]

**ga·lac·to·pho·ri·tis** (gă-lak′tō-fō-rī′tis) inflammation of the milk ducts. [galacto- + G. *phoros*, carrying, + -itis, inflammation]

**gal·ac·toph·o·rous** (gal-ak-tof′ŏ-rŭs) conveying milk.

**ga·lac·to·poi·e·sis** (gă-lak′tō-poy-ē′sis) milk production. [galacto- + G. *poiēsis*, forming]

**ga·lac·to·poi·et·ic** (gă-lak′tō-poy-et′ik) pertaining to galactopoiesis.

**ga·lac·tor·rhea** (gă-lak-tō-rē′ă) **1.** a flow of milk from the breasts other than normal lactation. **2.** any white discharge from a nipple. SYN lactorrhea. [galacto- + G. *rhoia*, a flow]

**ga·lac·tor·rhoea [Br.]** SEE galactorrhea.

**ga·lac·to·sae·mia [Br.]** SEE galactosemia.

**ga·lac·tos·a·mine** (gă-lak-tō-sam′ēn) the 2-amino-2-deoxy derivative of galactose, in which the NH$_2$ replaces the 2-OH group; the D-isomer occurs in various mucopolysaccharides, notably of chondroitin sulfuric acid and of B blood group substance; usually found as the *N*-acetyl derivative.

**ga·lac·tos·am·i·no·gly·can** (gă-lak′tōs-am-i-nō-glī′kan) SEE mucopolysaccharide.

**ga·lac·tose (Gal)** (gă-lak′tōs) an aldohexose found (in D form) as a constituent of lactose, cerebrosides, gangliosides, mucoproteins, etc., in galactoside or galactosyl combination; an epimer of D-glucose.

**ga·lac·tose cat·a·ract** a neonatal cataract associated with intralenticular accumulation of galactose alcohol. SEE galactosemia.

**ga·lac·to·se·mia** (gă-lak-tō-sē′mē-ă) an inborn error of galactose metabolism due to congenital deficiency of the enzyme galactosyl-1-phosphate uridyltransferase, resulting in tissue accumulation of galactose 1-phosphate; manifested by nutritional failure, hepatosplenomegaly with cirrhosis, cataracts, mental retardation, galactosuria, aminoaciduria, and albuminuria, which regress or disappear if galactose is removed from the diet. [galactose + G. *haima*, blood]

**ga·lac·tose-1-phos·phate** a phosphorylated derivative of galactose that is key in galactose metabolism; accumulates in certain types of galactosemia.

**α-D-ga·lac·to·sid·ase** (alfa-dē-gă-lak-tō-sīd′ās) an enzyme catalyzing the hydrolysis of α-D-galactosides to release free D-galactose. A deficiency of type A α-D-galactosidase is associated with Fabry disease.

**β-ga·lac·to·sid·ase** (beta-ga-lak′tō-si′dās) an enzyme that hydrolyzes the beta galactoside linkage in lactose-producing glucose and galactose; also hydrolyzes the chromogenic substrate IPTG (isopropylthiogalactoside) and thus is used as an indicator of fused genes and gene expression.

**β-D-ga·lac·to·sid·ase** a sugar-splitting enzyme that catalyzes the hydrolysis of lactose into D-glucose and D-galactose, and that of other β-D-galactosides; it also catalyzes galactotransferase reactions; a deficiency of β-D -galactosidase leads to problems in the intestinal digestion of lactose; used in the production of milk products for adults who do not have the intestinal enzyme; a defect of one isozyme of β-D-galactosidase is associated with Morquio syndrome type B. SYN lactase.

**ga·lac·to·side** (gă-lak′tō-sīd) a compound in which the H of the OH group on carbon-1 of galactose is replaced by an organic radical.

**ga·lac·to·sis** (gal-ak-tō'sis) formation of milk by the lacteal glands. [galacto- + G. *-osis,* condition]

**ga·lac·tos·u·ria** (gă-lak-tōs-yur'ē-ă) the excretion of galactose in the urine. [galactose + G. *ouron,* urine]

**ga·lac·to·syl** (gă-lak'tō-sil) a compound in which the –OH attached to carbon-1 of galactose is replaced by an organic radical.

**ga·lac·to·ther·a·py** (gă-lak'tō-thār'ă-pē) treatment of disease by means of an exclusive or nearly exclusive milk diet. SYN lactotherapy.

**Ga·lant re·flex** (gĕ-lahnt') a deep abdominal reflex in which there is a contraction of the abdominal muscles on tapping the anterior superior iliac spine.

**Ga·las·si pu·pil·lary phe·nom·e·non** (gah-lah' sē) SYN eye-closure pupil reaction.

**ga·lea** (gā'lē-ă) **1.** a structure shaped like a helmet. **2.** SYN epicranial aponeurosis. **3.** a form of bandage covering the head. **4.** SYN caul (1). [L. a helmet]

**Ga·le·az·zi frac·ture** (gah-lā-aht'sē) fracture of the shaft of the radius with dislocation of the distal radioulnar joint.

**ga·len·i·cals** (gā-len'i-kălz) **1.** herbs and other vegetable drugs, as distinguished from the mineral or chemical remedies. **2.** crude drugs and the tinctures, decoctions, and other preparations made from them, as distinguished from the alkaloids and other active principles. **3.** remedies prepared according to an official formula. [Claudius *Galen*]

**Gal·la·var·din phe·nom·e·non** (gah-lah-vardăn) dissociation between the noisy and musical elements of the ejection murmur of aortic stenosis, the musical element being better heard at the left sternal border and at the cardiac apex while the noisy element is better heard at the aortic area; projection of the aortic stenotic murmur to the low left sternal edge.

**gall·blad·der** (gawl'blad-er) a pear-shaped receptacle on the inferior surface of the liver, in a hollow between the right lobe and the quadrate lobe; it serves as a storage reservoir for bile. SYN vesica biliaris [TA], cholecyst, cholecystis.

**Gal·le·go dif·fer·en·ti·at·ing so·lu·tion** (gahyă-gō) a dilute solution of formaldehyde and acetic acid used in a modified Gram stain to differentiate and enhance the basic fuchsin binding to Gram-negative microorganisms.

**Gal·lie trans·plant** (gāl'ē) narrow strips of the femoral fascia lata used for suture material.

**gal·li·um (Ga)** (gal'ē-ŭm) a rare metal, atomic no. 31, atomic wt. 69.723. [L. *Gallia,* France]

**gal·li·um-67** a cyclotron-produced radionuclide with a half-life of 3.260 days and major gamma ray emissions; as a tumor- and inflammation-localizing radiotracer.

**gal·li·um-68** a positron emitter with a radioactive half-life of 1.130 hours.

**gal·lon** (găl'ŭn) a measure of U.S. liquid capacity containing 4 quarts, 231 cubic inches, or 8.3293 pounds of distilled water at 20° C; it is the equivalent of 3.785412 liters. The British imperial gallon contains 277.4194 cubic inches. [O.Fr. *galon*]

**gal·lop, gal·lop rhy·thm** (gal'op) a triple cadence to the heart sounds due to an abnormal third or fourth heart sound being heard in addition to the first and second sounds; sometimes indicative of serious disease. SYN cantering rhythm, Traube bruit.

**gall·stone** (gal'stōn) a concretion in the gallbladder or a bile duct, composed chiefly of a mixture of cholesterol, calcium bilirubinate, and calcium carbonate, occasionally as a pure stone composed of just one of these substances. SYN cholelith.

**gal·lus ad·e·no·like vi·rus** SYN GAL virus.

**Gal·ton law** (gahl'tŏn) in a population mating at random, the progeny of a parent with an extreme value for a measurable phenotype will tend on average to have values nearer the population mean than in the extreme parent.

**Gal·ton sys·tem of clas·si·fi·ca·tion of fin·ger·prints** (gahl'tŏn) a system of classification based on the variations in the patterns of the ridges, which are grouped into arches, loops, and whorls. SEE ALSO dermatoglyphics.

**Gal·ton whis·tle** (gahl'tŏn) a cylindrical whistle, attached to a compressible bulb, with a screw attachment that changes the frequency; used to test the hearing.

**gal·van·ic skin re·sponse (GSR)** a measure of changes in emotional arousal recorded by attaching electrodes to any part of the skin and recording changes in moment-to-moment perspiration and related autonomic nervous system activity.

**gal·va·nom·e·ter** (gal'vă-nom'ĕ-ter) an instrument for measuring the strength of an electric current.

**GAL vi·rus** a virus with characteristics of adenovirus, not known to be associated with natural disease. SYN gallus adenolike virus.

**Gam·bi·an try·pan·o·so·mi·a·sis** (gam-bē-ăn) a chronic disease of humans caused by *Trypanosoma brucei gambiense* in Africa; characterized by splenomegaly, drowsiness, an uncontrollable urge to sleep, and the development of psychotic changes; basal ganglia and cerebellar involvement commonly lead to chorea and athetosis; the terminal phase of the disease is characterized by wasting, anorexia, and emaciation that gradually leads to coma and death, usually from intercurrent infection. SYN chronic trypanosomiasis.

**game·keep·er's thumb** rupture of the volar ligament at the first metacarpophalangeal joint due to forceful abduction of the thumb while extended.

**gam·ete** (gam'ēt) **1.** one of two haploid cells undergoing karyogamy. **2.** any germ cell, whether oocyte or sperm. [G. *gametēs,* husband; *gametē,* wife]

**ga·mete in·tra·fal·lop·i·an trans·fer (GIFT)** placement of the oocyte and sperm into the ampulla of the fallopian tube; a form of assisted reproduction.

△**ga·met·o-** a gamete. [G. *gametēs,* husband, *gametē,* wife, fr. *gameō,* to marry]

**ga·me·to·cide** (gă-mē'tō-sīd) an agent destructive of gametes, specifically the malarial gametocytes. [gameto- + L. *caedo,* to kill]

**ga·me·to·cyte** (gă-mē'tō-sīt) a cell capable of dividing to produce gametes, e.g., a spermatocyte or oocyte. [gameto- + G. *kytos,* cell]

**ga·me·to·gen·e·sis** (gam'ĕ-tō-jen'ĕ-sis) the process of formation and development of gametes. [gameto- + G. *genesis,* production]

**gam·ma** (γ) (gă'mă) **1.** third letter in the Greek alphabet. **2.** CHEMISTRY the third in a series, the fourth carbon in an aliphatic acid, or position 2 removed from the α position in the benzene ring.

**3.** symbol for $10^{-4}$ gauss. **4.** For terms with the prefix γ, see the specific term.

**gam·ma an·gle** the angle formed between a line joining the fixation point to the center of the eye and the optic axis.

🔲**gam·ma cam·er·a** any one of several scintigraphic cameras that record simultaneously counts from the entire operative field of view. See page B12. SYN scintillation camera.

**gam·ma fi·bers** nerve fibers that have a conduction rate of about 20 m/sec.

**Gam·ma·her·pes·vir·i·nae** (gam′a-her′pez-vir′ĭ-nē) a subfamily of Herpesviridae containing Epstein-Barr virus and others that cause lymphoproliferation.

**gam·ma knife** a minimally invasive radiosurgical system used in the treatment of benign and malignant intracranial neoplasms and arteriovenous malformations.

**gam·mop·a·thy** (gă-mop′ă-thē) a primary disturbance in immunoglobulin synthesis.

**Gam·na dis·ease** (gahm′nă) a form of chronic splenomegaly characterized by conspicuous thickening of the capsule and the presence of multiple, small, rustlike, brown foci (Gamna-Gandy bodies), which contain iron; this condition may be observed in fibrocongestive splenomegaly, sickle cell disease, and some examples of hemochromatosis.

**gam·o·gen·e·sis** (gam-ō-jen′ĕ-sis) SYN sexual reproduction. [G. *gamos,* marriage, + *genesis,* production]

**gan·glia** (gang′glē-ă) plural of ganglion.

**gan·glia of au·to·nom·ic plex·us·es** autonomic ganglia lying in plexuses of autonomic fibers, e.g., the celiac and inferior mesenteric ganglia of the sympathetic, and the small parasympathetic ganglia of the myenteric plexus. SYN ganglia plexuum autonomicorum.

**gan·gli·al** (gang′glē-ăl) SYN ganglionic.

**gan·glia plex·u·um au·to·no·mi·co·rum** SYN ganglia of autonomic plexuses.

**gan·glia of sym·pa·thet·ic trunk** the clusters of postganglionic neurons located at intervals along the sympathetic trunks, including the superior cervical, middle cervical, and cervicothoracic (stellate) ganglion, the thoracic, lumbar, and sacral ganglia, and the ganglion impar. SYN ganglia trunci sympathici, paravertebral ganglia.

**gan·gli·ate, gan·gli·at·ed** (gang′glē-āt, gang′glē-ā-ted) having ganglia. SYN ganglionated.

**gan·gli·at·ed nerve** a sympathetic nerve.

**gan·glia trun·ci sym·pa·thi·ci** SYN ganglia of sympathetic trunk.

**gan·gli·ec·to·my** (gang-glē-ek′tō-mē) SYN ganglionectomy.

**gan·gli·form** (gang′glē-fōrm) having the form or appearance of a ganglion. SYN ganglioform.

**gan·gli·i·tis** (gang-glē-ī′tis) SYN ganglionitis.

**gan·gli·o·blast** (gang′glē-ō-blast) an embryonic cell from which develop ganglion cells. [ganglion + G. *blastos,* germ]

**gan·gli·o·cyte** (gang′glē-ō-sīt) SYN ganglion cell.

**gan·gli·o·cy·to·ma** (gang′glē-ō-sī-tō′mă) a rare lesion that contains neuronal (ganglion) cells in a sparse glial stoma. SYN central ganglioneuroma. [ganglion + G. *kytos,* cell, + *-oma,* tumor]

**gan·gli·o·form** (gang′glē-ō-fōrm) SYN gangliform.

**gan·gli·o·gli·o·ma** (gang′glē-ō-glē-ō′mă) a rare tumor consisting of a glioma component and an atypical neuronal (ganglion) cell component; in younger patients often associated with seizures.

**gan·gli·ol·y·sis** (gang-glē-ol′i-sis) the dissolution or breaking up of a ganglion.

**gan·gli·o·ma** (gang-glē-ō′mă) SYN ganglioneuroma.

**gan·gli·on,** pl. **gan·glia, gan·gli·ons** (gang′glē-on, gang′glē-ă, gang′glē-onz) [TA] **1.** an aggregation of nerve cell bodies located in the peripheral nervous system. SYN neuroganglion. **2.** a cyst containing mucopolysaccharide-rich fluid within a fibrous capsule ; usually attached to a tendon sheath in the hand, wrist, or foot, or connected with the underlying joint. SYN myxoid cyst, synovial cyst. [G. a swelling or knot]

**gan·gli·on·at·ed** (gang′glē-ō-nā′ted) SYN gangliate.

**gan·gli·on cell** a neuron the cell body of which is located outside the limits of the brain and spinal cord, hence forming part of the peripheral nervous system; ganglion cells are either 1) the pseudounipolar cells of the sensory spinal and cranial nerves (sensory ganglia), or 2) the peripheral multipolar motor neurons innervating the viscera (visceral or autonomic ganglia). SYN gangliocyte.

**gan·gli·on cer·vi·co·thor·a·ci·cum** [TA] SYN cervicothoracic ganglion.

**gan·gli·on cyst** collection of fluid or benign tumor mass within tendons of the wrist or ankle, most commonly on the dorsal aspect of the wrist.

**gan·gli·on·ec·to·my** (gang′glē-ō-nek′tō-mē) excision of a ganglion. SYN gangliectomy. [ganglion + G. *ektomē,* excision]

**gan·gli·o·neu·ro·blas·to·ma** (gang′lē-ō-noor-ō-blas-tō′ma) a tumor of mixed cellular type, with elements of neuroblastoma and ganglioneuroma.

**gan·glio·neu·ro·ma** (gang′glē-ō-noo-rō′mă) a benign neoplasm composed of mature ganglionic neurons, in varying numbers, scattered singly or in clumps within a relatively abundant and dense stroma of neurofibrils and collagenous fibers; usually found in the posterior mediastinum and retroperitoneum, sometimes in relation to the adrenal glands. SYN ganglioma. [ganglion + G. *neuron,* nerve, + *-oma,* tumor]

**gan·gli·on·ic** (gang-glē-on′ik) relating to a ganglion. SYN ganglial.

**gan·gli·on·ic block·ade** inhibition of nerve impulse transmission at autonomic ganglionic synapses by drugs such as nicotine or hexamethonium.

**gan·gli·on·ic block·ing a·gent** an agent that impairs the passage of impulses in autonomic ganglia.

**gan·gli·on·ic branch·es of max·il·lary nerve** the ganglionic branches, two short sensory branches of the maxillary nerve in the pterygopalatine fossa, the fibers of which pass through the pterygopalatine ganglion without synapse. SYN nervi pterygopalatini [TA].

**gan·gli·on·ic branch of in·ter·nal ca·rot·id ar·tery** branch to trigeminal ganglion; a small branch of the cavernous part of the internal carotid artery to the trigeminal ganglion.

**gan·gli·on im·par** the most inferior, unpaired ganglion of the sympathetic trunk; inconstant. SYN coccygeal ganglion, Walther ganglion.

**gan·gli·on in·fe·ri·us ner·vi va·gi** [TA] SYN inferior ganglion of vagus nerve.

**gan·gli·on·i·tis** (gang′glē-ō-nī′tis) **1.** inflamma-

g
a

tion of a lymphatic ganglion. **2.** inflammation of a nerve ganglion. SYN gangliitis.

**gan•gli•o•nos•to•my** (gang'glē-ō-nos'tō-mē) making an opening into a ganglion (2). [ganglion + G. *stoma*, mouth]

**gan•gli•o•ple•gic** (gang'glē-ō-plē'jik) a pharmacologic compound that paralyzes an autonomic ganglion, usually for a relatively short period of time. [ganglion + G. *plēgē*, stroke, shock]

**gan•gli•o•side** (gang'glē-ō-sīd) a glycosphingolipid chemically similar to cerebrosides but containing one or more sialic acid residues; found principally in nerve tissue, spleen, and thymus; $G_{M1}$ accumulates in generalized gangliosidosis; $G_{M2}$ accumulates in Tay-Sachs disease.

**gan•gli•o•si•do•sis** (gang'glē-ō-si-dō'sis) any disease characterized, in part, by the abnormal accumulation within the nervous system of specific gangliosides, e.g., $G_{M2}$ gangliosidosis, Tay-Sachs disease, caused by hexosaminidase A enzyme deficiency with accumulation of $G_{M2}$ ganglioside.

**gan•grene** (gang'grēn) **1.** necrosis due to obstruction, loss, or diminution of blood supply; it may be localized to a small area or involve an entire extremity or organ (such as the bowel), and may be wet or dry. SYN mortification. **2.** extensive necrosis from any cause, e.g., gas gangrene. [G. *gangraina*, an eating sore, fr. *graō*, to gnaw]

**gan•gre•nous** (gang'grĕ-nŭs) relating to or affected with gangrene. SYN mortified.

**gan•gre•nous sto•ma•ti•tis** stomatitis characterized by necrosis of oral tissue. SEE noma.

**Gan•ser syn•drome** (gahn'sĕr) a psychoticlike condition, without the symptoms and signs of a traditional psychosis, occurring typically in prisoners who feign insanity; e.g., such a person, when asked to multiply 6 by 4, will give 23 as the answer, or will call a key a lock.

**Gant clamp** (gant) a right-angled clamp used in hemorrhoidectomy.

**gap 1.** a hiatus or opening in a structure. **2.** an interval or discontinuity in any series or sequence. **3.** (G) a period in the cell cycle.

**gap 1** in the somatic cell cycle, the gap that follows mitosis and is followed by synthesis in preparation for the next cycle.

**gap 2** in the somatic cell cycle, a pause between completion of synthesis and the onset of cell division.

**gap junc•tion 1.** an intercellular junction having a 2-nm gap between apposed cell membranes; the gap contains subunits in the form of polygonal lattices; it occurs in epithelia, between certain nerve cells, and in smooth and cardiac muscle. SEE ALSO synapse. **2.** areas of increased electrochemical communication between myometrial cells which aid in the propagation of the contractions of labor. SYN nexus.

**gap$_0$ period, gap$_0$ phase** phase of a cell no longer in the cell cycle and thus at least temporarily incapable of division.

**gap phe•nom•e•non** a short period in the cycle of the atrioventricular or intraventricular conduction allowing passage of an impulse which at other times would be blocked in transit.

**Gard•ner-Di•a•mond syn•drome** (gărd'nĕr dī'mŏnd) SYN autoerythrocyte sensitization syndrome.

**Gard•ner•el•la** (gard'ner-el'ă) a genus of facultatively anaerobic, oxidase- and catalase-negative,

non–spore-forming, nonencapsulated, nonmotile, pleomorphic bacteria with Gram-variable rods.

**Gard•ner•el•la va•gi•na•lis** a species that is the etiologic agent of bacterial vaginosis.

**Gard•ner syn•drome** (gărd'nĕr) multiple polyposis predisposing to carcinoma of the colon; also multiple tumors, osteomas of the skull, epidermoid cysts, and fibromas; autosomal dominant inheritance, caused by mutation in the adenomatous polyposis coli gene (APC) on chromosome 5q. This disorder is allelic to familial adenomatous polyposis.

**gar•gle** (gar'gl) **1.** to rinse the fauces with fluid through which expired breath is forced to produce a bubbling effect while the head is held far back. **2.** a medicated fluid used for gargling; a throat wash. [O. Fr. fr. L. *gurgulio*, gullet, windpipe]

**Ga•ri•el pes•sa•ry** (găr-ē-el') a hollow inflatable rubber pessary made in the form of a ring or a pear.

**Gar•land tri•an•gle** (găr'lănd) a triangular area of relative resonance in the lower back near the spine, found on the same side as a pleural effusion.

**Gar•ré dis•ease** (gah-rā') SYN sclerosing osteitis

**Gar•ré os•te•o•my•e•li•tis** (gah-rā') chronic osteomyelitis with proliferative periostitis. A focal gross thickening of the periosteum with peripheral reactive bone formation resulting from mild infection.

**Gart•ner cyst** (gahrt'nĕr) a cyst of the principal duct in the vestigial structures of the paroöphoron in the cervix or anterolateral vaginal wall, corresponding to the sexual portion of mesonephros in the male.

**Gärt•ner meth•od** (gärt'nĕr) a method of measuring venous pressure, based upon Gärtner vein phenomenon; with the patient sitting erect, a vein is selected on the back of the hand, which is held dependent, well below the level of the right atrium, and then is raised slowly; when the vein is observed to collapse, the distance between its level and that of the atrium is measured with a millimeter rule; this distance gives the venous pressure in millimeters of blood; thus the vein itself is used as a manometer communicating with the right atrium; highly inaccurate, especially in elderly subjects.

**Gärt•ner to•nom•e•ter** (gärt'nĕr) an apparatus for estimating the blood pressure by noting the force, expressed by the height of a column of mercury, needed to arrest pulsation in a finger encircled by a compressing ring.

**Gärt•ner vein phe•nom•e•non** (gärt'nĕr) fullness of the veins of the arm and hand held below heart level and collapse at a certain variable distance above that level. An unreliable test for venous pressure.

**gas 1.** fluid, like air, capable of indefinite expansion but convertible by compression and cold into a liquid and, eventually, a solid. **2.** in clinical practice, a liquid entirely in its vapor phase at 1 atmosphere of pressure because ambient temperature is above its boiling point. [coined by J.B. van Helmont, Flemish chemist, 1577–1644]

**gas ab•scess** an abscess containing gas caused by *Enterobacter aerogenes*, *Escherichia coli*, or other gas-forming microorganisms.

**gas ba•cil•lus** SYN *Clostridium perfringens*.

**gas chro•ma•tog•ra•phy** a chromatographic procedure in which the mobile phase is a mixture of gases or vapors, which are separated by their differential adsorption on a stationary phase.

**gas·e·ous** (gas'ē-ŭs) of the nature of gas.

**gas gan·grene** gangrene occurring in a wound infected with various anaerobic sporeforming bacteria, especially *Clostridium perfringens* and *C. novyi*, which cause crepitation of the surrounding tissues, due to gas liberated by bacterial fermentation, and constitutional septic symptoms.

**Gas·kell clamp** (gas'kel) an instrument for crushing the atrioventricular bundle in experimental animals and thus producing heart block.

**gas·liq·uid chro·ma·tog·ra·phy (GLC)** gas chromatography, with the stationary phase being liquid rather than solid.

**gas·o·met·ric** (gas-ō-met'rik) relating to gasometry.

**gas·om·e·try** (gas-om'ĕ-trē) measurement of gases; determination of the relative proportion of gases in a mixture.

**gas per·i·to·ni·tis** inflammation of the peritoneum accompanied by an intraperitoneal accumulation of gas.

**Gas·ser (Gas·se·rio)** (gahs'ĕr, gahs-ĕr'ī-ō), Johann L., Austrian anatomist, 1723–1765. SEE gasserian.

**gas·ser·i·an** (ga-ser'ē-an) relating to or described by Johann L. Gasser.

**gas·sing** (gas'ing) poisoning by irrespirable or otherwise noxious gases.

**gas·ter** (gas'ter) [TA] SYN stomach. [G. *gastēr*, belly]

**gas·trad·e·ni·tis** (gas'trad-ĕ-nī'tis) inflammation of the glands of the stomach. [gastr- + G. *adēn*, gland, + -*itis*, inflammation]

**gas·trec·ta·sis, gas·trec·ta·sia** (gas-trek'tă-sis, gas-trek-tā'zē-ă) dilation of the stomach. [gastr- + G. *ektasis,* extension]

**gas·trec·to·my** (gas-trek'tō-mē) excision of a part or all of the stomach. [gastr- + G. *ektomē,* excision]

**gas·tric** (gas'trik) relating to the stomach.

**gas·tric a·nal·y·sis** measurement of pH and acid output of stomach contents; basal acid output can be determined by collecting the overnight gastric secretion or by a 1-hr collection; maximal acid output is determined following injection of histamine; output is measured by titration with a strong base.

**gas·tric ar·ter·ies** arteries supplying the stomach along the lesser curvature.

**gas·tric by·pass** high division of the stomach, anastomosis of the small upper pouch of the stomach to the jejunum, and closure of the distal part of the stomach that is retained; used for treatment of morbid obesity.

**gas·tric di·ges·tion** that part of digestion, chiefly of the proteins, carried on in the stomach by the enzymes of the gastric juice. SYN peptic digestion.

**gas·tric feed·ing** giving of nutriment directly into the stomach by means of a tube inserted via the nasopharynx and esophagus or directly through the abdominal wall.

**gas·tric fis·tu·la** a fistulous tract from the stomach to the abdominal wall.

**gas·tric glands** branched tubular glands lying in the mucosa of the fundus and body of the stomach; such glands contain parietal cells that se-

crete hydrochloric acid, zymogen cells that produce pepsin, and mucous cells.

**gas·tric in·di·ges·tion** SYN dyspepsia.

**gas·tric in·hib·i·to·ry pol·y·pep·tide (GIP), gas·tric in·hib·i·to·ry pep·tide (GIP)** a peptide hormone, secreted by the stomach, that stimulates insulin release as part of the digestive process; GIP inhibits the secretion of acids and of pepsin.

**gas·tric sta·pling** partitioning of the stomach by rows of staples; used to treat morbid obesity.

**gas·tric tet·a·ny** tetany associated with a gastric disorder, especially with loss of HCl by vomiting.

**gas·tric ver·ti·go** vertigo symptomatic of disease of the stomach.

**gas·trin·o·ma** (gas-tri-nō'mă) a gastrin-secreting tumor associated with the Zollinger-Ellison syndrome.

**gas·trins** (gas'trinz) hormones secreted in the pyloric-antral mucosa of the mammalian stomach that stimulate secretion of HCl by the parietal cells of the gastric glands; a competitive inhibitor of gastrins is cholecystokinin. [G. *gastēr*, stomach, + -in]

**gas·tri·tis** (gas-trī'tis) inflammation, especially mucosal, of the stomach. [gastr- + G. -*itis*, inflammation]

△**gas·tro-, gastr-** the stomach, abdomen. [G. *gastēr*, the belly]

**gas·tro·a·nas·to·mo·sis** (gas'trō-an-as-tō-mō' sis) anastomosis of the cardiac and antral segments of the stomach, for relief from marked hour-glass contraction of the stomach. SYN gastrogastrostomy.

**gas·tro·car·di·ac** (gas'trō-kar'dē-ak) relating to both the stomach and the heart.

**gas·tro·cele** (gas'trō-sēl) hernia of a portion of the stomach. [gastro- + G. *kēlē*, hernia]

**gas·troc·ne·mi·us** (gas-trok-nē'mē-ŭs) SYN gastrocnemius muscle. [G. *gastroknēmia*, calf of the leg, fr. *gaster* (*gastr-*), belly, + *knēmē*, leg]

**gas·troc·ne·mi·us mus·cle** origin, by two heads (lateral and medial) from the lateral and medial condyles of the femur; *insertion*, with soleus by tendo calcaneus into lower half of posterior surface of calcaneus; *action*, plantar flexion of foot; *nerve supply*, tibial. SYN musculus gastrocnemius [TA], gastrocnemius.

**gas·tro·co·lic** (gas'trō-kol'ik) relating to the stomach and the colon.

**gas·tro·co·lic re·flex** a mass movement of the contents of the colon, frequently preceded by a similar movement in the small intestine, that sometimes occurs immediately following the entrance of food into the stomach.

**gas·tro·co·li·tis** (gas'trō-kō-lī'tis) inflammation of both stomach and colon.

**gas·tro·co·los·to·my** (gas'trō-kō-los'tō-mē) establishment of a communication between stomach and colon. [gastro- + G. *kōlon,* colon, + *stoma,* mouth]

**gas·tro·du·o·de·nal** (gas'trō-doo'ō-dē'năl) relating to the stomach and duodenum.

**gas·tro·du·o·de·nal ar·tery** origin, hepatic; terminal *branches*, right gastroepiploic, superior pancreaticoduodenal. SYN arteria gastroduodenalis [TA].

**gas·tro·du·o·de·ni·tis** (gas'trō-doo-ō-dē-nī'tis) inflammation of both stomach and duodenum.

**gas·tro·du·o·de·nos·co·py** (gas'trō-doo-ō-dĕ-nos′kŏ-pē) visualization of the interior of the stomach and duodenum by a gastroscope. [gastro- + duodenum, + G. *skopeō*, to view]

**gas•tro•du•o•de•nos•to•my** (gas′trō-doo-ō-dĕ-nos′tō-mē) establishment of a communication between the stomach and the duodenum. [gastro- + duodenum + G. *stoma*, mouth]

**gas•tro•en•ter•ic** (gas′trō-en-ter′ik) SYN gastrointestinal.

**gas•tro•en•ter•i•tis** (gas′trō-en-ter-ī′tis) inflammation of the mucous membrane of both stomach and intestine. SYN enterogastritis. [gastro- + G. *enteron*, intestine, + -*itis*, inflammation]

**gas•tro•en•ter•i•tis vi•rus type A** SYN epidemic gastroenteritis virus.

**gas•tro•en•ter•i•tis vi•rus type B** SYN *Rotavirus.*

**gas•tro•en•ter•o•co•li•tis** (gas′trō-en′ter-ō-kō-lī′tis) inflammatory disease involving the stomach and intestines. [gastro- + G. *enteron*, intestine, + *kōlon*, colon, + -*itis*, inflammation]

**gas•tro•en•ter•ol•o•gist** (gas′trō-en-ter-ol′ō-jist) a specialist in gastroenterology.

**gas•tro•en•ter•ol•o•gy** (gas′trō-en-ter-ol′ō-jē) the medical specialty concerned with the function and disorders of the gastrointestinal tract, including stomach, intestines, and associated organs. [gastro- + G. *enteron*, intestine, + *logos*, study]

**gas•tro•en•ter•op•a•thy** (gas′trō-en-ter-op′ă-thē) any disorder of the alimentary canal. [gastro- + G. *enteron*, intestine, + *pathos*, suffering]

**gas•tro•en•ter•o•plas•ty** (gas′trō-en-ter-ō-plas′tē) operative repair of defects in the stomach and intestine. [gastro- + G. *enteron*, intestine, + *plassō*, to form]

**gas•tro•en•ter•op•to•sis** (gas′trō-en-ter-ō-tō′sis) downward displacement of the stomach and a portion of the intestine. [gastro- + G. *enteron*, intestine, + *ptōsis*, a falling]

**gas•tro•en•ter•os•to•my** (gas′trō-en-ter-os′tō-mē) establishment of a new opening between the stomach and the intestine, either anterior or posterior to the transverse colon. [gastro- + G. *enteron*, intestine, + *stoma*, mouth]

**gas•tro•en•ter•ot•o•my** (gas′trō-en-ter-ot′ō-mē) section into both stomach and intestine. [gastro- + G. *enteron*, intestine, + *tomē*, incision]

**gas•tro•ep•i•plo•ic** (gas′trō-ep′i-plō′ik) relating to the stomach and the greater omentum (epiploon).

**gas•tro•ep•i•plo•ic ar•ter•ies** arteries which supply the stomach and greater omentum as they course along the greater curvature of the stomach. SYN gastro-omental arteries.

**gas•tro•e•soph•a•ge•al** (gas′trō-ē-sof′ă-jē′ăl) relating to both stomach and esophagus. [gastro- + G. *oisophagos*, gullet (esophagus)]

**gas•tro•e•soph•a•ge•al her•nia** a hiatal hernia into the thorax.

**gas•tro•e•soph•a•ge•al re•flux dis•ease (GERD)** a syndrome of chronic or recurrent epigastric or retrosternal pain, accompanied by varying degrees of belching, nausea, cough, or hoarseness, due to reflux of acid gastric juice into the lower esophagus; results from malfunction of the lower esophageal sphincter (LES) and disordered gastric motility; may lead to peptic esophagitis, ulceration, stricture, or Barrett esophagus.

**gas•tro•e•soph•a•gi•tis** (gas′trō-ē-sof-ă-jī′tis) inflammation of the stomach and esophagus.

**gas•tro•e•soph•a•gos•to•my** (gas′trō-ē-sof-ă-

gos′tō-mē) SYN esophagogastrostomy. [gastro- + G. *oisophagos*, gullet (esophagus), + *stoma*, mouth]

**gas•tro•gas•tros•to•my** (gas′trō-gas-tros′tō-mē) SYN gastroanastomosis.

**gas•tro•ga•vage** (gas-trō-gă-vahzh′) SYN gavage (1).

**gas•tro•gen•ic** (gas-trō-jen′ik) deriving from or caused by the stomach.

**gas•tro•he•pat•ic** (gas′trō-he-pat′ik) relating to the stomach and the liver. [gastro- + G. *hēpar* (*hēpat-*), liver]

**gas•tro•il•e•ac re•flex** opening of the ileocolic valve induced by entrance of food into the stomach.

**gas•tro•il•e•i•tis** (gas′trō-il-ē-ī′tis) inflammation of the alimentary canal in which the stomach and ileum are primarily involved.

**gas•tro•il•e•os•to•my** (gas′trō-il-ē-os′tō-mē) a surgical joining of stomach to ileum; a technical error in which the ileum instead of jejunum is selected for the site of a gastrojejunostomy.

**gas•tro•in•tes•ti•nal (GI)** (gas′trō-in-tes′tin-ăl) relating to the stomach and intestines. SYN gastroenteric.

**gas•tro•in•tes•ti•nal au•to•nom•ic nerve tu••mor** benign or malignant tumor of stomach and small intestine histogenetically related to myenteric plexus; may be familial and related to gastrointestinal neuronal dysplasia.

**gas•tro•in•tes•ti•nal stro•mal tu•mor** benign or malignant tumor composed of unclassifiable spindle cells; immunohistochemically distinct from smooth muscle and Schwann cell tumors.

**gas•tro•in•tes•ti•nal tract (GI tract)** the stomach, small intestine, and large intestine; often used as a synonym of digestive tract.

**gas•tro•je•ju•no•co•lic** (gas′trō-jē-joo′nō-kol′ik) referring to the stomach, jejunum, and colon.

**gas•tro•je•ju•nos•to•my** (gas′trō-jē-joo-nos′tō-mē) establishment of a direct communication between the stomach and the jejunum. [gastro- + jejunum G. *stoma*, mouth]

**gas•tro•li•e•nal** (gas-trō-lī′ē-năl) SYN gastrosplenic. [gastro- + L. *lien*, spleen]

**gas•tro•lith** (gas′trō-lith) a concretion in the stomach. [gastro- + G. *lithos*, stone]

**gas•tro•li•thi•a•sis** (gas′trō-li-thī′ă-sis) presence of one or more calculi in the stomach. [gastro- + G. *lithos*, stone + -*iasis*, condition]

**gas•trol•y•sis** (gas-trol′i-sis) division of perigastric adhesions. [gastro- + G. *lysis*, loosening]

**gas•tro•ma•la•cia** (gas′trō-mă-lā′shē-ă) softening of the walls of the stomach. [gastro- + G. *malakia*, softness]

**gas•tro•meg•a•ly** (gas′trō-meg′ă-lē) **1.** enlargement of the stomach. **2.** enlargement of the abdomen. [gastro- + G. *megas* (*megal-*), large]

**gas•tro•myx•or•rhea** (gas′trō-mik-sō-rē′ă) excessive secretion of mucus in the stomach. [gastro- + G. *myxa*, mucus, + *rhoia*, a flow]

**gas•tro•oe•so•pha•ge•al [Br.]** SEE gastroesophageal.

**gas•tro•o•men•tal ar•ter•ies** SYN gastroepiploic arteries.

**gas•tro•o•men•tal ar•ter•ies** arteries that supply the stomach and greater omentum as they course along the greater curvature of the stomach.

**gas•tro•pa•ral•y•sis** (gas′trō-pă-ral′i-sis) paralysis of the muscular coat of the stomach.

**gas•tro•pa•re•sis** (gas-trō-pă-rē′sis, gas-trō-par′ĕ-sis) a slight degree of gastroparalysis. [gastro- + G. *paresis*, a letting go, paralysis]

**gas·tro·path·ic** (gas-trō-path'ik) denoting gastropathy.

**gas·trop·a·thy** (gas-trop'ă-thē) any disease of the stomach. [gastro- + G. *pathos*, disease]

**gas·tro·pex·y** (gas'trō-pek-sē) attachment of the stomach to the abdominal wall or diaphragm. [gastro- + G. *pēxis*, fixation]

**gas·tro·phren·ic** (gas'trō-fren'ik) relating to the stomach and the diaphragm. [gastro- + G. *phrēn*, diaphragm]

**gas·tro·plas·ty** (gas'trō-plas-tē) operative treatment of a defect in the stomach or lower esophagus which utilizes the stomach wall for the reconstruction. [gastro- + G. *plastos*, formed]

**gas·tro·pli·ca·tion** (gas'trō-pli-kā'shŭn) an operation for reducing the size of the stomach by suturing a longitudinal fold with the peritoneal surfaces in apposition. SYN gastrorrhaphy (2). [gastro- + L. *plico*, to fold]

**gas·tro·pto·sis, gas·tro·pto·sia** (gas-trō-tō'sis, gas-trō-tō'sē-ă) downward displacement of the stomach. [gastro- + G. *ptosis*, a falling]

**gas·tro·pul·mo·nary** (gas-trō-pŭl'mŏ-ner-ē) SYN pneumogastric.

**gas·tro·py·lor·ec·to·my** (gas'trō-pī-lōr-ek'tō-mē) SYN pylorectomy.

**gas·tro·py·lor·ic** (gas'trō-pī-lōr'ik) relating to the stomach as a whole and to the pylorus.

**gas·tror·rha·gia** (gas-trō-rā'jē-ă) hemorrhage from the stomach. [gastro- + G. *rhēgnymi*, to burst forth]

**gas·tror·rha·phy** (gas-trōr'ă-fē) 1. suture of a perforation of the stomach. 2. SYN gastroplication. [gastro- + G. *rhaphē*, a stitching]

**gas·tror·rhea** (gas-trō-rē'ă) excessive secretion of gastric juice or of mucus (gastromyxorrhea) by the stomach. [gastro- + G. *rhoia*, a flow]

**gas·tros·chi·sis** (gas-tros'ki-sis) a defect in the abdominal wall resulting from rupture of the amniotic membrane during physiological gut-loop herniation or, later, owing to delayed umbilical ring closure; usually accompanied by protrusion of viscera. [gastro- + G. *schisis*, a fissure]

**gas·tro·scope** (gas'trō-skōp) an endoscope for inspecting the inner surface of the stomach. [gastro- + G. *skopeō*, to examine]

**gas·tro·scop·ic** (gas-trō-skop'ik) relating to gastroscopy.

**gas·tros·co·py** (gas-tros'kŏ-pē) inspection of the inner surface of the stomach through an endoscope.

**gas·tro·spasm** (gas'trō-spazm) spasmodic contraction of the walls of the stomach.

**gas·tro·splen·ic** (gas-trō-splen'ik) relating to the stomach and the spleen. SYN gastrolienal.

**gas·tro·stax·is** (gas'trō-stak'sis) oozing of blood from the mucous membrane of the stomach. [gastro- + G. *staxis*, trickling]

**gas·tro·ste·no·sis** (gas-trō-ste-nō'sis) diminution in size of the cavity of the stomach. [gastro- + G. *stenōsis*, narrowing]

**gas·tros·to·la·vage** (gas-tros'tō-lă-vahzh') lavage of the stomach through a gastric fistula.

**gas·tros·to·my** (gas-tros'tō-mē) establishment of a new opening into the stomach. [gastro- + G. *stoma*, mouth]

**gas·trot·o·my** (gas-trot'ō-mē) incision into the stomach. [gastro- + G. *tomē*, incision]

**gas·tro·to·nom·e·try** (gas'trō-tō-nom'ĕ-trē) the measurement of intragastric pressure. [gastro- + G. *tonos*, tension, + *metron*, measure]

**gas·tro·tro·pic** (gas-trō-trop'ik) affecting the stomach. [gastro- + G. *tropikos*, turning]

**gas·tru·la** (gas'troo-lă) the embryo in the stage of development following the blastula; in the human embryo, the absence of yolk allows for a rapid, direct "putting in place" of the germ layers (ectoderm and endoderm), which are derived from the pluripotential embryonic disc. [Mod. L. dim. of G. *gastēr*, belly]

**gas·tru·la·tion** (gas-troo-lā'shŭn) transformation of the blastula into the gastrula; the development and invagination of the embryonic germ layers.

**gate-con·trol the·o·ry** a theory to explain the mechanism of pain; small-fiber afferent stimuli, particularly pain, entering the substantia gelatinosa can be modulated by large-fiber afferent stimuli and descending spinal pathways so that their transmission to ascending spinal pathways is blocked (gated).

**gat·ed ra·di·o·nu·clide an·gi·o·car·di·og·ra·phy** radionuclide angiocardiography using cardiac gating to combine images from several cardiac cycles to improve the quality of the images of separate phases (e.g., systole and diastole).

**gate·keep·er** (gāt'kēp-er) a health professional, typically a physician or nurse, who has the first encounter with a patient and who thus controls the patient's entry into the health care system.

**gat·ing** (gāt'ing) 1. in a biological membrane, the opening and closing of a channel, believed to be associated with changes in integral membrane proteins. 2. a process in which electrical signals are selected by a gate, which passes such signals only when the gate pulse is present to act as a control signal, or passes only the signals that have certain characteristics.

**gat·ing mech·a·nism** 1. occurrence of the maximum refractory period among cardiac conducting cells approximately 2 mm proximal to the terminal Purkinje fibers in the ventricular muscle; gating mechanism may be a cause of ventricular aberration, bidirectional tachycardia, and concealed extrasystoles; 2. a mechanism by which painful impulses may be blocked from entering the spinal cord. Cf. gate-control theory.

**Gauch·er cells** (gō-shā') large, finely and uniformly vacuolated cells derived from the reticuloendothelial system, and found especially in the spleen, lymph nodes, liver, and bone marrow of patients with Gaucher disease; Gaucher cells contain kerasin (a cerebroside), which accumulates as a result of a genetically determined absence of the enzyme glucosylceramidase.

**Gauch·er dis·ease** (gō-shā') a lysosomal storage disease resulting from glycocerebroside accumulation due to a genetic deficiency of glucocerebrosidase; may occur in adults but occurs most severely in infants; marked by hepatosplenomegaly, regression of neurologic maturation, and characteristic histiocytes (Gaucher cells) in the viscera.

**gauge** (gāj) a measuring device.

**gaunt·let ban·dage** a figure-of-8 bandage covering the hand and fingers.

**Gauss** (gows), Johann K.F., German physicist, 1777–1855. SEE gauss.

**gauss** (G) (gows) a unit of magnetic field intensity, equal to $10^{-4}$ tesla. [J.K.F. *Gauss*]

g
a

**gaus·si·an** (gows'ē-ăn) relating to or described by Johann K.F. Gauss.

**gaus·sian dis·tri·bu·tion** (gows'ē-ăn) the statistical distribution of members of a population around the population mean. In a gaussian distribution, 68.2% of values fall within ± 1 standard deviation (SD); 95.4% fall within ± 2 SD of the mean; and 99.7% fall within ± 3 SD of the mean. SYN bell-shaped curve, normal distribution.

**Gauss sign** (gows) marked mobility of the uterus in the early weeks of pregnancy.

**gauze** (gawz) a bleached cotton cloth of plain weave, used for dressings, bandages, and absorbent sponges; petrolatum gauze is saturated with petrolatum. [Fr. *gaze*, fr. Ar. *gazz*, raw silk]

**ga·vage** (gă-vahzh') **1.** forced feeding by stomach tube. SYN gastrogavage. **2.** therapeutic use of a high-potency diet administered by stomach tube. [Fr. *gaver*, to gorge fowls]

**gay** (gā) **1.** a homosexual, especially male. **2.** denoting a homosexual individual or the male homosexual lifestyle. SEE ALSO lesbian.

**gay bow·el syn·drome** gastrointestinal discomfort experienced by homosexual males; includes abdominal pain, cramps, bloating, flatulence, nausea, vomiting, or diarrhea caused by enteric bacteria, viruses, fungi, zooparasites, or trauma.

**Gay-Lus·sac e·qua·tion** (gā-loo-sahk) the overall chemical equation for alcoholic fermentation; $C_6H_{12}O_6 = 2CO_2 + 2CH_3CH_2OH$.

**Gay-Lus·sac law** (gā-loo-sahk) SYN Charles law.

**gaze** (gāz) the act of looking steadily at an object.

**G-band·ing stain** a chromosome-staining technique used in human cytogenetics to identify individual chromosomes, which produces characteristic bands; it utilizes acetic acid, proteolytic enzymes, salts, heat, detergents, or urea, and finally Giemsa stain; chromosome bands appear similar to those fluorochromed by Q-banding stain.

**GB vi·rus·es** members of the family Flaviviridae; GBV-A and GBV-B have been isolated from tamarins infected with human viral agents; GBV-C is a human pathogen related to hepatitis G virus.

**G cells** enteroendocrine cells that secrete gastrin, found primarily in the mucosa of the pyloric antrum of the stomach.

**G-CSF** granulocyte colony-stimulating factor.

**Gd** gadolinium.

**Ge** germanium.

**Gei·gel re·flex** (gī'gĕl) in the female, a contraction of the muscular fibers at the upper edge of the Poupart ligament on gently stroking the inner side of the thigh; analogue of the cremasteric reflex in males.

**gel** (jel) **1.** a jelly, or the solid or semisolid phase of a colloidal solution. **2.** to form a gel or jelly; to convert a sol into a gel. [Mod. L. *gelatum*]

**gel·a·tin** (jel'ă-tin) a derived protein formed from the collagen of tissues by boiling in water; it swells up when put in cold water, but dissolves only in hot water; used as a hemostat, plasma substitute, and protein food adjunct in malnutrition. [L. *gelo*, pp. *gelatus*, to freeze, congeal]

**ge·lat·i·nize** (jĕ-lat'i-nīz) **1.** to convert into gelatin. **2.** to become gelatinous.

**ge·lat·i·nous** (jĕ-lat'i-nŭs) **1.** pertaining to or characteristic of gelatin. **2.** jellylike or resembling gelatin.

**gel·a·tin·ous drop·like cor·ne·al dys·tro·phy**

a bilateral, autosomal recessive condition characterized by mulberrylike elevated amyloid deposits involving the epithelium and anterior corneal stroma.

**ge·lat·i·nous sub·stance** the apical part of the posterior horn (dorsal horn; posterior gray column) of the gray matter of the spinal cord, composed largely of very small nerve cells; its gelatinous appearance is due to its very low content of myelinated nerve fibers.

**ge·la·tion** (jĕ-lā'shŭn) COLLOIDAL CHEMISTRY the transformation of a sol into a gel.

**gel dif·fu·sion pre·cip·i·tin tests** precipitin tests in which the immune precipitate forms in a gel medium (usually agar) into which one or both reactants have diffused; generally classified in two types, in one dimension, and in two dimensions.

**Gé·li·neau syn·drome** (zhā-lē-nō') SYN narcolepsy.

**Gé·ly su·ture** (zhā-lē') a cobbler's suture used in closing intestinal wounds.

**Ge·mel·la** (jĕ-mel'ă) a genus of motile, aerobic, facultatively anaerobic, coccoid bacteria (family Streptococcaceae) that occur singly or in pairs, with flattened adjacent sides. They are Gram-indeterminate but have a cell wall like that of Gram-positive bacteria, and are parasitic on mammals. The type species is *Gemella haemolysans*, which is found in bronchial secretions and in mucus from the respiratory tract. [L. dim. of *geminus*, twin]

**Ge·mel·la mor·bil·lor·um** a microaerophilic bacterium, formerly called *Streptococcus morbillorum*, that fails to produce β-hemolysis of blood agar and lacks distinguishing serogroup antigens; causes serious infections in some patients similar to those seen with viridans streptococci.

**gem·i·nate** (jem'i-nāt) occurring in pairs. [L. *gemino*, pp. *-atus*, to double, fr. *geminus*, twin]

**gem·i·na·tion** (jem-i-nā'shŭn) embryologic partial division of a primordium. For example, gemination of a single tooth germ results in two partially or completely separated crowns on a single root. [L. *geminatio*, a doubling]

**gem·ma·tion** (jem-ā'shŭn) a form of fission in which the parent cell does not divide, but puts out a small budlike process (daughter cell) with its proportionate amount of chromatin; the daughter cell then separates to begin independent existence. SYN budding. [L. *gemma*, a bud]

**gem·mule** (jem'yul) **1.** a small bud that projects from the parent cell, and finally becomes detached, forming a cell of a new generation. **2.** SYN dendritic spines. [L. *gemmula*, dim. of *gemma*, bud]

**△gen-** being born, producing, coming to be. [G. *genos*, birth]

**△-gen** suffix denoting "precursor of." SEE ALSO pro- (2).

**ge·na** (jē'nă) SYN cheek. [L.]

**ge·nal** (jē'năl) relating to the gena, or cheek.

**ge·nal glands** SYN buccal glands.

**gen·der** (jen'der) category to which an individual is assigned by self or others, on the basis of sex. Cf. sex, gender role.

**gen·der i·den·ti·ty** the sex role adopted by an individual; the degree to which an individual acts out a stereotypical masculine or feminine role in everyday behavior. Cf. gender role, sex role.

**gen·der role** the sex of a child assigned by a

parent; when opposite to the child's anatomical sex (e.g., due to genital ambiguity at birth or to the parents' strong wish for a child of the opposite sex), the basis is set for postpubertal dysfunctions. SEE sex role, sex reversal.

**gene** (jēn) a functional unit of heredity that occupies a specific place (locus) on a chromosome, is capable of reproducing itself exactly at each cell division, and directs the formation of an enzyme or other protein. The gene as a functional unit consists of a discrete segment of a giant DNA molecule containing the purine (adenine and guanine) and pyrimidine (cytosine and thymine) bases in the correct sequence to code the sequence of amino acids of a specific peptide. Protein synthesis is mediated by molecules of messenger-RNA formed on the chromosome with the gene acting as a template. The RNA then passes into the cytoplasm and becomes oriented on the ribosomes where it in turn acts as a template to organize a chain of amino acids to form a peptide. In organisms reproducing sexually, genes normally occur in pairs in all cells except gametes, as a consequence of the fact that all chromosomes are paired except the sex chromosomes (X and Y) of the male. SYN factor (3). [G. *genos,* birth]

**ge·ne·al·o·gy** (jē-nē-awl′ō-jē) **1.** heredity. **2.** the explicit assembly of the descent of a person or family; it may be of any length. [G. *genea,* descent, + *logos,* study]

**gene dos·age com·pen·sa·tion** the putative mechanism that adjusts the X-linked phenotypes of males and females to compensate for the haploid state in males and the diploid state in females. It is now largely ascribed to lyonization which compensates the mean of the dose but not its variance, which is greater in females.

**gene ex·pres·sion 1.** the detectable effect of a gene. **2.** appearance of an inherited trait; for many reasons, a gene may not be expressed at all.

**gene fam·i·ly** group of genes related by sequence similarity.

**gen·era** (jen′er-ă) plural of genus.

**gen·er·al ad·ap·ta·tion re·ac·tion** SEE general adaptation syndrome.

**gen·er·al ad·ap·ta·tion syn·drome** a term introduced by Hans Selye to describe marked physiological changes in various organ systems of the body, especially the pituitary-endocrine system, as a result of exposure to prolonged physical or psychological stress.

**gen·er·al anat·o·my** the study of gross and microscopic structures as well as of the composition of the body, its tissues and fluids.

**gen·er·al an·es·the·sia** loss of ability to perceive pain associated with loss of consciousness produced by intravenous or inhalation anesthetic agents.

**gen·er·al an·es·thet·ic** a compound that produces loss of sensation associated with loss of consciousness.

**gen·er·al du·ty nurse** nurse who accepts assignment to any unit of a hospital other than an intensive care unit.

**gen·er·al im·mu·ni·ty** immunity associated with widely diffused mechanisms that tend to protect the body as a whole, as compared with local immunity.

**gen·er·al·i·sa·tion [Br.]** SEE generalization.

**gen·er·al·is·ed [Br.]** SEE generalized.

**gen·er·al·ist** (jen′er-ăl-ist) a general physician or family physician; a physician trained to take care of the majority of nonsurgical diseases, sometimes including obstetrics.

**gen·er·al·i·za·tion** (jen′er-ăl-i-zā′shŭn) **1.** Rendering or becoming general, diffuse, or widespread, as when a primarily local disease becomes systemic. **2.** The reasoning by which a basic conclusion is reached, which applies to different items, each having some common factor.

**gen·er·al·ized** (jen′er-ă-līzd) involving the whole of an organ, as opposed to a focal or regional process.

**gen·er·al·ized an·a·phy·lax·is** the immediate response, involving smooth muscles and capillaries throughout the body, that follows injection of antigen (allergen). SEE ALSO anaphylactic shock. SYN systemic anaphylaxis.

**gen·er·al·ized anx·i·e·ty dis·or·der** chronic, repeated episodes of anxiety or dread accompanied by autonomic changes. SEE ALSO anxiety.

**gen·er·al·ized len·tig·i·no·sis** lentigines occurring singly or in groups from infancy onward.

**gen·er·al·i·zed plane xan·tho·ma·to·sis** widespread xanthomatosis associated with multiple myeloma, familial hyperlipoproteinemia, or less commonly with primary biliary cirrhosis or no underlying disease.

**gen·er·al·ized Schwartz·man phe·nom·e·non** (shwahrtz′măn) when both the primary injection of endotoxin-containing filtrate and the secondary injection are given intravenously 24 hours apart, the animal usually dies within 24 hours after the second inoculation. This reaction has no immunological basis.

**gen·er·al·ized ton·ic-clo·nic sei·zure, gen·er·al·ized ton·ic-clo·nic ep·i·lep·sy** a generalized seizure characterized by the sudden onset of tonic contraction of the muscles often associated with a cry or moan, and frequently resulting in a fall to the ground. The tonic phase of the seizure gradually gives way to clonic convulsive movements occurring bilaterally and synchronously before slowing and eventually stopping, followed by a variable period of unconsciousness and gradual recovery. SYN grand mal.

**gen·er·alized tu·ber·cu·lo·sis** SYN miliary tuberculosis.

**gen·er·al stim·u·lant** a stimulant that affects the entire body.

**gen·er·a·tion** (jen-er-ā′shŭn) **1.** SYN reproduction (2). **2.** a discrete stage in succession of descent; e.g., father, son, and grandson are three generations, respectively first, second, and third. It may not be a unique designation, e.g., the offspring of an uncle-niece marriage is in the third generation in the paternal line but the fourth in the maternal line. [L. *generatio,* fr. *genero,* pp. *-atus,* to beget]

**gen·er·a·tive** (jen′er-ă-tiv) pertaining to the process of generating.

**gen·er·a·tor** (jen′er-ā-ter) an apparatus for conversion of chemical, mechanical, atomic, or other forms of energy into electricity. [*generator,* a begetter, producer]

**ge·ner·ic** (jĕ-nār′ik) **1.** relating to or denoting a genus. **2.** general. **3.** characteristic or distinctive. [L. *genus* (*gener-*), birth]

**ge·ner·ic name 1.** CHEMISTRY a noun that indicates the class or type of a single compound; e.g., salt, saccharide (sugar), hexose, alcohol, aldehyde, lactone, acid, amine, alkane, steroid, vitamin. "Class" is more appropriate and more often used than is "generic." **2.** in the pharmaceutical and commercial fields, a misnomer for nonproprietary name. **3.** in the biologic sciences, the first part of the scientific name (Latin binary combination or binomial) of an organism; written with an initial capital letter and in italics. In bacteriology, the species name consists of two parts (comprising one name): the generic name and the specific epithet; in other biologic disciplines, the species name is regarded as being composed of two names: the generic name and the specific name.

**ge·ner·ic sub·sti·tu·tion** the dispensing of a chemically equivalent, less expensive drug in place of a brand-name product.

**gen·e·sis** (jen′ĕ-sis) an origin or beginning process; also used as combining form in suffix position. [G.]

**gene splic·ing** SYN splicing (1).

**gene ther·a·py** the process of inserting a gene into an organism to replace or repair gene function to treat a disease or genetic defect.

**ge·net·ic** (jĕ-net′ik) pertaining to genetics; genetical.

**ge·net·ic am·pli·fi·ca·tion** a process for producing an increase in pertinent genetic material, particularly for increasing the proportion of plasmid DNA to that of bacterial DNA. Includes the production of extrachromosomal copies of the genes for RNA.

**ge·net·ic as·so·ci·a·tion** the occurrence together in a population, more often than can be readily explained by chance, of two or more traits of which at least one is known to be genetic.

**ge·net·ic code** the genetic information carried by the specific DNA molecules of the chromosomes; specifically, the system whereby particular combinations of three consecutive nucleotides in a DNA molecule control the insertion of one particular amino acid in equivalent places in a protein molecule.

**ge·net·ic de·ter·mi·nant** any antigenic determinant or identifying characteristic, particularly those of allotypes.

**gen·et·ic ep·i·de·mi·ol·o·gy** the branch of epidemiology that studies the role of genetic factors and their interactions with environmental factors in the occurrence of disease in various populations.

**ge·net·ic fe·male 1.** an individual with a normal female karyotype, including two X chromosomes; **2.** an individual whose cell nuclei contain Barr sex chromatin bodies, which are normally absent in males.

**ge·net·ic fit·ness** in a phenotype, the mean number of surviving offspring that it generates in its lifetime, usually expressed as a fraction or percentage of the average genetic fitness of the population.

**ge·net·i·cist** (jĕ-net′i-sist) a specialist in genetics.

**ge·net·ic le·thal** a disorder that prevents effective reproduction by those affected.

**ge·net·ic load** the aggregate of more or less harmful genes that are carried, mostly hidden, in the genome and may be transmitted to descendants and cause disease.

**ge·net·ic psy·chol·o·gy** a science dealing with the evolution of behavior and the relation to each other of the different types of mental activity.

**ge·net·ics** (jĕ-net′iks) **1.** the branch of science concerned with the means and consequences of transmission and generation of the components of biologic inheritance. **2.** the genetic features and constitution of any single organism or set of organisms. [G. *genesis*, origin or production]

**ge·net·o·tro·phic** (jĕ-net-ō-trof′ik) relating to inherited individual distinctions in nutritional requirements. [G. *genesis*, origin, + *trophē*, nourishment]

**ge·ni·al, ge·ni·an** (jĕ-nī′ăl, jĕ-nī′an) SYN mental (2). [G. *geneion*, chin]

**ge·ni·al tu·ber·cle** SYN mental spine.

△**-ge·nic** producing, forming; produced, formed by. [G. *genos*, birth]

**ge·nic·u·la** (je-nik′yu-lă) plural of geniculum.

**ge·nic·u·lar** (je-nik′yu-lăr) commonly used to mean genual.

**ge·nic·u·lar ar·ter·ies** arteries contributing to the articular network of the knee.

**ge·nic·u·late** (je-nik′yu-lāt) **1.** bent like a knee. **2.** referring to the geniculum of the facial nerve, denoting the ganglion there present. **3.** denoting the lateral or medial geniculate body. [L. *geniculo*, pp. -*atus*, to bend the knee, fr. *genu*, knee]

**ge·nic·u·late bod·y** SEE lateral geniculate body, medial geniculate body.

**ge·nic·u·late gan·gli·on** a ganglion of the nervus intermedius fibers conveyed by the facial nerve, located within the facial canal at the genu of the canal and containing the sensory neurons innervating the taste buds on the anterior two-thirds of the tongue and a small area on the external ear.

**ge·nic·u·late neu·ral·gia** a severe paroxysmal lancinating pain deep in the ear, on the anterior wall of the external meatus, and on a small area just in front of the pinna. SYN Hunt neuralgia, neuralgia facialis vera.

**ge·nic·u·lum,** pl. **ge·nic·u·la** (je-nik′yu-lŭm, je-nik′yu-lă) **1.** a small genu or angular kneelike structure. **2.** a knotlike structure. [L. dim. of *genu*, knee]

**ge·ni·o·glos·sus mus·cle** one of the paired lingual muscles; *origin*, mental spine of the mandible; *insertion*, lingual fascia beneath the mucous membrane and epiglottis; *action*, depresses and protrudes the tongue; *nerve supply*, hypoglossal. SYN musculus genioglossus [TA].

**ge·ni·o·hy·oid mus·cle** *origin*, mental spine of mandible; *insertion*, body of hyoid bone; *action*, draws hyoid forward, or depresses jaw when hyoid is fixed; *nerve supply*, fibers from ventral primary rami of first and second cervical spinal nerves accompanying hypoglossal. SYN musculus geniohyoideus [TA].

**ge·ni·on** (jĕ-nī′on) the tip of the mental spine, a point in craniometry. [G. *geneion*, chin]

**ge·ni·o·plas·ty** (jĕ-nī-ō-plas-tē) SYN mentoplasty. [G. *geneion*, chin, cheek, + *plastos*, formed]

**gen·i·tal** (jen′i-tăl) **1.** relating to reproduction or generation. **2.** relating to the primary female or male sex organs or genitals. **3.** relating to or characterized by genitality. [L. *genitalis*, pertaining to reproduction, fr. *gigno*, to bring forth]

**gen·i·tal am·bi·gu·i·ty** incomplete development of fetal genitalia as a result of excessive androgen action on a female fetus or inadequate amounts of androgen in a male fetus. SYN ambiguous genitalia.

**gen·i·tal cord** one of a pair of mesenchymal ridges bulging into the caudal part of the celom of a young embryo and containing the mesonephric and paramesonephric ducts.

**gen·i·tal cor·pus·cles** special encapsulated nerve endings found in the skin of the genitalia and nipples. SYN corpuscula genitalia [TA].

**gen·i·tal fur·row** a groove on the genital tubercle in the embryo, appearing toward the end of the second month.

**gen·i·tal her·pes** herpetic lesions on the penis of the male or on the cervix, perineum, vagina, or vulva of the female, caused by herpes simplex virus type 2. See page B3. SYN herpes genitalis.

**gen·i·ta·lia** (jen′i-tā′lē-ă) the organs of reproduction or generation, external and internal. SYN genitals. [L. neut. pl. of *genitalis*, genital]

**gen·i·tal·i·ty** (jen-i-tal′i-tē) PSYCHOANALYSIS a term referring to the genital components of sexuality (i.e., the penis and vagina), as opposed, for example, to orality and anality.

**gen·i·tal phase** in psychoanalytic personality theory, the final stage of psychosexual development, occurring during puberty, in which the individual's psychosexual development is so organized that sexual gratification can be achieved from genital-to-genital contact and the capacity exists for a mature affectionate relationship with another individual. SEE ALSO phallic phase.

**gen·i·tals** (jen′i-tălz) SYN genitalia. [see genitalia]

**gen·i·tal tract** the genital passages of the urogenital apparatus.

**gen·i·tal wart** SYN condyloma acuminatum.

**gen·i·to·fem·o·ral** (jen′i-tō-fem′ŏ-răl) relating to the genitalia and the thigh; denoting the genitofemoral nerve.

**gen·i·to·fem·o·ral nerve** arises from the first and second lumbar nerves, passes distad along the anterior surface of psoas major muscle and divides into genital and femoral branches. SYN nervus genitofemoralis [TA].

**gen·i·to·u·ri·nary (GU)** (jen′i-tō-yu′ri-nar-ē) relating to the organs of reproduction and urination. SYN urogenital.

**gen·i·to·uri·nary surgeon** SYN urologist.

**gen·o·copy** (jen′ō-kop-e) a genotype at one locus that produces a phenotype which at some levels of resolution is indistinguishable from that produced by another genotype; e.g., two types of elliptocytosis that are genocopies of each other, but are distinguished by the fact that one is linked to the Rh blood group locus and the other is not.

**ge·no·der·ma·to·sis** (jen′ō-der-mă-tō′sis) a skin condition of genetic origin.

**ge·nome** (je′nōm, jē-nom) **1.** a complete set of chromosomes derived from one parent, the haploid number of a gamete. **2.** the total gene complement of a set of chromosomes found in higher life forms (the haploid set in a eukaryotic cell), or the functionally similar but simpler linear arrangements found in bacteria and viruses. SEE ALSO Human Genome Project. [gene + chromosome]

**ge·nom·ic** (jě-nōm′ik) relating to a genome.

**ge·nom·ic clone** a cell with a vector containing a fragment of DNA from a different organism.

**ge·nom·ic im·print·ing** epigenetic process that leads to inactivation of paternal or maternal allele of certain genes susceptible to epigenetic regulation; accounts, among others, for the Angelman and Prader-Willi syndromes.

**gen·om·ics** (jen-ōm-′ks) study of the structure of the genome of particular organisms, including mapping and sequencing.

**ge·no·spe·cies** (jē′nō-spē-sēz, jen′o-spē-sēz) a group of organisms in which interbreeding is possible, as evidenced by genetic transfer and recombination.

**ge·note** (jē′nōt) MICROBIAL GENETICS an element of recombination in which one of the pair is not a complete chromosome; commonly used as a suffix (e.g., endogenote, exogenote, F genote). [gene + G. -ōtēs, toponymic suffix]

**ge·no·tox·ic** (jē-nō-toks′ik) denoting a substance that by damaging DNA may cause mutation or cancer. [gene + toxic]

**gen·o·type** (jen′ō-tīp) **1.** the genetic constitution of an individual. **2.** gene combination at one specific locus or any specified combination of loci. [G. *genos*, birth, descent, + *typos*, type]

**gen·o·typ·i·cal** (jen-ō-tip′i-kăl) relating to the genotype.

**gen·tian·o·phil, gen·tian·o·phile** (jen′shŭn-o-fil, jen′shŭn-o-fil) staining readily with gentian violet. [gentian + G. *philos*, fond]

**gen·tian·o·pho·bic** (jen′shŭn-ō-fō′bik) not taking a gentian violet stain, or taking it poorly. [gentian + G. *phobos*, fear]

**gen·tian vi·o·let** an unstandardized dye mixture of violet rosanilins.

**gen·ti·o·bi·ose** a disaccharide containing two D-glucopyranose molecules linked β-1,6; a structural moiety in many compounds (amygdalin). SYN amygdalose.

**gen·u, gen. ge·nus, pl. gen·ua** (jē′noo, jē′nŭs, jen′oo-ă; jē′nŭs; jen′ū-ă) [TA] **1.** the joint between the thigh and the leg. SYN knee (1). SEE ALSO knee joint, geniculum. **2.** any structure of angular shape resembling a flexed knee. [L.]

**gen·u·al** (jen′yu-ăl) relating to the knee. [L. *genu*, knee]

**gen·u·cu·bi·tal po·si·tion** SYN knee-elbow position.

**gen·u·pec·to·ral po·si·tion** SYN knee-chest position.

**gen·u re·cur·va·tum** hyperextension of the knee, the lower limb having a forward curvature.

**ge·nus, pl. gen·era** (jē′nŭs, jen′er-ă) in natural history classification, the taxonomic level of division between the family, or tribe, and the species; a group of species alike in the broad features of their organization but different in detail, and incapable of fertile mating. [L. birth, descent]

**gen·u val·gum** a deformity marked by lateral angulation of the leg in relation to the thigh. SYN knock-knee, tibia valga.

**gen·u va·rum** a deformity marked by medial angulation of the leg in relation to the thigh; an outward bowing of the lower extremities. SYN bowleg, bow-leg, tibia vara.

**geo-** the earth, soil. [G. *gē*, earth]

**ge·ode** (jē′ōd) a cystlike space (or spaces) with or without an epithelial lining, observed radiologically in subarticular bone, usually in arthritic disorders. [Fr., fr. L. *geodes*, precious stone, fr. G. *gē*, earth, + -ōdēs, appearance]

**ge·o·graph·ic in·for·ma·tion sys·tem** a computer-based system that combines cartographic capabilities with electronic data processing to rapidly produce customized maps for use in epidemiologic studies.

**ge·o·graph·ic ker·a·ti·tis** keratitis with coalescence of superficial lesions in herpes keratitis.

**ge·o·graph·ic re·tin·al a·tro·phy** a pattern of well-demarcated retinal pigment epithelial atrophy associated with choriocapillary layer and photoreceptor atrophy leading to vision loss.

**ge·o·graph·ic tongue** idiopathic, asymptomatic erythematous circinate macules, often bounded peripherally by a white band, as a result of atrophy of the filiform papillae; with time the lesions resolve, coalesce, and change in distribution; frequently associated with fissured tongues. SYN glossitis areata exfoliativa, lingua geographica, pityriasis linguae.

**ge·o·met·ric isom·er·ism** a form of isomerism displayed by unsaturated or ring compounds where free rotation about a bond (usually a carbon-carbon bond) is restricted. Cf. cis-, trans-.

**ge·o·met·ric mean** the mean calculated as the antilogarithm of the arithmetic mean of the logarithms of the individual values; it can also be calculated as the *n*th root of the product of *n* values.

**ge·o·met·ric sense** one or other of two directions along a curve in which something is moving, e.g., clockwise or counterclockwise.

**ge·o·met·ric un·sharp·ness** SYN penumbra.

**ge·o·pha·gia, ge·oph·a·gism, ge·oph·a·gy** (jē-ō-fā′jē-ă, jē-of′ă-jizm, jē-of′ă-jē) the practice of eating dirt or clay. SYN dirt-eating. [geo- + G. *phagō*, to eat]

**ge·ot·ri·cho·sis** (jē′ō-tri-kō′sis) an opportunistic systemic hyalohyphomycosis caused by *Geotrichum candidum;* ascribed symptoms are diverse and suggestive of secondary or mixed infections. [geo- + G. *thrix,* hair, + *-osis,* condition]

**ge·phy·rin** (je-fir′in) a protein in the ataxia telangiectasia mutation–related family, essential for glycine receptor clustering on neuronal membranes.

**GERD** gastroesophageal reflux disease.

**Ger·dy fon·ta·nelle** (zher-dē′) SYN sagittal fontanelle.

**ger·i·at·ric** (jer-ē-at′rik) relating to old age or to geriatrics.

**ger·i·at·rics** (jer-ē-at′riks) the branch of medicine concerned with the medical problems and care of the aged. [G. *gēras,* old age, + *iatrikos,* healing]

**Ger·li·er dis·ease** (zher-lē-ā′) SYN vestibular neuronitis.

**germ** (jerm) **1.** a microbe; a microorganism. **2.** a primordium; the earliest trace of a structure within an embryo. [L. *germen,* sprout, bud, germ]

**ger·ma·ni·um (Ge)** (jer-mān′ē-ŭm) a metallic element, atomic no. 32, atomic wt. 72.61. [L. *Germania,* Germany]

**Ger·man mea·sles** (jer-měn) SYN rubella.

**Ger·man mea·sles vi·rus** (jer-měn) SYN rubella virus.

**germ cell** SYN sex cell.

**ger·mi·ci·dal** (jer-mi-sī′dăl) SYN germicide (1).

**ger·mi·cide** (jer′mi-sīd) **1.** destructive to germs or microbes. SYN germicidal. **2.** an agent with this action. [germ + L. *caedo,* to kill]

**ger·mi·nal** (jer′mi-năl) relating to a germ or, in botany, to germination.

**ger·mi·nal ar·ea, ar·e·a ger·mi·na·ti·va** the place in the blastoderm where the embryo begins to be formed.

**ger·mi·nal cell** a cell from which other cells proliferate.

**ger·mi·nal disk, germ disk** the point in a telolecithal oocyte where the embryo begins to be formed.

**ger·mi·nal ep·i·the·li·um** a cuboidal layer of peritoneal epithelium covering the gonads, once thought to be the source of germ cells.

**ger·mi·nal lo·cal·i·za·tion** determination in very young embryos of the presumptive areas for specific organs or structures.

**ger·mi·nal pole** SYN animal pole.

**ger·mi·no·ma** (jer-mi-nō′mă) a neoplasm of the germinal tissue of gonads, mediastinum, or pineal region such as seminoma. [L. *germen,* bud, + *-oma,* tumor]

**germ line** a collection of haploid cells derived from the specialized cells of the primitive gonad.

**germ mem·brane, ger·mi·nal mem·brane** SYN blastoderm.

△**gero-, ger·ont-, ger·onto-** old age. SEE ALSO presby-. [G. *gerōn,* old man]

**ger·o·der·ma** (jer-ō-der′mă) **1.** the atrophic skin of the aged. **2.** any condition in which the skin is thinned and wrinkled, resembling the integument of old age. [gero- + G. *derma,* skin]

**ger·o·don·tics, ger·o·don·tol·o·gy** (jer-ō-don′tiks, jer-ō-don-tol′ō-jē) SYN dental geriatrics. [gero- + G. *odous,* tooth]

**ge·ron·tal** (jer-on′tăl) relating to old age.

**ger·on·tol·o·gist** (jer-on-tol′ō-jist) one who specializes in gerontology.

**ger·on·tol·o·gy** (jer-on-tol′ō-jē) the scientific study of the process and problems of aging. [geronto- + G. *logos,* study]

**ger·on·tox·on** (jer′on-tok′son) SYN arcus cornealis. [geronto- + G. *toxon,* bow]

**Ge·ro·ta cap·sule** (gā-rō′tah) SYN renal fascia.

**Ge·ro·ta fas·cia** (gā-rō′tah) SYN renal fascia.

**Ge·ro·ta meth·od** (gā-rō′tah) injection of the lymphatics with a dye that is soluble in chloroform or ether but not in water; alkannin, red sulfide of mercury, and Prussian blue are said to be suitable for this purpose.

**ges·ta·gen** (jes′tă-jen) any of several gestagenic substances, which are usually steroid hormones.

**ge·stalt, ge·stalt phe·nom·e·non** (gě-stahlt′) a perceived entity so integrated as to constitute a functional unit with properties not derivable from its parts. SEE ALSO gestaltism. [Ger. shape]

**ge·stalt·ism, ge·stalt psy·chol·o·gy** (gě-stahlt′izm) the theory in psychology that the objects of mind come as complete forms or configurations which cannot be split into parts; e.g., a square is perceived as such rather than as four discrete lines. [see gestalt]

**ge·stalt ther·a·py** a type of psychotherapy, used with individuals or groups, that emphasizes treatment of the person as a whole: the individual's biological component parts and their organic functioning, perceptual configuration, and interrelationships with the external world.

**ges·ta·tion** (jes-tā′shŭn) SYN pregnancy. [L. *gestatio,* from *gesto,* pp. *gestatus,* to bear]

**ges·ta·tion·al age** the age of a fetus expressed in elapsed time since conception or conception; usually measured from the first day of the last normal menstrual period.

**ges·ta·tion·al di·a·be·tes** carbohydrate intolerance during pregnancy usually resolving after delivery.

**ges·ta·tion·al e·de·ma** a generalized and excessive accumulation of fluid in the tissues of greater than 1+ pitting after 12 hours' bed rest, or of a weight gain of 5 pounds or more in 1 week due to the influence of pregnancy.

**ges·ta·tion·al hy·per·ten·sion** hypertension during pregnancy in a previously normotensive woman or aggravation of hypertension during pregnancy in a hypertensive woman. SYN pregnancy-induced hypertension.

**ges·ta·tion·al pro·tein·u·ria** the presence of proteinuria during or under the influence of pregnancy in the absence of hypertension, edema, renal infection, or known intrinsic renovascular disease.

**ges·ta·tion·al ring** the white ring identified by pulse echosonography that signals an early stage of pregnancy.

**ges·ta·tion·al sac** cystic structure of early pregnancy that represents the amnionic sac, fluid, and placenta.

**ges·to·sis**, pl. **ges·to·ses** (jes-tō′sis, jes-tō′sēz) any disorder of pregnancy. [L. *gesto,* to carry, to bear, + G. *-osis,* condition]

**Gey so·lu·tion** (gē) a salt solution usually used in combination with naturally occurring body substances (e.g., blood serum, tissue extracts) and/or more complex chemically defined nutritive solutions for culturing animal cells.

**GFR** glomerular filtration rate.

**G$_{M1}$ gan·gli·o·si·do·sis** three forms exist: infantile, generalized; juvenile; and adult; gangliosidosis characterized by accumulation of a specific monosialoganglioside, G$_{M1}$; due to deficiency of G$_{M1}$-β-galactosidase.

**G$_{M2}$ gan·gli·o·si·do·sis** one of the hereditary metabolic disorders; several forms exist, including Tay-Sachs disease, Sandhoff disease, AV variant and adult onset; characterized by accumulation of a specific metabolite, G$_{M2}$ ganglioside, due to deficiency of hexosaminidase A or B, or G$_{M2}$ activator factor.

**GH** growth hormone.

**GHB** γ-hydroxybutyrate.

**Ghon tu·ber·cle** (gon) calcification seen in pulmonary parenchyma (usually midlung) resulting from earlier, usually childhood, infection with tuberculosis; sometimes confused with a combination of parenchymal lesion and calcified lymph node, which is properly termed a Ranke complex.

**ghost cell 1.** a dead cell in which the outline remains visible, but without other cytoplasmic structures or stainable nucleus; **2.** an erythrocyte after loss of its hemoglobin.

**ghost cor·pus·cle** SYN achromocyte.

**GHRF, GH-RF** growth hormone-releasing factor.

**GHRH, GH-RH** growth hormone-releasing hormone.

**GHz** gigahertz, equal to one billion ($10^9$) hertz; used in ultrasound.

**GI** gastrointestinal; Gingival Index.

**gi·ant ax·o·nal neu·rop·a·thy** a rare disorder beginning at or after the third year of life, and presenting clinically with kinky hair, progressive clumsiness, muscle weakness and atrophy, sensory loss, and areflexia.

**gi·ant cell** a cell of large size, often with many nuclei.

**gi·ant cell ar·te·ri·tis** SYN temporal arteritis.

**gi·ant cell car·ci·no·ma** a malignant epithelial neoplasm characterized by unusually large anaplastic cells.

**gi·ant cell fi·bro·ma** a tumor of the oral mucosa composed of fibrous connective tissue with large stellate and multinucleate fibroblasts. Cf. giant cell granuloma.

**gi·ant cell gli·o·blas·to·ma mul·ti·for·me** a histologic form of glioblastoma with large, often multinucleated, bizarre, tumor cells.

**gi·ant cell gran·u·lo·ma** a non-neoplastic lesion characterized by a proliferation of granulation tissue containing numerous multinucleated giant cells; it occurs on the gingiva and alveolar mucosa (occasionally on other soft tissues) where it presents as a soft red-blue hemorrhagic nodular swelling; it also occurs within the mandible or maxilla as a unilocular or multilocular radiolucency. Identical bony lesions may be seen in hyperparathyroidism and cherubism. SEE ALSO giant cell tumor of bone. Cf. giant cell fibroma.

**gi·ant cell my·e·lo·ma** SYN giant cell tumor of bone.

**gi·ant cell tu·mor of bone** a soft, reddish-brown, sometimes malignant, osteolytic tumor composed of multinucleated giant cells and ovoid or spindle-shaped cells, occurring most frequently in an end of a long tubular bone of young adults. SYN giant cell myeloma, osteoclastoma.

**gi·ant cell tu·mor of ten·don sheath** a nodule arising commonly from the flexor sheath of the fingers and thumb; composed of fibrous tissue, lipid- and hemosiderin-containing macrophages, and multinucleated giant cells. SYN localized nodular tenosynovitis.

**gi·ant con·dy·lo·ma** a large type of condyloma acuminatum found in the anus, vulva, or preputial sac of the penis of middle-aged, uncircumcised men; it tends to extend deeply and recur.

**gi·ant·ism** (jī′an-tizm) SYN gigantism.

**gi·ant pap·il·lary con·junc·tiv·i·tis** conjunctival inflammation characterized by large papillae and associated with sensitization to antigenic material present on the surface of a contact lens.

**gi·ant ur·ti·car·ia** SYN angioedema.

***Gi·ar·dia*** (jē-ar′dē-ă) a genus of flagellates that parasitize the small intestine of human beings, domestic and wild mammals, and birds. [Alfred *Giard,* Fr. biologist, 1846–1908]

**gi·ar·di·a·sis** (jē-ar-dī′ă-sis) infection with the protozoan parasite *Giardia lamblia,* sometimes asymptomatic but often manifested by diarrhea, dyspepsia, and malabsorption.

**gib·bous** (gib′ŭs) humped; humpbacked; denoting a sharp angle in the flexion of the spine. [L. *gibbosus*]

**Gibbs the·o·rem** (gibz) substances that lower the surface tension of the pure dispersion medium tend to collect in its surface, whereas substances that raise the surface tension tend to remain out of the surface film.

**gib·bus** (gib′ŭs) extreme kyphosis, hump, or hunch; a deformity of spine in which there is a sharply angulated segment, the apex of the angle being posterior. [L. a hump]

**Gib·ney boot** (gib′nē) adhesive tape treatment of a sprained ankle or similar condition, applied in a basket-weave fashion under the sole of the foot and around the back of the lower leg.

**Gib·ney fix·a·tion ban·dage** (gib′nē) herring-

g
i

bone strapping of the foot and leg for sprain of the ankle.

**Gib·son ban·dage** (gib'sŏn) a bandage, resembling a Barton bandage, for stabilizing fracture of the mandible.

**Gib·son mur·mur** (gib'sŏn) SYN machinery murmur.

**Gi·em·sa stain** (gēm'se) compound of methylene blue-eosin and methylene blue used for demonstrating Negri bodies, *Tunga* species, spirochetes and protozoans, and differential staining of blood smears; also used for chromosomes, sometimes after hydrolyzing the cytologic preparation in hot hydrochloric acid, and for showing chromosome G bands.

**Gier·ke dis·ease** (gēr'kē) SYN type 1 glycogenosis.

**Gif·ford re·flex** (gi'fŏrd) SYN eye-closure pupil reaction.

**GIFT** gamete intrafallopian transfer.

△**gi·ga-** (G) prefix used in the SI and metric systems to signify one billion (10⁹). [G. *gigas,* giant]

**gi·gan·tism** (jī'gan-tizm) a condition of abnormal size or overgrowth of the entire body or of any of its parts. SYN giantism. [G. *gigas,* giant]

△**gi·gan·to-** huge, gigantic. [G. *gigas,* one of the race of giants]

**gi·gan·to·mas·tia** (jī-gan'tō-mas'tē-ă) massive hypertrophy of the breast. [giganto- + G. *mastos,* breast]

**Gig·li saw** (jē'lyē) a hand-held wire saw for use in craniotomy.

**GIH** growth hormone-inhibiting hormone.

**Gil·bert dis·ease** (zhēl'bār) SYN familial nonhemolytic jaundice.

**Gil·christ dis·ease** (gil'krist) SYN blastomycosis.

**Gilles de la Tou·rette syn·drome** (zhēl dĕ lah too-ret') SYN Tourette syndrome.

**Gil·les·pie syn·drome** (gĭ-les'pē), syndrome of congenital absence of the iris, mental retardation, and cerebellar ataxia; etiology unknown.

**Gil·li·am op·er·a·tion** (gile'ăm) an operation for retroversion of the uterus by suturing round ligaments to abdominal wall fascia.

**Gil·lies op·er·a·tion** (gil'ēz) a technique for reducing fractures of the zygoma and the zygomatic arch through an incision in the temporal region above the hairline.

**gin·gi·va,** gen. and pl. **gin·gi·vae** (jin'ji-vă, jin'ji-vē) [TA] the dense fibrous tissue, covered by mucous membrane, that envelops the alveolar processes of the upper and lower jaws and surrounds the necks of the teeth. SYN gum (2). [L.]

**gin·gi·val** (jin'ji-văl) relating to the gums.

**gin·gi·val ab·scess** an abscess confined to the gingival soft tissue.

**Gin·gi·val In·dex (GI)** an index of periodontal disease based upon the severity and location of the lesion.

**gin·gi·val line** the position of the margin of the gingiva in relation to the teeth in the dental arch. SYN gum line.

**gin·gi·val mar·gin 1.** the most coronal portion of the gingiva surrounding the tooth; **2.** the edge of the free gingiva.

**gin·gi·val mas·sage** mechanical stimulation of the gingiva by rubbing or pressure.

**Gin·gi·val-Per·i·o·don·tal In·dex (GPI)** an index of gingivitis, gingival irritation, and advanced periodontal disease.

**gin·gi·val sul·cus** the space between the surface of the tooth and the free gingiva.

**gin·gi·vec·to·my** (jin-ji-vek'tō-mē) surgical resection of unsupported gingival tissue. SYN gum resection. [gingiva + G. *ektomē,* excision]

**gin·gi·vi·tis** (jin-ji-vī'tis) inflammation of the gingiva. [gingiva + G. *-itis,* inflammation]

△**gin·gi·vo-** the gingivae, the gums of the mouth. [L. *gingiva*]

**gin·gi·vo·glos·si·tis** (jin'ji-vō-glos-sī'tis) inflammation of both the tongue and gingival tissues. SEE ALSO stomatitis.

**gin·gi·vo·lin·guo·ax·i·al** (jin'ji-vō-ling'gwō-ak' sē-ăl) referring to the point angle formed by the gingival, lingual, and axial walls of a cavity.

**gin·gi·vo·os·se·ous** (jin'ji-vō-os'ē-ŭs) referring to the gingiva and its underlying bone.

**gin·gi·vo·plas·ty** (jin'ji-vō-plas-tē) a surgical procedure that reshapes and recontours the gingival tissue in order to attain esthetic, physiologic, and functional form.

**gin·gi·vo·sis** (jin-ji-vō'sis) SYN chronic desquamative gingivitis.

**gin·gi·vo·sto·ma·ti·tis** (jin'ji-vō-stō'mă-tī'tis) inflammation of the gingiva and other oral mucous membranes. [gingivo- + G. *stoma,* mouth, + *-itis,* inflammation]

**gin·gly·form** (jing'gli-fōrm, ging-gli-fōrm) SYN ginglymoid. [G. *ginglymos,* a hinge joint, + L. *forma,* form]

**gin·glym·o·ar·thro·di·al** (jing'gli-mō-ar-thrō' dē-ăl, ging-gli-mō-ar-thrō'dē-ăl) denoting a joint having the form of both ginglymus and arthrodia, or hinge joint and sliding joint.

**gin·gly·moid** (jing'gli-moyd, ging-gli-moyd) relating to or resembling a hinge joint. SYN ginglyform. [G. *ginglymos,* a hinge joint, + *eidos,* resembling]

**gin·gly·moid joint** SYN hinge joint.

**gin·gly·mus** (jing'gli-mŭs, ging-gli-mŭs) SYN hinge joint. [G. *ginglymos*]

*Gink·go bil·o·ba* a tall ornamental deciduous tree of the family Ginkgoaceae with distinctive bilobed fan-shaped leaves; female trees bear edible seeds surrounded by a fleshy covering that when ripe smells strongly of butyric acid; native to China, but extinct in the wild, surviving only in cultivation; extracts of the leaves contain ginkgoheterosides and terpene lactones and are used medicinally in cerebral and peripheral vascular disease.

**GIP** gastric inhibitory polypeptide; gastric inhibitory peptide.

**Gi·rard re·a·gent** (jir-ărd') the hydrazine of betaine chloride, used to extract ketonic steroids by forming water-soluble hydrazones with them.

**gir·dle** (ger'dl) a belt; a zone. A structure that has the form of a belt or girdle. SYN cingulum (1) [TA]. [A.S. *gyrdel*]

**gir·dle an·es·the·sia** anesthesia distributed as a band encircling the trunk.

**gir·dle sen·sa·tion** SYN zonesthesia.

**GI tract** gastrointestinal tract.

**gla·bel·la** (glă-bel'ă) **1.** a smooth prominence, most marked in the male, on the frontal bone above the root of the nose. **2.** the most forward projecting point of the forehead in the midline at the level of the supraorbital ridges. SYN mesophryon. SEE ALSO antinion. SYN intercilium. [L. *glabellus,* hairless, smooth, dim. of *glaber*]

**gla·brous, gla·brate** (glā'brŭs, glā'brāt) smooth

or hairless; denoting areas of the body where hair does not normally grow, i.e., palms or soles. [L. *glaber,* smooth]

**gland** an organized aggregation of cells functioning as a secretory or excretory organ. SYN glandula (1). [L. *glans,* acorn]

**glan•des** (glan′dēz) plural of glans.

**glan•di•lem•ma** (glan-di-lem′ă) the capsule of a gland. [L. *glandula,* gland, + G. *lemma,* sheath]

**glands of the fe•male u•re•thra** numerous mucous glands in the wall of the female urethra.

**glands of the male u•re•thra** numerous mucous glands in the wall of the penile urethra.

**glan•du•la,** pl. **glan•du•lae** (glan′dyu-lă, glan′dyu-lē) **1.** SYN gland. **2.** SYN glandule. [L. gland, dim. of *glans,* acorn]

**glan•du•lae ce•ru•mi•no•sae** [TA] **1.** SYN ceruminous glands. **2.** tubuloalveolar glands of the external auditory meatus believed to be modified apocrine sweat glands; they secrete cerumen.

**glan•du•lar** (glan′dyu-lăr) relating to a gland. SYN glandulous.

**glan•du•lar ep•i•the•li•um** epithelium composed of secretory cells.

**glan•dule** (glan′dyul) a small gland. SYN glandula (2). [L. *glandula*]

**glan•du•lous** (glan′dyu-lŭs) SYN glandular.

**glans,** pl. **glan•des** (glanz, glan′dēz) a conical acorn-shaped structure. [L. acorn]

**glans cli•to•ri•dis** [TA] SYN glans of clitoris.

**glans of clit•o•ris** a small mass of highly sensitized erectile tissue capping the body of the clitoris. SYN glans clitoridis [TA].

**glans pe•nis** [TA] the conical expansion of the corpus spongiosum which forms the head of the penis.

**glan•u•lar** (glan′yu-lar) pertaining to the glans penis. [irreg. fr. *glans,* by analogy with *glandular*]

**Glanz•mann throm•bas•the•nia** (glahnts′měn) a hemorrhagic diathesis characterized by normal or prolonged bleeding time, normal coagulation time, defective clot retraction, normal platelet count but morphologic or functional abnormality of platelets; several kinds of platelet abnormalities have been described; caused by defect in platelet membrane glycoprotein IIb-IIIa complex; autosomal recessive inheritance, caused by mutation in the platelet-membrane glycoprotein IIb-IIIa complex gene (ITGA2B) on chromosome 17.

**gla•se•ri•an fis•sure** (glă-sē′rē-ăn) SYN petrotympanic fissure.

**Glas•gow Co•ma Scale** (glas′gō) a standard measure of thesystematic tool used to assess level of consciousness and the reaction to stimuli in a neurologically impaired patient based on using three categories; eye opening, verbal responseperformance, and motor responsiveness. Three number scores are added together. The lowest scores predict poorer outcomes. SYN outcome score. [Glasgow, Scotland]

**Glas•gow sign** (glas′gō) a systolic murmur heard over the brachial artery in aneurysm of the aorta.

**glass** a transparent substance composed of silica and oxides of various bases. [A.S. *glaes*]

**glass•es** (glas′ez) **1.** SYN spectacles. **2.** lenses for correcting refractive errors in the eyes.

**glass i•o•no•mer ce•ment** a dental cement produced by mixing calcium aluminosilicate glass

with an aqueous solution of polyacrylic acid. [ion + -mer (1)]

**glas•sy mem•brane 1.** the basement membrane present between the stratum granulosum and the theca interna of a vesicular ovarian follicle; it becomes very prominent in large atretic follicles; **2.** the basement membrane and associated connective tissue of the hair follicle. SYN hyaline membrane (2).

**glau•co•ma** (glaw-kō′mă) a disease of the eye characterized by increased intraocular pressure and excavation and atrophy of the optic nerve; produces defects in the visual field and may result in blindness. See this page. [G. *glaukōma,* opacity of the crystalline lens, fr. *glaukos,* bluish green]

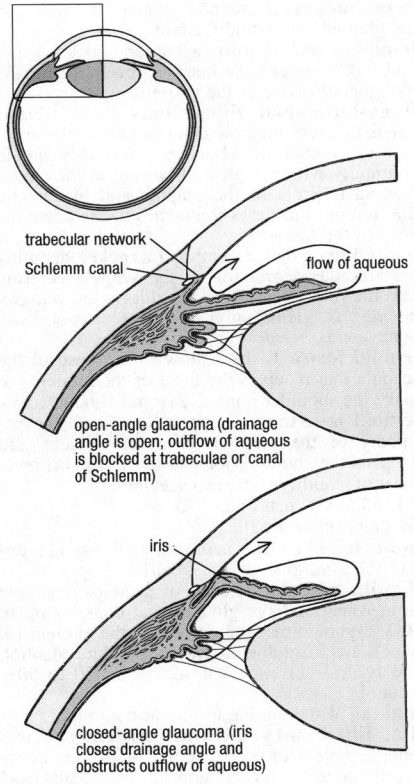

trabecular network
Schlemm canal
flow of aqueous

open-angle glaucoma (drainage angle is open; outflow of aqueous is blocked at trabeculae or canal of Schlemm)

iris

closed-angle glaucoma (iris closes drainage angle and obstructs outflow of aqueous)

**glaucoma**

**glau•co•ma•tous** (glaw-kō′mă-tŭs) relating to glaucoma.

**glau•co•ma•tous cat•a•ract** a nuclear opacity usually seen in absolute glaucoma.

**glau•co•ma•tous cup** a deep depression of the optic disk combined with optic atrophy; caused by glaucoma. See page B15. SYN glaucomatous excavation.

**glau•co•ma•tous ex•ca•va•tion** SYN glaucomatous cup.

**glau•co•ma•tous ha•lo 1.** a yellowish white ring surrounding the optic disk, indicating atrophy of the choroid in glaucoma; **2.** a halo surrounding lights, caused by corneal edema in glaucoma.

**GLC** gas-liquid chromatography.

**Glc, GlcA, GlcN, GlcNAc, GlcUA** symbols for the radicals of D-glucose, gluconic and glucuronic acid, glucosamine, *N*-acetylglucosamine, and glucuronic acid, respectively.

**Glea·son tu·mor grade** (glē′sŏn) a classification of adenocarcinoma of the prostate by evaluation of the pattern of glandular differentiation; the tumor grade, known as Gleason score, is the sum of the dominant and secondary patterns, each numbered on a scale of 1 to 5.

**Glenn op·er·a·tion** (glen) anastomosis between the superior vena cava and the right main pulmonary artery to increase pulmonary blood flow as a palliative correction for tricuspid atresia.

**gle·no·hu·mer·al** (glē′nō-hyu′mer-ăl) relating to the glenoid cavity and the humerus.

**gle·no·hu·mer·al joint** a ball-and-socket synovial joint between the head of the humerus and the glenoid cavity of the scapula.

**gle·no·hu·mer·al lig·a·ments** three fibrous bands that reinforce the anterior part of the articular capsule of the shoulder joint; they are in continuity with the glenoid labrum at the supraglenoid tubercle of the scapula and blend with the fibrous capsule as it attaches to the anatomic neck of the humerus.

**gle·noid** (glen′oyd) resembling a socket; denoting the articular depression of the scapula entering into the formation of the shoulder joint. [G. *glēnoeidēs*, fr. *glēnē*, pupil of eye, socket of joint, honeycomb, + *eidos*, appearance]

**gle·noid fos·sa 1.** the hollow in the head of the scapula that receives the head of the humerus to make the shoulder joint; **2.** SYN mandibular fossa.

**gle·noid la·brum** soft tissue lip around the periphery of the glenoid fossa that widens and deepens the shoulder joint to aid in the achievement of stability. SEE ALSO acetabulum.

**glia** (glī′ă) SYN neuroglia. [G. glue]

**glia cells** SEE neuroglia.

**gli·a·cyte** (glī′ă-sīt) a neuroglia cell. SEE neuroglia. [G. *glia*, glue, + *kytos*, cell]

**gli·a·din** (glī′ă-din) a class of protein, separable from wheat and rye glutens, that contains up to 40% L-glutamine; a member of the prolamins, which are insoluble in water, absolute alcohol, and neutral solvents, but soluble in 50 to 90% alcohol.

**gli·al** (glī′ăl) pertaining to glia or neuroglia.

**gli·al fib·ril·la·ry a·cid·ic pro·tein** a cytoskeletal protein of 51 kd found in fibrous astrocytes; stains for this protein are frequently used to assist in the differential diagnosis of neurologic lesions.

**glide·wire** (glīd′wīr) a hydrophilic or lubricated guidewire, generally used in the urinary tract. SEE ALSO guidewire.

**glid·ing joint** SYN plane joint.

△**glio-** glue, gluelike (relating specifically to the neuroglia). [G. *glia*, glue]

**gli·o·blast** (glī′ō-blast) an early neural cell developing, like the neuroblast, from the early ependymal cell of the neural tube; gives rise to neuroglial and ependymal cells, astrocytes, and oligodendrocytes. SEE ALSO spongioblast. [glio- + G. *blastos*, germ]

**gli·o·blas·to·ma multiforme** (glī′ō-blas-tō′mă mul-tē-fōr-mē) a glioma consisting chiefly of un-

differentiated anaplastic cells of glial origin that show marked nuclear pleomorphism, necrosis, and vascular endothelial proliferation; frequently, tumor cells are arranged radially about an irregular focus of necrosis; these neoplasms grow rapidly, invade extensively, and occur most frequently in the cerebrum of adults. SYN grade IV astrocytoma. [G. *glia*, glue, + *blastos*, germ, + *-oma*, tumor]

**gli·o·ma** (glī-ō′mă) any neoplasm derived from one of the various types of cells that form the interstitial tissue of the brain, spinal cord, pineal gland, posterior pituitary gland, and retina. [G. *glia*, glue, + *-oma*, tumor]

**gli·o·ma·to·sis** (glī-ō-mă-tō′sis) neoplastic growth of neuroglial cells in the brain or spinal cord; the term is used especially with reference to a relatively large neoplasm or to multiple foci. SYN neurogliomatosis.

**gli·o·ma·tous** (glī-ō′mă-tŭs) pertaining to or characterized by a glioma.

**gli·o·neu·ro·ma** (glī′ō-noo-rō′mă) a ganglioneuroma derived from neurons, with numerous glial cells and fibers in the matrix.

**gli·o·sar·co·ma** (glī′ō-sar-kō′mă) a glioblastoma multiforme with an associated malignant mesenchymal component. Sometimes used as a term for a malignant neoplasm derived from connective tissue (e.g., that associated with blood vessels in the brain) in which there are proliferating glial cells.

**gli·o·sis** (glī-ō′sis) overgrowth of the astrocytes in an area of damage in the brain or spinal cord.

**GLIP** glucagonlike insulinotropic peptide.

**Glis·son cap·sule** (glis′en) SYN fibrous capsule of liver.

**Glis·son cir·rho·sis** (glis′en) chronic perihepatitis with thickening and subsequent contraction, resulting in atrophy and deformity of the liver.

**Gln** glutamine or its acyl radical, glutaminyl.

**glob·al** (glō′băl) complete, generalized, overall, or total.

**glob·al a·pha·sia** in which all aspects of speech and communication are severely impaired. At best, patients can understand or speak only a few words or phrases; they cannot read or write. SYN mixed aphasia, total aphasia.

**glob·al bur·den of dis·ease** mathematical measure of loss of healthy life years due to disabling diseases in a country's population. SEE ALSO disability-adjusted life years.

**glo·bal warm·ing** (glō′bal warm′ing) an overall increase in the world's temperatures; could present a risk of malaria epidemics in the highland areas of tropical Africa by driving malaria transmission uphill into these populated areas.

**glo·bi** (glō′bī) **1.** plural of globus. **2.** brown bodies sometimes found in the granulomatous lesions of leprosy.

**glo·bin** (glō′bin) the protein of hemoglobin; α-globin and β-globin represent the two types of chains found in adult hemoglobin. SYN hematohiston.

**glo·bo·side** (glō′bō-sīd) a glycosphingolipid isolated from kidney and erythrocytes; accumulates in individuals with Sandhoff disease.

**glo·bo·tri·a·o·syl·cer·a·mide** (glō′bō-trī-ă-ō-sil-ser-a-mīd) a sphingolipid containing three sugar moieties that accumulates in individuals with Fabry disease.

**glob·ule** (glob′yul) **1.** a small spherical body of

any kind. **2.** a fat droplet in milk. [L. *globulus,* dim. of *globus,* a ball]

**glob•u•lin** (glob′yu-lin) name for a family of proteins precipitated from plasma by ammonium sulfate. Globulins may be further fractionated by solubility, electrophoresis, ultracentrifugation, and other separation methods into many subgroups, the main groups being α-, β-, and γ-globulin; these differ with respect to their content of physiologically important factors. Among the latter are immunoglobulins, lipoproteins, glucoor mucoproteins, and metal-binding and metal-transporting proteins. [L. *globulus,* globule]

β$_{1C}$ **glob•u•lin** the third component (C3) of complement. SEE component of complement.

β$_{1E}$ **glob•u•lin** the fourth component (C4) of complement. SEE component of complement.

β$_{1F}$ **glob•u•lin** the fifth component (C5) of complement. SEE component of complement.

**glob•u•li•nu•ria** (glob′yu-lin-yur′ē-ă) the excretion of globulin in the urine, usually, if not always, in association with serum albumin.

**glo•bus,** pl. **glo•bi** (glō′bŭs, glō′bī) **1.** a round body; ball. **2.** SEE globi. [L.]

**glo•bus hys•ter•i•cus** difficulty in swallowing; a sensation as of a ball in the throat or as if the throat were compressed; a symptom of conversion disorder.

**glo•bus pal•li•dus** [TA] the inner and lighter gray portion of the lentiform nucleus. SEE ALSO paleostriatum. SYN pallidum.

**glo•mal** (glō′măl) relating to or involving a glomus.

**glo•man•gi•o•ma** (glō-man-jē-ō′mă) a variant of glomus tumor, characterized by multiple tumors resembling cavernous hemangioma.

**glo•man•gi•o•sis** (glō-man-jē-ō′sis) the occurrence of multiple complexes of small vascular channels, each resembling a glomus.

**glo•mec•to•my** (glō-mek′tō-mē) excision of a glomus tumor. [L. *glomus* + G. *ektomē,* cutting out]

**glom•era** (glom′er-ă) plural of glomus.

**glo•mer•u•lar** (glo-mār′yu-lăr) relating to or affecting a glomerulus or the glomeruli.

**glo•mer•u•lar cap•sule** the expanded beginning of a nephron composed of an inner and outer layer: the visceral layer consists of podocytes which surround a tuft of capillaries (glomerulus); the parietal layer is simple squamous epithelium which becomes cuboidal at the tubular pole. SYN Bowman capsule, malpighian capsule (1).

**glo•mer•u•lar cyst** cyst formed by dilation of Bowman capsule, found in rare cases of congenital polycystic kidneys.

**glo•mer•u•lar fil•tra•tion rate (GFR)** the volume of water filtered out of the plasma through glomerular capillary walls into Bowman capsules per unit time; it is considered to be equivalent to inulin clearance.

**glo•mer•u•lar ne•phri•tis** SYN glomerulonephritis.

**glom•er•ule** (glom′er-yul) SYN glomerulus.

**glo•mer•u•li•tis** (glo-mer′yu-lī′tis) inflammation of a glomerulus, specifically of the renal glomeruli, as in glomerulonephritis.

**glo•mer•u•lo•ne•phri•tis** (glo-mer′yu-lō-nef-rī′tis) renal disease characterized by inflammatory changes in glomeruli which are not the result of infection of the kidneys. SYN glomerular nephri-

tis. [glomerulus + G. *nephros,* kidney, + -*itis,* inflammation]

**glo•mer•u•lop•a•thy** (glo-mer-yu-lop′ă-thē) glomerular disease of any type. [glomerulus + G. *pathos,* suffering]

**glo•mer•u•lo•sa cell** a cell of the zona glomerulosa of the adrenal cortex that is the source of aldosterone; the cells are arranged in spherical or oval groups.

**glo•mer•u•lo•scle•ro•sis** (glo-măr′yu-lō-sklĕ-rō′sis) hyaline deposits or scarring within the renal glomeruli, a degenerative process occurring in association with renal arteriosclerosis or diabetes. [glomerulus + G. *sklērōsis,* hardness]

**glo•mer•u•lus,** pl. **glo•mer•u•li** (glo-mer′yu-lŭs, glo-mer′-yu-lī) **1.** a plexus of capillaries. **2.** a tuft formed of capillary loops at the beginning of each nephric tubule in the kidney; this tuft with its capsule (Bowman capsule) constitutes the corpusculum renis (malpighian body). **3.** the twisted secretory portion of a sweat gland. **4.** a cluster of dendritic ramifications and axon terminals forming a complex synaptic relationship and surrounded by a glial sheath. SYN glomerule. [Mod. L. dim. of L. *glomus,* a ball of yarn]

**glo•mus,** pl. **glom•era** (glō′mŭs, glom′er-ă) **1.** a small globular body. **2.** a highly organized arteriolovenular anastomosis forming a tiny nodular focus in the nailbed, pads of the fingers and toes, ears, hands, and feet and many other organs of the body. The anastomosis is convoluted and richly innervated and drains into a periglomic vein and then into one of the veins of the skin. The glomus functions as a shunt or bypass regulating mechanism in the flow of blood, temperature, and conservation of heat in the part as well as in the indirect control of the blood pressure and other functions of the circulatory system. [L. *glomus,* a ball]

**glo•mus ju•gu•la•re tu•mor** SYN chemodectoma.

**glo•mus tu•mor** an unusual vascular neoplasm composed of specialized pericytes, usually in nodular masses, which occurs almost exclusively in the skin; it is exquisitely tender and may be so painful that patients voluntarily immobilize an extremity. SEE ALSO glomangioma.

**glo•mus tym•pan•i•cum tu•mor** a glomus tumor arising on the medial wall of the middle ear.

**glos•sa** (glos′ă) SYN tongue (1). [G.]

**glos•sal** (glos′ăl) SYN lingual (1).

**glos•sal•gia** (glos-al′jē-ă) SYN glossodynia. [gloss- + G. *algos,* pain]

**glos•sec•to•my** (glo-sek′tō-mē) resection or amputation of the tongue. SYN lingulectomy (1). [gloss- + G. *ektomē,* excision]

*Glos•si•na* (glo-sī′nă) a genus of bloodsucking Diptera (tsetse flies) confined to Africa; they serve as vectors of the trypanosomes that cause African sleeping sickness. [G. *glōssa,* tongue]

**glos•si•tis** (glo-sī′tis) inflammation of the tongue. [gloss- + G. -*itis,* inflammation]

**glos•si•tis ar•e•a•ta ex•fo•li•a•ti•va** SYN geographic tongue.

△**glos•so-, gloss-** language; corresponds to L. *linguo-.* Cf. linguo-. [G. *glōssa,* tongue]

**glos•so•cele** (glos′ō-sēl) protrusion of the tongue from the mouth, owing to its excessive size. SEE ALSO macroglossia. [glosso- + G. *kēlē,* tumor, hernia]

**glos•so•dyn•ia** (glos′ō-din′ē-ă) a condition characterized by burning or painful tongue. SYN burning tongue, glossalgia. [glosso- + G. *odynē*, pain]

**glos·so·ep·i·glot·tic, glos·so·ep·i·glot·tid·e·an** (glos'ō-ep-i-glot'ik, glos'ō-ep-i-glo-tid'ē-an) relating to the tongue and the epiglottis.

**glos·so·hy·al** (glos-ō-hī'ăl) SYN hyoglossal.

**glos·so·la·lia** (glos-ō-lā'lē-ă) rarely used term for unintelligible jargon or babbling. [glosso- + G. *lalia*, talk, chat]

**glos·sop·a·thy** (glos-op'ă-thē) a disease of the tongue. [glosso- + G. *pathos*, suffering]

**glos·so·pha·ryn·ge·al** (glos'ō-fă-rin'jē-ăl) relating to the tongue and the pharynx.

**glos·so·pha·ryn·ge·al breath·ing** respiration unaided by the usual primary muscles of respiration; the air is forced into the lungs by use of the tongue and muscles of the pharynx.

**glos·so·pha·ryn·ge·al nerve [CN IX]** ninth cranial nerve that emerges from the rostral end of the medulla and passes through the jugular foramen to supply sensation including taste to the pharynx and posterior third of the tongue; it also carries somatic motor fibers to the stylopharyngeus muscle and secretomotor presynaptic parasympathetic fibers to the otic ganglion for innervation of the parotid gland. SYN nervus glossopharyngeus [CN IX] [TA], ninth cranial nerve [CN IX].

**glos·so·plas·ty** (glos'ō-plas-tē) plastic surgery of the tongue. [glosso- + G. *plastos*, formed]

**glos·sor·rha·phy** (glo-sōr'ă-fē) suture of a wound of the tongue. [glosso- + G. *rhaphē*, suture]

**glos·so·spasm** (glos'ō-spazm) spasmodic contraction of the tongue.

**glos·sot·o·my** (glo-sot'ō-mē) any cutting operation on the tongue, usually to obtain access to further reaches of the pharynx. [glosso- + G. *tomē*, incision]

**glos·so·trich·ia** (glos-ō-trik'ē-ă) SYN hairy tongue. [glosso- + G. *thrix*, hair]

**glot·tal** (glot'ăl) relating to the glottis.

**glot·tal at·tack** excessive glottal closure prior to phonation resulting in loud and sudden voice onset. SYN coup de glotte.

**glot·tal fry** vocal fold vibration in the lowest part of the pitch range, characterized by a creaky, pulsed type of phonation. SYN gravel voice.

**glot·tal·iz·a·tion** (glot'al-ĭ-zā'shŭn) SYN vocal fry.

**glot·tic** (glot'ik) relating to (1) the tongue or (2) the glottis.

**glot·tis,** pl. **glot·ti·des** (glot'is, glot'i-dēz) [TA] the vocal apparatus of the larynx, consisting of the vocal folds of mucous membrane investing the vocal ligament and vocal muscle on each side, the free edges of which are the vocal cords, and of a median fissure, the rima glottidis. [G. *glōttis*, aperture of the larynx]

**glot·ti·tis** (glo-tī'tis) inflammation of the glottic portion of the larynx.

**glove an·es·the·sia** loss of sensation in the distal upper extremity, i.e., the hand and fingers.

**glov·er's su·ture** a continuous suture in which each stitch is passed through the loop of the preceding one.

**GLP-1** glucagonlike peptide.

**Glu** glutamic acid or its acyl radical, glutamyl.

**glu·ca·gon** (gloo'kă-gon) a hormone produced by pancreatic alpha cells. Parenteral administration of 0.5 to 1 mg results in prompt mobilization of hepatic glycogen, thus elevating blood glucose concentration. It is used in the treatment of glycogen storage disease (von Gierke's) and hypoglycemia, particularly hypoglycemic coma due to exogenously administered insulin. [glucose + G. *agō*, to lead]

**glu·ca·gon·like in·su·lin·o·trop·ic pep·tide (GLIP)** an insulinotropic substance originating in the gastrointestinal tract and released into the circulation following ingestion of a meal containing glucose.

**glu·ca·gon·like pep·tide (GLP-1)** a gut hormone that slows gastric emptying and stimulates insulin secretion. It may become useful in the future in the treatment of noninsulin-dependent diabetes mellitus, perhaps administered by patch, inhaler, or buccal pellet formulation.

**glu·ca·gon·o·ma** (gluˈkă-gon-ōˈmă) a glucagon-secreting tumor, usually derived from pancreatic islet cells.

**glu·can** (gloo'kan) a polyglucose; e.g., callose, cellulose, starch amylose, glycogen amylose.

**1,4-α-D-glu·can-branch·ing en·zyme** amylo-(1,4→1,6)-transglucosylase; or transglucosidase; an enzyme in muscle and in plants (Q enzyme) that cleaves α-1,4 linkages in glycogen or starch, transferring the fragments into α-1,6 linkages, creating branches in the polysaccharide molecules; in plants, it converts amylose to amylopectin; this enzyme is deficient in individuals with glycogen storage disease type IV.

**1,4-α-D-glu·can 6-α-D-glu·co·syl·trans·fer·ase, α-glu·can-branch·ing gly·co·syl·trans·fer·ase** a glucosyltransferase that transfers an α-glucosyl residue in a 1,4-α-glucan to the primary hydroxyl group of glucose in a 1,4-α-glucan.

**4-α-Dβ-glucanotransferase** a 4-glycosyltransferase which converts maltodextrins into amylose and glucose by transferring parts of 1,4-glucan chains to new 4-positions on glucose or other 1,4-glucans.

△**glu·co-** glucose. SEE ALSO glyco-. [G. *gleukos*, sweet new wine, sweetness]

**glu·co·cer·e·bro·side** (gloo-kō-ser'ĕ-brō-sīd) SYN glucosylceramide.

**glu·co·cor·ti·coid** (gloo-kō-kōr'ti-koyd) **1.** any steroid-like compound capable of promoting hepatic glycogen deposition and of exerting a clinically useful anti-inflammatory effect. Cortisol is the most potent of the naturally occurring glucocortocoids most semisynthetic glucocorticoids are cortisol derivatives. **2.** denoting this type of biological activity. SYN glycocorticoid.

**glu·co·fu·ra·nose** (gloo-kō-foor'ă-nōs) glucose in furanose form.

**glu·co·gen·e·sis** (gloo-kō-jen'ĕ-sis) formation of glucose. [gluco- + G. *genesis*, production]

**glu·co·gen·ic** (gloo-kō-jen'ik) giving rise to or producing glucose.

**glu·co·ki·nase** (gloo-kō-kī'nās) phosphotransferase that catalyzes the conversion of D-glucose and ATP D-glucose 6-phosphate and ADP; the liver enzyme has a higher $K_m$ value for D-glucose than does hexokinase.

**glu·co·ki·net·ic** (gloo'kō-ki-net'ik) tending to mobilize glucose; usually evidenced by a reduction of the glycogen stores in the tissues to produce an increase in the concentration of glucose circulating in the blood.

**glu•co•lip•ids** (gloo-kō-lip′idz) glycosphingolipids that contain D-glucose.

**glu•co•ne•o•gen•e•sis** (gloo′kō-nē-ō-jen′ĕ-sis) the formation of glucose from noncarbohydrates, such as protein or fat. Cf. glyconeogenesis.

**glu•con•ic ac•id** (gloo-kon′ik as′id) the hexonic (aldonic) acid derived from glucose by oxidation of the –CHO group to –COOH.

**glu•co•pro•tein** (gloo-kō-prō′tēn) a glycoprotein in which the sugar is glucose.

**glu•co•pyr•a•nose** (gloo-kō-pir′ă-nōs) glucose in its pyranose form.

**glu•co•san** (gloo′kō-san) a polysaccharide yielding glucose upon hydrolysis; e.g., callose, cellulose, glycogen, starch, dextrins.

**glu•cose** (gloo′kōs) a dextrorotatory monosaccharide found in the free form in fruits and other parts of plants, and in combination in glucosides, glycogen, disaccharides, and polysaccharides (starch cellulose); the chief source of energy in human metabolism, the final product of carbohydrate digestion, and the principal sugar of the blood; insulin is required for the use of glucose by cells; in diabetes mellitus the level of glucose in the blood is excessive, and it also appears in the urine. SYN D-glucose.

**D-glu•cose (G, Glc)** (dē-gloo′kōs) SYN glucose.

**glu•cose-de•pen•dent in•su•lin•o•tro•pic po•-ly•pep•tide** an insulinotropic substance originating in the gastrointestinal tract and released into the circulation following ingestion of a meal containing glucose.

**glu•cose ox•i•dase meth•od** a highly specific method for measurement of glucose in serum or plasma by reaction with glucose oxidase, in which gluconic acid and hydrogen peroxide are formed.

**glu•cose 6-phos•phate** an ester of glucose with phosphoric acid; made in the course of glucose metabolism by mammalian and other cells; a normal constituent of resting muscle.

**glu•cose-6-phos•phate de•hy•dro•gen•ase de•-fi•cien•cy** congenital deficiency of glucose-6-phosphate dehydrogenase, an enzyme important for maintaining cellular concentrations of reduced nucleotides. It can cause a variety of anemias including favism, primaquine sensitivity and other drug sensitivity anemias, anemia of the newborn, and chronic nonspherocytic hemolytic anemia.

**glu•cose trans•port max•i•mum** the maximal rate of reabsorption of glucose from the glomerular filtrate; it amounts to approximately 320 mg/min in humans.

**α-glucosidase inhibitor** an oral agent that aids in the control of diabetes mellitus by delaying the absorption of glucose from the digestive system.

**glu•co•si•dase in•hib•i•tors** agents such as acarbose which reduce gastrointestinal absorption of carbohydrates. This group of drugs has been known popularly as "starch blockers". They lower plasma glucose levels and tend to cause weight loss. A limiting side effect is flatulence.

**glu•co•si•das•es** (gloo′kō-sid-ās-ez) enzymes that hydrolyze glucosides.

**glu•co•side** (gloo′kō-sīd) a compound of glucose with an alcohol or other R–OH compound involving loss of the H atom of the 1-OH (hemiacetal) group of the glucose, yielding a –C–O–R link from the C-1 of the glucose; a glycoside of glucose.

**glu•co•sin•o•lates** a group of secondary plant metabolites occurring in cruciferous plants, especially *Brassica* vegetables (such as cabbage); hydrolyzed into wide range of biologically active compounds, including isothiocyanates, which show anticarcinogenic activity.

**glu•cos•u•ria** (gloo-kōs-yur′ē-ă) the urinary excretion of glucose, usually in enhanced quantities. SYN glycosuria (1), glycuresis (1). [glucose + G. *ouron,* urine]

**glu•co•syl•cer•a•mide** (gloo′kō-sil-ser′ă-mīd) a neutral glycolipid containing equimolar amounts of fatty acid, glucose, and sphingosine (or a derivative thereof); accumulates in individuals with Gaucher disease. SYN glucocerebroside.

**glu•co•syl•trans•fer•ase** (gloo′kō-sil-trans′fer-ās) any enzyme transferring glucosyl groups from one compound to another.

**glu•cu•ro•nate** (gloo-kyur′ō-nāt) a salt or ester of glucuronic acid.

**glu•cu•ron•ic ac•id** (gloo-kyur-on′ik as′id) the uronic acid of glucose in which C-6 is oxidized to a carboxyl group; the D-isomer detoxicates or inactivates various substances (e.g., benzoic acid, phenol, camphor, and the female sex hormones), the glucuronides so formed being excreted in the urine.

**β-D-glu•cu•ron•i•dase** (beta-dē-gloo-kyur-on′i-dās) an enzyme catalyzing the hydrolysis of various β-D-glucuronides, liberating free D-glucuronic acid and an alcohol; a deficiency of this enzyme is associated with Sly syndrome.

**β-*d*-glu•cu•ron•i•dase de•fi•cien•cy** a rare deficiency of β-*d*-glucuronidase; an autosomal recessive disorder with several allelic forms, characterized by abnormal mucopolysaccharide metabolism leading to progressive mental deterioration, splenic and hepatic enlargement, and dysostosis multiplex.

**glu•cu•ro•nide, glu•cu•ro•no•side** (gloo-kyur′on-īd, gloo-koo-ron′ō-sīd) a glycoside of glucuronic acid; many foreign chemicals, as well as catabolic products of normal body constituents (e.g., steroid hormones), are commonly excreted in the urine as D-glucuronides, the conjugation taking place in the liver.

**glue-sniff•ing** (gloo′snif-ing) inhalation of fumes from plastic cements; the solvents, which include toluene, xylene, and benzene, induce central nervous system stimulation followed by depression.

**glu•ta•mate** (gloo′tă-māt) a salt or ester of glutamic acid.

**glu•tam•ic ac•id (E, Glu)** (gloo-tam′ik as′id) an amino acid that occurs in proteins; the sodium salt is monosodium glutamate. Cf. glutamate.

**glu•tam•ic-ox•a•lo•a•ce•tic trans•am•i•nase (GOT)** SYN aspartate aminotransferase.

**glu•tam•ic-py•ru•vic trans•am•i•nase (GPT)** SYN alanine aminotransferase.

**glu•ta•min•ase** (gloo-tam′in-ās) an enzyme in kidney and other tissues that catalyzes the hydrolysis of L-glutamine to ammonia and L-glutamic acid; an important enzyme for urinary ammonia formation.

**glu•ta•mine (Gln, Q)** (gloo′tă-mēn) the δ-amide of glutamic acid, derived by oxidation from proline in the liver or by the combination of glutamic acid with ammonia; the L-isomer is present in proteins and in blood and other tissues, and is an important source of urinary ammonia.

g
l

**glu·tam·i·nyl (Glx, Gln, Q)** (gloo-tam′i-nil) the acyl radical of glutamine.

**glu·tam·o·yl** (gloo-tam′ō-il) the radical of glutamic acid from which both α- and δ-hydroxyl groups have been removed.

**glu·tam·yl (Glx, E, Glu)** (gloo-tam′il) the radical of glutamic acid from which either the α- or the δ-hydroxyl group has been removed.

**glu·ta·ral·de·hyde** high-level disinfectant. EPA-registered as a sterilant/disinfectant chemical.

**glu·tar·ic ac·id** (gloo-tar′ik as′id) an intermediate in tryptophan catabolism; accumulates in glutaric acidemia.

**glu·ta·thi·one (GSH)** (gloo-tă-thī′ōn) **1.** γ-L-glutamyl-L-cysteinylglycine; glutathione has a wide variety of roles in a cell. A deficiency of glutathione can cause hemolysis with oxidative stress. **2.** the principal low molecular weight thiol compound of living plant cells; used in the course of intermediary metabolism as a donor of thiol (SH) groups; essential for detoxification of acetaminophen.

**glu·te·al** (gloo′tē-ăl) relating to the buttocks. [G. *gloutos,* buttock]

**glu·te·al fold, glu·te·al fur·row** a prominent fold that marks the upper limit of the thigh and the lower limit of the buttock; it coincides with the lower border of the gluteus maximus muscle.

**glu·ten** (gloo′tĕn) the insoluble protein (prolamines) constituent of wheat and other grains; a mixture of gliadin, glutenin, and other proteins; the presence of gluten allows flour to rise. [L. *gluten,* glue]

**glu·ten a·tax·ia** ataxia resulting from immunologic damage to cerebellulm, posterior spinal columns, and periperal nerves in gluten-senstive individuals.

**glu·ten en·ter·op·a·thy** SYN celiac disease.

**glu·ten-free di·et** elimination of all wheat, rye, barley, and oat gluten from the diet; treatment for gluten-sensitive enteropathy. SEE celiac disease.

**glu·te·o·fem·o·ral** (gloo′tē-ō-fem′ō-răl) relating to the buttock and the thigh.

**glu·te·us max·i·mus mus·cle** *origin,* ilium behind posterior gluteal line, posterior surface of sacrum and coccyx, and sacrotuberous ligament; *insertion,* iliotibial band of fascia lata (superficial three-quarters) and gluteal ridge (deep inferior one-quarter) of femur; *action,* extends thigh, especially from the flexed position, as in climbing stairs or rising from a sitting position; *nerve supply,* inferior gluteal. SYN musculus gluteus maximus [TA].

**glu·te·us me·di·us mus·cle** *origin,* ilium between anterior and posterior gluteal lines; *insertion,* lateral surface of greater trochanter; *action,* abducts and rotates thigh; *nerve supply,* superior gluteal. SYN musculus gluteus medius [TA].

**glu·te·us mi·ni·mus mus·cle** *origin,* ilium between anterior and inferior gluteal lines; *insertion,* greater trochanter of femur; *action,* abducts thigh; *nerve supply,* superior gluteal. SYN musculus gluteus minimus [TA].

**glu·ti·nous** (gloo′tin-ŭs) sticky.

**glu·ti·tis** (gloo-tī′tis) inflammation of the muscles of the buttock. [G. *gloutos,* buttock, + *-itis,* inflammation]

**Glx** glutaminyl; glutamyl.

**Gly** glycine or its acyl radical, glycyl.

**gly·cae·mia [Br.]** SEE glycemia.

**gly·can** (glī′kan) SYN polysaccharide.

**gly·ca·ted he·mo·glo·bin** any one of four hemoglobin A fractions to which glucose and related monosaccharides bind; concentrations are increased in the erythrocytes of patients with diabetes mellitus. The glycated hemoglobin levels change slowly and can be used as a retrospective index of glucose control over the previous 8-10 weeks in such patients. SYN glycohemoglobin.

**gly·ce·mia** (glī-sē′mē-ă) the presence of glucose in the blood. [G. *glykys,* sweet, + *haima,* blood]

**gly·ce·mic in·dex** any of various measures of the rise in blood glucose level after ingestion of carbohydrate.

**glyc·er·al·de·hyde** (glis-er-al′dĕ-hīd) a triose and the simplest optically active aldose; the dextrorotatory isomer is taken as the structural reference point for all D compounds, the levorotatory isomer for all L compounds.

**gly·cer·ic ac·id** (gli-ser′ik as′id, glis′er-ik as′id) the fatty acid analog of glycerol; occurs particularly in the form of phosphorylated derivatives, as an intermediate in glycolysis.

**L-gly·cer·ic ac·i·du·ria** excretion of L-glyceric acid in the urine; a primary metabolic error due to deficiency of D-glyceric dehydrogenase resulting in excretion of L-glyceric and oxalic acids, leading to the clinical syndrome of oxalosis with frequent formation of oxalate renal calculi.

**glyc·er·i·das·es** (glis′er-ĭ-dās-ez) general term for enzymes catalyzing the hydrolysis of glycerol esters (glycerides); e.g., triacylglycerol lipase.

**glyc·er·ide** (glis′er-id, glis′-īd) an ester of glycerol.

**glyc·er·ol, glyc·er·in** (glis′er-ol, glis′er-in) a sweet oily fluid obtained by the saponification of fats and fixed oils; used as a solvent, as a skin emollient, by injection or in the form of suppository for constipation, orally to reduce ocular tension, and as a vehicle and sweetening agent.

**gly·cer·ol de·hy·dra·tion test** transient hearing improvement in some persons with Ménière disease after an oral glycerol dose resulting in an osmotic diuresis.

**glyc·er·yl** (glis′er-il) the trivalent radical, $C_3H_5''$, of glycerol; often used in error for glycero- or glycerol.

**gly·cine (G, Gly)** (glī′sēn) the simplest amino acid; a major component of gelatin and silk fibroin; used as a nutrient and dietary supplement, and in solution for irrigation.

**gly·cine am·i·di·no·trans·fer·ase** an enzyme catalyzing the transfer of an amidine group from L-arginine to glycine, forming guanidinoacetate and L-ornithine; an important reaction in creatine synthesis; it can also act on canavanine.

**gly·ci·nu·ria** (glī-sin-yur′ē-ă) the excretion of glycine in the urine. [glycine + G. *ouron,* urine]

△**gly·co-** combining form denoting relationship to sugars (e.g., glycogen), or to glycine (e.g., glycocholate). SEE ALSO gluco-. [G. *glykys,* sweet]

**gly·co·ca·lyx** (glī-kō-kā′liks) a PAS-positive filamentous coating on the apical surface of certain epithelial cells, composed of carbohydrate moieties of proteins that protrude from the free surface of the plasma membrane. [glyco- + G. *kalyx,* husk, shell]

**gly·co·cho·late** (glī-kō-kō′lāt) a salt or ester of glycocholic acid.

**gly·co·cho·lic ac·id** (glī-kō-kō′lik as′id) *N*-cholylglycine; one of the major bile acid conjugates, formed by condensation of the —COOH group of cholic acid and the amino group of glycine; water-soluble and a powerful detergent.

**gly·co·con·ju·gates** (glī-kō-kon′jŭ-gātz) a general class of sugar-containing macromolecules of the body including glycolipids, glycoproteins, and proteoglycans.

**gly·co·cor·ti·coid** (glī′kō-kōr′ti-koyd) SYN glucocorticoid.

**gly·co·gen** (glī′kō-jen) a glucosan of high molecular weight, resembling amylopectin in structure (with $\alpha$(1,4 linkages) but even more highly branched ($\alpha$(1,6 linkages), found in most of the tissues of the body, especially those of the liver and muscle; as the principal carbohydrate reserve, it is readily converted into glucose.

**gly·co·gen·e·sis** (glī-kō-jen′ĕ-sis) formation of glycogen from D-glucose by means of glycogen synthase and dextrin dextranase; the first enzyme catalyzes formation of a polyglucose with $\alpha$-1,4 links from UDP glucose, the second cleaves fragments from one chain and transfers them to an $\alpha$-1,6 linkage in another. [glyco- + G. *genesis,* production]

**gly·co·ge·net·ic** (glī′kō-jĕ-net′ik) glycogenic (2); relating to glycogenesis.

**gly·co·gen gran·ule** glycogen occurring in cells as beta granules which average about 300 Å in diameter, or as alpha granules which are aggregates measuring 900 Å of smaller particles.

**gly·co·gen load·ing** SYN carbohydrate loading.

**gly·co·gen·ol·y·sis** (glī′kō-jĕ-nol′i-sis) the hydrolysis of glycogen to glucose.

**gly·co·ge·no·sis** (glī′kō-jĕ-nō′sis) any glycogen deposition disease characterized by accumulation of glycogen of normal or abnormal chemical structure in tissue; there may be enlargement of the liver, heart, or striated muscle, including the tongue, with progressive muscular weakness. SYN dextrinosis.

**gly·co·gen su·per·com·pen·sa·tion** SYN carbohydrate loading.

**gly·co·he·mo·glob·in** (glī′ko-hē′mō-glō-bin) SYN glycated hemoglobin.

**gly·col·al·de·hyde** (glī-kol-al′dĕ-hīd) the simplest (2-carbon) sugar; the aerobic deamination product of ethanolamine.

**gly·col·ic ac·id** (glī-kol′ik as′id) an intermediate in the interconversion of glycine and ethanolamine.

**gly·col·ic ac·i·du·ria** excessive excretion of glycolic acid in the urine; a primary metabolic defect due to deficiency of 2-hydroxy-3-oxoadipate carboxylase, resulting in excretion of glycolic and oxalic acids, leading to the clinical syndrome of oxalosis.

**gly·co·lip·id** (glī-kō-lip′id) a lipid with one or more covalently attached sugars.

**gly·co·lyl** (glī′kō-lil) the acyl radical of glycolic acid, replacing acetyl in some sialic acids; the products are called *N*-glycolylneuraminic acids.

**gly·col·y·sis** (glī-kol′i-sis) the energy-yielding conversion of D-glucose to lactic acid (instead of pyruvate oxidation products) in various tissues, notably muscle, when sufficient oxygen is not available; since molecular oxygen is not consumed in the process, this is frequently referred to as "anaerobic glycolysis" [glyco- + G. *lysis,* a loosening]

**gly·co·lyt·ic** (glī-kō-lit′ik) relating to glycolysis.

**gly·co·ne·o·gen·e·sis** (glī′kō-nē-ō-jen′ĕ-sis) the formation of glycogen from noncarbohydrates,

such as protein or fat, by conversion of the latter to D-glucose. SEE ALSO glycogenesis. Cf. gluconeogenesis. [glyco- + G. *neos,* new, + *genesis,* production]

**gly·co·pe·nia** (glī-kō-pē′nē-ă) a deficiency of any or all sugars in an organ or tissue. [glyco- + G. *penia,* poverty]

**gly·co·pep·tide** (glī-kō-pep′tīd) a compound containing sugar(s) linked to amino acids (or peptides), with the latter preponderant, as in bacterial cell walls. Cf. peptidoglycan.

**gly·co·phil·ia** (glī-kō-fil′ē-ă) a condition in which there is a distinct tendency to develop hyperglycemia, even after the ingestion of a relatively small quantity of glucose. [glyko- + G. *phileō,* to love]

**gly·co·pro·tein** (glī-kō-prō′tēn) 1. one of a group of protein-carbohydrate compounds (conjugated proteins), among which the most important are the mucins, mucoid, and amyloid. 2. sometimes restricted to proteins containing small amounts of carbohydrate, in contrast to mucoids or mucoproteins. SEE ALSO mucoprotein.

**gly·co·pty·a·lism** (glī-kō-tī′ă-lizm) SYN glycosialia. [glyco- + G. *ptyalon,* saliva]

**gly·cor·rha·chia** (glī-kō-rā′kē-ă, glī-kō-rak-ē-ă) presence of sugar in the cerebrospinal fluid. [glyco- + G. *rhachis,* spine]

**gly·cor·rhea** (glī-kō-rē′ă) a discharge of sugar from the body, as in glucosuria, especially in unusually large quantities. [glyco- + G. *rhoia,* a flow]

**gly·co·se·cre·to·ry** (glī′kō-sē-krē′tō-rē) causing or involved in the secretion of glycogen.

**gly·co·si·a·lia** (glī′kō-sī-al′ē-ă, glī′kō-sī-ā′lē-ă) the presence of sugar in the saliva. SYN glycoptyalism. [glyco- + G. *sialon,* saliva]

**gly·co·si·a·lor·rhea** (glī′kō-sī′ă-lō-rē′ă) an excessive secretion of saliva that contains sugar. [glyco- + G. *sialon,* saliva, + *rhoia,* a flow]

**gly·co·side** (glī′kō-sīd) condensation product of a sugar with any other radical involving the loss of the H of the hemiacetal or hemiketal OH of the sugar, leaving the O of this OH as the link.

**gly·co·sphing·o·lip·id** (glī′kō-sfing-gō-lip′id) a ceramide linked to one or more sugars via the terminal OH group; included as glycosphingolipids are cerebrosides, gangliosides, and ceramide oligosaccharides (oligoglycosylceramides). The prefix glyc- may be replaced by gluc-, galact-, lact-, etc.

**gly·co·stat·ic** (glī-kō-stat′ik) indicating the property of certain extracts of the anterior hypophysis that permits the body to maintain its glycogen stores in muscle, liver, and other tissues.

**gly·cos·ur·ia** (glī-kōs-yur′ē-ă) 1. SYN glucosuria. 2. urinary excretion of carbohydrates. SYN glycuresis (2). [glyco- + G. *ouron,* urine]

**gly·co·syl** (glī′kō-sil) the radical resulting from detachment of the OH of the hemiacetal or hemiketal of a saccharide. Cf. glycoside.

**gly·co·syl·at·ed he·mo·glo·bin** any one of four hemoglobin A fractions ($A_{Ia1}$, $A_{Ia2}$, $A_{Ib}$, or $A_{Ic}$) to which D-glucose and related monosaccharides bind; concentrations are increased in the erythrocytes of patients with diabetes mellitus and can be used as a retrospective index of glucose control over time in such patients.

**gly·co·sy·la·tion** (glī′kō-si-lā′shŭn) formation of linkages with glycosyl groups, as between D-glucose and the hemoglobin chain to form the frac-

g
l

tion hemoglobin $A_{Ic}$, whose level rises in association with the raised blood D-glucose concentration in poorly controlled or uncontrolled diabetes mellitus. SEE ALSO glycosylated hemoglobin.

**gly·co·syl·trans·fer·ase** (glī'kō-sil-trans'fer-ās) any enzyme (EC subclass 2.4) transferring glycosyl groups from one compound to another.

**gly·co·tro·pic fac·tor** a principle in extracts of the anterior lobe of the hypophysis that raises the blood sugar and antagonizes the action of insulin; purified pituitary growth hormone produces an identical effect. SYN insulin-antagonizing factor.

**glyc·u·re·sis** (glī-kyu-rē'sis) **1.** SYN glucosuria. **2.** SYN glycosuria (2). [glyco- + G. *ourēsis*, urination]

**gly·cu·ron·ate** (glī-kyur'on-āt) a salt or ester of a glycuronic acid.

**glyc·yl (Gly)** (glī'sil) the acyl radical of glycine.

**GM-CSF** granulocyte-macrophage colony-stimulating factor.

**GMP** guanylic acid.

**gnat** (nat) a midge; general term applied to several species of minute insects, including species of *Simulium* (buffalo gnat) and *Hippelates* (eye gnat). [A.S. *gnaet*]

**gnath·ic** (nath'ik) relating to the jaw or alveolar process. [G. *gnathos*, jaw]

**gnath·i·on** (nath'ē-on) the most inferior point of the mandible in the midline. In cephalometrics, it is the midpoint between the most anterior and inferior point on the bony chin, measured at the intersection of the mandibular baseline and the nasion-pogonion line. [G. *gnathos*, jaw]

△**gnatho-, gnath-** the jaw. [G. *gnathos*]

**gnath·o·dy·nam·ics** (nath'ō-dī-nam'iks) the study of the relationship of the magnitude and direction of the forces developed by and upon the components of the masticatory system during function. [gnatho- + G. *dynamis*, power]

**gnath·o·dy·na·mom·e·ter** (nath'ō-dī-nă-mom'ĕ-ter) a device for measuring biting pressure. [gnatho- + dynamometer]

**gnath·o·log·ic·al** (nath-ō-loj'i-kăl) pertaining to gnathodynamics.

**gnath·o·plas·ty** (nath'ō-plas-tē) plastic surgery of the jaw. [gnatho- + G. *plastos*, formed]

*Gna·thos·to·ma* (nă-thos'tō-mă) a genus of spiruroid nematode worms (family Gnathostomatidae) characterized by several rows of cuticular spines about the head and by multiple-host aquatic life cycles; it includes pathogenic parasites of cats, cattle, and swine. [gnatho- + G. *stoma*, mouth]

**gno·sia** (nō'sē-ă) the perceptive faculty enabling one to recognize the form and the nature of persons and things; the faculty of perceiving and recognizing. [G. *gnōsis*, knowledge]

**gno·to·bi·ol·o·gy** (nō'tō-bī-ol'ō-jē) the study of animals in the absence of contaminating microorganisms; i.e., of "germ-free" animals. [G. *gnotos*, known, + *bios*, life, + *logos*, study]

**gno·to·bi·o·ta** (nō'tō-bī-ō'tă) living colonies or species, assembled from pure isolates. [G. *gnotos*, known, + Mod. L. *biota*, fr. G. *bios*, life]

**gno·to·bi·ot·ic** (nō'tō-bī-ot'ik) denoting germ-free or formerly germ-free organisms in which the composition of any associated microbial flora, if present, is fully defined. [see gnotobiota]

**GnRH** gonadotropin-releasing hormone.

**gob·let cell** an epithelial cell that becomes distended with a large accumulation of mucous se-

cretory granules at its apical end, giving it the appearance of a goblet. SYN beaker cell.

**Gog·gia sign** (gō'jē-ah) the fibrillation of the biceps muscle, when pinched and tapped, is confined to a limited area in cases of debilitating disease, whereas in health it is general.

**goi·ter** (goy'ter) a chronic enlargement of the thyroid gland, not due to a neoplasm, occurring endemically in certain localities, especially regions where glaciation occurred and the soil is low in iodine, and sporadically elsewhere. SYN struma. [Fr. from L. *guttur*, throat]

**goi·tre [Br.]** SEE goiter.

**goi·tro·gen·ic** (goy-trō-jen'ik) causing goiter.

**goi·trous** (goy'trŭs) denoting or characteristic of a goiter.

**gold (Au)** a yellow metallic element, atomic no. 79, atomic wt. 196.96654; [198]Au (half-life of 2.694 days) is used in the treatment of certain tumors and in imaging. SYN aurum.

**Gold·blatt hy·per·ten·sion** (gōld'blat) increased blood pressure following obstruction of blood flow to one kidney.

**Gold·blatt kid·ney** (gōld'blat) a kidney whose arterial blood supply has been compromised, as a consequence of which arterial (renovascular) hypertension develops.

**gol·den hour** term used to describe the maximum amount of time from injury to definitive care for a trauma victim.

**Gold·flam dis·ease** (gōlt'flahm) SYN myasthenia gravis.

**Gold·mann ap·pla·na·tion to·nom·e·ter** (gōld'mahn) an applanation tonometer that flattens only 3 mm$^2$ of cornea, used with a slitlamp.

**Gold·mann-Fa·vre syn·drome** (gōld'mahn fahv'rĕ) an autosomal recessive, progressive vitreotapetoretinal degeneration.

**Gold·schei·der test** (gōlt'shī-dĕr) determination of the temperature sense by touching the skin with a sharp-pointed metallic rod heated to varying degrees.

**Gold·stein toe sign** (gōld'stīn) increased space between the great toe and its neighbor, seen in Down syndrome, occasionally in cretinism, and as a normal variant.

**Gol·gi ap·pa·ra·tus** (gōl'jē) a membranous system of cisternae and vesicles located between the nucleus and the secretory pole or surface of a cell; concerned with the investment and intracellular transport of membrane-bounded secretory proteins.

**Gol·gi cells** (gōl'jē) SEE Golgi type I neuron, Golgi type II neuron.

**Gol·gi-Maz·zo·ni cor·pus·cle** (gōl'jē mats'zō'nē) an encapsulated sensory nerve ending similar to a pacinian corpuscle but simpler in structure.

**Gol·gi os·mi·o·bi·chro·mate fix·a·tive** (gōl'jē) an osmic-bichromate mixture used to demonstrate nerve cells and their processes.

**Gol·gi stain** (gōl'jē) any of several methods for staining nerve cells, nerve fibers, and neuroglia using fixation and hardening in formalin-osmic-dichromate combinations for various times, followed by impregnation in silver nitrate.

**Gol·gi ten·don or·gan** (gōl'jē) a proprioceptive sensory nerve ending embedded among the fibers of a tendon, often near the musculotendinous junction; it is activated by any increase of tension in the tendon, caused either by active contraction or passive stretch of the corresponding muscle. SYN neurotendinous spindle.

**Gol·gi type I neu·ron** (gōl′jē) nerve cells whose long axons leave the gray matter of which they form a part.

**Gol·gi type II neu·ron** (gōl′jē) nerve cells with short axons which ramify in the gray matter.

**gom·i·to·li** (gō-mē′tō-lē) intricately coiled and looped capillary vessels present largely in the upper infundibular stem of the stalk of the pituitary gland; they make up a portion of the pituitary portal circulation. [It. *gomitolo,* coil]

**Go·mo·ri al·de·hyde fuch·sin stain** (gō-mō′rē) a stain used to demonstrate beta cells of the pancreas, storage form of thyrotrophic hormone in beta cells of the anterior pituitary, hypophysial neurosecretory substance, mast cells, granules, elastic fibers, sulfated mucins, and gastric chief cells.

**Go·mo·ri chrome al·um he·ma·tox·y·lin-phlox·ine stain** (gō-mō′rē) a technique used to demonstrate cytoplasmic granules, after Bouin or formalin-Zenker fixatives, using oxidized hematoxylin plus phloxine; in the pancreas, beta cells are blue, alpha and delta cells are red, and zymogen granules are red to unstained; in the pituitary, alpha cells are pink, beta cells and chromophobes are gray-blue, and nuclei are purple to blue.

**Go·mo·ri meth·en·a·mine-sil·ver stain** (gō-mō′rē) techniques for 1) *argentaffin cells:* a method using a methenamine-silver solution in combination with gold chloride, sodium thiosulfate, and safranin O; argentaffin granules appear brown-black against a green background; 2) *urates:* warm sections are treated directly with a hot methenamine-silver solution to produce a blackening of urates; 3) *fungi:* see Grocott-Gomori methenamine-silver stain; 4) *melanin,* which reduces silver nitrate.

**Go·mo·ri non·spe·cif·ic ac·id phos·pha·tase stain** (gō-mō′rē) a method in which formalin-fixed frozen sections are incubated in a substrate containing sodium β-glycerophosphate and lead nitrate at pH 5.0; the insoluble lead phosphate produced is treated with ammonium sulfide to give a black lead sulfide.

**Go·mo·ri non·spe·cif·ic al·ka·line phos·pha·tase stain** (gō-mō′rē) a calcium-cobalt sulfide method using frozen sections or cold acetone- or formalin-fixed paraffin sections, plus sodium β-glycerophosphate as a substrate at pH 9.0–9.5 with Mg$^{2+}$ as activator; calcium ions precipitate the liberated phosphate, cobalt salt replaces the calcium phosphate, and ammonium sulfide converts the product to a black cobalt sulfide.

**Go·mo·ri one-step tri·chrome stain** (gō-mō′rē) a connective tissue stain that uses hematoxylin and a dye mixture containing chromotrope 2R and light green or aniline blue; muscle fibers appear red, collagen is green (or blue if aniline blue is used), and nuclei are blue to black.

**Go·mo·ri sil·ver im·preg·na·tion stain** (gō-mō′rē) a reliable method for reticulin, as an aid in the diagnosis of neoplasm and early cirrhosis of the liver; the staining solution employs silver nitrate, potassium hydroxide, and ammonia water carefully prepared to avoid having silver precipitate.

**Gom·pertz law** (gom′pĕrtz) the proportional relationship of mortality to age; after age 35–40, the increase in mortality with age tends to be logarithmic.

**gom·pho·sis** (gom-fō′sis) [TA] a form of fibrous joint in which a peglike process fits into a hole, as the root of a tooth into the socket in the alveolus. [G. *gomphos,* bolt, nail, + *-osis,* condition]

**go·nad** (gō′nad) an organ that produces sex cells; a testis or an ovary. [Mod. L. fr. G. *gonē,* seed]

**go·nad·al** (gō-nad′ăl) relating to a gonad.

**go·nad·al cords** columns of germinal and follicle cells penetrating centripetally into the embryonic ovarian or testicular cortex.

**go·nad·al dys·gen·e·sis** defective gonadal development; types include gonadal aplasia or agenesis, rudimentary gonads, congenitally defective gonads, and true hermaphroditism.

**go·nad·al ridge** an elevation of thickened mesothelium and underlying mesenchyme on the ventromedial border of the embryonic mesonephros; the primordial germ cells become embedded in it, establishing it as the primordium of the testis or ovary.

**go·nad·ec·to·my** (gō-nad-ek′tō-mē) excision of ovary or testis. [gonado- + G. *ektomē,* excision]

△**gonado-, gonad-** the gonads. [G. *gonē,* seed]

**go·nad·o·blas·to·ma** (gō-nad-ō-blas-tō′ma) benign neoplasm composed of germ cells, sex cord, stromal cells; appears in cases of mixed or pure gonadal dysgenesis; usually small (1–3 cm) and partially calcified, but may give rise to malignant germ-cell tumors, most often seminoma/dysgerminoma or embryonal.

**go·nad·o·crins** (gō-nad′ō-krinz) peptides that stimulate release of both follicle-stimulating hormone and luteinizing hormone from the pituitary; found in ovarian follicular fluid in rats. [gonad + G. *krinō,* to secrete]

**go·nad·o·lib·er·in** (gō′nad-ō-lib′er-in) 1. a hypothalamic substance causing the release of gonadotropin. SYN gonadotropin-releasing factor, gonadotropin-releasing hormone. 2. a decapeptide from pig hypothalami that induces release of both lutropin and follitropin in constant proportions and thus acts as both luliberin and folliberin. SYN luteinizing hormone/follicle-stimulating hormone-releasing factor. [gonad + L. *libero,* to free, + -in]

**gon·a·dop·athy** (gon-ă-dop′ă-thē) disease affecting the gonads. [gonado- + G. *pathos,* suffering]

**go·nad·o·rel·in hy·dro·chlo·ride** (gō-nad-ō-rel′ in hī-drō-klor-īd) a gonadotropin-releasing hormone obtained from sheep, pigs, or other animals and used to evaluate the functional capacity of the gonadotrophs of the anterior pituitary. [*go-nado*tropin-*rele*asing + -in]

**go·nad·o·troph** (gō-nad′ō-trōf, gon′ă-dō-trōf) an endocrine cell of the adenohypophysis that affects certain cells of the ovary or testis.

**go·nad·o·tro·phic** (gō′nad-o-trōf′ik, gon′ă-dō-trōf′ik) SYN gonadotropic. [gonado- + G. *trophē,* nourishment]

**go·nad·o·tro·phin** (gō′nad-ō-trō′fin, gon′ă-dō-trō′fin) SYN gonadotropin (1).

**go·nad·o·tro·pic** (gō′nad-ō-trōp′ik, gon′ă-dō-trōp′ik) 1. descriptive of or relating to the actions of a gonadotropin. 2. promoting the growth and/or function of the gonads. SYN gonadotrophic. [gonado- + G. *tropē,* a turning]

**go·nad·o·tro·pin, go·nad·o·tro·pic hor·mone** (gō′nad-ō-trō′pin) 1. a hormone capable of promoting gonadal growth and function; such ef-

g
0

fects, as exerted by a single hormone, usually are limited to discrete functions or histologic components of a gonad, such as stimulation of follicular growth or of androgen formation; most gonadotropins exert their effects in both sexes, although the effect of a given gonadotropin will differ in males and females. SYN gonadotrophin. **2.** any hormone that stimulates gonadal function. **3.** any substance that has the combined effects of follicle-stimulating hormone and luteinizing hormone.

**go·nad·o·tro·pin-re·leas·ing fac·tor** SYN gonadoliberin (1).

**go·nad·o·tro·pin-re·leas·ing hor·mone (GnRH)** SYN gonadoliberin (1).

**gon·a·duct** (gon'ă-dŭkt) **1.** SYN seminal duct. **2.** SYN uterine tube. [gonado- + duct]

**go·nal·gia** (gō-nal'jē-ă) pain in the knee. [G. *gony,* knee, + *algos,* pain]

**gon·an·gi·ec·to·my** (gon-an-jē-ek'tō-mē) SYN vasectomy. [G. *gonē,* seed. + *angeion,* vessel, + *ektome,* excision, + -y]

**gon·ar·thri·tis** (gon-ar-thrī'tis) inflammation of the knee joint. [G. *gony,* knee, + *arthron,* joint, + -*itis,* inflammation]

**gon·ar·throt·o·my** (gon-ar-throt'ō-mē) incision into the knee joint. [G. *gony,* knee, + *arthron,* joint, + *tomē,* incision]

**gon·e·cyst, gon·e·cys·tis** (gon'ĕ-sist, gon-ĕ-sis' tis) SYN seminal vesicle. [G. *gonē,* seed, + *kystis,* bladder]

**go·nia** (gō'nē-ă) plural of gonion.

△**go·nio-** angle. [G. *gōnia*]

**go·ni·om·e·ter** (gō-nē-om'ĕ-ter) **1.** an instrument for measuring angles. **2.** an appliance for the static test of labyrinthine disease, which consists of a plank, one end of which may be raised to any desired height; as one end of the plank is gradually raised, the point at which a patient loses balance is noted. **3.** a calibrated device designed to measure the arc or range of motion of a joint. SYN arthrometer, flexometer. [G. *gōnia,* angle, + *metron,* measure]

**go·ni·om·e·tre [Br.]** SEE goniometer.

**go·ni·on,** pl. **go·nia** (gō'nē-on, gō'nē-ă) [TA] the lowest posterior and most outward point of the angle of the mandible. In cephalometrics, it is measured by bisecting the angle formed by the tangents to the lower and the posterior borders of the mandible; when the angles of both sides of the mandible appear on the lateral radiograph, a point midway between the right and left side is used. [G. *gōnia,* an angle]

**go·ni·o·punc·ture** (gō'nē-ō-pŭnk-cher) an operation for congenital glaucoma in which a puncture is made in the filtration angle of the anterior chamber.

**go·ni·o·scope** (gō'nē-ō-skōp) a lens designed to study the angle of the anterior chamber of the eye. [G. *gōnia,* angle, + *skopeō,* to examine]

**go·ni·os·co·py** (gō-nē-os'kŏ-pē) examination of the angle of the anterior chamber of the eye with a gonioscope or with a contact prism lens.

**go·ni·o·syn·ech·ia** (gō'nē-ō-si-nek'ē-ă) adhesion of the iris to the posterior surface of the cornea in the angle of the anterior chamber; associated with angle-closure glaucoma. [G. *gōnia,* angle, + *synechis,* holding together]

**go·ni·ot·o·my** (gō-nē-ot'ō-mē) surgical opening of the trabecular meshwork in congenital glaucoma. [G. *gōnia,* angle, + *tomē,* incision]

**gon·o·cele** (gon'ō-sēl) a cystic lesion of the epididymis or rete testis, resulting from obstruction and containing secretions from the testis. [G. *gonē,* seed, + *kēlē,* tumor]

**go·no·coc·cae·mia [Br.]** SEE gonococcemia.

**gon·o·coc·cal** (gon'ō-kok'ăl) relating to the gonococcus. SYN gonococcic.

**gon·o·coc·cal ar·thri·tis** joint space infection in humans caused by disseminated *Neisseria gonorrhoeae;* characteristically monarticular, but may be polyarticular.

**gon·o·coc·cal con·junc·ti·vi·tis** a type of hyperacute, purulent conjunctivitis.

**gon·o·coc·ce·mia** (gon'ō-kok-sē'mē-ă) the presence of gonococci in the circulating blood. [gonococcus + G. *haima,* blood]

**gon·o·coc·cic** (gon'ō-kok'sik) SYN gonococcal.

**gon·o·coc·cus,** pl. **gon·o·coc·ci** (gon-ō-kok'ŭs, gon-ō-kok'sī) SYN *Neisseria gonorrhoeae.* See page B3. [G. *gonē,* seed, + *kokkos,* berry]

**gon·o·phore, gon·oph·o·rus** (gon'ō-fōr, gō-nof' ŏ-rŭs) any structure serving to store up or conduct the sexual cells; oviduct, spermatic duct, uterus, or seminal vesicle; an accessory generative organ. [G. *gonē,* seed, + *phoros,* bearing]

**gon·or·rhea** (gon-ō-rē'ă) a contagious catarrhal inflammation of the genital mucous membrane, transmitted chiefly by coitus and due to *Neisseria gonorrhoeae;* may involve the lower or upper genital tract, especially the urethra, endocervix, and uterine tubes, or spread to the peritoneum and rarely to the heart, joints, or other structures by way of the bloodstream. [G. *gonorrhoia,* fr. *gonē,* seed, + *rhoia,* a flow]

**gon·or·rhe·al** (gon-ō-rē'ăl) relating to gonorrhea.

**gon·or·rhe·al oph·thal·mia** acute purulent conjunctivitis due to *Neisseria gonorrhoeae.*

**go·nor·rhoea [Br.]** SEE gonorrhea.

**gon·or·rhoe·al [Br.]** SEE gonorrheal.

**go·ny·camp·sis** (gon-ē-kamp'sis) ankylosis or any abnormal curvature of the knee. [G. *gony,* knee, + *kampsis,* a bending or curving]

**Good·ell sign** (gud'el) softening of the cervix and vagina as being usually indicative of pregnancy.

**Good·e·nough draw-a-man test** (gud-ĕ-nuf') a brief test for assessing an individual's level of intelligence based on how accurately drawn and how many elements are included when a child or adult is given a pencil and sheet of white paper and asked to draw a man. Also called the Goodenough draw-a-person test and, in its current form, the Goodenough-Harris drawing test.

**Good·pas·ture stain** (gud'pas-cher) a stain for Gram-negative bacteria, using aniline fuchsin.

**Good·pas·ture syn·drome** (gud'pas-cher) glomerulonephritis of the anti-basement membrane type associated with or preceded by hemoptysis; the nephritis usually progresses rapidly to produce death from renal failure, and the lungs at autopsy show extensive hemosiderosis or recent hemorrhage.

**Gop·a·lan syn·drome** (gō'pah-lahn) severe discomfort of the feet associated with elevated skin temperature and excessive sweating.

**gor·get** (gōr'jet) a director or guide with wide groove for use in lithotomy.

**Gor·lin sign** (gōr'lin) unusual ease in touching the tip of the nose with the tongue; seen in Ehlers-Danlos syndrome.

**Gor·lin syn·drome** (gōr'lin) SYN basal cell nevus syndrome.

**gos·er·e·lin** (gos'er-ĕ-lin) a synthetic decapeptide agonist analogue of the LHRH (GnRH). It inhibits pituitary gonadotropin secretion and is used in the treatment of prostate cancer, breast cancer, endometriosis, and for thinning the endometrium before endometrial ablation or resection.

**Gos·se·lin frac·ture** (gos-la') v-shaped fracture of distal end of tibia.

**GOT** glutamic-oxaloacetic transaminase.

**gouge** (gowj) a strong, curved chisel used in operations on bone.

**Gould su·ture** (goold) an intestinal mattress suture in which each loop is invaginated in such a way that the tissue at the loop is bulged out, becoming convex instead of concave.

**Gou·ley cath·e·ter** (goo'lē) a solid curved steel instrument grooved on its inferior surface so that it can be passed over a guide through a urethral stricture.

**gout** (gowt) a disorder of purine metabolism, occurring especially in men, characterized by a raised but variable blood uric acid level and severe recurrent acute arthritis of sudden onset resulting from deposition of crystals of sodium urate in connective tissues and articular cartilage; most cases are inherited, resulting from a variety of abnormalities of purine metabolism. See this page. [L. *gutta,* drop]

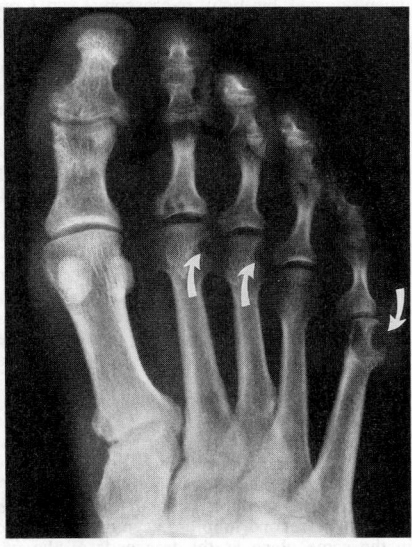

**gout:** detailed view of foot shows para-articular punched out lesions in the distal metatarsals (white arrows)

**gou·ty** (gow'tē) relating to or characteristic of gout.

**gou·ty ar·thri·tis** inflammation of the joints in gout.

**gou·ty to·phus** a deposit of uric acid and urates in periarticular fibrous tissue, cartilage of the external ear, or kidney, in gout.

**Gow·ers syn·drome** (gow'ĕrz) syndrome consisting of palpitation, chest pain, respiratory difficulties, and disturbances in gastric motility; once attributed to vagal stimulation, now considered psychogenic (anxiety neurosis).

**Gow·ers tract** (gow'ĕrz) SYN anterior spinocerebellar tract.

**GPI** Gingival-Periodontal Index.

**G protein dis·eases** a widely variant group of diseases resulting from mutations in G proteins; these include endocine adenomas, cholera, and nightblindness.

**GPT** glutamic-pyruvic transaminase.

**gr** grain (3).

**graaf·i·an fol·li·cle** (grah'fē-ăn) SYN vesicular ovarian follicle.

**grac·ile fas·cic·u·lus** the smaller medial subdivision of the posterior funiculus.

**gra·cile lob·ule** the anterior portion of the posteroinferior lobule of the cerebellum, the posterior portion being the semilunar lobule inferior; the two are continuous with the tuber of the vermis. SYN lobulus paramedianus [TA].

**grac·ile nu·cle·us** the medial one of the three nuclei of the dorsal column, the other two being the cuneate nucleus and the accessory cuneate nucleus, which corresponds to the clava; it receives dorsal-root fibers conveying sensory innervation of the leg, and lower trunk, and projects, by way of the medial lemniscus, to the ventral nucleus posterior nucleus of the thalamus.

**grac·i·lis mus·cle** *origin,* ramus of pubis near symphysis; *insertion,* shaft of tibia below medial tuberosity (see pes anserinus); *action,* adducts thigh, flexes knee, rotates leg medially; *nerve supply,* obturator. SYN musculus gracilis [TA].

**grade** (grād) 1. a rank, division, or level on the scale of a value system. 2. in cancer pathology, a classification of the degree of malignancy or differentiation of tumor tissue; e.g., well, moderately well, or poorly differentiated, and undifferentiated or anaplastic. 3. in exercise testing, the measurement of a vertical rise or fall as a percent of the horizontal distance traveled. [L. *gradus,* step]

**gra·ded ex·er·cise test (GXT)** multistage exercise testing (usually on treadmill or bicycle ergometer) in which exercise intensity is progressively increased (graded) through levels that bring the test subject to a self-imposed fatigue level.

**grade I as·tro·cy·to·ma** solid or cystic astrocytoma of high differentiation or low grade.

**grade II as·tro·cy·to·ma** astrocytoma of low to intermediate grade.

**grade III as·tro·cy·to·ma** astrocytoma of intermediate grade. SEE ALSO glioblastoma multiforme.

**grade IV as·tro·cy·to·ma** SYN glioblastoma multiforme.

**Gra·de·ni·go syn·drome** (grah-dĕ-nē'gō) a syndrome consisting of otorrhea, headache, diplopia, and retroorbital pain in petrositis due to an epidural abscess at the apex of the anterior surface of the petrous pyramid causing compression of the abducens nerve in Dorello canal and irritation of the trigeminal ganglion.

**gra·di·ent** (grā'dē-ent) rate of change of temperature, pressure, or other variable as a function of distance, time, etc.

**grad·i·ent-re·called ac·qui·si·tion in the stea·dy state (GRASS)** a type of gradient echo sequence with free induction decay sampling in magnetic resonance imaging; also called "fast imaging with steady-state precession." This family of sequences is faster than spin echo techniques, and is used for magnetic resonance angiography and cardiac imaging.

**grad·u·at·ed** (grad′yu-āt′ed) **1.** marked by lines or in other ways to denote capacity, degrees, percentages, etc. **2.** divided or arranged in levels, grades, or successive steps.

**grad·u·at·ed te·not·o·my** partial incisions of the tendon of an eye muscle for correction of strabismus.

**Grae·fe knife** (grā′fĕ) a narrow-bladed knife used in making a section of the cornea.

**Grae·fe op·er·a·tion** (grā′fĕ) **1.** removal of cataract by a limbal incision with capsulotomy and iridectomy. Both operations were landmarks in the field of ophthalmic surgery; **2.** iridectomy for glaucoma.

**Grae·fe sign** (grā′fĕ) in Grave disease, lag of the upper eyelid as it follows the rotation of the eyeball downward. SYN von Graefe sign.

**Graf·fi vi·rus** (grah′fē) a type C mouse myeloleukemia virus from filtrates of transplantable tumors; possibly related to Gross virus.

**graft 1.** any free (unattached) tissue or organ for transplantation. **2.** to transplant such structures. SEE ALSO flap, implant, transplant. [A.S. *graef*]

**graft ver·sus host dis·ease** an incompatibility reaction (which may be fatal) in a subject (host) of low immunological competence (deficient lymphoid tissue) who has been the recipient of immunologically competent lymphoid tissue from a donor who lacks at least one antigen possessed by the recipient host; the reaction, or disease, is the result of action of the transplanted cells against those host tissues that possess the antigen not possessed by the donor.

**graft ver·sus host re·ac·tion (GVHR)** clinical and histologic changes of graft versus host disease occurring in a specific organ.

**Gra·ham law** (grā′ăm) the relative rapidity of diffusion of two gases varies inversely as the square root of their densities, i.e., their molecular weights.

**Gra·ham Steell mur·mur** (grā′ăm stēl) an early diastolic murmur of pulmonic insufficiency secondary to pulmonary hypertension, as in mitral stenosis and various congenital defects associated with pulmonary hypertension. SYN Steell murmur.

**grain** (grān) **1.** cereal plants, such as corn, wheat, or rye, or a seed of one of them. **2.** a minute, hard particle of any substance, as of sand. **3. (gr)** a unit of weight, $\frac{1}{60}$ dram (apoth. or troy), $\frac{1}{437.5}$ avoirdupois ounce, $\frac{1}{480}$ troy ounce, $\frac{1}{5760}$ troy pound, $\frac{1}{7000}$ avoirdupois pound; the equivalent of 0.064799 gram. [L. *granum*]

**Gram** (grahm), Hans C.J., Danish bacteriologist, 1853–1938. SEE Gram stain.

**gram (g)** a unit of weight in the metric or centesimal system, the equivalent of 15.432358 grains or 0.03527 avoirdupois ounce.

△-**gram** a recording, usually by an instrument. Cf. -graph. [G. *gramma*, character, mark]

**gram cal·o·rie** SYN small calorie.

**gram-cen·ti·me·ter** the energy exerted, or work done, when a mass of 1 g is raised a height of 1 cm; equal to $9.807 \times 10^{-5}$ joules or newton-meters.

**Gram-chro·mo·trope stain** (gram) a modified

trichrome stain for microsporidian spores that combines Gram-stain reagents in the procedure.

**gram e·qui·va·lent 1.** the weight in grams of an element that combines with or replaces 1 gram of hydrogen; **2.** the atomic or molecular weight in grams of an atom or group of atoms involved in a chemical reaction divided by the number of electrons donated, taken up, or shared by the atom or group of atoms in the course of that reaction; **3.** the weight of a substance contained in 1 liter of 1 normal solution; a variant of (1). SYN equivalent (5).

**Gram i·o·dine** (gram) a solution containing iodine and potassium iodide, used in Gram stain.

**gram-i·on** the weight in grams of an ion that is equal to the sum of the atomic weights of the atoms making up the ion.

**gram-me·ter** a unit of energy equal to 100 gram-centimeters.

**gram-mol·e·cule** the amount of a substance with a mass in grams equal to its molecular weight; e.g., a gram-molecule of hydrogen weighs 2.016 g, that of water 18.015 g.

**Gram-neg·a·tive** (gram) refers to the inability of a bacterium to resist decolorization with alcohol after being treated with Gram crystal violet. However, following decolorization, these bacteria can be readily counterstained with safranin, imparting a pink or red color to the bacterium when viewed by light microscopy. SEE Gram stain.

**Gram-pos·i·tive** (gram) refers to the ability of a bacterium to resist decolorization with alcohol after being treated with Gram crystal violet stain, imparting a violet color to the bacterium when viewed by light microscopy. SEE Gram stain.

**Gram stain** (gram) a method for differential staining of bacteria; smears are fixed by flaming, stained in a solution of crystal violet, treated with iodine solution, rinsed, decolorized, and then counterstained with safranin O; Gram-positive organisms stain purple-black and Gram-negative organisms stain pink; useful in bacterial taxonomy and identification, and also in indicating fundamental differences in cell wall structure.

**grand·daugh·ter cyst** a tertiary cyst sometimes developed within a daughter cyst, as in the hydatid cyst of *Echinococcus*.

**grand mal** (grahn mahl) SYN generalized tonic-clonic seizure.

**Gran·ger line** (grān′jĕr) on lateral skull radiographs, the line produced by the groove of the optic chiasm or sulcus prechiasmaticus.

**gran·ny knot** a double knot in which the free ends of the second loop are asymmetric and not in the same plane as the free ends of the first loop.

**gran·u·lar** (gran′yu-lăr) **1.** composed of or resembling granules or granulations. **2.** particles with strong affinity for nuclear stains, seen in many bacterial species.

**gran·u·lar cell tu·mor** a microscopically specific, generally benign tumor, often involving peripheral nerves in skin, mucosa, or connective tissue, derived from Schwann cells; the abundant cytoplasm contains lysosomal granules, the cells infiltrate between adjacent tissues although growth is slow, and adjacent surface epithelium may show hyperplasia.

**gran·u·lar con·junc·ti·vi·tis** SYN trachomatous conjunctivitis.

**gran·u·lar cor·ne·al dys·tro·phy** an autosomal dominant disorder characterized by hyaline deposits in the corneal stroma.

**gran·u·lar cor·tex** SEE cerebral cortex.

**gran·u·lar en·do·plas·mic re·tic·u·lum** endoplasmic reticulum in which ribosomal granules are applied to the cytoplasmic surface of the cisternae; involved in the synthesis and secretion of protein via membrane-bound vesicles to the extracellular space. SYN ergastoplasm.

**gran·u·lar leu·ko·cyte** any one of the polymorphonuclear leukocytes, especially a neutrophilic leukocyte. SEE ALSO granulocyte, basophilic leukocyte, eosinophilic leukocyte.

**gran·u·lar oph·thal·mia** SYN trachoma.

**gran·u·lar pits** pits on the inner surface of the skull, along the course of the superior sagittal sinus, in which are lodged the arachnoidal granulations.

**gra·nu·la·tio**, pl. **gran·u·la·ti·o·nes** (gran-yu-lā′shē-ō, gran-yu-lā′-shē-o′nēz) SYN granulation. [L.]

**gran·u·la·tion** (gran′yu-lā′shŭn) **1.** formation into grains or granules; the state of being granular. **2.** a granular mass in or on the surface of any organ or membrane; or one of the individual granules forming the mass. **3.** the formation of minute, rounded, fleshy connective tissue projections on the surface of a wound, ulcer, or inflamed tissue surface during healing; one of the fleshy granules composing this surface. SEE ALSO granulation tissue. **4.** PHARMACY the formation of crystals by constant agitation of a supersaturated solution of a salt. SYN granulatio. [L. *granulatio*]

**gran·u·la·ti·o·nes ar·ach·noi·de·a·les** [TA] SYN arachnoid granulations. SEE ALSO arachnoid villi.

**gran·u·la·tion tis·sue** vascular connective tissue forming granular projections on the surface of a healing wound, ulcer, or inflamed surface. SEE ALSO granulation.

**gran·ule** (gran′yul) **1.** a grainlike particle; a granulation; a minute discrete mass. **2.** a very small pill, usually gelatin or sugar coated, containing a drug to be given in a small dose. **3.** a colony of the bacterium or fungus causing a disease or simply colonizing the tissues of the patient. In immunocompromised patients the differentiation is difficult. **4.** a small particle that can be seen by electron microscopy; contains stored material. [L. *granulum*, dim. of *granum*, grain]

**gran·ule cells 1.** small nerve cell bodies in the external and internal granular layers of the cerebral cortex; **2.** small nerve cell bodies in the granular layer of the cerebellar cortex.

⌂**gran·u·lo-** granular, granules. [L. *granulum*, a small grain.]

**gran·u·lo·cyte** (gran′yu-lō-sīt) a mature granular leukocyte, including neutrophilic, acidophilic, and basophilic types of polymorphonuclear leukocytes, i.e., respectively, neutrophils, eosinophils, and basophils. [granulo- + G. *kytos*, cell]

**gran·u·lo·cyte col·o·ny-stim·u·lat·ing fac·tor (G-CSF)** glycoproteins that are synthesized by a variety of cells and are involved in growth and differentiation of hematopoietic stem cells. SEE ALSO colony-stimulating factors.

**gran·u·lo·cyte-mac·ro·phage col·o·ny-stim·u·lat·ing fac·tor (GM-CSF)** a glycoprotein secreted by macrophages or bone stromal cells that functions as a growth factor for myeloid progeni-

tor cells such as granulocytes, macrophages, and eosinophils. SEE ALSO colony-stimulating factors.

**gran·u·lo·cyt·ic leu·ke·mia** a form of leukemia characterized by an uncontrolled proliferation of myelopoietic cells in the bone marrow and in extramedullary sites, and the presence of large numbers of immature and mature granulocytic forms in various tissues (and organs) and in the circulating blood. The predominant cell is usually of the neutrophilic series, but, in a few instances, eosinophilic or basophilic granulocytes, or even megakaryocytes, may represent the chief form. SYN myelocytic leukemia, myelogenic leukemia, myelogenous leukemia, myeloid leukemia.

**gran·u·lo·cyt·ic sar·co·ma** a malignant tumor of immature myeloid cells, frequently subperiosteal, associated with or preceding granulocytic leukemia. SEE ALSO chloroma. SYN myeloid sarcoma.

**gran·u·lo·cyt·ic se·ries** the cells in the several stages of development in the bone marrow leading to the mature granulocyte of the circulation, e.g., myeloblasts, different stages of the myelocyte, granulocytes.

**gran·u·lo·cy·to·pe·nia** (gran′yu-lō-sī-tō-pē′nē-ă) less than the normal number of granular leukocytes in the blood. SYN granulopenia. [granulocyte + G. *penia*, poverty]

**gran·u·lo·cy·to·poi·e·sis** (gran′yu-lō-sī′tō-poy-ē′sis) SYN granulopoiesis.

**gran·u·lo·cy·to·poi·et·ic** (gran′yu-lō-sī′tō-poy-et′ik) SYN granulopoietic. [granulocyte + G. *poieō*, to make]

**gran·u·lo·cy·to·sis** (gran′yu-lō-sī-tō′sis) a condition characterized by more than the normal number of granulocytes in the circulating blood or in the tissues.

**gran·u·lo·ma** (gran-yu-lō′mă) term applied to nodular inflammatory lesions, usually small or granular, firm, persistent, and containing compactly grouped modified phagocytes such as epithelioid cells, giant cells, and other macrophages. SEE ALSO granulomatosis. [granulo- + G. *-oma*, tumor]

**gran·u·lo·ma in·gui·na·le** a specific granuloma, classified as a sexually transmitted disease and caused by *Calymmatobacterium granulomatis* observed in macrophages as Donovan bodies; the ulcerating granulomatous lesions occur in the inguinal regions and on the genitalia. SYN donovanosis, granuloma venereum, ulcerating granuloma of pudenda.

**gran·u·lo·ma mul·ti·for·me** a chronic granulomatous annular eruption of the skin on the upper body in older adults in central Africa; of unknown cause.

**gran·u·lo·ma·to·sis** (gran′yu-lō-mă-tō′sis) any condition characterized by multiple granulomas.

**gran·u·lom·a·tous** (gran-yu-lōm′ă-tŭs) having the characteristics of a granuloma.

**gran·u·lom·a·tous co·li·tis** changes, identical to those of regional enteritis, involving the colon.

**gran·u·lom·a·tous en·ceph·a·lo·my·e·li·tis** an encephalomyelitis in which granulomas occur.

**gran·u·lom·a·tous en·ter·i·tis** SYN regional enteritis.

**gran·u·lom·a·tous in·flam·ma·tion** a form of proliferative inflammation SEE ALSO granuloma.

**gran·u·lo·ma tro·pi·cum** SYN yaws.

g
r

**gran·u·lo·ma ve·ne·re·um** SYN granuloma inguinale.

**gran·u·lo·mere** (gran'yu-lō-mēr) the central part of a blood platelet. SYN chromomere (2). [granulo- + G. *meros*, a part]

**gran·u·lo·pe·nia** (gran'yu-lō-pē'nē-ă) SYN granulocytopenia.

**gran·u·lo·plas·tic** (gran'yu-lō-plas'tik) forming granules.

**gran·u·lo·poi·e·sis** (gran'yu-lō-poy-ē'sis) production of granulocytes. In adults, granulocytes are produced chiefly in the red bone marrow of flat bones. SYN granulocytopoiesis. [granulo- (cyte) + G. *poiēsis*, a making]

**gran·u·lo·poi·et·ic** (gran'yu-lō-poy-et'ik) pertaining to granulopoiesis. SYN granulocytopoietic.

**gran·u·lo·sa cell** a cell of the membrana granulosa lining the vesicular ovarian follicle that becomes a luteal cell of the corpus luteum after ovulation.

**gran·u·lo·sa cell tu·mor** a benign or malignant tumor of the ovary arising from the membrana granulosa of the ovarian (graafian) follicle and frequently secreting estrogen. SYN folliculoma (1).

**gran·u·lo·sis** (gran-yu-lō'sis) a mass of minute granules of any character.

△**-graph 1.** something written, as in monograph, radiograph. **2.** the instrument for making a recording, as in kymograph. Cf. -gram. [G. *graphō*, to write]

**graph·an·es·the·sia** (graf'an-es-thē'zē-ă) tactual inability to recognize figures or letters written on the skin; may be due to spinal cord or brain disease. [G. *graphē*, writing + *anaisthēsia*, fr. an-priv. + *aisthēsis*, perception]

**graph·or·rhea** (graf-ō-rē'ă) rarely used term for the writing of long lists of meaningless words, associated with a schizophrenic disorder. [grapho- + G. *rhoia*, flow]

△**-graphy** a writing, a description. [G. *graphō*, to write]

**grasp·ing re·flex, grasp re·flex** an involuntary flexion of the fingers to tactile or tendon stimulation on the palm of the hand, producing an uncontrollable grasp; physiologic in the newborn, otherwise usually associated with frontal lobe lesions. Cf. darwinian reflex.

**GRASS** gradient-recalled acquisition in the steady state.

**Gras·set phe·nom·e·non** (grah-sā') in organic paralysis of the lower extremity, the supine patient can raise either limb separately, but not both together.

**Gras·set sign** (grah-sā') normal contraction of the sternocleidomastoid muscle on the paralyzed side in cases of hemiplegia.

**grat·tage** (gră-tazh') scraping or brushing an ulcer or surface with sluggish granulations to stimulate the healing process. [Fr. scraping]

**grave** (grāv) denoting symptoms of a serious or dangerous character. [L. *gravis*, heavy, grave]

**grav·el** (grav'l) small concretions, usually of uric acid, calcium oxalate, or phosphates, formed in the kidney and passed through the ureter, bladder, and urethra. [M.E., fr. O.Fr.]

**gra·vel voice** SYN glottal fry.

**Graves dis·ease** (grāvz) **1.** toxic goiter characterized by diffuse hyperplasia of the thyroid gland, a form of hyperthyroidism; exophthalmos is a common, but not invariable, concomitant; **2.** thyroid dysfunction and all or any of its clinical associations; **3.** an organ-specific autoimmune disease of the thyroid gland. SEE thyrotoxicosis, Hashimoto thyroiditis, goiter, myxedema. SYN Parry disease.

**Graves oph·thal·mop·a·thy** (grāvz) exophthalmos caused by increased water content of retroocular orbital tissues; associated with thyroid disease, usually hyperthyroidism. SYN Graves orbitopathy.

**Graves op·tic neu·rop·a·thy** (grāvz) visual dysfunction due to optic nerve compression in Graves orbitopathy.

**Graves or·bi·top·a·thy** (grāvz) SYN Graves ophthalmopathy.

**grav·id** SYN pregnant.

**grav·i·da** (grav'i-dă) a pregnant woman. Gravida followed by a roman numeral or preceded by a Latin prefix (primi-, secundi-, etc.) designates the number of pregnancies; e.g., **gravida I**, primigravida: a woman in her first pregnancy; **gravida II**, secundigravida: a woman in her second pregnancy. Also, gravida (or G) 1, 2, etc. Cf. para. [L. *gravidus* (adj.), fem. *gravida*, fr. *gravis*, heavy]

**gra·vid·ic** (grav-id'ik) relating to pregnancy or a pregnant woman.

**gra·vid·i·ty** (gră-vid'i-tē) the number of pregnancies (complete or incomplete) experienced by a woman. [L. *graviditas*, pregnancy]

**grav·id uter·us** the condition of the uterus in pregnancy.

**grav·i·met·ric** (grav-i-met'rik) relating to or determined by weight.

**grav·i·re·cep·tor** (grav'i-rē-sep'terz) a highly specialized receptor organ and nerve ending in the inner ear, joints, tendons, and muscles that give the brain information about body position, equilibrium, direction of gravitational forces, and the sensation of "down" or "up." [L. *gravis*, heavy, + receptor]

**grav·i·ta·tion·al in·se·cu·ri·ty** overreaction to changes in head position in relation to gravity; fear or strong emotional response to situations that normally require only a balance reaction.

**grav·i·ta·tion·al ul·cer** a chronic ulcer of the leg with impaired healing because of the incompetence of the valves of varicose veins; the venous return stagnates and creates hypoxemia. SEE ALSO varicose ulcer.

**grav·i·ty** (grav'i-tē) the attraction toward the earth that makes any mass exert downward force or have weight. [L. *gravitas*]

**grav·i·ty con·cen·tra·tion** a method of separating parasites from debris through gravity sedimentation of fecal suspensions.

**gray (Gy)** (grā) the SI unit of absorbed dose of ionizing radiation, equivalent to 1 J/kg of tissue; 1 Gy = 100 rad. [Louis H. *Gray*, British radiologist, 1905–1965]

**gray cat·a·ract** a cataract of gray color, usually seen in senile, mature, or cortical cataract.

**gray col·umns** the three somewhat ridge-shaped masses of gray matter (anterior, posterior, and lateral columns) that extend longitudinally through the center of each lateral half of the spinal cord; in transverse sections these columns appear as gray horns and are therefore commonly called ventral or anterior, dorsal or posterior, and lateral horn, respectively. SYN columnae griseae [TA].

**gray de·gen·er·a·tion** degeneration of the white substance of the spinal cord, the fibers of which lose their myelin sheaths and become darker in color.

**gray fi·bers** SYN unmyelinated fibers.

**gray hep·a·ti·za·tion** the second stage of hepatization in pneumonia, when the exudate is beginning to degenerate prior to breaking down; the color is a yellowish gray or mottled.

**gray in·du·ra·tion** a condition occurring in lungs during and after pneumonic processes in which there is failure of resolution; there is an increase in fibrous tissue but usually not a prominent degree of pigmentation, unless chronic passive congestion is also present.

**gray lit·er·a·ture** reports containing data, e.g., on health and disease in a population, that are unpublished or have limited distribution. Examples include local health department reports and masters' and doctoral dissertations lodged in university libraries.

**gray mat·ter** those regions of the brain and spinal cord that are made up primarily of the cell bodies and dendrites of nerve cells rather than myelinated axons. SYN substantia grisea [TA], gray substance.

**gray-scale ul·tra·so·nog·ra·phy** the display of the ultrasound echo amplitude or signal intensity as different shades of gray, improving image quality compared to the obsolete black-and-white presentation.

**gray sub·stance** SYN gray matter.

**gray syn·drome, gray ba·by syn·drome** gray appearance of an infant at birth and during the neonatal period which can be caused by transplacental toxic effects of the drug chloramphenicol taken by the mother during late pregnancy; the syndrome may be fatal.

**great ad·duc·tor mus·cle** SYN adductor magnus muscle.

**great au·ric·u·lar nerve** arises from the ventral primary rami of the second and third cervical spinal nerves, supplies the skin of part of the auricle, adjacent portion of the scalp, and that overlying the angle of the jaw; it also innervates the parotid sheath, conveying from it the pain fibers stimulated by stretching of the sheath during parotitis (mumps). SYN nervus auricularis magnus [TA].

**great car·di·ac vein** begins at the apex of the heart (anastomose with the middle cardiac vein), runs first with the anterior interventricular artery as it ascends the anterior interventricular groove, then turns to the left as it approaches or reaches the coronary groove to run with the circumflex branch of the left coronary artery; it merges with the oblique vein of the left atrium to form the coronary sinus.

**great ce·re·bral vein of Ga·len** (gā′len) a large, unpaired vein formed by the junction of the two internal cerebral veins in the caudal part of the tela choroidea of the third ventricle; it passes caudally between the splenium of the corpus callosum and the pineal gland, curving dorsally to merge with the inferior sagittal sinus to form the straight sinus.

**great·er a·lar car·ti·lage** one of a pair of cartilages that form the tip of the nose. It consists of a medial crus that extends into the nasal septum with its fellow of the opposite side, and a lateral crus that forms the anterior part of the wing of the nose.

**great·er cur·va·ture of stom·ach** the border of the stomach to which the greater omentum is attached.

**great·er mult·ang·u·lar bone** SYN trapezium.

**great·er o·men·tum** a peritoneal fold passing from the greater curvature of the stomach to the transverse colon, hanging like an apron in front of the intestines. SYN caul (2), cowl, velum (3).

**great·er pal·a·tine ca·nal** the canalis formed between the maxilla and palatine bones; it transmits the descending palatine artery and the greater palatine nerve. SYN pterygopalatine canal.

**great·er pal·a·tine fo·ra·men** an opening in the posterolateral corner of the hard palate opposite the last molar tooth, marking the lower end of the pterygopalatine canal.

**great·er pal·a·tine nerve** a branch of the pterygopalatine ganglion that passes downward through the greater palatine canal to supply the mucosa and glands of the hard palate, and the anterior part of the soft palate. SYN nervus palatinus major [TA].

**great·er pel·vis** the expanded portion of the pelvis above the brim. SYN false pelvis.

**great·er pos·te·ri·or rec·tus mus·cle of head** SYN rectus capitis posterior major muscle.

**great·er splanch·nic nerve** uppermost of the abdominopelvic splanchnic which arises from the fifth or sixth to the ninth or tenth thoracic sympathetic ganglia in the thorax and passes downward along the bodies of the thoracic vertebrae, penetrating the diaphragm to join the celiac plexus; conveys presynaptic sympathetic fibers to the celiac ganglia, and visceral afferent fibers from the celiac plexus. SYN nervus splanchnicus major [TA].

**great·er su·pra·cla·vi·cu·lar fos·sa** a depressed area above the middle of the clavicle, lateral to the sternocleidomastoid muscle, overlying the omoclavicular triangle, a subdivision of the posterior triangle of the neck.

**great·er tro·chan·ter** a strong process at the proximal and lateral part of the shaft of the femur, overhanging the root of the neck; it gives attachment to the gluteus medius and minimus, piriformis, obturator internus and externus, and gemelli muscles. SYN trochanter major [TA].

**great·er ves·tib·u·lar gland** one of two mucoid-secreting tubuloalveolar glands on either side of the lower part of the vagina, the equivalent of the bulbourethral glands in the male; ensheathed with vestibular bulbs by ischiocavernosus muscles; contraction of which causes secretion into vestibule of vagina. SYN Bartholin gland.

**great·er wing of sphe·noid bone** strong squamous processes extending in a broad superolateral curve from the body of the sphenoid bone. The greater wing presents these surfaces (facies): 1) cerebral surface: forms anterior 1/3 of the floor of the lateral portion of the middle cranial fossa; 2) temporal surface: forms the deepest portion of the temporal fossa; 3) infratemporal surface, forms the "roof" of the infratemporal fossa; 4) orbital surface: forms posterolateral wall of orbit. The greater wing forms the inferior border of the supraorbital fissure, and is perforated at its root by the foramina rotundum ovale and spinosum and the pterygoid canal.

g
r

**great fo•ra•men** SYN foramen magnum.

**great seg•men•tal med•ul•la•ry ar•tery** largest of the medullary arteries that supply the spinal cord by anastomosing with the anterior (longitudinal) spinal artery; it arises from a lower intercostal or upper lumbar artery (on the left side about 65% of the time) supplying most of the blood to the lower two-thirds of the anterior spinal artery. SEE medullary arteries of brain.

**great toe I** the first digit of the foot.

**Green•field fil•ter** (grēn'fēld) a multistrutted spring-styled filter usually placed in the inferior vena cava to prevent venous emboli from reaching the pulmonary circulation from the lower extremity.

**green•stick frac•ture** the bending of a bone with incomplete fracture involving the convex side of the curve only.

**Greig ce•pha•lo•po•ly•syn•dac•ty•ly syn••drome** (greg) an autosomal dominant disorder characterized by polysyndactyly of the hands and feet, macrocephaly, frontal bossing, hypertelorism, and flat nasal bridge; caused by mutation in the GLI3 gene on chromosome 7p13.

**grenz ray** (grents rā) very soft x-rays, closely allied to the ultraviolet rays in their wavelength (i.e., long) and in their biologic action upon tissues; they are produced by a specially built vacuum tube with a hot cathode operating from a transformer delivering not more than 8 kw. [Ger. *Grenze*, borderline, boundary]

**Grey Tur•ner sign** (grā ter'ner) local areas of discoloration about the umbilicus and in the region of the loins, in acute hemorrhagic pancreatitis and other causes of retroperitoneal hemorrhage.

**grid 1.** a chart with horizontal and perpendicular lines for plotting curves. **2.** X-RAY IMAGING a device formed of lead strips for preventing scattered radiation from reaching the x-ray film. [M.E. *gridel*, fr. L. *craticula*, lattice]

**Grid•ley stain** (grid'lē) a silver staining method for reticulum.

**Grid•ley stain for fun•gi** (grid'lē) a method for fixed tissue sections based on Bauer chromic acid leucofuchsin stain with the addition of Gomori aldehyde fuchsin stain and metanil yellow as counterstains; against a yellow background, hyphae, conidia, yeast capsules, elastin, and mucin appear in different shades of blue to purple.

**grief** (grēf) a normal emotional response to an external loss; distinguished from a depressive disorder since it usually subsides after a reasonable time.

**Grie•sing•er dis•ease** (grē'zing-er) bilious typhoid of Griesinger, a severe form of louse-borne relapsing fever caused by *Borrelia recurrentis* and causing high fever, epistaxis, dyspnea, intense jaundice, purpura, and splenomegaly.

**Grie•sing•er sign** (grē'zing-er) erythema and edema over the posterior part of the mastoid process due to septic thrombosis of the mastoid emissary vein and indicating thrombophlebitis of the sigmoid sinus.

**grind•ing** (grīnd'ing) SYN abrasion (3).

**grind•ing-in** a term used to denote the act of correcting occlusal disharmonies by grinding the natural or artificial teeth.

**grip** SYN influenza.

**grippe** (grip) SYN influenza. [Fr. *gripper*, to seize]

**gris•tle** (gris'l) SYN cartilage. [A.S.]

**Grit•ti op•er•a•tion** (grē'tē) SYN Gritti-Stokes amputation.

**Grit•ti-Stokes am•pu•ta•tion** (grē'tē stōkz) supracondylar amputation of the femur, the patella being preserved and applied to the end of the bone, its articular cartilage being removed so as to obtain union. SYN Gritti operation.

**Groc•co sign** (grok'ō) **1.** acute dilation of the heart following a muscular effort, described in Graves disease; also occurring in various forms of myocardiopathy; **2.** extension of the liver dullness several centimeters to the left of the midspinal line in cases of enlargement of that organ.

**Groc•co tri•an•gle** (grok'ō) a triangular patch of dullness at the base of the chest alongside the spinal column, on the side opposite a pleural effusion.

**gro•cer's itch** a vesicular dermatitis seen in grocers and bakers who handle sugar or flour; caused by a mite of the genus *Glycophagus*.

**Groe•nouw cor•ne•al dys•tro•phy** (grer'nō) **1.** a granular type of corneal dystrophy, with autosomal dominant inheritance, caused by mutation in the transforming growth factor, beta-induced, gene (TGFB1) encoding keratoepithelin on chromosome 5q; **2.** a progressive macular type of corneal dystrophy, characterized by punctate opacities and episodes of photophobia, corneal erosion, and foreign body sensation; autosomal recessive inheritance.

**groin** (groyn) **1.** SYN inguinal region. **2.** sometimes used to indicate just the crease in the junction of the thigh with the trunk.

**groove** (groo-v) a narrow elongated depression or furrow on any surface. SEE ALSO sulcus.

**groove of nail ma•trix** SYN sulcus matricis unguis.

**gross** coarse or large; large enough to be visible to the naked eye.

**gross anat•o•my** general anatomy, so far as it can be studied without the use of the microscope; commonly used to denote the study of anatomy by dissection of a cadaver. SYN macroscopic anatomy.

**Gross vi•rus** (grōs) the first strain of mouse leukemia virus isolated.

**ground bun•dles** SYN fasciculi proprii.

**ground-glass pat•tern** radiographic or CT appearance of hazy opacity which does not obscure underlying anatomic detail.

**ground la•mel•la** SYN interstitial lamella.

**ground state** the normal, inactivated state of an atom from which, on activation, the singlet, triplet, and other excited states are derived.

**ground sub•stance** the amorphous material in which structural elements occur; in connective tissue, it is composed of proteoglycans, plasma constituents, metabolites, water, and ions present between cells and fibers.

**group** (groop) **1.** a number of similar or related objects. **2.** in chemistry, a radical.

**group ag•glu•ti•na•tion** agglutination by antibodies specific for minor (group) antigens common to several microorganisms, each of which possesses its own major specific antigen.

**group ag•glu•ti•nin** an immune agglutinin specific for a group antigen. SYN cross-reacting agglutinin.

**group an·ti·gens** antigens that are shared by related genera of microorganisms.

**group A strep·to·coc·cal nec·ro·tiz·ing fas·ci·i·tis** a complication of infection with GAS (group A streptococci) in which the bacteria attack and destroy muscle tissue.

**group mod·el HMO** a physician practice group that contracts to be providers solely to that HMO's subscribers.

**group prac·tice** the cooperative practice of medicine by a group of physicians, each of whom as a rule specializes in some particular field; such a group often shares a common suite of consulting rooms, laboratories, staff, equipment, etc.

**Gro·ver dis·ease** (grō′ver) SYN transient acantholytic dermatosis.

**grow·ing pains** aching pains, frequently felt at night, in the limbs of growing children; attributed variously to growth, rheumatic state, faulty posture, fatigue, or ill-defined psychic causes.

**growth** (grōth) the increase in size of a living being or any of its parts occurring in the process of development.

**growth hor·mone (GH)** SYN somatotropin.

**growth hor·mone-in·hib·it·ing hor·mone (GIH)** SYN somatostatin.

**growth hor·mone-pro·duc·ing ad·e·no·ma** an adenoma that produces the clinical picture of gigantism or acromegaly, although a third of the cells have no granules or are a mixture of acidophils and chromophobes; some tumors may secrete both growth hormone and prolactin; often an acidophil or eosinophil adenoma.

**growth hor·mone-re·leas·ing fac·tor (GHRF, GH-RF)** SYN somatoliberin.

**growth hor·mone-re·leas·ing hor·mone (GHRH, GH-RH)** SYN somatoliberin.

**growth-on·set di·a·be·tes** SYN insulin-dependent diabetes mellitus.

**growth rate** absolute or relative growth increase, expressed per unit of time.

**Gru·ber meth·od** (groo′ber) a modification of the Politzer method in which the patient does not swallow, but says "hoc" at the instant of compression of the bag.

**gru·mous** (groo′mŭs) thick and lumpy, as clotting blood. [L. *grumus,* a little heap]

**Gru·nert spur** (groo′nert) epithelial outgrowth of the dilator muscle of the pupil at the junction of the iris and the ciliary body; part of the origin of the iris dilator muscle.

**Gryn·feltt tri·an·gle** (grin′felt) a triangular space bounded above by the end of the last rib and the serratus posterior inferior muscle, anteriorly by the internal oblique, and posteriorly by the quadratus lumborum; lumbar hernia occurs in this space. SYN Lesshaft triangle.

**gry·po·sis** (gri-pō′sis) an abnormal curvature. [G. *grypos,* hooked, + *-osis,* condition]

**GSH** glutathione.

**GSR** galvanic skin response.

**GSSG** glutathione disulfide.

**GTP** guanosine 5′-triphosphate.

**GU** genitourinary.

**Guan·a·ri·to vi·rus** (gwahn-ah-rē-tō) a species of Arenavirus causing Venezuelan hemorrhagic fever. [after municipality in Venezuela where all initial cases of Venezuelan hemorrhagic fever were confirmed]

**gua·nase** (gwahn′ās) SYN guanine deaminase.

**gua·ni·di·no·ac·e·tate** *N*-**meth·yl·trans·fer·-ase** the enzyme catalyzing the transfer of a methyl group from *S*-adenosyl-L-methionine ("active methionine") to guanidinoacetate (glycocyamine), forming creatine and *S*-adenosyl-L-homocysteine.

**gua·nine (G)** (gwahn′ēn, gwahn′in) one of the two major purines (the other being adenine) occurring in all nucleic acids.

**gua·nine de·am·i·nase** a deaminase of the liver that catalyzes the hydrolysis of guanine into xanthine and ammonia; the first step in purine degradation. SYN guanase.

**gua·nine de·ox·y·ri·bo·nu·cle·o·tide** SYN deoxyguanylic acid.

**gua·nine ri·bo·nu·cle·o·tide** SYN guanylic acid.

**gua·no·sine (G, Guo)** (gwahn′ō-sēn, gwahn′ō-sin) a major constituent of RNA and of guanine nucleotides.

**gua·no·sine 5′-tri·phos·phate (GTP)** an immediate precursor of guanine nucleotides in RNA; similar to ATP; has a crucial role in microtubule formation.

**gua·nyl·ic ac·id (GMP)** (gwă-nil′ik as′id) a major component of ribonucleic acids. SYN guanine ribonucleotide.

**guard·ing** (gard′ing) a spasm of muscles to minimize motion or agitation of sites affected by injury or disease.

**gu·ber·nac·u·lum** (goo′ber-nak′yu-lŭm) **1.** a fibrous cord connecting two structures. **2.** a mesenchymal column of tissue that connects the fetal testis to the developing scrotum; it appears to play a role in testicular descent. SYN gubernaculum testis [TA]. [L. a helm]

**gu·ber·nac·u·lum den·tis** a connective tissue band uniting the tooth sac with the gum.

**gu·ber·nac·u·lum tes·tis** [TA] SYN gubernaculum (2).

**Gub·ler syn·drome** (goo-blā′) a form of alternating hemiplegia characterized by contralateral hemiplegia and ipsilateral facial paralysis.

**Gué·neau de Mus·sey point** (gā-nō′ dŭ mŭ-sā′) a point, painful on pressure, at the junction of a line prolonging the left border of the sternum and a horizontal line at the level of end of the bony portion of the tenth rib; it is present in cases of diaphragmatic pleurisy.

**Gué·rin frac·ture** (gā-rah′) a fracture of the facial bones in which there is a horizontal fracture at the base of the maxillae above the apices of the teeth.

**guide** (gīd) **1.** to lead in a set course. **2.** any device or instrument by which another is led into its proper course, e.g., a grooved director, a catheter guide. [M.E., fr. O.Fr. *guier,* to show the way, fr. Germanic]

**gui·ded tis·sue re·gen·er·a·tion** regeneration of tissue directed by the physical presence and/or chemical activities of a biomaterial; often involves placement of barriers to exclude one or more cell types during healing or regeneration of tissue.

**guide·line** (gīd′līn) **1.** a marking in the form of a line that serves as a guide or reference. **2.** a rule or directive outlining a policy or procedure.

**guide·wire** (gīd′wīr) a long and flexible fine spring used to introduce and position an intravascular angiographic catheter (see Seldinger technique).

**Guil·lain-Bar·ré syn·drome** (gē-yă′ bă-rā′) a self-limiting demyelinating syndrome related to

g
u

autoimmune dysfunction, surgical complication, some vaccines, Hodgkin disease, and some types of drug reactions. Motor and/or sensory dysfunction begins in the extremities and moves proximally, sometimes leading to respiratory failure, before function is restored within weeks or months. SYN Landry paralysis, Landry syndrome.

**guil·lo·tine** (gil′ŏ-tēn, gē′ō-tēn) an instrument in the shape of a metal ring through which runs a sliding knifeblade, used in cutting off an enlarged tonsil. [Fr. an instrument for execution by decapitation]

**gul·let** (gŭl′et) SYN throat (1). [L. *gula*, throat]

**Gull·strand slit·lamp** (gul′strand) SYN slitlamp.

**gum** (gŭm) **1.** the dried exuded sap from a number of trees and shrubs, forming an amorphous brittle mass; it usually forms a mucilaginous solution in water. [L. *gummi*] **2.** SYN gingiva. [A.S. *goma*, jaw]

**gum line** SYN gingival line.

**gum·ma**, pl. **gum·ma·ta**, **gum·mas** (gŭm′ă, gŭm′ă-tă, gŭm′ăz) an infectious granuloma that is characteristic of tertiary syphilis. Gummas are characterized by an irregular central portion that is firm, sometimes partially hyalinized, and consisting of coagulative necrosis in which "ghosts" of structures may be recognized; a poorly defined middle zone of epithelioid cells, with occasional multinucleated giant cells; and a peripheral zone of fibroblasts and numerous capillaries, with infiltrated lymphocytes and plasma cells. SYN syphiloma. [L. *gummi*, gum, fr. G. *kommi*]

**gum·ma·tous** (gŭm′ă-tŭs) pertaining to or characterized by the features of a gumma.

**gum re·sec·tion** SYN gingivectomy.

**Gunn cross·ing sign** (gŭn) retinal arteriovenous crossing with venous compression in hypertensive disease.

**Gunn dots** (gŭn) minute, highly glistening, white or yellowish specks usually seen in the posterior part of the fundus; nonpathologic.

**Gunn sign** (gŭn) **1.** compression of the underlying vein at arteriovenous crossings seen ophthalmoscopically in arteriolar sclerosis; **2.** on alternate stimulation with light, the pupil of an eye with optic nerve transmission defect constricts poorly or even dilates when stimulated (a relative afferent pupillary defect). SYN Marcus Gunn sign.

**Gunn syn·drome** (gŭn) SYN jaw-winking syndrome.

**gun·stock de·for·mi·ty** a form of cubitus varus resulting from condylar fracture at the elbow in which the axis of the extended forearm is not continuous with that of the arm but is displaced toward midline.

**Guo** guanosine.

**gur·gling rale** coarse sound heard over large cavities or over trachea nearly filled with secretions.

**gur·ney** (ger′nē) a stretcher or cot with wheels used to transport hospital patients. [Scottish *gurn*, to grimace in pain; Sir Goldsworthy *Gurney*, British physician and inventor, 1793–1875]

**gush·er** (gush′er) an abundant flow of fluid.

**Gus·sen·bau·er su·ture** (gŭ′sen-baw′er) a figure-of-8 suture for the intestine, resembling the Czerny-Lembert suture but not including the mucous membrane.

▪ **gus·ta·tion** (gŭs-tā′shŭn) **1.** the act of tasting. **2.** the sense of taste. See this page. [L. *gustatio*, fr. *gusto*, pp. *-atus*, to taste]

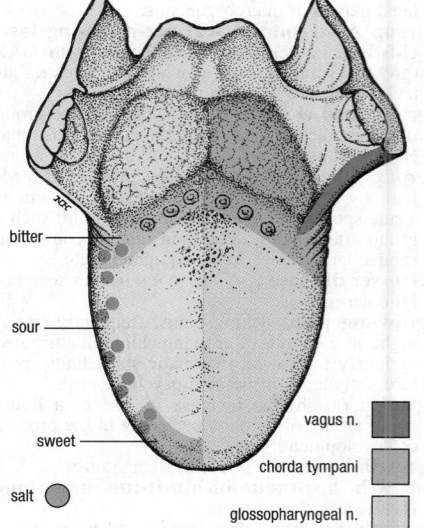

**gustation:** regions of taste perception and their gustatory nerves

**gus·ta·to·ry** (gŭs′tă-tōr-ē) relating to gustation, or taste.

**gus·ta·to·ry ag·no·sia** inability to classify or identify a tastant, even though the ability to distinguish between or recognize tastants may be normal; may be general, partial, or specific.

**gus·ta·tory au·ra** epileptic aura characterized by illusions or hallucinations of taste. SEE ALSO aura (1).

**gus·ta·to·ry cells** SYN taste cells.

**gus·ta·to·ry hy·per·hi·dro·sis** excessive sweating of the lips, nose, and forehead after eating certain foods.

**gus·ta·to·ry rhi·nor·rhea** watery nasal discharge associated with stimulation of the sense of taste.

**gut 1.** SYN intestine. **2.** embryonic digestive tube. **3.** abbreviated term for catgut. SEE ALSO suture.

**Guth·rie test** (gŭth′rē) bacterial inhibition assay for direct measurement of serum phenylalanine; in widespread use for detection of phenylketonuria in the newborn.

**gut·ta·per·cha** (gut′ă-per′chă) the coagulated, purified, dried, milky juice of trees of the genera *Palaguium* and *Payena* (family Sapotaceae); used as a filling material in dentistry, especially to fill root canals in endodontics, and in the manufacture of splints and electrical insulators; a solution is used as a substitute for collodion, as a protective, and to seal incised wounds. Solid at room temperature and soft and plastic when heated.

**gut·ta·per·cha points** cones of a gutta percha compound used for filling root canals in conjunction with a cement, paste, or plastic.

**gut·tate** (gŭt′tāt) of the shape of, or resembling, a drop, characterizing certain cutaneous lesions.

**gut·ter dys·tro·phy of cor·nea** a marginal furrow usually inferiorly about 1 mm from the limbus; and sometimes bilateral. SYN keratoleptynsis (1).

**gut·ter frac·ture** a long, narrow, depressed fracture of the skull.

**gut·ter wound** a tangential wound that makes a furrow without perforating the skin.

**Guttman scale** (goot′mahn) a measurement scale that ranks response categories to a question with each unit representing an increasingly strong expression of an attribute such as pain or disability.

**gut·tur·al** (gŭt′er-ăl) relating to the throat.

**Guy·on am·pu·ta·tion** (gē-yon′) amputation above the malleoli, a modification of Syme amputation.

**Guy·on ca·nal** (gē-yon′) the superficial canal between the flexor retinaculum of the hand and flexor carpi ulnaris through which pass the ulnar nerve and vasculature between forearm and hand.

**Guy·on sign** (gē-yon′) **1.** ballottement of the kidney in cases of nephroptosis, especially when there is also a renal tumor; **2.** the hypoglossal nerve lies directly upon the external carotid artery, whereby this vessel may be distinguished from the internal carotid when ligation is necessary.

**Guy·on tun·nel syn·drome** (gē-yon′) entrapment or compression of the ulnar nerve within Guyon canal as the ulnar nerve passes into the wrist.

**GVHR** graft versus host reaction.

**GXT** graded exercise test.

**Gy** gray (unit of absorbed radiation).

**Gym·no·din·i·um** (jim-nō-din′ē-um) genus of marine dinoflagellates that includes the unicellular organism that causes red tide.

**Gym·no·din·i·um bre·ve** a species of microscopic algae that causes red tide; it produces a toxin that affects the central nervous system of fish, paralyzing and killing them.

**gym·no·phal·loi·des** (jim-nō-fal-oy′dēz) small trematode (family Gymnophallidae) normally found in birds; often reported in human intestine in Korea; the intermediate host is presumed to be a marine oyster or clam.

**Gym·no·phal·loi·des se·o·i** trematode found in inhabitants of an island southwest of Korean peninsula; infection produces vague intestinal symptoms; it is a human parasite under natural conditions, not accidental infections, and bivalves are intermediate hosts.

**GYN** gynecology.

△**gyn-, gy·ne-, gy·ne·co-, gy·no-** female. [G. *gynē,* woman]

**gy·nae-** [Br.] SEE gyne-.

**gy·nae·co-** [Br.] SEE gyneco-.

**gy·nae·coid** [Br.] SEE gynecoid.

**gy·nae·co·log·ic** [Br.] SEE gynecologic.

**gy·nae·co·lo·gist** [Br.] SEE gynecologist.

**gy·nae·col·o·gy** [Br.] SEE gynecology.

**gy·nae·co·mas·tia** [Br.] SEE gynecomastia.

**gy·nae·pho·bia** [Br.] SEE gynephobia.

**gy·nan·drism** (ji-nan′drizm, gī′nan-drizm) a developmental abnormality characterized by hypertrophy of the clitoris and union of the labia majora, simulating in appearance the penis and scrotum. SEE hermaphroditism. [gyn- + G. *anēr* (*andr-*), man]

**gy·nan·dro·blas·to·ma** (ji-nan′drō-blas-tō′mă, gī-nan′drō-blas-tō′mă) **1.** SYN arrhenoblastoma. **2.** a rare variety of arrhenoblastoma of the ovary, containing granulosa or theca cell elements and

producing simultaneous androgenic and estrogenic effects.

**gy·nan·droid** (gī-nan′droyd, jĭ-nan′droyd) an individual exhibiting gynandrism. [gyn- + G. *anēr* (*andr-*), man, + *eidos,* resemblance]

**gy·nan·dro·mor·phism** (gī-nan-drō-mōr′fizm, jĭ-nan-drō-mōr′fizm) **1.** an abnormal combination of male and female characteristics. **2.** the presence of male and female sex chromosome complements in different tissues; sex chromosome mosaicism. [gyn- + G. *anēr* (*andr-*), a male human, + *morphē,* form]

**gy·nan·dro·mor·phous** (gī-nan-drō-mōr′fŭs, jĭ-nan-drō-mōr′fŭs) having both male and female characteristics.

**gy·ne·cic** (gī-nē′sik, jĭ-nē′sik) pertaining to or associated with women.

**gy·ne·coid** (gī′nĕ-koyd, jin′ĕ-koyd) **1.** resembling a woman in form and structure. **2.** OBSTETRICS referring to the shape of the normal female pelvis. [gyneco- + G. *eidos,* resemblance]

**gy·ne·coid o·be·si·ty** obesity with fat excess mainly in the femoral-gluteal region (pear shape).

**gy·ne·coid pel·vis** the normal female pelvis.

**gy·ne·co·log·ic** (gī′nĕ-kō-loj′ik, jin′ĕ-kō-loj′ik) relating to gynecology.

**gy·ne·col·o·gist** (gī′nĕ-kol′ō-jist, jĭ-nĕ-kol′ō-jist) a physician specializing in gynecology.

**gy·ne·col·o·gy** (GYN) (gī-nĕ-kol′ō-jē, jin-ĕ-kol′ō-jē) the medical specialty concerned with diseases of the female genital tract, as well as endocrinology and reproductive physiology of the female. [gyneco- + G. *logos,* study]

**gy·ne·co·ma·stia, gy·ne·co·mas·ty** (gī′nĕ-kō-mas′tē-ă, jin′ĕ-kō-mas′tē-ă; gī′nĕ-kō-mas′tē, jin-ĕ-kō-mas′tē) excessive development of the male mammary glands, due mainly to ductal proliferation with periductal edema; frequently secondary to increased estrogen levels, but mild gynecomastia may occur in normal adolescence. [gyneco- + G. *mastos,* breast]

**gy·ne·pho·bia** (gī-nĕ-fō′bē-ă, jin-ĕ-fō′bē-ă) morbid fear of women or of the female sex. [gyne- + G. *phobos,* fear]

**gy·no·gen·e·sis** (gī-nō-jen′ĕ-sis, jin-ō-jen′ĕ-sis) oocyte development activated by a sperm, but to which the male gamete contributes no genetic material. [gyno- + G. *genesis,* production]

**gy·no·plas·tics** SEE gynoplasty.

**gy·no·plas·ty** (gī′nō-plas-tiks) reparative or plastic surgery of the female genital organs. [gyno- + G. *plassō,* to form]

**gy·rate** (jī′rāt) **1.** of a convoluted or ring shape. **2.** to revolve. [L. *gyro,* pp. *gyratus,* to turn round in a circle, *gyrus*]

**gy·rec·to·my** (jī-rek′tō-mē) excision of a cerebral gyrus. [G. *gyros,* ring, + *ektomē,* excision]

**gy·ri** (jī′rī) plural of gyrus. [L.]

**Gy·ro·mi·tra es·cu·len·ta** (gī-rō-mē′tră es-kyu-len′tă) a species of mushroom that may produce a monomethylhydrazine toxin which causes nausea, diarrhea, and other symptoms; in severe cases death may occur.

**gy·rose** (jī′rōs) marked by irregular curved lines like the surface of a cerebral hemisphere. [G. *gyros,* circle]

**gy·ro·spasm** (jī′rō-spazm) spasmodic rotary movements of the head. [G. *gyros,* circle, + *spasmos,* spasm]

**gy·rus,** gen. and pl. **gy·ri** (jī′rŭs, jī′rī) one of the prominent rounded elevations that form the cerebral hemispheres, each consisting of an exposed superficial portion and a portion hidden from view in the wall and floor of the sulcus. [L. fr. G. *gyros,* circle]

**gy·rus for·ni·ca·tus 1.** SYN fornicate gyrus. **2.** used previously to refer to the entire limbic system.

# H

**H** hyperopia or hyperopic; horizontal; Hauch; henry, unit of electrical inductance; hydrogen; the Fraunhofer line at $\lambda$ 3968 due to calcium; histidine; magnetic field strength; heroin.

*H* enthalpy, heat content, in the equation for free energy.

**h** hecto-; height; hour.

*h* Planck constant; $h = h/2\pi$.

**H$^+$** hydrogen ion, the proton.

**$^1$H** hydrogen-1.

**$^2$H** hydrogen-2.

**haar·schei·be tu·mor** SYN trichodiscoma. [Ger. *Haar*, hair, + *Scheibe*, disk]

**Haa·se rule** (hah'sĕ) the length of the fetus in centimeters, divided by 5, is the duration of pregnancy in months, i.e., the age of the fetus.

**ha·be·na**, pl. **ha·be·nae** (hă-bē'nă, hă-bē'nē) **1.** a frenum or restricting fibrous band. **2.** a restraining bandage. **3.** SYN habenula (2). [L. strap]

**hab·e·nal, ha·be·nar** (hab'ē-năl, hă-bē'năr) relating to a habena.

**ha·ben·u·la**, pl. **ha·ben·u·lae** (ha-ben'yu-lă, ha-ben'yu-lă-lē) [TA] **1.** SYN frenulum. **2.** in neuroanatomy, the term originally denoted the stalk of the pineal gland (pineal habenula; pedunculus of pineal body), but gradually came to refer to a neighboring group of nerve cells with which the pineal gland was believed to be associated, the habenular nucleus. Currently, the TA term refers exclusively to this circumscript cell mass in the caudal and dorsal aspect of the dorsal thalamus, embedded in the posterior end of the medullary stria from which it receives most of its afferent fibers. By way of the retroflex fasciculus (habenulointerpeduncular tract) it projects to the interpeduncular nucleus and other paramedian cell groups of the midbrain tegmentum. Despite its proximity to the pineal stalk, no habenulopineal fiber connection is known to exist. It is a part of the epithalamus. SYN habena (3). [L.]

**ha·ben·u·lar** (hă-ben'yu-lăr) relating to a habenula, especially the stalk of the pineal body.

**Ha·ber syn·drome** (hah'ber) a permanent flushing and telangiectasia of the cheeks, nose, forehead, and chin, with prominent follicular openings, small papules with scaling, and minute pitted areas; occasionally accompanied by scaly and keratotic lesions of the trunk.

**hab·it 1.** an act, behavioral response, practice, or custom established in one's repertoire by frequent repetition of the same act. SEE ALSO addiction. **2.** a basic variable in the study of conditioning and learning used to designate a new response learned either by association or by being followed by a reward or reinforced event. SEE conditioning, learning. [L. *habeo*, pp. *habitus*, to have]

**hab·it cough** a persistent cough due to a tic or to psychological causes.

**hab·it spasm** SYN tic.

**ha·bit·u·al a·bor·tion** a condition in which a woman has had three or more consecutive, spontaneous abortions.

**ha·bit·u·al cen·tric** SYN centric occlusion.

**ha·bit·u·al pitch** central tendency of pitch, or fundamental frequency, most often used by an individual. Voice strain or vocal pathology may result when the habitual pitch is significantly dif-ferent from the optimal pitch. SEE optimal pitch. SYN modal frequency, modal pitch.

**ha·bit·u·a·tion** (ha-bit-choo-ā'shŭn) **1.** the process of forming a habit, referring generally to psychological dependence on the continued use of a drug to maintain a sense of well-being, which can result in drug addiction. **2.** the method by which the nervous system reduces or inhibits responsiveness during repeated stimulation.

**hab·i·tus** (hab'i-tŭs) the physical characteristics of a person. [L. habit]

**HACEK group** a group of Gram-negative bacteria that includes *Haemophilus* spp., *Actinobacillus actinomycetemcomitans*, *Cardiobacterium hominis*, *Eikenella corrodens*, and *Kingella kingae*. Bacteria in this group have in common a culture requirement of an enhanced carbon dioxide atmosphere and ability to infect human heart valves.

**Ha·der·up den·tal no·men·cla·ture** (hah'dĕr-ŭp) **1.** European system of identifying teeth by use of a number for each permanent tooth and a + or − sign to indicate the position of each tooth, e.g., 6 + is the upper right first permanent molar. **2.** a system for deciduous teeth analogous to the permanent one in which a 0 is added before the tooth number, e.g., 03+ is the upper right deciduous canine.

**Haeck·el gas·trea the·o·ry** (hek'ĕl) that the two-layered gastrula is the ancestral form of all multicellular animals.

**Haeck·el law** (hek'ĕl) SYN recapitulation theory.

**haem [Br.]** SEE heme.

△**haem-** SEE hem-.

**hae·ma- [Br.]** SEE hema-.

**hae·ma·chrome [Br.]** SEE hemachrome.

**haemacyte [Br.]** SYN erythrocyte.

**hae·ma·cyt·o·me·ter [Br.]** SEE hemacytometer.

**hae·mad·sorp·tion [Br.]** SEE hemadsorption.

**hae·mag·glu·ti·na·tion [Br.]** SEE hemagglutination.

**hae·mag·glu·tin·in [Br.]** SEE hemagglutinin.

**hae·mag·glu·tin·in-pro·tease [Br.]** SEE hemag-glutinin-protease.

**hae·ma·go·gic [Br.]** SEE hemagogic.

**hae·mal [Br.]** SEE hemal.

**haem·an·al·y·sis [Br.]** SEE hemanalysis.

**hae·man·giec·ta·sis [Br.]** SEE hemangiectasis.

**hae·man·gi·o- [Br.]** SEE hemangio-.

**hae·man·gi·o·blast [Br.]** SEE hemangioblast.

**hae·man·gi·o·blas·to·ma [Br.]** SEE hemangio-blastoma.

**haem·an·gio·en·do·the·lio·blas·to·ma [Br.]** SEE hemangioendothelioblastoma.

**haem·an·gio·en·do·the·lio·ma [Br.]** SEE hemangioendothelioma.

**hae·man·gi·o·ma [Br.]** SEE hemangioma.

**hae·man·gi·o·ma·to·sis [Br.]** SEE hemangiomatosis.

**haem·an·gio·per·i·cy·to·ma [Br.]** SEE hemangiopericytoma.

**haem·ar·thro·sis [Br.]** SEE hemarthrosis.

**hae·ma·sta·tic [Br.]** SEE hemostatic.

**hae·mat- [Br.]** SEE hemat-.

**hae·ma·tem·e·sis [Br.]** SEE hematemesis.

**hae·ma·ti·dro·sis [Br.]** SEE hematidrosis.

**hae·ma·tin [Br.]** SEE hematin.

**hae·ma·tin·o·me·ter [Br.]** SYN hemoglobinometry.

**hae·ma·to-** [Br.] SEE hemato-.
**hae·ma·to·cele** [Br.] SEE hematocele.
**hae·mat·o·che·zia** [Br.] SEE hematochezia.
**hae·ma·to·col·po·me·tra** [Br.] SEE hematocolpometra.
**hae·ma·to·col·pos** [Br.] SEE hematocolpos.
**hae·ma·to·crit** [Br.] SEE hematocrit.
**hae·ma·to·cry·a** (hē-mă-tok′rē-ă) cold-blooded vertebrates. [hemato- + G. *kryos,*cold]
**hae·ma·to·cry·al** [Br.] SYN poikilothermic.
**hae·ma·to·cys·tis** [Br.] SEE hematocystis.
**hae·ma·to·ge·ne·sis** [Br.] SYN hemopoiesis.
**hae·ma·to·ge·nic** [Br.] SEE hematogenic.
**hae·ma·to·ge·nous** [Br.] SYN hemopoiesis.
**hae·ma·toid** [Br.] SEE hematoid.
**hae·ma·tol·o·gist** [Br.] SEE hematologist.
**hae·ma·to·log·y** [Br.] SEE hematology.
**hae·ma·to·ma** [Br.] SEE hematoma.
**hae·mat·o·me·tra** [Br.] SEE hematometra.
**hae·ma·to·my·e·lia** [Br.] SEE hematomyelia.
**hae·ma·to·pa·tho·lo·gy** [Br.] SEE hematopathology.
**hae·ma·to·phi·lin·a** (hē-mă-tō-fil-ī′nă) a division of Cheiroptera that includes bloodsucking (vampire) bats [hemato- + G. *philos,*fond]
**haem·at·o·plast** [Br.] SEE hematoplast.
**haem·a·to·plas·tic** [Br.] SEE hematoplastic.
**haem·a·to·poi·e·sis** [Br.] SEE hematopoiesis.
**haem·a·to·poi·et·ic** [Br.] SEE hematopoietic.
**hae·ma·to·por·phyr·in** [Br.] SEE hematoporphyrin.
**haem·a·top·sia** [Br.] SYN hemophthalmia.
**hae·ma·to·sal·pinx** [Br.] SEE hematosalpinx.
**hae·mat·o·sin** [Br.] SEE hematosin.
**hae·mat·o·sis** [Br.] SEE hematosis.
**hae·ma·to·sta·tic** [Br.] SEE hematostatic.
**hae·ma·to·thor·ax** [Br.] SEE hemothorax.
**haem·a·tox·y·lin** [Br.] SEE hematoxylin.
**hae·mat·o·zoon** [Br.] SEE hematozoon.
**hae·ma·tu·ria** [Br.] SEE hematuria.
**haem·e·ryth·rin** [Br.] SEE hemerythrin.
**hae·mic** [Br.] SYN hematic.
**hae·min** [Br.] SEE hemin.
**hae·mo-** [Br.] SEE hemo-.
**haem·o·bil·ia** [Br.] SEE hemobilia.
**hae·mo·chro·ma·to·sis** [Br.] SEE hemochromatosis.
**hae·mo·chrome** [Br.] SYN hemochromogen.
**hae·mo·chro·mo·gen** [Br.] SEE hemochromogen.
**hae·mo·chro·mo·me·ter** [Br.] SYN hemoglobinometry.
**hae·mo·cla·sis** [Br.] SEE hemoclasis.
**hae·mo·cla·stic** [Br.] SEE hemoclastic.
**haem·o·co·el** [Br.] SEE hemocele.
**hae·mo·con·cen·tra·tion** [Br.] SEE hemoconcentration.
**haem·o·cy·an·in** [Br.] SEE hemocyanin.
**hae·mo·cyte** [Br.] SEE hemocyte.
**hae·mo·cy·to·blast** [Br.] SEE hemocytoblast.
**hae·mo·cy·to·ly·sis** [Br.] SEE hemocytolysis.
**haem·o·cy·to·ma** [Br.] SEE hemocytoma.
**hae·mo·cy·to·me·ter** [Br.] SEE hemocytometer.
**hae·mo·cy·to·tryp·sis** [Br.] SEE hemocytotripsis.
**haem·o·di·a·fil·tra·tion** [Br.] SEE hemodiafiltration.
**hae·mo·di·a·ly·ser** [Br.] SEE hemodialyzer.
**hae·mo·di·a·ly·sis** [Br.] SEE hemodialysis.
**hae·mo·di·lu·tion** [Br.] SEE hemodilution.
**haem·o·dy·na·mics** [Br.] SEE hemodynamics.

**hae·mo·dy·na·mo·me·ter** [Br.]
**hae·mo·fil·tra·tion** [Br.] SEE hemofiltration.
**hae·mo·glo·bin** [Br.] SEE hemoglobin.
**hae·mo·glo·bi·nae·mia** [Br.] SEE hemoglobinemia.
**hae·mo·glo·bi·no·ly·sis** [Br.] SEE hemoglobinolysis.
**haem·o·glo·bin·o·metry** [Br.] SEE hemoglobinometry.
**hae·mo·glo·bi·no·path·y** [Br.] SEE hemoglobinopathy.
**haem·o·glo·bins** [Br.] SEE hemoglobin.
**hae·mo·glo·bi·nur·ia** [Br.] SEE hemoglobinuria.
**hae·mo·gram** [Br.] SEE hemogram.
**haem·o·lymph** [Br.] SEE hemolymph.
**hae·mo·ly·sate** [Br.] SEE hemolysate.
**haem·o·ly·sin** [Br.] SEE hemolysin.
**hae·mo·ly·sis** [Br.] SEE hemolysis.
**hae·mo·ly·tic** [Br.] SEE hemolytic.
**haem·on·chia·sis** [Br.] SEE hemonchiasis.
*Hae·mon·chus* (hē-mong′kŭs) an economically important genus of nematodes (family Nematostrongylidae) that parasitize the abomasum of cattle, sheep, goats, and other ruminants, causing anemia; human infection occasionally occurs.
**hae·mon·ec·tin** [Br.] SEE hemonectin.
**haem·o·par·a·site** [Br.] SEE hemoparasite.
**hae·mo·pa·tho·lo·gy** [Br.] SYN hematopathology.
**hae·mo·pa·thy** [Br.] SEE hemopathy.
**hae·mo·per·fu·sion** [Br.] SEE hemoperfusion.
**hae·mo·per·i·car·di·um** [Br.] SEE hemopericardium.
**hae·mo·pe·ri·to·ne·um** [Br.] SEE hemoperitoneum.
**haem·o·pex·in** [Br.] SEE hemopexin.
**haem·o·phag·o·cyte** [Br.] SEE hemophagocyte.
**hae·mo·phi·lia** [Br.] SEE hemophilia.
**hae·mo·phi·li·ac** [Br.] SEE hemophiliac.
**hae·mo·phil·i·oid** [Br.] SEE hemophilioid.
*Hae·moph·i·lus* (hē-mof′i-lŭs) a genus of aerobic to facultatively anaerobic, nonmotile, minute, Gram-negative, rod-shaped cells that sometimes form threads and are pleomorphic. These organisms are strictly parasitic, growing best, or only, on media containing blood. They may or may not be pathogenic. They occur in various lesions and secretions, as well as in normal respiratory tracts, of vertebrates. The type species is *Haemophilus influenzae*. [G. *haima,* blood, + *philos,* fond]
*Hae·moph·i·lus ae·gyp·ti·us* a bacterial species that causes acute or subacute infectious conjunctivitis in warm climates. SYN Koch-Weeks bacillus.
*Hae·moph·i·lus du·crey·i* a species which causes soft chancre (chancroid). SYN Ducrey bacillus.
*Hae·moph·i·lus in·flu·en·zae* a species found in the respiratory tract that causes acute respiratory infections including pneumonia, acute conjunctivitis, bacterial meningitis, and purulent meningitis in children, rarely in adults; originally considered to be the cause of influenza, it is the type species of the genus *Haemophilus*. SYN Pfeiffer bacillus, Weeks bacillus.
*Hae·moph·i·lus in·flu·en·zae* **type b** the most virulent serotype (there are six, a–f, based on antigenic typing of the polysaccharide capsule); species responsible for meningitis and respiratory infections in young children.

*Hae·moph·i·lus in·flu·en·zae* **type B vac·cine** a conjugate of oligosaccharides of the capsular antigen of *H. influenzae* type B and diphtheria CRM protein.

*Hae·mo·phil·us pa·ra·trop·i·cal·is* a relatively nonpathogenic bacterial species that has been associated with human infection, including cases of endocarditis.

*Hae·mo·phil·us seg·nis* a usually saprophytic bacterial species that occasionally causes endocarditis, meningitis, and other infections in humans.

**hae·moph·thal·mia [Br.]** SEE hemophthalmia.

**hae·mo·plas·tic [Br.]** SYN hemopoietic.

**hae·mo·pneu·mo·tho·rax [Br.]** SEE hemopneumothorax.

**hae·mo·poi·e·sis [Br.]** SEE hemopoiesis.

**hae·mo·poi·e·tic [Br.]** SEE hemopoietic.

**hae·mop·ty·sis [Br.]** SEE hemoptysis.

**hae·mor·he·o·lo·gy [Br.]** SEE hemorheology.

**hae·mor·rhage [Br.]** SEE hemorrhage.

**hae·mor·rha·gic [Br.]** SEE hemorrhagic.

**hae·mor·rha·gins [Br.]** SEE hemorrhagins.

**hae·mor·rhoid [Br.]** SEE hemorrhoid.

**hae·mor·rhoi·dal [Br.]** SEE hemorrhoidal.

**hae·mor·rhoi·dec·to·my [Br.]** SEE hemorrhoidectomy.

**hae·mo·si·de·rin [Br.]** SEE hemosiderin.

**hae·mo·si·de·ro·sis [Br.]** SEE hemosiderosis.

**hae·mo·sper·mia [Br.]** SEE hemospermia.

*Hae·mo·spor·i·na* (hē-mō-spō-rī-′nǎ) a suborder of Coccidia (class Sporozoea); heteroxenous, with sporogony in bloodsucking insects and merogony in vertebrates including humans; includes the genus *Plasmodium*.

**hae·mo·sta·sis [Br.]** SEE hemostasis.

**hae·mo·stat [Br.]** SEE hemostat.

**hae·mo·stat·ic [Br.]** SEE hemostatic.

**hae·mo·the·ra·py [Br.]** SEE hemotherapy.

**hae·mo·tho·rax [Br.]** SEE hemothorax.

**hae·mo·tox·ic [Br.]** SEE hemotoxic.

**hae·mo·tox·in [Br.]** SEE hemotoxin.

**hae·mo·tym·pan·um [Br.]** SEE hemotympanum.

**haem·pro·tein [Br.]** SEE heme protein.

**Haff·kine vac·cine** (hahf′kīn) **1.** a killed culture of *Vibrio cholerae* in two strengths, a weaker one for the initial inoculation and a stronger one for the second inoculation 7–10 days after the first; **2.** a killed plague bacillus (*Yersinia pestis*) vaccine.

**haf·ni·um (Hf)** (haf′nē-ŭm) a rare chemical element, atomic no. 72, atomic wt. 178.49. [L. *Hafnia*, Copenhagen]

**Hage·man fac·tor** (hā′gě-mǎn) SYN factor XII.

**H ag·glu·ti·nin 1.** an agglutinin that is formed as the result of stimulation by, and which reacts with, the thermolabile antigen(s) in the flagella of motile strains of microorganisms; **2.** see ABO blood group, Blood Groups appendix.

**Hag·lund dis·ease** (hahg′loond) an abnormal prominence of the posterior superior lateral aspect of the os calcis.

**hahn·i·um** (hahn′ē-ŭm) name proposed for the artificially made element 105. [Otto *Hahn*, Ger. physical chemist and Nobel laureate, 1879–1968]

**Hai·din·ger brush·es** (hī′ding-ěr) the perception of two dark yellowish brushes or sheaves radiating about 5 degrees from the point of fixation when an evenly illuminated surface, such as the blue sky, is viewed through a polarizing lens.

**hair** (hār) **1.** one of the fine, keratinized filamen-tous epidermal growths arising from the skin of the body of mammals except the palms, soles, and flexor surfaces of the joints; the full length and texture of hair varies markedly in different body sites. **2.** one of the fine, hairlike processes of the auditory cells of the labyrinth, and of other sensory cells, called auditory hair, sensory hair, etc. SYN thrix. [A.S. *haer*]

**HAIR-AN syn·drome** hyperandrogenism, insulin resistance, and acanthosis nigricans; virilization in pubertal girls associated with markedly elevated insulin levels and normal levels of luteinizing hormone and follicle-stimulating hormone. [*hyper*androgenism, *i*nsulin *r*esistance, *ac*anthosis *n*igricans]

**hair ball** SYN trichobezoar.

**hair cell** sensory epithelial cells present in the spiral organ (organ of Corti), in the maculae and cristae of the membranous labyrinth of the ear, and in taste buds; they are characterized by having long stereocilia or kinocilia (or both) which, with the light microscope, appear as fine hairs. SEE ALSO taste cells.

**hair fol·li·cle** a tube-like invagination of the epidermis from which the hair shaft develops and into which the sebaceous glands open; the follicle is lined by a cellular inner and outer root sheath of epidermal origin and is invested with a fibrous sheath derived from the dermis. SYN folliculus pili [TA].

**hair·line frac·ture** a fracture without separation of the fragments, the line of break being hairlike, as seen sometimes in the skull. SYN capillary fracture.

**hair pa·pil·la** SYN papilla pili.

**hair·pin ves·sels** atypical blood vessels that double back on themselves, seen on colposcopy of the cervix; their presence indicates early invasive cervical cancer. SYN corkscrew vessels.

**hair root** the part of a hair that is embedded in the hair follicle, its lower succulent extremity capping the dermal papilla pili in the deep bulbous portion of the follicle.

**hair whorls** a spiral arrangement of the hairs, as at the crown of the head.

**hairy** (hār′ē) **1.** of or resembling hair. **2.** covered with hair. SEE ALSO hirsutism. SYN pilar, pilary, pileous, pilose.

**hairy cell** medium-sized leukocytes that have features of reticuloendothelial cells and multiple cytoplasmic projections (hairs) on the cell surface, but which may be a variety of B lymphocyte; they are found in hairy cell leukemia.

**hairy cell leu·ke·mia** a rare, usually chronic disorder characterized by proliferation of hairy cells in reticuloendothelial organs and blood.

**hairy leu·ko·pla·kia** a white lesion appearing on the tongue or buccal mucosa of immunocompromised patients; the lesion appears raised, with a corrugated or "hairy" surface. It has been associated with Epstein-Barr virus.

**hairy mole** SYN nevus pilosus.

**hairy ton·gue** a tongue with abnormal elongation of the filiform papillae, resulting in a thickened furry appearance. SYN glossotrichia, trichoglossia.

**ha·la·tion** (hǎ-lā′shŭn) blurring of the visual image by glare.

**Hal·dane ef·fect** (hawl′dān) the promotion of carbon dioxide dissociation by oxygenation of hemoglobin.

**Hale col·loi·dal iron stain** (hāl) a stain used to distinguish acid mucopolysaccharides such as hyaluronic acid; may be combined with PAS to also visualize carbohydrate-containing proteins and glycoproteins.

**half and half nail** division of the nail by a transverse line into a proximal dull white part and a distal pink or brown part; seen in uremia.

**half-life** (haf′līf) **1.** the period in which the radioactivity or number of atoms of a radioactive substance decreases by half; similarly applied to any substance whose quantity decreases exponentially with time. Cf. half-time. **2.** time required for the serum concentration of a drug to decline by 50%.

**half-time** (haf′tīm) the time, in a first-order chemical (or enzymic) reaction, for half of the substance (substrate) to be converted or to disappear. Cf. half-life.

**half-val·ue la·yer (HVL)** the thickness of a specific absorber (e.g., aluminum), that will reduce the intensity of a beam of radiation to one-half its initial value. SEE ALSO filter.

**half·way house** (haf′wā hows) a facility for individuals who no longer require the complete facilities of a hospital or institution but are not yet prepared to return to independent living.

**hal·ide** (hal′īd) a salt of a halogen.

**hal·i·to·sis** (hal-i-tō′sis) a foul odor of the breath. [L. *halitus,* breath, + G. *-osis,* condition]

**hal·i·tus** (hal′i-tŭs) any exhalation, as of a breath or vapor. [L., fr. *halo,* to breathe]

**Hallé point** (ah-lē′) a point at the intersection of a horizontal line touching the anterior superior spine of the ilium and a perpendicular line drawn from the spine of the pubis; here the ureter can be most readily palpated.

**Hal·ler arch·es** (hahl′ĕr) SEE lateral arcuate ligaments, medial arcuate ligaments.

**Hal·ler cir·cle** (hahl′ĕr) **1.** SYN vascular circle of optic nerve. **2.** SYN areolar venous plexus.

**Hal·ler·vor·den-Spatz syn·drome** (hah′lĕr-fōr′dĕn-shpahtz) a disorder characterized by dystonia with other extrapyramidal dysfunctions appearing in the first two decades of life; associated with large amounts of iron in the globus pallidus and substantia nigra.

**Hall·gren syn·drome** (hahl′grĕn) vestibulocerebellar ataxia, pigmentary retinal dystrophy, congenital deafness, and cataract.

**hal·lu·cal** (hal′ŭ-kăl) relating to the hallux.

**hal·lu·ci·na·tion** (ha-loo′si-nā′shŭn) the subjective perception of an object or event when no such stimulus or situation is present; may be visual, auditory, olfactory, gustatory, or tactile. [L. *alucinor,* to wander in mind]

**hal·lu·ci·no·gen** (ha-loo′si-nō-jen) a mind-altering chemical, drug, or agent, that elicits optical or auditory hallucinations, depersonalization, perceptual disturbances, and disturbances of thought processes. [L. *alucinor,* to wander in mind, + G. *-gen,* producing]

**hal·lu·ci·no·gen·ic** (ha-loo′si-nō-jen′ik) SYN psychedelic.

**hal·lu·ci·no·sis** (ha-loo-si-nō′sis) a syndrome, usually of organic origin (e.g., alcoholic hallucinosis characterized by more or less persistent hallucinations).

**hal·lux,** pl. **hal·lu·ces** (hal′ŭks, hal′ŭ-sēz) [TA] the great toe; the first digit of the foot. [a Mod. L. form for L. *hallex* (*hallic*-), great toe]

**hal·lux do·lo·ro·sus** a condition, usually associated with flatfoot, in which walking causes severe pain in the metatarsophalangeal joint of the great toe.

**hal·lux flex·us** hammer toe involving the first toe.

**hal·lux ri·gi·dus** a condition in which there is stiffness in the first metatarsophalangeal joint; the joint may be the site of osteoarthritis.

**hal·lux val·gus** a deviation of the tip of the great toe, or main axis of the toe, toward the outer or lateral side of the foot.

**hal·lux var·us** deviation of the main axis of the great toe to the inner side of the foot away from its neighbor.

**ha·lo** (hā′lō) **1.** a reddish yellow ring surrounding the optic disk, due to a widening of the scleral ring making the deeper structures visible. **2.** an annular flare of light surrounding a luminous body or a depigmented ring around a mole. SEE halo nevus. **3.** SYN areola (4). **4.** a circular metal band used in a halo cast or halo brace, attached to the skull with pins. [G. *halōs,* threshing floor on which oxen trod a circle; the halo round the sun or moon]

**ha·lo ef·fect 1.** the effect (usually beneficial) that the manner, attention, and caring of a provider have on a patient during a medical encounter, regardless of what medical procedure or services the encounter involves; **2.** the influence upon an observation of the observer's perception of the characteristics of the individual observed (other than the characteristics under study) or the influence of the observer's recollection or knowledge of findings on a previous occasion.

**hal·o·gen** (hal′ō-jen) one of the chlorine group (fluorine, chlorine, bromine, iodine, astatine) of elements; halogens form monobasic acids with hydrogen, and their hydroxides (fluorine forms none) are also monobasic acids. [G. *hals,* salt, + *-gen,* producing]

**hal·o·gen·o·der·ma** (hal-ō-jen′ō-der-mă) dermatosis caused by ingestion or injection of halogens, most notably bromides and iodides. [halogen + G. *derma,* skin]

**ha·lom·e·ter** (hal-om′ĕ-ter) an instrument used to measure the diffraction halo of a red blood cell; based on the premise that the halo of the large erythrocyte of pernicious anemia is smaller than that of the normal cell; the hazy colorless halo of normal size is characteristic of secondary anemia.

**ha·lo ne·vus** a benign, sometimes multiple, melanocytic nevus in which involution occurs with a central brown mole surrounded by a uniformly depigmented zone or halo. SYN Sutton nevus.

**hal·o·phil, hal·o·phile** (hal′ō-fil, hal-ō-fīl) a microorganism whose growth is enhanced by or dependent on a high salt concentration. [G. *hals,* salt, + *philos,* fond]

**hal·o·phil·ic** (hal-ō-fil′ik) requiring a high concentration of salt for growth.

**ha·lo sign** elevation of the subcutaneous fat layer over the fetal skull in a dead or dying fetus; said to be the most common radiologic sign of fetal death.

**Hal·sted law** (hal′sted) transplanted tissue will grow only if there is a lack of that tissue in the host.

**Hal·sted op·er·a·tion** (hal′sted) **1.** an operation

for the radical correction of inguinal hernia; **2.** SYN radical mastectomy.

**Hal•sted su•ture** (hal′sted) a suture placed through the subcuticular fascia; used for exact skin approximation.

**ha•mar•tia** (ham-ar′shē-ă) a localized developmental disturbance characterized by abnormal arrangement and/or combinations of the tissues normally present in the area. [G. *hamartion,* a bodily defect]

**ham•ar•to•blas•to•ma** (ha-mar′tō-blas-tō′mă) a malignant neoplasm of undifferentiated anaplastic cells thought to be derived from a hamartoma. [hamartoma + blastoma]

**ham•ar•to•ma** (ham-ar-tō′mă) a focal malformation that resembles a neoplasm, grossly and even microscopically, but results from faulty development, with a disproportion or abnormal mixture of tissue elements normally present at the site; develops and grows at virtually the same rate as normal tissue, and is not likely to compression or invade adjacent structures (in contrast to a neoplasm). [G. *hamartion,* a bodily defect, + *-oma,* tumor]

**ham•ar•tom•a•tous** (ham-ar-tō′mă-tŭs) relating to hamartoma.

**ha•mate** SEE hamate bone.

**ha•mate bone** the bone on the medial (ulnar) side of the distal row of the carpus; it articulates with the fourth and fifth metacarpal, triquetral, lunate, and capitate. SYN os hamatum [TA], unciform bone.

**Ham•bur•ger law** (hahm′boor-gĕr) albumins and phosphates pass from red corpuscles to serum and chlorides pass from serum to cells when blood is acid; the reverse occurs when blood is alkaline.

**Ham•bur•ger phe•nom•e•non** (hahm′boor-gĕr) SYN chloride shift.

**Ham•il•ton an•xi•e•ty ra•ting scale** (ham′il-ton) a list of specific symptoms used as a measure of severity of anxiety.

**Ham•il•ton de•pres•sion ra•ting scale** (ham′il-ton) a list of specific symptoms used as a measure of severity of depression.

**Ham•man mur•mur** (ham′ăn) a crunching precordial sound synchronous with the heartbeat; heard in mediastinal emphysema; also known as Hamman crunch.

**Ham•man-Rich syn•drome** (ham′ăn-rich) SYN idiopathic pulmonary fibrosis.

**Ham•man sign** (ham′ăn) a crunching, rasping sound, synchronous with heart beat, heard over the precordium and sometimes at a distance from the chest in mediastinal emphysema.

**Ham•man syn•drome** (ham′ăn) spontaneous mediastinal emphysema, resulting from rupture of alveoli.

**ham•mer** (ham′er) SYN malleus.

**Ham•mer•schlag meth•od** (hah′mer-shlahg) a hydrometric method of determining the specific gravity of the blood by allowing a drop of blood to fall into each of a series of tubes containing mixtures of chloroform and benzene of known graded specific gravities; the specific gravity of that mixture in which the drop remains exactly suspended, neither rising nor falling, corresponds to the specific gravity of the blood sample.

**ham•mer toe** permanent flexion at the midphalangeal joint of one or more of the toes.

**Ham•mond dis•ease** (ham′ŏnd) SYN athetosis.

**Hamp•ton hump** (hamp′ton) a juxtapleural pulmonary soft tissue density on a chest radiograph, convex toward the hilum, usually at the costophrenic angle; described as a manifestation of pulmonary infarction, due to pulmonary embolism.

**ham•string** one of the tendons bounding the popliteal space on either side; the **medial hamstring** comprises the tendons of the semimembranosus and semitendinosus, gracilis, and sartorius muscles; the **lateral hamstring** is the tendon of the biceps femoris muscle. Hamstring muscles (a) have origin from the ischial tuberosity, (b) act across (at) both the hip and knee joints (producing extension and flexion, respectively), and (c) are innervated by the tibial portion of the sciatic nerve. The medial hamstring contributes to medial rotation of the leg at the flexed knee joint, while the lateral hamstring contributes to lateral rotation.

**ham•string ten•don** SEE hamstring.

**Ham test** (ham) SYN acidified serum test.

**ham•u•lar** (ham′yu-lăr) hook-shaped; unciform. [L. *hamulus, q.v.*]

**ham•u•lus,** gen. and pl. **ham•u•li** (ham′yu-lŭs, ham′yu-lī) any hooklike structure. SYN hook (2). [L. dim. of *hamus,* hook]

**Han•cock am•pu•ta•tion** (han′kok) amputation of the foot through the astragalus (talus).

**hand** the portion of the upper limb distal to the radiocarpal joint, comprising the wrist, palm, and fingers. SYN manus [TA]. [A.S.]

**hand•ed•ness** (hand′ed-nes) preference for the use of one hand, most commonly the right, associated with dominance of the opposite cerebral hemisphere; may also be the result of training or habit.

**hand-foot-and-mouth dis•ease** an exanthematous eruption of small, pearl-gray vesicles of the fingers, toes, palms, and soles, accompanied by painful vesicles and ulceration of the buccal mucous membrane and the tongue and by slight fever; the disease lasts 4 to 7 days, and is usually caused by Coxsackie virus type A-16, but other types have been identified.

**hand•i•cap** (hand′i-kap) **1.** a physical, mental, or emotional condition that interferes with an individual's normal functioning. **2.** reduction in a person's capacity to fulfill a social role as a consequence of an impairment, inadequate training for the role, or other circumstances. SEE ALSO disability. [fr. *hand in cap* (game)]

**hand•ling** use of the therapist's hands in a trained manner on parts of the patient's body to decrease the frequency of abnormal patterns of movement and to increase the occurrence of automatic normal movement.

**Hand-Schül•ler-Chris•tian dis•ease** (hand-shēl′ĕr-kris′chen) the chronic disseminated form of Langerhans cell histiocytosis. The classic triad of signs consists of diabetes insipidus, exophthalmus, and bony lesions composed of histiocytes. SYN Christian disease (1), Christian syndrome, Schüller syndrome.

**hand•shapes** (hand′shāps) manual symbols of speech sounds used in cued speech.

**hang•man's frac•ture** a fracture of the cervical spine through the pedicles of C-2; may be associated with an anterior dislocation of the C-2 vertebral body with respect to C-3.

**hang•nail** (hang′nāl) a loose triangular tag of skin

attached at the proximal portion in the medial or lateral nail fold.

**Hanks so•lu•tion** (hanks) a salt solution usually used in combination with naturally occurring body substances (e.g., blood serum, tissue extracts) and/or more complex chemically defined nutritive solutions for culturing animal cells; two variations contain $CaCl_2$, $MgSO_4 \cdot 7H_2O$, $KCl$, $KH_2PO_4$, $NaHCO_3$, $NaCl$, $Na_2HPO_4 \cdot 2H_2O$, and D-glucose.

**Han•no•ver ca•nal** (hahn'ō-vĕr) the potential space between the ciliary zonule and the vitreous body.

**Han•sen ba•cil•lus** (hahn'sĕn) SYN *Mycobacterium leprae.*

**Han•sen dis•ease** (hahn'sĕn) SYN leprosy.

**Han•ta•vi•rus** (han'tä-vī-rŭs) a genus of Bunyaviridae responsible for pneumonia and hemorrhagic fevers. Four members of the genus are recognized thus far: Hantaan, Puumala, Seoul, and Prospect Hill. The first three of these are known human pathogens; Hantaan virus causes Korean hemorrhagic fever. Various rodent species are the asymptomatic carriers of these viruses, which are shed in saliva, urine, and feces. Human infection is direct, or by the respiratory route from contaminated specimens; person-to-person spread has not been demonstrated. In 1992 this virus was isolated from patients in Arizona and New Mexico. Affected persons may have a mild to fatal course. The most seriously ill have hemorrhagic fevers accompanied by renal failure and sometimes respiratory collapse.

**han•ta•vi•rus pul•mo•na•ry syn•drome** a febrile disease caused by several species of Hantavirus (Andes, Bayou, Black Creek Canal, New York, and Sin Nombre viruses) in North and South America and characterized by thrombocytopenia, leukocytosis, and capillary leakage in the lungs, with death due to shock and cardiac complications.

**H an•ti•gen 1.** the antigen in the flagella of motile bacteria; SEE ALSO O antigen (1). **2.** the chemical precursor of antigens of the ABO blood group locus.

**HA-P** hemagglutinin-protease

**haph•al•ge•sia** (haf-al-jē'zē-ă) pain or an extremely disagreeable sensation caused by the merest touch. SYN Pitres sign (1). [G. *haphē,* touch, + *algēsis,* sense of pain]

△**hap•lo-** simple, single. [G. *haplous*]

**hap•loid** (hap'loyd) denoting the number of chromosomes in sperm or ova, which is half the number in somatic (diploid) cells; the haploid number in normal human beings is 23. [G. *haplos,* simple, + *eidos,* appearance]

**hap•lo•pro•tein** (hap-lō-prō'tēn) the functional complex between an apoprotein and the prosthetic group that together are responsible for biological activity.

**hap•lo•scope** an instrument for presenting separate views to each eye so that they may be seen as one.

**hap•lo•scop•ic** (hap-lō-skop'ik) relating to a haploscope.

**hap•lo•type** (hap'lō-tīp) **1.** the genetic constitution of an individual with respect to one member of a pair of allelic genes; individuals are of the same haplotype (but of different genotypes) if alike with respect to one allele of a pair but different with respect to the other allele of a pair.

**2.** IMMUNOGENETICS that portion of the phenotype determined by a set of closely linked genes inherited from one parent (i.e., genes located on one of the pair of chromosomes). The human major histocompatability complex comprises 4 recognized loci (A, B, C, and D) for which there are more than 50 alleles. Similarly, the allotypic markers (antigens) of the immunoglobulin subclasses IgG1, IgG2, IgG3, and IgA2 occur in combinations and are inherited as units almost always unchanged in transmission; the alleles that control these various haplotypes are not linked to those controlling the antigens of the κ type L chains. [haplo- + G. *typos,* impression, model]

**hap•ten** a molecule that is incapable, alone, of causing the production of antibodies but can, however, combine with a larger antigenic molecule called a carrier. SYN incomplete antigen, partial antigen. [G. *haptō,* to fasten, bind]

**hap•tics** (hap'tiks) the science concerned with the tactile sense. [G. *haptō,* to grasp, touch]

**hap•to•glo•bin** (hap-tō-glō'bin) a group of $α_2$-globulins in human serum, so called because of their ability to combine with hemoglobin; variant types form a polymorphic system, with α- and β-polypeptide chains controlled by separate genetic loci. [G. *haptō,* to grasp, + hemoglobin]

**Ha•ra•da-Ito pro•ce•dure** (hah-rah'dah-ē'tō) a procedure designed to correct ocular extorsion due to fourth nerve palsy by selectively tightening the anterior fibers of the superior oblique tendon.

**Ha•ra•da-Mo•ri fil•ter pa•per strip cul•ture** (hah-rah'dah-mō'rē) a combination of filter paper, fecal specimen, and tap water placed in a centrifuge tube; provides an environment for nematode eggs to hatch and larvae to develop.

**Ha•ra•da syn•drome, Ha•ra•da dis•ease** (hahrah'dah, hah-rah'dah) bilateral retinal edema, uveitis, choroiditis, and retinal detachment, with temporary or permanent deafness, graying of the hair (poliosis), and alopecia; related to the Vogt-Koyanagi syndrome and sympathetic ophthalmia.

**hard chan•cre** SYN chancre.

**hard corn** the usual form of corn over a toe joint. SYN heloma durum.

**hard dru•sen** type of exudative or typical drusen that appear ophthalmoscopically as discrete, yellow nodules characterized histopathologically by well-defined accumulations of hyaline material in the inner and outer collagenous zones of Bruch membrane.

**hard•en•ing** (har'den-ing) **1.** a condition of lessened reactions to allergens from repeated or prolonged nontherapeutic exposure, similar to hyposensitization. **2.** any procedure in tissue preparation for examinations, such as sectioning for microscopy, that renders the tissue firmer.

**hard pal•ate 1.** the anterior part of the palate, consisting of the bony palate covered above by the mucous membrane of the floor of the nasal cavity and below by the mucoperiosteum of the roof of the mouth which contains the palatine vessels, nerves, and mucous glands; **2.** CEPHALOMETRICS a line connecting the anterior and posterior nasal spines to represent the position of the bony palate.

**hard pulse** a pulse that strikes forcibly against the tip of the finger and is with difficulty compressed, suggesting hypertension.

**hard tu•ber•cle** a tubercle lacking necrosis.

**hard ul•cer** SYN chancre.

**Har•dy-Rand-Rit•ter test** (har'dē-rand-rit'er) a test for color vision deficiency using pseudoisochromatic cards. These excellent cards have not been reprinted by the American Optical Co. since the plates were accidentally destroyed in 1965.

**Har•dy-Wein•berg law** (har'dē vīn'bĕrg) if mating occurs at random with respect to any one autosomal locus in a population in which the gene frequencies are equal in the two sexes, and the factors tending to change gene frequencies (mutation, differential selection, migration) are either absent or negligible, then in one generation the probabilities of all possible genotypes will on average equal the same proportions as if the genes were assembled at random. The law does not apply to two or more loci jointly, nor to X-linked traits where the initial gene frequencies differ in the two sexes.

**hare•lip** (hār'lip) SYN cleft lip.

**har•le•quin fe•tus** a severe form of collodion baby in a newborn, usually premature; a form of ichthyosiform erythroderma characterized by encasement of the body in grayish brown, often fissured plaques resembling plates of armor, and by grotesque deformity of the face, hands, and feet; usually fatal within a few days.

**har•mon•ic mean** the mean calculated as the number of values being averaged, divided by the sum of their reciprocals.

**har•mon•ic su•ture** SYN plane suture.

**har•mo•ni•ous cor•re•spon•dence** a type of anomalous retinal correspondence in which the angle of the visual direction of the two retinas is equal to the objective angle of strabismus.

**har•mo•ni•ous ret•i•nal cor•re•spon•dence** a type of anomalous retinal correspondence in which the angle of the visual direction of the two retinas is equal to the objective angle of strabismus.

**Har•ris he•ma•tox•y•lin** (har'is) an alum type of hematoxylin similar to Delafield hematoxylin, but which uses chemical ripening to produce oxidation of hematoxylin for immediate use.

**Har•ri•son groove** (har'ĭ-son) a deformity of the ribs which results from the pull of the diaphragm on ribs weakened by rickets or other softening of the bone.

**Hart•mann cu•rette** (hahrt'măn) a curette, cutting on the side, for the removal of adenoids.

**Hart•mann op•er•a•tion** (hahrt'măn) resection of the sigmoid colon beginning at or just above the peritoneal reflexion and extending proximally, with closure of the rectal stump and end-colostomy.

**Hart•mann so•lu•tion** (hahrt'măn) SYN lactated Ringer solution.

**Hart•man so•lu•tion** (hahrt'măn) a solution used to desensitize dentin in dental operations; contains thymol, ethyl alcohol, and diethyl ether.

**Hart•nup dis•ease, Hart•nup syn•drome** (hahrt'nŭp) a congenital metabolic disorder consisting of aminoaciduria due to a defect in renal tubular absorption of neutral α-amino acids and urinary excretion of tryptophan derivatives, because defective intestinal absorption leads to bacterial degradation of unabsorbed tryptophan in the gut; characterized by a pellagra-like, light-sensitive skin rash with temporary cerebellar ataxia.

**har•vest** to obtain cells or tissues for grafting or transplantation, from either a donor or the patient.

**Ha•shi•mo•to thy•roid•i•tis** (hah-shē-mō'tō) diffuse infiltration of the thyroid gland with lymphocytes, resulting in diffuse goiter, progressive destruction of the parenchyma, and hypothyroidism.

**hash•ish** (hash-ēsh') a form of cannabis that consists largely of resin from the flowering tops and sprouts of cultivated female hemp plants of the species *Cannabis sativa;* contains the highest concentration of cannabinols among preparations derived from cannabis. [Ar. hay]

**Has•sall bod•ies, Has•sall con•cen•tric cor•pus•cle** (has'ĕl) SYN thymic corpuscle.

**Has•son can•nu•la** (has'ĕn) a laparoscopic instrument for open (rather than blind needle insufflation) placement of the initial port. The Hasson has a blunt-tipped obturator instead of a sharp trocar and a balloon on the distal portion of the sheath to hold it in place.

**hatch•ing flask** a flask painted a dark color, so that only a small area of dechlorinated water at the top is exposed to light in simulation of pond water conditions, which stimulates hatching of any live schistosome eggs in fresh stool and urine sediment added to the flask; the released miracidium larvae will be searching for appropriate snail intermediate hosts.

**Hauch (H)** (howkh) a term used to designate the flagellar antigen of bacteria. SEE ALSO H antigen. [Ger. breath]

**haus•tral** (haw'străl) relating to a haustrum.

**haus•tra•tion** (haw-strā'shŭn) **1.** the process of formation of a haustrum. **2.** an increase in prominence of the haustra.

**haus•trum,** pl. **haus•tra** (haw'strŭm, haw'stră) [TA] one of a series of saccules or pouches, so called because of a fancied resemblance to the buckets on a water wheel. [L. a machine for drawing water, fr. *haurio,* pp. *haustus,* to draw up, drink up]

**HAV** hepatitis A virus.

**Ha•ver•hill fe•ver** (hav'ĕr-hil) an infection by *Streptobacillus moniliformis* marked by initial chills and high fever (gradually subsiding), by arthritis usually in the larger joints and spine, and by a rash occurring chiefly over the joints and on the extensor surfaces of the extremities. SYN erythema arthriticum epidemicum. [*Haverhill*, MA, where an epidemic occurred in 1926]

**ha•ver•si•an** (ha-ver'zhăn) relating to Clopton Havers and the various osseous structures described by him.

**ha•ver•si•an ca•nals** (ha-vĕr'zhăn) vascular canals that run longitudinally in the center of haversian systems of compact osseous tissue.

**ha•ver•si•an la•mel•la** (ha-vĕr'zhăn) SYN concentric lamella.

**ha•ver•si•an spac•es** (ha-vĕr'zhăn) spaces in bone formed by the enlargement of haversian canals.

**ha•ver•si•an sys•tem** (ha-vĕr'zhăn) SYN osteon.

**HA1 vi•rus** SYN hemadsorption virus type 1. SEE parainfluenza viruses.

**HA2 vi•rus** SYN hemadsorption virus type 2. SEE parainfluenza viruses.

**Haw•kins im•pinge•ment sign** (haw'kinz) pain produced by forced internal rotation of the humerus in 90° of abduction.

**h**
**a**

**Ha·yem so·lu·tion** (ah'yahn) a blood diluent used prior to counting red blood cells.

**hay fe·ver** a form of atopy characterized by an acute irritative inflammation of the mucous membranes of the eyes and upper respiratory passages accompanied by itching and profuse watery secretion, followed occasionally by bronchitis and asthma; the episode recurs annually at the same or nearly the same time of the year, in spring, summer, or late summer and autumn, caused by an allergic reaction to the pollen of trees, grasses, weeds, flowers, etc.

**Hay·flick lim·it** (hā'flik) the limit of human cell division in subcultures; such cells typically divide only about 50 times before dying out.

**Hay·garth nodes** (hā-garth') exostoses from the margins of the articular surfaces and from the periosteum and bone in the neighborhood of the joints of the fingers, leading to ankylosis and associated with lateral deflection of the fingers toward the ulnar side, which occur in rheumatoid arthritis.

**Hb** hemoglobin.

**Hb A** hemoglobin A.

**HB$_c$Ab** antibody to the hepatitis B core antigen.

**HB$_c$Ag** hepatitis B core antigen.

**HB$_s$Ag** hepatitis B surface antigen.

**H band** the paler area in the center of the A band of a striated muscle fiber, comprising the central portion of thick (myosin) filaments that are not overlapped by thin (actin) filaments.

**Hb C** hemoglobin C.

**HBE** His bundle electrogram.

**HBe, HB$_e$Ag** hepatitis B e antigen.

**Hb F** hemoglobin F.

**HBIG** hepatitis B immune globulin.

**Hb S** hemoglobin S; sickle cell hemoglobin.

**HBV** hepatitis B virus.

**HCFA** Health Care Financing Administration.

**HCPCS** Health Care Financing Administration Common Procedures Coding System.

**HCS** human chorionic somatomammotropic hormone.

**Hct** hematocrit.

**HCV** hepatitis C virus.

**HDL** high density lipoprotein. SEE lipoprotein.

**HDV** hepatitis D virus.

**He** helium.

**head** (hed) **1.** the upper or anterior extremity of the animal body, containing the brain and the organs of sight, hearing, taste, and smell. **2.** the upper, anterior, or larger extremity, expanded or rounded, of any body, organ, or other anatomic structure. **3.** the rounded extremity of a bone. **4.** that end of a muscle that is attached to the less movable part of the skeleton. [A.S. *heáfod*]

**head·ache** (hed'āk) pain in various parts of the head, not confined to the area of distribution of any nerve. SEE ALSO cephalodynia. SYN cephalalgia, encephalalgia.

**Head ar·e·as** (hed) areas of skin exhibiting reflex hyperesthesia and hyperalgesia due to visceral disease.

**head cap** SYN acrosomal cap.

**head-drop·ping test** a test used in the diagnosis of disease of the extrapyramidal or striatal system (e.g., parkinsonism, Wilson disease); with the patient supine and relaxed, the examiner briskly lifts the head with the right hand and then allows it to drop upon the palm of the left hand; the head of a normal person drops suddenly like

a dead weight, whereas, in striatal disease the head falls slowly, gently, and almost hesitantly.

**Head lines, Head zones** (hed, hed) bands of cutaneous hyperesthesia associated with acute or chronic inflammation of the viscera.

**heal** (hēl) **1.** to restore to health, especially to cause an ulcer or wound to cicatrize or unite. **2.** to become well, to be cured; to cicatrize or close, said of an ulcer or wound. [A.S. *healan*]

**heal·ing** (hēl'ing) **1.** restoring to health; promoting the closure of wounds and ulcers. **2.** the process of a return to health. **3.** closing of a wound. SEE ALSO union.

**heal·ing by first in·ten·tion** healing by fibrous adhesion, without suppuration or granulation tissue formation. SYN primary adhesion, primary union.

**heal·ing by sec·ond in·ten·tion** delayed closure of two granulating surfaces. SYN secondary adhesion, secondary union.

**heal·ing by third in·ten·tion** the slow filling of a wound cavity or ulcer by granulations, with subsequent cicatrization.

**health** (helth) **1.** the state of the organism when it functions optimally without evidence of disease or abnormality. **2.** a state characterized by anatomical, physiological, and psychological integrity, ability to perform personally valued family, work, and community roles; ability to deal with physical, biological, psychological and social stress; a feeling of well-being; and freedom from the risk of disease and untimely death. **3.** complete physical, mental, and social well-being, not just the absence of disease, as defined by the World Health Organization. [A.S. *haelth*]

**Health Ca·na·da** Canadian government agency that develops national health policy, enforces national health regulations, and promotes disease prevention.

**Health Care Fi·nanc·ing Ad·mi·ni·stra·tion (HCFA)** agency of the U.S. Department of Health and Human Services that manages the federal health care programs of Medicare and Medicaid.

**Health Care Fi·nanc·ing Ad·mi·ni·stra·tion Com·mon Pro·ce·dures Co·ding Sys·tem (HCPCS)** the alphanumeric coding system for reporting outpatient health care services for Medicare beneficiaries.

**health care pro·vi·der** general term for any institution or member of the health care team providing health care. SEE ALSO doctor, physician, nurse.

**health in·for·ma·tics** the practice and technology of collecting, storing, and analyzing healthcare data electronically and transferring data between computer systems.

**health in·for·ma·tion ma·nage·ment (HIM)** collection and analysis of health care data in order to provide information for health care decisions involving patient care, institutional management, health care policies and planning, and research; formerly known as medical records management. SEE ALSO record.

**health in·for·ma·tion sys·tem** combination of vital and health statistical data from multiple sources, used to derive information about the health needs, health resources, use of health services, and outcomes of use by the people in a defined region or jurisdiction.

**Health In·sur·ance Por·ta·bil·i·ty and Ac··**

**count·a·bil·i·ty Act (HIPAA)** federal legislation designed to preserve health insurance coverage for workers, and their families, when they change or lose their jobs.

**health main·te·nance or·ga·ni·za·tion (HMO)** a comprehensive prepaid system of health care with emphasis on the prevention and early detection of disease, and continuity of care. HMOs may be nonprofit or profit-making ventures, and along with preferred provider organizations (PPOs) and managed care plans have begun to dominate the health care market. HMOs generally offer a package of services; however, the choice of physician is frequently limited to those working within the HMO. SEE ALSO managed care, preferred provider organization.

**Health Plan Em·ploy·er Da·ta and In·for·ma·tion Set (HEDIS)** a set of standardized measures for comparing of health plans; developed and maintained by the National Committee for Quality Assurance (NCQA).

**health re·cord** formerly known as the medical record; a comprehensive record containing all the information in the medical record but also covering all aspects of the patient's physical, mental, and social health.

**health-re·la·ted phy·si·cal fit·ness** components of physical fitness (most commonly, aerobic fitness, body composition, abdominal muscular strength and endurance, and lower back and hamstring flexibility) that are associated with some aspect of overall good health or disease prevention.

**Health Re·sour·ces and Ser·vi·ces Ad·mi·ni·stra·tion (HRSA)** a federal agency responsible for managing national data banks, such as the National Practitioner Data Bank, as well as other health care programs.

**health risk ap·prais·al** a method of describing an individual's chance of falling ill or dying of a specified condition, based on actuarial calculations that allow for known exposure to risk; expressed as expected age at which death or disease will occur, and intended as a way of drawing an individual's attention to the probable consequences of risk behavior.

**healthy** (helth'ē) well; in a state of normal functioning; free from disease.

**Hea·ney op·er·a·tion** (hē'nē) technique for vaginal hysterectomy.

**hear·ing** (hēr'ing) the ability to perceive sound; the sensation of sound as opposed to vibration. SYN -acousis (2), audition.

**hear·ing aid** (hēr'ing ād) an electronic amplifying device designed to bring sound more effectively into the ear; it consists of a microphone, amplifier, and receiver. SYN hearing instrument.

**Hear·ing Han·di·cap In·ven·tory for the El·der·ly (HHIE-S)** screening test that uses a communication scale to determine if older adults have difficulty hearing and understanding speech.

**hear·ing im·pair·ment, hear·ing loss** a reduction in the ability to perceive sound; may range from slight inability to complete deafness. SEE ALSO deafness.

**hear·ing in·stru·ment** SYN hearing aid.

**hearing protector** occlusive devices for the external auditory canal made of pliable material or fluid (usually glycerin)-filled ear muffs for protection against noise-induced hearing loss.

**heart** (hart) a hollow muscular organ which receives the blood from the veins and propels it into the arteries. It is divided by a musculomembranous septum into two halves—right or venous and left or arterial—each of which consists of a receiving chamber (atrium) and an ejecting chamber (ventricle). See this page and A26. SYN cor [TA], coeur. [A.S. *heorte*]

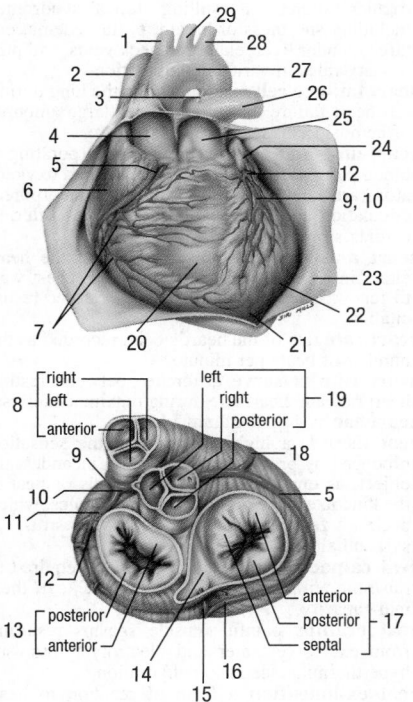

**human heart:** (top) a ventral view with pericardium opened (bottom) transverse section at the level of the valves: (1) brachiocephalic trunk, (2) superior vena cava, (3) ligamentum arteriosum, (4) ascending aorta, (5) right coronary a., (6) right atrium, (7) cardiac veins, (8) cusps of pulmonary valve, (9) anterior descending branch, (10) left coronary a. (11) circumflex branch, (12) great cardiac v., (13) cusps of mitral valve, (14) valve and ostium of coronary sinus, (15) middle cardiac v., (16) posterior interventricular branch, (17) cusps of tricuspid valve, (18) right marginal branch, (19) cusps of aortic valve, (20) right ventricle, (21) cardiac apex, (22) left ventricle, (23) pericardium, (24) left atrium, (25) pulmonary trunk, (26) left pulmonary a. (27) aortic arch, (28) left subclavian a., (29) left common carotid a.

**heart at·tack** SYN myocardial infarction.

**heart·beat** (hart'bēt) a single complete cycle of contraction and dilation of heart muscle.

**heart·burn** (hart'bern) SYN pyrosis.

**heart cham·ber re·mo·del·ing** an architectural change in any cardiac chamber (usually one or both ventricles) due to a pathologic or normal (neonatal) stimulus.

**heart fail·ure 1.** inadequacy of the heart so that as a pump it fails to maintain the circulation of blood, with the result that congestion and edema develop in the tissues; SYN cardiac insufficiency, congestive heart failure, myocardial insufficiency. SEE ALSO forward heart failure, backward heart failure, right ventricular failure, left ventricular failure. **2.** resulting clinical syndromes including shortness of breath, pitting edema, enlarged tender liver, engorged neck veins, and pulmonary rales in various combinations.

**heart fail·ure cell** macrophage in the lung during left heart failure that often carries large amounts of hemosiderin. SEE ALSO siderophore.

**heart-lung ma·chine** a device incorporating a blood pump (artificial heart) and a blood oxygenator (artificial lung) to provide extracorporeal circulation and oxygenation of the blood during cardiac surgery.

**heart mas·sage** rhythmic massage of the heart either in an open chest or through the chest wall to renew failed circulation during cardiac resuscitation.

**heart rate** rate of the heart's beat, recorded as the number of beats per minute.

**heart rate re·serve** difference between resting heart rate and heart rate during maximal exercise.

**heart sac** SYN pericardium.

**heat** (hēt) **1.** a high temperature; the sensation produced by proximity to fire or an incandescent object, as opposed to cold. The basis of heat is the kinetic energy of atoms and molecules, which becomes zero at absolute zero. **2.** SYN estrus. **3.** SYN enthalpy. [A.S. *haete*]

**heat ca·pac·i·ty** the quantity of heat required to raise the temperature of a system 1°C. SYN thermal capacity.

**heat cramps** painful muscle spasms resulting from excessive water and electrolyte loss. SEE hyperthermia. SEE ALSO dehydration.

**heat ex·haus·tion** a form of reaction to heat, marked by prostration, weakness, and collapse, resulting from severe dehydration.

**heat-la·bile** (hēt'lā'bīl) destroyed or altered by heat.

**heat lamp** a lamp that emits infrared light and produces heat; used to apply topical heat to the skin.

**heat rash** SYN miliaria rubra.

**heat stress in·dex** measure of environment's potential to cause heat injury; based on ambient air temperature and relative humidity.

**heat·stroke, heat stroke** (hēt'strōk) a severe and often fatal illness produced by exposure to excessively high temperatures, especially when accompanied by marked exertion; characterized by headache, vertigo, confusion, hot dry skin, and a slight rise in body temperature; in severe cases, very high fever, vascular collapse, and coma develop.

**heat ur·ti·car·ia** SYN cholinergic urticaria.

**heav·y chain** a polypeptide chain of high molecular weight determining the class and subclass of an immunoglobulin.

**heav·y chain dis·ease** a term used for a group of diseases, the paraproteinemias, characterized by production of homogeneous immunoglobulins or fragments, and associated with malignant disorders of the plasmacytic and lymphoid cell series.

**he·be·phre·nia** (hē-bĕ-frē'nē-ă, heb'ē-frē'nē-ă) a syndrome characterized by shallow and inappropriate affect, giggling, and silly, regressive behavior and mannerisms; a subtype of schizophrenia now renamed disorganized schizophrenia. [G. *hēbē*, puberty, + *phrēn*, the mind]

**he·be·phren·ic** (hē-bĕ-frēn'ik, heb-ē-frēn'ik) relating to or characterized by hebephrenia.

**he·be·phren·ic schiz·o·phre·nia** SYN disorganized schizophrenia.

**Heb·er·den nodes** (hē'bĕr-dĕn) exostoses about the size of a pea or smaller, found on the terminal phalanges of the fingers in osteoarthritis, which are enlargements of the tubercles at the articular extremities of the distal phalanges. SYN tuberculum arthriticum (1).

**he·bet·ic** (hē-bet'ik) pertaining to youth. [G. *hēbētikos*, youthful, fr. *hēbē*, youth]

**he·bi·at·rics** (hē-bē-at'riks) SYN adolescent medicine. [G. *hēbē*, youth, + *iatrikos*, relating to medicine]

**He·bra pru·ri·go** (hā'brah) a severe form of chronic dermatitis with secondary infection in which there are constantly recurring, intensely itchy papules and nodules, often associated with atopy.

**hec·a·ter·o·mer·ic** (hek'ă-ter-ō-mer'ik) denoting a spinal neuron whose axon divides and gives off processes to both sides of the cord; usually the same as a heteromeric neuron. [G. *hekateros*, each of two, + *meros*, part]

△**hec·to- (h)** prefix used in the SI and metric systems to signify one hundred ($10^2$). [G. *hekaton*, one hundred]

**hec·to·me·ter** (hek'tō-mē-ter) one hundred meters.

**hec·to·me·tre [Br.]** SEE hectometer.

**HEDIS** Health Plan Employer Data and Information Set.

**hed·ro·cele** (hed'rō-sēl) prolapse of the intestine through the anus. [G. *hedra*, a seat, the fundament, + *kēlē*, hernia]

**heel** (hēl) **1.** SYN calx (2). **2.** SYN distal end. [A.S. *hēla*]

**heel bone** SYN calcaneus (1).

**heel pad** an encapsulated body of fat beneath the plantar surface of the calcaneus, which cushions during weight bearing and walking.

**heel spur** an abnormal bony growth on the calcaneus. SYN bone spur, calcaneal spur.

**heel ten·don** SYN tendo calcaneus.

**Heer·fordt dis·ease** (hār'fort) SYN uveoparotid fever.

**He·gar di·la·tors** (hā'gahr) a series of cylindrical bougies of graduated sizes used to dilate the cervical canal.

**He·gar sign** (hā'gahr) softening and compressibility of the lower segment of the uterus in early pregnancy (about the seventh week) which, on bimanual examination, is felt by the finger in the vagina as though the neck and body of the uterus were separated, or connected by only a thin band of tissue.

**Hegg·lin a·nom·a·ly** (heg'lin) a disorder in which neutrophils and eosinophils contain basophilic structures known as Döhle or Amato bodies and in which there is faulty maturation of platelets, with thrombocytopenia; autosomal dominant inheritance.

**Hegg·lin syn·drome** (heg'lin) dissociation between electromechanical systole ($QS_2$ interval) and electrical systole (QT interval) so that the second heart tone (SII) is recorded before the end of the T wave; described by Hegglin as an energy-dynamic cardiac insufficiency during diabetic coma and other metabolic disorders.

**Hei·den·hain a·zan stain** (hī′dĕn-hīn) a technique using azocarmine B or G followed by aniline blue to stain nuclei and erythrocytes red, muscle orange, glia fibrils reddish, mucin blue, and collagen and reticulum dark blue. [*azo*carmine + *ani*line blue]

**Hei·den·hain iron he·ma·tox·y·lin stain** (hī′dĕn-hīn) an iron alum hematoxylin stain used for staining muscle striations and mitotic structures blue-black.

**Hei·den·hain law** (hī′dĕn-hīn) glandular secretion is always accompanied by an alteration in the structure of the gland.

**height (h)** (hīt) vertical measurement.

**height of con·tour** the line encircling a tooth or other structure at its greatest bulge or diameter with respect to a selected axis.

**Heil·bron·ner thigh** (hīl′bron-ĕr) in cases of organic paralysis, flattening and broadening of the thigh, when the patient lies supine on a hard mattress; absent in hysterical paralysis.

**Heim·lich ma·neu·ver** (hīm′lik) a procedure to expel an obstructing bolus of food from the throat by placing a fist on the abdomen between the navel and the costal margin, grasping the fist with the other hand, and thrusting it inward and upward so as to drive the diaphragm upward, forcing air up the trachea to dislodge the obstruction. See this page.

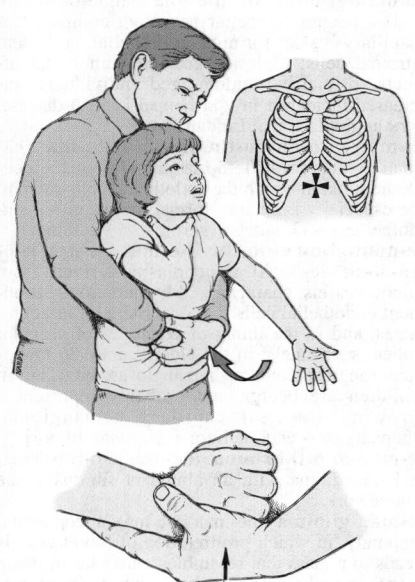

**Heimlich maneuver:** bottom image shows view from above

**Heinz-Ehr·lich bod·y** (hīnts-er′lik) SYN Ehrlich inner body. See page B2.

**HeLa** (hē′lă) referring to cells of the first continu-

ously cultured (human cervical) carcinoma strain. [*H*enrietta *La*cks (d. 1951), whose cervical carcinoma was the source of the cell line]

**hel·i·cal** (hel′i-kăl) **1.** relating to a helix. SYN helicine (2). **2.** SYN helicoid. [G. *helix,* a coil]

**hel·i·ces** (hel′i-sēz) plural of helix.

**hel·i·cine** (hel′i-sēn) **1.** coiled. **2.** SYN helical (1). [G. *helix,* a coil]

**Hel·i·co·bac·ter** (hel′i-kō-bak′ter) a genus of helical, curved, or straight microaerophilic bacteria with rounded ends and numerous sheathed flagella (unipolar or bipolar and lateral) with terminal bulbs. Form nonpigmented, translucent colonies, 1–2 mm in diameter. Catalase and oxidase positive. Found in gastric mucosa of ferrets and primates, including human beings. Some species are associated with gastric and peptic ulcers and predispose to gastric carcinoma. The type species is *Helicobacter pylori.*

**Hel·i·co·bac·ter ci·na·e·di** a bacterial species associated with cases of proctitis and colitis in homosexual men.

**Hel·i·co·bac·ter fen·nel·li·ae** a bacterial species reported associated with proctitis and colitis in homosexual men.

**Hel·i·co·bac·ter heil·man·ni·i** species observed in gastric mucosa. This agent has a low prevalence (less than 1% of patients), has not been cultured in vitro, and is of unknown pathogenic significance.

**Hel·i·co·bac·ter py·lo·ri** a recently identified species that produces urease and is associated with several gastroduodenal diseases including gastritis and peptic ulcer. The type species of the genus *Helicobacter.*

**hel·i·coid** (hel′i-koyd) resembling a helix. SYN helical (2). [G. *helix,* a coil, + *eidos,* resemblance]

**hel·i·co·pod gait** a gait, seen in some conversion reactions or hysterical disorders, in which the feet describe half circles. SYN helicopodia.

**hel·i·co·po·dia** (hel′i-kō-pō′dē-ă) SYN helicopod gait. [G. *helix,* a coil, + *pous,* foot]

**hel·i·co·tre·ma** (hel′i-kō-trē′mă) a semilunar opening at the apex of the cochlea through which the scala vestibuli and the scala tympani of the cochlea communicate with one another. [G. *helix,* a spiral, + *trēma,* a hole]

**he·li·en·ceph·a·li·tis** (hē-lē-en-sef-ă-lī′tis) inflammation of the brain following sunstroke. [G. *helios,* sun, + *enkephalos,* brain, + *-itis,* inflammation]

**he·li·um (He)** (hē′lē-ŭm) a gaseous element present in minute amounts in the atmosphere (0.000524% of dry volume); atomic no. 2, atomic wt. 4.002602; used as a diluent of medicinal gases, particularly oxygen [G. *hēlios,* the sun]

**he·li·um ther·a·py** the use of a helium-gas mixture (usually helium and oxygen) in the management of obstruction of the airways; the density of helium is much lower than that of either air or oxygen; as a result, the gaseous mixture will move past an airway obstruction more easily.

**he·lix,** pl. **hel·i·ces** (hē′liks, hel′i-sēz) [TA] **1.** the margin of the auricle; a folded rim of cartilage forming the upper part of the anterior, the superior, and the greater part of the posterior edges of the auricle. **2.** a line in the shape of a coil (or a spring, or the threads on a bolt), each point being equidistant from a straight line that is the axis of the cylinder in which each point of the helix lies.

h
e

USAGE NOTE: Often mistakenly applied to a spiral. [L. fr. G. *helix,* a coil]

**Hel·lin law** (hel'in) twins occur once in 89 births, triplets once in $89^2$, and quadruplets once in $89^3$. If the frequency of twins in a population is *p*, the frequency of triplets is $p^2$, and the frequency of quadruplets is $p^3$.

**Hel·ly fix·a·tive** (hel-ē) a combination of potassium dichromate, mercuric chloride, formaldehyde, and distilled water, used as a microanatomic fixative for cytoplasmic granules and nuclear staining; has the same disadvantages as Zenker fixative.

**Helm·holtz en·er·gy (A)** (helm'hōlts) energy equivalent to the internal energy minus the entropy contribution (TS).

**hel·minth** an intestinal vermiform parasite, primarily nematodes, cestodes, trematodes, and acanthocephalans. [G. *helmins,* worm]

**hel·min·tha·gogue** (hel-minth'ă-gog) SYN anthelmintic (1). [G. *helmins,* worm, + *agōgos,* leading]

**hel·min·them·e·sis** (hel-min-them'ě-sis) the vomiting or expulsion through the mouth of intestinal worms. [G. *helmins,* a worm, + *emesis,* vomiting]

**hel·min·thi·a·sis** (hel-min-thī'ă-sis) the condition of having intestinal vermiform parasites.

**hel·min·tho·ma** (hel-min-thō'mă) a discrete nodule of granulomatous inflammation (including the healed stage) caused by a helminth or its products. [G. *helmins,* worm, + *-oma,* tumor]

*Hel·min·tho·spo·ri·um* (hel-min-thō-spōr'ē-ŭm) a saprobic fungus, often isolated in clinical laboratories.

**he·lo·ma** (hē-lō'mă) SYN clavus. [G. *hēlos,* nail, + *-oma,* tumor]

**he·lo·ma du·rum** SYN hard corn.

**he·lo·ma mol·le** SYN soft corn.

**he·lot·o·my** (hē-lot'ō-mē) surgical treatment of corns. [heloma + G. *tomē,* cutting]

**help·er cells** SYN T helper cells.

**help·er vi·rus** a virus whose replication renders it possible for a defective virus or a virusoid (also present in the host cell) to develop into a fully infectious agent.

⊿**hem-, hem·a-** blood. SEE ALSO hemat-, hemato-, hemo-. [G. *haima*]

**he·ma·chrome** (hē'mă-krōm) the coloring matter of the blood, hemoglobin or hematin. [hema- + G. *chrōma,* color]

**he·ma·cyte** (hē'mă-sīt) SYN erythrocyte.

**he·ma·cy·tom·e·ter** (hē'mă-sī-tom'ě-ter, hem'ă-sī-tom'ě-ter) SYN hemocytometer.

**he·mad·sorp·tion** (hē'mad-sōrp-shŭn, hem'ad-sōrp-shŭn) a phenomenon manifested by an agent or substance adhering to or being adsorbed on the surface of a red blood cell.

**he·mad·sorp·tion vi·rus type 1** parainfluenza virus type 3. SEE parainfluenza viruses. SYN HA1 virus.

**he·mad·sorp·tion vi·rus type 2** parainfluenza virus type 1. SEE parainfluenza viruses. SYN HA2 virus.

**he·mag·glu·ti·na·tion** (hē-mă-gloo'ti-nā'shŭn) the agglutination of red blood cells; may be immune (as a result of specific antibody to red blood cell antigens or other antigens which coat the red blood cells), or nonimmune (as in hemagglutination caused by viruses or other microbes).

**he·mag·glu·ti·nin** (hē'mă-gloo'ti-nin, hem-ă-gloo'ti-nin) a substance, antibody or other, that causes hemagglutination.

**he·mag·glu·tin·in·pro·te·ase (HA-P)** a cytotoxic enzyme produced by Vibrio cholerae that alters epithelial structure and barrier function.

**he·ma·gog·ic** (hē-mă-goj'ik, hem-ă-) promoting a flow of blood.

**he·mal** (hē'măl) **1.** relating to the blood or blood vessels. **2.** referring to the ventral side of the vertebral bodies or their precursors, where the heart and great vessels are located, as opposed to neural (2). [G. *haima,* blood]

**he·mal·um** (hē-mal'ŭm, hem-al'ŭm) a solution of hematoxylin and alum used as a nuclear stain in histology, especially with eosin as a counterstain.

**he·ma·nal·y·sis** (hē-mă-nal'ĭ-sis, hem-a-nal'ĭ-sis) analysis of the blood; an examination of blood, especially with reference to chemical methods. [G. *haima,* blood, + analysis]

⊿**he·man·gi-** blood vessel. [G. *haima,* blood + *angeion,* vessel]

**he·man·gi·ec·ta·sis, he·man·gi·ec·ta·sia** (hē-man-jē-ek'tăsis, he-man-jē-ek'tăsis; hē-man-jē-ek-tā'zē-ă, he-man-jē-ek-tā'zē-ă) dilation of blood vessels. [G. *haima,* blood, + *angeion,* vessel, + *ektasis,* a stretching]

⊿**he·man·gi·o-** the blood vessels. [G. *haima,* blood, + *angeion,* vessel]

**he·man·gi·o·blast** (he-man'jē-ō-blast) a primordial embryonic cell of mesodermal origin producing cells from which are derived vascular endothelium, reticuloendothelial elements, and blood-forming cells of all types. [hemangio- + G. *blastos,* germ]

**he·man·gi·o·blas·to·ma** (he-man'jē-ō-blas-tō'mă) a benign cerebellar neoplasm composed of capillary vessel-forming endothelial cells and stromal cells; a slowly growing tumor that affects, primarily, middle-aged individuals; increased incidence in von Hippel-Lindau disease. SYN angioblastoma, Lindau tumor.

**he·man·gi·o·en·do·the·li·o·blas·to·ma** (hē-man'jē-ō-en-dō-thē'lē-ō-blas-tō'mă) hemangioendothelioma in which the endothelial cells seem to be especially immature forms. [hemangio- + endothelium + G. *blastos,* germ, + *-oma,* tumor]

**he·man·gi·o·en·do·the·li·o·ma** (he-man'jē-ō-en-dō-thē-lē-ō'mă) a neoplasm derived from blood vessels, characterized by numerous prominent endothelial cells that occur singly, in aggregates, and as the lining of congeries of vascular tubes or channels; in the elderly, may be malignant (angiosarcoma or hemangiosarcoma), but in children are benign and probably represent a growing stage of capillary hemangioma. [hemangio- + endothelium + G. *-oma,* tumor]

**he·man·gi·o·fi·bro·ma** (he-man'jē-ō-fī-brō'mă) a hemangioma with an abundant fibrous tissue framework.

**he·man·gi·o·ma** (he-man'jē-ō'mă) a congenital anomaly, in which proliferation of blood vessels leads to a mass that resembles a neoplasm; it can occur anywhere in the body but is most frequently noticed in the skin and subcutaneous tissues. SEE ALSO nevus. [hemangio- + G. *-oma,* tumor]

**he·man·gi·o·ma·to·sis** (he-man'jē-ō-mă-tō'sis) a condition in which there are numerous hemangiomas.

**he·man·gi·o·per·i·cy·to·ma** (he-man'jē-ō-per'i-sī-tō'mă) an uncommon vascular, usually benign, neoplasm composed of round and spindle cells that are derived from the pericytes and surround endothelium-lined vessels. [hemangio- + pericyte + G. -oma, tumor]

**he·man·gi·o·sar·co·ma** (he-man'jē-ō-sar-kō'mă) a rare malignant neoplasm characterized by rapidly proliferating, extensively infiltrating, anaplastic cells derived from blood vessels and lining irregular blood-filled or lumpy spaces.

**he·ma·po·phys·is** (hē-mă-pŏf'ĭ-sis) the sternal extremity of a rib with its cartilage, representing the second element in each half of a hemal arch. [hem- + apophysis]

**he·mar·thro·sis** (hē'mar-thrō'sis, hem'ar-thrō'sis) blood in a joint. [G. *haima*, blood, + *arthron*, joint]

△**he·mat-** blood. SEE ALSO hem-, hemato-, hemo-. [G. *haima* (*haimat-*)]

**he·ma·te·in** (hēm-ă-tē'in) an oxidation product of hematoxylin.

**he·ma·tem·e·sis** (hē-mă-tem'ĕ-sis, hem-ă-tem'ĕ-sis) vomiting of blood. [hemat- + G. *emesis*, vomiting]

**he·mat·en·ceph·a·lon** (hē'mat-en-sef'ă-lon, hem'at-en-sef'ă-lon) SYN cerebral hemorrhage. [hemat- + G. *enkephalos*, brain]

**he·mat·ic** (hē-mat'ik) 1. relating to blood. SYN hemic. 2. SYN hematinic (2). SYN haemic.

**he·ma·ti·dro·sis** (hē'mat-i-drō'sis, hem'at-i-drō'sis) excretion of blood or blood pigment in the sweat; an extremely rare disorder. SYN hemidrosis (1). [hemat- + G. *hidrōs*, sweat]

**hem·a·tin** (hē'mă-tin, hem'ă-tin) heme in which the iron is Fe(III) (Fe$^{3+}$); the prosthetic group of methemoglobin. SYN ferriheme, hematosin, oxyheme, oxyhemochromogen.

**hem·a·tin chlo·ride** SYN hemin.

**he·ma·ti·ne·mia** (hē'mă-ti-nē'mē-ă, hem'ă-ti-nē'mē-ă) the presence of heme in the circulating blood. [hematin + G. *haima*, blood]

**hem·a·tin·ic** (hē-mă-tin'ik, hem-a-tin'ik) 1. improving the condition of the blood. 2. an agent that increases the number of erythrocytes and/or the hemoglobin concentration of the blood. SYN hematic (2).

△**he·ma·to-** combining form denoting blood. SEE ALSO hem-, hemat-, hemo-. [G. *haima* (*haimat-*)]

**he·ma·to·blast** (hēmă-t'ō-blast) a primordial, undifferentiated form of blood cell from which erythroblasts, lymphoblasts, myeloblasts, and other immature blood cells are derived; in normal bone marrow, present only in small numbers and difficult to identify in smears, since hematoblasts are fragile and easily disintegrated. [hemato- + G. *blastos*, germ]

**he·ma·to·cele** (hē-ma-t'ō-sēl) 1. SYN hemorrhagic cyst. 2. effusion of blood into a canal or a cavity of the body. 3. swelling due to effusion of blood into the tunica vaginalis testis. [hemato- + G. *kēlē*, tumor]

**hem·a·to·ceph·a·ly** (hē'mă-tō-sef'ă-lē, hem'ă-tō-sef'ă-lē) intracranial effusion of blood, commonly in a fetus. [hemato- + G. *kephalē*, head]

**he·ma·to·che·zia** (hē-mat'ō-kē'zē-ă) passage of bloody stools, in contradistinction to melena, or tarry stools. [hemato- + G. *chezō*, to go to stool]

**he·ma·to·chy·lu·ria** (hē'mă-tō-kīl-yur'ē-ă) presence of blood as well as chyle in the urine. [hemato- + G. *chylos*, juice, + *ouron*, urine]

**he·ma·to·col·po·me·tra** (hē'mă-tō-kol'pō-mē'tră) accumulation of blood in the uterus and va-

gina resulting from an imperforate hymen or other lower vaginal obstruction. [hemato- + G. *kolpos*, vagina, + *mētra*, womb]

**he·ma·to·col·pos** (hē'mă-tō-kol'pos, hem'ă-tō-kol'pos) an accumulation of menstrual blood in the vagina in consequence of imperforate hymen or other obstruction. SYN retained menstruation. [hemato- + G. *kolpos*, vagina]

**he·mat·o·crit (Hct)** (hē-mat'ō-crit) percentage of the volume of a blood sample occupied by cells. Cf. plasmacrit. [hemato- + G. *krinō*, to separate]

**he·ma·to·cyst** (hē-mat'ō-sist) SYN hemorrhagic cyst.

**he·ma·to·cys·tis** (hē'mă-tō-sis'tis, hem'ă-tō-sis'tis) an effusion of blood into the bladder. [hemato- + G. *kystis*, bladder]

**he·ma·to·gen·e·sis** (hē'mă-tō-jen'ĕ-sis, hem'ă-tō-jen'ĕ-sis) SYN hemopoiesis. [hemato- + G. *genesis*, production]

**he·ma·to·gen·ic, he·ma·tog·e·nous** (hē'mă-tō-jen'ik, hem'ă-tō-jen'ik, hē'mă-tō-jen'ik; hem-ă-toj'en-ŭs) 1. SYN hemopoietic. 2. pertaining to anything produced from, derived from, or transported by the blood.

**he·ma·tog·e·nous jaun·dice** SYN hemolytic jaundice.

**he·ma·tog·e·nous me·tas·ta·sis** SEE metastasis.

**he·ma·to·his·ton** (hē'mă-tō-his'tŏn, hem'ă-tō-his'tŏn) SYN globin.

**he·ma·toid** (hē'mă-toyd, hem'ă-toyd) resembling blood. [hemato- + G. *eidos*, resemblance]

**he·ma·toi·din** (hē-mă-toy'din) a pigment derived from hemoglobin which contains no iron but is closely related to or similar to bilirubin. Hematoidin is formed intracellularly, presumably within reticuloendothelial cells, but is often found extracellularly after 5 to 7 days in foci of previous hemorrhage. SYN hemolutein. [hemato- + G. *eidos*, resemblance, + -in]

**he·ma·tol·o·gist** (hē-mă-tol'ō-jist, hem-ă-tol'ō-jist) a physician trained and experienced in hematology, i.e., skilled in performing diagnostic examinations of blood and bone marrow, or in treatment of such diseases, or both.

**he·ma·tol·o·gy** (hē-mă-tol'ō-jē, hem-ă-tol'ō-jē) the medical specialty that pertains to the anatomy, physiology, pathology, symptomatology, and therapeutics related to the blood and blood-forming tissues. [hemato- + G. *logos*, study]

**he·ma·to·lymph·an·gi·o·ma** (hē'mă-tō-limf'an-jē-ō'mă) a congenital anomaly consisting of numerous, closely packed, variably sized lymphatic vessels and larger channels, in association with a moderate number of blood vessels of a similar type.

**he·ma·tol·y·sis** (hē-mă-tol'ĭ-sis, hem-ă-tol'ĭ-sis) SYN hemolysis.

**he·ma·to·lyt·ic** (hē-mat'ō-lit'ik) SYN hemolytic.

**he·ma·to·ma** (hē-mă-tō'mă, hem-ă-tō'mă) a localized mass of extravasated blood that is relatively or completely confined within an organ or tissue, a space, or a potential space; the blood is usually clotted, and, depending on how long it has been there, may manifest various degrees of organization and decolorization. [hemato- + G. *-oma*, tumor]

**he·ma·to·me·tra** (hē'mă-tō-mē'tră, hem'ă-tō-mē'tră) a collection or retention of blood in the uterine cavity. SYN hemometra. [hemato- + G. *mētra*, uterus]

**he·ma·tom·e·try** (hē-mă-tom'ĕ-trē, hem-ă-tom'

h
e

ĕ-trē) examination of the blood in order to determine any or all of the following: 1) the total number, types, and relative proportions of various blood cells; 2) the number or proportion of other formed elements; 3) the percentage of hemoglobin. In some instances, hematometry is used to include a determination of blood pressure. [hemato- + G. *metron,* measure]

**he·mat·om·pha·lo·cele** (hē'mat-om-fal'ō-sēl, hem'at-om-fal'ō-sēl) umbilical hernia into which an effusion of blood has taken place. [hemato- + G. *omphalos,* umbilicus, + *kēlē,* hernia]

**he·ma·to·my·e·lia** (hē'mă-tō-mī'ē-lē-ă) hemorrhage into the substance of the spinal cord; it is usually a posttraumatic lesion but may also be encountered in instances of spinal cord capillary telangiectases. SYN hematorrhachis interna, myelapoplexy, myelorrhagia. [hemato- + G. *myelos,* marrow]

**he·ma·to·my·e·lo·pore** (hē'mă-tō-mī'ĕ-lō-por) formation of porosities in the spinal cord as a result of hemorrhages. [hemato- + G. *myelos,* marrow, + *poros,* a pore]

**he·ma·to·pa·thol·o·gy** (hē'mă-tō-path-ol'ō-jē, hem'ă-tō-path-ol'ō-jē) the division of pathology concerned with diseases of the blood and of hemopoietic and lymphoid tissues. SYN haemopathology, hemopathology. [hemato- + G. *pathos,* suffering, + *logos,* study]

**he·ma·to·plast** (hē'mă-tō-plast) [Br.]

**he·ma·to·plas·tic** (hē'mă-tō-plas'tik, hem'ă-tō-plas'tik) SYN hemopoietic. [hemato- + G. *plassō,* to form]

**he·ma·to·poi·e·sis** (hē'mă-tō-poy-ē'sis, hem'ă-tō-poy-ē'sis) SYN hemopoiesis.

**he·ma·to·poi·et·ic** (hē'mă-tō-poy-et'ik) SYN hemopoietic.

**he·ma·to·poi·et·ic gland** a blood-forming organ, such as the spleen.

**he·ma·to·poi·et·ic growth fac·tor (HGF)** any of several glycoproteins that regulate the survival, self-renewal, proliferation, and differentiation of hematopoietic progenitor cells. There are two nomenclature groups: interleukins (IL) and colony-stimulating factors (CSF).

**he·ma·to·poi·et·ic sys·tem** the blood-making organs; in the embryo at different ages these are the yolk sac, liver, thymus, spleen, lymph nodes, and bone marrow; after birth they are principally the bone marrow, spleen, thymus, and lymph nodes.

**he·ma·to·por·phy·rin** (hē'mă-tō-pōr'fi-rin, hem'ă-tō-pōr'fi-rin) a porphyrin resulting from the decomposition of hemoglobin; chemical composition is that of heme with the iron removed and the two vinyl groups hydrated to hydroxyethyl. SYN hemoporphyrin.

**he·ma·top·sia** (hē-mă-top'sē-ă, hem-ă-top'sē-ă) SYN hemophthalmia. [hemato- + G. *opsis,* vision]

**he·ma·tor·rha·chis** (hē-mă-tōr'ă-kis, hem-ă-tōr'ă-kis) a spinal hemorrhage. SYN hemorrhachis. [hemato- + G. *rhachis,* spine]

**he·ma·tor·rha·chis ex·ter·na** hemorrhage into the spinal canal external to the cord, either within or outside the dura.

**he·ma·tor·rha·chis in·ter·na** SYN hematomyelia.

**he·ma·to·sal·pinx** (hē'mă-tō-sal'pinks, hem'ă-tō-sal'pinks) collection of blood in a tube, often associated with a tubal pregnancy. SYN hemosalpinx. [hemato- + G. *salpinx,* a trumpet]

**hem·a·to·sin** (hē-mă-tō'sĭn) SYN hematin.

**hem·a·to·sis** (hē-mă-tō'sis) oxygenation of venous blood in the lungs.

**he·ma·to·sper·mat·o·cele** (hē'mă-tō-sper'mă-tō-sēl, hem'ă-tō-sper'mă-tō-sēl) a spermatocele that contains blood.

**he·ma·to·stat·ic** (hē'mă-tō-stat'ik, hem'ă-tō-stat'ik) **1.** variant of hemostatic. **2.** due to stagnation or arrest of blood flow.

**he·ma·to·stax·is** (hē'mă-tō-stak'sis, hem'ă-tō-stak'sis) spontaneous bleeding due to a disease of the blood. [hemato- + G. *staxis,* a dripping]

**he·ma·tos·te·on** (hē-mă-tos'tē-on, hem-ă-tos'tē-on) bleeding in the medullary cavity of a bone. [hemato- + G. *osteon,* bone]

**hem·a·to·ther·ma** (hē-mă-tō-ther'mă) the warm-blooded vertebrates (birds and mammals). [hemato- + G. *thermos,* warm]

**he·ma·to·therm·al** (hē-mă-tō-ther'măl) [Br.] SYN homeothermic.

**he·ma·to·tox·in** (hē'mă-tō-toks'in, hem'ă-tō-toks'in) SYN hemotoxin.

**he·ma·to·tro·pic** (hē'mă-tō-trop'ik, hem'ă-tō-trop'ik) SYN hemotropic.

**he·ma·tox·y·lin** (hē-mă-toks'i-lin) [CI 75290] a crystalline compound containing the coloring matter of *Haematoxylon campechianum* (logwood), from which it is obtained by extraction with ether. It is used as a dye in histology, especially for cell nuclei and chromosomes, muscle cross-striations, and enterochromaffin cells, and as an indicator (red to yellow at pH 0.0 to 1.0, yellow to violet at pH 5.0 to 6.0).

**he·ma·tox·y·lin and e·o·sin stain** the most generally useful staining method for tissues; nuclei are stained a deep blue-black with hematoxylin, and cytoplasm is stained pink after counterstaining with eosin, usually in water.

**hem·a·to·zo·on** (hē-mă-tō-zō'ŏn) SYN hemozoon.

**he·ma·tu·ria** (hē-măt-yur'ē-ă) any condition in which the urine contains blood or red blood cells. [hemato- + G. *ouron,* urine]

**heme** (hēm) **1.** the porphyrin chelate of iron in which the iron is Fe(II) ($Fe^{2+}$); the oxygen-carrying, color-furnishing, prosthetic group of hemoglobin. **2.** iron complexed with nonporphyrins but related tetrapyrrole structures (e.g., biliverdin heme). SYN reduced hematin. [G. *haima,* blood]

**heme pro·tein** any protein containing an iron-porphyrin (heme) prosthetic group resembling that of hemoglobin.

**hem·er·a·lo·pia** (hem'er-al-ō'pē-ă) inability to see as distinctly in a bright light as in reduced illumination; seen in patients with impaired cone function. SYN day blindness. [G. *hēmera,* day, + *alaos,* obscure, + *ōps,* eye]

**hem·eryth·rin** (hē-mĕ-rith'-'rĭn) any of several iron-containing, oxygen-binding circulatory proteins in certain invertebrates, with molecular weights similar to that of hemoglobin but lacking porphyrin groups. [hem- +G. *erythros,* red, + in]

△**hemi-** one-half. Cf. semi-. [G.]

**hem·i·ac·e·tal** (hem'ē-as'e-tăl) CH(OH)OR', a product of the addition of an alcohol to an aldehyde (an acetal is formed by the addition of an alcohol to a hemiacetal). In the aldose sugars, the hemiacetal formation is internal and labile, brought about by the 4-OH or 5-OH attack on the carbonyl O, yielding the furanose or pyranose structures; the hemiacetal forms of the sugars are involved in all polysaccharides, as glycosyls or glycosides. SEE ALSO hemiketal, acetal.

**hem·i·a·geu·sia** (hem′ē-ă-goo′zē-ă) loss of taste from one side of the tongue. [hemi- + G. *a-* priv. + *geusia,* taste]

**he·mi·a·naes·the·sia [Br.]** SEE hemianesthesia.

**hem·i·an·al·ge·sia** (hem′ē-an′al-jē′zē-ă) analgesia affecting one side of the body.

**hem·i·an·en·ceph·a·ly** (hem′ē-an-en-sef′ă-lē) anencephaly on one side only, or involving one side much more extensively than the other.

**hem·i·an·es·the·sia** (hem′ē-an-es-thē′zē-ă) anesthesia on one side of the body. SYN unilateral anesthesia.

**hem·i·a·no·pia** (hem′ē-ă-nō′pē-ă) loss of vision for one half of the visual field of one or both eyes.

**hem·i·an·os·mia** (hem′ē-an-oz′mē-ă) loss of the sense of smell on one side. [hemi- + G. *an-* priv. + *osmē,* smell]

**hem·i·a·prax·ia** (hem′ē-ă-prak′sē-ă) apraxia affecting one side of the body.

**hem·i·a·tax·ia** (hem′ē-ă-tak′sē-ă) ataxia affecting one side of the body.

**hem·i·ath·e·to·sis** (hem′ē-ath′ĕ-tō′sis) athetosis affecting one hand, or one hand and foot, only.

**hem·i·at·ro·phy** (hem-ē-at′rō-fē) atrophy of one lateral half of a part or of an organ, as the face or tongue.

**hem·i·az·y·gos vein** formed by the merger of the left ascending lumbar vein with the left subcostal vein or a communication from the inferior vena cava, it pierces the left crus of the diaphragm, ascends along the left side of the bodies of the lower thoracic vertebrae, opposite the eighth vertebra, crosses the midline behind the aorta, thoracic duct, and esophagus, and empties into the azygos vein, sometimes in common with the accessory hemiazygos vein.

**hem·i·bal·lis·mus** (hem-ē-bal-iz′mŭs) ballism involving one side of the body. [hemi- + G. *ballismos,* jumping about]

**hem·i·block** (hem′ē-blok) arrest of the impulse in one of the two main divisions of the left branch of the bundle of His; i.e., in either the anterior (superior) division or the posterior (inferior) division.

**he·mic** (hē′mik) SYN hematic (1).

**hem·i·car·dia** (hem-ē-kar′dē-ă) **1.** either lateral half, including atrium and ventricle, of the heart. **2.** a congenital malformation of the heart in which only two of the usual four chambers are formed. [hemi- + G. *kardia,* heart]

**hem·i·cen·trum** (hem′ē-sen′trŭm) one of the two lateral halves of the body of the vertebra. [hemi- + G. *kentron,* center]

**hem·i·ceph·a·lal·gia** (hem′ē-sef′ă-lal′jē-ă) the unilateral headache characteristic of migraine. SYN hemicrania (2). [hemi- + G. *kephalē,* head, + *algos,* pain]

**hem·i·ce·pha·lia** (hem-ē-se-fā′lē-ă) congenital failure of the cerebrum to develop normally; usually the cerebellum and basal ganglia are represented at least in rudimentary form. [hemi- + G. *kephalē,* head]

**hem·i·cho·rea** (hem′ē-kōr-ē′ă) chorea involving the muscles on one side only.

**he·mic mur·mur** SYN anemic murmur.

**hem·i·col·ec·to·my** (hem′ē-kō-lek′tō-mē) re-

moval of the right or left side of the colon. [hemi- + G. *kolon,* colon, + *ektomē,* excision]

**hem·i·cor·po·rec·to·my** (hem′ē-kōr-pō-rek′tō-mē) surgical removal of the lower half of the body, including the lower extremities, bony pelvis, genitalia, and various of the pelvic contents including the lower part of the rectum to the anus. [hemi- + L. *corpus,* body, + G. *ektomē,* excision]

**hem·i·cra·nia** (hem-ē-krā′nē-ă) **1.** SYN migraine. **2.** SYN hemicephalalgia. [hemi- + G. *kranion,* skull]

**hem·i·cra·ni·o·sis** (hem′ē-krā-nē-ō′sis) enlargement of one side of the cranium.

**hem·i·des·mo·somes** (hem-ē-des′mō-sōmz) half desmosomes that occur on the basal surface of the stratum basale of stratified squamous epithelium.

**hem·i·di·a·pho·re·sis** (hem′ē-dī-ă-fō-rē′sis) diaphoresis, or sweating, on one side of the body. SYN hemidrosis (2), hemihidrosis.

**hem·i·dro·sis** (hem-i-drō′sis) **1.** SYN hematidrosis. **2.** SYN hemidiaphoresis.

**hem·i·dys·es·the·sia** (hem′ē-dis-es-thē′zē-ă) dysesthesia affecting one side of the body.

**hem·i·dys·tro·phy** (hem-ē-dis′trō-fē) underdevelopment of one lateral half of the body. [hemi- + G. *dys-,* ill, + *trophē,* nourishment, growth]

**hem·i·ec·tro·me·lia** (hem′ē-ek-trō-mē′lē-ă) defective development of the limbs on one side of the body. [hemi- + ectromelia]

**hem·i·fa·cial** (hem-ē-fā′shăl) pertaining to one side of the face.

**he·mi·fa·cial spasm** a facial nerve disorder, with onset in late adult life, characterized by episodes of irregular, sometimes painful, myoclonic contractions of various facial muscles; triggered by voluntary or reflex movements of the face, spasm typically begins in the orbicularis oculi muscle and then spreads; occasionally a sequela of Bell palsy, but more often the result of proximal compression of the facial nerve by an aberrant blood vessel or neoplasm.

**hem·i·gas·trec·to·my** (hem′ē-gas-trek-tō-mē) excision of the distal one-half of the stomach.

**hem·i·glos·sec·to·my** (hem′ē-glos-ek′tō-mē) surgical removal of one-half of the tongue. [hemi- + G. *glōssa,* tongue, + *ektomē,* excision]

**hem·i·glos·si·tis** (hem′ē-glos-ī′tis) a vesicular eruption on one side of the tongue and the corresponding inner surface of the cheek, probably herpetic. [hemi- + G. *glōssa,* tongue, + *-itis,* inflammation]

**hem·i·gna·thia** (hem-ē-nath′ē-ă) defective development of one side of the mandible. [hemi- + G. *gnathos,* jaw]

**hem·i·hi·dro·sis** (hem′ē-hī-drō′sis) SYN hemidiaphoresis.

**hem·i·hyp·al·ge·sia** (hem′ē-hī-pal-je′zē-ă) hypalgesia affecting one side of the body.

**hem·i·hy·per·es·the·sia** (hem′ē-hī′per-es-thē′zē-ă) hyperesthesia, or increased tactile and painful sensibility, affecting one side of the body.

**hem·i·hy·per·to·nia** (hem′ē-hī-per-tō′nē-ă) exaggerated muscular tonicity on one side of the body. [hemi- + G. *hyper,* over, + *tonos,* tone]

**hem·i·hy·per·tro·phy** (hem′ē-hī-per′trō-fē) muscular or osseous hypertrophy of one side of the face or body.

**hem·i·hyp·es·the·sia** (hem′ē-hip-es-thē′zē-ă) di-

h
e

minished sensibility in one side of the body. [hemi- + G. *hypo,* under, + *aesthēses,* sensation]

**hem•i•hy•po•to•nia** (hem′ē-hī-pō-tō′nē-ă) partial loss of muscular tonicity on one side of the body. [hemi- + G. *hypo,* under, + *tonos,* tone]

**hem•i•ke•tal** (hem′ē-kē-tăl) C(R′)(OH)OR″, a product of the addition of an alcohol to a ketone. In the ketose sugars, the hemiketal formation is from an attack by an internal OH on the ketone carbonyl leading to intramolecular cyclization (furanose or pyranose); the hemiketal forms of the sugars are involved in polysaccharide formation, as glycosyls or glycosides. SEE ALSO hemiacetal, ketal.

**hem•i•lam•i•nec•to•my** (hem′ē-lam-i-nek′tō-mē) removal of a portion of a vertebral lamina, usually performed for exploration of, access to, or decompression of the intraspinal contents. [hemi- + L. *lamina,* layer, + G. *ektomē,* excision]

**hem•i•lar•yn•gec•to•my** (hem′ē-lar-in-jek′tō-mē) excision of one lateral half of the larynx. [hemi- + G. *larnyx* (*laryng-*), larynx, + *ektomē,* excision]

**hem•i•lat•er•al** (hem-ē-lat′er-ăl) relating to one lateral half.

**he•min** (hēm′in) chloride of heme in which $Fe^{2+}$ has become $Fe^{3+}$. Hemin crystals are called Teichmann crystals. SYN hematin chloride.

**hem•i•pa•re•sis** (hem-ē-pa-rē′sis, hem-ē-par′ĕ-sis) weakness affecting one side of the body.

**hem•i•pel•vec•to•my** (hem′ē-pel-vek′tō-mē) amputation of an entire leg together with the os coxae. SYN interpelviabdominal amputation, Jaboulay amputation. [hemi- + L. *pelvis,* basin (pelvis), + G. *ektomē,* excision]

**hem•i•ple•gia** (hem-ē-plē′jē-ă) paralysis of one side of the body. [hemi- + G. *plēgē,* a stroke]

**hem•i•ple•gic** (hem-ē-plē′jik) relating to hemiplegia.

**hem•i•ple•gic gait** gait in which the leg is stiff, without flexion at knee and ankle, and with each step is rotated away from the body, then towards it, forming a semicircle. SYN spastic gait.

**hem•i•sen•so•ry** (hem′ē-sen′sōr-ē) loss of sensation on one side of the body. Cf. hemianesthesia.

**hem•i•spasm** (hem′ē-spazm) a spasm affecting one or more muscles of one side of the face or body.

**hem•i•sphere** (hem′i-sfēr) half of a spherical structure. SYN cerebral hemisphere (1). SYN hemisphericum. [hemi- + G. *sphaira,* ball, globe]

**hem•i•sphere of cer•e•bel•lum HII–HX** the large part of the cerebellum lateral to the vermis cerebelli. SYN hemispherium (2).

**hem•i•spher•i•cum** (hem′i-sfēr′ē-kŭm) SYN hemisphere.

**hem•i•sphe•ri•um** (hem′i-sfēr′ē-ŭm) **1.** SYN cerebral hemisphere. **2.** SYN hemisphere of cerebellum HII–HX. [G. *hemisphairion*]

**hem•i•sys•to•le** (hem-ē-sis′tō-lē) contraction of the left ventricle following every second atrial contraction only, so that there is but one pulse beat to every two heart beats.

**hem•i•tho•rax** (hem-ē-thō′raks) one side of the thorax.

**hem•i•trun•cus** (hem′ē-trunk′us) a variant truncus arteriosus in which only one pulmonary artery originates from the truncal artery.

**hem•i•ver•te•bra** (hem-ē-ver′tĕ-bră) a congenital defect of the vertebral column in which one side of a vertebra fails to develop completely.

**hem•i•zy•gos•i•ty** (hem′i-zī-gos′i-tē) the state of being hemizygous.

**hem•i•zy•gote** (hem-i-zī′gōt) an individual hemizygous with respect to one or more specified loci; e.g., a normal male is a hemizygote with respect to the gene for all X-linked or Y-linked genes in his genome. [hemi- + G. *zygōtos,* yoked]

**hem•i•zy•got•ic** (hem′i-zī-got′ik) SYN hemizygous.

**hem•i•zy•gous** (hem-i-zī′gŭs) having unpaired genes in an otherwise diploid cell; males are normally hemizygous for genes on both sex chromosomes. SYN hemizygotic.

⚠ **he•mo-** combining form denoting blood. SEE ALSO hem-, hemat-, hemato-. [G. *haima*]

**he•mo•bil•ia** (hē-mō-bil′ē-ă) the presence of blood in the bile.

**he•mo•blast** (hēm′ō-blast) SYN hemocytoblast.

**he•mo•blas•to•sis** (hē′mō-blas-tō′sis) a proliferative condition of the hematopoietic tissues in general.

**he•mo•cath•e•re•sis** (hē′mō-kath-e-rē′sis) destruction of the blood cells, especially of erythrocytes (hemocytocatheresis). [hemo- + G. *kathairesis,* destruction]

**he•mo•cath•e•re•tic** (hē′mō-kath-ĕ-ret′ik) pertaining to or characterized by hemocatheresis.

**Hem•oc•cult test** a qualitative test for occult blood in stool based upon detecting the peroxidase activity of hemoglobin; a test kit can be used at home and the specimen mailed to a laboratory for evaluation.

**hem•o•cele** (hē′mō-sēl) the system of interconnected spaces within the bodies of arthropods containing blood or hemolymph [hemo- + G. *koilōma,* cavity]

**he•mo•cho•ri•al pla•cen•ta** the type of placenta, as in humans and some rodents, in which maternal blood is in direct contact with the chorion.

**he•mo•chro•ma•to•sis** (hē′mō-krō-mă-tō′sis) a disorder of iron metabolism characterized by excessive absorption of ingested iron, saturation of iron-binding protein, and deposition of hemosiderin in tissue, particularly in the liver, pancreas, and skin; cirrhosis of the liver, diabetes (bronze diabetes), bronze pigmentation of the skin, and, eventually heart failure may occur; also can result from administration of large amounts of iron orally, by injection, or in forms of blood transfusion therapy. [hemo- + G. *chrōma,* color, + *-osis,* condition]

**he•mo•chrome** (hē′mō-krōm) SYN hemochromogen.

**he•mo•chro•mo•gen** (hē-mō-krō′mō-jen) any compound in which 1 mol of ferro- or ferriporphyrin is combined with 2 mol of a nitrogenous base or protein. SYN haemochrome, hemochrome. [hemo- + G. *chrōma,* color, + *-gen,* producing]

**he•mo•cla•sis, he•mo•cla•sia** (hē-mok′lă-sis, hē′mō-klā′zē-ă) rupture, dissolution (hemolysis), or other type of destruction of red blood cells. [hemo- + G. *klasis,* a breaking]

**he•mo•clas•tic** (hē′mō-klas′tik) pertaining to hemoclasis.

**he•mo•con•cen•tra•tion** (hē′mō-kon-sen-trā′shŭn) decrease in the volume of plasma in relation to the number of red blood cells; increase in the concentration of red blood cells in the circulating blood.

**he•mo•co•nia** (hē-mō-kō′nē-ă) small refractive particles in the circulating blood, probably lipid material associated with fragmented stroma from red blood cells. [hemo- + G. *konis,* dust]

**he•mo•co•ni•o•sis** (hē′mō-kō-nē-ō′sis) a condition in which there is an abnormal concentration of hemoconia in the blood.

**he•mo•cy•a•nin** (hē-mō-sī′ă-nin) an oxygen-carrying pigment in some molluscs, crustacea, and arthropods; contains copper rather than heme; used as an experimental antigen. [hemo- + G. *kyanos,* blue material, + -in]

**he•mo•cyte** (hē′mō-sīt) any cell or formed element of the blood. [hemo- + G. *kytos,* a hollow (cell)]

**he•mo•cy•to•blast** (hē′mō-sī′tō-blast) a blood cell derived from embryonic mesenchyme, characterized by basophilic cytoplasm and a relatively large nucleus with a spongy, loose network of chromatin and several nucleoli; mitochondria are extremely fine and delicate. Hemocytoblasts represent the primitive stem cells of the monophyletic theory of the origin of blood and have the potentiality of developing into erythroblasts, young forms of the granulocytic series, megakaryocytes, etc. SYN hemoblast. [hemo- + G. *kytos,* cell, + *blastos,* germ]

**he•mo•cy•to•ca•ther•e•sis** (hē′mō-sī′tō-kă-ther′ē-sis) hemolysis, or other type of destruction of red blood cells. [hemo- + G. *kytos,* a hollow (cell), + *kathairesis,* destruction]

**he•mo•cy•tol•y•sis** (hē′mō-sī-tol′i-sis) the dissolution of blood cells, including hemolysis. [hemo- + G. *kytos,* cell, + *lysis,* dissolution]

**he•mo•cy•to•ma** (hē-mō-sī-tō′mă) [hemo- + G. *kytos,* cell, + -oma]

**he•mo•cy•tom•e•ter** (hē′mō-sī-tom′ĕ-ter) an apparatus for estimating the number of blood cells in a quantitatively measured volume of blood; it consists of a glass pipette with an ampulla for collecting and diluting the blood, and a counting chamber marked in squares. SYN hemacytometer. [hemo- + G. *kytos,* cell, + *metron,* measure]

**he•mo•cy•tom•e•try** (hē′mō-sī-tom′ĕ-trē) the counting of red blood cells.

**he•mo•cy•to•trip•sis** (hē′mō-sī-tō-trip′sis) fragmentation or disintegration of blood cells by means of mechanical trauma, e.g., compression between hard surfaces. [hemo- + G. *kytos,* + *tripsis,* a grinding]

**he•mo•di•a•fil•tra•tion** (hē-mō-dī-ă-fil-trā′shŭn) a combination of hemodialysis for diffusion of smaller molecular weight solutes with hemofiltration for convective transport of those of larger molecular weight

**he•mo•di•ag•no•sis** (hē′mō-dī-ag-nō′sis) diagnosis by means of examination of the blood.

**he•mo•di•al•y•sis** (hē′mō-dī-al′i-sis) dialysis of soluble substances and water from the blood by diffusion through a semipermeable membrane; separation of cellular elements and colloids from soluble substances is achieved by pore size in the membrane and rates of diffusion.

**he•mo•di•a•lyz•er** (hē-mō-dī′ă-lī-zer) a machine for hemodialysis in acute or chronic renal failure; toxic substances in the blood are removed by exposure to dialyzing fluid across a semipermeable membrane. SYN artificial kidney.

**he•mo•di•lu•tion** (hē′mō-di-loo′shŭn) increase in the volume of plasma in relation to red blood cells; reduced concentration of red blood cells in the circulation.

**he•mo•dy•nam•ic** (hē′mō-dī-nam′ik) relating to the physical aspects of the blood circulation.

**he•mo•dy•nam•ics** (hē′mō-dī-nam′iks) the study of the dynamics of the blood circulation. [hemo- + G. *dynamis,* power]

**he•mo•dy•na•nom•e•ter** (hē-mō-dī-nă-mŏm′-ĕ-ter) SYN sphygmomanometer. [hemo- + *dynamis,* power, + *metron,* measurement]

**he•mo•en•do•the•li•al pla•cen•ta** the type of placenta, as in rabbits, in which the trophoblast becomes so attenuated that, by light microscopy, maternal blood appears to be separated from fetal blood only by the endothelium of the chorionic capillaries.

**he•mo•fil•tra•tion** (hē′mō-fil-trā′shŭn) a process, similar to hemodialysis, by which blood is dialyzed using ultrafiltration and simultaneous reinfusion of physiologic saline solution.

**he•mo•flag•el•late** (hē-mō-flaj′ĕ-lāts) protozoan flagellates that are parasitic in the blood; they include the genera *Leishmania* and *Trypanosoma,* several species of which are important pathogens. [hemo- + L. *flagellum,* dim. of *flagrum,* a whip]

**he•mo•fus•cin** (hē-mō-fyoos′in) a brown pigment derived from hemoglobin that occurs in urine occasionally along with hemosiderin, usually indicative of increased red blood cell destruction; occurs also in the liver with hemosiderin in cases of hemochromatosis.

**he•mo•gen•e•sis** (hē-mō-jen′ĕ-sis) SYN hemopoiesis.

**he•mo•gen•ic** (hē-mō-jen′ik) SYN hemopoietic.

**he•mo•glo•bin (Hb)** (hē-mō-glō′bin) the red respiratory protein of erythrocytes, consisting of approximately 3.8% heme and 96.2% globin, with a molecular weight of 64,450, which as oxyhemoglobin ($HbO_2$) transports oxygen from the lungs to the tissues where the oxygen is readily released and $HbO_2$ becomes Hb. When Hb is exposed to certain chemicals, its normal respiratory function is blocked; e.g., the oxygen in $HbO_2$ is easily displaced by carbon monoxide, thereby resulting in the formation of fairly stable carboxyhemoglobin (HbCO), as in asphyxiation resulting from inhalation of exhaust fumes from gasoline engines. When the iron in Hb is oxidized from the ferrous to ferric state, as in poisoning with nitrates and certain other chemicals, a nonrespiratory compound, methemoglobin (MetHb), is formed.

**he•mo•glo•bin A (Hb A)** normal adult hemoglobin, consisting of two variants, designated Hb A (by far the more prevalent) and Hb $A_2$.

**he•mo•glo•bin Bart** a Hb homotetramer (all four polypeptides identical) of formula $\gamma_4$, found in the early embryo and in α-thalassemia 2; not effective in oxygen transport; does not display a Bohr effect.

**he•mo•glo•bin C (Hb C)** an abnormal hemoglobin that affects the physical properties of erythrocytes, causing hemolytic anemia; often found in persons also having sickle cell disease or thalassemia.

**he•mo•glo•bi•ne•mia** (hē′mō-glo-bi-nē′mē-ă) the presence of free hemoglobin in the blood plasma, as when intravascular hemolysis occurs.

**he•mo•glo•bin F (Hb F)** normal fetal hemoglobin; production is greatly reduced after infancy except in certain congenital or acquired hematologic disorders.

**he·mo·glo·bi·nol·y·sis** (hē′mō-glō-bi-nol′i-sis) destruction or chemical splitting of hemoglobin. [hemoglobin + G. *lysis,* dissolution]

**hem·o·glob·in·o·me·try** (hē-mō-glō-bi-nom′ĕ-trē) measurement of the hemoglobin concentration of the blood syn haematinometer, haemochromometer.

**he·mo·glo·bi·nop·a·thy** (hē′mō-glō-bi-nop′ă-thē) a disorder or disease caused by or associated with the presence of hemoglobins in the blood. [hemoglobin + G. *pathos,* disease]

**he·mo·glo·bi·no·phil·ic** (hē′mō-glō′bi-nō-fil′ik) denoting certain microorganisms that cannot be cultured except in the presence of hemoglobin. [hemoglobin + G. *phileō,* to love]

**he·mo·glo·bin S (Hb S)** an abnormal hemoglobin that renders erythrocytes subject to sickling and hemolysis at reduced oxygen tension; makes up 70–100% of hemoglobin in persons with sickle cell anemia. syn sickle cell hemoglobin.

**he·mo·glo·bi·nu·ria** (hē′mō-glō-bin-yur′ē-ă) the presence of hemoglobin in the urine, including certain closely related pigments formed from slight alteration of the hemoglobin molecule; indicative of intravascular hemolysis or of bleeding into the urinary tract, with hemolysis there. The urine may be reddish yellow to dark red. [hemoglobin + G. *ouron,* urine]

**he·mo·glo·bi·nu·ric** (hē′mō-glō-bin-yur′ik) relating to or marked by hemoglobinuria.

**he·mo·glo·bi·nu·ric ne·phro·sis** acute oliguric renal failure associated with hemoglobinuria, due to massive intravascular hemolysis.

**he·mo·gram** (hē′mō-gram) a complete detailed record of the findings in a thorough examination of the blood, especially with reference to the numbers, proportions, and morphologic features of the formed elements. [hemo- + G. *gramma,* a drawing]

**he·mo·his·ti·o·blast** (hē′mō-his′tē-ō-blast) a primitive mesenchymal cell believed to be capable of developing into all types of blood cells, including monocytes, and into histiocytes. syn Ferrata cell. [hemo- + G. *histion,* web, + *blastos,* germ]

**he·mo·lith** (hē′mō-lith) a concretion in the wall of a blood vessel. [hemo- + G. *lithos,* stone]

**he·mo·lu·tein** (hē-mō-loo′tē-ĭn) syn hematoidin. [hemo- + L. *luteus,* yellow, + -in]

**he·mo·lymph** (hē′mō-limf) **1.** blood and lymph, considered together. **2.** the nutrient fluid of certain invertebrates.

**he·mol·y·sate** (hē-mol′i-sāt) preparation resulting from the lysis of erythrocytes.

**he·mol·y·sin** (hē-mol′i-sin) **1.** any substance elaborated by a living agent and capable of causing lysis of red blood cells and liberation of their hemoglobin. syn erythrocytolysin, erythrolysin. **2.** a sensitizing that combines with red blood cells of the antigenic type that stimulated formation of the hemolysin, so that complement fixes with the antibody-cell union and causes dissolution of the cells.

**he·mo·ly·sin·o·gen** (hē′mō-lī-sin′ō-jen) the antigenic material in red blood cells that stimulates the formation of hemolysin.

**he·mo·ly·sin u·nit, he·mo·lyt·ic u·nit** the smallest quantity (highest dilution) of inactivated immune serum (hemolysin) that will sensitize the standard suspension of erythrocytes so that the standard complement will cause complete hemolysis.

**he·mol·y·sis** (hē-mol′i-sis) alteration, dissolution, or destruction of red blood cells in such a manner that hemoglobin is liberated into the medium in which the cells are suspended. syn erythrocytolysis, erythrolysis, hematolysis. [hemo- + G. *lysis,* destruction]

**he·mo·lyt·ic** (hē-mō-lit′ik) destructive to blood cells, resulting in liberation of hemoglobin. syn hematolytic, hemotoxic (2), hematotoxic, hematoxic.

▣ **he·mo·lyt·ic a·ne·mia** any anemia resulting from an increased rate of erythrocyte destruction. See page B2.

**he·mo·lyt·ic dis·ease of new·born** syn erythroblastosis fetalis.

**he·mo·lyt·ic jaun·dice** jaundice resulting from increased production of bilirubin from hemoglobin as a result of any process (toxic, genetic, or immune) causing increased destruction of erythrocytes. syn hematogenous jaundice.

**he·mo·ly·tic plaque as·say** syn Jerne plaque assay.

**he·mo·lyt·ic sple·no·meg·a·ly** splenomegaly associated with congenital hemolytic jaundice.

**α-hemolytic strep·to·coc·ci** streptococci that form a green variety of reduced hemoglobin in the area of the colony on a blood agar medium. see also *Streptococcus viridans.*

**β-he·mo·lyt·ic strep·to·coc·ci** those that produce active hemolysins (O and S) which cause a zone in the blood agar medium in the area of the colony; β-hemolytic streptococci are divided into groups (A to O) on the basis of cell wall C carbohydrate (see Lancefield classification); Group A includes strains that cause human infections such as streptococcal pharyngitis, impetigo, erysipelas, otitis media, and wound infections, and that can stimulate production of autoimmune globulins that cause acute rheumatic fever and acute glomerulonephritis. The more than 20 extracellular substances elaborated by strains of β-hemolytic streptococci include erythrogenic toxin (elaborated only by lysogenic strains), deoxyribonuclease (streptodornase), hemolysins (streptolysins O and S), hyaluronidase, and streptokinase.

**he·mo·lyt·ic u·re·mic syn·drome** hemolytic anemia and thrombocytopenia occurring with acute renal failure. In children, characterized by sudden onset of gastrointestinal bleeding, hematuria, oliguria, and microangiopathic hemolytic anemia in association with intestinal infection by *Shigella, Salmonella,* or *E. coli* srain O157:H7; in adults, associated with complications of pregnancy following normal delivery, or associated with oral contraceptive use or with infection.

**he·mo·lyze** (hē′mō-līz) to produce hemolysis or liberation of the hemoglobin from red blood cells.

**he·mo·me·di·as·ti·num** (hē′mō-mē-dē-ă-stī′nŭm) blood in the mediastinum.

**he·mo·me·tra** (hē-mō-mē′tră) syn hematometra.

**he·mon·chi·a·sis** (hē-mong-kī′a-sĭs) infestation with nematodes of the genus *Haemonchus.*

**he·mo·nec·tin** (hē-mō-nek′tin) an extracellular protein found in bone marrow matrix that promotes adhesion and differentiation of cells in the granulocyte line. [hemo- + L. *necto,* to fasten, + -in]

**he·mo·pa·ra·site** (hē-mō-păr'ă-sīt) a parasite that inhabits the bloodstream of the host.

**he·mo·pa·thol·o·gy** (hē'mō-pa-thol'ō-jē) SYN hematopathology.

**he·mop·a·thy** (hē-mop'ă-thē) any abnormal condition or disease of the blood or hemopoietic tissues. [hemo- + G. *pathos*, suffering]

**he·mo·per·fu·sion** (hē'mō-per-fyu'zhŭn) passage of blood through columns of adsorptive material, such as activated charcoal, to remove toxic substances from the blood. [hemo- + L. *perfusio*, to pass through]

**he·mo·per·i·car·di·um** (hē'mō-per'i-kar'dē-ŭm) blood in the pericardial sac.

**he·mo·per·i·to·ne·um** (hē'mō-per-i-tō-nē'ŭm) blood in the peritoneal cavity.

**he·mo·pex·in** (hēm-ō-peks'in) a serum protein related to β-globulins, important in binding heme and porphyrins, preventing excretion, and perhaps regulating heme in drug metabolism. [hemo- + G. *pēxis*, fixation, + -in]

**he·mo·phag·o·cyte** (hē-mō-fa'gō-sīt) a cell that engulfs and destroys blood cells, especially erythrocytes.

**he·mo·phil, he·mo·phile** (hē'mō-fil, hē'mō-fīl) a microorganism growing preferably in media containing blood. [hemo- + G. *philos*, fond]

**he·mo·phil·ia** (hē-mō-fil'ē-ă) an inherited disorder of blood coagulation characterized by a permanent tendency to hemorrhages, spontaneous or traumatic, due to a defect in the blood coagulating mechanism. [hemo- + G. *philos*, fond]

**he·mo·phil·ia A** hemophilia due to deficiency of factor VIII, occurring almost exclusively in males, and characterized by prolonged clotting time, decreased formation of thromboplastin, and diminished conversion of prothrombin. SYN classic hemophilia.

**he·mo·phil·ia B** a clotting disorder resembling hemophilia A, caused by hereditary deficiency of factor IX. SYN Christmas disease.

**he·mo·phil·i·ac** (hē-mō-fil'ē-ak) a person suffering from hemophilia.

**he·mo·phil·ic** (hē-mō-fil'ik) relating to hemophilia.

**he·mo·phi·li·oid** (hē-m-fil'e-ōyd) resembling hemophilia but not due to deficiency of factor VIII.

**he·mo·pho·re·sis** (hē'mō-fō-rē'sis) blood convection or irrigation of tissues. [hemo- + G. *phoreō*, to bear]

**he·moph·thal·mia, he·moph·thal·mus** (hē-mof-thal'mē-ah, hē-mof-thal'mŭs) a blood-filled eye. SYN haematopsia, hematopsia. [hemo- + G. *ophthalmos*, eye]

**he·mo·plas·tic** (hē-mō-plas'tik) SYN hemopoietic.

**he·mo·pneu·mo·per·i·car·di·um** (hē'mō-noo'mō-per-i-kar'dē-ŭm) the occurrence of blood and air in the pericardium. SYN pneumohemopericardium. [hemo- + G. *pneuma*, air, + pericardium]

**he·mo·pneu·mo·tho·rax** (hē'mō-noo-mō-thō'raks) accumulation of air and blood in the pleural cavity. SYN pneumohemothorax. [hemo- + G. *pneuma*, air, + thorax]

**he·mo·poi·e·sis** (hē'mō-poy-ē'sis) the process of formation and development of the various types of blood cells and other formed elements. SYN haematogenesis, haematogenous, hematogenesis, hematopoiesis, hemogenesis, sanguification. [hemo- + G. *poiēsis*, a making]

**he·mo·poi·et·ic** (hē'mō-poy-et'ik) pertaining to or related to the formation of blood cells. SYN

haemoplastic, hematogenic (1), hematogenous, hematoplastic, hematopoietic, hemogenic, hemoplastic, sanguifacient.

**he·mo·por·phy·rin** (hē-mō-pōr'fi-rin) SYN hematoporphyrin.

**he·mo·pre·cip·i·tin** (hē'mō-prē-sip'i-tin) an antibody that combines with and precipitates soluble antigenic material from erythrocytes.

**he·mo·pro·tein** (hē-mō-prō'tēn) protein linked to a metal-porphyrin compound (e.g., cytochromes, myoglobin, catalase).

**he·mop·ty·sis** (hē-mop'ti-sis) the spitting of blood derived from the lungs or bronchial tubes as a result of pulmonary or bronchial hemorrhage. [hemo- + G. *ptysis*, a spitting]

**he·mor·he·o·lo·gy** (hē'mō-rē-ol-ŏ-jē) the science of the flow of blood in relation to the pressures, flow, volumes, and resistances in blood vessels, especially with respect to blood viscosity and red blood cell deformation in the microcirculation. [hemo- + G. *rheos,*flow, + *logos,* study]

**he·mor·rha·chis** (hē-mōr'ă-kis) SYN hematorrhachis.

**hem·or·rhage** (hem'ŏ-rij) **1.** an escape of blood through ruptured or unruptured vessel walls. **2.** to bleed. [G. *haimorrhagia*, fr. *haima,* blood, + *rhēgnymi,* to burst forth]

**hem·or·rhag·ic** (hem-ŏ-raj'ik) relating to or marked by hemorrhage.

**hem·or·rhag·ic as·ci·tes** bloody or blood-stained serous fluid, frequently resulting from metastatic carcinoma, in the peritoneal cavity.

**hem·or·rhag·ic co·li·tis** abdominal cramps and bloody diarrhea, without fever, attributed to a self-limited infection by a strain of *Escherichia coli.*

**hem·or·rhag·ic cyst** a cyst containing blood or resulting from the encapsulation of a hematoma. SYN blood cyst, hematocele (1), hematocyst.

**hem·or·rhag·ic cys·ti·tis** bladder inflammation with macroscopic hematuria. Generally the result of a chemical or other traumatic insult to the bladder (chemotherapy, radiation therapy).

**hem·or·rhag·ic dis·ease of the new·born** a syndrome characterized by spontaneous internal or external bleeding accompanied by hypoprothrombinemia, slightly decreased platelets, and markedly elevated bleeding and clotting times, usually occurring between the third and sixth days of life and effectively treated with vitamin K.

**hem·or·rhag·ic en·do·vas·cu·li·tis** endothelial and medial hyperplasia of placental blood vessels with thrombosis, fragmentation, and diapedesis of red blood cells resulting in stillbirth or fetal developmental disorders.

**hem·or·rhag·ic fe·ver** a syndrome that occurs in infections by a number of different viruses. Some types of hemorrhagic fever are tick-borne, others mosquito-borne, and some seem to be zoonoses; clinical manifestations are high fever, scattered petechiae, gastrointestinal tract and other organ bleeding, hypotension, and shock; kidney damage may be severe, especially in Korean hemorrhagic fever and neurologic signs may appear, especially in the Argentinean-Bolivian types. Four types of hemorrhagic fever are transmissible person-to-person: Lassa fever, Ebola fever, Marburg virus disease, and Crimean-Congo hemorrhagic fever. SEE ALSO epidemic hemorrhagic fever.

h
e

**hem·or·rhag·ic fe·ver with re·nal syn·drome** SYN epidemic hemorrhagic fever.

**hem·or·rhag·ic in·farct** an infarct red in color from infiltration of blood from collateral vessels into the necrotic area.

**hem·or·rhag·ic mea·sles** a severe form in which the eruption is dark in color due to effusion of blood into affected areas of the skin.

**hem·or·rhag·ic plague** the hemorrhagic form of bubonic plague.

**hem·or·rhag·ic shock** hypovolemic shock resulting from acute hemorrhage, characterized by hypotension, tachycardia, pale, cold, and clammy skin, and oliguria.

**hem·or·rhag·ins** (hem-ŏ-raj′inz, hem-ŏ-rā′jins) toxins found in certain venoms and poisonous material from some plants, e.g., rattlesnake venom and ricin; hemorrhagins cause degeneration and lysis of endothelial cells in capillaries and small vessels, thereby resulting in numerous small hemorrhages in the tissues. [hemorrhage + -in]

**hem·or·rhoid** (hem′ŏ-royd) one of the tumors or varices constituting hemorrhoids.

**hem·or·rhoi·dal** (hem-ŏ-roy′dăl) relating to hemorrhoids.

**hem·or·rhoid·ec·to·my** (hem′ŏ-roy-dek′tō-mē) surgical removal of hemorrhoids; usually accomplished by excision of hemorrhoidal tissues by sharp dissection, or by application of elastic ligature at the base of the hemorrhoidal bundles to produce ischemic necrosis and ultimate ablation of the hemorrhoidectomy. [hemorrhoids + G. *ektomē,* excision]

**hem·or·rhoids** (hem′ŏ-roydz) a varicose condition of the external or internal rectal veins causing painful swellings at the anus. SYN piles. [G. *haimorrhois,* pl. *haimorrhoides,* veins likely to bleed, fr. *haima,* blood, + *rhoia,* a flow]

**he·mo·sal·pinx** (hē′mō-sal′pinks) SYN hematosalpinx.

**he·mo·sid·er·in** (hē-mō-sid′er-in) a yellow or brown protein produced by phagocytic digestion of hematin; found in most tissues, especially in the liver; but with a higher content, as stains blue with Perl Prussian blue stain. [hemo- + G. *sidēros,* iron, + -in]

**he·mo·sid·er·o·sis** (hē′mō-sid-er-ō′sis) accumulation of hemosiderin in tissue, particularly in liver and spleen. SEE hemochromatosis. [hemosiderin + -osis, condition]

**he·mo·sper·mia** (hē′mō-sper′mē-ă) the presence of blood in the seminal fluid. [hemo- + G. *sperma,* seed]

**he·mo·sta·sis** (hē′mō-stā-sis) 1. the arrest of bleeding. 2. the arrest of circulation in a part. 3. stagnation of blood. [hemo- + G. *stasis,* a standing]

**he·mo·stat** (hē′mō-stat) 1. any agent that arrests, chemically or mechanically, the flow of blood from an open vessel. 2. an instrument for arresting hemorrhage by compression of the bleeding vessel.

**he·mo·stat·ic** (hē-mō-stat′ik) 1. arresting the flow of blood within the vessels. 2. SYN antihemorrhagic.

**he·mo·stat·ic for·ceps** a forceps with a catch for locking the blades, used for seizing the end of a blood vessel to control hemorrhage.

**he·mo·tach·o·me·ter** an instrument for measuring the flow of blood in arteries.

**he·mo·tach·o·met·ry** making blood flow measurements.

**he·mo·ther·a·py, he·mo·ther·a·peu·tics** (hē′mō-thār′ă-pē, hē-mō-thār-ă-pyu′tiks) treatment of disease by the use of blood or blood derivatives, as in transfusion.

**he·mo·tho·rax** (hē-mō-thōr′aks) blood in the pleural cavity.

**he·mo·tox·ic, he·ma·to·tox·ic, he·ma·tox·ic** (hē-mō-tok′sik; hē′mă-tō-toks′ik, hem′ă-tō-toks′ ik; hē-mă-toks′ik, hem-ă-toks′ik) 1. causing blood poisoning. 2. SYN hemolytic.

**he·mo·tox·in** (hē-mō-tok′sin) any substance that causes destruction of red blood cells, including various hemolysins; usually used with reference to substances of biologic origin, in contrast to chemicals. SYN hematotoxin.

**he·mo·troph, he·mot·ro·phe** (hēm′ō-trof) the nutritive materials supplied to the embryos of placental mammals through the maternal bloodstream. Cf. embryotroph. [hemo- + G. *trophē,* food]

**he·mo·tro·pic** (hē-mō-trop′ik) pertaining to the mechanism by which a substance in or on blood cells, especially the erythrocytes, attracts phagocytic cells; the latter change direction and migrate toward the hemotropic cells. SYN hematotropic. [hemo- + G. *tropos,* direction (or *tropē,* a turning)]

**he·mo·tym·pa·num** (hē′mō-tim′pă-nŭm) the presence of blood in the middle ear.

**hem·ox·im·e·ter** (hēm-oks-im′ĕ-ter) SYN oximeter.

**hem·ox·im·e·try** (hē-mok-sim′ĕ-trē) spectrophotometric analysis of blood for determination of the saturation of oxyhemoglobin and of dyshemoglobins (for example, carboxyhemoglobin and methemoglobin).

**he·mo·zo·on** (hē-mō-zō′ŏn) a parasitic animal that resides in the blood of the host. SYN hematozoon. [hemo- + G. *zōon,* animal]

**Hen·der·son·Has·sel·balch e·qua·tion** (hen′ dĕr-sŏn has′ĕl-bawlk) a formula relating the pH value of a solution to the $pK_a$ value of the acid in the solution and the ratio of the acid and the conjugate base concentrations: pH = $pK_a$ + log ([A⁻]/[HA]) where [A⁻] is the concentration of the conjugate base and [HA] is the concentration of the protonated acid.

*Hen·der·son·u·la tor·u·loi·de·a* (hen-der-sō-nyu′lă tōr-yu-loy′dē-ă) a species of black yeast capable of producing chronic infections of the nails as well as of the skin of the feet.

**Hend·ra vi·rus** (hen′dră) SYN equine morbillivirus. [from Hendra, the suburb of Brisbane, Australia, where it was first isolated]

**Hen·le an·sa** (hen′lē) SYN nephronic loop.

**Hen·le glands** (hen-lē) formerly considered accessory lacrimal glands, these epithelial invaginations are located near the fornices in the medial part of the palpebral conjunctiva; they open on the conjunctiva surface. SYN Baumgarten glands.

**Hen·le lay·er** (hen′lē) the outer layer cells of the inner root sheath of the hair follicle.

**Henle loop** (hen′lē) SYN nephronic loop.

**Hen·le re·ac·tion** (hen′lē) dark brown staining of the medullary cells of the adrenal bodies when treated with the salts of chromium, the cortical cells remaining unstained.

**Hen·le sheath** (hen′lē) SYN endoneurium.

**Hen·ne·bert sign** (hen'ĕ-bert) nystagmus produced by pressure applied to a sealed external auditory canal; may be seen in labyrinthine fistula or with intact tympanic membrane in syphilitic involvement of the otic capsule.

**He·noch pur·pu·ra** (hĕ'nawk) SYN Henoch-Schönlein purpura.

**He·noch-Schön·lein pur·pu·ra** (hĕ'nawk-shern'līn) an eruption of nonthrombocytopenic purpuric lesions due to dermal leukocytoclastic vasculitis with IgA in vessel walls associated with joint pain and swelling, colic, and passage of bloody stools, and occurring characteristically in young children; glomerulonephritis may occur during an initial episode or develop later. SYN anaphylactoid purpura (2), Henoch purpura, Schönlein purpura.

**Hen·ry** (hen'rē), William, British chemist, 1775–1837. SEE Henry law.

**hen·ry (H)** (hen'rē) the unit of electrical inductance, when 1 volt is induced by a change in current of 1 ampere/sec. [Joseph *Henry*]

**Hen·ry law** (hen'rē) at equilibrium, at a given temperature, the amount of gas dissolved in a given volume of liquid is directly proportional to the partial pressure of that gas in the gas phase (this only holds for gases that do not react chemically with the solvent).

**Hen·sen cell** (hen'sĕn) one of the supporting cells in the organ of Corti, immediately to the outer side of the cells of Deiters.

**Hen·sen node** (hen'sĕn) SYN primitive node.

**He·pad·na·vi·ri·dae** (hep-ad-nă-vir'ĭ-dē) a family of DNA-containing viruses. The principal genus *Hepadnavirus* is associated with hepatitis B. [*hepa*titis + DNA + virus]

**he·par**, gen. **hep·a·tis** (hē'par, hē'pah-tis) [TA] SYN liver, liver. [L. borrowed fr. G. *hēpar*, gen. *hēpatos*, the liver]

**hep·a·rin** (hep'ă-rin) an anticoagulant that is a component of various tissues (especially liver and lung) and mast cells. Its principal active constituent is a glycosaminoglycan composed of D-glucuronic acid and D-glucosamine. In conjunction with a serum protein cofactor (the so-called heparin cofactor), heparin acts as an antithrombin and an antiprothrombin by preventing platelet agglutination and consequent thrombus formation.

**hep·a·rin·ize** (hep'ă-rin-īz) to perform therapeutic administration of heparin.

**hep·a·rin lock** an indwelling venous catheter used when intravenous infusions or withdrawal of venous blood for testing must be performed repeatedly over an extended period; between uses it is filled with the anticoagulant heparin.

**hep·at-, hep·at·i·co-, hep·ato-** the liver. [G. *hēpar* (*hēpat-*)]

**hep·a·ta·tro·phia, hep·a·tat·ro·phy** (hep'ă-tă-trō'fē-ă, hep-ă-tat'rō-fē) atrophy of the liver.

**hep·a·tec·to·my** (hep-ă-tek'tō-mē) removal of the liver, whole or in part. [hepat- + G. *ektomē*, excision]

**he·pa·tic** (he-pat'ik) relating to the liver. [G. *hēpatikos*]

**he·pa·tic ad·e·no·ma** a benign tumor of the liver, usually occurring in women in association with lengthy oral contraceptive use.

**he·pa·tic bran·ches of an·te·ri·or va·gal trunk** branches of the anterior and posterior vagal trunks distributed to the liver.

**he·pa·tic co·ma** coma that occurs with advanced hepatic insufficiency and portal-systemic shunts, caused by elevated blood ammonia levels; characteristic findings include asterixis in the precoma stage and paroxysms of bilaterally synchronous triphasic waves on EEG examination.

**he·pa·tic duct** SEE common hepatic duct.

**he·pa·tic en·ceph·a·lop·a·thy 1.** SYN portal-systemic encephalopathy. **2.** SYN Reye syndrome.

**he·pa·tic flex·ure** SYN right colic flexure.

**he·pa·tic lob·ule** SYN lobules of liver.

**he·pat·i·co·do·chot·o·my** (he-pat'i-kō-dō-kot'ō-mē) combined hepaticotomy and choledochotomy.

**he·pat·i·co·du·o·de·nos·to·my** (he-pat'i-kō-doo'ō-de-nos'tō-mē) establishment of a communication between the hepatic ducts and the duodenum. [hepatico- + duodenostomy]

**he·pat·i·co·en·ter·os·to·my** (he-pat'i-kō-en-ter-os'tō-mē) establishment of a communication between the hepatic ducts and the intestine. [hepatico- + enterostomy]

**he·pat·i·co·gas·tros·to·my** (he-pat'i-kō-gas-tros'tō-mē) establishment of a communication between the hepatic duct and the stomach. [hepatico- + gastrostomy]

**he·pat·i·co·li·thot·o·my** (he-pat'i-kō-li-thot'ō-mē) removal of a stone from a hepatic duct. [hepatico- + G. *lithos*, stone, + *tomē*, a cutting]

**he·pat·i·co·lith·o·trip·sy** (he-pat'i-kō-lith'ō-trip-sē) the crushing or fragmentation of a biliary calculus in the hepatic duct. [hepatico- + G. *lithos*, stone, + *tripsis*, a rubbing]

**he·pat·i·cos·to·my** (he-pat-i-kos'tō-mē) establishment of an opening into the hepatic duct. [hepatico- + G. *stoma*, mouth]

**he·pat·i·cot·o·my** (he-pat-i-kot'ō-mē) incision into the hepatic duct. [hepatico- + G. *tomē*, incision]

**he·pa·tic por·phyr·ia** a category of porphyria that includes porphyria cutanea tarda, variegate porphyria, and coproporphyria.

**he·pa·tic por·tal vein** SYN portal vein.

**he·pa·tic veins** drain the liver; they collect blood from the central veins and terminate in three large veins opening into the inferior vena cava below the diaphragm and several small inconstant veins entering the vena cava at more inferior levels.

**hep·a·tit·ic** (hep-ă-tit'ik) relating to hepatitis.

**hep·a·ti·tis** (hep-ă-tī'tis) inflammation of the liver; usually from a viral infection, but sometimes from toxic agents. [hepat- + G. *-itis*, inflammation]

**hep·a·ti·tis A** SYN viral hepatitis type A.

**hep·a·ti·tis A vi·rus (HAV)** an RNA virus, the causative agent of viral hepatitis type A. SYN infectious hepatitis virus.

**hep·a·ti·tis B** SYN viral hepatitis type B.

**hep·a·ti·tis B core an·ti·gen (HB$_c$Ab, HB$_c$Ag)** the antigen found in the core of the Dane particle (which is the complete virus) and also in hepatocyte nuclei in hepatitis B infections.

**hep·a·ti·tis B e an·ti·gen (HBe, HB$_e$Ag)** an antigen, or group of antigens, associated with hepatitis B infection and distinct from the surface antigen (HB$_s$Ag) and the core antigen (HB$_c$Ag). Its presence indicates that the virus is replicating and the individual is potentially infectious.

**hep·a·ti·tis B im·mune glo·bu·lin (HBIG)** a high-titer passive immune globulin directed

h
e

against type B hepatitis virus (HBV). Passive immunity to type B hepatitis can be conferred by administration of this immune serum globulin. It is recommended for those exposed to fluids from persons infected with HBV.

**hep·a·ti·tis B sur·face an·ti·gen (HB$_s$Ag)** antigen of the small (20 nm) spherical and filamentous forms of hepatitis B antigen, and a surface antigen of the larger (42 nm) Dane particle (complete infectious hepatitis B virus). SEE ALSO hepatitis B e antigen.

**hep·a·ti·tis B vi·rus (HBV)** a DNA virus, the causative agent of viral hepatitis type B. SYN serum hepatitis virus.

**hep·a·ti·tis C** a viral hepatitis, usually mild but often progressing to a chronic stage; the most prevalent type of post-transfusion hepatitis.

**hep·a·ti·tis C vi·rus (HCV)** a non-A, non-B RNA virus causing posttransfusion hepatitis.

**hep·a·ti·tis D vi·rus, hep·a·ti·tis del·ta vi·rus (HDV)** a small "defective" RNA virus that requires the presence of hepatitis B virus for replication. The clinical course is variable but is usually more severe than other hepatitides. SYN delta agent.

**hep·a·ti·tis E** a viral hepatitis occurring chiefly in the tropics; transmitted by the fecal-oral route, it does not become chronic or lead to a carrier state, but has a higher mortality than hepatitis A, particularly in pregnancy.

**hep·a·ti·tis E vi·rus (HEV)** an RNA virus that is the principal cause of enterically transmitted, waterborne, or epidemic non-A, non-B hepatitis occurring primarily in Asia and Africa.

**hep·a·ti·tis F** a disease caused by an as yet poorly characterized DNA virus.

**hep·a·ti·tis G** a disease caused by an RNA virus similar to hepatitis virus.

**hep·a·ti·tis G vi·rus (HGV)** an RNA virus related to the hepatitis C virus, and which may cause co-infection with that agent.

**hep·a·ti·za·tion** (hep′ă-ti-zā′shŭn) conversion of a loose tissue into a firm mass like the substance of the liver macroscopically, denoting especially such a change in the lungs in the consolidation of pneumonia.

**he·pa·to·blas·to·ma** (hep′ă-tō-blas-tō′mă) a malignant neoplasm occurring in young children, primarily in the liver, composed of tissue resembling embryonal or fetal hepatic epithelium, or mixed epithelial and mesenchymal tissues.

**he·pa·to·car·ci·no·ma** (hep′ă-tō-kar-si-nō′mă) SYN malignant hepatoma.

**he·pa·to·cele** (hep′ă-tō-sēl, he-pat′ō-sēl) protrusion of part of the liver through the abdominal wall or the diaphragm. [hepato- + G. *kēlē,* hernia]

**he·pa·to·cel·lu·lar car·ci·no·ma** SYN malignant hepatoma.

**he·pa·to·cel·lu·lar jaun·dice** jaundice resulting from diffuse injury or inflammation or failure of function of the liver cells, usually referring to viral or toxic hepatitis.

**he·pa·to·chol·an·gi·o·je·ju·nos·to·my** (hep′ă-tō-kō-lan′jē-ō-jē-joo-nos-tō-mē) union of the hepatic duct to the jejunum. [hepato- + G. *cholē,* bile, + *angeion,* vessel, + jejunostomy]

**he·pa·to·chol·an·gi·os·to·my** (hep′ă-tō-kō-lan-jē-os′tō-mē) creation of an opening into the common bile duct to establish drainage.

**he·pa·to·chol·an·gi·tis** (hep′ă-tō-kō-lan-jī′tis) inflammation of the liver and biliary tree.

**he·pa·to·cys·tic** (hep′ă-tō-sis′tik) relating to the gallbladder, or to both liver and gallbladder. [hepato- + G. *kystis,* bladder]

**he·pa·to·cyte** (hep′ă-tō-sīt) a parenchymal liver cell.

**he·pa·to·en·ter·ic** (hep′ă-tō-en-tĕr′ik) relating to the liver and the intestine. [hepato- + G. *enteron,* intestine]

**hep·a·to·fu·gal** (hep′ă-tō-fyu′găl) away from the liver, usually referring to portal blood flow.

**he·pa·to·gas·tric** (hep′ă-tō-gas′trik) relating to the liver and the stomach.

**he·pa·to·gen·ic, he·pa·tog·e·nous** (hep-ă-tō-jen′ik, hep-ă-toj′en-ŭs) of hepatic origin; formed in the liver.

**he·pa·tog·e·nous jaun·dice** jaundice resulting from disease of the liver, as distinguished from that due to blood changes.

**he·pa·tog·ra·phy** (hep-ă-tog′ră-fē) radiography of the liver. [hepato- + G. *graphē,* a writing]

**he·pa·toid** (hep′ă-toyd) resembling or like the liver. [hepato- + G. *eidos,* resemblance]

**he·pa·to·jug·u·lar re·flux** an elevation of venous pressure visible in the jugular veins and measurable in the veins of the arm, produced in active or impending congestive heart failure by firm pressure with the flat hand over the liver.

**he·pa·to·len·tic·u·lar de·gen·er·a·tion 1.** a familial disorder characterized by copper deposition in the liver, causing chronic hepatitis and eventually cirrhosis; degeneration of the lenticular (pallidal and putaminal) nuclei, and marked hyperplasia of astrocytes in the cerebral cortex, cerebellum, basal ganglia, and brainstem nuclei; plasma levels of ceruloplasmins and copper are decreased, urinary excretion of copper is increased, and the amounts of copper in the liver, brain, and kidneys is high; clinical features include deposition of golden brown pigment in the cornea (Kayser-Fleischer rings), dysphasia and dysarthria, rigidity, and a coarse resting tremor, which increases when the limbs are outstretched ("wing-beating" tremor). **2.** SYN Wilson disease (1).

**he·pa·to·lith** (hep′ă-tō-lith) a concretion in the liver. [hepato- + G. *lithos,* stone]

**he·pa·to·li·thec·to·my** (hep′ă-tō-li-thek′tō-mē) removal of a calculus from the liver. [hepato- + G. *lithos,* stone, + *ektomē,* excision]

**he·pa·to·li·thi·a·sis** (hep′ă-tō-li-thī′ă-sis) presence of calculi in the liver. [hepato- + G. *lithiasis,* presence of a calculus]

**he·pa·tol·o·gy** (hep-ă-tol′ō-jē) the branch of medicine concerned with diseases of the liver. [hepato- + G. *logos,* study]

**he·pa·tol·y·sin** (hep-ă-tol′i-sin) a cytolysin that destroys parenchymal cells of the liver.

**he·pa·to·ma** (hep-ă-tō′mă) SEE malignant hepatoma. [hepato- + G. *-oma,* tumor]

**he·pa·to·meg·a·ly, he·pa·to·me·ga·lia** (hep′ă-tō-meg′ă-lē, hep′ă-tō-mĕ-gā′lē-ă) enlargement of the liver. SYN megalohepatia. [hepato- + G. *megas,* large]

**he·pa·to·mel·a·no·sis** (hep′ă-tō-mel′ă-nō′sis) heavy pigmentation of the liver. [hepato- + G. *melas,* black, + *-osis,* condition]

**he·pa·tom·pha·lo·cele** (hep′ă-tom-fal′ō-sēl, hep-ă-tom′fă-lō-sēl) umbilical hernia with involvement of the liver. [hepato- + omphalocele]

**he·pa·to·neph·ric** (hep′ă-tō-nef′rik) SYN hepato-renal.

**he·pa·to·pan·cre·at·ic am·pul·la** the dilation within the major duodenal papilla that normally receives both the common bile duct and the main pancreatic duct.

**he·pa·to·path·ic** (hep′ă-tō-path′ik) damaging the liver.

**he·pa·top·a·thy** (hep-ă-top′ă-thē) disease of the liver. [hepato- + G. *pathos,* suffering]

**hep·a·to·pet·al** (hepă-top′ĕ-tal) toward the liver, usually referring to the normal direction of portal blood flow.

**he·pa·to·pex·y** (hep′ă-tō-pek-sē) anchoring of the liver to the abdominal wall. [hepato- + G. *pēxis,* fixation]

**he·pa·to·pneu·mon·ic** (hep′ă-tō-noo-mon′ik) relating to the liver and the lungs. SYN hepatopulmonary. [hepato- + G. *pneumonikos,* pulmonary]

**he·pa·to·por·tal** (hep′ă-tō-pōr′tăl) relating to the portal system of the liver.

**he·pa·to·pul·mo·nary** (hep′ă-tō-pŭl′mŏ-ner-ē) SYN hepatopneumonic.

**he·pa·to·re·nal** (hep-ă-tō-rē′năl) relating to the liver and the kidney. SYN hepatonephric. [hepato- + L. *renalis,* renal, fr. *renes,* kidneys]

**he·pa·to·re·nal syn·drome, hep·a·to·ne·pho·ric syn·drome** the occurrence of acute renal failure in patients with disease of the liver or biliary tract.

**he·pa·tor·rha·phy** (hep-ă-tōr′ă-fē) suture of a wound of the liver. [hepato- + G. *rhaphē,* a suture]

**he·pa·tor·rhex·is** (hep′ă-tō-rek′sis) rupture of the liver. [hepato- + G. *rhēxis,* rupture]

**he·pa·tos·co·py** (hep-ă-tos′kŏ-pē) examination of the liver. [hepato- + G. *skopeō,* to examine]

**he·pa·to·sple·ni·tis** (hep′ă-tō-splē-nī′tis) inflammation of the liver and spleen.

**he·pa·to·sple·nog·ra·phy** (hep′ă-tō-splē-nog′ră-fē) the use of a contrast medium to outline or depict the liver and spleen radiographically.

**he·pa·to·splen·o·meg·a·ly** (hep′ă-tō-splē-nō-meg′ă-lē) enlargement of the liver and spleen. [hepato- + G. *splēn,* spleen, + *megas,* large]

**he·pa·to·sple·nop·a·thy** (hep′ă-tō-splē-nop′ă-thē) disease of the liver and spleen.

**he·pa·tot·o·my** (hep-ă-tot′ō-mē) incision into the liver. [hepato- + G. *tomē,* incision]

**he·pa·to·tox·ae·mia [Br.]** SEE hepatotoxemia.

**he·pa·to·tox·e·mia** (hep′ă-tō-tok-sē′mē-ă) autointoxication assumed to be due to improper functioning of the liver. [hepato- + G. *toxikon,* poison, + *haima,* blood]

**he·pa·to·tox·ic** (hep′ă-tō-tok′sik) relating to an agent that damages the liver, or pertaining to any such action.

**he·pa·to·tox·in** (hep′ă-tō-tok′sin) a toxin that is destructive to parenchymal cells of the liver.

**hept-** seven. [G. *hepta,* seven]

△**hep·ta-** prefix denoting seven. Cf. septi-, sept-. [G. *hepta*]

**hep·tose** (hep′tōs) a sugar with seven carbon atoms in its molecule; e.g., sedoheptulose.

**herd** a group of people or animals in a given area. [O.E. *heord*]

**herd im·mu·ni·ty** the resistance to invasion and spread of an infectious agent in a group or community, based on the resistance to infection of a high proportion of individual members of the group.

**herd in·stinct** tendency or inclination to band together with and share the customs of others of

a group, and to conform to the opinions and adopt the views of the group.

**he·red·i·tary** (hĕ-red′i-ter-ē) transmissible from parent to offspring by information encoded in the parental germ cell. [L. *hereditarius;* fr. *heres* (*hered-*), an heir]

**he·red·i·tary be·nign te·lan·giec·ta·sia** an autosomal dominant disorder in which the face, upper trunk, and arms develop telangiectasias.

**he·red·i·tary cer·e·bel·lar a·tax·ia 1.** a disease of later childhood and early adult life, marked by ataxic gait, hesitating and explosive speech, nystagmus, and sometimes optic neuritis. **2.** collective term for a number of hereditary disorders in which cerebellar signs are the most prominent finding.

**he·red·i·tary cho·rea** SYN Huntington chorea.

**he·red·i·tary club·bing** simple hereditary clubbing of the digits without associated pulmonary or other progressive disease.

**he·red·i·tary deaf·ness** SEE hereditary hearing impairment.

**he·red·i·tary hear·ing im·pair·ment** hearing impairment occurring in syndromic forms (in which there are other anomalies in addition to the hearing impairment) and nonsyndromic forms (in which hearing impairment is the only unusual finding) with autosomal dominant and recessive, X-linked, and mitochondrial modes of transmission; may be congenital, of early onset in childhood, or late onset in mid-life and advanced age.

**he·red·i·tary non·po·lyp·o·sis co·lo·rec·tal can·cer** an autosomal dominant predisposition to cancer of the colon and rectum.

**he·red·i·tary pro·gress·ive ar·thro·oph·thal··mop·a·thy** a skeletal dysplasia associated with multiple dysplasia of the epiphyses, overtubulation of long bones with metaphyseal widening, flattened vertebral bodies, pelvic bone abnormalities, hypermobility of joints, cleft palate, progressive myopia, retinal detachment, and deafness. Autosomal dominant inheritance caused by mutation in either the COL2A1 gene on 12q, COL11A1 gene on 1p or COL11A2 gene on 6p. SYN Stickler syndrome.

**he·red·i·tary sphe·ro·cy·to·sis** a congenital defect of spectrin, the main component of the erythrocyte cell membrane, which becomes abnormally permeable to sodium, resulting in thickened and almost spherical erythrocytes that are fragile and susceptible to spontaneous hemolysis, with decreased survival in the circulation; results in chronic anemia with reticulocytosis, episodes of mild jaundice due to hemolysis, and acute crises with gallstones, fever, and abdominal pain. SYN familial jaundice, spherocytic anemia.

**he·red·i·tary spi·nal a·tax·ia** sclerosis of the posterior and lateral columns of the spinal cord, occurring in children and marked by ataxia in the lower extremities, extending to the upper, followed by paralysis and contractures. SEE ALSO spinocerebellar ataxia.

**he·red·i·ty** (hĕ-red′i-tē) **1.** the transmission of characters from parent to offspring by information encoded in the parental germ cells. **2.** genealogy. [L. *hereditas,* inheritance, fr. *heres* (*hered-*), heir]

△**he·redo-** heredity. [L. *heres,* an heir]

**Her·ing-Breu·er re·flex** (her′ing-broi′ĕr) the effects of afferent impulses from the pulmonary vagi in the control of respiration, e.g., inflation of the lungs arrests inspiration, with expiration then ensuing, while deflation of the lungs brings on inspiration.

**Her•ing law** (her'ing) states that paired agonist muscles from each eye operating in the same field of gaze receive equal innervation while paired antagonist muscles receive equal inhibition.

**Her•ing test** (her'ing) a test of binocular vision; the subject looks through an apparatus having at its far end a thread near which a small sphere is dropped; with binocular vision the observer recognizes the location of the sphere in front of or behind the thread; with monocular vision this is not possible.

**Her•ing the•o•ry of col•or vi•sion** (her'ing) that there are three opponent visual processes: blue-yellow, red-green, and white-black.

**her•i•ta•bil•i•ty** (her'i-tă-bil'i-tē) **1.** PSYCHOMETRICS a statistical term used to denote the extent of variance of an individual's total score or response which is attributable to a presumed genetic component, in contrast to an acquired component. **2.** GENETICS a statistical term used to denote the proportion of phenotypic variance due to variance in genotypes that is genetically determined, denoted by the traditional symbol $h^2$. [see heredity]

**Her•mann fix•a•tive** (her'man) a hardening fixative of glacial acetic acid, osmic acid, and platinum chloride.

**her•maph•ro•dite** (her-maf'rō-dīt) an individual with hermaphroditism. [G. *Hermaphroditos,* the son of *Hermēs,* Mercury, + *Aphroditē,* Venus]

**her•maph•ro•dit•ism** (her-maf'rō-dīt-izm) the presence in one individual of both ovarian and testicular tissue; i.e., true hermaphroditism.

**her•met•ic** (her-met'ik) airtight; denoting a vessel closed or sealed in such a way that air can neither enter it nor issue from it.

**her•nia** (her'nē-ă) protrusion of a part or structure through the tissues normally containing it. SYN rupture (1). [L. rupture]

**her•nia knife** a slender bladed knife, with short cutting edge, for dividing the constricting tissues at the mouth of the hernial sac. SYN herniotome.

**her•ni•al** (her'nē-ăl) relating to hernia.

**her•ni•al sac** the peritoneal envelope of a hernia.

**her•ni•at•ed** (her'nē-ā-ted) denoting any structure protruded through a hernial opening.

**🔒 her•ni•at•ed disk** protrusion of a degenerated or fragmented intervertebral disk into the intervertebral foramen with potential compression of a nerve root or into the spinal canal with potential compression of the cauda equina in the lumbar region or the spinal cord at higher levels. See page 445 and B11. SYN protruded disk, ruptured disk.

**her•ni•a•tion** (her-nē-ā'shŭn) protrusion of an anatomic structure (e.g., intervertebral disk) from its normal anatomic position.

△**her•ni•o-** a hernia. [L. *hernia,* rupture]

**her•ni•oid** (her'nē-oyd) resembling hernia. [hernio- + G. *eidos,* resemblance]

**her•ni•o•plas•ty** (her'nē-ō-plas-tē) SYN herniorrhaphy. [hernio- + G. *plastos,* formed]

**her•ni•or•rha•phy** (her'nē-ōr'ă-fē) surgical repair of a hernia. SYN hernioplasty. [hernio- + G. *rhaphē,* a seam]

**her•ni•o•tome** (her'nē-ō-tōm) SYN hernia knife.

**her•ni•ot•o•my** (her-nē-ot'ō-mē) surgical division of the constriction or strangulation of a hernia, often followed by herniorrhaphy. [hernio- + G. *tomē,* a cutting]

**he•ro•ic** (hē-rō'ik) denoting an aggressive, daring procedure in a dangerously ill patient which may endanger the patient but which also has a possibility of being successful, whereas lesser action would result in failure. [G. *hērōikos,* pertaining to a hero]

**her•o•in (H)** (her'ō-in) an alkaloid prepared from morphine by acetylation; formerly used for the relief of cough. Except for research, its use in the United States is prohibited by federal law because of its potential for abuse.

**her•pan•gi•na** (her-pan'ji-nă, herp-an-jī'nă) a disease caused by types of coxsackievirus and marked by vesiculopapular lesions around the fauces that break down to form grayish yellow ulcers. [G. *herpēs,* vesicular eruption, + L. *angina,* quinsy, fr. *ango,* to strangle]

**her•pes** (her'pēz) a papular, vesicular, or ulcerative eruption of skin or mucous membranes caused by local infection with herpesvirus 1 or 2 (herpes simplex) or by reactivation of the varicella-zoster virus. SYN serpigo (2). [G. *herpēs,* a spreading skin eruption, shingles, fr. *herpō,* to creep]

**her•pes gen•i•tal•is** SYN genital herpes.

**her•pes ges•ta•tio•nis** a polymorphous, bullous eruption beginning in the second or third trimester of pregnancy, flaring about the time of delivery, and subsequently resolving.

**her•pes i•ris 1.** SYN erythema iris. **2.** SYN erythema multiforme.

**🔒 her•pes sim•plex** a variety of infections caused by herpesvirus types 1 and 2; type 1 infections are marked most commonly by the eruption of one or more groups of vesicles on the vermilion border of the lips or at the external nares, type 2 by such lesions on the genitalia; both types often are recrudescent and reappear during other febrile illnesses or even physiologic states such as menstruation. See this page. SYN Simplexvirus.

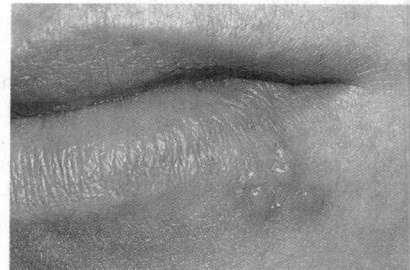

**recurrent herpes simplex** (labialis): a cluster of virus-laden vesicles.

**her•pes sim•plex en•ceph•a•li•tis** the most common acute encephalitis, caused by HSV-1; affects persons of any age; preferentially involves the inferomedial portions of the temporal lobe and the orbital portions of the frontal lobes; pathologically, severe hemorrhagic necrosis is present along with, in the acute stages, intranuclear eosinophilic inclusion bodies in the neurons and glial cells.

**her·pes sim·plex vi·rus (HSV)** SEE herpes simplex.

**her·pes·vi·rus, her·pes vi·rus** (her′pēz-vī′rŭs) any virus belonging to the family Herpesviridae.

**Her·pes·vi·rus sai·mi·ri** the cause of an ubiquitous infection of squirrel monkeys, which is highly oncogenic when injected into other monkey species.

**her·pes zos·ter** an infection caused by varicella-zoster virus, characterized by an eruption of groups of vesicles on one side of the body following the course of a nerve, due to inflammation of ganglia and dorsal nerve roots; the condition is self-limited but may be accompanied by or followed by severe postherpetic pain. See page B3. SYN shingles, zona (2), zoster.

**her·pes zos·ter oti·cus** a painful varicella virus infection presenting with a vesicular eruption on the pinna, with or without facial nerve paralysis. SYN Ramsay Hunt syndrome (2).

**her·pes zos·ter vi·rus** SYN varicella-zoster virus.

**her·pet·ic** (her-pet′ik) **1.** relating to or characterized by herpes. **2.** relating to or caused by a herpetovirus or herpesvirus.

**her·pet·ic ker·a·ti·tis** inflammation of the cornea (or cornea and conjunctiva) due to herpes simplex virus. SYN herpetic keratoconjunctivitis.

**her·pet·ic ker·a·to·con·junc·ti·vi·tis** SYN herpetic keratitis.

**her·pet·ic whit·low** painful herpes simplex virus infection of a finger from direct inoculation of the unprotected perionychial fold, often accompanied by lymphangitis and regional adenopathy, lasting up to several weeks; most common in physicians, dentists, and nurses as a result of exposure to the virus in a patient's mouth.

**her·pet·i·form** (her-pet′i-fōrm) resembling herpes.

**her·pet·i·form aph·thae** a variant of oral aphthae, of unknown etiology, characterized by up to several dozen ulcers, 2-3 mm in diameter, organized in a clustered herpetiform distribution.

**Herr·mann syn·drome** (her′mahn) a multisystem disorder beginning in late childhood or early adolescence, with photomyoclonus and hearing loss followed by diabetes mellitus, progressive dementia, pyelonephritis, and glomerulonephritis; progressive sensorineural hearing loss is of later onset; probably autosomal dominant inheritance with incomplete penetrance.

**her·sage** (ār-sahzh′) separating the individual fibers of a nerve trunk. [Fr. (from L. *hirpex*, a large rake), a harrowing]

**Hers dis·ease** (ārz) SYN type 6 glycogenosis.

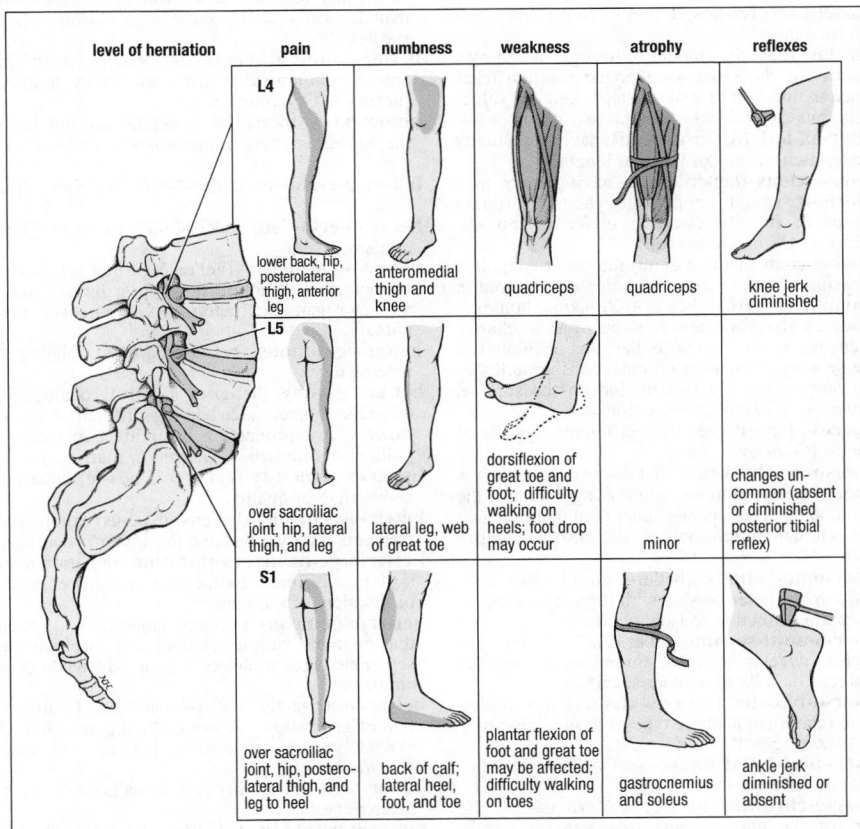

| level of herniation | pain | numbness | weakness | atrophy | reflexes |
|---|---|---|---|---|---|
| **L4** | lower back, hip, posterolateral thigh, anterior leg | anteromedial thigh and knee | quadriceps | quadriceps | knee jerk diminished |
| **L5** | over sacroiliac joint, hip, lateral thigh, and leg | lateral leg, web of great toe | dorsiflexion of great toe and foot; difficulty walking on heels; foot drop may occur | minor | changes uncommon (absent or diminished posterior tibial reflex) |
| **S1** | over sacroiliac joint, hip, posterolateral thigh, and leg to heel | back of calf; lateral heel, foot, and toe | plantar flexion of foot and great toe may be affected; difficulty walking on toes | gastrocnemius and soleus | ankle jerk diminished or absent |

**intervertebral disc herniation:** areas of herniation shown in purple

h
e

**Hert·wig sheath** (hĕrt'vik) the merged outer and inner epithelial layers of the enamel organ which extends beyond the region of the anatomical crown and initiates formation of dentin in the root of a developing tooth; it atrophies as the root is formed, and any of the cells that persist are called Malassez epithelial rests.

**Hertz** (herts), Heinrich R., German physicist, 1857–1894. SEE hertz.

**hertz (Hz)** (herts) a unit of frequency equivalent to 1 cycle per second. [H.R. *Hertz*]

**Herx·hei·mer re·ac·tion** (hĕrks'hīm-ĕr) a systemic inflammatory reaction affecting skin, mucous membrane, nervous system, or viscera occurring after antimicrobial treatment of treponemal disease (syphilis, Lyme disease); believed to be due to a rapid release of treponemal antigen with an associated allergic reaction in the patient. SYN Jarisch-Herxheimer reaction.

**hes·i·tan·cy** (hez'i-tăn-sē) an involuntary delay or inability in starting the urinary stream.

**hes·i·tant** (hez'ĭ-tant) term used to descibe the state of RNA polymerase when it is susceptible to pause, arrest, or termination signals. SEE ALSO overdrive, antitermination.

**Hes·sel·bach her·nia** (hes'ĕl-bahk) hernia with diverticula through the cribriform fascia, presenting a lobular outline.

**Hes·sel·bach tri·an·gle** (hes'ĕl-bahk) SYN inguinal triangle.

**Hess law** (hes) the amount of heat generated by a reaction is the same whether the reaction takes place in one step or several steps; i.e., $\Delta H$ values (and thus $\Delta G$ values) are additive.

**het·er·ax·i·al** (het-er-ak'sē-ăl) having mutually perpendicular axes of unequal length.

**het·er·e·cious** (het-er-ē'shŭs) having more than one host; said of a parasite passing different stages of its life cycle in different animals. [heter- + G. *oikion*, home]

**het·er·e·cism** (het'er-ē-sizm) the occurrence, in a parasite, of two cycles of development passed in two different hosts. [heter- + G. *oikion*, home]

**het·er·es·the·sia** (het-er-es-thē'zē-ă) a change occurring in the degree (either plus or minus) of the sensory response to a cutaneous stimulus as the latter crosses a certain line on the surface. [heter- + G. *aisthēsis*, sensation]

△**het·er·o-, het·er-** the other, different; opposite of homo- [G. *heteros*, other]

**het·er·o·ag·glu·ti·nin** (het'er-ō-ă-gloo'ti-nin) a form of hemagglutinin, one that agglutinates the red blood cells of species other than that in which the heteroagglutinin occurs. SEE ALSO hemagglutinin.

**het·er·o·an·ti·body** (het'er-ō-an'ti-bod-ē) antibody that is heterologous with respect to antigen, in contradistinction to isoantibody.

**het·er·o·an·ti·se·rum** (het'er-ō-an'ti-sē-rŭm) antiserum developed in one animal species against antigens or cells of another species.

**het·er·o·blas·tic** (het-er-ō-blas'tik) developing from more than a single type of tissue. [hetero- + G. *blastos*, germ]

**het·er·o·cel·lu·lar** (het'er-ō-sel'yu-lăr) formed of cells of different kinds.

**het·er·o·chro·ma·tin** (het'er-ō-krō'mă-tin) the part of the chromonema that remains tightly coiled and condensed during interphase and thus stains readily.

**het·er·o·chro·mia** (het-er-ō-krō'mē-ă) a differ-

ence in coloration in two structures which are normally alike in color. [hetero- + G. *chrōma*, color]

**het·er·o·chro·mic u·ve·i·tis** anterior uveitis and depigmentation of the iris. SYN Fuchs uveitis.

**het·er·o·chro·mo·some** (het'er-ō-krō'mō-sōm) SYN allosome.

**het·er·o·chro·mous** (het'er-ō-krō'mŭs) having an abnormal difference in coloration.

**het·er·o·chro·nia** (het-er-ō-krō'nē-ă) origin or development of tissues or organs at an unusual time or out of the regular sequence. Cf. synchronia. [hetero- + G. *chronos*, time]

**het·er·o·chron·ic** (het-er-ō-kron'ik) SYN heterochronous.

**het·er·och·ro·nous** (het-er-ok'rō-nŭs) relating to heterochronia. SYN heterochronic.

**het·er·o·crine** (het'er-ō-krin) denoting the secretion of two or more kinds of material. [hetero- + G. *krinō*, to separate]

**het·er·o·cy·to·tro·pic** (het'er-ō-sī'tō-trop'ik) having an affinity for cells of a different species. [hetero- + G. *kytos*, cell, + *tropē*, a turning toward]

**het·er·o·cy·to·tro·pic an·ti·bod·y** a cytotropic antibody (chiefly of the IgG class) similar in activity to homocytotropic antibody, but having an affinity for cells of a different species rather than for cells of the same or a closely related species.

**het·er·o·dont** (het'er-ō-dont) having teeth that are morphologically different, as in humans. [hetero- + G. *odous*, tooth]

**het·er·od·ro·mous** (het-er-ōd'rŏ-mŭs) moving in the opposite direction. [hetero- + G. *dromos*, running]

**het·er·o·e·rot·ic** (het'er-ō-ĕ-rot'ik) SYN alloerotic.

**het·er·o·er·o·tism** (het'er-ō-ār'ō-tizm) SYN alloerotism.

**het·er·o·ga·met·ic** (het'er-ō-gă-met'ik) having sex gametes of contrasting types; human males are heterogametic. [hetero- + G. *gametikos*, connubial]

**het·er·og·a·mous** (het-er-og'ă-mŭs) relating to heterogamy.

**het·er·og·a·my** (het-er-og'ă-mē) 1. conjugation of unlike gametes. 2. bearing different types of flowers. 3. reproduction by indirect methods of pollination. [hetero- + G. *gamos*, marriage]

**het·er·o·ge·ne·i·ty** (het'er-ō-jĕ-nē'i-tē) heterogeneous state or quality.

**het·er·o·ge·neous** (het'er-ō-jē'nē-ŭs) comprising elements with various and dissimilar properties.

**het·er·o·ge·neous ra·di·a·tion** radiation consisting of different frequencies, various energies, or a variety of particles.

**het·er·o·ge·neous sys·tem** CHEMISTRY a system that contains various distinct and mechanically separable parts or phases; e.g., a suspension or an emulsion.

**het·er·o·gen·e·sis** (het'er-ō-jen'ĕ-sis) 1. alternation of generations. 2. SYN asexual generation. 3. SYN spontaneous generation. [hetero- + G. *genesis*, production]

**het·er·o·ge·net·ic** (het'er-ō-jĕ-net'ik) relating to heterogenesis.

**het·er·o·ge·net·ic an·ti·gen** an antigen which is possessed by a variety of phylogenetically unrelated species; e.g., the various organ- or tissue-specific antigens, the alpha- and beta-crystalline protein of the lens of the eye, and Forssman antigen.

**het·er·o·ge·net·ic par·a·site** a parasite whose life cycle involves an alternation of generations.

**het·er·o·ge·ne·ic** (het′er-ō-jen′ik, het′er-ō-jĕ-nē′ik) having different gene constitutions, especially in diverse species.

**het·er·o·gen·ic, het·er·o·ge·ne·ic en·ter·o·bac·te·ri·al an·ti·gen** SYN common antigen.

**het·er·og·e·nous** (het-er-oj′ĕ-nŭs) of foreign origin. Commonly confused with heterogeneous.

**het·er·o·gon·ic life cy·cle** free-living stage of life cycle of an organism (e.g., *Strongyloides stercoralis*) that also has a parasitic stage.

**het·er·o·graft** (het′er-ō-graft) SYN xenograft.

**het·er·o·ki·ne·sis** (het′er-ō-ki-nē′sis) differential distribution of X and Y chromosomes during meiotic cell division. [hetero- + G. *kinēsis*, movement hetero- + G. *kinēsis*, movement]

**het·er·o·la·lia** (het′er-ō-lā′lē-ă) the habitual substitution of meaningless or inappropriate words for those intended; a form of aphasia. SYN heterophemia, heterophemy. [hetero- + G. *lalia*, speech]

**het·er·o·lat·er·al** (het′er-ō-lat′er-ăl) SYN contralateral. [hetero- + L. *latus*, side]

**het·er·ol·o·gous** (het-er-ol′ŏ-gŭs) **1.** pertaining to cytologic or histologic elements occurring where they are not normally found. SEE ALSO xenogeneic. **2.** derived from an animal of a different species; thus the serum of a horse is heterologous for a rabbit. [hetero- + G. *logos*, ratio, relation]

**het·er·ol·o·gous graft** SYN xenograft.

**het·er·ol·o·gous stim·u·lus** a stimulus that acts upon any part of the sensory apparatus or nerve tract.

**het·er·ol·o·gous tu·mor** a tumor composed of a tissue unlike that from which it springs.

**het·er·ol·o·gous twins** SYN dizygotic twins.

**het·er·ol·y·sis** (het-er-ol′i-sis) dissolution or digestion of cells or protein components from one species by a lytic agent from a different species. [hetero- + G. *lysis*, a loosening]

**het·er·o·lyt·ic** (het′er-ō-lit′ik) pertaining to heterolysis or to the effect of a heterolysin.

**het·er·o·mer·ic** (het′er-ō-mār′ik) **1.** having a different chemical composition. **2.** denoting spinal neurons that have processes passing over to the opposite side of the cord. [hetero- + G. *meros*, part]

**het·er·o·met·a·pla·sia** (het′er-ō-met-ă-plā′zē-ă) tissue transformation resulting in production of a tissue foreign to the part where produced.

**het·er·o·met·ric au·to·reg·u·la·tion** intrinsic regulation of the strength of cardiac contraction as a function of diastolic fiber length (volume), independent of afterload, autonomic nerves, and other extrinsic influences. Heterometric autoregulation is also known as the length-tension relationship, the relationship of end diastolic volume to end diastolic pressure, Starling law of the heart, and the Frank-Starling mechanism.

**het·er·o·me·tro·pia** (het′er-ō-me-trō′pē-ă) a condition in which the refraction is different in the two eyes. [hetero- + G. *metron*, measure, + *ōps*, eye]

**het·er·o·mor·pho·sis** (het′er-ō-mōr-fō′sis) **1.** development of one tissue from a tissue of another kind or type. **2.** embryonic development of tissue or an organ inappropriate to its site. [hetero- + G. *morphōsis*, a molding]

**het·er·o·mor·phous** (het′er-ō-mōr′fŭs) differing from the normal form.

**het·er·on·o·mous** (het-er-on′ō-mŭs) **1.** different from the type; abnormal. **2.** subject to the direction or control of another; not self-governing. [hetero- + G. *nomos*, law]

**het·er·on·o·my** (het-er-on′ō-mē) the condition or state of being heteronomous. [hetero- + G. *nomos*, law]

**het·er·op·a·thy** (het′er-op′ă-thē) **1.** abnormal sensitivity to stimuli. **2.** SYN allopathy. [hetero- + G. *pathos*, suffering]

**het·er·oph·a·gy** (het-er-of′ă-jē) digestion within a cell of a substance phagocytized from without. [hetero- + G. *phagō*, to eat]

**het·er·o·phe·mia, het·er·o·phe·my** (het′er-ō-fē′mē-ă, het-er-of′ĕ-mē) SYN heterolalia. [hetero- + G. *phēmē*, a speech]

**het·er·o·phil, het·er·o·phile** (het′er-ō-fil, het′er-ō-fīl) **1.** the neutrophilic leukocyte. **2.** pertaining to heterogenetic antigens occurring in different species or to antibodies directed against such antigens. [hetero- + G. *philos*, fond]

**het·er·o·pho·nia** (het′er-ō-fō′nē-ă) **1.** the change of voice at puberty. **2.** any abnormality in the voice sounds. [hetero- + G. *phōnē*, voice]

**het·er·o·pho·ria** (het′er-ō-fō′rē-ă) a tendency for deviation of the eyes from parallelism, prevented by binocular vision. [hetero- + G. *phora*, movement]

**het·er·oph·thal·mus** (het′er-of-thal′mŭs) a seldom-used term for a difference in the appearance of the two eyes, usually due to heterochromia iridis. [hetero- + G. *ophthalmos*, eye]

**het·er·o·phy·i·a·sis** (het′er-ō-fī-ī′ă-sis) infection with a heterophyid trematode, particularly *Heterophyes heterophyes*.

**het·er·o·pla·sia** (het′er-ō-plā′zē-ă) **1.** development of cytologic and histologic elements that are not normal for the organ or part in question, as the growth of bone in a site where there is normally fibrous connective tissue. **2.** malposition of tissue or a part that is otherwise normal, as a ureter that develops at the lower pole of a kidney. [hetero- + G. *plasis*, a forming]

**het·er·o·plas·tic** (het′er-ō-plas′tik) **1.** pertaining to or manifesting heteroplasia. **2.** relating to heteroplasty.

**het·er·o·ploid** (het′er-ō-ployd) relating to heteroploidy.

**het·er·o·ploi·dy** (het′er-ō-ploy′dē) the state of a cell possessing some number of complete haploid sets other than the normal. [hetero- + G. *ploides*, in form]

**het·er·o·pyk·no·sis** (het′er-ō-pik-nō′sis) any state of variable density or condensation, usually in different chromosomes or between different regions of the same chromosome; a region may be attenuated (negative heteropyknosis) or accentuated (positive heterpyknosis). [hetero- + G. *pyknos*, dense]

**het·er·o·pyk·not·ic** (het′er-ō-pik-not′ik) relating to or characterized by heteropyknosis.

**het·er·o·re·cep·tor** (het′er-ō-rē-sep′ter) a site on a neuron that binds a modulatory neuroregulator other than that released by the neuron. [hetero- + receptor]

**het·er·o·sex·u·al** (het′er-ō-seks′yu-ăl) **1.** a person whose sexual orientation is toward persons of the opposite sex. **2.** relating to or characteristic

h
e

of heterosexuality. **3.** one whose interests and behavior are characteristic of heterosexuality.

**het•er•o•sex•u•al•i•ty** (het'er-ō-seks-yu-al'i-tē) erotic attraction, predisposition, or activity, including sexual congress between persons of the opposite sex.

**het•er•o•sug•ges•tion** (het'er-ō-sŭg-jes'chŭn) hypnotic suggestion received from another person; opposed to autosuggestion.

**het•er•o•tax•ia** (het'er-ō-taks'ē-ă) abnormal arrangement of organs or parts of the body in relation to each other. [hetero- + G. *taxis,* arrangement]

**het•er•o•tax•ic** (het-er-ō-taks'ik) abnormally placed or arranged.

**het•er•o•to•nia** (het'er-ō-tō'nē-ă) abnormality or variation in tension or tonus. [hetero- + G. *tonos,* tension]

**het•er•o•to•pia** (het-er-ō-tō'pē-ă) **1.** SYN ectopia. **2.** NEUROPATHOLOGY displacement of gray substance (matter), typically into the deep cerebral white substance (matter). [hetero- + G. *topos,* place]

**het•er•o•top•ic** (het-er-ō-top'ik) **1.** SYN ectopic (1). **2.** relating to heterotopia (2). [hetero- + *topos,* place, + suffix *-ic,* pertaining to]

**het•er•ot•o•pous** (het-er-ot'ō-pŭs) heterotopic, especially in reference to teratomas composed of tissues that are out of place in the region where found.

**het•er•o•trans•plan•ta•tion** (het'er-ō-tranz-plan-tā'shŭn) transfer of a heterograft (xenograft).

**het•er•o•tri•cho•sis** (het'er-ō-tri-kō'sis) a condition characterized by hair growth of variegated color. [hetero- + G. *trichōsis,* growth of hair]

**het•er•o•troph** (het'er-ō-trof) a microorganism that obtains its carbon, as well as its energy, from organic compounds. SEE ALSO autotroph. [hetero- + G. *trophē,* nourishment]

**het•er•o•tro•phic** (het'er-ō-tro-fik) **1.** relating to or exhibiting the properties of heterotrophy. **2.** relating to a heterotroph.

**het•er•o•tro•pia, het•er•ot•ro•py** (het'er-ō-trō'pē-ă, het-er-ot'rō-pē) SYN strabismus. [hetero- + G. *tropē,* a turning]

**het•er•o•trop•ic preg•nan•cies** pregnancies occurring simultaneously in different sites, e.g., intrauterine and ampullary.

**het•er•o•typ•ic** (het'er-ō-tip'ik) of a different or unusual type or form.

**het•er•o•typ•i•cal chro•mo•some** SYN allosome.

**het•er•o•typ•ic cor•tex** SYN allocortex.

**het•er•o•xan•thine** (het'er-ō-zan'thin) 7-methylxanthine; one of the alloxuric bases in urine, representing end products of purine metabolism.

**het•er•ox•e•nous** (het-er-oks'ē-nŭs) SYN digenetic (1). [hetero- + G. *xenos,* stranger]

**het•er•ox•e•nous par•a•site** a parasite that has more than one obligatory host in its life cycle.

**het•er•o•zy•gos•i•ty, het•er•o•zy•go•sis** (het'er-ō-zī-gos'i-tē, het'er-ō-zī-gō'sis) the state of being heterozygous. [hetero- + G. *zygon,* a yoke]

**het•er•o•zy•gote** (het'er-ō-zī'gōt) a heterozygous individual. [hetero- + G. *zygotos,* yoked]

**het•er•o•zy•gous** (het'er-ō-zī'gŭs) having different allelic genes at one locus or (by extension) many loci; heterotic.

**Heub•ner ar•te•ri•tis** (hoib'nĕr) inflammation of arteries within the circle of Willis secondary to chronic basal meningitis from tubercle bacillus

or a gungus such as *Cryptococcus, Histoplasma,* or *Coccidiodes.*

**HEV** hepatitis E virus.

△**hex•a-, hex-** six. [G. *hex*]

**hex•ad** (heks'ad) a sexivalent element or radical.

**hex•a•dac•ty•ly, hex•a•dac•tyl•ism** (hek'să-dak'ti-lē, hek'să-dak'til-izm) the presence of six fingers or six toes on one or both hands or feet. [hexa- + G. *daktylos,* finger]

**Hex•ad•no•vi•rus** (hecks'ad-nō-vī-rŭs) a genus in the family Hepadnaviridae, which is the cause of hepatitis B.

**hex•a•mer** (hek'să-mer) **1.** SEE virion. **2.** a complex or compound containing six subunits or moieties. [hexa- + G. *meros,* part]

**hex•ane** (hek'sān) a saturated hydrocarbon, $C_6H_{14}$, of the paraffin series.

**hex•a•ploi•dy** (heks'ă-ploy-dē) SEE polyploidy.

**hex•i•tol** (heks'i-tol) the polyol (sugar alcohol) obtained on the reduction of a hexose (e.g., D-sorbitol).

**hex•o•ki•nase** (heks-ō-kī'nās) a phosphotransferase present in yeast, muscle, brain, and other tissues that catalyzes the phosphorylation of D-glucose and other hexoses to form D-glucose 6-phosphate (or other hexose 6-phosphate) (phosphate is transferred from ATP, which is converted to ADP); the first step in glycolysis; a deficiency of hexokinase can result in hemolytic anemia and impaired glycolysis.

**hex•o•ki•nase meth•od** the most specific method for measuring glucose in serum or plasma, involving hexokinase, ATP, glucose 6-phosphate NADP, and glucose 6-phosphate dehydrogenase.

**hex•one ba•ses, his•tone ba•ses** the α-amino acids arginine, histidine, and lysine, which are basic by virtue of the presence in the side chains of a guanidine, imidazole, and amine group, respectively.

**hex•os•a•mine** (hek'sō-sam'ēn) the amine derivative ($NH_2$ replacing OH) of a hexose; e.g., glucosamine.

**hex•os•a•min•i•dase** (hek'sō-sa-min'i-dās) general term for enzymes cleaving *N*-acetylhexose residues from ganglioside-like oligosaccharides.

**hex•o•sans** (hek'sō-sanz) polysaccharides with the general formula $(C_6H_{10}O_5)_x$ which, on hydrolysis, yield hexoses; included are glucosans (glucans), mannans, galactans, and fructosans (fructans).

**hex•ose** (hek'sōs) a monosaccharide containing six carbon atoms in the molecule ($C_6H_{12}O_6$); D-glucose is the principal hexose in nature.

**hex•ose phos•pha•tase** an enzyme catalyzing the hydrolysis of a hexose phosphate to a hexose (e.g., glucose-6-phosphatase).

**hex•u•lose** (heks'yu-lōs) SYN ketohexose.

**hex•yl** (hek'sil) the radical of hexane, $CH_3(CH_2)_4CH_2^-$.

**Hey am•pu•ta•tion** (hā) amputation of the foot in front of the tarsometatarsal joint.

**Hey•er-Pu•denz valve** (hā'er-poo'dens) a valve used in the shunting procedure for hydrocephaly; consisting of a catheter-valve system in which the ventricular catheter leads the cerebrospinal fluid into a one-way pump through which the cerebrospinal fluid passes down the distal catheter into the right atrium of the heart.

**Hey her•nia** (hā) SYN Cooper hernia.

**Hf** hafnium.

**HFV** high-frequency ventilation.

**Hg** mercury (hydrargyrum).

**HGE** human granulocytic ehrlichiosis.

**HGF** hematopoietic growth factor.

**HGSIL** high-grade squamous intraepithelial lesion.

**HGV** hepatitis G virus.

**HHIE-S** Hearing Handicap Inventory for the Elderly.

**hi·a·tal** (hī-ā′tăl) relating to a hiatus.

**hi·a·tal her·nia, hi·a·tus her·ni·a** hernia of a part of the stomach through the esophageal hiatus of the diaphragm. See this page.

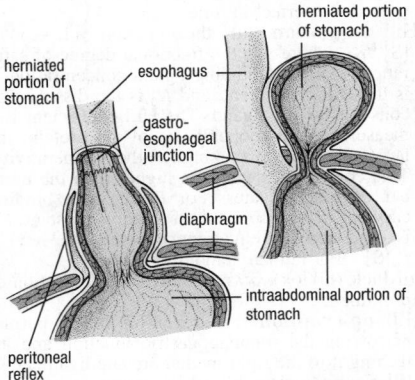

herniated portion of stomach

herniated portion of stomach

esophagus

gastro-esophageal junction

diaphragm

intraabdominal portion of stomach

peritoneal reflex

**sliding esophageal and paraesophageal hernias:** in sliding esophageal hernias (left) the upper stomach and cardio-esophageal junction slide in and out of thorax; in para-esophageal hernias (right) all or part of the stomach pushes through diaphragm next to gastroesophageal junction

**hi·a·tus,** pl. **hi·a·tus** (hī-ā′tŭs) an aperture, opening, or foramen. [L. an aperture, fr. *hio,* pp. *hiatus,* to yawn]

**hi·a·tus of ca·nal of less·er pe·tro·sal nerve** the small opening in the petrous bone lateral to the hiatus of facial canal that gives passage to the lesser petrosal nerve.

**hi·ber·no·ma** (hī′ber-nō′mă) a rare benign neoplasm consisting of brown fat that resembles the fat in certain hibernating animals. [L. *hibernus,* pertaining to winter, + G. *-ōma,* tumor]

**hic·cup, hic·cough** (hik′ŭp) a diaphragmatic spasm causing a sudden inhalation which is interrupted by a spasmodic closure of the glottis, producing a noise.

**hi·drad·e·ni·tis** (hī-drad′ĕ-nī′tis) inflammation of the sweat glands. [G. *hidrōs,* sweat, + *adēn,* gland, + *-itis,* inflammation]

**hi·drad·e·ni·tis sup·pu·ra·ti·va** chronic suppurative folliculitis of apocrine sweat-gland–bearing skin producing abscesses or sinuses with scarring.

**hi·drad·e·no·ma** (hī-drad-ĕ-nō′mă) a benign neoplasm derived from epithelial cells of sweat glands. [G. *hidrōs,* sweat, + *adēn,* gland, + *-oma,* tumor]

△**hi·dro-, hidr-** sweat, sweat glands. Cf. sudor-. [G. *hidrōs*]

**hi·dro·cys·to·ma** (hī′drō-sis-tō′mă) a cystic form of hidradenoma, usually apocrine. SYN syringo-

cystoma. [hidro- + G. *kystis,* bladder, + *-ōma,* tumor]

**hi·dro·poi·e·sis** (hī′drō-poy-ē′sis) the formation of sweat. [hidro- + G. *poiēsis,* formation]

**hi·dros·che·sis** (hī-dros′kē-sis, hid-ros′) suppression of sweating. [hidro- + G. *schesis,* a checking]

**hi·dro·sis** (hī-drō′sis) the production and excretion of sweat. [G. *hidrōs,* sweat, + *-osis,* condition]

**hi·drot·ic** (hī-drot′ik) relating to or causing hidrosis.

**hi·er·ar·chy** (hī-ĕ-rar′kē) **1.** any system of persons or things ranked one above the other. **2.** in psychology and psychiatry, an organization of habits or concepts in which simpler components are combined to form increasingly complex integrations. [G. *hierarchia,* rule or power of the high priest]

**high-dose-rate brachyther·a·py** high-dose brachytherapy over time.

**high en·do·the·li·al post·cap·il·lary ven·ules** venules in the lymph nodes, tonsils, and Peyer patches that have a high-walled endothelium through which blood lymphocytes migrate into the lymphatic parenchyma.

**high en·e·ma** an enema instilled high up into the colon. SYN enteroclysis (1).

**high-en·er·gy com·pounds** classically, a group of phosphoric esters whose hydrolysis takes place with a standard free energy change of −5 to −15 kcal/mol (or −20 to −63 kJ/mol) (in contrast to −1 to −4 kcal/mol, or −4 to −17 kJ/mol) for simple phosphoric esters like glucose 6-phosphate or α-glycerophosphates, thus being capable of driving energy-consuming reactions in living cells or reconstituted cell-free systems; adenosine 5′-triphosphate, with respect to the β- and γ-phosphates, is the best known and is regarded as the immediate energy source for most metabolic syntheses. Other examples include acid anhydrides, phosphoric esters of enols, phosphamic acid (R–NH–PO$_3$H$_2$) derivatives, acyl thioesters (e.g., of coenzyme A), sulfonium compounds (R$_3$–S$^+$), and aminoacyl esters of ribosyl moieties. SEE ALSO high-energy phosphates.

**high-en·er·gy phos·phate bond** SEE high-energy phosphates.

**high-en·er·gy phos·phates** those phosphate esters and phosphoanhydrides that, on hydrolysis, yield an unusually large amount of energy; e.g., nucleotide polyphosphates such as ATP, enol phosphates such as phospho*enol*pyruvate. SEE ALSO high-energy compounds.

**high·er or·der preg·nan·cy** a pregnancy that has three fetuses (triplets) or more.

**high·est in·ter·cos·tal vein** drains the first intercostal space into either the vertebral or the brachiocephalic vein.

**high-fi·ber di·et** a diet high in the nondigestible part of plants, which is fiber. Fiber is found in fruits, vegetables, whole grains, and legumes. Insoluble fiber increases stool bulk, decreases transit time of food in the bowel, and decreases constipation and the risk of colon cancer. Soluble fiber delays absorption of glucose, which helps to control blood sugar in diabetes mellitus, and delays absorption of lipids, which helps to control hyperlipidemia. Recommended in treatment of diverticular disease of the colon.

**high-fre·quen·cy cur·rent** an alternating electric current having a frequency of 10,000 or more cycles per second; it produces no muscular contractions and does not affect the sensory nerves.

**high-fre·quen·cy hear·ing im·pair·ment** selective loss of hearing for high frequencies, usually associated with sensory damage; common in acoustic trauma and noise-induced hearing loss.

**high-fre·quen·cy trans·duc·tion** specialized transduction in which the donor bacterium contains not only the transducing, defective probacteriophage but also nondefective prophage that serves as "helper" virus, enabling most of the defective prophage particles to develop sufficiently to function as transducing agents.

**high-fre·quen·cy ven·ti·la·tion (HFV)** a technique of positive-pressure ventilation in which breathing frequency is above normal and tidal volume is below normal. The ventilatory pattern is similar to that of an animal panting.

**high-grade squa·mous in·tra·e·pi·the·li·al le·sion (HSIL, HGSIL)** term used in the Bethesda system for reporting cervical/vaginal cytologic diagnosis to describe a spectrum of noninvasive cervical epithelial abnormalities, including moderate and severe dysplasia, carcinoma in situ, and cervical intraepithelial neoplasia grades 2 and 3. SEE ALSO Bethesda system, ASCUS, atypical glandular cells of undetermined significance, low-grade squamous intraepithelial lesion.

**high mo·lec·u·lar weight ki·nin·o·gen (HMWK)** a plasma protein of 110,000 molecular weight that normally exists in plasma in a 1:1 complex with prekallikrein. The complex is a cofactor in the activation of coagulation factor XII. The product of this reaction, XIIa, in turn activates prekallikrein to kallikrein.

**High·more body** (hī′mōr) SYN mediastinum testis.

**high-per·for·mance liq·uid chro·ma·tog·ra·phy (HPLC)** a chromatographic technology used to separate and quantitate mixtures of substances in solution. The technique is used to measure organic compounds including steroid hormones, pesticides and poisons, toxic and carcinogenic compounds, and drugs. SYN high-pressure liquid chromatography.

**high-pres·sure li·quid chro·ma·to·gra·phy (HPLC)** SYN high-performance liquid chromatography.

**high-res·o·lu·tion com·put·ed to·mog·ra·phy (HRCT)** computed tomography with narrow collimation to reduce volume-averaging and an edge-enhancing reconstruction algorithm to sharpen the image, sometimes with a restricted field of view to minimize the size of pixels in the region imaged; used particularly for lung imaging.

**high risk re·gis·ter (HRR)** AUDIOLOGY checklist of conditions known to exhibit a higher-than-normal prevalence of hearing loss. Conditions include: familial history of hearing loss, congenital infections, craniofacial anomalies, low birth weight, hyperbilirubinemia, ototoxic medications, bacterial meningitis, severe CNS depression at birth. SEE screening.

**high-step·page gait** a gait in which the foot is raised high to avoid catching a drooping foot and brought down suddenly in a flapping manner; often seen in peroneal nerve palsy (i.e., footdrop) and tabes.

**hi·la** (hī′lă) plural of hilum.

**hi·lar** (hī′lăr) pertaining to a hilum.

**hi·li·tis** (hī-lī′tis) inflammation of the lining membrane of any hilus.

**Hill cri·ter·ia of e·vi·dence** (hil) a set of epidemiologic criteria that help to indicate whether a statistically significant relationship obtained in epidemiologic and other studies is a causal relationship. The criteria are consistency, specificity, strength, dose-response relationship, temporality, biologic plausibility, coherence, and capability of experimental confirmation. Temporality is the only absolute criterion: the putative cause must precede the effect in time.

**Hill e·qua·tion** (hil) the equation $y(1 - y) = [S]^n/K_d$, where $y$ is the fractional degree of saturation, [S] is the binding ligand concentration, $n$ is the Hill coefficient, and $K_d$ is the dissociation constant for the ligand. The Hill coefficient is a measure of the cooperativity of the protein; the larger the value, the higher the cooperativity. This coefficient cannot be higher than the number of binding sites. For the oxygen binding curve of hemoglobin, an association constant, $K_a$, is used and the equation becomes $y/(1 - y) = K_a[S]^n$. For human hemoglobin, $n = 2.5$.

**hil·lock** (hil′lok) ANATOMY any small elevation or prominence.

**Hill op·er·a·tion** (hil) repair of hiatus hernia; narrowing the esophagogastric junction and attaching it to the right medial arcuate ligament.

**Hill-Sachs le·sion** (hil-saks) an articular cartilage defect on the posterior aspect of the humeral head, often caused by injury to the humeral head by the rim of the glenoid fossa after anterior glenohumeral dislocation.

**Hill sign** (hil) in aortic insufficiency, greater systolic blood pressure in the legs than in the arms; normal arterial systolic pressure in the leg is 10–20 mm of Hg above that in the arm, whereas in aortic insufficiency the difference may be 60–100 mm of Hg.

**Hil·ton law** (hil′tŏn) the nerve supplying a joint supplies also the muscles which move the joint and the skin covering the articular insertion of those muscles.

**Hil·ton meth·od** (hil′tŏn) division of the nerves supplying a part, for the relief of pain in ulcers.

**hi·lum,** pl. **hi·la** (hī′lŭm, hī′lă) [TA] **1.** the part of an organ where the nerves and vessels enter and leave. SYN porta (1). **2.** a depression or slit resembling the hilum in the olivary nucleus of the brain. [L. a small bit or trifle]

**hi·lus** (hī′lŭs) hilum. [an Eng. variant of L. *hilum*]

**hi·lus cells** cells in the hilus of the ovary that produce androgens; they are thought to be the ovarian counterpart of the interstitial cells of the testis.

**HIM** health information management.

**hind·brain** (hīnd′brān) SYN rhombencephalon.

**hind·foot val·gus** eversion of the calcaneus relative to the tibia. SYN rearfoot pronation.

**hind·foot va·rus** inversion of the calcaneus relative to the tibia. SYN rearfoot supination.

**hind·gut** (hīnd′gŭt) **1.** the caudal or terminal part of the embryonic gut. **2.** the left part of transverse colon, descending and sigmoid colon, rectum, and superior part of anal canal.

**hind·wa·ter** (hīnd′wah-ter) colloquialism for amniotic fluid *in utero* behind the presenting part of the fetus.

**hinged flap** a turnover flap transferred by lifting it over on its pedicle as if the pedicle were a hinge.

**hinge joint** a uniaxial joint in which a broad, transversely cylindrical convexity on one bone fits into a corresponding concavity on the other, allowing of motion in one plane only. SYN ginglymoid joint, ginglymus.

**hinge re•gion 1.** that part of a tRNA structure that is deformed, bending a "cloverleaf" (two-dimensional) model to form an "L" model (crystal form, as seen by electron microscopy); **2.** in an immunoglobulin, a short sequence of amino acids that lies between two longer sequences and allows the latter to bend about the former.

**hip 1.** the lateral prominence of the pelvis from the waist to the thigh. **2.** the joint between femur and pelvis; **3.** colloquially, the head, neck, and greater trochanter of femur, as in the in the phrases "hip fracture" and "hip replacement." [A.S. *hype*]

**HIPAA** Health Insurance Portability and Accountability Act.

**hip bone** a large flat bone formed by the fusion of the ilium, ischium, and pubis (in the adult), constituting the lateral half of the pelvis; it articulates with its fellow anteriorly, with the sacrum posteriorly, and with the femur laterally. SYN coxa (1), innominate bone.

**hip joint** the ball-and-socket synovial joint between the head of the femur and the acetabulum. SYN coxa (2).

**hip•po•cam•pal** (hip-ō-kam′păl) relating to the hippocampus.

**hip•po•cam•pal sul•cus** a shallow groove between the dentate gyrus and the parahippocampal gyrus; the remains of a fissure extending deep into the hippocampus between Ammon horn and the dentate gyrus which becomes obliterated during fetal development.

**hip•po•cam•pus** (hip-ō-kam′pŭs) [TA] the complex, internally convoluted structure that forms the medial margin of the cerebral hemisphere, bordering the choroid fissure of the lateral ventricle, and composed of two gyri (Ammon horn and the dentate gyrus), together with their white matter, the alveus and fimbria hippocampi. In humans the hippocampus is confined to the temporal lobe by the massive development of the corpus callosum. The hippocampus forms part of the limbic system. Its major afferent connections are with the entorhinal area of the parahippocampal gyrus, and transparent septum; by way of the fornix it projects to the septum, anterior nucleus of the thalamus, and mammillary body. [G. *hippocampos*, seahorse]

**hip•po•crat•ic** (hip-ŏ-krat′ik) relating to, described by, or attributed to Hippocrates.

**hip•po•crat•ic face** (hĭ-pŏ-krat′ik) SYN hippocratic facies.

**hip•po•crat•ic fa•ci•es** (hĭ-pŏ-krat′ik) a pinched expression of the face, with sunken eyes, concavity of cheeks and temples, relaxed lips, and leaden complexion; observed in one close to death after severe and prolonged illness. SYN hippocratic face.

**hip•po•crat•ic fin•gers** (hĭ-pŏ-krat′ik) SEE clubbing.

**hip•po•crat•ic nails** (hĭ-pŏ-krat′ik) the coarse curved nails capping clubbed digits (hippocratic fingers).

**Hip•po•crat•ic Oath** (hĭ-pŏ-krat′ik) an oath taken by physicians about to enter the practice of their profession, which, though usually attributed to Hippocrates of Cos, is probably an ancient oath of the Asclepiads.

**hip•po•crat•ic suc•cus•sion sound** (hĭ-pŏ-krat′ik) a splashing sound elicited by shaking a patient with hydro- or pyopneumothorax, the physician's ear being applied to the chest.

**hip poin•ter** contusion of the iliac crest.

**hip•pus** (hip′ŭs) intermittent pupillary dilation and constriction, independent of illumination, convergence, or psychic stimuli. [G. *hippos*, horse, from a fancied suggestion of galloping movements]

**hir•cus**, gen. and pl. **hir•ci** (her′kŭs, her′sī) **1.** the odor of the axillae. **2.** one of the hairs growing in the axillae. **3.** SYN tragus (1). [L. he-goat]

**Hirsch•berg meth•od** (hĕrsh′bĕrg) a method of measuring the amount of deviation of a strabismic eye, by observing the reflection of a light fixated by the straight eye on the cornea of the deviating eye.

**Hirsch•berg test** (hĕrsh′bĕrg) a test of binocular motor alignment by which a penlight is shone at the eyes and the position of the light reflex on the cornea observed, allowing an estimate of the amount of deviation, if present.

**Hirsch•feld ca•nals** (hĕrsh′fĕld) SYN interdental canals.

**Hirsch•sprung dis•ease** (hĕrsh′sproong) SYN congenital megacolon.

**hir•sute** (her-soot′) relating to or characterized by hirsutism. [L. *hirsutus*, shaggy]

**hir•su•tism** (her′soo-tizm) presence of excessive bodily and facial terminal hair, in a male pattern, especially in women; may be present in normal adults as an expression of an ethnic characteristic or may develop in children or adults as the result of androgen excess due to tumors or drugs, or nonandrogenetic drugs. [L. *hirsutus*, shaggy]

**hir•u•di•cide** (hi-roo′di-sīd) an agent that kills leeches. [L. *hirudo*, leech, + *caedo*, to kill]

**hir•u•din** (hir′oo-din) an antithrombin substance extracted from the salivary glands of the leech that has the property of preventing coagulation of the blood. [L. *hirudo*, leech]

**Hir•u•din•ea** (hir′oo-din′ē-ă) the leeches, a class of worms with flat, segmented bodies, a sucker at the posterior end, and often a smaller sucker at the anterior end; they are predatory on invertebrate tissues, or feed on blood and tissue exudates of vertebrates. [L. *hirudo*, leech]

*Hir•u•do* (hi-roo′dō) a genus of leeches; previously used in medicine. [L. leech]

**His** (hiz), Wilhelm, Sr., Swiss anatomist and embryologist in Germany, 1831–1904. SEE His line.

**His** (hiz), Wilhelm, Jr., German physician, 1863–1934. SEE His bundle electrogram.

**His** histidine.

**His-** histidyl.

**-His** histidino.

**His bun•dle** (hiz) SYN atrioventricular bundle.

**His bun•dle e•lec•tro•gram (HBE)** (hiz) an electrogram recorded from the His bundle, either in the experimental animal or in man during cardiac catheterization.

**His line** (hiz) a line extending from the tip of the anterior nasal spine (acanthion) to the hindmost point on the posterior margin of the foramen magnum (opisthion), dividing the face into an upper and a lower, or dental part.

**Hiss stain** (his) a stain for demonstrating the capsules of microorganisms, using gentian violet or basic fuchsin followed by a copper sulfate wash.

**His·ta·log test** (his′tă-log) a test for measurement of maximal production of gastric acidity or anacidity; it is similar to the histamine test, but uses Histalog (betazole hydrochloride), an analogue of histamine.

**his·ta·mi·nae·mia [Br.]** SEE histaminemia.

**his·ta·mine** (his′tă-mēn) a depressor amine derived from histidine and present in ergot and in animal tissues. It is a powerful stimulant of gastric secretion, a constrictor of bronchial smooth muscle and a vasodilator (capillaries and arterioles) that causes a fall in blood pressure. Histamine is liberated in the skin as a result of injury. When pricked into the skin in high dilution, it causes the triple response.

**his·ta·mine-fast** indicating the absence of the normal response to histamine, especially in speaking of true gastric anacidity.

**his·ta·mi·ne·mia** (his′tă-mi-nē′mē-ă) the presence of histamine in the circulating blood. [histamine + G. *haima*, blood]

**his·ta·mine-re·leas·ing fac·tor** a lymphokine produced from antigen-stimulated lymphocytes that induces the release of histamine from basophils.

**his·ta·mine test** a test for maximal production of gastric acidity or anacidity; after preliminary administration of an antihistamine, histamine acid phosphate is injected subcutaneously, followed by analysis of gastric contents. SEE ALSO Histalog test.

**his·ta·min·ic head·ache** SYN cluster headache.

**his·ta·mi·nu·ria** (his′tă-min-yu′rē-ă) the excretion of histamine in the urine. [histidine + G. *ouron*, urine]

**his·ti·dase** (his′ti-dās) SYN histidine ammonia-lyase.

**his·ti·dine (His, H)** (his′ti-dēn) the L-isomer is a basic amino acid found in most proteins.

**his·ti·dine am·mo·ni·a·ly·ase** an enzyme catalyzing deamination of L-histidine; this enzyme is absent or deficient in individuals with histidinemia. SYN histidase.

**his·ti·dine de·car·box·yl·ase** an enzyme catalyzing the decarboxylation of L-histidine to histamine and $CO_2$; it plays a role in constriction of bronchial smooth muscle.

**his·ti·dino (-His, −His)** (his′ti-din-ō) the radical of histidine produced by removal of a hydrogen from a nitrogen atom.

**his·ti·di·nu·ria** (his′ti-din-yur′ē-ă) excretion of considerable amounts of histidine in the urine; frequently observed in later months of pregnancy, and in histidinemia.

**his·ti·dyl (His-)** (his′ti-dil) the acyl radical of histidine.

△**his·tio-** tissue, especially connective tissue. [G. *histion*, web]

**his·ti·o·blast** (his′tē-ō-blast) a tissue-forming cell. SYN histoblast. [histio- + G. *blastos*, germ]

**his·ti·o·cyte** (his′tē-ō-sīt) a macrophage present in connective tissue. SYN histocyte. [histio- + G. *kytos*, cell]

**his·ti·o·cy·to·ma** (his′tē-ō-sī-tō′mă) a tumor composed of histiocytes. [histio- + G. *kytos*, cell, + *-ōma*, tumor]

**his·ti·o·cy·to·sis** (his′tē-ō-sī-tō′sis) a generalized multiplication of histiocytes. SYN histocytosis.

**his·ti·o·cy·to·sis X** proliferation of Langerhans cells of undetermined clinical type, possibly Hand-Schüller-Christian disease, Letterer-Siwe disease, and eosinophilic granuloma.

**his·ti·o·gen·ic** (his′tē-ō-jen′ik) SYN histogenous.

△**his·to-** tissue. [G. *histos*, web (tissue)]

**his·to·blast** (his′tō-blast) SYN histioblast.

**his·to·chem·is·try** (his′tō-kem′is-trē) SYN cytochemistry.

**his·to·com·pat·i·bil·i·ty** (his′tō-kom-pat-i-bil′i-tē) a state of immunologic similarity (or identity) that permits successful homograft transplantation.

**his·to·com·pa·ti·bil·i·ty com·plex** a family of fifty or more genes on the sixth human chromosome that code for cell surface proteins and play a role in the immune response. Histocompatibility genes control the production of proteins on the outer membranes of tissue and blood cells, especially lymphocytes, that are vital elements in cell-cell recognition. The proteins also determine the level and type of immune response, and may serve other biochemical or immunologic functions. In the case of allografts, it is necessary to determine whether donor and recipient possess compatible sets of proteins (histocompatibility antigens), to minimize the likelihood of rejection. Histocompatibility testing (HLA tissue typing) provides this information.

**his·to·com·pat·i·bil·i·ty test·ing** a testing system for HLA antigens, of major importance in transplantation.

**his·to·cyte** (his′tō-sīt) SYN histiocyte.

**his·to·cy·to·sis** (his′tō-sī-tō′sis) SYN histiocytosis.

**his·to·dif·fer·en·ti·a·tion** (his′tō-dif-er-en-shē-ā′shun) the morphologic appearance of tissue characteristics during development.

**his·to·gen·e·sis** (his-tō-jen′ĕ-sis) the origin of a tissue; the formation and development of the tissues of the body. [histo- + G. *genesis*, origin]

**his·to·ge·net·ic** (his-tō-jĕ-net′ik) relating to histogenesis.

**his·tog·e·nous** (his-toj′ĕ-nŭs) formed by the tissues; e.g., the histogenous cells in an exudate arising from proliferation of the fixed tissue cells. SYN histiogenic. [histo- + G. *-gen*, producing]

**his·toid** (his′toyd) **1.** resembling in structure one of the tissues of the body. **2.** the histologic structure of a neoplasm derived from and consisting of a single, relatively simple type of neoplastic tissue that closely resembles the normal. [histo- + G. *eidos*, resemblance]

**his·toid lep·ro·sy** a form of lepromatous leprosy with lesions microscopically resembling dermatofibromas or other spindle-celled tumors.

**his·to·in·com·pat·i·bil·i·ty** (his′tō-in′kom-pat-i-bil′i-tē) a state of immunologic dissimilarity of tissues sufficient to cause rejection of a homograft when tissue is transplanted from one individual to another; implies a difference in histocompatibility genes in donor and recipient.

**his·to·log·ic, his·to·log·i·cal** (his-tō-loj′ik, his-tō-loj-i-kăl) pertaining to histology.

**his·to·log·ic ac·com·mo·da·tion** change in shape of cells to meet altered physical conditions, as the flattening of cuboidal cells in cysts as a result of pressure.

**his·tol·o·gist** (his-tol'ō-jist) one who specializes in the science of histology. SYN microanatomist.

**his·tol·o·gy** (his-tol'ō-jē) the science concerned with the minute structure of cells, tissues, and organs in relation to their function. SEE ALSO microscopic anatomy. SYN microanatomy. [histo- + G. *logos,* study]

**his·tol·y·sis** (his-tol'i-sis) disintegration of tissue. [histo- + G. *lysis,* dissolution]

**his·to·ma** (his-tō'mă) a benign neoplasm in which the cytologic and histologic elements are closely similar to those of normal tissue from which the neoplastic cells are derived. [histo- + G. *-oma,* tumor]

**his·to·met·a·plas·tic** (his'tō-met-ă-plas'tik) exciting tissue metaplasia.

**his·tom·o·ni·a·sis** (hi-stom'ō-nī'ă-sis) a disease chiefly affecting turkeys, caused by *Histomonas meleagridis* and characterized by ulcerative and necrotic lesions of the liver and cecum, acute onset, and a high mortality rate. It is transmitted inside the eggs of the nematode *Heterakis gallinae,* which is primarily responsible for maintaining and spreading the infection. SYN blackhead (2).

**his·tone** (his'tōn) one of a number of simple proteins (often found in the cell nucleus) that contains a high proportion of basic amino acids, are soluble in water, dilute acids, and alkalies, and are not coagulable by heat.

**his·to·nu·ria** (his-tōn-yur'ē-ă) the excretion of histone in the urine, as observed in certain instances of leukemia, febrile illnesses, and wasting diseases. [histone + G. *ouron,* urine]

**his·to·path·o·gen·e·sis** (his'tō-path-ō-jen'ĕ-sis) abnormal embryonic development or growth of tissue. [histogenesis + pathogenesis]

**his·to·pa·thol·o·gy** (his'tō-pa-thol'ō-jē) the science or study dealing with the cytologic and histologic structure of abnormal or diseased tissue.

**his·to·phys·i·ol·o·gy** (his'tō-fiz-ē-ol'ŏ-jē) the microscopic study of tissues in relation to their functions.

*His·to·plas·ma cap·su·la·tum* (his-tō-plaz'mă kap-soo-lā'tŭm) a dimorphic fungus species that causes histoplasmosis; its ascomycetous state is *Ajellomyces capsulatum.* The organism's natural habitat is soil fertilized with bird and bat droppings, where it grows as a mold, fragments of which, following inhalation, produce the primary pulmonary infection; within the mammalian host, inhaled mycelial fragments grow as uninuclear yeasts that reproduce by budding. [histo- + G. *plasma,* something formed]

**his·to·plas·min** (his'tō-plas'min) an antigenic extract of *Histoplasma capsulatum,* used in immunological tests for the diagnosis of histoplasmosis; also used in skin test surveys of populations to determine the geographic distribution of the fungus and to predict those that are endemic for histoplasmosis.

**his·to·plas·mo·ma** (his'tō-plaz-mō'mă) an infectious granuloma caused by *Histoplasma capsulatum.*

**his·to·plas·mo·sis** (his'tō-plaz-mō'sis) a widely distributed infectious disease caused by *Histoplasma capsulatum* and occurring frequently in epidemics; usually acquired by inhalation of spores of the fungus in soil dust and manifested by a primary benign pneumonitis; occasionally, the primary disease progresses to produce local-

ized lesions in lung, such as pulmonary cavitation, or the typical disseminated disease of the reticuloendothelial system which is manifested by fever, emaciation, splenomegaly, and leukopenia.

**his·tor·rhex·is** (his-tō-rek'sis) breakdown of tissue by some agency other than infection. [histo- + G. *rhēxis,* rupture]

**his·to·tome** (his'tō-tōm) SYN microtome. [histo- + G. *tomē,* cut]

**his·tot·o·my** (his-tot'ō-mē) SYN microtomy.

**his·to·tope** (his'tō-tōp) that part of the Class II major histocompatibility molecule that interacts with the T cell receptor. [histo- + -tope]

**his·to·tox·ic** (his-tō-tok'sik) relating to poisoning of the respiratory enzyme system of the tissues.

**his·to·tox·ic an·ox·ia** poisoning of the respiratory enzyme systems of the tissues, as in the inhibition of cytochrome oxidase by cyanides; owing to the inability of tissue cells to utilize oxygen, its tension in arterial and capillary blood is usually greater than normal.

**his·to·tro·phic** (his-tō-trof'ik) providing nourishment for or favoring the formation of tissue. [histo- + G. *trophē,* nourishment]

**his·to·tro·pic** (his-tō-trop'ik) attracted toward the tissues; denoting certain parasites, stains, and chemical compounds. [histo- + G. *tropikos,* turning]

**hitch·hik·er's thumb** malposition of the thumb, which, as a result of shortness of the first metacarpal, stands at right angles to the radial border of the hand and in the same place as it; a characteristic sign of diastrophic dwarfism.

**hit·ting the wall** abrupt decline in the ability to maintain the desired intensity of endurance exercise performance; associated with accumulation of blood lactate and depletion of liver and muscle glycogen reserves. SYN bonking.

**HIV** human immunodeficiency virus.

**HIV-1** human immunodeficiency virus-1.

**hives** (hīvz) **1.** SYN urticaria. **2.** SYN wheal.

**HIV was·ting syn·drome** SYN wasting syndrome.

**hK3** human glandular kallikrein 3.

**HL-7** Health Level 7, a medical informatics standard that facilitates communication among different digital systems.

**HLA com·plex** the major histocompatibility complex in humans.

**HLA typ·ing** tests done in order to determine if a patient has antibodies against a potential donor's HLA antigens. The presence of antibodies means that a graft will be rejected.

**HMB-45** an antibody to a premelanosome glycoprotein found to be present in melanomas and other tumors derived from melanocytes.

**HME** human monocytic ehrlichiosis.

**HMG CoA-re·duc·tase in·hib·i·tors** drugs that interfere with the biosynthesis of cholesterol; used to treat hyperlipidemia.

**HMO** hypothetical mean organism; health maintenance organization.

**HMWK** high molecular weight kininogen.

**Ho** holmium.

**Hoag·land sign** (hōg'lănd) eyelid edema in infectious mononucleosis.

**hoarse** (hōrs) having a rough, harsh voice. [A.S. *hās*]

**hob·nail cell** cell characteristic of a clear cell adenocarcinoma; a round expansion of clear cy-

h
o

toplasm projects into the lumen of neoplastic tubules, but the basal part of the cell containing the nucleus is narrow.

**hob·nail liv·er** in Laënnec cirrhosis, the contraction of scar tissue and hepatic cellular regeneration which causes a nodular appearance of the liver's surface.

**Ho·bo·ken nod·ules** (hō′bō-kĕn) gross dilation on the outer surface of the umbilical arteries. SEE ALSO Hoboken valves.

**Ho·bo·ken valves** (hō′bō-kĕn) the flangelike protrusions into the lumen of the umbilical arteries where they are twisted or kinked in their course through the umbilical cord.

**Hodge pes·sa·ry** (hoj) a double-curve oblong pessary employed for the correction of retrodeviations of the uterus.

**Hodg·kin dis·ease** (hoj′kin) a disease marked by chronic enlargement of the lymph nodes, often local at the onset and later generalized, together with enlargement of the spleen and often of the liver, no pronounced leukocytosis, and commonly anemia and continuous or remittent (Pel-Ebstein) fever; considered to be a malignant neoplasm of lymphoid cells of uncertain origin (Reed-Sternberg cells), associated with inflammatory infiltration of lymphocytes and eosinophilic leukocytes and fibrosis; can be classified into lymphocytic predominant, nodular sclerosing, mixed cellularity, and lymphocytic depletion type; a similar disease occurs in domestic cats.

**Hodg·son dis·ease** (hoj′son) dilation of the arch of the aorta associated with insufficiency of the aortic valve.

**Hof·fa op·er·a·tion** (hawf′ă) in congenital dislocation of the hip, a rarely used operation consisting of hollowing out the acetabulum and reduction of the head of the femur after severing the muscles inserted into the upper portion of the bone.

**Hoff·mann mus·cu·lar at·ro·phy** (hawf′mahn) SYN spinal muscular atrophy, type I.

**Hoff·mann phe·nom·e·non** (hawf′mahn) excessive irritability of the sensory nerves to electrical or mechanical stimuli in tetany.

**Hoff·mann sign, Hoff·mann re·flex** (hawf′mahn) 1. in latent tetany mild mechanical stimulation of the trigeminal nerve causes severe pain; 2. flexion of the terminal phalanx of the thumb and of the second and third phalanges of one or more of the fingers when the volar surface of the terminal phalanx of the fingers is flicked. SYN digital reflex.

**Hof·mei·ster op·er·a·tion** (hawf′mī-stĕr) partial gastrectomy with closure of a portion of the lesser curvature and retrocolic anastomosis of the remainder to the jejunum.

**Hog·ben num·ber** (hog′ben) unique personal identifying number constructed by using a sequence of digits for birth date, sex, birthplace, and other identifiers; invented by and named for Lancelot Hogben, British mathematician; Hogben numbers are the basis for identification numbers in many primary care facilities and are used in many record linkage systems.

**hol·an·dric** (hol-an′drik) related to genes located on the Y chromosome. [G. *holos,* entire, + *aner,* human male]

**hol·an·dric gene** SYN Y-linked gene.

**ho·lism** (hō′lizm) 1. the principle that an organism, or one of its actions, is not equal to merely the sum of its parts but must be perceived or studied as a whole. 2. the approach to the study of a psychological phenomenon through the analysis of a phenomenon as a complete entity in itself. [G. *holos,* entire]

**ho·lis·tic** (hō-lis′tik) pertaining to the characteristics of holism or holistic psychologies.

**ho·lis·tic med·i·cine** an approach to medical care that emphasizes the study of all aspects of a person's health, especially that a person should be considered as a unit, including psychological as well as social and economic influences on health status.

**Hol·len·horst plaques** (hol′en-horst) glittering, orange-yellow, atheromatous emboli in the retinal arterioles that contain cholesterin crystals and originate in the carotid artery or great vessels.

**hol·low** (hol′ō) a concavity or depression.

**hol·low bone** SYN pneumatic bone.

**hol·low-ca·thode lamp** a lamp consisting of a metal cathode and an inert gas that can emit a line spectrum of specific wavelength; used in atomic absorption spectrophotometry.

**Holmes-Ad·ie pu·pil** (hōmz-ā′dē) SYN Adie syndrome.

**Holmes-Ad·ie syn·drome** (hōmz-ā′dē) SYN Adie syndrome.

**Holmes-Rahe ques·tion·naire** (hōlmz rā) a survey to measure, in life change units, the stressfulness of various life events such as an acute illness, bankruptcy, death of a loved one, etc.

**Holmes stain** (hōmz) a silver nitrate staining method for nerve fibers.

**Holm·gren wool test** (hōm′grĕn) a test for color blindness, in which the subject matches variously colored skeins of wool.

**hol·mi·um (Ho)** (hol′mē-ŭm) an element of the lanthanide group, atomic no. 67, atomic wt. 164.93032. [L. *Holmia,* for Stockholm]

⚠ **holo-** whole, entire, complete. [G. *holos*]

**hol·o·blas·tic** (hol-ō-blas′tik) denoting the involvement of the entire ovum in cleavage. [holo- + G. *blastos,* germ]

**hol·o·cord** (hol′ō-kōrd) relating to the entire spinal cord, extending from the cervico-medullary junction to the conus medullaris.

**hol·o·crine** (hol′ō-krin) SEE holocrine gland. [holo- + G. *krinō,* to separate]

**hol·o·crine gland** a gland whose secretion consists of disintegrated cells of the gland itself, e.g., a sebaceous gland, in contrast to a merocrine gland.

**hol·o·di·a·stol·ic** (hol′ō-dī-ă-stol′ik) relating to or occupying the entire diastolic period.

**hol·o·en·dem·ic** (hol′ō-en-dem′ik) endemic in the entire population.

**hol·o·en·zyme** (hol-ō-en′zīm) a complete enzyme, i.e., apoenzyme plus coenzyme, cofactor, metal ion, and/or prosthetic group.

**hol·o·gram** (hol′ō-gram) a three-dimensional image produced by wavefront reconstruction and recorded on a photographic plate. [holo- + G. *gramma,* something written]

**hol·o·gyn·ic** (hol-ō-jin′ik) related to characters manifest only in females. [holo- + G. *gynē,* woman]

**hol·o·pros·en·ceph·a·ly** (hol′ō-pros-en-sef′ă-lē) failure of the forebrain or prosencephalon to divide into hemispheres or lobes; cyclopia occurs in the severest form. It is often accompanied by a deficit in midline facial development. [holo- + G. *prosō*, forward, + *enkephalos*, brain]

**hol·o·ra·chis·chi·sis** (hol'ō-ră-kis'ki-sis) spina bifida of the entire spinal column. [holo- + G. *rhachis*, spine, + *schisis*, fissure]

**hol·o·sys·tol·ic** (hol'ō-sis-tol'ik) SYN pansystolic.

**Hol·ter mon·i·tor** (hōl'ter) a technique for long-term, continuous recording of electrocardiographic signals on magnetic tape for scanning and selection of significant but fleeting changes that might otherwise escape notice.

**Holt·house her·nia** (hōlt'houz) inguinal hernia with extension of the loop of intestine along Poupart ligament.

**Ho·mans sign** (hō'mĕnz) pain in the calf when the ankle is slowly and gently dorsiflexed (with the knee bent), indicative of incipient or established thrombosis in the veins of the leg.

**hom·ax·i·al** (hō-mak'sē-ăl) having all the axes alike, as a sphere. [G. *homos*, the same, + axis]

△**ho·me·o-** the same, alike. SEE ALSO homo- (1). [G. *homoios*, similar]

**ho·me·o·met·ric au·to·reg·u·la·tion** intrinsic regulation of strength of cardiac contraction in response to influences that do not depend on change in fiber length, i.e., the Frank-Starling mechanism, (e.g., the Anrep effect in which strength increases in response to increased afterload, and the Bowditch staircase effect (treppe) in which strength increases in response to increased heart rate) and do not depend on extrinsic regulation (e.g., in which strength increases in response to sympathetic nerve stimulation or norepinephrine).

**ho·me·o·mor·phous** (hō'mē-ō-mōr'fŭs) of similar shape, but not necessarily of the same composition. [homeo- + G. *morphē*, shape]

**ho·me·o·path** (hō'mē-ō-path) SYN homeopathist.

**ho·me·o·path·ic** (hō'mē-ō-path'ik) **1.** relating to homeopathy. SYN homeotherapeutic (1). **2.** denoting an extremely small dose of a pharmacological agent, such as might be used in homeopathy; more generally, a dose believed to be too small to produce the effect usually expected from that agent. Cf. pharmacologic (2), physiologic (4). [homeo- + G. *pathos*, disease]

**ho·me·op·a·thist** (hō-mē-op'ă-thist) a medical practitioner of homeopathy. SYN homeopath.

**ho·me·op·a·thy** (hō-mē-op'ă-thē) a system of therapy developed by Samuel Hahnemann based on the "law of infinitesimal doses" in *similia similibus curantur* (likes are cured by likes), which holds that a medicinal substance that can evoke certain symptoms in healthy individuals may be effective in the treatment of illnesses having symptoms closely resembling those produced by the substance. [homeo- + G. *pathos*, suffering]

**ho·me·o·pla·sia** (hō'mē-ō-plā'zē-ă) the formation of new tissue of the same character as that already existing in the part. [homeo- + G. *plasis*, a molding]

**ho·me·o·plas·tic** (hō'mē-ō-plas'tik) relating to or characterized by homeoplasia.

**ho·me·o·sta·sis** (hō'mē-ō-stā'sis) **1.** the state of equilibrium (balance between opposing pressures) in the body with respect to various functions and to the chemical compositions of the fluids and tissues. **2.** the processes through which such bodily equilibrium is maintained. [homeo- + G. *stasis*, a standing]

**ho·me·o·stat·ic** (hō'mē-ō-stat'ik) relating to homeostasis.

**ho·me·o·ther·a·peu·tic** (hō'mē-ō-thār-ă-pyu'tik) **1.** SYN homeopathic (1). **2.** relating to homeotherapy.

**ho·me·o·ther·a·py, ho·me·o·ther·a·peu·tics** (hō'mē-ō-thār'ă-pē, hō'mē-ō-thār-ă-pyu'tiks) treatment or prevention of a disease using the principles of homeopathy.

**ho·me·o·ther·mic** pertaining to, or having the essential characteristic of homeotherms. SYN hematothermal.

△**ho·mo- 1.** combining form meaning the same, alike; opposite of hetero-. SEE ALSO homeo-. **2.** CHEMISTRY prefix used to indicate insertion of one more carbon atom in a chain. [G. *homos*, the same]

**ho·mo·bi·o·tin** (hō-mō-bī'ō-tin) a compound resembling biotin except for the substitution of an oxygen atom for the sulfur and the presence of an additional $CH_2$ group in the side chain; an active biotin antagonist.

**ho·mo·blas·tic** (hō-mō-blas'tik) developing from a single type of tissue. [homo- + G. *blastos*, germ]

**ho·mo·car·no·sine** (hō-mō-kar'nō-sēn) a constituent of the brain formed from L-histidine and γ-aminobutyric acid.

**ho·mo·car·no·sin·o·sis** (hō-mō-kar'nō-sēn-ō-sis) an inborn error in metabolism in which homocarnosine levels are elevated, particularly in the cerebral spinal fluid.

**ho·mo·cit·rul·li·nu·ria** (hō-mō-sit'ru-lēn-yur'ē-ă) an inherited disorder associated with elevated urinary levels of homocitrulline.

**ho·mo·cys·te·ine** (hō-mō-sis'tē-ēn) a homolog of cysteine, produced by the demethylation of methionine, and an intermediate in the biosynthesis of L-cysteine from L-methionine via L-cystathionine.

**ho·mo·cys·tine** (hō-mō-sis'tēn) the disulfide resulting from the mild oxidation of homocysteine; an analog of cystine.

**ho·mo·cys·ti·ne·mia** (hō'mō-sis-ti-nē'mē-ă) presence of an excess of homocystine in the plasma, as in homocystinuria.

**ho·mo·cy·to·tro·pic** (hō'mō-sī'tō-trop'ik) having an affinity for cells of the same or a closely related species. [homo- + G. *kytos*, cell, + *trope*, a turning toward]

**ho·mo·cy·to·tro·pic an·ti·bod·y** antibody of the IgE class that has an affinity for tissues (notably mast cells) of the same or a closely related species and that, upon combining with specific antigen, triggers the release of pharmacological mediators of anaphylaxis from the cells to which it is attached. SYN reaginic antibody.

**ho·mo·dont** (hō'mō-dont) having teeth that are morphologically of the same type, as in the alligator. [homo- + G. *odous*, tooth]

**ho·mo·ga·met·ic** (hō'mō-gă-met'ik) producing only one type of gamete with respect to sex chromosomes; in humans and most animals, the female is homogametic. SYN monogametic. [homo- + G. *gametikos*, connubial]

**ho·mog·a·my** (hō-mog'ă-mē) similarity of husband and wife in a specific trait. [homo- + G. *gamos*, marriage]

**ho·mo·ge·neous** (hō-mō-jē'nē-ŭs) of uniform structure or composition throughout. [homo- + G. *genos*, race]

**ho·mo·ge·neous ra·di·a·tion** radiation consisting of a narrow band of frequencies, the same energy, or a single type of particle.

**ho·mo·ge·neous sys·tem** CHEMISTRY a system whose parts cannot be mechanically separated, and is therefore uniform throughout and possesses in every part identically physical properties; e.g., a solution of sodium chloride in water.

**ho·mo·gen·e·sis** (hō-mō-jen′ĕ-sis) production of offspring similar to the parents, in contrast to heterogenesis. [homo- + G. *genesis*, production]

**ho·mog·e·nous** (hō-moj′ĕ-nŭs) having a structural similarity because of descent from a common ancestor. Commonly confused with homogeneous. [homo- + G. *genos*, family, kind]

**ho·mo·gen·tis·ic ac·id** (hō′mō-jen-tis′ik as′id) an intermediate in L-phenylalanine and L-tyrosine catabolism; if made alkaline, it oxidizes rapidly in air to a quinone that polymerizes to a melanin-like material; elevated levels are observed in individuals having alcaptonuria. SYN alcapton, alkapton.

**ho·mo·gon·ic life cy·cle** parasitic stage of life cycle of an organism (e.g., *Strongyloides stercoralis*) that also has a free-living stage.

**ho·mo·graft** (hō′mō-graft) SYN allograft rejection.

**ho·mo·lat·er·al** (hō-mō-lat′er-ăl) SYN ipsilateral. [homo- + L. *latus*, side]

**ho·mol·o·gous** (hō-mol′ō-gŭs) Corresponding or alike in certain critical attributes. **1.** BIOLOGY denoting organs or parts corresponding in evolutionary origin and similar to some extent in structure, but not necessarily similar in function. **2.** CHEMISTRY denoting a single chemical series, differing by fixed increments. **3.** GENETICS denoting chromosomes or chromosome parts identical with respect to their construction and genetic content. **4.** IMMUNOLOGY denoting serum or tissue derived from members of a single species, or an antibody with respect to the antigen that produced it. [see homologue]

**ho·mol·o·gous chro·mo·somes** members of a single pair of chromosomes.

**ho·mol·o·gous graft** SYN allograft.

**ho·mol·o·gous re·com·bi·na·tion** the exchange of corresponding stretches of DNA between two sister chromosomes.

**ho·mol·o·gous stim·u·lus** a stimulus that acts only on the nerve terminations in a special sense organ.

**ho·mol·o·gous tu·mor** a tumor composed of tissue of the same sort as that from which it springs.

**ho·mol·y·sin** (hō-mol′i-sin) a sensitizing hemolytic antibody (hemolysin) formed as the result of stimulation by an antigen derived from an animal of the same species. [homo- + hemolysin]

**ho·mol·y·sis** (hō-mol′i-sis) lysis of red blood cells by a homolysin and complement.

**ho·mo·mor·phic** (hō-mō-mōr′fik) denoting two or more structures of similar size and shape. [homo- + G. *morphē*, shape, appearance]

**ho·mon·o·mous** (hō-mon′ō-mŭs) denoting parts, having similar form and structure, arranged in a series, as the fingers or toes. [G. *homonomos*, under the same laws, fr. *homos*, same, + *nomos*, law]

**ho·mon·y·mous** (hō-mon′i-mŭs) having the same name or expressed in the same terms, e.g., the corresponding halves (right or left, superior or inferior) of the retinas. [G. *homōnymous*, of the same name, fr. *onyma*, name]

**ho·mon·y·mous im·ag·es** double images produced by stimuli arising from points proximal to the horopter.

**ho·mo·phil** (hō′mō-fil) denoting an antibody that reacts only with the specific antigen which induced its formation. [homo- + G. *philos*, fond]

**ho·mo·pho·bia** (hō-mō-fō′bē-ă) irrational fear of homosexual feelings, thoughts, behaviors, or persons.

**ho·mo·plas·tic** (hō-mō-plas′tik) similar in form and structure, but not in origin. [homo- + G. *plastos*, formed]

**ho·mo·plas·tic graft** SYN allograft.

**ho·mo·plas·ty** (hō′mō-plas′tē) repair of a defect by a homograft.

**ho·mo·pol·y·mer** (hō-mō-pol′i-mer) a polymer composed of a series of identical radicals; e.g., polylysine, poly(adenylic acid), polyglucose.

**hom·or·gan·ic** (hom-ōr-gan′ik) produced by the same organs, or by homologous organs.

**ho·mo·ser·ine** (hō-mō-ser′ēn) a hydroxyamino acid differing from serine in the possession of an additional $CH_2$ group; formed in the conversion of L-methionine to L-cysteine.

**ho·mo·sex·u·al** (hō-mō-seks′yu-ăl) **1.** relating to or characteristic of homosexuality. **2.** one whose interests and behavior are characteristic of homosexuality. SEE gay, lesbian.

**ho·mo·sex·u·al·i·ty** (hō′mō-seks-yu-al′i-tē) erotic attraction, predisposition, or activity, including sexual congress, between individuals of the same sex, especially past puberty.

**ho·mo·sex·u·al pan·ic** an acute, severe attack of anxiety based on unconscious conflicts regarding homosexuality.

**ho·mo·ton·ic** (hō-mō-ton′ik) of uniform tension or tonus.

**ho·mo·top·ic** (hō-mō-top′ik) pertaining to or occurring at the same place or part of the body. [homo- + G. *topos*, place]

**ho·mo·type** (hō′mō-tīp) any part or organ of the same structure or function as another, especially as one on the opposite side of the body. [homo- + G. *typos*, type]

**ho·mo·typ·ic, ho·mo·typ·i·cal** (hō-mō-tip′ik, hō-mō-tip′i-kăl) of the same type or form; corresponding to the other one of two paired organs or parts.

**ho·mo·va·nil·lic ac·id (HVA)** (hō′mō-vă-nil′ik as′id) a phenol found in human urine; produced through the methylation of homoprotocatechuic acid on the *meta*-OH group.

**ho·mo·zy·gos·i·ty, ho·mo·zy·go·sis** (hō′mō-zī-gos′i-tē, hō′mō-zī-gō′sis) the state of being homozygous. [homo- + G. *zygon*, yoke]

**ho·mo·zy·gote** (hō-mō-zī′gŏt) a homozygous individual. [homo- + G. *zygōtos*, yoke]

**ho·mo·zy·gous** (hō-mō-zī′gŭs) having identical genes at one or more loci.

**ho·mo·zy·gous by de·scent** possessing two genes at a given locus that are descended from a single source, as may occur in consanguineous mating.

**ho·mun·cu·lus** (hō-mŭngk′yu-lŭs) the figure of a human sometimes superimposed on pictures of the surface of the brain to represent the motor or sensory regions of the body represented there. [L. dim. of *homo*, man]

**hon·ey·comb lung** the radiological and gross appearance of the lungs resulting from interstitial fibrosis and cystic dilation of bronchioles and distal air spaces; a sequel of any of several diseases, including eosinophilic granuloma and sarcoidosis.

**hon·ey·comb pat·tern** dense, slightly irregular circular shadows, most common next to the pleura at the lung base, on chest radiographs or CT; caused by chronic interstitial fibrosis of diverse causes.

**Hong Kong in·flu·en·za** influenza caused by a serotype of influenza virus type A and first identified in Hong Kong.

**hook** (huk) **1.** an instrument curved or bent near its tip, used for fixation of a part or traction. **2.** SYN hamulus. [A.S. *hōk*]

**Hooke law** (huk) the stress applied to stretch or compress a body is proportional to the strain, or change in length thus produced, so long as the limit of elasticity of the body is not exceeded.

**hook·worm** (huk′werm) common name for bloodsucking nematodes, chiefly members of the genera *Ancylostoma* (the Old World hookworm), *Necator*, and *Uncinaria*, and including the species *A. caninum* (dog hookworm) and *N. americanus* (New World hookworm).

**hook·worm dis·ease** SEE ancylostomiasis, necatoriasis.

**Hoo·ver signs** (hoo′vĕr) **1.** a subject lying supine, when asked to raise one leg, involuntarily creates counterpressure with the heel of the other leg; if this leg is paralyzed, whatever muscular power is preserved in it will be exerted in this way; or if the patient attempts to lift a paralyzed leg, counterpressure will be made with the other heel, whether any movement occurs in the paralyzed limb or not; not present in hysteria or malingering; **2.** a modification in the movement of the costal margins during respiration, caused by a flattening of the diaphragm; suggestive of empyema or other intrathoracic condition causing a change in the contour of the diaphragm.

**Hop·kins rod-lens tel·e·scope** (hop′kinz) an endoscopic telescope in which the air-containing spaces between the conventional series of lenses are replaced with glass rods with polished ends separated by small "air-lenses." This system transmits more light, yields greater magnification and provides greater depth and breadth of field than conventional lens systems.

**Hop·mann pap·il·lo·ma** (hop′mahn) a papillomatous overgrowth of the nasal mucous membrane.

**hor·de·o·lum** (hōr-dē′ō-lŭm) a suppurative inflammation of a gland of the eyelid. [Mod. L., *hordeolus*, a sty in the eye, dim. of *hordeum*, barley]

**hor·de·o·lum ex·ter·num** inflammation of the sebaceous gland of an eyelash. SYN sty, stye.

**hor·i·zon·tal fis·sure of cer·e·bel·lum** horizontal fissure that divides the ansiform lobule into its major parts, crus I (superior semilunar lobule) and crus II (inferior semilunar lobule).

**hor·i·zon·tal heart** description of the heart's electrical position; recognized in the electrocardiogram when the electrical axis lies between −30° and +30°.

**hor·i·zon·tal la·ryn·gec·tomy** SYN partial laryngectomy.

**hor·i·zon·tal max·il·la·ry frac·ture** a horizon-

tal fracture at the base of the maxillae above the apices of the teeth. SYN Le Fort I fracture.

**hor·i·zon·tal o·ver·lap** the projection of the upper anterior and/or posterior teeth beyond their antagonists in a horizontal direction. SYN overjet, overjut.

**hor·i·zon·tal plane** plane parallel and relative to the horizon; in the anatomic position, horizontal planes are transverse planes; in the supine or prone positions, horizontal planes are frontal (coronal planes).

**hor·i·zon·tal tear** a tear of articular cartilage roughly perpendicular to the long axis of the bone.

**hor·i·zon·tal trans·mis·sion** transmission of infectious agents from an infected individual to a susceptible contemporary, in contradistinction to vertical transmission.

**hor·mo·nal** (hōr-mōn′ăl) pertaining to hormones.

**hor·mo·nal gin·gi·vi·tis** gingivitis in which the host response to bacterial plaque is presumably exacerbated by hormonal alterations occurring during puberty, pregnancy, oral contraceptive use, or menopause. SYN pregnancy gingivitis.

**hor·mone** (hōr′mōn) a chemical substance, formed in a tissue or organ and carried in the blood, that stimulates or inhibits the growth or function of one or more other tissues or organs. [G. *hormōn*, pres. part. of *hormaō*, to rouse or set in motion]

**hor·mone re·place·ment therapy (HRT)** SYN estrogen replacement therapy.

**hor·mo·no·gen·e·sis** (hōr′mō-nō-jen′ĕ-sis) the formation of hormones. SYN hormonopoiesis.

**hor·mo·no·gen·ic** (hōr′mō-nō-jen′ik) pertaining to the formation of a hormone. SYN hormonopoietic.

**hor·mo·no·poi·e·sis** (hōr′mō-nō-poy-ē′sis) SYN hormonogenesis. [hormone + G. *poiēsis*, production]

**hor·mo·no·poi·et·ic** (hōr′mō-nō-poy-et′ik) SYN hormonogenic.

**horn** (hōrn) any structure resembling a horn in shape. SYN cornu (1). [A.S.]

**Hor·ner pu·pil** constricted pupil due to impairment of sympathetic nerve innervation of the dilator muscle of the pupil. SEE ALSO Horner syndrome.

**Hor·ner syn·drome** (hor′nĕr) ptosis, miosis, and anhidrosis on the side of a sympathetic palsy. Enophthalmos is more apparent than real. The affected pupil is visibly slow to dilate in dim light; due to a lesion of the cervical sympathetic chain or its central pathways.

**Hor·ner teeth** (hor′nĕr) incisor teeth having a horizontal, hypoplastic groove.

**Hor·ner-Tran·tas dots** (hor′ner-trahn′tahs) evanescent white cellular infiltrates occurring in the bulbar form of vernal keratoconjunctivitis.

**horn·y** (hōrn′ē) of the nature or structure of horn. SYN corneous, keratic, keratinous (2), keratoid (1), keroid.

**horn·y la·yer** SYN stratum corneum epidermidis.

**horse·rad·ish per·ox·i·das·es** an enzyme used in immunohistochemistry to label the antigen-antibody complex.

**horse·shoe fis·tu·la** an anal fistula partially encircling the anus and opening at both extremities on the cutaneous surface.

**horse·shoe kid·ney** union of the lower or occasionally the upper ends of the two kidneys by a band of tissue extending across the midline.

**Hor·te·ga cells** (ōr-tē'gă) SYN microglia.

**Hor·te·ga neu·rog·lia stain** (ōr-tē'gă) one of several silver carbonate methods to demonstrate astrocytes, oligodendroglia, and microglia.

**Hor·ton ar·te·ri·tis** (hōr'tŏn) SYN temporal arteritis.

**Hor·ton head·ache** (hōr'tŏn) SYN cluster headache.

**hose** thin, form-fitting leg covering; in medicine, used in the treatment of circulatory problems.

**hos·pice** (hos'pis) an institution that provides a centralized program of palliative and supportive services to dying persons and their families, in the form of physical, psychological, social, and spiritual care; such services are provided by an interdisciplinary team of professionals and volunteers who are available at home and in specialized inpatient settings. [L. *hospitium*, hospitality, lodging, fr. *hospes*, guest]

**hos·pi·tal** (hos'pi-tăl) an institution for the treatment, care, and cure of the sick and wounded, for the study of disease, and for the training of physicians, nurses, and allied health personnel. [L. *hospitalis*, for a guest, fr. *hospes* (*hospit-*), a host, a guest]

**hos·pi·tal-based phy·si·cian** SYN hospitalist (1).

**hos·pit·a·li·sa·tion [Br.]** SEE hospitalization.

**hos·pi·tal·ist** (hos'pit-al-ist) **1.** a physician whose professional activities are performed chiefly within a hospital, e.g., anesthesiologists, emergency department physicians, intensivists (intensive care specialists), pathologists, and radiologists. SYN hospital-based. **2.** a primary care physician (not a house officer) who assumes responsibility for the observation and treatment of hospitalized patients and returns them to the care of their private physicians when they are discharged from the hospital. [hospital + -ist]

**hos·pi·tal·i·za·tion** (hos'pi-tăl-i-zā'shŭn) confinement in a hospital as a patient for diagnostic study and treatment.

**hos·pi·tal rec·ord** the medical record generated during hospitalization, containing a history and physical examination report, physicians' progress notes and treatment orders, notes of nurses' observations and treatments administered, reports of laboratory tests, x-ray and other diagnostic studies, surgical procedures, consultants' opinions, and a discharge summary or autopsy record.

**host** the organism in or on which a parasite lives, deriving its body substance or energy from the host. [L. *hospes*, a host]

**host cell** a cell (e.g., a bacterium) in which a vector can be propagated.

**hot flash, hot flush** colloquialism for one of the vasomotor symptoms of the climacteric that may involve the whole body as a flash of heat; also used interchangeably with hot flush.

**hot nod·ule** a thyroid nodule with a much higher uptake of radioactive iodine than the surrounding parenchyma; usually benign but sometimes causing hyperthyroidism.

**hot spot** a region in a gene in which there is a putatively high rate of mutation.

**hot-wire flow-mea·sur·ing de·vice** a device used to measure flow; it relies on the effect of convective cooling as a stream of air passes over a small heated filament (thermistor).

**hour·glass con·trac·tion** constriction of the

middle portion of a hollow organ, such as the stomach or the gravid uterus.

**hour·glass mur·mur** one in which there are two areas of maximum loudness decreasing to a point midway between the two.

**hour·glass stom·ach** a condition in which there is a central constriction of the wall of the stomach dividing it into two cavities, cardiac and pyloric.

**house·maid's knee** an adventitious occupational bursitis occurring over the tibial tuberosity, the area of contact when kneeling; not to be confused with infrapatellar bursitis.

**house of·fi·cer** an intern or resident employed by a hospital to provide service to patients while receiving training in a medical specialty.

**house staff** physicians and surgeons in specialty training at a hospital who care for the patients under the direction and responsibility of the attending staff.

**Hous·ton-Har·ris syn·drome** (hyu'ston-har'is) SYN achondrogenesis type IA.

**How·ell-Jol·ly bod·ies** (how'el-zhō-lē') spherical or ovoid eccentrically located granules, approximately 1 μm in diameter, occasionally observed in the stroma of circulating erythrocytes after splenectomy or in megaloblastic or severe hemolytic anemia.

**Howship la·cu·nae** (how'ship) tiny depressions, pits, or irregular grooves in bone that is being resorbed by osteoclasts. SYN resorption lacunae.

**HPLC** high-pressure liquid chromatography; high-performance liquid chromatography.

**HPV** human papilloma virus.

**HR con·duc·tion time** SEE intraventricular conduction.

**HRCT** high-resolution computed tomography.

**HRR** high risk register.

**HRSA** Health Resources and Services Administration.

**HRT** hormone replacement therapy.

**Hruby lens** (rū'bē) a non–contact lens mounted on a slitlamp used for evaluating the retina.

**HSIL** high-grade squamous intraepithelial lesion.

**HSV** herpes simplex virus.

**5-HT** 5-hydroxytryptamine.

**Ht** total hyperopia.

**HTLV** human T-cell lymphoma/leukemia virus.

**HTLV-I** t-cell lymphotrophic virus type I; human lymphotropic virus, type 1.

**HTLV-II** t-cell lymphotrophic virus type II; human lymphotropic virus, type 2.

**HTLV-III** human T-cell lymphotropic virus type III. SEE human immunodeficiency virus.

**Hüc·kel rule** (hek-kĕl) the number of depolarized electrons in an aromatic ring is equal to $4n + 2$ where $n$ is 0 or any positive integer; L-tyrosine, L-phenylalanine, L-tryptophan, and L-histidine (when the imidazole ring is deprotonated) obey this rule.

**Hue·ter ma·neu·ver** (hē'tĕr) pressing the patient's tongue downward and forward with the left forefinger in passing a stomach tube.

**Hüf·ner equa·tion** (huf'ner) an equation expressing the relationship between myoglobin dissociation and oxygen partial pressure: $([MBO_2]/[Mb]) = (K \times pO_2)$.

**Hull tri·ad** (hul) the association of diastolic gallop, anasarca, and small pulse pressure.

**hum** (hŭm) a low continuous murmur. [echoic]

**hu·man an·ti·he·mo·phil·ic fac·tor** a lyophilized concentrate of factor VIII, obtained from fresh normal human plasma; used as a hemostatic agent in hemophilia.

**hu·man ca·lor·i·me·ter** a device to measure the heat output of the human body during various levels of physical exertion. It consists of a chamber with closed air circulation and a means of comparing the temperature of water entering a coil completely surrounding the subject with the temperature of water leaving the coil. See this page.

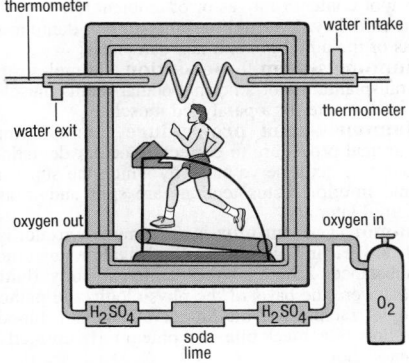

**human calorimeter**

**hu·man cho·ri·on·ic go·nad·o·tro·pin** SEE chorionic gonadotropin.

**β-hu·man cho·ri·on·ic go·nad·o·tro·pin** a 145-amino acid subunit unique to HCG, which has the same α-chain as FSH, LH, and TSH. Pregnancy tests specific for β-HCG are more sensitive since there is no confusion with other gonadotropins secreted by the pituitary.

**hu·man cho·ri·on·ic so·ma·to·mam·mo·tro·pic hor·mone (HCS)** SYN human placental lactogen.

**hu·man com·mu·ni·ca·tion** the production and reception of oral, written, signed, or gestured information among human beings; involves the use of symbols known as language received through the auditory, tactile, proprioceptive, and visual systems and generated through voice and speech, writing, manual signs, and gestures; communication among humans may at times involve the vestibular, olfactory, and gustatory senses.

**hu·man dip·loid cell vac·cine** an iodinated virus vaccine used for protection against rabies vaccine usually prepared in the human diploid cell WI-38.

**hu·man e·o·sin·o·phil·ic en·ter·i·tis** segmental eosinophilic inflammation of the gastrointestinal tract in humans; suspect etiologic agent is *Ancylostoma caninum;* laboratory indicators are eosinophilia and increased IgE.

**hu·man gam·ma glob·u·lin** a preparation of the proteins of liquid human plasma, containing the antibodies of normal adults; it is obtained from pooled liquid human plasma from a number of donors.

**hu·man ge·net·ics** the study of the genetic aspects of humans as a species. Cf. medical genetics.

**Hu·man Ge·nome Pro·ject** a comprehensive effort by molecular biologists worldwide to map the human genome, which consists of about 100,000 genes, or 3 billion DNA base pairs. The wholesale sequencing of the genome would not be possible without the automated method of gene sequencing, invented by Leroy Hood.

**hu·man glan·du·lar kal·l·ikrein 3 (hK3)** SYN prostate-specific antigen.

**hu·man gran·u·lo·cyt·ic ehr·lich·i·o·sis (HGE)** a febrile disease causing headache and myalgia and sometimes involving the respiratory, digestive, and central nervous systems; caused by *Ehrlichia phagocytophaga,* which is transmitted by ixodid ticks; laboratory findings include leukopenia, thrombocytopenia, and inclusion bodies (morulae) in neutrophils.

**hu·man her·pes·vi·rus 1** herpes simplex virus, type 1. SEE herpes simplex.

**hu·man her·pes·vi·rus 2** herpes simplex virus, type 2. SEE herpes simplex.

**hu·man her·pes·vi·rus 3** SYN varicella-zoster virus.

**hu·man her·pes·vi·rus 4** SYN Epstein-Barr virus.

**hu·man her·pes·vi·rus 5** SYN cytomegalovirus.

**hu·man her·pes·vi·rus 6** a herpesvirus found in certain lymphoproliferative disorders, and associated with roseola (exanthema subitum).

**hu·man her·pes·vi·rus 8** a linear double-stranded DNA virus that induces Kaposi sarcoma (KS) in immunodeficient persons. DNA sequences unique to this virus are regularly found in KS specimens from HIV-negative persons as well. The virus is also associated with several uncommon lymphoproliferative syndromes in AIDS patients, including multicentric Castleman disease and primary effusion lymphoma (body cavity–based lymphoma).

**hu·man im·mu·no·de·fi·cien·cy vi·rus-2** a virus, found primarily in West Africa, which causes a less virulent form of AIDS and is more closely related to Simian virus strains.

**hu·man im·mu·no·de·fi·cien·cy vi·rus (HIV)** human T-cell lymphotropic virus type III; a cytopathic retrovirus that is the etiologic agent of acquired immunodeficiency syndrome (AIDS). See page 460. SYN lymphadenopathy-associated virus.

**hu·man in·su·lin** a protein that has the normal structure of insulin produced by the human pancreas, prepared by recombinant DNA techniques and by semisynthetic processes.

**hu·man in·ter·leu·kin-11** a drug that increases the number of blood platelets; useful in ameliorating severe thrombocytopenia resulting from cancer chemotherapy. SYN recombinant human interleukin-11, recombinant interleukin-11.

**hu·man leuko·cyte an·ti·gen** any of several members of a system consisting of the gene products of at least four linked loci (A, B, C, and D) and a number of subloci on the sixth human chromosome that have been shown to have a strong influence on human allotransplantation, transfusions in refractory patients, and certain disease associations; more than 50 alleles are recognized, most of which are at loci HLA-A and HLA-B; autosomal dominant inheritance.

**hu·man men·o·pau·sal go·nad·o·tro·pin** a hormone of pituitary originally obtained from the urine of postmenopausal women now produced

h
u

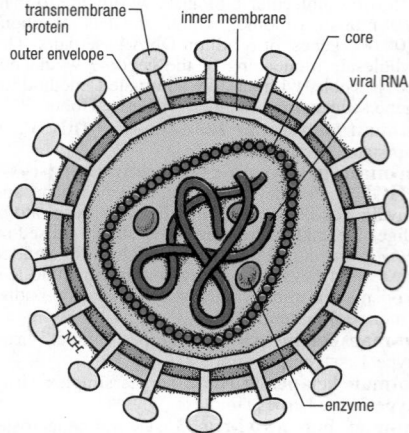

transmembrane protein — inner membrane — core — outer envelope — viral RNA — enzyme

**human immunodeficiency virus** (HIV)

synthetically; used to induce ovulation. SEE ALSO menotropins.

**hu•man mo•no•cy•tic ehr•lich•i•o•sis (HME)** a febrile disease caused by *Ehrlichia chaffeensis* and transmitted by the Lone Star tick (*Amblyomma americanum*); similar to human granulocytic ehrlichiosis, except that inclusions are found in monocytes.

**hu•man pap•il•lo•ma vi•rus (HPV)** DNA virus of the genus *Papillomavirus;* certain types cause cutaneous and genital warts in humans, including verruca vulgaris and condyloma acuminatum; other types are associated with severe cervical intraepithelial neoplasia and anogenital and laryngeal carcinomas. Over 70 types have been characterized on the basis of DNA relatedness. SYN infectious papilloma virus.

**hu•man pla•cen•tal lac•to•gen** lactogen isolated from human placentas; its biological activity mimics that of somatotropin and prolactin; secreted into maternal circulation; deficiency during pregnancy leads to abnormal intrauterine and postnatal growth. SYN chorionic growth hormone-prolactin, human chorionic somatomammotropic hormone, placental growth hormone.

**hu•man plas•ma pro•tein frac•tion** a solution of selected proteins derived from the plasma of human donors, containing 4.5 to 5.5 g of protein per 100 ml, of which 83 to 90% is albumin and the remainder is α- and β-globulins; used as a blood volume supporter.

**hu•man T-cell lym•pho•ma/leu•ke•mia vi•rus (HTLV)** a group of viruses (subfamily Oncovirinae, family Retroviridae) that are lymphotropic with a selective affinity for the helper/inducer cell subset of T lymphocytes and that are associated with adult T-cell leukemia and lymphoma.

**hu•mec•tant** (hyu-mek′tănt) an agent that promotes retention of moisture; a substance added to a powder, e.g., a dentifrice, to prevent hardening on exposure to air. [L. *humectus,* moist, fr. *humor,* moisture]

**hu•mer•al** (hyu′mer-ăl) relating to the humerus.
**hu•mer•al joint** SYN shoulder joint.
**hu•mer•o•ra•di•al** (hyu′mer-ō-rā′dē-ăl) relating

to both humerus and radius; denoting especially the ratio of length of one to the other.
**hu•mer•o•scap•u•lar** (hyu′mer-ō-skap′yu-lăr) relating to both humerus and scapula.
**hu•mer•o•ul•nar** (hyu′mer-ō-ŭl′năr) relating to both humerus and ulna; denoting especially the ratio of length of one to the other.
**hu•mer•us,** gen. and pl. **hu•meri** (hyu′mer-ŭs, hyu′mer-ī) [TA] the bone of the arm, articulating with the scapula above and the radius and ulna below. [L. shoulder]
**hu•mid•i•fi•er** a device for increasing the water vapor content of a gas or of ambient air.
**hu•mid•i•ty** (hyu-mid′i-tē) moisture or dampness, as of the air. [L. *humiditas,* dampness]
**Hum•mels•heim op•er•a•tion** (humel-shīm) transplantation of a normal ocular rectus muscle, to substitute for a paralyzed muscle.
**Hum•mels•heim pro•ce•dure** (humel-shīm) surgical procedure to correct an ocular deviation due to a sixth nerve palsy by which the superior and inferior rectus tendons are split and transferred laterally.
**hu•mor,** gen. **hu•mor•is** (hyu′mer, hyu-mōr′is) **1.** any clear fluid or semifluid hyaline anatomic substance. **2.** one of the elemental body fluids that were the basis of the physiologic and pathologic teachings of the hippocratic school: blood, yellow bile, black bile, and phlegm. [L. correctly, *umor,* liquid]
**hu•mor•al** (hyu′mōr-ăl) relating to a humor in any sense.
**hu•mor•al hy•per•cal•ce•mia of be•nig••nan•cy** hypercalcemia induced by parathyroid hormonelike protein of benign tumor.
**hu•mor•al im•mu•ni•ty** immunity associated with circulating antibodies, in contradistinction to cellular immunity.
**hu•mor•al reg•u•la•tor** a substance whose action is a result of contact with targets for activity through blood or body fluids.
**hump** (hŭmp) a rounded protuberance or bulge.
**hump•back** (hŭmp′bak) nonmedical term for kyphosis or gibbus.
**hun•ger** (hŭn′ger) **1.** a desire or need for food. **2.** any appetite, strong desire, or craving. [A.S.]
**hun•ger con•trac•tions** strong contractions of the stomach associated with hunger pains.
**hun•ger pain** cramp in the epigastrium associated with hunger.
**Hung meth•od** (hŭng) SYN Wilson method.
**Hun•ner ul•cer** (hŭn′ĕr) a focal and often multiple lesion involving all layers of the bladder wall in chronic interstitial cystitis; the surface epithelium is destroyed by inflammation and the initially pale lesion cracks and bleeds with distension of the bladder.
**Hun•ter ca•nal** (hun′ter) SYN adductor canal.
**Hun•ter op•er•a•tion** (hun′ter) ligation of an artery proximal and distal to an aneurysm.
**Hun•ter syn•drome** (hun′ter) an error of mucopolysaccharide metabolism characterized by deficiency of iduronate sulfatase, with excretion of dermatan sulfate and heparan sulfate in the urine; clinically similar to Hurler syndrome but distinguished by less severe skeletal changes, no corneal clouding, and X-linked recessive inheritance; caused by mutation in the iduronate sulfatase gene (IDS) on chromosome Xq.
**Hun•ter-Thomp•son dwarf•ism** (hun′ter-tom′son) a severe form of acromesomelic dwarfism,

characterized by shortening of the distal segments of the limbs; the lower limbs are more severely affected than the upper limbs; often associated with dislocations of elbows, knees, and hips. Autosomal recessive inheritance, caused by mutations in the cartilage-derived morphogenetic protein 1 (CDMP1) gene on chromosome 20q.

**hun·ting re·sponse** alternating vasodilatation and vasoconstriction in one or more extremities during application of ice or generalized hypothermia.

**Hun·ting·ton cho·rea** (hun'ting-tŏn) a neurodegenerative disorder, with onset usually in the third or fourth decade, characterized by chorea and dementia; pathologically, there is bilateral marked atrophy of the putamen and the head of the caudate nucleus. Autosomal dominant inheritance with complete penetrance, caused by mutation associated with trinucleotide repeat expansion in the Huntington gene (HD) on chromosome 4p. SYN hereditary chorea.

**Hunt neu·ral·gia** (hunt) SYN geniculate neuralgia.

**Hunt par·a·dox·ic phe·nom·e·non** (hunt) in dystonia musculorum deformans, if an attempt is made at plantar flexion of the foot when the foot is in dorsal spasm the only response is an increase of the extensor, or dorsal, spasm; if, however, the patient is told to extend the foot that is already in a state of strong dorsal flexion, there will be a sudden movement of plantar flexion; the same phenomenon, *mutatis mutandis*, is observed when there is a condition of strong plantar flexion.

**Hunt syn·drome** (hunt) **1.** an intention tremor beginning in one extremity, gradually increasing in intensity, and subsequently involving other parts of the body; **2.** facial paralysis, otalgia, and herpes zoster resulting from viral infection of the seventh cranial nerve and geniculate ganglion; **3.** a form of juvenile paralysis agitans associated with primary atrophy of the pallidal system. SYN Ramsay Hunt syndrome (1).

**Hur·ler syn·drome** (hĕr'lĕr) mucopolysaccharidosis in which there is a deficiency of α-L-iduronidase, an accumulation of an abnormal intracellular material, and excretion of dermatan sulfate and heparan sulfate in the urine; with severe abnormality in development of skeletal cartilage and bone, with dwarfism, kyphosis, deformed limbs, limitation of joint motion, spadelike hand, corneal clouding, hepatosplenomegaly, mental retardation, and gargoyle-like facies.

**Hurst dis·ease** (hĕrst) SYN acute necrotizing hemorrhagic encephalomyelitis.

**Hürth·le cell ad·e·no·ma** (hērt'lĕ) an uncommon type of thyroid tumor characterized by abundant eosinophilic cytoplasm containing numerous mitochondria. Often malignant with widespread metastases; rarely takes up radioiodine. SYN oncocytic adenoma.

**Hürth·le cell car·ci·no·ma** (hērt'lĕ) SYN Hürthle cell tumor. SYN oncocytic carcinoma, oxyphilic carcinoma.

**Hürth·le cell tu·mor** (hērt'lĕ) a neoplasm of the thyroid gland composed of polyhedral acidophilic cells, thought by some to be oncocytes; it may be benign or malignant, the behavior of the latter depending on the general microscopic pattern, whether follicular, papillary, or undifferen-

tiated. SEE ALSO Hürthle cell adenoma. SYN Hürthle cell carcinoma.

**Hutch·in·son cres·cen·tic notch** (huch'in-son) the semilunar notch on the incisal edge of Hutchinson teeth, encountered in congenital syphilis.

**Hutch·in·son fa·ci·es** (huch'in-son) the peculiar facial expression produced by the drooping eyelids and motionless eyes in external ophthalmoplegia.

**Hutch·in·son freck·le** (huch'in-son) SYN lentigo maligna.

**Hutch·in·son-Gil·ford dis·ease** (huch'in-sŏn-gil'ford) SYN progeria.

**Hutch·in·son in·ci·sors** (huch'in-son) SYN Hutchinson teeth.

**Hutch·in·son pu·pil** (huch'in-son) dilation of the pupil on the side of the lesion as part of a third nerve palsy; often due to herniation of the uncus of the temporal lobe through the tentorial notch.

**Hutch·in·son teeth** (huch'in-son) the incisors of congenital syphilis in which the incisal edge is notched and narrower than the cervical area giving a screwdriver appearance. SEE ALSO Hutchinson crescentic notch. SYN Hutchinson incisors.

**Hutch·in·son tri·ad** (huch'in-son) parenchymatous keratitis, labyrinthine disease, and Hutchinson teeth, significant of congenital syphilis.

**Hux·ley lay·er** (huks'lē) a layer of cells interposed between Henle layer and the cuticle of the inner root sheath of the hair follicle.

**Huy·gens prin·ci·ple** (hī-jenz) used in ultrasound technology; the principle that any wave phenomenon can be analyzed as the sum of many simple sources properly chosen with regard to phase and amplitude.

**HVA** homovanillic acid.

**HV con·duc·tion time** SEE intraventricular conduction.

**HV in·ter·val** the time from the initial deflection of the His bundle (H) potential and the onset of ventricular activity (normally 35–45 msec).

**HVL** half-value layer.

**hy·a·lin** (hī'ă-lin) a clear, eosinophilic, homogeneous substance occurring in degeneration; e.g., in arteriolar walls in arteriolar sclerosis and in glomerular tufts in diabetic glomerulosclerosis. [G. *hyalos*, glass]

**hy·a·line** (hī'ă-lin) transparent or colorless. SYN hyaloid. [G. *hyalos*, glass]

**hy·a·line bod·ies** homogeneous eosinophilic inclusions in the cytoplasm of epithelial cells; in renal tubules, hyaline bodies represent droplets of protein reabsorbed from the lumen. SEE ALSO Mallory bodies, drusen.

**hy·a·line car·ti·lage** cartilage having a frosted-glass appearance, with interstitial substance containing fine collagen fibers.

**hy·a·line de·gen·er·a·tion** a group of degenerative processes that affect various cells and tissues, resulting in rounded masses ("droplets") or broad bands of substances that are homogeneous, translucent, refractile, and acidophilic; may occur in the collagen of old fibrous tissue, smooth muscle of arterioles or the uterus, and as droplets in parenchymal cells.

**hy·a·line mem·brane 1.** the thin, clear basement membrane beneath certain epithelia; **2.** SYN glassy membrane (2).

**hy·a·line tu·ber·cle** a form of fibrous tubercle in

which the cellular fibrous tissue and collagenous fibers become altered and merged into a fairly homogeneous, acellular, deeply acidophilic, firm mass.

**hy·a·lin·i·za·tion** (hī'ă-lin-i-zā'shŭn) the formation of hyalin.

**hy·a·li·no·sis** (hī'ă-li-nō'sis) hyaline degeneration, especially that of relatively extensive degree.

**hy·a·lin·ur·ia** (hī-ă-lin-yur'ē-ă) the excretion of hyalin or casts of hyaline material in the urine. [hyalin + G. *ouron,* urine]

**hy·a·li·tis** (hī-ă-lī'tis) SYN vitreitis.

△**hy·al·o-, hy·al-** glassy, hyalin; vitreous. Cf. vitreo-. [G. *hyalos,* glass]

**hy·al·o·gens** (hī-al'ō-jenz) substances similar to mucoids that are found in many animal structures (e.g., cartilage, vitreous humor, hydatid cysts) and yield sugars on hydrolysis.

**hy·a·lo·hy·pho·my·co·sis** (hī'ă-lō-hī'fō-mī-kō' sis) an infection caused by a fungus with hyaline (colorless) mycelia in tissue, usually with a decrease in body resistance due to surgery, indwelling catheters, steroid therapy, or immunosuppressive drugs or cytotoxins. [hyalo- + G. *hyphē,* web, + *mykēs,* fungus, + *-osis,* condition]

**hy·a·loid** (hī'ă-loyd) SYN hyaline. [hyalo- + G. *eidos,* resemblance]

**hy·a·loid ar·tery** the terminal branch of the primordial ophthalmic artery, which forms in the embryo an extensive ramification in the primary vitreous and a vascular tunic around the lens; by 8½ months, these vessels have atrophied almost completely, but a few persistent remnants are evident entoptically as muscae volitantes. SYN arteria hyaloidea [TA].

**hy·a·loid bod·y** SYN vitreous body.

**hy·a·loid fos·sa** a depression on the anterior surface of the vitreous body in which lies the lens.

**hy·al·o·mere** (hī'ă-lō-mēr) the clear periphery of a blood platelet. [hyalo- + G. *meros,* part]

**hy·a·lo·pha·gia, hy·a·loph·a·gy** (hī'ă-lō-fā'jē-ă, hī-ă-lof'ă-jē) the eating or chewing of glass. [hyalo- + G. *phagō,* to eat]

**hy·al·o·plasm, hy·a·lo·plas·ma** (hī'ă-lō-plazm, hī'ă-lō-plaz'mă) the protoplasmic fluid substance of a cell. [hyalo- + G. *plasma,* thing formed]

**hy·a·lo·sis** (hī-ă-lō'sis) degenerative changes in the vitreous body. [hyalo- + G. *-osis,* condition]

**hy·al·o·some** (hī-al'ō-sōm) an oval or round structure within a cell nucleus that stains faintly but otherwise resembles a nucleolus. [hyalo- + G. *sōma,* body]

**hy·al·u·ro·nate** (hī-ăl-yur'on-āt) a salt or ester of hyaluronic acid.

**hy·al·u·ron·ic ac·id** (hī'ăl-yur-on'ik as'id) a mucopolysaccharide forming a gelatinous material in the tissue spaces and acting as a lubricant and shock absorbant; it is hydrolyzed by hyaluronidase.

**H-Y an·ti·gen** an antigen factor, dependent on the Y chromosome, responsible for the differentiation of the human embryo into the male phenotype by inducing the initially bipotential embryonic gonad to develop into a testis; in the absence of this antigen, the indifferent gonad develops into an ovary.

**hy·brid** (hī'brid) **1.** an individual (plant or animal) whose parents are different varieties of the same species or belong to different but closely allied species. **2.** fused tissue culture cells, as in a

hybridoma. [L. *hybrida,* offspring of a tame sow and a wild boar, fr. G. *hybris,* violation, wantonness]

**hy·brid·i·sa·tion [Br.]** SEE hybridization.

**hy·brid·i·za·tion** (hī'brid-i-zā'shŭn) **1.** the process of breeding a hybrid. **2.** crossing over between related but nonallelic genes. **3.** the specific reassociation of complementary strands of polynucleic acids; e.g., the formation of a DNA-RNA hybrid.

**hy·brid·o·ma** (hī-brid-ō'mă) a tumor of hybrid cells used in the production *in vitro* of specific monoclonal antibodies; produced by fusion of an established tissue culture line of lymphocyte tumor cells and specific antibody-producing cells. [G. *hybris,* violation, wantonness, + *-ōma,* tumor]

**hy·dan·to·in** (hī-dan'tō-in) a crystalline heterocyclic compound derived from urea and from allantoin; the NH–CH₂–CO group is prototypical of α-amino acids.

**hy·da·tid** (hī'da-tid) **1.** SYN hydatid cyst. **2.** a vesicular structure resembling an *Echinococcus* cyst. [G. *hydatis,* a drop of water, a hyatid]

**hy·da·tid cyst** a cyst formed in the liver by the larval stage of *Echinococcus,* chiefly in ruminants; two morphological forms caused by *Echinococcus granulosus* are found in humans: the unilocular hydatid cyst and the osseous hydatid cyst; a third form in humans is the alveolar hydatid cyst, caused by *Echinococcus multilocularis.* SYN echinococcus cyst, hydatid (1).

**hy·da·tid dis·ease** infection with larvae of the tapeworm *Echinococcus.*

**hy·da·tid frem·i·tus** SYN hydatid thrill.

**hy·da·tid·i·form** (hī-da-tid'i-fōrm) having the form or appearance of a hydatid.

**hy·da·tid·i·form mole, hy·da·tid mole** a vesicular or polycystic mass resulting from the proliferation of the trophoblast, with hydropic degeneration and avascularity of the chorionic villi.

**hy·da·tid·o·cele** (hī-da-tid'ō-sēl) a cystic mass composed of one or more hydatids formed in the scrotum. [hydatid + G. *kēlē,* tumor]

**hy·da·ti·do·ma** (hī'da-ti-dō'mă) a benign neoplasm in which there is prominent formation of hydatids. [hydatid + G. *-oma,* tumor]

**hy·da·tid·o·sis** (hī'da-ti-dō'sis) the morbid state caused by the presence of hydatid cysts.

**hy·da·ti·dos·to·my** (hī'da-ti-dos'tō-mē) surgical evacuation of a hydatid cyst. [hydatid + G. *stoma,* mouth]

**hy·da·tid thrill** the peculiar trembling or vibratory sensation felt on palpation of a hydatid cyst. SYN Blatin syndrome, hydatid fremitus.

**hy·drae·mia [Br.]** SEE hydremia.

**hy·dram·ni·os, hy·dram·ni·on** (hī-dram'nē-os, hī-dram'nē-on) presence of an excessive amount of amniotic fluid, usually over 2,000 mL. [G. *hydōr,* water, + amnion]

**hy·dran·en·ceph·a·ly** (hī'dran-en-sef'ă-lē) absence of cerebral hemispheres, which have been replaced by fluid-filled sacs, lined by leptomeninges. The skull and its brain cavities are normal. [hydr- + G. *an-* priv. + *enkephalos,* brain]

**hy·drar·gyr·ia, hy·drar·gy·rism** (hī-drar-jir'ē-ă, hī-drar'jir-izm) SYN mercury poisoning. [L. *hydrargyrum,* mercury]

**hy·drar·thro·di·al** (hī-drar-thrō'dē-ăl) relating to hydrarthrosis.

**hy·drar·thro·sis** (hī-drar-thrō'sis) effusion of a

serous fluid into a joint cavity. [hydr- + G. *arthron*, joint]

**hy•drase** (hī'drās) former name for hydratase.

**hy•dra•tase** (hī'dră-tās) certain hydro-lyases (EC class 4.2.1) catalyzing hydration-dehydration.

**hy•drate** (hī'drāt) an aqueous solvate (in older terminology, a hydroxide); a compound crystallizing with one or more molecules of water.

**hy•dra•tion** (hī-drā'shŭn) **1.** chemically, the addition of water; differentiated from hydrolysis, where the union with water is accompanied by a splitting of the original molecule and the water molecule. **2.** clinically, the taking in of water; used commonly in the sense of reduced hydration or dehydration.

**hy•dre•mia** (hī-drē'mē-ă) a condition in which the blood volume is increased as a result of an increase in the water content of plasma. [hydr- + G. *haima*, blood]

**hy•dren•ceph•a•lo•cele** (hī-dren-sef'ă-lō-sēl) protrusion, through a defect in the skull, of brain substance expanded into a sac containing fluid. SYN hydrocephalocele, hydroencephalocele. [hydr- + G. *enkephalos*, brain, + *kēlē*, tumor]

**hy•dren•ceph•a•lo•me•nin•go•cele** (hī'dren-sef'ă-lō-me-ning'gō-sēl) protrusion, through a defect in the skull, of a sac containing meninges, brain substance, and cerebrospinal fluid.

**hy•dric** (hī'drik) relating to hydrogen in chemical combination.

**hy•dride** (hī'drīd) a negatively charged hydrogen (i.e., H:⁻) or a compound of hydrogen in which it assumes a formal negative charge.

⌂**hy•dro-, hydr-** **1.** water, watery. **2.** containing or combined with hydrogen. **3.** a hydatid. [G. *hydōr*, water]

**hy•droa** (hī-drō'ă) any bullous eruption. [hydro + G. *ōon*, egg]

**hy•droa vac•ci•ni•for•me** a recurrent eruption of erythema evolving to umbilicated bullae, occurring on exposure to the sun and affecting chiefly male children with resolution before adult life.

**hy•dro•cal•y•co•sis** (hī'drō-kal-i-kō'sis) a usually symptomless anomaly of the renal calix that is dilated from obstruction of the infundibulum; usually discovered incidentally at pyelography or autopsy; may become infected. [hydro- + G. *kalyx*, cup of a flower]

**hy•dro•car•bon** (hī-drō-kar'bŏn) a compound containing only hydrogen and carbon.

**hy•dro•cele** (hī'drō-sēl) a collection of serous fluid in a sacculated cavity; specifically, such a collection in the space of the tunica vaginalis testis, or in a separate pocket along the spermatic cord. [hydro- + G. *kēlē*, hernia]

**hy•dro•ce•lec•to•my** (hī'drō-sē-lek'tō-mē) excision of a hydrocele. [hydrocele + G. *ektomē*, excision]

**hy•dro•ce•phal•ic** (hī'drō-se-fal'ik) relating to or suffering from hydrocephalus.

**hy•dro•ceph•a•lo•cele** (hī-drō-sef'ă-lō-sēl) SYN hydrencephalocele.

**hy•dro•ceph•a•loid** (hī-drō-sef'ă-loyd) **1.** resembling hydrocephalus. **2.** a condition in infants suffering from diarrhea or other debilitating disease, in which there is dehydration and general symptoms resembling those of hydrocephalus without, however, any abnormal accumulation of cerebrospinal fluid.

**hy•dro•ceph•a•lus** (hī-drō-sef'ă-lŭs) a condition marked by an excessive accumulation of cerebro-

spinal fluid resulting in dilation of the cerebral ventricles and raised intracranial pressure; may also result in enlargement of the cranium and atrophy of the brain. SYN hydrocephaly. [hydro- + G. *kephalē*, head]

**hy•dro•ceph•a•lus ex vac•u•o** hydrocephalus due to loss or atrophy of brain tissue; less commonly associated with raised intracranial pressure.

**hy•dro•ceph•a•ly** (hī-drō-sef'ă-lē) SYN hydrocephalus.

**hy•dro•chlo•ric ac•id** (hī-drō-klōr'ik as'id) the acid of gastric juice. The gas and the concentrated solution are strong irritants.

**hy•dro•chlo•ride** (hī-drō-klōr'īd) a compound formed by the addition of a hydrochloric acid molecule to an amine or related substance.

**hy•dro•cho•le•re•sis** (hī'drō-kō-ler-ē'sis) increased output of a watery bile of low specific gravity, viscosity, and solid content. [hydro- + G. *cholē*, bile, + *hairesis*, a taking]

**hy•dro•cho•le•ret•ic** (hī'drō-kō-ler-et'ik) pertaining to hydrocholeresis.

**hy•dro•col•loid** (hī-drō-kol'oyd) a gelatinous colloid in unstable equilibrium with its contained water, useful in dentistry for impressions because of its dimensional stability under controlled conditions.

**hy•dro•col•po•cele, hy•dro•col•pos** (hī-drō-kol'pō-sēl, hī-drō-kol'pos) accumulation of mucus or other nonsanguineous fluid in the vagina. [hydro- + G. *kolpos*, bosom (vagina)]

**hy•dro•cor•ti•sone** (hī-drō-kōr'ti-sōn) a steroid hormone secreted by the adrenal cortex and the most potent of the naturally occurring glucocorticoids in humans. SYN cortisol.

**hy•dro•cyst** (hī'drō-sist) a cyst with clear, watery contents. [hydro- + G. *kystis*, bladder]

**hy•dro•en•ceph•a•lo•cele** (hī'drō-en-sef'ă-lō-sēl) SYN hydrencephalocele.

**hy•dro•gel** (hī'drō-jel) a colloid in which the particles are in the external or dispersion phase and water in the internal or dispersed phase.

**hy•dro•gen (H)** (hī'drō-jen) **1.** a gaseous element, atomic no. 1, atomic wt. 1.00794. **2.** the molecular form of the element, $H_2$. SYN dihydrogen. [hydro- + G. -*gen*, producing]

**hy•dro•gen-1** ($^1H$) the common hydrogen-1 isotope, making up 99.985% of the hydrogen-1 atoms occurring in nature.

**hy•dro•gen-2** ($^2H$) the isotope of hydrogen-2 of atomic weight 2; the less common stable isotope of hydrogen-2 making up 0.015% of the hydrogen-2 atoms occurring in nature. SYN deuterium.

**hy•dro•gen-3** a hydrogen isotope of atomic weight 3; weakly radioactive, emitting beta particles to become the stable helium-3; half-life, 12.32 years. SYN tritium.

**hy•dro•gen•ase** (hī'drō-je-nās, hī-droj'ĕ-nās) any enzyme that removes a hydride ion (or H:⁻) from NADH (or NADPH) or adds hydrogen to ferricytochrome or to ferredoxin.

**hy•dro•gen•a•tion** (hī'drō-jĕ-nā'shŭn, hī-droj'ĕ-nā-shŭn) addition of hydrogen to a compound, especially to an unsaturated fat or fatty acid; thus, soft fats or oils are solidified or "hardened."

**hy•dro•gen bond** a bond arising from the sharing of a hydrogen atom, covalently bound to an electronegative element (e.g., N or O), with another electronegative element (e.g., N, O, or a halogen).

h
y

**hy·dro·gen chlo·ride** a very soluble gas which, in solution, forms hydrochloric acid.

**hy·dro·gen do·nor** a metabolite from which hydrogen is removed (by a dehydrogenase system) and transferred by a hydrogen carrier to another metabolite, which is thus reduced.

**hy·dro·gen ex·po·nent** the logarithm of the hydrogen ion concentration in blood or other fluid; its negative is the pH of that fluid.

**hy·dro·gen ion (H⁺)** a hydrogen atom minus its electron and therefore carrying a unit positive charge (i.e., a proton); in water, it combines with a water molecule to form hydronium ion, $H_3O^+$.

**hy·dro·gen pump** molecular mechanism for acid secretion from gastric parietal cells based on the activity of a $H^+$-$K^+$-ATPase.

**hy·dro·gen trans·port** the transfer of hydrogen from one metabolite (hydrogen donor) to another (hydrogen acceptor) through the action of an enzyme system; the donor is thus oxidized and the acceptor reduced.

**hy·dro·ki·net·ic** (hī′drŏ-ki-net′ik) pertaining to the motion of fluids and the forces giving rise to such motion.

**hy·dro·las·es** (hī′drŏ-lās-ez) enzymes (EC class 3) cleaving substrates with addition of $H_2O$ at the point of cleavage.

**hy·dro·ly·as·es** (hī-drŏ-lī′ăs-ĕz) a class of lyases (EC class 4.2.1) comprising enzymes removing H and OH as water, leading to formation of new double bonds within the affected molecule.

**hy·drol·y·sate** (hī-drol′ĭ-sāt) a solution containing the products of hydrolysis.

**hy·drol·y·sis** (hī-drol′ĭ-sis) a chemical process whereby a compound is cleaved into two or more simpler compounds with the uptake of the H and OH parts of a water molecule on either side of the chemical bond cleaved; hydrolysis is effected by the action of acids, alkalies, or enzymes. Cf. hydration. [hydro- + G. *lysis,* dissolution]

**hy·dro·lyt·ic** (hī-drŏ-lit′ik) referring to or causing hydrolysis.

**hy·dro·ma** (hī-drŏ′mă) SYN hygroma.

**hy·dro·me·nin·go·cele** (hī′drŏ-men-ing′gō-sēl) protrusion of the meninges of brain or spinal cord through a defect in the skull or vertebral column, the sac so formed containing cerebrospinal fluid. [hydro- + G. *mēninx,* membrane, + *kēlē,* hernia]

**hy·drom·e·ter** (hī-drom′ĕ-ter) an instrument for determining the specific gravity of a liquid. [hydro- + G. *mēron,* measure]

**hy·dro·me·tra** (hī-drŏ-mē′tră) accumulation of thin mucus or other watery fluid in the cavity of the uterus. [hydro- + G. *mētra,* uterus]

**hy·dro·met·ric** (hī-drŏ-met′rik) relating to hydrometry or the hydrometer.

**hy·dro·me·tro·col·pos** (hī′drŏ-mē-trŏ-kol′pos) distention of uterus and vagina by fluid other than blood or pus. [hydro- + G. *mētra,* uterus, + *kolpos,* bosom (vagina)]

**hy·drom·e·try** (hī-drom′ĕ-trē) determination of the specific gravity of a fluid by means of a hydrometer.

**hy·dro·mi·cro·ceph·a·ly** (hī′drŏ-mī-krŏ-sef′ă-lē) microcephaly associated with an increased amount of cerebrospinal fluid.

**hy·dro·my·e·lia** (hī-drŏ-mī-ē′lē-ă) an increase of fluid in the dilated central canal of the spinal cord, or in congenital cavities elsewhere in the cord substance. [hydro- + G. *myelos,* marrow]

**hy·dro·my·e·lo·cele** (hī-drŏ-mī′ĕ-lō-sēl) protrusion of a portion of the spinal cord, thinned out into a sac distended with cerebrospinal fluid, through a spina bifida. [hydro- + G. *myelos,* marrow, + *kēlē,* tumor, hernia]

**hy·dro·my·o·ma** (hī′drŏ-mī-ō′mă) a leiomyoma that contains cystlike foci of proteinaceous fluid; hydromyomas occur more frequently in leiomyomas of the uterus, as a result of degenerative changes. [hydro- + G. *mys,* muscle, + *-oma,* tumor]

**hy·dro·ne·phro·sis** (hī′drŏ-ne-frō′sis) dilation of the pelvis and calices of one or both kidneys resulting from obstruction to the flow of urine. SYN pelvocaliectasis, uronephrosis. [hydro- + G. *nephros,* kidney, + *-osis,* condition]

**hy·dro·ne·phrot·ic** (hī′drŏ-ne-frot′ik) relating to hydronephrosis.

**hy·dro·per·i·car·di·tis** (hī′drŏ-per-i-kar-dī′tis) pericarditis with a large serous effusion.

**hy·dro·per·i·car·di·um** (hī′drŏ-per-i-kar′dē-ŭm) a noninflammatory accumulation of fluid in the pericardial sac.

**hy·dro·per·i·to·ne·um, hy·dro·per·i·to·nia** (hī′drŏ-per-i-tō-nē′ŭm, hī′drŏ-per-i-tō′nē-ă) SYN ascites. [hydro- + peritoneum]

**hy·dro·phil·ia** (hī-drŏ-fil′ē-ă) a tendency of the blood and tissues to absorb fluid. [hydro- + G. *philos,* fond]

**hy·dro·phil·ic** (hī-drŏ-fil′ik) denoting the property of attracting or associating with water molecules, possessed by polar radicals or ions, as opposed to hydrophobic (2).

**hy·dro·pho·bia** (hī-drŏ-fō′bē-ă) SYN rabies. [hydro- + G. *phobos,* fear]

**hy·dro·pho·bic** (hī-drŏ-fōb′ik) **1.** relating to or suffering from hydrophobia. **2.** lacking an affinity for water molecules, as opposed to hydrophilic.

**hy·drop·ic de·gen·er·a·tion** SYN cloudy swelling.

**hy·dro·pneu·ma·to·sis** (hī-drŏ-noo-mă-tō′sis) combined emphysema and edema; the presence of liquid and gas in tissues. [hydro- + G. *pneuma,* breath, spirit]

**hy·dro·pneu·mo·go·ny** (hī′drŏ-noo-mō′gō-nē) injection of air into a joint to determine the amount of effusion. [hydro- + G. *pneuma,* air, + *gony,* knee]

**hy·dro·pneu·mo·per·i·car·di·um** (hī-drŏ-noo′mō-per-i-kar′dē-ŭm) the presence of a serous effusion and of gas in the pericardial sac. SYN pneumohydropericardium. [hydro- + G. *pneuma,* air, + pericardium]

**hy·dro·pneu·mo·per·i·to·ne·um** (hī-drŏ-noo′mō-per-i-tō-nē′ŭm) the presence of gas and serous fluid in the peritoneal cavity. SYN pneumohydroperitoneum. [hydro- + G. *pneuma,* air, + peritoneum]

**hy·dro·pneu·mo·tho·rax** (hī′drŏ-noo-mō-thōr′aks) the presence of both gas and fluids in the pleural cavity. SYN pneumohydrothorax. [hydro- + G. *pneuma,* air, + thorax]

**hy·drops** (hī′drops) an excessive accumulation of clear, watery fluid in any of the tissues or cavities of the body; synonymous, according to its character and location, with ascites, anasarca, or edema. [G. *hydrōps*]

**hy·dro·py·o·ne·phro·sis** (hī′drŏ-pī′ō-ne-frō′sis) presence of purulent urine in the pelvis and calices of the kidney following obstruction of the ureter. [hydro- + G. *pyon,* pus, + nephrosis]

**hy·dror·rhea** (hī-drō-rē′ă) a profuse discharge of watery fluid from any part of the body. [hydro- + G. *rhoia,* flow]

**hy·dro·sal·pinx** (hī-drō-sal′pinks) accumulation of serous fluid in the uterine tube, often an end result of pyosalpinx. [hydro- + G. *salpinx,* trumpet]

**hy·dro·sar·co·cele** (hī-drō-sar′kō-sēl) a chronic swelling of the testis complicated with hydrocele. [hydro- + G. *sarx,* flesh, + *kēlē,* tumor]

**hy·dro·stat·ic** (hī-drō-stat′ik) relating to the pressure of fluids or to their properties when in equilibrium.

**hy·dro·sta·tic weigh·ing** SYN underwater weighing.

**hy·dro·sy·rin·go·my·e·lia** (hī′drō-sĭ-rin′gō-mī-ē′lē-ă) SYN syringomyelia. [hydro- + G. *hydōr,* water, + *syrinx,* a tube, + *myelos,* marrow]

**hy·dro·tax·is** (hī-drō-tak′sis) the movement of cells or organisms in relation to water. [hydro- + G. *taxis,* arrangement]

**hydrotherapy** (hī-drō-thār′ă-pē) the external application of water as a liquid, solid, or vapor for therapeutic purposes. [hydro- + G. *therapeia,* therapy]

**hy·dro·thi·o·ne·mia** (hī′drō-thī-ō-nē′mē-ă) the presence of hydrogen sulfide in the circulating blood. [hydro- + G. *theion,* sulfur, + *haima,* blood]

**hy·dro·thi·on·ur·ia** (hī′drō-thī-ōn-yur′ē-ă) the excretion of hydrogen sulfide in the urine. [hydro- + G. *theion,* sulfur, + *ouron,* urine]

**hy·dro·tho·rax** (hī-drō-thōr′aks) presence of fluid in one or both pleural cavities, usually resulting from cardiac failure.

**hy·drot·ro·pism** (hī-drot′rō-pizm, hī-drō-trō′pizm) the property in growing organisms of turning toward a moist surface (**positive hydrotropism**) or away from a moist surface (**negative hydrotropism**). [hydro- + G. *tropos,* a turning]

**hy·dro·tu·ba·tion** (hī′drō-too-bā′shŭn) injection of a liquid medication or saline solution through the cervix into the uterine cavity and uterine tubes for dilation and/or treatment of the tubes.

**hy·dro·u·re·ter** (hī′drō-yur′ē-ter) distention of the ureter with urine, due to blockage from any cause.

**hy·dro·va·ri·um** (hī-drō-va′rē-ŭm) a collection of fluid in the ovary.

**hy·drox·ide** (hī-drok′sīd) a compound containing a potentially ionizable hydroxyl group; particularly a compound that liberates $OH^-$ upon dissolving in water.

△**hy·drox·y-** prefix indicating addition or substitution of the –OH group to or in the compound whose name follows. SEE ALSO oxa-, oxo-, oxy-.

**hy·drox·y·ap·a·tite** (hī-drok′sē-ap-ă-tīt) a natural mineral structure resembling the crystal lattice of bones and teeth; used in chromatography of nucleic acids; also found in pathologic calcifications.

γ**-hy·drox·y·bu·ty·rate (GHB)** (gam′ă-hī-drok′sē- byu′tir-āt) a naturally occurring short-chain fatty acid, a metabolite of γ-aminobutyric acid (GABA) found in all body tissues, with the highest concentration in the brain; it affects levels of GABA, dopamine, 5-hydroxytryptamine, and acetylcholine, and may itself be a neurotransmitter; accumulation of GHB in people with an in-

herited disorder in the metabolism of GABA causes ataxia and mental retardation. Synthetic GHB, formerly used in anesthesia and in the treatment of narcolepsy and alcohol withdrawal, has been banned by the Food and Drug Administration because of severe neurologic, cardiovascular, respiratory, and gastrointestinal side effects. SYN 4-hydroxybutyrate.

**4-hy·drox·y·bu·ty·rate** SYN γ-hydroxybutyrate.

**17-hy·drox·y·cor·ti·co·ste·roid test** a test, dependent on the Porter-Silber reaction, that is used as a measure of adrenocortical function and is performed on urine. Low values are seen in Addison disease and hypopituitarism; high values are seen in Cushing syndrome and extreme stress.

**hy·drox·yl** (hī-drok′sil) the radical, –OH.

**11-hy·drox·y·lase de·fi·cien·cy** a type of congenital adrenal hyperplasia, with various manifestations, including hypertensive types and salt-wasting varieties.

**21-hy·drox·y·lase de·fi·ci·en·cy** one form of congenital adrenal hyperplasia, with variable presentations, including simple virilizing, salt-wasting, and nonclassic types.

**hy·drox·y·las·es** (hī-drok′si-lā-sez) enzymes catalyzing formation of hydroxyl groups by addition of an oxygen atom, hence oxidizing the substrate.

**hy·drox·y·phen·yl·u·ria** (hī-drok′sē-fen-il-yur′ē-ă) urinary excretion of tyrosine and phenylalanine, as a result of ascorbic acid deficiency; occurs notably in those premature infants who lack this vitamin.

**21-hy·drox·y·pro·ges·ter·one** SYN deoxycorticosterone.

**3β-hy·drox·y·ste·roid sul·fa·tase** (thē-beta-hī-drok′sē-stēr′ōid sul-fă-tāse) an enzyme, found in most mammalian tissues, that is capable of hydrolyzing the sulfate ester bonds of a variety of sulfated sterols; a deficiency of this enzyme will result in X-linked ichthyosis.

**5-hy·drox·y·tryp·ta·mine (5-HT)** (fīv-hī-drok-sē-trip′tă-mēn) SYN serotonin.

**hy·giene** (hī′jēn) **1.** the science of health and its maintenance. **2.** cleanliness that promotes health and well being, especially of a personal nature. [G. *hygieinos,* healthful, fr. *hygiēs,* healthy]

**hy·gien·ic** (hī-jen′ik, hī-jē-en′ik) healthful; relating to hygiene; tending to maintain health.

**hy·gien·ist** (hī-jē′nist, hī′jē-en-ist) one who is skilled in the science of health and its maintenance.

△**hy·gro-, hygr-** moisture, humidity; opposite of xero-. [G. *hygros,* moist]

**hy·gro·ma** (hī-grō′mă) a cystic swelling containing a serous fluid. SYN hydroma. [hygro- + G. *-oma,* tumor]

**hy·grom·e·try** (hī-grom′ĕ-trē) SYN psychrometry.

**hy·gro·scop·ic** (hī-grō-skop′ik) denoting a substance capable of readily absorbing and retaining moisture; e.g., NaOH, $CaCl_2$.

**hy·gro·scop·ic con·den·ser hu·mid·i·fi·er** a passive humidification device that works by collecting heat and moisture on exhalation and returning it to inhaled gas SYN artificial nose.

**hy·men** (hī′men) [TA] a thin membranous fold, highly variable in appearance, which partly occludes the ostium of the vagina prior to its rupture, which may occur for a variety of reasons. It is frequently absent, even in virgins, although remnants are commonly present as hymenal tags (caruncula). [G. *hymēn,* membrane]

**hy·men·al** (hī'men-ăl) relating to the hymen. US-AGE NOTE: Often misspelled hymeneal, or so mispronounced.

**hy·me·nec·to·my** (hī-me-nek'tō-mē) excision of the hymen. [G. *hymēn,* membrane, + *ektomē,* excision]

**hy·me·ni·tis** (hī-me-nī'tis) inflammation of the hymen.

**hy·me·nol·o·gy** (hī-mĕ-nol'ō-jē) the branch of anatomy and physiology concerned with the membranes of the body. [G. *hymēn,* membrane, + *logos,* study]

**hy·men·ot·o·my** (hī-me-not'ō-mē) surgical division of a hymen. [G. *hymēn,* membrane, + *tomē,* incision]

**hy·o·ep·i·glot·tic** (hī'ō-ep-i-glot'ik) relating to the hyoid bone and the epiglottis; denoting the elastic hyoepiglottic ligament connecting the two structures.

**hy·o·glos·sal** (hī'ō-glos'ăl) relating to the hyoid bone and the tongue. SYN glossohyal.

**hy·o·glos·sal mem·brane** posterior widening of the lingual septum connecting the root of the tongue to the hyoid bone; the inferior fibers of the genioglossus are attached to it and by this means to the upper anterior body of the hyoid bone near the midline.

**hy·o·glos·sal mus·cle** SYN hyoglossus muscle.

**hy·o·glos·sus mus·cle** *origin,* body and greater horn of hyoid bone; *insertion,* side of the tongue; *action,* retracts and pulls down side of tongue; *nerve supply,* motor by hypoglossal, sensory by lingual. SYN musculus hyoglossus [TA], hyoglossal muscle.

**hy·oid** (hī'oyd) U-shaped or V-shaped; denoting the os hyoideum and the apparatus hyoideus. [G. *hyoeidēs,* shaped like the letter upsilon, υ]

**hy·oid arch** the second visceral, or pharyngeal (branchial in fish), arch; the second postoral arch in the pharyngeal (branchial in fish) arch series.

**hy·oid bone** a U-shaped bone lying between the mandible and the larynx, suspended from the styloid processes by slender stylohyoid ligaments.

⌂**hyp-** variation of the prefix hypo-, often used before a vowel. Cf. sub-.

**hyp·a·cu·sis** (hī'pă-koo'sis) hearing impairment of a conductive or neurosensory nature. SYN hypoacusis. [hypo- + G. *akousis,* hearing]

**hyp·aes·the·sia [Br.]** SEE hypesthesia.

**hyp·al·bu·mi·ne·mia** (hip-ăl-byu-mi-nē'mē-ă) SYN hypoalbuminemia. [G. *hypo,* under, + albuminemia]

**hyp·al·ge·sia** (hip-al-jē'zē-ă) decreased sensibility to pain. SYN hypoalgesia. [G. *hypo,* under, + *algēsis,* sense of pain]

**hyp·al·ge·sic, hyp·al·get·ic** (hip-ăl-jē'sik, hip-ăljet'ik) relating to hypalgesia; having diminished sensitiveness to pain.

⌂**hy·per-** excessive, above normal; opposite of hypo-. [G. *hyper,* above, over]

**hy·per·ab·duc·tion syn·drome 1.** diminution or loss of distal upper extremity pulses on hyperabduction of the limb. **2.** one of the forerunners of thoracic outlet syndrome, in which the subclavian or axillary artery in the brachial plexus was thought to be compressed, either in the costoclavicular space or beneath the pectoralis minor tendon, during hyperabduction of the limb. SYN Wright syndrome.

**hy·per·a·cid·i·ty** (hī'pĕr-a-sid'i-tē) an abnormally high degree of acidity, as of the gastric juice.

**hy·per·ac·tiv·i·ty** (hī'pĕr-ak-tiv'i-tē) **1.** SYN superactivity. **2.** general restlessness or excessive movement such as that characterizing children with attention deficit disorder or hyperkinesis.

**hy·per·a·cu·sis, hy·per·a·cu·sia** (hī'pĕr-ă-koo'sis, hī'pĕr-ă-koo-'sē-ă) abnormal acuteness of hearing due to increased irritability of the auditory apparatus. [hyper- + G. *akousis,* a hearing]

**hy·per·ad·e·no·sis** (hī'pĕr-ad-ĕ-nō'sis) glandular enlargement, especially of the lymphatic glands. [hyper- + G. *adēn,* gland, + *-ōsis,* condition]

**hy·per·ad·i·po·sis, hy·per·ad·i·pos·i·ty** (hī'pĕr-ad-i-pō'sis, hī'pĕr-ad-i-pos'i-tē) an extreme degree of adiposis or fatness.

**hy·per·aes·the·sia [Br.]** SEE hyperesthesia.

**hy·per·al·do·ste·ron·ism** (hī'pĕr-al-dos'ter-on-izm) SYN aldosteronism.

**hy·per·al·ge·sia** (hī-pĕr-al-jē'zē-ă) extreme sensitivity to painful stimuli. [hyper- + G. *algos,* pain]

**hy·per·al·ge·sic, hy·per·al·get·ic** (hī'pĕr-al-jē'sik, hī'pĕr-al-jet'ik) relating to hyperalgesia.

**hy·per·al·i·men·ta·tion** (hī'pĕr-al'i-men-tā'shŭn) administration or consumption of nutrients beyond minimum normal requirements, in an attempt to replace nutritional deficiencies.

**hy·per·am·y·la·se·mia** (hī'pĕr-am'i-lā-sē'mē-ă) elevated serum amylase, usually seen as one of the manifestations of acute pancreatitis. [hyper- + amylase, + G. *haima,* blood]

**hy·per·an·a·ki·ne·sia, hy·per·an·a·ki·ne·sis** (hī'pĕr-an-ă-ki-nē'zē-ă, hī'pĕr-an-ă-ki-nē'sis) excessive to-and-fro movement, as of the stomach or intestine. [hyper- + G. *anakinēsis,* to-and-fro movement]

**hy·per·a·phia** (hī'pĕr-ā'fē-ă) extreme sensitivity to touch. [hyper- + G. *haphē,* touch]

**hy·per·aph·ic** (hī-pĕr-af'ik) marked by hyperaphia.

**hy·per·bar·ic** (hī-pĕr-bar'ik) **1.** pertaining to pressure of ambient gases greater than 1 atmosphere. **2.** concerning solutions, more dense than the diluent or medium; e.g., in spinal anesthesia, a hyperbaric solution has a density greater than that of spinal fluid. [hyper- + G. *baros,* weight]

**hy·per·bar·ic cham·ber** a chamber providing pressures greater than atmospheric, commonly used to treat decompression sickness and to provide hyperbaric oxygenation.

**hy·per·bar·ic ox·y·gen, high pres·sure ox·y·gen** oxygen at a pressure greater than 1 atmosphere.

**hy·per·bar·ic ox·y·gen ther·a·py** treatment in which oxygen is provided in a sealed chamber at an ambient pressure greater than 1 atmosphere.

**hy·per·bar·ism** (hī-pĕr-bar'izm) disturbances in the body resulting from the pressure of ambient gases at greater than 1 atmosphere; e.g., nitrogen narcosis, oxygen toxicity, bends. [hyper- + G. *baros,* weight]

**hy·per·bi·li·ru·bi·nae·mia [Br.]** SEE hyperbilirubinemia.

**hy·per·bil·i·ru·bi·ne·mia** (hī'pĕr-bil'i-roo-bi-nē'mē-ă) an abnormally large amount of bilirubin in the circulating blood, resulting in clinically apparent icterus or jaundice when the concentration is sufficient.

**hy·per·cal·cae·mia [Br.]** SEE hypercalcemia.

**hy·per·cal·ce·mia** (hī′per-kal-sē′mē-ă) an abnormally high concentration of calcium compounds in the circulating blood; commonly used to indicate an elevated concentration of calcium ions in the blood. SYN calcaemia, calcemia.

**hy·per·cal·ci·u·ria** (hī′pĕr-kal-sē-yu′rē-ă) excretion of abnormally large amounts of calcium in the urine.

**hy·per·cap·nia** (hī-pĕr-kap′nē-ă) abnormally increased arterial carbon dioxide tension. SYN hypercarbia. [hyper- + G. *kapnos,* smoke, vapor]

**hy·per·cap·nic a·cid·o·sis** SYN respiratory acidosis.

**hy·per·car·bia** (hī-pĕr-kar′bē-ă) SYN hypercapnia.

**hy·per·cat·a·bol·ism** (hī′pĕr-kă-tab′ō-lizm) an increase in basal metabolic rate and in breakdown of muscle and adipose tissue as a result of injury, metabolic stress, or sepsis. SEE ALSO catabolism.

**hy·per·ce·men·to·sis** (hī′pĕr-sē-men-tō′sis) excessive deposition of secondary cementum on the root of a tooth, which may be caused by localized trauma or inflammation, excessive tooth eruption, or osteitis deformans, or may occur idiopathically. [hyper- + L. *caementum,* a rough quarry stone, + *-osis,* condition]

**hy·per·chlor·ae·mia [Br.]** SEE hyperchloremia.

**hy·per·chlor·e·mia** (hī-pĕr-klō-rē′mē-ă) an abnormally large concentration of chloride ions in the circulating blood.

**hy·per·chlor·hy·dria** (hī′pĕr-klōr-hī′drē-ă) presence of an excessive amount of hydrochloric acid in the stomach. SYN chlorhydria. [hyper- + chlorhydric (acid)]

**hypercholesteraemia [Br.]** SYN hypercholesterolemia.

**hy·per·cho·les·ter·e·mia** (hī′pĕr-kō-les′ter-ē′mē-ă) SYN hypercholesterolemia.

**hy·per·cho·les·ter·ol·ae·mia [Br.]** SEE hypercholesterolemia.

**hy·per·cho·les·ter·ol·e·mia** (hī′pĕr-kō-les′ter-ol-ē′mē- ă) the presence of an abnormally large amount of cholesterol in the blood. SYN hypercholesteraemia, hypercholesteremia.

**hy·per·cho·lia** (hī-pĕr-kō′lē-ă) a condition in which an abnormally large amount of bile is formed in the liver. [hyper- + G. *cholē,* bile]

**hy·per·chro·ma·sia** (hī-pĕr-krō-mā′zē-ă) SYN hyperchromatism.

**hy·per·chro·mat·ic** (hī′pĕr-krō-mat′ik) **1.** abnormally highly colored, excessively stained, or overpigmented. SYN hyperchromic (1). **2.** showing increased chromatin. [hyper- + G. *chrōma,* color]

**hy·per·chro·ma·tism** (hī′pĕr-krō′mă-tizm) **1.** excessive pigmentation. **2.** increased staining capacity, especially of cell nuclei for hematoxylin. **3.** an increase in chromatin in cell nuclei. SYN hyperchromasia, hyperchromia. [hyper- + G. *chrōma,* color]

**hy·per·chro·mia** (hī-pĕr-krō′mē-ă) SYN hyperchromatism.

**hy·per·chro·mic** (hī-pĕr-krōm′ik) **1.** SYN hyperchromatic (1). **2.** denoting increased light absorption.

**hy·per·chro·mic a·ne·mia, hy·per·chro··mat·ic a·ne·mi·a** anemia characterized by a decrease in the ratio of the weight of hemoglobin to the volume of the erythrocyte, i.e., the mean cor-

puscular hemoglobin concentration is less than normal.

**hy·per·chy·lia** (hī-pĕr-kī′lē-ă) excessive secretion of gastric juice. [hyper- + G. *chylos,* juice]

**hy·per·chy·lo·mi·cro·ne·mia** (hī′pĕr-kī′lō-mī-krō-nē′mē-ă) increased plasma concentrations of chylomicrons.

**hy·per·cor·ti·coid·ism** (hī′pĕr-kōr′ti-koyd-izm) excessive secretion of one or more steroid hormones of the adrenal cortex; sometimes used also to designate the state produced by therapeutic administration of large quantities of steroids having glucocorticoid activity, e.g., hydrocortisone. SEE ALSO Cushing syndrome.

**hy·per·cry·aes·the·sia [Br.]** SEE hypercryesthesia.

**hy·per·cry·al·ge·sia** (hī′pĕr-krī-al-jē′zē-ă) SYN hypercryesthesia. [hyper- + G. *kryos,* cold, + *algēsis,* the sense of pain]

**hy·per·cry·es·the·sia** (hī′pĕr-krī-es-thē′zē-ă) extreme sensibility to cold. SYN hypercryalgesia. [hyper- + G. *kryos,* cold, + *aisthēsis,* sensation]

**hy·per·cu·pre·mia** (hī′pĕr-koo-prē′mē-ă) an abnormally high level of plasma copper. [hyper- + L. *cuprum,* copper, + G. *haima,* blood]

**hy·per·cy·a·not·ic** (hī′pĕr-sī-ă-not′ik) marked by extreme cyanosis.

**hy·per·cy·the·mia** (hī′pĕr-sī-thē′mē-ă) the presence of an abnormally high number of red blood cells in the circulating blood. SYN hypererythrocythemia. [hyper- + G. *kytos,* cell, + *haima,* blood]

**hy·per·cy·to·sis** (hī′pĕr-sī-tō′sis) any condition in which there is an abnormal increase in the number of cells in the circulating blood or the tissues; frequently used synonymously with leukocytosis.

**hy·per·di·crot·ic** (hī′pĕr-dī-krot′ik) pronouncedly dicrotic.

**hy·per·ech·o·ic** denoting a region in an ultrasound image in which the echoes are stronger than normal or than surrounding structures. **1.** ULTRASONOGRAPHY pertaining to material that produces echoes of higher amplitude or density than the surrounding medium.

**hy·per·ek·plex·ia** (hī′pĕr-ek-pleks′ē-ă) a hereditary disorder in which there are pathologic startle responses, i.e., protective reactions to unanticipated, potentially threatening, stimuli of any type, particularly auditory; the stimuli induce often widespread and violent sudden contractions of the head, neck, spinal, and sometimes limb musculature, resulting in involuntary shouting, jerking, jumping, and falling; autosomal dominant and recessive inheritance forms, with the responsible gene localized to chromosome 5q; probably the result of lack of inhibitory neurotransmitters, glycine, or GABA. SYN kok disease, startle disease. [hyper- + G. *ekplēxia,* sudden shock, fr. *ekplēssō,* to startle]

**hy·per·em·e·sis** (hī-pĕr-em′ĕ-sis) excessive vomiting. [hyper- + G. *emesis,* vomiting]

**hy·per·e·met·ic** (hī′pĕr-ĕ-met′ik) marked by excessive vomiting.

**hy·per·e·mia** (hī-pĕr-ē′mē-ă) the presence of an increased amount of blood in a part or organ. SEE ALSO congestion. [hyper- + G. *haima,* blood]

**hy·per·e·mic** (hī-pĕr-ē′mik) denoting hyperemia.

**hy·per·en·ceph·a·ly** (hī′pĕr-en-sef′ă-lē) a fetal developmental deficiency of the neurocranium, exposing the poorly formed brain. [hyper- + G. *enkephalos,* brain]

**hy·per·en·dem·ic dis·ease** (hī'pĕr-en-dem'ik di-zēz') a disease that is constantly present at a high incidence and/or prevalence rate and affects all age groups equally.

**hy·per·e·o·sin·o·phil·ia** (hī'pĕr-ē-ō-sin-ō-fil'ē-ă) a greater degree of increase in the number of eosinophilic granulocytes in the circulating blood or the tissues than would be expected in the disease or condition causing the increase.

**hy·per·e·o·sin·o·phil·ic syn·drome** persistent peripheral eosinophilia with later infiltration into bone marrow, heart, and other organ systems; accompanied by nocturnal sweating, coughing, anorexia and weight loss, itching and various skin lesions, and symptoms of Löffler endocarditis.

**hy·per·er·ga·sia** (hī-pĕr-er-gā'zē-ă) increased or excessive functional activity. [hyper- + G. *ergasia,* work]

**hy·per·er·gia** (hī'pĕr-er'jē-ă) an allergic hypersensitivity. SYN hypergia.

**hy·per·er·gic** (hī-pĕr-er'jik) relating to hyperergia. SYN hypergic.

**hy·per·e·ryth·ro·cy·the·mia** (hī'pĕr-ē-rith'rō-sī-thē 'mē-ă) SYN hypercythemia.

**hy·per·es·o·pho·ria** (hī'pĕr-es-ō-fō'rē-ă) a tendency of one eye to deviate upward and inward, prevented by binocular vision. [hyper- + G. *esō,* inward, + *phora,* movement]

**hy·per·es·the·sia** (hī'pĕr-es-thē'zē-ă) abnormal acuteness of sensitivity to touch, pain, or other sensory stimuli. SYN oxyesthesia. [hyper- + G. *aisthēsis,* sensation]

**hy·per·es·thet·ic** (hī'pĕr-es-thet'ik) marked by hyperesthesia.

**hy·per·ex·o·pho·ria** (hī'pĕr-ek-sō-fō'rē-ă) a tendency of one eye to deviate upward and outward, prevented by binocular vision. [hyper- + G. *exō,* outward, + *phora,* movement]

**hy·per·ex·ten·sion** (hī'pĕr-eks-ten'shŭn) extension of a limb or part beyond the normal limit.

**hy·per·ex·ten·sion-hy·per·flex·ion in·ju·ry** violence to the body causing the unsupported head to move rapidly backward and forward resulting in hyperextension and hyperflexion of the neck; does not imply any specific resultant trauma or pathology.

**hy·per·fer·re·mia** (hī'pĕr-fer-ē'mē-ă) high serum iron level; found in hemochromatosis.

**hy·per·fi·brin·o·ge·ne·mia** (hī'pĕr-fī-brin'ō-jĕ-nē 'mē-ă) an increased level of fibrinogen in the blood. SYN fibrinogenemia.

**hy·per·fi·bri·nol·y·sis** (hī'pĕr-fī-brin-ol'i-sis) markedly increased fibrinolysis, as in subdural hematomas.

**hy·per·flex·ion** (hī-pĕr-flek'shŭn) flexion of a limb or part beyond the normal limit.

**hy·per·frac·tion·a·ted ra·di·a·tion** smaller fractions of a dose of radiation given more frequently than daily.

**hy·per·func·tion·al oc·clu·sion** occlusal stress of tooth or teeth exceeding normal physiologic demands.

**hy·per·gal·ac·to·sis** (hī'pĕr-ga-lak-tō'sis) excessive secretion of milk. [hyper- + G. *gala,* milk, + *-ōsis,* condition]

**hy·per·gam·ma·glo·bu·li·nae·mia [Br.]** SEE hypergammaglobulinemia.

**hy·per·gam·ma·glob·u·lin·e·mia** (hī'pĕr-gam-ă-glob'yu-li-nē' mē-ă) an increased concentration of γ-globulins in the plasma.

**hy·per·gen·e·sis** (hī-pĕr-jen'ē-sis) excessive development or redundant production of parts or organs of the body. [hyper- + G. *genesis,* production]

**hy·per·ge·net·ic** (hī-pĕr-jĕ-net'ik) relating to hypergenesis.

**hy·per·gen·i·tal·ism** (hī-pĕr-jen'i-tăl-izm) abnormal overdevelopment of genitalia.

**hy·per·geu·sia** (hī-pĕr-goo'sē-ă) abnormal acuteness of the sense of taste. SYN oxygeusia. [hyper- + G. *geusis,* taste]

**hy·per·gia** (hī-pĕr'jē-ă) SYN hyperergia.

**hy·per·gic** (hī-pĕr'jik) SYN hyperergic.

**hy·per·glan·du·lar** (hī-pĕr-glan'dyŭ-lăr) characterized by overactivity or increased size of a gland.

**hy·per·glob·u·lin·e·mia** (hī'pĕr-glob'yu-lin-ē' mē-ă) an abnormally high concentration of globulins in the circulating blood plasma.

**hy·per·gly·cae·mia [Br.]** SEE hyperglycemia.

**hyperglycemia** (hī'pĕr-glī-sē'mē-ă) an abnormally high concentration of glucose in the blood, a feature of diabetes mellitus. [hyper- + G. *glykys,* sweet, + *haima,* blood]

**hy·per·glyc·er·i·de·mia** (hī'pĕr-glis'er-i-dē'mē-ă) elevated plasma concentration of glycerides; normal if transiently present after absorption of a meal containing lipids, abnormal if a persistent state.

**hy·per·gly·ci·ne·mia** (hī'pĕr-glī-si-nē'mē-ă) elevated plasma glycine concentration.

**hy·per·gly·ci·nu·ria** (hī'pĕr-glī-sin-yur'ē-ă) enhanced urinary excretion of glycine.

**hy·per·gly·co·gen·ol·y·sis** (hī'pĕr-glī'kō-jĕ-nol' i-sis) excessive glycogenolysis. [hyper- + glycogen + G. *lysis,* loosening]

**hy·per·gly·cor·rha·chia** (hī'pĕr-glī-kō-rak'ē-ă) excessive sugar in the cerebrospinal fluid. [hyper- + G. *glykys,* sweet, + *rhachis,* spine]

**hy·per·gly·co·su·ria** (hī'pĕr-glī-kōs-yu'rē-ă) persistent excretion of unusually large amounts of glucose in the urine.

**hy·per·go·nad·ism** (hī-pĕr-gō'nad-izm) a clinical state resulting from enhanced secretion of gonadal hormones.

**hy·per·go·nad·o·tro·pic** (hī'pĕr-gō'nă-dō-trop' ik) indicating an increased production or excretion of gonadotropic hormones.

**hy·per·go·nad·o·tro·pic eu·nuch·oid·ism** eunuchoidism of gonadal origin, commonly accompanied by enhanced levels of pituitary gonadotropins in the blood and urine, as in Klinefelter syndrome.

**hy·per·he·mo·glo·bi·ne·mia** (hī'pĕr-hē'mō-glō-bi-nē'mē-ă) an unusually large amount of hemoglobin in the circulating blood plasma.

**hy·per·hi·dro·sis** (hī'pĕr-hī-drō'sis) excessive or profuse sweating. SYN hyperidrosis, polyhidrosis, polyidrosis. [hyper- + hidrosis]

**hy·per·hy·dra·tion** (hī'pĕr-hī-drā'shŭn) excess water content of the body.

**hy·per·i·dro·sis** (hī'pĕr-i-drō'sis) SYN hyperhidrosis.

**hy·per-IgM syn·drome** an X-linked immunodeficiency disorder with very low serum concentrations of IgG and IgA with a normal or a markedly elevated concentration of polyclonal IgM; affected boys develop recurrent bacterial infections in the 1st or 2nd year of life.

**hy·per·im·mu·no·glob·u·lin E syn·drome** an immunodeficiency disorder characterized by high levels of plasma IgE concentrations, a leukocyte chemotactic defect, and recurrent staphylococcal infections of the skin, upper respiratory tract, and other sites.

**hy·per·in·fec·tion** (hī′pĕr-in-fek′shŭn) infection by very large numbers of organisms as a result of immunologic deficiency.

**hy·per·in·su·lin·ae·mia [Br.]** SYN hyperinsulinism.

**hy·per·in·su·li·ne·mia** (hī′pĕr-in′sŭ-lin-ē-mē-ă) SYN hyperinsulinism.

**hy·per·in·su·lin·ism** (hī′pĕr-in′sŭ-lin-izm) increased levels of insulin in the plasma due to increased secretion of insulin by the beta cells of the pancreatic islets. SYN hyperinsulinaemia, hyperinsulinism.

**hy·per·in·vo·lu·tion** (hī′pĕr-in′vō-loo′shŭn) SYN superinvolution.

**hy·per·i·so·ton·ic** (hī′pĕr-ī-sō-ton′ik) SYN hypertonic.

**hy·per·ka·lae·mia [Br.]** SEE hyperkalemia.

**hy·per·ka·le·mia** (hī′pĕr-kă-lē′mē-ă) a greater than normal concentration of potassium ions in the circulating blood. SYN hyperpotassemia. [hyper- + Mod. L. *kalium,* potash, + G. *haima,* blood]

**hy·per·ka·le·mic pe·ri·od·ic pa·ral·y·sis** a form of periodic paralysis in which the serum potassium level is elevated during attacks; onset occurs in infancy, attacks are frequent but relatively mild, and myotonia is often present.

**hy·per·ker·a·tin·i·za·tion** (hī′pĕr-ker′at-i-ni-zā′shŭn) SYN hyperkeratosis.

**hy·per·ker·a·to·sis** (hī′pĕr-ker-ă-tō′sis) thickening of the horny layer of the epidermis or mucous membrane. SEE ALSO keratoderma, keratosis. SYN hyperkeratinization.

**hy·per·ke·to·ne·mia** (hī′pĕr-kē′tō-nē′mē-ă) elevated concentrations of ketone bodies in the blood.

**hy·per·ke·ton·u·ria** (hī′pĕr-kē′tōn-yur′ē-ă) increased urinary excretion of ketonic compounds.

**hy·per·ki·ne·mia** (hī′pĕr-ki-nē′mē-ă) increased circulation rate; increased volume flow through the circulation; supernormal cardiac output. [hyper- + G. *kineō,* to move, + *haima,* blood]

**hy·per·ki·ne·sis, hy·per·ki·ne·sia** (hī′pĕr-ki-nē′sis, hī′pĕr-ki-nē′zē-ă) **1.** excessive motility. **2.** excessive muscular activity. SYN supermotility. [hyper- + G. *kinēsis,* motion]

**hy·per·ki·net·ic** (hī′pĕr-ki-net′ik) pertaining to or characterized by hyperkinesia.

**hy·per·ki·net·ic dys·arth·ria** dysarthria associated with disorders of the extrapyramidal motor system resulting in involuntary movements of the articulatory and respiratory systems that cause variations in voice loudness and rate, and interruptions in ongoing speech. SEE ALSO extrapyramidal motor system, myoclonus, athetosis, Gilles de la Tourette syndrome.

**hy·per·ki·net·ic syn·drome** a condition marked by pathologically excessive energy seen sometimes in young children with brain injury, mental illness, and attention deficit disorder, and in epileptics; hypermotility and emotional instability are the chief characteristics; distractibility, inattention, and lack of shyness and of fear are common accompaniments.

**hy·per·leu·ko·cy·to·sis** (hī′pĕr-loo′kō-sī-tō′sis)

an increase in the number and proportion of leukocytes in the circulating blood or the tissues greater than that ordinarily observed in most instances of leukocytosis.

**hy·per·li·pae·mia [Br.]** SEE hyperlipemia.

**hy·per·li·pe·mia** (hī′pĕr-li-pē′mē-ă) hyperlipemia is associated with a deficiency of δ-aminoadipic semialdehyde synthase. SEE ALSO lipemia. [hyper- + G. *lipos,* fat, + *haima,* blood]

**hy·per·lip·i·dae·mia [Br.]** SYN lipemia.

**hy·per·lip·id·e·mia** (hī′pĕr-lip-i-dē′mē-ă) SYN lipemia.

**hy·per·lip·oi·de·mia** (hī′pĕr-lip-oy-dē′mē-ă) SYN lipemia.

**hy·per·li·po·pro·tei·nae·mia [Br.]** SEE hyperlipoproteinemia.

**hy·per·lip·o·pro·tein·e·mia** (hī′pĕr-lip′ō-prō′tē-in-ē′ă) an increase in the lipoprotein concentration of the blood.

**hy·per·lith·ur·ia** (hī′pĕr-lith-yur′ē-ă) an excessive excretion of uric (lithic) acid in the urine.

**hy·per·lu·cent** (hī′pĕr-loo′sent) a region on a chest film showing greater than normal film blackening from increased transmission of x-rays. [hyper- + L. *lucens,* shining, fr. *luceo,* to shine]

**hy·per·lu·cent lung** the radiographic finding that a lung or portion thereof is less dense than normal, as from air trapping by a bronchial foreign body, asymmetric emphysema, or decreasing blood flow.

**hy·per·ly·si·nae·mia [Br.]** SEE hyperlysinemia.

**hy·per·ly·si·ne·mia** a metabolic disorder characterized by mental retardation, convulsions, anemia, and asthenia; associated with an abnormal increase of the amino acid lysine in the circulating blood due to a deficiency of lysine-ketoglutarate reductase. One variant is associated with a deficiency of α-aminoadipic semialdehyde synthase, resulting in hyperlysinemia and saccharopinemia. SYN lysinemia.

**hy·per·ly·sin·ur·ia** (hī′pĕr-lī-sin-yur′ē-ă) the presence of abnormally high concentrations of lysine in the urine; a form of aminoaciduria that occurs in cystinuria, hepatolenticular degeneration, and the Fanconi syndrome.

**hy·per·mag·ne·sae·mia [Br.]** SEE hypermagnesemia.

**hy·per·mag·ne·se·mia** (hī′pĕr-mag-nĕ-sē′mē-ă) an abnormally large concentration of magnesium in the blood serum.

**hy·per·mas·tia** (hī-pĕr-mas′tē-ă) **1.** SYN polymastia. **2.** excessively large breasts. [hyper- + G. *mastos,* breast]

**hy·per·ma·ture cat·a·ract** a cataract in which the lens cortex becomes liquid, with the nucleus gravitating within the capsule (Morgagni cataract).

**hy·per·men·or·rhea** (hī′pĕr-men-ō-rē′ă) excessively prolonged or profuse menses. SYN menorrhagia, menostaxis. [hyper- + G. *mēn,* month, + *rhoia,* flow]

**hy·per·me·nor·rhoea [Br.]** SEE hypermenorrhea.

**hy·per·me·tab·o·lism** (hī′pĕr-me-tab′ŏ-lizm) heat production by the body above normal, as in thyrotoxicosis.

**hy·per·me·tria** (hī-pĕr-mē′trē-ă) ataxia characterized by overreaching a desired object or goal; usually seen with cerebellar disorders. Cf. hypometria. [hyper- + G. *metron,* measure]

h
y

**hy·per·me·tro·pia** (hī′pĕr-me-trō′pē-ă) SYN hyperopia. [hyper- + G. *metron*, measure, + *ōps*, eye]

**hy·per·mo·tor sei·zure** seizure characterized by automatisms involving predominantly proximal limb muscles and producing marked limb displacement.

**hy·per·my·o·to·nia** (hī′pĕr-mī-ō-tō′nē-ă) extreme muscular tonus. [hyper- + G. *mys*, muscle, + *tonos*, tension]

**hy·per·my·ot·ro·phy** (hī′pĕr-mī-ot′rō-fē) muscular hypertrophy. [hyper- + G. *mys*, muscle, + *trophē*, nourishment]

**hy·per·na·sal·i·ty** speech produced with excessive resonance in the nasal cavity, often due to dysfunction of the soft palate. SYN hyperrhinophonia.

**hy·per·na·trae·mia [Br.]** SEE hypernatremia.

**hy·per·na·tre·mia** (hī′pĕr-nă-trē′mē-ă) an abnormally high plasma concentration of sodium ions. [hyper- + natrium, + G. *haima*, blood]

**hy·per·na·tre·mic en·ceph·a·lop·a·thy** subarachnoid and subdural effusions in infants with hypernatremic dehydration.

**hy·per·ne·o·cy·to·sis** (hī′pĕr-nē′ō-sī-tō′sis) hyperleukocytosis in which there are considerable numbers of immature and young cells (especially in the granulocytic series). [hyper- + G. *neos*, new, + *kytos*, cell, + *-osis*, condition]

**hy·per·no·ea [Br.]** SEE hypernoia.

**hy·per·noia** (hī-pĕr-noy′ă) great rapidity of thought; excessive mental activity or imagination, as seen in the manic phase of bipolar disorder. [hyper- + G. *noeō*, to think]

**hy·per·on·cot·ic** (hī′pĕr-on-kot′ik) indicating an oncotic pressure higher than normal, e.g., of blood plasma.

**hy·per·o·nych·ia** (hī′pĕr-ō-nik′ē-ă) hypertrophy of the nails. [hyper- + G. *onyx, (onych-)*, nail]

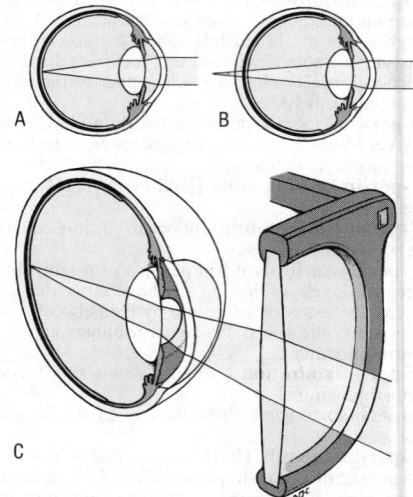**hy·per·o·pia (H)** (hī-pĕr-ō′pē-ă) longsightedness; that optical condition in which only convergent rays can be brought to focus on the retina. See this page. SYN farsightedness, hypermetropia. [hyper- + G. *ōps*, eye]

**hy·per·o·pic (H)** (hī-pĕr-ō′pik) pertaining to hyperopia.

**hy·per·o·pic a·stig·ma·tism** astigmatism in which one meridian is hyperopic and the one at a right angle to it is without a refractive error.

**hy·per·or·chi·dism** (hī-pĕr-ōr′ki-dizm) increased size or functioning of the testes. [hyper- + G. *orchis*, testis]

**hy·per·or·tho·cy·to·sis** (hī′pĕr-ōr′thō-sī-tō′sis) hyperleukocytosis in which the relative percentages of the various types of white blood cells are within the normal range. [hyper- + G. *orthos*, correct, + *kytos*, cell, + *-osis*, condition]

**hy·per·os·mia** (hī-pĕr-oz′mē-ă) an exaggerated or abnormally acute sense of smell. [hyper- + G. *osmē*, sense of smell]

**hy·per·os·mo·lal·i·ty** (hī′pĕr-oz-mō-lal′i-tē) increased concentration of a solution expressed as osmoles of solute per kilogram of serum water.

**hy·per·os·mo·lar (hy·per·gly·cem·ic) non··ke·tot·ic co·ma** a complication seen in diabetes mellitus in which marked hyperglycemia occurs (such as levels over 800 mg/dL), causing osmotic shifts in water in brain cells and resulting in coma. It can be fatal or lead to permanent neurologic damage. Ketoacidosis does not occur.

**hy·per·os·mo·lar·i·ty** (hī′pĕr-oz-mō-lar′i-tē) an

**hyperopia:** (A) normal (20/20) vision, light rays focus sharply on retina; (B) hyperopic (farsighted) vision, light rays from close objects come to sharp focus behind the retina; (C) hyperopia corrected by eyeglasses with convex lenses

increase in the osmotic concentration of a solution expressed as osmoles of solute per liter of solution.

**hy·per·os·mot·ic** (hī′pĕr-oz-mot′ik) **1.** having an osmolality greater than another fluid, ordinarily assumed to be plasma or extracellular fluid. **2.** relating to increased osmosis.

**hy·per·os·te·oi·do·sis** (hī′pĕr-os-tē-oy-dō′sis) excessive formation of osteoid, as seen in rickets and osteomalacia.

**hy·per·os·to·sis** (hī′pĕr-os-tō′sis) **1.** hypertrophy of bone. **2.** SYN exostosis. [hyper- + G. *osteon*, bone, + *-osis*, condition]

**hy·per·o·var·i·an·ism** (hī′pĕr-ō-var′ē-an-izm) sexual precocity in young girls due to premature development of ovaries accompanied by the secretion of ovarian hormones. SYN true precocious puberty.

**hy·per·ox·al·u·ria** (hī′pĕr-ok-săl-yur′ē-ă) presence of an unusually large amount of oxalic acid or oxalates in the urine. SYN oxaluria.

**hy·per·ox·ia** (hī-pĕr-ok′sē-ă) **1.** an increased amount of oxygen in tissues and organs. **2.** a greater oxygen tension than normal.

**hy·per·ox·y·gen·is·ed [Br.]**

**hy·per·ox·y·gen·iz·ed** (hī-pĕr-oks′ĭ-jĕn-īzd) combined with a large amount of oxygen.

**hy·per·par·a·sit·ism** (hī-pĕr-par′ă-sīt-izm) a condition in which a secondary parasite develops within a previously existing parasite.

**hy·per·par·a·thy·roid·ism** (hī′pĕr-par-ă-thī′royd-izm) a condition due to an increase in the secretion of the parathyroids, causing elevated serum calcium, decreased serum phosphorus, and increased excretion of both calcium and phosphorus, calcium stones and sometimes generalized osteitis fibrosa cystica.

**hy·per·pep·sin·ia** (hī′pĕr-pep-sin′ē-ă) an excess of pepsin in the gastric juice.

**hy·per·per·i·stal·sis** (hī′pĕr-per-i-stahl′sis) excessive rapidity of the passage of food through the stomach and intestine.

**hy·per·phe·nyl·al·a·ni·nae·mia [Br.]** SEE hyperphenylalaninemia.

**hy·per·phen·yl·al·a·ni·ne·mia** (hī′pĕr-fen′il-al-ă-ni-nē′ mēă) the presence of abnormally high blood levels of phenylalanine in newborn infants associated with phenylketonuria, maternal phenylketonuria, or transient deficiency of phenylalanine hydroxylase or *p*-hydroxyphenylpyruvic acid oxidase.

**hy·per·pho·ne·sis** (hī′pĕr-fō-nē′sis) an increase in the percussion sound or of the voice sound in auscultation. [hyper- + G. *phōnēsis,* a sounding]

**hy·per·pho·ria** (hī-pĕr-fō′rē-ă) a tendency of the visual axis of one eye to deviate upward, prevented by binocular vision. [hyper- + G. *phora,* motion]

**hy·per·phos·pha·tae·mia [Br.]** SEE hyperphosphatemia.

**hy·per·phos·pha·te·mia** (hī′pĕr-fos-fă-tē′mē-ă) abnormally high concentration of phosphates in the circulating blood.

**hy·per·phos·phat·ur·ia** (hī′pĕr-fos-făt-yur′ē-ă) an increased excretion of phosphates in the urine.

**hy·per·pig·men·ta·tion** (hī′pĕr-pig-men-tā′shŭn) an excess of pigment in a tissue or part.

**hy·per·pi·tu·i·ta·rism** (hī′pĕr-pi-too′i-tă-rizm) excessive production of anterior pituitary hormones, especially growth hormone; may result in gigantism or acromegaly.

**hy·per·pla·sia** (hī-pĕr-plā′zē-ă) an increase in number of cells in a tissue or organ, excluding tumor formation, whereby the bulk of the part or organ may be increased. SEE ALSO hypertrophy. [hyper- + G. *plasis,* a molding]

**hy·per·plas·tic** (hī-pĕr-plas′tik) relating to hyperplasia.

**hy·per·plas·tic gin·gi·vi·tis** gingivitis of long-standing duration in which the gingiva becomes enlarged and firm due to proliferation of fibrous connective tissue.

**hy·per·plas·tic pol·yp** a benign small sessile polyp of the large bowel showing lengthening and cystic dilation of mucosal glands; also applied to non-neoplastic gastric mucosal polyps. SYN metaplastic polyp.

**hy·per·plas·tic pulp·i·tis** hyperplastic granulation tissue growing out of the exposed pulp chamber of a grossly decayed tooth.

**hy·per·pnea** (hī-pĕr-nē′ă) breathing that is deeper and more rapid than is normal at rest. [hyper- + G. *pnoē,* breathing]

**hy·perp·noea [Br.]** SEE hyperpnea.

**hy·per·po·lar·i·za·tion** (hī′pĕr-pō′lăr-i-zā′ shŭn) an increase in polarization of membranes of nerves or muscle cells; the reverse change from that associated with excitatory action.

**hy·per·po·ne·sis** (hī′pĕr-pō-nē′sis) exaggerated activity within the motor portion of the nervous system. [hyper- + G. *ponos,* toil]

**hy·per·po·tas·se·mia** (hī′pĕr-pō-tas-ē′mē-ă) SYN hyperkalemia.

**hy·per·pre·be·ta·lip·o·pro·tein·e·mia** (hī′pĕr-prē-bā′tă-lip-ō-prō′tēn-ē′mē-ă) increased concentrations of pre-β-lipoproteins in the blood.

**hy·per·pro·in·su·li·ne·mia** (hī′pĕr-prō-in′sŭl-i-

nē′mēă) elevated plasma levels of proinsulin or proinsulin-like material.

**hy·per·pro·lac·ti·nae·mia [Br.]** SEE hyperprolactinemia.

**hy·per·pro·lac·ti·ne·mia** (hī′pĕr-prō-lak-ti-nē′mē-ă) elevated levels of prolactin in the blood; a normal physiological reaction during lactation, but pathological otherwise; often due to physical or emotional stress or rapid weight loss, sometimes to pituitary adenoma; amenorrhea is usually present.

**hy·per·pro·li·nae·mia [Br.]** SEE hyperprolinemia.

**hy·per·pro·li·ne·mia** (hī′per-prō-tē-in-ē′mē-ă) a metabolic disorder characterized by enhanced plasma proline concentrations and urinary excretion of proline, hydroxyproline, and glycine; autosomal recessive inheritance. Type I hyperprolinemia is associated with a deficiency of proline oxidase and renal disease; Type II hyperprolinemia is associated with a deficiency of Δ-pyrroline-5-carboxylate dehydrogenase, mental retardation, and convulsions and is caused by mutation in the δ-pyrroline 5 carboxylate gene (P5CD) on 1p.

**hy·per·pro·tein·e·mia** (hī′pĕr-prō′tēn-ē′mē-ă) an abnormally large concentration of protein in plasma.

**hy·per·pro·te·o·sis** (hī′pĕr-prō-tē-ō′sis) the condition due to an excessive amount of protein in the diet.

**hy·per·py·ret·ic** (hī′pĕr-pī-ret′ik) relating to hyperpyrexia. SYN hyperpyrexial.

**hy·per·py·rex·ia** (hī′pĕr-pī-rek′sē-ă) extremely high fever. [hyper- + G. *pyrexis,* feverishness]

**hy·per·py·rex·i·al** (hī′pĕr-pī-rek′sē-ăl) SYN hyperpyretic.

**hy·per·re·ac·tive ma·lar·i·ous sple·no·meg·a·ly** a syndrome characterized by persistent splenomegaly, exceptionally high serum IgM and malaria antibody levels, and hepatic sinusoidal lymphocytosis. SYN tropical splenomegaly syndrome.

**hy·per·re·flex·ia** (hī′pĕr-rē-flek′sē-ă) a condition in which the deep tendon reflexes are exaggerated.

**hy·per·res·o·nance** (hī-pĕr-rez′ō-nans) **1.** an extreme degree of resonance. **2.** resonance increased above the normal, and often of lower pitch, on percussion of an area of the body; occurs in the chest due to overinflation of the lung as in emphysema or pneumothorax and in the abdomen over a distended bowel.

**hy·per·rhi·no·pho·nia** SYN hypernasality.

**hy·per·sal·i·va·tion** (hī′pĕr-sal-i-vā′shŭn) increased salivation.

**hy·per·sen·si·tiv·i·ty** (hī′pĕr-sen-si-tiv′i-tē) abnormal sensitivity, a condition in which there is an exaggerated response by the body to the stimulus of a foreign agent. SEE allergy.

**hy·per·sen·si·tiv·i·ty pneu·mo·ni·tis** chronic progressive form of pneumonia with wheezing, dyspnea, diffuse infiltrates seen on radiographs; occurs following exposure to any of a variety of antigens, sometimes occupational and many names are given to cases with known types of exposure (such as farmer's lung, maple bark stripper's lung, chicken plucker's lung, bagassosis, byssinosis, humidifier lung, etc.); can progress to irreversible interstitial fibrotic disease with restrictive pattern on pulmonary function,

h
y

but in early disease most manifestations are reversible if offending antigen is identified and removed from environment.

**hy·per·sen·si·ti·za·tion** (hī'pĕr-sen'si-ti-zā'shŭn) the immunological process by which hypersensitivity is induced.

**hy·per·som·nia** (hī-pĕr-som'nē-ă) a condition in which sleep periods are excessively long, but the person responds normally in the intervals; distinguished from somnolence. [hyper- + L. *somnus,* sleep]

**hy·per·splen·ism** (hī-pĕr-splēn'izm) any condition in which the cellular components of the blood or platelets are removed at an abnormally high rate by the spleen.

**hy·per·sthe·nia** (hī-pĕr-sthē'nē-ă) excessive tension or strength. [hyper- + G. *sthenos,* strength]

**hy·per·sthen·ic** (hī-pĕr-sthen'ik) 1. pertaining to or marked by hypersthenia. 2. pertaining to a habitus characterized by marked overdevelopment of skeletal muscle.

**hy·per·sthen·u·ria** (hī'pĕr-sthen-yu'rē-ă) excretion of urine of unusually high specific gravity and concentration of solutes, resulting usually from loss or deprivation of water. [hyper- + G. *sthenos,* strength, + *ouron,* urine]

**hy·per·tel·or·ism** (hī-pĕr-tel'ōr-izm) abnormal distance between two paired organs. [hyper- + G. *tēle,* far off, + *horizō,* to separate, fr. *horos,* a boundary]

**hy·per·ten·sion** (hī'pĕr-ten'shŭn) high blood pressure; generally established guidelines are values of more than 140 mmHg systolic, or more than 90 mmHg diastolic blood pressure. Despite many discrete and inherited but rare forms that have been identified, the evidence is that for the most part blood pressure is a multifactorial, perhaps galtonian trait. [hyper- + L. *tensio,* tension]

**hy·per·ten·sive** (hī-pĕr-ten'siv) 1. marked by an increased blood pressure. 2. denoting a person suffering from high blood pressure.

**hy·per·ten·sive ar·te·ri·op·a·thy** arterial degeneration resulting from hypertension.

**hy·per·ten·sive ar·te·ri·o·scle·ro·sis** progressive increase in muscle and elastic tissue of arterial walls, resulting from hypertension; in long-standing hypertension, elastic tissue forms numerous concentric layers in the intima and there is replacement of muscle by collagen fibers and hyaline thickening of the intima of arterioles; such changes can develop with increasing age in the absence of hypertension and may then be referred to as senile arteriosclerosis.

**hy·per·ten·sive ret·i·nop·a·thy** a retinal condition occurring in accelerated vascular hypertension, marked by arteriolar constriction, flame-shaped hemorrhages, cotton-wool patches, star-figure edema at the macula, and papilledema.

**hy·per·ten·sive up·per e·so·pha·ge·al sphinc·ter** SYN cricopharyngeal achalasia.

**hy·per·ten·sor** (hī-pĕr-ten'ser) SYN pressor.

**hy·per·the·co·sis** (hī'pĕr-thē-kō'sis) diffuse hyperplasia of the theca cells of the graafian follicles.

**hy·per·the·lia** (hī-pĕr-thē'lē-ă) SYN polythelia. [hyper- + G. *thēlē,* nipple]

**hy·per·ther·mal·ge·sia** (hī'pĕr-ther-măl-jē'zē-ă) extreme sensitiveness to heat. [hyper- + G. *thermē,* heat, + *algēsis,* pain]

**hy·per·ther·mia** (hī-pĕr-ther'mē-ă) therapeutically induced hyperpyrexia. [hyper- + G. *thermē,* heat]

**hy·per·throm·bi·nae·mia** [Br.] SEE hyperthrombinemia.

**hy·per·throm·bi·ne·mia** (hī'pĕr-throm-bi-nē' mē-ă) an abnormal increase of thrombin in the blood, frequently resulting in a tendency to intravascular coagulation.

**hy·per·thy·mic** (hī-pĕr-thī'mik) 1. pertaining to hyperthymia. 2. pertaining to hyperthymism.

**hy·per·thy·roid·ism** (hī-pĕr-thī'royd-izm) an abnormality of the thyroid gland in which secretion of thyroid hormone is usually increased and is no longer under regulatory control of hypothalamic-pituitary centers; characterized by a hypermetabolic state, usually with weight loss, tremulousness, elevated plasma levels of thyroxin and/or triiodothyronine; often associated with exophthalmos (Graves disease).

**hy·per·thy·rox·i·nae·mia** [Br.] SEE hyperthyroxinemia.

**hy·per·thy·rox·i·ne·mia** (hī'pĕr-thī-rok-si-nē' mē-ă) an elevated thyroxine concentration in the blood.

**hy·per·to·nia** (hī-pĕr-tō'nē-ă) extreme tension of the muscles or arteries. SYN hypertonicity (1). [hyper- + G. *tonos,* tension]

**hy·per·ton·ic** (hī-pĕr-ton'ik) 1. having a greater degree of tension. SYN spastic (1). 2. having a greater osmotic pressure than a reference solution, which is ordinarily assumed to be blood plasma or interstitial fluid; more specifically, refers to a fluid in which cells shrink. SYN hyperisotonic.

**hy·per·to·nic·i·ty** (hī'pĕr-tō-nis'i-tē) 1. SYN hypertonia. 2. an increased effective osmotic pressure of body fluids.

**hy·per·tri·cho·sis** (hī'pĕr-tri-kō'sis) growth of hair in excess of the normal. SEE ALSO hirsutism. [hyper- + G. *trichōsis,* being hairy]

**hy·per·tri·gly·ce·ri·dae·mia** [Br.] SEE hypertriglyceridemia.

**hy·per·tri·glyc·er·i·de·mia** (hī'pĕr-trī-glis'er-i-dē'mē-ă) elevated triglyceride concentration in the blood.

**hy·per·tro·phic** (hī-pĕr-trof'ik) relating to or characterized by hypertrophy.

**hy·per·tro·phic ar·thri·tis** SYN osteoarthritis.

**hy·per·tro·phic car·di·o·my·o·pa·thy** cardiac hypertrophy of unknown cause, possibly genetic, with impairment of left ventricular filling, emptying, or both. SEE ALSO sudden death.

**hy·per·tro·phic pul·mo·nary os·te·o·ar·throp·a·thy** expansion of the distal ends, or the entire shafts, of the long bones, sometimes with erosions of the articular cartilages and thickening and villous proliferation of the synovial membranes, and frequently clubbing of fingers; the disorder occurs in chronic pulmonary disease, in heart disease, and occasionally in other acute and chronic disorders. SYN Bamberger-Marie disease.

**hy·per·tro·phic py·lor·ic ste·no·sis** muscular hypertrophy of the pyloric sphincter, associated with projectile vomiting beginning in the second or third week of life, usually in males. SYN congenital pyloric stenosis.

**hy·per·tro·phic rhi·ni·tis** chronic rhinitis with permanent thickening of the mucous membrane.

**hy·per·tro·phy** (hī-pĕr'trō-fē) general increase in bulk of a part or organ, due to increase in size, but not in number, of the individual tissue elements. SEE ALSO hyperplasia. [hyper- + G. *trophē,* nourishment]

**hy·per·tro·pia** (hī′pĕr-trō′pē-ă) an ocular deviation with one eye higher than the other. [hyper- + G. *tropē,* a turn]

**hy·per·u·ri·cae·mia [Br.]** SEE hyperuricemia.

**hy·per·u·ri·ce·mia** (hī′pĕr-yu-rē-sē′mē-ă) enhanced blood concentrations of uric acid.

**hy·per·u·ri·ce·mic** (hī′pĕr-yu-ri-sē′mik) relating to or characterized by hyperuricemia.

**hy·per·val·i·ne·mia** (hī′pĕr-val-i-nē′mē-ă) abnormally high plasma concentrations of valine, a common finding in maple syrup urine disease.

**hy·per·vas·cu·lar** (hī′pĕr-vas′kyu-ler) abnormally vascular; containing an excessive number of blood vessels. [hyper- + L. *vas,* a vessel]

**hy·per·ven·ti·la·tion** (hī′pĕr-ven-ti-lā′shŭn) increased alveolar ventilation relative to metabolic carbon dioxide production, so that alveolar carbon dioxide pressure decreases to below normal.

**hy·per·ven·ti·la·tion tet·a·ny** tetany caused by forced overbreathing, due to a reduction in $CO_2$ in the blood.

**hy·per·vi·ta·min·o·sis** (hī′pĕr-vī′tă-mi-nō′sis) a condition resulting from the ingestion of an excessive amount of a vitamin preparation, symptoms varying according to the particular vitamin.

**hy·per·vo·lae·mia [Br.]** SEE hypervolemia.

**hy·per·vo·le·mia** (hī′pĕr-vō-lē′mē-ă) abnormally increased volume of blood. SYN plethora (1), repletion (1). [hyper- + L. *volumen,* volume, + G. *haima,* blood]

**hy·per·vo·le·mic** (hī′pĕr-vō-lē′mik) pertaining to or characterized by hypervolemia.

**hyp·es·the·sia** (hi-p-es-thē′zē-ă) diminished sensitivity to stimulation. SYN hypoesthesia. [G. *hypo,* under, + *aisthēsis,* feeling]

**hy·pha,** pl. **hy·phae** (hī′fă, hī′fē) a branching tubular cell characteristic of the filamentous fungi (molds). Intercommunicating hyphae constitute a mycelium, the visible colony on natural substrates or artificial laboratory media. [G. *hyphē,* a web]

**hy·phae·ma [Br.]** SEE hyphema.

**hy·phae·mia [Br.]** SYN hypovolemia.

**hyp·he·do·nia** (hip-hē-dō′nē-ă) a habitually lessened or attenuated degree of pleasure from that which should normally give great pleasure. [G. *hypo,* under, + *hēdonē,* pleasure]

**hy·phe·ma** (hī-fē′mă) blood in the anterior chamber of the eye. See this page and B15. [G. *hyphaimos,* suffused with blood]

**hy·phe·mia** (hī-fē′mē-ă) SYN hypovolemia. [hypo- + G. *haima,* blood]

**hyp·na·gog·ic** (hip-nă-goj′ik) denoting a transitional state, related to the hypnoidal, preceding sleep; applied also to various hallucinations that may manifest themselves at that time. SEE ALSO hypnoidal. [hypno- + G. *agōgos,* leading]

**hyp·na·gog·ic hal·lu·cin·a·tion** a common symptom in narcolepsy characterized by vivid, dreamlike perceptions occurring with sleep onset. Often these perceptions involve fearful situations that are described as realistic and include visual, tactile, and auditory hallucinations.

**hyp·na·gogue** (hip′nă-gog) an agent that induces sleep. [hypno- + G. *agōgos,* leading]

**hyp·nap·a·gog·ic** (hip-nap-ă-goj′ik) denoting a state similar to the hypnagogic, through which the mind passes in coming out of sleep; denoting

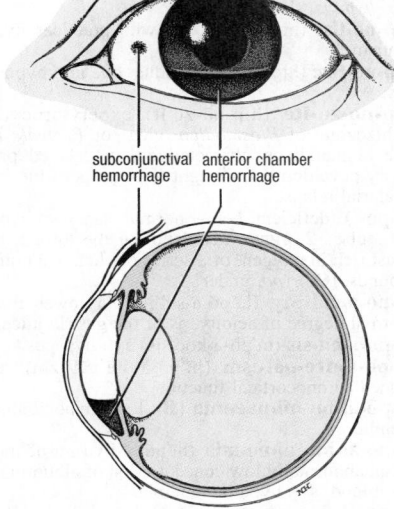

**hyphema** (anterior chamber hemorrhage) and subconjunctival hemorrhage

also hallucinations experienced at such time. [hypno- + G. *apo,* from, + *agōgos,* leading]

△**hyp·no-, hypn-** sleep, hypnosis. [G. *hypnos,*]

**hyp·no·a·nal·y·sis** (hip′nō-ă-nal′i-sis) psychoanalysis or other psychotherapy which employs hypnosis as an adjunctive technique.

**hyp·no·gen·e·sis** (hip-nō-jen′ĕ-sis) the induction of sleep or of the hypnotic state. [hypno- + G. *genesis,* production]

**hyp·no·gen·ic, hyp·nog·e·nous** (hip-nō-jen′ik, hip-noj′ĕ-nŭs) **1.** relating to hypnogenesis. **2.** an agent capable of inducing a hypnotic state. SEE hypnosis.

**hyp·no·gen·ic spot** a pressure-sensitive point on the body of certain susceptible persons, which, when pressed, causes the induction of sleep.

**hyp·noi·dal** (hip-noy′dăl) resembling hypnosis; denoting the subwaking state, a mental condition intermediate between sleeping and waking. SEE ALSO hypnagogic. [hypno- + G. *eidos,* resemblance]

**hyp·no·pom·pic hal·lu·ci·na·tion** vivid hallucinations that occur when wakening from sleep; occurs with narcolepsy, but grouped with hypnagogic hallucination.

**hyp·no·sis** (hip-nō′sis) an artificially induced trancelike state, resembling somnambulism, in which the subject is highly susceptible to suggestion and responds readily to the commands of the hypnotist. SEE ALSO mesmerism. [G. *hypnos,* sleep, + -*osis,* condition]

**hyp·no·ther·a·py** (hip-nō-thār′ă-pē) **1.** psychotherapeutic treatment by means of hypnotism. **2.** treatment of disease by inducing a trance-like sleep.

**hyp·not·ic** (hip-not′ik) **1.** causing sleep. **2.** an agent that promotes sleep. **3.** relating to hypnotism. [G. *hypnōtikos,* causing one to sleep]

h
y

**hyp·no·tism** (hip′nō-tizm) **1.** the process or act of inducing hypnosis. SYN somnipathy (2). **2.** the practice or study of hypnosis. SEE mesmerism. [G. *hypnos*, sleep]

**hyp·no·tist** (hip′nō-tist) one who practices hypnotism.

**hyp·no·tize** (hip′nō-tīz) to induct one into hypnosis.

**hyp·no·zo·ite** (hip-nō-zō′īt) exoerythrocytic schizozoite of *Plasmodium vivax* or *P. ovale* in the human liver, characterized by delayed primary development; thought to be responsible for malarial relapse.

⌂**hy·po- 1.** deficient, below normal. SEE ALSO hyp-. Cf. sub-. **2.** CHEMISTRY denoting the lowest, or least rich in oxygen, of a series of chemical compounds. [G. *hypo*, under]

**hy·po·a·cid·i·ty** (hī′pō-a-sid′i-tē) a lower than normal degree of acidity, as of the gastric juice.

**hy·po·a·cu·sis** (hī′pō-ă-koo′sis) SYN hypacusis.

**hy·po·a·dre·nal·ism** (hī′pō-ă-drē′năl-izm) reduced adrenocortical function.

**hy·po·al·bu·mi·nae·mia [Br.]** SEE hypoalbuminemia.

**hy·po·al·bu·mi·ne·mia** (hī′pō-al-byu-mi-nē′mē-ă) an abnormally low concentration of albumin in the blood. SYN hypalbuminemia.

**hy·po·al·do·ster·on·u·ria** (hī′pō-al-dos′ter-on-yur′ē-ă) abnormally low levels of aldosterone in the urine.

**hy·po·al·ge·sia** (hī-pō-al-jē′zē-ă) SYN hypalgesia. [hypo- + G. *algēsis*, a sense of pain]

**hy·po·az·ot·u·ria** (hī′pō-az-ōt-yur′ē-ă) excretion of abnormally small quantities of nonprotein nitrogenous material (especially urea) in the urine. [hypo- + Fr. *azote*, nitrogen, + G. *ouron*, urine]

**hy·po·bar·ic** (hī-pō-bar′ik) **1.** pertaining to pressure of ambient gases below 1 atmosphere. **2.** with respect to solutions, less dense than the diluent or medium; e.g., in spinal anesthesia, a hypobaric solution has a density lower than that of spinal fluid. [hypo- + G. *baros*, weight]

**hy·po·bar·ism** (hī-pō-bar′izm) dysbarism resulting from decreasing barometric pressure on the body without hypoxia; gas in body cavities tends to expand, and gases dissolved in body fluids tend to come out of solution as bubbles. Cf. decompression sickness.

**hy·po·ba·rop·a·thy** (hī′pō-ba-rop′ă-thē) sickness produced by reduced barometric pressure. [hypo- + G. *baros*, weight, + *pathos*, suffering]

**hy·po·bet·a·lip·o·pro·tein·ae·mia [Br.]** SEE hypobetalipoproteinemia.

**hy·po·be·ta·lip·o·pro·tein·e·mia** (hī′pō-bā′tă-lip′ō-prō′tēn-ē′mē-ă) abnormally low levels of β-lipoproteins in the plasma occasionally with acanthocytosis and neurological signs. SEE ALSO abetalipoproteinemia.

**hy·po·blast** (hī′pō-blast) SYN endoderm. [hypo- + G. *blastos*, germ]

**hy·po·blas·tic** (hī-pō-blas′tik) relating to or derived from the hypoblast.

**hy·po·cal·cae·mia [Br.]** SEE hypocalcemia.

**hy·po·cal·ce·mia** (hī′pō-kal-sē′mē-ă) abnormally low levels of calcium in the circulating blood; commonly denotes subnormal concentrations of calcium ions.

**hy·po·cal·ci·fi·ca·tion** (hī′pō-kal-si-fi-kā′shŭn) deficient calcification of bone or teeth.

**hy·po·cap·nia** (hī-pō-kap′nē-ă) abnormally decreased arterial carbon dioxide tension. SYN hypocarbia. [hypo- + G. *kapnos*, smoke, vapor]

**hy·po·car·bia** (hī-pō-kar′bē-ă) SYN hypocapnia.

**hy·po·chlo·rae·mia [Br.]** SEE hypochloremia.

**hy·po·chlor·e·mia** (hī′pō-klō-rē′mē-ă) an abnormally low level of chloride ions in the circulating blood.

**hy·po·chlor·hy·dria** (hī′pō-klōr-hī′drē-ă) presence of an abnormally small amount of hydrochloric acid in the stomach.

**hy·po·chlor·u·ria** (hī′pō-klōr-yu′rē-ă) excretion of abnormally small quantities of chloride ions in the urine.

**hy·po·cho·les·te·ro·lae·mia [Br.]** SEE hypocholesterolemia.

**hy·po·cho·les·ter·ol·e·mia** (hī′pō-kō-les′ter-ol-ē′mē-ă) the presence of abnormally small amounts of cholesterol in the circulating blood.

**hy·po·chon·dria** (hī-pō-kon′drē-ă) SYN hypochondriasis.

**hy·po·chon·dri·ac** (hī-pō-kon′drē-ak) **1.** a person with a somatic overconcern, including morbid attention to the details of bodily functioning and exaggeration of any symptoms no matter how insignificant. **2.** a person manifesting hypochondriasis. **3.** beneath the ribs; relating to the hypochondrium.

**hy·po·chon·dri·a·cal** (hī′pō-kon-drī′ă-kăl) relating to or suffering from hypochondriasis.

**hy·po·chon·dri·a·cal mel·an·cho·lia** melancholia with many associated physical complaints, often with little basis in fact.

**hy·po·chon·dri·ac re·gion** the region on each side of the abdomen covered by the costal cartilages; it is lateral to the epigastric region.

**hy·po·chon·dri·a·sis** (hī′pō-kon-drī′ă-sis) a morbid concern about one's own health and exaggerated attention to any unusual bodily or mental sensations; a delusion that one is suffering from some disease for which no physical basis is evident. SYN hypochondria. [fr. hypochondrium, regarded as the site of hypochondria, + G. *-iasis*, condition]

**hy·po·chon·dro·pla·sia** (hī′pō-kon-drō-plā′zē-ă) dwarfism similar to achondroplasia, not evident until mid-childhood; the skull and facies are normal. [hypo- + G. *chondros*, cartilage, + *plasis*, a molding]

**hy·po·chro·ma·sia** (hī′pō-krō-mā′zē-ă) SYN hypochromia.

**hy·po·chro·mat·ic** (hī′pō-krō-mat′ik) containing a small amount of pigment, or less than the normal amount for the individual tissue. SYN hypochromic (1). [hypo- + G. *chrōma*, color]

**hy·po·chro·ma·tism** (hī-pō-krō′mă-tizm) **1.** the condition of being hypochromatic. **2.** SYN hypochromia.

**hy·po·chro·mia** (hī-pō-krō′mē-ă) an anemic condition in which the percentage of hemoglobin in the red blood cells is less than the normal range. SYN hypochromasia, hypochromatism (2). [hypo- + G. *chrōma*, color]

**hy·po·chro·mic** (hī-pō-krō′mik) **1.** SYN hypochromatic. **2.** denoting decrease in light absorption with a shift in λ inferior to a lower wavelength.

**hy·po·chro·mic a·ne·mia** anemia characterized by a decrease in the ratio of the weight of hemoglobin to the volume of the erythrocyte, i.e., the mean corpuscular hemoglobin concentration is less than normal.

**hy·po·cone** (hī′pō-kōn) 1. The distolingual cusp of human upper molars. 2. A cusp appearing late in the evolution of the molars. SYN talon. [hypo- + G. *kōnos,* pine cone]

**hypoconid** (hī-pō-kon′id) 1. The distobuccal cusp of human lower molars. 2. One of the cusps that comprises the talonid of the molars. [hypocone + id (2)]

**hy·po·con·u·lid** (hī-pō-kon-yu′lid) 1. The distal cusp of the lower molars. 2. One of the cusps of the talonid. [hypo- + Mod. L. dim. of L. *conus,* cone]

**hy·po·cor·ti·coid·ism** (hī-pō-kōr′ti-koyd-izm) SYN adrenocortical insufficiency.

**hy·po·cu·pre·mia** (hī′pō-koo-prē′mē-ă) reduced copper content of the blood; found in Wilson disease because ceruloplasmin is depressed, even though serum albumin-attached copper is increased. [hypo- + L. *cuprum,* copper, + G. *haima,* blood]

**hy·po·cy·cloi·dal** (hī′pō-sī-kloy′dăl) a tricyclic motion used by mechanical tomography units to optimize blurring and reduce artifacts. [hypo- + G. *kuklos,* circle, + *-oeidēs,* appearance]

**hy·po·cy·thae·mia [Br.]** SEE hypocythemia.

**hy·po·cy·the·mia** (hī′pō-sī-thē′mē-ă) hypocytosis of the circulating blood, such as that observed in aplastic anemia. [hypo- + G. *kytos,* cell, + *haima,* blood]

**hy·po·dac·ty·ly, hy·po·dac·tyl·ia, hy·po·dac·tyl·ism** (hī′pō-dak′ti-lē, hī′pō-dak-til′ē-ă, hī′pō-dak′til-izm) a condition of having fewer than the normal complement of digits. [hypo- + G. *daktylos,* finger]

**hy·po·der·mic** (hī′pō-der′mik) SYN subcutaneous.

**hy·po·der·mic sy·ringe** a small syringe with a barrel (which may be calibrated), perfectly matched plunger, and tip; used with a hollow needle for subcutaneous injections and for aspiration.

**hy·po·der·mic tab·let** a compressed or molded tablet that dissolves completely in water to form an injectable solution.

**hy·po·der·mis** (hī-pō-der′mis) SYN superficial fascia.

**hy·po·der·moc·ly·sis** (hī′pō-der-mok′li-sis) subcutaneous injection of a saline or other solution. [hypo- + G. *derma,* skin, + *klysis,* a washing out]

**hy·po·dip·sia** (hī-pō-dip′sē-ă) a reduced sense of thirst; a physiologic condition, perhaps caused by hypertonicity of body fluids; loosely, oligodipsia. [hypo- + G. *dipsa,* thirst]

**hy·po·don·tia** (hī-pō-don′shē-ă) a condition of having fewer than the normal complement of teeth, either congenital or acquired. SYN oligodontia. [hypo- + G. *odous,* tooth]

**hy·po·dy·nam·ic** (hī′pō-dī-nam′ik) possessing or exhibiting subnormal power or force.

**hy·po·ec·cri·sis** (hī′pō-ek′ri-sis) reduced excretion of waste matter. [hypo- + G. *eccrisis,* separation]

**hy·po·ec·crit·ic** (hī′pō-ĕ-krit′ik) characterized by hypoeccrisis.

**hy·po·ech·o·ic** (hī′pō-ē-kō′ik) pertaining to a region in an ultrasound image in which the echoes are weaker or fewer than normal or in the surrounding regions. [hypo- + echo + -ic]

**hy·po·es·o·pho·ria** (hī′pō-es-ō-fō′rē-ă) a tendency of the visual axis of one eye to deviate downward and inward, prevented by binocular vision. [hypo- + G. *eso,* within, + *phoros,* bearing]

**hy·po·es·the·sia** (hī′pō-es-thē′zē-ă) SYN hypesthesia.

**hy·po·ex·o·pho·ria** (hī′pō-ek-sō-fō′rē-ă) a tendency of the visual axis of one eye to deviate downward and outward, prevented by binocular vision. [hypo- + G. *exo,* without, + *phoros,* bearing]

**hy·po·fer·re·mia** (hī′pō-fer-ē′mē-ă) a deficiency of iron in the circulating blood.

**hy·po·fi·bri·no·ge·nae·mia [Br.]** SEE hypofibrinogenemia.

**hy·po·fi·brin·o·ge·ne·mia** (hī′pō-fī-brin′ō-jĕ-nē′mē-ă) abnormally low concentration of fibrinogen in the circulating blood plasma.

**hy·po·frac·tion·a·ted ra·di·a·tion** larger fractions of a dose of radiation given less frequently than daily.

**hy·po·fron·tal·i·ty** (hī′pō-fron-tal′i-tē) a decrease in the neuronal activity of various areas of the frontal lobes, arising from various causes and associated with a number of clinical symptoms or disorders.

**hy·po·func·tion** (hī′pō-fŭnk-shŭn) reduced, low, or inadequate function.

**hy·po·ga·lac·tia** (hī′pō-ga-lak′shē-ă) less than normal milk secretion. [hypo- + G. *gala,* milk]

**hy·po·ga·lac·tous** (hī′pō-ga-lak′tŭs) producing or secreting a less than normal amount of milk.

**hy·po·gam·ma·glob·u·lin·ae·mia [Br.]** SEE hypogammaglobulinemia.

**hy·po·gam·ma·glob·u·lin·e·mia** (hī′pō-gam′ă-glob′yu-li-nē′mē-ă) decreased gamma fraction of serum globulin; associated with increased susceptibility to pyogenic infections.

**hy·po·gan·gli·o·no·sis** (hī′pō-gang-lē-on-ō′sis) a reduction in the number of ganglionic nerve cells.

**hy·po·gas·tric** (hī-pō-gas′trik) relating to the hypogastrium.

**hy·po·gas·tric nerve** one of the two nerve trunks (right and left) which lead from the superior hypogastric plexus into the pelvis to join the inferior hypogastric plexuses. SYN nervus hypogastricus [TA].

**hy·po·gas·tros·chi·sis** (hī′pō-gas-tros′ki-sis) congenital fissure of the anterior abdominal wall in the hypogastric region. [hypogastrium + G. *schisis,* cleaving]

**hy·po·gen·e·sis** (hī′pō-jen′ĕ-sis) congenital defect of growth with underdevelopment of parts or organs of the body. [hypo- + G. *genesis,* origin]

**hy·po·ge·net·ic** (hī′pō-jĕ-net′ik) relating to hypogenesis.

**hy·po·gen·i·tal·ism** (hī-pō-jen′i-tăl-izm) partial or complete failure of maturation of the genitalia; commonly, a consequence of hypogonadism.

**hy·po·geu·sia** (hī-pō-goo′zē-ă) blunting of the sense of taste. [hypo- + G. *geusis,* taste]

**hy·po·glos·sal** (hī-pō-glos′ăl) 1. below the tongue. 2. relating to the twelfth cranial nerve, nervus hypoglossus. [L. *hypoglossus* fr. hypo- + *glossus,* tongue]

**hy·po·glos·sal ca·nal** the canal through which the hypoglossal nerve emerges from the skull. SYN canalis hypoglossalis [TA], anterior condyloid foramen.

**hy·po·glos·sal nerve [CN XII]** arises from an oblong nucleus in the medulla and emerges by several root filaments between the pyramid and

h
y

the olive via the preolivary groove; it passes through the hypoglossal canal, then courses downward and forward to supply the intrinsic and four of five extrinsic muscles of the tongue. SYN nervus hypoglossus [CN XII] [TA], twelfth cranial nerve [CN XII].

**hy·po·glos·sal nu·cle·us** the motor nucleus innervating the intrinsic and four of the five extrinsic muscles of the tongue; it is located in the medulla oblongata near the midline, immediately beneath the floor of the inferior recess of the rhomboid fossa.

**hy·po·glot·tis** (hī′pō-glot′is) the undersurface of the tongue. [G. *hypoglōssis*, or *-glōttis*, undersurface of tongue, fr. *hypo*, under, + *glōssa*, tongue]

**hy·po·gly·cae·mia [Br.]** SEE hypoglycemia.

**hy·po·gly·cae·mic [Br.]** SEE hypoglycemic.

**hy·po·gly·ce·mia** (hī′pō-glī-sē′mē-ă) an abnormally small concentration of glucose in the circulating blood.

**hy·po·gly·ce·mic** (hī′pō-glī-sē′mik) pertaining to or characterized by hypoglycemia.

**hy·po·gly·ce·mic co·ma** a metabolic encephalopathy caused by hypoglycemia; usually seen in diabetics, and due to exogenous insulin excess.

**hy·po·gly·co·gen·ol·y·sis** (hī′pō-glī′kō-jĕ-nol′i-sis) deficient glycogenolysis.

**hy·po·gly·cor·rhach·ia** (hī′pō-glī-kō-rak′ē-ă) depressed concentration of glucose in the cerebrospinal fluid; a characteristic of bacterial, fungal, and tuberculous meningitis. [hypo- + G. *glykys*, sweet, + *rhachis*, spine]

**hy·pog·na·thous** (hī′pō-nath′ŭs, hī-pog′na-thŭs) having an abnormally small lower jaw. [hypo- + G. *gnathos*, jaw]

**hy·po·go·nad·ism** (hī′pō-gō′nad-izm) inadequate gonadal function, as manifested by deficiencies in gametogenesis and/or the secretion of gonadal hormones.

**hy·po·go·nad·o·tro·pic** (hī′pō-gon′ă-dō-trop′ik) indicating inadequate secretion of gonadotropins and its consequences.

**hy·po·hi·dro·sis** (hī′pō-hi-drō′sis) diminished perspiration.

**hy·po·hi·drot·ic** (hī′pō-hi-drot′ik) characterized by diminished sweating.

**hy·po·hy·dra·tion** decrease in body water content. New steady-state condition of decreased water content.

**hy·po·ka·lae·mia [Br.]** SEE hypokalemia.

**hy·po·ka·le·mia** (hī′pō-ka-lē′mē-ă) the presence of an abnormally small concentration of potassium ions in the circulating blood; occurs in familial periodic paralysis and in potassium depletion due to excessive loss from the gastrointestinal tract or kidneys. The changes of hypokalemia may include vacuolation of renal tubular epithelial cytoplasm with impairment of urinary concentrating power and acidification, flattening of the T wave of the electrocardiogram, and muscle weakness. SYN hypopotassemia. [hypo- + Mod. L. *kalium*, potassium, + G. *haima*, blood]

**hy·po·ka·le·mic pe·ri·od·ic pa·ral·y·sis** periodic paralysis in which the serum potassium level is low during attacks; attacks may be precipitated by cold, high carbohydrate meal, or alcohol, may last hours to days, and may cause respiratory paralysis.

**hy·po·ki·ne·sis, hy·po·ki·ne·sia** (hī′pō-ki-nē′sis, hī′pō-ki-nē′zē-ă) diminished or slow move-

ment. SYN hypomotility. [hypo- + G. *kinēsis,* movement]

**hy·po·ki·net·ic** (hī′pō-ki-net′ik) relating to or characterized by hypokinesis.

**hy·po·ki·ne·tic dys·arth·ria** dysarthria associated with disorders of the extrapyramidal motor system resulting in reduction and rigidity of movement, causing monotony of pitch and loudness, reduced stress, and imprecise enunciation of consonants. SEE ALSO extrapyramidal motor system, parkinsonian dysarthria.

**hy·po·ley·dig·ism** (hī-pō-lī′dig-izm) subnormal secretion of androgens by the interstitial (Leydig) cells of the testes.

**hy·po·lip·o·pro·tein·ae·mia [Br.]** SEE hypolipoproteinemia.

**hy·po·lip·o·pro·tein·e·mia** (hī-pō-li-pō-prō-tē-ne′mē-ă) [Br.] an abnormally low level of lipoprotein in plasma.

**hy·po·mag·nes·ae·mia [Br.]** SEE hypomagnesemia.

**hy·po·mag·ne·se·mia** (hī′pō-mag-nē-sē′mē-ă) subnormal blood serum concentration of magnesium.

**hy·po·mas·tia** (hī′pō-mas′tē-ă) atrophy or congenital smallness of the breasts. [hypo- + G. *mastos,* breast]

**hy·po·me·lia** (hī-pō-mē′lē-ă) general term for hypoplasia of some or all parts of one or more limbs. [hypo- + G. *melos,* limb]

**hy·po·men·or·rhea** (hī′pō-men-ō-rē′ă) diminution of the flow or a shortening of the duration of menstruation. [hypo- + G. *mēn,* month, + *rhoia,* flow]

**hy·po·me·nor·rhoea [Br.]** SEE hypomenorrhea.

**hy·po·mere** (hī′pō-mēr) **1.** the portion of the myotome that extends ventrolaterally to form body-wall muscle, innervated by the primary anterior ramus of a spinal nerve. **2.** somatic and splanchnic layers of the lateral mesoderm that give rise to the lining of the celom. [hypo- + G. *meros,* part]

**hy·po·me·tab·o·lism** (hī′pō-me-tab′ō-lizm) reduced metabolism.

**hy·po·me·tria** (hī-pō-mē′trē-ă) ataxia characterized by underreaching an object or goal; seen with cerebellar disease. Cf. hypermetria. [hypo- + G. *metron,* measure]

**hy·pom·ne·sia** (hī-pō-nē′zē-ă) impaired memory. [hypo- + G. *mnēmē,* memory]

**hy·po·morph** (hī′pō-mōrf) **1.** a person whose standing height is short in proportion to sitting height, owing to shortness of the limbs. Cf. endomorph. **2.** a mutant gene that causes a partial decrease in the activity controlled by the gene. [hypo- + G. *morphē,* form]

**hy·po·mo·til·i·ty** (hī′pō-mō-til′i-tē) SYN hypokinesis.

**hy·po·mo·tor sei·zure** seizure characterized by complete or partial arrest of ongoing motor activity in a patient whose level of consciousness cannot be determined accurately (e.g., newborns, infants, mentally retarded patients).

**hy·po·my·e·li·na·tion, hy·po·my·e·lin·o·gen·e·sis** (hī′pō-mī′ĕ-lin-ā-shŭn, hī′pō-mī′ĕ-lin-ō-jen′ĕ-sis) defective formation of myelin in the spinal cord and brain; the basis for a number of demyelinating diseases.

**hy·po·my·o·to·nia** (hī′pō-mī-ō-tō′nē-ă) a condition of diminished muscular tonus. [hypo- + G. *mys* (*myo-*) muscle, + *tonos,* tension]

**hy·po·myx·ia** (hī′pō-mik′sē-ă) a condition in which the secretion of mucus is diminished. [hypo- + G. *myxa*, mucus]

**hy·po·na·sal·i·ty** insufficient nasal resonance during speech, usually due to obstruction of the nasal tract. SYN hyporhinophonia.

**hy·po·na·trae·mia [Br.]** SEE hyponatremia.

**hy·po·na·tre·mia** (hī′pō-nă-trē′mē-ă) abnormally low concentrations of sodium ions in the circulating blood. [hypo- + natrium, + G. *haima*, blood]

**hy·po·ne·o·cy·to·sis** (hī′pō-nē′ō-sī-tō′sis) leukopenia associated with the presence of immature and young leukocytes (especially in the granulocytic series). [hypo- + G. *neos*, new, + *kytos*, cell, + *-osis*, condition]

**hy·po·nych·i·al** (hī′pō-nik′ē-ăl) **1.** SYN subungual. **2.** relating to the hyponychium.

**hy·po·nych·i·um** (hī′pō-nik′ē-ŭm) the epithelium of the nail bed, particularly its proximal part in the region of the nailroot and lunula, forming the nail matrix. [hypo- + G. *onyx*, nail]

**hy·pon·y·chon** (hī-pon′i-kon) an ecchymosis beneath a fingernail or toenail. [hypo- + G. *onyx*, nail]

**hy·po·or·tho·cy·to·sis** (hī′pō-ōr′thō-sī-tō′sis) leukopenia in which the relative numbers of the various types of white blood cells are within the normal ranges. [hypo- + G. *orthos*, correct, + *kytos*, cell, + *-osis*, condition]

**hy·po·pan·cre·a·tism** (hī′pō-pan′krē-ă-tizm) a condition of diminished activity of digestive enzyme secretion by the pancreas.

**hy·po·par·a·thy·roid·ism** (hī′pō-par-ă-thī′roydizm) a condition due to diminution or absence of the secretion of the parathyroid hormones, with low serum calcium, tetany, and sometimes increased bone density. SEE ALSO pseudohypoparathyroidism.

**hy·po·pha·lan·gism** (hī′pō-fă-lan′jizm) congenital absence of one or more of the phalanges of a finger or toe.

**hy·po·pha·ryn·ge·al di·ver·tic·u·lum** SYN pharyngoesophageal diverticulum.

**hy·po·phar·ynx** (hī′pō-far′inks) SYN laryngopharynx.

**hy·po·pho·ne·sis** (hī′pō-fō-nē′sis) in percussion or auscultation, a sound that is diminished or fainter than usual. [hypo- + G. *phōnēsis*, a sounding]

**hy·po·pho·ria** (hī′pō-fō′rē-ă) a tendency of the visual axis of one eye to deviate downward, prevented by binocular vision. [hypo- + G. *phora*, motion]

**hy·po·phos·phos·pha·tae·mia [Br.]** SEE hypophosphatemia.

**hy·po·phos·pha·ta·sia** (hī′pō-fos′fă-tā′zē-ă) an abnormally low content of alkaline phosphatase in the circulating blood.

**hy·po·phos·pha·te·mia** (hī′pō-fos-fă-tē′mē-ă) abnormally low concentrations of phosphates in the circulating blood.

**hy·po·phos·phat·ur·ia** (hī′pō-fos′făt-yur′ē-ă) reduced urinary excretion of phosphates.

**hy·poph·y·sec·to·my** (hī′pof-i-sek′tō-mē) surgical removal of the hypophysis or pituitary gland.

**hy·po·phys·e·o·priv·ic** (hī′pō-fiz′ē-ō-priv′ik) SYN hypophysioprivic.

**hy·po·phys·e·o·tro·pic** (hī′pō-fiz′ē-ō-trop′ik) SYN hypophysiotropic.

**hy·po·phy·si·al** (hī′pō-fiz′ē-ăl) relating to a hypophysis.

**hy·po·phy·si·al ca·chex·ia** SYN Simmonds disease, panhypopituitarism.

**hy·po·phy·si·al fos·sa** fossa of the sphenoid bone housing the pituitary gland. SEE ALSO sella turcica.

**hy·po·phy·si·al syn·drome** SYN dystrophia adiposogenitalis.

**hy·po·phys·i·o·priv·ic** (hī′pō-fiz′ē-ō-priv′ik) pertaining to absence or depressed function of the pituitary gland. SYN hypophyseoprivic. [hypophysis + L. *privus*, deprived of]

**hy·po·phys·i·o·sphe·noi·dal syn·drome** neoplastic invasion of the base of the skull in the region of the sphenoidal sinus, often with destruction of the dorsum sellae.

**hy·po·phys·i·o·tro·pic** (hī′pō-fiz′ē-ō-trop′ik) denoting a stimulatory hormone that acts on the pituitary gland (hypophysis). SYN hypophyseotropic.

**hy·poph·y·sis** (hī-pof′i-sis) [TA] an unpaired compound gland suspended from the base of the hypothalamus by a short extension of the infundibulum, the infundibular or pituitary stalk. The hypophysis consists of two major subdivisions: 1) the neurohypophysis, comprising the infundibulum and its bulbous termination, the neural part or infundibular process (posterior lobe), which is composed of neuroglia-like pituicytes, blood vessels, and unmyelinated nerve fibers of the hypothalamohypophyseal tract whose cell bodies reside in the supraoptic and paraventricular nuclei of the hypothalamus, and convey to the lobe for storage and release the neurosecretory hormones oxytocin and antidiuretic hormone; 2) the adenohypophysis, comprising the larger distal part, a sleevelike extension of this lobe (infundibular part) which invests the infundibular stalk, and a thin intermediate part (poorly developed in humans) between the anterior and posterior lobes; the anterior lobe consists of cords of cells of several different types interspersed with capillaries of the hypothalamohypophysial portal system; secretion of somatotropins, prolactin, thyroid-stimulating hormone, gonadotropins, adrenal corticotropin, and other related peptides in the adenohypophysis is regulated by releasing and inhibiting factors elaborated by neurons in the hypothalamus which are taken up by a primary plexus of capillaries in the median eminence and transported via portal vessels in the infundibular part and infundibular stem to a secondary plexus of capillaries in the distal part. SEE ALSO hypothalamus. SYN pituitary gland. [G. an undergrowth]

**hy·poph·y·si·tis** (hī-pof-i-sī′tis) inflammation of the hypophysis.

**hy·po·pi·e·sis** (hī′pō-pī-ē′sis) SYN hypotension (1). [hypo- + G. *piesis*, pressure]

**hy·po·pig·men·ta·tion** (hī′pō-pig-men-tā′shŭn) deficiency of cutaneous melanin relative to surrounding skin. SEE albinism. [hypo- + pigmentation]

**hy·po·pi·tu·i·ta·rism** (hī′pō-pi-too′i-tă-rizm) a condition due to diminished activity of the anterior lobe of the hypophysis, with inadequate secretion of one or more anterior pituitary hormones.

**hy·po·pla·sia** (hī′pō-plā′zē-ă) **1.** underdevelopment of a tissue or organ, usually due to a decrease in the number of cells. **2.** atrophy due to destruction of some of the elements and not merely to their general reduction in size. [hypo- + G. *plasis,* a molding]

**hy•po•plas•tic** (hī′pō-plas′tik) pertaining to or characterized by hypoplasia.

**hy•po•plas•tic a•ne•mia** progressive nonregenerative anemia resulting from greatly depressed, inadequately functioning bone marrow; as the process persists, aplastic anemia may occur.

**hy•pop•nea** (hī-pop′nē-ă) breathing that is shallower, and/or slower, than normal. SYN oligopnea. [hypo- + G. *pnoē,* breathing]

**hy•pop•noea [Br.]** SEE hypopnea.

**hy•pop•o•sia** (hī′pō-pō′sē-ă) hypodipsia, with emphasis on reduced tendency to drink rather than on the reduced sensation of thirst. [hypo- + G. *posis,* drinking]

**hy•po•po•tas•se•mia** (hī′pō-pō-ta-sē′mē-ă) SYN hypokalemia.

**hy•po•prax•ia** (hī-pō-prak′sē-ă) deficient activity. [hypo- + G. *praxis,* action, + *-ia,* condition]

**hy•po•pro•tein•ae•mia [Br.]** SEE hypoproteinemia.

**hy•po•pro•tein•e•mia** (hī′pō-prō-tēn-e′mē-ă) abnormally small amounts of total protein in the blood.

**hy•po•pro•throm•bi•nae•mia [Br.]** SEE hypoprothrombinemia.

**hy•po•pro•throm•bin•e•mia** (hī′pō-prō-throm′bin-ē′mē-ă) abnormally small amounts of prothrombin in the circulating blood.

**hy•pop•ty•a•lism** (hī′pō-tī′ă-lizm) SYN hyposalivation. [hypo- + G. *ptyalon,* saliva]

**hy•po•py•on** (hī-pō′pi-on) the presence of leukocytes in the anterior chamber of the eye. [hypo- + G. *pyon,* pus]

**hy•po•re•flex•ia** (hī′pō-rē-flek′sē-ă) a condition in which the deep tendon reflexes are weakened.

**hy•po•ren•i•ne•mia** (hī′pō-ren-i-nē′mē-ă) low levels of renin in the circulating blood.

**hy•po•ren•i•nem•ic** (hī′pō-ren-i-nē′mik) denoting or characterized by hyporeninemia.

**hy•po•rhi•no•pho•nia** SYN hyponasality.

**hy•po•ri•bo•fla•vin•o•sis** (hī′pō-rī′bō-flā-vi-nō′sis) NUTRITION a condition produced by a deficiency of riboflavin in the diet, characterized by cheilosis and magenta tongue and usually associated with other manifestations of B vitamin deficiency. A more correct term than the more commonly used ariboflavinosis.

**hy•po•sal•i•va•tion** (hī′pō-sal′i-vā′shŭn) reduced salivation. SYN hypoptyalism.

**hy•po•scle•ral** (hī-pō-sklēr′ăl) beneath the sclerotic coat of the eyeball.

**hy•po•sen•si•tiv•i•ty** (hī′pō-sen-si-tiv′i-tē) a condition of subnormal sensitivity, in which the response to a stimulus is unusually delayed or lessened in degree.

**hy•pos•mia** (hī-poz′mē-ă) diminished sense of smell. [hypo- + G. *osmē,* smell]

**hy•po•so•ma•to•tro•pism** (hī′pō-sō′mă-tō-trō′pizm) a state characterized by deficient secretion of pituitary growth hormone (somatotropin).

**hy•po•spa•di•ac** (hī′pō-spā′dē-ak) relating to hypospadias.

**hy•po•spa•di•as** (hī′pō-spā′dē-ăs) a developmental anomaly characterized by a defect on the ventral surface of the penis so that the urethral meatus is more proximal than normal; may be associated with chordee; also, a similar defect in the

female in which the urethra opens into the vagina. Cf. epispadias. SYN urogenital sinus anomaly. [hypo- + G. *spaō,* to tear or gouge]

**hy•po•sphyg•mia** (hī′pō-sfig′mē-ă) abnormally low blood pressure with sluggishness of the circulation. [hypo- + G. *sphyxis,* pulse]

**hy•po•splen•ism** (hī′pō-splēn′izm) absent or reduced splenic function, usually due to surgical removal, congenital aplasia, tumor replacement, or splenic vascular accident.

**hy•pos•ta•sis** (hi-pos′tă-sis) **1.** formation of a sediment at the bottom of a liquid. **2.** SYN hypostatic congestion. **3.** the phenomenon whereby the phenotype that would ordinarily be manifested at one locus is obscured by the genotype at another epistatic locus. [G. *hypo-stasis,* a standing under, sediment]

**hy•po•stat•ic** (hī-pō-stat′ik) **1.** Sedimentary; resulting from a dependent position. **2.** relating to hypostasis.

**hy•po•stat•ic con•ges•tion** congestion due to pooling of venous blood in a dependent part. SYN hypostasis (2).

**hy•po•stat•ic ec•ta•sia** dilation of a blood vessel, usually a vein, in a dependent portion of the body, as in varicose veins of the leg.

**hy•po•stat•ic pneu•mo•nia** pneumonia resulting from infection developing in the dependent portions of the lungs due to decreased ventilation of those areas, with resulting failure to drain bronchial secretions; occurs primarily in the aged or those debilitated by disease who lie in the same position for long periods.

**hy•po•sthe•nia** (hī′pos-thē′nē-ă) weakness. SEE asthenia. [hypo- + G. *sthenos,* strength]

**hy•po•sthen•ic** (hī-pos-then′ik) **1.** weak. **2.** pertaining to a slender habitus, with under development of skeletal muscle.

**hy•pos•then•ur•ia** (hī′pos-thěn-yur′ē-ă) excretion of urine of low specific gravity, due to inability of the renal tubules to produce concentrated urine; also occurs following excessive water ingestion in diabetes insipidus. [hypo- + G. *sthenos,* strength, + *ouron,* urine]

**hy•po•sto•mia** (hī′pō-stō′mē-ă) a form of microstomia in which the oral opening is a small vertical slit. [hypo- + G. *stoma,* mouth]

**hy•po•tel•or•ism** (hī-pō-tel′ŏr-izm) abnormal closeness of eyes. [hypo- + G. *tēle,* far off, + *horizō,* to separate, fr. *horos,* boundary]

**hy•po•ten•sion** (hī′pō-ten′shŭn) **1.** subnormal arterial blood pressure. SYN hypopiesis. **2.** reduced pressure or tension of any kind. [hypo- + L. *tensio,* a stretching]

**hy•po•ten•sive** (hī′pō-ten′siv) characterized by low blood pressure or causing reduction in blood pressure.

**hy•po•tha•lam•ic in•fun•dib•u•lum** the apical portion of the tuber cinereum extending into the stalk of the hypophysis.

**hy•po•thal•a•mo•hy•po•phy•si•al por•tal sys•tem** SYN portal hypophysial circulation.

**hy•po•thal•a•mus** (hī′pō-thal′ă-mŭs) [TA] the ventral and medial region of the diencephalon forming the walls of the ventral half of the third ventricle; it is delineated from the thalamus by the hypothalamic sulcus, lying medial to the internal capsule and subthalamus, continuous with the precommissural septum anteriorly and with the mesencephalic tegmentum and central gray substance posteriorly. Its ventral surface is marked by, from before backward, the optic chiasma, the unpaired infundibulum, which extends by way of the infundibular stalk into the posterior lobe of the hypophysis, and the paired mammillary bodies. The nerve cells of the hypothalamus are grouped into the supraoptic paraventricular, lateral preoptic, lateral hypothalamic, tuberal, anterior hypothalamic, ventromedial, dorsomedial, arcuate, posterior hypothalamic, and premammillary nuclei and the mammillary body. It has afferent fiber connections with the mesencephalon, limbic system, cerebellum, and efferent fiber connections with the same structures and with the posterior lobe of the hypophysis; its functional connection with the anterior lobe of the hypophysis is established by the hypothalamohypophysial portal system. The hypothalamus is prominently involved in the functions of the autonomic nervous system and, through its vascular link with the anterior lobe of the hypophysis, in endocrine mechanisms; it also appears to play a role in neural mechanisms underlying moods and motivational states. SEE ALSO hypophysis. [hypo- + thalamus]

**hy·po·the·nar** (hī′pō-thē′nar, hī-poth′ĕ-nar) **1.** [TA] SYN hypothenar eminence. **2.** denoting any structure in relation with the hypothenar eminence or its underlying collective components. [hypo- + G. *thenar,* the palm]

**hy·po·the·nar em·i·nence** the fleshy mass at the medial side of the palm. SYN hypothenar (1).

**hy·po·ther·mal** (hī-pō-ther′măl) denoting hypothermia.

**hy·po·ther·mia** (hī′pō-ther′mē-ă) a body temperature significantly below 98.6°F (37°C). [hypo- + G. *thermē,* heat]

**hy·poth·e·sis** (hī-poth′ĕ-sis) a conjecture cast in a form that is amenable to confirmation or refutation by experiment and the assembly of data; not to be confused with assumption, postulation, or unfocused speculation. SEE ALSO postulate, theory. [G. foundation, assumption fr. *hypotithēmi,* to lay down]

**hy·po·thet·i·cal mean or·ga·nism (HMO)** a hypothetical organism whose characters are the means of the positive characters of the organisms which belong to the same taxon as the HMO, as opposed to the calculated mean organism.

**hy·po·throm·bi·nae·mia [Br.]** SEE hypothrombinemia.

**hy·po·throm·bi·ne·mia** (hī′pō-throm-bin-ē′mē-ă) abnormally small amounts of thrombin in the circulating blood.

**hy·po·thy·mia** (hī′pō-thī′mē-ă) depression of spirits; the "blues." [hypo- + G. *thymos,* mind, soul]

**hy·po·thy·mic** (hī-pō-thē′mik) denoting or characteristic of hypothymia.

**hy·po·thy·roid** (hī′pō-thī′royd) marked by reduced thyroid function.

**hy·po·thy·roid·ism** (hī′pō-thī′royd-izm) diminished production of thyroid hormone, leading to clinical manifestations of thyroid insufficiency, including low metabolic rate, tendency to weight gain, somnolence and sometimes myxedema. [hypo- + G. *thyreoeidēs,* thyroid]

**hy·po·to·nia** (hī′pō-tō′nē-ă) **1.** reduced tension in any part, as in the eyeball. **2.** relaxation of the arteries. **3.** a condition in which there is a diminution or loss of muscular tonicity, in consequence of which the muscles may be stretched

beyond their normal limits. SYN hypotonicity (1). [hypo- + G. *tonos,* tone]

**hy·po·ton·ic** (hī-pō-ton′ik) **1.** having a lesser degree of tension. **2.** having a lesser osmotic pressure than a reference solution, ordinarily plasma or interstitial fluid.

**hy·po·to·nic·i·ty** (hī′pō-tō-nis′i-tē) **1.** SYN hypotonia. **2.** a decreased effective osmotic pressure.

**hy·po·tri·cho·sis** (hī′pō-tri-kō′sis) a less than normal amount of hair on the head and/or body. [hypo- + G. *trichōsis,* hairiness]

**hy·po·tri·gly·cer·i·dae·mia [Br.]** SEE hypotriglyceridemia.

**hy·po·tri·gly·cer·i·de·mia** (hī-pō-trī-glis-er-ĭ-dē-mē-ă) abnormally low level of triglyceride in plasma

**hy·po·tro·pia** (hī-pō-trō′pē-ă) an ocular deviation with one eye lower than the other. [hypo- + G. *tropē,* turn]

**hy·po·tym·pa·not·o·my** (hī′pō-tim-pă-not′ō-mē) surgical extirpation, without sacrifice of hearing, of small tumors confined to the lower tympanic cavity. [hypo- + G. *tympanon,* tympanum, + *tomē,* incision]

**hy·po·tym·pa·num** (hī′pō-tim′pă-nŭm) the lower part of the tympanic cavity.

**hy·po·ur·i·cae·mia [Br.]** SEE hypouricemia.

**hy·po·u·ri·ce·mia** (hī′pō-yu-ri-sē′mē-ă) reduced blood concentration of uric acid.

**hy·po·u·ri·cu·ria** (hī′pō-yu′ri-kyu′rē-ă) reduced excretion of uric acid in the urine.

**hy·po·ven·ti·la·tion** (hī′pō-ven-ti-lā′shŭn) reduced alveolar ventilation relative to metabolic carbon dioxide production, so that alveolar carbon dioxide pressure increases above normal.

**hy·po·vi·ta·min·o·sis** (hī′pō-vī′tă-min-ō′sis) insufficiency of one or more vitamins in the diet; manifested first by depletion of tissue levels, then by functional changes, and finally by appearance of morphologic lesions. Cf. avitaminosis.

**hy·po·vo·lae·mia [Br.]** SEE hypovolemia.

**hy·po·vo·le·mia** (hī′pō-vō-lē′mē-ă) a decreased amount of blood in the body. SYN hyphaemia, hyphemia. [hypo- + L. *volumen,* volume, + G. *haima,* blood]

**hy·po·vo·le·mic** (hī′pō-vō-lē′mik) pertaining to or characterized by hypovolemia.

**hy·po·vo·le·mic shock** shock caused by a reduction in volume of blood, as from hemorrhage or dehydration.

**hy·po·vo·lia** (hī-pō-vō′lē-ă) diminished water content or volume of a given compartment; e.g., extracellular hypovolia. [hypo- + L. *volumen,* volume]

**hy·po·xae·mia [Br.]** SEE hypoxemia.

**hy·po·xan·thine** (hī-pō-zan′thin) a purine present in the muscles and other tissues, formed during purine catabolism by deamination of adenine; elevated in molybdenum-cofactor deficiency.

**hy·pox·e·mia** (hī-pok-sē′mē-ă) subnormal oxygenation of arterial blood, short of anoxia. [hypo- + oxygen, + G. *haima,* blood]

**hy·pox·ia** (hī-pok′sē-ă) decrease below normal levels of oxygen in inspired gases, arterial blood, or tissue, short of anoxia. [hypo- + oxygen]

**hy·pox·ic** (hī-pok′sik) denoting or characterized by hypoxia.

**hy·pox·ic hy·pox·ia** hypoxia resulting from a defective mechanism of oxygenation in the lungs.

h
y

**hy·pox·ic ne·phro·sis** acute oliguric renal failure following hemorrhage, burns, shock, or other causes of hypovolemia and reduced renal blood flow;.

**hyp·sa·rhyth·mia, hyp·sar·rhyth·mia** (hip'să-ridh'mē-ă) the abnormal and characteristically chaotic electroencephalogram in patients with infantile spasms. [G. *hypsi*, high, + *a-* priv. + *rhythmos*, rhythm]

**hyp·so·dont** (hip'sō-dont) having long teeth, in some animals both the crown or body of the tooth is elongated while in others     there is a marked elongation of the cusps. [hypso- + G. *odous*, tooth]

**Hyrtl loop** (hĕr'tĕl) a communicating loop between the right and left hypoglossal nerves, lying between the geniohyoid and genioglossus muscles or in the substance of the geniohyoid; it is found in about one in ten persons.

**hys·ter·al·gia** (his'ter-al'jē-ă) pain in the uterus. SYN hysterodynia, metrodynia. [hystero- + G. *algos*, pain]

**hys·ter·a·tre·sia** (his'ter-ă-trē'zē-ă) atresia of the uterine cavity, usually resulting from inflammatory endocervical adhesions.

**hys·ter·ec·to·my** (his-ter-ek'tō-mē) removal of the uterus; unless otherwise specified, usually denotes complete removal of the uterus (corpus and cervix). [hystero- + G. *ektomē*, excision]

**hys·ter·e·sis** (his-ter-ē'sis) **1.** failure of either one of two related phenomena to keep pace with the other; or any situation in which the value of one depends upon whether the other has been increasing or decreasing. Cf. allosterism. **2.** the lag of a magnetic effect behind its cause. **3.** the temperature differential that exists when a substance melts at one temperature and solidifies at another. **4.** a type of cooperativity in enzyme-catalyzed reactions in which the degree of cooperativity is associated with a slow conformational change of the enzyme. Cf. allosterism. [G. *hysterēsis*, a coming later]

**hys·ter·eu·ry·sis** (his-ter-yu'rē-sis) dilation of the lower segment and cervical canal of the uterus. [hystero- + G. *eurynō*, to dilate, fr. *eurys*, wide]

**hys·te·ria** (his-ter'ē-ă) a somatoform disorder in which there is an alteration or loss of physical functioning that suggests a physical disorder such as paralysis of an arm or disturbance of vision, but that is instead apparently an expression of a psychological conflict or need. [G. *hystera*, womb, from the original notion of womb-related disturbances in women]

**hys·ter·i·cal, hys·ter·ic** (his-ter'i-kăl, his-ter'ik) relating to or characterized by hysteria.

**hys·ter·i·cal blind·ness** loss of vision or blurring of vision following a highly traumatic event.

**hys·ter·i·cal joint** a simulation of joint disease, with symptoms of pain, possibly swelling, and impairment of motion.

**hys·ter·i·cal psy·cho·sis 1.** a psychotic disturbance with predominantly hysterical symptoms; **2.** a mental disorder resembling conversion hysteria but of psychotic severity; **3.** a brief reactive psychosis, often culture bound.

**hys·ter·ics** (his-ter'iks) an expression of emotion accompanied often by crying, laughing, and screaming.

△**hys·tero-, hys·ter- 1.** the uterus. SEE ALSO metr-, utero-. [G. *hystera*, womb (uterus)] **2.** hysteria.

[G. *hystera*, womb (uterus)] **3.** later, following. [G. *hysteros*, later]

**hys·ter·o·cat·a·lep·sy** (his'ter-ō-kat'ă-lep-sē) hysteria with cataleptic manifestations.

**hys·ter·o·cele** (his'ter-ō-sēl) **1.** an abdominal or perineal hernia containing part or all of the uterus. **2.** protrusion of uterine contents into a weakened, bulging area of uterine wall. [hystero- + G. *kēlē*, hernia]

**hys·ter·o·clei·sis** (his'ter-ō-klī'sis) operative occlusion of the uterus. [hystero- + G. *kleisis*, closure]

**hys·ter·o·dyn·ia** (his'ter-ō-din'ē-ă) SYN hysteralgia. [hystero- + G. *odynē*, pain]

**hys·ter·o·ep·i·lep·sy** (his'ter-ō-ep'i-lep-sē) hysterical convulsions.

**hys·ter·o·gen·ic, hys·ter·og·en·ous** (his-ter-ō-jen'ik, his-ter-oj'ĕ-nŭs) causing hysterical symptoms or reactions. [hysteria + G. *-gen*, producing]

**hys·ter·o·gram** (his'ter-ō-gram) **1.** x-ray examination of the uterus, usually using a contrast medium. **2.** a recording of the strength of uterine contractions.

**hys·ter·o·graph** (his'ter-ō-graf) apparatus for recording the strength of uterine contractions.

**hys·ter·og·ra·phy** (his'ter-og'ră-fē) **1.** radiographic examination of the uterine cavity filled with a contrast medium. **2.** graphic procedure used to record uterine contractions. [hystero- + G. *graphō*, to write]

**hys·ter·oid** (his'ter-oyd) resembling or simulating hysteria. [hystero- + G. *eidos*, resemblance]

**hys·ter·ol·y·sis** (his-ter-ol'i-sis) breaking up of adhesions between the uterus and neighboring parts. [hystero- + G. *lysis*, dissolution]

**hys·ter·om·e·ter** (his-ter-om'ĕ-ter) a graduated sound for measuring the depth of the uterine cavity. SYN uterometer. [hystero- + G. *metron*, measure]

**hys·ter·o·my·o·ma** (his'ter-ō-mī-ō'mă) a myoma of the uterus. [hystero- + G. *mys*, muscle, + *-oma*, tumor]

**hys·ter·o·my·o·mec·to·my** (his'ter-ō-mī-ō-mek'tō-mē) operative removal of a uterine myoma. [hysteromyoma + G. *ektomē*, excision]

**hys·ter·o·my·ot·o·my** (his'ter-ō-mī-ot'ō-mē) incision into the muscles of the uterus. [hystero- + G. *mys*, muscle, + *tomē*, incision]

**hys·ter·o·o·oph·o·rec·to·my** (his'ter-ō-ō'of-ō-rek'tō-mē) surgical removal of the uterus and ovaries. [hystero- + G. *ōon*, egg, + *phoros*, bearing, + *ektomē*, excision]

**hys·ter·op·a·thy** (his-ter-op'ă-thē) any disease of the uterus. [hystero- + G. *pathos*, suffering]

**hys·ter·o·pex·y** (his'ter-ō-pek-sē) fixation of a displaced or abnormally movable uterus. SYN uterofixation, uteropexy. [hystero- + G. *pēxis*, fixation]

**hys·ter·o·plas·ty** (his'ter-ō-plas-tē) SYN uteroplasty.

**hys·ter·or·rha·phy** (his-ter-ōr'ă-fē) sutural repair of a lacerated uterus. [hystero- + G. *rhaphē*, suture]

**hys·ter·or·rhex·is** (his'ter-ō-rek'sis) rupture of the uterus. [hystero- + G. *rhēxis*, rupture]

**hys·ter·o·sal·pin·gec·to·my** (his'ter-ō-sal-pin-jek'tō-mē) operation for the removal of the uterus and one or both uterine tubes. [hystero- + G. *salpinx*, a trumpet, + *ektomē*, excision]

**hys·ter·o·sal·pin·gog·ra·phy** (his'ter-ō-sal-ping-gog'ră-fē) radiography of the uterus and uterine tubes after the injection of radiopaque material. SYN hysterotubography, metrosalpingography, uterosalpingography, uterotubography. [hystero- + G. *salpinx*, a trumpet, + *graphō*, to write]

**hys·ter·o·sal·pin·go·o·oph·o·rec·to·my** (his′ter-ō-sal-ping′gō-ō-of-ō-rek′tō-mē) excision of the uterus, oviducts, and ovaries. [hystero- + G. *salpinx*, trumpet, + *ōon*, egg, + *phoros*, bearing, + *ektomē*, excision]

**hys·ter·o·sal·pin·gos·to·my** (his′ter-ō-sal-ping-gos′tō-mē) operation to restore patency of a uterine tube. [hystero- + G. *salpinx*, trumpet, + *stoma*, mouth]

**hys·ter·o·scope** (his′ter-ō-skōp) an endoscope used in direct visual examination of the uterine cavity. SYN metroscope, uteroscope. [hystero- + G. *skopeō*, to view]

**hys·ter·os·co·py** (his-ter-os′kŏ-pē) visual instrumental inspection of the uterine cavity. SYN uteroscopy.

**hys·ter·o·spasm** (his′ter-ō-spazm) spasm of the uterus.

**hys·ter·ot·o·my** (his-ter-ot′ō-mē) incision of the uterus. SYN uterotomy. [hystero- + G. *tomē*, incision]

**hys·ter·o·trach·e·lec·to·my** (his′ter-ō-trak-el-ek′tō-mē) removal of the cervix uteri. [hystero- + G. *trachēlos*, neck, + *ektomē*, excision]

**hys·ter·o·trach·e·lo·plas·ty** (his′ter-ō-trak′ĕ-lō-plas-tē) plastic surgery of the cervix uteri. [hystero- + G. *trachēlos*, neck, + *plastos*, formed, shaped]

**hys·ter·o·tra·che·lor·rha·phy** (his′ter-ō-trak-ĕ-lōr′ă-fē) sutural repair of a lacerated cervix uteri. [hystero- + G. *trachēlos*, neck, + *rhaphē*, a seam]

**hys·ter·o·trach·e·lot·o·my** (his′ter-ō-trak-ĕ-lot′ō-mē) incision of the cervix uteri. [hystero- + G. *trachēlos*, neck, + *tomē*, incision]

**hys·ter·o·tu·bog·ra·phy** (his′ter-ō-too-bog′ră-fē) SYN hysterosalpingography.

**Hz** hertz.

# I

ι (ī-ō′ta) iota. SEE iota.

**I 1.** iodine; luminous intensity or radiant intensity; ionic strength (in mol/L); isoleucine; inosine. **2.** intensity of electrical current, expressed in amperes. **3.** as a subscript, symbol for inspired gas. **4.** designation for I blood group (see Blood Groups appendix).

△**-ia** condition, used in formation of names of many diseases. Cf. -ism. [G. *-ia*, an ancient noun-forming suffix]

**IAP** intermittent acute porphyria.

△**-ia•sis** a condition or state, especially an unhealthy one. [G. suffix forming nouns from verbs]

**iat•ric** (ī-at′rik) pertaining to medicine or to a physician or healer. [G. *iatros*, physician]

△**iat•ro-** physicians, medicine, treatment. Cf. medico-. [G. *iatros*, physician]

**iat•ro•gen•ic** (ī-at-rō-jen′ik) denoting response to medical or surgical treatment, induced by the treatment itself; usually used for unfavorable responses. [iatro- + G. *-gen*, producing]

**iat•ro•gen•ic pneu•mo•thor•ax** pneumothorax caused by a medical procedure, most often central venous catheter insertion, thoracentesis, or transbronchial and transthoracic lung biopsy.

**iat•ro•gen•ic trans•mis•sion** transmission of infectious agents due to medical interference (e.g., transmission by contaminated needles).

**I band** a light band on each side of the Z line of striated muscle fibers, comprising a region of the sarcomere where thin (actin) filaments are not overlapped by thick (myosin) filaments.

△**-ic 1.** suffix denoting of, pertaining to. **2.** chemical suffix denoting an element in a compound in one of its highest valencies. Cf. -ous (1). **3.** suffix indicating an acid. [L. *-icus*, fr. G. *-ikos*]

**ICAO stan•dard at•mos•phere** the standard atmosphere adopted by the International Civil Aviation Organization, used for calibrating altimeters and for expressing hypobaric chamber pressures in terms of equivalent altitude.

**ic•co•somes** (ī′kō-sōmz) beaded cytoplasmic structure on follicular dendrite cells; thought to be a repository for antigens. [*immune complex coated* + -*some*]

**ICD** International Classification of Diseases.

**ICDA** *International Classification of Diseases, Adapted for Use in the United States.*

**Ice•land dis•ease** SYN epidemic neuromyasthenia.

**I cell** a cultured skin fibroblast containing membrane-bound inclusions; characteristic of mucolipidosis II. SEE ALSO immunocyte. SYN inclusion cell.

**ice pick head•ache** SYN idiopathic stabbing headache.

**ICF 1.** intracellular fluid. **2.** intermediate care facility

**ichor** (ī′kōr) rarely used term for a thin watery discharge from an ulcer or unhealthy wound. [G. *ichōr*, serum]

**ichor•hae•mia [Br.]** SYN ichorrhemia.

**icho•roid** (ī′kō-royd) denoting a thin purulent discharge. [G. *ichōr*, serum, + *eidos*, resemblance]

**ichor•ous** (ī′kōr-ŭs) relating to or resembling ichor.

**ichor•rhea** (ī′kō-rē′ă) a profuse ichorous discharge. [G. *ichōr*, serum, + *rhoia*, a flow]

**ichor•rhe•mia** (ī-kō-rē′mē-ă) sepsis resulting from infection accompanied by an ichorous discharge. SYN ichorhaemia.

**ich•thy•ism** (ik′thē-izm) poisoning by eating stale or otherwise unfit fish. [G. *ichthys*, fish]

△**ich•thyo-** fish. [G. *ichthys*]

**ich•thy•oid** (ik′thē-oyd) fish-shaped. [ichthyo- + G. *eidos*, resemblance]

**ich•thy•o•si•form e•ryth•ro•der•ma** SYN congenital ichthyosiform erythroderma.

**ich•thy•o•sis** (ik-thē-ō′sis) congenital disorders of keratinization characterized by noninflammatory dryness and scaling of the skin, often associated with other defects and with abnormalities of lipid metabolism; distinguishable genetically, clinically, microscopically, and by epidermal cell kinetics. [ichthyo- + G. *-osis*, condition]

**ich•thy•ot•ic** (ik-thē-ot′ik) relating to ichthyosis.

**ich•thy•o•tox•ism** (ik′thē-ō-tok′sizm) poisoning by fish. [ichthyo- + G. *toxikon*, poison]

**ICP** intracranial pressure.

△**-ics** organized knowledge, practice, treatment. [-ic + -s]

**ICSH** interstitial cell-stimulating hormone.

**ic•tal** (ik′tăl) relating to or caused by a stroke or seizure. [L. *ictus*, a stroke]

**ic•ter•ic** (ik-ter′ik) relating to or marked by jaundice. [G. *ikterikos*, jaundiced]

△**ictero-** icterus. [G. *ikteros*, jaundice]

**ic•ter•o•gen•ic** (ik′ter-ō-jen′ik) causing jaundice. [ictero- + G. *-gen*, producing]

**ic•ter•o•hem•or•rha•gic fe•ver** infection with the variety of *Leptospira interrogans* serotype known as icterohemorrhagiae, characterized by fever, jaundice, hemorrhagic lesions, azotemia, and central nervous system manifestations.

**ic•ter•o•hep•a•ti•tis** (ik′ter-ō-hep-ă-tī′tis) inflammation of the liver with jaundice as a prominent symptom. [ictero- + G. *hēpar*, liver, + *-itis*, inflammation]

**ic•ter•oid** (ik′ter-oyd) yellow-hued, or seemingly jaundiced. [ictero- + G. *eidos*, resemblance]

**ic•ter•us** (ik′ter-ŭs) SYN jaundice. [G. *ikteros*]

**ic•ter•us gra•vis** jaundice associated with high fever and delirium; seen in severe hepatitis and other diseases of the liver with severe functional failure. SYN malignant jaundice.

**ic•ter•us ne•o•na•to•rum** icterus in the newborn; sometimes normal, but can be induced or accentuated by excessive hemolysis, sepsis, neonatal hepatitis, or congenital atresia of the biliary system. SYN jaundice of the newborn, physiologic icterus, physiologic jaundice.

**ic•tus** (ik′tŭs) **1.** a stroke or attack. **2.** a beat. [L.]

**ic•tus cor•dis** SYN apex beat.

**ICU** intensive care unit.

**ICU psy•cho•sis** psychotic episode(s) occurring within 24 hours after entering the ICU in individuals with no previous history of psychosis; related to sleep deprivation, overstimulation and time spent on life support systems.

**id 1.** PSYCHOANALYSIS one of three components of the psychic apparatus in the freudian structural framework, the other two being the ego and superego. It is completely in the unconscious realm, is unorganized, is the reservoir of psychic energy or libido, and is under the influence of the primary processes. **2.** the total of all psychic energy available from the innate biologic hungers, appetites, bodily needs, drives and impulses, in a newborn infant. [L. *id,* that]

⌂**-id 1.** a state of sensitivity of the skin in which a part remote from the primary lesion reacts ("-id reaction") to the pathogen, giving rise to a secondary inflammatory lesion; the lesion manifesting the reaction is designated by the use of -id as a suffix. [G. *-eidēs,* resembling, through Fr. *-ide*] **2.** small, young specimen. [G. *-idion,* a diminutive ending]

**IDDM** insulin-dependent diabetes mellitus.

⌂**-ide 1.** suffix denoting the more electronegative element in a binary chemical compound. **2.** suffix (in a sugar name) indicating substitution for the H of the hemiacetal OH; e.g., glycoside.

**IDEA** Individuals with Disabilities Education Act.

**idea** (ī-dē′ă) any mental image or concept. [G. semblance]

**ide•al** (ī-dēl′) a standard of perfection.

**idea of ref•er•ence** the misinterpretation that other people's statements or acts or neutral objects in the environment are directed toward one's self when, in fact, they are not.

**ide•a•tion** (ī-dē-ā′shŭn) the formation of ideas or thoughts.

**ide•a•tion•al** (ī-dē-ā′shŭn-ăl) relating to ideation.

**i•den•ti•cal twins** SYN monozygotic twins.

**iden•ti•fi•ca•tion** (ī-den′ti-fi-kā′shŭn) **1.** act or process of determining classification or nature of. **2.** a sense of oneness, or psychic continuity with another person or group; one of the freudian defense mechanisms common to everyone whereby anxiety regarding one's personal identity or worth is dissipated via the mechanism of perceiving oneself as having characteristics in common with a person in the public eye, or in childhood identifying with a more powerful person such as a parent. [Mediev. L. *identicus,* fr. L. *idem,* the same, + *facio,* to make]

**iden•ti•ty** (ī-den′ti-tē) the sum of characteristics by which a person is recognized (by self and others).

**i•den•ti•ty cri•sis** a disorientation concerning one's sense of self, values, and role in society, often of acute onset and related to a particular and significant event in one's life.

**i•den•ti•ty dis•or•der** a mental disorder of childhood or adolescence in which one suffers severe distress regarding one's ability to reconcile aspects of the self into a coherent acceptable sense of self.

⌂**ideo-** ideas; ideation Cf. idio-. [G. *idea,* form, notion]

**ide•o•ki•net•ic a•prax•ia, i•de•o•mo•tor a•prax•i•a** a form of apraxia in which simple acts are incapable of being performed, presumably because the connections between the cortical centers that control volition and the motor cortex are interrupted.

**ide•ol•o•gy** (ī-dē-ol′ō-jē, id-ē-ol′ō-jē) the composite system of ideas, beliefs, and attitudes that constitutes an individual's or group's organized view of others. [ideo- + G. *logos,* study]

⌂**id•io-** private, distinctive, peculiar to. Cf. ideo-. [G. *idios,* one's own]

**id•i•o•gram** (id′ē-ō-gram) **1.** SYN karyotype. **2.** diagrammatic representation of chromosome morphology characteristic of a species or population. [idio- + G. *gramma,* something written]

**id•i•o•het•er•o•ag•glu•ti•nin** (id′ē-ō-het′er-ō-ă-gloo′tin-in) an idioagglutinin occurring in the blood of one animal, but capable of combining with the antigenic material from another species. [idio- + G. *heteros,* another, + agglutinin]

**id•i•o•het•er•o•ly•sin** (id′ē-ō-het-er-ol′i-sin) an idiolysin occurring in the blood of one species, but capable of hemolyzing red blood cells of another species.

**id•i•o•i•so•ag•glu•ti•nin** (id′ē-ō-ī′sō-ă-gloo′tin-in) an idioagglutinin occurring in the blood of a certain species, capable of agglutinating cells from animals of the same species. [idio- + G. *isos,* equal, + agglutinin]

**id•i•o•i•sol•y•sin** (id′ē-ō-ī-sol′i-sin) an idiolysin occurring in the blood of an animal of a certain species, capable of hemolyzing red blood cells from animals of the same species.

**id•i•ol•y•sin** (id-ē-ol′i-sin) a lysin that occurs naturally in the blood of a person or an animal, without the injection of a stimulating antigen or the passive transfer of antibody.

**id•i•o•mus•cu•lar con•trac•tion** SYN myoedema.

**id•i•o•path•ic** (id′ē-ō-path′ik) denoting a disease of unknown cause. SYN agnogenic. [idio- + G. *pathos,* suffering]

**id•i•o•path•ic al•do•ste•ron•ism** SYN primary aldosteronism.

**id•i•o•path•ic hy•per•cal•ce•mia of in•fants** persistent hypercalcemia of unknown cause in very young children, associated with osteosclerosis, renal insufficiency, and sometimes hypertension.

**id•i•o•path•ic hy•per•tro•phic sub•a•or•tic ste•no•sis** left ventricular outflow obstruction due to hypertrophy, usually congenital, of the ventricular septum.

**id•i•o•path•ic neu•ral•gia** nerve pain not due to any apparent cause.

**id•i•o•path•ic pul•mo•nary fi•bro•sis (IPF)** subacute form also called Hamman-Rich syndrome; an acute to chronic inflammatory process of the lungs, the healing stage of diffuse alveolar damage or acute interstitial pneumonia, either idiopathic or associated with collagen-vascular diseases. SYN cryptogenic fibrosing alveolitis, Hamman-Rich syndrome.

**id•i•o•path•ic stab•bing head•ache** brief repetitive sharp pains in the temporal-parietal area of the head. SYN ice pick headache.

**id•i•o•path•ic sub•glot•tic ste•no•sis** narrowing of the infraglottic lumen, of unknown cause; apparently occurring only in women.

**id•i•o•path•ic throm•bo•cy•to•pe•nic pur•pu•ra (ITP)** a systemic illness characterized by extensive ecchymoses and hemorrhages from mucous membranes and very low platelet counts; resulting from destruction in the spleen of platelets to which an autoimmune globulin is bound; childhood cases, which often follow viral infection, are mild and transitory; in adults, bleeding may be recurrent and severe. SYN immune thrombocytopenic purpura, purpura hemorrhagica, thrombopenic purpura.

**id•i•op•a•thy** (id-ē-op′ă-thē) an idiopathic disease. [idio- + G. *pathos,* suffering]

**id•i•o•phren•ic** (id′ē-ō-fren′ik) relating to, or originating in, the mind or brain alone, not reflex or secondary. [idio- + G. *phrēn,* mind]

**id•i•o•syn•cra•sy** (id′ē-ō-sin′kră-sē) **1.** an individual mental, behavioral, or physical character-

i
d

istic or peculiarity. **2.** PHARMACOLOGY an abnormal reaction to a drug, sometimes specified as genetically determined. [G. *idiosynkrasia,* fr. *idios,* one's own, + *synkrasis,* a mixing together]

**id•i•o•syn•crat•ic** (id′ē-ō-sin-krat′ik) relating to or marked by an idiosyncrasy.

**id•i•ot-sa•vant** (ē-dē-ō′ sah-vahn′) a person of low general intelligence who possesses an unusual facility in performing certain mental tasks of which most normal persons are incapable. [Fr.]

**id•i•o•type** (id′ē-ō-tīp) a determinant that confers on an immunoglobulin molecule an antigenic "individuality" and is frequently a unique attribute of a given antibody in a given animal. [idio- + G. *typos,* model]

**id•i•o•typic an•ti•bod•y** an antibody that binds to an idiotope of another antibody.

**id•i•o•ven•tric•u•lar** (id-ē-ō-ven-trik′yu-lăr) pertaining to or associated with the cardiac ventricles alone.

**id•i•o•ven•tric•u•lar rhythm** a slow independent ventricular rhythm under control of an ectopic ventricular center. SYN ventricular rhythm.

**id re•ac•tion** an allergic manifestation of candidiasis, the dermatophytoses, and other mycoses characterized by itching, vesicular lesions that appear in response to superficial infections that are distant from the id reaction itself. SEE ALSO dermatophytid, -id (1).

**IEP** individualized education program.

**IF** initiation factor; intrinsic factor.

**IFN** interferon.

**Ig** immunoglobulin.

**IgA** immunoglobulin A.

**IgD** immunoglobulin D.

**IgE** immunoglobulin E.

**IGF** insulin-like growth factors.

**IgG** immunoglobulin G.

**IgM** immunoglobulin M.

**ig•ni•punc•ture** (ig′ni-pŭngk-cher) the original procedure of closing a retinal separation by transfixation with cautery. [L. *ignis,* fire, + puncture]

**IL** interleukin.

**IL-3** interleukin-3.

**IL-4** interleukin-4.

**IL-5** interleukin-5.

**IL-6** interleukin-6.

**IL-7** interleukin-7.

**IL-8** interleukin-8.

**IL-9** interleukin-9.

**IL-10** interleukin-10.

**IL-11** interleukin-11.

**IL-12** interleukin-12.

**IL-13** interleukin-13.

**IL-14** interleukin-14.

**IL-15** interleukin-15.

**IL-16** interleukin-16.

**IL-17** interleukin-17.

**IL-18** interleukin-18.

**ILA** insulin-like activity.

**il•e•ac** (il′ē-ak) **1.** relating to ileus. **2.** relating to the ileum.

**il•e•al** (il′ē-ăl) of or pertaining to the ileum.

**il•e•al ar•ter•ies** *origin,* superior mesenteric; *distribution,* ileum; *anastomoses,* other branches of superior mesenteric. SYN arteriae ileales [TA].

**il•e•al or•i•fice** the opening of the terminal ileum into the large intestine at the transition between the cecum and the ascending colon. SYN ileocecal valve, ileocolic vein, ostium ileale.

**il•e•al u•re•ter** SYN ureteroileoneocystostomy.

**il•e•al veins** SEE jejunal and ileal veins.

**il•e•ec•to•my** (il-ē-ek′tō-mē) removal of the ileum. [ileum + G. *ektomē,* excision]

**il•e•i•tis** (il-ē-ī′tis) inflammation of the ileum.

⌂**ileo-** the ileum; bottom of the small intestine. [New L. *ileum,* groin]

**i•le•o•cae•cal [Br.]** SEE ileocecal.

**i•le•o•cae•cos•to•my [Br.]** SEE ileocecostomy.

**il•e•o•ce•cal** (il′ē-ō-sē′kăl) relating to both ileum and cecum.

**il•e•o•ce•cal or•i•fice** SEE ileal orifice.

**il•e•o•ce•cal valve** SYN ileal orifice. SYN ileocolic valve.

**il•e•o•ce•cos•to•my** (il′ē-ō-sē-kos′tō′mē) anastomosis of the ileum to the cecum. SYN cecoileostomy.

**il•e•o•co•lic** (il′ē-ō-kol′ik) relating to the ileum and the colon.

**il•e•o•co•lic ar•tery** *origin,* superior mesenteric, often by a common trunk with the right colic; *distribution,* terminal part of ileum, cecum, vermiform appendix, and ascending colon; *anastomoses,* right colic and ileal. SYN arteria ileocolica [TA].

**il•e•o•co•lic valve** SYN ileocecal valve.

**il•e•o•co•lic vein** SYN ileal orifice.

**il•e•o•co•li•tis** (il′ē-ō-kō-lī′tis) inflammation of both ileum and colon.

**il•e•o•co•los•to•my** (il′ē-ō-kō-los′tō-mē) establishment of a new communication between the ileum and the colon. [ileo- + colostomy]

**il•e•o•cys•to•plas•ty** (il′ē-ō-sis′tō-plas-tē) surgical reconstruction of the bladder involving the use of an isolated intestinal segment to augment bladder capacity. [ileo- + G. *kystis,* bladder, + *plastos,* formed]

**il•e•o•il•e•os•to•my** (il′ē-ō-il-ē-os′tō-mē) **1.** establishment of a communication between two segments of the ileum. **2.** the opening so established. [ileum + ileum + G. *stoma,* mouth]

**il•e•o•je•ju•ni•tis** (il′ē-ō-je-joo-nī′tis) a chronic inflammatory condition involving the jejunum and of the ileum.

**il•e•o•pexy** (il′ē-ō-pek′sē) surgical fixation of ileum. [ileo- + G. *pēxis,* fixation]

**il•e•o•proc•tos•to•my** (il′ē-ō-prok-tos′tō-mē) establishment of a communication between the ileum and the rectum. [ileo- + G. *prōktos,* anus (rectum), + *stoma,* mouth]

**il•e•or•rha•phy** (il′ē-ōr′ă-fē) suturing the ileum. [ileo- + G. *rhaphē,* suture]

**il•e•o•sig•moid•os•to•my** (il′ē-ō-sig′moyd-os′tō-mē) establishment of a communication between the ileum and the sigmoid colon. [ileo- + sigmoid, + G. *stoma,* mouth]

**il•e•os•to•my** (il′ē-os′tō-mē) establishment of a fistula through which the ileum discharges directly to the outside of the body. See page 485. [ileo- + G. *stoma,* mouth]

**il•e•ot•o•my** (il′ē-ot′ō-mē) incision into the ileum. [ileo- + G. *tomē,* incision]

**il•e•um** (il′ē-ŭm) [TA] the third portion of the small intestine, about 3.6 m (12 ft) in length, extending from the jejunum to the ileocecal opening. [L. fr. G. *eileō,* to roll up, twist]

**il•e•us** (il′ē-ŭs) mechanical, dynamic, or adynamic obstruction of the bowel; may be accompanied by severe colicky pain, abdominal distention, vomiting, absence of passage of stool, and often

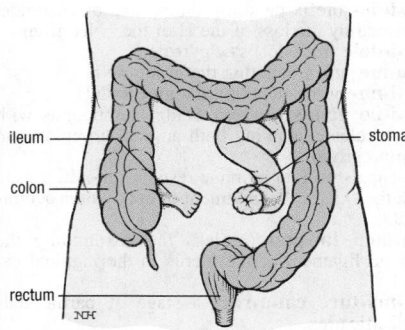

**ileostomy:** stoma opens on anterior abdominal wall

fever and dehydration. [G. *eileos,* intestinal colic, from *eilō,* to roll up tight]

**il·e·us sub·par·ta** obstruction of the large bowel by pressure of the pregnant uterus.

**il·i·ac** (il′ē-ak) relating to the ilium.

**il·i·ac bone** SYN ilium.

**il·i·ac co·lon** that portion of the descending colon which occupies the left iliac fossa, between the crest of the left ilium and the pelvic brim.

**il·i·ac crest** the long, curved upper border of the wing of the ilium.

**il·i·ac mus·cle** SYN iliacus muscle.

**il·i·a·cus mus·cle** *origin,* iliac fossa; *insertion,* tendon of psoas, anterior surface of lesser trochanter, and capsule of hip joint; *action,* flexes thigh and rotates it medially; *nerve supply,* lumbar plexus. SYN musculus iliacus [TA], iliac muscle.

⌂**il·io-** the ilium; top of hip bone. [L. *ilium*]

**il·i·o·coc·cyg·e·al** (il′ē-ō-kok-sij′ē-ăl) relating to the ilium and the coccyx.

**il·i·o·coc·cyg·e·al mus·cle** SYN iliococcygeus muscle.

**il·i·o·coc·cyg·e·us mus·cle** the posterior part of the levator ani arising from the tendinous arch of the levator ani muscle and inserting on the anococcygeal ligament and coccyx. SYN musculus iliococcygeus [TA], iliococcygeal muscle.

**il·i·o·cos·ta·lis cer·vi·cis mus·cle** *origin,* angles of upper six ribs; *insertion,* transverse processes of middle cervical vertebrae; *action,* extends, abducts, and rotates cervical vertebrae; *nerve supply,* dorsal branches of upper thoracic nerves.

**il·i·o·cos·ta·lis lum·bo·rum mus·cle** *origin,* with erector spinae; *insertion,* the angles of lower six ribs; *action,* extends, abducts, and rotates lumbar vertebrae; *nerve supply,* dorsal branches of thoracic and lumbar nerves. SYN lumbar iliocostal muscle.

**il·i·o·cos·ta·lis mus·cle** the lateral division of the erector spinae, having three subdivisions: iliocostalis lumborum musculus, iliocostalis thoracis musculus, and iliocostalis cervicis musculus. SYN musculus iliocostalis [TA], iliocostal muscle.

**il·i·o·cos·tal mus·cle** SYN iliocostalis muscle.

**il·i·o·fem·o·ral** (il′ē-ō-fem′ŏ-răl) relating to the ilium and the femur.

**il·i·o·fem·o·ral lig·a·ment** a triangular ligament attached by its apex to the anterior inferior spine of the ilium and rim of the acetabulum, and by its base to the anterior intertrochanteric line of the femur; the strong medial band is attached to the lower part of the intertrochanteric line; the strong lateral part is fixed to the tubercle at the upper part of this line; the bands diverge, forming a Y-like figure with a weak area between; among the strongest of ligaments, it limits extension at the hip joint. SYN ligamentum iliofemorale [TA], Y-shaped ligament.

**il·i·o·fem·o·ral tri·an·gle** SYN Bryant triangle.

**il·i·o·hy·po·gas·tric nerve** arises from the first lumbar nerve; it supplies the abdominal muscles and the skin of the lower part of the anterior abdominal wall. SYN nervus iliohypogastricus [TA].

**il·i·o·in·gui·nal** (il′ē-ō-ing′gwi-năl) relating to the iliac region and the groin.

**il·i·o·in·gui·nal nerve** arises from the first lumbar nerve, passes through the inguinal canal and superficial inguinal ring to supply the skin of the upper medial thigh, mons pubis, and scrotum or labium majus. SYN nervus ilioinguinalis [TA].

**il·i·o·lum·bar** (il-ē-ō-lŭm′băr) relating to the iliac and the lumbar regions.

**il·i·o·lum·bar ar·tery** *origin,* internal iliac; *distribution,* pelvic muscles and bones; *anastomoses,* deep circumflex iliac, lumbar. SYN arteria iliolumbalis [TA].

**il·i·o·lum·bar vein** accompanying the artery of the same name, anastomosing with the lumbar and deep circumflex iliac veins, and emptying into the internal iliac vein. SYN vena iliolumbalis [TA].

**il·i·o·pec·tin·e·al** (il′ē-ō-pek-tin′ē-ăl) relating to the ilium and the pubis.

**il·i·o·pec·tin·e·al line** SYN linea terminalis.

**il·i·o·pso·as mus·cle** a compound muscle, consisting of the iliacus musculus and psoas major musculus. SYN musculus iliopsoas [TA].

**il·i·o·pu·bic tract** thickened inferior margin of the transversalis fascia seen as a fibrous band running parallel and posterior (deep) to the inguinal ligament, contributing to the posterior wall of the inguinal canal as it bridges the external iliacfemoral vessels from the iliopectineal arch to the superior pubic ramus. It marks the inferior edge of the deep inguinal ring and the medial margin of the femoral canal. Seen only when the inguinal region is viewed from its internal aspect, it is a useful landmark in laparoscopy of this region, as for repair of inguinal herniae. SYN tractus iliopubicus [TA].

**il·i·o·tib·i·al band fric·tion syn·drome** a painful condition affecting the hip, thigh, or knee; produced by irritation of the iliotibial tract as it glides over the greater trochanter, anterior superior iliac spine, Gerdy tubercle, or the lateral femoral condyle; sometimes associated with a snapping or grating sensation.

**il·i·o·tib·i·al band syn·drome** a syndrome of knee pain that may result from inflammation due to mechanical friction of the iliotibial band and the lateral femoral epicondyle.

**il·i·o·tib·i·al tract** a fibrous reinforcement of the fascia lata on the lateral surface of the thigh, extending from the crest of the ilium to the lateral condyle of the tibia.

**il·i·o·tro·chan·ter·ic** (il′ē-ō-trō-kan-ter′ik) relating to the ilium and the great trochanter of the femur.

**il·i·o·tro·chan·ter·ic lig·a·ment** the lateral

strong band of the Y-shaped iliofemoral ligament; it is attached below to the tubercle at the upper part of the intertrochanteric line.

**il•i•um**, pl. **il•ia** (il'ē-ŭm, il'ē-ă) [TA] the broad, flaring portion of the hip bone, distinct at birth but later becoming fused with the ischium and pubis; it consists of a body, which joins the pubis and ischium to form the acetabulum and a broad thin portion, called the ala or wing. SYN iliac bone. [L. groin, flank]

**Il•i•zar•ov tech•nique** (il'iz-ah-rof) a method of promoting controlled osteogenesis to lengthen bone and correct angular and rotational deformities, in which gradually increasing force is applied to the apposed fragments of a surgically divided bone by an external fixation frame (Ilizarov device).

**ill•ness** (il'nes) SYN disease (1).

**il•lu•sion** (i-loo'zhŭn) a false perception; the mistaking of something for what it is not. [L. *illusio,* fr. *il- ludo,* pp. *-lusus,* to play at, mock]

**il•lu•sion•al** (i-loo'zhŭn-ăl) relating to or of the nature of an illusion.

**IM** internal medicine.

**im•age** (im'ij) **1.** representation of an object made by the rays of light emanating or reflected from it. **2.** representation produced by x-rays, ultrasound, tomography, thermography, radioisotopes, etc. **3.** to produce such a representation. [L. *imago,* likeness]

**im•age am•pli•fi•er** a device for converting a low light level fluoroscopic image to one that can be seen by the eye in a lighted environment; usually consists of an electronic light amplifier chained to a television tube.

**im•ag•e•ry** (im'ij-rē) a technique in behavior therapy in which the client or patient is conditioned to substitute pleasant fantasies to counter the unpleasant feelings associated with anxiety.

**imag•ing** (im'ă-jing) production of a clinical image using x-rays, ultrasound, computed tomography, magnetic resonance, radionuclide scanning, or thermography; especially, cross-sectional imaging, such as ultrasonography, CT, or MRI. [see image]

**ima•go**, pl. **imag•ines** (i-mā'gō, i-maj'i-nēz) **1.** the last stage of an insect after it has completed all its metamorphoses through the egg, larva, and pupa; the adult insect form. **2.** SYN archetype (2). [L. image]

**im•bal•ance** (im-bal'ans) **1.** lack of equality between opposing forces. **2.** lack of equality in some aspect of binocular vision, such as muscle balance or image size. [L. *in-* neg. + *bi-lanx* (*-lanc-*), having two scales, fr. *bis,* twice, + *lanx,* dish, scale of a balance]

**im•bi•bi•tion** (im-bi-bish'ŭn) **1.** absorption of fluid by a solid body without resultant chemical change in either. **2.** taking up of water by a gel. [L. *im-bibo,* to drink in (*in + bibo*)]

**im•bri•cate, im•bri•cat•ed** (im'bri-kāt, im'bri-kā-ted) overlapping like shingles. [L. *imbricatus,* covered with tiles]

**im•bri•ca•tion** (im'bri-kā'shŭn) the operative overlapping of layers of tissue in the closure of wounds or the repair of defects.

**im•id•a•zole** (im-id-az'ōl) a five-membered heterocyclic compound occurring in L-histidine and other biologically important compounds.

**im•ide** (im'īd) the radical or group, =NH, attached to two –CO– groups.

△**im•i•do-** prefix denoting the radical of an imide, formed by the loss of the H of the =NH group.

**im•i•dole** (im'i-dōl) SYN pyrrole.

△**-im•ine** suffix denoting the group =NH.

△**im•i•no-** prefix denoting the group =NH.

**im•i•no ac•ids** (im'i-nō as'idz) compounds with molecules containing both an acid group and an imino group.

**im•i•qui•mod** an immune response modifier used on the skin in the treatment of condyloma acuminata.

**Im•lach fat-pad** (im'lak) fat surrounding the round ligament of the uterus in the inguinal canal.

**im•ma•ture cat•a•ract** a stage of partial lens opacification.

**im•me•di•ate al•ler•gy** a type I allergic reaction; so called because in a sensitized subject the reaction becomes evident usually within minutes after contact with the allergen (antigen), reaches its peak within an hour or so, then rapidly recedes. SEE ALSO immediate reaction, anaphylaxis. Cf. delayed allergy.

**im•me•di•ate aus•cul•ta•tion, di•rect aus•cul•ta•tion** auscultation by application of the ear to the surface of the body.

**im•me•di•ate den•ture** a complete or partial denture constructed for insertion immediately following the removal of natural teeth.

**im•me•di•ate en•er•gy sys•tem** intramuscular non-aerobic energy system comprised of high-energy phosphates ATP and PCr; powers all-out physical effort for up to 6 to 8 seconds.

**im•me•di•ate flap** SYN direct flap.

**im•me•di•ate per•cus•sion** the striking of the part under examination directly with the finger or a plessor, without the intervention of another finger or plessimeter.

**im•me•di•ate re•ac•tion** local or generalized immune response that begins within a few minutes to about an hour after exposure to an antigen to which the individual has been sensitized. SEE ALSO skin test, wheal-and-erythema reaction.

**im•me•di•ate trans•fu•sion** SYN direct transfusion.

**im•mer•sion** (i-mer'zhŭn) **1.** the placing of a body under water or other liquid. **2.** MICROSCOPY filling the space between the objective lens and the top of the cover glass with a fluid, such as water or oil, to reduce spherical aberration and increase effective numerical aperture. [L. *immergo,* pp. *-mersus,* to dip in (*in + mergo*)]

**im•mer•sion foot** a condition resulting from prolonged exposure to damp and cold; the extremity is initially cold and anesthetic, but on rewarming becomes hyperemic, paresthetic, and hyperhidrotic; recovery is often slow.

**im•mer•sion ob•jec•tive** a high power objective used with a drop of oil between the lens and the specimen on the slide, allowing a greater numerical aperture; similar lenses are available for use with water as the immersing liquid.

**im•mis•ci•ble** (i-mis'i-bl) incapable of mutual solution; e.g., oil and water. [L. *immisceo,* to mix in (*in + misceo*)]

**im•mis•sion** (im-ish'in) environmental concentration of a pollutant, resulting from a combination of emissions and dispersals; often synonymous with exposure. [L. *immissio,* introduction, fr. *im-mitto,* to introduce]

**im•mit•tance** (i-mit'ans) AUDIOLOGY a general

term describing measurements of tympanic membrane impedance, compliance, or admittance. SYN admittance. [L. *immitto*, to send in]

**im·mo·bil·is·a·tion [Br.]** SEE immobilization.

**im·mo·bil·i·ty** (im-ō-bil'i-tē) the absence of movement, or inability to move.

**im·mo·bil·i·za·tion** (im-ō-bĭ-lĭ-zā-shŭn) the act or process of fixing or rendering immobile

**im·mo·bi·lize** (im-ō'bi-līz) to render fixed or incapable of moving. [L. *in-* neg. + *mobilis*, movable]

**im·mor·tal·i·sa·tion [Br.]** SEE immortalization.

**im·mor·tal·i·za·tion** (im-ō'bi-līzā'shŭn) conferring on normal cells cultured *in vitro* the property of an infinite lifespan, as from spontaneous mutation, by exposure to chemical carcinogens, or by viral infection.

**im·mov·a·ble joint** SYN fibrous joint.

**im·mune** (im-yun') **1.** free from the possibility of acquiring a given infectious disease; resistant to an infectious disease. **2.** pertaining to cell-mediated or humoral immunity, whereby an organism is so altered by previous contact with an antigen that it responds quickly and upon specifically subsequent contact; also to reactions *in vitro* with antibody-containing serum from such sensitized organisms. [L. *immunis*, free from service, fr. *in*, neg., + *munus* (*muner-*), service]

**im·mune ad·her·ence** the binding of antigen-antibody complexes or cells coated with antibodies or complement to cells bearing the appropriate complement or Fc receptors.

**im·mune ad·sorp·tion 1.** removal of antibody from antiserum by use of specific antigen. **2.** removal of antigen by specific antiserum.

**im·mune com·plex** antigen combined with specific antibody, to which complement may also be fixed, and which may precipitate or remain in solution. Frequently associated with autoimmune disease.

**im·mune com·plex dis·ease** an immunologic category of diseases evoked by the deposition of antigen-antibody or antigen-antibody-complement complexes on cell surfaces, with subsequent development of vasculitis; nephritis is common. Most of the connective tissue diseases, may belong in this immunologic category; immune complex diseases can also occur during a variety of diseases of known etiology, such as subacute bacterial endocarditis. SEE ALSO autoimmune disease.

**im·mune e·lec·tron mi·cros·co·py** electron microscopy of biological specimens to which specific antibody has been bound.

**im·mune pa·ral·y·sis** the induction of tolerance due to injection of large amounts of antigen. The antigen is poorly metabolized and the paralysis remains only during the persistence of the above. SYN immunologic paralysis.

**im·mune re·ac·tion** antigen-antibody reaction indicating a certain degree of resistance.

**im·mune re·sponse 1.** any response of the immune system to an antigen including antibody production and/or cell-mediated immunity; **2.** the response of the immune system to an antigen (immunogen) that leads to the condition of induced sensitivity; the immune response to the initial antigenic exposure (primary immune response) is detectable, as a rule, only after a lag period of from several days to two weeks; the immune response to a subsequent stimulus (secondary immune response) by the same antigen is more rapid than in the case of the primary immune response.

**im·mune re·sponse genes** genes in the HLA-D region of the histocompatibility complex of human chromosome 6 which control the immune response to specific antigens.

**im·mune se·rum** SYN antiserum.

**im·mune sur·veil·lance** a theory that the immune system destroys tumor cells which are constantly arising during the life of the individual. SYN immunological surveillance.

**im·mune sys·tem** an intricate complex of interrelated cellular, molecular, and genetic components which provides a defense (immune response) against foreign organisms or substances and aberrant native cells.

**im·mune throm·bo·cy·to·pe·nic pur·pu·ra** SYN idiopathic thrombocytopenic purpura.

**im·mu·ni·fa·cient** (im'yu-ni-fā'shent) making immune after a specific disease. [L. *immunis*, exempt, + *faciens*, making, pr. part. of *facio*]

**im·mu·ni·ty** (im-yu'ni-tē) the status or quality of being immune (1). SYN insusceptibility. [L. *immunitas* (see immune)]

**im·mu·ni·za·tion** protection of susceptible individuals from communicable diseases by administration of a living modified agent, a suspension of killed organisms, or an inactivated toxin. SEE ALSO vaccination.

**im·mu·nize** (im'yu-nīz) to render immune.

△**im·mu·no-** immune, immunity. [L. *immunis*, immune]

**im·mu·no·ad·ju·vant** (im'yu-nō-ad'joo-vant) SEE adjuvant (2).

**im·mu·no·as·say** (im'yu-nō-as'ā) detection and assay of substances by serological (immunological) methods. SEE ALSO radioimmunoassay, radioimmunoelectrophoresis, immunologic pregnancy test. SYN immunochemical assay.

**im·mu·no·blast** (im'yu-nō-blast) an antigenically stimulated lymphocyte; a large cell with well-defined basophilic cytoplasm, a large nucleus with prominent nuclear membrane, distinct nucleoli, and clumped chromatin. [immuno- + G. *blastos*, germ]

**im·mu·no·blot, im·mu·no·blot·ting** (i'myu-nō-blot') process by which antigens can be separated by electrophoresis and blotted to nitrocellulose sheets, where they bind and are subsequently identified by staining with labeled antibodies. SEE ALSO Western blot analysis.

**im·mu·no·chem·i·cal as·say** SYN immunoassay.

**im·mu·no·com·pe·tence** (im'yu-nō-kom'pĕ-tens) the ability to produce a normal immune response.

**im·mu·no·com·pe·tent** (im'yu-nō-kom'pĕ-tent) possessing the ability to mount a normal immune response.

**im·mu·no·com·pro·mised** (im'yu-nō-kom'pro-mīzd) denoting an individual whose immunologic mechanism is deficient either because of an immunodeficiency disorder or because it has been rendered so by immunosuppressive agents.

**im·mu·no·con·glu·ti·nin** (im'yu-nō-kon-gloo'ti-nin) an autoantibody-like immunoglobulin (IgM) formed by an organism against its own complement, following injection of complement-containing complexes or sensitized bacteria.

**im·mu·no·cyte** (im'yu-nō-sīt) an immunologically competent leukocyte capable of producing

i
m

antibodies or reacting in cell-mediated immunity reactions. SEE ALSO I cell. [immuno- + G. *kytos*, cell]

**im·mu·no·cy·to·ad·her·ence** (i'myu-nō-sī'tō-ad-her'ens) a method for determining cell surface properties, in which immunoglobulin or receptors on the surface of one cell population cause cells with corresponding molecular configurations on their surface to adhere in rosettes around the cells.

**im·mu·no·cy·to·chem·is·try** (im'yu-nō-sī-tō-kem'is-trē) the study of cell constituents by immunologic methods, such as the use of fluorescent antibodies.

**im·mu·no·de·fi·cien·cy** (im'yu-nō-dē-fish'en-sē) a condition resulting from a defective immune mechanism; may be *primary* (due to a defect in the immune mechanism itself) or *secondary* (dependent upon another disease process). SYN immunologic deficiency.

**im·mu·no·de·fi·cient** (im'yu-nō-dē-fish'ent) lacking in some essential function of the immune system.

**im·mu·no·dif·fu·sion** (im'yu-nō-di-fyu'zhŭn) a technique of study of antigen-antibody reactions by observing precipitates formed by combination of specific antigen and antibodies which have diffused in a gel in which they have been separately placed.

**im·mu·no·e·lec·tro·pho·re·sis** (im'yu-nō-ē-lek'trō-fō-rē'sis) a kind of precipitin test in which the components of one group of immunological reactants are first separated on the basis of electrophoretic mobility, the separated components then being identified on the basis of precipitates formed by reaction with components of the other group of reactants.

**im·mu·no·en·hance·ment** (im'yu-nō-en-hans'ment) IMMUNOLOGY the potentiating effect of specific antibody in establishing and in delaying rejection of a tumor allograft. SYN immunologic enhancement.

**im·mu·no·en·hanc·er** (im'yu-nō-en-hans'er) any specific or nonspecific substance that increases the degree of the immune response.

**im·mu·no·flu·o·res·cence** (im'yu-nō-floor-es'ens) an immunohistochemical technique using labeling of antibodies by fluorescent dyes to identify bacterial, viral, or other antigenic material specific for the labeled antibody; the binding of antibody can be determined microscopically by the application of ultraviolet rays to the preparation. SEE ALSO fluorescent antibody technique.

**im·mu·no·flu·o·res·cent stain** stain resulting from combination of fluorescent antibody with antigen specific for the antibody portion of the fluorochrome complex.

**im·mu·no·gen** (im'yu-nō-jen) SYN antigen.

**im·mu·no·ge·net·ics** (im'yu-nō-jĕ-net'iks) the study of the genetics of transplantation and tissue rejection, histochemical loci, immunologic response, immunoglobulin structure, and immunosuppression.

**im·mu·no·gen·ic** (im'yu-nō-jen'ik) SYN antigenic.

**im·mu·no·ge·nic·i·ty** (im'yu-nō-jĕ-nis'i-tē) SYN antigenicity.

**im·mu·no·glob·u·lin (Ig)** (im'yu-nō-glob'yu-lin) one of a class of structurally related proteins, each consisting of two pairs of polypeptide chains, one pair of light (L) [low molecular weight] chains ($\kappa$ or $\lambda$), and one pair of heavy (H) chains ($\gamma$, $\alpha$, $\delta$, and $\varepsilon$), all four linked together by disulfide bonds. On the basis of the structural and antigenic properties of the H chains, Igs are classified (in order of relative amounts present in normal human serum) as IgG (7 S in size, 80%), IgA (10 to 15%), IgM (19 S, a pentamer of the basic unit, 5 to 10%), IgD (less than 0.1%), and IgE (less than 0.01%). All of these classes are homogeneous and susceptible to amino acid sequence analysis. Each class of H chain can associate with either $\kappa$ or $\lambda$ L chains. Subclasses of Igs, based on differences in the H chains, are referred to as IgG1, etc.

When split by papain, IgG yields three pieces: the Fc piece, consisting of the C-terminal portion of the H chains, with no antibody activity but capable of fixing complement, and crystallizable; and two identical Fab pieces, carrying the antigen-binding sites and each consisting of an L chain bound to the remainder of an H chain.

Antibodies are Igs, and all Igs probably function as antibodies. However, Ig refers not only to the usual antibodies, but also to a great number of pathological proteins classified as myeloma proteins, which appear in multiple myeloma along with Bence Jones proteins, myeloma globulins, and Ig fragments.

From the amino acid sequences of Bence Jones proteins, it is known that all L chains are divided into a region of variable sequence ($V_L$) and one of constant sequence ($C_L$), each comprising about half the length of the L chain. The constant regions of all human L chains of the same type ($\kappa$ or $\lambda$) are identical except for a single amino acid substitution, under genetic controls. H chains are similarly divided, although the $V_H$ region, while similar in length to the $V_L$ region, is only one-third or one-fourth the length of the $C_H$ region. Binding sites are a combination of $V_L$ and $V_H$ protein regions. The large number of possible combinations of L and H chains make up the "libraries" of antibodies of each individual.

**im·mu·no·glob·u·lin do·mains** structural units of immunoglobulin heavy or light chains that are composed of approximately 110 amino acids. Light chains of an immunoglobulin are composed of one constant domain and one variable domain. Heavy chains are composed of either three or four constant domains and one variable domain.

**im·mu·no·his·to·chem·is·try** (im'yu-nō-his'tō-kem'is-trē) demonstration of specific antigens in tissues by the use of markers that are either fluorescent dyes or enzymes.

**im·mu·no·log·i·cal mech·a·nism** the groups of cells (chiefly lymphocytes and cells of the reticuloendothelial system) that function in establishing active acquired immunity (induced sensitivity, allergy).

**im·mu·no·log·i·cal pa·ral·y·sis** lack of specific antibody production after exposure to large doses of the antigen; immunological paralysis disappears when the antigen is eliminated.

**im·mu·no·log·i·cal sur·veil·lance** SYN immune surveillance.

**im·mu·no·log·ic com·pe·tence** capability of mounting an immunologic response.

**im·mu·no·log·ic de·fi·cien·cy** SYN immunodeficiency.

**im·mu·no·log·ic en·hance·ment** SYN immuno-enhancement.

**im·mu·no·log·ic mech·a·nism** the groups of cells (chiefly lymphocytes and cells of the reticuloendothelial system) that function in establishing active acquired immunity (induced sensitivity, allergy).

**im·mu·no·log·i·c pa·ral·y·sis** SYN immune paralysis.

**im·mu·no·log·ic preg·nan·cy test** a general term for tests for detection of increased human chorionic gonadotropin in plasma or urine by immunologic techniques including latex particle agglutination, hemagglutination inhibition, radioimmunoassay, and radioreceptor assays.

**im·mu·no·log·ic tol·er·ance** lack of immune response to antigen. Theories of tolerance induction include clonal deletion and clonal anergy. In clonal deletion, the actual clone of cells is eliminated whereas in clonal anergy the cells are present but nonfunctional.

**im·mu·nol·o·gist** (im-yu-nol'ō-jist) a specialist in the science of immunology.

**im·mu·nol·o·gy** (im'yu-nol'ō-jē) 1. the science concerned with the various phenomena of immunity, induced sensitivity, and allergy. 2. study of the structure and function of the immune system. [immuno- + G. *logos*, study]

**im·mu·no·mod·u·la·to·ry** (im'yu-nō-mod'yu-la-to-rē) 1. capable of modifying or regulating one or more immune functions. 2. an immunological adjustment, regulation, or potentiation.

**im·mu·no·per·ox·i·dase tech·nique** an immunologic test that utilizes antibodies chemically conjugated to the enzyme peroxidase.

**im·mu·no·phil·in** (im'yu-nō-fil-in) any of several high-affinity receptor proteins in the cytoplasm that combine with immunosuppressant drugs leading to rotamase inhibition and, in T cells, thus to interruption of cell activation. [*immune* + G. *philos*, fond, + in]

**im·mu·no·po·ten·ti·a·tion** (im'yu-nō-pō-ten-shē-ā'shŭn) enhancement of the immune response by increasing its rate or prolonging its duration.

**im·mu·no·po·ten·ti·a·tor** (im'yu-nō-pō-ten'shē-ā-tŏr) any substance which on inoculation enhances or augments an immune response.

**im·mu·no·pro·lif·er·a·tive dis·or·ders** disorders in which there is a continuing proliferation of cells of the immunocyte complex associated with autoallergic disturbances and immunoglobulin abnormalities, such as in chronic lymphocytic leukemia, "macroglobulinemias," and multiple myeloma.

**im·mu·no·ra·di·o·met·ric as·say** a procedure in which an unknown antigen binds to an excess of antibody that has a radioactive label. The unbound antibody is removed in a subsequent step. The amount of antigen present is directly proportional to the amount of measured radioactivity.

**im·mu·no·re·ac·tive** (im'yu-nō-rē-ak'tiv) denoting or exhibiting immunoreaction.

**im·mu·no·sor·bent** (im'yu-nō-sōr'bent) an antibody (or antigen) used to remove specific antigen (or antibody) from solution or suspension.

**im·mu·no·sup·pres·sant** (im'yu-nō-sŭ-pres'ant) an agent that induces immunosuppression. SYN immunosuppressive (2).

**im·mu·no·sup·pres·sion** (im'yu-nō-sŭ-presh'ŭn) prevention or interference with the development of immunologic response; may reflect natural immunologic unresponsiveness (tolerance), may be artificially induced by chemical, biological, or physical agents, or may be caused by disease.

**im·mu·no·sup·pres·sive** (im'yu-nō-sŭ-pres'iv) 1. denoting or inducing immunosuppression. 2. SYN immunosuppressant.

**im·mu·no·sur·veil·lance** (im'yu-nō-ser-vā'lance) theory that holds that the immune system eliminates tumor cells that arise spontaneously.

**im·mu·no·ther·a·py** (im'ū-nō-thār'ă-pē) originally, therapeutic administration of serum or immune globulin containing preformed antibodies produced by another individual; currently, immunotherapy includes nonspecific systemic stimulation, adjuvants, active specific immunotherapy, and adoptive immunotherapy. New forms of immunotherapy include the use of monoclonal antibodies. SYN biologic immunotherapy.

This method has been widely adopted in oncology, particularly in cases that fail to respond to other treatment. Immunotherapy seeks to boost immune system function, as with the administration of interferons and interleukin-2, or to attack cancerous cells directly, as with the injection of monoclonal antibodies. Various immunotherapeutic techniques have also been used in the treatment of AIDS. In addition, a number of alternative medical practices are claimed to enhance immune function, and various over-the-counter substances have gained popularity for this supposed property.

**im·mu·no·trans·fu·sion** (im'yu-nō-trans-fyu'zhŭn) an indirect transfusion in which the donor is first immunized by injections of antigen from microorganisms isolated from the recipient; later, the donor's blood is collected, defibrinated, and then administered to the patient; the latter is thus passively immunized by antibody formed in the donor.

**IMP** inosine 5'-monophosphate.

**im·pact·ed** (im-pak'ted) wedged or pressed closely so as to be immovable.

**im·pact·ed fe·tus** a fetus which, because of its large size or narrowing of the pelvic canal, has become wedged and incapable of spontaneous advance or recession.

**im·pact·ed frac·ture** a fracture in which one of the fragments is driven into the cancellous tissue of the other fragment.

**im·pact·ed tooth 1.** a tooth whose normal eruption is prevented by adjacent teeth or bone; **2.** a tooth that has been driven into the alveolar process or surrounding tissue as a result of trauma.

**im·pact fac·tor** mathematical expression of frequency with which a particular medical journal's original articles are cited in other medical journals.

**im·pair·ment** (im-pār'ment) any loss or abnormality of psychological, physiological or anatomical structure or function.

**im·ped·ance** (im-pē'dăns) 1. opposition to flow of gases, liquids, or electrical current. 2. resistance of an acoustic system to being set in motion.

**im·pe·dance match·ing** the force delivered through the mechanical advantages of the tympanic ossicles and the area ratio of the tympanic membrane to the oval window to overcome the acoustic impedance between the ambient air and the fluid in the inner ear.

i
m

**im·per·fect fun·gus** a fungus in which the means of sexual reproduction is not yet recognized; these fungi generally reproduce by means of conidia.

**im·per·fect stage** a mycological term used to describe the asexual life cycle phase of a fungus.

**im·per·fo·rate** (im-per'fŏr-āt) SYN atretic.

**im·per·fo·rate a·nus 1.** SYN anal atresia. **2.** SYN ectopic (1).

**im·per·fo·ra·tion** (im-per-fŏr-ā'shŭn) condition of being atretic, occluded, or closed. [L. *im-* neg. + *per-foro*, pp. *-atus*, to bore through]

**im·per·me·a·ble** (im-per'mē-ă-bl) not permitting the passage of liquids, gases, or heat through a membrane or other structure. [L. *im- permeabilis*, not to be passed through]

**im·pe·tig·i·nous** (im-pe-tij'i-nŭs) relating to impetigo.

🔲 **im·pe·ti·go** (im-pe-tī'gō) a contagious superficial pyoderma, caused by *Staphylococcus aureus* or Group A streptococci, that begins with a superficial flaccid vesicle which ruptures and forms a thick yellowish crust, most commonly occurring on the faces of children. See page B6. SYN impetigo contagiosa, impetigo vulgaris. [L. a scabby eruption, fr. *im-peto* (*inp-*), to rush upon, attack]

**im·pe·ti·go con·ta·gi·o·sa** SYN impetigo.

**im·pe·ti·go her·pet·i·for·mis** a rare pyoderma, occurring most commonly in the third trimester of pregnancy as an eruption of small closely aggregated pustules accompanied by severe constitutional symptoms and fetal death.

**im·pe·ti·go ne·o·na·to·rum 1.** SYN dermatitis exfoliativa infantum. **2.** SYN bullous impetigo of newborn.

**im·pe·ti·go vul·ga·ris** SYN impetigo.

**im·pinge·ment sign** pain in patients with rotator cuff tendinitis or tears within the subacromial space elicited by provocative physical examination maneuvers.

**im·pingement syn·drome** chronic shoulder pain and disability due to trauma to the rotator cuff (particularly the supraspinatus tendon) by surrounding bony processes and ligaments, such as occurs during performance of overhead work.

**im·pinge·ment test** diagnostic test in which local anesthetic is injected into the subacromial space of a patient with impingement signs; relief of pain following the injection during provocative maneuvers is helpful in confirming the subacromial space as the source of the symptoms.

**im·plant 1.** (im-plant') to graft or insert. **2.** (im' plant) material inserted or grafted into tissues. SEE ALSO graft, transplant. **3.** DENTISTRY a graft or insert set in or onto the alveolar recess prepared for its insertion. SEE ALSO implant denture. **4.** ORTHOPAEDICS a metallic or plastic device employed in joint reconstruction. [L. *im-*, in, + *planto*, pp. *-atus*, to plant, fr. *planta*, a sprout, shoot]

**im·plan·ta·tion** (im-plan-tā'shŭn) **1.** attachment of the fertilized ovum (blastocyst) to the endometrium, and its subsequent embedding in the compact layer, occurring 6 or 7 days after fertilization of the ovum in humans. **2.** the process of placing a device or substance within the body, e.g., placement of a saline-filled device beneath the breast mound. **3.** insertion of a natural tooth into an artificially constructed alveolus. **4.** tissue grafting. SEE ALSO transplantation.

**im·plant den·ture** a denture that receives its sta-

bility and retention from a substructure which is partially or wholly implanted under the soft tissues of the denture basal seat.

**im·plant·ed su·ture** passage of a pin through each lip of the wound parallel to the line of incision, the pins then being looped together with sutures.

**im·plo·sion** (im-plō'shŭn) **1.** a sudden collapse, as of an evacuated vessel, in which there is a bursting inward rather than outward as in explosion. **2.** a type of behavior therapy, similar to flooding, during which the patient is given massive exposure to extreme anxiety-arousing stimuli.

**im·po·tence, im·po·ten·cy** (im'pŏ-tens, im'pŏ-ten-sē) **1.** weakness; lack of power. **2.** inability of the male to achieve and/or maintain penile erection and thus engage in copulation; a manifestation of neurological, vascular, or psychological dysfunction. [L. *impotentia*, inability, fr. *in-* neg. + *potentia*, power]

**im·preg·nate** (im-preg'nāt) **1.** to fertilize or fecundate; to cause to conceive. **2.** to permeate or saturate with another substance. SEE ALSO saturate. [L. *im-*, in, + *praegnans*, with child]

**im·pres·sio,** pl. **im·pres·si·o·nes** (im-pres'ē-ō, im-pres-ē-ō'nēz) [TA] SYN impression. [L.]

**im·pres·sion** (im-presh'ŭn) **1.** a mark seemingly made by pressure of one structure or organ on another, seen especially in cadaveric dissections. See also *groove* for the various impressions of the lungs, e.g., descending aorta, subclavian artery, and vena cavae. **2.** an effect produced upon the mind by some external object acting through the organs of sense. **3.** an imprint or negative likeness; especially, the negative form of the teeth and/or other tissues of the oral cavity, made in a plastic material that becomes relatively hard or set while in contact with these tissues, made in order to reproduce a positive form or cast of the recorded tissues; classified, according to the materials of that they are made, as reversible and irreversible hydrocolloid impression, modeling plastic impression, plaster impression, and wax impression. SYN impressio [TA]. [L. *impressio,* fr. *im- primo*, pp. *-pressus*, to press upon]

**im·print·ing** a particular kind of learning characterized by its occurrence in the first few hours of life, and which determines species-recognition behavior.

**im·pulse** (im'pŭls) **1.** a sudden pushing or driving force. **2.** a sudden, often unreasoning, determination to perform some act. **3.** the action potential of a nerve fiber. [L. *im-pello*, pp. *-pulsus*, to push against, impel (*inp-*)]

**im·pulse con·trol dis·or·der** a class of mental disorders characterized by impulse to resist an impulse to perform some act harmful to oneself or to others; includes pathological gambling, pedophilia, kleptomania, pyromania, trichotillomania, intermittent and isolated explosive disorders.

**im·pul·sion** (im-pŭl'shŭn) an abnormal urge to perform a certain activity.

**im·pul·sive** (im-pŭl'siv) relating to or actuated by an impulse, rather than controlled by reason or careful deliberation.

**im·pul·sive ob·ses·sion** an obsession accompanied by action, sometimes becoming a mania.

**im·pure flut·ter** mixture of atrial flutter (FF) waves and fibrillation (ff) waves in the electrocardiogram. SYN flitter, flutter-fibrillation.

**IMV** intermittent mandatory ventilation.

**In** indium; inulin.

⚠**in-** **1.** not, akin to G. *a-, an-* or Eng. *un-*. **2.** in, within, inside. **3.** very; appears as im- before b, p, or m. [L.]

**in·ac·ti·vate** (in-ak'ti-vāt) to destroy the biological activity or the effects of an agent or substance.

**in·ac·ti·vat·ed po·li·o·vi·rus vac·cine** SEE poliovirus vaccine (1).

**in·ac·tive re·pres·sor** a repressor that cannot combine with an operator gene until it has combined with a corepressor (usually a product of a protein pathway); after activation, the repressor arrests production of the proteins controlled by the operator gene; a homeostatic mechanism for regulation of repressible enzyme systems. SYN aporepressor.

**in·ad·e·quate per·son·al·i·ty** a personality disorder, characterized by personal and social ineptness plus emotional and physical instability, which renders the individual unable to cope with the normal vicissitudes of life.

**in·ad·e·quate stim·u·lus** a stimulus too weak to evoke a response.

**in·an·i·mate** (in-an'i-māt) not alive. [L. *in-* neg. + *anima*, breath, soul]

**in·a·ni·tion** (in'ă-nish'ŭn) severe weakness and wasting as occurs from lack of food, defect in assimilation, or neoplastic disease. [L. *inanis*, empty]

**in·ap·pe·tence** (in-ap'ĕ-tens) lack of desire or of craving. [L. *in-* neg. + *ap-peto*, pp. *-petitus*, to strive after, long for (*adp-*)]

**in·ar·tic·u·late** (in-ar-tik'yu-lit) **1.** not articulate in the form of intelligible speech. **2.** unable to satisfactorily express oneself in words.

**in·as·sim·i·la·ble** (in-ă-sim'il-ă-bl) not assimilable; not capable of undergoing assimilation. SEE assimilation.

**in·born** (in'bōrn) implanted during development *in utero*. In the specific context of inborn error of metabolism, it connotes a genetic disruption of an enzyme. SEE inborn errors of metabolism. SYN innate.

**in·born er·rors of me·tab·o·lism** a group of disorders, each of which involves a disorder of a single unique enzyme, genetic in origin and operating from birth; effects are ascribable to accumulation of the substrate on which the enzyme normally acts (e.g., phenylketonuria), to deficiency of the product of the enzyme (e.g., albinism), or to forcing metabolism through an auxiliary pathway (e.g., oxaluria).

**in·bred** denoting populations (groups, genetic lines, etc.) descended over several generations almost exclusively from a small set of ancestors, and hence having a high rate of consanguinity.

**in·breed·ing** (in'brēd-ing) **1.** mating between organisms that are genetically more closely related than organisms selected at random from the population. **2.** a practice of mating animals that are closely related.

**in·car·cer·at·ed** (in-kar'ser-ā-ted) confined; imprisoned; trapped. [L. *in*, in, + *carcero*, pp. *-atus*, to imprison, fr. *carcer*, prison]

**in·car·cer·at·ed her·nia** SYN irreducible hernia.

**in·cen·tive spi·ro·me·ter** a device used in bronchial hygiene therapy that provides the patient with visual or other feedback during efforts to achieve a predetermined respiratory flow or volume; useful in increasing inspiratory volume, improving inspiratory muscle performance, maintaining airway patency, and preventing or reversing atelectasis.

**in·cest** (in'sest) **1.** sexual relations between persons closely related by blood, especially between parents and their children, and between siblings. **2.** the crime of sexual relations between persons related by blood, where such cohabitation is prohibited by law. [L. *incestus*, unchaste, fr. *in-*, not, + *castus*, chaste]

**in·ces·tu·ous** (in-ses'choo-ŭs) **1.** pertaining to incest. **2.** guilty of incest.

**in·ci·dence** (in'si-dens) **1.** the number of specified new events, e.g., persons falling ill with a specified disease, during a specified period in a specified population. **2.** OPTICS intersection of a ray of light with a surface. [L. *incido*, to fall into or upon, to happen]

**in·ci·dent·a·lo·ma** (in'sĭ-den-tă-lō'mă) mass lesion, usually of the adrenal gland, noted fortuitously during computerized tomographic examinations performed for other reasons. [incidental + *-oma*, tumor]

**in·ci·den·tal par·a·site** a parasite that normally lives on a host other than its present host. SYN accidental parasite.

**in·ci·dent com·mand sys·tem** SYN incident management system.

**in·ci·dent ma·nage·ment sys·tem** a nationally recognized system of unified command and control for dealing with mass-casualty or disaster incidents. SYN incident command system.

**in·ci·dent point** the point at which a light ray enters an optical system.

**in·ci·sal** (in-sī'zăl) cutting; relating to the cutting edges of the incisor and canine teeth. [L. *incido*, pp. *-cisus*, to cut into]

**in·ci·sal guide an·gle** the angle formed with the horizontal plane by drawing a line in the sagittal plane between incisal edges of the maxillary and mandibular central incisors when the teeth are in centric occlusion.

**in·cise** (in-sīz') to cut with a knife.

**in·cised wound** a clean cut, as by a sharp instrument.

▯**in·ci·sion** (in-sizh'ŭn) a cut; a surgical wound; a division of the soft parts made with a knife. See page 492. [L. *incisio*]

**in·ci·sion·al her·nia** hernia occurring through a surgical incision or scar.

▯**in·ci·sion bi·op·sy** removal of only a part of a lesion by incising into it. See page 117.

**in·ci·sive** (in-sī'siv) **1.** cutting; having the power to cut. **2.** relating to the incisor teeth.

**in·ci·sive bone** SYN os incisivum.

**in·ci·sive ca·nal, in·ci·sor ca·nal** one of several bony canals leading from the floor of the nasal cavity into the incisive fossa on the palatal surface of the maxilla; they convey the nasopalatine nerves and branches of the greater palatine arteries which anastomose with the septal branch of the sphenopalatine artery. SYN canalis incisivus [TA].

**in·ci·sive ca·nal cyst** a cyst in or near the incisive canal, arising from proliferation of epithelial remnants of the nasopalatine duct; the most common maxillary development cyst.

**in·ci·sive fo·ra·men** one of several (usually four) openings of the incisive canals into the incisive fossa.

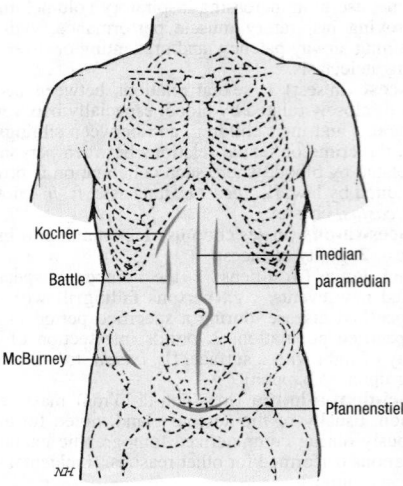

Kocher

Battle

McBurney

median

paramedian

Pfannenstiel

ЛН

**surgical incisions**

**in·ci·sive pa·pil·la** a slight elevation of the mucosa at the anterior extremity of the raphe of the palate.

**in·ci·sor** (in-sī′zŏr) one of the cutting teeth, incisor teeth, four in number in each jaw at the apex of the dental arch. [L. *incido,* to cut into]

**in·ci·sor tooth** a tooth with a chisel-shaped crown and a single conical tapering root; there are four of these teeth in the anterior part of each jaw, in both the deciduous and the permanent dentitions. SYN dens incisivus [TA].

**in·ci·su·ra,** pl. **in·ci·su·rae** (in′sī-soo′ră, in′si-soo′rē) [TA] SYN notch. [L. a cutting into]

**in·ci·sure** (in-sī′zhoor) SYN notch. [L. *incisura*]

**in·cli·na·tion** (in-kli-nā′shŭn) 1. a leaning or sloping. 2. DENTISTRY deviation of the long axis of a tooth from the perpendicular. SYN version (3). [L. *inclinatio,* a leaning]

**in·clu·sion** (in-kloo′zhŭn) 1. any foreign or heterogeneous substance contained in a cell or in any tissue or organ, not introduced as a result of trauma. 2. the process by which a foreign or heterogeneous structure is misplaced in another tissue. [L. *inclusio,* a shutting in, fr. *in-cludo,* pp. *-clusis,* to close in]

**in·clu·sion bod·ies** distinctive structures frequently formed in the nucleus or cytoplasm (occasionally in both locations) in cells infected with certain filtrable viruses, observed especially in nerve, epithelial, or endothelial cells.

**in·clu·sion bod·y dis·ease** SYN cytomegalic inclusion disease.

**in·clu·sion cell** SYN I cell.

**in·clu·sion con·junc·ti·vi·tis** a follicular conjunctivitis caused by *Chlamydia trachomatis.*

**in·com·pat·i·bil·i·ty** (in′kom-pat-i-bil′i-tē) 1. the quality of being incompatible. 2. a means of classifying bacterial plasmids; two plasmids are incompatible if they cannot coexist in one host cell.

**in·com·pat·i·ble** (in-kom-pat′i-bl) 1. not suitable to be combined or mixed with another substance. 2. denoting persons who are unable to associate with one another without anxiety and conflict. 3.

having genotypes that put progeny at high risk of severe recessive disorders or that promote harmful maternal-fetal reaction. [L. *in-* neg., + *con-,* with, + *patior,* pp. *passus,* to suffer, tolerate]

**in·com·pe·tence, in·com·pe·ten·cy** (in-kom′petens, in-kom′pĕ-ten-sē) 1. the quality of being incompetent or incapable of performing the allotted function, especially failure of cardiac or venous valves to close completely. SYN insufficiency (2). 2. FORENSIC PSYCHIATRY the inability to distinguish right from wrong or to manage one's affairs. [L. *in-,* neg. + *com-peto,* strive after together]

**in·com·pe·tent cer·vi·cal os** a defect in the strength of the internal os allowing premature dilation of the cervix.

**in·com·plete a·bor·tion** abortion in which part of the products of conception have been passed but part (usually the placenta) remains in the uterus.

**in·com·plete an·ti·bod·y** 1. SYN univalent antibody. 2. SYN serum agglutinin.

**in·com·plete an·ti·gen** SYN hapten.

**in·com·plete fis·tu·la** SYN blind fistula.

**in·com·plete foot pre·sen·ta·tion** SEE breech presentation.

**in·con·stant** (in-kon′stant) 1. irregular. 2. ANATOMY denoting a structure, such as an artery, or nerve, that may or may not be present.

**in·con·ti·nence** (in-kon′ti-nens) 1. inability to prevent the discharge of any of the excretions, especially of urine or feces. 2. lack of restraint of the appetites, especially sexual. SYN incontinentia. [L. *in-continentia,* fr. *in-* neg. + *con-tineo,* to hold together, fr. *teneo,* to hold]

**in·con·ti·nent** (in-kon′ti-nent) denoting incontinence.

**in·con·ti·nen·tia** (in-kon′ti-nen′shē-ă) SYN incontinence. [L.]

**in·co·or·di·na·tion** (in-kō-ōr-di-nā′shŭn) SYN ataxia. [L. *in-* neg. + coordination]

**in·crease** (in′krēs) any growth in quantity.

**in·cre·ment** (in′kre-ment) a change in the value of a variable; usually an increase, with "decrement" applied to a decrease, though "increment" can also correctly be applied to both. [L. *incrementum,* increase]

**in·cre·tin** generic term for all insulinotropic substances originating in the gastrointestinal tract that are released into the circulation by meals containing glucose. One is glucose-dependent insulinotropic polypeptide, which is released into the circulation from crypt cells in the proximal duodenum and jejunum after meals containing glucose or long-chain fatty acids. Another is proglucagon-derived polypeptide, cleavage product of glucagon, which is further processed into glucagonlike peptide-1 and then to glucagonlike insulinotropic peptide.

**in·cre·tion** (in-krē′shŭn) the functional activity of an endocrine gland. [in- + secretion]

**in·crus·ta·tion** (in′krŭs-tā′shŭn) 1. formation of a crust or a scab. 2. a coating of some adventitious material or an exudate; a scab. [L. *in-crusto,* pp. *-atus,* to incrust, fr. *crusta,* crust]

**in·cu·ba·tion** (in′kyu-bā′shŭn) 1. maintaining controlled environmental conditions to favor growth or development of microbial or tissue cultures. 2. maintenance of an artificial environment for an infant, usually a premature or hypoxic one, by providing proper temperature, humidity, and, usually, oxygen. **3.** the development, without sign or symptom, of an infection from the time the infectious agent gains entry until the appearance of the first signs or symptoms. [L. *incubo,* to lie on]

**in·cu·ba·tion pe·ri·od 1.** time interval between invasion of the body by an infecting organism and the appearance of the first sign or symptom it causes; SYN incubative stage, latent period (2), latent stage, prodromal stage. **2.** in a disease vector, the period between entry of the disease organism and the time at which the vector is capable of transmitting the disease to another human host.

**in·cu·ba·tive stage** SYN incubation period (1).

**in·cu·ba·tor** (in'kyu-bā'tōr) **1.** a container in which controlled environmental conditions may be maintained; e.g., for culturing microorganisms. **2.** an apparatus for maintaining an infant (usually premature) in an environment of proper oxygenation, humidity, and temperature.

**in·cu·bus** (in'koo-bŭs) **1.** originally, an evil spirit that lay upon and oppressed sleeping persons; especially, a male spirit that copulated with sleeping women. Cf. succubus. **2.** SYN nightmare. [L. fr. *incubo,* to lie on]

**in·cu·dal** (in'koo-dăl) relating to the incus.

**in·cu·dec·to·my** (in-koo-dek'tō-mē) removal of the incus of the tympanum. [incus + G. *ektomē,* excision]

**in·cu·des** (in-koo'dēz) plural of incus. [L.]

**in·cu·do·sta·pe·di·al** (in-koo'dō-stā-pē'dē-ăl) relating to the incus and the stapes; denoting the articulation between the incus and the stapes in the middle ear.

**in·cur·va·tion** (in'ker-vā'shŭn) an inward curvature; a bending inward.

**in·cus,** gen. **in·cu·dis,** pl. **in·cu·des** (ing'kŭs, in-koo'dis, in-koo'dēz) [TA] the middle of the three ossicles in the middle ear; it has a body and two limbs or processes (long crus and short crus); at the tip of the long crus is a small knob, the lenticular process which articulates with the head of the stapes. SYN anvil. [L. anvil]

**in·cy·clo·duc·tion** (in-sī-klō-dŭk'shŭn) a cyclo-duction in which the upper pole of the cornea is rotated inward (medially). [in- + cyclo- + L. *duco,* pp. *ductus,* to lead]

**in·cy·clo·pho·ria** (in-sī'klō-fō'rē-ă) a cyclopho-ria in which the 12 o'clock position in the iris tends to twist medially. [L. in- + cyclo- + G. *phora,* a carrying]

**in·cy·clo·tro·pia** (in-sī-klō-trō'pē-ă) a cyclotro-pia in which the upper poles of the corneas are rotated inward (medially) to each other. [in- + cyclo- + G. *trope,* a turning]

**in·de·pen·dent liv·ing mo·del** service delivery model that identifies the consumer as the decision maker regarding health care and other daily living needs upon presentation of choices by health care providers.

**in·de·pen·dent prac·tice as·soc·i·a·tion** an association of independent physicians or small groups of physicians formed for the purpose of contracting with one or more managed health care organizations. Member physicians provide medical services for HMO patients in their own offices and are allowed to maintain private practices. SEE ALSO managed care, health maintenance organization.

**in·de·pen·dent prac·tice as·so·ci·a·tion**

**HMO** arrangement by which physician providers are paid by the HMO on a fee-for-service basis for each patient seen, as negotiated with the HMO

**in·dex,** gen. **in·di·cis,** pl. **in·di·ces, in·dex·es** (in'deks, in-di-sis, in'di-sēz, in'dek-sĕz) **1.** [TA] SYN index finger. **2.** a guide, standard, indicator, symbol, or number denoting the relation in respect to size, capacity, or function, of one part or thing to another. SEE ALSO quotient, ratio. **3.** a core or mold used to record or maintain the relative position of a tooth or teeth to one another and/or to a cast. **4.** a guide, usually made of plaster, used to reposition teeth, casts, or parts. **5.** in epidemiology, a rating scale. [L. one that points out, an informer, the forefinger, an index, fr. *in-dico,* pp. *-atus,* to declare]

**in·dex case** SYN proband.

**in·dex ex·ten·sor mus·cle** SYN extensor indicis muscle.

**in·dex fin·ger** the second finger (the thumb being counted as the first). SYN index (1).

**in·di·can·i·dro·sis** (in'di-kan-i-drō'sis) excretion of indican in the sweat. [indican + G. *hidrōs,* sweat]

**in·di·can·u·ria** (in'di-kan-yu'rē-ă) an increased urinary excretion of indican, a derivative of indol formed chiefly in the intestine when protein is putrefied; indol is also formed during the putre-faction of protein in other sites.

**in·di·ca·tion** (in-di-kā'shŭn) the basis or rationale for using a particular treatment or diagnostic test; may be furnished by a knowledge of the cause (**causal indication**), by the symptoms present (**symptomatic indication**), or by the nature of the disease (**specific indication**). [L. fr. *in-dico,* pp. *-atus,* to point out, fr. *dico,* to proclaim]

**in·di·ca·tor** (in'di-kā-ter) **1.** in chemical analysis, a substance that changes color within a certain definite range of pH or oxidation potential, or in any way renders visible the completion of a chemical reaction; e.g., litmus, phenolsulfon-phthalein. **2.** an isotope that is used as a tracer. **3.** the labeled substance whose distribution between reactants of a system is used to determine the amount of analyte present. [L. one that points out]

**in·di·ces** (in'di-sēz) alternative plural of index.

**in·dif·fer·ent go·nad** the primordial organ in an embryo before its differentiation into testis or ovary.

**in·dif·fer·ent tis·sue** undifferentiated, nonspecialized, embryonic tissue.

**in·di·ges·tion** (in-di-jes'chŭn) nonspecific term for a variety of symptoms resulting from a failure of proper digestion and absorption of food in the alimentary tract.

**in·di·rect cal·o·rim·e·try** determination of heat production of an oxidation reaction by measuring uptake of oxygen and/or liberation of carbon di-oxide and nitrogen excretion.

**in·di·rect Coombs test** (koomz) a test routinely performed in cross-matching blood or in the investigation of transfusion reaction: test for patient's serum is incubated with a suspension of donor erythrocytes; if specific antibodies are present, they become attached to the antigen in the donor cells; after a washing with saline, Coombs antihuman globulin is added; agglutination at this point indicates that antibodies present

i
n

in the original test serum had indeed become attached to donor erythrocytes.

**in·di·rect frac·ture** a fracture, especially of the skull, that occurs at a point not at the site of impact.

**in·di·rect he·mag·glu·ti·na·tion test** SYN passive hemagglutination.

**in·di·rect im·mu·no·flu·o·res·cence** fluorescence microscopy of normal tissue after application of the patient's serum, to detect antibodies to normal tissue components (autoantibodies). SEE ALSO fluorescent antibody technique.

**in·di·rect lar·yn·gos·co·py** inspection of the larynx by means of a reflected image on a mirror.

**in·di·rect nu·cle·ar di·vi·sion** SYN mitosis.

**in·di·rect oph·thal·mo·scope** an instrument designed to visualize the interior of the eye, with the instrument at arm's length from the subject's eye and the observer viewing an inverted image through a convex lens located between the instrument and the subject's eye.

**in·di·rect re·act·ing bil·i·ru·bin** the fraction of serum bilirubin which has not been conjugated with glucuronic acid in the liver cell; so called because it reacts with the Ehrlich diazo reagent only when alcohol is added; increased levels are found in hepatic disease and hemolytic conditions.

**in·di·rect trans·fu·sion** transfusion into a patient of blood previously obtained from a donor and stored in a suitable container.

**in·di·rect vi·sion** SYN peripheral vision.

**in·di·um (In)** (in′dē-ŭm) a metallic element, atomic no. 49, atomic wt. 114.82. [*indigo*, because of its blue line in the spectrum]

**in·di·vid·u·al·ized ed·u·ca·tion pro·gram (IEP)** an education program tailored to a particular individual with a disability, whose provision is mandated by law. SEE ALSO Individuals with Disabilities Education Act.

**in·di·vid·u·al psy·chol·o·gy** a theory of human behavior emphasizing humans' social nature, strivings for mastery, and drive to overcome, by compensation, feelings of inferiority.

**In·di·vid·u·als with Dis·a·bil·i·ties Ed·u·ca·tion Act (IDEA)** federal law (Public Law 94-142, enacted in 1975 and subsequently amended) guaranteeing all students with disabilities, ages 3 through 21, the right to a free and appropriate public education designed to meet their individual needs. SEE ALSO individualized education program.

**in·di·vid·u·a·tion** (in′di-vid-yu-ā′shŭn) **1.** development of the individual from the specific. **2.** JUNGIAN PSYCHOLOGY the process by which one's personality is differentiated, developed, and expressed. **3.** regional activity in an embryo as a response to an organizer.

**in·di·vid·u·a·tion field** the field within which an organizer can bring about the rearrangement of primordial tissues in such a manner that a complete embryo is formed.

**in·do·cy·a·nine green** (in-dō-sī′ă-nēn) a tricarbocyanine dye that binds to serum albumin and is used in blood volume determinations and in liver function tests.

**in·do·cy·an·ine green an·gi·o·gra·phy** a test for studying choroidal vasculature by which indocyanine green dye, which absorbs infrared light at 805 nm and emits at 835 nm, is injected

intravenously and photographed as it flows through the retinal and choroidal vessels.

**in·dol·ac·e·tu·ria** (in′dōl-as-ĕt-yur′ē-ă) excretion of an appreciable amount of indoleacetic acid in the urine; a manifestation of Hartnup disease.

**in·dol·a·mine** (in-dol′ă-mēn) an indole or indole derivative containing a primary, secondary, or tertiary amine group.

**in·dole** (in′dōl) **1.** 2,3-benzopyrrole; basis of many biologically active substances (e.g., serotonin, tryptophan); formed in degradation of tryptophan. SYN ketole. **2.** any of many alkaloids containing the indole (1) structure.

**in·do·lent** (in′dō-lent) inactive; sluggish; painless or nearly so, said of a morbid process. [L. *in*-neg. + *doleo*, pr. p. *dolens* (-*ent*-), to feel pain]

**in·do·lent bu·bo** a painless, chronic enlargement of an inguinal node.

**in·dol·ic ac·ids** (in-dōl′ik as′idz) metabolites of L-tryptophan formed within the body or by intestinal microorganisms.

**in·dox·yl** (in-dok′sil) the radical of 3-hydroxyindole; a product of intestinal bacterial degradation of indoleacetic acid; increased amounts are excreted in in the urine in phenylketonuria.

**in·dox·yl·u·ria** (in-dok-sil-yu′rē-ă) the excretion of indoxyl, especially indoxyl sulfate, in the urine; indoxyluria may be associated with indicanuria, inasmuch as hydrolysis of indican results in formation of indoxyl.

**in·duced a·bor·tion** abortion brought on deliberately by drugs or mechanical means.

**in·duced en·zyme, in·duc·i·ble en·zyme** an enzyme that can be detected in a growing culture of a microorganism, after the addition of a particular substance (inducer) to the culture medium, but not prior to the addition.

**in·duced eryth·ro·cy·the·mia** SYN blood doping.

**in·duced hy·po·ten·sion, con·trolled hy·po·ten·sion** deliberate acute reduction of arterial blood pressure to reduce operative blood loss by pharmacologic means during anesthesia and surgery.

**in·duc·er** (in-doos′er) a molecule, usually a substrate of a specific enzyme pathway, that combines with and deactivates an active repressor (produced by a regulator gene); this allows an operator gene previously repressed to activate the structural genes controlled by it to resume enzyme production.

**in·duc·tance** (in-dŭk′tans) the coefficient of electromagnetic induction; the unit of inductance is the henry. [see induction]

**in·duc·tion** (in-dŭk′shŭn) **1.** production or causation. **2.** production of an electric current or magnetic state in a body by electricity or magnetism in another body close to the first body. **3.** the period from the start of anesthesia to the establishment of a depth of anesthesia adequate for a surgical procedure. **4.** EMBRYOLOGY the influence exerted by an organizer or evocator on the differentiation of adjacent cells or on the development of an embryonic structure. **5.** a modification imposed on the offspring by the action of environment on the germ cells of one or both parents. **6.** MICROBIOLOGY a change from probacteriophage to vegetative phage, which may occur spontaneously or after stimulation by certain physical and chemical agents. **7.** ENZYMOLOGY the process of increasing the amount or the activity of a protein. SEE ALSO inducer. **8.** a stage in the process of hypnosis. **9.** causal analysis; a method of reasoning in which an inference is made from one or more specific observations to a more general statement. Cf. deduction. [L. *inductio,* a leading in]

**in•duc•tion pe•ri•od** the period required for a specific agent to produce a disease; the interval from the causal action of a factor to initiation of disease; the interval between an initial injection of antigen and the appearance of demonstrable antibodies in the blood.

**in•duc•tor** (in-dŭk'ter) **1.** that which brings about induction. **2.** EMBRYOLOGY an evocator or an organizer.

**in•du•rat•ed** (in'doo-rāt-ed) hardened, usually used with reference to soft tissues becoming extremely firm but not as hard as bone. [L. *in-duro,* pp. *-duratus,* to harden, fr. *durus,* hard]

**in•du•ra•tion** (in-doo-rā'shŭn) **1.** the process of becoming extremely firm or hard, or having such physical features. **2.** a focus or region of indurated tissue. SYN sclerosis (1). [L. *induratio* (see indurated)]

**in•du•ra•tive** (in'doo-ră-tiv) pertaining to, causing, or characterized by induration.

**in•du•si•um,** pl. **in•du•sia** (in-doo'zē-ŭm, in-doo'zē-ă) **1.** a membranous layer or covering. **2.** the amnion. [L. a woman's undergarment, fr. *induo,* to put on]

**in•du•si•um gris•e•um** [TA] a thin layer of gray matter on the dorsal surface of the corpus callosum in which the medial and lateral longitudinal striae lie embedded. The indusium griseum is a rudimentary component of the hippocampus, continuous caudally around the splenium of the corpus callosum with the fasciolar gyrus, a slender convolution in turn continuous with the dentate gyrus of the hippocampus; rostrally the indusium griseum curves around the genu and rostrum of the corpus callosum and extends ventralward to the olfactory trigone as the tenia tecta or rudimentum hippocampi, hidden in the depth of the posterior parolfactory sulcus that marks the anterior border of the subcallosal gyrus or precommissural septum.

**in•dus•tri•al dis•ease** a morbid condition resulting from exposure to an agent discharged by a commercial enterprise into the environment. Cf. occupational disease.

**in•dus•tri•al hear•ing loss** SYN noise-induced hearing loss.

**in•dus•tri•al hy•giene** practices adopted by an industrial concern to minimize occupation-related disease and/or injury.

**in•dwell•ing cath•e•ter** a catheter left in place in the bladder, usually a balloon catheter.

**in•e•bri•ant** (in-ē'brē-ant) **1.** making drunk; intoxicating. **2.** an intoxicant, such as alcohol. SEE inebriation.

**in•e•bri•a•tion** (in-ē-brē-ā'shŭn) intoxication, especially by alcohol. SEE inebriant. [L. *in-,* intensive + *ebrietas,* drunkenness]

*In•er•mi•cap•si•fer* (in-er-mi-cap'si-fer) genus of tapeworm (order Cyclophyllidae) first recognized in humans in 1935; an arthropod is thought to be involved in transmission (rodent to human, human to human).

*In•er•mi•cap•si•fer ma•da•gas•car•i•en•sis* cestode often seen as human infection in Cuba in children 1–3 yrs old, causing vague intestinal symptoms; suspected arthropod vector; proglottids, eggs, and egg capsules resemble those of *Raillietina* spp.

**in•ert** (in-ert') **1.** slow in action; sluggish; inactive. **2.** devoid of active chemical properties, as the inert gases. **3.** denoting a drug or agent having no pharmacologic or therapeutic action. [L. *iners,* unskillful, sluggish, fr. *in,* neg. + *ars,* art]

**in•ert gas•es** SYN noble gases.

**in•er•tia** (in-er'shē-ă, in-er'shăh) **1.** the tendency of a physical body to oppose any force tending to move it from a position of rest or to change its uniform motion. **2.** denoting inactivity or lack of force, lack of mental or physical vigor, or sluggishness of thought or action. [L. want of skill, laziness]

**in•er•tia time** the interval elapsing between the reception of the stimulus from a nerve and the contraction of the muscle.

**in•fan•cy** (in'fan-sē) babyhood; the earliest period of extrauterine life; roughly, the first year of life.

**in•fant** a child under the age of 1 year; more specifically, a newborn baby. [L. *infans,* not speaking]

**in•fan•ti•cide** (in-fan'ti-sīd) **1.** the killing of an infant. **2.** one who murders an infant. [infant + L. *caedo,* to kill]

**in•fan•tile** (in'făn-tīl) **1.** relating to, or characteristic of, infants or infancy. **2.** denoting childish behavior.

**in•fan•tile ac•ro•pus•tu•lo•sis** a recurrent papulopustular and crusting pruritic eruption, usually in black children.

**in•fan•tile au•tism** a severe emotional disturbance of childhood characterized by qualitative impairment in reciprocal social interaction and in communication, language, and social development. SYN Kanner syndrome.

**in•fan•tile ec•ze•ma** eczema in infants; the clinical appearance varies according to the dominant causative mechanism, e.g., contact-type hypersensitivity, candidiasis, atopy, seborrhea, or a combination including intertrigo and diaper dermatitis.

**in•fan•tile hy•po•thy•roid•ism** can be due to endemic congenital goiter; nonendemic cases are usually due to defective thyroidal embryogenesis, defective hypothalamic-pituitary function, congenital defects in thyroid hormone synthesis or action, or intrauterine exposure to goitrogenic agents.

**in•fan•tile neu•ro•ax•o•nal dys•tro•phy** a rare, familial disorder of early childhood manifested as progressive psychomotor deterioration, increased reflexes, Babinski sign, hypotonia and progressive blindness.

**in•fan•tile os•te•o•ma•la•cia, ju•ve•nile os•te•o•ma•la•cia** SYN rickets.

**in•fan•tile pu•ru•lent con•junc•ti•vi•tis** SYN ophthalmia neonatorum.

**in•fan•tile scur•vy** a cachectic condition in infants, resulting from malnutrition and marked by pallor, fetid breath, coated tongue, diarrhea, and subperiosteal hemorrhages; probably a combination of scurvy and rickets due to combined deficiency of vitamins C and D. SYN Barlow disease, osteopathia hemorrhagica infantum.

**in•fan•tile sex•u•al•i•ty** PSYCHOANALYSIS the body of theories concerning psychosexual development in infants and children; encompasses the

i
n

overlapping oral, anal, and phallic phases during the first five years of life.

**in·fan·tile spinal mus·cu·lar at·ro·phy** transmitted as autosomal recessive on chromosome 5q. Progressive dysfunction of the anterior horn cells in the spinal cord and brainstem cranial nerves with profound weakness and bulbar dysfunction occurring in the first two years of life. Three groups, based on age of clinical onset, are recognized.

**in·fan·ti·lism** (in-fan′ti-lizm) **1.** a state marked by slow development of mind and body. **2.** childishness, as characterized by a temper tantrum of an adolescent or adult. **3.** underdevelopment of the sexual organs.

**in·fant mor·tal·i·ty rate** a measure of the rate of deaths of liveborn infants before their first birthday; the numerator is the number of infants under one year of age born alive in a defined region during a calendar year who die before they are one year old; the denominator is the total number of live births.

**in·farct** (in′farkt) an area of necrosis resulting from a sudden insufficiency of arterial or venous blood supply. SYN infarction (2). [L. *in-farcio,* pp. *-fartus (-ctus,* an incorrect form), to stuff into]

**in·farc·tion** (in-fark′shŭn) **1.** sudden insufficiency of arterial or venous blood supply due to emboli, thrombi, vascular torsion, or pressure that produces a macroscopic area of necrosis; the heart, brain, spleen, kidney, intestine, lung, and testes are likely to be affected, as are tumors, especially of the ovary or uterus. **2.** SYN infarct.

**in·farc·tus my·o·car·dii** SYN myocardial infarction.

**in·fect** (in-fekt′) **1.** to enter, invade, or inhabit another organism, causing infection or contamination. **2.** to dwell internally, endoparasitically, as opposed to externally (infest). [L. *in-ficio,* pp. *-fectus,* to dip into, dye, corrupt, infect, fr. *in + facio,* to make]

**in·fect·ed a·bor·tion** a septic complication of an abortion.

**in·fec·tion** (in-fek′shŭn) invasion of the body with organisms that have the potential to cause disease.

**in·fec·tion-ex·haus·tion psy·cho·sis** a psychosis following an acute infection, shock, or chronic intoxication; begins as delirium followed by pronounced mental confusion with hallucinations and unsystematized delusions, and sometimes stupor.

**in·fec·tion im·mu·ni·ty** the paradoxical immune status in which resistance to reinfection coincides with the persistence of the original infection.

**in·fec·tion trans·mis·sion pa·ra·me·ter** the proportion of total possible contacts between infectious cases and susceptibles that lead to new infections. SEE ALSO serial interval, mass action principle.

**in·fec·tious** (in-fek′shŭs) **1.** capable of being transmitted by infection, with or without actual contact. **2.** SYN infective. **3.** denoting a disease due to the action of a microorganism.

**in·fec·tious bo·vine ker·a·to·con·junc·ti·vi·tis** a disease of cattle caused by the bacterium *Moraxella bovis* and characterized by blepharospasm, conjunctivitis, lacrimation, and corneal opacity and ulceration. SYN pinkeye (2).

**in·fec·tious crys·tal·line ker·a·to·pa·thy** fern-like, needle-shaped deposits that may be seen in bacterial keratitis, particularly that due to α-hemolytic streptococci.

**in·fec·tious dis·ease, in·fec·tive dis·ease** a disease resulting from the presence and activity of a microbial agent.

**in·fec·tious ec·ze·ma·toid der·ma·ti·tis** an inflammatory reaction of skin adjacent to the site of a pyogenic infection; thought to be due to a local sensitization to the resident organisms.

**in·fec·tious en·do·car·di·tis, in·fec·tive en·do·car·di·tis** endocarditis due to infection by microorganisms.

**in·fec·tious hep·a·ti·tis vi·rus** SYN hepatitis A virus.

**in·fec·tious mon·o·nu·cle·o·sis** an acute febrile illness caused by the Epstein-Barr virus; frequently spread by saliva transfer; characterized by fever, sore throat, enlargement of lymph nodes and spleen, lymphocytosis with abnormal lymphocytes similar to monocytes, and heterophil antibody in serum.

**in·fec·tious·ness** (in-fek′shŭs-nes) the state or quality of being infectious.

**in·fec·tious pap·il·lo·ma vi·rus** SYN human papilloma virus.

**in·fec·tive** (in-fek′tiv) capable of transmitting an infection. SYN infectious (2).

**in·fec·tive em·bo·lism** SYN pyemic embolism.

**in·fec·tiv·i·ty** (in-fek-tiv′i-tē) **1.** the characteristic of a disease agent that embodies capability of entering, surviving in, and multiplying in a susceptible host. **2.** the proportion of exposures in defined circumstances that result in infection.

**in·fe·ri·or** (in-fē′rē-ōr) **1.** situated below or directed downward. **2.** ANATOMY situated nearer the soles of the feet in relation to a specific reference point; opposite of superior. **3.** less useful or of poorer quality. See page APP 89. [L. lower]

**in·fe·ri·or al·ve·o·lar ar·tery** origin, 1st part of maxillary artery; *distribution,* through mandibular foramen/canal to lower teeth and chin; *branches,* artery to mylohyoid, mental artery, dental arteries.

**in·fe·ri·or al·ve·o·lar nerve** one of the terminal branches of the mandibular, it enters the mandibular canal to be distributed to the lower teeth, periosteum, and gingiva of the mandible; a branch, the mental nerve, passes through the mental foramen to supply the skin and mucosa of the lower lip and chin. SYN nervus alveolaris inferior [TA].

**in·fe·ri·or ba·sal vein** tributary to the common basal vein draining the medial and posterior part of the inferior lobe in each lung.

**in·fe·ri·or cer·e·bel·lar pe·dun·cle** large paired bundles of nerve fibers which develop on the dorsolateral surfaces of the upper medulla, extend under the lateral recesses of the rhomboid fossa and curve dorsally into the cerebellum medial to the middle cerebellar peduncle; composed of a larger (lateral) bundle, the restiform body, and a small (medial) bundle, the juxtarestiform body. Fibers forming this composite bundle originate from spinal neurons and medullary relay nuclei. The largest constituent (restiform body) is crossed fibers from the inferior olive; it also contains the dorsal spinocerebellar tract and cerebellar projections from the lateral reticular nucleus, the accessory cuneate nucleus, the paramedian reticular nuclei and the perihypoglossal nuclei. Vestibulocerebellar fibers are placed medially in the inferior cerebellar peduncle and are usually separately identified as the juxtarestiform body.

**in·fe·ri·or ce·re·bral veins** numerous cerebral veins that drain the undersurface of the cerebral hemispheres and empty into the cavernous and transverse sinuses.

**in·fe·ri·or con·stric·tor mus·cle of phar·ynx** *origin*, outer surfaces of thyroid (thyropharyngeal part) and cricoid (cricopharyngeal part, musculus cricopharyngeus; superior or upper esophageal sphincter muscle) cartilages; *insertion*, pharyngeal raphe in the posterior portion of wall of pharynx; *action*, narrows lower part of pharynx in swallowing, the cricopharyngeal part has a sphincteric function for the esophagus, allowing some voluntary control of eructation and reflux; *nerve supply*, pharyngeal plexus.

**in·fe·ri·or ep·i·gas·tric vein** corresponds to the artery of the same name and empties into the external iliac vein just proximal to the inguinal ligament.

**in·fe·ri·or ex·ten·sor ret·i·nac·u·lum** a Y-shaped ligament restraining the extensor tendons of the foot distal to the ankle joint.

**in·fe·ri·or fib·u·lar ret·i·nac·u·lum** broad thickened band of deep fascia overlying fibularis longus and brevis tendons as they pass along the lateral margin of the foot, anchoring the tendons and their associated bursae in place; it is a lateral continuation of the stem of the Y-shaped inferior extensor retinaculum which attaches to the fibular trochlea of the calcaneus (which intervenes between the two tendons) and then continues to attach to the inferolateral aspect of the calcaneous. SYN inferior peroneal retinaculum.

**in·fe·ri·or gan·gli·on of glos·so·pha·ryn·ge·al nerve** the lower of two sensory ganglions on the glossopharyngeal nerve as it traverses the jugular foramen.

**in·fe·ri·or gan·gli·on of va·gus nerve** a large sensory ganglion of the vagus, anterior to the internal jugular vein. SYN ganglion inferius nervi vagi [TA].

**in·fe·ri·or ge·mel·lus mus·cle** *origin*, tuberosity of ischium; *insertion*, tendon of musculus obturator internus; *action*, rotates thigh laterally; *nerve supply*, sacral plexus.

**in·fe·ri·or·i·ty** (in-fēr-ē-ōr'i-tē) the condition or state of being or feeling inadequate or inferior, especially relative to one's peers or to others similarly situated.

**in·fe·ri·or·i·ty com·plex** a sense of inadequacy which is expressed in extreme shyness, diffidence, or timidity, or as a compensatory reaction in exhibitionism or aggressiveness.

**in·fe·ri·or la·bi·al vein** a tributary of the facial vein draining the lower lip.

**in·fe·ri·or lin·gu·lar (bronchopulmonary) seg·ment [S V]** of the four bronchopulmonary segments that typically comprise the superior lobe of the left lung, the most inferior, supplied by the inferior lingular bronchus [B V] and inferior lingular segmental (pulmonary) artery; corresponds approximately in position to the medial [S V] segment of the middle lobe of the right lung; the lingula is a feature of this part of the left lung.

**in·fe·ri·or lon·gi·tu·di·nal fas·cic·u·lus** a well-marked bundle of long association fibers running the whole length of the occipital and temporal lobes of the cerebrum, in part parallel with the inferior horn of the lateral ventricle. SYN fasciculus longitudinalis inferior [TA].

**in·fe·ri·or mac·u·lar ar·te·ri·ole** *origin*, central artery of retina; *distribution*, inferior part of macula. SYN arteriola macularis inferior [TA].

**in·fe·ri·or med·ul·lary ve·lum** a thin sheet of white matter, hidden by the cerebellar tonsil, attached along the peduncle of the flocculus and, at or near the midline, to the nodulus of the vermis; it is continuous caudally with the epithelial lamina and choroid plexus of the fourth ventricle.

**in·fe·ri·or nas·al con·cha 1.** a thin, spongy, bony plate with curved margins, on the lateral wall of the nasal cavity, separating the middle from the inferior meatus; it articulates with the ethmoid, lacrimal, maxilla, and palate bones; **2.** the above bony plate and its thick mucoperiosteum containing an extensive cavernous vascular bed for heat exchange.

**in·fe·ri·or ob·lique mus·cle** *origin*, orbital plate of maxilla lateral to the lacrimal groove; *insertion*, sclera between the superior and lateral recti; *action*, primary, extorsion; secondary, elevation and abduction; *nerve supply*, oculomotor (inferior branch). SYN musculus obliquus inferior [TA].

**in·fe·ri·or ol·i·vary nu·cle·us** a large aggregate of small densely packed nerve cells arranged in folded laminae shaped like a purse with the opening (hilum) directed medially. It corresponds in position to the oliva, projects to all parts of the contralateral half of the cerebellar cortex by way of the olivocerebellar tract, and is the only source of cerebellar climbing fibers. Its afferent connections include fibers from the spinal cord, the dentate nucleus and motor cortex, but its major input appears to be the central tegmental tract originating from multiple nuclei at midbrain levels.

**in·fe·ri·or pal·pe·bral (ar·te·ri·al) arch** formed by the medial palpebral artery, which communicates with a branch of the lacrimal artery along the tarsal margin.

**in·fe·ri·or pel·vic ap·er·ture** the lower opening of the true pelvis, bounded anteriorly by the pubic arch, laterally by the rami of the ischium and the sacrotuberous ligament on either side, and posteriorly by these ligaments and the tip of the coccyx.

**in·fe·ri·or per·o·ne·al re·tin·a·cu·lum** SYN inferior fibular retinaculum.

**in·fe·ri·or pu·bic ra·mus** inferior extension from body of pubic bone that meets with the ramus of the ischium to form the ischiopubic ramus.

**in·fe·ri·or rec·tal nerves** several branches of the pudendal nerve that pass to the external and sphincter anoderm and skin of the anal region. SYN nervi rectales inferiores [TA].

**in·fe·ri·or rec·tus mus·cle** *origin*, inferior part of the common tendinous ring; *insertion*, inferior part of sclera of the eye; *action*, primary, depression; secondary, adduction and extorsion; *nerve supply*, oculomotor (inferior branch). SYN musculus rectus inferior [TA].

**in·fe·ri·or renal seg·ment** portion of the kidney exclusively supplied by the inferior segmental (renal) artery.

**in·fe·ri·or seg·ment** a delimited part or section

i
n

of an organ or other structure that lies at the lowest level (nearest the feet) compared with the other similar parts or sections.

**in·fe·ri·or tem·po·ral line** the lower of two curved lines on the parietal bone; it marks the outer limit of attachment of the temporalis muscle.

**in·fe·ri·or tem·po·ral re·ti·nal ar·te·ri·ole** the branch of the central artery of the retina that passes laterally below the macula to supply the lower lateral or temporal part of the retina.

**in·fe·ri·or tem·po·ral sul·cus** the sulcus on the basal aspect of the temporal lobe that separates the fusiform gyrus from the inferior temporal gyrus on its lateral side.

**in·fe·ri·or tha·lam·ic pe·dun·cle** a large fiber bundle emerging from the anterior part of the thalamus in the ventral direction, in part joining the medial fibers of the internal capsule, in other part curving laterally around the medial margin of the capsule into the innominate substance. Many of its fibers establish a reciprocal connection of the mediodorsal nucleus of the thalamus with the orbital gyri of the frontal lobe, but numerous other fibers constitute a conduction system from the amygdala and olfactory cortex to the mediodorsal nucleus. SEE ALSO ansa peduncularis.

**in·fe·ri·or thal·a·mo·stri·ate veins** veins draining the thalamus and striate body exiting the anterior perforated substance; tributary to the basal vein. SYN striate veins.

**in·fe·ri·or ve·na ca·va (IVC)** receives the blood from the lower limbs and the greater part of the pelvic and abdominal organs; it begins at the level of the fifth lumbar vertebra on the right side by the merger of the right and left common iliac veins, pierces the diaphragm at the level of the eighth thoracic vertebra, and empties into the posteroinferior aspect of the right atrium of the heart. SYN postcava.

**in·fer·til·i·ty** (in-fer-til′i-tē) diminished or absent ability to produce offspring; does not imply sterility. [L. *in-* neg. + *fertilis,* fruitful]

**in·fest** (in-fest′) to dwell on or in a host as a parasite. [L. *infesto,* pp. *-atus,* to attack]

**in·fes·ta·tion** parasitization of a host; usually refers to multicellular parasites (worms, arthropods).

**in·fib·u·la·tion** (in-fib-yu-la′shŭn) closure of the vaginal vestibule by creating a fusion of the labia majora; typically done after excision of the labia minora and clitoris and incision of the labia majora to create raw surfaces that can be surgically joined by pinning so that they will eventually grow together; done for cultural, not medical, reasons. SEE ALSO female circumcision. [L. *infibulo,* to pin or clasp together, to join surgically (Celsus), fr. *in-* + *fibula,* pin, clasp]

**in·fil·trate** (in-fil′trāt) **1.** to perform or undergo infiltration. **2.** SYN infiltration (2). **3.** infiltration (1) in the lung as inferred from appearance of a localized, ill-defined opacity on a chest radiograph. [L. *in* + Mediev. L. *filtro,* pp. *-atus,* to strain through felt, fr. *filtrum,* felt]

**in·fil·tra·tion** (in′fil-trā′shŭn) **1.** the act of permeating or penetrating into a substance, cell, or tissue; said of gases, fluids, or matter held in solution. **2.** the gas, fluid, or dissolved matter that has entered any substance, cell, or tissue. SYN infiltrate (2). **3.** injection of solution into tissues,

as in infiltration anesthesia. **4.** extravasation of solutions intended for intravascular injection.

**in·fil·tra·tion an·es·the·sia** anesthesia produced by injection of local anesthetic solution directly into an area that is painful or about to be operated upon.

**in·fi·nite dis·tance** the limit of distant vision, the rays entering the eyes from an object at that point being practically parallel.

**in·firm** (in-ferm′) weak or feeble because of old age or disease. [L. *in-firmus,* fr. *in-* neg. + *firmus,* strong]

**in·fir·ma·ry** (in-fer′mă-rē) a clinic or small hospital, especially in a school or college. [L. *infirmarium;* see infirm]

**in·fir·mi·ty** (in-fer′mi-tē) a weakness; an abnormal, more or less disabling, condition of mind or body. [see infirm]

**in·flam·ma·tion** (in-flă-mā′shŭn) a fundamental, stereotyped complex of cytologic and chemical reactions that occur in affected blood vessels and adjacent tissues in response to an injury or abnormal stimulation caused by a physical, chemical, or biologic agent. [L. *inflammo,* pp. *-atus,* fr. *in,* in, + *flamma,* flame]

**in·flam·ma·to·ry** (in-flam′ă-tōr-ē) pertaining to, characterized by, causing, resulting from, or becoming affected by inflammation.

**in·flam·ma·to·ry car·ci·no·ma** carcinoma of the breast presenting with edema, hyperemia, tenderness, and rapid enlargment of the breast; microscopically, there is extensive invasion of dermal lymphatics by the carcinoma.

**in·flam·ma·tory lin·e·ar ver·ru·cous ep·i·der·mal ne·vus** rare pruritic confluent scaly erythematous papules in linear array, usually appearing in early childhood on a limb and resolving before adulthood.

**in·flam·ma·to·ry lymph** a faintly yellow, usually coagulable fluid (i.e., euplastic lymph) that collects on the surface of an acutely inflamed membrane or cutaneous wound.

**in·flam·ma·to·ry pap·il·lary hy·per·pla·sia** closely arranged papules of the palatal mucosa underlying an ill-fitting denture.

**in·flam·ma·to·ry pseu·do·tu·mor** a tumorlike mass in the lungs or other sites, composed of fibrous or granulation tissue infiltrated by inflammatory cells.

**in·flam·ma·to·ry rheu·ma·tism** rheumatoid arthritis or other cause of joint inflammation.

**in·fla·tion** (in-flā′shŭn) distention by a fluid or gas. SYN vesiculation (2). [L. *inflatio,* fr. *in-flo,* pp. *-flatus,* to blow into, inflate]

**in·flec·tion, in·flex·ion** (in-flek′shŭn) an inward bending. [L. *in-flecto,* pp. *-flexus,* to bend]

**in·flu·en·za** (in-floo-en′ză) an acute infectious respiratory disease, caused by influenza viruses, which attacks the respiratory epithelial cells and produces a catarrhal inflammation; characterized by sudden onset, chills, fever of short duration, severe prostration, headache, muscle aches, and a cough that usually is dry until secondary infection occurs. The disease commonly occurs in epidemics, sometimes in pandemics; strain-specific immunity develops, but mutations in the virus are frequent, and the immunity usually does not protect against antigenically different strains. SYN flu, grip, grippe. [It. influence (of planets or stars), fr. L. *influentia,* fr. *in-fluo,* to flow in]

**in•flu•en•zal** (in-floo-en'zăl) relating to, marked by, or resulting from influenza.

**in•flu•en•zal pneu•mo•nia 1.** pneumonia complicating influenza; **2.** pneumonia due to *Haemophilus influenzae.*

**In•flu•en•za vi•rus** (in-floo-en'ză-vī-rŭs) the family of Orthomyxoviridae contains 3 genera: Influenzavirus A, B; Influenzavirus C; and "Thogoto-like viruses." Each type of virus has a stable nucleoprotein group antigen common to all strains of the type, but distinct from that of the other types; the genome is negative-sense single-stranded RNA in 6–8 segments; each also has a mosaic of surface antigens (hemagglutinin and neuraminidase) that characterize the strains and that are subject to variations of two kinds: 1) a rather continual drift that occurs independently within the hemagglutinin and neuraminidase antigens; 2) after a period of years, a sudden shift (notably in type A virus of human origin) to a different hemagglutinin or neuraminidase antigen. The sudden major shifts are the basis of subdivisions of type A virus of human origin, which occur following infection of the animal host with 2 different strains at the same time, resulting in a hybrid virus. Strain notations indicate type, geographic origin, year of isolation, and, in the case of type A strains, the characterizing subtypes of hemagglutinin and neuraminidase antigens (e.g., A/Hong Kong/1/68 (H$_3$ N$_2$); B/Hong Kong/5/72).

*In•flu•en•za•vi•rus* (in-floo-en'ză-vī-rŭs) the genus of Orthomyxoviridae that comprises influenza viruses types A and B.

**in•for•ma•tics** (in-fōr-mat'iks) **1.** the study of information and ways to process and handle it, especially by means of information technology, i.e., computers and other electronic devices for rapid transfer, processing, and analysis of large amounts of data. **2.** the science of arranging and organizing the results of genomic and functional genomic studies. SEE ALSO bioinformatics. [*infor-ma*tion + -ics]

**in•for•ma•tion the•o•ry** BEHAVIORAL SCIENCES a system for studying the communication process through the detailed analysis, often mathematical, of all aspects of the process including the encoding, transmission, and decoding of signals; not concerned in any direct sense with the meaning of a message.

**in•formed con•sent** voluntary consent given by a person or a responsible proxy (e.g., a parent) for participation in a study, immunization program, or treatment regimen, after being informed of the purpose, methods, procedures, benefits, and risks. The essential criteria of informed consent are that the subject has both knowledge and comprehension, that consent is freely given without duress or undue influence, and that the right of withdrawal at any time is clearly communicated to the subject.

**in•for•mo•fers** (in-fōr'mō-fers) name suggested for the protein particles that appear when RNA is removed from nucleoprotein particles. [*informa-tion* + -fer]

**in•for•mo•somes** (in-fōr'mō-sōmz) name suggested for the bodies composed of messenger (informational) RNA and protein that are found in the cytoplasm of animal cells. [*informa*tion + G. *sōma,* body]

△**in•fra-** a position below the part denoted by the word to which it is joined. [L. below]

**in•fra•bulge** (in'fră-bŭlj) **1.** that portion of the crown of a tooth gingival to the height of contour. **2.** that area of a tooth where the retentive portion of a clasp of a removable partial denture is placed.

**in•fra•cla•vic•u•lar fos•sa** a triangular depression bounded by the clavicle and the adjacent borders of the deltoid and pectoralis major muscles.

**in•fra•clu•sion** (in-fră-kloo'zhŭn) the state wherein a tooth has failed to erupt to the maxillomandibular plane of interdigitation. SYN infraocclusion, infraversion (3).

**in•frac•tion** (in-frak'shŭn) a fracture; especially one without displacement. [L. *infractio,* a breaking, fr. *infringere,* to break]

**in•fra•di•an** (in-frā'dē-ăn) relating to biologic variations or rhythms occurring in cycles less frequent than every 24 hours. Cf. circadian, ultradian. [infra- + L. *dies,* day]

**in•fra•mam•il•lary** (in-fră-mam'ĭ-lār-ē) relating to that which is situated below a nipple.

**in•fra•mar•gin•al** (in-fră-mar'ji-năl) below any margin or edge.

**in•fra•max•il•lary** (in-fră-mak'si-lā-rē) SYN mandibular.

**in•fra•nod•al ex•tra•sys•to•le** SYN ventricular extrasystole.

**in•fra•oc•clu•sion** (in'fră-ŏ-kloo'zhŭn) SYN infraclusion.

**in•fra•or•bit•al ar•tery** *origin,* third part of maxillary; *distribution,* upper canine and incisor teeth, inferior rectus and inferior oblique muscles, lower eyelid, lacrimal sac, maxillary sinus, and upper lip; *anastomoses,* branches of ophthalmic, facial, superior labial, transverse facial, and buccal. SYN arteria infraorbitalis [TA].

**in•fra•or•bit•al ca•nal** a canal running beneath the orbital margin of the maxilla from the infraorbital groove, in the floor of the orbit, to the infraorbital foramen; it transmits the infraorbital artery and nerve. SYN canalis infraorbitalis [TA].

**in•fra•or•bit•al fo•ra•men** the external opening of the infraorbital canal, on the anterior surface of the body of the maxilla.

**in•fra•or•bit•al nerve** the continuation of the maxillary nerve after it has entered the orbit, via the infraorbital fissure, traversing the infraorbital canal to reach the face; it supplies the mucosa of the maxillary sinus, the upper incisors, canine and premolars, the upper gums, the inferior eyelid and conjunctiva, part of the nose and the superior lip. SYN nervus infraorbitalis [TA].

**in•fra•psy•chic** (in-fră-sī'kik) denoting ideas or actions originating below the level of consciousness.

**in•fra•red** (in'fră-red) that portion of the electromagnetic spectrum with wavelengths between 770 and 1000 nm.

**in•fra•red mi•cro•scope** a microscope that is equipped with infrared transmitting optics and that measures the infrared absorption of minute samples with the aid of photoelectric cells; images may be observed with image converters or television.

**in•fra•son•ic** (in'fră-son'ik) denoting those frequencies that lie below the range of human hearing. [infra- + L. *sonus,* sound]

**in•fra•spi•na•tus bur•sa** the bursa located between the tendon of the infraspinatus and the capsule of the shoulder joint.

**in·fra·spi·na·tus mus·cle** *origin*, infraspinous fossa of scapula; *insertion*, middle facet of greater tubercle of humerus; *action*, extends arm and rotates it laterally; *nerve supply*, suprascapular (from fifth to sixth cervical spinal nerves). SYN musculus infraspinatus [TA].

**in·fra·tem·por·al ap·proach** surgical approach to the base of the skull and its contents from inferior to the temporal bone.

**in·fra·tem·po·ral crest** a rough ridge marking the angle of union of the temporal and infratemporal surfaces of the greater wing of the sphenoid bone.

**in·fra·tem·po·ral fos·sa** the cavity on the side of the skull bounded laterally by the zygomatic arch and ramus of the mandible, medially by the lateral pterygoid plate, anteriorly by the zygomatic process of the maxilla, posteriorly by the articular tubercle of the temporal bone and the posterior border of the lateral pterygoid plate, and above by the squama of the temporal bone and the infratemporal crest on the greater wing of the sphenoid bone.

**in·fra·troch·le·ar nerve** a terminal branch of the nasociliary nerve running beneath the pulley of the superior oblique muscle to the front of the orbit, and supplying the skin of the eyelids and root of the nose. SYN nervus infratrochlearis [TA].

**in·fra·ver·sion** (in'frǎ-ver'shǔn) 1. a turning (version) downward. 2. PHYSIOLOGICAL OPTICS rotation of both eyes downward. 3. SYN infraclusion.

**in·fun·dib·u·la** (in-fǔn-dib'yu-lǎ) plural of infundibulum.

**in·fun·dib·u·lar** (in-fǔn-dib'yu-lǎr) relating to an infundibulum.

**in·fun·dib·u·lar stalk** SYN infundibular stem.

**in·fun·dib·u·lar stem** the neural component of the pituitary stalk that contains nerve tracts passing from the hypothalamus to the pars nervosa. SYN infundibular stalk.

**in·fun·dib·u·lec·to·my** (in'fǔn-dib'yu-lek'tō-mē) excision of an infundibulum, especially of hypertrophied ventricular septal myocardium encroaching on the ventricular outflow tract. [infundibulum + G. *ektomē*, excision]

**in·fun·dib·u·lo·fol·lic·u·li·tis** (in-fǔn-dib'yu-lō-fo-lik'yu-lī'tis) inflammation of the follicular infundibulum, the superficial part of the hair follicle above the opening of the sebaceous gland.

**in·fun·dib·u·lo·ma** (in-fǔn-dib'yu-lō'mǎ) a pilocytic astrocytoma arising in the neurohypophysis of the pituitary. [infundibulum + G. *-oma*, tumor]

**in·fun·dib·u·lum**, pl. **in·fun·dib·u·la** (in-fǔn-dib'yu-lǔm, in-fǔn-dib'yu-lǎ) 1. a funnel or funnel-shaped structure or passage. 2. SYN infundibulum of uterine tube. 3. the expanding portion of a calyx as it opens into the pelvis of the kidney. 4. SYN arterial cone. 5. termination of a bronchiole in the alveolus. 6. termination of the cochlear canal beneath the cupola. 7. the funnel-shaped, unpaired prominence of the base of the hypothalamus behind the optic chiasm, enclosing the infundibular recess of the third ventricle and continuous below with the stalk of the hypophysis. 8. the contact surface indentation in the incisor and cheek teeth of a horse. SYN mark (2). [L. a funnel]

**in·fun·di·bu·lum tu·bae ute·ri·nae** [TA] SYN infundibulum of uterine tube.

**in·fun·dib·u·lum of uter·ine tube** the funnel-like expansion of the abdominal extremity of the uterine (fallopian) tube. SYN infundibulum tubae uterinae [TA], infundibulum (2).

**in·fu·sion** (in-fyu'zhŭn) 1. the process of steeping a substance in water, either cold or hot (below the boiling point), in order to extract its soluble principles. 2. a medicinal preparation obtained by steeping the crude drug in water. 3. the introduction of fluid other than blood, e.g., saline solution, into a vein. [L. *infusio*, fr. *in-fundo*, pp. *-fusus*, to pour in]

**in·fu·sion-as·pi·ra·tion drain·age** a type of drainage in which antibiotics are continuously infused into a cavity at the same time fluid is being drained (aspirated) from the cavity.

**In·gel·fin·ger rule** (ing-el-fing'er) a principle developed by Franz Ingelfinger for use in the editorial offices of the *New England Journal of Medicine*, stating that original articles submitted for publication will be reviewed on the understanding that the same information will not be submitted for publication elsewhere during the period of review; has been adopted by many other peer-reviewed medical journals.

**in·ges·ta** (in-jes'tǎ) solid or liquid nutrients taken into the body. [pl. of L. *ingestum*, ntr. pp. of *in-gero*, *-gestus*, to carry in]

**in·ges·tion** (in-jes'chŭn) 1. introduction of food and drink into the stomach. 2. incorporation of particles into the cytoplasm of a phagocytic cell by invagination of a portion of the cell membrane as a vacuole. [L. *in-gero*, to carry in]

**in·ges·tive** (in-jes'tiv) relating to ingestion.

**in·gra·ves·cent** (in-grǎ-ves'ent) increasing in severity. [L. *ingravesco*, to grow heavier, fr. *gravis*, heavy]

**in·grown hair** hair that grows at more acute angles than is normal, and in all directions; it incompletely clears the follicle, turns back in, and causes pseudofolliculitis.

**in·grown na·il** a toenail, one edge of which is overgrown by the nailfold, producing a pyogenic granuloma; due to faulty trimming of the toenails or pressure from a tight shoe.

**in·gui·nal** (ing'gwi-nǎl) relating to the groin.

**in·gui·nal ca·nal** the obliquely directed passage through the layers of the lower abdominal wall that transmits the spermatic cord in the male and the round ligament in the female. SYN canalis inguinalis [TA].

**in·gui·nal falx** common tendon of insertion of the transversus and internal oblique muscles into the crest and tubercle of the pubis and iliopectineal line; it is frequently largely muscular rather than aponeurotic and may be poorly developed; forms posterior wall of medial inguinal canal. SYN falx inguinalis [TA].

🔲 **in·gui·nal her·nia** a hernia at the inguinal region: direct inguinal hernia involves the abdominal wall between the deep epigastric artery and the edge of the rectus muscle; indirect inguinal hernia involves the internal inguinal ring and passes into the inguinal canal. See page 501.

**in·gui·nal lig·a·ment** a fibrous band formed by the thickened inferior border of the aponeurosis of the external oblique muscle that extends from the anterior superior spine of the ilium to the pubic tubercle, bridging muscular and vascular

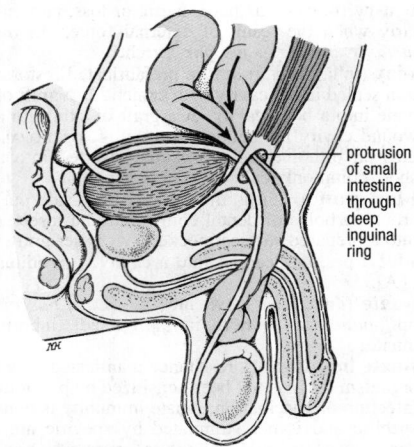

protrusion of small intestine through deep inguinal ring

**indirect inguinal hernia**

lacunae; forms the floor of the inguinal canal; gives origin to the lowermost fibers of internal oblique and transversus abdominis muscles. SYN ligamentum inguinale [TA].

**in·gui·nal re·gion** the topographical area of the inferior abdomen related to the inguinal canal, lateral to the pubic region. SYN groin (1).

**in·gui·nal tri·an·gle** the triangular area in the lower abdominal wall bounded by the inguinal ligament below, the border of the rectus abdominis medially and the inferior epigastric vessels (lateral umbilical fold) laterally. It is the site of direct inguinal hernia. SYN trigonum inguinale [TA], Hesselbach triangle, inguinal trigone.

**in·gui·nal tri·gone** SYN inguinal triangle.

**in·gui·no·cru·ral** (ing′gwi-nō-kroo′răl) relating to the groin and the thigh.

**in·gui·no·dyn·ia** (ing′gwi-nō-din′ē-ă) rarely used term for pain in the groin. [L. *inguen* (*inguin*-), groin, + G. *odynē*, pain]

**in·gui·no·la·bi·al** (ing′gwi-nō-lā′bē-ăl) relating to the groin and the labium.

**in·gui·no·per·i·to·ne·al** (ing′gwi-nō-per′i-tō-nē′ăl) relating to the groin and the peritoneum.

**in·gui·no·scro·tal** (ing′gwi-nō-skrō′tăl) relating to the groin and the scrotum.

**INH** isonicotinic acid hydrazide.

**in·hal·ant** (in-hā′lant) **1.** that which is inhaled; a remedy given by inhalation. **2.** a drug (or combination of drugs) with high vapor pressure, carried by an air current into the nasal passage, where it produces its effect. **3.** group of products consisting of finely powdered or liquid drugs that are carried to the respiratory passages by the use of special devices such as low pressure aerosol containers. SYN insufflation (2). SEE ALSO inhalation, aerosol. [see inhalation]

**in·ha·la·tion** (in-hă-lā′shŭn) **1.** the act of drawing in the breath. SYN inspiration. **2.** drawing a medicated vapor in with the breath. **3.** a solution of a drug or combination of drugs for administration as a nebulized mist intended to reach the respiratory tree. [L. *in-halo*, pp. *-halatus*, to breathe at or in]

**in·ha·la·tion an·es·the·sia** general anesthesia resulting from breathing of anesthetic gases or vapors.

**in·ha·la·tion an·es·thet·ic** a gas or a liquid with sufficient vapor pressure to produce general anesthesia when breathed.

**in·hale** (in-hāl′) to draw in the breath. SYN inspire.

**in·hal·er** (in-hāl′er) **1.** SYN respirator (1). **2.** an apparatus for administering medicines by inhalation.

**in·her·ent** (in-her′ent) occurring as a natural part or consequence; intrinsic. [L. *inhaerens*, sticking to, adhering]

**in·her·i·tance** (in-her′i-tans) **1.** characters or qualities that are transmitted from parent to offspring by coded cytological data; that which is inherited. **2.** cultural or legal endowment. **3.** the act of inheriting. [L. *heredito*, inherit, fr. *heres* (*hered*-), an heir]

**in·her·it·ed** (in-her′it-ed) derived from a preformed genetic code present in the parents. Contrast with acquired.

**in·her·it·ed char·ac·ter** a single attribute of an animal or plant that is transmitted at one locus from generation to generation in accordance with Mendel laws. SEE gene.

**in·hib·it** (in-hib′it) to curb or restrain.

**in·hi·bi·tion** (in-hi-bish′ŭn) **1.** depression or arrest of a function. SEE ALSO inhibitor. **2.** PSYCHOANALYSIS the restraining of instinctual or unconscious drives or tendencies, especially if they conflict with one's conscience or with societal demands. **3.** PSYCHOLOGY the gradual attenuation, masking, and extinction of a previously conditioned response. [L. *in-hibeo*, pp. *-hibitus*, to keep back, fr. *habeo*, to have]

**in·hib·i·tor** (in-hib′i-ter) **1.** an agent that restrains or retards physiologic, chemical, or enzymatic action. **2.** a nerve, stimulation of which represses activity. SEE ALSO inhibition.

**in·hib·i·to·ry** (in-hib′i-tōr-ē) restraining; tending to inhibit.

**in·hib·i·to·ry fi·bers** nerve fibers that inhibit the activity of the nerve cells with which they have synaptic connections, or of the effector tissue (smooth muscle, heart muscle, glands) in which they terminate.

**in·hib·i·to·ry nerve** a nerve conveying impulses that diminish functional activity in a part.

**in·hib·i·to·ry ob·ses·sion** an obsession involving an impediment to action, usually representing a phobia.

**in·hib·i·to·ry post·syn·ap·tic po·ten·tial** the change in potential produced in the membrane of the next neuron when an impulse which has an inhibitory influence arrives at the synapse; it is a local change in the direction of hyperpolarization; the frequency of discharge of a given neuron is determined by the extent to which impulses that lead to excitatory postsynaptic potentials predominate over those that cause inhibitory postsynaptic potentials.

**in·i·on** (in′ē-on) a point located on the external occipital protuberance at the intersection of the midline with a line drawn tangent to the uppermost convexity of the right and left superior nuchal lines. [G. nape of the neck]

**in·i·tial as·sess·ment** the first assessment of a prehospital patient following scene size-up to determine the presence of immediately life-threatening conditions. Also used to determine if the patient needs medical care and to establish further treatment and transport priorities.

**in·i·ti·a·ting a·gent** SEE initiation.

**in·i·ti·at·ing co·don** the trinucleotide AUG (or sometimes GUG) that codes for the first amino acid in protein sequences, formylmethionine; the latter is often removed post-transcriptionally.

**in·i·ti·a·tion** (i-ni-shē-ā′shŭn) **1.** the first stage of tumor induction by a carcinogen; subtle alteration of cells by exposure to a carcinogenic agent so that they are likely to form a tumor upon subsequent exposure to a promoting agent (promotion). **2.** starting point of replication or translation in macromolecule biosynthesis. **3.** start of chemical or enzymatic reaction.

**in·i·ti·a·tion co·don** a specific mRNA sequence (usually AUG, but sometimes GUG) that is the signal for the addition of fMet-tRNA and the beginning of translation.

**in·i·ti·a·tion fac·tor (IF)** one of several soluble proteins involved in the initiation of protein or RNA synthesis.

**in·i·tis** (in-ī′tis) **1.** inflammation of fibrous tissue. **2.** SYN myositis. [G. *is* (*in-*), fiber, + *-itis*, inflammation]

**in·ject** (in-jekt′) to introduce into the body; denoting a fluid forced beneath the skin or into a blood vessel. [L. *injicio*, to throw in]

**in·ject·ed** (in-jek′ted) **1.** denoting a fluid introduced into the body. **2.** denoting a surface whose blood vessels are visibly dilated.

**in·jec·tion 1.** introduction of a medicinal substance or nutrient material into the subcutaneous tissue (subcutaneous or hypodermic injection), the muscular tissue (intramuscular injection), a vein (intravenous injection), an artery (intraarterial injection), the rectum (rectal injection or enema), the vagina (vaginal injection or douche), the urethra, or other canals or cavities of the body. **2.** an injectable pharmaceutical preparation. **3.** congestion or hyperemia. See this page. [L. *injectio*, a throwing in, fr. *in-jicio*, to throw in]

**in·ju·ry** (in′jer-ē) damage, harm, or loss, particularly when the result of external force. [L. *injuria*, fr. in- neg. + *jus (jur-)*, right]

**in·lay** (in′lā) **1.** DENTISTRY a prefabricated restoration sealed in the cavity with cement. **2.** a graft of bone into a bone cavity. **3.** a graft of skin into a wound cavity for epithelialization. **4.** ORTHOPAEDICS an orthomechanical device inserted into a shoe; commonly called an "arch support."

**in·lay graft** a skin graft wrapped (raw side out) around a bolus of dental compound and inserted into a prepared surgical pocket. SYN Esser graft.

**in·let** a passage leading into a cavity. SYN aditus [TA].

**in·nate** (i′nāt, i-nāt′) SYN inborn. [L. *in-nascor*, pp. *-natus,* to be born in, pp. as adj. inborn, innate]

**in·nate im·mu·ni·ty** resistance manifested by an organism that has not been sensitized by previous infection or vaccination; innate immunity is nonspecific and is not stimulated by specific antigens. SEE ALSO self. SYN natural immunity, nonspecific immunity.

**in·ner·va·tion** (in′er-vā′shŭn) the supply of nerve fibers functionally connected with a part. See this page. [L. *in,* in, + *nervus,* nerve]

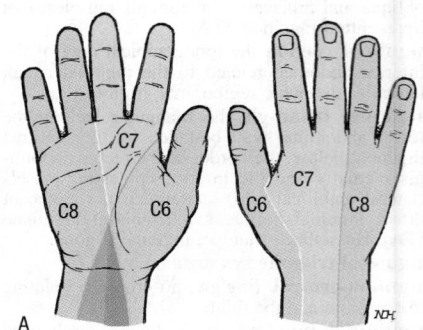

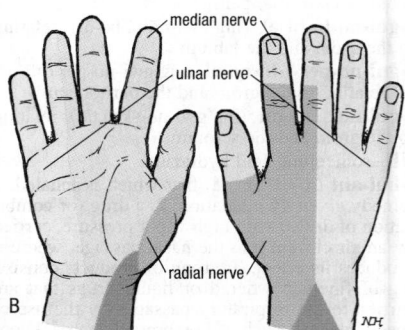

**innervation of the hand and wrist:** (A) segmental dermatomes, (B) cutaneous nerve distribution

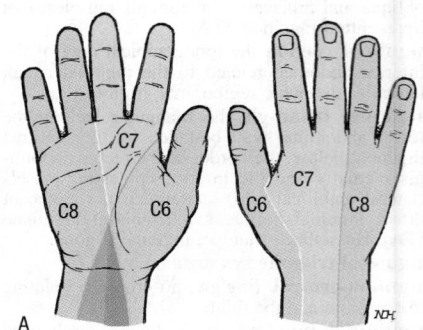

**injection**

**in·nid·i·a·tion** (i-nid-ē-ā′shŭn) the growth and multiplication of abnormal cells in location to which they have been transported by means of lymph or the blood stream, or both. SEE ALSO metastasis. [L. *in,* in, + *nidus,* nest]

**in·no·cent** (in'ō-sent) **1.** not apparently harmful. **2.** free from moral wrong. [L. *innocens* (*-ent-*), fr. *in*, neg., + *noceo*, to injure]

**in·no·cent mur·mur** SYN functional murmur.

**in·noc·u·ous** (i-nok'yu-ŭs) harmless. [L. *innocuus*]

**in·nom·i·nate** (i-nom'i-nāt) SYN anonyma. [L. *innominatus*, fr. *in-* neg. + *nomen* (*nomin-*), name]

**in·nom·i·nate ar·tery** obsolete term for brachiocephalic trunk.

**in·nom·i·nate bone** SYN hip bone.

**in·nom·i·nate veins** SYN brachiocephalic veins.

**INO** internuclear ophthalmoplegia.

**Ino** inosine.

**in·oc·u·la·bil·i·ty** (i-nok'yu-lă-bil'i-tē) the quality of being inoculable.

**in·oc·u·la·ble** (i-nok'yu-lă-bl) **1.** transmissible by inoculation. **2.** susceptible to a disease transmissible by inoculation.

**in·oc·u·late** (i-nok'yu-lāt) **1.** to introduce the agent of a disease or other antigenic material into the subcutaneous tissue or a blood vessel, or through an abraded or absorbing surface for preventive, curative, or experimental purposes. **2.** to implant microorganisms or infectious material into or upon culture media. **3.** to communicate a disease by transferring its virus. [L. *inoculo*, pp. *-atus*, to ingraft]

**in·oc·u·la·tion** (i-nok-yu-lā'shŭn) introduction into the body of the causative organism of a disease.

**in·oc·u·lum** (i-nok'yu-lŭm) the microorganism or other material introduced by inoculation.

**in·op·er·a·ble** (in-op'er-ă-bl) denoting that which cannot be operated upon, or cannot be corrected or removed by an operation.

**in·or·gan·ic** (in-ōr-gan'ik) **1.** not organic; not formed by living organisms. **2.** SEE inorganic compound. **3.** not containing carbon.

**in·or·gan·ic ac·id** an acid made up of molecules not containing organic radicals; e.g., HCl, $H_2SO_4$, $H_3PO_4$.

**in·or·gan·ic chem·is·try** the science concerned with compounds not involving carbon-containing molecules.

**in·or·gan·ic com·pound** a compound in which the atoms or radicals consist of elements other than carbon and are typically held together by electrostatic forces rather than by covalent bonds; often are capable of dissociation into ions in polar solvents (e.g., $H_2O$). Cf. organic compound.

**in·or·gan·ic or·tho·phos·phate ($P_i$, $P_1$)** any ion or salt form of phosphoric acid.

**in·os·a·mine** (in-ōs'ă-mēn) an inositol in which an –OH group is replaced by an –$NH_2$ group.

**in·os·co·py** (in-os'kŏ-pē) the microscopic examination of biologic materials (e.g., tissue, sputum, clotted blood) after dissecting or chemically digesting the fibrillary elements and strands of fibrin. [ino- + G. *skopeō*, to look at]

**in·o·se·mia** (in-ō-sē'mē-ă) the presence of inositol in the circulating blood. [inose + G. *haima*, blood]

**in·o·sine (I, Ino)** (in'ō-sēn) a nucleoside formed by the deamination of adenosine.

**in·o·sine 5′-mon·o·phos·phate (IMP)** SYN inosinic acid.

**in·o·sine 5′-tri·phos·phate (ITP)** inosine with triphosphoric acid esterified at its 5′ position;

participates in a number of enzyme-catalyzed reactions.

**in·o·sin·ic ac·id** (in-ō-sin'ik as'id) a mononucleotide found in muscle and other tissues; a key intermediate in purine biosynthesis; also produced in relatively high levels in muscle. SYN inosine 5′-monophosphate.

**in·o·si·tol** (in-ō'si-tōl) a member of the vitamin B complex.

*myo*-**in·o·si·tol** a constituent of various phosphatidylinositols and the most widely distributed form of inositol found in microorganisms, higher plants, and animals.

**in·o·si·tu·ria** (in'ō-sīt-yur'ē-ă) the excretion of inositol in the urine. [inositol + G. *ouron*, urine]

**in·o·tro·pic** (in-ō-trop'ik) influencing the contractility of muscular tissue. [ino- + G. *tropos*, a turning]

**in·pa·tient** patient who receives food and is assigned a bed in a health care facility while undergoing diagnosis and treatment.

**in·quest** (in'kwest) a legal inquiry into the cause of sudden, violent, or mysterious death. [L. *in*, in, + *quaero*, pp. *quaesitus*, to seek]

**INR** international normalized ratio.

**in·sane** (in-sān') **1.** of unsound mind; severely mentally impaired; deranged; crazy. **2.** relating to insanity. [L. *in-* neg. + *sanus*, sound, sane]

**in·san·i·tary** (in-san'i-tār-ē) injurious to health, usually in reference to an unclean or contaminated environment. SYN unsanitary. [L. *in-* neg. + *sanus*, sound]

**in·san·i·ty** (in-san'i-tē) **1.** a nonmedical term referring to severe mental illness or psychosis. **2.** LAW that degree of mental illness which negates the individual's legal responsibility or capacity. [L. *in-* neg. + *sanus*, sound]

**in·scrip·tion** (in-skrip'shŭn) **1.** the main part of a prescription; that which indicates the drugs and the quantity of each to be used in the mixture. **2.** a mark, band, or line. [L. *inscriptio*]

**in·sec·ti·cide** (in-sek'ti-sīd) an agent that kills insects. [insect + L. *caedō*, to kill]

**in·se·cu·ri·ty** (in-sē-kyur'i-tē) a feeling of unprotectedness and helplessness.

**in·sem·i·na·tion** (in-sem-i-nā'shŭn) deposit of seminal fluid within the vagina, normally during coitus. SYN semination. [L. *in-semino*, pp. *-atus*, to sow or plant in, fr. *semen*, seed]

**in·se·nes·cence** (in-sĕ-nes'ens) the process of growing old. [L. *insenesco*, to begin to grow old]

**in·sen·si·ble** (in-sen'si-bl) **1.** SYN unconscious. **2.** not appreciable by the senses. [L. *in-sensibilis*, fr. *in*, neg. + *sentio*, pp. *sensus*, to feel]

**in·sen·si·ble per·spi·ra·tion** perspiration that evaporates before it is perceived as moisture on the skin; the term sometimes includes evaporation from the lungs.

**in·ser·tion** (in-ser'shŭn) **1.** a putting in. **2.** the attachment of a muscle to the more movable part of the skeleton, as distinguished from origin. **3.** DENTISTRY the intraoral placing of a dental prosthesis. **4.** intrusion of fragments of any size from molecular to cytogenetic into the normal genome. [L. *insertio*, a planting in, fr. *insero*, *-sertus*, to plant in]

**in·ser·tion·al mu·ta·gen·e·sis** mutation caused by insertion of new genetic material into a normal gene, particularly of retroviruses into chromosomal DNA.

**in·ser·tion se·quen·ces** discrete DNA sequences

**i**
**n**

which are repeated at various sites on a bacterial chromosome, certain plasmids, and bacteriophages; insertion sequences can move from one site to another on the chromosome, to another plasmid in the same bacterium, or to a bacteriophage.

**in•sid•i•ous** (in-sid′ē-ŭs) treacherous; stealthy; denoting a disease that progresses gradually with inapparent symptoms. [L. *insidiosus,* cunning, fr. *insidiae* (pl.), an ambush]

**in•sight** (in′sīt) self-understanding as to the motives and reasons behind one's own actions or those of another's.

**in•sol•u•ble** (in-sol′yu-bl) not soluble.

**in•som•nia** (in-som′nē-ă) inability to sleep, in the absence of external impediments, such as noise, a bright light, etc., during the period when sleep should normally occur; may vary in degree from restlessness or disturbed slumber to a curtailment of the normal length of sleep or to absolute wakefulness. [L. fr. *in-* priv. + *somnus,* sleep]

**in•som•ni•ac** (in-som′nē-ak) **1.** a sufferer from insomnia. **2.** exhibiting, tending toward, or producing insomnia.

**in•sorp•tion** (in-sōrp′shŭn) movement of substances from the lumen of the gut into the blood. [L. *in,* in, + *sorbeo,* to suck]

**in•sper•sion** (in-sper′shŭn) sprinkling with a fluid or a powder. [L. *inspersio,* fr. *in-spergo,* pp. *-spersus,* to scatter upon, fr. *spargo,* to scatter]

**in•spi•ra•tion** (in-spi-rā′shŭn) SYN inhalation (1). [L. *inspiratio,* fr. *in-spiro,* pp. *-atus,* to breathe in]

**in•spi•ra•to•ry** (in-spī′ră-tō-rē) relating to or timed during inhalation.

**in•spi•ra•to•ry ca•pac•i•ty** the volume of air that can be inspired after a normal expiration; it is the sum of the tidal volume and the inspiratory reserve volume. SYN complementary air.

**in•spi•ra•to•ry re•serve vol•ume (IRV)** the maximal volume of air that can be inspired after a normal inspiration; the inspiratory capacity less the tidal volume. SYN complemental air.

**in•spi•ra•to•ry stri•dor** a crowing sound during the inspiratory phase of respiration due to pathology involving the epiglottis or larynx.

**in•spire** (in-spīr′) SYN inhale.

**in•spired gas (I)** (in-spīrd′) (gas symbol subscript I) **1.** any gas that is being inhaled; **2.** specifically, that gas after it has been humidified at body temperature.

**in•spis•sate** (in-spis′āt) to perform or undergo inspissation.

**in•spis•sa•tion** (in-spi-sā′shŭn) **1.** the act of thickening or condensing, as by evaporation or absorption of fluid. **2.** an increased thickening or diminished fluidity. [L. *in,* intensive, + *spisso,* pp. *-atus,* to thicken]

**in•sta•bil•i•ty** (in-stă-bil′i-tē) **1.** the state of being unstable, or lacking stability. **2.** the abnormal tendency of a joint to subluxate or dislocate with normal activities and stresses. SEE ALSO laxity.

**in•star** (in′stahr) any of the successive nymphal or larval stages in the metamorphosis of insects. [L. form]

**in•step** the arch, or highest part of the dorsum of the foot. SEE ALSO tarsus.

**in•stil•la•tion** (in-sti-lā′shŭn) dropping of a liquid on or into a part. [L. *instillatio,* fr. *in-stillo,* pp. *-atus,* to pour in by drops, fr. *stilla,* a drop]

**in•stinct** (in′stinkt) **1.** an enduring disposition or

tendency to act in an organized and biologically adaptive manner. **2.** the unreasoning impulse to perform some purposive action without an immediate consciousness of the end to which that action may lead. **3.** PSYCHOANALYTIC THEORY the forces assumed to exist behind the tension caused by the needs of the id. [L. *instinctus,* impulse]

**in•stinc•tive, in•stinc•tu•al** (in-stink′tiv, in-stink′choo-ăl) relating to instinct.

**In•sti•tu•tion•al Re•view Board (IRB)** the standing committee in a hospital or other facility that is charged with responsibility for ensuring the safety and well-being of human subjects involved in research.

**in•stru•ment** (in′stroo-ment) a tool or implement. [L. *instrumentum*]

**in•stru•men•tar•i•um** (in′stroo-men-tār′ē-ŭm) a collection of instruments and other equipment for an operation or for a medical procedure.

**in•su•date** (in′soo-dāt) fluid swelling within an arterial wall (ordinarily serous), differing from an exudate in that it does not come to lie extramurally. [L. *in,* in, + *sudo,* pp. *-atus,* to sweat]

**in•suf•fi•cien•cy** (in-sŭ-fish′en-sē) **1.** lack of completeness of function or power. **2.** SYN incompetence (1). [L. *in-,* neg. + *sufficientia,* fr. *sufficio* to suffice]

**in•suf•flate** (in-sŭf′lāt) to blow air, gas, or fine powder into a cavity. [L. *in-sufflo,* to blow on or into]

**in•suf•fla•tion** (in-sŭf-lā′shŭn) **1.** the act or process of insufflating. **2.** SYN inhalant (3).

**in•suf•fla•tion an•es•the•sia** maintenance of inhalation anesthesia by delivery of anesthetic gases or vapors directly to the airway of a spontaneously breathing patient.

**in•su•la,** gen. and pl. **in•su•lae** (in′soo-lă, in′soo-lē) **1.** an oval region of the cerebral cortex overlying the extreme capsule, lateral to the lenticular nucleus, buried in the depth of the fissura lateralis cerebri (sylvian fissure). SYN island of Reil. **2.** SYN island. **3.** any circumscribed body or patch on the skin. [L. island]

**in•su•lar** (in′soo-lăr) relating to any insula, especially the island of Reil.

**in•su•lar gy•ri** the short gyri of insula and long gyrus of insula.

**in•su•lin** (in′sŭ-lin) a polypeptide hormone, secreted by beta cells in the islets of Langerhans, that promotes glucose utilization, protein synthesis, and the formation and storage of neutral lipids; available in a variety of preparations including genetically engineered human insulin, which is presently favored, insulin is used parenterally in the treatment of diabetes mellitus. [L. *insula,* island, + -in]

**in•su•li•nae•mia [Br.]** SEE insulinemia.

**in•su•lin-an•tag•o•niz•ing fac•tor** SYN glycotropic factor.

**in•su•lin-de•pen•dent di•a•be•tes mel•li•tus (IDDM)** severe diabetes mellitus, often brittle, usually of abrupt onset during the first two decades of life but can develop at any age; characterized by polydipsia, polyuria, increased appetite, weight loss, low plasma insulin levels, and episodic ketoacidosis; immune-mediated destruction of pancreatic B cells; insulin therapy and dietary regulation are necessary. SYN growth-onset diabetes, juvenile-onset diabetes, type I diabetes.

**in•su•lin•e•mia** literally, insulin in the circulating

blood; usually connotes abnormally large concentrations of insulin in the circulating blood.

**in·su·lin-like ac·tiv·i·ty (ILA)** a measure of substances, usually in plasma, that exert biologic effects similar to those of insulin in various bioassays; sometimes used as a measure of plasma insulin concentrations; always gives higher values than immunochemical techniques for the measurement of insulin.

**in·su·lin-like growth fac·tors (IGF)** peptides whose formation is stimulated by growth hormone. These peptides bring about peripheral tissue effects of that hormone and have high (about 70%) homology to human insulin.

**in·su·lin·o·gen·e·sis** (in′sŭ-lin-ō-jen′ĕ-sis) production of insulin. [insulin + G. *genesis*, production]

**in·su·lin·o·gen·ic, in·su·lo·gen·ic** (in′sŭ-lin-ō-jen′ik, in′sŭ-lō-jen′ik) relating to insulinogenesis.

**in·su·li·no·ma** (in′sŭ-li-nō′mă) an islet cell adenoma that secretes insulin. SYN insuloma.

**in·su·lin re·cep·tor sub·strate-1 (IRS-1)** a cytoplasmic protein that is a direct substrate of the activated insulin receptor kinase. Insulin exposure results in its rapid phosphorylation at multiple tyrosine residues. Its phosphorylated sites associate with high affinity to certain cellular proteins. IRS-1 thus acts as an adaptor molecule that links the receptor kinase to various cellular activities regulated by insulin. IRS-1 is also phosphorylated after stimulation by insulinlike growth factor-1 and several interleukins.

**in·su·lin re·sis·tance** diminished effectiveness of insulin in lowering blood sugar levels; arbitrarily defined as requiring 200 units or more of insulin per day to prevent hyperglycemia or ketosis; usually due to insulin binding by antibodies, but abnormalities in insulin receptors on cell surfaces also occur; associated with obesity, ketoacidosis, infection, and certain rare conditions.

**in·su·lin shock** severe hypoglycemia produced by administration of insulin, manifested by sweating, tremor, anxiety, vertigo, and diplopia, followed by delirium, convulsions, and collapse.

**in·su·li·tis** (in′sŭ-li′tis) inflammation of the islands of Langerhans, with lymphocytic infiltration which may result from viral infection and be the initial lesion of insulin-dependent diabetes mellitus. [L. *insula,* island, + *-itis,* inflammation]

**in·su·lo·ma** (in-sŭ-lō′mă) SYN insulinoma. [L. *insula,* island, + *-oma,* tumor]

**in·sult** (in′sŭlt) an injury, attack, or trauma. [LL. *insultus,* fr L. *insulto,* to spring upon]

**in·sus·cep·ti·bil·i·ty** (in′sŭ-sep′ti-bil′i-tē) SYN immunity. [L. *suscipio,* pp. *-ceptus,* to take upon one, fr. *sub,* under, + *capio,* to take]

**in·te·gra·tion** (in-tĕ-grā′shŭn) **1.** the state of being combined, or the process of combining, into a complete and harmonious whole. **2.** PHYSIOLOGY the process of building up, as by accretion, anabolism, etc. **3.** MATHEMATICS the process of ascertaining a function from its differential. **4.** MOLECULAR BIOLOGY a recombination event in which a genetic element is inserted. [L. *integro,* pp. *-atus,* to make whole, fr. *integer,* whole]

**in·teg·ri·ty** (in-teg′ri-tē) soundness or completeness of structure; a sound or unimpaired condition.

**in·teg·u·ment** (in-teg′yu-ment) **1.** the enveloping membrane of the body; includes, in addition to the epidermis and dermis, all of the derivatives of the epidermis, e.g., hairs, nails, sudoriferous and sebaceous glands, and mammary glands. **2.** the rind, capsule, or covering of any body or part. SYN integumentum commune [TA], tegument. [L. *integumentum,* a covering, fr. *in-tego,* to cover]

**in·teg·u·men·ta·ry** (in-teg-yu-men′tă-rē) relating to the integument. SEE ALSO cutaneous, dermal.

**in·teg·u·men·tum com·mune** (in-teg-yu-men′ tŭm kō-moo′nē) [TA] SYN integument.

**in·tel·lec·tu·al·i·za·tion** (in-te-lek′choo-ăl-i-zā′ shŭn) an unconscious defense mechanism in which reasoning, logic, or focusing on and verbalizing intellectual minutiae is used in an attempt to avoid confrontation with an objectionable impulse, affect, or interpersonal situation. [L. *intellectus,* perception, discernment]

**in·tel·li·gence** (in-tel′i-jens) **1.** an individual's aggregate capacity to act purposefully, think rationally, and deal effectively with the environment, especially in meeting challenges and solving problems. **2.** PSYCHOLOGY an individual's relative standing on two quantitative indices, measured intelligence and effectiveness of adaptive behavior; a quantitative score or similar index on both indices constitutes the operational definition of intelligence. [L. *intelligentia*]

**in·tel·li·gence quo·tient (IQ)** the psychologist's index of intelligence as one part of a two-part determination, the other part being an index of adaptive behavior. IQ is ordinarily expressed as a ratio between the person's score on a given test and the score which the average individual of comparable age attained on the same test.

**in·ten·si·ty** (in-ten′si-tē) marked tension; great activity; often used simply to denote a measure of the degree or amount of some quality. [L. *intendo,* pp. *-tensus,* to stretch out]

**in·ten·sive care u·nit (ICU)** a hospital facility for provision of intensive nursing and medical care of critically ill patients, characterized by high quality and quantity of continuous nursing and medical supervision and by use of sophisticated monitoring and resuscitative equipment; may be organized for the care of specific patient groups, e.g., neonatal or newborn ICU, neurological ICU, pulmonary ICU. SYN critical care unit.

**in·ten·tion** (in-ten′shŭn) **1.** an objective. **2.** SURGERY a process or operation. [L. *intentio,* a stretching out; intention]

**in·ten·tion spasm** a spasmodic contraction of the muscles occurring when a voluntary movement is attempted.

**in·ten·tion-to-treat an·al·y·sis** method of analyzing results of a randomized controlled trial that includes in the analysis all the cases that should have received a treatment regimen but for whatever reason did not do so. All cases allocated to each arm of the trial are analyzed together as representing that treatment arm, whether or not they received or completed the prescribed regimen.

**in·ten·tion trem·or** a tremor that occurs during the performance of precise voluntary movements, caused by disorders of the cerebellum or its connections. SYN volitional tremor (2).

**inter-** among, between. [L. *inter,* between]

**in·ter·ac·tion** (int′er-ak′shŭn) **1.** the reciprocal action between two entities in a common envi-

i
n

ronment, as in chemical interaction, ecological interaction, and social interaction. **2.** the effects when two entities concur that would not be observed with either in isolation. **3.** STATISTICS, PHARMACOLOGY, QUANTITATIVE GENETICS the phenomenon that the combined effects of two causes differ from the sum of the effects separately (as in synergism and antagonism). **4.** independent operation of two or more causes to produce or prevent an effect. **5.** STATISTICS the necessity for a product term in a linear model.

**in·ter·al·ve·o·lar sep·tum 1.** the tissue intervening between two adjacent pulmonary alveoli; it consists of a close-meshed capillary network covered on both surfaces by very thin alveolar epithelial cells; **2.** one of the bony partitions between the tooth sockets.

**in·ter·arch dis·tance 1.** the vertical distance between the maxillary and mandibular arches under conditions of vertical dimensions which must be specified; **2.** the vertical distance between maxillary and mandibular ridges.

**in·ter·ar·y·te·noid fold** the soft tissue between the arytenoid cartilages.

**in·ter·a·tri·al block** SYN intraatrial block.

**in·ter·a·tri·al con·duc·tion time** SYN intraatrial conduction time (2).

**in·ter·a·tri·al sep·tum** the wall between the atria of the heart. SYN septum interatriale [TA].

**in·ter·au·ral** (in-ter-aw′ral) referring to differences between ears, particularly temporal events occurring in or emanating from the ears.

**in·ter·au·ral at·ten·u·a·tion** the reduction in intensity the head provides sound presented to one ear canal before it gets to the other ear; for air conduction, the reduction approximates 35 dB, but for bone conduction, it is only about 10 dB.

**in·ter·body** (in′ter-bod′ē) between the bodies of two adjacent vertebrae.

**in·ter·ca·dence** (in-ter-kā′dens) the occurrence of an extra beat between two regular pulse beats. [inter- + L. *cado,* pr. p. *cadens* (-*ent*-), to fall]

**in·ter·ca·dent** (in-ter-kā′dent) irregular in rhythm; characterized by intercadence.

**in·ter·ca·lary** (in-ter′kă-ler-ē, in-ter-kal′er-ē) **1.** occurring between two others; as in a pulse tracing, an upstroke interposed between two normal pulse beats. **2.** in fungi, located in a hypha or between hyphal segments, not at a hyphal terminus. [L. *intercalarius,* concerning an insertion]

**in·ter·ca·lat·ed** (in-ter′kă-lā-ted) interposed; inserted between two others. [L. *intercalatus*]

**in·ter·ca·lat·ed disk** a histologic feature of cardiac muscle, occurring at the junction of two myocardial cells; site of intercellular passage of ions and electrical impulses.

**in·ter·ca·lat·ed ducts** the minute ducts of glands, such as the salivary and the pancreas, that lead from the acini; they are lined by low cuboidal cells.

**in·ter·cap·il·lary glo·mer·u·lo·scle·ro·sis** SYN diabetic glomerulosclerosis.

**in·ter·ca·pit·u·lar veins** connect the dorsal and palmar veins in the hand, or the dorsal and plantar veins in the foot.

**in·ter·ca·rot·id bod·y** SYN carotid body.

**in·ter·car·pal joints** the synovial joints between the carpal bones. SYN carpal joints (1).

**in·ter·car·pal lig·a·ments** three sets of short fibrous bands that bind together the two rows of carpal bones; according to their location they are named dorsal intercarpal ligament (ligamentum intercarpalia dorsalia), interosseous intercarpal ligament (ligamentum intercarpalia interossea), and palmar intercarpal ligament (ligamentum intercarpalia palmaria).

**in·ter·cav·er·nous si·nus·es** the anterior and posterior anastomoses between the cavernous sinuses, passing anterior and posterior to the hypophysis and forming, with the cavernous sinuses, the circular sinus (1).

**in·ter·cel·lu·lar bridg·es** slender cytoplasmic strands connecting adjacent cells; in histological sections the bridges are shrinkage artifacts; true bridges with cytoplasmic confluence exist between incompletely divided germ cells. SYN cell bridges, cytoplasmic bridges.

**in·ter·cel·lu·lar can·a·lic·u·lus** one of the fine channels between adjoining secretory cells, such as those between serous cells in salivary glands.

**in·ter·cil·i·um** (in-ter-sil′ē-ŭm) SYN glabella. [inter- + L. *cilium,* eyelid]

**in·ter·cos·tal mem·branes** the membranous layers between ribs.

**in·ter·cos·tal nerves** ventral primary rami of the thoracic nerves. SYN nervi intercostales [TA].

**in·ter·cos·tal space** an interval between the ribs, occupied by intercostal muscles, veins, arteries and nerves.

**in·ter·cos·to·brach·i·al nerves** lateral cutaneous branches of the second and third intercostal nerves which pass to the skin of the medial side of the arm. SYN nervi intercostobrachiales [TA].

**in·ter·course** (in′ter-kōrs) communication or dealings between or among people. [L. *intercursus,* a running between]

**in·ter·cri·co·thy·rot·o·my** (in-ter-krī′kō-thī-rot′ ō-mē) SYN cricothyrotomy.

**in·ter·crines** (in′ter-krīnz) SYN chemokines. [inter- + G. *krinō,* to separate, secrete]

**in·ter·cross** (in′ter-kros) a mating between two individuals both heterozygous at a specified locus or loci.

**in·ter·cur·rent** (in-ter-ker′ent) intervening; said of a disease attacking a person who already has another disease. [inter- + L. *curro,* pr. p. *currens* (-*ent*-), to run]

**in·ter·cus·pal po·si·tion** SYN centric occlusion.

**in·ter·cus·pa·tion** (in′ter-kŭs-pā′shŭn) **1.** the cusp-to-fossa relation of the maxillary and mandibular posterior teeth to each other. **2.** the interlocking or fitting together of the cusps of opposing teeth. SYN interdigitation (4).

**in·ter·den·tal** (in-ter-den′tăl) **1.** between the teeth. **2.** denoting the relationship between the proximal surfaces of the teeth of the same arch. [inter- + L. *dens,* tooth]

**in·ter·den·tal ca·nals** canals that extend vertically through alveolar bone between roots of mandibular and maxillary incisor and maxillary bicuspid teeth. SYN Hirschfeld canals.

**in·ter·den·tal pa·pil·la** the gingiva that fills the interproximal space between two adjacent teeth.

**in·ter·den·tal sep·tum** the bony portion separating two adjacent teeth in a dental arch.

**in·ter·den·tal splint** a splint for a fractured jaw, consisting of two metal or acrylic resin bands wired to the teeth of the upper and lower jaws, respectively, and then fastened together to keep the jaws immovable.

**in·ter·den·ti·um** (in-ter-den′shē-ŭm) the interval between any two contiguous teeth.

**in·ter·dig·it** (in-ter-dij′it) that part of the hand or foot lying between any two adjacent fingers or toes.

**in·ter·di·gi·ta·ting re·tic·u·lum cell** an antigen-presenting cell in the paracortex of lymph nodes, interacting with T lymphocytes.

**in·ter·dig·i·ta·tion** (in′ter-dij-i-tā′shŭn) **1.** the mutual interlocking of toothed or tonguelike processes. **2.** the processes thus interlocked. **3.** infoldings or plicae of adjacent cell or plasma membranes. **4.** SYN intercuspation (2). [inter- + L. *digitus,* finger]

**in·ter·dis·ci·pli·nary** (in-ter-dis′i-pli-nār-ē) denoting the overlapping interests of different fields of medicine and science. [inter- + L. *disciplina,* instruction, teaching]

**in·ter·face** (in′ter-fās) **1.** a surface that forms a common boundary of two bodies. **2.** the boundary between regions of different radiopacity, acoustic, or magnetic resonance properties; the projection of the interface between tissues of different such properties on an image.

**in·ter·fa·cial ca·nals** intercellular spaces occurring in relation to intercellular attachments by desmosomes in stratified squamous epithelium, generally resulting from shrinkage of an artifact of fixation.

**in·ter·fer·ence** (in-ter-fēr′ens) **1.** the coming together of waves in various media in such a way that the crests of one series correspond to the hollows of the other, the two thus neutralizing each other; or so that the crests of the two series correspond, thus increasing the excursions of the waves. **2.** collision within the myocardium of two waves of excitation at the junction of territories controlled by each, as is seen in A-V dissociation. **3.** also, in A-V dissociation, the disturbance of the regular rhythm of the ventricles by a conducted impulse from the atria, e.g., by a ventricular capture (interference beat). **4.** the condition in which infection of a cell by one virus prevents superinfection by another virus, or in which superinfection prevents effects which would result from infection by either virus alone, even though both viruses persist. [inter- + L. *ferio,* to strike]

**in·ter·fer·on** (IFN) (in-ter-fēr′on) a class of small protein and glycoprotein cytokines (15–28 kD) produced by T cells, fibroblasts, and other cells in response to viral infection and other biological and synthetic stimuli. Interferons bind to specific receptors on cell membranes; their effects include inducing enzymes, suppressing cell proliferation, inhibiting viral proliferation, enhancing the phagocytic activity of macrophages, and augmenting the cytotoxic activity of T lymphocytes. Interferons are divided into five major classes (alpha, beta, gamma, tau, and omega) and several subclasses (indicated by Arabic numerals and letters) on the basis of physicochemical properties, cells of origin, mode of induction, and antibody reactions. [interfere + -on]

**in·ter·fer·on alpha 2b** a water-soluble protein (MW 19,271) secreted by cells infected by virus; used to treat hairy cell leukemia, malignant melanoma, condylomata acuminata, AIDS-related Kaposi sarcoma, and chronic hepatitis C.

**in·ter·fer·on be·ta 1b** a purified protein containing 165 amino acids (MW approximately 18,500) with antiviral and immunomodulatory effects, used in the treatment of relapsing-remitting multiple sclerosis to reduce the frequency of clinical exacerbations.

**in·ter·fer·on o·me·ga** a form of interferon known as interferon-alpha-2.

**in·ter·fer·on tau** an interferon secreted by bovine conceptus, with potent antiretroviral activity; in experimental use. SYN trophoblast interferon, trophoblastin.

**in·ter·fer·on type I** antiviral interferons, including interferon-alpha; and interferon-beta.

**in·ter·fer·on type II** immune interferon, interferon-gamma.

**in·ter·glo·bu·lar den·tin** imperfectly calcified matrix of dentin situated between the calcified globules near the dentinal periphery.

**in·ter·ic·tal** (in-ter-ik′tăl) the period between convulsions. [inter- + L. *ictus,* stroke]

**in·ter·im den·ture** a dental prosthesis to be used for a short time for reasons of esthetics, mastication, occlusal support, or convenience, or to condition the patient to accept an artificial substitute for missing natural teeth until more definite prosthetic dental treatment can be provided. SYN temporary denture.

**in·ter·ki·ne·sis** (in′ter-ki-nē′sis) period between the first and second divisions of meiosis; comparable to interphase of mitosis. [inter- + G. *kinēsis,* movement]

**in·ter·lam·i·nar jel·ly** the gelatinous material between ectoderm and endoderm that serves as the substrate on which mesenchymal cells migrate.

**in·ter·leu·kin** (IL) (in-ter-loo′kin) the name given to a group of multifunctional cytokines once their amino acid structure is known. They are synthesized by lymphocytes, monocytes, macrophages, and certain other cells. SEE ALSO lymphokine, cytokine. [inter- + *leuko*cyte + -in]

**in·ter·leu·kin-1** a cytokine, derived primarily from mononuclear phagocytes, which enhances the proliferation of T helper cells and growth and differentiation of B cells.

**in·ter·leu·kin-2** a cytokine derived from T helper lymphocytes that causes proliferation of T lymphocytes and activated B lymphocytes.

**in·ter·leu·kin-3** (IL-3) a cytokine derived from monocytes, fibroblasts, and endothelial cells that increases production of monocytes. SYN multicolony-stimulating factor.

**in·ter·leu·kin-4** (IL-4) a cytokine derived from T4 lymphocytes that causes differentiation of B lymphocytes. SYN B cell differentiating factor.

**in·ter·leu·kin-5** (IL-5) a cytokine derived from T lymphocytes that causes activation of B lymphocytes and differentiation of eosinophils.

**in·ter·leu·kin-6** (IL-6) a cytokine derived from fibroblasts, macrophages, and tumor cells that increases synthesis and secretion of immunoglobulins by B lymphocytes. SYN B cell stimulatory factor 2.

**in·ter·leu·kin-7** (IL-7) a cytokine derived from bone marrow cells that causes proliferation of B and T lymphocytes.

**in·ter·leu·kin-8** (IL-8) a cytokine derived from endothelial cells, fibroblasts, keratinocytes, macrophages, and monocytes which causes chemotaxis of neutrophils and T cell lymphocytes. SYN anionic neutrophil-activating peptide, monocyte-derived neutrophil chemotactic factor, neutrophil-activating factor.

**in·ter·leu·kin-9** (IL-9) a cytokine derived from

i
n

T cells which causes growth and proliferation of T cells.

**in·ter·leu·kin-10 (IL-10)** a cytokine derived from helper T cell lymphocytes, B cell lymphocytes, and monocytes that inhibits gamma-interferon (IFNγ) secretion by T cell lymphocytes and it inhibits mononuclear cell inflammation.

**in·ter·leu·kin-11 (IL-11)** a cytokine derived from bone marrow stromal cells (endothelial cells, macrophages, and preadipocytes) which stimulates increased plasma concentrations of acute phase proteins.

**in·ter·leu·kin-12 (IL-12)** a cytokine derived from B lymphocytes, T lymphocytes, and macrophages that induces gamma-interferon (IFNγ) gene expression in T lymphocytes and NK cells.

**in·ter·leu·kin-13 (IL-13)** a cytokine derived from helper T cell lymphocytes that inhibits mononuclear cell inflammation.

**in·ter·leu·kin-14 (IL-14)** a cytokine derived from T cells which stimulates B cell proliferation and inhibits Ig secretion.

**in·ter·leu·kin-15 (IL-15)** a cytokine derived from T cells which stimulates T cell proliferation and NK cell activation.

**in·ter·leu·kin-16 (IL-16)** a cytokine made by T cells that is a potent chemotactant for CD4$^+$ T cells.

**in·ter·leu·kin-17 (IL-17)** a proinflammatory cytokine made by T cells.

**in·ter·leu·kin-18 (IL-18)** a cytokine made by macrophages; a potent inducer of interferon-γ by T cells and NK cells.

**in·ter·lo·bar duct** a duct draining the secretion of the lobe of a gland and formed by the junction of a number of interlobular ducts.

**in·ter·lo·bar veins of kid·ney** veins that parallel the interlobar arteries, receive blood from arcuate veins, and terminate in the renal vein.

**in·ter·lo·bi·tis** (in′ter-lō-bī′tis) inflammation of the pleura separating two pulmonary lobes.

**in·ter·lob·u·lar ar·ter·ies** arteries that pass between lobules of an organ. SYN arteriae interlobulares [TA].

**in·ter·lob·u·lar duct** any duct leading from a lobule of a gland and formed by the junction of the fine ducts draining the acini.

**in·ter·lob·u·lar em·phy·se·ma** interstitial emphysema in the connective tissue septa between the pulmonary lobules.

**in·ter·lob·u·lar pleu·ri·sy** inflammation limited to the pleura in the sulci between the pulmonary lobes.

**in·ter·lob·u·lar veins of kid·ney** parallel the interlobular arteries and drain the peritubular capillary plexus, emptying into the arcuate veins.

**in·ter·lob·u·lar veins of liv·er** terminal branches of the portal vein that course in the portal canals between the conceptual liver lobules and empty into the liver sinusoids.

**in·ter·max·il·lary bone** SYN os incisivum.

**in·ter·max·il·lary su·ture** the line of union of the two maxillae.

**in·ter·me·di·ary nerve** a root of the facial nerve containing sensory fibers for taste from the anterior two-thirds of tongue whose cell bodies are located in the geniculate ganglion and presynaptic parasympathetic autonomic fibers whose cell bodies are located in the superior salivatory nucleus, i.e., the fibers eventually conveyed via the chorda tympani branch of the facial nerve to the lingual nerve. SYN nervus intermedius [TA], intermediate nerve.

**in·ter·me·di·ate** (in′ter-mē′dē-it) **1.** between two extremes; interposed; intervening. **2.** a substance formed in the course of chemical reactions that then proceeds to participate rapidly in further reactions, so that at any given moment it is present in minute concentrations only; such substances, when appearing in the course of the reactions involved in metabolism, are metabolic intermediates. **3.** DENTISTRY a cement base. **4.** an element or organ between right and left (or lateral and medial) structures. SYN intermedius.

**in·ter·me·di·ate ba·sil·ic vein** medial branch of the median antebrachial vein which joins the basilic vein.

**in·ter·me·di·ate care fa·cil·i·ty (ICF)** institutional setting where services are provided that do not require the level of care provided in a hospital or skilled-nursing facility. SEE nursing facility.

**in·ter·me·di·ate ce·phal·ic vein** lateral branch of the median antebrachial vein that joins the cephalic vein near the elbow.

**in·ter·me·di·ate cu·ne·i·form bone** a bone of the distal row of the tarsus; it articulates with the medial and lateral cuneiform, navicular, and second metatarsal bones. SYN wedge bone.

**in·ter·me·di·ate heart** description of the heart's electrical axis when this is directed at approximately between +30° and +60°.

**in·ter·me·di·ate host, in·ter·me·di·ar·y host 1.** one in which larval or developmental stages occur; **2.** a host through which a microorganism can pass or which contains an asexual stage of a parasite.

**in·ter·me·di·ate nerve** SYN intermediary nerve.

**in·ter·me·di·ate sa·cral crest** crests formed by the fusion of articular processes of all the sacral vertebrae. SYN articular crest.

**in·ter·me·di·ate trait** a measurable trait in which there is some evidence of the operation of a simple major cause, but in which the variation within the putative categories is such as to cause overlap and hence ambiguity in classification of any particular reading.

**in·ter·me·di·ate vas·tus mus·cle** SYN vastus intermedius muscle.

**in·ter·me·di·o·lat·er·al nu·cle·us** the cell column that forms the lateral horn of the spinal gray matter. Extending from the first thoracic through the second lumbar segment, the column contains the autonomic motor neurons that give rise to the preganglionic fibers of the sympathetic system.

**in·ter·me·di·o·me·di·al fron·tal branch of cal·lo·so·mar·gin·al ar·tery** branch of middle portion of callosomarginal artery to anterosuperior portion of medial aspect of frontal lobe of cerebrum.

**in·ter·me·di·o·me·di·al nu·cle·us** a small group of scattered visceral motor neurons immediately ventral to the thoracic nucleus in the thoracic and upper two lumbar segments of the spinal cord; considered to receive visceral afferent fibers at all spinal levels.

**in·ter·me·di·us** (in-ter-mē′dē-ŭs) SYN intermediate. [L.]

**in·ter·men·stru·al pain 1.** pelvic discomfort occurring approximately at the time of ovulation, usually at the midpoint of the menstrual cycle; **2.** SYN mittelschmerz.

**in·ter·met·a·car·pal joint** the synovial joints

between the bases of the second, third, fourth, and fifth metacarpal bones.

**in·ter·met·a·tar·sal joint** the synovial joints between the bases of the five metatarsal bones.

**in·ter·mit·tent** (in-ter-mit′ent) marked by intervals of complete quietude between two periods of activity.

**in·ter·mit·tent a·cute por·phyr·ia (IAP)** porphyria caused by hepatic overproduction of δ-aminolevulinic acid, with greatly increased urinary excretion of it and of porphobilinogen, due to a deficiency of porphobilinogen deaminase; characterized by intermittent acute attacks of hypertension, abdominal colic, psychosis, and polyneuropathy, but with no photosensitivity; exacerbation caused by ingestion of certain drugs (e.g., barbiturates). SYN acute intermittent porphyria, acute porphyria.

**in·ter·mit·tent clau·di·ca·tion** a condition caused by ischemia of the muscles; characterized by attacks of lameness and pain, brought on by walking, chiefly in the calf muscles; however, the condition may occur in other muscle groups. SYN Charcot syndrome, myasthenia angiosclerotica.

**in·ter·mit·tent com·pres·sion 1.** a neurodevelopmental treatment technique to facilitate contraction by applying pressure directly to the muscles surrounding a joint requiring better stabilization; SYN pressure tapping. **2.** a treatment procedure that employs intermittent external pressure to reduce edema in an extremity.

**in·ter·mit·tent cramp 1.** SYN tetany. **2.** SYN benign tetanus.

**in·ter·mit·tent ex·plo·sive dis·or·der** an uncommon disorder that begins in early childhood, characterized by repeated acts of violent, aggressive behavior in otherwise normal persons that is markedly out of proportion to the event that provokes it.

**in·ter·mit·tent man·da·to·ry ven·ti·la·tion (IMV)** a mode of mechanical ventilation in which the patient can trigger spontaneous breaths between preset mandatory breaths.

**in·ter·mit·tent pos·i·tive pres·sure breath·ing (IPPB)** SYN controlled mechanical ventilation.

**in·ter·mit·tent pos·i·tive pres·sure ven·ti·la·tion (IPPV)** SYN controlled mechanical ventilation.

**in·ter·mit·tent tet·a·nus** SYN tetany.

**in·ter·mus·cu·lar sep·tum** a term applied to aponeurotic sheets separating various muscles of the limbs; these are anterior and posterior crural, lateral and medial femoral, lateral and medial humeral.

**in·tern** (in′tern) an advanced student or recent graduate undertaking further education by assisting in the medical or surgical care of hospital patients, with supervision and instruction; formerly, one who resided within the institution. [F. *interne*, inside]

**in·ter·nal** (in-ter′năl) away from the surface. USAGE NOTE: Often incorrectly used to mean medial. [L. *internus*]

**in·ter·nal ad·he·sive per·i·car·di·tis** SYN concretio cordis.

**in·ter·nal au·di·to·ry veins** SYN labyrinthine veins.

**in·ter·nal base of skull** the interior aspect of the skull base on which the brain rests; the floor of the cranial cavity. SEE ALSO base of skull.

**in·ter·nal branch of trunk of ac·ces·so·ry nerve** branch of the accessory nerve trunk that carries fibers from the cranial root and that unites with the vagus nerve in the jugular foramen. SEE ALSO accessory nerve [CN XI].

**in·ter·nal cap·sule** a massive layer (8 to 10 mm thick) of white matter separating the caudate nucleus and thalamus (medial) from the more laterally situated lentiform nucleus (globus pallidus and putamen). It consists of 1) fibers ascending from the thalamus to the cerebral cortex that compose, among others, the visual, auditory, and somatic sensory radiations, and 2) fibers descending from the cerebral cortex to the thalamus, subthalamic region, midbrain, hindbrain, and spinal cord. The internal capsule is the major route by which the cerebral cortex is connected with the brainstem and spinal cord. Laterally and superiorly it is continuous with the corona radiata which forms a major part of the white matter of the cerebral hemisphere; caudally and medially it continues, much reduced in size, as the crus cerebri which contains, among others, the pyramidal tract. On horizontal section it appears in the form of a V opening out laterally; the V's obtuse angle is called genu (knee); its anterior and posterior limbs, respectively, the crus anterior and crus posterior. SYN capsula interna [TA].

**in·ter·nal ca·rot·id nerve** the cephalic arterial ramus conveying postsynaptic sympathetic fibers from the superior cervical ganglion to the internal carotid artery to form the internal carotid plexus. SYN nervus caroticus internus [TA].

**in·ter·nal ce·phal·ic ver·sion** version performed by means of one hand within the vagina. SEE ALSO cephalic version.

**in·ter·nal ce·re·bral veins** paired veins passing caudally near the midline in the tela choroidea of the third ventricle, formed by the union of the choroid vein, thalamostriate (terminal) vein, and vein of septum pellucidum, and uniting caudally so as to form the great cerebral vein. SYN venae internae cerebri [TA].

**in·ter·nal ear** SEE ear.

**in·ter·nal en·er·gy (U, U)** energy of a system measured by the heat absorbed from the system's surroundings and the amount of work done on the system by its surroundings.

**in·ter·nal fis·tu·la** a fistula between hollow viscera.

**in·ter·nal fix·a·tion** stabilization of fractured bony parts by direct fixation to one another with surgical wires, screws, pins, rods, plates, or methylmethacrylate.

**in·ter·nal hem·or·rhage** bleeding into organs or cavities of the body. SYN concealed hemorrhage.

**in·ter·nal il·i·ac ar·tery** *origin*, common iliac; *branches*, iliolumbar, lateral sacral, obturator, superior gluteal, inferior gluteal, umbilical, superior vesical, inferior vesical, middle rectal, and internal pudendal.

**in·ter·nal il·i·ac vein** runs from the upper border of the greater sciatic notch to the brim of the pelvis where it joins the external iliac vein to form the common iliac vein; it drains most of the territory supplied by the internal iliac artery.

**in·ter·nal in·ter·cos·tal mus·cle** each arises from lower border of rib and passes obliquely downward and backward to be inserted into upper border of rib below; *action*, contract during expiration, also maintain tension in the intercostal spaces to resist mediolateral movement; *nerve supply*, intercostal.

**in·ter·nal·i·za·tion** (in-ter'năl-i-zā'shŭn) adopting as one's own the standards and values of another person or society.

**in·ter·nal·ized ho·mo·pho·bia** homophobia occurring in a homosexual person, often associated with self-loathing, self-censure, and self-censorship.

**in·ter·nal med·i·cine (IM)** the branch of medicine concerned with nonsurgical diseases in adults, but not including diseases limited to the skin or to the nervous system.

**in·ter·nal ob·lique mus·cle** *origin*, iliac fascia deep to lateral part of inguinal ligament, anterior half of crest of ilium, and lumbar fascia; *insertion*, tenth to twelfth ribs and sheath of rectus; some of the fibers from inguinal ligament terminate in the conjoint tendon; *action*, diminishes capacity of abdomen, flexes lumbar vertebral column (bends thorax forward); *nerve supply*, lower thoracic. SYN musculus obliquus internus abdominis [TA].

**in·ter·nal ob·tu·ra·tor mus·cle** SYN obturator internus muscle.

**in·ter·nal oc·cip·i·tal crest** a ridge running from the internal occipital protuberance to the posterior margin of the foramen magnum, giving attachment to the falx cerebelli.

**in·ter·nal oph·thal·mop·a·thy** any disease of the internal structures of the eyeball.

**in·ter·nal oph·thal·mo·ple·gia** SYN ophthalmoplegia interna.

**in·ter·nal phase** the particles contained in a colloid solution.

**in·ter·nal po·dal·ic ver·sion** maneuver to deliver the fetus by inserting a hand into the uterine cavity, grasping one or both feet, and drawing them through the cervix; rarely indicated today except for the delivery of a second twin.

**in·ter·nal pu·den·dal ar·tery** *origin*, internal iliac; *branches*, inferior rectal, perineal, posterior scrotal (or labial), urethral, artery of bulb of penis (or of vestibule), deep artery of penis (or clitoris), dorsal artery of penis (or clitoris).

**in·ter·nal pu·den·dal vein** a tributary of the internal iliac vein that accompanies the internal pudendal artery as a single or double vessel. It drains the perineum.

**in·ter·nal rep·re·sen·ta·tion** term used by neurolinguistic programming to denote the way people use mental imagery (visual, auditory, or kinesthetic) to encode experience, the composite of which comprises their internal and external reality.

**in·ter·nal res·pi·ra·tion** SYN tissue respiration.

**in·ter·nal trac·tion** a pulling force created by using one of the cranial bones, above the point of fracture, for anchorage.

**in·ter·nal u·re·thral or·i·fice** the internal opening or orifice of the urethra, at the anterior and inferior angle of the trigone.

**in·ter·na·sal su·ture** line of union between the two nasal bones.

**In·ter·na·tion·al Clas·si·fi·ca·tion of Dis·eas·es (ICD)** the classification of specific conditions and groups of conditions determined by an internationally representative expert committee that advises the World Health Organization,

which publishes the complete list in a periodically revised book, the *Manual of the International Statistical Classification of Diseases, Injuries and Causes of Death*. The Tenth Revision (ICD-10) came into use in 1992; it has 20 chapters, each with a hierarchical arrangement of subdivisions (rubrics); some chapters are etiological, some relate to body systems, some to classes of conditions, some to procedures.

**In·ter·na·tion·al Clas·si·fi·ca·tion of Health Prob·lems in Pri·ma·ry Care** a classification of diseases, conditions and problems arranged for use in primary care where diagnostic precision is seldom possible.

**In·ter·na·tion·al Clas·si·fi·ca·tion of Im·pair·ments, Dis·a·bil·i·ties and Hand·i·caps** a WHO-sponsored numerical taxonomy of the impairments, disabilities and handicaps consequent upon injury and disease.

**in·ter·na·tion·al nor·mal·ized ra·tio (INR)** the prothrombin time ratio that would have been obtained if a standard reagent had been used in a prothrombin time determination; the prothrombin time ratio is expressed as the patient prothrombin time divided by the mean of the prothrombin time reference interval; the prothrombin time ratio is obtained for a working reagent in the laboratory through use of a parameter designated the international sensitivity index. SEE ALSO international sensitivity index.

**In·ter·na·tion·al Pho·ne·tic Al·pha·bet (IPA)** system of orthographic symbols devised for representing speech sounds; can be used for any language or to represent the sounds of disordered speech.

**in·ter·na·tion·al sen·si·ti·vi·ty in·dex (ISI)** the slope of the line of best fit relating the log prothrombin time obtained with a standard reagent to the log prothrombin time obtained with the working reagent for both normal persons and patients who receive stable oral anticoagulant therapy; the standard reagents used for this value assignment are reference preparations calibrated against the World Health Organization standard reagent. SEE ALSO international normalized ratio.

**In·ter·na·tion·al Sys·tem of U·nits (SI)** a system of measurements, based on the metric system, adopted at the 11th General Conference on Weights and Measures of the International Organization for Standardization (1960) to cover both the coherent units (basic, supplementary, and derived units) and the decimal multiples and submultiples of these units formed by use of prefixes proposed for general international scientific and technological use. SI proposes seven basic units: meter (m), kilogram (kg), second (s), ampere (A), Kelvin (K), candela (cd), and mole (mol) for the basic quantities of length, mass, time, electric current, temperature, luminous intensity, and amount of substance; supplementary units proposed include the radian (rad) for plane angle and steradian (sr) for solid angle; derived units (e.g., force, power, frequency) are stated in terms of the basic units (e.g., velocity is in meters per second, $m/s^{-1}$). Multiples (prefixes) in descending order are: exa- (E, $10^{18}$), peta- (P, $10^{15}$), tera- (T, $10^{12}$), giga- (G, $10^9$), mega- (M, $10^6$), kilo- (k, $10^3$), hecto- (h, $10^2$), deca- (da, $10^1$), deci- (d, $10^{-1}$), centi- (c, $10^{-2}$), milli- (m, $10^{-3}$), micro- (μ, $10^{-6}$), nano- (n, $10^{-9}$), pico- (p, $10^{-12}$), femto- (f, $10^{-15}$), atto- (a, $10^{-18}$). The prefix zepto (z) has been proposed for $10^{-21}$. Those involving a multiple of $10^3$ are recommended; compounds of these are not recommended (e.g., mμ for n). [Fr. *Système International d'Unités*]

**in•ter•na•tion•al u•nit** the amount of a substance, such as a drug, hormone, vitamin, enzyme, etc., that produces a specific effect as defined by an international body and accepted internationally. SYN unit (4).

**in•ter•neu•ro•nes [Br.]** SEE interneurons.

**in•ter•neu•rons** (in′ter-noo′ronz) combinations or groups of neurons between sensory and motor neurons that govern coordinated activity.

**in•tern•ist** (in-ter′nist, in′ter-nist) a physician trained in internal medicine.

**in•ter•nod•al seg•ment** the portion of a myelinated nerve fiber between two successive nodes. SYN internode.

**in•ter•node** (in′ter-nōd) SYN internodal segment.

**in•ter•nu•cle•ar** (in-ter-noo′klē-ăr) between nerve cell groups in the brain or retina.

**in•ter•nu•cle•ar oph•thal•mo•ple•gi•a (INO)** ophthalmoplegia in lesions of the medial longitudinal fasciculus, with failure of adduction in horizontal gaze but with retention of convergence.

**in•ter•nun•ci•al** (in-ter-nun′sē-ăl) **1.** indicating a neuron functionally interposed between two or more other neurons. **2.** acting as a medium of communication between two organs. [L. *inter-nuntius* (or *-nuncius*), a messenger between two parties, fr. *inter*, between, + *nuncius*, a messenger]

**in•ter•nun•ci•al neu•ron** a neuron interposed between and connecting two other neurons.

**in•ter•ob•serv•er er•ror** the differences in interpretation by two or more individuals making observations on the same phenomenon.

**in•ter•oc•clu•sal dis•tance 1.** the vertical distance between the opposing occlusal surfaces, assuming rest relation unless otherwise designated; **2.** SYN freeway space.

**in•ter•o•cep•tive** (in′ter-ō-sep′tiv) relating to the sensory nerve cells innervating the viscera (thoracic, abdominal and pelvic organs, and the cardiovascular system), their sensory end organs, or the information they convey to the spinal cord and the brain. [inter- + L. *capio,* to take]

**in•ter•o•cep•tor** (in′ter-ō-sep′ter) one of the various forms of small sensory end organs (receptors) situated within the walls of the respiratory and gastrointestinal tracts or in other viscera. [inter- + L. *capio,* to take]

**in•ter•os•se•ous car•ti•lage** SYN connecting cartilage.

**in•ter•pa•ri•e•tal su•ture** SYN sagittal suture.

**in•ter•par•ox•ys•mal** (in′ter-par-ok-siz′măl) occurring between successive paroxysms of a disease.

**in•ter•pe•dun•cu•lar fos•sa** deep depression on the inferior surface of the mesencephalon, between the crura cerebri, the floor of which is formed by the posterior perforated substance.

**in•ter•pe•dun•cu•lar nu•cle•us** a median, unpaired, ovoid cell group at the base of the midbrain tegmentum between the cerebral peduncles; it receives the retroflex fasciculus from the habenula, and projects to the raphe region (raphe nuclei) and periaqueductal gray substance of the midbrain.

**in•ter•pel•vi•ab•dom•i•nal am•pu•ta•tion** SYN hemipelvectomy.

**in•ter•pha•lan•ge•al** (in′ter-fă-lan′jē-ăl) between two phalanges; denoting the finger or toe joints.

**in•ter•pha•lan•ge•al joints of hand** the hinge synovial joints between the phalanges of the fingers.

**in•ter•phase** (in′ter-fāz) the stage between two successive divisions of a cell nucleus in which the biochemical and physiologic functions of the cell are performed and replication of chromatin occurs.

**in•ter•phy•let•ic** (in′ter-fī-let′ik) denoting the transitional forms between two kinds of cells during the course of metaplasia. [inter- + G. *phylē,* tribe]

**in•ter•pleu•ral space** SYN mediastinum (2).

**in•ter•po•lat•ed ex•tra•sys•to•le** a ventricular extrasystole which, instead of being followed by a compensatory pause, is sandwiched between two consecutive sinus cycles.

**in•ter•pre•ta•tion** (in-ter-pre-tā′shŭn) **1.** PSYCHO-ANALYSIS the characteristic therapeutic intervention of the analyst. **2.** CLINICAL PSYCHOLOGY drawing inferences and formulating the meaning in terms of the psychological dynamics inherent in an individual's responses to psychological tests or during psychotherapy.

**in•ter•prox•i•mal** (in-ter-prok′si-măl) between adjoining surfaces.

**in•ter•prox•i•mal space** the space between adjacent teeth in a dental arch; it is divided into the embrasure occlusal to the contact area, and the septal space gingival to the contact area.

**in•ter•pu•bic disk** the disk of fibrocartilage that unites the pubic bones at the pubic symphysis.

**in•ter•ra•dic•u•lar space** the space between the roots of multirooted teeth.

**in•ter•rupt•ed su•ture** a single stitch fixed by tying ends together.

**in•ter•sec•tio,** pl. **in•ter•sec•ti•o•nes** (in′ter-sek′ shē-ō, in′ter-sek-shē-ō′nēz) SYN intersection. [L.]

**in•ter•sec•tion** (in′ter-sek-shŭn) the site of crossing of two structures. SYN intersectio.

**in•ter•seg•men•tal vein** a vein receiving blood from adjacent bronchopulmonary segments; it emerges from the inferior margin of a segment to become a tributary of a branch of a pulmonary vein.

**in•ter•space** (in′ter-spās) any space between two similar objects, such as a costal interspace or interval between two ribs.

**in•ter•spi•na•les mus•cles** the paired muscles between spinous processes of adjacent vertebrae; subdivided into cervical, thoracic, and lumbar muscles. SYN musculi interspinales [TA], interspinal muscles.

**in•ter•spi•nal mus•cles** SYN interspinales muscles.

**in•ter•spi•nal plane** a horizontal plane passing through the anterior superior iliac spines; it marks the boundary between the lateral and umbilical regions superiorly and the inguinal and pubic regions inferiorly.

**in•ter•stice,** pl. **in•ter•stic•es** (in-tĕr′stĭs, in-ter′ stĭs-ēz) SYN interstitium. [L. *interstitium,* fr. *sisto,* to stand]

**in•ter•sti•tial** (in-ter-stish′ăl) **1.** relating to spaces or interstices in any structure. **2.** relating to spaces within a tissue or organ, but excluding such spaces as body cavities or potential space. Cf. intracavitary.

**in•ter•sti•tial cells 1.** cells between the seminiferous tubules of the testis that secrete testosterone; SYN Leydig cells. **2.** cells derived from the theca interna of atretic follicles of the ovary; they resemble luteal cells and are an important source of estrogens; **3.** pineal cells similar to glial cells with long processes.

**in·ter·sti·tial cell-stim·u·lat·ing hor·mone** SYN lutropin.

**in·ter·sti·tial cys·ti·tis** a chronic inflammatory condition of unknown etiology involving the mucosa and muscularis of the bladder, resulting in reduced bladder capacity, pain relieved by voiding, and severe bladder irritative symptoms. SEE ALSO Hunner ulcer.

**▣in·ter·sti·tial dis·ease** a disease occurring chiefly in the connective-tissue framework of an organ, the parenchyma suffering secondarily. See page B13.

**in·ter·sti·tial em·phy·se·ma 1.** presence of air in the pulmonary tissues consequent upon rupture of the air cells; **2.** presence of air or gas in the connective tissue.

**in·ter·sti·tial flu·id** the fluid in spaces between the tissue cells, constituting about 16% of the weight of the body; closely similar in composition to lymph.

**in·ter·sti·tial gas·tri·tis** inflammation of the stomach involving the submucosa and muscle coats.

**in·ter·sti·tial growth** growth from a number of different centers within an area; in contrast with appositional growth, it can occur only when the materials involved are nonrigid.

**in·ter·sti·tial her·nia** a hernia in which the protrusion is between any two of the layers of the abdominal wall.

**in·ter·sti·tial ker·a·ti·tis** an inflammation of the corneal stroma, often with neovascularization.

**in·ter·sti·tial la·mel·la** one of the lamellae of partially resorbed osteons occurring between newer, complete osteons. SYN ground lamella.

**in·ter·sti·tial ne·phri·tis** a form of nephritis in which the interstitial connective tissue is chiefly affected.

**in·ter·sti·tial neu·ri·tis** inflammation of the connective tissue framework of a nerve. SYN Eichhorst neuritis.

**in·ter·sti·tial plas·ma cell pneu·mo·nia** SYN *Pneumocystis carinii* pneumonia.

**in·ter·sti·tial preg·nan·cy** SYN intramural pregnancy.

**in·ter·sti·tial tis·sue** SYN connective tissue.

**in·ter·stit·i·um** (in-ter-stish′ē-ŭm) a small area, space, or gap in the substance of an organ or tissue. SEE ALSO connective tissue. SYN interstice. [L.]

**in·ter·tar·sal** (in-ter-tar′săl) denoting the articulations of the tarsal bones with each other.

**in·ter·tar·sal joints** the synovial joints which unite the tarsal bones. SYN tarsal joints.

**in·ter·trans·ver·sar·ii mus·cles** the paired muscles between transverse processes of adjacent vertebrae; there are anterior and posterior muscles in the cervical region; lateral and medial muscles in the lumbar region; and single muscles in the thoracic region. SYN musculi intertransversarii [TA], intertransverse muscles.

**in·ter·trans·verse mus·cles** SYN intertransversarii muscles.

**in·ter·tri·go** (in-ter-trī′gō) irritant dermatitis occurring between folds or juxtaposed surfaces of the skin, as between the scrotum and the thigh, caused by friction, sweat retention, moisture, warmth, and concomitant overgrowth of resident microorganisms. [L. a galling of the skin, fr. *inter,* between, + *tero,* to rub]

**in·ter·tro·chan·ter·ic crest** the rounded ridge that connects the greater and lesser trochanters of the femur posteriorly and marks the junction of the neck and shaft of the bone.

**in·ter·tro·chan·ter·ic frac·ture** fracture of the proximal femur located in the metaphyseal bone in the region between the greater and lesser trochanters.

**in·ter·tro·chan·ter·ic line** a rough line that separates the neck and shaft of the femur anteriorly; it passes downward and medially from the greater trochanter to the lesser trochanter and continues into the medial lip of the linea aspera. SYN linea intertrochanterica [TA].

**in·ter·tu·ber·cu·lar sheath** the extension of the synovial membrane of the shoulder joint downward in the intertubercular groove to surround the tendon of the long head of the biceps.

**in·ter·u·re·ter·ic fold** a fold of mucous membrane extending from the orifice of the ureter of one side to that of the other side. SYN plica intereuterica [TA].

**in·ter·val** (in′ter-văl) a time or space between two periods or objects; a break in continuity. [L. *inter-vallum,* space between breastworks in a camp, an interval, fr. *vallum,* a rampart, wall]

**in·ter·val train·ing** application of highly structured exercise with rest intervals using "supermaximum" effort to overload the specific systems of energy transfer; allows performance of inordinately high exercise intensities with relatively minimal fatigue.

**in·ter·ve·nous tu·ber·cle** the slight projection on the wall of the right atrium between the orifices of the venae cavae.

**in·ter·ven·tion** (in-ter-ven′shŭn) an action or ministration that produces an effect or that is intended to alter the course of a pathologic process. [L. *inter-ventio,* a coming between, fr *intervenio,* to come between]

**in·ter·ven·tric·u·lar fo·ra·men** the short, often slitlike passage that, on both the left and right side, connects the third brain ventricle (of the diencephalon) with the lateral ventricles (of the cerebral hemispheres); the passage is bounded anteriomedially by the column of fornix and posterolaterally by the anterior pole of the thalamus. SYN porta (2).

**in·ter·ven·tric·u·lar sep·tal branch·es of left-right cor·o·nary ar·te·ry** the interventricular septal branches; branches of the anterior and posterior interventricular arteries distributed to the muscle of the interventricular septum.

**in·ter·ven·tric·u·lar sep·tum** the wall between the ventricles of the heart.

**in·ter·ver·te·bral disk** a disk interposed between the bodies of adjacent vertebrae. It is composed of an outer fibrous part (anulus fibrosus) that surrounds a central gelatinous mass (nucleus pulposus).

**in·ter·ver·te·bral vein** one of numerous veins accompanying the spinal nerves through the intervertebral foramina, draining spinal cord and vertebral venous plexuses, and emptying in the neck into the vertebral vein, in the thorax into the intercostal veins, in the lumbar and sacral regions into the lumbar and sacral veins.

**in·ter·vil·lous la·cu·na** one of the blood spaces in the placenta into which the chorionic villi project.

**in·ter·vil·lous spac·es** the spaces containing maternal blood, located between placental villi; they are lined with syncytiotrophoblast.

**in·tes·ti·nal** (in-tes′ti-năl) relating to the intestine.

**in·tes·ti·nal a·nas·to·mo·sis** SYN enteroenterostomy.

**in·tes·ti·nal an·gi·na** SYN abdominal angina.

**in·tes·ti·nal ar·ter·ies** SEE ileal arteries, jejunal arteries.

**in·tes·ti·nal a·tre·sia** an obliteration of the lumen of the small intestine, with the ileum involved in 50% of cases and the jejunum and duodenum next in frequency; most frequent cause of intestinal obstruction in the newborn; etiology may be related to a failure of recanalization during early development or to some impairment of blood supply during intrauterine life.

**in·tes·ti·nal di·ges·tion** that part of digestion carried on in the intestine; it affects all the foodstuffs: starches, fats, and proteins.

**in·tes·ti·nal em·phy·se·ma** SYN pneumatosis cystoides intestinalis.

**in·tes·ti·nal fis·tu·la** a tract leading from the lumen of the small intestine to the exterior. SYN fecal fistula.

**in·tes·ti·nal fol·li·cles** SYN intestinal glands.

**in·tes·ti·nal glands** the tubular glands in the mucous membrane of the small and large intestines. SYN crypts of Lieberkühn, intestinal follicles, Lieberkühn glands.

**in·tes·ti·nal vil·li** projections (0.5 to 1.5 mm in length) of the mucous membrane of the intestine; they are leaf-shaped in the duodenum and become shorter, more finger-shaped, and sparser in the ileum.

**in·tes·tine** (in-tes′tin) **1.** the digestive tube passing from the stomach to the anus. It is divided primarily into the intestinum tenue (small intestine) and the intestinum crassum (large intestine). **2.** inward; inner. See this page. SYN intestinum [TA], gut (1). [L. *intestinum*]

**in·tes·ti·num**, pl. **in·tes·ti·na** (in-tes-tī′nŭm, in-tes′ti-nă) [TA] SYN bowel. SYN intestine. [L. *intestinus,* internal, neuter, as noun, the entrails, fr. *intus,* within]

**in-the-ca·nal hear·ing aid** hearing aid that is placed in the external auditory canal but is still visible.

**in-the-ear hear·ing aid** hearing aid that fits into the shell of the ear.

**in·ti·ma** (in′ti-mă) innermost. SEE tunica intima. [L. fem. of *intimus,* inmost]

**in·ti·mal** (in′ti-măl) relating to the intima or inner coat of a vessel.

**in·ti·mi·tis** (in-ti-mī′tis) inflammation of an intima, as in endangiitis. [intima + G. *-itis,* inflammation]

**in·toe** (in′tō) medial deviation of the axis of the foot. SYN metatarsus varus.

**in·tol·er·ance** (in-tol′er-ăns) abnormal metabolism, excretion, or other disposition of a given substance; term often used to indicate impaired utilization or disposal of dietary constituents.

**in·tor·sion** (in-tōr′shŭn) conjugate rotation of the

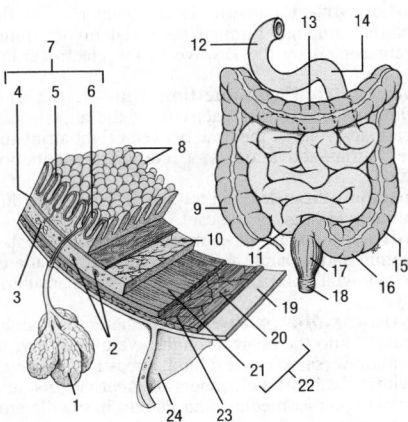

**intestines:** (bottom) diagram of four main layers of the wall of the digestive tube below the diaphragm: mucosa, submucosa, muscularis, and serosa; (top) anterior view of the intestines; (1) gland outside gut but developing from it (liver), (2) blood vessels, (3) gland in submucosa, (4) muscularis mucosae, (5) epithelium, (6) lamina propria, (7) mucous membrane, (8) villi, (9) ascending colon, (10) submucosa, (11) ileum, (12) duodenum, (13) transverse colon, (14) jejunum, (15) descending colon, (16) sigmoid, (17) rectum, (18) anus, (19) serosa, (20) circular muscle, (21) longitudinal muscle, (22) muscularis, (23) myenteric plexus, (24) mesentery

upper poles of each cornea inward. [L. *in-torqueo,* pp. *tortus,* to twist]

**in·tor·tor** (in-tōr′tŏr) a muscle that turns a part medialward. SEE ALSO invertor.

**in·tox·a·tion** (in-tok-sā′shŭn) poisoning, especially by the toxic products of bacteria or poisonous animals, other than alcohol. [L. *in,* in, + G. *toxikon,* poison]

**in·tox·i·cant** (in-tok′si-kant) **1.** having the power to intoxicate. **2.** an intoxicating agent, such as alcohol.

**in·tox·i·ca·tion** (in-tok-si-kā′shŭn) **1.** SYN poisoning. **2.** temporary acute alcoholism. [L. *in,* in, + G. *toxikon,* poison]

**in·tra-** inside, within; opposite of extra-. SEE ALSO endo-, ento-. [L. within]

**in·tra-a·or·tic bal·loon** SEE intraaortic balloon pump.

**intraaortic bal·loon pump** an externally actuated and intermittently inflatable balloon placed into the descending aorta and that, on activation during diastole, augments blood pressure and organ perfusion by its pulsatile thrust; then, on deflation, decreases the cardiac work with each systole—the so-called counterpulsation principle—by reducing cardiac afterload.

**in·tra·ar·tic·u·lar frac·ture** fracture occurring through the articular surface into the joint.

**in·tra-a·tri·al block** impaired conduction through the atria, manifested by widened and often notched P waves in the electrocardiogram. SYN interatrial block.

i
n

**in·tra·a·tri·al con·duc·tion** conduction of the cardiac impulse through the atrial myocardium, represented by the P wave in the electrocardiogram.

**in·tra·a·tri·al con·duc·tion time 1.** the total duration of electrical activity of the atria in one cardiac cycle; **2.** the time between right atrial and left atrial activation. SYN interatrial conduction time.

**in·tra·au·ric·u·lar** (in'tră-aw-rik'yu-lăr) within an auricle (e.g., of the ear).

**in·tra·cap·su·lar lig·a·ments** ligaments located within and separate from the articular capsule of a synovial joint. SYN ligamenta intracapsularia [TA].

**in·tra·car·di·ac cath·e·ter** a catheter that can be passed into the heart through a vein or artery, to withdraw samples of blood, measure pressures within the heart's chambers or great vessels, and inject contrast media; used mainly in the diagnosis and evaluation of congenital, rheumatic, and coronary artery lesions and to evaluate systolic and diastolic cardiac function. SYN cardiac catheter.

**in·tra·cath·e·ter** (in'tră-kath'e-ter) a plastic tube, usually attached to the puncturing needle, inserted into a blood vessel for infusion, injection, or pressure monitoring.

**in·tra·cav·i·tary** (in'tră-cav'i-tār-ē) within an organ or body cavity.

**in·tra·cel·lu·lar can·a·lic·u·lus** a fine canal formed by invagination of the cell membrane into the cytoplasm of a cell, such as those of the parietal cells of the stomach.

**in·tra·cel·lu·lar flu·id (ICF)** the fluid within the tissue cells, constituting about 30 to 40% of the body weight. SYN intracellular water.

**in·tra·cel·lu·lar tox·in** SYN endotoxin.

**in·tra·cel·lu·lar wa·ter** SYN intracellular fluid.

**in·tra·cor·ne·al im·plants** inserts placed within corneal pockets to alter the refractive power of the eye.

**in·tra·cor·po·re·al** (in'tră-kōr-po'rē-ăl) **1.** within the body. **2.** within any structure anatomically styled a corpus. [intra- + L. *corpus,* body]

**in·tra·cra·ni·al cav·i·ty** SYN cranial cavity.

**in·tra·cra·ni·al hem·or·rhage** escape of blood within the cranium due to loss of integrity of vascular channels, frequently forming a hematoma.

**in·tra·cra·ni·al pres·sure (ICP)** pressure within the cranial cavity.

**in·tra·crine** (in'tră-krin) denoting self-stimulation through cellular production of a factor that acts within the cell. [intra- + G. *krinō,* to separate, secrete]

**in·trac·ta·ble** (in'trak'tă-bl) **1.** SYN refractory (1). **2.** SYN obstinate (1). [L. *in-tractabilis,* fr. *in-* neg. + *tracto,* to draw, haul]

**in·tra·cu·ta·ne·ous re·ac·tion, in·tra·der·mal re·ac·tion** a reaction following the injection of antigen into the skin of a sensitive subject, such as in the case of the tuberculin test.

**in·tra·cy·to·plas·mic sperm in·jec·tion** a procedure in which a single sperm cell is injected into the oocyte during in vitro fertilization.

**in·trad** (in'trăd) toward the inner part.

**intradermal in·jec·tion** an injection into the corium, or substance of the skin.

**in·tra·der·mal ne·vus** a nevus in which nests of melanocytes are found in the dermis, but not at the epidermal-dermal junction; benign pigmented nevi in adults are most commonly intradermal.

**in·tra·der·mal test** SYN skin test.

**in·tra·em·bry·on·ic** (in'tră-em-brē-on'ik) within the embryonic body; referring to the portion of the umbilical vein within the embryo. Cf. extraembryonic.

**in·tra·fi·lar** (in'tră-fī'lăr) lying within the meshes of a network. [intra- + L. *filum,* thread]

**in·tra·fu·sal** (in'tră-fyu'săl) applied to structures within the muscle spindle.

**in·tra·fu·sal fi·bers** muscle fibers present within a neuromuscular spindle.

**in·tra·he·pa·tic cho·le·sta·sis of preg·nan·cy** intrahepatic cholestasis with centrilobular bile staining without inflammatory cells or proliferation of mesenchymal cells; clinically characterized by pruritus and/or icterus; of unknown cause but associated with high estrogen levels. SYN cholestasis of pregnancy, recurrent jaundice of pregnancy.

**in·tra·lig·a·men·ta·ry preg·nan·cy** pregnancy within the broad ligament.

**in·tra·lob·u·lar duct** a duct that lies within a lobule of a gland.

**in·tra·med·ul·lary trans·fu·sion** transfusion, most commonly in infants, into the medullary cavity of a long bone, usually the femur or tibia.

**in·tra·mu·ral he·ma·to·ma** a hematoma in the wall of a structure, such as the bowel or bladder, usually resulting from trauma.

**in·tra·mu·ral preg·nan·cy** development of the fertilized ovum in the uterine portion of the uterine tube. SYN interstitial pregnancy.

**in·tra·na·sal an·es·the·sia 1.** insufflation anesthesia in which an inhalation anesthetic is added to inhaled air passing through the nose or nasopharynx; **2.** anesthesia of nasal passages by infiltration and topical application of local anesthetic solution to nasal mucosa.

**in·tra·ob·serv·er er·ror** the differences in interpretation by an individual making observations of the same phenomenon at different times.

**in·tra·oc·u·lar pres·sure** the pressure of the intraocular fluid (usually measured in millimeters of mercury) with a manometer.

**in·tra·o·ral an·es·the·sia 1.** insufflation anesthesia in which an inhalation anesthetic is added to inhaled air passing through the mouth; **2.** regional anesthesia of the mouth and associated structures when local anesthetic solutions are used by topical application to oral mucosa, by local infiltration, or as nerve blocks.

**in·tra·pa·ri·e·tal sul·cus** a horizontal sulcus extending back from the postcentral sulcus over some distance, then dividing perpendicularly into two branches so as to form, with the postcentral sulcus, a figure H. It divides the parietal lobe into superior and inferior parietal lobules.

**in·tra·pa·rot·id plex·us of fa·cial nerve** the diverging branches of the facial nerve passing through the substance of the parotid gland, connected by numerous looped anastomoses. SYN pes anserinus (1).

**in·tra·par·tum** (in'tră-par'tŭm) during labor and delivery or childbirth. Cf. antepartum, postpartum. [intra- + L. *partus,* childbirth]

**in·tra·par·tum hem·or·rhage** hemorrhage occurring in the course of normal labor and delivery.

**in·tra·psy·chic** (in'tră-sī'kik) denoting the psychological dynamics that occur inside the mind without reference to the individual's exchanges with other persons or events.

**in·tra·seg·men·tal bron·chi** branches of segmental bronchi to the bronchopulmonary segments of the lungs. SYN bronchi intrasegmentales.

**in·tra·tho·ra·cic air·way ob·struc·tion** form of airway obstruction in which the site of airway narrowing is below the thoracic inlet. It can be variable (e.g., reduction in expiratory but not inspiratory flows) or fixed (reduction in both inspiratory and expiratory flows).

**in·tra·u·ter·ine am·pu·ta·tion** SYN congenital amputation.

**in·tra·u·ter·ine de·vic·es (IUD), in·tra·u·ter·ine con·tra·cep·tive de·vic·es (IUCD)** pieces of plastic or metal of various shapes (e.g., coil, loop, bow) inserted into the uterus to exert a contraceptive effect.

**in·tra·u·ter·ine frac·ture** a fracture of one or more bones of a fetus occurring before birth.

**in·tra·u·ter·ine growth re·tar·da·tion** SYN fetal growth restriction.

**in·tra·u·ter·ine in·sem·i·na·tion (IUI)** placement of sperm that have been washed of seminal fluid directly into the uterus to bypass the cervix.

**in·tra·vas·cu·lar lig·a·ture** balloon occlusion of the feeding vessels of a cerebral arteriovenous malformation.

**in·tra·ve·nous an·es·the·sia** general anesthesia produced by injection of central nervous system depressants into the venous circulation.

**in·tra·ve·nous an·es·thet·ic** a compound that produces anesthesia when injected intravenously.

**in·tra·ve·nous bo·lus** a relatively large volume of fluid or dose of a drug or test substance given intravenously and rapidly to hasten or magnify a response; in radiology, rapid injection of a large dose of contrast medium to increase opacification of blood vessels.

**in·tra·ve·nous chol·an·gi·og·ra·phy** cholangiography of bile ducts opacified by hepatic secretion of an intravenously injected contrast medium.

**in·tra·ve·nous drip** the slow but continuous introduction of solutions intravenously, a drop at a time.

**in·tra·ve·nous re·gion·al an·es·the·sia** regional anesthesia by intravenous injection of local anesthetic solution distal to an occlusive tourniquet in an extremity previously exsanguinated by pressure or gravity. SYN Bier method (1).

**in·tra·ve·nous u·rog·ra·phy, ex·cre·to·ry u·rog·ra·phy** radiography of kidneys, ureters, and bladder following injection of contrast medium into a peripheral vein. See this page.

**in·tra·ven·tric·u·lar block, I-V block** delayed conduction within the ventricular conducting system or myocardium, including bundle-branch block, peri-infarction blocks, the fascicular blocks, excitation, and the Wolff-Parkinson-White (pre-excitation) syndrome.

**in·tra·ven·tric·u·lar con·duc·tion** conduction of the cardiac impulse through the ventricular myocardium, represented by the QRS complex in the electrocardiogram. SYN ventricular conduction.

**in·tra·vi·tal stain** a stain which is taken up by living cells after parenteral administration, e.g., intravenously or subcutaneously.

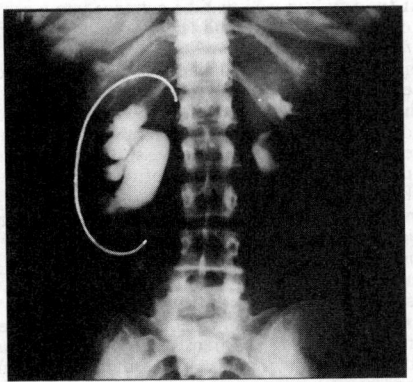

**urography:** intravenous urogram showing retention of a large amount of contrast medium in the right renal pelvis indicating hydronephrosis due to ureteral obstruction

**in·tra vi·tam** (in′trä vī′tăm) during life. [L. *vita*, life]

**in·trin·sic** (in-trin′sik) **1.** belonging entirely to a part. **2.** ANATOMY denoting those muscles whose origin and insertion are both within the structure under consideration, distinguished from the extrinsic muscles which have their origin outside of the structure under consideration; applied especially to the limbs but also to the ciliary muscle as distinguished from the recti and other orbital muscles which are outside the eyeball. SYN essential (6). [L. *intrinsecus*, on the inside]

**in·trin·sic co·ag·u·la·tion path·way** a part of the coagulation pathway that is activated by contact of coagulation proteins with negatively charged surfaces. All components are within the blood stream and include factors XII, XI, IX, VII, HMWK, and prekallikrein. The activated partial thromboplastin time tests for abnormalities in this pathway.

**in·trin·sic dys·men·or·rhea** SYN primary dysmenorrhea.

**in·trin·sic fac·tor (IF)** a relatively small mucoprotein secreted by the neck cell of the gastric glands and required for adequate absorption of vitamin $B_{12}$; deficiency results in pernicious anemia.

**in·trin·sic PEEP** SYN auto-positive-end-expiratory-pressure.

**in·trin·sic re·flex** a reflex muscular contraction elicited by the application of a stimulus, usually stretching, to the muscle itself as opposed to a muscular contraction caused by an extrinsic stimulus, e.g., skin, as in the abdominal skin reflexes.

**in·trin·sic sphinc·ter** a thickening of the circular fibers of the muscular coat of an organ.

**in·tro-** inwardly, into; opposite of extra-. Cf. intra-. [L. *intro*, into]

**in·tro·duc·er** (in-trō-doos′er) an instrument, such as a catheter, needle, or endotracheal tube, for introduction of a flexible device. [L. *intro-duco*, to lead into, introduce]

**in·tro·flec·tion, in·tro·flex·ion** (in′trō-flek′shŭn) a bending inward. [intro- + L. *flecto*, pp. *flectus*, to bend]

**in·tro·i·tus** (in-trō′i-tŭs) the entrance into a canal or hollow organ, as the vagina. [L. entrance, fr. *intro-eo,* to go into]

**in·tro·ject** (in′trō-jekt) the dynamically endowed, enduring internal representation of an object.

**in·tro·jec·tion** (in-trō-jek′shŭn) a psychological defense mechanism involving appropriation of an external happening and its assimilation by the personality, making it a part of the self. [intro- + L. *jacto,* to throw]

**in·tro·mis·sion** (in-trō-mish′ŭn) the insertion or introduction of one part into another. [intro- + L. *mitto,* to send]

**in·tro·mit·tent** (in-trō-mit′ent) conveying or sending into a body or cavity.

**in·tron** (in′tron) a portion of DNA that lies between two exons, is transcribed into RNA, but does not appear in that RNA after maturation, and so is not expressed (as protein) in protein synthesis. [inter- + -on]

**in·tro·spec·tion** (in-trō-spek′shŭn) looking inward; self-scrutinizing; contemplating one's own mental processes. [intro- + L. *specto,* to look at, inspect]

**in·tro·spec·tive** (in-trō-spek′tiv) relating to introspection.

**in·tro·sus·cep·tion** (in′trō-sŭs-sep′shŭn) SYN intussusception.

**in·tro·ver·sion** (in-trō-ver′zhŭn) **1.** the turning of a structure into itself. SEE ALSO intussusception, invagination. **2.** a trait of preoccupation with oneself, as practiced by an introvert. Cf. extraversion. [intro- + L. *verto,* pp. *versus,* to turn]

**in·tro·vert 1.** (in′trō-vert) one who tends to be unusually shy, introspective, self-centered, and avoids becoming concerned with or involved in the affairs of others. Cf. extrovert. **2.** (in-trō -vert′) to turn a structure into itself.

**in·tu·bate** (in′too-bāt) to perform intubation.

**in·tu·ba·tion** (in-too-bā′shŭn) insertion of a tubular device into a canal, hollow organ, or cavity; specifically, passage of an oro- or nasotracheal tube for anesthesia or for control of pulmonary ventilation. [L. *in,* in, + *tuba,* tube]

**in·tu·i·tive stage** PSYCHOLOGY a stage of development, usually occurring between 4 and 7 years of age, in which the most prominent aspects of the stimuli to which a child is exposed, rather than any form of logical thought, determine the child's thought processes.

**in·tu·mesce** (in-too-mes′) to swell up; to enlarge. [L. *in-tumesco,* to swell up, fr. *tumeo,* to swell]

**in·tu·mes·cence** (in-too-mes′ens) **1.** SYN enlargement. **2.** the process of enlarging or swelling; used to describe the spinal enlargements.

**in·tu·mes·cent** (in-too-mes′ent) enlarging; becoming enlarged or swollen.

**in·tu·mes·cen·tia** (in-too-mes-sen′shē-ă) SYN enlargement. [Mod. L.]

**in·tus·sus·cep·tion** (in′tŭs-sŭ-sep′shŭn) **1.** the taking up or receiving of one part within another, especially the enfolding of one segment of the intestine within another. SEE ALSO introversion, invagination. **2.** the incorporation of new material in the growth of the cell wall. SYN introsusception. [L. *intus,* within, + *sus-cipio,* to take up, fr. *sub* + *capio,* to take]

**in·tus·sus·cep·tive** (in′tŭs-sŭ-sep′tiv) relating to or characterized by intussusception.

**in·tus·sus·cep·tum** (in′tŭs-sŭ-sep′tŭm) the inner segment in an intussusception; that part of the bowel which is received within the other part.

**in·tus·sus·cip·i·ens** (in′tŭs-sŭ-sip′ē-enz) the portion of the bowel, in intussusception, which receives the other portion. [L. *intus,* within, + *sus-cipiens,* pr. p. of *suscipio,* to take up]

**in·u·lin (In)** (in′yu-lin) a fructose polysaccharide from the rhizome of *Inula* and other plants; used by intravenous injection to determine the rate of glomerular filtration. Cf. inulin clearance.

**in·u·lin clear·ance** an accurate measure of the rate of filtration through the renal glomeruli, because inulin filters freely with water and is neither excreted nor reabsorbed through tubule walls. Inulin is not a normal constituent of plasma and must be infused continously to maintain a steady plasma concentration and a steady rate of urinary excretion during the measurement.

**in·unc·tion** (in-ŭngk′shŭn) administration of a drug in ointment form by rubbing to cause absorption of the active ingredient. [L. *inunctio,* an anointing, fr. *inunguo,* pp. *-unctus,* to smear on]

**in·vag·i·nate** (in-vaj′i-nāt) to ensheathe, infold, or insert a structure within itself or another. [L. *in,* in, + *vagina,* a sheath]

**in·vag·i·na·tion** (in-vaj′i-nā′shŭn) **1.** the ensheathing, enfolding, or insertion of a structure within itself or another. **2.** the state of being invaginated. SEE ALSO introversion, intussusception.

**in·va·lid** (in′vă-lid) **1.** weak; sick. **2.** a person partially or completely disabled. [L. *in-* neg. + *validus,* strong]

**in·va·sive** (in-vā′siv) **1.** denoting or characterized by invasion. **2.** denoting a procedure requiring insertion of an instrument or device into the body through the skin or a body orifice for diagnosis or treatment.

**in·ven·to·ry** (in′ven-tōr-ē) a detailed, often descriptive, list of items.

**in·ver·sion** (in-ver′zhŭn) **1.** a turning inward, upside down, or in any direction contrary to the existing one. **2.** conversion of a disaccharide or polysaccharide by hydrolysis into a monosaccharide; specifically, the hydrolysis of sucrose to D-glucose and D-fructose; so called because of the change in optical rotation. **3.** alteration of a DNA molecule made by removing a fragment, reversing its orientation, and putting it back into place. **4.** heat-induced transition of silica, in which the quartz tridymite or cristobalite changes its physical properties as to thermal expansion. See page APP 91. [L. *inverto,* pp. *-versus,* to turn upside down, to turn about]

**in·ver·sion of the uter·us** a turning of the uterus inside out, usually following childbirth.

**in·ver·te·brate** (in-ver′tĕ-brāt) **1.** not possessed of a spinal or vertebral column. **2.** any animal that has no spinal column.

**in·ver·tor** (in-ver′ter) a muscle that inverts or causes inversion or turns a part, such as the foot, inward. [see inversion]

**in·vert sug·ar** a mixture of equal parts of D-glucose and D-fructose produced by hydrolysis of sucrose (inversion).

**in·vet·er·ate** (in-vet′er-āt) long seated; firmly established; said of a disease or of confirmed habits. [L. *in-vetero,* pp. *-atus,* to render old, fr. *vetus,* old]

**in·vis·ca·tion** (in-vis-kā′shŭn) **1.** smearing with mucilaginous matter. **2.** the mixing of the food, during mastication, with the buccal secretions. [L. *in*, in, on, + *viscum*, birdlime]

**in·vo·lu·crum**, pl. **in·vo·lu·cra** (in-vō-loo′krŭm, in-vō-loo′kră) **1.** an enveloping membrane, e.g., a sheath or sac. **2.** the sheath of new bone that forms around a sequestrum. [L. a wrapper, fr. *involvo*, to roll up]

**in·vol·un·tary** (in-vol′ŭn-tār-ē) **1.** independent of the will; not volitional. **2.** contrary to the will. [L. *in-* neg. + *voluntarius*, willing, fr. *volo*, to wish]

**in·vol·un·tary mus·cles** muscles not ordinarily under control of the will; except in the case of the heart, they are smooth (nonstriated) muscles, innervated by the autonomic nervous system.

**in·vo·lu·tion** (in-vō-loo′shŭn) **1.** return of an enlarged organ to normal size. **2.** turning inward of the edges of a part. **3.** PSYCHIATRY mental decline associated with advanced age. SYN catagenesis. [L. *in-volvo*, pp. *-volutus*, to roll up]

**in·vo·lu·tion·al** (in-vō-loo′shŭn-ăl) relating to involution.

**in·vo·lu·tion·al de·pres·sion** depression or psychosis first occurring in the involutional years (40 to 55 for women, 50 to 65 for men).

**in·vo·lu·tion·al mel·an·cho·lia** a depressive disorder of middle life, commonly associated with the climacteric.

**in·volved field** in radiation treatment, the area of the tumor itself.

**io·dide** (ī′ō-dīd) negative ion of iodine, I⁻.

**i·o·dide ac·ne** a follicular eruption on the face, trunk, and extremities, due to injection or ingestion of iodide in a hypersensitive individual. SEE ALSO iododerma.

**io·di·nate** (ī′ō-di-nāt) to treat or combine with iodine.

**io·di·nat·ed** ¹³¹I hu·man se·rum al·bu·min a sterile, buffered, isotonic solution prepared to contain not less than 10 mg of radioiodinated normal human serum albumin per ml, and adjusted to provide not more than 1 mCi of radioactivity per ml; used as a diagnostic aid in the measurement of blood volume and cardiac output.

**io·di·nat·ed** ¹²⁵I se·rum al·bu·min a sterile, buffered, isotonic solution prepared to contain not less than 10 mg of radioiodinated normal human serum albumin per ml, and adjusted to provide not more than 1 mCi of radioactivity per ml; used as a diagnostic aid in determining blood volume and cardiac output.

**io·dine (I)** (ī′ō-dīn, ī′ō-dēn) a nonmetallic chemical element, atomic no. 53, atomic wt. 126.90447; used as a catalyst, reagent, tracer, constituent of radiographic contrast media, topical antiseptic, therapy in thyroid disease, antidote for alkaloidal poisons, and in certain stains and solutions. [G. *iōdēs*, violet-like, fr. *ion*, a violet, + *eidos*, form]

**i·o·dine-fast** denoting hyperthyroidism unresponsive to iodine therapy, which develops frequently in most cases so treated.

**i·o·dine stain** a stain to detect amyloid, cellulose, chitin, starch, carotenes, and glycogen, and to stain amebas by virtue of their glycogen; feces and other wet preparations are stained directly with Lugol iodine solution; smears are treated with Schaudinn fixative and then stained with alcoholic iodine, followed by Heidenhain iron hematoxylin.

**io·din·o·phil, io·din·o·phile** (ī-ō-din′ō-fil, ī-ō-

din′ō-fīl) **1.** staining readily with iodine. SYN iodinophilous. **2.** any histologic element that stains readily with iodine. [iodine + G. *philos*, fond]

**io·din·oph·i·lous** (ī-ō-din-of′i-lŭs) SYN iodinophil (1).

**io·dism** (ī′ō-dizm) a condition marked by coryza, an acneform eruption, weakness, salivation, and foul breath, caused by the continuous administration of iodine or one of the iodides.

**io·dize** (ī′ō-dīz) to treat or impregnate with iodine.

**io·do·der·ma** (ī-ō′dō-der′mă) an eruption of follicular papules and pustules, or a granulomatous lesion, caused by iodine toxicity or sensitivity.

**io·do·met·ric** (ī-ō′dō-met′rik) relating to iodometry.

**io·dom·e·try** (ī-ō-dom′ĕ-trē) analytical techniques involving titrations in which iodine is either formed or consumed, the sudden appearance or disappearance of iodine marking the end point. [iodine + G. *metron*, measure]

**io·do·phil·ia** (ī-ō′dō-fil′ē-ă) an affinity for iodine, as manifested by some leukocytes in certain conditions. [iodine + G. *phileō*, to love]

**io·do·phor** (ī′ō′dō-fōr) any compound in which iodine is combined with an organic carrier; an intermediate-level disinfectant registered with the EPA as hospital disinfectant with tuberculocidal action. Available in topical antiseptics and hard-surface disinfectant form. [io- + G. *phoros*, carrying]

**io·dop·sin** (ī-ō-dop′sin) a visual pigment, composed of 11-*cis*-retinal bound to an opsin, found in the cones of the retina. SYN visual violet. [G. *ion*, violet, + *ōps*, eye, + -in]

**io·do·ther·a·py** (ī′ō-dō-thār′ă-pē) treatment with iodine.

**io·du·ria** (ī-ō-dyu′rē-ă) urinary excretion of iodine.

**ion** (ī′on) an atom or group of atoms carrying an electric charge by virtue of having gained or lost one or more electrons. Ions charged with negative electricity (anions) travel toward a positive pole (anode); those charged with positive electricity (cations) travel toward a negative pole (cathode). Ions may exist in solid, liquid, or gaseous environments, although those in liquid (electrolytes) are more common and familiar. [G. *iōn*, going]

**i·on chan·nel dis·or·ders** a number of diseases, mostly inherited and episodic in nature, caused by dysfunction of the calcium, chloride, potassium, or sodium channels of nerve or muscle; the inherited myotonias and periodic paralyses are included in this category; there is usually dominant inheritance, with the primary defect due to mutations of gene encoding on locus 7q32, 17q, or 1q31-32. SYN channelopathies.

**ion ex·change** (ī′on eks-chanj′) SEE anion exchange, cation exchange, ion exchange chromatography.

**i·on ex·change chro·ma·tog·ra·phy** chromatography in which cations or anions in the mobile phase are separated by electrostatic interactions with the stationary phase. SEE ALSO anion exchange, cation exchange.

**i·on-ex·change res·in** SEE anion exchange, cation exchange, ion exchange chromatography.

**ion·ic** (ī-on′ik) relating to an ion.

**i·on·ic strength (I)** symbolized as $\Gamma/2$ or I and set equal to $0.5\Sigma m_i z_i^2$, where $m_i$ equals the molar concentration and $z_i$ the charge of each ion present in solution; if molar concentrations ($c_i$) are used instead of molality (and the solution is dilute), then $I = 0.5(1/\rho_o)\Sigma c_i z_i^2$ where $\rho_o$ is the density of the solvent; a number of biochemically important events (e.g., protein solubility and rates of enzyme action) vary with the ionic strength of a solution.

**ion·i·za·tion** (ī'on-i-zā'shŭn) **1.** dissociation into ions, occurring when an electrolyte is dissolved in water or certain liquids or when molecules are subjected to electrical discharge or ionizing radiation. **2.** production of ions as a result of interaction of radiation with matter. **3.** SYN iontophoresis.

**i·on·i·za·tion cham·ber** a chamber for detecting ionization of the enclosed gas; used for determining intensity of ionizing radiation.

**ion·ize** (ī'on-īz) to separate into ions; to dissociate atoms or molecules into electrically charged atoms or radicals.

**i·on·iz·ing ra·di·a·tion** corpuscular (e.g., neutrons, electrons) or electromagnetic (e.g., x-ray, gamma) radiation of sufficient energy to ionize the irradiated material.

**ion·o·phore** (ī-on'ō-fōr) a compound or substance that forms a complex with an ion and transports it across a membrane. [ion + G. *phore,* a bearer]

**ion·o·pho·re·sis** (ī-on'ō-fōr-ē'sis) SYN electrophoresis. [ion + G. *phorēsis,* a carrying]

**ion·o·pho·ret·ic** (ī-on'ō-fōr-et'ik) SYN electrophoretic.

**ion·to·pho·re·sis** (ī-on'tō-fōr-ē'sis) the introduction, by means of electric current, of ions of soluble substances into tissue for therapeutic purposes. SYN ionization (3). [ion + G. *phorēsis,* a carrying]

**ion·to·pho·ret·ic** (ī-on'tō-fōr-et'ik) relating to iontophoresis.

**io·pro·mide** (ī-ō'prō-mid) a monomeric, nonionic, water-soluble, low osmolar radiographic contrast medium for intravenous urography or angiography.

**i·o·ta** (ι) (ī-ōt'a) **1.** the ninth letter in the Greek alphabet. **2.** CHEMISTRY denotes the ninth in a series, or the ninth atom from a carboxyl group or other functional group. **3.** a tiny or minute amount.

**IPA** International Phonetic Alphabet; isopropyl alcohol.

**ip·e·cac·u·a·nha** (ip-ě-kak-hwan'ǎ) the dried root of *Uragoga (Cephaelis) ipecacuanha* (family Rubiaceae), a shrub of Brazil and other parts of South America; contains emetine, cephaeline, emetamine, ipecacuanhic acid, psychotrine, and methylpsychotrine; has expectorant, emetic, and antidysenteric properties. [native Brazilian word]

**IPF** idiopathic pulmonary fibrosis.

**i·po·date** a radiographic contrast medium, given orally as the sodium or, more often, the calcium salt, for opacification of the gallbladder and central biliary tree.

*Ip·o·mo·ea* (ī-pō-mē'ǎ) a plant genus of the family *Convolvulaceae.*

**IPPB** intermittent positive pressure breathing.

**IPPV** intermittent positive pressure ventilation.

**ip·si·lat·er·al** (ip-si-lat'er-ăl) on the same side, with reference to a given point, e.g., a dilated pupil on the same side as an extradural hema-

toma. SYN homolateral. [L. *ipse,* same, + *latus (later-),* side]

**IQ** intelligence quotient.

**IR** infrared.

**Ir** iridium.

**IRB** Institutional Review Board.

**ir·i·dal** (ī'ri-dăl, ir'i-dăl) relating to the iris. SYN iridial, iridian, iridic.

**ir·i·dec·to·my** (ir'i-dek'tō-mē) **1.** excision of a portion of the iris. **2.** the hole in the iris produced by a surgical iridectomy. [irido- + G. *ektomē,* excision]

**ir·i·den·clei·sis** (ir'i-den-klī'sis) the incarceration of a portion of the iris by corneoscleral incision in glaucoma to effect filtration between the anterior chamber and subconjunctival space. [irido- + G. *enkleiō,* to shut in]

**ir·i·der·e·mia** (ir'i-der-ē'mē'ǎ, ī'rid-er-ē'mē'ǎ) condition wherein the iris is so rudimentary as to appear to be absent. Cf. aniridia. [irido- + G. *erēmia,* absence]

**ir·i·des** (ir'i-dēz) plural of iris. [G.]

**ir·i·de·sis** (i-rid'ě-sis, ī-rin-dē'sis) ligature of a portion of the iris brought out through an incision in the cornea. [irido- + G. *desis,* a binding together]

**ir·id·i·al, irid·i·an, ir·id·ic** (ī-rid'ē-al, ī-rid'ē-an, ī-rid'ik; ī-rid'ē-an; ī-rid'ik, i-rid'ik) SYN iridal.

**ir·id·i·um (Ir)** (i-rid'ē-ŭm) a white, silvery metallic element, atomic no. 77, atomic wt. 192.22; [192]Ir is a radioisotope that has been used in the interstitial treatment of certain tumors. [L. *iris,* rainbow]

**ir·i·do-, ir·id-** the iris. [G. *iris (irid-),* rainbow]

**ir·i·do·a·vul·sion** (ir'i-dō-ă-vŭl'shŭn) avulsion, or tearing away, of the iris.

**ir·i·do·cele** (ir'i-dō-sēl) herniation of a portion of the iris through a corneal defect. [irido- + G. *kēlē,* hernia]

**ir·i·do·cho·roid·i·tis** (ir'i-dō-kō-roy-dī'tis) inflammation of both iris and choroid.

**ir·i·do·col·o·bo·ma** (ir'i-dō-ko-lō-bō'mǎ) a coloboma or congenital defect of the iris. [irido- + G. *kolobōma,* coloboma]

**ir·i·do·cor·ne·al an·gle** the acute angle between the iris and the cornea at the periphery of the anterior chamber of the eye. SYN angulus iridocornealis [TA], angle of iris, filtration angle.

**ir·i·do·cor·ne·al en·do·the·li·al syn·drome** syndrome of glaucoma, iris atrophy, decreased corneal endothelium, anterior peripheral synechia, and multiple iris nodules. SYN Cogan-Reese syndrome, iris-nevus syndrome.

**ir·i·do·cor·ne·al mes·en·chy·mal dys·gen·e·sis** dysgenesis of cornea and iris, producing pupillary anomalies, posterior embryotoxon, and secondary glaucoma, resulting in part from anomalous development of the ocular mesenchyme.

**ir·i·do·cy·clec·to·my** (ir'i-dō-sī-klek'tō-mē) removal of the iris and ciliary body for excision of a tumor. [irido- + G. *kyklos,* circle (ciliary body), + *ektomē,* excision]

**ir·i·do·cy·cli·tis** (ir'i-dō-sī-klī'tis) inflammation of both iris and ciliary body. SEE ALSO iritis, uveitis. [irido- + G. *kyklos,* circle (ciliary body), + -*itis,* inflammation]

**ir·i·do·cy·clo·cho·roid·i·tis** (ir'i-dō-sī'klō-kō-royd-ī'tis) inflammation of the iris, involving the ciliary body and the choroid.

**ir·i·do·cys·tec·to·my** (ir'i-dō-sis-tek'tō-mē) an operation for making an artificial pupil when posterior synechiae follow extracapsular extraction of cataract. [irido- + G. *kystis*, bladder (capsule), + *ektomē*, excision]

**ir·i·do·di·al·y·sis** (ir'i-dō-dī-al'i-sis) a colobomatous defect of the iris caused by its separation from the scleral spur. [irido- + G. *dialysis*, loosening]

**ir·i·do·di·la·tor** (ir'i-dō-dī-lā'ter) causing dilation of the pupil; applied to the musculus dilator pupillae.

**ir·i·do·do·ne·sis** (ir'i-dō-dō-nē'sis) agitated motion of the iris. [irido- + G. *doneō*, to shake to and fro]

**ir·i·do·ki·net·ic** (ir'i-dō-ki-net'ik) relating to the movements of the iris. SYN iridomotor.

**ir·i·do·ma·la·cia** (ir'i-dō-mă-lā'shē-ă) degenerative softening of the iris. [irido- + G. *malakia*, softness]

**ir·i·do·mes·o·di·al·y·sis** (ir'i-dō-mes'ō-dī-al'i-sis) separation of adhesions around the inner margin of the iris. [irido- + G. *mesos*, middle, + *dialysis*, loosening]

**ir·i·do·mo·tor** (ir'i-dō-mō'tŏr) SYN iridokinetic.

**ir·i·do·pa·ral·y·sis** (ir'i-dō-pă-ral'i-sis) SYN iridoplegia.

**ir·i·dop·a·thy** (ir-i-dop'ă-thē) pathologic lesions in the iris.

**ir·i·do·ple·gia** (ir'i-dō-plē'jē-ă) paralysis of the musculus sphincter iridis. SYN iridoparalysis. [irido- + G. *plēgē*, stroke]

**ir·i·dop·to·sis** (ir'i-dop-tō'sis) prolapse of the iris. [irido- + G. *ptōsis*, a falling]

**ir·i·dor·rhex·is** (ir'i-dō-rek'sis) deliberate, surgical tearing of the iris from the scleral spur in order to increase the breadth of a coloboma. [irido- + G. *rhēxis*, rupture]

**ir·i·dos·chi·sis** (ir-i-dos'ki-sis) separation of the anterior layer of the iris from the posterior layer; ruptured anterior fibers float in the aqueous humor. [irido- + G. *schisma*, cleft]

**ir·i·do·scle·rot·o·my** (ir'i-dō-skle-rot'ō-mē) an incision involving both sclera and iris. [irido- + sclera, + G. *tomē*, incision]

**ir·i·dot·o·my** (ir-i-dot'ō-mē) transverse division of some of the fibers of the iris, forming an artificial pupil. [irido- + G. *tomē*, incision]

**IRI/G ra·tio** the ratio of immunoreactive insulin to serum or plasma glucose.

**iris**, pl. **ir·i·des** (ī'ris, ir'i-dēz) [TA] the anterior division of the vascular tunic of the eye, a diaphragm, perforated in the center (the pupil), attached peripherally to the scleral spur; it is composed of stroma and a double layer of pigmented retinal epithelium from which are derived the sphincter and dilator muscles of the pupil. [G. rainbow, the iris of the eye]

**iris-ne·vus syn·drome** SYN iridocorneal endothelial syndrome.

**iris pit** coloboma affecting the stroma of the iris with pigment epithelium intact.

**iris spat·u·la** a flat surgical instrument used for repositioning an iris that has prolapsed through a wound.

**irit·ic** (ī-rit'ik) relating to iritis.

**iri·tis** (ī-rī'tis) inflammation of the iris. SEE ALSO iridocyclitis, uveitis.

**IR·MA** immunoradiometric assay.

**iron (Fe)** (ī'rn) a metallic element, atomic no. 26, atomic wt. 55.847, that occurs in the heme of hemoglobin, myoglobin, transferrin, ferritin, and iron-containing porphyrins, and is an essential component of enzymes such as catalase, peroxidase, and the various cytochromes; its salts are used medicinally. [A.S. *iren*]

**iron-59** an iron isotope; a gamma and beta emitter with a half-life of 44.51 days; used as tracer in study of iron metabolism, determination of blood volume, and in blood transfusion studies.

**iron de·fi·cien·cy a·ne·mia** hypochromic microcytic anemia characterized by low serum iron, increased serum iron-binding capacity, decreased serum ferritin, and decreased marrow iron stores.

**iron fil·ings** small packets of *Paragonimus* spp. eggs that can be seen in the sputum; the egg clumps tend to be yellow-brown.

**iron line** deposition of iron in the corneal epithelium.

**iron lung** SYN Drinker respirator.

**iron-stor·age dis·ease** the storage of excess iron in the parenchyma of many organs, as in idiopathic hemochromatosis or transfusion hemosiderosis.

**ir·ra·di·ate** (i-rā'dē-āt) to apply radiation from a source to a structure or organism. [see irradiation]

**ir·ra·di·a·tion** (i-rā-dē-ā'shŭn) **1.** the subjective enlargement of a bright object seen against a dark background. **2.** exposure to the action of electromagnetic radiation (e.g., heat, light, x-rays). **3.** the spreading of nervous impulses from one area in the brain or cord, or from a tract, to another tract. SEE ALSO radiation. [L. *ir-radio*, (*in-r*), pp. *-radi-atus*, to beam forth]

**ir·ra·tion·al** (i-rash'ŭn-ăl) not rational; unreasonable (contrary to reason) or unreasoning (not exercising reason). [L. *irrationalis*, without reason]

**ir·re·duc·i·ble** (ir-rē-doo'si-bl) **1.** not reducible; incapable of being made smaller. **2.** CHEMISTRY incapable of being made simpler, or of being replaced, hydrogenated, or reduced in positive charge.

**ir·re·duc·i·ble her·nia** a hernia that cannot be reduced without operation. SYN incarcerated hernia.

**ir·reg·u·lar a·stig·ma·tism** astigmatism in which different parts of the same meridian have different degrees of curvature.

**ir·reg·u·lar bone** one of a group of bones having peculiar or complex forms, e.g., vertebrae, many of the skull bones.

**ir·reg·u·lar den·tin, ir·ri·ta·tion den·tin** SYN tertiary dentin.

**ir·re·sus·ci·ta·ble** (ir'rē-sŭs'i-tă-bl) incapable of being revived.

**ir·re·vers·i·ble pulp·i·tis** inflammation of the dental pulp from which the pulp is unable to recover; clinically, may be asymptomatic or characterized by pain which persists after thermal stimulation.

**ir·ri·gate** (ir'i-gāt) to perform irrigation. [L. *ir-rigo*, pp. *-atus*, to irrigate, fr. *in*, on, + *rigo*, to water]

**ir·ri·ta·bil·i·ty** (ir'i-tă-bil'i-tē) the property inherent in protoplasm of reacting to a stimulus. [L. *irritabilitas*, fr. *irrito*, pp. *-atus*, to excite]

**ir·ri·ta·ble** (ir'i-tă-bl) **1.** capable of reacting to a stimulus. **2.** tending to react immoderately to a stimulus. Cf. excitable.

**ir·ri·ta·ble bow·el syn·drome, ir·ri·ta·ble co·lon** a condition characterized by gastrointestinal signs and symptoms including constipation, diarrhea, gas and bloating, all in the absence of organic pathology. Associated with uncoordinated and inefficient contractions of the large intestine. SYN spastic colon.

**ir·ri·tant** (ir′i-tant) **1.** irritating; causing irritation. **2.** any agent with this action.

**ir·ri·tant con·tact der·ma·ti·tis** skin reactions ranging from erythema and scaling to necrotic burns resulting from nonimmunologic damage by chemicals in contact with the skin immediately or repeatedly.

**ir·ri·ta·tion** (ir-i-tā′shŭn) **1.** inflammatory reaction of the tissues to an injury. **2.** the normal response of nerve or muscle to a stimulus. **3.** the evocation of a normal or exaggerated reaction in the tissues by the application of a stimulus. [L. *irritatio*]

**ir·ri·ta·tion fi·bro·ma** a slow-growing nodule on the oral mucosa, composed of fibrous tissue covered by epithelium, resulting from mechanical irritation by dentures, fillings, cheek biting, etc.

**ir·ri·ta·tive** (ir-i-tā′tiv) causing irritation.

**ir·rup·tion** (i-rŭp′shŭn) act or process of breaking through to a surface. [L. *irruptio*, fr. *irrumpo*, to break in]

**IRS-1** insulin receptor substrate-1.

**IRV** inspiratory reserve volume.

**Ir·vine-Gass syn·drome** (ir′vīn-gas) macular edema, aphakia, and vitreous humor adherent to incision for cataract extraction.

**Isaacs syn·drome, Isaacs-Mer·tons syn·-drome** (ī′zaks mār′tĕns) a rare disorder resulting from abnormal, spontaneous muscle activity of neural origin, manifested as continuous muscle stiffness and delayed relaxation after exercise, often accompanied by pain, cramps, fasciculations, hyperhydrosis, and muscle hypertrophy (on EMG, manifests as myokymia). Isaac syndrome usually begins in the lower extremities but can affect abdominal, upper extremity, vocal, and respiratory muscles; it is most often sporadic, although autosomal dominant inheritance has been reported. Probably an autoimmune disease, with antibodies against the potassium channels of peripheral nerves.

**is·aux·e·sis** (ī-sawk-zē′sis) growth of parts at the same rate as growth of the whole. [G. *isos*, even, + *auxēsis*, increase]

**is·chae·mia [Br.]** SEE ischemia.

**is·chae·mic [Br.]** SEE ischemic.

**is·che·mia** (is-kē′mē-ă) local anemia due to mechanical obstruction (mainly arterial narrowing) of the blood supply. [G. *ischō*, to keep back, + *haima*, blood]

**is·che·mic** (is-kē′mik) relating to or affected by ischemia.

**is·che·mic con·trac·ture of the left ven·tri·cle** irreversible contraction of the left ventricle of the heart as a complication seen in the early period of cardiopulmonary bypass and now avoided by appropriate cardioplegic solutions. SYN stone heart.

**is·che·mic heart dis·ease** a general term for diseases of the heart caused by insufficient blood supply to myocardium, e.g., atherosclerotic coronary artery disease, angina pectoris, unstable angina, and myocardial infarction.

**is·che·mic hy·pox·ia** tissue hypoxia characterized by tissue oligemia and caused by arterial or arteriolar obstruction or vasoconstriction.

**is·che·mic ne·cro·sis** necrosis caused by hy-

poxia resulting from local deprivation of blood supply, as by infarction.

**is·chia** (is′kē-ă) plural of ischium.

**is·chi·ad·ic** (is-kē-ad′ik) SYN sciatic (1).

**is·chi·al** (is′kē-ăl) SYN sciatic (1).

**is·chi·al bone** SYN ischium.

**is·chi·al bur·sa** the bursa between the gluteus maximus muscle and the tuberosity of the ischium.

**is·chi·al bur·si·tis** inflammation of the bursa overlying the ischial tuberosity of the pelvis.

**is·chi·al·gia** (is-kē-al′jē-ă) **1.** pain in the hip; specifically, the ischium. SYN ischiodynia. **2.** rarely used term for sciatica. [G. *ischion*, hip, + *algos*, pain]

**is·chi·al spine** a pointed process from the posterior border of the ischium on a level with the lower border of the acetabulum; gives attachment to the sacrospinous ligament; the pudendal nerve passes dorsal to the ischial spine, which is palpable per vaginam or per rectum, and thus is used as a target for the needle-tip in administering a pudendal nerve block.

**is·chi·at·ic** (is-kē-at′ik) SYN sciatic (1).

**is·chi·at·ic her·nia** a hernia through the sacrosciatic foramen.

**is·chi·o-** ischium. [G. *ischion*, a hip-joint, haunch (ischium)]

**is·chi·o·cap·su·lar** (is-kē-ō-kap′soo-lăr) relating to the ischium and the capsule of the hip joint; denoting that part of the capsule which is attached to the ischium.

**is·chi·o·cav·ern·ous mus·cle** *origin*, ramus of ischium; *insertion*, corpus cavernosum penis (or clitoridis); *action*, compresses the crus of the penis (or clitoris) forcing blood in its sinuses into the distal part of the corpus cavernosum; *nerve supply*, perineal. SYN musculus ischiocavernosus [TA].

**is·chi·o·cele** (is′kē-ō-sēl) SYN sciatic hernia. [ischio- + G. *kēlē*, hernia]

**is·chi·o·coc·cyg·e·al** (is-kē-ō-kok-sij′ē-ăl) relating to the ischium and the coccyx.

**is·chi·o·dyn·ia** (is′kē-ō-din′ē-ă) SYN ischialgia (1). [ischio- + G. *odynē*, pain]

**is·chi·o·fem·o·ral** (is-kē-ō-fem′ŏ-răl) relating to the ischium, or hip bone, and the femur, or thigh bone.

**is·chi·o·fib·u·lar** (is′kē-ō-fib′yu-lăr) relating to or connecting the ischium and the fibula.

**is·chi·o·ni·tis** (is′kē-ō-nī′tis) inflammation of the ischium.

**is·chi·o·tib·i·al** (is′kē-ō-tib′ē-ăl) relating to or connecting the ischium and the tibia.

**is·chi·o·ver·te·bral** (is-kē-ō-ver′tĕ-brăl) relating to the ischium and the vertebral column.

**is·chi·um**, gen. **is·chii**, pl. **is·chia** (is′kē-ŭm, is-kē-ī, is′kē-ă) [TA] the lower and posterior part of the hip bone, distinct at birth but later becoming fused with the ilium and pubis; it consists of a body, where it joins the ilium and superior ramus of the pubis to form the acetabulum, and a ramus joining the inferior ramus of the pubis. SYN ischial bone. [Mod. L. fr. G. *ischion*, hip]

**is·chu·ria** (is-kyu′rē-ă) retention or suppression of urine. [G. *ischō*, to keep back, + *ouron*, urine]

**Ish·i·ha·ra test** (ish′ē-hah′rah) a test for color vision deficiency that utilizes a series of pseudoisochromatic plates on which numbers or letters are printed in dots of primary colors surrounded by dots of other colors; the figures are discernible by individuals with normal color vision.

**ISI** international sensitivity index.

**is·land** (ī′land) ANATOMY any isolated part, separated from the surrounding tissues by a groove, or marked by a difference in structure. SYN insula (2). [A.S. *īgland*]

**is·land flap** a flap in which the pedicle consists solely of the supplying artery and vein(s), sometimes including a nerve.

**is·land of Reil** (rīl) SYN insula (1).

**is·let** (ī′let) a small island.

**is·let cell** one of the cells of the pancreatic islets.

**is·let cell tu·mor** an endocrine tumor composed of cells equivalent or related to those in the normal islet of Langerhans; may be benign or malignant; usually hormonally active; comprises insulinomas, glucagonomas, vipomas, somatostatinomas, gastrinomas, pancreatic polypeptide-secreting tumor, and multihormonal or hormonally inactive pancreatic islet cell tumors.

**is·lets of Lan·ger·hans** (lahn′gĕr-hahnz) cellular masses varying from a few to hundreds of cells lying in the interstitial tissue of the pancreas; they are the source of insulin and glucagon. See this page.

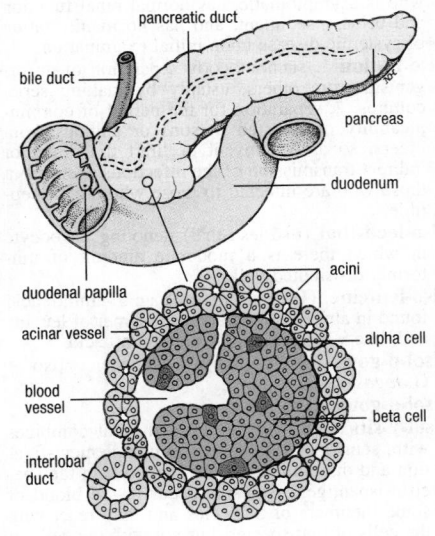

pancreatic duct

bile duct

pancreas

duodenum

acini

duodenal papilla

acinar vessel

alpha cell

blood vessel

beta cell

interlobar duct

**pancreatic islet**

△**-ism 1.** a medical condition or a disease resulting from or involving some specified thing. **2.** a practice, doctrine. Cf. -ia, -ismus. [G. *-isma*, *-ismos*, noun-forming suffix]

△**-is·mus** 1. for -ism; customarily used to imply spasm, contraction. [L. fr. G. *-ismos*, suffix forming nouns of action]

△**iso- 1.** prefix meaning equal, like. **2.** CHEMISTRY prefix indicating "isomer of" (isomerism); e.g., isocyanate vs. cyanate. **3.** IMMUNOLOGY prefix designating sameness with respect to species; in recent years, the meaning has shifted to sameness with respect to genetic constitution of individuals. [G. *isos*, equal]

**iso·ag·glu·ti·na·tion** (ī′sō-ă-gloo-ti-nā′shŭn) agglutination of red blood cells as a result of the

reaction between an isoagglutinin and specific antigen in or on the cells. SYN isohemagglutination. [iso- + L. *ad*, to, + *gluten*, glue]

**iso·ag·glu·ti·nin** (ī′sō-ă-gloo′ti-nin) an isoantibody that causes agglutination of cells of genetically different members of the same species. SYN isohemagglutinin.

**iso·ag·glu·tin·o·gen** (ī′sō-ă-gloo-tin′ō-jen) an isoantigen that induces agglutination of the cells to which it is attached upon exposure to its specific isoantibody.

**iso·am·y·lase** (ī-sō-am′il-ās) a hydrolase that cleaves 1,6-α-D-glucosidic branch linkages in glycogen, amylopectin, and their β-limit dextrins; part of the complex known as debranching enzyme.

**iso·an·ti·body** (ī′sō-an′ti-bod-ē) **1.** an antibody that occurs only in some individuals of a species and reacts specifically with a particular foreign isoantigen. **2.** sometimes used as a synonym of alloantibody. [G. *isos*, equal]

**iso·an·ti·gen** (ī′sō-an′ti-jen) **1.** an antigenic substance that occurs only in some individuals of a species, such as the blood group antigens of humans. **2.** sometimes used as a synonym of alloantigen.

**iso·bar** (ī′sō-bar) **1.** one of two or more nuclides having the same total number of protons plus neutrons, but with different distribution. **2.** the line on a map connecting points of equal barometric pressure. [iso- + G. *baros*, weight]

**iso·bar·ic** (ī-sō-bar′ik) **1.** having equal weights or pressures. **2.** with respect to solutions, having the same density as the diluent or medium.

**iso·cap·nia** (ī-sō-kap′nē-ă) a state in which the arterial carbon dioxide pressure remains constant or unchanged. [iso- + G. *kapnos*, vapor]

**iso·cel·lu·lar** (ī′sō-sel′yu-lăr) composed of cells of equal size or of similar character. [iso- + L. *cellula*, dim. of *cella*, a storeroom]

**iso·chro·mat·ic** (ī-sō-krō-mat′ik) **1.** of uniform color. **2.** denoting two objects of the same color. [iso- + G. *chrōma*, color]

**iso·chro·mat·o·phil, iso·chro·mat·o·phile** (ī′sō-krō-mat′ō-fil, ī′sō-krō-mat′ō-fīl) having an equal affinity for the same dye; said of cells or tissues. [iso- + G. *chrōma*, color, + *philos*, fond]

**iso·chro·mo·some** (ī′sō-krō′mō-sōm) a chromosomal aberration that arises as a result of transverse rather than longitudinal division of the centromere during meiosis; two daughter chromosomes are formed, each lacking one chromosome arm but with the other doubled.

**iso·chro·nia** (ī-sō-krō′nē-ă) **1.** the state of having the same chronaxie. **2.** agreement, with respect to time, rate, or frequency, between processes. [iso- + G. *chronos*, time]

**isoch·ro·nous** (ī-sok′rŏ-nŭs) occurring during the same time.

**iso·ci·trate** (ī-sō-sit′rāt) a salt or ester of isocitric acid.

**iso·cit·rate de·hy·dro·gen·ase** one of two enzymes that catalyze the conversion of *threo*-D$_s$-isocitrate to α-ketoglutarate (2-oxoglutarate) and $CO_2$.

**iso·cit·ric ac·id** (ī-sō-sit′rik as′id) an intermediate in the tricarboxylic acid cycle.

**iso·co·ria** (ī-sō-kō′rē-ă) equality in the size of the two pupils. [iso- + G. *korē*, pupil]

**iso·cor·tex** (ī-sō-kōr′teks) O. and C. Vogt's term for the larger part of the mammalian cerebral cortex, distinguished from the allocortex by being composed of a larger number of nerve cells arranged in six layers. SEE ALSO cerebral cortex.

**iso·cy·tol·y·sin** (ī′sō-sī-tol′i-sin) a cytolysin that reacts with the cells of certain other animals of the same species, but not with the cells of the individual that formed the isocytolysin.

**iso·dem·o·graph·ic map** diagrammatic method of displaying countries or administrative jurisdictions within a country in two-dimensional maps with each area directly proportional to the population density of the country or jurisdiction. [iso- + G. *dēmos*, people, + *graphō*, to write + -ic]

**iso·dense** (ī′sō-dens) denoting a tissue having a radiopacity (radiodensity) similar to that of another or adjacent tissue.

**iso·dose** area of equivalent radiation dose. [iso- + dose]

**iso·dy·nam·ic** (ī′sō-dī-nam′ik) **1.** of equal force or strength. **2.** relating to foods or other materials that liberate the same amount of energy on combustion. [iso- + G. *dynamis*, force]

**iso·e·lec·tric line** the baseline of the electrocardiogram.

**iso·e·lec·tric pe·ri·od** the period occurring in the electrocardiogram between the end of the S wave and the beginning of the T wave during which electrical forces neutralize each other so that there is no difference in potential under the two electrodes. SYN abnormal ST segment.

**iso·e·lec·tric point (pI)** the pH at which an amphoteric substance, such as protein or an amino acid, is electrically neutral.

**iso·en·er·get·ic** (ī′sō-en-er-jet′ik) exerting equal force; equally active.

**iso·en·zyme** (ī-sō-en′zīm) one of a group of enzymes that catalyze the same reaction but may be differentiated by variations in physical properties, such as isoelectric point, electrophoretic mobility, kinetic parameters, or modes of regulation. SYN isozyme.

**iso·e·ryth·rol·y·sis** (ī′sō-ĕ-rith-rol′i-sis) destruction of erythrocytes by isoantibodies. [iso- + erythrocyte = G. *lysis*, dissolution]

**iso·ga·mete** (ī-sō-gam′ēt) **1.** one of two or more similar cells that conjugate or fuse and subsequently divide, resulting in reproduction. **2.** a gamete of the same size as the gamete with which it unites. [iso- + G. *gametēs* or *gametē*, husband or wife]

**isog·a·my** (ī-sog′ă-mē) conjugation between two equal gametes or two individual cells alike in all respects. [iso- + G. *gamos*, marriage]

**iso·ge·ne·ic, iso·gen·ic** (ī′sō-jĕ-nē′ik, ī-sō-jen′ik) SYN syngeneic.

**iso·ge·ne·ic graft** SYN syngraft.

**isog·e·nous** (ī-soj′ĕ-nŭs) of the same origin, as in development from the same tissue or cell. [iso- + G. *genos*, family, kind]

**iso·graft** (ī′sō-graft) SYN syngraft.

**iso·hae·mag·glut·in·in [Br.]** SEE isohemagglutinin.

**iso·he·mag·glu·ti·na·tion** (ī′sō-hē′mă-gloo′ti-nā′shŭn) SYN isoagglutination. [iso- + G. *haima*, blood, + L. *ad*, to, + *gluten*, glue]

**iso·he·mag·glu·ti·nin** (ī′sō-hē′mă-gloo′ti-nin) SYN isoagglutinin.

**iso·he·mo·ly·sin** (ī′sō-hē-mol′i-sin) an isolysin that reacts with red blood cells.

**iso·he·mol·y·sis** (ī′sō-hē-mol′i-sis) dissolution of red blood cells as a result of the reaction between

an isolysin (isohemolysin) and specific antigen in or on the cells. [iso- + G. *haima*, blood, + *lysis*, dissolution]

**iso·im·mu·ni·za·tion** (ī′sō-im′yu-nī-zā′shŭn) development of a significant titer of specific antibody as a result of antigenic stimulation with material contained on or in the red blood cells of another individual of the same species.

**iso·late** (ī′sō-lāt) **1.** to separate, to set apart from others; that which is so treated. **2.** to free of chemical contaminants. **3.** PSYCHOANALYSIS to separate experiences or memories from the affects pertaining to them. **4.** GROUP PSYCHOTHERAPY an individual who is not responded to by others in the group. **5.** viable organisms separated on a single occasion from a field sample in experimental hosts, culture systems, or stabilates. **6.** a population that for geographic, linguistic, cultural, social, religious, or other reasons is subject to little or no gene flow. [It. *isolare*; Mediev. L. *insulo*, pp. -*atus*, to insulate, fr. L. *insula*, island]

**iso·lat·ed ex·plo·sive dis·or·der** a disorder of impulse control characterized by a single episode of failure to resist a violent, externally directed act that has a harmful impact on others.

**iso·lat·ed pro·tein·u·ria** proteinuria in a patient who is asymptomatic, has normal renal function and urinary sediment, and has no manifestation of systemic disease upon initial examination.

**iso·la·tion 1.** MICROBIOLOGY separation of an organism from others, usually by making serial cultures. **2.** separation for the period of communicability of infected persons or animals from others, so as to prevent or limit the direct or indirect transmission of the infectious agent from those who are infected to those who are susceptible.

**iso·lec·i·thal** (ī-sō-les′i-thăl) denoting an oocyte in which there is a moderate amount of uniformly distributed yolk.

**iso·leu·cine (I)** (ī-sō-loo′sēn) an L-amino acid found in almost all proteins; an isomer of leucine and, like it, a dietary essential amino acid.

**isol·o·gous** (ī-sol′ō-gŭs) SYN syngeneic. [iso- + G. *logos*, ratio]

**isol·o·gous graft** SYN syngraft.

**isol·y·sin** (ī-sol′i-sin) an antibody that combines with, sensitizes, and results in complement-fixation and dissolution of cells that contain the specific isoantigen; isolysins occur in the blood of some members of a species and they react with the cells of that species, but not with the cells of the individual (or the same type) in which the isolysins are naturally formed.

**isol·y·sis** (ī-sol′i-sis) lysis or dissolution of cells as a result of the reaction between an isolysin and specific antigen in or on the cells. SEE ALSO isohemolysis. [iso- + G. *lysis*, dissolution]

**iso·lyt·ic** (ī-sō-lit′ik) pertaining to, characterized by, or causing isolysis.

**iso·malt·ose** (ī-sō-mal′tōs) a disaccharide in which two glucose molecules are attached by an $\alpha1,6$ link, rather than an $\alpha1,4$ link as in maltose.

**iso·mer** (ī′sō-mer) **1.** one of two or more substances displaying isomerism. Cf. stereoisomer. **2.** one of two or more nuclides having the same atomic and mass numbers but differing in energy states for a finite period of time. [iso- + G. *meros*, part]

**isom·er·ase** (ī-som′er-ās) a class of enzymes (EC

class 5) catalyzing the conversion of a substance to an isomeric form.

**iso·mer·ic** (ī-sō-mār′ik) relating to or characterized by isomerism.

**isom·er·ism** (ī-som′er-izm) the existence of a chemical compound in two or more forms that are identical with respect to percentage composition but differ as to the positions of one or more atoms within the molecules, and also in physical and chemical properties.

**isom·er·i·za·tion** (ī-som′er-ī-zā′shŭn) a process in which one isomer is formed from another, as in the action of isomerases.

**iso·met·ric** (ī-sō-met′rik) **1.** of equal dimensions. **2.** PHYSIOLOGY denoting the condition when the ends of a contracting muscle are held fixed so that contraction produces increased tension at a constant overall length. Cf. auxotonic, isotonic (3), isovolumic. [iso- + G. *metron,* measure]

**iso·met·ric con·trac·tion** force development at constant length. Cf. isotonic contraction.

**iso·met·ric ex·er·cise** exercise consisting of muscular contractions without movement of the involved parts of the body.

**iso·met·ric pe·ri·od of car·di·ac cy·cle** that period in which the muscle fibers do not shorten although the cardiac muscle is excited and the pressure in the ventricles rises, extending from the closure of the atrioventricular valves to the opening of the semilunar valves (isovolumic constriction) or the reverse (isovolumic relaxation). SYN isovolumic period.

**iso·me·tro·pia** (ī′sō-me-trō′pē-ă) equality in refraction in the two eyes. [iso- + G. *metron,* measure, + ōps (ōp-), eye]

**iso·mor·phic** (ī-sō-mōr′fik) SYN isomorphous.

**iso·mor·phism** (ī-sō-mōr′fizm) similarity of form between two or more organisms or between parts of the body. [iso- + G. *morphē,* shape]

**iso·mor·phous** (ī-sō-mōr′fŭs) having the same form or shape, or being morphologically equal. SYN isomorphic.

**isop·a·thy** (ī-sop′ă-thē) treatment of disease by means of the causal agent or a product of the same disease; or treatment of a diseased organ by an extract of a similar organ from a healthy animal. SEE ALSO homeopathy. [iso- + G. *pathos,* suffering]

**iso·per·i·stal·tic a·nas·to·mo·sis** an anastomosis allowing flow of contents in the same and normal direction.

**isoph·a·gy** (ī-sof′ă-jē) SYN autolysis. [iso- + G. *phagō,* to eat]

**iso·phane in·su·lin** SYN NPH insulin.

**iso·plas·tic** (ī-sō-plas′tik) SYN syngeneic. [iso- + G. *plassō,* to form]

**iso·plas·tic graft** SYN syngraft.

**iso·pre·cip·i·tin** (ī′sō-prē-sip′i-tin) an antibody that combines with and precipitates soluble antigenic material in the plasma or serum, or in an extract of the cells, from another member, but not all members, of the same species. [iso- + precipitin]

**iso·prene** (ī′sō-prēn) an unsaturated five-carbon hydrocarbon with a branched chain, the basis for the formation of isoprenoids (terpenes, carotenoids, and rubber). Fat-soluble vitamins either are isoprenoid or have isoprenoid side chains; steroids are synthesized via isoprenoid intermediates.

**iso·pre·noids** (ī-sō-prēn′oydz) polymers whose

carbon skeletons consist in whole or in large part of isoprene units joined end to end.

**isop·ter** (ī-sop′ter) a line of equal retinal sensitivity in the visual field. [iso- + G. *optēr,* observer]

**isor·rhea** (ī-sō-rē′ă) equality of intake and output of water; maintenance of water equilibrium. [iso- + G. *rhoia,* a flow]

**isos·best·ic point** in applied spectroscopy, a wavelength at which absorbance of two substances, one of which can be converted into the other, is the same.

**iso·sex·u·al** (ī-sō-seks′yu-ăl) **1.** relating to the existence of characteristics or feelings of both sexes in one person. **2.** descriptive of an individual's somatic characteristics, or of internal processes, that are consonant with the sex of that individual.

**isos·mot·ic** (ī′sos-mot′ik) having the same total osmotic pressure or osmolality as another fluid (ordinarily intracellular fluid); such a fluid is not isosmotic if it includes solutes that freely permeate cell membranes.

*Isos·po·ra* (ī-sos′pō-ră) a genus of coccidia parasitizing chiefly mammals. [iso- + G. *sporos,* seed]

**isos·po·ri·a·sis** (ī-sos-pō-rī′ă-sis) disease caused by infection with a species of *Isospora,* such as *I. belli* of humans; human disease usually is mild except in cases of immunosuppression, as in AIDS, where it may cause an intractable diarrhea.

**isos·the·nu·ria** (ī-sos′then-yur′ē-ă) a state in chronic renal disease in which the kidney cannot form urine with a higher or a lower specific gravity than that of protein-free plasma; specific gravity of the urine becomes fixed around 1.010, irrespective of the fluid intake. [iso- + G. *sthenos,* strength, + *ouron,* urine]

**iso·ther·mal** (ī-sō-ther′măl) having the same temperature. [iso- + G. *thermē,* heat]

**iso·tone** (ī′sō-tōn) one of several nuclides having the same number of neutrons in their nuclei. [iso- + G. *tonos,* stretching, tension]

**iso·to·nia** (ī-sō-tō′nē-ă) a condition of tonic equality in which tension or osmotic pressure in two substances or solutions is the same. [iso- + G. *tonos,* tension]

**iso·ton·ic** (ī-sō-ton′ik) **1.** relating to isotonicity or isotonia. **2.** having equal tension; denoting solutions possessing the same osmotic pressure; more specifically, limited to solutions in which cells neither swell nor shrink. Thus, a solution that is isosmotic with intracellular fluid will not be isotonic if it includes solute, such as urea, that freely permeates cell membranes. **3.** PHYSIOLOGY denoting the condition when a contracting muscle shortens against a constant load, as when lifting a weight. Cf. auxotonic, isometric (2).

**iso·ton·ic con·trac·tion** shortening at constant force development. Cf. isometric contraction.

**iso·to·nic·i·ty** (ī-sō-tō-nis′i-tē) **1.** the quality of possessing and maintaining a uniform tone or tension. **2.** the property of a solution in being isotonic.

**iso·tope** (ī′sō-tōp) one of two or more nuclides that are chemically identical, having the same number of protons, yet differ in mass number, since their nuclei contain different numbers of neutrons; individual isotopes are named with the inclusion of their mass number in the superior position ($^{12}C$) and the atomic number (nuclear

i
s

protons) in the inferior position ($_6$C). [iso- + G. *topos*, part, place]

**iso·to·pic** (ī-sō-top'ik) of identical chemical composition but differing in some physical property, such as atomic weight.

**iso·tro·pic, isot·ro·pous** (ī-sō-trop'ik, ī-sot'rō-pŭs) having properties which are the same in all directions. [iso- + G. *tropē*, a turn]

**iso·type** (ī'sō-tīp) an antigenic determinant (marker) that occurs in all members of a subclass of an immunoglobulin class. [iso- + G. *typos*, model]

**iso·typ·ic** (ī-sō-tip'ik) pertaining to an isotype.

**iso·vol·u·mic** (ī'sō-vol-yu'mik) occurring without an associated alteration in volume, as when, in early ventricular systole, the muscle fibers initially increase their tension without shortening so that ventricular volume remains unaltered. SEE ALSO isometric.

**iso·vol·u·mic per·i·od** SYN isometric period of cardiac cycle.

**iso·zyme** (ī'sō-zīm) SYN isoenzyme.

**isth·mec·to·my** (is-mek'tō-mē) excision of the midportion of the thyroid. [G. *isthmos*, isthmus, + *ektomē*, excision]

**isth·mic, isth·mi·an** (is'mik, is'mē-an) denoting an anatomic isthmus.

**isth·mo·pa·ral·y·sis** (is'mō-pă-ral'i-sis) paralysis of the velum pendulum palati and the muscles forming the anterior pillars of the fauces. SYN isthmoplegia. [G. *isthmos*, isthmus, + paralysis]

**isth·mo·ple·gia** (is'mō-plē'jē-ă) SYN isthmoparalysis. [G. *isthmos*, isthmus, + *plēgē*, stroke]

**isth·mus**, pl. **isth·mi, isth·mus·es** (is'mŭs, is'mī, is'mŭs-ez) [TA] **1.** a constriction connecting two larger parts of an organ or other anatomic structure. **2.** a narrow passage connecting two larger cavities. **3.** the narrowest portion of the brainstem at the junction between midbrain and hindbrain. [G. *isthmos*]

**isth·mus of au·di·to·ry tube** the narrowest portion of the auditory tube at the junction of the cartilaginous and bony portions. SYN isthmus tubae auditivae [TA].

**isth·mus tu·bae au·di·ti·vae** [TA] SYN isthmus of auditory tube.

**itch 1.** a peculiar irritating sensation in the skin that arouses the desire to scratch. SYN pruritus (2). **2.** common name for scabies. [A.S. *gikkan*]

**itch·ing** an uncomfortable sensation of irritation of the skin or mucous membranes which causes scratching or rubbing of the affected parts. SYN pruritus (1).

△**-ite 1.** of the nature of, resembling. **2.** a salt of an acid that has the termination -ous. **3.** COMPARATIVE ANATOMY a suffix denoting an essential portion of the part to the name of which it is attached. SEE ALSO -ites. [G. *-itēs*, fem. *-itis*]

**iter** (ī'ter) a passage leading from one anatomic part to another. SEE ALSO canaliculus. [L. *iter* (*itiner*-), a way, journey]

**it·er·al** (ī'ter-ăl) relating to an iter.

△**-ites** adjectival suffix to nouns, corresponding to L. *-alis, -ale*, or *-inus, -inum*, or Eng. -y, -like, or the hyphenated nouns; the adjective so formed is used without the qualified noun. SEE ALSO -ite. [G. *itēs*, m., or *-ites*, n.]

△**-it·i·des** plural of -itis.

△**-it·is** SEE -ites. [G. fem. of *-ites*]

**Ito ne·vus** (ē'tō) pigmentation of skin innervated by lateral branches of the supraclavicular nerve and the lateral cutaneous nerve of the arm, due to scattered, heavily pigmented, dendritic melanocytes in the dermis.

**ITP** idiopathic thrombocytopenic purpura; inosine 5'-triphosphate.

**IUCD** intrauterine contraceptive devices.

**IUD** intrauterine devices.

**IUI** intrauterine insemination.

**$^{131}$I up·take test** a test of thyroid function in which $^{131}$I-iodide is given orally; after 24 hours, the amount present in the thyroid gland is measured and compared with normal values.

**IVC** inferior vena cava.

**Ive·mark syn·drome** (ē'vĕ-mahrk) SYN polysplenia.

**Ivor Lew·is es·o·pha·gec·to·my** (ī'vōr-loo'is) commonly used approach for esophagectomy via laparotomy and right thoracotomy, with intrathoracic anastomosis.

**IVU** intravenous urogram; preferred to intravenous pylogram (IVP). SEE intravenous urography.

*Ix·o·des* (ik-sō'dēz) a genus of hard ticks (family Ixodidae), many species of which are parasitic on humans and animals; they are characterized by an anal groove surrounding the anus anteriorly, absence of eyes and festoons, and marked sexual dimorphism; about 40 species have been described from North America. [G. *ixōdēs*, sticky, like bird-lime, fr. *ixos*, mistletoe, + *eidos*, form]

*Ix·o·des re·di·kor·zev·i* a Eurasian species that has caused human toxicosis in Israel.

*Ix·o·des sca·pu·lar·is* the black-legged or shoulder tick, a species found in the southern and eastern United States; the primary vector of Lyme disease in the United States.

**ix·o·di·a·sis** (ik-sō-dī'ă-sis) skin lesions caused by the bites of certain ixodid ticks.

**ix·od·ic** (ik-sod'ik) relating to or caused by ticks.

**ix·o·did** (ik'sŏ-did) common name for members of the family Ixodidae.

**Ix·od·i·dae** (ik-sod'i-dē) a family of ticks, the so-called hard ticks, genera of which transmit many important human and animal diseases and cause tick paralysis.

**J** joule; electric current density.

**J** flux (4).

**Ja·bou·lay am·pu·ta·tion** (zhah′boo-lā′) SYN hemipelvectomy.

**jack·et** (jak′et) **1.** a fixed bandage applied around the body in order to immobilize the spine. **2.** DENTISTRY an artificial crown composed of fired porcelain or acrylic resin. [M.E., fr. O.Fr. *jaquet*, dim. of *jaque*, tunic, fr. *Jacques*, nickname of Fr. peasants.]

**jack·so·ni·an sei·zure, jack·so·ni·an ep·i·lep·sy** (jak-sō′nē-ăn) a seizure originating in or near the rolandic neocortex, which clinically involves one part of the body; seizure spread is accompanied by progressive spread to other parts of the body on the same side; may become generalized.

**Jack·son law** (jak′son) loss of mental functions due to disease retraces in reverse order its evolutionary development.

**Jack·son mem·brane** (jak′son) a thin vascular membrane or veillike adhesion, covering the anterior surface of the ascending colon from the cecum to the right flexure; it may cause obstruction by kinking of the bowel.

**Jack·son rule** (jak′son) after an epileptic attack, simple and quasiautomatic functions are less affected and more rapidly recovered than the more complex ones.

**Jack·son sign** (jak′son) during quiet respiration the movement of the paralyzed side of the chest may be greater than that of the opposite side, while in forced respiration the paralyzed side moves less than the other.

**Ja·cob·son re·flex** (jā′kob-son) flexion of the fingers elicited by tapping the flexor tendons over the wrist joint or the lower end of the radius.

**jac·ti·ta·tion** (jak-ti-tā′shŭn) extreme restlessness or tossing about from side to side. [L. *jactatio*, a tossing, fr. *jacto*, pp. *-atus*, to throw]

**Jae·ger test types** (yā′gĕr) type of different sizes used for testing the acuity of near vision.

**Jahn·ke syn·drome** (yahn′kĕ) Sturge-Weber syndrome without glaucoma.

**Ja·net test** (zhah-nā′) a test for functional or organic anesthesia; the patient (with eyes closed) is told to say "yes" or "no" on feeling (or not) the touch of the examiner's finger; in the case of functional anesthesia the patient may say "no" when an anesthesia area is touched, but will say nothing, being unaware that he is touched, in cases of organic anesthesia.

**Jane·way le·sion** (jān′wā) one of the stigmata of infectious endocarditis: irregular, erythematous, flat, painless macules on the palms, soles, thenar and hypothenar eminences of the hands, tips of the fingers, and plantar surfaces of the toes.

**jan·i·ceps** (jan′i-seps) conjoined twins having their two heads fused together, with the faces looking in opposite directions. SEE conjoined twins. [L. *Janus*, a Roman deity having two faces, + *caput*, head]

**Jan·sen op·er·a·tion** (yahn′sen) an operation for frontal sinus disease; the lower wall and lower portion of the anterior wall are removed and the mucous membrane is curetted away.

**Ja·nus green B** (jan′us) [CI 11050] diethyl-safraninazodimethylaniline chloride; a basic dye used in histology and to stain mitochondria supravitally.

**Jap·a·nese B en·ceph·a·li·tis** (jap′ah-nēz) an epidemic encephalitis or encephalomyelitis of Japan, Siberian Russia, and other parts of Asia; due to the Japanese B encephalitis virus (genus *Flavivirus*) and transmitted by mosquitoes; can occur as a symptomless, subclinical infection but may cause an acute meningoencephalomyelitis.

**Jap·a·nese B en·ceph·a·li·tis vi·rus** (jap′ah-nēz) a virus of the genus *Flavivirus* (group B arbovirus) normally present in humans, especially in children, as an inapparent infection, but may cause febrile response and sometimes encephalitis.

**Jap·a·nese spot·ted fev·er** (jap′ah-nēz) a febrile disease caused by the bacterium *Rickettsia japonica* and characterized by headache and exanthema; found in Japan.

**jar·gon** (jar′gŏn) **1.** language or terminology peculiar to a specific field, profession, or group. **2.** SYN paraphasia. [Fr. gibberish]

**jar·gon a·pha·sia** SYN paragrammatism.

**Ja·risch-Herx·hei·mer re·ac·tion** (yah′rish herks′hī-mer) SYN Herxheimer reaction.

**Jar·man score** (jar′man) index of social and medical deprivation, used mainly by family doctors, especially in the U.K.

**Jar·vik ar·ti·fi·cial heart** (jahr′vik) a pneumatic artificial heart.

**jaun·dice** (jawn′dis) a yellowish staining of the integument, sclerae, and deeper tissues and the excretions with bile pigments, which are increased in the plasma. SYN icterus. [Fr. *jaune*, yellow]

**jaun·dice of the new·born** SYN icterus neonatorum.

**jaw 1.** one of the two bony structures, in which the teeth are set, forming the framework of the mouth. **2.** common name for either the maxilla or the mandible. [A.S. *ceōwan*, to chew]

**jaw bone** SYN mandible.

**Ja·wor·ski bod·ies** (yĕ-vor′skē) mucous shreds in the gastric contents in hyperchlorhydria.

**jaw re·flex** a spasmodic contraction of the temporal muscles following a downward tap on the loosely hanging mandible.

**jaw wink·ing** a paradoxical movement of eyelids associated with movements of the jaw.

**jaw-wink·ing syn·drome** an increase in the width of the palpebral fissures during chewing, sometimes with a rhythmic elevation of the upper lid when the mouth is open and ptosis when the mouth is closed. SYN Gunn syndrome, Marcus Gunn phenomenon, Marcus Gunn syndrome.

**JCAHO** Joint Commission on Accreditation of Healthcare Organizations.

**J chain** a glycopeptide disulfide that is bonded to polymeric IgA and IgM; its function is to ensure correct polymerization of the subunits of IgA and IgM. [joining]

**je·ju·nal** (je-joo′năl) relating to the jejunum.

**je·ju·nal ar·ter·ies** *origin*, superior mesenteric; *distribution*, jejunum; *anastomoses*, by a series of arches with each other and with ileal arteries. SYN arteriae jejunales [TA].

**je·ju·nal and il·e·al veins** drain the jejunum and ileum; they terminate in the superior mesenteric vein.

**je·ju·nec·to·my** (je-joo-nek'tō-mē) excision of all or a part of the jejunum. [jejunum + G. *ektomē*, excision]

**je·ju·ni·tis** (je-joo-nī'tis) inflammation of the jejunum.

△**je·ju·no-, je·jun-** the jejunum, jejunal. [L. *jejunus*, empty]

**je·ju·no·co·los·to·my** (je-joo-nō-kō-los'tō-mē) establishment of a communication between the jejunum and the colon. [jejuno- + colon + G. *stoma*, mouth]

**je·ju·no·il·e·al** (je-joo'nō-il'ē-ăl) relating to the jejunum and the ileum.

**je·ju·no·il·e·al by·pass, je·ju·no·il·e·al shunt** anastomosis of the upper jejunum to the terminal ileum for treatment of morbid obesity. SYN bowel bypass.

**je·ju·no·il·e·i·tis** (je-joo'nō-il-ē-ī'tis) inflammation of the jejunum and ileum.

**je·ju·no·il·e·os·to·my** (je-joo'nō-il-ē-os'tō-mē) establishment of a new communication between the jejunum and the ileum. [jejuno- + ileum + G. *stoma*, mouth]

**je·ju·no·je·ju·nos·to·my** (je-joo'nō-je-joo-nos'tō-mē) an anastomosis between two portions of jejunum. [jejuno- + jejuno- + G. *stoma*, mouth]

**je·ju·no·plas·ty** (je-joo'nō-plas-tē) a corrective surgical procedure on the jejunum. [jejuno- + G. *plastos*, molded]

**je·ju·nos·to·my** (je-joo-nos'tō-mē) operative establishment of an opening from the abdominal wall into the jejunum, usually with creation of a stoma on the abdominal wall. [jejuno- + G. *stoma*, mouth]

**je·ju·not·o·my** (je-joo-not'ō-mē) incision into the jejunum. [jejuno- + G. *tomē*, incision]

**je·ju·num** (jĕ-joo'nŭm) [TA] the portion of small intestine, about 8 feet in length, between the duodenum and the ileum. The jejunum is distinct from the ileum in being more proximal, of larger diameter with a thicker wall, having larger, more highly developed plicae circulares, being more vascular (redder in appearance), with the jejunal arteries forming fewer tiers of arterial arcades and longer vasa recta. [L. *jejunus*, empty]

**jel·ly** (jel'ē) 1. a semisolid tremulous compound usually containing some form of gelatin in aqueous solution. 2. SYN jellyfish. [L. *gelo*, to freeze]

**jel·ly·fish** (jel'ē-fish) marine coelenterates, including some poisonous species; toxin is injected into the skin by nematocysts on the tentacles, causing linear wheals. SYN jelly (2).

**Jen·dras·sik ma·neu·ver** (yen-drah'sik) a method of emphasizing the patellar reflex: the subject hooks the hands together by the flexed fingers and pulls against them with all possible strength.

**Jen·ner stain** (jen'ĕr) a methylene blue eosinate similar to Wright stain but differing in not using polychromed methylene blue; used for staining of blood smears.

**Jen·sen dis·ease** (yen'sĕn) SYN retinochoroiditis juxtapapillaris.

**jerk** 1. a sudden pull. 2. SYN deep reflex.

**jerk·y nys·tag·mus** nystagmus in which there is a slow drift of the eyes in one direction, followed by a rapid recovery movement, always described in the direction of the recovery movement; it usually arises from labyrinthine or neurologic lesions or stimuli.

**Jer·ne plaque as·say** (yed'nĕ) an assay that enumerates individual antibody-forming cells. SYN hemolytic plaque assay.

**jer·sey finger** (jŭr'zē fing'ger) avulsion of the flexor digitorum profundus tendon from the distal phalanx due to abrupt passive extension of the actively flexed finger.

**jet** a region of very high blood velocity immediately downstream of a vessel stenosis.

**jet lag** an imbalance of the normal circadian rhythm resulting from subsonic or supersonic travel through a number of time zones and leading to fatigue, irritability, and functional disturbances.

**jet neb·u·liz·er** an atomizer that uses an air or gas stream to change a liquid into small particles.

**Jeune syn·drome** (zhoon) SYN asphyxiating thoracic dystrophy.

**jew·el·ler's for·ceps** a small thumb forceps with very fine pointed blades, used to grasp tissues in microsurgical procedures.

**Jew·ett and Strong stag·ing** (joo'ĕt and strong) staging of bladder carcinoma: O, noninvasive; A, with submucosal invasion; B, with muscle invasion; C, with invasion of perivascular fat; D, with lymph node metastasis.

**JH virus** human rhinovirus strain 1A. [*Johns Hopkins University*, where first isolated]

**jig·ger** common name for *Tunga penetrans*. SEE ALSO chigoe.

**Jo·bert de Lam·bal·le su·ture** (zhō-bār' dŭ-lam-bahl') an interrupted intestinal suture, used for invaginating the margins of the intestines in circular enterorrhaphy.

**Jo·cas·ta com·plex** (jō-kas'tă) a mother's libidinous fixation on a son. [*Jocasta*, mother and wife of Oedipus]

**jock itch** SYN tinea cruris.

**Jod-Ba·se·dow phe·nom·e·non** (yod-bah'ze-dō) induction of thyrotoxicosis in a previously euthyroid individual as a result of exposure to large quantities of iodine; occurs most often in areas of endemic iodine-deficient goiter and in patients with multinodular goiter; also can develop following use of iodine-containing agents for diagnostic studies.

**Jof·froy re·flex** (zhof'rwah') twitching of the glutei muscles when firm pressure is made on the nates, in cases of spastic paralysis.

**Jof·froy sign** (zhof'rwah') disorder of the arithmetical faculty (the person being unable to do simple sums in addition or multiplication) in the early stages of organic brain disease.

**John·son meth·od** (jon'son) SYN chloropercha method.

▌**joint** (joynt) in anatomy, the place of union, usually more or less movable, between two or more bones. Joints between skeletal elements exhibit a great variety of form and function, and are classified into three general morphologic types: fibrous joints; cartilaginous joints; and synovial joints. See page 527. SYN arthrosis (1), articulation (1), junctura (1). [L. *junctura*; fr. *jungo*, pp. *junctus*, to join]

**joint cap·sule** SYN articular capsule.

**Joint Com·mis·sion on Ac·cre·di·ta·tion of Health·care Or·ga·ni·za·tions (JCAHO)** an independent nonprofit organization that evaluates and accredits health care organizations and programs in the United States.

**joint ef·fu·sion** increased fluid in synovial cavity of a joint.

**joint ex·ten·sion** SYN close-packed position.

**joints of foot** joints including the talocrural, intertarsal, tarsometatarsal, intermetatarsal, metatarsophalangeal and interphalangeal joints.

**joints of hand** these joints include the radiocarpal or wrist joint; intercarpal, carpometacarpal, intermetacarpal; metacarpophalangeal and interphalangeal joints.

**Jones I test** (jōnz) SYN primary dye test.

**Jones II test** (jōnz) SYN secondary dye test.

**Jones cri·ter·ia** (jōnz) criteria (proposed by T.D. Jones in 1944 and modified in 1965) used to make the diagnosis of rheumatic fever. There are five major criteria: carditis, polyarthritis, chorea, erythema marginatum, and subcutaneous nodules; minor criteria include fever, arthralgia, elevated erythrocyte sedimentation rate or C reactive protein, and prolonged PR interval on ECG. Diagnosis requires evidence of recent group A β-hemolytic streptococcal infection, plus two major and one minor criteria, or one major and two minor criteria; revised Jones criteria allow the diagnosis when indolent carditis or chorea exists with no other cause, or in patients with a previous history of rheumatic fever who have one major or two minor criteria in association with a recent streptococcal infection.

**Jones frac·ture** (jōnz) transverse stress fracture of the proximal shaft of the fifth metatarsal.

**Jones·ia den·i·tri·fi·cans** a species of motile, Gram-positive bacteria formerly classified as *Listeria denitrificans;* the only member of the genus *Jonesia.*

**Jones test** (jōnz) SYN fluorescein instillation test.

**Jones trans·fer** (jōnz) surgical procedure to treat claw deformities of the great toe in which the extensor hallucis longus tendon is transferred to the neck of the metatarsal; can also be used to correct claw deformities of the lesser toes.

**Jou·bert syn·drome** (zhoo-bār') agenesis of the cerebellar vermis, characterized clinically by attacks of tachypnea or prolonged apnea, abnormal eye movements, ataxia, and mental retardation.

**Joule** (jool), James P., British physicist, 1818–1889. SEE joule.

**joule (J)** (jool, jowl) a unit of energy; the heat generated, or energy expended, by an ampere flowing through an ohm for 1 second; equal to $10^7$ ergs and to a newton-meter. It is an approved multiple of the SI fundamental unit of energy, the erg, and is intended to replace the calorie (4.184 J). [J.P. *Joule*]

**Joule equiv·a·lent (J)** (jool) the dynamic equivalent of heat; the amount of work converted to heat that will raise the temperature of 1 pound of water 1°F is 778 foot-pounds; in metric units, 1 calorie, which raises 1 gram of water 1°C, equals $4.184 \times 10^7$ dyne-centimeters, which equals 4.184 joules.

**J point** the point marking the end of the QRS complex and the beginning of the ST segment in the electrocardiogram.

**Ju·det view** (zhŭ-dā') view consisting of two oblique radiographic projections centered on the hip in question, tilted 45° medially or laterally from a true anteroposterior direction; useful for fractures or deformities of the acetabulum.

**judg·ment** ability to evaluate the positive and negative aspects of a behavior or situation and act or react appropriately.

**ju·ga** (joo'gă) plural of jugum.

**ju·gal** (joo'găl) **1.** connecting; yoked. **2.** relating to the zygomatic bone. [L. *jugalis,* yoked together, fr. *jugum,* a yoke]

**ju·gal bone** SYN zygomatic bone.

**ju·ga·le** (joo-gā'lē) a craniometric point at the union of the temporal and frontal processes of the zygomatic bone. SYN jugal point.

**ju·gal point** SYN jugale.

**jug·u·lar** (jŭg'yu-lar) **1.** relating to the throat or neck. **2.** relating to the jugular veins. **3.** a jugular vein. [L. *jugulum,* throat]

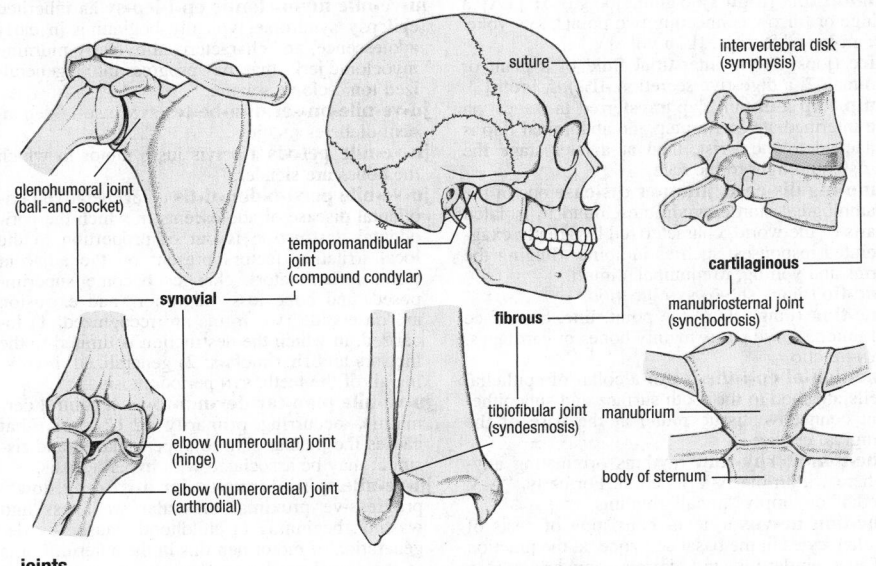

**joints**

**jug·u·lar fo·ra·men** a passage between the petrous portion of the temporal bone and the jugular process of the occipital, sometimes divided into two by the intrajugular processes; it contains the internal jugular vein, inferior petrosal sinus, the glossopharyngeal, vagus, and accessory nerves, and meningeal branches of the ascending pharyngeal and occipital arteries.

**jug·u·lar fos·sa** an oval depression near the posterior border of the petrous portion of the temporal bone, medial to the styloid process, in which lies the beginning of the internal jugular vein (jugular bulb);

**jug·u·lar gland** SYN signal lymph node.

**jug·u·lar glo·mus** a microscopic collection of chemoreceptor tissue in the adventitia of the jugular bulb; a tumor of this glomus may cause paralysis of the vocal cords, attacks of dizziness, blackouts, and nystagmus.

**jug·u·lar nerve** a communicating branch between the superior cervical ganglion of the sympathetic nerve, the superior ganglion of the vagus nerve, and the inferior ganglion of the glossopharyngeal nerve. SYN nervus jugularis [TA].

**jug·u·lar pulse** the venous pulse as observed in the jugular veins of the neck, usually the deep jugular veins.

**jug·u·lo·di·gas·tric lymph node** a prominent lymph node in the deep lateral cervical group lying below the digastric muscle and anterior to the internal jugular vein; it receives lymphatic drainage from the pharynx, palatine tonsil, and tongue.

**jug·u·lo·o·mo·hy·oid lymph node** a lymph node of the lateral deep cervical group that lies above the intermediate tendon of the omohyoid muscle and anterior to the internal jugular vein; it receives lymphatic drainage from the submental, submandibular, and deep anterior cervical nodes; its efferent vessels go to other deep lateral cervical nodes.

**ju·gum**, pl. **ju·ga** (joo′gŭm, joo′gă) **1.** [TA] a ridge or furrow connecting two points. SYN yoke. **2.** a type of forceps. [L. a yoke]

**juice** (joos) **1.** the interstitial fluid of a plant or animal. **2.** a digestive secretion. [L. *jus*, broth]

**jump flap** a distant flap transferred in stages via an intermediate carrier; e.g., an abdominal flap is attached to the wrist, then at a later stage the wrist is brought to the face.

**jump·ing dis·ease, jump·er dis·ease** one of the pathological startle syndromes found in isolated parts of the world, characterized by greatly exaggerated responses, such as jumping, flinging the arms and yelling, to minimal stimuli.

**junc·tio** (jŭngk′shē-ō) SYN junction.

**junc·tion** (jŭngk′shŭn) the point, line, or surface of union of two parts, mainly bones or cartilages. SYN junctio.

**junc·tion·al ep·i·the·li·um** a collar of epithelial cells attached to the tooth surface and subepithelial connective tissue found at the base of the gingival crevice.

**junc·tion·al rhy·thm** rhythms originating anywhere within the A-V junction. Formerly, "A-V nodal" or simply "nodal" rhythms.

**junc·tion ne·vus** a nevus consisting of nests of melanocytes in the basal cell zone, at the junction of the epidermis and dermis, appearing as a slightly raised, small, flat, nonhairy pigmented (brown or black) tumor.

**junc·tu·ra**, pl. **junc·tu·rae** (jŭngk-too′ră, jŭngk-too′rē) **1.** [TA] SYN joint. **2.** the point, line, or surface of union of two parts, mainly bones or cartilages. SYN juncture. [L. a joining]

**junc·ture** (jŭngk′cher) SYN junctura (2).

**jung·i·an** (yung′ē-an) the psychological system or the psychoanalytic form of treatment deriving from it; developed by Carl Gustav Jung.

**jung·i·an psy·cho·a·nal·y·sis** (yoong′ē-ăn) the theory of psychopathology and the practice of psychotherapy, according to the principles of C. G. Jung, which emphasized human beings' symbolic nature, and differs from freudian psychoanalysis especially in placing less significance upon instinctual (sexual) urges. SYN analytical psychology.

**junk DNA** that portion of DNA which is not transcribed and expressed, comprising about 90% of the 3 billion base pairs of the human genome; its function is not known. SYN selfish DNA.

**Jur·kat cells** a line of T cells often employed in immunologic research, originally derived from a Burkitt lymphoma.

**ju·ve·nile ar·thri·tis, ju·ve·nile rheu·ma·toid ar·thri·tis** chronic arthritis beginning in childhood, most cases of which are pauciarticular, i.e., affecting few joints. Several patterns of illness have been identified: in one subset, primarily affecting girls, iritis is common and antinuclear antibody is usually present; another subset, primarily affecting boys, frequently includes spinal arthritis resembling ankylosing spondylitis; some cases are true rheumatoid arthritis beginning in childhood and characterized by the presence of rheumatoid factor and destructive deforming joint changes, often undergoing remission at puberty. SEE ALSO Still disease.

**ju·ve·nile cat·a·ract** a soft cataract occurring in a child or young adult.

**ju·ve·nile cell** SYN metamyelocyte.

**ju·ve·nile my·o·clon·ic ep·i·lep·sy** an inherited epilepsy syndrome typically beginning in early adolescence, and characterized by early morning myoclonic jerks that may progress into a generalized tonic-clonic seizure.

**ju·ve·nile-on·set di·a·be·tes** SYN insulin-dependent diabetes mellitus.

**ju·ve·nile pel·vis** a pelvis justo minor in which the bones are slender.

**ju·ve·nile per·i·o·don·ti·tis** a degenerative periodontal disease of adolescents in which the periodontal destruction is out of proportion to the local irritating factors present on the adjacent teeth; inflammatory changes become superimposed, and bone loss, migration, and extrusion are observed. Two forms are recognized: 1) localized, in which the destruction is limited to the incisors and first molars; 2) generalized, involving all of the teeth. SYN periodontosis.

**ju·ve·nile plan·tar der·ma·to·sis** a painful dermatitis, occurring primarily in children, that causes the plantar skin to appear glazed and fissured; may be associated with hyperhidrosis.

**ju·ve·nile spin·al mus·cu·lar a·tro·phy** slowly progressive proximal muscular weakness and wasting, beginning in childhood, caused by degeneration of motor neurons in the anterior horns of the spinal cord; onset usually between 2 and 17 years of age; usually autosomal recessive inheritance.

**jux•ta•crine** (juks′tă-krin) a mode of hormone action that requires the cell producing the effector to be in direct contact with the cell containing the appropriate receptor. [L. *juxta*, close to, + G. *krinō*, to separate]

**jux•ta•ep•i•phys•i•al** (jŭks′tă-ep-i-fiz′ē-ăl) close to or adjoining an epiphysis.

**jux•ta-e•soph•a•ge•al pul•mo•nary lymph nodes, jux•ta-e•soph•a•ge•al lymph nodes** several nodes of the posterior mediastinal group located along either side of the esophagus; they receive lymph from both the esophagus and the lungs.

**jux•ta•glo•mer•u•lar** (jŭks′tă-glŏ-mer′yu-lăr) close to or adjoining a renal glomerulus.

**jux•ta•glo•mer•u•lar cells** cells located at the vascular pole of the renal corpuscle that secrete renin and form a component of the juxtaglomerular complex; they are modified smooth muscle cells primarily of the afferent arteriole of the renal glomerulus.

**jux•ta•glo•mer•u•lar cell tu•mor** a tumor of juxtaglomerular cell origin usually presenting with symptoms of secondary aldosteronism, including severe diastolic hypertension, which appears to be due to tumor-produced renin. The histologic appearance resembles that of a hemangiopericytoma.

**jux•ta•glo•mer•u•lar gran•ules** osmophilic secretory granules present in the juxtaglomerular cells, thought to contain renin.

**jux•tal•lo•cor•tex** (jŭks′tă-lō-kōr′teks) collective term for regions of the cerebral cortex between the isocortex and the allocortex.

**jux•ta•po•si•tion** (jŭks-tă-pō-zish′ŭn) a position side by side. SEE ALSO apposition, contiguity. [L. *juxta*, near to, + *positio*, a placing, fr. *pono*, pp. *positus*, to place]

j
u

# K

κ kappa. SEE kappa.

**k** 1. potassium (kalium); kelvin; lysine. **2.** OPTICS the coefficient of scleral rigidity. **3.** in contact lens fitting, the radius of curvature of the flattest meridian of the apical cornea. **4.** kilo-.

$^{39}$**K** potassium-39.

*k* rate constants.

**Kai·ser·ling fix·a·tive** (kī′zĕr-ling) a method of preserving histologic and pathologic specimens without altering the color, by immersing them in an aqueous solution of potassium nitrate, potassium acetate, and formalin.

△**kak-, kak·o-** SEE caco-.

△**kal-, kali-** potassium; sometimes improperly written as *kalio*-. [L. *kalium,* potassium]

**ka·la azar** (kah′lah ah-zahr′) SYN visceral leishmaniasis. [Hind. *kala,* black, + *azar,* poison]

**ka·le·mia** (kă-lē′mē-ă) the presence of potassium in the blood.

**ka·li·o·pe·nia** (kā′lē-ō-pē′nē-ă) insufficiency of potassium in the body. [Mod. L. *kalium,* potassium, + G. *penia,* poverty]

**ka·li·o·pe·nic** (kā′lē-ō-pē′nik) relating to kaliopenia.

**ka·li·um (k)** (kā′lē-ŭm) SYN potassium. [Mod. L. fr. Ar. *qali,* potash]

**ka·li·u·re·sis** (kā′lē-yu-rē′sis) SYN kaluresis.

**ka·li·u·ret·ic** (kā′lē-yu-ret′ik) SYN kaluretic.

**kal·lak** (kah-lak′) a pustular dermatitis observed among Eskimos. [Eskimo word meaning skin disease]

**kal·li·kre·in** (kal-i-krē′in) a group of enzymes (e.g., plasma, tissue, pancreatic, urinary, submandibular kallikrein) that can convert kininogen by proteolysis to bradykinin or kallidin; trypsin and plasmin can also effect the conversion; plasma kallikrein activates the Hageman factor and acts on kininogen. Tissue kallikrein is a serine endopeptidase that can generate kallidin from kininogen. SYN kininogenase, kininogenin.

**kal·u·re·sis** (kal-yu-rē′sis) the increased urinary excretion of potassium. SYN kaliuresis. [Mod. L. *kalium,* potassium, + G. *ourēsis,* urination]

**kal·u·ret·ic** (kal-yu-ret′ik) relating to, causing, or characterized by kaluresis. SYN kaliuretic.

**Kan·ner syn·drome** (kah′nĕr) SYN infantile autism.

**ka·od·ze·ra** (kah′od-ze′rā) a disease prevalent in Zimbabwe (formerly Rhodesia), similar to sleeping sickness, caused by *Trypanosoma rhodesiense.* SEE ALSO Rhodesian trypanosomiasis.

**ka·o·lin clot·ting time (KCT)** a sensitive test of platelet-poor plasma for detecting lupus anticoagulants in mixtures of plasmas taken from patients and from control groups; kaolin initiates clotting via the contact factors and subsequently involves the other factors in the intrinsic pathway of coagulation.

**ka·o·lin·o·sis** (kā′ō-lin-ō′sis) pneumonoconiosis caused by the inhalation of clay dust.

**Kap·lan-Mei·er a·nal·y·sis** (kap′lăn-mī′ĕr) a method of calculating survival of a patient population in which the increments are the actual survival times of the patients.

**Kap·lan-Mei·er es·ti·mate** (kap′lăn-mī′ĕr) nonparametric method of compiling life tables or survival tables that combines calculated probabilities of survival with estimates to allow for censored (missing) observations; used mainly in survival studies of cancer and similar long-term diseases.

🔲**Ka·po·si sar·co·ma** (kah-pō′sē) a multifocal malignant neoplasm of primitive vasoformative tissue, occurring in the skin and sometimes in lymph nodes or viscera, consisting of spindle cells and irregular small vascular spaces frequently infiltrated by hemosiderin-pigmented macrophages and extravasated red cells; clinically manifested by cutaneous lesions consisting of reddish-purple to dark-blue macules, plaques, or nodules; seen most commonly in men over 60 years of age and, in AIDS patients, as an opportunistic disease associated with human herpes virus 8 infection. See page B7.

**Ka·po·si var·i·cel·li·form e·rup·tion** (kah-pō′sē) a rare complication of either herpes simplex or vaccinia superimposed on atopic dermatitis, with generalized vesicles and vesicopapules and high fever.

**kap·pa** (κ) (kap′a) **1.** the 10th letter in the Greek alphabet. **2.** in chemistry, denotes the position of a substituent located on the 10th atom from the carboxyl or other functional group. **3.** a measure of the degree of nonrandom agreement between observers or measurements of the same categorical variable.

**kap·pa an·gle** the angle between the pupillary axis and the visual axis; it is positive when the pupillary axis is nasal to the visual axis, and negative when the pupillary axis is temporal to the visual axis.

**Kar·nof·sky sca·le** (kahr-nof′skē) a performance scale for rating a person's usual activities; used to evaluate a patient's progress after a therapeutic procedure.

**Kar·ta·ge·ner syn·drome** (kahr-tăg′ĕ-nĕr) complete situs inversus associated with bronchiectasis and chronic sinusitis associated with ciliary dysmotility and impaired ciliary mucus transport in the respiratory epithelium; autosomal recessive inheritance with variable penetrance. The mechanism of the reversal of laterality remains an enigma, but it appears to be strictly an abolition (indifference) of laterality rather than a true reversal.

**Kar·vo·nen meth·od** method of determining the training heart rate by adding to the resting heart rate a given percentage (60–85%) of the heart rate range (the difference between resting heart rate and maximal heart rate).

△**kar·yo-** nucleus. Cf. nucleo-. [G. *karyon,* nucleus]

**kar·y·o·cyte** (kar′ē-ō-sīt) a young, immature normoblast. [karyo- + G. *kytos,* cell]

**kar·y·o·gam·ic** (kar-ē-ō-gam′ik) relating to or marked by karyogamy.

**kar·y·og·a·my** (kar-ē-og′ă-mē) fusion of the nuclei of two cells, as occurs in fertilization or true conjugation. [karyo- + G. *gamos,* marriage]

**kar·y·o·gen·e·sis** (kar-ē-ō-jen′ē-sis) formation of the nucleus of a cell. [karyo- + G. *genesis,* production]

**kar·y·o·gen·ic** (kar-ē-ō-jen′ik) relating to karyogenesis; forming the nucleus.

**kar·y·ol·o·gy** (kar′ē-ol′o-jē) the branch of cytology that deals with the study of the cell nucleus, its organelles, structures, and functions. [karyo + -logy]

**kar·y·ol·y·sis** (kar-ē-ol′i-sis) destruction of the nucleus of a cell by swelling, with the loss of affinity of its chromatin for basic dyes. [karyo- + G. *lysis,* dissolution]

**kar·y·o·lyt·ic** (kar′ē-ō-lit′ik) relating to karyolysis.

**kar·y·o·mor·phism** (kar′ē-ō-mōr′fizm) **1.** development of the nucleus of a cell. **2.** denoting the nuclear shapes of cells, especially leukocytes. [karyo- + G. *morphē,* form]

**kar·y·on** (kar′ē-on) SYN nucleus (1). [G. *karyon,* a nut, kernel]

**kar·y·o·phage** (kar′ē-ō-fāj) an intracellular parasite that feeds on the host nucleus. [karyo- + G. *phagō,* to devour]

**kar·y·o·plast** (kar′ē-ō-plast) a cell nucleus surrounded by a narrow band of cytoplasm and a plasma membrane. [karyo- + G. *plastos,* formed]

**kar·y·o·pyk·no·sis** (kar′ē-ō-pik-nō′sis) cytologic characteristics of the superficial or cornified cells of stratified squamous epithelium in which there is shrinkage of the nuclei and condensation of the chromatin into structureless masses. [karyo- + G. *pyknos,* thick, crowded, + *-osis,* condition]

**kar·y·or·rhex·is** (kar-ē-ō-rak′sis) fragmentation of the nucleus whereby its chromatin is distributed irregularly throughout the cytoplasm; a stage of necrosis usually followed by karyolysis. [karyo- + G. *rhexis,* rupture]

**kar·y·o·some** (kar′ē-ō-sōm) a mass of chromatin often found in the interphase cell nucleus representing a more condensed zone of chromatin filaments. [karyo- + G. *sōma,* body]

**kar·y·o·type** (kar′ē-ō-tīp) the chromosome characteristics of an individual cell or of a cell line, usually presented as a systematized array of metaphase chromosomes from a photomicrograph of a single cell nucleus arranged in pairs in descending order of size and according to the position of the centromere. SYN idiogram (1). [karyo- + G. *typos,* model]

**Ka·sai op·er·a·tion** (kah′sī) SYN portoenterostomy.

**Ka·so·ker·o vi·rus** (kah′sō-ker′ō) a virus of the family Bunyaviridae causing a febrile disease in humans characterized by headache, abdominal pain, diarrhea, severe myalgia, and arthralgia. [after the Kasokero Cave in Uganda where the virus was first isolated from bats]

**Kas·ten flu·o·res·cent Feul·gen stain** (kahs′ten floo-res′ent foil′gĕn stān) a fluorescent modification of the Feulgen stain, utilizing any one of a variety of fluorescent basic dyes to which $SO_2$ is added; the brilliant fluorescence makes this method unusually sensitive and adaptable to cytofluorometric quantification of DNA.

**Kas·ten flu·o·res·cent PAS stain** (kahs′ten floo-res-ent pas stān) a fluorescent modification of the periodic acid-Schiff stain for polysaccharides which uses one of Kasten fluorescent Schiff reagents.

**Kas·ten flu·o·res·cent Schiff re·a·gents** (kahs′ ten floo-res-ent shif re-āj′ent) fluorescent analogs of Schiff reagent that are fluorescent basic dyes lacking acidic side groups and containing one or more primary amine groups; used in cytochemical detection of DNA in Kasten fluorescent Feulgen stain, polysaccharides in Kasten fluorescent PAS stain, and proteins in the ninhydrin-Schiff stain; such analogs include acriflavine, auramine O, and flavophosphine N.

**Kast syn·drome** (kăst) SYN Maffucci syndrome.

**kat** katal.

△**ka·ta-** alternative spelling for cata-; down. [G. *kata,* down]

**kat·al** (kat) (kat′ăl) unit of catalytic activity equal to one mole of product formed (or substrate consumed) per second, as of the amount of enzyme that catalyzes transformation of one mole of substrate per second.

**kath·ex·is** a rare disorder characterized by bone marrow retention of myeloid elements leading to severe peripheral neutropenia; neutrophils have a distinctly abnormal appearance; Gm-CSF levels are undetectable and administration of this substance is therapeutically effective. SYN myelokathexis.

**Ka·wa·sa·ki dis·ease, Ka·wa·sa·ki syn··drome** (kah′wah-sah′kē) a systemic vasculitis of unknown origin that occurs primarily in children under 8 years of age. Symptoms include a fever lasting more than 5 days, polymorphic rash, erythematous, dry, cracking lips; conjunctival injection, swelling of the hands and feet, irritability, adenopathy, and a perineal desquamative rash. Approximately 20% of untreated patients may develop coronary artery aneurysms. As the child recovers from the illness, thrombocytosis and peeling of the fingertips occur.

**Kay·ser-Flei·scher ring** (kī′zĕr-flī-shĕr) a greenish yellow pigmented ring encircling the cornea just within the corneoscleral margin, seen in hepatolenticular degeneration, due to copper deposited in Descemet membrane.

**Ka·zan·ji·an op·er·a·tion** (kah-zahn′jē-ăn) surgical extension of the vestibular sulcus of edentulous ridges to increase their height and to improve denture retention.

**kc** kilocycle.

**kcal** kilogram calorie; kilocalorie.

**K cells** SYN killer cells.

**KCT** kaolin clotting time.

**Kearns-Sayre syn·drome** (kernz-sār) a form of chronic progressive external ophthalmoplegia with associated cardiac conduction defects, short stature, and hearing loss; a sporadically ocurring mitochondrial myopathy presenting in childhood.

**Keat·ing-Hart meth·od** (kēt′ing-hahrt) fulguration in the treatment of external cancer or of the field of operation after the removal of a malignant growth.

**Keen op·er·a·tion** (kēn) removal of sections of the posterior branches of the spinal nerves to the affected muscles, and of the spinal accessory nerve, as a cure for torticollis.

**Keg·el ex·er·cis·es** (keg′ĕl) alternate contraction and relaxation of perineal muscles for treatment of urinary stress incontinence.

**Kehr sign** (kār) pain referred to the left border, due to splenic rupture.

**Kel·ly op·er·a·tion** (kel′ē) **1.** correction of retroversion of the uterus by plication of uterosacral ligaments. **2.** correction of urinary stress incontinence by vaginally placing sutures beneath the bladder neck.

**Kel·ly rec·tal spec·u·lum** (kel′ē) a tubular speculum with obturator for rectal examination.

**ke·loid** (kē′loyd) a nodular, firm, often linear mass of hyperplastic scar tissue, consisting of irregularly distributed bands of collagen; occurs in the dermis, usually after trauma, surgery, a burn, or severe cutaneous disease. See page B5.

k
e

[G. *kēlē*, a tumor (or *kēlis*, a spot), + *eidos*, appearance]

**ke•loi•do•sis** (kē'loy-dō'sis) multiple keloids.

**ke•lo•plas•ty** (kē'lō-plas-tē) operative removal of a scar or keloid. [keloid + G. *plastos*, formed]

**Kel•vin** (kel'vin), Lord William Thomson, Scottish physicist, 1824–1907. SEE kelvin, Kelvin scale.

**kel•vin (k)** a unit of thermodynamic temperature equal to $\frac{1}{273.16}$ of the thermodynamic temperature of the triple point of water. SEE ALSO Kelvin scale. [Lord *Kelvin*]

**Kel•vin scale** (kel'vin) temperature scale in which the triple point of water is assigned the value of 273.16 K; °C = K − 273.15. SYN absolute scale.

**Kemp ech•o** (kemp) phenomenon noted by David Kemp in 1978, i.e., that otoacoustic emissions are generated in the normal cochlea either spontaneously or in response to acoustic stimulation. SEE ALSO otoacoustic emission.

**Ken•dall** SEE Abell-Kendall method.

**Ken•ne•dy dis•ease** (ke'ne-dē) an X-linked recessive disorder characterized by progressive spinal and bulbar muscular atrophy; associated features include distal degeneration of sensory axons, and signs of endocrine dysfunction, including diabetes mellitus, gynecomastia, and testicular atrophy. SYN X-linked recessive bulbospinal neuronopathy.

**Ken•ne•dy syn•drome** (ke'ne-dē) ipsilateral optic atrophy with central scotoma and contralateral choked disk or papilledema, caused by a meningioma of the ipsilateral optic nerve. SYN Foster Kennedy syndrome.

**Ken•ny-Caf•fey syn•drome** (ken'ē-kāf'ē) a disorder characterized by intermittent hypocalcemia (associated with abnormalities in parathyroid hormone secretion) and bone and eye abnormalities; autosomal dominant and autosomal recessive forms exist.

△**ke•no-** SEE ceno- (3). [G. *kenos,* empty]

**Kent bun•dle** (kent) **1.** SYN atrioventricular bundle. **2.** a muscle fiber bundle occurring occasionally as an accessory conducting pathway between the atria and the ventricles, associated with Wolff-Parkinson-White syndrome.

**Ker•an•del sign** (ker-ahn-del') delayed sensation to pain indicative of African trypanosomiasis.

**ker•a•tan sul•fate** (ker'ă-tan) a type of sulfated mucopolysaccharide found in cartilage, bone, connective tissue, the cornea, aorta, and in the intervertebral disks; accumulates in Morquio syndrome. SYN keratosulfate.

**ker•a•tec•to•my** (ker-ă-tek'tō-mē) an operation done to change the refraction of the cornea; a crescentic piece of corneal stroma is removed and the resultant corneal wound is sutured. This steepens the cornea and increases its power in that axis. [kerato- + G. *ektomē,* excision]

**ke•rat•ic** (ke-rat'ik) SYN horny. [G. *keras* (*kerat-*), horn]

**ke•rat•ic pre•cip•i•tates** inflammatory cells on the corneal endothelium.

**ker•a•tin** (ker'ă-tin) a scleroprotein or albuminoid present in hair and nails; it contains a relatively large amount of sulfur, is insoluble in gastric juice, and is sometimes used for coating tablets that are intended to be dissolved only in the intestine. SYN cytokeratin. [G. *keras (kerat-),* horn, + -in]

**ker•a•tin•as•es** (ker'ă-tin-ās-ez) hydrolases catalyzing the hydrolysis of keratin.

**ker•a•tin•i•za•tion** (ker'ă-tin-i-zā'shŭn) keratin formation or development of a horny layer; may also apply to premature formation of keratin. SYN cornification.

**ke•rat•i•no•cyte** (ke-rat'i-nō-sīt) a cell of the living epidermis and certain oral epithelium that produces keratin in the process of differentiating into the dead and fully keratinized cells of the stratum corneum.

**ke•rat•i•no•some** (ke-rat'i-nō-sōm) a granule located in the upper layers of the stratum spinosum of certain stratified squamous epithelia. SYN membrane-coating granule.

**ke•rat•i•nous** (ke-rat'i-nŭs) **1.** relating to keratin. **2.** SYN horny.

**ke•rat•i•nous cyst** an epithelial cyst containing keratin.

**ker•a•tin pearl** a focus of central keratinization within concentric layers of abnormal squamous cells; seen in squamous cell carcinoma. SYN epithelial pearl.

**ker•a•ti•tis** (ker'ă-tī'tis) inflammation of the cornea. SEE ALSO keratopathy. [kerato- + G. *-itis,* inflammation]

△**ker•a•to-, ke•rat-** **1.** the cornea. **2.** horny tissue or cells. SEE ALSO cerat-, cerato-. [G. *keras,* horn]

▯**ker•a•to•ac•an•tho•ma** (ker'ă-tō-ak'an-thō'mă) a rapidly growing, umbilicated tumor, usually occurring on exposed areas of the skin, which invades the dermis but remains localized and usually resolves spontaneously. See page B7. [kerato- + G. *akantha,* thorn, +-*oma,* tumor]

**ker•a•to•cele** (ker'ă-tō-sēl) hernia of Descemet membrane through a defect in the outer layers of the cornea. [kerato- + G. *kēlē,* hernia]

**ker•a•to•con•junc•ti•vi•tis** (ker'ă-tō-kon-jŭngk'ti-vī'tis) inflammation of the conjunctiva and of the cornea.

**ker•a•to•con•junc•ti•vi•tis sic•ca** a chronic mucopurulent conjunctivitis, sometimes leading to corneal ulceration and scarring, due to deficit of the aqueous component of tears.

**ker•a•to•co•nus** (ker'ă-tō-kō'nŭs) a conical protrusion of the cornea caused by thinning of the stroma; usually bilateral. SEE ALSO Fleischer ring, Munson sign. SYN conical cornea. [kerato- + G. *kōnos,* cone]

**ker•a•to•cyst** (ker'ă-tō-sist) odontogenic cyst derived from remnants of the dental lamina and appearing as a unilocular or multilocular radiolucency which may produce jaw expansion; associated with the bifid rib basal cell nevus syndrome.

**ker•a•to•cyte** (ker'ă-tō-sīt) **1.** the fibroblastic stromal cell of the cornea. **2.** a variety of poikilocyte that owes its abnormal shape to fragmentation occurring as the cell flows through damaged small vessels. SYN schistocyte.

**ker•a•to•der•ma** (ker'ă-tō-der'mă) **1.** any horny superficial growth. **2.** a generalized thickening of the horny layer of the epidermis. [kerato- + G. *derma,* skin]

**ker•a•to•der•ma plan•ta•re sul•ca•tum** hyperkeratosis and fissure formation on the soles. SYN cracked heel.

**ker•a•to•ec•ta•sia** (ker'ă-tō-ek-tā'zē-ă) a bulging forward of the cornea.

**ker•a•to•ep•i•the•li•o•plas•ty** (ker'ă-tō-ep-i-thē'lē-ō-plas-tē) a surgical procedure for the repair of persistent corneal epithelial defects. Corneal epithelium is removed and small pieces of donor cornea, with epithelium attached, are placed at the corneoscleral limbus. [kerato- + epithelio- + G. *plastos*, formed]

**ker·a·tog·e·nous** (ker-ă-toj'ĕ-nŭs) causing a growth of cells that produce keratin and result in the formation of horny tissue, such as fingernails, scales, and feathers

**ker·a·tog·e·nous mem·brane** SYN nail bed.

**ker·a·to·glo·bus** (ker-ă-tō-glō'bŭs) congenital anomaly consisting of an enlarged anterior segment of the eye. SYN megalocornea. [kerato- + L. *globus*, ball]

**ker·a·to·hy·a·lin, ker·a·to·hy·a·lin gran·ules** (ker'ă-tō-hī'ă-lin) the substance in the large basophilic granules of the stratum granulosum of the epidermis. [kerato- + hyalin]

**ker·a·toid** (ker'ă-toyd) **1.** SYN horny. **2.** resembling corneal tissue. [kerato- + G. *eidos*, resemblance]

**ker·a·toid ex·an·the·ma** a symptom occurring in the secondary stage of yaws: patches of fine, light colored, furfuraceous desquamation, scattered irregularly over limbs and trunk.

**ker·a·to·lep·tyn·sis** (ker-ă-tō-lep-tin'sis) **1.** SYN gutter dystrophy of cornea. **2.** an operation for removing the surface of the cornea and replacement by bulbar conjunctiva for cosmetic reasons. [kerato- + G. *leptynsis*, a making thin]

**ker·a·to·leu·ko·ma** (ker'ă-tō-loo-kō'mă) a white corneal opacity. [kerato- + G. *leukos*, white, + -*ōma*, growth]

**ker·a·tol·y·sis** (ker-ă-tol'i-sis) **1.** separation or loosening of the horny layer of the epidermis. **2.** a disease characterized by a shedding of the epidermis recurring at more or less regular intervals. [kerato- + G. *lysis*, loosening]

**ker·a·to·lyt·ic** (ker'ă-tō-lit'ik) relating to keratolysis.

**ker·a·to·ma** (ker-ă-tō'mă) **1.** SYN callosity. **2.** a horny tumor. [kerato- + G. -*oma*, tumor]

**ker·a·to·ma·la·cia** (ker'ă-tō-mă-lā'shē-ă) dryness with ulceration and perforation of the cornea occurring in cachectic children; results from severe vitamin A deficiency. [kerato- + G. *malakia*, softness]

**ker·a·tome** (ker'ă-tōm) a knife used for incising the cornea. SYN keratotome.

**ker·a·tom·e·ter** (ker-ă-tom'ĕ-ter) an instrument for measuring the curvature of the anterior corneal surface. SYN ophthalmometer. [kerato- + G. *metron*, measure]

**ker·a·tom·e·try** (ker-ă-tom'ĕ-trē) measurement of the radii of corneal curvature.

**ker·a·to·mi·leu·sis** (ker-ă-tō-mil-oo'sis) surgical alteration of refractive error by changing the shape of a deep layer of the cornea: the anterior lamella is peeled back, frozen, and recurved on its back surface on a lathe; or, some of the corneal stroma can be removed from the bed with a laser or a knife. [fr. G. *keras* (*kerat*-), horn, cornea, + *smileusis*, carving]

**ker·a·to·path·ia** (ker'ă-tō-path'ē-ă) SYN keratopathy.

**ker·a·to·path·ia gut·ta·ta** wartlike endothelial excrescence on the posterior surface of the cornea.

**ker·a·top·a·thy** (ker-ă-top'ă-thē) any corneal disease, damage, dysfunction, or abnormality. SYN keratopathia. [kerato- + G. *pathos*, suffering, disease]

**ker·a·to·pha·kia** (ker'ă-tō-fak'ē-ă) implantation of a donor cornea or plastic lens within the corneal stroma to modify refractive error. [kerato- + G. *phakos*, lens]

**ker·a·to·plas·ty** (ker'ă-tō-plas-tē) any surgical modification of the cornea; the removal of a portion of the cornea containing an opacity and the insertion in its place of a piece of cornea of the same size and shape removed from elsewhere. SYN corneal graft. [kerato- + G. *plassō*, to form]

**ker·a·to·pros·the·sis** (ker'ă-tō-pros-thē'sis) replacement of the central area of an opacified cornea by plastic. [kerato- + G. *prosthesis*, addition]

**ker·a·to·rhex·is, ker·a·tor·rhex·is** (ker'ă-tō-rek'sis) rupture of the cornea, due to trauma or perforating ulcer. [kerato- + G. *rhēxis*, a bursting]

**ker·a·to·scle·ri·tis** (ker'ă-tō-skle-rī'tis) inflammation of both cornea and sclera.

**ker·a·to·scope** (ker'ă-tō-skōp) an instrument marked with lines or circles by means of which the corneal reflex can be observed. SYN Placido da Costa disk. [kerato- + G. *skopeō*, to examine]

**ker·a·tos·co·py** (ker-ă-tos'kŏ-pē) **1.** examination of the reflections from the anterior surface of the cornea in order to determine the character and amount of corneal astigmatism. **2.** a term first applied by Cuignet to his method of retinoscopy. [kerato- + G. *skopeō*, to examine]

**ker·a·tose** (ker'ă-tōs) keratotic, relating to or marked by keratosis.

**ker·a·to·sis**, pl. **ker·a·to·ses** (ker-ă-tō'sis, ker-ă-tō'sēz) any lesion on the epidermis marked by the presence of circumscribed overgrowths of the horny layer. [kerato- + G. -*osis*, condition]

**ker·a·to·sis fol·lic·u·la·ris** a familial eruption, beginning usually in childhood, in which keratotic papules originating from both follicles and interfollicular epidermis of the trunk, face, scalp, and axillae become crusted and verrucous; often intensely pruritic. SYN Darier disease.

**ker·a·to·sul·fate** (ker'ă-tō-sŭl-fāt) SYN keratan sulfate.

**ker·a·to·tome** (ker'ă-tō-tōm) SYN keratome.

**ker·a·tot·o·my** (ker'ă-tot'ō-mē) **1.** any incision through the cornea. **2.** an operation making a partial thickness incision into the cornea to flatten it and reduce its refractive power in that meridian. [kerato- + G. *tomē*, incision]

**Kerck·ring folds** (kerk'ring) SYN circular folds of small intestine.

**Kerck·ring valves** (kerk'ring) SYN circular folds of small intestine.

**ke·ri·on** (kē'rē-on) a granulomatous secondarily infected lesion complicating fungal infection of the hair; typically, a raised boggy lesion. [G. *kērion*, honeycomb; a skin disease, fr. *kēros*, beeswax]

**Ker·ley B lines** (ker'lē) fine peripheral septal lines.

**ker·nic·ter·us** (ker-nik'ter-ŭs) yellow staining and degenerative lesions in basal ganglia associated with high levels of unconjugated bilirubin in infants; may occur with hemolytic disorder such as Rh or ABO erythroblastosis or G6PD deficiency as well as with neonatal sepsis or Crigler-Najjar syndrome; characterized by opisthotonus, high-pitched cry, lethargy, and poor sucking, as well as abnormal or absent Moro reflex, and loss of upward gaze; later consequences include deafness, cerebral palsy, other sensorineural deficits, and mental retardation. SYN bilirubin encephalopathy, nuclear jaundice. [Ger. *Kern,* kernel (nucleus), + *Ikterus,* jaundice]

**Ker·nig sign** (ker′nig) when a subject is supine and the thigh is flexed to a right angle with the axis of the trunk, complete extension of the leg on the thigh is impossible; present in various forms of meningitis.

**Ker·no·han notch** (kĕr′nĕ-han) a notch in the cerebral peduncle caused by displacement of the brainstem against the incisura of the tentorium by a transtentorial herniation.

**ker·oid** (ker′oyd) SYN horny. [G. *keroeidēs,* hornlike]

**Kes·ten·baum num·ber** (kes′tĕn-bawm) the difference between the two pupil diameters when each eye is measured in bright light with the other eye tightly covered; an indicator of the relative afferent pupillary defect in patients with two innervated irises.

**Kes·ten·baum pro·ce·dure** (kes′tĕn-bawm) surgical procedure on the extraocular muscles indicated for patients with torticollis associated with nystagmus.

**Kes·ten·baum sign** (kes′tĕn-bawm) a decrease in the number of arterioles crossing optic disk margins as a sign of optic neuritis.

**ke·tal** (kē′tăl) a hydrated ketone in which both hydroxyl groups are esterified with alcohols.

△**ke·to-** combining form denoting a compound containing a ketone group; replaced by oxo- in systematic nomenclature. [Ger.]

**ke·to ac·id** (kē′tō as′id) an acid containing a ketone group (–CO–) in addition to the acid group(s).

**ke·to·ac·i·do·sis** (kē′tō-as-i-dō′sis) acidosis, as in diabetes or starvation, caused by the enhanced production of ketone bodies.

**ke·to·ac·i·du·ria** (kē′tō-as-id-yur′ē-ă) excretion of urine having an elevated content of ketonic acids.

**ke·to·gen·e·sis** (kē-tō-jen′ĕ-sis) metabolic production of ketones or ketone bodies.

**ke·to·gen·ic** (kē-tō-jen′ik) giving rise to ketone bodies in metabolism.

**ke·to·gen·ic di·et** a high-fat, low-carbohydrate, and normal protein diet causing ketosis.

**ke·to·hep·tose** (kē-tō-hep′tōs) a seven-carbon sugar possessing a ketone group.

**ke·to·hex·ose** (kē-tō-heks′ōs) a six-carbon sugar possessing a ketone group; e.g., fructose. SYN hexulose.

**ke·tol** (kē′tol) a ketone that has an OH group near the CO group.

**ke·tole** (kē′tōl) SYN indole (1).

**ke·tole group** carbons 1 and 2 of a 2-ketose (HOCH$_2$CO–).

**ke·to·lyt·ic** (kē-tō-lit′ik) causing the dissolution of ketone or acetone substances, referring usually to oxidation products of glucose and allied substances.

**ke·to·nae·mia [Br.]** SEE ketonemia.

**ke·tone** (kē′tōn) a substance with the carbonyl group linking two carbon atoms; the most important in medicine and the simplest in chemistry is dimethyl ketone (acetone).

**ke·tone bo·dy** one of a group of ketones that includes acetoacetic acid, β-hydroxybutyric acid, and acetone; high levels are found in tissues and body fluids in ketosis. SYN acetone body.

**ke·to·ne·mia** (kē-tō-nē′mē-ă) the presence of recognizable concentrations of ketone bodies in the plasma. [ketone + G. *haima,* blood]

**ke·ton·u·ria** (kē-tōn-yu′rē-ă) enhanced urinary excretion of ketone bodies.

**ke·tose** (kē′tōs) a carbohydrate containing the characteristic carbonyl group of the ketones.

**ke·to·sis** (kē-tō′sis) enhanced production of ketone bodies, as in diabetes mellitus or starvation. [ketone + *-osis,* condition]

**17-ke·to·ste·roids** (sev-en-tēn-kē-tō-stēr′oydz) any steroid with a ketone group on C-17; commonly used to designate urinary metabolites of androgenic and adrenocortical hormones that possess this structural feature. SYN 17-oxosteroids.

**ke·to·tic** (kē′tot-ik) pertaining to ketone bodies; presence of acidosis due to excess ketone body production such as occurs in uncontrolled insulin-dependent diabetes.

**key-in-lock ma·neu·ver** a method by which obstetrical forceps are used to rotate the fetal head.

**kg** kilogram.

🔳 **kid·ney** (kid′nē) one of the two organs that excrete the urine. The kidneys are bean-shaped organs (about 11 cm long, 5 cm wide, and 3 cm thick) lying on either side of the vertebral column, posterior to the peritoneum, about opposite the twelfth thoracic and first three lumbar vertebrae. See this page. SYN ren [TA]. [A.S. *cwith,* womb, belly, + *neere,* kidney (L. *ren,* G. *nephros*)]

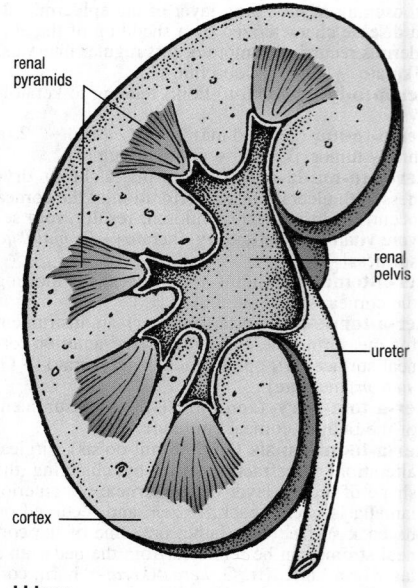

renal
pyramids

renal
pelvis

ureter

cortex

**kidney**

**Kiel clas·si·fi·ca·tion** (kēl) classification of non-Hodgkin lymphoma into low-grade malignancy (lymphocytic, lymphoplasmacytoid, centrocytic, and centroblastic-centrocytic types) and high-grade malignancy (centroblastic, lymphoblastic of Burkitt or convoluted cell, and immunoblastic types).

**Kien·böck dis·ease** (kēn'berk) osteonecrosis of the lunate bone resulting from unknown etiolgy, although can occur after trauma.

**Kien·böck dis·lo·ca·tion** (kēn'berk) dislocation of semilunar bone.

**Kier·nan space** (kēr'nĕn) interlobular space in the liver.

**Kies·sel·bach ar·ea** (kē'sĕl-bahk) an area on the anterior portion of the nasal septum rich in capillaries (Kiesselbach plexus) and often the seat of epistaxis. SYN Little area.

**Ki·ku·chi dis·ease** (kē-koo'chē) necrotizing lymphadenitis of unknown etiology, most often encountered in young women in Japan but also in other parts of the world; lymph node enlargement, associated with fever, subsides spontaneously.

**kill·er cells** cytotoxic cells involved in antibody-dependent cell-mediated immune responses. SYN K cells, null cells (1), T cytotoxic cells.

**Kil·li·an bun·dle** (kil'ē-ăn) SEE inferior constrictor muscle of pharynx.

**Kil·li·an op·er·a·tion** (kil'ē-ăn) an operation for frontal sinus disease in which the entire anterior wall is removed and the mucous membrane is curetted away; the ethmoid cells are removed through an opening in the nasal process of the maxillary bone, and the upper portion of the medial wall of the orbit is removed as well.

**Kil·li·an tri·an·gle** (kil'ē-ăn) the triangular-shaped area of the cervical esophagus, bordered by the oblique fibers of the inferior constrictor muscle of the pharynx and the transverse fibers of the cricopharyngeus muscle, through which Zenker diverticulum occurs.

△**ki·lo- (k)** prefix used in the SI and metric systems to signify one thousand ($10^3$). [French fr. G. *chilioi,* one thousand]

**kil·o·cal·o·rie (kcal)** (kil'ō-kal-ō-rē) SYN large calorie.

**kil·o·cy·cle (kc)** (kil'ō-sī-kl) one thousand cycles per second.

**kil·o·gram (kg)** (kil'ō-gram) the SI unit of mass, 1000 g; equivalent to 15,432.358 gr, 2.2046226 lb. avoirdupois, or 2.6792289 lb. troy.

**kil·o·gram cal·o·rie (kcal)** SYN large calorie.

**kil·o·gram-me·ter** the energy exerted, or work done, when a mass of 1 kg is raised a height of 1 m; equal to 9.80665 J in the SI system.

**kil·o·gram-met·re [Br.]** SEE kilogram-meter.

**kil·o·volt (kv)** (kil'ō-vōlt) a unit of electrical potential, potential difference, or electromotive force, equal to $10^3$ volts. [kilo + volt]

**kil·o·volt peak (kVp)** the highest voltage applied across an X-ray tube; it influences the penetrating power of the X-ray beam.

**Kim·mel·stiel-Wil·son syn·drome, Kim·mel·stiel-Wil·son dis·ease** (kim'ĕl-shtīl-wil'sŏn, kim'ĕl-shtīl-wil'sŏn) nephrotic syndrome and hypertension in diabetics, associated with diabetic glomerulosclerosis.

**ki·naes·the·sia [Br.]** SEE kinesthesia.

**ki·naes·thes·is [Br.]** SEE kinesthesis.

**ki·na·naes·the·sia [Br.]** SEE kinanesthesia.

**kin·an·es·the·sia** (kin-an-es-thē'zē-ă) a disturbance of deep sensibility in which there is inability to perceive either direction or extent of movement, the result being ataxia. [G. *kinēsis,* motion, + *an-* priv. + *aisthēsis,* sensation]

**ki·nase** (kī'nās) **1.** an enzyme catalyzing the conversion of a proenzyme to an active enzyme. **2.**

an enzyme catalyzing the transfer of phosphate groups to form triphosphates (e.g., ATP).

**kin·dred** an aggregate of genetically related persons; distinguished from pedigree, which is a stylized representation of a kindred. [O.E. *kynrēde,* fr. *cyn,* kin, + *rēde,* condition]

**kin·e·mat·ic chain** a combination of several joints linking several limb segments together during a specific movement or posture.

**kin·e·mat·ics** (kin-ĕ-mat'iks) PHYSIOLOGY the science concerned with movements of the parts of the body. [G. *kinēmatica,* things that move]

**kin·e·mat·ic vis·cos·i·ty** (v, υ) a measure used in studies of fluid flow; the dynamic viscosity, μ, in poises divided by the density of the material; units: stokes.

**kin·e·plas·tics** (kin'ĕ-plas-tiks) SYN cineplastic amputation.

**kin·e·sal·gia, ki·ne·si·al·gia** (kin-ĕ-sal'jē-ă, ki-nē-sē-al'jē-ă) pain caused by muscular movement. [G. *kinēsis,* motion, + *algos,* pain]

△**kin·e·si-, kin·e·si·o-, ki·ne·so-** motion. [G. *kinēsis*]

**ki·ne·sia** (ki-nē'sē-ă) SYN motion sickness. [G. *kinēsis,* movement]

**ki·ne·si·at·rics** (ki-nē'sē-at'riks) SYN kinesitherapy. [G. *kinēsis,* movement, + *iatrikos,* relating to medicine]

**ki·ne·sics** (ki-nē'siks) the study of nonverbal, bodily motion in communication.

**ki·ne·sim·e·ter** (kin-ĕ-sim'ĕ-ter) an instrument for measuring the extent of a movement. SYN kinesiometer. [G. *kinēsis,* movement, + *metron,* measure]

**ki·ne·si·ol·o·gy** (ki-nē-sē-ol'ō-jē) the science or the study of movement, and the active and passive structures involved. [G. *kinēsis,* movement, + *-logos,* study]

**ki·ne·si·om·e·ter** (ki-nē-sē-om'ĕ-ter) SYN kinesimeter.

**ki·ne·sis** (ki-nē'sis) motion; as a termination, used to denote movement or activation, particularly the kind induced by a stimulus. [G.]

**ki·ne·si·ther·a·py** (ki-nē-si-thār'ă-pē) physical therapy involving motion and range of motion exercises. SEE movement. SYN kinesiatrics.

**kin·es·the·sia, kin·es·the·sis** (kin'es-thē'zē-ă, kin-ĕs-the'sis) **1.** the sense perception of movement; the muscular sense. **2.** an illusion of moving in space. [G. *kinēsis,* motion, + *aisthēsis,* sensation]

**kin·es·the·si·om·e·ter** (kin'es-thē'zē-om'ĕ-ter) an instrument for determining the degree of muscular sensation. [kinesthesia, + G. *metron,* measure]

**kin·es·thet·ic** (kin-es-thet'ik) relating to kinesthesia.

**kin·es·thet·ic a·ware·ness** SYN body scheme.

**kin·es·thet·ic sense** SYN myesthesia.

**ki·net·ic** (ki-net'ik) relating to motion or movement. [G. *kinētikos,* of motion, fr. *kinētos,* moving]

**ki·net·ic en·er·gy** the energy of motion.

**ki·net·ics** (ki-net'iks) the study of motion, acceleration, or rate of change.

△**ki·ne·to-** motion. [G. *kinētos,* moving, movable]

**ki·ne·to·car·di·o·gram** (ki-net'ō-kar'dē-ō-gram) one type of graphic recording of the vibrations of the chest wall produced by cardiac activity.

**ki·ne·to·car·di·o·graph** (ki-net'ō-kar'dē-ō-graf) a device for recording precordial impulses due to

k
i

cardiac movement; the absolute displacement of a point on the chest wall is recorded relative to a fixed reference point above the recumbent patient.

**ki·ne·to·chore** (ki-net′ō-kōr) the structural portion of the chromosome to which microtubules attach. Cf. centromere. [kineto- + G. *chōra,* space]

**ki·ne·to·gen·ic** (ki-net-ō-jen′ik) causing or producing motion.

**ki·ne·to·plast** (ki-net′ō-plast) an intensely staining extranuclear DNA structure found in parasitic flagellates near the base of the flagellum. Electron micrographs show it to be part of a single giant mitochondrion filling most of the cytoplasm of amastigote flagellates. SEE ALSO parabasal body. [kineto- + G. *plastos,* formed]

***Kin·gel·la*** (kin-jel′ah) newly recognized member of the family Neisseriaceae; a Gram-negative coccus with a requirement of enhanced carbon dioxide for recovery in culture.

***Kin·gel·la in·do·log·e·nes*** a species that causes eye infections or endocarditis (when prosthetic heart valves are present) in humans.

***Kin·gel·la kin·gae*** a species that causes endocarditis in humans. SEE HACEK group.

**ki·nin** (kī′nin) one of a number of differing substances having pronounced physiological effects. Some are polypeptides, formed in blood in various pathological processes, that stimulate visceral smooth muscle but relax vascular smooth muscle, thus producing vasodilation. [G. *kineō,* to move, + -in]

**ki·nin·o·gen** (kī-nin′ō-jen) the globulin precursor of a (plasma) kinin.

**ki·nin·o·ge·nase** (kī-nin′ō-jĕ-nās) SYN kallikrein.

**ki·nin·o·gen·in** (kī-nin′ō-jen-in) SYN kallikrein.

**kink** an angulation, bend, or twist.

**kin·ky-hair dis·ease** an inborn error of copper metabolism with onset within a few weeks of birth; manifested by short, sparse, poorly pigmented kinky hair; failure to thrive; development of seizures; spasticity; and progressive mental deterioration leading to death. X-linked recessive inheritance due to a defect of copper transport, caused by mutation in the Menkes gene (MNK), which encodes a copper-transporting ATPase on Xq. SYN Menkes syndrome.

△**ki·no-** movement. [G. *kineō,* to move]

**ki·no·cil·i·um** (kī-nō-sil′ē-ŭm) a cilium, usually motile, having nine peripheral double microtubules and two single central ones. [kino- + cilium]

**kin·ship** the state of being genetically related.

**Kirk am·pu·ta·tion** (kĭrk) amputation at the lower end of the femur, using the tendon of the quadriceps extensor to cover the end of the bone.

**Kirsch·ner wire** (kirsh′nĕr) an apparatus for skeletal traction in long bone fracture or for fracture fixation.

**Kisch re·flex** (kish) closure of the eye in response to stimulation of the skin at the depth of the external auditory meatus.

**kis·sing punc·ta** a condition in which the upper punctum is apposed to the lower punctum when the eyes are open.

**Ki·ta·sa·to ba·cil·lus** (kit-ah-sah′tō) SYN *Yersinia pestis.*

**Kjel·land for·ceps** (kyel′ĕnd) an obstetrical forceps having a sliding lock, and little pelvic curve.

**Kjer op·tic at·ro·phy** (kyer) SYN dominant optic atrophy.

***Kleb·si·el·la*** (kleb-sē-el′ă) a genus of aerobic, facultatively anaerobic, nonmotile, nonsporeforming bacteria (family Enterobacteriaceae) containing Gram-negative, encapsulated rods which occur singly, in pairs, or in short chains. These organisms produce acetylmethylcarbinol and lysine decarboxylase or ornithine decarboxylase. They do not usually liquefy gelatin. Citrate and glucose are ordinarily used as sole carbon sources. These organisms may or may not be pathogenic. They occur in the respiratory, intestinal, and urogenital tracts of man as well as in soil, water, and grain. The type species is *Klebsiella pneumoniae.* [E. *Klebs*]

***Kleb·si·el·la ox·y·to·ca*** a species characterized by its ability to produce indole. Clinically it resembles *Klebsiella pneumoniae;* however, nosocomial strains exhibit a greater propensity to develop antibiotic resistance.

***Kleb·si·el·la pneu·mo·ni·ae*** a species found in soil and water, on grain, and in the intestinal tract of humans and other animals; it also occurs in association with several pathologic conditions, urinary tract infections, sputum, feces, and metritis in mares; capsular types 1, 2, and 3 of this organism may be causative agents in pneumonia; organisms previously identified as nonmotile strains of *Aerobacter aerogenes* are now placed in this species; it is the type species of *Klebsiella.* SYN Friedländer bacillus.

**Klei·hau·er-Bet·ke tech·nique** (klī′haw-er-bet′kĕ) procedure used to determine the concentration of fetal cells in maternal circulation.

**Klei·hau·er stain** (klī′haw-ĕr) a combination of aniline blue and Biebrich scarlet red used for detection of fetal cells in the maternal blood.

**klep·to·ma·nia** (klep-tō-mā′nē-ă) a disorder of impulse control characterized by a morbid tendency to steal. [G. *kleptō,* to steal, + *mania,* insanity]

**klep·to·ma·ni·ac** (klep-tō-mā′nē-ak) a person exhibiting kleptomania.

**Kline·fel·ter syn·drome** (klīn′fel-tĕr) a chromosomal anomaly with chromosome count 47, XXY sex chromosome constitution; patients are male in development but have seminiferous tubule dysgenesis, elevated urinary gonadotropins, gynecomastia, and eunuchoid habitus. SYN XXY syndrome.

**Klump·ke pal·sy, Klump·ke pa·ral·y·sis** (kloomp-kē) a type of brachial birth palsy in which there is paralysis of the muscles of the distal forearm and hand (all ulnar innervated muscles, plus more distal radial and median-innervated muscles), due to a lesion of the lower trunk of the brachial plexus, or of the C8 and T1 cervical roots.

**Knapp streaks** (nahp) SYN angioid streaks.

**Knapp stri·ae** (nahp) SYN angioid streaks.

**knee** (nē) **1.** SYN genu (1). **2.** any structure of angular shape resembling a flexed knee. [A.S. *cneōw*]

**knee-ank·le-foot orth·o·sis** an orthosis extending from the upper portion of the thigh, crossing the knee and ankle, and terminating at the toes; designed to control knee and ankle motion.

**knee-cap** (nē′kap) SYN patella.

**knee-chest po·si·tion** a prone posture resting on the knees and upper part of the chest, assumed for gynecologic or rectal examination. SYN genupectoral position.

**knee com·plex** the tibiofemoral joint, the patellofemoral joint, and related musculature and connective tissue. SEE ALSO patellofemoral joint.

**knee dis·ar·tic·u·la·tion am·pu·ta·tion** SYN Callander amputation.

**knee-el·bow po·si·tion** a prone position resting on the knees and elbows, assumed for gynecologic or rectal examination or operation. SYN genucubital position.

**knee-jerk re·flex** SYN patellar reflex.

**knee joint** a compound condylar synovial joint consisting of the joint between the condyles of the femur and the condyles of the tibia, articular menisci (semilunar cartilages) being interposed, and the articulation between femur and patella.

**knee pre·sen·ta·tion** SEE breech presentation.

**knee re·flex** SYN patellar reflex.

**knife,** pl. **knives** (nīf, nīvz) a cutting instrument used in surgery and dissection. [M.E. *knif,* fr. A.S. *cnif,* fr. O. Norse *knīfr*]

**knit·ting** (nit′ing) nonmedical term denoting the process of union of the fragments of a broken bone or of the edges of a wound. [M.E., *knitten,* to knot, fr. A.S. *cnyttan*]

**knob** (nob) a protuberance; a mass; a nodule.

**knock-knee** (nok′nē) SYN genu valgum.

**knock-out** (nok′out) a genetically engineered organism in which the genome has been altered by site-directed recombination so that a gene is deleted.

**knock·out mouse** a mouse from whose genome a single gene has been artificially deleted.

**Knoop the·o·ry** (noop) that the catabolism of fatty acids occurs in stages in each of which there is a loss of two carbon atoms as a result of oxidation at the β-carbon atom, e.g.,

**knot** (not) **1.** a compact intertwining of two or more cords or cord-like structures in such a way that they cannot spontaneously become separated; or a similar twining or infolding of a single cord on itself. **2.** ANATOMY, PATHOLOGY a node, ganglion, or circumscribed swelling suggestive of a knot. [A.S. *cnotta*]

**Knott tech·nique** (not) concentration procedure using blood and dilute formalin; designed to detect microfilaria.

**knuck·le** (nŭk′l) **1.** a joint of a finger when the fist is closed, especially a metacarpophalangeal joint. **2.** a kink or loop of intestine, as in a hernia. [M.E. *knokel*]

**knuck·le pads 1.** an autosomal dominant trait, in which thick pads of skin appear over the proximal phalangeal joints; occasionally associated with leukonychia and deafness or Dupuytren contracture; **2.** calluses of the knuckles formed as a result of occupational or self-inflicted trauma.

**Knud·sen hy·po·the·sis** (nood′sĕn) an explanation for the bilateral (and earlier) occurrence of hereditary retinoblastoma; if one tumor suppressor gene is mutated by inheritance, only one somatic mutation is needed inactivate the other allele. In the sporadic form, two mutations, which inactivate each allele, are necessary.

**Kob·ber·ling-Dun·ni·gan syn·drome** (kob′ĕrling-dun′i-găn) SYN familial partial lipodystrophy.

**Ko·belt tu·bules** (kō′bĕlt) remnants of the mesonephric tubules in the female, contained within the epoöphoron.

**Koch ba·cil·lus** (kahk) SYN Mycobacterium tuberculosis.

**Ko·cher in·ci·sion** (kō′kĕr) an incision several inches below and parallel with the right costal margin.

**Ko·cher sign** (kō′kĕr) in Graves disease, on upward gaze, the globe lags behind the movement of the upper eyelid.

**Koch law** (kahk) SYN Koch postulate.

**Koch old tu·ber·cu·lin** (kahk) SEE tuberculin (1).

**Koch phe·nom·e·non** (kahk) **1.** the phenomenon of infection immunity; living tubercle bacilli (*Mycobacterium tuberculosis*) do not cause reinfection when inoculated into tuberculous guinea pigs (i.e., the animals are "immune" to reinfection) even though the original infections continue to develop and eventually cause death of the animals; **2.** rise of temperature and increase of the local lesion, in a tuberculous subject, following an injection of tuberculin.

**Koch pos·tu·late** (kahk) to establish the specificity of a pathogenic microorganism, it must be present in all cases of the disease, inoculations of its pure cultures must produce disease in animals, and from these it must be again obtained and be propagated in pure cultures. SYN Koch law.

**Koch tri·an·gle** (kahk) a triangular area of the wall of the right atrium of the heart, which marks the approximate situation of the atrioventricular node.

**Koch-Weeks ba·cil·lus** (kahk-wēks) SYN Haemophilus aegyptius.

**Kock pouch** (kŏk) a continent ileostomy with a reservoir and valved opening fashioned from doubled loops of ileum.

**Köhler dis·ease** (kĕr′lĕr) osteonecrosis of the tarsal navicular bone or of the patella.

**koi·lo·cyte** (koy′lō-sīt) a squamous cell, often binucleated, showing a perinuclear halo; characteristic of condyloma acuminatum. [G. *koilos,* hollow, + *kytos,* cell]

**koi·lo·cy·to·sis** (koy′lō-sī-tō′sis) perinuclear vacuolation. SEE ALSO koilocyte. [G. *koilos,* hollow, + *kytos,* cell, + -*osis,* condition]

**koi·lo·nych·ia** (koy-lō-nik′ē-ă) a malformation of the nails in which the outer surface is concave; often associated with iron deficiency or softening by occupational contact with oils. SYN spoon nail. [G. *koilos,* hollow, + *onyx* (*onych-*), nail]

**kok dis·ease** SYN hyperekplexia.

**Ko·ko·skin stain** (kō-kŏs′kin) a modified trichrome stain for microsporidian spores in which heat is used to shorten the staining times.

**Koll·mann di·la·tor** (kawl′mahn) a metallic expandable instrument used to dilate urethral strictures.

△**kolp-** SEE colpo-.

**ko·lyt·ic** (kō-lit′ik) denoting an inhibitory action. [G. *kolyō,* to hinder]

**Kom·mer·ell di·ver·tic·u·lum** (kŏm′ĕr-ĕl) not a true diverticulum, but a bulblike swelling at the origin of the left subclavian artery due to a remnant of the left fourth aortic arch; associated vascular ring compression syndromes involve persistent right aortic arch; the left subclavian artery may pass behind the esophagus; the diverticulum may be large enough to compress the trachea and esophagus even after the vascular ring has been divided and may need to be resected or affixed to the chest wall or vertebral fascia.

k
o

**Kon·do·le·on op·er·a·tion** (kon-dō'lā-ĕn) excision of strips of subcutaneous connective tissue for the relief of elephantiasis.

**ko·ni·o·cor·tex** (kō'nē-ō-kōr'teks) regions of the cerebral cortex characterized by a particularly well developed inner granular layer (layer 4); this type of cerebral cortex is represented by the primary sensory area 17 of the visual cortex, areas 1 to 3 of the somatic sensory cortex, and area 41 of the auditory cortex. SEE ALSO cerebral cortex. [G. *konis*, dust, + L. *cortex*, bark]

**kon·zo** (kon'zō) a cyanide-caused upper motor neuron disease manifested principally as spastic paraplegia, seen in Africa, and resulting from the consumption of improperly prepared cassava roots, which contain high concentrations of cyanogenetic glucosides. [Yaka, tired legs]

**Kop·lik spots** (kop'lik) small red spots on the buccal mucous membrane, in the center of each of which may be seen, in a strong light, a minute bluish white speck; they occur early in measles (morbilli), before the skin eruption, and are regarded as a pathognomonic sign of the disease.

△**kop·ro-** SEE copro-.

**Ko·re·an hem·or·rhag·ic fe·ver, Ko·re·an hem·or·rhag·ic fe·ver vi·rus** (kōr'ē-en) a form of epidemic hemorrhagic fever caused by the Hantaan virus.

**Ko·rot·koff sounds** (kĕ-rot-kof') sounds heard during blood pressure determination. Sounds originating within the blood passing through the vessel or produced by a vibrating motion of the arterial wall.

**Ko·rot·koff test** (kĕ-rot-kof') a test of collateral circulation; while the artery above an aneurysm is compressed, the blood pressure in the distal circulation is estimated; if it is fairly high, the collateral circulation is good.

**Kor·sa·koff syn·drome** (kor-sĕ-kŏf) an alcohol amnestic syndrome characterized by confusion and severe impairment of memory, especially for recent events, for which the patient compensates by confabulation; typically encountered in chronic alcoholics; delirium tremens may precede the syndrome, and Wernicke syndrome often coexists; the precise pathogenesis is uncertain, but direct toxic effects of alcohol are probably less important than severe nutritional deficiencies often associated with chronic alcoholism. SYN amnestic syndrome (1), polyneuritic psychosis.

**Kr** krypton.

**Kras·ke op·er·a·tion** (krahs'kĕ) removal of the coccyx and excision of the left wing of the sacrum to afford approach for resection of the rectum for cancer or stenosis.

**krau·ro·sis vul·vae** (kraw-rō'sis vŭl'vē) atrophy and shrinkage of the epithelium of the vagina and vulva, often accompanied by a chronic inflammatory reaction in the deeper tissues, as in lichen sclerosus. [G. *krauros*, dry, brittle]

**Krau·se end bulb** (krou'zĕ) nerve terminals in skin, mouth, conjunctiva, and other parts, consisting of a laminated capsule of connective tissue enclosing the terminal, branched, convoluted ending of an afferent nerve fiber; generally believed to be sensitive to cold.

**Krebs cy·cle** (krebz) SYN tricarboxylic acid cycle.

**Krebs-Hen·se·leit cy·cle, Krebs or·ni·thine cy·cle, Krebs u·re·a cy·cle** (krebz-hen-sĕl-īt) SYN urea cycle.

**kri·ging** (krī'jing) a method first used in the earth sciences to smooth data from spatially scattered point measurements, used in geographic epidemiology. [D. G. *Krige*, South African engineer]

**Krim·sky test** (krim'skē) a test of binocular motor alignment by which a penlight is shone at the eyes and the position of the light reflex centered with a prism, thus indicating the amount of deviation.

**krin·gle** (kring'gl) a structural motif or domain seen in certain proteins in which a fold of large loops is stabilized by disulfide bonds; an important structural feature in blood coagulation factors. [Ger. *Kringel*, curl]

**Kro·nec·ker stain** (krō'nek-ĕr) a 5% sodium chloride stain rendered faintly alkaline with sodium carbonate, used in the examination of fresh tissues under the microscope.

**Krö·nig isth·mus** (krĕr'nig) the narrow straplike portion of the resonant field that extends over the shoulder, connecting the larger areas of resonance over the pulmonary apex in front and behind.

**Krönig steps** (krĕr'nig) extension of the lower part of the right border of absolute cardiac dullness in hypertrophy of the right heart.

**Kru·ken·berg am·pu·ta·tion** (kroo'kĕn-berg) a cineplastic amputation at the carpus with the distal end of the forearm used to create a fork-like stump; especially valuable in the blind because the stump has proprioception.

**Kru·ken·berg spin·dle** (kroo'kĕn-berg) a vertical fusiform area of melanin pigmentation on the posterior surface of the central cornea.

**Kru·ken·berg tu·mor** (kroo'kĕn-berg) a metastatic carcinoma of the ovary, usually bilateral and secondary to a mucous carcinoma of the stomach, which contains signet-ring cells filled with mucus.

**Kru·ken·berg veins** (kroo'kĕn-berg) SYN central veins of liver.

**Kru·se brush** (kroo'sĕ) a bunch of fine platinum wires attached to a holder; used in bacteriological work to spread material over the surface of a culture medium.

△**kry·mo-, kry·o-** SEE crymo-, cryo-.

**kryp·ton (Kr)** (krip'ton) one of the inert gases, present in small amounts in the atmosphere (1.14 ppm by dry volume); atomic no. 36, atomic wt. 83.80; $^{85}$Kr has been used in studies of cardiac abnormalities. [G. *kryptos,* concealed]

**kryp·ton la·ser** laser used for ophthalmic procedures, particularly retinal photocoagulation in the presence of vitreous hemorrhage, consisting of photons in the red (647 nm) spectrum.

**KTP la·ser** laser in the blue-green to green (532 nm) spectrum, used for hemostasis; produced by doubling the frequency of an Nd:YAG laser by passing the beam through a KTP crystal. [*K* (potassium) *T*itanyl *P*hosphate]

**Küh·ne fi·ber** (kē'nĕ) artificial muscle fiber made by filling the intestine of an insect with a growth of myxomycetes; used to demonstrate the contractility of protoplasm.

**Küh·ne meth·yl·ene blue** (kē'nĕ) methylene blue in absolute alcohol and phenol solution.

**Küh·ne phe·nom·e·non** (kē'nĕ) when a constant current is passed through a muscle, an undulation is seen to pass from the positive to the negative pole.

**Küh·ne plate** (kē'nĕ) the endplate of a motor nerve fiber in a muscle spindle.

**Kuhnt spac·es** (koont) shallow diverticula or recesses between the ciliary body and ciliary zonule that open into the posterior chamber of the eye.

**Kupf·fer cells** (koop'fĕr) phagocytic cells of the mononuclear phagocyte series found on the luminal surface of the hepatic sinusoids.

**Kür·stei·ner ca·nals** (kĕr-shtīn'ĕr) a fetal complex of vesicular, canalicular, and glandlike structures derived from parathyroid or thymus; normally remain rudimentary but may persist postnatally as cystic structures.

**Kurtz·ke mul·ti·ple scle·ro·sis dis·a·bil·i·ty scale** (kertz'kĕ) SYN expanded disability status scale.

**ku·ru** (koo'roo) a progressive, fatal form of spongiform encephalopathy, endemic in New Guinea and caused by prions. Transmission is believed to occur through ritual cannibalism. SEE prion. [native dialect, to shiver from fear or cold]

**Kuss·maul res·pi·ra·tion** (koos'mawl) deep, rapid respiration characteristic of diabetic or other causes of acidosis.

**Kuss·maul sign** (koos'mawl) in constrictive pericarditis, a paradoxical increase in venous distention and pressure or failure to collapse during inspiration; seen occasionally in effusive-constrictive pericarditis when tamponading pericardial fluid overlies a constricting epicardium.

**kv** kilovolt.

**Kveim an·ti·gen** (kvīm) a saline suspension of human sarcoid tissue prepared from the spleen of an individual with active sarcoidosis; used in the Kveim test.

**Kveim test** (kvīm) an intradermal test for the detection of sarcoidosis, done by injecting Kveim antigen (obtained from spleens of persons with sarcoidosis) and examining skin biopsies after three and six weeks; a positive test is indicated by typical nodules showing evidence of sarcoid tissue.

**kVp** (**kil·o·volt peak**) kilovolt peak, the highest instantaneous energy across an x-ray tube, corresponding to the highest energy x-rays emitted.

**kwa·shi·or·kor** (kwah-shē-ōr'kōr) a disease seen in African children one to three years old, due to dietary deficiency, particularly of protein; characterized by marked hypoalbuminemia, anemia, edema, pot belly, depigmentation of the skin, loss of hair or change in hair color to red, and bulky stools containing undigested food. [Native, red boy or displaced child]

△**ky-** for words beginning thus and not found below, see cy-.

**ky·ma·tism** (kī'mă-tizm) SYN myokymia. [G. *kyma*, wave]

**ky·mo·gram** (kī'mō-gram) the graphic curve made by a kymograph.

**ky·mo·graph** (kī'mō-graf) an instrument for recording wavelike motions or modulation; it consists of a drum revolved by clockwork and covered smoked paper upon which the curve is inscribed by writing point. [G. *kyma*, wave, + *graphō*, to record]

**ky·mog·ra·phy** (kī-mog'ră-fē) use of the kymograph.

**kyn·u·ren·ic ac·id** (kin-yu-rē'nik as'id) a product of the metabolism of L-tryptophan; appears in urine in pyridoxine deficiency.

**kyn·u·ren·ine** (kin-yu'rĕ-nēn) a product of the metabolism of L-tryptophan, excreted in the urine.

**ky·phos** (kī'fos) a hump, the convex prominence in kyphosis.

**ky·pho·sco·li·o·sis** (kī'fō-skō-lē-ō'sis) kyphosis combined with scoliosis; congestive heart failure is a late complication.

**ky·pho·sis** (kī-fō'sis) **1.** an anteriorly concave curvature of the vertebral column, such as occurs normally in the thoracic and sacral regions. **2.** an abnormal exaggeration of the normal forward (flexion) curvature of the thoracic spine. See page 923. [G. *kyphōsis*, hump-back, fr. *kyphos*, bent, hump-backed]

**ky·phot·ic** (kī-fot'ik) relating to or suffering from kyphosis.

**ky·phot·ic pel·vis** backward curvature of the lumbar spine causing contraction of pelvic measurements.

△**ky·to-** SEE cyto-.

k
y

# L

Λ, λ lambda.

*L* linking number.

l liter.

△l- prefix indicating a chemical compound to be structurally (sterically) related to L-glyceraldehyde. Cf. D-.

△l- levorotatory. Cf. *d*-. [L. *laevus,* on the left-hand side]

**La** lanthanum.

**La·band syn·drome** (lă-band′) fibromatosis of the gingivae associated with hypoplasia of the distal phalanges, nail dysplasia, joint hypermotility, and sometimes hepatosplenomegaly; autosomal dominant inheritance.

**la·bel 1.** to incorporate into a compound a substance that is readily detected, such as a radionuclide, whereby its metabolism can be followed or its physical distribution detected. **2.** the substance so incorporated.

**la belle in·dif·fér·ence** (lah bel an-dif-er-ahns′) a naive, inappropriate lack of emotion or concern for the perceptions by others of one's disability, typically seen in persons with conversion hysteria. [Fr.]

**la·bia** (lā′bē-ă) plural of labium.

**la·bi·al** (lā′bē-ăl) **1.** relating to the lips or any labium. **2.** toward a lip. **3.** one of the letters formed by means of the lips. [L. *labium,* lip]

**la·bi·al branch·es of men·tal nerve** branches of mental nerve to lower lip.

**la·bi·al her·nia** hernia through the canal of Nuck.

**la·bi·al splint** an appliance of plastic, metal, or in combination, made to conform to the outer aspect of the dental arch and used in the management of jaw and facial injuries.

**la·bile** (lā′bīl, lā′-bil) unstable; unsteady, not fixed; denoting: **1.** an adaptability to alteration or modification, i.e., relatively easily changed or rearranged. **2.** constituents of serum affected by increases in heat. **3.** an electrode that is kept moving over the surface during the passage of an electric current. **4.** PSYCHOLOGY free and uncontrolled mood or behavioral expression of the emotions. **5.** easily removable; e.g., a labile hydrogen atom. [L. *labilis,* liable to slip, fr. *labor,* pp. *lapsus,* to slip]

**la·bil·i·ty** (lă-bil′i-tē) the state of being labile.

△**la·bi·o-** the lips. SEE ALSO cheilo-. [L. *labium,* lip]

**la·bi·o·cer·vi·cal** (lā′bē-ō-ser′vi-kăl) relating to a lip and a neck; specifically, to the labial or buccal surface of the neck of a tooth. [labio- + L. *cervix,* neck]

**la·bi·o·cho·rea** (lā-bē-ō-kōr-ē′ă) a chronic spasm of the lips, interfering with speech. [labio- + G. *choreia,* dance]

**la·bi·o·cli·na·tion** (lā′bē-ō-kli-nā′shŭn) inclination of position more toward the lips than is normal; said of a tooth.

**la·bi·o·den·tal** (lā-bē-ō-den′tăl) relating to the lips and the teeth; denoting certain letters the sound of which is formed by both lips and teeth. [labio- + L. *dens,* tooth]

**la·bi·o·gin·gi·val** (lā′bē-ō-jin′ji-văl) relating to the point of junction of the labial border and the gingival line on the distal or mesial surface of an incisor tooth.

**la·bi·o·graph** (lā′bē-ō-graf) an instrument for recording the movements of the lips in speaking. [labio- + G. *graphō,* to record]

**la·bi·o·men·tal** (lā′bē-ō-men′tăl) relating to the lower lip and the chin. [labio- + L. *mentum,* chin]

**la·bi·o·na·sal** (lā′bē-ō-nā′săl) **1.** relating to the upper lip and the nose, or to both lips and the nose. **2.** denoting a letter which is both labial and nasal in the production of its sound.

**la·bi·o·pal·a·tine** (lā′bē-ō-pal′ă-tīn) relating to the lips and the palate.

**la·bi·o·place·ment** (lā′bē-ō-plās′ment) positioning (e.g., of a tooth) more toward the lips than normal.

**la·bi·o·plas·ty** (lā′bē-ō-plas-tē) plastic surgery of a lip. [labio- + G. *plastos,* formed]

**la·bi·o·ver·sion** (lā′bē-ō-ver-zhŭn) malposition of an anterior tooth from the normal line of occlusion toward the lips.

**la·bi·um,** gen. **la·bii,** pl. **la·bia** (lā′bē-ŭm, lā′bē-ī, lā′bē-ă) [TA] **1.** SYN lip. **2.** any lip-shaped structure. [L.]

**la·bi·um ma·jus** one of two rounded folds of integument forming the lateral boundaries of the pudendal cleft. The labia majora are the female homolog of the scrotum.

**la·bi·um mi·nus** one of two narrow longitudinal folds of mucous membrane enclosed in the pudendal cleft within the labia majora; posteriorly, they gradually merge into the labia majora and join to form the frenulum labiorum pudendi (fourchette); anteriorly, each labium divides into two portions which unite with those of the opposite side in front of the glans clitoridis to form the prepuce.

**la·bor** (lā′bŏr) the process of expulsion of the fetus and the placenta from the uterus. The stages of labor are: **first stage,** beginning with the onset of uterine contractions through the period of dilation of the os uteri; **second stage,** the period of expulsive effort, beginning with complete dilation of the cervix and ending with expulsion of the infant; **third stage,** or **placental stage,** the period beginning at the expulsion of the infant and ending with the completed expulsion of the placenta and membranes. [L. toil, suffering]

**lab·o·ra·tory** (lab′ŏ-ră-tō-rē) a place equipped for the performance of tests, experiments, and investigative procedures and for the preparation of reagents, therapeutic chemical materials, and so on. [Mediev. L. *laboratorium,* a workplace, fr. L. *laboro,* pp. *-atus,* to labor]

**lab·o·ra·tory di·ag·no·sis** a diagnosis made by a chemical, microscopic, microbiologic, immunologic, or pathologic study of secretions, discharges, blood, or tissue.

**la·bor curve** SYN partogram.

**la·bor pains** rhythmical uterine contractions which under normal conditions increase in intensity, frequency, and duration, culminating in vaginal delivery of the infant.

**la·bour [Br.]** SEE labor.

**la·brum,** pl. **la·bra** (lā′brŭm, lā′bră) [TA] **1.** a lip. **2.** a lip-shaped structure. [L.]

**lab·y·rinth** (lab′i-rinth) any of several anatomic structures with numerous intercommunicating cells or canals. **1.** the internal or inner ear, composed of the semicircular ducts, vestibule, and cochlea. **2.** any group of communicating cavities, as in each lateral mass of the ethmoid bone. **3.** a group of communicating culture tubes used for separating motile from nonmotile microorganisms.

**lab·y·rin·thec·to·my** (lab-ĭ-rin-thek′tō-mē) excision of the labyrinth; a destructive operation to destroy labyrinthine function. [labyrinth + G. *ektomē*, excision]

**lab·y·rin·thine** (lab-ĭ-rin′thin) relating to any labyrinth.

**lab·y·rin·thine ar·tery** internal acoustic meatal branch, a branch of the basilar artery that enters the labyrinth through the internal acoustic meatus.

**lab·y·rin·thine fis·tu·la** a fistula between a fluid-filled compartment of the inner ear and another fluid-filled compartment in the inner ear (internal) or a space external to the inner ear as the middle ear or mastoid air cells or subarachnoid space (external); it may result in auditory and vestibular disturbances, depending on its location.

**lab·y·rin·thine nys·tag·mus** SYN vestibular nystagmus.

**lab·y·rin·thine veins** one or more veins accompanying the labyrinthine artery; they drain the internal ear, pass out through the internal acoustic meatus, and empty into the transverse sinus or the inferior petrosal sinus. SYN internal auditory veins.

**lab·y·rin·thine ver·ti·go** SYN Ménière disease.

**lab·y·rin·thi·tis** (lab′ĭ-rin-thī′tis) inflammation of the labyrinth (the internal ear), sometimes accompanied by vertigo and deafness. SYN otitis interna.

**lab·y·rin·thot·o·my** (lab-ĭ-rin-thot′ō-mē) incision into the labyrinth. [labyrinth + G. *tomē*, incision]

**lac·er·at·ed** (las′er-ā-ted) torn; rent; having a ragged edge. [L. *lacero*, pp. *-atus*, to tear to pieces]

**lac·er·a·tion** (las-er-ā′shŭn) 1. a torn or jagged wound caused by blunt trauma; incorrectly applied to a cut. 2. the process or act of tearing the tissues. [L. *lacero*, pp. *-atus*, to tear to pieces]

**la·cer·tus** (lă-ser′tŭs) 1. the muscular part of the upper limb from shoulder to elbow. 2. a fibrous band, bundle, or slip related to a muscle. [L.]

**Lach·man test** (lock′man) a maneuver to detect deficiency of the anterior cruciate ligament; with the knee flexed 20 to 30°, the tibia is displaced anteriorly relative to the femur; a soft endpoint or greater than 4 mm displacement is positive (abnormal).

**lac·ri·mal** (lak′ri-măl) relating to the tears, their secretion, the secretory glands, and the drainage apparatus. [L. *lacrima*, a tear]

**lac·ri·mal ap·pa·ra·tus** consisting of the lacrimal gland, the lacrimal lake, the lacrimal canaliculi, the lacrimal sac, and the nasolacrimal duct.

**lac·ri·mal ar·tery** *origin*, ophthalmic; *distribution*, lacrimal gland, lateral and superior rectus muscles, superior eyelid, forehead, and temporal fossa. SYN arteria lacrimalis [TA].

**lac·ri·mal bone** an irregularly rectangular thin plate, forming part of the medial wall of the orbit behind the frontal process of the maxilla; it articulates with the inferior nasal concha, ethmoid, frontal, and maxillary bones.

**lac·ri·mal can·a·lic·u·lus** a curved canal beginning at the lacrimal punctum in the margin of each eyelid near the medial commissure and run-

ning transversely medially to empty with its fellow into the lacrimal sac.

**lac·ri·mal ca·run·cle** a small reddish body at the medial angle of the eye, containing modified sebaceous and sweat glands.

**lac·ri·mal fold** a fold of mucous membrane guarding the lower opening of the nasolacrimal duct. SYN plica lacrimalis [TA].

**lac·ri·mal fos·sa** a hollow in the orbital plate of the frontal bone, formed by the overhanging margin and zygomatic process, lodging the lacrimal gland.

**lac·ri·mal gland** the gland that secretes tears; it consists of 6–12 separate compound tubuloalveolar serous glands, located in the upper lateral part of the orbit, and is partially divided into a smaller palpebral part and a larger orbital part by the aponeurosis of the levator palpebrae muscle.

**lac·ri·mal lake** the small cistern-like area of the conjunctiva at the medial angle of the eye, in which the tears collect after bathing the anterior surface of the eyeball and the conjunctival sac. SYN lacus lacrimalis [TA].

**lac·ri·mal nerve** a branch of the ophthalmic nerve supplying sensory fibers to the lateral part of the upper eyelid, conjunctiva, and lacrimal gland. The secretomotor fibers of the latter were conveyed to the lacrimal nerve by the communicating branch of the zygomatic nerve (a branch of the maxillary nerve). SYN nervus lacrimalis [TA].

**lac·ri·mal pa·pil·la** a slight projection from the margin of each eyelid near the medial commissure, in the center of which is the lacrimal punctum (opening of the lacrimal duct).

**lac·ri·mal punc·tum** the minute circular opening of the lacrimal canaliculus, on the margin of each eyelid near the medial commissure.

**lac·ri·mal sac** the upper portion of the nasolacrimal duct into which empty the two lacrimal canaliculi. SYN saccus lacrimalis [TA], dacryocyst, tear sac.

**lac·ri·mal vein** drains the lacrimal gland, passing posteriorly through the orbit with the lacrimal artery to empty into the superior ophthalmic vein.

**lac·ri·ma·tion** (lak′ri-mā′shŭn) the secretion of tears, especially in excess. [L. *lacrimatio*]

**lac·ri·ma·tor** (lak′ri-mā-ter) an agent (such as tear gas) that irritates the eyes and produces tears. [L. *lacrima*, tear]

**lac·ri·ma·to·ry** (lak′ri-mă-tō-rē) causing lacrimation.

**lac·ri·mo·gus·ta·to·ry re·flex** chewing of food causing secretion of tears. SEE ALSO crocodile tears syndrome.

**lac·ri·mot·o·my** (lak-ri-mot′ō-mē) the operation of incising the lacrimal duct or sac. [L. *lacrima*, tear, + G. *tomē*, incision]

△**lact-, lac·ti-, lac·to-** milk. SEE ALSO galacto-. [L. *lac, lactis*]

**lac·tac·i·do·sis** (lak-tas-i-dō′sis) acidosis due to increased lactic acid.

**lact·a·cid ox·y·gen debt** slow phase of recovery oxygen consumption used to reconvert some lactate accumulated during exhaustive exercise to glycogen; also supports the high level of physiologic function and the metabolic-stimulating effects of an elevated core temperature from the preceding exercise. SYN lactic acid oxygen debt.

**lac·tam, lac·tim** (lak′tam, lak′tim) contractions

of "lactoneamine" and "lactoneimine," and applied to the tautomeric forms –NH–CO– and –N=C(OH)–, respectively, observed in many purines, pyrimidines, and other substances.

**β-lac·tam** a cyclical unit found in the molecular structure of penicillins and cephalosporins.

**β-lac·ta·mase** (beta-lak'tă-mās) an enzyme that brings about the hydrolysis of a β-lactam (as penicillin to penicilloic acid); found in most staphylococcus strains that are naturally resistant to penicillin.

**β-lac·tam·ase in·hib·i·tors** drugs such as clavulanic acid, which are used to inhibit bacterial β-lactamases; often used with a penicillin or cephalosporin to overcome drug resistance.

**lac·tase** (lak'tās) SYN β-D-galactosidase.

**lac·tate** (lak'tāt) **1.** a salt or ester of lactic acid. **2.** to produce milk in the mammary glands.

**lac·tate de·hy·dro·gen·ase (LDH)** name for four enzymes. The first two transfer H to ferricytochrome *c;* the last two transfer it to NAD⁺, in catalyzing the oxidation of lactate to pyruvate; the isozyme distribution of heart and muscle lactate dehydrogenase is of diagnostic use in myocardial infarction.

**lac·tate de·hy·dro·gen·ase vi·rus** an arterivirus present perhaps as a "passenger" in various transplantable mouse tumors; the virus may cause a life-long infection and be recognized by elevated plasma lactate dehydrogenase.

**lac·tat·ed Ring·er so·lu·tion** (ring'ĕr) a solution containing NaCl, sodium lactate, CaCl₂(dihydrate), and KCl in distilled water; used for the same purposes as Ringer solution. SYN Hartmann solution.

**lac·tate par·a·dox** reduced capacity for lactate production by skeletal muscle during exercise at altitude despite reduction in arterial PO₂; related to an altitude-induced reduction in the glucose-mobilizing hormone epinephrine during exercise.

**lac·tate thresh·old** a point, during exercise of increasing intensity, when a measurable increase in venous blood lactate levels occurs in conjunction with an exponential increase in respiratory frequency. SYN onset of blood lactate accumulation.

**lac·ta·tion** (lak-tā'shŭn) **1.** production of milk. **2.** period following birth during which milk is secreted in the breasts. [L. *lactatio,* suckle]

**lac·ta·tion a·men·or·rhea** physiological suppression of menses while nursing.

**lac·te·al** (lak'tē-ăl) **1.** relating to or resembling milk; milky. **2.** a lymphatic vessel that conveys chyle from the intestine. SYN chyle vessel, lacteal vessel.

**lac·te·al ves·sel** SYN lacteal (2).

**lac·tic ac·id** a normal intermediate in the fermentation (oxidation, metabolism) of sugar.

**lac·tic ac·i·de·mia** (lak'tik-as-i-dē'mē-ă) the presence of dextrorotatory lactic acid in the circulating blood. [lactic acid + G. *haima,* blood]

**lac·tic a·cid ox·y·gen debt** SYN lactacid oxygen debt.

**lac·tif·er·ous** (lak-tif'er-ŭs) yielding milk. SYN lactigerous. [lacti- + L. *fero,* to bear]

**lac·tif·er·ous ducts** one of the ducts, numbering 15–20, which drain the lobes of the mammary gland; they open at the nipple. SYN galactophore, mammillary ducts, milk ducts.

**lac·tif·er·ous si·nus** a circumscribed spindle-shaped dilation of the lactiferous duct just before

it enters the nipple. In nursing mothers this dilation stores a droplet of milk which is expressed by compression as the infant begins to suckle; this is thought to encourage continual suckling while the let-down reflex ensues.

**lac·tig·e·nous** (lak-tij'ĕ-nŭs) producing milk. [lacti- + -*gen,* producing]

**lac·tig·er·ous** (lak-tij'er-ŭs) SYN lactiferous. [lacti- + L. *gero,* to carry]

***Lac·to·ba·cil·lus*** (lak-tō-bă-sil'ŭs) a genus of microaerophilic or anaerobic, non–spore-forming, ordinarily nonmotile bacteria containing Gram-positive rods which vary from long and slender cells to short coccobacilli; chains are commonly produced. These organisms are found in dairy products, the effluents of grain and meat products, water, sewage, beer, wine, fruits and fruit juices, pickled vegetables, and in sourdough and mash, and are part of the normal flora of the mouth, intestinal tract, and vagina of many warm-blooded animals, including humans; rarely are they pathogenic. The type species is *Lactobacillus delbrueckii.* [lacto- + bacillus]

**lac·to·ba·cil·lus** (lak-tō-bă-sil'ŭs) a vernacular term used to refer to any member of the genus *Lactobacillus.*

**lac·to·cele** (lak'tō-sēl) SYN galactocele. [lacto- + G. *kēlē,* tumor]

**lac·to·gen** (lak'tō-jen) an agent that stimulates milk production or secretion. [lacto- + G. *-gen,* producing]

**lac·to·gen·e·sis** (lak-tō-jen'ĕ-sis) milk production. [lacto- + G. *genesis,* production]

**lac·to·gen·ic** (lak-tō-jen'ik) pertaining to lactogenesis.

**lac·to·gen·ic hor·mone** SYN prolactin.

**lac·to·glob·u·lin** (lak-tō-glob'yu-lin) the globulin present in milk; it makes up 50 to 60% of bovine whey protein.

**lac·tone** (lak'tōn) an intramolecular organic anhydride formed from a hydroxyacid by the loss of water between an –OH and a –COOH group; a cyclic ester.

**lac·to·phen·ol cot·ton blue stain** a solution consisting of phenol crystals, glycerol, lactic acid, and distilled water to which cotton blue or crystal violet is added; used as a stain in mycology.

**lac·tor·rhea** (lak-tō-rē'ă) SYN galactorrhea. [lacto- + G. *rhoia,* a flow]

**lac·tose** (lak'tōs) a disaccharide present in milk, obtained from cow's milk and used in food for infants and convalescents and in pharmaceutical preparations; large doses act as an osmotic diuretic and as a laxative. SYN milk sugar.

**lac·tos·u·ria** (lak'tōs-yu'rē-ă) excretion of lactose (milk sugar) in the urine; a common finding during pregnancy and lactation, and in newborn, especially premature, babies. [lactose + G. *ouron,* urine, + -ia]

**lac·to·ther·a·py** (lak-tō-thār'ă-pē) SYN galactotherapy.

**la·cu·na,** pl. **la·cu·nae** (lă-koo'nă, la-koo'nē) **1.** a small space, cavity, or depression. **2.** a gap or defect. **3.** an abnormal space between strata or between the cellular elements of the epidermis. **4.** SYN corneal space. [L. a pit, dim. of *lacus,* a hollow, a lake]

**la·cu·na mag·na** a recess on the roof of the fossa navicularis of the penis, formed by a fold of mucous membrane, the valve of the navicular fossa.

**la·cu·nar** (lă-koo'năr) relating to a lacuna.

**la·cu·nar am·ne·sia, lo·cal·ized am·ne·sia** amnesia in reference to isolated events.

**la·cu·nar lig·a·ment** a curved fibrous band that passes horizontally backward from the medial end of the inguinal ligament to the pectineal line; it forms the medial boundary of the femoral ring. SYN ligamentum lacunare [TA].

**la·cu·nule** (lă-koo'nyul) a very small lacuna. [Mod. L. *lacunula,* dim. of L. *lacuna*]

**la·cus,** pl. **la·cus** (lā'kŭs) a small collection of fluid. SYN lake (1). [L. lake]

**la·cus la·cri·ma·lis** [TA] SYN lacrimal lake.

**la·cus se·mi·na·lis** the vault of the vagina after insemination. SYN seminal lake.

**LAD** leukocyte adhesion deficiency.

**Ladd band** (lad) a peritoneal attachment of an incompletely rotated cecum, found in malrotation of the intestine; may cause obstruction of the duodenum.

**lad·der splint** a flexible splint consisting of two stout parallel wires with finer cross wires.

**Ladd op·er·a·tion** (lad) division of Ladd band to relieve duodenal obstruction in malrotation of the intestine.

**La·dy Win·der·mere syn·drome** (lā'dē win' der-mēr) nontuberculous mycobacterial pulmonary disease in a frail, elderly woman, often with pectus excavatum or scoliosis. [named for the main character in Oscar Wilde's play, *Lady Windermere's Fan*]

**La·ën·nec cir·rho·sis** (lah-ĕ-nek') cirrhosis in which normal liver lobules are replaced by small regeneration nodules, sometimes containing fat, separated by a fairly regular framework of fine fibrous tissue strands (hobnail liver); usually due to chronic alcoholism. Can cause severe impairment of liver function, portal hypertension with ascites and esophageal varices, and life-threatening complications.

**la·e·trile** (lā'ĕ-tril) an allegedly antineoplastic drug consisting chiefly of amygdalin derived from apricot pits; its antitumor effect is unproven.

**laev-** SEE levo-.

**lae·vo- [Br.]** SEE levo-.

**lae·vo·car·dia [Br.]** SEE levocardia.

**lae·vo·do·pa [Br.]** SEE levodopa.

**lae·vo·ro·ta·tion [Br.]** SEE levorotation.

**lae·vo·ro·ta·to·ry [Br.]** SEE levorotatory.

**La·fo·ra bod·y** (lah-fō'rah) an intraneural intracytoplasmic inclusion body composed of acid mucopolysaccharides, seen in familial myoclonus epilepsy.

**la·ge·na,** pl. **la·ge·nae** (lă-jē'nă, lă-jē-nē) **1.** SYN cupular cecum of the cochlear duct. **2.** one of the three parts of the membranous labyrinth of the inner ear of lower vertebrates; in mammals, the lagena becomes the cochlea. [L. flask]

**lag·ging** retarded or diminished ventilatory movement of the affected side of the chest due to pleural disease with muscle splinting or collapse of a lung.

**lake** (lāk) **1.** SYN lacus. **2.** to cause blood plasma to become red as a result of the release of hemoglobin from erythrocytes. SEE ALSO lacuna. [A.S. *lacu,* fr. L. *lacus,* lake]

**La·ki-Lor·and fac·tor** (lah'kī-lōr'ănd) SYN factor XIII.

**la·ky** (lā'kē) pertaining to the transparent bright red appearance of blood serum or plasma, developing as a result of hemoglobin being released from destroyed red blood cells.

**lal·ling** (lal'ing) a form of stammering in which the speech is almost unintelligible. [G. *laleō,* to chatter]

**lal·o·che·zia** (lal-ō-kē'zē-ă) emotional discharge gained by uttering indecent or filthy words. [G. *lalia,* speech, + *chezō,* to relieve oneself]

**la·lo·ple·gia** (la-lō-plē'jē-ă) paralysis of the muscles concerned in the mechanism of speech. [G. *lalia,* speech, + *plēgē,* a stroke]

**La·maze meth·od** (lă-mahz') a technique of psychoprophylactic preparation for childbirth, designed to minimize the pain of labor.

**lambda** ($\Lambda$, $\lambda$) (lam'dă) **1.** the 11th letter of the Greek alphabet. **2.** symbol ($\lambda$) for Avogadro number; wavelength; radioactive constant; Ostwald solubility coefficient; molar conductivity of an electrolyte ($\Lambda$). **3.** CHEMISTRY the position of a substituent located on the 11th atom from the carboxyl or other functional group ($\lambda$). **4.** the craniometric point at the junction of the sagittal and lambdoid sutures.

**lamb·doid** (lam'doyd) resembling the Greek letter lambda, as does the lambdoid suture. [lambda + G. *eidos,* resemblance]

**lamb·doid su·ture** line of union between the occipital and the parietal bones.

**Lam·bert law** (lam'bert) **1.** each layer of equal thickness absorbs an equal fraction of the light that traverses it. **2.** the illumination of a surface on which the light falls normally from a point source is inversely proportional to the square of the distance from the source.

**Lambl ex·cres·cence** (lam'bl) a small pointed projection from the edge of an aortic cusp, of unknown significance.

*Lamb·lia in·tes·ti·na·lis* (lam'blē-ă in-tes-ti-nā' lis) old term for *Giardia lamblia,* still frequently used, especially by protozoologists in the former Soviet Union.

**Lam·bri·nu·di op·er·a·tion** (lahm-brē-noo'dē) a form of triple arthrodesis done in such a manner as to prevent foot-drop such as occurs in poliomyelitis.

**la·mel·la,** pl. **la·mel·lae** (lă-mel'ă, lă-mel'ē) **1.** a thin sheet or layer, such as occurs in compact bone. **2.** a preparation in the form of a medicated gelatin disk, used as a means of making local applications to the conjunctiva in place of solutions. SYN discus [TA], disk (2). [L. dim. of *lamina,* plate, leaf]

**lam·el·lar** (lam'ĕ-lăr, lă-mel'ăr) **1.** arranged in thin plates or scales. **2.** relating to lamellae.

**lam·el·lar bone** the normal type of adult mammalian bone, whether cancellous or compact, composed of parallel lamellae in the former and concentric lamellae in the latter.

**lam·el·lar cat·a·ract** a cataract in which the opacity is limited to the cortex. SYN zonular cataract.

**lam·el·lat·ed cor·pus·cles** small oval bodies in the skin of the fingers, in the mesentery, tendons, and elsewhere, formed of concentric layers of connective tissue with a soft core in which the axon of a nerve fiber runs, splitting up into a number of fibrils that terminate in bulbous enlargements; they are sensitive to pressure. SYN corpuscula lamellosa [TA], pacinian corpuscles.

l
a

la•mel•li•po•di•um, pl. la•mel•li•po•dia (lă-mel-i-pō'dē-ŭm, lă-mel-i-pō'dē-ă) a cytoplasmic veil produced on all sides of migrating polymorphonuclear leukocytes.

lam•i•na, pl. lam•i•nae (lam'i-nă, lam'i-nē) thin plate or flat layer. SEE ALSO layer, stratum. [L]

lam•i•na ar•cus ver•te•brae [TA] SYN lamina of vertebral arch.

lam•i•na ba•sa•lis cho•roi•de•ae [TA] the transparent, nearly structureless inner layer of the choroid in contact with the pigmented layer of the retina. SYN basal layer of choroid, Bruch membrane, vitreous lamella, vitreous membrane (3).

lam•i•na cho•roid•o•ca•pil•la•ris [TA] SYN choriocapillary layer.

lam•i•na cri•bro•sa os•sis eth•moi•da•lis [TA] SYN cribriform plate of ethmoid bone.

lam•i•na cri•bro•sa scler•ae the portion of the sclera through which pass the fibers of the optic nerve.

lam•i•na fus•ca of scle•ra an exceedingly delicate layer of loose, pigmented connective tissue on the inner surface of the sclera, connecting it with the choroid.

lam•i•na•gram (lam'i-nă-gram) an image made by laminagraphy.

lam•i•na•graph (lam'i-nă-graf) a device for laminagraphy; a laminagram.

lam•i•nag•ra•phy, lami•nog•ra•phy (lam'i-nahg'ră-fē, lam'i-nog-ră-fē) radiographic technique in which the images of tissues above and below the plane of interest are blurred out by movement of the x-ray tube and film holder, to show a specific area more clearly. SEE ALSO tomography. [lamina + G. graphē, a writing]

lam•i•na of lens one of a series of concentric layers composed of the lens fibers that make up the substance of the lens.

lam•i•na lim•i•tans an•ter•i•or cor•ne•ae SYN anterior elastic lamina of cornea.

lam•i•na lim•i•tans pos•ter•i•or cor•ne•ae SYN posterior elastic lamina of cornea.

lam•i•na me•dul•la•ris me•di•a•lis [TA] SEE medullary laminae of thalamus.

lam•i•na me•dul•la•ris me•di•a•lis nu•clei len•ti•for•mis [TA] SYN medial medullary lamina of lentiform nucleus.

lam•i•na of mes•en•ce•phal•ic tec•tum the roofplate of the mesencephalon formed by the quadrigeminal bodies. SYN tectum of midbrain.

lam•i•na mul•ti•for•mis [TA] SYN multiform layer of cerebral cortex.

lam•i•na pro•pria the layer of connective tissue underlying the epithelium of a mucous membrane.

lam•i•nar (lam'i-nar) 1. arranged in plates or laminae. 2. relating to any lamina.

lam•i•nar flow the relative motion of elements of a fluid along smooth parallel paths, which occurs at lower values of Reynolds number.

lam•i•nat•ed clot a clot formed in a succession of layers such as occurs in an aneurysm.

lam•i•nat•ed ep•i•the•li•um SYN stratified epithelium.

lam•i•na of ver•te•bral arch the flattened posterior portion of the vertebral arch extending between the pedicles and the midline, forming the dorsal wall of the vertebral foramen; the spinous process extends from the midline junction

of right and left laminae. SYN lamina arcus vertebrae [TA], neurapophysis.

lam•i•na vis•ce•ra•lis [TA] SYN visceral layer.

lam•i•nec•to•my (lam'i-nek'tō-mē) excision of a vertebral lamina; commonly used to denote removal of the posterior arch. [L. lamina, layer, + G. ektomē, excision]

lam•i•ni•tis (lam-i-nī'tis) inflammation of any lamina.

lam•i•not•o•my (lam'i-not'ō-mē) an operation on one or more vertebral laminae. SYN rachiotomy. [L. lamina, layer, + G. tomē, incision]

lamp illuminating device; source of light. SEE ALSO light.

Lan•cas•ter red green test (lan'kas-tĕr) test to measure ocular deviations in various fields of gaze in adult patients with acquired strabismus and diplopia by placing a red filter over the right eye and a green filter over the left eye followed by alignment by the patient of a red or green light with light of opposite color projected by the examiner.

lance (lans) 1. to incise a part, as an abscess or boil. 2. a lancet. [L. lancea, a slender spear]

Lance•field clas•si•fi•ca•tion (lans'fēld) a serologic classification dividing hemolytic streptococci into groups (A to O) based on precipitation tests for group-specific carbohydrate substances. Group A contains strains pathogenic for humans.

lan•cet (lan'set) a surgical knife with a short, wide, sharp-pointed, two-edged blade. [Fr. lancette]

lan•ci•nat•ing (lan'si-nāt'ing) denoting a sharp cutting or tearing pain. [L. lancino, pp. -atus, to tear]

Lan•ci•si sign (lahn-chē'zē) a large systolic jugular venous wave caused by tricuspid regurgitation replacing the normal negative systolic trough ("x" descent).

Lan•dau-Kleff•ner syn•drome (lan'dow-kleffner) childhood disorder characterized by generalized and psychomotor seizures associated with acquired aphasia; multifocal spikes and spike and wave discharges in the electroencephalogram. SYN acquired epileptic aphasia.

Lan•dol•fi sign (lan-dolf'ē) in aortic insufficiency, systolic contraction and diastolic dilation of the pupil.

Lan•dry pa•ral•y•sis, Lan•dry syn•drome (lah-drā', lah-drā') SYN Guillain-Barré syndrome.

land•scape e•co•lo•gy the study of the reciprocal effects of spatial pattern on ecologic processes.

Lane band (lān) a congenital band on the distal ileum that may extend into the right iliac fossa causing stasis. SYN Lane kink.

Lane kink SYN Lane band.

Lan•gen•beck tri•an•gle (lahng'ĕn-bek) a triangle formed by lines drawn from the anterior superior iliac spine to the surface of the greater trochanter and to the surgical neck of the femur; a penetrating wound in this area probably involves the joint.

Lan•gen•dorff meth•od (lahng'ĕn-dōrf) perfusion of the isolated mammalian heart by carrying fluid under pressure into the sectioned aorta, and thus into the coronary system.

Lan•ger•hans cell his•ti•o•cy•to•sis (lahng'ĕr-hahnz) a set of closely related disorders unified by a common proliferating element, the Langerhans cell. Three overlapping clinical syndromes are recognized: a single site disease (eosinophilic granuloma), a multifocal unisystem process (Hand-Schuller-Christian syndrome), and a multifocal, multisystem histiocytosis (Letter-Siwe syndrome.) Formerly this process was known as histiocytosis X.

**Lan·ger·hans cells** (lahng′ĕr-hahnz) **1.** dendritic clear cells in the epidermis, containing distinctive granules but lacking tonofilaments, melanosomes, and desmosomes; they carry surface receptors for immunoglobulin (Fc) and complement (C3), and are believed to be antigen fixing and processing cells of monocytic origin; active participants in cutaneous delayed hypersensitivity. **2.** cells seen in eosinophilic granuloma and lymphoma of the lungs.

**Lan·ger-Sal·di·no syn·drome** (lahng′er-sahl-dē′nō) SYN achondrogenesis type II.

**Lang·hans cells** (lahng′hahnz) **1.** multinucleated giant cells seen in tuberculosis and other granulomatous diseases; the nuclei are arranged in an arciform manner at the periphery of the cells; SYN Langhans-type giant cells. **2.** SYN cytotrophoblastic cells.

**Lang·hans-type gi·ant cells** (lahng′hahnz) SYN Langhans cells (1).

**lan·guage** (lang′gwij) the use of spoken, manual, written, and other symbols to express, represent, or receive communication. [L. *lingua*]

**lan·guage board** SYN communication board.

**lan·tha·nides** (lan′thă-nīdz) those elements with atomic numbers 57–71 which closely resemble one another chemically and were once difficult to separate from one another. [*lanthanum,* first element of the series]

**lan·tha·num (La)** (lan′thă-nŭm) a metallic element, atomic no. 57, atomic wt. 138.9055; first of the rare earth elements (lanthanides). [G. *lanthanō,* to lie hidden]

**la·nu·gi·nous** (lă-noo′ji-nŭs) covered with lanugo.

**la·nu·go** (lă-noo′gō) fine, soft, lightly pigmented fetal hair with minute shafts and large papillae; it appears toward the end of the third month of gestation. SYN lanugo hair. [L. down, wooliness, from *lana,* wool]

**la·nu·go hair** SYN lanugo.

**LAO** left anterior oblique position. In chest radiography, used to assess the size of the left atrium and ventricle.

△**lap·a·ro-** the loins (less properly, the abdomen in general). [G. *lapara,* flank, loins]

**lap·a·ro·cele** (lap′ă-rō-sēl) SYN abdominal hernia. [laparo- + G. *kēlē,* hernia]

**lap·a·ro·en·do·scop·ic** (lap′ă-rō-en-dō-skop′ik) having to do with the introduction of a laparoscope into the abdominal cavity for a variety of intracavitary procedures.

**lap·a·ror·rha·phy** (lap′ă-rōr′ă-fē) SYN celiorrhaphy.

**lap·a·ro·scope** (lap′ă-rō-skōp) an endoscope for examining the peritoneal cavity. SYN peritoneoscope. [laparo- + G. *skopeō,* to view]

**lap·a·ro·scop·ic-as·sis·ted vag·i·nal hys·ter·ec·to·my** vaginal hysterectomy in which the ovarian pedicle, broad ligament, and uterosacral ligaments are surgically severed using laparoscopic instruments and the procedure completed through a colpotomy done in the typical fashion.

**lap·a·ro·scop·ic cho·le·cys·tot·o·my** minimally invasive surgical technique for removal of the gallbladder that uses a laparoscope for visualiza-

tion of the gallbladder and placement of instruments into the abdominal cavity through trocars.

**lap·a·ro·scop·ic knot** a knot placed intracorporally through a laparoscopic instrument. The knot itself may be tied extracorporally and passed into the body through a cannula or the knot may be both placed and tied intracorporally.

**lap·a·ro·scop·ic ne·phrec·to·my** removal of a kidney by percutaneous endoscopic technique.

**lap·a·ro·scop·ic uter·o·sa·cral nerve ab·la·tion** laparoscopic transection via laser (usually KTP or argon) of the uterosacral nerves for the treatment of primary dysmenorrhea.

**lap·a·ros·co·py** (lap-ă-ros′kŏ-pē) examination of the contents of the peritoneum with a laparoscope. The abdomen is first inflated with carbon dioxide, and the laparoscope passed through a small incision in the abdominal wall. The device is frequently used to view the female reproductive organs, in particular where endometriosis or pelvic inflammatory disease is suspected. Fitted with grasping and cutting tools, the laparoscope can perform minor surgery and take tissue samples for biopsy. SEE ALSO peritoneoscopy.

**lap·a·rot·o·my** (lap′ă-rot′ō-mē) **1.** incision into the loin. **2.** SYN celiotomy. [laparo- + G. *tomē,* incision]

**lap·a·rot·o·my pad** a pad made from several layers of gauze folded into a rectangular shape; used as a sponge or packing material in surgery. SYN abdominal pad.

**La·picque law** (lah-pēk′) the chronaxie is inversely proportional to the diameter of an axon.

**lap·i·ni·za·tion** (lap′i-ni-zā′shŭn) serial passage of a virus or vaccine in rabbits. [Fr. *lapin,* rabbit]

**lap·i·nized** (lap′i-nīzd) denoting viruses which have been adapted to develop in rabbits by serial transfers in this species. [Fr. *lapin,* rabbit]

**La·place for·ceps** (lah-plahs′) a forceps for approximating intestines during surgical anastomosis.

**La·place law** (lah-plahs′) the equilibrium relationship between transmural pressure difference ($\Delta P$), wall tension ($T$), and radius of curvature ($R$) in a concave surface; for a sphere: $\Delta P = 2T/R$; for a cylinder: $\Delta P = T/R$.

**la·quer stain for al·co·hol·ic hy·a·lin** (lă′kĕr) a combination of Altmann aniline-acid fuchsin stain with a Masson trichrome stain which, on a gray-brown background, stains alcoholic hyalin red, collagen green, and nuclei brown.

**large cal·o·rie (C)** the quantity of energy required to raise the temperature of 1 kg of water from 14.5° to 15.5°C; it is 1000 times the value of the small calorie. SYN kilocalorie, kilogram calorie.

**large cell car·ci·no·ma** an anaplastic carcinoma, particularly bronchogenic, composed of cells which are much larger than those in oat cell carcinoma of the lung.

**large cell lym·pho·ma** lymphoma composed of large mononuclear cells of undetermined type.

**large in·tes·tine** the portion of the digestive tube extending from the ileocecal valve to the anus; it comprises the cecum, colon, rectum, and anal canal.

**La·ron-type dwarf·ism** (lah-ron′) dwarfism associated with deficiency of somatomedin C (insulin-like growth factor I) or abnormalities in receptor activity.

**La·ro·yen·ne op·er·a·tion** (lah-rō-yahn′) punc-

l
a

ture of Douglas pouch to evacuate the pus and to secure drainage in cases of pelvic suppuration.

**Lar·rey am·pu·ta·tion** (lah-rā′) amputation at the shoulder joint.

**Lar·son-Jo·hans·son dis·ease** (lahr′son-yōhahn′son) inflammation or partial avulsion of the lower pole of the patella due to traction forces. SEE ALSO Osgood-Schlatter disease.

**lar·va**, pl. **lar·vae** (lar′vă, lar′vē) **1.** the wormlike developmental stage or stages of an insect or helminth. **2.** the second stage in the life cycle of a tick; the stage which hatches from the egg and, following engorgement, molts in the nymph. **3.** the young of fishes or amphibians which often differ in appearance from the adult. [L. a mask]

**lar·va cur·rens** (lar′vă kŭr′enz) cutaneous larva migrans caused by rapidly moving larvae of *Strongyloides stercoralis* (up to 10 cm/hr), typically extending from the anal area down the upper thighs and observed as a rapidly progressing linear urticarial trail. [L. *larva,* mask + *currens,* racing]

**lar·val** (lar′văl) **1.** relating to larvae. **2.** SYN larvate.

**lar·va mi·grans** (lar′vă mī′granz) a larval worm, typically a nematode, that wanders for a period in the host tissues but does not develop to the adult stage; this usually occurs in abnormal hosts that inhibit normal development of the parasite. [L. *larva,* mask, + *migro,* to transfer, migrate]

**lar·vate** (lar′vāt) masked or concealed; applied to a disease with undeveloped, absent, or atypical symptoms. SYN larval (2). [L. *larva,* mask]

**lar·vi·cid·al** (lar-vi-sī′dăl) destructive to larvae.

**lar·vi·cide** (lar′vi-sīd) an agent that kills larvae. [larva + L. *caedo,* to kill]

**la·ryn·ge·al** (lă-rin′jē-ăl) relating in any way to the larynx.

**la·ryn·ge·al pap·il·lo·ma·to·sis** multiple squamous papillomas of the larynx in young children, usually due to infection by the human papilloma virus, which may be transmitted at birth from maternal condylomata.

**la·ryn·ge·al prom·i·nence** the projection on the anterior portion of the neck formed by the thyroid cartilage of the larynx; serves as an external indication of the level of the fifth cervical vertebra.

**la·ryn·ge·al ste·no·sis** narrowing or stricture of any or all areas of the larynx; may be congenital or acquired.

**la·ryn·ge·al syn·co·pe** a paroxysmal neurosis characterized by attacks of coughing, with unusual sensations, as of tickling, in the throat, followed by a brief period of unconsciousness.

**lar·yn·ge·al ven·tri·cle** the recess in each lateral wall of the larynx between the vestibular and vocal folds and into which the laryngeal sacculus opens. SYN Morgagni sinus (3).

**la·ryn·ge·al web** congenital anomaly consisting of mucous membrane–covered connective tissue between the vocal cords located ventrally and extending dorsally for varying distances; it causes airway obstruction and hoarse cry in the newborn.

**lar·yn·gec·to·mee** (lar-in-jek′tō-mē) a person who has had a laryngectomy.

**la·ryn·gec·to·my** (lar′in-jek′tō-mē) excision of the larynx. [laryngo- + G. *ektomē,* excision]

**la·ryn·ges** (lă-rin′jēz) plural of larynx. [L.]

**lar·yn·gis·mus** (lar-in-jiz′mŭs) a spasmodic nar-

rowing or closure of the rima glottidis. [L. fr. G. *larynx,* + *-ismos,* -ism]

**lar·yn·gis·mus stri·du·lus** a spasmodic closure of the glottis, lasting a few seconds, followed by a noisy inspiration. Cf. laryngitis stridulosa. SYN pseudocroup.

**lar·yn·git·ic** (lar-in-jit′ik) relating to or caused by laryngitis.

**lar·yn·gi·tis** (lar-in-jī′tis) inflammation of the mucous membrane of the larynx. [laryngo- + G. *-itis,* inflammation]

**lar·yn·gi·tis sic·ca** laryngitis characterized by dryness and crusting of the mucous membrane of the larynx.

**lar·yn·gi·tis stri·du·lo·sa** catarrhal inflammation of the larynx in children, accompanied by night attacks of spasmodic closure of the glottis, causing inspiratory stridor.

△**la·ryn·go-, la·ryng-** the larynx. [G. *larynx*]

**la·ryn·go·cele** (lă-ring′gō-sēl) an air sac communicating with the larynx through the ventricle, often bulging outward into the tissue of the neck, especially during coughing. [laryngo- + G. *kēlē,* hernia]

**la·ryn·go·fis·sure** (lă-ring′gō-fish′er) operative opening into the larynx, generally through the midline, commonly done for the excision of early carcinoma or the correction of laryngostenosis. SYN thyrotomy (2).

**lar·yn·gol·o·gy** (lar′ing-gol′ō-jē) the branch of medical science concerned with the larynx; the specialty of diseases of the larynx. [laryngo- + G. *logos,* study]

**la·ryn·go·pa·ral·y·sis** (lă-ring′gō-pă-ral′i-sis) paralysis of the laryngeal muscles. SYN laryngoplegia.

**la·ryn·go·pha·ryn·ge·al** (lă-ring′gō-fă-rin′jē-ăl) relating to both larynx and pharynx or to the laryngopharynx.

**la·ryn·go·phar·yn·gec·to·my** (lă-ring′gō-far′in-jek′tō-mē) resection or excision of both larynx and pharynx.

**la·ryn·go·phar·yn·gi·tis** (lă-ring′gō-far-in-jī′tis) inflammation of the larynx and pharynx.

**la·ryn·go·phar·ynx** (lă-ring′gō-far-ingks) the part of the pharynx lying below the aperture of the larynx and behind the larynx; it extends from the vestibule of the larynx to the esophagus at the level of the inferior border of the cricoid cartilage. SYN hypopharynx.

**la·ryn·go·plas·ty** (lă-ring′gō-plas-tē) reparative or plastic surgery of the larynx. [laryngo- + G. *plassō,* to form]

**la·ryn·go·ple·gia** (lă-ring′gō-plē′jē-ă) SYN laryngoparalysis. [laryngo- + G. *plēgē,* stroke]

**la·ryn·go·pto·sis** (lă-ring-gō-tō′sis) an abnormally low position of the larynx; may occur as a normal variant at birth or with aging. [laryngo- + G. *ptōsis,* a falling]

**la·ryn·go·scope** (lă-ring′gō-skōp) any of several types of hollow tubes, equipped with electrical lighting, used in examining or operating upon the interior of the larynx through the mouth. [laryngo- + G. *skopeō,* to inspect]

**la·ryn·go·scop·ic** (lă-ring′gō-skop′ik) relating to laryngoscopy.

**lar·yn·gos·co·py** (lar′ing-gos′kŏ-pē) inspection of the larynx by means of the laryngoscope.

**la·ryn·go·spasm** (lă-ring′gō-spazm) spasmodic closure of the glottic aperture.

**la·ryn·go·ste·no·sis** (lă-ring′gō-stĕ-nō′sis) stricture or narrowing of the lumen of the larynx. [laryngo- + G. *stenōsis,* a narrowing]

**lar·yn·gos·to·my** (lar'ing-gos'tō-mē) the establishment of a permanent opening from the neck into the larynx. [laryngo- + G. *stoma,* mouth]

**lar·yn·got·o·my** (lar-ing-got'ō-mē) a surgical incision of the larynx. [laryngo- + G. *tomē,* incision]

**la·ryn·go·tra·che·al** (lă-ring'gō-trā'kē-ăl) relating to both larynx and trachea.

**la·ryn·go·tra·che·i·tis** (lă-ring'gō-trā-kē-ī'tis) inflammation of both larynx and trachea.

**la·ryn·go·tra·che·o·bron·chi·tis** (lă-ring'gō-trā' kē-ō-brong-kī'tis) an acute respiratory infection involving the larynx, trachea, and bronchi. SEE croup.

**la·ryn·go·trach·e·o·e·so·pha·ge·al cleft** absence of fusion of the musculature or cricoid cartilaginous laminae of varying severity: type 1, submucous cleft of the interarytenoid muscles (known also as occult posterior laryngeal cleft or submucous laryngeal cleft); type 2, partial cricoid cleft (known also as partial posterior laryngeal cleft); type 3, total cricoid cleft (known also as laryngotracheoesophageal cleft or total cricoid cleft); and type 4, extension of the cleft into the esophagus.

**lar·yn·go·tra·che·o·plas·ty** (lar-ing'gō-trā'kē-ō-plas'tē) operation to repair subglottic stenosis.

⊞ **lar·ynx,** pl. **la·ryn·ges** (lar'ingks, lă-rin'jēz) [TA] the organ of voice production; the part of the respiratory tract between the pharynx and the trachea; it consists of a framework of cartilages and elastic membranes housing the vocal folds and the muscles which control the position and tension of these elements. See this page. [Mod. L. fr. G.]

**lase** (lāz) to cut, divide, or dissolve a substance, or to treat an anatomical structure, with a laser beam.

**Lasègue sign** (lah-seg') when a subject is supine with hip flexed and knee extended, dorsiflexion of the ankle causing pain or muscle spasm in the posterior thigh indicates lumbar root or sciatic nerve irritation.

**Lasègue syn·drome** (lah-seg') in conversion hysteria, inability to move an anesthetic limb, except under control of the sight.

**la·ser** (lā'zer) **1.** (noun) a device that concentrates high energies into an intense narrow beam of nondivergent monochromatic electromagnetic radiation; used in microsurgery, cauterization, and for a variety of diagnostic purposes. **2.** (verb) to treat a structure with a laser beam. [acronym coined from *l*ight *a*mplification by *s*timulated *e*mission of *r*adiation]

**la·ser-as·sis·ted in si·tu ker·a·to·mi·leu·sis (LASIK)** a refractive procedure to correct myopia by which a flap of cornea is made, excimer laser ablation of corneal stoma is performed, and the flap laid back in position.

**la·ser plume** the production of smoke with laser ablation; can cause respiratory difficulty for surgical team. [L. *pluma,* feather]

**Lash ca·sein hy·dro·ly·sate-se·rum me·di·um** (lash) used to detect the presence of *Trichomonas vaginalis.*

**Lash op·er·a·tion** (lash) removal of a wedge of the internal cervical os with suturing of the internal os into a tighter canal structure.

**LASIK** laser-assisted in situ keratomileusis.

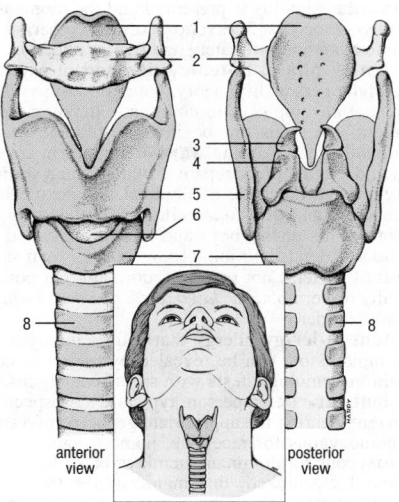

**the laryngeal cartilages:** (1) epiglottis, (2) hyoid bone, (3) corniculate cartilage, (4) arytenoid cartilage, (5) thyroid cartilage, (6) cricothyroid ligament, (7) cricoid cartilage, (8) trachea

**Las·sa fe·ver** a severe form of epidemic hemorrhagic fever which is highly fatal. It was first recognized in Lassa, Nigeria, is caused by the Lassa virus, a member of the Arenaviridae family, and is characterized by high fever, sore throat, severe muscle aches, skin rash with hemorrhages, headache, abdominal pain, vomiting, and diarrhea; the multimammate rat *Mastomys natalensis* serves as reservoir, but person-to-person transmission also is common.

**Las·sa vi·rus** an arenavirus that causes Lassa fever, an acute febrile disease with a high mortality.

**las·si·tude** (las'i-tood) a sense of weariness. [L. *lassitudo,* fr. *lassus,* weary]

**la·tah** (lah'tah) one of the pathological startle syndromes. A culture-bound disorder characterized by an exaggerated physical response to being startled or to unexpected suggestion, the subjects involuntarily uttering cries or executing movements in response to command or in imitation of what they hear or see in others. SEE ALSO jumping disease. [Malay, ticklish]

**late au·di·to·ry-e·voked re·sponse** response of the auditory cortex to acoustic stimulation.

**late dum·ping syn·drome** syndrome in patients who have had ablation of the pyloric sphincter mechanism; associated with flushing, sweating, dizziness, weakness, and vasomotor collapse 2–3 hours after a meal and caused by hypoglycemia resulting from the rapid absorption of a large carbohydrate load, which then stimulates insulin release. SEE ALSO dumping syndrome.

**late lu·te·al phase dys·phor·ia** SYN premenstrual syndrome.

**la·ten·cy** (lā'ten-sē) **1.** the state of being latent. **2.** in conditioning, or other behavioral experiments, the period of apparent inactivity between the time the stimulus is presented and the moment a response occurs. **3.** PSYCHOANALYSIS the period of time from approximately age five to puberty.

**la•ten•cy phase, la•ten•cy pe•ri•od** in psychoanalytic personality theory, the period of psychosexual development in children, extending from about age 5 to the beginning of adolescence around age 12, during which the apparent cessation of sexual preoccupation stems from a strong, aggressive blockade of libidinal and sexual impulses in an effort to avoid oedipal relationships; during this phase, boys and girls are inclined to choose friends and join groups of their own sex.

**la•tent** (lā′tent) not manifest, dormant, but potentially discernible. [L. *lateo*, pres. p. *latens* (-ent-), to lie hidden]

**la•tent al•ler•gy** allergy that causes no signs or symptoms but can be revealed by means of certain immunologic tests with specific allergens.

**la•tent car•ri•er** a person, typically a prospective parent, bearing the appropriate genotype of a trait (homozygous for recessive, homozygous or heterozygous for dominant, hemizygous or homozygous for X-linked) that manifests the trait only under certain conditions, e.g., age, an environmental insult, etc.

**la•tent con•tent** the hidden, unconscious meaning of thoughts or actions, especially in dreams or fantasies.

**la•tent di•a•be•tes** a mild form of diabetes mellitus in which the patient has no overt symptoms, but displays abnormal responses to certain diagnostic procedures, such as an elevated fasting blood glucose concentration or reduced glucose tolerance. SYN chemical diabetes.

**la•tent gout** hyperuricemia without symptoms of gout. Often used synonymously with interval gout.

**la•tent hy•per•o•pia** the difference between total and manifest hyperopia.

**la•tent im•age** the undeveloped image on an exposed x-ray film; it becomes visible after chemical processing.

**la•tent learn•ing** that learning which is not evident to the observer at the time it occurs, but which is inferred from later performance in which learning is more rapid than would be expected without the earlier experience.

**la•tent mem•brane pro•tein** gene product of Epstein-Barr virus.

**la•tent nys•tag•mus** jerky nystagmus that is brought out by covering one eye. The fast phase is always away from the covered eye.

**la•tent pe•ri•od 1.** the period elapsing between the application of a stimulus and the response, e.g., contraction of a muscle; **2.** SYN incubation period (1).

**la•tent re•flex** a reflex which must be considered normal but which usually appears only under some pathologic circumstance that lowers its threshold.

**la•tent schiz•o•phre•nia** a preexisting susceptibility for developing overt schizophrenia under strong emotional stress.

**la•tent stage** SYN incubation period (1).

**lat•er•ad** (lat′er-ad) toward the side. [L. *latus*, side, + *ad*, to]

▪ **lat•er•al** (lat′er-ăl) **1.** on the side. **2.** farther from the median or midsagittal plane. **3.** DENTISTRY a position either right or left of the midsagittal plane. **4.** a radiograph made with the film in the sagittal plane; especially, the second view of a chest series. See page APP 89. [L. *lateralis*, lateral, fr. *latus*, side]

**lat•er•al ab•er•ra•tion** in spherical aberration, the distance between paraxial focus of central rays on the optic axis.

**lat•er•al ap•er•ture of fourth ven•tri•cle** one of the two lateral openings of the fourth ventricle into the subarachnoid space (the lateral cerebellomedullary cistern) at the cerebellopontine angle. SYN apertura lateralis ventriculi quarti [TA].

**lat•er•al ar•cu•ate lig•a•ments** a thickening of the fascia of the quadratus lumborum muscle between the transverse process of the first lumbar vertebra and the twelfth rib on either side that gives attachment to a portion of the diaphragm (one of the Haller arches).

**lat•er•al ba•sal (bronchopulmonary) seg•ment [S IX]** of the four bronchopulmonary segments of the inferior lobes of the right or left lung that contact the diaphragm, the one lying farthest to the right in the right lung, and farthest to the left in the left lung, supplied by the lateral basal segmental bronchi [B IX] and lateral basal segmental (pulmonary) artery.

**lat•er•al branch•es of ar•tery of tu•ber cin•er•e•um** branches arising from the lateral aspect of the artery of tuber cinereum.

**lat•er•al branch•es of pon•tine ar•ter•ies** longer branches of the basilar artery extending across the inferior surface of the pons to reach the lateral aspects.

**lat•er•al car•ti•lage of nose** the cartilage located in the lateral wall of the nose above the alar cartilage. SYN cartilago nasi lateralis [TA].

**lat•er•al ce•re•bral sul•cus** the deepest and most prominent of the cortical fissures, extending from the anterior perforated substance first laterally at the deep incisure between the frontal and temporal lobes, then back and slightly upward over the lateral aspect of the cerebral hemisphere, with the superior temporal gyrus as its lower bank, the insula forming its greatly expanded floor. Two short side branches, the ramus anterior and ramus ascendens, divide the inferior frontal gyrus into an orbital part, triangular part, and opercular part.

**lat•er•al col•umn** a slight protrusion of the gray matter of the spinal cord into the lateral funiculus of either side, especially marked in the thoracic region where it encloses preganglionic motor neurons of the sympathetic division of the autonomic nervous system; it corresponds to the lateral horn appearing in transverse sections of the spinal cord. SEE ALSO gray columns.

**lat•er•al cord of brach•i•al plex•us** in the brachial plexus, the bundle of nerve fibers, formed by the anterior divisions of the superior and middle trunks that lies lateral to the axillary artery. This cord gives off the lateral pectoral nerve and terminates by dividing into the musculocutaneous nerve and the lateral root of the median nerve.

**lat•er•al cu•ne•i•form bone** a bone of the distal row of the tarsus; it articulates with the intermediate cuneiform, cuboid, navicular, and second, third, and fourth metatarsal bones. SYN wedge bone.

**lat•er•al ep•i•con•dy•li•tis** SYN tennis elbow.

**lat•er•al folds** ventral foldings of the lateral margins of the embryonic disk, the development of which establishes the definitive embryonic body form.

**lat•er•al fu•nic•u•lus** the lateral white column of the spinal cord between the lines of exit and entrance of the anterior and posterior nerve roots.

**lat•er•al ge•nic•u•late bo•dy** the lateral one of a pair of small oval masses that protrude slightly from the posteroinferior aspects of the thalamus; its main (dorsal) subdivision serves as a processing station in the major pathway from the retina to the cerebral cortex, receiving fibers from the optic tract and giving rise to the geniculocalcarine radiation to the visual cortex in the occipital lobe. SYN corpus geniculatum laterale [TA].

**lat•er•al her•maph•ro•dit•ism** a form in which a testis is present on one side and an ovary on the other.

**lat•er•al hu•mer•al ep•i•con•dy•li•tis** SYN tennis elbow.

**lat•er•al•i•ty** (lat-er-al′i-tē) referring to a side of the body or of a structure; specifically, the dominance of one side of the brain or the body.

**lat•er•al lon•gi•tu•di•nal stria** a thin longitudinal band of nerve fibers accompanied by gray matter, near each outer edge of the upper surface of the corpus callosum under cover of the cingulate gyrus.

**lat•er•al med•ul•lary branch•es of (in•tra••cra•ni•al part of) ver•te•bral ar•te•ry** minute branches of the vertebral artery (or its larger branches) that course laterally along the ventral aspect of the medulla oblongata.

**lat•er•al me•nis•cus** attached to the lateral border of the upper articular surface of the tibia.

**lat•er•al na•sal branch of fa•cial ar•te•ry** branch of facial artery to the side of the nose (ala and dorsum); anastomoses with its contralateral partner, as well as the septal and alar branches of the superior labial, the dorsal nasal branch of the ophthalmic, and the infraorbital branch of the maxillary artery.

**lat•er•al oc•cip•i•tal ar•tery** one of the terminal branches of the posterior cerebral artery; it supplies, by several named branches, the lateral portions of the temporal lobe.

**lat•er•al pinch** OCCUPATIONAL THERAPY pinch between the tip pad of the thumb and the lateral surface of the index finger at the proximal interphalangeal (PIP) joints.

**lat•er•al plate** a nonsegmented mass of mesoderm on the lateral periphery of the embryonic disk.

**lat•er•al rec•tus mus•cle** *origin*, lateral part of the common tendinous ring that bridges superior orbital fissure; *insertion*, lateral part of sclera of eye; *action*, abduction; *nerve supply*, abducens. SYN musculus rectus lateralis [TA], abducens oculi.

**lat•er•al rec•tus mus•cle of the head** SYN rectus capitis lateralis muscle.

**lat•er•al re•cum•bent po•si•tion** SYN Sims position.

**lat•er•al sa•cral veins** several veins that receive the drainage of the sacral venous plexus and sacral intervertebral veins, then accompany the corresponding artery and empty into the internal iliac vein on each side.

**lat•er•al tar•sal strip pro•ce•dure** a procedure designed to correct lower eyelid malposition due to horizontal lid laxity by shortening it at the lateral canthal end.

**lat•er•al vas•tus mus•cle** SYN vastus lateralis muscle.

**lat•er•al ven•tri•cle** a cavity shaped somewhat like a horseshoe in conformity with the general shape of the hemisphere; each lateral ventricle communicates with the third ventricle through the interventricular foramen of Monro, and expands from there forward into the frontal lobe as the anterior horn as well as caudally over the thalamus as the central part or cella media which, behind the thalamus, curves ventrally and laterally, then forward into the temporal lobe as the inferior horn; from the apex of the curve a variably sized posterior horn extends back into the white matter of the occipital lobe. The large choroid plexus of the lateral ventricle invades the cella media and the inferior horn (but not the anterior and posterior horn) from the medial side.

**late rick•ets** SYN osteomalacia.

△**lat•ero-** lateral, to one side. [L. *lateralis*, lateral, fr. *latus*, side]

**lat•er•o•de•vi•a•tion** (lat′er-ō-dē-vē-ā′shŭn) a bending or a displacement to one side. [latero- + L. *devio*, to turn aside, fr. *via*, a way]

**lat•er•o•duc•tion** (lat′er-ō-dŭk′shŭn) a drawing to one side; denoting a movement of a limb or turning of the eyeball away form the midline. [latero- + L. *duco*, pp. *ductus*, to lead]

**lat•er•o•flex•ion, lat•er•o•flec•tion** (lat′er-ō-flek′shŭn) a bending or curvature to one side. [latero- + L. *flecto*, pp. *flexus*, to bend]

**lat•er•o•tor•sion** (lat′er-ō-tōr′shŭn) a twisting to one side; denoting rotation of the eyeball around its anteroposterior axis, so that the top part of the cornea turns away from the sagittal plane. [latero- + L. *torsio*, a twisting]

**lat•er•o•tru•sion** (lat′er-ō-troo′zhŭn) the outward thrust given by the muscles of mastication to the rotating mandibular condyle during movement of the mandible. [latero- + L. *trudo*, pp. *trusus*, to thrust]

**lat•er•o•ver•sion** (lat′er-ō-ver′zhŭn) version to one side or the other, denoting especially a malposition of the uterus. [latero- + L. *verto*, pp. *versus*, to turn]

**late sys•to•le** SYN prediastole.

**la•tex** (lā′teks) **1.** an emulsion or suspension produced by some seed plants; it contains suspended microscopic globules of natural rubber. **2.** similar synthetic materials such as polystyrene, polyvinyl chloride, etc. [L. liquid]

**lath•y•rism** (lath′i-rizm) a disease occurring in Ethiopia, Algeria, and India, characterized by various nervous manifestations, tremors, spastic paraplegia, and paresthesias; prevalent in districts where vetches, khasari (*Lathyrus sativus*), and allied species form the main food. [L. *lathyrus*, vetch]

**la•tis•si•mus dor•si mus•cle** *origin*, spinous processes of lower five or six thoracic and the lumbar vertebrae, median ridge of sacrum, and outer lip of iliac crest; *insertion*, with teres major into posterior lip of bicipital groove of humerus; *action*, adducts arm, rotates it medially, and extends it; *nerve supply*, thoracodorsal. SYN musculus latissimus dorsi [TA].

**lat•i•tude** (la′ti-tood) the range of light or x-ray exposure acceptable with a given photographic emulsion. [L. *latitudo*, width, fr. *latus*, wide]

***La•tro•dec•tus*** (lat-rō-dek′tŭs) a genus of relatively small spiders, the widow spiders, capable of inflicting highly poisonous, neurotoxic, painful bites. [L. *latro*, servant, robber, + G. *dēktēs*, a biter]

**LATS** long-acting thyroid stimulator.

**la•tus**, gen. **la•te•ris**, pl. **la•te•ra** (lā′tŭs, lat′er-is, lat′er-ă) [TA] the side of the body between the pelvis and the ribs. SYN flank. [L. broad]

**Latz•ko ce•sar•e•an sec•tion** (lahtz′kō) a cesarean section in which the uterus is entered by paravesical blunt dissection without entering the peritoneal cavity.

**Lau•gi•er her•nia** (lō-zhē-ā′) a hernia passing through an opening in the lacunar ligament.

**Laurence-Moon syn•drome** (law′rĕns-moon) disorder characterized by mental retardation, pigmentary retinopathy, hypogenitalism, and spastic paraplegia; autosomal recessive inheritance. This syndrome is to be distinguished from Bardet-Biedl; in the past, the two syndromes have been lumped together under the designation of Laurence-Moon-Bardet-Biedl syndrome.

**Lau•rer ca•nal** (lăw-rer) a tube originating on the surface of the ootype of trematodes, directed dorsally to or near the surface; it may have originally served as a vagina or possibly as a reservoir of excess shell material.

**Lauth ca•nal** (lōt) SYN scleral venous sinus.

**Lauth vi•o•let** (lōt) SYN thionine.

**LAV** lymphadenopathy-associated virus.

**la•vage** (lă-vahzh′) the washing out of a hollow cavity or organ by copious injections and rejections of fluid. [Fr. from L. *lavo*, to wash]

**law 1.** a principle or rule. **2.** a statement of a sequence or relation of phenomena that is invariable under the given conditions. SEE ALSO principle, rule, theorem. [A.S. *lagu*]

**law of con•ti•gu•i•ty** when two ideas or psychologically perceived events have once occurred in close association they are likely to so occur again, the subsequent occurrence of one tending to elicit the other; this law figures prominently in modern theories of conditioning and learning.

**law of ex•ci•ta•tion** a motor nerve responds, not to the absolute value, but to the alteration of value from moment to moment, of the electric current; i.e., rate of change of intensity of the current is a factor in determining its effectiveness.

**law of the heart** the energy liberated by the heart when it contracts is a function of the length of its muscle fibers at the end of diastole.

**law of in•de•pen•dent as•sort•ment** different hereditary factors assort independently when the gametes are formed; traits at linked loci are an exception. SYN Mendel second law.

**law of par•tial pres•sures** SYN Dalton law.

**law of re•ferred pain** pain arises only from irritation of nerves which are sensitive to those stimuli that produce pain when applied to the surface of the body.

**law of re•frac•tion** for two given media, the sine of the angle of incidence bears a constant relation to the sine of the angle of refraction. SYN Descartes law, Snell law.

**law•ren•ci•um (Lr)** (law-ren′sē-ŭm) an artificial transplutonium element; atomic no. 103; atomic wt. 262.11. [E.O. *Lawrence*, U.S. physicist and Nobel laureate, 1901–1958]

**law of seg•re•ga•tion** factors that affect development retain their individuality from generation to generation, do not become contaminated when

mixed in a hybrid, and become sorted out from one another when the next generation of gametes is formed. SYN Mendel first law.

**law of sim•i•lars** SEE similia similibus curantur.

**lax•a•tive** (lak′să-tiv) any oral agent that promotes the expulsion of feces, including harsh stimulant laxatives (senna, bisacodyl), saline laxatives (magnesium citrate), stool softeners (docusate sodium), bulking laxatives (psyllium, methylcellulose), and lubricants (mineral oil). [L. *laxativus*, fr. *laxo*, pp. *-atus*, to slacken, relax]

**lax•i•ty** (lăks′ĭ-tē) looseness or freedom of movement in a joint, normal or excessive. SEE ALSO instability. [L. *laxitas*, looseness]

**lay•er** (lā′er) a sheet of one substance lying on another and distinguished from it by a difference in texture or color or by not being continuous with it. SEE ALSO stratum, lamina.

**LCAT de•fi•cien•cy** a rare condition characterized by corneal opacities, hemolytic anemia, proteinuria, renal insufficiency, and premature atherosclerosis, and very low levels of lecithin cholesterol acyltransferase (LCAT) activity; results in accumulation of unesterfied cholesterol in plasma and tissues.

**LD** lethal dose.

**LDH** lactate dehydrogenase.

**LDL** low density lipoprotein. See lipoprotein.

**L-do•pa** SYN levodopa.

**L dos•es** a group of terms that indicate the relative activity or potency of diphtheria toxin; the L doses are different from the minimal lethal dose and minimal reacting dose, inasmuch as the latter two represent the direct effects of toxin, whereas the L doses pertain to the combining power of toxin with specific antitoxin. ["L" for L. *limes*, limit, boundary]

**LE, L.E.** left eye; lupus erythematosus.

**leach•ing** (lēch′ing) removal of the soluble constituents of a substance by running water through it. [A.S. *leccan*, to wet]

**lead** (lēd) **1.** an electrical conductor carrying current or intermittent signals between an organ or tissue and an electrical or electronic device. **2.** the tracing obtained from a particular combination of electrode positions.

**lead (Pb)** (led) a metallic element, atomic no. 82, atomic wt. 207.2; occurs in nature as an oxide or one of the salts, but chiefly as the sulfide, or galena; $^{210}$Pb (half-life equal to 22.6 years) has been used in the treatment of certain eye conditions. SYN plumbum.

**lead en•ceph•a•lop•a•thy, lead en•ceph•a•li•tis** a metabolic encephalopathy, caused by the ingestion of lead compounds and seen particularly in early childhood; it is characterized pathologically by extensive cerebral edema, status spongiosus, neurocytolysis, and some reactive inflammation; clinical manifestations include convulsions, delirium, and hallucinations. SEE ALSO lead poisoning.

**lead poi•son•ing** acute or chronic intoxication by lead or any of its salts; symptoms of **acute lead poisoning** usually are those of acute gastroenteritis in adults or encephalopathy in children; **chronic lead poisoning** is manifested chiefly by anemia, constipation, colicky abdominal pain, neuropathy with paralysis, especially wrist-drop involving the extensor muscles of the forearm, bluish lead line of the gums, and interstitial nephritis; saturnine gout, convulsions, and coma may occur. SYN plumbism.

**lean bo·dy mass** SYN fat-free body mass.

**Lear com·plex** (lēr) a father's libidinous fixation on a daughter. [*Lear,* Shakespearean character]

**learned drive** SYN motive (1).

**learned help·less·ness** a laboratory model of depression involving both classical (respondent) and instrumental (operant) conditioning techniques; application of unavoidable shock is followed by failure to cope in situations where coping might otherwise be possible.

**learn·ing** (lern'ing) generic term for the relatively permanent change in behavior that occurs as a result of practice. SEE ALSO conditioning, memory.

**learn·ing dis·a·bil·i·ty** a disorder in one or more of the basic cognitive and psychological processes involved in understanding or using written or spoken language; may be manifested in age-related impairment in the ability to read, write, spell, speak, or perform mathematical calculations.

**least con·fu·sion cir·cle** in the configuration of rays emerging from a spherocylindrical lens system, the place where diverging rays of the lens first forming a line image are balanced by converging rays of the second lens.

**leath·er-bot·tle stom·ach** marked thickening and rigidity of the stomach wall, with reduced capacity of the lumen although often without obstruction; nearly always due to scirrhous carcinoma, as in linitis plastica.

**Le·ber he·red·i·tary op·tic at·ro·phy** (lā'bĕr) degeneration of the optic nerve and papillomacular bundle with resulting loss of central vision and blindness, progressive for several weeks, then usually becoming stationary with permanent central scotoma; the age of onset is variable, most often in the third decade; more males than females are affected. Mitochondrial or cytoplasmic inheritance via the maternal lineage, caused by mutation in the mitochondrial gene(s) acting autonomously or in association with each other.

**Le·ber id·i·o·path·ic stel·late ret·i·nop·a·thy** (la-ber) SEE neuroretinitis.

**LE cell** a polymorphonuclear leukocyte containing an amorphous round body; formed in vitro in the blood of patients with systemic lupus erythematosus, or by the action of the patient's serum on normal leukocytes. SYN lupus erythematosus cell.

**LE cell test** *in vitro* incubation of blood or bone marrow of patients with systemic lupus erythematosus, or action of their serum on normal leukocytes, causes formation of characteristic LE cells. SYN lupus erythematosus cell test.

**Le Cha·te·li·er law** (lĕ-shah-tĕl-yā') if external factors such as temperature and pressure disturb a system in equilibrium, adjustment occurs in such a way that the effect of the disturbing factors is reduced to a minimum.

**lec·i·thal** (les'i-thăl) having a yolk or pertaining to the yolk of any egg; used especially as a suffix. [G. *lekithos,* egg yolk]

**lec·i·thin** (les'i-thin) traditional term for phospholipids that on hydrolysis yield two fatty acid molecules and a molecule each of glycerophosphoric acid and choline. Lecithins are found in nervous tissue, especially in the myelin sheaths, in egg yolk, and as essential constituents of animal and vegetable cells. [G. *lekithos,* egg yolk]

**lec·i·thi·nase** (les'i-thi-nās) SYN phospholipase.

**lec·i·thin/sphin·go·my·e·lin ra·tio** a ratio used to determine fetal pulmonary maturity, found by testing the amniotic fluid; when the lungs are mature, lecithin exceeds sphingomyelin by 2 to 1.

**lec·i·tho·blast** (les'i-thō-blast) one of the cells proliferating to form the yolk-sac endoderm. [G. *lekithos,* egg yolk, + *blastos,* germ]

**Le·cler·ci·a** (le-kler'sē-a) a genus in the family Enterobacteriaceae that resembles the genus *Escherichia,* but is separable by metabolic and genetic classification. Isolated from the feces of humans and animals, it has been recovered clinically from blood, sputum, urine, and wounds; its degree of pathogenicity is unclear.

**lec·tin** (lek'tin) a protein of primarily plant (usually seed) origin that binds to glycoproteins on the surface of cells causing agglutination, precipitation, or other phenomena resembling the action of specific antibody; lectins include plant agglutinins (phytoagglutinins, phytohemagglutinins), plant precipitins, and perhaps certain animal proteins; some have mitogenic properties. [L. *lego,* pp. *lectum,* to select, + -in]

**lec·tin gly·co·his·to·chem·is·try** technique for measuring the endogenous ligands for specific sugar moieties, such as peanut agglutinin, wheat germ agglutinin, and gorse seed agglutinin, in characterization of surface epithelium.

**lec·tin path·way mol·e·cule** the binding of mannose-binding protein to bacterial carbohydrates resulting in activation of the complement pathway.

**ledge** (lej) in anatomy, a structure resembling a ledge. SEE ALSO lamina.

**leech** (lēch) **1.** a bloodsucking aquatic annelid worm (genus *Hirudo*) sometimes used in medicine and plastic surgery for local withdrawal of blood. **2.** to treat medically by applying leeches. [A.S. *laece,* a physician; a leech, because of its therapeutic use]

**LEEP** loop electrocautery excision procedure.

**Le Fort am·pu·ta·tion** (lĕ-for') a modification of Pirogoff amputation; the calcaneus is sawed through horizontally instead of vertically so that the patient steps on the same part of the heel as before.

**Le Fort I frac·ture** (lĕ-for') SYN horizontal maxillary fracture. See this page.

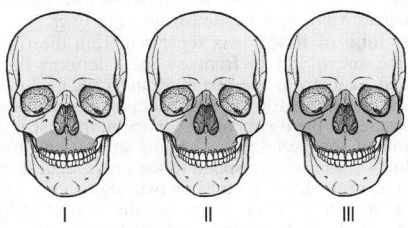

I    II    III

**Le Fort** classification of horizontal maxillary fractures

**left atri·um of heart** atrium of the left side of the heart which receives the blood from the pulmonary veins. SYN atrium cordis sinistrum [TA], atrium pulmonale, atrium sinistrum cordis.

**left bun·dle of a·tri·o·ven·tric·u·lar bun·dle** the left limb or branch of the atrioventricular bundle that separates from the atrioventricular bundle just below the membranous portion of the interventricular septum to descend the septal wall of the left ventricle and begins to ramify subendocardially.

**left col·ic flex·ure** the bend at the junction of the transverse and descending colon. SYN flexura coli sinistra [TA], splenic flexure.

**left-foot·ed** SYN sinistropedal.

**left gas·tric ar·tery** *origin*, celiac; *distribution*, cardia of stomach at lesser curvature, abdominal part of the esophagus, and, frequently, a portion of the left lobe of the liver via an aberrant left hepatic branch; *anastomoses*, esophageal, right gastric.

**left gas·tric vein** arises from a union of veins from both surfaces of the cardia of the stomach and an esophageal tributary from the cardiac portion of the esophagus; it runs in the lesser omentum and empties into the portal vein. SEE ALSO esophageal veins.

**left-hand·ed** denoting the habitual or more skillful use of the left hand for writing and for most manual operations. SYN sinistromanual.

**left heart** the left atrium and left ventricle.

**left heart by·pass** any procedure that shunts blood returning from the pulmonary circulation to the systemic circulation without passing through the left heart. This is used during cardiac surgery and in severe left heart failure or cardiogenic shock.

**left he·pa·tic duct** the duct that drains bile from the left half of the liver, including the quadrate lobe and the left part of the caudate lobe.

**left lat·er·al di·vi·sion of liv·er** the portion of the liver that lies to the left of the approximately vertical plane of the left hepatic vein and includes the left posterior and anterior lateral segments (hepatic segments II and III); it corresponds to the left anatomic lobe of the liver, and so is demarcated externally by the falciform ligament on the diaphragmatic surface and by the fissures for the ligamentum venosum and ligamentum teres on the viscera surface. SYN divisio lateralis sinistra hepatis [TA].

**left liv·er** portion of the liver receiving blood from the left branches of the hepatic artery and portal vein, and from which bile is drained via the left hepatic duct; the plane of the middle hepatic vein separates left from right liver.

**left lobe of liv·er** it is separated from the right lobe above and in front by the falciform ligament, and from the quadrate and caudate lobes by the fissure for the ligamentum teres and the fissure for the ligamentum venosum; the distribution of the portal vein, hepatic artery, and bile ducts does not correspond to the gross lobar divisions of the liver. It contains two segments, superior and inferior. SYN lobus hepatis sinister [TA].

**left me·di·al di·vi·sion of liv·er** the portion of the liver that lies between the approximately vertical planes of the left and middle hepatic veins and includes the left medial segment (hepatic segment IV); on the diaphragmatic surface, it is approximately the left third of the anatomic right lobe of the liver; on the visceral surface, its infe-

rior portion corresponds to the quadrate lobe. SYN divisio medialis sinistra hepatis [TA].

**left pul·mo·na·ry ar·te·ry** the shorter of the two terminal branches of the pulmonary trunk, it pierces the pericardium to enter the hilum of the left lung. Its branches accompany the segmental and subsegmental bronchi. Branches to the superior lobe (rami lobi superioris [TA]) are apical (ramus apicalis [TA]), anterior ascending (ramus anterior ascendens [TA]), anterior descending (ramus anterior descendens [TA]), posterior (ramus posterior [TA]), and lingular (ramus lingularis [TA]), the last having inferior and superior branches (rami lingulares inferior et superior [TA]). Branches to the inferior lobe (rami lobi inferioris [TA]) are the superior branch of the inferior lobe (ramus superior lobi inferior [TA]) and the medial (medialis), anterior, lateral (lateralis) and posterior basal branches (rami basalis [TA]).

**left-to-right shunt** a diversion of blood from the left side of the heart to right (as through a septal defect), or from the systemic circulation to the pulmonary (as through a patent ductus arteriosus).

**left um·bil·i·cal vein** returns the blood from the placenta to the fetus; traversing the umbilical cord, it enters the fetal body at the umbilicus and passes thence into the liver, where it is joined by the portal vein; its blood then flows by way of the ductus venosus and the inferior vena cava to the right atrium. SYN vena umbilicalis [TA].

**left ven·tri·cle** the lower chamber on the left side of the heart that receives the arterial blood from the left atrium and drives it by the contraction of its walls into the aorta.

**left-ven·tric·u·lar as·sist de·vice** mechanical pump inserted at some point in the circulation to parallel the activity of the left ventricle and thereby reduce its load.

**left ven·tric·u·lar e·jec·tion time (LVET)** the time measured clinically from onset to incisural notch of the carotid or other pulse; properly the time of ejection of blood from the left ventricle beginning with aortic valve opening and ending with aortic valve closure.

**left ven·tric·u·lar fail·ure** congestive heart failure manifested by signs of pulmonary congestion and edema.

**left ven·tri·cu·lar vol·ume re·duc·tion sur·gery** operation in which the volume of a dilated, nonaneurysmal left ventricle is reduced by myocardial resection to improve ventricular geometry and mechanical function and thereby treat endstage congestive heart failure. SYN Battista operation, partial left ventriculectomy, reduction left ventriculoplasty.

**leg 1.** the segment of the inferior limb between the knee and the ankle; commonly used to mean the entire inferior limb. **2.** a structure resembling a leg. SYN crus (1) [TA].

**le·gal blind·ness** generally, visual acuity of less than 6/60 or 20/200 using Snellen test types, or visual field restriction to 20° or less in the better eye; the criteria used to define legal blindness vary.

**le·gal med·i·cine** SYN forensic medicine.

**Le·gen·dre sign** (lĕ-zhā-dr′) in facial hemiplegia of central origin, when the examiner raises the lids of the actively closed eyes the resistance is less on the affected side.

⌂**-le•gia** reading, as distinguished from the G. derivatives, *-lexis* and *-lexy*, which signify speech, from G. *legō*, to say. [L. *lego*, to read]

*Le•gion•el•la* (lē-jŭ-nel'lă) a genus of aerobic, motile, non-acid-fast, non-encapsulated, Gram-negative bacilli; they are water-dwelling and air-borne-spread, and are pathogenic for humans. The type species is *Legionella pneumophila*.

*Le•gion•el•la boze•man•ii* a species that causes human pneumonia.

*Le•gion•el•la mic•da•dei* a species that causes Pittsburgh pneumonia, a variant of Legionnaires disease. Accounts for approximately 60% of *Legionella* pneumonias other than those caused by *Legionella pneumophila*. SYN Pittsburgh pneumonia agent.

**Le•gion•naires dis•ease** (lē-jŭ-nārz) an acute infectious disease, caused by *Legionella pneumophila*, with prodromal influenzalike symptoms and a rapidly rising high fever, followed by severe pneumonia and production of usually nonpurulent sputum, and sometimes mental confusion, hepatic fatty changes, and renal tubular degeneration. It has a high case-fatality rate; acquired from contaminated water, usually by aerosolization rather than from transmitted from person-to-person. [American *Legion* convention, 1976, at which many delegates were infected]

**Leigh dis•ease** (lē) subacute encephalomyelopathy affecting infants, causing seizures, spasticity, optic atrophy, and dementia; the genetic causation is heterogeneous; may be associated with deficiency of cytochrome c oxidase or NADH-ubiquinone oxidoreductase or other enzymes involved in energy metabolism. Autosomal recessive, X-linked recessive and mitochondrial inheritance have been described; mutations have been identified in the surfeit-1 gene (SURF) on chromosome 9, in a mtDNA-encoded subunit of ATP synthase, in the X-linked E1-alpha subunit of pyruvate dehydrogenase, and in several subunits of mitochondrial complex I.

**Lei•ner dis•ease** (lī'nĕr) SYN erythroderma desquamativum.

⌂**lei•o-** smooth. [G. *leios*]

**lei•o•der•mia** (lī-ō-der'mē-ă) smooth, glossy skin. [leio- + G. *derma*, skin]

**lei•o•my•o•fi•bro•ma** (lī-ō-mī'ō-fī-brō'mă) SYN fibroleiomyoma.

**lei•o•my•o•ma** (lī'ō-mī-ō'mă) a benign neoplasm derived from smooth (nonstriated) muscle. [leio- + G. *mys*, muscle, + *-oma*, tumor]

**lei•o•my•o•ma cu•tis** cutaneous eruption of multiple small painful nodules composed of smooth muscle fibers; derived from arrector muscles of hair. SYN dermatomyoma.

**lei•o•my•o•ma•to•sis** (lī'ō-mī'ō-mă-tō'sis) the state of having multiple leiomyomas throughout the body.

**lei•o•my•o•ma•to•sis per•i•to•ne•a•lis dis•sem•i•na•ta** a benign condition characterized by multiple small nodules on abdominal and pelvic peritoneum grossly mimicking disseminated ovarian cancer but with histologic characteristics of benign myoma; often associated with recent pregnancy.

**lei•o•my•o•sar•co•ma** (lī'ō-mī'ō-sar-kō'mă) a malignant neoplasm derived from smooth (nonstriated) muscle. [leio- + myosarcoma]

**Leish•man-Don•o•van bod•y** (lēsh'măn-don'ĕ-văn) the intracytoplasmic, nonflagellated

leishmanial form of certain intracellular parasites, such as species of *Leishmania* or the intracellular form of *Trypanosoma cruzi*. SYN amastigote.

*Leish•man•ia* (lēsh-man'ē-ă) a genus of digenetic, asexual, protozoan flagellates that occur as amastigotes in the macrophages of vertebrate hosts, and as promastigotes in invertebrate hosts and in cultures. [W. B. *Leishman*]

**leish•man•ia**, pl. **leish•man•i•ae** (lēsh-man'ē-ă) a member of the genus *Leishmania*.

**leish•man•i•a•sis** (lēsh'mă-nī'ă-sis) infection with a species of *Leishmania* resulting in a group of diseases traditionally divided into four major types: 1) visceral leishmaniasis (kala azar); 2) Old World cutaneous leishmaniasis; 3) New World cutaneous leishmaniasis; 4) mucocutaneous leishmaniasis. SEE tropical diseases.

**Leish•man stain** (lēsh'măn) a polychromed eosin-methylene blue stain used in the examination of blood films.

**Lem•bert su•ture** (lahm-bār') the second row of the Czerny-Lembert intestinal suture; an inverting suture for intestinal surgery, used either as a continuous suture or interrupted suture, producing serosal apposition and including the collagenous submucosal layer but not entering the lumen of the intestine.

*Le•min•or•el•la* (lem'in-ŏ-rel'ă) a genus in the family Enterobacteriaceae containing two species, *Leminorella grimontii* and *Leminorella richardii*, that have been isolated from clinical material, primarily from fecal samples; its clinical importance is unclear.

**lem•mo•blast** (lem'ō-blast) in an embryo, a cell of neural crest origin capable of forming a cell of the neurilemma sheath. [G. *lemma*, husk, + *blastos*, germ]

**lem•mo•cyte** (lem'ō-sīt) one of the cells of the neurolemma. [G. *lemma*, husk, + *kytos*, cell]

**lem•nis•cus**, pl. **lem•nis•ci** (lem-nis'kŭs,lem-nis'ī) a bundle of nerve fibers ascending from sensory relay nuclei to the thalamus. SYN fillet (1). [L. from G. *lēmniskos*, ribbon or fillet]

**lem•on sign** (lĕm'on) the ultrasound finding of frontal bone scalloping associated with Arnold-Chiari malformation.

**Len•drum phlox•ine-tar•tra•zine stain** (len' drŭm) a stain for demonstrating acidophilic inclusion bodies, which appear red on a yellow background; nuclei stain blue, but Negri bodies do not stain.

**Le•nèg•re syn•drome** (lĕ-neg'rĕ) isolated damage of the cardiac conduction system as a result of a sclerodegenerative lesion; characterized ordinarily as idiopathic fibrosis of the atrioventricular nodal, His bundle, or bundle branches with corresponding conduction block(s).

**length** (length, lenth) linear distance between two points.

**Len•nert lym•pho•ma** (len'ĕrt) malignant lymphoma with a high proportion of diffusely scattered epithelioid cells, tonsillar involvement, and an unpredictable course.

**Len•nox-Gas•taut syn•drome, Len•nox syn•drome** (len'oks-gahs-tō', len'ŏks) a generalized myoclonic astatic epilepsy in children, with mental retardation, resulting from various cerebral afflictions such as perinatal hypoxia, cerebral hemorrhage, encephalitides, maldevelopment or metabolic disorders of the brain; characterized by

l
e

tal retardation, resulting from various cerebral afflictions such as perinatal hypoxia, cerebral hemorrhage, encephalitides, maldevelopment or metabolic disorders of the brain; characterized by multiple seizure types (generalized tonic, atonic, myoclonic, tonic-clonic, and atypical absence) and background slowing and slow spike and wave pattern on EEG; patients are usually mentally retarded or developmentally delayed.

**lens** (lenz) **1.** a transparent material with one or both surfaces having a concave or convex curve; acts upon electromagnetic energy to cause convergence or divergence of light rays. **2.** [TA] the transparent biconvex cellular refractive structure lying between the iris and the vitreous humor, consisting of a soft outer part (cortex) with a denser part (nucleus), and surrounded by a basement membrane (capsule); the anterior surface has a cuboidal epithelium, and at the equator the cells elongate to become lens fibers. [L. a lentil]

**lens cap·sule** the capsule enclosing the lens of the eye.

**lens·ec·to·my** (len-zek'tō-mē) removal of the lens of the eye by an infusion-aspiration cutter; often done by puncture incision through the pars plana in the course of vitrectomy. [lens + G. *ektomē,* excision]

**lens pits** the paired depressions formed in the superficial ectoderm of the embryonic head as the lens placodes sink in toward the optic cup; the external openings of the pits are closed as the lens vesicles are formed.

**lens stars 1.** SYN radii of lens. **2.** congenital cataracts with opacities along the suture lines of the lens; may be anterior or posterior, or both.

**lens ves·i·cle** in the embryo, the ectodermal invagination that forms opposite the optic cup; it is the primordium of the lens of the eye.

**len·ti·co·nus** (len-ti-kō'nŭs) conical projection of the anterior or posterior surface of the lens of the eye, occurring as a developmental anomaly. [lens + L. *conus,* cone]

**len·tic·u·lar** (len-tik'yu'lăr) **1.** relating to or resembling a lens of any kind. **2.** of the shape of a lentil. [L. *lenticula,* a lentil]

**len·tic·u·lar a·stig·ma·tism** astigmatism due to defect in the curvature, position, or index of refraction of the lens.

**len·tic·u·lar loop** the pallidal efferent fibers curving around the medial border of the internal capsule.

**len·tic·u·lar nu·cle·us** the large cone-shaped mass of gray matter forming the central core of the cerebral hemisphere. The convex base of the cone, oriented laterally and rostrally, is formed by the putamen which together with the caudate nucleus composes the striatum; the apical part, oriented medially and caudally, consists of the two segments of the globus pallidus. The nucleus is ventral and lateral to the thalamus and caudate nucleus, from which it is separated by the internal capsule, and together with the caudate nucleus composes the striate body.

**len·tic·u·lar pro·cess of in·cus** a knob at the tip of the long limb of the incus, which articulates with the stapes. SYN orbiculare.

**len·tic·u·lo·pap·u·lar** (len-tik'yu-lō-pap'yu-lăr) indicating an eruption with dome-shaped or lens-shaped papules.

**len·ti·form** (len'ti-fōrm) lens-shaped.

**len·tig·i·no·sis** (len-tij-i-nō'sis) presence of len-

tigenes in very large numbers or in a distinctive configuration.

**len·ti·glo·bus** (len-ti-glō'bŭs) rare congenital anomaly with a spheroid elevation on the posterior surface of the lens of the eye. [lens + L. *globus,* sphere]

**len·ti·go,** pl. **len·tig·i·nes** (len-tī'gō, len-tij'i-nēz) a brown macule resembling a freckle except that the border is usually regular, and microscopic proliferation of rete ridges is present; scattered melanocytes are seen in the basal cell layer. SEE ALSO junction nevus. SYN lentigo simplex. [L. fr. *lens* (*lent-*), a lentil]

🔳 **len·ti·go ma·lig·na** a brown or black mottled, irregularly outlined, slowly enlarging lesion resembling a lentigo in which there are increased numbers of scattered atypical melanocytes in the epidermis, usually occurring on the face of older persons; after many years the dermis may be invaded and the lesion is then termed lentigo maligna melanoma. See page B7. SYN Hutchinson freckle.

**len·ti·go sim·plex** SYN lentigo.

**le·o·nine fa·cies** SYN leontiasis.

**le·on·ti·a·sis** (lē-on-tī'ă-sis) a leonine appearance due to ridges and furrows on the forehead and cheeks of patients with advanced lepromatous leprosy. SYN leonine facies. [G. *leōn* (*leont-*), lion]

**LEOPARD syn·drome** a hereditary syndrome consisting of *l*entigines (multiple), *e*lectrocardiographic abnormalities, *o*cular hypertelorism, *p*ulmonary stenosis, *a*bnormalities of genitalia, *r*etardation of growth, and *d*eafness (sensorineural).

**Le·o·pold ma·neu·vers** (lā'ĕ-pōld) four maneuvers employed to determine fetal position: 1) determination of what is in the fundus; 2) evaluation of the fetal back and extremities; 3) palpation of the presenting part above the symphysis; 4) determination of the direction and degree of flexion of the head.

**lep·er** (lep'er) a person who has leprosy. [G. *lepra*]

**le·pid·ic** (lĕ-pid'ik) relating to scales or a scaly covering layer. [G. *lepis* (*lepid-*), scale, rind]

**lep·o·thrix** (lep'ō-thriks) SYN trichomycosis axillaris. [G. *lepos,* rind, husk, + *thrix,* hair]

**lep·re·chaun·ism** (lep'rĕ-kawn-izm) congenital dwarfism characterized by extreme growth retardation, endocrine disorders, and emaciation, with elfin facies and large low-set ears. [Irish *leprechaun,* elf]

**lep·rid** early cutaneous lesion of leprosy. [G. *lepra,* leprosy, + *-id* (1)]

**le·pro·ma** (lĕ-prō'mă) a discrete focus of granulomatous inflammation, caused by *Mycobacterium leprae.* [G. *lepros,* scaly, + *-oma,* tumor]

**lep·rom·a·tous** (lep-rō'mă-tŭs) pertaining to, or characterized by, the features of a leproma.

🔳 **lep·rom·a·tous lep·ro·sy** a form of leprosy in which nodular cutaneous lesions are infiltrated, have ill-defined borders, and are bacteriologically positive. See page B3.

**lep·ro·min** (lep'rō-min) an extract of tissue infected with *Mycobacterium leprae* used in skin tests to classify the stage of leprosy. SEE ALSO test.

**lep·ro·min test** a test utilizing an intradermal injection of a lepromin, to classify the stage of leprosy. It differentiates tuberculoid leprosy, in which there is a positive delayed reaction at the injection site, from lepromatous leprosy, in which there is no reaction.

**lep•ro•sar•i•um** (lep′rō-sar′ē-ŭm) a hospital especially designed for the care of those suffering from leprosy, especially those who need expert care.

**lep•ro•stat•ic** (lep-rō-stat′ik) **1.** inhibiting to the growth of *Mycobacterium leprae*. **2.** an agent having this action.

**lep•ro•sy** (lep′rō-sē) **1.** a chronic granulomatous infection caused by *Mycobacterium leprae* affecting the cooler body parts, especially the skin, peripheral nerves, and testes. Leprosy is classified into two main types, lepromatous and tuberculoid, representing extremes of immunologic response. **2.** a name used in the Bible to describe various cutaneous diseases, especially those of a chronic or contagious nature, which probably included psoriasis and leukoderma. SYN Hansen disease. [G. *lepra*, from *lepros*, scaly]

△-**lep•sis, -lep•sy** a seizure. [G. *lēpsis*]

**lep•tin** (lep′tin) a helical protein secreted by adipose tissue and acting on a receptor site in the ventromedial nucleus of the hypothalamus to curb appetite and increase energy expenditure as body fat stores increase. Leptin levels are 40% higher in women, and show a further 50% rise just before menarche, later returning to baseline levels; levels are lowered by fasting and increased by inflammation. [G. leptos, thin, + -in]

△**lep•to-** light, thin, frail. [G. *leptos,* slender, delicate, weak]

**lep•to•ceph•a•lous** (lep-tō-sef′ă-lŭs) having an abnormally tall, narrow cranium. [lepto- + G. *kephalē*, head]

**lep•to•ceph•a•ly** (lep-tō-sef′ă-lē) a malformation characterized by an abnormally tall, narrow cranium. [lepto- + G. *kephalē,* head]

**lep•to•cyte** (lep′tō-sīt) SYN target cell. [lepto- + G. *kytos,* cell]

**lep•to•cy•to•sis** (lep′tō-sī-tō′sis) the presence of leptocytes in the circulating blood, as seen in thalassemia and after splenectomy.

**lep•to•dac•ty•lous** (lep-tō-dak′ti-lŭs) having slender fingers. [lepto- + G. *daktylos,* finger]

**lep•to•me•nin•ge•al** (lep′tō-me-nin′jē-ăl) pertaining to the leptomeninges.

**lep•to•me•nin•ges,** sing. **lep•to•me•ninx** (lep-tō-me-nin′jēz, lep′tō-mē′ninks) the two delicate layers of the meninges, the arachnoid mater and pia mater considered together. SEE ALSO arachnoid, pia mater. SYN pia-arachnoid, piarachnoid. [lepto- + G. *mēninx,* pl. *mēninges,* membrane]

**lep•to•men•in•gi•tis** (lep′tō-men-in-jī′tis) inflammation of leptomeninges. SEE ALSO arachnoiditis. SYN pia-arachnitis.

**lep•to•so•mat•ic, lep•to•som•ic** (lep′tō-sō-mat′ ik, lep′tō-sō′mik) having a slender, light, or thin body. [lepto- + G. *sōma,* body]

***Lep•to•spi•ra*** (lep′tō-spī′ră) a genus of aerobic bacteria containing thin, tightly coiled organisms 6 to 20 μm in length. Associated with icterohemorrhagic fever. [lepto- + G. *speira,* a coil]

**lep•to•spi•ral jaun•dice** jaundice associated with infection by various species of *Leptospira*.

**lep•to•spi•ro•sis** (lep′tō-spī-rō′sis) infection with *Leptospira interrogans*.

**lep•to•spi•ru•ria** (lep′tō-spīr-yu′rē-ă) presence of species of the genus *Leptospira* in the urine, as a result of leptospirosis in the renal tubules.

**lep•to•tene** (lep′tō-tēn) early stage of prophase in

meiosis in which the chromosomes contract and become visible as long filaments well separated from each other. [lepto- + G. *tainia,* band, tape]

***Lep•to•trich•ia*** (lep-tō-trik′ē-ă) a genus of anaerobic, nonmotile bacteria containing Gram-negative, straight or slightly curved rods, with one or both ends rounded or pointed. These organisms occur in the oral cavity of humans. The type species is *Leptotrichia buccalis.* [lepto- + G. *thrix,* hair]

***Lep•to•trom•bid•i•um*** (lep′tō-trom-bid′ē-ŭm) an important genus of trombiculid mites, which includes all of the vectors of scrub typhus (tsutsugamushi disease).

***Lep•to•trom•bid•i•um ak•a•mu•shi*** one of two species, the other being *Leptotrombidium deliensis* (*T. deliensis*), implicated in the transmission of *Rickettsia tsutsugamushi,* agent of tsutsugamushi disease in the Orient.

**Le•riche op•er•a•tion** (lĕ-rēsh′) SYN periarterial sympathectomy.

**Le•riche syn•drome** (lĕ-rēsh′) aortoiliac occlusive disease producing distal ischemic symptoms and signs.

**Le•ri sign** (lā-rē′) voluntary flexion of the elbow is impossible in a case of hemiplegia when the wrist on that side is passively flexed.

**Ler•mo•yez syn•drome** (ler-mwah-yā′) increasing hearing loss and tinnitus preceding an attack of vertigo, after which the hearing improves. Variant of Mèniére disease.

**LES** lower esophageal sphincter.

**les•bi•an** (lez′bē-ăn) **1.** a female homosexual or a female homosexual lifestyle. **2.** one who practices lesbianism. SEE ALSO gay.

**les•bi•an•ism** (lez′bē-ăn-izm) homosexuality between women. SYN sapphism. [G. *lesbios,* relating to the island of Lesbos]

**le•sion** (lē′zhŭn) **1.** a wound or injury. **2.** a pathologic change in the tissues. **3.** one of the individual points or patches of a multifocal disease. See page 556. [L. *laedo,* pp. *laesus,* to injure]

**less•er a•lar car•ti•lag•es** the two to four cartilaginous plates of the wing of the nose posterior to the greater alar cartilage.

**less•er cur•va•ture of stom•ach** the right border of the stomach to which the lesser omentum is attached.

**less•er o•men•tum** a peritoneal fold passing from the margins of the porta hepatis and the bottom of the fissure of the ductus venosus to the lesser curvature of the stomach and to the upper border of the duodenum for a distance of about 2 cm beyond the gastroduodenal pylorus.

**less•er pa•la•tine ca•nals** canals located in the posterior part of the palatine bone.

**less•er pal•a•tine fo•ram•i•na** openings on the hard palate of palatine canals that pass vertically through the tuberosity of the palatine bone and transmit the smaller palatine nerves and vessels. SYN foramina palatina minora [TA].

**less•er pal•a•tine nerves** usually two, these nerves emerge through the lesser palatine foramina and supply the mucosa and glands of the soft palate and uvula; they are branches of the pterygopalatine ganglion and contain postsynaptic parasympathetic and sensory fibers of the maxillary nerve. SYN nervi palatini minores [TA].

**less•er pel•vis** the cavity of the pelvis below the brim or superior aperture.

**less•er splanch•nic nerve** one of the abdominopelvic splanchnic nerves arising in the thorax from the last two thoracic sympathetic ganglia and passing through the diaphragm to the aorticorenal ganglion; conveys presynaptic sympathetic fibers and visceral afferent fibers. SYN nervus splanchnicus minor [TA].

**Less•er tri•an•gle** (lā′zär) the space between the bellies of the digastric muscle and the hypoglossal nerve.

**less•er tro•chan•ter** a pyramidal process project-

ing from the medial and proximal part of the shaft of the femur at the line of junction of the shaft and the neck; it receives the insertion of the psoas major and iliacus (iliopsoas) muscles.

**less•er ves•tib•u•lar glands** a number of minute mucous glands opening on the surface of the vestibule between the orifices of the vagina and urethra.

**less•er wing of sphe•noid bone** one of a bilateral pair of triangular, pointed plates extending

**primary lesions**

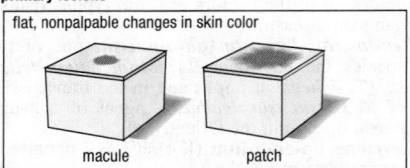

**secondary lesions**

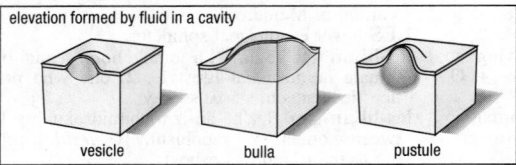

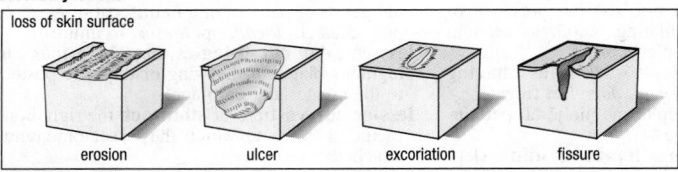

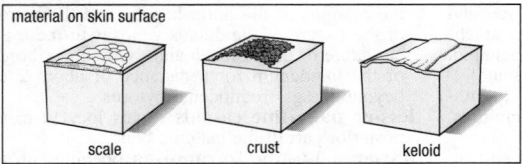

**vascular lesions**

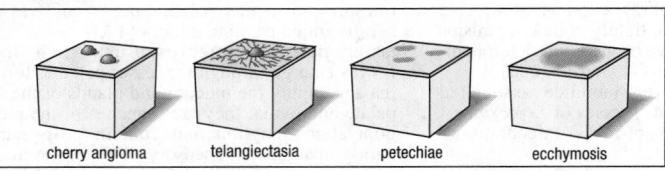

**lesions:** types of primary, secondary, and vascular lesions

laterally from the anterolateral body of the sphenoid bone. Forming the posteriormost portion of the floor of the anterior cranial fossa, their sharp posterior edge forms the sphenoidal ridge separating anterior and middle cranial fossae. The medial end of the lesser wing attaches to the body by means of two pedicles, thus forming the optic canal. The wing itself forms the superior margin of the supraorbital fissure. SYN ala minor ossis sphenoidalis [TA].

**Less·haft tri·an·gle** (les′hahft) SYN Grynfeltt triangle.

**LET** leukocyte esterase test.

**le·thal** (lē′thăl) pertaining to or causing death; denoting especially the causal agent. [L. *letalis*, fr. *letum*, death]

**le·thal dose (LD)** the dose of a chemical or biologic preparation (e.g., a bacterial exotoxin or a suspension of bacteria) that is likely to cause death; it varies in relation to the type of animal and the route of administration; when followed by a subscript (generally "$LD_{50}$" or median lethal dose), it denotes the dose likely to cause death in a certain percentage (e.g., 50%) of the test animals; median lethal dose is $LD_{50}$, absolute lethal dose is $LD_{100}$, and minimal lethal dose is $LD_{05}$.

**le·thal fac·tor** SEE genetic lethal.

**le·thal gene** a gene that produces a genotype that leads to death of the organism before reproduction is possible or that precludes reproduction; for a recessive gene the homozygous or hemizygous state is lethal.

**le·thal mu·ta·tion** a mutant trait that leads to a phenotype incompatible with effective reproduction.

**leth·ar·gy** (leth′ar-jē) a state of deep and prolonged unconsciousness, resembling profound slumber, from which one can be aroused but into which one immediately relapses. [G. *lēthargis*, drowsiness]

**LETS** *l*arge, *e*xternal *t*ransformation-*s*ensitive fibronectin.

△**leuc-, leuco-** white; white blood cell. SEE leuko-, leuk-. [G. *leukos*, white]

**leu·cae·mia [Br.]** SEE leukemia.

**leu·ca·phe·re·sis [Br.]** SEE leukapheresis.

**leu·cine** (loo′sēn) the L-isomer is one of the amino acids of proteins; a nutritionally essential amino acid.

**leu·cin·u·ria** (loo-sin-yu′rē-ă) the excretion of leucine in the urine.

**leu·co·cid·in [Br.]** SEE leukocidin.

**leu·co·cyte [Br.]** SEE leukocyte.

**leu·co·cy·tic [Br.]** SEE leukocytic.

**leu·co·cy·to·ly·sis [Br.]** SEE leukocytolysis.

**leu·co·cy·to·ma [Br.]** SEE leukocytoma.

**leu·co·cy·to·pe·nia [Br.]** SEE leukopenia.

**leu·co·cy·to·sis [Br.]** SEE leukocytosis.

**leu·co·der·ma [Br.]** SEE leukoderma.

**leu·co·dy·stro·phy [Br.]** SEE leukodystrophy.

**leu·co·en·ce·pha·li·tis [Br.]** SEE leukoencephalitis.

**leu·co·en·ce·pha·lo·pa·thy [Br.]** SEE leukoencephalopathy.

**leu·co·e·ryth·ro·bla·sto·sis [Br.]** SEE leukoerythroblastosis.

**leu·co·kin·in·ase [Br.]** SEE leukokininase.

**leu·co·ma [Br.]** SEE leukoma.

**leu·co·ny·chia [Br.]** SEE leukonychia.

**leu·co·pe·nia [Br.]** SEE leukopenia.

**leu·co·pla·kia [Br.]** SEE leukoplakia.

**leu·co·poi·e·sis [Br.]** SEE leukopoiesis.

**leu·cor·rhoea [Br.]** SEE leukorrhea.

**leu·co·sis [Br.]** SEE leukosis.

**leu·co·to·my [Br.]** SEE leukotomy.

**leu·co·tri·ene [Br.]** SEE leukotrienes.

**Leu·det tin·ni·tus** (lŭ-dā′) a dry spasmodic click, audible also through the otoscope, heard in catarrhal inflammation of the eustachian tube; caused by reflex spasm of the tensor palati muscle.

**leu·kae·mia [Br.]** SEE leukemia.

**leu·kae·mic [Br.]** SEE leukemia.

**leu·kae·mo·gen·e·sis [Br.]** SEE leukemogenesis.

**leuk·a·phe·re·sis** (loo′kă-fĕ-rē′sis) a procedure, analogous to plasmapheresis, in which leukocytes are removed from the withdrawn blood and the remainder of the blood is retransfused into the donor. [leuko- + G. *aphairesis*, a withdrawal]

**leu·ke·mia** (loo-kē′mē-ă) progressive proliferation of abnormal leukocytes found in hemopoietic tissues, other organs, and usually in the blood in increased numbers. Leukemia is classified by the dominant cell type, and by duration from onset to death. This occurs in *acute leukemia* within a few months in most cases, and is associated with acute symptoms including severe anemia, hemorrhages, and slight enlargement of lymph nodes or the spleen. The duration of *chronic leukemia* exceeds one year, with a gradual onset of symptoms of anemia or marked enlargement of spleen, liver, or lymph nodes. [leuko- + G. *haima*, blood]

**leu·ke·mia cu·tis** yellow-brown, red, blue-red, or purple, sometimes nodular lesions associated with diffuse infiltration of leukemic cells in the skin.

**leu·ke·mia in·hib·i·tory fac·tor** a lymphokine that inhibits the migration of neutrophils.

**leu·ke·mic** (loo-kē′mik) pertaining to, or having the characteristics of, any form of leukemia.

**leu·ke·mic ret·i·nop·a·thy** appearance of the retina in all types of leukemia, characterized by engorgement and tortuosity of veins, scattered hemorrhages, and edema of the retina and disk.

**leu·ke·mid** (loo-kem′id) any nonspecific type of cutaneous lesion that is associated with leukemia but is not a localized accumulation of leukemic cells; e.g., petechiae, vesicles, wheals, bullae, hematomas, and the lesions of exfoliative dermatitis and herpes zoster. [leuko- + G. *haima*, blood, + *id* (1)]

**leu·ke·mo·gen** (loo-kē′mō-jen) any substance or entity considered to be a causal factor in the occurrence of leukemia.

**leu·ke·mo·gen·e·sis** (loo-kē-mō-jen′ĕ-sis) the causation (or induction), development, and progression of a leukemic disease. [leukemia + G. *genesis*, production]

**leu·ke·mo·gen·ic** (loo-kē-mō-jen′ik) pertaining to the causation, induction, and development of leukemia; manifesting the ability to cause leukemia.

**leu·ke·moid** (loo-kē′moyd) resembling leukemia in various signs and symptoms, especially with reference to changes in the circulating blood. SEE ALSO leukemoid reaction. [leukemia + G. *eidos*, resemblance]

**leu·ke·moid re·ac·tion** leukocytosis similar to that occurring in leukemia, but not the result of leukemic disease. Leukemoid reactions are sometimes observed as a feature of infectious

l
e

disease (tuberculosis, diphtheria), intoxication (eclampsia, mustard gas poisoning), malignant neoplasms, and acute hemorrhage or hemolysis.

△**leuko-, leuk-** white; white blood cells. For some words beginning thus, see leuc- and leuco-. [G. *leukos*, white]

**leu·ko·ag·glu·ti·nin** (loo′kō-ă-gloo′ti-nin) an antibody that agglutinates white blood cells.

**leu·ko·blast** (loo′kō-blast) an immature white blood cell that is transitional between the lymphoidocyte and the promyelocyte; the cytoplasm is polychromatophilic, the nuclear chromatin is thicker, and the nucleoli less distinct. [leuko- + G. *blastos*, germ]

**leu·ko·blas·to·sis** (loo′kō-blas-tō′sis) a general term for the abnormal proliferation of leukocytes, especially that occurring in myelocytic and lymphocytic leukemia.

**leu·ko·ci·din** (loo-kos′i-din) a heat-labile substance that is elaborated by many strains of *Staphylococcus aureus, Streptococcus pyogenes,* and pneumococci and manifests a destructive action on leukocytes, with or without lysis of the cells. [leukocyte + L. *caedo,* to kill]

**leu·ko·co·ria, leu·ko·ko·ria** (loo-kō-kō′rē-ă, loo-kō-kō′rē-ă) reflection from a white mass within the eye giving the appearance of a white pupil. SYN leukokoria. [*leuko-* white, + G. *korē,* pupil]

**leu·ko·cyte** (loo′kō-sīt) a type of cell formed in the myelopoietic, lymphoid, and reticular portions of the reticuloendothelial system in various parts of the body, and normally present in those sites and in the circulating blood. Under various abnormal conditions, the total number of leukocytes may be increased or decreased or their relative proportions altered, and they may appear in other tissues and organs. Leukocytes represent three lines of development from primitive elements: myeloid, lymphoid, and monocytic series. On the basis of features observed with various methods of staining with polychromatic dyes, cells of the myeloid series are frequently termed granular leukocytes, or granulocytes; because the cytoplasmic granules of lymphocytes and monocytes are smaller and frequently not clearly visualized with routine methods, these cells are sometimes termed nongranular or agranular leukocytes. Granulocytes are commonly known as polymorphonuclear leukocytes (also polynuclear or multinuclear leukocytes), because in a mature cell the nucleus is divided into two to five rounded or ovoid lobes that are connected with thin strands or small bands of chromatin; they consist of three distinct types: neutrophils, eosinophils, and basophils, named on the basis of the staining reactions of the cytoplasmic granules. Cells of the lymphocytic series are smaller than other leukocytes and have relatively large, darkly staining, eccentrically placed nuclei. Cells of the monocytic series are usually larger than the other leukocytes, and are characterized by a relatively abundant, slightly opaque, pale blue or blue-gray cytoplasm that contains many fine reddish-blue granules. Monocytes are usually indented, reniform, or shaped similarly to a horseshoe, but are sometimes rounded or ovoid; their nuclei are usually large and centrally placed and, even when eccentrically located, are completely surrounded by at least a small band of cytoplasm. SYN white blood cell. [leuko- + G. *kytos,* cell]

**leu·ko·cyte ad·he·sion de·fi·cien·cy (LAD)** an inherited disorder in which there is a defective CD18 adherence complex that disturbs leukocyte chemotaxis. It is characterized by recurrent bacterial infections and impaired wound healing.

**leu·ko·cyte es·ter·ase test (LET)** a chemical test for the presence of lysed or intact white blood cells in urine, performed with a dipstick as part of routine urinalysis; serves as an adjunct to microscopic examination of urinary sediment, and used to screen asymptomatic persons for urinary tract infection, especially chlamydial urethritis.

**leu·ko·cyt·ic** (loo-kō-sit′ik) pertaining to or characterized by leukocytes.

**leu·ko·cy·to·blast** (loo-kō-sī′tō-blast) a nonspecific term for any immature cell from which a leukocyte develops, including lymphoblast, myeloblast, and the like. [leukocyte + G. *blastos,* germ]

**leu·ko·cy·toc·la·sis** (loo′kō-sī-tok′lă-sis) karyorrhexis of leukocytes. [leuko- + G. *kytos,* cell, + *klasia,* a breaking]

**leu·ko·cy·to·clas·tic vas·cu·li·tis** cutaneous acute vasculitis characterized clinically by palpable purpura, especially of the legs, and histologically by exudation of the neutrophils and sometimes fibrin around dermal venules, with nuclear dust and extravasation of red cells; may be limited to the skin or involve other tissues as in Henoch-Schönlein purpura. SEE ALSO cutaneous vasculitis. [G. *leukos,* white, + *kytos,* cell, + *klastos,* broken, fr. *klao,* to break]

**leu·ko·cy·to·gen·e·sis** (loo′kō-sī-tō-jen′ĕ-sis) the formation and development of leukocytes. [leukocyte + G. *genesis,* production]

**leu·ko·cy·tol·y·sin** (loo′kō-sī-tol′i-sin) any substance (including lytic antibody) that causes dissolution of leukocytes. SYN leukolysin.

**leu·ko·cy·tol·y·sis** (loo′kō-sī-tol′i-sis) dissolution or lysis of leukocytes. [leukocyte + G. *lysis,* dissolution]

**leu·ko·cy·to·lyt·ic** (loo′kō-sī-tō-lit′ik) pertaining to, causing, or manifesting leukocytolysis.

**leu·ko·cy·to·ma** (loo′kō-sī-tō′mă) a fairly well circumscribed, nodular, dense accumulation of leukocytes. [leukocyte + G. *-oma,* tumor]

**leu·ko·cy·to·pe·nia** (loo′kō-sī-tō-pē′nē-ă) SYN leukopenia.

**leu·ko·cy·to·pla·nia** (loo′kō-sī-tō-plā′nē-ă) movement of leukocytes from the lumens of blood vessels, through serous membranes, or in the tissues. [leukocyte + G. *plane,* a wandering]

**leu·ko·cy·to·poi·e·sis** (loo′kō-sī-tō-poy-ē′sis) SYN leukopoiesis. [leukocyte + G. *poiēsis,* a making]

**leu·ko·cy·to·sis** (loo′kō-sī-tō′sis) an abnormally large number of leukocytes; a white blood cell count of 10,000 or more per cu mm. Most examples of leukocytosis represent a disproportionate increase in the neutrophils, and the term is frequently synonymous with neutrophilia. [leukocyte + G. *-osis,* condition]

**leu·ko·cy·to·tac·tic** (loo′kō-sī-tō-tak′tik) pertaining to, characterized by, or causing leukocytotaxia. SYN leukotactic.

**leu·ko·cy·to·tax·ia** (loo-kō-sī-tō-tak′sē-ă) **1.** the active ameboid movement of leukocytes, especially the neutrophilic granulocytes, either toward (**positive leukocytotaxia**) or away from (**negative leukocytotaxia**) certain microorganisms as well as various substances formed in inflamed tissue. **2.** the property of attracting or repelling leukocytes. SYN leukotaxia, leukotaxis. [leukocyte + G. *taxis,* arrangement]

**leu·ko·cy·to·tox·in** (loo'kō-sī-tō-tok'sin) any substance that causes degeneration and necrosis of leukocytes, including leukolysin and leukocidin. SYN leukotoxin. [leukocyte + G. *toxikon,* poison]

**leu·ko·cy·tu·ria** (loo'kō-sīt-yu'rē-ă) the presence of leukocytes in urine that is recently voided or collected by means of a catheter. [leukocyte + G. *ouron,* urine]

**leu·ko·der·ma** (loo-kō-der'mă) an absence of pigment, partial or total, in the skin. SYN leukopathia, leukopathy. [leuko- + G. *derma,* skin]

**leu·ko·dys·tro·phy** (loo-kō-dis'trō-fē) term for a group of white matter diseases, some familial, characterized by progressive cerebral deterioration in early life and primary absence or degeneration of the myelin of the central and peripheral nervous systems; probably related to a defect in lipid metabolism; the adult type of Pelizaeus-Merzbacher disease is inherited as an autosomal dominant trait. [leuko- + G. *dys,* bad, + *trophē,* nourishment]

**leu·ko·e·de·ma** (loo'kō-e-dē'mă) a bluish-white opalescence of the buccal mucosa which becomes the normal mucosal color on stretching the tissue; may be considered a normal anatomic variation.

**leu·ko·en·ceph·a·li·tis** (loo'kō-en-sef-ă-lī'tis) encephalitis restricted to the white matter.

**leu·ko·en·ceph·a·lop·a·thy** (loo'kō-en-sef-ă-lop'ă-thē) white matter changes first described in children with leukemia, associated with radiation and chemotherapy injury, often associated with methotrexate; pathologically characterized by diffuse reactive astrocytosis with multiple areas of necrotic foci without inflammation. [leuko- + G. *enkephalos,* brain, + *pathos,* suffering]

**leu·ko·e·ryth·ro·blas·to·sis** (loo'kō-ě-rith'rō-blas-tō'sis) any anemic condition resulting from space-occupying lesions in the bone marrow; the blood contains immature cells of the granulocytic series and nucleated red blood cells. SYN myelophthisic anemia, myelopathic anemia.

**leu·ko·ki·nin·ase** (loo-kō-kī'nĭ-nās) an enzyme that cleaves tuftsin to release leukokinin.

**leu·kol·y·sin** (loo-kol'i-sin) SYN leukocytolysin.

**leu·ko·ma** (loo-kō'mă) a dense white opacity of the cornea. [G. whiteness, a white spot in the eye, fr. *leukos,* white]

**leu·ko·ma·tous** (loo-kō'mă-tŭs) denoting leukoma.

**leu·ko·my·e·lop·a·thy** (loo'kō-mī'ĕ-lop'ă-thē) any disease involving the white matter or the conducting tracts of the spinal cord. [leuko- + G. *myelos,* marrow, + *pathos,* suffering]

**leu·ko·nych·ia** (loo-kō-nik'ē-ă) the occurrence of white spots, streaks, or patches under the nails, due to the presence of air bubbles between the nail and its bed. [leuko- + G. *onyx (onych-),* nail]

**leu·ko·path·ia, leu·kop·a·thy** (loo-kō-path'ē-ă, loo-kop'ă-thē) SYN leukoderma. [leuko- + G. *pathos,* disease]

**leu·ko·pe·de·sis** (loo'kō-pē-dē'sis) the movement of white blood cells (especially polymorphonuclear leukocytes) through the walls of capillaries and into the tissues. [leuko- + G. *pēdēsis,* a leaping]

**leu·ko·pe·nia** (loo-kō-pē'nē-ă) any condition in which the number of leukocytes in the circulating blood is less than normal, the lower limit of which is generally regarded as 4000–5000 per cu mm. SYN leukocytopenia. [leuko(cyte) + G. *penia,* poverty]

**leu·ko·pe·nic** (loo-kō-pē'nik) pertaining to leukopenia.

**leu·ko·pe·nic in·dex** a significant decrease in the white blood count after ingestion of food to which a patient is hypersensitive, a count made during the normal fasting state being used as the basis for evaluation of the postprandial count.

**leu·ko·pe·nic leu·ke·mia** a form of lymphocytic, granulocytic, or monocytic leukemia in which the number of white blood cells in the normal range or slightly depressed.

**leu·ko·pla·kia** (loo-kō-plā'kē-ă) a white patch of oral mucous membrane which cannot be wiped off and cannot be diagnosed clinically; biopsy may show malignant or premalignant changes. See this page. [leuko- + G. *plax,* plate]

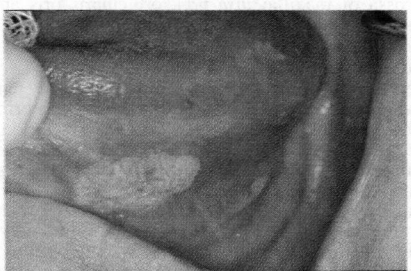
**leukoplakia:** with mild epithelial dysplasia

**leu·ko·pla·kia vul·vae** a clinical term for hyperkeratotic white patches of the vulvar epithelium; biopsy is necessary for specific diagnosis.

**leu·ko·poi·e·sis** (loo'kō-poy-ē'sis) formation and development of the various types of white blood cells. SYN leukocytopoiesis. [leuko- + G. *poiēsis,* a making]

**leu·ko·poi·et·ic** (loo'kō-poy-et'ik) pertaining to or characterized by leukopoiesis, as manifested by portions of the bone marrow and reticuloendothelial and lymphoid tissues, which form (respectively) the granulocytes, monocytes, and lymphocytes.

**leu·kor·rha·gia** (loo-kō-rā'jē-ă) SYN leukorrhea. [leuko- + G. *rhēgnymi,* to burst forth]

**leu·kor·rhea** (loo-kō-rē'ă) discharge from the vagina of a white or yellowish viscid fluid. SYN leukorrhagia. [leuko- + G. *rhoia,* flow]

**leu·ko·sis** (loo-kō'sis) abnormal proliferation of one or more of the leukopoietic tissues; the term includes myelosis, certain forms of reticuloendotheliosis, and lymphadenosis.

**leu·ko·tac·tic** (loo-kō-tak'tik) SYN leukocytotactic.

**leu·ko·tax·ia** (loo-kō-tak'sē-ă) SYN leukocytotaxia.

**leu·ko·tax·ine** (loo-kō-tak'sēn) a cell-free nitrogenous material prepared from injured, acutely degenerating tissue and from inflammatory exudates.

**leu·ko·tax·is** (loo-kō-tak'sis) SYN leukocytotaxia.

**leu·kot·ic** (loo-kot'ik) pertaining to, characterized by, or manifesting leukosis.

**leu·kot·o·my** (loo-kot'ō-mē) incision into the white matter of the frontal lobe of the brain. [leuko- + G. *tomē,* a cutting]

**leu·ko·tox·in** (loo-kō-tok'sin) SYN leukocytotoxin.

**leu·ko·trich·ia** (loo-kō-trik'ē-ă) whiteness of the hair. [leuko- + G. *thrix,* hair]

**leu·ko·tri·enes (LT)** (loo-kō-trī'ēnz) products of eicosanoid metabolism with physiologic roles in inflammation and allergic reactions.

**LEU M1** the epitope for a monoclonal antibody generated to the human histiocytic cell line that localizes to neutrophils, adherent monocytes, and a subgroup of activated T cells.

**le·va·tor** (le-vā'ter) **1.** a surgical instrument for prying up the depressed part in a fracture of the skull. **2.** one of several muscles whose action is to raise the part into which it is inserted. [L. a lifter, fr. *levo,* pp. *-atus,* to lift, fr. *levis,* light]

**le·va·tor an·gu·li o·ris mus·cle** *origin,* canine fossa of maxilla; *insertion,* orbicularis oris and skin at angle of mouth; *action,* raises angle of mouth; *nerve supply,* facial. SYN musculus levator anguli oris [TA].

**le·va·tor ani mus·cle** formed by pubococcygeus and iliococcygeus muscles; *origin,* posterior body of pubis, tendinous arch of the levator ani, and spine of ischium; *insertion,* anococcygeal ligament, sides of the lower part of the sacrum and of coccyx; *action,* resists prolapsing forces and draws the anus upward following defecation; supports the pelvic viscera; *nerve supply,* nerve to levator ani (fourth sacral spinal nerve). SYN musculus levator ani [TA].

**le·va·tor la·bii su·pe·ri·o·ris a·lae·que na·si mus·cle** *origin,* root of nasal process of maxilla; *insertion,* wing of nose and orbicularis oris muscle of upper lip; *action,* elevates upper lip and wing of nose; *nerve supply,* facial. SYN musculus levator labii superioris alaeque nasi [TA].

**le·va·tor la·bii su·pe·ri·o·ris mus·cle** *origin,* maxilla below infraorbital foramen; *insertion,* orbicularis oris of upper lip; *action,* elevates upper lip; *nerve supply,* facial. SYN musculus levator labii superioris [TA].

**le·va·tor mus·cle of thy·roid gland** a fasciculus occasionally passing from the thyrohyoid muscle to the isthmus of the thyroid gland. SYN musculus levator glandulae thyroideae [TA].

**le·va·tor pal·pe·brae su·pe·ri·o·ris mus·cle** *origin,* orbital surface of the lesser wing of the sphenoid, above and anterior to the optic canal; *insertion,* skin of eyelid, tarsal plate, and orbital walls, by medial and lateral expansions of the aponeurosis of insertion; *action,* raises the upper eyelid; *nerve supply,* oculomotor. SYN musculus levator palpebrae superioris [TA], elevator muscle of upper eyelid.

**le·va·tor pros·ta·tae mus·cle** in the male, the most medial fibers of the levator ani (pubococcygeus) muscle that extend from the pubis into the fascia of the prostate. SYN musculus levator prostatae [TA].

**le·va·tor scap·u·lae mus·cle** *origin,* from posterior tubercles of transverse processes of four upper cervical vertebrae; *insertion,* into superior angle of scapula; *action,* raises the scapula; *nerve supply,* dorsal scapular nerve. SYN musculus levator scapulae [TA], elevator muscle of scapula.

**le·va·tor ve·li pa·la·ti·ni mus·cle** *origin,* apex of petrous portion of temporal bone and lower part of cartilaginous auditory (eustachian) tube; *insertion,* aponeurosis of soft palate; *action,* raises soft palate; through the expansion of its fleshy belly during contraction, it helps to "push" open the auditory tube; *nerve supply,* pharyngeal plexus (cranial root of accessory nerve). SYN musculus levator veli palatini [TA], elevator muscle of soft palate.

**lev·el** (lev'el) any rank, position, or status in a graded scale of values.

**lev·el of con·scious·ness** the degree of a subject's differing levels of alertness and awareness of self and environment, varying from. Examples: wakefulness, lethargic, to coma. A decrease is often measured by the Glasgow Coma Scale, improves. Is used for uniformity in of assessment by more than one observer as a way of standardizing subjective assessment data. SEE ALSO Glasgow Coma Scale.

**lev·el-de·pen·dent fre·quen·cy re·sponse** one of several strategies used in hearing aids to alter the balance in amplification between high- and low-frequency sounds.

**Le·vey-Jen·nings chart** (lē-vē-jen'ings) SYN quality control chart.

**Le·vin tube** (lĕ-vin') a tube introduced through the nose into the upper alimentary canal, to facilitate intestinal decompression.

△**le·vo-** left, toward or on the left side. [L. *laevus*]

**le·vo·car·dia** (lē-vō-kar'dē-ă) situs inversus of the other viscera but with the heart normally situated on the left; congenital cardiac lesions are commonly associated. [levo- + G. *kardia,* heart]

**le·vo·do·pa** (lē-vō-dō-pă) the biologically active form of dopa; an antiparkinsonian agent that is converted to dopamine. SYN L-dopa.

**le·vo·duc·tion** (lē-vō-dŭk'shŭn) turning of one eye to the left. [levo- + L. *duco,* pp. *ductus,* to lead]

**le·vo·ro·ta·tion** (lē-vō-rō-tā'shŭn) **1.** a turning or twisting to the left; in particular, the counterclockwise twist given the plane of plane-polarized light by solutions of certain optically active substances. **2.** SYN sinistrotorsion. [levo- + L. *roto,* to turn]

**le·vo·ro·ta·to·ry** (lē-vō-rō'tă-tōr-ē) denoting levorotation, or crystals or solutions capable of causing it; as a chemical prefix, usually abbreviated *l-* or (−). Cf. dextrorotatory.

**le·vo·tor·sion** (lē-vō-tōr'shŭn) **1.** SYN sinistrotorsion. **2.** rotation of the upper pole of the cornea of one or both eyes to the left. [levo- + L. *torsio,* a twisting]

**le·vo·ver·sion** (lē'vō-ver'zhŭn) **1.** version toward the left. **2.** conjugate turning of both eyes to the left. [levo- + L. *verto,* pp. *versus,* to turn]

**Lev·ret for·ceps** (lĕv-rā') a modification of the Chamberlen forceps, curved to correspond to the curve of the birth canal.

**Lev syn·drome** (lev) bundle branch block in a patient with normal myocardium and normal coronary arteries resulting from fibrosis or calcification including the conducting system; affects the membranous septum, the apex of the muscular septum, and often the mitral and aortic valve rings.

**Lew·is** (loo'is), Ivor. SEE Ivor Lewis esophagectomy.

**Lew·is ac·id** (loo'is) an acid that is an electron pair acceptor.

**Lew·is base** (loo'is) a base that is an electron-pair donor.

**Le·wy bod·y de·men·tia** (lā'vē) SYN diffuse Lewy body disease.

**lex·i·cal** (leks'ĭ-kal) denoting the vocabulary of speech or language.

△**-lex·is, -lexy** suffixes that properly relate to speech, although often confused with -legia (Latin -*lego*, to read) and thus erroneously employed to relate to reading. [G. *lexis*, word, speech, from *legō*, to say]

**Ley·den neu·ri·tis** (lī'dĕn) fatty degeneration of the fibers of the affected nerve.

**Ley·dig cells** (lī'dig) SYN interstitial cells (1).

**Leydig cell tu·mor** (lī'dig) a testicular and, less commonly, ovarian neoplasm composed of Leydig cells, usually benign but may be malignant; may secrete androgens or estrogens.

**LFT** left frontotransverse position; liver function test.

**LGSIL** low-grade squamous intraepithelial lesion.

**Lher·mitte sign** (lār-mēt') sudden electric-like shocks extending down the spine on flexing the head.

**Li** lithium.

**li·ber·ins** (lib'er-ins) SYN releasing factors. [L. *libero*, to free, + -in]

**li·bid·i·nous** (li-bid'i-nŭs) lascivious; invested with or arousing sexual desire or energy. [L. *libidinosus*, fr. *libido* (*libidin*-), pleasure, desire]

**li·bi·do** (li-bē'dō, li-bī'dō) 1. conscious or unconscious sexual desire. 2. any passionate interest or form of life force. 3. in jungian psychology, synonymous with psychic energy. [L. lust]

**Lib·man-Sacks en·do·car·di·tis, Lib·man-Sacks syn·drome** (lib'mĕn sāks) verrucous endocarditis sometimes associated with disseminated lupus erythematosus. SYN atypical verrucous endocarditis, nonbacterial verrucous endocarditis.

**lice** (līs) plural of louse.

**li·censed prac·ti·cal nurse** a nurse who has graduated from an accredited school of practical (vocational) nursing, and has been licensed by public authority after passing a qualifying examination.

**li·chen** (lī'ken) a discrete flat papule or an aggregate of papules giving a patterned configuration resembling lichens growing on rocks. [G. *leichēn*, lichen; a lichen-like eruption]

🔲 **li·chen·i·fi·ca·tion** (lī'ken-i-fi-kā'shŭn) leathery induration and thickening of the skin with hyperkeratosis, caused by scratching in atopic or chronic contact dermatitis. See page B5. [lichen + L. *facio*, to make]

**li·chen myx·e·de·ma·to·sus** a lichenoid eruption of papules or plaques of mucinous edema due to deposit of glycosaminoglycans in the skin and fibroblast proliferation, in the absence of endocrine disease. SYN papular mucinosis.

**li·chen·oid** (lī'kĕ-noyd) 1. resembling lichen. 2. accentuation of normal skin markings observed in cases of chronic eczema. 3. microscopically resembling lichen planus.

**li·chen·oid der·ma·to·sis** any chronic skin eruption, characterized by induration and thickening of the skin with accentuation of the skin markings.

**li·chen·oid ker·a·to·sis** a solitary benign papule or plaque, with microscopic features resembling lichen planus, occurring on sun-exposed or unexposed skin.

**li·chen pla·nus, li·chen ru·ber pla·nus** eruption of flat-topped, shiny, violaceous papules on flexor surfaces, male genitalia, and buccal mucosa of unknown cause; may form linear groups. Spontaneous resolution is common after months to years.

**li·chen scle·ro·sus et a·tro·phi·cus** a chronic eruption, seen chiefly in the anogenital region, consisting of white atrophic papules which may be discrete or confluent and may contain a central depression or a black keratotic plug.

**li·chen scrof·u·lo·so·rum** small asymptomatic lichen papules on the trunk of children with tuberculosis. SYN papular tuberculid.

**li·chen stri·a·tus** a self-limited papular eruption occurring primarily in children (more commonly in females); the lesions are arranged in linear groups and usually occur on one extremity.

**li·chen ur·ti·ca·tus** SYN papular urticaria.

**lid** SYN eyelid.

**lie** (lī) relationship of the long axis of the fetus to that of the mother.

**Lie·ber·kühn glands** (le'ber-kēn) SYN intestinal glands.

**Lie·ber·mei·ster rule** (lē'bēr-mīs'tĕr) in adult febrile tachycardia, about eight pulse beats correspond to an increase of 1°C.

**Lie·big the·o·ry** (lē'big) theory that the hydrocarbons that oxidize readily and burn are aliments that produce the greatest quantity of animal heat.

**lie de·tec·tor** SYN polygraph (2).

**li·en** (lī'en) [TA] SYN spleen. [L.]

△**li·en-, li·e·no-** the spleen. SEE spleno-. [L. *lien*]

**li·en ac·ces·so·ri·us** SYN accessory spleen.

**li·e·nal** (lī'ĕ-năl) SYN splenic.

**li·e·nal ar·tery** SYN splenic artery.

**li·en mo·bi·lis** SYN floating spleen.

**li·en·ter·ic** (lī-en-ter'ik) relating to, or marked by, lientery.

**li·en·ter·ic di·ar·rhea** diarrhea in which undigested food appears in the stools.

**li·en·tery** (lī'en-ter-ē) passage of undigested food in the stools. [G. *leienteria*, fr. *leios*, smooth, + *enteron*, intestine]

**life** 1. the quality or condition proper to living beings; the state of existence characterized by such functions as metabolism, growth, reproduction, adaptation, and response to stimuli. 2. living organisms such as animals and plants. [A.S. *life*]

**life e·vents** occurrences in one's daily life, some of which act as stressors.

**life in·stinct** the instinct of self-preservation and sexual procreation; the basic urge toward preservation of the species.

**life-span de·vel·op·ment** development and mastery (or loss) of differing biologic, intellectual, behavioral, and social skills in different epochs of the life-span from the prenatal through the gerontological periods of growth.

**life stress** events or experiences that produce severe strain, e.g., failure on the job, marital separation, loss of a love object.

**life-style** habits and customs influenced by the lifelong process of socialization, including social use of alcohol and tobacco, dietary habits, and exercise, all of which have important implications for health.

**life ta·ble** a representation of the probable years of survivorship of a defined population of subjects.

**lig·a·ment** (lig'ă-ment) **1.** a band or sheet of fibrous tissue connecting two or more bones, cartilages, or other structures, or serving as support for fasciae or muscles. **2.** a fold of peritoneum supporting any of the abdominal viscera. **3.** any structure resembling a ligament though not performing the function of such. **4.** the cordlike remains of a fetal vessel or other structure that has lost its original lumen. SYN ligamentum. [L. *ligamentum,* a band, bandage]

**lig·a·men·ta in·tra·cap·su·lar·ia** [TA] SYN intracapsular ligaments.

**lig·a·men·ta sus·pen·so·ria mam·mae** [TA] SYN suspensory ligaments of breast.

**lig·a·ment of head of fe·mur** a flattened ligament that passes from the fovea in the head of the femur to the borders of the acetabular notch (transverse acetabular ligament); the ligament does not contribute to the integrity of the joint or control movements there. SYN ligamentum capitis femoris [TA], round ligament of femur.

**lig·a·men·to·pex·is, lig·a·men·to·pexy** (lig'ă-men-tō-pek'sis, lig'ă-men'tō-pek-sē) shortening of any ligament of the uterus. [ligament + G. *pēxis,* fixation]

**lig·a·men·tous** (lig'ă-men'tŭs) relating to or of the form or structure of a ligament.

**lig·a·men·tum,** pl. **lig·a·men·ta** (lig'ă-men'tŭm, lig'ă-men'tă) SYN ligament. [L. a band, tie, fr. *ligo,* to bind]

**lig·a·men·tum ca·pi·tis fem·o·ris** [TA] SYN ligament of head of femur.

**lig·a·men·tum cor·a·co·ac·ro·mi·ale** [TA] SYN coracoacromial ligament.

**lig·a·men·tum cor·a·co·cla·vi·cu·la·re** [TA] SYN coracoclavicular ligament.

**lig·a·men·tum cos·to·cla·vi·cu·la·re** [TA] SYN costoclavicular ligament.

**lig·a·men·tum cos·to·trans·ver·sa·ri·um** [TA] SYN costotransverse ligament.

**lig·a·men·tum cru·ci·a·tum an·te·ri·us** [TA] SYN anterior cruciate ligament.

**lig·a·men·tum cru·ci·a·tum pos·te·ri·us** [TA] SYN posterior cruciate ligament.

**lig·a·men·tum del·toi·de·um** SYN deltoid ligament.

**lig·a·men·tum fal·ci·for·me hep·a·tis** [TA] SYN falciform ligament of liver.

**lig·a·men·tum il·i·o·fem·o·ra·le** [TA] SYN iliofemoral ligament.

**lig·a·men·tum in·gui·na·le** [TA] SYN inguinal ligament.

**lig·a·men·tum la·cu·na·re** [TA] SYN lacunar ligament.

**lig·a·men·tum la·tum uter·i** [TA] SYN broad ligament of the uterus.

**lig·a·men·tum lon·gi·tu·di·na·le** [TA] SYN longitudinal ligament.

**lig·a·men·tum lum·bo·cos·ta·le** [TA] SYN lumbocostal ligament.

**lig·a·men·tum nu·chae** [TA] a sagittal ligamentous band at the back of the neck, formed of thickened supraspinous ligaments; it extends from the external occipital protuberance to the posterior border of the foramen magnum crani-

ally, and to the seventh cervical spinous process caudally. SYN nuchal ligament.

**lig·a·men·tum pa·tel·lae** [TA] SYN patellar ligament.

**lig·a·men·tum pec·ti·ne·a·le** [TA] SYN pectineal ligament.

**lig·a·men·tum phre·ni·co·co·li·cum** [TA] SYN phrenicocolic ligament.

**lig·a·men·tum pul·mo·na·le** [TA] SYN pulmonary ligament.

**lig·a·men·tum splen·o·re·na·le** [TA] SYN splenorenal ligament.

**lig·a·men·tum sus·pen·so·ri·um o·va·rii** [TA] SYN suspensory ligament of ovary.

**lig·a·men·tum te·res hep·a·tis** [TA] SYN round ligament of liver.

**lig·a·men·tum te·res uter·i** [TA] SYN round ligament of uterus.

**lig·a·men·tum trans·ver·sum ge·nus** [TA] SYN transverse ligament of knee.

**lig·a·men·tum tra·pe·zoi·de·um** [TA] SYN trapezoid ligament.

**lig·a·men·tum vo·ca·le** [TA] SYN vocal ligament.

**lig·and** (lig'and, lī'gand) **1.** an organic molecule attached to a central metal ion by multiple coordinate bonds. **2.** an organic molecule attached to a tracer element, e.g., a radioisotope. **3.** a molecule that binds to a macromolecule, e.g., a ligand binding to a receptor. **4.** the analyte in competitive binding assays, such as radioimmunoassay. [L. *ligo,* to bind]

**lig·and-bind·ing site** the site on the surface of a protein that binds a ligand; equivalent to the active site if the ligand is the substrate of an enzyme.

**li·gase** (lī'gās) generic term for enzymes (EC class 6) catalyzing the joining of two molecules coupled with the breakdown of a pyrophosphate bond in ATP or a similar compound. SEE ALSO synthetase.

**li·gase chain re·ac·tion** a technique for target amplification of DNA in which DNA ligase is used to join two complementary oligonucleotide probes that have bound to a target sequence in vitro. The ligation product is used as a template for ligation of complementary oligonucleotides that, through repeated enzymatic processing, allow for logarithmic accumulation of products that can be used to determine the presence of the target of interest.

**li·gate** (lī'gāt) to apply a ligature. [L. *ligo,* pp. *-atus,* to bind]

**li·ga·tion** (lī-gā'shŭn) **1.** application of a ligature. **2.** the act of binding or annealing. [L. *ligatio,* fr. *ligo,* to bind]

**lig·a·ture** (lig'ă-cher) **1.** a thread, wire, fillet, or the like, tied tightly around a blood vessel, the pedicle of a tumor, or other structure to constrict it. **2.** ORTHODONTICS a wire or other material used to secure an orthodontic attachment or tooth to an archwire. [L. *ligatura,* a band or tie, fr. *ligo,* to tie]

**light** (līt) that portion of electromagnetic radiation to which the retina is sensitive. SEE ALSO lamp. [A.S. *leōht*]

**light ad·ap·ta·tion** the visual adjustment occurring under increased illumination in which the retinal sensitivity to light is reduced. SEE ALSO light-adapted eye. SYN photopic adaptation.

**light-a·dapt·ed eye** an eye that has been exposed

to light, with bleaching of rhodopsin (visual purple) and insensitivity to low illumination. SYN photopic eye.

**light chain** a polypeptide chain with low molecular weight, as the κ or λ chains in immunoglobulin.

**light chain-re·lat·ed am·y·loi·do·sis** a form of primary amyloidosis in which the fibrillar amyloid deposits are derived from the light chains of immunoglobulin; seen in B-lymphocyte and plasma-cells dyscrasias.

**light·en·ing** (līt'en-ing) sensation of decreased abdominal distention during the later weeks of pregnancy following the descent of the fetal head into the pelvic inlet.

**light re·flex 1.** SYN pupillary reflex. **2.** a red glow reflected from the fundus of the eye when a light is cast upon the retina, as in retinoscopy; **3.** SYN Politzer luminous cone, Wilde triangle. SYN pyramid of light.

**light sleep** SYN dysnystaxis.

**light treat·ment** SYN phototherapy.

**Li·kert scale** (lī'kert) ordinal scale of responses to a question or statement, ordered in hierarchical sequence from strongly negative to strongly positive. Used mainly in behavioral sciences and psychiatry.

**Lil·lie al·lo·chrome con·nec·tive tis·sue stain** (lil'ē) a procedure using PAS, hematoxylin, picric acid, and methyl blue; used for distinction between basement membrane and reticulin, and for demonstration of arteriosclerotic lesions.

**Lil·lie az·ure-e·o·sin stain** (lil'ē) a stain in which an azure eosinate solution is used to stain bacteria and rickettsiae in tissues.

**Lil·lie fer·rous iron stain** (lil'ē) a method using potassium ferrocyanide in acetic acid that demonstrates melanins as a deep green color; lipofuscins and heme pigments are unreactive.

**Lil·lie sul·fu·ric ac·id Nile blue stain** (lil'ē) a technique for showing fatty acids when present in high concentrations.

**limb** (lim) **1.** an extremity; a member; an arm or leg. SYN member. **2.** a segment of any jointed structure. SEE ALSO leg. [A.S. *lim*]

**limb bud** an ectodermally covered mesenchymal outgrowth on the embryonic trunk giving rise to either the upper limb or lower limb.

**limb-gir·dle mus·cu·lar dys·tro·phy** one of the less well-defined types of muscular dystrophy. Characterized by weakness and wasting, usually symmetrical, of the pelvic girdle muscles, the shoulder girdle muscles, or both, but not the facial muscles. Muscle pseudohypertrophy, heart involvement, and mental retardation are absent. Variable inheritance.

**lim·bic** (lim'bik) **1.** relating to a limbus. **2.** relating to the limbic system.

**lim·bic sys·tem** collective term denoting a heterogeneous array of brain structures at or near the edge (limbus) of the medial wall of the cerebral hemisphere, in particular the hippocampus, amygdala, and fornicate gyrus; the term is often used so as to include also the interconnections of these structures, as well as their connections with the septal area, the hypothalamus, and a medial zone of mesencephalic tegmentum. By way of the latter connections, the limbic system exerts an important influence upon the endocrine and autonomic motor systems; its functions also appear to affect motivational and mood states.

**limb lead** one of the three standard leads (leads I, II, III) or one of the unipolar limb leads (aVR, aVL, aVF).

**lim·bus**, pl. **lim·bi** (lim'bŭs, lim'bī) [TA] the edge, border, or fringe of a part. [L. a border]

**lim·bus of cor·nea** the margin of the cornea overlapped by the sclera.

**lime** (līm) **1.** an alkaline earth oxide occurring in grayish white masses (quicklime); on exposure to the atmosphere it becomes converted into calcium hydrate and calcium carbonate (air-slaked lime); direct addition of water to calcium oxide produces calcium hydrate (slaked lime). SYN calx (1). **2.** fruit of the lime tree, *Citrus medica*, which is a source of ascorbic acid and acts as an antiscorbutic agent. [O.E. *līm*, birdlime]

**li·men**, pl. **lim·i·na** (li'men, lim'i-nă) [TA] entrance; the external opening of a canal or space, such as limen insulae. SYN threshold (4). [L.]

**li·men in·su·lae** [TA] the band of transition between the anterior portion of the gray matter of the insula and the anterior perforated substance; it is formed by a narrow strip of olfactory cortex along the lateral side of the lateral olfactory stria.

**li·men na·si** [TA] a ridge marking the boundary between the nasal cavity proper and the vestibule.

**li·mes** (lī'mēz) a boundary, limit, or threshold. SEE ALSO L doses. [L.]

**lim·i·nal** (lim'i-năl) **1.** pertaining to a threshold. **2.** pertaining to a stimulus just strong enough to excite a tissue, e.g., nerve or muscle. [L. *limen* (*limin-*), a threshold]

**lim·it** a boundary or end. [L. *limes*, boundary]

**lim·i·ted neck dis·sec·tion** SYN functional neck dissection.

**limiting decision** an understanding of self achieved as a result of response to a significant or traumatic event. SEE ALSO Time-Line therapy.

**lim·it test·ing** OCCUPATIONAL THERAPY attempts to approach or exceed established boundaries or guidelines for purposes of challenge or control.

**limp** a lame walk with a yielding step; asymmetrical gait. SEE ALSO claudication.

**Lin·dau tu·mor** (lin'dou) SYN hemangioblastoma.

**Lind·ner bod·ies** (lind'nĕr) initial bodies resembling inclusion bodies found in scrapings of epithelial cells infected with trachoma.

**line** (līn) **1.** a long, narrow mark or a strand of material. In anatomy, any linear mark or streak distinguished from adjacent tissues by color, texture, or elevation. SEE ALSO line. **2.** a strain of cells or organisms derived from a single ancestor or precursor. **3.** a section of tubing supplying fluid or conducting impulses for monitoring equipment; e.g., intravenous line, arterial line. SYN linea [TA]. [L. *linea*, a linen thread, a string, line, fr. *linum*, flax]

**lin·e·a**, gen. and pl. **lin·e·ae** (lin'ē-ă, lin'ē-ē) [TA] SYN line. [L.]

**lin·e·a al·ba** [TA] a fibrous band running vertically the entire length of the center of the anterior abdominal wall, receiving the attachments of the oblique and transverse abdominal muscles. SYN white line (1).

**lin·e·a a·no·cu·ta·nea** [TA] SYN pectinate line.

**lin·e·ae a·tro·phi·cae** SYN striae cutis distensae.

**lin·e·a ep·i·phys·i·a·lis** [TA] SYN epiphysial line.

**lin·e·a in·ter·tro·chan·te·ri·ca** [TA] SYN intertrochanteric line.

**line ang·le** an angle formed by the junction of two surfaces of a tooth or two surfaces of a cavity preparation.

**lin·ea nig·ra** the linea alba in pregnancy, which then becomes pigmented.

**lin·e·ar** (lin'ē-ăr) pertaining to or resembling a line.

**lin·e·ar ac·cel·er·a·tor** a device imparting high velocity and energy to atomic and subatomic particles; an important device for radiation therapy.

**lin·e·ar am·pli·fi·ca·tion** a hearing aid circuit in which all frequencies receive equivalent amplification.

**lin·e·ar at·ro·phy** SYN striae cutis distensae.

**lin·e·ar frac·ture** a fracture running parallel with the long axis of the bone. SYN fissured fracture.

**lin·e·ar·i·ty** (lin-ē-ar'ĭ-tē) a relationship between two quantities whereby a change in one causes a directly proportional change in the other. [L. *linearis,* linear, fr. *linea,* line]

**lin·e·ar scler·o·der·ma** localized scleroderma with band-like lesions of skin with induration, atrophy, hyper- or hypopigmentation, which may be disfiguring with extension into underlying tissues and joint contractures. Involvement of the forehead and scalp has been called coup de Sabre.

**lin·ea sem·i·lu·na·ris** [TA] the slight groove in the external abdominal wall parallel to the lateral edge of the rectus sheath. SYN semilunar line.

**lin·ea ster·na·lis** [TA] SYN sternal line.

**lin·ea ter·mi·na·lis** [TA] an oblique ridge on the inner surface of the ilium and continued on the pubis, which forms the lower boundary of the iliac fossa; it separates the true from the false pelvis. SYN iliopectineal line, terminal line.

**line of de·mar·ca·tion** a zone of inflammatory reaction separating a gangrenous area from healthy tissue.

**line of fix·a·tion** a line joining the object (or point of fixation) with the fovea.

**lines of Blasch·ko** (blash'kō) a pattern of distribution of skin lesions or pigmentary anomalies; linear on the extremities, S-shaped curves on the abdomen, and V-shaped on the back, thought to result from genetic mosaicism and the interplay of transverse clonal proliferation and longitudinal growth and flexion of the embryo.

**line spec·trum** an emission spectrum of elements in which the emitted light bands cover a very narrow range of energies.

**lin·gua,** gen. and pl. **lin·guae** (ling'gwă, ling'gwē) [TA] **1.** SYN tongue (1). **2.** SYN tongue (2). [L. tongue]

**lin·gua ge·o·gra·phi·ca** SYN geographic tongue.

**lin·gual** (ling'gwăl) **1.** relating to the tongue or any tongue-like part. SYN glossal. **2.** next to or toward the tongue.

**lin·gual ar·tery** *origin,* external carotid; *distribution,* runs along under surface of tongue, terminates as deep lingual artery; *branches,* suprahyoid and dorsal lingual branches and sublingual artery.

**lin·gual fol·li·cles** collections of lymphoid tissue in the mucosa of the pharyngeal part of the tongue posterior to the terminal sulcus collectively forming the lingual tonsil. SYN folliculi linguales [TA].

**lin·gual fren·u·lum** a fold of mucous membrane extending from the floor of the mouth to the midline of the undersurface of the tongue.

**lin·gual goi·ter** a tumor of thyroid tissue involving the embryonic rudiment at the base of the tongue.

**lin·gual gy·rus** a relatively short horizontal convolution on the inferomedial aspect of the occipital and temporal lobes, demarcated from the lateral occipitotemporal or fusiform gyrus by the deep collateral sulcus, from the cuneus by the calcarine sulcus; its anterior extreme abuts the isthmus of the parahippocampal gyrus; the medial or upper strip of the gyrus forming the lower bank of the calcarine sulcus corresponds to the inferior half of the striate area or primary visual cortex and represents the contralateral upper quadrant of the binocular field of vision.

**lin·gual nerve** one of the branches of the mandibular nerve, passing medially to the lateral pterygoid muscle, between the medial pterygoid and the mandible, and beneath the mucous membrane of the floor of the mouth to the side of the tongue over the anterior two-thirds of which it is distributed; it supplies also the mucous membrane of the floor of the mouth. It passes close to the lingual side of the roots of the second and third lower molar teeth and is endangered during tooth extractions. SYN nervus lingualis [TA].

**lin·gual pa·pil·la 1.** one of numerous variously shaped projections of the mucous membrane of the dorsum of the tongue; **2.** the lingual portion of the gingiva filling the interproximal space between adjacent teeth; in molar and premolar areas, there may be separate lingual and buccal interdental papillae. SEE ALSO interdental papilla.

**lin·gual ton·sil** a collection of lymphoid follicles on the posterior or pharyngeal portion of the dorsum of the tongue. SYN tonsilla lingualis [TA].

**lin·gual vein** receives blood from the tongue, sublingual and submandibular glands, and muscles of the floor of the mouth; empties into the internal jugular or the facial vein.

**lin·gua nig·ra** SYN black tongue.

**lin·gui·form** (ling'gwi-fōrm) tongue-shaped.

**lin·gu·la,** pl. **lin·gu·lae** (ling'gyu-lă, ling'gyu-lē) [TA] **1.** a term applied to several tongue-shaped processes, particularly that of the cerebellum and of the upper lobe of the left lung. **2.** when not qualified, the lingula of cerebellum. [L. dim. of *lingua,* tongue]

**lin·gu·lar** (ling'gyu-lăr) pertaining to any lingula.

**lin·gu·lec·to·my** (ling'gyu-lek'tō-mē) **1.** SYN glossectomy. **2.** excision of the lingular portion of the upper lobe of the left lung.

△**lin·guo-** the tongue. [L. *lingua*]

**lin·guo·clu·sion** (ling-gwō-kloo'zhŭn) displacement of a tooth toward the interior of the dental arch, or toward the tongue.

**lin·guo·pap·il·li·tis** (ling'gwō-pap'i-lī'tis) small painful ulcers involving the papillae on the tongue margins.

**lin·guo·ver·sion** (ling'gwō-ver-zhŭn) malposition of a tooth lingual to the normal position.

**lin·i·ment** (lin'i-ment) a liquid preparation for external use; frequently applied by friction to the skin. [L., fr. *lino,* to smear]

**li·ni·tis** (li-nī'tis, lī-nī'tis) inflammation of cellular tissue, specifically of the perivascular tissue of the stomach. [G. *linon,* flax, linen cloth, + *-itis,* inflammation]

**li·ni·tis plas·ti·ca** infiltrating scirrhous carcinoma, causing extensive thickening of the wall of the stomach; often called leather-bottle stomach.

**link·age** (lingk′ij) **1.** a chemical covalent bond. **2.** the relationship between syntenic loci sufficiently close that the respective alleles are not inherited independently by the offspring; a characteristic of loci, not genes.

**link·age dis·e·qui·lib·ri·um** a state involving two loci in which the probability of a joint gamete is not equal to the product of the probabilities of the constituent genes. The difference between these quantities is the increase of the disequilibrium; there are many causes of the disequilibrium.

**link·age mark·er** a locus at which there is a high probability of heterozygotes (indispensible state for linkage analysis), but in itself perhaps of no clinical interest.

**linked** said of two genetic loci that exhibit genetic linkage.

**link·er** a fragment of synthetic DNA containing a restriction site that may be used for splicing genes.

**link·ing num·ber** (*L*) a property of a long biopolymer (such as duplex DNA) equal to the number of twists (related to the frequency of turns around the central axis of the helix) plus the writhing number.

**lip 1.** one of the two muscular folds with an outer mucosa having a stratified squamous epithelial surface layer that bound the mouth anteriorly. **2.** any liplike structure bounding a cavity or groove. SYN labium (1) [TA]. [A.S. *lippa*]

**li·pae·mia** [Br.] SEE lipemia.

**li·pase** (lī′pās) any fat-splitting or lipolytic enzyme; a carboxylesterase.

**lip·ec·to·my** (lip-ek′tō-mē) surgical removal of fatty tissue, as in cases of adiposity. [lipo- + G. *ektomē*, excision]

**lip·e·de·ma** (lip′e-dē′mă) chronic swelling, usually of the lower extremities, particularly in middle-aged women, caused by the widespread even distribution of subcutaneous fat and fluid. [lipo- + G. *oidēma*, swelling]

**li·pe·de·ma·tous al·o·pe·cia** alopecia with itching, soreness, or redness of the scalp in black women; the scalp is thickened and soft, subcutaneous fat is increased, and the hair is sparse and short.

**li·pe·mia** (lip-ē′mē-ă) the presence of an abnormally high concentration of lipids in the circulating blood. SYN hyperlipidaemia, hyperlipidemia, hyperlipoidemia, lipidaemia, lipidemia, lipoidemia. [lipid + G. *haima*, blood]

**li·pe·mia re·ti·na·lis** a creamy appearance of the retinal blood vessels that occurs when the lipids of the blood exceed 5%.

**li·pe·mic** (li-pē′mik) relating to lipemia.

**lip·id** (lip′id) "fat-soluble," an operational term describing a solubility characteristic, not a chemical substance, i.e., denoting substances extracted from animal or vegetable cells by nonpolar solvents; included in the heterogeneous collection of materials thus extractable are fatty acids, glycerides and glyceryl ethers, phospholipids, sphingolipids, long-chain alcohols and waxes, terpenes, steroids, and "fat-soluble" vitamins such as A, D, and E. [G. *lipos*, fat]

**lipid A** the glycolipid component of lipopolysaccharide responsible for its endotoxic activity.

**lip·i·dae·mia** [Br.] SYN lipemia.

**lip·i·de·mia** (lip′i-dē′mē-ă) SYN lipemia.

**lip·id gran·u·lo·ma·to·sis, lip·oid gran·u·lo··ma·to·sis** SYN xanthomatosis.

**lip·i·do·sis**, pl. **lip·i·do·ses** (lip-i-dō′sis, lip-i-dō′sēz) hereditary abnormality of lipid metabolism that results in abnormal amounts of lipid deposition; classification is based on the responsible enzymatic deficiency and type of lipid involved. Such enzymatic activity takes place in the lysosomes, and the abnormal products appear as lysosomal storage diseases. Sphingolipidoses make up the largest portion of recognized lipidoses, including abnormal metabolism of gangliosides, ceramides, and cerebrosides. [lipid + G. *-ōsis*, condition]

**lip·id pneu·mo·nia, lip·oid pneu·mo·ni·a** pulmonary condition marked by inflammatory and fibrotic changes in the lungs due to the inhalation of various oily or fatty substances, particularly liquid petrolatum, or resulting from accumulation in the lungs of endogenous lipid material, either cholesterol from obstructive pneumonitis or following fracture of a bone; phagocytes containing lipid are usually present.

△**lipo-, lip-** fatty, lipid. [G. *lipos*, fat]

**lip·o·ar·thri·tis** (lip′ō-ar-thrī′tis) inflammation of the periarticular fatty tissues of the knee. [lipo- + arthritis]

**lip·o·ate** (lip′ō-āt) a salt or ester of lipoic acid.

**lip·o·ate a·ce·tyl·trans·fer·ase** SYN dihydrolipoamide acetyltransferase.

**lip·o·at·ro·phy** (lip-ō-at′rō-fē) loss of subcutaneous fat, which may be total, congenital, and associated with hepatomegaly, excessive bone growth, and insulin-resistant diabetes. [G. *lipos*, fat, + *a-*, priv. + *trophē*, nourishment]

**lip·o·blast** (lip′ō-blast) an embryonic fat cell. [lipo- + G. *blastos*, germ]

**lip·o·blas·to·ma** (lip′ō-blas-tō′mă) **1.** SYN liposarcoma. **2.** a benign subcutaneous tumor composed of embryonal fat cells separated into distinct lobules, occurring usually in infants.

**lip·o·blas·to·ma·to·sis** (lip′ō-blas-tō-mă-tō′sis) a diffuse form of lipoblastoma that infiltrates locally but does not metastasize.

**lip·o·cer·a·tous** (lip-ō-ser′ă-tŭs) SYN adipoceratous.

**lip·o·cere** (lip′ō-sēr) SYN adipocere. [lipo- + L. *cera*, wax]

**lip·o·chrome** (lip′ō-krōm) **1.** a pigmented lipid, e.g., lutein, carotene. **2.** more specifically, yellow pigments that seem to be identical to carotene and xanthophyll and are frequently found in the serum, skin, adrenal cortex, corpus luteum, and arteriosclerotic plaques, as well as in the liver, spleen, and adipose tissue. **3.** the pigment produced by certain bacteria. [lipo- + G. *chroma*, color]

**lip·o·crit** (lip′ō-krit) an apparatus and procedure for separating and volumetrically analyzing the amount of lipid in blood or other body fluid. [lipo- + G. *krinō*, to separate]

**lip·o·cyte** (lip′ō-sīt) SYN fat-storing cell. [lipo- + G. *kytos*, cell]

**lip·o·der·moid** (lip-ō-der′moyd) congenital, yellowish-white, fatty, benign tumor located subconjunctivally. [lipo- + dermoid]

**lip·o·dys·tro·phy** (lip-ō-dis′trō-fē) defective metabolism of fat. [lipo- + G. *dys-*, bad, difficult, + *trophē*, nourishment]

**lip·o·e·de·ma** (lip′ō-e-dē′mă) edema of subcutaneous fat, causing painful swellings, especially of the legs in women. SYN cellulite (2).

**lip·o·fi·bro·ma** (lip'ō-fī-brō'mă) a benign neoplasm of fibrous connective tissue, with conspicuous numbers of adipose cells.

**lip·o·fus·cin** (lip-ō-fyoos'in) brown pigment granules representing lipid-containing residues of lysosomal digestion and considered one of the aging or "wear and tear" pigments; found in liver, kidney, heart muscle, adrenal, and ganglion cells.

**lip·o·fus·ci·no·sis** (lip'ō-fyus-i-nō'sis) abnormal storage of any one of a group of fatty pigments.

**lip·o·gen·e·sis** (lip-ō-jen'ĕ-sis) the production of fat, either fatty degeneration or fatty infiltration; also applied to the normal deposition of fat or to the conversion of carbohydrate or protein to fat. SYN adipogenesis. [lipo- + G. *genesis,* production]

**lip·o·gen·ic** (lip-ō-jen'ik) relating to lipogenesis. SYN adipogenic, adipogenous, lipogenous.

**li·pog·e·nous** (li-poj'ĕ-nŭs) SYN lipogenic.

**lip·o·gran·u·lo·ma** (lip'ō-gran-yu-lō'mă) a nodule or focus of granulomatous inflammation (usually of the foreign-body type) in association with lipid material deposited in tissues, e.g., after the injection of certain oils. SEE ALSO paraffinoma.

**lip·o·gran·u·lo·ma·to·sis** (lip'ō-gran'yu-lō-mă-tō'sis) **1.** presence of lipogranulomas. **2.** local inflammatory reaction to necrosis of adipose tissue.

**lip·oid** (lip'oyd) **1.** resembling fat. **2.** former term for lipid. SYN adipoid. [lipo- + G. *eidos,* appearance]

**lip·oi·de·mia** (lip-oy-dē'mē-ă) SYN lipemia.

**lip·oid gran·u·lo·ma** granuloma characterized by aggregates or accumulations of fairly large mononuclear phagocytes that contain lipids.

**lip·oid ne·phro·sis** idiopathic nephrotic syndrome occurring most commonly in children, in which glomeruli show minimal changes with no thickening of the basement membranes, fat vacuoles in the tubular epithelium, and fusion of glomerular foot processes.

**lip·oi·do·sis** (lip-oy-do'sis) presence of anisotropic lipoids in the cells.

**lip·oid the·o·ry of nar·co·sis** that narcotic efficiency parallels the coefficient of partition between oil and water, and that lipoids in the cell and on the cell membrane absorb the drug because of this affinity.

**lip·o·in·jec·tion** (lip-ō-in-jek'shŭn) augmentation of tissue with fat cells after atrophy, as in vocal cord paralysis or scarring.

**li·pol·y·sis** (li-pol'i-sis) the splitting up (hydrolysis), or chemical decomposition, of fat. [lipo- + G. *lysis,* dissolution]

**lip·o·lyt·ic** (lip-ō-lit'ik) relating to or causing lipolysis.

**li·po·ma** (li-pō'mă) a benign neoplasm of adipose tissue, composed of mature fat cells. [lipo- + G. *-oma,* tumor]

**li·po·ma·toid** (li-pō'mă-toyd) resembling a lipoma, frequently said of accumulations of adipose tissue that is not thought to be neoplastic.

**lip·o·ma·to·sis** (lip'ō-mă-tō'sis) SYN adiposis.

**li·po·ma·tous** (li-pō'mă-tŭs) pertaining to or manifesting the features of lipoma, or characterized by the presence of a lipoma (or lipomas).

**li·po·ma·tous in·fil·tra·tion** nonencapsulated

adipose tissue forming a lipoma-like mass, usually in the cardiac interatrial septum where it may cause arrhythmia and sudden death.

**lip·o·me·nin·go·cele** (lip'ō-mĕ-ning'gō-sēl) a lipoma of the cauda equina associated with a spina bifida. [lipo- + G. *mēninx,* membrane, + *kēlē,* tumor]

**lip·o·pe·nia** (lip-ō-pē'nē-ă) an abnormally small amount, or a deficiency, of lipids in the body. [lipo- + G. *penia,* poverty]

**lip·o·phage** (lip'ō-fāj) a cell that ingests fat. [G. *lipos,* fat, + *phagō,* to eat]

**lip·o·phag·ic** (lip-ō-fā'jik) relating to lipophagy.

**lip·oph·a·gy** (lip-of'ă-jē) ingestion of fat by a lipophage. [lipo- + G. *phagō,* to eat]

**lip·o·phil** (lip'ō-fil) a substance with lipophilic (hydrophobic) properties. [lipo- + G. *philos,* fond of]

**lip·o·phil·ic** (lip-ō-fil'ik) capable of dissolving, of being dissolved in, or of absorbing lipids.

**lip·o·pol·y·sac·cha·ride** (lip'ō-pol'ē-sak'ă-rīd) a compound or complex of lipid and carbohydrate; the lipopolysaccharide (endotoxin) released from the cell walls of Gram-negative organisms that produces septic shock.

**lip·o·pro·tein** (lip-ō-prō'tēn) complexes or compounds containing lipid and protein. Almost all the lipids in plasma are present as lipoproteins and are therefore transported as such. Plasma lipoproteins are characterized by their flotation constants as chylomicra, very low density (VLDL), intermediate density (IDL), low density (LD), high density (HDL), very high density (VHDL). They range in molecular weight from 175,000 to $1 \times 10^9$. Levels of lipoproteins are important in assessing the risk of cardiovascular disease.

$\alpha_1$**-lip·o·pro·tein** a lipoprotein fraction of relatively low molecular weight, high density, rich in phospholipids, and found in the $\alpha_1$-globulin fraction of human plasma.

$\beta_1$**-lip·o·pro·tein** a lipoprotein fraction of relatively high molecular weight, low density, rich in cholesterol, and found in the $\beta$-globulin fraction of human plasma.

**lip·o·pro·tein (a)** a lipoprotein consisting of an LDL particle to which a large glycoprotein, apolipoprotein (a), is covalently bonded. Elevation of the concentration in serum has been identified as a risk factor for coronary artery disease.

Elevation of plasma lipoprotein (a) above 30 mg/dL is a strong independent risk factor for coronary artery disease and possibly for stroke. A unique feature of lipoprotein (a) is the structural similarity of its nonlipid moiety, apolipoprotein (a), to plasminogen. This similarity allows it to bind to endothelium and to proteins of cellular membranes. It inhibits fibrinolysis by competing for plasminogen binding sites and also favors lipid deposition and stimulates smooth muscle cell proliferation. Niacin and estrogen lower Lp(a), but HMG-CoA reductase inhibitors, fibrates, and bile acid sequestrants do not.

**lip·o·pro·tein li·pase** an enzyme that hydrolyzes one fatty acid from a triacylglycerol; its activity is enhanced by heparin and inactivated by heparinase. SEE ALSO clearing factors.

**lip·o·sar·co·ma** (lip'ō-sar-kō'mă) a malignant neoplasm of adults that occurs especially in the retroperitoneal tissues and the thigh; planes composed of well-differentiated fat cells, or may be dedifferentiated, either myxoid, round celled, or pleomorphic; recurrences are common, and dedifferentiated liposarcomas metastasize to the lungs or serosal surfaces. SYN lipoblastoma (1). [lipo- + *sarx*, flesh, + *-oma*, tumor]

**li·po·sis** (li-pō'sis) **1.** SYN adiposis. **2.** fatty infiltration, neutral fats being present in the cells. [lipo- + G. *-osis*, condition]

**lip·o·sol·u·ble** (lip-ō-sol'yu-bl) fat-soluble.

**lip·o·suc·tion** (lip'ō-sŭk-shŭn) method of removing unwanted subcutaneous fat using percutaneously placed suction tubes.

**lip·o·suc·tion·ing** (lip'ō-sŭk'shŭn-ing) removal of fat by high vacuum pressure; used in body contouring.

**lip·o·tro·phic** (lip-ō-trof'ik) relating to lipotrophy.

**li·pot·ro·phy** (li-pot'rō-fē) an increase of fat in the body. [lipo- + G. *trophē*, nourishment]

**lip·o·tro·pic** (lip-ō-trop'ik) **1.** pertaining to substances preventing or correcting excessive fat deposits in liver such as occurs in choline deficiency. **2.** relating to lipotropy.

**lip·o·tro·pic hor·mone, lip·o·tro·pic pi·tu·i·tar·y hor·mone** SYN lipotropin.

**lip·o·tro·pin** (li-pō-trō'pin) a pituitary hormone mobilizing fat from adipose tissue. SYN lipotropic hormone, lipotropic pituitary hormone.

**li·pot·ro·py** (li-pot'rō-pē) **1.** affinity of basic dyes for fatty tissue. **2.** prevention of accumulation of fat in the liver. **3.** affinity of nonpolar substances for each other. [lipo- + G. *tropē*, turning]

**lip·o·vac·cine** (lip'ō-vak-sēn) a vaccine having a vegetable oil as a solvent.

**li·pox·i·dase** (li-poks'i-dās) SYN lipoxygenase.

**li·pox·y·ge·nase** (li-poks'ē-jě-nās) an enzyme that catalyzes the oxidation of unsaturated fatty acids with $O_2$ to yield hydroperoxides of the fatty acids. SYN lipoxidase.

**lip·ping** (lip'ing) the formation of a liplike structure, as at the articular end of a bone in osteoarthritis.

**lip read·ing** SYN speech reading.

**lip re·flex** a pouting movement of the lips provoked in young infants by tapping near the angle of the mouth.

**li·pu·ria** (li-pyu'rē-ă) presence of lipids in the urine. SYN adiposuria. [lipo- + G. *ouron*, urine]

**li·pur·ic** (li-pyu'rik) pertaining to lipuria.

**liq·ue·fa·cient** (lik'wē-fā'shent) **1.** making liquid; causing a solid to become liquid. **2.** denoting a resolvent supposed to cause the resolution of a solid tumor by liquefying its contents. [L. *liquefacio*, pres. p. *-faciens*, to make fluid, fr. *liqueo*, to be liquid]

**liq·ue·fac·tion** (lik-wě-fak'shŭn) the act of becoming liquid; change from a solid to a liquid form. [see liquefacient]

**liq·ue·fac·tive ne·cro·sis** a type of necrosis characterized by dull, opaque, partly or completely fluid remains of tissue. It is observed in abscesses and frequently in infarcts of the brain.

**li·ques·cent** (li-kwes'ent) becoming or tending to become liquid. [L. *liquesco*, to become liquid]

**liq·uid** (lik'wid) **1.** an inelastic substance, like water, that is neither solid nor gaseous and in which the molecules are relatively free to move with respect to each other yet still are restricted by intermolecular forces. **2.** flowing like water. [L. *liquidus*]

**liq·uid-liq·uid chro·ma·tog·ra·phy** chromatography in which both the moving phase and the stationary (or reverse-moving) phase are liquids, as in countercurrent distribution.

**liq·uid scin·til·la·tor** a liquid with the properties of a scintillator, in which the substance whose radioactivity is to be measured can be dissolved, to be placed in a well counter.

**li·quor**, gen. **li·quor·is**, pl. **li·quo·res** (lik'er, līk'wor; lik-wōr'is; lik'wō'rēs) **1.** any liquid or fluid. **2.** a term used for certain body fluids. **3.** the pharmacopeial term for any aqueous solution (not a decoction or infusion) of a nonvolatile substance and for aqueous solutions of gases. SEE ALSO solution. [L.]

**li·quor am·nii** SYN amnionic fluid.

**Lisch nod·ule** (lish) iris hamartomas typically seen in type 1 neurofibromatosis.

**Lis·franc am·pu·ta·tion** (lis-frahngk') amputation of the foot at the tarsometatarsal joint, the sole being preserved to make the flap.

**Lis·franc in·ju·ry** (lis-frahngk') disruption of the tarsometatarsal joint, with or without an associated fracture.

**lisp·ing** mispronunciation of the sibilants *s* and *z*.

**lis·pro in·su·lin** (lĭs'prō) a modified version of natural human insulin, synthesized by a genetically programmed strain of nonpathogenic *Escherichia coli*, in which the amino acids lysine (Lys) and proline (Pro) near the end of the B chain are transposed. This chemical alteration yields an insulin with a much faster onset of action, which reaches its peak effect earlier than regular insulin. [Lys + Pro]

**lis·sen·ce·pha·lia** (lis'en-sě-fā'lē-ă) SYN agyria. [G. *lissos*, smooth, + *enkephalos*, brain]

**lis·sen·ce·phal·ic** (lis'en-sě-fal'ik) pertaining to, or characterized by, lissencephalia.

**lis·sive** (lis'iv) having the property of relieving muscle spasm without causing flaccidity. [G. *lissos*, smooth]

**lis·so·sphinc·ter** (lis'ō-sfingk'ter) a sphincter of smooth musculature. [G. *lissos*, smooth, + sphincter]

***Lis·te·ria*** (lis-tēr-ē-ă) a genus of aerobic to microaerophilic, motile, bacteria (family Corynebacteriaceae) containing small, coccoid, Gram-positive rods; found in the feces of humans and other animals, on vegetation, and in silage, and parasitic on poikilothermic and warm-blooded animals, including humans. The type species is *Listeria monocytogenes*. [Joseph Lister]

**lis·te·ri·o·sis** (lis-tēr'ē-ō'sis) a sporadic disease of animals and humans, particularly those who are immunocompromised or pregnant, caused by the bacterium, *Listeria monocytogenes*. [fr. organism *Listeria*]

**lis·ter·ism** (lis'ter-izm) SYN Lister method.

**Lis·ter meth·od** (lis'těr) antiseptic surgery, as first advocated by Lister in 1867; the operation was performed under a cloud of diluted carbolic acid spray, the instruments were dipped in a carbolic solution before use, and the wound was dressed with a thick layer of carbolized gauze; from this was developed the present practice of aseptic surgery. SYN listerism.

**Lis·ting law** (lis'ting) when the eye leaves one object and fixes upon another, it revolves about an axis perpendicular to a plane cutting both the former and the present lines of vision.

Listing 568 livor

**Lis•ting re•duced eye** (lis'ting) a representation that simplifies calculations of retinal imagery: radius of anterior refracting surface, 5.1 mm; total length, 20 mm; distance of nodal point to retina, 15 mm.

**li•ter (l)** (lē'ter) a measure of capacity of 1000 cubic centimeters or 1 cubic decimeter; equivalent to 1.056688 quarts (U.S., liquid). [Fr., fr. G. *litra,* a pound]

**lith•a•gogue** (lith'ă-gog) causing the dislodgment or expulsion of calculi, especially urinary calculi. [litho- + G. *agōgos,* drawing forth]

**li•thec•to•my** (li-thek'tō-mē) SYN lithotomy. [litho- + G. *ektomē,* excision]

**li•thi•a•sis** (li-thī'ă-sis) formation of calculi of any kind, especially of biliary or urinary calculi. [litho- + G. *-iasis,* condition]

**lith•i•um (Li)** (lith'ē-ŭm) an element of the alkali metal group, atomic no. 3, atomic wt. 6.941. Many salts have clinical applications. [Mod. L. fr. G. *lithos,* a stone]

⌂**litho-, lith-** a stone, calculus, calcification. [G. *lithos*]

**lith•o•clast** (lith'ō-klast) SYN lithotrite. [litho- + G. *klastos,* broken]

**lith•o•gen•e•sis, li•thog•e•ny** (lith-ō-jen'ĕ-sis, lith-oj'ĕ-nē) formation of calculi. [litho- + G. *genesis,* production]

**lith•o•gen•ic** (lith-ō-jen'ik) promoting the formation of calculi.

**lith•og•e•nous** (lith-oj'ĕ-nŭs) calculus-forming.

**li•thol•a•paxy** (li-thol'ă-pak-sē) the operation of crushing a stone in the bladder and washing out the fragments through a catheter. [litho- + G. *lapaxis,* an emptying out]

**li•thol•y•sis** (li-thol'i-sis) the dissolution of urinary calculi. [litho- + G. *lysis,* dissolution]

**lith•o•lyt•ic** (lith-ō-lit'ik) **1.** tending to dissolve calculi. **2.** an agent having such properties. [litho- + G. *lysis,* dissolution]

**lith•o•ne•phri•tis** (lith'ō-ne-frī'tis) interstitial nephritis associated with calculus formation.

**lith•o•pe•di•on, lith•o•pe•di•um** (lith-ō-pē'dē-on, lith-ō-pē'dēŭm) a retained fetus, usually extrauterine, that has become calcified. [litho- + G. *paidion,* small child]

**li•thot•o•my** (li-thot'ō-mē) cutting for stone; a cutting operation for the removal of a calculus, especially a vesical calculus. SYN lithectomy. [litho- + G. *tomē,* incision]

**li•thot•o•my po•si•tion** a supine position with buttocks at the end of the operating table, the hips and knees being fully flexed with feet strapped in position.

**lith•o•trip•sy** (lith'ō-trip-sē) the crushing of a stone in the renal pelvis, ureter, or bladder, by mechanical force or sound waves. SYN lithotrity. [litho- + G. *tripsis,* a rubbing]

**lith•o•trip•tic** (lith-ō-trip'tik) **1.** relating to lithotripsy. **2.** an agent that effects the dissolution of a calculus.

**lith•o•trip•tos•co•py** (lith'ō-trip-tos'kŏ-pē) crushing of a stone in the bladder under direct vision by use of a lithotriptoscope. [litho- + G. *tribō,* to rub, crush, + *skopeō,* to view]

**lith•o•trite** (lith'ō-trīt) a mechanical instrument used to crush a urinary calculus in lithotripsy. SYN lithoclast. [litho- + L. *tero,* pp. *tritus,* to rub]

**li•thot•ri•ty** (li-thot'ri-tē) SYN lithotripsy.

**lith•u•re•sis** (lith'yu-rē'sis) the passage of gravel in the urine. [litho- + G. *ourēsis,* urination]

**lit•mus** (lit'mŭs) a blue coloring matter obtained from *Roccella tinctorial* and other lichens, the principal component of which is azolitmin; used as an indicator (reddened by acids and turned blue again by alkalies). [Dutch *lakmoes*]

**lit•ter** (lit'er) **1.** a stretcher or portable couch for moving the sick or injured. **2.** a group of animals of the same parents, born at the same time. [Fr. *litière;* fr. *lit,* bed]

**lit•tle ACTH** the conventional ACTH molecule when contrasted with big ACTH.

**Lit•tle ar•ea** (lit'ĕl) SYN Kiesselbach area.

**Lit•tle League el•bow** inflammation of the medial epicondyle of the humerus due to overuse or cumulative trauma, as in athletics. SYN medial epicondylitis.

**Lit•tle League shoul•der** fracture of the growth plate of the humeral head in the adolescent, resulting from repetitive rotational stresses during the act of pitching a baseball.

**lit•tle toe [V]** fifth digit of the foot.

**Lit•tré glands** (lē'trĕ) SYN urethral glands of male.

**Lit•tré her•nia** (lē'trĕ) **1.** SYN parietal hernia. **2.** hernia of Meckel diverticulum.

**Litz•mann ob•liq•ui•ty** (litz'mĕn) inclination of the fetal head so that the biparietal diameter is oblique in relation to the plane of the pelvic brim, the posterior parietal bone presenting to the parturient canal. SYN posterior asynclitism.

**live•born in•fant** the product of a live birth; an infant who shows evidence of life after birth.

**li•ve•do** (li-vē'dō) a bluish discoloration of the skin, either in limited patches or general. [L. lividness, fr. *liveo,* to be black and blue]

**liv•e•doid** (liv'ĕ-doyd) pertaining to or resembling livedo.

**liv•e•doid der•ma•ti•tis** a reddish blue mottled condition of the skin due to affection of the cutaneous vascular apparatus.

**li•ve•do re•tic•u•la•ris** a persistent purplish network-patterned discoloration of the skin caused by dilation of capillaries and venules due to stasis or changes in underlying blood vessels including hyalinization.

**liv•er** (liv'er) the largest gland of the body, lying beneath the diaphragm in the right hypochondrium and upper part of the epigastrium; it is of irregular shape and weighs from 1 to 2 kg, or about 1/40 the weight of the body. It secretes the bile and is also of great importance in both carbohydrate and protein metabolism. SYN hepar [TA]. [A.S. *lifer*]

**liv•er ac•i•nus** the smallest functional unit of the liver, comprising all of the liver parenchyma supplied by a terminal branch of the portal vein and hepatic artery.

**liv•er spot** SYN senile lentigo.

**live vac•cine** vaccine prepared from living, attenuated organisms.

**liv•id** having a black and blue or a leaden or ashy gray color, as in discoloration from a contusion, congestion, or cyanosis. [L. *lividus,* being black and blue]

**li•vid•i•ty** (li-vid'i-tē) the state of being livid.

**living will** legal document used to indicate one's preference to die rather than be sustained artificially if sick or injured beyond the prospect of recovery. SEE advance directive. SYN durable power of attorney (2).

**li•vor** (lī'vōr) the livid discoloration of the skin on

the dependent parts of a corpse. [L. a black and blue spot]

**LM** licentiate in midwifery.

**lm** lumen (2).

**LMA** left mentoanterior position.

**LMP** left mentoposterior position.

**LMRP** Local Medical Review Policy.

**LMT** left mentotransverse position.

**LNPF** lymph node permeability factor.

**load** (lōd) **1.** a departure from normal body content, as of water, salt, or heat; positive loads are quantities in excess of the normal; negative loads are quantities in deficit. **2.** the quantity of a measurable entity borne by an object or organism. [M.E. *lode*, fr. A.S. lād,]

**load-and-shift ma·neu·ver** a test of shoulder instability in which the humeral head is pushed against the glenoid and moved anteriorly and posteriorly.

**load·ing** (lōd′ing) administration of a substance for the purpose of testing metabolic function or of rapidly achieving therapeutic levels of a drug.

***Loa loa*** (lō′ă lō′ă) the African eye worm, a species of the family Onchocercidae that is the causal agent of loiasis. Humans are the only known definitive host, and parasites are transmitted by *Chrysops* flies; infective larvae from the latter require 3 years or more to mature in humans, and the adult forms may persist in humans for as long as 17 years. SEE ALSO loiasis.

**lo·bar** (lō′bar) relating to any lobe.

**lo·bar pneu·mo·nia** pneumonia affecting one or more lobes, or part of a lobe, of the lung in which the consolidation is virtually homogeneous; commonly due to infection by *Streptococcus pneumoniae;* sputum is scanty and usually of a rusty tint from altered blood.

**lo·bate** (lō′bāt) **1.** divided into lobes. **2.** lobe-shaped; denoting a bacterial colony with a deeply undulate margin.

**lobe** (lōb) **1.** one of the subdivisions of an organ or other part, bounded by fissures, connective tissue, septa, or other structural demarcations. **2.** a rounded projecting part, as the lobe of the ear. SEE ALSO lobule. **3.** one of the larger divisions of the crown of a tooth, formed from a distinct point of calcification. SYN lobus. [G. *lobos*, lobe]

**lo·bec·to·my** (lō-bek′tō-mē) excision of a lobe of any organ or gland. [G. *lobos*, lobe, + *ektomē*, excision]

**lo·bi** (lō′bī) plural of lobus. [L.]

**lo·bi·tis** (lō-bī′tis) inflammation of a lobe.

**lo·bot·o·my** (lō-bot′ō-mē) **1.** incision into a lobe. **2.** division of one or more nerve tracts in a lobe of the cerebrum. [G. *lobos*, lobe, + *tomē*, a cutting]

**lo·bu·lar** (lob′yu-lăr) relating to a lobule.

**lo·bu·lar cap·il·lary he·man·gi·o·ma** SYN pyogenic granuloma.

**lob·u·lar glo·mer·u·lo·ne·phri·tis** SYN membranoproliferative glomerulonephritis.

**lob·u·late, lob·u·lat·ed** (lob′yu-lāt, lob′yu-lāt-ed) divided into lobules.

**lob·ule** (lob′yul) a small lobe or subdivision of a lobe. SYN lobulus [TA].

**lob·ules of ep·i·did·y·mis** the coiled portion of the efferent ductules that constitute the head of the epididymis; these join the ductus epididymidis. SYN lobuli epididymidis.

**lob·ules of liv·er** the conceptual polygonal histologic unit of the liver, consisting of masses of liver cells arranged around a central vein, a terminal branch of one of the hepatic veins; at the periphery are located preterminal and terminal branches of the portal vein, hepatic artery, and bile duct; in the human liver, hepatic lobules are distinguishable only when fibrous septa are present as a result of disease. SYN lobulus hepatis [TA], hepatic lobule.

**lob·u·li ep·i·did·y·mi·dis** SYN lobules of epididymis.

**lob·u·lus,** gen. and pl. **lob·u·li** (lob′yu-lŭs, lob′yu-lī) [TA] SYN lobule. [Mod. L. dim. of *lobus*, lobe]

**lob·u·lus hep·a·tis** [TA] SYN lobules of liver.

**lob·u·lus pa·ra·me·di·a·nus** [TA] SYN gracile lobule.

**lo·bus,** gen. and pl. **lo·bi** (lō′bŭs, lō′bī) SYN lobe. [LL. fr. G. *lobos*]

**lo·bus an·te·ri·or hy·po·phys·e·os** [TA] SYN adenohypophysis.

**lo·bus cau·da·tus** SYN posterior hepatic segment I. SYN caudate lobe.

**lo·bus hep·a·tis dex·ter** [TA] SYN right lobe of liver.

**lo·bus hep·a·tis sin·is·ter** [TA] SYN left lobe of liver.

**lo·bus pos·te·ri·or hy·po·phys·e·os** [TA] SYN neurohypophysis. SEE ALSO hypophysis.

**lo·bus tem·po·ra·lis** [TA] SYN temporal lobe.

**lo·cal** (lō′kăl) having reference or confined to a limited part; not general or systemic. [L. *localis*, fr. *locus*, place]

**lo·cal an·a·phy·lax·is** the immediate, transient kind of response that follows the injection of antigen (allergen) into the skin of a sensitized individual and is limited to the area surrounding the site of inoculation. SEE ALSO skin test.

**lo·cal an·es·the·sia** a general term referring to topical, infiltration, field block, or nerve block anesthesia but usually not to spinal or epidural anesthesia.

**lo·cal as·phyx·ia** stagnation of the circulation, sometimes resulting in local gangrene, especially of the fingers; one of the symptoms usually associated with Raynaud disease.

**lo·cal death** death of a part of the body or of a tissue by necrosis.

**lo·cal flap** a flap transferred to an adjacent area.

**lo·cal im·mu·ni·ty** a natural or acquired immunity to certain infectious agents, as manifested by an organ or a tissue, as a whole or in part.

**lo·cal·i·za·tion** (lō′kăl-i-zā′shŭn) **1.** limitation to a definite area. **2.** the reference of a sensation to its point of origin. **3.** the determination of the location of a morbid process.

**lo·cal·i·za·tion-re·lat·ed ep·i·lep·sy 1.** SYN myoclonus epilepsy. **2.** SYN focal epilepsy.

**lo·cal·ized** (lō′kăl-īzd) restricted or limited to a definite part.

**lo·cal·ized mu·ci·no·sis** SEE mucinosis.

**lo·cal·ized nod·u·lar ten·o·syn·o·vi·tis** SYN giant cell tumor of tendon sheath.

**lo·cal·ized scle·ro·der·ma** SYN morphea.

**lo·cal·iz·ing symp·tom** a symptom indicating clearly the seat of the morbid process.

**Lo·cal Med·i·cal Re·view Pol·i·cy (LMRP)** a guideline for making local medical coverage decisions in the absence of a specific Medicare statute, regulation, or national coverage policy, or as an adjunct to an existing national coverage

l
o

policy; devised by coverage contractors in consultation with the local medical community.

**lo·cal re·ac·tion** SYN focal reaction.

**lo·cal stim·u·lant** a stimulant whose action is confined to the part to which it is applied.

**lo·ca·tor** (lō′kā-ter) an instrument or apparatus for finding the position of a foreign object in tissue.

**lo·chia** (lō′kē-ă) discharge from the vagina of mucus, blood, and tissue debris, following childbirth. [G. neut. pl. of *lochios,* relating to childbirth, fr. *lochos,* childbirth]

**lo·chi·al** (lō′kē-ăl) relating to the lochia.

**lo·chi·o·me·tra** (lō-kē-ō-mē′tră) distention of the uterus with retained lochia. [G. *mētra,* womb]

**lo·chi·or·rhea, lo·chi·or·rha·gia** (lō-kē-ō-rē′ă, lō-kē-ō-rā′jē-ă) profuse flow of the lochia. [lochia + G. *rhoia,* a flow]

**lo·ci** (lō′sī) plural of locus.

**lock** (lŏk) **1.** an enclosing, fastening, or securing device. **2.** a mechanism which, when moved, permits or obstructs passage.

**locked-in syn·drome** basis pontis infarct resulting in tetraplegia, horizontal ophthalmoplegia, dysphagia, and facial diplegia with preserved consciousness; caused by basilar artery occlusion.

**locked knee** a condition in which the knee lacks full extension and flexion because of internal derangement, usually the result of a torn medial meniscus.

**locked twins** a form of malpresentation in which a breech twin and a vertex twin become locked at the chin during labor and attempted delivery.

**Locke so·lu·tion** (lok) a solution containing NaCl, CaCl$_2$, KCl, NaHCO$_3$, and D-glucose; used for irrigating mammalian heart and other tissues, in laboratory experiments; also used in combination with naturally occurring body substances (e.g., blood serum, tissue extracts) and/or more complex chemically defined nutritive solutions for culturing animal cells.

**lock·ing su·ture** a running suture in which the suture material is made to pass through the loop made from the previous stitch. SYN lock stitch.

**lock·jaw** (lok′jaw) SYN trismus.

**lock stitch** SYN locking suture.

**lo·co·mo·tor** (lō-kō-mō′ter) relating to locomotion, or movement from one place to another. [L. *locus,* place, + L. *moveo,* pp. *motus,* to move)

**loc·u·lar** (lok′yu-lăr) relating to a loculus.

**loc·u·late** (lok′yu-lāt) containing numerous loculi.

**loc·u·lat·ed pleu·ral ef·fu·sion** pleural effusion that is confined to one or more fixed pockets in the pleural space.

**loc·u·la·tion** (lok-yu-lā′shŭn) **1.** a loculate region in an organ or tissue, or a loculate structure formed between surfaces of organs or mucous or serous membranes. **2.** the process that results in the formation of a loculus or loculi.

**loc·u·lus,** pl. **loc·u·li** (lok′yu-lŭs, lok-yu-lī) a small cavity or chamber. [L. dim. of *locus,* place]

**lo·cus,** pl. **lo·ci** (lō′kŭs, lō′sī) **1.** a place; usually, a specific site. **2.** the position that a gene occupies on a chromosome. **3.** the position of a point, as defined by the coordinates on a graph. [L.]

**lo·cus of con·trol** a theoretical construct designed to assess a person's perceived control over personal behavior; classified as *internal* if the person feels in control of events, *external* if others are perceived to have that control.

**lod score** (lod skōr) a number used in genetic linkage studies; logarithm (base 10) of the odds in favor of genetic linkage. [*logarithm* + *odds*]

**Loeb de·cid·u·o·ma** (lōb) mass of decidual tissue produced in the uterus, in the absence of a fertilized ovum, by means of mechanical or hormonal stimulation.

**Loef·fler ba·cil·lus** (lĕrf′lĕr) SYN *Corynebacterium diphtheriae.*

**Loef·fler blood cul·ture me·di·um** (lĕrf′lĕr) a culture medium consisting of beef blood serum, sheep blood serum, and beef bouillon containing peptone, glucose, and sodium chloride; used for the isolation of *Corynebacterium diphtheriae.*

**Loef·fler caus·tic stain** (lĕrf′lĕr) a stain for flagella, utilizing an aqueous solution of tannin and ferrous sulfate with the addition of an alcoholic fuchsin stain.

**Loef·fler stain** (lĕrf′lĕr) a stain for flagella; the specimen is treated with a mixture of ferrous sulfate, tannic acid, and alcoholic fuchsin, then stained with aniline-water fuchsin or gentian violet made alkaline with sodium hydroxide solution.

**Loe·wen·thal re·ac·tion** (lĕr′vĕn-tahl) the agglutinative reaction in relapsing fever.

**Löf·fler en·do·car·di·tis** (lĕrf′lĕr) fibroplastic constrictive parietal endocarditis with eosinophilia, an endocarditis of obscure cause characterized by progressive congestive heart failure, multiple systemic emboli, and eosinophilia.

**Löf·fler pa·ri·e·tal fi·bro·plas·tic en·do·car·di·tis** (lĕrf′lĕr) sclerosis of the endocardium in the presence of a high eosinophil count.

**Löf·fler syndrome** (lĕrf′lĕr) SYN pulmonary eosinophilia.

**log·ag·no·sia** (log-ag-nō′sē-ă) SYN aphasia. [logo- + G. *agnosia,* ignorance]

**log·a·graph·ia** (log-ă-graf′ē-ă) SYN agraphia. [logo- + G. *a-* priv. + *graphō,* to write]

**log·am·ne·sia** (log-am-nē′zē-ă) SYN aphasia. [logo- + G. *amnēsia,* forgetfulness]

**Lo·gan bow** (lō′găn) heavy stainless steel wire bent in an arc and taped to both cheeks to protect a freshly repaired cleft lip.

**log·a·pha·sia** (log-ă-fā′zē-ă) aphasia of articulation. [logo- + G. *aphasia,* speechlessness]

**log·as·the·nia** (log-as-thē′nē-ă) SYN aphasia. [logo- + G. *astheneia,* weakness]

△**-lo·gia 1.** the study of the subject noted in the body of the word, or a treatise on the same; the English equivalent is -logy, or, with a connecting vowel, -ology. [G. *logos,* discourse, treatise] **2.** collecting or picking. [G. *legō,* to collect)

**Lo·gis·tic Or·gan Dys·func·tion Score** an evaluation method used in intensive care that rates the level of dysfunction of each organ system and among organ systems; includes evaluation of degree of dysfunction of cardiovascular, hepatic, hematologic, pulmonary, renal, and nervous systems.

△**logo-, log-** speech, words. [G. *logos,* word, discourse]

**log·o·ple·gia** (log-ō-plē′jē-ă) paralysis of the organs of speech. [logo- + G. *plēgē,* stroke]

**log·or·rhea** (log-ō-rē′ă) rarely used term for abnormal or pathologic talkativeness or garrulousness. [logo- + G. *rhoia,* a flow]

**lo·gor·rhoea [Br.]** SEE logorrhea.

**lo·go·spasm** SYN stuttering.

△**-lo·gy** SEE -logia. [G. *logos*, treatise, discourse]

**lo·i·a·sis** (lō-ī'ă-sis) a chronic disease caused by the filarial nematode *Loa loa*, with symptoms first occurring three to four years after a bite by an infected tabanid fly. When the larvae mature, the adult worms move about through connective tissue, frequently becoming visible beneath the skin and mucous membranes. The worms provoke hyperemia and exudation of fluid; the patient is annoyed by the "creeping" in the tissues and intense itching, as well as occasional pain, especially when the swelling is in the region of tendons and joints.

**loin** (loyn) the part of the side and back between the ribs and the pelvis. SYN lumbus. [Fr. *longe;* E. *lumbus*]

**lo·mus·tine** (lō-mŭs'tēn) 1-(2-chloroethyl)-3-cyclohexyl-1-nitrosourea; an antineoplastic agent.

**long-act·ing thy·roid stim·u·la·tor (LATS)** a substance, found in the blood of some hyperthyroid patients, that exerts a prolonged stimulatory effect on the thyroid gland; associated in plasma with the IgG (7S γ-globulin) fraction and seems to be an antibody or, perhaps, an immune complex.

**long ad·duc·tor mus·cle** SYN adductor longus muscle.

**long bone** one of the elongated bones of the extremities, consisting of a tubular shaft (diaphysis) and two extremities (epiphyses) usually wider than the shaft; the shaft is composed of compact bone surrounding a central medullary cavity. Cf. short bone.

**lon·gev·i·ty** (lon-jev'i-tē) duration of a particular life beyond the norm for the species.

**long ex·ten·sor mus·cle of toes** SYN extensor digitorum longus muscle.

**long flex·or mus·cle of great toe** SYN flexor hallucis longus muscle.

**long flex·or mus·cle of thumb** SYN flexor pollicis longus muscle.

**long flex·or mus·cle of toes** SYN flexor digitorum longus muscle.

**long gy·rus of in·su·la** the most posterior and longest of the slender straight gyri that compose the insula.

**lon·gis·si·mus ca·pi·tis mus·cle** *origin*, from transverse processes of upper thoracic and transverse and articular processes of lower and middle cervical vertebrae; *insertion*, into mastoid process; *action*, keeps head erect, draws it backward or to one side; *nerve supply*, dorsal primary rami of cervical spinal nerves. SYN musculus longissimus capitis [TA].

**lon·gis·si·mus cer·vi·cis mus·cle** *origin*, transverse processes of upper thoracic vertebrae; *insertion*, transverse processes of middle and upper cervical vertebrae; *action*, extends cervical vertebrae; *nerve supply*, dorsal primary rami of lower cervical and upper thoracic spinal nerves. SYN musculus longissimus cervicis [TA].

**lon·gis·si·mus tho·ra·cis mus·cle** *origin*, with iliocostalis and from transverse processes of lower thoracic vertebrae; *insertion*, by lateral slips into most or all of the ribs between angles and tubercles and into tips of transverse processes of upper lumbar vertebrae, and by medial slips into accessory processes of upper lumbar and transverse processes of thoracic vertebrae;

*action*, extends vertebral column; *nerve supply*, dorsal primary rami of thoracic and lumbar spinal nerves. SYN musculus longissimus thoracis [TA], thoracic longissimus muscle.

**lon·gi·tu·di·nal** (lon'ji-too'di-năl) 1. running lengthwise; in the direction of the long axis of the body or any of its parts. 2. studied over a period of time, diachronic; contrast with cross-sectional or synchronic, which give equivalent results only under certain strict conditions of stability and equilibrium. [L. *longitudo,* length]

**lon·gi·tu·di·nal ab·er·ra·tion** in spherical aberration, the distance separating the focus of paraxial and peripheral rays on the optic axis.

**lon·gi·tu·di·nal dis·so·ci·a·tion** dissociation between parallel chambers of the heart, as between one atrium and the other or between one ventricle and the other, in contrast to dissociation between atria and ventricles.

**lon·gi·tu·di·nal frac·ture** a fracture involving the bone in the line of its axis.

**lon·gi·tu·di·nal lie** that relationship in which the long axis of the fetus is longitudinal and roughly parallel to the long axis of the mother; the presenting part may be either the head or the breech.

**lon·gi·tu·di·nal lig·a·ment** one of two extensive fibrous bands running the length of the vertebral column: the anterior longitudinal ligament and the posterior longitudinal ligament. SYN ligamentum longitudinale [TA].

**lon·gi·tu·di·nal pon·tine fas·cic·u·li** the massive bundles of corticofugal fibers passing longitudinally through the ventral part of pons; they are composed of corticopontine, corticobulbar, and corticospinal fibers.

**longitudinal pontine fibers** SEE longitudinal pontine fasciculi.

**lon·gi·tu·di·nal re·lax·a·tion** MAGNETIC RESONANCE IMAGING the return of the magnetic dipoles of the hydrogen nuclei (magnetization vector) to equilibrium parallel to the magnetic field, after they have been flipped 90°; varies in rate in different tissues, taking up to 15 seconds for water. SEE T1.

**lon·gi·tu·di·nal sec·tion** a cross section attained by slicing in any plane parallel to the long or vertical axis, actually or through imaging techniques, the body or any part of the body or anatomic structure. Longitudinal sections include, but are not limited to, median, sagittal, and coronal sections.

**lon·gi·tu·di·nal tear** a tear of articular cartilage roughly parallel to the long axis of the bone.

**long le·va·to·res cos·ta·rum mus·cles** *insertion*, the second rib below their origin; *action*, raise ribs; *nerve supply*, intercostal.

**Long·mire op·er·a·tion** (long'emīr) intrahepatic cholangiojejunostomy with partial hepatectomy for biliary obstruction.

**long mus·cle of head** SYN longus capitis muscle.

**long mus·cle of neck** SYN longus colli muscle.

**long QT syn·dromes** any of several congenital and acquired diseases in which the electrocardiographic QT interval is longer than established measurements for age and sex; the presence of long QT intervals presages arrhythmias and sudden death. SEE ALSO QT interval.

**long ra·di·al ex·ten·sor mus·cle of wrist** SYN extensor carpi radialis longus muscle.

**long slow dis·tance train·ing** SYN continuous training.

1
0

**long-term care fa·ci·li·ty** SYN nursing facility.

**long-term mem·o·ry (LTM)** that phase of the memory process considered the permanent storehouse of information which has been registered, encoded, passed into the short-term memory, coded, rehearsed, and finally transferred and stored for future retrieval; material and information retained in LTM underlies cognitive abilities.

**long tho·rac·ic nerve** arises from the fifth, sixth, and seventh cervical nerves (roots of brachial plexus), descends the neck behind the brachial plexus, and is distributed to the serratus anterior muscle; it is somewhat unusual in that it courses on the superficial aspect of the muscle it supplies; its paralysis results in "winged scapula." SYN nervus thoracicus longus [TA].

**lon·gus ca·pi·tis mus·cle** *origin*, anterior tubercles of transverse processes of third to sixth cervical vertebrae; *insertion*, basilar process of occipital bone; *action*, twists or flexes neck anteriorly; *nerve supply*, cervical plexus. SYN musculus longus capitis [TA], long muscle of head.

**lon·gus col·li mus·cle** medial part: *origin*, the bodies of the third thoracic to the fifth cervical vertebrae; *insertion*, the bodies of the second to fourth cervical vertebrae; superolateral part: *origin*, the anterior tubercles of the transverse processes of the third to fifth cervical vertebrae; *insertion*, the anterior tubercle of the atlas; inferolateral part: *origin*, the bodies of the first to third thoracic vertebrae; *insertion*, the anterior tubercles of the transverse processes of the fifth and sixth cervical vertebrae; *action*, for all three parts, twist neck and flex neck anteriorly; *nerve supply*, for all three parts, ventral primary rami of cervical spinal nerves (cervical plexus). SYN musculus longus colli [TA], long muscle of neck.

**loop** (loop) **1.** a sharp curve or complete bend in a vessel, cord, or other elongate body, forming an oval or circular ring. SEE ALSO ansa. **2.** a wire (usually of platinum or nichrome) fixed into a handle at one end and bent into a circle at the other, rendered sterile by flaming, and used to transfer microorganisms. [M.E. *loupe*]

**loop di·u·ret·ic** a class of diuretic agents (e.g., furosemide, ethacrynic acid) that act by inhibiting reabsorption of sodium and chloride, not only in the proximal and distal tubules but also in Henle loop.

**loop e·lec·tro·cau·tery ex·ci·sion pro·ce·dure (LEEP)** electrocautery excisional biopsy of abnormal cervical tissue.

**loop elec·tro·sur·gi·cal ex·ci·sion pro·ce·dure** SYN loop excision.

**loop ex·ci·sion** a diagnostic and therapeutic gynecological surgical technique for removing dysplastic cells from the cervix with a small wire loop. SYN loop electrosurgical excision procedure.

**loops of spi·nal nerves** loops of the spinal nerves, connecting ventral primary rami of the spinal nerves. SYN ansae nervorum spinalium.

**loose as·so·ci·a·tions** a manifestation of a thought disorder whereby the patient's responses do not relate to the interviewer's questions or one paragraph, sentence, or phrase is not logically connected to those that occur before or after.

**loos·en·ing of as·so·ci·a·tions** a manifestation of a severe thought disorder characterized by the lack of an obvious connection between one thought or phrase and the next, or with the response to a question.

**loose-packed po·si·tion** resting position of a joint; position of least strain.

**loph·o·dont** (lof'ō-dont) having the crowns of the molar teeth formed in transverse or longitudinal crests or ridges, as in the herbivores. [G. *lophos*, ridge, + *odous*, tooth]

**lor·do·sco·li·o·sis** (lōr'dō-skō-lē-ō'sis) combined backward and lateral curvature of the spine. [G. *lordos*, bent back, + *skoliōsis*, crookedness, fr. *skolios*, bent, aslant]

**lor·do·sis** (lōr-dō'sis) [TA] **1.** a normal anteriorly convex curvature of the vertebral column. **2.** an abnormal anteriorly convex curvature of the spine, usually lumbar. [G. *lordōsis*, a bending backward]

**lor·do·sis cer·vi·cis** [TA] SYN cervical lordosis.

**lor·do·sis col·li** SYN cervical lordosis.

**lor·do·sis lum·ba·lis** [TA] SYN lumbar lordosis.

**lor·dot·ic** (lōr-dot'ik) pertaining to or marked by lordosis.

**lor·dot·ic po·si·tion** a radiographic position with exaggerated lumbar lordotic curve, allowing x-ray examination of the lung apices without the clavicles being superimposed.

**Lo·schmidt num·ber** (lō'shmit) the number of molecules in 1 cm$^3$ of ideal gas at 0°C and 1 atm of pressure; Avogadro number divided by 22,414 (i.e., $2.6868 \times 10^{19}$ cm$^{-3}$).

**LOT** left occipitotransverse position.

**lo·tion** (lō'shŭn) a class of liquid suspensions or dispersions intended for external application. [L. *lotio*, a washing, fr. *lavo*, to wash]

**loud·ness dis·com·fort lev·el** the intensity at which sound, particularly speech, causes discomfort.

**Lou Geh·rig dis·ease** (loo ger'ig) SYN amyotrophic lateral sclerosis.

**Lou·is an·gle, Lud·wig an·gle** (loo-ē', lood'vig) SYN sternal angle.

**loupe** (loop) a magnifying lens. [Fr.]

**louse**, pl. **lice** (lows, līs) common name for members of the ectoparasitic insect orders Anoplura (sucking lice) and Mallophaga (biting lice). [A.S. *lūs*]

**Lo·vi·bond an·gle** (lŏv'ĭ-bond) the angle made at the meeting of the proximal nail fold and the nail plate when viewed from the radial aspect; normally, less than 180° but exceeding this in clubbing of the fingers.

**Lö·wen·berg for·ceps** (lĕr'vĕn-berg) forceps with short curved blades ending in rounded grasping extremities devised for the removal of adenoid growths in the nasopharynx.

**low·er air·way** the portion of the respiratory tract that extends from the subglottis to and including the terminal bronchioles.

**low·er e·soph·a·ge·al sphinc·ter (LES)** musculature of the gastroesophageal junction that is tonically active except during swallowing.

**low·er ex·trem·i·ty** SYN lower limb.

**low·er limb** the hip, thigh, leg, ankle, and foot. SYN lower extremity.

**low·er mo·tor neu·ron** the final motor neurons that innervate skeletal muscles; distinguished from upper motor neurons of the motor cortex that contribute to the pyramidal or corticospinal tract. SEE ALSO motor neuron.

**low·est splanch·nic nerve** one of the abdominopelvic splanchnic nerves arising in the thorax and penetrating the diaphragm to supply presynaptic sympathetic fibers for the renal plexus; often combined with the lesser splanchnic nerve, but occasionally existing as an independent nerve. SYN nervus splanchnicus imus [TA].

**low-fre·quen·cy trans·duc·tion** specialized transduction in which only a small portion of the prophage particles, because of their defectiveness, are able to develop sufficiently to serve as effective transducing agents.

**low-grade squa·mous in·tra·ep·i·the·li·al le·sion (LGSIL, LSIL)** term used in the Bethesda system for reporting cervical/vaginal cytologic diagnosis to describe a spectrum of noninvasive cervical epithelial abnormalities; these lesions include the cellular changes associated with human papilloma virus cytopathologic effect and mild dysplasia (cervical intraepithelial neoplasia grade 1). SEE ALSO Bethesda system, reactive changes, ASCUS, atypical glandular cells of undetermined significance.

**low-mo·lec·u·lar weight pro·tein** a gene product that is a component of a proteosome.

**low os·mo·lar con·trast agent** nonionic water-soluble radiographic contrast material. SYN low osmolar contrast medium, nonionic contrast agent.

**low os·mo·lar con·trast me·di·um** SYN low osmolar contrast agent.

**low-pu·rine di·et** a diet low in precursors of purines (such as tissues rich in cells with abundant nuclei, as in liver, glandular meats, etc.) to minimize formation of uric acid. Useful in treatment of patients with gout or urate-containing renal calculi.

**low-salt di·et** a diet with restricted amounts of sodium chloride, and other sodium salts, necessary in the treatment of some cases of hypertension, heart failure, and other syndromes characterized by fluid retention and/or edema formation.

**low-ten·sion glau·co·ma** optic nerve atrophy and excavation with typical field defects of glaucoma but without abnormal increase in intraocular pressure. SYN normal-tension glaucoma.

**low-tone hearing loss** inability to hear low notes or frequencies.

**lox·os·ce·lism** (lok-sos'ĕ-lizm) illness produced by the brown recluse spider, *Loxosceles reclusus;* characterized by gangrenous slough at the site of the bite, nausea, malaise, fever, hemolysis, and thrombocytopenia.

**loz·enge** (loz'enj) SYN troche. [Fr. *losange,* fr. *lozangé,* rhombic]

**LPO** left posterior oblique, a radiographic position in which the left posterior side of the body part being examined is closest to the film.

**Lr** lawrencium.

**Lr dose, $L_r$ dose** the limes reacting dose of diphtheria toxin, i.e., the smallest amount of toxin that, when mixed with one unit of antitoxin and injected intracutaneously in the shaved skin of a susceptible guinea pig, yields a minimal, positive reaction and inflammation localized to the region of the injection; the L ,d. closely approximates the L $_0$d., as would be expected, inasmuch as the slight excess of unneutralized toxin results in a reaction.

**LSA** left sacroanterior position.

**LSD training** SYN continuous training.

**L selectin** cell surface receptor produced by leukocytes.

**L shell** the next lowest energy level of electrons in the atom, after the K shell.

**LSIL** low-grade squamous intraepithelial lesion.

**LSP** left sacroposterior position.

**LST** left sacrotransverse position.

**LT** leukotrienes, usually followed by another letter with a subscript number; e.g., $LTA_4$, $LTC_4$.

**LTM** long-term memory.

**Lu** lutetium.

**Lu·barsch crys·tals** (loo'bahrsh) intracellular crystals in the testis resembling sperm crystals.

**lu·cid·i·ty** (loo-sid'i-tē) the quality or state of being lucid.

**lu·cif·u·gal** (loo-sif'yu-găl) avoiding light. [L. *lux,* light, + *fugio,* to flee from]

**Lu·cio lep·ro·sy** (loo'syō) an acute form occurring in pure diffuse lepromatous leprosy and presenting irregularly shaped, intensely erythematous, tender plaques, especially of the legs, with tendency to ulceration and scarring.

**lu·cip·e·tal** (loo-sip'i-tăl) seeking light. [L. *lux,* light, + *peto,* to seek]

**Luc·ké vi·rus** (luk'ā) a herpesvirus associated with Lucké carcinoma.

**Luc op·er·a·tion** (look) SYN Caldwell-Luc operation.

**Lud·wig an·gi·na** (lood'vig) cellulitis, usually of odontogenic origin, bilaterally involving the submaxillary, sublingual, and submental spaces, resulting in painful swelling of the floor of the mouth, elevation of the tongue, dysphasia, dysphonia, and (at times) compromise of the airway. [W.F. Ludwig]

**Ludwig gan·gli·on** (lood'vig) a small collection of parasympathetic nerve cells in the interatrial septum.

**Lu·er sy·ringe** (loo'ĕr) a glass syringe with a metal tip and locking device to secure the needle; used for hypodermic and intravenous injections and phlebotomy.

**lu·es** (loo'ēz) a plague or pestilence; specifically, syphilis. [L. pestilence]

**lu·et·ic** (loo-et'ik) SYN syphilitic.

**lu·et·ic mask** a dirty brownish yellow pigmentation, blotchy in character, resembling that of chloasma, occurring on the forehead, temples, and sometimes the cheeks in patients with tertiary syphilis.

**Luft dis·ease** (looft) a metabolic disease due to relative uncoupling of phosphorylation in skeletal muscle causing myopathy and general hypermetabolism; a mitochondial myopathy.

**Luft po·tas·si·um per·man·ga·nate fix·a·tive** (looft) a fixative useful in electron microscopy for cytologic preservation of lipoprotein complexes in membranes and myelin, because of its oxidative properties.

**Lu·gol i·o·dine so·lu·tion** (loo-gol') an iodine-potassium iodide solution used as an oxidizing agent, for removal of mercurial fixation artifacts, and also in histochemistry and to stain amebas.

**lu·lib·er·in** (loo-lib'er-in) a decapeptide hormone from the hypothalamus that stimulates the anterior pituitary to release both follicle-stimulating hormone and luteinizing hormone. SYN luteinizing hormone-releasing hormone. [luteinizing hormone + L. *libero,* to free, + -in]

**lum·ba·go** (lŭm-bā'gō) pain in mid and lower

l
u

back; a descriptive term not specifying cause. SYN lumbar rheumatism. [L. fr. *lumbus,* loin]

**lum·bar** (lŭm′bar) relating to the loins, or the part of the back and sides between the ribs and the pelvis. [L. *lumbus,* a loin]

**lum·bar ar·tery** *origin,* abdominal aorta; one of four or five pairs; *distribution,* lumbar vertebrae, muscles of back, abdominal wall; *anastomoses,* intercostal, subcostal, superior and inferior epigastric, deep circumflex iliac, and iliolumbar. SYN arteriae lumbales [TA].

**lum·bar flex·ure** the normal ventral curve of the vertebral column in the lumbar region.

**lum·bar her·nia** a protrusion between the last rib and the iliac crest where the aponeurosis of the transversus muscle is covered only by the latissimus dorsi.

**lum·bar il·i·o·cos·tal mus·cle** SYN iliocostalis lumborum muscle.

**lum·bar·i·za·tion** (lŭm′bar-i-zā′shŭn) a congenital anomaly of the lumbosacral junction characterized by development of the first sacral vertebra as a lumbar vertebra resulting in six lumbar vertebrae instead of five.

**lum·bar lor·do·sis** the normal, anteriorly convex curvature of the lumbar segment of the vertebral column; a secondary curvature, acquired postnatally as the upright posture is assumed when one learns to walk. SYN lordosis lumbalis [TA].

**lum·bar nerves [L1–L5]** five bilaterally paired spinal nerves emerging from the lumbar portion of the spinal cord; the first four nerves enter into the formation of the lumbar plexus, the fourth and fifth into that of the sacral plexus. SYN nervi lumbales [TA].

**lum·bar plex·us 1.** a nervous plexus, formed by the ventral rami of the first four lumbar nerves; it lies in the substance of the psoas muscle; **2.** a lymphatic plexus formed of about twenty lymph nodes and connecting vessels situated along the lower portion of the aorta and the common iliac vessels.

**lum·bar punc·ture** a puncture into the subarachnoid space of the lumbar region to obtain spinal fluid for diagnostic or therapeutic purposes. SYN rachicentesis, rachiocentesis, spinal tap.

**lum·bar rheu·ma·tism** SYN lumbago.

**lum·bar rib** an occasional rib articulating with the transverse process of the first lumbar vertebra.

**lum·bar splanch·nic nerves** branches from the lumbar sympathetic trunks that pass anteriorly to convey presynaptic sympathetic fibers to, and visceral afferents from, the celiac, intermesenteric, aortic, and superior hypogastric plexuses. SYN nervi splanchnici lumbales [TA].

**lum·bar tri·an·gle** an area in the posterior abdominal wall bounded by the edges of the latissimus dorsi and external oblique muscles and the iliac crest; herniations occasionally occur here. SYN Petit lumbar triangle, trigonum lumbale.

**lum·bar vein** veins accompanying the lumbar arteries, which drain the posterior body wall and the lumbar vertebral venous plexuses, and terminate anteriorly as follows: the first and second in the ascending lumbar vein, the third and fourth in the inferior vena cava, and the fifth in the iliolumbar vein; all communicate via the ascending lumbar veins.

**lum·bar ver·te·brae L1–L5** the vertebrae, usu-ally five in number, located in the lumbar region of the back. SYN vertebrae lumbales [L1–L5].

**lum·bi** (lŭm′bī) plural of lumbus. [L.]

**lum·bo·cos·tal** (lŭm′bō-kos′tăl) **1.** relating to the lumbar and the hypochondriac regions. **2.** relating to the lumbar vertebrae and the ribs; denoting a ligament connecting the first lumbar vertebra with the neck of the twelfth rib. [L. *lumbus,* loin, + *costa,* rib]

**lum·bo·cos·tal lig·a·ment** a strong band that unites the twelfth rib with the tips of the transverse processes of the first and second lumbar vertebrae. SYN ligamentum lumbocostale [TA].

**lum·bo·cos·to·ab·dom·i·nal tri·an·gle** an irregular area bounded by the serratus posterior inferior, obliquus externus, obliquus internus, and erector spinae muscles.

**lum·bo·in·gui·nal** (lŭm′bō-ing′gwi-năl) relating to the lumbar and the inguinal regions. [L. *lumbus,* loin, + *inguen* (*inguin-*), groin]

**lum·bo·sa·cral** (lŭm′bō-sā′krăl) relating to the lumbar vertebrae and the sacrum. SYN sacrolumbar.

**lum·bri·cal mus·cles of foot** four intrinsic muscles of the foot; *origin,* first: from tibial side of tendon to second toe of flexor digitorum longus; second, third, and fourth: from adjacent sides of all four tendons of this musculus; *insertion,* tibial side of extensor tendon on dorsum of each of the four lateral toes; *action,* flex the proximal and extend the middle and distal phalanges; *nerve supply,* lateral (second to fourth lumbricals) and medial (first lumbrical) plantar. SYN musculus lumbricalis pedis [TA].

**lum·bri·cal mus·cles of hand** four intrinsic muscles of the hand; *origin,* the two lateral: from the radial side of the tendons of the flexor digitorum profundus going to the index and middle fingers; the two medial: from the adjacent sides of the second and third, and third and fourth tendons; *insertion,* radial side of extensor tendon on dorsum of each of the four fingers; *action,* flexes metacarpophalangeal joint and extends the proximal and distal interphalangeal joint; *nerve supply,* the two radial muscles by the median, the two ulnar muscles by the ulnar. SYN musculus lumbricalis manus [TA].

**lum·bri·ci·dal** (lŭm-bri-sī′dăl) destructive to lumbricoid (intestinal) worms.

**lum·bri·cide** (lŭm′bri-sīd) an agent that kills lumbricoid (intestinal) worms. [L. *lumbricus,* worm, + *caedo,* to kill]

**lum·bri·coid** (lŭm′bri-koyd) denoting or resembling a roundworm, especially *Ascaris lumbricoides.* SEE ALSO vermiform. [L. *lumbricus,* earthworm, + G. *eidos,* resemblance]

**lum·bri·co·sis** (lŭm′bri-kō′sis) infection with round intestinal worms.

**lum·bus,** gen. and pl. **lum·bi** (lŭm′bŭs, lŭm′bī) SYN loin. [L.]

**lu·men,** pl. **lu·mi·na, lu·mens** (loo′men, loo′min-ă, loo′menz) **1.** the space in the interior of a tubular structure, such as an artery or the intestine. **2.** (**lm**) the unit of luminous flux; the luminous flux emitted in a unit solid angle of 1 steradian by a uniform point source of light having a luminous intensity of 1 candela. [L. light, window]

**lu·mi·nal** (loo′mi-năl) relating to the lumen of a blood vessel or other tubular structure. SYN luminalis.

**lu·mi·na·lis** SYN luminal.

**lu·mi·nance** (loo′mi-năns) the brightness of an object, expressed as the luminous flux per unit solid angle per unit projected area, measured in lamberts or in candelas per square meter. [L. *lumino*, to light up, fr. *lumen*, light]

**lu·mi·nes·cence** (loo-mi-nes′ens) emission of light from a body as a result of a chemical reaction. [L. *lumen*, light]

**lu·mi·nif·er·ous** (loo-mi-nif′er-ŭs) producing or conveying light. [L. *lumen*, light, + *fero*, to carry]

**lu·mi·no·phore** (loo-mi-nŏ-for′) an atom or atomic grouping in an organic compound that increases its ability to emit light. [L. *lumen*, light, + G. *phoros*, bearing]

**lu·mi·nous** (loo′mi-nŭs) emitting light, with or without accompanying heat. [L. *lumen*, light]

**lu·mi·nous in·ten·si·ty (I)** the luminous flux per unit solid angle in a given direction. SYN radiant intensity.

**lu·mi·rho·dop·sin** (loo′mi-rō-dop′sin) an intermediate between rhodopsin and all-*trans*-retinal plus opsin during bleaching of rhodopsin by light; formed from bathorhodopsin and converted to metarhodopsin. [L. *lumen*, light, + G. *rhodon*, rose, + *opsis*, vision]

**lump·ec·to·my** (lŭm-pek′tō-mē) removal of either a benign or malignant lesion from the breast, with preservation of surrounding tissue. [lump + G. *ektomē*, excision]

**lu·nar** (loo′ner) **1.** relating to the moon or to a month. **2.** resembling the moon in shape, especially a half moon. SYN lunate (1), semilunar. SEE ALSO crescentic. **3.** relating to silver (the moon was the symbol of silver in alchemy). [L. *luna*, moon]

**lu·nate** (loo′nāt) **1.** SYN lunar (2). **2.** relating to the lunate bone.

**lu·nate bone** one of the proximal row in the carpus between the scaphoid and triquetral; it articulates with the radius, scaphoid, triquetral, hamate, and capitate.

**lung** (lŭng) one of a pair of viscera occupying the pulmonary cavities of the thorax, the organs of respiration in which aeration of the blood takes place. As a rule, the right lung is slightly larger than the left and is divided into three lobes (an upper, a middle, and a lower or basal), while the left has but two lobes (an upper and a lower or basal). Each lung is irregularly conical in shape, presenting a blunt upper extremity (the apex), a concave base following the curve of the diaphragm, an outer convex surface (costal surface), an inner or mediastinal surface (mediastinal surface), a thin and sharp anterior border, and a thick and rounded posterior border. See page 576. SYN pulmo [TA]. [A.S. *lungen*]

**lung com·pli·ance** the change in lung volume per unit change in transpulmonary pressure; may be static or dynamic.

**lung vol·ume re·duc·tion sur·gery** procedure whereby nonfunctional lung tissue in emphysema patients is removed, allowing more room in the thoracic cavity for relatively healthy tissue and thus theoretically improving lung function. SEE ALSO emphysema.

**lung·worms** (lŭng′wermz) nematodes that inhabit the air passages of animals.

**lu·nu·la,** pl. **lu·nu·lae** (loo′nyu-lă, loo′nyu-lē) **1.** the pale arched area at the proximal portion of

the nail plate. **2.** a small semilunar structure. [L. dim. of *luna*, moon]

**lu·nule 1.** SYN lunule of nail. **2.** a small semilunar structure.

**lu·nule of nail** the pale arched area at the proximal portion of the nail plate. SYN lunule (1).

**lu·pi·form** (loo′pi-fōrm) SYN lupoid.

**lu·poid** (loo′poyd) resembling lupus. SYN lupiform. [L. *lupus* + G. *eidos,* resemblance]

**lu·poid hep·a·ti·tis** jaundice with evidence of liver cell damage and positive antinuclear antibody or LE cell tests, but without evidence of systemic lupus erythematosus.

**lu·poid sy·co·sis** a papular or pustular inflammation of the hair follicles of the beard, followed by punctuate scarring and loss of the hair.

**lu·pous** (loo′pŭs) relating to lupus.

**lu·pus** (loo′pŭs) a term originally used to depict erosion (as if gnawed) of the skin, now used with modifying terms designating the various diseases listed below. [L. wolf]

**lu·pus an·ti·co·ag·u·lant** antiphospholipid antibody causing elevation in partial thromboplastin time; associated with venous and arterial thrombosis.

**lu·pus band test** a direct immunofluorescent technique for demonstrating a band of immunoglobulins at the dermal-epidermal junction of the skin of patients with lupus erythematosus.

**lu·pus er·y·the·ma·to·sus (LE, L.E.)** an illness which may be characterized by skin lesions alone or systemic (disseminated) with antinuclear antibodies present and usually involvement of vital structures. SEE ALSO discoid lupus erythematosus, systemic lupus erythematosus. See page B6.

**lu·pus er·y·the·ma·to·sus cell** SYN LE cell.

**lu·pus er·y·the·ma·to·sus cell test** SYN LE cell test.

**lu·pus er·y·the·ma·to·sus pro·fun·dus** a subcutaneous panniculitis with deep-seated, firm, rubbery nodules, usually of the face; may occur in systemic and localized lupus erythematosus.

**lu·pus li·ve·do** persistent cyanotic lesions on the extremities, associated with the cutaneous manifestations of Raynaud disease.

**lu·pus mil·i·a·ris dis·se·mi·na·tus fa·ci·ei** a milletlike papular eruption of the face associated with a (histopathologically) tuberculoid perifollicular infiltration but probably related to rosacea rather than tuberculous infection.

**lu·pus ne·phri·tis** glomerulonephritis occurring in some patients with systemic lupus erythematosus, characterized by hematuria and a progressive course culminating in renal failure.

**lu·pus per·nio** sarcoid lesions, clinically resembling frostbite and microscopically resembling lupus vulgaris, involving ears, cheeks, nose, hands, and fingers.

**lu·pus vul·ga·ris** cutaneous tuberculosis with characteristic nodular lesions on the face, particularly about the nose and ears.

**LUQ** left upper quadrant (of abdomen).

**lus·i·tropic** (loos-ē-trō′pik) relating to lusitropy.

**lus·it·ropy** (loos-it′trō-pē) relaxation functions of cardiac muscle and chambers.

**lu·te·al** (loo′tē-ăl) relating to the corpus luteum; luteal cells, luteal hormone, etc. [L. *luteus*, saffron-yellow]

**lu·te·al cell, lu·te·in cell** a cell of the corpus luteum of the ovary that is derived from the granulosa cells of the preovulatory follicle; it secretes progesterone and estrogen.

**lu·te·al phase** that portion of the menstrual cycle extending from the time of formation of the corpus luteum to the onset of menses, usually 14 days in length; **short luteal phase**, a period of 10 days or less between ovulation and the onset of menses, frequently associated with infertility.

**lu·te·in** (loo′tē-in) **1.** the yellow pigment in the corpus luteum, in the yolk of eggs, or any lipochrome. **2.** SYN xanthophyll. [L. *luteus,* saffron-yellow]

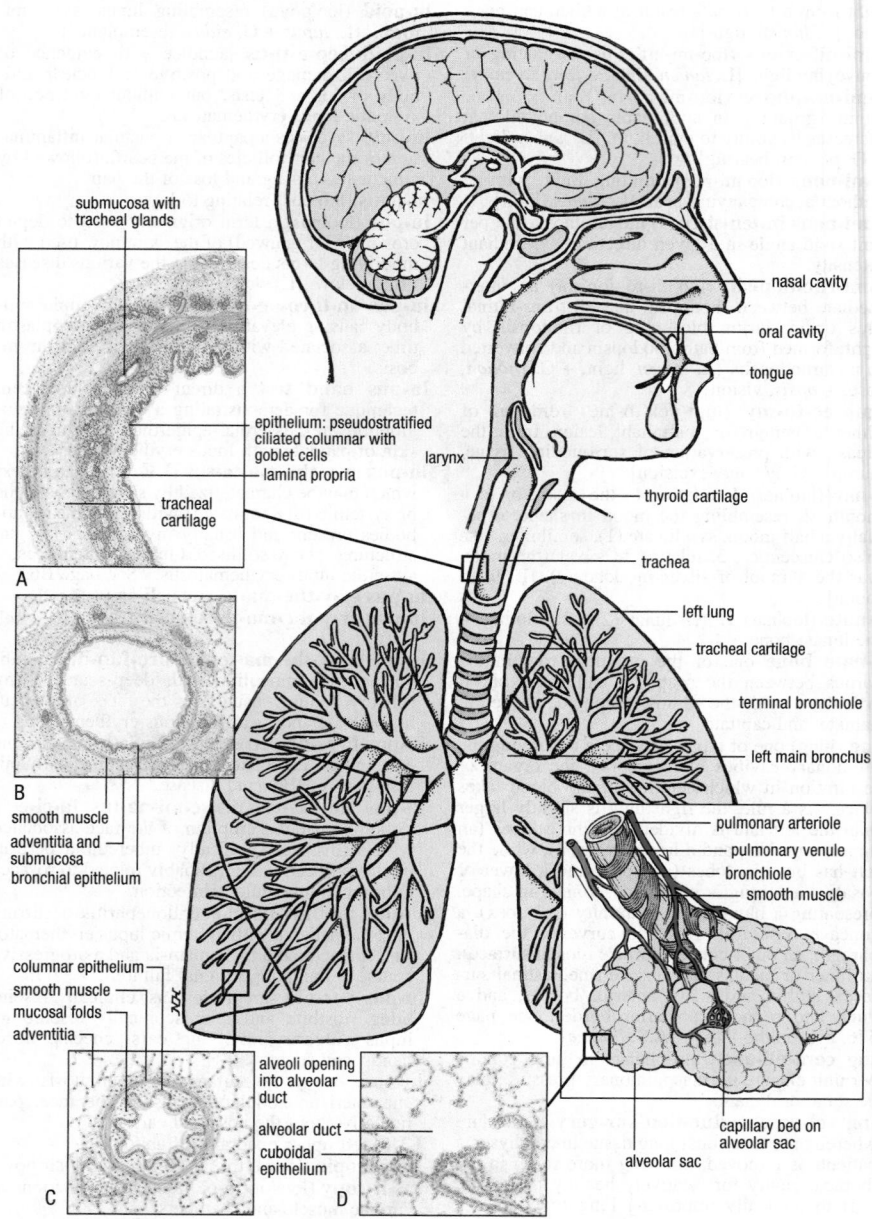

submucosa with
tracheal glands

epithelium: pseudostratified
ciliated columnar with
goblet cells
lamina propria

larynx

tracheal
cartilage

A

smooth muscle
adventitia and
submucosa
bronchial epithelium

B

columnar epithelium
smooth muscle
mucosal folds
adventitia

alveoli opening
into alveolar
duct

alveolar duct
cuboidal
epithelium

C

D

nasal cavity

oral cavity

tongue

thyroid cartilage

trachea

left lung

tracheal cartilage

terminal bronchiole

left main bronchus

pulmonary arteriole
pulmonary venule
bronchiole
smooth muscle

capillary bed on
alveolar sac

alveolar sac

**lungs and respiratory anatomy:** (A) trachea (panoramic, transverse sections); (B) intrapulmonary bronchus; (C) terminal bronchiole; (D) respiratory bronchiole with alveoli

**lu·te·in·i·za·tion** (loo'tē-in-i-zā'shŭn) transformation of the mature ovarian follicle and its theca interna into a corpus luteum after ovulation.

**lu·te·in·ized un·rup·tured fol·li·cle** a follicle that has undergone luteinization without prior rupture; once thought to cause infertility but now believed to occur equally often in fertile and infertile women.

**lu·te·i·niz·ing hor·mone** SYN lutropin.

**lu·te·i·niz·ing hor·mone/fol·li·cle-stim·u·lat·-ing hor·mone-re·leas·ing fac·tor** SYN gonadoliberin (2).

**lu·te·i·niz·ing hor·mone-re·leas·ing fac·tor** former name for luteinizing hormone-releasing hormone.

**lu·te·i·niz·ing hor·mone-re·leas·ing hor·-mone** SYN luliberin.

**Lu·tem·ba·cher syn·drome** (loo'tĕm-bahk'ĕr) a congenital cardiac abnormality consisting of a defect of the interatrial septum, mitral stenosis, and enlarged right atrium.

**lu·te·o·hor·mone** (loo'tē-ō-hōr'mōn) SYN progesterone.

**lu·te·ol·y·sis** (loo-tē-ol'i-sis) degeneration or destruction of ovarian luteinized tissue.

**lu·te·o·lyt·ic** (loo-tē-ō-lit'ik) promoting or characteristic of luteolysis.

**lu·te·o·ma** (loo-tē-ō'mă) an ovarian tumor of granulosa or theca-lutein cell origin, producing progesterone effects on the uterine mucosa.

**lu·te·o·pla·cen·tal shift** the change in site of production of the estrogen and progesterone essential for human pregnancy from the corpus luteum to the placenta; after the sixth week of pregnancy, a human placenta can produce enough of these hormones to prevent abortion despite ovariectomy.

**lu·te·o·tro·pic, lu·te·o·tro·phic** (loo'tē-ō-trop'ik, loo'tē-ō-trof'ik) having a stimulating action on the development and function of the corpus luteum.

**lu·te·o·tro·pic hor·mone** SYN luteotropin.

**lu·te·o·tro·pin** (loo'tē-ō-trō'pin) an anterior pituitary hormone whose action maintains the function of the corpus luteum. SYN luteotropic hormone.

**lu·te·ti·um (Lu)** (loo-tē'shē-ŭm) a rare earth element; atomic no. 71, atomic wt. 174.967. [L. *Lutetia*, Paris]

**lu·tro·pin** (loo'trō-pin) a glycoprotein hormone that stimulates the final ripening of an ovarian follicle, its secretion of progesterone, its rupture to release the egg, and the conversion of the ruptured follicle into the corpus luteum. SYN interstitial cell-stimulating hormone, luteinizing hormone.

**Lutz-Splen·do·re-Al·mei·da dis·ease** (loots-splen-dō'rä-ahl-mā'dah) SYN paracoccidioidomycosis.

**lux** (lŭks) a unit of light or illumination; the reception of a luminous flux of 1 lumen per square meter of surface. SYN candle-meter, meter-candle. [L. light]

**lux·a·tion** (lŭk-sā'shŭn) **1.** SYN dislocation. **2.** DENTISTRY the dislocation or displacement of the condyle in the temporomandibular fossa, or of a tooth from the alveolus. [L. *luxatio*]

**Lux·ol fast blue** (luk'sahl) name for a group of closely related copper phthalocyanine dyes used as stains (with PAS, PTAH, hematoxylin, silver nitrate, etc.) for myelin in nerve fibers.

**LVET** left ventricular ejection time.

**ly·ase** (lī'ās) class name for enzymes removing groups nonhydrolytically (EC class 4); prefixes such as "hydro-," "ammonia-," etc., are used to indicate the type of reaction. Trivial names for lyases include synthases, decarboxylases, aldolases, dehydratases. Cf. synthase, synthetase.

**ly·can·thro·py** (lī-kan'thrō-pē) the morbid delusion that one is a wolf. [G. *lykos*, wolf, + *anthrōpos*, man]

**ly·co·pene** (lī'kō-pēn) the red pigment of the tomato the parent substance from which all natural carotenoid pigments are derived.

**ly·co·pe·ne·mia** (lī'kō-pĕ-nē'mē-ă) a condition in which there is a high concentration of lycopene in the blood, producing carotenoid-like yellowish pigmentation of the skin; found in persons who consume excessive amounts of tomatoes or tomato juice, or lycopene-containing fruits and berries. [lycopene + G. *haima*, blood]

**ly·co·per·do·no·sis** (lī'kō-per-don-ō'sis) a persisting pneumonitis following inhalation of spores of the puffballs *Lycoperdon pyriforme* and *L. bovista*.

**Ly·ell syn·drome** (lī'ĕl) SYN toxic epidermal necrolysis.

**Lyme ar·thri·tis** (līm) the arthritic manifestation of Lyme disease.

**Lyme dis·ease** (līm) an inflammatory disorder typically occurring during the summer months and caused by *Borrelia burgdorferi*, a spirochete transmitted by *Ixodes scapularis* in the eastern U.S. and *I. pacificus* in the western U.S.; the characteristic skin lesion, erythema chronicum migrans, usually is preceded or accompanied by fever, malaise, fatigue, headache, and stiff neck; neurologic or cardiac manifestations, or arthritis (Lyme arthritis) may occur weeks to months later. Dogs, horses, and cattle are also affected. See page B3. [Lyme, CT, where first observed]

**lymph** (limf) a clear, transparent, sometimes faintly yellow and slightly opalescent fluid that is collected from the tissues throughout the body, flows in the lymphatic vessels, through the lymph nodes, and is eventually added to the venous blood circulation. Lymph consists of a clear liquid portion, varying numbers of white blood cells (chiefly lymphocytes), and a few red blood cells. [L. *lympha*, clear spring water]

**lym·phad·e·nec·to·my** (lim-fad-ĕ-nek'tō-mē) excision of lymph nodes. [lymphadeno- + G. *ektomē*, excision]

**lym·phad·e·ni·tis** (lim'fad'ĕ-nī'tis) inflammation of a lymph node or lymph nodes. [lymphadeno- + G. *-itis*, inflammation]

△**lym·pha·de·no-, lym·pha·den-** the lymph nodes. [L. *lympha*, spring water, + G. *adēn*, gland]

**lym·phad·e·nog·ra·phy** (lim-fad'ĕ-nog'ră-fē) radiographic visualization of lymph nodes after injection of a contrast medium; lymphography. [lymphadeno- + G. *graphō*, to write]

**lym·phad·e·noid** (lim-fad'ĕ-noyd) relating to, or resembling, or derived from a lymph node. [lymphadeno- + G. *eidos*, resemblance]

**lym·phad·e·nop·a·thy** (lim-fad-ĕ-nop'ă-thē) any disease process affecting a lymph node or lymph nodes. [lymphadeno- + G. *pathos*, suffering]

l
y

**lymph·ad·e·nop·a·thy-as·so·ci·at·ed vi·rus (LAV)** SYN human immunodeficiency virus.

**lym·phad·e·no·sis** (lim-fad'ĕ-nō'sis) the basic underlying proliferative process that results in enlargement of lymph nodes, as in lymphocytic leukemia and certain inflammations. [lymphadeno- + G. -osis, condition]

**lym·phan·gi·al** (lim-fan'jē-ăl) relating to a lymphatic vessel.

**lym·phan·gi·ec·ta·sis, lym·phan·gi·ec·ta·sia** (lim-fan'jē-ek'tă-sis, lim-fan'jē-ek-tā'zē-a) dilation of the lymphatic vessels, the basic process that may result in the formation of a lymphangioma. SYN lymphectasia. [lymphangio- + G. ektasis, a stretching]

**lym·phan·gi·ec·tat·ic** (lim-fan'jē-ek-tat'ik) relating to or characterized by lymphangiectasis.

**lym·phan·gi·ec·to·my** (lim-fan'jē-ek'tō-mē) excision of a lymph channel. [lymphangio- + G. ektomē, excision]

**lym·phan·gi·i·tis** (lim-fan'jē-ī'tis) SYN lymphangitis.

△**lym·phan·gio-, lym·phan·gi-** the lymphatic vessels. [L. lympha, spring water, + G. angeion, vessel]

**lym·phan·gi·o·en·do·the·li·o·ma** (lim-fan'jē-ō-en'dō-thē-lē-ō'mă) a neoplasm consisting of irregular groups of endothelial cells, and intubate structures that are thought to be derived from lymphatic vessels. [lymphangio- + endothelium + -oma, tumor]

**lym·phan·gi·og·ra·phy** (lim-fan'jē-og'ră-fē) radiographic demonstration of lymphatics and lymph nodes following the injection of a contrast medium; lymphography. [lymphangio- + G. graphō, to write]

**lym·phan·gi·ol·o·gy** (lim-fan-jē-ol'ō-jē) the branch of medical science concerned with the lymphatic vessels. SYN lymphology. [lymphangio- + G. logos, study]

**lym·phan·gi·o·ma** (lim-fan'jē-ō'mă) a well-circumscribed nodule of lymphatic vessels that are usually greatly dilated and are lined with normal endothelial cells; lymphoid tissue is usually present in the peripheral portions of the lesions, which are present at birth or shortly therafter, and probably represent anomalous development of lymphatic vessels (rather than true neoplasms); they occur most frequently in the neck and axilla. [lymphangio- + G. -oma, tumor]

**lym·phan·gi·o·phle·bi·tis** (lim-fan'jē-ō-flĕ-bī'tis) inflammation of the lymphatic vessels and veins.

**lym·phan·gi·o·plas·ty** (lim-fan'jē-ō-plas-tē) surgical alteration of lymphatic vessels. [lymphangio- + G. plastos, formed]

**lym·phan·gi·o·sar·co·ma** (lim-fan'jē-ō-sar-kō'mă) a malignant neoplasm derived from the endothelial cells of lymphatic vessels, usually developing in the arm several years after radical mastectomy.

**lym·phan·gi·ot·o·my** (lim-fan'jē-ot'ō-mē) incision of lymphatic vessels. [lymphangio- + G. tomē, incision]

**lym·phan·gi·tis** (lim-fan-jī'tis) inflammation of the lymphatic vessels. SYN lymphangiitis. [lymphangio- + G. -itis, inflammation]

**lym·pha·phe·re·sis** (lim'fă-fĕ-rē'sis) SYN lymphocytapheresis.

**lym·phat·ic** (lim-fat'ik) **1.** pertaining to lymph. **2.** a vascular channel that transports lymph. **3.** sometimes used to pertain to a sluggish or phlegmatic characteristic. [L. lymphaticus, frenzied; Mod. L. use, of or for lymph]

**lym·phat·ic duct** one of the two large lymph channels, right lymphatic duct or thoracic duct.

**lym·phat·ic fil·a·ri·a·sis gran·u·lo·ma** granulomatous lesion often found surrounding dead microfilariae.

**lym·phat·ic leu·ke·mia** SYN lymphocytic leukemia.

**lym·phat·ic node** SEE lymph node.

**lym·phat·i·cos·to·my** (lim-fat-i-kos'tō-mē) making an opening into a lymphatic duct. [lymphatic + G. stoma, mouth]

**lym·phat·ic plex·us** a plexus of lymphatic capillaries, usually without valves, that opens into one or more larger lymphatic vessels.

**lym·phat·ic si·nus** the channels in a lymph node crossed by a reticulum of cells and fibers and bounded by littoral cells; there are subcapsular, trabecular, and medullary sinuses.

**lym·phat·ic tis·sue, lym·phoid tis·sue** a three-dimensional network of reticular fibers and cells the meshes of which are occupied in varying degrees of density with lymphocytes; there is nodular, diffuse, and loose lymphatic tissue. SYN adenoid tissue.

**lym·pha·ti·tis** (lim-fă-tī'tis) inflammation of the lymphatic vessels or lymph nodes. [lymphatic + G. -itis, inflammation]

**lym·pha·tol·y·sis** (lim'fă-tol'i-sis) destruction of the lymphatic vessels or lymphoid tissue, or both. [lymphatic + G. lysis, dissolution]

**lym·pha·to·lyt·ic** (lim'fă-tō-lit'ik) pertaining to or characterized by lymphatolysis.

**lymph cap·il·lary** the beginning of the lymphatic system of vessels; it is lined with a highly attenuated endothelium with poorly developed basement membrane and a lumen of variable caliber. SEE lacteal (2).

**lymph cor·pus·cle, lym·phat·ic cor·pus·cle, lym·phoid cor·pus·cle** a mononuclear type of leukocyte formed in lymph nodes and other lymphoid tissue, and also in the blood.

**lymph drain·age** SYN manual lymph drainage.

**lym·phec·ta·sia** (lim-fek-tā'zē-ă) SYN lymphangiectasis. [lymph + G. ektasis, a stretching]

**lymph·e·de·ma** (limf'e-dē'mă) swelling (especially in subcutaneous tissues) as a result of obstruction of lymphatic vessels or lymph nodes and the accumulation of large amounts of lymph in the affected region. [lymph + G. oidēma, a swelling]

**lym·phe·mia** (lim-fē'mē-ă) the presence of unusually large numbers of lymphocytes or their precursors, or both, in the circulating blood. [lymph(ocyte) + G. haima, blood]

**lymph fol·li·cle, lym·phat·ic fol·li·cle** one of the spherical masses of lymphoid cells, frequently having a more lightly staining center. SYN folliculus lymphaticus, lymph nodule, nodulus lymphaticus.

**lymph gland** SYN lymph node.

**lymph node** one of numerous round, oval, or bean-shaped bodies located along the course of lymphatic vessels, varying greatly in size (1–25 mm in diameter) and usually presenting a depressed area, the hilum, on one side through which blood vessels enter and efferent lymphatic vessels emerge. The structure consists of a fibrous capsule and internal trabeculae supporting lymphoid tissue and lymph sinuses; lymphoid tissue is arranged in nodules in the cortex and cords in the medulla of a node, with afferent vessels entering at many points of the periphery. SYN nodus lymphaticus [TA], nodus lymphoideus [TA], lymph gland, lymphoglandula, lymphonodus.

**lymph node per·me·a·bil·i·ty fac·tor (LNPF)** a substance, released by lymphocytes when stimulated or damaged, that increases capillary permeability and the accumulation of mononuclear cells.

**lymph nod·ule** SYN lymph follicle.

△**lym·pho-, lymph-** lymph. [L. *lympha*, spring water]

**lym·pho·blast** (lim′fō-blast) an immature cell that matures into a lymphocyte and is characterized by more abundant cytoplasm than in a lymphocyte, a nucleus in which the chromatin is finer than in a lymphocyte (but coarser than in a myeloblast), and one or two prominent nucleoli. SYN lymphocytoblast. [lympho- + G. *blastos*, germ]

**lym·pho·blas·tic** (lim-fō-blas′tik) pertaining to the production of lymphocytes.

**lym·pho·blas·tic leu·ke·mia** acute lymphocytic leukemia in which the abnormal cells are chiefly (or almost totally) blast forms of the lymphocytic series, or in which unusually large numbers of the immature forms occur in association with adult lymphocytes.

**lym·pho·blas·tic lym·pho·ma** a diffuse lymphoma in children, with supradiaphragmatic distribution and T lymphocytes having convoluted nuclei; many patients develop acute lymphoblastic leukemia.

**lym·pho·blas·to·ma** (lim-fō-blas-tō′mă) a form of malignant lymphoma in which the chief cells are lymphoblasts. [lymphoblast + G. *-oma*, tumor]

**lym·pho·blas·to·sis** (lim′fō-blas-tō′sis) the presence of lymphoblasts in the peripheral blood; sometimes used as a synonym for acute lymphocytic leukemia. [lymphoblast + G. *-osis*, condition]

**lym·pho·cy·ta·phe·re·sis** (lim′fō-sī-tă-fĕ-rē′sis) separation and removal of lymphocytes from the withdrawn blood, with the remainder of the blood retransfused into the donor. SYN lymphapheresis. [lymphocyte + G. *aphairesis*, a withdrawal]

🔲**lym·pho·cyte** (lim′fō-sīt) a white blood cell formed in lymphatic tissue throughout the body (e.g., lymph nodes, spleen, thymus, tonsils, Peyer patches, and sometimes in bone marrow) and in normal adults making up approximately 22–28% of the total number of leukocytes in the circulating blood. Lymphocytes are generally small (7–8 μm), but larger forms are frequent (10–20 μm); with Wright (or a similar) stain, the nucleus is deeply colored (purple-blue), and is composed of dense aggregates of chromatin within a sharply defined nuclear membrane; the nucleus is usually round, but may be slightly indented, and is eccentrically situated within a relatively small amount of light blue cytoplasm that ordinarily contains no granules; especially in larger forms, the cytoplasm may be fairly abundant and include several bright red-violet fine granules; in contrast to granules of the myeloid series of cells, those in lymphocytes do not yield a positive oxidase or peroxidase reaction. Lymphocytes are divided into 2 principal groups, termed T and B cells, based on their surface molecules as well as function. Natural killer cells, which are large granular lymphocytes, represent a small percentage of the lymphocyte population. See page B1. [lympho- + G. *kytos*, call]

**lym·pho·cy·thae·mia [Br.]** SEE lymphocytosis.

**lym·pho·cy·the·mia** (lim′fō-sī-thē′mē-ă) SYN lymphocytosis.

**lym·pho·cyt·ic** (lim-fō-sit′ik) pertaining to or characterized by lymphocytes.

**lym·pho·cyt·ic ad·e·no·hy·poph·y·si·tis** a diffuse lymphocytic infiltration of the adenohypophysis, often related to pregnancy; probably a disturbance in the immune system.

**lym·pho·cyt·ic cho·ri·o·men·in·gi·tis** meningitis that usually occurs in young adults during the fall and winter months. Caused by a virus carried by the common house mouse. SEE ALSO lymphocytic choriomeningitis virus.

**lym·pho·cyt·ic cho·ri·o·men·in·gi·tis vi·rus** an RNA virus that causes lymphocytic choriomeningitis; infection may be inapparent, but sometimes the virus causes influenzalike disease, meningitis, or, rarely, meningoencephalomyelitis.

**lym·pho·cy·tic hy·po·phy·si·tis** an acute anterior pituitary lymphocytic reaction characterized clinically by signs and symptoms of anterior pituitary insufficiency; probably an autoimmune disorder because antipituitary antibodies are present in the serum.

**lym·pho·cyt·ic leu·ke·mia** a variety of leukemia characterized by an uncontrolled proliferation and conspicuous enlargement of lymphoid tissue in various sites (e.g., lymph nodes, spleen, bone marrow, lungs), and the occurrence of increased numbers of cells of the lymphocytic series in the blood. SYN lymphatic leukemia.

**lym·pho·cyt·ic se·ries, lym·phoid se·ries** the cells at various states in the development in lymphoid tissue of the mature lymphocytes, e.g., lymphoblasts, young lymphocytes, mature lymphocytes.

**lym·pho·cy·to·blast** (lim-fō-sī′tō-blast) SYN lymphoblast. [lymphocyte + G. *blastos*, germ]

**lym·pho·cy·to·ma** (lim′fō-sī-tō′mă) a circumscribed nodule or mass of mature lymphocytes, grossly resembling a neoplasm. [lymphocyte + G. *-oma*, tumor]

**lym·pho·cy·to·pe·nia** (lim′fō-sī-tō-pē′nē-ă) SYN lymphopenia.

**lym·pho·cy·to·poi·e·sis** (lim′fō-sī-tō-poy-ē′sis) the formation of lymphocytes. [lymphocyte + G. *poiēsis*, a making]

**lym·pho·cy·to·sis** (lim′fō-sī-tō′sis) a form of leukocytosis in which there is an actual or relative increase in the number of lymphocytes. SYN lymphocythemia.

**lym·pho·duct** (lim′fō-dŭkt) a lymphatic vessel. [lympho- + L. *ductus*, a leading]

**lym·pho·ep·i·the·li·o·ma** (lim′fō-ep-i-thē-lē-ō′mă) a poorly differentiated radiosensitive squamous cell carcinoma involving lymphoid tissue in the region of the tonsils and nasopharynx; metastasizes early to cervical lymph nodes. [lympho- + epithelium + *-oma*, tumor]

**lym·pho·gen·ic** (lim-fō-jen′ik) SYN lymphogenous (1).

**lym·phog·e·nous** (lim-foj′ĕ-nŭs) **1.** originating

from lymph or the lymphatic system. SYN lymphogenic. 2. producing lymph.

**lym·phog·e·nous me·tas·ta·sis** SEE metastasis.

**lym·pho·glan·du·la** (lim-fō-glan'dyu-lă) SYN lymph node.

**lym·pho·gran·u·lo·ma** (lim'fō-gran-yu-lō'mă) old nonspecific term used with reference to a few basically dissimilar diseases in which the pathologic processes result in granulomas or granulomalike lesions, especially in various groups of lymph nodes (which then become conspicuously enlarged).

**lym·pho·gran·u·lo·ma ve·ne·re·um, ve·ne·re·al lymph·o·gran·u·lo·ma** (lim'fō-gran-yu-lō'mă ve-nē'rē-ŭm) a sexually transmitted infection usually caused by *Chlamydia trachomatis*, and characterized by a transient genital ulcer and inguinal adenopathy in the male; in the female, perirectal lymph nodes are involved and rectal stricture is a common occurrence. SYN tropical bubo.

**lym·phog·ra·phy** (lim-fog'ră-fē) visualization of lymphatics (lymphangiography), lymph nodes (lymphadenography), or both by radiography following the intra-lymphatic injection of a contrast medium, usually an iodized oil. [lympho- + *graphō*, to write]

**lym·pho·his·ti·o·cy·to·sis** (lim'fō-his'tē-ō-sī-tō'sis) proliferation or infiltration of lymphocytes and histiocytes.

**lym·phoid** (lim'foyd) 1. resembling lymph or lymphatic tissue, or pertaining to the lymphatic system. 2. SYN adenoid (1). [lympho- + G. *eidos*, appearance]

**lym·phoi·dec·to·my** (lim-foy-dek'tō-mē) excision of lymphoid tissue. [lymphoid + G. *ektomē*, excision]

**lym·pho·kine** (lim'fō-kīnz) hormonelike peptide, released by activated lymphocytes, that mediates immune response; a cytokine obtained from lymphocytes. [*lympho*cyte + G. *kineō*, to set in motion]

**lym·pho·ki·ne·sis** (lim'fō-ki-nē'sis) 1. circulation of lymph in the lymphatic vessels and through the lymph nodes. 2. movement of endolymph in the semicircular canals of the inner ear. [lympho- + G. *kinēsis*, movement]

**lym·phol·o·gy** (lim-fol'ō-jē) SYN lymphangiology. [lympho- + G. *logos*, study]

**lym·pho·ma** (lim-fō'mă) any neoplasm of lymphoid tissue; in general use, synonymous with malignant lymphoma. [lympho- + G. *-oma*, tumor]

**lym·pho·ma·toid** (lim-fō'mă-toyd) resembling a lymphoma.

**lym·pho·ma·toid pol·y·po·sis** multifocal mantle cell lymphoma, producing numerous lymphoid polyps in the intestines.

**lym·pho·ma·to·sis** (lim'fō-mă-tō'sis) any condition characterized by the occurrence of multiple, widely distributed sites of involvement with lymphoma.

**lym·pho·ma·tous** (lim-fō'mă-tŭs) pertaining to or characterized by lymphoma.

**lym·pho·myx·o·ma** (lim'fō-mik-sō'mă) a soft nonmalignant neoplasm that contains lymphoid tissue in a matrix of loose, areolar connective tissue. [lympho- + G. *myxa*, mucus, + *-oma*, tumor]

**lym·pho·no·dus** SYN lymph node.

**lym·phop·a·thy** (lim-fop'ă-thē) any disease of

the lymphatic vessels or lymph nodes. [lympho- + G. *pathos*, suffering]

**lym·pho·pe·nia** (lim-fō-pē'nē-ă) a reduction, relative or absolute, in the number of lymphocytes in the circulating blood. SYN lymphocytopenia. [lympho- + G. *penia*, poverty]

**lym·pho·plas·ma·cel·lu·lar dis·or·ders** term used to refer to a group of disorders including plasmacytoma, multiple myeloma, lymphoplasmacytic lymphoma, MALT lymphoma, and amyloidosis.

**lym·pho·plas·ma·phe·re·sis** (lim'fō-plaz'mă-fĕ-rē'sis) separation and removal of lymphocytes and plasma from the withdrawn blood, with the remainder of the blood retransfused into the donor. [lymphocyte + plasma + G. *aphairesis*, a withdrawal]

**lym·pho·poi·e·sis** (lim-fō-poy-ē'sis) the formation of lymphatic tissue. [lympho- + G. *poiēsis*, a making]

**lym·pho·poi·et·ic** (lim-fō-poy-et'ik) pertaining to or characterized by lymphopoiesis.

**lym·pho·re·tic·u·lo·sis** (lim'fō-rĕ-tik-yu-lō'sis) proliferation of the reticuloendothelial cells (macrophages) of the lymph glands.

**lym·phor·rhea, lym·phor·rha·gia** (lim-fō-rē'ă, lim-fō-rā'jē-ă) an escape of lymph on the surface from ruptured, torn, or cut lymphatic vessels. [lympho- + G. *rhoia*, a flow]

**lym·phor·rhoid** (lim'fō-royd) a dilation of a lymph channel, resembling a hemorrhoid. [lymph + *-rrhoid*, tending to leak, on the analogy of *hemorrhoid*]

**lym·phos·ta·sis** (lim-fos'tă-sis) obstruction of the normal flow of lymph. [lympho- + G. *stasis*, a standing still]

**lym·pho·tax·is** (lim-fō-tak'sis) the exertion of an effect that attracts or repels lymphocytes. [lympho- + G. *taxis*, orderly arrangement]

**lym·pho·tox·ic·i·ty** (lim'fō-tok-sis'i-tē) toxicity to lymphocytes.

**lym·pho·tox·in** (lim'fō-tok-sin) a lymphokine that lyses or damages many cell types.

**lymph ves·sels** the vessels that convey the lymph; they anastomose freely with each other. SYN vasa lymphatica.

**Lynch syn·drome** (linch) type I, familial colorectal cancer, generally occurring at an early age; type II, familial colorectal cancer occurring at an early age in conjunction with female genital cancer or cancers at other sites proximal to the bowel.

**lyo-** dissolution. SEE ALSO lyso-. [G. *lyō*, to loosen, dissolve]

**Ly·on hy·poth·e·sis** (lī'on) SYN lyonization.

**ly·on·i·za·tion** (lī'on-i-zā'shŭn) the normal phenomenon that wherever there are two or more haploid sets of X-linked genes in each cell all but one of the genes are inactivated apparently at random and have no phenotypic expression. Its randomness explains the more variable expressivity of X-linked traits in women than in men. SEE ALSO gene dosage compensation. SYN Lyon hypothesis, X-inactivation. [M. *Lyon*]

**ly·o·phil, ly·o·phile** (lī'ō-fil, lī'ō-fīl) a substance that is lyophilic.

**ly·o·phil·ic** (lī-ō-fil'ik) COLLOID CHEMISTRY denoting a dispersed phase having a pronounced affinity for the dispersion medium; when the dispersed phase is lyophilic, the colloid is usually a reversible one. SYN lyotropic. [lyo- + G. *phileō*, to love]

**ly·oph·i·li·za·tion** (lī-of'i-li-zā'shŭn) the process of isolating a solid substance from solution by freezing the solution and evaporating the ice under vacuum. SYN freeze-drying.

**ly·o·phobe** (lī'ō-fōb) a substance that is lyophobic.

**ly·o·pho·bic** (lī-ō-fo'bik) COLLOID CHEMISTRY denoting a dispersed phase having but slight affinity for the dispersion medium; when the dispersed phase is lyophobic, the colloid is usually an irreversible one. [lyo- + G. *phobos*, fear]

**ly·o·tro·pic** (lī-ō-trop'ik) SYN lyophilic. [lyo- + G. *tropē*, a turning]

**Lys** lysine, or its radicals in peptides.

**ly·sate** (lī'sāt) material produced by the destructive process of lysis.

**lyse** (līz) to break up, to disintegrate, to effect lysis. SYN lyze.

**ly·se·mia** (lī-sē'mē-ă) disintegration or dissolution of red blood cells and the occurrence of hemoglobin in the circulating plasma and in the urine. [lyso- + G. *haima*, blood]

**ly·sin** (lī'sin) **1.** a complement-fixing antibody that acts destructively on cells and tissues; the various types are designated in accordance with the form of antigen that stimulates the production of the lysin, e.g., hemolysin, bacteriolysin. **2.** any substance that causes lysis.

**ly·si·nae·mia [Br.]** SYN hyperlysinemia.

**ly·sine** (k, Lys) (lī'sēn) a nutritionally essential α-amino acid found in many proteins; distinguished by an ε-amino group.

**ly·sin·o·gen** (lī-sin'ō-jen) an antigen that stimulates the formation of a specific lysin.

**ly·si·no·gen·ic** (lī'si-nō-jen'ik) having the property of a lysinogen.

**ly·sin·u·ria** (lī-si-nyu'rē-ă) the presence of lysine in the urine.

**ly·sis** (lī'sis) **1.** destruction of red blood cells, bacteria, and other structures by a specific lysin, usually referred to by the structure destroyed (e.g., hemolysis, bacteriolysis, nephrolysis); may be due to a direct toxin or an immune mechanism, such as antibody reacting with antigen on the surface of a target cell, usually by binding and activation of a series of proteins in the blood with enzymatic activity (complement system). **2.** gradual subsidence of the symptoms of an acute disease, a form of the recovery process, as distinguished from crisis. [G. dissolution or loosening]

**ly·sis of ad·he·sions** surgical division of postinflammatory or postoperative adhesions, particularly abdominal (peritoneal) adhesions.

△**ly·so-, lys-** lysis, dissolution. SEE ALSO lyo-. [G. *lysis*, a loosening]

**ly·so·gen** (lī'sō-jen) **1.** that which is capable of inducing lysis. **2.** a bacterium in the state of lysogeny. [lysin + G. *-gen*, producing]

**ly·so·gen·e·sis** (lī-sō-jen'ĕ-sis) the production of lysins.

**ly·so·gen·ic** (lī-sō-jen'ik) **1.** causing or having the

power to cause lysis, as the action of certain antibodies and chemical substances. **2.** pertaining to bacteria in the state of lysogeny.

**ly·so·gen·ic bac·te·ri·um 1.** a bacterium in the symbiotic condition in which its genome includes the genome (probacteriophage) of a temperate bacteriophage; in occasional instances the probacteriophage dissociates from the bacterial genome, develops into vegetative bacteriophage, and then matures, causing lysis of the respective host bacterium and release into the culture medium of infective temperate bacteriophage; **2.** formerly, a pseudolysogenic bacterial strain, i.e., a "carrier" strain of bacteriophage of low infectivity.

**ly·so·ge·nic·i·ty** (lī'sō-jĕ-nis'i-tē) the property of being lysogenic.

**ly·sog·e·ny** (lī-soj'ĕ-nē) the phenomenon by which a bacterium is infected by a temperate bacteriophage whose DNA is integrated into the bacterial genome and replicates along with the bacterial DNA but remains latent or unexpressed; triggering of the lytic cycle may occur spontaneously or by certain agents and will result in the production of bacteriophage and lysis of the bacterial cell.

**ly·so·ki·nase** (lī-sō-kī'nās) term proposed for activator agents (e.g., streptokinase, urokinase, staphylokinase) that produce plasmin by indirect or multiple-stage action on plasminogen.

**ly·so·so·mal dis·ease** a disease due to inadequate functioning of a lysosomal enzyme; most such diseases are associated with a storage disease.

**ly·so·some** (lī'sō-sōm) a cytoplasmic membrane-bound vesicle measuring 5–8 nm (primary lysosome) and containing a wide variety of glycoprotein hydrolytic enzymes active at an acid pH; serves to digest exogenous material, such as bacteria, as well as effete organelles of the cells. [lyso- + G. *soma*, body]

**ly·so·type** (li'so-tīp) a type within a bacterial species determined by its reaction to specific phages. [lyso + type]

**ly·so·zyme** (lī'sō-zīm) an enzyme destructive to cell walls of certain bacteria; present in tears, egg white, and some plant tissues; used in the prevention of caries and in the treatment of infant formulas. SYN muramidase.

**lys·sa** (lis'ă) **1.** a cartilage in the tongue of the dog. **2.** old term for rabies. [G. *madness*]

**Lys·sa·vi·rus** (lis'ă-vī-rŭs) a genus of viruses (family Rhabdoviridae) that includes the rabies virus group.

***Lyth·o·glyph·op·sis*** (lith-ō-glif-op'sis) a genus of amphibious freshwater operculate snails of the family Hydrobiidae (subfamily Hydrobiinae; subclass Prosobranchiata). In the Mekong River delta, *Lythoglyphopsis aperta* serves as an intermediate host of the blood fluke, *Schistosoma mekongi.*

**lyt·ic** (lit'ik) pertaining to lysis; used colloq. as an abbreviation for osteolytic.

**lyze** (līz) SYN lyse.

l
y

# M

μ mu. SEE mu.
μμ micromicro-; micromicron.
μΩ microhm.
μC microcoulomb.
μCi microcurie.
μg microgram.
μl, μL microliter.
μM micromolar.
μm micrometer.
μmol micromole.
μmol/L micromolar.
μV microvolt.
M molarity.
$M_r$ molecular weight ratio or relative molecular mass.
mμ millimicron.
mM millimolar ($10^{-3}$ M).
M moles per liter (also written M or *M*).
⌂m- meta- (3).
MA mental age.
ma, mA milliampere.
Mac·chi·a·vel·lo stain (ma′chē-ah′ve′lō) a basic fuchsin-citric acid-methylene blue sequence in smears which produces red staining of rickettsiae and inclusion bodies, with nuclei staining blue.
Mac·Con·key a·gar (mĕ-kong-kē′) medium containing peptone, lactose, bile salts, neutral red, and crystal violet, used to identify Gram-negative bacilli and characterize them according to their status as lactose fermenters. Fermenters appear as red colonies while nonfermenters are colorless.
mac·er·ate (mas′er-āt) to soften by steeping or soaking. [see maceration]
mac·er·a·tion (mas-er-ā′shŭn) 1. softening by the action of a liquid. 2. softening of tissues after death by nonputrefactive (sterile) autolysis; seen especially in the stillborn, with bullous separation of the epidermis. [L. *macero*, pp. -*atus*, to soften by soaking]
Mac·ew·en sign (mĕ-kyu-ĕn) percussion of the skull gives a cracked-pot sound in cases of hydrocephalus.
Mac·ew·en tri·an·gle (mĕ-kyu-ĕn) SYN supra-meatal triangle.
Ma·cha·do-Jo·seph dis·ease (mĕ-ka′dō-jō′sef) a rare form of hereditary ataxia, characterized by onset in early adult life of progressive spinocerebellar and extrapyramidal disease with external ophthalmoplegia, rigidity, dystonia, and often peripheral amyotrophy; found predominantly in people of Azorean ancestry; autosomal dominant inheritance, caused by a trinucleotide repeat expansion mutation in the Machado-Joseph gene (MJD1) on 14q. [Surnames of two families studied in major descriptions of the disease.]
Mach band (mahk) a relatively bright or dark band perceived in a zone where the luminance increases or decreases rapidly.
Mach ef·fect (mahk) the appearance of a light or dark line on a radiograph where there is a concave or convex interface in the subject, a physiological optical form of edge enhancement.
ma·chine (mă-shēn′) any mechanical apparatus or device. [L. *machina*, contrivance]
ma·chin·ery mur·mur the long "continuous" rumbling murmur of patent ductus arteriosus. SYN Gibson murmur.
Mac·ken·zie am·pu·ta·tion (mĕ-ken′zē) a mod-

ification of Syme amputation at the ankle joint, the flap being taken from the inner side.
Mac·leod syn·drome (mĕ-klowd′) SYN unilateral lobar emphysema.
Mac·Neal tet·ra·chrome blood stain (mĕk-nēl) a stain for blood smears composed of a mixture of methylene blue, azure A, methylene violet, and eosin Y.
mac·ren·ceph·a·ly, mac·ren·ce·pha·lia (mak′ren-sef′ă-lē, mak′ren-sĕ-fā′lē-ă) hypertrophy of the brain; the condition of having a large brain. [macro- + G. *enkephalos*, brain]
⌂mac·ro-, macr- large, long. SEE ALSO mega-, megalo-. [G. *makros*]
mac·ro·ad·e·no·ma (mak′rō-ad-ĕ-nō′mă) a pituitary adenoma larger than 10 mm in diameter.
mac·ro·am·y·lase (mak-rō-am′i-lās) a form of serum amylase in which the enzyme is joined to a globulin.
mac·ro·am·y·la·se·mia (mak′rō-am′i-lā-sē′mē-ă) a form of hyperamylasemia, in which a portion of serum amylase exists as macroamylase. [macroamylase + G. *haima*, blood]
mac·ro·bi·ot·ic (mak′rō-bī-ot′ik) 1. long-lived. 2. tending to prolong life.
mac·ro·bi·ot·ic di·et a diet claimed to promote longevity, often by promoting an emphasis on natural foods and restrictions on noncereal foods, as well as liquids.
mac·ro·blast (mak′rō-blast) a large erythroblast. [macro- + G. *blastos*, germ]
mac·ro·car·dia (mak-rō-kar′dē-ă) SYN cardiomegaly.
mac·ro·ce·phal·ic, mac·ro·ceph·a·lous (mak′rō-se-fal′ik, mak′rō-sef′ă-lŭs) SYN megacephalic. [macro- + G. *kephalē*, head]
mac·ro·ceph·a·ly, mac·ro·ce·pha·lia (mak-rō-sef′ă-lē, mak′rō-sĕ-fā′lē-ă) SYN megacephaly. [macro- + G. *kephalē*, head]
mac·ro·chei·lia, mac·ro·chi·li·a (mak-rō-kī′lē-ă) 1. abnormally enlarged lips. 2. cavernous lymphangioma of the lip, a condition of permanent swelling resulting from the presence of greatly distended lymphatic spaces. [macro- + G. *cheilos*, lip]
mac·ro·chei·ria, mac·ro·chi·ri·a (mak-rō-kī′rē-ă) a condition characterized by abnormally large hands. SYN megalocheiria, megalochiria. [macro- + G. *cheir*, hand]
mac·ro·co·lon (mak′rō-kō′lon) a sigmoid colon of unusual length; a variety of megacolon.
mac·ro·cor·nea (mak-rō-kōr′nē-ă) an abnormally large cornea.
mac·ro·cra·ni·um (mak-rō-krā′nē-ŭm) an enlarged skull, especially the bones containing the brain, as seen in hydrocephalus; the face appears relatively small in comparison.
mac·ro·cry·o·glob·u·li·ne·mia (mak′rō-krī-ō-glob′yu-lin-ē′mē-ă) the presence of cold-precipitating macroglobulins in the peripheral blood; such macrocryoglobulins are often called cold hemagglutinins.
mac·ro·cyte (mak′rō-sīt) a large erythrocyte, such as those observed in pernicious anemia. [macro- + G. *kytos*, a hollow (cell)]
ma·cro·cy·thae·mia [Br.] SEE macrocythemia.
mac·ro·cy·the·mia (mak′rō-sī-thē′mē-ă) the occurrence of unusually large numbers of macro-

cytes in the circulating blood. SYN macrocytosis. [macrocyte + G. *haima*, blood]

**mac·ro·cyt·ic a·ne·mia** any anemia in which the average size of circulating erythrocytes is greater than normal, i.e., the mean corpuscular volume is 94 cu μm or more (normal range, 82 to 92 cu μm), including such syndromes as pernicious anemia, sprue, celiac disease, macrocytic anemia of pregnancy, anemia of diphyllobothriasis, and others.

**mac·ro·cy·to·sis** (mak'rō-sī-tō'sis) SYN macrocythemia. See page B2. [macrocyte + G. *-osis*, condition]

**mac·ro·don·tia, mac·ro·don·tism** (mak-rō-don'shē-ă, mak-rō-don'tizm) a condition in which a single tooth, pairs of teeth, or the entire dentition is disproportionately large. SYN megadontism, megalodontia.

**mac·ro·ele·ments** (mak'rō-el'ě-ments) inorganic nutrients needed in relatively high daily amounts (i.e., more than 100 mg per day) e.g., calcium, phosphorus, sodium, etc.

**mac·ro·ga·mete** (mak-rō-gam'ēt) the female element in anisogamy; it is the larger of the two sex cells, with more reserve material, and usually nonmotile. [macro- + G. *gametē*, wife]

**mac·ro·ga·me·to·cyte** (mak'rō-gă-mē'tō-sīt) the female gametocyte or mother cell producing the female or macrogamete among fungi or protozoa that undergo anisogamy.

**mac·ro·gen·i·to·so·mia** (mak'rō-jen'i-tō-sō'mē-ă) excessive bodily and genital development. [macro- + L. *genitalis*, genital, + G. *sōma*, body]

**ma·crog·lia** (ma-krog'lē-ă) SYN astrocyte. [macro- + G. *glia*, glue]

**ma·cro·glo·bu·li·nae·mia [Br.]** SEE macroglobulinemia.

**mac·ro·glob·u·lin·e·mia** (mak'rō-glob'yu-li-nē'mē-ă) increased levels of macroglobulins in the blood.

**mac·ro·glos·sia** (mak-rō-glos'ē-ă) enlargement of the tongue, either developmental or due to a neoplasm or vascular hamartoma. SYN megaloglossia. [macro- + G. *glōssa*, tongue]

**mac·ro·gna·thia** (mak-rō-nā'thē-ă) enlargement or elongation of the jaw. [macro- + G. *gnathos*, jaw]

**mac·ro·lide** (mak'rō-līd) a natural lactone, whose ring is large, usually of 14–20 atoms; several antibiotics, including erythromycin, are macrolides. They inhibit protein biosynthesis.

**mac·ro·mas·tia, mac·ro·ma·zia** (mak-rō-mas'tē-a, mak'rō-mā'zē-ă) abnormally large breasts. SEE ALSO hypermastia (2). [macro- + G. *mastos*, breast]

**mac·ro·me·lia** (mak-rō-mē'lē-ă) abnormal size of one or more of the limbs. SYN megalomelia. [macro- + G. *melos*, limb]

**mac·ro·mol·e·cule** (mak-rō-mol'ě-kyul) a molecule of colloidal size; e.g., proteins, polynucleic acids, polysaccharides.

**mac·ro·mon·o·cyte** (mak-rō-mon'ō-sīt) an unusually large monocyte.

**mac·ro·my·e·lo·blast** (mak-rō-mī'ě-lō-blast) an abnormally large myeloblast.

**mac·ro·nor·mo·blast** (mak-rō-nōr'mō-blast) 1. a large normoblast. 2. a large, incompletely hemoglobiniferous, nucleated red blood cell with a "cart-wheel" nucleus.

**mac·ro·nu·cle·us** (mak-rō-noo'klē-ŭs) 1. a nucleus that occupies a relatively large portion of the cell, or the larger nucleus where two or more are present in a cell. 2. the larger of the two nuclei in ciliates, which governs vegetative metabolic functions and not reproduction. SEE ALSO micronucleus (2).

**mac·ro·nu·tri·ent** (mak-rō-noo'trē-ent) nutrients required in the greatest amount; e.g., carbohydrates, protein, fats.

**mac·ro·nych·ia** (mak-rō-nik'ē-ă) abnormally large fingernails or toenails. [macro- + G. *onyx*, nail]

**mac·ro·pe·nis** (mak-rō-pē'nis) an abnormally large penis.

**mac·ro·phage** (mak'rō-fāj) any mononuclear, actively phagocytic cell arising from monocytic stem cells in the bone marrow; these cells are widely distributed and vary in morphology and motility; most are large, long-lived cells with nearly round nuclei and abundant endocytic vacuoles, lysosomes, and phagolysosomes. Phagocytic activity is typically mediated by serum recognition factors, including certain immunoglobulins and components of the complement system, but also may be nonspecific for some inert materials and bacteria, as in the case of alveolar macrophages; macrophages also are involved in both the production of antibodies and in cell-mediated immune responses, participate in presenting antigens to lymphocytes, and secrete a variety of immunoregulatory molecules. [macro- + G. *phagō*, to eat]

**mac·ro·phage col·o·ny-stim·u·lat·ing fac·tor (M-CSF)** a glycoprotein growth factor that causes the committed cell line to proliferate and mature into macrophages. SEE ALSO colony-stimulating factors.

**mac·ro·po·dia** (mak-rō-pō'dē-ă) abnormally large feet. SYN megalopodia. [macro- + G. *pous*, foot]

**mac·ro·pol·y·cyte** (mak-rō-pol'ē-sīt) an unusually large polymorphonuclear neutrophilic leukocyte that contains a multisegmented nucleus (e.g., 8, 10, or more lobes); frequently observed pernicious anemia and certain other forms of anemia. [macro- + G. *polys*, many, + *kytos*, cell]

**mac·ro·pro·so·pia** (mak'rō-prō-sō'pē-ă) a condition in which the face is too large in proportion to the size of the cranial vault. [macro- + G. *prosōpon*, face]

**mac·ro·rhin·ia** (mak-rō-rin'ē-ă) excessive size of the nose, either congenital or pathologic. [macro- + G. *rhis* (*rhin-*), nose]

**mac·ro·scop·ic** (mak-rō-skop'ik) 1. of a size visible with the naked eye or without the use of a microscope. 2. relating to macroscopy.

**mac·ro·scop·ic a·nat·o·my** SYN gross anatomy.

**ma·cros·co·py** (mă-kros'kŏ-pē) examination of objects with the naked eye. [macro- + G. *skopeō*, to view]

**mac·ro·sig·moid** (mak-rō-sig'moyd) enlargement or dilation of the sigmoid colon.

**mac·ro·so·mia** (mak-rō-sō'mē-ă) abnormally large size of the body. [macro- + G. *sōma*, body]

**mac·ro·sto·mia** (mak-rō-stō'mē-ă) abnormally large size of the mouth resulting from failure of fusion between the maxillary and mandibular prominences of the embryonic face. [macro- + G. *stoma*, mouth]

**mac·ro·tia** (mak-rō'shē-ă) congenital enlargement of the auricle, particularly the pinna. [macro- + G. *ous*, ear]

m
a

**mac·ro·trau·ma** tissue damage resulting from a single injury.

**mac·u·la**, pl. **mac·u·lae** (mak′yu-lă, mak′yu-lē) **1.** a small spot, perceptibly different in color from the surrounding tissue. **2.** a small, discolored patch or spot on the skin, neither elevated above nor depressed below the skin's surface. SEE ALSO spot. SYN macule, spot (1). [L. a spot]

**mac·u·la ad·he·rens** SYN desmosome.

**mac·u·la a·tro·phi·ca** an atrophic glistening white spot on the skin.

**mac·u·la ce·ru·lea** a bluish stain on the skin caused by the bites of fleas or lice, seen especially in pediculosis pubis. SYN blue spot (1).

**mac·u·la cor·ne·ae** a moderately dense opacity of the cornea.

**mac·u·la cri·bro·sa**, pl. **mac·u·lae cri·bro·sae** [TA] one of three areas on the wall of the vestibule of the labyrinth, marked by numerous foramina giving passage to nerve filaments supplying portions of the membranous labyrinth; **macula cribrosa inferior**, located in the posterior bony ampulla for passage of posterior ampullary nerve fibers; **macula cribrosa media**, area near the base of the cochlea through which the saccular nerve fibers pass; **macula cribrosa superior**, perforated area above the elliptical recess for passage of the utriculoampullary nerve fibers; **macula cribrosa quarta**, a name sometimes applied to the opening for the cochlear nerve.

**mac·u·la den·sa** a closely packed group of densely staining cells in the distal tubular epithelium of a nephron, in direct apposition to the juxtaglomerular cells; they may function as either chemoreceptors or as baroreceptors feeding information to the juxtaglomerular cells.

**mac·u·lae a·cus·ti·cae** SEE macula of saccule, macula of utricle.

**mac·u·la fla·va** a yellowish spot at the anterior extremity of the rima glottidis where the two vocal folds join.

**mac·u·lar, mac·u·late** (mak′yu-lăr, mak′yu-lāt) **1.** relating to or marked by macules. **2.** denoting the central retina, especially the macula retinae.

**mac·u·lar am·y·loi·do·sis** a localized form of amyloidosis cutis characterized by pruritic symmetrical brown reticulated macules, especially on the upper back; microscopically, amyloid is deposited as small subepidermal globules.

**mac·u·lar ar·ter·ies** SEE inferior macular arteriole, superior macular arteriole.

**ma·cu·lar cor·ne·al dys·tro·phy** an autosomal recessive disorder characterized by glycosaminoglycan deposits in the corneal stroma.

**mac·u·lar dys·tro·phy** a group of disorders involving predominantly the posterior portion of the ocular fundus, due to degeneration in the sensory layer of the retina, retinal pigment epithelium, Bruch membrane, choroid, or a combination of these tissues.

**ma·cu·la of ret·i·na** an oval area of the sensory retina, 3 by 5 mm, temporal to the optic disk corresponding to the posterior pole of the eye; at its center is the central fovea, which contains only retinal cones. SYN macula retinae [TA].

**mac·u·la ret·i·nae** [TA] SYN macula of retina.

**mac·u·lar lep·ro·sy** a form of tuberculoid leprosy in which the lesions are small, hairless, and dry, and are erythematous in light skin and hypopigmented or copper-colored in dark skin.

**mac·u·lar retinal dys·tro·phy** a group of disor-ders involving predominantly the posterior portion of the ocular fundus, due to degeneration in the sensory layer of the retina, retinal pigment epithelium, Bruch membrane, choroid, or a combination of these tissues. SEE Stargardt disease, Best disease.

**mac·u·la of sac·cule** the oval neuroepithelial sensory receptor in the anterior wall of the saccule; hair cells of the neuroepithelium support the statoconial membrane and have terminal arborizations of vestibular nerve fibers around their bodies.

**mac·u·la of u·tri·cle** the neuroepithelial sensory receptor in the inferolateral wall of the utricle; hair cells of the neuroepithelium support the statoconial membrane and have terminal arborizations of vestibular nerve fibers around their bodies; sensitive to linear acceleration in the longitudinal axis of the body and to gravitational influences.

🔲 **mac·ule** (mak′yul) SYN macula. See page B4. [L. *macula*, spot]

**mac·u·lo·ce·re·bral** (mak′yu-lō-ser′ĕ-brăl) relating to the macula lutea and the brain; denoting a type of nervous disease marked by degenerative lesions in both the retina and the brain.

**mac·u·lo·er·y·the·ma·tous** (mak′yu-lō-er-i-them′ă-tŭs) denoting lesions that are erythematous and macular, covering wide areas.

**mac·u·lo·pap·ule** (mak′yu-lō-pap′yul) a lesion with a flat base surrounding a papule in the center.

**mac·u·lop·a·thy** (mak-yu-lop′ă-thē) any pathological condition of the macula lutea.

**mad·a·ro·sis** SYN alopecia adnata.

**Mad·dox rod** (mad′ĕks) a glass rod, or a series of parallel glass rods, that converts the image of a light source into a streak of light perpendicular to the axis of the rod. The position of this streak in relation to the image of the light source seen by the fellow eye indicates the presence and amount of heterophoria.

**Ma·de·lung de·for·mi·ty** (mah′dĕ-loong) a distal radioulnar subluxation due to a relative deficiency of axial growth of the medial side of the distal radius, which, as a consequence, is abnormally inclined proximally and ulnarwards.

**Ma·de·lung neck** (mah′dĕ-loong) multiple symmetric lipomatosis (Madelung disease) confined to the neck.

**Mad Hat·ter syn·drome** gastrointestinal and central nervous system manifestations of chronic mercury poisoning, including stomatitis, diarrhea, ataxia, tremor, hyperreflexia, sensorineural impairment, and emotional instability; previously seen in workers in lead manufacturing who put mercury-containing materials in their mouths to make them more pliable. [fr. char. in *Alice in Wonderland*]

**Mad·u·ra boil** (mad′yu-rah) SYN mycetoma (1).

**Mad·u·rel·la** (mad′yu-rel′ă) a genus of fungi including a number of species that cause mycetoma. [*Madura*, India]

**ma·du·ro·my·co·sis** (mad′yu-rō-mī-kō′sis) SYN mycetoma (1). [*Madura*, India, + mycosis]

**Maf·fuc·ci syn·drome** (mĕ-foo′chē) enchondromas of the limbs in association with venous and lymphaticovenous malformation; propensity to develop other benign or malignant tumors. SYN Kast syndrome.

**Ma·gen·die law** (mah-zhah-dē′) SYN Bell law.

**mag•got** (mag′ot) a fly larva or grub.

**Ma•gill for•ceps** (mĕ-gil′), a bent blunt forceps used to facilitate nasotracheal intubation.

**mag•ma** (mag′mă) **1.** a soft mass left after extraction of the active principles. **2.** a salve or thick paste. [G. a soft mass or salve, fr. *massō,* to knead]

**Mag•nan sign** (mah-nyah′) paresthesia in the psychosis of cocaine addicts, who imagine they have a foreign body, in the shape of a powder or fine sand, under the skin, and that it is constantly changing its position.

**Mag•nan trom•bone move•ment** (mah-nyah′) an involuntary forward and back movement of the tongue when it is drawn out of the mouth; may be seen in several basal ganglia disorders.

**mag•ne•si•um (Mg)** (mag-nē′zē-ŭm) an alkaline earth element, atomic no. 12, atomic wt. 24.3050, that oxidizes to magnesia; a bioelement; many salts have clinical applications. [Mod. L. fr. G. *Magnēsia,* a region in Thessaly]

**mag•net 1.** a body that has the property of attracting particles of iron, cobalt, nickel, or any of various metallic alloys and that when freely suspended tends to assume a definite direction between the magnetic poles of the earth (magnetic polarity). **2.** a bar or horseshoe-shaped piece of iron or steel that has been made magnetic by contact with another magnet or, as in an electromagnet, by passage of electric current around a metallic (iron) core. **3.** an electromagnet built in a cylindrical configuration to accommodate a patient in its core, for magnetic resonance imaging. [G. *magnēs*]

🔳**mag•net•ic res•o•nance i•mag•ing (MRI)** a diagnostic modality in which the magnetic nuclei (especially protons) of a patient are aligned in a strong, uniform magnetic field, absorb energy from tuned radiofrequency pulses, and emit radiofrequency signals as their excitation decays. These signals, which vary in intensity according to nuclear abundance and molecular chemical environment, are converted into sets of tomographic images by using field gradients in the magnetic field, which permits 3-dimensional localization of the point sources of the signals. Unlike conventional radiography or computed tomography, MRI does not expose patients to ionizing radiation. See page B11.

**mag•ni•fi•ca•tion** (mag′ni-fi-kā′shŭn) **1.** the seeming increase in size of an object viewed under the microscope; when written, this increased size is expressed by a figure preceded by ×, indicating the number of times its diameter is enlarged. **2.** the increased amplitude of a tracing, as of a muscular contraction, caused by the use of a lever with a long writing arm. [L. *magnifico,* pp. *-atus,* to magnify]

**mag•ni•fi•ca•tion ra•di•og•ra•phy** radiography using a microfocal x-ray tube and increased subject-film distance to provide magnification of the subject without loss of sharpness or increase in radiation exposure.

**mag•ni•tude i•mage** in magnetic resonance imaging, an image formed from the amplitude of the signal, distinct from the phase information. SEE ALSO magnetic resonance imaging.

**mag•no•cel•lu•lar** (mag′nō-sel′yu-lăr) composed of cells of large size. [L. *magnus,* large, + cellular]

**MAI** *Mycobacterium avium-intracellulare.* SEE

ALSO *Mycobacterium avium-intracellulare complex.*

**mAi** milliampere-impulse.

**main•stream aer•o•sol** a system for administering an aerosol that directs the mainstream of inspired airflow through the aerosol generator.

**main•stream•ing** (mān′strēm-ing) providing the least restrictive environment (socially, physically, and educationally) for individuals with chronic disabilities by introducing them into the natural environment rather than segregating them into homogeneous groups living in sheltered environments under constant supervision.

**main•tain•er** (mān-tā′ner) a device utilized to hold or keep teeth in a given position.

**main•te•nance** (mān′ten-ans) **1.** a therapeutic regimen intended to preserve benefit. Cf. compliance (2), adherence (2). **2.** the extent to which the patient continues good heath practices without supervision, incorporating them into a general life-style. Cf. compliance. [M.E., fr O.Fr., fr. Mediev. L. *manuteneo,* to hold in the hand]

**Mai•son•neuve frac•ture** (mā′zō-noov′) spiral fracture of the neck of the fibula resulting from violent external rotation of the ankle.

**ma•jor ag•glu•ti•nin** immune agglutinin present in greatest quantity in an antiserum and evoked by the most dominant of a mosaic of antigens. SYN chief agglutinin.

**ma•jor his•to•com•pat•i•bil•i•ty com•plex (MHC)** a group of linked loci, collectively termed H-2 complex in the mouse and HLA complex in humans, that codes for cell-surface histocompatibility antigens and is the principal determinant of tissue type and transplant compatibility.

**ma•jor sal•i•vary glands** a category of salivary glands that includes the three largest glands of the oral cavity that also secrete most of the saliva: the parotid, submandibular, and sublingual glands.

**ma•jor sub•lin•gual duct** the duct that drains the anterior portion of the sublingual gland; it opens at the sublingual papilla.

**mal** (mahl) a disease or disorder. [Fr., Sp. fr. L. *malum,* an evil]

△**mal-** ill, bad; opposite of eu-. Cf. dys-, caco-. [L. *malus,* bad]

**ma•la** (mā′lă) **1.** SYN cheek. **2.** SYN zygomatic bone. [L. cheek bone]

**mal•ab•sorp•tion** (mal-ab-sōrp′shŭn) imperfect, inadequate, or otherwise disordered gastrointestinal absorption.

**mal•ab•sorp•tion syn•drome** a state characterized by diverse features such as diarrhea, weakness, edema, lassitude, weight loss, poor appetite, protuberant abdomen, pallor, bleeding tendencies, paresthesias, and muscle cramps, caused by any of several conditions in which there is ineffective absorption of nutrients, e.g., sprue, gluten-induced enteropathy, gastroileostomy, tuberculosis, and certain fistulas.

**ma•la•cia** (mă-lā′shē-ă) a softening or loss of consistency and contiguity in any of the organs or tissues. Also used as a combining form in the suffix position. SYN mollities (2). SYN malacosis. [G. *malakia,* a softness]

**mal•a•co•pla•kia, mal•a•ko•pla•kia** (mal′ă-kō-plā′kē-ă, mal′a-kō-plā′kē-a) rare lesion in the mucosa of the urinary bladder characterized by mottled yellow and gray soft nodules that consist of macrophages and calcospherites (Michaelis-Guttmann bodies). [malaco- + G. *plax,* plate, plaque]

**mal·a·co·sis** (mal'ă-kō'sis) SYN malacia.

**mal·a·cot·ic** (mal'ă-kot'ik) pertaining to or characterized by malacia.

**mal·ad·just·ment** (mal-ad-jŭst'ment) in the mental health professions, an inability to cope with the problems and challenges of everyday living. [mal- + *adjust,* fr. O.Fr. *adjuster,* fr. L.L. *adjuxto,* to put close to, + -ment]

**mal·a·dy** (mal'ă-dē) a disease or illness. [Fr. *maladie,* illness]

**mal·aise** (mă-lāz') a feeling of general discomfort or uneasiness, an "out-of-sorts" feeling, often the first indication of an infection or other disease. [Fr. discomfort]

**mal·a·lign·ment** (mal-ă-līn'ment) displacement of a tooth or teeth from a normal position in the dental arch.

**ma·lar** (mā'lăr) relating to the mala, the cheek or cheek bones.

**ma·lar bone** SYN zygomatic bone.

**ma·lar·ia** (mă-lār'ē-ă) a disease caused by the presence of the sporozoan *Plasmodium* in red blood cells, usually transmitted by the bite of an infected female mosquito of the genus *Anopheles* that previously sucked blood from a person with malaria. Human infection begins with the exoerythrocytic cycle in liver parenchyma cells, followed by a series of erythrocytic schizogenous cycles repeated at regular intervals; production of gametocytes in other red cells provides future gametes for another mosquito infection; characterized by episodic severe chills and high fever, prostration, occasionally fatal termination. SEE tropical diseases. SEE ALSO *Plasmodium.* SYN *swamp fever (2).* [It. *malo* (fem. *mala),* bad, + *aria,* air, referring to the old theory of the miasmatic origin of the disease]

**ma·lar·i·ae ma·lar·ia** a malarial fever with paroxysms that recur every 72 hours or every fourth day, reckoning the day of the paroxysm as the first; due to the schizogony and release of merozoites from infected cells, with invasion of new red blood corpuscles by *Plasmodium malariae.* SYN quartan malaria.

**ma·lar·i·al** (mă-lār'ē-ăl) pertaining to or affected with malaria.

**ma·lar·i·al cres·cent** the male or female gametocyte(s) of *Plasmodium falciparum,* whose presence in human red blood cells is diagnostic of falciparum malaria. SYN crescent (3).

**ma·lar·i·o·ther·a·py** (ma-lar-ē-ō-thār'a-pē) SYN therapeutic malaria.

**Ma·las·sez ep·i·the·li·al rests** (mahl'ah-sā) epithelial remains of Hertwig root sheath in the periodontal ligament.

**Ma·las·sez·ia** (mal-ă-sā'zē-ă) a genus of fungi (family Cryptococcaceae) of low pathogenicity that lack the ability to synthesize medium-chain and long-chain fatty acids and require for growth an exogenous supply of these lipids as can be found in the skin. [L. C. *Malassez*]

**Ma·las·sez·ia pach·y·der·ma·tis** a fungus occasionally isolated from skin lesions of humans and animals; a rare cause of fungemia in patients receiving intravenous lipids.

**mal·as·sim·i·la·tion** (mal'ă-sim-i-lā'shŭn) rarely used term for incomplete or faulty assimilation; malabsorption.

**ma·late** (mal'āt) a salt or ester of malic acid.

**ma·late de·hy·dro·gen·ase** any enzyme that catalyzes the dehydrogenation of malate to oxaloacetate. At least six are known; one is an enzyme in the tricarboxylic acid cycle.

**mal·ax·a·tion** (mal'ak-sā'shŭn) **1.** formation of ingredients into a mass for pills and plasters. **2.** a kneading process in massage. [L. *malaxo,* pp. *-atus,* to soften]

**mal del pin·to** SYN pinta.

**mal de mer** SYN seasickness.

**male** (māl) **1.** ZOOLOGY denoting the sex to which those belong that produce spermatozoa; an individual of that sex. **2.** SYN masculine. [L. *masculus,* fr. *mas,* male]

🔲 **male pat·tern al·o·pe·cia** the most common form of androgenic alopecia, seen in men as receding frontal and bilateral triangular temple hair lines, and a balding patch on the vertex, which may progress to complete alopecia. See page 357.

**mal·e·rup·tion** (mal-ē-rŭp'shŭn) faulty eruption of teeth.

**mal·for·ma·tion** (mal-fōr-mā'shŭn) failure of proper or normal development; more specifically, a primary structural defect that results from a localized error of morphogenesis; e.g., cleft lip. Cf. deformation.

**mal·func·tion** (mal-fŭnk'shŭn) disordered, inadequate, or abnormal function.

**Mal·gai·gne her·nia** (mahl-gen'yĕ) infantile inguinal hernia prior to the descent of the testis.

**Mal·gai·gne lux·a·tion** (mahl-gen'yĕ) SYN nursemaid's elbow.

**Mal·her·be cal·ci·fy·ing ep·i·the·li·o·ma** (mahl-ārb') SYN pilomatrixoma.

**mal·ic ac·id** (mal'ik as'id) hydroxysuccinic acid; found in apples and various other tart fruits; an intermediate in the tricarboxylic acid cycle, the glyoxylate cycle, and in a shuttle system.

**ma·lig·nan·cy** (mă-lig'nan-sē) the property or condition of being malignant.

**ma·lig·nant** (mă-lig'nănt) **1.** Resistant to treatment; occurring in severe form and frequently fatal; tending to become worse. **2.** in reference to a neoplasm, having the properties of locally invasive and destructive growth and metastasis. [L. *maligno,* pres. p. *-ans (ant-),* to do anything maliciously]

**ma·lig·nant a·ne·mia** SYN pernicious anemia.

**ma·lig·nant bu·bo** the enlarged lymph node associated with bubonic plague.

**ma·lig·nant cil·i·ary ep·i·the·li·o·ma** malignant hyperplasia of ciliary epithelium with frequent involvement of the pigmented layer.

**ma·lig·nant dys·ker·a·to·sis** dyskeratosis that may occur in precancerous or malignant lesions.

**ma·lig·nant ex·ter·nal oti·tis** a life-threatening *Pseudomonas* osteomyelitis of the temporal bone in elderly diabetics that begins with ear pain and swelling of and discharge from the external auditory canal. SYN *Pseudomonas* osteomyelitis.

**ma·lig·nant fi·brous his·ti·o·cy·to·ma** a deeply situated tumor, especially on the extremities of adults, frequently recurring after surgery and metastasizing to the lungs; shows partial fibroblastic and histiocytic differentiation with a variable storiform pattern, myxoid areas, and giant cells.

**ma·lig·nant gran·u·lo·ma** SYN midline lethal granuloma.

**ma·lig·nant he·pa·to·ma** a carcinoma derived

from parenchymal cells of the liver. SYN hepatocarcinoma, hepatocellular carcinoma.

**ma·lig·nant his·ti·o·cy·to·sis** a rapidly fatal form of lymphoma, characterized by fever, jaundice, pancytopenia, and enlargement of the liver, spleen, and lymph nodes; the affected organs show focal necrosis and hemorrhage, with proliferation of histiocytes and phagocytosis of red blood cells.

**ma·lig·nant hy·per·ten·sion** severe hypertension that runs a rapid course, causing necrosis of arteriolar walls in kidney and retina, hemorrhages, and death most frequently due to uremia or rupture of a cerebral vessel.

**ma·lig·nant hy·per·ther·mia** rapid onset of extremely high fever with muscle rigidity, precipitated by exogenous agents in genetically susceptible persons, especially by halothane or succinylcholine.

**ma·lig·nant jaun·dice** SYN icterus gravis.

**ma·lig·nant lym·pho·ma** general term for malignant neoplasms of lymphoid and reticuloendothelial tissues which present as solid tumors composed of cells that appear primitive or resemble lymphocytes, plasma cells, or histiocytes. Lymphomas appear most frequently in lymph nodes, spleen, or other normal sites of lymphoreticular cells. Lymphomas are classified by cell type, degrees of differentiation, and nodular or diffuse pattern; Hodgkin disease and Burkitt lymphoma are special forms.

**ma·lig·nant mel·a·no·ma** SYN melanoma. See page B7.

**ma·lig·nant mel·a·no·ma in si·tu** a melanoma limited to the epidermis and composed of nests of atypical melanocytes and scattered single cells extending into the upper epidermis; local excision is curative although the lesion, if untreated, may soon invade the dermis. Malignant lentigo may be considered a slowly progressive type of malignant melanoma in situ.

**ma·lig·nant neph·ro·scle·ro·sis** the renal changes in malignant hypertension; subcapsular petechiae, necrosis in the walls of scattered afferent glomerular arterioles, and red blood cells and casts in the urine, with uremia as a common termination.

**ma·lig·nant ter·tian ma·lar·ia** SYN falciparum malaria.

**ma·lig·nant tu·mor** a tumor that invades surrounding tissues, is usually capable of producing metastases, may recur after attempted removal, and is likely to cause death of the host unless adequately treated. SEE ALSO cancer.

**ma·ling·er** (mă-ling′er) to engage in malingering.

**ma·ling·er·er** (mă-ling′er-er) one who engages in malingering.

**mal·in·ter·dig·i·ta·tion** (mal′in-ter-dij′i-tā′shŭn) faulty intercuspation of teeth.

**mal·le·a·ble** (mal′ē-ă-bl) capable of being shaped by being beaten or by pressure; a property of certain metals such as gold and silver. [L. *malleus*, a hammer]

**mal·le·ar folds** two ligamentous bands, anterior and posterior, making folds on the tympanic side of the tympanic membrane extending from each extremity of the tympanic notch to the malleolar prominence; they mark the boundary between the tense and the flaccid portions of the tympanic membrane.

**mal·le·o·in·cu·dal** (mal′ē-ō-ing′koo-dăl) relating to the malleus and the incus in the tympanum.

**mal·le·o·lar** (mă-lē′ō-lăr) relating to one or both malleoli.

**mal·le·o·lar stria** a bright line seen through the membrana tympani, produced by the attachment of the manubrium of the malleus.

**mal·le·o·lus,** pl. **mal·le·o·li** (ma-lē′ō-lŭs, mă-lē′ō-lī) [TA] a rounded bony prominence such as those on either side of the ankle joint. [L. dim. of *malleus,* hammer]

**mal·le·ot·o·my** (mal′ē-ot′ō-mē) **1.** division of the malleus. [malleus + G. *tomē,* incision] **2.** division of the ligaments holding the malleoli in apposition in order to permit their separation in certain cases of clubfoot. [malleolus + G. *tomē,* incision]

**mal·let fin·ger 1.** flexion deformity of a distal phalanx due to avulsion of the extensor tendon by forceful passive flexion of the phalanx **2.** SYN baseball finger.

**mal·le·us,** gen. and pl. **mal·lei** (mal′ē-ŭs, mal′ē-ī) the largest of the three auditory ossicles, resembling a club rather than a hammer; it is regarded as having a head, below which is the neck, and from this diverge the handle or manubrium, and the slender, anterior process; from the base of the manubrium the short lateral process arises. The manubrium and lateral process are firmly attached to the tympanic membrane, and the head articulates with a saddle-shaped surface on the body of the incus. SYN hammer. [L. a hammer]

**Mall for·mu·la** (mahl) a formula for determining the age (in days) of a human embryo; calculated as the square root of its length (measured from vertex to breech) in millimeters multiplied by 100.

**Mal·lo·ry an·i·line blue stain** (mal′ĕ-rē) SYN Mallory trichrome stain.

**Mal·lo·ry bod·ies** (mal′ĕ-rē) large, poorly defined accumulations of eosinophilic material in the cytoplasm of damaged hepatic cells in certain forms of cirrhosis and marked fatty change especially due to alcoholism.

**Mal·lo·ry col·la·gen stain** (mal′ĕ-rē) one of a number of staining methods using phosphomolybdic or phosphotungstic acid with an acid stain, such as aniline blue, or with hematoxylin for connective tissue staining.

**Mal·lo·ry io·dine stain** (mal′ĕ-rē) amyloid appears red-brown after Gram iodine, then violet and blue after flooding with dilute sulfuric acid.

**Mal·lo·ry phlox·ine stain** (mal′ĕ-rē) a technique based on retention of phloxine by hyaline after overstaining and then decolorizing with lithium carbonate, used in combination with alum hematoxylin to give nuclear staining; hyaline appears red, older hyaline is pink to colorless, amyloid is pale pink, and nuclei are blue-black.

**Mal·lo·ry phos·pho·tung·stic ac·id he·ma·tox·y·lin stain** (mal′ĕ-rē) SYN phosphotungstic acid hematoxylin.

**Mal·lo·ry stain for ac·ti·no·my·ces** (mal′ĕ-rē) a stain using alum hematoxylin, followed by eosin; immersion in Ehrlich aniline crystal violet stain, and Weigert iodine solution; mycelia stain blue and clubs stain red.

**Mal·lo·ry stain for he·mo·fuch·sin** (mal′ĕ-rē) sections are stained sequentially in alum hematoxylin and basic fuchsin; the lipofuchsin-like pigment and ceroid stain bright red, nuclei stain blue, while melanin and hemosiderin appear unstained in their natural browns.

**Mal·lo·ry tri·chrome stain** (mal'ĕ-rē) a method especially suitable for studying connective tissue; sections are stained in acid fuchsin, aniline blue-orange G solution, and phosphotungstic acid; fibrils of collagen are blue; fibroglia, neuroglia, and muscle fibers are red; and fibrils of elastin are pink or yellow. SYN Mallory aniline blue stain, Mallory triple stain.

**Mal·lo·ry tri·ple stain** (mal'ĕ-rē) SYN Mallory trichrome stain.

**Mal·lo·ry-Weiss le·sion** (mal'ĕ-rē-wīs) laceration of the gastric cardia, as seen in the Mallory-Weiss syndrome. SYN Mallory-Weiss tear.

**Mal·lo·ry-Weiss syn·drome** (mal'ĕ-rē-wīs) laceration of the lower end of the esophagus associated with bleeding, or penetration into the mediastinum, with subsequent mediastinitis; caused usually by severe retching and vomiting.

**Mal·lo·ry-Weiss tear** (mal'ĕ-rē-wīs) SYN Mallory-Weiss lesion.

**mal mo·ra·do** (mal mō-rā'dō) purplish skin discoloration seen in acute attacks of onchodermatitis caused by *Onchocerca volvulus* in Central America. [Sp. *mal,* disease, + *morado,* purple]

**mal·nu·tri·tion** (mal-noo-trish'ŭn) faulty nutrition resulting from malabsorption, poor diet, or overeating.

**mal·oc·clu·sion** (mal-ō-kloo'zhŭn) **1.** any deviation from a physiologically acceptable contact of opposing dentitions. **2.** any deviation from an ideal occlusion.

**ma·lon·di·al·de·hyde-mod·i·fied low-den··si·ty lip·o·pro·tein** LDL molecule with aldehyde-substituted lysine residue(s) in the apoprotein moiety, resulting from oxidative reaction accompanying prostaglandin synthesis and platelet aggregation.

**ma·lo·nic ac·id** (mă-lō'nik as'id) a dicarboxylic acid of importance in intermediary metabolism; an inhibitor of succinate dehydrogenase.

**mal·o·nyl-CoA** the condensation product of malonic acid and coenzyme A, an intermediate in fatty acid biosynthesis.

**mal·pi·ghi·an** (mahl-pig'ē-an) described by or attributed to Marcello Malpighi.

**mal·pi·ghi·an bod·ies** (mahl-pig'ē-ăn) SYN splenic lymph follicles.

**mal·pi·ghi·an cap·sule** (mahl-pig'ē-ăn) **1.** SYN glomerular capsule. **2.** a thin fibrous membrane enveloping the spleen and continued over the vessels entering at the hilus.

**mal·pi·ghi·an pyr·a·mid** (mahl-pig'ē-ăn) SYN renal pyramid.

**mal·pi·ghi·an stig·mas** (mahl-pig'ē-ăn) the points of entrance of the smaller veins into the larger veins of the spleen.

**mal·pi·ghi·an stra·tum** (mahl-pig'ē-ăn) the living layer of the epidermis comprising the stratum basale, stratum spinosum, and stratum granulosum.

**mal·po·si·tion** (mal-pō-zish'ŭn) SYN dystopia.

**mal·prac·tice** (mal-prak'tis) mistreatment of a patient through ignorance, carelessness, neglect, or criminal intent.

**mal·pre·sen·ta·tion** (mal'prē-sen-tā'shŭn) faulty presentation of the fetus; presentation of any part other than the occiput.

**mal·ro·ta·tion** (mal-rō-tā'shŭn) failure during embryonic development of normal rotation of all

or part of an organ or system such as the primordial gut or kidney.

**MALT** mucosa-associated lymphoid tissue.

**mal·tese cross** a tetrad formation of the early ringlike parasites within the red blood cell seen in babesiosis.

**MALToma** B-cell lymphoma of mucosa-associated lymphoid tissue. SYN extranodal marginal zone lymphoma.

**mal·tose** (mawl-tōs) a disaccharide formed in the hydrolysis of starch and consisting of two D-glucose residues.

**ma·lum** (mā'lŭm) a disease. [L. an evil]

**mam·il·la·tion** (mam-i-lā'shŭn) **1.** a nipple-like projection. **2.** the condition of being mamillated.

**mam·ma**, gen. and pl. **mam·mae** (mam'ă, mam' ē) [TA] SYN breast. SEE ALSO mammary gland. [L.]

**mam·mal·gia** (mă-mal'jē-ă) SYN mastodynia. [L. *mamma,* breast, + G. *algos,* pain]

**mam·ma·plas·ty** (mam'ă-plas-tē) plastic surgery of the breast to alter its shape, size, or position, or all of these. SYN mammoplasty, mastoplasty. [L. *mamma,* breast, + G. *plastos,* formed]

**mam·ma·ry** (mam'ă-rē) relating to the breasts.

**mam·ma·ry duct ec·ta·sia** dilation of mammary ducts by lipid and cellular debris in older women; rupture of ducts may result in granulomatous inflammation and infiltration by plasma cells. SEE ALSO plasma cell mastitis.

**mam·ma·ry fold** SYN mammary ridge.

**mam·ma·ry gland** the compound alveolar apocrine secretory gland that forms the breast. It consists of 15–24 lobes, each consisting of many lobules, separated by adipose tissue and fibrous septa; the parenchyma of the resting gland consists of ducts; the alveoli develop only during pregnancy.

**mam·ma·ry ridge** bandlike thickening of ectoderm in the embryo extending on either side from just below the axilla to the inguinal region; in human embryos, the mammary glands arise from primordia in the thoracic part of the ridge. SYN mammary fold, milk line.

**mam·mec·to·my** (ma-mek'tō-mē) SYN mastectomy. [L. *mamma,* breast, + *ektomē,* excision]

**mam·mi·form** (mam'i-fōrm) resembling a breast; breast-shaped. SYN mammose (1). [L. *mamma,* breast, + *forma,* form]

⚠**mam·mil-, mam·mil·li-** the mamillae. SEE ALSO mammil-. Cf. thelo-. [L. *mammilla (mamilla),* nipple]

⚠**mam·mil-, mam·mil·li-** the mamillae. SEE ALSO mammil-. Cf. thelo-. [L. *mamilla,* nipple]

**mam·mil·la**, pl. **mam·mil·lae** (mă-mil'ă, mă-mil'ē) **1.** a small rounded elevation resembling the female breast. **2.** SYN nipple. [L. nipple]

**mam·mil·la·plas·ty** (ma-mil'ă-plas-tē) plastic surgery of the nipple and areola. SYN theleplasty. [L. *mammilla,* nipple, + G. *plastos,* formed]

**mam·mil·la·re** (mam-i-lā'rē) SYN mammillary. [L.]

**mamm·il·lar·ia** SEE mammillary body.

**mam·mil·lary** (mam'i-lār-ē) relating to or shaped like a nipple. SYN mammillare.

**mam·mil·lary bo·dy** a small, round, paired cell group that protrudes into the interpeduncular fossa from the inferior aspect of the hypothalamus. It receives hippocampal fibers through the fornix and projects fibers to the anterior thalamic nuclei and into the brainstem tegmentum. SYN corpus mammillare [TA].

**mam·mil·lary ducts** SYN lactiferous ducts.

**mam·mil·lary line** a vertical line passing through the nipple on either side. SYN nipple line.

**mam·mil·late, mam·mil·lat·ed** (mam'i-lāt, mam'i-lāt'ed) studded with nipple-like projections.

**mam·mil·la·tion** (mam-i-lā'shŭn) **1.** a nipple-like projection. **2.** the condition of being mamillated.

**mam·mil·li·form** (mă-mil'i-fōrm) nipple-shaped. [L. *mamilla*, nipple, + *forma*, form]

**mam·mil·li·tis** (mam-i-lī'tis) inflammation of the nipple. [L., *mamilla*, nipple, + G. *-itis*, inflammation]

⚠**mam·mo-** the breasts. Cf. masto-. [L. *mamma*, breast]

🗎**mam·mo·gram** (mam'ō-gram) the record produced by mammography. See page B14.

🗎**mam·mog·ra·phy** (ma-mog'ră-fē) imaging examination of the breast by means of x-rays, ultrasound, and nuclear magnetic resonance; used for screening and diagnosis of breast disease. See page B14. [mammo- + G. *graphō*, to write]

*Mam·mo·mon·o·ga·mus* (mam'ō-mon-og'ă-mus) genus of syngamid trematode (family Syngamidae) found in the respiratory system of ruminants and occasionally reported in humans; worms usually joined together in a Y-shaped formation.

*Mam·mo·mon·o·ga·mus la·ryn·ge·us* (mam'ō-mon-og'ă-mus la-ryn-gē-ŭs) nematode found in upper respiratory tract of some mammals; approximately 100 human cases, most from Caribbean islands; worm is red to reddish-brown; copulating male and female present a Y shape; life cycle not known.

**mam·mo·plas·ty** (mam'ō-plas-tē) SYN mammaplasty. [mammo- + G. *plastos*, formed]

**mam·mose** (mam'mōs) **1.** SYN mammiform. **2.** having large breasts.

**mam·mo·so·ma·to·troph cell ade·no·ma** a rare prolactin- and growth hormone–producing pituitary adenoma composed of ultrastructurally monomorphic cells with both somatotrophic and lactotrophic differentiation.

**mam·mot·o·my** (ma-mot'ō-mē) SYN mastotomy. [mammo- + G. *tomē*, incision]

**mam·mo·tro·pic, mam·mo·tro·phic** (mam-ō-trop'ik, mam-ō-trof'ik) having a stimulating effect upon the development, growth, or function of the mammary glands. [mammo- + G. *tropos*, a turning]

**man·aged care** an arrangement whereby a third-party payer (e.g., insurance company, government, or corporation) mediates between physicians and patients, negotiating fees for service and overseeing the types of treatment given. The third-party payer requires second opinions and precertification review for patients requiring hospital admission, negotiates wholesale prices with physicians, and carries out cost-containment measures, including auditing hospitals and reviewing claims. SEE health maintenance organization. SEE ALSO capitation.

**Man·ches·ter op·er·a·tion** (man'chĕs-tĕr) a vaginal operation for prolapse of the uterus, consisting of cervical amputation and parametrial fixation (cardinal ligaments) anterior to the uterus. SYN Fothergill operation. [*Manchester, England*]

**man·da·to·ry breath** during mechanical ventilation a mandatory breath is one that is either initiated (triggered) or terminated (cycled) by some preset mechanism in the ventilator rather than by the patient.

**man·di·ble** (man'di-bl) a U-shaped bone, forming the lower jaw, articulating by its upturned extremities with the temporal bone on either side. SYN jaw bone, mandibula, submaxilla.

**man·dib·u·la,** pl. **man·dib·u·lae** (man-dib'yu-lă, man-dib'yu-lē) SYN mandible. [L. a jaw, fr. *mando*, pp. *mansus*, to chew]

**man·dib·u·lar** (man-dib'yu-lăr) relating to the lower jaw. SYN inframaxillary, submaxillary (1).

**man·dib·u·lar arch** the first postoral arch in the pharyngeal (branchial in fish) arch series. SYN mandibular process.

**man·dib·u·lar car·ti·lage** a cartilage bar in the first pharyngeal arch (mandibular arch) that forms a temporary supporting structure in the embryonic mandible; the cartilaginous primordia of the malleus and incus develop from its proximal end, and it also gives rise to the sphenomandibular and anterior malleolar ligaments. SYN Meckel cartilage.

**man·di·bu·lar for·a·men** an opening on the medial surface of the ramus of the mandible through which the inferior alveolar artery, vein, and nerve pass to supply the lower teeth. SYN foramen mandibulae [TA].

**man·dib·u·lar fos·sa** a deep hollow in the squamous portion of the temporal bone at the root of the zygoma, in which rests the condyle of the mandible. SYN glenoid fossa (2).

**man·dib·u·lar joint** SYN temporomandibular joint.

**man·dib·u·lar lymph node** one of the facial lymph nodes located by the facial artery near the point it crosses the mandible.

**man·dib·u·lar nerve [CN V3]** the third division of the trigeminal nerve formed by the union of sensory fibers from the trigeminal ganglion and the motor root of the trigeminal nerve in the foramen ovale, through which the nerve emerges; its branches are: meningeal, masseteric, deep temporal, lateral and medial pterygoid, buccal, auriculotemporal, lingual, and inferior alveolar; its sensory fibers are distributed to the auricle, external acoustic meatus, tympanic membrane, temporal region, cheek, skin overlying the mandible (except its angle), anterior 2/3 of tongue, floor of mouth, lower teeth, and gingiva; its motor fibers innervate all the muscles of mastication plus the mylohyoid, anterior belly of the digestive, and the tensores veli palati and tympani. SYN nervus mandibularis [CN V3] [TA].

**man·dib·u·lar pro·cess** SYN mandibular arch.

**man·dib·u·lo·ac·ral dys·pla·sia** an autosomal recessive disorder characterized by dental crowding, acro-osteolysis, stiff joints, and atrophy of the skin of the hands and feet; clavicles are hypoplastic, cranial sutures are wide, and multiple wormian bones are present.

**man·dib·u·lo·fa·cial** (man-dib'yu-lō-fā'shăl) relating to the mandible and the face.

**man·dib·u·lo·fa·cial dys·os·to·sis** a variable syndrome of malformations primarily of derivatives of the first branchial arch; characterized by palpebral fissures sloping outward and downward with notches or colobomas in the outer third of the lower lids, bony defects or hypoplasia of malar bones and zygoma, hypoplasia of the mandible, macrostomia with high or cleft palate and malposition and malocclusion of teeth, lowset malformed external ears, atypical hair growth, and occasional pits or clefts between mouth and ear.

**man•dib•u•lo-oc•u•lo•fa•cial** (man-dib'yu-lō-ok'yu-lō-fā'shăl) relating to the mandible and the orbital part of the face.

**man•drel, man•dril 1.** the shaft or spindle to which a tool is attached and by means of which it is rotated. **2.** SYN mandrin. **3.** DENTISTRY an instrument used in a handpiece to hold a disk, stone, or cup used for grinding, smoothing, or finishing. [G. *mandra,* a stable; the bed in which a ring's stone is set]

**man•drin** a stiff wire or stylet inserted in the lumen of a soft catheter to give it shape and firmness while passing through a hollow tubular structure. SYN mandrel (2), mandril. [Fr. *mandrin,* mandrel]

**ma•neu•ver** (mă-noo'ver) a planned movement or procedure. [Fr. *manoeuvre,* fr. L. *manu operari,* to work by hand]

**man•ga•nese (Mn)** (mang'gă-nēz) a metallic element resembling and often associated, in ores, with iron; atomic no. 25, atomic wt. 54.94; manganous salts are sometimes used in medicine. [Mod. L. *manganesium, manganum,* an altered form of *magnesium*]

**mange** (mānj) a cutaneous disease of domestic and wild animals caused by any one of several genera of skin-burrowing mites; in humans, mite infestations are usually referred to as scabies. [Fr. *manger,* to eat]

**ma•nia** (mā'nē-ă) an emotional disorder characterized by euphoria or irritability, increased psychomotor activity, rapid speech, flight of ideas, decreased need for sleep, distractibility, grandiosity, and poor judgment; usually occurs in bipolar disorder. SEE manic-depressive. [G. frenzy]

⚠-**man•ia** an abnormal love for, or morbid impulse toward, some specific object, place, or action. [G. frenzy]

**ma•ni•a•cal** (mă-nī'ă-kăl) relating to or characterized by mania. SYN manic.

**man•ic** (man'ik, mā'nik) SYN maniacal.

**man•ic-de•pres•sive 1.** pertaining to a manic-depressive psychosis (bipolar disorder). **2.** one suffering from such a disorder.

**man•ic-de•pres•sive psy•cho•sis** SYN bipolar disorder.

**man•ic ep•i•so•de** manifestation of a major mood disorder in which there is a distinct period during which the predominant mood of the individual is either elevated, expansive, or irritable, and there are associated symptoms of the excited or manic phase of the bipolar disorder. SEE affective disorder, endogenous depression.

**man•i•cy, man•i•cky** (man'i-sē, man'i-kē) behavior characteristic of the manic phase of bipolar disorder.

**man•i•fes•ta•tion** (man'i-fes-tā'shŭn) the display or disclosure of characteristic signs or symptoms of an illness. [L. *manifestus,* caught in the act]

**man•i•fest con•tent** those elements of fantasy and dreams which are consciously available and reportable.

**man•i•fest hy•per•o•pia** hyperopia for which accommodation can compensate. SYN facultative hyperopia.

**man•i•fest•ing het•er•o•zy•gote** an organism heterozygous for what is ordinarily a recessive condition, which, as a result of special mechanisms (such as lyonization, allelic exclusion, or a deletion in the homologous chromosome), has phenotypic manifestations.

**man•ner•ism** (man'er-izm) a peculiar or unusual characteristic mode of movement, action, or speech.

**Mann•kopf sign** (mahn'kopf) acceleration of the pulse when a painful point is pressed upon.

**Mann meth•yl blue-e•o•sin stain** (man) a stain useful for anterior pituitary and viral inclusion bodies; a mixture of the two dyes stains alpha cell granules red, beta cell granules dark blue, chromophobes gray to pink, colloid red, erythrocytes orange-red, and collagen fibers blue; this method is also useful for enterochromaffin, goblet, Paneth, and pancreatic islet cells; Negri bodies appear red while their nuclei and central granules are blue.

**man•nose** (man'ōs) an aldohexose obtained from various plant sources (i.e., from mannans).

**man•nose-bind•ing pro•tein** a protein involved in innate immunity that can bind mannosylated microorganisms and activate the complement pathway.

**ma•noeu•vre [Br.]** SEE maneuver.

**ma•nom•e•ter** (mă-nom'ĕ-ter) an instrument for measuring the pressure of gases or liquids. [G. *manos,* thin, scanty, + *metron,* measure]

**man•o•met•ric** (man-ō-met'rik) relating to a manometer.

**ma•nom•e•try** (mă-nom'ĕ-trē) measurement of the pressure of gases by means of a manometer. [see manometer]

**Man•son schis•to•so•mi•a•sis** (man'sĕn) SYN schistosomiasis mansoni.

**man•tle** (man'tl) **1.** a covering layer. **2.** SYN pallium.

**man•tle cell lym•pho•ma** a clinically and biologically distinct B-cell neoplasm with a recurring acquired genetic abnormality, the t(11;14) translocation, and a heterogeneous histologic appearance that may lead to confusion with reactive or other neoplastic lymphoproliferative disorders.

**man•tle ra•di•o•ther•a•py** radiotherapy with protection of uninvolved radiosensitive structures or organs.

**Man•toux test** (mahn-too') SEE tuberculin test.

**man•u•al Eng•lish** a means of communicating in English with a person with profound hearing impairment by a combination of signs, finger spelling, and gestures.

**man•u•al lymph drain•age** a massage technique intended to promote the absorption of interstitial fluid by stimulating flow in lymphatic channels. SYN lymph drainage.

**man•u•al ven•ti•la•tion** intermittent manual compression of a gas-filled reservoir bag to force gases into a patient's lungs and thus maintain oxygenation and carbon dioxide elimination during apnea or hypoventilation.

**man•u•al vis•u•al meth•od** a method for the education of deaf children that emphasizes the role of vision in communication and the early and consistent use of ASL or other national sign languages. SEE ALSO oral auditory method, combined methods, total communication.

**ma·nu·bri·um**, pl. **ma·nu·bria** (mă-noo′brē-ŭm, mă-noo′brē-ă) the portion of the sternum or of the malleus that represents the handle. [L. handle]

**ma·nu·bri·um of mal·le·us** the handle of the malleus; the portion that extends downward, inward, and backward from the neck of the malleus; it is embedded throughout its length in the tympanic membrane.

**ma·nu·bri·um of ster·num** the upper segment of the sternum, a flattened, roughly triangular bone, occasionally fused with the body of the sternum, forming with it a slight angle, the sternal angle.

**ma·nus**, gen. and pl. **ma·nus** (mā′nŭs) [TA] SYN hand. [L.]

**map** a representation of a region or structure; e.g., of a stretch of DNA.

**map·ping func·tion** LINKAGE ANALYSIS a formula that converts the recombination fraction (which is on the probability scale) into map distance (in morgans).

**Ma·ra·ñón sign** (mahr-ahn-yōn′) in Graves disease, a vasomotor reaction following stimulation of the skin over the throat.

**ma·ran·tic** (mă-ran′tik) SYN marasmic. [G. *marantikos*, wasting]

**ma·ras·mic** (mă-raz′mik) relating to or suffering from marasmus. SYN marantic.

**ma·ras·mus** (mă-raz′mŭs) cachexia, especially in young children, primarily due to prolonged dietary deficiency of protein and calories. SYN Parrot disease (2). [G. *marasmos*, withering]

**Mar·burg dis·ease** (mahr′berg) infection with an unusual rhabdovirus composed of RNA and lipid, tentatively assigned to the family of Filoviridae. Virus is "pantropic" and affects most organ systems. The disease is characterized by a prominent rash and hemorrhages in many organs and is often fatal. First seen in Marburg, Germany, among laboratory workers exposed to African green monkeys. Some person-to-person spread has been observed. Attempts to isolate virus should be done only in high-security laboratories. SYN Marburg virus disease.

**Mar·burg vi·rus** (mahr′berg) an RNA-containing virus, genus *Filovirus*, first recognized at Marburg University (Germany), where it was the cause of a highly fatal hemorrhagic fever among laboratory workers and handlers of green monkeys.

**Mar·burg vi·rus dis·ease** (mahr′berg) SYN Marburg disease.

**Mar·chand adre·nal** (mahr′shahnd) a small collection of accessory adrenal tissue in the broad ligament of the uterus or in the testis.

**Mar·chand wan·der·ing cell** (mahr′shahnd) a cell of the mononuclear phagocyte system.

**march frac·ture** a stress fracture in the shaft of a metatarsal bone, often due to prolonged marching in military recruits unaccustomed to such activity.

**march he·mo·glo·bi·nu·ria** a form occurring after marathon races, protracted marching, or heavy physical exercise.

**Mar·chi·a·fa·va-Big·na·mi dis·ease** (mahr′kē-ă-fah′vah-bēn-yah′mē) a disorder characterized by demyelination of the corpus callosum and cortical laminar necrosis involving the frontal and temporal lobes. Occurs predominantly in chronic alcoholics, particularly wine drinkers.

**Mar·chi fix·a·tive** (mahr′kē) a mixture of Müller fixative with osmium tetroxide, with potassium chlorate substituted for the potassium dichromate of Müller fixative for better results; used to demonstrate degenerating myelin. SEE ALSO Marchi stain.

**Mar·chi re·ac·tion** (mahr′kē) failure of the myelin sheath of a nerve to blacken when submitted to the action of osmic acid.

**Mar·chi stain** (mahr′kē) a staining method in which the specimen is hardened for 8–10 days in a modified Müller fixative, followed by immersion for 1–3 weeks in the same with the addition of osmic acid; fat and degenerating nerve fibers stain black.

**Mar·cus Gunn phe·nom·e·non, Mar·cus Gunn syn·drome** (mahr′kĕs-gun) SYN jaw-winking syndrome.

**Mar·cus Gunn sign** (mahr′kĕs-gun) SYN Gunn sign.

**Ma·rek dis·ease vi·rus** (mar′ek) SYN avian neurolymphomatosis virus.

**ma·re·no·strin** SYN pyrin.

**Ma·rey law** (mah-rā′) the pulse rate varies inversely with the blood pressure; i.e., the pulse is slow when the pressure is high; an expression of baroreceptor reflex influences on heart rate.

**mar·fan·oid** (mar′fan-oyd) a term used of those whose phenotype bears a superficial resemblance to that of Marfan syndrome.

**Mar·fan syn·drome** (mahr-fahn′) a connective tissue multisystemic disorder characterized by skeletal changes (arachnodactyly, long limbs, joint laxity, pectus), cardiovascular defects (aortic aneurysm which may dissect, mitral valve prolapse), and ectopia lentis; autosomal dominant inheritance, caused by mutation in the fibrillin-1 gene (FBN1) on chromosome 15q.

**mar·gin** (mar′jin) a boundary, edge, or border, as of a surface or structure. SEE ALSO border. SYN margo [TA]. [L. *margo*, border, edge]

**mar·gi·nal** (mar′ji-năl) relating to a margin.

**marginal ridge** 1. An elevation of enamel that forms the proximal boundaries of the occlusal surface of premolars and molars. 2. An elevation on the mesial and distal portions of the lingual surface and, occasionally, the labial surface of incisors.

**mar·gi·nal ten·to·ri·al branch of in·ter·nal ca·rot·id ar·tery** a small branch from the cavernous part of the internal carotid artery to the free margin of the tentorium.

**mar·gi·nal zone** a zone between the red and white pulp of the spleen containing numerous macrophages and a rich plexus of sinusoids supplied by white pulp arterioles carrying blood-borne antigens.

**mar·gi·nal zone lym·pho·ma** a heterogeneous group of neoplasms originating from the B-cell–rich zones of the lymph nodes, spleen, or extranodal lymphoid tissue. Those tumors originating from mucosa-associated lymphoid tissue (MALT), most often in the stomach, intestines, salivary glands, and lungs, are called MALTomas.

**mar·gin·a·tion** (mar′ji-nā′shŭn) a phenomenon that occurs during the relatively early phases of inflammation; as a result of dilation of capillaries and slowing of the bloodstream, leukocytes tend to occupy the periphery of the cross-sectional

m
a

lumen and adhere to the endothelial cells that line the vessels.

**mar·gi·no·plas·ty** (mar′ji-nō-plas-tē) plastic surgery of the tarsal border of an eyelid.

**mar·gin of safe·ty** the margin between the minimal therapeutic dose and the minimal toxic dose of a drug.

**mar·go**, gen. **mar·gi·nis**, pl. **mar·gi·nes** (mar′ gō, mar′ji-nis, mar′ji-nēz) [TA] SYN margin, border. [L.]

**margo orbitalis** [TA] SYN orbital margin.

**mar·i·jua·na** (mar-i-wah′nǎ) popular name for the dried flowering leaves of *Cannabis sativa*, which are smoked as cigarettes, "joints," or "reefers." In the U.S. marijuana includes any part of, or any extracts from, the female plant. Alternative spellings are mariguana, marihuana. SEE ALSO cannabis. [fr. Sp. *Maria Juana*, Mary Jane]

**Mar·ine-Len·hart syn·drome** (mah′rēn-len-hahrt) toxic multinodular goiter.

**Ma·ri·nes·co suc·cu·lent hand** (mah-rē-nes′kō) edema of the hand with coldness and lividity of the skin, observed in syringomyelia.

**Mar·i·on dis·ease** (mah-rē-aw′) a congenital obstruction of the posterior urethra.

**Mar·i·otte ex·per·i·ment** (mah-rē-ot′) an experiment in which one looks fixedly with one eye (the other being closed) at a black dot on a card, on which is also marked a black cross; as the card is moved to or from the eye, at a certain distance the cross becomes invisible but appears again as the card is moved further; this proves the absence of photoreceptors where the optic nerve enters the eye.

**Mar·i·otte law** (mah-rē-ot′) SYN Boyle law.

**Mar·jo·lin ul·cer** (mahr′zhō-lā′) well-differentiated but aggressive squamous cell carcinoma occurring in cicatricial tissue at the epidermal edge of a sinus draining underlying osteomyelitis.

**mark 1.** any spot, line, or other figure on the cutaneous or mucocutaneous surface, visible through difference in color, elevation, or other peculiarity. **2.** SYN infundibulum (8). [A.S. *mearc*]

**mark·er 1.** a device used to make a mark or to indicate measurement. **2.** a characteristic or factor by which a cell or molecule can be recognized or identified. **3.** a locus containing two or more alleles that, being harmless, are common and therefore yield high frequencies of heterozygotes which facilitate linkage analysis.

**mark·er trait** a trait that may be of little importance in itself but which by association, linkage, or other means facilitates the detection, anticipation, or understanding of a disease or (for genetic diseases) the localization of the causative gene on the karyotype.

**marker X syndrome** SYN fragile X syndrome.

**mar·mo·rat·ed** (mar′mō-rā-ted) denoting a condition in which the appearance of the skin is streaked like marble. SEE ALSO cutis marmorata. [L. *marmoratus*, marbled]

**Mar·quis re·a·gent** (mar-kē′) a solution of formaldehyde in sulfuric acid used in color tests for formaldehyde.

**mar·row** (mar′ō) **1.** a highly cellular hematopoietic connective tissue filling the medullary cavities and spongy epiphyses of bones that becomes predominantly fatty with age, particularly in the long bones of the limbs. **2.** any soft gelatinous or

fatty material resembling the marrow of bone. SEE ALSO medulla. [A.S. *mearh*]

**mar·row-mes·en·chyme con·nec·tions** uninterrupted continuations between bone marrow and mesenchyme of fetal and newborn middle ears.

**Mar·shall ob·lique vein** (mar′shĕl) SYN oblique vein of left atrium.

**mar·su·pi·al·i·za·tion** (mar-soo′pē-ăl-i-zā′shŭn) exteriorization of a cyst or other such enclosed cavity by resecting the anterior wall and suturing the cut edges of the remaining wall to adjacent edges of the skin, thereby creating a pouch. [L. *marsupium*, pouch]

**Mar·te·gi·a·ni ar·ea** (mahr-tĕ-jē′anē) SYN Martegiani funnel.

**Mar·te·gi·a·ni fun·nel** (mahr-tĕ-jē′anē) the funnel-shaped dilation on the optic disk that indicates the beginning of the hyaloid canal. SYN Martegiani area.

**Mar·tin ban·dage** (mar′tin) a roller bandage of soft rubber used to provide compression to a limb in the treatment of varicose veins or ulcers.

**Mar·tin-Bell syn·drome** (mar′tin-bel) SYN fragile X syndrome.

**Mar·ti·not·ti cell** (mahr-tĭ-nōt′ē) a small multipolar nerve cell with short branching dendrites scattered through various layers of the cerebral cortex; its axon ascends toward the surface of the cortex.

**Mar·tin tube** (mar′tin) a drainage tube with a cross piece near the extremity to keep it from slipping out of a cavity.

**Mar·to·rell syn·drome** (măr-tō-rel′) SYN aortic arch syndrome.

**Mar·y·land co·ma scale** SEE coma scale.

**mA-s** milliampere-second.

**mas·cu·line** (mas′kyu-lin) relating to or marked by the characteristics of the male sex or gender. SYN male (2). [L. *masculus*, male, fr. *mas*, male]

**mas·cu·line pel·vis 1.** a pelvis justo minor in which the bones are large and heavy; **2.** a slight degree of funnel-shaped pelvis in the woman, in which the shape approximates that of the male pelvis.

**mas·cu·line uter·us** SYN prostatic utricle.

**mas·cu·lin·i·ty** (mas-kyu-lin′i-tē) the qualities and characteristics of a male.

**mas·cu·lin·i·za·tion** (mas′kyu-lin-i-zā′shŭn) the condition marked by the attainment of male characteristics, such as facial hair, either physiologically as part of male maturation, or pathologically by individuals of either sex. [L. *masculus*, male]

**mas·cu·li·nize** (mas′kyu-li-nīz) to confer the qualities or characteristics peculiar to the male.

**mask 1.** any of a variety of disease states producing alteration or discoloration of the skin of the face. **2.** the expressionless appearance seen in certain diseases; e.g., Parkinson facies. **3.** a facial bandage. **4.** a shield designed to cover the mouth and nose for maintenance of aseptic conditions. **5.** a device designed to cover the mouth and nose for administration of inhalation anesthetics, oxygen, or other gases.

**masked vi·rus** a virus ordinarily occurring in the host in a noninfective state, but which may be activated and demonstrated by special procedures such as blind passage in experimental animals.

**mask·ing 1.** the use of noise of any kind to interfere with the audibility of another sound. For any given intensity, low pitched tones have a greater masking effect than those of a high pitch. **2.** AUDIOLOGY the use of a noise applied to one ear while testing the hearing acuity of the other ear. **3.** the hiding of smaller rhythms in the brain wave record by larger and slower ones whose wave form they distort. **4.** DENTISTRY an opaque covering used to camouflage the metal parts of a prosthesis. **5.** RADIOGRAPHY superimposition of an altered positive image on the original negative to produce an enhanced copy photographically.

**mask·ing di·lem·ma** a problem encountered in establishing the bone conduction thresholds in severe bilateral conductive hearing loss, in which the amount of masking of the nontest ear exceeds the interaural attenuation so that enough masking is too much masking.

**mask·ing lev·el dif·fer·ence** a technique of comparing threshold responses with masking noise presented in phase and out of phase with the test signal; release from masking is normal and indicates an intact brainstem auditory pathway.

**mask·like face** SYN Parkinson facies.

**mask of preg·nan·cy** SYN melasma.

**Mas·low hi·er·ar·chy** (maz-lō) a ranking of needs which humans presumably fills successively in the order of lowest to highest: physiological needs, love and belonging, self-esteem, and self-actualization.

**mas·och·ism** (mas′ō-kizm) **1.** passive algolagnia; a form of perversion, often sexual in nature, in which a person experiences pleasure in being abused, humiliated, or maltreated. Cf. sadism. **2.** a general orientation in life that personal suffering relieves guilt and leads to a reward. [Leopold von Sacher-*Masoch,* Austrian novelist, 1836–1895]

**mas·o·chist** (mas′ō-kist) the passive party in the practice of masochism.

**mas·o·chis·tic per·son·al·i·ty** a personality disorder in which the individual accepts exploitation and sacrifices self-interest while at the same time feeling morally superior or feigning moral superiority, attempting to elicit sympathy, and inducing guilt in others.

**ma·son lung** silicosis occurring in stone masons.

**MASS** *m*itral valve prolapse, *a*ortic anomalies, *s*keletal changes, and *s*kin changes.

**mass 1.** a lump or aggregation of coherent material. **2.** in pharmacy, a soft solid preparation containing an active medicinal agent, of such consistency that it can be divided into small pieces and rolled into pills. **3.** one of the seven fundamental quantities in the SI system; its unit is the kilogram, defined as the mass of the international prototype of the kilogram, which is made of platinum-iridium and kept at the International Bureau of Weights and Measures. SYN massa. [L. *massa,* a dough-like mass]

**mas·sa,** gen. and pl. **mas·sae** (mas′să, mas′sē) SYN mass. [L.]

**mass ac·tion prin·ci·ple** the fundamental principle in epidemic theory: the incidence of an infectious disease is determined by the product of the current prevalence and the number of susceptibles in the population. SEE ALSO serial interval, infection transmission parameter.

**mas·sage** (mă-sahzh′) a method of manipulation of the body by rubbing, pinching, kneading, or tapping. [Fr. from G. *massō,* to knead]

**mas·sage the·ra·py** a collection of modalities that have the intention of improving health through the medium of human touch and the manipulation of soft tissues. SEE ALSO bodywork. SYN massotherapy, myotherapy.

**mas·se·ter·ic ar·tery** *origin,* maxillary; *distribution,* deep surface of masseter muscle; *anastomoses,* branches of transverse facial and masseteric branches of facial. SYN arteria masseterica [TA].

**mas·se·ter·ic nerve** a muscular branch of the mandibular nerve passing through the mandibular notch to the medial surface of the masseter muscle; which it supplies, and the temporomandibular joint. SYN nervus massetericus [TA].

**mas·se·ter mus·cle** *origin,* superficial part: inferior border of the anterior two-thirds of the zygomatic arch; deep part: inferior border and medial surface of the zygomatic arch; *insertion,* lateral surface of ramus and coronoid process of the mandible; *action,* elevates mandible (closes jaw); *nerve supply,* masseteric branch of mandibular division of trigeminal. SYN musculus masseter [TA].

**mass hys·te·ria 1.** simultaneous identical physical and/or emotional symptoms among a group of individuals; **2.** a socially contagious frenzy of irrational behavior in a group of people as a reaction to an event. SYN mass sociogenic illness.

**Mas·son ar·gen·taf·fin stain** (mah-saw′) a stain used to stain enterochromaffin granules brown-black.

**Mas·son-Fon·tan·a am·mo·ni·a·c sil·ver stain** (mah-saw′-fon-tah′nă) a stain used to demonstrate melanin and argentaffin granules.

**Mas·son tri·chrome stain** (mah-saw′) original composition for multicolored tissue preparations including ponceau de xylidine, acid fuchsin, iron alum hematoxylin, and either aniline blue or fast green FCF; chromatin stains black, cytoplasm is in shades of red, granules of eosinophils and mast cells are deep red, erythrocytes are black, elastic fibers are red, and collagen fibers and mucus are dark blue (aniline blue) or green (fast green FCF); modifications substitute other dyes, such as Biebrich scarlet red and wool green stain.

**mas·sothe·ra·py** SYN massage therapy.

**mass per·i·stal·sis** forcible peristaltic movements of short duration, occurring only three or four times a day, which move the contents of the large intestine from one division to the next, as from the ascending to the transverse colon.

**mass so·ci·o·gen·ic ill·ness** SYN mass hysteria.

**MAST** military antishock trousers.

**mast·ad·e·ni·tis** (mast′ad-ĕ-nī′tis) SYN mastitis. [masto- + G. *adēn,* gland, + -*itis,* inflammation]

**mast·ad·e·no·ma** (mast′ad-ĕ-nō′mă) an adenoma of the breast. [masto- + G. *adēn,* gland, + -*ōma,* tumor]

***Mast·ad·e·no·vi·rus*** (mast-ad′ĕ-nō-vī′rŭs) a genus of adenoviruses with over 40 antigenic types (species) being infective for humans. They cause respiratory infections in children, epidemic acute respiratory disease in military recruits, epidemic follicular conjunctivitis in adults, and epidemic keratoconjunctivitis; many infections are inapparent. [G. *mastos,* breast, hence mammal, + adenovirus]

**mas·tal·gia** (mas-tal′jē-ă) SYN mastodynia. [masto- + G. *algos,* pain]

**mas·tat·ro·phy, mas·ta·tro·phia** (mas-tat′rō-fē, mast-ă-trō′fē-ă) atrophy or wasting of the breasts. [masto- + atrophy]

**mast cell** a connective tissue cell that contains coarse, basophilic, metachromatic granules; secretes heparin and histamine. SYN mastocyte.

**mast cell leu·ke·mia** SYN basophilic leukemia.

**mas·tec·to·my** (mas-tek'tō-mē) excision of the breast. SYN mammectomy. [masto- + G. *ektomē*, excision]

**mas·ter pa·tient in·dex (MPI)** database of all patients ever treated at a health care facility.

**mas·ti·cate** (mas'ti-kāt) to chew; to perform mastication.

◫**mas·ti·ca·tion** (mas-ti-kā'shŭn) the process of chewing food in preparation for deglutition and digestion; the act of grinding or comminuting with the teeth. See this page. [L. *mastico*, pp. *-atus*, to chew]

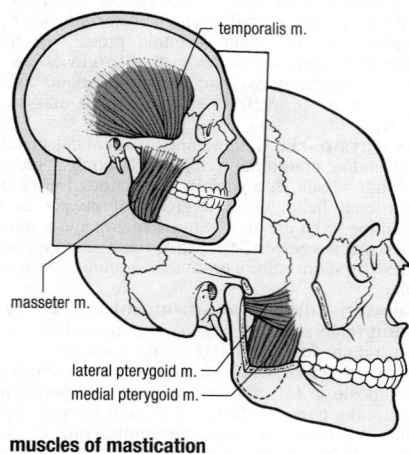

- temporalis m.
- masseter m.
- lateral pterygoid m.
- medial pterygoid m.

**muscles of mastication**

**mas·ti·ca·to·ry** (mas'ti-kǎ-tō-rē) relating to mastication.

**mas·ti·ca·to·ry force** SYN force of mastication.

**mas·ti·gote** (mas'ti-gōt) an individual flagellate. [G. *mastix*, a whip]

**mas·ti·tis** (mas-tī'tis) inflammation of the breast. SYN mastadenitis. [masto- + G. *-itis*, inflammation]

**mast leu·ko·cyte** SYN basophilic leukocyte.

△**mas·to-, mast-** the breast; the mastoid. Cf. mammo-, mazo-. [G. *mastos*]

**mas·to·cyte** (mas'tō-sīt) SYN mast cell.

**mas·to·cy·to·ma** (mas'tō-sī-tō'mǎ) a fairly well-circumscribed accumulation or nodular focus of mast cells, grossly resembling a neoplasm. [mastocyte + G. *-oma*, tumor]

**mas·to·cy·to·sis** (mas'tō-sī-tō'sis) abnormal proliferation of mast cells in a variety of tissues; may be systemic, involving a variety of organs, or cutaneous (urticaria pigmentosa). [mastocyte + G. *-osis*, condition]

**mas·to·dyn·ia** (mas-tō-din'ē-ǎ) pain in the breast. SYN mammalgia, mastalgia. [masto- + G. *odynē*, pain]

**mas·toid** (mas'toyd) **1.** resembling a breast; breast-shaped. **2.** relating to the mastoid process, antrum, cells, etc. [masto- + G. *eidos*, resemblance]

**mas·toid air cells** numerous small intercommunicating cavities in the mastoid process of the temporal bone that empty into the mastoid or tympanic antrum.

**mas·toid an·trum** a cavity in the petrous portion of the temporal bone, communicating posteriorly with the mastoid cells and anteriorly with the epitympanic recess of the middle ear via the aperture of the mastoid antrum.

**mas·toid bone** SYN mastoid process.

**mas·toid can·a·lic·u·lus** the canal that extends from the jugular fossa laterally through the mastoid process. It transmits the auricular branch of the vagus.

**mas·toid cor·tex** the plate of bone on the lateral surface of the mastoid process of the temporal bone.

**mas·toid·ec·to·my** (mas'toy-dek'tō-mē) hollowing out of the mastoid process by curretting, gouging, drilling, or otherwise removing the bony partitions forming the mastoid cells. [mastoid (process) + G. *ektomē*, excision]

**mas·toid fo·ra·men** an opening at the posterior portion of the mastoid process, transmitting the mastoid branch of the occipital artery to the dura and an emissary vein to the sigmoid sinus.

◫**mas·toid·i·tis** (mas-toy-dī'tis) inflammation of any part of the mastoid process. See this page.

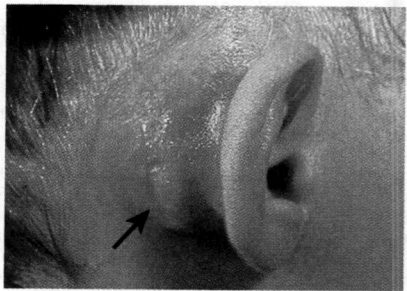

**mastoiditis:** ruptured retroauricular abscess

**mas·toid pro·cess** the nipplelike projection of the petrous part of the temporal bone. SYN mastoid bone.

**mas·ton·cus** (mas-tong'kŭs) a tumor or swelling of the breasts. [masto- + G. *onkos*, mass]

**mas·to·oc·cip·i·tal** (mas'tō-ok-sip'i-tǎl) relating to the mastoid portion of the temporal bone and to the occipital bone, denoting the suture uniting them.

**mas·to·pa·ri·e·tal** (mas'tō-pa-rī'ĕ-tǎl) relating to the mastoid portion of the temporal bone and to the parietal bone, denoting the suture uniting them.

**mas·top·a·thy** (mas-top'ǎ-thē) any disease of the breasts. [masto- + G. *pathos*, suffering]

**mas·to·pexy** (mas'tō-pek-sē) plastic surgery to affix sagging breasts in a more elevated and normal position, often with some improvement in shape. [masto- + G. *pēxis*, fixation]

**mas·to·pla·sia** (mas-tō-plā'zē-ǎ) enlargement of the breast. [masto- + G. *plasis*, a molding]

**mas·to·plas·ty** (mas'tō-plas-tē) SYN mammaplasty. [masto- + G. *plastos*, formed]

**mas·top·to·sis** (mas-top-tō'sis) ptosis or sagging of the breast. [masto- + G. *ptōsis*, a falling]

**mas·tor·rha·gia** (mas-tō-rā'jē-ǎ) hemorrhage

from a breast. [masto- + G. *rhḗgnymi*, to burst forth]

**mas·to·squa·mous** (mas'tō-skwā'mŭs) relating to the mastoid and the squamous portions of the temporal bone.

**mas·tot·o·my** (mas-tot'ō-mē) incision of the breast. SYN mammotomy. [masto- + G. *tomē*, incision]

**mas·tur·bate** (mas'ter-bāt) to practice masturbation. [L. *masturbari*, pp. *masturbatus*]

**mas·tur·ba·tion** self-stimulation of the genitals for erotic pleasure, often resulting in orgasm.

**MAT** multifocal atrial tachycardia.

**matched groups** a method of experimental control in which subjects in one group are matched on a one-to-one basis with subjects in other groups concerning all organism variables (e.g., age, sex, height, weight) that the experimenter believes could influence the variable being investigated.

**match·ing** the process of making a study group and a comparison group in an epidemiological study comparable with respect to extraneous or confounding factors such as age, sex, weight, etc.

**ma·ter** (mā'ter, mah'ter) the "sheltering" coverings of the central nervous system. SEE arachnoid mater, dura mater, pia mater. [L. mother]

**ma·te·ria** (mă-tē'rē-ă) substance or matter. [L. substance]

**ma·te·ria al·ba** accumulation or aggregation of microorganisms, desquamated epithelial cells, blood cells, and food debris loosely adherent to surfaces of plaques, teeth, gingiva, or dental appliances. [L. white matter]

**ma·te·ri·al** (mă-tēr'ē-ăl) of which something is made or composed; the constituent element of a substance. [L. *materialis*, fr. *materia*, substance]

**ma·te·ria med·i·ca 1.** that aspect of medical science concerned with the origin and preparation of drugs, their doses, and their mode of administration; **2.** any agent used therapeutically. SEE ALSO pharmacognosy, pharmacology. [L. medical matter]

**ma·ter·nal** (mă-ter'năl) relating to or derived from the mother. [L. *maternus*, fr. *mater*, mother]

**ma·ter·nal death rate** the number of maternal deaths occurring as the direct result of the reproductive process per 100,000 live births. SYN maternal mortality ratio.

**ma·ter·nal dys·to·cia** dystocia caused by an abnormality or physical problem in the mother.

**maternal-fe·tal med·i·cine** a subspecialty of obstetrics/gynecology devoted to the study of the obstetrical, medical, and surgical complications of pregnancy.

**maternal morbidity** medical complications in a woman caused by pregnancy, labor, or delivery.

**ma·ter·nal mor·tal·i·ty ra·tio** SYN maternal death rate.

**ma·ter·nal pla·cen·ta** SYN pars uterina placentae.

**ma·ter·ni·ty** (mă-ter'ni-tē) motherhood. [see maternal]

**mat·ing** (māt'ing) the pairing of male and female for the purpose of reproduction.

**mat·ri·cal** (mat'ri-kăl) relating to any matrix.

**ma·tri·ces** (mā'tri-sēz) plural of matrix. [L.]

**mat·ri·cide** (mat'ri-sīd) **1.** the killing of one's mother. **2.** one who commits such an act. [L. *mater*, mother, + *caedo*, to kill]

**mat·ri·lin·e·al** (mat-ri-lin'ē-ăl) denoting descent

through the female line. [L. *mater*, mother, + *linea*, line]

**ma·trix**, pl. **ma·tri·ces** (mā'triks; mā'tri-sēz, mat'ri-sēz) **1.** the formative portion of a tooth or a nail. **2.** the intercellular substance of a tissue. **3.** a surrounding substance within which something is contained or embedded. **4.** a mold in which anything is cast or swaged; a counterdie; a specially shaped instrument, plastic material, or metal strip used for holding and shaping the material used in filling a tooth cavity. **5.** a rectangular array of numbers or symbol quantities that simplify the execution of linear operations of tedious complexity; the theory of matrices is widely used in solving simultaneous equations and in population genetics. [L. womb; female breeding animal]

**ma·trix band** a metal or plastic band secured around the crown of a tooth to confine restorative material to be adapted into a prepared cavity.

**ma·trix cal·cu·lus** a yellowish-white to light tan urinary calculus containing calcium salts in an organic matrix and usually associated with chronic infection.

**ma·trix me·tal·lo·pro·tein·ase** a subfamily of endopeptidases that hydrolyze extracellular proteins, especially collagens and elastin. By regulating the integrity and composition of the extracellular matrix, these enzymes play a pivotal role in the control of signals elicited by matrix molecules that regulate cell proliferation, differentiation, and death.

**ma·trix un·guis** SYN nail bed.

**mat·ter** SYN substance. SEE ALSO substance. [L. *materies*, substance]

**mat·tress su·ture** a suture utilizing a double stitch that forms a loop about the tissue on both sides of a wound, producing eversion of the edges when tied.

**mat·u·ra·tion** (mat-yu-rā'shŭn) **1.** achievement of full development or growth. **2.** developmental changes that lead to maturity. **3.** processing of a macromolecule; e.g., posttranscriptional modification of RNA or posttranslational modification of proteins. [L. *maturatio*, a ripening, fr. *maturus*, ripe]

**mat·u·ra·tion ar·rest** cessation of complete differentiation of cells at an immature stage; in spermatogenic maturation arrest, the seminiferous tubules contain spermatocytes, but no spermatozoa develop.

**mat·u·ra·tion in·dex** an index indicating the degree of maturation attained by the vaginal epithelium as adjudged by the cell types being exfoliated; serves as an objective means of evaluating hormonal secretion or response; represents the percentage of parabasal cells/intermediate cells /superficialis, in that order; "shift to the left" indicates more immature cells on the surface (atrophy), while "shift to the right" indicates more mature epithelium.

**ma·ture** (mă-choor') **1.** ripe; fully developed. **2.** to ripen; to become fully developed. [L. *maturus*, ripe]

**ma·ture bac·te·ri·o·phage** the complete, infective form of bacteriophage.

**ma·ture cat·a·ract** a cataract in which both the nucleus and cortex are opaque.

**ma·tu·ri·ty** (mă-choor'i-tē) a state of full development or completed growth.

**ma·tu·ri·ty-on·set di·a·be·tes** non-insulin-dependent diabetes mellitus.

**Mau·rer dots** (mow′rer) finely granular precipitates or irregular cytoplasmic particles that usually occur diffusely in red blood cells infected with the trophozoites of *Plasmodium falciparum*, occasionally those of *P. malariae;* rarely observed in *P. falciparum* blood smears because its trophozoites seldom are seen in peripheral blood.

**Mau·ri·ac syn·drome** (mō′rē-ahk′) dwarfism with obesity and hepatosplenomegaly in children with poorly controlled diabetes mellitus.

**Mau·ri·ceau ma·neu·ver** (mō-rē-sō′) a method of assisted breech delivery in which the infant's body is astraddle the right forearm, and the middle finger of the right hand is in the fetal mouth to maintain flexion while traction is made upon the shoulders by the other hand.

**Mauth·ner sheath** (mowt′ner) SYN axolemma.

**max·il·la**, gen. and pl. **max·il·lae** (mak-sil′ă, mak-sil′ē) [TA] an irregularly shaped bone, supporting the superior teeth and taking part in the formation of the orbit, hard palate, and nasal cavity. [L. jawbone]

**max·il·lary** (mak′si-lār-ē) relating to the maxilla, or upper jaw.

**max·il·lary ar·tery** *origin*, external carotid; *branches*, deep auricular, anterior tympanic, middle meningeal, inferior alveolar, masseteric, deep temporal, buccal, posterior superior alveolar, infraorbital, descending palatine, artery of pterygoid canal, sphenopalatine. SYN arteria maxillaris [TA].

**max·il·lary gland** SYN submandibular gland.

**max·il·lary nerve [CN V2]** the second division of the trigeminal nerve, passing from the trigeminal ganglion in the middle cranial fossa through the foramen rotundum into the pterygopalatine fossa, where it gives off ganglionic branches to the pterygopalatine ganglion and continues forward to give off the zygomatic nerve and enter the orbit, where it continues as the infraorbital nerve. Its sensory fibers are distributed to the skin and conjunctiva of the lower eyelid; the skin and mucosa of the upper lip and cheek; the palate, upper teeth and gingiva; the maxillary sinus; wings of the nose; and posterior/interior nasal cavity. SYN nervus maxillaris [CN V2] [TA].

**max·il·lary pro·cess** a thin plate of irregular form projecting from the middle of the upper border of the inferior concha, articulating with the maxilla bone and partly closing the orifice of the maxillary sinus.

**max·il·lary si·nus** the largest of the paranasal sinuses occupying the body of the maxilla, communicating with the middle meatus of the nose.

**max·il·lary vein** the posterior continuation of the pterygoid plexus; it joins the superficial temporal vein to form the retromandibular vein.

**max·il·lo·den·tal** (mak-sil′ō-den′tăl) relating to the upper jaw and its associated teeth.

**max·il·lo·fa·cial** (mak-sil′ō-fā′shăl) pertaining to the jaws and face, particularly with reference to specialized surgery of this region.

**max·il·lo·man·dib·u·lar** (mak-sil′ō-man-dib′yu-lăr) relating to the upper and lower jaws.

**max·il·lot·o·my** (mak-si-lot′ō-mē) surgical sectioning of the maxilla to allow movement of all or a part of the maxilla into the desired position. [maxilla + G. *tomē,* incision]

**max·i·mal dose** the largest amount of a drug or physical procedure that an adult can take with safety.

**max·i·mal oxy·gen con·sump·tion** highest amount of oxygen an individual can consume during maximal exercise of several minutes' duration. SYN aerobic capacity, aerobic power, maximal oxygen uptake, $VO_{2max}$.

**max·i·mal oxy·gen up·take** SYN maximal oxygen consumption.

**max·i·mal thy·mec·tomy** SYN extended thymectomy.

**Max·i·mow stain for bone mar·row** (maks-ē-mŏv) an alum-hematoxylin and azure II-eosin stain used to distinguish granulated leukocytes, mast cells, and cartilage.

**max·i·mum** (mak′si-mŭm) the greatest amount, value, or degree attained or attainable. [L. neuter of *maximus,* greatest]

**max·i·mum breath·ing ca·pac·i·ty (MBC)** SYN maximum voluntary ventilation.

**max·i·mum ex·pi·ra·tory pres·sure (MEP)** the maximum pressure within the alveoli that occurs during a forceful expiration; the measurement is made when the lungs are full.

**max·i·mum in·spi·ra·tory pres·sure (MIP)** the maximum pressure within the alveoli that occurs during inspiration; the measurement of MIP provides a global assessment of inspiratory muscle function.

**max·i·mum in·ten·si·ty pro·jec·tion (MIP)** a computerized image display method used in MR angiography and helical computed tomography; a series of slices are combined with display of the brightest pixel on any slice at each location, and suppression of the background; simulates a projection angiogram.

**max·i·mum per·mis·si·ble dose (MPD)** defined by the International Commission on Radiological Protection as the greatest dose of radiation which, in the light of present knowledge, is not expected to cause detectable bodily injury to a person at any time during his lifetime. This dose has been reduced with each Commission report. The MPD is given in terms of acute or chronic exposure of the whole body or of organs, systems, or regions of the body, and differs for persons who are occupationally exposed versus the public at large.

**max·i·mum pow·er out·put** the greatest sound resulting from amplification that the instrument can produce; an indication of hearing aid performance.

**max·i·mum ve·loc·i·ty ($V_{max}$) 1.** the maximum rate of an enzyme-catalyzed reaction that can be achieved by progressively increasing the substrate concentration at a given enzyme concentration; in cases of substrate inhibition, $V_{max}$ is an extrapolated value in the absence of such inhibition; **2.** the maximum initial rate of shortening of a myocardial fiber that can be obtained under zero load; used to evaluate the contractility of the fiber.

**max·i·mum vol·un·tary ven·ti·la·tion (MVV)** the volume of air breathed when an individual breathes as deeply and as quickly as possible for a given time. SYN maximum breathing capacity.

**May·er he·mal·um stain** (mī′yer) a progressive nuclear stain also used as a counterstain.

**May·er mu·ci·car·mine stain** (mī′yer) SEE mucicarmine.

**May·er mu·ci·he·ma·te·in stain** (mī′yer) SEE mucihematein.

**May·er pes·sa·ry** (mī'yer) SYN Dumontpallier pessary.

**May·er re·flex** (mī'yer) SYN basal joint reflex.

**Mayo op·er·a·tion** (mā'ō) an operation for the radical cure of umbilical hernia; the neck of the sac is exposed by two elliptical incisions, the gut is returned to the abdomen, the sac and adherent omentum are cut away, and the fascial edges of the opening are overlapped with mattress sutures.

**Mayo-Rob·son point** (ma'ō-rob'son) a point just above and to the right of the umbilicus, where tenderness on pressure exists in disease of the pancreas.

**Mayo-Rob·son po·si·tion** (ma'ō-rob'son) a supine position with a thick pad under the loins, causing a marked lordosis in this region; used in operations on the gallbladder.

**Mayo stand** (ma'ō) a removable instrument tray set on a movable stand that is positioned over or adjacent to a surgical site; it provides a place for sterile instruments and supplies used during surgery.

**May-White syn·drome** (mā-whīt) progressive myoclonus epilepsy with lipomas, deafness, and ataxia; probably a familial form of mitochondrial encephalomyopathy.

⌂**ma·zo-** the breast. SEE ALSO masto-. [G. *mazos*]

**Mb** myoglobin.

**M band** SYN M line.

**MBC** maximum breathing capacity.

**MbCO** myoglobin in combination with CO.

**MbO₂** oxymyoglobin.

**mc** for millicurie.

**Mc·Ar·dle dis·ease** (mě-kahr'děl) SYN type 5 glycogenosis.

**Mc·Ar·dle-Schmid-Pear·son dis·ease** (mě-kahr'děl-shmid-pēr'son) SYN type 5 glycogenosis.

**Mc·Bur·ney in·ci·sion** (měk-ber'nē) an incision parallel with the course of the external oblique muscle, one or two inches cephalad to the anterior superior spine of the ilium.

**Mc·Bur·ney point** (měk-ber'nē) a site one-third the distance from the anterior superior iliac spine (ASIS) to the umbilicus that with deep palpation produces rebound tenderness indicating appendicitis. SEE ALSO appendicitis.

**Mc·Bur·ney sign** (měk-ber'nē) tenderness at site two-thirds of the distance between the umbilicus and the anterior-superior iliac spine; seen in appendicitis.

**Mc·Call cul·do·plas·ty pro·ce·dure** (měk-kǎl') method of supporting the vaginal cuff during a vaginal hysterectomy by attaching the uterosacral and cardinal ligaments to the peritoneal surface with suture material that, when tied, draws toward the midline, helping to close off the cul-de-sac.

**Mc·Car·ey-Kauf·mann me·dia** (měk-kar'ē-kawf-mahn) a culture solution used for storage of enucleated eyes for corneal transplantation.

**Mc·Car·thy re·flex·es** (me-kahr'thē) SYN spino-adductor reflex.

**Mc·Cune-Al·bright syn·drome** (měk-kyoon' awl'brīt) polyostotic fibrous dysplasia with irregular brown patches of cutaneous pigmentation and endocrine dysfunction, especially precocious puberty in girls. SEE ALSO pseudohypoparathyroidism. SYN Albright disease, Albright syndrome (1).

**Mc·Don·ald ma·neu·ver** (měk-don'ěld) measurement of uterus from the upper border of the symphysis to a line tangential to the fundus over the abdomen with a tape to determine the height of the uterus; each centimeter approximately corresponds to the gestational age in weeks from 20–34 weeks' gestation.

**Mc·Goon tech·nique** (mě-goon) plastic reconstruction of an incompetent mitral valve, when the incompetence is due to rupture of chordae to the posterior leaflet, by plication of the redundant leaflet.

**MCH** mean corpuscular hemoglobin.

**MCHC** mean corpuscular hemoglobin concentration.

**mCi** millicurie.

**Mc·Ku·sick met·a·phys·e·al dys·pla·sia** (měk-kyoo'sik) SYN cartilage-hair hypoplasia.

**Mc·Mur·ray test** (měk-mur'ē) rotation of the tibia on the femur to determine injury to meniscal structures.

**Mc·Ne·mar test** (měk-ne'mar) a form of chi-square test for matched paired data.

**MCP** metacarpophalangeal.

**Mc·Ro·berts ma·neu·ver** (mǐk-rob'ertz) maneuver to reduce a fetal shoulder dystocia by flexion of the maternal hips.

**M-CSF** macrophage colony-stimulating factor.

**MCV** mean corpuscular volume.

**McVay op·er·a·tion** (měk-vā') repair of inguinal and femoral hernias by suture of the transversus abdominis muscle and its associated fasciae (transversus layer) to the pectineal ligament.

**MD** methyldichloroarsine.

**Md** mendelevium.

**MDF** myocardial depressant factor.

**MDI** metered-dose inhaler.

**MDS** minimum data set.

**ME** myalgic encephalomyelitis.

**mead·ow der·ma·ti·tis, mead·ow grass der·ma·ti·tis** a photoallergic reaction to contact with a plant containing furocoumarin; often occurs after sunbathing. SYN phytophlyctodermatitis.

**Mead·ows syn·drome** (me'dōz) cardiomyopathy developing during pregnancy or the puerperium.

**meal** (mēl) **1.** the food consumed at regular intervals or at a specified time. **2.** ground flour from a grain.

**mean** (mēn) a statistical measurement of central tendency or average of a set of values, usually assumed to be the arithmetic mean unless otherwise specified. [M.E., *mene* fr. O.Fr., fr. L. *medianus*, in the middle]

**mean cal·o·rie** one hundredth of the energy required to raise the temperature of 1 g of water from 0°C to 100°C.

**mean cor·pus·cu·lar he·mo·glo·bin (MCH)** the hemoglobin content of the average red cell, calculated from the hemoglobin therein and the red cell count, in erythrocyte indices.

**mean cor·pus·cu·lar he·mo·glo·bin con·cen·tra·tion (MCHC)** the average hemoglobin concentration in a given volume of packed red cells, calculated from the hemoglobin therein and the hematocrit, in erythrocyte indices.

**mean cor·pus·cu·lar vol·ume (MCV)** the average volume of red cells, calculated from the hematocrit and the red cell count, in erythrocyte indices.

**mea·sles** (mē'zlz) **1.** an acute exanthematous disease, caused by measles virus and marked by fever and other constitutional disturbances, a catarrhal inflammation of the respiratory mucous

**m**
**e**

membranes, and a generalized maculopapular eruption of a dusky red color; the eruption occurs early on the buccal mucous membrane in the form of Koplik spots; incubation period is from 10 to 12 days. SYN morbilli, rubeola. **2.** a disease of swine caused by the presence of *Cysticercus cellulosae*, the measle or larva of *Taenia solium*, the pork tapeworm. **3.** a disease of cattle caused by the presence of *Cysticercus bovis*, the measle or larva of *Taenia saginata*, the beef tapeworm. [D. *maselen*]

**mea·sles vi·rus** an RNA virus of the genus *Morbillivirus* that causes measles and is transmitted via the respiratory tract; possesses hemagglutinating, hemadsorbing, and hemolyzing properties. SYN rubeola virus.

**measurement** determination of a dimension or quantity.

**me·a·tal** (mē-ā′tăl) relating to a meatus.

△**me·a·to-** meatus. [L. *meatus*, passage]

**me·a·to·plas·ty** (mē′ă-tō-plas-tē) plastic surgery of a meatus or canal, e.g., the external auditory meatus or the urethral meatus.

**me·a·tor·rha·phy** (mē-ă-tŏr′ă-fē) closing by suture of the wound made by performing a meatotomy. [meato- + G. *rhaphē*, suture]

**me·a·tos·co·py** (mē-ă-tos′kŏ-pē) inspection, usually instrumental, of any meatus, especially of the meatus of the urethra. [meato- + G. *skopeō*, to view]

**me·a·tot·o·my** (mē-ă-tot′ō-mē) an incision made to enlarge a meatus, e.g., of the urethra or ureter. [meato- + G. *tomē*, incision]

**me·a·tus**, pl. **me·a·tus** (mē-ā′tŭs) a passage or channel, especially the external opening of a canal. [L. a going, a passage, fr. *meo*, pp. *meatus*, to go, pass]

**meatus acusticus** SYN acoustic meatus.

**meatus nasi** SYN nasal meatus.

**me·chan·i·cal** (mĕ-kan′i-kăl) **1.** performed by means of some apparatus, not manually. **2.** explaining phenomena in terms of mechanics. **3.** automatic. [G. *mechanikos*, relating to a machine, fr. *mēchanē*, a contrivance, machine]

**me·chan·i·cal an·ti·dote** a substance that prevents the absorption of a poison.

**me·chan·i·cal dys·men·or·rhea** dysmenorrhea due to obstruction of discharge of menstrual blood, as in cervical stenosis. SYN obstructive dysmenorrhea.

**me·chan·i·cal ef·fi·ci·en·cy** the ratio of work output to work input, expressed as a percentage.

**me·chan·i·cal il·e·us** obstruction of the bowel due to some mechanical cause, e.g., volvulus, gallstone, adhesions.

**me·chan·i·cal jaun·dice** SYN obstructive jaundice.

**me·chan·i·cal vec·tor** a vector that conveys pathogens to a susceptible individual without essential biological development of the pathogens in the vector, as in the transfer of septic organisms on the feet or mouth parts of the housefly.

**me·chan·i·cal ven·ti·la·tion** the use of an automatic mechanical device to perform all or part of the work the body must produce to breathe. SEE ALSO ventilator.

**me·chan·ics** (mĕ-kan′iks) the science of the action of forces in promoting motion or equilibrium. SEE mechanical.

**mech·a·nism** (mek′ă-nizm) **1.** an arrangement or grouping of the parts of anything that has a definite action. **2.** the means by which an effect is obtained. **3.** the chain of events in a particular process. **4.** the detailed description of a reaction pathway. [G. *mēchanē*, a contrivance]

**me·chan·o·e·lec·tric trans·duc·tion** the conversion of mechanical energy to electric energy by sensory cells such as auditory and vestibular hair cells.

**mech·a·no·re·cep·tor** (mek′ă-nō-rē-sep′tŏr) a receptor which responds to mechanical pressure or distortion; e.g., receptors in the carotid sinuses, touch receptors in the skin.

**Mec·kel car·ti·lage** (mek′el) SYN mandibular cartilage.

**Mec·kel di·ver·tic·u·lum** (mek′el) the remains of the yolk stalk of the embryo, which, when persisting abnormally as a blind sac or pouch in the adult, is located on the ileum a short distance above the cecum; it may be attached to the umbilicus and, if the lining includes gastric mucosa, peptic ulceration and bleeding can occur.

**Mec·kel scan** (mek′el) use of technetium-99m pertechnetate in a scan of the gastric mucosa to detect ectopic gastric mucosa in Meckel diverticulum; the pertechnetate anion is secreted by epithelial cells in the gastric mucosa.

**me·co·ni·um** (mē-kō′nē-ŭm) the first intestinal discharges of the newborn infant, greenish in color and consisting of epithelial cells, mucus, and bile. [L., fr. G. *mēkōnion*, dim. of *mēkōn*, poppy]

**me·co·ni·um as·pi·ra·tion** intrauterine aspiration by the fetus of amniotic fluid contaminated by meconium resulting from fetal hypoxic distress.

**me·co·ni·um as·pi·ra·tion syn·drome** SYN fetal aspiration syndrome.

**me·co·ni·um il·e·us** intestinal obstruction in the fetus and newborn following inspissation of meconium and caused by lack of trypsin; associated with cystic fibrosis.

**me·co·ni·um per·i·to·ni·tis** peritonitis caused by intestinal perforation in the fetus or newborn; associated with congenital obstruction or fibrocystic disease of the pancreas.

**me·co·ni·um plug** a plug of thick, inspissated meconium that may cause intestinal obstruction.

**me·di·a** (mē′dē-ă) **1.** SYN tunica media. **2.** plural of medium. [L. fem. of *medius*, middle]

📘**me·di·al** (mē′dē-ăl) relating to the middle or center; nearer to the median or midsagittal plane. See page APP 89. [L. *medialis*, middle]

**me·di·al ar·cu·ate lig·a·ments** one of Haller arches; a tendinous thickening of the psoas fascia that extends from the body of the first lumbar vertebra to its transverse process on either side. A portion of the diaphragm arises from it.

**me·di·al col·lat·er·al lig·a·ment** a broad, flat band attached superiorly to the medial condyle of the femur and inferiorly to the medial condyle of the tibia; stabilizes the knee joint medially, resisting valgus stress. SYN tibial collateral ligament.

**me·di·al cu·ne·i·form bone** the largest of the three cuneiform bones, the medial bone of the distal row of the tarsus, articulating with the intermediate cuneiform, navicular, and first and second metatarsal bones. SYN wedge bone.

**me·di·al epi·con·dy·li·tis** SYN Little League elbow.

**me·di·al fore·brain bun·dle** a fiber system

coursing longitudinally through the lateral zone of the hypothalamus, connecting the latter reciprocally with the midbrain tegmentum and with various components of the limbic system; it also carries fibers from norepinephrine-containing and serotonin-containing cell groups in the brainstem to the hypothalamus and cerebral cortex, as well as dopamine-carrying fibers from the substantia nigra to the caudate nucleus and putamen.

**me·di·al ge·nic·u·late bo·dy** the medial one of a pair of prominent cell groups in the posteroinferior parts of the thalamus; it functions as the last of a series of processing stations along the auditory conduction pathway to the cerebral cortex, receiving the brachium of the inferior colliculus and giving rise to the auditory radiation to the auditory cortex in the superior temporal gyrus.

**med·i·al·i·za·tion** (mēd-ē-al-ĭ-zā′shŭn) an operation to move a part toward the midline, such as the arytenoid cartilage or vocal cord, in vocal cord paralysis.

**me·di·al lig·a·ment** the bundle of fibers strengthening the medial part of the articular capsule of the temporomandibular joint.

**me·di·al med·ul·la·ry la·mi·na of len·ti·form nu·cle·us** a fiber layer separating the medial and lateral segments of the globus pallidus. SYN lamina medullaris medialis nuclei lentiformis [TA].

**me·di·al me·nis·cus** attached to the medial border of the upper articular surface of the tibia.

**me·di·al oc·cip·i·tal ar·tery** one of the terminal branches of the posterior cerebral artery; it is distributed, by several named branches, to the posterior corpus callosum and the medial and superolateral portions of the occipital lobe including the visual cortex.

**me·di·al rec·tus mus·cle** *origin*, medial part of the anulus tendineus communis; *insertion*, medial part of sclera of the eye; *action*, adduction; *nerve supply*, oculomotor. SYN musculus rectus medialis [TA].

**me·di·al vas·tus mus·cle** SYN vastus medialis muscle.

**me·di·an** (mē′dē-an) **1.** central; middle; lying in the midline. **2.** the middle value in a set of measurements; like the mean, a measure of central tendency. [L. *medianus*, middle]

**me·di·an an·te·brach·i·al vein** it begins at the base of the dorsum of the thumb, curves around the radial side, ascends the middle of the forearm, and just below the bend of the elbow divides into the intermediate basilic and intermediate cephalic veins; sometimes it divides lower down, one branch going to the basilic vein, the other to the intermediate vein of the elbow.

**me·di·an ap·er·ture of fourth ven·tri·cle** the large midline opening in the posterior inferior part of the roof of the fourth ventricle, connecting the ventricle with the posterior cerebellomedullary cistern. SYN apertura mediana ventriculi quarti [TA].

**me·di·an ar·tery** *origin*, anterior interosseous; *distribution*, accompanies median nerve to palm; *anastomoses*, branches of superficial palmar arch. SYN arteria mediana, comitant artery of median nerve.

**me·di·an cu·bi·tal vein** passes across the anterior aspect of the elbow from the cephalic vein to the basilic vein; commonly this vein is replaced by intermediate basilic and intermediate cephalic

veins. The median cubital vein is often used for venipuncture.

**me·di·an ef·fec·tive dose (ED₅₀)** SEE effective dose.

**me·di·an groove of tongue** median groove or median longitudinal raphe of tongue; raphe linguae; a slight longitudinal depression running forward on the dorsal surface of the tongue from the foramen cecum.

**me·di·an nerve** formed by the union of medial and lateral roots from the medial and lateral cords of the brachial plexus, respectively; it supplies all the muscles in the anterior compartment of the forearm with the exception of the flexor carpi ulnaris and ulnar half of the flexor digitorum profundus; it passes through the carpal tunnel to supply the thenar muscles (except adductor pollicis and the deep head of flexor pollicis brevis) via its recurrent thenar branch; its sensory fibers are distributed to the skin of the palmar and distal dorsal aspects of the radial 3-1/2 digits and adjacent palm. The median nerve is most commonly injured through compression in carpal tunnel syndrome, resulting in a loss of ability to oppose the thumb ("ape hand") and loss of sensation over the radial portion of the hand. SYN nervus medianus [TA].

⊞**me·di·an plane** a vertical plane through the midline of the body that divides the body into right and left halves. See page APP 88. SYN midsagittal plane.

**me·di·an rhi·nos·co·py** inspection of the roof of the nasal cavity and openings of the posterior ethmoid cells and sphenoidal sinus by means of a long-bladed nasal speculum or nasopharyngoscope.

**me·di·an rhom·boid glos·si·tis** an asymptomatic, ovoid or rhomboid, macular or mamillated, erythematous lesion with papillary atrophy on the dorsum of the tongue just anterior to the circumvallate papillae; thought to represent a persistent tuberculum impar.

**me·di·an sa·cral crest** an unpaired crest formed by the fused spinous processes of the upper four sacral vertebrae.

**me·di·an sa·cral vein** an unpaired vein accompanying the middle sacral artery receiving blood from the sacral venous plexus and emptying into the left common iliac vein.

**me·di·an sec·tion** a cross section obtained by slicing in the median plane, actually or through imaging techniques, the body or any part of the body which occupies or crosses the median plane or by slicing any generally symmetrical anatomic structure, such as a finger or a cell, in its midline. Since actual sectioning the median plane results in a right and a left half, an anatomical median section may be a two-dimensional view of the cut surface on the medial aspect of either half.

**me·di·as·ti·nal** (mē′dē-as-tī′năl) relating to the mediastinum.

**me·di·as·ti·nal em·phy·se·ma** deflection of air, usually from a ruptured emphysematous bleb in the lung, into the mediastinal tissue.

**me·di·as·ti·nal fi·bro·sis** fibrosis that may obstruct the superior vena cava, pulmonary arteries, veins, or bronchi; most common cause is histoplasmosis; less commonly tuberculosis or unknown.

**me·di·as·ti·nal space** SYN mediastinum (2).

**me·di·as·ti·nal veins** several small veins from

**m**
**e**

the mediastinum emptying into the brachiocephalic veins or the superior vena cava.

**me·di·as·ti·ni·tis** (mē'dē-as-ti-nī'tis) inflammation of the cellular tissue of the mediastinum.

**me·di·as·ti·nog·ra·phy** (mē'dē-as-ti-nog'ră-fē)
radiography of the mediastinum. [mediastinum +
G. *graphō*, to write]

**me·di·as·tin·o·per·i·car·di·tis** (me'dē-as'tin-ō-
per'i-kar-dī'tis) inflammation of the pericardium
and of the surrounding mediastinal cellular tissue.

**me·di·as·tin·o·scope** (mē-dē-as'tin'ō-skōp) an
endoscope for inspection of mediastinum through
a suprasternal incision.

**me·di·as·ti·nos·co·py** (mē'dē-as-ti-nos'kŏ-pē)
exploration of the mediastinum through a suprasternal incision, for biopsy of paratracheal lymph
nodes. [mediastinum + G. *skopeō*, to view]

**me·di·as·ti·not·o·my** (mē'dē-as-ti-not'ō-mē) incision into the mediastinum. [mediastinum + G.
*tomē*, incision]

**me·di·as·ti·num** (me'dē-as-tī'nŭm) [TA] **1.** a
septum between two parts of an organ or a cavity. **2.** the median partition of the thoracic cavity,
covered by the mediastinal part of the parietal
pleura and containing all the thoracic viscera and
structures except the lungs. It is divided arbitrarily into two major divisions: a superior mediastinum (mediastinum superius [TA]), which lies
directly superior to a horizontal plane intersecting the sternal angle and approximately the T4–5
intervertebral disk, and an inferior mediastinum
(mediastinum inferius [TA]) inferior to that
plane; the latter is, in turn, subdivided in 3 parts:
a middle mediastinum (mediastinum medium
[TA]), which is coterminous with the pericardial
sac containing the heart, a nearly potential anterior mediastinum (mediastinum anterius [TA])
lying in front, and a posterior mediastinum (mediastinum posterius [TA]) behind, containing the
esophagus, descending aorta, and thoracic duct.
SYN interpleural space, mediastinal space. [Mod.
L. a middle septum, fr. Mediev. L. *mediastinus*,
medial, fr. L. *mediastinus*, a lower servant, fr.
*medius*, middle]

**me·di·as·ti·num tes·tis** [TA] a mass of fibrous
tissue continuous with the tunica albuginea, projecting into the testis from its posterior border.
SYN Highmore body.

**me·di·ate 1.** (mē'dē-it) situated between; intermediate. **2.** (mē'dē-āt) to effect something by means
of an intermediary substance, as in complement-
mediated phagocytosis. [L. *mediatus*, fr. *medio*,
pp. *-atus*, to divide in the middle]

**me·di·ate aus·cul·ta·tion** auscultation performed with the use of a stethoscope.

**me·di·ate per·cus·sion** percussion effected by
the intervention of a finger or a plessimeter between the striking finger or plessor and the part
percussed.

**me·di·a·tor com·plex** co-activation proteins involved in RNA polymerase transcription of DNA
segments.

**med·i·ca·ble** (med'i-kă-bl) treatable, with hope
of a cure.

**Med·i·caid** program established under Title XIX
of the Social Security Act, which provides
health insurance to poor people; it is funded
jointly by the state and federal governments. Formerly known as medical assistance. SEE ALSO
Medicare.

**med·i·cal** (med'i-kăl) **1.** relating to medicine or
the practice of medicine. SYN medicinal (2). **2.**
SYN medicinal (1). [L. *medicalis*, fr *medicus*,
physician]

**med·i·cal as·sis·tant** a person who supports a
physician by performing clerica, administrative,
and routine technical tasks.

**med·i·cal di·a·ther·my** diathermy of mild degree causing no destruction of tissue.

**med·i·cal di·rec·tor** 1) A physician designated
by an EMS system or service to provide medical
control. Advanced level prehospital providers
usually function under the medical license of the
medical director. 2) A physician designated by
an educational program or institution to provide
medical oversight of an EMS education program
or course.

**med·i·cal ge·net·ics** the study of the etiology,
pathogenesis, and natural history of human diseases which are at least partially genetic in origin. Cf. clinical genetics, human genetics.

**med·i·cal psy·chol·o·gy** the branch of psychology concerned with the application of psychologic principles to the practice of medicine; the
application of clinical psychology or clinical
health psychology, usually in a hospital setting.

**med·i·cal rec·ord** SEE record (1).

**med·i·cal tran·scrip·tion·ist** an individual who
performs machine transcription of physician-dic-
tated medical records; a certified medical transcriptionist (CMT) has satisfied the requirements
for certification by the American Association for
Medical Transcription (AAMT).

**Med·i·care** federally managed health insurance
plan covering Americans over age 65 and Amer-
cans under age 65 who have certain disabilities;
established by a 1965 amendment to the Social
Security Act. SEE ALSO Medicaid.

**med·i·cate** (med'i-kāt) **1.** to treat disease by the
giving of drugs. **2.** to impregnate with a medicinal substance. [L. *medico*, pp. *-atus*, to heal]

**med·i·ca·tion** (med-i-kā'shŭn) **1.** the act of medi-
cating. **2.** a medicinal substance, or medicament.

**me·dic·i·nal** (mĕ-dis'i-năl) **1.** relating to medicine having curative properties. SYN medical (2).
**2.** SYN medical (1).

**med·i·cine** (med'i-sin) **1.** a drug. **2.** the art of
preventing, diagnosing, and treating disease; the
science concerned with disease in all its relations. **3.** the study and treatment of general diseases or those affecting the internal parts of the
body, especially those not usually requiring surgical intervention. [L. *medicina*, fr. *medicus*,
physician (see medicus)]

△**med·i·co-** medical. Cf. iatro-. [L. *medicus*, physi-
cian]

**med·i·co·chi·rur·gi·cal** (med'i-kō-kī-rŭr'ji-kăl)
relating to both medicine and surgery, or to both
physicians and surgeons. [medico- G.
*cheirourgia*, surgery]

**med·i·co·le·gal** (med'i-kō-lē'găl) relating to both
medicine and the law. SEE ALSO forensic medicine. [medico- + L. *legalis*, legal]

△**me·dio-, me·di-** middle, median. [L. *medius*]

**me·di·o·car·pal** (mē'dē-ō-kar'păl) SYN midcar-
pal.

**me·di·o·dor·sal** (mē'dē-ō-dōr'săl) relating to the
median plane and the dorsal plane.

**me·di·o·lat·er·al** (mē'dē-ō-lat'er-ăl) relating to
the median plane and a side.

**me·di·o·ne·cro·sis** (mē′dē-ō-ne-krō′sis) necrosis of a tunica media.

**me·di·o·tar·sal am·pu·ta·tion** SYN Chopart amputation.

**Med·i·ter·ra·ne·an ery·the·ma·tous fe·ver** a form of Mediterranean spotted fever that causes skin redness; its course and other symptoms may be similar to those of Mediterranean exanthematous fever. SEE *Rickettsia conorii*.

**Med·i·ter·ra·ne·an ex·an·them·a·tous fe·ver** an affection occurring sporadically in the Mediterranean littoral marked by a severe chill with abrupt rise of temperature, pains in the joints, tonsillitis, diarrhea, vomiting, and, on the third to fifth day, a rash of elevated nonconfluent macules beginning on the thighs and spreading to the entire body; lasts from ten days to two weeks and then disappears by rapid lysis without desquamation; probably caused by *Rickettsia conorii*, like Boutonneuse fever.

**Med·i·ter·ra·ne·an spot·ted fe·ver** tick-borne infection with *Rickettsia conorii* seen in Africa, Europe, the Middle East, and India and known by different names in different areas, e.g., Marseilles fever, Crimean fever, Indian tick typhus, and Kenya fever. Two forms are Mediterranean exanthematous fever, which manifests as skin eruptions, and Mediterranean erythematous fever, which manifests as skin redness. SEE *Rickettsia conorii*.

**me·di·um**, pl. **me·dia** (mē′dē-ŭm, mē′dē-ă) **1.** a means; that through which an action is performed. **2.** a substance through which impulses or impressions are transmitted. **3.** SYN culture medium. **4.** the liquid holding a substance in solution or suspension. [L. neuter of *medius,* middle]

**MED·LARS** Medical Literature Analysis and Retrieval System, a computerized index system of the U.S. National Library of Medicine.

**MED·LINE** [MEDLARS-on-line] a computer-based telephone linkage to MEDLARS for rapid provision of medical bibliographies and other information.

**me·dul·la**, pl. **me·dul·lae** (me-dŭl′ă, me-dŭl′ē) any soft marrow-like structure, especially in the center of a part. SEE ALSO medulla oblongata. SYN substantia medullaris (1). [L. marrow, fr. *medius,* middle]

**me·dul·la of hair shaft** the central axis of some hairs, containing a column of large vacuolated and keratinized cells; the medullary portion is surrounded by the cortex.

**me·dul·la of lymph node** the central portion of a node consisting of cordlike masses of lymphocytes, plasma cells, and macrophages in a stroma of reticular fibers separated by lymph sinuses; it reaches the surface of the node at the hilum.

**me·dul·la ob·lon·ga·ta** [TA] the most caudal subdivision of the brainstem, continuous with the spinal cord, extending from the lower border of the decussation of the pyramid to the pons; its ventral surface resembles that of the spinal cord except for the bilateral prominence of the inferior olive; the dorsal surface of its upper half forms part of the floor of the fourth ventricle. Motor nuclei of the medulla oblongata include the hypoglossal nucleus, the dorsal motor nucleus, inferior salivatory nucleus, and the nucleus ambiguus; sensory nuclei include the nuclei of the posterior column (gracile and cuneate), the cochlear and vestibular nuclei, the mid and caudal

portions of the spinal trigeminal nucleus, and the nucleus of the solitary tract. SEE ALSO medulla. SYN myelencephalon, oblongata.

**me·dul·lar** (med-yul′ăr) SYN medullary.

**med·ul·lary** (med′ŭ-lār-ē, mĕ-dul′er-ē, med′yū-lār-ē) relating to the medulla or marrow. SYN medullar.

**med·ul·lary ar·ter·ies of brain** branches of the cortical arteries that penetrate to and supply the white matter of the cerebrum.

**med·ul·lary car·ci·no·ma** a malignant neoplasm, comparatively soft and brainlike in consistency, that consists chiefly of neoplastic epithelial cells, with only a scant amount of fibrous stroma.

**med·ul·lary car·ci·no·ma of breast** a subtype of breast carcinoma composed of sheets of large epithelial cells surrounded by scant fibrous stroma; it is soft and well circumscribed and has a better prognosis than invasive ductal carcinoma.

**med·ul·lary car·ci·no·ma of thy·roid** a malignant thyroid neoplasm composed of calcitonin producing C-cells and amyloid rich stroma; it may be sporadic or familial; the familial form may be part of the multiple endocrine neoplasia syndrome, type 2A and 2B.

**med·ul·lary cav·i·ty** the marrow cavity in the shaft of a long bone.

**med·ul·lary cone** the tapering lower extremity of the spinal cord. SYN conus medullaris [TA].

**med·ul·la·ry la·mi·nae of thal·am·us** layers of myelinated fibers that appear on transverse sections of the thalamus; the lamina medullaris lateralis [TA] (external medullary lamina) marks the ventral and lateral borders of the thalamus and delimits it from the subthalamus and reticular nucleus of thalamus; the lamina medullaris medialis [TA] (internal medullary lamina) is interposed between the mediodorsal and ventral nuclei of the thalamus and encloses the intralaminar nuclei (centromedian, paracentral, and central lateral nuclei).

**med·ul·lary mem·brane** SYN endosteum.

**med·ul·lary plate** SYN neural plate.

**med·ul·lary pyr·a·mid** SYN renal pyramid.

**med·ul·lary ray** the center of the renal lobule, which has the shape of a small, steep pyramid, consisting of straight tubular parts; these may be either ascending or descending limbs of the nephronic loop or collecting tubules. SYN Ferrein pyramid.

**med·ul·lary space** the central cavity and the cellular intervals between the trabeculae of bone, filled with marrow.

**med·ul·lary sponge kid·ney** cystic disease of the renal pyramids associated with calculus formation and hematuria; differs from cystic disease of the renal medulla in that renal failure does not usually develop.

**med·ul·lary striae of fourth ven·tri·cle** slender fascicles of fibers extending transversely below the ependymal floor of the ventricle from the median sulcus to enter the inferior cerebellar peduncle. They arise from the arcuate nuclei on the ventral surface of the medullary pyramid.

**med·ul·lary stria of thal·a·mus** a narrow, compact fiber bundle that extends along the line of attachment of the roof of the third ventricle to the thalamus on each side and terminates posteriorly in the habenular nucleus. It is composed of fibers

**m**
**e**

originating in the septal area, the anterior perforated substance, the lateral preoptic nucleus, and the medial segment of the globus pallidus.

**med·ul·lary sub·stance 1.** the lipid material present in the myelin sheath of nerve fibers; **2.** medulla of bones and other organs. SYN substantia medullaris (2).

**me·dul·la spi·na·lis** SYN spinal cord.

**med·ul·lat·ed** (med′ŭ-lā-ted) **1.** having a medulla or medullary substance. **2.** SYN myelinated.

**med·ul·lec·to·my** (med-ŭ-lek′tō-mē) excision of any medullary substance. [medulla + G. *ektomē*, excision]

**med·ul·li·za·tion** (med′ŭ-li-zā′shŭn) enlargement of the medullary spaces in rarefying osteitis.

⌂**med·ul·lo-** medulla. Cf. myel-. [L. *medulla*]

**me·dul·lo·ar·thri·tis** (med-ŭ-lō-ar-thrī′tis) inflammation of the cancellous articular extremity of a long bone.

**me·dul·lo·blas·to·ma** (med′ŭ-lō-blas-tō′mă) a tumor consisting of neoplastic cells that resemble the undifferentiated cells of the primitive medullary tube; medulloblastomas are usually located in the vermis of the cerebellum, comprise approximately 3% of all intracranial neoplasms, and occur most frequently in children.

**me·dul·lo·ep·i·the·li·o·ma** (me′dŭ-lō-ep′ĭ-thē-lē-ō′mă) a rare, primitive, rapidly growing intracranial neoplasm thought to originate from the cells of the embryonic medullary canal. [medullo- + epithelium + -oma, tumor]

**Me·du·sa head** (me-doo′sa) SYN caput medusae.

**Mees line** (māz) a horizontal white band of the nails seen in chronic arsenical poisoning, and occasionally in leprosy.

⌂**me·ga- 1.** large, oversize; opposite of micro-. SEE ALSO macro-, megalo-. **2.** prefix used in the SI and metric systems to signify one million ($10^6$). [G. *megas*, big]

**meg·a·bac·te·ri·um** (meg′ă-bak-tēr′ē-ŭm) a bacterium of unusually large size.

**me·ga·blad·der** (meg′ă-blad-er) SYN megacystis.

**meg·a·ce·phal·ic** (meg′ă-se-fal′ik) relating to or characterized by megacephaly. SYN macrocephalic, macrocephalous, megacephalous.

**meg·a·ceph·a·lous** (meg-ă-sef′ă-lŭs) SYN megacephalic.

**meg·a·ceph·a·ly** (meg-ă-sef′ă-lē) a condition, either congenital or acquired, in which the head is abnormally large; usually applied to an adult skull with a capacity of over 1450 ml. SYN macrocephaly, macrocephalia, megalocephaly, megalocephalia. [mega- + G. *kephalē*, head]

**meg·a·co·lon** (meg′ă-kō′lon) a condition of extreme dilation and hypertrophy of the colon.

**meg·a·cy·cle** (meg′ă-sī-kl) one million cycles per second.

**meg·a·cys·tic syn·drome** a combination of a large smooth thin-walled bladder, vesicoureteral regurgitation, and dilated ureters.

**meg·a·cys·tis** (meg′ă-sis-tis) pathologically large bladder in children. SYN megabladder, megalocystis. [mega- + *kystis*, bladder]

**meg·a·dac·ty·ly, meg·a·dac·tyl·ia, meg·a·dac·tyl·ism** (meg-ă-dak′ti-lē, meg-ă-dak-til′ē-ă) condition characterized by enlargement of one or more digits (fingers or toes). SYN dactylomegaly. [mega- + G. *daktylos*, digit]

**meg·a·don·tism** (meg-ă-don′tizm) SYN macrodontia.

**meg·a·e·soph·a·gus** (meg′ă-ē-sof′ă-gŭs) great enlargement of the lower portion of the esophagus, as seen in patients with achalasia and Chagas disease.

**meg·a·hertz (MHz)** (meg′ă-hertz) one million hertz.

**meg·a·kar·y·o·blast** (meg-ă-kar′ē-ō-blast) the precursor of a megakaryocyte.

**meg·a·kar·y·o·cyte** (meg-ă-kar′ē-ō-sīt) a large cell with a multilobed nucleus. megakaryocytes are normally present in bone marrow, not in the circulating blood, and give rise to blood platelets. SYN megalokaryocyte. [mega- + G. *karyon*, nut (nucleus), + *kytos*, hollow vessel (cell)]

**megakaryocyte growth and development factor** SYN thrombopoietin.

**meg·a·kar·y·o·cyt·ic leu·ke·mia** an unusual form of myelopoietic disease that is characterized by uncontrolled proliferation of megakaryocytes in the bone marrow, and sometimes by the presence of megakaryocytes in the blood.

**meg·al·gia** (meg-al′jē-ă) very severe pain. [mega- + G. *algos*, pain]

⌂**me·ga·lo-, me·gal-** large; opposite of micro-. SEE ALSO macro-, mega-. [G. *megas* (*megal-*)]

**meg·a·lo·blast** (meg′ă-lō-blast) a large, nucleated, embryonic type of cell that is a precursor of erythrocytes in an abnormal erythropoietic process observed in pernicious anemia; a megaloblast's four stages of development are as follows: 1) promegaloblast, 2) basophilic megaloblast, 3) polychromatic megaloblast, 4) orthochromatic megaloblast. SEE ALSO erythroblast. [megalo- + G. *blastos*, + germ, sprout]

**meg·a·lo·blas·tic a·ne·mia** any anemia in which there is a predominant number of megaloblastic erythroblasts, and relatively few normoblasts, among the hyperplastic erythroid cells in the bone marrow (as in pernicious anemia).

**meg·a·lo·car·dia** (meg′ă-lō-kar′dē-ă) SYN cardiomegaly. [megalo- + G. *kardia*, heart]

**meg·a·lo·ceph·a·ly, meg·a·lo·ce·pha·lia** (meg′ă-lō-sef′ă-lē, meg′ă-lō-sĕ-fā′lē-ă) SYN megacephaly.

**meg·a·lo·chei·ria, meg·a·lo·chi·ria** (meg′ă-lō-kī′rē-ă) SYN macrocheiria. [megalo- + G. *cheir*, hand]

**meg·a·lo·cor·nea** (meg′ă-lō-kōr′nē-ă) SYN keratoglobus.

**meg·a·lo·cys·tis** (meg′ă-lō-sis′tis) SYN megacystis. [megalo- + G. *kystis*, bladder]

**meg·a·lo·cyte** (meg′ă-lō-sīt) a large (10 to 20 μm) nonnucleated red blood cell. [megalo- + G. *kytos*, cell]

**meg·a·lo·don·tia** (meg′ă-lō-don′shē-ă) SYN macrodontia.

**meg·a·lo·en·ce·phal·ic** (meg′ă-lō-en′sě-fal′ik) denoting an abnormally large brain.

**meg·a·lo·en·ceph·a·lon** (meg′ă-lō-en-sef′ă-lon) an abnormally large brain. [megalo- + G. *enkephalos*, brain]

**meg·a·lo·en·ceph·a·ly** (meg′ă-lō-en-sef′ă-lē) abnormal largeness of the brain. [megalo- + G. *enkephalon*, brain]

**meg·a·lo·en·ter·on** (meg′ă-lō-en′ter-on) abnormal largeness of the intestine. SYN enteromegaly, enteromegalia. [megalo- + G. *enteron*, intestine]

**meg·a·lo·gas·tria** (meg′ă-lō-gas′trē-ă) abnormally large size of the stomach. [megalo- + G. *gastēr*, stomach]

**meg·a·lo·glos·sia** (meg′ă-lō-glos′sē-ă) SYN macroglossia. [megalo- + G. *glōssa*, tongue]

**meg·a·lo·he·pat·ia** (meg′ă-lo-he-pat′ē-ă) SYN hepatomegaly.

**meg·a·lo·kar·y·o·cyte** (meg′ă-lō-kar′ē-ō-sīt) SYN megakaryocyte.

**meg·a·lo·ma·nia** (meg′ă-lō-mā′nē-ă) **1.** a delusion of greatness; belief that one is Christ, God, Napoleon, a prince, ace athlete in all divisions of sport, etc. **2.** morbid verbalized overevaluation of oneself or of some aspect of oneself. [megalo- + G. *mania*, frenzy]

**meg·a·lo·ma·ni·ac** (meg′ă-lō-mā′nē-ak) a person exhibiting megalomania.

**meg·a·lo·me·lia** (meg′ă-lō-mē′lē-ă) SYN macromelia.

**meg·a·loph·thal·mos** (meg′ă-lof-thal′mos) abnormal largeness of the eyeball. [megalo- + G. *ophthalmos*, eye]

**meg·a·lo·po·dia** (meg′ă-lō-pō′dē-ă) SYN macropodia. [megalo- + G. *pous*, foot]

**meg·a·lo·sple·nia** (meg′ă-lō-splē′nē-ă) SYN splenomegaly.

**meg·a·lo·syn·dac·ty·ly, meg·a·lo·syn·dac·tyl·ia** (meg′ă-lō-sin-dak′ti-lē, meg′ă-lō-sin-dak-til′ē-ă) condition of webbed or fused fingers or toes of large size. [megalo- + G. *syn*, together, + *daktylos*, finger]

**meg·a·lo·u·re·ter** (meg′ă-lō-yu-rē′ter) an enlarged, dilated ureter.

**△-meg·aly** large. [G. *megas (megal-)*]

**me·ga·oe·so·pha·gus [Br.]** SEE megaesophagus.

**megapoietin** (meg′ă-poy′ĕ-tin) SYN thrombopoietin. [mega- + G. *poiētēs*, maker, + -in]

**meg·a·rec·tum** (meg-ă-rek′tŭm) extreme dilation of the rectum.

**meg·a·volt** (meg′ă-vōlt) one million volts.

**mei·bo·mi·an** (mī-bō′mē-an) attributed to or described by Meibom.

**mei·bo·mi·an cyst** (mī-bō′mē-ăn) SYN chalazion.

**mei·bo·mi·an glands** (mī-bō′mē-ăn) SYN tarsal glands.

**mei·bo·mi·tis, mei·bo·mi·a·ni·tis** (mī′bō-mī′tis, mī-bō′mē-ă-nī′tis) inflammation of the meibomian glands.

**Mei·ge dis·ease** (mezh′ĕ) autosomal dominant lymphedema with onset at about the age of puberty.

**Meigs syn·drome** (megz) fibromyoma of the ovary associated with hydroperitoneum and hydrothorax.

**△meio-** for words beginning thus and not found here, see mio-.

**mei·o·sis** (mī-ō′sis) a special process of cell division comprising two nuclear divisions in rapid succession that result in four gametocytes, each containing half the number of chromosomes found in somatic cells. [G. *meiōsis*, a lessening]

**mei·ot·ic** (mī-ot′ik) pertaining to meiosis.

**Meis·cher syn·drome** (mī′sher) SYN cheilitis granulomatosa.

**Meiss·ner cor·pus·cle** (mīs′ner) SYN tactile corpuscle.

**△mel-, me·lo-** **1.** limb. [G. *melos*] **2.** a cheek. [G. *mēlon*] **3.** honey, sugar. SEE ALSO meli-. [L. *mel, mellis*, G. *meli, melitos*] **4.** sheep. [G. *mēlon*]

**me·lae·na [Br.]** SEE melena.

**me·lag·ra** (mĕ-lag′ră) rheumatic or myalgic pains in the arms or legs. [G. *melos*, limb, + *agra*, seizure]

**me·lal·gia** (mĕ-lal′jē-ă) pain in a limb; specifi-cally, burning pain in the feet extending up the leg and even to the thigh. [G. *melos*, a limb, + *algos*, pain]

**△mel·an-, mel·an·o-** black, extreme darkness of hue. [G. *melas*]

**mel·an·cho·lia** (mel-an-kō′lē-ă) **1.** a severe form of depression marked by anhedonia, insomnia, psychomotor changes, and guilt. **2.** a symptom occurring in other conditions, marked by depression of spirits and by a sluggish and painful process of thought. SYN melancholy. [melan- + G. *cholē*, bile. See humoral *doctrine*]

**mel·an·chol·ic** (mel-an-kol′ik) **1.** relating to or characteristic of melancholia. **2.** denoting a temperament characterized by irritability and a pessimistic outlook. **3.** a person who is exhibiting melancholia.

**mel·an·choly** (mel′an-kol-ē) SYN melancholia.

**mel·an·e·de·ma** (mel′an-e-dē′mă) SYN anthracosis. [melan- + G. *oidēma*, swelling]

**mel·a·nif·er·ous** (mel-ă-nif′er-ŭs) containing melanin or other black pigment. [melan- (melanin) + L. *ferro*, to carry]

**mel·a·nin** (mel′ă-nin) any of the dark brown to black pigments that occur in the skin, hair, pigmented coat of the retina, and medulla and zona reticularis of the adrenal gland. [G. *melas (melan-)*, black]

**mel·a·nism** (mel′ă-nizm) unusually marked, diffuse melanin pigmentation of body hair and skin (usually not affecting the iris). SEE ALSO melanosis.

**△melano-** SEE melan-.

**mel·a·no·ac·an·tho·ma** (mel′ă-nō-ak-an-thō′mă) a seborrheic keratosis with melanin pigmentation associated with proliferation of intraepidermal melanocytes. [melano- + G. *akantha*, thorn, + suffix -ōma, tumor]

**mel·a·no·blast** (mel′ă-nō-blast) a cell derived from the neural crest, which matures into a melanocyte. [melano- + G. *blastos*, germ, sprout]

**mel·a·no·cyte** (mel′ă-nō-sīt) a pigment-producing cell located in the basal layer of the epidermis with branching processes by means of which melanosomes are transferred to epidermal cells, resulting in pigmentation of the epidermis. [melano- + G. *kytos*, cell]

**mel·a·no·cyte-stim·u·lat·ing hor·mone** SYN melanotropin.

**mel·a·no·cy·to·ma** (mel′ă-nō-sī-tō′mă) **1.** a pigmented tumor of the uveal stroma. **2.** usually benign melanoma of the optic disk, appearing in markedly pigmented individuals as a small deeply pigmented tumor at the edge of the disk, sometimes extending into the retina and choroid. [megalo- + cyto- + G. -oma; tumor]

**mel·a·no·der·ma** (mel′ă-nō-der′mă) **1.** an abnormal darkening of the skin by deposition of excess melanin. **2.** hyperpigmentation of the skin by melanin or deposition of dark metallic substances such as silver and iron. [melano- + G. *derma*, skin]

**mel·a·no·der·ma·ti·tis** (mel′ă-nō-der-mă-tī′tis) excessive deposit of melanin in an area of dermatitis.

**mel·a·no·der·mic** (mel′ă-nō-der′mik) relating to or marked by melanoderma.

**mel·a·no·gen** (mĕ-lan′ō-jen, mel′ă-nō-jen) a colorless substance that may be converted into melanin. [melanin + G. -gen, producing]

**mel·a·no·gen·e·sis** (mel′ă-nō-jen′ĕ-sis) formation of melanin. [melanin + G. *genesis,* production]

**mel•a•no•glos•sia** (mel'ă-nō-glos'ē-ă) SYN black tongue. [melano- + G. *glōssa,* tongue]

**mel•a•noid** (mel'ă-noyd) a dark pigment, resembling melanin, formed from glucosamines in chitin.

**mel•a•no•leu•ko•der•ma** (mel'ă-nō-loo-kō-der'mă) marbled, or marmorated, skin. [melano- + G. *leukos,* white, + *derma,* skin]

**mel•a•no•leu•ko•der•ma col•li** SYN syphilitic leukoderma.

**mel•an•o•li•ber•in** (mel'ă-nō-lib'er-in) a hexapeptide similar to oxytocin; it stimulates the release of melanotropin. SYN melanotropin-releasing factor, melanotropin-releasing hormone. [melanotropin + L. *libero,* to free, + -in]

**mel•a•no•ma** (mel'ă-nō'mă) a malignant neoplasm, derived from cells that are capable of forming melanin, arising most commonly in the skin or in the eye, and, rarely, in the mucous membranes of the genitalia, anus, oral cavity, or other sites; occurs mostly in adults and may originate *de novo* or from a pigmented nevus or lentigo maligna. Melanomas frequently metastasize widely; regional lymph nodes, skin, liver, lungs, and brain are likely to be involved. SYN malignant melanoma. [melano- + G. *-ōma,* tumor]

**mel•a•no•ma•to•sis** (mel'ă-nō-mă-tō'sis) a condition characterized by numerous, widespread lesions of melanoma. [melanoma + G. *-osis,* condition]

**mel•a•no•nych•ia** (mel'ă-nō-nik'ē-ă) black pigmentation of the nails. [melano- + G. *onyx* (*onych*-), nail]

**mel•a•no•phage** (mel'ă-nō-fāj, mĕ-lan'ō-fāj) a histiocyte that has phagocytized melanin. [melano- + G. *phagō,* to eat]

**mel•a•no•pla•kia** (mel'ă-nō-plā'kē-ă) the occurrence of pigmented patches on the tongue and buccal mucous membrane. [melano- + G. *plax,* plate, plaque]

**mel•a•no•sis** (mel-ă-nō'sis) abnormal dark brown or brown-black pigmentation of various tissues or organs, as the result of melanin or, in some situations, other substances that resemble melanin to varying degrees; e.g., melanosis of the skin may occur in widespread metastatic melanoma, sunburn, during pregnancy, and as a result of chronic infections. [melano- + G. *-osis,* condition]

**mel•a•no•sis co•li** melanosis of the large intestinal mucosa due to accumulation of pigment of uncertain composition within macrophages in the lamina propria.

**mel•a•no•some** (mel'ă-nō-sōm) the generally oval pigment granule (0.2 by 0.6 μm) produced by melanocytes. [melano- + G. *sōma,* body]

**mel•an•o•sta•tin** inhibits synthesis and release of melanotropin. SYN melanotropin release-inhibiting hormone. [melanotropin + G. *states,* stationary, + -in]

**mel•a•not•ic** (mel'ă-not'ik) **1.** pertaining to the presence, normal or pathologic, of melanin. **2.** relating to or characterized by melanosis.

**mel•a•not•ic car•ci•no•ma** obsolete term for melanoma.

**mel•a•not•ic neu•ro•ec•to•der•mal tu•mor of in•fan•cy** a benign neoplasm of neuroectodermal origin that most often involves the anterior max-

illa of infants in the first year of life. It presents clinically as a rapidly growing blue-black lesion producing a destructive radiolucency; histologically, it is characterized by small, round, undifferentiated tumor cells interspersed with larger polyhedral melanin-producing cells arranged in an alveolar configuration.

**mel•a•no•troph** (mel'ă-nō-trōf) a cell of the intermediate lobe of the hypophysis that produces melanotropin. [melano- + G. *trophē,* nourishment]

**mel•a•no•tro•phin** (mel'ă-nō-trō'fin) SYN melanotropin. [melano- + G. *trophē,* nourishment, + -in]

**me•la•no•tro•pin** (mel'ă-nō-trōp-in) a polypeptide hormone secreted by the intermediate lobe of the hypophysis in humans (in neurohypophysis in certain other species) which causes dispersion of melanin by melanophores, resulting in darkening of the skin, presumably by promoting melanin synthesis; this effect is readily demonstated in some lower vertebrates, such as frogs and fish; α-melanotropin is an *N*-acetylated peptide with 13 amino acids; β-melanotropin has 22 amino acids. SYN melanocyte-stimulating hormone, melanotrophin.

**melanotropin release-inhibiting hormone (MIH)** SYN melanostatin.

**mel•a•no•tro•pin-re•leas•ing fac•tor** SYN melanoliberin.

**mel•a•no•tro•pin-re•leas•ing hor•mone (MRH)** SYN melanoliberin.

**mel•a•nu•ria** (mel-ă-nyu'rē-ă) the excretion of urine of a dark color, resulting from the presence of melanin or other pigments or from the action of phenol and other coal tar derivatives. [melano- + G. *ouron,* urine]

**mel•a•nu•ric** (mel-ă-nyu'rik) pertaining to or characterized by melanuria.

**MELAS** *m*itochondrial myopathy, *e*ncephalopathy, *l*actic *a*cidosis, and *s*trokelike episodes. One of the mitochondrial disorders, this condition is usually hereditary, with a mutation at the mitochondrial genome at locus 3243.

**me•las•ma** (mĕ-laz'mă) a patchy or generalized pigmentation of the skin. SEE ALSO chloasma. SYN mask of pregnancy. [G. a black color, a black spot]

**me•las•ma grav•i•dar•um** chloasma occurring in pregnancy.

**mel•a•ton•in** (mel-ă-tōn'in) a substance formed by the pineal gland that appears to depress gonadal function; a precursor is serotonin, melatonin is rapidly metabolized and is taken up by all tissues; it is involved in circadian rhythms. [melanophore + G. *tonos,* stretching, + -in]

**me•le•na** (me-lē'nă) passage of dark-colored, tarry stools, due to the presence of blood altered by the intestinal juices. Cf. hematochezia. [G. *melaina,* fem. of *melas,* black]

**Me•le•ney ul•cer** (mĕ-lē'nē) undermining ulcer of the skin and subcutaneous tissues caused by a synergistic infection by microaerophilic nonhemolytic streptococci and aerobic hemolytic staphylococci.

△**me•li-** honey, sugar. SEE ALSO mel- (3). [G. *meli*]

**me•li•tis** (mē-lī'tis) inflammation of the cheek. [G. *mēlon,* cheek, + *-itis,* inflammation]

**Mel•nick-Need•les os•te•o•dys•plas•ty** (mel'nik-nēd'lz) a generalized skeletal dysplasia with prominent forehead and small mandible; radiographically, there are irregular ribbonlike constrictions of the ribs and tubular bones; probably X-linked. Autosomal dominant and recessive inheritance have also been suggested. SYN osteodysplasty.

**mel·o·plas·ty** (mel′ō-plas-tē) plastic surgery of the cheek. [melo- + G. *plastos*, formed]

**mel·o·rhe·os·to·sis** (mel′ō-rē-os-tō′sis) rheostosis confined to the long bones. [G. *melos*, limb, + *rheos*, stream, + *osteon*, bone, + -*ōsis*]

**me·lo·tia** (me-lō′shē-ă) congenital displacement of the auricle onto the cheek. [G. *mēlon*, cheek, + *ous*, ear]

**melt** denature, used to describe RNA polymerase action in decoupling DNA base pairs.

**melt·ing point (Tm) 1.** the temperature at which a solid becomes a liquid; **2.** the temperature at which 50% of a macromolecule becomes denatured.

**Melt·zer law** (melt′zĕr) all living functions are continually controlled by two opposite forces: augmentation or action on the one hand, and inhibition on the other.

**mem·ber** SYN limb (1). [L. *membrum*]

**mem·bra** (mem′bră) [TA] plural of membrum. [L.]

**mem·bra·na,** gen. and pl. **mem·bra·nae** (mem-brā′nă, mem-brā′nē) [TA] SYN biomembrane. [L.]

**mem·bra·na ad·ven·ti·tia** SYN decidua capsularis.

**mem·bra·na de·cid·u·a** SYN deciduous membrane.

**mem·bra·na pu·pil·la·ris** [TA] SYN pupillary membrane.

**mem·bra·na re·tic·u·la·ris** [TA] SYN reticular membrane.

**mem·bra·na se·ro·sa 1.** SYN serosa, chorion. **2.** SYN serosa (2).

**mem·bra·na syn·o·vi·a·lis** [TA] SYN synovial membrane.

**mem·bra·na tec·to·ria duc·tus co·chle·a·ris** [TA] SYN tectorial membrane of cochlear duct.

**mem·bra·na tym·pa·ni** [TA] SYN tympanic membrane.

**mem·bra·na tym·pa·ni se·cun·dar·ia** [TA] SYN secondary tympanic membrane.

**mem·bra·na vit·el·li·na 1.** the membrane enveloping the yolk; specifically, the thickened cell membrane of large-yolked oocyte. SYN ovular membrane. **2.** sometimes used to designate the zona pellucida of a mammalian oocyte. SYN yolk membrane.

**mem·bra·na vi·trea** [TA] SYN posterior limiting layer of cornea.

**mem·brane** (mem′brān) **1.** a thin sheet or layer of pliable tissue, serving as a covering or envelope, the lining of a cavity, a partition or septum, or a connection between two structures. **2.** SYN biomembrane. [L. *membrana*, a skin or membrane that covers parts of the body, fr. *membrum*, a member]

**mem·brane bone** a bone that develops embryologically within a membrane of vascularized primordial mesenchymal tissue without prior formation of cartilage.

**mem·brane-coat·ing gran·ule** SYN keratinosome.

**mem·brane ex·pan·sion the·o·ry** that adsorption of anesthetics into membranes so alters membrane volume and/or configuration that

membrane function is affected in such a way as to produce anesthesia.

**mem·brane po·ten·tial** the potential inside a cell membrane, measured relative to the fluid just outside; it is negative under resting conditions and becomes positive during an action potential.

**mem·brane rup·ture** rupture of the amnionic sac allowing the amnionic fluid to escape through the vagina.

**mem·brane strip·ping** separation of gestational membranes from the lower uterine segment by insertion of a finger through the cervical os, to initiate the Ferguson reflex or prostaglandin release from the decidua and hasten labor.

**mem·bra·ni·form** (mem-brā′ni-fōrm) of the appearance or character of a membrane. SYN membranoid.

**mem·bra·no·car·ti·lag·i·nous** (mem′bră-nō-kar-ti-laj′i-nŭs) **1.** partly membranous and partly cartilaginous. **2.** derived from both a mesenchymal membrane and cartilage; denoting certain bones.

**mem·bra·noid** (mem′bră-noyd) SYN membraniform.

**mem·bra·no·pro·lif·er·a·tive glo·mer·u·lo·ne·phri·tis** chronic glomerulonephritis characterized by mesangial cell proliferation, increased lobular separation of glomeruli, thickening of glomerular capillary walls and increased mesangial matrix, and low serum levels of complement; occurs mainly in older children, with a variably slow progressive course, episodes of hematuria or edema, and hypertension. SYN lobular glomerulonephritis.

**mem·bra·nous** (mem′bră-nŭs) relating to or of the form of a membrane.

**mem·bra·nous am·pul·lae of the sem·i·cir·cu·lar ducts** a nearly spherical enlargement of one end of each of the three semicircular ducts, anterior, posterior, and lateral, where they connect with the utricle. Each contains a neuroepithelial crista ampullaris. SYN ampulla membranacea.

**mem·bra·nous cat·a·ract** a secondary cataract composed of the remains of the thickened capsule and degenerated lens fibers.

**mem·bra·nous dys·men·or·rhea** dysmenorrhea accompanied by an exfoliation of the menstrual decidua.

**mem·bra·nous glo·mer·u·lo·ne·phri·tis** glomerulonephritis characterized by diffuse thickening of glomerular capillary basement membranes, due in part to subepithelial deposits of immunoglobulins separated by spikes of basement membrane material, and clinically by an insidious onset of the nephrotic syndrome and failure of disappearance of proteinuria; the disease is most commonly idiopathic but may be secondary to malignant tumors, drugs, infections, or systemic lupus erythematosus.

**mem·bra·nous lab·y·rinth** a complex arrangement of communicating membranous canaliculi and sacs, filled with endolymph and surrounded by perilymph, suspended within the cavity of the bony labyrinth; its chief divisions are the cochlear labyrinth and the vestibular labyrinth.

**mem·bra·nous lar·yn·gi·tis** a form in which there is a pseudomembranous exudate on the vocal cords.

**mem·bra·nous os·si·fi·ca·tion** intramembranous ossification, development of osseous tissue

m
e

within mesenchymal tissue without prior cartilage formation, such as occurs in the frontal and
parietal bones.

**mem·brum**, pl. **mem·bra** (mem′brŭm, mem′bră)
a limb; a member. [L. member]

**mem·o·ry** (mem′ŏ-rē) **1.** general term for the recollection of that which was once experienced or
learned. **2.** the mental information processing
system that receives (registers), modifies, stores,
and retrieves informational stimuli; composed of
three stages: encoding, storage, and retrieval. [L.
*memoria*]

**mem·o·ry B cells** B lymphocytes that mediate
immunologic memory; these allow for enhanced
immunologic reaction when an immunologically
competent organism is reexposed to an antigen.

**mem·ory T cells** T lymphoctyes that mediate
immunologic memory; these allow for enhanced
immunologic reaction when an immunologically
competent organism is reexposed to an antigen.

**MEN** multiple endocrine neoplasia.

**MEN1** multiple endocrine neoplasia 1.

**men·ac·me** (me-nak′mē) the period of menstrual
activity in a woman's life. [G. *mēn*, month, +
*akmē*, prime]

**Me·nan·gle vi·rus** (men′ang-ĕl) a virus of the
family Paramyxoviridae causing infection in
pigs, humans, and fruit bats in Australia; human
infection has resulted in an influenzalike illness
with rash. [named after the location in Australia
of the laboratory where it was first isolated]

**men·a·quin·one-6** hexaprenylmenaquinone;
prenylmenaquinone-6; 2-methyl-3-hexaprenyl-
1,4-naphthoquinone; isolated from putrified fish
meal; potency is about 60% of that of phylloquinone (vitamin $K_1$). SYN vitamin $K_2$, vitamin
$K_2(30)$.

**men·ar·che** (me-nar′kē) establishment of the
menstrual function; the time of the first menstrual period. [G. *mēn*, month, + *archē*, begin-
ning]

**Men·del-Bech·te·rew re·flex** (men′del-bek-ter′
yev) SYN Bechterew-Mendel reflex.

**Men·de·lé·eff law** (men′de-lā′ĕf) the properties
of elements are periodical functions of their
atomic weights; i.e., if the elements are arranged
in the order of their atomic weights, every element in the series will be related in respect to its
properties to the eighth in order before or after it.

**men·de·le·vi·um (Md)** (men-dĕ-lē′vē-ŭm) an element, atomic no. 101, atomic wt. 258.1, prepared in 1955 by bombardment of einsteinium
with alpha particles. [*D. Mendeléeff*]

**Men·del first law** (men′dĕl) SYN law of segregation.

**men·de·li·an** (men-dē′lē-ăn) attributed to or described by Gregor Mendel; usually referring to
the behavior and the mechanism of the genetic
transmission of single-locus traits.

**men·de·li·an in·her·i·tance** (men-dē′lē-ăn) inheritance in which stable and undecomposable
characters controlled entirely or overwhelmingly
by a single genetic locus are transmitted over
many generations. SEE law of segregation, law of
independent assortment.

**Men·de·li·an In·her·i·tance in Man (MIM)** a
standard, comprehensive, regularly updated reference source for traits in humans that have been
shown to be mendelian or that are thought on
reasonable grounds to be so. Each entry has a
six-digit catalog number. Those securely estab-

lished (by molecular biology or by extensive
clinical studies) are marked with an asterisk.

**Men·del in·step re·flex** (men′dĕl) the foot being
firmly supported on its inner side, a sharp tap on
the dorsal tendons causes extension of the second
to the fifth toes.

**Men·del second law** (men′dĕl) SYN law of independent assortment.

**Men·del·sohn ma·neu·ver** (men-dĕl-sŏn) during a swallow, maintenance of the larynx for a
few seconds at the highest position in the neck by
voluntary muscular contraction. This laryngeal
elevation results in wider and longer esophageal
opening, and is a therapeutic technique for management of swallowing disorders.

**Mé·né·trier dis·ease, Mé·né·trier syn·drome**
(mā-nā-trē-ār′, mā-nā-trē-ār′) gastric mucosal hyperplasia, either mucoid or glandular; the latter
type may be associated with the Zollinger-
Ellison syndrome.

**Men·ge pes·sa·ry** (meng′gĕ) a ring pessary with
a central horizontal bar into which a detachable
handle is inserted.

**Mé·ni·è·re dis·ease, Mé·ni·è·re syn·drome**
(měn-yer′, měn-yer′) an affection characterized
clinically by vertigo, nausea, vomiting, tinnitus,
and progressive hearing loss due to hydrops of
the endolymphatic duct. SYN auditory vertigo,
labyrinthine vertigo.

**me·nin·ge·al** (mě-nin′jē-ăl, men′in-jē′ăl) relating
to the meninges.

**me·nin·ge·al veins** accompany the meningeal arteries; they communicate with venous sinuses
and diploic veins and drain into regional veins
outside the cranial vault.

**me·nin·ge·or·rha·phy** (mě-nin′jē-ōr′ă-fē) suture
of the cranial or spinal meninges or of any membrane. [G. *mēninx* (*mēning*-), membrane, + *rhaphē*, suture]

**me·nin·ges** (mě-nin′jēz) plural of meninx.

**me·nin·gi·o·ma** (mě-nin′jē-ō′mă) a benign, encapsulated neoplasm of arachnoidal origin, occurring most frequently in adults; most frequent
form consists of elongated, fusiform cells in
whorls and pseudolobules with psammoma bodies frequently present; meningiomas tend to occur along the superior sagittal sinus, along the
sphenoid ridge, or in the vicinity of the optic
chiasm; in addition to meningothelial meningioma, angiomatous, chondromatous, osteomatous,
lipomatous, melanotic, fibroblastic and transitional varieties are recognized. [mening- + G.
-*oma*, tumor]

**me·nin·gism** (men′in-jizm, mě-nin′jizm) a condition in which the symptoms simulate meningitis,
but in which no actual inflammation of these
membranes is present.

**men·in·git·ic** (men′in-jit′ik) relating to or characterized by meningitis.

**men·in·git·ic streak** a line of redness resulting
from drawing a point across the skin, especially
notable in cases of meningitis. SYN Trousseau
spot.

**men·in·gi·tis**, pl. **men·in·git·i·des** (men-in-jī′
tis, men-in-jit′i-dēz; men-in-jit′i-dēz) inflammation of the membranes of the brain or spinal cord.
SEE ALSO arachnoiditis, leptomeningitis. SYN cerebrospinal meningitis. [mening- + G. *itis*, in-
flammation]

⌂**me·nin·go-, me·ning-** the meninges. [G. *mēninx*,
membrane]

**me•nin•go•cele** (men′ing-gŏ-sēl) protrusion of the membranes of the brain or spinal cord through a defect in the skull or vertebral column. [meningo- + G. *kēlē,* tumor]

**me•nin•go•coc•cal men•in•gi•tis** an acute infectious disease affecting children and young adults, caused by *Neisseria meningitidis;* characterized by nasopharyngeal catarrh, headache, vomiting, convulsions, stiffness in the neck (nuchal rigidity), photophobia, constipation, cutaneous hyperesthesia, a purpuric or herpetic eruption, and the presence of Kernig sign. Fulminant form may cause Waterhouse-Friderichsen syndrome.

**me•nin•go•coc•ce•mia** (mĕ-ning′gō-kok-sē′mē-ă) presence of meningococci (*N. meningitidis*) in the circulating blood.

**me•nin•go•coc•cus**, pl. **me•nin•go•coc•ci** (mĕ-ning′gō-kok′ŭs, mĕ-ning′gō-kok′sī) SYN *Neisseria meningitidis.* [meningo- + G. *kokkos,* berry]

**me•nin•go•cor•ti•cal** (mĕ-ning′gō-kōr′ti-kăl) relating to the meninges and the cortex of the brain.

**me•nin•go•cyte** (mĕ-ning′gō-sīt) a mesenchymal epithelial cell of the subarachnoid space; it may become a macrophage. [meningo- + G. *kytos,* cell]

**me•nin•go•en•ceph•a•li•tis** (mĕ-ning′gō-en-sef′ăl-ī′tis) an inflammation of the brain and its membranes. SYN cerebromeningitis, encephalomeningitis. [meningo- + G. *enkephalos,* brain, + *-itis,* inflammation]

**me•nin•go•en•ceph•a•lo•cele** (mĕ-ning′gō-en-sef′ă-lō-sēl) a protrusion of the meninges and brain through a congenital defect in the cranium, usually in the frontal or occipital region. SYN encephalomeningocele. [meningo- + G. *enkephalos,* brain, + *kēlē,* hernia]

**me•nin•go•en•ceph•a•lo•my•e•li•tis** (mĕ-ning′gō-en-sef′ă-lō-mī-ĕ-lī′tis) inflammation of the brain and spinal cord together with their membranes. [meningo + G. *enkephalos,* brain, + *myelos,* marrow, + *-itis,* inflammation]

**me•nin•go•en•ceph•a•lop•a•thy** (mĕ-ning′gō-en-sef-ă-lop′ă-thē) disorder affecting the meninges and the brain. SYN encephalomeningopathy. [meningo- + G. *enkephalos,* brain, + *pathos,* suffering]

**me•nin•go•my•e•li•tis** (mĕ-ning′gō-mī′ĕ-lī′tis) inflammation of the spinal cord and of its enveloping arachnoid and pia mater, and less commonly also of the dura mater. [meningo- + G. *myelos,* marrow, + *-itis,* inflammation]

**me•nin•go•my•e•lo•cele** (mĕ-ning-gō-mī′ĕ-lō-sēl) protrusion of the spinal cord and its membranes through a defect in the vertebral column. SYN myelocystomeningocele, myelomeningocele. [meningo- + G. *myelos,* marrow, + *kēlē,* tumor]

**me•nin•go•ra•dic•u•lar** (mĕ-ning′gō-ra-dik′yu-lăr) relating to the meninges covering cranial or spinal nerve roots. [meningo- + L. *radix,* root]

**me•nin•go•ra•dic•u•li•tis** (mĕ-ning′gō-ra-dik-yu-lī′tis) inflammation of the meninges and roots of the nerves.

**me•nin•gor•rha•chid•i•an** (mĕ-ning′gō-ra-kid′ē-an) relating to the spinal cord and its membranes. [meningo- + G. *rhachis,* spine]

**me•nin•gor•rha•gia** (mĕ-ning′gō-rā′jē-ă) hemorrhage into or beneath the cerebral or spinal meninges. [meningo- + G. *rhēgnymi,* to burst forth]

**men•in•go•sis** (men′ing-gō′sis) membranous union of bones, as in the skull of the newborn. [meningo- + G. *-ōsis,* condition]

**me•nin•go•vas•cu•lar** (mĕ-ning′gō-vas′kyu-lăr) concerning the blood vessels in the meninges; or the meninges and blood vessels.

**me•ninx**, gen. **me•nin•gis**, pl. **me•nin•ges** (mē′ninks, men′ingks, mĕ-nin′jēz) any membrane; specifically, one of the membranous coverings of the brain and spinal cord. SEE ALSO arachnoidea, dura mater, pia mater. [Mod. L. fr. G. *mēninx,* membrane]

**men•is•cec•to•my** (men′i-sek′tō-mē) excision of a meniscus, usually from the knee joint. [G. *mēniskos,* crescent (meniscus) + *ektomē,* excision]

**me•nis•ci** (mĕ-nis′sī) plural of meniscus.

**men•is•ci•tis** (men′i-sī′tis) inflammation of a fibrocartilaginous meniscus. [G. *mēniskos,* crescent (meniscus), + *-itis,* inflammation]

**me•nis•cus**, pl. **me•nis•ci** (mĕ-nis′kŭs, mĕ-nis′sī) **1.** SYN meniscus lens. **2.** a crescent-shaped structure. **3.** a crescent-shaped fibrocartilaginous structure of the knee, the acromio- and sternoclavicular and the temporomandibular joints. [G. *mēniskos,* crescent]

**me•nis•cus lens** a lens having a spherical concave curve on one side and a spherical convex curve on the other. SYN meniscus (1).

**me•nis•cus sign** SYN crescent sign.

**Men•kes syn•drome** (meng′kĕs) SYN kinky-hair disease.

**meno-** the menses, menstruation. [G. *mēn,* month]

**men•o•me•tror•rha•gia** (men′ō-mē-trō-rā′jē-ă) irregular or excessive bleeding during menstruation and between menstrual periods. [meno- + G. *mētra,* uterus, + *rhēgnymi,* to burst forth]

**men•o•pau•sal** (men′ō-paw-zăl) associated with or occasioned by the menopause.

**men•o•pause** (men′ō-pawz) permanent cessation of the menses; termination of the menstrual life. [meno- + G. *pausis,* cessation]

**men•or•rha•gia** (men-ō-rā′jē-ă) SYN hypermenorrhea. [meno- + G. *rhēgnymi,* to burst forth]

**men•or•rhal•gia** (men-ō-ral′jē-ă) SYN dysmenorrhea. [meno- + G. *algos,* pain]

**me•nos•che•sis** (me-nos′ke-sis, men-ō-skē′sis) suppression of menstruation. [meno- + G. *schesis,* retention]

**men•o•stax•is** (men-ō-stak′sis) SYN hypermenorrhea. [meno- + G. *staxis,* a dripping]

**men•o•tro•pins** (men-ō-trō′pinz) extract of postmenopausal urine containing primarily the follicle-stimulating hormone. SEE ALSO human menopausal gonadotropin, urofollitropin.

**men•ses** (men′sēz) a periodic physiologic hemorrhage, occurring at approximately 4-week intervals, and having its source from the uterine mucous membrane; usually the bleeding is preceded by ovulation and predecidual changes in the endometrium. SEE ALSO menstrual cycle. SYN emmenia, menstrual period. [L. pl. of *mensis,* month]

**men•stru•al** (men′stroo-ăl) relating to the menses. SYN emmenic. [L. *menstrualis*]

**men•stru•al cy•cle** the period in which an ovum matures, is ovulated, and enters the uterine lumen via the uterine tube; ovarian hormonal secretions effect endometrial changes such that, if fertilization occurs, nidation will be possible; in the absence of fertilization, ovarian secretions wane, the endometrium sloughs, and menstruation begins; this cycle lasts an average of 28 days, with day 1 of the cycle designated as that day on which menstrual flow begins.

**men·stru·al mo·li·mi·na** SYN premenstrual syndrome.

**men·stru·al pe·ri·od** SYN menses.

**men·stru·ate** (men′stroo-āt) to undergo menstruation. [L. *menstruo*, pp. *-atus*, to be menstruant]

**men·stru·a·tion** (men-stroo-ā′shŭn) cyclic endometrial shedding and discharge of a bloody fluid from the uterus during the menstrual cycle. SEE menstruate.

**men·stru·um**, pl. **men·strua** (men′stroo-ŭm, men′stroo-ă) old term for solvent. [Mediev. L. menstrual fluid, thought to possess certain solvent properties, ntr. of L. *menstruus,* monthly]

**men·tal 1.** relating to the mind. [L. *mens* (*ment-*), mind] **2.** relating to the chin. SYN genial, genian. [L. *mentum,* chin]

**men·tal age (MA)** a measure, expressed in years and months, of a child's intelligence relative to age norms as determined by testing with the Stanford-Binet intelligence scale.

**men·tal ar·tery** *distribution,* chin; the terminal branch of the inferior alveolar; *anastomoses,* inferior labial artery. SYN arteria mentalis [TA].

**men·tal branch of in·fe·ri·or al·ve·o·lar ar·tery** *distribution,* chin; the terminal branch of the inferior alveolar; *anastomoses,* inferior labial artery.

**men·tal dis·ease** SEE mental illness.

**men·tal dis·or·der** a psychological syndrome or behavioral pattern associated with either subjective distress or objective impairment. SEE ALSO mental illness, behavior disorder.

**men·tal fo·ra·men** the anterior opening of the mandibular canal on the body of the mandible lateral to and above the mental tubercle giving passage to the mental artery and nerve.

**men·tal health** emotional, behavioral, and social maturity or normality; the absence of a mental or behavioral disorder; a state of psychological well-being in which the individual has achieved a satisfactory integration of instinctual drives acceptable to both self and social milieu; an appropriate balance of love, work, and leisure pursuits.

**men·tal hy·giene** the science and practice of maintaining and restoring mental health; a branch of early twentieth century psychiatry that has become an interdisciplinary field including subspecialities in psychology, nursing, social work, law, and other professions.

**men·tal ill·ness 1.** a broadly inclusive term, generally denoting one or all of the following: 1) a disease of the brain, with predominant behavioral symptoms; 2) a disease of the "mind" or personality, evidenced by abnormal behavior, as in hysteria or schizophrenia; **2.** any psychiatric illness listed in *Current Medical Information and Terminology* of the American Medical Association or in the *Diagnostic and Statistical Manual of Mental Disorders* of the American Psychiatric Association. SEE ALSO behavior disorder.

**men·tal im·age** a picture of an object not present, produced in the mind by memory or imagination.

**men·ta·lis mus·cle** *origin,* incisor fossa of mandible; *insertion,* skin of chin; *action,* raises and wrinkles skin of chin, thus elevating the lower lip; *nerve supply,* facial. SYN musculus mentalis [TA].

**men·tal·i·ty** (men-tal′i-tē) the functional attributes of the mind; mental activity.

**men·tal nerve** a branch of the inferior alveolar nerve, arising in the mandibular canal and passing through the mental foramen to the chin and lower lip. SYN nervus mentalis [TA].

**men·tal point** SYN pogonion.

**men·tal re·tar·da·tion** subaverage general intellectual functioning that originates during the developmental period and is associated with impairment in adaptive behavior. Mental retardation classification requires assignment of an index for performance relative to a person's peers on two interrelated criteria: measured intelligence (IQ) and overall socioadaptive behavior. In general an IQ of 70 or below indicates mental retardation.

**men·tal sco·to·ma** absence of insight into, or inability to comprehend, items relative to a subject whose content is highly emotional to the individual. SYN blind spot (2).

**men·tal spine** a slight projection, sometimes two, in the middle line of the posterior surface of the body of the mandible, giving attachment to the geniohyoid muscle (below) and the genioglossus (above). SYN genial tubercle.

**men·tal sym·phy·sis** the fibrocartilaginous union of the 2 halves of the mandible in the fetus; it becomes an osseous union during the first year.

**men·to·an·te·ri·or po·si·tion** a cephalic presentation of the fetus with its chin pointing to the right (**right mentoanterior, RMA**) or to the left (**left mentoanterior, LMA**) acetabulum of the mother.

**men·to·plas·ty** (men′tō-plas-tē) plastic surgery of the chin, whereby its shape or size is altered. SYN genioplasty. [L. *mentum,* chin, + G. *plastos,* formed]

**men·to·pos·te·ri·or po·si·tion (MP)** a cephalic presentation of the fetus with its chin pointing to the right (**right mentoposterior, RMP**) or to the left (**left mentoposterior, LMP**) sacroiliac articulation of the mother.

**men·to·trans·verse po·si·tion** a cephalic presentation of the fetus with its chin pointing to the right (**right mentotransverse, RMT**) or to the left (**left mentotransverse, LMT**) iliac fossa of the mother.

**men·tum,** gen. **men·ti** (men′tŭm, men-tī) SYN chin. [L.]

**MEP** maximum expiratory pressure.

**me·phit·ic** (me-fit′ik) foul, poisonous, or noxious. [L. *mephitis,* a noxious exhalation]

**mEq, meq** milliequivalent.

△**-mer 1.** chemical suffix attached to a prefix such as mono-, di-, poly-, tri-, etc., to indicate the smallest unit of a repeating structure; e.g., polymer. **2.** suffix denoting a member of a particular group; e.g., isomer, enantiomer.

**me·ral·gia** (me-ral′jē-ă) pain in the thigh; specifically, meralgia paresthetica. [G. *mēros,* thigh, + *algos,* pain]

**me·ral·gia par·a·es·thet·i·ca** tingling, formication, itching, and other forms of paresthesia in the outer side of the lower part of the thigh in the area of distribution of the lateral femoral cutaneous nerve; there may be pain, but the skin is usually hypesthetic to the touch. SYN Bernhardt disease.

**M:E ra·tio** the ratio of myeloid to erythroid precursors in bone marrow; normally it varies from

2:1 to 4:1; an increased ratio is found in infections, chronic myelogenous leukemia, or erythroid hypoplasia; a decreased ratio may mean a depression of leukopoiesis or normoblastic hyperplasia depending on the overall cellularity of the bone marrow.

**mer·cap·tan** (mer-kap'tan) **1.** a class of substances in which the oxygen of an alcohol has been replaced by sulfur (e.g., cysteine). **2.** DENTISTRY a class of elastic impression compounds sometimes referred to as rubber base materials.

⌂**mer·cap·to-** prefix indicating the presence of a thiol group, –SH.

**mer·cap·tu·ric ac·id** (mer-kap-tyur'ik as'id) a condensation product of L-cysteine with aromatic compounds, such as bromobenzene; formed in the liver and excreted in the urine.

**Mer·ci·er sound** (mer-sē-ā') a catheter the beak of which is short and bent almost at a right angle.

**mer·cu·ri·al** (mer-kyu'rē-ăl) **1.** relating to mercury. **2.** any salt of mercury used medicinally. **3.** having the characteristic of rapid, changing moods.

**mer·cu·ri·a·lism** (mer-kyu'rē-ă-lizm) SYN mercury poisoning.

**mer·cu·ric** (mer-kyu'rik) denoting a salt of mercury in which the ion of the metal is bivalent.

**mer·cu·rous** (mer-kyu'rŭs) denoting a salt of mercury in which the ion of the metal is univalent.

**mer·cu·ry (Hg)** (mer'kyu-rē) a dense liquid metallic element, atomic no. 80, atomic wt. 200.59; used in thermometers, barometers, manometers, and other scientific instruments; some salts and organic mercurials are used medicinally; [197]Hg (half-life of 2.672 days) and [203]Hg (half-life of 46.61 days) have been used in brain and renal scanning. [L. *Mercurius,* Mercury, the god of trade, messenger of the gods; in Mediev. L., quicksilver, mercury]

**mer·cu·ry poi·son·ing** a disease usually caused by the ingestion of mercury or mercury compounds, which are toxic in relation to their ability to produce mercuric ions; usually **acute mercury poisoning** is associated with ulcerations of the stomach and intestine and toxic changes in the renal tubules; anuria and anemia may occur; usually **chronic mercury poisoning** is a result of industrial poisoning and causes gastrointestinal or central nervous system manifestations including stomatitis, diarrhea, ataxia, tremor, hyperreflexia, sensorineural impairment, and emotional instability (Mad Hatter syndrome). SYN hydrargyria, hydrargyrism, mercurialism.

⌂**mere-, mero-** part; also indicating one of a series of similar parts. SEE ALSO -mer. [G. *mēros,* share]

**Mer·en·din·o tech·nique** (mer-en-dē'nō) plastic reconstruction of an incompetent mitral valve using heavy sutures to narrow the anulus in the region of the medial commissure.

**Me·re·to·ja syn·drome** (mā-rā-tō'yah) a familial form of systemic amyloidosis with lattice, corneal dystrophy, cranial and peripheral nerve palsies, protruding lips, masklike facies, and floppy ears.

**me·rid·i·an** (mĕ-rid'ē-an) **1.** a line encircling a globular body at right angles to its equator and touching both poles, or the half of such a circle extending from pole to pole. **2.** ACUPUNCTURE the lines connecting different anatomical sites. [L.

*meridianus,* pertaining to midday, on the south side, southern]

**me·rid·i·o·nal** (mĕ-rid'ē-ŏ-năl) relating to a meridian.

**me·rid·i·o·nal ab·er·ra·tion** an aberration produced in the plane of a single meridian of a lens.

**me·rid·i·o·nal am·bly·op·ia** amblyopia due to an uncorrected, large astigmatism during the amblyogenic period of visual development.

**me·rid·i·o·nal fi·bers of ciliary muscle** the longitudinal fibers of the ciliary muscle. SYN fibrae meridionales muscularis ciliaris [TA].

**Mer·kel cor·pus·cle** (mer'kel) SYN tactile meniscus.

**Mer·kel tac·tile cell** (mer'kel) SYN tactile meniscus.

**Mer·kel tac·tile disk** (mer'kel) SYN tactile meniscus.

*Mer·mis* (mer'mis) genus of long, opaque nematodes; larval stages passed in the hemocylic cavity of insects, particularly grasshoppers, while adults are free-living in the soil. Accidental ingestion by humans causes infection.

*Mer·mis ni·gres·cens* nematode species found in soil that deposits eggs on above-ground plants; normal host is the grasshopper; has been recovered from alimentary and urogenital tracts of humans but infections are rare.

**mer·o·an·en·ceph·a·ly** a type of anencephaly in which the brain and cranium are present in rudimentary form. [mero- + G. *an-,* priv. + *enkephalos,* brain]

**mer·o·crine gland** a gland that releases only an acellular secretory product, in contrast to a holocrine gland.

**mer·o·di·a·stol·ic** (mer'ō-dī-ă-stol'ik) partially diastolic; relating to a part of the diastole of the heart. [mero- + diastole]

**mer·o·gen·e·sis** (mer-ō-jen'ĕ-sis) **1.** reproduction by segmentation. **2.** cleavage of an oocyte. [mero- + G. *genesis,* origin]

**mer·o·ge·net·ic, mer·o·gen·ic** (mer-ō-jĕ-net'ik, mer-ō-jen'ik) relating to merogenesis.

**me·rog·o·ny** (mĕ-rog'ō-nē) **1.** the incomplete development of an oocyte that has been disorganized. **2.** a form of asexual schizogony, typical of sporozoan protozoa, in which the nucleus divides several times before the cytoplasm divides; the schizont divides to form merozoites in this asexual phase of the life cycle. [mero- + G. *gonē,* generation]

**mer·o·me·lia** (mer-ō-mē'lē-ă) partial absence of a free limb (exclusive of girdle); e.g., hemimelia, phocomelia. [mero- + G. *melos,* a limb]

**mer·o·mi·cro·so·mia** (mer'ō-mī'krō-sō'mē-ă) abnormal smallness of some portion of the body; local dwarfism. [mero- + G. *mikros,* small, + *sōma,* body]

**mer·o·my·o·sin** (mer-ō-mī'ō-sin) a subunit of the tryptic digestion of myosin; two types are produced, H-meromyosin and L-meromyosin.

**me·ros·mia** (me-roz'mē-ă) a condition in which the perception of certain odors is wanting; analogous to color blindness. [mero- + G. *osmē,* smell]

**mer·o·sys·tol·ic** (mer'ō-sis-tol'ik) partially systolic; relating to a portion of the systole of the heart. [mero- + systole]

**me·rot·o·my** (me-rot'ō-mē) the procedure of cutting into parts, as the cutting of a cell into separate parts to study their capacity for survival and development. [mero- + G. *tomē,* incision]

m
e

**mer•o•zo•ite** (mer-ō-zō′īt) the motile infective stage of sporozoan protozoa that results from schizogony or a similar type of asexual reproduction. Merozoites are responsible for the vast reproductive powers of sporozoan parasites. [mero- + G. *zōon,* animal]

**me•ro•zy•gote** (mē-rō-zī′gōt) MICROBIAL GENETICS an organism that, in addition to its own original genome (endogenote), contains a fragment (exogenote) of a genome from another organism; the relatively small size of the exogenote permits a diploid condition for only a limited region of the endogenote. [mero- + *zygōtos,* yoked]

**MERRF** *m*yoclonic *e*pilepsy with *r*agged *r*ed *f*iber myopathy. One of the mitochondrial disorders, this condition is caused by a point mutation of the mitochondria genome locus 8344, where transfer RNA is coded.

**me•sad** (mē′zad, mē′sad) passing or extending toward the median plane of the body or of a part. SYN mesiad. [G. *mesos,* middle, + L. *ad,* to]

**mes•an•gi•al** (mes-an′jē-ăl) referring to the mesangium.

**mes•an•gi•al ne•phri•tis** glomerulonephritis with an increase in glomerular mesangial cells or matrix, or mesangial deposits.

**mes•an•gi•al pro•lif•er•a•tive glo•mer•u•lo•ne•phri•tis** glomerulonephritis characterized clinically by the nephrotic syndrome and histologically by diffuse glomerular increases in endocapillary and mesangial cells and in mesangial matrix; in some cases, there are mesangial deposits of IgM and complement.

**mes•an•gi•um** (mes-an′jē-ŭm) a central part of the renal glomerulus between capillaries; mesangial cells are phagocytic and for the most part separated from capillary lumina by endothelial cells. [mes- + G. *angeion,* vessel]

**mes•a•or•ti•tis** (mes-ā-ōr-tī′tis) inflammation of the middle or muscular coat of the aorta. [mes- + aortitis]

**mes•ar•ter•i•tis** (mes-ar-ter-ī′tis) inflammation of the middle (muscular) coat of an artery. [mes- + arteritis]

**me•sat•i•pel•lic, me•sat•i•pel•vic** (mē-sat′i-pel′ik, mē-sat′i-pel′vik) denoting an individual with a pelvic index between 90 and 95; the superior strait has a round appearance, the transverse diameter exceeding the anteroposterior by 1 cm or less. [G. *mesatos,* midmost, + *pellis,* a bowl (pelvis)]

**mes•ax•on** (mez-ak′son) the plasma membrane of the neurolemma that is folded in to surround a nerve axon. In electron micrographs this double layer resembles a membrane in appearance.

**mes•ec•to•derm** (mez-ek′tō-derm) **1.** cells in the area around the dorsal lip of the blastopore where mesoderm and ectoderm undergo a process of separation. **2.** that part of the mesenchyme derived from ectoderm, especially from the neural crest in the cephalic region in very young embryos. [mes- + ectoderm]

**mes•en•ce•phal•ic** (mez-en′se-fal′ik) relating to the mesencephalon.

**mes•en•ce•phal•ic flex•ure** SYN cephalic flexure.

**mes•en•ce•phal•ic teg•men•tum** that major part of the substance of the mesencephalon or midbrain that extends from the substantia nigra to the level of the cerebral aqueduct. SYN tegmentum (2).

**mes•en•ceph•a•li•tis** (mez′en-sef′ă-lī′tis) inflammation of the midbrain (mesencephalon).

**mes•en•ceph•a•lon** (mez-en-sef′ă-lon) [TA] that part of the brainstem developing from the middle of the three primary cerebral vesicles of the embryo. In the adult, the mesencephalon is characterized by the unique conformation of its roof plate, the lamina of the mesencephalic tectum, composed of the bilaterally paired superior and inferior colliculi, and by the massive paired prominence of the crus cerebri at its ventral surface. Prominent cell groups of the mesencephalon include the motor nuclei of the trochlear and oculomotor nerves, the red nucleus, and the substantia nigra. SYN midbrain. [mes- + G. *enkephalos,* brain]

**mes•en•ceph•a•lot•o•my** (mez′en-sef′ă-lot′ō-mē) **1.** the sectioning of any structure in the midbrain, especially of the spinothalamic tracts for the relief of intractable pain or the cerebral peduncle for dyskinesias. **2.** a mesencephalic spinothalamic tractotomy. [mesencephalon + G. *tomē,* incision]

**me•sen•chy•mal** (mē-seng′ki-măl, mez-eng-kī′măl) relating to the mesenchyme.

**mes•en•chyme** (mez′en-kīm) **1.** an aggregation of mesenchymal cells. **2.** primordial embryonic connective tissue consisting of mesenchymal cells, usually stellate in form, supported in interlaminar jelly. [mes- + G. *enkyma,* infusion]

**mes•en•chy•mo•ma** (mez′en-kī-mō′mă) a neoplasm in which there is a mixture of mesenchymal derivatives, other than fibrous tissue. A **benign mesenchymoma** may contain foci of vascular, muscular, adipose, osteoid, osseous, and cartilaginous tissue. A **malignant mesenchymoma** may also occur as a similar mixture of two or more types of mesenchymal cells that are malignant.

**mes•en•ter•ic** (mez-en-ter′ik) relating to the mesentery.

**mes•en•ter•i•o•pexy** (mes′en-ter-ē-ō-pek′sē) fixation or attachment of a torn or incised mesentery. SYN mesopexy. [mesentery + G. *pēxis,* fixation]

**mes•en•ter•i•or•rha•phy** (mez′en-ter-ē-ōr′ă-fē) suture of the mesentery. SYN mesorrhaphy. [mesentery + G. *rhaphē,* suture]

**mes•en•ter•i•pli•ca•tion** (mez′en-ter-i-pli-kā′shŭn) reducing redundancy of a mesentery by making one or more tucks in it. [mesentery + L. *plico,* pp. *-atus,* to fold]

**mes•en•ter•i•tis** (mez′en-ter-ī′tis) inflammation of the mesentery.

**mes•en•te•ri•um** (mez′en-ter′ē-ŭm) SYN mesentery, mesentery. [Mod. L.]

**me•sen•ter•o•ax•i•al vol•vu•lus** a type of gastric volvulus in which the axis of twist is parallel to the line of the gastric mesentery.

**mes•en•tery** (mes′en-ter-ē) **1.** a double layer of peritoneum attached to the abdominal wall and enclosing in its fold a portion or all of one of the abdominal viscera, conveying to it its vessels and nerves. **2.** the fan-shaped fold of peritoneum encircling the greater part of the small intestines (jejunum and ileum) and attaching it to the posterior abdominal wall at the root of the mesentery (radix mesenterii). SYN mesenterium. [Mod. L. *mesenterium,* fr. G. *mesenterion,* fr. G. *mesos,* middle, + *enteron,* intestine]

**me•si•ad** (mē′zē-ad, mes′ē-ad) SYN mesad.

**me·si·al** (mē′zē-ăl, mes′ē-ăl) toward the median plane following the curvature of the dental arch, in contrast to distal (2). SYN proximal (2). [G. *mesos,* middle]

**me·si·al an·gle** the angle formed by the meeting of the mesial with the labial (or buccal) or lingual surface of a tooth.

**me·si·al oc·clu·sion 1.** occlusion in which the mandibular teeth articulate with the maxillary teeth in a position anterior to normal; SYN mesio-occlusion. **2.** SYN mesioclusion.

**⌂me·sio-** mesial (especially in dentistry). [G. *mesos,* middle]

**me·si·o·buc·cal** (mē′zē-ō-bŭk′ăl) relating to the mesial and buccal surfaces of a tooth; denoting especially the angle formed by the junction of these two surfaces.

**me·si·o·cer·vi·cal** (mē′zē-ō-ser′vi-kăl) **1.** relating to the line angle of a cavity preparation at the junction of the mesial and cervical walls. **2.** pertaining to the area of a tooth at the junction of the mesial surface and the cervical region.

**me·si·o·clu·sion** (mē′zē-ō-kloo′zhŭn) a malocclusion in which the mandibular arch articulates with the maxillary arch in a position mesial to normal; in Angle classification, a Class III malocclusion. SYN mesial occlusion (2).

**me·si·o·dens** (mē′zē-ō-denz) a supernumerary tooth located in the midline of the anterior maxillae, generally between the maxillary central incisor teeth. [mesio- + L. *dens,* tooth]

**me·si·o·dis·tal** (mē′zē-ō-dis′tăl) denoting the plane or diameter of a tooth cutting its mesial and distal surfaces.

**me·si·o·gin·gi·val** (mē′zē-ō-jin′ji-văl) relating to the angle formed by the junction of the mesial surface with the gingival line of a tooth.

**me·si·o·la·bi·al** (mē′zē-ō-lā′bē-ăl) relating to the mesial and labial surfaces of a tooth; denoting especially the angle formed by their junction.

**me·si·o·lin·gual** (mē′zē-ō-ling′gwăl) relating to the mesial and lingual surfaces of a tooth; denoting especially the angle formed by their junction.

**me·si·o·lin·guo·oc·clu·sal** (mē′zē-ō-ling′gwō-ŏ-klōo′săl) denoting the angle formed by the junction of the mesial, lingual, and occlusal surfaces of a premolar or molar tooth.

**me·si·o·lin·guo·pul·pal** (mē′zē-ō-ling′gwō-pŭl′păl) relating to the angle denoting the junction of the mesial, lingual, and pulpal surfaces in a tooth cavity preparation.

**me·sio·oc·clu·sal** (mē′zē-ō-ō-kloo′zăl) denoting the angle formed by the junction of the mesial and occlusal surfaces of a premolar or molar tooth.

**me·sio·oc·clu·sion** (mē′zē-ō-ō-kloo′zhŭn) SYN mesial occlusion (1).

**me·si·o·ver·sion** (mē′zē-ō-ver-zhŭn) malposition of a tooth mesial to normal, in an anterior direction following the curvature of the dental arch.

**mes·mer·ism** (mes′mer-izm) a system of therapeutics from which were developed hypnotism and therapeutic suggestion. [F.A. *Mesmer,* Austrian physician, 1734–1815]

**⌂meso-, mes-** **1.** middle, mean, intermediate. **2.** a mesentery, mesentery-like structure. **3.** a prefix denoting a compound, containing more than one chiral center, having an internal plane of symmetry; such compounds do not exhibit optical activity (e.g., *meso*-cystine). [G. *mesos*]

**mes·o·ap·pen·dix** (mez′ō-ă-pen′diks) [TA] the short mesentery of the appendix lying behind the terminal ileum, in which the appendicular artery courses.

**mes·o·bi·lane** (mez-ō-bī′lān) a reduced mesobilirubin with no double bonds between the pyrrole rings and, consequently, colorless. SEE ALSO bilirubinoids. SYN mesobilirubinogen.

**mes·o·bil·i·ru·bin** (mez′ō-bil-i-roo′bin) a compound differing from bilirubin only in that the vinyl groups of bilirubin are reduced to ethyl groups. SEE ALSO bilirubinoids.

**mes·o·bil·i·ru·bin·o·gen** (mez′ō-bil-i-roo-bin′ō-jen) SYN mesobilane.

**mes·o·blast** (mez′ō-blast) SYN mesoderm. [meso- + G. *blastos,* germ]

**mes·o·blas·te·ma** (mez′ō-blas-tē′mă) all the cells collectively which constitute the early undifferentiated mesoderm. [meso- + G. *blastēma,* a sprout]

**mes·o·blas·tem·ic** (mez′ō-blas-tē′mik) relating to or derived from the mesoblastema.

**mes·o·blas·tic** (mez′ō-blas′tik) relating to or derived from the mesoderm.

**mes·o·car·dia** (mez′ō-kar′dē-ă) **1.** atypical position of the heart in a central position in the chest, as in early embryonic life. **2.** plural of mesocardium. [meso- + G. *kardia,* heart]

**mes·o·car·di·um,** pl. **mes·o·car·dia** (mez-ō-kar′dē-ŭm) the double layer of splanchnic mesoderm supporting the embryonic heart in the pericardial cavity. It disappears before birth. [meso- + G. *kardia,* heart]

**mes·o·ca·val shunt 1.** anastomosis of the side of the superior mesenteric vein to the proximal end of the divided inferior vena cava, for control of portal hypertension; **2.** H-shunt anastomosis of the inferior vena cava to the superior mesenteric vein, using a synthetic conduit or autologous vein.

**mes·o·ce·cal** (mez′ō-sē′kăl) relating to the mesocecum.

**mes·o·ce·cum** (mez′ō-sē′kŭm) part of the mesocolon, supporting the cecum, that occasionally persists when the ascending colon becomes retroperitoneal during fetal life. [meso- + cecum]

***Mes·o·ces·toi·des*** (mez-ō-ses-toy′dēz) tapeworm genus found in carnivorous mammals, such as foxes; mites probably intermediate hosts; few human cases identified in Japan, the United States, and China.

**mes·o·col·ic** (mez′ō-kol′ik) relating to the mesocolon.

**mes·o·co·lon** (mez′ō-kō′lon) the fold of peritoneum attaching the colon to the posterior abdominal wall; ascending mesocolon (mesocolon ascendens [TA]), transverse mesocolon (mesocolon transversum [TA]), descending mesocolon (mesocolon descendens [TA]), and sigmoid mesocolon (mesocolon sigmoideum [TA]) correspond to the respective divisions of the colon; the ascending and descending portions are usually fused to the peritoneum of the posterior abdominal wall, but can be mobilized. [meso- + *kolon,* colon]

**mes·o·co·lo·pexy** (mez′ō-kō′lō-pek-sē) an operation for shortening the mesocolon, for correction of undue mobility and ptosis. SYN mesocoloplication. [meso- + G. *kolon,* colon, + *pēxis,* fixation]

**mes·o·co·lo·pli·ca·tion** (mes′ō-kō′lō-pli-kā′shŭn) SYN mesocolopexy. [meso- + G. *kolon,* colon, + L. *plico,* pp. -*atus,* to fold]

**mes·o·cord** (mez′ō-kŏrd) a fold of amnion that

sometimes binds a segment of the umbilical cord to the placenta.

**mes·o·derm** (mez'ō-derm) the middle of the three primary germ layers of the embryo (the others being ectoderm and endoderm); mesoderm is the origin of all connective tissues, all musculature, blood, cardiovascular and lymphatic systems, most of the urogenital system, and the lining of the pericardial, pleural, and peritoneal cavities. SYN mesoblast. [meso- + G. *derma*, skin]

**mes·o·der·mic** (mez-ō-der'mik) relating to the mesoderm.

**mes·o·du·o·de·nal** (mez'ō-doo-ō-dē'năl) relating to the mesoduodenum.

**mes·o·du·o·de·num** (mez'ō-doo'ō-dē'nŭm) the mesentery of the duodenum.

**mes·o·ep·i·did·y·mis** (mez-ō-ep-i-did'i-mis) an occasional fold of the tunica vaginalis binding the epididymis to the testis. [meso- + epididymis]

**mes·o·gas·ter** (mez-ō-gas'ter) SYN mesogastrium.

**mes·o·gas·tric** (mez-ō-gas'trik) relating to the mesogastrium.

**mes·o·gas·tri·um** (mez-ō-gas'trē-ŭm) in the embryo, the mesentery of the dilated portion of the alimentary canal that is the future stomach; it gives rise to the greater omentum and consequently is involved in the formation of the omental bursa. The spleen and body of the pancreas develop within it, and thus the splenorenal and gastrosplenic ligaments are derivatives of the (dorsal) mesogastrium. SYN mesogaster. [meso- + G. *gastēr* stomach]

**mes·o·gen·ic** (mez-ō-jen'ik) denoting a virus capable of inducing lethal infection in embryonic hosts, after a short incubation period, and an inapparent infection in immature and adult hosts. [meso- + G. -*gen*, producing]

**me·sog·lia** (me-sog'lē-ă) neuroglial cells of mesodermal origin. SEE ALSO microglia. SYN mesoglial cells. [meso- + G. *glia*, glue]

**me·sog·li·al cells** SYN mesoglia.

**mes·o·glu·te·al** (mez'ō-gloo'tē-ăl) relating to the musculus gluteus medius.

**mes·o·il·e·um** (mez-ō-il'ē-ŭm) the mesentery of the ileum.

**mes·o·je·ju·num** (mez'ō-je-joo'nŭm) the mesentery of the jejunum.

**mes·o·lym·pho·cyte** (mez-ō-lim'fō-sīt) a mononuclear leukocyte of medium size, probably a lymphocyte, with a deeply staining nucleus of large size but relatively smaller than that in most lymphocytes. [meso- + lymphocyte]

**mes·o·me·lia** (mez-ō-mē'lē-ă) the condition of having abnormally short arms and legs. [meso- + G. *melos*, limb]

**mes·o·mel·ic dwarf·ism** dwarfism with shortness of the forearms and legs.

**mes·o·mere** (mez'ō-mēr) **1.** a blastomere of a size intermediate between a macromere and a micromere. **2.** the zone between an epimere and a hypomere. [meso- + G. *meros*, part]

**mes·o·met·a·neph·ric car·ci·no·ma** SYN mesonephroma.

**mes·o·me·tri·um** (mez'ō-mē'trē-ŭm) [TA] the broad ligament of the uterus, below the mesosalpinx. [meso- + G. *mētra*, uterus]

**mes·o·morph** (mez'ō-mōrf) a constitutional body type or build (biotype or somatotype) in which tissues that originate from the mesoderm prevail; from the morphological standpoint, there is a balance between trunk and limbs. SEE ALSO hypo-

morph, ectomorph, endomorph. [meso- + G. *morphē*, form]

**mes·o·mor·phic** (mez-ō-mōrf'ik) relating to a mesomorph.

**me·son** (mez'on, mē'zon, mes'on) an elementary particle having a rest mass intermediate in value between the mass of an electron and that of a proton. [G. neuter of *mesos*, middle]

**mes·o·neph·ric** (mez-ō-nef'rik) relating to the mesonephros.

**mes·o·neph·ric duct** a duct in the embryo draining the mesonephric tubules; in the male it becomes the ductus deferens; in the female it becomes vestigial. SYN wolffian duct.

**mes·o·neph·ric fold** SYN mesonephric ridge.

**mes·o·neph·ric ridge** a ridge which, in early human embryos, comprises the entire urogenital ridge; however, later in development a more medial genital ridge, the potential gonad, is demarcated from it. SEE ALSO urogenital ridge. SYN mesonephric fold.

**mes·o·neph·roi** (mez'ō-nef'roy) plural of mesonephros.

**mes·o·ne·phro·ma** (mez'ō-ne-frō'mă) a rare malignant neoplasm of the ovary and corpus uteri, thought to originate in mesonephric structures that become misplaced in ovarian tissue during embryonic development. SYN clear cell carcinoma, mesometanephric carcinoma. [mesonephros + -*oma*, tumor]

**mes·o·neph·ros**, pl. **mes·o·neph·roi** (mez'ō-nef'ros, mez'ō-nef'roy) one of three excretory organs appearing in the evolution of vertebrates; in life forms with a metanephros, the mesonephros is located between the regressing pronephros and the metanephros, cephalic to the latter. In young mammalian embryos, the mesonephros is well developed and briefly functional until establishment of the metanephros, the definitive kidney; in older embryos, the mesonephros undergoes regression as an excretory organ, but its duct system is retained in the male as the epididymis and ductus deferens. SYN wolffian body. [meso- + G. *nephros*, kidney]

**mes·o·neu·ri·tis** (mez'ō-noo-rī'tis) inflammation of a nerve or of its connective tissue without involvement of its sheath.

**mes·o·pexy** (mez'ō-pek-sē) SYN mesenteriopexy.

**mes·o·phil, mes·o·phile** (mez'ō-fil, mez'ō-fīl) a microorganism with an optimum temperature between 25°C and 40°C, but growing within the limits of 10°C and 45°C. [meso- + G. *philos*, fond]

**mes·o·phil·ic** (mez'ō-fil'ik) pertaining to a mesophil.

**mes·o·phle·bi·tis** (mez'ō-flě-bī'tis) inflammation of the middle coat of a vein. [meso- + phlebitis]

**me·soph·ry·on** (mez-of'ri-on) SYN glabella (2). [meso- + Gr. *ophrys*, eyebrow]

**mes·o·por·phy·rins** (mez-ō-pōr'fi-rinz) porphyrin compounds resembling the protoporphyrins except that the vinyl side chains of the latter are reduced to ethyl side chains; e.g., mesobilane.

**me·sor·chi·al** (mez-ōr'kē-ăl) relating to the mesorchium.

**me·sor·chi·um** (mez-ōr'kē-ŭm) **1.** in the fetus, a fold of tunica vaginalis testis supporting the mesonephros and the developing testis. **2.** in the adult, a fold of tunica vaginalis testis between the testis and epididymis. [meso- + G. *orchis*, testis]

**mes·o·rec·tum** (mez-ō-rek'tŭm) the peritoneal

investment of the rectum, covering the upper part only.

**mes·or·rha·phy** (mez-ōr′ă-fē) SYN mesenteriorrhaphy.

**mes·o·sal·pinx** (mez′ō-sal′pinks) [TA] the part of the broad ligament investing the uterine (fallopian) tube. [meso- + G. *salpinx*, trumpet]

**mes·o·sig·moid** (mez′ō-sig′moyd) sigmoid mesocolon. SEE mesocolon.

**mes·o·sig·moid·i·tis** (mes′ō-sig-moy-dī′tis) inflammation of the mesosigmoid.

**mes·o·sig·moid·o·pexy** (mez-ō-sig-moy′dō-peksē) surgical fixation of the mesosigmoid.

**mes·o·some** (mes′ō-sōm) a convoluted membranous body formed by involution of the plasma membranes of certain bacteria; it functions in cellular respiration and septum formation. [meso + G. *soma*, body]

**mes·o·ten·di·ne·um** (mez′ō-ten-din′ē-ŭm) SYN mesotendon.

**mes·o·ten·don** (mez′ō-ten′dŏn) the synovial layers that pass from a tendon to the wall of a tendon sheath in certain places where tendons lie within osteofibrous canals. In most instances, the mesotendon degenerates, leaving only the vincula. SYN mesotendineum.

**mes·o·the·lia** (mez-ō-thē′lē-ă) plural of mesothelium.

**mes·o·the·li·al** (mez-ō-thē′lē-ăl) relating to the mesothelium.

**mes·o·the·li·o·ma** (mez′ō-thē-lē-ō′mă) a rare malignant neoplasm, derived from the lining cells of the pleura and peritoneum, which grows as a thick sheet covering the viscera. [mesothelium + G. *-oma*, tumor]

**mes·o·the·li·um**, pl. **mes·o·the·lia** (mez-ō-thē′lē-ŭm, mez-ō-thē′lē-ă) a single layer of flattened cells forming an epithelium that lines serous cavities; e.g., peritoneum, pleura, pericardium. [meso- + epithelium]

**mes·o·tym·pan·um** (mez-ō-tim′pan-um) the portion of the middle ear medial to the tympanic membrane.

**mes·o·va·ri·um**, pl. **mes·o·va·ria** (mezō′varē-ŭm, mezō′varē-ă) a short peritoneal fold connecting the anterior border of the ovary with the posterior layer of the broad ligament of the uterus. [meso- + L. *ovarium*, ovary]

**mes·sen·ger RNA (mRNA)** the RNA reflecting the exact nucleoside sequence of the genetically active DNA and carrying the "message" of the latter, coded in its sequence, to the cytoplasmic areas where protein is made in amino acid sequences specified by the mRNA, and hence primarily by the DNA; viral RNA is considered to be natural messenger RNA.

**MET** muscle energy technique.

**MET** metabolic equivalent.

⌂**meta- 1.** after, subsequent to, behind, or hindmost. Cf. post-. **2.** CHEMISTRY an italicized prefix denoting joint, action sharing. **3. (m-)** CHEMISTRY an italicized prefix denoting compound formed by two substitutions in the benzene ring separated by one carbon atom, i.e., linked to the first and third, second and fourth, etc., carbon atoms of the ring. For terms beginning with *meta-*, or *m-*, see the specific name. [G. after, between, over]

**met·a·a·nal·y·sis** (met′ă-ă-nal′i-sis) the process of using statistical methods to combine the results of different studies; systematic, organized,

and structured evaluation of a problem using information, commonly in the form of statistical tables, from a number of different studies of a problem.

**met·a·anal·y·sis** (met′ă-ă-nal′i-sis) systematic process for finding, evaluating, and combining the results of sets of data from different scientific studies. SEE ALSO analysis.

**me·tab·a·sis** (mĕ-tab′ă-sis) rarely used term for a change of any kind in symptoms or course of a disease. [G. a passing over, change, fr. *metabainō*, to pass over]

**met·a·bi·o·sis** (met′ă-bī-ō′sis) dependence of one organism on another for its existence. SEE ALSO commensalism, mutualism, parasitism. [meta- + G. *biōsis*, way of life]

**met·a·bi·sul·fite test** a test for sickle cell hemoglobin (Hb S); deoxygenation of cells containing Hb S is enhanced by addition of sodium metabisulfite to the blood, causing sickling visible on a slide; certain other abnormal hemoglobins (Hb $C_{Harlem}$ and Hb I) also sickle in this test.

**met·a·bol·ic** (met-ă-bol′ik) relating to metabolism.

**met·a·bol·ic ac·i·do·sis** decreased pH and bicarbonate concentration in the body fluids caused either by the accumulation of acids or by abnormal losses of fixed base from the body, as in diarrhea or renal disease.

**met·a·bol·ic al·ka·lo·sis** an alkalosis associated with an increased arterial bicarbonate concentration, resulting from an excessive intake of alkaline materials or an excessive loss of acid in the urine or through persistent vomiting; the base excess and standard bicarbonate are both elevated. SEE ALSO compensated alkalosis.

**met·a·bol·ic co·ma** coma resulting from diffuse failure of neuronal metabolism, caused by such abnormalities as intrinsic disorders of neuron or glial cell metabolism, or extracerebral disorders that produce intoxication or electrolyte imbalances.

**met·a·bol·ic cra·ni·op·a·thy** SYN Morgagni syndrome.

**met·a·bol·ic en·ceph·a·lo·pa·thy** encephalopathy characterized by memory loss, vertigo, and generalized weakness, due to metabolic brain disease including hypoxia, ischemia, hypoglycemia, or secondary to other organ failure such as liver or kidney.

**met·a·bol·ic e·quiv·a·lent (MET)** the oxygen cost of energy expenditure measured at supine rest (1 MET = 3.5 ml $O_2$ per kg of body weight per minute); multiples of MET are used to estimate the oxygen cost of activity.

**met·a·bol·ic mu·ci·no·sis** SEE mucinosis.

**me·tab·o·lism** (mĕ-tab′ō-lizm) **1.** the sum of the chemical and physical changes occurring in tissue, consisting of anabolism, those reactions that convert small molecules into large, and catabolism, those reactions that convert large molecules into small, including both endogenous large molecules as well as biodegradation of xenobiotics. **2.** often incorrectly used as a synonym for anabolism or catabolism. [G. *metabolē*, change]

**me·tab·o·lite** (mĕ-tab′ō-līt) any product (foodstuff, intermediate, waste product) of metabolism, especially of catabolism.

**me·tab·o·lize** (mĕ-tab′ō-līz) to undergo the chemical changes of metabolism.

**me·tab·o·re·cep·tors** (mĕ-tab′ō-rē-sep′terz) pe-

m
e

ripheral afferent nerve endings that respond to metabolites (lactate, $CO_2$, pH) produced by active muscle. [*metabo*lism + receptor]

**met·a·car·pal** (met′ă-kar′păl) **1.** relating to the metacarpus. **2.** any one of the metacarpal bones (I–V).

**met·a·car·pal [I–V]** five long bones (numbered I to V, beginning with the bone on the radial or thumb side) forming the skeleton of the metacarpus or palm; they articulate with the bones of the distal row of the carpus and with the five proximal phalanges. SYN ossa metacarpi.

**met·a·car·pec·to·my** (met′ă-kar-pek′tō-mē) excision of one or all of the metacarpals. [metacarpus + G. *ektomē,* excision]

**met·a·car·po·pha·lan·ge·al (MCP)** (met′ă-kar′ pō-fă-lan′jē-ăl) relating to the metacarpus and the phalanges; denoting the articulations between them.

**met·a·car·po·pha·lan·ge·al joint** the spheroid synovial joints between the heads of the metacarpals and the bases of the proximal phalanges.

**met·a·car·pus,** pl. **met·a·car·pi** (met′ă-kar′pŭs, met′ă-kar′pī) [TA] the five bones of the hand between the carpus and the phalanges. [meta- + G. *karpos,* wrist]

**met·a·cen·tric** (met-ă-sen′trik) having the centromere about equidistant from the extremities, said of a chromosome. [meta- + G. *kentron,* circle]

**met·a·cen·tric chro·mo·some** a chromosome with a centrally placed centromere that divides the chromosome into two arms of approximately equal length.

**met·a·cer·ca·ria,** pl. **met·a·cer·ca·ri·ae** (met′ă-ser-kar′ē-ă, met′ă-ser-kar′ē-ē) the post-cercarial encysted stage in the life history of a fluke, prior to transfer to the definitive host. Some cercariae attach themselves to vegetation, form metacercaria, and are ingested by herbivores; others encyst in muscles of fish or crayfish. [meta- + G. *kerkos,* tail]

**met·a·chro·ma·sia** (met′ă-krō-mā′zē-ă) **1.** the condition in which a cell or tissue component takes on a color different from the dye solution with which it is stained. SYN metachromatism (2). **2.** a change in the characteristic color of certain basic thiazine dyes, such as toluidine blue, when the dye molecules are bound to tissue polyanionic polymers. [meta- + G. *chrōma,* color]

**met·a·chro·mat·ic** (met′ă-krō-mat′ik) denoting cells or dyes that exhibit metachromasia. SYN metachromophil, metachromophile.

**met·a·chro·mat·ic bod·ies** concentrated deposits consisting primarily of polymetaphosphate and occurring in many bacteria as well as in algae, fungi, and protozoa; m. bodies differ in staining properties from the surrounding protoplasm. SEE metachromasia.

**met·a·chro·mat·ic leu·ko·dys·tro·phy** a metabolic disorder, usually of infancy, characterized by myelin loss, accumulation of metachromatic lipids (galactosyl sulfatidates) in the white matter of the central and peripheral nervous systems, progressive paralysis, and mental retardation; psychosis and dementia are seen in adults.

**met·a·chro·mat·ic stain** a stain, such as methylene blue, thionine, or azure A, that interacts chemically with certain histologic or cytologic structures, yielding a color different from that of the stain.

**met·a·chro·ma·tism** (met-ă-krō′mă-tizm) **1.** any color change, whether natural or produced by basic aniline dyes. **2.** SYN metachromasia (1). [meta- + G. *chrōma,* color]

**met·a·chro·mo·phil, met·a·chro·mo·phile** (met-ă-krō′mō-fil, met-ă-krō′mō-fīl) SYN metachromatic. [meta- + G. *chrōma,* color, + *philos,* fond]

**met·a·cone** (met′ă-kōn) **1.** The distobuccal cusp of human upper molars. **2.** A cusp derived from the protocone in the evolutionary history of the molars. [meta- + G. *chronos,* time]

**met·a·co·nid** (met-ă-kon′id) **1.** The mesiolingual cusp of human lower molars. **2.** A cusp derived from the protoconid in the evolutionary history of the molars.

**met·a·her·pet·ic ker·a·ti·tis** a postinfectious corneal inflammation in herpetic keratitis leading to epithelial erosion; not due to virus replication.

**met·a·ki·ne·sis, met·a·ki·ne·sia** (met′ă-ki-nē′ sis, met′ă-ki-nē′sē-ă) moving apart; the separation of the two chromatids of each chromosome and their movement to opposite poles in the anaphase of mitosis. [meta- + G. *kinēsis,* movement]

**met·al** (met′ăl) one of the electropositive elements, either amphoteric or basic, characterized by luster, malleability, ductility, the ability to conduct electricity and heat, and the tendency to lose rather than gain electrons in chemical reactions. [L. *metallum,* a mine, a mineral, fr. G. *metallon,* a mine, pit]

△**me·tal·lo-** metal, metallic. [see metal]

**me·tal·lo·en·zyme** (mĕ-tal-ō-en′zīm) an enzyme containing a metal (ion) as an integral part of its active structure; e.g., cytochromes (Fe, Cu), aldehyde oxidase (Mo), catechol oxidase (Cu), carbonic anhydrase (Zn).

**me·tal·lo·por·phy·rin** (mĕ-tal-ō-pōr′fi-rin) a combination of a porphyrin with a metal, e.g., Fe (hematin), Mg (as in chlorophyll), Cu (in hemocyanin), Zn.

**me·tal·lo·pro·tein** (mĕ-tal-ō-prō′tēn) a protein with a tightly bound metal ion or ions; e.g., hemoglobin.

**me·tal·lo·pro·tein·ase** (met′a-lō-prō′tēn-āz) a family of protein-hydrolyzing endopeptidases that contain zinc ions as part of the active structure.

**me·tal·lo·thi·o·nein** (mĕ-tal-ō-thī′ō-nēn) a small protein, rich in cysteinyl residues, that is synthesized in the liver and kidney in response to the presence of divalent ions (zinc, mercury, cadmium, copper, etc.) and that binds these ions tightly; of importance in ion transport and detoxification.

**met·a·mer** (met′ă-mer) an entity that is similar to, but ultimately differentiable from, another entity. [meta- + -mer]

**met·a·mere** (met′ă-mēr) one of a series of homologous segments in the body. SEE ALSO somite. [meta- + G. *meros,* part]

**met·a·mer·ic** (met-ă-mer′ik) relating to or showing metamerism, or occurring in a metamere.

**met·a·mer·ic ner·vous sys·tem** that part of the nervous system which innervates body structures developed in ontogeny from the segmentally arranged somites or, in the head region, pharyngeal (branchial in fish) arches. The term implies reference to the neural mechanisms intrinsic to the spinal cord and brainstem (represented by the sensory nuclei, motoneuronal cell groups, and their associated interneurons in the reticular formation); by strict definition it should exclude the autonomic nervous system.

**me·tam·er·ism** (me-tam′er-izm) a pattern of anatomic structure exhibiting serial repetition of homologous structures, as vertebrae, ribs, intercostal muscles, and spinal nerves.

**met·a·mor·phop·sia** (met′ă-mōr-fop′sē-ă) distortion of visual images. [meta- + G. *morphē,* shape, + *opsis,* vision]

**met·a·mor·pho·sis** (met-ă-mōr′fŏ-sis) **1.** a change in form, structure, or function. **2.** transition from one developmental stage to another. SYN transformation (1). [G. *meta,* beyond, over, + *morphē,* form]

**met·a·mor·phot·ic** (met′ă-mōr-fot′ik) relating to or marked by metamorphosis.

**met·a·my·el·o·cyte** (met-ă-mī′el-ō-sīt) a transitional form of myelocyte with nuclear construction that is intermediate between the mature myelocyte (myelocyte C of Sabin) and the two-lobed granular leukocyte. SYN juvenile cell. [meta- + G. *myelos,* marrow, + *kytos,* cell]

**met·a·neph·ric duct** the slender tubular portion of the metanephric diverticulum; the primordium of the epithelial lining of the ureter.

**met·a·neph·ro·gen·ic, met·a·ne·phrog·e·nous** (met′ă-nef-rō-jen′ik, met-ă-nĕ-froj′ĕ-nŭs) applied to the more caudal part of the intermediate mesoderm, which, under the inductive action of the metanephric diverticulum, has the potency to form metanephric tubules. [meta- + G. *nephros,* kidney, + *-gen,* producing]

**met·a·neph·ros,** pl. **met·a·neph·roi** (met-ă-nef′ros, met-ă-nef′roy) the most caudally located of the three excretory organs appearing in the evolution of the vertebrates (the others being the pronephros and the mesonephros); in mammalian embryos, the metanephros develops caudal to the mesonephros during its regression, becoming the permanent kidney. [meta- + G. *nephros,* kidney]

**met·a·phase** (met′ă-fāz) the stage of mitosis or meiosis in which the chromosomes become aligned on the equatorial plate of the cell separating the centromeres. In mitosis and in the second meiotic division, the centromeres of each chromosome divide, and the two daughter centromeres are directed toward opposite poles of the cell; in the first division of meiosis, the centromeres do not divide, but the centromeres of each pair of homologous chromosomes become directed toward opposite poles. [meta- + G. *phasis,* an appearance]

**met·a·phy·se·al fi·brous cor·ti·cal de·fect** a small fibrous cortical defect located in the metaphysis of a long bone.

**met·a·phy·si·al dys·os·to·sis** a rare developmental abnormality of the skeleton in which metaphyses of tubular bones are expanded by deposits of cartilage.

**met·a·phy·si·al dys·pla·sia** an abnormality that occurs when new bone at the metaphyses of long bones fails to undergo remodeling to the normal tubular structure; the ends of long bones appear to be expanded and porotic, with thin cortex; there may be an associated overgrowth of cranial bones (craniometaphysial dysplasia).

**me·taph·y·sis,** pl. **me·taph·y·ses** (mĕ-taf′i-sis, mĕ-taf′i-sēz) a conical segment between the epiphysis and diaphysis of a long bone. [meta- + G. *physis,* growth]

**met·a·pla·sia** (met-ă-plā′zē-ă) abnormal transformation of an adult, fully differentiated tissue of one kind into a differentiated tissue of another kind; an acquired condition, in contrast to heteroplasia. [G. *metaplasis,* transformation]

**met·a·plasm** (met′ă-plazm) SYN cell inclusions (1). [meta- + G. *plasma,* something formed]

**met·a·plas·tic** (met-ă-plas′tik) pertaining to metaplasia or metaplasis.

**met·a·plas·tic a·ne·mia** pernicious anemia in which the various formed elements in the blood are changed, e.g., multisegmented, unusually large neutrophils (macropolycytes), immature myeloid cells, bizarre platelets.

**met·a·plas·tic car·ci·no·ma** a carcinoma in which some of the tumor cells are spindle shaped, suggesting a sarcoma, or in which the stroma shows foci of bone or cartilage.

**met·a·plas·tic os·si·fi·ca·tion** the formation of irregular foci of bone (sometimes including bone marrow) in various soft structures, such as the muscles, lungs, brain, and other sites where osseous tissue is abnormal.

**met·a·plas·tic pol·yp** SYN hyperplastic polyp.

**met·a·psy·chol·o·gy** (met′ă-sī-kol′ō-jē) **1.** a systematic attempt to discern and describe what lies beyond the empirical facts and laws of psychology, such as the relations between body and mind, or concerning the place of the mind in the universe. **2.** PSYCHOANALYSIS psychology concerning the fundamental assumptions of the freudian theory of the mind, which entail five points of view: 1) dynamic, concerning psychologic forces; 2) economic, concerning psychologic energy; 3) structural, concerning psychologic configurations; 4) genetic, concerning psychologic origins; 5) adaptive, concerning psychologic relations with the environment. [G. *meta,* beyond, transcending, + psychology]

**met·ar·ter·i·ole** (met′ar-tēr′ē-ōl) one of the small peripheral blood vessels between the arterioles and the true capillaries that contain scattered groups of smooth muscle fibers in their walls. [meta- + arteriole]

**met·a·ru·bri·cyte** (met-ă-roo′bri-sīt) orthochromatic normoblast. SEE normoblast.

**me·tas·ta·sis,** pl. **me·tas·ta·ses** (mĕ-tas′tă-sis, mĕ-tas′tă-sēz) **1.** the shifting of a disease or its local manifestations, from one part of the body to another, as in mumps when the symptoms referable to the parotid gland subside and the testis becomes affected. **2.** the spread of a disease process from one part of the body to another, as in the appearance of neoplasms in parts of the body remote from the site of the primary tumor; results from dissemination of tumor cells by the lymphatics or blood vessels or by direct extension through serous cavities or subarachnoid or other spaces. **3.** transportation of bacteria from one part of the body to another, through the bloodstream (hematogenous metastasis) or through lymph channels (lymphogenous metastasis). [G. a removing, fr. *meta,* in the midst of, + *stasis,* a placing]

**me·tas·ta·size** (mĕ-tas′tă-sīz) to pass into or invade by metastasis.

**met·a·stat·ic** (met-ă-stat′ik) relating to metastasis.

**met·a·stat·ic ab·scess** a secondary abscess formed, at a distance from the primary focus, as a

me
e

result of the transportation of pyogenic bacteria by the lymph or bloodstream.

**met·a·stat·ic cal·ci·fi·ca·tion** calcification occurring in nonosseous, viable tissue in hypercalcemia.

**met·a·tar·sal** (met′ă-tar′săl) relating to the metatarsus or to one of the metatarsal bones.

**met·a·tar·sal ar·tery** one of four dorsal or four plantar arteries coursing in relation to the metatarsal bones, each dividing distally into a medial and a lateral digital artery, serving the dorsal or plantar aspects of adjacent sides of two toes.

**met·a·tar·sal (bones) [I–V]** the five long bones numbered I to V beginning with the bone on the medial side forming the skeleton of the anterior portion of the foot, articulating posteriorly with the three cuneiform and the cuboid bones, anteriorly with the five proximal phalanges. SYN ossa metatarsi.

**met·a·tar·sal·gia** (met′ă-tar-sal′jē-ă) pain in the forefoot in the region of the heads of the metatarsals. [meta- + G. *algos*, pain]

**met·a·tar·sec·to·my** (met′ă-tar-sek′tō-mē) excision of the metatarsus. [metarsus + G. *ektomē*, excision]

**met·a·tar·so·pha·lan·ge·al (MTP)** (met′ă-tar′ sō-fă-lan′jē-ăl) relating to the metatarsal bones and the phalanges; denoting the articulations between them.

**met·a·tar·so·pha·lan·ge·al joints** the spheroid synovial joints between the heads of the metatarsals and the bases of the proximal phalanges of the toes.

**met·a·tar·sus,** pl. **me·ta·tar·si** (met′ă-tar′sŭs, met′ă-tar′sī) the distal portion of the foot between the instep and the toes, having as its skeleton the five long bones (metatarsal bones) articulating posteriorly with the cuboid and cuneiform bones and distally with the phalanges. [meta- + G. *tarsos*, tarsus]

**met·a·tar·sus la·tus** deformity caused by sinking down of the transverse arch of the foot.

**met·a·tar·sus var·us** fixed deformity in which the forepart of the foot is rotated on the long axis of the foot, so that the plantar surface faces the midline of the body. SYN intoe.

**met·a·thal·a·mus** (met′ă-thal′ă-mŭs) the most caudal and ventral part of the thalamus, composed of the medial and lateral geniculate bodies. [meta- + G. *thalamos*, thalamus]

**me·tath·e·sis** (me-tath′ĕ-sis) **1.** transfer of a pathologic product (e.g., a calculus) from one place to another where it causes less inconvenience or injury, when it is not possible or expedient to remove it from the body. **2.** CHEMISTRY a double decomposition, wherein a compound, A-B, reacts with another compound, C-D, to yield A-C + B-D, or A-D + B-C. [meta- + G. *thesis*, a placing]

**met·a·troph·ic** (met-ă-trof′ik) denoting the ability to undertake anabolism or to obtain nourishment from varied sources, i.e., both nitrogenous and carbonaceous organic matter. [meta- + G. *trophē*, nourishment]

**Met·a·zoa** (met-ă-zō′ă) a subkingdom of the kingdom Animalia, including all multicellular animal organisms in which the cells are differentiated and form tissues; distinguished from the subkingdom Protozoa, or unicellular animal organisms. [meta- + G. *zōon*, animal]

**met·a·zo·o·no·sis** (met′ă-zō-ō-nō′sis) a zoonosis that requires both a vertebrate and an invertebrate

host to complete the life cycle of the causative organism. [meta- + G. *zōon*, animal, + *nosos*, disease]

**Metch·ni·koff the·o·ry** (mech′nĭ-kof) the phagocytic theory, according to which the body is protected against infection by the leukocytes and other cells that engulf and destroy the invading microorganisms.

**met·en·ce·phal·ic** (met′en-se-fal′ik) relating to the metencephalon.

**met·en·ceph·a·lon** (met′en-sef′ă-lon) the anterior of the two major subdivisions of the rhombencephalon (the posterior being the myelencephalon or medulla oblongata), composed of the pons and the cerebellum. [meta- + G. *en-kephalos*, brain]

**Me·te·ni·er sign** (me-ten-yā′) easy eversion of the upper eyelid in Ehlers-Danlos syndrome.

**me·te·or·ism** (mē′tē-ŏ-rizm) SYN tympanites. [G. *meteōrismos*, a lifting up]

**me·te·or·o·tro·pic** (mē′tē-ōr-ō-trop′ik) denoting diseases affected in their incidence by the weather. [G. *meteōra*, things high in the air, + G. *tropos*, a turning]

**me·ter** (mē′ter) **1.** the fundamental unit of length in the SI and metric systems, equivalent to 39.37007874 inches. Defined to be the length of path traveled by light in a vacuum in $1/299792458$ sec. **2.** a device for measuring the quantity of that which passes through it. [Fr. *metre*; G. *metron*, measure]

**me·ter an·gle** the amount of convergence required to view binocularly an object 1 meter distant and exerting 1 diopter of accommodation.

**me·ter-can·dle** (mē′ter-kan′dl) SYN lux.

**metered-dose inhaler (MDI)** a device consisting of a canister, propellant, drug, and mouthpiece (or other patient adjunct) that delivers a known dose of drug as an aerosol with each actuation. See this page.

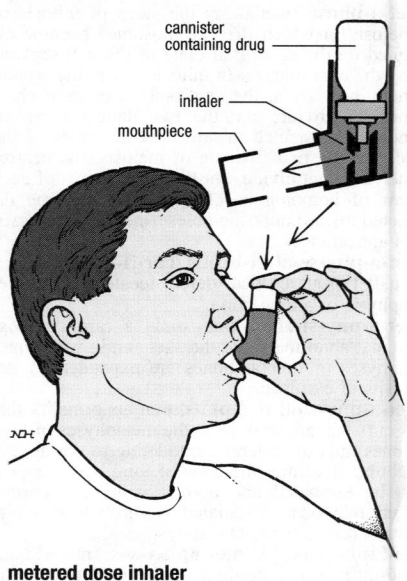

cannister containing drug

inhaler

mouthpiece

**metered dose inhaler**

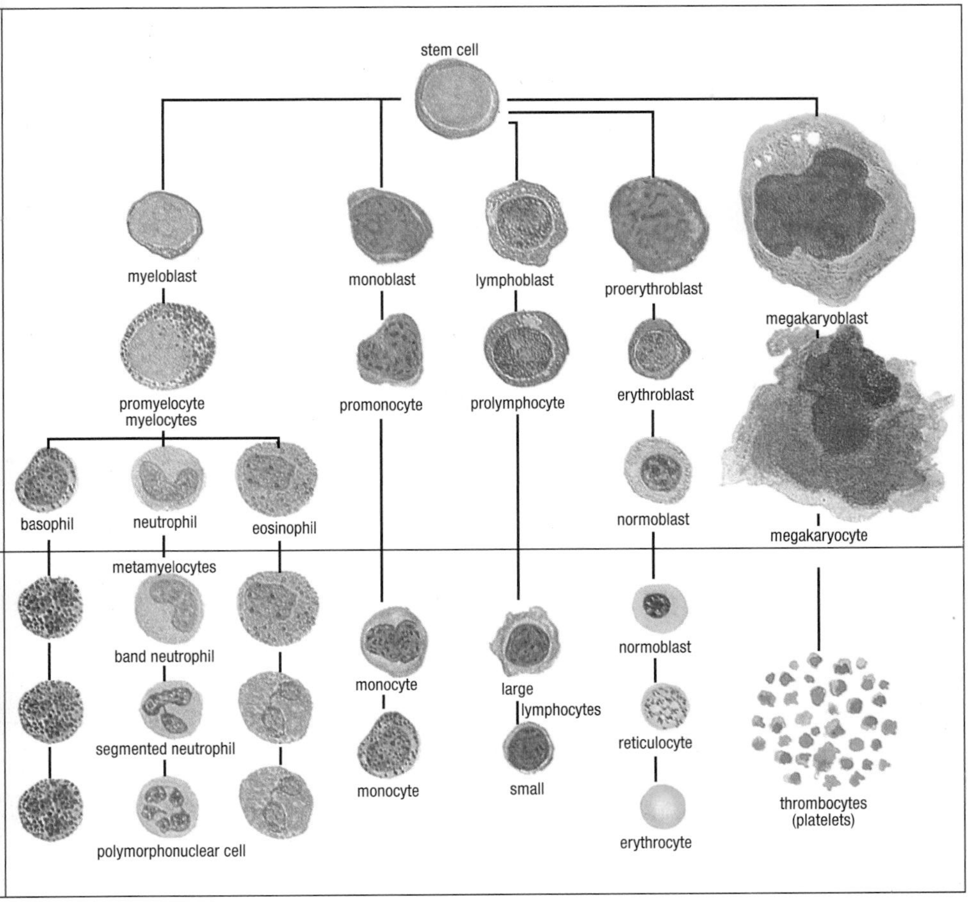

stem cell

myeloblast

monoblast

lymphoblast

proerythroblast

megakaryoblast

promyelocyte
myelocytes

promonocyte

prolymphocyte

erythroblast

basophil  neutrophil  eosinophil

normoblast

megakaryocyte

metamyelocytes

band neutrophil

monocyte

large
lymphocytes

normoblast

segmented neutrophil

monocyte

small

reticulocyte

thrombocytes
(platelets)

polymorphonuclear cell

erythrocyte

Images

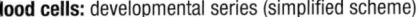
**lood cells:** developmental series (simplified scheme)

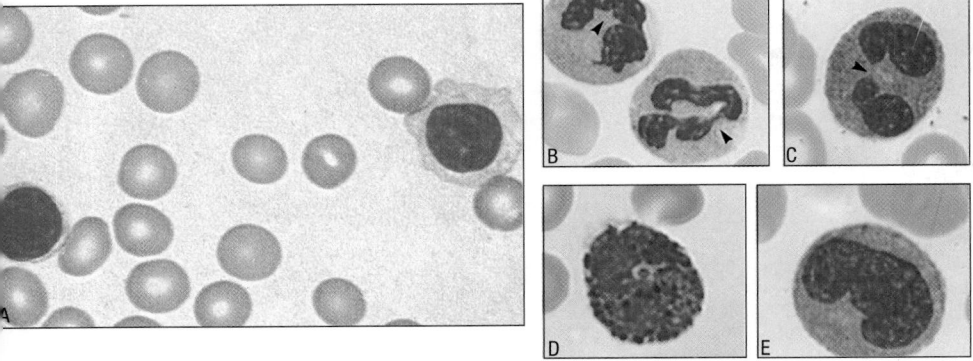

**lood cells:** (A) stained smear of normal blood showing a small **lymphocyte** (left) and a large lymphocyte (right); (B) **neutrophils** owing a somewhat granular cytoplasm and lobulated nuclei (arrows); (C) **eosinophils** with large pink granules and sausage- aped nuclei (arrow); (D) **basophil** with dense, dark, large granules; (E) **monocyte** characterized by large size, acentric, kidney- aped nucleus, and lack of specific granules

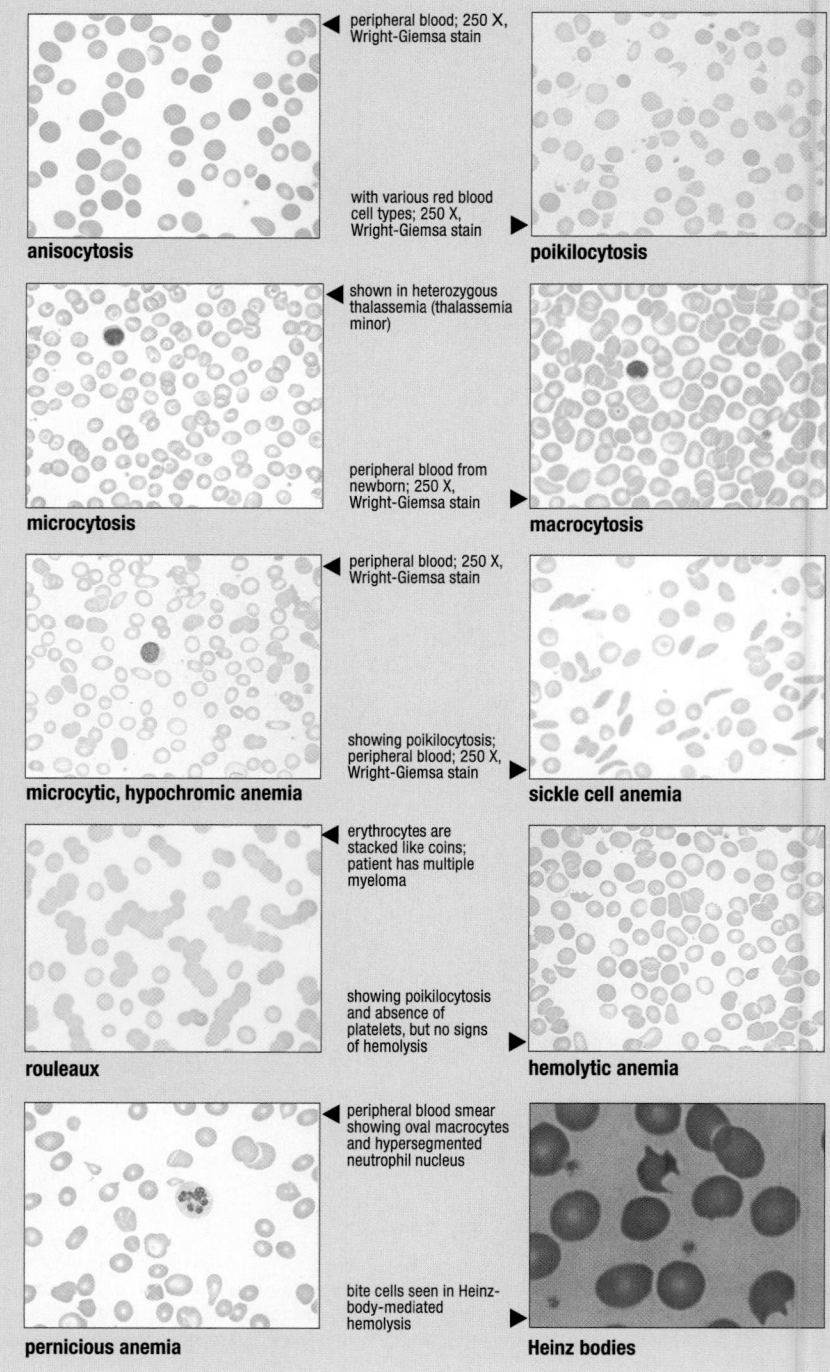

peripheral blood; 250 X, Wright-Giemsa stain

**anisocytosis**

with various red blood cell types; 250 X, Wright-Giemsa stain

**poikilocytosis**

shown in heterozygous thalassemia (thalassemia minor)

**microcytosis**

peripheral blood from newborn; 250 X, Wright-Giemsa stain

**macrocytosis**

peripheral blood; 250 X, Wright-Giemsa stain

**microcytic, hypochromic anemia**

showing poikilocytosis; peripheral blood; 250 X, Wright-Giemsa stain

**sickle cell anemia**

erythrocytes are stacked like coins; patient has multiple myeloma

**rouleaux**

showing poikilocytosis and absence of platelets, but no signs of hemolysis

**hemolytic anemia**

peripheral blood smear showing oval macrocytes and hypersegmented neutrophil nucleus

**pernicious anemia**

bite cells seen in Heinz-body-mediated hemolysis

**Heinz bodies**

## *bacteria and bacterial diseases*

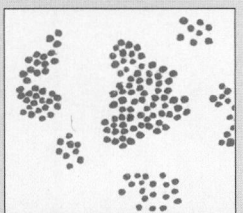

**staphylococci**

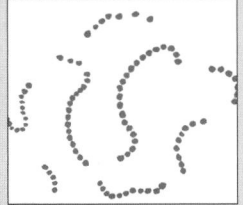

**streptococci**

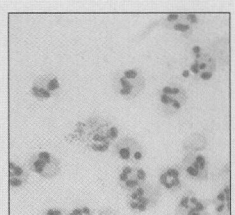

**gonococci**

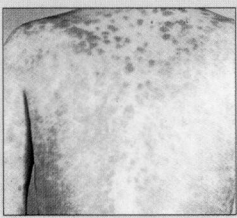

**lepromatous leprosy**

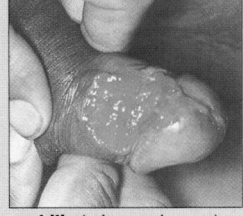

**syphilis** (primary chancre)

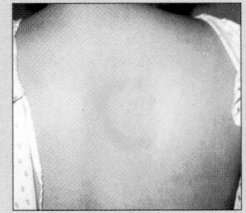

**Lyme disease** (erythema chronicum migrans)

## *viruses and viral diseases*

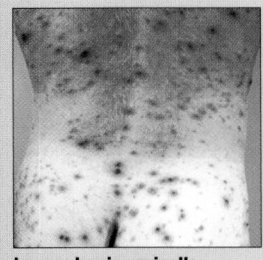

**hemorrhagic varicella** (chicken pox)

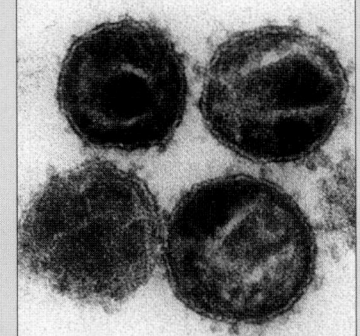

**AIDS virus**

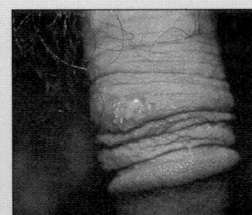

**genital herpes** (HSV-2)

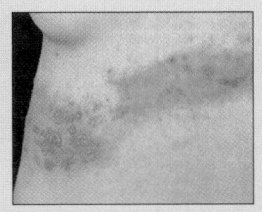

**herpes zoster**

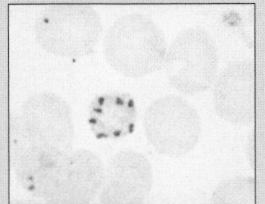

**condylomata acuminata** (genital warts)

## *parasites and parasitic diseases*

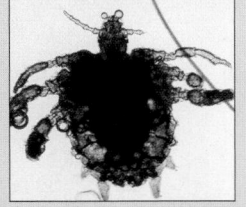

***Plasmodium malariae:*** schizonts in erythrocyte

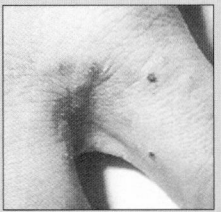

***Pthirus pubis*** (adult female)

**scabies**

Images

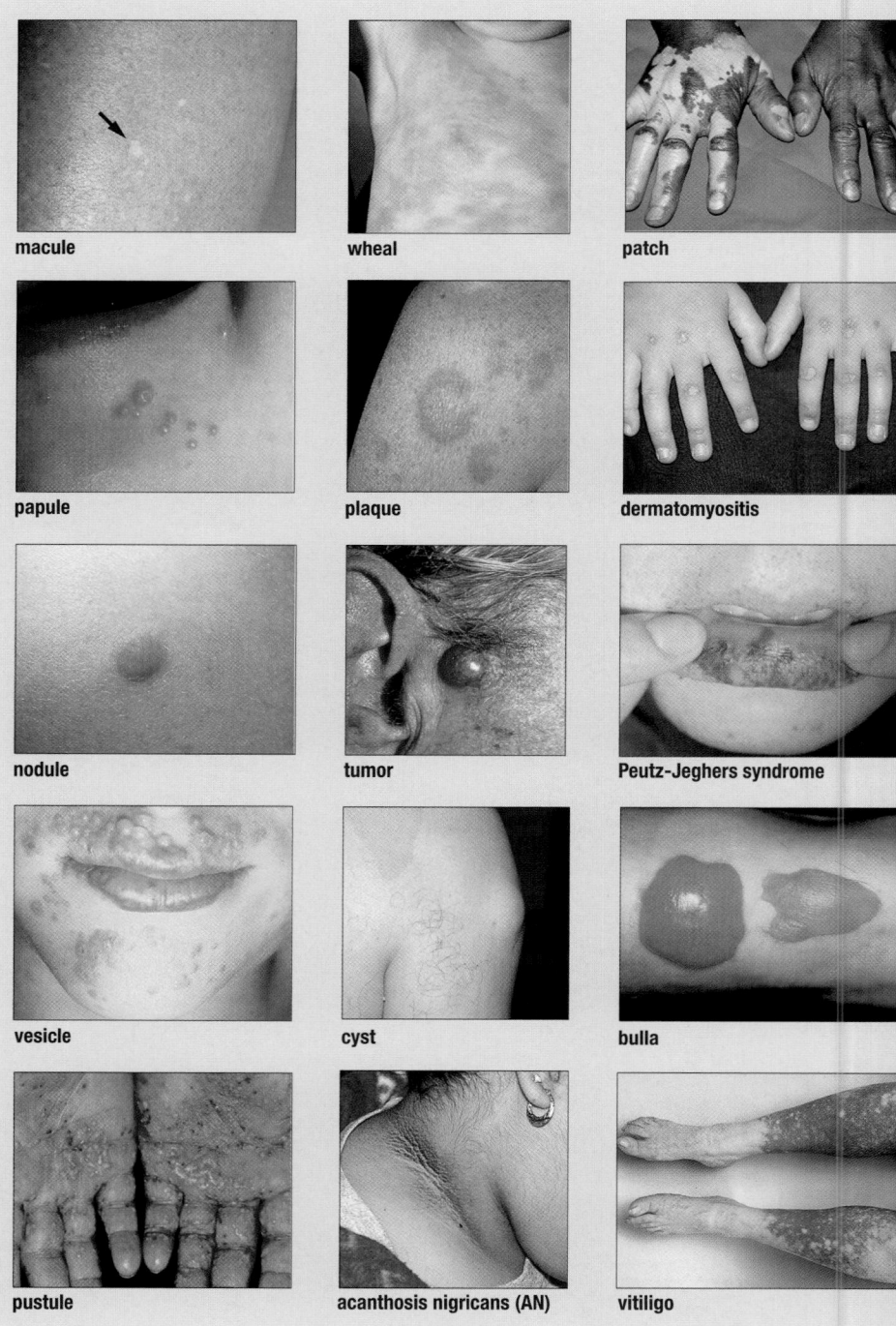

macule

wheal

patch

papule

plaque

dermatomyositis

nodule

tumor

Peutz-Jeghers syndrome

vesicle

cyst

bulla

pustule

acanthosis nigricans (AN)

vitiligo

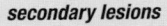
*secondary lesions*

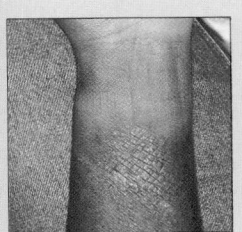
**lichenification**

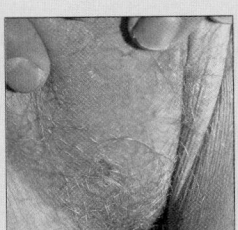
**erosion**

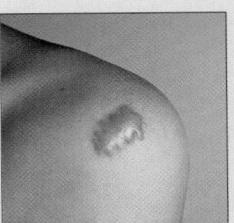
**keloid**

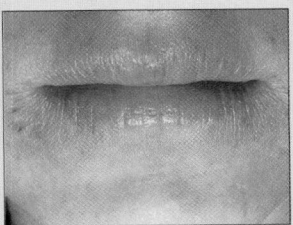
**fissure**

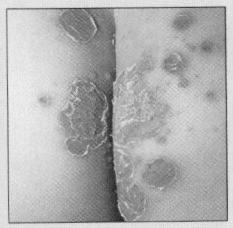
**scale**

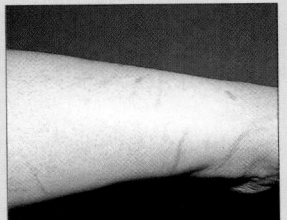
**excoriation**

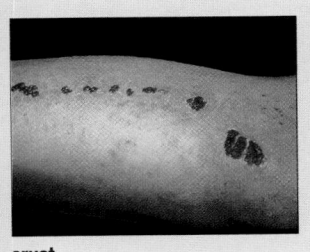
**crust**

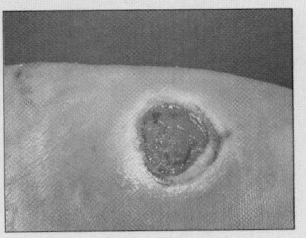
**ulcer**

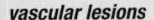
*vascular lesions*

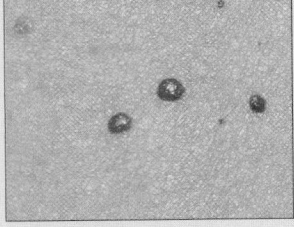
**cherry angiomata**

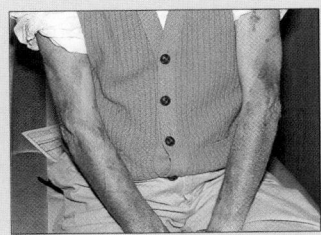
**ecchymosis**

**telangiectasia**

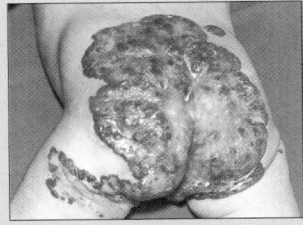
**cavernous hemangioma**

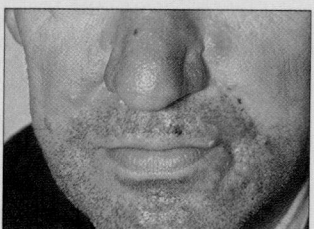

rosacea

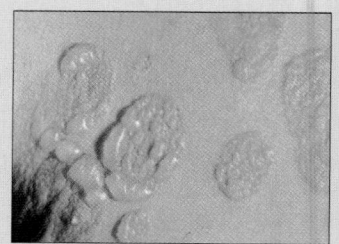

dermatitis herpetiformis

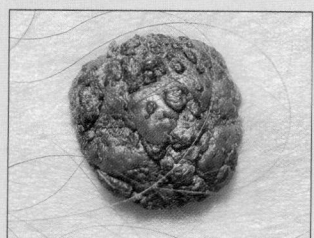

seborrheic keratosis

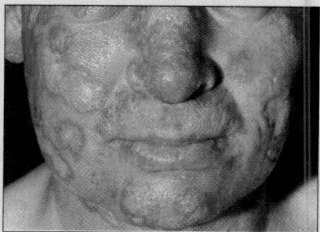

lupus erythematosus

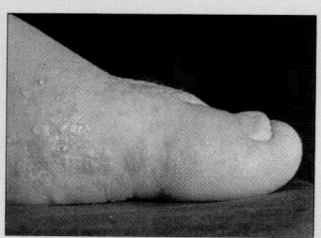

tinea pedis

**actinic keratoses:** ▶
numerous keratoses
over the scalp
induced by chronic
ultraviolet exposure

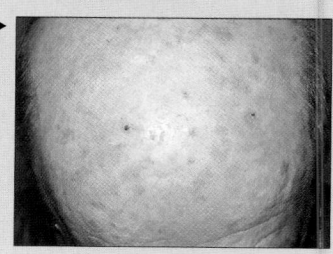

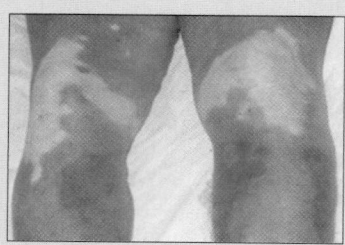

purpura fulminans

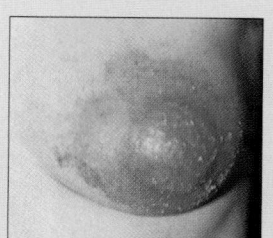

tinea corporis (ringworm)

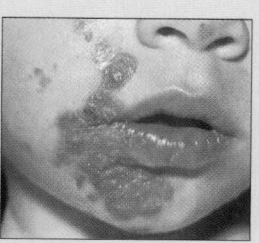

impetigo

Paget disease of nipple

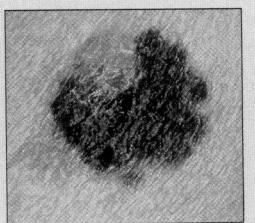

**malignant melanoma:** showing uneven pigmentation

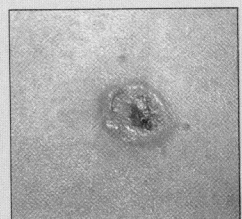

**basal cell carcinoma**

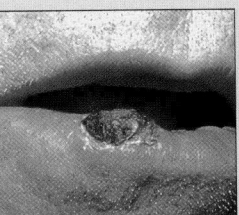

**squamous cell carcinoma**

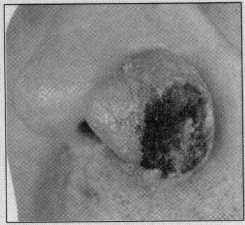

**keratoacanthoma:** of the nose

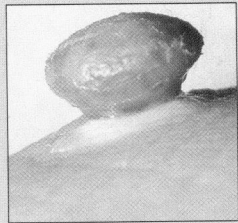

**pyogenic granuloma**

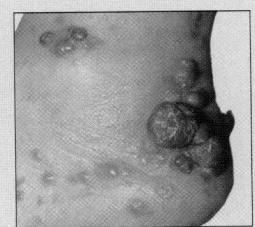

**Kaposi sarcoma**

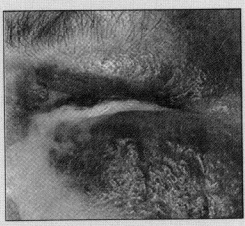

**angiosarcoma:** on left side of face

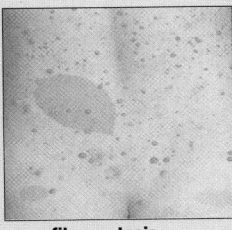

**neurofibromatosis**

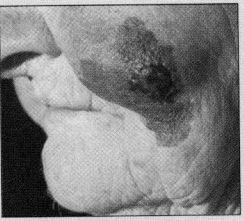

**lentigo maligna melanoma**

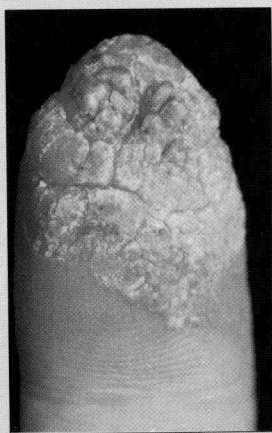

**Bowen disease:** squamous cell carcinoma in situ on fingertip

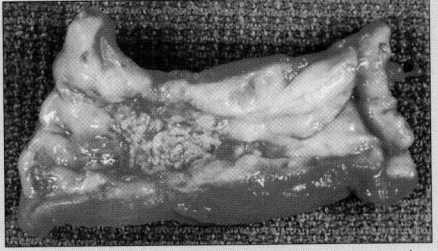

**ulcerative squamous cell carcinoma:** of the esophagus

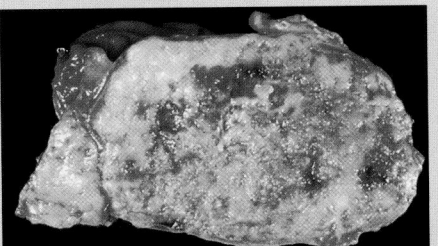

**benign tumor of stomach**

Images

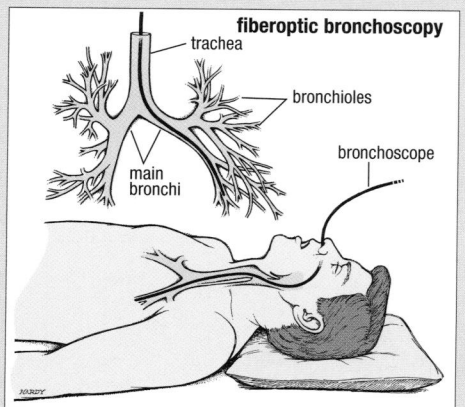

**fiberoptic bronchoscopy**

trachea

bronchioles

main bronchi

bronchoscope

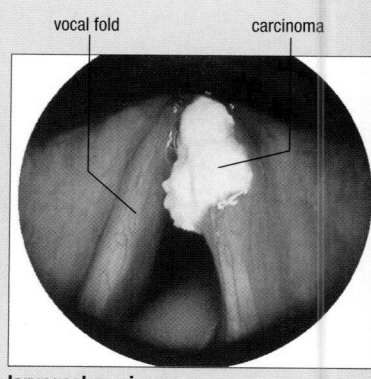

vocal fold

carcinoma

**laryngeal carcinoma**

**bronchoscopy** is the examination of the respiratory apparatus with a flexible bronchoscope for diagnostic or treatment purposes; the bronchoscope is introduced nasally and slowly led down the trachea until the desired level is reached; the photographs on this page were taken with a camera that attaches to the examiner's end of the instrument

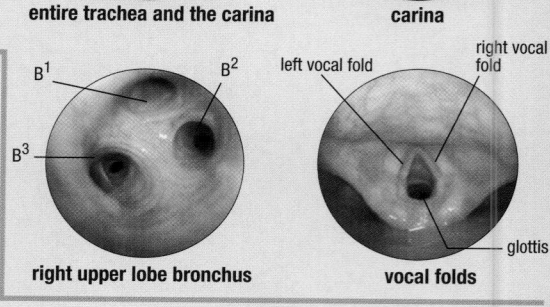

carina

carina

left main bronchus

right main bronchus

**entire trachea and the carina**

**carina**

**esophagogastroduodenoscopy** is the examination of the esophagus, stomach, and upper small intestine using a flexible esophagogastroduodenoscope; fiberoptics in the instrument conduct bright, cool light along a curved path, allowing illumination of tissues and structures within the body; the scope often contains small instruments such as biopsy snares

$B^1$   $B^2$

$B^3$

left vocal fold

right vocal fold

glottis

**right upper lobe bronchus**

**vocal folds**

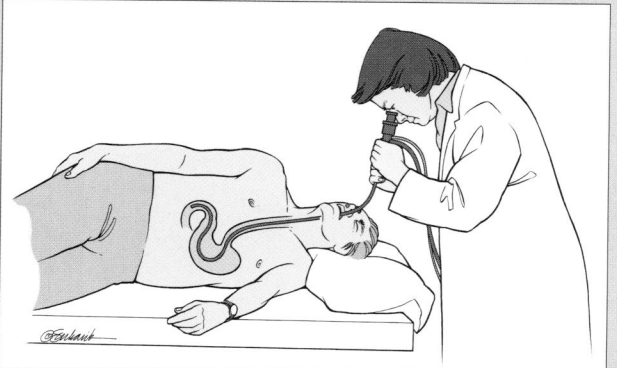

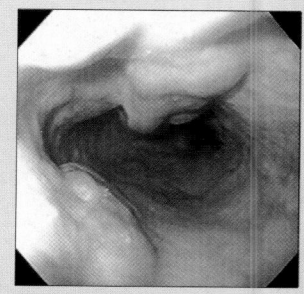

**esophageal varices**

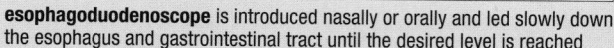
**esophagoduodenoscope** is introduced nasally or orally and led slowly down the esophagus and gastrointestinal tract until the desired level is reached

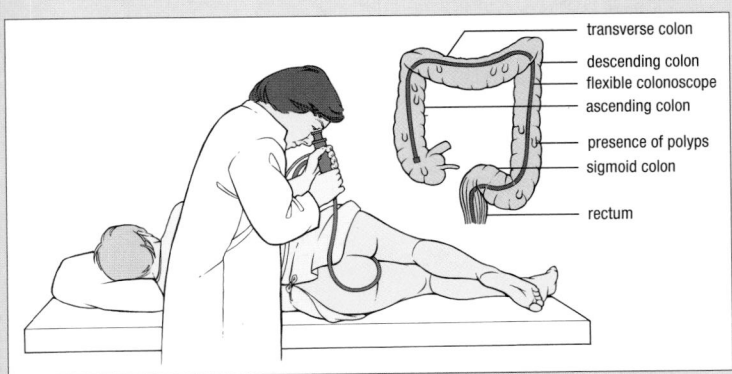

- transverse colon
- descending colon
- flexible colonoscope
- ascending colon
- presence of polyps
- sigmoid colon
- rectum

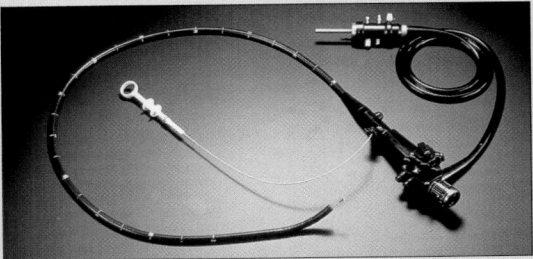

**colonoscope**

**colonoscopy** is the examination and diagnosis of conditions of the colon; the flexible colonoscope passes through the rectum and sigmoid colon into the descending, transverse, and ascending colon (above); small instruments can be passed through the colonoscope and used to perform minor operative procedures; the images below were taken by a camera attached to the colonoscope

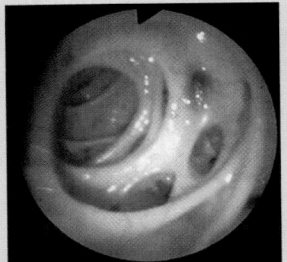

**diverticulosis**

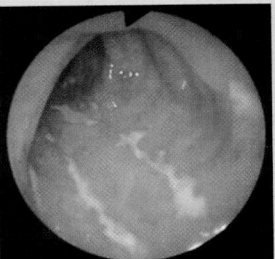

**ulcerative colitis**

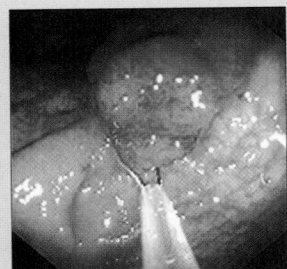

**colon polypectomy**

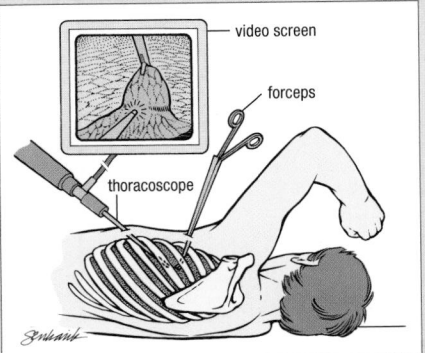

- video screen
- forceps
- thoracoscope

**thoracoscopy** is a diagnostic procedure in which the pleural cavity is examined with an endoscope (left); small incisions are made into the pleural cavity in an intercostal space; the use of fiberoptic instruments and miniature video equipment permits visualization of thoracic structures; tissue can be excised for biopsy, and treatment of some thoracic conditions can be conducted

Images

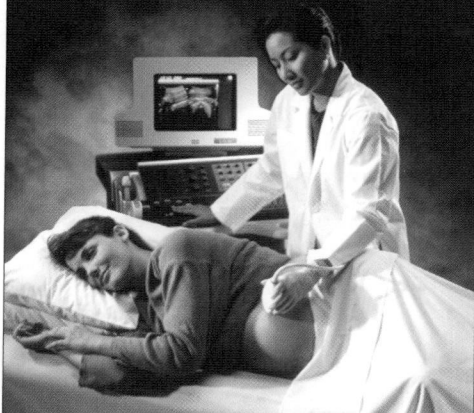

**obstetrical sonography** performed on pregnant woman

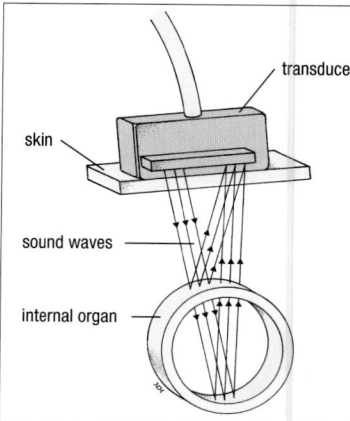

**principle of sonography**

during **sonography** (above), energy in the form of sound waves is reflected off internal organs or, during pregnancy, the fetus, and is transformed into an image on a TV-type monitor; in the case of obstetrical sonography (top left), an ultrasound image of the pregnant uterus is created in order to determine fetal development

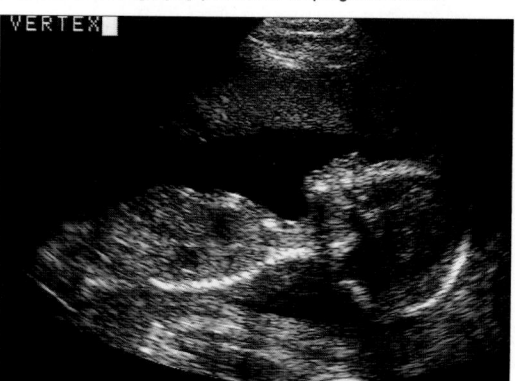

**fetus in breech position:** sagittal view

**echocardiography** is the use of ultrasound in the investigation of the heart and great vessels and diagnosis of vascular lesions

during **Doppler sonography,** an instrument emits an ultrasonic beam into the body; the ultrasound reflected from moving structures changes its frequency (Doppler effect); Doppler sonography is often used in diagnosing peripheral vascular and cardiac disease

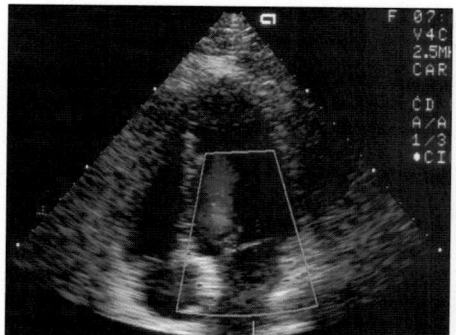

**echocardiogram:** normal, two-dimensional, apical four-chamber view

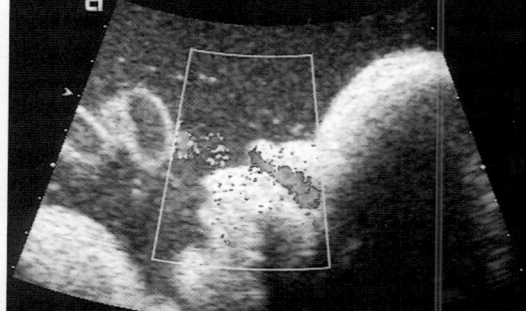

**Doppler flow sonogram** showing the flow of amniotic fluid into the nasal cavity of the fetus

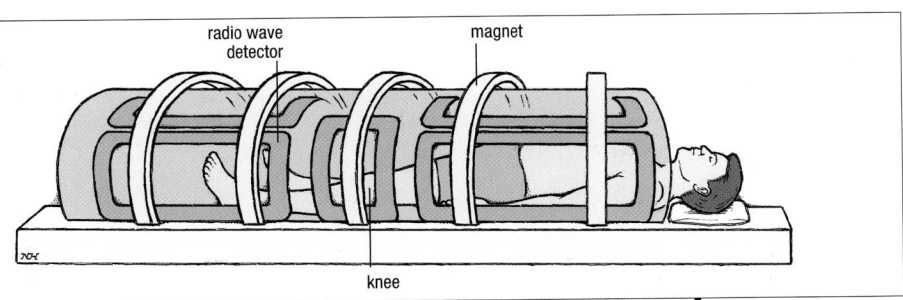

radio wave detector

magnet

knee

**magnetic resonance imaging (MRI)** is a nonionizing (non-x-ray) technique using magnetic fields and radio frequency waves to visualize anatomic structures; it is useful in detecting joint, tendon, and vertebral disorders; the patient is positioned within a magnetic field (above) as radio wave signals are conducted through the selected body part; energy is absorbed by tissues and then released

computer processes the released energy and formulates image

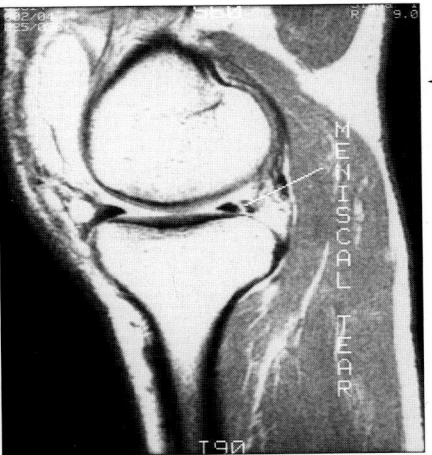

**magnetic resonance image** of knee (lateral view) identifying a torn meniscus

Images

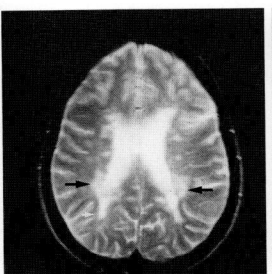

**multiple sclerosis:** contiguous T2-weighted MR images, showing areas of ventricular plaques of high signal (arrows)

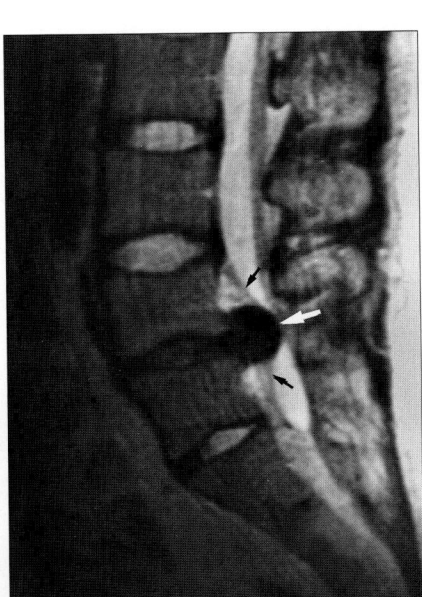

**herniated nucleus pulposus:** sagittal MRI showing a large posterior herniation (arrows) at the L4 disc space; note the posterior displacement of the thecal space (small arrows)

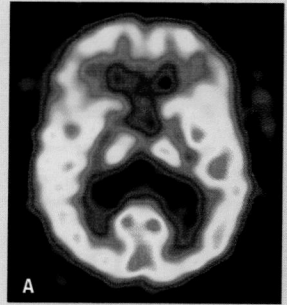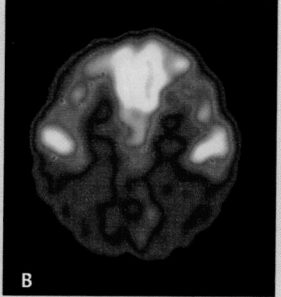

**A** **B**

warm colors (red and yellow) indicate a higher rate of metabolism and brain activity in the **normal brain** (A) when compared to the brain of a patient with **Alzheimer disease** (B)

**nuclear medicine** imaging is a diagnostic imaging technique using injected or ingested radioactive isotopes and a gamma camera for determining size, shape, location, and function of various body parts

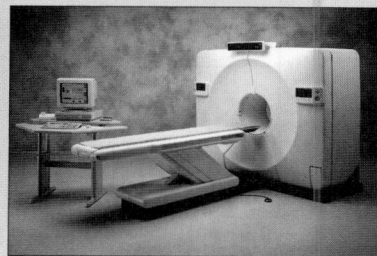

**positron emission tomography** (PET) combines nuclear medicine and computed tomography to produce images of brain anatomy and corresponding physiology; it is used to study conditions such as stroke, Alzheimer disease (above left), epilepsy, metabolic brain disorders, and chemistry of neural function

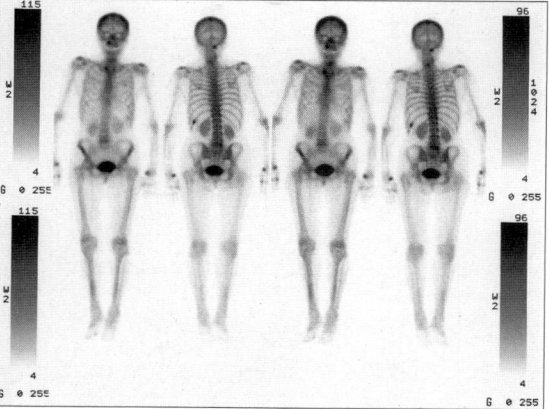

◀ **bone scan:** nuclear scan of bone tissue to detect abnormalities such as tumors and malignancies; left is an example of a full-body bone scan

**nuclear lung scan** is used ▶ to detect abnormalities of perfusion (blood flow) or ventilation (respiration), commonly called V̇/Q̇ (ventilation/perfusion) scan; (A) gamma-camera used to produce lung scan; in this patient a posterior lung scan shows an embolus in the right lung; ventilation scan (B) shows a normal pattern; absence of blood flow to the right lung is apparent on perfusion scan (C)

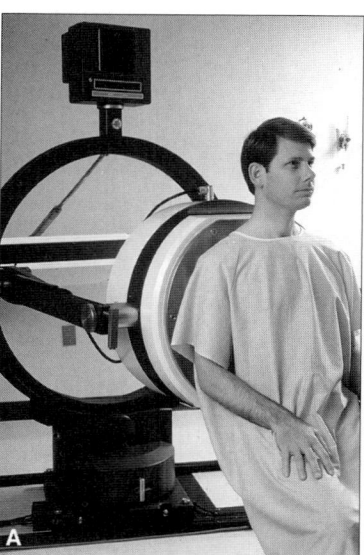

**A**

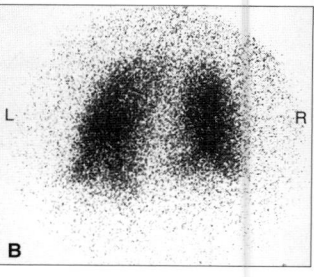

**B**

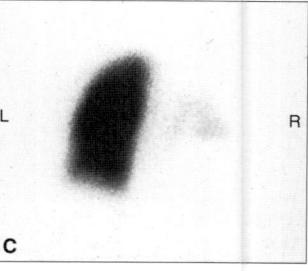

**C**

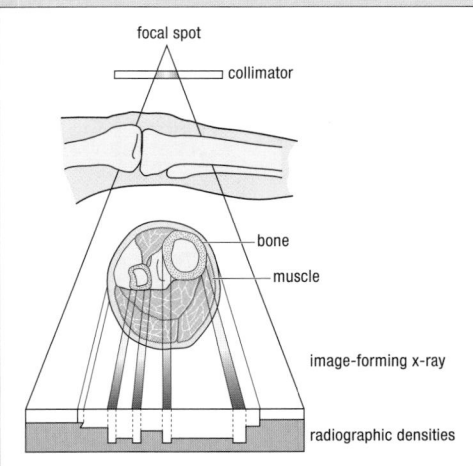

focal spot

collimator

bone

muscle

image-forming x-ray

radiographic densities

**radiography** or **roentgenography** is the examination of any part of the body for diagnostic purposes by means of x-rays, with the record of findings usually impressed upon a photographic film

◀ **x-rays** pass through body parts, with denser structures absorbing more x-rays and consequently appearing as lighter areas on the radiograph

as shown in the graphic above, differential absorption of x-rays depends on the composition of various tissues; denser tissue (such as bone) absorbs more x-rays, less dense tissue (such as subcutaneous fat) transmits more x-rays; greater absorption produces less darkening while lesser absorption produces more darkening; the resultant radiographic image is essentially a "shadowgram"

the **plain chest radiology** images on this page show various pathological conditions of the chest and respiratory system

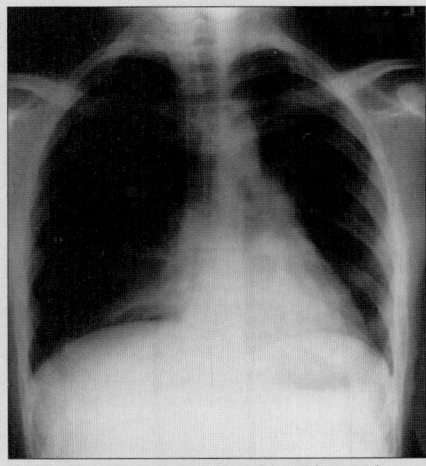

**right-sided pneumothorax:** with evidence of mediastinal shift (tension)

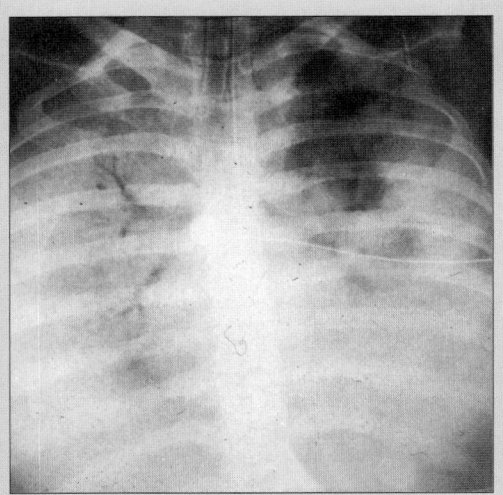

**adult respiratory distress syndrome (ARDS)**

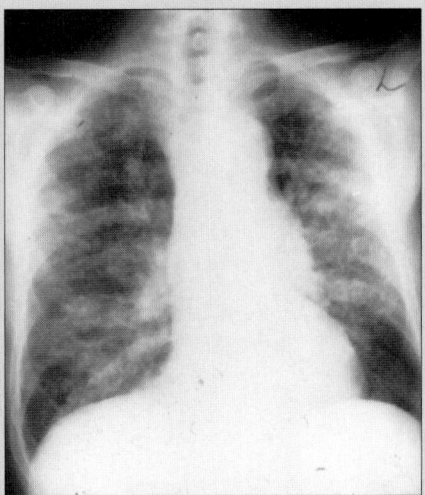

**interstitial lung disease**

Images

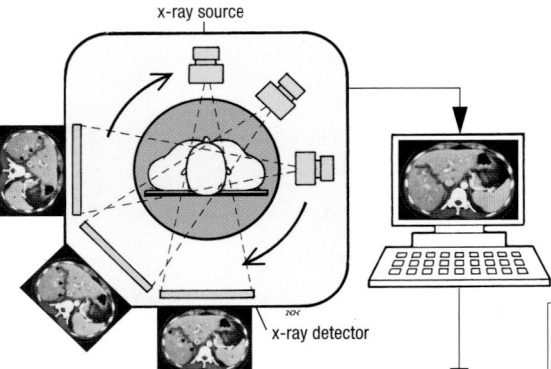

**computed tomography (CT)** is a radiologic procedure using a machine called a scanner to examine a body site by taking a series of cross-sectional images one slice at a time in a full-circle rotation; a computer then calculates and converts the rates of absorption and density of the x-rays into a picture on a screen

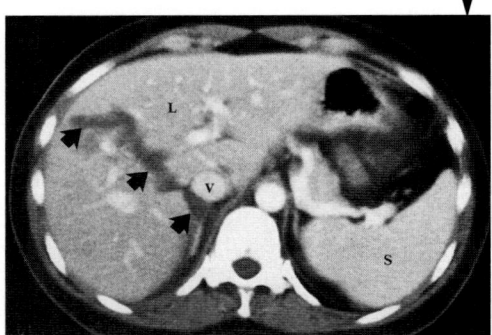

**CT scan** of patient involved in a motor vehicle accident demonstrates a jagged laceration (arrows) extending from posterior to inferior vena cava (V) through right lobe of the liver (L); (S), spleen

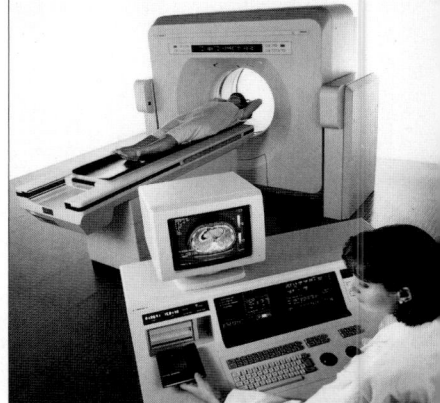

**computed tomography apparatus**

**mammography** is the imaging examination of the breast by means of x-rays, ultrasound, and nuclear magnetic resonance, used for the screening and diagnosis of breast disease; x-ray mammography has proved to have the greatest efficacy for detecting occult breast cancer

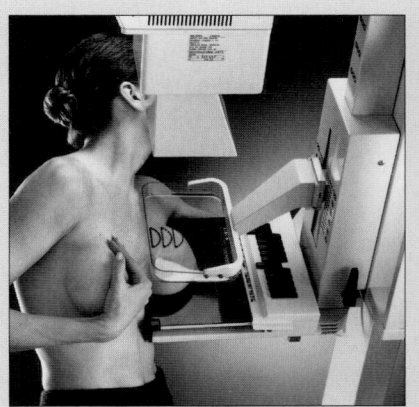

patient positioning for a MLO view

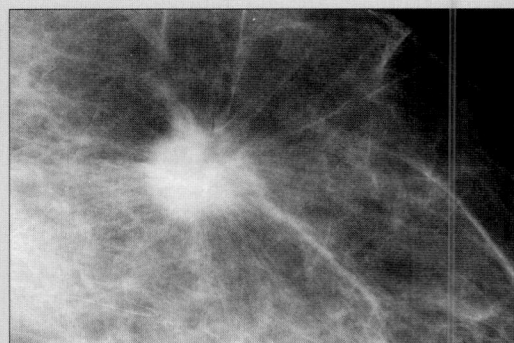

**classic breast carcinoma:** this spiculated breast mass is an infiltrating duct carcinoma

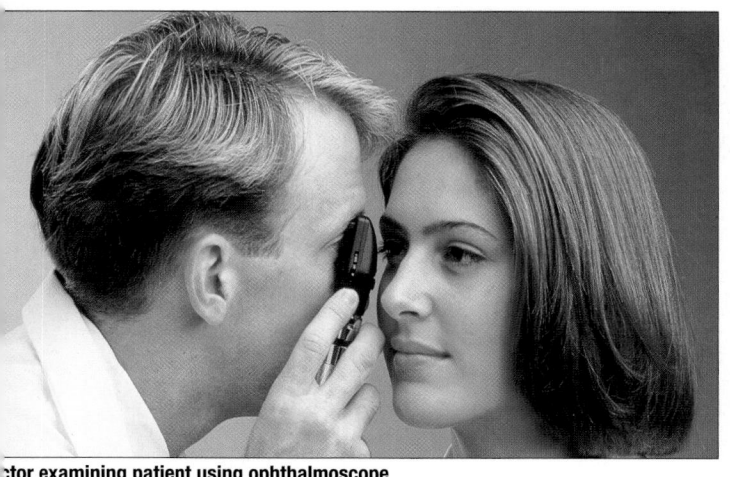

doctor examining patient using ophthalmoscope

ophthalmoscope

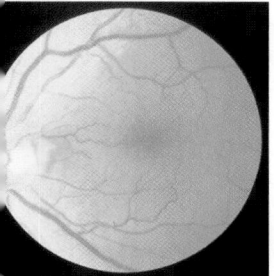

normal fundus

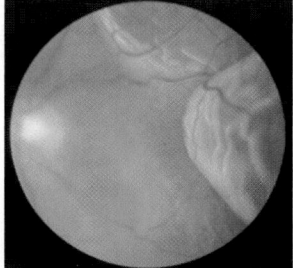

retinal detachment

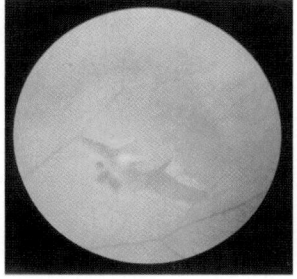

retinal tear

Images

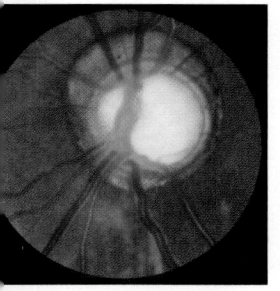

glaucomatous cupping of disc

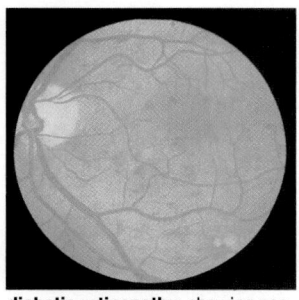

**diabetic retinopathy:** showing neo-vascularization

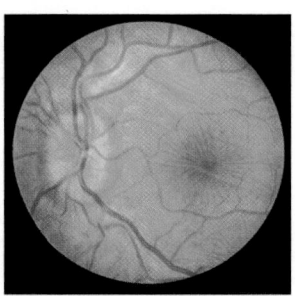

**papilledema:** with conspicuous retinal folding

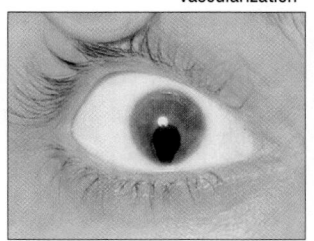

coloboma

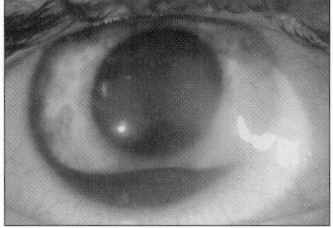

hyphema

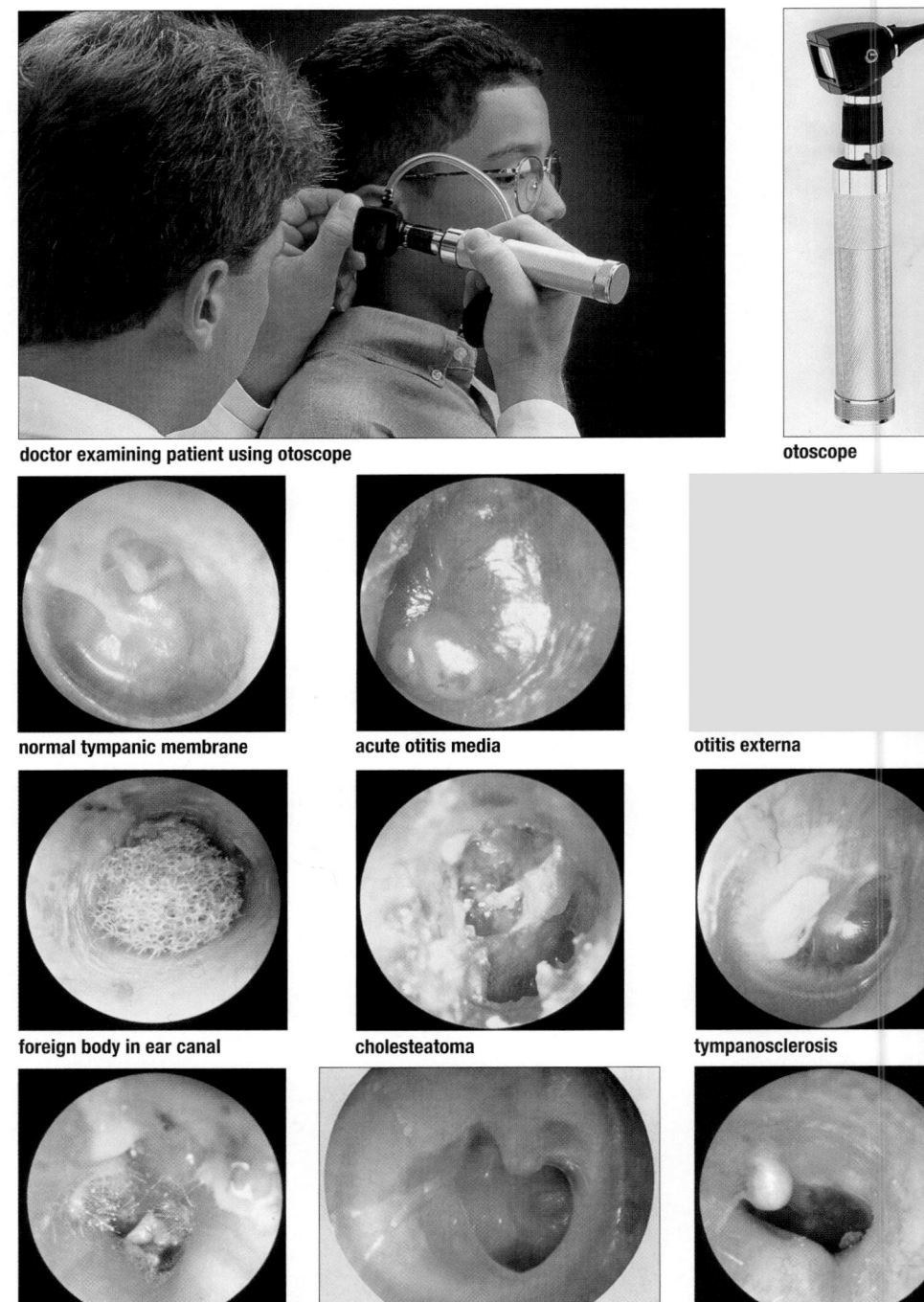

doctor examining patient using otoscope

otoscope

normal tympanic membrane

acute otitis media

otitis externa

foreign body in ear canal

cholesteatoma

tympanosclerosis

otomycosis

perforation

exostosis

**met·es·trus, met·es·trum** (met-es′trŭs, met-es′ trŭm) the period between estrus and diestrus in the estrous cycle. [meta- + estrus]

⚠**meth-, metho-** chemical prefixes usually denoting a methyl, methoxy group.

**met·hae·mal·bu·min [Br.]** SEE methemalbumin.

**met·hae·mo·glo·bin [Br.]** SEE methemoglobin.

**met·hae·mo·glo·bi·nae·mia [Br.]** SEE methemoglobinemia.

**met·hae·mo·glo·bi·nu·ria [Br.]** SEE methemoglobinuria.

**meth·ane** (meth′ān) an odorless gas produced by the decomposition of organic matter; explosive when mixed with 7 or 8 volumes of air, constituting then the firedamp in coal mines.

**meth·an·o·gen** (meth-an′ō-jen) any methane-producing bacterium of the family Methanobacteriaceae.

**meth·a·nol** (meth′ă-nol) SYN methyl alcohol.

**metHb** methemoglobin.

**met·hem·al·bu·min** (met′hēm-al-byu′min) an abnormal compound formed in the blood as a result of heme combining with plasma albumin.

**met·hem·al·bu·mi·ne·mia** (met′hēm-al-byu-min-ē′mē-ă) the presence of methemalbumin in the circulating blood, indicative of hemoglobin breakdown; found in some patients with blackwater fever or paroxysmal nocturnal hemoglobinuria.

**met·he·mo·glo·bin (metHb)** (met-hē-mō-glō′ bin) a transformation product of oxyhemoglobin because of the oxidation of the normal $Fe^{2+}$ to $Fe^{3+}$, thus converting ferroprotoporphyrin to ferriprotoporphyrin; useless for respiration; found in sanguineous effusions and in the circulating blood after poisoning with acetanilid, potassium chlorate, and other substances.

**met·he·mo·glo·bi·ne·mia** (met-hē′mō-glō-bi-nē′ mē-ă) the presence of methemoglobin in the circulating blood. [methemoglobin + G. *haima*, blood]

**met·he·mo·glo·bi·nu·ria** (met-hē′mō-glō-bin-yu′rē-ă) the presence of methemoglobin in the urine. [methemoglobin + G. *ouron*, urine]

**meth·e·na·mine sil·ver stain** a stain used for cysts of *Pneumocystis carinii*.

**me·thi·o·nine** (me-thī′ō-nēn) a nutritionally essential amino acid and the most important natural source of "active methyl" groups in the body, hence usually involved in methylations *in vivo*.

**meth·od** (meth′ŏd) the mode or manner or orderly sequence of events of a process or procedure. SEE ALSO fixative, operation, procedure, stain, technique. [G. *methodos*; fr. *meta*, after, + *hodos*, way]

⚠**meth·oxy-** chemical prefix denoting substitution of a methoxyl group.

**me·thox·yl** (me-thok′sil) the group, $-OCH_3$.

**meth·yl** (meth′il) the radical, $-CH_3$. [G. *methy*, wine, + *hylē*, wood]

**meth·yl al·co·hol** a flammable, toxic, mobile liquid, used as an industrial solvent, antifreeze, and in chemical manufacture; ingestion may result in severe acidosis, visual impairment, and other effects on the central nervous system. SYN methanol.

**meth·yl·a·tion** (meth-i-lā′shŭn) addition of methyl groups; in histochemistry, used to esterify carboxyl groups and remove sulfate groups by treating tissue sections with hot methanol in the presence of hydrochloric acid; the net effect being to reduce tissue basophilia and abolish metachromasia.

**meth·yl·di·chlo·ro·ar·sine (MD)** (meth′il-dī-klōr-ō-ar′sēn) a vesicant; irritating to the respiratory tract; produces lung and eye injury; has been used in certain military operations.

**meth·yl·ene** (meth′i-lēn) the radical, $-CH_2-$.

**meth·yl·ene blue** [CI 52015] a basic dye easily oxidized to azure, with dye mixtures; used in histology and microbiology, to stain intestinal protozoa in wet mount preparations, to track RNA and RNase in electrophoresis, and as an antidote for methemoglobinemia; its redox indicator properties are useful in milk bacteriology.

**meth·yl green** [CI 42585] a basic triphenylmethane dye used as a chromatin stain and, in combination with pyronin, for differential staining of RNA (red) and DNA (green); also used as a tracking dye for DNA in electrophoresis.

**meth·yl·ol** (meth′i-lol) hydroxymethyl; the radical, $-CH_2OH$.

**meth·yl·pen·tose** (meth-il-pen′tōs) a hexose (a 6-deoxyhexose) in which carbon-6 is part of a methyl group; e.g., rhamnose, fucose.

**meth·yl·trans·fer·ase** (meth-il-trans′fer-ās) any enzyme transferring methyl groups from one compound to another. SYN transmethylase.

**metMb** metmyoglobin.

**met·my·o·glo·bin (metMb)** (met′mī-ō-glō′bin) myoglobin in which the ferrous ion of the heme prosthetic group is oxidized to ferric ion.

**me·ton·y·my** (mĕ-ton′i-mē) imprecise or circumscribed labeling of objects or events, characteristic of the language disturbance of schizophrenics; e.g., the patient speaks of having had a "menu" rather than a "meal." [meta- + G. *onyma*, name]

**me·top·ic** (me-tō′pik, me-top′ik) relating to the forehead or anterior portion of the cranium. [G. *metōpon*, forehead]

**me·top·ic su·ture** a persistent frontal suture, sometimes discernible a short distance above sutura frontonasalis.

**met·o·po·plas·ty** (met′ŏ-pō-plas-tē, me-top′ō-plas-tē) plastic surgery of the skin or bone of the forehead. [G. *metōpon*, forehead, + *plastos*, formed]

⚠**metr-, met·ra-, met·ro-** the uterus. SEE ALSO hystero- (1), utero-. [G. *mētra*]

**me·tra** (mē′tră) SYN uterus. [G. uterus]

**me·tra·to·nia** (mē-tră-tō′nē-ă) atony of the uterine walls after childbirth. [metra- + G. *a-* priv. + *tonos*, tension]

**me·trat·ro·phy, me·tra·tro·phia** (mē-trat′rō-fē, mē-tră-trō′fē-ă) uterine atrophy. [metra-atrophy]

**me·tria** (mē′trē-ă) pelvic cellulitis or other inflammatory affection in the puerperal period. [G. *mētra*, uterus]

**met·ric** (met′rik) quantitative; relating to measurement. SEE metric system. [G. *metrikos*, fr. *metron*, measure]

**met·ric sys·tem** a system of weights and measures, universal for scientific use, based upon the meter, the gram, and the liter.

**me·tri·tis** (mē-trī′tis) inflammation of the uterus. [G. *mētra*, uterus, + *-itis*, inflammation]

**me·tro·cyte** (mē′trō-sīt) SYN mother cell. [G. *mētēr*, mother, + *kytos*, a hollow (cell)]

**me·tro·dyn·ia** (mē-trō-dī′nē-ă) SYN hysteralgia. [metro- + G. *odynē*, pain]

**me·tro·fi·bro·ma** (mē′trō-fī-brō′mă) a fibroma of the uterus.

**me·tro·lym·phan·gi·tis** (mē'trō-lim-fan-jī'tis) inflammation of the uterine lymphatics. [metro- + lymphangitis]

**me·tro·pa·ral·y·sis** (mē'trō-pă-ral'i-sis) flaccidity or paralysis of the uterine muscle during or immediately after childbirth. [metro- + paralysis]

**me·tro·path·ia** (mē-trō-path'ē-ă) SYN metropathy. [L.]

**me·tro·path·ia hem·or·rha·gi·ca** abnormal, excessive, often continuous uterine bleeding due to persistence and exaggeration of the follicular phase of the menstrual cycle; the endometrium is the seat of glandular hyperplasia with cyst formation.

**me·tro·path·ic** (mē-trō-path'ik) relating to or caused by uterine disease.

**me·trop·a·thy** (mē-trop'ă-thē) any disease of the uterus, especially of the myometrium. SYN metropathia. [metro- + G. *pathos,* suffering]

**me·tro·per·i·to·ni·tis** (mē'trō-per-i-tō-nī'tis) inflammation of the uterus involving the peritoneal covering. SYN perimetritis. [metro- + peritonitis]

**me·tro·phle·bi·tis** (mē'trō-flē-bī'tis) inflammation of the uterine veins usually following childbirth. [metro- + G. *phleps,* vein, + *-itis,* inflammation]

**met·ro·plas·ty** (met'rō-plas-tē, mē'trō-plas-tē) SYN uteroplasty.

**me·tror·rha·gia** (mē-trō-rā'jē-ă) any irregular, acyclic bleeding from the uterus between periods. [metro- + G. *rhēgnymi,* to burst forth]

**me·tror·rhea** (mē'trō-rē'ă) discharge of mucus or pus from the uterus. [metro- + G. *rhoia,* a flow]

**me·tro·sal·pin·gi·tis** (mē'trō-sal-pin-jī'tis) inflammation of the uterus and of one or both fallopian tubes. [metro- + G. *salpinx,* trumpet (oviduct), + *-itis,* inflammation]

**me·tro·sal·pin·gog·ra·phy** (mē'trō-sal-pin-gog'ră-fē) SYN hysterosalpingography. [metro- + G. *salpinx,* tube, + *graphō,* to write]

**me·tro·scope** (mē'trō-skōp) SYN hysteroscope. [metro- + G. *skopeō,* to view]

**me·tro·stax·is** (mē-trō-stak'sis) small but continuous hemorrhage of the uterine mucous membrane. [metro- + G. *staxis,* a dripping]

**me·tro·ste·no·sis** (mē'trō-ste-nō'sis) a narrowing of the uterine cavity. [metro- + G. *stenōsis,* a narrowing]

**Mev** 1 million electron-volts.

**Mexican hat cell** SYN target cell.

**Mey·en·burg com·plex** (mī'ĕn-berg) clusters of small bile ducts occurring in polycystic livers, separate from the portal areas.

**Mey·en·burg dis·ease** (mī'ĕn-berg) SYN relapsing polychondritis.

**Mey·er line** (mī'er) a line through the axis of the big toe and passing the midpoint of the heel in a normal foot.

**Mey·nert cells** (mī'nert) solitary pyramidal cells found in the cortex in the region of the calcarine fissure.

**Mg** magnesium.

**mg** milligram.

**MGUS** monoclonal gammopathy of unknown significance.

**MHC** major histocompatibility complex.

**mho** (mō) SYN siemens. [*ohm* reversed]

**MHz** megahertz.

**MI** myocardial infarction.

**Mi·bel·li an·gi·oker·a·to·ma** (mē-bel'ē) a small

telangiectatic papule occurring commonly on the extremities in adolescent girls.

**Mi·bel·li dis·ease** (mē-bel'ē) SYN porokeratosis.

**Mi·chae·lis con·stant** (mĭ-kā'lis) **1.** the true dissociation constant for the enzyme-substrate binary complex in a single-substrate rapid equilibrium enzyme-catalyzed reaction (usually symbolized by $K_s$); **2.** the concentration of the substrate at which half the true maximum velocity of an enzyme-catalyzed reaction is achieved.

**Mi·chae·lis-Men·ten hy·poth·e·sis** (mĭ-kā'lis-men'tĕn) that a complex is formed between an enzyme and its substrate (the O'Sullivan-Tompson hypothesis), which complex then decomposes to yield free enzyme and the reaction products (Brown hypothesis), the latter rate determining the overall rate of substrate-product conversion.

**Mi·chel mal·for·ma·tion** (mē-shel') hypoplasia of the petrous pyramid and aplasia of the inner ear.

**Mi·chel spur** (mē-shel') epithelial outgrowth of the dilator muscle of the pupil at the peripheral border of the sphincter; part of the insertion of the dilator muscle onto the iris sphincter.

**mi·cra·cou·stic** (mī'kră-koo'stik) **1.** relating to faint sounds. **2.** magnifying very faint sounds so as to make them audible. SYN microcoustic. [micro- + G. *akoustikos,* relating to hearing, fr. *akouō,* to hear]

**mi·cren·ceph·a·ly** (mī-kren-sef'ă-lē) abnormal smallness of the brain. SYN microencephaly. [micro- + G. *enkephalos,* brain]

⚠**mi·cro-, micr-** **1.** prefixes denoting smallness. **2.** (μ) prefix used in the SI and metric systems to signify one-millionth ($10^{-6}$) of such unit. **3.** CHEMISTRY prefix to terms denoting chemical procedures or analyses that use minimal quantities of substance to be examined; specimen materials and reagents. **4.** microscopic; opposite of macro-, megalo-. [G. *mikros,* small]

**mi·cro·ab·scess** (mī'krō-ab'ses) a very small circumscribed collection of leukocytes in solid tissues.

**mi·cro·ad·e·no·ma** (mī'krō-ad-ĕ-nō'mă) a pituitary adenoma less than 10 mm in diameter.

**mi·cro·aer·o·phil, mi·cro·aer·o·phile** (mī-krō-ār'ō-fil, mī'krō-ār-ō-fīl) **1.** an aerobic bacterium that requires oxygen, but less than is present in the air, and grows best under modified atmospheric conditions. **2.** relating to such an organism. SYN microaerophilic. [micro- + G. *aēr,* air, + *philos,* fond]

**mi·cro·aer·o·phil·ic** (mī'krō-ār-ō-fil'ik) SYN microaerophil (2).

**mi·cro·ag·gre·gate** (mī'krō-ăg'rē-gāt) small aggregates (20–120 microns) composed of fibrin, degenerating platelets, white cells, or cellular debris which form in blood stored in the refrigerator 5 or more days. Microaggregate filters can be used to filter out the microaggregates during administration of the blood unit.

**mi·cro·al·bu·mi·nu·ria** (mī'krō-al-byu-min-yu'rē-ă) a slight increase in urinary albumin excretion that can be detected using immunoassays but not using conventional urine protein measurements; an early marker for renal disease in patients with diabetes. [micro- + albuminuria]

**mi·cro·a·nas·to·mo·sis** (mī'krō-ă-nas-tō-mō'sis) anastomosis of minute structures performed under a surgical microscope.

**mi·cro·a·nat·o·mist** (mī′krō-ă-nat′ŏ-mist) SYN histologist.

**mi·cro·a·nat·o·my** (mī′krō-ă-nat′ŏ-mē) SYN histology.

**mi·cro·an·eu·rysm** (mī′krō-an′yu-rizm) focal dilation of retinal capillaries occurring in diabetes mellitus, retinal vein obstruction, and absolute glaucoma, or of arteriolocapillary junctions in many organs in thrombotic thrombocytopenic purpura.

**mi·cro·an·gi·og·ra·phy** (mī′krō-an-jē-og′ră-fē) radiography of the finer vessels of an organ after the injection of a contrast medium and enlargement of the resulting radiograph. [micro- + angiography]

**mi·cro·an·gi·o·path·ic he·mo·lyt·ic a·ne·mia** hemolysis due to narrowing or obstruction of small blood vessels usually due to inflammation, causing fragmentation and distortion in the shape of red blood cells.

**mi·cro·an·gi·op·a·thy** (mī′krō-an-jē-op′ă-thē) SYN capillaropathy.

**mi·cro-As·trup meth·od** (mī-krō-as′trŭp) an interpolation technique for acid-base measurement, based on pH and the use of the Siggaard-Andersen nomogram.

**mi·crobe** (mī′krōb) any very minute organism, including both microscopic and ultramicroscopic organisms (spirochetes, bacteria, rickettsiae, and viruses). These organisms are considered to form a biologically distinctive group, in that the genetic material is not surrounded by a nuclear membrane, and mitosis does not occur during replication. [Fr., fr. G. *mikros*, small, + *bios*, life]

**mi·cro·bi·al** (mī-krō′bē-ăl) relating to a microbe or to microbes.

**mi·cro·bi·ci·dal** (mī-krō′bi-sī′dăl) destructive to microbes. SYN microbicide (1).

**mi·cro·bi·cide** (mī-krō′bi-sīd) **1.** SYN microbicidal. **2.** an agent destructive to microbes; a germicide; an antiseptic. [microbe + L. *caedo*, to kill]

**mi·cro·bi·o·log·ic** (mī′krō-bī-ō-loj′ik) relating to microbiology.

**mi·cro·bi·ol·o·gist** (mī′krō-bī-ol′ō-jist) one who specializes in the science of microbiology.

**mi·cro·bi·ol·o·gy** (mī′krō-bī-ol′ō-jē) the science concerned with microorganisms, including fungi, protozoa, bacteria, and viruses. [Fr. *microbiologie*]

**mi·cro·blast** (mī′krō-blast) a small, nucleated red blood cell. [micro- + G. *blastos*, sprout, germ]

**mi·cro·bleph·a·ron** (mī′krō-blef′ă-ron) eyelids with abnormal vertical shortness. [micro + G. *blepharon*, eyelid + *ia*, condition]

**mi·cro·body** (mī′krō-bod-ē) SYN peroxisome.

**mi·cro·bra·chia** (mī-krō-brā′kē-ă) abnormal smallness of the arms. [micro- + G. *brachiōn*, arm]

**mi·cro·cal·ci·fi·ca·tions** (mī′krō-kal-si-fi-kā′ shŭns) calcifications less than 1 mm in diameter as seen on mammography; often associated with malignant lesions. [micro- + calcification]

**mi·cro·car·dia** (mī-krō-kar′dē-ă) abnormal smallness of the heart. [micro- + G. *kardia*, heart]

**mi·cro·cen·trum** (mī-krō-sen′trŭm) SYN cytocentrum. [micro- + G. *kentron*, center]

**mi·cro·ce·phal·ic** (mī′krō-sĕ-fal′ik) having a small head. SYN nanocephalous, nanocephalic.

**mi·cro·ceph·a·ly** (mī-krō-sef′ă-lē) abnormal smallness of the head; applied to a skull with a

capacity below 1350 ml. Usually associated with mental retardation. SYN nanocephaly. [micro- + G. *kephalē*, head]

**mi·cro·chei·lia, mi·cro·chi·li·a** (mī-krō-kī′lē-ă) smallness of the lips. [micro- + G. *cheilos*, lip]

**mi·cro·chei·ria, mi·cro·chi·ri·a** (mī-krō-kī′rē-ă) smallness of the hands. [micro- + G. *cheir*, hand]

**mi·cro·chem·is·try** (mī-krō-kem′is-trē) the use of chemical procedures involving minute quantities or reactions not visible to the unaided eye.

**micro·chim·er·ism** (mī-krō-kim′er-izm) the presence of donor cells in a graft recipient, or of fetal cells remaining in maternal circulation, which can be detected by molecular methods but not by flow cytometry.

**mi·cro·cin·e·ma·tog·ra·phy** (mī′kro-sin-ĕ-mă-tog′ră-fē) the application of moving pictures taken through magnifying lenses to the study of an organ or system in motion; e.g., the circulation in living embryos. [micro- + G. *kinēma*, movement, + *graphō*, to write]

**mi·cro·cir·cu·la·tion** (mī′krō-sir-kyu-lā′shŭn) passage of blood in the smallest vessels, namely arterioles, capillaries, and venules.

**Mi·cro·coc·ca·ce·ae** (mī′krō-kok-ā′sē-ē) a family of bacteria containing Gram-positive spherical cells which occur singly or in pairs, tetrads, packets, irregular masses, or even chains. Freeliving, saprophytic, parasitic, and pathogenic species occur. The type genus is *Micrococcus*.

**mi·cro·coc·ci** (mī′krō-kok′sī) plural of micrococcus.

**Mi·cro·coc·cus** (mī′krō-kok-ŭs) a genus of Micrococcaceae containing Gram-positive, spherical cells that occur in irregular masses, never in packets. Some species are motile or produce motile mutants. These organisms are saprophytic, facultatively parasitic, or parasitic but are not truly pathogenic. The type species is *Micrococcus luteus*. [micro- + G. *kokkos*, berry]

**mi·cro·coc·cus**, pl. **mi·cro·coc·ci** (mī′krō-kok′ ŭs, mī′krō-kok′sī) a vernacular term used to refer to any member of the genus *Micrococcus*.

**mi·cro·co·lon** (mī′krō-kō-lon) a small-caliber unused colon, seen in the neonate on radiographic contrast enema; usually a consequence of intestinal atresia or meconium ileus.

**mi·cro·co·ria** (mī-krō-kō′rē-ă) a congenitally small pupil with an inability to dilate. [micro- + G. *korē*, pupil]

**mi·cro·cor·nea** (mī′krō-kōr′nē-ă) an abnormally small cornea.

**mi·cro·cou·lomb** (μC) (mī-krō-koo′lom) one-millionth of a coulomb.

**mi·cro·cou·stic** (mī′krō-koo′stik) SYN micracoustic.

**mi·cro·cu·rie** (μCi) (mī′krō-kyu′rē) one-millionth of a curie; a quantity of any radionuclide with $3.7 \times 10^4$ disintegrations per second.

**mi·cro·cyst** (mī′krō-sist) a tiny cyst, frequently of such dimensions that a magnifying lens or microscope is required for observation.

**mi·cro·cyte** (mī′krō-sīt) a small (5 μm or less) non-nucleated red blood cell. SYN microerythrocyte. [micro- + G. *kytos*, cell]

**mi·cro·cy·thae·mia [Br.]** SEE microcythemia.

**mi·cro·cy·the·mia** (mī′krō-sī-thē′mē-ă) the presence of many microcytes in the circulating blood. SYN microcytosis. [microcyte + G. *haima*, blood]

▊**mi·cro·cyt·ic a·ne·mia** any anemia in which the

average size of circulating erythrocytes is smaller than normal, i.e., the mean corpuscular volume is 80 cu μm or less (normal range, 82 to 92 cu μm). See page B2.

**ℹ mi•cro•cy•to•sis** (mī′krō-sī-tō′sis) SYN microcythemia. See page B2. [microcyte + G. *-osis,* condition]

**mi•cro•dac•ty•ly** (mī-krō-dak′ti-le) smallness or shortness of the fingers or toes. [micro- + G. *dactylos,* finger, toe]

**mi•cro•di•al•y•sis** a method of studying extracellular fluid composition and response to exogenous agents, utilizing a tiny tubular probe with a dialysis membrane and fluid flow rates of 1–3 μL/min, inserted into tissues.

**mi•cro•dis•sec•tion** (mī′krō-di-sek′shŭn) dissection of tissues under a microscope or magnifying glass, usually done by teasing the tissues apart by means of needles.

**mi•cro•don•tia, mi•cro•don•tism** (mī-krō-don′shē-ă, mī-krō-don′tizm) a condition in which a single tooth, or pairs of teeth, or the whole dentition, is disproportionately small. [micro- + G. *odous,* tooth]

**mi•cro•en•ceph•a•ly** (mī′krō-en-sef′ă-le) SYN micrencephaly.

**mi•cro•e•ryth•ro•cyte** (mī′krō-ĕ-rith′rō-sīt) SYN microcyte.

**mi•cro•fi•bril** (mī-krō-fī′brĭl) a very small fibril having an average diameter of 13 nm; it may be a bundle of still smaller microfilaments.

**mi•cro•fil•a•ment** (mī-krō-fil′ă-ment) the finest filamentous element of the cytoskeleton, having a diameter of about 5 nm and consisting primarily of actin. SEE ALSO actin filament.

**mi•cro•fil•a•re•mia** (mī′krō-fil-ă-rē′mē-ă) infection of the blood with microfilariae.

**mi•cro•fi•lar•ia,** pl. **mi•cro•fi•lar•i•ae** (mī′krō-fi-lar′ē-ă, mī′krō-fi-lar′ē-ē) term for embryos of filarial nematodes in the family Onchocercidae. SEE *Filaria.*

**mi•cro•ga•mete** (mī-krō-gam′ēt) the male element in anisogamy, or conjugation of cells of unequal size; it is the smaller of the two cells and actively motile. [micro- + G. *gametēs,* husband]

**mi•cro•ga•me•to•cyte** (mī-krō-gam′ĕ-tō-sīt) the mother cell producing the microgametes, or male elements of sexual reproduction in sporozoan protozoans and fungi.

**mi•cro•gas•tria** (mī-krō-gas′trē-ă) smallness of the stomach. [micro- + G. *gastēr,* stomach]

**mi•cro•gen•ia** (mī-krō-jēn′ē-ă) abnormal smallness of the chin resulting from underdevelopment of the mental symphysis. [micro- + G. *geneion,* chin]

**mi•cro•gen•i•tal•ism** (mī-krō-jen′i-tal-izm) abnormal smallness of the external genital organs.

**mi•cro•glan•du•lar ad•e•no•sis** adenosis of the breast in which irregular clusters of small tubules are present in adipose or fibrous tissues, resembling tubular carcinoma but lacking stromal fibroblastic proliferation.

**mi•crog•lia** (mī-krog′lē-ă) small neuroglial cells, possibly of mesodermal origin, which may become phagocytic, in areas of neural damage or inflammation. SYN Hortega cells. [micro- + G. *glia,* glue]

**mi•crog•li•a•cyte** (mī-krōg′lē-ă-sīt) a cell, especially an embryonic cell, of the microglia. [micro- + G. *glia,* glue, + *kytos,* cell]

**mi•cro•glos•sia** (mī-krō-glos′ē-ă) smallness of the tongue. [micro- + G. *glōssa,* tongue]

**mi•cro•gna•thia** (mī-krō-nā′thē-ă, mī-krog-nath′ē-ă) abnormal smallness of the jaws, especially of the mandible. [micro- + G. *gnathos,* jaw]

**mi•cro•gram** (μg) (mī′krō-gram) one-millionth of a gram.

**mi•cro•graph** (mī′krō-graf) SYN photomicrograph. [micro- + G. *graphō,* to write]

**mi•cro•gy•ria** (mī-krō-jī′rē-ă) abnormal narrowness of the cerebral convolutions. [micro- + G. *gyros,* convolution]

**mi•cro•he•mat•o•crit con•cen•tra•tion** the centrifugation of whole, anticoagulated blood, using microhematocrit tubes, to obtain a buffy coat layer containing white blood cells; blood films for staining can be prepared from this layer of cells and examined for the presence of parasites (trypanosomes and intracellular leishmaniae).

**mi•cro•he•pat•ia** (mī-krō-he-pat′ē-ă) abnormal smallness of the liver. [micro- + G. *hepar* (*hepat-*), liver]

**mi•crohm** (μΩ) (mī′krōm) one-millionth of an ohm.

**mi•cro•in•cis•ion** (mī-krō-in-sizh′ŭn) an incision made with the aid of a microscope.

**mi•cro•in•va•sion** (mī′krō-in-vā′zhŭn) invasion of tissue immediately adjacent to a carcinoma in situ, the earliest stage of malignant neoplastic invasion.

**mi•cro•kat•al** (mī′krō-kat′ăl) one-millionth of a katal.

**mi•cro•li•ter** (μl, μL, λ) (mī′krō-lē-ter) one-millionth of a liter.

**mi•cro•lith** (mī′krō-lith) a minute calculus, usually multiple and constituting a coarse sand called gravel. [micro- + G. *lithos,* stone]

**mi•cro•li•thi•a•sis** (mī-krō-li-thī′ă-sis) the formation, presence, or discharge of minute concretions, or gravel.

**mi•cro•ma•nip•u•la•tion** (mī′krō-mă-nip′yu-lā′shŭn) dissection, stimulation, and other mechanical operations performed on minute structures under the microscope.

**mi•cro•me•lia** (mī-krō-mē′lē-ă) condition of having disproportionately short or small limbs. SEE ALSO achondroplasia. SYN nanomelia. [micro- + G. *melos,* limb]

**mi•cro•mel•ic dwarf•ism** dwarfism with abnormally short or small limbs.

**mi•cro•mere** (mī′krō-mēr) a blastomere of small size; e.g., one of the blastomeres at the animal pole of an amphibian egg. [micro- + G. *meros,* a part]

**mi•cro•me•tas•ta•sis** (mī′krō-mĕ-tas′tă-sis) a stage of metastasis when the secondary tumors are too small to be clinically detected, as in micrometastatic disease.

**mi•cro•met•a•stat•ic** (mī′krō-met-ă-stat′ik) denoting or characterized by micrometastasis, as in micrometastatic disease.

**mi•crom•e•ter** (μm) (mī-krom′ĕ-ter) **1.** one-millionth of a meter; formerly called micron. **2.** a device for measuring various objects in an accurate and precise manner. In medicine and biology, the term is usually used with reference to a glass slide or lens that is accurately marked for measuring microscopic forms. [micro- + G. *metron,* measure]

**mi•crom•e•try** (mī-krom′ĕ-trē) measurement of

objects with some type of micrometer and a microscope.

**⌂mi·cro·mi·cro-** (μμ) prefix formerly used to signify one-trillionth ($10^{-12}$); now pico-.

**mi·cro·mi·cron** (μμ) (mī-krō-mī'kron) former term for picometer.

**mi·cro·mo·lar** (μM, μmol/L) (mī-krō-mō'lar) denoting a concentration of $10^{-6}$ mole per liter ($10^{-6}$ M or 1 μM).

**mi·cro·mole** (μmol) (mī'krō-mōl) one-millionth of a mole.

**mi·cro·my·e·lia** (mī'krō-mī-ē'lē-ă) abnormal smallness or shortness of the spinal cord. [micro- + G. *myelos*, marrow]

**mi·cro·my·el·o·blast** (mī-krō-mī'el-ō-blast) a small myeloblast, often the predominating cell in myeloblastic leukemia.

**mi·cro·my·el·o·blas·tic leu·ke·mia** a form of myelocytic leukemia in which relatively large proportions of micromyeloblasts are found in the circulating blood and in bone marrow and other tissues.

**mi·cron** (μ) (mī'kron) former term for micrometer.

**mi·cro·nod·u·lar** (mī'krō-nod'yu-lăr) characterized by the presence of minute nodules; denoting a somewhat coarser appearance than that of a granular tissue or substance. [G. *mikros*, small]

**mi·cro·nu·cle·us** (mī-krō-noo'klē-ŭs) **1.** a small nucleus in a large cell, or the smaller nuclei in cells that have two or more such structures. **2.** the smaller of the two nuclei in ciliates dividing mitotically and bearing specific inheritable material. SEE ALSO macronucleus (2).

**mi·cro·nu·tri·ents** (mī-krō-noo'trē-ents) essential food factors required in only small quantities by the body; e.g., vitamins, trace minerals.

**mi·cro·nych·ia** (mī-krō-nik'ē-ă) abnormal smallness of nails. [micro- + G. *onyx*, nail]

**mi·cro·oph·thal·mia trans·crip·tion fac·tor gene** gene that when mutated causes Waardenburg syndrome type 2 and Tietz syndrome in at least some subsets of families with these autosomal dominant inherited syndromes.

**mi·cro·or·gan·ism** (mī'krō-ōr'gan-izm) a microscopic organism (plant or animal).

**mi·cro·pa·thol·o·gy** (mī'krō-pa-thol'ō-jē) the microscopic study of disease changes. [micro- + G. *pathos*, suffering, + *logos*, study]

**mi·cro·pe·nis** (mī-krō-pē'nis) abnormally small penis. SYN microphallus.

**mi·cro·phage** (mī'krō-fāj) a polymorphonuclear leukocyte that is phagocytic. SEE ALSO phagocyte. [micro- + phag(ocyte)]

**mi·cro·phal·lus** (mī-krō-fal'ŭs) SYN micropenis.

**mi·cro·pho·to·graph** (mī-krō-fō'tō-graf) a minute photograph of any object, as distinguished from a photomicrograph.

**mi·croph·thal·mia** (mī'krof-thal'mē-ă) SYN microphthalmos.

**mi·croph·thal·mos** (mī'krof-thal'mos) abnormal smallness of the eye. SYN microphthalmia. [micro + G. *ophthalmos*, eye]

**mi·cro·pleth·ys·mog·ra·phy** (mī'krō-pleth-iz-mog'ră-fē) the technique of measuring minute changes in the volume of a part as a result of blood flow into or out of it.

**mi·cro·po·dia** (mī-krō-pō'dē-ă) abnormal smallness of the feet. [micro- + G. *pous*, foot]

**mi·crop·sia** (mī-krop'sē-ă) perception of objects as smaller than they are. [micro- + G. *opsis*, sight]

**mi·cro·punc·ture** (mī'krō-pŭnk-cher) a puncture made with the aid of a microscope.

**mi·cro·re·frac·tom·e·ter** (mī'krō-rē-frak-tom'ĕ-ter) a refractometer used in the study of blood cells.

**mi·cro·res·pi·rom·e·ter** (mī'krō-res-pi-rom'ĕ-ter) an apparatus for measuring the utilization of oxygen by small particles of isolated tissues or cells or particles of cells.

**mi·cro·scope** (mī'krō-skōp) an instrument that gives an enlarged image of an object or substance that is minute or not visible with the naked eye; usually the term denotes a compound microscope; for low magnifications the term simple microscope, or magnifying glass, is used. [micro- + G. *skopeō*, to view]

**mi·cro·scop·ic, mi·cro·scop·i·cal** (mī-krō-skop'ik, mī-krō-skop'i-kăl) **1.** of minute size; visible only with the aid of the microscope. **2.** relating to a microscope.

**mi·cro·scop·ic a·nat·o·my** the branch of anatomy in which the structure of cells, tissues, and organs is studied with the light microscope. SEE ALSO histology.

**mi·cro·scop·ic pol·y·an·gi·i·tis** systemic, nongranulomatous small-vessel vasculitis, associated with glomerulonephritis, pulmonary capillaritis, palpable purpura, and antineutrophil cytoplasmic autoantibodies.

**mi·cros·co·py** (mī-kros'kŏ-pē) investigation of minute objects by means of a microscope. SEE ALSO microscope.

**mi·cro·some** (mī'krō-sōm) one of the small spherical vesicles derived from the endoplasmic reticulum after disruption of cells and ultracentrifugation. [micro- + G. *sōma*, body]

**mi·cro·so·mia** (mī-krō-sō'mē-ă) abnormal smallness of body, as in dwarfism or as in a fetus. SYN nanocormia. [micro- + G. *sōma*, body]

**mi·cro·spec·tro·pho·tom·e·try** (mī'krō-spek-trō-fō-tom'ĕ-trē) a technique for characterizing and quantitating nucleoproteins in single cells or cell organelles by their natural absorption spectra (ultraviolet) or after binding stoichiometrically in selective cytochemical staining reactions, as in the Feulgen stain for DNA.

**mi·cro·spec·tro·scope** (mī-krō-spek'trō-skōp) an instrument for observing the optical spectrum of microscopic objects.

**mi·cro·sphe·ro·cy·to·sis** (mī'krō-sfēr'ō-sī-tō'sis) a condition of the blood seen in hemolytic icterus in which small spherocytes are predominant; the red blood cells are smaller and more globular than normal.

**mi·cro·sphyg·my** (mī'krō-sfig'mē) a circumstance in which the pulse is difficult to discern manually. [micro- + G. *sphygmos*, pulse]

**mi·cro·sple·nia** (mī-krō-sple'nē-ă) abnormal smallness of the spleen.

*Mi·cros·po·rum* (mī-kros'pŏ-rŭm, mī-krō-spō'rŭm) a genus of pathogenic fungi causing dermatophytosis. [micro- + G. *sporos*, seed]

**mi·cro·steth·o·scope** (mī-krō-steth'ō-skōp) a stethoscope that amplifies the sounds heard.

**mi·cro·sto·mia** (mī-krō-stō'mē-ă) smallness of the oral aperture. [micro- + G. *stoma*, mouth]

**mi·cro·sur·gery** (mī-krō-ser'jer-ē) surgical procedures performed under the magnification of a surgical microscope.

m
i

**mi•cro•su•ture** (mī-krō-soo′cher) tiny caliber suture material, often 9-0 or 10-0, with an attached needle of corresponding size, for use in microsurgery.

**mi•cro•sy•ringe** (mī′krō-si-rinj′) a hypodermic syringe that has a micrometer screw attached to the piston, whereby accurately measured minute quantities of fluid may be injected.

**mi•cro•tia** (mī-krō′shē-ă) smallness of the external ear with a blind or absent external auditory meatus. [micro- + G. *ous,* ear]

**mi•cro•tome** (mī′krō-tōm) an instrument for making sections of biological tissue for examination under the microscope. SYN histotome.

**mi•crot•o•my** (mī-krot′ō-mē) the making of thin sections of tissues for examination under the microscope. SYN histotomy. [micro- + G. *tomē,* incision]

**mi•cro•trau•ma** a minor or microscopic lesion due to injury, which may become significant if often repeated.

*Mi•cro•trom•bid•i•um* (mī′krō-trom-bid′ē-ŭm) a genus of chigger or harvest mites that cause severe itching from the presence of the larval stage (chigger) in the skin. [micro- + Mod. L. *trombidium,* a timid one]

**mi•cro•tu•bule** (mī-krō-too′byul) a cylindrical cytoplasmic element that occurs widely in the cytoskeleton of plant and animal cells; microtubules increase in number during mitosis and meiosis, where they may be related to movement of the chromosomes or chromatids on the nuclear spindle during nuclear division. See this page.

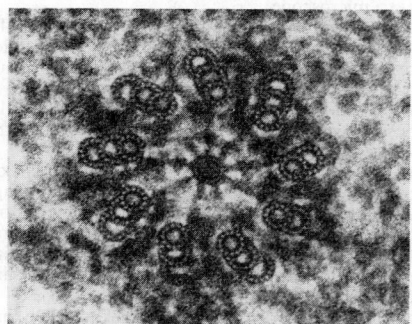

**microtubules:** electron micrograph ( X 330,000) of a centriole in transverse section; nine triplet microtubules are arranged around an axial cartwheel-like structure

**mi•cro•vil•lus,** pl. **mi•cro•vil•li** (mī-krō-vil′ŭs, mī-krō-vil′ī) one of the minute projections of cell membranes greatly increasing surface area; microvilli form the striated or brush borders of certain cells.

**mi•cro•volt (μV)** (mī′krō-vōlt) one-millionth of a volt.

**mi•cro•waves** (mī′krō-wāvz) that portion of the radio wave spectrum of shortest wavelength, including the region with wavelengths of 1 mm to 30 cm (1000 to 300,000 megacycles per second).

**mi•crox•y•phil** (mī-krok′si-fil) a multinuclear oxyphil leukocyte. [micro- + G. *oxys,* acid, + *philos,* fond]

**mi•cro•zo•on** (mī-krō-zō′on) a microscopic form of the animal kingdom; a protozoon. [micro- + G. *zōon,* animal]

**mi•crur•gi•cal** (mī-krer′ji-kăl) relating to procedures performed on minute structures under a microscope. [micro- + G. *ergon,* work]

**mic•tion** (mik′shŭn) SYN urination.

**mic•tu•rate** (mik′choo-rāt) SYN urinate. [see micturition]

**mic•tu•rat•ing cys•to•u•re•thro•gram** SYN voiding cystourethrogram.

**mic•tu•ri•tion** (mik-choo-rish′ŭn) **1.** SYN urination. **2.** the desire to urinate. **3.** frequency of urination. [L. *micturio,* to desire to make water]

**MID** minimal infecting dose.

△**mid-** middle. [A.S. *mid, midd*]

**mid•bo•dy** (mid′bod′ē) a dense stalk of residual interzonal spindle fibers (microtubules) and actin-containing filaments that is formed during anaphase of mitosis and connects daughter cells during telophase; midbodies are frequently observed between spermatids.

**mid•brain** (mid′brān) SYN mesencephalon.

**mid•car•pal** (mid′kar-păl) **1.** relating to the central part of the carpus. **2.** denoting the articulation between the two rows of carpal bones. SYN mediocarpal.

**mid•dle** denoting an anatomic structure that is between two other similar structures or that is midway in position.

**mid•dle car•di•ac vein** begins at the apex of the heart, anastomoses with the great cardiac vein, and ascends within the posterior interventricular sulcus to the coronary sinus.

**mid•dle cer•e•bel•lar pe•dun•cle** the largest of three paired cerebellar peduncles, composed mainly of fibers that originate in the pontine nuclei, cross the midline in the ventral part of pons, and emerge on the opposite side as a massive bundle arching dorsally along the lateral side of the pontine tegmentum into the cerebellum; its fibers are distributed chiefly to the cortex of the cerebellar hemisphere.

**mid•dle col•ic ar•tery** *origin,* superior mesenteric; *distribution,* transverse colon; *anastomoses,* right and left colic.

**mid•dle con•stric•tor mus•cle of phar•ynx** *origin,* stylohyoid ligament, lesser cornu of the hyoid bone (chondropharyngeal part) and greater cornu of the hyoid bone (ceratopharyngeal part); *insertion,* pharyngeal raphe in the posterior wall of the pharynx; *action,* narrows pharynx in the act of swallowing; *nerve supply,* pharyngeal plexus.

**mid•dle ear** SEE ear.

**mid•dle-ear ef•fu•sion** a condition in which the air in the middle ear has been replaced with serous or mucoid fluid as a consequence of otitis media. SYN serous otitis media.

**mid•dle fos•sa ap•proach** surgical approach to the cerebellopontine angle through that portion of the floor of the middle cranial fossa that is the anterior surface of the petrous pyramid of the temporal bone.

**mid•dle ge•nic•u•lar ar•tery** *origin,* popliteal; *distribution,* synovial membrane and cruciate ligaments of knee joint.

**mid•dle la•ten•cy re•sponse** a response to acoustic stimulation recorded from the auditory cortex of the brain.

**mid•dle mac•u•lar ar•ter•i•ole** an arteriole supplying the part of the retina between the optic disk and the macula.

**mid•dle me•nin•ge•al veins** the venae comitantes of the middle meningeal artery that empty into the pterygoid plexus.

**mid•dle na•sal con•cha 1.** the middle thin, spongy, bony plate with curved margins, part of the ethmoidal labyrinth, projecting from the lateral wall of the nasal cavity and separating the superior meatus from the middle meatus; **2.** the above bony plate and its thick mucoperiosteum containing a cavernous vascular bed for heat exchange.

**mid•dle rec•tal lymph node** a lymph node along the middle rectal artery that receives afferents from the pararectal nodes and sends efferents to the internal iliac nodes.

**mid•dle tem•po•ral vein** it arises near the lateral angle of the eye and joins the superficial temporal veins to form the retromandibular vein.

**midge** (midj) the smallest of the biting flies, in the genus *Culicoides;* swarms may attack humans and other animals; vectors of filarial infections. [O.E. *mycg*]

**mid•gut** (mid′gŭt) **1.** the central portion of the digestive tube; the distal duodenum, small intestine, and proximal colon. **2.** the portion of the embryonic gut tract between the foregut and the hindgut which originally is open to the yolk sac.

**mid•life cri•sis** a point in a sequence of events during the middle years of life at which certain trends of prior and subsequent events in one's life are pondered, generally involving an aggregate of personal, career, or sexual dissatisfactions.

**mid•line le•thal gran•u•lo•ma** destruction of the nasal septum, hard palate, lateral nasal walls, paranasal sinuses, skin of the face, orbit and nasopharynx by an inflammatory infiltrate with atypical lymphocytic and histiocytic cells; presumably a hypersensitivity response to an unidentified antigen in most cases. SYN malignant granuloma.

**mid•line my•e•lot•o•my** section of the midline transverse fibers of the spinal cord for the treatment of intractable pain. SYN commissurotomy (2).

**mid•riff** (mid′rif) SYN diaphragm (1). [A.S. *mid,* middle, + *hrif,* belly]

▣ **mid•sag•it•tal plane** SYN median plane. See page APP 88.

**mid•tar•sal** (mid′tar′săl) relating to the middle of the tarsus.

**mid•wife** (mid′wīf) a person qualified to practice midwifery, having specialized training in obstetrics and child care. [A.S. *mid,* with, + *wif,* wife]

**mid•wife•ry** (mid′wif′rē, mid′wīf′rē) independent care of essentially normal, healthy women and infants by a midwife, antepartally, intrapartally, postpartally, and/or obstetrically in a hospital, birth center, or home setting, and including normal delivery of the infant, with medical consultation, collaborative management, and referral of cases in which abnormalities develop; strong emphasis is placed on educational preparation of parents for childbearing and childrearing, with an orientation toward childbirth as a normal physiological process requiring minimal intervention.

**Mie•scher e•las•to•ma** (mē′sher) circinate groups of hyperkeratotic papules that become

dislodged, leaving a small bloody depression; associated with pseudoxanthoma elasticum.

**Mie•scher gran•u•lo•ma** (mē′sher) SYN actinic granuloma.

**Mie•scher tube** (mē′sher) an elongate fusiform or cylindrical body forming the encapsulated cystic intramuscular stage of the protozoan *Sarcocystis.*

**mi•graine** (mī′grān) a symptom complex occurring periodically and characterized by pain in the head (usually unilateral), vertigo, nausea and vomiting, photophobia, and scintillating appearances of light. Classified as classic migraine, common migraine, cluster headache, hemiplegic migraine, ophthalmoplegic migraine, and ophthalmic migraine. SYN hemicrania (1), sick headache. [through O. Fr., fr. G. *hēmi- krania,* pain on one side of the head, fr. *hēmi-,* half, + *kranion,* skull]

**mi•graine head•ache** SEE migraine.

**mi•graine-re•lat•ed ves•tib•u•lop•a•thy** a disorder characterized by movement-associated disequilibrium, unsteadiness, space and motion discomfort, and vertigo before onset of headache.

**mi•grat•ing ab•scess** SYN perforating abscess.

**mi•gra•tion** (mī-grā′shŭn) **1.** passing from one part to another, said of certain morbid processes or symptoms. **2.** SYN diapedesis. **3.** movement of a tooth or teeth out of normal position. **4.** movement of molecules during electrophoresis. [L. *migro,* pp. *-atus,* to move from place to place]

**MIH** melanotropin release-inhibiting hormone.

**Mi•ku•licz aph•thae** (mē′koo-lich) SYN aphthae major.

**Mi•ku•licz dis•ease** (mē′koo-lich) benign swelling of the lacrimal, and usually also of the salivary, glands due to infiltration of and replacement of the normal gland structure by lymphoid tissue. SEE ALSO Mikulicz syndrome, Sjögren syndrome.

**Mi•ku•licz drain** (mē′koo-lich) a drain made of several strings of gauze held together by a single layer of gauze.

**Mi•ku•licz op•er•a•tion** (mē′koo-lich) excision of bowel in two stages: 1) exteriorizing the diseased area, suturing efferent and afferent limbs together, and closing the abdomen around them, after which the diseased part is excised; 2) at a later time, cutting the spur with an enterotome and closing the stoma extraperitoneally.

**Mi•ku•licz syn•drome** (mē′koo-lich) the symptoms characteristic of Mikulicz disease occurring as a complication of some other disease, such as lymphoma, leukemia, or uveoparotid fever.

**Miles op•er•a•tion** (mīlz) combined abdominoperineal resection for carcinoma of the rectum.

**mil•ia** (mil′ē-ă) plural of milium.

**mil•i•a•ria** (mil-ē-ār′ē-ă) an eruption of minute vesicles and papules due to retention of fluid at the orifices of sweat glands. SYN miliary fever (2). [L. *miliarius,* relating to millet, fr. *milium,* millet]

**mil•i•a•ria ru•bra** an eruption of papules and vesicles at the orifices of sweat glands, accompanied by redness and inflammatory reaction of the skin. SYN heat rash, prickly heat, strophulus, tropical lichen, lichen tropicus.

**mil•i•a•ry** (mil′ē-ar-ē) **1.** resembling a millet seed in size (about 2 mm). **2.** marked by the presence of nodules of millet seed size on any surface. [see miliaria]

m
i

**mil·i·a·ry ab·scess** one of a number of minute collections of pus, widely disseminated throughout an area or the whole body.

**mil·i·a·ry em·bo·lism** embolism occurring simultaneously in a number of capillaries.

**mil·i·a·ry fe·ver 1.** an infectious disease characterized by profuse sweating and the production of sudamina, occurring formerly in severe epidemics; **2.** SYN miliaria.

**mil·i·a·ry pat·tern** a chest radiographic pattern of fine, rounded opacities, typical of hematogenous dissemination of tuberculosis.

**miliary tuberculosis** general dissemination of tubercle bacilli in the blood, resulting in the formation of miliary tubercles in various organs and tissues, and occasionally producing symptoms of profound toxemia. SYN generalized tuberculosis.

**mi·lieu** (mē-lyu′) **1.** surroundings; environment. **2.** PSYCHIATRY the social setting of the mental patient, e.g., the family setting or a hospital unit. [Fr. *mi,* fr. L. *medius,* middle, + *lieu,* fr. L. *locus,* place]

**mil·ieu ther·a·py** psychiatric treatment employing manipulation of the social environment for the benefit of the patient.

**mil·i·tary an·ti·shock trou·sers (MAST)** SYN pneumatic antishock garment.

**mil·i·um,** pl. **mil·ia** (mil′ē-ŭm, mil′ē-ă) a small subepidermal keratin cyst, usually multiple and therefore commonly referred to in the plural. SYN whitehead (1). [L. millet]

**milk 1.** a white liquid, containing proteins, sugar, and lipids, secreted by the mammary glands after childbirth, and serving for the nourishment of the infant. **2.** any whitish milky fluid; e.g., the juice of the coconut or a suspension of various metallic oxides. **3.** a pharmacopeial preparation that is a suspension of insoluble drugs in a water medium; distinguished from gels mainly in that the suspended particles of milk are larger. **4.** SYN strip (1). [A.S. *meolc*]

**milk·al·ka·li syn·drome** a chronic disorder of the kidneys, reversible in its early stages, induced by ingestion of large amounts of calcium and alkali in the therapy of peptic ulcer; can progress to renal failure. SYN Burnett syndrome.

**milk crust** SYN crusta lactea.

**milk den·ti·tion** SYN deciduous tooth.

**milk ducts** SYN lactiferous ducts.

**milk fe·ver 1.** a slight elevation of temperature following childbirth, said to be due to the establishment of the secretion of milk, but probably the same as absorption fever; **2.** an afebrile metabolic disease, occurring shortly after parturition in dairy cattle, characterized by hypocalcemia and manifested by loss of consciousness and general paralysis.

**milk line** SYN mammary ridge.

**Milk·man syn·drome** (milk′man) osteomalacia with multiple pseudofractures, usually bilateral and symmetrical, may develop true pathologic fractures.

**milk sug·ar** SYN lactose.

**milk tooth** SYN deciduous tooth.

**Mil·ler-Ab·bott tube** (mil′ĕr-a′bŏt) a tube with two lumens, one ending in a small collapsible balloon and the other in a metallic tip with numerous perforations; used for intestinal decompression. SYN Abbott tube.

**Mil·ler chem·i·co·par·a·sit·ic the·o·ry** (mil′ĕr) that dental caries is caused by microorganisms of the mouth fermenting dietary carbohydrates and producing acids that demineralize the teeth.

**mill·er's asth·ma** asthma caused by flour or grain allergens.

△**mil·li-** prefix used in the SI and metric systems to signify one-thousandth ($10^{-3}$). [L. *mille,* one thousand]

**mil·li·am·pere (ma, mA)** (mil′ē-am′pēr) one thousandth of an ampere.

**mil·li·am·pere-im·pulse (mAi)** SYN milliampere-second.

**mil·li·am·pere-sec·ond (mA-s)** a radiologic unit denoting the product of the number of electrons applied to the cathode of the X-ray tube multiplied by the exposure time in seconds; it directly determines the amount of X-ray energy produced. SYN milliampere-impulse.

**mil·li·cu·rie (mc, mCi)** (mil′i-kyu′rē) a unit of radioactivity equivalent to $3.7 \times 10^7$ disintegrations per second.

**mil·li·e·quiv·a·lent (mEq, meq)** (mil′i-ē-kwiv′ă-lent) one-thousandth equivalent; $10^{-3}$ mole divided by valence.

**mil·li·gram (mg)** (mil′i-gram) one-thousandth of a gram.

**mil·li·li·ter (ml, mL)** (mil′i-lē-ter) one-thousandth of a liter.

**mil·li·me·ter (mm)** (mil′i-mē-ter) one-thousandth of a meter.

△**mil·li·mi·cro-** prefix formerly used to signify one-billionth ($10^{-9}$); now nano-.

**mil·li·mi·cron (mμ)** (mil′i-mī-kron) former term for nanometer.

**mil·li·mole (mmol)** (mil′i-mōl) one-thousandth of a gram-molecule.

**mil·li·sec·ond (ms, msec)** (mil′i-sek′ŏnd) one-thousandth of a second.

**mil·li·volt (mV)** (mil′i-vōlt) one thousandth of a volt.

**mil·pho·sis** (mil-fō′sis) loss of eyelashes. [G. *milphōsis*]

**Mil·roy dis·ease** (mil′roy) the congenital type of autosomal dominant lymphedema.

**MIM** Mendelian Inheritance in Man.

**mi·me·sis** (mi-mē′sis, mī-mē′sis) **1.** hysterical simulation of organic disease. **2.** the symptomatic imitation of one organic disease by another. [G. *mimēsis,* imitation, fr. *mimeomai,* to mimic]

**mi·met·ic** (mi-met′ik, mī-met′ik) relating to mimesis. [G. *mimētikos,* imitative]

**mim·ic** (mim′ik) to imitate or simulate. [G. *mimikos,* imitating, fr. *mimos,* a mimic]

**MIM num·ber** the catalog assignment for a mendelian trait in the MIM system. If the initial digit is 1, the trait is deemed autosomal dominant; if 2, autosomal recessive; if 3, then X-linked.

**Mi·na·ma·ta dis·ease** (min-ah-mah′tah) a neurologic disorder caused by methyl mercury intoxication; first described in the inhabitants of Minamata Bay, Japan, resulting from their eating fish contaminated with mercury industrial waste. Characterized by peripheral sensory loss, tremors, dysarthria, ataxia, and both hearing and visual loss.

**mind 1.** the organ or seat of consciousness and higher functions of the human brain, such as cognition, reasoning, willing, and emotion. **2.** the organized totality of all mental processes and psychic activities, with emphasis on the relatedness of the phenomena. [A.S. *gemynd*]

**min·er·al** (min'er-ăl) any homogeneous inorganic material usually found in the earth's crust. [L. *mineralis,* pertaining to mines, fr. *mino,* to mine]

**min·er·al·o·cor·ti·coid** (min'er-al-ō-kōr'ti-koyd) one of the steroids of the adrenal cortex that influence salt (sodium and potassium) metabolism.

**min·er·al wa·ter** water that contains appreciable amounts of certain salts, which give it therapeutic properties.

**min·er's lung 1.** SYN anthracosis. **2.** SYN black lung.

**min·i·lap·a·rot·o·my** (min'ē-lap-ă-rot'ō-mē) technique for sterilization by surgical ligation of the uterine tubes, performed through a small suprapubic incision.

**min·im 1.** a fluid measure, $\frac{1}{60}$ of a fluidram; in the case of water, about one drop. **2.** smallest; least; the smallest of several similar structures. [L. *minimus,* least]

**min·i·mal brain dys·func·tion** SEE attention deficit disorder.

**min·i·mal dose** the smallest amount of a drug or physical procedure that will produce a desired physiologic effect in an adult.

**min·i·mal in·fect·ing dose (MID)** the smallest quantity of infectious material regularly producing infection; usually expressed as I.D.$_{50}$, the quantity causing infection in 50% of a suitable series of animals or cells (cell cultures).

**min·i·mal le·thal dose (MLD, mld) 1.** the minimal dose of a toxic substance or infectious agent that is lethal, as assayed in various experimental animals; when followed by a subscript (generally "MLD$_{50}$"), denotes the minimal dose that is lethal to a certain percentage (e.g., 50%) of animals so assayed; **2.** lD$_{05}$. SEE lethal dose.

**min·i·mal re·act·ing dose (MRD, mrd)** the minimal dose of a toxic substance causing a reaction, as manifested in the skin of a series of susceptible test animals; the assay is based on the development of a characteristic, minimal but definite, "standard," focal inflammation.

**min·i·mum data set (MDS)** smallest number of data that can be collected and still positively identify the patient.

**mi·ni·thor·a·cot·omy** any thoracotomy involving less muscle division than the classic posterolateral thoracotomy.

**Min·ne·so·ta Multiphasic Per·son·al·i·ty In·ven·to·ry (MMPI)** SYN Minnesota multiphasic personality inventory test.

**Min·ne·so·ta mul·ti·pha·sic per·son·al·i·ty in·ven·to·ry test** (min-ĕ-sō'tă) a questionnaire type of psychological test for ages 16 and over, with 550 true-false statements coded in 4 validity and 10 personality scales which may be administered in both an individual or group format. SYN Minnesota Multiphasic Personality Inventory.

**mi·nor** (mī'ner) smaller; lesser; denoting the smaller of two similar structures. [L.]

**mi·nor ag·glu·ti·nin** immune agglutinin present in an antiserum in lesser concentration than the major agglutinin. SYN partial agglutinin.

**mi·nor his·to·com·pat·i·bil·ity com·plex** genes outside of MHC that are present on various chromosomes that encode antigens contributing to graft rejection.

**mi·nor hys·te·ria** a mild form of hysteria characterized chiefly by subjective pains, nervousness, undue sensitiveness, and sometimes episodes of emotional excitement, but without paralysis or other such symptoms.

**mi·nor sal·i·vary glands** the smaller, largely mucous-secreting, exocrine glands of the oral cavity, consisting of the labial, buccal, molar, lingual, and palatine glands.

**mi·nor sub·lin·gual ducts** 8–20 small ducts of the sublingual salivary gland that open into the mouth on the surface of the sublingual fold; a few join the submandibular ducts. SYN Rivinus ducts, Walther ducts.

**min·ute ven·ti·la·tion** SYN minute volume.

**min·ute vol·ume** the volume of any gas or fluid moved per minute; e.g., cardiac output or the respiratory minute volume. SYN minute ventilation.

△**mio-** less. [G. *meiōn*]

**mi·o·sis** (mī-ō'sis) **1.** contraction of the pupil. **2.** incorrect alternative spelling for meiosis. [G. *meiōsis,* a lessening]

**mi·o·sphyg·mia** (mī'ō-sfig'mē-ă) condition in which pulse beats are fewer than heart beats. [mio- + G. *sphygmos,* pulse]

**mi·ot·ic** (mī-ot'ik) **1.** relating to or characterized by contraction of the pupil. **2.** an agent that causes the pupil to contract.

**MIP** maximum inspiratory pressure; maximum intensity projection.

**mire** (mēr) one of the test objects in the ophthalmometer; its image (also called a mire), mirrored on the corneal surface, is measured to determine the radii of curvature of the cornea. [L. *miror,* pp. *-atus,* to wonder at]

**Mi·riz·zi syn·drome** (mir-its'ē) benign obstruction of the hepatic ducts due to spasm and/or fibrous scarring of surrounding connective tissue; often associated with a stone in the cystic duct and chronic cholecystitis.

**mir·ror** (mir'ŏr) a polished surface reflecting the rays of light reflected from objects in front of it. [Fr. *miroir,* fr. L. *miror,* to wonder at]

**mir·ror-im·age cell 1.** a cell whose nuclei have identical features and are placed in the cytoplasm in similar fashion; **2.** a binucleate form of Reed-Sternberg cell often found in Hodgkin disease; the twin nuclei are disposed in relation to an imaginary plane between them like a single nucleus together with its image in a mirror.

**mir·ror speech** a reversal of the order of syllables in a word, analogous to mirror writing.

**mir·ya·chit** (mir-yah'chit) a nervous affection observed in Siberia. SEE jumping disease.

**mis·an·dry** (mis'an-drē) aversion to or hatred of men. [G. *miseō,* to hate, + *anēr, andros,* male]

**mis·an·thro·py** (mis-an'thrō-pē) aversion to and hatred of human beings. [G. *miseō,* to hate, + *anthrōpos,* man]

**mis·car·riage** (mis-kar'ij) spontaneous expulsion of the products of pregnancy before the middle of the second trimester.

**misc·e·ge·na·tion** (mis'e-jĕ-nā'shŭn) marriage or interbreeding of individuals of different races. [L. *misceo,* to mix, + *genus,* descent, race]

**mis·ci·ble** (mis'i-bĕl) capable of being mixed and remaining so after the mixing process ceases. [L. *misceo,* to mix]

**mis·di·ag·no·sis** (mis'dī-ag-nō'sis) a wrong or mistaken diagnosis.

**mi·sog·a·my** (mi-sog'ă-mē) aversion to marriage. [G. *miseō,* to hate, + *gamos,* marriage]

**mi·sog·y·ny** (mi-soj'i-nē) aversion to or hatred of women. [G. *miseō,* to hate, + *gynē,* woman]

**mis·o·pe·dia, mis·op·e·dy** (mis-ō-pē'dē-ă, mis-op'ĕ-dē) aversion to or hatred of children. [G. *miseō,* to hate, + *pais (paid-),* child]

**missed a·bor·tion** abortion in which the fetus dies but is retained *in utero* for two months or longer.

**missed la·bor** brief uterine contractions which do not lead to labor and expulsion of the infant, but which cease, resulting in the indefinite retention of the fetus (usually lifeless).

**mis·sense mu·ta·tion** a mutation in which a base change or substitution results in a codon that causes insertion of a different amino acid into the growing polypeptide chain, giving rise to an altered protein. [mis-sense by analogy with non-sense]

**Mitch·ell dis·ease** (mich'ĕl) SYN erythromelalgia.

**Mitch·ell pro·ce·dure** (mich'ĕl) surgical procedure to correct a hallux valgus by combining a bunionectomy and soft tissue correction of the first metatarsophalangeal joint with an osteotomy of the proximal portion of the first metatarsal.

**Mitch·ell treat·ment** (mich'ĕl) treatment of mental illness by rest, nourishing diet, and a change of environment.

**mite** (mīt) a minute arthropod of the order Acarina, a vast assemblage of parasitic and (primarily) free-living organisms. A few are of medical importance as vectors or intermediate hosts of pathogenic agents, by directly causing dermatitis or tissue damage, or by causing blood or tissue fluid loss. [A.S.]

**mite ty·phus** SYN tsutsugamushi disease.

**mith·ri·da·tism** (mith'ri-dā'tizm, mith-rid'ă-tizm) immunity against the action of a poison produced by small and gradually increasing doses of the same. [*Mithridates,* King of Pontus (132–63 B.C.), supposedly an unsuccessful suicide (by poison) because of repeated small doses taken to become invulnerable to assassination by poison]

**mi·ti·ci·dal** (mī-ti-sī'dăl) destructive to mites.

**mi·ti·cide** (mī'ti-sīd) an agent destructive to mites. [mite + L. *caedo,* to kill]

**mit·i·gate** (mit'i-gāt) SYN palliate. [L. *mitigo,* pp. *-atus,* to make mild or gentle, fr. *mitis,* mild, + *ago,* to do, make]

**mi·to·chon·dria** (mī-tō-kon'drē-ă) plural of mitochondrion.

**mi·to·chon·dri·al** (mī-tō-kon'drē-ăl) relating to mitochondria.

**mi·to·chon·dri·al bi·o·gen·e·sis** the process by which mitochondria increase their ability to make adenosine triphosphate by synthesizing additional respiratory enzyme complexes.

**mi·to·chon·dri·al chro·mo·some** the DNA component of mitochondria, the chief function of which is synthesis of adenosine triphosphate and the management of cellular energy.

**mi·to·chon·dri·al dis·or·ders** a group of diverse hereditary disorders caused by genetic mutation of mitochrondrial DNA; includes ragged red fiber myopathy; progressive external ophthalmoplegia; Leigh syndrome; myoclonic epilepsy with ragged red fiber myopathy (MERRF); mitochondrial myopathy, encephalopathy, lactacidosis, and stroke (MELAS); and Lieber optic neuropathy.

**mi·to·chon·dri·on**, pl. **mi·to·chon·dria** (mī-tō-kon'drē-on, mī-tō-kon'drē-ă) an organelle of the cell cytoplasm consisting of two sets of membranes, a smooth continuous outer coat and an inner membrane arranged in tubules or more often in folds that form platelike double membranes called cristae; mitochondria are the principal energy source of the cell and contain the cytochrome enzymes of terminal electron transport and the enzymes of the citric acid cycle, fatty acid oxidation, and oxidative phosphorylation. See this page. [G. *mitos,* thread, + *chondros,* granule, grits]

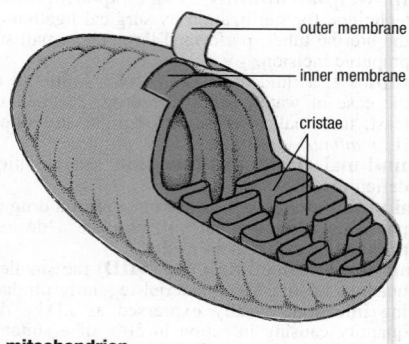

**mitochondrion**

**mi·to·gen** (mī'tō-jen) a substance that stimulates mitosis and lymphocyte transformation; includes not only lectins such as phytohemagglutinins and concanavalin A, but also substances from streptococci (associated with streptolysin S) and from strains of α-toxin-producing staphylococci. [mitosis + G. *-gen,* producing]

**mi·to·gen·e·sis** (mī-tō-jen'ĕ-sis) the induction of mitosis in a cell. [mitosis + G. *genesis,* origin]

**mi·to·ge·net·ic** (mī'tō-jĕ-net'ik) pertaining to the factor or factors promoting cell mitosis.

**mi·to·gen·ic** (mī-tō-jen'ik) causing mitosis or transformation.

**mi·to·sis**, pl. **mi·to·ses** (mī-tō'sis, mī-tō'sēz) the usual process of somatic reproduction of cells consisting of a sequence of modifications of the nucleus (prophase, prometaphase, metaphase, anaphase, telophase) that result in the formation of two daughter cells with exactly the same chromosome and DNA content as that of the original cell. SEE ALSO cell cycle. SYN indirect nuclear division. [G. *mitos,* thread]

**mi·tot·ic** (mī-tot'ik) relating to or marked by mitosis.

**mi·tot·ic fig·ure** the microscopic appearance of a cell undergoing mitosis; a cell of which the chromosomes are visible by the light microscope.

**mi·tot·ic rate** the proportion of cells in a tissue that are undergoing mitosis, expressed as a mitotic index or, roughly, as the number of cells in mitosis in each microscopic high-power field in tissue sections.

**mi·tot·ic spin·dle** the fusiform figure characteristic of a dividing cell; it consists of microtubules (spindle fibers), some of which become attached to each chromosome at its centromere and appear to be involved in chromosomal movement; other microtubules (continuous fibers) pass from pole to pole. SYN nuclear spindle.

**mi·tral** (mī'trăl) **1.** relating to the mitral or bicuspid valve. **2.** shaped like a bishop's miter; denoting a structure resembling the shape of a headband or turban. [L. *mitra*, a coif or turban]

**mi·tral in·suf·fi·cien·cy** SEE valvular regurgitation.

**mi·tral·i·za·tion** (mī'tră-li-zā'shŭn) straightening of the left heart border on a chest radiograph due to prominence of the left atrial appendage or the pulmonary outflow tract; an unreliable indication of mitral valve disease.

**mi·tral mur·mur** a murmur produced at the mitral valve, either obstructive or regurgitant.

**mi·tral or·i·fice** an atrioventricular opening which leads from the left atrium into the left ventricle of the heart.

**mi·tral ste·no·sis (MS)** pathologic narrowing of the orifice of the mitral valve.

**mi·tral valve** the valve closing the orifice between the left atrium and left ventricle of the heart; its two cusps are called anterior and posterior. SYN bicuspid valve.

**mi·tral valve pro·lapse** excessive retrograde movement of one or both mitral valve leaflets into the left atrium during left ventricular systole, often allowing mitral regurgitation; responsible for the click-murmur of Barlow syndrome, and rarely may be due to rheumatic carditis, a connective tissue disorder such as Marfan syndrome or ruptured chorda tendinea ("flail mitral leaflet").

**Mit·su·o phe·nom·e·non** (mit-soo'ō) restoration of the normal color of the fundus with dark adaptation in Oguchi disease.

**mit·tel·schmerz** (mit'ĕl-shmertz) abdominal pain occurring at the time of ovulation, resulting from irritation of the peritoneum by bleeding from the ovulation site. SYN intermenstrual pain (2). [Ger. Mittelschmerz, middle + pain]

**Mit·ten·dorf dot** (mit'ĕn-dorf) a small dot visible on the posterior aspect of the lens capsule on ophthalmologic examination that represents a remnant of the primitive hyaloid vascular system.

**mixed ag·glu·ti·na·tion re·ac·tion** immune agglutination in which the aggregates contain cells of two different kinds but with common antigenic determinants; when used to identify isoantigens, the test cells are exposed to appropriate isoantibody, washed, and then mixed with indicator erythrocytes that combine with free sites on the test cell-attached isoantibody.

**mixed ag·glu·ti·na·tion test** SEE mixed agglutination reaction.

**mixed a·pha·sia** SYN global aphasia.

**mixed a·stig·ma·tism** astigmatism in which one meridian is hyperopic while the one at a right angle to it is myopic.

**mixed con·nec·tive-tis·sue dis·ease** disease with overlapping features of various systemic connective-tissue diseases and with serum antibodies to nuclear ribonucleoprotein.

**mixed ex·pired gas** one or more complete breaths of expired gas coming thoroughly mixed from the dead space and the alveoli.

**mixed gland 1.** a gland that contains both serous and mucous secretory units; **2.** a gland that is both exocrine and endocrine, e.g., the pancreas.

**mixed hear·ing loss** combination of conductive and sensorineural hearing loss.

**mixed leu·ke·mia, mixed cell leu·ke·mi·a** granulocytic leukemia with occurrence in the

blood of increased numbers of cells in the myeloid series (i.e., neutrophilic, eosinophilic, and basophilic granulocytes).

**mixed lym·pho·cyte cul·ture** SEE mixed lymphocyte culture test.

**mixed lym·pho·cyte cul·ture test** a test for histocompatibility of HL-A antigens in which donor and recipient lymphocytes are mixed in culture; the degree of incompatibility is indicated by the number of cells that have undergone transformation and mitosis, or by the uptake of radioactive isotope-labeled thymidine.

**mixed nerve** a nerve containing both afferent and efferent fibers.

**mixed pa·ral·y·sis** combined motor and sensory paralysis.

**mixed tu·mor** a tumor composed of two or more varieties of tissue.

**mix·ture** (miks'cher) **1.** a mutual incorporation of two or more substances, without chemical union, the physical characteristics of each of the components being retained. A **mechanical mixture** is a mixture of particles or masses distinguishable as such under the microscope or in other ways; a **physical mixture** is a more intimate mixture of molecules, as in the case of gases and many solutions. **2.** CHEMISTRY a mingling together of two or more substances without the occurrence of a reaction by which they would lose their individual properties, i.e., without permanent gain or loss of electrons. **3.** PHARMACY a preparation, consisting of a liquid holding an insoluble medicinal substance in suspension by means of acacia, sugar, or some other viscid material. [L. *mixtura* or *mistura*]

*Mi·ya·ga·wa·nel·la* (mē'ă-gah'wă-nel'ă) formerly considered a genus of Chlamydiaceae, but now synonymous with *Chlamydia*. [Y. *Miyagawa*]

**ml, mL** milliliter.

**MLD, mld** minimal lethal dose.

**MLD** manual lymph drainage.

**M line** a fine line in the center of the A band of the sarcomere of striated muscle myofibrils. SYN M band.

**mm** millimeter.

**M-mode** a diagnostic ultrasound presentation of the temporal changes in echoes in which the depth of echo-producing interfaces is displayed along one axis with time (T) along the second axis; motion (M) of the interfaces toward and away from the transducer is displayed.

**M-mode echocardiography** SEE M-mode.

**mmol** millimole.

**MMPI** Minnesota Multiphasic Personality Inventory.

**Mn** manganese.

**M'Nagh·ten rule** (mĕk-naw'tĕn) the classic English test of criminal responsibility (1843): "to establish a defense on the ground of insanity, it must be clearly proved that, at the time of committing the act, the party accused was laboring under such a defect of reasoning, from disease of the mind, as not to know the nature and quality of the act he was doing, or if he did know it, that he did not know he was doing what was wrong."

**mne·men·ic, mne·mic** (nē-men'ik, nē'mik) relating to memory.

**mne·mon·ic** (nē-mon'ik) SYN anamnestic (1).

**mne·mon·ics** (nē-mon'iks) the art of improving

m
n

the memory; a system for aiding the memory. [G. *mnēmonikos,* mnemonic, pertaining to memory]

**Mo** molybdenum.

**mo•bile end** for a given movement, the end of a bone that moves in response to muscle activity or gravity while the other end of the bone (the fixed end) is held stationary (as a consequence of attachment or muscular fixation). SYN punctum mobile.

**mo•bi•li•za•tion** (mō'bi-li-zā'shŭn) **1.** making movable; restoring the power of motion in a joint. **2.** the act or the result of the act of mobilizing; exciting a hitherto quiescent process into physiologic activity. [see mobilize]

**Mo•bitz block** (mō'bitz) second degree atrioventricular block in which there is a ratio of two or more atrial deflections (P waves) to ventricular responses.

**Mö•bi•us sign** (mer'bē-ăs, mō'bē-us) impairment of ocular convergence in Graves disease.

**Mö•bi•us syn•drome** (mer'bē-ăs, mō'bē-us) a developmental bilateral facial paralysis usually associated with oculomotor or other neurological disorders.

**mo•dal fre•quen•cy** SYN habitual pitch.

**mo•dal•i•ty** (mō-dal'i-tē) **1.** a form of application or employment of a therapeutic agent or regimen. **2.** various forms of sensation, e.g., touch, vision, etc.. [Mediev. L. *modalitas,* fr. L. *modus,* a mode]

**mo•dal pitch** SYN habitual pitch.

**mode** (mōd) in a set of measurements, that value which appears most frequently. [L. *modus,* a measure, quantity]

**mod•el** (mod'ĕl) **1.** a representation of something, often idealized or modified to make it conceptually easier to understand. **2.** something to be imitated. **3.** in dentistry, a cast. **4.** a mathematical representation of a particular phenomenon. **5.** an animal that is used to mimic a pathologic condition. [It. *midello,* fr. L. *modus,* measure, standard]

**mod•el•ing** (mod'ĕl-ing) **1.** LEARNING THEORY the acquiring and learning of a new skill by observing and imitating that behavior being performed by another individual. **2.** BEHAVIOR MODIFICATION a treatment procedure whereby the therapist or another significant person presents (models) the target behavior which the learner is to imitate. **3.** a continuous process by which a bone is altered in size and shape during its growth by resorption and formation of bone at different sites and rates.

**mod•i•fi•ca•tion** (mod'i-fi-kā'shŭn) **1.** a nonhereditary change in an organism; e.g., one that is acquired from its own activity or environment. **2.** a chemical or structural alteration in a molecule.

**mod•i•fied acid-fast stain** a stain for coccidia (*Cryptosporidium, Cyclospora, Isospora*) in which the decolorizer is a very dilute acid (1–3% sulfuric acid); less likely to remove too much dye.

**mod•i•fied rad•i•cal mas•tec•to•my** excision of the entire breast including the nipple, areola, and overlying skin, as well as the lymphatic-bearing tissue in the axilla with preservation of the pectoral muscles.

**mod•i•fied rad•i•cal mas•toid•ec•to•my** an operation for the management of cholesteatoma that lies lateral to the remnant of the tympanic membrane and middle-ear ossicles; involves exentera-

tion of the remaining air cells of the mastoid process and removal of the posterior and superior walls of the external auditory canal to open the mastoid and attic of the middle ear to the outside and preserve hearing.

**mod•i•fied tri•chrome stain** a stain developed from the Wheatley modification of the Gomori trichrome stain using 10 times the amount of chromotrope 2R dye for microsporidian spores, which stain pink to red.

**mod•i•fi•er** (mod'ĭ-fī'er) that which alters or limits.

**mo•di•o•lus,** pl. **mo•di•o•li** (mō-dī'ō-lŭs, mō-dī'ō-lī) **1.** the central cone-shaped core of spongy bone about which turns the spiral canal of the cochlea. **2.** SYN modiolus labii. [L., the nave of a wheel]

**mo•di•o•lus la•bii** a point near the corner of the mouth where several muscles of facial expression converge. SYN modiolus (2).

**mod•u•la•tion** (mod-yu-lā'shŭn) **1.** the functional and morphologic fluctuation of cells in response to changing environmental conditions. **2.** systematic variation in a characteristic (e.g., frequency, amplitude) of a sustained oscillation to code additional information. **3.** a change in the kinetics of an enzyme or metabolic pathway. **4.** the regulation of the rate of translation of mRNA by a modulating codon. [L. *modulor,* to measure off properly]

**mod•u•la•tor** that which regulates or adjusts.

**mo•du•lus** (mod'yu-lŭs) a coefficient expressing the magnitude of a physical property by a numerical value. [L. dim. of *modus,* a measure, quantity]

**Mohs che•mo•sur•gery** (mōz) a technique for removal of skin tumors with a minimum of normal tissue, by prior necrosis with zinc chloride paste, mapping of the tumor site, and excision and microscopic examination of frozen section of thin horizontal layers of tissue, until all of the tumor is removed. The preliminary step of chemical necrosis may be omitted.

**Mohs fresh tis•sue che•mo•sur•gery tech•nique** (mōz) chemosurgery in which superficial cancers are excised after fixation in vivo.

**moi•e•ty** (moy'i-tē) **1.** originally a half; now, loosely, a portion of something. **2.** functional group. [M.E. *moite,* a half]

**moist gan•grene** SYN wet gangrene.

**moist rale** a bubbling rale caused by air mixing with a fluid exudate in the bronchial tubes or a cavity.

**Mo•ko•la vi•rus** (mō-krō'lah) a rabies-related virus of the genus *Lyssavirus,* which has caused fatal neurological disease.

**mol** mole (4).

**mo•lal** (mō'lăl) denoting 1 mol of solute dissolved in 1000 g of solvent; such solutions provide a definite ratio of solute to solvent molecules. Cf. molar (4).

**mo•lal•i•ty** (mō-lal'i-tē) moles of solute per kilogram of solvent; the molarity is equal to mρ/(1 + mM), where m is the molality, ρ is the density of the solution, and M is the molar mass of the solute. Cf. molarity.

**mo•lar** (mō'lăr) **1.** denoting a grinding, abrading, or wearing away. [L. *molaris,* relating to a mill, millstone] **2.** SYN molar tooth. **3.** massive; relating to a mass; not molecular. [L. *moles,* mass] **4.** denoting a concentration of 1 gram-molecular weight (1 mol) of solute per liter of solution, the common unit of concentration in chemistry. Cf. molal. **5.** denoting specific quantity, e.g., molar volume (volume of 1 mol).

**mo·lar ab·sorp·tion co·ef·fi·cient** (ε) absorbance (of light) per unit path length (usually the centimeter) and per unit of concentration (moles per liter); a fundamental unit in spectrophotometry. SYN absorbancy index (2), absorptivity (2).

**mo·lar·i·ty** (M) (mō-lar′i-tē) moles per liter of solution (mol/L). Cf. molality.

**mo·lar tooth** a tooth having a somewhat quadrangular crown with four or five cusps on the grinding surface; the root is bifid in the lower jaw, but there are three conical roots in the upper jaw; there are six molars in each jaw, three on either side behind the premolars in the permanent dentition; in the deciduous dentition there are but four molars in each jaw, two on either side behind the canines. SYN dens molaris [TA], molar (2).

**mold** (mōld) **1.** a filamentous fungus, generally a circular colony that may be cottony, wooly, etc., or glabrous, but with filaments not organized into large fruiting bodies, such as mushrooms. **2.** a shaped receptacle into which wax is pressed or fluid plaster is poured in making a cast. **3.** to shape a mass of plastic material according to a definite pattern. **4.** to change in shape; denoting especially the adaptation of the fetal head to the pelvic canal. **5.** the term used to specify the shape of an artificial tooth (or teeth).

**mole** (mōl) **1.** SYN nevus (2). **2.** SYN nevus pigmentosus. [A.S. *māēl* (L. *macula*), a spot] **3.** an intrauterine mass formed by the degeneration of the partly developed products of conception. [L. *moles,* mass] **4. (mol)** in the SI system, the unit of amount of substance, defined as that amount of a substance containing as many "elementary entities" as there are atoms in 0.0120 kg of carbon-12; "elementary entities" may be atoms, molecules, ions, or any describable entity or defined mixture of entities and must be specified when this term is used; in practical terms, the mole is $6.0221367 \times 10^{23}$ "elementary entities." SEE ALSO Avogadro number.

**mo·lec·u·lar** (mō-lek′yu-lăr) relating to molecules.

**mo·lec·u·lar bi·ol·o·gy** study of phenomena in terms of molecular interactions; it differs from biochemistry in that it emphasizes chemical interactions involved in the replication of DNA, its "transcription" into RNA, and its "translation" into or expression in protein.

**mo·lec·u·lar dis·ease** a disease in which the manifestations are due to alterations in molecular structure and function.

**mo·lec·u·lar epi·de·mi·ol·o·gy** the use in epidemiologic studies of techniques of molecular biology such as DNA typing.

**mo·lec·u·lar move·ment** SYN brownian movement.

**mo·lec·u·lar ro·ta·tion** one-hundredth of the product of the specific rotation of an optically active compound and its molecular weight.

**mo·lec·u·lar weight (mol wt, MW)** the sum of the atomic weights of all the atoms constituting a molecule; the mass of a molecule relative to the mass of a standard atom, now $^{12}$C (taken as 12.000). Relative molecular mass ($M_r$) is the mass relative to the dalton and has no units. SEE

ALSO atomic weight. SYN molecular weight ratio, relative molecular mass.

**mo·lec·u·lar weight ra·tio ($M_r$)** SYN molecular weight.

**mol·e·cule** (mol′ĕ-kyul) the smallest possible quantity of a di-, tri-, or polyatomic substance that retains the chemical properties of the substance. [Mod. L. *molecula,* dim. of L. *moles,* mass]

**mo·li·men,** pl. **mo·lim·i·na** (mō-lī′men, mol-lim′i-nă) an effort; laborious performance of a normal function. [L. an endeavor]

**Mol·la·ret men·in·gi·tis** (mol-lah-rā′) a recurrent aseptic meningitis; febrile illness accompanied by headaches, malaise, meningeal signs, and cerebrospinal fluid monocytes.

**Moll glands** (mol) SYN ciliary glands.

**mol·li·ti·es** (mō-lish′ē-ēz) **1.** characterized by a soft consistency. **2.** SYN malacia. [L. *mollis,* soft]

**Mol·lusc·i·pox·vi·rus** (mol′lusk-′e-poks-vī-rŭs) a genus in the family Poxviridae; causes localized wartlike skin lesions.

**mol·lus·cous** (mo-lŭs′kŭs) relating to or resembling molluscum.

**mol·lus·cum** (mo-lŭs′kŭm) a disease marked by the occurrence of soft rounded tumors of the skin. [L. *molluscus,* soft]

**mol·lus·cum con·ta·gi·o·sum** a contagious disease of the skin caused by intranuclear proliferation of a virus of the family Poxviridae and characterized by the appearance of small, pearly, umbilicated papular epidermal growths. In adults it typically occurs on or near the genitals and is sexually transmitted.

**Mo·lo·ney test** (mĕ-lō′nē) a test to detect a high degree of sensitivity to diphtheria toxoid; more than a minimal local reaction to toxoid given intradermally indicates that prophylactic toxoid should be administered in fractional doses at suitable intervals.

**Mo·lo·ney vi·rus** (mĕ-lō′nē) a lymphoid leukemia retrovirus of mice, in the family Retroviridae, isolated originally during propagation of S 37 mouse sarcoma.

**molt** (mōlt) to cast off feathers, hair, or cuticle; to undergo ecdysis. [L. *muto,* to change]

**mol wt** molecular weight.

**mo·lyb·den·ic, mo·lyb·de·nous** (mō-lib′den-ik, mō-lib′den-ŭs) relating to molybdenum.

**mo·lyb·de·num (Mo)** (mō-lib′dĕ-nŭm) a silvery white metallic element, atomic no. 42, atomic wt. 95.94; a bioelement found in a number of proteins (e.g., xanthine oxidase). SEE molybdenum target tube. [G. *molybdaina,* a piece of lead; a metal, prob. galena, fr. *molybdos,* lead]

**mo·lyb·de·num tar·get tube** an x-ray tube with an anode surface made of molybdenum instead of tungsten, used in mammography.

**mo·nad** (mō′nad, mon′ad) **1.** a univalent element or radical. **2.** a unicellular organism. **3.** in meiosis, the single chromosome derived from a tetrad after the first and second maturation divisions. [G. *monas,* the number one, unity]

**Mo·na·kow syn·drome** (mō-nah′kof) contralateral hemiplegia, hemianesthesia, and homonomous hemianopsia due to occlusion of the anterior choroidal artery.

**mon·ar·thric** (mon-ar′thrik) SYN monarticular.

**mon·ar·thri·tis** (mon-ar-thrī′tis) arthritis of a single joint.

**mon·ar·tic·u·lar** (mon-ar-tik′yu-lăr) relating to a single joint. SYN monarthric.

**mon·as·ter** (mon-as′ter) the single star figure at the end of prophase in mitosis. [mono- + G. *astēr*, star]

**mon·ath·e·to·sis** (mon-ath-ĕ-tō′sis) athetosis affecting one hand or foot.

**mon·a·tom·ic** (mon-ă-tom′ik) **1.** relating to or containing a single atom. **2.** SYN monovalent (1).

**mon·au·ral** (mon-aw′răl) pertaining to one ear. [mono- + L. *auris*, ear]

**Mön·cke·berg ar·te·ri·o·scle·ro·sis** (merng′kĕ-berk) arterial sclerosis involving the peripheral arteries, especially of the legs of older people, with deposition of calcium in the medial coat (pipestem arteries) but with little or no encroachment on the lumen. SYN Mönckeberg calcification, Mönckeberg degeneration, Mönckeberg sclerosis.

**Mön·cke·berg cal·ci·fi·ca·tion** (merng′kĕ-berk) SYN Mönckeberg arteriosclerosis.

**Mön·cke·berg de·gen·er·a·tion** (merng′kĕ-berk) SYN Mönckeberg arteriosclerosis.

**Mön·cke·berg scler·o·sis** (merng′kĕ-berk) SYN Mönckeberg arteriosclerosis.

**Mon·di·ni dys·pla·sia** (mon-dē′nē) congenital anomaly of osseous and membranous labyrinth characterized by aplastic cochlea, and deformity of the vestibule and semicircular canals with partial or complete loss of auditory and vestibular function; may be associated with spontaneous cerebrospinal fluid otorrhoea resulting in meningitis.

**Mon·di·ni hear·ing im·pair·ment** (mon-dē′nē) the hearing impairment resulting from the structural aberration of Mondini dysplasia.

**Mon·dor dis·ease** (mon′dor) thrombophlebitis of the thoracoepigastric vein of the breast and chest wall.

**mon·es·thet·ic** (mon-es-thet′ik) relating to a single sense or sensation. [mono- + G. *aisthēsis*, sense perception]

**Mon·ge dis·ease** (mon-gĕ) SYN chronic mountain sickness.

**mon·go·li·an** (mon-gō′lē-ăn) relating to a member of the Mongolian race.

**mon·go·li·an spot** any of a number of dark-bluish or mulberry-colored rounded or oval spots on the sacral region due to the ectopic presence of scattered melanocytes in the dermis. These congenital lesions are frequent in black, Native American, and Asian children from 2 to 12 years, after which time they gradually recede; they do not disappear on pressure and are sometimes mistaken for bruises from child abuse. SYN blue spot (2).

**mo·nil·e·thrix** (mō-nil′ĕ-thriks) an inherited trichodystrophy in which brittle hairs show a series of constrictions, usually without a medulla. SYN beaded hair, moniliform hair. [L. *monile*, necklace, + G. *thrix*, hair]

**Mo·nil·i·a** (mo-nil′ē-ă) generic term for a group of fungi that are commonly known as fruit molds; the sexual state is *Neurospora*. A few closely related pathogenic organisms formerly classified in this genus are now properly termed *Candida*. [L. *monile*, necklace]

**mo·nil·i·al** (mō-nil′ē-ăl) pertaining to the genus *Candida* (formerly grouped with the genus *Monilia*).

**mon·i·li·a·sis** (mō-ni-lī′ă-sis) SYN candidiasis.

**mo·nil·i·form** (mo-nil′i-fōrm) shaped like a string of beads or beaded necklace. [L. *monile*, necklace, + *forma*, appearance]

**mo·nil·i·form hair** SYN monilethrix.

**Mo·nil·i·for·mis** (mo-nil-i-fōr′mis) a genus of thorny-headed worms. A few infections in humans have been reported. [L. *monile*, necklace, + *forma*, appearance]

**mo·nil·i·id** (mō-nil′ē-id) minute macular or papular lesions occurring as an allergic reaction to monilial infection.

**mon·i·tor** (mon′i-ter) a device that displays and/or records specified data for a given series of events, operations, or circumstances. [L., one who warns, fr. *moneo*, pp. *monitum*, to warn]

△**mono-, mon-** the participation or involvement of a single element or part. Cf. uni-. [G. *monos*, single]

**mon·o·a·me·lia** (mon-ō-ă-mē′lē-ă) absence of one limb.

**mon·o·am·ide** (mon-ō-am′īd, mon-ō-am′-id) a molecule containing one amide group.

**mon·o·am·ine** (mon-ō-am′īn, mon-ō-am′in) a molecule containing one amine group.

**mon·o·am·ine hy·poth·e·sis** the classical theory of the neurochemical basis of depression linking it to a deficiency of at least one of three monoamine neurotransmitters, norepinephrine, serotonin, or dopamine.

**mon·o·am·ine oxi·dase in·hib·i·tor** any of several antidepressants that inhibit enzymatic breakdown of monoamine neurotransmitters of the sympathetic/adrenergic system; not used as first-line therapy because of the risk of hypertensive crisis after consumption of foods or beverages containing pressor amines, including cheese, chocolate, beer, and wine.

**mon·o·am·i·ner·gic** (mon′ō-am-i-ner′jik) referring to nerve cells or fibers that transmit nervous impulses by the medium of a catecholamine or indolamine. [monoamine + G. *ergon*, work]

**mon·o·am·ni·ot·ic twins** twins within a common amnion; such twins are monovular in origin and may be conjoined.

**mon·o·ba·sic** (mon-ō-bā′sik) denoting an acid with only one replaceable hydrogen atom, or only one replaced hydrogen atom.

**mon·o·blast** (mon′ō-blast) an immature cell that develops into a monocyte. [mono- + G. *blastos*, germ]

**mon·o·cho·rea** (mon′ō-kō-rē′ă) chorea affecting the head alone or only one extremity.

**mon·o·cho·ri·on·ic** (mon′ō-kōr-ē-on′ik) relating to or having a single chorion; denoting monovular twins.

**mon·o·cho·ri·on·ic di·am·ni·on·ic pla·cen·ta** SEE twin placenta.

**mon·o·chro·mat·ic** (mon′ō-krō-mat′ik) **1.** having but one color. **2.** indicating a light of a single wavelength. **3.** relating to or characterized by monochromatism.

**mon·o·chro·mat·ic ab·er·ra·tion** a defect in an optical image arising because of the nature of lenses; the main types are spherical, coma, curvature, and distortion aberration, and astigmatism of oblique pencils.

**mon·o·chro·mat·ic ra·di·a·tion** light rays or ionizing radiation of a very narrow band of wavelengths (ideally, of a single wavelength). Cf. characteristic radiation.

**mon·o·chro·ma·tism** (mon-ō-krō′mă-tizm) **1.**

the state of having or exhibiting only one color. **2.** SYN achromatopsia. [mono- + G. *chrōma,* color]

**mon·o·chro·mat·o·phil, mon·o·chro·mat·o·phile** (mon'ō-krō-mat'ō-fil, mon'ō-krō-mat'ō-fīl) **1.** taking only one stain. **2.** a cell or any histologic element staining with only one kind of dye. [mono- + G. *chrōma,* color, + *philos,* fond]

**mon·o·clo·nal** (mon-ō-klō'năl) IMMUNOCHEMISTRY pertaining to a protein from a single clone of cells, all molecules of which are the same.

**mon·o·clo·nal an·ti·bo·dy** an antibody produced by a clone or genetically homogeneous population of hybrid cells i.e., hybridoma; hybrid cells are cloned to establish cell lines producing a specific antibody that is chemically and immunologically homogeneous; a mainstay of immunological research and medical diagnosis. SEE ALSO cluster of differentiation.

**mon·o·clo·nal gam·mop·athy of un·de·ter·mined sig·ni·fi·cance** a paraproteinemia (an abnormal gammaglobulin, typically with λ light chain component) of less than 3 g/100 ml, which at the time of discovery, is without apparent cause; specifically, there is no evidence of multiple myeloma or other malignant disorders. SYN benign monoclonal gammopathy.

**mon·o·clo·nal gam·mop·athy of un·known sig·ni·fi·cance (MGUS)** a gammopathy diagnosed by electrophoresis of serum of asymptomatic elderly persons who have no other evidence of plasma cell neoplasia; in 20% of cases it evolves into plasma cell malignancy.

**mon·o·clo·nal im·mu·no·glob·u·lin** a homogeneous immunoglobulin resulting from the proliferation of a single clone of plasma cells and which, during electrophoresis of serum, appears as a narrow band or "spike"; it is characterized by heavy chains of a single class and subclass, and light chains of a single type. SYN paraprotein (2).

**mon·o·crot·ic** (mon'ō-krot'ik) denoting a pulse the curve of which presents no notch or subsidiary wave in its descending line. [mono- + G. *krotos,* a beat]

**mon·oc·ro·tism** (mon-ok'rō-tizm) the state in which the pulse is monocrotic. [mono- + G. *krotos,* a beat]

**mo·noc·u·lar** (mon-ok'yu-lăr) relating to, affecting, or visible by one eye only. [mono- + L. *oculus,* eye]

**mo·noc·u·lar di·plo·pia** a double image or an extra ghost image produced in one eye, almost always by an aberration of the ocular media.

**mon·o·cyte** (mon'ō-sīt) a relatively large mononuclear leukocyte (16 to 22 μm in diameter), that normally constitutes 3 to 7% of the leukocytes of the circulating blood, and is normally found in lymph nodes, spleen, bone marrow, and loose connective tissue. In stained smears monocytes have abundant pale blue or blue-gray cytoplasm that contains numerous fine red-blue granules and vacuoles; the nucleus is usually indented, or slightly folded. See page B1. [mono- + G. *kytos,* cell]

**mon·o·cyte che·mo·a·ttrac·tant pro·tein** a cytokine involved in monocyte migration.

**mon·o·cyte-de·rived neu·tro·phil che·mo·tac·tic fac·tor** SYN interleukin-8.

**mon·o·cyt·ic leu·ke·mia** a form of leukemia characterized by large numbers of cells that can be definitely identified as monocytes, in addition to larger, apparently related cells formed from the uncontrolled proliferation of the reticuloendothelial tissue. The disease runs an acute or subacute course in older persons, and is characterized by swelling of gums, oral ulceration, bleeding in skin or mucous membranes, secondary infection, and splenomegaly.

**mon·o·cy·toid cell** a cell that resembles a monocyte but is nonphagocytic.

**mon·o·cy·to·pe·nia** (mon'ō-sī-tō-pē'nē-ă) diminution in the number of monocytes in the circulating blood. [mono- + G. *kytos,* cell, + *penia,* poverty]

**mon·o·cy·to·sis** (mon'ō-sī-tō'sis) an abnormal increase in the number of monocytes in the circulating blood.

**mon·o·dac·ty·ly, mon·o·dac·tyl·ism** (mon-ō-dak'ti-lē, mon-ō-dak'ti-lizm) the presence of a single finger on the hand, or a single toe on the foot. [mono- + G. *daktylos,* digit]

**mon·o·fix·a·tion syn·drome** a small-angle strabismus (fewer than 10 prism diopters) with central fixation by the preferred eye, central suppression of the deviating eye, and binocular fusion of peripheral vision

**mon·o·ga·met·ic** (mon'ō-gă-met'ik) SYN homogametic.

**mo·nog·a·my** (mon-og'ă-mē) the marriage or mating system in which each partner has but one mate. [mono- + G. *gamos,* marriage]

**mon·o·gen·e·sis** (mon-ō-jen'ĕ-sis) **1.** the production of similar organisms in each generation. **2.** the production of young by one parent only, as in nonsexual generation and parthenogenesis. **3.** the process of parasitizing a single host, in which the entire life cycle of the parasite is passed. [mono- + G. *genesis,* origin, production]

**mon·o·ge·net·ic** (mon'ō-jĕ-net'ik) relating to monogenesis. SYN monoxenous.

**mon·o·gen·ic** (mon-ō-jen'ik) relating to a hereditary disease or syndrome, or to an inherited characteristic, controlled by alleles at a single genetic locus.

**mo·nog·e·nous** (mŏ-noj'ĕ-nŭs) asexually produced, as by fission, gemmation, or sporulation.

**mon·o·hy·dric al·co·hol** an alcohol containing one OH group.

**mon·o·lay·ers** (mon-ō-lā'erz) **1.** films, one molecule thick, formed on water by certain substances, such as proteins and fatty acids, characterized by molecules containing some atom groupings that are soluble in water and other atom groupings that are insoluble in water. **2.** a confluent sheet of cells, one cell deep, growing on a surface in a cell culture.

**mon·o·loc·u·lar** (mon-ō-lok'yu-lăr) having one cavity or chamber. SYN unicameral, unicamerate. [mono- + L. *loculus,* a small place]

**mon·o·ma·nia** (mon-ō-mā'nē-ă) an obsession or abnormal enthusiasm for a single idea or subject; a psychosis marked by limitation of symptoms to a certain group, as the delusion in paranoia. [mono- + G. *mania,* frenzy]

**mon·o·mel·ic** (mon-ō-mel'ik) relating to one limb. [mono- + G. *melos,* limb]

**mon·o·mer** (mon'ō-mer) **1.** the molecular unit that, by repetition, constitutes a large structure or polymer. **2.** the protein structural unit of a virion capsid. SEE virion. **3.** the protein subunit of a protein composed of several loosely associated

**m**
**0**

such units, usually noncovalently bound together. [mono- + -mer]

**mon·o·mer·ic** (mon-ō-mer′ik) **1.** consisting of a single component. **2.** GENETICS relating to a hereditary disease or characteristic controlled by genes at a single locus. **3.** consisting of monomers. [mono- + G. *meros*, part]

**mon·o·mor·phic** (mon-ō-mōr′fik) of one shape; unchangeable in shape. [mono- + G. *morphē*, shape]

**mon·o·my·o·ple·gia** (mon′ō-mī′ō-plē′jē-ă) paralysis limited to one muscle. [mono- + G. *mys*, muscle, + *plēgē*, a stroke]

**mon·o·my·o·si·tis** (mon′ō-mī-ō-sī′tis) inflammation of a single muscle.

**mon·o·neu·ral, mon·o·neu·ric** (mon′ō-noo′răl, monō-noo′rik) **1.** having only one neuron. **2.** supplied by a single nerve.

**mon·o·neu·ral·gia** (mon′ō-noo-ral′jă) pain along the course of one nerve.

**mon·o·neu·ri·tis** (mon′ō-noo-rī′tis) inflammation of a single nerve.

**mon·o·neu·rop·a·thy** (mon′ō-noo-rop′ă-thē) disorder involving a single nerve.

**mon·o·nu·cle·ar** (mon-ō-noo′klē-ăr) having only one nucleus; used especially in reference to blood cells.

**mon·o·nu·cle·ar phag·o·cyte sys·tem** a widely distributed family of both free and fixed macrophages derived from bone marrow precursor cells by way of monocytes; their substantial phagocytic activity is mediated by immunoglobulin and the serum complement system. In both connective and lymphoid tissue, they may occur as free and fixed macrophages; in the sinusoids of the liver, as Kupffer cells; in the lung, as alveolar macrophages; and in the nervous system, as microglia.

**mon·o·nu·cle·o·sis** (mon′ō-noo-klē-ō′sis) presence of abnormally large numbers of mononuclear leukocytes in the circulating blood, especially with reference to forms that are not normal.

**mon·o·nu·cle·o·tide** (mon-ō-noo′klē-ō-tīd) SYN nucleotide.

**mon·o·ox·y·ge·na·ses** (mon-ō-ok′si-jĕ-nā-sez) oxidoreductases that induce the incorporation of one atom of oxygen from $O_2$ into the substance being oxidized.

**mon·o·pa·re·sis** (mon′o-pa-rē′sis, mon′o-par′ĕ-sis) paresis affecting a single extremity or part of an extremity.

**mon·o·par·es·the·sia** (mon′ō-par-es-thē′zē-ă) paresthesia affecting a single region only.

**mon·o·path·ic** (mon-ō-path′ik) relating to a monopathy.

**mo·nop·a·thy** (mon-op′ă-thē) **1.** a single uncomplicated disease. **2.** a local disease affecting only one organ or part. [mono- + G. *pathos*, suffering]

**mon·o·pha·sia** (mon-ō-fā′zē-ă) inability to speak other than a single word or sentence. [mono- + G. *phasis*, speech]

**mon·o·pha·sic** (mon-ō-fā′zik) **1.** marked by monophasia. **2.** occurring in or characterized by only one phase or stage. **3.** fluctuating from the baseline in one direction only.

**mon·oph·thal·mos** (mon-of-thal′mos) failure of outgrowth of a primary optic vesicle with absence of ocular tissues; the remaining eye is often maldeveloped. [mono- + G. *ophthalmos*, eye]

**mon·o·phy·let·ic** (mon′ō-fī-let′ik) **1.** having a single cell type of origin; derived from one line of descent, in contrast to polyphyletic. **2.** HEMATOLOGY relating to monophyletism. [mono- + G. *phylē*, tribe]

**mon·o·ple·gia** (mon-ō-plē′jē-ă) paralysis of one limb. [mono- + G. *plēgē*, a stroke]

**mon·o·po·dia** (mon-ō-pō′dē-ă) fetal malformation in which sirenomelia is accompanied by fusion of the feet into a single structure. [mono- + G. *pous*, foot]

**mon·o·po·lar cau·tery** electrocautery by high frequency electrical current passed from a single electrode, where the cauterization occurs, the patient's body serving as a ground.

**mon·or·chid·ic, mon·or·chid** (mon-ōr-kid′ik, mon-ōr′kid) **1.** having only one testis. **2.** having apparently only one testis, the other being undescended.

**mon·or·chism** (mon′ōr-kizm) a condition in which only one testis is apparent, the other being absent or undescended. [mono- + G. *orchis*, testis]

**mon·o·sac·cha·ride** (mon-ō-sak′ă-rīd) a carbohydrate that cannot form any simpler sugar by simple hydrolysis; e.g., pentoses, hexoses.

**mon·o·so·mia** (mon-ō-sō′mē-ă) in conjoined twins, a condition in which the trunks are completely merged although the heads remain separate. SEE conjoined twins. [mono- + G. *sōma*, body]

**mon·o·so·mic** (mon-ō-sō′mik) relating to monosomy.

**mon·o·so·my** (mon′ō-sō-mē) absence of one chromosome of a pair of homologous chromosomes. [see monosome]

**mon·o·spasm** (mon′ō-spazm) spasm affecting only one muscle or group of muscles, or a single extremity.

**mon·o·stot·ic** (mon-os-tot′ik) involving only one bone. [mono- + G. *osteon*, bone]

**mon·o·stra·tal** (mon-ō-strā′tăl) composed of a single layer. [mono- + L. *stratum*, layer]

**mon·o·symp·to·mat·ic** (mon′ō-simp-tō-mat′ik) denoting a disease or morbid condition manifested by only one marked symptom.

**mon·o·sy·nap·tic** (mon′ō-si-nap′tik) referring to direct neural connections not involving an intermediary neuron.

**mon·o·ther·mia** (mon-ō-ther′mē-ă) evenness of bodily temperature; absence of an evening rise in body temperature. [mono- + G. *thermē*, heat]

**mo·not·ri·chous** (mŏ-not′ri-kŭs) denoting a microorganism possessing a single flagellum or cilium.

**mon·o·va·lence, mon·o·va·len·cy** (mon-ō-vā′lens, mon-ō-vā′len-sē) a combining power (valence) equal to that of a hydrogen atom. SYN univalence, univalency.

**mon·o·va·lent** (mon-ō-vā′lent) **1.** having the combining power (valence) of a hydrogen atom. SYN monatomic (2), univalent. **2.** pertaining to a monovalent (specific) antiserum to a single antigen or organism.

**mon·o·xe·nic cul·ture** culture of parasites grown in association with a single known microbiota.

**mon·ox·e·nous** (mon-oks′ē-nŭs) SYN monogenetic. [mono- + G. *xenos*, stranger]

**mon·ox·ide** (mon-ok′sīd) any oxide having only one atom of oxygen; e.g., CO.

**mon·o·zy·got·ic, mon·o·zy·gous** (mon-ō-zī-got′ ik, mon-ō-zī′gŭs) SYN unigerminal. SEE monozy-gotic twins. [mono- + G. *zygōtos,* yoked]

**mon·o·zy·got·ic twins** twins resulting from a single fertilized ovum that at an early stage of development becomes separated into independ-ently growing cell aggregations giving rise to two individuals of the same sex and identical genetic constitution. SYN enzygotic twins, identi-cal twins.

**Mon·ro doc·trine** (měn-rō′) a doctrine that states that the cranial cavity is a closed rigid box and that therefore a change in the quantity of intra-cranial blood can occur only through the dis-placement of or replacement by cerebrospinal fluid.

**mons,** gen. **mon·tis,** pl. **mon·tes** (monz, mon′tis, mon′tēz) an anatomical prominence or slight ele-vation above the general level of the surface. [L. a mountain]

**mons pu·bis** the prominence caused by a pad of fatty tissue over the symphysis pubis in the fe-male.

**Mon·teg·gia frac·ture** (mon-tej′ē) fracture of the proximal ulna with dislocation of the head of the radius.

**Mon·te·vi·deo unit** (mon′tě-vī-dā′ō) a unit of uterine contraction intensity in labor, defined as the peak pressure achieved by the contraction minus the baseline tone. [from Montevideo, Ar-gentina, where developed]

**Mont·gom·ery fol·li·cles** (mont-gum′ěr-ē) SYN areolar glands.

**Mont·gom·ery tu·ber·cles** (mont-gum′ěr-ē) ele-vated reddened areolar glands, usually associated with pregnancy.

**mon·tic·u·lus,** pl. **mon·tic·u·li** (mon-tik′yu-lŭs, mon-tik′yu-lī) 1. any slight rounded projection above a surface. 2. the central portion of the superior vermis forming a projection on the sur-face of the cerebellum; its anterior and most prominent portion is called the culmen, its posterior sloping portion, the declive. [L. dim. of *mons,* mountain]

**mood** (mood) the pervasive feeling, tone, and in-ternal emotional state which, when impaired, can markedly influence virtually all aspects of a per-son's behavior or perception of external events.

**mood-con·gru·ent hal·lu·ci·na·tion** hallucina-tion in which the content is mood appropriate.

**mood-in·con·gru·ent hal·lu·ci·na·tion** halluci-nation that is not consistent with external stimuli; content is not consistent with either manic or depressed mood.

**mood sta·bil·i·zing agent** a functional category of drugs used to normalize mood, particularly by damping mood swings (e.g., lithium and some anticonvulsants such as carbamazepine and val-proic acid).

**mood swing** oscillation of a person's emotional feeling tone between euphoria and depression.

**moon face** the round, usually red face, with large jowls, seen in Cushing disease or in exogenous hyperadrenocorticalism.

**Moon mo·lars** (moon) small dome-shaped first molar teeth occurring in congenital syphilis.

**Moore light·ning streaks** (moor) photopsia manifested by vertical flashes of light, seen usu-ally on the temporal side of the affected eye, caused by the involutional shrinkage of vitreous humor.

**Moore meth·od** (moor) treatment of aneurysm by the introduction of silver or zinc wire into the sac to induce fibrin deposition.

**Moo·ren ul·cer** (mō′rěn) chronic inflammation of the peripheral cornea that slowly progresses centrally with corneal thinning and sometimes perforation.

*Mor·ax·el·la* (mōr′ak-sel′ă) a genus of obligately aerobic nonmotile bacteria containing Gram-neg-ative coccoids or short rods which usually occur in pairs. They are parasitic on the mucous mem-branes of man and other mammals. [V. *Morax*]

**mor·bid** (mōr′bid) 1. diseased or pathologic. 2. PSYCHOLOGY abnormal or deviant. [L. *morbidus,* ill, fr. *morbus,* disease]

**mor·bid·i·ty** (mōr-bid′i-tē) 1. a diseased state. 2. the ratio of sick to well in a community. SEE ALSO morbidity rate. 3. the frequency of the appear-ance of complications following a surgical proce-dure or other treatment.

**mor·bid·i·ty rate** the proportion of patients with a particular disease during a given year per given unit of population.

**mor·bid o·be·si·ty** obesity sufficient to prevent normal activity or physiologic function, or to cause the onset of a pathologic condition.

**mor·bif·ic** (mōr-bif′ik) SYN pathogenic. [L. *mor-bus,* disease, + *facio,* to make]

**mor·bil·li** (mōr-bil′ī) SYN measles (1). [Mediev. L. *morbillus,* dim. of L. *morbus,* disease]

**mor·bil·li·form** (mōr-bil′i-fōrm) resembling measles (1). [see morbilli]

*Mor·bil·li·vi·rus* (mōr-bil′i-vī′rŭs) a genus in the family Paramyxoviridae, including measles, ca-nine distemper, and bovine rinderpest viruses.

**mor·bus** (mōr′bŭs) SYN disease (1). [L. disease]

**mor·cel·lat·ed neph·rec·tomy** removal of a kidney in pieces.

**mor·cel·la·tion** (mōr-se-lā′shŭn) division into and removal of small pieces, as of a tumor. [Fr. *morceler,* to subdivide]

**mor·cel·la·tion op·er·a·tion** vaginal hysterec-tomy in which the uterus is removed in multiple pieces after being split or partitioned.

**mor·dant** (mōr′dant) 1. a substance capable of combining with a dye and the material to be dyed, thereby increasing the affinity or binding of the dye. 2. to treat with a mordant. [L. *mordeo,* to bite]

**Mo·rel ear** (mō-rel′) a large, misshapen, out-standing auricle, with obliterated grooves and thinned edges.

**mor·gag·ni·an cyst** SYN vesicular appendages of epoophoron.

**Mor·ga·gni cat·a·ract** (mōr-gah′nyē) a hyper-mature cataract in which the nucleus gravitates within the capsule.

**Mor·ga·gni col·umns** (mōr-gah′nyē) SYN anal columns.

**Mor·ga·gni dis·ease** (mōr-gah′nyē) SYN Adams-Stokes syndrome.

**Mor·gag·ni for·a·men her·nia** (mōr-gah′nyē) a congenital anterior, retrosternal hernia of abdom-inal contents, most often only omentum but occa-sionally stomach, usually through the right retro-sternal Morgagni foramen, through which the in-ternal mammary artery passes to become the su-perior epigastric artery; often asymptomatic. SYN parasternal hernia.

**Mor·ga·gni glob·ules** (mōr-gah′nyē) vesicles

beneath the capsule and between lens fibers in early cataract.

**Mor·ga·gni pro·lapse** (mōr-gah′nyē) chronic inflammation of Morgagni ventricle.

**Mor·ga·gni ret·i·nac·u·lum** (mōr-gah′nyē) SYN frenulum of ileal orifice.

**Mor·ga·gni si·nus** (mōr-gah′nyē) **1.** SYN anal sinuses (1). **2.** SYN prostatic utricle. **3.** SYN laryngeal ventricle.

**Mor·ga·gni syn·drome** (mōr-gah′nyē) hyperostosis frontalis interna in elderly women, with obesity and neuropsychiatric disorders of uncertain cause; at least sometimes familial. SYN metabolic craniopathy.

**Mor·gan** (mōr′găn), Harry de R., British physician, 1863–1931.

**mor·gan** (mōr′găn) the standard unit of genetic distance on the genetic map: the distance between two loci such that on average one crossing over will occur per meiosis; for working purposes, the centimorgan (0.01 M) is used. [T.H. Morgan, U.S. geneticist, 1866–1945]

*Mor·gan·el·la* (mōr′gan-el′ah) a genus of Gramnegative, facultatively anaerobic, chemoorganotrophic, straight rods that are motile by peritrichous flagella. Found in feces of human beings, other animals, and reptiles. Can cause opportunistic infections of the blood, respiratory tract, wounds, and urinary tract.

*Mor·gan·el·la mor·ga·ni·i* type (and only) species of the genus *Morganella.*

**morgue** (mōrg) **1.** a building where unidentified dead are kept pending identification before burial. **2.** a building or room in a hospital or other facility where the dead are kept pending autopsy, burial, or cremation. SYN mortuary (2). [Fr.]

**mo·ria** (mōr′ē-ă) **1.** rarely used term denoting foolishness or dullness of comprehension. **2.** rarely used term for a mental state marked by frivolity, joviality, an inveterate tendency to jest, and inability to take anything seriously.

**mor·i·bund** (mōr′i-bŭnd) dying; at the point of death. [L. *moribundus,* dying, fr. *morior,* to die]

**Mör·ner test** (mer′ner) **1.** for cysteine, which gives a brilliant purple color with sodium nitroprusside; **2.** for tyrosine, which gives a green color on boiling with sulfuric acid containing formaldehyde.

**morn·ing af·ter pill** an oral drug that, when taken by a woman within 2–3 days after intercourse, reduces the probability that she will become pregnant. SYN emergency hormonal contraception.

**morn·ing sick·ness** the nausea and vomiting of early pregnancy. SYN nausea gravidarum.

**Mo·ro reflex** (mo′rō) SYN auropalpebral reflex.

**mor·phea** (mōr-fē′ă) cutaneous lesion(s) characterized by indurated, slightly depressed plaques of thickened dermal fibrous tissue, of a whitish or yellowish white color surrounded by a pinkish or purplish halo. SYN localized scleroderma. [G. *morphē,* form, figure]

**mor·phine** (mōr′fēn, mōr-fēn′) the major phenanthrene alkaloid of opium, which contains 9–14% of anhydrous morphine. It produces a combination of depression and excitation in the central nervous system and some peripheral tissues; predominance of either central stimulation or depression depends upon the species and dose; repeated administration leads to the development of tolerance, physical dependence, and (if

abused) psychic dependence. Used as an analgesic, sedative, and anxiolytic. [L. *Morpheus,* god of dreams or of sleep]

**mor·phine sul·fate (MS)** morphine used for formulation of tablets as well as solutions for parenteral, epidural, or intrathecal injection to relieve pain.

△**mor·pho-, morph-** form, shape, structure. [G. *morphē*]

**mor·phoea [Br.]** SEE morphea.

**mor·pho·gen·e·sis** (mōr-fō-jen′ĕ-sis) **1.** differentiation of cells and tissues in the early embryo that establishes the form and structure of the various organs and parts of the body. **2.** the ability of a molecule or group of molecules (particularly macromolecules) to assume a certain shape. [morpho- + G. *genesis,* production]

**mor·pho·ge·net·ic** (mōr′fō-jĕ-net′ik) relating to morphogenesis.

**mor·pho·ge·net·ic move·ment** the streaming of cells in the early embryo to form tissues or organs.

**mor·pho·log·ic** (mōr-fō-loj′ik) relating to morphology.

**mor·phol·o·gy** (mōr-fol′ō-jē) the science concerned with the configuration or the structure of animals and plants. [morpho- + G. *logos,* study]

**mor·pho·met·ric** (mōr′fō-met′rik) pertaining to morphometry.

**mor·phom·e·try** (mōr-fom′ĕ-trē) the measurement of the form of organisms or their parts. [morpho- + G. *metron,* measure]

**mor·pho·sis** (mōr-fō′sis) mode of development of a part. [G. formation, act of forming]

**mors,** gen. **mor·tis** (mōrz, mōr′tis) SYN death. [L.]

**mor·tal** (mōr′tăl) **1.** pertaining to or causing death. **2.** destined to die. [L. *mortalis,* fr. *mors,* death]

**mor·tal·i·ty** (mōr-tal′i-tē) **1.** the state of being mortal. **2.** SYN death rate. **3.** a fatal outcome. [L. *mortalitas,* fr. *mors* (*mort-*), death]

**mor·tal·i·ty rate** SYN death rate.

**mor·tar** (mōr′tăr) a vessel with rounded interior in which crude drugs and other substances are crushed or bruised by means of a pestle. [L. *mortarium*]

**mor·ti·fi·ca·tion** (mōr′ti-fi-kā′shŭn) SYN gangrene (1). [L. *mors* (*mort-*), death, + *facio,* to make]

**mor·ti·fied** (mōr′ti-fīd) SYN gangrenous.

**mor·tise joint** SYN ankle joint.

**Mor·ton neu·ral·gia** (mōr′tŏn) neuralgia of an interdigital nerve, usually the anastomotic branch between the medial and lateral plantar nerves, resulting from compression of the nerve by the metatarsophalangeal joint.

**Mor·ton syn·drome** (mōr′tŏn) congenital shortening of the first metatarsal causing metatarsalgia.

**Mor·ton toe** (mōr′tŏn) metatarsal pain caused by compression of sensory nerves by the metatarsal heads, sometimes with neuroma formation.

**mor·tu·ary** (mōr′tyu-ār-ē) **1.** relating to death or to burial. **2.** SYN morgue. [L. *mortuus,* dead, part. adj. fr. *morior,* pp. *mortuus,* to die]

**mor·u·la** (mōr′yŭ-lă) the solid mass of blastomeres resulting from the early cleavage divisions of the zygote. [Mod. L. dim. of L. *morus,* mulberry]

**mor·u·la·tion** (mōr-yŭ-lā'shŭn) formation of the morula.

**Mor·van cho·rea** (mōr-vah') SYN myokymia.

**Mor·van dis·ease** (mōr-vah') SYN syringomyelia.

**mo·sa·ic** (mō-zā'ik) **1.** inlaid; resembling inlaid work. **2.** the juxtaposition in an organism of genetically different tissues; it may occur normally (as in lyonization, *q.v.*), or pathologically, as an occasional phenomenon. [Mod. L. *mosaicus, musaicus*, pertaining to the Muses, artistic]

**mo·sa·ic in·her·i·tance** inheritance in which the paternal influence is dominant in one group of cells and the maternal in another. Cf. lyonization.

**mo·sa·i·cism** (mō-zā'i-sizm) condition of being mosaic (2).

**mo·sa·ic pat·tern** on high-resolution CT scans of the lungs, a pattern of brighter and darker regions corresponding to differences in perfusion or aeration; found in some cases of chronic thromboembolism or of bronchiolitis obliterans. Cf. oligemia.

**mo·sa·ic wart** plantar growth of numerous closely aggregated warts forming a mosaic appearance, frequently caused by human papilloma virus type 2.

**Mos·ler sign** (mōz'lĕr) tenderness over the sternum in a patient with acute myeloblastic anemia.

**mos·qui·to**, pl. **mos·qui·toes** (mŭs-kē'tō, mŭs-kē'tōs) a blood-sucking dipterous insect of the family Culicidae. *Aedes, Anopheles, Culex, Mansonia*, and *Stegomyia* are the genera containing most of the species involved in the transmission of protozoan and other disease-producing parasites. [Sp. dim. of *mosca*, fly, fr. L. *musca*, a fly]

**Mos·so er·go·graph** (mos'ō) an instrument consisting of pulleys, weights, and a recording lever, which is used to obtain a graphic record of flexion of a finger, hand, or arm.

**Mos·so sphyg·mo·ma·nom·e·ter** (mos'ō) an apparatus for measuring the blood pressure in the digital arteries.

**Moss tube** (mos) **1.** a triple-lumen, nasogastric, feeding-decompression tube that utilizes a gastric balloon to occlude the cardioesophageal junction, with simultaneous esophageal aspiration and intragastric feeding; **2.** a double-lumen, gastric lavage tube that provides continuous delivery of saline via a small bore, with simultaneous aspiration of fluid and some particles via a large bore.

**Mo·tais op·er·a·tion** (mō-tā') transplantation of the middle third of the tendon of the superior rectus muscle of the eyeball into the upper lid, between the tarsus and skin, to supplement the action of the levator muscle in ptosis.

**mote** (mōt) a small particle; a speck. [A.S. *mot*]

**moth·er** (mŭdh'er) **1.** the female parent. **2.** any cell or other structure from which other similar bodies are formed. [A.S. *mōdor*]

**moth·er cell** a cell that, by division, gives rise to two or more daughter cells. SYN metrocyte.

**moth·er cyst** a hydatid cyst from the inner, or germinal, layer, from which secondary cysts containing scoleces (daughter cysts) are developed; occurs most frequently in the liver, but may be found in other organs and tissue. SYN parent cyst.

**moth·er yaw** a large granulomatous lesion, considered to be the initial lesion in yaws, most commonly present on the hand, leg, or foot. SYN buba madre, frambesioma.

**mo·tile** (mō'til) **1.** having the power of spontaneous movement. **2.** denoting the type of mental imagery in which one learns and recalls most readily that which has been felt. Cf. audile. **3.** a person having such mental imagery. [see motion]

**mo·til·i·ty** (mō-til'i-tē) the power of spontaneous movement.

**mo·tion sick·ness** the syndrome of pallor, nausea, weakness, and malaise, which may progress to vomiting and incapacitation, caused by stimulation of the semicircular canals during travel or motion as on a boat, plane, train, car, swing, or rotating amusement ride. SYN kinesia.

**mo·tive** (mō'tiv) **1.** an acquired predisposition, need, or specific state of tension within an individual which arouses, maintains, and directs behavior toward a goal. SYN learned drive. **2.** the reason attributed to or given by an individual for a behavioral act. Cf. instinct. [L. *moveo*, to move, to set in motion]

**mo·to·fa·cient** (mō-tō-fā'shent) causing motion; denoting the second phase of muscular activity in which actual movement is produced. [L. *motus*, motion, + *facio*, to make]

**mo·to·neu·ron** (mō'tō-noo'ron) SYN motor neuron.

**mo·to·neu·ro·ne [Br.]** SEE motor neuron.

**mo·tor** (mō'ter) **1.** ANATOMY, PHYSIOLOGY denoting those neural structures that, by the impulses generated and transmitted by them cause muscle fibers or pigment cells to contract, or glands to secrete. SEE ALSO motor cortex, motor endplate, motor neuron. **2.** PSYCHOLOGY denoting the overt reaction of an organism to a stimulus (motor response). [L. a mover, fr. *moveo*, to move]

**mo·tor a·pha·sia** SYN expressive aphasia. SYN Broca aphasia.

**mo·tor ar·ea** SYN motor cortex.

**mo·tor a·tax·ia** ataxia developing upon attempting to perform coordinated muscular movements.

**mo·tor cor·tex** the region of the cerebral cortex most immediately influencing movements of the face, neck, trunk, arms, and leg; its effects upon the motor neurons innervating the skeletal musculature are mediated by the pyramidal tract. SYN excitable area, motor area, Rolando area.

**mo·tor de·cus·sa·tion** SYN pyramidal decussation.

**mo·tor end·plate** the large and complex endformation by which the axon of a motor neuron establishes synaptic contact with a striated muscle fiber (cell).

**mo·tor fi·bers** nerve fibers that transmit impulses that activate effector cells, e.g., in muscle or gland tissue.

**mo·tor im·age** the image of body movements.

**mo·tor nerve** an efferent nerve conveying an impulse that excites muscular contraction; motor nerves in the autonomic nervous system also elicit secretions from glandular epithelia.

**mo·tor neu·ron** a nerve cell in the spinal cord, rhombencephalon, or mesencephalon characterized by an axon that leaves the central nervous system to establish a functional connection with an effector (muscle or glandular) tissue; **somatic motor neurons** directly synapse with striated muscle fibers by motor endplates; **visceral motor neurons** or **autonomic motor neurons** (preganglionic motor neurons), by contrast, innervate smooth muscle fibers or glands only by the intermediary of a second, peripheral, neuron (postganglionic or ganglionic motor neuron) located in an autonomic ganglion. SEE ALSO motor end-

m
0

plate, autonomic division of nervous system. SYN motoneuron.

**mo·tor neu·ron dis·ease** a general term including progressive spinal muscular atrophy (infantile, juvenile, and adult), amyotrophic lateral sclerosis, progressive bulbar paralysis, and primary lateral sclerosis; frequently a familial disease.

**mo·tor pa·ral·y·sis** loss of the power of muscular contraction.

**mo·tor plate** a motor endplate.

**mo·tor point** a point on the skin where the application of an electrical stimulus, via an electrode, will cause the contraction of an underlying muscle.

**mo·tor speech cen·ter** SYN Broca center.

**mo·tor u·nit** a single somatic motor neuron and the group of muscle fibers innervated by it.

**mo·tor ur·gen·cy** urgency from overactive detrusor function.

**MOTT** term used to describe mycobacteria other than *Mycobacterium tuberculosis*, *M. bovis*, and *M. africanum*, (*M. tuberculosis* complex).

**mot·tled e·nam·el** alterations in enamel structure due to excessive fluoride ingestion during tooth formation.

**mot·tling** (mot'ling) an area of skin composed of macular lesions of varying shades or colors. [E. *motley*, variegated in color]

**mound·ing** (mownd'ing) SYN myoedema.

**mount** (mownt) **1.** to prepare for microscopic examination. **2.** to climb on for purposes of copulation.

**moun·tain sick·ness** SYN altitude sickness.

**mouse** (mows) a small rodent belonging to the genus *Mus*.

**mouse-tooth for·ceps** a forceps with one or two fine points at the tip of each blade, fitting into hollows between the points on the opposite blade.

**mouth** (mowth) **1.** SYN oral cavity. **2.** the opening, usually the external opening, of a cavity or canal. SEE OS (2), ostium, orifice, stoma (2). See this page. [A.S. *mūth*]

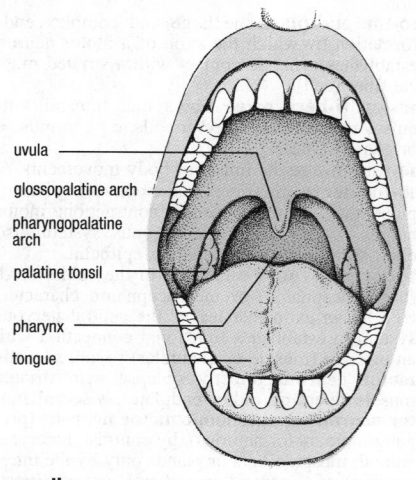

uvula
glossopalatine arch
pharyngopalatine arch
palatine tonsil
pharynx
tongue

**mouth**

**mouth-to-mouth res·pi·ra·tion** a method of artificial ventilation involving an overlap of the patient's mouth (and nose in small children) with the operator's mouth to inflate the patient's lungs by blowing, followed by an unassisted expiratory phase brought about by elastic recoil of the patient's chest and lungs; repeated 12 to 16 times a minute; where the nose is not covered by the operator's mouth, the nostrils must be closed by pinching.

**mouth-to-mouth re·sus·ci·ta·tion** mouth-to-mouth respiration employed as part of emergency cardiopulmonary resuscitation.

**mouth·wash** a medicated liquid used for cleaning the mouth and treating disorders of the oral mucosa.

**mov·a·ble joint** SYN synovial joint.

**mov·a·ble spleen** SYN floating spleen.

**move·ment** (moov'ment) **1.** active change of position or location; said of the entire body or of one or more of its members or parts. **2.** SYN stool. **3.** SYN defecation. [L. *moveo*, pp. *motus*, to move]

**move·ment econ·o·my** SYN exercise economy.

**move·ment sys·tem 1.** a physiologic system that functions to produce motion of the whole body or of its component parts. **2.** the functional interaction of structures that contribute to the act of moving.

**Mow·ry col·loi·dal iron stain** a stain used for demonstrating acid mucopolysaccharides.

**MP** mentoposterior position.

**MPD** maximum permissible dose.

**MPI** master patient index.

**MRD, mrd** minimal reacting dose.

**MRF** melanotropin-releasing factor.

**MRH** melanotropin-releasing hormone.

**MRI** magnetic resonance imaging. See page B11.

**mRNA** messenger RNA. See entries under ribonucleic acid.

**MS** multiple sclerosis; morphine sulfate; mitral stenosis.

**ms** millisecond.

**msec** millisecond.

**M shell** the lowest energy level at which electron transitions give rise to x-rays.

**MTP** metatarsophalangeal.

**mu** (myu) **1.** twelfth letter of the Greek alphabet (μ). **2.** micro- (2); micron; magnetic or electric dipole moment of a molecule; chemical potential; denotes the position of a substituent located on the 12th atom from the carboxyl or other functional group.

**Much ba·cil·lus** (mook) an alleged non–acid-fast granular form of the tubercle bacillus; not demonstrable by the Ziehl stain, but takes a modified Gram stain; it is said to be the form present in the tuberculous skin lesion.

**mu·ci-** mucous, mucin. SEE ALSO muco-. [L. *mucus*]

**mu·ci·car·mine** (mū-si-kar'mĭn) a red stain containing aluminum chloride and carmine; used to detect epithelial mucins and mucin-secreting adenocarcinomas; also used to demonstrate the capsule of *Cryptococcus neoformans* an dother fungi.

**mu·ci·form** (myu'si-fōrm) resembling mucus. SYN blennoid, mucoid (2).

**mu·ci·he·ma·te·in** (mū-si-hē'mă-tē-in) a violet-blue staining fluid containing aluminum chloride and hematein; used to detect connective tissue mucins.

**mu·ci·lage** (myu'si-lij) a pharmacopeial preparation consisting of a solution in water of the mucilaginous principles of vegetable substances; used as a soothing application to the mucous membranes and in the preparation of official and extemporaneous mixtures. [L. *mucilago*]

**mu·ci·lag·i·nous** (myu-sĭ-laj'ĭ-nŭs) resembling mucilage; i.e., adhesive, viscid, sticky.

**mu·cin** (myu'sin) a secretion containing carbohydrate-rich glycoproteins such as that from the goblet cells of the intestine, the submaxillary glands, and other mucous glandular cells; it is also present in the ground substance of connective tissue.

**mu·cin·ase** (myu'si-nās) any enzyme that hydrolyzes mucopolysaccharide substances (mucins). SYN mucopolysaccharidase.

**mu·cin·o·gen** (myu'sin-ō-jen) a glycoprotein that forms mucin through the imbibition of water. [mucin + G. *-gen,* producing]

**mu·ci·noid** (myu'si-noyd) **1.** SYN mucoid (1). **2.** resembling mucin.

**mu·ci·no·sis** (myu-si-nō'sis) a condition in which mucin is present in the skin in excessive amounts, or in abnormal distribution. Classified as metabolic mucinosis, secondary mucinosis, and localized mucinosis. [mucin + G. *-osis,* condition]

**mu·ci·nous** (myu'si-nŭs) relating to or containing mucin. SYN mucoid (3).

**mu·ci·nous car·ci·no·ma** a variety of adenocarcinoma in which the neoplastic cells secrete conspicuous quantities of mucin; the neoplasms are glistening, sticky, and gelatinoid in consistency. SYN colloid carcinoma.

⚠**mu·co-** mucous, mucous (mucous membrane). SEE ALSO muci-. [L. *mucus*]

**mu·co·cele** (myu'kō-sēl) a retention cyst of the salivary gland, lacrimal sac, paranasal sinuses, appendix, or gallbladder. Most common site is the lower lip lateral to the midline. [muco- + G. *kēlē,* tumor, hernia]

**mu·co·cil·i·ary** (myu-kō-sĭl'ē-ār-e) pertaining to ciliated columnar epithelium found in the bronchial tree to the level of the terminal bronchioles, and in the uterine tubes. SEE ciliary.

**mu·co·cil·i·ary clear·ance** the movement of the mucous covering of the respiratory epithelium by the beating of cilia: rapid, forward (effective) stroke and slow, return (recovery) stroke.

**mu·co·cil·i·ary clear·ance rate** velocity of movement of the mucus blanket over respiratory epithelium, usually expressed in mm/hr.

**mu·co·cil·i·ary trans·port** movement of mucus and mucoid fluid through the bronchial tree by the action of cilia.

**mu·co·cu·ta·ne·ous** (myu-kō-kyu-tā'nē-ŭs) relating to mucous membrane and skin; denoting the line of junction of the two at the nasal, oral, vaginal, and anal orifices.

**mu·co·cu·ta·ne·ous junc·tion** the site of transition from epidermis to the epithelium of a mucous membrane.

**mu·co·cu·ta·ne·ous leish·man·i·a·sis** a grave disease caused by *Leishmania braziliensis braziliensis,* endemic in Mexico and Central and South America. The organism does not invade the viscera, and the disease is limited to the skin and mucous membranes, the lesions resembling the sores of cutaneous leishmaniasis. The sores heal after a time, but some months or years later, fungating and eroding forms of ulceration may appear on the tongue and buccal or nasal mucosa. SEE ALSO espundia. SYN American leishmaniasis, nasopharyngeal leishmaniasis, New World leishmaniasis.

**mu·co·cu·ta·ne·ous lymph node syn·drome** SYN Kawasaki syndrome.

**mu·co·en·ter·i·tis** (myu'kō-en-ter-i'tis) **1.** inflammation of the intestinal mucous membrane. **2.** SYN mucomembranous enteritis.

**mu·co·ep·i·der·moid** (myu'kō-ep-i-der'moyd) denoting a mixture of mucus-secreting and epithelial cells, as in mucoepidermoid carcinoma.

**mu·coid** (myu'koyd) **1.** general term for a mucin, mucoprotein, or glycoprotein. SYN mucinoid (1). **2.** SYN muciform. **3.** SYN mucinous. [mucus + G. *eidos,* appearance]

**mu·coid de·gen·er·a·tion** a conversion of any of the connective tissues into a gelatinous or mucoid substance. SYN myxomatosis (1).

**mu·co·lyt·ic** (myu-kō-lit'ik) capable of dissolving, digesting, or liquefying mucus.

**mu·co·mem·bra·nous** (myu'kō-mem'bră-nŭs) relating to a mucous membrane.

**mu·co·mem·bra·nous en·ter·i·tis** a disorder of the intestinal mucous membrane characterized by constipation or diarrhea (sometimes alternating), colic, and the passage of pseudomembranous shreds or incomplete casts of the intestine. SYN mucoenteritis (2).

**mu·co·per·i·os·te·al** (myu'kō-per-ē-os'tē-ăl) relating to mucoperiosteum.

**mu·co·per·i·os·te·um** (myu'kō-per-ē-os'tē-ŭm) mucous membrane and periosteum so intimately united as to form practically a single membrane, as that covering the hard palate.

**mu·co·pol·y·sac·cha·ri·dase** (myu'kō-pol-ē-sak'ă-ri-dās) SYN mucinase.

**mu·co·pol·y·sac·cha·ride** (myu'kō-pol-ē-sak'ă-rīd) general term for a protein-polysaccharide complex obtained from proteoglycans and containing as much as 95% polysaccharide; mucopolysaccharides include the blood group substances. A more modern term is glycosaminoglycan.

**mu·co·pol·y·sac·cha·ri·do·sis,** pl. **mu·co·pol·y·sac·cha·ri·do·ses** (myu'kō-pol-ē-sak'ă-ri-dō'sis, myu'kō-pol-ē-sak'ă-rīd-ō-sēz) any of a group of lysosomal storage diseases that have in common a disorder in metabolism of mucopolysaccharides, as evidenced by excretion of various mucopolysaccharides in urine and infiltration of these substances into connective tissue, with resulting various defects of bone, cartilage, connective tissue, and other organs.

**mu·co·pol·y·sac·cha·ri·du·ria** (myu'kō-pol-ē-sak'ă-ri-dyu're-ă) the excretion of mucopolysaccharides in the urine.

**mu·co·pro·tein** (myu-kō-prō'tēn) general term for a protein-polysaccharide complex, usually implying that the protein component is the major part of the complex. Mucoproteins include the $\alpha_1$- and $\alpha_2$-globulins of serum.

**mu·co·pu·ru·lent** (myu-kō-pyur'ŭ-lent) pertaining to an exudate that is chiefly purulent (pus), but containing relatively conspicuous proportions of mucous material.

*Mu·cor* (myu'kōr) a genus of fungi (class Zygomycetes, family Mucoraceae), most species of

m
u

which are saprobic; several are pathogenic and may cause zygomycosis in humans.

**Mu·cor·al·es** (myu-kor-al′ez) an order of the fungal class Zygomycetes that contains all the species causing mucormycosis in humans. The genera include *Cunninghamella, Rhizopus, Absidia, Rhizomucor, Mucor, Apophysomyces, Saksenaea, Syncephalastrum,* and *Cokeromyces. Mortierella* species are included but are of doubtful pathogenicity for humans.

**mu·cor·my·co·sis** (myu′kōr-mī-kō′sis) SYN zygomycosis.

**mu·co·sa** (myu-kō′să) a mucous tissue lining various tubular structures, consisting of epithelium, lamina propria, and, in the digestive tract, a layer of smooth muscle. [L. fem. of *mucosus,* mucous]

**mu·co·sa-as·so·ci·at·ed lym·phoid tis·sue (MALT)** a class of lymphoid tissue comprising nodular aggregates found in association with the wet mucosal surfaces of the body such as those of the respiratory, digestive, and urinary systems.

**mu·co·sal** (myu-kō′săl) relating to the mucosa or mucous membrane.

**mu·co·sal wave** the movement of the mucous membrane of the vocal cord during phonation.

**mu·co·san·guin·e·ous, mu·co·san·guin·o·lent** (myu′kō-sang-gwin′ē-ŭs, myu′kō-sang-gwin′ō-lent) pertaining to an exudate or other fluid material that has a relatively high content of blood and mucus. [muco- + L. *sanguis,* blood]

**mu·co·sec·to·my** (myu-kō-sek′tō-me) excision of the mucosa, usually of the rectum prior to ileoanal anastomosis for treatment of ulcerative colitis. [mucosa + G. *ektomē,* excision]

**mu·co·se·rous** (myu-kō-sē′rŭs) pertaining to an exudate or secretion that consists of both mucus and serum or a watery component.

**mu·co·se·rous cells** glandular cells intermediate in histologic characteristics between serous and mucous cells

**mu·cous** (myu′kŭs) relating to mucus or a mucous membrane. [L. *mucosus,* mucous, fr. *mucus*]

**mu·cous cell** a cell secreting mucus; e.g., a goblet cell.

**mu·cous co·li·tis** an affection of the mucous membrane of the colon characterized by colicky pain, constipation or diarrhea (sometimes alternating), and passage of mucous or slimy pseudomembranous shreds and patches. SYN myxomembranous colitis.

**mu·cous con·nec·tive tis·sue** a type of connective tissue little differentiated beyond the mesenchymal stage; its ground substance of glycoproteins is abundant and contains fine collagenous fibers and fibroblasts; in its most characteristic form, it appears in the umbilical cord as Wharton jelly.

**mu·cous cyst** a retention cyst resulting from obstruction in the duct of a mucous gland.

**mu·cous gland** a gland that secretes mucus.

**mu·cous glands of au·di·to·ry tube** glands located principally near the pharyngeal end of the auditory tube.

**mu·cous plug** a mass of mucus and cells filling the cervical canal between periods or during pregnancy; a mass of mucous occluding a main or lobar bronchus.

**mu·cus** (myu′kŭs) the clear viscid secretion of the mucous membranes, consisting of mucin, epithe-

lial cells, leukocytes, and various inorganic salts suspended in water. [L.]

**mu·cus blan·ket** the mucous covering of respiratory epithelium.

**mud fe·ver** a leptospirosis caused by the *grippotyphosa* serovar of *Leptospira interrogans.*

**Muehr·cke line** (myūr′kē) a white line of the nail; lines occur serially, parallel with the lunula and separated from each other by normal pink areas; associated with hypoalbuminemia; the lines do not move outward with nail growth, but disappear when the serum albumin returns to normal.

**Muel·ler e·lec·tron·ic to·nom·e·ter** (myu-ler) a Schiötz type tonometer that electronically indicates the extent of corneal indentation; may also have an attached recorder for continuous pressure readings (tonography).

**Muel·ler-Hin·ton me·di·um** (myu′ler-hĭn′ton) an agar-based medium composed of beef infusion, casamino acids, and starch useful in the isolation of gonococci and meningococci; the recommended medium for antibacterial susceptibility tests for most common aerobic and facultatively anaerobic bacteria.

**MUGA** multiple-gated acquisition scan.

**mul·ber·ry mo·lar** a malformed molar with a crown resembling a mulberry, with hypoplasia, crenellations, and short cusps. It may be a manifestation of congenital syphilis but also occurs in other conditions.

**Mules op·er·a·tion** (myulz) evisceration of the eyeball followed by the insertion within the sclera of a spherical prosthesis to support an artificial eye.

**mule-spin·ner's can·cer** carcinoma of the scrotum or adjacent skin exposed to oil, observed in some workers in cotton-spinning mills.

**mu·li·e·bria** (moo′lē-ē′brē-ă) the female genital organs. [L. neut pl. of *muliebris,* relating to *mulier,* a woman]

**Mül·ler duct, mül·le·ri·an duct** (myu-ler) SYN paramesonephric duct.

**Mül·ler fix·a·tive** (myu-ler) a hardening fixative composed of potassium dichromate, sodium sulfate, and distilled water, similar to Regaud fixative.

**mül·le·ri·an in·hib·i·ting sub·stance** (myu-lā′rē-an) a 535-amino acid glycoprotein secreted by the Sertoli cells of the testis. It is related to inhibin.

**Mül·ler law** (myu-ler) each type of sensory nerve ending, however stimulated (electrically, mechanically), gives rise to its own specific sensation; moreover, each type of sensation depends not upon any special character of the different nerves but upon the part of the brain in which their fibers terminate.

**Mül·ler ma·neu·ver** (myu-ler) after a forced expiration, an attempt at inspiration is made with closed mouth and nose or closed glottis, whereby the negative pressure in the chest and lungs is made very subatmospheric; the reverse of Valsalva maneuver.

**Mül·ler sign** (myu-ler) in aortic insufficiency, rhythmical pulsatory movements of the uvula, synchronous with cardiac contractions; accompanied by swelling and redness of the velum palati and tonsils.

**Mül·ler tu·ber·cle** (myu-ler) a median protuberance projecting into the embryonic urogenital sinus from its dorsal wall; it is formed from the fused caudal ends of the paramesonephric ducts and is the first evidence of the embryonic uterus and vagina.

**mult·ang·u·lar bone** SEE trapezium, trapezoid bone.

⚠**mul·ti-** Many. SEE ALSO pluri-. Cf. poly-. [L. *multus,* much]

**mul·ti·ar·tic·u·lar** (mŭl'tē-ar-tik'yu-lăr) relating to or involving many joints. SYN polyarthric, polyarticular. [multi- + L. *articulus,* joint]

**mul·ti·ax·i·al joint** one in which movement occurs in a number of axes. SEE ball-and-socket joint. SYN polyaxial joint.

**mul·ti·col·o·ny-stim·u·lat·ing fac·tor** SYN interleukin-3.

**mul·ti·cus·pi·date** (mŭl-tē-kŭs'pi-dāt) **1.** having more than two cusps. **2.** a molar tooth with three or more cusps or projections on the crown.

**mul·ti·fac·to·ri·al in·her·i·tance** inheritance involving many factors, of which at least one is genetic but none is of overwhelming importance, as in the causation of a disease by multiple genetic and environmental factors.

**mul·ti·fid** (mŭl'tē-fid) divided into many clefts or segments. [L. *multifidus,* fr. *multus,* much, + *findo,* to cleave]

**mul·tif·i·dus mus·cle** *origin,* from the sacrum, sacroiliac ligament, mamillary processes of the lumbar vertebrae, transverse processes of thoracic vertebrae, and articular processes of last four cervical vertebrae; *insertion,* into the spinous processes of all the vertebrae up to and including the axis; *action,* rotates vertebral column; *nerve supply,* dorsal primary rami of spinal nerves. SYN musculus multifidus lumborum [TA], musculus multifidus [TA].

**mul·ti·fo·cal** (mŭl-tē-fō'kăl) relating to or arising from many foci.

**mul·ti·fo·cal atri·al tach·y·car·dia (MAT)** SYN atrial chaotic tachycardia.

**mul·ti·fo·cal lens** a lens with segments providing two or more powers; commonly, a trifocal lens.

**mul·ti·form** (mŭl'ti-fōrm) SYN polymorphic.

**mul·ti·for·mat cam·era** photographic or laser printer for recording a variable number of video images on a sheet of film, as in computed tomography or ultrasound.

**mul·ti·form lay·er of cerebral cortex** the innermost layer of the cerebral cortex, layer XI. SYN lamina multiformis [TA].

**mul·ti·grav·i·da** (mŭl-tē-grav'i-dă) a pregnant woman who has been pregnant one or more times previously. [multi- + L. *gravida,* pregnant]

**mul·ti·in·fec·tion** (mŭl'tē-in-fek'shŭn) mixed infection with two or more varieties of microorganisms developing simultaneously.

**mul·ti·lam·el·lar bo·dy** SYN cytosome (2).

**mul·ti·lo·bar, mul·ti·lo·bate, mul·ti·lobed** (mŭl-tē-lō'bar, mŭl-tē-lō'bāt, mŭl-tē-lōbd') having several lobes.

**mul·ti·lob·u·lar** (mŭl-tē-lob'yu-lăr) having many lobules.

**mul·ti·lo·cal** (mŭl-tē-lō'kăl) denoting traits with an etiology comprising effects of multiple genetic loci operating together and simultaneously.

**mul·ti·loc·u·lar** (mŭl-tē-lok'yu-lăr) many-celled; having many compartments or loculi.

**mul·ti·loc·u·lar cyst** a cyst containing several compartments formed by membranous septa.

**mul·ti·nod·u·lar, mul·ti·nod·u·late** (mŭl-tē-

nod'yu-lăr, mŭl-tē-nod'yu-lāt) having many nodules.

**mul·ti·nod·u·lar goi·ter** adenomatous goiter with several colloid nodules.

**mul·ti·nu·cle·ar, mul·ti·nu·cle·ate** (mŭl-tē-noo'klē-ăr, mŭl-tē-noo'klē-āt) having two or more nuclei. SYN polynuclear, polynucleate.

**mul·tip·a·ra** (mŭl-tip'ă-ră) a woman who has given birth at least two times to an infant, liveborn or not, weighing 500 g or more, or having an estimated length of gestation of at least 20 weeks. [multi- + L. *pario,* to bring forth, to bear]

**mul·ti·par·i·ty** (mŭl-tē-par'i-tē) condition of being a multipara.

**mul·tip·a·rous** (mŭl-tip'ă-rŭs) relating to a multipara.

**mul·ti·ple ego states** various psychological organizational states reflecting different personas or life experiences.

**mul·ti·ple en·do·crine de·fi·cien·cy syn·drome** acquired deficiency of the function of several endocrine glands, usually on an autoimmune basis.

**mul·ti·ple en·do·crine ne·o·pla·sia (MEN)** a group of disorders characterized by functioning tumors in more than one endocrine gland.

**mul·ti·ple en·do·crine ne·o·pla·sia 1 (MEN1)** syndrome characterized by tumors of the pituitary gland, pancreatic islet cells, and parathyroid glands and may be associated with Zollinger-Ellison syndrome; autosomal dominant inheritance, caused by mutation in the MEN1 gene on chromosome 11q. SYN Wermer syndrome.

**mul·ti·ple en·do·crine ne·o·pla·sia 2** syndrome associated with pheochromocytoma, parathyroid adenoma and medullary thyroid carcinoma; autosomal dominant inheritance, caused by mutation in the RET oncogene on chromosome 10q.

**mul·ti·ple en·do·crine ne·o·pla·sia 3** syndrome characterized by tumors found in MEN2, tall, thin habitus, prominent lips, and neuromas of the tongue and eyelids; autosomal dominant inheritance, caused by mutation in the RET oncogene on 10q. SYN multiple endocrine neoplasia 2B.

**mul·ti·ple en·do·crine ne·o·pla·sia 2B** SYN multiple endocrine neoplasia 3.

**mul·ti·ple ep·i·phys·i·al dys·pla·si·a (EDM)** a dominantly inherited abnormality of epiphyses characterized by difficulty in walking, pain and stiffness of joints, stubby fingers, and often dwarfism of short-limb type; on x-ray examination, the epiphyses are mottled and irregular; ossification centers are late in appearance and may be multiple, but the vertebrae are normal. There is also an autosomal recessive form. SYN dysplasia epiphysealis multiplex.

**mul·ti·ple fis·sion** division of the nucleus into a number of daughter nuclei, followed by division of the cell body into an equal number of daughter cells, each containing a nucleus.

**mul·ti·ple frac·ture 1.** fracture at two or more places in a bone; **2.** fracture of several bones occurring simultaneously.

**mul·ti·ple-ga·ted ac·qui·si·tion scan (MUGA)** a nuclear medicine cardiac blood pool study collected by multiple-gated acquisition; used for ejection fraction and wall motion assessment. SEE ALSO radionuclide ejection fraction.

**mul·ti·ple in·tes·ti·nal pol·yp·o·sis 1.** begins

m
u

usually in late childhood; polyps increase in numbers, causing symptoms of chronic colitis, and carcinoma of the colon almost invariably develops in untreated cases; autosomal dominant inheritance. In the Gardner syndrome there are extracolonic changes (desmoid tumors, etc.); **2.** hamartomatous polyposis of the small or large intestine, Peutz-Jeghers syndrome with melanin spots on the lips, less common; **3.** miscellaneous, rare, and doubtful occurrences.

**mul·ti·ple mark·er screen** use of two or more markers in the maternal serum to determine the relative risk of an abnormal fetus. SEE ALSO triple screen.

**mul·ti·ple mu·co·sal neu·ro·ma syn·drome** multiple submucosal neuromas or neurofibromas of the tongue, lips, and eyelids in young persons; sometimes associated with tumors of the thyroid or adrenal medulla, or with subcutaneous neurofibromatosis.

**mul·ti·ple my·e·lo·ma, my·e·lo·ma mul·ti·plex** an uncommon disease that occurs more frequently in men and is associated with anemia, hemorrhage, recurrent infections, and weakness. A malignant neoplasm that originates in bone marrow and involves chiefly the skeleton; characterized by numerous diffuse foci or nodular accumulations of abnormal or malignant plasma cells in the marrow of various bones and abnormal proteins in the serum and urine; the most frequent abnormalities in the metabolism of protein are Bence Jones proteinuria, an increase in monoclonal γ-globulin in the plasma, the formation of cryoglobulin, and a form of primary amyloidosis. SEE ALSO plasma cell myeloma. SYN plasma cell myeloma (1).

**mul·ti·ple my·o·si·tis** the occurrence of multiple foci of acute inflammation in the muscular tissue and overlying skin in various parts of the body, accompanied by fever and other signs of systemic infection. SEE ALSO dermatomyositis.

**mul·ti·ple neu·ri·tis** SYN polyneuropathy.

**mul·ti·ple per·son·al·i·ty** a dissociative disorder in which two or more distinct conscious personalities alternately prevail in the same person, without any personality being aware of the others.

**mul·ti·ple preg·nan·cy** condition of bearing two or more fetuses simultaneously. SYN polycyesis.

**mul·ti·ple punc·ture tu·ber·cu·lin test** a kind of tine test SEE tuberculin test.

**mul·ti·ple scle·ro·sis (MS)** common demyelinating disorder of the central nervous system, causing patches of sclerosis (plaques) in the brain and spinal cord; occurs primarily in young adults; clinical manifestations depend upon the location and size of the plaques; typical symptoms include visual loss, diplopia, nystagmus, dysarthria, weakness, paresthesias, bladder abnormalities, and mood alterations; characteristically, the symptoms show exacerbations and remissions. See page B11.

**mul·ti·ple stain** a mixture of several dyes each having an independent selective action on one or more portions of the tissue.

**mul·ti·ple sys·tem atro·phy** nonhereditary, neurodegenerative disease of unknown cause, characterized clinically by the development of parkinsonism, ataxia, autonomic failure, or pyramidal tract signs, in various combinations. Pathologically there are nerve cell loss, gliosis,

and the accumulation of abnormal tubular structures in the cytoplasm and nucleus of oligodendrocytes and neurons in the basal ganglion, cerebellum, and intermediolateral columns of the spinal cord; can present as predominantly parkinsonism, as predominantly ataxia, or as a combination of parkinsonism, ataxia, and autonomic failure; it is a relatively rapidly progressive and fatal disorder.

**mul·ti·ple vi·sion** SYN polyopia.

**mul·ti·pli·ca·tive di·vi·sion** reproduction by simultaneous division of a mother cell into a number of daughter cells. If the process occurs without fertilization of the mother cell, or encystment, the daughter cells are called merozoites; if they develop within a cyst, and usually after fertilization, they are called sporozoites.

**mul·ti·po·lar** (mŭl-tē-pō′lăr) having more than two poles; denoting a nerve cell in which the branches project from several points.

**mul·ti·po·lar cell** a nerve cell with a number of dendrites arising from the cell body.

**mul·ti·po·lar neu·ron** a neuron with several processes, usually an axon and three or more dendrites.

**mul·ti·sy·nap·tic** (mŭl′tē-si-nap′tik) SYN polysynaptic.

**mul·ti·va·lence, mul·ti·va·len·cy** (mŭl-tē-vā′lens, mŭl-tē-vā′len-sē) the state of being multivalent.

**mul·ti·va·lent** (mŭl-tē-vā′lent) **1.** CHEMISTRY having a combining power (valence) of more than one hydrogen atom. **2.** efficacious in more than one direction. **3.** an antisera specific for more than one antigen or organism. SYN polyvalent (1).

**mul·ti·va·lent vac·cine** SYN polyvalent vaccine.

**mum·mi·fi·ca·tion** (mŭm′i-fi-kā′shŭn) **1.** SYN dry gangrene. **2.** shrivelling of a dead, retained fetus. **3.** DENTISTRY treatment of inflamed dental pulp with fixative drugs (usually formaldehyde derivatives) in order to retain teeth so treated for relatively short periods; generally acceptable only for deciduous teeth. [mummy + L. *facio*, to make]

**mumps** (mŭmps) SYN epidemic parotiditis. [dialectic Eng. *mump*, a lump or bump]

**mumps skin test an·ti·gen** a suspension of killed mumps virus used to determine susceptibility to mumps or to confirm previous exposure.

**mumps vi·rus** a virus of the genus *Paramyxovirus* causing parotitis, sometimes with complications of orchitis, oophoritis, pancreatitis, meningoencephalitis and others, and transmitted by infectious salivary secretions. SYN epidemic parotitis virus.

**Mun·ro mi·cro·ab·scess** (mĕn-rō′) a microscopic collection of polymorphonuclear leukocytes found in the stratum corneum in psoriasis.

**Mun·ro point** (mĕn-rō′) a point at the right edge of the rectus abdominis muscle, between the umbilicus and the anterior superior spine of the ilium, where pressure elicits tenderness in appendicitis.

**Mun·son sign** (mŭn′son) in keratoconus, the extra bowing of the lower eyelid caused by the misshapen cornea as the eye rotates downward.

**mu·ral** (myu′răl) relating to the wall of any cavity. [L. *muralis*; fr. *murus*, wall]

**mu·ral en·do·car·di·tis** inflammation of the endocardium involving the walls of the chambers of the heart.

**mu·ral throm·bo·sis** the formation of a thrombus in contact with the endocardial lining of a cardiac chamber, or a large blood vessel, if not occlusive.

**mu·ral throm·bus** a thrombus formed on and attached to a diseased patch of endocardium, not on a valve or on one side of a large blood vessel. SEE ALSO parietal thrombus.

**mu·ram·i·dase** (myu-ram′i-dās) SYN lysozyme.

**mu·rine** (myu′rīn) relating to animals of the family Muridae. [L. *murinus,* relating to mice, fr. *mus* (*mur-*), a mouse]

**mu·rine ty·phus** a milder form of epidemic typhus caused by *Rickettsia typhi* and transmitted to humans by rat or mouse fleas. SYN endemic typhus.

**mur·mur** (mer′mer) an abnormal, usually periodic sound heard on auscultation of the heart or blood vessels. [L.]

**Mur·phy but·ton** (mer′fē) a device used for intestinal anastomosis; it consists of two round, hollow cylinders that insert into each end of the transected intestine; the intestine is secured to each of the components with a suture and the ends are brought into approximation and the two cylinders joined with a locking mechanism; the apparatus is degradable and within approximately 10 days dissolves and is sloughed into the lumen of the intestine. A modification of an obsolete metal device bearing the same name.

**Mur·phy drip** (mer′fē) SYN proctoclysis.

**Mur·phy per·cus·sion** (mer′fē) examination for dullness by striking the chest wall directly with the fingertips of one hand successively, beginning with the fifth finger.

**Mur·phy sign** (mer′fē) pain on palpation of the right subcostal area during inspiration frequently associated with acute cholecystitis.

**Mur·ray Val·ley en·ceph·a·li·tis** (mer′ē val′ē) a severe encephalitis with a high mortality rate occurring in the Murray Valley of Australia; the disease is most severe in children and is characterized by headache, fever, malaise, drowsiness or convulsions, and rigidity of the neck; extensive brain damage may result; it is caused by the Murray Valley encephalitis virus (genus *Flavivirus*). SYN Australian X disease.

*Mus·ca* (mŭs′kă) a genus of flies that includes the common housefly, *Musca domestica;* it breeds in filth and organic waste, and is involved in the mechanical transfer of numerous pathogens. [L. fly]

**mus·cae vol·i·tan·tes** (mŭs′sē vol-i-tan′tēs, mŭs′kē vol-i-tan′tēs) floaters; appearance of moving spots before the eyes, arising from remnants of the embryologic hyaloid vascular system in the vitreous humor. [L. pl. of *musca,* fly; pres. ppl. of *volito,* to fly to and fro]

**mus·ca·rine** (mŭs′kă-rēn, mŭs′kă-rin) a toxin with neurologic effects, first isolated from *Amanita muscaria* (fly agaric) and also present in some species of *Hebeloma* and *Inocybe*. It is a cholinergic substance whose pharmacologic effects include cardiac inhibition, vasodilation, salivation, lacrimation, bronchoconstriction, and gastrointestinal stimulation.

**mus·ca·rin·ic** (mŭs-kă-rin′ik) **1.** having a muscarine-like action, i.e., producing effects that resemble postganglionic parasympathetic stimulation. **2.** an agent that stimulates the postganglionic parasympathetic receptor. SEE ALSO muscarine, nicotinic.

**mus·cle** (mŭs′ĕl) a primary tissue, consisting predominantly of highly specialized contractile cells, which may be classified as skeletal muscle, cardiac muscle, or smooth muscle; microscopically, the latter is lacking in transverse striations characteristic of the other two types; one of the contractile organs of the body by which movements of the various organs and parts are effected; typical musculus is a mass of musculus fibers (venter or belly), attached at each extremity, by means of a tendon, to a bone or other structure; the more proximal or more fixed attachment is called the *origin,* the more distal or more movable attachment is the *insertion;* the narrowing part of the belly that is attached to the tendon of origin is called the caput or head. For gross anatomic description, see musculus. SYN musculus. [L. *musculus*]

**mus·cle-bound** (mŭs′ĕl-bownd) denoting a condition in which individual muscles are overdeveloped but dyssynergic in concerted action.

**mus·cle con·trac·tion heada·che** SYN tension headache.

**mus·cle en·er·gy tech·nique** a massage therapy modality that works to adjust proprioceptive activity and levels of resting tension through stretches and muscle contraction with resistance. SEE ALSO proprioceptive neuromuscular facilitation. SYN strain-counterstrain.

**mus·cle fi·ber** classification of muscle fiber based on contractile and metabolic characteristics. Slow-twitch (type I) fibers contract slowly and develop relatively low tension; they display high oxidative and low glycolytic capacity associated with endurance performance. Fast-twitch (type II) fibers have rapid speed of activation and develop high tension; they display low oxidative and high glycolytic capacity associated with strength and power performance. See page 642.

**mus·cle of heart** SYN cardiac muscle.

**mus·cle he·mo·glo·bin** SYN myoglobin.

**mus·cle plate** SYN myotome (2).

**mus·cles of au·di·to·ry os·si·cles** the musculus stapedius and musculus tensor tympani.

**mus·cle se·rum** the fluid remaining after the coagulation of muscle plasma and the separation of myosin.

**mus·cles of head** the muscles of expression, of mastication, and the suboccipital muscles in general.

**mus·cles of lar·ynx** the intrinsic muscles that regulate the length, position and tension of the vocal cords and adjust the size of the openings between the aryepiglottic folds, the ventricular folds, and the vocal folds. SYN musculi laryngis [TA].

**mus·cle-spar·ing thor·a·cot·omy** any type of thoracotomy that does not involve significant division of the latissimus dorsi muscle and the serratus anterior muscle.

**mus·cle spasm** SYN spasm.

**mus·cle tone 1.** the internal state of muscle-fiber tension within individual muscles and muscle groups. **2.** degree of muscle tension or resistance during rest or in response to stretching.

**mus·cle of tra·gus** SYN tragicus muscle.

**mus·cle of uvu·la** SYN uvular muscle.

**mus·cu·lar** (mŭs′kyu-lăr) **1.** relating to a muscle

or the muscles. **2.** having well-developed musculature.

**mus·cu·lar as·the·no·pia** asthenopia due to imbalance of the extrinsic ocular muscles.

**mus·cu·lar at·ro·phy** wasting of muscular tissue.

**mus·cu·lar coat** the muscular, usually middle,
layer of a tubular structure; for most of the gastrointestinal tract, it consists of an outer longitudinal layer of muscle and an inner circular layer.

**mus·cu·lar dys·tro·phy** a general term for a
number of hereditary, progressive degenerative
disorders affecting skeletal muscles, and often
other organ systems as well. SYN myodystrophy,
myodystrophia.

**mus·cu·lar en·du·rance** ability of muscles to
exert tension over an extended period.

**mus·cu·la·ris** (mŭs-kyu-lā′ris) the muscular coat
of a hollow organ or tubular structure. [Mod. L.
muscular]

**mus·cu·la·ris mu·co·sae** the thin layer of
smooth muscle found in most parts of the digestive tube located outside the lamina propria mucosae and adjacent to the tela submucosa.

**mus·cu·lar·i·ty** (mŭs′kyu-lar′i-tē) the state or
condition of having well developed muscles.

**mus·cu·lar pow·er** ability of muscles to produce
force at a given time.

**mus·cu·lar re·lax·ant** an agent that relaxes striated muscle; includes drugs acting at the brain
and/or spinal cord level or directly on muscle.

**mus·cu·lar sense** SYN myesthesia.

**mus·cu·lar tis·sue** a tissue characterized by the
ability to contract upon stimulation; its three varieties are skeletal, cardiac, and smooth. SEE muscle. SYN flesh (2).

**mus·cu·lar tri·an·gle** the triangle bounded by
the sternocleidomastoid muscle, the superior
belly of the omohyoid muscle, and the anterior
midline of the neck; the infrahyoid muscles occupy most of it. SYN trigonum musculare [TA].

**mus·cu·la·ture** (mŭs′kyu-lă-cher) the arrangement of the muscles in a part or in the body as a
whole.

**mus·cu·li ar·rec·to·res pi·lo·rum** [TA] SYN arrector muscle of hair.

**mus·cu·li in·ter·spi·na·les** [TA] SYN interspinales muscles.

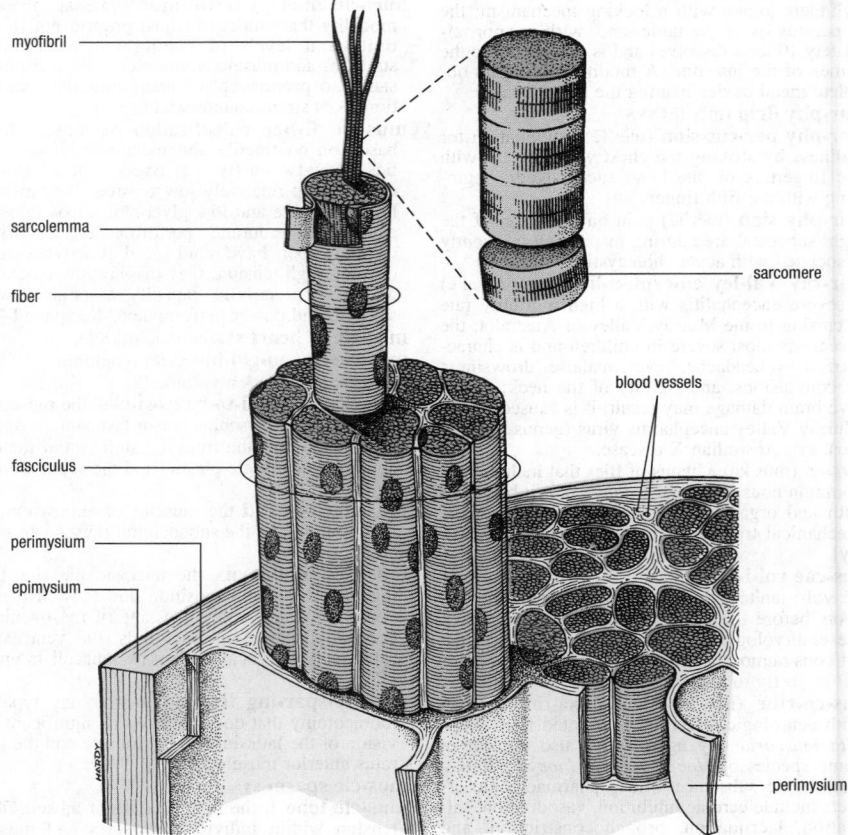

myofibril

sarcolemma

fiber

sarcomere

blood vessels

fasciculus

perimysium

epimysium

perimysium

**skeletal muscle:** diagram of the connective tissue components; the relationships between a muscle bundle
(fasciculus), a single muscle cell (fiber), and a myofibril also are indicated

**mus•cu•li in•ter•trans•ver•sa•rii** [TA] SYN intertransversarii muscles.

**mus•cu•li la•ryn•gis** [TA] SYN muscles of larynx.

**mus•cu•li pec•ti•na•ti** [TA] SYN pectinate muscles.

**mus•cu•li ro•ta•to•res** [TA] SYN rotatores muscles.

**mus•cu•lo•ap•o•neu•rot•ic** (mŭs′kyu-lō-ap′ō-noo-rot′ik) relating to muscular tissue and an aponeurosis of origin or insertion.

**mus•cu•lo•cu•ta•ne•ous** (mŭs′kyu-lō-kyu-tā′nē-ŭs) relating to both muscle and skin. SYN myocutaneous.

**mus•cu•lo•cu•ta•ne•ous nerve** arises from lateral cord of the brachial plexus, passes through the coracobrachialis muscle, and then downward between the brachialis and biceps, supplying these three muscles and being prolonged as the lateral cutaneous nerve of the forearm. SYN nervus musculocutaneus [TA].

**mus•cu•lo•mem•bra•nous** (mŭs′kyu-lō-mem′bră-nŭs) relating to both muscular tissue and membrane; denoting certain muscles, such as the occipitofrontalis, that are largely membranous.

**mus•cu•lo•phren•ic ar•tery** *origin*, the lateral terminal branch of internal thoracic; *distribution*, diaphragm and intercostal muscles; *anastomoses*, branches of pericardiacophrenic, inferior phrenic, and posterior intercostal arteries. SYN arteria musculophrenica [TA].

**mus•cu•lo•phren•ic veins** accompany the musculophrenic artery and drain blood from the upper abdominal wall and anterior portions of the lower intercostal spaces and the diaphragm.

**mus•cu•lo•skel•e•tal** (mŭs′kyu-lō-skel′ĕ-tăl) relating to muscles and to the skeleton, as, for example, the musculoskeletal system.

**mus•cu•lo•spi•ral pa•ral•y•sis** paralysis of the muscles of the forearm due to injury of the radial (musculospiral) nerve.

**mus•cu•lo•ten•di•nous** (mŭs′kyu-lō-ten′di-nŭs) relating to both muscular and tendinous tissues.

**mus•cu•lo•tro•pic** (mŭs′kyu-lō-trop′ik) affecting, acting upon, or attracted to muscular tissue.

**mus•cu•lo•tu•bal ca•nal** a canal beginning at the anterior border of the petrous portion of the temporal bone near its junction with the squamous portion, and passing to the tympanic cavity; it is divided by the cochleariform process into two semicanals: one for the auditory (eustachian) tube, the other for the tensor tympani muscle. SYN canalis musculotubarius [TA].

**mus•cu•lus**, gen. and pl. **mus•cu•li** (mŭs′kyu-lŭs, mŭs′-kyu-lī) muscle. For histologic description, see muscle. [L. a little mouse, a muscle, fr. *mus* (*mur*-), a mouse]

**mus•cu•lus ab•duc•tor hal•lu•cis** [TA] SYN abductor hallucis muscle.

**mus•cu•lus ad•duc•tor bre•vis** [TA] SYN adductor brevis muscle.

**mus•cu•lus ad•duc•tor hal•lu•cis** [TA] SYN adductor hallucis muscle.

**mus•cu•lus ad•duc•tor lon•gus** [TA] SYN adductor longus muscle.

**mus•cu•lus ad•duc•tor mag•nus** [TA] SYN adductor magnus muscle.

**mus•cu•lus ad•duc•tor pol•li•cis** [TA] SYN adductor pollicis muscle.

**mus•cu•lus an•co•ne•us** [TA] SYN anconeus muscle.

**mus•cu•lus an•ti•trag•i•cus** [TA] SYN antitragicus muscle.

**mus•cu•lus ar•ti•cu•la•ris cu•bi•ti** [TA] SYN articularis cubiti muscle.

**mus•cu•lus ar•ti•cu•la•ris ge•nus** [TA] SYN articularis genus muscle.

**mus•cu•lus ar•y•ep•i•glot•ti•cus** [TA] SYN aryepiglottic muscle.

**mus•cu•lus at•tol•lens au•rem, mus•cu•lus at•tol•lens au•ric•u•lam** SYN superior auricular muscle.

**mus•cu•lus at•tra•hens au•rem, mus•cu•lus at•tra•hens au•ric•u•lam** SYN anterior auricular muscle.

**mus•cu•lus bi•ceps bra•chii** [TA] SYN biceps brachii muscle.

**mus•cu•lus bi•ceps fem•o•ris** [TA] SYN biceps femoris muscle.

**mus•cu•lus bra•chi•a•lis** [TA] SYN brachialis muscle.

**mus•cu•lus bra•chi•o•ra•di•a•lis** [TA] SYN brachioradialis muscle.

**mus•cu•lus buc•ci•na•tor** [TA] SYN buccinator muscle.

**mus•cu•lus cap•i•tis pos•te•ri•or ma•jor** [TA] SYN rectus capitis posterior major muscle.

**mus•cu•lus cer•a•to•cri•coi•de•us** [TA] SYN ceratocricoid muscle.

**mus•cu•lus cil•i•ar•is** [TA] SYN ciliary muscle.

**mus•cu•lus coc•cyg•e•us** [TA] SYN coccygeus muscle.

**mus•cu•lus con•stric•tor phar•yn•gis su•pe•ri•or** [TA] SYN superior constrictor muscle of pharynx.

**mus•cu•lus cor•a•co•bra•chi•a•lis** [TA] SYN coracobrachialis muscle.

**mus•cu•lus cor•ru•ga•tor su•per•ci•lii** [TA] SYN corrugator supercilii muscle.

**mus•cu•lus cre•mas•ter** [TA] SYN cremaster muscle.

**mus•cu•lus cri•co•thy•roi•de•us** [TA] SYN cricothyroid muscle.

**mus•cu•lus del•toi•de•us** [TA] SYN deltoid muscle.

**mus•cu•lus de•pres•sor an•gu•li o•ris** [TA] SYN depressor anguli oris muscle.

**mus•cu•lus de•pres•sor la•bii in•fe•ri•o•ris** [TA] SYN depressor labii inferioris muscle.

**mus•cu•lus de•pres•sor sep•ti** [TA] SYN depressor septi muscle.

**mus•cu•lus de•pres•sor su•per•ci•lii** [TA] SYN depressor supercilii muscle.

**mus•cu•lus di•gas•tri•cus** [TA] SYN digastric muscle (2).

**mus•cu•lus di•la•ta•tor pu•pil•lae** [TA] SYN dilator pupillae muscle.

**mus•cu•lus di•la•ta•tor tu•bae** [TA] SYN dilator tubae muscle.

**mus•cu•lus ep•i•cra•ni•us** [TA] SYN epicranius muscle.

**mus•cu•lus e•rec•tor spi•nae** [TA] SYN erector spinae muscles.

**mus•cu•lus ex•ten•sor car•pi ra•di•a•lis brev•is** [TA] SYN extensor carpi radialis brevis muscle.

**mus•cu•lus ex•ten•sor car•pi ra•di•a•lis long•us** [TA] SYN extensor carpi radialis longus muscle.

**mus•cu•lus ex•ten•sor car•pi ul•na•ris** [TA] SYN extensor carpi ulnaris muscle.

m
u

**mus·cu·lus ex·ten·sor di·gi·ti mi·ni·mi** [TA] SYN extensor digiti minimi muscle.

**mus·cu·lus ex·ten·sor di·gi·to·rum** [TA] SYN extensor digitorum muscle.

**mus·cu·lus ex·ten·sor di·gi·to·rum bre·vis** [TA] SYN extensor digitorum brevis muscle.

**mus·cu·lus ex·ten·sor di·gi·to·rum lon·gus** [TA] SYN extensor digitorum longus muscle.

**mus·cu·lus ex·ten·sor hal·lu·cis bre·vis** [TA] SYN extensor hallucis brevis muscle.

**mus·cu·lus ex·ten·sor hal·lu·cis lon·gus** [TA] SYN extensor hallucis longus muscle.

**mus·cu·lus ex·ten·sor in·di·cis** [TA] SYN extensor indicis muscle.

**mus·cu·lus flex·or car·pi ra·di·a·lis** [TA] SYN flexor carpi radialis muscle.

**mus·cu·lus flex·or car·pi ul·na·ris** [TA] SYN flexor carpi ulnaris muscle.

**mus·cu·lus flex·or di·gi·ti mi·ni·mi bre·vis ma·nus** [TA] SYN flexor digiti minimi brevis muscle of hand.

**mus·cu·lus flex·or di·gi·ti mi·ni·mi bre·vis pe·dis** [TA] SYN flexor digiti minimi brevis muscle of foot.

**mus·cu·lus flex·or di·gi·to·rum bre·vis** [TA] SYN flexor digitorum brevis muscle.

**mus·cu·lus flex·or di·gi·to·rum lon·gus** [TA] SYN flexor digitorum longus muscle.

**mus·cu·lus flex·or di·gi·to·rum pro·fun·dus** [TA] SYN flexor digitorum profundus muscle.

**mus·cu·lus flex·or di·gi·to·rum su·per·fi·ci·a·lis** [TA] SYN flexor digitorum superficialis muscle.

**mus·cu·lus gas·troc·ne·mi·us** [TA] SYN gastrocnemius muscle.

**mus·cu·lus ge·ni·o·glos·sus** [TA] SYN genioglossus muscle.

**mus·cu·lus ge·ni·o·hy·oi·de·us** [TA] SYN geniohyoid muscle.

**mus·cu·lus glu·te·us max·i·mus** [TA] SYN gluteus maximus muscle.

**mus·cu·lus glu·te·us me·di·us** [TA] SYN gluteus medius muscle.

**mus·cu·lus glu·te·us mi·ni·mus** [TA] SYN gluteus minimus muscle.

**mus·cu·lus grac·i·lis** [TA] SYN gracilis muscle.

**mus·cu·lus hy·o·glos·sus** [TA] SYN hyoglossus muscle.

**mus·cu·lus il·i·a·cus** [TA] SYN iliacus muscle.

**mus·cu·lus il·i·o·coc·cyg·e·us** [TA] SYN iliococcygeus muscle.

**mus·cu·lus il·i·o·cos·ta·lis** [TA] SYN iliocostalis muscle.

**mus·cu·lus il·i·o·pso·as** [TA] SYN iliopsoas muscle.

**mus·cu·lus in·fra·spi·na·tus** [TA] SYN infraspinatus muscle.

**mus·cu·lus in·ter·os·se·us pal·mar·is**, pl. **mus·cu·li in·ter·os·se·i pal·ma·res** [TA] SYN palmar interosseous muscle.

**mus·cu·lus in·ter·os·se·us plan·tar·is**, pl. **mus·cu·li in·ter·os·se·i plan·tar·es** [TA] SYN plantar interosseous muscle.

**mus·cu·lus is·chi·o·cav·er·no·sus** [TA] SYN ischiocavernous muscle.

**mus·cu·lus la·tis·si·mus dor·si** [TA] SYN latissimus dorsi muscle.

**mus·cu·lus le·va·tor an·gu·li o·ris** [TA] SYN levator anguli oris muscle.

**mus·cu·lus le·va·tor ani** [TA] SYN levator ani muscle.

**mus·cu·lus le·va·tor glan·du·lae thy·roi·de·ae** [TA] SYN levator muscle of thyroid gland.

**mus·cu·lus le·va·tor la·bii su·pe·ri·o·ris** [TA] SYN levator labii superioris muscle.

**mus·cu·lus le·va·tor la·bii su·pe·ri·o·ris a·laeque na·si** [TA] SYN levator labii superioris alaeque nasi muscle.

**mus·cu·lus le·va·tor pal·pe·brae su·pe·ri·o·ris** [TA] SYN levator palpebrae superioris muscle.

**mus·cu·lus le·va·tor pro·sta·tae** [TA] SYN levator prostatae muscle.

**mus·cu·lus le·va·tor scap·u·lae** [TA] SYN levator scapulae muscle.

**mus·cu·lus le·va·tor ve·li pa·la·ti·ni** [TA] SYN levator veli palatini muscle.

**mus·cu·lus lon·gis·si·mus ca·pi·tis** [TA] SYN longissimus capitis muscle.

**mus·cu·lus lon·gis·si·mus cer·vi·cis** [TA] SYN longissimus cervicis muscle.

**mus·cu·lus lon·gis·si·mus tho·ra·cis** [TA] SYN longissimus thoracis muscle.

**mus·cu·lus lon·gus ca·pi·tis** [TA] SYN longus capitis muscle.

**mus·cu·lus lon·gus col·li** [TA] SYN longus colli muscle.

**mus·cu·lus lum·bri·ca·lis ma·nus**, pl. **mus·cu·li lum·bri·ca·les ma·nus** [TA] SYN lumbrical muscles of hand.

**mus·cu·lus lum·bri·ca·lis pe·dis**, pl. **mus·cu·li lum·bri·ca·les pe·dis** [TA] SYN lumbrical muscles of foot.

**mus·cu·lus mas·se·ter** [TA] SYN masseter muscle.

**mus·cu·lus men·ta·lis** [TA] SYN mentalis muscle.

**mus·cu·lus mul·tif·i·dus** [TA] SYN multifidus muscle.

**mus·cu·lus mul·ti·fi·dus lum·bo·rum** [TA] SYN multifidus muscle.

**mus·cu·lus my·lo·hy·oi·de·us** [TA] SYN mylohyoid muscle.

**mus·cu·lus na·sa·lis** [TA] SYN nasalis muscle.

**mus·cu·lus ob·li·qu·us ex·ter·nus ab·do·mi·nis** [TA] SYN external oblique muscle.

**mus·cu·lus ob·li·qu·us in·fe·ri·or** [TA] SYN inferior oblique muscle.

**mus·cu·lus ob·li·qu·us in·ter·nus ab·do·mi·nis** [TA] SYN internal oblique muscle.

**mus·cu·lus ob·li·qu·us su·pe·ri·or** [TA] SYN superior oblique muscle.

**mus·cu·lus ob·tu·ra·tor·i·us ex·ter·nus** [TA] SYN obturator externus muscle.

**mus·cu·lus ob·tu·ra·tor·i·us in·ter·nus** [TA] SYN obturator internus muscle.

**mus·cu·lus oc·cip·i·to·fron·ta·lis** [TA] SYN occipitofrontalis muscle.

**mus·cu·lus o·mo·hy·oi·de·us** [TA] SYN omohyoid muscle.

**mus·cu·lus op·po·nens di·gi·ti mi·ni·mi** [TA] SYN opponens digiti minimi muscle.

**mus·cu·lus op·po·nens pol·li·cis** [TA] SYN opponens pollicis muscle.

**mus·cu·lus or·bi·cu·la·ris oc·u·li** [TA] SYN orbicularis oculi muscle.

**mus·cu·lus or·bi·cu·la·ris o·ris** [TA] SYN orbicularis oris muscle.

**mus·cu·lus or·bi·ta·lis** [TA] SYN orbitalis muscle.

**mus·cu·lus pal·a·to·glos·sus** [TA] SYN palatoglossus muscle.

**mus·cu·lus pal·a·to·pha·ryn·ge·us** [TA] syn palatopharyngeus muscle.

**mus·cu·lus pa·pil·la·ris** [TA] syn papillary muscle.

**mus·cu·lus pec·ti·ne·us** [TA] syn pectineus muscle.

**mus·cu·lus pi·ri·for·mis** [TA] syn piriformis muscle.

**mus·cu·lus plan·tar·is** [TA] syn plantaris muscle.

**mus·cu·lus pleu·ro·e·soph·a·ge·us** [TA] syn pleuroesophageal muscle.

**mus·cu·lus pop·lit·e·us** [TA] syn popliteus muscle.

**mus·cu·lus pro·ce·rus** [TA] syn procerus muscle.

**mus·cu·lus pro·na·tor quad·ra·tus** [TA] syn pronator quadratus muscle.

**mus·cu·lus pro·na·tor te·res** [TA] syn pronator teres muscle.

**mus·cu·lus pu·bo·coc·cy·ge·us** [TA] syn pubococcygeus muscle.

**mus·cu·lus pu·bo·pros·ta·ti·cus** [TA] syn puboprostatic muscle.

**mus·cu·lus pu·bo·rec·ta·lis** [TA] syn puborectalis muscle.

**mus·cu·lus pu·bo·va·gi·na·lis** [TA] syn pubovaginalis muscle.

**mus·cu·lus pu·bo·ve·si·ca·lis** [TA] syn pubovesicalis muscle.

**mus·cu·lus py·ra·mi·da·lis** [TA] syn pyramidalis muscle.

**mus·cu·lus py·ra·mi·da·lis au·ric·u·lae** [TA] syn pyramidal auricular muscle.

**mus·cu·lus quad·ra·tus fem·o·ris** [TA] syn quadratus femoris muscle.

**mus·cu·lus quad·ra·tus la·bii su·pe·ri·o·ris** syn quadratus labii superioris muscle.

**mus·cu·lus quad·ra·tus lum·bo·rum** [TA] syn quadratus lumborum muscle.

**mus·cu·lus quad·ra·tus plan·tae** [TA] syn quadratus plantae muscle.

**mus·cu·lus quad·ri·ceps fem·o·ris** [TA] syn quadriceps femoris muscle.

**mus·cu·lus rec·to·coc·cyg·e·us** [TA] syn rectococcygeus muscle.

**mus·cu·lus rec·to·u·re·thra·lis** [TA] syn rectourethralis muscle.

**mus·cu·lus rec·to·u·te·ri·nus** [TA] syn rectouterine muscle.

**mus·cu·lus rec·to·ve·si·ca·lis** [TA] syn rectovesicalis muscle.

**mus·cu·lus rec·tus ab·do·mi·nis** [TA] syn rectus abdominis muscle.

**mus·cu·lus rec·tus ca·pi·tis an·te·ri·or** [TA] syn rectus capitis anterior muscle.

**mus·cu·lus rec·tus ca·pi·tis la·te·ra·lis** [TA] syn rectus capitis lateralis muscle.

**mus·cu·lus rec·tus fem·o·ris** [TA] syn rectus femoris muscle.

**mus·cu·lus rec·tus in·fe·ri·or** [TA] syn inferior rectus muscle.

**mus·cu·lus rec·tus la·te·ra·lis** [TA] syn lateral rectus muscle.

**mus·cu·lus rec·tus me·di·a·lis** [TA] syn medial rectus muscle.

**mus·cu·lus rec·tus su·pe·ri·or** [TA] syn superior rectus muscle.

**mus·cu·lus ri·so·ri·us** [TA] syn risorius muscle.

**mus·cu·lus sal·pin·go·pha·ryn·ge·us** [TA] syn salpingopharyngeus muscle.

**mus·cu·lus sar·to·ri·us** [TA] syn sartorius muscle.

**mus·cu·lus sem·i·mem·bra·no·sus** [TA] syn semimembranosus muscle.

**mus·cu·lus sem·i·spi·na·lis ca·pi·tis** [TA] syn semispinalis capitis muscle.

**mus·cu·lus sem·i·spi·na·lis cer·vi·cis** [TA] syn semispinalis cervicis muscle.

**mus·cu·lus sem·i·spi·na·lis tho·ra·cis** [TA] syn semispinalis thoracis muscle.

**mus·cu·lus sem·i·ten·di·no·sus** [TA] syn semitendinosus muscle.

**mus·cu·lus ser·ra·tus an·te·ri·or** [TA] syn serratus anterior muscle.

**mus·cu·lus so·le·us** [TA] syn soleus muscle.

**mus·cu·lus sphinc·ter duc·tus cho·led·o·chi** [TA] syn sphincter of common bile duct.

**mus·cu·lus sphinc·ter duc·tus pan·cre·a·ti·ci** [TA] syn sphincter of pancreatic duct.

**mus·cu·lus sphinc·ter pu·pil·lae** [TA] syn sphincter pupillae.

**mus·cu·lus sphinc·ter py·lo·ri·cus** [TA] syn pyloric sphincter.

**mus·cu·lus sphinc·ter ure·thrae** [TA] syn sphincter urethrae.

**mus·cu·lus sphinc·ter ve·si·cae** [TA] syn sphincter vesicae.

**mus·cu·lus spi·na·lis ca·pi·tis** [TA] syn spinalis capitis muscle.

**mus·cu·lus spi·na·lis cer·vi·cis** [TA] syn spinalis cervicis muscle.

**mus·cu·lus spi·na·lis tho·ra·cis** [TA] syn spinalis thoracis muscle.

**mus·cu·lus sple·ni·us ca·pi·tis** [TA] syn splenius capitis muscle.

**mus·cu·lus sple·ni·us cer·vi·cis** [TA] syn splenius cervicis muscle.

**mus·cu·lus sta·pe·di·us** [TA] syn stapedius muscle.

**mus·cu·lus ster·na·lis** [TA] syn sternalis muscle.

**mus·cu·lus ster·no·clei·do·mas·toi·de·us** [TA] syn sternocleidomastoid muscle.

**mus·cu·lus ster·no·hy·oi·de·us** [TA] syn sternohyoid muscle.

**mus·cu·lus ster·no·thy·roi·de·us** [TA] syn sternothyroid muscle.

**mus·cu·lus sty·lo·glos·sus** [TA] syn styloglossus muscle.

**mus·cu·lus sty·lo·hy·oi·de·us** [TA] syn stylohyoid muscle.

**mus·cu·lus sty·lo·pha·ryn·ge·us** [TA] syn stylopharyngeus muscle.

**mus·cu·lus sub·cla·vi·us** [TA] syn subclavius muscle.

**mus·cu·lus sub·cos·ta·lis,** pl. **mus·cu·li sub·cos·ta·les** [TA] syn subcostal muscle.

**mus·cu·lus sub·scap·u·la·ris** [TA] syn subscapularis muscle.

**mus·cu·lus su·pi·na·tor** [TA] syn supinator muscle.

**mus·cu·lus su·pra·spi·na·tus** [TA] syn supraspinatus muscle.

**mus·cu·lus sus·pen·so·ri·us du·o·de·ni** [TA] syn suspensory muscle of duodenum.

**mus·cu·lus tem·po·ra·lis** [TA] syn temporalis muscle.

**mus·cu·lus tem·po·ro·pa·ri·e·ta·lis** [TA] syn temporoparietalis muscle. SEE ALSO anterior auricular muscle, superior auricular muscle.

m
u

mus·cu·lus ten·sor fas·ci·ae la·tae [TA] SYN tensor fasciae latae muscle.

mus·cu·lus ten·sor tym·pa·ni [TA] SYN tensor tympani muscle.

mus·cu·lus ten·sor ve·li pa·la·ti·ni [TA] SYN tensor veli palati muscle.

mus·cu·lus te·res ma·jor [TA] SYN teres major muscle.

mus·cu·lus te·res mi·nor [TA] SYN teres minor muscle.

mus·cu·lus thy·ro·ar·y·te·noi·de·us [TA] SYN thyroarytenoid muscle.

mus·cu·lus thy·ro·ep·i·glot·ti·cus [TA] SYN thyroepiglottic muscle.

mus·cu·lus thy·ro·hy·oi·de·us SYN thyrohyoid muscle.

mus·cu·lus tib·i·al·is post·er·i·or [TA] SYN tibialis posterior muscle.

mus·cu·lus tib·i·o·fas·ci·a·lis an·te·ri·or,
mus·cu·lus tib·i·o·fas·ci·a·lis an·ti·cus SYN anterior tibiofascial muscle.

mus·cu·lus tra·che·a·lis [TA] SYN trachealis muscle.

mus·cu·lus tra·gi·cus [TA] SYN tragicus muscle.

mus·cu·lus trans·ver·so·spi·na·lis [TA] SYN transversospinalis muscle.

mus·cu·lus trans·ver·sus ab·do·mi·nis [TA] SYN transversus abdominis muscle.

mus·cu·lus trans·ver·sus lin·guae [TA] SYN transverse muscle of tongue.

mus·cu·lus trans·ver·sus men·ti [TA] SYN transversus menti muscle.

mus·cu·lus trans·ver·sus nu·chae [TA] SYN transversus nuchae muscle.

mus·cu·lus trans·ver·sus pe·ri·nei pro·fun·dus [TA] SYN deep transverse perineal muscle.

mus·cu·lus trans·ver·sus pe·ri·nei su·per·fi·ci·a·lis [TA] SYN superficial transverse perineal muscle.

mus·cu·lus trans·ver·sus tho·ra·cis [TA] SYN transversus thoracis muscle.

mus·cu·lus tra·pe·zi·us [TA] SYN trapezius muscle.

mus·cu·lus tri·ceps bra·chii [TA] SYN triceps brachii muscle.

mus·cu·lus tri·ceps su·rae [TA] SYN triceps surae muscle.

mus·cu·lus u·vu·lae [TA] SYN uvular muscle.

mus·cu·lus ver·ti·ca·lis lin·guae [TA] SYN vertical muscle of tongue.

mus·cu·lus vo·ca·lis [TA] SYN vocalis muscle.

mus·cu·lus zy·go·ma·ti·cus ma·jor [TA] SYN zygomaticus major muscle.

mush·room poi·son·ing SEE mycetism.

mu·si·co·ther·a·py (myu′sik-ō-thār′ă-pē) an adjunctive treatment of mental disorders by means of music.

Mus·set sign (moo-sā′) in incompetence of the aortic valve, rhythmic nodding of the head, synchronous with the heartbeat. SYN de Musset sign.

mus·si·ta·tion (mŭs-i-tā′shŭn) movements of the lips as if speaking, but without sound; observed in delirium and in semicoma. [L. mussito, to murmur constantly, fr. musso, pp. -atus, to mutter]

Mus·tard op·er·a·tion (mŭs′terd) correction, at the atrial level, of hemodynamic abnormality due to transposition of the great arteries by an intraatrial baffle to direct pulmonary venous blood through the tricuspid orifice into the right ventricle and the systemic venous blood through the mitral valve into the left ventricle.

mu·ta·gen (myu′tă-jen) any agent that promotes a mutation or causes an increase in the rate of mutational events, e.g., radioactive substances, x-rays, or certain chemicals. [L. muto, to change, + G. -gen, producing]

mu·ta·gen·e·sis (moo-tă-jen′ĕ-sis, myoo-tă-jen′e-sis) 1. production of genetic alterations by using chemicals or radiation. 2. production of a mutation.

mu·ta·gen·ic (myu-tă-jen′ik) promoting mutation.

mu·tant (myu′tant) 1. a phenotype in which a mutation is manifested. 2. a gene that is rare and usually harmful, in contrast to a wild-type gene, not necessarily generated recently.

mu·tant gene a gene that has been changed from an ancestral type, not necessarily in the current generation. SEE ALSO mutant, mutation.

mu·tase (myu′tās) any enzyme that catalyzes the apparent migration of groups within one molecule; sometimes the transfer is from one molecule to another.

mu·ta·tion (myu-tā′shŭn) 1. a change in the chemistry of a gene that is perpetuated in subsequent divisions of the cell in which it occurs; a change in the sequence of base pairs in the chromosomal molecule. 2. the sudden production of a species, as distinguished from variation. [L. muto, pp. -atus, to change]

mu·ta·tion rate the probability (or proportion) of progeny genes with a particular component of the genome not present in either biological parent; usually expressed as the number of mutants per generation occurring at one gene or locus.

mute (myut) 1. unable or unwilling to speak. 2. a person who does not have the faculty of speech. [L. mutus]

mu·tein (myu′tēn) a protein arising as a result of a mutation. [mutation + protein]

mu·ti·lat·ing ker·a·to·der·ma diffuse keratoderma of the extremities, with the development during childhood of constricting fibrous bands around the middle phalanx of the fingers or toes which may lead to spontaneous amputation.

mu·ti·la·tion (myu-ti-lā′shŭn) disfigurement or injury by removal or destruction of any conspicuous or essential part of the body. [L. mutilatio, fr. mutilo, pp. -atus, to maim]

mut·ism (myu′tizm) 1. the state of being silent. 2. organic or functional absence of the faculty of speech. [L. mutus, mute]

mu·ton (myu′ton) GENETICS the smallest unit of a chromosome in which alteration can be effective in causing a mutation. [mutation + -on]

mu·tu·al·ism (myu′tyu-ăl-izm) symbiotic relationship in which both species derive benefit. Cf. commensalism, metabiosis, parasitism.

mu·tu·al·ist (myu′tyu-ăl-ist) SYN symbion. [L. mutuus, in return, mutual]

mu·tu·al re·sis·tance SYN antagonism.

mV millivolt.

MVV maximum voluntary ventilation.

MW molecular weight.

my·al·gia (mī-al′jē-ă) muscular pain. SYN myodynia. [G. mys, muscle, + algos, pain]

my·al·gic en·ceph·a·lo·mye·li·tis SYN chronic fatigue syndrome.

my·as·the·nia (mī-as-thē′nē-ă) muscular weakness. [G. mys, muscle, + astheneia, weakness]

**my·as·the·nia an·gi·o·scle·ro·ti·ca** SYN intermittent claudication.

**my·as·the·nia gra·vis** disorder of neuromuscular transmission, marked by fluctuating weakness, especially of the oculofacial muscles and the proximal limb muscles; the weakness characteristically increases with activity; due to an immunological disorder. SYN Goldflam disease.

**my·as·then·ic** (mī′as-then′ik) relating to myasthenia.

**my·as·then·ic fa·ci·es** the facial expression in myasthenia gravis, caused by drooping of the eyelids and corners of the mouth, and weakness of the muscles of the face.

**my·as·then·ic syn·drome** a disorder of neuromuscular transmission marked primarily by limb and girdle weakness, absent deep tendon reflexes, dry mouth, and impotence; due to an immunological disorder; often, especially in males, a paraneoplastic syndrome linked to small cell carcinoma of the lung.

**my·a·to·nia, my·at·o·ny** (mī-ă-tō′nē-ă, mī-at′ō-nē) abnormal extensibility of a muscle. [G. *mys*, muscle, + *a* priv. + *tonos*, tone]

**my·a·to·nia con·gen·i·ta** SYN amyotonia congenita (1).

**my·ce·lia** (mī-sē′lē-ă) plural of mycelium.

**my·ce·li·an** (mī-sē′lē-an) pertaining to a mycelium.

**my·ce·li·um,** pl. **my·ce·lia** (mī-sē′lē-ŭm, mī-sē′lē-ă) the mass of hyphae making up a colony of fungi. [G. *mykēs*, fungus, + *hēlos*, nail, wart, excrescence on animal or plant]

△**my·cet-, my·ceto-** fungus. SEE ALSO myco-. [G. *mykēs*, fungus]

**my·cete** (mī′sēt) a fungus. [G. *mykēs*, fungus]

**my·ce·tism, my·ce·tis·mus** (mī′sē-tizm, mī′sē-tiz′mŭs) poisoning by certain species of mushrooms. [G. *mykēs*, fungus]

**my·ce·to·ge·net·ic, my·ce·to·gen·ic** (mī-sē′tō-jĕ-net′ik, mī-sē′tō-jen′ik) caused by fungi. [G. *mykēs*, fungus, + *gennētos*, begotten]

**my·ce·to·ma** (mī-sē-tō′mă) **1.** a chronic infection involving the feet and characterized by the formation of localized lesions with tumefactions and multiple draining sinuses. The exudate contains granules that may be yellow, white, red, brown, or black, depending upon the causative agent. actinomycotic mycetoma is caused by actinomycetes; eumycotic mycetoma is caused by true fungi. SYN Madura boil, maduromycosis. **2.** any tumor with draining sinuses produced by filamentous fungi.

**my·cid** (mī′sid) an allergic reaction to a remote focus of mycotic infection. [G. *mykēs*, fungus, + -id]

△**my·co-** fungus. SEE ALSO mycet-. [G. *mykēs*, fungus]

**my·co·bac·te·ria** (mī′kō-bak-tē′rē-ă) organisms belonging to the genus *Mycobacterium*.

**my·co·bac·te·ri·o·sis** (mī′kō-bak-tēr′ē-ō′sis) infection with mycobacteria.

*My·co·bac·te·ri·um* (mī′kō-bak-tēr′ē-ŭm) a genus of aerobic, nonmotile bacteria (family Mycobacteriaceae) containing Gram-positive, acid-fast, slender, straight or slightly curved rods; slender filaments occasionally occur, but branched forms rarely are produced. Parasitic and saprophytic species occur. A number of species are associated with infections in immunocompromised persons, especially those with

AIDS. The type species is *Mycobacterium tuberculosis*. It is the type genus of the family Mycobacteriaceae. [myco- + bacterium]

*My·co·bac·te·ri·um a·vi·um* a species causing tuberculosis in fowl and other birds. Recently linked to opportunistic infections in humans. SYN tubercle bacillus (3).

*My·co·bac·te·ri·um avi·um-in·tra·cel·lu·lare com·plex* an opportunistic agent of infection in persons with AIDS. Difficult to treat because *Mycobacterium* is resistant to many antibiotics. May also cause chronic lower respiratory tract infections.

*My·co·bac·te·ri·um bo·vis* a species that is the primary cause of tuberculosis in cattle; transmissible to humans and other animals, causing tuberculosis. SYN tubercle bacillus (2).

*My·co·bac·te·ri·um che·lo·nae* rapidly growing mycobacterium that causes sporadic infection following cardiothoracic surgery, peritoneal dialysis, and hemodialysis, augmentation mammaplasty, arthroplasty, and in immunocompromised patients.

*My·co·bac·te·ri·um kan·sa·si·i* a species causing a tuberculosis-like pulmonary disease; also found to cause infections (and usually lesions) in meninges, spleen, liver, pancreas, testes, hip joint, knee joint, finger, wrist, and lymph nodes.

*My·co·bac·te·ri·um lep·rae* a species that causes Hansen disease. SYN Hansen bacillus.

*My·co·bac·te·ri·um ma·ri·num* a species causing spontaneous tuberculosis in saltwater fish; it also occurs in other cold-blooded animals, in some swimming pools in which it may cause human cutaneous infection, irrigation canals and ditches, and ocean beaches.

*My·co·bac·te·ri·um scro·fu·la·ce·um* a species frequently associated with cervical adenitis in children.

*My·co·bac·te·ri·um tu·ber·cu·lo·sis* a species which causes tuberculosis in humans;it is the type species of the genus *Mycobacterium*. SYN Koch bacillus, tubercle bacillus (1).

*My·co·bac·te·ri·um vac·cae* a rapidly growing scotochromogenic, nonpathogenic species that is distributed widely in nature.

**my·co·der·ma·ti·tis** (mī′kō-der-mă-tī′tis) a nonspecific term used to designate an eruption of mycotic (fungus, yeast, mold) origin.

**my·col·o·gist** (mī-kol′ŏ-jist) a person specializing in mycology.

**my·col·o·gy** (mī-kol′ō-jē) the study of fungi: their identification, classification, edibility, cultivation, and biology, including pathogenicity. [myco- + G. *logos*, study]

**my·co·phage** (mī′kō-fāj) a virus whose host is a fungus. SEE ALSO mycovirus. [myco- + G. *phagō*, to eat]

*My·co·plas·ma* (mī′kō-plaz-mă) a genus of aerobic to facultatively anaerobic bacteria containing Gram-negative cells that do not possess a true cell wall but are bounded by a three-layered membrane. The cells are pleomorphic, and in liquid media appear as coccoid bodies, rings, or filaments. These organisms are found in humans and other animals and are parasitic to pathogenic. [myco- + G. *plasma*, something formed (plasm)]

**my·co·plas·ma,** pl. **my·co·plas·ma·ta** (mī′kō-plaz-mă, mī′kō-plaz′mah-tă) a vernacular term used to refer to any member of the genus *Mycoplasma*.

**m
y**

**My·co·plas·ma hom·i·nis** a species that is an agent of pelvic inflammatory disease and other genitourinary tract infections; can also cause chorioamnionitis and postpartum fever.

**my·co·plas·mal pneu·mo·nia** SYN primary atypical pneumonia.

**My·co·plas·ma my·coi·des** a bacterial species of which subspecies cause contagious pleuropneumonia in cattle, sheep, and goats; it is the type species of the genus *Mycoplasma*.

**My·co·plas·ma pha·ryn·gis** a species occurring as a commensal in the human oropharynx.

**My·co·plas·ma pneu·mo·ni·ae** a species causing primary atypical pneumonia in human beings. SYN Eaton agent.

**My·co·plas·ma·ta·les** (mī'kō-plaz'mă-tā'lēz) an order of Gram-negative bacteria containing cells which are bounded by a three-layered membrane but which do not possess a true cell wall. Pathogenic and saprophytic species occur. These organisms reproduce through the breaking up of branched filaments into coccoid, filterable elementary bodies. The order includes the so-called pleuropneumonia-like organisms (PPLO).

**my·co·sis**, pl. **my·co·ses** (mī-kō'sis, mī-kō'sēz) any disease caused by a fungus (filamentous or yeast). [myco- + G. *-osis,* condition]

🔲 **my·co·sis fun·goi·des** a chronic progressive lymphoma arising in the skin which initially simulates eczema or other inflammatory dermatoses; in advanced cases, ulcerated tumors and infiltrations of lymph nodes may occur. See this page.

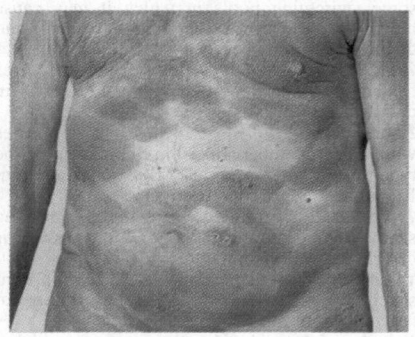

**mycosis fungoides**

**my·cot·ic** (mī-kot'ik) relating to or caused by a fungus.

**my·cot·ic an·eu·rysm** an aneurysm caused by the growth of fungi within the vascular wall, usually following impaction of a septic embolus; also used to refer to the growth of bacteria within the vascular wall of an aneurysm; may result from impaction of septic embolus or from primary infection of the vessel wall.

**my·co·tox·i·co·sis** (mī'kō-tok-si-kō'sis) poisoning due to the ingestion of preformed substances produced by the action of certain fungi on particular foodstuffs or ingestion of the fungi themselves; e.g., ergotism. [myco- + G. *toxikon,* poison, + *-osis,* condition]

**my·co·tox·in** (mī'kō-tok-sin) toxic compound produced by certain fungi; some are used for medicinal purposes; e.g., muscarine, psilocybin.

**my·co·vi·rus** (mī'kō-vī-rŭs) a virus that infects fungi.

**my·dri·a·sis** (mĭ-drī'ă-sis) dilation of the pupil. [G.]

**myd·ri·at·ic** (mĭ-drē-at'ik) **1.** causing mydriasis or dilation of the pupil. **2.** an agent that dilates the pupil.

**my·ec·to·my** (mī-ek'tō-mē) excision of all or part of a muscle. [G. *mys,* muscle, + *ektomē,* excision]

**my·ec·to·py, my·ec·to·pia** (mī-ek'tō-pē, mī-ek-tō'pē-ă) rarely used term for dislocation of a muscle. [G. *mys,* muscle, + *ektopos,* out of place]

△**my·el-, my·elo- 1.** the bone marrow. **2.** the spinal cord and medulla oblongata. Cf. medullo-. **3.** the myelin sheath of nerve fibers. [G. *myelos,* medulla, marrow]

**my·el·ap·o·plexy** (mī'el-ap'ō-plek'sē) SYN hematomyelia. [myel- + G. *apoplēxia,* apoplexy]

**my·el·a·te·lia** (mī'el-ă-tē'lē-ă) any developmental defect of the spinal cord. [myel- + G. *ateleia,* incompleteness]

**my·el·en·ceph·a·lon** (mī'el-en-sef'ă-lon) SYN medulla oblongata. [myel- + G. *enkephalos,* brain]

**my·e·lin** (mī'ě-lin) **1.** the lipoproteinaceous material of the myelin sheath, composed of alternating membranes of lipid and protein. **2.** droplets of lipid formed during autolysis and postmortem decomposition.

**my·e·li·nat·ed** (mī'ě-li-nāt-ed) having a myelin sheath. SYN medullated (2).

**my·e·li·na·tion** (mī'ě-li-nā'shŭn) the acquisition, development, or formation of a myelin sheath around a nerve fiber.

**my·e·li·nol·y·sis** (mī'ě-li-nol'i-sis) dissolution of the myelin sheaths of nerve fibers. [myelin + G. *lysis,* dissolution]

**my·e·lin sheath** the lipoproteinaceous envelope in vertebrates surrounding most axons of more than 0.5-μm diameter; it consists of a double plasma membrane wound tightly around the axon in a variable number of turns, and supplied by oligodendroglia cells (in the brain and spinal cord) or Schwann cells (in peripheral nerves).

**my·e·lit·ic** (mī-ě-lit'ik) relating to or affected by myelitis.

**my·e·li·tis** (mī-ě-lī'tis) **1.** inflammation of the spinal cord. **2.** inflammation of the bone marrow. [myel- + G. *-itis,* inflammation]

**my·e·lo·blast** (mī'ě-lō-blast) an immature cell in the granulocytic series, occurring normally in bone marrow but not in the blood. When stained, the cytoplasm is light blue and variable in amount; the nucleus deep purple-blue with finely divided, punctate, threadlike chromatin. A few light blue nucleoli in the nucleus generally disappear as the myeloblast matures into a promyelocyte and then a myelocyte. [myelo- + G. *blastos,* germ]

**my·e·lo·blas·te·mia** (mī'ě-lō-blas-tē'mē-ă) the presence of myeloblasts in the circulating blood. [myeloblast + G. *haima,* blood]

**my·e·lo·blas·tic leu·ke·mia** a form of granulocytic leukemia in which there are large numbers of myeloblasts in various tissues and in the blood. Used synonymously for acute granulocytic leukemia.

**my·e·lo·blas·to·ma** (mī'ě-lō-blas-tō'mă) a nodular focus or fairly well-circumscribed accumulation of myeloblasts, as sometimes observed in acute myeloblastic leukemia and chlorosis. [myeloblast + G. *-oma*, tumor]

**my•e•lo•blas•to•sis** (mī′ĕ-lō-blas-tō′sis) the presence of unusually large numbers of myeloblasts in the circulating blood, or tissues, or both (as in acute leukemia).

**my•e•lo•cele** (mī′ĕ-lō-sēl) **1.** protrusion of the spinal cord in spina bifida. [myelo- + G. *kēlē*, hernia] **2.** the central canal of the spinal cord. [G. *myelos*, marrow, + *koilia*, a hollow]

**my•e•lo•cyst** (mī′ĕ-lō-sist) any cyst (usually lined with columnar or cuboidal cells) that develops from a rudimentary medullary canal in the central nervous system. [myelo- + G. *kystis*, bladder]

**my•e•lo•cyst•ic** (mī′ĕ-lō-sist′ik) pertaining to or characterized by the presence of a myelocyst.

**my•e•lo•cys•to•cele** (mī′ĕ-lō-sis′tō-sēl) spina bifida containing spinal cord substance. [myelo- + G. *kystis*, bladder, + *kēlē*, tumor]

**my•e•lo•cys•to•me•ning•o•cele** (mī′ĕ-lō-sis′tō-mĕ-ning′gō-sēl) syn meningomyelocele. [myelo- + G. *kystis*, bladder, + *mēninx* (*mēning-*), membrane, + *kēlē*, hernia]

**my•e•lo•cyte** (mī′ĕ-lō-sīt) **1.** a young cell of the granulocytic series, occurring normally in bone marrow, but not in circulating blood. When stained, the cytoplasm is distinctly basophilic and more abundant than in myeloblasts or promyelocytes; numerous cytoplasmic granules are present in the more mature forms. The nucleus is regular in contour, i.e., not indented, and seems to be "buried" beneath the numerous cytoplasmic granules. **2.** a nerve cell of the gray matter of the brain or spinal cord. [myelo- + G. *kytos*, cell]

**my•e•lo•cy•the•mia** (mī′ĕ-lō-sī-thē′mē-ă) the presence of myelocytes in the circulating blood, especially in persistently large numbers (as in myelocytic leukemia). [myelocyte + G. *haima*, blood]

**my•e•lo•cyt•ic** (mī′ĕ-lō-sit′ik) pertaining to or characterized by myelocytes.

**my•e•lo•cyt•ic leu•ke•mia, my•e•lo•gen•ic leu•ke•mi•a, my•e•log•e•nous leu•ke•mi•a, my•e•loid leu•ke•mi•a** syn granulocytic leukemia.

**my•e•lo•cy•to•ma** (mī′ĕ-lō-sī-tō′mă) a nodular focus or fairly well-circumscribed, relatively dense accumulation of myelocytes, as in certain tissues of persons with myelocytic leukemia. [myelocyte + G. *-oma*, tumor]

**my•e•lo•cy•to•ma•to•sis** (mī′ĕ-lō-sī′tō-mă-tō′sis) a form of tumor involving chiefly the myelocytes.

**my•e•lo•cy•to•sis** (mī′ĕ-lō-sī-tō′sis) the occurrence of abnormally large numbers of myelocytes in the circulating blood, or tissues, or both. [myelocyte + G. *-osis*, condition]

**my•e•lo•dys•pla•sia** (mī′ĕ-lō-dis-plā′zē-ă) **1.** an abnormality in development of the spinal cord, especially the lower part of the cord. **2.** a disorder within the bone marrow, characterized by the proliferation of abnormal stem cells, that has the potential of developing into a specific type of leukemia. [myelo- + G. *dys-*, difficult, + *plasis*, a molding]

**my•e•lo•dys•plas•tic syn•drome** a primary, neoplastic, pluripotential stem-cell disorder characterized by peripheral blood cytopenias and prominent maturation abnormalities in the bone marrow. The disease evolves progressively and may transform into leukemia. Classified by the French-American-British (FAB) system into five groups. see also French-American-British classification system. syn chronic erythremic myelosis, preleukemia, smoldering leukemia.

**my•e•lo•fi•bro•sis** (mī′ĕ-lō-fī-brō′sis) fibrosis of the bone marrow, especially generalized, associated with myeloid metaplasia of the spleen and other organs, leukoerythroblastic anemia, and thrombocytopenia, although the bone marrow often contains many megakaryocytes. syn myelosclerosis.

**my•e•lo•gen•e•sis** (mī′ĕ-lō-jen′ĕ-sis) **1.** development of bone marrow. **2.** development of the central nervous system. **3.** formation of myelin around an axon.

**my•e•lo•ge•net•ic, my•e•lo•gen•ic** (mī′ĕ-lō-jĕ-net′ik, mī′ĕ-lō-jen′ik) **1.** relating to myelogenesis. **2.** produced by or originating in the bone marrow. syn myelogenous.

**my•e•log•e•nous** (mī-ĕ-loj′ĕ-nŭs) syn myelogenetic (2).

**my•e•lo•gone, my•e•lo•go•ni•um** (mī′ĕ-lō-gōn, mī′ĕ-lo-gō′nē-ŭm) an immature white blood cell of the myeloid series that is characterized by a large, deeply stained, reticulated nucleus and a scant amount of nongranular basophilic cytoplasm. [myelo- + G. *gonē*, seed]

**my•e•lo•gram** (mī′ĕ-lō-gram) radiographic contrast study of the spinal subarachnoid space and its contents.

**my•e•log•ra•phy** (mī′ĕ-log′ră-fē) radiography of the spinal cord and nerve roots after the injection of a contrast medium into the spinal subarachnoid space. [myelo- + G. *graphē*, a drawing]

**my•e•loid** (mī′ĕ-loyd) **1.** pertaining to, derived from, or manifesting certain features of the bone marrow. **2.** sometimes used with reference to the spinal cord. **3.** pertaining to certain characteristics of myelocytic forms, but not necessarily implying origin in the bone marrow. [myel- + -oid]

**my•e•loid met•a•pla•sia** a syndrome characterized by anemia, enlargement of the spleen, nucleated red blood cells and immature granulocytes in the blood, and foci of extramedullary hemopoiesis in the spleen and liver; may develop in the course of polycythemia rubra vera; there is a high incidence of development of myeloid leukemia.

**my•e•loi•do•sis** (mī′ĕ-loy-dō′sis) general hyperplasia of myeloid tissue.

**my•e•loid sar•co•ma** syn granulocytic sarcoma.

**my•e•loid se•ries** the granulocytic and the erythrocytic series.

**my•e•loid tis•sue** bone marrow consisting of the developmental and adult stages of erythrocytes, granulocytes, and megakaryocytes in a stroma of reticular cells and fibers, with sinusoidal vascular channels.

**my•e•lo•kath•ex•is** syn kathexis.

**my•e•lo•li•po•ma** (mī′ĕ-lō-li-pō′mă) nodular foci that are not neoplasms, but probably represent localized proliferation of reticuloendothelial tissue in the adrenal glands; foci of bone marrow containing erythropoietic or myeloid cells.

**my•e•lo•ma** (mī-ĕ-lō′mă) **1.** a tumor composed of cells derived from hemopoietic tissues of the bone marrow. **2.** a plasma cell tumor. [myelo- + G. *-oma*, tumor]

**my•e•lo•ma•la•cia** (mī′ĕ-lō-ma-lā′shē-ă) softening of the spinal cord. [myelo- + G. *malakia*, a softness]

m
y

**my•e•lo•ma•to•sis** (mī'ĕ-lō-mă-tō'sis) a disease characterized by the occurrence of myeloma in various sites.

**my•e•lo•me•ning•o•cele** (mī'ĕ-lō-mĕ-ning'gō-sēl) SYN meningomyelocele. [myelo- + G. *mēninx*, membrane, + *kēlē*, hernia]

**my•e•lo•mere** (mī'ĕ-lō-mēr) neuromere of the brain or spinal cord. [myelo- + G. *meros*, part]

**my•e•lo•neu•ri•tis** (mī'ĕ-lō-noo-rī'tis) SYN neuromyelitis.

**my•e•lon•ic** (mī-e-lon'ik) relating to the spinal cord. [G. *myelon*, fr. *myelos*, marrow]

**my•e•lo•path•ic** (mī'ĕ-lō-path'ik) relating to myelopathy.

**my•e•lop•a•thy** (mī-ĕ-lop'ă-thē) **1.** disorder of the spinal cord. **2.** a disease of the myelopoietic tissues. [myelo- + G. *pathos*, suffering]

**my•e•lop•e•tal** (mī-ĕ-lop'ĕ-tăl) proceeding in a direction toward the spinal cord; said of different nerve impulses. [myelo- + L. *peto*, to seek]

**my•e•lo•phthis•ic** (mī'ĕ-lō-tiz'ik, mī'ĕ-lō-thiz'ik) relating to or suffering from myelophthisis.

**my•e•lo•phthis•ic a•ne•mia, my•e•lo•path•ic a•ne•mi•a** SYN leukoerythroblastosis.

**my•e•loph•thi•sis** (mī'ĕ-lof'thi-sis, mī'ĕ-lō-tī'sis) **1.** wasting or atrophy of the spinal cord as in tabes dorsalis. **2.** replacement of hemopoietic tissue in the bone marrow by abnormal tissue, usually fibrous tissue metastatic carcinomas. SYN panmyelophthisis. [myelo- + G. *phthisis*, a wasting away]

**my•e•lo•plast** (mī'ĕ-lō-plast) any of the leukocytic series of cells in the bone marrow, especially young forms. [myelo- + G. *plastos*, formed]

**my•e•lo•poi•e•sis** (mī'ĕ-lō-poy-ē'sis) formation of the tissue elements of bone marrow, or any of the types of blood cells derived from bone marrow; or both processes. [myelo- + G. *poiēsis*, a making]

**my•e•lo•poi•et•ic** (mī'ĕ-lō-poy-et'ik) relating to myelopoiesis.

**my•e•lo•pro•lif•er•a•tive** (mī'ĕ-lō-prō-lif'er-ă-tiv) pertaining to or characterized by unusual proliferation of myelopoietic tissue.

**my•e•lo•pro•lif•er•a•tive syn•dromes** a group of conditions that result from a disorder in the rate of formation of cells of the bone marrow, including chronic granulocytic leukemia, erythremia, myelosclerosis, panmyelosis, and erythremic myelosis and erythroleukemia.

**my•e•lo•ra•dic•u•li•tis** (mī'ĕ-lō-ra-dik-yu-lī'tis) inflammation of the spinal cord and nerve roots. [myelo- + L. *radicula*, root, + G. *-itis*, inflammation]

**my•e•lo•ra•dic•u•lo•dys•pla•sia** (mī'ĕ-lō-ra-dik' yu-lō-dis-plā-zē-ă) congenital maldevelopment of the spinal cord and spinal nerve roots. [myelo- + L. *radicula*, root, + dysplasia]

**my•e•lo•ra•dic•u•lop•a•thy** (mī'ĕ-lō-ră-dik'yu-lop'ă-thē) disease involving the spinal cord and nerve roots. SYN radiculomyelopathy. [myelo- + L. *radicula*, root, + G. *pathos*, disease]

**my•e•lor•rha•gia** (mī'ĕ-lō-rā'jē-ă) SYN hematomyelia. [myelo- + G. *rhēgnymi*, to burst forth]

**my•e•lor•rha•phy** (mī-ĕ-lōr'ă-fē) suture of a wound of the spinal cord. [myelo- + G. *rhaphē*, a seam]

**my•e•lo•scle•ro•sis** (mī'ĕ-lō-skle-rō'sis) SYN myelofibrosis. [myelo- + G. *sklērōsis*, induration]

**my•e•lo•sis** (mī-ĕ-lō'sis) **1.** a condition characterized by abnormal proliferation of tissue or cellular elements of bone marrow, e.g., multiple myeloma, myelocytic leukemia, myelofibrosis. **2.** a condition in which there is abnormal proliferation of medullary tissue in the spinal cord, as in a glioma.

**my•e•lot•o•my** (mī-ĕ-lot'ō-mē) incision of the spinal cord. [myelo- + G. *tomē*, incision]

**my•e•lo•tox•ic** (mī'ĕ-lō-tok'sik) **1.** inhibitory, depressant, or destructive to one or more of the components of bone marrow. **2.** pertaining to, derived from, or manifesting the features of diseased bone marrow.

**my•en•ter•ic** (mī-en-ter'ik) relating to the myenteron.

**my•en•ter•ic plex•us** a plexus of unmyelinated fibers and postganglionic autonomic cell bodies lying in the muscular coat of the esophagus, stomach, and intestine; it communicates with the subserous and submucous plexusex, all subdivisions of the enteric plexus.

**my•en•ter•on** (mī-en'ter-on) the muscular coat, or muscularis, of the intestine. [G. *mys*, muscle, + *enteron*, intestine]

**my•es•the•sia** (mī-es-thē'zē-ă) the sensation felt in muscle when it is contracting; awareness of movement or activity in muscles or joints; sense of position or movement mediated in large part by the posterior columns and medial lemniscus. SEE ALSO bathyesthesia. SYN kinesthetic sense, muscular sense. [G. *mys*, muscle, + *aisthēsis*, sensation]

**my•i•a•sis** (mī-ī'ă-sis) any infection due to invasion of tissues or cavities of the body by larvae of dipterous insects. [G. *myia*, a fly]

**my•lo•hy•oid** (mī'lō-hī'oyd) relating to the molar teeth, or posterior portion of the lower jaw, and to the hyoid bone; denoting various structures. SEE nerve, muscle, region, sulcus. [G. *mylē*, a mill, in pl. *mylai*, molar teeth]

**my•lo•hy•oid mus•cle** *origin*, mylohyoid line of mandible; *insertion*, upper border of hyoid bone and raphe separating muscle from its fellow; *action*, elevates floor of mouth and the tongue, depresses jaw when hyoid is fixed; *nerve supply*, nerve to mylohyoid from mandibular division of trigeminal. SYN musculus mylohyoideus [TA].

**my•lo•hy•oid nerve** a small branch of the inferior alveolar nerve given off posteriorly just before the nerve enters the mandibular foramen, distributed to the anterior belly of the digastric muscle and to the mylohyoid muscle. SYN nervus mylohyoideus [TA].

△**myo-** muscle. [G. *mys*, muscle]

**my•o•ar•chi•tec•ton•ic** (mī'ō-ar'ki-tek-ton'ik) relating to the structural arrangement of muscle or of fibers in general. [myo- + G. *architektonikos*, relating to construction]

**my•o•blast** (mī'ō-blast) a primordial muscle cell with the potentiality of developing into a muscle fiber. SYN sarcoblast. [myo- + G. *blastos*, germ]

**my•o•blas•tic** (mī-ō-blas'tik) relating to a myoblast or to the mode of formation of muscle cells.

**my•o•blas•to•ma** (mī'ō-blas-tō'mă) a tumor of immature muscle cells. [myo- + G. *blastos*, germ, + *-oma*, tumor]

**my•o•bra•dia** (mī-ō-brā'dē-ă) sluggish reaction of muscle to stimulation. [myo- + G. *bradys*, slow]

**my•o•car•di•al** (mī-ō-kar'dē-ăl) relating to the myocardium.

**my·o·car·di·al de·pres·sant fac·tor (MDF)** a toxic factor in shock that impairs cardiac contractility.

**my·o·car·di·al in·farc·tion (MI)** infarction of an area of the heart muscle, usually as a result of occlusion of a coronary artery. SYN heart attack, infarctus myocardii.

**my·o·car·di·al in·suf·fi·cien·cy** SYN heart failure (1).

**my·o·car·di·o·graph** (mī'ō-kar'dē-ō-graf) an instrument composed of a tambour with recording lever attachment, by which a tracing is made of the movements of the heart muscle. [myo- + G. *kardia,* heart, + *graphō,* to record]

**my·o·car·di·op·a·thy** (mī'ō-kar-dē-op'ă-thē) SYN cardiomyopathy. [myocardium + G. *pathos,* suffering]

**my·o·car·di·tis** (mī'ō-kar-dī'tis) inflammation of the muscular walls of the heart.

**my·o·car·di·um,** pl. **my·o·car·dia** (mī-ō-kar' dē-ŭm, mī-ō-kar'dē-ă) the middle layer of the heart, consisting of cardiac muscle. [myo- + G. *kardia,* heart]

**my·o·cele** (mī'ō-sēl) 1. protrusion of muscle substance through a rent in its sheath. [myo- + G. *kēlē,* hernia] 2. the small cavity that appears in somites. [myo- + G. *koilia,* a cavity]

**my·o·cel·lu·li·tis** (mī'ō-sel-yu-lī'tis) inflammation of muscle and cellular tissue. [myo- + Mod. L. *cellularis,* cellular (tissue), + G. *-itis,* inflammation]

**my·o·ce·ro·sis** (mī'ō-sē-rō'sis) waxy degeneration of the muscles. [myo- + G. *kēros,* wax]

**my·o·clo·nia** (mī'ō-klō'nē-ă) any disorder characterized by myoclonus. [myo- + G. *klonos,* a tumult]

**my·o·clon·ic** (mī-ō-klon'ik) showing myoclonus.

**my·o·clon·ic a·stat·ic ep·i·lep·sy** a petit mal variant characterized by atonic (drop attacks) and tonic or tonic-clonic attacks in neurologically disabled (hemiplegic, ataxic, etc.) children with mental retardation; usually progresses in spite of medication.

**my·oc·lo·nus** (mī-ok'lō-nŭs, mī-ō-klo'nŭs) one or a series of shock like contractions of a group of muscles, of variable regularity, synchrony, and symmetry, generally due to a central nervous system lesion. [myo- + G. *klonos,* tumult]

**my·oc·lo·nus ep·i·lep·sy** a clinically diverse group of epilepsy syndromes, some benign, some progressive. Many are hereditary and all are characterized by the occurrence of myoclonus. Specific syndromes include cherry red spot myoclonus syndrome, ceroid lipofuscinosis, myoclonic epilepsy with ragged red fibers, and Baltic myoclonus. SYN localization-related epilepsy (1).

**my·oc·lo·nus mul·ti·plex** an ill-defined disorder marked by rapid and widespread muscle contractions. SYN polyclonia, polymyoclonus.

**my·o·cu·ta·ne·ous** (mī-ō-kyu-tā'nē-ŭs) SYN musculocutaneous. [myo- + L. *cutis,* skin]

**my·o·cyte** (mī'ō-sīt) a muscle cell. [myo- + G. *kytos,* cell]

**my·o·cy·tol·y·sis** (mī-ō-sī-tol'i-sis) dissolution of muscle fiber. [myo- + G. *kytos,* cell, + *lysis,* a loosening]

**my·o·cy·to·ma** (mī'ō-sī-tō'mă) a benign neoplasm derived from muscle.

**my·o·de·mia** (mī-ō-dē'mē-ă) fatty degeneration of muscle. [myo- + G. *dēmos,* tallow]

**my·o·dyn·ia** (mī'ō-din'ē-ă) SYN myalgia. [myo- + G. *odynē,* pain]

**my·o·dys·to·ny** (mī-ō-dis'tō-nē) a condition of slow relaxation, interrupted by a succession of slight contractions, following electrical stimulation of a muscle. [myo- + G. *dys-,* difficult, + *tonos,* tone, tension]

**my·o·dys·tro·phy, my·o·dys·tro·phia** (mī-ō-dis'trō-fē, mī'ō-dis-trō'fē-ă) SYN muscular dystrophy. [myo- + G. *dys-,* difficult, poor, + *trophē,* nourishment]

**my·o·e·de·ma** (mī'ō-e-dē'mă) a localized contraction of a degenerating muscle, occurring at the point of a sharp blow, independent of the nerve supply. SYN idiomuscular contraction, mounding. [myo- + G. *oidēma,* swelling]

**my·o·e·las·tic** (mī'ō-e-las'tik) pertaining to closely associated smooth muscle fibers and elastic connective tissue.

**my·o·en·do·car·di·tis** (mī-ō-en'dō-kar-dī'tis) inflammation of the muscular wall and lining membrane of the heart. [myo- + G. *endon,* within, + *kardia,* heart, + *-itis,* inflammation]

**my·o·ep·i·the·li·al** (mī'ō-ep-i-thē'lē-ăl) relating to myoepithelium.

**my·o·ep·i·the·li·o·ma** (mī'ō-ep-i-thē-lē-ō'mă) a benign tumor of myoepithelial cells. [myo- + epithelium, + G. *-ōma,* tumor]

**my·o·ep·i·the·li·um** (mī'ō-ep-i-the'lē-ŭm) spindle-shaped, contractile, smooth muscle-like cells of epithelial origin that are arranged longitudinally or obliquely around sweat glands and the secretory alveoli of the mammary gland; stellate myoepithelial cells occur around lacrimal and some salivary gland secretory units. [myo- + epithelium]

**my·o·fa·cial pain-dys·func·tion syn·drome** dysfunction of the masticatory apparatus related to spasm of the muscles of mastication precipitated by occlusal disharmony or alteration in vertical dimension of the jaws, and exacerbated by emotional stress; characterized by pain in the preauricular region, muscle tenderness, popping noise in the temporomandibular joint, and limitation of jaw motion. SYN temporomandibular joint pain-dysfunction syndrome, TMJ syndrome.

**my·o·fas·ci·al** (mī-ō-fash'ē-ăl) of or relating to the fascia surrounding and separating muscle tissue.

**my·o·fas·ci·tis** (mī'ō-fă-sī'tis) SYN myositis fibrosa.

**my·o·fi·bril** (mī-ō-fī'bril) one of the fine longitudinal fibrils occurring in a skeletal or cardiac muscle fiber and consisting of many regularly overlapped ultramicroscopic thick and thin myofilaments. [myo- + Mod. L. *fibrilla,* fibril]

**my·o·fi·bro·blast** (mī-ō-fī'brō-blast) a cell thought to be responsible for contracture of wounds; such cells have some characteristics of smooth muscle, such as contractile properties and fibrils, and are also believed to produce, temporarily, type III collagen.

**my·o·fi·bro·ma** (mī'ō-fī-brō'mă) a benign neoplasm that consists chiefly of fibrous connective tissue, with variable numbers of muscle cells forming portions of the neoplasm.

**my·o·fi·bro·sis** (mī'ō-fī-brō'sis) chronic myositis with diffuse hyperplasia of the interstitial connective tissue pressing upon and causing atrophy of the muscular tissue.

**my·o·fi·bro·si·tis** (mī'ō-fī-brō-sī'tis) inflammation of the perimysium.

**my·o·fil·a·ments** (mī-ō-fil'ă-ments) the ultramicroscopic threads of filamentous proteins making up myofibrils in striated muscle. Thick ones contain myosin and thin ones actin; thick and thin myofilaments also occur in smooth muscle fibers but are not regularly arranged in discrete myofibrils and thus do not impart a striated appearance to these cells.

**my·o·func·tion·al the·ra·py** SPEECH PATHOLOGY any technique used to promote normal patterns of tongue movement and swallowing; primarily used to ameliorate tongue thrust. SEE tongue thrust. SYN tongue thrust therapy.

**my·o·gen·e·sis** (mī-ō-jen'ĕ-sis) embryonic formation of muscle cells or fibers. [myo- + G. *genesis*, origin]

**my·o·ge·net·ic, my·o·gen·ic** (mī-ō-jĕ-net'ik, mī-ō-jen'ik) **1.** originating in or starting from muscle. **2.** relating to the origin of muscle cells or fibers. SYN myogenous.

**my·og·e·nous** (mī-oj'ĕ-nŭs) SYN myogenetic.

**my·o·glo·bin (MbO₂, Mb)** (mī-ō-glō'bin) the oxygen-transporting and storage protein of muscle, resembling blood hemoglobin in function but with a molecular weight approximately one-quarter that of hemoglobin. Serum levels of this protein are often measured to assist in diagnosing an acute myocardial infarction; it is released into the circulation within 2–4 hours after myocardial infarction, peaks at about 8–12 hours, and returns to normal after 18–24 hours. SEE ALSO oxymyoglobin. SYN muscle hemoglobin. [myo- + hemoglobin]

**my·o·glo·bi·nu·ria** (mī'ō-glō-bi-nyu're-ă) excretion of myoglobin in the urine; results from muscle degeneration, which releases myoglobin into the blood; occurs in certain types of trauma (crush syndrome), advanced or protracted ischemia of muscle, or as a paroxysmal process of unknown etiology.

**my·o·glob·u·lin** (mī-ō-glob'yu-lin) globulin present in muscle tissue.

**my·o·glob·u·li·nu·ria** (mī'ō-glob'yu-li-nyu'rē-ă) the excretion of myoglobulin in the urine.

**my·o·gram** (mī'ō-gram) the tracing made by a myograph. [myo- + G. *gramma*, a drawing]

**my·o·graph** (mī'ō-graf) a recording instrument by which tracings are made of muscular contractions. [myo- + G. *graphō*, to write]

**my·o·graph·ic** (mī-ō-graf'ik) relating to a myogram, or the record of a myograph.

**my·og·ra·phy** (mī-og'ră-fē) **1.** the recording of muscular movements by the myograph. **2.** a description of or treatise on the muscles.

**my·oid** (mī'oyd) **1.** resembling muscle. **2.** one of the fine, contractile, threadlike protoplasmic elements found in certain epithelial cells in lower animals. [myo- + G. *eidos*, appearance]

**my·oid cells** flattened smooth muscle-like cells of mesodermal origin that lie just outside the basal lamina of the seminiferous tubule. SYN peritubular contractile cells.

**my·o·kin·e·sim·e·ter** (mī'ō-kin-ĕ-sim'ĕ-ter) a device for registering the exact time and extent of contraction of the larger muscles of the lower extremity in response to electric stimulation. [myo- + G. *kinesis*, movement, + *metron*, measure]

**my·o·ky·mia** (mī-ō-kī'mē-ă) continuous involuntary quivering or rippling of muscles at rest, caused by spontaneous, repetitive firing of groups of motor unit potentials. SYN kymatism, Morvan chorea. [myo- + G. *kyma*, wave]

**my·o·li·po·ma** (mī'ō-li-pō'mă) a benign neoplasm that consists chiefly of fat cells (adipose tissue), with variable numbers of muscle cells forming portions of the neoplasm.

**my·ol·o·gy** (mī-ol'ō-jē) the branch of science concerned with the muscles and their accessory parts, tendons, aponeuroses, bursae, and fasciae. [myo- + G. *logos*, study]

**my·ol·y·sis** (mī-ol'i-sis) dissolution or liquefaction of muscular tissue, frequently preceded by degenerative changes such as infiltration of fat, atrophy, and fatty degeneration. [myo- + G. *lysis*, dissolution]

**my·o·ma** (mī-ō'mă) a benign neoplasm of muscular tissue. SEE ALSO leiomyoma, rhabdomyoma. [myo- + G. *-oma*, tumor]

**my·o·ma·la·cia** (mī'ō-mă-lā'shē-ă) pathologic softening of muscular tissue. [myo- + G. *malakia*, softness]

**my·o·ma·tous** (mī-ō'mă-tŭs) pertaining to or characterized by the features of a myoma.

**my·o·mec·to·my** (mī-ō-mek'tō-mē) operative removal of a myoma, specifically of a uterine myoma. [myoma + G. *ektomē*, excision]

**my·o·mel·a·no·sis** (mī'ō-melă-nō'sis) abnormal dark pigmentation of muscular tissue. SEE ALSO melanosis. [myo- + G. *melanōsis*, becoming black]

**my·o·mere** (mī'ō-mēr) SYN myotome (4). [myo- + G. *meros*, a part]

**my·om·e·ter** (mī-om'ĕ-ter) an instrument for measuring the extent of a muscular contraction. [myo- + G. *metron*, measure]

**my·o·me·tri·al** (mī-ō-mē'trē-ăl) relating to the myometrium.

**my·o·me·tri·tis** (mī'ō-mē-trī'tis) inflammation of the muscular wall of the uterus. [myo- + G. *mētra*, uterus, + *-itis*, inflammation]

**my·o·me·tri·um** (mī'ō-mē'trē-ŭm) the muscular wall of the uterus. [myo- + G. *mētra*, uterus]

**my·o·ne·cro·sis** (mī'ō-nĕ-krō'sis) necrosis of muscle.

**my·o·neme** (mī'ō-nēm) **1.** a muscle fibril. **2.** one of the contractile fibrils of certain protozoans; thought to function in an analogous fashion to metazoan muscle fibers. [myo- + G. *nēma*, thread]

**my·o·neu·ral** (mī-ō-noo'răl) relating to both muscle and nerve; denoting specifically the synapse of the motor neuron with striated muscle fibers: myoneural junction or motor endplate. SEE ALSO neuromuscular. [myo- + G. *neuron*, nerve]

**my·o·neu·ral block·ade** inhibition of nerve impulse transmission at myoneural junctions by a drug such as curare.

**my·o·neu·ral junc·tion** the synaptic connection of the axon of the motor neuron with a muscle fiber. SEE motor endplate.

**my·o·oe·de·ma [Br.]** SEE myoedema.

**my·o·pal·mus** (mī-ō-pal'mŭs) muscle twitching. [myo- + G. *palmos*, a quivering]

**my·o·pa·ral·y·sis** (mī-ō-pă-ral'i-sis) muscular paralysis.

**my·o·pa·re·sis** (mī-ō-pă-rē'sis, mī-ō-par'ē-sis) slight muscular paralysis.

**my·o·path·ic** (mī-ō-path'ik) denoting a disorder involving muscular tissue.

**my•op•a•thy** (mī-op′ă-thē) any abnormal condition or disease of the muscular tissues; commonly designates a disorder involving skeletal muscle. [myo- + G. *pathos,* suffering]

**my•o•per•i•car•di•tis** (mī′ō-per-i-kar-dī′tis) inflammation of the muscular wall of the heart and of the enveloping pericardium; also, perimyocarditis. [myo- + pericarditis]

**my•o•pia** (mī-ō′pē-ă) that optical condition in which only rays from a finite distance from the eye focus on the retina. See this page. SYN nearsightedness, shortsightedness. [G. fr. *myo,* to shut, + *ōps,* eye]

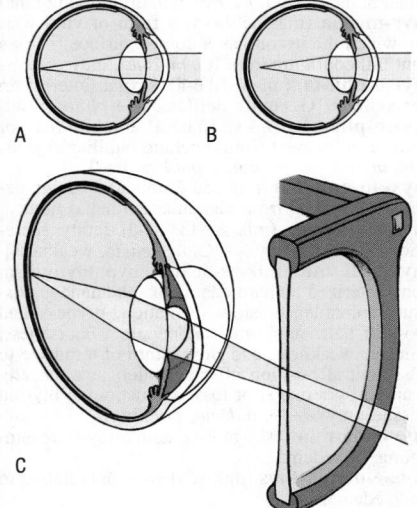

A      B

C

**myopia:** (A) normal (20/20) vision: light rays focus sharply on retina, (B) myopic (nearsighted) vision: light rays from a distance come to sharp focus in front of the retina, (C) myopia corrected by eyeglasses with concave lenses

**my•o•pic** (mī-op′ik, mī-ō′pik) relating to or suffering from myopia.

**my•o•pic a•stig•ma•tism** astigmatism in which one meridian is myopic and the one at a right angle to it is without refractive error.

**my•o•pic cres•cent** a white or grayish white crescentic area in the fundus of the eye located on the temporal side of the optic disk; caused by atrophy of the choroid, permitting the sclera to become visible.

**my•o•plasm** (mī′ō-plazm) the contractile portion of the muscle cell, as distinguished from the sarcoplasm. [myo- + G. *plasma,* a thing formed]

**my•o•plas•tic** (mī-ō-plas′tik) relating to the plastic surgery of the muscles, or to the use of muscular tissue in correcting defects.

**my•o•plas•ty** (mī′ō-plas-tē) plastic surgery of muscular tissue. [myo- + G. *plastos,* formed]

**my•or•rha•phy** (mī-ōr′ă-fē) suture of a muscle. [myo- + G. *rhaphē,* seam]

**my•or•rhex•is** (mī-ō-rek′sis) tearing of a muscle. [myo- + G. *rhēxis,* a rupture]

**my•o•sal•pinx** (mī′ō-sal′pingks) the muscular tunic of the uterine tube. [myo- + salpinx]

**my•o•sar•co•ma** (mī′ō-sar-kō′mă) a general term for a malignant neoplasm derived from muscular tissue. SEE ALSO leiomyosarcoma, rhabdomyosarcoma.

**my•o•scle•ro•sis** (mī′ō-skle-rō′sis) chronic myositis with hyperplasia of the interstitial connective tissue.

**my•o•sin** (mī′ō-sin) a globulin present in muscle; in combination with actin, it forms actomyosin; myosin forms the thick filaments in muscle.

**my•o•sin fil•a•ment** one of the contractile elements in skeletal, cardiac, and smooth muscle fibers; in skeletal muscle, the filament is about 10 nm thick and 1.5 μm long.

**my•o•sit•ic** (mī-ō-sit′ik) relating to myositis.

**my•o•si•tis** (mī-ō-sī′tis) inflammation of a muscle. SYN initis (2). [myo- + G. *-itis,* inflammation]

**my•o•si•tis fi•bro•sa** induration of a muscle through an interstitial growth of fibrous tissue. SYN myofascitis.

**my•o•si•tis os•sif•i•cans** ossification of inflammatory tissue within a muscle, usually at the site of a hematoma due to blunt trauma. See this page.

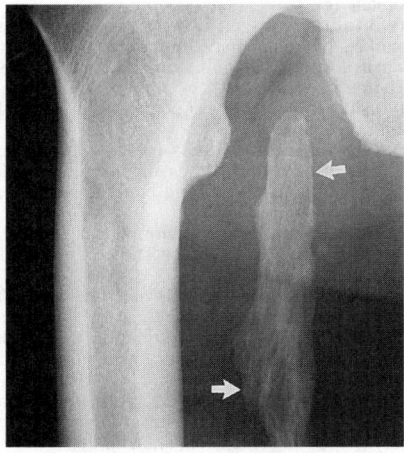

**myositis ossificans:** well-organized ossifying hematoma present in the adductor magnus muscle (arrows)

**my•o•spasm, my•o•spas•mus** (mī′ō-spazm, mī-ō-spaz′mŭs) spasmodic muscular contraction.

**my•o•tac•tic** (mī-ō-tak′tik) relating to the muscular sense. [myo- + L. *tactus,* a touching]

**my•ot•a•sis** (mī-ot′ă-sis) stretching of a muscle. [myo- + G. *tasis,* a stretching]

**my•o•tat•ic** (mī-ō-tat′ik) relating to myotasis.

**my•o•tat•ic con•trac•tion** a reflex contraction of a skeletal muscle that occurs as a result of stimulation of the stretch receptors in the muscle, i.e., as part of a myotatic reflex.

**my•o•tat•ic ir•ri•ta•bil•i•ty** the ability of a muscle to contract in response to the stimulus produced by a sudden stretching.

**my•o•tat•ic re•flex** tonic contraction of the mus-

m
y

cles in response to a stretching force, due to stimulation of muscle proprioceptors. SYN deep tendon reflex, stretch reflex.

**my·o·ten·o·si·tis** (mī'ō-te-nō-sī'tis) inflammation of a muscle with its tendon. [myo- + G. *tenōn,* tendon, + *-itis,* inflammation]

**my·o·te·not·o·my** (mī'ō-te-not'ō-mē) cutting through the principal tendon of a muscle, with division of the muscle itself in whole or in part. SYN tenomyotomy. [myo- + G. *tenōn,* tendon, + *tomē,* incision]

**my·o·the·ra·py** SYN massage therapy.

**my·o·tome** (mī'ō-tōm) 1. a knife for dividing muscle. 2. in embryos, that part of the somite that develops into skeletal muscle. SYN muscle plate. 3. all muscles derived from one somite and innervated by one segmental spinal nerve. 4. in primitive vertebrates, the muscular part of a metamere. SYN myomere. [myo- + G. *tomos,* a cut]

**my·ot·o·my** (mī-ot'ō-mē) 1. anatomy or dissection of the muscles. 2. surgical division of a muscle. [myo- + G. *tomē,* excision]

**my·o·to·nia** (mī-ō-tō'nē-ă) delayed relaxation of a muscle after a strong contraction, or prolonged contraction after mechanical stimulation (as by percussion) or brief electrical stimulation; due to abnormality of the muscle membrane, specifically the ion channels. [myo- + G. *tonos,* tension, stretching]

**my·o·to·nia con·gen·i·ta** a hereditary disease marked by momentary tonic spasms occurring when a voluntary movement is attempted. SYN Thomsen disease.

**my·o·ton·ic** (mī-ō-ton'ik) pertaining to or exhibiting myotonia.

**my·o·ton·ic chon·dro·dys·tro·phy** a rare congenital disease that causes myotonia, muscular hypertrophy, joint and long bone abnormalities, and weakness.

**my·o·ton·ic re·sponse** failure of muscle relaxation caused by repetitive discharge of muscle fiber action potentials.

**my·ot·o·noid** (mī-ot'ŏ-noyd) denoting a muscular reaction, naturally or electrically excited, characterized by slow contraction and, especially, slow relaxation. [myo- + G. *tonos,* tone, tension, + *eidos,* resemblance]

**my·ot·o·nus** (mī-ot'ŏ-nŭs) a tonic spasm or temporary rigidity of a muscle or group of muscles. [myo- + G. *tonos,* tension, stretching]

**my·ot·o·ny** (mī-ot'ŏ-nē) muscular tonus or tension. [myo- + G. *tonos,* tension]

**my·ot·ro·phy** (mī-ot'rō-fē) nutrition of muscular tissue. [myo- + G. *trophē,* nourishment]

**my·o·tube** (mī'ō-toob) a skeletal muscle fiber formed by the fusion of myoblasts during a developmental stage.

**my·rin·ga** (mĭ-ring'gă) SYN tympanic membrane. [Mod. L. drum membrane]

**myr·in·gec·to·my** (mir-in-jek'tō-mē) excision of the tympanic membrane. [myring- + G. *ektomē,* excision]

**myr·in·gi·tis** (mir-in-jī'tis) inflammation of the tympanic membrane. SYN tympanitis. [myring- + G. *-itis,* inflammation]

⚠**my·rin·go-, my·ring-** the membrana tympani. [Mod. L. *myringa*]

**my·rin·go·plas·ty** (mĭ-ring'gō-plas'tē) operative repair of a damaged tympanic membrane. [myringo- + G. *plassō,* to form]

**my·rin·go·scler·o·sis** (mĭ-ring'gō-skler-ō'sis)

formation of dense connective tissue in the tympanic membrane, usually not associated with hearing loss. [myringo- + sclerosis]

**my·rin·go·sta·pe·di·o·pexy** (mĭ-ring'gō-stā-pē'dē-ō-pek'sē) a technique of tympanoplasty in which the drum membrane or grafted drum membrane is brought into functional connection with the stapes. [myringo- + L. *stapes,* stirrup (stapes), + G. *pēxis,* fixation]

**myr·in·got·o·my** (mir-ing-got'ŏ-mē) paracentesis of the tympanic membrane. SYN tympanostomy, tympanotomy. [myringo- + G. *tomē,* excision]

**my·rinx** (mī'ringks, mir'ringks) SYN tympanic membrane. [Mod. L. *myringa,* drum membrane]

**myr·me·cia** (mĭr-mē'shē-ă) a form of viral wart in which the lesion has a domed surface (i.e., an ant hill configuration). [G. *murmex,* ant]

**my·so·phil·ia** (mī-sō-fil'ē-ă) sexual interest in excretions. [G. *mysos,* defilement, + *philos,* fond]

**my·so·pho·bia** (mī-sō-fō'bē-ă) morbid fear of dirt or defilement from touching familiar objects. [G. *mysos,* defilement, + *phobos,* fear]

**myx·ad·e·no·ma** (mik-sad-ĕ-nō'mă) a benign neoplasm derived from glandular epithelial tissue.

**myx·as·the·nia** (mik-sas-thē'nē-ă) faulty secretion of mucus. [myx- + G. *astheneia,* weakness]

**myx·e·de·ma** (mik-se-dē'mă) hypothyroidism characterized by hard edema of subcutaneous tissue, somnolence, slow mentation, dryness and loss of hair, subnormal temperature, hoarseness, muscle weakness, and slow return of a muscle to the neutral position after a tendon jerk; usually caused by removal or loss of functioning thyroid tissue. [myx- + G. *oidēma,* swelling]

**myx·e·de·ma·toid** (mik-sĕ-dem'ă-toyd) resembling myxedema.

**myx·e·dem·a·tous** (mik-sĕ-dem'ă-tŭs) relating to myxedema.

**myx·o·chon·dro·fi·bro·sar·co·ma** (mik'sō-kon'drō-fī'brō-sar-kō'mă) a malignant neoplasm derived from fibrous connective tissue in which there are foci of cartilaginous and myxomatous tissue. [myxo- + G. *chondros,* cartilage, + L. *fibra,* fiber, + G. *sarx,* flesh, + *-ōma,* tumor]

**myx·o·chon·dro·ma** (mik'sō-kon-drō'mă) a benign neoplasm of cartilaginous tissue in which the stroma resembles primitive mesenchymal tissue. [myxo- + G. *chondros,* cartilage, + *-ōma,* tumor]

**myx·o·cyte** (mik'sō-sīt) one of the stellate or polyhedral cells present in mucous tissue. [myxo- + G. *kytos,* cell]

**my·xo·e·de·ma [Br.]** SEE myxedema.

**myx·o·fi·bro·ma** (mik'sō-fī-brō'mă) a benign neoplasm of fibrous connective tissue that resembles primitive mesenchymal tissue. [myxo- + L. *fibra,* fiber, + G. *-ōma,* tumor]

**myx·o·fi·bro·sar·co·ma** (mik'sō-fī'brō-sar-kō'mă) a malignant fibrous histiocytoma with a predominance of myxoid areas that resemble primitive mesenchymal tissue. [myxo- + L. *fibra,* fiber, + G. *sarx,* flesh, + *-ōma,* tumor]

**myx·oid** (mik'soyd) resembling mucus. [myxo- + G. *eidos,* resemblance]

**myx·oid cyst** SYN ganglion (2).

**myx·o·li·po·ma** (mik'sō-li-pō'mă) a benign neoplasm of adipose tissue in which portions of the tumor resemble mucoid mesenchymal tissue. [myxo- + G. *lipos,* fat, + *-ōma,* tumor]

**myx·o·ma** (mik-sō'mă) a benign neoplasm de-

rived from connective tissue, consisting of polyhedral and stellate cells embedded in a soft mucoid matrix; occurs in bone, skin, and muscle;
when arising from cardiac muscle may encroach
on the cavity of an atrium. [myxo- + G. -ōma,
tumor]

**myx·o·ma·to·sis** (mik′sō-mă-tō′sis) **1.** SYN mucoid degeneration. **2.** multiple myxomas.

**myx·o·ma·tous** (mik-sō′mă-tŭs) **1.** pertaining to
or characterized by the features of a myxoma. **2.**
said of tissue that resembles primitive mesenchymal tissue.

**myx·o·mem·bra·nous co·li·tis** SYN mucous colitis.

**myx·o·pap·il·lary ep·en·dy·mo·ma** a slow-
growing ependymoma of the filum terminale, oc-

curring most often in young adults, consisting of
cuboidal cells in papillary arrangement around a
mucinous vascular core.

**myx·o·pap·il·lo·ma** (mik′sō-pap-i-lō′mă) a benign neoplasm of epithelial tissue in which the
stroma resembles primitive mesenchymal tissue.
[myxo- + L. *papilla*, a nipple, + G. -ōma, tumor]

**myx·o·poi·e·sis** (mik′sō-poy-ē′sis) mucus production. [myxo- + G. *poiēsis*, a making]

**myx·o·sar·co·ma** (mik′sō-sar-kō′mă) a sarcoma,
usually a liposarcoma or malignant fibrous histiocytoma, with an abundant component of myxoid tissue resembling primitive mesenchyme
containing connective tissue mucin. [myxo- + G.
*sarx*, flesh, + -ōma, tumor]

# N

ν nu. SEE nu.

**n** nano- (2); reaction order.

**N** normal concentration. SEE normal (3).

***n* 1.** the number in a scientific study. Sample size. **2.** refractive index.

**N$_A$** Avogadro number.

**NA** Nomina Anatomica.

**na·both·i·an cyst** (nĕ-bō'thē-ăn) a retention cyst that develops when a mucous gland of the cervix uteri is obstructed; of no pathologic significance. SYN nabothian follicle.

**na·both·i·an fol·li·cle** (nĕ-bō'thē-ăn) SYN nabothian cyst.

**na·cre·ous** (nā'krē-ŭs) lustrous, like mother-of-pearl; descriptive term for bacterial colonies. [Fr. *nacre,* mother-of-pearl]

**NAD** nicotinamide adenine dinucleotide.

**NAD⁺** nicotinamide adenine dinucleotide (oxidized form).

**NADH** nicotinamide adenine dinucleotide (reduced form).

**NADH de·hy·dro·gen·ase** an iron-sulfur–containing flavoprotein reversibly oxidizing NADH to NAD⁺; an inherited deficiency of this complex results in overwhelming acidosis.

**NADP** nicotinamide adenine dinucleotide phosphate.

**NADP⁺** nicotinamide adenine dinucleotide phosphate (oxidized form).

**NADPH** nicotinamide adenine dinucleotide phosphate (reduced form).

**Nae·ge·li syn·drome** (nā'gĕ-lē) reticular skin pigmentation, diminished sweating, hypodontia, and hyperkeratosis of the palms and soles.

**nae·vus [Br.]** SEE nevus.

**Naff·zi·ger op·er·a·tion** (naf'zig-ĕr) orbital decompression for severe malignant exophthalmos by removal of the lateral and superior orbital walls.

**Nä·ge·le ob·liq·ui·ty** (nah-gĕ-lē) inclination of the fetal head in cases of flat pelvis, so that the biparietal diameter is oblique in relation to the plane of the pelvic brim, the anterior parietal bone presenting to the parturient canal.

**Nä·ge·le pel·vis** (nah-gĕ-lĕ) an obliquely contracted or unilateral synostotic pelvis, marked by arrest of development of one lateral half of the sacrum, usually ankylosis of the sacroiliac joint on that side, rotation of the sacrum toward the same side, and deviation of the symphysis pubis to the opposite side.

**Nä·ge·le rule** (nah-gĕ-lē) determination of the estimated delivery date by adding 7 days to the first day of the last normal menstrual period, counting back 3 months, and adding 1 year.

**Na·gel test** (nah'gel) a test for color vision in which the observer determines the relative amounts of red and green necessary to match spectral yellow; an instrument called the Nagel anomaloscope is used.

**nail** (nāl) **1.** one of the thin, horny, translucent plates covering the dorsal surface of the distal end of each terminal phalanx of fingers and toes. A nail consists of corpus or body, the visible part, and radix or root at the proximal end concealed under a fold of skin. The under part of the nail is formed from the stratum germinativum of the epidermis, the free surface from the stratum lucidum, the thin cuticular fold overlapping the lunula representing the stratum corneum. **2.** a slender rod of metal, bone, or other solid substance, used in operations to fasten together the divided extremities of a broken bone. SYN unguis [TA], nail plate, onyx. [A.S. *naegel*]

**nail bed** the area of the corium on which the nail rests; it is extremely sensitive and presents numerous longitudinal ridges on its surface. SYN keratogenous membrane, matrix unguis.

**nail fold** the fold of skin overlapping the lateral and proximal margins of the nail.

**nail pits** small punctate depressions on the surface of the nail plate due to defective nail formation; seen in psoriasis and other disorders.

**nail plate** SYN nail.

**Nair buf·fered meth·y·lene blue stain** (nār) stain used to show nuclear detail of protozoan trophozoites when used at low pH (3.6–4.8).

**Na·ka·ni·shi stain** (nah-kah-nish-ē) a method for vital staining of bacteria in which a slide is treated with hot methylene blue solution until it acquires a sky-blue color, after which a drop of an emulsion of the bacteria is put on the cover glass and the latter laid on the slide; the bacteria are stained differentially, some parts more intensely than others.

**na·ked vi·rus** a virus consisting only of a nucleocapsid; i.e., one that does not possess an enclosing envelope.

**Nance-In·sley syn·drome** (nans-ins'lē) SYN chondrodystrophy with sensorineural deafness.

**Nance-Swee·ney chon·dro·dys·pla·sia** (nans-swē'nē) SYN chondrodystrophy with sensorineural deafness.

**nan·ism** (nan'izm) dwarfism. [G. *nanos;* L. *nanus,* dwarf]

△**nano-** **1.** dwarfism (nanism). **2. (n)** prefix used in the SI and metric systems to signify one-billionth ($10^{-9}$). [G. *nanos,* dwarf]

**nan·o·ceph·a·lous, nan·o·ce·phal·ic** (nan-ō-sef'ă-lŭs, nan-ō-se-fal'ik) SYN microcephalic.

**nan·o·ceph·a·ly** (nan-ō-sef'ă-lē) SYN microcephaly. [nano- + G. *kephalē,* head]

**nan·o·cor·mia** (nan-ō-kōr'mē-ă) SYN microsomia. [nano- + G. *kormos,* trunk]

**nan·o·gram (ng)** (nan'ō-gram) one-billionth of a gram ($10^{-9}$ g).

**nan·o·me·lia** (nan-ō-mē'lē-ă) SYN micromelia. [nano- + G. *melos,* limb]

**nan·o·me·ter (nm)** (năn-om'ĕ-ter) one-billionth of a meter ($10^{-9}$ m).

**nan·o·me·tre [Br.]** SEE nanometer.

**nape** (nāp) SYN nucha.

**naph·thol yel·low S** [CI 10316] an acid dye used as a stain for basic proteins in microspectrophotometry.

**nar·cis·sism** (nar-sis'izm, nar'si-sizm) **1.** sexual attraction toward one's own person. **2.** a state in which the individual interprets and regards everything in relation to himself or herself and not to other persons or things. SYN self-love. [*Narkissos,* G. myth. char.]

△**nar·co-** stupor, narcosis. [G. *narkoō,* to benumb, deaden]

**nar·co·a·nal·y·sis** (nar'kō-ă-nal'i-sis) psychotherapeutic treatment under light anesthesia. SYN narcosynthesis.

**nar·co·hyp·nia** (nar-kō-hip'nē-ă) a general

numbness sometimes experienced at the moment of waking. [narco- + G. *hypnos,* sleep]

**nar·co·hyp·no·sis** (nar′kō-hip-nō′sis) stupor or deep sleep induced by hypnosis. [narco- + G. *hypnos,* sleep]

**nar·co·lep·sy** (nar′kō-lep-sē) a sleep disorder that usually appears in young adulthood, consisting of recurring episodes of sleep during the day, and often disrupted nocturnal sleep; frequently accompanied by cataplexy, sleep paralysis, and hypnagogic hallucinations; a genetically determined disease. SYN Gélineau syndrome. [narco- + G. *lēpsis,* seizure]

**nar·co·sis** (nar-kō′sis) general and nonspecific reversible depression of neuronal excitability, produced by a number of physical and chemical agents, usually resulting in stupor rather than in anesthesia (with which narcosis was once synonymous). [G. a benumbing]

**nar·co·syn·the·sis** (nar-kō-sin′thĕ-sis) SYN narcoanalysis.

**nar·co·ther·a·py** (nar-kō-thār′ă-pē) psychotherapy conducted with the patient under the influence of a sedative or narcotic.

**nar·cot·ic** (nar-kot′ik) **1.** any drug derived from opium or opium-like compounds with potent analgesic effects associated with both significant alteration of mood and behavior and potential for dependence and tolerance. **2.** any drug, synthetic or naturally occurring, with effects similar to those of opium and opium derivatives. **3.** capable of inducing a state of stuporous analgesia. [G. *narkōtikos,* benumbing]

**nar·cot·ic block·ade** the use of drugs to inhibit the effects of narcotic substances, as with naloxone.

**nar·cot·ic re·ver·sal** the use of narcotic antagonists, such as naloxone, to terminate the action of narcotics.

**na·ris,** pl. **na·res** (nā′ris, nā′rēz) SYN nostril. [L.]

**NARP** *n*europathy, *a*taxia, *r*etinitis *p*igmentosa syndrome, one of the inherited mitochondrial disorders, caused by a point mutation resulting in the substitution of a single amino acid in the mitochondrial DNA at position 8993. A more severe expression of the same point mutation manifests clinically as Leigh disease.

**nar·row-an·gle glau·co·ma** SYN angle-closure glaucoma.

**nar·row·band** a limited band of sound frequencies, as opposed to the wideband of frequencies also known as white noise; used to mask hearing in the nontest ear in hearing measurement.

**na·sal** (nā′zăl) relating to the nose. SYN rhinal. [L. *nasus,* nose]

**na·sal bone** an elongated rectangular bone which, with its fellow, forms the bridge of the nose; it articulates with the frontal bone superiorly, the ethmoid and the frontal process of the maxilla posteriorly, and its fellow medially. SYN os nasale [TA].

**na·sal cap·sule** the cartilage around the developing nasal cavity of the embryo.

**na·sal cav·i·ty** the cavity on either side of the nasal septum, lined with ciliated respiratory mucosa, extending from the naris anteriorly to the choana posteriorly, and communicating with the paranasal sinuses through their orifices in the lateral wall, from which also project the three conchae; the cribriform plate, through which the olfactory nerves are transmitted, forms the roof; the floor is formed by the hard palate.

**na·sal crest** the midline ridge in the floor of the nasal cavity, formed by the union of the paired maxillae and palatine bones; the vomer attaches to the crest.

**na·sal emis·sion** SPEECH PATHOLOGY the sound of air forcefully flowing through the nose during speech (as opposed to nasal resonance), usually due to poor valving between the oral and nasal cavities, as in cleft palate. SEE hypernasality. SYN nasal escape, snorting.

**na·sal es·cape** SYN nasal emission.

**na·sa·lis mus·cle** compound muscle consisting of: a transverse part (pars transversa musculi nasalis [NA], musculus compressor naris) arising from the maxilla above the root of the canine tooth on each side and forming an aponeurosis across the bridge of the nose; and an alar part (pars alaris musculi nasalis [NA], musculus dilator naris) arising from the maxilla above the lateral incisor and attaching to the wing of the nose; the alar part dilates the nostril; *nerve supply,* facial. SYN musculus nasalis [TA], nasal muscle.

**na·sal me·a·tus** the three passages (inferior, middle, superior) in the nasal cavity formed by the projection of the conchae. SYN meatus nasi.

**na·sal mus·cle** SYN nasalis muscle.

**na·sal pits** the paired depressions formed when the nasal placodes come to lie below the general external contour of the developing face as a result of the rapid growth of the adjacent nasal elevations; the pits are the primordia of the rostral portions of the nasal chambers.

**na·sal point** SYN nasion.

**na·sal re·flex** sneezing caused by irritation of the nasal mucous membrane.

**na·sal sep·tal car·ti·lage** a thin cartilaginous plate located between vomer, perpendicular plate of the ethmoid, and nasal bones, and completing the nasal septum anteriorly.

**na·sal sep·tum** the wall dividing the nasal cavity into halves; it is composed of a central supporting skeleton covered on each side by a mucous membrane.

**na·sal spine of fron·tal bone** a projection from the center of the nasal part of the frontal bone, which lies between and articulates with the nasal bones and the perpendicular plate of the ethmoid.

**nasal spines** spina nasalis anterior, posterior, and ossis frontalis.

**nas·cent** (nas′ent, nā′sent) **1.** beginning; being born or produced. **2.** denoting the state of a chemical element at the moment it is set free from one of its compounds. [L. *nascor,* pres. p. *nascens,* to be born]

**na·si·on** (nā′zē-on) [TA] a point on the skull corresponding to the middle of the nasofrontal suture. SYN nasal point. [L. *nasus,* nose]

△**na·so-** the nose. [L. *nasus*]

**na·so·an·tral** (nā′zō-an′trăl) relating to the nose and the maxillary sinus.

**na·so·cil·i·ary nerve** a branch of the ophthalmic nerve in the superior orbital fissure, passing through the orbit, giving rise to the communicating branch to the ciliary ganglion, the long ciliary nerves, and the posterior and anterior ethmoidal nerves, and terminating as the infratrochlear and nasal branches, which supply the mucous membrane of the nose, the skin of the tip of the nose, and the conjunctiva. SYN nervus nasociliaris [TA].

**na·so·fron·tal** (nā-zō-frŭn′tăl) relating to the nose and forehead, or to the nasal cavity and frontal sinuses.

**na·so·fron·tal vein** located in the anterior medial part of the orbit that connects the superior ophthalmic vein with the angular vein.

**na·so·gas·tric** (nā-zō-gas′trik) pertaining to or involving the nasal passages and the stomach, as in nasogastric intubation.

**na·so·gas·tric tube** a stomach tube passed through the nose.

**na·so·la·bi·al** (nā-zō-lā′bē-ăl) relating to the nose and upper lip. [naso- + L. *labium,* lip]

**na·so·la·bi·al lymph node** one of the facial lymph nodes located near the junction of the superior labial and facial arteries.

**na·so·lach·ry·mal [Br.]** SEE nasolacrimal.

**na·so·lac·ri·mal** (nā-zō-lak′ri-măl) relating to the nasal and the lacrimal bones, or to the nasal cavity and the lacrimal ducts.

**na·so·lac·ri·mal ca·nal** the bony canal formed by the maxilla, lacrimal bone, and inferior concha, which transmits the nasolacrimal duct from the orbit to the inferior meatus of the nose. SYN canalis nasolacrimalis [TA].

**na·so·lac·ri·mal duct** the passage leading downward from the lacrimal sac on each side to the anterior portion of the inferior meatus of the nose, through which tears are conducted into the nasal cavity.

**na·so·oral** (nā-zō-ō′răl) relating to the nose and mouth.

**na·so·pal·a·tine** (nā′zō-pal′ă-tēn) relating to the nose and the palate.

**na·so·pal·a·tine nerve** a branch from the pterygopalatine ganglion, passing through the sphenopalatine foramen, crossing to and then down the nasal septum, and through the incisive foramen to supply the mucous membrane of the hard palate. SYN nervus nasopalatinus [TA].

**na·so·pha·ryn·ge·al** (nā′zō-fă-rin′jē-ăl) relating to the nose or nasal cavity and the pharynx.

**na·so·pha·ryn·ge·al car·ci·no·ma** a squamous cell carcinoma arising from the surface epithelium of the nasopharynx; three histologic variants are recognized: keratinizing, nonkeratinizing, and undifferentiated carcinoma.

**na·so·pha·ryn·ge·al leish·man·i·a·sis** SYN mucocutaneous leishmaniasis.

**na·so·pha·ryn·go·la·ryn·go·scope** (nā′zō-fa-ring′gō-lā-ring′gō-skōp) an instrument, often of fiberoptic type, used to visualize the upper airways and pharynx.

**na·so·pha·ryn·gos·co·py** (nā′zō-fa-ring-gos′kŏ-pē) examination of the nasopharynx by flexible or rigid optical instruments, or with a mirror. [nasopharynx + G. *skopeō,* to view]

**na·so·pha·rynx** (nā′zō-far′ingks) the part of the pharynx that lies above the soft palate; anteriorly it opens into the nasal cavity; inferiorly, it communicates with the oropharynx via the pharyngeal isthmus; laterally it communicates with tympanic cavities via auditory tubes. SYN epipharynx.

**na·so·si·nu·si·tis** (nā′zō-sī-nŭ-sī′tis) inflammation of the nasal cavities and of the accessory sinuses.

**na·so·tra·che·al tube** a tracheal tube inserted through the nasal passages.

**Nas·se law** (nah′sĕ) an early statement of the

pattern of X-linked recessive inheritance: hemophilia affects only boys but is transmitted through mothers and sisters.

**na·sus** (nā′sŭs) **1.** SYN external nose. **2.** SYN nose. [L.]

**na·tal** (nā′tăl) **1.** relating to birth. [L. *natalis,* fr. *nascor,* pp. *natus,* to be born] **2.** relating to the buttocks or nates. [L. *nates,* buttocks]

**na·tal·i·ty** (nā-tal′i-tē) the birth rate; the ratio of births to the general population. [see natal (1)]

**Na·tal sore** (nah-tahl′) lesion of cutaneous leishmaniasis.

**na·tal tooth** a deciduous tooth that is in the oral cavity at birth

**na·tes** (nā′tēz) [TA] SYN buttocks. [L. pl. of *natis*]

**na·ti·mor·tal·i·ty** (nā′ti-mōr-tal′i-tē) the perinatal death rate; the proportion of fetal and neonatal deaths to the general natality. [L. *natus,* birth, + *mortalitas,* fr. *mors,* death]

**Na·tion·al Com·mit·tee for Qual·i·ty As·su·rance (NCQA)** national independent nonprofit organization that evaluates managed care plans.

**Na·tion·al For·mu·lary** an official compendium formerly issued by the American Pharmaceutical Association but now published by the United States Pharmacopeial Convention for the purpose of providing standards and specifications that can be used to evaluate the quality of pharmaceuticals and therapeutic agents.

**na·trae·mia [Br.]** SEE natremia.

**na·tre·mia, na·tri·e·mia** (nā-trē′mē-ă, nā′trē-ē′mē-ă) the presence of sodium in the blood. [natrium, sodium, + G. *haima,* blood]

**na·trif·er·ic** (nā-trif′er-ik) tending to increase sodium transport. [natrium + L. *fero,* to carry]

**na·tri·um** (nā′trē-ŭm) SYN sodium. [Ar. *natrūm,* fr. G. *nitron,* carbonate of soda]

**na·tri·u·re·sis** (nā′trē-yu-rē′sis) urinary excretion of sodium; commonly designates enhanced sodium excretion, which may occur in certain diseases or as a result of the administration of diuretic drugs. [natrium + G. *ouron,* urine]

**na·tri·u·ret·ic** (nā′trē-yu-ret′ik) **1.** pertaining to or characterized by natriuresis. **2.** a substance that increases urinary excretion of sodium, usually as a result of decreased tubular reabsorption of sodium ions from glomerular filtrate.

*Nat·tras·sia man·gi·fe·rae* a dematiaceous mold, previously known as *Hendersonula toruloidea,* that causes onychomycosis and phaeohyphomycosis. *Scytalidium dimidiatum* is a synanamorph.

**nat·u·ral an·ti·bo·dy** SYN normal antibody.

**nat·u·ral dyes** dyes obtained from animals or plants.

**nat·u·ral im·mu·ni·ty, non·spe·cif·ic im·mu·ni·ty** SYN innate immunity.

**nat·u·ral kil·ler cell leu·ke·mia** a leukemia originating from cells of natural killer cell origin; often associated with the presence of monoclonal Epstein-Barr virus infecting tumor cells; usually indicates a leukemic subtype of poor prognosis.

**nat·u·ral kil·ler cells** large granular lymphocytes which do not express markers of either T or B cell lineage. These cells kill target cells using antibody-dependent cell-mediated cytotoxicity. NK cells can also use perforin to kill cells in the absence of antibody. Killing may occur without previous sensitization. SYN NK cells.

**nat·u·ral pitch** SYN optimal pitch.

**nat•u•ral se•lec•tion** "survival of the fittest," the principle that in nature those individuals best able to adapt to their environment will survive and reproduce, while those less able will die without progeny; and the genes carried by the survivors will increase in frequency. This principle is heuristic rather than rigorous since it cannot be tested, the outcome being tautologous with the empirical definition of fitness.

**na•tur•o•path•ic** (nā′choor-ō-path′ik) relating to or by means of naturopathy.

**na•tur•op•a•thy** (nā-choor-op′ă-thē) a system of therapeutics in which neither surgical nor medicinal agents are used, dependence being placed only on natural (nonmedicinal) forces.

**nau•sea** (naw′zē-ă, naw′zhă) a feeling of being sick at the stomach; an inclination to vomit. [L. fr. G. *nausia*, seasickness, fr. *naus*, ship]

**nau•sea grav•i•dar•um** SYN morning sickness.

**nau•se•ant** (naw′zē-ănt) **1.** nauseating; causing nausea. **2.** an agent that causes nausea.

**nau•se•ate** (naw′zē-āt) to cause an inclination to vomit.

**nau•se•at•ed** (naw′zē-ā-ted) affected with nausea. SYN sick (2).

**nau•seous** (naw′zē-ŭs, naw′shŭs) causing nausea.

**Nau•ta stain** (now′tah) a stain for degenerating axons, with which they appear as fragmented and swollen fibers.

**na•vel** (nā′vel) SYN umbilicus. [A.S. *nafela*]

**na•vic•u•lar** (nă-vik′yu-lăr) SYN scaphoid. [L. *navicularis*, relating to shipping]

**na•vic•u•lar ab•do•men** SYN scaphoid abdomen.

**na•vic•u•lar bone** a bone of the tarsus on the medial side of the foot articulating with the head of the talus, the three cuneiform bones, and occasionally the cuboid.

**na•vic•u•lar fos•sa of u•re•thra** the terminal dilated portion of the urethra in the glans penis.

**navigator echo** a method of respiratory gating used in magnetic resonance imaging to limit respiratory motion artifact; a signal is derived from the top of the diaphragm, and image data are collected only when it is in a selected range.

**Nb** niobium.

**NCQA** National Committee for Quality Assurance.

**Nd** neodymium.

**NDT** neurodevelopmental treatment.

**Nd:YAG laser** laser in the infrared spectrum (1064 nm), with a greater depth of penetration than other lasers. [*Nd* (neodymium) + *Y*ttrium-*A*luminum-*Garnet*]

**Ne** neon.

**near point** that point in conjugate focus with the retina when the eye exerts maximal accommodation.

**near•sight•ed•ness** (nēr′sīt-ed-nes) SYN myopia.

**ne•ar•thro•sis** (nē-ar-thrō′sis) a new joint; e.g., a pseudarthrosis arising in an ununited fracture, or an artificial joint resulting from a total joint replacement operation. SYN neoarthrosis. [G. *neos*, new, + *arthrōsis*, a jointing]

**neb•u•la**, pl. **neb•u•lae** (neb′yu-lă, neb′yu-lē) **1.** a translucent foglike opacity of the cornea. **2.** a spray. [L. fog, cloud, mist]

**neb•u•liz•er** (neb′yu-līz-er) a device used to disperse liquid medication in a mist of extremely fine particles; useful in delivering medication to deeper parts of the respiratory tract. SEE ALSO atomizer, vaporizer.

**Ne•ca•tor** (nē-kā′tŏr) a genus of nematode hookworms. Species include *Necator americanus*, the New World hookworm; the adults of this species attach to villi in the small intestine and suck blood, causing abdominal discomfort, diarrhea and cramps, anorexia, loss of weight, and hypochromic microcytic anemia. SEE ALSO *Ancylostoma*. [L. a murderer]

**ne•ca•to•ri•a•sis** (nē-kā-tō-rī′ă-sis) hookworm disease caused by *Necator*, the resulting anemia being usually less severe than that from ancylostomiasis.

**neck** (nek) **1.** part of body by which the head is connected to the trunk: it extends from the base of the cranium to the top of the shoulders. **2.** in anatomy, any constricted portion having a fancied resemblance to the neck of an animal. **3.** the germinative portion of an adult tapeworm which develops the segments or proglottids; the region of cestode segmentation behind the scolex. SYN cervix (1), collum. [A.S. *hnecca*]

**neck of glans** a constriction behind the corona of the glans penis.

**neck•lace** (nek′lăs) term used to describe a rash that encircles the neck.

**neck of pan•cre•as** segment of pancreas, approximately 2 cm long, connecting head and body of pancreas; it intervenes between the duodenum anteriorly and the junction of the splenic and superior mesenteric veins, forming the beginning of the portal vein, posteriorly. SYN collum pancreaticus [TA].

**neck of u•ri•nary blad•der** the lowest part of the bladder formed by the junction of the fundus and the inferolateral surfaces.

**ne•cro-, necr-** death, necrosis. [G. *nekros*, corpse]

**nec•ro•bi•o•sis** (nek′rō-bī-ō′sis) **1.** physiologic or normal death of cells or tissues as a result of changes associated with development, aging, or use. **2.** necrosis of a small area of tissue. SYN bionecrosis. [necro- + G. *biōs*, life]

**nec•ro•bi•o•sis li•poi•di•ca, nec•ro•bi•o•sis li•poi•di•ca di•a•be•ti•co•rum** a condition often associated with diabetes, in which one or more yellow, atrophic lesions develop on the legs.

**nec•ro•bi•ot•ic** (nek′rō-bī-ot′ik) pertaining to or characterized by necrobiosis.

**nec•ro•cy•to•sis** (nek′rō-sī-tō′sis) abnormal death of cells [necro- + G. *kytos*, cell, + -*osis*, condition]

**nec•ro•gen•ic** (nek-rō-jen′ik) relating to, living in, or having origin in dead matter. [necro- + G. *genesis*, origin]

**nec•ro•gen•ic wart** SYN postmortem wart.

**ne•crol•o•gy** (ně-krol′ō-jē) the science of the collection, classification, and interpretation of mortality statistics. [necro- + G. *logos*, study]

**nec•rol•y•sis** (ně-krol′i-sis) necrosis and loosening of tissue. [necro- + G. *lysis*, loosening]

**nec•ro•ma•nia** (nek-rō-mā′nē-ă) **1.** a morbid tendency to dwell with longing on death. **2.** a morbid attraction to dead bodies. [necro- + G. *mania*, frenzy]

**ne•croph•a•gous** (ně-krof′ă-gŭs) **1.** living on carrion. **2.** SYN necrophilous. [necro- + G. *phagō*, to eat]

**nec•ro•phil•ia, ne•croph•i•lism** (nek-rō-fil′ē-ă, ně-krof′i-lizm) **1.** a morbid fondness for being in the presence of dead bodies. **2.** the impulse to have sexual contact, or the act of such contact, with a dead body, usually of males with female corpses. [necro- + G. *phileō,* to love]

**ne·croph·i·lous** (ně-krof′i-lŭs) having a preference for dead tissue; denoting certain bacteria. SYN necrophagous (2). [necro- + G. *philos,* fond]

**nec·ro·pho·bia** (nek-rō-fō′bē-ă) morbid fear of corpses. [necro- + G. *phobos,* fear]

**ne·crop·sy** (nek′rop-sē) SYN autopsy. [necro- + G. *opsis,* view]

**ne·crose** (ně-krōs′) **1.** to cause necrosis. **2.** to become the site of necrosis.

**ne·cro·sis** (ně-krō′sis) pathologic death of one or more cells, or of a portion of tissue or organ, resulting from irreversible damage; earliest irreversible changes are mitochondrial, consisting of swelling and granular calcium deposits seen by electron microscopy; most frequent visible alterations are nuclear: pyknosis, shrunken and abnormally dark basophilic staining; karyolysis, swollen and abnormally pale basophilic staining; or karyorrhexis, rupture and fragmentation of the nucleus. After such changes, the outlines of individual cells are indistinct, and affected cells may become merged, sometimes forming a focus of coarsely granular, amorphous, or hyaline material. [G. *nekrōsis,* death, fr. *nekroō,* to make dead]

**nec·ro·sper·mia** (nek-rō-sper′mē-ă) a condition in which there are dead or immobile spermatozoa in the semen. [necro- + G. *sperma,* seed]

**ne·crot·ic** (ně-krot′ik) pertaining to or affected by necrosis.

**nec·rot·ic arach·ni·dism** systemic poisoning caused by spiders belonging to the genus *Loxosceles;* cutaneous necrosis develops at the bite site, with slow healing and possible disfigurement.

**ne·crot·ic cir·rho·sis** SYN postnecrotic cirrhosis.

**ne·crot·ic in·flam·ma·tion, nec·ro·tiz·ing in·· flam·ma·tion** an acute inflammatory reaction in which the predominant histologic change is rapid necrosis that occurs diffusely or extensively throughout the affected tissue.

**ne·crot·ic pulp** necrosis of the dental pulp which clinically does not respond to thermal stimulation; the tooth may be asymptomatic or sensitive to percussion and palpation. SYN dead pulp, nonvital pulp.

**nec·ro·tiz·ing ar·ter·i·o·li·tis** necrosis in the media of arterioles, characteristic of malignant hypertension. SYN arteriolonecrosis.

**nec·ro·tiz·ing en·ter·o·co·li·tis** extensive ulceration and necrosis of the ileum and colon in premature infants.

**nec·ro·tiz·ing ker·a·ti·tis** severe inflammation and destruction of corneal tissue that may be seen in response to herpes infection.

**nec·ro·tiz·ing ul·cer·a·tive gin·gi·vi·tis (NUG)** an acute or recurrent gingivitis of young and middle-aged adults characterized clinically by gingival erythema and pain, fetid odor, and necrosis and sloughing of interdental papillae and marginal gingiva which gives rise to a gray pseudomembrane; fever, regional lymphadenopathy, and other systemic manifestations also may be present. A fusiform bacillus and *Treponema vincentii* can be isolated from the gingival tissues in large numbers and are felt to play a significant but poorly defined role in the pathogenesis. SYN fusospirochetal gingivitis, trench mouth, ulcero-

membranous gingivitis, Vincent disease, Vincent infection.

**ne·crot·o·my** (ne-krot′ŏ-mē) **1.** SYN dissection. **2.** operation for the removal of a necrosed portion of bone (sequestrum). [necro- + G. *tomē,* cutting]

**ne·do·cro·mil** a nonbronchodilator, antiinflammatory, antiasthmatic drug that acts on the mast cells to inhibit the release of histamine.

**nee·dle** (nē′dl) **1.** a slender, solid, usually sharppointed instrument used for puncturing tissues, suturing, or passing a ligature around or through a vessel. **2.** a hollow needle used for injection, aspiration, biopsy, or to guide introduction of a catheter into a vessel or other space. **3.** to separate the tissues by means of one or two needles, in the dissection of small parts. **4.** to perform discission of a cataract by means of a knife needle. [M.E. *nedle,* fr. A.S. *nǣedl*]

**nee·dle bath** a bath in which water is projected forcibly against the body in many very fine jets.

⊞**nee·dle bi·op·sy** any method in which the specimen for biopsy is removed by aspirating it through an appropriate needle or trocar that pierces the skin, or the external surface of an organ. See page 117. SYN aspiration biopsy.

**nee·dle for·ceps** SYN needle-holder.

**nee·dle-hold·er, nee·dle-car·ri·er, nee·dle-driv·er** an instrument for grasping a needle in suturing. SYN needle forceps.

**nee·dling** (nēd′ling) discission of a soft or secondary cataract.

**NEEP** negative end-expiratory pressure.

**Neer im·pinge·ment sign** (nēr) pain produced by forceful maximum forward elevation of the upper extremity.

**ne·ga·tion** (ně-gā′shŭn) SYN denial.

**neg·a·tive** (neg′ă-tiv) **1.** not affirmative; refutative; not positive. **2.** MATHEMATICS having a value less than zero. **3.** PHYSICS, CHEMISTRY having an electric charge resulting from a gain or overabundance of electrons, hence able to donate (lose) electrons. **4.** MEDICINE denoting a response to a diagnostic maneuver or laboratory study that indicates the absence of the disease or condition tested for. [L. *negativus,* fr. *nego,* to deny]

**neg·a·tive ac·com·mo·da·tion** the decrease of accommodation that occurs when shifting from near vision to distance vision.

**neg·a·tive base ex·cess** a measure of metabolic acidosis; the amount of strong alkali that would have to be added per unit volume of whole blood to titrate it to pH 7.4 while at 37°C and at a carbon dioxide pressure of 40 mmHg.

**neg·a·tive con·ver·gence** the slight divergence of the visual axes when convergence is at rest, as when observing the far point or during sleep.

**neg·a·tive elec·trode** SYN cathode.

**neg·a·tive end-ex·pi·ra·to·ry pres·sure (NEEP)** a subatmospheric pressure at the airway at the end of expiration.

**neg·a·tive my·o·clon·ic seiz·ure** seizure characterized by abrupt, brief cessation of muscular activity, occasionally preceded by a single myoclonic contraction; term usually is applied to unilateral, distal muscles.

**neg·a·tive pres·sure ven·ti·la·tion** a mode of mechanical ventilation in which a positive transrespiratory pressure is generated by decreasing body surface pressure below the pressure at the airway opening.

**neg·a·tive sco·to·ma** a scotoma that appears as a blank or black patch in the visual field.

**neg·a·tive stain** stain forming an opaque or colored background against which the object to be demonstrated appears as a translucent or colorless area; in electron microscopy, an electron opaque material, such as phosphotungstic acid or sodium phosphotungstate, is used to give detail as to surface structure.

**neg·a·tive symp·tom** one of the deficit symptoms of schizophrenia that follow from diminished volition and executive function including inertia, anergia, lack of involvement with the environment, poverty of thought, social withdrawal, and blunted affect.

**neg·a·tiv·ism** (neg′ă-tiv-izm) a tendency to do the opposite of what one is requested to do, or to stubbornly resist for no apparent reason; seen in catatonic states and in toddlers.

**neg·a·tron** (neg′ă-tron) term used for an electron to emphasize its negative charge in contradistinction to the positive charge carried by the otherwise similar positron.

**ne·glect** in occupational therapy, the tendency to behave as if one side of the body and/or one side of space does not exist, with impairment of skilled or purposeful movements. There are two types of neglect: personal and spatial. SEE ALSO hemiapraxia.

**Ne·gri bo·dies** (nā′grē) eosinophilic, sharply outlined, pathognomonic inclusion bodies (2 to 10 μm in diameter) found in the cytoplasm of certain nerve cells containing the virus of rabies, especially in Ammon horn of the hippocampus.

*Neis·se·ria* (nī-se′rē-ă) a genus of aerobic to facultatively anaerobic bacteria containing Gram-negative cocci which occur in pairs with the adjacent sides flattened. [A. *Neisser*]

**neis·se·ria**, pl. **neis·se·ri·ae** (nī-se′rē-ă, nī-se′rē-ē) a vernacular term used to refer to any member of the genus *Neisseria*.

*Neis·se·ria gon·or·rhoe·ae* a species that causes gonorrhea and other infections in humans; the type species of the genus *Neisseria*. SYN gonococcus.

*Neis·se·ria me·nin·gi·ti·dis* a species found in the nasopharynx; the causative agent of meningococcal meningitis; virulent organisms are strongly Gram-negative and occur singly or in pairs; in the latter case the cocci are elongated and are arranged with long axes parallel and facing sides kidney-shaped; groups characterized by serologically specific capsular polysaccharides are designated by capital letters (the main serogroups being A, B, C, and D). SYN meningococcus.

**Né·la·ton cath·e·ter** (nā-lah-taw′) a flexible catheter of red rubber.

**Né·la·ton line** (nā-lah-taw′) a line drawn from the anterior superior iliac spine to the tuberosity of the ischium; normally the greater trochanter lies in this line, but in cases of iliac dislocation of the hip or fracture of the neck of the femur the trochanter is felt above the line.

**Nel·son syn·drome** (nel′son) a syndrome of hyperpigmentation, third nerve damage, and enlarging sella turcica caused by pituitary adenomas presumably present before adrenalectomy for Cushing syndrome but enlarging and symptomatic afterward. SYN postadrenalectomy syndrome.

**nem** a nutritional unit defined as 1 gram breast milk of specific nutritional components having a caloric value equivalent to ⅔ calorie. [Ger. *Nahrungseinheit Milch,* milk nutrition unit]

**nem·a·to·cyst** (nem′ă-tō-sist) a stinging cell of coelenterates consisting of a poison sac and a coiled barbed sting capable of being ejected and penetrating the skin of an animal on contact; of considerable consequence in large jellyfish and in the Portuguese man-of-war whose large numbers of these stinging cells can cause great pain and even death. [nemato- + G. *kystis,* bladder]

**Nem·a·to·da** (nem-ă-tō′dă) the roundworms, a large phylum that includes many of the helminths parasitic in man. Parasitic nematodes fall into two groups, the intestinal roundworms and the filarial roundworms of the blood, lymphatic tissues, and viscera. [nemat- + G. *eidos,* form]

**nem·a·tode** (nem′ă-tōd) a common name for any roundworm of the phylum Nematoda.

**nem·a·to·di·a·sis** (nem′ă-tō-dī′ă-sis) infection with nematode parasites.

**nem·a·toid** (nem′ă-toyd) **1.** resembling a thread. **2.** relating to nematodes.

△**neo-** new, recent. [G. *neos*]

**ne·o·ad·ju·vant** (nē-ō-ad′joo-vant) chemotherapy or radiation given before cancer surgery. [neo- + adjuvant]

**ne·o·an·ti·gens** (nē-ō-an′ti-jenz) SYN tumor antigens.

**ne·o·ar·thro·sis** (nē-ō-ar-thrō′sis) SYN nearthrosis.

**ne·o·blad·der** (nē′ō-blad′er) surgically constructed replacement for urinary bladder, usually using stomach or intestine.

**ne·o·blas·tic** (nē-ō-blas′tik) developing in or characteristic of new tissue. [neo- + G. *blastos,* germ, offspring]

**ne·o·cer·e·bel·lum** (nē′ō-ser-ĕ-bel′ŭm) [TA] the larger lateral portion of the cerebellar hemisphere, receiving its dominant input from the pontine nuclei which, in turn, are dominated by afferent nerves from the cerebral cortex; phylogenetically of more recent origin than the archicerebellum and paleocerebellum the neocerebellum reaches its largest development in humans and other primates.

**ne·o·cys·tos·to·my** (nē′ō-sis-tos′tō-mē) an operation in which the ureter is implanted into the bladder. [neo- + G. *kystis,* bladder, + *stoma,* mouth]

**ne·o·cyte** (nē′ō-sīt) a new cell; cell recently released into the peripheral blood from the bone marrow. SEE reticulocyte. [neo- + -cyte]

**ne·o·dym·i·um** (Nd) (nē-ō-dim′ē-ŭm) one of the rare earth elements; atomic no. 60, atomic wt. 144.24. [*neo-,* new, + G. *didymos,* twin (of lanthanum)]

**ne·o·gen·e·sis** (nē-ō-jen′ĕ-sis) SYN regeneration (1). [neo- + G. *genesis,* origin]

**ne·o·ge·net·ic** (nē′ō-je-net′ik) pertaining to or characterized by neogenesis.

**ne·o·ki·net·ic** (nē′ō-ki-net′ik) denoting one of the divisions of the motor system, the function of which is the transmission of isolated synergic movements of voluntary origin; it represents a more highly specialized form of movement than the paleokinetic function. [neo- + G. *kinētikos,* relating to movement]

**ne·ol·o·gism** (nē-ol′ō-jizm) a new word or phrase of the patient's own making often seen in schizophrenia (e.g., headshoe to mean hat), or an existing word used in a new sense; in psychiatry, such usages may have meaning only to the patient or be indicative of the underlying condition. [neo- + G. *logos,* word]

**ne•o•mem•brane** (nē-ō-mem'brān) SYN false membrane.

**ne•on (Ne)** (nē'on) an inert gaseous element in the atmosphere; atomic no. 10, atomic wt. 20.1797. [G. *neos,* new]

**ne•o•na•tal** (nē-ō-nā'tăl) relating to the period immediately succeeding birth and continuing through the first 28 days of life. SYN newborn. [neo- + L. *natalis,* relating to birth]

**ne•o•na•tal a•ne•mia** SYN erythroblastosis fetalis.

**ne•o•na•tal di•ag•no•sis** systematic evaluation of the newborn for evidence of disease or malformations, and the conclusion reached.

**ne•o•na•tal hep•a•ti•tis** hepatitis in the neonatal period due to a variety of causes, chiefly viral.

**ne•o•na•tal her•pes** herpes simplex virus type 1 or 2 infection transmitted from the mother to the newborn infant, often during passage through an infected birth canal.

**ne•o•na•tal hy•per•bil•i•ru•bi•ne•mia** serum bilirubin greater than 12.9 mg/dl (220 μol/L) or rising at a rate greater than 5 mg/dl per day; also applied to a nonphysiologic pattern of hyperbilirubinemia, i.e., jaundice in the first 24 hours of life or extending beyond the first week of life in term infants.

**ne•o•na•tal med•i•cine** SYN neonatology.

**ne•o•na•tal mor•tal•i•ty rate** the number of deaths in the first 28 days of life divided by the number of live births occurring in the same population during the same period of time.

**ne•o•na•tal tet•a•ny** hypocalcemic tetany occurring in neonates or young infants, due to transient functional hypoparathyroidism in consumption of cow's milk (high phosphorus content). SYN tetanism.

**ne•o•nate** (nē'ō-nāt) a newborn infant. SYN newborn. [neo- + L. *natus,* born, fr. *nascor,* to be born]

**ne•o•na•tol•o•gist** (nē'ō-nā-tol'ō-jist) one who specializes in neonatology.

**ne•o•na•tol•o•gy** (nē'ō-nā-tol'ō-jē) the pediatric subspecialty concerned with disorders of the neonate. SYN neonatal medicine. [neo- + L. *natus,* pp. born, + G. *logos,* theory]

**ne•o•neu•rot•i•za•tion** (nē-ō-noo-rot'ĭ-zā'shŭn) rarely observed phenomenon of return of facial motor function following deliberate transection of the facial nerve; believed to represent trigeminal reinnervation of the facial muscles.

**ne•o•pla•sia** (nē-ō-plā'zē-ă) the pathologic process that results in the formation and growth of a neoplasm. [neo- + G. *plasis,* a molding]

**ne•o•plasm** (nē'ō-plazm) an abnormal tissue that grows by cellular proliferation more rapidly than normal and continues to grow after the stimuli that initiated the new growth cease. Neoplasms show partial or complete lack of structural organization and functional coordination with the normal tissue, and usually form a distinct mass of tissue which may be either benign (benign tumor) or malignant (cancer). SYN tumor (2). [neo- + G. *plasma,* thing formed]

**ne•o•plas•tic** (nē-ō-plas'tik) pertaining to or characterized by neoplasia, or containing a neoplasm.

**ne•op•ter•in** (nē-op'tĕ-rin) a pteridine present in body fluids; elevated levels result from immune system activation, malignant disease, allograft rejection, and viral infections (especially as in AIDS). [neo- + G. *pteron,* wing, + -in]

**ne•o•stri•a•tum** (nē-ō-strī-ā'tŭm) the caudate nucleus and putamen considered as one and distinguished from the globus pallidus (paleostriatum).

**ne•o•thal•a•mus** (nē-ō-thal'ă-mŭs) the portion of the thalamus projecting to the neocortex.

**ne•o•vas•cu•lar•i•za•tion** (nē'ō-vas'kyu-lar-i-zā'shŭn) proliferation of blood vessels in tissue not normally containing them, or proliferation of blood vessels of a different kind than usual in tissue.

**ne•per (Np)** a unit for comparing the magnitude of two powers, usually in electricity or acoustics; it is one half of the natural logarithm of the ratio of the two powers. [fr. *neperus,* latinized form of (John) *Napier*]

**neph•e•lom•e•try** (nef-ĕ-lom'ĕ-trē) estimation of the number and size of particles in suspension by measurement of light scattered from a beam passed through the solution.

**ne•phral•gia** (ne-fral'jē-ă) pain in the kidney. [nephr- + G. *algos,* pain]

**ne•phrec•to•my** (ne-frek'tō-mē) removal of a kidney. [nephr- + G. *ektomē,* excision]

**neph•rel•co•sis** (nef-rel-kō'sis) ulceration of the mucous membrane of the pelvis or calices of the kidney. [nephr- + G. *helkōsis,* ulceration]

**neph•ric** (nef'rik) relating to the kidney. SYN renal.

**ne•phrit•ic** (ne-frit'ik) relating to or suffering from nephritis.

**ne•phrit•ic syn•drome** the clinical symptoms of acute glomerulonephritis, particularly hematuria, hypertension, and renal failure.

**ne•phri•tis,** pl. **ne•phrit•i•des** (ne-frī'tis, ne-frit'i-dēz) inflammation of the kidneys. [nephr- + G. *-itis,* inflammation]

**neph•rit•o•gen•ic** (nef'ri-tō-jen'ik) causing nephritis; said of conditions or agents. [nephritis + G. *genesis,* production]

⌂**ne•phro-, nephr-** the kidney. SEE ALSO reno-. [G. *nephros,* kidney]

**neph•ro•cal•ci•no•sis** (nef'rō-kal-si-nō'sis) a form of renal lithiasis characterized by diffusely scattered foci of calcification in the renal parenchyma; deposits of calcium phosphate, calcium oxalate monohydrate, and similar compounds are usually demonstrable radiologically. [nephro- + calcinosis]

**neph•ro•car•di•ac** (nef'rō-kar'dē-ak) SYN cardiorenal. [nephro- + G. *kardia,* heart]

**neph•ro•cele** (nef'rō-sēl) **1.** hernial displacement of a kidney. [nephro- + G. *kēlē,* hernia] **2.** in lower vertebrates, the developmental cavity connecting the myocele with the celom. [nephro- + G. *koilōma,* a hollow (celom)]

**neph•ro•cys•to•sis** (nef'rō-sis-tō'sis) formation of renal cysts. [nephro- + G. *kystis,* cyst, + -osis, condition]

**neph•ro•ge•net•ic, neph•ro•gen•ic** (nef'rō-jĕ-net'ik, nef'rō-jen'ik) developing into kidney tissue. [nephro- + G. *genesis,* origin]

**neph•ro•gen•ic di•a•be•tes in•sip•i•dus** diabetes insipidus due to inherited inability of the kidney tubules to respond to antidiuretic hormone.

**ne•phrog•e•nous** (ne-froj'ĕ-nŭs) developing from kidney tissue.

**neph•ro•gram** (nef′rō-gram) radiographic examination of the kidney after the intravenous injection of a water-soluble iodinated contrast material; also, the diffuse opacification of the renal parenchyma following such injection, an indication of renal blood flow and glomerular filtration. A persistent nephrogram indicates obstruction of kidney drainage.

**ne•phrog•ra•phy** (ne-frog′ră-fē) radiography of the kidney. [nephro- + G. *graphō*, to write]

**neph•roid** (nef′royd) kidney-shaped; resembling a kidney. SYN reniform. [nephro- + G. *eidos*, resemblance]

**neph•ro•li•thi•a•sis** (nef′rō-li-thī′ă-sis) presence of renal calculi. See this page.

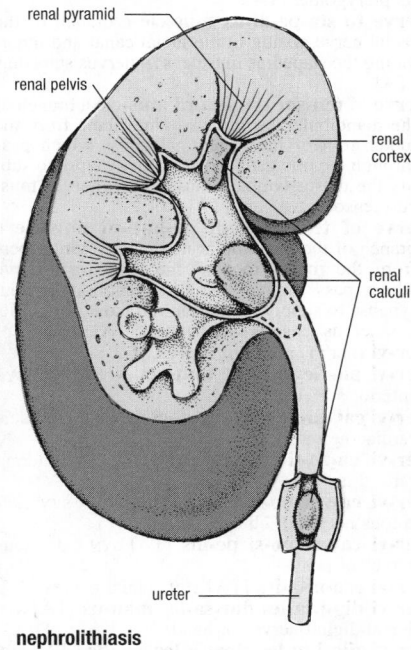

renal pyramid

renal pelvis

renal cortex

renal calculi

ureter

**nephrolithiasis**

**neph•ro•li•thot•o•my** (nef′rō-li-thot′ō-mē) incision into the kidney for the removal of a renal calculus. [nephro- + G. *lithos*, stone, + *tomē*, incision]

**ne•phrol•o•gy** (ne-frol′ō-jē) the branch of medical science concerned with medical diseases of the kidneys. [nephro- + G. *logos*, study]

**ne•phrol•y•sis** (ne-frol′i-sis) **1.** freeing of the kidney from inflammatory adhesions, with preservation of the capsule. **2.** destruction of renal cells. [nephro- + G. *lysis*, dissolution]

**neph•ro•lyt•ic** (nef-rō-lit′ik) pertaining to, characterized by, or causing nephrolysis. SYN nephrotoxic (2).

**ne•phro•ma** (ne-frō′mă) a tumor arising from renal tissue. [nephro- + G. *-oma*, tumor]

**neph•ro•meg•a•ly** (nef-rō-meg′ă-lē) extreme hypertrophy of one or both kidneys. [nephro- + G. *megas*, great]

**neph•ron** (nef′ron) a long convoluted tubular structure in the kidney, consisting of the renal corpuscle, the proximal convoluted tubule, the nephronic loop, and the distal convoluted tubule. [G. *nephros*, kidney]

**neph•ron•ic loop** the U-shaped part of the nephron extending from the proximal to the distal convoluted tubules, consisting of descending and ascending limbs, located in the medulla renalis and medullary ray. SYN Henle ansa, Henle loop.

**neph•ro•path•ia** (nef′rō-path′ē-ă) SYN nephropathy.

**ne•phrop•a•thy** (ne-frop′ă-thē) any disease of the kidney. SYN nephropathia, nephrosis (1). [nephro- + G. *pathos*, suffering]

**neph•ro•pexy** (nef′rō-pek-sē) operative fixation of a floating or mobile kidney. [nephro- + G. *pēxis*, fixation]

**neph•roph•thi•sis** (nef-rof′thĭ-sis, nef-rof′tĭ-sis) **1.** suppurative nephritis with wasting of the substance of the organ. **2.** tuberculosis of the kidney. [nephro- + G. *phthisis*, a wasting]

**neph•rop•to•sis, neph•rop•to•sia** (nef-rop-tō′sis, nef-rop-tō′sē-ă) prolapse of the kidney. [nephro- + G. *ptōsis*, a falling]

**neph•ro•py•o•sis** (nef′rō-pī-ō′sis) SYN pyonephrosis. [nephro- + G. *pyōsis*, suppuration]

**neph•ror•rha•phy** (nef-rōr′ă-fē) nephropexy by suturing the kidney. [nephro- + G. *rhaphē*, a suture]

**neph•ro•scle•ro•sis** (nef′rō-skle-rō′sis) induration of the kidney from overgrowth and contraction of the interstitial connective tissue. [nephro- + G. *sklērōsis*, hardening]

**neph•ro•scle•rot•ic** (nef′rō-skle-rot′ik) pertaining to or causing nephrosclerosis.

**neph•ro•scope** (nef′rō-skōp) an endoscope passed into the renal pelvis to view it. Route of access may be percutaneous, through a surgically exposed kidney, or retrograde via the ureter.

**ne•phro•sis** (ne-frō′sis) **1.** SYN nephropathy. **2.** degeneration of renal tubular epithelium. **3.** SYN nephrotic syndrome. [nephro- + G. *-osis*, condition]

**ne•phros•to•gram** (ne-fros′tō-gram) a radiograph of the kidney after opacification of the renal pelvis by injecting a contrast agent through a nephrostomy tube. [nephrostomy + G. *gramma*, writing]

**ne•phros•to•my** (ne-fros′tō-mē) establishment of an opening between the pelvis of the kidney through its cortex to the exterior of the body. [nephro- + G. *stoma*, mouth]

**ne•phros•to•my tube** a tube placed in the renal collecting system for drainage, diagnostic tests, or removal of calculi. May be placed through a percutaneous route or during an open surgical procedure.

**neph•rot•ic** (nef-rot′ik) relating to, caused by, or similar to nephrosis.

**neph•rot•ic syn•drome** a clinical state characterized by edema, albuminuria, decreased plasma albumin, doubly refractile bodies in the urine, and usually increased blood cholesterol; lipid droplets may be present in the cells of the renal tubules, but the basic lesion is increased permeability of the glomerular capillary basement membranes, of unknown cause or resulting from glomerulonephritis, diabetic glomerulosclerosis, systemic lupus erythematosus, amyloidosis, renal vein thrombosis, or hypersensitivity to various toxic agents. SYN nephrosis (3).

**neph•ro•to•mo•gram** (nef-rō-tō′mō-gram) a tomographic examination of the kidneys following the intravenous administration of water-soluble iodinated contrast material. [nephro- + G. *tomos*, a cutting + *gramma*, a writing]

**neph·ro·to·mog·ra·phy** (nef′rō-tō-mog′ră-fē) tomographic examination of the kidney.

**ne·phrot·o·my** (ne-frot′ō-mē) incision into the kidney. [nephro- + G. *tomē*, incision]

**neph·ro·tox·ic** (nef-rō-tok′sik) **1.** pertaining to nephrotoxin; toxic to renal cells. **2.** SYN nephrolytic.

**neph·ro·tox·ic·i·ty** (nef′rō-tok-sis′i-tē) the quality or state of being toxic to kidney cells.

**neph·ro·tox·in** (nef-rō-tok′sin) a cytotoxin that is specific for cells of the kidney.

**neph·ro·tro·phic** (nef-rō-trof′ik) SYN renotrophic.

**neph·ro·tro·pic** (nef-rō-trop′ik) SYN renotrophic.

**neph·ro·tu·ber·cu·lo·sis** (nef′rō-too-ber-kyu-lō′sis) tuberculosis of the kidney.

**neph·ro·u·re·ter·ec·to·my** (nef′rō-yu-rē′ter-ek′tō-mē) surgical removal of a kidney and its ureter. SYN ureteronephrectomy. [nephro- + ureter + G. *ektomē*, excision]

**neph·ro·u·re·ter·o·cys·tec·to·my** (nef′rō-yu-rē′ter-ō-sis-tek′tō-mē) removal of kidney, ureter, and part or all of the bladder. [nephro- + ureter + G. *kystis*, bladder, + *ektomē*, excision]

**Nep·tune gir·dle** (nep′toon) a wet pack applied around the abdomen.

**nep·tu·ni·um** (Np) (nep-too′nē-ŭm) a radioactive element; atomic no. 93; first element of the transuranian series (not found in nature); $^{237}$Np has a half-life of $2.14 \times 10^6$ years. [planet, *Neptune*]

**Néri sign** (nā′rē) in hemiplegia, the knee bends spontaneously when the leg is passively extended.

**Nernst e·qua·tion** (nernst) the equation relating the equilibrium potential of electrodes to ion concentrations; the equation relating the electrical potential and concentration gradient of an ion across a permeable membrane at equilibrium: $E = [RT / nF] [\ln (C_1/C_2)]$, where $E$ = potential, $R$ = absolute gas constant, $T$ = absolute temperature, $n$ = valence, $F$ = the Faraday, $\ln$ = the natural logarithm, and $C_1$ and $C_2$ are the ion concentrations on the two sides; in nonideal solutions, concentration should be replaced by activity. SEE ALSO activity (2).

**nerve** (nerv) a whitish cordlike structure composed of one or more bundles (fascicles) of myelinated or unmyelinated nerve fibers, or more often mixtures of both, coursing outside of the central nervous system, together with connective tissue within the fascicle and around the neurolemma of individual nerve fibers (endoneurium), around each fascicle (perineurium), and around the entire nerve and its nourishing blood vessels (epineurium), by which stimuli are transmitted from the central nervous system to a part of the body or the reverse. SYN nervus [TA]. [L. *nervus*]

**nerve a·vul·sion** the tearing away of a peripheral nerve at its point of origin from its parent nerve due to traction.

**nerve block** interruption of conduction of impulses in peripheral nerves or nerve trunks by injection of anesthetic.

**nerve block an·es·the·sia** conduction anesthesia in which local anesthetic solution is injected about nerves, nerve trunks, or nerve plexuses.

**nerve con·duc·tion** the transmission of an impulse along a nerve fiber.

**nerve de·com·pres·sion** release of pressure on a nerve trunk by the surgical excision of constricting bands or widening of a bony canal.

**nerve plex·us** a plexus formed by the interlacing of nerves by means of numerous communicating branches.

**nerve of pter·y·goid ca·nal** the nerve constituting the parasympathetic and sympathetic root of the pterygopalatine ganglion; it is formed in the region of the foramen lacerum by the union of the greater superficial petrosal and the deep petrosal nerves, and runs through the pterygoid canal to the pterygopalatine fossa. SYN nervus canalis pterygoidei [TA].

**nerve to sta·pe·di·us mus·cle** a branch of the facial nerve arising in the facial canal and innervating the stapedius muscle. SYN nervus stapedius [TA].

**nerve of ten·sor tym·pa·ni mus·cle** a branch of the mandibular nerve conveying fibers from the motor root of the trigeminal nerve which pass through the otic ganglion without synapse to supply the tensor tympani muscle. SYN nervus musculi tensoris tympani [TA].

**nerve of ten·sor ve·li pa·la·ti·ni mus·cle** a branch of the mandibular nerve conveying fibers from the motor root of the trigeminal nerve which pass through the otic ganglion without synapse to supply the tensor veli palatini muscle. SYN nervus tensoris veli palatini [TA].

**ner·vi** (ner′vī) plural of nervus. [L.]

**ner·vi au·ric·u·la·res an·te·ri·o·res** [TA] SYN anterior auricular nerves.

**ner·vi car·di·a·ci tho·ra·ci·ci** [TA] SYN thoracic cardiac nerves.

**ner·vi ca·ro·ti·ci ex·ter·ni** [TA] SYN external carotid nerves.

**ner·vi ca·ver·no·si cli·tor·i·dis** [TA] SYN cavernous nerves of clitoris.

**ner·vi ca·ver·no·si pe·nis** [TA] SYN cavernous nerves of penis.

**ner·vi cra·ni·a·les** [TA] SYN cranial nerves.

**ner·vi dig·i·ta·les dor·sa·les man·us** [TA] SYN dorsal digital nerves of hand.

**ner·vi dig·i·ta·les dor·sa·les pe·dis** [TA] SYN dorsal digital nerves of foot.

**ner·vi in·ter·cos·ta·les** [TA] SYN intercostal nerves.

**ner·vi in·ter·cos·to·bra·chi·a·les** [TA] SYN intercostobrachial nerves.

**ner·vi lum·ba·les** [TA] SYN lumbar nerves [L1–L5].

**ner·vi·mo·tor** (ner-vi-mō′ter) relating to a motor nerve. SYN neurimotor.

**ner·vi ol·fac·to·rii** [TA] SYN olfactory nerves [CN I].

**ner·vi pa·la·ti·ni mi·no·res** [TA] SYN lesser palatine nerves.

**ner·vi pe·ri·ne·al·es** [TA] SYN perineal nerves.

**ner·vi phren·i·ci ac·ces·so·rii** [TA] SYN accessory phrenic nerves.

**ner·vi pte·ry·go·pa·la·ti·ni** [TA] SYN ganglionic branches of maxillary nerve.

**ner·vi rec·ta·les in·fe·ri·o·res** [TA] SYN inferior rectal nerves.

**ner·vi sa·cra·les** [TA] SYN sacral nerves [S1–S5].

**ner·vi spi·na·les** [TA] SYN spinal nerves.

**ner·vi splanch·ni·ci lum·ba·les** [TA] SYN lumbar splanchnic nerves.

**ner·vi splanch·ni·ci sa·cra·les** [TA] SYN sacral splanchnic nerves.

**ner·vi tem·po·ra·les pro·fun·di** [TA] SYN deep temporal nerves.

**ner·vi ter·mi·na·les** [TA] SYN terminal nerves.

**ner·vi tho·ra·ci·ci [T1–12]** [TA] SYN thoracic nerves [T1–T12].

**ner·vi va·gi·na·les** [TA] SYN vaginal nerves.

**ner·von·ic ac·id** (ner-von'ik as'id) a 24-carbon straight-chain fatty acid unsaturated between C-15 and C-16; occurs in cerebrosides such as nervone.

**ner·vous** (ner'vŭs) **1.** relating to a nerve or the nerves. **2.** easily excited or agitated; suffering from mental or emotional instability; tense or anxious. **3.** formerly, denoting a temperament characterized by excessive mental and physical alertness, rapid pulse, excitability, often volubility, but not always fixity of purpose. [L. *nervosus*]

**ner·vous blad·der** a bladder condition in which there is a need to urinate frequently but with failure to empty the bladder completely.

**ner·vous break·down** nonmedical term for an emotional or mental illness; often a euphemism for a psychiatric disorder.

**ner·vous in·di·ges·tion** indigestion caused by emotional upsets or stress.

**ner·vous lobe of hy·poph·y·sis** the bulbous part of the neurohypophysis attached to the hypothalamus by the infundibulum. It is composed of pituicytes, blood vessels, and terminals of nerve fibers from the supraoptic and paraventricular nuclei.

**ner·vous·ness** (ner'vŭs-nes) a condition of being nervous (2).

**ner·vous sys·tem** the entire nerve apparatus, composed of a central part, the brain and spinal cord, and a peripheral part, the cranial and spinal nerves, autonomic ganglia, and plexuses.

**ner·vus,** gen. and pl. **ner·vi** (ner'vŭs, ner'vī) [TA] SYN nerve. [L.]

**ner·vus ab·du·cens [CN VI]** [TA] SYN abducent nerve [CN VI].

**ner·vus ac·ces·so·ri·us [CN XI]** [TA] SYN accessory nerve [CN XI].

**ner·vus al·ve·o·la·ris in·fe·ri·or** [TA] SYN inferior alveolar nerve.

**ner·vus a·no·coc·cyg·e·us** [TA] SYN anococcygeal nerve.

**ner·vus au·ric·u·la·ris mag·nus** [TA] SYN great auricular nerve.

**ner·vus au·ric·u·la·ris pos·te·ri·or** [TA] SYN posterior auricular nerve.

**ner·vus au·ric·u·lo·tem·po·ra·lis** [TA] SYN auriculotemporal nerve.

**ner·vus ax·il·la·ris** [TA] SYN axillary nerve.

**ner·vus buc·ca·lis** [TA] SYN buccal nerve.

**ner·vus ca·na·lis pte·ry·goi·dei** [TA] SYN nerve of pterygoid canal.

**ner·vus ca·ro·ti·cus in·ter·nus** [TA] SYN internal carotid nerve.

**ner·vus coc·cyg·e·us** [TA] SYN coccygeal nerve [Co].

**ner·vus dor·sa·lis cli·tor·i·dis** [TA] SYN dorsal nerve of clitoris.

**ner·vus dor·sa·lis pe·nis** [TA] SYN dorsal nerve of penis.

**ner·vus dor·sa·lis scap·u·lae** [TA] SYN dorsal scapular nerve.

**ner·vus fa·ci·a·lis [CN VII]** [TA] SYN facial nerve [CN VII].

**ner·vus fe·mo·ra·lis** [TA] SYN femoral nerve.

**ner·vus fron·ta·lis** [TA] SYN frontal nerve.

**ner·vus gen·i·to·fe·mo·ra·lis** [TA] SYN genitofemoral nerve.

**ner·vus glos·so·pha·ryn·ge·us [CN IX]** [TA] SYN glossopharyngeal nerve [CN IX].

**ner·vus hy·po·gas·tri·cus** [TA] SYN hypogastric nerve.

**ner·vus hy·po·glos·sus [CN XII]** [TA] SYN hypoglossal nerve [CN XII].

**ner·vus il·i·o·hy·po·gas·tri·cus** [TA] SYN iliohypogastric nerve.

**ner·vus il·i·o·in·gui·na·lis** [TA] SYN ilioinguinal nerve.

**ner·vus in·fra·or·bi·ta·lis** [TA] SYN infraorbital nerve.

**ner·vus in·fra·troch·le·a·ris** [TA] SYN infratrochlear nerve.

**ner·vus in·ter·me·di·us** [TA] SYN intermediary nerve.

**ner·vus in·ter·os·se·us an·te·bra·chii an·te··ri·or** [TA] SYN anterior interosseous nerve.

**ner·vus in·ter·os·se·us an·te·bra·chii pos·te··ri·or** [TA] SYN posterior interosseous nerve.

**ner·vus in·ter·os·se·us cru·ris** [TA] SYN crural interosseous nerve.

**ner·vus is·chi·a·di·cus** [TA] SYN sciatic nerve.

**ner·vus ju·gu·la·ris** [TA] SYN jugular nerve.

**ner·vus la·cri·ma·lis** [TA] SYN lacrimal nerve.

**ner·vus lin·gua·lis** [TA] SYN lingual nerve.

**ner·vus man·di·bu·la·ris [CN V3]** [TA] SYN mandibular nerve [CN V3].

**ner·vus mas·se·te·ri·cus** [TA] SYN masseteric nerve.

**ner·vus max·il·la·ris [CN V2]** [TA] SYN maxillary nerve [CN V2].

**ner·vus me·di·a·nus** [TA] SYN median nerve.

**ner·vus men·ta·lis** [TA] SYN mental nerve.

**ner·vus mus·cu·li ten·so·ris tym·pa·ni** [TA] SYN nerve of tensor tympani muscle.

**ner·vus mus·cu·lo·cu·ta·ne·us** [TA] SYN musculocutaneous nerve.

**ner·vus my·lo·hy·oi·de·us** [TA] SYN mylohyoid nerve.

**ner·vus na·so·cil·i·a·ris** [TA] SYN nasociliary nerve.

**ner·vus na·so·pal·a·ti·nus** [TA] SYN nasopalatine nerve.

**ner·vus ob·tu·ra·to·ri·us** [TA] SYN obturator nerve.

**ner·vus o·cu·lo·mo·to·ri·us [CN III]** [TA] SYN oculomotor nerve [CN III].

**ner·vus ol·fac·to·rii [CN I]** [TA] SYN olfactory nerves [CN I].

**ner·vus oph·thal·mi·cus [CN V1]** [TA] SYN ophthalmic nerve [CN V1].

**ner·vus op·ti·cus [CN II]** [TA] SYN optic nerve [CN II].

**ner·vus pal·a·ti·nus ma·jor** [TA] SYN greater palatine nerve.

**ner·vus phre·ni·cus** [TA] SYN phrenic nerve.

**ner·vus pte·ry·goi·de·us** [TA] SYN pterygoid nerve.

**ner·vus pu·den·dus** [TA] SYN pudendal nerve.

**ner·vus ra·di·a·lis** [TA] SYN radial nerve.

**ner·vus sac·cu·la·ris** [TA] SYN saccular nerve.

**ner·vus sa·phe·nus** [TA] SYN saphenous nerve.

**ner·vus splanch·ni·cus i·mus** [TA] SYN lowest splanchnic nerve.

**ner·vus splanch·ni·cus ma·jor** [TA] SYN greater splanchnic nerve.

**ner·vus splanch·ni·cus mi·nor** [TA] SYN lesser splanchnic nerve.

**ner·vus sta·pe·di·us** [TA] SYN nerve to stapedius muscle.

**ner·vus sub·cla·vi·us** [TA] SYN subclavian nerve.

**ner·vus sub·cos·ta·lis** [TA] SYN subcostal nerve.

**ner·vus sub·lin·gua·lis** [TA] SYN sublingual nerve.

**ner·vus sub·oc·cip·i·ta·lis** [TA] SYN suboccipital nerve.

**ner·vus su·pra·or·bi·ta·lis** [TA] SYN supraorbital nerve.

**ner·vus su·pra·scap·u·la·ris** [TA] SYN suprascapular nerve.

**ner·vus su·pra·troch·le·a·ris** [TA] SYN supratrochlear nerve.

**ner·vus su·ra·lis** [TA] SYN sural nerve.

**ner·vus ten·so·ris ve·li pa·la·ti·ni** [TA] SYN nerve of tensor veli palatini muscle.

**ner·vus tho·ra·ci·cus lon·gus** [TA] SYN long thoracic nerve.

**ner·vus tho·ra·co·dor·sa·lis** [TA] SYN thoracodorsal nerve.

**ner·vus tib·i·a·lis** [TA] SYN tibial nerve.

**ner·vus trans·ver·sus col·li** [TA] SYN transverse cervical nerve.

**ner·vus tri·gem·i·nus [CN V]** [TA] SYN trigeminal nerve [CN V].

**ner·vus troch·le·ar·is [CN IV]** [TA] SYN trochlear nerve [CN IV].

**ner·vus tym·pa·ni·cus** [TA] SYN tympanic nerve.

**ner·vus ul·na·ris** [TA] SYN ulnar nerve.

**ner·vus u·tri·cu·la·ris** [TA] SYN utricular nerve.

**ner·vus u·tri·cu·lo·am·pul·la·ris** [TA] SYN utriculoampullar nerve.

**ner·vus va·gus [CN X]** [TA] SYN vagus nerve [CN X].

**ner·vus ver·te·bra·lis** [TA] SYN vertebral nerve.

**ner·vus ves·ti·bu·lo·co·chle·a·ris [CN VIII]** [TA] SYN vestibulocochlear nerve [CN VIII].

**ner·vus zy·go·ma·ti·cus** [TA] SYN zygomatic nerve.

**nest** a group or collection of similar objects. SEE ALSO nidus. [A.S.]

**nest·ed pol·y·mer·ase chain re·ac·tion** use of the PCR in series, so that a specified piece of DNA is amplified, and then a portion contained within the first piece is amplified further; used where extremely low amounts of DNA are present, or where there are problems with background or contaminating DNA.

**net** SYN network (1).

**Neth·er·ton syn·drome** (neth′ĕr-tĕn) congenital ichthyosiform erythroderma or ichthyosis linearis circumscripta associated with bamboo hair, atopy, urticaria, intermittent aminoaciduria, and mental retardation; probably an autosomal recessive trait; frequently resolves or improves in adolescence.

**Net·tle·shop-Falls al·bin·ism** (net′ĕl-ship fahlz) SYN ocular albinism 1.

**net·work** (net′werk) **1.** a structure bearing a resemblance to a woven fabric. A network of nerve fibers or small vessels. SYN rete (1) [TA], net. SEE ALSO reticulum. **2.** the persons in a patient's environment, especially as significant for the course of the illness.

**net·work mod·el HMO** arrangement by which an HMO contracts with group practice physicians to be providers for HMO subscribers, with the physicians retaining the option to see other patients.

**Neu·feld cap·su·lar swell·ing** (noi-felt) increase in opacity and visibility of the capsule of capsulated organisms exposed to specific agglutinating anticapsular antibodies. SYN Neufeld reaction, quellung phenomenon, quellung reaction (1), quellung test.

**Neu·feld re·ac·tion** (noi-felt) SYN Neufeld capsular swelling.

**Neu·mann law** (noi′mahn) in compounds of analogous chemical constitution, the molecular heat, or the product of the specific heat and the atomic weight, is always the same.

⌂ **neur-, neuri-** nerve, nerve tissue, the nervous system. [G. neuron]

**neu·ral** (noor′ăl) **1.** relating to any structure composed of nerve cells or their processes, or that on further development will evolve into nerve cells. **2.** referring to the dorsal side of the vertebral bodies or their precursors, where the spinal cord is located, as opposed to hemal (2). [G. neuron, nerve]

**neu·ral arch** SYN vertebral arch.

**neu·ral crest** a band of neuroectodermal cells along either side of the line of closure of the embryonic neural groove; with the formation of the neural tube, these bands come to lie dorsolateral to the developing spinal cord and lateral to the brainstem, where they separate into clusters of cells that develop into, for example, spinal ganglion cells, autonomic ganglion cells, the chromaffin cells of the suprarenal (adrenal) medulla, Schwann cells, sensory ganglia of cranial nerves V, VII, VIII, IX, and X, part of the meninges, or integumentary pigment cells.

**neu·ral crest syn·drome** syndrome consisting of loss of pain sensibility, autonomic dysfunction, pupillary abnormalities, neurogenic anhidrosis, vasomotor instability, aplasia of dental enamel, meningeal thickening, hyperflexion, and a degree of albinism; may reflect developmental abnormalities of the neural crest.

**neu·ral folds** the elevated margins of the neural groove.

**neu·ral·gia** (noo-ral′jē-ă) pain of a severe, throbbing, or stabbing character in the course or distribution of a nerve. SYN neurodynia. [neur- + G. algos, pain]

**neu·ral·gia fa·ci·a·lis ve·ra** SYN geniculate neuralgia.

**neu·ral·gic** (noo-ral′jik) relating to, resembling, or of the character of, neuralgia.

**neu·ral·gic a·my·ot·ro·phy** a neurological disorder, of unknown cause, characterized by the sudden onset of severe pain, usually about the shoulder and often beginning at night, soon followed by weakness and wasting of various forequarter muscles, particularly shoulder girdle muscles; both sporadic and familial in occurrence with the former much more common; often preceded by some antecedent event, such as an upper respiratory infection, hospitalization, vaccination, or nonspecific trauma; usually attributed to a brachial plexus lesion, because the nerve fibers involved are most often derived from the upper trunk, but actually multiple proximal mononeuropathies. SYN shoulder-girdle syndrome.

**neu·ral groove** the gutter-like groove formed in the midline of the dorsal surface of the embryo by the progressive elevation of the lateral margins of the neural plate; the dorsal fusion of the margins results in the formation of the neural tube.

**neu·ral hear·ing loss** form of sensorineural hearing loss due to a lesion in the auditory division of the 8th cranial nerve.

**neu·ral plate** the unpaired neuroectodermal region on the dorsal surface of the early embryo that becomes the neural tube and neural crest. SYN medullary plate.

**neu·ral spine** the middle point of the neural arch of the typical vertebra, represented by the spinous process.

**neur·a·min·ic ac·id** (noor′ă-min′ik as′id) an aldol product of D-mannosamine and pyruvic acid. The *N*- and *O*-acyl derivatives of neuraminic acid are known as sialic acids and are constituents of gangliosides and of the polysaccharide components of muco- and glycoproteins from many tissues and secretions.

**neur·an·a·gen·e·sis** (noor′an-ă-jen′ĕ-sis) regeneration of a nerve. [neur- + G. *ana,* up, again, + *genesis,* origin]

**neur·a·poph·y·sis** (noor-ă-pof′i-sis) SYN lamina of vertebral arch. [neur- + G. *apophysis,* offshoot]

**neur·a·prax·ia** (noor-ă-prak′sē-ă) the mildest type of focal nerve lesion that produces clinical deficits; localized loss of conduction along a nerve without axon degeneration; caused by a focal lesion, usually demyelinating, and followed by a complete recovery. SEE ALSO axonotmesis. [neur- + G. a- priv. + *praxis,* action]

**neur·as·the·nia** (noor-as-thē′nē-ă) an ill-defined condition, commonly accompanying or following depression, characterized by vague fatigue believed to be brought on by psychological factors. [neur- + G. *astheneia,* weakness]

**neur·as·then·ic** (noor-as-then′ik) relating to, or suffering from, neurasthenia.

**neur·ax·is** (noo-rak′sis) the axial, unpaired part of the central nervous system: spinal cord, rhombencephalon, mesencephalon, and diencephalon, in contrast to the paired cerebral hemisphere, or telencephalon.

**neur·ec·ta·sis, neur·ec·ta·sia, neur·ec·ta·sy** (noo-rek′tă-sis, noor-ek-tā′zē-ă, noo-r-ek′tă-sē) the operation of stretching a nerve or nerve trunk. [neur- + G. *ektasis,* extension]

**neu·rec·to·my** (noo-rek′tō-mē) excision of a segment of a nerve. [neur- + G. *ektomē,* excision]

**neur·ec·to·pia, neur·ec·to·py** (noor-ek-tō′pē-ă, noor-ek′tō-pē) **1.** dislocation of a nerve trunk. **2.** a condition in which a nerve follows an anomalous course. [neur- + G. *ektopos,* fr. *ek,* out of, + *topos,* place]

**neur·en·ter·ic cysts** paravertebral cysts commonly connected to the meninges or a portion of the gastrointestinal tract that develop due to incomplete separation of endoderm from the notochord during early fetal life; often symptomatic.

**neu·rer·gic** (noo-rer′jik) relating to the activity of a nerve. [neur- + G. *ergon,* work]

**neur·ex·er·e·sis** (noor-ek-ser′ĕ-sis) tearing out or

evulsion of a nerve. [neur- + G. *exairesis,* a taking out, fr. *haireō,* to grasp, take]

**neu·ri·lem·ma** (noor-i-lem′ă) a cell that enfolds one or more axons of the peripheral nervous system; in myelinated fibers its plasma membrane forms the lamellae of myelin. SYN neurolemma, sheath of Schwann. [neuri + G. *lemma,* husk]

**neu·ri·lem·ma cells** SYN Schwann cells.

**neu·ri·le·mo·ma** (noor′i-lē-mō′mă) SYN schwannoma. [neurilemma + G. *-oma,* tumor]

**neu·ri·mo·tor** (noor-i-mō′ter) SYN nervimotor.

**neu·ri·no·ma** (noor-i-nō′mă) obsolete term for schwannoma.

**neu·rit·ic** (noo-rit′ik) relating to neuritis.

**neu·rit·ic plaque** SYN senile plaque.

**neu·ri·tis,** pl. **neu·ri·ti·des** (noo-rī′tis, noo-rit′i-dēz; noo-rit′i-dēz) **1.** inflammation of a nerve. **2.** SYN neuropathy. [neuri + G. *-itis,* inflammation]

△**neu·ro-** SEE neur-.

**neu·ro·an·as·to·mo·sis** (noor′ō-an-as-tō-mō′sis) surgical formation of a junction between nerves.

**neu·ro·a·nat·o·my** (noor′ō-ă-nat′ō-mē) the anatomy of the nervous system, usually specific to the central nervous system.

**neu·ro·ar·throp·a·thy** (noor′ō-ar-throp′ă-thē) a joint disorder caused by loss of joint sensation. SEE Charcot joint. [neuro- + G. *arthron,* joint, + *pathos,* suffering, disease]

**neu·ro·blast** (noor′ō-blast) an embryonic nerve cell. [neuro- + G. *blastos,* germ]

**neu·ro·blas·to·ma** (noor′ō-blas-tō′mă) a malignant neoplasm characterized by immature nerve cells of embryonic type, i.e., neuroblasts; the stroma is sparse and foci of necrosis and hemorrhage are not unusual. Neuroblastomas occur frequently in infants and children in the mediastinal and retroperitoneal regions; widespread metastases to the liver, lungs, lymph nodes, cranial cavity, and skeleton are very common.

**neu·ro·car·di·ac** (noor-ō-kar′dē-ak) **1.** relating to the nerve supply of the heart. **2.** relating to a cardiac neurosis. [neuro- + G. *kardia,* heart]

**neu·ro·chem·is·try** (noor-ō-kem′is-trē) the science concerned with the chemical aspects of nervous system structure and function.

**neu·ro·cho·ri·o·ret·i·ni·tis** (noor-ō-kōr′ē-ō-ret-in-ī′tis) inflammation of the choroid, the retina, and the optic nerve.

**neu·ro·cho·roi·di·tis** (noor′ō-kō-roy-dī′tis) inflammation of the choroid and the optic nerve.

**neu·roc·la·dism** (noo-rok′lă-dizm) the outgrowth of axons from the central stump to bridge the gap in a cut nerve. [neuro- + G. *klados,* a young branch]

**neu·ro·cra·ni·um** (noor-ō-krā′nē-ŭm) those bones of the skull enclosing the brain, as distinguished from the bones of the face. SYN braincase. [neuro- + G. *kranion,* skull]

**neu·ro·cris·top·a·thy** (noor′ō-kris-top′ă-thē) developmental anomaly of the neural crest manifested by abnormal development and tumors of the neural axis. [neuro- + L. *crista,* crest, + G. *pathos,* suffering]

**neu·ro·cyte** (noor′o-sīt) SYN neuron. [neuro- + G. *kytos,* cell]

**neu·ro·cy·tol·y·sis** (noor′ō-sī-tol′i-sis) destruction of neurons. [neuro- + G. *kytos,* cell, + *lysis,* dissolution]

**neu·ro·cy·to·ma** (noor′ō-sī-tō′mă) a tumor of neuronal differentiation usually intraventricular in location, consisting of sheets of cells with uniform nuclei and occasional perivascular pseudorosette formation. [neuro- + G. *kytos,* cell, + *-oma,* tumor]

**neu·ro·den·drite** (noor-ō-den'drīt) SYN dendrite (1).

**neu·ro·der·ma·ti·tis** (noor'ō-der-mă-tī'tis) a chronic lichenified skin lesion; loosely applied to atopic dermatitis. SYN neurodermatosis. [neuro- + G. *derma,* skin, + *-itis,* inflammation]

**neu·ro·der·ma·to·sis** (noor'ō-der-mă-tō'sis) SYN neurodermatitis.

**neu·ro·de·vel·op·men·tal treat·ment (NDT)** a therapeutic method involving hands-on intervention to facilitate normal movement patterns necessary for the acquisition of functional skills.

**neu·ro·dy·nam·ic** (noor'ō-dī-nam'ik) pertaining to nervous energy. [neuro- + G. *dynamis,* force]

**neu·ro·dyn·ia** (noor-ō-din'ē-ă) SYN neuralgia. [neuro- + G. *odynē,* pain]

**neu·ro·ec·to·derm** (noor-ō-ek'tō-derm) that central region of the early embryonic ectoderm that on further development forms the brain and spinal cord, and also evolves into the nerve cells and neurilemma or Schwann cells of the peripheral nervous system.

**neu·ro·ec·to·der·mal** (noor'ō-ek-tō-der'măl) relating to the neuroectoderm.

**neu·ro·en·ceph·a·lo·my·e·lop·a·thy** (noor'ō-en-sef'ă-lō-mī-ĕ-lop'ă-thē) disease of the brain, spinal cord, and nerves.

**neu·ro·en·do·crine** (noor-ō-en'dō-krin) **1.** pertaining to the anatomical and functional relationships between the nervous system and the endocrine apparatus. **2.** descriptive of cells that release a hormone into the circulating blood in response to a neural stimulus.

**neu·ro·en·do·crin·ol·o·gy** (noor-ō-en'dō-krin-ol'ō-jē) the specialty concerned with the anatomic and functional relationships between the nervous system and the endocrine apparatus.

**neu·ro·ep·i·the·li·al** (noor'ō-ep-i-thē'lē-ăl) relating to the neuroepithelium.

**neu·ro·ep·i·the·li·um** (noor'ō-ep-i-thē'lē-um) epithelial cells specialized for the reception of external stimuli, such as the hair cells of the inner ear, the receptor cells of the taste buds and the rods and cones of the retina.

**neu·ro·fi·bril** (noor-ō-fī'bril) a filamentous structure seen with the light microscope in the body, dendrites, axon, and sometimes synaptic endings of a nerve cell.

**neu·ro·fi·bril·lar** (noor-ō-fī'bri-lĕr) relating to neurofibrils.

**neu·ro·fi·bro·ma** (noor'ō-fī-brō'mă) a benign, encapsulated tumor resulting from proliferation of Schwann cells. SYN fibroneuroma.

**neu·ro·fi·bro·ma·to·sis** (noor'ō-fī-brō-mă-tō' sis) two distinct major hereditary disorders called type 1 and type 2. Type 1 (peripheral) neurofibromatosis, by far the more common, is characterized by patches of hyperpigmentation in both cutaneous and subcutaneous tumors. skin areas, present from birth, are called café-au-lait spots. The cutaneous and subcutaneous tumors, nerve sheath neoplasms called neurofibromas, can develop anywhere along the peripheral nerves. Neurofibromas can become quite large, causing disfigurement, eroding bone, and compressing peripheral nerves. SYN von Recklinghausen disease. Type 2 (central) neurofibromatosis has few cutaneous manifestations, and consists primarily of acoustic neuromas, causing deafness, often accompanied by other intracranial/paraspinal neoplasms, such as meningiomas and gliomas. See page B7.

**neu·ro·fil·a·ment** (noor-ō-fil'ă-ment) a class of intermediate filaments found in neurons.

**neu·ro·gang·li·on** (noor-ō-gang'lē-on) SYN ganglion (1).

**neu·ro·gen·e·sis** (noor-ō-jen'ĕ-sis) formation of the nervous system. [neuro- + G. *genesis,* production]

**neu·ro·gen·ic, neu·ro·ge·net·ic** (noor-ō-jen'ik, noor-ō-jĕ-net'ik) **1.** originating in, starting from, or caused by, the nervous system or nerve impulses. SYN neurogenous. **2.** relating to neurogenesis.

**neu·ro·gen·ic blad·der** SYN neuropathic bladder.

**neu·ro·gen·ic clau·di·ca·tion** claudication with neurologic injury, usually in association with lumbar spinal stenosis.

**neu·rog·e·nous** (noo-roj'ĕ-nŭs) SYN neurogenic (1).

**neu·rog·lia** (noo-rog'lē-ă) [TA] non-neuronal cellular elements of the central and peripheral nervous system; thought to have important metabolic functions. In central nervous tissue they include oligodendroglia cells, astrocytes, ependymal cells, and microglia cells. See this page. SYN glia, reticulum (2). [neuro- + G. *glia,* glue]

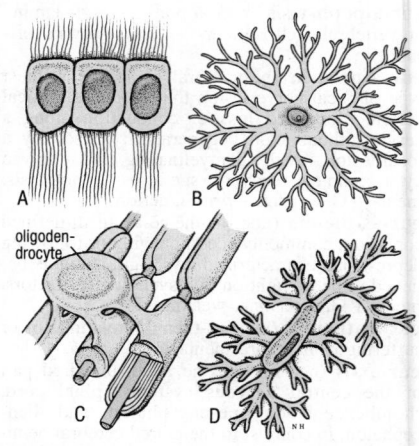

**neuroglia:** (A) ependymal cells, (B) astrocyte, (C) oligodendrocyte, (D) microglia

**neu·rog·li·a·cyte** (noo-rog'lē-ă-sīt) a neuroglia cell. SEE neuroglia. [neuro- + G. *glia,* glue, + *kytos,* cell]

**neu·rog·li·al, neu·rog·li·ar** (noo-rog'lē-ăl, noo-rog'l-lē-ăr) relating to neuroglia.

**neu·rog·li·o·ma·to·sis** (noo-rog'lē-ō-mă-tō'sis) SYN gliomatosis.

**neu·ro·gram** (noor'ō-gram) the imprint on the brain substance theoretically remaining after every mental experience, i.e., the engram or physical register of the mental experience, stimulation of which retrieves and reproduces the original experience, thereby producing memory. [neuro- + G. *gramma,* something written]

**neu·ro·his·tol·o·gy** (noor'ō-his-tol'ō-jē) the microscopic anatomy of the nervous system.

**neu·ro·hor·mone** (noor-ō-hōr′mōn) a hormone formed by neurosecretory cells and liberated by nerve impulses (e.g., norepinephrine).

**neu·ro·hy·po·phys·i·al** (noor′ō-hī-pō-fiz′ē-ăl) relating to the neurohypophysis.

**neu·ro·hy·poph·y·sis** (noor′ō-hī-pof′i-sis) [TA] a neuroendocrine structure suspended from the base of the hypothalamus. It is composed of the infundibulum and the posterior lobe of the hypophysis. SEE ALSO hypophysis. SYN lobus posterior hypophyseos [TA], posterior lobe of hypophysis. [neuro- + hypophysis]

**neu·roid** (noor′oyd) resembling a nerve; nervelike. [neuro- + G. eidos, resemblance]

**neu·ro·lem·ma** (noor-ō-lem′ă) SYN neurilemma. [neuro- + G. lemma, husk]

**neu·ro·lem·ma cells** SYN Schwann cells.

**neu·ro·lept·an·al·ge·sia** (noor′ō-lept-an-ăl-jē′zē-ă) an intense analgesic and amnesic state produced by administration of narcotic analgesics and neuroleptic drugs; unconsciousness may or may not occur, and cardiorespiratory function may be altered.

**neu·ro·lept·an·es·the·sia** (noor′ō-lept-an-es-thē′zē-ah) a technique of general anesthesia based upon intravenous administration of neuroleptic drugs, together with inhalation of a weak anesthetic with or without neuromuscular relaxants.

**neu·ro·lep·tic** (noor-ō-lep′tik) 1. any of a class of psychotropic drugs used to treast psychosis, particularly schizophrenia; includes the phenothiazine, thioxanthene, and butyrophenone derivatives and the dihydroindolones. SYN neuroleptic agent. SEE ALSO antipsychotic agent. 2. denoting a condition similar to that produced by such an agent. [neuro- + G. lēpsis, taking hold]

**neu·ro·lep·tic a·gent** SYN neuroleptic (1).

**neu·ro·lep·tic ma·lig·nant syn·drome** hyperthermia with extrapyramidal and autonomic disturbances which may result in death, following the use of neuroleptic agents.

**neu·ro·lin·guis·tic pro·gram·ming** a branch of cognitive-behavioral psychology employing specific techniques, that use language to access the unconscious in order to change a client's internal states or external behaviors.

**neu·rol·o·gist** (noo-rol′ō-jist) a specialist in the diagnosis and treatment of disorders of the neuromuscular system: the central, peripheral, and autonomic nervous systems, the neuromuscular junction, and muscle.

**neu·rol·o·gy** (noo-rol′ō-jē) the branch of medical science concerned with the various nervous systems (central, peripheral, and autonomic, plus the neuromuscular junction and muscle) and its disorders. [neuro- + G. logos, study]

**neu·rol·y·sin** (nŭ-rol′i-sin) an antibody causing destruction of ganglion and cortical cells, obtained by the injection of brain substance. SYN neurotoxin (1).

**neu·rol·y·sis** (noo-rol′i-sis) 1. destruction of nerve tissue. 2. freeing of a nerve from inflammatory adhesions. [neuro- + G. lysis, dissolution]

**neu·ro·lyt·ic** (noor-ō-lit′ik) relating to neurolysis.

**neu·ro·ma** (noo-ro′mă) general term for any neoplasm derived from cells of the nervous system, e.g., ganglioneuroma, neurilemoma, pseudoneuroma, and others. [neuro- + G. -oma, tumor]

**neu·ro·ma cu·tis** neurofibroma of the skin.

**neu·ro·ma·la·cia** (noor′ō-mă-lā′shē-ă) pathologic softening of nervous tissue. [neuro- + G. malakia, softness]

**neu·ro·ma tel·an·gi·ec·to·des** a neurofibroma with a conspicuous number of blood vessels, some of which have unusually large lumens (in proportion to the thickness of the walls).

**neu·ro·ma·to·sis** (noor′ō-mă-tō′sis) the presence of multiple neuromas, as in neurofibromatosis.

**neu·ro·mere** (noor′ō-mēr) elevations in the wall of the developing neural tube, especially the rhombencephalon/rhombomeres; that segment of the developing spinal cord to which dorsal and ventral roots are attached. [neuro- + G. meros, part]

**neu·ro·mus·cu·lar** (noor-ō-mŭs′kyu-lăr) referring to the relationship between nerve and muscle, in particular to the motor innervation of skeletal muscles and its pathology (e.g., neuromuscular disorders). SEE ALSO myoneural.

**neu·ro·mus·cu·lar spin·dle** a fusiform end organ in skeletal muscle in which afferent and a few efferent nerve fibers terminate; this sensory end organ is particularly sensitive to passive stretch of the muscle in which it is enclosed.

**neu·ro·my·as·the·nia** (noor′ō-mī-as-thē′nē-ă) obsolete term for muscular weakness due to a neurologic or psychologic disorder. [neuro- + G. mys, muscle, + a- priv. + sthenos, strength]

**neu·ro·my·e·li·tis** (noor′ō-mī-el-ī′tis) neuritis combined with spinal cord inflammation. SYN myeloneuritis. [neuro- + G. myelos, marrow, + -itis, inflammation]

**neu·ro·my·e·li·tis op·ti·ca** a demyelinating disorder consisting of a transverse myelopathy and optic neuritis. SYN Devic disease.

**neu·ro·my·op·a·thy** (noor′ō-mī-op′ă-thē) 1. a disorder of muscle due to impairment of its nerve supply. 2. simultaneous disorders of nerve and muscles. [neuro- + G. mys, muscle, + pathos, disease]

**neu·ron** (noor′on) [TA] the morphologic and functional unit of the nervous system, consisting of the nerve cell body with its the dendrites and axon. SYN neurocyte. 2. obsolete term for axon. See page 670. [G. neuron, a nerve]

**neu·ro·nal** (noor′ō-năl) pertaining to a neuron.

**neurone [Br.]** SEE neuron.

**neu·ro·ne·vus** (noor-ō-nē′vŭs) a variety of intradermal nevus in adults in which nests of atrophic nevus cells in the lower dermis are hyalinized and resemble nerve bundles.

**neu·ron·i·tis** (noor-ŏ-nī′tis) inflammatory disorder of the neuron.

**neu·ro·nop·a·thy** (noor-ō-nop′ă-thē) disorder, often toxic, of the neuron (1).

**neu·ron·o·phage** (noo-ron′ō-fāj) a phagocyte that ingests neuronal elements. SEE microglia. [neuron + G. phagō, to eat]

**neu·ron·o·pha·gia, neu·ro·noph·a·gy** (noor′on′ō-fā′jē-ă, noor-ō-nof′ă-jē) phagocytosis of nerve cells. [neuron + G. phagō, to eat]

**neu·ron-spe·ci·fic en·o·lase** an isoenzyme of enolase present in neurons and glial cells; stains for this enzyme are frequently used in the differential diagnosis of neuronal or neuroendocrine tumors.

**neu·roon·col·o·gy** (noor′ō-on-kol′ō-jē) the branch of medicine concerned with the direct and indirect effects of neoplasms on the nervous system, neuromuscular junction, and muscle. [neuro- + onco- + G. logos, study]

**neu·rooph·thal·mol·o·gy** (noor′ō-of-thal-mol′ō-jē) that branch of medicine concerned with the neurological aspects of the visual apparatus.

**neu·ro·otol·o·gy** (noor′ō-ō-tol′ō-jē) the branch of medicine concerned with the nervous system related to the auditory and vestibular systems.

**neu·ro·pa·ral·y·sis** (noor′ō-pă-ral′i-sis) paralysis resulting from disease of the nerve supplying the affected part.

**neu·ro·par·a·lyt·ic** (noor′ō-pară-lit′ik) denoting or characterized by neuroparalysis.

**neu·ro·par·a·lyt·ic ker·a·ti·tis** SYN neurotrophic keratitis.

**neu·ro·par·a·lyt·ic ker·a·top·a·thy** corneal inflammation or ulceration associated with dys-

function of the ophthalmic branch of the trigeminal nerve.

**neu·ro·path·ia** (noo-rō-path′ē-ă) SYN neuropathy.

**neu·ro·path·ia epi·dem·i·ca** hemorrhagic fever with renal complications; due to Puumala virus.

**neu·ro·path·ic** (noor-ō-path′ik) relating in any way to neuropathy.

**neu·ro·path·ic ar·throp·a·thy** SYN neuropathic joint.

**neu·ro·path·ic blad·der** any defective functioning of bladder due to impaired innervation, e.g., cord bladder, neuropathic bladder. SYN neurogenic bladder.

**neu·ro·path·ic joint** joint disease caused by diminished proprioceptive sensation, with gradual destruction of the joint by repeated subliminal

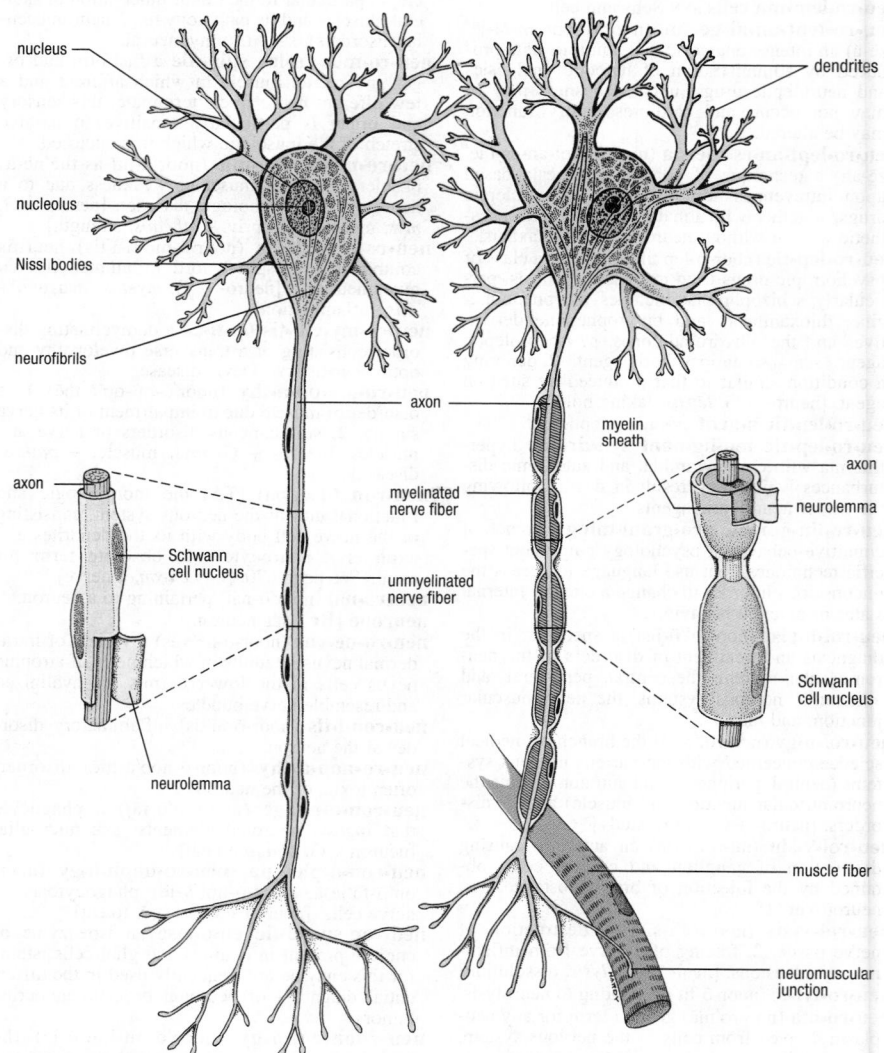

**typical efferent neurons:** (left) unmyelinated fiber, (right) myelinated fiber

injury, commonly associated with tabes dorsalis or diabetic neuropathy. SYN Charcot joint, neuropathic arthropathy.

**neu•ro•path•o•gen•e•sis** (noor'ō-path-ō-jen'ĕ-sis) the origin or causation of a disease of the nervous system. [neuro- + G. *pathos,* suffering, + *genesis,* origin]

**neu•ro•pa•thol•o•gy** (noor'ō-pa-thol'ō-jē) **1.** pathology of the nervous system. **2.** that branch of pathology concerned with the nervous system.

**neu•rop•a•thy** (noo-rop'ă-thē) **1.** any disorder affecting the nervous system. **2.** in contemporary usage, a disease involving the cranial nerves, or the peripheral or autonomic nervous systems. SYN neuritis (2), neuropathia. [neuro- + G. *pathos,* suffering]

**neu•ro•pep•tide** (noor-ō-pep'tīd) any of a variety of peptides found in neural tissue; e.g., endorphins, enkephalins.

**neu•ro•phar•ma•col•o•gy** (noor'ō-far'mă-kol'ō-jē) the study of drugs that affect neuronal tissue.

**neu•ro•phy•sins** (noor-ō-fiz'inz) a family of proteins synthesized in the hypothalamus as part of the large precursor protein that includes vasopressin and oxytocin in the neurosecretory granules; neurophysins function as carriers in the transport and storage of neurohypophysial hormones.

**neu•ro•phys•i•ol•o•gy** (noor'ō-fiz-ē-ol'ō-jē) physiology of the nervous system.

**neu•ro•pil, neu•ro•pile** (noor'ō-pil, noo'ō-pīl) the complex, feltlike net of axonal, dendritic, and glial arborizations that forms most of the gray matter of the central nervous system, and in which the nerve cell bodies lie embedded. [neuro- + G. *pilos,* felt]

**neu•ro•plasm** (noor'ō-plazm) the protoplasm of a nerve cell.

**neu•ro•plas•ty** (noor'ō-plas-tē) plastic surgery of the nerves. [neuro- + G. *plastos,* formed]

**neu•ro•ple•gic** (noor-ō-plē'jik) pertaining to paralysis due to nervous system disease. [neuro- + G. *plēgē,* a stroke]

**neu•ro•po•dia** (noor-ō-pō'dē-ă) SYN axon terminals. [pl. of *neuropodium* or *neuropodion,* fr. neuro- + G. *podion,* little foot]

**neu•ro•pore** (noor'ō-pōr) an opening in the embryo leading from the central canal of the neural tube to the exterior of the tube. [neuro- + G. *poros,* pore]

**neu•ro•psy•chi•a•try** (noor'ō-sī-kī'ă-trē) the specialty dealing with both organic and psychic disorders of the nervous system.

**neu•ro•psy•cho•log•ic dis•or•der** a disturbance of mental function due to brain trauma, associated with one of more of the following: neurocognitive, psychotic, neurotic, behavioral, or psychophysiologic manifestations, or mental impairment. SEE ALSO mental illness.

**neu•ro•psy•chop•a•thy** (noor'ō-sī-kop'ă-thē) an emotional illness of neurologic and/or functional origin.

**neu•ro•ra•di•ol•o•gy** (noor'rō-rā-dē-ol'ō-jē) the clinical subspecialty concerned with the diagnostic radiology of diseases of the central nervous system, head, and neck.

**neu•ro•reg•u•la•tor** (noor'ō-reg'yu-lā-ter) a chemical factor that exerts a modulatory effect on a neuron.

**neu•ro•ret•i•ni•tis** (noor'ō-ret-i-nī'tis) an inflammation affecting the optic nerve head and the posterior pole of the retina, with cells in the nearby vitreous, usually producing a macular star. SYN papilloretinitis.

**neu•ror•rha•phy** (noor-ōr'ă-fē) joining together, usually by suture, of the two parts of a divided nerve. SYN neurosuture. [neuro- + G. *rhaphē,* suture]

**neu•ro•sar•co•clei•sis** (noor'ō-sar-kō-klī'sis) an operation for the relief of neuralgia, consisting of resection of one of the walls of an osseous canal traversed by the nerve and transposition of the nerve into the soft tissues. [neuro- + G. *sarx,* flesh, + *kleisis,* closure]

**neu•ro•sar•coid•o•sis** (noor'ō-sar-koy-dō'sis) a granulomatous disease of unknown etiology involving the central nervous system, usually with concomitant systemic involvement.

**neu•ro•sci•ence** (noor-ō-sī'ens) the scientific discipline concerned with the development, structure, function, chemistry, pharmacology, clinical assessments, and pathology of the nervous system.

**neu•ro•se•cre•tion** (noor'ō-sē-krē'shŭn) the release of a secretory substance from the axon terminals of certain nerve cells in the brain into the circulating blood.

**neu•ro•se•cre•to•ry** (noor'ō-sē'krĕ-tōr-ē, noor'ō-sē-krē'tōr-ē) relating to neurosecretion.

**neu•ro•sis,** pl. **neu•ro•ses** (noo-rō'sis, noo-rō'sēz) **1.** a psychological or behavioral disorder in which anxiety is the primary characteristic; defense mechanisms or any of the phobias are the adjustive techniques which an individual learns in order to cope with this underlying anxiety. In contrast to the psychoses, persons with a neurosis do not exhibit gross distortion of reality or disorganization of personality. **2.** a functional nervous disease, or one for which there is no evident lesion. **3.** a peculiar state of tension or irritability of the nervous system; any form of nervousness. SYN neurotic disorder, psychoneurosis. [neuro- + G. *-osis,* condition]

**neu•ro•splanch•nic** (noor-ō-splangk'nik) SYN neurovisceral. [neuro- + G. *splanchnon,* a viscus]

*Neu•ros•po•ra* (noo-ros'pōr-ă) a genus of fungi grown in cultures and used in research in genetics and cellular biochemistry. [neuro- + G. *spora,* seed]

**neu•ro•sur•geon** (noo-rō-ser'jŭn) a surgeon specializing in operations on the nervous system.

**neu•ro•sur•gery** (noo-rō-ser'jer-ē) surgery of the nervous system.

**neu•ro•su•ture** (noo-rō-soo'cher) SYN neurorrhaphy.

**neu•ro•syph•i•lis** (noo-rō-sif'i-lis) infection of the central nervous system by *Treponema pallidum.*

**neu•ro•ten•di•nous** (noo-rō-ten'di-nŭs) relating to both nerves and tendons.

**neu•ro•ten•di•nous spin•dle** SYN Golgi tendon organ.

**neu•ro•ten•sin** (noo-rō-ten'sin) a 13-amino acid peptide neurotransmitter found in synapsomes in the hypothalamus, amygdala, basal ganglia, and dorsal gray matter of the spinal cord.

**neu•ro•the•ke•o•ma** (noo-rō-thē'kē-ō-mă) a benign myxoma of cutaneous nerve sheath origin. [neuro- + G. *thēkē,* box, sheath, + *-oma,* tumor]

**neu•rot•ic** (noo-rot'ik) relating to or suffering from a neurosis. SEE neurosis.

**neu·rot·ic dis·or·der** SYN neurosis.

**neu·rot·i·za·tion** (noo-rot′ĭ-zā′shŭn) the acquisition of nervous substance; the regeneration of a nerve.

**neu·rot·me·sis** a type of axon loss lesion resulting from focal peripheral nerve injury in which, at the lesion site, the nerve stroma is damaged to varying degrees, as well as the axon and myelin, which degenerate from that point distally. SEE axonotmesis, neurapraxia. [neuro- + G. *tmēsis*, a cutting]

**neu·rot·o·my** (noo-rot′ō-mē) operative division of a nerve. [neuro- + G. *tomē*, a cutting]

**neu·ro·ton·ic** (noo-rō-ton′ik) 1. relating to neurotony. 2. strengthening or stimulating impaired nervous action. 3. an agent that improves the tone or force of the nervous system.

**neu·ro·tox·ic** (noo-rō-tok′sik) poisonous to nervous substance.

**neu·ro·tox·in** (noo-rō-tok′sin) 1. SYN neurolysin. 2. any toxin that acts specifically on nervous tissue.

**neu·ro·trans·mit·ter** (noo-rō-trans-mit′er) any specific chemical agent released by a presynaptic cell, upon excitation, that crosses the synapse to stimulate or inhibit the postsynaptic cell. [neuro- + L. *transmitto*, to send across]

**neu·ro·trip·sy** (noo-r-ō-trip′sē) operative crushing of a nerve. [neuro- + G. *tripsis*, a rubbing]

**neu·ro·tro·phic** (noo-r-ō-trōf′ik) relating to neurotrophy.

**neu·ro·tro·phic ker·a·ti·tis** inflammation of the cornea after corneal anesthesia. SYN neuroparalytic keratitis.

**neu·rot·ro·phy** (noo-rot′rō-fē) nutrition and metabolism of tissues under nervous influence. [neuro- + G. *trophē*, nourishment]

**neu·ro·tro·pic** (noo-rō-trōp′ik) having an affinity for the nervous system.

**neu·rot·ro·py, neu·rot·ro·pism** (noo-rot′rō-pē, noo-rōt′rō-pizm) 1. affinity of basic dyes for nervous tissue. 2. the attraction of certain pathogenic microorganisms, poisons, and nutritive substances toward the nerve centers. [neuro- + G. *tropē*, a turning]

**neu·ro·tu·bule** (noo-rō′-too-byul) one of the microtubules, 10–20 nm in diameter, occurring in the cell body, dendrites, axon, and in some synaptic endings of neurons.

**neu·ro·vac·cine** (noo-rō-vak′sēn) a fixed or standardized vaccine virus of definite strength, obtained by continued passage through the brain of rabbits.

**neu·ro·vas·cu·lar** (noo-rō-vas′kyu-lăr) relating to both nervous and vascular systems; relating to the nerves supplying the walls of the blood vessels, the vasomotor nerves.

**neu·ro·vas·cu·lar bun·dle of Walsh** (walsh) the anatomic structure composed of capsular arteries and veins that provides the macroscopic landmark used during nerve-sparing radical pelvic surgery.

**neu·ro·vi·rus** (noo-rō-vī′rŭs) vaccine virus modified by means of passage into and growth in nervous tissue.

**neu·ro·vis·cer·al** (noo-rō-vis′er-ăl) referring to the innervation of the internal organs by the autonomic nervous system. SYN neurosplanchnic. [neuro- + L. *viscera*, the internal organs]

**neu·ru·la**, pl. **neu·ru·lae** (noo-rŭ-lă, noo-rŭ-lē) stage in embryonic development after the gas-trula state, in which the neural plate forms and closes to become the neural tube. [neur- + L. *-ulus*, small one]

**Neus·ser gra·nule** (noi′sĕr) a tiny basophilic granule sometimes observed in groups forming an indistinct zone about the nucleus of a leukocyte.

**neu·ter** (noo′ter) to sterilize a male or female animal surgically. [L. neither, i.e., neither male nor female]

**neu·tral** (noo′trăl) 1. exhibiting no positive properties; indifferent. 2. CHEMISTRY neither acid nor alkaline. [L. *neutralis*, fr. *neuter*, neither]

**neu·tral·i·sa·tion [Br.]** SEE neutralization.

**neu·tral·i·za·tion** (noo′trăl-i-zā′shŭn) 1. the change in reaction of a solution from acid or alkaline to neutral by the addition of just a sufficient amount of an alkaline or of an acid substance, respectively. 2. the rendering ineffective of any action, process, or potential.

**neu·tral·i·za·tion plate** a metal plate used for the internal fixation of a long bone fracture to neutralize the forces producing displacement.

**neu·tral·i·za·tion test** SYN protection test.

**neu·tra·liz·ing an·ti·bod·y** a form of antibody that reacts with an infectious agent (usually a virus) and destroys or inhibits its infectivity and virulence.

**neu·tral mu·ta·tion** a mutation with a negligible impact on genetic fitness.

**neu·tral oc·clu·sion** 1. an arrangement of teeth such that the maxillary and mandibular first permanent molars are in normal anteroposterior relation; SYN normal occlusion (2). 2. SYN neutroclusion.

**neu·tral stain** a compound of an acid stain and a basic stain, such as the eosinate of methylene blue, in which the anion and cation each contains a chromophore group.

**neu·tro-, neutr-** neutral. [L. *neutralis*, fr. *neuter*, neither]

**neu·tro·clu·sion** (noo-trō-kloo′zhŭn) a malocclusion in which there is a normal anteroposterior relationship between the maxilla and mandible; in Angle classification, a Class I malocclusion. SYN neutral occlusion (2). [neutro- + occlusion]

**neu·tron** (noo′tron) an electrically neutral particle in the nuclei of all atoms (except hydrogen-1) with a mass slightly larger than that of a proton; in isolation, it breaks down to a proton and an electron with a half-life of about 10.3 minutes. [L. *neuter*, neither]

**neu·tro·pe·nia** (noo-trō-pē′nē-ă) the presence of abnormally small numbers of neutrophils in the circulating blood. [neutrophil + G. *penia*, poverty]

**neu·tro·phil, neu·tro·phile** (noo′trō-fil, noo′trō-fīl) 1. a mature white blood cell in the granulocytic series, formed by bone marrow and released into the circulating blood, where they normally represent from 54% to 65% of the total number of leukocytes. When stained, neutrophils are characterized by: 1) a nucleus that is dark purple-blue and lobated; 2) a cytoplasm that is faintly pink and contains numerous fine pink or violet-pink granules. The precursors of neutrophils in order of increasing maturity, are: myeloblasts, promyelocytes, myelocytes, metamyelocytes, and band forms. SEE ALSO leukocyte, leukocytosis. 2. any cell or tissue that manifests no special affinity for acid or basic dyes, i.e., the cytoplasm stains approximately equally with either type of dye. See page B1. [neutro- + G. *philos*, fond]

**neu·tro·phil-ac·ti·va·ting fac·tor** SYN interleukin-8.

**neu·tro·phil-ac·ti·va·ting pro·tein** old term for interleukin-8.

**neu·tro·phil·ia** (noo-trō-fil'ē-ă) an increase of neutrophilic leukocytes in blood or tissues.

**neu·tro·phil·ic** (noo-trō-fil'ik) **1.** pertaining to or characterized by neutrophils, such as an exudate in which the predominant cells are neutrophilic granulocytes. **2.** characterized by a lack of affinity for acid or basic dyes, i.e., staining approximately equally with either type.

**neu·tro·phil·ic leu·ko·cyte** a neutrophilic granulocyte, the most frequent of the polymorphonuclear leukocytes, and also the most active phagocyte among the various types of white blood cells; when treated with Wright stain the fairly abundant cytoplasm is faintly pink, and numerous tiny pink or violet-pink granules are recognizable in the cytoplasm; the deeply stained blue nucleus is sharply distinguished from the cytoplasm and is distinctly lobated, with thin strands of chromatin connecting the three to five lobes.

**neu·tro·tax·is** (noo-trō-tak'sis) a phenomenon in which neutrophilic leukocytes are stimulated by a substance in such a manner that they are either attracted, and move toward it (**positive neutrotaxis**), or they are repelled, and move away from it (**negative neutrotaxis**). [neutrophil + G. *taxis*, arrangement]

**ne·vi** (nē'vī) plural of nevus. [L.]

**ne·void** (nē'voyd) resembling a nevus. SYN nevose (2), nevous. [L. *naevus*, mole (nevus), + G. *eidos*, resemblance]

**ne·vose, ne·vous** (nē'vōs, nē'vŭs) **1.** marked with nevi. **2.** SYN nevoid.

**ne·vus**, pl. **ne·vi** (nē'vŭs, nē'vī) **1.** a circumscribed malformation of the skin, especially one that is colored by hyperpigmentation or increased vascularity; a nevus may be predominantly epidermal, adnexal, melanocytic, vascular, or mesodermal, or a compound overgrowth of these tissues. **2.** a benign localized overgrowth of melanin-forming cells of the skin present at birth or appearing early in life. SYN mole (1). [L. *naevus*, mole, birthmark]

**ne·vus cell** the cell of a pigmented cutaneous nevus that differs from a normal melanocyte in that it lacks dendrites.

**ne·vus co·me·do·ni·cus, com·e·do ne·vus** congenital or childhood linear keratinous cystic invaginations of the epidermis, with failure of development of normal pilosebaceous follicles.

**ne·vus flam·me·us** a large congenital vascular nevus having a purplish color; it is usually found on the head and neck and persists throughout life. SYN port-wine mark, port-wine stain.

**ne·vus pig·men·to·sus** a benign pigmented melanocytic proliferation; raised or level with the skin, present at birth or arising early in life. SYN mole (2).

**ne·vus pi·lo·sus** a mole covered with an abundant growth of hair. SYN hairy mole.

**ne·vus spi·lus** a form of (flat) nevus pigmentosus.

**ne·vus u·ni·us la·te·ris** a congenital systematized linear nevus limited to one side of the body or to portions of the extremities on one side; lesions are often extensive, forming wave-like bands on the trunk and spiraling streaks on the extremities.

**ne·vus vas·cu·la·ris, ne·vus vas·cu·lo·sus** SYN capillary hemangioma.

**new·born** (noo'bōrn) SYN neonatal, neonate.

**New·com·er fix·a·tive** (noo'kŏm-ĕr) a fixative containing isopropanol, propionic acid, and dioxane, recommended as a substitute for Carnoy fixative in preservation of chromatin; also useful for fixing polysaccharides; small pieces of tissue must be used, although excessive shrinkage may still occur.

**New Hamp·shire rule** (noo-hămp'sher) pioneering American test of criminal responsibility (1871): "if the [criminal] act was the offspring of insanity, a criminal intent did not produce it."

**New·ton** (noo'tŏn), Sir Isaac, English physicist, 1642–1727. SEE newton, newtonian constant of gravitation.

**new·ton** (noo'tŏn) derived unit of force in the SI system, expressed as meters-kilograms per second squared ($m·kg·s^{-2}$); equivalent to $10^5$ dynes in the CGS system. [I. *Newton*]

**New·ton disk** (noo'tŏn) a disk on which are seven colored sectors, each occupying proportionally the same space as the corresponding primary color in the spectrum; when the disk is rapidly rotated it appears white.

**new·to·ni·an con·stant of grav·i·ta·tion (G)** (noo-tō'nē-an) a universal constant relating the gravitational force, $f$, attracting two masses, $m_1$ and $m_2$, toward each other when they are separated by a distance, $r$, in the equation: $f = G(m_1 m_2 / r^2)$; it has the value of $6.67259 \times 10^{-8}$ dyne $cm^2$ $g^{-2} = 6.67259 \times 10^{-11}$ $m^3$ $kg^{-1}$ $s^{-2}$ in SI units.

**New·ton law** (noo'tĕn) the attractive force between any two bodies is proportional to the product of their masses, and inversely proportional to the square of the distance between their centers.

**new·ton-me·ter** a unit of the MKS system, expressed as energy expended, or work done, by a force of 1 newton acting through a distance of 1 meter; equal to 1 joule = $10^7$ ergs.

**New World leish·man·i·a·sis** (noo-world) SYN mucocutaneous leishmaniasis.

**New York Heart As·so·ci·a·tion clas·si·fi·ca·tion** (noo-yŏrk) a functional classification to assess cardiovascular disability. Class I: cardiac disease without limitation of physical activity. Ordinary activity does not cause symptoms. Class II: cardiac disease with slight limitation of activity; comfortable at rest. Ordinary physical activity results in fatigue, palpitations, dyspnea or angina. Class III: cardiac disease producing marked limitation of activity: comfortable at rest. Less than ordinary physical activity causes symptoms. Class IV: cardiac disease resulting in inability to carry on any physical activity without discomfort. Symptoms may be present even at rest.

**New York vi·rus** (noo yŏrk) a species of Hantavirus in the United States causing hantavirus pulmonary syndrome.

**nex·ins** (neks'inz) proteins that bridge adjacent microtubule doublets of the axoneme of cilia and flagella. [L. *nexus*, a binding, fr. *necto*, to bind + -in]

**nex·us,** pl. **nex·us** (nek'sŭs) SYN gap junction. [L. interconnection]

**ng** nanogram.

**Ni** nickel.

**ni·a·cin** (nī'ă-sin) SYN nicotinic acid.

**ni·a·cin·a·mide** (nī'ă-sin-am'īd) SYN nicotinamide.

**nib** DENTISTRY the portion of a condensing instrument that comes into contact with the restorative material being condensed.

**niche** (nitch, nēsh) **1.** RADIOGRAPHY an eroded or ulcerated area, especially gastrointestinal or vascular, which can be detected when it fills with contrast medium. **2.** an ecological term for the position occupied by a species in a biotic community, particularly its relationships to various other competitor, predator, prey, and parasite species. [Fr.]

**nick·el (Ni)** (nik'l) a metallic bioelement, atomic no. 28, atomic wt. 58.6934, closely resembling cobalt and often associated with it. Protects ribosome structure against heat denaturation. A deficiency of nickel causes changes in the ultrastructure of the liver. [abbrev. fr. Ger. *kupfer-nickel,* name of copper-colored ore from which nickel was first obtained; *nickel,* the Ger. word for a dwarfish imp]

**nick·ing** (nik'ing) localized constrictions in retinal blood vessels.

**Nick pro·ce·dure** (nik) enlarges the aortic anulus by incising the noncoronary sinus and the roof of the left atrium.

**Ni·colle stain for cap·sules** (nē-kōl') stain in a mixture of a saturated solution of gentian violet in alcohol-phenol.

**nic·o·tin·a·mide** (nik-ō-tin'ă-mīd) the biologically active amide of nicotinic acid, used in the prevention and treatment of pellagra. SYN niacinamide.

**nic·o·tin·a·mide ad·e·nine di·nu·cle·o·tide (NAD)** ribosylnicotinamide 5′-phosphate (NMN) and adenosine 5′-phosphate (AMP) linked by the two phosphoric groups; binds as a coenzyme to proteins, serves in respiratory metabolism (hydrogen acceptor and donor). See also entries under NAD and NADP. SYN diphosphopyridine nucleotide.

**nic·o·tin·a·mide ad·e·nine di·nu·cle·o·tide phos·phate (NADP)** a coenzyme of many oxidases (dehydrogenases), in which the reaction $NADP^+ + 2H \leftrightarrow NADPH + H^+$ takes place; the third phosphoric group esterifies the 2′-hydroxyl of the adenosine moiety of NAD.

**nic·o·tin·a·mide mon·o·nu·cle·o·tide (NMN)** a condensation product of nicotinamide and ribose 5-phosphate, a precursor in the synthesis of $NAD^+$.

**nic·o·tine** (nik'ō-tēn) a poisonous volatile alkaloid derived from tobacco (*Nicotiana* spp.) and responsible for many of the effects of tobacco; it first stimulates (small doses), then depresses (large doses) at autonomic ganglia and myoneural junctions. Nicotine is an important tool in physiologic and pharmacologic investigation and is used as an insecticide and fumigant.

**nic·o·tin·ic** (nik-ō-tin'ik) relating to the stimulating action of acetylcholine and other nicotine-like agents on autonomic ganglia, adrenal medulla, and the motor end plate of striated muscle.

**nic·o·tin·ic ac·id** a part of the vitamin B complex; used in the prevention and treatment of pellagra, as a vasodilator, and as an HDL-raising agent. SYN niacin.

**nic·ti·ta·tion** (nik-ti-tā'shŭn) winking. [L. *nicto,* pp. *-atus,* to wink, fr. *nico,* to beckon]

**ni·dal** (nī'dăl) relating to a nidus, or nest.

**ni·da·tion** (nī-dā'shŭn) embedding of the early embryo in the uterine endometrium. [L. *nidus,* nest]

**NIDDM** non-insulin-dependent diabetes mellitus.

**ni·dus,** pl. **ni·di** (nī'dŭs, nī'dī) **1.** a nest. **2.** the nucleus or central point of origin of a nerve. **3.** a focus of infection. **4.** the coalescence of molecules or small particles that is the beginning of a crystal or similar solid deposit. **5.** the focus of reduced density at the center of an osteoid osteoma, on bone radiographs. [L. nest]

**ni·dus a·vis** a deep depression on each side of the inferior surface of the cerebellum, between the uvula and the biventral lobe, in which the tonsil rests. [L. bird's nest]

**Nie·mann-Pick C1 dis·ease (NPC)** (nē'mahn-pik) a rare inherited lipid storage disorder, affecting viscera and central nervous system, inherited as an autosomal recessive. There are two types of disease, with same clinical manifestations and biochemical abnormalities, resulting from abnormalities in two separate genes, NPC-1, the major locus, and NPC-2, the minor locus; then two types have identical clinical and biochemical phenotypes. Cells from NPC patients are defective in the esterification and release of cholesterol from lysosomes; lysosomal sequestration of LDL-derived cholesterol, including delayed down-regulation of LDL uptake and de novo synthesis occur.

**Nie·mann-Pick cell** (nē'mahn-pik) SYN Pick cell.

**Nie·mann sple·no·meg·a·ly** (nē'mahn) enlargement of spleen occurring in Niemann-Pick disease.

**night blind·ness** SYN nyctalopia.

**night·mare** (nīt'mār) a terrifying dream, as in which one is unable to cry for help or to escape from a seemingly impending evil. SYN incubus (2). [A.S. *nyht,* night, + *mara,* a demon]

**night soil** human feces used for fertilizer.

**night·stick frac·ture** fracture of the ulna due to a direct blow.

**night ter·rors** (nīt' tār'erz) a disorder allied to nightmare, occurring in children, in which the child awakes screaming with fright, the distress persisting for a time during a state of semiconsciousness. SYN pavor nocturnus.

**night vi·sion** SYN scotopic vision.

**nig·ra** (nī'gră) NEUROANATOMY the substantia nigra. [L. fr. *niger,* black]

**ni·gri·ti·es** (nī-grish'i-ēz) a black pigmentation. [L. blackness, fr. *niger,* black]

**ni·gro·sin, ni·gro·sine** (nī'grō-sin, nī'grō-sēn) [CI 50420] a mixture of blue-black aniline dyes used as a histologic stain for nervous tissue and as a negative stain for studying bacteria and spirochetes; also used to discriminate between live and dead cells in dye-exclusion staining.

**ni·gro·stri·a·tal** (nī'grō-strī-ā'tăl) referring to the efferent connection of the substantia nigra with the striatum. SEE substantia nigra.

**NIH** National Institutes of Health (U.S. Public Health Service).

**ni·hil·ism** (nī'i-lizm, nī'hi-lizm) **1.** PSYCHIATRY the delusion of the nonexistence of everything, especially of the self or part of the self. **2.** engagement in acts which are totally destructive to one's own purposes and those of one's group. [L. *nihil*, nothing]

**Ni·ki·fo·roff meth·od** (nē-kē′fē-rof) the fixing of blood films by immersion for 5 to 15 minutes in absolute alcohol, a mixture of equal parts of alcohol and ether, or pure ether.

**Ni·kol·sky sign** (nĭ-kol′skē) a peculiar vulnerability of the skin in pemphigus vulgaris; the apparently normal epidermis can be separated at the basal layer and rubbed off when pressed with a sliding motion.

**nil per os** [L.] nothing by mouth.

**nin·hy·drin** (nin-hī′drin) triketohydrindene, an analytic reagent that reacts with free amino acids to yield $CO_2$, $NH_3$, and an aldehyde, the $NH_3$ produced yielding a colored product. SEE ALSO ninhydrin reaction. [Ger. trade name, fr. the chemical name]

**nin·hy·drin re·ac·tion** a test for proteins, peptones, peptides, and amino acids possessing free carboxyl and α-amino groups that is based upon the reaction with triketohydrinene hydrate; a blue color reaction is used to quantitate free amino acids.

**ninth cra·ni·al nerve [CN IX]** SYN glossopharyngeal nerve [CN IX].

**ni·o·bi·um (Nb)** (nī-ō′bē-ŭm) a rare metallic element, atomic no. 41, atomic wt. 92.90638, usually found with tantalum. [*Niobe*, daughter of Tantalus]

**Ni·pah vi·rus** (ni-pah) a paramyxovirus that can cause fatal disease in humans, with features of encephalitis and meningitis; the virus spreads from swine to humans. [Nipah, Malaysia, where first human case detected, 1999]

**nip·ple** (nip′l) a wartlike projection at the apex of the breast on the surface of which the lactiferous ducts open; it is surrounded by a circular pigmented area, the areola. SYN mammilla (2), teat (1), thelium (3). [dim. of A.S. *neb*, beak, nose (?)]

**nip·ple line** SYN mammillary line.

**nip·ple shield** a cap or dome placed over the nipple to protect it during nursing.

**ni·sin** (nī′sin) a polypeptide antibiotic produced by *Streptococcus lactis;* active against certain streptococci, *Mycobacterium tuberculosis, Clostridium difficile*, and other bacteria.

**Nis·sen fun·do·pli·ca·tion** (nis′en) complete (360°) fundoplication; can be done via abdominal or thoracic approach; currently most often performed laparoscopically.

**Nis·sl bod·ies** (nis′ĕl) SYN Nissl substance.

**Nis·sl gran·ules** (nis′ĕl) SYN Nissl substance.

**Nis·sl stain** (nis′ĕl) **1.** a method for staining nerve cells with basic fuchsin; **2.** a method for staining aggregates of rough endoplasmic reticulum and ribosomes in neuronal cell bodies and dendrites with basic dyes such as cresyl violet (or cresyl echt violet), thionine, toluidin blue O, or methylene blue.

**Nis·sl sub·stance** (nis′ĕl) the material consisting of granular endoplasmic reticulum and ribosomes that occurs in nerve cell bodies and dendrites. SYN Nissl bodies, Nissl granules.

**nit 1.** the ovum of a body, head, or crab louse; it is attached to human hair or clothing by a layer of chitin. **2.** a unit of luminance; a luminous intensity of 1 candela per square meter of orthogonally projected surface. [A.S. *knitu*]

**Ni·ta·buch mem·brane, Ni·ta·buch stri·a, Ni·ta·buch lay·er** (nē′tah-boo-k) a layer of fibrin between the boundary zone of compact endometrium and the cytotrophoblastic shell in the placenta.

**ni·trate** (nī′trāt) a salt of nitric acid.

**ni·tric ac·id** (nī′trik as′id) a strong acid oxidant and corrosive.

**ni·tric ox·ide (NO)** a colorless, free-radical gas; it reacts rapidly with $O_2$ to form other nitrogen oxides (e.g., $NO_2$, $N_2O_3$, and $N_2O_4$) and ultimately is converted to nitrite ($NO_2^-$) and nitrate ($NO_3^-$). Physiologically, it is a naturally occurring vasodilator formed in endothelial cells, macrophages, neutrophils, and platelets, and a mediator of cell-to-cell communication formed in bone, brain, endothelium, granulocytes, pancreatic β-cells and peripheral nerves.

**ni·trid·a·tion** (nī-tri-dā′shŭn) formation of nitrides; formation of nitrogen compounds through the action of ammonia (analogous to oxidation).

**ni·tride** (nī′trīd) a compound of nitrogen and one other element; e.g., magnesium nitride, $Mg_3N_2$.

**ni·tri·fi·ca·tion** (nī′tri-fi-kā′shŭn) **1.** bacterial conversion of nitrogenous matter into nitrates. **2.** treatment of a material with nitric acid.

**ni·trile** (nī′tril) an alkyl cyanide. Individual nitriles are named for the acid formed on hydrolysis.

△**ni·tri·lo-** prefix indicating a tervalent nitrogen atom attached to three identical groups; e.g., nitrilotriacetic acid, $N(CH_2COOH)_3$.

**ni·trite** (nī′trīt) a salt of nitrous acid.

**ni·tri·tu·ria** (nī-trī-tyu′rē-ă) the presence of nitrites in the urine, as a result of the action of *Escherichia coli, Proteus vulgaris*, and other microorganisms that may reduce nitrates.

△**ni·tro-** prefix denoting the group –$NO_2$. [G. *nitron*, sodium carbonate.]

**ni·tro dyes** dyes in which the chromophore is -$NO_2$, which is so acidic that all dyes in this group are of the acid type.

**ni·tro·fu·ran·to·in** (nī′trō-foo-ran′tō-in) a nitrofuran compound (*O*-[5-nitrofurfurylideneamino]-hydantoin) with antimicrobial activity against a wide spectrum of Gram-positive and -negative bacteria.

**ni·tro·gen** (nī′trō-jen) **1.** a gaseous element, atomic no. 7, atomic wt. 14.00674; forms about 78.084% by volume of the dry atmosphere. **2.** the molecular form of nitrogen, $N_2$. **3.** pharmaceutical grade $N_2$, containing not less than 99.0% by volume of $N_2$; used as a diluent for medicinal gases, and for air replacement in pharmaceutical preparations. [L. *nitrum*, niter, + *-gen*, to produce]

**ni·tro·ge·nase** (nī′trō-jĕ-nās) a term for enzyme systems that catalyze the reduction of molecular nitrogen to ammonia in nitrogen-fixing bacteria with reduced ferredoxin and ATP.

**ni·tro·gen bal·ance** the difference between the total nitrogen intake by an organism and its total nitrogen loss. A normal, healthy adult has a zero nitrogen balance; the balance may become negative (more excreted than taken in).

**ni·tro·gen cy·cle** the series of events in which the nitrogen of the atmosphere is fixed, thus made available for plant and animal life, and is then returned to the atmosphere: nitrifying bacteria convert $N_2$ and $O_2$ to $NO_2^-$ and $NO_3^-$, the latter being absorbed by plants and converted to protein; if plants decay, the nitrogen is in part given up to the atmosphere and the remainder is converted by microorganisms to ammonia, nitrites, and nitrates; if the plants are eaten, the animals' excreta or bacterial decay return the nitrogen to the soil and air.

**ni•tro•gen dis•tri•bu•tion** SYN nitrogen partition.

**ni•tro•gen e•quiv•a•lent** the nitrogen content of protein; used in calculating the protein breakdown in the body from the nitrogen excreted in the urine, 1 g of nitrogen considered as having originated in 6.25 g of protein catabolized.

**ni•tro•gen group** five trivalent or quinquivalent elements whose hydrogen compounds are basic and whose oxyacids vary from monobasic to tetrabasic: nitrogen, phosphorus, arsenic, antimony, and bismuth.

**ni•tro•gen lag** the length of time after the ingestion of a given protein before the amount of nitrogen equal to that in the protein has been excreted in the urine.

**ni•tro•gen nar•co•sis 1.** narcosis produced by nitrogenous materials such as occurs in certain forms of uremia and hepatic coma; **2.** the stuporous condition characterized by disorientation and by loss of judgment and skill, attributed to an increased partial pressure of nitrogen in the inspired air of deepsea divers during underwater operations. Commonly referred to as "rapture of the deep."

**ni•trog•e•nous** (nī-troj′ĕ-nŭs) relating to or containing nitrogen.

**ni•tro•gen par•ti•tion** determination of the distribution of nitrogen in the urine among the various constituents. SYN nitrogen distribution.

**ni•tro•prus•side test** a qualitative test for cystinuria; following the addition of sodium cyanide to the urine, the further addition of nitroprusside produces a red-purple color if the cyanide has reduced any cystine present to cysteine.

⊘**ni•tro•so-** prefix denoting a compound containing nitrosyl. [L. *nitrosus*]

**S-nitrosohemoglobin** (es-nī-trō′sō-hē′mō-glō′bin) a compound formed by the binding of nitric oxide with hemoglobin; release and uptake of the nitric oxide group produce changes in vascular resistance and blood flow, which assist in oxygen homeostasis.

**ni•tro•syl** (nī′trō-sil) a univalent radical or atom group, –N=O, forming the nitroso compounds.

**ni•trous** (nī′trŭs) denoting a nitrogen compound containing one less atom of oxygen than the nitric compounds; one in which the nitrogen is present in its trivalent state.

**ni•trous ac•id** a standard biologic and clinical laboratory reagent.

**ni•trous ox•ide** a nonflammable, nonexplosive gas that will support combustion; widely used as a rapidly acting, rapidly reversible, nondepressant, and nontoxic inhalation analgesic to supplement other anesthetics and analgesics; its anesthetic potency is inadequate to provide surgical anesthesia.

**ni•tryl** (nī′tril) the radical –NO$_2$ of the nitro compounds.

**NK cells** SYN natural killer cells.

**nM** nanomolar ($10^{-9}$ M).

**nm** nanometer.

**NMN** nicotinamide mononucleotide.

**NMR** nuclear magnetic resonance.

**NNN me•di•um** agar slant overlaid with defibrinated rabbit blood used to detect the presence of leishmania or *Trypanosoma cruzi.*

**NO** nitric oxide.

**No** nobelium.

**No•ack syn•drome** (nō′ahk) SYN Pfeiffer syndrome.

**no•bel•i•um (No)** (nō-bel′ē-ŭm) an unstable transuranium element, atomic no. 102, prepared by bombardment of curium with carbon-12 nuclei and similar heavy ions on other elements of the transuranium series. [*Nobel* Institute for Physics and A.B. Nobel, Swedish inventor, 1833–1896]

**no•ble gas•es** elements in the zero group in the periodic series: helium, neon, argon, krypton, xenon, and radon. SYN inert gases.

**No•ble po•si•tion** (nō′bĕl) patient standing and bent slightly forward; useful for inspection of a swelling of the loin that may occur with pyelonephritis.

**No•ble stain** (nō′bĕl) a basic fuchsin-orange G staining technique for detection of viral inclusion bodies in fixed tissues.

*No•car•dia* (nō-kar′dē-ă) a genus of aerobic actinomycetes (family Nocardiaceae, order Actinomycetales), higher bacteria, containing weakly acid-fast, slender rods or filaments, frequently swollen and occasionally branched, forming a mycelium. Coccus or bacillary forms are produced by these organisms, which are mainly saprophytic but may be a cause of mycetoma or nocardiosis. [E. *Nocard*]

**no•car•dia,** pl. **no•car•di•ae** (nō-kar′dē-ă, nō-kar′dē-ē) a vernacular term used to refer to any member of the genus *Nocardia.*

*No•car•dia as•ter•oi•des* a species of aerobic, Gram-positive, partially acid-fast, branching organisms causing nocardiosis and possibly mycetoma in humans.

*No•car•dia ca•vi•ae* a species that causes mycetoma in humans.

*No•car•dia far•ci•ni•ca* a species causing bovine farcy; it is the type species of the genus *Nocardia.*

*No•car•dia med•i•ter•ra•nei* a species that produces rifamycin.

*Nocardia nova* a bacterial species commonly recovered from human infections.

*No•car•dia or•i•en•ta•lis* a species that produces vancomycin.

*No•car•dia oti•ti•dis•ca•vi•a•rum* a higher bacteria (formerly *Nocardia caviae*) living in soil and one of the causes of nocardiosis and actinomycetoma.

*No•car•dia trans•va•len•sis* an aerobic actinomycete; a cause of nocardiosis.

*No•car•di•op•sis* (nō-kar-dē-op′sis) a genus of higher bacteria living in soil that cause subacute or chronic pneumonia, subcutaneous infection, or disseminated disease, usually in immunosuppressed patients.

*No•car•di•op•sis das•son•vil•lei* an aerobic actinomycete, formerly *Nocardia dassonvillei;* a cause of actinomycetoma.

**no•car•di•o•sis** (nō-kar-dē-ō′sis) a generalized disease in humans and other animals caused by *Nocardia asteroides* and *N. brasiliensis* and characterized by primary pulmonary lesions which may be subclinical or chronic with hematogenous spread, and usually with involvement of the central nervous system.

**no•ce•bo** (nō-sē′bō) an unpleasant effect attributable to administration of a placebo. [L. I shall harm, fr. *noceo*, to harm, by analogy with *placebo*, I shall please]

△**no•ci-** hurt, pain, injury. [L. *noceo*]

**no•ci•cep•tive** (nō-si-sep′tiv) capable of appreciation or transmission of pain. [see nociceptor]

**no•ci•cep•tor** (nō-si-sep′ter) a peripheral nerve organ or mechanism for the reception and transmission of painful or injurious stimuli. [noci- + L. *capio*, to take]

**no•ci•fen•sor** (nō-si-fen′ser) denoting processes or mechanisms that act to protect the body from injury; specifically, a system of nerves in the skin and mucous membranes that react to adjacent injury by causing vasodilation. [noci- + L. *fendo* (only in compounds), to strike, ward off]

**no•ci-in•flu•ence** (nō′si-in′floo-ens) injurious or harmful influence.

**no•ci•per•cep•tion** (nō′si-per-sep′shŭn) the appreciation of injurious influences, referring to nerve centers. [noci- + perception]

△**noct-** nocturnal. SEE ALSO nycto-. [L. *nox*, night]

**noc•tu•ria** (nok-tyu′rē-ă) excessive urination at night. [noct- + G. *ouron*, urine]

**noc•tur•nal** (nok-ter′năl) pertaining to the hours of darkness; opposite of diurnal (1). [L. *nocturnus*, of the night]

**noc•tur•nal en•u•re•sis** urinary incontinence during sleep. SYN bed-wetting.

**noc•tur•nal my•oc•lo•nus** frequently repeated muscular jerks occurring at the moment of dropping off to sleep.

**no•dal** (nō′dăl) relating to any node.

**no•dal point** one of two points in a compound optical system so related that a ray directed toward the first point will appear to have passed through the second point parallel to its original direction. SYN axial point.

**nod•ding spasm 1.** in infants, a drop of the head on the chest due to loss of tone in the neck muscles as in epilepsia nutans, or to tonic spasm of anterior neck muscles as in West syndrome; **2.** in adults, a nodding of the head from clonic spasms of the sternomastoid muscles. SYN spasmus nutans (1).

**node** (nōd) **1.** a knob or nodosity; a circumscribed swelling. **2.** ANATOMY a circumscribed mass of differentiated tissue, especially a lymph node. SYN nodus. [L. *nodus*, a knot]

**node of Clo•quet** (klō-kā′) one of the deep inguinal lymph nodes located in or adjacent to the femoral canal; sometimes mistaken for a femoral hernia when enlarged.

**node of Ran•vi•er** (rahn-vyā′) SYN Ranvier node.

**no•di** (nō′dī) plural of nodus. [L.]

**no•dose** (nō′dōs) having nodes or knotlike swellings. SYN nodous, nodular, nodulate, nodulated, nodulous. [L. *nodosus*]

**no•dose rheu•ma•tism 1.** SYN rheumatoid arthritis. **2.** an acute or subacute articular rheumatism, accompanied by the formation of nodules on the tendons, ligaments, and periosteum in the neighborhood of the affected joints.

**no•dos•i•ty** (nō-dos′i-tē) **1.** a node; a knoblike or knotty swelling. **2.** the condition of being nodose. [L. *nodositas*]

**no•dous, nod•u•lar, nod•u•late, nod•u•lat•ed** (nō′dŭs, nod′yu-lăr, nod′yu-lāt, nod′yu-lā′ted) SYN nodose.

**nod•u•lar am•y•loi•do•sis** a localized form of amyloidosis in which amyloid occurs as masses or nodules beneath the skin or mucous membranes, e.g., in the larynx. SYN amyloid tumor, focal amyloidosis.

**nod•u•lar lep•ro•sy** SYN tuberculoid leprosy.

**nod•u•lar lym•pho•ma** malignant lymphoma arising from lymphoid follicular B cells which may be small or large, growing in a nodular pattern. SYN follicular lymphoma.

**nod•u•la•tion** (nod-yu-lā′shŭn) the formation or the presence of nodules.

🛈**nod•ule** (nod′yul) a small node. SEE ALSO nodule. See page B4. SYN nodulus (1). [L. *nodulus*, dim. of *nodus*, knot]

**nod•ule of sem•i•lu•nar valve** a nodule at the center of the free border of each semilunar valve at the beginning of the pulmonary artery and aorta.

**nod•u•lous** (nod′yu-lŭs) SYN nodose.

**no•du•lus,** pl. **no•du•li** (nod′yu-lŭs, nod′yu-lī) **1.** SYN nodule. **2.** the posterior extremity of the inferior vermis of the cerebellum, forming with the posterior medullary velum the central portion of the flocculonodular lobe. SYN nodulus vermis [TA]. [L. dim. of *nodus*]

**no•du•lus lym•pha•ti•cus** SYN lymph follicle.

**no•du•lus ver•mis** [TA] SYN nodulus.

**no•dus,** pl. **no•di** (nō′dŭs, nō′dī) SYN node. [L. a knot]

**no•dus lym•pha•ti•cus,** pl. **no•di lym•pha•ti•ci** (nō′dŭs lim′fat′ē-kus, nō′dī lim-fa′ti-sī) [TA] SYN lymph node. [lympho- + L. *nodus*, node]

**no•dus lym•phoid•e•us,** pl. **no•di lym•phoid•ei** [TA] SYN lymph node.

**noise** (noyz) **1.** unwanted sound, particularly complex sound that lacks a musical quality because the various frequencies of which it is composed are not whole or partial number multiples (harmonics) of each other. **2.** unwanted additions to a signal not arising at its source; e.g., the 60-cycle frequency wave in an electrocardiogram; largely eliminated from modern (post-1980) machines (includes visual noise on imaging studies). SEE signal-to-noise ratio. **3.** extraneous uncontrolled variables influencing the distribution of measurements in a set of data. [M.E., fr. O.Fr., fr. L.L. *nausea*, seasickness]

**noise-induced hearing loss** sensory hearing loss due to exposure to intense impulse or continuous sound. SYN boilermaker's hearing loss, industrial hearing loss, occupational hearing loss.

**noise pol•lu•tion** annoying or physiologically damaging environmental sound levels, as from automobile engines, industrial machinery, and amplified music.

**no•ma** (nō′mă) a gangrenous stomatitis with conspicuous necrosis and sloughing of tissue. Several organisms are usually found in the necrotic material, but fusiform bacilli, *Borrelia* organisms, staphylococci, and anaerobic streptococci are most frequently observed. SYN stomatonecrosis. [G. *nomē*, a spreading (sore)]

**no•men•cla•ture** (nō′men-klā-cher) a set system of names used in any science, as of anatomic structures, organisms, etc. [L. *nomenclatura*, a listing of names, fr. *nomen*, name, + *calo*, to proclaim]

**Nom•i•na An•a•tom•i•ca (NA)** (nom′i-nă an-ă-tom′i-kă, nō′mi-nă an′ă-tō′mi-kă) the modification of the Basle Nomina Anatomica or BNA system of anatomic terminology adopted in 1955 by the International Congress of Anatomists in Paris, France, and revised periodically thereafter; supplanted since 1997 by Terminologia Anatomica (TA).

**nom·i·nal a·pha·sia** SYN anomic aphasia. SYN amnestic aphasia, amnesic aphasia, anomia.

🔲 **nom·o·gram** (nŏm'ō-gram) a form of line chart showing scales for the variables involved in a particular formula in such a way that corresponding values for each variable lie in a straight line intersecting all the scales. See page APP 129-30. [G. *nomos,* law, + *gramma,* something written]

**no·mo·top·ic** (nō-mō-top'ik) relating to, or occurring at, the usual or normal place. [G. *nomos,* law, custom, + *topos,* place]

**non–A-E hep·a·ti·tis** an acute hepatitis not caused by any of the identified viral agents A through E.

**non·bac·te·ri·al ver·ru·cous en·do·car·di·tis** SYN Libman-Sacks endocarditis.

**non·com·mu·ni·cat·ing hy·dro·ceph·a·lus** SYN obstructive hydrocephalus.

**non·com·pet·i·tive in·hi·bi·tion** a type of enzyme inhibition in which the inhibiting compound does not compete with the natural substrate for the active site on the enzyme, but inhibits the reaction by combining with the enzyme-substrate complex, once the latter has been formed, and with the free enzyme.

**non com·pos men·tis** (non kom'pos men'tis) not of sound mind; mentally incapable of managing one's affairs. [L. *non,* not, + *compos,* participating, competent, + *mens,* gen. *mentis,* mind]

**non·con·ju·ga·tive plas·mid** a plasmid that cannot effect conjugation and self-transfer to another bacterium (bacterial strain); transfer depends upon mediation of another (and conjugative) plasmid.

**non·con·tained disk her·ni·at·ion** herniated disk material that comes directly in contact with the anterior epidural space through a complete defect in the posterior anulus fibrosus and posterior longitudinal ligament; of two main types: (1) extrusions, herniated material that is in continuity with the disk space, but extends completely into the epidural space and (2) sequestered, material that has lost continuity with the disk space and becomes a free fragment in the epidural space.

**non·co·va·lent bond** bond in which electrons are not shared between atoms; e.g., electrostatic bond, hydrogen bond.

**non·de·po·lar·iz·ing block** skeletal muscle paralysis unaccompanied by changes in polarity of the motor endplate, as occurs following administration of tubocurarine.

**non·dis·junc·tion** (non-dis-jŭnk'shŭn) failure of one or more pairs of chromosomes to separate at the meiotic stage of karyokinesis, with the result that both chromosomes are carried to one daughter cell and none to the other.

**non·e·lec·tro·lyte** (non-ē-lek'trō-līt) a substance with molecules that do not, in solution, dissociate to ions and therefore do not carry an electric current.

**non·es·sen·tial a·mi·no ac·ids** those amino acids that may be synthesized by an organism and are thus not required as such in its diet.

**non·fen·es·trat·ed for·ceps** obstetrical forceps without openings in the blades, thus facilitating rotation of the head.

**non·flu·en·cy** SYN dysfluency.

**non·flu·ent a·pha·sia** SYN expressive aphasia.

**non-Hodg·kin lym·pho·ma** a lymphoma other than Hodgkin disease, classified by Rappaport into a nodular or diffuse tumor pattern and by cell type; a working or international formulation separates such lymphomas into low, intermediate, and high grade malignancy and into cytologic subtypes reflecting follicular center cell or other origin.

**non·im·mune se·rum** a serum from a subject that is not immune; a serum that is free of antibodies to a given antigen.

**non-in·su·lin-de·pen·dent di·a·be·tes mel·li·tus (NIDDM)** an often mild form of diabetes mellitus of gradual onset, usually in obese individuals over age 35; absolute plasma insulin levels are normal to high, but relatively low in relation to plasma glucose levels; ketoacidosis is rare, but hyperosmolar coma can occur; responds well to dietary regulation and/or oral hypoglycemic agents, but diabetic complications and degenerative changes can develop.

**non·in·va·sive** (non-in-vā'siv) denoting a procedure that does not require insertion of an instrument or device through the skin or a body orifice for diagnosis or treatment.

**non·i·on·ic con·trast agent** SYN low osmolar contrast agent.

**non·i·so·lat·ed pro·tein·u·ria** proteinuria associated with other abnormalities.

**non·la·mel·lar bone** SYN woven bone.

**non·med·ul·lat·ed fi·bers** SYN unmyelinated fibers.

**non·ob·struc·tive jaun·dice** any jaundice in which the main biliary passages are not obstructed.

**non·or·al com·mu·ni·ca·tion** SYN augmentative and alternative communication.

**non·os·te·o·gen·ic fi·bro·ma** SYN fibrous cortical defect.

**non·ox·y·nol 9** (non'noks-ĭ-nol nīn) a group of compounds which are surface acting agents, used in spermicidal preparations such as contraceptive foam and diaphragm jelly.

**non·pa·ra·met·ric** (non-par'ă-met'rik) a group of statistical maneuvers that can be applied effectively to data nonnormal or non-Gaussian in distribution.

**non·pen·e·trance** (non-pen'ĕ-trans) the state in which a genetic trait, although present in the appropriate genotype, fails to manifest itself in the phenotype because of nongenetic mechanisms. Cf. hypostasis.

**non·pen·e·trant trait** a genetic trait that is not phenotypically manifest because of nongenetic factors; it therefore does not include recessivity, epistasis, hypostasis, or parastasis but does include environmental factors and pure random effects such as lyonization.

**non·pen·e·trat·ing wound** injury, especially within the thorax or abdomen, produced without disruption of the surface of the body.

**non·pit·ting e·de·ma** swelling of subcutaneous tissues which cannot be indented easily by compression. Usually due to metabolic abnormality, such as increased glycosaminoglycan content, like that which occurs in Graves disease (pretibial myxedema) or in early phase of scleroderma. SYN brawny edema.

**non·prop·o·si·tion·al speech** SYN automatic speech.

**non·pro·pri·e·tary name** (non-prō-prī′ĕ-tār-ē nām) a short name (often called a generic name) of a chemical, drug, or other substance that is not subject to trademark (proprietary) rights but is, in contrast to a trivial name, recognized or recommended by government agencies (e.g., Federal Food and Drug Administration) and by quasi-official organizations (e.g., U.S. Adopted Names Council) for general public use. Cf. trivial name, proprietary name, systematic name.

**non·pro·tein ni·tro·gen (NPN)** the nitrogen content of other than protein bodies; e.g., about one-half the nonprotein nitrogen in the blood is contained in urea.

**non-rap·id eye move·ment (NREM)** slow oscillation of the eyes during sleep.

**non·re·as·sur·ing fe·tal sta·tus** abnormal fetal heart rate or rhythm on electronic monitoring, suggesting fetal ischemia.

**non·re·breath·ing an·es·the·sia** a technique for inhalation anesthesia in which valves exhaust all exhaled air from the circuit.

**non·rig·id con·nec·tor** a connector or joint that is not rigid or solid. SYN stress-broken connector, stress-broken joint.

**non·se·cre·tor** (non-sē-krē′tŏr) an individual whose saliva does not contain antigens of the ABO blood group. SEE ALSO secretor.

**non·sense** as used in genetics, relating to a mutation that causes a sequence such that the growing peptide chain terminates, often after several incorrect amino acid residues are incorporated.

**non·sense trip·let 1.** a trinucleotide (codon) in which a base change to a termination codon results in premature termination of the growing polypeptide chain and, consequently, incomplete protein molecules; **2.** a termination codon.

**non·sex·u·al gen·er·a·tion** SYN asexual generation.

**non·shiv·er·ing ther·mo·gen·e·sis** thermogenesis resulting from the effects of the sympathetic nervous system neurotransmitters, epinephrine, and norepinephrine, acting to increase the cellular metabolic rate in skeletal muscle and other tissues, thereby increasing heat production. In a specialized form of adipose tissue, brown fat, the effect of the sympathetic neurotransmitters is to increase the rate of uncoupled oxidative phosphorylation by the mitochondria, which results in heat production without formation of ATP.

**non·spec·i·fic build·ing-re·lat·ed ill·ness·es** a heterogeneous group of work- or domicile-related symptoms without clear objective physical or laboratory findings. Cf. specific building-related illnesses.

**non·spe·cif·ic pro·tein** a protein substance that elicits a response not mediated by specific antigen-antibody reaction.

**non·ste·roi·dal an·ti·in·flam·ma·to·ry drug (NSAID)** drugs exerting anti-inflammatory (and also usually analgesic and antipyretic) actions; examples include aspirin, diclofenac, ibuprofen, and naproxen. A contrast is made with steroidal compounds (such as hydrocortisone or prednisone) exerting anti-inflammatory activity.

**non·sup·pres·si·ble in·su·lin·like ac·tiv·i·ty** plasma insulinlike activity not suppressed by antibodies to insulin and mostly present after pancreatectomy. Nonsuppressible insulinlike activity

is mostly the action of polypeptide insulinlike growth factors IGF-I and IGF-II.

**non·throm·bo·cy·to·pe·nic pur·pu·ra** SYN purpura simplex.

**non·tox·ic goi·ter** goiter not accompanied by hyperthyroidism.

**non·trop·i·cal sprue** sprue occurring in persons away from the tropics; usually called celiac disease; due to gluten-induced enteropathy.

**non·un·ion** (non′yun-yŭn) failure of normal healing of a fractured bone.

**non·va·lent** (non-vā′lent) having no valency; not capable of entering into chemical composition.

**non·ver·bal com·mu·ni·ca·tion** SYN augmentative and alternative communication.

**non·vi·a·ble** (non-vī′ă-bl) **1.** incapable of independent existence; often denoting a prematurely born fetus. **2.** denoting a microorganism or parasite incapable of metabolic or reproductive activity.

**non·vit·al pulp** SYN necrotic pulp.

**non-weight-bear·ing ex·er·cise** SYN weight-supported exercise.

**Noo·nan syn·drome** (noon′ăn) a syndrome found in both males and females, with a phenotype reminiscent of Turner syndrome; characterized by hypertelorism, downslanting of palpebral fissures, webbing of the neck, short stature, and congenital heart disease, especially pulmonary stenosis; normal chromosomal karyotype; autosomal dominant inheritance.

⚠**nor- 1.** chemical prefix denoting 1) elimination of one methylene group from a chain, the highest permissible locant being used; 2) contraction of a (steroid) ring in one $CH_2$ unit, the locant being the capital letter identifying the ring. Elimination of two methylene groups is denoted by the prefix dinor-; three groups, by trinor-, etc. **2.** chemical prefix denoting "normal," i.e., an unbranched chain of carbon atoms in aliphatic compounds, as opposed to branched with the same number of carbon atoms; e.g., norleucine, leucine.

**nor·a·dren·a·line** (nor-ă-dren′ă-lin) SYN norepinephrine.

**nor·ep·i·neph·rine** (nōr′ep-i-nef′rin) a catecholamine hormone, the postganglionic adrenergic mediator, acting on alpha and beta receptors; it is stored in chromaffin granules in the adrenal medulla and secreted in response to hypotension and physical stress; used pharmacologically as a vasopressor. SYN noradrenaline.

**nor·leu·cine** (nōr-loo′sin) α-amino-*n*-caproic acid; 2-aminohexanoic acid; an α-amino acid, not found in proteins; a deamination product of L-lysine, to which it is linked in collagens.

**nor·ma**, pl. **nor·mae** (nōr′mă, nōr′mē) SYN profile (1). [L. a carpenter's square]

**nor·mal** (nōr′măl) **1.** typical; usual; according to the rule or standard. **2.** BACTERIOLOGY nonimmune; untreated; denoting an animal, or the serum or substance contained therein, that has not been experimentally immunized against any microorganism or its products. **3.** denoting a solution containing 1 equivalent of replaceable hydrogen or hydroxyl per liter. **4.** PSYCHIATRY, PSYCHOLOGY denoting a level of effective functioning which is satisfactory to both the patient and the patient's social milieu. [L. *normalis*, according to pattern]

**nor·mal an·ti·bo·dy** antibody demonstrable in the serum or plasma of various persons or animals not known to have been stimulated by specific antigen, either artificially or as the result of naturally occurring contact. SYN natural antibody.

**nor·mal an·ti·tox·in** serum that is capable of neutralizing an equivalent quantity of a normal toxin solution.

**nor·mal con·cen·tra·tion (N)** SEE normal (3).

**nor·mal dis·tri·bu·tion** SYN gaussian distribution.

**nor·mal hu·man plas·ma** sterile plasma obtained by pooling approximately equal amounts of the liquid portion of citrated whole blood from eight or more adult humans who have been certified as free from any disease which is transmissible by transfusion, and treating it with ultraviolet irradiation to destroy possible bacterial and viral contaminants.

**nor·mal hu·man se·rum al·bu·min** a sterile preparation of serum albumin obtained by fractionating blood plasma proteins from healthy persons; used as a transfusion material and to treat edema due to hypoproteinemia.

**nor·ma·li·sa·tion [Br.]** SEE normalization.

**nor·ma·li·za·tion** (nōr′mal-i-zā′shun) **1.** making normal or according to the standard. **2.** reducing or strengthening of a solution to make it normal. **3.** adjusting one curve to another by multiplication of the points of the one by some arbitrary factor.

**nor·mal oc·clu·sion 1.** that arrangement of teeth and their supporting structure which is usually found in health and which approaches an ideal or standard arrangement; **2.** SYN neutral occlusion (1).

**nor·mal op·so·nin** that normally present in the blood without stimulation by a specific antigen; it is relatively thermolabile and reacts with various organisms.

**nor·mal pres·sure hy·dro·ceph·a·lus** a type of hydrocephalus developing usually in older people, due to failure of cerebrospinal fluid to be absorbed by the pacchionian granulations, and characterized clinically by progressive dementia, unsteady gait, urinary incontinence, and usually, a normal spinal fluid pressure.

**nor·mal range** SYN reference range.

**nor·mal se·rum** a nonimmune serum, usually with reference to a serum obtained prior to immunization.

**nor·mal so·lu·tion** SEE normal (3).

**nor·mal-ten·sion glau·co·ma** SYN low-tension glaucoma.

**nor·mal val·ues** a set of laboratory test values used to characterize apparently healthy individuals; now replaced by reference values.

△**nor·mo-** normal, usual. [L. *normalis*, according to pattern]

**nor·mo·blast** (nōr′mō-blast) a nucleated red blood cell, the immediate precursor of a normal erythrocyte in humans. Its four stages of development are: 1) pronormoblast, 2) basophilic normoblast, 3) polychromatic normoblast, and 4) orthochromatic normoblast SEE ALSO erythroblast. [normo- + G. *blastos*, sprout, germ]

**nor·mo·cap·nia** (nōr-mō-kap′nē-ă) a state in which the arterial carbon dioxide pressure is normal, about 40 mmHg. [normo- + G. *kapnos*, vapor]

**nor·mo·chro·mia** (nōr-mō-krō′mē-ă) normal color; referring to blood in which the amount of

hemoglobin in the red blood cells is normal. [normo- + G. *chrōma*, color]

**nor·mo·chro·mic a·ne·mia** any anemia in which the concentration of hemoglobin in the erythrocytes is within the normal range, i.e., the mean corpuscular hemoglobin concentration is from 32 to 36%.

**nor·mo·cyt·ic a·ne·mia** any anemia in which the erythrocytes are normal in size, i.e., the mean corpuscular volume ranges from 82 to 92 cu μm.

**nor·mo·cy·to·sis** (nōr′mō-sī-tō′sis) a normal state of the blood with regard to its component formed elements.

**nor·mo·gly·cae·mia [Br.]** SYN euglycemia.

**nor·mo·gly·ce·mia** (nōr′mō-glī-sē′mē-ă) SYN euglycemia.

**nor·mo·gly·ce·mic** (nōr′mō-glī-sē′mik) SYN euglycemic.

**nor·mo·ka·le·mia, nor·mo·ka·li·e·mia** (nōr′mō-kă-lē′mē-ă, nōr′mō-ka-lē-ē′mē-ă) a normal level of potassium in the blood.

**nor·mo·ka·le·mic pe·ri·od·ic pa·ral·y·sis** periodic paralysis in which the serum potassium level is within normal limits during attacks; there is often severe quadriplegia, usually improved by the administration of sodium salts;

**nor·mo·ten·sive** (nōr-mō-ten′siv) indicating a normal arterial blood pressure. SYN normotonic (2).

**nor·mo·ther·mia** (nōr-mō-ther′mē-ă) environmental temperature that does not cause increased or depressed activity of body cells. [normo- + G. *thermē*, heat]

**nor·mo·ton·ic** (nōr-mō-ton′ik) **1.** relating to or characterized by normal muscular tone. SYN eutonic. **2.** SYN normotensive.

**nor·mo·vol·e·mia** (nōr′mō-vol-ē′mē-ă) a normal blood volume. [normo- + volume, + G. *haima*, blood]

**Nor·rie dis·ease** (nor′ē) congenital bilateral masses of tissue arising from the retina or vitreous and resembling gliomas (pseudogliomas), usually with atrophy of iris and development of cataract; associated mental retardation and deafness; X-linked recessive inheritance, caused by mutation in the Norrie disease gene (NDP) on Xp.

**Nor·ris cor·pus·cle** (nor′is) a decolorized red blood cell that is invisible or almost invisible in the blood plasma, unless appropriately stained.

**North A·mer·i·can blas·to·my·co·sis** SEE blastomycosis.

**North·ern blot a·nal·y·sis** a procedure similar to the Southern blot analysis, used mostly to separate and identify RNA fragments; typically via transferring RNA fragments from an agarose gel to a nitrocellulose filter followed by detection with a suitable probe. [Coined to distinguish it from eponymic Southern blot a.]

**Nor·ton op·er·a·tion** (nor′tŏn) extraperitoneal cesarean section by a paravesical approach.

**Nor·walk vi·rus** a virus associated with acute viral gastroenteritis and probably belonging to the calicivirus group.

**Nor·wood op·er·a·tion** (nor′wud) operation performed in infants with subaortic stenosis and tricuspid atresia; the pulmonary artery is divided and both ends are attached to the aorta, the distal end via a prosthetic graft.

**nose** (nōz) that portion of the respiratory pathway above the hard palate; includes both the external nose and the nasal cavity. SYN nasus (2). [A.S. *nosu*]

**nose•bleed** (nōs'blēd) SYN epistaxis.

**nose•piece** (nōs'pēs) a microscope attachment, consisting of several objectives surrounding a central pivot.

⚠**no•so-** disease. SEE ALSO path-. [G. *nosos*]

**no•so•ac•u•sis** (nō-sō-ak-yu'sis) hearing loss due to disease, as opposed to aging. [noso- + G. *akousis,* hearing]

**nos•o•co•mi•al** (nos-ō-kō'mē-ăl) **1.** relating to a hospital. **2.** denoting a new disorder (not the patient's original condition) associated with being treated in a hospital, such as a hospital-acquired infection. [G. *nosokomeion,* hospital, fr. *nosos, disease,* + *komeō,* to take care of]

**nos•o•gen•ic** (nos-ō-jen'ik) SYN pathogenic.

**nos•o•log•ic** (nos-ō-loj'ik) relating to nosology.

**no•sol•o•gy** (nō-sol'ō-jē) **1.** the science of classification of diseases. **2.** classification of ill persons into groups, whatever the criteria for the classification, and agreement as to the boundaries of the groups. SYN nosonomy, nosotaxy. [noso- + G. *logos,* study]

**nos•o•ma•nia** (nos-ō-mā'nē-ă) an unfounded morbid belief that one is suffering from some special disease. [noso- + G. *mania,* insanity]

**no•son•o•my** (nō-son'ō-mē) SYN nosology. [noso- + G. *nomos,* law]

**nos•o•phil•ia** (nos-ō-fil'ē-ă) a morbid desire to be sick. [noso- + G. *phileō,* to love]

**nos•o•pho•bia** (nos-ō-fō'bē-ă) an inordinate dread and fear of disease. [noso- + G. *phobos,* fear]

**nos•o•poi•et•ic** (nos'ō-poy-et'ik) SYN pathogenic. [noso- + G. *poiēsis,* a making]

**nos•o•taxy** (nos'ō-tak-sē) SYN nosology. [noso- + G. *taxis,* arrangement]

**nos•tal•gia** (nos-tal'jē-ă) the longing to return home, to a former time in one's life, or to familiar people and surroundings. [G. *nostos,* a return (home), + *algos,* pain]

**nos•tril** (nos-tril) anterior opening to either side of the nasal cavity. SYN naris, praenaris, prenaris.

**nos•trum** (nos'trŭm) general term for a therapeutic agent, sometimes patented but usually of secret composition, offered to the general public as a specific remedy for any disease or class of diseases. [L. neuter of *noster,* our, "our own remedy"]

**no•tal** (nō'tăl) relating to the back. [G. *nōtos,* the back]

**no•tan•ce•pha•lia** (nō'tan-se-fā'lē-ă) congenital absence of the occipital bone. [G. *nōtos,* back, + *an-* priv. + *kephalē,* head]

**no•tan•en•ce•pha•lia** (nō'tan-en-se-fā'lē-ă) absence of the cerebellum. [G. *nōtos,* back, + *an-* priv. + *enkephalos,* brain]

**notch** **1.** an indentation at the edge of any structure. **2.** any short, narrow, V-shaped deviation, whether positive or negative, in a linear tracing. SYN incisura [TA], incisure.

**no•ten•ceph•a•lo•cele** (nō-ten-sef'ă-lō-sēl) malformation in the occipital portion of the cranium with protrusion of brain substance. [G. *nōtos,* back, + *enkephalos,* brain, + *kēlē,* hernia]

**Noth•na•gel syn•drome** (not'nah-gel) dizziness, staggering, and rolling gait, with irregular forms of oculomotor paralysis and often nystagmus, seen in cases of tumor of the midbrain.

**no•tice of non•cov•er•age** SYN advance beneficiary notice.

**no•ti•fi•a•ble dis•ease** a disease that, by statutory requirements, must be reported to public health or veterinary authorities. SYN reportable disease.

**no•to•chord** (nō'tō-kōrd) **1.** in primitive vertebrates, the primary axial supporting structure of the body, derived from the notochordal or head process of the early embryo; an important organizer for determining the final form of the nervous system and related structures. **2.** in embryos, the axial fibrocellular cord about which the vertebral primordia develop; vestiges of it persist in the adult as the nuclei pulposi of the intervertebral discs. [G. *nōtos,* back, + *chordē,* cord, string]

**no•to•chor•dal** (nō-tō-kōr'dăl) relating to the notochord.

**nour•ish•ment** (ner'ish-ment) a substance used to feed or to sustain life and growth of an organism.

**No•vy and Mac•Neal blood a•gar** (nō've and měk'nēl) a nutrient agar containing two volumes of defibrinated rabbit's blood; suitable for the cultivation of a number of trypanosomes.

**nox•ious** (nok'shŭs) injurious; harmful. [L. *noxius,* injurious, fr. *noceo,* to injure]

**Np** **1.** neptunium. **2.** neper.

**NPC** Niemann-Pick C1 disease.

**NPH in•su•lin** modified form of insulin composed of insulin, protamine, and zinc; an intermediately acting preparation used for the treatment of diabetes mellitus. SYN isophane insulin.

**NPN** nonprotein nitrogen.

**NPO, n.p.o.** *1. non per os* or *nil per os,* nothing by mouth.

**NREM** non-rapid eye movement.

**nRNA** nuclear RNA.

**NSAID** nonsteroidal anti-inflammatory drug.

**N ter•mi•nus** SEE amino-terminal.

**nu** (noo) **1.** thirteenth letter of the Greek alphabet (ν). **2.** kinematic viscosity; frequency; stoichiometric number. **3.** CHEMISTRY the position of a substituent located on the thirteenth atom from the carboxyl or other functional group.

**nu•cha** (noo'kă) the back of the neck. SYN nape. [Fr. *nuque*]

**nu•chal** (noo'kăl) relating to the nucha.

**nu•chal arm** situation in vaginal breech delivery during which one or both arms are found around the back of the neck, interfering with delivery.

**nu•chal cord** loop(s) of umbilical cord around the fetal neck, posing risk of intrauterine hypoxia, fetal distress, or death.

**nu•chal lig•a•ment** SYN ligamentum nuchae.

**nu•chal plane** the external surface of the squamous part of the occipital bone below the superior nuchal line, giving attachment to the muscles of the back of the neck.

**nu•chal rig•id•i•ty** impaired neck flexion resulting from muscle spasm (not actual rigidity) of the extensor muscles of the neck; usually attributed to meningeal irritation.

**nu•cle•ar** (noo'klē-er) relating to a nucleus, either cellular or atomic; in the latter sense, usually referring to radiation emanating from atomic nuclei (α, β, or γ) or to atomic fission.

**nu•cle•ar cat•a•ract** a cataract involving the nucleus.

**nu•cle•ar:cy•to•plas•mic ra•tio** the ratio of the volume of the cell's nucleus to the volume of the cytoplasm. In general, as blood cells mature, the N:C ratio decreases.

**nu·cle·ar en·ve·lope** the double membrane at the boundary of the nucleoplasm; it has regularly spaced pores covered by a disklike nuclear pore complex and a space or cisterna about 150 Å wide between the two layers; the outer membrane is continuous at intervals with the endoplasmic reticulum. SYN nuclear membrane.

**nu·cle·ar fac·tor-κB** a transcription factor associated with cytokine production.

**nu·cle·ar fam·i·ly** in genetics, two parents and their progeny in common.

**nu·cle·ar in·clu·sion bod·ies** SEE inclusion bodies.

**nu·cle·ar jaun·dice** SYN kernicterus.

**nu·cle·ar mag·net·ic res·o·nance (NMR)** the phenomenon in which certain atomic nuclei possessing a magnetic moment will precess around the axis of a strong external magnetic field, the frequency of precession being specific for each nucleus and the strength of the magnetic field; spinning nuclei induce their own oscillating magnetic fields and therefore emit electromagnetic radiation that can produce a detectable signal. NMR is used as a method of identifying covalent bonds and is applied clinically in magnetic resonance imaging.

**nu·cle·ar med·i·cine** the clinical discipline concerned with the diagnostic and therapeutic uses of radionuclides, excluding the therapeutic use of sealed radiation sources.

**nu·cle·ar med·i·cine tech·nol·o·gist** an individual skilled in injecting and following the course of radioisotopes in the diagnosing of disease.

**nu·cle·ar mem·brane** SYN nuclear envelope.

**nu·cle·ar oph·thal·mo·ple·gia** ophthalmoplegia due to a lesion of the nuclei of origin of the motor nerves of the eye.

**Nu·cle·ar Reg·u·la·tory Com·mis·sion** the U.S. federal commission supervising the use of radioactive by-product material for commercial and medical purposes; successor to the Atomic Energy Commission along with the U.S. Department of Energy.

**nu·cle·ar RNA (nRNA)** rNA found in nuclei, or associated with DNA, or with nuclear structures (nucleoli).

**nu·cle·ar spin·dle** SYN mitotic spindle.

**nu·cle·ar stain** a stain for cell nuclei, usually based on the binding of a basic dye to DNA or nucleohistone.

**nu·cle·ase** (noo′klē-ās) general term for enzymes that catalyze the hydrolysis of nucleic acid into nucleotides or oligonucleotides. Cf. exonuclease, endonuclease.

**nu·cle·ate** (noo′klē-āt) a salt of a nucleic acid.

**nu·cle·at·ed** (noo′klē-ā-ted) provided with a nucleus, a characteristic of all true cells.

**nu·cle·a·tion** (noo-klē-ā′shŭn) process of forming a nidus (4).

**nu·clei** (noo′klē-ī) plural of nucleus.

**nu·clei an·ter·i·or·es thal·a·mi** [TA] SYN anterior nuclei of thalamus.

**nu·cle·ic ac·id** (noo-klē′ik as′id) a family of macromolecules found in the chromosomes, nucleoli, mitochondria, and cytoplasm of all cells, and in viruses; in complexes with proteins, they are called nucleoproteins.

**nu·clei co·chle·a·res** [TA] the nucleus cochlea-

ris dorsalis and nucleus cochlearis ventralis, located on the dorsal and lateral surface of the inferior cerebellar peduncle, in the floor of the lateral recess of the rhomboid fossa. They receive the incoming fibers of the cochlear part of the vestibulocochlear nerve and are the major source of origin of the lateral lemniscus or central auditory pathway.

**nu·cle·i·form** (noo′klē-i-fōrm) shaped like or having the appearance of a nucleus. SYN nucleoid (1).

**nu·clei of or·i·gin** collections of motor neurons (forming a continuous column in the spinal cord, discontinuous in the medulla and pons) giving origin to the spinal and cranial motor nerves.

△**nu·cleo-, nucl-** nucleus, nuclear. SEE ALSO karyo-, caryo-. [L. *nucleus*]

**nu·cle·o·cap·sid** (noo′klē-ō-kap′sid) SEE virion.

**nu·cle·of·u·gal** (noo-klē-of′yu-găl) **1.** moving within the cell body in a direction away from the nucleus. **2.** moving in a direction away from a nerve nucleus; said of nerve transmission. [nucleo- + L. *fugio*, to flee]

**nu·cle·o·his·tone** (noo′klē-ō-his′tōn) a complex of histone and deoxyribonucleic acid, the form in which the latter is usually found in the nuclei of cells.

**nu·cle·oid** (noo′klē-oyd) **1.** SYN nucleiform. **2.** a nuclear inclusion body. **3.** SYN nucleus (2). [nucleo- + G. *eidos*, resemblance]

**nu·cle·o·lar** (noo-klē′ō-lăr) relating to a nucleolus.

**nu·cle·o·li** (noo-klē′ō-lī) plural of nucleolus.

**nu·cle·o·li·form** (noo-klē′ō-lē-fōrm) resembling a nucleolus. SYN nucleoloid.

**nu·cle·o·loid** (noo-klē′ō-loyd) SYN nucleoliform. [nucleolus + G. *eidos*, resemblance]

**nu·cle·o·lo·ne·ma** (noo-klē′ō-lō-nē′mă) the irregular network or rows of fine ribonucleoprotein granules or microfilaments forming most of the nucleolus. [nucleolus + G. *nēma*, thread]

**nu·cle·o·lus**, pl. **nu·cle·o·li** (noo-klē′ō-lŭs, noo-klē′ō-lī) a small rounded mass within the cell nucleus where ribonucleoprotein is produced. [L. dim of *nucleus*, a nut, kernel]

**nu·cle·on** (noo′klē-on) **1.** one of the subatomic particles of the atomic nucleus; i.e., either a proton or a neutron. **2.** slang term for specialist in nuclear medicine. [nucleus + -on]

**nu·cle·op·e·tal** (noo-klē-op′ĕ-tăl) **1.** moving in the cell body in a direction toward the nucleus. **2.** moving in a direction toward a nerve nucleus; said of a nervous impulse. [nucleo- + L. *peto*, to seek]

**nu·cle·o·phil, nu·cle·o·phile** (noo′klē-ō-fil, noo′klē-ō-fīl) **1.** the electron pair donor atom in a chemical reaction in which a pair of electrons is picked up by an electrophil. **2.** relating to a nucleophil. SYN nucleophilic (1). [nucleo- + G. *philos*, fond]

**nu·cle·o·phil·ic** (noo′klē-ō-fil′ik) **1.** SYN nucleophil (2). **2.** a reaction involving a nucleophile.

**nu·cle·o·plasm** (noo′klē-ō-plazm) the protoplasm of the nucleus of a cell.

**nu·cle·o·pro·tein** (noo′klē-ō-prō′tēn) a complex of protein and nucleic acid, the form in which essentially all nucleic acids exist in nature; chromosomes and viruses are largely nucleoprotein.

**nu·cle·or·rhex·is** (noo′klē-ō-rek′sis) fragmentation of a cell nucleus. [nucleo- + G. *rhēxis*, rupture]

**nu·cle·o·si·das·es** (noo'klē-ō-sī'dās-ez) enzymes that catalyze the hydrolysis or phosphorolysis of nucleosides, releasing the purine or pyrimidine base.

**nu·cle·o·side** (noo'klē-ō-sīd) a compound of a sugar (usually ribose or deoxyribose) with a purine or pyrimidine base.

**nu·cle·o·some** (noo'klē-ō-sōm) a localized aggregation of histone and DNA that is evident when chromatin is in the uncondensed stage. [nucleo- + G. *sōma*, body]

**nu·cle·o·ti·da·ses** (noo'klē-ō-tī-dās-ez) enzymes that catalyze the hydrolysis of nucleotides into phosphoric acid and nucleosides.

**nu·cle·o·tide** (noo'klē-ō-tīd) a combination of a (nucleic acid) purine or pyrimidine, one sugar (usually ribose or deoxyribose), and a phosphoric group. SYN mononucleotide.

**nu·cle·o·tid·yl·trans·fer·as·es** (noo'klē-ō-tī'dil-trans'fer-ās-ez) enzymes transferring nucleotide residues (nucleotidyls) from nucleoside di- or tri-phosphates into dimer or polymer forms.

**nu·cle·o·tox·in** (noo'klē-ō-tok'sin) a toxin acting upon the cell nuclei.

**nu·cle·us**, pl. **nu·clei** (noo'klē-ŭs, noo'klē-ī) **1.** in cytology, typically a rounded or oval mass of protoplasm within the cytoplasm of a plant or animal cell; it is surrounded by a nuclear envelope, which encloses euchromatin, heterochromatin, and one or more nucleoli and undergoes mitosis during cell division. SYN karyon. **2.** by extension, because of similar function, the genome of microorganisms (microbes), which is relatively simple in structure, lacks a nuclear membrane and does not undergo mitosis during replication. SYN nucleoid (3). SEE ALSO virion. **3.** in neuroanatomy, a group of nerve cell bodies in the brain or spinal cord that can be demarcated from neighboring groups on the basis of either differences in cell type or the presence of a surrounding zone of nerve fibers or cell-poor neuropil. **4.** any substance (e.g., foreign body, mucus, crystal) around which a urinary or other calculus is formed. **5.** the central portion of an atom (composed of protons and neutrons) where most of the mass and all of the positive charge are concentrated. **6.** a particle on which a crystal, droplet, or bubble forms. **7.** a characteristic arrangement of atoms in a series of molecules; e.g., the benzene nucleus is a series of aromatic compounds. [L. a little nut, the kernel, stone of fruits, the inside of a thing, dim. of *nux*, nut]

**nu·cle·us of the an·sa len·tic·u·lar·is** [TA] SEE dorsal hypothalamic area.

**nu·cle·us caer·u·le·us** [TA] a shallow depression, blue in the fresh brain, lying laterally in the most rostral portion of the rhomboidal fossa near the cerebral aqueduct; it lies near the lateral wall of the fourth ventricle and consists of about 20,000 melanin-pigmented neuronal cell bodies whose norepinephrine-containing axons have a remarkably wide distribution in the cerebral cortex, dorsal thalamus, amygdaloid complex and hippocampus, mesencephalic tegmentum, cerebellar nuclei and cortex, various nuclei in the pons and medulla, and the gray matter of the spinal cord.

**nu·cle·us den·ta·tus** [TA] SYN dentate nucleus of cerebellum.

**nu·cle·us of pos·ter·i·or com·mis·sure** [TA] a group of cells located immediately adjacent to the posterior commissure at the mesencephalon-diencephalon junction; may be divided into pars ventralis [TA] (ventral subdivision), pars dorsalis [TA] (dorsal subdivision), and pars interstitialis [TA] (interstitial subdivision).

**nu·cle·us of sol·i·tary tract** a slender cell column extending sagittally through the dorsal part of the medulla oblongata, beneath the floor of the rhomboid fossa, immediately lateral to the limiting sulcus. It is the visceral sensory (visceral afferent) nucleus of the brainstem, receiving the afferent fibers of the vagus, glossopharyngeal, and facial nerves by way of the solitary tract. The caudal two-thirds of the nucleus processes impulses originating in the pharynx, larynx, intestinal and respiratory tracts, and heart and large blood vessels; its rostral one-third receives impulses from the taste buds and is known as the rhombencephalic gustatory nucleus. SYN nucleus tractus solitarii [TA].

**nu·cle·us tract·us so·li·ta·rii** [TA] SYN nucleus of solitary tract.

**nu·clide** (noo'klīd) a particular (atomic) nuclear species with defined atomic mass and number. SEE ALSO isotope.

**NUG** necrotizing ulcerative gingivitis.

**null cells 1.** SYN killer cells. **2.** large granular lymphocytes that lack surface markers or membrane-associated proteins of either B or T lymphocytes.

**null hy·poth·e·sis** the statistical hypothesis that one variable has no association with another, or that experimental results do not differ from those that might be expected by the operation of chance alone.

**nul·li·grav·i·da** (nŭl-i-grav'i-dă) a woman who has never conceived a child. [L. *nullus*, none, + *gravida*, pregnant]

**nul·lip·a·ra** (nŭ-lip'ă-ră) a woman who has never borne children. [L. *nullus*, none, + *pario*, to bear]

**nul·li·par·i·ty** (nŭl-i-par'i-tē) condition of having borne no children.

**nul·lip·a·rous** (nŭl-ip'ă-rŭs) never having borne children.

**numb chin syn·drome** paresthesia and sensory loss affecting one side of the chin and lower lip, resulting from neoplastic infiltration of the ipsilateral mental nerve; common causes include multiple myeloma and breast or prostate carcinoma.

**num·ber** (nŭm'ber) **1.** a symbol expressive of a certain value or of a specific quantity determined by count. **2.** the place of any unit in a series.

**numb·ness** (nŭm'nes) indefinite term for abnormal sensation, including absent or reduced sensory perception as well as paresthesias.

**num·mu·lar** (nŭm'yu-ler) **1.** discoid or coin-shaped; denoting thick mucopurulent sputum, so called because of the disc shape assumed when it is flattened on the bottom of a sputum mug containing water or transparent disinfectant. **2.** arranged like stacks of coins, denoting the lining up of the red blood cells into rouleaux formation. [L. *nummulus*, small coin, dim. of *nummus*, coin]

**num·mu·lar ec·ze·ma** discrete, coin-shaped patches of eczema.

**num·mu·lar spu·tum** a thick, coherent mass expectorated in globular shape which does not run at the bottom of the cup but forms a discoid mass resembling a coin.

**nurse** (ners) **1.** one who is educated in the science

and art of nursing who has been trained under defined standards of education and is concerned with the assessment, diagnosis, treatment, and evaluation of human responses to actual or potential health problems. **2.** to breast feed. [O. Fr. *nourice,* fr. L. *nutrix,* wet-nurse, nurse, fr. *nutrio,* to suckle, to tend]

**nurse an·es·the·tist** a registered nurse with advanced training and certification in anesthesia.

**nurse·maid's el·bow** longitudinal subluxation of the radial head from the annular ligament. SYN Malgaigne luxation.

**nurse prac·ti·tion·er** (ners prak-tish′ŭ-ner) a registered nurse with advanced education in the primary care of particular groups of clients, who provides services, within the scope of nursing practice, in the areas of health promotion, disease prevention, therapy, rehabilitation, and support at all levels of the health care system.

**nurs·ing** (ner′sing) **1.** nursing is a discipline, profession, and an area of practice. As a discipline nursing is centred around knowledge development. Emphasis is placed on discovering, describing, extending, and modifying knowledge for professional nursing practice. As a profession, nursing has a social mandate to be responsible and accountable to the public it serves. Nursing is an integral part of the health care system, and as such encompasses the promotion of health, prevention of illness, and care of physically ill, mentally ill, and disabled people of all ages, in all health care and other community settings. Within this broad spectrum of health care, the phenomena of particular concern to nurses are individual, family, and group "responses to actual or potential health problems." The human responses range broadly from health restoring reactions to an individual episode of illness to the development of policy in promoting the long-term health of a population. **2.** feeding an infant at the breast; tending and caring for a child.

**nurs·ing au·dit** a method of evaluating nursing practice by reviewing records that document the care provided to patients.

**nurs·ing di·ag·no·sis** the process of assessing potential or actual health problems, including those pertaining to a family or community, that fall within the scope of nursing practice; also, a judgment or conclusion reached as a result of such assessment or derived from assessment data.

**nurs·ing fa·cil·i·ty** health care facility for patients who require long-term nursing or rehabilitation services; formerly known as a nursing home. SYN long-term care facility.

**nurs·ing his·to·ry** the gathering of information about the medical, psychological, social, and spiritual history of a patient as a basis for nursing diagnosis and the formulation of a care plan.

**nurs·ing home** former term for nursing facility. SEE nursing facility.

**nu·ta·tion** (noo-tā′shŭn) the act of nodding, especially involuntary nodding. [L. *annuo,* to nod]

**nu·tra·ceu·ti·cal** (noo′tră-soo′tĭ-kal) a product derived from a food that is marketed in the form of medicine and is demonstrated to have a physiologic benefit or to provide protection against chronic disease. [*nutr*ient + pharm*aceutical*]

⊞**nu·tri·ent** (noo′trē-ent) a constituent of food necessary for normal physiologic function. See this page. [L. *nutriens,* fr. *nutrio,* to nourish]

**nu·tri·ent ar·ter·ies of hu·mer·us** *origin,* deep brachial; *distribution,* the medullary cavity of the humerus.

**nu·tri·ent ar·tery** an artery of variable origin that supplies the medullary cavity of a long bone. SYN arteria nutricia [TA], nutrient vessel.

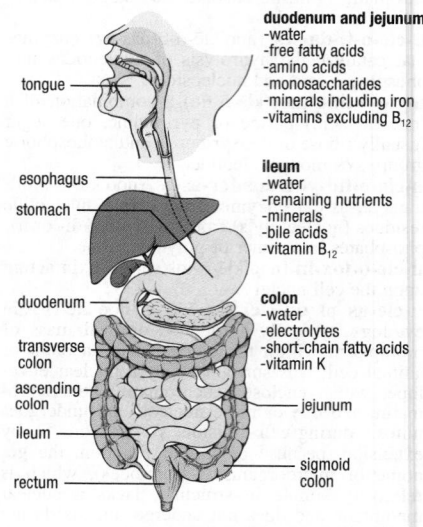

| | |
|---|---|
| tongue | **duodenum and jejunum**<br>-water<br>-free fatty acids<br>-amino acids<br>-monosaccharides<br>-minerals including iron<br>-vitamins excluding B₁₂ |
| esophagus | **ileum**<br>-water<br>-remaining nutrients |
| stomach | -minerals<br>-bile acids<br>-vitamin B₁₂ |
| duodenum | **colon**<br>-water<br>-electrolytes |
| transverse colon | -short-chain fatty acids<br>-vitamin K |
| ascending colon | jejunum |
| ileum | |
| rectum | sigmoid colon |

**nutrient absorption:** gastrointestinal tract sites

**nu·tri·ent ar·tery of fe·mur** one of two arteries, superior and inferior, arising from the first and third perforating arteries respectively (sometimes second and fourth). SYN arteria nutricia femoris [TA].

**nu·tri·ent ar·tery of fib·u·la** *origin,* peroneal (fibular); *distribution,* fibula. SYN arteria nutricia fibulae [TA].

**nu·tri·ent ca·nal** a canal in the shaft of a long bone or in other locations in irregular bones through which the nutrient artery enters a bone. SYN canalis nutricius [TA].

**nu·tri·ent fo·ra·men** the external opening of the nutrient canal in a bone.

**nu·tri·ent ves·sel** SYN nutrient artery.

⊞**nu·trit·ion** (noo-trish′ŭn) **1.** a function of living plants and animals, consisting in the taking in and metabolism of food material whereby tissue is built up and energy liberated. **2.** the study of the food and liquid requirements of human beings or animals for normal physiologic function, including energy, need, maintenance, growth, activity, reproduction, and lactation. See page APP 153. [L. *nutritio,* fr. *nutrio,* to nourish]

**nu·tri·tive** (noo′tri-tiv) **1.** pertaining to nutrition. **2.** capable of nourishing.

**nu·tri·tive e·qui·lib·ri·um** condition in which there is a perfect balance between intake and excretion of nutritive material, so that there is no increase or loss in weight.

**nu·tri·ture** (noo′tri-cher) state or condition of the nutrition of the body; state of the body with regard to nourishment. [L. *nutritura,* a nursing, fr. *nutrio,* to nourish]

**nyc·tal·gia** (nik-tal′jē-ă) denoting especially the osteocopic pains of syphilis occurring at night. [nyct- + G. *algos,* pain]

**nyc·ta·lo·pia** (nik-tă-lō′pē-ă) decreased ability to see in reduced illumination. Seen in patients with impaired rod function; often associated with a deficiency of vitamin A. SYN night blindness. [nyct- + G. *alaos,* obscure, + *ōps,* eye]

**nyc·ter·ine** (nik′ter-īn) **1.** by night. **2.** dark or obscure. [G. *nykterinos*]

△**nyc·to-, nyct-** night, nocturnal. SEE ALSO noct-. [G. *nyx*]

**nyc·to·hem·e·ral** (nik-tō-hē′mer-ăl) both daily and nightly. [nycto- + G. *hēmera,* day]

**nyc·to·phil·ia** (nik-tō-fil′ē-ă) preference for the night or darkness. SYN scotophilia. [nycto- + G. *philos,* fond]

**nyc·to·pho·bia** (nik-tō-fō′bē-ă) morbid fear of night or of the dark. SYN scotophobia. [nycto- + G. *phobos,* fear]

**nym·pha,** pl. **nym·phae** (nim′fă, nim′fē) one of the labia minora. [Mod. L., fr. G. *nymphē,* a bride]

**nym·phec·to·my** (nim-fek′tō-mē) surgical removal of hypertrophied labia minora. [nympha + G. *ektomē,* excision]

**nym·phi·tis** (nim-fī′tis) inflammation of the labia minora. [nympha + G. *-itis,* inflammation]

△**nym·pho-, nymph-** the nymphae (labia minora). [L. *nympha*]

**nym·pho·ma·nia** (nim-fō-mā′nē-ă) an insatiable impulse to engage in sexual behavior in a female; the counterpart of satyriasis in a male. [nympho- + G. *mania,* frenzy]

**nym·pho·ma·ni·a·cal** (nim′fō-mă-nī′ă-kăl) pertaining to, or exhibiting, nymphomania.

**nym·phon·cus** (nim-fong′kŭs) swelling or hypertrophy of one or both labia minora. [nympho- + G. *onkos,* tumor]

**nym·phot·o·my** (nim-fot′ō-mē) incision into the labia minora or the clitoris. [nympho- + G. *tomē,* incision]

**nys·tag·mic** (nis-tag′mik) relating to or suffering from nystagmus.

**nys·tag·mi·form** (nis-tag′mi-fōrm) SYN nystagmoid.

**nys·tag·mo·graph** (nis-tag′mō-graf) an apparatus for measuring the amplitude, periodicity, and velocity of ocular movements in nystagmus, by measuring the change in the resting potential of the eye as the eye moves. [nystagmus + G. *graphō,* to write]

**nys·tag·mog·ra·phy** (nis-tag-mog′ră-fē) the technique of recording nystagmus.

**nys·tag·moid** (nis-tag′moyd) resembling nystagmus. SYN nystagmiform. [nystagmus + G. *eidos,* resemblance]

**nys·tag·mus** (nis-tag′mŭs) rhythmical oscillation of the eyeballs, either pendular or jerky. See this page. [G. *nystagmos,* a nodding, fr. *nystazō,* to be sleepy, nod]

**nyx·is** (nik′sis) a pricking; paracentesis. [G.]

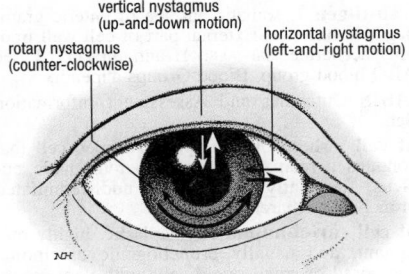

**nystagmus:** thicker arrows indicate the slower first phase

# O

**Ω, ω** omega. SEE omega.

**O 1.** oxygen; orotidine. **2.** opening (in formulas for electrical reactions). **3.** a blood group in the ABO system. See ABO blood group, Blood Groups appendix. **4.** an abbreviation derived from *ohne Hauch* (without a film), used as a designation for: 1) antigens that occur in the bacterial cell, in contrast to those in the flagella; 2) specific antibodies for such somatic antigens; 3) the agglutinative reaction between somatic antigen and its antibody.

**OA** occipitoanterior position.

**OAE** otoacoustic emission.

**O ag·glu·ti·nin 1.** an agglutinin that is formed as the result of stimulation by, and that reacts with, the relatively thermostable antigen(s) in the cell bodies of microorganisms; **2.** see ABO blood group, Blood Groups appendix.

**O an·ti·gen 1.** somatic antigen of enteric gram-negative bacteria. External part of cell wall lipopolysaccharide; SEE ALSO H antigen (1). **2.** see ABO blood group, Blood Groups appendix.

**OASIS** Outcomes and Assessment Information Set.

**oat cell** a short, bluntly spindle-shaped cell that contains a relatively large, hyperchromatic nucleus, frequently observed in undifferentiated bronchogenic carcinoma.

**oat cell car·ci·no·ma** an anaplastic, highly malignant, and usually bronchogenic carcinoma composed of small ovoid cells with very scanty cytoplasm; this carcinoma and small round cell carcinomas comprise over one-third of carcinomas of the lung. SYN small cell carcinoma (2).

**OB** obstetrics.

**ob·dor·mi·tion** (ob-dōr-mish'ŭn) numbness of an extremity, due to pressure on the sensory nerve. [L. *ob-dormio*, pp. *-itus*, to sleep]

**obe·li·ac** (ō-bē'lē-ak) relating to the obelion.

**obe·li·on** (ō-bē'lē-on) a craniometric point on the sagittal suture between the parietal foramina near the lambdoid suture. [G. *obelos*, a spit]

**Ober test** (ō'bĕr) test to evaluate a tight, contracted, or inflamed iliotibial tract; the patient lies on the uninvolved side and the involved hip is abducted by the examiner as the knee is flexed to 90°; the hip is allowed to adduct passively; the degree of abduction or the production of pain along the iliotibial tract can assist in identifying the location of the inflammation or contracture.

**obese** (ō-bēs') excessively fat. SYN corpulent. [L. *obesus*, fat, partic. adj., fr. *ob-edo*, pp. *-esus*, to eat away, devour]

**obe·si·ty** (ō-bē'si-tē) an abnormal increase of fat in the subcutaneous connective tissues. See this page. SYN adiposity (1), corpulence, corpulency.

**obex** (ō'beks) the point on the midline of the dorsal surface of the medulla oblongata that marks the caudal angle of the rhomboid fossa or fourth ventricle. It corresponds to a small, transverse medullary fold overhanging the calamus scriptorius. [L. barrier]

**OB/GYN** obstetrics and gynecology.

**ob·ject** (ob'jekt) **1.** anything to which thought or action is directed. **2.** in psychoanalysis, that

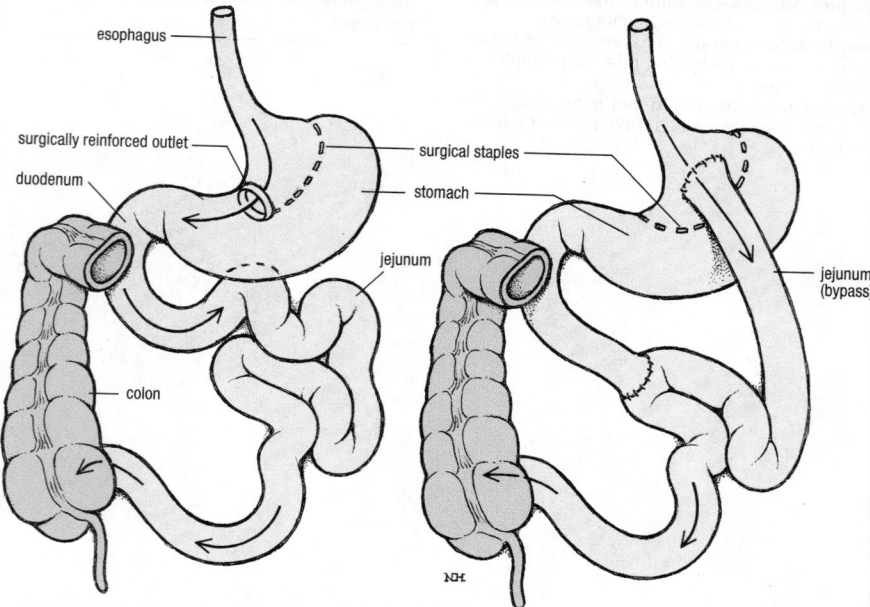

**surgical procedures to control morbid obesity:** (A) vertical banded gastroplasty, (B) gastric bypass (gastro-jejunostomy); in both procedures the reduction in gastric capacity leads to early satiety and thus favors consumption of smaller meals

through which an instinct can achieve its aim. **3.** in psychoanalysis, often used synonymously with person.

**ob·ject choice** PSYCHOANALYSIS the object (usually a person) upon which psychic energy is centered.

**ob·jec·tive** (ob-jek'tiv) **1.** the lens or lenses in the lower end of the body tube of a microscope. **2.** pertaining to facts, conditions, or phenomena as they actually exist, without distortion by personal viewpoint or prejudice; open to observation by oneself and by others. Cf. subjective. [L. *objicio,* pp. *-jectus,* to throw before]

**ob·jec·tive as·sess·ment da·ta** those facts that are observable and measurable by the nurse.

**ob·jec·tive sen·sa·tion** a sensation caused by a verifiable stimulus.

**ob·jec·tive symp·tom** a symptom that is evident to the observer.

**ob·ject re·la·tion·ship** BEHAVIORAL SCIENCES the emotional bond between an individual and another person (or between two groups), as opposed to the individual's or group's interest in self.

**OBLA** onset of blood lactate accumulation.

**ob·li·gate** (ob'li-gāt) without an alternative system or pathway. [L. *ob-ligo,* pp. *-atus,* to bind to]

**ob·li·gate aer·obe** an organism which cannot live or grow in the absence of oxygen.

**ob·li·gate an·aer·obe** an anaerobe that will grow only in the absence of free oxygen.

**ob·li·gate par·a·site** a parasite that cannot lead an independent nonparasitic existence, in contrast to facultative parasite.

**ob·lique** (ob-lēk') **1.** slanting; deviating from the perpendicular, horizontal, sagittal, or coronal plane of the body. **2.** RADIOGRAPHY a projection that is neither frontal nor lateral. [L. *obliquus*]

**ob·lique am·pu·ta·tion** amputation in which the line of section through an extremity is at other than a right angle; this yields an oval appearance to the cut surface (hence sometimes, though rarely, referred to as an oval amputation).

**ob·lique di·am·e·ter** a measurement across the pelvic inlet from the sacroiliac joint of one side to the opposite iliopectineal eminence.

**ob·lique fi·bers of mus·cu·lar la·yer of stom·ach** the smooth muscle fibers of the innermost layer of the muscular coat of the stomach; the fibers occur chiefly at the cardiac end of the stomach and spread over the anterior and posterior surfaces.

**ob·lique frac·ture** a fracture the line of which runs obliquely to the axis of the bone.

**ob·lique lie** that relationship in which the long axis of the fetus crosses the maternal axis at an angle other than a right angle.

**ob·lique ridge** a crest on the occlusal surface of upper molars comprising the distal cusp ridge of the mesiolingual cusp and the triangular ridge of the distobuccal cusp.

**ob·lique sec·tion** a diagonal cross section attained by slicing, actually or through imaging techniques, the body or any part of the body or anatomic structure, in any plane which does not parallel the longitudinal axis or intersect it at a right angle, i.e., which is neither longitudinal (vertical) nor transverse (horizontal).

**ob·lique vein of left a·tri·um** a small vein on the posterior wall of the left atrium that merges with the great cardiac vein to form the coronary

sinus; it is developed from the left common cardinal vein, and occasionally persists as a left superior vena cava. SYN Marshall oblique vein.

**ob·liq·ui·ty** (ob-lik'wi-tē) SYN asynclitism.

**ob·lit·er·a·tion** (ob-lit-er-ā'shŭn) **1.** blotting out, especially by filling of a natural space or lumen by fibrosis or inflammation. **2.** RADIOLOGY disappearance of the contour of an organ when the adjacent tissue has the same x-ray absorption. [L. *oblittero,* to blot out]

**o·blit·er·a·tive bron·chi·tis, bron·chi·tis ob·li·te·rans** fibrinous bronchitis in which the exudate is not expectorated but becomes organized, obliterating the affected portion of the bronchial tubes with consequent permanent collapse of affected portions of the lung.

**ob·lit·er·a·tive per·i·car·di·tis** complete obliteration of the pericardial cavity by postinflammatory adhesions.

**ob·lon·ga·ta** (ob-long-gā'tă) SYN medulla oblongata. [L. fem. of *oblongatus,* from *oblongus,* rather long]

**OBS** organic brain syndrome,

**ob·ses·sion** (ob-sesh'ŭn) a recurrent and persistent idea, thought, or impulse to carry out an act that is ego-dystonic, that is experienced as senseless or repugnant, and that the individual cannot voluntarily suppress. [L. *obsideo,* pp. *-sessus,* to besiege, fr. *sedeo,* to sit]

**ob·ses·sive-com·pul·sive** having a tendency to perform certain repetitive acts or ritualistic behavior to relieve anxiety, as in obsessive-compulsive neurosis (e.g., a compulsive, ritualistic need to wash one's hands many dozens of times per day).

**ob·ses·sive-com·pul·sive dis·or·der** a type of anxiety disorder whose essential feature is recurrent obsessions, persistent, intrusive ideas, thoughts, impulses or images, or compulsions (repetitive, purposeful, and intentional behaviors performed in response to an obsession) sufficiently severe to cause marked distress, be time-consuming, or interfere significantly with the individual's normal routine, occupational functioning, or usual social activities or relationships with others.

**ob·stet·ric, ob·stet·ri·cal** (ob-stet'rik, ob-stet'ri-kăl) relating to obstetrics.

**ob·stet·ri·cal bind·er** a supporting garment covering the abdomen from the ribs to the trochanters, tightly pinned at the back, affording support after childbirth or, rarely, during childbirth.

**ob·stet·ri·cal for·ceps** forceps used for grasping and applying traction to or for rotation of the fetal head; the blades are introduced separately into the genital canal, permitting the fetal head to be grasped firmly but with minimal compression, and are articulated after being placed in position.

**ob·stet·ri·cal hand** SYN accoucheur's hand.

**ob·stet·ric con·ju·gate** the shortest diameter through which the fetal head must pass in descending into the superior strait; as measured by x-ray, the distance from the promontory of the sacrum to a point on the inner surface of the symphysis a few millimeters below its upper margin.

**ob·stet·ri·c hand** SYN accoucheur's hand.

**ob·ste·tri·cian** (ob-stě-trish'ŭn) a physician specializing in the medical care of women during pregnancy and childbirth. [see obstetrics]

**ob·stet·ric pal·sy** a brachial plexus lesion sustained by an infant during delivery; three types are recognized: 1) upper plexus type, affecting the shoulder and upper arm (Erb palsy, by far the most common form); 2) total plexus type, involving the whole arm; 3) lower plexus type, involving the forearm and hand (Klumpke palsy). SYN obstetric paralysis.

**ob•stet•ric pa•ral•y•sis** SYN obstetric palsy.

**ob•stet•rics (OB)** (ob-stet′riks) the specialty of medicine concerned with the care of women during pregnancy, parturition, and the puerperium. [L. *obstetrix,* a midwife, fr. *ob-sto,* to stand before, denoting the position formerly taken by the midwife]

**ob•sti•nate** (ob′sti-năt) **1.** firmly adhering to one's own purpose, opinion, etc. even when wrong; not yielding to argument, persuasion, or entreaty. SYN intractable (2), refractory (2). **2.** SYN refractory (1). [L. *obstinatus,* determined]

**ob•sti•pa•tion** (ob-sti-pā′shŭn) intestinal obstruction; severe constipation. [L. *ob,* against, + *stipo,* pp. *-atus,* to crowd]

🛈 **ob•struc•tion** (ob-strŭk′shŭn) blockage or clogging, e.g., by occlusion or stenosis. See this page. [L. *obstructio*]

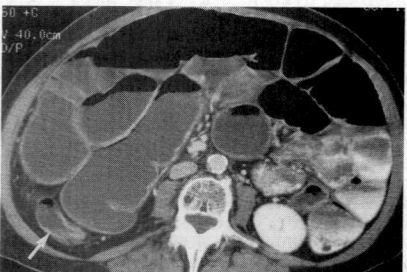

**small bowel obstruction:** CT demonstrates dilated fluid- and air-filled loops of small intestine; adhesions obstructing the distal ileum were found at surgery

**ob•struc•tive ap•nea, pe•riph•e•ral ap•ne•a** apnea either as the result of obstruction of the air passages or inadequate respiratory muscle activity.

**ob•struc•tive dys•men•or•rhea** SYN mechanical dysmenorrhea.

**ob•struc•tive hy•dro•ceph•a•lus** hydrocephalus secondary to a block in cerebrospinal fluid flow in the ventricular system or between the ventricular system and spinal canal. SYN noncommunicating hydrocephalus.

**ob•struc•tive jaun•dice** jaundice resulting from obstruction to the flow of bile into the duodenum, whether intra- or extrahepatic. SYN mechanical jaundice.

**ob•struc•tive mur•mur** a murmur caused by narrowing of one of the valvular orifices.

**ob•struc•tive sleep ap•nea** a disorder, first described in 1965, characterized by recurrent interruptions of breathing during sleep due to temporary obstruction of the airway by lax, excessively bulky, or malformed pharyngeal tissues (soft palate, uvula, and sometimes tonsils), with resultant hypoxemia and chronic lethargy.

**ob•struc•tive throm•bus** a thrombus due to ob-struction in the vessel from compression or other cause.

**ob•struc•tive u•rop•a•thy** any pathologic condition, anatomic or functional, of the urinary tract caused by obstruction.

**ob•struc•tive ven•ti•la•tory de•fect** slowing of airflow during forced ventilatory maneuvers, generally expiratory.

**ob•tund** (ob-tŭnd′) to dull or blunt, especially to blunt sensation or deaden pain. [L. *ob-tundo,* pp. *-tusus,* to beat against, blunt]

**ob•tu•rat•ing em•bo•lism** complete closing of the lumen of a vessel by an embolus.

**ob•tu•ra•tion** (ob-too-rā′shŭn) obstruction or occlusion. [see obturator]

**ob•tu•ra•tor** (ob′too-rā-tŏr) **1.** any structure that occludes an opening. **2.** denoting the obturator foramen, the obturator membrane, or any of several parts in relation to this foramen. **3.** a prosthesis used to close an opening of the hard palate, usually a cleft palate. **4.** the stylus or removable plug used during the insertion of many tubular instruments. [L. *obturo,* pp. *-atus,* to occlude or stop up]

**ob•tu•ra•tor ar•tery** *anastomoses,* iliolumbar, inferior epigastric, medial circumflex femoral; *origin,* anterior division of the internal iliac; *distribution,* ilium, pubis, obturator and adductor muscles; *branches,* pubic, acetabular, anterior, and posterior. SYN arteria obturatoria [TA].

**ob•tu•ra•tor branch of pu•bic branch of in•fe•ri•or epi•gas•tric vein** branch of the pubic branch of inferior epigastric artery that descends over the pelvic brim to anastomose with the pubic branch of the obturator artery; in 20–30% of people, this branch is larger than or replaces the obturator artery.

**ob•tu•ra•tor ca•nal** the opening in the superior part of the obturator membrane through which the obturator nerve and vessels pass from the pelvic cavity into the thigh. SYN canalis obturatorius [TA].

**ob•tu•ra•tor crest** a ridge that extends from the pubic tubercle to the acetabular notch, giving attachment to the pubofemoral ligament of the hip joint.

**ob•tu•ra•tor ex•ter•nus mus•cle** *origin,* lower half of margin of obturator foramen and adjacent part of external surface of obturator membrane; *insertion,* trochanteric fossa of greater trochanter; *action,* rotates thigh laterally; *nerve supply,* obturator. SYN musculus obturatorius externus [TA], external obturator muscle.

**ob•tu•ra•tor fo•ra•men** a large, oval or irregularly triangular aperture in the hip bone, the margins of which are formed by the pubis and the ischium; it is closed by the obturator membrane, except for a small opening for the passage of the obturator vessels and nerve. SYN foramen obturatum [TA].

**ob•tu•ra•tor her•nia** hernia through the obturator foramen.

**ob•tu•ra•tor in•ter•nus mus•cle** *origin,* pelvic surface of obturator membrane and margin of obturator foramen; *insertion,* passes out of pelvis through lesser sciatic foramen, in so doing, making a 90° turn to insert into the medial surface of greater trochanter; *action,* rotates thigh laterally; *nerve supply,* nerve to obturator internus (sacral plexus). SYN musculus obturatorius internus [TA], internal obturator muscle.

**ob·tu·ra·tor nerve** arises from the second, third, and fourth lumbar nerves in the psoas muscle, crosses the brim of the pelvis, and enters the thigh through the obturator canal; it supplies muscles of the medial compartment of the thigh (adductors of thigh at the hip joint) and terminates as the cutaneous branch of the obturator nerve, supplying a small area of medial thigh above knee. SYN nervus obturatorius [TA].

**ob·tu·ra·tor vein** formed by the union of tributaries draining the hip joint and the obturator and adductor muscles of the thigh; it enters the pelvis by the obturator canal as venae comitantes of the obturator artery and empties into the internal iliac vein.

**ob·tuse** (ob-toos′) **1.** dull in intellect; of slow understanding. **2.** blunt; not acute. [see obtund]

**ob·tu·sion** (ob-too′zhŭn) **1.** dullness of sensibility. **2.** a dulling or deadening of sensibility.

**Oc·cam ra·zor** the principle of scientific parsimony. William of Occam (14th century) stated it thus: "The assumptions introduced to explain a thing must not be multiplied beyond necessity."

**oc·cip·i·tal** (ok-sip′i-tăl) relating to the occiput; referring to the occipital bone or to the back of the head.

**oc·cip·i·tal ar·tery** *origin*, external carotid; *branches*, sternocleidomastoid, meningeal, auricular, occipital, mastoid, and descending. SYN arteria occipitalis [TA].

**oc·cip·i·tal bone** a bone at the lower and posterior part of the skull, consisting of three parts (basilar, condylar, and squamous), enclosing a large oval hole, the foramen magnum; it articulates with the parietal and temporal bones on either side, the sphenoid anteriorly, and the atlas below. SYN os occipitale [TA].

**oc·cip·i·tal ce·re·bral veins** the superior cerebral veins draining the occipital cortex and emptying into the superior sagittal sinus and the transverse sinus.

**oc·cip·i·tal·i·za·tion** (ok′sip′i-tăl-i-zā′shŭn) bony ankylosis between the atlas and occipital bone.

**oc·cip·i·tal lobe of cer·e·brum** the posterior, somewhat pyramid-shaped part of each cerebral hemisphere, demarcated by no distinct surface markings on the lateral convexity of the hemisphere from the parietal and temporal lobes, but sharply delineated from the parietal lobe by the parieto-occipital sulcus on the medial surface.

**oc·cip·i·tal lobe ep·i·lep·sy** a localization-related epilepsy where seizures originate from the occipital lobe. Symptoms commonly include visual abnormalities during seizures.

**oc·cip·i·tal pole of cer·e·brum** the most posterior promontory of each cerebral hemisphere; the apex of the occipital lobe.

**oc·cip·i·tal si·nus** an unpaired dural venous sinus commencing at the confluence of the sinuses and passing downward in the base of the falx cerebelli to the foramen magnum.

**oc·cip·i·tal vein** drains the occipital region and empties into the internal jugular vein or the suboccipital plexus.

△**oc·ci·pi·to-** the occiput, occipital structures. [L. *occiput*]

**oc·cip·i·to·an·te·ri·or po·si·tion (OA)** a cephalic presentation of the fetus with its occiput turned toward the right (**right occipitoanterior,** ROA) or to the left (**left occipitoanterior,** LOA) acetabulum of the mother.

**oc·cip·i·to·fa·cial** (ok-sip′i-tō-fā′shăl) relating to the occiput and the face.

**oc·cip·i·to·fron·tal** (ok-sip′i-tō-frŭn′tăl) **1.** relating to the occiput and the forehead. **2.** relating to the occipital and frontal lobe of the cerebral cortex and association pathways that interconnect these regions.

**oc·cip·i·to·fron·tal di·am·e·ter** the diameter of the fetal head from the external occipital protuberance to the most prominent point of the frontal bone in the midline.

**oc·cip·i·to·fron·ta·lis mus·cle** a part of musculus epicranius; the occipital belly (occipitalis muscle) arises from the occipital bone and inserts into the galea aponeurotica; the frontal belly (frontalis muscle) arises from the galea and inserts into the skin of the eyebrow and nose; *action*, to move the scalp; *nerve supply*, facial. SYN musculus occipitofrontalis [TA], occipitofrontal muscle.

**oc·cip·i·to·fron·tal mus·cle** SYN occipitofrontalis muscle.

**oc·cip·i·to·men·tal** (ok-sip′i-tō-men′tăl) relating to the occiput and the chin.

**oc·cip·i·to·men·tal di·am·e·ter** the diameter of the fetal head from the external occipital protuberance to the midpoint of the chin.

**oc·cip·i·to·pos·te·ri·or po·si·tion (OP)** a cephalic presentation of the fetus with its occiput turned toward the right (**right occipitoposterior,** ROP) or to the left (**left occipitoposterior,** LOP) sacroiliac joint of the mother.

**oc·cip·i·to·trans·verse po·si·tion** a cephalic presentation of the fetus with its occiput turned toward the right (**right occipitotransverse,** ROT) or to the left (**left occipitotransverse,** LOT) iliac fossa of the mother.

**oc·ci·put,** gen. **oc·cip·i·tis** (ok′si-put, ok-sip′i-tis) the back of the head. [L.]

**oc·clude** (ŏ-klood′) **1.** to close or bring together. **2.** to enclose, as in an occluded virus. [see occlusion]

**oc·clu·sal** (ŏ-kloo′zăl) **1.** pertaining to occlusion or closure. **2.** DENTISTRY pertaining to the contacting surfaces of opposing occlusal units (teeth or occlusion rims), or the masticating surfaces of the posterior teeth.

**oc·clu·sal a·nal·y·sis** a study of the relations of the occlusal surfaces of opposing teeth and their effect upon related structures. SYN bite analysis.

**oc·clu·sal equil·i·bra·tion** the modification of occlusal forms of teeth by grinding with the intent of equalizing occlusal stress, or producing simultaneous occlusal contacts, or of harmonizing cuspal relations.

**oc·clu·sal film** intraoral projection taken to provide a wider view of either the maxilla and palate or the mandible and floor of the mouth. See page 364.

**oc·clu·sal force** the result of muscular force applied on opposing teeth.

**oc·clu·sal im·bal·ance** an inharmonious relationship between the teeth of the maxilla and mandible during closing or functional movements of the jaw.

**oc·clu·sal po·si·tion** the relationship of the mandible and maxillae when the jaws are closed and the teeth are in maximum contact; it may or may not coincide with centric occlusion.

**oc·clu·sion** (ŏ-kloo′zhŭn) **1.** the act of closing or the state of being closed. **2.** in chemistry, the absorption of a gas by a metal or the inclusion of one substance within another (as in a gelatinous precipitate). **3.** any contact between the incising or masticating surfaces of the upper and lower teeth. **4.** the relationship between the occlusal surfaces of the maxillary and mandibular teeth when they are in contact. [L. *oc- cludo*, pp. *-clusus*, to shut up, fr. *ob.*, against, + *claudo*, to close]

**oc·clu·sive** (ŏ-kloo′siv) serving to close; denoting a bandage or dressing that closes a wound and excludes it from the air.

**oc·clu·sive dress·ing** a dressing that hermetically seals a wound.

**oc·clu·sive il·e·us** complete mechanical blocking of the intestinal lumen.

**oc·clu·sive men·in·gi·tis** leptomeningitis causing occlusion of the spinal fluid pathways.

**oc·cult** (ŏ-kŭlt′, ok′ŭlt) **1.** hidden; concealed; not manifest. **2.** denoting a disease or condition (bleeding, infection) that is clinically inapparent, though it may be inferred from indirect evidence or identified by special tests. SEE occult blood. **3.** ONCOLOGY a clinically unidentified primary tumor with recognized metastases. [L. *oc-culo*, pp. *-cultus*, to cover, hide]

**oc·cult blood** blood in the feces in amounts too small to be seen but detectable by chemical tests.

**oc·cult cho·roi·dal ne·o·vas·cu·l·ar·i·za·tion** area of leakage of undetermined source seen in the late phases of a retinal angiogram.

**oc·cult cleft pa·late** lack of closure in the bone of the hard palate or muscle of the soft palate, but with full closure of the overlying surface tissues. SYN submucous cleft palate.

**oc·cult frac·ture** a condition in which there are clinical signs of fracture but no x-ray evidence; after 3–4 weeks x-ray imaging shows new bone formation.

**oc·cult PEEP** SYN auto-positive-end-expiratory-pressure.

**oc·cult pos·te·ri·or la·ryn·ge·al cleft** SEE laryngotracheoesophageal cleft.

**oc·cu·pa·tion·al be·ha·vior** broadly, engagement in purposeful activity; such behavior has an organizing and integrating effect on psychological and social functioning; it is employed in occupational therapy to restore or maintain interest and self-confidence, overcome disability, or combat various features of physical or mental illness.

**oc·cu·pa·tion·al dis·ease** a morbid condition resulting from exposure to an agent during the usual performance of one's occupation. Cf. industrial disease.

**oc·cu·pa·tion·al hear·ing loss** SYN noise-induced hearing loss.

**oc·cu·pa·tion·al role** a function undertaken to provide the context for organizing one's time for work, play, and rest.

**occupational science** the study of the effects of occupation upon human behavior.

**oc·cu·pa·tion·al ther·a·py** therapeutic use of self-care, work, and recreational activities to increase independent function, enhance development, prevent disability and achieve optimum quality of life.

**Ochoa law** (ō′chō′ah) the content of the X-chromosome tends to be phylogenetically conserved.

**ochra·tox·in** (ō-kra-toks′in) a mycotoxin produced by *Aspergillus ochraceus* growing on stored cereal grains. Affects poultry and other animals fed the grain.

**ochra·tox·in A** ochratoxin produced by some species of *Aspergillus* and *Penicillium* that can contaminate cereal grains and feeds, primarily following improper storage; a potent carcinogen in rodents.

**o·chre co·don** the termination codon UAA.

**Och·ro·bac·trum** (ō-krō-bak′trum) a Gram-negative genus of bacteria similar to *Alcaligenes* and *Pseudomonas* spp. in their distribution in environmental and water sources and their culture characteristics. These have been isolated from a number of clinical sources and appear to be a cause of nosocomial bacteremia.

**ochrom·e·ter** (ō-krom′ĕ-ter) an instrument for determining the capillary blood pressure; one of two adjacent fingers is compressed by a rubber balloon until blanching of the skin occurs, after which the force necessary to accomplish this color change is read in millimeters of mercury. [G. *ōchros*, pale yellow, + *metron*, measure]

**ochro·no·sis** (o-kron-ō′sis) a condition observed in persons with alkaptonuria, characterized by pigmentation of the cartilages; may also affect the sclera, mucous membrane of the lips, and skin of the ears, face, and hands, and cause standing urine to be dark-colored and contain pigmented casts; pigmentation from oxidized homogentisic acid; cartilage degeneration results in osteoarthritis. [G. *ōchros*, pale yellow, + *nosos*, disease]

**ochro·not·ic** (ō-kron-ot′ik) relating to or characterized by ochronosis.

**oct-, octi-, octo-, octa-** eight. [G. *oktō*, L. *octo*]

**oc·ta·fluor·o·pro·pane** (ok′ta-floo-r′ō-prō-pān) a drug used for contrast enhancement during ultrasound imaging.

**oc·tan** (ok′tan) applied to fever, the paroxysms of which recur every eighth day, the day of a paroxysm being counted as the first in the computation. [L. *octo*, eight]

**oc·u·lar** (ok′yu-lăr) **1.** SYN ophthalmic. **2.** the eyepiece of a microscope, the lens or lenses at the observer end of a microscope, by means of which the image focused by the objective is viewed. [L. *oculus*, eye]

**oc·u·lar al·bi·nism** absence of pigment chiefly in the iris, choroid, and retinal pigment epithelium with deafness; X-linked inheritance.

**oc·u·lar al·bin·ism 1** type of ocular albinism characterized by depigmentation of the fundus and prominent choroidal vessels, nystagmus, and titubation; vision is usually impaired; caused by mutation in the OA1 gene on chromosome Xp; X-linked inheritance. SYN Nettleshop-Falls albinism.

**oc·u·lar al·bin·ism 2** type of ocular albinism characterized by hypoplasia of the fovea, marked impairment of vision, nystagmus, myopia, astigmatism, and protanomalous color blindness, in addition to albinism of the fundus. SYN Aland Island albinism, Forsius-Eriksson albinism.

**oc·u·lar al·bin·ism 3** type of ocular albinism characterized by impaired vision, translucent irides, congenital nystagmus, photophobia, albinotic fundi with hyperplasia of the fovea, and strabismus; caused by mutation in the pinkeye gene (P) on 6q; autosomal recessive inheritance.

**oc·u·lar cic·a·tri·cial pem·phi·goid** a chronic disease that produces adhesions and progressive cicatrization and shrinkage of the conjunctival, oral, and vaginal mucous membranes.

**oc·u·lar hu·mor** one of the two humors of the eye: aqueous and vitreous.

**oc·u·lar hy·per·tel·or·ism** increased width between the eyes due to an enlarged sphenoid bone; other congenital anomalies and mental retardation may be associated. SYN Opitz BBB syndrome, Opitz G syndrome.

**oc·u·lar·ist** (ok′yu-lăr-ist) one skilled in the design, fabrication, and fitting of artificial eyes and the making of prostheses associated with the appearance or function of the eyes. [L. *oculus*, eye]

**oc·u·lar lar·va mi·grans gran·u·lo·ma** eosinophilic granulomata found surrounding dead worms (generally, *Toxocara* spp.) in the eye; may mimic retinoblastoma.

**oc·u·lar ten·sion (Tn)** resistance of the tunics of the eye to deformation; it can be estimated digitally or measured by means of a tonometer.

**oc·u·lar ver·ti·go** dizziness attributed to refractive errors or imbalance of the extrinsic muscles.

**oc·u·li** (ok′yu-lī) plural of oculus. [L.]

**oc·u·list** (ok′yu-list) SYN ophthalmologist. [L. *oculus*, eye]

△**ocu·lo-** the eye, ocular. SEE ALSO ophthalmo-. [L. *oculus*]

**oc·u·lo·cu·ta·ne·ous** (ok′yu-lō-kyu-tā′nē-ŭs) relating to the eyes and the skin.

**oc·u·lo·dyn·ia** pain in the eyeball. [ophthalmo- + G. *algos*, pain]

**oc·u·lo·fa·cial** (ok-yu-lō-fā′shăl) relating to the eyes and the face.

**oc·u·log·ra·phy** (ok-yu-log′ră-fē) a method of recording eye position and movements. [oculo- + G. *graphē*, a writing]

**oc·u·lo·gy·ria** (ok′yu-lō-jī′rē-ă) the limits of rotation of the eyeballs. [oculo- + G. *gyros*, circle]

**oc·u·lo·gy·ric** (ok′yu-lō-jī′rik) referring to rotation of the eyeballs; characterized by oculogyria.

**oc·u·lo·mo·tor** (ok′yu-lō-mō′tŏr) pertaining to the oculomotor cranial nerve. [L. *oculomotorius*, fr. oculo- + L. *motorius*, moving]

**oc·u·lo·mo·tor nerve [CN III]** the third cranial nerve, it supplies all the extrinsic muscles of the eye, except the lateral rectus and superior oblique; it also supplies the levator palpebrae superioris and conveys presynaptic parasympathetic fibers to the ciliary ganglion for innervation of the ciliary muscle and sphincter pupillae; its origin is in the midbrain below the cerebral aqueduct; it emerges from the brain in the interpeduncular fossa, pierces the dura mater to the side of the posterior clinoid process, passes in the lateral wall of the cavernous sinus, and enters the orbit through the superior orbital fissure. SYN nervus oculomotorius [CN III] [TA], third cranial nerve [CN III].

**oc·u·lo·mo·tor nu·cle·us** the composite group of motor neurons innervating all of the external eye muscles except the musculus rectus lateralis and musculus obliquus superior, and including the musculus levator palpebrae superioris; the most rostral component of the nucleus is the Edinger-Westphal nucleus which innervates the musculi sphincter pupillae and ciliaris via the ciliary ganglion. The oculomotor nucleus lies in the rostral half of the midbrain, near the midline in the most ventral part of the central gray substance; fibers of the medial longitudinal fasciculus form its lateral borders.

**oc·u·lo·na·sal** (ok′yu-lō-nā′săl) relating to the eyes and the nose. [oculo- + L. *nasus*, nose]

**oc·u·lo·pha·ryn·ge·al dys·tro·phy** a dominantly inherited form of chronic progressive external ophthalmoplegia usually presenting in middle life or old age with chronic ptosis and/or difficulty swallowing. Many sufferers have French-Canadian ancestry.

**oc·u·lo·pleth·ys·mog·ra·phy** (ok′yu-lō-pleth-iz-mog′ră-fē) indirect measurement of the hemodynamic significance of internal carotid artery stenosis or occlusion by demonstration of an ipsilateral delay in the arrival of ocular pressure transmitted from branches of the ophthalmic artery. [oculo- + G. *plēthymos*, increase, + *graphē*, to write]

**oc·u·lo·pneu·mo·pleth·ys·mog·ra·phy** (ok′yu-lō-noo′mō-pleth-iz-mog′ră-fē) a method of bilateral measurement of ophthalmic artery pressure that reflects pressure and flow in the internal carotid artery. SEE oculoplethysmography.

**oc·u·lo·pu·pil·lary** (ok′yu-lō-pyu′pi-lār-ē) pertaining to the pupil of the eye.

**oc·u·lo·sym·pa·thet·ic** (ok′oo-lō-sim-pa-the′tik) pertaining to the sympathetic pathway to the eye, damage to which produces Horner syndrome.

**oc·u·lo·zy·go·mat·ic** (ok′yu-lō-zī-gō-mat′ik) relating to the orbit or its margin and the zygomatic bone.

**oc·u·lus**, gen. and pl. **oc·u·li** (ok′yu-lŭs, ok′yu-lī) [TA] SYN eye (1). [L.]

△**ocy-** SEE oxy-.

**OD** overdose; optical density (see absorbance).

**od** a force assumed to be exerted upon the nervous system by magnets. [G. *hodos*, way]

△**-odes** having the form of, resembling. [G. *eidos*, form, resemblance]

△**odont-, odonto-** a tooth, teeth. [G. *odous* (*odont-*)]

**odon·tal·gia** (ō-don-tal′jē-ă) SYN toothache. [odont- + G. *algos*, pain]

**odon·tal·gic** (ō-don-tal′jik) relating to or marked by toothache.

**odon·tec·to·my** (ō-don-tek′tō-mē) removal of teeth by the reflection of a mucoperiosteal flap and excision of bone from around the root or roots before the application of force to effect the tooth removal. [odont- + G. *ektomē*, excision]

**odon·to·blast** (ō-don′tō-blast) one of the dentin-forming cells, derived from mesenchyme of neural crest origin, lining the pulp cavity of a tooth. [odonto- + G. *blastos*, sprout, germ]

**o·don·to·blas·tic lay·er** a layer of connective tissue cells at the periphery of the dental pulp of the tooth.

**odon·to·blas·to·ma** (ō-don′tō-blas-tō′mă) **1.** a tumor composed of neoplastic epithelial and mesenchymal cells that may differentiate into cells able to produce calcified tooth substances. **2.** an odontoma in its early formative stage. [odontoblast + G. *-oma*, tumor]

**odon·to·clast** (ō-don′tō-klast) one of the osteoclastic cells believed to produce resorption of the roots of the deciduous teeth. [odonto- + G. *klastos*, broken]

**odon·to·dys·pla·sia** (ō-don′tō-dis-plā′zē-ă) a developmental disturbance of one or of several adjacent teeth, of unknown etiology, characterized by deficient formation of enamel and dentin which results in an abnormally large pulp chamber and imparts a ghostlike radiographic image to the teeth; such teeth exhibit delayed eruption into the oral cavity.

**odon·to·gen·e·sis** (ō-don-tō-jen'ĕ-sis) the process of development of the teeth. SYN odontogeny, odontosis. [odonto- + G. *genesis,* production]

**o·don·to·gen·ic cyst** a cyst derived from odontogenic epithelium. [odont- + G. *genos,* birth, origin, + suffix -*ic,* pertaining to]

**odon·to·gen·ic ke·ra·to·cyst** (ō-don-tō-jen'ik ker'atō-sist) a cyst of dental lamina origin with a high recurrence rate, a corrugated parakeratin surface, uniformly thin epithelium, and a palisaded basal layer. One manifestation of the basal cell nevus syndrome.

**odon·tog·e·ny** (ō-don-toj'ĕ-nē) SYN odontogenesis.

**odon·to·glyph·ics** (ō-don'tō-glĭf'iks) a method of classification of the molar grooves defined in an individually distinctive pattern like that of fingerprints. [odonto- + G. *glyphē,* carving]

**odon·toid** (ō-don'toyd) **1.** shaped like a tooth. **2.** relating to the toothlike odontoid process of the second cervical vertebra. [odont- + G. *eidos,* resemblance]

**odon·toid pro·cess of ep·i·stro·phe·us** SYN dens (2).

**odon·tol·o·gy** (ō-don-tol'ŏ-jē) the study of the teeth and their supporting structures. [odonto- + G. *logos,* study]

**odon·tol·y·sis** (ō-don-tol'i-sis) SYN erosion (3). [odonto- + G. *lysis,* dissolution]

**odon·to·ma** (ō-don-tō'mă) **1.** a tumor of odontogenic origin. **2.** a hamartomatous odontogenic tumor composed of enamel, dentin, cementum, and pulp tissue that may or may not be arranged in the form of a tooth. [odonto- + G. -*oma,* tumor]

**odon·to·neu·ral·gia** (ō-don'tō-noo-ral'jē-ă) facial neuralgia caused by a carious tooth.

**odon·ton·o·my** (ō-don-ton'ō-mē) dental nomenclature. [odonto- + G. *onoma,* name]

**odon·top·a·thy** (ō-don-top'ă-thē) any disease of the teeth or of their sockets. [odonto- + G. *pathos,* suffering]

**odon·to·plas·ty** (ō-dŏn'tō-plăs-tē) reshaping of a portion of a tooth; may be performed for therapeutic or cosmetic purposes. [odonto- + -plasty]

**odon·to·sis** (ō-don-tō'sis) SYN odontogenesis.

**odon·tot·o·my** (ō-don-tot'ō-mē) cutting into the crown of a tooth. [odonto- + G. *tomē,* incision]

**odor** (ō'dŏr) emanation from any substance that stimulates the olfactory cells in the organ of smell. SYN smell (3). [L.]

⚠**odyn-, odyno-** pain. [G. *odynē*]

**odyn·a·cu·sis** (ō-din'ă-koo'sis) hypersensitiveness of the organ of hearing, so that noises cause actual pain. [odyn- + G. *akouō,* to hear]

**ody·nom·e·ter** (ō-di-nom'ĕ-ter) SYN algesiometer. [odyno- + G. *metron,* measure]

**odyn·o·pha·gia** (ō-din-ō-fā'jē-ă) pain on swallowing. [odyno- + G. *phagō* to eat]

⚠**oe-** for words so beginning and not found here, see e-.

**oe·de·ma [Br.]** SEE edema.

**oe·de·ma·tous [Br.]** SEE edematous.

**oe·di·pal phase** in psychoanalysis, a stage in the psychosexual development of the child, characterized by erotic attachment to the parent of the opposite sex, repressed because of fear of the parent of the same sex; usually occurring between the ages of 3 and 6 years.

**oe·di·pism** (ed'i-pizm) **1.** self-infliction of injury to the eyes, usually an attempt at evulsion. **2.** manifestation of the Oedipus complex. [*Oedipus,* G. myth. char.]

**Oed·i·pus com·plex** a group of associated ideas, aims, instinctual drives, and fears in male children 3–6 years old: at the peak of the phallic phase of psychosexual development, the child's sexual interest is attached primarily to the mother and is accompanied by aggressive feelings toward the father; in psychoanalytic theory, it is replaced by the castration complex. [*Oedipus,* G. myth. char.]

**oe·nol·o·gy [Br.]** SEE enology.

**oe·no·man·ia [Br.]** SYN delirium tremens.

**oer·sted** (er'sted) a unit of magnetic field intensity; the magnetic field intensity that exerts a force of 1 dyne on unit magnetic pole; equal to $(1000/4\pi)$ A·m$^{-1}$. [Hans-Christian *Oersted,* Danish physicist, 1777–1851]

**oe·soph·a·ge·al [Br.]** SEE esophageal.

**oe·soph·a·gec·tas·ia [Br.]** SEE esophagectasia.

**oe·soph·a·gec·to·my [Br.]** SEE esophagectomy.

**oe·soph·a·gism [Br.]** SEE esophagism.

**oe·soph·a·gi·tis [Br.]** SEE esophagitis.

**oe·soph·a·go·car·di·o·plas·ty [Br.]** SEE esophagocardioplasty.

**oe·soph·a·go·cele [Br.]** SEE esophagocele.

**oe·soph·a·go·du·o·den·os·to·my [Br.]** SEE esophagoduodenostomy.

**oe·soph·a·go·en·ter·os·to·my [Br.]** SEE esophagoenterostomy.

**oe·soph·a·go·gas·tro·du·o·den·os·co·py [Br.]** SEE esophagogastroduodenoscopy.

**oe·soph·a·go·gas·tro·plas·ty [Br.]** SYN cardioplasty.

**oe·soph·a·go·plas·ty [Br.]** SEE esophagoplasty.

**oe·soph·a·go·scope [Br.]** SEE esophagoscope.

**oe·soph·a·go·scopy [Br.]** SEE esophagoscopy.

**oe·soph·a·go·spasm [Br.]** SEE esophagospasm.

**oe·soph·a·go·sten·o·sis [Br.]** SEE esophagostenosis.

**oe·soph·a·go·sto·mi·a·sis [Br.]** SEE esophagostomiasis.

***Oe·soph·a·gos·to·mum*** (ē-sof'ă-gos'tō-mum) a genus of nematodes (superfamily Strongyloidea) that parasitize the intestines of animals; larvae encyst in the intestinal wall.

**oe·soph·a·go·sto·my [Br.]** SEE esophagostomy.

**oe·soph·a·got·o·my [Br.]** SEE esophagotomy.

**oe·soph·a·gus [Br.]** SEE esophagus.

**oes·tra·di·ol [Br.]** SEE estradiol.

**oes·tri·ol [Br.]** SEE estriol.

**oes·tro·gen [Br.]** SEE estrogen.

**oes·tro·ne [Br.]** SEE estrone.

**oes·tru·al [Br.]** SYN estrous.

**oes·tru·a·tion [Br.]** SEE estruation.

**oes·trus [Br.]** SEE estrus.

**of·fi·cial** (ŏ-fish'ăl) authoritative; denoting a drug or a chemical or pharmaceutical preparation recognized as standard in the Pharmacopeia. [L. *officialis,* fr. *officium,* a favor, service, fr. *opus,* work, + *facio,* to do]

**of·fi·cial for·mu·la** a formula contained in the Pharmacopeia or the National Formulary.

**off la·bel in·di·ca·tion** use of a medication for a purpose other than that approved by the FDA.

**off-ver·ti·cal ro·ta·tion** rotation about an axis eccentric to the body.

**O·fu·ji dis·ease** (ō-foo'jē) SYN eosinophilic pustular folliculitis.

**Og·il·vie syn·drome** pseudoobstruction, predominantly of the colon, believed to be the result of motility disturbance; without physical obstruction.

**O·gi·no-Knaus rule** (ō-gē-nō-naws) the time in the menstrual period when conception is most likely to occur is at about midway between two menstrual periods; fertilization of the ovum is least likely just before or just after menstruation; the basis for the rhythm method of contraception.

**Og·ston line** (ŏg'stŏn) a line drawn from the adductor tubercle of the femur to the intercondylar notch; a guide to resection of the medial condyle for knock-knee.

**O·gu·chi dis·ease** (ō-goo'chē) a rare congenital nonprogressive night blindness with diffuse yellow or gray coloration of fundus; after two or three hours in total darkness, fundus resumes normal color; autosomal recessive inheritance, caused by mutation in either the arrestin gene (SAG) on 2q or the rhodopsin kinase gene (RHOK) on 13q.

**O·gu·ra op·er·a·tion** (ō-goo'rah) orbital decompression by removal of the floor of the orbit through an opening made in the supradental (canine) fossa.

**OHI-S** Simplified Oral Hygiene Index.

**Ohm** (ōm), Georgi S., German physicist, 1787–1854. SEE ohm.

**ohm** (Ω) (ōm) the practical unit of electrical resistance; the resistance of any conductor allowing 1 ampere of current to pass under the electromotive force of 1 volt. [G.S. *Ohm*]

**Ohm law** (ōm) in an electric current passing through a wire, the intensity of the current ($I$) in amperes equals the electromotive force ($E$) in volts divided by the resistance ($R$) in ohms: $I = E/R$.

**oh·ne Hauch** (ō'nă howch) term used to designate the nonspreading growth of nonflagellated bacteria on agar media; also applied to somatic agglutination. SEE ALSO O antigen. [Ger. without breath]

**Ohn·gren line** (ŏn'gren) a theoretical plane passing between the medial canthus of the eye and the angle of the mandible; used as an arbitrary dividing line in classifying localized tumors of the maxillary sinus; tumors above the line invade vital structures early and have a poorer prognosis, whereas those below the line have a more favorable prognosis.

**OI** osteogenesis imperfecta.

△**oi-** for words so beginning and not found here, see e-.

△**-oid** resemblance to, joined properly to words formed from G. roots; equivalent to Eng. -form. [G. *eidos*, form, resemblance]

**oid·i·o·my·cin** (ō-id'ē-ō-mī'sin) an antigen used to demonstrate cutaneous hypersensitivity in patients infected with *Candida;* one of a series of antigens used to demonstrate an immunocompromised patient's capacity to react to any cutaneous antigen. [oidium + G. *mykēs*, fungus, + -in]

**oil** an inflammable liquid, of fatty consistency and unctuous feel, that is insoluble in water, soluble or insoluble in alcohol, and freely soluble in ether. Oils are variously classified as animal, vegetable, and mineral oils according to their source; into fatty (fixed) and volatile oils; and into drying and nondrying (fatty) oils, the former becoming gradually thicker when exposed to the air and finally drying to a varnish, the latter not drying but liable to become rancid on exposure. Many of the oils, both fixed and volatile, are used in medicine. For individual oils, see the specific names.

**oil of vi·tri·ol** SYN sulphuric acid.

**oint·ment** (oynt'ment) a semisolid preparation usually containing medicinal substances and intended for external application. SYN salve, unguent. [O. Fr. *oignement;* L. *unguo,* pp. *unctus,* to smear]

**OKT cells** cells recognized by monoclonal antibodies to T lymphocyte antigens. Current usage favors CD designations. [*Ortho-Kung T* cell]

△**-ol** suffix denoting that a substance is an alcohol or a phenol.

**Old·field syn·drome** (ōld'fēld), familial polyposis of the colon.

**Old World leish·man·i·a·sis** SYN cutaneous leishmaniasis.

**o·le·ag·i·nous** (ō-lē-aj'i-nŭs) oily or greasy. [L. *oleagineus,* pertaining to *olea,* the olive tree]

**ole·ate** (ō'lē-āt) **1.** a salt of oleic acid. **2.** a pharmacopeial preparation consisting of a combination or solution of an alkaloid or metallic base in oleic acid, used as an inunction.

**olec·ra·non** (ō-lek'ră-non, ō'lē-krā'non) [TA] the prominent curved proximal extremity of the ulna, the upper and posterior surface of which gives attachment to the tendon of the triceps muscle, the anterior surface entering into the formation of the trochlear notch. SYN elbow bone, point of elbow. [G. the head or point of the elbow, fr. *ōlenē,* ulna, + *kranion,* skull, head]

**ole·fin** (ō'lē-fin) SYN alkene.

△**ol·eo-** oil. SEE ALSO eleo-. [L. *oleum*]

**El ol·fac·tion** (ol-fak'shŭn) **1.** the sense of smell. SYN smell (2). **2.** the act of smelling. See this page. SYN osphresis. [L. *ol- facio,* pp. *-factus,* to smell]

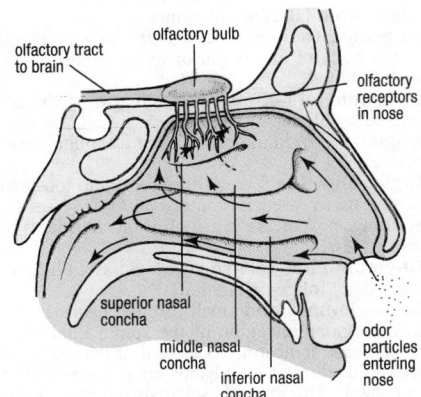

**olfactory nerves** (receptors in nose)

**ol·fac·to·ry** (ol-fak'tŏ-rē) relating to the sense of smell. SYN osphretic. [see olfaction]

**ol·fac·tory ag·no·sia** inability to classify or identify an odorant, although the ability to distinguish between or recognize odorants may be normal; may be general, partial, or specific.

**ol·fac·tory au·ra** epileptic aura characterized by

illusions or hallucinations of smell. SEE ALSO aura (1).

**ol·fac·to·ry bulb** the grayish expanded rostral extremity of the olfactory tract, lying on the cribriform plate of the ethmoid and receiving the olfactory filaments. SYN bulbus olfactorius [TA].

**ol·fac·to·ry ep·i·the·li·um** an epithelium of the pseudostratified type that contains olfactory, receptor, nerve cells whose axons extend to the olfactory bulb of the brain.

**ol·fac·to·ry fo·ra·men** one of the openings in the cribriform plate of the ethmoid bone, transmitting the olfactory nerves.

**ol·fac·to·ry glands** branched tubuloalveolar serous secreting glands (of Bowman) in the mucous membrane of the olfactory region of the nasal cavity.

**ol·fac·to·ry mem·brane** that part of the nasal mucosa having olfactory receptor cells and glands of Bowman.

**ol·fac·to·ry nerves [CN I]** collective term denoting the numerous olfactory filaments: slender fascicles each composed of the thin, unmyelinated axons of 8 to 12 of the bipolar olfactory receptor cells in the olfactory portion of the nasal mucosa; the olfactory filaments pass through the cribriform plate of the ethmoid bone and enter the olfactory bulb, where they terminate in synaptic contact with mitral cells, tufted cells, and granule cells. SYN nervi olfactorii [TA], nervus olfactorii [CN I] [TA], first cranial nerve [CN I].

**ol·fac·to·ry re·cep·tor cells** very slender nerve cells, with large nuclei and surmounted by six to eight long, sensitive cilia in the olfactory epithelium at the roof of the nose; they are the receptors for smell.

**ol·fac·to·ry sul·cus** the sagittal sulcus on the inferior or orbital surface of each frontal lobe of the cerebrum, demarcating the straight gyrus from the orbital gyri, and covered on the orbital surface by the olfactory bulb and tract.

**ol·ig·ae·mia [Br.]** SEE oligemia.

**ol·i·ge·mia** (ol-i-gē'mē-ă) a deficiency of blood in the body or any organ or tissue. [oligo- + G. *haima*, blood]

**ol·i·ge·mic** (ol-i-gē'mik) pertaining to or characterized by oligemia.

**ol·i·go** (ol'i-gō) in molecular genetics, oligonucleotide.

△**oli·go-, olig-** 1. a few, a little; too little, too few. 2. CHEMISTRY used in contrast to "poly-" in describing polymers; e.g., oligosaccharide. [G. *oligos*, few]

**ol·i·go·am·ni·os** (ol'i-gō-am'nē-os) SYN oligohydramnios. [oligo- + amnion]

**ol·i·go·clo·nal band** small discrete bands in the gamma globulin region of the spinal fluid electrophoresis, indicating local central nervous system production of IgG; bands are frequently seen in patients with multiple sclerosis but can also be found in other diseases of the central nervous system including syphilis, sarcoidosis, and chronic infection or inflammation.

**ol·i·go·cys·tic** (ol'i-gō-sis'tik) consisting of only a few cysts. [oligo- + G. *kystis*, bladder, cyst]

**ol·i·go·dac·ty·ly, ol·i·go·dac·tyl·ia** (ol'i-gō-dak'ti-lē, ol'i-gō-dak-til'ē-ă) presence of fewer than five digits on one or more limbs. [oligo- + G. *daktylos*, finger or toe]

**ol·i·go·den·dria** (ol'i-gō-den'drē-ă) SYN oligodendroglia.

**ⓘ ol·i·go·den·dro·cyte** (ol'i-gō-den'drō-sīt) a cell of the oligodendroglia. See this page.

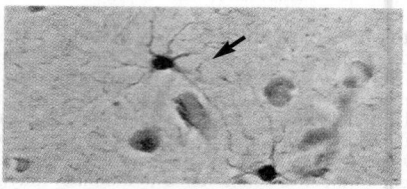

**oligodendrocyte** (arrow) in section of brain

**ol·i·go·den·drog·lia** (ol'ĭ-gō-den-drog'lē-ă) one of the three types of glia cells (the other two being macroglia or astrocytes, and microglia) that, together with nerve cells, compose the tissue of the central nervous system. Oligodendroglia cells are characterized by variable numbers of veillike or sheetlike processes that are wrapped each around individual axons to form the myelin sheath of nerve fibers in the central nervous system. SYN oligodendria. [oligo- + G. *dendron*, tree, + *glia*, glue]

**ol·i·go·den·dro·gli·o·ma** (ol'i-gō-den'drō-glī-ō'mă) a rare, slowly growing glioma derived from oligodendrocytes that occurs most frequently in the cerebrum of adult persons. [oligo- + G. *dendron*, tree, + glia, + -oma]

**ol·i·go·dip·sia** (ol'i-gō-dip'sē-ă) abnormal lack of thirst. SEE ALSO hypodipsia. [oligo- + G. *dipsa*, thirst]

**ol·i·go·don·tia** (ol'i-gō-don'shē-ă) SYN hypodontia. [oligo- + G. *odous*, tooth]

**ol·i·go·dy·nam·ic** (ol'i-gō-dī-nam'ik) active in very small quantity. [oligo- + G. *dynamis*, power]

**ol·i·go·ga·lac·tia** (ol'i-gō-gă-lak'shē-ă) slight or scant secretion of milk. [oligo- + G. *gala*, milk]

**ol·i·go-α1,6-glu·co·si·dase** a glucanohydrolase cleaving α-1,6 links in isomaltose and dextrins produced from starch and glycogen by α-amylase; secreted into the duodenum; a deficiency of this enzyme leads to defects in intestinal digestion of limit dextrins. SEE ALSO sucrose α-D-glucohydrolase.

**ol·i·go·hy·dram·ni·os** (ol'i-gō-hī-dram'nē-os) the presence of an insufficient amount of amniotic fluid (less than 300 ml at term). SYN oligoamnios. [oligo- + G. *hydōr*, water, + amnion]

**ol·i·go·men·or·rhea** (ol'i-gō-men-ō-rē'ă) scanty menstruation. [oligo- + menorrhea]

**ol·ig·o·men·or·rhoea [Br.]** SEE oligomenorrhea.

**ol·i·go·mer·i·sa·tion [Br.]** SEE oligomerization.

**o·li·go·mer·i·za·tion** (ol'i-gō-mer-ĭ-zā-shŭn) formation of oligomers from larger or smaller molecules.

**ol·i·go·mor·phic** (ol'i-gō-mōr'fik) presenting few changes of form; not polymorphic. [oligo- + G. *morphē*, form]

**ol·i·go·nu·cle·o·tide** (ol'i-gō-noo'klē-o-tīd) a compound made up of the condensation of a small number (typically fewer than twenty) of nucleotides. Cf. polynucleotide.

**ol·i·gop·nea** (ol'i-gop-nē'ă, ol'i-gop'nē-ă) SYN hypopnea. [oligo- + G. *pnoē*, breath]

**ol·i·go·pty·a·lism** (ol'i-gō-tī'ă-lizm, ol'i-gop-tī'a-lizm) a scanty secretion of saliva. [oligo- + G. *ptyalon*, saliva]

**ol·i·gor·ia** (ol-i-gōr′ē-ă) an abnormal indifference toward or dislike of persons or things. [G. *oligōria*, negligence, slight esteem, fr. *oligos*, little, + *ōra*, care, regard]

**ol·i·go·sac·cha·ride** (ol′i-gō-sak′ă-rīd) a compound made up of the condensation of a small number of monosaccharide units. Cf. polysaccharide.

**ol·i·go·sper·mia, ol·i·go·sper·ma·tism** (ol-i-gō-sper′mē-ă, ol-i-gō-sper′mă-tizm) a subnormal concentration of spermatozoa in the penile ejaculate. [oligo- + G. *sperma*, seed]

**ol·i·go·sy·nap·tic** (ol′i-gō-si-nap′tik) referring to neural conduction pathways that are interrupted by only a few synaptic junctions, i.e., made up of a sequence of only few nerve cells, in contrast to polysynaptic pathways. SYN paucisynaptic.

**ol·i·go·tro·phia, ol·i·got·ro·phy** (ol′i-gō-trō′fē-ă, ol-i-got′rō-fē) deficient nutrition. [oligo- + G. *trophē*, nourishment]

**ol·i·go·zo·o·sper·mia** (ol′i-gō-zō′ō-sperm′ē-ă) a subnormal concentration of spermatozoa in the penile ejaculate. [oligo- + G. *zōos*, living, + *sperma*, seed, semen, + -ia]

**ol·i·gu·ria** (ol-i-gyu′rē-ă) scanty urine production. [oligo- + G. *ouron*, urine]

**oli·va**, pl. **oli·vae** (ō-lī′vă, ō-lī′vē) [TA] a smooth oval prominence of the ventrolateral surface of the medulla oblongata lateral to the pyramidal tract, corresponding to the inferior olivary nucleus. SYN corpus olivare [TA], olive (1). [L.]

**ol·i·vary** (ol′i-ver-ē) **1.** relating to the oliva. **2.** relating to or shaped like an olive.

**ol·ive** (ol′iv) **1.** SYN oliva. **2.** common name for a tree of the genus *Olea* (family Oleaceae) or its fruit. [L. *oliva*]

**ol·i·vif·u·gal** (ol′i-vif′yu-găl) in a direction away from the olive. [oliva + L. *fugio*, to flee]

**ol·i·vip·e·tal** (ol′i-vip′ĕ-tăl) in a direction toward the olive. [oliva + L. *peto*, to seek]

**ol·i·vo·pon·to·cer·e·bel·lar** (ol′i-vō-pon′tō-ser-ĕ-bel′ar) relating to the olivary nucleus, basis pontis, and cerebellum.

**Ol·li·er graft** (ō-lē-ā′) a thin split-thickness graft, usually in small pieces. SYN Ollier-Thiersch graft.

**Ol·li·er the·o·ry** (ō-lē-ā′) a theory of compensatory growth; after resection of the articular extremity of a bone, the articular cartilage of the other bone entering into the structure of the joint takes on an increased growth.

**Ol·li·er-Thiersch graft** (ō-lē-ā′ tērsh) SYN Ollier graft.

**Olm·sted syn·drome** (ohlm′sted) congenital palmar, plantar, and periorificial keratoderma leading to flexion contractures and digital spontaneous amputation.

△**-ol·o·gy** SEE -logia.

△**-oma** a tumor or neoplasm. [G. -*ōma*]

△**-omata** plural of -oma.

**o·me·ga** (ō-mā′gă) **1.** twenty-fourth and last letter of the Greek alphabet (ω). **2.** Ohm.

**o·me·ga-ox·i·da·tion the·o·ry** that the oxidation of fatty acids commences at the $CH_3$ group, i.e., the terminal or omega-group; beta-oxidation then proceeds at both ends of the fatty acid chain.

**O·menn syn·drome** (ō′men) a rapidly fatal immunodeficiency disease characterized by erythroderma, diarrhea, repeated infections, hepatosplenomegaly, and leukocytosis with eosinophilia; autosomal recessive inheritance, caused by mutation in either the recombination activat-

ing gene 1 (RAG1) or the adjacent RAG2 gene on chromosome 11p.

**omen·tal** (ō-men′tăl) relating to the omentum. SYN epiploic.

**omen·tal ap·pen·dices** one of a number of little processes or sacs of peritoneum filled with adipose tissue and projecting from the serous coat of the large intestine, except the rectum; they are most evident on the transverse and sigmoid colon, being most numerous along the free tenia. SYN appendices omentales [TA].

**o·men·tal bur·sa** an isolated portion of the peritoneal cavity lying dorsal to the stomach and extending craniad to the liver and diaphragm and caudad into the greater omentum; it opens into the general peritoneal cavity at the epiploic foramen.

**o·men·tal flap** a segment of omentum, with its supplying blood vessels, transplanted either with an intact pedicle or as free tissue to a distant area and revascularized by arterial and venous anastomoses.

**omen·tal for·a·men** the passage, below and behind the portal hepatis, connecting the two sacs of the peritoneum; it is bounded anteriorly by the hepatoduodenal ligament and posteriorly by a peritoneal fold over the inferior vena cava.

**o·men·tal graft** a segment of omentum, with its supplying blood vessels, transplanted as a free flap to a distant area and revascularized by arterial and venous anastomoses.

**omen·tec·to·my** (ō-men-tek′tō-mē) resection or excision of the omentum. [omentum + G. *ektomē*, excision]

**omen·ti·tis** (ō-men-tī′tis) peritonitis involving the omentum. [L. *omentum* + G. -*itis*, inflammation]

△**omen·to-, oment-** the omentum. SEE ALSO epiplo-. [L. *omentum*]

**omen·to·fix·a·tion** (ō-men′tō-fik-sā′shŭn) SYN omentopexy.

**omen·to·pexy** (ō-men′tō-pek-sē) **1.** suture of the greater omentum to the abdominal wall to induce collateral portal circulation. **2.** suture of the omentum to another organ to increase arterial circulation. SEE ALSO omentoplasty. SYN omentofixation. [omento- + G. *pēxis*, fixation]

**omen·to·plas·ty** (ō-men′tō-plas-tē) use of the greater omentum to cover or fill a defect, augment arterial or portal venous circulation, absorb effusions, or increase lymphatic drainage. SEE ALSO omentopexy. [omento- + G. *plastos*, formed]

**omen·tor·rha·phy** (ō-men-tōr′ă-fē) suture of an opening in the omentum. [omento- + G. *rhaphē*, suture]

**omen·tum**, pl. **omen·ta** (ō-men′tŭm, ō-men′tă) [TA] a fold of peritoneum passing from the stomach to another abdominal organ. [L. the membrane that encloses the bowels]

**OML** orbitomeatal line.

**om·ni·fo·cal lens** a lens for near and distant vision in which the reading portion is a continuously variable curve.

**om·niv·o·rous** (om-niv′ŏ-rŭs) living on food of all kinds, upon both animal and vegetable food. [L. *omnis*, all, + *voro*, to eat]

△**omo-** the shoulder (sometimes including the upper arm). [G. *ōmos*, shoulder]

**o·mo·hy·oid mus·cle** formed of two bellies attached to intermediate tendon; *origin*, by inferior belly from upper border of scapula between superior angle and notch; *insertion*, by superior belly into hyoid bone; *action*, depresses hyoid; *nerve supply*, upper cervical spinal nerves through ansa cervicalis. SYN musculus omohyoideus [TA].

⌂**om•phal-**, **om•phalo-** the umbilicus, the navel. [G. *omphalos*, navel (umbilicus)]

**om•pha•lec•to•my** (om-fă-lek'tō-mē) excision of the umbilicus or of a neoplasm connected with it. [omphal- + G. *ektomē*, excision]

**om•phal•el•co•sis** (om'fal-el-kō'sis) ulceration at the umbilicus. [omphal- + G. *helkōsis*, ulceration]

**om•phal•ic** (om-fal'ik) SYN umbilical. [G. *omphalos*, umbilicus]

**om•pha•li•tis** (om-fă-lī'tis) inflammation of the umbilicus and surrounding parts.

**om•phal•o•cele** (om'fal-ō-sēl, om'fă-lō-sēl) congenital herniation of viscera into the base of the umbilical cord, with a covering membranous sac of peritoneum-amnion. SEE ALSO umbilical hernia. SYN exomphalos (3), exumbilication (3). [omphalo- + G. *kēlē*, hernia]

**om•pha•lo•en•ter•ic** (om'fă-lō-en-tār-ik) relating to the umbilicus and the intestine.

**om•pha•lo•mes•en•ter•ic** (om'fă-lō-mez-en-tār'ik) **1.** term denoting relationship of the midgut to the yolk sac. As the head and tail folds of the embryo continue to form, this relationship is diminished and is represented by a narrow yolk stalk or vitelline duct. **2.** relating to the vitelline duct.

**om•pha•lo•mes•en•ter•ic duct** SYN yolk stalk.

**om•pha•lo•phle•bi•tis** (om'fă-lō-fle-bī'tis) inflammation of the umbilical veins. [omphalo- + G. *phleps*, vein, + -*itis*, inflammation]

**om•pha•lor•rha•gia** (om'fă-lō-rā'jē-ă) bleeding from the umbilicus. [omphalo- + G. *rhēgnymi*, to burst forth]

**om•pha•lor•rhea** (om'fă-lō-rē'ă) a serous discharge from the umbilicus. [omphalo- + G. *rhoia*, flow]

**om•pha•lor•rhex•is** (om'fă-lō-rek'sis) rupture of the umbilical cord during childbirth. [omphalo- + G. *rhēxis*, rupture]

**om•pha•lo•site** (om'fă-lō-sīt) underdeveloped twin of allantoangiopagous twin; joined by umbilical vessels. [omphalo- + G. *sitos*, food]

**om•pha•lo•spi•nous** (om'fă-lō-spī'nŭs) denoting a line connecting the umbilicus and the anterior superior spine of the ilium, on which lies McBurney point.

**om•pha•lot•o•my** (om-fă-lot'ō-mē) cutting of the umbilical cord at birth. [omphalo- + G. *tomē*, incision]

**onan•ism** (ō'nan-izm) **1.** withdrawal of the penis before ejaculation, in order to prevent conception. **2.** incorrectly, masturbation. [*Onan*, son of Judah, who practiced it. Genesis 38:9]

**on•cho•cer•co•ma** (on'kō-ser-kō'ma) nodule containing adult worms of *Onchocera volvulus*. [*Onchocerca*, taxonomic term, + -oma]

⌂**on•co-**, **on•cho-** a tumor. [G. *onkos*, bulk, mass]

**on•co•cyte** (ong'kō-sīt) a large, granular, acidophilic tumor cell containing numerous mitochondria; a neoplastic oxyphil cell. [onco- + G. *kytos*, cell]

**on•co•cy•tic ade•no•ma** SYN Hürthle cell adenoma.

**on•co•cy•tic car•ci•no•ma** SYN Hürthle cell carcinoma.

**on•co•cyt•ic he•pa•to•cel•lu•lar tu•mor** SYN fibrolamellar liver cell carcinoma.

**on•co•fe•tal** (ong-kō-fē'tăl) relating to tumor-associated substances present in fetal tissue, as oncofetal antigens.

**on•co•fe•tal an•ti•gens** tumor-associated antigens present in fetal tissue but not in normal adult tissue, including α-fetoprotein and carcinoembryonic antigen.

**on•co•fe•tal mark•er** a tumor marker produced by tumor tissue and by fetal tissue of the same type as the tumor, but not by normal adult tissue from which the tumor arises.

**on•co•gene** (ong'kō-jēn) **1.** any of a family of genes which under normal circumstances code for proteins involved in cell growth or regulation (e.g., protein kinases, GTPases, nuclear proteins, growth factors) but may foster malignant processes if mutated or activated by contact with retroviruses. Oncogenes often work in concert to produce cancer, and their action may be exacerbated by retroviruses, jumping genes, or inherited genetic mutations. SEE antioncogene. **2.** found in certain DNA tumor viruses. It is required for viral replication. [onco- + gene]

**on•co•gen•e•sis** (ong-kō-jen'ě-sis) origin and growth of a neoplasm. [onco- + G. *genesis*, production]

**on•co•gen•ic** (ong-kō-jen'ik) SYN oncogenous.

**on•co•gen•ic vi•rus** a virus of one of the two groups of tumor-inducing viruses; the RNA tumor viruses, which are well defined and rather homogeneous, or the DNA viruses, which are more diverse. SYN tumor virus.

**on•cog•en•ous** (ong-koj'ě-nŭs) causing, inducing, or being suitable for the formation and development of a neoplasm. SYN oncogenic.

**on•col•o•gist** (ong-kol'ō-jist) a specialist in oncology.

**on•col•o•gy** (ong-kol'ō-jē) the study or science dealing with the physical, chemical, and biologic properties and features of neoplasms, including causation, pathogenesis, and treatment. [onco- + G. *logos*, study]

**on•col•y•sis** (ong-kol'i-sis) destruction of a neoplasm; sometimes used with reference to the reduction of any swelling or mass. [onco- + G. *lysis*, dissolution]

**on•co•lyt•ic** (ong-kō-lit'ik) pertaining to, characterized by, or causing oncolysis.

**on•cor•na•vi•rus•es** (ong-kōr'nă-vī'rŭs-ez) SYN Oncovirinae.

**on•co•sis** (ong-kō'sis) the formation of one or more neoplasms or tumors. [G. *onkōsis*, swelling, fr. *onkos*, bulk, mass]

**on•co•stat•in M** (onk'ō-stat'in em) an interleukin 6. [onco- + -stat + -in]

**on•cot•ic** (ong-kot'ik) relating to or caused by edema or any swelling (oncosis).

**on•cot•ic pres•sure** the osmotic pressure attributed to proteins and other macromolecules.

**on•cot•o•my** (ong-kot'ō-mē) rarely used term for incision of an abscess, cyst, or other tumor. [onco- + G. *tomē*, incision]

**on•co•tro•pic** (ong'kō-trop'ik) manifesting a special affinity for neoplasms or neoplastic cells. [onco- + G. *tropē*, a turning]

**On•co•vir•i•nae** (ong-kō-vir'i-nē) a subfamily of viruses (family Retroviridae) composed of the RNA tumor viruses that contain two identical plus stranded RNA molecules. SYN oncornaviruses.

**on•co•vi•rus** (ong′kō-vī′rŭs) any virus of the subfamily Oncovirinae. SEE ALSO oncogenic virus.

**On•dine curse** (on-dēn′) idiopathic central alveolar hypoventilation in which involuntary control of respiration is depressed, but voluntary control of ventilation is not impaired. [*Ondine*, char. in play by J. Giraudoux, based on Undine, Ger. myth. char.]

△**-one** suffix indicating a ketone (–CO–) group.

**one-car•bon frag•ment** the formyl or methyl group that takes part in transformylation or transmethylation reactions; by means of these reactions, a group containing a single carbon atom is added to a compound being biosynthesized, adding a methyl or hydroxymethyl group or closing a ring.

**onei•ric** (ō-nī′rik) **1.** pertaining to dreams. **2.** pertaining to the clinical state of oneirophrenia. [G. *oneiros*, dream]

**onei•rism** (ō-nī′rizm) a waking dream state. [G. *oneiros*, dream]

**onei•ro•dyn•ia** (ō-nī-rō-din′ē-ă) rarely used term for an unpleasant or painful dream. [G. *oneiros*, dream, + *odynē*, pain]

**onei•ro•phre•nia** (ō-nī-rō-frē′nē-ă) a state in which hallucinations occur, caused by such conditions as prolonged deprivation of sleep, sensory isolation, and a variety of drugs. [G. *oneiros*, dream, + *phrēn*, mind]

**onei•ros•co•py** (ō-nī-ros′kŏ-pē) the diagnosis of a patient's mental state by an analysis of the person's dreams. [G. *oneiros*, dream, + *skopeō*, to examine]

**on•go•ing as•sess•ment** repeat of the focused or rapid ed assessment of a prehospital patient to detect changes in condition and to judge the effectiveness of treatment before or during transport. Repeated every 5 minutes for an unstable patient and every 15 minutes for a stable patient.

△**-oni•um** suffix indicating a positively charged radical; e.g., ammonium, $NH_4^+$.

△**on•ko-** SEE onco-.

**on•lay** (on′lā) **1.** a metal cast restoration of the occlusal surface of a posterior tooth or the lingual surface of an anterior tooth, the entire surface of which is in dentin without side walls; retention in the anterior tooth is by pins and in the posterior by pins and/or boxes in retentive grooves in the buccal and lingual walls. **2.** a graft applied on the exterior of a bone.

**on-off phe•nom•e•non** a phase in the treatment of Parkinson disease with *l*-dopa, in which there is a rapid fluctuation of akinetic (off) and choreoathetotic (on) states.

**on•o•mat•o•ma•nia** (on′ō-mat-ō-mā′nē-ă) an abnormal impulse to dwell upon certain words and their supposed significance, or to frantically try to recall a particular word. [G. *onoma*, name, + *mania*, frenzy]

**on•o•mat•o•pho•bia** (on′ō-mat-ō-fō′bē-ă) abnormal dread of certain words or names because of their supposed significance. [G. *onoma*, name, + *phobos*, fear]

**on•set of blood lac•tate ac•cu•mu•la•tion (OBLA)** SYN lactate threshold.

**on-site mas•sage** SYN seated massage.

**on•to•gen•e•sis** (on-tō-jen′ĕ-sis) SYN ontogeny.

**on•to•ge•net•ic, on•to•gen•ic** (on′tō-jĕ-net′ik, on′tō-jen′ik) relating to ontogeny.

**on•tog•e•ny** (on-toj′ĕ-nē) development of the individual, as distinguished from phylogeny, which is evolutionary development of the species. SYN ontogenesis. [G. *ōn*, being, + *genesis*, origin]

**on•y•chal•gia** (on-i-kal′jē-ă) pain in the nails. [onycho- + G. *algos*, pain]

**on•y•cha•tro•phia, on•ych•at•ro•phy** (on′i-kă-trō′fē-ă, on-ik-at′rō-fē) atrophy of the nails. [onycho- + G. *atrophia*, atrophy]

**on•y•chaux•is** (on-i-kawk′sis) marked overgrowth of the fingernails or toenails. [onycho- + G. *auxē*, increase]

**on•y•chec•to•my** (on-i-kek′tō-mē) ablation of a toenail or fingernail. [onycho- + G. *ektomē*, excision]

**onych•ia** (ō-nik′ē-ă) inflammation of the matrix of the nail. SYN onychitis. [onycho- + G. *-ia*, condition]

**on•y•chi•tis** (on-i-kī′tis) SYN onychia.

△**ony•cho-, onych-** a finger nail, a toenail. [G. *onyx*, nail]

**on•y•choc•la•sis** (on-i-kok′lă-sis) breaking of the nails. [onycho- + G. *klasis*, breaking]

**on•y•cho•dys•tro•phy** (on′i-kō-dis′trō-fē) dystrophic changes in the nails occurring as a congenital defect or due to any illness or injury that may cause a malformed nail. [onycho- + G. *dys-*, bad, + *trophē*, nourishment]

**on•y•cho•graph** (on′i-kō-graf) an instrument for recording the capillary blood pressure as shown by the circulation under the nail. [onycho- + G. *graphō*, to write]

**on•y•cho•gry•po•sis** (on′i-kō-gri-pō′sis) enlargement with increased thickening and curvature of the fingernails or toenails. [onycho- + G. *grypōsis*, a curvature]

**on•y•cho•het•er•o•to•pia** (on′i-kō-het-er-ō-tō′pē-ă) abnormal placement of nails.

**on•y•choid** (on′i-koyd) resembling a fingernail in structure or form. [onycho- + G. *eidos*, resemblance]

**on•y•chol•y•sis** (on-i-kol′i-sis) loosening of the nails, beginning at the free border, and usually incomplete. [onycho- + G. *lysis*, loosening]

**on•y•cho•ma** (on-i-kō′mă) a tumor arising from the nail bed. [onycho- + G. *-ōma*, tumor]

**on•y•cho•ma•de•sis** (on′i-kō-mă-dē′sis) complete shedding of the nails, usually associated with systemic disease. [onycho- + G. *madēsis*, a growing bald, fr. *madaō*, to be moist, (of hair) fall off]

**on•y•cho•ma•la•cia** (on′i-kō-mă-lā′shē-ă) abnormal softness of the nails. [onycho- + G. *malakia*, softness]

**on•y•cho•my•co•sis** (on′i-kō-mī-kō′sis) very common fungus infections of the nails, causing thickening, roughness, and splitting, often caused by *Trichophyton rubrum* or *T. mentagrophytes*, *Candida* in the immunodeficient, and molds in the elderly. [onycho- + G. *mykēs*, fungus, + *-ōsis*, condition]

**on•y•cho•path•ic** (on′i-kō-path′ik) relating to or suffering from any disease of the nails.

**on•y•chop•a•thy** (on-i-kop′ă-thē) any disease of the nails. SYN onychosis. [onycho- + G. *pathos*, suffering]

**on•y•choph•a•gy, on•y•cho•pha•gia** (on-i-kof′ă-jē, on′i-kō-fā′jē-ă) habitual nailbiting. [onycho- + G. *phagō*, to eat]

**on•y•cho•plas•ty** (on′i-kō-plas-tē) a corrective or plastic operation on the nail matrix. [onycho- + G. *plastos*, formed, shaped]

**on·y·chor·rhex·is** (on′i-kō-rek′sis) abnormal brittleness of the nails with splitting of the free edge. [onycho- + G. *rhēxis,* a breaking]

**on·y·cho·schiz·ia** (on′i-kō-skiz′ē-ă) splitting of the nails in layers. [onycho- + G. *schizō,* to divide, + *-ia,* condition]

**on·y·cho·sis** (on-i-kō′sis) SYN onychopathy.

**on·y·chot·il·lo·ma·nia** (on′i-kot′i-lō-mā′nē-ă) a tendency to pick at the nails. [onycho- + G. *tillō,* to pluck, + *mania,* insanity]

**on·y·chot·o·my** (on-i-kot′ō-mē) incision into a toenail or fingernail. [onycho- + G. *tomē,* cutting]

**on·yx** (on′iks) SYN nail. [G. nail]

⌂**oo-** egg, ovary. SEE ALSO oophor-, ovario-, ovi-, ovo-. [G. *ōon,* egg. OO-]

**oo·cyst** (ō′ō-sist) the encysted form of the fertilized macrogamete, or zygote, in coccidian Sporozoea in which sporogonic multiplication occurs; results in the formation of sporozoites, infectious agents for the next stage of the sporozoan life cycle. [G. *ōon,* egg, + *kystis,* bladder]

**oo·cyte** (ō′ō-sīt) the female sex cell. When fertilized by a spermatozoon, an oocyte is capable of developing into a new individual of the same species; during maturation, the oocyte, like the spermatozoon, undergoes a halving of its chromosomal complement so that, at its union with the male gamete, the species number of chromosomes (46 in humans) is maintained; yolk contained in the ova of different species varies greatly in amount and distribution, which influences the pattern of the cleavage divisions. SYN ovum. [G. *ōon,* egg, + *kytos,* a hollow (cell)]

**oo·gen·e·sis** (ō-ō-jen′ĕ-sis) process of formation and development of the oocyte. SYN ovigenesis. [G. *ōon,* egg, + *genesis,* origin]

**oo·ge·net·ic** (ō-ō-jĕ-net′ik) producing oocytes (ova). SYN ovigenetic, ovigenic.

**oo·go·ni·um,** pl. **oo·go·nia** (ō-ō-gō′nē-ŭm, ō-ō-gō′nē-ă) 1. primordial germ cells; proliferate by mitotic division. 2. in fungi, the female gametangium bearing one or more oospores. [G. *ōon,* egg, + *gonē,* generation]

**oo·ki·ne·sis, oo·ki·ne·sia** (ō′ō-k′i-nē′sis, ō′ō-kī-nē′zē-ă) chromosomal movements of the egg during maturation and fertilization. [G. *ōon,* egg, + *kinēsis,* movement]

**oo·ki·nete** (ō′ō-k′i-nē′t) the motile zygote of the malarial organism that penetrates the mosquito stomach to form an oocyst under the outer gut lining; the contents of the oocyst subsequently divide to produce numerous sporozoites. [G. *ōon,* egg, + *kinētos,* motile]

**oo·lem·ma** (ō-ō-lem′ă) plasma membrane of the oocyte. [G. *ōon,* egg, + *lemma,* sheath]

⌂**ooph·or-, ooph·oro-** the ovary. SEE ALSO oo-, ovario-. [Mod. L. *oophoron,* ovary, fr. G. *ōophoros,* egg-bearing]

**ooph·o·rec·to·my** (ō-of-ōr-ek′tō-mē) SYN ovariectomy. [G. *ōon,* egg, + *phoros,* bearing, + *ektomē,* excision]

**ooph·or·i·tis** (ō-of-ōr-ī′tis) inflammation of an ovary. SYN ovaritis. [G. *ōon,* egg, + *phoros,* a bearing, + *-itis,* inflammation]

**ooph·or·o·cys·tec·to·my** (ō-of′ōr-ō-sis-tek′tō-mē) excision of an ovarian cyst.

**ooph·or·o·cys·to·sis** (ō-of′ōr-ō-sis-tō′sis) ovarian cyst formation.

**ooph·or·o·hys·ter·ec·to·my** (ō-of′ōr-ō-his-ter-ek′tō-mē) SYN ovariohysterectomy.

**ooph·or·on** (ō-of′ōr-on) SYN ovary. [G. *ōon,* egg, + *phoros,* bearing]

**ooph·or·o·pexy** (ō-of′ōr-ō-pek-sē) surgical fixation or suspension of an ovary. [oophoro- + G. *pēxis,* fixation]

**ooph·or·o·plas·ty** (ō-of′ōr-ō-plas-tē) plastic operation upon an ovary. [oophoro- + G. *plastos,* formed, shaped]

**ooph·or·os·to·my** (ō-of-ōr-os′tō-mē) SYN ovariostomy. [oophoro- + G. *stoma,* mouth]

**ooph·or·ot·o·my** (ō-of-ōr-ot′ō-mē) SYN ovariotomy. [oophoro- + G. *tomē,* incision]

**oo·plasm** (ō′ō-plazm) protoplasmic portion of the oocyte. [G. *ōon,* egg, + *plasma,* a thing formed]

**oo·tid** (ō′ō-tid) the nearly mature oocyte after the first meiotic division has been completed and the second initiated; in most higher mammals, the second meiotic division is not completed unless fertilization occurs. [G. *ōotidion,* a diminutive egg. See -id (2)]

**OP** occipitoposterior position.

**opac·i·fi·ca·tion** (ō-pas′i-fi-kā′shŭn) 1. the process of making opaque. 2. the formation of opacities. [L. *opacus,* shady]

**opac·i·ty** (ō-pas′i-tē) 1. a lack of transparency; an opaque or nontransparent area. 2. on a radiograph, a more transparent area is interpreted as an opacity to x-rays in the body. 3. mental dullness. [L. *opacitas,* shadiness]

**opal co·don** SYN umber codon.

**opal·es·cent den·tin** dentin usually associated with dentinogenesis imperfecta. It gives an unusual opalescent or translucent appearance to the teeth.

**opaque** (ō-pāk′) impervious to light; not translucent or only slightly so. Cf. radiopaque. [Fr. fr. L. *opacus,* shady]

**open-an·gle glau·co·ma** primary glaucoma in which the aqueous humor has free access to the trabecular meshwork. SYN simple glaucoma, glaucoma simplex.

**open bi·op·sy** biopsy requiring a surgical incision.

**open chain com·pound** SYN acyclic compound.

**open chest mas·sage** rhythmic manual compression of the ventricles of the heart with the hand inside the thoracic cavity.

**open cir·cuit meth·od** a method for measuring oxygen consumption and carbon dioxide production by collecting the expired gas over a known period of time and measuring its volume and composition.

**open-cir·cuit ni·tro·gen wash-out** a gas-dilution technique for measuring the functional residual capacity (FRC); the subject breathes 100% oxygen to wash out the resident nitrogen.

**open cir·cuit spi·rom·e·try** measurement of the volume and rate of respiratory air flow by a device into which the subject expels inspired room air.

**open com·e·do** a comedo with a wide opening on the skin surface capped with a melanin-containing blackened mass of epithelial debris. SYN blackhead (1).

**open dis·lo·ca·tion** a dislocation complicated by a wound opening from the surface down to the affected joint. SYN compound dislocation.

**open drain·age** drainage allowing air to enter.

**open drop an·es·the·sia** inhalation anesthesia by vaporization of a liquid anesthetic placed drop by drop on a gauze mask covering the mouth and nose.

**open flap** SYN flat flap.

**open frac•ture** fracture in which the skin is perforated and there is an open wound down to the fracture. SYN compound fracture.

**open head in•ju•ry** a head injury in which there is a loss of continuity of scalp or mucous membranes; the term is sometimes used to indicate a communication between the exterior and the intracranial cavity. SEE ALSO penetrating wound.

**open heart sur•gery** operative procedure(s) performed on or within the exposed heart, usually with cardiopulmonary bypass.

**open hos•pi•tal** a hospital where all physicians, not members of the regular staff, are permitted to send their patients and control their treatment.

**open•ing** (ō′pen-ing) a gap in or entrance to an organ, tube, or cavity. SEE ALSO aperture, fossa, ostium, orifice, pore.

**open•ing of ex•ter•nal a•cous•tic me•a•tus** the orifice of the external acoustic meatus in the tympanic portion of the temporal bone.

**open•ing of in•ter•nal a•cous•tic me•a•tus** the inner opening of the internal acoustic meatus on the posterior surface of the petrous part of the temporal bone.

**open•ing of pul•mo•na•ry trunk** the opening of the pulmonary trunk from the right ventricle, guarded by the pulmonary valve.

**open•ing snap** a sharp, high-pitched click in early diastole, usually best heard between the cardiac apex and the lower left sternal border, related to opening of the abnormal valve in cases of mitral stenosis.

**open-packed po•si•tion 1.** joint position in which contact between the articulating structures is minimal. **2.** SYN flexion.

**open pneu•mo•thor•ax** a free communication between the atmosphere and the pleural space either via the lung or through the chest wall. SYN sucking chest wound, sucking wound.

**open re•duc•tion of frac•tures** reduction by manipulation of bone, after incision in skin and muscle over the site of the fracture.

**open tu•ber•cu•lo•sis** pulmonary tuberculosis, tuberculous ulceration, or other form in which the tubercle bacilli are present in the excretions or secretions; in the lung, usually the result of cavity formation.

**open wound** a wound in which the tissues are exposed to the air.

**op•er•a•ble** (op′er-ă-bl) denoting a patient or condition on which a surgical procedure can be performed with a reasonable expectation of cure or relief.

**op•er•ant** (op′er-ănt) in conditioning, any behavior or specific response chosen by the experimenter; its frequency is intended to increase or decrease by the judicious pairing with it of a reinforcer when it occurs. SYN target response.

**op•er•ate** (op′er-āt) to perform a therapeutic procedure on the body with the hands or with instruments. [L. *operor*, pp. *-atus*, to work, fr. *opus*, work]

**op•er•at•ing mi•cro•scope** SYN surgical microscope.

**op•er•a•tion** (op-er-ā′shŭn) **1.** any surgical procedure. **2.** the act, manner, or process of functioning. SEE ALSO method, procedure, technique.

**Op•er•a•tion Re•store Trust (ORT)** a federal pilot program designed to combat fraud, waste, and abuse in the Medicare and Medicaid programs. ORT targets home health agencies, nursing homes, and durable medical equipment suppliers.

**op•er•a•tive** (op′er-ă-tiv) **1.** relating to, or effected by means of an operation. **2.** active or effective.

**op•er•a•tor** (op′er-ā-tor) **1.** one who performs an operation or operates equipment. **2.** GENETICS a sequence of DNA that interacts with a repressor of operon to control the expression of adjacent structural genes. SEE operator gene. **3.** a symbol representing a mathematical operation. [L. worker, fr. *operor*, to work]

**op•er•a•tor gene** a gene with the function of activating the production of messenger RNA by one or more adjacent structural loci; part of the feedback system for determining the rate of production of an enzyme.

**oper•cu•lar** (ō-per′kyu-lăr) relating to an operculum.

**oper•cu•li•tis** (ō-perk-yu-lī′tis) a pericoronitis originating under an operculum. [operculum + G. *-itis*, inflammation]

**oper•cu•lum** (ō-per′kyu-lŭm), gen. **oper•cu•li**, pl. **oper•cu•la** (ō-per′kyu-lī, ō-per′kyu-lă) **1.** anything resembling a lid or cover. **2.** [TA] ANATOMY the portions of the frontal, parietal, and temporal lobes bordering the lateral sulcus and covering the insula. **3.** mucus sealing the endocervical canal of the uterus after conception has taken place. **4.** PARASITOLOGY the lid or caplike cover of the shell opening of operculated freshwater snails in the subclass Prosobranchiata, and of the eggs of certain trematode and cestode parasites. **5.** the attached flap in the tear of retinal detachment. **6.** the mucosal flap partially or completely covering a partially erupted tooth. [L. cover or lid, fr. *operio*, pp. *opertus*, to cover]

**ophi•a•sis** (ō-fī′ă-sis) a form of alopecia areata in which the loss of hair occurs in bands along the scalp margin partially or completely encircling the head. [G., fr. *ophis*, snake]

**oph•ri•tis** (of-rī′tis) dermatitis in the region of the eyebrows. [G. *ophrys*, eyebrow, + *-itis*, inflammation]

**oph•ry•on** (of′rē-on) the point on the midline of the forehead just above the glabella (1). [G. *ophrys*, eyebrow]

**oph•ry•o•sis** (of-rē-ō′sis) spasmodic twitching of the upper portion of the orbicularis palpebrarum muscle causing a wrinkling of the eyebrow. [G. *ophrys*, eyebrow, + *-osis*, condition]

**oph•thal•mia** (of-thal′mē-ă) **1.** severe, often purulent, conjunctivitis. **2.** inflammation of the deeper structures of the eye. [G.]

**oph•thal•mia ne•o•na•to•rum** a conjunctival inflammation occurring within the first 10 days of life; causes include *Neisseria gonorrhoeae*, *Staphylococcus*, *Streptococcus pneumoniae*, and *Chlamydia trachomatis*. SYN infantile purulent conjunctivitis.

**oph•thal•mic** (of-thal′mik) relating to the eye. SYN ocular (1). [G. *ophthalmikos*]

**oph•thal•mic ar•tery** origin, internal carotid; branches, ciliary, central artery of retina, anterior meningeal, lacrimal, conjunctival, episcleral, supraorbital, ethmoidal, palpebral, dorsal nasal, and supratrochlear. SYN arteria ophthalmica [TA].

**oph•thal•mic nerve [CN V1]** a branch of the

trigeminal nerve that passes forward from the trigeminal ganglion in the lateral wall of the cavernous sinus, entering the orbit through the superior orbital fissure; through its branches, frontal, lacrimal, and nasociliary, it supplies sensation to the orbit and its contents, the anterior part of the nasal cavity, and the skin of the nose and forehead. SYN nervus ophthalmicus [CN V1] [TA].

**oph·thal·mic solution** sterile solution, free from foreign particles and suitably compounded and dispensed for instillation into the eye.

**oph·thal·mic ves·i·cle** in the embryo, one of the paired evaginations from the ventrolateral walls of the forebrain from which the sensory and pigment layers of the retina develop.

△**oph·thal·mo-, oph·thalm-** relationship to the eye. SEE ALSO oculo-. [G. *ophthalmos*]

**oph·thal·mo·dy·na·mom·e·ter** (of-thal'mō-dī-nă-mom'ĕ-ter) an instrument to measure the blood pressure in the retinal vessels. [ophthalmo- + G. *dynamis*, power, + *metron*, measure]

**oph·thal·mo·dy·na·mom·e·try** (of-thal'mō-dī-nă-mom'ĕ-trē) the measurement of blood pressure in the retinal vessels by means of an ophthalmodynamometer. [ophthalmo- + G. *dynamis*, power, + *metron*, measure]

**oph·thal·mo·lith** (of-thal'mō-lith) SYN dacryolith. [ophthalmo- + G. *lithos*, stone]

**oph·thal·mol·o·gist** (of-thal-mol'ō-jist) a specialist in ophthalmology. SYN oculist.

**oph·thal·mol·o·gy** (of-thal-mol'ō-jē) the medical specialty concerned with the eye, its diseases, and refractive errors. [ophthalmo- + G. *logos*, study]

**oph·thal·mo·ma·la·cia** (of-thal'mō-mă-lā'shē-ă) abnormal softening of the eyeball. [ophthalmo- + G. *malakia*, softness]

**oph·thal·mom·e·ter** (of-thal-mom'ĕ-ter) SYN keratometer. [ophthalmo- + G. *metron*, measure]

**oph·thal·mo·my·co·sis** (of-thal'mō-mī-kō'sis) any disease of the eye or its appendages caused by a fungus. [ophthalmo- + G. *mykēs*, fungus, + -*osis*, condition]

**oph·thal·mop·a·thy** (of-thal-mop'ă-thē) any disease of the eyes. [ophthalmo- + G. *pathos*, suffering]

**oph·thal·mo·ple·gia** (of-thal-mō-plē'jē-ă) paralysis of one or more of the ocular muscles. [ophthalmo- + G. *plēgē*, stroke]

**oph·thal·mo·ple·gia ex·ter·na** paralysis affecting one or more of the extrinsic eye muscles. SYN external ophthalmoplegia.

**oph·thal·mo·ple·gia in·ter·na** paralysis affecting only the sphincter muscle of the pupil and the ciliary muscle. SYN internal ophthalmoplegia.

**oph·thal·mo·ple·gic** (of-thal-mō-plē'jik) relating to or marked by ophthalmoplegia.

🔲**oph·thal·mo·scope** (of-thal'mō-skōp) a device for studying the interior of the eyeball through the pupil. See page B15. [ophthalmo- + G. *skopeō*, to examine]

**oph·thal·mo·scop·ic** (of'thal-mō-skop'ik) relating to examination of the interior of the eye.

🔲**oph·thal·mos·co·py** (of-thal-mos'kŏ-pē) examination of the fundus of the eye by means of the ophthalmoscope. See page B15.

**oph·thal·mo·vas·cu·lar** (of-thal'mō-vas'kyu-lăr) relating to the blood vessels of the eye.

△**-opia** vision. [G. *ōps*, eye]

**opi·ate** (ō'pē-āt) any preparation or derivative of opium.

**opi·ate re·cep·tors** regions of the brain which have the capacity to bind morphine; some, along the aqueduct of Sylvius and in the centromedian nucleus, are in areas related to pain, but others, as in the striatum, are not related.

**opi·o·cor·tin** (ō'pē-ō-kōr'tin) SYN opiomelanocortin.

**opi·oid** (ō'pē-oyd) a narcotic substance, either natural or synthetic.

**opi·oid ant·ag·on·ist** agents such as naloxone and naltrexone that have high affinity for opiate receptors but do not activate these receptors. These drugs block the effects of exogenously administered opioids such as morphine, heroin, meperidine, and methadone, or of endogenously released endorphins and enkephalins.

**opi·o·mel·a·no·cor·tin** a linear polypeptide of the pituitary gland that contains in its sequence the sequences of endorphins, MSH, ACTH, and the like, which are split off enzymically. SYN opiocortin.

**opis·the·nar** (ō-pis'thē-nar) dorsum of the hand. [G. back of the hand, from *opisthen*, behind, + *thenar*, palm of the hand]

**opis·thi·on** (ō-pis'thē-on) [TA] the middle point on the posterior margin of the foramen magnum, opposite the basion. [G. *opisthios*, posterior]

△**op·is·tho-** backward, behind, dorsal. [G. *opisthen*, at the rear, behind]

**op·is·thot·on·ic** (op-is-thot'ō-nik, ō-pis'thō-ton'ik) relating to or characterized by opisthotonos.

**op·is·thot·o·nos, op·is·thot·o·nus** (op-is-thot'ō-nŭs) a tetanic spasm in which the spine and extremities are bent with convexity forward, the body resting on the head and the heels. [opistho- + G. *tonos*, tension, stretching]

**O·pitz BBB syn·drome** (ō'pits) SYN ocular hypertelorism.

**O·pitz G syn·drome** (ō'pits) SYN ocular hypertelorism.

**Op·pen·heim dis·ease** (op'en-hīm) SYN amyotonia congenita.

**Op·pen·heim re·flex** (op'en-hīm) extension of the toes induced by scratching the inner side of the leg or by sudden flexion of the thigh on the abdomen and the leg on the thigh; a sign of cerebral irritation.

**op·po·nens di·gi·ti mi·ni·mi mus·cle** *origin*, hamulus of the hamate bone and transverse carpal ligament; *insertion*, shaft of fifth metacarpal; *action*, "cups" palm, drawing ulnar side of hand toward center of palm; *nerve supply*, ulnar. SYN musculus opponens digiti minimi [TA].

**op·po·nens pol·li·cis mus·cle** *origin*, ridge of trapezium and flexor retinaculum; *insertion*, anterior surface of the full length of the shaft of the first metacarpal bone; *action*, acts at carpometacarpal joint to "cup" palm, enabling one to oppose thumb to other fingers; *nerve supply*, median. SYN musculus opponens pollicis [TA].

**op·por·tun·is·tic** (op'ŏr-too-nis'tik) **1.** denoting an organism capable of causing disease only in a host whose resistance is lowered, e.g., by other diseases or by drugs. **2.** denoting a disease caused by such an organism.

**op·po·si·tion·al de·fi·ant dis·or·der** a disorder of childhood or adolescence characterized by a recurrent pattern of negativistic, hostile, and disobedient behavior toward authority figures.

**op·sin** the protein portion of the rhodopsin molecule; at least three separate opsins are located in cone cells.

**op·sin·o·gen** (op-sin′ō-jen) a substance that stimulates the formation of opsonin, such as the antigen contained in a suspension of bacteria used for immunization. SYN opsogen. [opsonin + -gen]

**op·si·u·ria** (op-sē-yu′rē-ă) a more rapid excretion of urine during fasting than after a full meal. [G. *opsi*, late, + *ouron*, urine]

**op·so·clo·nus** (op′sō-klō′nŭs) rapid, irregular, nonrhythmic movements of the eye in horizontal and vertical directions. [G. *ōps, ōpos*, eye, + *klonos*, confused motion]

**op·so·gen** (op′sō-jen) SYN opsinogen.

**op·so·ma·nia** (op′sō-mā′nē-ă) a longing for a particular article of diet, or for highly seasoned food. [G. *opson*, seasoning, + *mania*, frenzy]

**op·son·ic** (op-son′ik) relating to opsonins or to their utilization.

**op·son·ic in·dex** a value that indicates the relative content of opsonin in the blood of a person with an infectious disease, as evaluated *in vitro* in comparison with presumably normal blood; the opsonic index is calculated from the following equation: phagocytic index of normal serum ÷ phagocytic index of test serum = 1 ÷ $x$, where $x$ represents the opsonic index.

**op·so·nin** (op′sŏ-nin) a substance that binds to antigens, enhancing phagocytosis. [G. *opson,* boiled meat, provisions, fr. *hepsō*, to boil, + -in]

**op·so·ni·sa·tion [Br.]** SEE opsonization.

**op·son·i·za·tion** (op′sŏ-nī-zā′shŭn) the process by which bacteria are altered in such a manner that they are more readily and more efficiently engulfed by phagocytes.

**op·so·no·cy·to·pha·gic** (op′sŏ-nō-sī′tō-fā′jik) pertaining to the increased efficiency of phagocytic activity of the leukocytes in blood that contains specific opsonin. [opsonin + G. *kytos,* a hollow (cell), + *phagō*, to eat]

**op·so·nom·e·try** (op-sŏ-nom′ĕ-trē) determination of the opsonic index or the opsonocytophagic activity.

**op·tic, op·ti·cal** (op′tik, op′ti-kăl) relating to the eye, vision, or optics. [G. *optikos*]

**op·ti·c ac·tiv·i·ty** the ability of a compound in solution (one possessing no plane of symmetry, usually because of the presence of one or more asymmetric carbon atoms) to rotate the plane of polarized light.

**op·ti·cal ab·er·ra·tion** failure of rays from a point source to form a perfect image after traversing an optical system.

**op·ti·cal ac·tiv·i·ty** SEE optic activity.

**op·ti·cal den·si·ty (OD)** SYN absorbance.

**op·ti·cal im·age** an image formed by the refraction or reflection of light.

**op·ti·cal isom·er·ism** stereoisomerism involving the arrangement of substituents about an asymmetric atom or atoms (usually carbon) so that there is a difference in the behavior of the various isomers with regard to the extent of their rotation of the plane of polarized light. Cf. stereoisomerism.

**op·ti·cal ker·a·to·plas·ty** transplantation of transparent corneal tissue to replace a leukoma or scar that impairs vision.

**op·ti·cal ro·ta·tion** the change in the plane of polarization of polarized light of a given wavelength upon passing through optically active sub-

stances; measured in terms of specific rotation by polarimetry, an important tool in chemical structural work, especially on carbohydrates.

**op·tic atax·ia** an inability to guide the hand toward an object using visual information; seen in Balint syndrome.

**op·tic ax·is** the axis of the eye connecting the anterior and posterior poles; it usually diverges from the visual axis by five degrees or more.

**op·tic ca·nal** the short canal through the lesser wing of the sphenoid bone at the apex of the orbit that gives passage to the optic nerve and the ophthalmic artery. SYN canalis opticus [TA], optic foramen.

**op·tic cap·sule** the concentrated zone of mesenchyme around the developing optic cup; the primordium of the sclera of the eye.

**op·tic chi·asm** a flattened quadrangular body in front of the tuber cinereum and infundibulum, the point of crossing or decussation of the fibers of the optic nerves; most of the fibers cross to the opposite side, some run directly forward on each side without crossing, some pass transversely on the posterior surface between the two optic tracts and others pass transversely on the anterior surface between the two optic nerves. SYN optic decussation.

**op·tic cup** the double-walled cup formed by the invagination of the embryonic optic vesicle; its inner component becomes the neural layer of the retina; its outer layer, the pigmented layer.

**op·tic de·cus·sa·tion** SYN optic chiasm.

**op·ti·c den·si·ty** SYN absorbance.

**op·tic disk** an oval area of the ocular fundus devoid of light receptors where the axons of the retinal ganglion cell converge to form the optic nerve head. SYN discus nervi optici [TA], blind spot (3), optic papilla.

**op·tic fo·ra·men** SYN optic canal.

**op·ti·cian** (op-tish′an) one who practices opticianry.

**op·ti·cian·ry** (op-tish′an-rē) the professional practice of filling prescriptions for ophthalmic lenses, dispensing spectacles, and making and fitting contact lenses.

**op·tic isom·er·ism** SEE optical isomerism.

**op·tic nerve [CN II]** although classified as a cranial nerve, it is actually an extension of the forebrain; it conveys afferent fibers from the ganglion cells of the retina, it passes out of the orbit through the optic canal to the chiasm, where part of the fibers cross to the opposite side and pass through the optic tract to the geniculate bodies, superior colliculus, and the pretectum. SYN nervus opticus [CN II] [TA], second cranial nerve [CN II].

**op·tic neu·ri·tis** inflammation of the optic nerve. SEE ALSO neuromyelitis optica, retrobulbar neuritis, papillitis.

**op·ti·co·cil·i·a·ry** (op′ti-kō-sil′ē-ār-ē) relating to the optic and ciliary nerves.

**op·ti·co·pu·pil·lary** (op′ti-kō-pyu′pi-lār-ē) relating to the optic nerve and the pupil.

**op·tic pa·pil·la (p)** SYN optic disk.

**op·tic ra·di·a·tion** the massive, fanlike fiber system passing from the lateral geniculate body of the thalamus to the visual cortex; the fibers follow the retrolenticular and sublenticular limbs of the internal capsule into the corona radiata but they curve back along the lateral wall of the temporal and occipital horns of the lateral ventricle to the striate cortex on the medial surface and pole of the occipital lobe. SYN radiatio optica.

**op·tic ro·ta·tion** SEE optical rotation.

**op·ti·c ro·ta·to·ry dis·per·sion** the change in optic rotation with the wavelength of the incident monochromatic polarized light; the displacement of the former from zero within the absorption band is known as the cotton effect.

**op·tics** (op′tiks) the science concerned with the properties of light, its refraction and absorption, and the refracting media of the eye in that relation. [G. optikos, fr. ōps, eye]

**op·tic tract** the continuation of the optic nerve fibers beyond their hemidecussation in the optic chiasm; each of the two symmetrical optic tracts is composed of fibers originating from the temporal half of the retina of the ipsilateral eye and a nearly equal number of fibers from the nasal half of the contralateral retina; it forms a compact, somewhat flattened fiber band passing caudolaterally alongside the base of the hypothalamus and over the basal surface of the crus cerebri; most of its fibers terminate in the lateral geniculate body; a smaller number of fibers enter the brachium of the superior colliculus, to terminate in the superior colliculus and the pretectal region. SYN tractus opticus [TA].

**op·ti·mal pitch** the frequency of vocal fold movement that allows optimum resonance with least vocal effort for an individual. SEE ALSO habitual pitch, fundamental frequency. SYN natural pitch.

**op·ti·mum dose** the dose of a drug or radiation that will produce the desired effect with minimum likelihood of undesirable symptoms.

△**op·to-, op·ti·co-** optical; optic; ocular. [G. optikos, optical, from ōps, eye]

**op·to·coe·lia [Br.]** a cavity of the optic lobe of the brain in some animals.

**op·to·ki·net·ic nys·tag·mus** nystagmus induced by looking at moving visual stimuli.

**op·tom·e·ter** (op-tom′ĕ-ter) an instrument for determining the refraction of the eye. [opto- + G. metron, measure]

**op·tom·e·trist** (op-tom′ĕ-trist) one who practices optometry.

**op·tom·e·try** (op-tom′ĕ-trē) **1.** the profession concerned with the examination of the eyes and related structures to determine the presence of vision problems and eye disorders, and with the prescription and adaptation of lenses and other optical aids or the use of visual training for maximum visual efficiency. **2.** the use of an optometer.

**op·to·my·om·e·ter** (op′tō-mī-om′ĕ-ter) an instrument for determining the relative power of the extrinsic muscles of the eye. [opto- + G. mys, muscle, + metron, measure]

**ora**, pl. **orae** (ō′ră, ō′rē) an edge or a margin. [L.]

**ora** (ō′ră) plural of L. os, the mouth. [L.]

**or·ad** (ō′răd) **1.** in a direction toward the mouth. **2.** situated nearer the mouth in relation to a specific reference point; opposite of aborad. [L. os, mouth, + ad, to]

**or·al** (ōr′ăl) relating to the mouth. [L. os (or-), mouth]

**or·al a·prax·ia** reduced ability, due to cortical sensorimotor damage, to perform voluntary movements of the oral musculature, especially sequenced movements. Often occurs with apraxia of speech. SEE ALSO apraxia. SYN oral motor apraxia.

**or·al au·di·tory meth·od** an approach to the education of deaf children that emphasizes early auditory training, speech and speech reading, and early and consistent use of high quality amplification for residual hearing. SEE ALSO manual visual method, combined methods, total communication.

**or·al bi·ol·o·gy** that aspect of biology devoted to the study of biological phenomena associated with the oral cavity in health and disease (e.g., dental caries, mastication, periodontal disease).

**or·al cav·i·ty** the region consisting of the vestibulum oris, the narrow cleft between the lips and cheeks, and the teeth and gums, and the cavitas oris propria. SYN mouth (1).

**or·al con·tra·cep·tive** any orally effective preparation designed to prevent conception.

**or·al de·fen·sive·ness** overreaction to the tastes or textures of things placed in one's mouth.

**or·al hy·giene** the cleaning of the mouth by means of brushing, flossing, irrigating, massaging, or the use of other devices.

**oral·i·ty** (ōr-al′i-tē) FREUDIAN PSYCHOLOGY the psychic organization derived from, and characteristic of, the oral period of psychosexual development.

**or·al and max·il·lo·fa·cial sur·ge·ry** the dental specialty that includes the surgical correction of injuries and malformations of the midface, jaws, and dentition.

**or·al mo·tor aprax·ia** SYN oral apraxia.

**or·al pa·thol·o·gy** the branch of dentistry concerned with the etiology, pathogenesis, and clinical, gross, and microscopic aspects of oral and paraoral disease, including oral soft tissues, the teeth, jaws, and salivary glands.

**or·al phase** in psychoanalytic personality theory, the earliest stage in psychosexual development, lasting through the first 18 months of life, during which the oral zone is the center of the infant's needs, expression, gratification, and pleasurable erotic experiences; has a strong influence on the organization and development of the child's psyche.

**or·al po·li·o·vi·rus vac·cine** SEE poliovirus vaccine (2).

**or·al sur·geon** SYN dental surgeon.

**or·al sur·ge·ry** the branch of dentistry concerned with the diagnosis and surgical and adjunctive treatment of diseases, injuries, and deformities of the oral and maxillofacial region.

**or·al ves·ti·bule** that part of the mouth bounded anteriorly and laterally by the lips and the cheeks, posteriorly and medially by the teeth and/or gums, and above and below by the reflections of the mucosa from the lips and cheeks to the gums.

**or·ange wood** a soft wood used in dentistry for placement of bridges, crowns, etc. by biting pressure, also used as a burnishing point in the polishing of root surfaces.

**ora ser·ra·ta retinae** the serrated extremity of the optic part of the retina, located a little behind the ciliary body and marking the limits of the percipient portion of the membrane.

**or·bic·u·lar** (or-bik′yu-lăr) similar in form to an orb; circular in form. [L. orbiculus, a small disk, dim. of orbis, circle]

**or·bic·u·la·re** (ōr-bik-yu-lā′rē) SYN lenticular process of incus. [L., fr. *orbiculus,* a small disk]

**or·bi·cu·la·ris oc·u·li mus·cle** consists of three portions: orbital part, or external portion, which arises from frontal process of maxilla and nasal process of frontal bone, encircles aperture of orbit, and is inserted near origin; palpebral part, or internal portion, which arises from medial palpebral ligament, passes through each eyelid, and is inserted into lateral palpebral raphe; lacrimal part (tensor tarsi muscle, Duverney or Horner muscle) which arises from posterior lacrimal crest and passes across lacrimal sac to join palpebral portion; *action,* closes eye, wrinkles forehead vertically; *nerve supply,* facial. SYN musculus orbicularis oculi [TA].

**or·bi·cu·la·ris o·ris mus·cle** *origin,* by nasolabial band from septum of the nose, by superior incisive bundle from incisor fossa of maxilla, by inferior incisive bundle from lower jaw each side of symphysis; *insertion,* fibers surround mouth between skin and mucous membrane of lips and cheeks, and are blended with other muscles; *action,* closes lips; *nerve supply,* facial. SYN musculus orbicularis oris [TA].

**or·bi·cu·lus cil·i·ar·is** (ōr-bik′yu-lŭs sil-ē-ār′is) the darkly pigmented posterior zone of the ciliary body continuous with the retina at the ora serrata. SYN ciliary disk, ciliary ring, pars plana. [Mod. L.]

▯**or·bit** (ōr′bit) the bony cavity containing the eyeball and its adnexa; it is formed of parts of the frontal, maxillary, sphenoid, lacrimal, zygomatic, ethmoid, and palatine bones. See this page. SYN orbita [TA], orbital cavity.

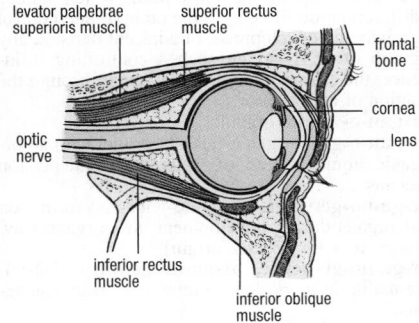

levator palpebrae superioris muscle   superior rectus muscle   frontal bone   cornea   lens   optic nerve   inferior rectus muscle   inferior oblique muscle

**orbit:** containing the eyeball and the ocular muscles

**or·bi·ta,** gen. **or·bi·tae** (ōr′bi-tă, ōr′bi-tē) [TA] SYN orbit. [L. a wheel-track, fr. *orbis,* circle]

**or·bi·tal** (ōr′bi-tăl) relating to the orbits.

**or·bi·tal cav·i·ty** SYN orbit.

**or·bi·tal cel·lu·li·tis** cellulitis that involves the tissue layers posterior to the orbital septum.

**or·bi·ta·le** (ōr-bi-tā′lē) CEPHALOMETRICS the lowermost point in the lower margin of the bony orbit that may be felt under the skin. [L. of an orbit]

**or·bi·tal gy·ri** a number of small, irregular convolutions occupying the concave inferior surface of each frontal lobe of the cerebrum.

**or·bi·ta·lis mus·cle** a rudimentary nonstriated muscle, crossing the infraorbital groove and

sphenomaxillary fissure, intimately united with the periosteum of the orbit. SYN musculus orbitalis [TA], orbital muscle.

**or·bi·tal mar·gin** the mostly sharp edge of the orbital opening which is the peripheral border of the base of the pyramid-shaped orbit. The superior half of the orbital rim is the supraorbital margin; the inferior half is the infraorbital margin. The frontal, maxillary, and zygomatic bones contribute to the orbital rim, which is generally strong to protect the orbital contents. Weak, potential fracture sites of the rim coincide with the sutures between the participating bones. SYN margo orbitalis [TA].

**or·bi·tal mus·cle** SYN orbitalis muscle.

**or·bi·tal plane** the orbital surface of the maxilla, lying perpendicular to the orbitomeatal plane at the orbitale.

**or·bi·tal pro·cess** the anterior and larger of the two processes at the upper extremity of the vertical plate of the palatine bone, articulating with the maxilla, ethmoid, and sphenoid bones.

**or·bi·tog·ra·phy** (ōr′bi-tog′ră-fē) radiographic evaluation of the orbit. [L. *orbita,* orbit, + G. *graphō,* to write]

**or·bi·to·mea·tal line (OML)** SYN base line.

**or·bi·to·mea·tal plane** a standard craniometric reference plane passing through the right and left porion and the left orbitale; drawn on the profile radiograph or photograph from the superior margin of the acoustic meatus to the orbitale.

**or·bi·to·na·sal** (ōr′bi-tō-nā′săl) relating to the orbit and the nose or nasal cavity.

**or·bi·to·nom·e·ter** (ōr′bi-tō-nom′ĕ-ter) an instrument that measures the resistance offered to pressing the eyeball backwards into its socket. [L. *orbita,* orbit, + G. *metron,* measure]

**or·bi·to·nom·e·try** (ōr′bi-tō-nom′ĕ-trē) measurement by means of the orbitonometer.

**or·bi·top·a·thy** disease of the orbit and its contents.

**or·bi·tot·o·my** (ōr-bi-tot′ō-mē) surgical incision into the orbit. [L. *orbita,* orbit, + *tomē,* a cutting]

*Or·bi·vi·rus* (ōr′bi-vī-rŭs) a genus of viruses of vertebrates that multiply in insects, including Colorado tick fever virus of man. [L. *orbis,* ring, + virus]

**or·ce·in** (ōr′sē-in) a natural dye derived from orcinol which is used in various histologic staining methods.

**orch·al·gia** (ork-al′jē-ă) SYN orchialgia.

⟡**or·chi-, or·chi·do-, or·chio-** the testes. [G. *orchis,* testis]

**or·chi·al·gia** (ōr-kē-al′jē-ă) pain in the testis. SYN orchalgia, testalgia. [orchi- + G. *algos,* pain]

**or·chi·dec·to·my** (ōr-ki-dek′tō-mē) SYN orchiectomy.

**or·chid·ic** (ōr-kid′ik) relating to the testis.

**or·chi·dom·e·ter** (ōr-ki-dom′ĕ-ter) **1.** a caliper device used to measure the size of testes. **2.** a set of sized models of testes for comparison of testicular development. [orchido- + G. *metron,* measure]

**or·chi·do·pexy** (ōr-kid′ō-peks-ē) SYN orchiopexy.

**or·chi·ec·to·my** (ōr-kē-ek′tō-mē) removal of one or both testes. SYN orchidectomy, testectomy. [orchi- + G. *ektomē,* excision]

**or·chi·ep·i·did·y·mi·tis** (ōr′kē-ep′i-did′i-mī′tis) inflammation of the testis and epididymis. [orchi- + epididymis, + G. *-itis,* inflammation]

**or•chi•o•cele** (ōr′kē-ō-sēl) a testis retained in the inguinal canal. [orchio- + G. *kēlē,* hernia, tumor]

**or•chi•op•a•thy** (ōr-kē-op′ă-thē) disease of a testis. [orchio- + G. *pathos,* suffering]

**or•chi•o•pexy** (ōr′kē-ō-pek′sē) surgical treatment of an undescended testicle by freeing it and implanting it into the scrotum. SYN cryptorchidopexy, orchidopexy. [orchio- + G. *pēxis,* fixation]

**or•chi•o•plas•ty** (ōr′kē-ō-plas-tē) surgical reconstruction of the testis. [orchio- + G. *plastos,* formed]

**or•chi•ot•o•my** (ōr-kē-ot′ō-mē) incision into a testis. [orchio- + G. *tomē,* incision]

**or•chis,** pl. **or•chis•es** (ōr′kis, ōr′ki-sēz) [TA] SYN testis. [G. testis, an orchid]

**or•chit•ic** (ōr-kit′ik) denoting orchitis.

**or•chi•tis** (ōr-kī′tis) inflammation of the testis. SYN testitis. [orchi- + G. *-itis,* inflammation]

**Ord** orotidine.

**or•der** (ōr′der) **1.** in biological classification, the division just below the class (or subclass) and above the family. **2.** in a reaction, the sum of the exponents of all the concentration terms in that reaction's rate expression. [L. *ordo,* regular arrangement]

**or•der•ly** (ōr′der-lē) an attendant in a hospital unit who assists in the care of patients.

**or•di•nate** (ōr′di-nāt) in a plane cartesian coordinate system, the vertical axis (*y*).

**orex•i•gen•ic** (ŏ-rek-si-jen′ik) appetite-stimulating.

**or•gan** (ōr′găn) any part of the body exercising a specific function, as of respiration, secretion, digestion. SYN organum [TA], organon. [L. *organum,* fr. G. *organon,* a tool, instrument]

**or•ga•na** (ōr′gă-nă) plural of organum.

**or•gan cul•ture** the maintenance or growth of tissues, organ primordia, or the parts or whole of an organ *in vitro* in such a way as to allow differentiation or preservation of the architecture or function.

**or•gan•elle** (or′gă-nel) one of the specialized parts of a protozoan or tissue cell; mitochondria, the Golgi apparatus, nucleus and centrioles, granular and agranular endoplasmic reticulum, vacuoles, microsomes, lysosomes, plasma membrane, and certain fibrils, as well as plastids of plant cells. SYN organoid (3). [G. *organon,* organ, + Fr. *-elle,* dim. suffix, fr. L. *-ella*]

**or•gan•ic** (ōr-gan′ik) **1.** relating to an organ. **2.** relating to or formed by an organism. **3.** organized; structural. **4.** SEE organic compound. [G. *organikos*]

**or•gan•ic ac•id** an acid made up of molecules containing organic radicals; e.g., acetic acid, citric acid, which contain the ionizable —COOH group.

**or•gan•ic brain syn•drome (OBS)** a constellation of behavioral or psychological signs and symptoms including problems with attention, concentration, memory, confusion, anxiety, and depression caused by transient or permanent dysfunction of the brain.

**or•gan•ic chem•is•try** that branch of chemistry concerned with covalently linked atoms, centering around carbon compounds of this type; originally, and still including, the chemistry of natural products.

**or•gan•ic com•pound** a compound composed of atoms (some of which are carbon) held together

by covalent (shared electron) bonds. Cf. inorganic compound.

**or•gan•ic con•trac•ture** contracture, usually due to fibrosis within the muscle that persists whether the subject is conscious or unconscious.

**or•gan•ic de•lu•sions** false beliefs experienced in the delirium associated with injury to the brain, organic change in the brain such as in Alzheimer syndrome, or cocaine or other drug intoxication.

**or•gan•ic dis•ease** a disease in which there are anatomical or pathophysiological changes in some bodily tissue or organ, in contrast to a disorder of psychogenic origin.

**or•gan•ic ev•o•lu•tion** SYN biologic evolution.

**or•gan•ic hear•ing im•pair•ment** deafness due to a pathologic process or an organic cause, as opposed to psychogenic hearing impairment.

**or•gan•ic men•tal dis•or•der** a psychological, cognitive, or behavioral abnormality associated with transient or permanent dysfunction of the brain, usually characterized by the presence of an organic mental syndrome.

**or•gan•ic mur•mur** a murmur caused by an organic lesion.

**or•gan•ic ver•ti•go** vertigo due to brain damage.

**or•ga•nism** (ōr′gă-nizm) any living individual, whether plant or animal, considered as a whole.

**or•ga•ni•za•tion** (ōr′gan-i-zā′shŭn) **1.** an arrangement of distinct but mutually dependent parts. **2.** the conversion of coagulated blood, exudate, or dead tissue into fibrous tissue.

**or•ga•nize** (ōr′gan-īz) to provide with, or to assume, a structure.

**or•ga•niz•er** (ōr′gan-ī-zer) **1.** a group of cells on the dorsal lip of the blastopore, which induce differentiation of cells in the embryo and control growth and development of adjacent parts. **2.** any group of cells having such a controlling influence, the effects being brought about through the action of an evocator.

**or•gan•o-** organ; organic. [G. *organon*]

**or•gan•o•gel** (ōr-gan′ō-jel) a hydrogel with an organic liquid instead of water as the dispersion means.

**or•ga•no•gen•e•sis** (ōr′gă-nō-jen′ĕ-sis) formation of organs during development. SYN organogeny. [organo- + G. *genesis,* origin]

**or•ga•no•ge•net•ic, or•ga•no•gen•ic** (ōr′gă-nō-jĕ-net′ik, ōr′gă-nō-jen′ik) relating to organogenesis.

**or•gan•og•e•ny** (ōr-gan-oj′ĕ-nē) SYN organogenesis.

**or•gan•oid** (ōr′gă-noyd) **1.** resembling in superficial appearance or in structure any of the organs or glands of the body. **2.** composed of glandular or organic elements, and not of a single tissue; pertaining to certain neoplasms that contain cytologic and histologic elements arranged in a pattern that closely resembles that of a normal organ. SEE ALSO histoid. **3.** SYN organelle. [organo- + G. *eidos,* resemblance]

**or•gan•oid tu•mor** a tumor of complex structure, glandular in origin, containing epithelium and connective tissue.

**or•gan•o•meg•a•ly** (ōr′gă-nō-meg′ă-lē) SYN visceromegaly.

**or•gan•o•mer•cur•i•al** (ōr-gan′ō-mer-kyu′rē-ăl) any organic mercurial compound; e.g., merbromin, thimerosal.

**or•ga•no•me•tal•lic** (ōr′gă-nō-me-tal′ik) denoting an organic compound containing one or more metallic atoms in its structure.

**or·ga·non**, pl. **or·ga·na** (ōr′gă-non, ōr′gă-nă) SYN organ. [G. organ]

**or·ga·no·phos·phate** (ōr-gă-nō-fos′fāt) phosphorus-containing organic compounds that phosphorylate cholinesterase and thus irreversibly inhibit it. Used as insecticides; have also been used as war gases.

**or·ga·no·tro·phic** (ōr′gă-nō-trof′ik) **1.** pertaining to the nourishment of an organ. **2.** pertaining to a microorganism that uses organic sources as a reducing power. [organo- + G. *trophē*, nourishment]

**or·ga·no·tro·pic** (ōr′gă-nō-trop′ik) pertaining to or characterized by organotropism.

**or·ga·not·ro·pism** (ōr-gă-not′rō-pizm) the special affinity of particular drugs, pathogens, or metastatic tumors for particular organs or their component parts. Cf. parasitotropism. [organo- + G. *tropē*, a turning]

**or·gan-spe·cif·ic** denoting or pertaining to a serum produced by the injection of the cells of a certain organ or tissue that, when injected into another animal, destroys the cells of the corresponding organ.

**or·gan-spe·cif·ic an·ti·gen** a heterogenetic antigen with organ specificity; e.g., in addition to species-specific antigen, kidney of one species contains antigen that is identical to that in kidney of other species. SYN tissue-specific antigen.

**or·ga·num**, pl. **or·ga·na** (ōr′gă-nŭm, ōr′gă-nă) [TA] SYN organ, organ. [L. tool, instrument]

**or·gasm** (ōr′gazm) the peak state of excitement in the sexual act. SYN climax (2). [G. *orgaō*, to swell, be excited]

**or·gas·mic**, **or·gas·tic** (ōr-gaz′mik, ōr-gas′tik) relating to, characteristic of, or tending to produce an orgasm.

**or·i·en·ta·tion** (ōr-ē-en-tā′shŭn) **1.** the recognition of one's temporal, spatial, and personal relationships and environment. **2.** the relative position of an atom with respect to one to which it is connected. [Fr. *orienter,* to set toward the East, fr. L. *sol oriens,* the rising sun]

*Ori·en·tia* (ōr-ē-en′shē-ă) a member of the bacterial family Rickettsiae.

*Ori·en·tia tsut·su·ga·mu·shi* the only member of its genus, this species is the causative agent of scrub typhus, transmitted by mites; formerly called *Rickettsia tsutsugamushi.*

**or·i·ent·ing re·flex** an aspect of attending in which an organism's initial response to a change or to a novel stimulus is such that the organism becomes more sensitive to the stimulation; e.g., dilation of the pupil of the eye in response to dim light. SYN orienting response.

**or·i·ent·ing re·sponse** SYN orienting reflex.

**or·i·fice** (or′i-fis) any aperture or opening. SYN orificium. [L. *orificium*]

**or·i·fi·cial** (ōr-i-fish′ăl) relating to an orifice of any kind.

**or·i·fi·ci·um**, pl. **or·i·fi·cia** (ōr-i-fish′ē-ŭm, ōr-i-fish′ē-ă) SYN orifice, orifice. [L.]

**or·i·gin** (ōr′i-jin) **1.** the less movable of two sites of attachment of a muscle; that which is attached to the more fixed part of the skeleton. **2.** the starting point of a cranial or spinal nerve. The former have two origins: the **ental origin, deep origin**, or **real origin**, the cell group in the brain or medulla whence the fibers of the nerve begin, and the **ectal origin, superficial origin**, or **apparent origin**, the point where the nerve emerges from the brain. [L. *origo,* source, beginning, fr. *orior,* to rise]

**Or·mond dis·ease** (or′mŏnd) SYN retroperitoneal fibrosis.

**Orn** ornithine or its radical.

**or·ni·thine (Orn)** (ōr′ni-thēn, ōr′ni-thin) the amino acid formed when L-arginine is hydrolyzed by arginase; an important intermediate in the urea cycle; elevated levels seen in certain defects of the urea cycle.

**or·ni·thi·nu·ria** (ōr′ni-thi-nyu′rē-ă) excretion of excessive amounts of ornithine in the urine.

*Or·ni·thod·o·ros* (ōr-ni-thod′ŏ-rŭs) a genus of soft ticks, several species of which are vectors of pathogens of various relapsing fevers. [G. *ornis* (*ornith-*), bird, + *doros,* a leather bag]

**or·ni·tho·sis** (ōr-ni-thō′sis) SYN psittacosis. [G. *ornis* (*ornith-*), bird, + -*osis,* condition]

**Oro** orotic acid or orotate.

△**oro- 1.** the mouth. [L. *os, oris,* mouth] **2.** obsolete alternative spelling is orrho-. SEE sero-. [G. *orrhos,* whey, serum]

**or·o·dig·i·to·fa·cial** (ōr′ō-dij′i-tō-fā′shăl) relating to the mouth, fingers, and face.

**or·o·fa·cial** (ōr-ō-fā′shăl) relating to the mouth and face.

**or·o·lin·gual** (ōr-ō-ling′gwăl) relating to the mouth and tongue.

**or·o·na·sal** (ōr-ō-nā′săl) relating to the mouth and nose.

**or·o·pha·ryn·ge·al** (ōr-ō-fă-rin′jē-ăl) relating to the oropharynx.

**or·o·phar·ynx** (ōr′ō-far′ingks) the portion of the pharynx that lies posterior to the mouth; it is continuous above with the nasopharynx via the pharyngeal isthmus and below with the laryngopharynx. [L. *os* (*or-*), mouth]

**Oro·pouche fever** (ōr-o′poosh) acute febrile illness caused by a species of Bunyavirus.

**or·o·so·mu·coid** (ōr′ō-sō-myu′koyd) increased plasma levels associated with inflammation.

**or·o·tate (Oro)** (ōr′ō-tāt) a salt or ester of orotic acid.

**orot·ic ac·id (Oro)** (ōr-ot′ik as′id) an important intermediate in the formation of the pyrimidine nucleotides; elevated in certain inherited defects of pyrimidine biosynthesis.

**orot·i·dine (O, Ord)** (ō-rot′i-dēn) Orotic acid-3-β-D-ribonucleoside; uridine-6-carboxylic acid; elevated in cases of orotidinuria.

**or·o·tra·che·al tube** a tracheal tube inserted through the mouth.

**O·ro·ya fe·ver** (ō-rō-yah) a generalized, acute, febrile, endemic, and systemic form of bartonellosis; marked by high fever, rheumatic pains, progressive, severe anemia, and albuminuria. SYN Carrión disease.

**or·phan dis·ease** a disease for which no treatment has been developed because of its rarity. SEE ALSO orphan products.

**or·phan drugs** SYN orphan products.

**or·phan pro·ducts** drugs, biologicals, and medical devices (including diagnostic *in vitro* tests) that may be useful in uncommon or rare diseases but which are not considered commercially viable. SYN orphan drugs.

**or·phan re·cep·tor** a nuclear receptor for which no ligand has yet been identified.

**or·phan vi·rus·es** viruses, such as the enteric

orphan viruses, which when originally found were not specifically associated with disease; a number of these have since been shown to be pathogenic.

**ORT** Operation Restore Trust.

**or•the•sis** (ōr-thē′sis) SYN orthosis. [ortho- + -esis, process]

**or•thet•ics** (ōr-thet′iks) SYN orthotics.

**Orth fix•a•tive** (orth) formalin added to Müller fixative, used for bringing out chromaffin, studying early degenerative processes and necrosis, and for demonstrating rickettsiae and bacteria.

△**or•tho-, orth-** 1. straight, normal, in proper order. 2. CHEMISTRY italicized prefix denoting that a compound has two substitutions on adjacent carbon atoms in a benzene ring. For terms beginning ortho- or o-, see the specific name. [Gr. orthos correct]

**or•tho•cho•rea** (ōr′thō-kōr-ē′ă) a form of chorea in which the spasms occur only or chiefly when the patient is in the erect posture.

**or•tho•chro•mat•ic** (ōr′thō-krō-mat′ik) denoting any tissue or cell that stains the color of the dye used, i.e., the same color as the dye solution with which it is stained. [ortho- + G. chrōma, color]

**or•tho•cy•to•sis** (ōr′thō-sī-tō′sis) a condition in which all of the cellular elements in the circulating blood are mature forms, irrespective of the proportions of various types and total numbers. [ortho- + G. kytos, cell, + -osis, condition]

**or•tho•de•ox•ia** fall in arterial blood oxygen upon assuming the upright posture.

**or•tho•don•tics** (ōr-thō-don′tiks) that branch of dentistry concerned with the correction and prevention of irregularities and malocclusion of the teeth. [ortho- + G. odous, tooth]

**or•tho•dont•ist** a dental specialist who practices orthodontics.

**or•tho•dro•mic** (ōr-thō-drō′mik) denoting the propagation of an impulse along an axon in the normal direction. Cf. antidromic. [ortho- + G. dromos, course]

**or•thog•na•thia** (ōr-thō-nath′ē-ă) the study of the causes and treatment of conditions related to malposition of the bones of the jaws. [ortho- + G. gnathos, jaw]

**or•thog•nath•ic, or•thog•na•thous** (ōr-thō-nath′ ik, ōr-thog′năthŭs) 1. relating to orthognathia. 2. having a face without projecting jaw, one with a gnathic index below 98. 3. having a normal relationship of the jaws. [ortho- + G. gnathos, jaw]

**or•tho•grade** (ōr′thō-grād) walking or standing erect; denoting the posture of human beings; opposed to pronograde. [ortho- + L. gradior, pp. gressus, to walk]

**or•tho•grade de•gen•er•a•tion** SYN wallerian degeneration.

**or•tho•ker•a•tol•o•gy** (ōr′thō-ker-ă-tol′ŏ-jē) a method of molding the cornea with contact lenses to improve unaided vision. [ortho- + G. keras, horn (cornea), + logos, science]

**or•tho•ker•a•to•sis** (ōr′thō-ker-ă-tō′sis) formation of an anuclear keratin layer, as in the normal epidermis. [ortho- + G. keras, horn, + -osis, condition]

**or•tho•me•chan•i•cal** (ōr-thō-mĕ-kan′i-kăl) pertaining to braces, prostheses, orthotic devices, and appliances. [ortho- + mechanical]

**or•tho•mo•lec•u•lar** (ōr′thō-mō-lek′yu-lăr) a therapeutic approach designed to provide an optimum molecular environment for body functions,

with particular reference to the optimum concentrations of substances normally present in the body.

**Or•tho•myx•o•vir•i•dae** (ōr′thō-mik-sō-vir′i-dē) the family of viruses that comprises the three groups of influenza viruses, types A, B, and C. The only recognized genus is *Influenzavirus*, which comprises the strains of virus types A and B, both of which are subject to mutation resulting in epidemics. Influenza virus type C differs from types A and B somewhat and probably belongs to a separate genus. SEE ALSO *Influenzavirus*.

**or•tho•pae•dic, or•tho•pe•dic** (ōr-thō-pē′dik) relating to orthopedics.

**or•tho•pae•dics, or•tho•pe•dics** (ōr-thō-pē′diks) the medical specialty concerned with the preservation, restoration, and development of form and function of the musculoskeletal system, extremities, spine, and associated structures by medical, surgical, and physical methods. [ortho- + G. pais (paid-), child]

**or•tho•pe•dic sur•gery** the branch of surgery that embraces the treatment of acute and chronic disorders of the musculoskeletal system, including injuries, diseases, dysfunction, and deformities (orig. deformities in children) in the extremities and spine. SEE ALSO orthopaedics.

**or•tho•per•cus•sion** (ōr′thō-per-kŭsh′ŭn) very light percussion of the chest, used to determine the size of the heart.

**or•tho•pho•ria** (ōr-thō-fōr′ē-ă) absence of heterophoria; the condition of binocular fixation in which the lines of sight meet at a distant or near point of reference in the absence of a fusion stimulus. [ortho- + G. phora, motion]

**or•tho•phor•ic** (ōr-thō-fōr′ik) pertaining to orthophoria.

**or•tho•phos•phate** (ōr-thō-fos′fāt) a salt or ester of orthophosphoric acid.

**or•tho•phos•phor•ic ac•id** (ōr′thō-fos-fōr′ik as′ id) phosphoric acid, $O=P(OH)_3$, distinguished by ortho- from meta- and pyrophosphoric acids.

**or•thop•nea** (ōr-thop-nē′ă, ōr-thop′nē-ă) discomfort in breathing that is brought on or aggravated by lying flat. Cf. platypnea. [ortho- + G. pnoē, a breathing]

**or•thop•ne•ic** (or′thop-ne′ik) relating to or characterized by orthopnea.

**or•thop•noea [Br.]** SEE orthopnea.

**or•thop•noe•ic [Br.]** SEE orthopneic.

*Or•tho•pox•vi•rus* (ōr-thō-poks′vī-rŭs) the genus of the family Poxviridae which comprises the viruses of alastrim, vaccinia, variola, cowpox, ectromelia, monkeypox, and rabbitpox.

**or•tho•psy•chi•a•try** (ōr′thō-sī-kī′ă-trē) a cross-disciplinary science combining child psychiatry, developmental psychology, pediatrics, and family care devoted to the discovery, prevention, and treatment of mental and psychological disorders in children and adolescents.

**or•thop•tic** (ōr-thop′tik) relating to orthoptics.

**or•thop•tics** (ōr-thop′tiks) the study and treatment of defective binocular vision, of defects in the action of the ocular muscles, or of faulty visual habits. [ortho- straightened + G. optikos, sight]

*Or•tho•re•o•vi•rus* (ōr-thō-rē′ō-vī-rus) a genus in the family Reoviridae associated with a variety of respiratory and enteric diseases, but its causal relationship is not proven.

**or•tho•scope** (ōr′thō-skōp) an instrument by

means of which one is able to draw the outlines of the various normas of the skull. [ortho- + G. *skopeō*, to view]

**or·tho·sis**, pl. **or·tho·ses** (ōr-thō′sis, ōr-thō′sēz) an external orthopedic appliance, as a brace or splint, that prevents or assists movement of the spine or the limbs. SYN orthesis. [G. *orthōsis*, a making straight]

**or·tho·stat·ic** (ōr-thō-stat′ik) relating to an erect posture or position.

**orth·o·sta·tic con·ges·tion** pooling of blood in lower parts of the body due to upright posture.

**or·tho·stat·ic hy·po·ten·sion** a form of low blood pressure that occurs in a standing posture.

**or·thot·ics** (ōr-thot′iks) the science concerned with the making and fitting of orthopaedic appliances. SYN orthetics.

**or·tho·tist** (or′thō-tist) a maker and fitter of orthopaedic appliances.

**or·thot·o·nos, or·thot·o·nus** (ōr-thot′ŏ-nos, ōr-thot′ŏ-nŭs) a form of tetanic spasm in which the neck, limbs, and body are held fixed in a straight line. [ortho- + G. *tonos*, tension]

**or·tho·top·ic** (ōr-thō-top′ik) in the normal or usual position. [ortho- + G. *topos*, place]

**or·tho·top·ic ure·ter·o·cele** a ureterocele entirely within the bladder.

**or·tho·tro·pic** (ōr-thō-trop′ik) extending or growing in a straight, especially a vertical, direction. [ortho- + G. *tropē*, a turn]

**Orth stain** (orth) a lithium carmine stain for nerve cells and their processes.

**Or·to·la·ni man·eu·ver** (or-tō-lah′nē) a maneuver for reduction of hip dislocation, using thigh flexion and abduction with anterior movement of the femoral head; reduction is accompanied by palpable reseating of the femoral head in the acetabulum.

**ORYX** a methodology that enables standardized outcome and performance measurement for health care organizations; established by the Joint Commission on Accreditation of Healthcare Organizations.

**Os** osmium.

**os**, gen. **o·ris**, pl. **ora** (os) **1.** [TA] the mouth. **2.** term applied sometimes to an opening into a hollow organ or canal, especially one with thick or fleshy edges. [L. mouth]

**os**, gen. **os·sis**, pl. **os·sa** (os, os′is, os′ă) [TA] SYN bone. For histological description, see specific types of bone. [L. bone]

△**os·che-, os·che·o-** the scrotum. [G. *osche*]

**os·che·al** (os′kē-ăl) SYN scrotal.

**os·che·i·tis** (os-kē-ī′tis) inflammation of the scrotum. [osche- + G. *-itis*, inflammation]

**os·che·o·hy·dro·cele** (os-kē-ō-hī′drō-sēl) scrotal hydrocele. [oscheo- + G. *hydōr*, water, + *kēlē*, tumor]

**os·che·o·plas·ty** (os′kē-ō-plas-tē) SYN scrotoplasty. [oscheo- + *plastos*, formed]

**os·cil·lat·ing vi·sion** SYN oscillopsia.

**os·cil·la·tion** (os-i-lā′shŭn) **1.** a to-and-fro movement. **2.** a stage in inflammation in which the accumulation of leukocytes in small vessels arrests the passage of blood and there is simply a to-and-fro movement at each cardiac contraction. [L. *oscillatio*, fr. *oscillo*, to swing]

**os·cil·la·to·ry po·ten·tial** the variable voltage in the positive deflection of the electroretinogram (B-wave) of the dark-adapted eye arising from amacrine cells.

**os·cil·lom·e·ter** (os-i-lom′ĕ-ter) an apparatus for measuring oscillations of any kind, especially those of the bloodstream in sphygmometry. [L. *oscillo*, to swing, + G. *metron*, measure]

**os·cil·lo·met·ric** (os′i-lō-met′rik) relating to the oscillometer or the records made by its use.

**os·cil·lom·e·try** (os-i-lom′ĕ-trē) the measurement of oscillations of any kind with an oscillometer.

**os·cil·lop·sia** (os-i-lop′sē-ă) the subjective sensation of oscillation of objects viewed. SYN oscillating vision. [L. *oscillo*, to swing, + G. *opsis*, vision]

**os·cu·lum**, pl. **os·cu·la** (os′kyu-lŭm, os′kyu-lă) a pore or minute opening. [L. dim. of *os*, mouth]

△**-ose 1.** CHEMISTRY a terminator usually indicating a carbohydrate. **2.** suffix appended to some Latin stems, with significance of the more common *-ous* (2). [L. *-osus*, full of, abounding] **3.** full of, having much of.

**Os·good-Schlat·ter dis·ease** (oz′good shlaht′er) inflammation or partial avulsion of the tibial apophysis due to traction forces. SYN Schlatter disease, Schlatter-Osgood disease.

**OSHA** Occupational Safety and Health Administration of the U.S. Department of Labor, responsible for establishing and enforcing safety and health standards in the workplace.

**os ha·ma·tum** [TA] SYN hamate bone.

**O shell** the outermost shell of electrons, so called because displacement of electrons causes an emission in the visible or optical range.

**os in·ci·si·vum** the anterior and inner portion of the maxilla, which in the fetus and sometimes in the adult is a separate bone; the incisive suture runs from the incisive canal between the lateral incisor and the canine tooth. SYN incisive bone, intermaxillary bone, premaxillary bone.

**os in·ter·met·a·tar·se·um** a supernumerary bone at the base of the first metatarsal, or between the first and second metatarsal bones, usually fused with one or the other or with the medial cuneiform bone.

△**-os·is**, pl. **-os·es** a process, condition, or state, usually abnormal or diseased colon; production of an abnormal substance, increase of a normal substance, or parasitic infestation. [G.]

**Os·ler dis·ease** (ōs′lĕr) SYN polycythemia vera.

**Os·ler node** (ōs′lĕr) a small, tender, nodular cutaneous lesion in the pads of fingers or toes, probably of immunopathic origin, characteristic of subacute bacterial endocarditis.

**Os·ler-Va·quez dis·ease** (ōs′ler vah-kāz′) SYN polycythemia vera.

**OSMED** otospondylomegaepiphyseal dysplasia.

**os·mic ac·id** (oz′mik as′id) a volatile caustic and strong oxidizing agent; colorless crystals, poorly soluble in water, but soluble in organic solvents; the aqueous solution is a fat and myelin stain and a general fixative for electron microscopy.

**os·mics** (oz′miks) the science of olfaction. [G. *osmē*, smell]

**os·mi·dro·sis** (oz-mi-drō′sis) SYN bromidrosis. [G. *osmē*, smell, + *hidrōs*, sweat]

**os·mi·um (Os)** (oz′mē-ŭm) a metallic element of the platinum group, atomic no. 76, atomic wt. 190.2. [G. *osmē*, smell, because of the strong odor of the tetroxide]

△**os·mo- 1.** osmosis. [G. *ōsmos*, impulsion] **2.** smell, odor. [G. *osmē*]

**os·mo·lal·i·ty** (os-mō-lal′i-tē) the concentration

of a solution expressed in osmoles of solute particles per kilogram of solvent.

**os•mo•lar** (os-mō′lăr) SYN osmotic.

**os•mo•lar•i•ty** (os-mō-lār′i-tē) the osmotic concentration of a solution expressed as osmoles of solute per liter of solution.

**os•mole** (os′mōl) the molecular weight of a solute, in grams, divided by the number of ions or particles into which it dissociates in solution.

**os•mom•e•try** (ŏz-mŏm′ĕ-trē) technique used to determine the number of solute particles in solution by measuring changes in a colligative property. [osmo- + -metry]

**os•mo•re•cep•tor** (os′mō-rē-sep′ter) **1.** a receptor in the central nervous system (probably the hypothalamus) that responds to changes in the osmotic pressure of the blood. [G. *osmos,* impulsion] **2.** a receptor that receives olfactory stimuli. [G. *osmē,* smell]

**os•mo•reg•u•la•to•ry** (os-mō-reg′yu-lă-tōr-ē) influencing the degree and rapidity of osmosis.

**os•mose** (os′mōs) to move through a membrane by osmosis.

**os•mo•sis** (os-mō′sis) the process by which solvent tends to move through a semipermeable membrane from a solution of lower to a solution of higher osmolal concentration of the solutes to which the membrane is relatively impermeable. [G. *ōsmos,* a thrusting, an impulsion]

**os•mot•ic** (os-mot′ik) relating to osmosis. SYN osmolar.

**os•mot•ic di•u•ret•ics** drugs, such as mannitol, which by their osmotic effects promote the elimination of water and electrolytes in the urine.

**os•mot•ic fra•gil•i•ty** the susceptibility of erythrocytes to hemolyze when exposed to increasingly hypotonic saline solutions. SYN fragility of the blood.

**os•mot•ic pres•sure** (Π) the pressure that must be applied to a solution to prevent the passage into it of solvent when solution and pure solvent are separated by a membrane permeable only to the solvent.

**os mult•ang•u•lum ma•jus** SYN trapezium.

**os na•sale** [TA] SYN nasal bone.

**os oc•ci•pi•ta•le** [TA] SYN occipital bone.

△**os•phre•sio-** odor; sense of smell. [G. *osphrēsis,* smell]

**os•phre•sis** (os-frē′sis) SYN olfaction. [G. *osphrēsis,* smell]

**os•phret•ic** (os-fret′ik) SYN olfactory.

**os•sa** (os′ă) plural of L. *os,* bone. [L.]

**os•sa cra•nii** [TA] SYN bones of skull.

**os•sa met•a•car•pi** SYN metacarpal [I–V].

**os•sa me•ta•tar•si,** pl. **os•sa me•ta•tar•sa•li•a** SYN metatarsal (bones) [I–V].

**os sca•phoi•de•um** SYN scaphoid bone.

**os•se•in, os•se•ine** (os′ē-in) SYN collagen. [L. *os,* bone]

△**os•seo-** bony. SEE ALSO ossi-, osteo-. [L. *osseus*]

**os•se•o•car•ti•lag•i•nous** (os′ē-ō-kar-ti-laj′i-nŭs) relating to, or composed of, both bone and cartilage. SYN osteocartilaginous.

**os•se•o•in•te•gra•tion** (os′ē-ō-in′tĕ-grā′shŭn) the direct attachment to bone of an inert, alloplastic material without intervening connective tissue, as with dental implants.

**os•se•o•mu•cin** (os′ē-ō-myu′sin) the ground substance of bony tissue.

**os•se•ous** (os′ē-ŭs) bony, of bone-like consistency or structure. SYN osteal. [L. *osseus*]

**os•se•ous hy•da•tid cyst** a morphological form of hydatid cyst caused by *Echinococcus granulosus* and found in the long bones or the pelvic arch of humans if the embryo is filtered out in bony tissue; in this site no limiting membrane forms and the cyst grows in an uncontrolled fashion, producing cancellous structures and inducing fracture, followed by spread to new sites.

**os•se•ous la•cu•na** a cavity in bony tissue occupied by an osteocyte.

**os•se•ous spi•ral lam•i•na** a double plate of bone winding spirally around the modiolus dividing the spiral canal of the cochlea incompletely into two, scala tympani and scala vestibuli; between the two plates of this lamina the fibers of the cochlear nerve reach the spiral organ (organ of Corti).

**os•se•ous tis•sue** a connective tissue, the matrix of which consists of collagen fibers and ground substance and in which are deposited calcium salts (phosphate, carbonate, and some fluoride) in the form of an apatite. SYN bone tissue.

△**os•si-** bone. SEE ALSO osseo-, osteo-. [L. *os*]

**os•si•cle** (os′i-kl) a small bone; specifically, one of the bones of the tympanic cavity or middle ear. SYN bonelet, ossiculum. [L. *ossiculum,* dim. of *os,* bone]

**os•sic•u•la** (ŏ-sik′yu-lă) plural of ossiculum. [L.]

**os•sic•u•la au•di•tus** [TA] SYN auditory ossicles.

**os•sic•u•lar** (ŏ-sik′yu-lăr) pertaining to an ossicle.

**os•sic•u•lar re•con•struc•tion** generic term denoting a number of surgical techniques to restore the continuity of the ossicular chain from the tympanic membrane to the oval window for sound pressure transmission and, thereby, improved hearing.

**os•sic•u•lec•to•my** (os′i-kyu-lek′tō-mē) removal of one or more of the ossicles of the middle ear. [L. *ossiculum,* ossicle, + G. *ektomē,* excision]

**os•si•cu•lot•o•my** (os′i-kyu-lot′ō-mē) division of one of the processes of the ossicles of the middle ear, or of a fibrous band causing ankylosis between any two ossicles. [L. *ossiculum,* ossicle, + G. *tomē,* incision]

**os•sic•u•lum,** pl. **os•sic•u•la** (ŏ-sik′yu-lŭm, ŏ-sik′yu-lă) SYN ossicle. [L. dim. of *os,* bone]

**os•sif•er•ous** (ŏ-sif′er-ŭs) containing or producing bone. [ossi- + L. *fero,* to bear]

**os•sif•ic** (o-sif′ik) relating to a change into, or formation of, bone.

**os•si•fi•ca•tion** (os′i-fi-kā′shŭn) **1.** the formation of bone. **2.** a change into bone. [L. *ossificatio,* fr. *os,* bone, + *facio,* to make]

**os•sif•ic cen•ter** SYN center of ossification.

**os•si•fy** (os′i-fī) to form bone or convert into bone. [ossi- + L. *facio,* to make]

**os•te•al** (os′tē-ăl) SYN osseous. [G. *osteon,* bone]

**os•te•al•gia** (os-tē-al′jē-ă) pain in a bone. SYN osteodynia. [osteo- + G. *algos,* pain]

**os•te•al•gic** (os-tē-al′jik) relating to or marked by bone pain.

**os•tec•to•my** (os-tek′tō-mē) **1.** surgical removal of bone. **2.** DENTISTRY resection of supporting osseous structure to eliminate periodontal pockets. [osteo- + G. *ektomē,* excision]

**os•te•in, os•te•ine** (os′tē-in) SYN collagen. [G. *osteon,* bone]

**os•te•it•ic** (os-tē-it′ik) relating to or affected by osteitis. SYN ostitic.

**os•te•i•tis** (os-tē-ī′tis) inflammation of bone. SYN ostitis. [osteo- + G. *-itis,* inflammation]

**os·te·i·tis de·for·mans** SYN Paget disease (1).

**os·te·i·tis fi·bro·sa cys·ti·ca** increased osteoclastic resorption of calcified bone with replacement by fibrous tissue, due to primary hyperparathyroidism or other causes of the rapid mobilization of mineral salts. SYN Recklinghausen disease of bone.

**os·te·i·tis pu·bis** (ŏs-tē-ī′tĭs pyu′bĭs) painful inflammation of the pubic bones near the midline, sometimes due to repeated overload of the adductor muscles or repetitive stress activities.

**os tem·po·ra·le** [TA] SYN temporal bone.

**os·tem·py·e·sis** (os′tem-pī-ē′sis) suppuration in bone. [osteo- + G. *empyēsis,* suppuration]

△**os·teo-, ost-, oste-** bone. SEE ALSO osseo-, ossi-. [G. *osteon*]

🔲 **os·te·o·ar·thri·tis** (os′tē-ō-ar-thrī′tis) arthritis characterized by erosion of articular cartilage, which becomes soft, frayed, and thinned with eburnation of subchondral bone and outgrowths of marginal osteophytes; pain and loss of function result; mainly affects weight-bearing joints, is more common in overweight and older persons. See this page. SYN degenerative joint disease, hypertrophic arthritis, osteoarthrosis.

**os·te·o·ar·throp·a·thy** (os′tē-ō-ar-throp′ă-thē) a disorder affecting bones and joints. [osteo- + G. *arthron,* joint, + *pathos,* suffering]

**os·te·o·ar·thro·sis** (os′tē-ō-ar-thrō′sis) SYN osteoarthritis. [osteo- + G. *arthron,* joint, + *-osis,* condition]

**os·te·o·blast** (os′tē-ō-blast) a bone-forming cell that is derived from mesenchyme (fibroblast) and forms an osseous matrix in which it becomes enclosed as an osteocyte. [osteo- + G. *blastos,* germ]

**os·te·o·blas·tic** (os′tē-ō-blas′tik) relating to the osteoblasts; describes any region of increased radiographic bone density, in particular, metastases that stimulate osteoblastic activity.

**os·te·o·blas·to·ma** (os′tē-ō-blas-tō′mă) an uncommon benign tumor of osteoblasts with areas of osteoid and calcified tissue, occurring most frequently in the spine of a young person.

**os·te·o·car·ti·lag·i·nous** (os′tē-ō-kar-ti-laj′i-nŭs) SYN osseocartilaginous.

**os·te·o·chon·dral frac·ture** fracture involving the articular cartilage and underlying bone.

**os·te·o·chon·dri·tis** (os′tē-ō-kon-drī′tis) inflammation of a bone and its cartilage. [osteo- + G. *chondros,* cartilage, + *-itis,* inflammation]

**os·te·o·chon·dri·tis dis·se·cans** complete or incomplete separation of a portion of joint cartilage and underlying bone, usually involving the knee, associated with epiphyseal aseptic necrosis.

**os·te·o·chon·dro·dys·tro·phy** (os′tē-ō-kon′drō-dis′trō-fē) SYN chondro-osteodystrophy.

🔲 **os·te·o·chon·dro·ma** (os′tē-ō-kon-drō′mă) a benign cartilaginous neoplasm that consists of a pedicle of normal bone covered with a rim of proliferating cartilage cells; multiple osteochondromas are inherited and referred to as hereditary multiple exostoses. See page 342. [osteo- + G. *chondros,* cartilage, + *-oma,* tumor]

**os·te·o·chon·dro·sar·co·ma** (os′tē-ō-kon′drō-sar-kō′mă) chondrosarcoma arising in bone. Sarcomas in bone containing foci of neoplastic cartilage as well as bone are classified as osteogenic

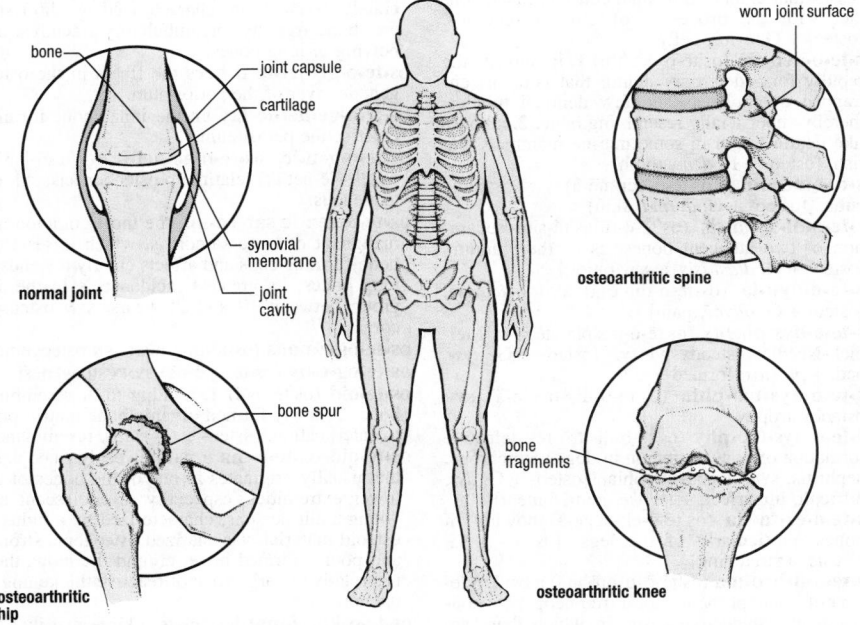

bone
joint capsule
cartilage
synovial membrane
joint cavity
**normal joint**

worn joint surface
**osteoarthritic spine**

bone spur
**osteoarthritic hip**

bone fragments
**osteoarthritic knee**

**osteoarthritis:** problems associated with osteoarthritis and some sites where they commonly occur

sarcomas. [osteo- + G. *chondros,* cartilage, + *sarx,* flesh, + *-oma,* tumor]

**os•te•o•chon•dro•sis** (os'tē-ō-kon-drō'sis) any of a group of disorders of one or more ossification centers in children, characterized by degeneration or aseptic necrosis followed by reossification; includes the various forms of epiphysial aseptic necrosis. [osteo- + G. *chondros,* cartilage, + *-osis,* condition]

**os•te•oc•la•sis, os•te•o•cla•sia** (os'tē-ok'lă-sis, os'tē-ō-klā'zē-ă) intentional fracture of a bone in order to correct deformity. [osteo- + G. *klasis,* fracture]

**os•te•o•clast** (os'tē-ō-klast) **1.** a large multinucleated cell, possibly of monocytic origin, with abundant acidophilic cytoplasm, functioning in the absorption and removal of osseous tissue. SYN osteophage. **2.** an instrument used to fracture a bone to correct a deformity. [osteo- + G. *klastos,* broken]

**os•te•o•clast ac•ti•vat•ing fac•tor** a lymphokine that stimulates bone resorption and inhibits bone-collagen synthesis.

**os•te•o•clas•tic** (os'tē-ō-klas'tik) pertaining to osteoclasts, especially with reference to their activity in the absorption and removal of osseous tissue.

**os•te•o•clas•to•ma** (os'tē-ō-klas-tō'mă) SYN giant cell tumor of bone.

**os•te•o•cra•ni•um** (os'tē-ō-krā'nē-ŭm) the cranium of the fetus after ossification of the membranous cranium has made it firm. [osteo- + G. *kranion,* skull]

**os•te•o•cys•to•ma** (os'tē-ō-sis-tō'mă) SYN solitary bone cyst.

**os•te•o•cyte** (os'tē-ō-sīt) a cell of osseous tissue that occupies a lacuna and has cytoplasmic processes that extend into canaliculi and make contact with the processes of other osteocytes. [osteo- + G. *kytos,* cell]

**os•te•o•den•tin** (os'tē-ō-den'tin) **1.** in humans the rapidly formed tertiary dentin that contains entrapped odontoblasts and few dentinal tubules, thereby superficially resembling bone. **2.** a bone-like dentin found in some marine mammals and fish. [osteo- + L. *dens,* tooth]

**os•te•o•der•mia** (os'tē-ō-der'mē-ă) SYN osteoma cutis. [osteo- + G. *derma,* skin]

**os•te•o•di•as•ta•sis** (os'tē-ō-dī-as'tă-sis) separation of two adjacent bones, as of the cranium. [osteo- + G. *diastasis,* a separation]

**os•te•o•dyn•ia** (os-tē-ō-din'ē-ă) SYN ostealgia. [osteo- + G. *odynē,* pain]

**os•te•o•dys•plas•ty** (os'tē-ō-dis'plas-tē) SYN Melnick-Needles osteodysplasty. [osteo- + G. *dys-,* bad, + *plastos,* formed]

**os•te•o•dys•tro•phia** (os'tē-ō-dis-trō'fē-ă) SYN osteodystrophy.

**os•te•o•dys•tro•phy** (os'tē-ō-dis'trō-fē) defective formation of bone; common in dogs with chronic nephritis. SYN osteodystrophia. [osteo- + G. *dys,* difficult, imperfect, + *trophē,* nourishment]

**os•te•o•ec•ta•sia** (os'tē-ō-ek-tā'zē-ă) bowing of bones, particularly of the legs. [osteo- + G. *ektasis,* a stretching]

**os•te•o•fi•bro•ma** (os'tē-ō-fī-brō'mă) a benign lesion of bone, probably not a true neoplasm, consisting of connective tissue in which there are small foci of osteogenesis.

**os•te•o•fi•bro•sis** (os'tē-ō-fī-brō'sis) fibrosis of bone, mainly involving red bone marrow.

**os•te•o•gen** (os'tē-ō-jen) a bone matrix-producing tissue or layer. [osteo- + G. *-gen,* producing]

**os•te•o•gen•e•sis** (os'tē-ō-jen'ĕ-sis) the formation of bone. SYN osteogeny, osteosis (2). [osteo- + G. *genesis,* production]

**os•te•o•gen•e•sis im•per•fec•ta (OI)** abnormal fragility and plasticity of bone, with recurring fractures on trivial trauma; variable associated features include deformity of long bones, blueness of sclerae, laxity of ligaments, and otosclerosis. SYN brittle bones.

**os•te•o•gen•e•sis im•per•fec•ta con•gen•i•ta** a severe form, with fractures occurring before or at birth.

**os•te•o•gen•e•sis im•per•fec•ta tar•da** a less severe form, with fractures occurring later in childhood.

**os•te•o•gen•e•sis im•per•fec•ta type I** a mild form characterized by blue sclerae, hearing loss, easy bruising, prepubertal bone fragility, and short stature.

**os•te•o•gen•e•sis im•per•fec•ta type II** a perinatal lethal form associated with stillbirth or lifespan less than 1 year; very fragile connective tissue, and radiographic findings of fractures in utero, large soft cranium, micromelia, tubular long bones, and beaded ribs.

**os•te•o•gen•e•sis im•per•fec•ta type III** a progressive deforming form with severe bone fragility, easy fractures, triangular facies with relative macrocephaly, skeletal deformities with scoliosis, bowing of limbs, dwarfism, and radiographic findings of metaphyseal flaring of long bones with sutural bone formation. Most cases are autosomal dominant disorders, but autosomal recessive inheritance has also been described.

**os•te•o•gen•e•sis im•per•fec•ta type IV** a moderately severe form, characterized by short stature, bone fragility, preambulatory fractures, and bowing of long bones.

**os•te•o•ge•net•ic fi•bers** the fibers in the osteogenetic layer of the periosteum.

**os•te•o•ge•net•ic lay•er** the inner bone-forming layer of the periosteum.

**os•te•o•gen•ic, os•te•o•ge•net•ic** (os'tē-ō-jen'ik, os'tē-ō-jĕ-net'ik) relating to osteogenesis. SYN osteogenous.

**os•te•o•gen•ic sar•co•ma** the most common and malignant of bone sarcomas, which arises from bone-forming cells and affects chiefly the ends of long bones; its greatest incidence is in the age group between 10 and 25 years. SYN osteosarcoma.

**os•te•og•e•nous** (os-tē-oj'ĕ-nŭs) SYN osteogenic.

**os•te•og•e•ny** (os-tē-oj'ĕ-nē) SYN osteogenesis.

**os•te•oid** (os'tē-oyd) **1.** relating to or resembling bone. **2.** newly formed organic bone matrix prior to calcification. [osteo- + G. *eidos,* resemblance]

**os•te•oid os•te•o•ma** a painful benign neoplasm that usually originates in one of the bones of the lower extremities, especially in adolescent and young adult persons; characterized by a nidus of osteoid material, vascularized osteogenic stroma, and poorly formed bone; around the nidus there is a relatively large zone of reactive thickening of the cortex.

**os•te•o•kin•e•mat•ics** (os-tē-o-kin-e-mat-iks) the study of the movement of bones associated with joints.

**os•te•ol•o•gy** (os'tē-ol'ŏ-jē) the anatomy of the

bones; the science concerned with the bones and their structure. [osteo- + G. *logos*, study]

**os·te·ol·y·sis** (os-tē-ol'i-sis) softening, absorption, and destruction of bony tissue, a function of the osteoclasts. [osteo- + G. *lysis*, dissolution]

**os·te·o·lyt·ic** (os-tē-ō-lit'ik) pertaining to, characterized by, or causing osteolysis.

**os·te·o·ma** (os-tē-ō'mă) a benign slow-growing mass of mature, predominantly lamellar bone, usually arising from the skull or mandible. [osteo- + G. *-oma*, tumor]

**os·te·o·ma cu·tis** cutaneous ossification in foci of degeneration in tumors or inflammatory lesions or rarely primary new bone formation with normal skin. SYN osteodermia, osteosis cutis.

**os·te·o·ma·la·cia** (os'tē-ō-mă-lā'shē-ă) a disease characterized by a gradual softening and bending of the bones with varying severity of pain; softening occurs because the bones contain osteoid tissue which has failed to calcify due to lack of vitamin D or renal tubular dysfunction. SYN adult rickets, late rickets. [osteo- + G. *malakia*, softness]

**os·te·o·ma·lac·ic** (os'tē-ō-mă-lā'sik) relating to, or suffering from, osteomalacia.

**os·te·o·ma·lac·ic pel·vis** a pelvic deformity in osteomalacia; the pressure of the trunk on the sacrum and lateral pressure of the femoral heads produce a pelvic aperture that is three-cornered or has the shape of a heart or a cloverleaf, while the pubic bone becomes beak shaped. SYN beaked pelvis.

**os·te·o·ma me·dul·la·re** an osteoma containing spaces that are filled (or partly filled) with various elements of bone marrow.

**os·te·o·ma spon·gi·o·sum** an osteoma that consists chiefly of cancellous bone tissue.

**os·te·o·ma·toid** (os-tē-ō'mă-toyd) an abnormal nodule or small mass of overgrowth of bone; lesions are not neoplasms but anomalous outpouchings of the cortex, and are more properly termed exostoses. [osteoma + G. *eidos*, appearance, form]

**os·te·o·mere** (os'tē-ō-mēr) one of the series of bone segments, such as the vertebrae. [osteo- + G. *meros*, a part]

**os·te·o·my·e·li·tis** (os'tē-ō-mī-ě-lī'tis) inflammation of the bone marrow and adjacent bone. SYN central osteitis (1). [osteo- + G. *myelos*, marrow, + *-itis*, inflammation]

**os·te·o·my·e·lo·dys·pla·sia** (os'tē-ō-mī'ě-lō-dis-plā'zē-ă) a disease characterized by enlargement of the marrow cavities of the bones, thinning of the osseous tissue, leukopenia, and irregular fever. [osteo- + G. *myelos*, marrow, + *dysplasia*]

**os·te·on, os·te·one** (os'tē-on, os'tē-ōn) a central canal containing blood capillaries and the concentric osseous lamellae around it occurring in compact bone. SYN haversian system. [G. *osteon*, bone]

**os·te·o·ne·cro·sis** (os'tē-ō-ne-krō'sis) the death of bone en mass, as distinguished from caries ("molecular death") or relatively small foci of necrosis in bone. [osteo- + G. *nekrōsis*, death]

**os·te·o·path** (os'tē-ō-path) SYN osteopathic physician.

**os·te·o·path·ia** (os'tē-ō-path'ē-ă) SYN osteopathy (1).

**os·te·o·path·ia he·mor·rhag·i·ca in·fan·tum** SYN infantile scurvy.

**os·te·o·path·ic** (os-tē-ō-path'ik) relating to osteopathy.

**os·te·o·path·ic med·i·cine** SYN osteopathy (2).

**os·te·o·path·ic phy·si·cian** a practitioner of osteopathy. SYN osteopath.

**os·te·op·a·thy** (os-tē-op'ă-thē) **1.** any disease of bone. SYN osteopathia. **2.** a school of medicine based upon a concept of the normal body as a vital machine capable, when in correct adjustment, of making its own remedies against infections and other toxic conditions; practitioners use the diagnostic and therapeutic measures of conventional medicine in addition to manipulative measures. SYN osteopathic medicine. [osteo- + G. *pathos*, suffering]

**os·te·o·pe·nia** (os'tē-ō-pē'nē-ă) **1.** decreased calcification or density of bone; a descriptive term applicable to all skeletal systems in which such a condition is noted; carries no implication about causality. **2.** reduced bone mass due to inadequate osteoid synthesis. [osteo- + G. *penia*, poverty]

**os·te·o·per·i·os·ti·tis** (os'tē-ō-per'ē-os-tī'tis) inflammation of the periosteum and of the underlying bone.

**os·te·o·pe·tro·sis** (os'tē-ō-pe-trō'sis) excessive formation of dense trabecular bone and calcified cartilage, especially in long bones, leading to obliteration of marrow spaces and to anemia, with myeloid metaplasia and hepatosplenomegaly, beginning in infancy and with progressive deafness and blindness. [osteo- + G. *petra*, stone, + *-osis*, condition]

**os·te·o·phage** (os'tē-ō-fāj) SYN osteoclast (1). [osteo- + G. *phagō*, to eat]

**os·te·o·phle·bi·tis** (os'tē-ō-fle-bī'tis) inflammation of the veins of a bone. [osteo- + G. *phleps*, vein, + *-itis*, inflammation]

**os·te·o·phy·ma** (os-tē-ō-fī'mă) SYN osteophyte. [osteo- + G. *phyma*, tumor]

**os·te·o·phyte** (os'tē-ō-fīt) a bony outgrowth or protuberance. SYN osteophyma. [osteo- + G. *phyton*, plant]

**os·te·o·plas·tic bone flap** vascularized tissue that includes living bone, usually with attached muscle and fascia, which can be attached by its pedicle or transferred by microvascular anastomosis from one site to another.

**os·te·o·plas·tic ob·lit·er·a·tion of the fron·tal si·nus** operation to remove the diseased contents, including the mucous membrane, of the frontal sinus and to obliterate the sinus with a free fat graft without altering the external contour of the sinus.

**os·te·o·plas·ty** (os'tē-ō-plas-tē) **1.** bone grafting; reparative or plastic surgery of the bones. **2.** DENTISTRY resection of osseous structure to achieve acceptable gingival contour. [osteo- + G. *plastos*, formed]

**os·te·o·poi·ki·lo·sis** (os'tē-ō-poy-ki-lō'sis) mottled or spotted bones caused by widespread foci of compact bone in the substantia spongiosa. [osteo- + G. *poikilos*, dappled, + *-osis*, condition]

**os·te·o·po·ro·sis** (os'tē-ō-pō-rō'sis) reduction in the quantity of bone or atrophy of skeletal tissue; occurs in postmenopausal women and elderly men, resulting in bone trabeculae that are scanty, thin, and without osteoclastic resorption. [osteo- + G. *poros*, pore, + *-osis*, condition]

**os·te·o·po·rot·ic** (os'tē-ō-pŏ-rot'ik) pertaining to,

characterized by, or causing a porous condition of the bones.

**os·te·o·pro·gen·i·tor cell** a mesenchymal cell that differentiates into an osteoblast. SYN preosteoblast.

**os·te·o·pro·teg·er·in** (os'tē-ō-prō-teg'er-in) a secreted protein that inhibits osteoclast differentiation.

**os·te·o·ra·di·ol·o·gy** the clinical subspecialty of diagnostic bone radiology.

**os·te·o·ra·di·o·ne·cro·sis** (os'tē-ō-rā'dē-ō-ne-krō'sis) necrosis of bone produced by ionizing radiation; may be planned or unplanned. [osteo- + radionecrosis]

**os·te·or·rha·phy** (os-tē-ōr'ă-fē) wiring together the fragments of a broken bone. SYN osteosuture. [osteo- + G. *rhaphē*, suture]

**os·te·o·sar·co·ma** (os'tē-ō-sar-kō'mă) SYN osteogenic sarcoma.

**os·te·o·scle·ro·sis** (os'tē-ō-skle-rō'sis) abnormal hardening or eburnation of bone. [osteo- + G. *sklērōsis*, hardness]

**os·te·o·scle·rot·ic** (os'tē-ō-skle-rot'ik) relating to, due to, or marked by hardening of bone substance.

**os·te·o·sis** (os-tē-ō'sis) **1.** a morbid process in bone. **2.** SYN osteogenesis. [osteo- + G. *-osis*, condition]

**os·te·o·sis cu·tis** SYN osteoma cutis.

**os·te·o·su·ture** (os-tē-ō-soo'cher) SYN osteorrhaphy.

**os·te·o·syn·the·sis** (os-tē-ō-sin'thē-sis) internal fixation of a fracture by means of a mechanical device, such as a pin, screw, or plate.

**os·te·o·throm·bo·sis** (os'tē-ō-throm-bō'sis) thrombosis in one or more of the veins of a bone.

**os·te·o·tome** (os'tē-ō-tōm) an instrument for use in cutting bone. [osteo- + G. *tomē*, incision]

**os·te·ot·o·my** (os-tē-ot'ō-mē) cutting a bone, usually by means of a saw or chisel. [osteo- + G. *tomē*, incision]

**os·te·o·tribe** (os'tē-ō-trīb) an instrument for crushing off bits of necrosed or carious bone. [osteo- + G. *tribō*, to bruise, to grind down]

**os·te·o·trite** (os'tē-ō-trīt) an instrument with conical or olive-shaped tip having a cutting surface, resembling a dental bur, used for the removal of carious bone. [osteo- + L. *tritus*, a grinding, a wearing off]

**os·tia** (os'tē-ă) plural of ostium. [L.]

**os·ti·al** (os'tē-ăl) relating to any orifice, or ostium.

**os·ti·tic** (os-tī'tik) SYN osteitic.

**os·ti·tis** (os-tī'tis) SYN osteitis.

**os·ti·um**, pl. **os·tia** (os'tē-ŭm, os'tē-ă) [TA] a small opening, especially one of entrance into a hollow organ or canal. [L. door, entrance, mouth]

**os·ti·um il·e·ale** SYN ileal orifice.

**os·to·mate** (os'tō-māt) term for one who has an ostomy. [L. *ostium*, mouth]

**os·to·my** (os'tō-mē) **1.** an artificial stoma or opening into the urinary or gastrointestinal canal, or the trachea. **2.** any operation by which a permanent opening is created between two hollow organs or between a hollow viscus and the skin externally, as in tracheostomy. [L. *ostium*, mouth]

**os tra·pe·zi·um** [TA] SYN trapezium.

**os tri·go·num** an independent ossicle sometimes present in the tarsus; usually it forms part of the talus, constituting the lateral tubercle of the posterior process. SYN triangular bone.

**Ost·wald sol·u·bil·i·ty co·ef·fi·cient (lambda)** (ost'wahld) the milliliter of gas dissolved per milliliter of liquid and per atmosphere (760 mmHg) partial pressure of the gas at any given temperature. This differs from Bunsen solubility coefficient ($\alpha$) in that the amount of dissolved gas is expressed in terms of its volume at the temperature of the experiment, instead of STPD. Thus, $\lambda = \alpha (1 + 0.00367t)$, where $t$ = temperature in degrees Celsius.

**os zy·go·ma·ti·cum** [TA] SYN zygomatic bone.

△**ot-** the ear. SEE ALSO auri-. [G. *ous*]

**otal·gia** (ō-tal'jē-ă) SYN earache. [ot- + G. *algos*, pain]

**otal·gic** (ō-tal'jik) **1.** relating to otalgia, or earache. **2.** a remedy for earache.

**oth·er·di·rect·ed** (odh'er-di-rek'ted) pertaining to a person readily influenced by the attitudes of others.

**otic** (ō'tik) relating to the ear. [G. *otikos*, fr. *ous*, ear]

**otic cap·sule** the cartilage capsule surrounding the internal ear mechanism; in the embryo it is cartilaginous at first but later becomes bony.

**otic gan·gli·on** an autonomic ganglion situated below the foramen ovale medial to the mandibular nerve; its postganglionic, parasympathetic fibers are distributed to the parotid gland.

**otic ves·i·cle** SYN auditory vesicle.

**oti·tic** (ō-tit'ik) relating to otitis.

**oti·tic ab·scess** a brain abscess, usually involving the temporal lobe or cerebellar hemisphere, secondary to suppuration of the middle ear.

**otit·ic men·in·gi·tis** infection of the meninges secondary to mastoiditis or otitis media.

**oti·tis** (ō-tī'tis) inflammation of the ear. [ot- + G. *-itis*, inflammation]

▯**oti·tis ex·ter·na** SYN swimmer's ear. See this page and B16.

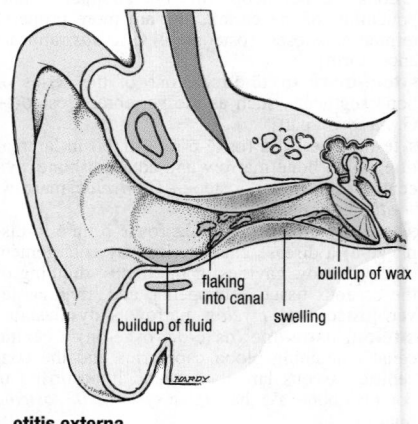

**otitis externa**

**oti·tis in·ter·na** SYN labyrinthitis.

▯**oti·tis me·dia** inflammation of the middle ear, or tympanum. See page 713 and B16.

△**oto-** the ear. SEE ALSO auri-. [G. *ous*]

**oto·a·cous·tic emis·sion (OAE)** sounds that issue from the external acoustic meatus as a result of vibrations originating within the cochlea. SEE ALSO Kemp echo.

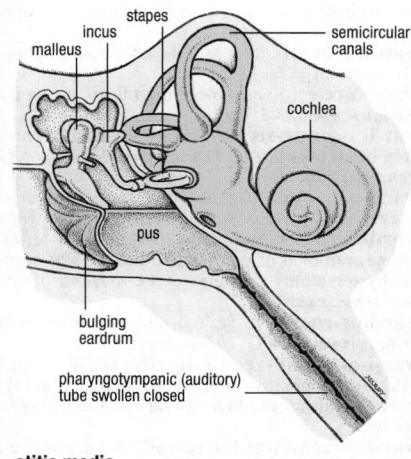

**otitis media**

**O
u**

**oto•ceph•a•ly** (ō-tō-sef′ă-lē) malformation characterized by markedly defective development of the lower jaw (micrognathia or agnathia) and the union or close approach of the ears (synotia) on the front of the neck. [oto- + G. *kephalē,* head]

**oto•co•nia,** sing. **oto•co•ni•um** (ō-tō-kō′nē-ă, ō-to-kō′nē-ŭm) syn statoliths.

**oto•cra•ni•al** (ō-tō-krā′nē-ăl) relating to the otocranium.

**oto•cra•ni•um** (ō′tō-krā′nē-ŭm) the bony case of the internal and middle ear, consisting of the petrous portion of the temporal bone. [oto- + G. *kranion,* cranium]

**oto•cyst** (ō′tō-sist) **1.** embryonic auditory vesicle. **2.** a balancing organ, analogous to the utricle of mammals, possessed by certain invertebrates and containing grains of calcareous material or of sand. [oto- + G. *kystis,* a bladder]

**oto•dyn•ia** (ō-tō-din′ē-ă) syn earache. [oto- + G. *odynē,* pain]

**oto•en•ceph•a•li•tis** (ō′tō-en-sef-ă-lī′tis) inflammation of the brain by extension of the process from the middle ear and mastoid cells. [oto- + G. *enkephalos,* brain, + *-itis,* inflammation]

**oto•gen•ic, otog•e•nous** (ō′tō-jen′ik, ō-toj′ĕ-nŭs) of otic origin; originating within the ear, especially from inflammation of the ear. [oto- + G. *-gen,* producing]

**oto•lar•yn•gol•o•gist** (ō′tō-lar-ing-gol′ŏ-jist) a physician who specializes in otolaryngology.

**oto•lar•yn•gol•o•gy** (ō′tō-lar-ing-gol′ŏ-jē) the combined specialties of diseases of the ear and larynx, often including upper respiratory tract and many diseases of the head and neck, tracheobronchial tree, and esophagus. [oto- + G. *larynx,* + *logos,* study]

**oto•lith•ic cri•sis** a sudden drop attack without loss of consciousness, vertigo, auditory disturbances, or autonomic manifestations.

**oto•lith•ic or•gans** the utricle and saccule of the inner ear that possess otoliths and respond to linear acceleration and deceleration, including gravity.

**oto•log•ic** (ō′tō-loj′ik) relating to otology.

**otol•o•gist** (ō-tol′ŏ-jist) a specialist in otology.

**otol•o•gy** (ō-tol′ŏ-jē) the branch of medical sci-

ence concerned with the study, diagnosis, and treatment of diseases of the ear and related structures. [oto- + G. *logos,* study]

**oto•mu•cor•my•co•sis** (ō-tō-myu′kōr-mī-kō′sis) mucormycosis of the ear.

△**-ot•o•my** see -tomy.

**oto•my•co•sis** (ō′tō-mī-kō′sis) an infection due to a fungus in the external auditory canal, usually unilateral, with scaling, itching, and pain as the primary symptoms. See page B16.

**otop•a•thy** (ō-top′ă-thē) any disease of the ear. [oto- + G. *pathos,* suffering]

**oto•pha•ryn•ge•al** (ō′tō-fa-rin′jē-ăl) relating to the middle ear and the pharynx.

**oto•plas•ty** (ō′tō-plas-tē) reparative or plastic surgery of the auricle of the ear. [oto- + G. *plastos,* formed]

**oto•rhi•no•lar•yn•gol•o•gy** (ō′tō-rī′nō-lar-ing-gol′ō-jē) the combined specialties of diseases of the ear, nose, and larynx; including diseases of related structures of the head and neck. see also otolaryngology. [oto- + G. *rhis,* nose, + *larynx,* larynx, + *logos,* study]

**otor•rhea** (ō-tō-rē′ă) a discharge from the ear. [oto- + G. *rhoia,* flow]

**oto•scle•ro•sis** (ō′tō-skle-rō′sis) a new formation of spongy bone about the stapes and fenestra vestibuli (ovalis), resulting in progressively increasing deafness, without signs of disease in the auditory tube or tympanic membrane. [oto- + G. *sklērōsis,* hardening]

**oto•scope** (ō′tō-skōp) an instrument for examining the drum membrane or auscultating the ear. See page B16. [oto- + G. *skopeō,* to view]

**otos•co•py** (ō-tos′kŏ-pē) inspection of the ear, especially of the drum membrane. See page B16. [oto- + G. *skopeō,* to view]

**oto•spon•dylome•ga•epi•phy•seal dysplasia** syn chondrodystrophy with sensorineural deafness.

**oto•spon•gi•o•sis** (ot-ō-spun-jē-ō′sis) a more accurately descriptive term for the pathologic changes in otosclerosis.

**otos•te•al** (ō-tos′tē-ăl) relating to the ossicles of the ear. [oto- + G. *osteon,* bone]

**oto•tox•ic** (ō′tō-tok′sik) having a toxic action upon the ear. [oto- + G. *toxikon,* poison]

**oto•tox•ic•i•ty** (ō-tō-tok-sis′i-te) the property of being ototoxic.

**Ot•to dis•ease** (ot′ō) a disease characterized by an inward bulging of the acetabulum into the pelvic cavity, resulting in protrusion of the femoral head; found in association with arthritis of the hip joints, usually rheumatoid arthritis.

**Ouch•ter•lo•ny tech•nique** (owk′ter-lōn-e) a technique in which both reaction partners (antigen and antibody) are allowed to diffuse to each other in a gel in a precipitation reaction.

**ounce** (owns) **1.** a weight containing 480 gr, or $\frac{1}{12}$ pound troy and apothecaries' weight, or $437\frac{1}{2}$ gr, $\frac{1}{16}$ pound avoirdupois. The apothecary oz (used in the USP) contains 8 dr and is equivalent to 31.10349 g; the avoirdupois oz is equivalent to 28.35 g. **2.** fluid ounce; United States: $\frac{1}{128}$ U.S. gallon (29.57 mL, 1.804 cu in). British Imperial System: the volume occupied by one avoirdupois ounce of distilled water at 62 degrees Fahrenheit (28.41 mL, 1.734 cu in). [L. *uncia,* the twelfth part (of a pound or foot) hence also inch]

△**-ous 1.** chemical suffix attached to the name of an

element in one of its lower valencies. Cf. -ic (1).
**2.** having much of. [L. *-osus,* full of, abounding]

**Out•comes and As•sess•ment In•for•ma•tion Set (OASIS)** a standard system used in home health care to measure service quality and patient satisfaction; use is mandated by the U.S. Department of Health and Human Services.

**out•come score** SYN Glasgow Coma Scale.

**out•let** (owt′let) an exit or opening of a passageway. SEE ALSO aperture.

**out•let for•ceps de•liv•ery** delivery by forceps applied to the fetal head when it has reached the perineal floor and is visible between contractions.

**out•pa•tient** (owt′pā′shent) a patient treated in a hospital dispensary or clinic instead of in a room or ward.

**out•pa•tient sur•gery** SYN ambulatory surgery.

**out•put** (owt′put) the quantity produced, ejected, or excreted of a specific entity in a specified period of time or per unit time, e.g., urinary sodium output; the opposite of intake or input.

**out•stand•ing ear** excessive protrusion of the ear from the head, usually due to failure of the antihelical fold to develop. SYN protruding ear.

**ova** (ō′vă) plural of ovum. [L.]

**oval am•pu•ta•tion 1.** amputation in which the flaps are obtained by oval incisions through the skin and muscle; **2.** rarely used term for oblique amputation.

**ov•al•bu•min** (ō-văl-byu′min) the chief protein occurring in the white of egg and resembling serum albumin; also found in phosphorylated form. SYN albumen, egg albumin.

**oval•o•cyte** (ō′văl-ō-sīt) SYN elliptocyte. [L. *ovalis,* oval, + G. *kytos,* cell]

**oval•o•cy•to•sis** (ō′vă-lō-sī-tō′sis) SYN elliptocytosis.

**oval win•dow** SYN fenestra vestibuli.

**ova and pa•ra•site ex•am•in•a•tion** a comprehensive review of a fecal specimen, using direct wet mounts, concentration wet mounts, and permanent stained smears, for the recovery and identification of protozoan and helmintic parasite stages such as trophozoites, cysts, oocysts, spores, eggs, and larvae.

**ovar•i•al•gia** (ō-var-ē-al′jē-ă) pain in an ovary. [ovario- + G. *algos,* pain]

**ovar•i•an** (ō-var′ē-an) relating to the ovary.

**ovar•i•an ar•tery** origin, aorta; *distribution,* ureter, ovary, ovarian ligament and uterine tube; *anastomoses,* uterine. SYN arteria ovarica [TA].

**ovar•i•an cy•cle** the normal sex cycle which includes development of an ovarian (graafian) follicle, rupture of the follicle with discharge of the ovum, and formation and regression of a corpus luteum.

**ovar•i•an cyst** a cystic tumor of the ovary, either non-neoplastic (follicle, lutein, germinal inclusion, or endometrial) or neoplastic.

**ovar•i•an fol•li•cle** one of the spheroidal cell aggregations in the ovary containing an oocyte.

**ovar•i•an fos•sa** a depression in the parietal peritoneum of the pelvis; it is bounded in front by the obliterated umbilical artery, and behind by the ureter and the uterine vessels; it lodges the ovary.

**ovar•i•an preg•nan•cy** development of an impregnated oocyte in an ovarian follicle. SYN ovariocyesis.

**ovar•i•ec•to•my** (ō-var-ē-ek′tō-mē) excision of one or both ovaries. SYN oophorectomy. [ovario- + G. *ektomē,* excision]

△**ovar•io-, ovari-** ovary. SEE ALSO oo-, oophor-. [L. *ovarium*]

**ovar•i•o•cele** (ō-var′ē-ō-sēl) hernia of an ovary. [ovario- + G. *kēlē,* hernia]

**ovar•i•o•cen•te•sis** (ō-var′ē-ō-sen-tē′sis) puncture of an ovary or an ovarian cyst. [ovario- + G. *kentēsis,* puncture]

**ovar•i•o•cy•e•sis** (ō-var′ē-ō-sī-ē′sis) SYN ovarian pregnancy. [ovario- + G. *kyēsis,* pregnancy]

**ovar•i•o•hys•ter•ec•to•my** (ō-var′ē-ō-his-ter-ek′tō-mē) removal of ovaries and uterus. SYN oophorohysterectomy. [ovario- + G. *hystera,* uterus, + *ektomē,* excision]

**ovar•i•or•rhex•is** (ō-var′ē-ō-rek′sis) rupture of an ovary. [ovario- + G. *rhēxis,* rupture]

**ovar•i•o•sal•pin•gec•to•my** (ō-var′ē-ō-sal-pin-jek′tō-mē) operative removal of an ovary and the corresponding oviduct. [ovario- + salpingectomy]

**ovar•i•o•sal•pin•gi•tis** (ō-var′ē-ō-sal-pin-jī′tis) inflammation of ovary and oviduct. [ovario- + salpingitis]

**ovar•i•os•to•my** (ō-var-ē-os′tō-mē) establishment of a temporary fistula for drainage of a cyst of the ovary. SYN oophorostomy. [ovario- + G. *stoma,* mouth]

**ovar•i•ot•o•my** (ō-var-ē-ot′o-mē) an incision into an ovary, e.g., a biopsy or a wedge excision. SYN oophorotomy. [ovario- + G. *tomē,* incision]

**ova•ri•tis** (ō-vă-rī′tis) SYN oophoritis.

**ovar•i•um,** pl. **ova•ria** (ō-var′ē-ŭm, ō-var′ă) [TA] SYN ovary. [Mod. L. fr. *ovum,* egg]

**ova•ry** (ō′vă-rē) one of the paired female reproductive glands containing the oocytes (ova) or germ cells; its stroma is a vascular connective tissue containing ovarian follicles, each enclosing an oocyte; surrounding this stroma is a denser layer called the tunica albuginea. SYN ovarium [TA], oophoron. [Mod. L. *ovarium,* fr. *ovum,* egg]

**over•anx•ious dis•or•der** a mental disorder of childhood or adolescence marked by excessive worrying and fearful behavior not related specifically to separation or due to recent stress.

**over•bite** (ō′ver-bīt) SYN vertical overlap.

**over•com•pen•sa•tion** (ō′ver-kom-pen-sā′shŭn) **1.** an exaggeration of personal capacity by which one overcomes a real or imagined inferiority. **2.** the process in which a psychologic deficiency inspires exaggerated correction. SEE compensation.

**over•cor•rec•tion** (ō′ver-kŏ-rek′shŭn) in behavior modification treatment programs, especially those involving mentally retarded individuals, overlearning the desired target behavior beyond the set criterion to assure that the behavior will continue to meet the established criterion when the post-learning decrements and forgetting occur.

**over•den•ture** (ō-ver-den′tyur) SYN overlay denture.

**over•de•ter•mi•na•tion** (ō′ver-dē-ter′min-ā′shŭn) PSYCHOANALYSIS ascribing the cause of a single behavioral or emotional reaction, mental symptom, or dream to the operation of two or more forces (e.g., ascribing an emotional outburst not only to the immediate precipitant but also to a lingering inferiority complex).

**over•dom•i•nance** (ō-ver-dom′i-năns) that state

in which the heterozygote has greater phenotype value and perhaps is more fit than the homozygous state for either of the alleles that it comprises. Cf. balanced polymorphism.

**over·dom·i·nant** (ō-ver-dom′i-nănt) denoting heterozygous states that exhibit overdominance.

**over·drive** (ō-ver-drīv′) an electrophysiologic pacing technique to exceed the rate of an abnormal pacemaker and so capture the territory controlled by that pacemaker (usually atrial).

**over·jet, over·jut** (ō′ver-jet, ō′ver-jŭt) SYN horizontal overlap.

**over·lap** (ō′ver-lap) 1. suturing of one layer of tissue above or under another to gain strength. 2. an extension or projection of one tissue over another.

**over·lay den·ture** a complete denture that is supported by both soft tissue and natural teeth that have been altered so as to permit the denture to fit over them. The altered teeth may have been fitted with short or long copings, locking devices, or connecting bars. SYN overdenture.

**overload principle** EXERCISE SCIENCE fundamental principle of training stating that exercise at an intensity above that normally attained will induce highly specific adaptations enabling the body to function more efficiently. Overload is applied by manipulating combinations of training frequency, intensity, and duration.

**over·rid·ing** (ō′ver-rī′ding) 1. slippage of the lower fragment of a broken long bone upward and alongside the proximal portion. 2. denoting a fetal head which is palpable above the symphysis because of cephalopelvic disproportion.

**over·shoot** (ō′ver-shoot) 1. any response to a step change in some factor that is greater than the steady-state response to the new level of that factor; common in systems in which inertia or a time lag in negative feedback outweighs any damping that may be present. 2. momentary reversal of the membrane potential of a cell (inside becoming positive rather than negative relative to the outside) during an action potential.

**overt ho·mo·sex·u·al·i·ty** homosexual inclinations consciously experienced and expressed in actual homosexual behavior.

**overtraining syndrome** a group of symptoms resulting from excessive physical training; includes fatigue, poor exercise performance, frequent upper-respiratory tract infections, general malaise, and loss of interest in high-level training. SYN burnout, staleness.

**overuse syndrome** injury caused by accumulated microtraumatic stress placed on a structure or body area.

**over·win·ter·ing** (ō′ver-win′ter-ing) persistence of an infectious agent in its vector for extended periods, such as the cooler winter months, during which the vector has no opportunity to be reinfected or to infect another host.

△**ovi-** egg. SEE ALSO oo-, ovo-. [L. *ovum*]

**ovi·ci·dal** (ō-vi-sī′dăl) causing death of the oocyte (ovum). [ovi- + L. *caedo*, to kill]

**ovi·du·cal** (ō-vi-doo′kăl) SYN oviductal.

**ovi·duct** (ō′vi-dŭkt) SYN uterine tube. [ovi- + L. *ductus*, a leading, fr. *duco*, pp. *ductus*, to lead]

**ovi·duc·tal** (ō-vi-dŭk′tăl) relating to a uterine tube. SYN oviducal.

**ovif·er·ous** (ō-vif′er-ŭs) carrying, containing, or producing oocytes (ova). [ovi- + L. *fero*, to carry]

**ovi·form** (ō′vi-fōrm) SYN ovoid (2).

**ovi·gen·e·sis** (ō-vi-jen′ĕ-sis) SYN oogenesis.

**ovi·ge·net·ic, ovi·gen·ic** (ō-vi-jĕ-net′ik, ō-vi-jen′ik) SYN oogenetic.

△**ovo-** egg. SEE ALSO oo-, ovi-. [L. *ovum*]

**ovoid** (ō′voyd) 1. an oval or egg-shaped form. 2. resembling an egg. SYN oviform. [ovo- + G. *eidos*, resemblance]

**ovo·plasm** (ō′vō-plazm) protoplasm of an unfertilized egg.

**ovo·sis·ton** (ō-vō-sis′ton) an oral contraceptive that consists of a mixture of a progestin and an estrogen.

**ovo·tes·tis** (ō′vō-tes′tis) gonad in which both testicular and ovarian components are present; a form of hermaphroditism.

**ovu·lar** (ov′yu-lăr) relating to an ovule.

**o·vu·lar mem·brane** SYN membrana vitellina (1).

**ovu·la·tion** (ov′yu-lā′shŭn) release of an oocyte from the ovarian follicle.

**ovu·la·to·ry** (ov′yu-lă-tō-rē) relating to ovulation.

**ovule** (ov′yul) 1. the oocyte (ovum) of a mammal, especially while still in the ovarian follicle. 2. a small beadlike structure resembling an ovule. SYN ovulum. [Mod. L. *ovulum*, dim. of L. *ovum*, egg]

**ovu·lo·cy·clic** (ov′yu-lō-sī′klik) denoting any recurrent phenomenon associated with and occurring at a certain time within the ovulatory cycle, as, for example, ovulocyclic porphyria.

**ovu·lum**, pl. **ovu·la** (ov′yu-lŭm, ov′yu-lă) SYN ovule.

**ovum**, gen. **ovi**, pl. **ova** (ō′vŭm, ō-vī, ō′vă) SYN oocyte. [L. egg]

**Ow·en lines** (ō′ĕn) accentuated incremental lines in the dentin thought to be due to disturbances in the mineralization process.

**Ow·ren dis·ease** (ō′ren) a congenital deficiency of factor V, resulting in prolongation of prothrombin time; bleeding and clotting times are consistently prolonged; autosomal recessive inheritance caused by mutation in the F5 gene on chromosome 1q.

△**oxa-** combining form inserted in names of organic compounds to signify the presence or addition of oxygen atom(s) in a chain or ring (as in ethers), not appended to either (as in ketones and aldehydes). SEE ALSO hydroxy-, oxo-, oxy-. [English *oxygen*]

**oxalaemia [Br.]** SEE oxalemia.

**ox·a·late** (ok′să-lāt) a salt of oxalic acid.

**ox·a·late cal·cu·lus** a urinary calculus of calcium oxalate.

**ox·a·le·mia** (ok-să-lē′mē-ă) the presence of an abnormally large amount of oxalate in the blood. [oxalate + G. *haima*, blood]

**ox·al·ic ac·id** (ok-sal′ik as′id) an acid found in many plants and vegetables; used as a hemostatic in veterinary medicine, but toxic when ingested by humans; also used in the removal of ink and other stains, and as a general reducing agent; salts of oxalic acid are found in renal calculi; accumulates in cases of primary hyperoxaluria.

**ox·a·lo·a·ce·tic ac·id** (ok′să-lō-ă-sē′tik as′id) a ketodicarboxylic acid and important intermediate in the tricarboxylic acid cycle.

**ox·a·lo·suc·cin·ic ac·id** (ok′să-lō-sŭk-sin′ik as′id) an enzyme-bound intermediate of the tricarboxylic acid cycle.

**ox·a·lu·ria** (ok-săl-yu′rē-ă) SYN hyperoxaluria. [oxalate + G. *ouron*, urine]

**ox·a·lyl·u·rea** (ok'să-lil-yu-rē'ă) the cyclic (end-to-end) amide anhydride of oxaluric acid; an oxidation product of uric acid.

**ox·a·zin dyes** similar to azin dyes except that one of the connecting N atoms is replaced by O.

**ox·a·zo·lid·i·nones** (oks'ă-zō-lid'i-nōnz) any of a new class of antibacterial antibiotics.

**ox heart** a very large heart, usually due to chronic hypertension or, more often, to aortic valve disease. SYN cor bovinum.

**ox·i·dant** (ok'si-dant) the substance that is reduced and that, therefore, oxidizes the other component of an oxidation-reduction system.

**ox·i·dase** (ok'si-dās) one of a group of enzymes that bring about organic reactions in which $O_2$ acts as an acceptor (of H or of electrons).

**ox·i·da·tion** (ok-si-dā'shŭn) **1.** combination with oxygen; increasing the valence of an atom or ion by the loss from it of hydrogen or of one or more electrons. **2.** BACTERIOLOGY the aerobic dissimilation of substrates with the production of energy and water; the transfer of electrons is accomplished via the respiratory chain, which utilizes oxygen as the final electron acceptor.

**ox·i·da·tion-re·duc·tion** any chemical oxidation or reduction reaction, which must, *in toto*, comprise both oxidation and reduction; the basis for calling all oxidative enzymes (formerly oxidases) oxidoreductases. Often shortened to "redox."

**ox·i·da·tive** (ok-si-dā'tiv) having the power to oxidize; denoting a process involving oxidation.

**ox·i·da·tive phos·pho·ryl·a·tion** formation of high energy phosphoric bonds from the energy released by the dehydrogenation (*i.e.*, oxidation) of various substrates.

**ox·ide** (ok'sīd) a compound of oxygen with another element or a radical.

**ox·i·dize** (ok'si-dīz) to combine or cause an element or radical to combine with oxygen or to lose electrons.

**ox·i·do·re·duc·tase** (ok'si-dō-rē-dŭk'tās) an enzyme (EC class 1) catalyzing an oxidation-reduction reaction. Trivial names for oxidoreductases include dehydrogenase, reductase, oxidase, oxygenase, peroxidase, and hydroxylase. SEE ALSO oxidase.

**ox·ime** (ok'sēm) a compound resulting from the action of hydroxylamine, $NH_2OH$, on a ketone or an aldehyde to yield the oxygen =N–OH attached to the former carbonyl carbon atom.

**ox·im·e·ter** (ok-sim'ĕ-ter) a laboratory instrument capable of measuring the concentration of oxyhemoglobin, reduced hemoglobin, carboxyhemoglobin, and methemoglobin in a sample of blood. SYN co-oximeter, hemoximeter.

**ox·im·e·try** (ok-sim'ĕ-trē) measurement with an oximeter of the oxygen saturation of hemoglobin in a sample of blood.

△**oxo-** prefix denoting addition of oxygen; used in place of keto- in systematic nomenclature. SEE ALSO hydroxy-, oxa-, oxy-.

**3-ox·o·ac·yl-ACP re·duc·tase** (thrē-ok'sō-as'il-ā-sē-pē rē-dŭk'tās) an enzyme of the fatty acid synthase complex.

**3-ox·o·ac·yl-ACP syn·thase** an enzyme participating in fatty acid synthesis.

**17-ox·o·ste·roids** (sev-en-tē-ok-sō-stēr'oydz) SYN 17-ketosteroids.

△**oxy- 1.** shrill; sharp, pointed; quick (incorrectly used for ocy-, from G. *ōkys*, swift). **2.** CHEMISTRY combining form denoting the presence of oxy-

gen, either added or substituted, in a substance. SEE ALSO hydroxy-, oxa-, oxo-. [G. *oxys*, keen]

**ox·y·ce·phal·ic, ox·y·ceph·a·lous** (ok-sē-se-fal'ik, ok-sē-sef'ă-lŭs) relating to or characterized by oxycephaly. SYN acrocephalic, acrocephalous.

**ox·y·ceph·a·ly** (ok-sē-sef'ă-lē) a type of craniosynostosis in which there is premature closure of the lambdoid and coronal sutures, resulting in an abnormally high, peaked, or cone-shaped skull. SYN acrocephaly, acrocephalia. [G. *oxys*, pointed, + *kephalē*, head]

**ox·y·chro·mat·ic** (ok'sē-krō-mat'ik) SYN acidophilic. [G. *oxys*, sour, acid, + *chrōma*, color]

**11-ox·y·cor·ti·coids** (e-lev-en-ok-sē-kōr'ti-koydz) corticosteroids bearing an alcohol or ketonic group on carbon-11; e.g., cortisone, cortisol.

**ox·y·es·the·sia** (ok'sē-es-thē'zē-ă) SYN hyperesthesia. [G. *oxys*, acute, + *aisthēsis*, sensation]

**ox·y·gen (O)** (ok'si-jen) **1.** a gaseous element, atomic no. 8, atomic wt. 15.9994 on basis of $^{12}C$ = 12.0000; an abundant and widely distributed chemical element, which combines with most of the other elements to form oxides and is essential to animal and plant life. **2.** the molecular form of oxygen, $O_2$. **3.** a medicinal gas that contains not less than 99.0%, by volume, of $O_2$. [G. *oxys*, sharp, acid and *genes*, forming]

**ox·y·gen af·fin·i·ty hy·pox·ia** hypoxia due to reduced ability of hemoglobin to release oxygen.

**ox·y·gen·ase** (ok'si-jĕ-nās) one of a group of enzymes (EC subclass 1.13) catalyzing direct incorporation of $O_2$ into substrates. Cf. dioxygenase, monooxygenases.

**ox·y·gen·ate** (ok'si-jĕ-nāt) to accomplish oxygenation.

**ox·y·gen·a·tion** (ok'si-jĕ-nā'shŭn) addition of oxygen to any chemical or physical system.

**ox·y·gen ca·pac·i·ty** the maximum quantity of oxygen that will combine chemically with the hemoglobin in a unit volume of blood; normally it amounts to 1.34 ml of $O_2$ per gm of Hb or 20 ml of $O_2$ per 100 ml of blood.

**ox·y·gen con·cen·tra·tor** an electrically powered device for oxygen delivery in the home; it uses a filtering mechanism to purify entrained ambient air.

**ox·y·gen con·sump·tion ($\dot{V}O_2$)** the volume of oxygen consumed by the body in one minute; it is reported in liters or ml per minute at STPD.

**ox·y·gen con·tent** the total amount of oxygen carried in the blood; it is equal to the amount of oxygen carried by the hemoglobin in the red blood cells plus the amount of oxygen dissolved in the plasma.

**ox·y·gen debt** the extra oxygen, taken in by the body during recovery from exercise, beyond the resting needs of the body; sometimes used as if synonymous with oxygen deficit.

**ox·y·gen def·i·cit** the difference between oxygen uptake of the body during early stages of exercise and during a similar duration in a steady state of exercise; sometimes considered as the formation of the oxygen debt.

**ox·y·gen-de·rived free rad·i·cals** an atom or atom group having an unpaired electron on an oxygen atom, typically derived from molecular oxygen. For example, one-electron reduction of $O_2$ produces the superoxide radical, $\bar{O}_2\cdot$; other examples include the hydroperoxyl radical (HOO·), the hydroxyl radical (HO·), and nitric oxide (NO·). These apparently have a role in reprofusion injury.

**ox•y•gen pulse ($\dot{V}O_2$ HR)** volume of oxygen consumed by the body per heartbeat.

**ox•y•gen tox•ic•i•ty** a body disturbance resulting from breathing high partial pressures of oxygen; characterized by visual and hearing abnormalities, unusual fatigue while breathing, muscular twitching, anxiety, confusion, incoordination, and convulsions.

**ox•y•geu•sia** (ok-sē-goo′sē-ă) SYN hypergeusia. [G. *oxys*, acute, + *geusis*, taste]

**ox•y•hae•mo•glo•bin [Br.]** SEE oxyhemoglobin.

**ox•y•heme** (ok′sē-hēm) SYN hematin.

**ox•y•he•mo•chro•mo•gen** (ok′sē-hēm′ō-krō′mō-jen) SYN hematin.

**ox•y•he•mo•glo•bin** (ok′sē-hē-mō-glō′bin) hemoglobin in combination with oxygen, the form of hemoglobin present in arterial blood, scarlet or bright red when dissolved in water.

**ox•y•he•mo•glo•bin dis•so•ci•a•tion curve** a graphic illustration of the relationship between oxygen saturation of hemoglobin and the partial pressure of arterial oxygen ($PaO_2$); the position and overall shape of this sigmoidal curve are affected by the hydrogen ion concentration (pH), body temperature, partial pressure of carbon dioxide ($PCO_2$), and organic phosphates.

**ox•y•my•o•glo•bin ($MbO_2$)** (ok′sē-mī-ō-glō′bin) myoglobin in its oxygenated form, analogous in structure to oxyhemoglobin. SEE ALSO myoglobin.

**ox•yn•tic** (ok-sin′tik) acid-forming, e.g., the parietal cells of the gastric glands. [G. *oxynō*, to sharpen, make sour, acid]

**ox•yn•tic cell** SYN parietal cell.

**ox•y•phil, ox•y•phile** (ok′si-fil, ok′si-fīl) **1.** oxyphil *cell*. **2.** SYN eosinophilic leukocyte. **3.** SYN oxyphilic. [G. *oxys*, sour, acid, + *philos*, fond]

**ox•y•phil cell** cell of the parathyroid gland that increase in number with age; the cytoplasm contains numerous mitochondria and stains with eosin. Similar cells, and tumors composed of them, are found in salivary glands and the thyroid; in the latter, also called Hürthle cell.

**ox•y•phil•ic** (ok-si-fil′ik) having an affinity for acid dyes; denoting certain cell or tissue elements. SYN oxyphil (3), oxyphile.

**ox•y•phil•ic car•ci•no•ma** SYN Hürthle cell carcinoma.

**ox•y•phil•ic leu•ko•cyte** SYN eosinophilic leukocyte.

**ox•y•pho•nia** (ok-si-fō′nē-ă) shrillness or high pitch of the voice. [G. *oxys*, sharp, + *phōnē*, voice]

**ox•y•ta•lan** (ok-sit′ă-lan) a type of connective tissue fiber found in the periodontal ligaments of a number of animals having the same ultrastructural features as immature elastin, i.e., microfilaments without the elastin. [G. *oxys*, acid, + *talas*, suffering, resisting; coined term probably intended to mean "resistant to acid hydrolysis"]

**ox•y•to•cia** (ok-si-tō′sē-ă) rapid parturition. [G. *okytokos*, swift birth]

**ox•y•to•cic** (ok-si-tō′sik) hastening childbirth.

**ox•y•to•cin** (ok-si-tō′sin) a nonapeptide neurohypophysial hormone that causes myometrial contractions at term and promotes milk release during lactation; used for the induction or stimulation of labor, in the management of postpartum hemorrhage and atony, and to relieve painful breast engorgement. [G. *oxytokos*, swift birth]

**ox•y•to•cin chal•lenge test** a contraction stress test accomplished by administration of intravenous dilute oxytocin solution to stimulate contractions. SYN contraction stress test.

**ox•y•u•ri•a•sis** (ok-si-yu-rī′ă-sis) infection with nematode parasites of the genus *Oxyuris*.

**ox•y•u•ri•cide** (ok′si-yu′ri-sīd) an agent that destroys pinworms. [oxyurid + L. *caedo*, to kill]

**ox•y•u•rid** (ok-si-yu′rid) common name for members of the family Oxyuridae. [see *Oxyuris*]

**Ox•y•u•ri•dae** (ok-si-yu′ri-dē) a family of parasitic nematodes found in the large intestine or cecum of vertebrates and the intestine of invertebrates, especially insects and millipedes.

***Ox•y•u•ris*** (ok′si-yu′ris) a genus of nematodes commonly called seatworms or pinworms (although the pinworm of humans is the closely related form, *Enterobius vermicularis*). [G. *oxys*, sharp, + *oura*, tail]

**-oyl** suffix denoting an acyl radical; -yl replaces -ic in acid names.

**ozae•na [Br.]** SEE ozena.

**oze•na** (ō-zē′nă) a disease characterized by intranasal crusting, atrophy, and fetid odor. [G. *ozaina*, a fetid polypus, fr. *ozō*, to smell]

**ozone** (ō′zōn) a powerful oxidizing agent; air containing a perceptible amount of $O_3$ formed by an electric discharge or by the slow combustion of phosphorus; also formed by the action of solar UV radiation on atmospheric $O_2$. [G. *ozō*, to smell]

# P

π, Π pi, SEE pi.
φ, Φ phi. SEE phi.
Ψ psi. SEE psi.
**p 1.** pupil; optic papilla. **2.** in polynucleotide symbolism, phosphoric ester or phosphate. **3.** pico-(2); momentum (in italics). **4.** CYTOGENETICS the short arm of a chromosome. [fr. Fr. *petit,* small]
**P₁** parental generation.
**P_{CO2}, pCO₂** partial pressure (tension) of carbon dioxide. SEE partial pressure.
**P_i** inorganic orthophosphate.
**p53** a tumor suppressor gene located on the short arm of chromosome 17 that encodes a nucleophosphoprotein that binds DNA and negatively regulates cell division; frequently measured as a marker of malignant diseases.
**Pa** pascal; protactinium.
**Paas dis·ease** (pahz) a familial skeletal deformation marked by coxa valga, double patella, shortening of the middle and terminal phalanges of fingers and toes, deformities of the elbows, scoliosis, and spondylitis deformans of the lumbar vertebrae; all these manifestations may be unilateral or bilateral.
**PABA** *p*-aminobenzoic acid.
**pac·chi·o·ni·an** (pahk-ē-ō′nē-an) attributed to or described by Antonio Pacchioni (1665–1726).
**pac·chi·o·ni·an bod·ies** (pahk′ē-ō′nē-ăn) SYN arachnoid granulations.
**pace·fol·low·er** (pās′fawl-ō-er) any cell in excitable tissue that responds to stimuli from a pacemaker.
**pace·ma·ker** (pās′mă-ker) **1.** biologically, any rhythmic center that establishes a pace of activity. **2.** an artificial regulator of rate activity. **3.** CHEMISTRY the substance whose rate of reaction sets the pace for a series of chain reactions. [L. *passus,* step, pace]
**pace·ma·ker lead** a wire transmitting impulses from an artificial pacemaker to the heart.
**Pa·che·co par·rot dis·ease vi·rus** (pa-chā′kō) a virus of the family Herpesviridae, possibly related to the virus of infectious laryngotracheitis.
**Pa·chon meth·od** (pah-sho′) cardiography carried out with the patient lying on the left side.
**Pa·chon test** (pah-shō) in a case of aneurysm, determination of the collateral circulation by estimation of the blood pressure.
△**pachy-** thick. [G. *pachys,* thick]
**pach·y·bleph·a·ron** (pak′ē-blef′ă-ron) thickening of the tarsal border of the eyelid. [pachy- + G. *blepharon,* eyelid]
**pach·y·ce·phal·ic, pach·y·ceph·a·lous** (pak′ē-se-fal′ik, pak′ē-sef′ă-lŭs) relating to or marked by pachycephaly.
**pach·y·ceph·a·ly** (pak-i-sef′ă-lē) abnormal thickness of the skull. [pachy- + G. *kephalē,* head]
**pach·y·chei·lia, pach·y·chi·li·a** (pak-i-kī′lē-ă) swelling or abnormal thickness of the lips. [pachy- + G. *cheilos,* lip]
**pach·y·chro·mat·ic** (pak′ē-krō-mat′ik) having a coarse chromatin reticulum.
**pach·y·dac·ty·ly** (pak-i-dak′ti-lē) enlargement of the fingers or toes, especially extremities; often seen in neurofibromatosis. [pachy- + G. *daktylos,* finger or toe]
**pach·y·der·ma** (pak-i-der′mă) abnormally thick

skin. SEE ALSO elephantiasis. [pachy- + G. *derma,* skin]
**pach·y·der·ma la·ryn·gis** a circumscribed connective tissue hyperplasia at the posterior commissure of the larynx.
**pach·y·der·mat·o·cele** (pak′ē-der-mat′ō-sēl) SYN cutis laxa. [pachy- + G. *derma,* skin, + *kēlē,* tumor]
**pach·y·der·mo·dac·ty·ly** digital swelling due to diffuse fibromatosis occurring on the proximal interphalangeal joints of the index, middle, and ring fingers (sometimes involving the fifth finger, rarely the thumb); a familial form exists.
**pach·y·glos·sia** (pak-i-glos′ē-ă) an enlarged thick tongue. [pachy- + G. *glōssa,* tongue]
**pach·y·gy·ria** (pak-i-jī′rē-ă) condition in which the convolutions of the cerebral cortex are abnormally large; there are fewer sulci than normal and the amount of brain substance may be increased. [pachy- + G. *gyros,* circle]
**pach·y·lep·to·men·in·gi·tis** (pak′i-lep′tō-men-in-jī′tis) inflammation of all the membranes of the brain or spinal cord. [G. *pachys,* thick, + *leptos,* thin, + *mēninx* (*mēning-*), membrane, + *-itis,* inflammation]
**pach·y·men·in·gi·tis** (pak′i-men′in-jī′tis) inflammation of the dura mater. SYN perimeningitis. [pachy- + G. *mēninx,* membrane, + *-itis,* inflammation]
**pach·y·me·nin·gop·a·thy** (pak′ē-mĕ-ning-gop′ă-thē) disease of the dura mater. [pachy- + G. *mēninx* (*mēning-*), membrane, + *pathos,* disease]
**pach·y·me·ninx** (pak′i-mē′ningks) [TA] the dura mater. [pachy- + G. *mēninx,* membrane]
**pa·chyn·sis** (pă-kin′sis) any pathologic thickening. [G. a thickening]
**pa·chyn·tic** (pă-kin′tic) relating to pachynsis.
**pach·y·o·nych·ia** (pak′ē-ō-nik′ē-ă) abnormal thickness of the fingernails or toenails. [pachy- + G. *onyx,* nail]
**pach·y·per·i·os·ti·tis** (pak′i-per′ē-ōs-tī′tis) proliferative thickening of the periosteum caused by inflammation. [pachy- + periostitis]
**pach·y·per·i·to·ni·tis** (pak′i-per′i-tō-nī′tis) inflammation of the peritoneum with thickening of the membrane. [pachy- + peritonitis]
**pach·y·pleu·ri·tis** (pak′ē-ploo-rī′tis) inflammation of the pleura with thickening of the membrane. [pachy- + pleura + G. *-itis,* inflammation]
**pach·y·sal·pin·gi·tis** (pak′ē-sal-pin-jī′tis) SYN chronic interstitial salpingitis.
**pach·y·sal·pin·go·o·va·ri·tis** (pak-i-sal′pin-gō-ō′va-rī′tis) chronic parenchymatous inflammation of the ovary and uterine (fallopian) tube. [pachy- + salpinx + Mod. L. *ovarium,* ovary, + G. *-itis,* inflammation]
**pach·y·so·mia** (pak-i-sō′mē-ă) pathologic thickening of the soft parts of the body, notably in acromegaly. [pachy- + G. *sōma,* body]
**pach·y·tene** (pak′i-tēn) the stage of prophase in meiosis in which pairing of homologous chromosomes is complete; longitudinal cleavage occurs in each chromosome to form two sister chromatids so that each homologous chromosome pair becomes a set of four intertwined chromatids. [pachy- + G. *tainia,* band, tape]
**pach·y·vag·i·nal·i·tis** (pak′i-vaj′i-năl-ī′tis) chronic inflammation with thickening of the tu-

nica vaginalis testis. [pachy- + Mod. L. (tunica) *vaginalis,* + G. *-itis,* inflammation]

**pach•y•vag•i•ni•tis** (pak'i-vaj'i-nī'tis) chronic vaginitis with thickening and induration of the vaginal walls. [pachy- + vagina + G. *-itis,* inflammation]

**pac•ing cath•e•ter** a cardiac catheter with one or more electrodes at its tip which can be used to artificially pace the heart.

**pa•ci•ni•an** (pa-sin'ē-an, pa-chin'ē-an) attributed to or described by Filippo Pacini (1812–1883).

**pa•ci•ni•an cor•pus•cles** (pa-sin'ē-an) SYN lamellated corpuscles.

**pack** (pak) **1.** to fill, stuff, or tampon. **2.** to enwrap or envelop the body in a sheet, blanket, or other covering. **3.** to apply a dressing or covering to a surgical site. **4.** the items used above. [M.E. *pak,* fr. Germanic]

**pack•er** (pak'er) **1.** an instrument for tamponing. **2.** SYN plugger.

**pack•ing** (pak'ing) **1.** filling a natural cavity, a wound, or a mold with some material. **2.** the material so used. **3.** the application of a pack.

**PA con•duc•tion time** SEE atrioventricular conduction.

**PACS** *p*icture *a*rchive and *c*ommunication *s*ystem, a computer network for digitized radiologic images and reports.

**pad 1.** a thin cushion of resilient or absorbent material applied to relieve pressure or absorb fluid. **2.** a more or less encapsulated body of fat or some other tissue serving to fill a space or act as a cushion in the body.

*Pae•cil•o•my•ces* (pē-sil-ō-mī'sēz) a genus of saprophytic deuteromycetous fungi whose conidia-bearing hyphae superficially resemble the penicilli of *Penicillium;* occasional opportunistic human pathogen causing pulmonary infection, keratitis, and endocarditis.

*Pae•ci•lo•my•ces li•la•ci•nus* a mold; a rare cause of paecilomycosis; has been implicated in human eye infections due to contaminated implanted intraocular lenses. SYN *Penicillium lilacinum.*

△**paed-** SEE ped-.

**paed•e•ras•ty [Br.]** SEE pederasty.

**pae•di- [Br.]** SEE pedi-.

**pae•di•a•tric [Br.]** SEE pediatric.

**pae•di•a•tri•cian [Br.]** SEE pediatrician.

**pae•di•a•trics [Br.]** SEE pediatrics.

**pae•do- [Br.]** SEE pedo-.

**pae•do•don•tia [Br.]** SYN pedodontics.

**pae•do•don•tics [Br.]** SEE pedodontics.

**pae•do•phil•ia [Br.]** SEE pedophilia.

**PAGE** polyacrylamide gel electrophoresis.

**Pa•gen•stech•er cir•cle** (pah-gen-stek-ěr) in the case of a freely movable abdominal tumor, the mass is moved throughout its entire range, its position at intervals being marked on the abdominal wall; when these points are joined, a circle is formed, the center of which marks the point of attachment of the tumor.

**Pa•get cell** (paj'ět) a relatively large, neoplastic epithelial cell (carcinoma cell) with a hyperchromatic nucleus and abundant palely staining cytoplasm; in Paget disease of the breast, such cells occur in neoplastic epithelium in the ducts and in the epidermis of the nipple, areola, and adjacent skin.

**◨Pa•get dis•ease** (paj'ět) **1.** a generalized skeletal disease, frequently familial, of older persons in which bone resorption and formation are both increased, leading to thickening and softening of bones (e.g., the skull), and bending of weight-bearing bones; SYN osteitis deformans. **2.** a disease of elderly women, characterized by an infiltrated, somewhat eczematous lesion surrounding and involving the nipple and areola, and associated with subjacent intraductal cancer of the breast and infiltration of the lower epidermis by malignant cells; **3.** SYN extramammary Paget disease. See page B6.

**pag•et•oid cells** atypical melanocytes resembling Paget cells, found in some cutaneous melanomas.

△**-pa•gus** conjoined twins, the first element of the word denoting the parts fused. SEE ALSO -didymus, -dymus. [G. *pagos,* something fixed, fr. *pēgnymi,* to fasten together]

**pain** (pān) **1.** an unpleasant sensation associated with actual or potential tissue damage, and mediated by specific nerve fibers to the brain where its conscious appreciation may be modified by various factors. **2.** term used to denote a painful uterine contraction occurring in childbirth. [L. *poena,* a fine, a penalty]

**pain•ful arc sign** pain elicited during active abduction of the upper extremity between 60° and 120°.

**pain•ful heel** a condition in which bearing weight on the heel causes pain of varying severity. SYN calcaneodynia, calcodynia.

**pain-plea•sure prin•ci•ple** PSYCHOANALYSIS the concept that one tends to seek pleasure and avoid pain; a term borrowed by experimental psychology to denote the same tendency of an animal in a learning situation. SYN pleasure principle.

**pain-spasm-is•che•mia cy•cle** SYN pain-spasm-pain cycle.

**pain-spasm-pain cy•cle** a self-perpetuating cycle in which skeletal muscle spasm causes local ischemia and pain, which exacerbate the spasm, which in turn exacerbates the pain. SEE ALSO fibromyalgia. SYN pain-spasm-ischemia cycle.

**PA in•ter•val** the time from onset of the P wave to the initial rapid deflection of the A wave in the His bundle electrogram (normally 25–45 msec); it represents the intraatrial conduction time.

**pair** (pār) two objects considered together because of similarity, for a common purpose, or because of some attracting force between them.

**pal•a•tal** (pal'ă-tăl) relating to the palate or the palate bone. SYN palatine.

**pal•a•tal re•flex, pal•a•tine re•flex** swallowing reflex induced by stimulation of the palate.

**pal•ate** (pal'ăt) the bony and muscular partition between the oral and nasal cavities. SYN palatum [TA]. [L. *palatum,* palate]

**pal•a•tine** (pal'ă-tīn) SYN palatal.

**pal•a•tine bone** an irregularly shaped bone posterior to the maxilla, which enters into the formation of the nasal cavity, the orbit, and the hard palate; it articulates with the maxilla, inferior nasal concha, sphenoid, and ethmoid bones, the vomer and its fellow of the opposite side.

**pal•a•tine pro•cess** in the embryo, medially directed shelves from the oral surface of the maxillae; they develop into the secondary palate after midline fusion.

**pal•a•tine ra•phe** a rather narrow, low elevation in the center of the hard palate that extends from the incisive papilla posteriorly over the entire length of the mucosa of the hard palate.

**pal•a•tine spines** the longitudinal ridges along the palatine grooves on the inferior surface of the palatine process of the maxilla.

**pal•a•tine ton•sil** a large, oval mass of lymphoid tissue embedded in the lateral wall of the oropharynx on either side between the pillars of the fauces. SYN tonsilla palatina [TA], tonsilla [TA], faucial tonsil, tonsil (2).

**pal•a•tine u•vu•la** a conical projection from the posterior edge of the middle of the soft palate, composed of connective tissue containing a number of racemose glands, and some muscular fibers (uvulae muscle).

**pal•a•tine vein** drains the palatine regions and empties into the facial vein.

**pal•a•ti•tis** (pal-ă-tī′tis) inflammation of the palate.

△**pal•a•to-** palate. [L. *palatum,* palate]

**pal•a•to•glos•sal** (pal′ă-tō-glos′ăl) relating to the palate and the tongue, or to the palatoglossus muscle.

**pal•a•to•glos•sal arch** one of a pair of ridges or folds of mucous membrane passing from the soft palate to the side of the tongue; it encloses the palatoglossus muscle and forms the anterior margin of the tonsillar fossa. Also demarcates the oral cavity from the isthmus of fauces.

**pal•a•to•glos•sus mus•cle** forms anterior pillar of tonsillar fossa; *origin,* oral surface of soft palate; *insertion,* side of tongue; *action,* raises back of tongue and narrows fauces; *nerve supply,* pharyngeal plexus (cranial root of accessory nerve). SYN musculus palatoglossus [TA].

**pal•a•tog•na•thous** (pal′ă-tog′nă-thŭs) having a cleft palate. [palato- + G. *gnathos,* jaw]

**pal•a•to•max•il•lary** (pal′ă-tō-mak′si-lār-ē) relating to the palate and the maxilla.

**pal•a•to•na•sal** (pal-ă-tō-nā′sal) relating to the palate and the nasal cavity.

**pal•a•to•pha•ryn•ge•al** (pal′ă-tō-fa-rin′jē-ăl) relating to palate and pharynx.

**pal•a•to•pha•ryn•ge•al arch** one of a pair of ridges or folds of mucous membrane which pass downward from the posterior margin of the soft palate to the lateral wall of the pharynx. It encloses the palatopharyngeus muscle and forms the posterior margin of the tonsillar fossa. It also demarcates the isthmus of the fauces from the oropharynx.

**pal•a•to•pha•ryn•ge•al mus•cle** SYN palatopharyngeus muscle.

**pal•a•to•pha•ryn•ge•us mus•cle** *origin,* soft palate; forms the posterior pillar of the fauces or tonsillar fossa; *insertion,* posterior border of thyroid cartilage and aponeurosis of pharynx; *action,* narrows fauces, depresses soft palate, elevates pharynx and larynx; *nerve supply,* pharyngeal plexus (cranial root of accessory nerve). SYN musculus palatopharyngeus [TA], palatopharyngeal muscle.

**pal•a•to•pha•ryn•gor•rha•phy** (pal′ă-tō-far′in-gōr′ă-fē) SYN staphylopharyngorrhaphy. [palato- + pharynx + G. *rhaphē,* suture]

**pal•a•to•plas•ty** (pal′ă-tō-plas-tē) surgery of the palate to restore form and function. SYN staphyloplasty, uranoplasty. [palato- + G. *plassō,* to form]

**pal•a•to•ple•gia** (pal′ă-tō-plē′jē-ă) paralysis of the muscles of the soft palate. [palato- + G. *plēgē,* stroke]

**pal•a•tor•rha•phy** (pal-ă-tōr′ă-fē) the surgical repair of a cleft palate. SYN staphylorrhaphy, uranorrhaphy. [palato- + G. *rhaphē,* suture]

**pal•a•tos•chi•sis** (pal-ă-tos′ki-sis) SYN cleft palate. [palato- + G. *schisis,* fissure]

**pa•la•tum,** pl. **pa•la•ti** (pă-lā′tŭm, pal′ă-tī) [TA] SYN palate. [L.]

△**paleo-, pale-** old, primitive, primary, early. [G. *palaios,* old, ancient]

**pa•le•o•cer•e•bel•lum** (pā′lē-ō-ser′ĕ-bel′ŭm) [TA] the portion of the cerebellum including most of the vermis and the adjacent zones of the cerebellar hemispheres rostral to the primary fissure, corresponding to the zone of distribution of the spinocerebellar tracts; in phylogenetic age, it is thought to be intermediate between the archicerebellum and the neocerebellum. SYN spinocerebellum [TA]. [paleo- + L. *cerebellum*]

**pa•le•o•cor•tex** (pā′lē-ō-kōr′teks) [TA] the phylogenetically oldest part of the cortical mantle of the cerebral hemisphere, represented by the olfactory cortex.

**pa•le•o•ki•net•ic** (pā′lē-ō-ki-net′ik) denoting the primitive motor mechanisms underlying muscular reflexes and automatic, stereotyped movements. [paleo- + G. *kinētikos,* relating to movement]

**pa•le•o•pa•thol•o•gy** (pā′lē-ō-pa-thol′ō-jē) the science of disease in prehistoric times as revealed in bones, mummies, and archaeologic artifacts. [paleo- + pathology]

**pa•le•o•stri•a•tal** (pā′lē-ō-strī-ā′tăl) relating to the paleostriatum.

**pa•le•o•stri•a•tum** (pā′lē-ō-strī-ā′tŭm) term denoting the globus pallidus and expressing the hypothesis that this component of the striate body developed earlier in evolution than the "neostriatum" or striatum (caudate nucleus and putamen) and that it is a diencephalic derivative. [paleo- + L. *striatum*]

**pa•le•o•thal•a•mus** (pā′lē-ō-thal′ă-mŭs) the intralaminar nuclei, believed to be the earliest components of the thalamus to have evolved; they lack reciprocal connections with the isocortex.

**pal•i•ki•ne•sia, pal•i•ci•ne•sia** (pal-i-ki-nē′zē-ă, pal-i-si-nē′zē-ă) involuntary repetition of movements. [G. *palin,* again, + *kinēsis,* movement]

**pal•i•la•lia** (pal-i-lā′lē-ă) SYN paliphrasia. [G. *palin,* again, + *lalia,* a form of speech]

**pal•in•drome** (pal′in-drōm) MOLECULAR BIOLOGY a self-complementary nucleic acid sequence; a sequence identical to its complementary strand, if both are "read" in the same 5′- to 3′ direction, or inverted repeating sequences running in opposite directions (but same 5′- to 3′- direction) on either side of an axis of symmetry; palindromes occur at sites of important reactions. [G. *palindromos,* a running back]

**pal•in•dro•mia** (pal-in-drō′mē-ă) a relapse or recurrence of a disease. [G. *palindromos,* a running back, + *-ia,* condition]

**pal•in•drom•ic** (pal-in-drōm′ik) recurring.

**pal•i•nop•sia** (pal-i-nop′sē-ă) abnormal recurring visual hallucinations. [G. *palin,* again, + *opsis,* vision]

**pal•i•phra•sia** (pal-i-frā′zē-ă) in speech, involuntary repetition of words or sentences. SEE ALSO echolalia. SYN palilalia. [G. *palin,* again, + *phrasis,* speech]

**pal•la•di•um** (Pd) (pă-lā′dē-ŭm) a metallic element resembling platinum, atomic no. 46, atomic wt. 106.42. [fr. the asteroid, Pallas; G. *Pallas,* goddess of wisdom]

**pal·laes·the·sia [Br.]** SEE pallesthesia.

**pall·an·es·the·sia** (pal′an-es-thē′zē-ă) absence of pallesthesia. SYN apallesthesia. [G. *pallō,* to quiver, + *anaisthēsia,* insensibility]

**pall·es·the·sia** (pal′es-thē′zē-ă) the appreciation of vibration, a form of pressure sense; most acute when a vibrating tuning fork is applied over a bony prominence. [G. *pallō,* to quiver, + *aisthēsis,* sensation]

**pall·es·thet·ic** (pal-es-thet′ik) pertaining to pallesthesia.

**pal·li·al** (pal′ē-ăl) relating to the pallium.

**pal·li·ate** (pal′ē-āt) to reduce the severity of; to relieve slightly. SYN mitigate. [L. *palliatus* (adj.), dressed in a *pallium,* cloaked]

**pal·li·a·tive** (pal′ē-ă-tiv) reducing the severity of; denoting the alleviation of symptoms without curing the underlying disease.

**pal·li·a·tive treat·ment** treatment to alleviate symptoms without curing the disease.

**pal·li·dal** (pal′i-dăl) relating to the pallidum.

**pal·li·dec·to·my** (pal′i-dek′tō-mē) excision or destruction of the globus pallidus, usually by stereotaxy. [pallidum + G. *ektomē,* excision]

**pal·li·do·an·sot·o·my** (pal′i-dō-an-sot′ō-mē) production of lesions in the globus pallidus and ansa lenticularis.

**pal·li·dot·o·my** (pal-i-dot′ō-mē) a destructive operation on the globus pallidus, done to relieve involuntary movements or muscular rigidity. [pallidum + G. *tomē,* incision]

**pal·li·dum** (pal′i-dŭm) SYN globus pallidus. [L. *pallidus,* pale]

**pal·li·um** (pal′ē-ŭm) [TA] the cerebral cortex with the subjacent white substance. SYN mantle (2). [L. cloak]

**pal·lor** (pal′ŏr) paleness, as of the skin. [L.]

**palm** (pahm) the flat of the hand; the flexor or anterior surface of the hand, exclusive of the thumb and fingers; the opposite of the dorsum. SYN palma [TA]. [L. *palma*]

**pal·ma,** pl. **pal·mae** (pah′mă, pah′mē) [TA] SYN palm, palm. [L.]

**pal·mar** (pah′măr) pertaining to the palm of the hand or the caudal aspect of the carpus on the forelimb of an animal. [L. *palmaris,* fr. *palma*]

**pal·mar arch 1.** deep palmar arch; the arterial arch located deep to the long flexor tendons in the hand, fomred by the radial artery and the deep palmar branch of the ulnar artery. SYN arcus palmaris profundus [TA]. **2.** superficial palmar arch; the arterial arch in the hand located superficial to the long flexor tendons, formed principally by the ulnar artery and usually completed by a communication with the superficial palmar branch of the radial artery. SYN arcus palmaris superficiales [TA]. SYN arcus palmaris.

**pal·mar in·ter·os·se·ous mus·cle** three muscles in the hand; *origin,* first: ulnar side of second metacarpal; second and third: radial sides of fourth and fifth metacarpals; *insertion,* first: into ulnar side of index; second and third: into radial sides of ring and little fingers; *action,* adducts fingers toward axis of middle finger; *nerve supply,* ulnar. SYN musculus interosseus palmaris [TA].

**pal·mar pinch** OCCUPATIONAL THERAPY pinch between the pad of the thumb and the pads of the index and middle fingers.

**pal·mar pso·ri·a·sis** patchy, hyperkeratotic psoriasis affecting contact points of the volar surface of fingers and palms, alone or with mild psoriasis elsewhere; believed to be an isomorphic response, it may affect one palm involved in a sport or occupation.

**pal·mar ra·di·o·car·pal lig·a·ment** a strong ligament that passes from the distal end of the radius to the proximal row of carpal bones on the anterior surface of the wrist joint.

**pal·mar ul·no·car·pal lig·a·ment** the fibrous band that passes from the ulnar styloid process to the carpal bones.

**pal·mate folds** the two longitudinal ridges, anterior and posterior, in the mucous membrane lining the cervix uteri, from which numerous secondary folds, or rugae, branch off. SYN plicae palmatae [TA].

**Pal·mer den·tal no·men·cla·ture** (pah′mer) **1.** a system of identifying permanent teeth by the use of a tooth number indicating the number of the tooth distally from the midline and a bracket to indicate the position, e.g., 6[underline along with vertical line to form a right angle to the right and below the number] is the upper right first permanent molar. **2.** a system for deciduous teeth analogous to the permanent one with letters substituted for numbers (A through E or a through e). SYN Zsigmondy dental nomenclature.

**palm·ic** (pah′mik) beating; throbbing; relating to a palmus.

**pal·mit·o·le·ic ac·id** (pal′mi-tō-lē′ik as′id) a monounsaturated 16-carbon acid; one of the common constituents of the triacylglycerols of human adipose tissue.

**pal·mus,** pl. **pal·mi** (pah′mŭs, pah′ī) **1.** SYN facial tic. **2.** rhythmical fibrillary contractions in a muscle. SEE ALSO jumping disease. **3.** the heart beat. [G. *palmos,* pulsation, quivering]

**pal·pa·ble** (pal′pă-bl) **1.** perceptible to touch; capable of being palpated. **2.** evident; plain. [see palpation]

**pal·pate** (pal′pāt) to examine by feeling and pressing with the palms of the hands and the fingers.

**pal·pa·tion** (pal-pā′shŭn) **1.** examination with the hands, feeling for organs, masses, or infiltration of a part of the body, feeling the heart or pulse beat, vibrations in the chest, etc. SYN touch (2). **2.** touching, feeling, or perceiving by the sense of touch. [L. *palpatio,* fr. *palpo,* pp. *-atus,* to touch, stroke]

**pal·pa·to·ry per·cus·sion** finger percussion in which attention is focused upon the resistance and reverberation of the tissues under the finger as well as upon the sound elicited.

**pal·pe·bra,** pl. **pal·pe·brae** (pal-pē′bră, pal-pē′brē) [TA] SYN eyelid. [L.]

**pal·pe·bral** (pal′pē-brăl) relating to an eyelid or the eyelids.

**pal·pe·bral ar·ter·ies** branches of the ophthalmic supplying the upper and lower eyelids, consisting of two sets, lateral and medial. SYN arteriae palpebrales [TA].

**pal·pe·bral fis·sure** SYN rima palpebrarum.

**pal·pe·bral veins** drain the superior eyelid posteriorly as tributaries of the superior ophthalmic vein.

**pal·pi·ta·tion** (pal-pi-tā′shŭn) forcible or irregular pulsation of the heart, perceptible to the patient, usually with an increase in frequency or force, with or without irregularity in rhythm. SYN trepidatio cordis. [L. *palpito,* to throb]

**pal•sy** (pawl′zē) paralysis or paresis. [a corruption of O. Fr. fr. L. and G. *paralysis*]

**PAM** potential acuity meter.

**pam•pin•i•form** (pam-pin′i-fōrm) having the shape of a tendril; denoting a vinelike structure. [L. *pampinus,* a tendril, + *forma,* form]

**pam•pin•i•form plex•us** a plexus formed, in the male, by veins from the testicle and epididymis, consisting of 8–10 veins lying in front of the ductus deferens and forming part of the spermatic cord; in the female the ovarian veins form this plexus between the layers of the broad ligament; in the male it is part of the thermoregulatory system of the testis, helping to keep the testis at a constant temperature slightly lower than the other body temperature.

△**pan-** all, entire (properly affixed to words derived from G. roots). SEE ALSO pant-. [G. *pas,* all]

**pan•a•cea** (pan-ă-sē′ă) a cure-all; a remedy claimed to be curative of all diseases. [G. *panakeia,* universal remedy, fr. Panacea, Aesculapius' daughter]

**pan•ag•glu•ti•nins** (pan-ă-gloo′ti-ninz) agglutinins that react with all human erythrocytes. [pan + L. *agglutino,* to glue]

**pan•an•gi•i•tis** (pan′an-jē-ī′tis) inflammation involving all the coats of a blood vessel. [pan- + angiitis]

**pan•ar•thri•tis** (pan-ar-thrī′tis) **1.** inflammation involving all the tissues of a joint. **2.** inflammation of all the joints of the body.

**pan•at•ro•phy** (pan-at′rō-fē) **1.** atrophy of all the parts of a structure. **2.** general atrophy of the body.

**pan•cake kid•ney** a disk-shaped organ produced by fusion of both poles of the contralateral kidney anlagen (primordia of the kidneys).

**pan•car•di•tis** (pan-kar-dī′tis) inflammation of all the structures of the heart.

**Pan•coast syn•drome** (pan′kōst) lower trunk brachial plexopathy and Horner syndrome due to malignant tumor in the region of the superior pulmonary sulcus.

**pan•co•lec•to•my** (pan′kō-lek′tō-mē) extirpation of the entire colon.

▊**pan•cre•as,** pl. **pan•cre•a•ta** (pan′krē-as, pan-krē-ā′tă) [TA] an elongated lobulated retroperitoneal gland extending from the duodenum to the spleen; it consists of a flattened head (caput) within the duodenal concavity, an elongated three-sided body extending transversely across the abdomen, and a tail in contact with the spleen. The gland secretes from its exocrine part pancreatic juice that is discharged into the intestine, and from its endocrine part the internal secretions, insulin and glucagon. See this page. [G. *pankreas,* the sweetbread, fr. *pas* (*pan*), all, + *kreas,* flesh]

△**pan•cre•at-, pan•cre•a•ti•co-, pan•cre•a•to-, pancreo-** the pancreas. [G. *pankreas,* pancreas]

**pan•cre•a•tal•gia** (pan′krē-ă-tal′jē-ă) pain arising from the pancreas or felt in or near the region of the pancreas. [pancreat- + G. *algos,* pain]

**pan•cre•a•tec•to•my** (pan′krē-ă-tek′tō-mē) excision of the pancreas. [pancreat- + G. *ektomē,* excision]

**pan•cre•at•ic** (pan-krē-at′ik) relating to the pancreas.

**pan•cre•at•ic cal•cu•lus** a concretion, usually

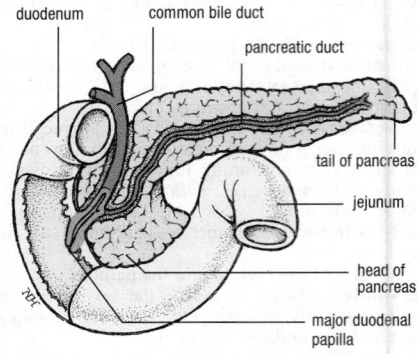

duodenum — common bile duct — pancreatic duct — tail of pancreas — jejunum — head of pancreas — major duodenal papilla

**pancreas** (and part of duodenum)

multiple, in the pancreatic duct, associated with chronic pancreatitis.

**pan•cre•at•ic cys•to•du•o•de•nos•to•my** surgical or endoscopic drainage of pancreatic pseudocyst into duodenum. SYN duodenocystostomy (3).

**pan•cre•at•ic di•ges•tion** digestion in the intestine by the enzymes of the pancreatic juice.

**pan•cre•at•ic duct** the excretory duct of the pancreas, which extends through the gland from tail to head, where it empties into the duodenum at the greater duodenal papilla. SYN Wirsung canal, Wirsung duct.

**pan•cre•at•i•co•du•o•de•nal** (pan-krē-at′i-kō-doo′ō-dē′năl) relating to the pancreas and the duodenum.

**pan•cre•at•i•co•du•o•de•nal veins** accompany the superior and inferior pancreaticoduodenal arteries, empty into the superior mesenteric or portal vein.

**pan•cre•at•ic veins** drain the pancreas and empty into the splenic vein and the superior mesenteric vein.

**pan•cre•a•ti•tis** (pan′krē-ă-tī′tis) inflammation of the pancreas.

**pan•cre•at•o•du•o•de•nec•to•my, pan•cre•at•i•co•duo•den•ec•to•my** (pan-krē-at′ō-doo-ō-dē-nek′tō-mē, pan-krē-at′ĭ-kō-doo-od′en-ek′ō-mē) excision of all or part of the pancreas together with the duodenum. SYN Whipple operation.

**pan•cre•at•o•du•o•de•nos•to•my** (pan-krē-at′ō-doo-ō-dē-nos′tō-mē, pan′krē-ă-tō-doo-ō-dē-nos′tō-mē) surgical anastomosis of a pancreatic duct, cyst, or fistula to the duodenum.

**pan•cre•at•o•gas•tros•to•my** (pan-krē-at′ō-gas-tros′tō-mē) surgical anastomosis of a pancreatic cyst or fistula to the stomach.

**pan•cre•a•to•gen•ic, pan•cre•a•tog•en•ous** (pan′krē-ă-tō-jen′ik, pan′krē-ă-toj′ĕ-nŭs) of pancreatic origin; formed in the pancreas. [pancreato- + G. *genesis,* origin]

**pan•cre•a•tog•ra•phy** (pan′krē-ă-tog′ră-fē) radiographic demonstration of the pancreatic ducts, after retrograde injection of radiopaque material into the distal duct. [pancreato- + G. *graphō,* to write]

**pan•cre•at•o•li•thec•to•my** (pan-krē-at′ō-li-thek′tō-mē) SYN pancreatolithotomy. [pancreato- + G. *lithos,* stone, + *ektomē,* excision]

**pan•cre•at•o•li•thi•a•sis** (pan-krē-at′ō-li-thī′ă-sis) stones in the pancreas, usually found in the pancreatic duct system.

**pan·cre·at·o·li·thot·o·my** (pan-krē-at′ō-li-thot′ō-mē) removal of a pancreatic concretion. SYN pancreatolithectomy. [pancreato- + G. *lithos,* stone, + *tomē,* incision]

**pan·cre·a·tol·y·sis** (pan′krē-ă-tol′i-sis) destruction of the pancreas. [pancreato- + G. *lysis,* dissolution]

**pan·cre·a·to·lyt·ic** (pan′krē-ă-tō-lit′ik) denoting pancreatolysis.

**pan·cre·a·top·a·thy** (pan′krē-ă-top′ă-thē) any disease of the pancreas. [pancreato- + G. *pathos,* suffering]

**pan·cre·a·to·re·nal syn·drome** acute renal failure occurring in a patient with severe acute pancreatitis; the mortality rate is high.

**pan·cre·a·tot·o·my** (pan′krē-ă-tot′ō-mē) incision of the pancreas. [pancreato- + G. *tomē,* incision]

**pan·cre·a·tro·pic** (pan′krē-ă-trop′ik) exerting an action on the pancreas. [pancreat- + G. *tropikos,* relating to a turning]

**pan·cre·li·pase** (pan-krē-lip′ās) a concentrate of pancreatic enzymes standardized for lipase content; a lipolytic used for substitution therapy.

**pan·cy·to·pe·nia** (pan′sī-tō-pē′nē-ă) pronounced reduction in the number of erythrocytes, all types of white blood cells, and the blood platelets in the circulating blood. [pan- + G. *kytos,* cell, + *penia,* poverty]

**pan·dem·ic** (pan-dem′ik) denoting a disease affecting or attacking the population of an extensive region, country, continent; extensively epidemic. [pan- + G. *dēmos,* the people]

**pan·en·ceph·a·li·tis** (pan′en-sef-ă-lī′tis) a diffuse inflammation of the brain.

**pan·en·do·scope** (pan-en′dō-skōp) an illuminated instrument for inspection of the interior of the urethra as well as the bladder by means of a Foroblique lens system. [pan- + G. *endon,* within, + *skopeō,* to view]

**pan·es·the·sia** (pan-es-thē′zē-ă) the sum of all the sensations experienced by a person at one time. SEE ALSO cenesthesia. [pan- + G. *aisthēsis,* sensation]

**pang** a sudden sharp, brief pain.

**pan·hy·po·pi·tu·i·tar·ism (PHP)** (pan-hī′pō-pi-too′i-tă-rizm) a state in which the secretion of all anterior pituitary hormones is inadequate or absent. SYN hypophysial cachexia.

**pan·ic** (pan′ik) extreme and unreasoning anxiety and fear, often accompanied by disturbed breathing, increased heart activity, vasomotor changes, sweating, and a feeling of dread. SEE anxiety. [fr. G. myth. char., *Pan*]

**pan·ic at·tack** sudden onset of intense apprehension, fear, terror, or impending doom accompanied by increased autonomic nervous system activity and by various constitutional disturbances, depersonalization, and derealization.

**pan·ic dis·or·der** recurrent panic attacks that occur unpredictably. SEE generalized anxiety disorder.

**pan·im·mu·ni·ty** (pan-i-myu′ni-tē) a general immunity to all infectious diseases.

**pan·lob·u·lar em·phy·se·ma** emphysema affecting all parts of the lobules, in part, or usually the whole, of the lungs, and usually associated with α₁-antiprotease deficiency emphysema.

**pan·my·e·loph·thi·sis** (pan′mī-ĕ-lof′thi-sis) SYN myelophthisis (2).

**pan·my·e·lo·sis** (pan′mī-ĕ-lō′sis) myeloid metaplasia with abnormal immature blood cells in the spleen and liver, associated with myelofibrosis. [pan- + G. *myelos,* marrow, + *-osis,* condition]

**Pan·ner dis·ease** (pahn′ĕr) epiphysial osteonecrosis of the capitellum of the humerus.

**pan·nic·u·lar her·nia** the escape of subcutaneous fat through a gap in a fascia or an aponeurosis. SYN fatty hernia.

**pan·nic·u·lec·to·my** (pa-nik-yu-lek′tō-mē) surgical excision of redundant panniculus adiposus, usually of the abdomen. [panniculus + G. *ektomē,* a cutting out]

**pan·nic·u·li·tis** (pă-nik′yū-lī′tis) inflammation of subcutaneous adipose tissue. [panniculus + G. *-itis,* inflammation]

**pan·nic·u·lus,** pl. **pan·nic·u·li** (pă-nik′yu-lŭs, pă-nik′yu-lī) [TA] a sheet or layer of tissue. [L. dim. of *pannus,* cloth]

**pan·ning** (pan′ing) use of plastic plates or surfaces coated with either antigen or antibody to separate or concentrate specific cells with appropriate receptors.

**pan·nus,** pl. **pan·ni** (pan′ŭs, pan′ī) A membrane of granulation tissue covering a normal surface: **1.** the articular cartilages in rheumatoid arthritis and in chronic granulomatous diseases such as tuberculosis; **2.** the cornea in trachoma. SEE ALSO corneal pannus. [L. cloth]

**pan·nus cras·sus** SEE corneal pannus.

**pan·nus sic·cus** SEE corneal pannus.

**pan·nus ten·u·is** SEE corneal pannus.

**pan·o·ram·ic ra·di·o·graph** a radiographic view of the maxillae and mandible extending from the left to the right glenoid fossae.

▣**pan·o·ram·ic x-ray film** DENTISTRY a radiograph taken to give a panoramic view of the entire upper and lower dental arch as well as the temporomandibular joints. See page 364.

**pan·o·ti·tis** (pan′ō-tī′tis) general inflammation of all parts of the ear; specifically, a disease which begins as an otitis interna, the inflammation subsequently extending to the middle ear and neighboring structures. [pan- + G. *ous,* ear, + *-itis,* inflammation]

**pan·si·nu·si·tis** (pan-sī-nŭ-sī′tis) inflammation of all the accessory sinuses of the nose on one or both sides.

**pan·sys·tol·ic** (pan′sis-tol′ik) lasting throughout systole, extending from first to second heart sound. SYN holosystolic.

**pan·sys·tol·ic mur·mur** a murmur occupying the entire systolic interval, from first to second heart sounds.

**pant** to breathe rapidly and shallowly. [Fr. *panteler,* to gasp]

△**pant-, pan·to-** entire. SEE ALSO pan-. [G. *pas,* all]

**pan·tal·gia** (pan-tal′jē-ă) pain involving the entire body. [pant- + G. *algos,* pain]

**pan·ta·loon her·nia** an inguinal hernia that involves both an indirect and a direct component.

**pan·to·mo·gram** (pan′tō-mō-gram) a panoramic radiographic record of the maxillary and mandibular dental arches and their associated structures, obtained by a pantomograph. [pan- + tomogram]

**pan·to·mo·graph** (pan′tō-mō-graf) a panoramic radiographic instrument that permits visualization of the entire dentition, alveolar bone, and contiguous structures on a single extraoral film.

**pan·to·mog·ra·phy** (pan-tō-mog′ră-fē) a method of radiography by which a radiograph (pantomogram) of the maxillary and mandibular dental arches and their contiguous structures may be obtained on a single film.

**pan·to·scop·ic tilt** an oblique astigmatism caused by slanting a spherical lens so that light rays strike the lens at a nonperpendicular angle, altering the spherical and cylindrical refractive power of the lens.

**pan·to·the·nate** (pan-tō-the′nāt) a salt or ester of pantothenic acid.

**pan·to·then·ic ac·id** (pan-tō-then′ik as′id) the β-alanine amide of pantoic acid. A growth substance widely distributed in plant and animal tissues, and essential for growth of a number of organisms; deficiency in diet causes a dermatitis in chicks and rats and achromotrichia in the latter; a precursor to coenzyme A.

**Pan·um ar·ea** (pah′noom) area in space surrounding the empirical horopter where single binocular vision is observed despite stimulation of noncorresponding retinal points.

**PAP** *per*oxidase *anti*peroxidase complex, 3′-phosphoadenosine 5′-phosphate. SEE PAP technique.

**Pa·pa·ni·co·la·ou stain** (pă-pĕ-nĭ-kō-lā′oo) a multichromatic stain used principally on exfoliated cytologic specimens and based on aqueous hematoxylin with multiple counterstaining dyes in 95% ethyl alcohol, giving great transparency and delicacy of detail; important in cancer screening, especially of gynecologic smears.

**pa·per chro·ma·tog·ra·phy** partition chromatography in which the moving phase is a liquid and the stationary phase is paper.

**pa·per mill work·er's dis·ease** extrinsic allergic alveolitis caused by moldy wood pulp containing spores of *Alternaria* fungi.

**pa·pil·la**, pl. **pa·pil·lae** (pă-pil′ă, pă-pil′ē) any small, nipplelike process. SYN teat (3). [L. a nipple, dim. of *papula*, a pimple]

**pa·pil·la of der·mis** the superficial projections of the dermis (corium) that interdigitate with recesses in the overlying epidermis; they contain vascular loops and specialized nerve endings, and are arranged in ridgelike lines best developed in the hand and foot. SYN dermal papillae.

**pa·pil·lae val·la·tae** SYN vallate papilla.

**pa·pil·la pi·li** a knoblike indentation of the bottom of the hair follicle, upon which the hair bulb fits like a cap; it is derived from the corium and contains vascular loops for the nourishment of the hair root. SYN hair papilla.

**pap·il·lary, pap·il·late** (pap′i-lār-ē, pap′-i-lāt) relating to, resembling, or provided with papillae.

**pap·il·lary ad·e·no·car·ci·no·ma** an adenocarcinoma containing finger-like processes of vascular connective tissue covered by neoplastic epithelium, projecting into cysts or the cavity of glands or follicles.

**pap·il·lary ad·e·no·ma of large in·tes·tine** SYN villous adenoma.

**pap·il·lary car·ci·no·ma** a malignant neoplasm characterized by the formation of numerous irregular finger-like projections of fibrous stroma covered with a layer of neoplastic epithelial cells.

**pap·il·lary cys·tic ad·e·no·ma** an adenoma in which the lumens of the acini are frequently distended by fluid, and the neoplastic epithelial elements tend to form irregular, fingerlike projections.

**pap·il·lary ducts** [TA] the largest straight excretory ducts in the kidney medulla and papillae

whose openings form the area cribrosa; they are a continuation of the collecting tubules. SYN Bellini ducts.

**pap·il·lary hi·drad·e·no·ma** a solitary benign tumor occurring in women usually in the labia majora, cystic and papillary, and composed of epithelium resembling that of apocrine glands. SYN apocrine adenoma.

**pap·il·lary mus·cle** one of the group of myocardial bundles which terminate in the chordae tendineae which attach to the cusps of the atrioventricular valves; each has an anterior and a posterior papillary muscle; the right ventricle sometimes has a septal papillary muscle. SYN musculus papillaris [TA].

**pap·il·lary sta·sis** obsolete term for papilledema.

**pap·il·lary tu·mor** SYN papilloma.

**pa·pil·la val·la·ta** [TA] SYN vallate papilla.

**pap·il·lec·to·my** (pap-i-lek′tō-mē) surgical removal of any papilla. [papilla + G. *ektomē*, excision]

🔲 **pa·pil·le·de·ma** (pă-pil-e-dē′mă) edema of the optic disk, often due to increased intracranial pressure. See page B15. SYN choked disk. [papilla + edema]

**pa·pil·li·form** (pă-pil′i-fōrm) resembling or shaped like a papilla.

**pap·il·li·tis** (pap-i-lī′tis) **1.** optic neuritis with swelling of the optic disk. **2.** inflammation of the renal papilla. [papilla + G. *-itis*, inflammation]

△ **pa·pil·lo-** a papilla, papillary. [L. *papilla*]

**pap·il·lo·ad·e·no·cys·to·ma** (pap′i-lō-ad′ĕ-nō-sis-tō′mă) a benign epithelial neoplasm characterized by glands or glandlike structures, formation of cysts, and finger-like projections of neoplastic cells covering a core of fibrous connective tissue.

**pap·il·lo·car·ci·no·ma** (pap′i-lō-kar-si-nō′mă) **1.** a papilloma that has become malignant. **2.** a carcinoma that is characterized by papillary, finger-like projections of neoplastic cells in association with cores of fibrous stroma as a supporting structure. [papilla + G. *karkinōma*, cancer]

**pa·pil·loe·de·ma** [Br.] SEE papilledema.

**pap·il·lo·ma** (pap-i-lō′mă) a circumscribed benign epithelial tumor projecting from the surrounding surface and consisting of villous or arborescent outgrowths of fibrovascular stroma covered by neoplastic cells. SYN papillary tumor, villoma. [papilla + G. *-oma*, tumor]

**pap·il·lo·ma·to·sis** (pap′i-lō-mă-tō′sis) **1.** the development of numerous papillomas. **2.** papillary projections of the epidermis forming a microscopically undulating surface.

**pap·il·lo·ma·tous** (pap-i-lō′mă-tŭs) relating to a papilloma.

*Pa·pil·lo·ma·vi·rus* (pap-i-lō′mă-vī-rŭs) a genus of viruses containing DNA and including the papilloma and wart viruses of humans and other animals, some of which are associated with induction of carcinoma. Over 70 types are known to infect humans and are differentiated by DNA homology.

**pap·il·lo·ret·i·ni·tis** (pap′i-lō-ret-i-nī′tis) SYN neuroretinitis.

**pap·il·lot·o·my** (pă-pi-lot′ō-mē) an incision into the major duodenal papilla. [papilla + G. *tomē*, incision]

*Pa·po·va·vir·i·dae* (pă-po′vă-vir′i-dē) a family of small, antigenically distinct viruses that replicate in nuclei of infected cells; most have oncogenic properties. The family includes the genera *Papillomavirus* and *Polyomavirus*. [*pa*pilloma + *pol*yoma + *vacuolating*]

**pa•po•va•vi•rus** (pă-pō′vă-vī′rŭs) any virus of the family Papovaviridae.

**Pap•pen•hei•mer bod•ies** (pahp′ĕn-hīm-ĕr) phagosomes, containing ferruginous granules, found in red blood cells in diseases such as sideroblastic anemia, hemolytic anemia, and sickle cell disease.

**PA pro•jec•tion** a radiographic study in which x-rays travel from posterior to anterior. SYN posteroanterior projection.

**Pap smear** (pap) a smear of vaginal or cervical cells obtained for cytological study.

**PAP tech•nique** (pap) an unlabeled antibody peroxidase method which reacts both with the rabbit antihorseradish peroxidase antibody and free horseradish peroxidase to form a soluble complex of peroxidase antiperoxidase or PAP; a uniquely sensitive immunohistochemical method that is applicable to paraffin-embedded tissues.

**Pap test** (pap) microscopic examination of cells exfoliated or scraped from a mucosal surface after staining with Papanicolaou stain; used especially for detection of cancer of the uterine cervix.

**pap•u•lar** (pap′yu-lăr) relating to papules.

**pap•u•lar mu•ci•no•sis** SYN lichen myxedematosus.

**pap•u•lar tu•ber•cu•lid** SYN lichen scrofulosorum.

**pap•u•lar ur•ti•car•ia** a sensitivity reaction to insect bites, especially human and pet fleas, seen mostly in young children as wheals followed by papules on exposed areas. SYN lichen urticatus.

**pap•u•la•tion** (pap-yu-lā′shŭn) the formation of papules.

**pap•ule** (pap′yul) a small, circumscribed, solid elevation on the skin. See page B4. [L. *papula*, pimple]

**pap•u•lo-** papule. [L. *papula*, papule]

**pap•u•lo•er•y•them•a•tous** (pap′yu-lō-er-i-them′ă-tŭs) denoting an eruption of papules on an erythematous surface.

**pap•u•lo•ne•crot•ic tu•ber•cu•lid** dusky-red papules followed by crusting and ulceration primarily on the extremities and predominantly in young adults with a deep focus of tuberculosis or with a history of preceding infection.

**pap•u•lo•pus•tu•lar** (pap′yu-lō-pŭs′tyu-lăr) denoting an eruption composed of papules and pustules.

**pa•pu•lo•sis** (pap-yu-lō′sis) the occurrence of numerous widespread papules.

**pap•u•lo•squa•mous** (pap′yu-lō-skwä′mŭs) denoting an eruption composed of both papules and scales. [papulo- + L. *squamosus*, scaly (squamous)]

**pap•u•lo•ve•sic•u•lar** (pap′yu-lō-ve-sik′yu-lăr) denoting an eruption composed of papules and vesicles.

**PAPVR** partial anomalous pulmonary venous return.

**pap•y•ra•ceous** (pap-i-rā′shŭs) like parchment or paper. [L. *papyraceus*, made of *papyrus*]

**par** a pair; specifically a pair of cranial nerves, e.g., par nonum, ninth pair, glossopharyngeal; par vagum, the vagus or tenth pair. [L. equal]

**para** (par′ă) a woman who has given birth to one or more infants. Para followed by a roman nu-

meral or preceded by a Latin prefix (primi-, secundi-, terti-, quadri-, etc.) designates the number of times a pregnancy has culminated in a single or multiple birth; e.g., **para I**, primipara; a woman who has given birth for the first time; **para II**, secundipara; a woman who has given birth for the second time to one or more infants. Cf. gravida. [L. *pario*, to bring forth]

**para- 1.** prefix denoting a departure from the normal. **2.** prefix denoting involvement of two like parts or a pair. **3.** adjacent, alongside, near, etc. **4.** CHEMISTRY an italicized prefix denoting two substitutions in the benzene ring arranged symmetrically, i.e., linked to opposite carbon atoms in the ring. For words beginning with *para-* or *p-*, see the specific name. [G. alongside of, near]

**par•a•a•or•tic bod•ies** small masses of chromaffin tissue found near the sympathetic ganglia along the aorta; they are more prominent during fetal life. The chromaffin cells secrete noradrenalin; chemoreceptive endings monitor levels of blood gases. SYN corpora para-aortica [TA], Zuckerkandl bodies.

**par•a•bal•lism** (par-ă-bal′izm) severe jerking movements of both legs. [para- + G. *ballismos*, jumping about]

**par•a•ba•sal bod•y** part of the giant mitochondrion of certain parasitic flagellates. The parabasal body plus the basal body were previously thought to comprise a kinetoplast, but kinetoplast is now restricted to part of the DNA giant mitochondrion.

**par•a•bi•o•sis** (par-ă-bī-ō′sis) **1.** fusion of whole eggs or embryos, as occurs in conjoined twins. **2.** surgical joining of the vascular systems of two organisms. [para- + G. *biōsis*, life]

**par•a•bi•ot•ic** (par-ă-bī-ot′ik) relating to, or characterized by, parabiosis.

**par•a•bu•lia** (par-ă-boo′lē-ă) perversion of volition or will in which one impulse is checked and replaced by another. [para- + G. *boulē*, will]

**par•a•ca•se•in** (par-ă-kā′sē-in) the compound produced by the action of rennin upon κ-casein, which precipitates with calcium ion as the insoluble curd.

**par•a•ce•nes•the•sia** (par′ă-sē-nes-thē′zē-ă) deterioration in one's sense of bodily well-being, i.e., of the normal functioning of one's organs. [para- + G. *koinos*, common, + *aisthēsis*, feeling]

**par•a•cen•te•sis** (par′ă-sen-tē′sis) the passage into a cavity of a trocar and cannula, needle, or other hollow instrument for the purpose of removing fluid; variously designated according to the cavity punctured. SYN tapping (2). [G. *parakentēsis*, a tapping for dropsy, fr. *para*, beside, + *kentēsis*, puncture]

**par•a•cen•tet•ic** (par-ă-sen-tet′ik) relating to paracentesis.

**par•a•cen•tral fis•sure** a curved fissure (sulcus) on the medial surface of the cerebral hemisphere, bounding the paracentral gyrus and separating it from the precuneus and the cingulate gyrus.

**par•a•cer•vi•cal** (par-ă-ser′vi-kăl) connective tissue adjacent to the uterine cervix.

**par•a•cer•vix** (par-ă-ser′viks) the connective tissue of the pelvic floor extending from the fibrous subserous coat of the cervix of the uterus laterally between the layers of the broad ligament.

**par•a•chol•er•a** (par-ă-kol′er-ă) a disease resembling Asiatic cholera but due to a vibrio specifically different from *Vibrio cholerae*.

**par·a·chor·dal** (par-ă-kōr′dăl) alongside the anterior portion of the notochord in the embryo; designating the bilateral cartilaginous bars that enter into the formation of the base of the skull. [para- + G. *chordē*, cord]

**par·a·chro·ma, par·a·chro·ma·to·sis** (par-ă-krō′mă, par-ă-krō-mă-tō′sis) abnormal coloration of the skin. [para- + G. *chrōma*, color]

**par·a·chute mi·tral valve** congenital deformity of the mitral valve characterized by the presence of a single papillary muscle from which the chordae tendineae of both valve leaflets divide; the condition often produces a stenosis as the combined result of the tugging action of the chordae tendineae on, and the subsequent narrowing between, the leaflets.

**par·a·chute re·flex** SYN startle reflex (1).

**par·a·ci·ca·tri·ci·al em·phy·se·ma** dilated terminal air spaces adjacent to a scar in the lung.

**par·a·coc·cid·i·o·i·dal gran·u·lo·ma** SYN paracoccidioidomycosis.

***Par·a·coc·cid·i·oi·des bra·sil·i·en·sis*** (par-ă-kok-sid-ē-oy′dēz bră-sil-ē-en′sis) a dimorphic fungus that causes paracoccidioidomycosis.

**par·a·coc·cid·i·oi·din** (par′ă-kok-sid-ē-oy′din) antigen prepared from the fungus, *Paracoccidioides brasiliensis;* used for demonstrating present or past infection and identifying endemic areas.

**par·a·coc·cid·i·oi·do·my·co·sis** (par′ă-kok-sid-ē-oy′dō-mī-kō′sis) a chronic mycosis characterized by primary pulmonary lesions with dissemination to many visceral organs, conspicuous ulcerative granulomas of the buccal and nasal mucosa with extensions to the skin, and generalized lymphangitis; caused by *Paracoccidioides brasiliensis.* SYN Almeida disease, Lutz-Splendore-Almeida disease, paracoccidioidal granuloma, South American blastomycosis.

**par·a·co·li·tis** (par′ă-kō-lī′tis) inflammation of the peritoneal coat of the colon.

**par·a·cone** (par′ă-kōn) **1.** the mesiobuccal cusp of human upper molars. **2.** a cusp arising from the protocone in the evolution of the molars. Thought to be the first cusp to arise rather than the protocone. [para- + G. *kōnos*, cone]

**par·a·con·id** (par-ă-kon′id) a cusp derived from the protoconid in the evolution of the molars; in humans it is very small or   nonexistent. [para-cone + -id (2)]

**par·a·crine** (par′ă-krin) relating to a kind of hormone function in which the effects of the hormone are restricted to the local environment. Cf. endocrine. [para- + G. *krinō*, to separate]

**par·a·cu·sis, par·a·cu·sia** (par′ă-koo′sis, par′ă-koo′sē-ă) **1.** impaired hearing. **2.** auditory illusions or hallucinations. [para- + G. *akousis*, hearing]

**par·a·cys·tic** (par-ă-sis′tik) alongside or near a bladder, specifically the urinary bladder. [para- + G. *kystis*, bladder]

**par·a·cys·ti·tis** (par′ă-sis-tī′tis) inflammation of the connective tissue and other structures about the urinary bladder. [para- + G. *kystis*, bladder, + -*itis*, inflammation]

**par·a·did·y·mis, pl. par·a·did·y·mi·des** (par′ă-did′i-mis, par′ă-di-dim′i-dēz) a small body sometimes attached to the front of the lower part of the spermatic cord above the head of the epididymis; the remnants of tubules of the mesonephros. SYN parepididymis. [para- + G. *didymos*, twin, in pl. *didymoi*, testes]

**par·a·dip·sia** (par-ă-dip′sē-ă) an abnormal desire to consume fluids, without regard to bodily need. [para- + G. *dipsa*, thirst]

**par·a·dox** (par′ă-doks) that which is apparently, though not actually, inconsistent with or opposed to the known facts in any case. [G. *paradoxos*, incredible, beyond belief, fr. *doxa*, belief]

**par·a·dox·i·cal con·trac·tion** a tonic contraction of the anterior tibial muscles when a sudden passive dorsal flexion of the foot is made.

**par·a·dox·i·cal di·a·phragm phe·nom·e·non** in pyopneumothorax, hydropneumothorax, and some cases of injury, the diaphragm on the affected side rises during inspiration and falls during expiration.

**par·a·dox·ical ex·ten·sor re·flex** SYN Babinski sign (1).

**par·a·dox·i·cal pulse** a reversal of the normal variation in the pulse volume with respiration, the pulse becoming weaker with inspiration and stronger with expiration; characteristic of cardiac tamponade and rare in constrictive pericarditis. So called because these changes are independent of changes in the cardiac rate as measured directly or by electrocardiogram. SYN pulsus paradoxus.

**par·a·dox·i·cal re·flex** any reflex in which the usual response is reversed or does not conform to the pattern characteristic of the particular reflex.

**par·a·dox·i·cal res·pi·ra·tion** deflation of the lung during inspiration and inflation of the lung during the phase of expiration; seen in the lung on the side of an open pneumothorax.

**par·a·dox·i·cal sleep** a deep sleep, with a brain wave pattern more like that of waking states than of other states of sleep, which occurs during rapid eye movement sleep.

**par·a·dox·i·cal vo·cal cord move·ment** adduction of the vocal cords on inspiration, resulting in stridor and airway obstruction.

**par·a·dox·ic pulse** an exaggeration of the normal variation in the systemic arterial pulse volume with respiration, becoming weaker with inspiration and stronger with expiration; characteristic of cardiac tamponade, rare in constrictive pericarditis; so called because these changes are independent of changes in the cardiac rate as measured directly or by electrocardiogram.

**par·a·dox·ic pu·pil·lary re·flex** constriction of pupils in darkness, the reverse of that expected.

**par·af·fi·no·ma** (par′ă-fi-nō′mă) a tumefaction, usually a granuloma, caused by the prosthetic or therapeutic injection of paraffin into the tissues. SEE ALSO lipogranuloma.

**par·a·fol·lic·u·lar cells** cells present between follicles or interspersed among follicular cells; they are rich in mitochondria and are believed to be the source of thyrocalcitonin.

**par·a·func·tion** (par′ă-fŭngk-shŭn) **1.** abnormal or disordered function. **2.** DENTISTRY movements of the mandible that are outside   normal function, e.g., bruxism. [para- + function]

**par·a·gan·glia** (par-ă-gang′glē-ă) plural of paraganglion.

**par·a·gan·gli·o·ma** (par′ă-gang-glē-ō′mă) a neoplasm usually derived from the chromoreceptor tissue of a paraganglion, such as the carotid body, or the medulla of the adrenal gland; the latter is usually termed a chromaffinoma or pheochromocytoma.

**par·a·gan·gli·on, pl. par·a·gan·glia** (par-ă-gang′glē-on, par-ă-gang′glē-ă) a small, roundish body containing chromaffin cells; a number of such bodies may be found retroperitoneally near the aorta and in organs such as the kidney, liver, heart, and gonads. SYN chromaffin body.

**par·a·geu·sia** (par-ă-goo′sē-ă) disordered or abnormal sense of taste. [para- + G. *geusis,* taste]

**par·a·geu·sic** (par-ă-goo′sik) relating to parageusia.

**par·a·glot·tic space** the space on each side of the glottis bounded laterally by the perichondrium of the thyroid cartilage and the cricothyroid membrane and posteriorly by the mucous membrane of the pyriform sinus; anterosuperiorly it extends into the preepiglottic space. It is an important route of transglottic and extralaryngeal spread of carcinoma of the larynx.

*Par·a·go·ni·mus* **gran·u·lo·ma** lesions caused by adult worms and eggs of the lung fluke trapped in the pulmonary parenchyma.

**par·a·gram·ma·tism** (par-ă-gram′ă-tizm) speech that is fluent but consists mainly of semantic and phonetic errors (paraphasias), so that the grammatical structure and meaning cannot be discerned. This disorder is typical of severe receptive aphasia. SYN jargon aphasia.

**par·a·graph·ia** (par-ă-graf′ē-ă) **1.** loss of the power of writing from dictation, although the words are heard and comprehended. **2.** writing one word when another is intended. [para- + G. *graphō,* to write]

**par·a·hip·po·cam·pal gy·rus** a long convolution on the medial surface of the temporal lobe, forming the lower part of the fornicate gyrus, extending from behind the splenium corporis callosi forward along the dentate gyrus of the hippocampus from which it is demarcated by the hippocampal fissure. The anterior extreme of the gyrus curves back upon itself, forming the uncus, the major location of the olfactory cortex.

**par·a·hor·mone** (par-ă-hōr′mōn) a substance, product of ordinary metabolism, not produced for a specific purpose, that acts like a hormone in modifying the activity of some distant organ; e.g., the action of carbon dioxide on the control of breathing.

**par·a·in·flu·en·za vi·rus·es** viruses of the genus *Paramyxovirus,* of four types: type 1 (hemadsorption virus type 2), which includes sendai virus, causes acute laryngotracheitis in children and occasionally adults; type 2 (croup-associated virus) is associated especially with acute laryngotracheitis or croup in young children and minor upper respiratory infections in adults; type 3 (hemadsorption virus type 1; shipping fever virus) has been isolated from small children with pharyngitis, bronchiolitis, and pneumonia, and causes occasional respiratory infection in adults; type 4 has been isolated from a very few children with minor respiratory illness.

**par·a·ker·a·to·sis** (par′-ker-ă-tō′sis) retention of nuclei in the cells of the stratum corneum of the epidermis, observed in many scaling dermatoses such as psoriasis and subacute or chronic dermatitis.

**par·a·ki·ne·sia, par·a·ki·ne·sis** (par′ă-ki-nē′zē-ă, par′ă-ki-nē′sis) any motor abnormality. [para- + G. *kinēsis,* movement]

**par·a·la·lia** (par-ă-lā′lē-ă) any speech defect; especially one in which one letter is habitually substituted for another. [para- + G. *lalia,* talking]

**par·a·lex·ia** (par-ă-lek′sē-ă) misapprehension of written or printed words, other meaningless words being substituted for them in reading. [para- + G. *lexis,* speech]

**par·al·ge·sia** (par-al-jē′zē-ă) painful paresthesia; any disorder or abnormality of the sense of pain. [para- + G. *algēsis,* the sense of pain]

**par·al·lac·tic** (par-ă-lak′tik) relating to a parallax.

**par·al·lax** (par′ă-laks) the apparent displacement of an object that follows a change in the position from which it is viewed. [G. alternately, fr. *par-allassō,* to make alternate, fr. *allos,* other]

**par·al·lax test** measurement of the deviation in strabismus by the alternate cover test combined with neutralization of the deviation using prisms.

**par·al·ler·gic** (par-ă-ler′jik) denoting an allergic state in which the body becomes predisposed to nonspecific stimuli following original sensitization with a specific allergen.

**par·a·lo·gia, pa·ral·o·gism, pa·ral·o·gy** (par-ă-lō′jē-ă, pă-ral′ō-jizm, pă-ral′ō-jē) false reasoning, involving self-deception. [G. *paralogia,* a fallacy, fr. *para,* beside, + *logos,* reason]

**pa·ral·y·sis,** pl. **pa·ral·y·ses** (pă-ral′i-sis, pă-ral′i-sēz) **1.** loss of power of voluntary movement in a muscle through injury to or disease of its nerve supply. **2.** loss of any function, as sensation, secretion, or mental ability. [G. fr. para- + *lysis,* a loosening]

**par·a·lyt·ic** (par-ă-lit′ik) relating to paralysis or suffering from paralysis.

**par·a·lyt·ic de·men·tia** dementia and paralysis resulting from a chronic syphilitic meningoencephalitis.

**par·a·lyt·ic il·e·us** SYN adynamic ileus.

**par·a·ly·zant** (pă-ral′i-zant) **1.** causing paralysis. **2.** any agent, such as curare, that causes paralysis.

**par·a·lyze** (par′ă-līz) to render incapable of movement.

*Par·a·me·ci·um* (par-ă-mē′shē-ŭm, par-ă-mē′sē-ŭm) an abundant genus of freshwater holotrichous ciliates, characteristically slipper-shaped and often large enough to be visible to the naked eye; commonly used for genetic and other studies. [G. *paramēkēs,* rather long, fr. *mēkos,* length]

**par·a·med·ic** SYN prehospital provider.

**par·a·med·i·cal** (par-ă-med′i-kăl) **1.** related to the medical profession in an adjunctive capacity, e.g., denoting allied health fields such as physical therapy, speech pathology, etc. **2.** relating to a paramedic.

**par·a·me·nia** (par-ă-mē′nē-ă) any disorder or irregularity of menstruation. [para- + G. *mēn,* month]

**par·a·mes·o·neph·ric duct** either of the two paired embryonic tubes extending along the mesonephros roughly parallel to the mesonephric duct and emptying into the cloaca; in the female, the upper parts of the ducts form the uterine tubes, while the lower parts fuse to form the uterus and part of the vagina; in the male, vestiges of the ducts form the prostatic utricle (vagina masculina) and the appendix testis. SYN Müller duct, müllerian duct.

**pa·ram·e·ter** (pă-ram′ĕ-ter) One of many dimensions or ways of measuring or describing an object or evaluating a subject: **1.** MATHEMATICS an arbitrary constant that can possess different values, each value defining other expressions. **2.**

STATISTICS a term used to define a characteristic of a population, in contrast to a sample from that population. **3.** PSYCHOANALYSIS any tactic, other than interpretation, used by the analyst to further the patient's progress. [para- + G. *metron*, measure]

**par·a·me·tri·al** (par-ă-mē′trē-ăl) pertaining to the parametrium.

**par·a·met·ric** (par-ă-met′rik) relating to the parametrium, or structures immediately adjacent to the uterus.

**par·a·me·trit·ic** (par′ă-me-trit′ik) relating to parametritis.

**par·a·me·tri·tis** (par′ă-me-trī′tis) inflammation of the tissue adjacent to the uterus, particularly in the broad ligament. SYN pelvic cellulitis. [parametrium + G. -*itis*, inflammation]

**par·a·me·tri·um**, pl. **par·a·me·tria** (par-ă-mē′ trē-ŭm, par-ă-mē′trē-ă) [TA] the connective tissue of the pelvic floor extending from the fibrous subserous coat of the supracervical portion of the uterus laterally between the layers of the broad ligament. [para- + G. *mētra*, uterus]

**par·a·mim·ia** (par-ă-mim′ē-ă) the use of gestures unsuited to the words which they accompany. [para- + G. *mimia*, imitation]

**par·am·ne·sia** (par-am-nē′zē-ă) false recollection, as of events that have never occurred. [para- + G. *amnēsia*, forgetfulness]

**par·am·y·loi·do·sis** (par-am′ĭ-loy-dō′sis) **1.** deposition in tissues of an amyloidlike protein in primary amyloidosis or in atypical amyloidosis of multiple myeloma. **2.** various hereditary amyloidoses (Portuguese amyloidosis, Indiana amyloidosis) characterized by progressive hypertrophic polyneuritis with sensory changes, ataxia, paresis, and muscle atrophy due to amyloid deposits in peripheral and visceral nerves.

**par·a·my·o·to·nia** (par′ă-mī-ō-tō′nē-ă) an atypical form of myotonia.

**Par·a·myx·o·vir·i·dae** (par-ă-mik′sō-vir′i-dē) a family of RNA-containing viruses. Three genera are recognized: *Paramyxovirus, Morbillivirus,* and *Pneumovirus,* all of which cause cell fusion and produce cytoplasmic eosinophilic inclusions.

***Par·a·myx·o·vi·rus*** (par-ă-miks′ō-vī-rŭs) a genus of viruses that includes Newcastle disease, mumps, and parainfluenza viruses (types 1 to 4).

**par·a·na·sal si·nus·es** the paired air-filled cavities in the bones of the face lined by mucous membrane continuous with that of the nasal cavity; these sinuses are the frontal, sphenoidal, maxillary, and ethmoidal.

**par·a·ne·o·pla·sia** (par′ă-nē-ō-plā′zē-ă) hormonal, neurological, hematological, and other clinical and biochemical disturbances associated with malignant neoplasms but not directly related to invasion by the primary tumor or its metastases.

**par·a·ne·o·plas·tic** (par′ă-nē-ō-plas′tik) relating to or characteristic of paraneoplasia.

**par·a·ne·o·plas·tic en·ceph·a·lo·my·e·lop·a·thy** an encephalomyelopathy as a remote effect of carcinoma, most often oat cell carcinoma of the lung.

**par·a·ne·o·plas·tic pem·phi·gus** painful mucosal erosions and polymorphous skin eruptions with biopsy findings resembling pemphigus vulgaris, associated with neoplasm and serum antibodies reactive with intercellular substance of all epithelia; usually rapidly fatal.

**par·a·ne·o·plas·tic syn·drome** a syndrome directly resulting from a malignant neoplasm, but not resulting from the presence of tumor cells in the affected parts.

**par·a·neph·ric** (par-ă-nef′rik) **1.** relating to the paranephros. **2.** SYN pararenal.

**par·a·neph·ros**, pl. **par·a·neph·roi** (par-ă-nef′ ros, par-ă-nef′roy) SYN suprarenal gland. [para- + G. *nephros*, kidney]

**par·a·noia** (par-ă-noy′ă) a disorder characterized by the presence of systematized delusions, often of a persecutory character involving being followed, poisoned, or harmed by other means, in an otherwise intact personality. SEE ALSO paranoid personality. [G. derangement, madness, fr. para- + *noeō*, to think]

**par·a·noid** (par′ă-noyd) **1.** relating to or characterized by paranoia. **2.** having delusions of persecution.

**par·a·noid per·son·al·i·ty** a personality disorder characterized by hypersensitivity, rigidity, unwarranted suspicion, jealousy, and a tendency to blame others and ascribe evil motives to them; though neither a neurosis nor psychosis, it interferes with the individual's ability to maintain interpersonal relationships.

**par·a·noid schiz·o·phre·nia** schizophrenia characterized predominantly by delusions of persecution and megalomania.

**par·a·no·mia** (par-ă-nō′mē-ă) a form of aphasia in which objects are called by the wrong names. [para- + G. *onoma*, name]

**par·a·nu·cle·ar** (par-ă-noo′klē-ăr) **1.** SYN paranucleate. **2.** outside, but near the nucleus.

**par·a·nu·cle·ate** (par′ă-noo′klē-āt) relating to or having a paranucleus. SYN paranuclear (1).

**par·a·nu·cle·us** (par-ă-noo′klē-ŭs) an accessory nucleus or small mass of chromatin lying outside, though near, the nucleus.

**par·a·op·er·a·tive** (par-ă-op′er-ă-tiv) SYN perioperative.

**par·a·pa·re·sis** (par-ă-pă-rē′sis) weakness affecting the lower extremities. [para- + paresis]

**par·a·pa·ret·ic** (par′ă-pă-ret′ik) **1.** relating to paraparesis. **2.** a person with paraparesis.

**par·a·per·i·to·ne·al her·nia** a vesical hernia in which only a part of the protruded organ is covered by the peritoneum of the sac.

**par·a·pha·ryn·ge·al ab·scess** an abscess lying lateral to the pharynx.

**par·a·pha·sia** (par-ă-fā′zē-ă) a symptom of aphasia in which speech is fluent but incorrect due to word and sound substitutions. SEE ALSO paragrammatism, receptive aphasia. SYN jargon (2). [para- + G. *phasis*, speech]

**par·a·pha·sic** (par-ă-fā′sik) relating to paraphasia.

**pa·ra·phia** (pa-rā′fē-ă) any disorder of the sense of touch. SYN parapsia, pseudesthesia (1). [para- + G. *haphē*, touch]

**par·a·phil·ia** (par-ă-fil′ē-ă) a mental disorder characterized by socially proscribed sexual practices. [para- + G. *philos*, loving]

**par·a·phi·mo·sis** (par′ă-fī-mō′sis) painful constriction of the glans penis by a phimotic foreskin, which has been retracted behind the corona. [para- + G. phimosis]

**par·a·plec·tic** (par-ă-plek′tik) SYN paraplegic. [G. *paraplēktikos*, paralyzed]

**par·a·ple·gia** (par-ă-plē′jē-ă) paralysis of both lower extremities and, generally, the lower trunk. [para- + *plēgē*, a stroke]

**par·a·ple·gic** (par-ă-plē′jik) relating to or suffering from paraplegia. SYN paraplectic.

**par·a·prax·ia** (par-ă-prak′sē-ă) a condition analogous to paraphasia and paragraphia in which there is a defective performance of purposive acts; e.g., slips of the tongue, or mislaying of objects. [para- + G. *praxis,* a doing]

**par·a·pro·tein** (par-a-prō′tēn) **1.** a monoclonal immunoglobulin of the blood plasma, produced by a clone of plasma cells arising from the abnormal rapid multiplication of a single cell. Paraprotein in serum may be seen in a variety of malignant, benign, or nonneoplastic diseases. **2.** SYN monoclonal immunoglobulin. [para + protein, fr. G. *protos,* first]

**par·a·pro·tein·ae·mia [Br.]** SEE paraproteinemia.

**par·a·pro·tein·e·mia** (par′ă-prō-tēn-ē′mē-ă) the presence of abnormal proteins in the blood.

**pa·rap·sia** (pă-rap′sē-ă) SYN paraphia. [para- + G. *hapsis,* touch]

**par·a·pso·ri·a·sis** (par′ă-sō-rī′ă-sis) a heterogenous group of skin disorders including pityriasis lichenoides and small and large plaque variants.

**par·a·psy·chol·o·gy** (par′ă-sī-kol′ō-jē) the study of extrasensory perception, such as thought transference (telepathy) and clairvoyance.

**par·a·re·flex·ia** (par′ă-rē-flek′sē-ă) a condition characterized by abnormal reflexes.

**par·a·re·nal** (par-ă-rē′năl) near or adjacent to the kidneys. SYN paranephric (2).

**par·a·ro·san·i·lin** (par′ă-rō-san′i-lin) [CI 42500] a biologic stain used in Schiff reagent to detect cellular DNA (Feulgen stain), mucopolysaccharides (PAS stain), and proteins (ninhydrin-Schiff stain).

**par·a·rhyth·mia** (par-ă-ridh′mē-ă) a cardiac dysrhythmia in which two independent rhythms coexist, but not as a result of A-V block; pararrhythmia thus includes parasystole and A-V dissociation (2), but not complete A-V block. [para- + G. *rhythmos,* rhythm]

**par·a·si·noi·dal** (par′ă-sī-noy′dăl) near a sinus, particularly a cerebral sinus.

**par·a·site** (par′ă-sīt) **1.** an organism that lives on or in another and draws its nourishment therefrom. **2.** in the case of a fetal inclusion or conjoined twins, the usually incomplete twin that derives its support from the more nearly normal autosite. [G. *parasitos,* a guest, fr. *para,* beside, + *sitos,* food]

**par·a·si·te·mia** (păr′ă-sī-tē′mē-ă) the presence of parasites in the circulating blood; used especially with reference to malarial and other protozoan forms, and microfilariae.

**par·a·sit·ic** (par-ă-sit′ik) **1.** relating to or of the nature of a parasite. **2.** denoting organisms that normally grow only in or on the living body of a host.

**par·a·sit·ic cyst** a cyst formed by the larva of a metazoan parasite, such as a hydatid or trichinal cyst.

**par·a·sit·i·ci·dal** (par′ă-sit-i-sī′dăl) destructive to parasites.

**par·a·sit·i·cide** (par-ă-sit′i-sīd) an agent that destroys parasites. [parasite + L. *caedo,* to kill]

**par·a·sit·ic mel·a·no·der·ma** excoriations and melanoderma caused by scratching the bites of the body louse, *Pediculus corporis.* SYN vagabond's disease, vagrant's disease.

**par·a·sit·ism** (par′ă-si-tizm) a symbiotic relationship in which one species (the parasite) benefits at the expense of the other (the host). Cf. mutualism, commensalism, symbiosis, metabiosis.

**par·a·si·tize** (par′ă-si-tīz) to invade as a parasite.

**par·a·si·to·gen·ic** (par′ă-sī-tō-jen′ik) **1.** caused by certain parasites. **2.** favoring parasitism. [parasite + G. *-gen,* producing]

**par·a·si·tol·o·gist** (par′ă-sī-tol′ō-jist) one who specializes in the science of parasitology.

**par·a·si·tol·o·gy** (par′ă-sī-tol′ō-jē) the branch of biology and of medicine concerned with all aspects of parasitism. [parasite + G. *logos,* study]

**par·a·sit·o·sis** (par′ă-sī-tō′sis) infestation or infection with parasites.

**par·a·si·to·tro·pic** (par′ă-sī-tō-trop′ik) pertaining to or characterized by parasitotropism.

**par·a·si·tot·ro·pism** (par′ă-sī-tot′rō-pizm) the special affinity of particular drugs or other agents for parasites rather than for their hosts, including microparasites that infect a larger parasite. Cf. organotropism. [parasite + G. *tropē,* a turning]

**par·a·som·nia** (par-ă-som′nē-ă) any dysfunction associated with sleep, e.g., somnambulism, pavor nocturnus, enuresis, or nocturnal seizures.

**par·a·sta·sis** (par-ă-stā′sis) **1.** a reciprocal relationship among causal mechanisms that can compensate for, or mask defects in, each other. **2.** GENETICS a relationship between non-alleles (classified by some as a form of epistasis). [G. standing shoulder to shoulder]

**par·a·ster·nal her·nia** SYN Morgagni foramen hernia.

**par·a·sym·pa·thet·ic** (par-ă-sim-pa-thet′ik) pertaining to a division of the autonomic nervous system. SEE autonomic division of nervous system.

**par·a·sym·pa·thet·ic gan·glia** those ganglia of the autonomic nervous system composed of cholinergic neurons receiving afferent fibers from preganglionic visceral motor neurons in either the brainstem or the middle sacral spinal segments (S2 to S4). SEE ALSO autonomic division of nervous system.

**par·a·sym·pa·thet·ic nerve** one of the nerves of the parasympathetic nervous system.

**par·a·sym·pa·tho·lyt·ic** (par-ă-sim′pă-thō-lit′ik) relating to an agent that annuls or antagonizes the effects of the parasympathetic nervous system; e.g., atropine.

**par·a·sym·pa·tho·mi·met·ic** (par-ă-sim′pă-thō-mi-met′ik) relating to drugs or chemicals having an action resembling that caused by stimulation of the parasympathetic nervous system. SEE ALSO cholinomimetic. [para- + G. *sympatheia,* sympathy, + *mimētikos,* imitative]

**par·a·sy·nap·sis** (par′ă-si-nap′sis) union of chromosomes side to side in the process of reduction. [para- + G. *synapsis,* a connection, junction]

**par·a·sy·no·vi·tis** (par′ă-si-nō-vī′tis) inflammation of the tissues immediately adjacent to a joint. [para- + synovitis]

**par·a·sys·to·le** (par-ă-sis′tō-lē) a second automatic rhythm existing simultaneously with normal sinus or other dominant rhythm, the parasystolic center being protected from the dominant rhythm's impulses so that its basic rhythm is undisturbed, although it may be manifest in the ECG only at various multiples of its basic periodicity. [para- + G. *systolē,* a contracting]

**par·a·tax·ic dis·tor·tion** an attitude toward another person based on a distorted evaluation, usually because of too close an identification of that person with emotionally significant figures in the patient's past life.

**par•a•ten•on** (par-ă-ten′on) the tissue, fatty or synovial, between a tendon and its sheath. [para- + G. *tenōn,* tendon]

**par•a•thy•roid** (par-ă-thī′royd) **1.** adjacent to the thyroid gland. **2.** SYN parathyroid gland.

**par•a•thy•roid•ec•to•my** (pa′ră-thī-roy-dek′to-mē) excision of the parathyroid glands. [parathyroid + G. *ektomē,* excision]

**par•a•thy•roid gland** one of two small paired endocrine glands, superior and inferior, usually found embedded in the connective tissue capsule on the posterior surface of the thyroid gland; they secrete parathyroid hormone, which regulates the metabolism of calcium and phosphorus. The parenchyma is composed of chief and oxyphilic cells arranged in anastomosing cords. Inadvertent removal of all parathyroid glands, as during thyroidectomy, produces tetany and death. SYN parathyroid (2).

**par•a•thy•roid hor•mone** a peptide hormone formed by the parathyroid glands; it maintains the serum calcium level by promoting intestinal absorption and renal tubular reabsorption of calcium, and release of calcium from bone to extracellular fluid.

**par•a•thy•roid hor•mone-re•late•d pep•tide (PTHrP)** a hormone that can be produced by tumors, especially of the squamous cell type; massive overproduction can lead to hypercalcemia and other manifestations of hyperparathyroidism. PTHrP exerts a biologic action similar to that of parathyroid hormone (PTH), acting via the same receptor, which is expressed in many tissues but most abundantly in kidney, bone, and growth plate cartilage. It apparently has significant actions during development, but it is uncertain whether PTHrP circulates at all or has any function in normal human adults. The structure of the gene for human PTHrP is more complex than that of PTH, and varying molecular forms exist, including proteins of 141, 139, and 173 amino acids, which share a significant homology with parathyroid hormone.

**par•a•thy•roid tet•a•ny** tetany due to lack of parathyroid function, spontaneous or following excision of the parathyroid glands.

**par•a•thy•ro•tro•pic, par•a•thy•ro•tro•phic** (par′ă-thī-rō-trōp′ik, par′ă-thī-rō-trof′ik) influencing the growth or activity of the parathyroid glands. [parathyroid + G. *tropē,* a turning; *trophē,* nourishment]

**par•a•tope** (par′a-tōp) that part of an antibody molecule composed of the variable regions of both the light and heavy chains that combine with the antigen. SYN antibody-combining site. [para- + -tope]

**par•a•ty•phoid fe•ver, par•a•ty•phoid** (par-ă-tī′foyd) an acute infectious disease with symptoms and lesions resembling those of typhoid fever, though milder in character; associated with the presence of the paratyphoid organism of which at least three varieties (types A, B, and C) have been described.

**par•a•um•bil•i•cal veins** arise from cutaneous veins around the umbilicus running along the round ligament of the liver, and terminating as accessory portal veins in its substance; they constitute a portocaval anastomosis and are subject

to varicosity during portal hypertension; varicose paraumbilical veins form the "caput medusae."

**par•a•u•re•thral ducts** inconstant ducts along the side of the female urethra that convey the mucoid secretion of Skene glands to the vestibule.

**par•a•vag•i•ni•tis** (par′ă-vaj-i-nī′tis) inflammation of the connective tissue alongside the vagina.

**par•a•ver•te•bral gan•glia** SYN ganglia of sympathetic trunk.

**par•ax•i•al** (par-ak′sē-ăl) by the side of the axis of any body or part.

**par•ax•on** (par-ak′son) a collateral branch of an axon. [para- + G. *axōn,* axis]

**pa•ren•chy•ma** (pă-reng′ki-mă) **1.** the distinguishing or specific cells of a gland or organ, contained in and supported by the connective tissue framework, or stroma. **2.** the endoplasm of a protozoan cell. [G. anything poured in beside, fr. *parencheō,* to pour in beside]

**pa•ren•chy•ma•ti•tis** (pă-reng′ki-mă-tī′tis) inflammation of the parenchyma or differentiated substance of a gland or organ.

**par•en•chym•a•tous** (par′eng-kim′ă-tŭs) relating to the parenchyma.

**par•en•chym•a•tous de•gen•er•a•tion** SYN cloudy swelling.

**par•en•chym•a•tous goi•ter** a form of goiter in which there is a great increase in the follicles with proliferation of the epithelium. SYN follicular goiter.

**par•en•chym•a•tous hem•or•rhage** bleeding into the substance of an organ.

**par•en•chym•a•tous neu•ri•tis** inflammation of the nervous substance proper, the axons, and myelin.

**pa•ren•tal gen•er•a•tion (P₁)** the parents of a mating, commonly experimental, involving contrasting genotypes; the original mating of a genetic experiment; parents of the $F_1$ generation.

**par•ent cyst** SYN mother cyst.

**par•en•ter•al** (pă-ren′ter-ăl) by some other means than through the gastrointestinal tract; referring particularly to the introduction of substances into an organism by intravenous, subcutaneous, intramuscular, or intramedullary injection. [para- + G. *enteron,* intestine]

**par•en•ter•ic fe•ver** one of a group of fevers clinically resembling typhoid and paratyphoid A and B, but caused by bacteria differing specifically from those of either of these diseases.

**Pa•ren•ti-Frac•ca•ro syn•drome** (pah-ren′tē-frah-kah′rō) SYN achondrogenesis type IB.

**par•ep•i•did•y•mis** (par′ep′i-did′i-mis) SYN paradidymis.

**pa•re•sis** (pă-rē′sis) **1.** partial or incomplete paralysis. **2.** a disease of the brain, syphilitic in origin, marked by progressive dementia, tremor, speech disturbances, and increasing muscular weakness; in a large proportion of cases there is a preliminary stage of irritability often followed by exaltation and delusions of grandeur. SYN Bayle disease. [G. a letting go, slackening, paralysis, fr. *paritēmi,* to let go]

**par•es•the•sia** (par-es-thē′zē-ă) an abnormal sensation, such as of burning, pricking, tickling, or tingling. [para- + G. *aisthēsis,* sensation]

**par•es•thet•ic** (par-es-thet′ik) relating to or marked by paresthesia; denoting numbness and tingling in an extremity which usually occurs on the resumption of the blood flow to a nerve following temporary pressure or mild injury.

**Pa·ré su·ture** (pah-rā′) the approximation of the edges of a wound by pasting strips of cloth to the surface and stitching them instead of the skin.

**pa·ret·ic** (pa-ret′ik) relating to or suffering from paresis.

**pa·reu·nia** (pa-roo′nē-ă) SYN coitus. [G. *pareunos,* lying beside, fr. *para,* beside, + *eunē,* a bed]

**par·i·es,** gen. **pa·ri·e·tis,** pl. **pa·ri·e·tes** (par′i-ēz, pā′rī-ēz; pă-rī′ě-tēz) SYN wall. [L. wall]

**pa·ri·e·tal** (pă-rī′ě-tăl) **1.** relating to the wall of any cavity. **2.** SYN somatic (1). **3.** SYN somatic (2). **4.** relating to the parietal bone.

**pa·ri·e·tal bone** a flat, curved bone of irregular quadrangular shape, at either side of the vault of the cranium; it articulates, with its fellow medially, with the frontal anteriorly, the occipital posteriorly, and the temporal and sphenoid inferiorly.

**pa·ri·e·tal cell** one of the cells of the gastric glands; it lies upon the basement membrane, covered by the chief cells, and secretes hydrochloric acid that reaches the lumen of the gland through fine intracellular and intercellular canals (canaliculi). SYN acid cell, oxyntic cell.

**pa·ri·e·tal fis·tu·la** a fistula, either blind or complete, opening on the wall of the thorax or abdomen.

**pa·ri·e·tal fo·ra·men** an inconstant foramen in the parietal bone occasionally found bilaterally near the sagittal margin posteriorly; when present it transmits an emissary vein to the superior sagittal sinus.

**pa·ri·e·tal her·nia** a hernia in which only a portion of the wall of the intestine is engaged. SYN Littré hernia (1), Richter hernia.

**pa·ri·e·tal lobe of cer·e·brum** the middle portion of each cerebral hemisphere, separated from the frontal lobe by the central sulcus, from the temporal lobe by the lateral sulcus in front and an imaginary line projected posteriorly, and from the occipital lobe only partially by the parietooccipital sulcus on its medial aspect.

**pa·ri·e·tal lymph nodes** the lymph nodes draining the walls of the abdomen or of the pelvis.

**pa·ri·e·tal throm·bus** an arterial thrombus adhering to one side of the wall of the vessel. SEE ALSO mural thrombus.

**pa·ri·e·tal wall** the body wall or the somatopleure from which it is formed.

△**parieto-** a wall (of the body, e.g., the abdominal wall); a parietal bone. [L. *paries,* wall]

**pa·ri·e·tog·ra·phy** (pa-rī′ē-tog′ră-fē) rarely used term for a radiographic examination of the wall of the stomach using a combination of pneumoperitoneum and intraluminal air and barium. [parieto- + G. *graphē,* a writing]

**pa·ri·e·to·oc·cip·i·tal** (pă-rī′ě-tō-ok-sip′i-tăl) relating to the parietal and occipital bones or to the parts of the cerebral cortex corresponding thereto.

**pa·ri·e·to·oc·cip·i·tal sul·cus** a very deep, almost vertically oriented fissure on the medial surface of the cerebral cortex, marking the border between the parietal lobe and the cuneus of the occipital lobe; its lower part curves forward and fuses with the anterior extent of the calcarine fissure (sulcus calcarinus); the great depth of this combined fissure causes a bulge in the medial

wall of the occipital horn of the lateral ventricle, the calcar avis.

**Pa·ri·naud con·junc·ti·vi·tis** (pah-rĭ-nō′) a chronic necrotic inflammation of the conjunctiva characterized by large, irregular, reddish follicles and regional lymphadenopathy.

**Pa·ri·naud oc·u·lo·glan·du·lar syn·drome** (pah-rĭ-nō′) unilateral conjunctival granuloma with preauricular adenopathy in tularemia, chancre, tuberculosis, and cat-scratch disease.

**Pa·ri·naud syn·drome, Pa·ri·naud oph·thal·mo·ple·gi·a** (pah-rĭ-nō′) paralysis of conjugate upward gaze with a lesion at the level of the superior colliculi; Bell phenomenon is present. SYN dorsal midbrain syndrome.

**par·i·ty** (par′i-tē) the condition of having given birth to an infant or infants, alive or dead; a multiple birth is considered as a single parous experience. [L. *pario,* to bear]

**Park an·eu·rysm** (pahrk) an arteriovenous aneurysm in which the brachial artery communicates with the brachial and median basilic veins.

**Parkes Web·er syn·drome** (pahrks vā′ber) concurrence of multiple congenital arteriovenous fistulae or arteriovenous malformations with capillary stain and lymphaticovenous anomalies in an enlarged limb.

**Par·kin·son dis·ease** (pahr′kin-sĕn) SYN parkinsonism (1).

**Par·kin·son fa·ci·es** (pahr′kin-sĕn) the expressionless or masklike facies characteristic of parkinsonism (1). SYN masklike face.

**par·kin·so·ni·an** (par-kin-sō′nē-an) relating to or the suffering from parkinsonism (1).

**par·kin·so·ni·an dys·arth·ri·a** a hypokinetic dysarthria associated with Parkinson disease, characterized by rigidity and reduced range of articulatory movements, monotony of pitch and loudness, reduced loudness, short rushes of speech, and rapid rate. SEE parkinsonism.

**par·kin·son·ism** (par′kin-son-izm) **1.** a neurological syndrome usually resulting from deficiency of the neurotransmitter dopamine as the consequence of degenerative, vascular, or inflammatory changes in the basal ganglia; characterized by rhythmical muscular tremors, rigidity of movement, festination, droopy posture, and masklike facies. SYN Parkinson disease. **2.** a syndrome similar to parkinsonism appearing as a side effect of certain antipsychotic drugs. [J. *Parkinson*]

**par·ol·fac·to·ry sul·ci** small sulci found in the parolfactory area, which is located immediately rostral to the lamina terminalis; they frequently consist of anterior and posterior sulci. SYN sulci paraolfactorii [TA].

**par·om·pha·lo·cele** (par-om′fă-lō-sēl) **1.** a tumor near the umbilicus. **2.** a hernia through a defect in the abdominal wall near the umbilicus. [para- + G. *omphalos,* umbilicus, + *kēlē,* tumor, hernia]

🔒**par·o·nych·i·a** (par-ō-nik′ē-ă) suppurative inflammation of the nail fold surrounding the nail plate; may be due to bacteria or fungi, most commonly staphylococci and streptococci. See page 732. [para- + G. *onyx,* nail]

**par·o·nych·i·al** (par-ō-nik′ē-ăl) relating to paronychia.

**par·o·öph·o·ron** (par-ō-of′ōr-on) remnants of the tubules and glomeruli of the lower part of the mesonephros appearing as a few scattered tubules in the broad ligament between the epoöph-

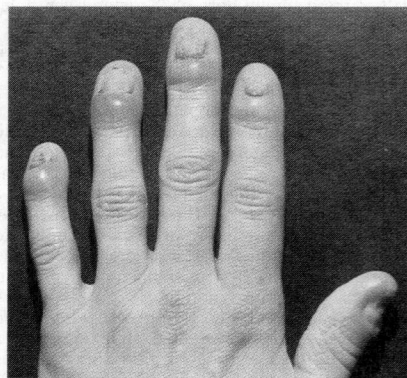

**paronychia:** chronic form

oron and the uterus. Its equivalent in the male is the paradidymis. [para- + oophoron, ovary]

**par·or·chid·i·um** (par-ōr-kid′ē-ŭm) SYN ectopia testis. SYN ectopia testis. [para- + G. *orchis, testis*]

**par·o·rex·ia** (par-ō-rek′sē-ă) an abnormal or disordered appetite. [para- + G. *orexis,* appetite]

**par·os·mia** (par-oz′mē-ă) any disorder of the sense of smell, especially subjective perception of nonexistent odors. [para + G. *osmē,* sense of smell]

**par·os·te·o·sis, par·os·to·sis** (par′os-tē-ō′sis, par-os-tō′sis) **1.** development of bone in an unusual location, as in the skin. **2.** abnormal or defective ossification. [para- + G. *osteon,* bone, + *-osis,* condition]

**pa·rot·ic** (pă-rot′ik) near or beside the ear. [para- + G. *ous,* ear]

**pa·rot·id** (pă-rot′id) situated near or beside the ear; denoting several structures in this neighborhood. Usually refers to the parotid salivary gland. [G. *parōtis (parōtid-),* the gland beside the ear, fr. *para,* beside, + *ous (ōt-),* ear]

**pa·rot·id duct** the duct of the parotid gland opening from the cheek into the vestibule of the mouth opposite the neck of the superior second molar tooth. SYN Stensen duct, Steno duct.

**pa·rot·i·dec·to·my** (pă-rot′i-dek′tō-mē) surgical removal of the parotid gland. [parotid + G. *ektomē,* excision]

**pa·rot·id gland** the largest of the salivary glands, one of two compound acinous glands situated inferior and anterior to the ear, on either side, extending from the angle of the jaw to the zygomatic arch and posteriorly to the sternocleidomastoid muscle; it is subdivided into a superficial part and a deep part by emerging branches of the facial nerve, and discharges through the parotid duct.

**pa·rot·i·di·tis** (pă-rot-i-dī′tis) inflammation of the parotid gland. SYN parotitis.

**pa·rot·id notch** the space between the ramus of the mandible and the mastoid process of the temporal bone.

**pa·rot·id pa·pil·la** the projection at the opening of the parotid duct into the vestibule of the mouth opposite the neck of the upper 2nd molar tooth.

**pa·rot·id veins** drain part of the parotid gland and empty into the retromandibular vein.

**par·o·ti·tis** (par-o-tī′tis) SYN parotiditis.

**par·ous** (par′ŭs) pertaining to parity. [L. *pario,* to bear]

**par·o·var·i·an** (par-ō-var′ē-an) **1.** relating to the paroöphoron. **2.** beside or in the neighborhood of the ovary.

**par·ox·ysm** (par′ok-sizm) **1.** a sharp spasm or convulsion. **2.** a sudden onset of a symptom or disease, especially one with recurrent manifestations such as the chills and rigor of malaria. [G. *paroxysmos,* fr. *paroxynō,* to sharpen, irritate, fr. *oxys,* sharp]

**par·ox·ys·mal** (par-ok-siz′măl) relating to or occurring in paroxysms.

**par·ox·ys·mal cold he·mo·glo·bin·u·ria (PCH)** an autoimmune hemolytic anemia characterized by hemolysis and subsequent hemoglobinuria upon exposure to cold. The hemolysis is caused by the Donath-Landsteiner antibody, which attaches to the red cell at temperatures below 15°C. Upon warming, the antibody dissociates from the cell, but the terminal complement components are activated, causing cell injury and hemolysis. SEE ALSO Donath-Landsteiner antibody.

**par·ox·ys·mal hy·per·ten·sion** SYN episodic hypertension.

**par·ox·ys·mal noc·tur·nal dysp·nea** acute dyspnea appearing suddenly at night, usually waking the patient after an hour or two of sleep; caused by pulmonary congestion that results from left-sided heart failure.

**par·ox·ys·mal noc·tur·nal he·mo·glo·bin·e·mia** an acquired hematopoietic stem cell disorder characterized by formation of defective platelets, granulocytes, erythrocytes, and possibly lymphocytes. The red cell abnormality causes complement-mediated intravascular lysis, which may be expressed in an irregular or even occult manner.

**par·ox·ys·mal noc·tur·nal he·mo·glo·bin·u·ria (PNH)** a hemolytic anemia in which the red cell membrane is abnormal, rendering the cell more susceptible to hemolysis by complement. The membrane defects include a lack of decay-accelerating factor (DAF) and C8 binding protein (C8bp) due to lack of glycosyl phosphatidyl inositol (GPI). GPI is a membrane glycolipid that attaches proteins to the cell membrane. Hemolysis is intravascular and intermittent, characterized by passage of reddish urine.

**par·ox·ys·mal tach·y·car·dia** recurrent attacks of tachycardia, with abrupt onset and often also abrupt termination, originating from an ectopic focus which may be atrial, A-V junctional, or ventricular.

**Par·rot dis·ease** (pah-rō′) **1.** pseudoparalysis in infants, due to syphilitic osteochondritis; **2.** SYN marasmus. **3.** SYN psittacosis.

**par·rot fe·ver** SYN psittacosis.

**par·rot's beak tear** an injury to articular cartilage resulting in the separation of a narrow, curved wedge resembling a parrot's beak.

**Par·ry dis·ease** (par′ē) SYN Graves disease.

**pars,** pl. **par·tes** (parz, par′tēz) a part; a portion. [L. *pars (part-)* a part]

**pars a·mor·pha** the part of the nucleolus that occupies irregular spaces in the nucleolonema and contains finely filamentous substance. SEE ALSO pars granulosa.

**pars gran·u·lo·sa** the granular and filamentous part of the nucleolonema of the nucleolus.

**pars in·ter·ar·tic·u·lar·is** the region between the superior and inferior articulating facets of a vertebra; frequently the site of fracture in spondylolysis.

**pars pla·na** SYN orbiculus ciliaris.

**pars-pla·ni·tis** (parz′plă-nī′tis) a clinical syndrome consisting of inflammation of the peripheral retina and/or pars plana, exudation into the overlying vitreous base, and edema of the optic disk and adjacent retina.

**pars tym·pan·i·ca** tympanic portion of the temporal bone, forming the greater part of the wall of the external acoustic meatus.

**pars u·te·ri·na pla·cen·tae** [TA] the part of the placenta derived from the uterine tissue. SEE ALSO placenta. SYN maternal placenta.

**part** a portion.

**par·the·no·gen·e·sis** (par′the-nō-jen′ĕ-sis) a form of nonsexual reproduction, or agamogenesis, in which the female reproduces its kind without fecundation by the male. [G. *parthenos,* virgin, + *genesis,* product]

**par·tial ag·glu·ti·nin** SYN minor agglutinin.

**par·tial an·om·a·lous pul·mo·na·ry ve·nous con·nec·tions** SEE anomalous pulmonary venous connections, total or partial.

**par·tial an·ti·gen** SYN hapten.

**par·tial cri·coid cleft** SEE laryngotracheoesophageal cleft.

**par·tial den·ture** a dental prosthesis which restores one or more, but not all, of the natural teeth and/or associated parts, and is supported by the teeth and/or the mucosa; it may be removable or fixed. SYN bridgework.

**par·tial lar·yn·gec·to·my** incomplete resection of the larynx in which the supraglottic portion is removed preserving the vocal cords. SYN horizontal laryngectomy, supraglottic laryngectomy.

**par·tial left ven·tric·u·lec·tomy** SYN left ventricular volume reduction surgery.

**par·tial pos·te·ri·or la·ryn·ge·al cleft** SEE laryngotracheoesophageal cleft.

**par·tial pres·sure** the pressure exerted by a single component of a mixture of gases, commonly expressed in mmHg or torr; for a gas dissolved in a liquid, the partial pressure is that of a gas that would be in equilibrium with the dissolved. In respiratory physiology, symbolized by P, followed by subscripts denoting location and/or chemical species (e.g., $P_{CO_2}$, $P_{O_2}$, $PA_{CO_2}$).

**par·tial re·breath·ing mask** a face mask and a reservoir bag permitting a portion of the exhaled gas to enter the bag for mixing with source gas.

**par·tial sei·zure** seizure characterized by localized cerebral ictal onset. The symptoms experienced are dependent on the cortical area of ictal onset or seizure spread.

**par·tial-thick·ness flap** SYN split-thickness flap.

**par·tial-thick·ness graft** SYN split-thickness graft.

**par·tial throm·bo·plas·tin time (PTT)** SEE activated partial thromboplastin time.

**par·tial vol·ume** the actual volume occupied by one species of molecule or particle in a solution; the reciprocal of the density of the molecule.

**par·ti·cle** (par′ti-kl) **1.** a very small piece or portion of anything. **2.** an elementary particle such as a proton or electron. [L. *particula,* dim. of *pars,* part]

**par·tic·u·late** (par-tik′yu-lāt) relating to or occurring in the form of fine particles; formed elements, discret e bodies, as contrasted with the surrounding liquid or semiliquid material; e.g., granules or mitochondria in cells.

**par·tic·u·late wear de·bris** microscopic particles produced by friction between articulating surfaces in a total joint replacement; debris can include particles of metal, polyethylene, and polymethylmethacrylate cement, and can induce osteolysis.

**par·ti·tion chro·ma·tog·ra·phy** the separation of similar substances by repeated divisions between two immiscible liquids, so that the substances, in effect, cross the partition between the liquids in opposite directions.

**par·to·gram** (par′tō-gram) graph of labor parameters of time and dilation with alert and action lines to prompt intervention if the curve deviates from expected. SYN Friedman curve, labor curve. [L. *partus,* childbirth, + -gram]

**par·tu·ri·ent** (par-too′rē-ent) relating to or in the process of childbirth. [L. *parturio,* to be in labor]

**par·tu·ri·ent ca·nal** SYN birth canal.

**par·tu·ri·om·e·ter** (par-too-r-ē-om′ĕ-ter) device for determining the force of the uterine contractions in childbirth. [L. *parturitio,* parturition, + G. *metron,* measure]

**par·tu·ri·tion** (par-too-r-ish′ŭn) SYN childbirth. [L. *parturitio,* fr. *parturio,* to be in labor]

**par·vo·cel·lu·lar** (par-vi-sel′yu-lăr) relating to or composed of cells of small size. [L. *parvus,* small, + Mod. L. *cellularis,* cellular]

**Par·vo·vir·i·dae** (par-vō-vir′i-dē) a family of small viruses containing single-stranded DNA. Three genera are recognized: *Parvovirus, Densovirus,* and *Dependovirus,* which includes the adeno-associated satellite virus.

**Par·vo·vi·rus** (par′vō-vī-rŭs) a genus of viruses that replicate autonomously in suitable cells. [L. *parvus,* small, + virus]

**Par·vo·vi·rus B19** a single-stranded DNA virus belonging to the family Parvoviridae; the cause of erythema infectiosum (fifth disease) and aplastic crises.

**Pas·cal** (pahs-kahl′), Blaise, French scientist, 1623–1662. SEE pascal, Pascal law.

**pas·cal (Pa)** (pas-kahl′) a derived unit of pressure or stress in the SI system, expressed in newtons per square meter; equal to $10^{-5}$ bar or 7.50062 × $10^{-3}$ torr. [B. *Pascal*]

**Pas·cal law** (pahs-kahl′) fluids at rest transmit pressure equally in every direction.

**Pas·sa·vant ridge** (pahs′ĕ-vahnt) a prominence on the posterior wall of the nasopharynx formed by contraction of the superior constrictor muscle of the pharynx during swallowing.

**Pas·sa·voy fac·tor** (pas-a-voy) a clotting factor of which congenital deficiency causes a moderate bleeding diathesis in which the activated partial thromboplastin time (APTT) is prolonged.

**pas·sive** (pas′iv) not active; submissive. [L. *passivus,* fr. *patior,* to endure]

**pas·sive-ag·gres·sive per·son·al·i·ty** a personality disorder in which aggressive feelings are manifested in passive ways, especially through mild obstructionism and stubbornness.

**pas·sive an·a·phy·lax·is** a reaction resulting from inoculation of antigen in an animal previously inoculated intravenously with specific antiserum from another animal, a latent period being required between the two inoculations. SYN antiserum anaphylaxis.

**pas•sive at•el•ec•ta•sis** the pulmonary collapse that occurs due to a space-occupying intrathoracic process such as pneumothorax or hydrothorax.

**pas•sive clot** a clot formed in an aneurysmal sac consequent to cessation or slowing of circulation.

**pas•sive con•ges•tion** congestion caused by obstruction or slowing of the venous drainage, resulting in partial stagnation of blood in the capillaries and venules.

**pas•sive he•mag•glu•ti•na•tion** agglutination in which erythrocytes, usually modified by treatment with chemicals, adsorb soluble antigen and then agglutinate in the presence of antiserum specific for the adsorbed antigen. SYN indirect hemagglutination test.

**pas•sive hy•per•e•mia** hyperemia due to an obstruction in the flow of blood from the affected part, the venous radicles becoming distended. SYN venous hyperemia.

**pas•sive im•mu•ni•ty** SEE acquired immunity.

**pas•sive move•ment** movement imparted to an organism or any of its parts by external agency; movement of any joint effected by the hand of another person, or by mechanical means, without participation of the subject.

**pas•siv•ism** (pas′iv-izm) an attitude of submission, particularly in sexual relations. [see passive]

**paste** (pāst) a soft semisolid of firmer consistency than pap but soft enough to flow slowly and not to retain its shape. [L. *pasta*]

**Pas•teur ef•fect** (pahs-toor′) the inhibition of fermentation by oxygen, first observed by Pasteur; either not observed, or only slightly observed, in malignant tumors.

*Pas•teu•rel•la* (pas-ter-el′ă) a genus of aerobic to facultatively anaerobic, nonmotile bacteria (family Brucellaceae) containing very small, Gram-negative, cocci or ellipsoidal to elongated rods which, with special methods, may show bipolar staining. These organisms are parasites of humans and other animals, including birds. The type species is *Pasteurella multocida*. [L. *Pasteur*]

**pas•teu•rel•la,** pl. **pas•teu•rel•lae** (pas-ter-el′ă, pas-ter-el′ē) a vernacular term used to refer to any member of the genus *Pasteurella*.

*Pas•teu•rel•la aero•ge•nes* a species found in swine that may cause human wound infections following pig bites.

*Pas•teu•rel•la mul•to•ci•da* a species that causes fowl cholera and hemorrhagic septicemia in warm-blooded animals and may infect dog or cat bites or scratches and cause cellulitis and septicemia in humans with chronic disease. Most common pathogen associated with cat and dog bites. It is the type species of the genus *Pasteurella*.

*Pas•teu•rel•la pseu•do•tu•ber•cu•lo•sis* SYN *Yersinia pseudotuberculosis.*

*Pasteurella "SP"* a rarely encountered organism of problematic taxonomy that can cause infection after a guinea pig bite; human infections are quite rare, probably because the bacterium is not widespread and is of low virulence.

**pas•teur•el•lo•sis** (pas′ter-ĕ-lō′sis) infection with bacteria of the genus *Pasteurella*.

**pasteurisation [Br.]** SEE pasteurization.

**pas•teur•i•za•tion** (pas′ter-i-zā′shŭn) the heating of milk, wines, fruit juices, etc., for about 30 minutes at 68°C (154.4°F), whereby living bacteria are destroyed but the flavor or bouquet is preserved; the spores are unaffected, but are kept from developing by immediately cooling the liquid to 10°C (50°F) or lower. SEE ALSO sterilization. [L. *Pasteur*]

**Pas•tia sign** (pahs′tē-ah) the presence of pink or red transverse lines at the bend of the elbow in the preeruptive stage of scarlatina; they persist through the eruptive stage and remain as pigmented lines after desquamation. SYN Thomson sign.

**pas•til, pas•tille** (pas′til, pas-tēl′) **1.** a small mass of benzoin and other aromatic substances to be burned for fumigation. **2.** SYN troche. [Fr. *pastille;* L. *pastillus,* a roll (of bread), dim. of *panis,* bread]

▯**patch 1.** a small circumscribed area differing in color or structure from the surrounding surface. **2.** in dermatology, a flat area greater than 1.0 cm in diameter. **3.** an intermediate stage in the formation of a cap on the surface of a cell. See page B4.

**patch test** a test of skin sensitiveness: a small piece of paper, tape, or a cup, wet with a dilute solution or suspension of test material, is applied to skin of the upper back or upper outer arm and after 48 hours the area previously covered is compared with the uncovered surface; an erythematous reaction with vesicles occurs if the substance causes contact allergy. SEE ALSO photopatch test.

**pa•tel•la,** gen. and pl. **pa•tel•lae** (pa-tel′ă, pa-tel′-ē) [TA] the large sesamoid bone that covers the anterior surface of the knee. It is formed in the tendon of the quadriceps femoris muscle and is attached to the tibia by the patellar tendon. SYN kneecap. [L. a small plate, the kneecap, dim. of *patina,* a shallow disk, fr. *pateo,* to lie open]

**pa•tel•la al•ta** term used to describe a somewhat more proximal position of the patella than anticipated when it is visualized on a lateral radiograph of the knee. [patella + L. *alta,* high]

**pa•tel•la ba•ja** term used to describe a somewhat more distal position of the patella than anticipated when it is visualized on a lateral radiograph of the knee. [patella + Sp. *baja,* low]

**pa•tel•lar** (pa-tel′ăr) relating to the patella.

**pa•tel•lar ap•pre•hen•sion sign** a physical finding in which forced lateral displacement of the patella produces anxiety and resistance in patients with a history of lateral patellar instability.

**pa•tel•lar lig•a•ment** a strong flattened fibrous band passing from the apex and adjoining margins of the patella to the tuberosity of the tibia. SYN ligamentum patellae [TA].

**pa•tel•lar re•flex** a sudden contraction of the anterior muscles of the thigh, caused by a smart tap on the patellar tendon while the leg hangs loosely at a right angle with the thigh. SYN knee reflex, knee-jerk reflex, quadriceps reflex.

**pat•el•lec•to•my** (pat′ĕ-lek′tō-mē) excision of the patella. [patella + G. *ektomē,* excision]

**pa•tel•li•form** (pa-tel′i-fōrm) of the shape of the patella.

**pa•tel•lo•ad•duc•tor re•flex** crossed adduction of the leg on tapping the quadriceps tendon.

**patellofemoral joint** the sliding articulation between the patella and the distal femur. SEE ALSO knee complex.

**pa•tel•lo•fem•or•al stress syn•drome** SYN runner's knee.

**pa·tel·lo·fem·or·al syn·drome** chronic knee pain due to failure of the patella to glide smoothly in its groove on the femur, as a result of structural misalignment or deviant traction by the quadriceps tendon. SEE ALSO chondromalacia patellae.

**pa·ten·cy** (pā'ten-sē) the state of being freely open or exposed.

**pa·tent** (pa'tent, pā'tent) open or exposed. SYN patulous. [L. *patens*, pres. p. of *pateo*, to lie open]

**pa·tent for·a·men ova·le** valvular incompetence of the foramen ovale of the heart; a condition contrasting with probe patency of the foramen ovale in that the valvula foraminis ovalis has abnormal perforations in it, or is of insufficient size to afford adequate valvular action at the foramen ovale prenatally, or effect a complete closure postnatally.

**pa·tent med·i·cine** a medicine, usually originally patented, advertised to the public.

△**path-, -path·y, patho-, path·ic** disease. [G. *pathos*, feeling, suffering, disease]

**path·er·gy** (path'er-jē) those reactions resulting from a state of altered activity, both allergic (immune) and nonallergic. [G. *pathos*, disease, + *ergon*, work]

**path·find·er** (path'fīn-der) a filiform bougie for introduction through a narrow stricture and to serve as a guide for the passage of a larger sound or catheter.

**path·o·bi·ol·o·gy** (path'ō-bī-ol'ō-jē) pathology with emphasis more on the biological than on the medical aspects.

**path·o·clis·is** (path-ō-klis'is) a specific tendency to sensitivity to special toxins; a tendency for toxins to attack certain organs. [patho- + G. *klisis*, bending, proneness]

**path·o·gen** (path'ō-jen) any virus, microorganism, or other substance causing disease. [patho- + G. *-gen*, to produce]

**path·o·gen·e·sis** (path-ō-jen'ĕ-sis) the pathologic, physiologic, or biochemical mechanism resulting in the development of a disease or morbid process. Cf. etiology. [patho- + G. *genesis*, production]

**path·o·gen·ic, path·o·ge·net·ic** (path-ō-jen'ik, path-ō-jĕ-net'ik) causing disease or abnormality. SYN morbific, nosogenic, nosopoietic.

**path·o·ge·nic·i·ty** (path'ō-jĕ-nis'i-tē) the condition or quality of being pathogenic, or the ability to cause disease.

**path·o·gen·ic oc·clu·sion** an occlusal relationship capable of producing pathologic changes in the supporting tissues.

**path·og·no·mon·ic** (path'og-nō-mon'ik) characteristic or indicative of a disease; denoting especially one or more typical symptoms, findings, or pattern of abnormalities specific for a given disease and not found in any other condition. [see pathognomy]

**path·og·no·mon·ic symp·tom** a symptom that, when present, points unmistakably to the presence of a certain definite disease.

**path·o·log·ic, path·o·log·i·cal** (path-ō-loj'ik, path-ō-loj'-i-kăl) **1.** pertaining to pathology. **2.** morbid or diseased; resulting from disease.

**path·o·log·i·cal a·nat·o·my** SYN anatomic pathology.

**path·o·log·ic cal·ci·fi·ca·tion** calcification occurring in excretory or secretory passages as calculi, and in tissues other than bone and teeth.

**path·o·log·ic frac·ture** a fracture occurring at a site weakened by preexisting disease, especially neoplasm or necrosis, of the bone.

**path·o·log·ic mod·el** an animal or animal stock that by inheritance or by artificial manipulation develops a disorder similar to some disease of interest and hence directly or by analogy furnishes evidence of its pathogenesis and may be used as a model for the study of preventive or therapeutic measures.

**path·o·log·ic my·o·pia** progressive myopia marked by fundus changes, posterior staphyloma, and subnormal corrected acuity.

**path·o·log·ic proteins** SEE paraprotein.

**path·o·log·ic re·trac·tion ring** a constriction located at the junction of the thinned lower uterine segment with the thick retracted upper uterine segment, resulting from obstructed labor; this is one of the classic signs of threatened rupture of the uterus. SYN Bandl ring.

**pa·thol·o·gist** (pa-thol'ō-jist) a specialist in pathology; a physician who performs, interprets, or supervises diagnostic tests, using materials removed from living or dead patients, and functions as a laboratory consultant to clinicians, or who conducts experiments or other investigations to determine the causes or nature of disease changes.

**pa·thol·o·gy** (pa-thol'ō-jē) the medical science, and specialty practice, concerned with all aspects of disease, but with special reference to the essential nature, causes, and development of abnormal conditions, as well as the structural and functional changes that result from the disease processes. [patho- + G. *logos*, study, treatise]

**path·o·mi·me·sis** (path'ō-mi-mē'sis) mimicry of a disease or dysfunction, whether intentional or unconscious. [patho- + G. *mimēsis*, imitation]

**path·o·phys·i·ol·o·gy** (path'ō-fiz-ē-ol'ō-jē) derangement of function seen in disease; alteration in function as distinguished from structural defects.

**pa·tho·sis** (pă-thō'sis) rarely used term for a state of disease, diseased condition, or disease entity. [patho- + G. *-osis*, condition]

**path·way** (path'wā) **1.** a collection of axons establishing a conduction route for nerve impulses from one group of nerve cells to another group or to an effector organ composed of muscle or gland cells. **2.** any sequence of chemical reactions leading from one compound to another; if taking place in living tissue, usually referred to as a biochemical pathway.

**pa·tient** (pā'shent) one who is suffering from disease, injury, abnormal state, or mental disorder. Cf. case (1). [L. *patiens*, pres. p. of *patior*, to suffer]

**pa·tient-con·trolled an·al·ge·sia (PCA), pa·tient-con·trolled an·es·the·sia** a method for control of pain based upon a pump for the constant intravenous or, less frequently, epidural infusion of a dilute narcotic solution that includes a mechanism for the self-administration at predetermined intervals of a predetermined amount of the narcotic solution should the infusion fail to relieve pain.

**Pat·rick test** (pat'rik) a test to determine the presence or absence of sacroiliac disease; with the patient supine, the hip and knee are flexed and the external malleolus is placed above the patella of the opposite leg; this can ordinarily be done without pain, but, on depressing the knee, pain is promptly elicited in sacroiliac disease.

**pat·ri·lin·e·al** (pat-ri-lin'ē-ăl) related to descent through the male line; inheritance of the Y chromosome is exclusively patrilineal. [L. *pater*, father, + *linea*, line]

**pat·tern** (pat'ern) **1.** a design. **2.** DENTISTRY a form used in making a mold, as for an inlay or partial denture framework.

**pat·tern dis·tor·tion am·bly·o·pia** amblyopia due to a blurred retinal image during the amblyogenic period of visual development.

**pat·terned al·o·pe·cia** SYN androgenic alopecia.

**pat·tern ret·i·nal dys·tro·phy** a spectrum of autosomal dominant diseases affecting the retinal pigment epithelium, leading to mild to moderate vision loss.

**pat·tern-sen·si·tive ep·i·lep·sy** a form of reflex epilepsy precipitated by viewing certain patterns.

**pat·u·lous** (pat'yu-lŭs) SYN patent. [L. *patulus*, fr. *pateo*, to lie open]

**pau·ci·ar·ti·cu·lar** (paw-sē-ar-tik'yu-lar) a joint condition in which only a few (>1, <5) joints are involved [L. *pauci*, few, + articular]

**pau·ci·bac·il·lary** (paw-sē-bas'i-lār-ē) made up of, or denoting the presence of, few bacilli.

**pau·ci·sy·nap·tic** (paw'sē-si-nap'tik) SYN oligosynaptic. [L. *paucus*, few, + synapse]

**Pau·li ex·clu·sion prin·ci·ple** (pawl'ē) the theory limiting the number of electrons in the orbit or shell of an atom; that it is not possible for any two electrons to have all four quantum numbers identical.

**pause** (pawz) temporary stop. [G. *pausis*, cessation]

**pause sig·nal** a DNA sequence that causes pausing of RNA polymerase transcription.

**Pau·tri·er mi·cro·ab·scess** (pō-trē-ā') a microscopic lesion in the epidermis, seen in mycosis fungoides; it is composed of the same type of atypical mononuclear cells as those that form the infiltrate in the corium.

**Pav·lov re·flex** (pahv'lof) SYN auriculopressor reflex.

**pav·or noc·tur·nus** (pā'vŏr nok-ter'nŭs) SYN night terrors. [L.]

**Payne op·er·a·tion** (pān) a jejunoileal bypass for morbid obesity utilizing end-to-side anastomosis of the upper jejunum to the terminal ileum, with closure of the proximal end of the bypassed intestine.

**Payr clamp** (pīr) a large, slightly curved clamp used in gastrectomy or enterectomy.

**Payr sign** (pīr) pain on pressure over the sole of the foot; a sign of thrombophlebitis.

**Pb** lead (plumbum).

**PBG** porphobilinogen.

**PCA** patient-controlled analgesia.

**pCa** a way of reporting calcium ion levels; equal to $-\log[Ca^{2+}]$.

**PCH** paroxysmal cold hemoglobinuria.

**PCIS** *patient care information system*, an interactive computer system used to store medical records in a hospital.

**P con·gen·i·ta·le** (pē-kon-jen-i-tā'lē) the P-wave pattern in the electrocardiogram seen in some cases of congenital heart disease, consisting of tall peaked P waves in leads I, II, aVF, and aVL

(usually largest in lead II) with predominant positivity of diphasic waves in V1–2.

**PCr** polymerase chain reaction.

**PCr** phosphocreatine.

**PCWP** pulmonary capillary wedge pressure.

**PD** phenyldichloroarsine.

**Pd** palladium.

**PDLL** poorly differentiated lymphocytic lymphoma.

**PEA** pulseless electrical activity.

**peak** (pēk) the top or upper limit of a graphic tracing or of any variable. [M.E. *peke*, *pike*, fr. Sp. *pico*, beak, fr. L. *picus*, magpie]

**peak ex·pi·ra·to·ry flow** the maximum flow at the outset of forced expiration, which is reduced in proportion to the severity of airway obstruction, as in asthma.

**peak flow·me·ter (PEFR)** a portable device for measuring and displaying the highest expiratory flow produced by a patient; it is commonly used to monitor pulmonary function in patients with a reversible disease of the airways.

**pearl** (perl) **1.** a concretion formed around a grain of sand or other foreign body within the shell of certain mollusks. **2.** one of a number of small, tough masses, such as mucus occurring in the sputum in asthma.

**Pearl in·dex** (pĕrl) the number of failures of a contraceptive method per 100 woman years of exposure.

**peau d'orange** (pō-dŏ-rahnj') a swollen pitted skin surface overlying carcinoma of the breast in which there is both stromal infiltration and lymphatic obstruction with edema. [Fr. orange peel]

**pec·cant** (pek'ant) unhealthy; producing disease. [L. *peccans* (*-ant-*), pres. p. of *pecco*, to sin]

**pec·ten** (pek'ten) **1.** a structure with comblike processes or projections. **2.** SYN anal pecten. [L. comb]

**pec·ten an·a·lis** SYN anal pecten.

**pec·ten·i·tis** (pek-ten-ī'tis) inflammation of the sphincter ani. [L. *pecten*, a comb, + G. *-itis*, inflammation]

**pec·ten·o·sis** (pek-ten-ō'sis) exaggerated enlargement of the pecten band.

**pec·ten pu·bis** the continuation on the superior ramus pubis of the linea terminalis, forming a sharp ridge.

**pec·ti·nate** (pek'ti-nāt) **1.** combed; comb-shaped. SYN pectiniform. **2.** in fungi, used to describe a particular type of branching hyphae in cultures of dermatophytes.

**pec·ti·nate line** the line between the simple columnar epithelium of the rectum and the stratified epithelium of the anal canal. SYN linea anocutanea [TA].

**pec·ti·nate mus·cles** prominent ridges of atrial myocardium located on the inner surface of much of the right atrium and both auricles. SYN musculi pectinati [TA].

**pec·ti·nate zone** the outer two-thirds of the basilar membrane of the cochlear duct. SYN zona pectinata.

**pec·tin·e·al** (pek-tin'ē-ăl) ridged; relating to the os pubis or to any comblike structure.

**pec·tin·e·al lig·a·ment** a thick, strong fibrous band that passes laterally from the lacunar ligament along the pectineal line of the pubis. SYN ligamentum pectineale [TA].

**pec·tin·e·al mus·cle** SYN pectineus muscle.

**pec·ti·ne·us mus·cle** *origin*, crest of pubis; *in-*

*sertion*, pectineal line of femur; *action*, adducts thigh and assists in flexion; *nerve supply*, obturator and femoral. SYN musculus pectineus [TA], pectineal muscle.

**pec•tin•i•form** (pek-tin′i-fōrm) SYN pectinate (1).

**pec•to•ral** (pek′tŏ-răl) relating to the chest. [L. *pectoralis*; fr. *pectus*, breast bone]

**pec•to•ral gir•dle** SYN shoulder girdle.

**pec•to•ral re•gion** the region of the chest demarcated by the outline of the pectoralis major muscle. SEE ALSO regions of chest.

**pec•to•ral veins** drain the pectoral muscles and empty directly into the subclavian vein.

**pec•to•ril•o•quy** (pek-tō-ril′ō-kwē) increased transmission of the voice sound through the pulmonary structures, so that it is clearly audible on auscultation of the chest; usually indicates consolidation of the underlying lung parenchyma. [L. *pectus*, chest, + *loquor*, to speak]

**pec•tus**, gen. **pec•to•ris**, pl. **pec•to•ra** (pek′tŭs, pek′tō-ris, pek′tō-ră) [TA] SYN chest. [L.]

**pec•tus ca•ri•na•tum** flattening of the chest on either side with forward projection of the sternum resembling the keel of a boat. SYN chicken breast, pigeon breast.

**pec•tus ex•ca•va•tum** a hollow at the lower part of the chest caused by a backward displacement of the xiphoid cartilage. SYN funnel breast, funnel chest.

△**ped-, pe•di-, pe•do-** 1. child. [G. *pais*, child] 2. foot, feet. [L. *pes*, foot]

**ped•al** (ped′ăl) relating to the feet, or to any structure called pes. [L. *pedalis*, fr. *pes* (*ped*-), a foot]

**ped•er•as•ty** (ped′er-as-tē) sexual relations between a man and a boy. [G. *paiderastia*; fr. *pais* (*paid*-), boy, + *eraō*, to long for]

**Pe•der•son spec•u•lum** (ped′er-son) a narrow flat speculum used to examine a vagina with a narrow introitus.

**pe•de•sis** (pē-dē′sis) SYN brownian movement. [G. *pēdēsis*, a leaping]

**pe•di•at•ric** (pē-dē-at′rik) relating to pediatrics. [G. *pais* (*paid*-), child, + *iatrikos*, relating to medicine]

**pe•di•at•ric den•tist** SYN pedodontist.

**pe•di•at•ric den•tis•try** the branch of dentistry concerned with the dental care and treatment of children.

**pe•di•a•tric•ian** (pē′dē-ă-trish′ăn) a specialist in pediatrics.

**pe•di•at•rics** (pē-dē-at′riks) the medical specialty concerned with the study and treatment of children in health and disease during development from birth through adolescence. [G. *pais* (*paid*-), child, + *iatreia*, medical treatment]

**ped•i•cel** (ped′i-sel) the secondary process of a podocyte, which helps form the visceral capsule of a renal corpuscle. SYN foot process, footplate (2), foot-plate. [Mod. L. *pedicellus*, dim. of L. *pes*, foot]

**ped•i•cel•late** (ped′i-sel-lāt) SYN pediculate.

**ped•i•cel•la•tion** (ped′i-sĕ-lā′shŭn) formation of a pedicle or peduncle.

**ped•i•cle** (ped′i-kl) 1. a constricted portion or stalk. SYN pediculus (1). 2. a stalk by which a nonsessile tumor is attached to normal tissue. SYN peduncle (2), pedunculus. 3. a stalk through which a flap receives nourishment until its transfer to another site results in the nourishment coming from that site. [L. *pediculus*, dim. of *pes*, foot]

**ped•i•cle flap 1.** a skin flap sustained by a blood-carrying stem from the donor site during transfer; **2.** PERIODONTAL SURGERY a flap used to increase the width of attached gingiva, or to cover a root surface, by moving the attached gingiva, which remains joined at one side, to an adjacent position and suturing the free end.

**pe•dic•u•lar** (pĕ-dik′yu-lăr) relating to pediculi, or lice. [L. *pedicularis*]

**pe•dic•u•late** (pĕ-dik′yu-lāt) not sessile, having a pedicle or peduncle. SYN pedicellate, pedunculate. [L. *pediculatus*]

**pe•dic•u•la•tion** (pĕ-dik′yu-lā′shŭn) infestation with lice. [L. *pediculus*, louse]

**pe•dic•u•li** (pĕ-dik′yu-lī) plural of pediculus. [L.]

**pe•dic•u•li•cide** (pĕ-dik′yu-li-sīd) an agent used to destroy lice. [L. *pediculus*, louse, + *caedo*, to kill]

**pe•dic•u•lo•sis** (pĕ-dik′yu-lō′sis) the state of being infested with lice. [L. *pediculus*, louse, + G. *-osis*, condition]

**pe•dic•u•lo•sis pu•bis** infestation with the pubic or crab louse, *Pthirus pubis*, especially in pubic hair, causing pruritus and maculae ceruleae.

**pe•dic•u•lous** (pĕ-dik′yu-lŭs) infested with lice.

***Pe•dic•u•lus*** (pĕ-dik′yu-lŭs) a genus of parasitic lice that live in the hair and feed periodically on blood. Important species include *Pediculus humanus* var. *capitis*, the head louse of man; *Pediculus humanus* var. *corporis* (also called *Pediculus corporis*), the body louse or clothes louse, which lives and lays eggs (nits) in clothing and feeds on the human body; and *Pediculus pubis*. [L.]

**pe•dic•u•lus**, pl. **pe•dic•u•li** (pĕ-dik′yu-lŭs, pĕ-dik′yu-lī) **1.** SYN pedicle (1). [L. pedicle] **2.** a louse. SEE *Pediculus*. [L.]

**ped•i•gree** (ped′i-grē) ancestral line of descent, especially as diagrammed on a chart to show ancestral history; used in genetics to analyze inheritance. [M.E. *pedegra* fr. O.Fr. *pie de grue*, foot of crane]

**ped•i•gree a•nal•y•sis** the formal study of the pattern of a trait in a pedigree to determine such properties as its mode of inheritance, age of onset, and variability in phenotype.

**pe•do•don•tics** (pē-dō-don′tiks) the branch of dentistry concerned with the dental care and treatment of children. SYN paedodontia. [G. *pais*, child, + *odous*, tooth]

**pe•do•don•tist** (pē-dō-don′tist) a dentist who practices pedodontics. SYN pediatric dentist.

**ped•o•dy•na•mom•e•ter** (ped′ō-dī-nă-mom′ĕ-ter) an instrument for measuring the strength of the leg muscles. [L. *pes* (*ped*-), foot, + G. *dynamis*, force, + G. *metron*, measure]

**pe•do•mor•phism** (pē-dō-mōr′fizm) description of adult behavior in terms appropriate to child behavior. [G. *pais* (*paid*), child, + *morphē*, form]

**pe•do•phil•ia** (pē-dō-fil′ē-ă) an abnormal sexual attraction to children in an adult. [G. *pais*, child, + *philos*, fond]

**pe•do•phil•ic** (pē-dō-fil′ik) relating to or exhibiting pedophilia.

**pe•dun•cle** (pe-dŭng′kl) **1.** in neuroanatomy, term loosely applied to a variety of stalklike connecting structures in the brain, composed either exclusively of white matter (e.g., cerebellar peduncle) or of white and gray matter (e.g., cerebral peduncle). **2.** SYN pedicle (2). [Mod. L. *pedunculus*, dim. of *pes*, foot]

p
e

**pe·dun·cu·lar** (pĕ-dŭng'kyu-lăr) relating to a pedicle or peduncle.

**pe·dun·cu·late** (pĕ-dŭng'kyu-lāt) SYN pediculate.

**pe·dun·cu·lot·o·my** (pe-dŭng'kyu-lot'ō-mē) 1. a total or partial section of a cerebral peduncle. 2. a mesencephalic pyramidal tractotomy. [peduncle + G. *tomē,* incision]

**pe·dun·cu·lus,** pl. **pe·dun·cu·li** (pe-dŭng'kyu-lŭs, pĕ-dŭng'kyu-lī) SYN pedicle (2). [Mod. L. dim. of *pes,* foot]

**PEEP** positive end-expiratory pressure.

**peep·ing tes·tis** an undescended testis that migrates back and forth at the internal inguinal ring.

**peer re·view** assessment of research proposals, manuscripts submitted for publication, or a physician's clinical practice by other physicians or scientists in the same field.

**peer-re·view or·gan·i·za·tion (PRO)** an organization that contracts with the Health Care Financing Administration (which pays for health care to Medicare patients) to review the need for and quality of care given to Medicare patients, and to monitor the accuracy of assigned DRGs submitted by the health care facility as the basis for reimbursement for services provided.

**PEFR** peak flowmeter.

**pegged tooth** a conical tooth whose sides converge from the cervical to the incisal region.

**Pel-Eb·stein fe·ver, Pel-Eb·stein dis·ease** (pel-eb'shtīn) the remittent fever common in Hodgkin disease.

**pe·li·o·sis** (pē-lē-ō'sis, pel-ē-ō'sis) SYN purpura. [G. *peliōsis,* a livid spot, livor]

**pe·li·o·sis hep·a·tis** the presence throughout the liver of blood-filled cavities which may become lined by endothelium or become organized; a feature of bacillary angiomatosis, caused by *Rochalimaea henselae* in immunocompromised persons.

**pel·la·gra** (pĕ-lag'ră, pĕ-lā'gră) an affection characterized by diarrhea, dermatitis, and dementia due to dietary deficiency of niacin. [It. *pelle,* skin, + *agra,* rough]

**pel·lag·rous** (pĕ-lag'rŭs) relating to or suffering from pellagra.

**Pel·le·gri·ni dis·ease** (pel-ĕ-grē'nē) a calcific density in the medial collateral ligament and/or bony growth on the medial aspect of the medial condyle of the femur.

**pel·let** (pel'et) 1. a pilule, or very small pill. 2. a small rod-shaped dosage form composed essentially of pure steroid hormones in compressed form, intended for subcutaneous implantation in body tissues; serves as a depot providing for the slow release of the hormone over an extended period of time. [Fr. *pelote;* L. *pila,* a ball]

**pel·li·cle** (pel'i-kl) 1. literally and nonspecifically, a thin skin. 2. a film or scum on the surface of a liquid. 3. cell boundary of sporozoites and merozoites among members of the protozoan subphylum Apicomplexa (Sporozoa), consisting of an outer unit membrane and an inner layer of two unit membranes. [L. *pellicula,* dim of *pellis,* skin]

**pel·lu·cid** (pe-loo'sid) allowing the passage of light. [L. *pellucidus*]

**pel·lu·cid mar·gi·nal cor·ne·al de·gen·er·a·tion** bilateral opacification and vascularization of the periphery of the cornea, progressing to formation of a gutter and ectasia.

**pel·lu·cid zone** SYN zona pellucida.

**pel·ta·tion** (pel-tā'shŭn) protection provided by inoculation with an antiserum or with a vaccine. [L. *pelta,* a light shield, fr. G. *peltē*]

△**pel·vi-, pel·vio-, pel·vo-** the pelvis. Cf. pyelo-. [L. *pelvis,* basin (pelvis)]

**pel·vic** (pel'vik) relating to a pelvis.

**pel·vic ax·is** a hypothetical curved line joining the center point of each of the four planes of the pelvis, marking the center of the pelvic cavity at every level. SYN plane of pelvic canal.

**pel·vic cav·i·ty** the space bounded at the sides by the bones of the pelvis, above by the superior aperture of the pelvis, and below by the pelvic diaphragm; it contains the pelvic viscera.

**pel·vic cel·lu·li·tis** SYN parametritis.

**pel·vic di·a·phragm, di·a·phragm of pel·vis** the paired levator ani and coccygeus muscles together with the fascia above and below them.

**pel·vic di·rec·tion** (pel'vik dī-rek'shŭn) the direction of the axis of the pelvis.

**pel·vi·ceph·a·lom·e·try** (pel'vi-sef-ă-lom'ĕ-trē) measurement of the female pelvic diameters in relation to those of the fetal head. [pelvi- + G. *kephalē,* head, + *metron,* measure]

**pel·vic fas·cia** general term for the fascia lining the pelvic cavity (fascia pelvis parietalis) and investing the pelvic viscera (fascia pelvis visceralis).

**pel·vic gan·glia** the parasympathetic ganglia scattered through the pelvic plexus on either side.

**pel·vic gir·dle** the bony ring formed by the hip bones and the sacrum, to which the lower limbs are attached.

**pel·vic in·flam·ma·to·ry dis·ease (PID)** acute or chronic inflammation in the organs of the female pelvic cavity, particular suppurative lesions of the upper genital tract; most commonly due to infection by *Chlamydia trachomatis* or *Neisseria gonorrhoeae,* which have ascended into the uterus, uterine tubes, or ovaries from the lower genital tract as a result of childbirth or surgical procedures. The chief symptoms are pelvic pain and fever; complications include abscess formation and generalized peritonitis. Scarring may cause tubal infertility and raise the risk of ectopic pregnancy.

**pel·vic per·i·to·ni·tis** generalized inflammation of the peritoneum surrounding the uterus and fallopian tubes. SYN pelviperitonitis.

**pel·vic plane of great·est di·men·sions** the plane extending from the middle of the posterior surface of the pubic symphysis to the junction of the second and third sacral vertebrae, and laterally passing through the ischial bones over the middle of the acetabulum.

**pel·vic plane of least di·men·sions** the plane that extends from the end of the sacrum to the inferior border of the pubic symphysis; it is bounded posteriorly by the end of the sacrum, laterally by the ischial spines, and anteriorly by the inferior border of the pubic symphysis.

**pel·vic pole** the breech end of the fetus.

**pel·vic ver·sion** version by means of which a transverse or oblique presentation is converted into a pelvic presentation by manipulating the buttocks of the fetus.

**pel·vi·fix·a·tion** (pel-vi-fik-sā'shŭn) surgical attachment of a floating pelvic organ to the wall of the pelvic cavity.

**pel·vi·li·thot·o·my** (pel'vi-li-thot'ō-mē) SYN pyelolithotomy. [pelvi- + G. *lithos*, stone, + *tomē*, incision]

**pel·vim·e·ter** (pel-vim′ĕ-ter) calipers for measuring the diameters of the pelvis.

**pel·vim·e·try** (pel-vim′ĕ-trē) measurement of the diameters of the pelvis. [pelvi- + G. *metron*, measure]

**pel·vi·o·plas·ty** (pel′vē-ō-plas-tē) **1.** symphysiotomy or pubiotomy for enlargement of the female pelvic outlet. **2.** SYN pyeloplasty. [pelvio- + G. *plastos*, formed]

**pel·vi·ot·o·my, pel·vit·o·my** (pel′vē-ot′ō-mē, pel′vit-ō-mē) **1.** SYN symphysiotomy. **2.** SYN pubiotomy. **3.** SYN pyelotomy. [pelvio- + G. *tomē*, incision]

**pel·vi·per·i·to·ni·tis** (pel-vē-per-i-tō-nī′tis) SYN pelvic peritonitis.

■**pel·vis**, pl. **pel·ves** (pel′vis, pel′vēz) [TA] **1.** the massive cup-shaped ring of bone, with its ligaments, at the lower end of the trunk, formed of the hip bone (the pubic bone, ilium, and ischium) on either side and in front, and of the sacrum and the coccyx posteriorly. **2.** any basinlike or cup-shaped cavity, as the pelvis of the kidney. See this page. [L. basin]

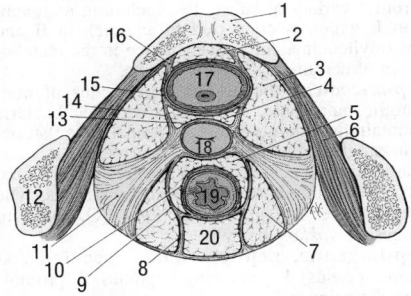

16 1 2 17 15 14 13 3 4 5 6 18 12 19 20 11 10 8 7 9

**pelvic spaces:** formed by firm connective tissue and ligaments surrounding the bladder, cervix, and rectum; (1) pubis symphysis, (2) prevesical space, (3) paravesical space, (4) vesicocervical space, (5) rectovaginal space, (6) obturator internus muscle, (7) pararectal space, (8) rectal pillar (posterior layer), (9) rectal pillar (anterior layer), (10) rectal fascia, (11) cardinal ligament, (12) ischium, (13) cervical fascia, (14) vesicouterine ligament, (15) bladder fascia, (16) pubovesical ligament, (17) bladder, (18) cervix, (19) rectum, (20) retrorectal space

**pel·vis jus·to ma·jor** a symmetrical pelvis with greater than normal measurements in all diameters.

**pel·vis jus·to mi·nor** a pelvis of the female type, but with all its diameters smaller than normal.

**pel·vi·ver·te·bral an·gle** the angle made by the pelvis as defined by the plane of the superior pelvic aperture with the general axis of the trunk or vertebral column.

**pel·vo·ca·li·ec·ta·sis** (pel′vō-kal-ē-ek-tā′sis) SYN hydronephrosis.

**pem·phi·goid** (pem′fi-goyd) **1.** resembling pemphigus. **2.** a disease resembling pemphigus but significantly distinguishable histologically (nona-

cantholytic) and clinically (generally benign course). [G. *pemphix*, blister, + *eidos*, resemblance]

**pem·phi·gus** (pem′fi-gŭs) **1.** auto-immune bullous diseases with acantholysis: pemphigus vulgaris, pemphigus foliaceus, pemphigus erythematosus, or pemphigus vegetans. **2.** a nonspecific term for blistering skin diseases. [G. *pemphix*, a blister]

**pem·phi·gus er·y·the·ma·to·sus** an eruption involving sun-exposed skin, especially the face; the lesions are scaling erythematous macules and blebs.

**pem·phi·gus fo·li·a·ceus** a generally chronic form of pemphigus in which extensive exfoliative dermatitis may be present in addition to the bullae.

**pem·phi·gus gan·gre·no·sus 1.** SYN dermatitis gangrenosa infantum. **2.** SYN bullous impetigo of newborn.

**pem·phi·gus vul·ga·ris** a serious form of pemphigus, occurring in middle age, in which cutaneous bullae and oral erosions may be localized a few months before becoming generalized; blisters break easily and are slow to heal; results from the action of autoimmune antibodies that localize to intercellular sites of stratified squamous epithelium.

**Pen·dred syn·drome** (pen′drĕd) characterized by congenital sensorineural hearing impairment with goiter (usually small) due to defective organic binding of iodine in the thyroid; afflicted individuals are usually euthyroid; autosomal recessive inheritance, caused by mutation in the Pendred syndrome gene (PDS) encoding pendrin on chromosome 7q.

**pen·du·lar nys·tag·mus** a nystagmus that has oscillations equal in speed and amplitude, usually arising from a visual disturbance.

**pe·nes** plural of penis.

**pen·e·trance** (pen′ĕ-trans) the frequency, expressed as a fraction or percentage, of individuals who are phenotypically affected, among persons of an appropriate genotype; factors affecting expression may be environmental, or due to purely random variation; contrasted with hypostasis where the condition has a genetic origin and therefore tends to cause correlation in relatives. [see penetration]

**pen·e·trat·ing wound** a wound with disruption of the body surface that extends into underlying tissue or into a body cavity.

△**-pe·nia** deficiency. [G. *penia*, poverty]

**pe·ni·cil·li·o·sis** invasive infection by a species of *Penicillium*.

***Pen·i·cil·li·um*** (pen-i-sil′ē-ŭm) a genus of fungi species of which yield various antibiotic substances and biologicals. [see penicillus]

***Pen·i·cil·li·um li·la·ci·num*** SYN *Paecilomyces lilacinus*.

**pen·i·cil·lus**, pl. **pe·ni·cil·li** (pen-i-sil′ŭs, pen-i-sil′ī) **1.** one of the tufts formed by the repeated subdivision of the minute arterial twigs in the spleen. **2.** in fungi, one of the branched conidiophores bearing chains of conidia in *Penicillium* species. [L. paint brush]

**pe·nile** (pē′nīl) relating to the penis.

**pe·nile pros·the·sis** device placed inside penis to correct erectile failure.

**pe·nile ra·phe** the continuation of the raphe of the scrotum onto the underside of the penis.

**pe·nis**, pl. **pe·nes** (pē'nis) [TA] the organ of copulation in the male; it is formed of three columns of erectile tissue, two arranged laterally on the dorsum (corpora cavernosa penis) and one median below (corpus spongiosum); the urethra traverses the latter; the extremity (glans penis) is formed by an expansion of the corpus spongiosum, and is more or less completely covered by a free fold of skin (preputium). SYN phallus. [L. tail]

**pe·nis·chi·sis** (pē-nis'ki-sis) a fissure of the penis resulting in an abnormal opening into the urethra, either above (epispadias), below (hypospadias), or to one side (paraspadias). [L. *penis* + G. *schisis*, fissure]

**pen·nate** (pen'āt) feathered; resembling a feather. SYN penniform. [L. *pennatus*, fr. *penna*, feather]

**pen·ni·form** (pen'i-fōrm) SYN pennate. [L. *penna*, feather, + *forma*, form]

**Pen·rose drain** (pen'rōz) a soft tube-shaped rubber drain.

△**pen·ta-** five. [G. *pente*, five]

**pen·tose** (pen'tōs) a monosaccharide containing five carbon atoms in the molecule.

**pen·tose phos·phate path·way** a secondary pathway for the oxidation of D-glucose (not occurring in skeletal muscle), generating reducing power (NADPH) in the cytoplasm outside the mitochondria and synthesizing pentoses and a few other sugars. This pathway is defective in certain inherited diseases, e.g., glucose-6-phosphate dehydrogenase deficiency. SYN Dickens shunt.

**pen·to·su·ria** (pen-tō-syu'rē-ă) the excretion of one or more pentoses in the urine.

**pen·tyl** (pen'til) **1.** SYN amyl. **2.** the $CH_3(CH_2)_3CH_2-$ moiety.

**pe·num·bra** RADIOLOGY the blurred margin of an image. SYN geometric unsharpness.

**pep·lo·mer** (pep'lō-mer) a part or subunit of the peplos of a virion, the assemblage of which produces the complete peplos, produced from the peplos by detergent treatment. [see peplos]

**pep·los** (pep'lōs) the coat or envelope of lipoprotein material that surrounds certain virions. [G. an outer garment worn by women]

**pep pills** colloquialism for tablets containing a central nervous system stimulant, especially amphetamine.

**pep·sin·o·gen** (pep-sin'ō-jen) a proenzyme formed and secreted by the chief cells of the gastric mucosa; the acidity of the gastric juice and pepsin itself remove 42 amino acid residues from pepsinogen to form active pepsin. SYN propepsin. [pepsin + G. *-gen*, producing]

**pep·tic** (pep'tik) relating to the stomach, to gastric digestion, or to pepsin A. [G. *peptikos*, fr. *peptō*, to digest]

**pep·tic cell** SYN zymogenic cell.

**pep·tic di·ges·tion** SYN gastric digestion.

**pep·tic ul·cer** an ulcer of the alimentary mucosa, usually in the stomach or duodenum, exposed to acid gastric secretion.

**pep·ti·dase** (pep'ti-dās) any enzyme capable of hydrolyzing one of the peptide links of a peptide; e.g., carboxypeptidases, aminopeptidases.

**pep·tide** (pep'tīd) a compound of two or more amino acids in which a carboxyl group of one is united with an amino group of another, with the elimination of a molecule of water, thus forming a peptide bond, $-CO-NH-$; i.e., a substituted amide.

**pep·tide an·ti·bi·ot·ic** antibiotic composed of peptides; the antibacterial action is based on the physical disruption of cell membranes.

**pep·tide bond** the common link ($-CO-NH-$) between amino acids in proteins, formed by elimination of $H_2O$ between the $-COOH$ of one amino acid and the $H_2N-$ of another.

**pep·ti·der·gic** (pep-ti-der'jik) referring to nerve cells or fibers that are believed to employ small peptide molecules as their neurotransmitter. [peptide + G. *ergon*, work]

**pep·ti·do·gly·can** (pep'ti-dō-glī'kan) a compound containing amino acids (or peptides) linked to sugars, with the latter preponderant. Cf. glycopeptide.

**pep·ti·doid** (pep'ti-doyd) a condensation product of two amino acids involving at least one condensing group other than the α-carboxyl or α-amino group; e.g., glutathione.

**pep·ti·do·lyt·ic** (pep'ti-dō-lit'ik) causing the cleavage or digestion of peptides. [peptide + G. *lytikos*, solvent]

**pep·ti·dyl di·pep·ti·dase A** (pep'ti-dil-di-pep-ti-dās ā) a hydrolase cleaving C-terminal dipeptides from a variety of substrates, including angiotensin I, which is converted to angiotensin II and histidylleucine. An important step in the metabolism of certain vasopressor agents.

***Pep·to·coc·cus*** (pep'tō-kok'ŭs) a genus of nonmotile, anaerobic, chemoorganotrophic bacteria containing Gram-positive, spherical cells that occur singly, in pairs, tetrads, or irregular masses, rarely in short chains. They are frequently found in association with pathologic conditions. The type species is *Peptococcus niger*. [G. *peptō*, to digest, + *kokkos*, berry]

**pep·to·gen·ic, pep·tog·e·nous** (pep-tō-jen'ik, pep-toj'ĕ-nŭs) **1.** producing peptones. **2.** promoting digestion.

**pep·tol·y·sis** (pep-tol'i-sis) the hydrolysis of peptones.

**pep·to·lyt·ic** (pep-tō-lit'ik) **1.** pertaining to peptolysis. **2.** denoting an enzyme or other agent that hydrolyses peptones.

**pep·tone** (pep'tōn) descriptive term applied to intermediate polypeptide products, formed in partial hydrolysis of proteins, that are soluble in water, diffusible, and not coagulable by heat; used in bacterial culture media.

**pep·ton·ic** (pep-ton'ik) relating to or containing peptone.

**pep·to·ni·za·tion** (pep'ton-i-zā'shŭn) conversion by enzymic action of native protein into soluble peptone.

***Pep·to·strep·to·coc·cus*** (pep'tō-strep-tō-kok'ŭs) a genus of nonmotile, anaerobic, chemoorganotrophic bacteria containing spherical to ovoid, Gram-positive cells that occur in pairs and short or long chains. These organisms are found in normal and pathologic female genital tracts and blood in puerperal fever, in respiratory and intestinal tracts of normal humans and other animals, in the oral cavity, and in pyogenic infections, putrefactive war wounds, and appendicitis; they may be pathogenic. The type species is *Peptostreptococcus anaerobius*. [G. *peptō*, to digest, + *streptos*, curved, + *kokkos*, berry]

△**per- 1.** through; denoting intensity. **2.** CHEMISTRY more or most, with respect to the amount of a given element or radical contained in a compound; the degree of substitution for hydrogen, as in peroxides, peroxy acids (e.g., hydrogen peroxide, peroxyformic acid). SEE ALSO peroxy-. [L. through, throughout, extremely]

**per·ac·id** (pĕr-as′id) an acid containing a peroxide group (–O–OH); e.g., peracetic acid.

**per·a·cute** (pĕr-ă-kyut′) very acute; said of a disease. [L. *peracutus,* very sharply]

**per an·um** (pĕr ā′nŭm) by or through the anus. [L.]

**per·cept** (pĕr′sept) **1.** that which is perceived; the complete mental image, formed by the process of perception, of an object or idea. **2.** CLINICAL PSYCHOLOGY a single unit of perceptual report, such as one of the responses to an inkblot in the Rorschach test. [L. *perceptum,* a thing perceived]

**per·cep·tion** (pĕr-sep′shun) the mental process of becoming aware of or recognizing an object or idea; primarily cognitive rather than affective or conative, although all three aspects are manifested. SYN esthesia.

**per·cep·tive** (pĕr-sep′tiv) relating to or having a higher than normal power of perception.

**per·cep·tive hear·ing im·pair·ment** former term for sensorineural deafness.

**per·cep·tiv·i·ty** (pĕr-sep-tiv′i-tē) the power of perception.

**per·cep·tu·al pro·ces·sing** the organization of sensory input into meaningful patterns.

**per·co·la·tion** (pĕr-kō-lā′shŭn) **1.** SYN filtration. **2.** extraction of the soluble portion of a solid mixture by passing a solvent liquid through it. **3.** passage of saliva or other fluids into the interface between tooth structure and restoration; sometimes induced by thermal changes. [L. *percolatio,* fr. per- + *colare,* to strain]

**per con·tig·u·um** (pĕr kon-tig′yu-ŭm) in contiguity; denoting the mode by which an inflammation or other morbid process spreads into an adjacent contiguous structure. [per- + L. *contiguus,* touching, fr. *tango,* to touch]

**per con·tin·u·um** (pĕr kon-tin′yu-ŭm) in continuity; continuous; denoting the mode by which an inflammation or other morbid process spreads from one part to another through continuous tissue. [per- + L. *continuus,* holding together, continuous, fr. *teneo,* to hold]

**per·cuss** (pĕr-kŭs′) to perform percussion.

**per·cus·sion** (pĕr-kŭsh′ŭn) **1.** a diagnostic procedure designed to determine the density of a part by the sound produced by tapping the surface with the finger or a plessor; performed primarily over the chest to determine presence of normal air content in the lungs and over the abdomen to evaluate air in the loops of intestine. **2.** a form of massage, consisting of repeated blows or taps of varying force. See this page. [L. *percussio,* fr. *per-cutio,* pp. -*cussus,* to beat, fr. *quatio,* to shake, beat]

**per·cus·sor** (pĕr-kŭs′er) SYN plessor.

**per·cu·ta·ne·ous** (pĕr-kyu-tā′nē-ŭs) denoting the passage of substances through unbroken skin, as in absorption by inunction; also passage through the skin by needle puncture, including introduction of wires and catheters by Seldinger technique.

**per·cu·ta·ne·ous trans·he·pa·tic chol·an·gi·og·ra·phy (PTHC)** contrast radiographic examination of biliary system performed by injection

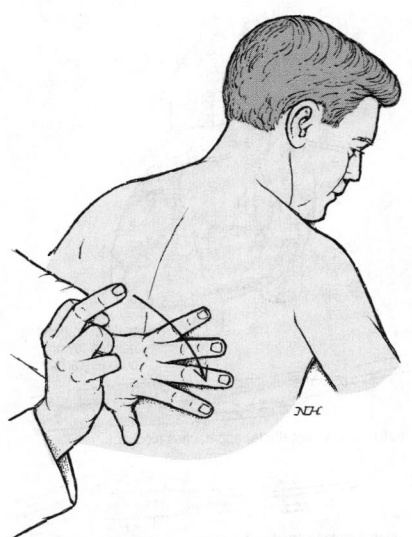

**percussion:** distal phalanx of left middle finger is pressed firmly against chest wall parallel with ribs; a short, quick blow is struck at the base of the distal phalanx of the middle finger with the tip of the middle finger of the right hand

through a percutaneously placed needle inserted into an intrahepatic bile duct.

**per·cu·ta·ne·ous trans·lu·mi·nal an·gi·o·plas·ty (PTA)** an operation for enlarging a narrowed vascular lumen by inflating and withdrawing through the stenotic region a balloon on the tip of an angiographic catheter; may include positioning of an intravascular stent. See page 742.

**per·en·ceph·a·ly** (pĕr-en-sef′ă-lē) a condition marked by one or more cerebral cysts. [G. *pēra,* a purse, a wallet, + *enkephalos,* brain]

**per·fect fun·gus** a fungus possessing both sexual and asexual means of reproduction, and in which both mating forms are recognized.

**per·fec·tion·ism** (pĕr-fek′shŭn-izm) a tendency to set rigid high standards of performance for oneself.

**per·fec·tion·is·tic per·so·na·li·ty** a personality characterized by rigidity, extreme inhibition, and excessive concern with conformity and adherence to often unique standards.

**per·fect stage** a mycological term used to describe the sexual life cycle phase of a fungus in which spores are formed after nuclear fusion.

**per·fo·rat·ed** (pĕr′fō-rāt-ed) pierced with one or more holes. [L. *perforatus,* fr. *per-foro,* pp. -*atus,* to bore through]

**per·fo·rat·ed ul·cer** an ulcer extending through the wall of an organ.

**per·fo·rat·ing ab·scess** an abscess that breaks down tissue barriers to enter adjacent areas. SYN migrating abscess, wandering abscess.

**per·fo·rat·ing ar·ter·ies** *origin,* arteria profunda femoris; *distribution,* as three or four vessels that pass through the aponeurosis of the adductor magnus to the posterior and anterior compartments of the thigh. SYN arteriae perforantes [TA].

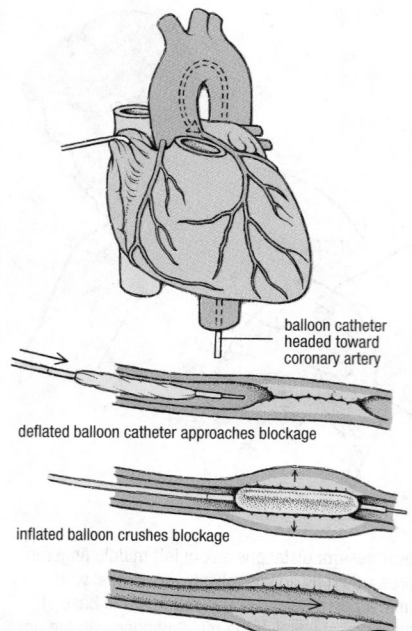

balloon catheter
headed toward
coronary artery

deflated balloon catheter approaches blockage

inflated balloon crushes blockage

catheter removed and circulation reestablished

**percutaneous transluminal angioplasty**

**per·fo·rat·ing fi·bers** bundles of collagenous fibers that pass into the outer circumferential lamellae of bone or the cementum of teeth.

**per·fo·rat·ing veins** accompany the perforating arteries from the profunda femoris artery; drain blood from the vastus lateralis and hamstring muscles and terminate in the profunda femoris vein.

**per·fo·rat·ing wound** a wound with an entrance and exit opening.

**per·fo·ra·tion** (pĕr-fō-rā′shŭn) abnormal opening in a hollow organ or viscus. SEE ALSO perforated. See page B16. SYN tresis.

**per·fo·rin** (pĕr′fōr-in) a protein found in the cytoplasmic granules of both T cytotoxic lymphocytes and natural killer cells, implicated in target cell lysis. [L. *per-foro*, to bore, pierce, + -in]

**per·for·mance** (pĕr-fōr-mans) organized patterns of behavior that are characteristic or expected of a person in a given situation.

**per·for·mance ar·e·as** activities of daily living, work or other productive activity, play, and leisure that determine a person's functional abilities and define human activity.

**per·for·mance com·po·nents** sensorimotor, cognitive, psychosocial, and psychological elements of functional performance required for successful engagement in performance areas and evaluated and addressed during intervention for the purpose of improving performance.

**per·for·mance con·text** the physical, social, and cultural features of the environment that influence performance of meaningful and purposeful life tasks of daily life.

**per·for·mance in·ten·si·ty** the improvement in

recognition of spoken words that occurs with increasing intensity of sound.

**per·fuse** (pĕr-fyus′) to force blood or other fluid to flow from the artery through the vascular bed of a tissue or to flow through the lumen of a hollow structure (e.g., an isolated renal tubule). [L. *perfusio*, fr. per- + *fusio*, a pouring]

**per·fu·sion** (pĕr-fyu′zhŭn) **1.** the act of perfusing. **2.** the flow of blood or other perfusate per unit volume of tissue, as in ventilation/perfusion ratio.

△**peri-** around, about, near. Cf. circum-. [G. around]

**per·i·ad·e·ni·tis** (per′ē-ad-ĕ-nī′tis) inflammation of the tissues surrounding a gland. [peri- + G. *adēn*, gland, + -itis, inflammation]

**per·i·ad·e·ni·tis mu·co·sa ne·cro·ti·ca re·cur·rens** SYN aphthae major.

**per·i·an·gi·tis** (per′ē-an-jī′tis) inflammation of the adventitia of a blood vessel or of the tissues surrounding it or a lymphatic vessel. SEE ALSO periarteritis, periphlebitis, perilymphangitis. SYN perivasculitis. [peri- + G. *angeion*, a vessel, + -itis, inflammation]

**per·i·a·or·ti·tis** (per′ē-ā-ōr-tī′tis) inflammation of the adventitia of the aorta and of the tissues surrounding it.

**per·i·ap·i·cal** (per-ē-ap′i-kăl) **1.** at or around the apex of a root of a tooth. **2.** denoting the periapex.

**per·i·ap·i·cal ce·ment·al dys·pla·sia** a benign, painless, non-neoplastic condition of the jaws which occurs almost exclusively in middle-aged black females; lesions are usually multiple, most frequently involve vital mandibular anterior teeth, surround the root apices, and are initially radiolucent (becoming more opaque as they mature).

**per·i·ap·i·cal cu·ret·tage 1.** removal of a cyst or granuloma from its pathologic bony crypt, utilizing a curette; **2.** the removal of tooth fragments and debris from sockets at the time of extraction or of bone sequestra subsequently.

**per·i·ap·i·cal film** intraoral radiographic projection taken to include tooth apices and surrounding alveolar bone. Film sizes 0–2 made be utilized. SEE periapical radiograph.

**per·i·ap·i·cal gran·u·lo·ma** a proliferation of granulation tissue surrounding the apex of a nonvital tooth and arising in response to pulpal necrosis. SYN apical granuloma, dental granuloma.

**per·i·ap·i·cal ra·di·o·graph** a radiograph demonstrating tooth apices and surrounding structures in a particular intraoral area.

**per·i·ap·pen·di·ce·al ab·scess** SYN appendiceal abscess.

**per·i·ap·pen·di·ci·tis** (per′ē-ă-pen-di-sī′tis) inflammation of the tissue surrounding the vermiform appendix.

**per·i·ar·te·ri·al plex·us** an autonomic plexus that accompanies an artery, surrounding it in a network of autonomic nerve fibers.

**per·i·ar·te·ri·al plex·us·es of co·ro·na·ry ar·te·ries** the continuation of the cardiac plexus onto the coronary arteries.

**per·i·ar·te·ri·al sym·pa·thec·to·my** sympathetic denervation by arterial decortication. SYN Leriche operation.

**per·i·ar·te·ri·tis** (per′ē-ar-ter-ī′tis) inflammation of the adventitia of an artery.

**per·i·ar·te·ri·tis no·do·sa** SYN polyarteritis nodosa.

**per·i·ar·thri·tis** (per′ē-ar-thrī′tis) inflammation of the parts surrounding a joint. [peri- + arthritis]

**per·i·ar·tic·u·lar ab·scess** an abscess surrounding a joint, not necessarily involving it.

**per·i·bron·chi·o·li·tis** (per′i-brong′kē-ō-lī′tis) inflammation of the tissues surrounding the bronchioles.

**per·i·bron·chi·tis** (per′i-brong-kī′tis) inflammation of the tissues surrounding the bronchi or bronchial tubes.

**per·i·car·dia** (per-i-kar′dē-ă) plural of pericardium.

**per·i·car·di·ac, per·i·car·di·al** (per-i-kar′dē-ak, per-i-kar′dē-ăl) **1.** surrounding the heart. **2.** relating to the pericardium.

**per·i·car·di·a·co·phren·ic ar·tery** *origin*, internal thoracic; *distribution*, pericardium, diaphragm, and pleura; *anastomoses*, musculophrenic, inferior phrenic, mediastinal and pericardial branches of the internal thoracic. SYN arteria pericardiacophrenica [TA].

**per·i·car·di·a·co·phren·ic veins** accompany the pericardiacophrenic artery and emptying into the brachiocephalic veins or superior vena cava.

**per·i·car·di·al cav·i·ty 1.** the potential space between the parietal and visceral layers of the serous pericardium; **2.** in the embryo, that part of the primary celom containing the heart; originally it is in open communication with the pericardioperitoneal cavities and indirectly, through them, with the peritoneal part of the celom.

**per·i·car·di·al de·com·pres·sion** SYN cardiac decompression.

**per·i·car·di·al ef·fu·sion** increased amounts of fluid within the pericardial sac, usually due to inflammation.

**per·i·car·di·al frem·i·tus** vibration in the chest wall produced by the friction of opposing roughened surfaces of the pericardium.

**per·i·car·di·al mur·mur** a friction sound, synchronous with the heart movements, heard in certain cases of pericarditis.

**per·i·car·di·al sym·phy·sis** adhesion between the parietal and visceral layers of the pericardium.

**per·i·car·di·al veins** several small veins from the pericardium emptying into the brachiocephalic veins or superior vena cava.

**per·i·car·di·cen·te·sis** (per-i-kar′dē-sen-tē′sis) needle drainage of the pericardium, usually accompanied by placement of an indwelling catheter for continuing drainage.

**per·i·car·di·ec·to·my** (per′i-kar-dē-ek′tō-mē) excision of a portion of the pericardium. [pericardium + G. *ektomē*, excision]

**per·i·car·di·ol·ogy** (per-ē-kar-dē-ol′ō-jē) the science or study of the pericardium, its physiology, and diseases.

**per·i·car·di·o·per·i·to·ne·al** (per-i-kar′dē-ō-per-i-tō-nē′ăl) relating to the pericardial and peritoneal cavities.

**per·i·car·di·o·phren·ic** (per-i-kar′dē-ō-fren′ik) relating to the pericardium and the diaphragm. [pericardium + G. *phrēn*, diaphragm]

**per·i·car·di·o·pleur·al** (per-i-kar′dē-ō-ploor′ăl) relating to the pericardial and pleural cavities.

**per·i·car·di·or·rha·phy** (per′i-kar-dē-ōr′ă-fē) suture of the pericardium. [pericardium + G. *rhaphē*, suture]

**per·i·car·di·os·to·my** (per′i-kar-dē-os′tō-mē) establishment of an opening into the pericardium. [pericardium + G. *stoma*, mouth]

**per·i·car·di·ot·o·my** (per′i-kar-dē-ot′ō-mē) incision into the pericardium. [pericardium + G. *tome*, incision]

**per·i·car·dit·ic** (per′i-kar-dit′ik) relating to pericarditis.

**per·i·car·di·tis** (per′i-kar-dī′tis) inflammation of the pericardium.

**per·i·car·di·tis ob·li·te·rans** inflammation of the pericardium leading to adhesion of the two layers, obliterating the sac. SEE ALSO adhesive pericarditis.

**per·i·car·di·tis with ef·fu·sion** pericardial inflammation producing excess pericardial fluid.

**per·i·car·di·um,** pl. **per·i·car·dia** (per-i-kar′dē-ŭm, per-i-kar′dē-ă) [TA] the fibroserous membrane, consisting of mesothelium and submesothelial connective tissue, covering the heart and beginnings of the great vessels. It is a closed sac having two layers: the visceral layer (epicardium), immediately surrounding the heart, and the outer parietal layer, forming the sac, composed of strong fibrous tissue, the fibrous pericardium, lined with the serous membrane, serous pericardium. SYN heart sac, theca cordis. [L. fr. G. *pericardion*, the membrane around the heart]

**per·i·cho·lan·gi·tis** (per′i-kō-lan-jī′tis) inflammation of the tissues around the bile ducts. [peri- + G. *cholē*, bile, + *angeion*, vessel, + *-itis*, inflammation]

**per·i·chon·dral, per·i·chon·dri·al** (per-i-kon′drăl, per-i-kon′drē-ăl) relating to the perichondrium.

**per·i·chon·dral bone** in the development of a long bone a collar or cuff of osseous tissue forms in the perichondrium of the cartilage model; the connective tissue membrane of this perichondral bone then becomes periosteum.

**per·i·chon·dri·tis** (per′i-kon-drī′tis) inflammation of the perichondrium.

**per·i·chon·dri·um** (per-i-kon′drē-ŭm) [TA] the dense, irregular connective tissue membrane around cartilage. [peri- + G. *chondros*, cartilage]

**per·i·chrome** (per′i-krōm) denoting a nerve cell in which the chromophil substance, or stainable material, is scattered throughout the cytoplasm. [peri- + G. *chrōma*, a color]

**per·i·co·li·tis** (per′i-kō-lī′tis) inflammation of the connective tissue or peritoneum surrounding the colon. SYN serocolitis.

**per·i·col·pi·tis** (per′i-kol-pī′tis) SYN perivaginitis. [peri- + G. *kolpos*, bosom (vagina), + *-itis*, inflammation]

**per·i·cor·o·ni·tis** (per-i-kōr-ŏ-nī′tis) inflammation around the crown of a tooth, usually a partially emerged one. [peri- + L. *corona*, crown, + G. *-itis*, inflammation]

**per·i·cra·ni·tis** (per′i-krā-nī′tis) inflammation of the pericranium.

**per·i·cra·ni·um** (per′i-krā′nē-ŭm) the periosteum of the skull. [peri- + G. *kranion*, skull]

**per·i·cys·tic** (per′i-sis′tik) **1.** surrounding the urinary bladder. **2.** surrounding the gallbladder. **3.** surrounding a cyst. SYN perivesical. [peri- + G. *kystis*, bladder]

**per·i·cys·ti·tis** (per′i-sis-tī′tis) inflammation of the tissues surrounding a bladder, especially the urinary bladder.

**per·i·cyte** (per′i-sīt) one of the slender mesenchymal-like cells found in close association with the outside wall of postcapillary venules; it is relatively undifferentiated and may become a fibroblast, macrophage, or smooth muscle cell. SYN adventitial cell. [peri- + G. *kytos,* cell]

**per·i·cyt·ic ven·ules** SYN postcapillary venules.

**per·i·den·tal mem·brane** SYN periodontal ligament.

**per·i·derm, per·i·der·ma** (per′i-derm, per-i-der′mă) the outermost layer of the epidermis of the embryo and fetus to the sixth month of intrauterine life; desquamated epitrichial cells are a considerable component of the vernix caseosa. SYN epitrichium. [peri- + G. *derma,* skin]

**per·i·des·mi·tis** (per′i-dez-mī′tis) inflammation of the connective tissue surrounding a ligament. [peri- + G. *desmos,* band, + *-itis,* inflammation]

**per·i·des·mi·um** (per-i-dez′mē-ŭm) the connective tissue membrane surrounding a ligament. [peri- + G. *desmion (desmos),* band]

**per·i·did·y·mi·tis** (per′i-did-i-mī′tis) inflammation of the perididymis.

**per·i·di·ver·tic·u·li·tis** (per′i-dī′ver-tik′yu-lī′tis) inflammation of the tissues around an intestinal diverticulum.

**per·i·du·o·de·ni·tis** (per′i-dū′ō-dē-nī′tis) inflammation around the duodenum.

**per·i·du·ral anes·the·sia** SYN epidural anesthesia.

**per·i·en·ceph·a·li·tis** (per′ē-en-sef-ă-lī′tis) inflammation of the cerebral membranes, particularly leptomeningitis or inflammation of the pia mater with involvement of the underlying cortex. [peri- + G. *enkephalos,* brain]

**per·i·en·ter·i·tis** (per′ē-en-ter-ī′tis) inflammation of the peritoneal coat of the intestine. SYN seroenteritis.

**per·i·e·soph·a·gi·tis** (per′ē-e-sof′ă-jī′tis) inflammation of the tissues surrounding the esophagus.

**per·i·fol·lic·u·li·tis** (per′i-fŏ-lik′yu-lī′tis) the presence of an inflammatory infiltrate surrounding hair follicles; frequently occurs in conjunction with folliculitis.

**per·i·gas·tri·tis** (per′i-gas-trī′tis) inflammation of the peritoneal coat of the stomach.

**per·i·glot·tis** (per-i-glot′is) the mucous membrane of the tongue. [G. *periglōttis,* covering of the tongue]

**per·i·hep·a·ti·tis** (pĕr′i-hep-ă-tī′tis) inflammation of the serous, or peritoneal, covering of the liver. [peri- + G. *hēpar,* liver, + *-itis,* inflammation]

**per·i-in·farc·tion block** an electrocardiographic abnormality associated with an old myocardial infarct and caused by delayed activation of the myocardium in the region of the infarct; characterized by an initial vector directed away from the infarcted region with the terminal vector directed toward it.

**per·i·je·ju·ni·tis** (per′i-jĕ-joo-nī′tis) inflammation around the jejunum.

**per·i·kar·y·on,** pl. **per·i·kar·ya** (per-i-kar′ē-on, per-i-kar′ē-ă) **1.** the cytoplasm around the nucleus, such as that of the cell body of nerve cells. **2.** the body of the odontoblast, excluding the dentinal fiber. **3.** the cell body of the nerve cell, as distinguished from its axon and dendrites. [peri- + G. *karyon,* kernel]

**per·i·ky·ma·ta** (per-i-kī′mă-tă) shallow, horizontal furrows on the enamel of a tooth where the

striae of Retzius meet the surface. [peri- + G. *kyma,* wave]

**per·i·lab·y·rin·thi·tis** (per′i-lab′ĭ-rin-thī′tis) inflammation of the parts about the labyrinth.

**per·i·lymph** (per′i-limf) the fluid contained within the osseous labyrinth, surrounding and protecting the membranous labyrinth; perilymph resembles extracellular fluid in composition (sodium is the predominant cation) and, via the perilymphatic duct, is in continuity with cerebrospinal fluid. SYN perilympha.

**per·i·lym·pha** (per′i-lim′fă) SYN perilymph. [peri- + L. *lympha,* a clear fluid (lymph)]

**per·i·lym·phan·gi·tis** (per′i-lim-fan-jī′tis) inflammation of the tissues surrounding a lymphatic vessel.

**per·i·lym·phat·ic** (per′i-lim-fat′ik) **1.** surrounding a lymphatic structure (node or vessel). **2.** the spaces and tissues surrounding the membranous labyrinth of the inner ear.

**per·i·lym·phat·ic duct** a fine canal connecting the perilymphatic space of the cochlea with the subarachnoid space. SYN aqueductus cochleae [TA].

**per·i·lym·pha·tic fis·tu·la** a fistula between the vestibule of the inner ear and the middle ear through which perilymph can leak, resulting in auditory and vestibular disturbances; common sites for perilymphatic fistula are the oval window through or around the footplate of the stapes or the round window through the round window membrane.

**per·i·lym·pha·tic gush·er** abnormal flow of perilymph when the footplate of the stapes is perforated; occurs in X-linked mixed deafness (DFN 3) due to a mutation of the POU3F4 gene and in other conditions.

**per·i·lym·phat·ic space** space between the bony and membranous portions of the labyrinth.

**per·i·men·in·gi·tis** (per′i-men-in-jī′tis) SYN pachymeningitis.

**pe·rim·e·ter** (pĕ-rim′ĕ-ter) **1.** a circumference, edge, or border. **2.** an instrument, usually half a circle or sphere, used to measure the field of vision. [G. *perimetros,* circumference, fr. *peri,* around, + *metron,* measure]

**per·i·met·ric** (per-i-met′rik) **1.** surrounding the uterus; relating to the perimetrium. SYN periuterine. [G. *peri,* around, + *mētra,* uterus] **2.** relating to the circumference of any part or area. [G. *perimetros,* circumference] **3.** relating to perimetry.

**per·i·me·trit·ic** (per-i-me-trit′ik) relating to or marked by perimetritis.

**per·i·me·tri·tis** (per′i-me-trī′tis) SYN metroperitonitis. [perimetrium + G. *-itis,* inflammation]

**per·i·me·tri·um,** pl. **per·i·me·tria** (per-i-mē′trē-ŭm, per-i-mē′trē-ă) [TA] the serous (peritoneal) coat of the uterus. [peri- + G. *mētra,* uterus]

**pe·rim·e·try** (pĕ-rim′ĕ-trē) **1.** the determination of the limits of the visual field. **2.** the mapping of the sensitivity contours of the visual field. [G. *perimetros,* circumference]

**per·i·mol·y·sis** (per-ĕ-mol′i-sis) decalcification of the teeth from exposure to gastric acid in individuals with chronic vomiting. [perimylolysis, fr. peri- + G. *mylos,* molar + *lysis,* loosening, dissolving, fr. *luō,* to loosen]

**per·i·my·e·li·tis** (per′i-mī-ĕ-lī′tis) SYN endosteitis.

**per·i·my·o·si·tis** (per′i-mī-ō-sī′tis) inflammation

of the loose cellular tissue surrounding a muscle. SYN perimysiitis (2), perimysitis.

**per·i·my·si·al** (per-i-mis′ē-ăl) relating to the perimysium; surrounding a muscle.

**per·i·my·si·i·tis, per·i·my·si·tis** (per′i-mis-ē-ī′tis, per′i-mī-sī′tis) **1.** inflammation of the perimysium. **2.** SYN perimyositis.

**per·i·my·si·um,** pl. **per·i·my·sia** (per-i-mis′ē-ŭm, per-i-mis′-ē-ă) the fibrous sheath enveloping each of the primary bundles of skeletal muscle fibers. [peri- + G. *mys,* muscle]

**per·i·na·tal** (per-i-nā′tăl) occurring during, or pertaining to, the periods before, during, or after the time of birth; i.e., before delivery from the 28th week of gestation through the first 7 days after delivery. [peri- + L. *natus,* pp. of *nascor,* to be born]

**per·i·na·tal med·i·cine** SYN perinatology.

**per·i·na·tol·o·gist** (per-i-nā-tol′ō-jist) an obstetrician who subspecializes in perinatology.

**per·i·na·tol·o·gy** (per-i-nā-tol′ō-jē) a subspecialty of obstetrics concerned with care of the mother and fetus during pregnancy, labor, and delivery, particularly when the mother and/or fetus are at a high risk for complications. SYN perinatal medicine.

**per·i·ne·al** (per′i-nē′ăl) relating to the perineum.

**per·i·ne·al ar·tery** *origin,* internal pudendal; *distribution,* superficial structures of the perineum; *anastomoses,* external pudendal arteries. SYN arteria perinealis [TA].

**per·i·ne·al fas·cia** fascia that intimately invests the superficial perineal muscles (ischiocavernosus, bulbospongiosus, and superficial transverse perineal muscles); anteriorly it is fused to the suspensory ligament of the penis/clitoris, and is continuous with the deep fascia covering the external oblique muscle of the abdomen and the rectus sheath. SYN superficial investing fascia of perineum.

**per·i·ne·al her·nia** a hernia protruding through the pelvic diaphragm.

**per·i·ne·al nerves** the superficial terminal branches of the pudendal nerve, supplying most of the muscles of the perineum (deep branch) as well as the skin of that region (superficial branch). SYN nervi perineales [TA].

**per·i·ne·al ra·phe** the central anteroposterior line of the perineum, most marked in the male, being continuous with the raphe of the scrotum.

**per·i·ne·al sec·tion** any cutting through the perineum, either lateral or median lithotomy or external urethrotomy.

⚠**per·i·neo-** the perineum. [L. fr. G. *perineos, perinaion*]

**per·i·ne·o·cele** (per-i-nē′ō-sēl) a hernia in the perineal region, either between the rectum and the vagina or the rectum and the bladder, or alongside the rectum. [perineo- + G. *kēlē,* hernia]

**per·i·ne·o·plas·ty** (per-i-nē′ō-plas-tē) plastic surgery of the perineum. [perineum + G. *plastos,* formed]

**per·i·ne·or·rha·phy** (per-i-nē-ōr′ă-fē) suture of the perineum, performed in perineoplasty. [perineum + G. *rhaphē,* a sewing]

**per·i·ne·o·scro·tal** (per-i-nē′ō-skrō′tăl) relating to the perineum and the scrotum.

**per·i·ne·os·to·my** (per-i-nē-os′tō-mē) urethrostomy through the perineum. [perineo- + G. *stoma,* mouth]

**per·i·ne·ot·o·my** (per-i-nē-ot′ō-mē) incision into

the perineum to facilitate childbirth. SEE ALSO episiotomy.

**per·i·ne·o·vag·i·nal** (per-i-nē′ō-vaj′i-năl) relating to the perineum and the vagina.

**per·i·neph·ri·al** (per′i-nef′rē-ăl) relating to the perinephrium.

**per·i·neph·ri·tis** (per′i-ne-frī′tis) inflammation of perinephric tissue.

**per·i·neph·ri·um,** pl. **per·i·neph·ria** (per′i-nef′rē-ŭm, per′i-nef′rē-ă) the connective tissue and fat surrounding the kidney. [peri- + G. *nephros,* kidney]

**per·i·ne·um,** pl. **per·i·nea** (pĕr′i-nē′ŭm, per′i-nē′ă) **1.** the area between the thighs extending from the coccyx to the pubis and lying below the pelvic diaphragm. **2.** the external surface of the central tendon of the perineum, lying between the vulva and the anus in the female and the scrotum and the anus in the male. [L. fr. G. *perineon, perinaion*]

**per·i·neu·ral an·es·the·sia** anesthesia produced by injection of an anesthetic agent around a nerve.

**per·i·neu·ri·al** (per′i-noo′rē-ăl) relating to the perineurium.

**per·i·neu·ri·tis** (per′i-noo-rī′tis) inflammation of the perineurium. SEE ALSO adventitial neuritis.

**per·i·neu·ri·um,** pl. **per·i·neu·ria** (per-i-noo′rē-ŭm, per′i-noo′-rē-ă) [TA] one of the supporting structures of peripheral nerve trunks, consisting of layers of flattened cells and collagenous connective tissue, which surround the nerve fasciculi and form the major diffusion barrier within the nerve; with the endoneurium and epineurium, composes the peripheral nerve stroma. [L. fr. peri- + G. *neuron,* nerve]

**pe·ri·od** (pēr′ē-od) **1.** a certain duration or division of time. **2.** one of the stages of a disease, e.g., period of incubation, period of convalescence. SEE ALSO stage, phase. **3.** colloquialism for menses. **4.** any of the horizontal rows of chemical elements in the periodic table. [G. *periodos,* a way round, a cycle, fr. *peri,* around, + *hodos,* way]

**pe·ri·od·ic** (pēr-ē-od′ik) **1.** recurring at regular intervals. **2.** denoting a disease with regularly recurring exacerbations or paroxysms.

**pe·ri·od·ic dis·ease** any condition or disease in which episodes tend to recur at regular intervals; many such cases are manifestations of familial Mediterranean fever; the cause of the periodicity is usually unknown.

**per·i·o·dic·i·ty** (pēr′ē-ō-dis′i-tē) tendency to recurrence at regular intervals.

**pe·ri·od·ic neu·tro·pe·nia** neutropenia recurring at regular intervals, in association with various types of infectious diseases.

**pe·ri·od·ic pa·ral·y·sis** term for a group of diseases characterized by recurring episodes of muscular weakness or flaccid paralysis without loss of consciousness, speech, or sensation; attacks begin when the patient is at rest, and there is apparent good health between attacks. SEE hyperkalemic periodic paralysis, hypokalemic periodic paralysis, normokalemic periodic paralysis.

**per·i·o·di·za·tion** sequenced program that varies training volume and intensity to optimize physiologic functional capacity and exercise performance by structuring training into time blocks of different duration (macrocycles, mesocycles).

Goal is to prevent staleness while peaking physiologically for competition.

**per·i·o·don·tal** (per'ē-ō-don'tăl) around a tooth. [peri- + G. *odous*, tooth]

**Per·i·o·don·tal Index (PI)** an index for the epidemiological classification of periodontal disease.

**per·i·o·don·tal lig·a·ment** the connective tissue that surrounds the tooth root and attaches it to its bony socket; it consists of fibers anchored in the cementum and extending into the alveolar bone; the tissues that surround and support the teeth, including the gingivae, cementum, periodontal ligament, and alveolar and supporting bone. SYN alveolodental ligament, alveolodental membrane, peridental membrane, periodontal membrane, periodontium (2).

**per·i·o·don·tal mem·brane** SYN periodontal ligament.

**Per·i·o·don·tal Screen·ing Rec·ord** a modified CPITN used primarily in the United States. SEE ALSO Community Periodontal Index of Treatment Needs.

**per·i·o·don·tia** (per'ē-ō-don'shē-ă) **1.** plural of periodontium. **2.** SYN periodontics.

**per·i·o·don·tics** (per'ē-ō-don'tiks) the branch of dentistry concerned with the study of the normal tissues and the treatment of abnormal conditions of the tissues immediately about the teeth. SYN periodontia (2). [peri- + G. *odous*, tooth]

**per·i·o·don·tist** (per'ē-ō-don'tist) a dentist who specializes in periodontics.

**per·i·o·don·ti·tis** (per'ē-ō-don-tī'tis) **1.** inflammation of the periodontium. **2.** a chronic inflammatory disease of the periodontium occurring in response to bacterial plaque on the adjacent teeth; characterized by gingivitis, destruction of the alveolar bone and periodontal ligament, apical migration of the epithelial attachment resulting in the formation of periodontal pockets, and ultimately loosening and exfoliation of the teeth. [periodontium + G. *-itis*, inflammation]

**per·i·o·don·ti·um**, pl. **per·i·o·don·tia** (per'ē-ō-don'shē-ŭm, per'ē-ō-don'shē-ă) **1.** all of the tissues that invest and support the teeth. **2.** SYN periodontal ligament. [L. fr. peri- + G. *odous*, tooth]

**per·i·o·don·to·cla·sia** (per'ē-ō-don-tō-klā'zē-ă) destruction of periodontal tissues, gingiva, pericementum, alveolar bone, and cementum. [periodontium + *klasis*, breaking]

**per·i·o·don·to·sis** (per'ē-ō-don-tō'sis) SYN juvenile periodontitis. [periodontium + G. *-osis*, condition]

**per·i·o·nych·ia** (per-ē-ō-nik'ē-ă) **1.** inflammation of the perionychium. **2.** plural of perionychium.

**per·i·o·nych·i·um**, pl. **per·i·o·nych·ia** (per-ē-ō-nik'ē-ŭm, per-ē-ō-nik'ē-ă) SYN eponychium (2). [peri- + G. *onyx*, nail]

**per·i·o·o·pho·ri·tis** (per'ē-ō-of'ō-rī'tis) inflammation of the peritoneal covering of the ovary. SYN periovaritis. [peri- + Mod. L. *oophoron*, ovary, + *-itis*, inflammation]

**per·i·o·o·pho·ro·sal·pin·gi·tis** (per'ē-ō-of'ō-rō-sal-pin-jī'tis) inflammation of the peritoneum and other tissues around the ovary and oviduct. SYN perisalpingoovaritis. [peri- + Mod. L. *oophoron*, ovary, + *salpinx*, trumpet, + *-itis*, inflammation]

**per·i·op·er·a·tive** (per-ē-op'er-ă-tiv) around the time of operation. SYN paraoperative.

**per·i·or·bit** (per-ē-ōr'bit) SYN periorbita.

**pe·ri·or·bi·ta** (perē-ōr'bi-tă) [TA] the periosteum of the orbit. SYN periorbit. [peri- + L. *orbita*, orbit]

**per·i·or·bi·tal** (per-ē-ōr'bi-tăl) **1.** relating to the periorbita. **2.** SYN circumorbital.

**per·i·or·bi·tal cel·lu·li·tis** SYN preseptal cellulitis.

**per·i·or·chi·tis** (per'ē-ōr-kī'tis) inflammation of the tunica vaginalis testis. [peri- + G. *orchis*, testis, + *-itis*, inflammation]

**pe·ri·os·tea** (per-ē-os'tē-ă) plural of periosteum.

**per·i·os·te·al** (per-ē-os'tē-ăl) relating to the periosteum.

**per·i·os·te·al bud** a vascular connective tissue bud from the perichondrium that invades the ossification center of the cartilaginous model of a developing long bone.

**per·i·os·te·al el·e·va·tor** an instrument used for separating the periosteum from the bone. SYN rugine (1).

**per·i·os·te·al graft** a graft of periosteum, usually placed on bare bone.

**per·i·os·te·i·tis** (per'ē-os-tē-ī'tis) SYN periostitis.

△**per·i·os·te·o-** the periosteum. [Mod. L. *periosteum*]

**per·i·os·te·o·ma** (per'ē-os'tē-ō'mă) a neoplasm derived from the periosteum. SYN periosteophyte.

**per·i·os·te·o·my·e·li·tis** (per-ē-os'tē-ō-mī-ĕ-lī'tis) inflammation of the entire bone, with the periosteum and marrow. [periosteo- + G. *myelos*, marrow, + *-itis*, inflammation]

**per·i·os·te·o·phyte** (per-ē-os'te-ō-fīt) SYN periosteoma. [periosteo- + G. *phyton*, growth]

**per·i·os·te·o·plas·tic am·pu·ta·tion** SYN subperiosteal amputation.

**per·i·os·te·o·sis** (per'ē-os-tē-ō'sis) the formation of a periosteoma. SYN periostosis.

**per·i·os·te·ot·o·my** (per'ē-os-tē-ot'ō-mē) the operation of cutting through the periosteum to the bone. [periosteo- + G. *tomē*, incision]

**per·i·os·te·um**, pl. **pe·ri·os·tea** (per-ē-os'tē-ŭm, per-ē-os'tē-ă) [TA] the thick fibrous membrane covering the entire surface of a bone except its articular cartilage. In young bones, it consists of two layers: an inner cellular layer that is osteogenic, forming new bone tissue, and an outer fibrous connective tissue layer conveying the blood vessels and nerves supplying the bone; in older bones, the osteogenic layer is reduced. SEE ALSO perichondral bone. [Mod. L. fr. G. *periosteon*, ntr. of adj. *periosteos*, around the bones, fr. *peri*, around, + *osteon*, bone]

**per·i·os·ti·tis** (per'ē-os-tī'tis) inflammation of the periosteum. SYN periosteitis.

**per·i·os·to·sis**, pl. **per·i·os·to·ses** (per'ē-os-tō'sis, per'ē-os-tō-sēz) SYN periosteosis.

**per·i·o·va·ri·tis** (per'ē-ō-vă-rī'tis) SYN perioophoritis.

**per·i·pach·y·men·in·gi·tis** (per'i-pak'ē-men-in-jī'tis) inflammation of the area between the dura and bony covering of the central nervous system. [peri- + pachymeninx (dura mater) + G. *-itis*, inflammation]

**per·i·pan·cre·a·ti·tis** (per'i-pan'krē-ă-tī'tis) inflammation of the peritoneal coat of the pancreas.

**pe·riph·e·rad** (pĕ-rif'ē-rad) in a direction toward the periphery. [G. *periphereia*, periphery, + L. *ad*, to]

**pe·riph·e·ral** (pĕ-rif'ē-răl) **1.** relating to or situated at the periphery. **2.** situated nearer the periphery of an organ or part of the body in relation to a specific reference point; opposite of central (centralis). SYN eccentric (3).

**pe·riph·e·ral fa·cial pa·ral·y·sis** SYN Bell palsy.

**pe·riph·e·ral ner·vous sys·tem** the peripheral part of the nervous system external to the brain and spinal cord from their roots to their peripheral terminations. This includes the ganglia, both sensory and autonomic and any plexuses through which the nerve fibers run. SEE ALSO autonomic division of nervous system. SYN peripheral part of nervous system.

**pe·riph·e·ral os·si·fy·ing fi·bro·ma** a reactive focal gingival overgrowth derived histogenetically from cells of the periodontal ligament and usually developing in response to local irritants (plaque and calculus) on associated teeth; consists microscopically of a hyperplastic cellular fibrous stroma supporting deposits of bone, cementum, or dystrophic calcification.

**pe·riph·e·ral part of ner·vous sys·tem** SYN peripheral nervous system.

**pe·riph·e·ral sco·to·ma** a scotoma outside of the central 30 degrees of the visual field.

**pe·riph·e·ral T-cell lym·pho·ma, un·spe·ci·fied** a heterogeneous group of T-cell neoplasms expressing typical T-cell markers such as CD2, CD3, CD5, and either T-cell α/β or γ/δ receptors.

**pe·riph·e·ral vi·sion** vision resulting from retinal stimulation beyond the macula. SYN indirect vision.

**pe·riph·e·ry** (pĕ-rif′ĕ-rē) 1. the part of a body away from the center; the outer part or surface. 2. SYN denture border. [G. *periphereia*, fr. *peri*, around, + *pherō*, to carry]

**per·i·phle·bi·tis** (per′i-fle-bī′tis) inflammation of the outer coat of a vein or of the tissues surrounding it. [peri- + G. *phleps*, vein, + -*itis*, inflammation]

**per·i·po·ri·tis** (per′i-pŏ-rī′tis) miliary papules and papulovesicles with staphylococcic infection; most frequently on the face and in infants. [peri- + G. *poros*, pore, + -*itis*, inflammation]

**per·i·proc·ti·tis** (per′i-prok-tī′tis) inflammation of the areolar tissue about the rectum. SYN perirectitis.

**per·i·pros·ta·ti·tis** (per′i-pros-tă-tī′tis) inflammation of the tissues surrounding the prostate.

**per·i·py·le·phle·bi·tis** (per-i-pī′lĕ-fle-bī′tis) inflammation of the tissues around the portal vein. [peri- + G. *pylē*, gate, + *phleps*, vein, + -*itis*, inflammation]

**per·i·rec·ti·tis** (per′i-rek-tī′tis) SYN periproctitis.

**per·i·rhi·zo·cla·sia** (per′ē-rī-zō-klā′zē-ă) inflammatory destruction of tissues immediately around the root of a tooth. [peri- + G. *rhiza*, root, -o- + *klasis*, destruction]

**per·i·sal·pin·gi·tis** (per-i-sal-pin-jī′tis) inflammation of the peritoneum covering the uterine tube. [peri- + G. *salpinx*, trumpet, + -*itis*, inflammation]

**per·i·sal·pin·go·ova·ri·tis** (per′i-sal-pin′gō-ō-vă-rī′tis) SYN perioophorosalpingitis. [peri- + G. *salpinx*, trumpet, + ovary + G. -*itis*, inflammation]

**per·i·sal·pinx** (per′i-sal′pingks) the peritoneal covering of the uterine tube. [peri- + G. *salpinx* (*salping*-), trumpet]

**per·i·scop·ic** (per′i-skop′ik) denoting that which gives the ability to see objects to one side as well

as in the direct axis of vision. [peri- + G. *skopeō*, to view]

**per·i·sig·moi·di·tis** (per′i-sig-moy-dī′tis) inflammation of the connective tissues surrounding the sigmoid flexure, giving rise to symptoms, referable to the left iliac fossa, similar to those of perityphlitis in the right iliac fossa.

**per·i·sper·ma·ti·tis** (per′i-sper-mă-tī′tis) inflammation of the tissues around the spermatic cord.

**per·i·splanch·ni·tis** (per′i-splangk-nī′tis) inflammation surrounding any viscus or viscera. [peri- + G. *splanchna*, viscera, + -*itis*, inflammation]

**per·i·sple·ni·tis** (per′i-sple-nī′tis) inflammation of the peritoneum covering the spleen.

**per·i·spon·dy·li·tis** (per-i-spon-di-lī′tis) inflammation of the tissues about a vertebra. [peri- + G. *spondylos*, vertebra, + -*itis*, inflammation]

**per·i·stal·sis** (per-i-stal′sis) the movement of the intestine or other tubular structure, characterized by waves of alternate circular contraction and relaxation of the tube by which the contents are propelled onward. SYN vermicular movement. [peri- + G. *stalsis*, constriction]

**per·i·stal·tic** (per-i-stal′tik) relating to peristalsis.

**pe·ris·to·le** (pĕ-ris′tō-lē) the tonic activity of the walls of the stomach whereby the organ contracts about its contents; contrasting with the peristaltic waves passing from the cardia toward the pylorus (peristalsis). [peri- + G. *stellō*, to contract]

**per·i·stol·ic** (per-i-stol′ik) relating to peristole.

**per·i·tec·to·my** (per′i-tek′tō-mē) 1. the removal of a paracorneal strip of the conjunctiva for the relief of corneal disease. 2. SYN circumcision (2). [peri- + G. *ektomē*, excision]

**pe·ri·ten·di·ne·um**, pl. **pe·ri·ten·di·nea** (per-i-ten-din′ē-ŭm, per-i-ten-din′ē-ē-ă) one of the fibrous sheaths surrounding the primary bundles of fibers in a tendon. [L. fr. peri- + G. *tenōn*, tendon]

**per·i·ten·di·ni·tis** (per′i-ten-di-nī′tis) inflammation of the sheath of a tendon. SYN peritenonitis, peritenontitis.

**peri·ten·on·itis** (per′ē-ten-on-ī′tiz) SYN peritendinitis.

**peri·ten·on·ti·tis** (per′i-ten-on-tī′tis) SYN peritendinitis.

**per·i·the·li·um**, pl. **per·i·the·lia** (per-i-thē′lē-ŭm, per-i-thē′lē-ă) the connective tissue that surrounds smaller vessels and capillaries. [peri- + G. *thēlē*, nipple]

**per·i·thy·roi·di·tis** (per′i-thī-roy-dī′tis) inflammation of the capsule or tissues surrounding the thyroid gland.

**pe·rit·o·my** (pĕ-rit′ō-mē) 1. a circumcorneal incision through the conjunctiva. 2. SYN circumcision (1). [G. *peritomē*, fr. *peri*, around, + *tomē*, incision]

**per·i·to·ne·al** (per′i-tō-nē′ăl) relating to the peritoneum.

**per·i·to·ne·al cav·i·ty** the interior of the peritoneal sac, normally only a potential space between the parietal and visceral layers of the peritoneum.

**per·i·to·ne·al di·al·y·sis** removal from the body of soluble substances and water by transfer across the peritoneum, utilizing a dialysis solution which is intermittently introduced into and removed from the peritoneal cavity.

**per·i·ton·e·al in·suf·fla·tion** the administration of a gas, usually carbon dioxide, within the peritoneal cavity to facilitate laparoendoscopic procedures.

⟳**per·i·to·neo-** the peritoneum. [L. *peritoneum*]

**per·i·to·ne·o·cen·te·sis** (per'i-tō-nē'ō-sen-tē'sis) paracentesis of the abdomen. [peritoneum + G. *kentēsis*, puncture]

**per·i·to·ne·oc·ly·sis** (per'i-tō-nē-ok'li-sis) irrigation of the abdominal cavity. [peritoneum, + G. *klysis*, a washing out]

**per·i·to·ne·o·per·i·car·di·al** (per'i-tō-nē'ō-per'i-kar'dē-ăl) relating to the peritoneum and the pericardium.

**per·i·to·ne·o·pexy** (per'i-tō-nē'ō-pek-sē) a suspension or fixation of the peritoneum. [peritoneum + G. *pēxis*, fixation]

**per·i·to·ne·o·plas·ty** (per'i-tō-nē'ō-plas-tē) loosening adhesions and covering the raw surfaces with peritoneum to prevent reformation. [peritoneum + G. *plastos*, formed]

**per·i·to·ne·o·scope** (per'i-tō-nē'ō-skōp) SYN laparoscope. [peritoneum + G. *skopeō*, to view]

**per·i·to·ne·os·co·py** (per'i-tō-nē-os'kŏ-pē) examination of the contents of the peritoneum with a peritoneoscope passed through the abdominal wall. SEE ALSO laparoscopy. SYN abdominoscopy, celioscopy, ventroscopy.

**per·i·to·ne·ot·o·my** (per'i-tō-nē-ot'ō-mē) incision of the peritoneum. [peritoneum + G. *tomē*, incision]

**per·i·to·ne·o·ve·nous shunt** a shunt, usually by a catheter, between the peritoneal cavity and the venous system.

**per·i·to·ne·um**, pl. **pe·ri·to·nea** (per'i-tō-nē'ŭm, per'i-tō-nē'-ă) [TA] the serous membrane, consisting of mesothelium and connective tissue, that lines the abdominal cavity and covers most of the viscera contained therein; it forms two sacs: the peritoneal (or greater) sac and the omental bursa (lesser sac) connected by the epiploic foramen. [Mod. L. fr. G. *peritonaion*, fr. *periteinō*, to stretch over]

**per·i·to·ne·um uro·gen·i·ta·le** SYN urogenital peritoneum.

**per·i·to·ni·tis** (per'i-tō-nī'tis) inflammation of the peritoneum.

**per·i·ton·sil·lar ab·scess** extension of tonsillar infection beyond the capsule with abscess formation usually above and behind the tonsil. SYN quinsy.

**per·i·ton·sil·li·tis** (per'i-ton'si-lī'tis) inflammation of the connective tissue above and behind the tonsil.

**pe·rit·ri·chal, pe·rit·ri·chate, per·i·trich·ic** (pe-rit'ri-kăl, pe-rit'ri-kāt, per-i-trik'ik) SYN peritrichous (2).

**pe·rit·ri·chous** (pe-rit'ri-kŭs) **1.** relating to cilia or other appendicular organs projecting from the periphery of a cell. **2.** having flagella uniformly distributed over a cell; used especially with reference to bacteria. SYN peritrichal, peritrichate, peritrichic. [peri- + G. *thrix*, hair]

**per·i·tu·bu·lar con·trac·tile cells** SYN myoid cells.

**per·i·u·re·ter·i·tis** (per'i-yu-rē'ter-ī'tis) inflammation of the tissues about a ureter. [peri- + ureter + G. *-itis*, inflammation]

**per·i·u·re·thri·tis** (per'i-yu-rē-thrī'tis) inflammation of the tissues about the urethra. [peri- + urethra + G. *-itis*, inflammation]

**per·i·u·ter·ine** (per'i-yu'ter-in) SYN perimetric (1).

**per·i·vag·i·ni·tis** (per'i-vaj-i-nī'tis) inflammation of the connective tissue around the vagina. SYN pericolpitis.

**per·i·vas·cu·li·tis** (per'i-vas-kyu-lī'tis) SYN periangitis.

**per·i·ves·i·cal** (per-i-ves'i-kăl) SYN pericystic. [peri- + L. *vesica*, bladder]

**per·i·vis·cer·i·tis** (per'i-vis-er-ī'tis) inflammation surrounding any viscus or viscera. [peri- + L. *viscera*, internal organs, + G. *-itis*, inflammation]

**per·ma·nent car·ti·lage** cartilage that is not replaced by bone.

⊟**per·ma·nent den·ti·tion** the adult dentition of 32 teeth, consisting in each quadrant of two incisors, one canine, two premolars, and three molars, in that order from the midline. See this page.

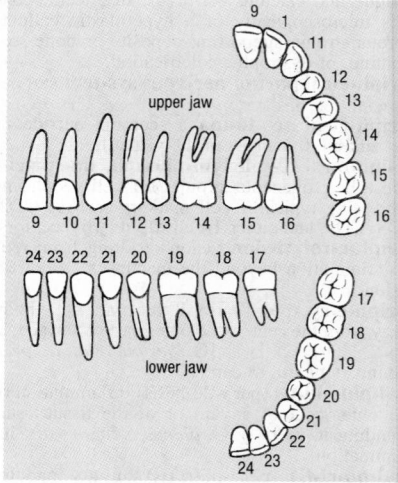

**permanent dentition, half view, left side** (numbering code, universal system of permanent teeth): central incisor 9, 24; lateral incisor 10, 23; canine 11, 22; first bicuspid 12, 21; second biscupid 13, 20; first molar 14, 19; second molar 15, 18; third molar 16, 17

**per·ma·nent stained smear exam·in·a·tion** microscopic review at oil immersion (1000×) magnification of fecal specimens stained with trichrome, iron-hematoxylin, and such stains; primarily used for protozoan trophozoites, cysts, oocysts, and spores.

**per·ma·nent thresh·old shift** the irreversible hearing loss that results from exposure to intense impulse or continuous sound, as opposed to the reversible temporary threshold shift that also results from such exposure.

**per·ma·nent tooth** one of the 32 teeth belonging to the second, or permanent, dentition; eruption of the permanent teeth begins from the 5th to the 7th year, and is not completed until the 17th to the 23rd year, when the last of the wisdom teeth appears. SYN dens permanens [TA], second tooth, secondary dentition.

**per·me·a·bil·i·ty** (per'mē-ă-bil'i-tē) the property of being permeable.

**per·me·a·bil·i·ty co·ef·fi·cient** a coefficient associated with simple diffusion through a membrane that is proportional to the partition coefficient and the diffusion coefficient and inversely proportional to membrane thickness.

**per·me·a·bil·i·ty con·stant** a measure of the ease with which an ion can cross a unit area of membrane driven by a 1.0 M difference in concentration; usually expressed in centimeters per second. Cf. permeability coefficient.

**per·me·a·ble** (per′mē-ă-bl) permitting the passage of substances (e.g., liquids, gases, heat), as through a membrane or other structure. SYN pervious. [L. *permeabilis* (see permeate)]

**per·me·ase** (per′mē-ās) any of a group of membrane-bound carriers (enzymes) that effect the transport of solute through a semipermeable membrane.

**per·me·ate** (per′mē-āt) 1. to pass through a membrane or other structure. 2. that which can so pass. [L. *permeo,* to pass through]

**per·me·a·tion** (per-mē-ā′shŭn) the process of spreading through or penetrating, as the extension of a malignant neoplasm by proliferation of the cells continuously along the blood vessels or lymphatics. [L. *per-meo,* pp. *-meatus,* to pass through]

**per·ni·cious** (per-nish′ŭs) destructive; harmful; denoting a disease of severe character and usually fatal without appropriate treatment. [L. *perniciosus,* destructive, fr. *pernicies,* destruction]

⊞ **per·ni·cious a·ne·mia** a chronic progressive anemia of older adults due to failure of absorption of vitamin $B_{12}$, usually resulting from a defect of the stomach accompanied by mucosal atrophy and associated with lack of secretion of "intrinsic" factor; characterized by numbness and tingling, weakness, and a sore smooth tongue, as well as dyspnea after slight exertion, faintness, pallor of the skin and mucous membranes, anorexia, diarrhea, loss of weight, and fever; laboratory studies usually reveal greatly decreased red blood cell counts, low levels of hemoglobin, numerous characteristically oval shaped macrocytic erythrocytes, and hypo- or achlorhydria, in association with a predominant number of megaloblasts and relatively few normoblasts in the bone marrow; the leukocyte count in peripheral blood may be less than normal, with relative lymphocytosis and hypersegmented neutrophils; a low level of vitamin $B_{12}$ is found in peripheral red blood cells; administration of vitamin $B_{12}$ results in a characteristic reticulocyte response, relief from symptoms, and an increase in erythrocytes, provided that pernicious anemia is not complicated by another disease. See page B2. SYN Addison anemia, malignant anemia.

**per·ni·cious vom·it·ing** uncontrollable vomiting.

△**pero-** maimed, malformed. [G. *pēros*]

**pe·ro·dac·ty·ly, pe·ro·dac·tyl·ia** (pē-rō-dak′ti-lē, pē-rō-dak-til′ē-ă) congenital deformity of fingers and toes. [pero- + G. *daktylos,* finger or toe]

**pe·ro·me·lia, pe·rom·e·ly** (pē-rō-mē′lē-ă, pĕ-rom′ĕ-lē) severe congenital malformations of limbs, including absence of hand or foot. [pero- + G. *melos,* limb]

**per·o·ne·al** (per-ō-nē′ăl) relating to the fibula, to the lateral side of the leg, or to the muscles there present. [L. *peroneus,* fr. G. *peronē,* fibula]

**per·o·ne·al ar·tery** origin, posterior tibial; dis-

*tribution,* soleus, tibialis posterior, flexor longus hallucis, peroneal muscles, inferior tibiofibular articulation, and ankle joint; *anastomoses,* anterior lateral malleolar, lateral tarsal, lateral plantar, dorsalis pedis. SYN arteria peronea [TA], fibular artery.

**per·o·ne·al mus·cu·lar at·ro·phy** a group of familial peripheral neuromuscular disorders, sharing the common feature of marked wasting of the distal parts of the extremities, particularly the peroneal muscle groups, resulting in "stork legs." SYN Charcot-Marie-Tooth disease.

**per·o·ne·al ret·i·nac·u·lum** superior and inferior fibrous bands retaining the tendons of the peroneus longus and brevis in position as they cross the lateral side of the ankle. SYN retinacula of peroneal muscles.

**per·o·ne·al veins** venae comitantes of the peroneal artery; they join the posterior tibial veins to enter the popliteal vein. SYN fibular veins.

**per·o·ne·us ter·ti·us mus·cle** origin, in common with musculus extensor digitorum longus; *insertion,* dorsum of base of fifth metatarsal bone; *nerve supply,* deep branch of peroneal; *action,* assists in dorsiflexion and eversion of foot. SYN third peroneal muscle.

**per·o·ral** (pĕr-ō′răl) through the mouth, denoting a method of medication or an approach. [L. *per,* through, + *os* (*or-*), mouth]

**per os (PO)** by or through the mouth, denoting a method of medication. [L.]

△**per·oxi-** SEE peroxy-.

**per·ox·i·das·es** (pĕr-ok′si-dās-ez) [EC subclass 1.11] enzymes in animal and plant tissues that catalyze the dehydrogenation (oxidation) of various substances in the presence of hydrogen peroxide, which acts as hydrogen acceptor, being converted to water in the process.

**per·ox·ide** (pĕr-ok′sīd) that oxide of any series that contains the greatest number of oxygen atoms.

**per·ox·i·some** (pĕr-ok′si-sōm) a membrane-bound organelle occurring in nearly all eukaryotic cells that often contains oxidative enzymes relating to the formation and degradation of $H_2O_2$. SYN microbody. [peroxide + G. *sōma,* body]

△**per·oxy-** prefix denoting the presence of an extra O atom, as in peroxides, peroxy acids.

**per·ox·yl** (pĕr-ok′sil) one of the free radicals presumed formed as a result of the bombardment of tissue by high-energy radiation.

**per pri·mam in·ten·ti·o·nem** (pĕr prī′mam in-ten-shē-ō′nem) by first intention. SEE healing by first intention. [L.]

**per rec·tum** (pĕr rek′tŭm) by or through the rectum, denoting a method of examination or treatment. [L.]

**per·salt** (pĕr′sawlt) CHEMISTRY any salt that contains the greatest possible amount of the acid radical.

**per·sev·er·a·tion** (pĕr-sev-er-ā′shŭn) 1. the constant repetition of a meaningless word or phrase. 2. the duration of a mental impression, measured by the rapidity with which one impression follows another as determined by the revolving of a two-colored disk. 3. CLINICAL PSYCHOLOGY the uncontrollable repetition of a previously appropriate or correct response, even though the repeated response has since become inappropriate or incorrect. [L. *persevero,* to persist]

**per·sis·tence** (pĕr-sis'tens) **1.** obstinate continuation of characteristic behavior. **2.** survival in spite of opposition or adverse environmental conditions. [L. *persisto,* to abide, stand firm]

**per·sis·tent an·te·ri·or hy·per·plas·tic pri·mary vit·re·ous** a unilateral congenital abnormality occurring in full-term infants; characterized by a retrolental fibrovascular membrane formed by persistent primary vitreous with remnants of the hyaloid artery and tunica vasculosa lentis; associated with leukokoria, microphthalmos, shallow anterior chamber, and elongated ciliary processes.

**per·sis·tent chron·ic hep·a·ti·tis** a benign chronic hepatitis that may follow acute viral hepatitis B or C or complicate bowel diseases; rarely progresses to cirrhosis, portal hypertension, or liver failure.

**per·sis·tent clo·a·ca** a condition in which the urorectal septum has failed to divide the cloaca of the embryo into rectal and urogenital portions.

**per·sis·tent pos·te·ri·or hy·per·plas·tic pri·mary vit·re·ous** a unilateral congenital anomaly in full-term infants; associated with a congenital retinal fold and a vitreous membranous stalk containing remnants of the hyaloid artery.

**per·sis·tent trun·cus ar·te·ri·o·sus** a congenital cardiovascular deformity resulting from failure of development of the spiral septum and consisting of a common arterial trunk opening out of both ventricles, the pulmonary arteries being given off from the ascending common trunk.

**per·sis·tent veg·e·ta·tive state (PVS)** vegetative state of prolonged duration (defined in different sources as duration of greater than 1 month, 1 year, or 2 years); usually permanent. SEE ALSO vegetative.

**per·so·na** (pĕr-sō'nă) a term that embodies the total constellation of physical, psychological, and behavioral attributes of each unique individual; in jungian psychology, the outer aspect of character, as opposed to anima (2); the assumed personality used to mask the true one. [L. *persona,* actor's mask; character, role, prob. fr. Etruscan]

**per·son·al e·qua·tion** a slight error in judgment, perceptual response, or action peculiar to the individual and so constant that it is usually possible to allow for it in accepting the person's statements or conclusions, thus arriving at approximate exactness.

**per·son·al·i·ty** (pĕr-sŏn-al'i-tē) **1.** the unique self; the organized system of attitudes and behavioral predispositions by which one feels, thinks, acts, and impresses and establishes relationships with others. **2.** an individual with a particular personality pattern.

**per·son·al·i·ty dis·or·der** general term for a group of behavioral disorders characterized by usually lifelong, ingrained, maladaptive patterns of deviant behavior, life style, and social adjustment that are different in quality from psychotic and neurotic symptoms; former designations for individuals with these personality disorders were psychopath and sociopath. SEE ALSO antisocial personality disorder.

**per·son·al·i·ty for·ma·tion** the life history associated with the development of individual patterns and of one's individuality.

**per·son·al·i·ty pro·file 1.** a method by which the results of psychological testing are presented

in graphic form; **2.** a vignette or brief personality description.

**per·son·al space** a term used in the behavioral sciences to denote the physical area immediately surrounding an individual who is in proximity to one or more others, whether known or unknown, and which serves as a body buffer zone in such interpersonal transactions.

**pers·pi·ra·tion** (pĕrs-pi-rā'shŭn) **1.** the excretion of fluid by the sweat glands of the skin. SYN diaphoresis, sudation, sweating. SEE ALSO sweat. **2.** all fluid loss through normal skin, whether by sweat gland secretion or by diffusion through other skin structures. **3.** the fluid excreted by the sweat glands; it consists of water containing sodium chloride and phosphate, urea, ammonia, ethereal sulfates, creatinine, fats, and other waste products; the average daily quantity is estimated at about 1500 g. SYN sudor. SEE ALSO sweat (1). [L. *per-spiro,* pp. *-atus,* to breathe everywhere]

**per·tac·tin** (pĕr-tak'tin) an antigenic material produced by *Bordetella pertussis* used to improve the effectiveness of pertussis vaccines. [*pert*ussis + act + -in]

**per·tech·ne·tate** (pĕr-tek-ne-tāt) anionic form of technetium used widely in nuclear scanning; $^{99m}$TcO4.

**Per·thes test** (per'tĕz) a test for patency of the deep femoral vein; with the patient standing, a tourniquet is applied above the knee; after walking, if the deep circulation is competent, the superficial varicosities remain unchanged; if the deep circulation is occluded, the legs become painful.

**Per·tik di·ver·tic·u·lum** (per'tik) an abnormally deep recessus pharyngeus.

**per tu·bam** (pĕr too'băm) through a tube. [L.]

**per·tus·sis** (pĕr-tŭs'is) an acute infectious inflammation of the larynx, trachea, and bronchi caused by *Bordetella pertussis;* characterized by recurrent bouts of spasmodic coughing that continues until the breath is exhausted, then ending in a noisy inspiratory stridor (the "whoop") caused by laryngeal spasm. SYN whooping cough. [L. *per,* very (intensive), + *tussis,* cough]

**Pe·ru·vi·an wart** (per-oo'vē-an) SYN verruga peruana.

**per·va·sive de·vel·op·men·tal dis·or·der** a class of mental disorders of infancy, childhood, or adolescence characterized by distortions in the development of the multiple basic psychological functions involved in the development of social skills and language.

**per vi·as na·tu·ra·les** (pĕr vī'as nach'er-ā'lēz) through the natural passages; e.g., denoting a normal delivery, as opposed to cesarean section, or the passage in stool of a foreign body instead of its surgical removal. [L.]

**per·vi·ous** (pĕr'vē-ŭs) SYN permeable. [L. *pervius,* fr. *per,* through, + *via,* a way]

**pes,** gen. **pe·dis,** pl. **pe·des** (pes, pē'dis, pe-dēz) [TA] **1.** SYN foot (1). **2.** any footlike or basal structure or part. **3.** talipes. In this sense, pes is always qualified by a word expressing the specific type. [L.]

**pes an·se·ri·nus 1.** SYN intraparotid plexus of facial nerve. **2.** the combined tendinous expansions of the sartorius, gracilis, and semitendinosus muscles at the medial border of the tuberosity of the tibia.

**pes cav·us** condition characterized by increased height of the foot's medial longitudinal arch.

**pes pla·nus** SYN talipes planus.

**pes·sa·ry** (pes′ă-rē) **1.** an appliance of varied form, introduced into the vagina to support the uterus or to correct any displacement. **2.** a medicated vaginal suppository. [L. *pessarium*, fr. G. *pessos*, an oval stone used in certain games]

**pest** SYN plague (2). [L. *pestis*]

**pes·ti·cide** (pes′ti-sīd) general term for an agent that destroys fungi, insects, rodents, or any other pest.

**pes·ti·lence** (pes′ti-lens) **1.** SYN plague (2). **2.** a virulent outbreak of any disease. [L. *pestilentia*]

**pes·ti·len·tial** (pes-ti-len′shăl) relating to or tending to produce a pestilence.

**pes·tle** (pes′l) an instrument in the shape of a rod with one rounded and weighted extremity, used for bruising, breaking, grinding, and mixing substances in a mortar. [L. *pistillum*, fr. *pinso*, or *piso*, to pound]

**PET** positron emission tomography.

△**pe·ta-** prefix used in the SI and metric systems to signify one quadrillion ($10^{15}$).

△**-pe·tal** seeking; movement toward the part indicated by the main portion of the word. [L. *peto*, to seek, strive for]

**pe·te·chi·ae**, sing. **pe·te·chia** (pe-tē′kē-ē, pe-tē′kē-ă) minute hemorrhagic spots, of pinpoint to pinhead size, in the skin, which are not blanched by diascopy. [Mod. L. form of It. *petecchie*]

**pe·te·chi·al** (pē-tē′kē-ăl) relating to, accompanied by, or characterized by petechiae.

**pe·te·chi·al hem·or·rhage** capillary hemorrhage into the skin that forms petechiae. SYN punctate hemorrhage.

**Pe·ters ovum** (pā′tĕrz) an ovum with a presumptive fertilization age of about 13 days; for many years, it was one of very few young human embryos recovered in good condition and its study furnished many facts regarding early embryonic changes.

**pet·i·o·late, pet·i·o·lat·ed** (pet′ē-ō-lāt, pet′ē-ō-lāt-ed) having a stem or pedicle. [L. *petiolus*]

**pe·ti·o·lus** (pe-tī′ō-lŭs) a stem or pedicle. [L. dim. of *pes* (foot), the stalk of a fruit]

**Pe·tit her·nia** (pĕ′tē) lumbar hernia, occurring in Petit triangle.

**Pe·tit her·ni·ot·o·my** (pĕ′tē) herniotomy without incision into the sac.

**Pe·tit lum·bar tri·an·gle** (pĕ′tē) SYN lumbar triangle.

**pe·tit mal** (pĕ-tē′) type of seizure. [Fr. small]

**Pe·tri dish cul·ture** (pē′trē) a combination of filter paper, fecal specimen, and tap water placed in a Petri dish; provides an environment for nematode eggs to hatch and larvae to develop.

**pet·ri·fac·tion** (pet-ri-fak′shŭn) fossilization, as in conversion into stone. [L. *petra*, rock + *facio*, to make]

**pé·tris·sage** (pā-trē-sazh′) a movement in massage that involves the lifting of tissues away from underlying structures, with the intention of improving elasticity and stimulating blood and lymph circulation. Includes kneading, skin rolling, and wringing. [Fr. kneading]

△**pet·ro-** stone; stonelike hardness. [L. *petra*, rock; G. *petros*, stone]

**pet·ro·mas·toid** (pet′rō-mas′toyd) relating to the petrous and the squamous portions of the tempo-

ral bone, which are usually united at birth by the petrosquamosal suture.

**pet·ro·oc·cip·i·tal** (pet′rō-ok-sip′i-tăl) denoting the cranial suture between the occipital bone and the petrous portion of the temporal.

**pet·ro·oc·cip·i·tal fis·sure** a fissure between the petrous part of the temporal bone and the basilar part of the occipital bone that extends anteromedially from the jugular foramen; includes the jugular foramen (at its posterior end).

**pe·tro·sa**, pl. **pe·tro·sae** (pe-trō′să, pe-trō′-sē) the petrous portion of the temporal bone. [L. fr. *petra*, rock]

**pe·tro·sal** (pe-trō′săl) relating to the petrosa. SYN petrous (2).

**pet·ro·si·tis** (pet-rō-sī′tis) an inflammation involving the petrous portion of the temporal bone and its air cells.

**pet·ro·sphe·noid** (pet′rō-sfē′noyd) relating to the petrous portion of the temporal bone and to the sphenoid bone.

**pet·ro·squa·mo·sal, pet·ro·squa·mous** (pet′rō-skwā-mō′săl, pet′rō-skwā′mŭs) relating to the petrous and the squamous portions of the temporal bone.

**pet·ro·tym·pan·ic fis·sure** a fissure between the tympanic and petrous portions of the temporal bone; it transmits the chorda tympani nerve through a small patent portion, the anterior canaliculus of the chorda tympani. SYN glaserian fissure.

**pet·rous** (pet′rŭs, pē′trŭs) **1.** of stony hardness. **2.** SYN petrosal. [L. *petrosus*, fr. *petra*, a rock]

**pet·rous part of in·ter·nal ca·rot·id ar·tery** the part of the internal carotid artery in the carotid canal; its branches are carotidotympanic arteries and the artery of the pterygoid canal.

**pet·rous part of tem·po·ral bone** the part of the temporal bone that contains the structures of the inner ear and the second part of the internal carotid artery; in antenatal life it appears as a separate ossification center.

**Petz·val sur·face** (pets′vahl) the curved image plane upon which any extended linear object is focused by a lens; it is curved toward the edges of a convex lens and away from the edges of a concave lens. SEE barrel distortion, pincushion distortion.

**pex·is** (pek′sis) fixation of substances in the tissues. [G. *pēxis*, fixation]

△**-pexy** fixation, usually surgical. [G. *pēxis*, fixation]

**Pey·er patch·es** (pi′ĕr) collections of many lymphoid follicles closely packed together, forming oblong elevations on the mucous membrane of the small intestine.

**Pey·ro·nie dis·ease** (pā-rō-nē′) a disease in which plaques or strands of dense fibrous tissue surrounding the corpus cavernosum of the penis cause penile bending and pain on erection; sometimes associated with Dupuytren contracture.

**Pey·rot tho·rax** (pā-rō′) an obliquely oval deformity of the chest in cases of a very large pleural effusion.

**PF** platelet factor 4.

**Pfan·nen·stiel in·ci·sion** (fahn′ĕn-shtēl, fan-en-stēl) an incision made transversely, and through the external sheath of the recti muscles, about an inch above the pubes, the muscles being separated at the midline in the direction of their fibers.

**Pfeif·fer ba·cil·lus** (fī'fĕr) SYN *Haemophilus influenzae.*

**Pfeif·fer phe·nom·e·non** (fī'fĕr) the alteration and complete disintegration of cholera vibrios when introduced into the peritoneal cavity of an immunized guinea pig, or into that of a normal one if immune serum is injected at the same time; extended to include bacteriolysis in general.

**Pfeif·fer syn·drome** (fī'fĕr) variable syndactyly of the digits; craniosynostosis is a variable feature. SYN Noack syndrome.

**PFT** pulmonary function test.

**pg** picogram.

**P-gly·co·pro·tein** (pē-glī-kō-prō'tēn) protein associated with tumor multidrug resistance; acts as energy-requiring efflux pump for many classes of natural products and chemotherapeutic drugs.

**Ph** phenyl.

**pH** symbol for the negative logarithm of the $H^+$ ion concentration (measured in moles per liter); a solution with pH 7.00 is neutral at 22°C, one with a pH of more than 7.0 is alkaline, and one with a pH lower than 7.00 is acid. At a temperature of 37°C, neutrality is at a pH value of 6.8. [p (power or potency) of $H^+$]

**PHA** phytohemagglutinin.

△**pha·co-** 1. lens-shaped, relating to a lens; 2. birthmark; as in phacomatosis. [G. *phakos,* lentil (lens), anything shaped like a lentil]

**phac·o·an·a·phy·lax·is** (fak'ō-an-ă-fī-lak'sis) hypersensitivity to protein of the lens of the eye.

**phac·o·cele** (fak'ō-sēl) hernia of the lens of the eye through the sclera. [phaco- + G. *kēlē,* hernia]

**phac·o·e·mul·si·fi·ca·tion** (fak'ō-ē-mŭl-si-fi-kā'shŭn) a method of emulsifying and aspirating a cataract with a low frequency ultrasonic needle.

**phac·o·er·y·sis** (fak-ō-er'i-sis) extraction of the lens of the eye by means of a suction cup called the erysophake. [phaco- + G. *erysis,* pulling, drawing off]

**phac·o·gen·ic glau·co·ma** SYN phacomorphic glaucoma.

**pha·coid** (fak'oyd) of lentil shape. [phaco- + G. *eidos,* resemblance]

**pha·col·y·sis** (fă-kol'i-sis) operative breaking down and removal of the lens. [phaco- + G. *lysis,* dissolution]

**pha·co·lyt·ic** (fak-ō-lit'ik) characterized by or referring to phacolysis.

**pha·co·ma** (fa-kō'mă) a hamartoma found in phacomatosis; often refers to a retinal hamartoma in tuberous sclerosis. SYN phakoma. [phaco- + G. *-oma,* tumor]

**pha·co·ma·la·cia** (fak'ō-mă-lā'shē-ă) softening of the lens, as may occur in hypermature cataract. [phaco- + G. *malakia,* softness]

**phac·o·ma·to·sis** (fak'ō-mă-tō'sis) a generic term for a group of hereditary diseases characterized by hamartomas involving multiple tissues; e.g., von Hippel-Lindau disease, neurofibromatosis, Sturge-Weber syndrome, tuberous sclerosis. SYN phakomatosis. [Van der Hoeve's coinage fr. G. *phakos,* mother-spot]

**phac·o·mor·phic glau·co·ma** secondary glaucoma caused by either excessive size or spherical shape of the lens. SYN phacogenic glaucoma.

**phac·o·scope** (fak'ō-skōp) an instrument in the form of a dark chamber for observing the changes in the lens during accommodation. [phaco- + G. *skopeō,* to view]

△**phae·o-** SEE pheo-.

**phae·o·chro·mo·cy·to·ma** [Br.] SEE pheochromocytoma.

**phae·o·hy·pho·my·co·sis** (fē'ō-hī'fō-mī-kō'sis) a group of superficial and deep infections caused by fungi that form pigmented hyphae and yeastlike cells in tissue. [G. *phaios,* dusky, + *hyphē,* web, + mycosis]

**phage** (fāj) SYN bacteriophage.

△**-phage, -phag·ia, -phagy** eating, devouring. [G. *phagō,* to eat]

**phag·e·de·na** (faj-ĕ-dē'nă) an ulcer that rapidly spreads peripherally, destroying the tissues as it increases in size. [G. *phagedaina,* a canker]

**phag·e·den·ic** (faj-ĕ-den'ik) relating to or having the characteristics of phagedena.

**phag·e·den·ic ul·cer** a rapidly spreading ulcer attended by the formation of extensive sloughing.

△**phag·o-** eating, devouring. [G. *phagō,* to eat]

**phag·o·cyte** (fag'ō-sīt) a cell possessing the property of ingesting bacteria, foreign particles, and other cells. Phagocytes are divided into two general classes: 1) microphages, polymorphonuclear leukocytes that ingest chiefly bacteria; 2) macrophages, mononucleated cells (histiocytes and monocytes) that are largely scavengers, ingesting dead tissue and degenerated cells. [phago- + G. *kytos,* cell]

**phag·o·cyt·ic** (fag-ō-sit'ik) relating to phagocytes or phagocytosis.

**phag·o·cyt·ic in·dex** the average number of bacteria observed in the cytoplasm of polymorphonuclear leukocytes after mixing and incubating, at 37°C, 1) a suspension of washed, presumably normal leukocytes, 2) the serum to be tested for opsonin, and 3) a young culture of microorganisms that are causing disease in the patient.

**phag·o·cyt·ic pneu·mo·no·cyte** an alveolar phagocyte containing hemosiderin, carbon, or other foreign particles.

**phag·o·cy·tin** (fag-ō-sī'tin) a very labile bactericidal substance that may be isolated from polymorphonuclear leukocytes.

**phag·o·cy·tize** (fag'ō-si-tīz) SYN phagocytose.

**phag·o·cy·tol·y·sis** (fag'ō-sī-tol'i-sis) 1. destruction of phagocytes, or leukocytes, occurring in the process of blood coagulation or as the result of the introduction of certain antagonistic foreign substances into the body. 2. a spontaneous breaking down of the phagocytes, preliminary to the liberation of complement. [phagocyte + G. *lysis,* dissolution]

**phag·o·cy·to·lyt·ic** (fag'ō-sī-tō-lit'ik) relating to phagocytolysis.

**phag·o·cy·tose** (fagŏ-sī'tōz) to perform phagocytosis, denoting the action of phagocytic cells. SYN phagocytize.

**phag·o·cy·to·sis** (fag'ō-sī-tō'sis) the process of ingestion and digestion by cells of solid substances, e.g., other cells, bacteria, bits of necrotic tissue, foreign particles. SEE ALSO endocytosis. [phagocyte + G. *-osis,* condition]

**phag·o·ly·so·some** (fag-ŏ-lī'sō-sōm) a body formed by union of a phagosome or ingested particle with a lysosome having hydrolytic enzymes.

**phag·o·some** (fag'ŏ-sōm) a vesicle that forms around a particle (bacterial or other) within the phagocyte that engulfed it, separates from the cell membrane, and then fuses with and receives the contents of cytoplasmic granules (lysosomes), thus forming a phagolysosome in which digestion of the engulfed particle occurs. [phago- + G. *sōma*, body]

**phag·o·type** (fag'ŏ-tīp) MICROBIOLOGY a subdivision of a species distinguished from other strains therein by sensitivity to a certain bacteriophage or set of bacteriophages. [phago- + G. *typos*, type]

**pha·kic eye** an eye containing the natural lens.

△**pha·ko-** for words so beginning and not listed here, see phaco-.

**pha·ko·ma** (fa-kō'mă) SYN phacoma.

**phak·o·ma·to·sis** (fak'ō-mă-tō'sis) SYN phacomatosis.

**pha·lan·ge·al** (fă-lan'jē-ăl) relating to a phalanx.

**phal·an·gec·to·my** (făl-an-jek'tō-mē) excision of one or more of the phalanges of hand or foot. [phalang- + G. *ektomē*, excision]

**pha·lanx**, gen. **pha·lan·gis**, pl. **pha·lan·ges** (fā'langks, fă-langks'; fă-lan'jis; fă-lan'-jēz) [TA] **1.** one of the long bones of the digits, 14 in number for each hand or foot, two for the thumb or great toe, and three each for the other four digits; designated as proximal, middle, and distal, beginning from the metacarpus. **2.** one of a number of cuticular plates, arranged in several rows, on the surface of the spiral organ (of Corti), which are the heads of the outer row of pillar cells and of phalangeal cells. [L. fr. G. *phalanx* (-*ang*-), line of soldiers, bone between two joints of the fingers and toes]

**Pha·len ma·neu·ver** (fā'lĕn) maneuver in which the wrist is maintained in volar flexion; paresthesia occurring in the distribution of the median nerve within 60 sec may be indicative of carpal tunnel syndrome.

△**phall-, phal·li-, phal·lo-** the penis. [G. *phallos*]

**phal·lec·to·my** (fal-ek'tō-mē) surgical removal of the penis. [phall- + G. *ektomē*, excision]

**phal·lic** (fal'ik) **1.** relating to the penis. **2.** PSYCHOANALYSIS relating to the penis, especially during the phases of infantile psychosexuality. SEE ALSO phallic phase. [G. *phallos*, penis]

**phal·lic phase** in psychoanalytic personality theory, the stage in psychosexual development, occurring when a child is between 2 and 6 years of age, during which interest, curiosity, and pleasurable experiences are centered around the penis in boys and the clitoris in girls. SEE ALSO genital phase.

**phal·lo·camp·sis** (fal-ō-kamp'sis) curvature of the erect penis. SEE ALSO chordee. [phallo- + G. *kampsis*, a bending]

**phal·lo·dyn·ia** (fal-ō-din'ē-ă) pain in the penis. [phallo- + G. *odynē*, pain]

**phal·loi·din** (fă-loy'din) best known of the toxic cyclic peptides produced by the poisonous mushroom, *Amanita phalloides;* closely related to amanitin.

**phal·lo·plas·ty** (fal'ō-plas-tē) surgical reconstruction of the penis. [phallo- + G. *plastos*, formed]

**phal·lot·o·my** (fal-ot'ō-mē) surgical incision into the penis. [phallo- + G. *tomē*, a cutting]

**phal·lus**, pl. **phal·li** (fal'ŭs, fal'ī) SYN penis. [L.; G. *phallos*]

**phan·ta·sia** (fan-tā'zē-ă) SYN fantasy. [G. appearance]

**phan·tasm** (fan'tazm) the mental imagery produced by fantasy. SYN phantom (1). [G. *phantasma*, an appearance]

**phan·tas·ma·go·ria** (fan-taz-mă-gōr'ē-ă) a fantastic sequence of haphazardly associative imagery.

**phan·tom** (fan'tŏm) **1.** SYN phantasm. **2.** a model, especially a transparent one, of the human body or any of its parts. **3.** RADIOLOGY a mechanical or computer-originated model for predicting irradiation dosage deep in the body. [G. *phantasma*, an appearance]

**phan·tom cor·pus·cle** SYN achromocyte.

**phan·tom limb, phan·tom limb pain** the sensation that an amputated limb is still present, often associated with painful paresthesia. SYN pseudesthesia (3).

**phan·tom tu·mor** accumulation of fluid in the interlobar spaces of the lung, secondary to congestive heart failure, radiologically simulating a neoplasm.

**phar·ma·ceu·tic, phar·ma·ceu·ti·cal** (far-mă-soo'tik, far-mă-soo'tikăl) relating to pharmacy or to pharmaceutics. [G. *pharmakeutikos*, relating to drugs]

**phar·ma·ceu·ti·cal care** the responsible provision of drug therapy for the purpose of achieving definite outcomes that improve a patient's quality of life.

**phar·ma·ceu·tics** (far-mă-soo'tiks) **1.** SYN pharmacy (1). **2.** the science of pharmaceutical systems, i.e., preparations, dosage forms, etc.

**phar·ma·cist** (far'mă-sist) one who is licensed to prepare and dispense drugs and compounds and is knowledgeable concerning their properties. [G. *pharmakon*, a drug]

△**phar·ma·co-** drugs. [G. *pharmakon*, medicine]

**phar·ma·co·di·ag·no·sis** (far'mă-kō-dī-ag-nō'sis) use of drugs in diagnosis.

**phar·ma·co·dy·nam·ic** (far'mă-kō-dī-nam'ik) relating to drug action, particularly at the receptor level.

**phar·ma·co·dy·nam·ics** (far'mă-kō-dī-nam'iks) the study of uptake, movement, binding, and interactions of pharmacologically active molecules at their tissue site(s) of action. [pharmaco- + G. *dynamis*, force]

**phar·ma·co·ec·o·nom·ics** science dealing with the description and analysis of the costs of drug therapy to health care systems and society.

**pharm·a·co·ep·i·de·mi·ol·o·gy** the application of epidemiologic knowledge, methods, and reasoning to the study of the effects and uses of pharmacologic treatments in a defined time, space, and population. SEE epidemiology, pharmacology.

**phar·ma·co·ge·net·ics, phar·ma·co·gen·om·ics** (far'mă-kō-jĕ-net'iks, far'mă-kō-jēn-om'iks) the study of genetically determined variations in responses to drugs in humans or in laboratory organisms.

**phar·ma·cog·no·sy** (far-mă-kog'nō-sē) a branch of pharmacology concerned with the physical characteristics and botanical and animal sources of crude drugs. [pharmaco- + G. *gnōsis*, knowledge]

**phar·ma·co·ki·net·ic** (far'mă-kō-ki-net'ik) relating to the disposition of drugs in the body (i.e., their absorption, distribution, metabolism, and elimination).

**phar·ma·co·ki·net·ics** (far'mă-kō-ki-net'iks) study of the movement of drugs within biological systems, as affected by absorption, distribution, metabolism, and excretion; particularly the rates of such movements. [pharmaco- + G. *kinēsis*, movement]

**phar·ma·co·log·ic, phar·ma·co·log·i·cal** (far′mă-kō-loj′ik, far′mă-kō-loj′i-kăl) **1.** relating to pharmacology or to the composition, properties, and actions of drugs. **2.** PHYSIOLOGY a dose of a chemical agent that is so much larger or more potent than would occur naturally that it might have qualitatively different effects. Cf. homeopathic (2), physiologic (4).

**phar·ma·col·o·gist** (far-mă-kol′ō-jist) a specialist in pharmacology.

**phar·ma·col·o·gy** (far-mă-kol′ō-jē) the science concerned with drugs, their sources, appearance, chemistry, actions, and uses. [pharmaco- + G. *logos*, study]

**Phar·ma·co·pe·ia, Phar·ma·co·poe·i·a** (far′mă-kō-pē′ă) a work containing monographs of therapeutic agents, standards for their strength and purity, and their formulations. The various national pharmacopeias are referred to by abbreviations, of which the most frequently encountered are *USP*, the Pharmacopeia of the United States of America (United States Pharmacopeia); and *BP*, British Pharmacopoeia. [G. *pharmakopoiia*, fr. *pharmakon*, a medicine, + *poieo*, to make]

**phar·ma·co·pe·ial** (far′mă-kō-pē′ăl) relating to the Pharmacopeia; denoting a drug in the list of the Pharmacopeia. SEE ALSO official.

**phar·ma·co·pe·ial gel** a suspension, in a water medium, of an insoluble drug in hydrated form wherein the particle size approaches or attains colloidal dimensions.

**phar·ma·co·poe·ial [Br.]** SEE pharmacopeial.

**phar·ma·co·ther·a·py** (far′mă-kō-thār′ă-pē) treatment of disease by means of drugs. SEE ALSO chemotherapy. [pharmaco- + G. *therapeia*, therapy]

**phar·ma·cy** (far′mă-sē) **1.** the practice of preparing and dispensing drugs and the delivery of pharmaceutical care. SYN pharmaceutics (1). **2.** a drugstore. [G. *pharmakon*, drug]

**phar·ma·ki·ne·tics** the mathematical characterization of the disposition of a drug in the body over time. Used to help understand and interpret blood levels and to adjust dosage and interval for maximum therapeutic results and minimum toxic effects.

**pha·ryn·ge·al** (fă-rin′jē-ăl) relating to the pharynx. [Mod. L. *pharyngeus*]

**pha·ryn·ge·al arch** typically, six arches in vertebrates; in the lower vertebrates, they bear gills; in the higher vertebrates, they appear transiently and give rise to specialized structures in the head and neck. SYN branchial arch.

**pha·ryn·ge·al bur·sa** a cystic notochordal remnant found inconstantly in the posterior wall of the nasopharynx at the lower end of the pharyngeal tonsil.

**pha·ryn·ge·al cleft** the pharyngeal ectodermal grooves of human embryos, which are imperforate, rudimentary homologues of gill clefts in fishes.

**pha·ryn·ge·al flap** flap of tissue placed to reduce the size of the opening between the oral and nasal cavities, to mitigate insufficient velar closure. SEE ALSO hypernasality, cleft palate.

**pha·ryn·ge·al groove** the ectodermal groove between two pharyngeal arches in the embryo.

**pha·ryn·ge·al o·pen·ing of au·di·to·ry tube** an opening in the upper part of the nasopharynx about 1.2 cm behind the posterior extremity of the inferior concha on each side.

**pha·ryn·ge·al re·flex 1.** SYN swallowing reflex. **2.** SYN vomiting reflex.

**pha·ryn·ge·al ton·sil** a collection of more or less closely aggregated lymphoid nodules on the posterior wall and roof of the nasopharynx; when hypertrophic these are called adenoids.

**pha·ryn·ge·al veins** several veins from the pharyngeal venous plexus emptying into the internal jugular vein.

**phar·yn·gec·to·my** (far′in-jek′tō-mē) resection of the pharynx. [pharyng- + G. *ektomē*, excision]

**phar·yn·ges** (fă-rin′jēz) plural of pharynx.

**phar·yn·gis·mus** (far-in-jiz′mŭs) spasm of the muscles of the pharynx. SYN pharyngospasm.

**phar·yn·git·ic** (far-in-jit′ik) relating to pharyngitis.

**phar·yn·gi·tis** (far-in-jī′tis) inflammation of the mucous membrane and underlying parts of the pharynx. [pharyng- + G. *-itis*, inflammation]

△**pha·ryn·go-, pha·ryng-** the pharynx. [Mod. L. fr. G. *pharynx*]

**pha·ryn·go·cele** (fă-rin′gō-sēl) a diverticulum from the pharynx. [pharyngo- + G. *kēlē*, hernia]

**pha·ryn·go·con·junc·ti·val fe·ver** a disease characterized by fever, pharyngitis, and conjunctivitis, and caused by adenoviruses, often type 3 but occasionally other types.

**pha·ryn·go·ep·i·glot·tic, pha·ryn·go·ep·i·glot·tid·e·an** (fă-rin′gō-ep′i-glot′ik, fă-rin′gō-ep′i-glo-tid′ē-an) relating to the pharynx and the epiglottis.

**pha·ryn·go·e·soph·a·ge·al** (fă-rin′gō-ē-sof′ă-jē′ă l) relating to the pharynx and the esophagus.

**pha·ryn·go·e·soph·a·ge·al di·ver·tic·u·lum** most common diverticulum of the esophagus; arises between the inferior pharyngeal constrictor and the crico-pharyngeus muscle. SYN hypopharyngeal diverticulum, Zenker diverticulum.

**pha·ryn·go·glos·sal** (fă-rin′gō-glos′ăl) relating to the pharynx and the tongue.

**pha·ryn·go·la·ryn·ge·al** (fă-rin′gō-lă-rin′jē-ăl) relating to both the pharynx and the larynx.

**pha·ryn·go·lar·yn·gi·tis** (fă-rin′gō-lar-in-jī′tis) inflammation of both the pharynx and the larynx.

**pha·ryn·go·lith** (fă-rin′gō-lith) a concretion in the pharynx. [pharyngo- + G. *lithos*, stone]

**pha·ryn·go·my·co·sis** (fă-rin′gō-mī-kō′sis) invasion of the mucous membrane of the pharynx by fungi. [pharyngo- + G. *mykēs*, a fungus]

**pha·ryn·go·na·sal** (fă-rin′gō-nā′săl) relating to the pharynx and the nasal cavity.

**pha·ryn·go·plas·ty** (fă-rin′gō-plas-tē) plastic surgery of the pharynx. [pharyngo- + G. *plastos*, formed]

**pha·ryn·go·ple·gia** (fă-rin′gō-plē′jē-ă) paralysis of the muscles of the pharynx. [pharyngo- + G. *plēgē*, stroke]

**pha·ryn·go·scope** (fă-rin′gō-skōp) an instrument like a laryngoscope, used for inspection of the mucous membrane of the pharynx. [pharyngo- + G. *skopeō*, to view]

**phar·yn·gos·co·py** (far′in-gos′kŏ-pē) inspection and examination of the pharynx. [pharyngo- + G. *skopeō*, to view]

**pha·ryn·go·spasm** (fă-rin′gō-spazm) SYN pharyngismus.

**pha·ryn·go·ste·no·sis** (fă-rin′gō-ste-nō′sis) stricture of the pharynx. [pharyngo- + G. *stenōsis,* a narrowing]

**phar·yn·got·o·my** (far'in-got'ŏ-mē) any cutting operation upon the pharynx either from without or from within. [pharyngo- + G. *tomē,* incision]

**pha·ryn·go·tym·pan·ic (auditory) tube** a tube leading from the tympanic cavity to the nasopharynx; it consists of an osseous (posterolateral) portion at the tympanic end, and a fibrocartilaginous (anteromedial) portion at the pharyngeal end; where the two portions join, in the region of the sphenopetrosal fissure, is the narrowest portion of the tube (isthmus); the auditory tube enables equalization of pressure within the tympanic cavity with ambient air pressure, referred to commonly as "popping of the ears." SYN salpinx (2) [TA], tuba auditiva [TA], auditory tube, eustachian tube, tuba auditoria.

**phar·ynx,** gen. **pha·ryn·gis,** pl. **pha·ryn·ges** (far'ingks, fă-rin'jis, fă-rin'jēz) [TA] the upper expanded portion of the digestive tube, between the esophagus below and the mouth and nasal cavities above and in front. [Mod. L. fr. G. *pharynx* (*pharyng-*), the throat, the joint opening of the gullet and windpipe]

**phase** (fāz) **1.** a stage in the course of change or development. **2.** a homogeneous, physically distinct, and separable portion of a heterogeneous system; e.g., oil, gum, and water are three phases of an emulsion. **3.** the time relationship between two or more events. **4.** a particular part of a recurring time pattern or wave form. SEE ALSO stage, period. [G. *phasis,* an appearance]

**phase I block** inhibition of nerve impulse transmission across the myoneural junction associated with depolarization of the motor endplate, as in the muscle paralysis produced by succinylcholine.

**phase II block** inhibition of nerve impulse transmission across the myoneural junction unaccompanied by depolarization of the motor endplate, as in the muscle paralysis produced by tubocurarine.

**phase im·age** a magnetic resonance image showing only phase shift information, to detect motion.

**phase mi·cro·scope, phase-con·trast mi·cro·scope** a specially constructed microscope that has a special condenser and objective containing a phase-shifting ring whereby small differences in index of refraction are made visible as intensity or contrast differences in the image; particularly useful for examining structural details in transparent specimens such as living or unstained cells and tissues.

**PH con·duc·tion time** SEE atrioventricular conduction.

**Phem·is·ter graft** (fem'is-tĕr) an autogenous onlay bone graft used in treating delayed union of fractures.

⚠ **phen-, phe·no-** **1.** appearance. **2.** CHEMISTRY combining form denoting derivation from benzene (phenyl-). [fr. G. *phainō,* to appear, show forth]

**phen·ac·e·tur·ic ac·id** (fĕ-nas-ĕt-yur'ik as'id) an end product of the metabolism of phenylated fatty acids with even numbers of carbon atoms. SYN phenylaceturic acid.

**phe·no·copy** (fē'nō-kop'ē) **1.** a set of clinical and laboratory characteristics that would ordinarily warrant the diagnosis of a specific genetic abnor-

mality, but are of environmental rather than genetic etiology. **2.** a condition of environmental etiology that mimics one usually of genetic etiology. [G. *phainō,* to display, + copy]

**phe·nol co·ef·fi·cient** SYN Rideal-Walker coefficient.

**phe·nol·u·ria** (fē-nol-yu're-ă) the excretion of phenols in the urine.

**phe·nom·e·non,** pl. **phe·nom·e·na** (fĕ-nom'ĕ-non, fĕ-nom'ĕ-nă) **1.** a symptom; an occurrence of any sort, whether ordinary or extraordinary, in relation to a disease. **2.** any unusual fact or occurrence. [G. *phainomenon,* fr. *phainō,* to cause to appear]

**phe·no·type** (fē'nō-tīp) manifestation of a genotype or the combined manifestation of several different genotypes. The discriminating power of the phenotype in identifying the genotype depends on its level of subtlety; thus special methods of detecting carriers distinguish them from normal subjects from whom they are inseparable on simple physical examination. Phenotype is the immediate cause of genetic disease and object of genetic selection. [G. *phainō,* to display, + *typos,* model]

**phe·no·typ·ic** (fē'nō-tip'ik, fen-ō-tip'ik) relating to phenotype.

**phe·no·typ·ic val·ue** QUANTITATIVE GENETICS the metrical quantity of some trait associated with a particular phenotype.

**phe·no·zy·gous** (fē'nō-zī'gŭs, fe-noz'i-gŭs) having a narrow cranium as compared with the width of the face, so that when the skull is viewed from above, the zygomatic arches are visible. [G. *phainō,* to show, + *zygon,* yoke]

**phen·yl (Ph, Φ)** (fen'il) the univalent radical, $C_6H_5-$, of benzene.

**phen·yl·a·ce·tic ac·id** (fen'il-ă-sē'tik as'id) an abnormal product of phenylalanine catabolism, appearing in the urine of individuals with phenylketonuria.

**phen·yl·a·ce·tur·ic ac·id** (fen'il-as-ĕt-yur'ik as'id) SYN phenaceturic acid.

**phen·yl·al·a·nin·ase** (fen-il-al'ă-nin-ās) phenylalanine 4-monooxygenase.

**phen·yl·al·a·nine (F)** (fen-il-al'ă-nēn) one of the common amino acids in proteins; a nutritionally essential amino acid.

**phen·yl·al·a·nine 4-mon·o·ox·y·gen·ase** an enzyme that catalyzes the oxidation of L-phenylalanine to L-tyrosine; a deficiency results in phenylketonuria.

**phen·yl·di·chlo·ro·ar·sine (PD)** (fen'il-dī-klōr-ō-ar'sēn) a toxic liquid that has been used as a blister and vomiting agent by certain military and police organizations; it was first used in a limited manner in World War I.

**phen·yl·hy·dra·zine he·mol·y·sis** (fen'il-hī'dră-zin) an *in vitro* test for G6PD deficiency; hemolysis resulting from *in vitro* addition of phenylhydrazine to blood with red cells which are deficient in glucose-6-phosphate dehydrogenase (G6PD), with the appearance of Heinz-Ehrlich bodies.

**phen·yl·ke·to·nu·ria (PKU)** (fen'il-kē'tō-nyu'rē-ă) congenital deficiency of phenylalanine 4-monooxygenase or occasionally of dihydropherine reductase or of dihydrobiopterin synthetase; it causes inadequate formation of L-tyrosine, elevation of serum L-phenylalanine, urinary excretion of phenylpyruvic acid and other derivatives, and accumulation of phenylalanine and its metabolites, which can produce brain damage resulting in severe mental retardation, often with seizures, other neurologic abnormalities such as retarded myelination, and deficient melanin formation leading to hypopigmentation of the skin and eczema. Cf. hyperphenylalaninemia. SYN Folling disease. [phenyl + ketone + G. *ouron,* urine]

**phen·yl·lac·tic ac·id** (fen-il-lak'tik as'id) a product of phenylalanine catabolism, appearing prominently in the urine in individuals with phenylketonuria.

**phe·nyl·py·ru·vic ac·id** (fen'il-pī-roo'vik as'id) the transaminated product of the action of phenylalanine aminotransferase; elevated in the urine in individuals with phenylketonuria.

**phen·yl·thi·o·hy·dan·to·in** (fen'il-thī'ō-hī-dan'tō-in) the compound formed from an amino acid in the Edman method of protein degradation, in which phenylisothiocyanate reacts with the amino moiety of the N-terminal amino acid to form a phenylthiocarbamoyl peptide or protein, on which weak acids act to release the phenylthiohydantoin containing the N-terminal amino acid.

△**pheo- 1.** prefix denoting the same substituents on a phorbin or phorbide (porphyrin) residue as are present in chlorophyll, excluding any ester residues and Mg. **2.** combining form meaning gray, dark-colored. [G. *phaios,* dusky]

**phe·o·chrome** (fē'ō-krōm) **1.** SYN chromaffin. **2.** staining darkly with chromic salts. [G. *phaios,* dusky, + *chrōma,* color]

**phe·o·chro·mo·cyte** (fē-ō-krō'mō-sīt) a chromaffin cell of a sympathetic paraganglion, medulla of an adrenal gland, or of a pheochromocytoma. [pheochrome + G. *kytos,* cell]

**phe·o·chro·mo·cy·to·ma** (fē'ō-krō'mō-sī-tō'mă) a functional chromaffinoma, usually benign, derived from adrenal medullary tissue cells and characterized by the secretion of catecholamines, resulting in hypertension, which may be paroxysmal and associated with attacks of palpitation, headache, nausea, dyspnea, anxiety, pallor, and profuse sweating. SEE ALSO paraganglioma.

**phe·re·sis** (fe-rē'sis) a procedure in which blood is removed from a donor, separated, and a portion retained, with the remainder returned to the donor. SEE ALSO leukapheresis, plateletpheresis, plasmapheresis. [G. *aphairesis,* a taking away, a withdrawal]

**pher·o·mones** (fer'ō-mōnz) a type of ectohormone secreted by an individual and perceived by a second individual of the same species, thereby producing a change in the sexual or social behavior of that individual. [G. *pherō,* to carry, + *hormaō,* to excite, stimulate]

**phi** (φ, Φ) (fī) **1.** the 21st letter of the Greek alphabet (φ). **2.** phenyl; potential energy; magnetic flux (Φ). **3.** plane angle; volume fraction; quantum yield; the dihedral angle of rotation about the N–C$_\alpha$ bond associated with a peptide bond (φ).

*Phi·a·loph·o·ra* (fī-ă-lof'ō-ră) a genus of fungi of which at least two species, *Phialophora verrucosa* and *Phialophora dermatitidis,* cause chromoblastomycosis. [G. *phialē,* a broad, flat vessel, + *phoreō,* to carry]

△**-phil, -phile, -phil·ic, -phil·ia** affinity for, craving for. [G. *philos,* fond, loving; *phileō,* to love]

🔲**Phi·la·del·phia chro·mo·some** an abnormal minute chromosome. Formed by a rearrangement of chromosomes 9 and 22; found in cultured leukocytes of many patients with chronic granulocytic leukemia. See this page.

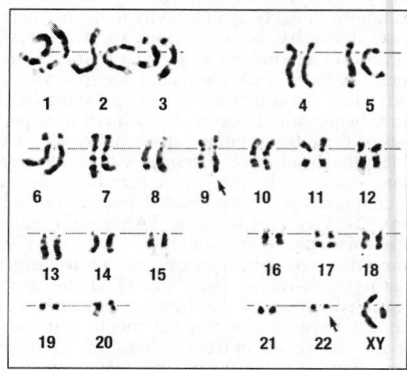

**Philadelphia chromosome translocation:** karyotype from a patient with chronic granulocytic leukemia showing the Philadelphia chromosome (number 22) translocation, t(9:22)(q34;q11)

**Phil·lips cath·e·ter** (fil'ips) a catheter with a filiform guide for the urethra.

**Phil·lip·son re·flex** (fil'ip-son) a contraction of the extensors of the knee when the extensors of the opposite knee are inhibited.

**phil·trum,** pl. **phil·tra** (fil'trŭm, fil'-tră) **1.** a philter or love potion. **2.** [TA] the infranasal depression; the groove in the midline of the upper lip. [L., fr. G. *philtron,* a love-charm, depression on upper lip, fr. *phileō,* to love]

**phi·mo·sis,** pl. **phi·mo·ses** (fī-mō'sis, fī-ō-sēz) narrowness of the opening of the prepuce, preventing its being drawn back over the glans. [G. a muzzling, fr. *phimos,* a muzzle]

**phi·mot·ic** (fī-mot'ik) pertaining to phimosis.

**phleb·ec·ta·sia** (fleb-ek-tā'zē-ă) dilation of the veins. SYN venectasia. [phlebo- + G. *ektasis,* a stretching]

**phle·bec·to·my** (fle-bek'tō-mē) excision of a segment of a vein, performed sometimes for the cure of varicose veins. SEE ALSO strip (2). SYN venectomy. [phlebo- + G. *ektomē,* excision]

**phle·bit·ic** (fle-bit'ik) relating to phlebitis.

**phle·bi·tis** (fle-bī'tis) inflammation of a vein. [phlebo- + G. *-itis,* inflammation]

△**phle·bo-, phleb-** vein [G. *phleps*]

**phleb·o·cly·sis** (flĕ-bok'li-sis) intravenous injection of an isotonic solution of dextrose or other substances in quantity. [phlebo- + G. *klysis,* a washing out]

**phleb·o·gram** (fleb'ō-gram) a tracing of the jugular or other venous pulse. SYN venogram (2). [phlebo- + G. *gramma,* something written]

**phleb·o·graph** (fleb'ō-graf) a venous sphygmograph; an instrument for making a tracing of the venous pulse. [phlebo- + G. *graphō,* to write]

**phle·bog·ra·phy** (fle-bog'ră-fē) **1.** the recording of the venous pulse. **2.** SYN venography. [phlebo- + G. *graphē,* a writing]

**phleb·o·lith** (fleb'ō-lith) a calcific deposit in a

venous wall or thrombus; commonly seen on abdominal radiographs in the lower pelvic region. [phlebo- + G. *lithos*, stone]

**phleb·o·li·thi·a·sis** (fleb′ō-li-thī′ă-sis) the formation of phleboliths.

**phle·bo·ma·nom·e·ter** (fleb′ō-mă-nom′ĕ-ter) a manometer for measuring venous blood pressure.

**phleb·o·phle·bos·to·my** (fleb′ō-fle-bos′tō-mē) SYN venovenostomy.

**phleb·o·plas·ty** (fleb′ō-plas-tē) repair of a vein. [phlebo- + G. *plastos*, formed]

**phle·bor·rha·phy** (fle-bōr′ă-fē) suture of a vein. [phlebo- + G. *rhaphē*, seam]

**phleb·o·scle·ro·sis** (fleb′ō-skle-rō′sis) fibrous hardening of the walls of the veins. SYN venosclerosis. [phlebo- + G. *sklērōsis*, hardening]

**phle·bos·ta·sis** (fle-bos′tă-sis) **1.** abnormally slow motion of blood in veins, usually with venous distention. **2.** treatment of congestive heart failure by compressing proximal veins of the extremities with tourniquets. SYN venostasis. [phlebo- + G. *stasis*, a standing still]

**phleb·o·ste·no·sis** (fleb′ō-stĕ-nō′sis) narrowing of the lumen of a vein from any cause. [phlebo- + G. *stenōsis*, a narrowing]

**phleb·o·throm·bo·sis** (fleb′ō-throm-bō′sis) thrombosis, or clotting, in a vein without primary inflammation. [phlebo- + thrombosis]

**phle·bot·o·mist** (fle-bot′ō-mist) an individual trained and skilled in phlebotomy.

**phle·bot·o·mize** (fle-bot′ō-mīz) **1.** to draw blood from. **2.** to achieve iron overload reduction by repeated removal of blood, as in hemochromatosis.

***Phle·bot·o·mus*** (fle-bot′ō-mŭs) a genus of very small bloodsucking sandflies of the subfamily Phlebotominae, family Psychodidae. [phlebo- + G. *tomos*, cutting]

**phle·bot·o·my** (fle-bot′ō-mē) incision into a vein for the purpose of drawing blood. SYN venesection, venotomy. [phlebo- + G. *tomē*, incision]

**phlegm** (flem) **1.** abnormal amounts of mucus, especially as expectorated from the mouth. **2.** one of the four humors of the body, according to the ancient Greek humoral doctrine. [G. *phlegma*, inflammation]

**phleg·ma·sia** (fleg-mā′zē-ă) obsolete term for inflammation, especially when acute and severe. [G. fr. *phlegma*, inflammation]

**phleg·mat·ic** (fleg-mat′ik) relating to the heavy one of the four ancient Greek humors (see phlegm), and therefore calm, apathetic, unexcitable. [G. *phlegmatikos*, relating to phlegm]

**phleg·mon** obsolete term for an acute suppurative inflammation of the subcutaneous connective tissue.

**phleg·mon·ous** (fleg′mon-ŭs) denoting phlegmon.

**phleg·mon·ous ab·scess** circumscribed suppuration characterized by intense surrounding inflammatory reaction which produces induration and thickening of the affected area.

**phlo·ri·zin gly·cos·ur·ia, phlo·rid·zin gly··cos·ur·i·a** the presence of sugar in the urine after the experimental administration of phlorizin, which results in a lower renal threshold for glucose reabsorption of glucose.

**phlyc·te·na,** pl. **phlyc·te·nae** (flik-tē′nă, flik-tē′nē) a small vesicle, especially one of a number of small blisters following a first degree burn. [G. *phlyktaina*, a blister made by a burn]

**phlyc·te·nar** (flik′tĕ-năr) relating to or marked by the presence of phlyctenae.

**phlyc·te·noid** (flik′tĕ-noyd) resembling a phlyctena. [G. *phlyktaina*, blister, + *eidos*, resemblance]

**phlyc·ten·u·la,** pl. **phlyc·ten·u·lae** (flik-ten′yu-lă) a small red nodule of lymphoid cells, with ulcerated apex, occurring in the conjunctiva. SYN phlyctenule. [Mod. L. dim. of G. *phlyktaina*, blister]

**phlyc·ten·u·lar** (flik-ten′yu-lăr) relating to a phlyctenula.

**phlyc·ten·u·lar ker·a·ti·tis** an inflammation of the corneal conjunctiva with the formation of small red nodules of lymphoid tissue (phlyctenulae) near the corneoscleral limbus.

**phlyc·ten·ule** (flik′ten-yul) SYN phlyctenula.

**phlyc·ten·u·lo·sis** (flik-ten′yu-lō′sis) a nodular hypersensitive affection of corneal and conjunctival epithelium due to endogenous toxin.

**pho·bia** (fō′bē-ă) any objectively unfounded morbid dread or fear that arouses a state of panic. The word is used as a combining form in many terms expressing the object that inspires the fear. [G. *phobos*, fear]

**pho·bic** (fō′bik) pertaining to or characterized by phobia.

**pho·bo·pho·bia** (fō-bō-fō′bē-ă) morbid dread of developing some phobia. [G. *phobos*, fear]

**pho·co·me·lia, pho·com·e·ly** (fō-kō-mē′lē-ă, fō-kom′ĕ-lē) defective development of arms or legs, or both, so that the hands and feet are attached close to the body, resembling the flippers of a seal. [G. *phōkē*, a seal, + *melos*, extremity]

**phon** (fōn) a unit of loudness of sound.

**pho·nal** (fō′năl) relating to sound or to the voice. [G. *phōnē*, voice]

**phon·as·the·nia** (fō-nas-thē′nē-ă) difficult or abnormal voice production, the enunciation being too high, too loud, or too hard. [phon- + G. *astheneia*, weakness]

**pho·na·tion** (fō-nā′shŭn) the utterance of sounds by means of vocal folds. [G. *phōnē*, voice]

**pho·na·tory** (fō′nă-tōr-ē) relating to phonation.

**pho·neme** (fō′nēm) the smallest sound unit which, in terms of the phonetic sequences of sound, controls meaning. [G. *phōnēma*, a voice]

**pho·nen·do·scope** (fō-nen′dō-skōp) a stethoscope that intensifies the auscultatory sounds by means of two parallel resonating plates, one resting on the patient's chest or attached to a stethoscope tube, the other vibrating in unison with it. [phon- + G. *endon*, within, + *skopeō*, to view]

**pho·net·ic** (fō-net′ik) relating to speech or to the voice. SEE ALSO phonic. [G. *phōnētikos*]

**pho·net·ic ba·lance** that property by which a group of words used in the measurement of hearing has the various phonemes occurring at approximately the same frequency at which they occur in ordinary conversation in that language; phonetically balanced word lists are used in determining the discrimination score.

**pho·net·ics** (fō-net′iks) the science of speech and of pronunciation.

**pho·ni·at·rics** (fō-nē-at′riks) a branch of medicine concerned with the diagnosis and treatment of voice and speech disorders. [phon- + G. *iatrikos*, of the healing art]

**phon·ic** (fon′ik, fō′nik) relating to sound or to the voice. SEE ALSO phonetic.

⌂**pho·no-, phon-** sound, speech, or voice sounds. [G. *phōnē*]

**pho·no·an·gi·og·ra·phy** (fō′nō-an-jē-og′ră-fē) recording and analysis of the audible frequency-intensity components of the bruit of turbulent arterial blood flow through a stenotic lesion. [phono- + G. *angeion*, vessel, + *graphō*, to write]

**pho·no·car·di·o·gram** (fō-nō-kar′dē-ō-gram) a record of the heart sounds made by means of a phonocardiograph.

**pho·no·car·di·o·graph** (fō-nō-kar′dē-ō-graf) an instrument, utilizing microphones, amplifiers, and filters, for graphically recording the heart sounds, which are displayed on an oscilloscope or analog tracing.

**pho·no·car·di·og·ra·phy** (fō′nō-kar-dē-og′ră-fē) 1. recording of the heart sounds with a phonocardiograph. 2. the science of interpreting phonocardiograms. [phono- + G. *kardia*, heart, + *graphō*, to record]

**pho·no·cath·e·ter** (fō-nō-kath′ĕ-ter) a cardiac catheter with diminutive microphone housed in its tip, for recording sounds and murmurs from within the heart and great vessels.

**pho·no·gram** (fō′nō-gram) a graphic curve depicting the duration and intensity of a sound. [phono- + G. *gramma*, diagram]

**pho·nom·e·ter** (fō-nom′ĕ-ter) an instrument for measuring the pitch and intensity of sounds. [phono- + G. *metron*, measure]

**pho·no·my·oc·lo·nus** (fō′nō-mī-ok′lō-nŭs) clonic spasms of muscles in response to aural stimuli. [phono- + G. *mys*, muscle, + *klonos*, tumult]

**pho·nop·a·thy** (fō-nop′ă-thē) any disease of the vocal organs affecting speech. [phono- + G. *pathos*, suffering]

**pho·no·pho·re·sis** (fō-nō-fōr-e′sĭs) introduction of anti-inflammatory drugs through the skin by the use of ultrasound. SEE ALSO iontophoresis. [phono- + G. *phorēsis*, a carrying]

**pho·no·pho·tog·ra·phy** (fō′nō-fō-tog′ră-fē) the recording on a moving photographic plate of the movements imparted to a diaphragm by sound waves. [phono- + photography]

**pho·nop·sia** (fō-nop′sē-ă) a condition in which the hearing of certain sounds gives rise to a subjective sensation of color. [phono- + G. *opsis*, vision]

**pho·no·re·cep·tor** (fō′nō-rē-sep′ter) a receptor for sound stimuli.

**pho·re·sis** (fōr′ē-sis, fō-rē′sis) 1. SYN electrophoresis. 2. a biological association in which one organism is transported by another. [G. *phorēsis*, a being borne]

**phor·ia** (fōr′ē-ă) the relative directions assumed by the eyes during binocular fixation of a given object in the absence of an adequate fusion stimulus. SEE cyclophoria, esophoria, exophoria, heterophoria, hyperphoria, hypophoria, orthophoria. [G. *phora*, a carrying, motion]

⌂**pho·ro-, phor-** carrying, bearing; a carrier, a bearer; phobia. [G. *phoros*, carrying, bearing]

⌂**phos-** light. [G. *phōs*]

**phos·gene** (fos′jēn) carbonic dichloride, COCl₂; a colorless liquid below 8.2°C, but an extremely poisonous gas at ordinary temperatures; more than 80% of World War I chemical agent fatalities were caused by phosgene.

⌂**phosph-, phos·pho-, phos·phor-, phos·phoro-** prefixes indicating the presence of phosphorus in a compound. See phospho- for specific usage of that prefix. [G. *phōs*, light; *phoros*, carrying]

**phos·pha·tae·mia [Br.]** SEE phosphatemia.

**phos·pha·tase** (fos′fă-tās) any of a group of enzymes (EC sub-subclass 3.1.3) that liberate inorganic phosphate from phosphoric esters.

**phos·phate** (fos′fāt) 1. a salt or ester of phosphoric acid. 2. the trivalent ion, PO₄³⁻.

**phos·phate di·a·be·tes** excessive secretion of phosphate in the urine due to a defect in tubular reabsorption; usually part of a more generalized abnormality, such as Fanconi syndrome.

**phos·pha·te·mia** (fos-fă-tē′mē-ă) an abnormally high concentration of inorganic phosphates in the blood. [phosphate + G. *haima*, blood]

**phos·phat·ic** (fos-fat′ik) relating to or containing phosphates.

**phos·phat·i·dyl·glyc·er·ol** (fos-fă-tī′dĭl-glis′ĕr-ol) a constituent in human amniotic fluid that denotes fetal lung maturity when present in the last trimester.

**phos·pha·tu·ria** (fos-fă-tyu′rē-ă) excessive excretion of phosphates in the urine. [phosphate + G. *ouron*, urine]

**phos·phene** (fos′fēn) sensation of light produced by mechanical or electrical stimulation of the peripheral or central optic pathway of the nervous system. [G. *phōs*, light, + *phainō*, to show]

**phos·phide** (fos′fīd) a compound of phosphorus with valence −3; e.g., sodium phosphide, Na₃P.

⌂**phos·pho-** prefix for *O*-phosphono-, which may replace the suffix phosphate; e.g., glucose phosphate is *O*-phosphonoglucose or phosphoglucose. SEE ALSO phosph-.

**3′-phos·pho·aden·o·sine 5′-phos·phate (PAP)** (thrē-fos′fō-a-den′ō-sēn fīv fos-fāt) a product in sulfuryl transfer reactions.

**phos·pho·am·i·dase** (fos-fō-am′i-dās) an enzyme catalyzing the hydrolysis of phosphorus-nitrogen bonds.

**phos·pho·am·ides** (fos-fō-am′īdz) amides of phosphoric acid (phosphoramidic acids) and their salts or esters.

**phos·pho·cre·a·tine** (fos-fō-krē′ă-tēn) a phosphagen; a compound of creatine with phosphoric acid; a source of energy in the contraction of vertebrate muscle, its breakdown furnishing phosphate for the resynthesis of ATP from ADP by creatine kinase. SYN creatine phosphate, *N*ᵂ-phosphonocreatine.

**phos·pho·di·es·ter·as·es** (fos′fō-dī-es′ter-ās-ez) enzymes (EC sub-subclass 3.1.4) cleaving phosphodiester bonds, such as those in cAMP or between nucleotides in nucleic acids, liberating smaller poly- or oligonucleotide units or mononucleotides but not inorganic phosphate.

**phos·pho·e·nol·pyr·u·vic ac·id** (fos′fō-ē′nol-pī-roo′vik as′id) the phosphoric ester of pyruvic acid in the latter's enol form; an intermediate in the conversion of glucose to pyruvic acid and an example of a high energy phosphate ester.

**6-phos·pho·D-glu·co·no-δ-lac·tone** an intermediate in the pentose phosphate pathway that is synthesized from D-glucose 6-phosphate.

**phos·pho·glyc·er·ides** (fos-fō-glis′er-īdz) acylglycerol and diacylglycerol phosphates; constituents of nerve tissue, and involved in fat transport and storage.

**phos·pho·li·pase** (fos-fō-lip′ās) an enzyme that catalyzes the hydrolysis of a phospholipid. SYN lecithinase.

**phos·pho·lip·id** (fos-fō-lip′id) a lipid containing phosphorus, thus including the lecithins and other phosphatidyl derivatives, sphingomyelin, and plasmalogens; the basic constituents of biomembranes.

**phos·pho·mu·tase** (fos-fō-myu′tās) one of a number of enzymes that catalyze intramolecular transfer of phosphate.

**phos·pho·ne·cro·sis** (fos-fō-ne-krō′sis) necrosis of the osseous tissue of the jaw, as a result of poisoning by inhalation of phosphorus fumes, occurring especially in persons with prolonged occupational exposure. [phosphorus + G. *nekrōsis*, death (necrosis)]

**N<sup>ω</sup>-phosphonocreatine** SYN phosphocreatine.

**phos·pho·pro·tein** (fos-fō-prō′tēn) a protein containing phosphoryl groups attached directly to the side chains of some of its constituent amino acids.

**phos·phor** (fos′fōr) a chemical substance that transforms incident electromagnetic or radioactive energy into light, as in scintillation radioactivity determinations or radiographic intensifying screens or image amplifiers. [G. *phōs*, light, + *phoros*, bearing]

△**phos·phor-, phos·phoro-** SEE phosph-.

**phos·pho·res·cence** (fos-fō-res′ens) the quality or property of emitting light without active combustion or the production of heat, generally as the result of prior exposure to radiation, which persists after the inciting cause is removed. [G. *phōs*, light, + *phoros*, bearing]

**phos·pho·res·cent** (fos′fō-res′ent) having the property of phosphorescence.

**5-phos·pho-α-D-ri·bo·syl 1-py·ro·phos·phate (PRPP)** 5-phosphoribosyl 1-diphosphate; D-Ribose carrying a phosphate group on ribose carbon-5 and a pyrophosphate group on ribose carbon-1; an intermediate in the formation of the pyrimidine and purine nucleotides as well as NAD⁺.

**phos·phor·ic ac·id** (fos-fōr′ik as′id) a strong acid of industrial importance; dilute solutions have been used as urinary acidifiers and as dressings to remove necrotic debris. In dentistry, it comprises about 60% of the liquid used in zinc phosphate and silicate cements; solutions are used for conditioning enamel surfaces prior to applications of various types of resins.

**phos·phor·ism** (fos′fōr-izm) chronic poisoning with phosphorus.

**phos·pho·rol·y·sis** (fos-fō-rol′i-sis) a reaction analogous to hydrolysis except that the elements of phosphoric acid, rather than of water, are added in the course of splitting a bond.

**phos·pho·rous** (fos′fōr-ŭs, fos-fōr′ŭs) **1.** relating to, containing, or resembling phosphorus. **2.** referring to phosphorus in its lower (+3) valence state.

**phos·pho·rus** (fos′fōr-ŭs) a nonmetallic chemical element, atomic no. 15, atomic wt. 30.973762, occurring extensively in nature, always in chemical combination; the elemental form is extremely poisonous, causing intense inflammation and fatty degeneration; repeated inhalation of phosphorus fumes may cause necrosis of the jaw (phosphonecrosis). [G. *phōsphoros*, fr. *phōs*, light, + *phoros*, bearing]

**phos·pho·rus-32** radioactive phosphorus isotope; beta emitter with half-life of 14.28 days; used as tracer in metabolic studies and in the treatment of certain diseases of the osseous and hematopoietic systems.

**phos·phor·y·lase** (fos-fōr′i-lās) a phosphorylated enzyme cleaving poly(1,4-α-D-glucosyl)$_n$ with inorganic phosphate to form poly(1,4-α- D-glucosyl)$_{n-1}$ and α-D-glucose 1-phosphate.

**phos·phor·y·lase phos·pha·tase** an enzyme catalyzing the conversion of one phosphorylase *a* into two phosphorylase *b*, with the release of four phosphates.

**phos·pho·ryl·a·tion** (fos′fōr-i-lā′shŭn) addition of phosphate to an organic compound, such as glucose to produce glucose monophosphate, through the action of a phosphotransferase (phosphorylase) or kinase.

**phos·pho·sug·ar** (fos-fō-shug′er) a phosphorylated saccharide; any sugar containing an alcoholic group esterified with phosphoric acid.

**phos·pho·tung·stic ac·id (PTA)** (fos-fō-tŭng′ stik as′id) a mixture of phosphoric and tungstic acids, approximately 24 $WO_3$, 2 $H_3PO_4$, 48 $H_2O$; a protein precipitant and reagent for arginine, lysine, histidine, and cystine; used with hematoxylin for nuclear and muscle staining; also used in electron microscopy as a stain for collagen and as a negative stain.

**phos·pho·tung·stic ac·id he·ma·tox·y·lin (PTAH)** a stain with broad application in cytology and histology; nuclei, mitochrondria, fibrin, neuroglial fibrils, and cross-striations of skeletal and cardiac muscle stain blue; cartilage ground substance, bone reticulum, and elastin appear in shades of yellow-orange and brownish red; also useful for demonstrating abnormal or diseased astrocytes, often in combination with periodic acid-Schiff stain and Luxol fast blue. SYN Mallory phosphotungstic acid hematoxylin stain.

**pho·tal·gia** (fō-tal′jē-ă) light-induced pain, especially of the eyes. SYN photodynia. [phot- + G. *algos*, pain]

**pho·tic** (fō′tik) relating to light.

**pho·tic driv·ing** a normal EEG phenomenon whereby the frequency of the activity recorded over the parieto-occipital regions is time-locked to the flash frequency during photic stimulation.

**photi·c-sneeze re·flex** SYN photoptarmosis.

**pho·tism** (fō′tizm) production of a sensation of light or color by a stimulus to another sense organ, such as of hearing, taste, or touch.

△**pho·to-, phot-** light. [G. *phōs* (*phōt-*)]

**pho·to·ab·la·tion** (fō′tō-ab-lā′shun) the process of photoablative decomposition of tissue by laser light, e.g., in photorefractive keratectomy.

**pho·to·a·ging** (fō′tō-āj′ing) damage from years of sun exposure, particularly wrinkling of skin. [photo- + aging]

**pho·to·bi·ot·ic** (fō′tō-bī-ot′ik) living or flourishing only in the light. [photo- + G. *bios*, life]

**pho·to·cat·a·lyst** (fō-tō-kat′ă-list) a substance that helps bring about a light-catalyzed reaction; e.g., chlorophyll. [photo- + G. *katalysis*, dissolution (catalysis)]

**pho·to·chem·i·cal** (fō-tō-kem′i-kăl) denoting chemical changes caused by or involving light.

**pho·to·che·mo·ther·a·py** (fō′tō-kem-ō-ther′ă-pē, fō′tō-kē-mō-ther′ă-pē) SYN photoradiation.

**pho·to·chro·mic lens** a light-sensitive spectacle lens that reduces light transmission in sunlight and increases transmission in reduced light.

**pho·to·co·ag·u·la·tion** (fō′tō-kō-ag′yu-lā′shŭn) a method by which a beam of electromagnetic energy is directed to a desired tissue under visual control; localized coagulation results from absorption of light energy and its conversion to heat or conversion of tissue to plasma (atoms stripped of electrons). [photo- + L. *coagulo,* pp. *-atus,* to curdle]

**pho·to·co·ag·u·la·tor** (fō'tō-kō-ag'yu-lā'ter, fō' tō-kō-ag'yu-lā'tŏr) the apparatus used in photocoagulation.

**pho·to·der·ma·ti·tis** (fō'tō-der-mă-tī'tis) dermatitis caused or elicited by exposure to sunlight; may be phototoxic or photoallergic, and can result from topical application, ingestion, inhalation, or injection of mediating phototoxic or photoallergic material. SEE ALSO photosensitization. SYN actinic dermatitis, actinodermatitis. [photo- + G. *derma,* skin, + *-itis,* inflammation]

**pho·to·de·tec·tor** (fō'-tō-dĕ-tĕk-tŏr) a device in a spectrophotometer that responds to photons in a manner usually proportional to the number of photons striking its light-sensitive surface.

**pho·to·dis·tri·bu·tion** (fō'tō-dis-tri-byu'shŭn) areas on the skin that receive the greatest amount of exposure to sunlight, and which are involved in eruptions due to photosensitivity.

**pho·to·dy·nam·ic sen·si·ti·za·tion** the action by which certain substances, notably fluorescing dyes (acridine, eosin, methylene blue, rose bengal) absorb visible light and emit the energy at wavelengths that are deleterious to microbes or other organisms in the dye-containing suspension, or selectively destroy cancer cells sensitized by intravenous porphyrin and exposed to red laser light. SYN photosensitization (2).

**pho·to·dy·na·mic ther·a·py** SYN photoradiation.

**pho·to·dyn·ia** (fō-tō-din'ē-ă) SYN photalgia. [photo- + G. *odynē,* pain]

**pho·to·e·lec·tric** (fō'tō-ē-lek'trik) denoting electronic or electric effects produced by the action of light.

**pho·to·flu·o·rog·ra·phy** (fō'tō-floor-og'ră-fē) miniature radiographs made by contact photography of a fluoroscopic screen, formerly used in mass radiographic examination of the lungs. SYN fluorography. [photo- + L. *fluor,* a flow, + G. *graphē,* a writing]

**pho·to·gas·tro·scope** (fō'tō-gas'trō-skōp) an instrument for taking photographs of the interior of the stomach. [photo- + G. *gastēr,* stomach, + *skopeō,* to view]

**pho·to·gen·ic, pho·tog·e·nous** (fō-tō-jen'ik, fō-toj'ĕ-nŭs) denoting or capable of photogenesis.

**pho·to·gen·ic ep·i·lep·sy** a form of reflex epilepsy precipitated by light.

**pho·to·in·ac·ti·va·tion** (fō'tō-in-ak-ti-vā'shŭn) inactivation by light; e.g., as in the treatment of herpes simplex by local application of a photoactive dye followed by exposure to a fluorescent lamp.

**pho·to·lu·mi·nes·cent** (fō'tō-loo-mi-nes'ent) having the ability to become luminescent upon exposure to visible light. [photo- + L. *lumen,* light]

**pho·tol·y·sis** (fō-tol'i-sis) decomposition of a chemical compound by the action of light. [photo- + G. *lysis,* dissolution]

**pho·to·lyt·ic** (fō-tō-lit'ik) pertaining to photolysis.

**pho·to·mi·cro·graph** (fō'tō-mī'krō-graf) an enlarged photograph of an object viewed with a microscope, as distinguished from microphoto-

graph. SYN micrograph. [photo- + G. *mikros,* small, + *graphē,* a record]

**pho·to·mi·crog·ra·phy** (fō'tō-mī-krog'ră-fē) the production of a photomicrograph.

**pho·to·my·oc·lo·nus** (fō'tō-mī-ok'lō-nŭs) clonic spasms of muscles in response to visual stimuli. [photo- + G. *mys,* muscle, + *klonos,* confused motion]

**pho·ton** (γ) (fō'ton) PHYSICS a corpuscle of energy or particle of light; a quantum of light or other electromagnetic radiation.

**pho·to·patch test** a test of contact photosensitization: after application of a patch with the suspected sensitizer for 48 hours to two sites, if there is no reaction, one area is exposed to a weak erythema dose of sunlight or ultraviolet light; if positive, a more severe reaction with vesiculation develops at the exposed patch area than the nonexposed skin patch site.

**pho·to·per·cep·tive** (fō'tō-per-sep'tiv) capable of both receiving and perceiving light.

**pho·to·pho·bia** (fō-tō-fō'bē-ă) morbid dread and avoidance of light. Although often an expression of undue anxiety about the eyes, photosensitivity and photalgia, past or present, should be considered. [photo- + G. *phobos,* fear]

**pho·to·pho·bic** (fō-tō-fō'bik) relating to or suffering from photophobia.

**pho·toph·thal·mia** (fō'tof-thal'mē-ă) keratoconjunctivitis caused by ultraviolet energy, as in snow blindness, exposure to an ultraviolet lamp, arc welding, or the short circuit of a high-tension electric current. SEE ALSO photoretinopathy. [photo- + G. *ophthalmos,* eye]

**pho·to·pia** (fō-tō'pē-ă) SYN photopic vision. [photo- + G. *opsis,* vision]

**pho·top·ic** (fō-top'ik) pertaining to photopic vision.

**pho·top·ic ad·ap·ta·tion** SYN light adaptation.

**pho·top·ic eye** SYN light-adapted eye.

**pho·top·ic vi·sion** vision when the eye is light-adapted. SEE light adaptation, light-adapted eye. SYN photopia.

**pho·top·sia** (fō-top'sē-ă) a subjective sensation of lights, sparks, or colors due to electrical or mechanical stimulation of the ocular system. SYN photopsy. [photo- + G. *opsis,* vision]

**pho·top·sin** (fō-top'sin) the protein moiety (opsin) of the pigment (iodopsin) in the cones of the retina.

**pho·top·sy** (fō-top'sē) SYN photopsia.

**pho·to·ptar·mo·sis** (fō'tō-tar-mō'sis) reflex sneezing that occurs when bright light stimulates the retina. SYN photic-sneeze reflex. [photo- + G. *ptarmos,* a sneezing, + *-osis,* condition]

**pho·to·ra·di·a·tion, pho·to·ra·di·a·tion ther·a·py** (fō'tō-rā-dē-ā'shŭn) treatment of cancer by intravenous injection of a photosensitizing agent, such as hematoporphyrin, followed by exposure to visible light of superficial tumors or of deep tumors by a fiberoptic probe. SYN photochemotherapy, photodynamic therapy.

**pho·to·re·ac·tion** (fō'tō-rē-ak'shŭn) a reaction caused or affected by light; e.g., a photochemical reaction, photolysis, photosynthesis, phototropism, thymine dimer formation.

**pho·to·re·ac·ti·va·tion** (fō'tō-rē-ak-ti-vā'shŭn) activation by light of something or of some process previously inactive or inactivated.

**pho·to·re·cep·tive** (fō'tō-rē-sep'tiv) functioning as a photoreceptor.

**pho·to·re·cep·tor** (fō′tō-rē-sep′tŏr) a receptor that is sensitive to light, e.g., a retinal rod or cone. [photo- + L. *re-cipio,* pp. *-ceptus,* to receive, fr. *capio,* to take]

**pho·to·re·cep·tor cells** rod and cone cells of the retina.

**pho·to·ret·i·ni·tis** (fō′tō-ret′i-nī′tis) SEE photoretinopathy.

**pho·to·ret·i·nop·a·thy** (fō′tō-ret′i-nop′ă-thē) a macular burn from excessive exposure to sunlight or other intense light (e.g., the flash of a short circuit); characterized subjectively by reduced visual acuity. [photo- + retina, + G. *pathos,* suffering]

**pho·to·scan** (fō′tō-skan) SYN scintiscan.

**pho·to·sen·si·ti·sa·tion [Br.]** SEE photosensitization.

**pho·to·sen·si·ti·za·tion** (fō′tō-sen-si-ti-zā′shŭn) **1.** sensitization of the skin to light, usually due to the action of certain drugs, plants, or other substances; may occur shortly after administration of the drug (phototoxic sensitivity), or may occur only after a latent period of days to months (photoallergic sensitivity, or photoallergy). **2.** SYN photodynamic sensitization.

**pho·to·sta·ble** (fō′tō-stā-běl) not subject to change upon exposure to light.

**pho·to·steth·o·scope** (fō-tō-steth′ō-skōp) device that converts sound into flashes of light; used for continuous observation of the fetal heart.

**pho·to·syn·the·sis** (fō-tō-sin′thě-sis) **1.** the compounding or building up of chemical substances under the influence of light. **2.** the process by which green plants, using chlorophyll and the energy of sunlight, produce carbohydrates from water and carbon dioxide, liberating molecular oxygen in the process. [photo- + G. *synthesis,* a putting together]

**pho·to·tax·is** (fō-tō-tak′sis) reaction of living protoplasm to the stimulus of light, involving bodily motion of the whole organism toward **(positive phototaxis)** or away from **(negative phototaxis)** the stimulus. Cf. phototropism. [photo- + G. *taxis,* orderly arrangement]

**phototherapeutic keratectomy (PTK)** ablation of diseased corneal tissue using an excimer laser.

**pho·to·ther·a·py** (fō-tō-ther′ă-pē) treatment of disease by means of light rays. SYN light treatment.

**pho·to·tim·er** (fō-tō-tīm′ěr) an electronic device in radiography that measures the radiation that has passed through the patient and terminates the x-ray exposure when it is sufficient to form an image.

**pho·to·tox·ic·it·y** (fō-tō-tok-sis′i-tē) the condition resulting from an overexposure to ultraviolet light, or from the combination of exposure to certain wavelengths of light and a phototoxic substance. SEE ALSO photosensitization. [photo- + G. *toxikon,* poison]

**pho·tot·ro·pism** (fō-to′trō-pizm) movement of a part of an organism toward **(positive phototropism)** or away from **(negative phototropism)** the stimulus of light. Cf. phototaxis. [photo- + G. *tropē,* a turning]

**pho·tu·ria** (fō-tyu′rē-ă) the passage of phosphorescent urine. [photo- + G. *ouron,* urine]

**PHP** panhypopituitarism.

**phre·nal·gia** (fre-nal′jē-ă) **1.** SYN psychalgia (1). **2.** pain in the diaphragm. [phren- + G. *algos,* pain]

**phre·net·ic** (frě-net′ik) **1.** frenzied; maniacal. **2.** an individual exhibiting such behavior. [G. *phrenitikos,* frenzied]

△**-phre·nia 1.** the diaphragm. **2.** the mind. SEE phreno-. [G. *phrēn,* the diaphragm, mind, heart (as seat of emotions)]

**phren·ic** (fren′ik) **1.** SYN diaphragmatic. **2.** relating to the mind.

**phren·i·cec·to·my** (fren-i-sek′tō-mē) exsection of a portion of the phrenic nerve, to prevent reunion such as may follow phrenicotomy. SYN phrenicoexeresis. [phreni- + G. *ektomē,* excision]

**phren·ic gan·glia** several small autonomic ganglia contained in the plexuses accompanying the inferior phrenic arteries.

**phren·i·cla·sia** (fren-i-klā′zē-ă) crushing of a section of the phrenic nerve to produce a temporary paralysis of the diaphragm. SYN phrenicotripsy. [phreni- + G. *klasis,* a breaking away]

**phren·ic nerve** arises from the cervical plexus, chiefly from the fourth cervical nerve, passes downward in front of the anterior scalene muscle and enters the thorax between the subclavian artery and vein behind the sternoclavicular articulation; it then passes in front of the root of the lung to the diaphragm; it is mainly the motor nerve of the diaphragm but sends sensory fibers to the mediastinal parietal pleura, the pericardium, the diaphragmatic pleura and peritoneum, and branches (phrenicoabdominales branches) that communicate with branches from the celiac plexus. SYN nervus phrenicus [TA].

**phren·i·co·ab·dom·i·nal branches of phren·ic nerve** terminal branches of phrenic nerve providing motor innervation of diaphragm and sensory innervation to the diaphragm and the diaphragmatic pleura and peritoneum.

**phren·i·co·col·ic** (fren′i-kō-kol′ik) relating to the diaphragm and the colon.

**phren·i·co·col·ic lig·a·ment** a triangular fold of peritoneum attached to the left flexure of the colon and to the diaphragm, on which rests the inferior pole or extremity of the spleen. SYN ligamentum phrenicocolicum [TA].

**phren·i·co·ex·er·e·sis** (fren′i-kō-ek-ser′ě-sis) SYN phrenicectomy. [phrenico- + G. *exairesis,* a taking out, fr. *haireō,* to take, grasp]

**phren·i·co·gas·tric** (fren′i-kō-gas′trik) relating to the diaphragm and the stomach.

**phren·i·co·he·pa·tic** (fren′i-kō-he-pa′tik) relating to the diaphragm and the liver.

**phren·i·co·pleur·al fas·cia** the thin layer of endothoracic fascia intervening between the diaphragmatic pleura and the diaphragm.

**phren·i·cot·o·my** (fren-i-kot′ō-mē) section of the phrenic nerve in order to induce unilateral paralysis of the diaphragm, which is then pushed up by the abdominal viscera and exerts compression upon a diseased lung. [phrenico- + G. *tomē,* incision]

**phren·i·co·trip·sy** (fren′i-kō-trip′sē) SYN phreniclasia. [phrenico- + G. *tripsis,* a rubbing]

△**phreno-, phren-, phre·ni-, phren·i·co-** the diaphragm; the mind; the phrenic nerve. [G. *phrēn,* diaphragm, mind, heart (as seat of emotions)]

**phren·o·car·dia** (fren-ō-kar′dē-ă) precordial pain and dyspnea of psychogenic origin, often a symptom of anxiety neurosis. SEE cardiac neurosis. [phreno- + G. *kardia,* heart]

**phren·o·ple·gia** (fren-ō-plē′jē-ă) paralysis of the diaphragm. [phreno- + G. *plēgē*, stroke]

**phren·op·to·sia** (fren-op-tō′sē-ă) an abnormal sinking down of the diaphragm. [phreno- + G. *ptōsis*, a falling]

**phryn·o·der·ma** (frin-ō-der′mă) a follicular hyperkeratotic eruption thought to be due to deficiency of vitamin A. [G. *phrynos*, toad, + *derma*, skin]

**Phthi·rus** (thī′rŭs) SEE *Pthirus*. [L. *phthir;* G. *phtheir*, a louse]

**phy·co·my·co·sis** (fī′kō-mī′kō-sis) SYN zygomycosis.

**phy·lax·is** (fī-lak′sis) protection against infection. [G. a guarding, protection]

**phyl·lo·qui·none** (fil-ō-kwin′ōn) 2-methyl-3-phytyl-1,4-naphthoquinone; 3-phytyl-menaquinone; isolated from alfalfa; also prepared synthetically; major form of vitamin K found in plants. SYN vitamin $K_1$, vitamin $K_1$(20).

△**phy·lo-** tribe, race; a taxonomic phylum. [G. *phylon*, tribe]

**phy·lo·gen·e·sis** (fī-lō-jen′ĕ-sis) SYN phylogeny. [phylo- + G. *genesis*, origin]

**phy·lo·ge·net·ic, phy·lo·gen·ic** (fī′lō-jĕ-net′ik, fī′lō-jen′ik) relating to phylogenesis.

**phy·log·e·ny** (fī-loj′ĕ-nē) the evolutionary development of one's species, as distinguished from ontogeny, development of the individual. SYN phylogenesis.

**phy·lum,** pl. **phy·la** (fī′lŭm, fī′lă) a taxonomic division below the kingdom and above the class. [Mod. L. fr. G. *phylon*, tribe]

**phy·ma** (fī′mă) a nodule or small rounded tumor of the skin. [G. a tumor]

**phy·ma·to·sis** (fī-mă-tō′sis) the growth or the presence of phymas or small nodules in the skin.

*Phy·sal·ia* a genus of the invertebrate phylum Cnidaria that includes the Portuguese man-of-war.

*Phy·sal·ia phy·sa·lis* the Portuguese man-of-war, a jellyfishlike animal consisting of a complex colony of individual members that can inflict extremely painful stings. SYN Portuguese man-of-war.

**phy·sal·i·form** (fi-sal′i-fōrm) like a bubble or small bleb. [G. *physallis*, bladder, bubble, + L. *forma*, form]

**phys·a·lis** (fis′ă-lis) a vacuole in a giant cell found in certain malignant neoplasms, such as chordoma. [G. *physallis*, a bladder]

**phys·e·al** (fiz′ē-ăl) pertaining to the physis, or growth cartilage area, separating the metaphysis and the epiphysis.

**phys·i·at·rics** (fiz-ē-at′riks) **1.** old term for physical therapy. **2.** rehabilitation management. [G. *physis*, nature, + *iatrikos*, healing]

**phys·i·a·trist** (fiz-ī′ă-trist) a physician who specializes in physical medicine.

**phys·i·a·try** (fi-zī′ă-trē) SYN physical medicine.

**phys·i·cal** (fiz′i-kăl) relating to the body, as distinguished from the mind. [Mod. L. *physicalis,* fr. G. *physikos*]

**phys·i·cal ac·tiv·i·ty** any body movement produced by muscles that results in energy expenditure. SEE exercise.

**phys·i·cal agent** a form of acoustical, aqueous, electrical, mechanical, thermal, or light energy applied to living tissues in a systematic manner to alter physiological processes, in conjunction with or for therapeutic purposes. SEE modality.

**phys·i·cal al·ler·gy** excessive response to factors in the environment such as heat or cold.

**phys·i·cal con·di·tion·ing** systematic use of regular physical activity to induce functional and structural adaptations that enhance energy capacity and exercise performance.

**phys·i·cal di·ag·no·sis** a diagnosis made by means of physical examination of the patient, or the process of a physical examination.

**phys·i·cal fit·ness** a set of attributes relating to one's ability to perform physical activity. SEE health-related physical fitness.

**phys·i·cal map** a map of a stretch of DNA with ordered landmarks a known distance from each other; the ultimate physical map would be the base sequence of the entire chromosome.

**phys·i·cal med·i·cine** the study and treatment of disease mainly by mechanical and other physical methods. SYN physiatry.

**phys·i·cal sign** a sign that is evident on inspection or elicited by auscultation, percussion, or palpation.

**phys·i·cal ther·a·pist** a practitioner of physical therapy.

**phys·i·cal ther·a·py (PT) 1.** treatment of pain, disease, or injury by physical means; SYN physiotherapy. **2.** the health profession concerned with promotion of health, with prevention of physical disabilities, with evaluation and rehabilitation of persons disabled by pain, disease, or injury, and with treatment by physical therapeutic measures as opposed to medical, surgical, or radiologic measures.

**phy·si·cian** (fi-zish′ŭn) **1.** a doctor; a person who has been educated, trained, and licensed to practice the art and science of medicine. **2.** a practitioner of medicine, as contrasted with a surgeon. [Fr. *physicien,* a natural philosopher]

**phy·si·cian-as·sis·ted su·i·cide** voluntary termination of one's own life by administration of a lethal substance with the direct or indirect assistance of a physician. Physician-assisted suicide is to be distinguished from the withholding or discontinuance of life-support measures in terminal or vegetative states so that the patient dies of the underlying illness, and from administration of narcotic analgesics in terminal cancer, which may indirectly hasten death. SEE ALSO end-of-life care, advance directive.

**physician office laboratory (POL)** clinical laboratory located in a physician's office for on-site testing of specimens from patients seen by the physician.

**Phy·sick pouch·es** (fiz′ik) proctitis with mucous discharge and burning pain, involving especially the sacculations between the rectal valves.

**phys·i·co·chem·i·cal** (fiz′i-kō-kem′i-kăl) relating to the field of physical chemistry.

**phys·ics** (fiz′iks) the branch of science concerned with the phenomena of matter and energy and their interactions.

△**phys·io-, physi-** 1. physical, physiological. 2. natural, relating to physics. [G. *physis,* nature]

**phys·i·o·gen·ic** (fiz′ē-ō-jen′ik) related to or caused by physiologic activity. [physio- + G. *genesis,* origin]

**phys·i·og·no·my** (fiz-ē-og′nō-mē) **1.** the physical appearance of one's face, countenance, or habitus, especially regarded as an indication of character. **2.** estimation of one's character and mental qualities by a study of the face and other external bodily features. [physio- + G. *gnōmōn,* a judge]

**phys·i·o·log·ic, phys·i·o·log·i·cal** (fiz-ē-ō-loj′ik, fiz-ē-ō-loj′i-kăl) **1.** relating to physiology. **2.** normal, as opposed to pathologic; denoting the various vital processes. **3.** denoting something that is apparent from its functional effects rather than from its anatomic structure; e.g., a physiologic sphincter. **4.** denoting a dose of a hormone, neurotransmitter, or other naturally occurring agent that is within the range of concentrations or potencies that would occur naturally. Cf. homeopathic (2), pharmacologic (2).

**phys·i·o·log·i·cal drives** those drives such as hunger and thirst which stem from the biological needs of an organism.

**phys·i·o·log·ic an·ti·dote** an agent that produces systemic effects contrary to those of a given poison.

**phys·i·o·log·i·c chem·is·try** SYN biochemistry.

**phys·i·o·log·ic con·ges·tion** SYN functional congestion.

**phys·i·o·log·ic dead space** the sum of anatomic and alveolar dead space; the dead space calculated when the carbon dioxide pressure in systemic arterial blood is used instead of that of alveolar gas in Bohr equation; it is a virtual or apparent volume that takes into account the impairment of gas exchange because of uneven distributions of lung ventilation and perfusion.

**phys·i·o·log·ic ho·me·o·sta·sis** SYN Bernard-Cannon homeostasis.

**phys·i·o·log·ic hy·per·tro·phy** temporary increase in size of an organ or part to provide for a natural increase of function.

**phys·i·o·log·ic ic·ter·us** SYN icterus neonatorum.

**phys·i·o·log·ic jaun·dice** SYN icterus neonatorum.

**phys·i·o·log·ic leu·ko·cy·to·sis** any form of leukocytosis that is associated with apparently normal situations and that is not directly related to a pathologic condition.

**phys·i·o·log·ic oc·clu·sion** occlusion in harmony with functions of the masticatory system.

**phys·i·o·log·ic rest po·si·tion** the usual position of the mandible when the patient is resting comfortably in the upright position and the condyles are in a neutral unstrained position in the mandibular fossae. SYN postural position, postural resting position.

**phys·i·o·log·ic re·trac·tion ring** a ridge on the inner uterine surface at the boundary line between the upper and lower uterine segment that occurs in the course of normal labor.

**phys·i·o·log·ic sa·line** an isotonic aqueous solution of salts, containing 0.9% sodium chloride.

**phys·i·o·log·ic sco·to·ma** the negative scotoma in the visual field, corresponding to the optic disk. SYN blind spot (1).

**phys·i·o·log·ic sphinc·ter** a section of a tubular structure that acts as if it has a band of circular muscle to constrict it, although no such specialized structure can be found on morphologic examination. SYN radiologic sphincter.

**phys·i·o·log·ic u·nit 1.** the ultimate (hypothetical) vital unit of protoplasm, as conceived by Spencer; **2.** the smallest division of an organ that will perform its function; e.g., the uriniferous tubule.

**phys·i·ol·o·gist** (fiz-ē-ol′ō-jist) a specialist in physiology.

**phys·i·ol·o·gy** (fiz-ē-ol′ō-jē) the science concerned with the normal vital processes of animal and vegetable organisms, especially as to how things normally function in the living organism rather than to their anatomical structure, their biochemical composition, or how they are affected by drugs or disease. [L. or G. *physiologia,* fr. G. *physis,* nature, + *logos,* study]

**phys·i·o·ther·a·peu·tic** (fiz′ē-ō-thār-ă-pyu′tik) pertaining to physical therapy.

**phys·i·o·ther·a·pist** (fiz′ē-ō-thār′ă-pist) a physical therapist. SEE physical therapy (2).

**phys·i·o·ther·a·py** (fiz′ē-ō-thār′ă-pē) SYN physical therapy (1). [physio- + G. *therapeia,* treatment]

**phy·sique** (fi-zēk′) constitutional type; the physical or bodily structure; the "build." [Fr.]

△**physo- 1.** tendency to swell or inflate. **2.** relation to air or gas. [G. *physaō,* to inflate, distend]

**phy·so·cele** (fi′sō-sēl) **1.** a circumscribed swelling due to the presence of gas. **2.** a hernial sac distended with gas. [physo- + G. *kēlē,* tumor, hernia]

**phy·so·me·tra** (fi-sō-mē′tră) distention of the uterine cavity with air or gas. [physo- + G. *mētra,* uterus]

**phy·so·py·o·sal·pinx** (fi′sō-pī-ō-sal′pingks) pyosalpinx accompanied by a formation of gas in a uterine (fallopian) tube. [physo- + G. *pyon,* pus, + *salpinx,* trumpet]

△**phyto-, phyt-** plants. [G. *phyton,* a plant]

**phy·to·ag·glu·ti·nin** (fi′tō-ă-gloo′ti-nin) a lectin that causes agglutination of erythrocytes or of leukocytes.

**phy·to·be·zoar** (fi-tō-bē′zōr) a gastric concretion formed of vegetable fibers, with the seeds and skins of fruits, and sometimes starch granules and fat globules. SYN food ball. [phyto- + bezoar]

**phy·to·chem·i·cal** a biologically active but nonnutrient substance found in plants; includes antioxidants and phytosterols. SYN bioactive non-nutrient, phytoprotectant.

**phy·to·der·ma·ti·tis** (fi′tō-der-mă-tī′tis) dermatitis caused by various mechanisms including mechanical and chemical injury, allergy, or photosensitization (phytophotodermatitis) at skin sites previously exposed to plants.

**phy·to·hae·mag·glu·tin·in [Br.]** SEE phytohemagglutinin.

**phy·to·hem·ag·glu·ti·nin (PHA)** (fi′tō-hēm-ă-gloo′ti-nin) a phytomitogen from plants that agglutinates red blood cells. The term is commonly used specifically for the lectin obtained from the red kidney bean (*Phaseolus vulgaris*) which is also a mitogen. SYN phytolectin.

**phy·toid** (fi′toyd) resembling a plant; denoting an animal having many of the biologic characteristics of a vegetable. [G. *phytōdēs,* fr. *phyton,* plant, + *eidos,* resemblance]

**phy·tol** (fi′tol) an unsaturated primary alcohol derived from the hydrolysis of chlorophyll; a constituent of vitamins E and $K_1$.

**phy·to·lec·tin** (fi-tō-lek′tin) SYN phytohemagglutinin.

**phy·to·mi·to·gen** (fi-tō-mī′tō-jen) a mitogenic lectin causing lymphocyte transformation accompanied by mitotic proliferation of the resulting blast cells identical to that produced by antigenic stimulation; e.g., phytohemagglutinin, concanavalin A.

**phy·to·phlyc·to·der·ma·ti·tis** (fī'tō-flik'tō-der-mă-ti'tis) SYN meadow dermatitis. [phyto- + G. *phlyktaina,* blister, + dermatitis]

**phy·to·pho·to·der·ma·ti·tis** (fī'tō-fō'tō-der-mă-tī'tis) phytodermatitis resulting from photosensitization.

**phy·to·pro·tec·tant** SYN phytochemical.

**phy·to·tox·ic** (fī-tō-tok'sik) **1.** poisonous to plant life. **2.** pertaining to a phytotoxin.

**phy·to·tox·in** (fī-tō-tok'sin) a substance similar in its properties to an extracellular bacterial toxin. [phyto- + G. *toxikon,* poison]

**PI** Periodontal Index.

**pI** the pH value for the isoelectric point of a given substance.

**pi** (π, Π) (pī) **1.** the 16th letter of the Greek alphabet (π, Π). **2.** osmotic pressure (Π). **3.** MATHEMATICS symbol for the product of a series (Π). **4.** symbol for the ratio of the circumference of a circle to its diameter (approximately 3.14159265) (π).

**pia** (pī'ă, pē'ă) SYN pia mater. [L. fem. of *pius,* tender]

**pia-a·rach·ni·tis** (pī'ă-ă-rak-nī'tis) SYN leptomeningitis.

**pia-a·rach·noid** (pī'ă-ă-rak'noyd, pē'ă-ă-rak' noyd) SYN leptomeninges.

**pi·al** (pī'al, pē'al) relating to the pia mater.

**pia mat·er** (pī'ă mā'ter, pē'ă mah'ter) [TA] a delicate vasculated fibrous membrane firmly adherent to the glial capsule of the brain (**pia mater cranialis [encephali]** [TA]) and spinal cord (**pia mater spinalis** [TA] or **membrana limitans gliae**); following exactly the outer markings of the cerebrum and also the ependymal lining circumference of the choroid membranes and plexus, it invests the cerebellum but not so intimately as it does the cerebrum, not dipping down into all the smaller sulci. The pia mater and the arachnoid are collectively called leptomeninges, as distinguished from dura mater or pachymeninx. SYN pia. [L. tender, affectionate mother, mistransl. of Arabic *umm raqīqah,* delicate covering or protection]

**pia ma·ter en·ceph·a·li** [TA] SYN cranial pia mater.

**pi·an** (pē-an', pī'an) SYN yaws.

**pi·a·rach·noid** (pī'ă-rak'noyd) SYN leptomeninges.

**pi·ca** (pī'kă, pē'kă) an appetite for substances not fit as food or of no nutritional value; clay, dried paint, starch. [L. *pica,* magpie]

**Pic·chi·ni syn·drome** (pǐ-chē'nē) a form of polyserositis involving the three great serosae in contact with the diaphragm, sometimes also the meninges, tunica vaginalis testis, synovial sheaths, and bursae, caused by the presence of a trypanosome.

**Pick at·ro·phy** (pik) circumscribed atrophy of the cerebral cortex.

**Pick bod·ies** (pik) intracytoplasmic argentophilic neuronal inclusion bodies seen in Pick disease.

**Pick cell** (pik) a relatively large mononuclear cell with foamlike cytoplasm that contains numerous droplets of sphingomyelin; such cells are widely distributed in the spleen and other tissues in patients with Niemann-Pick disease. SYN Niemann-Pick cell.

**Pick dis·ease** (pik) progressive circumscribed cerebral atrophy; a rare type of cerebrodegenerative disorder manifested primarily as dementia, in which there is striking atrophy of portions of the frontal and temporal lobes. [F. Pick]

**Pick·les chart** (pik'elz) day-by-day plots of new cases of infectious disease used to demonstrate the progress of an epidemic in a small, relatively isolated population.

**pick·wick·i·an syn·drome** (pik-wik'ē-ăn) a combination of severe, grotesque obesity, somnolence, and general debility, theoretically resulting from hypoventilation induced by the obesity; hypercapnia, pulmonary hypertension and cor pulmonale can result. [after the "fat boy" in Dickens's *Pickwick Papers*]

△**pi·co-** **1.** small. **2.** (p) prefix used in the SI and metric systems to signify one-trillionth ($10^{-12}$). SYN bicro-. [It. *piccolo*]

**pi·co·gram (pg)** (pī'kō-gram) one-trillionth of a gram.

**pi·co·ka·tal (pkat)** (pī'kō-kat'ăl) one trillionth of a katal ($10^{-12}$ katal).

**pi·com·e·ter (pm)** (pī'kō-mē-ter) one-trillionth of a meter. SYN bicron.

**pi·co·mole (pmol)** (pē'kō-mōl) one-trillionth of a mole ($10^{-12}$ mole).

**Pi·cor·na·vir·i·dae** (pi-kōr-nă-vir'i-dē) a family of very small viruses having a core of single-stranded RNA. Numerous species (including the polioviruses, coxsackieviruses, and echoviruses) are included in the family. There are four accepted genera: Enterovirus, Rhinovirus, Cardiovirus, and Aphthovirus. [It. *piccolo,* very small, + RNA + -viridae]

**pi·cor·na·vi·rus** (pi-kōr-nă-vī'rŭs) a virus of the family Picornaviridae.

**pic·ro·car·mine stain, pic·ro·car·mine** (pik-rō-kar'min, pik-rō-kar'mēn) a red crystalline powder derived from a solution of carmine, ammonia, and picric acid which is evaporated, leaving the powder (soluble in water); it produces excellent staining of keratohyaline granules.

**PID** pelvic inflammatory disease.

**Pid·gin Sign Eng·lish (PSE)** (pij'in sīn in-glīsh') a system of communication that is a manual representation of English in which American Sign Language signs are used in English word order; there are no inflectional signs, and finger spelling is used for proper names.

**pie·bald eye·lash** an isolated bundle of white eyelashes among normally pigmented eyelashes.

**pie·bald·ism** (pī'bawld-izm) SYN piebaldness.

**pie·bald·ness** (pī'bawld-ness) patchy absence of the pigment of scalp hair, giving a streaked appearance; patches of vitiligo may be present in other areas due to absence of melanocytes. May be associated with neurological defects or eye changes. SYN piebald skin, piebaldism.

**pie·bald skin** SYN piebaldness.

**pie·dra** (pē-ā'dră) a fungus disease of the hair characterized by the formation of numerous waxy, small, firm, nodular masses on the hair shaft. [Sp. a stone]

**Pi·erre Rob·in syn·drome** (pyăr' rō-bah') micrognathia and abnormal smallness of the tongue, often with cleft palate, severe myopia, congenital glaucoma, and retinal detachment. SYN Robin syndrome.

**pi·e·ses·the·sia** (pī-ē-ses-thē'zē-ă) SYN pressure sense. [G. *piesis,* pressure, + *aisthēsis,* sensation]

**pi·e·sim·e·ter, pi·e·som·e·ter** (pī-ĕ-sim'ĕ-ter,

pī-ĕ-som′ĕ-ter) an instrument for measuring the pressure of a gas or a fluid. [G. *piesis*, pressure]

**pi•e•zo•gen•ic ped•al pap•ule** pressure-induced papules of the heel, occurring probably as a result of herniation of fat tissue.

**PIF** prolactin-inhibiting factor.

**pi•geon breast** SYN pectus carinatum.

**pig•ment 1.** any coloring matter, as that of the red blood cells, hair, iris, etc., or the stains used in histologic or bacteriologic work, or that in paints. **2.** a medicinal preparation for external use, applied to the skin like paint or coloring agents used in paints. [L. *pigmentum*, paint]

**pig•men•tary** (pig′men-tār-ē) relating to a pigment.

**pig•men•tary ret•i•nop•a•thy** SYN retinitis pigmentosa.

**pig•men•ta•tion** (pig-men-tā′shŭn) coloration, either normal or pathologic, of the skin or tissues resulting from a deposit of pigment.

**pig•ment dis•per•sion syn•drome** increased resistance to flow of aqueous humor through the pupil from the anterior chamber to the posterior chamber, leading to posterior bowing of the peripheral iris against the zonules; a possible mechanism for pigmentary glaucoma.

**pig•ment•ed** (pig′men-ted) colored as the result of a deposit of pigment.

**pig•ment•ed lay•er of ret•i•na** the outer layer of the retina, consisting of pigmented epithelium.

**pig•ment•ed vil•lo•nod•u•lar syn•o•vi•tis** diffuse outgrowths of synovial membrane of a joint, usually the knee, composed of synovial villi and fibrous nodules infiltrated by hemosiderin- and lipid-containing macrophages and multinucleated giant cells; the condition may be inflammatory, although recurrence is likely to follow incomplete removal.

**pig•ment•ed vil•lo•nod•u•lar ten•o•syn•o•vi•tis** SYN villous tenosynovitis.

**pig•men•to•ly•sin** (pig-men-tol′i-sin) an antibody causing destruction of pigment. [L. *pigmentum*, pigment, + G. *lysis*, a loosening]

**pig•men•tum ni•grum** (pig-men′tŭm nī′grŭm) melanin of the choroid coat of the eye.

**pig•tail cath•e•ter** an angiographic catheter with a tightly curled end to reduce the impact of the injectant on the vessel wall.

**PIH** prolactin-inhibiting hormone.

**pi•lar, pi•la•ry** (pī′lăr, pil′ă-rē) SYN hairy. [L. *pilus*, hair]

**pi•lar cyst** a common cyst of the skin and subcutis which contains sebum and keratin, and is lined by pale-staining stratified epithelial cells derived from follicular trichilemma.

**pi•lar tu•mor of scalp** a benign solitary tumor of the scalp in elderly women that may ulcerate.

**pile** (pīl) **1.** a series of plates of two different metals imposed alternately one on the other, separated by a sheet of material moistened with a dilute acid solution, used to produce a current of electricity. [L. *pila*, pillar] **2.** an individual hemorrhoidal tumor. SEE hemorrhoids. [L. *pila*, ball]

**pi•le•ous** (pī′lē-ŭs) SYN hairy. [L. *pilus*, hair]

**pi•le•ous gland** a sebaceous gland emptying into the hair follicle.

**piles** (pīlz) SYN hemorrhoids. [L. *pila*, a ball]

**pi•li** (pī′lī) plural of pilus. [L.]

**pi•li tor•ti** a condition in which many hair shafts are twisted on the long axis, congenital or acquired as a result of distortion of the follicles

from a scarring inflammatory process, mechanical stress, or cicatrizing alopecia; the hair shafts resemble spangles in reflected light, are brittle, and break at varying lengths with many areas appearing bald with a dark stubble; as a developmental defect it can be manifested in such syndromes as Björnstad, Crandall, and Menkes. SYN twisted hairs.

**pill 1.** a small globular mass of soluble material containing a medicinal substance to be swallowed; colloquially, any solid dosage form of oral medicine including tablets and capsules. **2.** the Pill; colloquial term for an oral contraceptive. [L. *pilula*; dim. of *pila*, ball]

**pil•lar** (pil′ăr) a structure or part having a resemblance to a column or pillar. [L. *pila*]

**pil•lars of fau•ces** SEE palatoglossal arch, palatopharyngeal arch.

**pil•lars of for•nix** the columna fornicis and crus fornicis.

**pil•low splint** a splint that is inflatable or that is made from unusually bulky fabric.

**pill-roll•ing** (pil′rōl′ing) a circular movement of the opposed tips of the thumb and the index finger appearing as a form of tremor in paralysis agitans.

**pill-roll•ing trem•or** resting tremor of the thumb and fingers seen in Parkinson disease.

△**pilo-** hair. [L. *pilus*]

**pi•lo•be•zoar** (pī-lō-bē′zōr) SYN trichobezoar. [pilo- + bezoar]

**pi•lo•cys•tic** (pī′lō-sis′tik) denoting a dermoid cyst containing hair. [pilo- + G. *kystis*, bladder]

**pi•lo•cy•tic as•tro•cy•to•ma** a slowly growing astrocytoma composed histologically of elongated astrocytes; often located in the optic chiasm region of the third ventricle, hypothalamus, or cerebellum, predominantly in younger individuals.

**pi•lo•e•rec•tion** (pī′lō-ē-rek′shŭn) erection of hair due to action of arrectores pilorum muscles.

**pi•loid** (pī′loyd) hairlike; resembling hair. [pilo- + G. *eidos*, resemblance]

**pi•lo•jec•tion** (pī-lō-jek′shŭn) process of shooting shafts of stiff mammalian hair into a saccular aneurysm in the brain in order to produce thrombosis. [pilo- + injection]

**pi•lo•ma•trix•o•ma** (pī′lō-mā-trik-sō′mă) a benign solitary hair follicle tumor containing cells resembling basal cell carcinoma and areas of epithelial necrosis. SYN Malherbe calcifying epithelioma. [pilo- + matrix + G. *-oma*, tumor]

**pi•lo•mo•tor** (pī′lō-mō′ter) moving the hair; denoting the arrectores pilorum muscles of the skin and the postganglionic sympathetic nerve fibers innervating these small smooth muscles. [pilo- + L. *motor*, mover]

**pi•lo•mo•tor re•flex** contraction of the smooth muscle of the skin resulting in "gooseflesh" caused by mild application of a tactile stimulus or by local cooling.

**pi•lo•ni•dal** (pī-lō-nī′dăl) denoting the presence of hair in a dermoid cyst or in a sinus opening on the skin. [pilo- + L. *nidus*, nest]

**pi•lo•ni•dal si•nus** a fistula or pit in the sacral region, communicating with the exterior, containing loose, broken-off body hairs which may act as a foreign body producing chronic inflammation.

**pi•lose** (pī′lōs) SYN hairy. [L. *pilosus*]

**pi•lo•se•ba•ceous** (pī′lō-sē-bā′shŭs) relating to

the hair follicles and sebaceous glands. [pilo- + L. *sebum,* suet]

**pi·lus,** pl. **pi·li** (pī'lŭs, pī'lī) **1.** one of the fine, keratinized filamentous epidermal growths arising from the skin of the body of mammals except the palms, soles, and flexor surfaces of the joints; the full length and texture of the hair varies markedly in different body sites. **2.** a fine filamentous appendage, somewhat analogous to the flagellum, that occurs on some bacteria. SYN fimbria (2). SEE ALSO conjugative plasmid. [L.]

**pi·mel·ic ac·id** (pĭ-mel'ĭk as'id) an intermediate in the oxidation of oleic acid in some microorganisms; a precursor of biotin.

△**pi·me·lo-** fat, fatty. [G. *pimelē,* soft fat, lard, fr. *piar,* fat]

**pim·ple** (pim'pl) a papule or small pustule; usually meant to denote an inflammatory lesion of acne.

**PIN** prostatic intraepithelial neoplasia.

**pin** rod used in surgical treatment of bone fractures. SEE ALSO nail. [O.E. *pinn,* fr. L. *pinna,* feather]

**Pi·nard ma·neu·ver** (pē-nahr') in management of a frank breech presentation, pressure on the popliteal space is made by the index finger while the other three fingers flex the leg while sliding it along the other thigh as the foot of the flexed leg is brought down and out.

**pince·ment** (pans-mon') a pinching manipulation in massage. [Fr. pinching]

**pin·cer nail** transverse overcurvature of the nail that increases distally, causing the lateral borders of the nail to pinch the soft tissue with resulting tenderness; may result from a developmental anomaly or subungual exostosis.

**pinch** OCCUPATIONAL THERAPY grip between fingers at the most distal joints. See this page.

**pinch graft** small bits of skin, of partial or full thickness, removed from a healthy area and seeded in a site to be covered.

**pin·cush·ion dis·tor·tion** irregular image produced when axial magnification is greater than peripheral magnification. SEE Petzval surface.

**pin·e·al** (pīn'ē-ăl) **1.** shaped like a pine cone. SYN piniform. **2.** pertaining to the pineal body. [L. *pineus,* relating to the pine, *pinus*]

**pin·e·al bod·y** a small, unpaired, flattened body, shaped somewhat like a pine cone, attached at its anterior pole to the region of the posterior and habenular commissures, and lying in the depression between the two superior colliculi below the splenium of the corpus callosum; it is a glandular structure, composed of follicles containing epithelioid cells and lime concretions called brain sand; despite its attachment to the brain, it appears to receive nerve fibers exclusively from the peripheral autonomic nervous system. It produces melatonin. SYN corpus pineale [TA], conarium, pineal gland.

**pin·e·al·ec·to·my** (pīn'ē-ă-lek'tō-mē) removal of the pineal body. [pineal + G. *ektomē,* excision]

**pin·e·al gland** SYN pineal body.

**pin·e·a·lo·cyte** (pīn-ē'al-ō-sīt) a cell of the pineal body with long processes ending in bulbous expansions. Pinealocytes receive a direct innervation from sympathetic neurons that form recognizable synapses. [pineal + G. *kytos,* cell]

**pin·e·a·lo·ma** (pīn'ē-ă-lō'mă) a term that has been variably used to designate germ cell tumors,

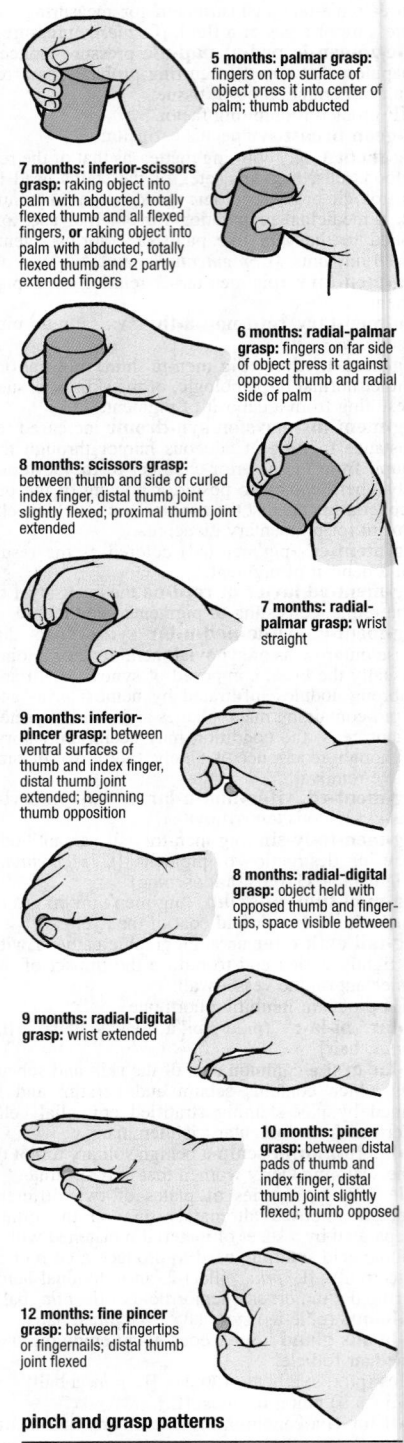

**5 months: palmar grasp:** fingers on top surface of object press it into center of palm; thumb abducted

**7 months: inferior-scissors grasp:** raking object into palm with abducted, totally flexed thumb and all flexed fingers, **or** raking object into palm with abducted, totally flexed thumb and 2 partly extended fingers

**6 months: radial-palmar grasp:** fingers on far side of object press it against opposed thumb and radial side of palm

**8 months: scissors grasp:** between thumb and side of curled index finger, distal thumb joint slightly flexed; proximal thumb joint extended

**7 months: radial-palmar grasp:** wrist straight

**9 months: inferior-pincer grasp:** between ventral surfaces of thumb and index finger, distal thumb joint extended; beginning thumb opposition

**8 months: radial-digital grasp:** object held with opposed thumb and fingertips, space visible between

**9 months: radial-digital grasp:** wrist extended

**10 months: pincer grasp:** between distal pads of thumb and index finger, distal thumb joint slightly flexed; thumb opposed

**12 months: fine pincer grasp:** between fingertips or fingernails; distal thumb joint flexed

**pinch and grasp patterns**

pineocytomas and pineoblastomas of the pineal gland. [pineal + G. *-oma,* tumor]

**pin·e·al stalk** the attachment of the pineal body to the roof of the third ventricle; it contains the pineal recess of the third ventricle.

**Pi·nel sys·tem** (pē-něl´) the abolition of forcible restraint in the treatment of the mental hospital patient.

**pin·e·o·blas·to·ma** (pīn´ē-ō-blas-tō´mǎ) a poorly differentiated tumor of the pineal gland consisting of small cells with a scant amount of cytoplasms and often forming pseudorosettes. [pineal + G. *blastos,* germ, + *-oma,* tumor]

**pin·guec·u·la, pin·guic·u·la** (ping-gwek´yu-lǎ ping-gwik´yu-lǎ) a yellowish accumulation of connective tissue that thickens the conjunctiva; occurs in the aged. [L. *pinguiculus,* fattish, fr. *pinguis,* fat]

**pin·hole pu·pil** an extremely constricted pupil.

**pin·i·form** (pin´i-fōrm) SYN pineal (1). [L. *pinus,* pine, + *forma,* form]

**pink dis·ease** acrodynia (2).

**pink·eye** (pink´ī) **1.** SYN acute contagious conjunctivitis. **2.** SYN infectious bovine keratoconjunctivitis. **3.** in horses, a form of equine viral arteritis.

**pin·na,** pl. **pin·nae** (pin´ǎ, pin´ē) **1.** SYN auricle (1). **2.** a feather, wing, or fin. [L. *pinna* or *penna,* a feather, in pl. a wing]

**pin·nal** (pin´ǎl) relating to the pinna.

**pin·o·cyte** (pin´ō-sīt) a cell that exhibits pinocytosis. [G. *pineō,* to drink, + *kytos,* cell]

**pin·o·cy·to·sis** (pin´ō-sī-tō´sis) the cellular process of actively engulfing liquid, a phenomenon in which minute incuppings or invaginations are formed in the surface of the cell membrane and close to form fluid-filled vesicles; it resembles phagocytosis. [pinocyte + G. *-osis,* condition]

**pin·o·some** (pin´ō-sōm) a fluid-filled vacuole formed by pinocytosis. [G. *pineō,* to drink, + *sōma,* body]

**Pins sign** (pins) SYN Ewart sign.

**Pins syn·drome** (pins) dullness, diminution of vocal fremitus and of the vesicular murmur, and a slight distant blowing sound, heard in the posteroinferior region of the chest on the left side, in cases of pericardial effusion; there is sometimes also a fine rale in this region, but all the adventitious auscultatory signs disappear when the patient assumes the genupectoral position.

**pint** (pīnt) a measure of quantity (U.S. liquid), containing 16 fluid ounces, 28.875 cubic inches; 473.1765 cc. An imperial pint contains 20 British fluid ounces, 34.67743 cubic inches; 568.2615 cc.

**pin·ta** (pin´tǎ, pēn´tǎ) a disease caused by a spirochete, *Treponema carateum,* and characterized by a small primary papule followed by an enlarging plaque and disseminated secondary macules of varying color called pintids that finally become white. SYN mal del pinto. [Sp. painted]

**pin·worm** (pin´werm) a member of the genus *Enterobius* or related nematodes causing intestinal parasitism in a large variety of vertebrates, including man (*Enterobius vermicularis,* the human pinworm). SYN seatworm.

**Pi·per for·ceps** (pī´pěr) obstetrical forceps used to facilitate delivery of the head in breech presentation.

**pi·pette, pi·pet** (pī-pet´, pī-pet´) a graduated tube (marked in ml) used to transport a definite vol-

ume of a gas or liquid in laboratory work. [Fr. dim. of *pipe,* pipe]

**pir·i·form** (pir´i-fōrm) pear-shaped. [L. *pirum,* pear, + *forma,* form]

**pi·ri·for·mis mus·cle** *origin,* margins of pelvic sacral foramina and greater sciatic notch of ilium; *insertion,* upper border of greater trochanter; *action,* rotates thigh laterally; *nerve supply,* nerve to piriformis (sciatic plexus). SYN musculus piriformis [TA], piriform muscle.

**pir·i·form mus·cle** SYN piriformis muscle.

**pir·i·form neu·ron lay·er** the layer of Purkinje cells between the molecular and granular layers of the cerebellar cortex.

**Pi·ro·goff am·pu·ta·tion** (pīr´ō-gof) amputation of the foot; the lower articular surfaces of the tibia and fibula are sawed through and the ends covered with a portion of the os calcis which has also been sawed through from above posteriorly downward and forward.

**Pir·quet test** (pir-kā´) a cutaneous tuberculin test. SEE tuberculin test.

**pis·i·form** (pis´i-fōrm) pea-shaped or pea-sized. [L. *pisum,* pea, + *forma,* appearance]

**pis·i·form bone** a small bone resembling a pea in size and shape, in the proximal row of the carpus, lying on the anterior surface of the triquetral, with which it articulates; it gives insertion to the tendon of the flexor carpi ulnaris muscle.

**pit 1.** any natural depression on the surface of the body, such as the axilla. Cf. dimple. **2.** one of the pinhead-sized depressed scars following the pustule of acne or chickenpox (pockmark). **3.** a depression in the enamel surface of a tooth due to faulty or incomplete calcification or formed at the confluent point of two or more lobes of enamel. **4.** to indent, as by pressure of the finger on the edematous skin; to become indented, said of the edematous tissues when pressure is made with the fingertip. [L. *puteus*]

**pit-1** a nuclear binding transcriptional factor found in many cells in normal human pituitary glands and expressed in a large percentage of pituitary adenomas, in particular those positive for growth hormone, or thyrotropin.

**pitch** auditory perception of tone on a scale ranging from low to high, based on the frequency of vibration of the object emitting the tone. For the human voice, pitch relates to frequency of vibration of the vocal folds. SEE voice, frequency.

**pitch wart** a precancerous keratotic epidermal tumor, common among workers in pitch and coal tar derivatives.

**pith 1.** the center of a hair. **2.** the spinal cord and medulla oblongata. **3.** to pierce the medulla of an animal with a sharp instrument introduced at the base of the skull. [A.S. *pitha*]

**pith·e·coid** (pith´ě-koyd) resembling an ape. [G. *pithēkos,* ape, + *eidos,* resemblance]

**Pi·tres sign** (pē´trě) **1.** SYN haphalgesia. **2.** diminished sensation in the testes and scrotum in tabes dorsalis.

**pit·ted ker·a·tol·y·sis** noninflammatory Gram-positive bacterial infection of the plantar surfaces producing small depressions in the stratum corneum, associated frequently with humidity and hyperhidrosis.

**pit·ting** DENTISTRY the formation of well defined, relatively deep depressions in a surface, usually used in describing defects in surfaces (often golds, solder joints, or amalgam). It may arise from a variety of causes, although the clinical occurrence is often associated with corrosion. SEE ALSO pitting edema, nail pits.

**pit·ting e·de·ma** edema that retains for a time the indentation produced by pressure.

**Pitts·burgh pneu·mo·nia** (pits'berg) a variant of Legionnaires disease caused by *Legionella micdadei*.

**Pitts·burgh pneu·mo·nia a·gent** SYN *Legionella micdadei*.

**pi·tu·i·cyte** (pi-too'i-sīt) the primary cell of the posterior lobe of the pituitary gland, a fusiform cell closely related to neuroglia. [pituitary + G. *kytos,* cell]

**pi·tu·i·cy·to·ma** (pi-too'i-sī-tō'mă) a rare gliogenous neoplasm derived from pituicytes, occurring in the posterior lobe of the pituitary gland and characterized by cells with small nuclei and long processes that form a network of cytoplasmic material, in which droplets of fat may be demonstrated. [pituicyte + G. *-oma,* tumor]

**pi·tu·i·tar·ism** (pi-too'i-tār-izm) pituitary dysfunction. SEE hyperpituitarism, hypopituitarism.

**pi·tu·i·tary** (pi-too'i-tār-ē) relating to the pituitary gland (hypophysis). [L. *pituita,* phlegm]

**pi·tu·i·tary ca·chex·ia** SYN Simmonds disease.

**pi·tu·i·tary di·ver·tic·u·lum** a tubular outgrowth of ectoderm from the stomodeum of the embryo; it grows dorsad toward the infundibulum of the diencephalon, around which it forms a cup-like mass, giving rise to the pars distalis and pars juxtaneuralis of the hypophysis. SYN Rathke pocket, Rathke pouch.

**pi·tu·i·tary dwarf·ism** a rare form of dwarfism caused by the absence of a functional anterior pituitary gland; may be present at birth or develop during early childhood.

**pi·tu·i·tary dys·to·pia** failure of union of neurohypophysis and adenohypophysis.

**pi·tu·i·tary gi·gan·tism** a form of gigantism caused by hypersecretion of pituitary growth hormone; a rare disorder commonly the result of a pituitary adenoma.

**pi·tu·i·tary gland** SYN hypophysis.

**pi·tu·i·tary go·nad·o·tro·pic hor·mone** SYN anterior pituitary gonadotropin.

**pi·tu·i·tary growth hor·mone** SYN somatotropin.

**pi·tu·i·tary myx·e·de·ma** myxedema resulting from inadequate secretion of the thyrotropic hormone; commonly occurs in association with inadequate secretion of other anterior pituitary hormones.

**pi·tu·i·tary stalk** a process comprising the tuberal part investing the infundibular stem that attaches the hypophysis to the tuber cinereum at the base of the brain.

**pit·y·ri·a·sic** (pit-i-rī'ă-sik) relating to or suffering from pityriasis.

**pit·y·ri·a·sis** (pit-i-rī'ă-sis) a dermatosis marked by branny desquamation. [G. fr. *pityron,* bran, dandruff]

**pit·y·ri·a·sis al·ba** patchy hypopigmentation of the skin resulting from mild dermatitis.

**pit·y·ri·a·sis lin·guae** SYN geographic tongue.

**pit·y·ri·a·sis ro·sea** a self-limited eruption of macules or papules involving the trunk and less frequently extremities, scalp, and face; the lesions are usually oval and follow the crease lines of the skin; the onset is frequently preceded by a single larger scaling lesion known as the herald patch.

**pit·y·ri·a·sis ru·bra** SYN exfoliative dermatitis.

**pit·y·ri·a·sis ru·bra pi·la·ris** an uncommon chronic pruritic eruption of the hair follicles, which become firm, red, surmounted with a horny plug, and often confluent to form scaly plaques.

**pit·y·ri·a·sis ver·si·col·or** SYN tinea versicolor.

**pit·y·roid** (pit'i-royd) SYN furfuraceous. [G. *pityrōdēs,* branlike, fr. *pityron,* bran, + *eidos,* resemblance]

*Pit·y·ro·spo·rum* (pit-i-ros'pō-rŭm, pit'i-rō-spō'rŭm) a genus of fungi found in dandruff and seborrheic dermatitis. [G. *pityron,* bran, + *sporos,* seed]

**PIVKA** protein induced by vitamin K absence.

**piv·ot joint** a synovial joint in which a section of a cylinder of one bone fits into a corresponding cavity on the other. SYN rotary joint, rotatory joint, trochoid joint.

**pix·el** (pik'sel) a contraction for picture element, a two-dimensional representation of a volume element (voxel) in the display of the CT or MR image, usually 512 by 512 or 256 by 256 pixels respectively.

**PJ in·ter·val** the time elapsing from the beginning of the P wave to the end of the QRS complex (J for junction between QRS and T wave) in the electrocardiogram.

**PK** pyruvate kinase.

**$pK_a$** the negative decadic logarithm of the ionization constant ($K_a$) of an acid; equal to the pH value at which equal concentrations of the acid and conjugate base forms of a substance (often a buffer) are present.

**pkat** picokatal.

**PKU** phenylketonuria.

**pla·ce·bo** (plă-sē'bō) **1.** a medicinally inactive substance given as a medicine for its suggestive effect. **2.** an inert compound identical in appearance to material being tested in experimental research, which may or may not be known to the physician and/or patient, administered to distinguish between drug action and suggestive effect of the material under study. [L. I will please, future of *placeo*]

**place cod·ing** frequency coding as determined by the activation of the spiral organ (organ of Corti) from the base to the apex of the cochlea in a gradation with higher frequencies transmitted from near the base and lower frequencies from near the apex.

**pla·cen·ta** (plă-sen'tă) organ of metabolic interchange between fetus and mother. It has a portion of embryonic origin, derived from the outermost embryonic membrane (chorion frondosum or villous chorionic sac), and a maternal portion formed by a modification of the part of the uterine mucosa (decidua basalis) in which the chorionic vesicle is implanted. Within the placenta, the chorionic villi, with their contained capillaries carrying blood of the embryonic circulation, are exposed to maternal blood in the intervillous spaces in which the villi lie; no direct mixing of fetal and maternal blood occurs, but the intervening tissue (the placental membrane) is sufficiently thin to permit the absorption of nutritive materials, oxygen, and some harmful substances, like viruses, into the fetal blood and the release of carbon dioxide and nitrogenous waste from it.

At term, the human placenta is disk-shaped, about 4 cm in thickness and 18 cm in diameter, and averages about one-sixth to one-seventh the weight of the fetus; its fetal surface is smooth, being formed by the adherent amnion, with the umbilical cord normally attached near its center; the maternal surface of a detached placenta is rough because of the torn decidual tissue adhering to the chorion and shows lobular elevations called cotyledons or lobes. See this page. [L. a cake]

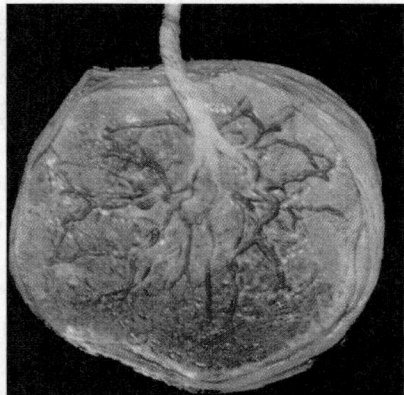

placenta: amniotic surface, with umbilical cord

**pla·cen·ta ac·cre·ta** the abnormal adherence of the chorionic villi to the myometrium, associated with partial or complete absence of the decidua basalis and, in particular, the stratum spongiosum.

**pla·cen·ta cir·cum·val·la·ta** a cup-shaped placenta with raised edges, having a thick, round, white, opaque ring around its periphery; a portion of the decidua separates the margin of the placenta from its chorionic plate; the remainder of the chorionic surface is normal in appearance, but the fetal vessels are limited in their course across the placenta by the ring. SEE ALSO placenta marginata, placenta reflexa.

**pla·cen·ta fe·nes·tra·ta** a placenta in which there are areas of thinning, sometimes extending to entire absence of placental tissue.

**pla·cen·ta in·cre·ta** a form of placenta accreta in which the chorionic villi invade the myometrium.

**pla·cen·tal** (pla-sen′tăl) relating to the placenta.

**pla·cen·tal bar·ri·er** SYN placental membrane.

**pla·cen·tal cir·cu·la·tion** the circulation of blood through the placenta during intrauterine life, serving the needs of the fetus for aeration, absorption, and excretion; also, maternal circulation through the intervillous space of the placenta.

**pla·cen·tal dys·to·cia** retention or difficult delivery of the placenta.

**pla·cen·tal growth hor·mone** SYN human placental lactogen.

**pla·cen·tal mem·brane** the semipermeable layer of fetal tissue separating the maternal from the fetal blood in the placenta; composed of: 1) endothelium of the fetal vessels in the chorionic villi, 2) stromata of the villi, 3) cytotrophoblast

(negligible after the fifth month of gestation), and 4) syncytiotrophoblast covering the villi; the placental membrane acts as a selective membrane regulating passage of substances from the maternal to the fetal blood. SYN placental barrier.

**pla·cen·tal pre·sen·ta·tion** SYN placenta previa.

**pla·cen·tal trans·fu·sion syn·drome** in utero transfusion of blood from one twin to the other such that the donor becomes anemic and growth retarded and the recipient becomes polycythemic and develops hydrops. SEE ALSO twin-twin transfusion.

**pla·cen·ta mar·gi·na·ta** a placenta with raised edges, less pronounced than the placenta circumvallata. SEE ALSO placenta reflexa.

**pla·cen·ta mem·bra·na·cea** an abnormally thin placenta covering an unusually large area of the uterine lining.

**pla·cen·ta pre·via** the condition in which the placenta is implanted in the lower segment of the uterus, extending to the margin of the internal os of the cervix or partially or completely obstructing the os. SYN placental presentation.

**pla·cen·ta re·flexa** an anomaly of the placenta in which the margin is thickened so as to appear turned back upon itself. SEE ALSO placenta circumvallata, placenta marginata.

**pla·cen·ta spu·ria** a mass of placental tissue which has no vascular connection with the main placenta.

**plac·en·ta·tion** (plas-en-tā′shŭn) the structural organization and mode of attachment of fetal to maternal tissues in the formation of the placenta.

**plac·en·ti·tis** (plas-en-tī′tis) inflammation of the placenta.

**plac·en·to·ma** (plas-en-tō′mă) SYN deciduoma.

**Pla·ci·do da Cos·ta disk** (plah′sē-dō dah kōs′ tah) SYN keratoscope.

**plac·ode** (plak′ōd) local thickening in the embryonic ectoderm layer; the cells of the placode ordinarily constitute a primordial group from which a sense organ or ganglion develops. [G. *plakōdēs*, fr. *plax*, anything flat or broad, + *eidos*, like]

**pla·fond** (plă-fon′) a ceiling, especially the ceiling of the ankle joint, i.e., the articular surface of the distal end of the tibia. [Fr. ceiling]

△**pla·gio-** oblique, slanting. [G. *plagios*]

**pla·gi·o·ce·phal·ic** (plā′jē-ō-se-fal′ik) relating to or marked by plagiocephaly.

**pla·gi·o·ceph·a·ly** (plā′jē-ō-sef′ă-lē) an asymmetric craniostenosis due to premature closure of the lambdoid and coronal sutures on one side; characterized by an oblique deformity of the skull. SYN asynclitism of the skull. [G. *plagios*, oblique, + *kephalē*, head]

**plague** (plāg) **1.** any disease of wide prevalence or of excessive mortality. **2.** an acute infectious disease caused by *Yersinia pestis* and marked by high fever, toxemia, prostration, a petechial eruption, lymph node enlargement, and pneumonia, or hemorrhage from the mucous membranes; primarily a disease of rodents, transmitted to humans by fleas that have bitten infected animals. In humans the disease takes one of four clinical forms: bubonic *plague*, septicemic *plague*, pneumonic *plague*, or ambulant *plague*. SYN pest, pestilence (1). [L. *plaga*, a stroke, injury]

**plain film** a radiograph made without use of a contrast medium.

**pla·na** (plā′nă) plural of planum. [L.]

**plan of care** SYN careplan.

**Planck con·stant (h)** (plahngk) a constant, $6.6260755 \times 10^{-34}$ J · s (joule-seconds) or $6.6260755 \times 10^{-27}$ erg-seconds = $6.6260755 \times 10^{-34}$ J Hz$^{-1}$ (joule per hertz).

**Planck the·o·ry** (plahngk) SYN quantum theory.

⊞**plane** (plān) **1.** a flat surface. SEE planum. **2.** an imaginary surface formed by extension through any axis or two definite points in reference especially to craniometry and to pelvimetry. See page APP 88. [L. *planus,* flat]

**plane joint** a synovial joint in which the opposing surfaces are nearly planes and in which there is only a slight, gliding motion, as in the intermetacarpal joints. SYN arthrodia, arthrodial joint, gliding joint.

**plane of pel·vic ca·nal** SYN pelvic axis.

**plane su·ture** a simple firm apposition of two smooth surfaces of bones, without overlap, as seen in the lacrimomaxillary suture. SYN harmonic suture.

**pla·nig·ra·phy** (pla-nig′ră-fē) SYN tomography. [L. *planum,* plane, + G. *graphē,* a writing]

**plan·ing** (plān′ing) SYN dermabrasion.

△**pla·no-, plan-, pla·ni- 1.** a plane; flat, level. [L. *planum,* plane; *planus,* flat] **2.** wandering. [G. *planos,* roaming]

**pla·no·cel·lu·lar** (plā-nō-sel′yu-lăr) relating to or composed of flat cells. [L. *planus,* flat, + cellular]

**pla·no·con·cave** (plā′nō-kon′kāv) flat on one side and concave on the other; denoting a lens of that shape.

**pla·no·con·cave lens** a lens that is flat on one side and concave on the other.

**pla·no·con·vex** (plā′nō-kon′veks) flat on one side and convex on the other; denoting a lens of that shape.

**pla·no·con·vex lens** a lens that is flat on one side and convex on the other.

**pla·nog·ra·phy** (pla-nog′ră-fē) SYN tomography.

**pla·no·val·gus** (plā-nō-val′gŭs) a condition in which the longitudinal arch of the foot is flattened and everted. [plano- + L. *valgus,* turned outward]

**plan·ta,** gen. and pl. **plan·tae** (plan′tă, plan′tē) [TA] SYN sole. [L.]

**plan·tal·gia** (plan-tal′jē-ă) pain on the plantar surface of the foot over the plantar fascia. [L. *planta,* sole of foot, + G. *algos,* pain]

**plan·tar** (plan′tăr) relating to the sole of the foot or the caudal aspect of the tarsus on the hindlimb of an animal. [L. *plantaris*]

**plan·tar arch 1.** the arterial arch formed by the lateral plantar artery running across the bases of the metatarsal bones and anastomosing with the dorsalis pedis artery; **2.** either of two bony arches of the foot, longitudinal arch or transverse arch.

**plan·tar cal·ca·ne·o·na·vic·u·lar lig·a·ment** a dense fibroelastic ligament that extends from the sustentaculum tali to the plantar surface of the navicular bone; it supports the head of the talus.

**plan·tar fas·ci·i·tis** inflammation of the fascia of the plantar surface of the foot, usually at the calcaneal attachment.

**plan·tar fi·bro·ma·to·sis** nodular fibroblastic proliferation in plantar fascia of one or both feet; rarely associated with contracture. SYN Dupuytren disease of the foot.

**plan·tar·flex·ion** (plăn-tăr-flĕk′shŭn) extension of the ankle, pointing of the foot and toes.

**plan·tar in·ter·os·se·ous mus·cle** three intrinsic muscles of foot; *origin,* the medial side of the third, fourth, and fifth metatarsal bones; *insertion,* corresponding side of proximal phalanx of the same toes; *action,* adducts three lateral toes; *nerve supply,* lateral plantar. SYN musculus interosseus plantaris [TA].

**plan·tar·is mus·cle** *origin,* lateral supracondylar ridge; *insertion,* medial margin of tendo achilles and deep fascia of ankle; *action,* traditionally described as plantar flexion of foot; many investigators now believe the plantaris muscle to be primarily a proprioceptive organ; *nerve supply,* tibial nerve. SYN musculus plantaris [TA], plantar muscle.

**plan·tar me·ta·tar·sal ar·te·ry** one of four branches of the plantar arterial arch that divide into plantar digital arteries to supply the toes. SYN arteria metatarsalis plantaris [TA].

**plan·tar mus·cle** SYN plantaris muscle.

**plan·tar re·flex** the response to tactile stimulation of the ball of the foot, normally plantar flexion of the toes; the pathologic response is Babinski sign (1).

**plan·tar space** one of four areas between fascial layers in the foot, where pus may be confined when the foot is infected.

**plan·tar wart** an often painful wart on the sole; usually caused by human papilloma virus type 1. SYN verruca plantaris.

**plan·ti·grade** (plan′ti-grād) walking with the entire sole and heel of the foot on the ground, as in man and bears. [L. *planta,* sole, + *gradior,* to walk]

**pla·num,** pl. **pla·na** (plā′nŭm, plā′nă) [TA] a plane or flat surface. SEE ALSO plane. [L. plane]

⊞**plaque** (plak) **1.** a patch or small differentiated area on a body surface (e.g., skin, mucosa, or arterial endothelium) or on the cut surface of an organ such as the brain. **2.** an area of clearing in a flat confluent growth of bacteria or tissue cells. **3.** a sharply defined zone of demyelination characteristic of multiple sclerosis. **4.** SEE dental plaque. See page B4. [Fr. a plate]

△**-pla·sia** formation (especially of cells). SEE plasma-. [G. *plassō,* to form]

**plasm** (plazm) SYN plasma.

**plas·ma** (plaz′mă) **1.** the fluid (noncellular) portion of the circulating blood, as distinguished from the serum obtained after coagulation. SYN blood plasma. **2.** the fluid portion of the lymph. **3.** a "fourth state of matter" in which, owing to elevated temperature (*ca.* $10^6$ degrees), atoms have broken down to form free electrons and more or less stripped nuclei; produced in the laboratory in connection with hydrogen fusion (thermonuclear) research. SYN plasm. [G. something formed]

△**plas·ma-, plasmat-, plas·mat·o-, plas·mo-** formative, organized; plasma. [G. *plasma,* something formed]

**plas·ma ac·cel·er·a·tor glob·u·lin** SYN factor V.

**plas·ma·blast** (plaz′mă-blast) precursor of the plasma cell. [plasma + G. *blastos,* germ]

**plas·ma cell** an ovoid cell with an eccentric nucleus having chromatin arranged like a clock face or spokes of a wheel; the cytoplasm is strongly basophilic because of the abundant RNA in its endoplasmic reticulum; plasma cells are derived from B lymphocytes and are active in the formation of antibodies. SYN plasmacyte.

**plas·ma cell leu·ke·mia** an unusual disease characterized by leukocytosis and other signs and symptoms that are suggestive of leukemia, in association with diffuse infiltrations and aggregates of plasma cells in the spleen, liver, bone marrow, and lymph nodes, and plasma cells in the blood.

**plas·ma cell mas·ti·tis** a condition of the breasts characterized by tumorlike indurated masses containing numerous plasma cells, usually resulting from mammary duct ectasia; although clinically resembling malignant disease (attachment to skin and enlargement of axillary lymph nodes), it is not neoplastic.

**plas·ma cell my·e·lo·ma 1.** SYN multiple myeloma. **2.** plasmacytoma of bone, which is usually a solitary lesion and not associated with the occurrence of Bence Jones protein or other disturbances in the metabolism of protein (as observed in multiple myeloma).

**plas·ma·crit** (plaz′mă-krit) a measure of the percentage of the volume of blood occupied by plasma, in contrast to a hematocrit. [plasma + G. *krinō*, to separate]

**plas·ma·crit test** a serologic screening method for syphilis; heparinized blood is centrifuged in a capillary tube and the plasma thus separated with cardiolipin antigen. The presence of flocculation should not be regarded as conclusively diagnostic, but a negative result excludes the likelihood of syphilis.

**plas·ma·cyte** (plaz′mă-sīt) SYN plasma cell.

**plas·ma·cy·to·ma** (plaz′mă-sī-tō′mă) a discrete, presumably solitary mass of neoplastic plasma cells in bone or in one of various extramedullary sites; in humans, such lesions are probably the initial phase of developing plasma cell myeloma. [plasmacyte + G. *-oma*, tumor]

**plas·ma·cy·to·sis** (plaz′mă-sī-tō′sis) **1.** presence of plasma cells in the circulating blood. **2.** presence of unusually large proportions of plasma cells in the tissues or exudates. [plasmacyte + G. *-osis*, condition]

**plas·ma fi·bro·nec·tin** a circulating $\alpha_2$-glycoprotein that functions as an opsonin, mediating reticuloendothelial and macrophage clearance of fibrin microaggregates, collagen debris, and bacterial particulates, protecting microvascular perfusion and lymphatic drainage.

**plas·ma·kin·ins** (plaz′mă-kīn′inz) a group of highly active oligopeptides found in sera that act upon smooth muscle of blood vessels, uterus, bronchi, etc.; e.g., bradykinin, kallidin.

**plas·ma·lem·ma** (plaz-mă-lem′ă) SYN cell membrane. [plasma + G. *lemma*, husk]

**plas·mal·o·gens** (plaz-mal′ō-jenz) generic term for glycerophospholipids in which the glycerol moiety bears a 1-alkenyl or 1-alkyl ether group.

**plas·ma mem·brane** SYN cell membrane.

**plas·ma·phe·re·sis** (plaz′mă-fĕ-rē′sis) removal of whole blood from the body, separation of its cellular elements by centrifugation, and reinfusion of them suspended in saline or some other plasma substitute, thus depleting the body's own plasma without depleting its cells. [plasma + G. *aphairesis*, a withdrawal]

**plas·ma·phe·ret·ic** (plaz′mă-fĕ-ret′ik) relating to plasmapheresis.

**plas·ma pro·teins** dissolved proteins (more than

100) of blood plasma, mainly albumins and globulins (normally 6 to 8 g/100 ml); they hold fluid in blood vessels by osmosis and include antibodies and blood-clotting proteins.

**plas·ma re·nin ac·tiv·i·ty (PRA)** estimation of renin in plasma by measuring the rate of formation of angiotensin I or II.

**plas·ma throm·bo·plas·tin an·te·ced·ent (PTA)** SYN factor XI.

**plas·mat·ic** (plaz-mat′ik) relating to plasma. SYN plasmic.

**plas·mic** (plaz′mik) SYN plasmatic.

**plas·mid** (plaz′mid) a genetic particle physically separate from the chromosome of the host cell (chiefly bacterial) that can stably function and replicate; not essential to the basic functioning of the cell. SYN extrachromosomal element, extrachromosomal genetic element. [cyto*plasm* + -id]

**plas·min** (plaz′min) an enzyme hydrolyzing peptides and esters of L-arginine and L-lysine, and converting fibrin to soluble products; plasmin is responsible for the dissolution of blood clots. SYN fibrinase (2), fibrinolysin.

**plas·min·o·gen** (plaz-min′ō-jen) a precursor of plasmin. There is an autosomal dominant deficiency of plasminogen that may promote thrombosis. SEE plasmin.

**plas·min·o·gen ac·ti·va·tor** a proteinase that converts plasminogen to plasmin by cleavage of a single (usually Arg-Val) bond in the former. SYN urokinase.

**plas·mo·dia** (plaz-mō′-dē-ă) plural of plasmodium. [L.]

**plas·mo·di·al** (plaz-mō′dē-ăl) **1.** relating to a plasmodium. **2.** relating to any species of the genus *Plasmodium.*

***Plas·mo·di·um*** (plaz-mō′dē-ŭm) a genus of the protozoan family Plasmodiidae, blood parasites of vertebrates; includes the causal agents of malaria, with an asexual cycle occurring in liver and red blood cells of vertebrates and a sexual cycle in mosquitoes, the latter cycle resulting in the production of large numbers of infective sporozoites in the salivary glands of the vector, which are transmitted when the mosquito bites and draws blood. [Mod. L. from G. *plasma,* something formed, + *eidos,* appearance]

**plas·mo·di·um,** pl. **plas·mo·dia** (plaz-mō′dē-ŭm, plaz-mō′-dē-ă) a protoplasmic mass containing several nuclei, resulting from multiplication of the nucleus with cell division. [Mod. L. fr. G. *plasma,* something formed, + *eidos,* appearance]

***Plas·mo·di·um fal·cip·a·rum*** *Laverania falciparum,* a species that is the causal agent of falciparum (malignant tertian) malaria; infected erythrocytes are normal or contracted in size and are likely to contain basophilic granules and red dots (Maurer clefts or dots); multiple infection is extremely frequent and causes bouts of fever somewhat irregularly since the parasites' cycles of multiplication are usually asynchronous.

⬛ ***Plas·mo·di·um ma·lar·i·ae*** a species that is the causal agent of quartan malaria; infected erythrocytes are normal or slightly contracted in size, usually with no stippling (the two most important characteristics that distinguish it from *Plasmodium vivax*), although extremely fine Ziemann dots may be observed; multiple infection is extremely rare, thus bouts of fever occur fairly regularly at 72-hour intervals. See page B3.

***Plas·mo·di·um o·va·le*** a species that is the agent

of the least common form of human malaria; Schüffner dots are abundant and appear early, host cells are normal or only slightly enlarged, and only about 8 to 10 grapelike merozoites are produced; fever is tertian (every 48 hours), and relapses are infrequent.

**Plas•mo•di•um vi•vax** a species that is the most common malarial parasite of human beings except in west Africa; affected red blood cells are pale, enlarged, and contain Schüffner dots in the later stages of growth; causes bouts of fever fairly regularly at 48-hour intervals; but multiple infection is common.

**plas•mog•a•my** (plaz-mog′ă-mē) union of two or more cells with preservation of the individual nuclei; formation of a plasmodium. [plasmo- + G. *gamos,* marriage]

**plas•mol•y•sis** (plaz-mol′i-sis) **1.** dissolution of cellular components. **2.** shrinking of plant cells by osmotic loss of cytoplasmic water. [plasmo- + G. *lysis,* dissolution]

**plas•mo•lyt•ic** (plaz-mō-lit′ik) relating to plasmolysis.

**plas•mon** (plaz′mon) the total of the extrachromosomal genetic properties of the eukaryotic cell cytoplasm. [cyto*plasm* + -on]

**plas•mor•rhex•is** (plaz-mō-rek′sis) the splitting open of a cell from the pressure of the protoplasm.

**plas•mos•chi•sis** (plaz-mos′ki-sis) the splitting of protoplasm into fragments. [plasmo- + G. *schisis,* a cleaving]

**plas•mo•tro•pic** (plaz-mō-trōp′ik) pertaining to or manifesting plasmotropism.

**plas•mot•ro•pism** (plaz-mo′trō-pizm) a condition in which the bone marrow, spleen, and liver are sites for the destruction of the erythrocytes, as opposed to destruction in the circulating blood. [plasmo- + G. *tropē,* a turning]

**plas•ter 1.** a solid preparation which can be spread when heated, and which becomes adhesive at the temperature of the body; used to keep the edges of a wound in apposition, to protect raw surfaces, and, when medicated, to redden or blister the skin or to apply drugs to the surface to obtain their systemic effects. **2.** DENTISTRY colloquialism for plaster of Paris. [L. *emplastrum;* G. *emplastron,* plaster or mold]

**plas•ter ban•dage** a roller bandage impregnated with plaster of Paris and applied moist; used to make a rigid dressing for a fracture or diseased joint.

**plas•tic** (plas′tik) **1.** capable of being formed or molded. **2.** a material that can be shaped by pressure or heat to the form of a cavity or mold. [G. *plastikos,* relating to molding]

**plas•tic en•ve•lope cul•ture** simplified method for transport and culture of specimens for the diagnosis of infection with *Trichomonas vaginalis;* liquid culture medium is examined microscopically through the envelope, so pipette sampling of the medium is not required.

**plas•tic•i•ty** (plas-tis′i-tē) the capability of being formed or molded; the quality of being plastic.

**plas•tic pleu•ri•sy** SYN dry pleurisy.

**plas•tic sur•gery** the surgical specialty or procedure concerned with the restoration, construction, reconstruction, or improvement in the shape and appearance of body structures that are missing, defective, damaged, or misshapen.

**plas•tid** (plas′tid) **1.** one of the differentiated structures in cytoplasm of plant cells where photosynthesis or other cellular processes are carried on; plastids contain DNA and are self-replicating. SYN trophoplast. **2.** one of the granules of foreign or differentiated matter in cells: food particles, fat, waste material, chromatophores, and trichocysts. **3.** a self-duplicating virus-like particle that multiplies within a host cell, such as kappa particles in certain paramecia. [G. *plastos,* formed, + -id]

△-**plas•ty** molding, shaping or the result thereof, as of a surgical procedure. [G. *plastos,* formed, shaped]

**plate** (plāt) **1.** in anatomy, a thin, relatively flat, structure. **2.** a metal bar perforated for screws applied to a fractured bone to maintain the ends in apposition. **3.** the agar layer within a Petri dish or similar vessel. **4.** to form a very thin layer of a bacterial culture by streaking it on the surface of an agar plate (usually within a Petri dish) to isolate individual organisms from which a colonial clone will develop. **5.** any one of the horizontal perforated plates that comprise the fractionating component of a column in fractional distillation (or, the theoretic equivalent of such a plate). [O.Fr. *plat,* a flat object, fr. G. *platys,* flat, broad]

**pla•teau pres•sure** the equilibrium pressure between airways and alveoli in a patient-ventilator system; it is considered to be at least a close approximation of alveolar pressure.

**pla•teau pulse** a slow, sustained pulse.

**plate•let** (plāt′let) an irregularly shaped disklike cytoplasmic fragment of a megakaryocyte that is shed in the marrow sinus and subsequently found in the peripheral blood where it functions in clotting. A platelet contains granules in the central part (granulomere) and, peripherally, clear protoplasm (hyalomere), but no definite nucleus; is about one-third to one-half the size of an erythrocyte. SYN blood disk, elementary particle (1), thrombocyte, thromboplastid (1). [see plate]

**plate•let-ac•ti•vat•ing fac•tor** SYN platelet-aggregating factor.

**plate•let-ag•gre•gat•ing fac•tor** phospholipid mediator of platelet aggregation, inflammation, and anaphylaxis. Produced in response to specific stimuli by a variety of cell types, including neutrophils, basophils, platelets, and endothelial cells. Several molecular species of PAF have been identified which vary in the length of the *O*-alkyl side chain. It is an important mediator of bronchoconstriction. SYN platelet-activating factor.

**plate•let fac•tor 4 (PF)** a cationic polypeptide synthesized by megakaryocytes and contained in platelet alpha granules; these granules, released when platelets are activated, neutralize the anticoagulant activity of heparin.

**plate•let fac•tor 3** a blood coagulation factor derived from platelets; chemically, a phospholipid lipoprotein that acts with certain plasma thromboplastin factors to convert prothrombin to thrombin.

**plate•let neu•tra•li•za•tion pro•ce•dure (PNP)** a procedure based on the ability of platelets to bypass the effect of a lupus anticoagulant by correcting prolonged coagulation times in various phospholipid-dependent test systems; the disrupted platelet membranes in the freeze-thawed platelet suspension neutralize phospholipid antibodies in the plasma of patients with lupus anti-coagulant; after mixing the patient plasma with the freeze-thawed platelet suspension, the activated partial thromboplastin time will be corrected when compared with the original baseline activated partial thromboplastin time.

**plate·let·phe·re·sis** (plāt'let-fĕ-rē'sis) removal of blood from a donor with replacement of all blood components except platelets. [platelet + G. *aphairesis,* a withdrawal]

**plate·let tis·sue fac·tor** SYN thromboplastin.

**plate·like at·el·ec·ta·sis** SYN subsegmental atel-ectasis.

**plat·i·num (Pt)** (plat'i-nŭm) a metallic element, atomic no. 78, atomic wt. 195.08, used for making small parts for chemical apparatus because of its resistance to acids; in powdered form (**platinum black**) it is an important catalyst in hydrogenation. A derivative, cisplatin, is used as an antineoplastic agent. [Mod. L., originally *platina,* fr. Sp. *plata,* silver]

△**platy-** width; flatness. [G. *platys,* flat, broad]

**plat·y·ba·sia** (plat-i-bā'sē-ă) a developmental anomaly of the skull or an acquired softening of the skull bones that allows the floor of the posterior cranial fossa to bulge upward in the region about the foramen magnum. [*platy-* + G. *basis,* ground]

**plat·y·ceph·a·ly** (plat-i-sef'ă-lē) flatness of the skull, a condition in which the vertical cranial index is below 70. [platy- + G. *kephalē,* head]

**plat·y·hel·minth** (plat-i-hel'minth) common name for any flatworm of the phylum Platyhel-minthes; any cestode (tapeworm) or trematode (fluke). [platy- + G. *helmins,* worm]

**Plat·y·hel·min·thes** (plat'i-hel-min'thēz) a phylum of flatworms that are bilaterally symmetric, flattened, and acelomate. Parasitic species of medical importance are in the subclass Cestoda (the true tapeworms) of the class Cestoidea, and in the subclass Digenea (the digenetic flukes) of the class Trematoda.

**plat·y·pel·lic pel·vis** flat oval pelvis, in which the transverse diameter is more than 3 cm longer than the anteroposterior diameter.

**plat·y·pel·loid pel·vis** simple flat pelvis.

**pla·typ·nea** (plă-tip'nē-ă) difficulty in breathing when erect, relieved by recumbency. Cf. orthopnea. [platy- + G. *pnoē,* a breathing]

**pla·typ·noea [Br.]** SEE platypnea.

**pla·tys·ma** [TA] SYN platysma muscle.

**pla·tys·ma mus·cle** *origin,* subcutaneous layer and fascia covering pectoralis major and deltoid at level of first or second rib; *insertion,* lower border of mandible, risorius and platysma of opposite side; *action,* depresses lower lip, forms ridges in skin of neck and upper chest when jaws are "clenched", denoting stress, anger; *nerve supply,* cervical branch of facial. SYN platysma [TA].

**plat·y·spon·dyl·ia, plat·y·spon·dyl·i·sis** (plat-i-spon-dil'ē-ă, plat'i-spon-dil'i-sis) flatness of the bodies of the vertebrae. [platy- + G. *spondylos,* vertebra]

**play ther·a·py** a type of therapy used with children in which they can express or reveal their problems and fantasies by playing with dolls or other toys, drawing, etc.

**plea·sure prin·ci·ple** SYN pain-pleasure principle.

**pled·get** (plej'et) a tuft of wool, cotton, or lint.

△**-ple·gia** paralysis. [G. *plēgē,* stroke]

△**plei·o-** rarely used alternative spelling for pleo-.

**plei·o·tro·pic** (plī-ō-trōp'ik) denoting, or characterized by, pleiotropy.

**plei·o·tro·pic gene** a gene that has multiple, apparently unrelated, phenotypic manifestations. SYN polyphenic gene.

**plei·ot·ro·py, plei·o·tro·pia** (plī-ot'rō-pē, plī'ō-trō'pē-ă) production by a single mutant gene of apparently unrelated multiple effects at the clinical or phenotypic level. [pleio- + G. *tropos,* turning]

△**pleo-** More. [G. *pleiōn*]

**ple·o·cy·to·sis** (plē'ō-sī-tō'sis) presence of more cells than normal, often denoting leukocytosis and especially lymphocytosis or round cell infiltration. [pleo- + G. *kytos,* cell, + -*ōsis,* condition]

**ple·o·mas·tia, ple·o·ma·zia** (plē-ō-mas'tē-ă, plē-ō-mā'zē-ă) SYN polymastia. [pleo- + G. *mastos,* breast]

**ple·o·mor·phic** (plē-ō-mōr'fik) **1.** SYN polymorphic. **2.** among fungi, having two or more spore forms; also used to describe a sterile mutant dermatophyte resulting from degenerative changes in culture.

**ple·o·mor·phic li·po·ma** SYN atypical lipoma.

**ple·o·mor·phism** (plē-ō-mōr'fizm) SYN polymorphism. [pleo- + G. *morphē,* form]

**ple·o·mor·phous** (plē-ō-mōr'fŭs) SYN polymorphic.

**ple·o·nasm** (plē'ō-nazm) excess in number or size of parts. [G. *pleonasmos,* exaggeration, excessive, fr. *pleiōn,* more]

**ple·on·os·te·o·sis** (plē'on-os-tē-ō'sis) superabundance of bone formation. [pleo- + G. *osteon,* bone, + -*osis,* condition]

△**pless-, ples·si-** a striking, especially percussion. [G. *plēssō,* to strike]

**ples·sim·e·ter** (ple-sim'ĕ-ter) an oblong flexible plate used in mediate percussion by being placed against the surface and struck with the plessor. SYN pleximeter, plexometer. [G. *plēssō,* to strike, + *metron,* measure]

**ples·sor** (ples'er) a small hammer, usually with soft rubber head, used to tap the part directly, or with a plessimeter, in percussion of the chest or other part. SYN percussor, plexor. [G. *plēssō,* to strike]

**pleth·o·ra** (pleth'ō-ră) **1.** SYN hypervolemia. **2.** an excess of any of the body fluids. SYN repletion (2). [G. *plēthōrē,* fullness, fr. *plēthō,* to become full]

**pleth·o·ric** (ple-thōr'ik, pleth'ŏ-rik) relating to plethora. SYN sanguine (1), sanguineous (2).

**ple·thys·mo·graph** (plĕ-thiz'mō-graf) a device for measuring and recording changes in volume of a part, organ, or whole body. [G. *plēthysmos,* increase, + *graphō,* to write]

**pleth·ys·mog·ra·phy** (pleth-iz-mog'ră-fē) measuring and recording changes in volume of an organ or other part of the body by a plethysmograph. [G. *plēthysmos,* increase, + *graphē,* a writing]

**pleth·ys·mom·e·try** (pleth-iz-mom'ĕ-trē) measuring the fullness of a hollow organ or vessel, as of the pulse. [G. *plēthysmos,* increase, + *metron,* measure]

△**pleur-, pleu·ro-, pleu·ra-** rib, side, pleura. [G. *pleura;* a rib, the side]

**pleu·ra,** gen. and pl. **pleu·rae** (ploor'ă, plūr'ē) [TA] the serous membrane enveloping the lungs and lining the walls of the pleural cavity. [G. *pleura*, a rib, pl. the side]

**pleu·ral** (ploor'ăl) relating to the pleura.

**pleu·ral cav·i·ty** the potential space between the parietal and visceral layers of the pleura. SYN pleural space.

**pleu·ral ef·fu·sion** increased amounts of fluid within the pleural cavity, usually due to inflammation.

**pleu·ral flu·id** the thin film of fluid between the visceral and parietal pleurae.

**pleu·ral frem·i·tus** vibration in the chest wall produced by the rubbing together of inflamed opposing surfaces of the pleura.

**pleu·ral space** SYN pleural cavity.

**pleu·ral tap** SYN thoracentesis.

**pleur·a·poph·y·sis** (ploor'ă-pof'i-sis) a rib, or the process on a cervical or lumbar vertebra corresponding thereto. [pleur- + G. *apophysis*, process, offshoot]

**pleur·ec·to·my** (ploo-rek'tō-mē) excision of pleura, usually parietal. [pleur- + G. *ektomē*, excision]

**pleu·ri·sy** (ploor'i-sē) inflammation of the pleura. SYN pleuritis. [L. *pleurisis*, fr. G. *pleuritis*]

**pleu·ri·sy with ef·fu·sion** pleurisy accompanied by serous exudation. SYN serous pleurisy.

**pleu·rit·ic** (ploo-rit'ik) pertaining to pleurisy.

**pleu·rit·ic rub** a friction sound produced by the rubbing together of inflamed surfaces of the parietal and visceral pleurae.

**pleu·ri·tis** (ploo-rī'tis) SYN pleurisy. [G. fr. *pleura*, side, + -*itis*, inflammation]

**pleu·ro·cele** (ploor'ō-sēl) SYN pneumonocele. [pleuro- + G. *kēlē*, hernia]

**pleu·ro·cen·te·sis** (ploor'ō-sen-tē'sis) SYN thoracentesis. [pleuro- + G. *kentēsis*, puncture]

**pleu·ro·cen·trum** (plūr'ō-sen'trŭm) one of the lateral halves of the body of a vertebra. [pleuro- + G. *kentron*, center]

**pleu·roc·ly·sis** (ploor-ok'li-sis) washing out of the pleural cavity. [pleuro- + G. *klysis*, a washing out]

**pleu·rod·e·sis** (ploor-od'e-sis) the creation of a fibrous adhesion between the visceral and parietal layers of the pleura, obliterating the pleural cavity; it is performed surgically by abrading the pleura or by inserting a sterile irritant into the pleural canal in cases of recurrent spontaneous pneumothorax, malignant pleural effusion, and chylothorax. [pleuro- + G. *desis*, a binding together]

**pleu·ro·dyn·ia** (ploor-ō-din'ē-ă) 1. pleuritic pain in the chest. 2. a painful affection of the tendinous attachments of the thoracic muscles, usually of one side only. SYN costalgia. [pleuro- + G. *odynē*, pain]

**pleu·ro·e·soph·a·ge·al mus·cle** muscular fasciculi, arising from the mediastinal pleura, which reinforce musculature of esophagus. SYN musculus pleuroesophageus [TA].

**pleu·ro·gen·ic** (ploor-ō-jen'ik) of pleural origin; beginning in the pleura. SYN pleurogenous (1). [pleuro- + G. -*gen*, producing]

**pleu·rog·e·nous** (ploor-oj'ě-nŭs) 1. SYN pleurogenic. 2. in fungi, denoting spores or conidia developed on the sides of a conidiophore or hypha.

**pleu·rog·ra·phy** (ploor-og'ră-fē) radiography of the pleural cavity after injecting contrast medium. [pleuro- + G. *graphō*, to write]

**pleu·ro·hep·a·ti·tis** (ploor'ō-hep-ă-tī'tis) hepatitis with extension of the inflammation to the neighboring portion of the pleura. [pleuro- + G. *hēpar*, liver, + -*itis*, inflammation]

**pleu·ro·lith** (ploor'ō-lith) a concretion in the pleural cavity. [pleuro- + G. *lithos*, stone]

**pleu·rol·y·sis** (ploor-ol'i-sis) locating pleural adhesions by the aid of an endoscope and then dividing them with the electric cautery. [pleuro- + G. *lysis*, dissolution]

**pleu·ro·per·i·car·di·al** (ploor'ō-per-i-kar'dē-ăl) relating to both pleura and pericardium.

**pleu·ro·per·i·car·di·tis** (ploor'ō-per-i-kar-dī'tis) combined inflammation of the pericardium and of the pleura. [pleuro- + pericardium + G. -*itis*, inflammation]

**pleu·ro·per·i·to·ne·al** (ploor'ō-per-i-tō-nē'ăl) relating to both pleura and peritoneum.

**pleu·ro·per·i·to·ne·al shunt** a surgically implanted catheter for transport of fluid from a pleural space into the peritoneal cavity, where it is absorbed; used mainly for treatment of malignant pleural effusions.

**pleu·ro·pneu·mo·nec·to·my** surgical resection of an entire lung along with the parietal pleura; formerly used mainly for destroyed lung due to tuberculosis; currently, a method of treating malignant mesothelioma.

**pleu·ro·pneu·mo·nia-like or·ga·nisms (PPLO)** the original name given to a group of bacteria which did not possess cell walls; these organisms, isolated from man and other animals, soil, and sewage, are now assigned to the order Mycoplasmatales.

**pleu·ro·pul·mo·nary** (ploor-ō-pul'mŏ-ner-ē) relating to the pleura and the lungs.

**pleu·rot·o·my** (ploo-rot'ō-mē) SYN thoracotomy. [pleuro- + G. *tomē*, incision]

**pleu·ro·ve·nous shunt** a surgically implanted catheter for transport of fluid from a pleural space into the venous system; rarely used, mainly for treatment of malignant pleural effusions.

**pleu·ro·vis·cer·al** (ploor'ō-vis'er-ăl) SYN visceropleural.

**plex·al** (plek'săl) relating to a plexus.

**plex·ect·o·my** (plek-sek'tō-mē) surgical excision of a plexus. [plexus + G. *ektomē*, excision]

**plex·i·form** (plek'si-fōrm) weblike, or resembling or forming a plexus. [plexus + L. *forma*, form]

**plex·i·form neu·ro·fi·bro·ma** a type of neurofibroma, representing an anomaly rather than a true neoplasm, in which the proliferation of Schwann cells occurs from the inner aspect of the nerve sheath; seen most frequently in neurofibromatosis. SYN plexiform neuroma.

**plex·i·form neu·ro·ma** SYN plexiform neurofibroma.

**plex·im·e·ter** (plek-sim'i-ter) SYN plessimeter. [G. *plēxis*, stroke]

**plex·i·tis** (plek-sī'tis) inflammation of a plexus.

**plex·o·gen·ic** (plek'sō-jen-ik) giving rise to weblike or plexiform structures. [plexus + G. -*gen*, producing]

**plex·om·e·ter** (plek-som'ě-ter) SYN plessimeter.

**plex·op·a·thy** (pleks-op'a-thē) disorder involving one of the major peripheral neural plexuses: cervical, brachial, or lumbosacral. [plexus + G. *pathos*, disease]

**plex·or** (plek'ser) SYN plessor. [G. *plēxis*, a stroke]

**plex·us**, pl. **plex·us**, **plex·us·es** (plek'sŭs, plek' sŭs) [TA] a network or interjoining of nerves and blood vessels or of lymphatic vessels. [L. a braid]

**plex•us ce•li•a•cus** [TA] SYN celiac plexus.

**pli•ca,** gen. and pl. **pli•cae** (plī′kă, plī′sē) **1.** [TA] one of several anatomical structures in which there is a folding over of the parts. **2.** SYN false membrane. SEE ALSO fold. [Mod. L. a plait or fold]

**pli•ca ar•y•ep•i•glot•ti•ca** [TA] SYN aryepiglottic fold.

**pli•cae cir•cu•la•res in•tes•ti•ni te•nuis** [TA] SYN circular folds of small intestine.

**pli•cae pal•ma•tae** [TA] SYN palmate folds.

**pli•ca in•ter•u•re•te•ri•ca** [TA] SYN interureteric fold.

**pli•ca la•cri•ma•lis** [TA] SYN lacrimal fold.

**pli•ca se•mi•lu•nar•is con•junc•ti•vae** [TA] SYN semilunar conjunctival fold.

**pli•ca spi•ra•lis duc•tus cys•ti•ci** [TA] SYN spiral fold of cystic duct.

**pli•cate** (plī′kāt) folded; pleated; tucked.

**pli•ca•tion** (plī-kā′shŭn, pli-kā′shŭn) a folding or putting together in pleats; specifically, an operation for reducing the size of a hollow viscus by taking folds or tucks in its walls. [L. *plico,* pp. *-atus,* to fold]

**pli•ca ves•ti•bu•la•ris** [TA] SYN vestibular fold.

**pli•ca vo•ca•lis** [TA] SYN vocal fold.

**pli•cot•o•my** (plī-kot′ō-mē) division of the plica mallearis. [plica + G. *tomē,* incision]

△**-ploid** multiple in form; its combinations are used both adjectivally and substantively of a (specified) multiple of chromosomes. [G. *-plo-,* -fold, + *-ides,* in form; L. *-ploïdeus*]

**ploi•dy** (ploy′dē) the number of haploid sets in a cell. Gametes normally contain one; autosomal cells two. SEE ALSO polyploidy. [-ploid + *-y,* condition]

**plot** (plot) a graphical representation.

**plug** (plŭg) any mass filling a hole or closing an orifice.

**plug•ger** a dental instrument used for condensing gold (foil), amalgam, or any plastic material in a cavity, operated by hand or by mechanical means. SYN packer (2).

**plum•bism** (plŭm′bizm) SYN lead poisoning. [L. *plumbum,* lead]

**plum•bum** (plŭm′bŭm) SYN lead. [L.]

**Plum•mer-Vin•son syn•drome** (plum′er-vin′son) iron deficiency anemia, dysphagia, esophageal web, and atrophic glossitis.

△**plu•ri-** several, more. SEE ALSO multi-, poly-. [L. *plus, pluris*]

**plu•ri•glan•du•lar** (ploo-ri-glan′dyu-lăr) denoting several glands or their secretions. SYN polyglandular.

**plu•rip•o•tent, plu•ri•po•ten•tial** (ploo-rip′ō-tent, ploo′rē-pō-ten′shăl) **1.** having the capacity to affect more than one organ or tissue. **2.** not fixed as to potential development.

**plu•to•ni•um (Pu)** (ploo-tō′nē-ŭm) a transuranium artificial radioactive element, atomic no. 94, atomic wt. 244.064. The best-known α-emitting isotope is $^{239}$Pu (half-life 24,110 years) which, like $^{235}$U, is fissionable and can be used in atomic bombs and nuclear power plants; $^{238}$Pu (half-life 87.74 years) is used as an energy source in pacemakers. Pu ions are bone seekers; ingestion is a radiation hazard as with radium and radiostrontium. [planet, *Pluto*]

**ply•o•met•ric train•ing** exercise training that exploits the stretch-recoil characteristics of skeletal muscle and neurologic modulation through the stretch or myotatic reflex; used by athletes who require specific, powerful movements (e.g., in football, volleyball, sprinting, and basketball).

**Pm** promethium.

**pM** picomolar ($10^{-12}$ M).

**pm** picometer.

**P mit•ra•le** (pē mī-trā′lē) broad, notched P waves in several or many leads of the electrocardiogram with a prominent late negative component to the P wave in lead $V_1$; it is characteristic of overload of the left atrium such as occurs in disease of the mitral valve. SYN P sinistrocardiale.

**PML** progressive multifocal leukoencephalopathy.

**pmol** picomole.

**PMS** premenstrual syndrome.

△**-pnea** breath, respiration. [G. *pneō,* to breathe]

△**pne•o-** combining form denoting breath or respiration. SEE ALSO pneum-, pneumo-. [G. *pneō,* to breathe]

△**pneum-, pneu•ma-, pneumat-, pneu•mato-** presence of air or gas, the lungs, or breathing. SEE ALSO pneo-, pneumo-. [G. *pneuma, pneumatos,* air, breath]

**pneu•marth•ro•gram** (noo-marth′rō-gram) film records of pneumarthrography.

**pneu•marth•rog•ra•phy** (noo-marth-rog′ră-fē) radiographic examination of a joint following the introduction of air, with or without another contrast medium. SYN pneumoarthrography. [G. *pneuma,* air, + *arthron,* joint, + *graphō,* to write]

**pneu•mar•thro•sis** (noo-mar-thrō′sis) presence of air in a joint. [G. *pneuma,* air, + *arthron,* joint, + *-osis,* condition]

**pneu•mat•ic** (noo-mat′ik) **1.** relating to air or gas, or to a structure filled with air. **2.** relating to respiration. [G. *pneumatikos*]

**pneu•mat•ic an•ti•shock gar•ment** an inflatable suit used to apply pressure to the peripheral circulation, thus reducing blood flow and fluid exudation into tissues, to maintain central blood flow in the presence of shock. SYN military anti-shock trousers.

**pneu•mat•ic bone** a bone that is hollow or contains many air cells, such as the mastoid process of the temporal bone. SYN hollow bone.

**pneu•ma•tic di•la•tor** any of a variety of catheters fitted with distal balloons that can be inflated to desired pressures for overcoming obstructions in hollow viscera; most often used to rupture the lower esophageal sphincter to treat achalasia.

**pneu•mat•ic o•tos•co•py** inspection of the ear with a device capable of varying air pressure against the eardrum. Imparting movement to the tympanic membrane suggests normal middle ear compliance; the lack of movement indicates either increased impedance or eardrum perforation.

**pneu•mat•ic to•nom•e•ter** a recording applanation tonometer operated by compressed gas.

**pneu•ma•ti•za•tion** (noo′mă-ti-zā′shŭn) the development of air cells such as those of the mastoid and ethmoidal bones. [G. *pneuma,* air]

**pneu•ma•to•car•dia** (noo′mă-tō-kar′dē-ă) presence of air bubbles or gas in the blood of the heart; produced by air embolism.

**pneu•ma•to•cele** (noo′mă-tō-sēl) **1.** an emphysematous or gaseous swelling. **2.** SYN pneumono-cele. **3.** a thin-walled cavity within the lung, one of the characteristic sequelae of staphylococcus pneumonia. [G. *pneuma*, air, + *kēlē*, tumor, hernia]

**pneu•ma•tor•rha•chis** (noo-mă-tōr′ă-kis) SYN pneumorrhachis. [G. *pneuma*, air, + *rhachis*, spine]

**pneu•ma•to•sis** (noo-mă-tō′sis) abnormal accumulation of gas in any tissue or part of the body. [G. a blowing out]

**pneu•ma•to•sis cys•toi•des in•tes•ti•na•lis** a condition of unknown cause characterized by the occurrence of gas cysts in the intestinal mucous membrane; may produce intestinal obstruction. SYN intestinal emphysema.

**pneu•ma•tu•ria** (noo-mă-tyu′rē-ă) the passage of gas or air from the urethra during or after urination, resulting from decomposition of bladder urine or, more commonly, from an intestinal fistula. [G. *pneuma*, air, + *ouron*, urine]

⚠**pneu•mo-, pneu•mon-, pneu•mo•no-** the lungs, air or gas, respiration, or pneumonia. SEE ALSO aer-, pneo-, pneum-. [G. *pneumōn, pneumonos,* lung]

**pneu•mo•ar•throg•ra•phy** (noo′mō-ar-throg′ră-fē) SYN pneumarthrography.

**pneu•mo•car•di•al** (noo′mō-kar′dē-ăl) SYN cardiopulmonary.

**pneu•mo•cele** (noo′mō-sēl) SYN pneumonocele.

**pneu•mo•cen•te•sis** (noo′mō-sen-tē′sis) SYN pneumonocentesis.

**pneu•mo•ceph•a•lus** (noo-mō-sef′ă-lŭs) presence of air or gas within the cranial cavity. [G. *pneuma*, air, + *kephalē*, head]

**pneu•mo•coc•cal** (noo-mō-kok′ăl) pertaining to or containing the pneumococcus.

**pneu•mo•coc•ce•mia** (noo′mō-kok-sē′mē-ă) the presence of pneumococci in the blood. [pneumococcus + G. *haima*, blood]

**pneu•mo•coc•ci•dal** (noo′mō-kok-sī′dăl) destructive to pneumococci. [pneumococcus + L. *caedo*, to kill]

**pneu•mo•coc•co•sis** (noo′mō-kok-ō′sis) rarely used term for infection with pneumococci.

**pneu•mo•coc•co•su•ria** (noo′mō-kok-o-syu′rē-ă) the presence of pneumococci or their specific capsular substance in the urine. [pneumococcus + G. *ouron*, urine]

**pneu•mo•coc•cus,** pl. **pneu•mo•coc•ci** (noo-mō-kok′ŭs, noo′mō-kok′sī) SYN *Streptococcus pneumoniae.* [G. *pneumōn*, lung, + *kokkos*, berry (coccus)]

**pneu•mo•co•ni•o•sis,** pl. **pneu•mo•co•ni•o•ses** (noo′mō-kō-nē-ō′sis, noo′mō-kō-nē-ō′-sēz) inflammation commonly leading to fibrosis of the lungs caused by the inhalation of dust in various occupations; characterized by pain in the chest, cough with little or no expectoration, dyspnea, reduced thoracic excursion, sometimes cyanosis, and fatigue after slight exertion; degree of disability depends on the types of particles inhaled, as well as the level of exposure to them. [G. *pneumōn*, lung, + *konis*, dust, + *-osis*, condition]

**pneu•mo•cra•ni•um** (noo-mō-krā′nē-ŭm) air present between the cranium and the dura mater; the term is commonly used to indicate extradural or subdural air. [G. *pneuma*, air, + *-o-* + *kranion*, skull]

*Pneu•mo•cys•tis ca•ri•nii* (noo-mō-sis′tis kă-rī′nē-ī) the microorganism that causes interstitial

plasma cell pneumonia in immunodeficient persons, particularly those with AIDS. [G. *pneuma*, air, breathing, + *kystis*, bladder, pouch]

*Pneu•mo•cys•tis ca•ri•nii* **pneu•mo•nia** pneumonia resulting from infection with *Pneumocystis carinii*, frequently seen in the immunologically compromised, such as persons with AIDS, or steroid-treated individuals, the elderly, or premature or debilitated babies. Throughout the alveolar walls and pulmonary septa there is a diffuse infiltration of mononuclear inflammatory cells, chiefly plasma cells and macrophages, as well as a few lymphocytes. Helmet-shaped organisms can be demonstrated in sputum and tissue specimens with silver stains. Patients may be only slightly febrile (or even afebrile), but are likely to be extremely weak, dyspneic, and cyanotic. This is a major cause of morbidity among patients with AIDS. SYN interstitial plasma cell pneumonia, pneumocystosis.

**pneu•mo•cys•tog•ra•phy** (noo′mō-sis-tog′ră-fē) radiography of the bladder following injection of air. [G. *pneuma*, air, + *kystis*, bladder, + *graphō*, to write]

**pneu•mo•cys•to•sis** (noo′mō-sis-tō′sis) SYN *Pneumocystis carinii* pneumonia.

**pneu•mo•der•ma** (noo-mō-der′mă) SYN subcutaneous emphysema. [G. *pneuma*, air, + *-o-* + *derma*, skin]

**pneu•mo•dy•nam•ics** (noo′mō-dī-nam′iks) the mechanics of respiration. [G. *pneuma*, breath, + *dynamis*, force]

**pneu•mo•gas•tric** (noo-mō-gas′trik) relating to the lungs and the stomach. SYN gastropulmonary. [G. *pneumōn*, lung, + *gastēr*, stomach]

**pneu•mo•gas•tric nerve** SYN vagus nerve [CN X].

**pneu•mo•gram** (noo′mō-gram) **1.** the record or tracing made by a pneumograph. **2.** radiographic record of pneumography. [G. *pneumōn*, lung, + *gramma*, a drawing]

**pneu•mo•graph** (noo′mō-graf) generic term for any device that records respiratory excursions from movements on the body surface. [G. *pneumōn*, lung, + *graphō*, to write]

**pneu•mog•ra•phy** (noo-mog′ră-fē) **1.** examination with a pneumograph. **2.** a general term indicating radiography after injection of air. SYN pneumoradiography. [G. *pneumōn*, lung, + *graphō*, to write]

**pneu•mo•he•mo•per•i•car•di•um** (noo′mō-hē-mō-per-i-kar′dē-ŭm) SYN hemopneumopericardium.

**pneu•mo•he•mo•thor•ax** (noo′mō-hē-mō-thōr′aks) SYN hemopneumothorax.

**pneu•mo•hy•dro•me•tra** (noo′mō-hī-drō-mē′tră) the presence of gas and serum in the uterine cavity. [G. *pneuma*, air, + *hydōr* (*hydr-*), water, + *mētra*, uterus]

**pneu•mo•hy•dro•per•i•car•di•um** (noo′mō-hī′drō-per-i-kar′dē-ŭm) SYN hydropneumopericardium.

**pneu•mo•hy•dro•per•i•to•ne•um** (noo′mō-hī-drō-per-i-tō-nē′ŭm) SYN hydropneumoperitoneum.

**pneu•mo•hy•dro•thor•ax** (noo-mō-hī-drō-thōr′aks) SYN hydropneumothorax.

**pneu•mo•lith** (noo′mō-lith) a calculus in the lung. [G. *pneumōn*, lung, + *lithos*, stone]

**pneu•mo•li•thi•a•sis** (noo-mō-li-thī′ă-sis) formation of calculi in the lungs.

**pneu·mo·me·di·as·ti·num** (noo′mō-mē′dē-ă-stī′nŭm) escape of air into mediastinal tissues, usually from interstitial emphysema or from a ruptured pulmonary bleb. [G. *pneuma*, air, + mediastinum]

**pneu·mo·my·e·log·ra·phy** (noo′mō-mī′ĕ-log′rǎ-fē) rarely used radiographic examination of spinal canal after injection of air or gas into the subarachnoid space. [G. *pneuma*, air, + *myelos*, marrow, + *graphō*, to write]

**pneu·mo·nec·to·my** (noo′mō-nek′tō-mē) removal of all pulmonary lobes from a lung in one operation. [G. *pneumōn*, lung, + *ektomē*, excision]

🔲**pneu·mo·nia** (noo-mō′nē-ă) inflammation of the lung parenchyma characterized by consolidation of the affected part, the alveolar air spaces being filled with exudate, inflammatory cells, and fibrin. Most cases are due to infection by bacteria or viruses, a few to inhalation of chemicals or trauma to the chest wall, and a small minority to rickettsiae, fungi, and yeasts. Distribution may be lobar, segmental, or lobular; when lobular and associated with bronchitis, it is termed bronchopneumonia. SEE ALSO pneumonitis. See this page. [G. fr. *pneumōn*, lung, + *-ia*, condition]

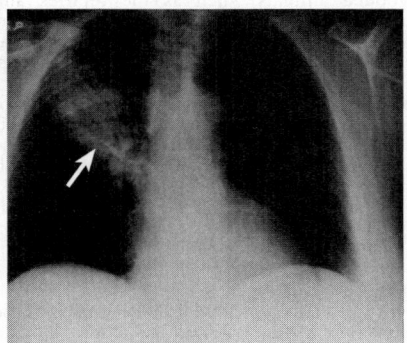

**lobar pneumonia:** chest radiograph showing pulmonary infiltrates (arrow) in upper lobe of right lung

**pneu·mon·ic** (noo-mon′ik) 1. SYN pulmonary. 2. relating to pneumonia.

**pneu·mon·ic plague** a rapidly progressive and frequently fatal form of plague in which there are areas of pulmonary consolidation, with chill, pain in the side, bloody expectoration, and high fever.

**pneu·mo·ni·tis** (noo-mō-nī′tis) inflammation of the lungs. SEE ALSO pneumonia. SYN pulmonitis. [G. *pneumōn*, lung, + *-itis*, inflammation]

**pneu·mo·no·cele** (noo-mōn′ō-sēl) protrusion of a portion of the lung through a defect in the chest wall. SYN pleurocele, pneumatocele (2), pneumocele.

**pneu·mo·no·cen·te·sis** (noo′mō-nō-sen-tē′sis) rarely used term for paracentesis of the lung. SYN pneumocentesis. [G. *pneumōn*, lung, + *kentēsis*, puncture]

**pneu·mo·no·coc·cal** (noo′mō-nō-kok′ăl) relating to or associated with *Streptococcus pneumoniae*.

**pneu·mo·no·cyte** (noo′mō-nō-sīt) nonspecific term referring to cells lining alveoli in the respi-

ratory part of the lung. [G. *pneumōn*, lung, + *kytos*, cell]

**pneu·mo·no·pexy** (noo′mō-nō-pek-sē) fixation of the lung by suturing the costal and pulmonary pleurae or otherwise causing adhesion of the two layers. [G. *pneumōn*, lung, + *pēxis*, fixation]

**pneu·mo·nor·rha·phy** (noo-mō-nōr′ă-fē) suture of the lung. [G. *pneumōn*, lung, + *rhaphē*, suture]

**pneu·mo·not·o·my** (noo-mō-not′ō-mē) incision of the lung. SYN pneumotomy. [G. *pneumōn*, lung, + *tomē*, incision]

**pneu·mo·or·bi·tog·ra·phy** (noo′mō-ōr′bi-tog′rǎ-fē) radiographic visualization of the orbital contents following injection of a gas, usually air.

**pneu·mo·per·i·car·di·um** (noo′mō-per-i-kar′dē-ŭm) presence of gas in the pericardial sac. [G. *pneuma*, air, + pericardium]

**pneu·mo·per·i·to·ne·um** (noo′mō-per-i-tō-nē′ŭm) presence of air or gas in the peritoneal cavity as a result of disease, or produced artificially in the abdomen to achieve exposure during laparoscopy and laporoscopic surgery for treatment of pulmonary or intestinal tuberculosis, bronchiectasis, tuberculous empyema, and certain other conditions. [G. *pneuma*, air, + peritoneum]

**pneu·mo·per·i·to·ni·tis** (noo′mō-per-i-tō-nī′tis) inflammation of the peritoneum with an accumulation of gas in the peritoneal cavity. [G. *pneuma*, air, + peritonitis]

**pneu·mo·pleu·ri·tis** (noo′mō-ploo-rī′tis) pleurisy with air or gas in the pleural cavity. [G. *pneuma*, air, + pleur- + *-itis*, inflammation]

**pneu·mo·py·e·log·ra·phy** (noo′mō-pī-ĕ-log′rǎ-fē) radiography of the kidney after air or gas has been injected into the renal pelvis. [G. *pneuma*, air, + *pyelos*, pelvis, + *graphō*, to write]

**pneu·mo·py·o·thor·ax** (noo′mō-pī-ō-thōr′aks) SYN pyopneumothorax.

**pneu·mo·ra·di·og·ra·phy** (noo′mo-rā-dǐ-og′rǎ-fē) SYN pneumography (2).

**pneu·mo·ret·ro·per·i·to·ne·um** (noo′mō-ret′rō-per-i-tō-nē′ŭm) escape of air into the retroperitoneal tissues.

**pneu·mor·rha·chis** (noo-mō-rā′kis) the presence of gas in the spinal canal. SYN pneumatorrhachis. [G. *pneuma*, air, + *rhachis*, spinal column]

**pneu·mo·tach·o·gram** (noo-mō-tak′ō-gram) a recording of respired gas flow as a function of time, produced by a pneumotachograph. [G. *pneuma*, air, + *tachys*, swift, + *gramma*, something written]

**pneu·mo·tach·o·graph** (noo-mō-tak′ō-graf) an instrument for measuring the instantaneous flow of respiratory gases. SYN pneumotachometer.

**pneu·mo·ta·chom·e·ter** (noo′mō-tă-kom′ĕ-ter) SYN pneumotachograph. [G. *pneuma*, air, + -o- + *tachys*, swift, + *metron*, measure]

🔲**pneu·mo·thor·ax** (noo-mō-thōr′aks) the presence of air or gas in the pleural cavity. See page B13. [G. *pneuma*, air, + thorax]

**pneu·mot·o·my** (noo-mot′ō-mē) SYN pneumonotomy.

**PNF** proprioceptive neuromuscular facilitation.

**PNH** paroxysmal nocturnal hemoglobinuria.

**PNP** platelet neutralization procedure.

**PNPB** positive-negative pressure breathing.

**PO** per os.

**Po** polonium.

**pock** (pok) the specific pustular cutaneous lesion of smallpox. [A.S. *poc*, a pustule]

**pock·et** (pok′et) 1. a cul-de-sac or pouchlike cavity. **2.** a diseased gingival attachment; a space between the inflamed gum and the surface of a tooth, limited apically by an epithelial attachment. **3.** to enclose within a confined space, as the stump of the pedicle of an ovarian or other abdominal tumor between the lips of the external wound. **4.** a collection of pus in a nearly closed sac. **5.** to approach the surface at a localized spot, as with the thinned out wall of an abscess which is about to rupture. [Fr. *pochette*]

**pock·et do·si·me·ter** small ionization chamber that provides an immediate reading of radiation exposure. SEE ALSO film badge.

**pock·et·ed cal·cu·lus** SYN encysted calculus.

**pock·mark** (pok′mark) the small depressed scar left after the healing of the smallpox pustule.

△**pod-, po·do-** foot, foot-shaped. Cf. ped-. [G. *pous, podos*]

**po·dag·ra** (pō-dag′ră) severe pain in the foot, especially that of typical gout in the great toe. [G. fr. *pous,* foot, + *agra,* a seizure]

**po·dal·gia** (pō-dal′jē-ă) pain in the foot. SYN pododynia, tarsalgia. [pod- + G. *algos,* pain]

**po·dal·ic** (pō-dal′ik) relating to the foot. [G. *pous* (*pod*-), foot]

**po·dal·ic ver·sion** a manual procedure that results in a podalic extraction.

**pod·ar·thri·tis** (pod-ar-thrī′tis) inflammation of any of the tarsal or metatarsal joints. [pod- + arthritis]

**pod·e·de·ma** (pod-e-dē′mă) edema of the feet and ankles.

**po·di·a·tric** (pō-dī′ă-trik) relating to podiatry.

**po·di·a·tric med·i·cine** SYN podiatry.

**po·di·a·trist** (pō-dī′ă-trist) a practitioner of podiatry. SYN chiropodist. [pod- + G. *iatros,* physician]

**po·di·a·try** (pō-dī′ă-trē) the specialty concerned with the diagnosis and/or medical, surgical, mechanical, physical, and adjunctive treatment of the diseases, injuries, and defects of the human foot. SYN chiropody, podiatric medicine. [pod- + G. *iatreia,* medical treatment]

**pod·o·cyte** (pod′ō-sīt) an epithelial cell of the visceral layer of Bowman capsule in the renal corpuscle, attached to the outer surface of the glomerular capillary basement membrane by cytoplasmic foot processes (pedicels); believed to play a role in the ultrafiltration of blood. [podo- + G. *kytos,* a hollow (cell)]

**pod·o·dy·na·mom·e·ter** (pod′ō-dī′nă-mom′ĕ-ter) an instrument for measuring the strength of the muscles of the foot or leg. [podo- + G. *dynamis,* force, + *metron,* measure]

**pod·o·dyn·ia** (pod-ō-din′ē-ă) SYN podalgia. [podo- + G. *odynē,* pain]

**pod·o·gram** (pod′ō-gram) an imprint of the sole of the foot, showing the contour and the condition of the arch, or an outline tracing. [podo- + G. *gramma,* written]

**pod·o·mech·a·no·ther·a·py** (pod-ō-mek′ă-nō-thār′ă-pē) treatment of foot conditions with mechanical devices; e.g., arch supports, orthoses.

**poe·ci·lia** livebearing fish including guppy and molly. Species used in cancer, neurologic, and physiologic research.

**po·go·ni·on** (pō-gō′ni-on) in craniometry, the most anterior point on the mandible in the midline; the most anterior, prominent point on the chin. SYN mental point. [G. dim. of *pōgōn,* beard]

**pOH** the negative logarithm of the $OH^-$ concentration (in moles per liter).

△**-poi·e·sis** production; producing. [G. *poiēsis,* a making]

△**poi·ki·lo-** irregular, varied. [G. *poikilos,* many colored, varied]

**poi·ki·lo·blast** (poy′ki-lō-blast) a nucleated red blood cell of irregular shape. [poikilo- + G. *blastos,* germ]

**poi·ki·lo·cyte** (poy′ki-lō-sīt) a red blood cell of irregular shape. [poikilo- + G. *kytos,* cell]

**poi·ki·lo·cy·thae·mia [Br.]** SYN poikilocytosis.

**poi·ki·lo·cy·the·mia** (poy′ki-lō-sī-thē′mē-ă) SYN poikilocytosis. [poikilocyte + G. *haima,* blood]

⚑**poi·ki·lo·cy·to·sis** (poy′ki-lō-sī-tō′sis) the presence of poikilocytes in the peripheral blood. See page B2. SYN poikilocythaemia, poikilocythemia. [poikilocyte + G. *-osis,* condition]

**poi·ki·lo·der·ma** (poy′ki-lō-der′mă) a variegated hyperpigmentation and telangiectasia of the skin, followed by atrophy. [poikilo- + G. *derma,* skin]

**poi·ki·lo·ther·mic, poi·ki·lo·ther·mal, poi·ki·lo·ther·mous** (poy′ki-lō-ther′mic, poy′ki-lō-ther′măl, poy′ki-lō-ther-mŭs) **1.** varying in temperature according to the temperature of the surrounding medium; denoting the so-called cold-blooded animals, such as the reptiles and amphibians, and the plants. **2.** capable of existence and growth in mediums of varying temperatures. SYN haematocryal. [poikilo- + G. *thermē,* heat]

**point** (poynt) **1.** SYN punctum. **2.** a sharp end or apex. **3.** a slight projection. **4.** a stage or condition reached, as the boiling point **5.** to become ready to open, said of an abscess or boil the wall of which is becoming thin and is about to break. **6.** in mathematics, a dimensionless geometric element. **7.** a location or position on a graph, plot, or diagram. **9.** decimal point. [Fr.; L. *punctum,* fr. *pungo,* pp. *punctus,* to pierce]

**point A** SYN subspinale.

**point an·gle** the junction of three surfaces of the crown of a tooth, or of the walls of a cavity.

**point B** SYN supramentale.

**point of care tes·ting** performance of clinical laboratory testing at the site of patient care rather than in a laboratory, and often by nonlaboratorians. SYN bedside testing.

**point of el·bow** SYN olecranon.

**point ep·i·dem·ic** an epidemic where a pronounced clustering of cases of disease occurs within a very short period of time (within a few days or even hours) due to exposure of persons or animals to a common source of infection such as food or water.

**point of fix·a·tion** the point on the retina at which the rays coming from an object regarded directly are focused.

**poin·til·lage** (pwan-tē-yazh′) a massage manipulation with the tips of the fingers. [Fr. dotting, stippling]

**point mu·ta·tion** a mutation that involves a single nucleotide; it may consist of loss of a nucleotide, substitution of one nucleotide for another, or the insertion of an additional nucleotide.

**point of os·si·fi·ca·tion** SYN center of ossification.

**poise** (poyz, pwahz) in the CGS system, the unit of viscosity equal to 1 dyne-second per square centimeter and to 0.1 pascal-second. [J. *Poiseuille*]

**Poi·seu·il·le law** (pwah-swē′) in laminar flow, the volume of a homogeneous fluid passing per unit time through a capillary tube is directly proportional to the pressure difference between its ends and to the fourth power of its internal radius, and inversely proportional to its length and to the viscosity of the fluid.

**Poi·seu·il·le space** (pwah-swē′) SYN still layer.

**Poi·seu·il·le vis·cos·i·ty co·ef·fi·cient** (pwah-swē′) an expression of the viscosity as determined by the capillary tube method; the coefficient $\eta = (\pi Pr^4/8vl)$, where $P$ is the pressure difference between the inlet and outlet of the tube, $r$ the radius of the tube, $l$ its length, and $v$ the volume of liquid delivered in the time $t$. If volume is in cubic centimeters, time is in seconds, and $l$ and $r$ are in centimeters, then $\eta$ will be in poise.

**poi·son** (poy′zŭn) any substance, either taken internally or applied externally, that is injurious to health or dangerous to life. [Fr., fr. L. *potio, potion, draught*]

**poi·son·ing** (poy′zŏn-ing) 1. the administering of poison. 2. the state of being poisoned. SYN intoxication (1).

**poi·son·ous** (poy′zŭn-ŭs) characterized by, having the characteristics of, or containing a poison. SYN toxic (1), venenous.

**pok·er spine** stiff spine resulting from widespread joint immobility or overwhelming muscle spasm as might occur in osteomyelitis of a vertebra or a rheumatoid spondylitis.

**POL** physician office laboratory.

**Po·land syn·drome** (pō′lĕnd) an anomaly consisting of absence of the pectoralis major and minor muscles, ipsilateral breast hypoplasia, and absence of two to four rib segments.

**po·lar** (pō′lăr) 1. relating to a pole. 2. having poles, said of certain nerve cells having one or more processes. [Mod. L. *polaris*, fr. *polus*, pole]

**po·lar bod·y** one of two small cells formed by the first and second meiotic division of oocytes; the first is usually released just before ovulation, the second not until discharge of the oocyte from the ovary.

**po·lar cat·a·ract** a capsular cataract limited to an area of the anterior or posterior pole of the lens.

**po·lar·i·ty** (pō-lar′i-tē) 1. the property of having two opposite poles, as that possessed by a magnet. 2. the possession of opposite properties or characteristics. 3. the direction or orientation of positivity relative to negativity. 4. the direction along a polynucleotide chain; or any biopolymer, or macro-structure (e.g., microtubules). [Mod. L. *polaris*, polar]

**po·lar·i·ty ther·a·py** a bodywork modality that blends Eastern and Western medical traditions; employs gentle touch, rocking movements and other noninvasive therapies as well as nutritional counseling and exercise; said to restore energetic balance, reduce pain, and improve overall health. SEE ALSO five element theory.

**po·lar·i·za·tion** (pō′lăr-i-zā′shŭn) 1. ELECTRICITY coating of an electrode with a thick layer of hydrogen bubbles, with the result that the flow of current is weakened or arrested. 2. a change effected in a ray of light passing through certain media, whereby the transverse vibrations occur in one plane only, instead of in all planes as in an ordinary light ray. 3. development of differences

in potential between two points in living tissues, as between the inside and outside of a cell wall.

**po·lar·ized light** in which, as a result of reflection or transmission through certain media, the vibrations are all in one plane, transverse to the ray, instead of in all planes.

**po·lar star** SYN daughter star.

**po·lar tem·por·al ar·te·ry** *origin:* anterior temporal branch of middle cerebral artery; *distribution:* superomedial aspect of temporal lobe, extending to the temporal pole, of cerebrum. SYN arteria polaris temporalis [TA].

**pole** (pōl) 1. one of the two points at the extremities of the axis of any organ or body. 2. either of the two points on a sphere at the greatest distance from the equator. 3. one of the two points in a magnet or an electric battery or cell having extremes of opposite properties; the negative pole is a cathode, the positive pole an anode. 4. either end of a spindle. 5. either of the differentiated zones at opposite ends of an axis in a cell, organ, or organism. SYN polus [TA]. [L. *polus*, the end of an axis, pole, fr. G. *polos*]

**po·lice·man** (pō-lēs′man) an instrument, usually a rubber-tipped rod, for removing solid particles from a glass container.

**po·lio** (pō′lē-ō) abbreviated term for poliomyelitis.

△**po·lio-** gray; gray matter (substantia grisea). [G. *polios*]

**po·li·o·clas·tic** (pō′lē-ō-klas′tik) destructive to gray matter of the nervous system. [polio- + G. *klastos*, broken]

**po·li·o·dys·tro·phia** (pō′lē-ō-dis-trō′fē-ă) SYN poliodystrophy.

**po·li·o·dys·tro·phia ce·re·bri pro·gres·si·va in·fan·ti·lis** familial progressive spastic paresis of extremities with progressive mental deterioration, with development of seizures, blindness and deafness, beginning during the first year of life, and with destruction and disorganization of nerve cells of the cerebral cortex.

**po·li·o·dys·tro·phy** (pō′lē-ō-dis′trō-fē) wasting of the gray matter of the nervous system. SYN poliodystrophia. [polio- + G. *dys-*, bad, + *trophē*, nourishment]

**po·li·o·en·ceph·a·li·tis** (pō′lē-ō-en-sef′ă-lī′tis) inflammation of the gray matter of the brain, either of the cortex or of the central nuclei; as contrasted to inflammation of the white matter. [polio- + G. *enkephalos*, brain, + *-tis*, inflammation]

**po·li·o·en·ceph·a·lo·me·nin·go·my·e·li·tis** (pō′lē-ō-en-sef′ă-lō-mĕ-nin′gō-mī-ĕ-lī′tis) inflammation of the gray matter of the brain and spinal cord and of the meningeal covering of the parts. [polio- + G. *enkephalos*, brain, + *mēninx*, membrane, + *myelon*, marrow, + *-itis*, inflammation]

**po·li·o·en·ceph·a·lo·my·e·li·tis** (pō′lē-ō-en-sef′ă-lō-mī′ĕ-lī′tis) SYN poliomyeloencephalitis.

**po·li·o·en·ceph·a·lop·a·thy** (pō′lē-ō-en-sef′ă-lop′ă-thē) any disease of the gray matter of the brain. [polio- + G. *enkephalos*, brain, + *pathos*, suffering]

**po·li·o·my·e·li·tis** (pō′lē-ō-mī′ĕ-lī′tis) an inflammatory process involving the gray matter of the cord. [polio- + G. *myelos*, marrow, + *-itis*, inflammation]

**po·li·o·my·e·li·tis vi·rus** the picornavirus (genus *Enterovirus*) causing poliomyelitis in humans;

the route of infection is the alimentary tract, but the virus may enter the bloodstream and nervous system, sometimes causing paralysis of the limbs and, rarely, encephalitis; many infections are inapparent; serologic types 1, 2, and 3 are recognized, type 1 being responsible for most paralytic poliomyelitis and most epidemics. SYN poliovirus hominis.

**po·li·o·my·e·lo·en·ceph·a·li·tis** (pō'lē-ō-mī'ĕ-lō-en-sef'ă-lī'tis) acute anterior poliomyelitis with pronounced cerebral signs. SYN polioencephalomyelitis. [polio- + G. *myelon,* marrow, + *enkephalos,* brain, + *-itis,* inflammation]

**po·li·o·my·e·lop·a·thy** (pō'lē-ō-mī'ĕ-lop'ă-thē) any disease of the gray matter of the spinal cord. [polio- + G. *myelon,* marrow, + *pathos,* suffering]

**po·li·o·sis** (po-lē-ō'sis) a patchy absence or lessening of melanin in hair of the scalp, brows, or lashes, due to lack of pigment in the epidermis; it occurs in several hereditary syndromes but may be caused by inflammation, irradiation, or infection such as herpes zoster. [G., fr. *polios,* gray]

**po·li·o·vi·rus hom·i·nis** (pō'lē-ō-vī'rŭs hom'i-nis) SYN poliomyelitis virus.

**po·li·o·vi·rus vaccine 1.** inactivated poliovirus vaccine (IPV), an aqueous suspension of inactivated strains of poliomyelitis virus (types 1, 2, and 3) used by injection; **2.** oral poliovirus vaccine (OPV), an aqueous suspension of live, attenuated strains of poliomyelitis virus (types 1, 2, and 3) given orally for active immunization against poliomyelitis.

**Po·lit·zer bag** (pol'it-zĕr) a pear-shaped rubber bag used for forcing air through the auditory tube by the Politzer method.

**pol·itz·er·i·za·tion** (pol'it-zer-i-zā'shŭn) inflation of the auditory tube and middle ear by the Politzer method.

**Po·lit·zer lu·mi·nous cone** (pol'it-zĕr) SYN light reflex (3).

**pol·len** (pol'en) microspores of seed plants carried by wind or insects prior to fertilization; important in the etiology of hay fever and other allergies. [L. fine dust, fine flour]

**pol·lex,** gen. **pol·li·cis,** pl. **pol·li·ces** (pol'eks, pol'i-sis, pol'i-sēz) [TA] SYN thumb. [L.]

**pol·li·ci·za·tion** (pol'i-si-zā'shŭn) construction of a substitute thumb. [L. *pollex,* thumb, + *-ize,* to make like, + *-ation,* state]

**pol·li·no·sis, pol·le·no·sis** (pol-i-nō'sis, pol-ĕ-nō'sis) hay fever excited by the pollen of various plants. [L. *pollen,* pollen, + G. *-osis,* condition]

**pol·lu·tant** (pŏ-loo'tănt) an undesired contaminant that results in pollution.

**pol·lu·tion** (pŏ-loo'shŭn) rendering unclean or unsuitable by contact or mixture with an undesired contaminant. [L. *pollutio,* fr. *pol-luo,* pp. *-lutus,* to defile]

**po·lo·ni·um (Po)** (pō-lō'nē-ŭm) a radioactive element, atomic no. 84, isolated from pitchblende; the longest-lived isotope is $^{209}$Po (half-life 102 years); $^{210}$Po is radium F (half-life 138.38 days), the only readily accessible isotope. [L. fr. *Polonia,* Poland, native country of Marie Curie, who, with her husband Pierre, discovered the substance]

**po·lus,** pl. **po·li** (pō'lŭs, pō-lī) [TA] SYN pole. [L. pole]

△**poly-** **1.** many; multiplicity. Cf. multi-, pluri-. **2.**

CHEMISTRY prefix meaning "polymer of," as in polypeptide, polysaccharide, polynucleotide; often used with symbols, as in poly(A) for poly-(adenylic acid), poly(Lys) for poly(L-lysine). [G. *polys,* much, many]

**pol·y·ac·ry·la·mide gel e·lec·tro·pho·re·sis (PAGE)** separation of proteins or nucleic acids on the basis of both size and charge in a gel formed by cross-linking of acrylamide.

**pol·y·ad·e·ni·tis** (pol'ē-ad-ĕ-nī'tis) inflammation of many lymph nodes, especially with reference to the cervical group.

**pol·y·ad·e·nop·a·thy** (pol'ē-ad-ĕ-nop'ă-thē) adenopathy affecting many lymph nodes.

**Pól·ya gas·trec·to·my, Pól·ya op·er·a·tion** (pōl'yah) operation in which a portion of the stomach is removed and a retrocolic gastrojejunostomy is constructed in an end-to-side fashion to the entire cut end of the stomach.

**pol·y·a·mine** (pol-ē-am'ēn) class name for substances of the general formula $H_2N(CH_2)_nNH_2$, $H_2N(CH_2)_nNH(CH_2)_nNH_2$, $H_2N(CH_2)_nNH$-$(CH_2)_nNH(CH_2)_nNH_2$, where n = 3, 4, or 5. Many polyamines arise by bacterial action on protein; many are normally occurring body constituents of wide distribution, or are essential growth factors for microorganisms. [G. *polys,* much, many + amine]

**pol·y(a·mine)** (pol-ē-ă-mēn) a polymer of an amine. SEE poly- (2).

**pol·y·an·gi·i·tis** (pol'ē-an-jē-ī'tis) inflammation of many blood vessels involving more than one type of vessel, e.g., arteries and veins, or arterioles and capillaries.

**pol·y·an·i·on** (pol-ē-an'ī-on) anionic sites on proteoglycans in the renal glomeruli that restrict filtration of anionic molecules and facilitate filtration of cationic proteins; loss of polyanion may cause albuminuria in lipoid nephrosis.

**pol·y·ar·ter·i·tis** (pol'ē-ar-ter-ī'tis) simultaneous inflammation of a number of arteries.

**pol·y·ar·ter·i·tis no·do·sa** segmental inflammation, with infiltration by eosinophils, and necrosis of medium-sized or small arteries, most common in males, with varied symptoms related to involvement of arteries in the kidneys, muscles, gastrointestinal tract, and heart. SYN periarteritis nodosa.

**pol·y·ar·thric** (pol-ē-ar'thrik) SYN multiarticular.

**pol·y·ar·thri·tis** (pol'ē-ar-thrī'tis) simultaneous inflammation of several joints. [poly- + G. *arthron,* joint, + *-itis,* inflammation]

**pol·y·ar·tic·u·lar** (pol-ē-ar-tik'yu-lăr) SYN multiarticular. [poly- + L. *articulus,* joint]

**pol·y·ax·i·al joint** SYN multiaxial joint.

**pol·y·ba·sic** (pol-ē-bās'ik) having more than one replaceable hydrogen atom, denoting an acid with a basicity greater than 1.

**pol·y·blast** (pol'ē-blast) one of a group of ameboid, mononucleated, wandering phagocytic cells found in inflammatory exudates. [poly- + G. *blastos,* germ]

**pol·y·chon·dri·tis** (pol'ē-kon-drī'tis) a widespread disease of cartilage. [poly- + G. *chondros,* cartilage, + *-itis,* inflammation]

**pol·y·chro·ma·sia** (pol'ē-krō-mā'zē-ă) SYN polychromatophilia.

**pol·y·chro·mat·ic** (pol-ē-krō-mat'ik) multicolored.

**pol·y·chro·mat·ic cell** a primitive erythrocyte in bone marrow, with basophilic material as well as hemoglobin (acidophilic) in the cytoplasm. SYN polychromatophil cell.

**pol·y·chro·mat·ic ra·di·a·tion** radiation containing gamma rays of many different energies; in diagnostic radiology, typically bremsstrahlung.

**pol·y·chro·mat·o·cyte** (pol'ē-krō-mat'ō-sīt) SYN polychromatophil (2).

**pol·y·chro·ma·to·phil, pol·y·chro·ma·to·phile** (pol-ē-krō'mă-tō-fil, pol-ē-krō'mă-tō-fīl) **1.** staining readily with acid, neutral, and basic dyes; denoting certain cells, especially certain red blood cells. SYN polychromatophilic. **2.** a young or degenerating erythrocyte that manifests acid and basic staining affinities. SYN polychromatocyte. [poly- + G. *chrōma*, color, + *phileō*, to love]

**pol·y·chro·ma·to·phil cell** SYN polychromatic cell.

**pol·y·chro·ma·to·phil·ia** (pol-ē-krō'mă-tō-fil'ē-ă) **1.** a tendency of certain cells, such as the red blood cells in pernicious anemia, to stain with basic and also acid dyes. **2.** condition characterized by the presence of many red blood cells that have an affinity for acid, basic, or neutral stains. SYN polychromasia.

**pol·y·chro·ma·to·phil·ic** (pol-ē-krō'mă-tō-fil'ik) SYN polychromatophil (1).

**pol·y·chro·me·mia** (pol-ē-krō-mē'mē-ă) an increase in the total amount of hemoglobin in the blood.

**pol·y·clin·ic** (pol-ē-klin'ik) a dispensary for the treatment and study of diseases of all kinds. [poly- + G. *klinē*, bed]

**pol·y·clo·nal** (pol-ē-klō'năl) IMMUNOCHEMISTRY pertaining to proteins from more than a single clone of cells, in contradistinction to monoclonal.

**pol·y·clo·nal gam·mop·a·thy** a gammopathy in which there is a heterogeneous increase in immunoglobulins involving more than one cell line; may be caused by any of a variety of inflammatory, infectious, or neoplastic disorders.

**pol·y·clo·nia** (pol'ē-klō'nē-ă) SYN myoclonus multiplex. [poly- + G. *klonos*, tumult]

**pol·y·co·ria** (pol-ē-kō'rē-ă) the presence of two or more pupils in one iris. [poly- + G. *korē*, pupil]

**pol·y·crot·ic** (pol-ē-krot'ik) relating to or marked by polycrotism.

**po·lyc·ro·tism** (pol-ik'rō-tizm) a condition in which the sphygmographic tracing shows several upward breaks in the descending wave. [poly- + G. *krotos*, a beat]

**pol·y·cy·e·sis** (pol'ē-sī-ē'sis) SYN multiple pregnancy. [poly- + G. *kyēsis*, pregnancy]

**pol·y·cys·tic** (pol-ē-sis'tik) composed of many cysts.

**pol·y·cys·tic kid·ney, pol·y·cys·tic dis·ease of kid·neys** a progressive disease characterized by formation of multiple cysts of varying size scattered diffusely throughout both kidneys, resulting in compression and destruction of kidney parenchyma, usually with hypertension, gross hematuria, and uremia.

**pol·y·cys·tic liv·er** gradual cystic dilation of intralobular bile ducts (Meyenburg complexes) that fail to involute in embryonic development of the liver; associated with polycystic kidneys and occasionally with cystic involvement of the pancreas, lungs, and other organs.

**pol·y·cys·tic ova·ry** enlarged cystic ovaries pearl

white in color, with thickened tunica albuginea, characteristic of the Stein-Leventhal syndrome; clinical features are abnormal menses, obesity, and evidence of masculinization, such as hirsutism.

**pol·y·cys·tic ova·ry syn·drome** a condition commonly characterized by hirsutism, obesity, menstrual abnormalities, infertility, and enlarged ovaries; thought to reflect excessive androgen secretion of ovarian origin.

**pol·y·cy·thae·mia [Br.]** SEE polycythemia.

**pol·y·cy·the·mia** (pol'ē-sī-thē'mē-ă) an increase above the normal in the number of red cells in the blood. SYN erythrocythaemia, erythrocythemia. [poly- + G. *kytos,* cell, + *haima,* blood]

**pol·y·cy·the·mia hy·per·to·ni·ca** polycythemia associated with hypertension, but without splenomegaly. SYN Gaisböck syndrome.

**pol·y·cy·the·mia ru·bra** SYN polycythemia vera.

**pol·y·cy·the·mia ve·ra** a chronic form of polycythemia of unknown cause; characterized by bone marrow hyperplasia, an increase in blood volume as well as in the number of red cells, redness or cyanosis of the skin, and splenomegaly. SYN erythraemia, erythremia, Osler disease, Osler-Vaquez disease, polycythemia rubra, Vaquez disease.

**pol·y·dac·ty·ly** (pol-ē-dak'ti-lē) presence of more than five digits on hand or foot. [poly- + G. *daktylos,* finger]

**pol·y·dip·sia** (pol-ē-dip'sē-ă) excessive thirst that is relatively prolonged. [poly- + G. *dipsa,* thirst]

**pol·y·dys·pla·sia** (pol'ē-dis-plā'zē-ă) tissue development abnormal in several respects. [poly- + G. *dys-,* bad, + *plasis,* a molding]

**poly·en·do·crin·op·a·thy** (pol'ē-en'dō-krǐn-op'ă-thē) a disease usually caused by insufficiency of multiple endocrine glands. SEE multiple endocrine deficiency syndrome.

**pol·y·e·no·ic ac·ids** (pol-ē-en'ik as'idz) fatty acids with more than one double bond in the carbon chain; e.g., linoleic, linolenic, and arachidonic acids.

**pol·y·er·gic** (pol-ē-er'jik) capable of acting in several different ways. [poly- + G. *ergon,* work]

**pol·y·es·the·sia** (pol-ē-es-thē'zē-ă) a disorder of sensation in which a single touch or other stimulus is felt as several. [poly- + G. *aisthēsis,* sensation]

**pol·y·ga·lac·tia** (pol'ē-gă-lak'shē-ă) excessive secretion of breast milk, especially at the weaning period. [poly- + G. *gala,* milk]

**pol·y·ga·lac·tu·ro·nase** (pol'ē-gă-lak'too-ron-ās) pectin depolymerase; an enzyme catalyzing the random hydrolysis of 1,4-α-D-galactosiduronic linkages in pectate and other galacturonans.

**pol·y·gene** (pol'ē-jēn) one of many genes that contribute to the phenotypic value of a measurable phenotype.

**pol·y·gen·ic** (pol-ē-jen'ik) relating to a hereditary disease or normal characteristic controlled by the added effects of genes at multiple loci.

**pol·y·glan·du·lar** (pol-ē-glan'dyu-lăr) SYN pluriglandular.

**pol·y·graph** (pol'ē-graf) **1.** an instrument to obtain simultaneous tracings from several different sources; e.g., radial and jugular pulse, apex beat of the heart, phonocardiogram, electrocardiogram. The ECG is nearly always included for timing. **2.** an instrument for recording changes in respiration, blood pressure, galvanic skin re-

**p**
**o**

sponse, and other physiological changes while the subject is interviewed or asked to give associations to relevant and irrelevant words; the physiological changes are presumed to be emotional reactions, and thus whether the person is telling the truth. SYN lie detector. [poly- + G. *graphō*, to write]

**pol·y·gy·ria** (pol-ē-jī′rē-ă) condition in which the brain has an excessive number of convolutions. [poly- + G. *gyros*, circle, gyre]

**pol·y·hi·dro·sis** (pol′ē-hī-drō′sis) SYN hyperhidrosis.

**pol·y·hy·dram·ni·os** (pol′ē-hī-dram′nē-os) excess amount of amniotic fluid. [poly- + G. *hydōr*, water, + amnion]

**pol·y·hy·dric** (pol-ē-hī′drik) containing more than one hydroxyl group, as in polyhydric alcohols and polyhydric acids.

**pol·y·i·dro·sis** (pol′ē-i-drō′sis) SYN hyperhidrosis.

**pol·y·lep·tic** (pol-ē-lep′tik) denoting a disease occurring in many paroxysms, e.g., malaria, epilepsy. [poly- + G. *lēpsis*, a seizing]

**pol·y·mas·tia** (pol-ē-mas′tē-ă) in humans, a condition in which more than two breasts are present. SYN hypermastia (1), pleomastia, pleomazia. [poly- + G. *mastos*, breast]

**pol·y·me·lia** (pol-ē-mē′lē-ă) a developmental defect in which there are supernumerary limbs or parts of limbs. [poly- + G. *melos*, limb]

**pol·y·men·or·rhea** (pol-ē-men-ō-rē′ă) occurrence of menstrual cycles of greater than usual frequency. [poly- + G. *mēn*, month, + *rhoia*, flow]

**pol·y·men·or·rhoea [Br.]** SEE polymenorrhea.

**pol·y·mer** (pol′i-mer) a substance of high molecular weight, made up of a chain of repeated units sometimes called "mers." [see -mer (1)]

**pol·y·mer·ase** (po-lim′er-ās) general term for any enzyme catalyzing a polymerization, as of nucleotides to polynucleotides, thus belonging to EC class 2, the transferases.

**pol·y·mer·ase chain re·ac·tion (PCr)** (po-lim′er-ās) an enzymatic method for the repeated copying and amplification of the two strands of DNA of a particular gene sequence. It is widely used in the detection of HIV.

**pol·y·me·ria** (pol-ē-mēr′ē-ă) condition characterized by an excessive number of parts, limbs, or organs of the body. [poly- + G. *meros*, part]

**pol·y·mer·ic** (pol-i-mer′ik) **1.** having the properties of a polymer. **2.** relating to or characterized by polymeria. **3.** rarely used synonym for polygenic.

**po·lym·er·i·sa·tion [Br.]** SEE polymerization.

**po·lym·er·i·za·tion** (po-lim′er-i-za′shŭn) a reaction in which a high-molecular-weight product is produced by successive additions to or condensations of a simpler compound.

**po·lym·er·ize** (pol′i-mer-īz, po-lim′er-īz) to bring about polymerization.

**pol·y·mor·phic** (pol-ē-mōr′fik) occurring in more than one morphologic form. SYN multiform, pleomorphic (1), pleomorphous, polymorphous. [G. *polymorphos*, multiform]

**pol·y·mor·phic gen·e·tic mark·er** inherited characteristic that occurs within a given population as two or more traits.

**pol·y·mor·phism** (pol-ē-mōr′fizm) occurrence in more than one form; existence in the same spe-

cies or other natural group of more than one morphologic type. SYN pleomorphism.

**pol·y·mor·pho·cel·lu·lar** (pol-ē-mōr′fō-sel′yu-lăr) relating to or formed of cells of several different kinds. [G. *polymorphos*, multiform, + L. *cellula*, cell]

**pol·y·mor·pho·nu·cle·ar** (pol′ē-mōr-fō-noo′klē-ăr) having nuclei of varied forms; denoting a variety of leukocyte. [G. *polymorphos*, multiform, + L. *nucleus*, kernel]

**pol·y·mor·pho·nu·cle·ar leu·ko·cyte, pol·y·nu·cle·ar leu·ko·cyte** common term for granulocyte or granulocytic leukocyte; the term includes basophilic, eosinophilic, and neutrophilic leukocytes, but is usually used especially with reference to the neutrophilic leukocytes.

**pol·y·mor·phous** (pol-ē-mōr′fŭs) SYN polymorphic.

**pol·y·mor·phous light e·rup·tion** a common pruritic papular eruption appearing in a few hours and lasting up to several days on skin exposed to shortwave ultraviolet light; subepidermal edema and deep perivascular lymphocytic infiltration is seen microscopically.

**pol·y·mor·phous low-grade car·ci·no·ma of sal·i·vary glands** a low-grade malignant tumor of salivary glands showing several histologic patterns, such as cribriform, ductal, and papillary growth. SYN terminal duct carcinoma.

**pol·y·my·al·gia** (pol′ē-mī-al′jē-ă) pain in several muscle groups. [poly- + G. *mys*, muscle, + *algos*, pain]

**pol·y·my·oc·lo·nus** (pol′ē-mī-ok′lō-nŭs) SYN myoclonus multiplex.

**pol·y·my·o·si·tis** (pol′ē-mī-ō-sī′tis) inflammation of a number of voluntary muscles simultaneously. [poly- + G. *mys*, muscle, + *-itis*, inflammation]

**pol·y·ne·sic** (pol-i-nē′sik) occurring in many separate foci; denoting certain forms of inflammation or infection. [poly- + G. *nēsos*, island]

**pol·y·neu·ral** (pol-ē-noo′răl) relating to, supplied by, or affecting several nerves. [poly- + G. *neuron*, nerve]

**pol·y·neu·ral·gia** (pol′ē-noo-ral′jē-ă) neuralgia of several nerves simultaneously.

**pol·y·neu·rit·ic psy·cho·sis** SYN Korsakoff syndrome.

**pol·y·neu·ri·tis** (pol′ē-noo-rī′tis) SYN polyneuropathy (2).

**pol·y·neu·rop·a·thy** (pol′ē-nū-rop′ă-thē) **1.** a disease process involving a number of peripheral nerves (literal sense). **2.** a nontraumatic generalized disorder of peripheral nerves, affecting the distal fibers most severely, with proximal shading (e.g., the feet are affected sooner or more severely than the hands), and typically symmetrically; most often affects motor and sensory fibers almost equally, but can involve either one solely or very disproportionately; classified as axon degenerating (axonal), or demyelinating; many causes, particularly metabolic and toxic; familial or sporadic in nature. SYN polyneuritis. SYN multiple neuritis. [poly- + G. *neuron*, nerve, + *pathos*, disease]

**pol·y·nu·cle·ar, pol·y·nu·cle·ate** (pol-ē-noo′klē-ăr, pol-ē-noo′klē-āt) SYN multinuclear.

**pol·y·nu·cle·o·ti·dase** (pol′ē-noo′klē-ō-ti′dās) enzyme catalyzing the hydrolysis of polynucleotides to oligonucleotides or to mononucleotides.

**pol·y·nu·cle·o·tide** (pol-ē-noo′klē-ō-tīd) a linear

polymer containing an indefinite (usually large) number of nucleotides, linked from one ribose (or deoxyribose) to another via phosphoric residues. Cf. oligonucleotide.

**pol·y·o·don·tia** (pol-ē-ō-don′shē-ă) presence of supernumerary teeth. [poly- + G. *odous*, tooth]

**pol·y·on·co·sis, pol·y·on·cho·sis** (pol′ē-ong-kō′sis) formation of multiple tumors. [poly- + G. *onkos*, tumor, + -*osis*, condition]

**pol·y·o·nych·ia** (pol-ē-ō-nik′ē-ă) presence of supernumerary nails on fingers or toes. [poly- + G. *onyx*, nail]

**pol·y·o·pia, pol·y·op·sia** (pol′ē-ō′pē-ă, pol′ē-op′sē-ă) the perception of several images of the same object. SYN multiple vision. [poly- + G. *ōps*, eye]

**pol·y·or·chism, pol·y·or·chid·ism** (pol-ē-ōr′kizm, pol-ē-ōr′kid-izm) presence of one or more supernumerary testes. [poly- + G. *orchis*, testis]

**pol·y·os·tot·ic** (pol′ē-os-tot′ik) involving more than one bone. [poly- + G. *osteon*, bone]

**pol·y·o·tia** (pol-ē-ō′shē-ă) presence of a supernumerary auricle on one or both sides of the head. [poly- + G. *ous*, ear]

**pol·y·ov·u·lar** (pol-ē-ō′vyu-lăr) containing more than one ovum.

**pol·y·ov·u·la·tory** (pol-ē-ō′vyu-lă-tōr-ē) discharging several ova in one ovulatory cycle.

**▣ pol·yp** (pol′ip) a general descriptive term used with reference to any mass of tissue that bulges or projects outward or upward from the normal surface level, thereby being macroscopically visible as a hemispheroidal, spheroidal, or irregular moundlike structure growing from a relatively broad base or a slender stalk; polyps may be neoplasms, foci of inflammation, degenerative lesions, or malformations. See this page. SYN polypus. [L. *polypus;* G. *polypous,* contr. fr. G. *polys,* many, + *pous,* foot]

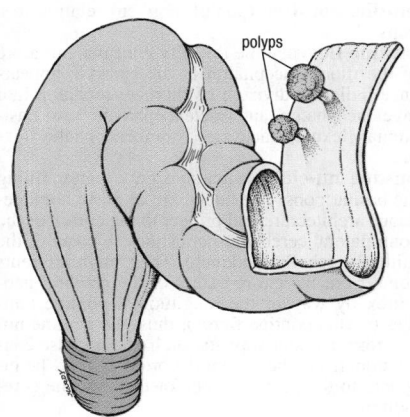

**polyps:** in sigmoid colon

**▣ pol·y·pec·to·my** (pol-i-pek′tō-mē) excision of a polyp. See page B9. [polyp + G. *ektomē*, excision]

**pol·y·pep·tide** (pol-ē-pep′tīd) a peptide formed by the union of an indefinite (usually large) number of amino acids by peptide links (–NH–CO–).

**pol·y·pha·gia** (pol-ē-fā′jē-ă) excessive eating; gluttony. [poly- + G. *phagō*, to eat]

**pol·y·phar·ma·cy** (pol-ē-far′mă-sē) the administration of many drugs at the same time.

**pol·y·phen·ic gene** SYN pleiotropic gene.

**pol·y·pho·bia** (pol-ē-fō′bē-ă) morbid fear of many things; a condition marked by the presence of many phobias. [poly- + G. *phobos*, fear]

**pol·y·phra·sia** (pol-ē-frā′zē-ă) extreme talkativeness. SEE logorrhea. [poly- + G. *phrasis*, speech]

**pol·y·phy·let·ic** (pol′ē-fī-let′ik) **1.** derived from more than one source, or having several lines of descent, in contrast to monophyletic. **2.** HEMATOLOGY relating to polyphyletism.

**po·ly·pi** (pol′i-pī) plural of polypus.

**pol·y·plas·tic** (pol-ē-plas′tik) **1.** formed of several different structures. **2.** capable of assuming several forms. [poly- + G. *plastikos*, plastic]

**pol·yp·loid** (pol′ē-ployd) characterized by or pertaining to polyploidy.

**pol·y·ploi·dy** (pol′ē-ploy′dē) the state of a cell nucleus containing three or more haploid sets. Cells containing three, four, five, or six multiples are referred to, respectively, as triploid, tetraploid, pentaploid, hexaploid, etc. [poly- + G. *ploidēs*, in form]

**pol·yp·nea** (pol-ip-nē′ă) SYN tachypnea. [poly- + G. *pnoia*, breath]

**pol·yp·oid** (pol′i-poyd) resembling a polyp in gross features. [polyp + G. *eidos*, resemblance]

**po·lyp·or·ous** (pol-ip′ōr-ŭs) SYN cribriform. [poly- + G. *poros*, pore]

**pol·yp·o·sis** (pol′i-pō′sis) presence of several polyps. [polyp + G. -*osis*, condition]

**pol·y·pous** (pol′i-pŭs) pertaining to, manifesting the gross features of, or characterized by the presence of a polyp or polyps.

**pol·yp·tych·i·al** (pol-ē-tik′ē-ăl) folded or arranged so as to form more than one layer. [G. *polyptychos,* having many folds or layers, fr. poly- + *ptychē,* fold or layer]

**pol·y·pus,** pl. **po·ly·pi** (pol′i-pŭs, pol′i-pī) SYN polyp. [L.]

**pol·y·ra·dic·u·li·tis** (pol′ē-ra-dik′yu-lī′tis) SYN polyradiculopathy.

**pol·y·ra·dic·u·lo·my·op·a·thy** (pol′ē-ra-dik′yu-lō-mī-op′ă-thē) coexisting polyradiculopathy and myopathy.

**pol·y·ra·dic·u·lo·neu·rop·a·thy** (pol-ē-ra-dik′yu-lō-noo-rop′ă-thē) coexisting polyradiculopathy and polyneuropathy.

**pol·y·ra·dic·u·lop·a·thy** (pol-ē-ra-dik′yu-lop′ă-thē) diffuse root involvement; seen with, among other disorders, diabetic neuropathy (diabetic polyradiculopathy). SYN polyradiculitis.

**pol·y·ri·bo·somes** (pol-ē-rī′bō-sōmz) two or more ribosomes connected by a molecule of messenger RNA. SYN polysomes.

**pol·y·sac·char·ide** (pol-ē-sak′ă-rīd) a carbohydrate containing a large number of saccharide groups; e.g., starch. Cf. oligosaccharide. SYN glycan.

**pol·y·sac·cha·ride con·ju·gat·ed vac·cine** a vaccine made from the capsular polysaccharide of the microorganism conjugated with a protein such as the *Haemophilus influenzae* type B vaccine against meningitis.

**pol·y·ser·o·si·tis** (pol′ē-sēr-ō-sī′tis) chronic inflammation with effusions in several serous cavities resulting in fibrous thickening of the serosa and constrictive pericarditis. SYN Bamberger disease (2), Concato disease. [poly- + L. *serum,* serum, + G. -*itis,* inflammation]

**pol·y·si·nu·si·tis** (pol'ē-sī-nŭ-sī'tis) simultaneous inflammation of two or more sinuses.

**pol·y·somes** (pol'ē-sōmz) SYN polyribosomes.

**pol·y·so·mia** (pol-ē-sō'mē-ă) fetal malformation involving two or more imperfect and partially fused bodies. [poly- + G. *sōma*, body]

**pol·y·so·mic** (pol-ē-sō'mik) pertaining to or characterized by polysomy.

**pol·y·som·no·gram** (pol-ē-som'nō-gram) the recorded physiologic function(s) obtained in polysomnography. [poly- + L. *somnus*, sleep, + G. *gramma*, diagram]

**pol·y·som·nog·ra·phy** (pol'ē-som-nog'ră-fē) simultaneous and continuous monitoring of relevant normal and abnormal physiological activity during sleep. [poly- + L. *somnus*, sleep, + G. *graphō*, to write]

**pol·y·so·my** (pol-ē-sō'mē) state of a cell nucleus in which a specific chromosome is represented more than twice. Cells containing three, four, or five homologous chromosomes are referred to, respectively, as trisomic, tetrasomic, or pentasomic. Cf. polyploidy. [poly- + G. *sōma*, body (chromosome)]

**pol·y·sper·mia, pol·y·sper·mism** (pol-ē-sper' mē-ă, pol-ē-sper'mizm) **1.** SYN polyspermy. **2.** an abnormally profuse spermatic secretion.

**pol·y·sper·my** (pol'ē-sper-mē) the entrance of more than one spermatozoon into the oocyte. SYN polyspermia (1), polyspermism.

**pol·y·sple·nia** a condition in which splenic tissue is divided into nearly equal masses or totally absent; congenital heart disease and malposition and maldevelopment of abdominal organs are common; may be related to situs inversus. Most cases are sporadic, although some suggest autosomal recessive inheritance. SYN Ivemark syndrome.

**pol·y·stich·ia** (pol-ē-stik'ē-ă) arrangement of the eyelashes in two or more rows. [poly- + G. *stichos*, row]

**pol·y·sym·brach·y·dac·ty·ly** (pol'ē-sim-brak-ē-dak'ti-lē) malformation of the hand or foot in which the shortened digits are syndactylous and polydactylous. [poly- + symbrachydactyly]

**pol·y·syn·ap·tic** (pol'ē-si-nap'tik) referring to neural pathways formed by a chain of a large number of synaptically connected nerve cells, as distinguished from oligosynaptic conduction systems. SYN multisynaptic.

**pol·y·syn·dac·ty·ly** (pol'ē-sin-dak'ti-lē) syndactyly of several fingers or toes.

**pol·y·ten·di·ni·tis** (pol'ē-ten-di-nī'tis) inflammation of several tendons.

**pol·y·the·lia** (pol-ē-thē'lē-ă) presence of supernumerary nipples, either on the breast or elsewhere on the body. SYN hyperthelia. [poly- + G. *thēlē*, nipple]

**pol·y·to·mog·ra·phy** (pol-i-tō-mog'ră-fē) body section radiography using a machine designed to effect complex motion; images a thinner tissue plane compared to simple linear or circular tomography.

**pol·y·trich·ia** (pol-ē-trik'ē-ă) excessive hairiness. [poly- + G. *thrix (trich-*), hair]

**pol·y·u·ria** (pol-ē-yu'rē-ă) excessive excretion of urine resulting in profuse micturition. [poly- + G. *ouron*, urine]

**pol·y·va·lent** (pol-ē-vā'lent) **1.** SYN multivalent. **2.** pertaining to a polyvalent antiserum.

**pol·y·va·lent al·ler·gy** allergic response mani-

fested simultaneously for several or numerous specific allergens.

**pol·y·va·lent se·rum** an antiserum obtained by inoculating an animal with several antigens or species or strains of bacteria.

**pol·y·va·lent vac·cine** a vaccine prepared from cultures of two or more strains of the same species or microorganism. SYN multivalent vaccine.

**po·made ac·ne** acne commonly found on the forehead and temples of black males after repeated application of hair creams.

**POMC** pro-opiomelanocortin.

**Pom·er·oy op·er·a·tion** (pom'er-ōy) excision of a ligated portion of the fallopian tubes.

**Pom·pe dis·ease** (pom'pĕ) SYN type 2 glycogenosis.

**POMR** problem-oriented medical record.

**pon·ceau de xy·li·dine** (pon-sō' dĕ zī'li-dēn) [CI-16151] a monoazo acid dye originally employed as a red histologic counterstain in Masson trichrome stain.

**Pon·fick shad·ow** (pon'fik) SYN achromocyte.

**pons** (ponz) **1.** [TA] in neuroanatomy, the pons varolii or pons cerebelli; that part of the brainstem between the medulla oblongata caudally and the mesencephalon rostrally, composed of the basilar part of pons and the tegmentum of pons. On the ventral surface of the brain the basilar part of pons, the white pontine protuberance, is demarcated from both the medulla oblongata and the mesencephalon by distinct transverse grooves. **2.** any bridgelike formation connecting two more or less disjoined parts of the same structure or organ. [L. bridge]

**pon·tic** (pon'tik) an artificial tooth on a fixed or removable partial denture; it replaces the lost natural tooth, restores its functions, and usually occupies the space previously occupied by the natural crown.

**pon·tile, pon·tine** (pon'tīl, pon'tēn) relating to a pons.

**pon·tine flex·ure** the dorsally concave curvature of the rhombencephalon in the embryo; appearance indicates division of rhombencephalon into myelencephalon and metencephalon. SYN basicranial flexure, transverse rhombencephalic flexure.

**pon·tine nu·clei** the massive gray matter filling the basilar pons. The nuclei are of fairly homogeneous architecture and project to the cortex of the contralateral cerebellar hemisphere by way of the middle cerebellar peduncle. Their main afferents come from the entire extent of the cerebral neocortex by way of the longitudinal pontine bundles (corticopontine fibers); thus, the pontine nuclei form a major way-station in the impulse conduction from the cerebral cortex of one hemisphere to the posterior lobe of the opposite cerebellum.

**pon·to·cer·e·bel·lar fi·bers** fibers arising from the nuclei of the basilar pons and primarily crossing the midline (there is a modes uncrossed projection), centering the cerebellum via the middle cerebellar peduncle and terminating as mossy fibers in the cerebellar cortex.

**pon·to·med·ul·lary groove** the transverse groove on the ventral aspect of the brainstem that demarcates the pons from the medulla oblongata; from its bottom the sixth, seventh, and eighth cranial nerves emerge.

**pool** (pool) **1.** a collection of blood or other fluid

in any region of the body; pool of blood results from dilation and retardation of the circulation in the capillaries and veins of the part. **2.** a combination of resources. [A.S. *pōl*]

**Pool phe·nom·e·non** (pool) **1.** in tetany, spasm of both the quadriceps and calf muscles when the extended leg is flexed at the hip; SYN Schlesinger sign. **2.** in tetany, contraction of the arm muscles following the stretching of the brachial plexus by elevation of the arm above the head with the forearm extended, resembles the contraction resulting from stimulation of the ulnar nerve.

**poor·ly dif·fer·en·ti·at·ed lym·pho·cyt·ic lym·pho·ma (PDLL)** a B-cell lymphoma with nodular or diffuse lymph node or bone marrow involvement by large lymphoid cells.

**pop·lit·e·al** (pop-lit'ē-ăl, pop-li-tē'ăl) relating to the popliteal fossa.

**pop·lit·e·al ar·tery** continuation of femoral artery in the popliteal space, bifurcating (at the lower border of the popliteus muscle as it passes deep to the arcus tendineus of the soleus muscle) into the anterior and posterior tibial arteries; *branches*, lateral and medial superior genicular, middle genicular, lateral and medial inferior genicular, and sural arteries. SYN arteria poplitea [TA].

**pop·lit·e·al fos·sa** the diamond-shaped space posterior to the knee joint bounded superficially by the diverging biceps femoris and semimembranosus muscles above and inferiorly by the two heads of the gastrocnemius muscle; deeply, the fossa is bound superiorly by the diverging supracondylar lines of the femur and the soleal line of the tibia inferiorly. Contents: tibial nerve, popliteal artery, vein, fat.

**pop·lit·e·al groove** a groove on the lateral condyle of the femur between the epicondyle and the articular margin. Its anterior end gives origin to the popliteus muscle; its posterior end lodges the tendon of the muscle when the knee is fully flexed.

**pop·lit·e·al mus·cle** SYN popliteus muscle.

**pop·lit·e·al vein** formed at the lower border of the popliteus muscle by the union of the anterior and posterior tibial veins, ascends through the popliteal space where it receives the lesser saphenous vein and passes through the adductor hiatus, entering the adductor canal as the femoral vein.

**pop·li·te·us mus·cle** *origin*, lateral condyle of femur; *insertion*, posterior surface of tibia above oblique line; *action*, from the fully extended and "locked" position, rotates the femur medially, on the fixed (planted) tibial plateau about 5°, "unlocking" the knee to enable flexion to occur; *nerve supply*, tibial. SYN musculus popliteus [TA], popliteal muscle.

**pop·u·la·tion** (pop-yu-lā'shŭn) statistical term denoting all the objects, events, or subjects in a particular class. Cf. sample (1). [L. *populus,* a people, nation]

**pop·u·la·tion ge·net·ics** the study of genetic influences on the components of cause and effect in the somatic characteristics of populations.

**POR** problem-oriented medical record.

**pore** (pōr) **1.** an opening, hole, perforation, or foramen. A pore, meatus, or foramen. **2.** SYN sweat pore. [G. *poros,* passageway]

**por·en·ce·pha·lia** (pōr'en-se-fā'lē-ă) SYN porencephaly.

**por·en·ce·phal·ic** (pōr'en-se-fal'ik) relating to or characterized by porencephaly. SYN porencephalous.

**por·en·ceph·a·li·tis** (pōr'en-sef-ă-lī'tis) chronic inflammation of the brain with the formation of cavities in the organ's substance. [G. *poros,* pore, + *enkephalos,* brain, + *-itis,* inflammation]

**por·en·ceph·a·lous** (pōr-en-sef'ă-lŭs) SYN porencephalic.

**por·en·ceph·a·ly** (pōr-en-sef'ă-lē) the occurrence of cavities in the brain substance, communicating usually with the lateral ventricles. SYN porencephalia. [G. *poros,* pore, + *enkephalos,* brain]

**po·ri** (pō'rī) plural of porus.

**PORN** progressive outer retinal necrosis.

**po·ro·ker·a·to·sis** (pō'rō-ker-ă-tō'sis) a rare dermatosis in which there is a thickening of the stratum corneum with an annular keratotic rim or cornoid lamella surrounding progressive centrifugal atrophy; cutaneous carcinoma has been reported to arise in the lesions. SYN Mibelli disease. [G. *poros,* pore, + keratosis]

**po·ro·ma** (pō-rō'mă) **1.** SYN callosity. **2.** SYN exostosis. **3.** induration following a phlegmon. **4.** a tumor of cells lining the skin openings of sweat glands. [G. *pōrōma,* callus, fr. *pōros,* stone]

**po·ro·sis,** pl. **po·ro·ses** (pō-rō'sis, pō-rō'sēz) a porous condition. SYN porosity (1). [L. *porosus,* porous]

**po·ros·i·ty** (pō-ros'i-tē) **1.** SYN porosis. **2.** a perforation. [G. *poros,* pore]

**po·rous** (pō'rŭs) having openings that pass directly or indirectly through the substance.

**por·pho·bi·lin** (pōr'fō-bī'lin) general term denoting intermediates between the monopyrrole, porphobilinogen, and the cyclic tetrapyrrole of heme (a porphin derivative).

**por·pho·bi·lin·o·gen (PBG)** (pōr'fō-bī-lin'ō-jen) a porphyrin precursor of porphyrinogens, porphyrins, and heme; found in the urine in large quantities in cases of acute or congenital porphyria.

**por·phyr·ia** (pōr-fir'ē-ă) a group of disorders involving heme biosynthesis, characterized by excessive excretion of porphyrins or their precursors; may be inherited or may be acquired, as from the effects of certain chemical agents (e.g., hexachlorobenzene).

**por·phyr·ia cu·ta·nea tar·da** familial or sporadic porphyria characterized by liver dysfunction and photosensitive cutaneous lesions, with hyperpigmentation and scleroderma-like changes in the skin, and increased excretion of uroporphyrin; caused by a deficiency of uroporphyrinogen decarboxylase induced in sporadic cases by chronic alcoholism. SYN symptomatic porphyria.

**por·phy·rin·o·gens** (pōr-fi-rin'ō-jenz) intermediates in the biosynthesis of heme; certain porphyrinogens are elevated in certain porphyrias.

**por·phy·rins** (pōr'fi-rinz) pigments widely distributed throughout nature (e.g., heme, bile pigments, cytochromes) consisting of four pyrroles joined in a ring (porphin) structure.

**por·phy·ri·nu·ria** (pōr'fir-i-nyu'rē-ă) excretion of porphyrins and related compounds in the urine. SYN purpurinuria.

*Por·phy·ro·mo·nas* (pōr'fir-ō-mōn'as) a genus of small anaerobic Gram-negative nonmotile cocci and usually short rods that produce smooth, gray to black pigmented colonies, the size of which varies with the species. In humans, they are found as part of the normal flora in the orophar-

p
o

ynx, including gingival crevices, and in the vaginal and intestinal tracts. The type species is *Porphyromonas asaccharolytica*.

**Por·phyr·o·mo·nas a·sac·char·o·ly·ti·ca** a species that rarely causes infections independently but is an important component of mixed infections associated with oral, genitourinary, and intra-abdominal abscesses, as well as in infections associated with impaired circulation and diabetic gangrene.

**port** (port) SYN portal.

**por·ta**, pl. **por·tae** (pōr′tă, pōr′tē) **1.** SYN hilum (1). **2.** SYN interventricular foramen. [L. gate]

**por·ta·ca·val** (pōr′tă-kā′văl) concerning the portal vein and the inferior vena cava.

**por·ta·ca·val shunt 1.** surgical anastomosis between portal and systemic veins; **2.** surgical anastomosis between the portal vein and the vena cava, as in an Eck fistula.

**por·ta hep·a·tis** [TA] a transverse fissure on the visceral surface of the liver between the caudate and quadrate lobes, lodging the portal vein, hepatic artery, hepatic nerve plexus, hepatic ducts, and lymphatic vessels. SYN caudal transverse fissure, portal fissure.

**por·tal** (pōr′tăl) **1.** relating to any porta or hilus, specifically to the porta hepatis and the portal vein. **2.** the point of entry into the body of a pathogenic microorganism. SYN port. [L. *portalis,* pertaining to a porta (gate)]

**por·tal ca·nals** connective tissue spaces in the substance of the liver that are occupied by preterminal ramifications of the bile ducts, portal vein, and hepatic artery, as well as nerves and lymphatics.

**por·tal cir·cu·la·tion 1.** circulation of blood to the liver from the small intestine, the right half of the colon, and the spleen via the portal vein; sometimes specified as the hepatic portal circulation; **2.** more generally, any part of the systemic circulation in which blood draining from the capillary bed of one structure flows through a larger vessel(s) to supply the capillary bed of another structure before returning to the heart; e.g., the hypothalamohypophysial portal system.

**por·tal fis·sure** SYN porta hepatis.

**por·tal hy·per·ten·sion** elevation of pressure in the hepatic portal circulation due to cirrhosis or other fibrotic change in liver tissue; when pressure exceeds 10 mmHg, a collateral circulation may develop to maintain venous return from structures drained by the portal vein; engorgement of collateral veins can lead to esophageal varices and, less often, caput medusae.

**por·tal hy·po·phy·si·al cir·cu·la·tion** a capillary network that carries hormones from the hypothalamus to their sites of action in the anterior hypophysis. SEE portal circulation, hypophysis, hypothalamus. SYN hypothalamohypophysial portal system.

**por·tal lob·ule of liv·er** a conceptual unit of the liver, emphasizing its exocrine function in bile secretion, which comprises a roughly triangular shaped cross-sectional area with a portal canal at its center and three or more venae centrales hepatis at its periphery.

**por·tal sys·tem** a system of vessels in which blood, after passing through one capillary bed, is conveyed through a second capillary network, as in the hepatic portal system in which blood from the intestines passes through the liver sinusoids.

**por·tal-sys·tem·ic en·ceph·a·lop·a·thy** an encephalopathy associated with cirrhosis of the liver, attributed to the passage of toxic nitrogenous substances from the portal to the systemic circulation; cerebral manifestations may include coma. SYN hepatic encephalopathy (1).

**por·tal tri·ad** branches of the portal vein, hepatic artery, and the biliary ducts bound together in the perivascular fibrous capsule or portal tract as they ramify within the substance of the liver. SYN triad (3).

**por·tal vein** a wide short vein formed by the superior mesenteric and splenic vein posterior to the neck of the pancreas, ascending in front of the inferior vena cava, and dividing at the right end of the porta hepatis into right and left branches, which ramify within the liver. SYN vena portae hepatis [TA], hepatic portal vein.

**por·tio**, pl. **por·ti·o·nes** (pōr′shē-ō, pōr′shē-ō′ nēz) [TA] a part. [L. portion]

**por·tion** (pōr′shun) part or division.

△**por·to-** portal. [L. *porta,* gate]

**por·to·bil·i·o·ar·te·ri·al** (pōr′tō-bil′ē-ō-ar-tēr′ē-ăl) relating to the portal vein, biliary ducts, and hepatic artery, which have similar distributions.

**por·to·en·ter·os·to·my** (pōr′tō-en-ter-os′tō-mē) an operation for biliary atresia in which a Roux-en-Y loop of jejunum is anastomosed to the hepatic end of the divided extravascular portal structures, including rudimentary bile ducts. SYN Kasai operation.

**por·to·gram** (pōr′tō-gram) radiographic record of portography. [porto- + G. *gramma,* a writing]

**por·to·ra·phy** (pōr-tog′ră-fē) delineation of the portal circulation by roentgenograms, using radiopaque material, usually introduced into the spleen or into the portal vein at operation. [porto- + G. *graphō,* to write]

**por·to·sys·tem·ic** (pōr′tō-sis-tem′ik) relating to connections between the portal and systemic venous systems.

**Por·tu·guese man-of-war** SYN *Physalia physalis.*

**port-wine mark, port-wine stain** SYN nevus flammeus.

▪**po·si·tion** (pŏ-zish′ŭn) **1.** an attitude, posture, or place occupied. **2.** posture or attitude assumed by a patient for comfort and to facilitate the performance of diagnostic, surgical, or therapeutic procedures. **3.** in obstetrics, the relation of an arbitrarily chosen portion of the fetus to the right or left side of the mother; with each presentation there may be a right or left position; the fetal occiput, chin, and sacrum are the determining points of position in vertex, face, and breech presentations, respectively. Cf. presentation. See page APP 87-97. [L. *positio,* a placing, position, fr. *pono,* to place]

**po·si·tion·al nys·tag·mus** nystagmus occurring only when the head is in a particular position.

**po·si·tion·al ver·ti·go** vertigo occurring with a change in body position.

**po·si·tion ef·fect** a change in the phenotypic expression of one or more genes due to a change in its physical location with respect to other genes; may result from change in chromosome structure or from crossing-over.

**po·si·tion sense** SYN posture sense.

**pos·i·tive** (poz′i-tiv) **1.** affirmative; definite; not negative. **2.** MATHEMATICS having a value more than zero. **3.** PHYSICS, CHEMISTRY having an electric charge resulting from a loss or deficit of electrons, hence able to attract or gain electrons. **4.** MEDICINE denoting a response to a diagnostic maneuver or laboratory study that indicates the presence of the disease or condition tested for. [L. *positivus,* settled by arbitrary agreement, fr. *pono,* pp. *positus,* to set, place]

**pos·i·tive ac·com·mo·da·tion** increased refractivity of the eye that occurs when shifting from the distance to a near object.

**pos·i·tive con·ver·gence** inward deviation of the visual axes even when convergence is at rest, as in cases of convergent squint.

**pos·i·tive end-ex·pi·ra·to·ry pres·sure (PEEP)** a technique used in respiratory therapy in which airway pressure greater than atmospheric pressure is achieved at the end of exhalation by introduction of a mechanical impedance to exhalation.

**pos·i·tive-neg·a·tive pres·sure breath·ing (PNPB)** inflation of the lungs with positive pressure and deflation with negative pressure by an automatic ventilator.

**pos·i·tive pre·ssure ven·ti·la·tion (PPV)** a mode of mechanical ventilation in which a positive transrespiratory pressure is generated by increasing airway opening pressure above body surface pressure.

**pos·i·tive sco·to·ma** a scotoma that is perceived as a black spot within the field of vision.

**pos·i·tive stain** direct binding of a dye with a tissue component to produce contrast; in electron microscopy, heavy metals like uranyl and lead salts are used to bind to selective cell constituents to produce increased density to the electron beam, i.e., contrast.

**pos·i·tive symp·tom** one of the acute or florid symptoms of schizophrenia, including hallucinations, delusions, thought disorder, loose associations, ambivalence, or affective lability.

**pos·i·tron** ($\beta^+$) (poz'i-tron) a subatomic particle of mass and charge equal to the electron but of opposite (i.e., positive) charge.

**▣ pos·i·tron e·mis·sion to·mog·ra·phy (PET)** tomographic images formed by computer analysis of photons detected from annihilation of positrons emitted by radionuclides incorporated into biochemical substances; the images, often quantitated with a color scale, show the uptake and distribution of the substances in the tissue, permitting analysis and localization of metabolic and physiological function. See page B12.

**po·so·log·ic** (pō-sō-loj'ik) relating to posology.

**po·sol·o·gy** (pō-sol'ō-jē) the branch of pharmacology and therapeutics concerned with a determination of the dosages of drugs; the science of dosage. [G. *posos,* how much, + *logos,* study]

**△ post-** after, behind, posterior; opposite of anti-. Cf. meta-. [L. *post*]

**post·a·dre·nal·ec·to·my syn·drome** SYN Nelson syndrome.

**post·au·ri·cu·lar in·ci·sion** an incision parallel and a few millimeters posterior to the retroauricular fold, made to gain access to the mastoid cortex.

**post·ax·i·al** (pōst-ak'sē-ăl) **1.** posterior to the axis of the body or any limb, the latter being in the anatomical position. **2.** denoting the portion of a limb bud that lies caudal to the axis of the limb: the ulnar aspect of the upper limb and the fibular aspect of the lower limb.

**post·bra·chi·al** (pōst'brā'kē-ăl) on or in the posterior part of the upper arm.

**post·cap·il·lary ven·ules** the microvasculature immediately following the capillaries, ranging in size from 10 to 50 μm, and characterized by investment of pericytes; they are the site of extravasation of blood cells, are particularly sensitive to histamine, and are believed to be important in blood-interstitial fluid exchanges. SYN pericytic venules.

**post·ca·va** (pōst'kā'vă) SYN inferior vena cava.

**post·ca·val** (pōst'kā'văl) relating to the inferior vena cava.

**post·cen·tral ar·ea** the cortex of the postcentral gyrus.

**post·cen·tral gy·rus** the anterior convolution of the parietal lobe, bounded in front by the central sulcus (fissure of Rolando) and posteriorly by the interparietal sulcus.

**post·cen·tral sul·cus** the sulcus that demarcates the postcentral gyrus from the superior and inferior parietal lobules.

**post·ci·bal** (pōst-sī'băl) after a meal or the taking of food. [L. *cibum,* food]

**post·co·i·tal** (pōst-kō'i-tăl) after coitus.

**post·coi·tal con·tra·cep·tion** SYN emergency hormonal contraception.

**post·coi·tal test** a test on cervical mucus about time of ovulation to evaluate its receptivity to sperm.

**post·co·i·tus** (pōst-kō'i-tŭs) the time immediately after coitus.

**post·com·mis·sur·ot·o·my syn·drome** SYN postpericardiotomy syndrome.

**post·con·cu·ssion syn·drome** delayed postconcussion signs such as headaches, blurred vision inability to concentrate, nausea, irritability, and change of character.

**post·cor·dial** (pōst'kōr'jăl) posterior to the heart. [L. *cor (cord-),* heart]

**post·cos·tal a·nas·to·mo·sis** longitudinal anastomosis of intersegmental arteries giving rise to the vertebral artery.

**post·cu·bi·tal** (pōst'kyu'bi-tăl) on or in the posterior or dorsal part of the forearm.

**post·date preg·nan·cy** a pregnancy of more than 294 days or 42 completed weeks. SYN prolonged pregnancy.

**post·duc·tal** (pōst-dŭk'tăl) relating to that part of the aorta distal to the aortic opening of the ductus arteriosus.

**▣ pos·te·ri·or** (pos-tēr'ē-ŏr) **1.** after, in relation to time or space. **2.** HUMAN ANATOMY denoting the back surface of the body. Often used to indicate the position of one structure relative to another, i.e., nearer the back of the body. SYN dorsal (2). **3.** near the tail or caudal end of certain embryos. **4.** a substitute for caudal in quadrupeds; in veterinary anatomy, posterior is used only to denote some structures of the head. See page APP 89. [L. comparative of *posterus,* following]

**pos·ter·i·or a·pha·sia** SYN receptive aphasia.

**pos·te·ri·or arch of at·las** the posterior arch of the atlas, which connects the lateral masses of the atlas posteriorly, forming the posterior wall of the vertebral canal at this level.

**pos·te·ri·or a·syn·cli·tism** SYN Litzmann obliquity.

**pos·te·ri·or au·ric·u·lar nerve** the first extracranial branch of the facial nerve, it passes behind the ear, supplying the posterior auricular muscle and intrinsic muscles of the auricle and, through its occipital branch, innervating the occipital belly of the occipitofrontalis muscle. SYN nervus auricularis posterior [TA].

**pos•te•ri•or ble•pha•ri•tis** inflammation of eyelid margins characterized by inspissation and occlusion of tarsal glands orifices.

**pos•te•ri•or ce•re•bral com•mis•sure** a thin band of white matter, crossing from side to side beneath the habenula of the pineal body and over the aditus ad aqueductum cerebri; it is largely composed of fibers interconnecting the left and right pretectal region and related cell groups of the midbrain; dorsally, it marks the junction of the diencephalon and mesencephalon. SYN commissura posterior cerebri [TA].

**pos•te•ri•or cham•ber of eye•ball** the ringlike space, filled with aqueous humor, between the iris anteriorly and the lens and ciliary body posteriorly.

**pos•te•ri•or col•umn** the pronounced, dorsolaterally oriented ridge of gray matter in each lateral half of the spinal cord, corresponding to the posterior or dorsal horn appearing in transverse sections of the cord. SYN posterior column of spinal cord (1).

**pos•te•ri•or col•umn of spi•nal cord 1.** SYN posterior column. **2.** in clinical parlance, the term often refers to the posterior funiculus of the spinal cord.

**pos•ter•i•or com•part•ment of thigh** posterior portion of the space enclosed by the fascia lata, separated from the medial and anterior compartments by the posterior and lateral intermuscular septa, respectively; contains the hamstring muscles (extensor of the thigh at the hip joint and flexors of the leg at the knee joint) and the short head of the biceps; all innervated by the sciatic nerve (the former by the tibial nerve portion, the latter by the fibular nerve portion).

**pos•te•ri•or cord of bra•chi•al plex•us** in the brachial plexus, the bundle of nerve fibers, formed by the posterior divisions of the upper, middle and lower trunks that lies posterior to the axillary artery; it gives rise to the upper and lower subscapular and thoracodorsal nerves, and ends by dividing into the axillary, and radial nerves.

**pos•ter•i•or cor•ne•al dys•tro•phy** opacification with primary involvement of the endothelium of the cornea.

**pos•te•ri•or cru•ci•ate lig•a•ment** the strong fibrous cord that extends from the posterior intercondylar area of the tibia to the anterior part of the lateral surface of the medial condyle of the femur. SYN ligamentum cruciatum posterius [TA].

**pos•ter•i•or e•las•tic la•mi•na of cor•nea** a delicate hyaline membrane lying between the substantia propria of the cornea and the corneal endothelium. SYN Descemet membrane, lamina limitans posterior corneae.

**pos•te•ri•or em•bry•o•tox•on** a developmental abnormality marked by a prominent white ring of Schwalbe and iris strands that partially obscure the chamber angle.

**pos•te•ri•or fo•cal point** the point of a compound optical system where parallel rays entering the system are focused.

**pos•ter•i•or fos•sa ap•proach** surgical approach

to the cerebellopontine angle through the mastoid process of the temporal bone.

**pos•te•ri•or fu•nic•u•lus** posterior white column of the spinal cord, the large wedge-shaped fiber bundle lying between the posterior gray column and the posterior median septum, and composed largely of dorsal root fibers.

**pos•ter•i•or glan•du•lar branch of su•per•i•or thy•roid ar•tery** branch of superior thyroid artery that descends to supply the apical portion of the ipsilateral lobe of the thyroid, continuing along the posterior border of the gland to anastomose with the inferior thyroid artery.

**pos•te•ri•or he•pa•tic seg•ment I** a small lobe of the liver situated posteriorly between the sulcus for the vena cava and the fissure for the ligamentum venosum. SYN lobus caudatus, Spigelius lobe.

**pos•te•ri•or horn** the posterior or occipital division of the lateral ventricle of the brain, extending backward into the occipital lobe; the posterior gray column of the spinal cord as appearing in cross section. SYN cornu posterius.

**pos•te•ri•or in•ter•cos•tal veins** drain the intercostal spaces posteriorly; those of the first intercostal space drain into the brachiocephalic veins; from spaces 2–3 they drain into right and left superior intercostal veins; from the 4th to the 11th spaces on the right they are tributaries of the azygos vein; on the left they empty into either the hemiazygos or accessory hemiazygos veins. SYN venae intercostales [TA].

**pos•te•ri•or in•ter•os•se•ous nerve** the deep terminal branch of the radial nerve, arises in the cubital region, penetrating and supplying the supinator and continuing with the posterior interosseous artery to supply all the extensor muscles in the forearm. SYN nervus interosseus antebrachii posterior [TA].

**pos•ter•i•or la•bi•al bran•ches of in•ter•nal per•i•ne•al ar•tery** branches of the perineal artery to the posterior portion of the labium majus.

**pos•te•ri•or la•bi•al branch•es of per•i•ne•al ar•te•ry** superficial branches of the perineal artery supplying the posterior portions of the labia majora and minora.

**pos•te•ri•or la•bi•al com•mis•sure** a slight fold uniting the labia majora posteriorly in front of the anus.

**pos•te•ri•or la•bi•al veins** pass posteriorly from the labia majora and minora to the internal pudendal veins.

**pos•te•ri•or lac•ri•mal crest** a vertical ridge on the orbital surface of the lacrimal bone which, together with the anterior lacrimal crest, bounds the fossa for the lacrimal sac.

**pos•ter•i•or la•ryn•ge•al cleft** laryngotracheoesophageal cleft (type 2 or 3).

**pos•ter•i•or leu•ko•en•ceph•a•lo•path•y syn••drome** a reversible clinicoradiologic syndrome characterized by confusion, headaches, seizures, cortical blindness, and other visual abnormalities, emesis, and motor signs, associated with MRI or CT evidence of bilateral white matter edema involving the parietal-occipital cerebral regions.

**pos•te•ri•or lim•it•ing lay•er of cor•nea** a transparent homogeneous acellular layer between the substantia propria and the endothelial layer of the cornea; considered to be a highly developed basement membrane. SYN membrana vitrea [TA], vitreous membrane (1).

**pos·te·ri·or lobe of hy·poph·y·sis** SYN neurohypophysis.

**pos·te·ri·or na·sal spine** the sharp posterior extremity of the nasal crest of the hard palate.

**pos·te·ri·or neph·rec·to·my** retroperitoneal removal of a kidney through an incision in the posterior lumbar muscles, usually with the patient in a prone position.

**pos·ter·i·or pol·y·mor·phous cor·ne·al dys·tro·phy** an autosomal dominant condition characterized by vesicular and linear abnormalities of the corneal endothelium; occasionally leads to corneal edema.

**pos·ter·i·or ra·mus of la·ter·al ce·re·bral sul·cus** the long, posteriorly-directed continuation of the lateral cerebral sulcus which extends between the temporal lobe inferiorly and the parietal lobe superiorly, its termination surrounded by the supramarginal gyrus.

**pos·ter·i·or ra·mus of spi·nal nerve** the smaller, posteriorly directed major terminal branch (with the anterior ramus) of all 31 pairs of mixed spinal nerves, formed at the intervertebral foramen and turning abruptly posteriorly to divide into lateral and medial branches, both of which will supply the deep (true) muscles of the back. The medial branch (rami medialis [TA]) of the dorsal primary ramus also supplies articular branches to the zygapophyseal joints and the periosteum of the vertebral arch. In the neck and upper back, the medial branch continues through the deep and superficial back muscles to supply overlying skin; in the lower back, the lateral branch does this. Terminologia Anatomica lists posterior rami (rami dorsales) for each group of spinal nerves: 1) cervical (nervorum cervicalium [TA]), 2) thoracic (nervorum thoracicorum [TA]), 3) lumbar (nervorum lumbalium [TA]), 4) sacral (nervorum sacralium [TA]), and 5) coccygeal (nervi coccygei [TA]).

**pos·te·ri·or rhi·nos·co·py** inspection of the nasopharynx and posterior portion of the nasal cavity by means of the rhinoscope, or with a nasopharyngoscope. SEE ALSO nasopharyngoscopy.

**pos·te·ri·or rhi·zot·o·my** section of posterior spinal root. SYN Dana operation.

**pos·te·ri·or sag·it·tal di·am·e·ter** distance from the sacrococcygeal junction to the middle of an imaginary line running between the left and right ischial tuberosities.

**pos·te·ri·or scle·ri·tis** inflammation, often mononocular, of the sclera adjacent to the optic nerve, with frequent extension to the retina and choroid.

**pos·ter·i·or seg·ment of eye·ball** the large space between the lens and the retina; it is filled with the vitreous body.

**pos·te·ri·or spi·no·cer·e·bel·lar tract** a compact bundle of heavily myelinated, thick fibers at the periphery of the dorsal half of the lateral funiculus of the spinal cord, originating in the ipsilateral thoracic nucleus (column of Clarke) and ascending by way of the inferior cerebellar peduncle. Terminals end as mossy fibers in the granular layer of the cortex of the cerebellar vermis. The bundle conveys largely proprioceptive information originating from the annulospiral nerve endings surrounding muscle spindles and from Golgi tendon organs.

**pos·te·ri·or staph·y·lo·ma** a bulging near the posterior pole of the eyeball due to degenerative changes in severe myopia. SYN Scarpa staphyloma.

**pos·te·ri·or tem·po·ral branch of mid·dle ce·re·bral ar·te·ry** a branch of the insular part (M2 segment) of the middle cerebral artery distributed to the cortex of the posterior part of the temporal lobe.

**pos·te·ri·or tooth** any of the premolar and molar teeth.

**pos·ter·i·or ur·e·thral valves** anomalous folds occurring at the level of the seminal colliculus. SYN Amussat valvula.

**pos·te·ri·or vein of left ven·tri·cle** arises on the diaphragmatic surface of the heart near the apex, runs to the left and parallel to the posterior interventricular sulcus, and empties in the coronary sinus.

**pos·te·ri·or ves·tib·u·lar branch of ves·tib·u·lo·coch·le·ar ar·te·ry** *origin:* terminal branch, with cochlear branch, of vestibulocochlear artery; *distribution:* utricle and (especially ampulla of) posterior semicircular duct.

△ **pos·ter·o-** posterior; at the back of. [L. *posterior*]

**pos·ter·o·an·te·ri·or** (pos′ter-ō-an-tēr′ē-ŏr) a term denoting the direction of view or progression, from posterior to anterior, through a part.

**pos·ter·o·an·ter·i·or pro·jec·tion** SYN PA projection.

**pos·ter·o·ex·ter·nal** (pos′ter-ō-ek-ster′năl) SYN posterolateral.

**pos·ter·o·in·ter·nal** (pos′ter-ō-in-ter′năl) SYN posteromedial.

**pos·ter·o·lat·er·al** (pos′ter-ō-lat′ě-răl) behind and to one side, specifically to the outer side. SYN posteroexternal.

**pos·ter·o·lat·er·al sul·cus** a longitudinal furrow on either side of the posterior median sulcus of the spinal cord marking the line of entrance of the posterior nerve roots. SYN dorsolateral sulcus.

**posterola·ter·al thor·a·cot·o·my** thoracotomy, involving division of the latissimus dorsi muscle and the serratus anterior muscle.

**pos·ter·o·me·di·al** (pos′ter-ō-mē′dē-ăl) behind and to the inner side. SYN posterointernal.

**pos·ter·o·me·di·an** (pos′ter-ō-mē′dē-an) occupying a central position posteriorly.

**pos·ter·o·su·pe·ri·or** (pos′ter-ō-soo-pē′rē-ŏr) situated behind and at the upper part.

**post·es·trus, post·es·trum** (pōst-es′trŭs, pōst-es′trŭm) the period in the estrus cycle following estrus; characterized by the growth of the corpus luteum and physiologic changes related to the production of progesterone.

**post·ex·tra·sys·tol·ic pause** the somewhat prolonged cycle immediately following an extrasystole.

**post·ex·tra·sys·tol·ic T wave** the modified T wave of the beat immediately following an extrasystole.

**post·gan·gli·on·ic** (pōst′gang-glē-on′ik) distal to or beyond a ganglion; referring to the unmyelinated nerve fibers originating from cells in an autonomic ganglion.

**post·gas·trec·to·my syn·drome** SYN dumping syndrome.

**post·hep·a·tit·ic cir·rho·sis** SYN active chronic hepatitis.

**pos·thi·o·plas·ty** (pos′thē-ō-plas-tē) surgical reconstruction of the prepuce. [G. *posthion*, dim. form of *posthē*, prepuce, + *plastos*, formed]

**pos•thi•tis** (pos-thī'tis) inflammation of the prepuce. [G. *posthē*, prepuce, + *-itis*, inflammation]

**post•hyp•not•ic** (pōst-hip-not'ik) following hypnotism; denoting an act suggested during hypnosis that is to be carried out at some time after the hypnotized subject is awakened.

**post•hyp•not•ic sug•ges•tion** suggestion given to a subject who is under hypnosis for certain actions to be performed after he or she is "awakened" from the hypnotic trance.

**post•ic•tal** (pōst-ik'tăl) following a seizure, e.g., epileptic.

**post-lumbar puncture syndrome** SYN spinal headache.

**post•ma•lar•ia neur•o•lo•gic syn•drome** a self-limited central nervous system disorder that develops soon after recovery from a severe bout of falciparum malaria, characterized principally by an acute state of confusion or psychosis, generalized convulsions, or both, lasting 1–10 days and associated with negative blood smears for malaria parasite; linked to preceding mefloquine therapy.

**post•ma•ture, post-term in•fant, post•ma•ture in•fant** (pōst-mă-tyur') referring to a fetus that remains in the uterus longer than the normal gestational period; i.e., longer than 42 weeks (288 days) in humans, which puts the child at risk because of inadequate placental function. The infant usually shows wrinkled skin, sometimes more serious abnormalities.

**post•men•o•pau•sal** (pōst-men-ō-paw'săl) relating to the period following the menopause.

**post•mor•tem** (pōst-mōr'tem) **1.** pertaining to or occurring during the period after death. **2.** colloquialism for autopsy (1). [post- + L. acc. case of *mors* (*mort-*), death]

**post•mor•tem de•liv•ery** extraction of the fetus after the death of its mother.

**post•mor•tem li•ve•do, post•mor•tem li•vid•i•ty** a purple coloration of dependent parts, except in areas of contact pressure, appearing within one half to two hours after death, as a result of gravitational movement of blood within the vessels.

**post•mor•tem ri•gid•i•ty** SYN rigor mortis.

**post•mor•tem wart** a tuberculous warty growth (tuberculosis cutis verrucosa) on the hand of one who performs postmortem examinations. SYN anatomic wart, dissection tubercle, necrogenic wart, verruca necrogenica.

**post•na•sal** (pōst'nā'săl) **1.** posterior to the nasal cavity. **2.** relating to the posterior portion of the nasal cavity.

**post•na•sal drip** term sometimes used to describe sensation of excessive mucoid or mucopurulent discharge from the posterior nares.

**post•na•tal** (pōst-nā'tăl) occurring after birth. [L. *natus*, birth]

**post•ne•crot•ic cir•rho•sis, post-ne•crot•ic cir•rho•sis** cirrhosis characterized by necrosis involving whole hepatic lobules, with collapse of the reticular framework to form large scars; regeneration nodules are also large; may follow viral or toxic necrosis, or develop as a result of ischemic necrosis. SYN necrotic cirrhosis.

**post•op•er•a•tive** (pōst-op'er-ă-tiv) following an operation.

**post•o•ral** (pos-tō'răl) in the posterior part of, or posterior to, the mouth. [L. *os* (*or-*), mouth]

**post•par•tum** (pōst-par'tŭm) after childbirth. Cf. antepartum, intrapartum. [L. *partus*, birth (noun), fr. *pario*, pp. *partus*, to bring forth]

**post•par•tum a•to•ny** atony of the uterine walls after childbirth.

**post•par•tum blues** mood disturbance (including insomnia, weepiness, depression, anxiety, and irritability) experienced by up to 50% of women the first week postpartum; apparently precipitated by progesterone withdrawal.

**post•par•tum hem•or•rhage** hemorrhage from the birth canal in excess of 500 ml after a vaginal delivery or 1000 ml after a cesarean delivery during the first 24 hours after birth.

**post•par•tum psy•cho•sis** an acute mental disorder with depression in the mother following childbirth.

**post•per•i•car•di•ot•o•my per•i•car•di•tis** a syndrome characterized by fever, substernal chest pain, and pericardial rub following cardiac surgery.

**post•per•i•car•di•ot•o•my syn•drome** pericarditis, with or without fever and often in repeated episodes, weeks to months after cardiac surgery. SYN postcommissurotomy syndrome.

**post•po•li•o•my•e•li•tis syn•drome** SYN postpolio syndrome.

**post•po•lio syn•drome** a progressive weakness and deterioration in the muscles of an individual previously affected by poliomyelitis. It usually affects the muscles most heavily impacted by the disease, but may affect others as well. SYN postpoliomyelitis syndrome.

**post•pran•di•al** (pōst-pran'dē-ăl) following a meal. [L. *prandium*, breakfast]

**post•pu•ber•al, post•pu•ber•tal** (pōst-pyu'ber-ăl, pōst-pyu'ber-tăl) SYN postpubescent.

**post•pu•bes•cent** (pōst-pyu-bes'ent) subsequent to the period of puberty. SYN postpuberal, postpubertal.

**post•re•mal cham•ber of eye•ball** the large space between the lens and the retina; it is filled with the vitreous body. SYN camera postrema, camera vitrea.

**post•sphyg•mic** (pōst-sfig'mik) occurring after the pulse wave. [G. *sphygmos*, pulse]

**post–steady state** any period of time, particularly in an enzyme-catalyzed reaction, after the steady-state interval; e.g., when the rate of product formation is declining in an enzyme-catalyzed reaction.

**post•syn•ap•tic mem•brane** that part of the plasma membrane of a neuron or muscle fiber with which an axon terminal forms a synaptic junction.

**post•tib•i•al** (pōst'tib'ē-ăl) posterior to the tibia; situated in the posterior portion of the leg.

**post•trans•plant lymph•o•pro•li•fer•a•tive dis•ease** a complication of organ transplantation in children; characterized by a mononucleosislike syndrome, tonsillar enlargement, and Epstein-Barr virus seroconversion.

**post•trau•mat•ic** (pōst-traw-mat'ik) occurring after trauma, and, by implication, caused by it.

**post•trau•mat•ic de•lir•i•um** delirium caused by a structural traumatic brain injury.

**post•trau•mat•ic de•men•tia** dementia caused by traumatic brain injury.

**post•trau•mat•ic ep•i•lep•sy** a convulsive state following and causally related to head injury, with brain damage either manifested clinically or ascertained by special examinations such as computed tomography.

**post·trau·mat·ic head·ache** headache following trauma to the head or neck.

**post·trau·mat·ic stress dis·or·der** development of characteristic symptoms following a psychologically traumatic event that is generally outside the range of usual human experience; symptoms include numbed responsiveness to environmental stimuli, a variety of autonomic and cognitive dysfunctions, and dysphoria.

**post·trau·mat·ic syn·drome** a clinical disorder that often follows head injury, characterized by headache, dizziness, neurasthenia, hypersensitivity to stimuli, and diminished concentration.

**pos·tu·late** (pos′tyu-lăt) a proposition that is taken as self-evident or assumed without proof as a basis for further analysis. SEE ALSO hypothesis, theory. [L. *postulo*, pp. *-atus*, to demand]

**pos·tur·al** (pos′tyu-răl) relating to or affected by posture.

**pos·tur·al a·lign·ment** maintenance of biomechanical integrity among body parts.

**pos·tur·al con·trac·tion** maintenance of muscular tension (usually isometric) sufficient to maintain posture.

**pos·tur·al drain·age** drainage used in bronchiectasis and lung abscess. The patient's body is positioned so that the trachea is inclined downward and below the affected chest area. See this page.

**pos·tur·al po·si·tion, pos·tur·al rest·ing po·si·tion** SYN physiologic rest position.

**pos·tur·al sway re·sponse** the body sway induced by vestibular stimulation.

**pos·tur·al syn·co·pe** syncope upon assuming an upright position; caused by failure of normal vasoconstrictive mechanisms.

**pos·tur·al ver·ti·go** **1.** SYN benign positional vertigo. **2.** light-headedness that appears particularly in elderly people with change of position,

usually from lying or sitting to standing; due to orthostatic hypotension.

**pos·ture** (pos′pos′cher) the position of the limbs or the carriage of the body as a whole. [L. *positura*, fr. *pono*, pp. *positus*, to place]

**pos·ture sense** the ability to recognize the position in which a limb is passively placed, with the eyes closed. SYN position sense.

**pos·tur·og·ra·phy** (pos-tyur-og′ra-fē) SYN dynamic posturography. [posture + G. *graphō*, to write]

**post·vac·ci·nal en·ceph·a·lo·my·e·li·tis** a severe type of encephalomyelitis that can follow the rabies vaccination.

**post·val·var, post·val·vu·lar** (pōst-val′văr, pōst-val′vyū-lăr) relating to a position distal to the pulmonary or aortic valves.

**po·ta·ble** (pō′tă-bl) drinkable; fit to drink. [L. *potabilis*, fr. *poto*, to drink]

**Po·tain sign** (pō-tā′) in dilation of the aorta, dullness on percussion extending from the manubrium sterni toward the second intercostal space and the third costal cartilage on the right, the upper limit extending from the base of the sternum in the segment of a circle to the right.

**po·tas·si·um (k)** (pō-tas′ē-ŭm) an alkaline metallic element, atomic no. 19, atomic wt. 39.0983, occurring abundantly in nature but always in combination; its salts are used medicinally. For organic potassium salts not listed below, see the name of the anion. SYN kalium. [Mod. L., fr. Eng. potash (fr. pot + ashes) + *-ium*]

**po·tas·sium-39** ($^{39}$K) most abundant, nonradioactive isotope of potassium; accounts for 93.1% of natural potassium.

**po·tas·si·um spar·ing di·u·ret·ics** diuretic agents that retain potassium; examples are triamterene and amiloride. Used in hypertension and in congestive heart failure.

**po·ten·cy** (pō′ten-sē) **1.** power, force, or strength; the condition or quality of being potent. **2.** specifically, sexual potency. **3.** in therapeutics, the

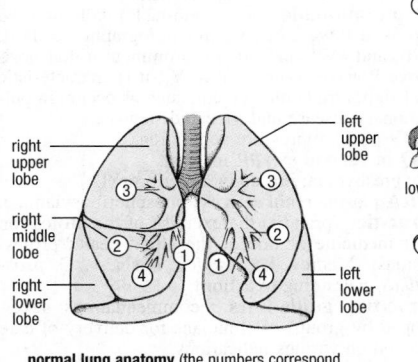

right upper lobe
right middle lobe
right lower lobe
left upper lobe
left lower lobe

**normal lung anatomy** (the numbers correspond to the areas to be drained with postural drainage)

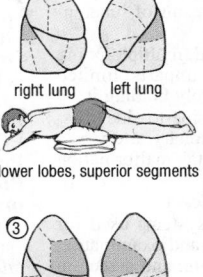

lateral view
right lung   left lung
lower lobes, superior segments
lower lobes, anterior basal segment

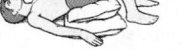

upper lobes, anterior segment

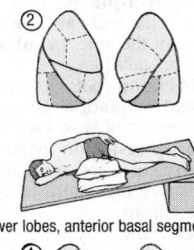

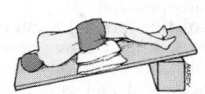

lower lobes, lateral basal segment

**postural drainage:** usually bronchi of the lower and middle lobes empty most effectively when the head is down; gravity helps drain secretions from smaller bronchial airways to the main bronchi and trachea, from which the patient is able to cough up secretions; this procedure is most effective in the early morning

relative pharmacological activity of a compound. [L. *potentia,* power]

**po•tent** (pō'tent) **1.** possessing force, power, strength. **2.** indicating the ability of a primitive cell to differentiate. **3.** possessing sexual potency.

**po•ten•tial** (pō-ten'shăl) **1.** capable of doing or being, although not yet doing or being; possible, but not actual. **2.** a state of tension in an electric source enabling it to do work under suitable conditions; in relation to electricity, potential is analogous to the temperature in relation to heat. [L. *potentia,* power, potency]

**po•ten•tial a•cu•i•ty me•ter (PAM)** instrument used to project an image such as Snellen test types through a cataractous lens onto the retina in order to predict likely visual function if the cataract were removed.

**po•ten•tial en•er•gy** the energy, existing in a body by virtue of its position or state of existence, which is not being exerted at the time.

**po•ten•ti•a•tion** (pō-ten'shē-ā'shŭn) interaction between two or more drugs or agents resulting in a pharmacologic response greater than the sum of individual responses to each drug or agent.

**po•tion** (pō'shŭn) a draft or large dose of liquid medicine. [L. *potio, potus,* fr. *poto,* to drink]

**Pott ab•scess** (pot) tuberculous abscess of the spine.

**Pott an•eu•rysm** (pot) SYN aneurysmal varix.

**Pott cur•va•ture** (pot) SYN angular curvature.

**Pott dis•ease** (pot) SYN tuberculous spondylitis.

**Pot•ter-Buck•y di•a•phragm** SYN Bucky diaphragm.

**Pot•ter syn•drome** (pot'ĕr) renal agenesis with hypoplastic lungs and associated neonatal respiratory distress, hemodynamic instability, acidosis, cyanosis, edema, and characteristic (Potter) facies; death usually occurs from respiratory insufficiency, which develops before uremia.

**Pott frac•ture** (pot) fracture of the lower part of the fibula and of the malleolus of the tibia, with lateral displacement of the foot.

**Pott par•a•ple•gia** (pot) paralysis of the lower part of the body and the extremities, due to pressure on the spinal cord as the result of tuberculous spondylitis.

**Potts clamp** (pots) a fine-toothed, multiple-point, vascular fixation clamp that imparts limited trauma to the vessel while securely holding it.

**Potts op•er•a•tion** (pots) direct side-to-side anastomosis between aorta and pulmonary artery as a palliative procedure in congenital malformation of the heart.

**pouch** (powch) a pocket or cul-de-sac.

**pouch cul•ture** plastic culture systems used for transport of specimens, culture, and examination chambers for the isolation, growth, and detection of *Trichomonas vaginalis.*

**pou•drage** (poo-drahzh') **1.** powdering. **2.** SYN talc operation. [F.]

**poul•tice** (pōl'tis) a soft magma or mush prepared by wetting various powders or other absorbent substances with oily or watery fluids, sometimes medicated, and usually applied hot to the surface; it exerts an emollient, relaxing, or stimulant, counterirritant effect upon the skin and underlying tissues. [L. *puls (pult-),* a thick pap; G. *poltos*]

**pound** (pownd) a unit of weight, containing 12 ounces, apothecaries' weight, or 16 ounces, av-

oirdupois; equivalent to 2.2046 kg. [A.S. *pund;* L. *pondus,* weight]

**Pow•as•san en•ceph•a•li•tis** an acute disease of children varying clinically from undifferentiated febrile illness to encephalitis; caused by the Powassan virus and transmitted by ixodid ticks.

**pow•der 1.** a dry mass of minute separate particles of any substance. **2.** PHARMACEUTICS a homogeneous dispersion of finely divided, relatively dry, particulate matter consisting of one or more substances. **3.** a single dose of a powdered drug, enclosed in an envelope of folded paper. **4.** to reduce a solid substance to a state of very fine division. [Fr. *poudre* fr. L. *pulvis*]

**pow•er 1.** OPTICS the refractive vergence of a lens. **2.** PHYSICS, ENGINEERING the rate at which work is done.

**pox** (poks) **1.** an eruptive disease, usually qualified by a descriptive prefix; e.g., smallpox, cowpox, chickenpox. See the specific term. **2.** an eruption, first papular then pustular, occurring in chronic antimony poisoning. **3.** archaic or colloquial term for syphilis. [var. of pl. *pocks*]

**Pox•vir•i•dae** (poks-vir'i-dē) a family of large complex viruses, with a marked affinity for skin tissue, that are pathogenic for man and other animals. a number of genera are recognized including: *Orthopoxvirus, Avipoxvirus, Capripoxvirus, Leporipoxvirus,* and *Parapoxvirus.*

**pox•vi•rus** (poks'vī-rŭs) any virus of the family Poxviridae.

**PP** pyrophosphate.

**PPCA** proserum prothrombin conversion accelerator.

**PPLO** pleuropneumonia-like organisms.

**ppm** parts per million.

**PPO** 2,5-diphenyloxazole, a liquid scintillator; preferred provider organization.

**PPPPPP** a mnemonic of 6 Ps designating the symptom complex of acute arterial occlusion. [*p*ain, *p*allor, *p*araesthesia, *p*ulselessness, *p*aralysis, *p*rostration]

**PPS** postpolio syndrome.

**PPS** prospective payment system.

**P pul•mo•na•le** (pē-pul-mō-nā'lē) tall, narrow, peaked P waves in electrocardiographic leads II, III, and aVF, and often a prominent initial positive P wave component in $V_1$; it is characteristic of right atrial enlargement, such as occurs in pulmonary disease and tricuspid stenosis.

**PPV** positive pressure ventilation.

**PQ in•ter•val** SYN PR interval.

**Pr** presbyopia; praseodymium; propyl.

**PRA** plasma renin activity; phosphoribosylamine.

**prac•tice** (prak'tis) the exercise of the profession of medicine or one of the allied health professions. [Mediev. L. *practica,* business, G. *praktikos,* pertaining to action]

**prac•tice guide•lines** recommendations developed by groups of clinicians for delivery of care based on various indications.

**prac•ti•tion•er** (prak-tish'ŭn-er) a person who practices medicine or one of the allied health care professions.

⌂**prae-** SEE pre-.

**prae•ca•va [Br.]** SEE precava.

**prae•com•mis•sure [Br.]** SYN anterior commissure.

**prae•cor•a•coid [Br.]** anterior part of coracoid in shoulder girdle of reptiles and amphibians.

**prae•cor•d•ia [Br.]** SEE precordia.

**prae·cor·di·al [Br.]** SEE precordial.
**prae·co·rnu [Br.]** SYN anterior horn.
**prae·nar·is [Br.]** SYN nostril.
**prae·na·sal [Br.]** SEE prenasal.
**prag·ma·tism** (prag′mă-tizm) a philosophy emphasizing practical applications and consequences of beliefs and theories, that the meaning of ideas or things is determined by the testability of the idea in real life. [G. *pragma* (*pragmat-*), thing done]
**Prague ma·neu·ver** (prahg) a technique for delivery of the fetus in breech position when the fetal occiput is posterior; one hand of the operator delivers the shoulders, while making pressure above the symphysis pubis with the other hand.
**Prague pel·vis** (prahg) SYN spondylolisthetic pelvis.
**pran·di·al** (pran′dē-ăl) relating to a meal. [L. *prandium*, breakfast]
**pra·se·o·dym·i·um (Pr)** (prā-sē-ō-dim′ē-ŭm) an element of the lanthanide or "rare earth" group; atomic no. 59, atomic wt. 140.90765. [G. *prasios*, leekgreen, fr. *prason*, a leek, + *didymos*, twin]
**Pratt symp·tom** (prat) rarely used term for rigidity in the muscles of an injured limb, which precedes the occurrence of gangrene.
**prax·is** (prăk′sĭs) OCCUPATIONAL THERAPY conception and planning of a motor act in response to an environmental demand. [G., practice, activity]
**PRE** progressive-resistance exercise.
△**pre-** anterior; before (in time or space). SEE ALSO ante-, pro- (1). [L. *prae*]
**pre·ag·o·nal** (prē-ag′ō-năl) immediately preceding death. [pre- + G. *agōn*, struggle (agony)]
**pre·an·es·thet·ic** (prē-an-es-thet′ik) before anesthesia.
**pre·au·ri·cu·lar pit** SYN preauricular sinus.
**pre·au·ri·cu·lar sinus** sinus tract or pit in preauricular skin, resulting from developmental defect of the first and second pharyngeal (branchial) arches. SYN preauricular pit.
**pre·au·to·mat·ic pause** a temporary pause in cardiac activity before an automatic pacemaker escapes. SEE ALSO escape.
**pre·ax·i·al** (prē-ak′sē-ăl) **1.** anterior to the axis of the body or a limb, the latter being in the anatomical position. **2.** denoting the portion of a limb bud that lies cranial to the axis of the limb: the radial aspect of the upper limb and the tibial aspect of the lower limb.
**pre·can·cer** (prē-kan′ser) a lesion from which a malignant neoplasm is believed to develop in a significant number of instances, and which may or may not be recognizable clinically or by microscopic changes in the affected tissue.
**pre·can·cer·ous** (prē-kan′ser-ŭs) pertaining to any lesion that is interpreted as precancer. SYN premalignant.
**pre·cap·il·lary** (prē-kap′i-lār-ē) preceding a capillary; an arteriole or venule.
**pre·car·ti·lage** (prē-kar′ti-lij) a closely packed aggregation of mesenchymal cells just prior to their differentiation into embryonic cartilage.
**pre·ca·va** (prē-kā′vă) SYN superior vena cava.
**pre·cen·tral ar·ea** the cortex of the precentral gyrus.
**pre·cen·tral gy·rus** bounded posteriorly by the central sulcus and anteriorly by the precentral sulcus.
**pre·cen·tral sul·cus** an interrupted fissure ante-

rior to and in general parallel with the central sulcus, marking the anterior border of the precentral gyrus.
**pre·cip·i·ta·ble** (prē-sip′i-tă-bl) capable of being precipitated.
**pre·cip·i·tant** (prē-sip′i-tant) anything causing a precipitation from a solution.
**pre·cip·i·tate** (prē-sip′i-tāt) **1.** to cause a substance in solution to separate as a solid. **2.** a solid separated out from a solution or suspension; a floc or clump, such as that resulting from the mixture of a specific antigen and its antibody. **3.** accumulation of inflammatory cells on the corneal endothelium in uveitis (keratic precipitates). [L. *praecipito*, pp. *-atus*, to cast headlong]
**pre·cip·i·tate la·bor** very rapid labor ending in delivery of the fetus.
**pre·cip·i·ta·tion** (prē-sip-i-tā′shŭn) **1.** the process of formation of a solid previously held in solution or suspension in a liquid. **2.** the phenomenon of clumping of proteins in serum produced by the addition of a specific precipitin. [see precipitate]
**pre·cip·i·tin** (prē-sip′i-tin) an antibody that under suitable conditions combines with and causes its specific and soluble antigen to precipitate from solution.
**pre·cip·i·tin·o·gen** (prē-sip-i-tin′ō-jen) **1.** an antigen that stimulates the formation of specific precipitin when injected into an animal body. **2.** a precipitable soluble antigen. [precipitin + G. *-gen*, producing]
**pre·cip·i·tin test** an *in vitro* test in which antigen is in soluble form and precipitates when it combines with added specific antibody in the presence of an electrolyte. SEE ALSO gel diffusion precipitin tests.
**pre·ci·sion** (prē-sĭ′zhun) **1.** the quality of being sharply defined or stated; one measure of precision is the number of distinguishable alternatives to a measurement. **2.** STATISTICS the inverse of the variance of a measurement or estimate. **3.** reproducibility of a quantifiable result; an indication of the random error.
**pre·clin·i·cal** (prē-klin′i-kăl) **1.** before the onset of disease. **2.** a period in medical education before the student becomes involved with patients and clinical work.
**pre·co·cious** (prē-kō′shŭs) developing unusually early or rapidly. [L. *praecox*, premature]
**pre·co·cious pu·ber·ty** condition in which pubertal changes begin at an unexpectedly early age.
**pre·coc·i·ty** (prē-kos′i-tē) unusually early or rapid development of mental or physical traits. [see precocious]
**pre·cog·ni·tion** (prē-kog-nish′ŭn) advance knowledge, by means other than the normal senses, of a future event; a form of extrasensory perception. [L. *praecogito*, to ponder before]
**pre·col·lag·e·nous fi·bers** immature, argyrophilic fibers.
**pre·com·mis·sure** (prē-kom′ĭ-sher) SYN anterior commissure.
**pre·con·cep·tu·al stage** PSYCHOLOGY the stage of development in an infant's life, prior to actual conceptual thinking, in which sensorimotor activity predominates.
**pre·con·scious** (prē-kon′shŭs) PSYCHOANALYSIS one of the three divisions of the psyche, the other two being the conscious and unconscious; in-

**p**
**r**

cludes all ideas, thoughts, past experiences, and other memory impressions that with effort can be consciously recalled. Cf. foreconscious.

**pre·con·vul·sive** (prē-kon-vŭl'siv) denoting the stage in an epileptic paroxysm preceding convulsions (e.g., aura).

**pre·cor·dia** (prē-kōr'dē-ă) the epigastrium and anterior surface of the lower part of the thorax. [L. *praecordia* (ntr. pl. only), the diaphragm, the entrails, fr. *prae*, before, + *cor* (*cord-*), heart]

**pre·cor·di·al** (prē-kōr'dē-ăl) relating to the precordia.

**pre·cor·di·al leads** SYN chest leads.

**pre·cor·di·um** (prē-kōr'dē-ŭm) singular of precordia.

**pre·cor·nu** (prē-kor'nū) SYN anterior horn.

**pre·cos·tal anas·to·mo·sis** (prē-kos-tal a-nas-tō-mō-sis) longitudinal anastomosis of intersegmental arteries in the embryo that gives rise to the thyrocervical and costocervical trunks.

**pre·cu·ne·ate** (prē-koo'nē-āt) relating to the precuneus.

**pre·cu·ne·us** (prē-koo'nē-ŭs) a division of the medial surface of each cerebral hemisphere between the cuneus and the paracentral lobule; it lies above the subparietal sulcus and is bounded anteriorly by the marginal part of the cingulate sulcus and posteriorly by the parietooccipital sulcus. SYN quadrate lobe (3). [pre- + L. *cuneus*, a wedge]

**pre·cur·sor** (prē-ker'ser) that which precedes another or from which another is derived, applied especially to a physiologically inactive substance that is converted to an active enzyme, vitamin, hormone, etc., or to a chemical substance that is built into a larger structure in the course of synthesizing the latter. [L. *praecursor*, fr. *prae-*, pre- + *curro*, to run]

**pre·cur·so·ry car·ti·lage** SYN temporary cartilage.

**pre·de·cid·u·al** (prē-dē-sid'yu-ăl) relating to the premenstrual or secretory phase of the menstrual cycle.

**pre·den·tin** (prē-den'tin) the organic fibrillar matrix of the dentin before its calcification.

**pre·De·sce·met cor·ne·al dys·tro·phy** opacification with primary involvement of the posterior stroma of the cornea.

**pre·di·a·be·tes** (pre'dī-ă-bē'tēz) a state of potential diabetes mellitus, with normal glucose tolerance but with an increased risk of developing diabetes, (e.g., family history).

**pre·di·as·to·le** (prē-dī-as'tō-lē) the interval in the cardiac rhythm immediately preceding diastole. SYN late systole.

**pre·di·a·stol·ic** (prē-dī-ă-stol'ik) late systolic, relating to the interval preceding cardiac diastole.

**pre·dic·tive val·ue** an expression of the likelihood that a given test result correlates with the presence or absence of disease. A positive predictive value is the ratio of patients with the disease who test positive to the entire population of individuals with a positive test result; a negative predictive value is the ratio of patients without the disease who test negative to the entire population of individuals with a negative test.

**pre·di·ges·tion** (prē-dī-jes'chŭn) the artificial initiation of digestion of proteins (proteolysis) and starches (amylolysis) before they are eaten.

**pre·dis·pose** (prē'dis-pōz) to render susceptible.

**pre·dis·po·si·tion** (prē'dis-pō-zish'ŭn) a condition of special susceptibility to a disease.

**pre·duc·tal** (prē-dŭk'tăl) relating to that part of the aorta proximal to the aortic opening of the ductus arteriosus.

**pre·e·clamp·sia** (prē-ē-klamp'sē-ă) development of hypertension with proteinuria or edema, or both, due to pregnancy or the influence of a recent pregnancy; it usually occurs after the 20th week of gestation, but may develop before this time in the presence of trophoblastic disease. [pre- + G. *eklampsis*, a shining forth (eclampsia)]

**pre·ep·i·glot·tic space** the space anterior to the epiglottis that is bounded anteriorly by the thyrohyoid membrane and the superior parts of the lamina of the thyroid cartilage, superiorly by the hyoepiglottic ligament and inferiorly by the thyroepiglottic ligament; laterally it extends into the paraglottic spaces. Carcinoma of the infrahyoid portion of the epiglottis often extends into the preepiglottic space.

**pre·ex·ci·ta·tion** (prē'ek-sī-tā'shŭn) premature activation of part of the ventricular myocardium by an impulse that travels by an anomalous path and so avoids physiological delay in the atrioventricular junction; an intrinsic part of the Wolff-Parkinson-White syndrome.

**pre·ex·ci·ta·tion syn·drome** SYN Wolff-Parkinson-White syndrome.

**pre·ferred pro·vi·der or·ga·ni·za·tion (PPO)** a health care organization that negotiates set rates of reimbursement with participating health care providers for services to insured clients. This is a type of prospective payment system. SEE health maintenance organization.

**pre·fron·tal ar·ea** SEE frontal cortex.

**pre·gan·gli·on·ic** (prē'gang-glē-on'ik) situated proximal to or preceding a ganglion; referring specifically to the preganglionic motor neurons of the autonomic nervous system (located in the spinal cord and brainstem) and the preganglionic, myelinated nerve fibers by which they are connected to the autonomic ganglia.

**preg·nan·cy** (preg'nan-sē) the state of a female after conception and until the termination of the gestation. SYN gestation. [L. *praegnans* (*praegnant-*), pregnant, fr. *prae*, before, + *gnascor*, pp. *natus*, to be born]

**preg·nan·cy gin·gi·vi·tis** SYN hormonal gingivitis.

**preg·nan·cy-in·duced hy·per·ten·sion** SYN gestational hypertension.

**preg·nane** (preg'nān) parent hydrocarbon of the progesterones, pregnane alcohols, ketones, and several adrenocortical hormones.

**preg·nane·di·ol** (preg-nān-dī'ol) the chief steroid metabolite of progesterone; it is biologically inactive and occurs as pregnanediol glucuronate in the urine.

**preg·nane·di·one** (preg-nān-dī'ōn) a metabolite of progesterone, formed in relatively small quantities, that occurs in 5α and 5β isomeric forms.

**preg·nane·tri·ol** (preg-nān-trī'ol) a urinary metabolite of 17-hydroxyprogesterone and a precursor in the biosynthesis of cortisol; its excretion is enhanced in certain diseases of the adrenal cortex and following administration of corticotropin.

**preg·nant** denoting a gestating female. SYN gravid. [see pregnancy]

**pre·hen·sile** (prē-hen'sil) adapted for taking hold

of or grasping. [L. *prehendo,* pp. -*hensus,* to lay hold of, seize]

**pre•hen•sion** (prē-hen′shŭn) the act of grasping, or taking hold of.

**pre•hor•mone** (prē-hōr′mōn) a glandular secretory product, having little or no inherent biological potency, that is converted peripherally to an active hormone. Cf. prohormone.

**pre•hos•pi•tal care** assessment, stabilization, and care of a medical emergency or trauma victim, including transport to the appropriate receiving facility.

**pre•hos•pi•tal care re•port** a written report completed by a prehospital provider, which contains demographic and medical information as well as a record of the treatment and transport of a patient. A copy of the prehospital care report is often left at the receiving facility as a medical reference and for inclusion in the patient's medical record.

**pre•hos•pi•tal pro•vi•der** one who provides care in case of medical emergency or trauma, most often an emergency medical technician (EMT) or paramedic. SYN emergency medical technician, paramedic.

**pre•ic•tal** (prē-ik′tăl) occurring before a seizure or stroke. [pre- + L. *ictus,* a stroke]

**pre•in•duc•tion** (prē-in-dŭk′shŭn) a modification in the third generation resulting from the action of environment on the germ cells of one or both individuals of the grandparental generation. An effect from the action of environment on the germ cells of progenitors upon their grandchildren. [L. *prae,* before, + *inductio,* a bringing in, fr. *induco,* to lead in]

**pre•in•farc•tion an•gi•na** SYN unstable angina.

**pre•kal•li•kre•in** (prē-kal-ĭ-krē′in) a plasma glycoprotein which in complex with kininogen serves as a cofactor in the activation of factor XII. Prekallikrein also serves as the proenzyme for plasma kallikrein. SYN Fletcher factor.

**pre•lam•i•nar branch of spi•nal branch of dor•sal branch of pos•te•ri•or in•ter•cos•tal ar•te•ry** *origin:* spinal artery in intervertebral foramen; *distribution:* to anterior surface of laminae and ligamenta flava of thoracic vertebrae and the anterior aspects of the zygapophysial joints.

**pre•leu•ke•mia** SYN myelodysplastic syndrome.

**pre•load** (prē′lōd) **1.** the load to which a muscle is subjected before shortening. **2.** SYN ventricular preload.

**pre•log•i•cal think•ing** a concrete type of thinking, characteristic of children and primitives, to which schizophrenic persons sometimes regress.

**pre•ma•lig•nant** (prē-mă-lig′nănt) SYN precancerous.

**pre•ma•ture** (prē-mă-toor′) **1.** occurring before the usual or expected time. **2.** denoting an infant born less than 37 weeks (8-1/2 months) after conception. [L. *praematurus,* too early, fr. *prae-,* pre- + *maturus,* ripe (mature)]

**pre•ma•ture birth** birth of an infant after viability has been achieved with gestation of at least 20 weeks or birth weight of at least 500 g, but before 37 weeks.

**pre•ma•ture de•liv•er•y** birth of a fetus before its proper time. SEE ALSO premature birth.

**pre•ma•ture e•jac•u•la•tion** during sexual intercourse, too rapid achievement of climax and ejaculation in the male relative to his own or his partner's wishes.

**pre•ma•ture la•bor** onset of labor before the 37th completed week of pregnancy dated from the last normal menstrual period.

**pre•ma•ture mem•brane rup•ture** rupture of the membranes before the onset of labor.

**pre•ma•ture men•o•pause** failure of cyclic ovarian function before age 40. SYN premature ovarian failure.

**pre•ma•ture ovar•i•an fail•ure** SYN premature menopause.

**pre•ma•ture sys•to•le** SYN extrasystole.

**pre•ma•tu•ri•ty** (prē-mă-toor′i-tē) **1.** the state of being premature. **2.** DENTISTRY deflective occlusal contact.

**pre•max•il•lary bone** SYN os incisivum.

**pre•med•i•ca•tion** (prē′med-i-kā′shŭn) **1.** administration of drugs before induction of general anesthesia to allay apprehension, produce sedation, and facilitate the administration of anesthetic. **2.** drugs used for such purposes.

**pre•men•stru•al** (prē-men′stroo-ăl) relating to the period of time preceding menstruation.

**pre•men•stru•al dys•phor•ic dis•or•der 1.** a pervasive pattern occurring during the last week of the luteal phase in most menstrual cycles for at least a year and remitting within a few days of the onset of the follicular phase, with some combination of depressed mood, mood lability, marked anxiety, or irritability; various specific physical symptoms; and significant functional impairment; the symptoms are comparable in severity to those seen in a major depressive episode, distinguishing this disorder from the far more common premenstrual syndrome. SEE ALSO premenstrual syndrome. **2.** a specified set of criteria in the DSM, proposed for the purpose of further research.

**pre•men•stru•al syn•drome (PMS)** in some women of reproductive age, the regular monthly experience of physiological and emotional distress, usually during the several days preceding menses; characterized by nervousness, depression, fluid retention, and weight gain. SYN late luteal phase dysphoria, menstrual molimina, premenstrual tension.

**pre•men•stru•al ten•sion** SYN premenstrual syndrome.

**pre•men•stru•um** (prē-men′stroo-ŭm) the few days preceding menstruation. [pre- + L. *menstruum,* ntr. of *menstruus,* monthly, pertaining to menstruation]

**pre•mo•lar** (prē-mō′lăr) **1.** anterior to a molar tooth. **2.** the permanent teeth that replace the deciduous molars. **3.** often referred to (incorrectly) as a bicuspid. SYN bicuspid (2).

**pre•mo•lar tooth** a tooth usually having two tubercles or cusps on the grinding surface and a flattened root, single in the lower jaw and upper second premolar, and furrowed in the upper first premolar. There are four premolars in each jaw, two on either side between the canine and the molars; there are no premolars in the deciduous dentition. SYN dens premolaris [TA], bicuspid tooth.

**pre•mon•o•cyte** (prē-mon′ō-sīt) an immature monocyte not normally seen in the circulating blood. SYN promonocyte.

**pre•mor•bid** (prē-mōr′bid) preceding the occurrence of disease. [pre- + L. *morbidus,* ill, fr. *morbus,* disease]

**pre•mu•ni•tion** (pre-moo-nish′ŭn) a state of existing resistance of a host to infection or reinfection with a parasite; used especially in malaria epidemiology. [L. *praemunitio,* fortification in advance, fr. *prae-,* + *munio,* to fortify]

**pre·mu·ni·tive** (prē-moo'ni-tiv) relating to premunition.

**pre·my·e·lo·blast** (prē-mī'ě-lō-blast) the earliest recognizable precursor of the myeloblast.

**pre·my·e·lo·cyte** (prē-mī'ě-lō-sīt) SYN promyelocyte.

**pre·nar·es**

**prenaris,** pl. **pre·nar·es** (prē-nā'ris) SYN nostril.

**pre·na·sal** (prē-nā'zǎl) in front of the nose.

**pre·na·tal** (prē-nā'tǎl) preceding birth. SYN antenatal. [pre- + L. *natus,* born]

**pre·na·tal di·ag·no·sis** diagnosis utilizing procedures available for the recognition of diseases and malformations *in utero,* and the conclusion reached.

**pre·ne·o·plas·tic** (prē'nē-ō-plas'tik) preceding the formation of any neoplasm, benign or malignant. [pre- + G. *neos,* new, + *plastikos,* formative]

**Pren·tice rule** (pren'tis) each centimeter of decentration of a lens results in 1 prism diopter of deviation of light for each diopter of lens power.

**pre·op·er·a·tive** (prē-op'er-ǎ-tiv) preceding an operation.

**pre·os·te·o·blast** (prē-os'tē-ō-blast) SYN osteoprogenitor cell.

**pre·ox·y·gen·a·tion** (prē'ok-sě-jě-nā'shŭn) denitrogenation with 100% oxygen prior to induction of general anesthesia.

**prep** (prep) to prepare the skin or other body surface for an operative procedure, usually by cleaning and application of antiseptic solutions. [slang for preparation or prepare]

**pre·pan·cre·at·ic ar·te·ry** *origin:* arises from dorsal pancreatic artery as its left terminal branch; *distribution:* often double, it runs between the neck and uncinate process of the pancreas to form an arterial arch (arcade) with the anterior superior pancreaticodoudenal artery. SYN arteria prepancreatica [TA].

**pre·pa·tel·lar bur·sa** a bursa between the skin and the lower part of the patella.

**pre·pa·tent pe·ri·od** PARASITOLOGY the period equivalent to the incubation period of microbial infections; it is biologically different, however, because the parasite is undergoing developmental stages in the host.

**pre·pon·der·ance** (prē-pon'der-ans) quality of outweighing, or exceeding in extent or importance.

**pre·po·ten·tial** (prē-pō-ten'shǎl) a gradual rise in potential between action potentials as a phasic swing in electric activity of the cell membrane, which establishes its rate of automatic activity, as in the ureter or cardiac pacemaker.

**pre·psy·chot·ic** (prē-sī-kot'ik) **1.** relating to the period before the onset of psychosis. **2.** denoting a potential for a psychotic episode, one that appears imminent under continued stress.

**pre·pu·ber·al, pre·pu·ber·tal** (prē-pyu'ber-ǎl, prē-pyu'ber-tǎl) before puberty.

**pre·pu·bes·cent** (prē-pyu-bes'ent) immediately prior to the commencement of puberty.

**pre·puce** (prē'pyus) the free fold of skin that covers more or less completely the glans penis. SYN preputium [TA], foreskin. [L. *praeputium,* foreskin]

**pre·puce of clit·o·ris** the external fold of the labia minora, forming a cap over the clitoris.

**pre·pu·ti·al** (pre-pyu'shē-ǎl) relating to the prepuce.

**pre·pu·ti·al cal·cu·lus** a calculus occurring beneath the foreskin.

**pre·pu·ti·al glands** sebaceous glands of the corona glandis and inner surface of the prepuce, which produce an odoriferous substance called smegma.

**pre·pu·ti·ot·o·my** (prē-pyu'shē-ot'ō-mē) incision of prepuce. [preputium + G. *tomē,* incision]

**pre·pu·ti·um,** pl. **pre·pu·tia** (prē-pyu'shē-ŭm, prē'pyu-shē-ǎ) [TA] SYN prepuce. [L. *praeputium*]

**pre·py·lor·ic vein** a tributary of the right gastric vein that passes anterior to the pylorus at its junction with the duodenum.

**pre·sac·ral fascia** layer of endopelvic fascia passing between sacrum and rectum, forming the anterior boundary of the presacral (retrorectal) fascial space, in which the hypogastric nervous plexus is embedded.

**pre·sa·cral neu·rec·to·my, pre·sa·cral sym··pa·thec·to·my** cutting of the presacral nerve to relieve severe dysmenorrhea. SYN Cotte operation.

△**pres·by-, pres·byo-** old age. SEE ALSO gero-. [G. *presbys,* old man]

**pres·by·a·cu·sis, pres·by·a·cu·si·a** (prez'bē-ǎ-koo'sis) loss of ability to perceive or discriminate sounds as a part of the aging process; the pattern and age of onset may vary. [presby- + G. *akousis,* hearing]

**pres·by·a·sta·sis** (prez'bǐ-ǎ-stā'sis) impairment of vestibular function associated with aging. [presby- + G. *a-* priv. + *stasis,* standing]

**pres·by·o·pia (Pr)** (prez-bē-ō'pē-ǎ) the physiologic loss of accommodation in the eyes in advancing age, said to begin when the near point has receded beyond 22 cm (9 inches). [presby- + G. *ōps,* eye]

**pres·by·op·ic** (prez'bē-op'ik) relating to or suffering from presbyopia.

**pre·scribe** (prē-skrīb') to give directions, either orally or in writing, for the preparation and administration of a remedy to be used in the treatment of any disease. [L. *prae-scribo,* pp. *-scriptus,* to write before]

**pre·scrip·tion** (prē-skrip'shŭn) **1.** a written formula for the preparation and administration of any remedy. **2.** a medicinal preparation compounded according to formulated directions, consisting of four parts: 1) *superscription,* consisting of the word *recipe,* take, or its sign, ℞; 2) *inscription,* the main part of the prescription, containing the names and amounts of the drugs ordered; 3) *subscription,* directions for mixing the ingredients and designation of the form (pill, powder, solution, etc.) in which the drug is to be made; 4) *signature,* directions to the patient regarding the dose and times of taking the remedy. [L. *praescriptio;* see prescribe]

**pre·se·nile** (prē-sē'nīl) prior to the usual onset of senility.

**pre·se·nile de·men·tia, de·men·ti·a pre·se·-ni·lis 1.** dementia of Alzheimer disease developing before age 65; **2.** SYN Alzheimer disease.

**pre·se·nil·i·ty** (prē-sě-nil'i-tē) premature old age; the condition of an individual, not old in years, who displays the physical and mental characteristics of old age but not to the extent of senility. [pre- + L. *senilis,* old]

**pre·sent** (prē-zent′) **1.** to precede or appear first at the os uteri, said of the part of the fetus first felt during examination. **2.** to appear for examination, treatment, etc., said of a patient. [L. *praesens* (*-sent-*), pres. p. of *prae-sum,* to be before, be at hand]

**pre·sen·ta·tion** (prē′zen-tā′shŭn) that part of the fetus presenting at the superior strait of the maternal pelvis; occiput, chin, and sacrum are, respectively, the determining points in vertex, face, and breech presentation. SEE ALSO position (3), present. [see present]

**pre·sep·tal cell·u·li·tis** infection involving the superficial tissue layers anterior to the orbital septum. SYN periorbital cellulitis.

**pre·ser·va·tive** (prē-zer′vă-tiv) a substance added to food products or to an organic solution to prevent chemical change or bacterial action.

**pre·so·mite** (prē-sō′mīt) relating to the embryonic stage before the appearance of somites (before day 19 in the human).

**pre·sphyg·mic** (prē-sfig′mik) preceding the pulse beat; denoting a brief interval following the filling of the ventricles with blood before their contraction forces open the semilunar valves, corresponding to the isovolumic contraction period. [pre- + G. *sphygmos,* pulse]

**pres·sor** (pres′er) exciting to vasomotor activity; producing increased blood pressure; denoting afferent nerve fibers which, when stimulated, excite vasoconstrictors which increase peripheral resistance. SYN hypertensor. [L. *premo,* pp. *pressus,* to press]

**pres·sor a·mine** SYN pressor base.

**pres·sor base 1.** one of several products of intestinal putrefaction believed to cause functional hypertension when absorbed; **2.** any alkaline substance that raises blood pressure. SYN pressor amine.

**pres·so·re·cep·tive** (pres′ō-rē-sep′tiv) capable of detecting or responding to changes in pressure, especially changes of blood pressure. SYN pressosensitive.

**pres·so·re·cep·tor** (pres′ō-rē-sep′ter) SYN baroreceptor.

**pres·sor fi·bers** sensory nerve fibers whose stimulation causes vasoconstriction and rise of blood pressure.

**pres·sor nerve** an afferent nerve, stimulation of which excites a reflex vasoconstriction, thereby raising the blood pressure.

**pres·so·sen·si·tive** (pres-ō-sen′si-tiv) SYN pressoreceptive.

**pres·sure** (presh′ŭr) **1.** a stress or force acting in any direction against resistance. **2.** (P, frequently followed by a subscript indicating location) in physics and physiology, the force per unit area exerted by a gas or liquid against the walls of its container or that would be exerted on a wall immersed at that spot in the middle of a body of fluid. The pressure can be considered either relative to some reference pressure, such as that of the ambient atmosphere (gauge pressure), or in absolute terms (relative to a perfect vacuum). [L. *pressura,* fr. *premo,* pp. *pressus,* to press]

**pres·sure al·o·pe·cia** loss of hair over a circumscribed area usually on the posterior scalp, resulting from the continuous pressure on the occiput

in a lengthy operative procedure, or unconsciousness following a drug overdose.

**pres·sure con·trolled ven·ti·la·tion** a mode of mechanical ventilation in which the ventilator delivers a preset pressure waveform; the resultant tidal volume and inspiratory flow depend on the shape of the pressure waveform and respiratory system resistance and compliance.

**pres·sure dress·ing** a dressing by which pressure is exerted on the area covered to prevent the collection of fluids in the underlying tissues; most commonly used after skin grafting and in the treatment of burns.

**pres·sure e·pi·phy·sis** a secondary center of ossification in the articular end of a long bone.

**pres·sure pa·ral·y·sis** paralysis due to compression of a nerve, nerve trunk, or spinal cord.

**pres·sure point** a cutaneous locus having pressure-sensitive elements that, when compressed, produce a sensation of pressure.

**pres·sure pulse dif·fer·en·ti·a·tion** the processing of a pressure pulse signal so that the output depends upon the rate of change of the input, yielding dP/dt (pressure) or, for noninvasively recorded pulses, dD/dt (rate of change of displacement).

**pres·sure re·ver·sal** cessation of anesthesia by hyperbaric pressure; of major importance in understanding the mode of action of anesthetics.

**pres·sure sense** the faculty of discriminating various degrees of pressure on the surface. SYN baraesthesia, baresthesia, piesesthesia.

**pres·sure sore** SYN decubitus ulcer.

**pres·sure sta·sis** SYN traumatic asphyxia.

**pres·sure sup·port ven·ti·la·tion (PSV)** a mode of mechanical ventilation in which spontaneous breaths are patient-triggered, pressure-limited, and flow-cycled.

**pres·sure tap·ping** SYN intermittent compression (1).

**pres·sure ul·cer** SYN decubitus ulcer.

**pres·sure ven·ti·la·tor** a device designed to deliver inspired gas into the lungs until a preset level of pressure is reached.

**pres·sure-vol·ume in·dex** method of evaluating the cerebrospinal fluid hydrodynamics.

**pres·sure wave·form** a graphic representation of intravascular or intracardiac pressure related to phases of the cardiac cycle, displayed on an oscilloscope monitor or paper copy.

**pre-steady state** those conditions and the time interval prior to establishment of steady state.

**pre·sumed oc·u·lar his·to·plas·mo·sis** subretinal neovascularization in the macular region associated with chorioretinal atrophy and pigment proliferation adjacent to the optic disk, and peripheral chorioretinal atrophy ("histo-spots").

**pre·sup·pu·ra·tive** (prē-sŭp′yu-rā-tiv) denoting an early stage in an inflammation prior to the formation of pus.

**pre·syn·ap·tic** (prē′si-nap′tik) pertaining to the area on the proximal side of a synaptic cleft.

**pre·syn·ap·tic mem·brane** that part of the plasma membrane of an axon terminal that faces the plasma membrane of the neuron or muscle fiber with which the axon terminal establishes a synaptic junction. SEE ALSO synapse.

**pre·sys·to·le** (prē-sis′tō-lē) that part of diastole immediately preceding systole.

**pre·sys·tol·ic** (prē-sis-tol′ik) late diastolic, relating to the interval immediately preceding systole.

**pre·sys·tol·ic gal·lop** gallop rhythm in which the gallop sound is an audible fourth heart sound due to forceful ventricular filling.

**pre·sys·tol·ic mur·mur** a murmur heard at the end of ventricular diastole (during atrial systole if in sinus rhythm), usually due to obstruction at one of the atrioventricular orifices.

**pre·sys·tol·ic thrill** a thrill immediately preceding the ventricular contraction, that is sometimes felt on palpation over the apex of the heart.

**pre·tar·sal** (prē-tar'săl) denoting the anterior, or inferior, portion of the tarsus.

**pre·term in·fant** an infant with gestational age of less than 37 completed weeks (259 completed days).

**pre·term mem·brane rup·ture** rupture of fetal membranes before term (<37 weeks gestation).

**pre·tib·i·al fe·ver** a mild disease first observed among military personnel at Fort Bragg, North Carolina, characterized by fever, moderate prostration, splenomegaly, and a rash on the anterior aspects of the legs; due to the *autumnalis* serovar of *Leptospira interrogans*. SYN Fort Bragg fever.

**pre·tib·i·al myx·e·de·ma** SYN circumscribed myxedema.

**prev·a·lence** (prev'ă-lens) the number of cases of a disease existing in a given population at a specific period of time (*period prevalence*) or at a particular moment in time (*point prevalence*).

**pre·ven·tive** (prē-ven'tiv) SYN prophylactic (1). [L. *prae-venio*, pp. *-ventus*, to come before, prevent]

**pre·ven·tive den·tis·try** a philosophy and method of dental practice which seeks to prevent the initiation, progression, and recurrence of dental caries.

**pre·ven·tive med·i·cine** the branch of medical science concerned with the prevention of disease and with promotion of physical and mental health, through study of the etiology and epidemiology of disease processes.

**pre·ver·te·bral gan·glia** the sympathetic ganglia (celiac, aorticorenal, superior and inferior mesenteric) lying in front of the vertebral column, as distinguished from the ganglia of the sympathetic trunk (paravertebral ganglia); these ganglia occur mostly around the origin of the major branches of the abdominal aorta; all are in the abdominopelvic cavity, concerned with innervation of abdominopelvic viscera.

**pre·ver·te·bral lay·er of cer·vi·cal fa·scia** the part of the cervical fascia that covers the bodies of the cervical vertebrae and the muscles attaching to them and to the anterior parts of their transverse processes.

**pre·vi·us** (prē'vē-ŭs) obstructing; denoting anything blocking the passages in childbirth. [L. *prae*, before, + *via*, way]

*Pre·vo·tel·la* (prev'ō-tel'ah) genus of Gram-negative, nonmotile, nonsporeforming, obligately anaerobic, chemoorganotrophic, and pleomorphic rods; contains many species previously classified in the genus Bacteroides.

*Pre·vo·tel·la bi·vi·a* the species of *Prevotella* in highest concentration in the human vaginal tract.

*Pre·vo·tel·la den·ti·co·la* a bacterial species found in the human mouth; a cause of infections of the oral cavity and adjacent structures.

*Pre·vo·tel·la he·par·i·no·ly·ti·ca* a bacterial species associated with human periodontal disease.

*Pre·vo·tel·la in·ter·me·di·a* a species found in gingival crevices, especially associated with gingivitis, and other oral infections.

*Pre·vo·tel·la mel·a·nin·o·ge·ni·ca* a species found in the mouth, feces, infections of the mouth, soft tissue, respiratory tract, urogenital tract, and the intestinal tract. Implicated in periodontal disease; seen in aspiration pneumonitis. The type species of *Prevotella*. SYN *Bacteroides melaninogenicus*.

**PRF** prolactin-releasing factor.

**PRH** prolactin-releasing hormone.

**pri·a·pism** (prī'ă-pizm) persistent erection of the penis, accompanied by pain and tenderness, resulting from a pathologic condition rather than sexual desire.

**Price-Jones curve** (prīs-jōnz) a distribution curve of the measured diameters of red blood cells.

**prick·le cell** one of the cells of the stratum spinosum of the epidermis; so called because of shrinkage artifacts that occur in histological preparations, resulting in intercellular bridges at points of desmosomal adhesion.

**prick·le cell lay·er** SYN stratum spinosum epidermidis.

**prick·ly heat** SYN miliaria rubra.

**pri·mal** (prī'măl) **1.** first or primary. **2.** SYN primordial (2).

**pri·mal scene** PSYCHOANALYSIS the actual or fantasized observation by a child of sexual intercourse, particularly between its parents.

**pri·mary** (prī'mār-ē) **1.** the first or foremost, as a disease or symptoms to which others may be secondary or occur as complications. **2.** relating to the first stage of growth or development. SEE primordial. [L. *primarius*, fr. *primus*, first]

**pri·mary ad·he·sion** SYN healing by first intention.

**pri·mary a·dre·no·cor·ti·cal in·suf·fi·cien·cy** adrenocortical insufficiency caused by disease, destruction, or surgical removal of the adrenal cortices.

**pri·mary al·co·hol** an alcohol characterized by the univalent radical, —CH$_2$OH.

**pri·mary al·do·ste·ron·ism** an adrenocortical disorder caused by excessive secretion of aldosterone and characterized by headaches, nocturia, polyuria, fatigue, hypertension, potassium depletion, hypokalemic alkalosis, hypervolemia, and decreased plasma renin activity; may be associated with small benign adrenocortical adenomas. SYN Conn syndrome, idiopathic aldosteronism.

**pri·mary amen·or·rhea** amenorrhea in which the menses have never occurred.

**pri·mary amine** SEE amine.

**pri·mary am·y·loi·do·sis** amyloidosis not associated with other recognized disease. Tends to involve arterial walls and mesenchymal tissues in the tongue, lungs, intestinal tract, skin, skeletal muscle, and myocardium; the amyloid frequently does not manifest the usual affinity for Congo red, and sometimes provokes a foreign-body type of inflammatory reaction.

**pri·mary an·es·thet·ic** the compound that contributes most to loss of sensation when a mixture of anesthetics is administered.

**pri·mary at·el·ec·ta·sis** nonexpansion of the lungs after birth, found in all stillborn infants and in liveborn infants who die before respiration is established.

**pri·mary a·typ·i·cal pneu·mo·nia** an acute

systemic disease with involvement of the lungs, caused by *Mycoplasma pneumoniae* and marked by high fever, cough, relatively few physical signs, and scattered densities on x-rays; usually associated with development of cold agglutinins and antibodies to the bacteria. SYN atypical pneumonia, mycoplasmal pneumonia.

**pri•mary brain ves•i•cle** SYN cerebral vesicle.

**pri•mary care** health care services such as family practice, internal medicine, obstetrics/gynecology, or pediatrics that are the first point of health care for a patient in an ambulatory setting.

**pri•mary care phy•si•cian** physician in family practice, internal medicine, obstetrics/gynecology, or pediatrics who is a patient's first contact for health care in an ambulatory setting. SEE ALSO health care provider.

**pri•mary com•plex** the typical lesions of primary pulmonary tuberculosis, consisting of a small peripheral focus of infection, with hilar or paratracheal lymph node involvement.

**pri•mary de•men•tia** dementia occurring independently as a mental disorder.

**pri•mary den•tin** dentin which forms until the root is completed.

**pri•mary den•ti•tion** SYN deciduous tooth.

**pri•mary de•vi•a•tion** the ocular deviation seen in paralysis of an ocular muscle when the nonparalyzed eye is used for fixation.

**pri•mary di•ges•tion** digestion in the alimentary tract.

**pri•mary dis•ease** a disease that arises spontaneously and is not associated with or caused by a previous disease, injury, or event, but which may lead to a secondary disease.

**pri•mary dye test** assessment of lacrimal drainage following the fluorescein instillation test by attempting to recover fluorescein dye beneath the inferior turbinate using a swab. SYN Jones I test.

**pri•mary dys•men•or•rhea** dysmenorrhea due to a functional disturbance and not due to inflammation, new growths, or anatomic factors. SYN essential dysmenorrhea, functional dysmenorrhea, intrinsic dysmenorrhea.

**pri•mary fis•sure of cer•e•bel•lum** the deepest fissure of the cerebellum; demarcates the division of anterior and posterior lobes of the cerebellum; second to appear embryologically.

**pri•mary gain** interpersonal, social, or financial advantages from the conversion of emotional stress directly into illness (e.g., hysterical blindness or paralysis). Cf. secondary gain.

**pri•mary he•mo•chro•ma•to•sis** a specific inherited metabolic defect with increased absorption and accumulation of iron on a normal diet.

**pri•mary hem•or•rhage** hemorrhage immediately after an injury or operation, as distinguished from intermediate or secondary hemorrhage.

**pri•mary her•pet•ic gin•gi•vo•sto•ma•ti•tis** SYN primary herpetic stomatitis.

**pri•mary her•pet•ic sto•ma•ti•tis** first infection of oral tissues with herpes simplex virus; characterized by gingival inflammation, vesicles, and ulcers. SYN primary herpetic gingivostomatitis.

**pri•mary im•mune re•sponse** SEE immune response.

**pri•mary lat•er•al scle•ro•sis** considered by many to be a subgroup of motor neuron disease; a slowly progressive degenerative disorder of the motor neurons of the cerebral cortex, resulting in widespread weakness on an upper motor neuron basis; spasticity, hyperreflexia, and Babinski signs are present, but not fasciculation potentials, nor any electrodiagnostic evidence of a lower motor neuron lesion.

**pri•mary ly•so•somes** lysosomes produced at the Golgi apparatus where hydrolytic enzymes are incorporated; they fuse with phagosomes or pinosomes to become secondary lysosomes.

**pri•mary non•dis•junc•tion** nondisjunction occurring in a previously normal cell.

**pri•mary nur•sing** a way of providing nursing services for inpatients whereby one nurse plans the care of specific patients for a period of 24 hours. The primary nurse provides direct care to those patients when on duty and is responsible for directing and supervising their care by means of care plans, conferences, and referrals, in collaboration with other health care team members.

**pri•mary oo•cyte** an oocyte during its growth phase and before it completes the first maturation division.

**pri•mary ovar•i•an fol•li•cle** an ovarian follicle before the appearance of an antrum; marked by developmental changes in the oocyte and follicular cells so that the latter form one or more layers of cuboidal or columnar cells; the follicle becomes surrounded by a sheath of stroma, the theca.

**pri•mary pro•cess** PSYCHOANALYSIS the mental process directly related to the functions of the primitive life forces associated with the id and characteristic of unconscious mental activity; marked by unorganized, illogical thinking and by the tendency to seek immediate discharge and gratification of instinctual demands. Cf. secondary process.

**pri•mary pro•gres•sive a•pha•sia** a degenerative disorder of which the early major symptom is an aphasia that increases in severity and (usually) eventually includes dementia.

**pri•mary pul•mo•nary lob•ule** SYN pulmonary acinus.

**pri•mary se•nile de•men•tia** SYN Alzheimer disease.

**pri•mary sex char•ac•ters** the sex glands, testes or ovaries, and the accessory sex organs.

**pri•mary sper•ma•to•cyte** the spermatocyte derived by a growth phase from a spermatogonium, and that undergoes the first division of meiosis.

**pri•mary stut•ter•ing** a pattern of dysfluency characterized by easy repetitions of words or parts of words, unaccompanied by signs of anxiety; may be a precursor of more severe stuttering.

**pri•mary syph•i•lis** the first stage of syphilis SEE syphilis.

**pri•mary tooth** SYN deciduous tooth.

**pri•mary tu•ber•cu•lo•sis** first infection by *Mycobacterium tuberculosis*, typically seen in children but also occurs in adults, characterized in the lungs by the formation of a primary complex consisting of small peripheral pulmonary focus with spread to hilar or paratracheal lymph nodes; may cavitate or heal with scarring or may progress.

**pri•mary un•ion** SYN healing by first intention.

**pri•mate** (prī′māt) an individual of the order Primates. [L. *primus,* first]

**pri•mi•grav•i•da** (prī-mi-grav′i-dă) SEE gravida.

[L. fr. *primus,* first, + *gravida,* a pregnant woman]

**pri·mip·a·ra** (prī-mip′ă-ră) a woman who has given birth for the first time. SEE para. [L. fr. *primus,* first, + *pario,* to bring forth]

**pri·mi·par·i·ty** (prī-mi-par′i-tē) condition of being a primipara.

**pri·mip·a·rous** (prī-mip′ă-rŭs) denoting a primipara.

**prim·i·tive** (prim′i-tiv) SYN primordial (2). [L. *primitivus,* fr. *primus,* first]

**prim·i·tive groove** the median depression in the primitive streak flanked by the primitive ridges.

**prim·i·tive gut** a flat sheet of intraembryonic endoderm that becomes a tubular gut due to the folding of embryonic body—head, tail and lateral body folds. SYN primordial gut.

**prim·i·tive knot** SYN primitive node.

**prim·i·tive node** a local thickening of the blastoderm at the cephalic end of the primitive streak of the embryo. SYN Hensen node, primitive knot.

**prim·i·tive streak** an ectodermal ridge in the midline at the caudal end of the embryonic disk from which arises the intraembryonic mesoderm; achieved by inward and then lateral migration of cells; in human embryos, it appears on day 15 and gives a cephalocaudal axis to the developing embryo.

**pri·mor·dia** (prī-mōr′dē-ă) plural of primordium.

**pri·mor·di·al** (prī-mōr′dē-ăl) **1.** relating to a primordium. **2.** relating to a structure in its first or earliest stage of development. SYN primal (2), primitive.

**pri·mor·di·al gut** a flat sheet of intraembryonic endoderm that will change into a tubular gut due to the folding of embryonic body—head, tail and lateral body folds. SYN primitive gut.

**pri·mor·di·al ovar·i·an fol·li·cle** a follicle in which the primary oocyte is surrounded by a single layer of flattened follicular cells.

**pri·mor·di·um** (prī-mōr′dē-ŭm) an aggregation of cells in the embryo indicating the first trace of an organ or structure. SYN anlage (1). [L. origin, fr. *primus,* first, + *ordior,* to begin]

**prin·ceps,** pl. **prin·ci·pes** (prin′seps, prin′si-pēz) principal. ANATOMY term used to distinguish the largest or most important of several arteries. [L. chief, fr. *primus,* first, + *capio,* to take, choose]

**prin·ceps pol·li·cis ar·te·ry** origin, radial (deep palmar (arterial) arch); *distribution,* palmar surface and sides of thumb; *anastomoses,* arteries on dorsum of thumb.

**prin·ci·pal di·ag·no·sis** diagnosis found, after testing and study, to be the main reason for the patient's need for health care services.

**prin·ci·pal op·tic ax·is** a line passing through the center of the lens of a refracting system at right angles to its surface.

**prin·ci·pal point** one of two points on an optic axis so related that an object at one is exactly imaged at the other without magnification, minification, or inversion.

**prin·ci·ple** (prin′si-pl) **1.** a general or fundamental doctrine or tenet. SEE ALSO law, rule, theorem. **2.** the essential ingredient in a substance, especially one that gives it its distinctive quality or effect. [L. *principium,* a beginning, fr. *princeps,* chief]

**PR in·ter·val** in the electrocardiogram, the time elapsing between the beginning of the P wave and the beginning of the next QRS complex; it

corresponds to the a-c interval of the venous pulse and is normally 0.12–0.20 sec. SYN PQ interval.

**Prinz·met·al an·gi·na** a form of angina pectoris, characterized by pain that is not precipitated by cardiac work, is of longer duration, is usually more severe, and is associated with unusual electrocardiographic manifestations including elevated ST segments in leads that are ordinarily depressed in typical angina, and usually without reciprocal ST changes; occurring at night in bed in EKG leads in which ST segment depression occurs in typical angina. SYN angina inversa, variant angina pectoris, variant angina.

**pri·on** (prī′on) SYN prion protein. [proteinaceous infectious particle]

**pri·on pro·tein** small, infectious proteinaceous particle, of non-nucleic acid composition; the causative agent of four spongiform encephalopathies in humans: kuru, Creutzfeldt-Jakob disease, Gerstmann-Straussler-Scheinker syndrome, and fatal familial insomnia. The gene encoding for the PrP is found on chromosome 20. SYN prion.

**prism** (prizm) a transparent solid, with sides that converge at an angle, that deflects a ray of light toward the thickest portion (the base) and splits white light into its component colors; in spectacles, a prism corrects ocular muscle imbalance. [G. *prisma*]

**pris·ma,** pl. **pris·ma·ta** (priz′mă, priz′mah-tă) a structure resembling a prism. [G. something sawed, a prism]

**pris·m bar** a graduated series of prism bars mounted on a frame and used in ocular diagnosis.

**pri·sm di·op·ter** the unit of measurement of the deviation of light in passing through a prism, being a deflection of 1 cm at a distance of 1 m.

**pri·va·cy** (prī′vă-sē) **1.** being apart from others; seclusion; secrecy. **2.** especially in psychiatry and clinical psychology, respect for the confidential nature of the therapist-patient relationship.

**pri·vate du·ty nurse 1.** a nurse who is not a member of a hospital staff, but is hired on a fee-for-service basis to care a patient; **2.** a nurse who specializes in the care of patients with diseases of a particular class, e.g., surgical cases, tuberculosis, children's diseases.

**pri·vate hos·pi·tal 1.** a hospital similar to a group hospital except that it is controlled by a single practitioner or by the practitioner and the associates in his or her office; **2.** a hospital operated for profit.

**priv·i·leged site** an anatomic area lacking lymphatic drainage, such as the brain, cornea, and hamster cheek pouch, in which heterologous tumors may grow because the host does not become sensitized.

**PRN** pro re nata

**PRO** peer-review organization.

**Pro** proline or its radicals.

△**pro- 1.** before, forward. SEE ALSO ante-, pre-. **2.** CHEMISTRY prefix indicating precursor of. SEE ALSO -gen. [L. and G. *pro*]

**pro·ac·cel·er·in** (prō-ak-sel′er-in) SYN factor V.

**pro·ac·ro·so·mal gran·ules** small carbohydrate-rich granules appearing in vesicles of the Golgi apparatus of spermatids; they coalesce into a single acrosomal granule contained within an acrosomal vesicle.

**pro·ac·ti·va·tor** (prō-ak′ti-vā-ter) a substance that, when chemically split, yields a fragment (activator) capable of rendering another substance enzymatically active.

**prob·a·bil·i·ty 1.** a measure, ranging from zero to 1, of the degree of belief in a hypothesis or statement. **2.** the limit of the relative frequency of an event in a sequence of N random trials as N approaches infinity.

**pro·bac·te·ri·o·phage** (prō-bak-tēr'ē-ō-fāj) the stage of a temperate bacteriophage in which the genome is incorporated in the genetic apparatus of the bacterial host. SYN prophage.

**pro·band** (prō'band) HUMAN GENETICS the patient or member of the family that brings a family under study. SYN index case. [L. *probo,* to test, prove]

**probe** (prōb) **1.** a slender rod of flexible material, with blunt bulbous tip, used for exploring sinuses, fistulas, other cavities, or wounds. **2.** a device or agent used to detect or explore a substance; e.g., a molecule used to detect the presence of a specific fragment of DNA or RNA or of a specific bacterial colony. **3.** to enter and explore, as with a probe. [L. *probo,* to test]

**probe sy·ringe** a syringe with an olive-shaped tip, used in treatment of diseases of the lacrimal passages.

**pro·bi·o·sis** (prō-bī-o-ō'sis) an association of two organisms that enhances the life processes of both. Cf. antibiosis (1), symbiosis, mutualism. [pro- + G. *biōsis,* life]

**pro·bi·ot·ic** (prō-bī-ot'ik) relating to probiosis.

**prob·lem-o·ri·ent·ed med·i·cal rec·ord (POR, POMR)** a medical record model designed to organize patient information by the presenting problem. The record includes the patient database, problem list, plan of care, and progress notes in an accessible format.

**pro·cap·sid** (prō-kap'sid) a protein shell lacking a virus genome.

**pro·car·box·y·pep·ti·dase** (prō'kar-bok-sē-pep'ti-dās) inactive precursor of a carboxypeptidase.

**pro·car·y·ote** (pro-kar'ē-ōt) SYN prokaryote. [pro- + G. *karyon,* kernel, nut]

**pro·car·y·ot·ic** (prō'kar-ē-ot'ik) SYN prokaryotic.

**pro·ce·dure** (prō-sē'jŭr) act or conduct of diagnosis, treatment, or operation. SEE ALSO method, operation, technique.

**pro·ce·lia** (prō-sē'lē-ă) a lateral ventricle of the brain; the hollow of the prosencephalon. SYN procoele. [pro- + G. *koilos,* hollow]

**pro·cen·tri·ole** (prō-sen'trē-ōl) the early phase in development *de novo* of centrioles or basal bodies from the centrosphere; procentrioles form in relation to deuterosomes (procentriole organizers).

**pro·ce·phal·ic** (prō-se-fal'ik) relating to the anterior part of the head. [pro- + G. *kephalē,* head]

**pro·ce·rus mus·cle** *insertion,* into frontalis; *action,* assists frontalis; *origin,* from membrane covering bridge of nose; *nerve supply,* branch of facial. SYN musculus procerus [TA].

**pro·cess** (pros'es) **1.** in anatomy, a projection or outgrowth. SYN processus [TA]. **2.** a method or mode of action used in the attainment of a certain result. **3.** a natural progression, development, or sequence of events, as in the progress of a disease. SEE processus. **4.** a pathologic condition or disease. **5.** in dentistry, a series of operations that convert a wax pattern, such as that of a denture base, into a solid denture base of another

material. [L. *processus,* an advance, progress, process, fr. *pro-cedo,* pp. *-cessus,* to go forward]

**pro·ces·sing** the activity of effecting a series of changes in something so as to achieve a particular result.

**pro·ces·sor** (pră'ses-sŏr) a device that converts one form of energy into another form of energy or one form of material into another form of material.

**pro·ces·sus,** pl. **pro·ces·sus** (prō-ses'ŭs) [TA] SYN process (1). [L. see process]

**pro·ces·sus ar·ti·cu·la·ris** [TA] SYN articular process.

**pro·ces·sus cli·noi·de·us an·te·ri·or** [TA] SYN anterior clinoid process.

**pro·ces·sus fal·ci·for·mis** [TA] SYN falciform process.

**pro·ces·sus va·gi·na·lis of per·i·to·ne·um** a peritoneal diverticulum in the embryonic lower anterior abdominal wall that traverses the inguinal canal; in the male it forms the tunica vaginalis testis and normally loses its connection with the peritoneal cavity; a persistent processus vaginalis in the female is known as the canal of Nuck.

**pro·ces·sus xi·phoi·de·us** [TA] SYN xiphoid process.

**pro·chon·dral** (prō-kon'drăl) denoting a developmental stage prior to the formation of cartilage. [pro- + G. *chondros,* cartilage]

**pro·chy·mo·sin** (prō-kī'mō-sin) the precursor of chymosin. SYN prorennin, renninogen, rennogen.

**pro·ci·den·tia** (pros-i-den'shē-ă) a sinking down or prolapse of any organ or part. [L. a falling forward, fr. *procido,* to fall forward]

**procoele** (prō'sēl) SYN procelia.

**pro·coel·ia [Br.]** SEE procelia.

**pro·col·la·gen** (prō-kol'ă-jen) soluble precursor of collagen formed by fibroblasts and other cells in the process of collagen synthesis.

**pro·con·ver·tin** (prō-kon-ver'tin) SYN factor VII.

**pro·cre·ate** (prō'krē-āt) to beget; to produce by the sexual act. [L. *pro-creo,* pp. *-creatus,* to beget]

**pro·cre·a·tion** (prō-krē-ā'shŭn) SYN reproduction (2).

**pro·cre·a·tive** (prō'krē-ā-tiv) having the power to beget or procreate.

**proc·tal·gia** (prok-tal'jē-ă) pain at the anus, or in the rectum. SYN proctodynia, rectalgia. [proct- + G. *algos,* pain]

**proc·ta·tre·sia** (prok-tă-trē'zē-ă) SYN anal atresia. [proct- + G. *a-* priv. + *trēsis,* a boring]

**proc·tec·to·my** (prok-tek'tō-mē) surgical resection of the rectum. SYN rectectomy. [proct- + G. *ektomē,* excision]

**proc·ti·tis** (prok-tī'tis) inflammation of the mucous membrane of the rectum. SYN rectitis. [proct- + G. *-itis,* inflammation]

△**proct·o-, proct-** anus; (more frequently) rectum; Cf. recto-. [G. *prōktos*]

**proc·to·cele** (prok'tō-sēl) prolapse or herniation of the rectum. SYN rectocele. [procto- + G. *kēlē,* tumor]

**proc·to·cly·sis** (prok-tok'li-sis) slow, continuous administration of saline solution by instillation into the rectum and sigmoid colon. SYN Murphy drip. [procto- + G. *klysis,* a washing out]

**proc·to·coc·cy·pexy** (prok-tō-kok'si-pek-sē) suture of a prolapsing rectum to the tissues anterior to the coccyx. SYN rectococcypexy. [procto- + G. *kokkyx,* coccyx, + *pēxis,* fixation]

**proc•to•co•lec•to•my** (prok'tō-kō-lek'tō-mē) surgical removal of the rectum together with part or all of the colon. [procto- + G. *kolon,* colon, + *ektomē,* excision]

**proc•to•co•lo•nos•co•py** (prok'tō-kō'lō-nos'kō-pē) inspection of the interior of the rectum and colon. [procto- + G. *kolon,* colon, + *skopeō,* to view]

**proc•to•col•po•plas•ty** (prok'tō-kol'pō-plas-tē) surgical closure of a rectovaginal fistula. [procto- + G. *kolpos,* bosom (vagina), + *plastos,* formed]

**proc•to•cys•to•plas•ty** (prok'tō-sis'tō-plas-tē) surgical closure of a rectovesical fistula. [procto- + G. *kystis,* bladder, + *plastos,* formed]

**proc•to•cys•tot•o•my** (prok'tō-sis-tot'ō-mē) incision into the bladder from the rectum. [procto- + G. *kystis,* bladder, + *tomē,* incision]

**proct•o•dae•um [Br.]** SEE proctodeum.

**proc•to•de•al** (prok'tō-dē-ăl) relating to the proctodeum.

**proc•to•de•um,** pl. **proc•to•dea** (prok-tō-dē'ŭm, prok'tō-dē'ă) **1.** an ectodermally lined depression under the root of the tail, adjacent to the terminal part of the embryonic hindgut; at its bottom, proctodeal ectoderm and cloacal endoderm form the cloacal plate. When this epithelial plate ruptures, the anal and urogenital external orifices are established. SYN anal pit. **2.** terminal portion of the insect alimentary canal. [L. fr. G. *prōktos,* anus + *hodaios,* on the way, fr. *hodos,* a way]

**proc•to•dyn•ia** (prok'tō-din'ē-ă) SYN proctalgia. [procto- + G. *odynē,* pain]

**proc•to•log•ic** (prok-tō-loj'ik) relating to proctology.

**proc•tol•o•gist** (prok-tol'ō-jist) a specialist in proctology.

**proc•tol•o•gy** (prok-tol'ō-jē) surgical specialty concerned with the anus and rectum and their diseases. [procto- + G. *logos,* study]

**proc•to•pa•ral•y•sis** (prok'tō-pa-ral'i-sis) paralysis of the anus, leading to incontinence of feces.

**proc•to•pexy** (prok'tō-pek-sē) surgical fixation of a prolapsing rectum. SYN rectopexy. [procto- + G. *pēxis,* fixation]

**proc•to•plas•ty** (prok'tō-plas-tē) plastic surgery of the anus or rectum. SYN rectoplasty. [procto- + G. *plastos,* formed]

**proc•to•ple•gia** (prok'tō-plē'jē-ă) paralysis of the anus and rectum occurring with paraplegia. [procto- + G. *plēgē,* stroke]

**proc•top•to•sia, proc•top•to•sis** (prok-top-tō'sē-ă, prok-top-tō'sis) prolapse of the rectum and anus. [procto- + G. *ptōsis,* a falling]

**proc•tor•rha•phy** (prok-tōr'ă-fē) repair by suture of a lacerated rectum or anus. [procto- + G. *rhaphē,* suture]

**proc•tor•rhea** (prok-tō-rē'ă) a mucoserous discharge from the rectum. [procto- + G. *rhoia,* a flow]

**proc•to•scope** (prok'tō-skōp) a rectal speculum. SYN rectoscope. [procto- + G. *skopeō,* to view]

**proc•tos•co•py** (prok-tos'kŏ-pē) visual examination of the rectum and anus, as with a proctoscope.

**proc•to•sig•moi•dec•to•my** (prok'tō-sig-moy-dek'tō-mē) excision of the rectum and sigmoid colon. [procto- + sigmoid, + G. *ektomē,* excision]

**proc•to•sig•moi•di•tis** (prok'tō-sig-moy-dī'tis)

inflammation of the sigmoid colon and rectum. [procto- + sigmoid + G. *-itis,* inflammation]

**proc•to•sig•moi•dos•co•py** (prok'tō-sig-moy-dos'kŏ-pē) direct inspection through a sigmoidoscope of the rectum and sigmoid colon. [procto- + sigmoid + G. *skopeō,* to view]

**proc•to•spasm** (prok'tō-spazm) **1.** spasmodic stricture of the anus. **2.** spasmodic contraction of the rectum. [procto- + G. *spasmos,* spasm]

**proc•to•ste•no•sis** (prok'tō-stĕ-nō'sis) stricture of the rectum or anus. SYN rectostenosis. [procto- + G. *stenōsis,* a narrowing]

**proc•tos•to•my** (prok-tos'tō-mē) the formation of an artificial opening into the rectum. SYN rectostomy. [procto- + G. *stoma,* mouth]

**proc•tot•o•my** (prok-tot'ō-mē) an incision into the rectum. SYN rectotomy. [procto- + G. *tomē,* incision]

**proc•to•tre•sia** (prok-tō-trē'zē-ă) operation for correction of an imperforate anus. [procto- + G. *trēsis,* a boring]

**proc•to•val•vot•o•my** (prok'tō-val-vot'ō-mē) incision of rectal valves.

**pro•cur•sive ep•i•lep•sy** a psychomotor attack initiated by whirling or running.

**pro•dro•mal** (prō-drō'măl, prod'rō'măl) relating to a prodrome. SYN prodromic, prodromous.

**pro•dro•mal stage** SYN incubation period (1).

**pro•dro•mal symp•tom** an early symptom of a disease.

**pro•drome** (prō'drōm) an early or premonitory symptom of a disease. [G. *prodromos,* a running before, fr. pro- + *dromos,* a running, a course]

**pro•dro•mic, pro•dro•mous** (prō-drō'mik, prod'rō-mik; prō-drō-mŭs) SYN prodromal.

**pro•drug** (prō'drŭg) a class of drugs, the pharmacologic action of which results from conversion by metabolic processes within the body (biotransformation).

**pro•duct** (prod'ŭkt) **1.** anything produced or made, either naturally or artificially. **2.** MATHEMATICS the result of multiplication. [L. *productus,* fr. *pro-duco,* pp. *-ductus,* to lead forth]

**pro•duc•tive** (prō-dŭk'tiv) producing or capable of producing; denoting especially an inflammation leading to the production of new tissue with or without an exudate. [see product]

**pro•duct•ive cough** a cough accompanied by expectoration.

**pro•en•zyme** (prō-en'zīm) the precursor of an enzyme, requiring some change (usually the hydrolysis of an inhibiting fragment that masks an active grouping) to render it active; e.g., pepsinogen, trypsinogen, profibrinolysin. SYN zymogen.

**pro•e•ryth•ro•blast** (prō-ĕ-rith'rō-blast) SYN pronormoblast.

**pro•e•ryth•ro•cyte** (prō-ĕ-rith'rō-sīt) the precursor of an erythrocyte; an immature red blood cell with a nucleus.

**pro•es•tro•gen** (prō-es'trō-jen) a substance that acts as an estrogen only after it has been metabolized in the body to an active compound.

**pro•es•trus** (prō-es'trŭs) the period preceding estrus, characterized by heightened follicular activity and estrogen production. [pro- + estrus]

**Pro•fe•ta law** (prō'fe-tah) the subject of congenital syphilis is immune to the acquired disease.

**pro•fi•bri•nol•y•sin** (prō'fī-bri-nol'i-sin) SEE plasmin.

**pro•fi•cien•cy sam•ples** samples sent to a laboratory as unknowns to allow an external assessment of laboratory performance, a frequent practice as part of proficiency testing programs to ensure the laboratory is generating correct results. SEE ALSO proficiency testing.

**pro·fi·cien·cy test·ing** a program in which specimens of quality control material are periodically sent to members of a group of laboratories for analysis, with each laboratory's results compared with those of its peers. SEE ALSO proficiency samples.

**pro·file** (prō'fīl) **1.** an outline or contour, especially one representing a side view of the human head. SYN norma. **2.** a summary, brief account, or record. [It. *profilo,* fr. L. *pro,* forward, + *filum,* thread, line (contour)]

**pro·fun·da bra·chii ar·tery** *origin,* brachial; *distribution,* humerus and muscles and integument of arm; *anastomoses,* posterior circumflex humeral, radial recurrent, recurrent interosseous, ulnar collateral, i.e., articular vascular network of elbow. SYN deep artery of arm.

**pro·fun·da fem·o·ris ar·tery** *origin,* femoral; *branches,* lateral circumflex femoral, medial circumflex femoral, terminating in three or four perforating arteries.

**pro·gas·trin** (prō-gas'trin) precursor of gastric secretion in the mucous membrane of the stomach.

**pro·ge·nia** (prō-jē'nē-ă) SYN prognathism. [pro- + L. *gena,* cheek]

**pro·gen·i·tor** (prō-jen'i-ter) a precursor, ancestor; one who begets. [L.]

**prog·e·ny** (proj'ě-nē) offspring; descendants. [L. *progenies,* fr. *progigno,* to beget]

**pro·ge·ria** (prō-jēr'ē-ă) a condition in which normal development in the first year is followed by gross retardation of growth, with a senile appearance characterized by dry wrinkled skin, total alopecia, and birdlike facies; genetics unclear. SYN Hutchinson-Gilford disease. [pro- + G. *gēras,* old age]

**pro·ges·ta·tion·al** (prō'jes-tā'shŭn-ăl) **1.** favoring pregnancy; conducive to gestation; capable of stimulating the uterine changes essential for implantation and growth of a fertilized ovum. **2.** referring to progesterone, or to a drug with progesterone-like properties.

**pro·ges·ta·tion·al hor·mone** SYN progesterone.

**pro·ges·ter·one** (ap'op-tō-sis) 4-pregnene-3,20-dione; an antiestrogenic steroid, believed to be the active principle of the corpus luteum, isolated from the corpus luteum and placenta or synthetically prepared; used to correct abnormalities of the menstrual cycle, as a contraceptive, and to control habitual abortion. SYN corpus luteum hormone, luteohormone, progestational hormone.

**pro·gest·er·one chal·lenge test** administration of a progestational agent in case of amenorrhea to detect the presence of an estrogen-primed endometrium.

**pro·gest·er·one re·cep·tor** intracellular receptor for progesterone; often over-expressed in breast cancer.

**pro·ges·tin** (prō-jes'tin) **1.** a hormone of the corpus luteum. **2.** generic term for any substance, natural or synthetic, that effects some or all of the biological changes produced by progesterone. [pro- + gestation + -in]

**pro·ges·to·gen** (prō-jes'tō-jen) **1.** any agent capable of producing biological effects similar to those of progesterone; most progestogens are ste-

roids like the natural hormones. **2.** a synthetic derivative from testosterone or progesterone that has some of the physiologic activity and pharmacologic effects of progesterone; progesterone is antiestrogenic, whereas some progestogens have estrogenic or androgenic properties in addition to progestational activity. [pro- + gestation + G. *-gen,* producing]

**pro·glos·sis** (prō-glos'is) the anterior portion, or tip, of the tongue. [pro- + G. *glōssa,* tongue]

**pro·glot·tid** (prō-glot'id) one of the segments of a tapeworm, containing the reproductive organs. SYN proglottis. [pro- + G. *glōssa,* tongue]

**pro·glot·tis,** pl. **pro·glot·ti·des** (prō-glot'is, prō-glot'i-dēz) SYN proglottid.

**prog·nath·ic** (prog-nath'ik, prog-nā'thik) **1.** having a projecting jaw; having a gnathic index above 103. **2.** denoting a forward projection of either or both of the jaws relative to the craniofacial skeleton. SYN prognathous. [pro- + G. *gnathos,* jaw]

**prog·na·thism** (prog'nă-thizm) the condition of being prognathic; abnormal forward projection of one or of both jaws beyond the established normal relationship with the cranial base; the mandibular condyles are in their normal rest relationship to the temporomandibular joints. SYN progenia.

**prog·na·thous** (prog'nă-thŭs) SYN prognathic.

**prog·no·sis** (prog-nō'sis) a forecast of the probable course and/or outcome of a disease. [G. *prognōsis,* fr. *pro,* before, + *gignōskō,* to know]

**prog·nos·tic** (prog-nos'tik) **1.** relating to prognosis. **2.** a symptom upon which a prognosis is based, or one indicative of the likely outcome. [G. *prognōstikos*]

**prog·nos·ti·cate** (prog-nos'ti-kāt) to give a prognosis.

**prog·nos·ti·cian** (prog-nos-tish'ŭn) one skilled in prognosis.

**pro·gram 1.** a formal set of procedures for conducting an activity. **2.** an ordered list of instructions directing a computer to carry out a desired sequence of operations required to solve a problem.

**pro·gram·ma·ble hear·ing aid** multichannel hearing aid that can use more than one level-dependent frequency response strategy.

**pro·grammed cell death** SYN apoptosis.

**pro·gram·ming** (prō'gram-ing) sequential instruction; a method of training in discrete segments.

**pro·gran·u·lo·cyte** (prō-gran'yu-lō-sīt) SYN promyelocyte.

**pro·gress·ive** (prō-gres'iv) going forward; advancing; denoting the course of a disease, especially, when unqualified, an unfavorable course.

**pro·gres·sive bul·bar pa·ral·y·sis** progressive weakness and atrophy of the muscles of the tongue, lips, palate, pharynx, and larynx; most often caused by motor neuron disease. SYN bulbar paralysis.

**pro·gres·sive cat·a·ract** a cataract in which the opacification process progresses to involve the entire lens.

**pro·gres·sive chor·oi·dal a·tro·phy** SYN choroideremia.

**pro·gres·sive hy·per·tro·phic pol·y·neu·rop·a·thy** SYN Dejerine-Sottas disease.

**pro·gres·sive mul·ti·fo·cal leu·ko·en·ceph·a·lop·a·thy** (PML) a rare, subacute, afebrile disease characterized by areas of demyelinization surrounded by markedly altered neuroglia, including inclusion bodies in glial cells; it occurs usually in individuals with AIDS, leukemia, lymphoma, or other debilitating diseases, or in those who have been receiving immunosuppressive treatment. Caused by JC virus, a human polyoma virus.

**pro·gres·sive mus·cu·lar at·ro·phy** SYN amyotrophic lateral sclerosis.

**pro·gres·sive out·er ret·i·nal ne·cro·sis (PORN)** a viral syndrome occurring in AIDS patients, caused by herpesvirus and characterized by destruction of peripheral retina.

**pro·gres·sive-re·sis·tance ex·er·cise (PRE)** the practical application of the overload principle in order to improve muscular strength and size. Resistance is gradually and continually increased to keep pace with strength gains as training progresses.

**pro·gres·sive stain·ing** a procedure in which staining is continued until the desired intensity of coloring of tissue elements is attained.

**pro·gres·sive tap·e·to·chor·oi·dal dys·tro·phy** SYN choroideremia.

**pro·hor·mone** (prō-hōr'mōn) an intraglandular precursor of a hormone; e.g., proinsulin. Cf. prehormone.

**pro·in·su·lin** (prō-in'sŭ-lin) a single-chain precursor of insulin.

**pro·jec·tile vom·it·ing** expulsion of the contents of the stomach with great force.

🔲**pro·jec·tion** (prō-jek'shŭn) **1.** a pushing out; an outgrowth or protuberance. **2.** the referring of a sensation to the object producing it. **3.** a defense mechanism by which a repressed complex in the individual is denied and conceived as belonging to another person, as when faults which the person tends to commit are perceived in or attributed to others. **4.** the conception by the consciousness of a mental occurrence belonging to the self as of external origin. **5.** localization of visual impressions in space. **6.** NEUROANATOMY the system or systems of nerve fibers by which a group of nerve cells discharges its nerve impulses ("projects") to one or more other cell groups. **7.** the image of a three-dimensional object on a plane, as in a radiograph. **8.** RADIOGRAPHY a standard x-ray study, named by body part, position, the direction of the x-ray beam through the body part, or eponym. See page APP 96-7. [L. *projectio;* fr. *pro- jicio,* pp. *-jectus,* to throw before]

**pro·jec·tion an·gi·o·gram** a digital angiogram, such as in computed tomography or magnetic resonance imaging, reconstructed by computer to appear as does a radiographic angiogram.

**pro·jec·tion fi·bers** nerve fibers connecting the cerebral cortex with other centers in the brain or spinal cord; fibers arising from cells in the central nervous system that pass to distant loci.

**pro·jec·tive i·den·ti·fi·ca·tion** a defensive attribution of one's own psychic processes to another person.

**pro·kar·y·ote** (prō-kar'ē-ōt) a member of the superkingdom Prokaryotae; an organism consisting of a single cell, or a precellular organism, which lacks a nuclear membrane, paired organized chromosomes, a mitotic mechanism for cell division, microtubules, and mitochondria. SEE ALSO eukaryote. SYN procaryote.

**pro·kar·y·ot·ic** (prō'kar-ē-ot'ik) pertaining to or characteristic of a prokaryote. SYN procaryotic.

**pro·la·bi·um** (prō-lā'bē-ŭm) **1.** the exposed carmine margin of the lip. **2.** the isolated central soft-tissue segment of the upper lip in the embryonic state and in an unrepaired bilateral cleft palate. [pro- + L. *labium,* lip]

**pro·lac·tin** (prō-lak'tin) a protein hormone of the anterior lobe of the hypophysis that stimulates the secretion of milk and possibly, during pregnancy, breast growth. SYN lactogenic hormone. [pro- + L. *lac, lact-,* milk, + -in]

**pro·lac·tin-in·hib·it·ing fac·tor (PIF)** SYN prolactostatin.

**pro·lac·tin-in·hib·it·ing hor·mone (PIH)** SYN prolactostatin.

**pro·lac·ti·no·ma** (prō-lak-ti-nō'mă) SYN prolactin-producing adenoma.

**pro·lac·tin-pro·duc·ing ad·e·no·ma** a pituitary adenoma composed of prolactin-producing cells; it gives rise to symptoms of nonpuerperal amenorrhea and galactorrhea (Forbes-Albright syndrome) in women and to impotence in men. SYN prolactinoma.

**pro·lac·tin-re·leas·ing fac·tor (PRF)** SYN prolactoliberin.

**pro·lac·tin-re·leas·ing hor·mone** SYN prolactoliberin.

**pro·lac·to·lib·er·in** (prō-lak-tō-lib'er-in) a substance of hypothalamic origin that stimulates the release of prolactin. SYN prolactin-releasing factor, prolactin-releasing hormone. [prolactin + L. *libero,* to free, + -in]

**pro·lac·to·stat·in** (prō-lak-tō-stat'in) a substance of hypothalamic origin capable of inhibiting the synthesis and release of prolactin. SYN prolactin-inhibiting factor, prolactin-inhibiting hormone. [prolactin + G. *stasis,* standing still, + -in]

**pro·lapse** (prō-laps') **1.** to sink down, said of an organ or other part. **2.** a sinking of an organ or other part, especially its appearance at a natural or artificial orifice. SEE ALSO procidentia, ptosis. [L. *prolapsus,* a falling]

**pro·lapse of um·bil·i·cal cord** presentation of part of the umbilical cord ahead of the fetus; it may cause fetal death due to compression of the cord between the presenting part of the fetus and the maternal pelvis.

**pro·lapse of the uter·us** downward movement of the uterus due to laxity and atony of the muscular and fascial structures of the pelvic floor, usually resulting from injuries of childbirth or advanced age.; prolapse occurs in three forms. SEE **first degree prolapse, second degree prolapse, third degree prolapse**.

**pro·lec·tive** (prō'lek-tiv) pertaining to data collected by planning in advance proportional mortality ratio. Number of deaths from a given cause in a specified period, per 100 or per 1000 total deaths. [pro- + L. *lego,* pp. *lectum,* to gather]

**pro·lep·sis** (prō-lep'sis) recurrence of the paroxysm of a periodical disease at regularly shortening intervals. [G. *prolēpsis,* anticipation]

**pro·lep·tic** (prō-lep'tik) relating to prolepsis.

**pro·li·dase** (prō'li-dās) SYN proline dipeptidase.

**pro·lif·er·ate** (prō-lif'ě-rāt) to grow and increase in number by means of reproduction of similar forms. [L. *proles,* offspring, + *fero,* to bear]

**pro·lif·er·at·ing cell nu·cle·ar ant·i·gen** a nuclear nonhistone protein with a molecular weight of 36 kd that plays a role in the initiation of cell proliferation by augmenting DNA polymerase; stains for proliferating cell nuclear antigen in tumors correlate with grade and mitotic activity.

**pro·lif·er·a·tion** (prō-lif-ĕ-rā'shŭn) growth and reproduction of similar cells.

**pro·lif·er·a·tive, pro·lif·er·ous** (prō-lif'er-ă-tiv, prō-lif-er-ŭs) increasing the numbers of similar forms.

**pro·lif·er·a·tive in·flam·ma·tion** an inflammatory reaction in which the distinguishing feature is an increase in the number of tissue cells, especially the reticuloendothelial macrophages, rather than of cells exuded from blood vessels.

**pro·lif·er·a·tive ret·i·nop·a·thy** neovascularization of the retina extending into the vitreous humor. SYN retinitis proliferans.

**pro·lig·er·ous** (prō-lij'er-ŭs) germinating; producing offspring. [L. *proles,* offspring, + *gero,* to bear]

**pro·li·nase** (prō'li-nās) SYN prolyl dipeptidase.

**pro·line (Pro)** (prō'lēn) an amino acid found in proteins, especially the collagens.

**pro·line di·pep·ti·dase** an enzyme cleaving aminoacyl-L-proline bonds in dipeptides containing a C-terminal prolyl residue; a deficiency of this enzyme results in hyperimidodipeptiduria. SYN prolidase.

**pro·line im·i·no·pep·ti·dase** [EC 3.4.11.5] a hydrolase cleaving L-proline residues from the N-terminal position in peptides.

**pro·longed preg·nan·cy** SYN postdate pregnancy.

**pro·lyl** (prō'lil) the acyl radical of proline.

**pro·lyl di·pep·ti·dase** an enzyme cleaving L-prolyl-amino acid bonds in dipeptides containing N-terminal prolyl residues. SYN prolinase.

**pro·mas·ti·gote** (prō-mas'ti-gōt) the flagellate stage of a trypanosomatid protozoan in which the flagellum arises from a kinetoplast in front of the nucleus and emerges from the anterior end of the organism; usually an extracellular phase, as in the insect intermediate host (or in culture) of *Leishmania* parasites. [pro- + G. *mastix,* whip]

**pro·meg·a·lo·blast** (prō-meg'ă-lō-blast) the earliest of four maturation stages of the megaloblast. SEE erythroblast.

**pro·met·a·phase** (prō-met'ă-fāz) the stage of mitosis or meiosis in which the nuclear membrane disintegrates and the centrioles reach the poles of the cell, while the chromosomes continue to contract.

**pro·me·thi·um (Pm)** (prō-mē'thē-ŭm) a radioactive element of the rare earth series, atomic no. 61; [145]Pm has the longest known half-life (17.7 years). [*Prometheus,* a Titan of G. myth who stole fire to give to mortals]

**prom·i·nence** (prom'i-nens) ANATOMY tissues or parts that project beyond a surface. SYN prominentia. [L. *prominentia*]

**prom·i·nent heel** a condition marked by a tender swelling on the os calcis due to a thickening of the periosteum or fibrous tissue covering the back of the os calcis.

**prom·i·nen·tia**, pl. **prom·i·nen·ti·ae** (prom-i-nen'shē-ă, prom-i-nen'shē-ē) SYN prominence. [L. fr. *promineo,* to jut out, be prominent]

**PROMM** proximal myotonic myopathy.

**pro·mon·o·cyte** (prō-mon'ō-sīt) SYN premonocyte.

**prom·on·to·ry** (prom'on-tō-rē) an eminence or

projection. A projection of a part. [L. *promontorium*]

**prom·on·tory flush** SYN Schwartze sign.

**pro·mot·er** (prō-mō'ter) **1.** CHEMISTRY a substance that increases the activity of a catalyst. **2.** MOLECULAR BIOLOGY a DNA sequence at which RNA polymerase binds and initiates transcription.

**pro·mot·ing a·gent** SEE promotion.

**pro·mo·tion** (prō-mō'shŭn) stimulation of tumor induction, following initiation, by a promoting agent which may of itself be noncarcinogenic.

**pro·my·e·lo·cyte** (prō-mī'ĕ-lō-sīt) **1.** the developmental stage of a granular leukocyte between the myeloblast and myelocyte, when a few specific granules appear in addition to azurophilic ones. **2.** a large uninuclear cell occurring in the circulating blood of persons with myelocytic leukemia. SYN premyelocyte, progranulocyte. [pro- + G. *myelos,* marrow, + *kytos,* cell]

**pro·na·si·on** (prō-nā'zē-on) the point of the angle between the septum of the nose and the surface of the upper lip, found at the point where a tangent applied to the nasal septum meets the upper lip. [pro- + L. *nasus,* nose]

**pro·nate** (prō'nāt) **1.** to assume, or to be placed in, a prone position. **2.** to perform pronation of the forearm or foot. [L. *pronatus,* fr. *prono,* pp. *-atus,* to bend forward, fr. *pronus,* bent forward]

■ **pro·na·tion** (prō-nā'shŭn) the condition of being prone; the act of assuming or of being placed in a prone position. See page APP 91.

**pro·na·tor** (prō-nā'ter, prō-nā'tōr) a muscle which turns a part into the prone position. SEE muscle. [L.]

**pro·na·tor quad·ra·tus mus·cle** *origin,* distal fourth of anterior surface of ulna; *insertion,* distal fourth of anterior surface of radius; *action,* pronates forearm; *nerve supply,* anterior interosseous. SYN musculus pronator quadratus [TA].

**pro·na·tor syn·drome** entrapment of the median nerve in the forearm between the heads of the pronator teres muscle.

**pro·na·tor te·res mus·cle** *origin,* superficial (humeral) head (ulnar) from the common flexor origin on the medial epicondyle of the humerus, deep (ulnar) head from the medial side of the coronoid process of the ulna; *insertion,* middle of the lateral surface of the radius; *action,* pronates forearm; *nerve supply,* median. SYN musculus pronator teres [TA].

**pro·na·tor te·res syn·drome** entrapment or compression of the median nerve in the proximal forearm, usually where the nerve passes between the two heads of the pronator teres muscle.

**prone** (prōn) **1.** denoting the position of the body when lying face downward. **2.** the position of hand or foot with volar surface downward. [L. *pronus,* bending down or forward]

**pro·neph·ros,** pl. **pro·neph·roi** (prō-nef'ros, prō-nef'roy) **1.** the definitive excretory organ of primitive fishes. **2.** in the embryos of higher vertebrates, a vestigial structure consisting of a series of tortuous tubules emptying into the cloaca by way of the primary nephric duct; in the human embryo, the pronephros is a very rudimentary and temporary structure, followed by the mesonephros and still later by the metanephros. [pro- + G. *nephros,* kidney]

**pro·nor·mo·blast** (prō-nōr'mō-blast) the earliest of four stages in development of the normoblast.

SEE ALSO erythroblast. SYN proerythroblast, rubriblast.

**pro•nu•cle•us,** pl. **pro•nu•clei** (prō-noo′klē-ŭs, prō-noo′klē-ī) **1.** one of a pair of nuclei undergoing fusion in karyogamy. **2.** EMBRYOLOGY the nuclear material of the head of the spermatozoon (male pronucleus) or of the oocyte (female pronucleus), after the oocyte has been penetrated by the spermatozoon; each pronucleus normally carries a haploid set of chromosomes, so that the merging of the pronuclei in fertilization reestablishes the diploidy.

**pro•opi•o•mel•a•no•cor•tin (POMC)** (prō-ō′ pē-ō-mel′ă-nō-kōr′tin) a large molecule found in the anterior and intermediate lobes of the pituitary gland, the hypothalamus, and other parts of the brain as well as in the lungs, gastrointestinal tract, and placenta; the precursor of ACTH, CLIP, β-LPH, γ-MSH, β-endorphin, and met-enkephalin.

**pro•o•tic** (prō-ō′tik) in front of the ear. [pro- + G. *ous,* ear]

**prop•a•gate** (prop′ă-gāt) **1.** to reproduce; to generate. **2.** to move along a fiber, e.g., propagation of the nerve impulse. [L. *propago,* pp. *-atus,* to generate, reproduce]

**prop•a•ga•tion** (prop-ă-gā′shŭn) the act of propagating.

**prop•a•ga•tive** (prop-ă-gā′tiv) relating to or concerned in propagation; denoting the sexual part of an animal or plant as distinguished from the soma.

**pro•pane** (prō′pān) one of the alkane series of hydrocarbons.

**pro•par•a•thy•roid hor•mone** the immediate precursor of parathyroid hormone.

**pro•pep•sin** (prō-pep′sin) SYN pepsinogen.

**pro•per•din** (prō-per′din) a group of proteins involved in resistance to infection that participate, in conjunction with other factors, in an alternate pathway to the activation of the terminal components of complement. SEE ALSO properdin system, component of complement. [pro- + L. *perdo,* to destroy]

**pro•per•din fac•tor A** a component of the properdin system; a hydrazine-sensitive β₁-globulin now known to be C3 (third component of complement).

**pro•per•din fac•tor B** a normal serum protein and a component of the properdin system.

**pro•per•din fac•tor D** a normal serum α-globulin required in the properdin system.

**pro•per•din fac•tor E** a serum protein required for activation of C3 (third component of complement) by cobra venom factor. SEE ALSO properdin system.

**pro•per•din sys•tem** an immunological system that is the alternative pathway for complement, composed of several distinct proteins that react in a serial manner and activate C3 (third component of complement); the system can be activated, in the absence of specific antibody, by bacterial endotoxins, and a variety of polysaccharides and lipopolysaccharides.

**pro•phage** (prō′fāj) SYN probacteriophage.

**pro•phase** (prō′fāz) the first stage of mitosis or meiosis, consisting of linear contraction and increase in thickness of the chromosomes (each composed of two chromatids) accompanied by migration of the two daughter centrioles and their

asters toward the poles of the cell. [G. *prophasis,* from *prophainō,* to foreshadow]

**pro•phy•lac•tic** (prō-fi-lak′tik) **1.** preventing disease; relating to prophylaxis. SYN preventive. **2.** an agent that acts to prevent a disease. [G. *prophylaktikos;* see prophylaxis]

**pro•phy•lac•tic treat•ment** the institution of measures designed to protect a person from an attack of a disease to which he or she has been, or is liable to be, exposed.

**pro•phy•lax•is,** pl. **pro•phy•lax•es** (prō-fi-lak′ sis, prō-fi-lak′sēz) prevention of disease or of a process that can lead to disease. [Mod. L. fr. G. *pro-phylassō,* to guard before, take precaution]

**pro•pi•o•nate** (prō′pē-ō-nāt) a salt or ester of propionic acid.

*Pro•pi•on•i•bac•te•ri•um* (prō-pē-on-i-bak-tēr′ē-ŭm) a genus of nonmotile, nonsporeforming, anaerobic to aerotolerant bacteria containing Grampositive rods which are usually pleomorphic, diphtheroid, or club-shaped with one end rounded, the other tapered or pointed. The cells usually occur singly, in pairs, in V and Y configurations, short chains, or clumps. These organisms occur in dairy products, on human skin, and in the intestinal tracts of humans and other animals. They may be pathogenic. The type species is *Propionibacterium freudenreichii.*

**pro•pi•on•ic ac•id** (prō-pē-on′ik as′id) methylacetic acid; ethylformic acid; found in sweat.

**pro•por•tion•ate dwarf•is•m** dwarfism characterized by a symmetric shortening of the limbs and trunk; generally results from chemical, endocrine, nutritional, or nonosseous abnormalities.

**pro•po•si•tion•al speech** intellectual, rational use of language for specific communication goals. SEE automatic speech.

**pro•pos•i•tus,** pl. **pro•po•si•ti** (prō′poz′i-tŭs, prō′poz′i-tī) **1.** proband distinguished by sex. **2.** a premise; an argument. [L. fr. *propono,* pp. *-positus,* to lay out, propound]

**pro•pri•e•tary med•i•cine** a medicinal compound the formula and mode of manufacture of which are the property of the maker.

**pro•pri•e•tary name** (prō-prī′ĕ-tār-ē nām) the protected brand name or trademark, registered with the U.S. Patent Office, under which a manufacturer markets a product. It is written with a capital initial letter, if appropriate, and is often further distinguished by a superscript R in a circle (®). Cf. generic name, nonproprietary name. [L. *proprietarius*]

**pro•pri•o•cep•tion** (prō-prē-ō-sep′shun) a sense or perception, usually at a subconscious level, of the movements and position of the body and especially its limbs, independent of vision; this sense is gained primarily from input from sensory nerve terminals in muscles and tendons (muscle spindles) and the fibrous capsule of joints combined with input from the vestibular apparatus. SEE ALSO exteroceptor.

**pro•pri•o•cep•tive** (prō′prē-ō-sep′tiv) capable of receiving stimuli originating in muscles, tendons, and other internal tissues. [L. *proprius,* one's own, + *capio,* to take]

**pro•pri•o•cep•tive mech•a•nism** the mechanism of sense of position and movement, by which muscular movements can be adjusted to a great degree of accuracy and equilibrium maintained.

**pro•pri•o•cep•tive neu•ro•mus•cu•lar fa•cil•i•ta•tion (PNF)** a massage technique using passive muscle stretching and resisted muscular contractions to reduce resting tension mediated by Golgi tendon organs and muscle spindles. SEE ALSO muscle energy technique.

**pro·pri·o·cep·tive sen·si·bil·i·ty** SEE proprioceptive.

**pro·pri·o·cep·tor** (prō'prē-ō-sep'ter) one of a variety of sensory end organs (such as the muscle spindle and Golgi tendon organ) in muscles, tendons, and joint capsules.

**prop·to·sis** (prop-tō'sis) SYN exophthalmos. [G. *proptōsis*, a falling forward]

**prop·tot·ic** (prop-tot'ik) referring to proptosis.

**pro·pul·sion** (prō-pŭl'shŭn) the tendency to fall forward; responsible for the festination in paralysis agitans. [G. *pro-pello*, pp. *-pulsus*, to drive forth]

**pro·pyl (Pr)** (prō'pil) the alkyl radical of propane, $CH_3CH_2CH_2-$.

**pro·pyl al·co·hol** ethylcarbinol; a solvent for resins and cellulose esters.

**pro·py·lene** (prō'pi-lēn) methylethylene; a gaseous olefinic hydrocarbon.

**pro re na·ta (PRN)** (prō rē nā'tă) as the occasion arises; as necessary. [L.]

**pro·ren·nin** (prō-rēn'in) SYN prochymosin.

**pro·ru·bri·cyte** (prō-roo'bri-sīt) basophilic normoblast. SEE erythroblast. [pro- + rubricyte]

**pro·se·cre·tin** (prō-sē-krē'tin) unactivated secretin.

**pro·sect** (prō-sekt') to dissect a cadaver or any part, that it may serve for a demonstration of anatomy before a class. [L. *pro-seco*, pp. *-sectus*, to cut]

**pro·sec·tor** (prō'sek'ter) one who prosects, or prepares the material for a demonstration of anatomy before a class.

**pros·en·ceph·a·lon** (pros-en-sef'ă-lon) the anterior primitive cerebral vesicle and the most rostral of the three primary brain vesicles of the embryonic neural tube; it subdivides to form the diencephalon and telencephalon. SYN forebrain. [G. *prosō*, forward, + *enkephalos*, brain]

**pro·se·rum pro·throm·bin con·ver·sion ac·cel·er·a·tor (PPCA)** SYN factor VIII.

**pros·o·dem·ic** (pros-ō-dem'ik) denoting a disease that is transmitted directly from person to person. [G. *prosō*, forward, + *dēmos*, people]

**pros·o·dy** (proz'ŏ-dē) the varying rhythm, stress, and frequency of speech that aids meaning transmission.

**pros·o·pag·no·sia** (pros'ō-pag-nō'sē-ă) difficulty in recognizing familiar faces. [prosop- + G. *a*-priv. + *gnōsis*, recognition]

**pros·o·pal·gia** (pros-ō-pal'jē-ă) SYN trigeminal neuralgia. [prosop- + G. *algos*, pain]

**pros·o·pal·gic** (pros-ō-pal'jik) relating to or suffering from trigeminal neuralgia.

**pros·o·pla·sia** (pros-ō-plā'zē-ă) progressive transformation, such as the change of cells of the salivary ducts into secreting cells. SEE cytomorphosis. [G. *prosō*, forward, + *plasis*, a molding]

**⟳pro·sopo-, pro·sop-** the face. SEE ALSO facio-. [G. *prosōpon*]

**pros·o·po·di·ple·gia** (pros'ō-pō-dī-plē'jē-ă) paralysis affecting both sides of the face. [prosopo- + diplegia]

**pros·o·po·neu·ral·gia** (pros'ō-pō-noo-ral'jē-ă) SYN trigeminal neuralgia.

**pros·o·po·ple·gia** (pros'ō-pō-plē'jē-ă) SYN facial paralysis. [prosopo- + G. *plēgē*, stroke]

**pros·o·po·ple·gic** (pros'ō-pō-plē'jik) relating to, or suffering from, facial paralysis.

**pros·o·pos·chi·sis** (pros-ō-pos'ki-sis) congenital facial cleft from mouth to the inner canthus of the eye. [prosopo- + G. *schisis*, fissure]

**pros·o·po·spasm** (pros'ō-pō-spazm) SYN facial tic. [prosopo- + G. *spasmos*, spasm]

**pros·pec·tive pay·ment sys·tem (PPS)** arrangement mandated by the Tax Equity and Fiscal Responsibility Act of 1982 (TEFRA) to control Medicare costs; payment for services provided to a Medicare patient is fixed and adjusted annually by the Health Care Financing Administration (HCFA); payment is based on assigned diagnosis-related groups (DRGs).

**pros·ta·no·ic ac·id** (pros'tă-nō-ik as'id) the 20-carbon acid that is the skeleton of the prostaglandins.

**pros·ta·ta** (pros'tah-tă) [TA] SYN prostate. [Mod. L. from G. *prostatēs*, one standing before]

**pros·ta·tal·gia** (pros-tă-tal'jē-ă) a rarely used term for pain in the area of the prostate gland. [prostat- + G. *algos*, pain]

**pros·tate** (pros'tāt) a chestnut-shaped body, surrounding the beginning of the urethra in the male, that consists of two lateral lobes connected anteriorly by an isthmus and posteriorly by a middle lobe lying above and between the ejaculatory ducts. In structure, the prostate consists of 30 to 50 compound tubuloalveolar glands between which is abundant stroma consisting of collagen and elastic fibers and many smooth muscle bundles. The secretion of the glands is a milky fluid that is discharged by excretory ducts into the prostatic urethra at the time of the emission of semen. USAGE NOTE: Often mispronounced prostrate, and so misspelled. SYN prostata [TA], prostate gland.

**pros·ta·tec·to·my** (pros-tă-tek'tō-mē) removal of a part or all of the prostate. [prostat- + G. *ektomē*, excision]

**pros·tate gland** SYN prostate.

**pros·tate-spe·cif·ic an·ti·gen (PSA)** a single chain 31 kilodalton glycoprotein with 240 amino acid residues and 4 carbohydrate side chains that is a kallikrein protease; found in normal seminal fluid and produced by the prostatic epithelial cells. Elevated levels of PSA in blood serum are associated with prostatic enlargement and prostatic adenocarcinoma, and this allows early detection of cancer in many cases. In about 70% of cases, the rise is due to a cancerous condition. Thus, some studies have suggested that PSA testing may supplement an older test for prostatic acid phosphatase (PAP), previously a fairly reliable gauge of metastatic prostate cancer. However, because no large-scale clinical studies have been completed, the medical and economic value of PSA testing remains uncertain. SYN human glandular kallikrein 3.

**pros·tat·ic** (pros-tat'ik) relating to the prostate.

**pros·tat·ic cal·cu·lus** a concretion formed in the prostate gland, composed chiefly of calcium carbonate and phosphate (corpora amylacea).

**pros·tat·ic duc·tules, pros·tat·ic ducts** about 20 minute canals that receive the prostatic secretion from the glandular tubules and discharge it through openings on either side of the urethral crest in the posterior wall of the urethra. SYN ductuli prostatici [TA].

**p**
**r**

**pros•tat•ic flu•id** succus prostaticus; a whitish secretion that is one of the constituents of semen.

**pros•tat•ic in•tra•ep•i•the•li•al ne•o•pla•si•a (PIN)** dysplastic changes involving glands and ducts of the prostate which may be a precursor of adenocarcinoma; low grade (PIN 1), mild dysplasia with variation in nuclear size and shape and irregular cell spacing; high grade (PIN 2 and 3), moderate to severe dysplasia with nucleomegaly, nucleolomegaly, and irregular cell spacing.

**pros•tat•ic mas•sage 1.** manual expression of prostatic secretions by digital rectal technique; **2.** the emptying of prostatic sinuses and ducts by repeated downward compression maneuvers; used in the treatment of various congestive and inflammatory prostatic conditions.

**pros•tat•ic si•nus** the groove on either side of the urethral crest in the prostatic part of the urethra into which the prostatic ducts open.

**pros•tat•ic utri•cle** a minute pouch in the prostate opening on the summit of the seminal colliculus, the analogue of the uterus and vagina in the female. SYN utriculus prostaticus [TA], masculine uterus, Morgagni sinus (2), vesica prostatica.

**pros•ta•tism** (pros'tă-tizm) a syndrome, occurring mostly in older men, usually caused by enlargement of the prostate gland and manifested by irritative (nocturia, frequency, decreased voided volume, sensory urgency, and urgency incontinence) and obstructive (hesitancy, decreased stream, terminal dribbling, double voiding, and urinary retention) symptoms.

**pros•ta•ti•tis** (pros-tă-tī'tis) inflammation of the prostate. [prostat- + G. -itis, inflammation]

△**pros•ta•to-, pros•tat-** the prostate gland. [Med. L. prostata fr. G. prostatēs, one who stands before, protects]

**pros•ta•to•cys•ti•tis** (pros'tă-tō-sis-tī'tis) inflammation of the prostate and the bladder; cystitis by extension of inflammation from the prostatic urethra. [prostato- + G. kystis, bladder, + -itis, inflammation]

**pros•ta•to•li•thot•o•my** (pros'tă-tō-li-thot'ō-mē, pros-tat'ō-li-thot'ō-mē) incision of the prostate for removal of a calculus. [prostato- + G. lithos, stone, + tomē, incision]

**pros•ta•to•meg•a•ly** (pros'tă-tō-meg'ă-lē) enlargement of the prostate gland. [prostato- + G. megas, large]

**pros•ta•tor•rhea** (pros'tă-tō-rē'ă) an abnormal discharge of prostatic fluid. [prostato- + G. rhoia, a flow]

**pros•ta•tor•rhoea [Br.]** SEE prostatorrhea.

**pros•ta•tot•o•my** (pros'tă-tot'ō-mē) an incision into the prostate. [prostato- + G. tomē, incision]

**pros•ta•to•ve•sic•u•lec•to•my** (pros'tă-tō-ve-sik'yu-lek'tō-mē) surgical removal of the prostate gland and seminal vesicles.

**pros•ta•to•ve•sic•u•li•tis** (pros'tă-tō-ve-sik'yu-lī'tis) inflammation of the prostate gland and seminal vesicles.

**pros•the•sis,** pl. **pros•the•ses** (pros'thē-sis, pros'thē-sēz) fabricated substitute for a diseased or missing part of the body. [G. an addition]

**pros•thet•ic** (pros-thet'ik) **1.** relating to a prosthesis or to an artificial part. **2.** SEE prosthetic group.

**pros•thet•ic group** a non-amino acid compound attached to a protein, often in a reversible fashion, that confers new properties upon the conjugated protein thus produced. SEE ALSO coenzyme.

**pros•thet•ics** (pros-thet'iks) the art and science of

making and adjusting artificial parts of the human body.

**pros•the•tist** (pros'the-tist) one skilled in constructing and fitting prostheses.

**pros•thi•on** (pros'thē-on) the most anterior point on the maxillary alveolar process in the midline. SYN alveolar point. [G. ntr. of prosthios, foremost]

**pros•tho•don•tics** (pros-thō-don'tiks) the science of and art of providing suitable substitutes for the coronal portions of teeth, or for one or more lost or missing teeth and their associated parts, in order that impaired function, appearance, comfort, and health of the patient may be restored. [L. prosthodontia, fr. G. prosthesis + odous (odont-), tooth]

**pros•tho•don•tist** (pros-thō-don'tist) a dentist engaged in the practice of prosthodontics.

**pros•tra•tion** (pros-trā'shŭn) a marked loss of strength, as in exhaustion. [L. pro-sterno, pp. -stratus, to strew before, overthrow]

△**prot-** SEE proteo-, proto-.

**prot•ac•tin•i•um (Pa)** (prō-tak-tin'ē-ŭm) a radioactive element, atomic no. 91, atomic wt. 231.03588, formed in the decay of uranium and thorium; its longest-lived isotope, $^{231}$Pa, has a half-life of 32,500 years. [G. prōtos, first]

**prot•a•mine** (prō'tă-mēn) any of a class of proteins found in fish spermatozoa in combination with nucleic acid; neutralizes anticoagulant action of heparin.

**pro•ta•no•pia** (prō'tă-nō'pē-ă) a form of dichromatism characterized by absence of the red-sensitive pigment in cones, decreased luminosity for long wavelengths of light, and confusion in recognition of red and green. [G. prōtos, first, + a-priv. + ōps (ōp-) eye]

**pro•te•an** (prō'tē-an) changeable in form; having the power to change body form, like the ameba. [G. Prōteus, a god having the power to change his form]

**pro•te•ase** (prō'tē-ās) descriptive term for proteolytic enzymes, both endopeptidases and exopeptidases; enzymes that hydrolyze (break) polypeptide chains.

**pro•te•ase in•hib•i•tor** a class of synthetic drug used in the treatment of HIV infection, with a mode of action different from those of previously used antiretroviral agents including nucleoside analogs.

**pro•tec•tion test** a test to determine the antimicrobial activity of a serum by inoculating a susceptible animal with a mixture of the serum and the virus or other microbe being tested. SYN neutralization test.

**pro•tec•tive la•ryn•ge•al re•flex** closure of the glottis to prevent entry of foreign substances into the respiratory tract.

**pro•tec•tor** a cover or shield. [L.L. protectus from pp. protegere, to protect, to cover over]

**pro•tein** (prō'tēn) macromolecules consisting of long sequences of α-amino acids [H$_2$N–CHR–COOH] in peptide (amide) linkage (elimination of H$_2$O between the α-NH$_2$ and α-COOH of successive residues). Protein is three-fourths of the dry weight of most cell matter and is involved in structures, hormones, enzymes, muscle contraction, immunological response, and essential life functions. The amino acids involved are generally the 20 α-amino acids (glycine, L-alanine, etc.) recognized by the genetic code. Cross-links yielding globular forms of protein are often effected through the –SH groups of two sulfur-containing L-cysteinyl residues, as well as by noncovalent forces (hydrogen bonds, lipophilic attractions, etc.). [G. *prōtos*, first, + -in]

**pro•tein•a•ceous** (prō′tē-nā′shŭs) resembling a protein; possessing, to some degree, the physicochemical properties characteristic of proteins.

**pro•tein in•duced by vit•a•min K ab•sence (PIVKA)** nonfunctional protein precursors of the prothrombin group of coagulation factors (Factors II, VII, IX, X). They are synthesized in the liver in the absence of vitamin K and lack the carboxyl (COOH⁻) group needed to bind the factor to a phospholipid surface.

**pro•tein ki•nase C** any of a number of cytoplasmic calcium-activated kinases involved in numerous processes, including hormonal binding, platelet activation, and tumor promotion.

**pro•tein-los•ing en•ter•op•a•thy** increased fecal loss of serum protein, especially albumin, causing hypoproteinemia.

**pro•tein me•tab•o•lism** decomposition and synthesis of protein in the tissues.

**pro•tein•o•sis** (pro-tē-nō′sis) a state characterized by disordered protein formation and distribution, particularly as manifested by the deposition of abnormal proteins in tissues. [protein + G. *-osis*, condition]

**pro•tein p53** a multifunctional protein that modulates gene transcription and controls DNA repair, apoptosis, and the cell cycle.

**pro•tein S** a vitamin K-dependent antithrombotic protein that functions as a cofactor with activated protein C.

**pro•tein•u•ria** (prō-tē-nyu′rē-ă) **1.** presence of urinary protein in concentrations greater than 0.3 g in a 24-hour urine collection or in concentrations greater than 1 g/l in a random urine collection on two or more occasions at least 6 hours apart; specimens must be clean-voided midstream or obtained by catheterization. **2.** SYN albuminuria. [protein + G. *ouron*, urine]

⌂**pro•teo-, prot-** protein.

**pro•te•o•gly•can ag•gre•gate** a large aggregation of proteoglycans noncovalently bound to a long molecule of hyaluronic acid; involved in cross-linking the collagen fibrils of cartilage matrix.

**pro•te•o•gly•cans** (prō′tē-ō-glī′kanz) glycoaminoglycans (mucopolysaccharides) bound to protein chains in covalent complexes; occur in the extracellular matrix of connective tissue.

**pro•te•o•lip•ids** (prō′tē-ō-lip′idz) a class of lipid-soluble proteins found in brain tissue, insoluble in water but soluble in chloroform-methanol-water mixtures.

**pro•te•ol•y•sis** (prō-tē-ol′i-sis) the decomposition of protein; primarily via the hydrolysis of peptide bonds, both enzymatically and nonenzymatically. [proteo- + G. *lysis*, dissolution]

**pro•te•o•lyt•ic** (prō′tē-ō-lit′ik) relating to or effecting proteolysis.

**pro•te•o•met•a•bol•ic** (prō′tē-ō-met′ă-bol′ik) relating to the metabolism of proteins.

**pro•te•ose** (prō′tē-ōs) a nondescript mixture of intermediate products of proteolysis between protein and peptone.

**pro•te•o•some** (prō′tē-ō-sōm) a cluster of genes that encode components of the cell cytosolic proteolytic complex, a set of proteins thought to be involved in cellular processing and transport of peptides in the formation of the major histocompatibility complex class I molecules. [proteo- + G. *sōma*, body]

**Pro•te•us** (prō′tē-ŭs) a genus of motile, peritrichous, nonsporeforming, aerobic to facultatively anaerobic bacteria containing Gram-negative rods. Coccoid forms, filaments, and spheroplasts occur under certain conditions. The metabolism is fermentative, producing acid. *Proteus* occurs primarily in fecal matter and in putrefying materials. [G. *Prōteus*, a sea god, who had the power to change his form]

*Pro•te•us mor•ga•ni•i* a species found in the intestinal canal and in normal and diarrheal stools.

*Pro•te•us vul•ga•ris* the type species of the genus *Proteus*, found in putrefying materials and in abscesses; certain strains are agglutinated by the serum of persons with typhus and other rickettsial diseases (Weil-Felix reaction). SEE ALSO Weil-Felix reaction.

**pro•throm•bin** (prō-throm′bin) a glycoprotein formed and stored in the parenchymal cells of the liver and present in blood in a concentration of approximately 20 mg/100 ml. In the presence of thromboplastin and calcium ion, prothrombin is converted to thrombin, which in turn converts fibrinogen to fibrin, this process resulting in coagulation of blood; a deficiency of prothrombin leads to impaired blood coagulation.

**pro•throm•bin ac•cel•er•a•tor** SYN factor V.

**pro•throm•bin•ase** (prō-throm′bi-nās) SYN factor X.

**pro•throm•bin frag•ment 1.2 (F1.2)** a peptide released when prothrombin is cleaved by factor Xa. This fragment binds to phospholipid via calcium and interacts with factor Va. Elevated plasma levels of F1.2 have been described in patients with thrombosis or prethrombotic states.

**pro•throm•bin test** a quantitative test for prothrombin in the blood based on the clotting time of oxalated blood plasma in the presence of thromboplastin and calcium chloride; measures the integrity of the extrinsic and common pathways of coagulation. SEE ALSO prothrombin time. SYN Quick test.

**pro•throm•bin time (PT)** the time required for clotting after thromboplastin and calcium are added in optimal amounts to blood of normal fibrinogen content; if prothrombin is diminished, the clotting time increases; used to evaluate the extrinsic clotting system. SEE ALSO prothrombin test.

**pro•tist** (prō′tist) a member of the kingdom Protista.

**Pro•tis•ta** (prō-tis′ta) a kingdom of both plantlike and animal-like eucaryotic unicellular organisms, either in the form of solitary organisms, e.g., protozoa, or colonies of cells lacking true tissues. [G. ntr. pl. of *prōtistos*, the first of all]

⌂**pro•to-, prot-** the first in a series; the highest in rank (properly prefixed to words derived from G. roots). [G. *prōtos*, first]

**pro•to•col** (prō′tō-kol) **1.** a precise and detailed plan for the study of a biomedical problem or for a regimen of therapy, especially cancer chemotherapy. **2.** a record of findings in an experiment or investigation, especially an autopsy.

**pro•to•cone** (prō′tō-kōn) **1.** The mesiolingual cusp of human upper molars. **2.** Formerly thought to be the first upper molar cusp to develop evolutionarily. [proto- + G. *kōnos,* cone]

**pro•to•con•id** (prō-tō-kon'id) **1.** the mesiobuccal cusp of human lower molars. **2.** the first lower molar cusp to develop evolutionarily. [protocone + -id (2)]

**Pro•toc•tis•ta** (prō-tok-tis'tă) a kingdom of eukaryotes incorporating the algae and the protozoans that comprise the presumed ancestral stocks of the fungi, plant, and animal kingdoms; they lack the developmental pattern stemming from a blastula, typical of animals, the pattern of embryo development typical of plants, and development from spores as in the fungi. Included are the nucleated algae and seaweeds, the flagellated water molds, slime molds and slime nets, and the protozoa; unicellular, colonial, and multicellular organisms are included, but the complex development of tissues and organs of plants and animals is absent. [G. *prōtos,* the first, + *ktizō,* to create]

**pro•to•di•a•stol•ic** (prō'tō-dī-ă-stol'ik) early diastolic, relating to the beginning of cardiac diastole.

**pro•to•di•a•stol•ic gal•lop** gallop rhythm in which the gallop sound is an abnormal third heart sound.

**pro•to•du•o•de•num** (prō'tō-doo-ō-dē'nŭm) the first part of the duodenum, which extends from the pylorus as far as the major duodenal papilla and develops from the caudal foregut of the embryo; it has no plicae circulares and is the seat of the duodenal glands.

**pro•ton** (prō'ton) the positively charged unit of the nuclear mass; protons form part (or in hydrogen-1 the whole) of the nucleus of the atom around which the negative electrons revolve. [G. ntr. of *prōtos,* first]

**pro•ton pump** molecular mechanism for the net transport of protons across a membrane; usually involves the activity of an ATPase.

**pro•ton pump in•hib•i•tor** an agent that blocks the transport of hydrogen ions into the stomach and hence is useful in the treatment of gastric hyperacidity, as observed in ulcer disease.

**pro•to•nymph** (prō'tō-nimf) in mites, the second instar.

**pro•to•on•co•gene** (prō-tō-on'kō-jēn) a gene in the normal human genome that appears to have a role in normal cellular physiology and is involved in regulation of normal cell growth or proliferation; as a result of somatic mutations, these genes may become oncogenic; products of proto-oncogenes may have important roles in normal cellular differentiation.

**pro•to•path•ic** (prō-tō-path'ik) denoting a supposedly primitive set or system of peripheral sensory nerve fibers conducting a low order of pain and temperature sensibility which is poorly localized. Cf. epicritic. [proto- + G. *pathos,* suffering]

**pro•to•path•ic sen•si•bil•i•ty** SEE protopathic.

**pro•to•plasm** (prō'tō-plazm) **1.** living matter, the substance of which animal and vegetable cells are formed. SEE ALSO cytoplasm, nucleoplasm. **2.** the total cell material, including cell organelles. Cf. cytoplasm, cytosol, hyaloplasm. [proto- + G. *plasma,* thing formed]

**pro•to•plas•mic as•tro•cyte** one form of astrocyte, found mainly in gray matter, having few fibrils and numerous branching processes.

**pro•to•plast** (prō'tō-plast) a bacterial cell from which the rigid cell wall has been completely removed; the bacterium loses its characteristic form. [proto- + G. *plastos,* formed]

**pro•to•por•phyr•ia** (prō'tō-pōr-fir'ē-ă) enhanced fecal excretion of protoporphyrin.

**pro•to•sty•lid** (prō-tō-stī'lid) an accessory cusp found on the buccal surface of the mesiobuccal cusp of lower molars, ranging from a small groove to a cusp rivaling the mesiobuccal cusp in size. [proto- + G. *stylis, -idos,* mast, spar]

**pro•to•troph** (prō'tō-trof, prō-to-trōf) a bacterial strain that has the same nutritional requirements as the wild-type strain from which it was derived. [proto- + G. *trophē,* nourishment]

**pro•to•type** (prō'tō-tīp) the primitive form; the first form to which subsequent individuals of the class or species conform. [proto- + G. *typos,* type]

**pro•to•ver•te•bra** (prō'tō-ver'tĕ-bră) the caudal half of each sclerotomal concentration, which is the primordium of the centrum of a vertebra. SYN provertebra.

**Pro•to•zoa** (prō-tō-zō'ă) formerly considered a phylum, now regarded as a subkingdom of the animal kingdom, including all of the so-called acellular or unicellular forms. They consist of a single functional cell unit or aggregation of nondifferentiated cells, loosely held together and not forming tissues. [proto- + G. *zōon,* animal]

**pro•to•zo•al** (prō-tō-zō'ăl) SYN protozoan (2).

**pro•to•zo•an** (prō-tō-zō'an) **1.** a member of the phylum Protozoa. SYN protozoon. **2.** relating to protozoa. SYN protozoal.

**pro•to•zo•i•a•sis** (prō'tō-zō-ī'ă-sis) infection with protozoans.

**pro•to•zo•ol•o•gy** (prō'tō-zō-ol'ō-jē) the science concerned with all aspects of the biology and human interest in protozoa. [protozoa + G. *logos,* study]

**pro•to•zo•on,** pl. **pro•to•zoa** (prō-tō-zō'on, prō-tō-zō'ă) SYN protozoan (1).

**pro•to•zo•o•phage** (prō-tō-zō'ō-fāj) a phagocyte that ingests protozoa. [protozoa + G. *phagō,* to eat]

**pro•trac•tion** (prō-trak'shŭn) DENTISTRY the extension of teeth or other maxillary or mandibular structures into a position anterior to normal. [see protractor]

**pro•trac•tor** (prō-trak'ter) a muscle drawing a part forward, as antagonistic to a retractor. [L. *pro-traho,* pp. *-tractus,* to draw forth]

**pro•trud•ed disk** SYN herniated disk.

**pro•trud•ing ear** SYN outstanding ear.

**pro•tru•sion** (prō-troo'zhŭn) **1.** the state of being thrust forward or projected. **2.** DENTISTRY a position of the mandible forward from centric relation. [L. *protrusio*]

**pro•tru•sive oc•clu•sion** occlusion which results when the mandible is protruded forward from centric position.

**pro•tu•ber•ance** (prō-too'ber-ans) a swelling or knoblike outgrowth. A bulging, swelling, or protruding part. SYN protuberantia. [Mod. L. *protuberantia*]

**pro•tu•ber•ant ab•do•men** unusual or prominent convexity of the abdomen, due to excessive subcutaneous fat, poor muscle tone, or an increase in intra-abdominal content.

**pro•tu•be•ran•tia** (prō-too-ber-an'shē-ă) SYN protuberance. SEE ALSO protuberance, prominence, eminence. [Mod. L. fr. *protubero,* to swell out, fr. *tuber,* a swelling]

**proud flesh** exuberant granulation tissue on the surface of a wound.

**Proust space** (proost) SYN rectovesical pouch.

**pro·ver·te·bra** (prō-ver'tĕ-bră) SYN protovertebra.

*Pro·vi·den·cia* (prov'i-den'sē-ă) a genus of motile, peritrichous, nonsporeforming, aerobic or facultatively anaerobic bacteria containing Gram-negative rods. These organisms occur particularly in urinary tract infections and in small outbreaks and sporadic cases of diarrheal disease.

*Pro·vi·den·cia al·ca·li·fa·ci·ens* a species found in extraintestinal sources, particularly in urinary tract infections; it has also been isolated from small outbreaks and sporadic cases of diarrheal disease; it is the type species of the genus *Providencia.*

*Pro·vi·den·cia rett·ger·i* species that is found in chicken cholera and human gastroenteritis.

*Pro·vi·den·cia stu·ar·ti·i* a species isolated from urinary tract infections and from small outbreaks and sporadic cases of diarrheal disease.

**pro·vi·der** (prō-vī'der) a person or agency that supplies goods or services, particularly medical or paramedical services. [L. *pro-videre*]

**pro·vi·rus** (prō-vī'rŭs) the precursor of an animal virus; theoretically analogous to the prophage in bacteria, the provirus being integrated in the nucleus of infected cells.

**prox·i·mad** (prok'si-mad) in a direction toward a proximal part, or toward the center; not distad. [L. *proximus,* nearest, next, + *ad,* to]

⊞**prox·i·mal** (prok'si-măl) **1.** nearest the trunk or the point of origin, said of part of a limb, of an artery or a nerve, etc., so situated. **2.** SYN mesial. **3.** DENTAL ANATOMY denoting the surface of a tooth in relation with its neighbor, whether mesial or distal, i.e., nearer to or farther from the anteroposterior median plane. See page APP 89. [Mod. L. *proximalis,* fr. L. *proximus,* nearest, next]

**prox·i·mal deep in·gui·nal lymph node** one of the deep inguinal lymph nodes located in or adjacent to the femoral canal; sometimes mistaken for a femoral hernia when enlarged. SYN Rosenmüller gland, Rosenmüller node.

**prox·i·mal my·o·ton·ic my·o·path·y (PROMM)** an autosomal dominant, multisystem disorder, with onset in young adult life, characterized by proximal myotonia and weakness, muscle pain, baldness, cataracts, cardiac conduction disturbances, and testicular atrophy. In contrast to myotonic dystrophy, features of this disorder do not include facial weakness and ptosis, distal limb weakness and wasting, and trinucleotide repeat expansion at the gene loci for myotonic dystrophy.

**prox·i·mal sple·nor·e·nal shunt** anastomosis of the proximal end of the cut splenic vein to the side of the left renal vein for control of portal hypertension; this is considered a central or complete visceral venous shunt.

**prox·i·mate** (prok'si-māt) immediate; next; proximal.

△**prox·i·mo-, prox·i-, prox-** proximal. [L. *proximus,* nearest, next (to)]

**prox·i·mo·a·tax·ia** (prok'si-mō-ă-tak'sē-ă) ataxia or lack of muscular coordination in the

proximal portions of the extremities, i.e., arms and thighs. Cf. acroataxia. [proximo- + ataxia]

**pro·zone** (prō'zōn) a phenomenon in which visible agglutination and precipitation do not occur in mixtures of specific antigen and antibody because of antibody excess.

**PRPP** 5-phospho-α-D-ribosyl 1-pyrophosphate.

**PR seg·ment** that part of the electrocardiographic curve between the end of the P wave and the beginning of the QRS complex.

**pru·rig·i·nous** (proo-rij'i-nŭs) relating to or suffering from prurigo. [L. *pruriginosus,* having the itch]

**pru·ri·go** (proo-rī'gō) a chronic disease of the skin marked by a persistent eruption of papules that itch intensely. [L. itch, fr. *prurio,* to itch]

**pru·ri·go mi·tis** a mild form of a chronic dermatitis characterized by recurring, intensely itching papules and nodules, probably atopic.

**pru·ri·go no·du·la·ris** an eruption of hard nodules (Picker nodules) in the skin caused by rubbing and accompanied by intense itching.

**pru·ri·go sim·plex** a mild form of prurigo having a pronounced tendency to relapse.

**pru·rit·ic** (proo-rit'ik) relating to pruritus.

**pru·rit·ic ur·ti·car·i·al pap·ules and plaques of preg·nan·cy (PUPPP)** intensely pruritic papulovesicles that begin on the abdomen in the third trimester and spread peripherally, resolves rapidly after delivery and does not affect the fetus.

**pru·ri·tus** (proo-rī'tŭs) **1.** SYN itching. **2.** SYN itch (1). [L. an itching, fr. *prurio,* to itch]

**pru·ri·tus ani** itching at the anus; may be associated with seborrheic dermatitis, candidosis, or external hemorrhoids, or occur in systemic disease.

**pru·ri·tus gra·vi·dar·um** severe pruritus without associated rash occurring during pregnancy secondary to intrahepatic cholestasis and bile salt retention.

**pru·ri·tus se·ni·lis, se·nile pru·ri·tus** itching associated with dryness of the skin in the aged.

**pru·ri·tus vul·vae** itching of the external female genitalia, caused by seborrheic dermatitis, allergy to local contactants, senile atrophy of the vulva, or systemic disease.

**Prus·sian blue** [CI 77510] SYN Berlin blue.

**PSA** prostate-specific antigen.

△**psammo-** sand. [G. *psammos*]

**psam·mo·ma** (sa-mō'mă) obsolete term for psammomatous meningioma or meningioma. [psammo- + G. *-oma,* tumor]

**psam·mo·ma bo·dies 1.** mineralized bodies occurring in the meninges, choroid plexus, and in certain meningiomas; composed usually of a central capillary surrounded by concentric whorls of meningocytes in various stages of hyaline change and mineralization; can also occur in benign and malignant epithelial tumors (often papillary) or with chronic inflammation; **2.** SYN corpora arenacea. **3.** SYN calcospherite.

**psam·mo·ma·tous me·nin·gi·o·ma** a firm cellular neoplasm derived from fibrous tissue of the meninges, choroid plexus, and certain other structures associated with the brain, characterized by the formation of multiple, discrete, concentrically laminated, calcareous bodies (psammoma bodies); most of these neoplasms are histologically benign, but may lead to severe symptoms as a result of compressing the brain. SYN Virchow psammoma.

**psam•mous** (sam′ŭs) sandy. [G. *psammos*, sand]

**PSA vel•o•ci•ty** a measure of the rapidity of change in a person's PSA level.

**PSE** Pidgin Sign English.

**P se•lec•tin** cell surface receptor present on endothelium that is involved with neutrophil migration into inflamed tissue.

**pseud•a•graph•ia** (soo-dă-graf′ē-ă) partial agraphia in which one can do no original writing, but can copy correctly. SYN pseudoagraphia. [pseud- + G. *a-* priv. + *graphō,* to write]

***Pseud•al•les•che•ria boy•dii*** (sood′al-es-kē′rē-ă boy′dē-ī) a species of fungus that causes eumycotic mycetoma and pseudallescheriasis; its conidial (asexual) state is *Scedosporium apiospermum.*

**pseud•al•les•che•ri•a•sis** (sood′al-es-kē′ri-ă-sis) a variety of clinical diseases resulting from infection with *Pseudallescheria boydii;* e.g., pulmonary colonization, fungoma, and invasive pneumonitis, as well as mycotic keratitis, endophthalmitis, endocarditis, meningitis, sinusitis, brain abscesses, cutaneous and subcutaneous infections, and disseminated systemic infections.

**pseud•an•ky•lo•sis** (soo-dang′ki-lō′sis) SYN fibrous ankylosis.

**pseud•ar•thro•sis** (soo-dar-thrō′sis) a new, false joint arising at the site of an ununited fracture. SYN false joint, pseudoarthrosis. [pseud- + G. *arthrōsis,* a joint]

**pseud•es•the•sia** (soo-des-thē′zē-ă) 1. SYN paraphia. 2. a subjective sensation not arising from an external stimulus. 3. SYN phantom limb. [pseud- + G. *aisthēsis,* sensation]

⚠**pseu•do-** (psi), **pseud-** false (often used about a deceptive resemblance). [G. *pseudēs*]

**pseu•do•a•graph•ia** (soo′dō-ă-graf′ē-ă) SYN pseudagraphia.

**pseu•do•al•lel•ic** (sū′dō-ă-le′lik) relating to pseudoallelism.

**pseu•do•al•lel•ism** (soo-dō-ă-lē′lizm) relationship of two or more loci that are difficult to distinguish from a single locus by classical genetic analysis.

**pseu•do•a•ne•mia** (soo′dō-ă-nē′mē-ă) pallor of the skin and mucous membranes without the blood changes of anemia. SYN false anemia.

**pseu•do•ar•thro•sis** (soo′dō-ar-thrō′sis) SYN pseudarthrosis.

**pseu•do•bul•bar** (soo-dō-bŭl′bar) denoting a supranuclear paralysis of the bulbar nerves.

**pseu•do•bul•bar pal•sy** spastic paralysis of the bulbar musculature due to bilateral impairment of corticobulbar upper motor neuron fibers.

**pseu•do•bul•bar pa•ral•y•sis** paralysis of the lips and tongue, simulating progressive bulbar paralysis, but due to supranuclear lesions with bilateral involvement of the upper motor neurons; characterized by speech and swallowing difficulties, emotional instability, and spasmodic, mirthless laughter.

**pseu•do•car•ti•lage** (soo-dō-kar′ti-lij) SYN chondroid tissue (1).

**pseu•do•cast** (soo′dō-kast) SYN false cast.

**pseu•do•chan•cre** (soo-dō-shang′ker) a nonspecific indurated sore, usually located on the penis, resembling a chancre.

**pseu•do•cho•rea** (soo-dō-kōr-ē′ă) a spasmodic disorder or extensive tic resembling chorea.

**pseu•do•chro•mes•the•sia** (soo′dō-krō-mes-thē′zē-ă) 1. an anomaly in which each vowel in the printed word is seen as colored. SEE ALSO photism. 2. SYN color hearing. [pseudo- + G. *chrōma,* color, + *aisthēsis,* sensation]

**pseu•do•co•arc•ta•tion** (soo′dō-kō-ark-tā′shŭn) distortion, often with slight narrowing, of the aortic arch at the level of insertion of the ligamentum arteriosum.

**pseu•do•cop•ro•sta•sis** (soo-dō-cop-rō-stā′sis) VETERINARY MEDICINE impaction of feces in the colon due to an external blockage of the anus, usually due to matted hair covering the anus. [pseudo- + coprostasis]

**pseu•do•croup** (soo-dō-kroop′) SYN laryngismus stridulus.

**pseu•do•cryp•tor•chism** (soo-dō-krip′tōr-kizm) a condition in which the testes descend to the scrotum but intermittently retreat into the inguinal canal. [pseudo- + G. *kryptos,* hidden, + *orchis,* testis]

**pseu•do•cy•e•sis** (soo′dō-sī-ē′sis) SYN false pregnancy. [pseudo- + G. *kyēsis,* pregnancy]

**pseu•do•cyl•in•droid** (soo-dō-sil′in-droyd) a shred of mucus or other substance in the urine resembling a renal cast.

**pseu•do•cyst** (soo′dō-sist) 1. an accumulation of fluid in a cystlike loculus, but without an epithelial or other membranous lining. SYN adventitious cyst. 2. a cyst whose wall is formed by a host cell and not by a parasite. 3. a mass of 50 or more *Toxoplasma* bradyzoites, found within a host cell, frequently in the brain; a true cyst enclosed in its own membrane within the host cell that may rupture to release particles that form new cysts. [pseudo- + G. *kystis,* bladder]

**pseu•do•de•men•tia** (soo′dō-dē-men′shē-ă) a condition resembling dementia but usually due to a depressive disorder rather than brain dysfunction.

**pseu•do•diph•the•ria** (soo′dō-dif-thēr′ē-ă) SYN diphtheroid (1).

**pseu•do•dom•i•nance** (soo-dō-dom′ĭ-nans) SYN quasidominance.

**pseu•do•e•de•ma** (soo′dō-e-dē′mă) a puffiness of the skin not due to a fluid accumulation. [pseudo- + G. *oidēma,* a swelling (edema)]

**pseu•do•ex•fol•i•a•tion syn•drome** a condition, often leading to glaucoma, in which deposits on the surface of the lens resemble exfoliation of the lens capsule.

**pseu•do•ex•fol•i•a•tive glau•co•ma** glaucoma occurring in association with widespread deposition of cellular organelles on the lens capsule, ocular blood vessels, iris, and ciliary body.

**pseu•do•fol•lic•u•li•tis** (soo′dō-fo-lik-yu-lī′tis) erythematous follicular papules or, less commonly, pustules resulting from close shaving of curly hair; tips of growing hairs reenter the skin producing ingrown hairs; pseudofolliculitis of the beard area is very common in blacks.

**pseu•do•frac•ture** (soo-dō-frak′cher) a condition in which a radiograph shows formation of new bone with thickening of periosteum at site of an injury to bone.

**pseu•do•gan•gli•on** (soo-dō-gang′glē-on) a localized thickening of a nerve trunk having the appearance of a ganglion.

**pseu•do•geu•ses•the•sia** (soo′dō-gyu-ses-thē′zē-ă) SYN color taste. [pseudo- + G. *geusis,* taste, + *aisthēsis,* sensation]

**pseu·do·geu·sia** (soo-dō-gyu′sē-ă) a subjective taste sensation not produced by an external stimulus. [pseudo- + G. *geusis*, taste]

**pseu·do·gout** (soo′dō-gowt) acute episodes of synovitis caused by deposits of calcium pyrophosphate crystals rather than urate crystals as in true gout; associated with articular chondrocalcinosis.

**pseu·do-Grae·fe phe·nom·e·non** (grā′fĕ) retraction of the upper eyelid on downward movement of the eyes.

**pseu·do·hae·ma·tu·ria [Br.]** SEE pseudohematuria.

**pseu·do·he·ma·tu·ria** (soo′dō-hem-ă-too′rē-ă) a red pigmentation of urine caused by certain foods or drugs, and thus not actually hematuria. SYN false hematuria.

**pseu·do·her·maph·ro·dite** (soo′dō-her-maf′rō-dīt) an individual exhibiting pseudohermaphroditism.

**pseu·do·her·maph·ro·dit·ism** (soo′dō-her-maf′rō-dī-tizm) a state in which the individual is of an unambiguous gonadal sex (i.e., possesses either testes or ovaries) but has ambiguous external genitalia. SYN false hermaphroditism.

**pseu·do·hy·per·kal·e·mia** (soo′dō-hī′per-kal-ē′mē-ă) a spurious elevation of the serum concentration of potassium occurring when potassium is released in vitro from cells in a blood sample collected for a potassium measurement. This may be a consequence of disease (i.e., myeloproliferative disorders with marked leukocytosis or thrombocytosis) or as a result of improper collection technique with in vitro hemolysis. [pseudo- + G. *hyper*, above + L. *kalium*, potassium, G. *haima*, blood]

**pseu·do·hy·per·par·a·thy·roid·ism** (soo′dō-hī′per-par-ă-thī′roy-dizm) hypercalcemia in a patient with a malignant neoplasm in the absence of skeletal metastases or primary hyperparathyroidism; believed to be due to formation of parathyroid-like hormone by nonparathyroid tumor tissue.

**pseu·do·hy·per·tro·phic** (soo′dō-hī-per-trōf′ik) relating to or marked by pseudohypertrophy.

**pseu·do·hy·per·tro·phy** (soo′dō-hī-per′trō-fē) increase in size of an organ or a part, due not to increase in size or number of the specific functional elements but to that of some other tissue, fatty or fibrous.

**pseu·do·hy·po·a·cu·sis** (soo′dō-hī′pō-ă-koo′sis) apparent loss of hearing without an organic disorder or with insufficient pathological evidence to explain the extent of the loss; usually due to conversion disorder or malingering.

**pseu·do·hy·po·na·tre·mia** (soo′dō-hī-pō-nă-trē′mē-ă) a low serum sodium concentration due to volume displacement by massive hyperlipidemia or hyperproteinemia; also used to describe the low serum sodium concentration which may occur with high blood glucose.

**pseu·do·hy·po·par·a·thy·roid·ism** (soo′dō-hī′pō-par-ă-thī′roid-izm) a disorder resembling hypoparathyroidism, with high serum phosphate and low calcium levels, but with normal or elevated serum parathyroid hormone levels; due to lack of end-organ responsiveness to parathyroid hormone.

**pseu·do·ic·ter·us** (soo-dō-ik′ter-ŭs) yellowish discoloration of the skin not due to bile pigments, as in Addison disease. SYN pseudojaundice.

**pseu·do·i·so·chro·mat·ic** (soo′dō-ī-sō-krō-mat′ik) apparently of the same color; denoting certain charts containing colored spots mixed with figures printed in confusion colors; used in testing for color vision deficiency.

**pseu·do·jaun·dice** (soo-dō-jawn′dis) SYN pseudoicterus.

**pseu·do·lo·gia** (soo-dō-lō′jē-ă) pathological lying in speech or writing. [pseudo- + G. *logos*, word]

**pseu·do·lo·gia phan·tas·ti·ca** a fantastic account of a patient's exploits, which the patient appears to believe.

**pseu·do·lym·pho·ma** (soo′dō-lim-fō′mă) a benign infiltration of lymphoid cells or histiocytes that microscopically resembles a malignant lymphoma.

**pseu·do·ma·lig·nan·cy** (soo′dō-mă-lig′nan-sē) a benign tumor that appears, clinically or histologically, to be a malignant neoplasm. SEE ALSO pseudotumor.

**pseu·do·ma·nia** (soo-dō-mā′nē-ă) **1.** a factitious mental disorder. **2.** a mental disorder in which the patient falsely claims to have committed a crime. **3.** generally, the morbid impulse to falsify or lie, as in pseudologia.

**pseu·do·mem·brane** (soo-dō-mem′brān) SYN false membrane.

**pseu·do·mem·bra·nous** (soo-dō-mem′bră-nŭs) relating to or marked by the presence of a false membrane.

**pseu·do·mem·bra·nous bron·chi·tis** SYN fibrinous bronchitis.

**pseu·do·mem·bra·nous co·li·tis** SYN pseudomembranous enterocolitis.

**pseu·do·mem·bra·nous en·ter·i·tis** SYN pseudomembranous enterocolitis.

**pseu·do·mem·bra·nous en·ter·o·co·li·tis** enterocolitis with the formation and passage of pseudomembranous material, due to infection by *Clostridium difficile;* it is commonly a sequel to prolonged antibiotic therapy. SYN pseudomembranous colitis, pseudomembranous enteritis.

**pseu·do·mem·bra·nous gas·tri·tis** gastritis characterized by the formation of a false membrane.

**pseu·do·mem·bra·nous in·flam·ma·tion** a form of exudative inflammation that involves mucous and serous membranes; large quantities of fibrin in the exudate result in a tenacious membrane-like covering that is adherent to the underlying acutely inflamed tissue.

**pseu·do·mo·nad** (soo-dō-mō′nad) a vernacular term used to refer to any member of the genus *Pseudomonas.*

*Pseu·do·mo·nas* (soo-dō-mō′nas) a genus of motile, polar-flagellate, non–spore-forming, strictly aerobic bacteria (family Pseudomonadaceae) containing straight or curved, but not helical, Gram-negative rods that occur singly. The metabolism is respiratory, never fermentative. They occur commonly in soil and in freshwater and marine environments. Some species are plant pathogens. Others are involved in human infections. The type species is *Pseudomonas aeruginosa.* [pseudo- + G. *monas,* unit, monad]

*Pseu·do·mo·nas mal·lei* SYN *Burkholderia mallei.*

*Pseu·do·mo·nas* os·te·o·mye·li·tis SYN malignant external otitis.

**pseudomonilethrix** (soo′dō-mō-nil′ĕ-thriks) a

nodal trichodystrophy similar to monilethrix but with fractures within the nodal swellings; autosomal dominant inheritance with late onset.

**pseu·do·myx·o·ma** (soo′dō-mik-sō′mǎ) a gelatinous mass resembling a myxoma but composed of epithelial mucus.

**pseu·do·myx·o·ma pe·ri·to·nei** the accumulation of large quantities of mucoid or mucinous material in the peritoneal cavity, either as a result of rupture of a mucocele of the appendix, or rupture of benign or malignant cystic neoplasms of the ovary.

**pseu·do·ne·o·plasm** (soo-dō-nē′ō-plazm) SYN pseudotumor.

**pseu·do·os·te·o·ma·la·cic pel·vis** an extreme degree of rachitic pelvis, resembling the puerperal osteomalacic pelvis, in which the pelvic canal is obstructed by a forward projection of the sacrum, and an approximation of the acetabula.

**pseu·do·pap·il·le·de·ma** (soo′dō-pap-il-e-dē′mǎ) anomalous elevation of the optic disk; seen in severe hyperopia and optic nerve drusen.

**pseu·do·pa·ral·y·sis** (soo′dō-pǎ-ral′i-sis) apparent paralysis due to voluntary inhibition of motion because of pain, to incoordination, or other cause, but without actual paralysis. SYN pseudoparesis (1).

**pseu·do·par·a·ple·gia** (soo′dō-par-ă-plē′jē-ă) apparent paralysis in the lower extremities, in which the tendon and skin reflexes and the electrical reactions are normal; the condition is sometimes observed in rickets.

**pseu·do·pa·re·sis** (soo′dō-pa-rē′sis) 1. SYN pseudoparalysis. 2. a condition marked by the pupillary changes, tremors, and speech disturbances suggestive of early paresis, in which, however, the serologic tests are negative.

**pseu·do·pe·lade** (soo′dō-pĕ-lahd′) a scarring type of alopecia; usually occurs in scattered irregular patches; of uncertain cause. [pseudo- + Fr. *pelade,* disease that causes sporadic falling of hair]

**pseu·do·plate·let** (soo-dō-plāt′let) any of the fragments of neutrophils which may be mistaken for platelets, especially in peripheral blood smears of leukemic patients.

**pseu·do·pod** (soo′dō-pod) SYN pseudopodium.

**pseu·do·po·di·um,** pl. **pseu·do·po·dia** (soo-dō-pō′dē-ŭm, soo-dō-pō′-dē-ă) a temporary protoplasmic process, put forth by an ameboid stage or amebic protozoan for locomotion or for prehension of food. SYN pseudopod. [pseudo- + G. *pous,* foot]

**pseu·do·pol·yp** (soo-dō-pol′ip) a projecting mass of granulation tissue, large numbers of which may develop in ulcerative colitis; may become covered by regenerating epithelium.

**pseu·do·preg·nan·cy** (soo-dō-preg′nan-sē) 1. SYN false pregnancy. 2. a condition in which symptoms resembling those of pregnancy are present, but which is not pregnancy.

**pseu·do·pte·ryg·i·um** (soo′dō-tě-rij′ē-ŭm) adhesion of the conjunctiva to the cornea, occurring after injury.

**pseu·do·p·to·sis** (soo-dō-tō′sis) a condition resembling an inability to elevate the eyelid, due to blepharophimosis, blepharochalasis, or some other affection. SYN false blepharoptosis. [pseudo- + G. *ptōsis,* a falling]

**pseu·do·re·ac·tion** (soo′dō-rē-ak′shŭn) a false

reaction; one not due to specific causes in a given test.

**pseu·do·rick·ets** (soo-dō-rik′ets) SYN renal rickets.

**pseu·do·ro·sette** (soo′dō-rō-zet′) perivascular radial arrangement of neoplastic cells around a small blood vessel. SEE rosette (2).

**pseu·do·scar·la·ti·na** (soo′dō-skar-lă-tē′nă) erythema with fever, due to causes other than *Streptococcus pyogenes.*

**pseu·dos·mia** (soo-doz′mē-ă) subjective sensation of an odor that is not present. [pseudo- + G. *osmē,* smell]

**pseu·do·stra·bis·mus** (soo′dō-stra-biz′mŭs) the appearance of strabismus caused by epicanthus, abnormality in interorbital distance, or corneal light reflex not corresponding to the center of the pupil. [pseudo- + G. *strabismos,* a squinting]

**pseu·do·strat·i·fied ep·i·the·li·um** an epithelium that gives a superficial appearance of being stratified because the cell nuclei are at different levels, but in which all cells reach the basement membrane,.

**pseu·do·tu·mor** (soo′dō-too-mer) 1. an enlargement of nonneoplastic character which clinically resembles a true neoplasm so closely as to often be mistaken for such. 2. a condition, commonly associated with obesity in young females, of cerebral edema with narrowed small ventricles but with increased intracranial pressure and frequently papilledema. SYN pseudoneoplasm.

**pseu·do·tu·mour [Br.]** SEE pseudotumor.

**pseu·do·u·ri·dine (Ψ, Q)** (soo-dō-yu′ri-dēn) 5-β-D-ribosyluracil; a naturally occurring isomer of uridine found in transfer ribonucleic acids; unique in that the ribosyl is attached to carbon (C-5) rather than to nitrogen; excreted in urine.

**pseu·do·xan·tho·ma elas·ti·cum** (soo′dō-zan-thō′mă e-las′ti-kŭm) an inherited disorder of connective tissue characterized by yellowish plaques on the neck, axillae, abdomen, and thighs, associated with angioid streaks of the retina and similar elastic tissue degeneration and calcification in arteries.

**psi** (sī) 1. the 23rd letter of the Greek alphabet (ψ). 2. pseudouridine; pseudo-; psychology; wave function; the dihedral angle of rotation about the $C_1$–$C_\alpha$ bond associated with a peptide bond.

**psi** pounds per square inch.

**P sin·is·tro·car·di·a·le** (pē sin-is-trō-kar-dē-ā′lē) SYN P mitrale.

**psi phe·nom·e·non** a phenomenon that includes both psychokinesis and extrasensory perception; the extrasensory mental processes involved in the alleged ability to send or receive telepathic messages.

**psit·ta·co·sis** (sit-ă-kō′sis) an infectious disease in psittacine birds and humans caused by the bacterium *Chlamydia psittaci.* Avian infections are mainly inapparent or latent, although acute disease does occur; human infections may result in mild disease with a flulike syndrome or in severe disease, with symptoms of bronchopneumonia. SYN ornithosis, Parrot disease (3), parrot fever. [G. *psittakos,* a parrot, + *-osis,* condition]

**pso·as ab·scess** an abscess, usually tuberculous, originating in tuberculous spondylitis and extending through the iliopsoas muscle to the inguinal region.

**pso·rel·co·sis** (sō-rel-kō′sis) cutaneous ulceration

resulting from scabies. [G. *psōra,* itch, + *helkōsis,* ulceration]

**pso·ri·a·sic** (sō-rī'ă-sik) SYN psoriatic.

**pso·ri·a·si·form** (sō-rī'ă-si-fōrm) resembling psoriasis.

**pso·ri·a·sis** (sō-rī'ă-sis) a common inherited condition characterized by the eruption of reddish, silvery-scaled maculopapules, predominantly on the elbows, knees, scalp, and trunk. [G. *psōriasis,* fr. *psōra,* the itch]

**pso·ri·at·ic** (sō-rē-at'ik) relating to psoriasis. SYN psoriasic.

**pso·ri·at·ic ar·thri·tis** the concurrence of psoriasis and polyarthritis, resembling rheumatoid arthritis but thought to be a specific disease entity, seronegative for rheumatoid factor and often involving the digits. SYN arthropathia psoriatica.

**PSR** Periodontal Screening Record.

**PSV** pressure support ventilation.

**psy·chal·gia** (sī-kal'jē-ă) **1.** distress attending a mental effort, noted especially in melancholia. SYN phrenalgia (1). **2.** SYN psychogenic pain. [psych- + G. *algos,* pain]

**psy·cha·tax·ia** (sī-kă-tak'sē-ă) mental confusion; inability to fix one's attention or to make any continued mental effort. [psych- + G. *ataxia,* confusion]

**psy·che** (sī'kē) term for the subjective aspects of the mind, self, soul; the psychological or spiritual as distinct from the bodily nature of persons. [G. mind, soul]

**psy·che·del·ic** (sī-kě-del'ik) **1.** pertaining to a category of drugs with mainly central nervous system action, said to be the expansion or heightening of consciousness, e.g., LSD, hashish, mescaline. **2.** a hallucinogenic substance, visual display, music, or other sensory stimulus having such action. SYN hallucinogenic. [psyche- + G. *dēloō,* to manifest]

**psy·chi·at·ric** (sī-kē-at'rik) relating to psychiatry.

**psy·chi·a·tric re·hab·i·li·ta·tion** service and support provided, with limited professional intervention, to assist persons with long-term psychiatric disabilities in self-directed, self-satisfying functional life tasks.

**psy·chi·a·trist** (sī-kī'ă-trist) a physician who specializes in psychiatry.

**psy·chi·a·try** (sī-kī'ă-trē) the medical specialty concerned with the diagnosis and treatment of mental disorders. [psych- + G. *iatreia,* medical treatment]

**psy·chic** (sī'kik) **1.** relating to the phenomena of consciousness, mind, or soul. **2.** a person supposedly endowed with the power of communicating with spirits. [G. *psychikos*]

**psy·chic trau·ma** an upsetting experience precipitating or aggravating an emotional or mental disorder.

△**psy·cho-, psych-, psy·che-** the mind; mental; psychological. [G. *psychē,* soul, mind]

**psy·cho·ac·tive** (sī-kō-ak'tiv) possessing the ability to alter mood, anxiety, behavior, cognitive processes, or mental tension; usually applied to pharmacologic agents.

**psy·cho·a·nal·y·sis** (sī'kō-ă-nal'i-sis) **1.** a method of psychotherapy, originated by Freud, designed to bring preconscious and unconscious material to consciousness primarily through the analysis of transference and resistance. SYN psychoanalytic therapy. SEE ALSO freudian psychoanalysis. **2.** a method of investigating total mental life, conscious and unconscious, of a person with a mental disorder, employing interpretation of resistance and transference, free association, and dream analysis. **3.** an integrated body of observations and theories on personality development, motivation, and behavior. **4.** a school of psychotherapy, as in jungian or freudian psychoanalysis. [psycho- + analysis]

**psy·cho·an·a·lyst** (sī-kō-an'ă-list) a psychotherapist, usually a psychiatrist or clinical psychologist, trained in psychoanalysis and employing its methods in the treatment of emotional disorders.

**psy·cho·an·a·lyt·ic** (sī'kō-an-ă-lit'ik) pertaining to psychoanalysis.

**psy·cho·an·a·lyt·ic psy·chi·a·try** psychiatric theory and practice emphasizing the principles of psychoanalysis. SYN dynamic psychiatry.

**psy·cho·an·a·lyt·ic ther·a·py** SYN psychoanalysis (1).

**psy·cho·bi·ol·o·gy** (sī'kō-bī-ol'ō-jē) the study of the interrelationships of the biology and psychology in cognitive functioning, including intellectual, memory, and related neurocognitive processes.

**psy·cho·di·ag·no·sis** (sī'kō-dī-ag-nō'sis) **1.** any method used to discover the factors which underlie behavior, especially maladjusted or abnormal behavior. **2.** a subspecialty within clinical psychology that emphasizes the use of psychological tests and techniques for assessing psychopathology.

**psy·cho·dra·ma** (sī'kō-drah-mā) a method of psychotherapy in which patients act out their personal problems by spontaneously enacting without rehearsal diagnostically specific roles in dramatic performances put on before their patient peers.

**psy·cho·dy·nam·ics** (sī'kō-dī-nam'iks) the systematized study and theory of the psychological forces that underlie human behavior, emphasizing the interplay between unconscious and conscious motivation and the functional significance of emotion. SEE ALSO role-playing. [psycho- + G. *dynamis,* force]

**psy·cho·gen·e·sis** (sī-kō-jen'ĕ-sis) the origin and development of the psychic processes including mental, behavioral, emotional, personality, and related psychological processes. [psycho- + G. *genesis,* origin]

**psy·cho·gen·ic, psy·cho·ge·net·ic** (sī-kō-jen'ik, sī-kō-jĕ-net'ik) **1.** of mental origin or causation. **2.** relating to emotional and related psychological development or to psychogenesis.

**psy·cho·gen·ic deaf·ness** hearing loss without evidence of organic cause or malingering; often follows severe psychic shock. SYN functional deafness.

**psy·cho·gen·ic hear·ing im·pair·ment** hearing impairment without evidence of organic cause; often follows severe psychic shock. SYN functional hearing impairment.

**psy·cho·gen·ic pain** somatoform pain; pain which is associated or correlated with a psychological, emotional, or behavioral stimulus. SYN psychalgia (2).

**psy·cho·gen·ic pain dis·or·der** a disorder in which the principal complaint is pain that is out of proportion to objective findings and that is related to psychological factors.

**psy·cho·gen·ic vom·it·ing** vomiting associated with emotional distress and anxiety.

**psy·cho·ki·ne·sis, psy·cho·ki·ne·sia** (sī'kō-ki-nē'sis, sī'kō-ki-nē'zē-ă) **1.** the influence of mind upon matter, as the use of mental "power" to move or distort an object. **2.** impulsive behavior. [psycho- + G. *kinēsis,* movement]

**psy·cho·lin·guis·tics** (sī'kō-ling-gwi'stiks) study of a host of psychological factors associated with speech, including voice, attitudes, emotions, and grammatical rules, that affect communication and understanding of language. [psycho- + L. *lingua,* tongue]

**psy·cho·log·ic, psy·cho·log·i·cal** (sī-kō-loj'ik, sī-kō-loj'i-kăl) **1.** relating to psychology. **2.** relating to the mind and its processes. SEE psychology.

**psy·chol·o·gist** (sī-kol'ō-jist) a specialist in psychology licensed to practice professional psychology (e.g., clinical psychologist), or qualified to teach psychology as a scholarly discipline (academic psychologist), or whose scientific specialty is a subfield of psychology (research psychologist).

**psy·chol·o·gy** (Ψ) (sī-kol'ō-jē) the profession (e.g., clinical psychology), scholarly discipline (academic psychology), and science (research psychology) concerned with the behavior of humans and animals, and related mental and physiological processes. [psycho- + G. *logos,* study]

**psy·cho·met·rics** (sī-kō-met'riks) SYN psychometry.

**psy·chom·e·try** (sī-kom'ĕ-trē) the discipline pertaining to psychological and mental testing, and to any quantitative analysis of an individual's psychological traits or attitudes or mental processes. SYN psychometrics. [psycho- + G. *metron,* measure]

**psy·cho·mo·tor** (sī-kō-mō'ter) **1.** relating to the psychological processes associated with muscular movement, and to the production of voluntary movements. **2.** relating to the combination of psychic and motor events, including disturbances. [psycho- + L. *motor,* mover]

**psy·cho·mo·tor ep·i·lep·sy** attacks with elaborate and multiple sensory, motor, and/or psychic components, the common feature being a clouding or loss of consciousness and amnesia for the event; clinical manifestations may take the form of automatisms, emotional outbursts, or motor or psychic disturbances. SEE ALSO procursive epilepsy. SYN psychomotor seizure.

**psy·cho·mo·tor sei·zure** SYN psychomotor epilepsy.

**psy·cho·neu·ro·sis** (sī'kō-noo-rō'sis) SYN neurosis.

**psy·cho·neu·rot·ic** (sī'kō-noo-rot'ik) pertaining to or suffering from psychoneurosis.

**psy·cho·path** (sī'kō-path) former designation for an individual with an antisocial type of personality disorder. SEE ALSO antisocial personality disorder, sociopath. [psycho- + G. *pathos,* disease]

**psy·cho·path·ic** (sī-kō-path'ik) relating to or characteristic of psychopathy.

**psy·cho·pa·thol·o·gy** (sī'kō-pă-thol'ō-jē) **1.** the science concerned with the pathology of the mind and behavior. **2.** the science of mental and behavioral disorders, including psychiatry and abnormal psychology. [psycho- + G. *pathos, disease,* + *logos,* study]

**psy·cho·phar·ma·ceu·ti·cals** (sī'kō-far-mă-sū'ti-kălz) drugs used in the treatment of emotional disorders.

**psy·cho·phar·ma·col·o·gy** (sī'kō-far'mă-kol'ō-jē) **1.** the use of drugs to treat mental and psychological disorders. **2.** the science of drug-behavior relationships. [psycho- + G. *pharmakon,* drug, + *logos,* study]

**psy·cho·phys·i·cal** (sī-kō-fiz'i-kăl) **1.** relating to the mental perception of physical stimuli. SEE psychophysics. **2.** SYN psychosomatic.

**psy·cho·phys·ics** (sī-kō-fiz'iks) the science of the relation between the physical attributes of a stimulus and the measured, quantitative attributes of the mental perception of that stimulus.

**psy·cho·phys·i·o·log·ic** (sī'kō-fiz-ē-ō-loj'ik) **1.** pertaining to psychophysiology. **2.** denoting a psychosomatic illness. **3.** denoting a somatic disorder with significant emotional or psychological etiology.

**psy·cho·phys·i·ol·o·gy** (sī'kō-fiz-ē-ol'ō-jē) the science of the relation between psychological and physiological processes.

**psy·cho·sen·so·ry, psy·cho·sen·so·ri·al** (sī'kō-sen'sōr-ē, sī'kō-sen-sōr'ē-ăl) **1.** denoting the mental perception and interpretation of sensory stimuli. **2.** denoting a hallucination which by effort the mind is able to distinguish from reality.

**psy·cho·sex·u·al** (sī-kō-seks'yu-ăl) pertaining to the relationships among the emotional, mental physiologic, and behavioral components of sex or sexual development.

**psy·cho·sex·u·al de·vel·op·ment** maturation and development of the psychic and behavioral phases of sexuality from birth to adult life through the oral, anal, phallic, latency, and genital phases.

**psy·cho·sex·u·al dys·func·tion, sex·u·al dys·func·tion** a disturbance of sexual functioning, e.g., impotence, premature ejaculation, anorgasmia, presumed to be of psychological rather than physical etiology.

**psy·cho·sis,** pl. **psy·cho·ses** (sī-kō'sis, sī'kō-sēz) **1.** a mental and behavioral disorder causing gross distortion or disorganization of a person's mental capacity, affective response, and capacity to recognize reality, communicate, and relate to others to the degree of interfering with the person's capacity to cope with the ordinary demands of everyday life. **2.** generic term for any of the so-called insanities, the most common forms being the schizophrenias. **3.** a severe emotional and behavioral disorder. SYN psychotic disorder. [G. an animating]

**psy·cho·so·cial** (sī-kō-sō'shăl) involving both psychological and social aspects; e.g., age, education, marital history.

**psy·cho·so·mat·ic** (sī'kō-sō-mat'ik) pertaining to the influence of the mind or higher functions of the brain (emotions, fears, desires, etc.) upon the functions of the body, especially in relation to bodily disorders or disease. SEE psychophysiologic. SYN psychophysical (2). [psycho- + G. *sōma,* body]

**psy·cho·so·mat·ic dis·or·der, psy·cho·phys·i·o·log·ic dis·or·der** a disorder characterized by physical symptoms of psychic origin, usually involving a single organ system innervated by the autonomic nervous system; physiological and organic changes stem from a sustained disturbance.

**psy·cho·so·mat·ic med·i·cine** the study and treatment of diseases, disorders, or abnormal states in which psychological processes resulting in physiological reactions are believed to play a prominent role.

**psy·cho·so·mi·met·ic** (sī-kō′sō-mi-met′ik) SYN psychotomimetic.

**psy·cho·stim·u·lant** (sī-kō-stim′yu-lant) an agent with antidepressant or mood-elevating properties.

**psy·cho·sur·gery** (sī-kō-ser′jer-ē) the treatment of mental disorders by operation upon the brain, e.g., lobotomy.

**psy·cho·ther·a·peu·tics** (sī′kō-thār-ă-pyū′tiks) SYN psychotherapy.

**psy·cho·ther·a·pist** (sī-kō-thār′ă-pist) a person, usually a psychiatrist or clinical psychologist, professionally trained and engaged in psychotherapy. Currently, the term is also applied to social workers, nurses, and others whose state licensing practice acts include psychotherapy.

**psy·cho·ther·a·py** (sī-kō-thār′ă-pē) treatment of emotional, behavioral, personality, and psychiatric disorders based primarily upon verbal or nonverbal communication and interventions with the patient, in contrast to treatments utilizing chemical and physical measures. SEE psychoanalysis, psychiatry, psychology, therapy. SYN psychotherapeutics. [psycho- + G. *therapeia*, treatment]

**psy·chot·ic** (sī-kot′ik) relating to or affected by psychosis.

**psy·chot·ic dis·or·der** SYN psychosis.

**psy·chot·o·gen·ic** (sī-kot-ō-jen′ik) capable of inducing psychosis; particularly referring to drugs of the LSD series and similar substances.

**psy·chot·o·mi·met·ic** (sī-kot′ō-mi-met′ik) **1.** a drug or substance that produces psychological and behavioral changes resembling those of psychosis; e.g., LSD. **2.** denoting such a drug or substance. SYN psychosomimetic. [psychosis + G. *mimetikos*, imitative]

**psy·cho·tro·pic** (sī-kō-trōp′ik) capable of affecting the mind, emotions, and behavior; denoting drugs used in the treatment of mental illnesses. [psycho- + G. *trope̅*, a turning]

△**psy·chro-** cold. SEE ALSO cryo-, crymo-. [G. *psychros*]

**psy·chro·al·gia** (sī-krō-al′jē-ă) a painful sensation of cold. [psychro- + G. *algos*, pain]

**psy·chrom·e·try** (sī-krom′ĕ-trē) the calculation of relative humidity and water vapor pressures from wet and dry bulb temperatures and barometric pressure; whereas relative humidity is the value ordinarily employed, the vapor pressure is the measurement of physiological significance. SYN hygrometry. [psychro- + G. *metron*, measure]

**psy·chro·phile, psy·chro·phil** (sī′krō-fīl) an organism which grows best at a low temperature (0 to 32°C; 32 to 86°F), with optimum growth occurring at 15 to 20°C (59 to 68°F). [psychro- + G. *phileo̅*, to love]

**psy·chro·phil·ic** (sī-krō-fil′ik) pertaining to a psychrophile. [psychro- + G. *phileo̅*, to love]

**psy·chro·phore** (sī′krō-fōr) a double catheter through which cold water is circulated to apply cold to the urethra or another canal or cavity. [psychro- + G. *phoros*, bearing]

**PT** physical therapy or physical therapist; prothrombin time.

**Pt** platinum.

**PTA** plasma thromboplastin antecedent; phosphotungstic acid; percutaneous transluminal angioplasty.

**PTAH** phosphotungstic acid hematoxylin.

△**pter-, ptero-** wing; feather. [G. *pteron*, wing, feather]

**pter·i·on** (tē′rē-on) [TA] a craniometric point in the region of the sphenoid fontanelle, at the junction of the greater wing of the sphenoid, the squamous portion of the temporal, the frontal, and the parietal bones; it intersects the course of the anterior division of the middle meningeal artery. [G. *pteron*, wing]

**pte·ryg·i·um** (tĕ-rij′ē-ŭm) **1.** a triangular patch of hypertrophied bulbar subconjunctival tissue, extending from the medial canthus to the border of the cornea or beyond, with apex pointing toward the pupil. **2.** forward growth of the cuticle over the nail plate, seen most commonly in lichen planus. **3.** an abnormal skin web. [G. *pterygion*, anything like a wing, a disease of the eye, dim. of *pteryx*, wing]

△**pter·y·go-** wing-shaped, usually relating to the pterygoid process. [G. *pteryx, pterygos*, wing]

**pter·y·goid** (ter′i-goyd) wing-shaped; resembling a wing; a term applied to various anatomical parts relating to the sphenoid bone. [G. *pteryx* (*pteryg-*), wing, + *eidos*, resemblance]

**pter·y·goid ca·nal** an opening through the base of the medial pterygoid process of the sphenoid bone through which pass the artery, vein, and nerve of the pterygoid canal. SYN canalis pterygoideus [TA].

**pter·y·goid nerve** one of two motor branches, lateral and medial, of the mandibular nerve, supplying the lateral and medial pterygoid muscles with fibers of the motor root of the trigeminal nerve. SYN nervus pterygoideus [TA].

**pter·y·goid pro·cess** a long process extending downward from the junction of the body and greater wing of the sphenoid bone on either side; it is formed of two plates (lateral and medial), united anteriorly but separated below to form the pterygoid notch; the pterygoid fossa is formed by the divergence of these two plates posteriorly.

**pter·y·go·man·dib·u·lar** (ter′i-gō-man-dib′yu-lăr) relating to the pterygoid process and the mandible.

**pter·y·go·max·il·lary** (ter′i-gō-mak′si-lār-ē) relating to the pterygoid process and the maxilla.

**pte·ry·go·men·in·ge·al ar·te·ry** *origin:* maxillary or middle meningeal artery; *distribution:* traverses foramen ovale to enter cranial cavity, where it supplies the trigeminal ganglion, dura mater, and bone of the floor of the middle cranial fossa; however, its main distribution is extracranially to the pterygoid and tensor tympani muscles, the sphenoid bone, and the mandibular nerves and its otic ganglion. SYN arteria pterygomeningealis [TA].

**pter·y·go·pal·a·tine** (ter′i-gō-pal′ă-tīn) relating to the pterygoid process and the palatine bone.

**pter·y·go·pal·a·tine ca·nal** SYN greater palatine canal.

**pter·y·go·pal·a·tine gan·gli·on** a small parasympathetic ganglion in the upper part of the pterygopalatine fossa whose postsynaptic fibers supply the lacrimal, nasal, palatine and pharyngeal glands.

**PTHC** percutaneous transhepatic cholangiography.

■*Pthir·us* (thī′rŭs) a genus of lice formerly grouped in the genus *Pediculus*. The main species is *Pthirus pubis*, the crab or pubic louse, a parasite that infests the pubes and adjacent hairy parts of the body. Often incorrectly spelled *Phthirus* or *Phthirius*. See page B3. [irreg. fr. G. *phtheir*, louse]

**PTHrP** parathyroid hormone-related peptide.

**PTK** phototherapeutic keratectomy.

**pto·maine** (tō'mān) an indefinite term applied to poisonous substances, e.g., toxic amines, formed in the decomposition of protein by the decarboxylation of amino acids by bacterial action. [G. *ptōma*, a corpse]

**ptosed** (tōst) SYN ptotic.

**pto·sis**, pl. **pto·ses** (tō'sis, tō'sēz) **1.** a sinking down or prolapse of an organ. **2.** SYN blepharoptosis. [G. *ptōsis*, a falling]

△**-pto·sis** a sinking down or prolapse of an organ. [G. *ptōsis*, a falling]

**pto·tic** (tot'ik) relating to or marked by ptosis. SYN ptosed.

**PTT** partial thromboplastin time.

**pty·a·lec·ta·sis** (tī'ă-lek'tă-sis) SYN sialectasis. [ptyal- + G. *ektasis*, a stretching out]

**pty·a·lism** (tī'al-izm) SYN sialism. [G. *ptyalismos*, spitting]

**pty·a·lo·cele** (tī'ă-lō-sēl) SYN ranula (2).

**Pu** plutonium.

**pu·bar·che** (pyu-bar'kē) onset of puberty, particularly as manifested by the appearance of pubic hair. [puberty + G. *archē*, beginning]

**pu·ber·al, pu·ber·tal** (pyu'ber-ăl, pyu'ber-tăl) relating to puberty.

**pu·ber·ty** (pyu'ber-tē) sequence of events by which a child becomes a young adult, characterized by the beginning of gametogenesis, secretion of gonadal hormones, development of secondary sexual characteristics and reproductive functions; sexual dimorphism is accentuated. In girls, the first signs of puberty may be evident at age 8 with the process largely completed by age 16; in boys, puberty commonly begins at ages 10–12 and is largely completed by age 18. Ethnic and geographic factors may influence the time at which various events typical of puberty occur. [L. *pubertas*, fr. *puber*, grown up]

**pu·bes** (pyu'bēz) **1.** [TA] the area above the external genitals where hair growth signals puberty. **2.** one of the pubic hairs; the hair of the pubic region. USAGE NOTE: Often incorrectly called pubis. [L. *pubes*, the hair on the genitals; the genitals]

**pu·bes·cence** (pyu-bes'ens) **1.** the approach of the age of puberty or sexual maturity. [L. *pubesco*, to attain puberty] **2.** presence of downy or fine, short hair. [L. *pubes*, pubic hair]

**pu·bes·cent** (pyu-bes'ent) pertaining to pubescence.

**pu·bic** (pyu'bik) relating to the pubes or to the pubic bone.

**pu·bic an·gle** SYN subpubic angle.

**pu·bic arch** the arch formed by the symphysis, bodies and inferior rami of the pubic bones. SEE ALSO subpubic angle.

**pu·bic bone** the anteroinferior portion of the hip bone, distinct at birth but later becoming fused with the ilium and ischium; it consists of a body, which articulates with its fellow at the symphysis pubis, and two rami; the superior ramus enters into the formation of the acetabulum, and the inferior ramus fuses with the ramus of the ischium to form the ischiopubic ramus.

**pu·bic crest** the rough anterior border of the

body of the pubis, continuous laterally with the pubic tubercle.

**pu·bic re·gion** the lower central region of the abdomen below the umbilical region.

**pu·bic sym·phy·sis** the firm fibrocartilaginous joint between the two pubic bones.

**pu·bi·ot·o·my** (pyu-bē-ot'ō-mē) severance of the pubic bone a few centimeters lateral to the symphysis, in order to increase the capacity of a contracted pelvis sufficiently to permit the passage of a living child. SYN pelviotomy (2), pelvitomy. [L. *pubis*, pubic bone, + G. *tomē*, incision]

**pu·bis** (pyu'bis) official alternate term for os pubis, the pubic bone.

**pub·lic health** the art and science of community health, concerned with statistics, epidemiology, hygiene, and the prevention and eradication of epidemic diseases; an effort organized by society to promote, protect, and restore the people's health; public health is a social institution, a service, and a practice.

△**pu·bo-** pubic, pubes. [L. *pubes*]

**pu·bo·coc·cy·ge·al mus·cle** SYN pubococcygeus muscle.

**pu·bo·coc·cy·ge·us mus·cle** fibers of the levator ani, arising from the pelvic surface of the body of the pubis and adjacent tendinous arch of obturator fascia, attaching to the coccyx. SYN musculus pubococcygeus [TA], pubococcygeal muscle.

**pu·bo·pros·tat·ic** (pyu'bō-pros-tat'ik) relating to the pubic bone and the prostate.

**pu·bo·pros·tat·ic mus·cle** smooth muscle fibers within the puboprostatic ligament. SYN musculus puboprostaticus [TA].

**pu·bo·rec·tal** (pyu'bō-rek'tăl) relating to the pubic bone and the rectum.

**pu·bo·rec·ta·lis mus·cle** the medial part of the musculus levator ani (pubococcygeus muscle) that passes from the body of the pubis around the anus to form a muscular sling at the level of the anorectal junction; it contracts to increase the perineal flexure during a peristalsis to maintain fecal continence and relaxes to allow defecation. SYN musculus puborectalis [TA], puborectal muscle.

**pu·bo·rec·tal mus·cle** SYN puborectalis muscle.

**pu·bo·va·gi·na·lis mus·cle** in the female, the most medial fibers of the levator ani (pubococcygeus) muscle that extend from the pubis into the lateral walls of the vagina. SYN musculus pubovaginalis [TA], pubovaginal muscle.

**pu·bo·vag·i·nal mus·cle** SYN pubovaginalis muscle.

**pu·bo·ves·i·cal** (pyu'bō-ves'i-kăl) relating to the pubic bone and the bladder.

**pu·bo·ves·i·ca·lis mus·cle** smooth muscle fibers within the pubovesical ligament in the female. SYN musculus pubovesicalis [TA], pubovesical muscle.

**pu·bo·ves·i·cal mus·cle** SYN pubovesicalis muscle.

**Pucht·ler-Sweat stain for base·ment mem·branes** (pukt-ler-swet) a staining method using resorcin-fuchsin and nuclear fast red solutions after Carnoy fixative; basement membranes are gray to black and nuclei pink to red.

**Pucht·ler-Sweat stain for he·mo·glo·bin and he·mo·sid·er·in** (pukt-ler-swet) a complex staining method in which, on a yellow background, hemoglobin is stained red, hemosiderin blue to green and elastic fibers are pink.

**Pucht·ler-Sweat stains** (pukt-ler-swet) SEE Puchtler-Sweat stain for basement membranes, Puchtler-Sweat stain for hemoglobin and hemosiderin.

**pu·den·dal** (pyu-den′dăl) relating to the external genitals. SYN pudic.

**pu·den·dal ca·nal** the space within the obturator internus fascia lining the lateral wall of the ischiorectal fossa that transmits the pudendal vessels and nerves. SYN canalis pudendalis [TA].

**pu·den·dal cleft** the cleft between the labia majora.

**pu·den·dal nerve** formed by fibers from the ventral primary rami of the second, third, and fourth sacral spinal nerves; it exits the pelvis via the greater sciatic foramen, passes posterior to the sacrospinous ligament, and accompanies the internal pudendal artery into the perineum via the lesser sciatic foramen; it gives off inferior rectal nerves, then courses through the pudendal canal in the lateral wall of the ischiorectal fossa, terminating as the dorsal nerve of the penis or the clitoris. SYN nervus pudendus [TA].

**pu·den·dum**, pl. **pu·den·da** (pyu-den′dŭm, pyu-den′dă) the external genitals, especially the female genitals (vulva). Used also in the plural. [L. ntr. of *pudendus,* particip. adj. of *pudeo,* to feel ashamed]

**pu·dic** (pyu′dik) SYN pudendal. [L. *pudicus,* modest]

**pu·er·pera**, pl. **pu·er·per·ae** (pyu-er′per-ă, pyu-er′per-ē) a woman who has just given birth. [L., fr. *puer,* child, + *pario,* to bring forth]

**pu·er·per·al** (pyu-er′per-ăl) relating to the puerperium, or period after childbirth. SYN puerperant (1).

**pu·er·per·al ec·lamp·sia** convulsions and coma associated with hypertension, edema, or proteinuria occurring in a woman following delivery.

**pu·er·per·al fe·ver** postpartum sepsis with a rise in temperature after the first 24 hours following delivery, but before the eleventh postpartum day. SYN childbed fever.

**pu·er·per·al sep·ti·ce·mia** a severe bloodstream infection resulting from an obstetric delivery or procedure.

**pu·er·per·al tet·a·nus** tetanus occurring during the puerperium from infection of the obstetric wound.

**pu·er·per·ant** (pyu-er′per-ant) **1.** SYN puerperal. **2.** a puerpera.

**pu·er·pe·ri·um**, pl. **pu·er·pe·ria** (pyu-er-pēr′ē-ŭm, pyu-er-pēr′ē-ă) period from the termination of labor to complete involution of the uterus, usually defined as 42 days. [L. childbirth, fr. *puer,* child, + *pario,* to bring forth]

**Pues·tow pro·ce·dure** (pyoo′stō) longitudinal pancreaticojejunostomy for treatment of chronic pancreatitis.

***Pu·lex*** (pyu′leks) a genus of fleas (family Pulicidae, order Siphonaptera). [L. flea]

**Pul·frich phe·no·me·non** (pŭlf′rik) the binocular perception that an small target oscillating in the frontal plane is moving in an elliptical path seen when one eye is covered by a filter or in the presence of a unilateral optic neuropathy.

**pu·lic·i·cide, pu·li·cide** (pyu-lis′ĭ-sīd, pyū′li-sīd) a chemical agent destructive to fleas. [L. *pulex* (*pulic-*), flea, + *caedo,* to kill]

**pul·ley** (pŭl′ē) SEE trochlea.

**pul·mo**, gen. **pul·mo·nis**, pl. **pul·mo·nes** (pŭl′mō, pŭl-mō′nis, pŭl′mō′nēz) [TA] SYN lung. [L.]

**☖pul·mo-, pul·mon-, pul·mo·no-** the lungs. SEE ALSO pneum-, pneumo-. [L. *pulmo,* lung]

**pul·mo·a·or·tic** (pŭl′mō-ā-ōr′tik) relating to the pulmonary artery and the aorta.

**pul·mo·nary** (pŭl′mŏ-ner-ē) relating to the lungs, to the pulmonary artery, or to the aperture leading from the right ventricle into the pulmonary artery. SYN pneumonic (1), pulmonic. [L. *pulmonarius,* fr. *pulmo,* lung]

**pul·mo·nary ac·i·nus** that part of the airway consisting of a respiratory bronchiole and all of its branches. SYN primary pulmonary lobule.

**pul·mo·nary ad·e·no·ma·to·sis** a neoplastic disease in which the alveoli and distal bronchi are filled with mucus and mucus-secreting columnar epithelial cells; characterized by abundant, extremely tenacious sputum, chills, fever, cough, dyspnea, and pleuritic pain.

**pul·mo·nary al·ve·o·lar mi·cro·li·thi·a·sis** microscopic granules of calcium or bone disseminated throughout the lungs.

**pul·mo·nary al·ve·o·lar pro·tein·o·sis** a chronic progressive lung disease of adults, characterized by alveolar accumulation of granular proteinaceous material that is PAS-positive and lipid rich, with little inflammatory cellular exudate; the cause is unknown.

**pul·mo·nary al·ve·o·lus** one of the thin-walled saclike terminal dilations of the respiratory bronchioles, alveolar ducts, and alveolar sacs across which gas exchange occurs between alveolar air and the pulmonary capillaries. SYN alveolus (1) [TA], air cells (1), air vesicles, alveoli pulmonis, bronchic cells.

**pul·mo·nary ar·tery** SYN pulmonary trunk.

**pul·mo·nary ar·tery a·tre·sia** absence of one, usually the right, pulmonary artery.

**pul·mo·nary ar·tery cath·e·ter** SYN Swan-Ganz catheter.

**pul·mo·nary bleb** air-filled alveolar dilation less than 1 cm in diameter on the edge of the lung at the apex of upper lobe or superior segment of lower lobe; usually occurs in young people and can rupture, producing primary pneumothorax.

**pul·mo·nary cap·il·lary wedge pres·sure (PCWP)** the pressure obtained when a catheter is passed from the right side of the heart into pulmonary artery as far as it will go and "wedged" into an end artery. The pressure distal to the wedged catheter is an approximation of cardiac left atrial pressure. The pressure recorded with the balloon deflated is pulmonary artery pressure.

**⊞pul·mo·nary cir·cu·la·tion** the passage of blood from the right ventricle through the pulmonary artery to the lungs and back through the pulmonary veins to the left atrium. See page 820.

**pul·mo·na·ry col·lapse** secondary atelectasis due to bronchial obsturction, pleural effusion or pneumothorax, cardiac hypertrophy, or enlargement of other structures adjacent to the lungs.

**pul·mo·nary dys·ma·tu·ri·ty syn·drome** a respiratory disorder occurring in premature infants who are incapable of normal pulmonary ventilation and who often die of hypoxia after an illness of 6 to 8 weeks; the lungs contain widespread focal emphysematous blebs and the parenchyma has thickened alveolar walls.

**pul·mo·nary e·de·ma** edema of lungs usually

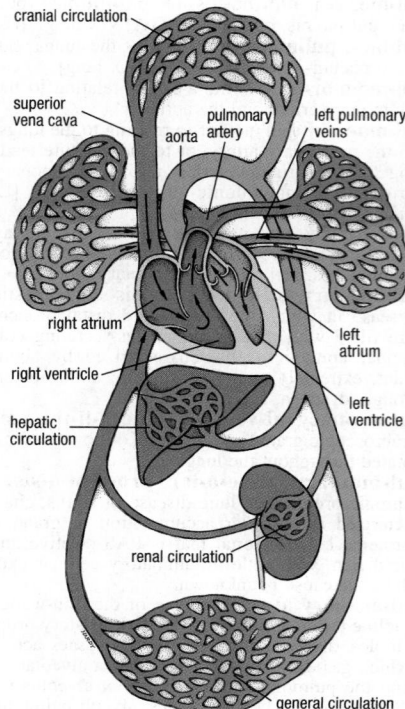

cranial circulation

superior vena cava

pulmonary artery

aorta

left pulmonary veins

right atrium

left atrium

right ventricle

left ventricle

hepatic circulation

renal circulation

general circulation

**pulmonary circulation:** through the lungs, from the right ventricle to the left atrium

**systemic circulation:** through the body, from the left ventricle to the right atrium

**red:** oxygenated blood

**blue:** deoxygenated blood

---

resulting from mitral stenosis or left ventricular failure.

**pul•mo•nary em•bo•lism** embolism of pulmonary arteries, most frequently by detached fragments of thrombus from a leg or pelvic vein, commonly when thrombosis has followed an operation or confinement to bed.

**pul•mo•nary em•phy•se•ma** SYN emphysema (2).

**pul•mo•nary e•o•sin•o•phil•ia** eosinophilic pulmonary infiltrates, often associated with parasitic migration; also associated with reactions to some antibiotics, to L-tryptophan, or to crack cocaine. SYN Löffler syndrome.

**pul•mo•nary func•tion tech•ni•cian** SYN pulmonary function technologist.

**pul•mo•nary func•tion tech•no•lo•gist** individual trained to perform pulmonary function tests for the diagnostic assessment and monitoring of cardiopulmonary disorders. SYN pulmonary function technician.

**pul•mo•nary func•tion test (PFT)** the assessment (from various breathing maneuvers) that provides information about airflow, lung volumes, and the diffusion of gas; the assessment of

airflow is made from spirometry, peak flow meters, and the body plethysmograph; the assessment of lung volumes requires the measurement of functional residual capacity and of slow vital capacity; the assessment of diffusing capacity is usually made by the single-breath carbon monoxide technique. Other PFTs include exercise, bronchial provocation, and pressure-volume assessment.

**pul•mo•nary ham•ar•to•ma** hamartoma of the lung, producing a coin lesion composed primarily of cartilage and bronchial epithelium. SYN adenochondroma.

**pul•mo•nary hy•per•ten•sion** hypertension in the pulmonary circuit; may be primary, or secondary to pulmonary or cardiac disease, e.g., fibrosis of the lung or mitral stenosis.

**pul•mo•nary in•suf•fi•cien•cy** SEE valvular regurgitation.

**pul•mo•nary lig•a•ment** two-layered fold formed as the pleura of the mediastinum is reflected onto the lung inferior to the root of the lung. SYN ligamentum pulmonale [TA].

**pul•mo•nary mur•mur, pul•mon•ic mur•mur** a murmur produced at the pulmonary orifice of the heart, either obstructive or regurgitant.

**pul•mo•nary plex•us** one of two autonomic plexuses, anterior and posterior, at the hilus of each lung, formed by cardiopulmonary splanchnic nerves of the sympathetic trunk and bronchial branches of the vagus nerve; from them various branches accompany the bronchi and arteries into the lung.

**pul•mo•nary ste•no•sis** narrowing of the opening into the pulmonary artery from the right ventricle.

**pul•mon•ary toi•let** cleansing of the trachea and bronchial tree.

**pul•mo•nary trunk** *origin,* right ventricle of heart; *distribution,* it divides into the right pulmonary artery and the left pulmonary artery, which enter the corresponding lungs and branch along with the segmental bronchi. SYN truncus pulmonalis [TA], arteria pulmonalis, pulmonary artery.

**pul•mo•nary valve** the valve at the entrance to the pulmonary trunk from the right ventricle; it consists of semilunar cusps (valvules) which are usually arranged in the adult in right anterior, left anterior, and posterior positions; however, they are named in accordance with their embryonic derivation; thus the posteriorly located cusp is designated as the left cusp, the right anteriorly located cusp is designated the right cusp and the left anteriorly positioned cusp is called the anterior cusp.

**pul•mo•nary vas•cu•lar re•sis•tance** the resistance to blood flow through the pulmonary circulation, which is largely influenced by the degree of tone or caliber of the pulmonary arteries and capillaries. Can be measured with the use of hemodynamic monitoring.

**pul•mo•nary ven•ti•la•tion** respiratory minute volume, i.e., the total volume of gas per minute inspired ($V_I$) or expired ($V_E$) expressed in liters per minute; differs from alveolar ventilation by including the exchange of dead space gas.

**pul•mon•ic** (pŭl-mon'ik) SYN pulmonary.

**pul•mo•ni•tis** (pŭl-mō-nī'tis) SYN pneumonitis.

**pulp** (pŭlp) **1.** a soft, moist, coherent solid. SYN

pulpa [TA]. **2.** SYN dental pulp. **3.** SYN chyme. [L. *pulpa*, flesh]

**pul•pa** (pŭl′pă) [TA] SYN pulp (1). [L. pulp]

**pul•pal** (pŭl′păl) relating to the pulp.

**pulp am•pu•ta•tion** SYN pulpotomy.

**pulp ca•nal** SYN root canal of tooth.

**pulp cav•i•ty** the central hollow of a tooth consisting of the crown cavity and the root canal; it contains the fibrovascular dental pulp and is lined throughout by odontoblasts.

**pulp cham•ber** that portion of the pulp cavity which is contained in the crown or body of the tooth.

**pulp•ec•to•my** (pŭl-pek′tō-mē) removal of the entire pulp structure of a tooth, including the pulp tissue in the roots. [L. *pulpa*, pulp, + G. *ektomē*, excision]

**pulp horn** a prolongation of the pulp extending toward the cusp of a tooth.

**pul•pi•fac•tion** (pŭl-pi-fak′shŭn) reduction to a pulpy condition. [L. *pulpa*, pulp, + *facio*, pp. *factus*, to make]

**pulp•i•tis** (pŭl-pī′tis) inflammation of the pulp of a tooth. [L. *pulpa*, pulp, + G. *-itis*, inflammation]

**pulp•ot•o•my** (pŭl-pot′ō-mē) removal of a portion of the pulp structure of a tooth, usually the coronal portion. SYN pulp amputation. [L. *pulpa*, pulp, + G. *tomē*, incision]

**pulp stone** SYN endolith.

**pulp test** SYN vitality test.

**pulpy** (pŭl′pē) in the condition of a soft, moist solid.

**pul•sate** (pŭl′sāt) to throb or beat rhythmically; said of the heart or an artery. [L. *pulso*, pp. *-atus*, to beat]

**pul•sa•tile** (pŭl′să-til) throbbing or beating.

**pul•sa•tion** (pŭl-sā′shŭn) a throbbing or rhythmical beating, as of the pulse or the heart. [L. *pulsatio*, a beating]

**ⓘpulse** (pŭls) palpable rhythmic expansion of an artery, produced by the increased volume of blood thrown into the vessel by the contraction of the heart. A pulse may also at times occur in a vein or a vascular organ, such as the liver. See page 822. SYN pulsus. [L. *pulsus*]

**pulse def•i•cit 1.** the absence of palpable pulse waves in a peripheral artery for one or more heart beats, as is often seen in atrial fibrillation; **2.** the number of such missing pulse waves (usually expressed as heart rate minus pulse rate per minute).

**pulsed las•er** a laser in which energy output is pulsed, allowing short bursts of high energy.

**pulse-field gel e•lec•tro•pho•re•sis** gel electrophoresis in which, after electrophoretic migration has begun, the current is briefly stopped and reapplied in a different orientation; allows for the purification of long DNA molecules.

**pulse gen•er•a•tor** a device that produces an electrical discharge with a regular or rhythmic wave form in which the electromotive force varies in a specific pattern in relation to time; e.g., in an electronic pacemaker, it produces an electric discharge at regular intervals, and these intervals may be modified by a sensory circuit which can reset the time-base for subsequent discharge on the basis of other electrical activity, such as that produced by spontaneous cardiac beating.

**pulse height an•a•lyz•er** electronic circuitry that determines the energy of scintillations recorded

by a detector, allowing use of a discriminator to select for photons of a specific type.

**pulse•less dis•ease** SYN Takayasu arteritis.

**pulse•less e•lec•tri•cal ac•ti•vi•ty (PEA)** SYN electromechanical dissociation.

**pulse ox•i•me•ter** a spectrophotometric device that noninvasively estimates saturation of arterial oxyhemoglobin ($SaO_2$) by use of selected wavelengths of light.

**pulse pres•sure** the variation in blood pressure occurring in an artery during the cardiac cycle; it is the difference between the systolic or maximum and diastolic or minimum pressures.

**pulse rate** rate of the pulse as observed in an artery; recorded as beats per minute.

**pulse se•quence** in magnetic resonance imaging, a series of changes in the induced magnetic field, which include the phase and frequency-encoding gradients and read-out functions.

**pulse wave** the progressive expansion of the arteries occurring with each contraction of the left ventricle of the heart.

**pulse wave du•ra•tion** the interval between onset of the leading edge and the end of the trailing edge of a pulse wave.

**pul•sion** (pŭl′shŭn) a pushing outward or swelling. [L. *pulsio*]

**pul•sion di•ver•tic•u•lum** a diverticulum formed by pressure from within, frequently causing herniation of mucosa through the muscularis.

**pul•sus** (pŭl′sŭs) SYN pulse. [L. a stroke, pulse]

**pul•sus al•ter•nans** SYN alternating pulse.

**pul•sus bi•gem•i•nus** SYN bigeminal pulse.

**pul•sus bis•fe•ri•ens** SYN bisferious pulse.

**pul•sus ce•ler** a pulse beat swift to rise and fall.

**pul•sus dif•fer•ens** a condition in which the pulses in the two radial or other corresponding arteries differ in strength.

**pul•sus par•a•dox•us** (pŭl′sŭs păr-ă-doks′ŭs) SYN paradoxical pulse.

**pul•sus tar•dus** a pulse with pathologically gradual upstroke typical of severe aortic stenosis. SEE ALSO plateau pulse.

**pul•sus tri•gem•i•nus** SYN trigeminal pulse.

**pul•ta•ceous** (pŭl-tā′shŭs) macerated; pulpy. [G. *poltos*, porridge]

**pul•vi•nar** (pŭl-vī′năr) [TA] the expanded posterior extremity of the thalamus which forms a cushionlike prominence overlying the geniculate bodies. [L. a couch made from cushions, fr. *pulvinus*, cushion]

**pump** (pŭmp) **1.** an apparatus for forcing a gas or liquid from or to any part. **2.** any mechanism for using metabolic energy to accomplish active transport of a substance.

**pumped las•er** a laser whose energy level is increased by the application of separate sources of electrons or photons, which may themselves be primary lasers.

**pump lung** SYN shock lung.

**pump-ox•y•gen•a•tor** (pŭmp-ok′si-je-nā′ter) a mechanical device that can substitute for both the heart (pump) and the lungs (oxygenator) during open heart surgery.

**ⓘpunch bi•op•sy** any method that removes a small cylindrical specimen for biopsy by means of a special instrument that pierces the organ directly or through the skin or a small incision in the skin. See page 117.

**punch•drunk syn•drome, punch•drunk** (pŭnch′drŭnk) a condition seen in boxers, often years after retirement, and presumably caused by repeated cerebral injury, characterized by weakness in the lower limbs, unsteadiness of gait, slowness of muscular movements, tremors of hands, dysarthria, and slow cerebration.

**punch grafts** small full-thickness grafts of the scalp, removed with a circular punch and transplanted to a bald area to grow hair.

**punc•ta** (pŭngk′tă) plural of punctum. [L.]

**punc•tate** (pŭngk′tāt) marked with points or dots differentiated from the surrounding surface by color, elevation, or texture. [L. *punctum,* a point]

**punc•tate hem•or•rhage** SYN petechial hemorrhage.

**punc•tate hy•a•lo•sis** a condition marked by minute opacities in the vitreous.

**punc•ti•form** (pŭngk′ti-fōrm) very small but not microscopic, having a diameter of less than 1 mm. [L. *punctum,* a point, + *forma,* shape]

**punc•tum**, gen. **punc•ti**, pl. **punc•ta** (pŭngk′ tŭm, pungk-tī, pŭngk′tă) **1.** the tip of a sharp process. **2.** a minute round spot differing in color or otherwise in appearance from the surrounding tissues. **3.** a point on the optic axis of an optical system. SEE ALSO point. SYN point (1). [L. a prick, point, pp. ntr. of *pungo,* to prick, used as noun]

**punc•tum ce•cum** the blind spot in the visual field corresponding to the location of the optic disk.

**punc•tum fix•a** SYN fixed end.

**punc•tum mo•bile** SYN mobile end.

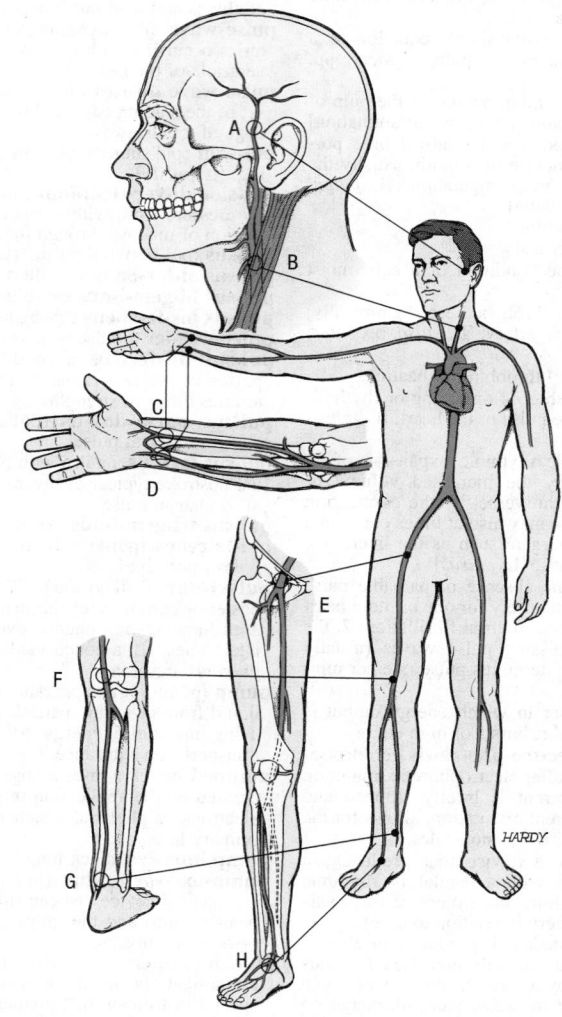

**peripheral pulses:** (A) temporal, (B) carotid, (C) radial, (D) ulnar, (E) femoral, (F) popliteal, (G) posterior tibial, (H) dorsalis pedis

**punc·tum vas·cu·lo·sum** one of the minute dots seen on section of the brain, due to small drops of blood at the cut extremities of the arteries.

**punc·ture** (pŭnk′cher) **1.** to make a hole with a small pointed object, such as a needle. **2.** a prick or small hole made with a pointed instrument. [L. *punctura,* fr. *pungo,* pp. *punctus,* to prick]

**punc·ture wound** a wound in which the opening is relatively small as compared to the depth, as produced by a narrow pointed object.

**PUO** pyrexia of unknown (or undetermined) origin.

**pu·pa,** pl. **pu·pae** (pyu′pă, pyu′pē) the stage of insect metamorphosis following the larva and preceding the imago. [L. *pupa,* doll]

**pu·pil (p)** (pyu′pĭl) the circular orifice in the center of the iris, through which light rays enter the eye. SYN pupilla [TA]. [L. *pupilla*]

**pu·pil·la,** pl. **pu·pil·lae** (pyu-pil′ă, pyū-pil′ē) [TA] SYN pupil. [L. dim. of *pupa,* a girl or doll]

**pu·pil·lary** (pyū′pi-lār-ē) relating to the pupil.

**pu·pil·lary block** increased resistance to flow of aqueous humor through the pupil from the posterior chamber to the anterior chamber, leading to anterior bowing of the peripheral iris over the trabecular meshwork and to angle-closure glaucoma.

**pu·pil·lary dis·tance** the distance between the center of each pupil; the major reference points in measuring for fitting of spectacle frames and lenses.

**pu·pil·lary mem·brane** remnants of the central portion of the anterior layer of the iris stroma (the iridopupillary lamina) which occludes the pupil in fetal life, and normally atrophies about the seventh month of gestation. Failure to regress is a rare cause of congenital blindness. SYN membrana pupillaris [TA], Wachendorf membrane (1).

**pu·pil·lary re·flex** change in diameter of the pupil as a reflex response to any type of stimulus; e.g., constriction caused by light. SYN light reflex (1).

**pu·pil·lar·y-skin re·flex** dilation of the pupil following scratching of the skin of the neck. SYN ciliospinal reflex.

△**pu·pil·lo-** the pupils. [L. *pupilla,* pupil]

**pu·pil·lom·e·ter** (pyu′pi-lom′ĕ-ter) an instrument for measuring and recording the diameter of the pupil. [pupillo- + G. *metron,* measure]

**pu·pil·lom·e·try** (pyu′pi-lom′ĕ-trē) measurement of the pupil.

**pu·pil·lo·mo·tor** (pyu′pĭ-lō-mō′ter) relating to the autonomic nerve fibers that supply the smooth muscle of the iris. [pupillo- + L. *motor,* mover]

**pu·pil·lo·sta·tom·e·ter** (pyu′pi-lō-stă-tom′ĕ-ter) an instrument for measuring the distance between the centers of the pupils. [pupillo- + G. *statos,* placed, + *metron,* measure]

**pu·pil·lo·to·nic pseu·do·stra·bis·mus** SYN Adie syndrome.

**PUPPP** *p*ruritic *u*rticarial *p*apules and *p*laques of pregnancy, an intensely pruritic, occasionally vesicular, eruption of the trunk and arms appearing in the third trimester of pregnancy; spontaneous involution occurs within 10 days of term.

**pure ab·sence** SYN simple absence.

**pure au·to·no·mic fail·ure** a degenerative, sporadic neurologic disorder of adult onset, manifested principally as orthostatic hypotension and syncope, with no neurologic defects other than autonomic nervous system dysfunction evident; probably caused by selective degeneration of neurons in the sympathetic ganglia, with denervation of smooth muscle vasculature and the adrenal glands. SYN Bradbury-Eggleston syndrome.

**pure cul·ture** in the ordinary bacteriologic sense, a culture consisting of the descendants of a single cell.

**pure tone** an audible tone that can be represented by a sine wave; an oscillation showing only one frequency of vibration, with no overtones or harmonics. SEE ALSO conduction, sine wave.

**pure tone au·di·o·gram** an audiogram in which the threshold for pure tone stimuli is charted in decibels of hearing level down the vertical axis, the horizontal axis being the frequency that is usually measured in octave steps from 125 Hz to 8 kHz. See this page.

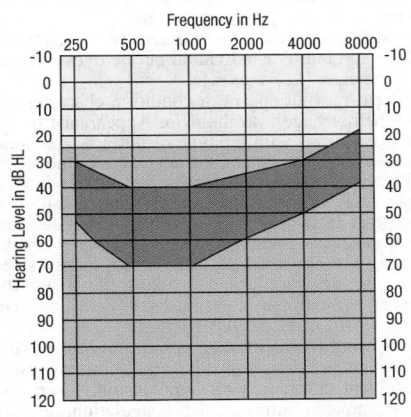

**pure tone audiogram:** yellow area indicates limits of normal hearing; dark green area illustrates the frequency and intensity of the English phonemes; dBHL=decibels (of) hearing loss

**pure-tone a·ver·age** average in decibels of the thresholds for pure tones at 500, 1000, and 2000 Hz.

**pur·ga·tion** (per-gā′shŭn) evacuation of the bowels with the aid of a purgative or cathartic. SYN catharsis (1). [L. *purgatio*]

**pur·ga·tive** (per′gă-tiv) an agent used for purging the bowels. SEE ALSO cathartic (2). [L. *purgativus,* purging]

**purge** (perj) **1.** to cause a copious evacuation of the bowels. **2.** a cathartic remedy. [L. *purgo,* to cleanse, fr. *purus,* pure, + *ago,* to do]

**pu·rine** (pyūr′ēn) the parent substance of adenine, guanine, and other naturally occurring purine "bases"; not known to exist as such in mammals.

**Pur·kin·je cell lay·er** (pĕr-kin′jē) the layer of large neuron cell bodies located at the interface of molecular and granular layers in the cerebellar cortex; dendrites of these cells fan outward into the molecular layer in a plane transverse to the folium. SYN Purkinje cells, Purkinje corpuscles.

**Pur·kin·je cells** (pĕr-kin′jē) SYN Purkinje cell layer.

**Pur·kin·je cor·pus·cles** (pĕr-kin'jē) SYN Purkinje cell layer.

**Pur·kin·je fi·bers** (pĕr-kin'jē) SYN subendocardial branches of atrioventricular bundles.

**Pur·kin·je fig·ures** (pĕr-kin'jē) shadows of the retinal vessels, seen as dark lines on a reddish field when a light enters the eye through the sclera and not the pupil.

**Pur·kin·je net·work** (pĕr-kin'jē) the network formed by Purkinje fibers beneath the endocardium.

**Pur·kin·je phe·nom·e·non** (pĕr-kin'jē) in the light-adapted eye, the region of maximal brightness is in the yellow; in the dark-adapted eye, the region of maximal brightness is in the green.

**Pur·kin·je-San·son im·a·ges** (pĕ-kin'jē san-son) the two images formed by the anterior and posterior surfaces of the cornea and the two images formed by the anterior and posterior surfaces of the lens. SYN Sanson images.

**Pur·mann meth·od** (pĕr'mahn) treatment of aneurysm by extirpation of the sac.

**pur·ple** (pĕr'pl) a color formed by a mixture of blue and red. For individual purple dyes see specific name. [L. *purpura*]

**pur·pu·ra** (pŭr'poo-ră) a condition characterized by hemorrhage into the skin. Appearance of the lesions varies with the type of purpura, the duration of the lesions, and the acuteness of the onset. The color is first red, gradually darkens to purple, fades to a brownish yellow, and usually disappears in two or three weeks; color of residual permanent pigmentation depends largely on the type of unabsorbed pigment of the extravasated blood; extravasations may occur also into the mucous membranes and internal organs. SYN peliosis. [L. fr. G. *porphyra*, purple]

**pur·pu·ra ful·mi·nans** a severe and rapidly fatal form of purpura hemorrhagica, occurring especially in children, with hypotension, fever, and disseminated intravascular coagulation, usually following an infectious illness. See page B6.

**pur·pu·ra hem·or·rha·gi·ca** SYN idiopathic thrombocytopenic purpura.

**pur·pu·ra se·ni·lis** the occurrence of petechiae and ecchymoses on the atrophic skin of the legs in aged and debilitated subjects.

**pur·pu·ra sim·plex** the eruption of petechiae or larger ecchymoses, usually unaccompanied by constitutional symptoms and not associated with systemic illness. SYN nonthrombocytopenic purpura.

**pur·pu·ric** (pŭr-poo'rik) relating to or affected with purpura.

**pur·pu·ri·nu·ria** (pĕr'pyu-ri-nyu'rē-ă) SYN porphyrinuria.

**purse-string in·stru·ment** an intestinal clamp with jaws at an angle to the handle; when closed across the bowel, large grooved interdigitating serrations allow passage of a straight needle and suture through each side to form a purse-string suture.

**purse-string su·ture** a continuous suture placed in a circular manner either for inversion (as for an appendiceal stump) or closure (as for a hernia).

**Purt·scher ret·i·nop·a·thy** (poor'cher) transient traumatic retinal angiopathy due to a sudden rise in venous pressure, as in compression of the body from seat belt injury; ocular fundi show large white patches associated with the retinal

veins about the disk or macula, hemorrhages, and retinal edema; thought to be due to fat embolism from bone marrow.

**pu·ru·lence, pu·ru·len·cy** (pyur'ŭ-lens, pyur'ŭ-len-sē; pyur'yu-lens; pyur'ŭ-lens-ē) the condition of containing or forming pus. [L. *purulentia*, a festering, fr. *pus* (*pur*-), pus]

**pu·ru·lent** (pyur'ŭ-lent, pyur'yu-lent) containing, consisting of, or forming pus.

**pu·ru·lent in·flam·ma·tion** an acute exudative inflammation in which polymorphonuclear leukocytes cause liquefaction of the affected tissues, focally or diffusely; the purulent exudate is frequently termed pus. SYN suppurative inflammation.

**pu·ru·lent oph·thal·mia** purulent conjunctivitis, usually of gonorrheal origin.

**pu·ru·lent pleu·ri·sy** pleurisy with empyema.

**pu·ru·lent syn·o·vi·tis** SYN suppurative arthritis.

**pu·ru·loid** (pyu'rŭ-loyd) resembling pus.

**pus** (pŭs) a fluid product of inflammation containing leukocytes and the debris of dead cells and tissue elements. [L.]

**pus·tu·lar** (pŭs'choo-lăr) relating to or marked by pustules.

**pus·tu·la·tion** (pŭs'choo-lā'shŭn) the formation or the presence of pustules.

**pus·tule** (pŭs'chool) a small, circumscribed elevation of the skin, containing purulent material. See page B4. [L. *pustula*]

**pus·tu·lo·sis** (pŭs-choo-lō'sis) **1.** an eruption of pustules. **2.** term occasionally used to designate acropustulosis. [L. *pustula*, pustule, + G. *-osis*, condition]

**pus·tu·lo·sis pal·mar·is et plan·tar·is** a sterile pustular eruption of the fingers and toes, variously attributed to dyshidrosis, pustular psoriasis, and unidentified bacterial infection. SYN acrodermatitis continua, acrodermatitis perstans, dermatitis repens.

**pu·ta·men** (pyu-tā'men) [TA] the outer, larger, and darker gray of the three portions into which the lenticular nucleus is divided by laminae of white fibers; it is connected with the caudate nucleus by bridging bands of gray substance that penetrate the internal capsule. Its histological structure is similar to that of the caudate nucleus; together they compose the striatum. SEE ALSO striate body. [L. that which falls off in pruning, fr. *puto*, to prune]

**Put·nam-Da·na syn·drome** (put'năm dā-nă) SYN subacute combined degeneration of the spinal cord.

**pu·tre·fac·tion** (pyu-tri-fak'shŭn) decomposition or rotting, the breakdown of organic matter usually by bacterial action, resulting in the formation of other substances of less complex constitution with the evolution of ammonia or its derivatives and hydrogen sulfide; characterized usually by the presence of toxic or malodorous products. SYN decay (2), decomposition. [L. *putre-facio*, pp. *-factus*, to make rotten]

**pu·tre·fac·tive** (pyu-tri-fak'tiv) relating to or causing putrefaction.

**pu·tre·fy** (pyu'tri-fī) to cause to become, or to become, putrid.

**pu·tres·cence** (pyu-tres'ens) the state of putrefaction.

**pu·tres·cent** (pyu-tres'ent) denoting, or in the process of, putrefaction. [L. *putresco*, to grow rotten, fr. *puter*, rotten]

**pu·tres·cine** (pyu-tres'ēn) a poisonous polyamine formed from the amino acid arginine during putrefaction; found in urine and feces.

**pu·trid** (pyu'trid) **1.** in a state of putrefaction. **2.** denoting putrefaction. [L. *putridus*]

**Put·ti-Platt op·er·a·tion** (poo'ti-plat) a procedure for recurrent dislocation of shoulder joint.

**Pu·u·ma·la vi·rus** (poo-oo-mah-lah vī'us) a species of Hantavirus found in Europe causing hemorrhagic fever with renal syndrome.

**PUVA** oral administration of *p*soralen and subsequent exposure to long wavelength ultraviolet light (*uv-a*); used to treat psoriasis.

**PVA fix·a·tive** schaudinn fixative using either a mercuric chloride, zinc sulfate, or copper sulfate base; contains polyvinyl alcohol plastic powder that is used as an adhesive for fecal specimens in the preparation of permanent smears for subsequent staining.

**PVS** persistent vegetative state.

**P wave** the first complex of the electrocardiogram, representing depolarization of the atria; if the P wave is retrograde or ectopic in axis or form, it is labeled P'.

**py·ae·mia [Br.]** SEE pyemia.

**py·ar·thro·sis** (pī-ar-thrō'sis) SYN suppurative arthritis. [G. *pyon*, pus, + *arthrōsis*, a jointing]

△ **pyc·no-** SEE pykno-.

**pyc·no·dys·o·sto·sis [Br.]** SEE pyknodysostosis.

**pyc·no·me·ter [Br.]** SEE pyknometer.

**py·e·lec·ta·sis, py·e·lec·ta·sia** (pī-ĕ-lek'tă-sis, pī-ĕ-lek-tā'zē-ă) dilation of the pelvis of the kidney. [pyel- + G. *ektasis*, extension]

**py·e·lit·ic** (pī-ĕ-lit'ik) relating to pyelitis.

**py·e·li·tis** (pī-ĕ-lī'tis) inflammation of the renal pelvis. [pyel- + G. -*itis*, inflammation]

△ **py·e·lo-, py·e·l-** pelvis, usually the renal pelvis. [G. *pyelos*, trough, tub, vat]

**py·e·lo·cal·i·ce·al** (pī'ĕ-lō-kal'i-sē'ăl) relating to the renal pelvis and calices.

**py·e·lo·cys·ti·tis** (pī-ĕ-lō-sis-tī'tis) inflammation of the renal pelvis and the bladder. [pyelo- + G. *kystis*, bladder, + -*itis*, inflammation]

**py·e·lo·flu·o·ros·co·py** (pī'ĕ-lō-floo-r-os'kŏ-pē) fluoroscopic examination of the renal pelves and ureters, following administration of contrast medium. [pyelo- + L. *fluo*, to flow, + G. *skopeō*, to view]

**py·el·o·gram** (pī'el-ō-gram) a radiograph or series of radiographs of the renal pelvis and ureter, following injection of contrast medium.

**py·e·log·ra·phy** (pī'ĕ-log'ră-fē) radiologic study of the kidney, ureters, and/or the bladder, performed with the aid of a contrast agent either injected intravenously, or directly through a ureteral or nephrostomy catheter or percutaneously. SYN pyeloureterography, ureteropyelography. [pyelo- + G. *graphō*, to write]

**py·e·lo·li·thot·o·my** (pī'ĕ-lō-li-thot'ō-mē) operative removal of a calculus from the kidney through an incision in the renal pelvis. SYN pelvilithotomy. [pyelo- + G. *lithos*, stone, + *tomē*, incision]

**py·e·lo·ne·phri·tis** (pī'ĕ-lō-ne-frī'tis) inflammation of the renal parenchyma, calices, and pelvis, particularly due to local bacterial infection. [pyelo- + G. *nephros*, kidney, + -*itis*, inflammation]

**py·e·lo·plas·ty** (pī'e-lō-plas-tē) surgical reconstruction of the kidney pelvis to correct an obstruction. SYN pelvioplasty (2). [pyelo- + G. *plastos*, formed]

**py·e·los·co·py** (pī-ĕ-los'kŏ-pē) fluoroscopic observation of the pelvis and calices of the kidney, and the ureter, after the injection through the ureter of a radiopaque solution. [pyelo- + G. *skopeō*, to view]

**py·e·los·to·my** (pī-ĕ-los'tō-mē) formation of an opening into the kidney pelvis to establish urinary drainage. [pyelo- + G. *stoma*, mouth]

**py·e·lot·o·my** (pī-ĕ-lot'ō-mē) incision into the pelvis of the kidney. SYN pelviotomy (3), pelvitomy. [pyelo- + G. *tomē*, incision]

**py·e·lo·u·re·ter·ec·ta·sis** (pī'ĕ-lō-yu-rē'ter-ek'tă-sis) dilation of kidney pelvis and ureter, seen in hydronephrosis due to obstruction in the lower urinary tract. [pyelo- + ureter + G. *ektasis*, a stretching]

**py·e·lo·u·re·ter·og·ra·phy** (pī'ĕ-lō-yu-rē'ter-og'ră-fē) SYN pyelography.

**py·e·lo·ve·nous** (pī'ĕ-lō-vē'nŭs) relating to the renal pelvis and renal veins. Denoting the passage of urine from the renal pelvis into the renal veins, because of increased intrapelvic pressure. [pyelo- + venous]

**py·e·lo·ve·nous back·flow** retrograde movement of fluid (urine or injected contrast materials) from renal pelvis into renal venous system. This occurs under conditions of distal obstruction or injection of solutions into renal collecting system.

**py·em·e·sis** (pī-em'ĕ-sis) the vomiting of pus. [G. *pyon*, pus, + *emesis*, vomiting]

**py·e·mia** (pī-ē'mē-ă) septicemia due to pyogenic organisms causing multiple abscesses. [G. *pyon*, pus, + *haima*, blood]

**py·e·mic** (pī-ē'mik) relating to or suffering from pyemia.

**py·e·mic ab·scess** a hematogenous abscess resulting from pyemia, septicemia, or bacteremia. SYN septicemic abscess.

**py·e·mic em·bo·lism** plugging of an artery by an embolus detached from a suppurating thrombus. SYN infective embolism.

**py·en·ceph·a·lus** (pī-en-sef'ă-lŭs) SYN pyocephalus. [G. *pyon*, pus, + *enkephalos*, brain]

**py·e·sis** (pī-ē'sis) SYN suppuration. [G. *pyon*, pus, + -*esis*, condition or process]

**pyg·my** (pig'mē) a physiologic dwarf; especially one of a race of similar people, such as the pygmies of central Africa. [G. *pygmaios*, dwarfish, fr. *pygmē*, fist, also a measure of length from elbow to knuckles]

**pyk·nic** (pik'nik) denoting a constitutional body type characterized by well-rounded external contours and ample body cavities; virtually synonymous with endomorphic. [G. *pyknos*, thick]

△ **pyk·no-, pyk-** thick, dense, compact. [G. *pyknos*]

**pyk·no·dys·os·to·sis** (pik-nō-dĭs-os-tō'sĭs) a familial dysmorphism characterized by short stature, delayed closure of the fontanels, and hypoplasia of the terminal phalanges; autosomal recessive inheritance. [pykno- + dys- + G. *osteon*, bone, + -*osis*, condition]

**pyk·nom·e·ter** (pik-nom'ĕ-ter) a flask of standard volume, used to determine the specific gravity of fluids by weighing; a standard flask for measuring and comparing the densities of liquids. [pykno- + G. *metron*, measure]

**pyk·no·mor·phous** (pik'nō-mōr'fŭs) denoting a cell or tissue that stains deeply because the stainable material is closely packed. [pykno- + G. *morphē*, form, shape]

**pyk·no·sis** (pik-nō'sis) a thickening or condensation; specifically, a condensation and reduction in size of the cell or its nucleus, usually associated with hyperchromatosis; nuclear pyknosis is a stage of necrosis. [pykno- + G. *-osis*, condition]

**pyk·not·ic** (pik-not'ik) relating to or characterized by pyknosis.

**py·le·phle·bi·tis** (pī'lē-fle-bī'tis) inflammation of the portal vein or any of its branches. [G. *pylē*, a gate, + *phleps*, vein, + *-itis*, inflammation]

**py·le·throm·bo·phle·bi·tis** (pī-lē-throm'bō-phle-bī'tis) inflammation of the portal vein with the formation of a thrombus. [G. *pylē*, gate, + *thrombos*, a clot, + *phleps*, vein, + *-itis*, inflammation]

**py·le·throm·bo·sis** (pī'lē-throm-bō'sis) thrombosis of the portal vein or its branches. [G. *pylē*, gate, + *thrombos*, a clot, + *-osis*, condition]

**py·lo·rec·to·my** (pī'lōr-ek'tō-mē) excision of the pylorus. SYN gastropylorectomy, pylorogastrectomy. [pylor- + G. *ektomē*, excision]

**py·lo·ri** (pī-lōr'ī) plural of pylorus. [L.]

**py·lor·ic** (pī-lōr'ik) relating to the pylorus.

**py·lor·ic an·trum** the initial portion of the pyloric part of the stomach, which may temporarily become partially or completely shut off from the remainder of the stomach during digestion by peristaltic contraction of the prepyloric "sphincter"; it is sometimes demarcated from the second part of the pyloric part of the stomach (pyloric canal) by a slight groove. SYN antrum (2).

**py·lor·ic ca·nal** the segment of the stomach that succeeds the antrum and ends at the gastroduodenal junction. SYN canalis pyloricus [TA].

**py·lor·ic cap** archaic term for duodenal cap.

**py·lor·ic con·stric·tion** a prominent fold of mucous membrane at the gastroduodenal junction overlying the pyloric sphincter.

**py·lor·ic glands** the coiled, tubular glands of the pylorus whose cells secrete mucus.

**py·lor·ic or·i·fice** the opening between the stomach and the superior part of the duodenum.

**py·lor·ic sphinc·ter** a thickening of the circular layer of the gastric musculature encircling the gastroduodenal junction. SYN musculus sphincter pyloricus [TA].

**py·lor·ic ste·no·sis** narrowing of the gastric pylorus, especially by congenital muscular hypertrophy or scarring resulting from a peptic ulcer. SEE ALSO hypertrophic pyloric stenosis.

**py·lor·ic vein** SYN right gastric vein.

**py·lo·ri·ste·no·sis** (pī-lōr'i-ste-nō'sis) stricture or narrowing of the orifice of the pylorus. SYN pylorostenosis. [pylor- + G. *stenōsis*, a narrowing]

△**py·lor·o-, py·lor-** the pylorus. [G. *pyloros*, gatekeeper]

**py·lo·ro·du·o·de·ni·tis** (pī-lōr'ō-doo'od-ĕ-nī'tis) inflammation involving the pyloric outlet of the stomach and the duodenum. [pyloro- + duodenitis]

**py·lo·ro·gas·trec·to·my** (pī-lōr'ō-gas-trek'tō-mē) SYN pylorectomy.

**py·lo·ro·my·ot·o·my** (pī-lōr'ō-mī-ot'ō-mē) longitudinal incision through the anterior wall of the pyloric canal to the level of the submucosa, to treat hypertrophic pyloric stenosis. SYN Fredet-Ramstedt operation, Ramstedt operation. [pyloro- + G. *mys*, muscle, + *tomē*, incision]

**py·lo·ro·plas·ty** (pī-lōr'ō-plas-tē) widening of the pyloric canal and any adjacent duodenal stricture by means of a longitudinal incision closed transversely. [pyloro- + G. *plastos*, formed]

**py·lo·ro·spasm** (pī-lōr'ō-spazm) spasmodic contraction of the pylorus.

**py·lo·ro·ste·no·sis** (pī-lōr'ō-stĕ-nō'sis) SYN pyloristenosis.

**py·lo·ros·to·my** (pī-lō-ros'tō-mē) establishment of a fistula from the abdominal surface into the stomach near the pylorus. [pyloro- + G. *stoma*, mouth]

**py·lo·rot·o·my** (pī-lō-rot'ō-mē) incision of the pylorus. [pyloro- + G. *tomē*, incision]

**py·lo·rus**, pl. **py·lo·ri** (pī-lōr'ŭs, pī-lōr'ī) [TA] **1.** a muscular or myovascular device to open (musculus dilator) and to close (musculus sphincter) an orifice or the lumen of an organ. **2.** the muscular tissue surrounding and controlling the aboral outlet of the stomach. [L. fr. G. *pylōros*, a gatekeeper, the pylorus, fr. *pylē*, gate, + *ouros*, a warder]

**py·lor·us-pre·serv·ing pan·cre·a·tic·o·du·o·de·nec·to·my** excision of all or part of the pancreas and the duodenum with preservation of the distal stomach and the innervated pylorus; usually limited to the head and neck of the pancreas and most often performed for pancreatic carcinoma.

△**pyo-** suppuration, accumulation of pus. [G. *pyon*, pus]

**py·o·cele** (pī'ō-sēl) an accumulation of pus in the scrotum. [pyo- + G. *kēlē*, tumor, hernia]

**py·o·ceph·a·lus** (pī'ō-sef'ă-lŭs) a purulent effusion within the cranium. SYN pyencephalus. [pyo- + G. *kephalē*, head]

**py·o·che·zia** (pī-ō-kē'zē-ă) a discharge of pus from the bowel. [pyo- + G. *chezō*, to defecate]

**py·o·coc·cus** (pī'ō-kok'ŭs) one of the cocci causing suppuration, especially *Streptococcus pyogenes*. [pyo- + G. *kokkos*, berry (coccus)]

**py·o·col·po·cele** (pī-ō-kol'pō-sēl) a vaginal tumor or cyst containing pus. [pyo- + G. *kolpos*, bosom (vagina), + *kēlē*, tumor, hernia]

**py·o·col·pos** (pī-ō-kol'pos) accumulation of pus in the vagina. [pyo- + G. *kolpos*, bosom (vagina)]

**py·o·cy·an·ic** (pī'ō-sī-an'ik) relating to blue pus or the organism that causes blue pus, *Pseudomonas aeruginosa*. [pyo- + G. *kyanos*, blue]

**py·o·cy·a·no·gen·ic** (pī'ō-sī'ă-nō-jen'ik) causing blue pus. [pyo- + G. *kyanos*, blue, + *-gen*, producing]

**py·o·cyst** (pī'ō-sist) a cyst with purulent contents. [pyo- + G. *kystis*, bladder]

**py·o·der·ma** (pī-ō-der'mă) any pyogenic infection of the skin; may be primary, as impetigo, or secondary to a previously existing condition. [pyo- + G. *derma*, skin]

**py·o·der·ma gan·gre·no·sum** a chronic, noninfective eruption of spreading, undermined ulcers showing central healing, with diffuse dermal neutrophil infiltration; often associated with ulcerative colitis.

**py·o·gen·e·sis** (pī'ō-jen'ĕ-sis) SYN suppuration. [pyo- + G. *genesis*, production]

**py·o·gen·ic, py·o·ge·net·ic** (pī-ō-jen'ik, pī'ō-jĕ-net'ik) pus-forming; relating to pus formation.

⊞**py·o·gen·ic gran·u·lo·ma, gran·u·lo·ma py·o·gen·i·cum** an acquired small rounded mass of highly vascular granulation tissue, frequently with an ulcerated surface, projecting from the skin or mucosa; histologically, the mass resembles a capillary hemangioma. See page B7. SYN lobular capillary hemangioma.

**py·o·hae·mo·thor·ax [Br.]** SEE pyohemothorax.

**py·o·he·mo·tho·rax** (pī′ō-hē-mō-thōr′aks) presence of pus and blood in the pleural cavity. [pyo- + G. *haima*, blood, + thorax]

**py·oid** (pī′oyd) resembling pus. [G. *pyōdēs*, fr. *pyon*, pus, + *eidos*, resemblance]

**py·o·me·tra** (pī-ō-mē′tră) accumulation of pus in the uterine cavity. [pyo- + G. *mētra*, uterus]

**py·o·me·tri·tis** (pī′ō-mē-trī′tis) inflammation of uterine musculature associated with pus in the uterine cavity. [pyo- + G. *mētra*, womb, + *-itis*, inflammation]

**py·o·my·o·si·tis** (pī′ō-mī-ō-sī′tis) abscesses, carbuncles, or infected sinuses lying deep in muscles. [pyo- + G. *mys*, muscle, + *-itis*, inflammation]

**py·o·ne·phri·tis** (pī-ō-ne-frī′tis) suppurative inflammation of the kidney. [pyo- + G. *nephros*, kidney, + *-itis*, inflammation]

**py·o·neph·ro·li·thi·a·sis** (pī′ō-nef′rō-li-thī′ă-sis) presence in the kidney of pus and calculi. [pyo- + G. *nephros*, kidney, + *lithos*, stone, + *-iasis*, condition]

**py·o·ne·phro·sis** (pī′ō-ne-frō′sis) distention of the pelvis and calices of the kidney with pus, usually associated with obstruction. SYN nephropyosis. [pyo- + G. *nephros*, kidney, + *-osis*, condition]

**pyo·ova·ri·um** (pī′-ō-ō-var′ē-ŭm) presence of pus in the ovary; an ovarian abscess.

**py·o·per·i·car·di·tis** (pī′ō-per-i-kar-dī′tis) suppurative inflammation of the pericardium.

**py·o·per·i·car·di·um** (pī′ō-per-i-kar′dē-ŭm) an accumulation of pus in the pericardial sac.

**py·o·per·i·to·ne·um** (pī′ō-per-i-tō-nē′ŭm) an accumulation of pus in the peritoneal cavity. [G. *pyon*, pus]

**py·o·per·i·to·ni·tis** (pī′ō-per-i-tō-nī′tis) suppurative inflammation of the peritoneum. [pyo- + peritonitis]

**py·o·phy·so·me·tra** (pī′ō-fī-sō-mē′tră) presence of pus and gas in the uterine cavity. [pyo- + G. *physa*, air, + *mētra*, uterus]

**py·o·pneu·mo·cho·le·cys·ti·tis** (pī′ō-noo′mō-kō′lē-sis-ī′tis) combination of pus and gas in an inflamed gallbladder caused by gas-producing organisms or by the entry of gas from the duodenum through the biliary tree. [pyo- + G. *pneuma*, air, + cholecystitis]

**py·o·pneu·mo·hep·a·ti·tis** (pī′ō-noo′mō-hep-ă-tī′tis) combination of pus and gas in the liver, usually in association with an abscess. [pyo- + G. *pneuma*, air, + hepatitis]

**py·o·pneu·mo·per·i·car·di·um** (pī′ō-noo′mō-per-i-kar′dē-ŭm) presence of pus and gas in the pericardial sac. [pyo- + G. *pneuma*, air, + pericardium]

**py·o·pneu·mo·per·i·to·ne·um** (pī′ō-noo′mō-per-i-tō-nē′ŭm) presence of pus and gas in the peritoneal cavity. [pyo- + G. *pneuma*, air, + peritoneum]

**py·o·pneu·mo·per·i·to·ni·tis** (pī′ō-noo′mō-per-i-tō-nī′tis) peritonitis with gas-forming organisms or with gas introduced from a ruptured bowel. [pyo- + G. *pneuma*, air, + peritonitis]

**py·o·pneu·mo·tho·rax** (pī′ō-noo-mō-thōr′aks) the presence of gas together with a purulent effusion in the pleural cavity. SYN pneumopyothorax. [pyo- + G. *pneuma*, air, + thorax]

**py·o·poi·e·sis** (pī′ō-poy-ē′sis) SYN suppuration. [pyo- + G. *poiēsis*, a making]

**py·o·poi·et·ic** (pī′ō-poy-et′ik) pus-producing.

**py·o·py·e·lec·ta·sis** (pī′ō-pī-ĕ-lek′tă-sis) dilation of the renal pelvis with pus-producing inflammation. [pyo- + G. *pyelos*, pelvis, + *ektasis*, a stretching]

**py·or·rhea** (pī-ō-rē′ă) a purulent discharge. [pyo- + G. *rhoia*, a flow]

**py·or·rhoea [Br.]** SEE pyorrhea.

**py·o·sal·pin·gi·tis** (pi′o-sal-pin-ji′tis) suppurative inflammation of the fallopian tube. [pyo- + salpingitis]

**py·o·sal·pin·go·ooph·o·ri·tis** (pī-ō-sal′pin-gō-ō-of′ō-rī′tis) suppurative inflammation of the fallopian tube and the ovary. [pyo- + G. *salpinx*, trumpet (tube), + oophoritis]

**py·o·sal·pinx** (pī-ō-sal′pingks) distention of a fallopian tube with pus. [pyo- + G. *salpinx*, trumpet (tube)]

**py·o·sis** (pī-ō′sis) SYN suppuration. [G.]

**py·o·tho·rax** (pī-ō-thōr′aks) empyema in a pleural cavity.

**py·o·u·ra·chus** (pī-ō-yu′ră-kŭs) a purulent accumulation in the urachus.

**py·o·u·re·ter** (pī-ō-yu-rē′ter) distention of a ureter with pus.

**pyr·a·mid** (pir′ă-mid) **1.** a term applied to a number of anatomic structures having a more or less pyramidal shape. SYN pyramis [TA]. **2.** an obsolete term denoting the petrous portion of the temporal bone. [G. *pyramis* (*pyramid-*), a pyramid]

**py·ram·i·dal** (pi-ram′i-dal) **1.** of the shape of a pyramid. **2.** relating to any anatomical structure called pyramid.

**py·ram·i·dal au·ric·u·lar mus·cle** an occasional prolongation of the fibers of the tragicus to the spina helicis. SYN musculus pyramidalis auriculae [TA], pyramidal muscle of auricle.

**py·ram·i·dal bone** SYN triquetral bone.

**py·ram·i·dal cat·a·ract** a cone-shaped, anterior polar cataract.

**py·ram·i·dal cells** neurons of the cerebral cortex which, in sections perpendicular to the cortical surface, exhibit a triangular shape with a long apical dendrite directed toward the surface of the cortex.

**py·ram·i·dal de·cus·sa·tion** the intercrossing of the bundles of the pyramidal tracts at the lower border region of the medulla oblongata. SYN decussatio pyramidum [TA], motor decussation.

**py·ram·i·dal frac·ture** a fracture of the midfacial skeleton with the principal fracture lines meeting at an apex at or near the superior aspect of the nasal bones.

**py·ra·mi·da·lis mus·cle** origin, crest of pubis; insertion, lower portion of linea alba; action, makes linea alba tense; nerve supply, subcostal. SYN musculus pyramidalis [TA], pyramidal muscle.

**py·ram·i·dal lobe of thy·roid gland** an inconstant narrow lobe of the thyroid gland that arises from the upper border of the isthmus and extends upward, sometimes as far as the hyoid bone; it marks the point of continuity with the thyroglossal duct.

**py·ram·i·dal mus·cle** SYN pyramidalis muscle.

**py·ram·i·dal mus·cle of au·ri·cle** SYN pyramidal auricular muscle.

**py·ram·i·dal ra·di·a·tion** corticospinal fibers

passing from the cortex into the pyramid. SYN radiatio pyramidalis.

**py·ram·i·dal tract** a massive bundle of fibers originating from pyramidal cells in the precentral motor and premotor area, and the postcentral gyrus. Fibers from these cortical regions descend through the internal capsule, the middle third of the crus cerebri, and the ventral part of the pons to emerge on the ventral surface of the medulla oblongata as the pyramis. Continuing caudally, most of the fibers cross to the opposite side in the pyramidal decussation and descend in the spinal cord as the lateral pyramidal tract, which distributes its fibers to interneurons of the spinal gray matter. Interruption of the pyramidal tract at or below its cortical origin causes impairment of movement in the opposite body-half, especially severe in the arm and leg and characterized by muscular weakness, spasticity and hyperreflexia, and a loss of discrete finger and hand movements. Babinski sign is associated with this condition of hemiplegia.

**pyr·a·mid of light** a triangular area at the anterior inferior part of the tympanic membrane, running from the umbo to the periphery, where there is seen a bright reflection of light. SYN cone of light, light reflex (3), red reflex.

**pyr·a·mid of me·dul·la ob·lon·ga·ta** an elongated, white prominence on the ventral surface of the medulla oblongata on either side along the anterior median fissure, corresponding to the pyramidal tract. SYN anterior pyramid, pyramis medullae oblongatae.

**pyr·a·mid sign** any of the symptoms indicating a morbid condition of the pyramidal tracts, such as the Babinski or Gordon sign, spastic spinal paralysis, foot clonus, etc.

**pyr·a·mid of ver·mis** a subdivision of the inferior vermis of the cerebellum between the tuber and the uvula.

**pyr·a·mis,** pl. **py·ra·mi·des** (pir'ă-mis, pi-ram'i-dēz) [TA] SYN pyramid (1). [Mod. L. fr. G. pyramid]

**pyr·a·mis me·dul·lae ob·lon·ga·tae** SYN pyramid of medulla oblongata.

**pyr·a·mis re·na·lis,** pl. **py·ra·mi·des re·na·les** SYN renal pyramid.

**pyr·a·nose** (pir'ă-nōs, pī'ră-nōs) a cyclic form of a sugar in which the oxygen bridge forms a pyran.

**py·ret·ic** (pī-ret'ik) SYN febrile. [G. pyretikos]

⚠ **py·re·to-** fever. SEE ALSO pyro- (1). [G. pyretos, fever, fr. pyr, fire]

**py·rex·ia** (pī-rek'sē-ă) SYN fever. [G. pyrexis, feverishness]

**py·rex·i·al** (pī-rek'sē-ăl) relating to fever.

**py·rex·ia of un·known or·i·gin** SYN fever of unknown origin.

**py·ri·din·i·um** a breakdown product of bone collagen, excreted in urine, and assayed as a measure of osteoclast activity; increased in disease states such as Paget disease, primary hyperparathyroidism, and osteoporosis.

**py·ri·din·o·line** hydroxypyridinium; a. breakdown product of bone collagen, assayed as is pyridinium to gauge osteoclastic activity.

**pyr·i·dox·al 5'-phos·phate** a coenzyme essential to many reactions in tissue, notably transaminations and amino acid decarboxylations.

**pyr·i·dox·a·mine** (pir-i-dok'să-mēn) the amine

of pyridoxine which has a similar physiologic action. SEE pyridoxine.

**4-pyr·i·dox·ic ac·id** (fōr-pir-i-dok'sik as'id) the principal product of the metabolism of pyridoxal, appearing in the urine.

**pyr·i·dox·ine** (pir-i-dok'sēn) the original vitamin $B_6$, which term now includes pyridoxal and pyridoxamine, associated with the utilization of unsaturated fatty acids. Deficiency may result in increased irritability, convulsions, and peripheral neuritis. The hydrochloride is used in pharmaceutical preparations; the chief form in vegetables.

**py·rim·i·dine** (pī-rim'i-dēn) a heterocyclic substance, the formal parent of several "bases" present in nucleic acids (uracil, thymine, cytosine) as well as of the barbiturates.

**py·rin** an abnormal neutrophil protein encoded by the MEFV gene in familial Mediterranean fever. SYN marenostrin.

⚠ **py·ro- 1.** fire, heat, or fever. SEE ALSO pyreto-. **2.** CHEMISTRY combining form denoting derivatives formed by removal of water (usually by heat) to form anhydrides. SEE ALSO anhydro-. [G. pyr, fire]

**py·ro·gen** (pī'rō-jen) a fever-inducing agent; pyrogens are produced by bacteria, molds, viruses, and yeasts, and commonly occur in distilled water. [pyro- + G. -gen, producing]

**py·ro·gen·ic** (pī-rō-jen'ik) causing fever.

**py·ro·glob·u·lins** (pī-rō-glob'yu-linz) serum proteins (immunoglobulins), usually associated with multiple myeloma or macroglobulinemia, which precipitate irreversibly when heated to 56°C.

**py·rol·y·sis** (pī-rol'i-sis) decomposition of a substance by heat. [pyro- + G. lysis, dissolution]

**py·ro·ma·nia** (pī-rō-mā'nē-ă) a morbid impulse to set fires. [pyro- + G. mania, frenzy]

**py·ro·nin** (pī'rō-nin) a fluorescent red basic xanthene dye, used in combination with methyl green for differential staining of RNA (red) and DNA (green); also used as a tracking dye for RNA in electrophoresis.

**py·ro·pho·bia** (pī-rō-fō'bē-ă) morbid dread of fire. [pyro- + G. phobos, fear]

**py·ro·phos·pha·tase** (pī-rō-fos'fă-tās) any enzyme cleaving a pyrophosphate bond between two phosphoric groups, leaving one on each of the two fragments. SYN diphosphatase.

**py·ro·phos·phate (PP)** (pī-rō-fos'fāt) a salt of pyrophosphoric acid; accumulates in cases of hypophosphatasia; sometimes referred to as inorganic pyrophosphate ($PP_i$).

**py·ro·sis** (pī-rō'sis) substernal pain or burning sensation, usually associated with regurgitation of acid-peptic gastric juice into the esophagus. SYN heartburn. [G. a burning]

**pyr·role** (pir'ōl) a heterocyclic compound found in many biologically important substances. SYN azole, imidole.

**pyr·rol·i·dine** (pi-rol'i-dēn) **1.** pyrrole to which four H atoms have been added; the structural basis of proline and hydroxyproline. **2.** a class of alkaloids containing a pyrrolidine (1) moiety or a pyrrolidine derivative.

**py·ru·vate** (pī'roo-vāt) a salt or ester of pyruvic acid.

**py·ru·vate ki·nase (PK)** phospho*enol*pyruvate kinase; a phosphotransferase catalyzing transfer of phosphate from phospho*enol*pyruvate to ADP, forming ATP and pyruvate; other nucleoside phosphates can participate in the reaction; a key step in glycolysis; a deficiency in pyruvate kinase will lead to hemolytic anemia.

**py•ru•vic ac•id** (pī-roo′vik as′id) an intermediate compound in the metabolism of carbohydrate; in thiamin deficiency, its oxidation is retarded and it accumulates in the tissues. SEE phosphoenolpyruvic acid.

**py•u•ria** (pī-yu′rē-ă) presence of pus in the urine when voided. [G. *pyon*, pus, + *ouron*, urine]

# Q

**Q** coulomb; quantity; quaternary; glutamine; glutaminyl; pseudouridine; coenzyme Q; electric charge; the second product formed in an enzyme-catalyzed reaction.

**Q̇** blood flow. SEE flow (3). [quantity + an overdot denoting the time derivative]

**Q$_{CO_2}$** symbol for the microliters STPD of $CO_2$ given off per milligram of tissue per hour.

**q 1.** CYTOGENETICS long arm of a chromosome (in contrast to p for the short arm). **2.** abbreviation for [L.] *quodque*, each, every. **3.** symbol for heat.

**QA** quality assurance.

**Q-an·gle** the angle formed by the line of traction of the quadriceps tendon on the patella and the line of traction of the patellar tendon on the tibial tubercle.

**Q-band·ing stain** a fluorescent stain for chromosomes which produces specific banding patterns for each pair of homologous chromosomes; the acridine dye derivative, quinacrine hydrochloride, or other derivatives like quinacrine mustard dihydrochloride produces a green-yellow fluorescence at pH 4.5 in chromosome segments rich in constitutive heterochromatin with deoxyadenylate-deoxythymidilate (A-T) bases of DNA; centromeric regions of human chromosomes 3, 4, and 13 are specifically stained, as are satellites of some acrocentric chromosomes and the end of the long arm of the Y chromosome.

**QC** quality control.

**Q fe·ver** a febrile disease characterized by headache and myalgia and sometimes pneumonitis or hepatitis; caused by *Coxiella burnetii;* the organism propagates in sheep and cattle, where it produces no symptoms; human infections occur as a result of contact not only with such animals but also with other infected humans, air and dust, wild reservoir hosts, and other sources. [*Q,* for "query," so named because etiologic agent was unknown]

**QH$_2$** ubiquinol.

**QNS** quantity not sufficient (amount of specimen submitted to laboratory is inadequate to perform test requested).

**QRB in·ter·val** the time between the onset of the Q wave of the QRS complex and the right bundle-branch potential (normally 15–20 msec).

**QR in·ter·val** the time elapsing from the onset of the QRS complex to the peak of the R or the final R wave; measures the time of onset of the intrinsicoid deflection if determined in an appropriate unipolar lead tracing.

**QRS com·plex** portion of electrocardiogram corresponding to the depolarization of ventricular myocardium.

**QS$_2$ in·ter·val** SYN electromechanical systole.

**Q-switched las·er** (quality-switched); a laser in which the quality, or energy storage capacity is altered between a very high and a low value.

**Q-T in·ter·val, QT in·ter·val** the time from Q wave (of QRS complex) to the end of the T wave as it can be measured on electrocardiogram; corresponds to ventricular systole.

**quack** (kwak) SYN charlatan. [Abbreviation of quacksalver, Dutch *quack*, to boast + *salf*, cream]

**qua·dran·gu·lar lob·ule** the main portion of the superior part of each hemisphere of the cerebellum, corresponding to the monticulus of the vermis; it is divided into two portions, the anterior and the posterior crescentic lobules, corresponding to the culmen and the declive of the vermis. SYN quadrate lobe (2).

**quad·rant** (kwah′drant) one quarter of a circle. ANATOMY roughly circular areas are divided for descriptive purposes into quadrants. The abdomen is divided into right upper and lower, and left upper and lower quadrants by a horizontal and a vertical line intersecting at the umbilicus. Quadrants of the ocular fundus (superior and inferior nasal, superior and inferior temporal) are demarcated by a horizontal and a vertical line intersecting at the optic disk. The tympanic membrane is divided into anterosuperior, anteroinferior, posterosuperior, and posteroinferior quadrants by a line drawn across the diameter of the drum in the axis of the handle of the malleus and another intersecting the first at right angles at the umbo. See this page. [L. *quadrans,* a quarter]

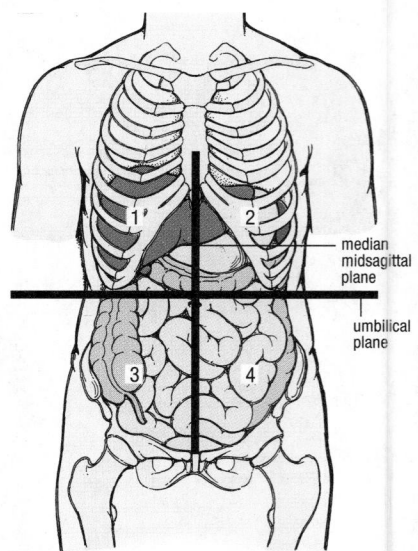

**quadrants:** (1) right upper, (2) left upper, (3) right lower, (4) left lower

**quad·rate** (kwah′drāt) having 4 equal sides; square. [L. *quadratus,* square]

**quad·rate lobe 1.** a lobe on the inferior surface of the liver located between the fossa for the gallbladder and the fissure for the ligamentum teres; **2.** SYN quadrangular lobule. **3.** SYN precuneus.

**quad·ra·tus fem·o·ris mus·cle** *insertion,* intertrochanteric ridge; *origin,* lateral border of tuberosity of ischium; *action,* rotates thigh laterally; *nerve supply,* nerve to quadratus femoris (sacral plexus). SYN musculus quadratus femoris [TA].

**quad·ra·tus la·bii su·pe·ri·or·is mus·cle** composed of three heads usually described as three separate muscles; they are the caput angulare or levator labii superioris alaeque nasi muscle; caput infraorbitale or levator labii superioris muscle; caput zygomaticum or zygomaticus minor muscle. SYN musculus quadratus labii superioris.

**quad•ra•tus lum•bo•rum mus•cle** *origin*, iliac crest, iliolumbar ligament, and transverse processes of lower lumbar vertebrae; *insertion*, twelfth rib and transverse processes of upper lumbar vertebrae; *action*, abducts trunk; *nerve supply*, ventral primary rami of upper lumbar spinal nerves. SYN musculus quadratus lumborum [TA].

**quad•ra•tus plan•tae mus•cle** *origin*, by two heads from the lateral and medial borders of the inferior surface of the calcaneus; *insertion*, tendons of flexor digitorum longus; *action*, assists long flexor; *nerve supply*, lateral plantar. SYN musculus quadratus plantae [TA].

△**quad•ri-** four. [L. *quattuor*]

**quad•ri•ba•sic** (kwah-dri-bā′sik) denoting an acid having four hydrogen atoms that are replaceable by atoms or radicals of a basic character.

**quad•ri•ceps** (kwah′dri-seps) having four heads; denoting a muscle of the thigh, quadriceps femoris muscle, and one of the calf, quadriceps surae muscle, or the combined gastrocnemius (with two heads), soleus, and plantaris, more commonly called triceps surae muscle, the plantaris being counted as a separate muscle. [L. fr. quadri- + *caput,* head]

**quad•ri•ceps fem•o•ris mus•cle** *origin*, by four heads: rectus femoris, vastus lateralis, vastus intermedius, and vastus medialis; *insertion*, patella, and thence by ligamentum patellae to tuberosity of tibia; *action*, extends leg; flexes thigh by action of rectus femoris; *nerve supply*, femoral. SYN musculus quadriceps femoris [TA], quadriceps muscle of thigh.

**quad•ri•ceps mus•cle of thigh** SYN quadriceps femoris muscle.

**quad•ri•ceps re•flex** SYN patellar reflex.

**quad•ri•gem•i•nal** (kwah′dri-jem′i-năl) fourfold. [quadri- + L. *geminus,* twin]

**quad•ri•gem•i•nal rhy•thm** a cardiac arrhythmia in which the heartbeats are grouped in fours, each usually composed of one sinus beat followed by three extrasystoles, but a repetitive group of four of any composition is quadrigeminal.

**quad•ri•ge•mi•num** (kwah′dri-jem′i-nŭm) one of the quadrigeminal bodies.

**quad•ri•pa•re•sis** (kwah′dri-pă-rē′sis) SYN tetraparesis.

**qua•dri•pe•dal ex•ten•sor re•flex** extension of the arm of a hemiplegic patient when turned prone as if on all fours. SYN Brain reflex.

**quad•ri•ple•gia** (kwah′dri-plē′jē-ă) paralysis of all four limbs. SYN tetraplegia. [quadri- + G. *plēgē,* stroke]

**quad•ri•ple•gic** (kwah′dri-plē′jik) pertaining to or afflicted with quadriplegia.

**quad•ri•va•lent** (kwah-dri-vā′lent) having the combining power (valency) of four. SYN tetravalent.

**quad•rup•let** (kwah′drŭp-let, kwă-droo′plet) one of four children born at one birth. [L. *quadruplus,* fourfold]

**qual•i•ta•tive a•nal•y•sis** determination of the nature, as opposed to the quantity, of each of the elements composing a substance.

**qual•i•ty as•sur•ance (QA)** an institutional program designed to assess the success of the total

organization in achieving its goals. SEE ALSO quality control.

**qual•i•ty con•trol (QC)** the control of laboratory analytical error by monitoring analytical performance with control sera and maintaining error within established limits around the mean control values, most commonly ±2 SD.

**qual•i•ty con•trol chart** a chart illustrating the allowable limits of error in laboratory test performance, the limits being a defined deviation from the mean of a control serum, most commonly ±2 SD. SYN Levey-Jennings chart.

**qual•i•ty of life** a patient's general well-being, including mental status, stress level, sexual function, and self-perceived health status.

**quan•tal ef•fect** an effect that can be expressed only in binary terms, as occurring or not occurring.

**quan•ti•le** (kwahn′tīl) division or distribution into equal, ordered subgroups; deciles are tenths, quartiles are quarters, quintiles are fifths, terciles are thirds, centiles are hundredths. [L. *quantum,* how much, + *-ilis,* adj. suffix]

**quan•ti•ta•tive a•nal•y•sis** determination of the amount, as well as the nature, of each of the elements composing a substance.

**Quant sign** (quahnt) a T-shaped depression in the occipital bone occurring in many cases of rickets, especially in infants lying constantly in bed with pressure on the occiput.

**quan•tum,** pl. **quan•ta** (kwahn′tŭm, kwahn′tă) **1.** a unit of radiant energy (ε) varying according to the frequency (ν) of the radiation. **2.** a certain definite amount. [L. how much]

**quan•tum the•o•ry** that energy can be emitted, transmitted, and absorbed only in discrete quantities (quanta), so that atoms and subatomic particles can exist only in certain energy states. SYN Planck theory.

**quan•tum yield** (φ) the number of molecules transformed (e.g., via a reaction) per quantum of light absorbed; the inverse of the quantum requirement.

**quar•an•tine** (kwar′an-tēn) the isolation of a person with a known or possible contagious disease. [It. *quarantina* fr. L. *quadraginta,* forty]

**quark** (qwark) a fundamental particle believed to be the primary constituent of all mesons and baryons; quarks have a charge that is a fraction of 1 electron charge and interact through electromagnetic and nuclear forces. Six varieties are thought to exist with the unusual names of up, down, strange, charmed, bottom, and top. [a word of indeterminate sense used by James Joyce in his novel *Finnegans Wake*]

**quart** (kwŏrt) **1.** a measure of fluid capacity; the fourth part of a gallon; the equivalent of 0.9468 liter. **2.** a dry measure holding a little more than the fluid measure. [L. *quartus,* fourth]

**quar•tan** (kwōr′tan) recurring every fourth day, including the first day of an episode in the computation, i.e., after a free interval of two days. SEE malariae malaria. [L. *quartanus,* relating to a fourth (thing)]

**quar•tan ma•lar•ia** SYN malariae malaria.

**quartz** (kwŏrts) a crystalline form of silicon dioxide used in chemical apparatus and in optical and electric instruments.

**quasi-con•tin•u•ous wave las•er** a laser whose output can be controlled in milliseconds or similarly small increments by electronic control.

q
u

**qua·si·dom·i·nance** (kwā-si-dom'i-nans) simulation by a recessive trait of the pedigree of dominant inheritance (i.e., recurrence in several generations) by repeated, and often occult, consanguineous matings. SYN pseudodominance.

**qua·si·dom·i·nant** (kwā-si-dom'i-nănt) denoting a trait in an inbred pedigree that exhibits quasidominance.

**qua·ter·na·ry (Q)** (kwah'ter-nār-ē, kwah-ter'nĕ-rē) **1.** denoting a chemical compound containing four elements. **2.** fourth in a series. **3.** relating to organic compounds in which some central atom is attached to four functional groups. **4.** referring to a level of structure of macromolecules in which more than one biopolymer is present. [L. *quaternarius,*, fr. *quaterni,* four each, fr. *quattuor,* four, + *-arius,* adj. suffix]

**Queck·en·stedt-Stook·ey test** (kwek'ĕn-shtet-stook'ē) compression of the jugular vein in a healthy person causes an increase in the pressure of the spinal fluid in the lumbar region within 10 to 12 seconds; when there is a block of subarachnoid channels, compression of the vein causes little or no increase of pressure in the cerebrospinal fluid.

**quel·lung phe·nom·e·non** SYN Neufeld capsular swelling.

**quel·lung re·ac·tion 1.** SYN Neufeld capsular swelling. **2.** if pneumococcal organisms, India ink, and specific antisera are mixed, the antibodies present in the sera will bind to the polysaccharide antigens of the pneumococcal capsule and the capsule will appear more opaque and swollen. [Ger. *Quellung,* swelling]

**quel·lung test** SYN Neufeld capsular swelling.

**quench·ing** (kwench'ing) **1.** the process of extinguishing, removing, or diminishing a physical property such as heat or light. **2.** in beta liquid scintillation counting, the shifting of the energy spectrum from a true to a lower energy; it is caused by a variety of interfering materials in the counting solution. **3.** the process of stopping a chemical or enzymatic reaction. [M. E. *quenchen,* fr. O.E. *ācwencan*]

**ques·tion·naire** (kwes-chŭn-ār') a list of questions submitted orally or in writing to obtain personal information or statistically useful data.

**quick** (kwik) **1.** pregnant with a child whose fetal movements are recognizable. **2.** a sensitive part, painful to touch. [A.S. *cwic,* living]

**quick·en·ing** (kwik'ĕn-ing) signs of life felt by the mother as a result of the fetal movements, usually noted from 16 to 20 weeks of pregnancy. [A.S. *cwic,* living]

**Quick test** (kwik) SYN prothrombin test.

**qui·es·cent** (kwī-es'ent) at rest or inactive.

**qui·et lung** the collapse of a lung during thoracic operations undertaken to facilitate surgical procedure through absence of lung movement.

**Quin·cke pulse** (kwing'kĕ) the capillary pulse as appreciated in the finger nails and toenails during aortic regurgitation; ebb and flow is seen.

**qui·nine** (kwī-nīn, kwin'īn) the most important of the alkaloids derived from cinchona; an antimalarial effective against the asexual and erythrocytic forms of the parasite, but having no effect on the exoerythrocytic (tissue) forms. It does not produce a radical cure of malaria produced by *Plasmodium vivax, P. malariae,* or *P. ovale,* but is used in the treatment of cerebral malaria and other severe attacks of malignant tertian malaria, and in malaria produced by chloroquine-resistant strains of *P. falciparum;* it is also used as an antipyretic, analgesic, sclerosing agent, stomachic, and oxytocic (occasionally), and in the treatment of atrial fibrillation, myotonia congenita, and other myopathies.

**quin·sy** (kwin'zē) SYN peritonsillar abscess. [M.E. *quinsie (quinesie),* a corruption of L. *cynanche,* sore throat]

**quin·tan** (kwin'tan) recurring every fifth day, including the first day of an episode in the computation, i.e., after a free interval of three days. [L. *quintus,* fifth]

**quin·tu·plet** (kwin-tŭp'let) one of five children born at one birth. [L. *quintuplex,* fivefold]

**quit tam action** a civil action brought by an informer, usually against an employer, for activities alleged to be fraudulent or illegal.

**quod·que (q)** each, every. [L.]

**quo·tid·i·an** (kwō-tid'ē-ăn) daily; occurring every day. SEE quotidian malaria. [L. *quotidianus,* daily, fr. *quot,* as many as, + *dies,* day]

**quo·tid·i·an ma·lar·ia** malaria in which the paroxysms occur daily; usually a double tertian malaria, in which there is an infection by two distinct groups of *Plasmodium vivax* parasites sporulating alternately every 48 hours.

**quo·tient** (kwo'shĕnt) the number of times one amount is contained in another. SEE ALSO index (2), ratio. [L. *quoties,* how often]

**Q wave** the initial deflection of the QRS complex when such deflection is negative (downward).

# R

ρ, P rho. SEE rho.

$R_f$, $R_F$ symbol denoting movement of a substance in paper chromatography relative to the solvent front; equal to the migration distance of a substance divided by the migration distance of the solvent front.

*R* abbreviation or symbol for (in italics) molar gas constant; one of two stereochemical designations in the Cahn, Ingold, and Prelog system; the third product formed in an enzyme-catalyzed reaction.

r racemic, occasionally used in naming compounds in place of the more common DL- or (±)-, as "r-alanine" (more often as the prefix rac-); roentgen; radius.

**Ra** radium.

**rab•bet•ing** (rab'et-ing) making congruous stepwise cuts on apposing bone surfaces for stability after impaction. [Fr. *raboter*, to plane]

**rab•id** relating to or suffering from rabies. [L. *rabidus*, raving, mad]

**ra•bies** (rā'bēz) highly fatal infectious disease transmitted by the bite of infected animals including dogs, cats, skunks, wolves, foxes, raccoons, and bats, and caused by a neurotropic lyssavirus that replicates in the central nervous system and the salivary glands. The symptoms are excitement, aggressiveness, and madness, followed by paralysis and death. Characteristic cytoplasmic inclusion bodies (Negri bodies) found in many of the neurons are an aid to rapid laboratory diagnosis. SYN hydrophobia. [L. rage, fury, fr. *rabio*, to rave, to be mad]

**ra•bies vi•rus** a large bullet-shaped virus of the genus *Lyssavirus*, in the family Rhabdoviridae, that is the causative agent of rabies.

△**rac-** prefix for racemic.

**rac•coon eyes** periorbital ecchymosis appearing several hours after delayed discoloration around the eyes from a fracture of the floor of the anterior cranial fossa.

**rac•e•mase** (rā'sē-mās) an enzyme capable of catalyzing racemization, i.e., inversions of asymmetric groups; when more than one center of asymmetry is present, "epimerase" is used.

**rac•e•mate** (rā'sē-māt) a racemic compound, or the salt or ester of such a compound. SEE ALSO racemic.

**ra•ceme** (rā-sēm') an optically inactive chemical compound. SEE ALSO racemic.

**ra•ce•mic (r)** (rā-sē'mik, rā-sem'ik) denoting a mixture of optically active compounds that is itself optically inactive, being composed of an equal number of dextro- and levorotatory substances, which are separable.

**rac•e•mi•za•tion** (rā'sē-mi-zā'shŭn) partial conversion of one enantiomorph into another (as an L-amino acid to the corresponding D-amino acid) so that the specific optical rotation is decreased, or even reduced to zero, in the resulting mixture.

**rac•e•mose** (ras'ĕ-mōs) branching, with nodular terminations; resembling a bunch of grapes. [L. *racemosus*, full of clusters]

**rac•e•mose an•eu•rysm** SYN cirsoid aneurysm.

**rac•e•mose gland** a gland that has the appearance of a bunch of grapes if viewed as a three-dimensional reconstruction; e.g., a compound acinous or alveolar gland.

△**ra•chi-, ra•chio-** the spine. [G. *rhachis*, spine, backbone]

**ra•chi•al** (rā'kē-ăl) SYN spinal.

**ra•chi•cen•te•sis** (rā-kē-sen-tē'sis) SYN lumbar puncture. [rachi- + G. *kentēsis*, puncture]

**ra•chid•i•al** (rā-kid'ē-ăl) SYN spinal.

**ra•chi•graph** (rā'kē-graf) a graph for recording the curves of the vertebrae. [rachi- + G. *graphō*, to write]

**ra•chil•y•sis** (ră-kil'i-sis) forcible correction of lateral curvature of the spine by lateral pressure against the convexity of the curve. [rachi- + G. *lysis*, a loosening]

**ra•chi•o•cen•te•sis** (rā-kē-ō-sen-tē'sis) SYN lumbar puncture. [rachio- + G. *kentēsis*, puncture]

**ra•chi•om•e•ter** (rā-kē-om'ĕ-ter) an instrument for measuring the curvature of the spine, natural or pathologic, of the spinal column. [rachio- + G. *metron*, measure]

**ra•chi•ot•o•my** (rā-kē-ot'ō-mē) SYN laminotomy. [rachio- + G. *tomē*, incision]

**ra•chis**, pl. **rach•i•des**, **ra•chis•es** (rā'kis, rā'ki-dēz, rā-kis'ēz) SYN vertebral column. [G. spine, backbone]

**ra•chis•chi•sis** (ră-kis'ki-sis) 1. embryologic failure of fusion of vertebral arches and neural tube with consequent exposure of neural tissue at surface; spina bifida cystica with myelocele or myeloschisis. 2. spinal dysraphism. [G. *rhachis*, spine, + *schisis*, division]

**ra•chit•ic** (ră-kit'ic) relating to or suffering from rickets (rachitis).

**ra•chit•ic pel•vis** a contracted and deformed pelvis, most commonly a flat pelvis, occurring from rachitic softening of the bones in early life.

**ra•chit•ic ro•sa•ry** a row of beading at the junction of the ribs with their cartilages, often seen in rachitic children.

**ra•chi•tis** (ră-kī'tis) SYN rickets. [G. *rhachitis*]

**rach•i•to•gen•ic** (ră-kit-ō-jen'ik) producing or causing rickets. [rachitis + G. *genesis*, production]

**rack•et am•pu•ta•tion** a circular or slightly oval amputation, in which a long incision is made in the axis of the limb.

**rad 1.** the unit for the dose absorbed from ionizing radiation, equivalent to 100 ergs per gram of tissue; 100 rad = 1 Gy. **2.** radian. **3.** racemic.

**ra•dar•ky•mog•ra•phy** (rā'dar-kī-mog'ră-fē) an obsolete procedure involving the video tracking of heart motion by means of image intensification and closed circuit television during fluoroscopy; enabled cardiac motion to be measured by reproducible linear graphic tracing.

**ra•dec•to•my** (rā-dek'tō-mē) SYN root amputation. [L. *radix*, root, + G. *ektomē*, excision]

**ra•di•a•bil•i•ty** (rā'dē-ă-bil'i-tē) the property of being radiable.

**ra•di•a•ble** (rā'dē-ă-bl) capable of being penetrated or examined by rays, especially by x-rays.

**ra•di•ad** (rā'dē-ad) in a direction toward the radial side.

**ra•di•al** (rā'dē-ăl) 1. relating to the radius (bone of the forearm), to any structures named from it, or to the radial or lateral aspect of the upper limb as compared to the ulnar or medial aspect. 2. relating to any radius. 3. radiating; diverging in all directions from any given center. SYN brachio- (2). [L. *radialis*, fr. *radius*, ray, lateral bone of the forearm]

**ra•di•al ar•tery** *origin*, brachial; *branches*, radial

recurrent, dorsal metacarpal, dorsal digital, princeps pollicis, radial index, palmar metacarpal, and muscular, carpal, and perforating. SYN arteria radialis [TA].

**ra·di·al col·lat·er·al ar·tery** the anterior terminal branch of the profunda brachii, anastomosing with the radial recurrent, forming part of the articular network of the elbow.

**ra·di·al flex·or mus·cle of wrist** SYN flexor carpi radialis muscle.

**ra·di·al growth phase** the early pattern of growth of cutaneous malignant melanoma, in which tumor cells spread laterally in the epidermis.

**ra·di·a·lis in·di·cis ar·tery** origin, radial; distribution, radial side of index finger.

**ra·di·al ker·a·tot·o·my** a keratotomy with radial incisions around a clear central zone. A form of refractive keratoplasty used in the treatment of myopia.

**ra·di·al nerve** arises from the posterior cord of the brachial plexus; it curves round the posterior surface of the humerus and passes down to the cubital fossa where it divides into its two terminal branches, the superficial branch and the deep branch; it supplies muscular and cutaneous branches to the posterior compartments of the arm and forearm. The radial nerve is most commonly injured by fractures of the middle third of the humerus, resulting in a loss of extension at the wrist ("wrist drop"). SYN nervus radialis [TA].

**ra·di·al re·cur·rent ar·tery** origin, radial; distribution, ascends around lateral side of elbow joint; anastomoses, radial collateral, interosseous recurrent.

**ra·di·al tun·nel syn·drome** pain in the lateral aspect of the elbow and forearm without motor or sensory deficits, resulting from compression of the radial nerve, at any of various sites along its course, as it passes the elbow and the proximal forearm.

**ra·di·al veins** venae comitantes of the radial artery continuing from those of the radial aspect of the deep palmar arch, draining into the venae comitantes of the brachial artery in the cubital fossa.

**ra·di·an (rad)** (rā′dē-ăn) a supplementary SI unit of plane angle. [L. radius, ray]

**ra·di·ant** (rā′dē-ant) **1.** giving out rays. **2.** a point from which light radiates to the eye.

**ra·di·ant in·ten·si·ty (I)** SYN luminous intensity.

**ra·di·ate** (rā′dē-āt) **1.** to spread out in all directions from a center. **2.** to emit radiation. [L. radio, pp. -atus, to shine]

**ra·di·ate crown** SYN corona radiata.

**ra·di·ate lig·a·ment of head of rib** the radiate, stellate, or anterior costovertebral ligament connecting the head of each rib to the bodies of the two vertebrae with which it articulates.

**ra·di·a·tio**, pl. **ra·di·a·ti·o·nes** (rā-dē-ā′shē-ō, rā′dē-ā′shē-ō′nēz) [TA] NEUROANATOMY a term applied to any one of the thalamocortical fiber systems that together compose the corona radiata of the cerebral hemisphere's white matter (e.g., optic radiation, acoustic radiation, etc.). SYN radiation (3). [L.]

**ra·di·a·tio a·cus·ti·ca** [TA] SYN acoustic radiation.

**ra·di·a·tio cor·po·ris cal·lo·si** [TA] SYN radiation of corpus callosum.

**ra·di·a·tion** (rā′dē-ā′shŭn) **1.** the act or condition of diverging in all directions from a center. **2.** the sending forth of light, short radio waves, ultraviolet or x-rays, or any other rays for treatment or diagnosis or for other purpose. Cf. irradiation (2). **3.** SYN radiatio. **4.** a ray. **5.** radiant energy or a radiant beam. [L. radiatio, fr. radius, ray, beam]

**ra·di·a·tion bi·ol·o·gy** science that studies the biological effects of ionizing radiation.

**ra·di·a·tion of cor·pus cal·lo·sum** the spreading out of the fibers of the corpus callosum in the centrum semiovale of each cerebral hemisphere. SYN radiatio corporis callosi [TA].

**ra·di·a·tion der·ma·to·sis** skin changes at the site of ionizing radiation, particularly erythema in the acute stage, temporary or permanent epilation, and chronic changes in the epidermis and dermis resembling actinic keratosis.

**ra·di·a·tion on·col·o·gy 1.** the medical specialty concerned with the use of ionizing radiation in the treatment of disease. **2.** the medical specialty of radiation therapy. **3.** the use of radiation in the treatment of neoplasms. SYN therapeutic radiology.

**ra·di·a·tion sick·ness** a systemic condition caused by substantial whole-body irradiation, seen after nuclear explosions or accidents, rarely after radiotherapy. Manifestations depend on dose, ranging from anorexia, nausea, vomiting, and mild leukopenia, to thrombocytopenia with hemorrhage, severe leukopenia with infection, anemia, central nervous system damage, and death.

**ra·di·a·tion ther·a·py** treatment with x-rays or radionuclides.

**ra·di·a·tio op·ti·ca** SYN optic radiation.

**ra·di·a·tio py·ra·mi·da·lis** SYN pyramidal radiation.

**rad·i·cal** (rad′i-kăl) **1.** CHEMISTRY a group of elements or atoms usually passing intact from one compound to another, but usually incapable of prolonged existence in a free state (e.g., methyl, $CH_3$); in chemical formulas, a radical is often distinguished by being enclosed in parentheses or brackets. **2.** thorough or extensive; relating or directed to the extirpation of the root or cause of a morbid process; e.g., a radical operation. **3.** denoting treatment by extreme, drastic, or innovative, as opposed to conservative, measures. **4.** SYN free radical. [L. radix (radic-), root]

**rad·i·cal hys·ter·ec·to·my** complete removal of the uterus, upper vagina, and parametrium.

**rad·i·cal mas·tec·to·my** excision of the entire breast including the nipple, areola, and overlying skin, as well as the pectoral muscles, lymphatic-bearing tissue in the axilla, and various other neighboring tissues. SYN Halsted operation (2).

**rad·i·cal neck dis·sec·tion** an operation for the removal of metastases to the lymph nodes of the neck in which all of the tissue is removed between the superficial and the deep cervical fascia from the mandible to the clavicle. SEE ALSO functional neck dissection.

**ra·di·ces** (rā-dī′sēz) plural of radix.

**rad·i·cle** (rad′i-kl) a rootlet or structure resembling one, as the radicle of a vein, a minute veinlet joining with others to form a vein, or the radicle of a nerve, a nerve fiber which joins others to form a nerve. [L. radicula, dim. of radix, root]

**rad·i·cot·o·my** (rad-i-kot'ō-mē) SYN rhizotomy. [L. *radix* (*radic-*), root, + G. *tomē*, incision]

**ra·dic·u·la** (ră-dik'yu-lă) a spinal nerve root. [L. dim of *radix*, root]

**ra·dic·u·lal·gia** (ra-dik'yu-lal'jē-ă) neuralgia due to irritation of the sensory root of a spinal nerve. [radicul- + G. *algos*, pain]

**ra·dic·u·lar** (ra-dik'yu-lăr) 1. relating to a radicle. 2. pertaining to the root of a tooth.

**ra·dic·u·lar fi·la** the small, individual fiber fascicles into which the roots of all of the spinal nerves and several cranial nerves (hypoglossus, vagus, oculomotorius) divide in fanlike fashion before entering or leaving the spinal cord or brainstem; the spinal dorsal root may divide into 8–12 such rootlets.

**ra·dic·u·lec·to·my** (ra-dik'yu-lek'tō-mē) SYN rhizotomy. [radicul- + G. *ektomē*, excision]

**ra·dic·u·li·tis** (ra-dik-yu-lī'tis) SYN radiculopathy. [radicul- + G. *-itis*, inflammation]

△**ra·di·cu·lo-, ra·di·cul-** radicle; radicular. [L. *radicula*, radicle, dim. of *radix*, root]

**ra·dic·u·lo·gang·li·o·ni·tis** (ra-dik'yu-lō-gang' glē-ō-nī'tis) involvement of roots and ganglia.

**ra·dic·u·lo·me·nin·go·my·e·li·tis** (ra-dik'yu-lō-mĕ-ning'gō-mī-ĕ-lī'tis) SYN rhizomeningomyelitis.

**ra·dic·u·lo·my·e·lop·a·thy** (ra-dik'yu-lō-mī'ĕ-lop'ă-thē) SYN myeloradiculopathy.

**ra·dic·u·lo·neu·rop·a·thy** (ra-dik'yu-lō-noo-rop'ă-thē) disease of the spinal nerve roots and nerves.

**ra·dic·u·lop·a·thy** (ra-dik'yu-lop'ă-thē) disorder of the spinal nerve roots. SYN radiculitis. [radiculo- + G. *pathos*, suffering]

**ra·di·ec·to·my** (rā-dē-ek'tō-mē) SYN root amputation. [L. *radix*, root, + G. *ektomē*, excision]

**ra·dii** (rā'dē-ī) plural of radius. [L.]

**ra·dii of lens** 9–12 faint lines on the anterior and posterior surfaces of the lens that radiate from the poles toward the equator; they mark the lines along which the ends of lens fibers abut. SYN lens stars (1), radii lentis.

**ra·dii len·tis** SYN radii of lens.

△**ra·di·o-** 1. radiation, chiefly (in medicine) gamma or x-ray. 2. SYN radioactive. 3. SYN radius. [L. *radius*, ray]

**ra·di·o·ac·tive** (rā'dē-ō-ak'tiv) possessing radioactivity. SYN radio- (2).

**ra·di·o·ac·tive con·stant (lambda)** SYN decay constant.

**ra·di·o·ac·tive iso·tope** an isotope with an unstable nuclear composition; such nuclei decompose spontaneously by emission of a nuclear electron (β particle) or helium nucleus (α particle) and radiation (γ rays), thus achieving a stable nuclear composition; used as tracers, and as radiation and energy sources. SEE half-life.

**ra·di·o·ac·tiv·i·ty** (rā'dē-ō-ak-tiv'i-tē) the property of some atomic nuclei of spontaneously emitting gamma rays or subatomic particles (alpha and beta rays).

**ra·di·o·al·ler·go·sor·bent test (RAST)** a radioimmunoassay test to detect IgE-bound allergens responsible for tissue hypersensitivity: the allergen is bound to insoluble material and the patient's serum is reacted with this conjugate; if the serum contains antibody to the allergen, it will be complexed to the allergen.

**ra·di·o·au·tog·ra·phy** (rā'dē-ō-aw-tog'ră-fē) SYN autoradiography.

**ra·di·o·bi·cip·i·tal** (rā'dē-ō-bī-sip'i-tăl) relating to the radius and the biceps muscle.

**ra·di·o·bi·ol·o·gy** (rā'dē-ō-bī-ol'ō-jē) the study of the biological effects of ionizing radiation upon living tissue. Cf. radiopathology.

**ra·di·o·car·di·o·gram** (rā'dē-ō-kar'dē-ō-gram) a graphic record of the concentration of injected radioisotope within the cardiac chambers.

**ra·di·o·car·di·og·ra·phy** (rā'dē-ō-kar-dē-og'ră-fē) the technique of recording or interpreting radiocardiograms.

**ra·di·o·car·pal** (rā'dē-ō-kar'păl) 1. relating to the radius and the bones of the carpus. 2. on the radial or lateral side of the carpus.

**ra·di·o·car·pal joint** SYN wrist joint.

**ra·di·o·chem·is·try** (rā'dē-ō-kem'is-trē) 1. the science of using radionuclides to synthesize labeled compounds for biochemical or biological research, or radiopharmaceuticals for clinical diagnostic studies. 2. the study of methods of labeling compounds with radionuclides.

**ra·di·o·cin·e·ma·tog·ra·phy** (rā'dē-ō-sĭ-nē-mă-tog'ră-fē) taking a motion picture of the movements of organs or other structures as revealed by x-ray fluoroscopic examination. [radio- + G. *kinēma*, motion, + *graphō*, to write]

**ra·di·o·cur·a·ble** (rā'dē-ō-kyur'ă-bl) curable by irradiation therapy.

**ra·di·o·dense** (rā'dē-ō-dens) SYN radiopaque.

**ra·di·o·den·si·ty** (rā'dē-ō-den'si-tē) SYN radiopacity.

**ra·di·o·der·ma·ti·tis** (rā'dē-ō-der-mă-tī'tis) dermatitis due to exposure to x-rays or gamma rays causing ionization of tissue water with changes resembling thermal injury.

**ra·di·o·di·ag·no·sis** (rā'dē-ō-dī-ag-nō'sis) diagnosis using x-rays; or, more broadly, diagnostic imaging, including radiology, ultrasound, and magnetic resonance.

**ra·di·o·fre·quen·cy** (rā'dē-o-frē'kwen-sē) 1. radiant energy of a certain frequency range; e.g., radio and television employ radiant energy having a frequency between $10^5$–$10^{11}$ Hz, while diagnostic x-rays have a frequency in the range of $3 \times 10^{18}$ Hz. 2. MAGNETIC RESONANCE IMAGING the energy applied to switch or create a gradient in the magnetic field.

**ra·di·o·graph** (rā'dē-ō-graf) a negative image on photographic film made by exposure to x-rays that have passed through matter or tissue. SYN roentgenogram, roentgenograph. [radio- + G. *graphō*, to write]

**ra·di·og·raph·er** (rā-dē-og'ră-fĕr) a technologist trained to position patients and take radiographs or perform other radiodiagnostic procedures.

**ra·di·o·gra·phic art·i·fact** blemish on a radiograph caused by heat, light, damaged screens, dust, or improper handling of the x-ray film.

**ra·di·o·gra·phic con·trast** the variation of the light and dark areas on a radiograph.

**ra·di·o·gra·phic den·si·ty** the amount of blackening on an x-ray film produced by the interaction of silver halide crystals with developing agents.

**ra·di·og·ra·phy** (rā'dē-ō-g'ră-fē) examination of any part of the body for diagnostic purposes by means of x-rays with the record of the findings usually impressed upon a photographic film. See page 836. SYN roentgenography.

**ra·di·o·im·mu·ni·ty** (rā'dē-ō-i-myu'ni-tē) lessened sensitivity to radiation.

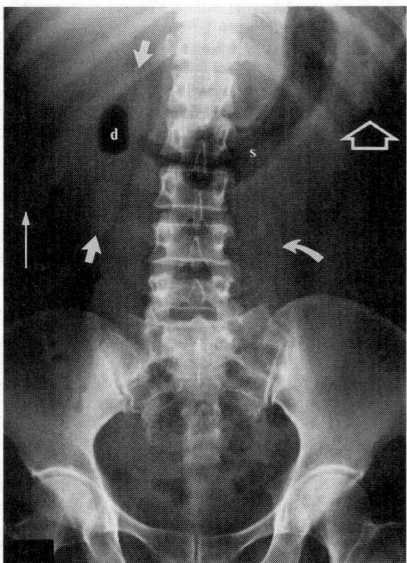

**plain film radiograph of abdomen:** showing how anatomic structures differ in their capacity to attenuate x-rays that pass through the patient; stomach (s), duodenum (d), right kidney (between short straight arrows), edge of liver (long straight arrow), edge of spleen (open arrow), left psoas muscle (curved arrow)

**ra·di·o·im·mu·no·as·say** (rā′dē-ō-im′u-nō-as′sā) an immunological (immunochemical) procedure that uses the competition between radioisotope-labeled antigen (hormone) or other substance and unlabeled antigen for antiserums, resulting in quantitation of the unlabeled antigen; any method for detecting or quantitating antigens or antibodies using radiolabeled reactants.

**ra·di·o·im·mu·no·dif·fu·sion** (rā′dē-ō-im′yu-nō-di-fyu′zhŭn) a method for the study of antigen-antibody reactions by gel diffusion using radioisotope-labeled antigen or antibody.

**ra·di·o·im·mu·no·elec·tro·pho·re·sis** (rā′dē-ō-im′yu-nō-ē-lek′trō-fō-rē′sis) immunoelectrophoresis in which the antigen or antibody is labeled with a radioisotope.

**ra·di·o·im·mu·no·pre·cip·i·ta·tion (RIP)** (rā′dē-ō-im′yu-nō-prē-sip-i-tā′shŭn) immunoprecipitation utilizing a radioisotope-labeled antibody or antigen.

**ra·di·o·im·mun·o·sor·bent test (RIST)** a competition test, performed *in vitro*, used to measure IgE specific for a particular antigen. Known amounts of radiolabeled IgE compete with the patient's unlabeled IgE to bind to a surface coated with anti-IgE. The reduction in radiolabeled IgE due to the presence of IgE in the patient's serum can be determined by comparison to known IgE standards; thus, the amount of the patient's total serum IgE can be determined.

**ra·di·o·i·so·tope** (rā′dē-ō-ī′sō-tōp) an isotope that changes to a more stable state by emitting radiation.

**ra·di·o·le·sion** (rā′dē-ō-lē′zhŭn) a lesion produced by ionizing radiation.

**ra·di·o·li·gand** (rā′dē-ō-lig′and) a molecule with a radionuclide tracer attached; usually used for radioimmunoassay procedures. [radio- + L. *ligandus*, that which is to be bound, fr. *ligo*, to bind]

**ra·di·o·log·ic, ra·di·o·log·i·cal** (rā-dē-ō-log′ik, rā-dē-ō-loj′i-kăl) pertaining to radiology.

**ra·di·o·log·i·cal a·nat·o·my** the study of bodily structure by radiography and other imaging methods.

**ra·di·o·log·ic dis·tor·tion** misrepresentation of the true size and shape of an object being radiographed (as in magnification, elongation, and foreshortening).

**ra·di·o·log·ic en·ter·oc·ly·sis** method of imaging the duodenum and small intestine by intubation of the duodenum and instillation of dilute barium; also known as small bowel enema.

**ra·di·o·log·ic sphinc·ter** SYN physiologic sphincter.

**ra·di·o·log·ic tech·no·lo·gist** an individual skilled in the use of ionizing radiation to produce diagnostic images.

**ra·di·ol·o·gist** (rā-dē-ol′ō-jist) a physician trained in the diagnostic and/or therapeutic use of x-rays and radionuclides, radiation physics, and biology; a diagnostic radiologist is also trained in diagnostic ultrasound and magnetic resonance imaging and applicable physics.

**ra·di·ol·o·gy** (rā-dē-ol′ō-jē) **1.** the science of high energy radiation and of the sources and the chemical, physical, and biologic effects of such radiation; the term usually refers to the diagnosis and treatment of disease. **2.** the scientific discipline of medical imaging using ionizing radiation, radionuclides, nuclear magnetic resonance, and ultrasound. SYN diagnostic radiology. [radio- + G. *logos*, study]

**ra·di·o·lu·cen·cy** (rā-dē-ō-loo′sen-sē) the state of being radiolucent.

**ra·di·o·lu·cent** (rā-dē-ō-loo′sent) relatively penetrable by x-rays or other forms of radiation. Cf. radiopaque. [radio- + L. *lucens*, shining]

**ra·di·om·e·ter** (rā-dē-om′ě-ter) a device for determining the penetrative power of x-rays. [radio- + G. *metron*, measure]

**ra·di·o·mi·met·ic** (rā′dē-ō-mi-met′ik) imitating the biologic effects of radiation, as in the case of chemicals such as nitrogen mustards. [radio- + G. *mimētikos*, imitative]

**ra·di·o·ne·cro·sis** (rā′dē-ō-ne-krō′sis) necrosis due to radiation; e.g., after excessive exposure to x- or gamma rays.

**ra·di·o·neu·ri·tis** (rā′dē-ō-noo-rī′tis) neuritis caused by prolonged or repeated exposure to x-rays or radium.

**ra·di·o·nu·clide** (rā′dē-ō-noo′klīd) an isotope of artificial or natural origin that exhibits radioactivity. Radionuclides are used in diagnostic imaging and cancer therapy.

**ra·di·o·nu·clide an·gi·o·car·di·og·ra·phy** the display, by means of a stationary scintillation camera device, of the passage of a bolus of a rapidly injected radiopharmaceutical.

**ra·di·o·nu·clide e·jec·tion frac·tion** a nuclear medicine study for determination of ejection fraction of either ventricle; supersedes multiple-gated acquisition scan in some centers. SEE ALSO multiple-gated acquisition scan.

**ra·di·o·nu·clide gen·er·a·tor** a column containing a large amount of a particular radionuclide (mother radionuclide) that decays down to a second radionuclide of shorter physical half-life; the daughter radionuclide is separated from the parent by the process of elution and affords a continuing supply of relatively short-lived radionuclides for laboratory use; the elution is loosely termed "milking" with the generator referred to as a "radioactive cow."

**ra·di·o·pac·i·ty** (rā′dē-ō-pas′i-tē) state of being radiopaque. SYN radiodensity.

**ra·di·o·paque** (rā-dē-ō-pāk′) exhibiting relative opacity to, or impenetrability by, x-rays or any other form of radiation. Cf. radiolucent. SYN radiodense. [radio- + Fr. opaque fr. L. *opacus*, shady]

**ra·di·o·pa·thol·o·gy** (rā′dē-ō-path-ol′ō-jē) a branch of radiology or pathology concerned with the effects of radiation on cells and tissues. Cf. radiobiology.

**ra·di·o·pel·vim·e·try** (rā′dē-ō-pel-vim′ĕ-trē) radiographic measurement of the pelvis. SEE pelvimetry.

**ra·di·o·phar·ma·ceu·ti·cal syn·o·vec·to·my** the treatment of abnormal synovial membranes by radiation derived from the instillation in the joint of a radiopharmaceutical, such as radiogold.

**ra·di·o·pro·tec·tant** (rā′dē-ō-prō-tek′tant) substance that prevents or lessens the effects of radiation.

**ra·di·o·re·cep·tor** (rā′dē-ō-rē-sep′ter) **1.** a receptor that normally responds to radiant energy such as light or heat. **2.** a receptor used as a binding agent for unlabeled and radiolabeled analyte in a type of competitive binding assay called radioreceptor assay.

**ra·di·o·re·sis·tant** (rā′dē-ō-rē-zis′tant) indicates cells or tissues that are less affected than average mammalian cells on exposure to radiation; when applied to neoplasms, indicates less susceptibility to damage from therapeutic radiation than the surrounding host tissues.

**ra·di·o·sen·si·tive** (rā′dē-ō-sen′si-tiv) readily affected by radiation. Cf. radioresistant.

**ra·di·o·sen·si·tiv·i·ty** (rā′dē-ō-sen-si-tiv′i-tē) the condition of being readily affected by radiant energy.

**ra·di·o·te·lem·e·try** (rā′dē-ō-tĕ-lem′ĕ-trē) SEE telemetry, biotelemetry.

**ra·di·o·ther·a·peu·tic** (rā′dē-ō-thār-ă-pyu′tik) relating to radiotherapy or to radiotherapeutics.

**ra·di·o·ther·a·peu·tics** (rā′dē-ō-thār-ă-pyu′tiks) the study and use of radiotherapeutic agents.

**ra·di·o·ther·a·pist** (rā′dē-ō-thār′ă-pist) one who practices radiotherapy or is versed in radiotherapeutics.

**ra·di·o·ther·a·py** (rā′dē-ō-thār′ă-pē) the medical specialty concerned with the use of electromagnetic or particulate radiation in the treatment of disease.

**ra·di·o·ther·my** (rā′dē-ō-ther′mē) diathermy effected by heat from radiant sources. [radio- + G. *thermē*, heat]

**ra·di·o·tox·ae·mia [Br.]** SEE radiotoxemia.

**ra·di·o·tox·e·mia** (rā′dē-ō-tok-sē′mē-ă) radiation sickness caused by the products of disintegration produced by the action of x-rays or other forms of radioactivity and by the depletion of certain cells and enzyme systems from the organism. [radio- + G. *toxikon*, poison, + *haima*, blood]

**ra·di·o·trans·par·ent** (rā′dē-ō-trans-par′ent) allowing relatively free transmission of radiant energy.

**ra·di·o·trop·ic** (rā′dē-ō-trop′ik) affected by radiation. [radio- + G. *tropē*, a turning]

**ra·di·sec·to·my** (rā-dē-sek′tō-mē) SYN root amputation. [L. *radix*, root, + G. *ektomē*, excision]

**ra·di·um (Ra)** (rā′dē-ŭm) a metallic element, atomic no. 88, extracted in very minute quantities from pitchblende; an alkaline earth metal with properties similar to those of barium. Its therapeutic action is similar to that of x-rays. [L. *radius*, ray]

**ra·di·us**, gen. and pl. **ra·dii** (rā′dē-ŭs, rā′dē-ī) **1.** [TA] the lateral and shorter of the two bones of the forearm. **2.** a straight line passing from the center to the periphery of a circle. SYN radio- (3). [L. spoke of a wheel, rod, ray]

**ra·dix**, gen. **ra·di·cis**, pl. **ra·di·ces** (rā′diks, rā-di′sis, rā-dī′sēz) [TA] **1.** SYN root (1). **2.** SYN root of tooth. **3.** the hypothetical size of the birth cohort in a life table, commonly 1,000 or 100,000. [L.]

**ra·dix cli·ni·ca den·tis** [TA] SYN clinical root of tooth.

**ra·don (Rn)** (rā′don) a gaseous radioactive element, atomic no. 86, resulting from the breakdown of radium; $^{222}$Rn is medically significant as an alpha-emitter with a half-life of 3.8235 days; it is used in the treatment of certain malignancies. Poorly ventilated homes in some parts of the country accumulate a dangerous amount of naturally occurring radon gas. [from radium]

**Rae·der par·a·tri·gem·i·nal syn·drome** (rā′der) a postganglionic Horner syndrome associated with trigeminal nerve dysfunction caused by involvement of the carotid sympathetic plexus, near Meckel cave.

**Rai·ney cor·pus·cles** (rān′ē) rounded, ovoidal, or sickle-shaped spores or bradyzoites, 12–16 by 4–9 μm, found within the elongated cysts (Miescher tubes) of the protozoan *Sarcocystis*.

**rale** (rahl) an extraneous sound heard on auscultation of breath sounds; used by some to denote rhonchus and by others for crepitation. [Fr. rattle]

**ral·ox·i·fene** (ral-ox′ī-fēn) a selective estrogen receptor modulator (SERM) that has estrogen-agonistic effects on bone and lipid metabolism but estrogen-antagonistic effects on breast and uterus; used in the prophylaxis of osteoporosis after menopause.

**ra·mal** (rā′măl) relating to a ramus.

**Ram·bourg chro·mic ac·id-phos·pho·tung·stic ac·id stain** (ram′berg) a stain for glycoproteins, used with an electron microscope, with which ultrathin tissue sections reveal complex carbohydrates in the same locations as shown by Rambourg periodic acid-chromic methenamine-silver stain.

**Ram·bourg pe·ri·od·ic ac·id-chro·mic meth·en·a·mine-sil·ver stain** (ram′berg) a stain for glycoproteins, used with an electron microscope, adapted from the Gomori-Jones periodic acid-methenamine-silver stain; it produces silver deposits in mature saccules of the Golgi apparatus, lysosomal vesicles, cell coat, and basement membranes.

**ra·mi** (rā′mī) plural of ramus. [L.]

**ram·i·fi·ca·tion** (ram′i-fi-kā′shŭn) the process of dividing into a branchlike pattern.

**ram•i•fy** (ram'i-fī) to split into a branchlike pattern. [L. *ramus*, branch, + *facio*, to make]

**ram•i•sec•tion** (ram-i-sek'shŭn) section of the rami communicantes of the sympathetic nervous system. [L. *ramus*, branch, + L. *sectio*, section]

**ram•i•tis** (ram-ī'tis) inflammation of a ramus. [L. *ramus*, branch, + G. *-itis*, inflammation]

**Ram•say Hunt syn•drome** (ram'sē-hunt) **1.** SYN Hunt syndrome. **2.** SYN herpes zoster oticus.

**Ram•stedt op•er•a•tion** (rahm'shtet) SYN pyloromyotomy.

**ram•u•lus**, pl. **ram•u•li** (ram'yu-lŭs, ram'yu-lī) a small branch or twig; one of the terminal divisions of a ramus. [L. dim. of *ramus*, a branch]

**ra•mus**, pl. **ra•mi** (rā'mŭs, rā'mī) **1.** [TA] SYN branch. **2.** one of the primary divisions of a nerve or blood vessel. SEE ALSO artery, nerve. **3.** a part of an irregularly shaped bone (less slender than a "process") that forms an angle with the main body (e.g., ramus of mandible). **4.** one of the primary divisions of a cerebral sulcus. [L.]

**ran•cid** (ran'sid) having a disagreeable odor and taste, usually characterizing fat undergoing oxidation or bacterial decomposition to more volatile odoriferous substances. [L. *rancidus*, stinking, rank]

**Ran•dall plaques** (ran'dal) mineral concentrations on renal papillae.

**ran•dom•i•sa•tion [Br.]** SEE randomization.

**ran•dom•i•za•tion** (ran-dŭm-ĭ-zā'shŭn) assignment of the subjects of experimental research to groups by chance.

**ran•dom mat•ing** a practice of mating in a population in which at some specified locus mating patterns occur with expected frequencies predicted by the product of the frequencies of the genotypes in the population.

**ran•dom pat•tern flap** a flap in which the pedicle blood supply is derived randomly from the network of vessels in the area, rather than from a single longitudinal artery as in an axial pattern flap.

**ran•dom sam•pling** a selection of elements by a formal randomizing device for purposes of inference about a population in such a way that the probability of each possible outcome may be precisely specified in advance; the inferences are necessarily stochastic.

**range** (rānj) a statistical measure of the dispersion or variation of values determined by the endpoint values themselves or the difference between them; e.g., in a group of children aged 6, 8, 9, 10, 13, and 16, the range would be from 6 to 16 or, alternately, 10 (16 minus 6). [O.Fr. *rang*, line fr. Germanic]

**range of ac•com•mo•da•tion** the distance between an object viewed with minimal refractivity of the eye and one viewed with maximal accommodation.

**range of mo•tion (ROM) 1.** the measured beginning and terminal angles, as well as the total degrees of motion, traversed by a joint moved by active muscle contraction or by passive movement. **2.** joint movement (active, passive, or a combination of both) carried out to assess, preserve, or increase the arc of joint motion.

**ra•nine** (rā'nīn) **1.** relating to the frog. **2.** relating to the undersurface of the tongue. [L. *rana*, a frog]

**Ran•kin clamp** (rank'in) a three-bladed clamp used in resection of colon.

**Ran•so•hoff sign** (ran'sō-hof) yellow pigmentation in the umbilical region in rupture of the common bile duct.

**ran•u•la** (ran'yu-lă) **1.** hypoglottis. **2.** any cystic tumor of the undersurface of the tongue or floor of the mouth, especially one of the floor of the mouth due to obstruction of the duct of the sublingual glands. SYN ptyalocele, sialocele, sublingual cyst. [L. tadpole, dim. of *rana*, frog]

**ran•u•lar** (ran'yu-lăr) relating to a ranula.

**Ran•vi•er node** (rahn-vē-ā') a short interval in the myelin sheath of a nerve fiber, occurring between segments of the myelin sheath; at the node, the axon is invested only by short, fingerlike cytoplasmic processes of the two neighboring Schwann cells or, in the central nervous system, oligodendroglia cells. SEE ALSO myelin sheath. SYN node of Ranvier.

**RAO** right anterior oblique, a radiographic position in which the right anterior part of the chest is closest to the film.

**Ra•oult law** (rah-ool') the vapor pressure of a solution of a nonvolatile nonelectrolyte is that of the pure solvent multiplied by the mole-fraction of the solvent in the solution.

**rape** (rāp) **1.** sexual intercourse by force, duress, intimidation, or without legal consent (as with a minor). **2.** the performance of such an act. [L. *rapio*, to seize, to drag away]

**ra•phe** (rā'fē) the line of union of 2 contiguous, bilaterally symmetrical structures. [G. *rhaphē*, suture, seam]

**ra•phe nu•clei** collective term denoting a variety of unpaired nerve cell groups in and along the median plane of the mesencephalic and rhombencephalic tegmentum: the nucleus centralis tegmenti superior, and the nucleus raphes dorsalis, nucleus raphes pontis, nucleus raphes magnus, nucleus raphes pallidus, and nucleus raphes obscurus. These nuclei include neurons characterized by their containing the neurotransmitter serotonin; their serotonin-carrying axons extend rostrally to the hypothalamus, septum, hippocampus, and cingulate gyrus and include projections to brainstem, cerebellum, and spinal cord.

**rap•id ca•ni•ti•es** whitening of hair overnight or over a few days; in the latter case, may be seen in alopecia areata, when surviving pigmented hairs are preferentially shed from gray hair.

**rap•id eye move•ments (REM)** symmetrical quick scanning movements of the eyes occurring many times during sleep in clusters for 5 to 60 minutes; associated with dreaming.

**ra•pid me•di•cal as•sess•ment** quick head-to-toe physical examination of an unresponsive prehospital medical patient to discover signs of disease or injury before transport.

**ra•pid trau•ma as•sess•ment** quick head-to-toe physical examination of an unresponsive prehospital trauma patient for the purpose of discovering and assessing injuries before transport.

**Ra•po•port-Leu•ber•ing shunt** (rap'ŏ-port-loo'ber-ing) a shunt of the glycolytic pathway in which 1,3 diphosphoglycerate (1,3-DPG) is converted to 2,3-DPG. 2,3-DPG enhances the release of oxygen from hemoglobin to the tissues.

**Ra•po•port test** (rap'ŏ-pōrt) a differential ureteral catheterization test used to evaluate suspected renovascular hypertension; urine specimens from each kidney are obtained by bilateral ureteral catheterization, and the tubular rejection fraction ratio is determined by measuring concentrations of sodium and creatinine in the urine from each kidney.

**rap•port** (rap-ōr′) **1.** a feeling of relationship, especially when characterized by emotional affinity. **2.** a conscious feeling of accord, trust, empathy, and mutual responsiveness between two or more persons (e.g., physician and patient) that fosters the therapeutic process. [Fr.]

**rare earths** SEE lanthanides.

**rar•e•fac•tion** (rār-ĕ-fak′shŭn) the process of becoming light or less dense; the condition of being light; opposed to condensation. [L. *rarus*, thin, scanty + *facio*, to make]

**RAS** reticular activating system.

**rash** lay term for a cutaneous eruption. [O. Fr. *rasche*, skin eruption, fr. L. *rado*, pp. *rasus*, to scratch, scrape]

**Ras•mus•sen an•eu•rysm** (rahs′mŭ-sĕn) aneurysmal dilation of a branch of a pulmonary artery in a tuberculous cavity, rupture of which may cause serious hemoptysis.

**Ras•mus•sen en•ceph•a•li•tis** (rahs′mŭ-sĕn) encephalitis in which antibodies to a stimulatory glutamate receptor in the CNS are found; perhaps autoimmune.

**ras on•co•gene** point mutations first described in rat sarcoma cells that can be shown to have transforming activity in culture as well as in tumorigenesis models in mice; the ras gene family is composed of three closely related genes on three different chromosomes; abnormalities have been identified in a variety of human tumors.

**ras•pa•to•ry** (ras′pă-tōr-ē) a surgical instrument used to smooth the edges of a divided bone. [L. *raspatorium*]

**RAST** radioallergosorbent test.

**Ras•tel•li op•er•a•tion** (rahs-tel′ē) for "anatomic" repair of transposition of the great arteries (ventriculoarterial discordance) with ventricular septal defect and left ventricular outflow tract obstruction; conduits are used to create left ventricular to aortic continuity and right ventricular to pulmonary artery continuity. All septal defects are obliterated, as are any previously constructed palliative shunts.

**rat** a rodent of the genus *Rattus*, involved in the spread of some diseases, including bubonic plague.

**rat-bite fe•ver** a single designation for two bacterial diseases associated with rat bites, one caused by *Streptobacillus moniliformis* (Haverhill fever), the other by *Spirillum minus* (sodoku); both diseases are characterized by relapsing fever, chills, headache, arthralgia, lymphadenopathy, and a maculopapular rash on the extremities.

**rate** (rāt) **1.** a measurement of an event or process in terms of its relation to some fixed standard; measurement is expressed as the ratio of one quantity to another (e.g., velocity, distance per unit time). **2.** a measure of the frequency of an event in a defined population; the components of a rate are: the numerator (number of events); the denominator (population at risk of experiencing the event); the specified time in which the events occur; and usually a multiplier, a power of 10, which makes it possible to express the rate as a whole number. [L. *ratum*, a reckoning (see ratio)]

**rate con•stants** (*k*) proportionality constants

equal to the initial rate of a reaction divided by the concentration of the reactant(s); e.g., in the reaction A → B + C, the rate of the reaction equals $-d[A]/dt = k_1[A]$. The rate constant $k_1$ is a unimolecular rate constant since there is only one molecular species reacting and has units of reciprocal time (e.g., $\sec^{-1}$). For the reverse reaction, B + C → A, the rate equals $-d[B]/dt = d[A]/dt = k_2[B][C]$. The rate constant $k_2$ is a bimolecular rate constant and has units of reciprocal concentration-time (e.g., $M^{-1} \sec^{-1}$).

**Rath•ke cleft cyst** (raht′kĕ) an intrasellar or suprasellar cyst lined by cuboidal epithelium derived from remnants of Rathke pouch.

**Rath•ke pock•et** (raht′kĕ) SYN pituitary diverticulum.

**Rath•ke pouch** (raht′kĕ) SYN pituitary diverticulum.

**Rath•ke pouch tu•mor** (raht′kĕ) SYN craniopharyngioma.

**ra•ting of per•ceived ex•er•tion (RPE)** subjective numerical rating (range 6–19) of exercise intensity based on how an individual feels in relation to level of physiologic stress. An RPE of 13 or 14 (exercise that feels "somewhat hard") coincides with an exercise heart rate of about 70% maximum. SYN Borg scale.

**ra•tio** (ra′shē-ō) an expression of the relation of one quantity to another (e.g., of a proportion or rate). SEE ALSO index (2), quotient. [L. *ratio* (*ration-*) a reckoning, reason, fr. *reor*, pp. *ratus*, to reckon, compute]

**ra•tion•al** (rash′ŭn-ăl) **1.** pertaining to reasoning or to the higher thought processes; based on objective or scientific knowledge, in contrast to empirical (1). **2.** influenced by reasoning rather than by emotion. **3.** having the reasoning faculties; not delirious or comatose. [L. *rationalis*, fr. *ratio*, reason]

**ra•tion•al for•mu•la** CHEMISTRY a formula that indicates the constitution as well as the composition of a substance.

**ra•tion•al•i•za•tion** (ra-shŭn-ăl-i-zā′shŭn) a psychoanalytic defense mechanism through which irrational behavior, motives, or feelings are made to appear reasonable. [L. *ratio*, reason]

**ra•tion•al ther•a•py** therapeutic procedures based on the premise that lack of information or illogical thought patterns are basic causes of a patient's difficulties.

**RAV** Rous-associated virus.

**ray** (rā) **1.** a beam of light, heat, or other form of radiation. The rays from radium and other radioactive substances are produced by a spontaneous disintegration of the atom; they are electrically charged particles or electromagnetic waves of extremely short wavelength. **2.** a part or branch that extends radially from a structure. [L. *radius*]

**Ray•naud phe•nom•e•non** (rā-nō′) spasm of the digital arteries, with blanching and numbness or pain of the fingers, often precipitated by cold. Fingers become variably red, white, and blue.

**Ray•naud sign** (rā-nō′) SYN acrocyanosis.

**Ray•naud syn•drome** (rā-nō′) idiopathic paroxysmal bilateral cyanosis of the digits due to arterial and arteriolar contraction; caused by cold or emotion. SEE ALSO Raynaud phenomenon.

**R-band•ing stain** a reverse Giemsa chromosome banding method that produces bands complementary to G-bands; induced by treatment with high temperature, low pH, or acridine orange staining; often used together with G-banding on human karyotype to determine whether there are deletions.

**rbc, RBC** red blood cell; red blood count.

**RBF** renal blood flow. SEE effective renal blood flow.

**RBRVS** Resource Based Relative Value Scale.

**RCP** respiratory care practitioner.

**RDA** recommended daily allowance.

**RDPA** right descending pulmonary artery.

**Re** rhenium.

△**re-** prefix meaning again or backward. [L.]

**re•act** (rē-akt′) to take part in or to undergo a chemical reaction. [Mod. L. *reactus*]

**re•ac•tance (X, *X*)** (rē-ak′tans) the weakening of an alternating electric current by passage through a coil of wire or a condenser.

**re•ac•tant** (rē-ak′tant) a substance taking part in a chemical reaction.

**re•ac•tion** (rē-ak′shŭn) **1.** the response of a muscle or other living tissue or organism to a stimulus. **2.** the color change effected in litmus and certain other organic pigments by contact with substances such as acids or alkalies; also the property that such substances possess of producing this change. **3.** in chemistry, the intermolecular action of two or more substances upon each other, whereby these substances are caused to disappear, new ones being formed in their place (chemical reaction). **4.** in immunology, action of an antibody on a specific antigen in vivo or in vitro, with or without the involvement of a complement or other components of the immunologic system. [L. *re-*, again, backward, + *actio,* action]

**re•ac•tion of de•gen•er•a•tion (DR)** the electrical reaction in a degenerated nerve and the muscles supplied by it; characterized by absence of response to both galvanic and faradic stimulus in the nerve and to faradic stimulus in the muscles.

**re•ac•tion for•ma•tion** in psychoanalysis, a postulated defense mechanism in which attitudes and behaviors that are adopted are the opposites of that which the individual would ordinarily be expected to express and actually feel at an unconscious level.

**re•ac•tion time** the interval between the presentation of a stimulus and the responsive reaction to it.

**re•ac•ti•vate** (rē-ak′ti-vāt) **1.** to render active again. **2.** in particular, of an inactivated immune serum to which normal serum (complement) is added.

**re•ac•tive air•ways dis•ease** SYN asthma.

**re•ac•tive chan•ges** term in the Bethesda classification system for reporting cervical/vaginal cytologic diagnosis that refers to changes benign in nature, associated with inflammation (including typical repair), atrophy with inflammation, radiation, an intrauterine device, and other nonspecific causes. SEE ALSO Bethesda system, AGUS, LSIL, HSIL.

**re•ac•tive de•pres•sion** a psychological state occasioned directly by an intensely sad external situation (frequently loss of a loved person), relieved by the removal of the external situation (e.g., reunion with a loved person).

**re•ac•tive hy•per•e•mia** hyperemia following the arrest and subsequent restoration of the blood supply to a part.

**re•ac•tiv•i•ty** (rē-ak-tiv′i-tē) **1.** the property of re-

acting, chemically or in any other sense. **2.** the process of reacting.

**read•ing** (rēd′ing) **1.** the perception and understanding of the meaning of visual symbols (e.g., letters or words) by the scanning of writing or print with the eyes. **2.** any of several alternative ways of interpreting symbols, such as Braille or the close observation of a speaker's facial movements.

**read•through** (rēd′throo) MOLECULAR BIOLOGY transcription of a nucleic acid sequence beyond its normal termination sequence.

**re•a•gent** (rē-ā′jent) any substance added to a solution of another substance to participate in a chemical reaction. [Mod. L. *reagens*]

**re•a•gin•ic an•ti•bo•dy** SYN homocytotropic antibody.

**REAL** Revised European-American Classification of Lymphoid Neoplasms. SEE REAL classification.

**REAL clas•si•fi•ca•tion** a classification of lymphoma first published in 1994 and based on the correlation of clinical features of lymphomas with their histopathology and immunophenotype and genotype of neoplastic cells; groups lymphoproliferative diseases into chronic leukemia/lymphoma, nodal or extranodal lymphoma, acute leukemia lymphoma, plasma cell disorders, and Hodgkin disease. [*R*evised *E*uropean-American /lymphoma classification]

**re•al•i•ty a•ware•ness** the ability to distinguish external objects as being different from oneself.

**re•al•i•ty prin•ci•ple** the concept that the pleasure principle in personality development is modified by the demands of external reality; the principle or force that compels the growing child to adapt to the demands of external reality.

**re•al•i•ty test•ing** in psychiatry and psychology, the ego function by which the objective or real world and one's subjectively sensed relationship to it are evaluated and appreciated; the ability to distinguish internal from external events.

**real-time e•cho•car•di•o•gra•phy** SYN two-dimensional echocardiography.

**ream•er** (rē′mer) a rotating finishing or drilling tool used to shape or enlarge a hole. [A.S. *ryman,* to widen]

**rear•foot pro•na•tion** SYN hindfoot valgus.

**rear•foot su•pi•na•tion** SYN hindfoot varus.

**re•bound phe•no•me•non 1.** SYN Stewart-Holmes sign. **2.** generally, any phenomenon in which a variable that has been displaced from its normal state by a disturbing influence temporarily deviates from normal in the opposite direction when the disturbing influence is suddenly removed, before finally stabilizing at its normal state.

**re•bound ten•der•ness** SYN Blumberg sign.

**re•breath•ing** (rē-brēdh′ing) inhalation of part or all of gases previously exhaled.

**re•breath•ing an•es•the•sia** a technique for inhalation anesthesia in which a portion or all of the gases that are exhaled are subsequently inhaled after carbon dioxide has been absorbed.

**re•breath•ing tech•nique** use of a breathing or anesthesia circuit in which exhaled air is subsequently inhaled either with or without absorption of $CO_2$ from the exhaled air.

**re•breath•ing vol•ume** the volume of exhaled gas reinhaled on inspiration as a result of the presence of a breathing apparatus; this volume is also referred to as instrument dead space.

**re·cal·ci·fi·ca·tion** (rē-kal'si-fi-kā'shŭn) restoration to the tissues of lost calcium salts.

**re·call** (rē'kawl) the process of remembering thoughts, words, and actions of a past event in an attempt to recapture actual happenings.

**re·call bi·as** systematic error due to differences in accuracy or completeness of recall to memory of past events or experiences.

**Ré·ca·mi·er op·er·a·tion** (rā-kĕ-myā') curettage of the uterus.

**re·ca·nal·i·za·tion** (rē-kan'ăl-i-zā'shŭn) **1.** restoration of a lumen in a blood vessel following thrombotic occlusion, by organization of the thrombus with formation of new channels. **2.** spontaneous restoration of the continuity of the lumen of any occluded duct or tube, as with postvasectomy recanalization.

**re·ca·pi·tu·la·tion the·o·ry** that individuals in their embryonic development pass through stages similar in general structural plan to the stages their species passed through in its evolution; more technically phrased, the theory that ontogeny is an abbreviated recapitulation of phylogeny. SYN Haeckel law.

**re·cep·tac·u·lum**, pl. **re·cep·tac·u·la** (rē'sep-tak'yu-lŭm, rē'sep-tak'yu-lă) a receptacle. SYN reservoir. [L. fr. *re-cipio,* pp. *-ceptus,* to receive, fr. *capio,* to take]

**re·cep·tive a·pha·sia** aphasia in which there is impairment in the comprehension of spoken and written words, associated with effortless, articulated, but paraphasic, speech and writing; malformed words, substitute words, and neologisms are characteristic. When severe, and speech is incomprehensible, it is called jargon aphasia. The patient often appears unaware of his deficit. The lesion typically includes portion of the superior temporal lobe. SYN fluent aphasia, posterior aphasia, sensory aphasia.

**re·cep·tor** (rē-sep'tŏr) **1.** a structural protein molecule on the cell surface or within the cytoplasm that binds to a specific factor, such as a drug, hormone, antigen, or neurotransmitter. **2.** C. Sherrington's term for any one of the various sensory nerve endings in the skin, deep tissues, viscera, and special sense organs. [L. receiver, fr. *recipio,* to receive]

**re·cep·tor pro·tein** an intracellular protein (or protein fraction) that has an affinity for a known stimulus to cellular activity, such as a steroid hormone or adenosine 3',5'-cyclic phosphate.

**re·cess** (rē'ses) a small hollow or indentation. SYN recessus [TA]. [L. *recessus*]

**re·ces·sion** (rē-sesh'ŭn) a withdrawal or retreating. SEE ALSO retraction. [L. *recessio* (see recessus)]

**re·ces·sive** (rē-ses'iv) **1.** drawing away; receding. **2.** GENETICS denoting a trait due to a particular allele that does not manifest itself in the presence of other alleles that generate traits dominant to it.

**re·ces·sive char·ac·ter** an inherited character expressed in the homozygous state only.

**re·ces·sive in·her·i·tance** SEE dominance of traits.

**re·ces·sive trait** SEE dominance of traits.

**re·ces·sus**, pl. **re·ces·sus** (rē-ses'sŭs) [TA] SYN recess. [L. a withdrawing, a receding]

**re·cid·i·va·tion** (rē-sid-i-vā'shŭn) relapse of a disease, a symptom, or a behavioral pattern such

as an illegal activity for which one was previously imprisoned. [L. *recidivus,* falling back, recurring, fr. *re- cido,* to fall back]

**re·cid·i·vism** (rē-sid'i-vizm) the tendency of an individual toward recidivation. [L. *recidivus,* recurring]

**re·cid·i·vist** (rē-sid'i-vist) a person who tends toward recidivation.

**rec·i·pe** (res'i-pē) **1.** the superscription of a prescription, usually indicated by the sign ℞. **2.** a prescription or formula. [L. imperative of *recipio,* to receive]

**re·cip·ro·cal forc·es** in dentistry, forces whereby the resistance of one or more teeth is utilized to move one or more opposing teeth.

**re·cip·ro·cal trans·fu·sion** an attempt to confer immunity by transfusing blood taken from a donor into a receiver suffering from the same affection, the balance being maintained by transfusing an equal amount from the receiver to the donor.

**re·cip·ro·cal trans·lo·ca·tion** translocation without demonstrable loss of genetic material.

**Reck·ling·hau·sen dis·ease of bone** (rek-ling-how-zen) SYN osteitis fibrosa cystica.

**Reck·ling·hau·sen tu·mor** (rek-ling-how-zen) SYN adenomatoid tumor.

**rec·li·na·tion** (rek-li-nā'shŭn) turning the cataractous lens over into the vitreous to displace it from the line of vision. [L. *reclino,* pp. *-atus,* to bend back]

**rec·og·ni·tion fac·tors** factors that effect "recognition" of target antigens by polymorphonuclear leukocytes; apparently the Fc portion of antibody molecules and the activated third component of complement (C3), for both of which phagocytes have receptor sites.

**re·com·bi·nant** (rē-kom'bi-nant) **1.** a progeny that has received chromosomal parts from different parental strains as a result of uncorrected crossing over. **2.** pertaining to or denoting such organisms. **3.** in linkage analysis, the change of coupling phase at two loci during meiosis. If two syntenic, nonallelic genes are inherited from the same parent, they must be in coupling.

**re·com·bi·nant DNA** altered DNA resulting from the insertion into the chain, by chemical, enzymatic, or biological means, of a sequence (a whole or partial chain of DNA) not originally (biologically) present in that chain.

**re·com·bi·nant hu·man in·ter·leu·kin-11 (rhIL-11)** SYN human interleukin-11. SYN rhIL-11.

**re·com·bi·nant in·ter·leu·kin-11** SYN human interleukin-11.

**re·com·bi·nant vec·tor** a vector into which a foreign DNA has been inserted. SYN vector (5).

**re·com·bi·na·tion** (rē-kom-bi-nā'shŭn) **1.** the process of reuniting of parts that had become separated. **2.** the reversal of coupling phase in meiosis as gauged by the resulting phenotype. SEE ALSO recombinant.

**rec·om·mend·ed dai·ly al·low·ance (RDA)** the amount of daily nutrient intake judged to be adequate for the maintenance of good nutrition in an average adult.

**re·con·struc·tion** (rē-cŏn-strŭk'shŭn) the computerized synthesis of one or more two-dimensional images from a series of x-ray projections in computed tomography, or from a large number of measurements in magnetic resonance imaging; several methods are used; the earliest was back-projection, and the most common is 2D Fourier transformation.

**re•con•struc•tive mam•ma•plas•ty** the making of a simulated breast by plastic surgery, to replace the appearance of one that has been removed.

**re•con•struc•tive sur•gery** SEE plastic surgery.

**rec•ord** (rek′erd) **1.** MEDICINE a chronologic written account that includes a patient's initial complaint(s) and medical history, the physician's physical findings, the results of diagnostic tests and procedures, and any therapeutic medications and/or procedures. **2.** DENTISTRY a registration of desired jaw relations in a plastic material or on a device to permit these relationships to be transferred to an articulator. [M.E. *recorden,* fr. O.Fr. *recorder,* fr. L. *re-cordor,* to remember, fr. *re-,* back, again, + *cor,* heart]

**re•cor•ded de•tail** the visible sharpness of features on a radiograph (for example, bone trabeculae or pulmonary markings).

**re•cru•des•cence** (rē-kroo-des′ens) resumption of a morbid process or its symptoms after a period of remission. [L. *re-crudesco,* to become raw again, break out afresh, fr. *crudus,* raw, harsh]

**re•cru•des•cent** (rē-kroo-des′ent) becoming active again, relating to a recrudescence.

**re•cru•des•cent ty•phus** SYN Brill-Zinsser disease.

**re•cruit•ment** (rē-kroot′ment) **1.** AUDIOLOGY the unequal reaction of the ear to equal steps of increasing intensity, measured in decibels, with greater than normal increment in perceived loudness. **2.** the bringing into activity of additional motor neurons, causing greater activity in response to increased duration of the stimulus applied to a given receptor or afferent nerve. SEE ALSO irradiation. **3.** the adding of parallel channels of flow in any system. [Fr. *recrutement,* fr. L. *re-cresco,* pp. *-cretus,* to grow again]

**rec•tal** (rek′tăl) relating to the rectum.

**rec•tal am•pul•la** a dilated portion of the rectum just above the anal canal.

**rec•tal an•es•the•sia** general anesthesia produced by instillation into the rectum of a solution containing a central nervous system depressant.

**rec•tal col•umns** SYN anal columns.

**rec•tal•gia** (rek-tal′jē-ă) SYN proctalgia.

**rec•tec•to•my** (rek-tek′tō-mē) SYN proctectomy.

**rec•ti•fy** (rek′ti-fī) **1.** to correct. **2.** to purify or refine by distillation; usually implies repeated distillations. [L. *rectus,* right, straight]

**rec•ti•tis** (rek-tī′tis) SYN proctitis.

△**rec•to-, rect-** the rectum. SEE ALSO procto-. [L. *rectum,* fr. *rectus,* straight]

**rec•to•cele** (rek′tō-sēl) SYN proctocele. [recto- + G. *kēlē,* tumor, hernia]

**rec•to•coc•cyg•e•al mus•cle** SYN rectococcygeus muscle.

**rec•to•coc•cyg•e•us mus•cle** a band of smooth muscle fibers passing from the posterior surface of the rectum to the anterior surface of second or third coccygeal segment. SYN musculus rectococcygeus [TA], rectococcygeal muscle.

**rec•to•coc•cy•pexy** (rek-tō-kok′si-pek-sē) SYN proctococcypexy.

**rec•to•pexy** (rek′tō-pek-sē) SYN proctopexy.

**rec•to•plas•ty** (rek′tō-plas-tē) SYN proctoplasty.

**rec•to•scope** (rek′tō-skōp) SYN proctoscope.

**rec•to•sig•moid** (rek′tō-sig′moyd) the rectum and

sigmoid colon considered as a unit; the term is also applied to the junction of the sigmoid colon and rectum.

**rec•to•ste•no•sis** (rek′tō-stě-nō′sis) SYN proctostenosis.

**rec•tos•to•my** (rek-tos′tō-mē) SYN proctostomy.

**rec•tot•o•my** (rek-tot′ō-mē) SYN proctotomy.

**rec•to•u•re•thra•lis mus•cle** smooth muscle fibers that pass forward from the longitudinal muscle layer of the rectum to the membranous urethra in the male. SYN musculus rectourethralis [TA].

**rec•to•u•ter•ine mus•cle** a band of fibrous tissue and smooth muscle fibers passing between the cervix of the uterus and the rectum in the rectouterine fold, on either side. SYN musculus rectouterinus [TA].

**rec•to•u•ter•ine pouch** a pocket formed by the deflection of the peritoneum from the rectum to the uterus. SYN excavatio rectouterina [TA], cul-de-sac (2).

**rec•to•vag•i•nal sep•tum** the fascial layer between the vagina and the lower part of the rectum.

**rec•to•ve•si•ca•lis mus•cle** smooth muscle fibers in the sacrogenital fold in the male; they correspond to musculus rectouterinus. SYN musculus rectovesicalis [TA], rectovesical muscle.

**rec•to•ves•i•cal mus•cle** SYN rectovesicalis muscle.

**rec•to•ves•i•cal pouch** a pocket formed by the deflection of the peritoneum from the rectum to the bladder in the male. SYN excavatio rectovesicalis [TA], Proust space.

**rec•to•ves•i•cal sep•tum** a fascial layer that extends superiorly from the central tendon of the perineum to the peritoneum between the prostate and rectum.

**rec•tum,** pl. **rec•tums, rec•ta** (rek′tŭm, rek′tŭmz, rek′tă) [TA] the terminal portion of the digestive tube, extending from the rectosigmoid junction to the anal canal. [L. *rectus,* straight, pp. of *rego,* to make straight]

**rec•tus ab•do•mi•nis mus•cle** muscle of ventral abdominal wall, flanking the linea alba, and characterized by tendinous intersections separating its length into multiple bellies; *origin,* crest and symphysis of the pubis; *insertion,* xiphoid process and fifth to seventh costal cartilages; *action,* flexes lumbar vertebral column, draws thorax downward toward pubis; *nerve supply,* thoracoabdominal nerves. SYN musculus rectus abdominis [TA], rectus muscle of abdomen.

**rec•tus ca•pi•tis an•te•ri•or mus•cle** *origin,* transverse process and lateral mass of atlas; *insertion,* basilar process of occipital bone; *action,* turns and inclines head forward; *nerve supply,* ventral primary ramus of first and second cervical spinal nerve. SYN musculus rectus capitis anterior [TA].

**rec•tus ca•pi•tis la•te•ra•lis mus•cle** *origin,* transverse process of atlas; *insertion,* jugular process of occipital bone; *action,* inclines head to one side; *nerve supply,* ventral primary ramus of first cervical spinal nerve. SYN musculus rectus capitis lateralis [TA], lateral rectus muscle of the head.

**rec•tus ca•pi•tis pos•te•ri•or ma•jor mus•cle** *origin,* spinous process of axis; *insertion,* middle of inferior nuchal line of occipital bone; *action,* rotates and draws head backward; *nerve supply,* dorsal branch of first cervical (suboccipital). SYN musculus capitis posterior major [TA], greater posterior rectus muscle of head.

**rec·tus ca·pi·tis pos·te·ri·or mi·nor mus·cle** *origin*, from posterior tubercle of atlas; *insertion*, medial third of inferior nuchal line of occipital bone; *action*, rotates head and draws it backward; *nerve supply*, dorsal branch of first cervical (suboccipital). SYN smaller posterior rectus muscle of head.

**rec·tus fe·mo·ris mus·cle** *origin*, anterior inferior spine of ilium and upper margin of acetabulum; *insertion*, via common tendon of quadriceps femoris into patella, and via patellar ligament to tibial tuberosity. SYN musculus rectus femoris [TA], rectus muscle of thigh.

**rec·tus mus·cle of ab·do·men** SYN rectus abdominis muscle.

**rec·tus mus·cle of thigh** SYN rectus femoris muscle.

**re·cum·bent** (rē-kŭm′bent) leaning; reclining; lying down. [L. *recumbo*, to lie back, recline, fr. *re-*, back, + *cubo*, to lie]

**re·cu·per·ate** (rē-koo′per-āt) to undergo recuperation. [L. *recupero* (or *recip-*), pp. *-atus*, to take again, recover]

**re·cur·rence** (rē-kŭr′ens) **1.** a return of the symptoms in the course of a disease, following improvement or remission. **2.** SYN relapse. **3.** appearance of a genetic trait in a relative of a proband. [L. *re-curro*, to run back, recur]

**re·cur·rence risk** risk that a disease will occur elsewhere in a pedigree, given that at least one member of the pedigree (the proband) exhibits the disease.

**re·cur·rent** (rē-kŭr′ent) **1.** ANATOMY turning back on itself. **2.** denoting symptoms or lesions reappearing after an intermission or remission.

**re·cur·rent a·bor·tion** the loss of 3 or more sequential pregnancies before 20 weeks of gestation.

**re·cur·rent aph·thous ul·cers** SYN aphtha (2).

**re·cur·rent her·pet·ic sto·ma·ti·tis** reactivation of herpes simplex virus infection, characterized by vesicles and ulceration limited to the hard palate and attached gingiva.

**re·cur·rent jaun·dice of preg·nan·cy** SYN intrahepatic cholestasis of pregnancy.

**re·cur·rent re·spir·a·tory pa·pil·lo·ma·to·sis** a disease of the respiratory tract caused by the human papilloma virus; characterized by rapid recurrence of papillomas after surgical removal, airway obstruction, and hoarseness to aphonia when the larynx is involved. SEE ALSO laryngeal papillomatosis.

**re·cur·rent ul·cer·a·tive sto·ma·ti·tis** SYN aphtha (2).

**re·cur·rent ul·nar ar·tery** *origin*, ulnar artery; *distribution*, two branches, anterior and posterior, pass medially in front of and behind the elbow joint; *anastomoses*, superior and inferior ulnar collateral, i.e., with articular vascular network of elbow. SYN arteria recurrens ulnaris [TA].

**re·cur·ring dig·i·tal fi·bro·ma of child·hood** multiple fibrous flesh-colored nodules on the extensor aspect of the terminal phalanges of adjacent digits of infants and young children that often recur after attempted excision, do not metastasize, and may spontaneously regress in two to three years; composed of spindle cells containing cytoplasmic inclusions believed to be derived from myofibrils.

**re·cur·va·tion** (rē-ker-vā′shŭn) a backward bending or flexure. [L. *re-curvus*, bent back]

**red blood cell (rbc, RBC)** SYN erythrocyte.

**red cor·pus·cle** SYN erythrocyte.

**red hep·a·ti·za·tion** the first stage of hepatization in which the exudate is blood-stained.

**red im·por·ted fire ant** SYN *Solenopsis invicta.*

**red in·du·ra·tion** a condition observed in lungs in which there is an advanced degree of acute passive congestion, or acute pneumonitis (sometimes termed interstitial pneumonia), or a similar pathologic process.

**re·din·te·gra·tion** (rē′din-tĕ-grā′shŭn) **1.** the restoration of lost or injured parts. **2.** restoration to health. **3.** the recalling of a whole experience on the basis only of some item or portion of the original stimulus or circumstances of the experience. [L. *red-integro*, pp. *-atus*, to make whole again, renew, fr. *integer*, untouched, entire]

**red mus·cle** slow-twitch muscle in which small dark "red" muscle fibers predominate; myoglobin is abundant and great numbers of mitochondria occur, characterized by slow, sustained (tonic) contraction. Contrast with white muscle.

**red neu·ral·gia** SYN erythromelalgia.

**red nu·cle·us** a large, well defined, somewhat elongated cell mass, of reddish-gray hue in the fresh brain, located in the rostral mesencephalic tegmentum. The nucleus receives a massive projection from the contralateral half of the cerebellum by way of the superior cerebellar peduncle, and an additional projection from the ipsilateral motor cortex. Projections from the anterior interposed nucleus and motor cortex to the red nucleus are somatopically organized. Its efferent connections are with the contralateral rhombencephalic reticular formation and spinal cord by way of the rubrobulbar and rubrospinal tracts. Rubrospinal fibers have somatotopic origin.

**red oil** [CI 26125] a weakly acid diazo oil-soluble dye, used in histologic demonstration of neutral fats.

**re·dox** (rēd′oks) contraction of reduction-oxidation.

**red pulp** splenic pulp seen grossly as a reddish brown substance, due to its abundance of red blood cells, consisting of splenic sinuses and the tissue intervening between them (splenic cords).

**red re·flex** SYN pyramid of light.

**red tide** a natural phenomenon resulting from higher than normal concentrations of the microscopic algae *Gymnodinium breve* in seawater. [When the causative organism is extremely concentrated, sea water can have a reddish-brown color.]

**re·duce** (rē-doos′) **1.** to perform reduction (1). **2.** CHEMISTRY to initiate reduction (2). [L. *re-duco*, to lead back, restore, reduce]

**re·duced hem·a·tin** SYN heme.

**re·duced he·mo·glo·bin** the form of Hb in red blood cells after the oxygen of oxyhemoglobin is released in the tissues.

**re·duc·i·ble** (rē-doos′i-bl) capable of being reduced.

**re·duc·i·ble her·nia** a hernia in which the contents of the sac can be returned to their normal location.

**re·duc·tant** (rē-dŭk′tant) the substance that is oxidized in the course of reduction.

r
e

**re•duc•tase** (rē-dŭk'tās) an enzyme that catalyzes a reduction; since all enzymes catalyze reactions in either direction, any reductase can, under the proper conditions, behave as an oxidase and vice versa, hence the term oxidoreductase.

**5α-reductase inhibitors** drugs that inhibit the action of 5α-reductase, resulting in lower levels of prostatic dihydrotestosterone, produced by the enzyme from testosterone as the primary androgen in the prostate.

**re•duc•tion** (rē-dŭk'shŭn) **1.** the restoration, by surgical or manipulative procedures, of a part to its normal anatomical relation. SYN repositioning. **2.** CHEMISTRY a reaction involving a gain of one or more electrons by a substance. [L. *reductio,* fr. *re-duco,* pp. *ductus,* to lead back]

**re•duc•tion of chro•mo•somes** the process during meiosis whereby one member of each homologous pair of chromosomes is distributed to a sperm or ovum; the diploid set of chromosomes (46 in humans) is thus reduced to the haploid set in each gamete; union of the sperm and ovum restores the diploid or somatic number in the one-cell zygote.

**re•duc•tion de•for•mi•ty** congenital absence or attenuation of one or more body parts; usually of the limbs or limb components.

**re•duc•tion left ven•tri•cu•lo•plas•ty** SYN left ventricular volume reduction surgery.

**re•duc•tion mam•ma•plas•ty** plastic surgery of the breast to reduce its size and (frequently) to improve its shape and position.

**re•du•pli•ca•tion** (rē'doo'pli-kā'shŭn) **1.** a redoubling. **2.** a duplication or doubling, as of the sounds of the heart in certain morbid states or the presence of two instead of a normally single part. **3.** a fold or duplicature. [L. *reduplicatio,* fr. *re-,* again, + *duplico,* to double, fr. *duplex,* two-fold]

**Red•u•vi•i•dae** (redj-ĕ-vī-ĕ-dē) a family of predatory insects, the assassin bugs; it includes the subfamily Triatominae, the kissing or cone-nosed bugs, whose type genus *Triatoma* includes species that are vectors of *Trypanosoma cruzi.*

**red, white, and blue sign** the contemporaneous occurrence of erythema, ischemia, and necrosis in a wound, as in loxoscelism.

**REE** resting energy expenditure.

**Reed-Frost mo•del** (rēd-frost) mathematical model of infectious disease transmission and herd immunity. The model gives the number of new cases of an infection that can be expected in a specified time in a closed, freely mixing population of immune and susceptible individuals, with varying assumptions about frequency of contact.

**Reed-Stern•berg cell** (rēd-stern'berg) large transformed lymphocytes, probably B cell in origin, generally regarded as pathognomonic of Hodgkin lymphoma; a typical cell has a pale-staining acidophilic cytoplasm and one or two large nuclei showing marginal clumping of chromatin and unusually conspicuous deeply acidophilic nucleoli; binucleate Reed-Sternberg cells frequently show a mirror-image form (mirror-image cell).

**reef•ing** (rēf'ing) surgically reducing the extent of a tissue by folding it and securing with sutures, as in plication.

**re•en•trant mech•a•nism** the probable basis of most arrhythmias, requiring at least three criteria:

1. a loop circuit, 2. unidirectional block, 3. slowed conduction.

**re•en•try** (rē-en'trē) return of the same impulse into a zone of heart muscle that it has recently activated, sufficiently delayed that the zone is no longer refractory, as seen in most ectopic beats, reciprocal rhythms, and most tachycardias.

**ref•er•ence range** the usual range of test values for a healthy population. SYN normal range.

**ref•er•ence val•ues** a set of laboratory test values obtained from an individual or group in a defined state of health; this term replaces normal values, since it is based on a defined state of health rather than on apparent health.

**re•ferred pain** pain at a site other than the actual location of trauma or disease.

**re•ferred sen•sa•tion** a sensation felt in one place in response to a stimulus applied in another.

**re•fine** (rē-fīn') to free from impurities.

**re•flec•tance** a measure of reflected acoustic energy as a function of immitance, as in middle ear impedance.

**re•flec•tance spec•tro•pho•to•me•try** a quantitative spectrophotometric technique in which light is reflected from the surface of a colorimetric reaction and is then used to measure the amount of the reaction product.

**re•flect•ed in•gui•nal lig•a•ment** a triangular fibrous band extending from the aponeurosis of the external oblique to the pubic tubercle of the opposite side.

**re•flec•tion** (rē-flek'shŭn) **1.** the act of reflecting. **2.** that which is reflected. **3.** PSYCHOTHERAPY a technique in which a patient's statements are repeated, restated, or rephrased in order that the patient will continue to explore and expound on emotionally significant content. [L. *reflexio,* bending back]

**re•flec•tion co•ef•fi•cient** (σ) a measure of the relative permeability of a particular membrane to a particular solute; calculated as the ratio of observed osmotic pressure to that calculated from van't Hoff law.

**re•flec•tor** (rē-flek'ter) any surface that reflects light, heat, or sound.

**re•flex** (rē'fleks) **1.** an involuntary reaction in response to a stimulus applied to the periphery and transmitted to the nervous centers in the brain or spinal cord. Most of the deep reflexes listed as subentries are stretch or myotatic reflexes, elicited by striking a tendon or bone, causing stretching, even slight, of the muscle which then contracts as a result of the stimulus applied to its proprioceptors. SEE ALSO phenomenon. **2.** a reflection. **3.** SYN consensual. [L. *reflexus,* pp. of *re-flecto,* to bend back]

**re•flex arc** the route followed by nerve impulses in the production of a reflex act, from the peripheral receptor organ through the afferent nerve to the central nervous system synapse and then through the efferent nerve to the effector organ.

**re•flex cough** a cough excited reflexly by irritation in some distant part, as the ear or the stomach.

**re•flex ep•i•lep•sy** seizures which are induced by peripheral stimulation; e.g., audiogenic, laryngeal, photogenic, or other stimulation.

**re•flex in•hi•bi•tion** a situation in which sensory stimuli decrease reflex activity.

**re•flex neu•ro•gen•ic blad•der** an abnormal

condition of urinary bladder function whereby the bladder is cut off from upper motor neuron control, but where the lower motor neuron arc is still intact.

**re·flex·o·gen·ic** (rē-flek-sō-jen′ik) causing a reflex.

**re·flex·o·graph** (rē-flek′sō-graf) an instrument for graphically recording a reflex. [reflex + G. *graphō*, to write]

**re·flex·o·lo·gy** a massage technique focusing on specific points, particularly on the feet, that are said to correspond via meridians to other organs or areas of the body; lesser points on hands and ears. SYN reflex zone therapy.

**re·flex·om·e·ter** (rē-flek-som′ĕ-ter) an instrument for measuring the force necessary to excite a reflex. [reflex + G. *metron*, measure]

**re·flex sym·pa·thet·ic dys·tro·phy (RSD)** diffuse persistent pain usually in an extremity often associated with vasomotor disturbances, trophic changes, and limitation or immobility of joints; frequently follows local injury. SEE ALSO causalgia.

**re·flex symp·tom** a disturbance of sensation or function in an organ or part more or less remote from the morbid condition giving rise to it; e.g., muscle spasm due to joint inflammation.

**re·flex zone ther·a·py** SYN reflexology.

**re·flux** (rē′flŭks) **1.** a backward flow. SEE ALSO regurgitation. **2.** CHEMISTRY to boil without loss of vapor because of the presence of a condenser that returns vapor as liquid. [L. *re-*, back, + *fluxus*, a flow]

**re·flux e·soph·a·gi·tis, pep·tic e·soph·a·gi·tis** inflammation of the lower esophagus from regurgitation of acid gastric contents, usually due to malfunction of the lower esophageal sphincter; symptoms include substernal pain, heartburn, and regurgitation of acid juice.

**re·flux o·ti·tis me·dia** otitis media caused by passage of nasopharyngeal secretions through the auditory tube.

**re·fract** (rē-frakt′) **1.** to change the direction of a ray of light. **2.** to detect an error of refraction and to correct it by means of lenses. [L. *refringo*, pp. *-fractus*, to break up]

**re·frac·tion** (rē-frak′shŭn) **1.** the deflection of a ray of light when it passes from one medium into another of different optical density; in passing from a denser into a rarer medium it is deflected away from a line perpendicular to the surface of the refracting medium; in passing from a rarer to a denser medium it is bent toward this perpendicular line. **2.** the act of determining the nature and degree of the refractive errors in the eye and correction of them by lenses. SYN refringence. [L. *refractio* (see refract)]

**re·frac·tion·ist** (rē-frak′shŭn-ist) a person trained to measure the refraction of the eye and to determine the proper corrective lenses.

**re·frac·tive** (rē-frak′tiv) **1.** pertaining to refraction. **2.** having the power to refract. SYN refringent.

**re·frac·tive in·dex** (*n*) the relative velocity of light in another medium compared to the velocity in air.

**re·frac·tive ker·a·to·plas·ty** any procedure in which the shape of the cornea is modified, with the intent of changing the refractive error of the eye; for example, if the cornea is flattened, the eye becomes less myopic. SEE keratophakia, keratomileusis, radial keratotomy.

**re·frac·tive ker·a·tot·o·my** modification of corneal curvature by means of corneal incisions to minimize hyperopia, myopia, or astigmatism. In this type of radial keratotomy surgery, performed by excimer laser, pie-shaped pieces of cornea are removed under local anesthetic. The resulting scar tissue formation reshapes the cornea.

**re·frac·tiv·i·ty** (rē-frak-tiv′i-tē) refractive power.

**re·frac·tom·e·ter** (rē-frak-tom′ĕ-ter) an instrument for measuring the degree of refraction in translucent substances, especially the ocular media. SEE refractive index. [refraction + G. *metron*, measure]

**re·frac·tom·e·try** (rē-frak-tom′ĕ-trē) **1.** measurement of the refractive index. **2.** use of a refractometer to determine the refractive error of the eye.

**re·frac·to·ry** (rē-frak′tōr-ē) **1.** resistant to treatment, as of a disease. SYN intractable (1), obstinate (2). **2.** SYN obstinate (1). [L. *refractarius*, fr. *refringo*, pp. *-fractus*, to break in pieces]

**re·frac·to·ry a·ne·mia** progressive anemia unresponsive to therapy other than transfusion.

**re·frac·to·ry pe·ri·od 1.** the period following effective stimulation, during which excitable tissue such as heart muscle and nerve fails to respond to a stimulus of threshold intensity (i.e., excitability is depressed); **2.** a period of temporary psychophysiologic resistance to further sexual stimulation which occurs immediately following orgasm.

**re·frac·to·ry state** subnormal excitability immediately following a response to previous excitation; the state is divided into absolute and relative phases.

**re·frac·ture** (rē-frak′ cher) breaking a bone that has united after a previous fracture. [re- + fracture]

**re·fresh** (rē-fresh′) **1.** to renew; to cause to recuperate. **2.** to perform revivification (2). [O. Fr. *re-frescher*]

**re·frig·er·ant** (rē-frij′er-ănt) **1.** cooling; reducing slight fever. **2.** an agent that gives a sensation of coolness or relieves feverishness. [L. *re-frigero*, pp. *-atus*, pr. p. *-ans*, to make cold, fr. *frigus* (*frigor-*), cold]

**re·frig·er·a·tion** (rē-frij′er-ā′shŭn) the act of cooling or reducing fever. [L. *refrigeratio* (see refrigerant)]

**re·frig·er·a·tion an·es·the·sia** SYN cryoanesthesia.

**re·frin·gence** (rē-frin′jens) SYN refraction.

**re·frin·gent** (rē-frin′jent) SYN refractive.

**Ref·sum dis·ease** (ref′soom) a rare degenerative disorder due to a deficiency of phytanic acid α-hydroxylase; clinically characterized by retinitis pigmentosa, ichthyosis, demyelinating polyneuropathy, deafness, and cerebellar signs; autosomal recessive inheritance caused by mutation in the gene encoding phytanoyl-CoA hydroxylase (PAHX or PAYH) on chromosome 10p. Infantile Refsum disease is an impaired peroxisomal function with accumulation of phytanic acid, pipecolic acid; autosomal recessive inheritance, caused by mutation in the PEX 1 gene on 7q.

**re·fu·sion** (rē-fyu′zhŭn) return of the circulation of blood which has been temporarily cut off by ligature of a limb. [L. *re-fundo*, pp. *-fusus*, to pour back]

**Re·gaud fix·a·tive** (rē-gō′) a fixative containing formaldehyde and sodium dichromate, used to preserve mitochondria but not fat; requires after-chroming and extensive washing.

**re·gen·er·a·tion** (rē′jen-er-ā′shŭn) **1.** reproduction or reconstitution of a lost or injured part. SYN neogenesis. **2.** a form of asexual reproduction; e.g., when a worm is divided into two or more parts, each segment is regenerated into a new individual. [L. *regeneratio* (see regenerate)]

**re·gen·er·a·tive pol·yp** a hyperplastic polyp of the gastric mucosa.

**reg·i·men** (rej′i-men) a program, including drugs, which regulates aspects of one's life-style for a hygienic or therapeutic purpose; a program of treatment; sometimes mistakenly called regime. [L. direction, rule]

**re·gio,** gen. **re·gi·o·nis,** pl. **re·gi·o·nes** (rē′jē-ō, rē′jē-ō′nis, rē′jē-ō′nēz) [TA] SYN region. [L.]

**re·gion** (rē′jŭn) **1.** an often arbitrarily limited portion of the surface of the body. SEE ALSO space, zone. **2.** a portion of the body having a special nervous or vascular supply, or a part of an organ having a special function. SEE ALSO area, space, spatium, zone. SYN regio [TA]. [L. *regio*]

**re·gion·al** (rē′jŭn-ăl) relating to a region.

**re·gion·al a·nat·o·my** my a method of anatomic study based on regions, parts, or divisions of the body (e.g., the foot or the inguinal region), emphasizing the relationships of structures (e.g., muscles, nerves, and arteries) within that area; distinguished from systemic anatomy. SYN topographic anatomy.

**re·gion·al an·es·the·sia** use of local anesthetic solution(s) to produce circumscribed areas of loss of sensation; a generic term including conduction, nerve block, spinal, epidural, field block, infiltration, and topical anesthesia. SYN conduction analgesia.

**re·gion·al en·ter·i·tis** a chronic enteritis, of unknown cause, involving the terminal ileum and less frequently other parts of the gastrointestinal tract; characterized by patchy deep ulcers that may cause fistulas, and narrowing and thickening of the bowel by fibrosis and lymphocytic infiltration, with noncaseating tuberculoid granulomas that also may be found in regional lymph nodes; symptoms include fever, diarrhea, cramping abdominal pain, and weight loss. SYN Crohn disease, distal ileitis, regional ileitis, terminal ileitis, granulomatous enteritis.

**re·gion·al gran·u·lom·a·tous lym·phad·e·ni·tis** SYN catscratch disease.

**re·gion·al hy·po·ther·mia** reduction of the temperature of an extremity or organ by external cold or perfusion with cold blood or solutions.

**re·gi·o·nes** (rē′jē-ō′nēz) plural of regio. [L.]

**re·gion of in·ter·est** in computed tomography or other computerized imaging, an interactively selected portion of the image, whose individual or average pixel values can be displayed numerically.

**re·gions of back** the topographical regions of the back of the trunk, including the vertebral region, sacral region, scapular region, infrascapular region, and lumbar region.

**re·gions of chest** the topographical divisions of the chest: presternal, mammary, inframammary, and axillary. SEE pectoral region.

**re·gions of face** the topographical subdivisions

of the face, including nasal, oral, mental, orbital, infraorbital, buccal, and zygomatic.

**re·gions of head** the topographical division of the cranium in relation to the bones of the cranial vault; the regions include frontal, parietal, occipital, and temporal.

**re·gions of low·er limb** the topographical divisions of the lower limb: gluteal, thigh (or femoral), knee, leg (or crural), ankle, and foot.

**re·gions of neck** the topographical subdivisions of the neck.

**re·gions of up·per limb** the topographic divisions of the upper limb: deltoid, arm, elbow, forearm, carpal region, and hand.

**reg·is·tered nurse** one who has graduated from an accredited nursing program and has been licensed by public authority to practice nursing; may have advanced skills acquired through clinical or master's or doctoral programs.

**reg·is·tra·tion** the reception of external stimuli; the capacity to perform this activity.

**reg·is·try** database on patients who share a particular characteristic; common registries include cancer, trauma, and implants; data are used to assess the quality of care, monitor trends, and do research.

**re·gres·sion** (rē-gresh′ŭn) **1.** a subsidence of symptoms. **2.** a relapse; a return of symptoms. **3.** any retrograde movement or action. **4.** a return to a more primitive mode of behavior due to an inability to function adequately at a more adult level. **5.** the tendency for offspring of exceptional parents to possess characteristics closer to those of the general population. **6.** an unconscious defense mechanism by which there occurs a return to earlier patterns of adaptation. **7.** the distribution of one random variable given particular values of other variables relevant to it, e.g., a formula for the distribution of weight as a function of height and chest circumference. [L. *regredior,* pp. *-gressus,* to go back]

**re·gres·sion a·nal·y·sis** the statistical method of finding the "best" mathematical model to describe one variable as a function of another.

**re·gres·sive** (rē-gres′iv) relating to or characterized by regression.

**re·gres·sive stain·ing** a type of staining in which tissues are overstained and the excess dye is then removed selectively until the desired intensity is obtained.

**reg·u·lar a·stig·ma·tism** astigmatism in which the curvature in each meridian is equal throughout its course, and the meridians of greatest and least curvature are at right angles to each other.

**reg·u·la·tion** (reg′yu-lā′shŭn) **1.** control of the rate or manner in which a process progresses or a product is formed. **2.** EXPERIMENTAL EMBRYOLOGY the power of a pregastrula embryo to continue approximately normal development after a part or parts have been manipulated or destroyed. [L. *regula,* a rule]

**reg·u·la·tor** (reg-yu-lā′tōr) a substance or process that controls another substance or process.

**reg·u·la·tor gene** a gene that produces a repressor substance that inhibits an operator gene when combined with it. It thus prevents production of a specific enzyme. When the enzyme is again in demand, a specific regulatory metabolite inhibits the repressor substance.

**reg·u·la·tory dis·or·der** a disorder, first evident in infancy and early childhood, characterized by a distinct behavioral pattern that presents with a sensory, sensorimotor, or organizational processing difficulty that interferes with the child's ability to maintain positive interaction and relationships and to make daily adaptation.

**reg·u·la·to·ry se·quence** any DNA sequence that is responsible for the regulation of gene expression, such as promoters and operators.

**reg·u·lon** (reg′yu-lon) a set of structural genes, all with the same gene regulation, whose gene products are involved in the same reaction pathway.

**re·gur·gi·tant** (rē-ger′ji-tant) regurgitating; flowing backward.

**re·gur·gi·tant mur·mur** a murmur due to leakage or backward flow at one of the valvular orifices of the heart.

**re·gur·gi·tate** (rē-ger′ji-tāt) **1.** to flow backward. **2.** to expel the contents of the stomach in small amounts, short of vomiting. [L. *re-,* back, + *gurgito,* pp. *-atus,* to flood, fr. *gurges* (*gurgit-*), a whirlpool]

**re·gur·gi·ta·tion** (rē-ger′ji-tā′shŭn) **1.** a backward flow, as of blood through an incompetent valve of the heart. **2.** the return of gas or small amounts of food from the stomach. [L. *regurgitatio* (see regurgitate)]

**re·gur·gi·ta·tion jaun·dice** jaundice due to biliary obstruction, the bile pigment having been conjugated and secreted by the hepatic cells and then reabsorbed into the bloodstream.

**re·ha·bil·i·ta·tion** (rē′hă-bil-i-tā′shŭn) spontaneous or therapeutic restoration, after disease, illness, or injury, of the ability to function in a normal or near normal manner. [L. *rehabilitare,* pp. *-tatus,* to make fit, fr. *re-* + *habilitas,* ability]

**re·hears·al** (rē-her′săl) a process associated with enhancing short-term and long-term memory wherein newly presented information, such as a name or a list of words, is repeated to oneself one or more times in order not to forget it.

**re·hy·dra·tion** (rē-hī-drā′shŭn) the return of water to a system after its loss.

**Rei·chel-Pól·ya stom·ach pro·ce·dure** (rī′kel-pōl′yah) retrocolic anastomosis of the full circumference of the open stomach to the jejunum.

**Rei·chert car·ti·lage** (rī-kĕrt) a cartilage in the mesenchyme of the second pharyngeal arch in the embryo, from which develop the stapes, the styloid processes, the stylohyoid ligaments, and the lesser cornua of the hyoid bone.

**Reid base line** (rēd) a line drawn from the inferior margin of the orbit to the auricular point (center of the orifice of the external acoustic meatus) and extending backward to the center of the occipital bone. Used as the zero plane in computed tomography.

**Reif·en·stein syn·drome** (rīf′en-stīn) partial androgen sensitivity; a familial form of male pseudohermaphroditism characterized by varying degrees of ambiguous genitalia or hypospadias, postpubertal development of gynecomastia, and infertility associated with seminiferous tubular sclerosis; cryptorchidism may be present, and Leydig cell hypofunction may lead to impotence in later years; chromosomal studies show 46,XY karyotype; X-linked recessive inheritance, caused by mutation in the androgen receptor gene (AR) on Xq.

**Rei·ki** (rā′kē) a trademarked bodywork modality based on an Eastern concept that the universe is composed of energy that can be influenced by human thought and action. Reiki is practiced through the laying on of hands and the conscious or subconscious direction of healing energy through the therapist to recipient. SEE ALSO chi.

**re·im·plan·ta·tion** (rē′im-plan-tā′shŭn) SYN replantation.

**re·in·fec·tion** (rē-in-fek′shŭn) a second infection by the same microorganism, after recovery from or during the course of a primary infection.

**re·in·force·ment** (rē-in-fōrs′ment) **1.** an increase of force or strength; denoting specifically the increased sharpness of the patellar reflex when the patient at the same time closes the fist tightly or pulls against the flexed fingers or contracts some other set of muscles. **2.** DENTISTRY a structural addition or inclusion used to give additional strength in function; e.g., bars in plastic denture base. **3.** CONDITIONING the totality of the process in which the conditioned stimulus is followed by presentation of the unconditioned stimulus which itself elicits the response to be conditioned. SEE ALSO reinforcer.

**re·in·forc·er** (rē-in-fōrs′er) in conditioning, a pleasant or satisfaction-yielding (**positive reinforcer**) or painful or unsatisfying (**negative reinforcer**), stimulus, object, or stimulus event that is obtained upon the performance of a desired or predetermined operant. SEE ALSO reinforcement (3). SYN reward.

**Rein·ke space** (rīn-kĕ) a potential space between the lamina propria and the external elastic lamina of the vocal fold. Edema in this space produces hoarseness in chronic inflammation.

**re·in·ner·va·tion** (rē-in-ner-vā′shŭn) restoration of nerve control of a paralyzed muscle or other effector organ by means of regrowth of nerve fibers, either spontaneously or after anastomosis.

**re·in·te·gra·tion** (rē′in-tĕ-grā′shŭn) in the mental health professions, the return to well-adjusted functioning following disturbances due to mental illness.

**Reis-Bück·lers cor·ne·al dys·trophy** (rīs-buk′lĕr) an autosomal dominant disorder of Bowman membrane of the cornea, characterized by a reticular haze and associated with recurrent corneal erosions.

**Reis·sei·sen mus·cles** (rīs-ī-sĕn) microscopic smooth muscle fibers in the smallest bronchial tubes.

**Reiss·ner mem·brane** (rīs-ner) SYN vestibular membrane.

**Rei·ter syn·drome** (rī-tĕr) the association of urethritis, iridocyclitis, mucocutaneous lesions, and arthritis, sometimes with diarrhea; one or more of these conditions may recur at intervals of months or years, but the arthritis may be persistent.

**re·jec·tion** (rē-jek′shŭn) **1.** the immunological response to incompatibility in a transplanted organ. **2.** a refusal to accept, recognize, or grant; a denial. **3.** elimination of small ultrasonic echoes from display. [L. *rejectio,* a throwing back]

**re·lapse** (rē′laps) return of the manifestations of a disease after an interval of improvement. SYN recurrence (2). [L. *re-labor,* pp. *-lapsus,* to slide back]

**re·laps·ing feb·rile nod·u·lar non·sup·pur·a·tive pan·nic·u·li·tis** nodular fat necrosis of a variety of possible causes. SYN Christian disease (2), Christian syndrome.

**re·laps·ing fe·ver** an acute infectious disease caused by any one of a number of strains of *Borrelia*, marked by febrile attacks lasting about six days and separated from each other by apyretic intervals of about the same length; the microorganism is found in the blood during the febrile periods but not during the intervals. There are two epidemiologic varieties: 1) the louseborne variety, occurring chiefly in Europe, northern Africa, and India, and caused by strains of *B. recurrentis;* 2) the tick-borne variety, occurring in Africa, Asia, and North and South America, caused by various species of *Borrelia*, each of which is transmitted by a different species of the soft tick, *Ornithodoros*.

**re·laps·ing pol·y·chon·dri·tis** a hereditary degenerative disease of cartilage producing a bizarre form of arthritis, with collapse of the ears, the cartilaginous portion of the nose, and the tracheobronchial tree; death may occur from chronic infection or suffocation because of loss of stability in the tracheobronchial tree. SYN Meyenburg disease.

**re·la·tion** (rē-lā′shŭn) **1.** an association or connection between or among people or objects. SEE ALSO relationship. **2.** DENTISTRY the mode of contact of teeth or the positional relationship of oral structures. [L. *relatio*, a bringing back]

**re·la·tion·ship** (rē-lā′shŭn-ship) the state of being related, associated, or connected.

**rel·a·tive ac·com·mo·da·tion** quantity of accommodation required for single binocular vision for any specified distance, or for any particular degree of convergence.

**rel·a·tive bi·o·log·ic ef·fec·tive·ness** a factor used to compare the biologic effect of absorbed doses of different types and energies of ionizing radiation. It is determined by the ratio of an absorbed dose of the particular radiation in question to the absorbed dose of a reference radiation required to produce an identical biologic effect in a specific organism, organ, or tissue.

**rel·a·tive hu·mid·i·ty** the actual amount of water vapor present in the air or in a gas, divided by the amount necessary for saturation at the same temperature and pressure; expressed as a percentage.

**rel·a·tive leu·ko·cy·to·sis** an increased proportion of one or more types of leukocytes in the circulating blood, without an actual increase in the total number of white blood cells.

**rel·a·tive mo·lec·u·lar mass** ($M_r$) SYN molecular weight.

**rel·a·tive pol·y·cy·the·mia** a relative increase in the number of red blood cells as a result of loss of the fluid portion of the blood.

**rel·a·tive sco·to·ma** a scotoma in which there is visual depression but not complete loss of light perception.

**rel·a·tive spec·i·fic·i·ty** the specificity of a medical screening test as determined by comparison with the same type of test (e.g., specificity of a new serological test to specificity of an established serological test).

**re·lax·ant** (rē-lak′sănt) **1.** relaxing; causing relaxation; reducing tension, especially muscular tension. **2.** an agent that reduces muscular tension or produces skeletal muscle paralysis, usually referred to as a muscle relaxant.

**re·lax·ant re·ver·sal** use of acetylcholinesterase inhibitors to terminate the action of nondepolarizing neuromuscular relaxants.

**re·lax·a·tion** (rē-lak-sā′shŭn) **1.** loosening, lengthening, or lessening of tension in a muscle. **2.** MAGNETIC RESONANCE IMAGING the decay in magnetization of tissue after the direction of the surrounding magnetic field is changed; the different rates of relaxation for individual nuclei and tissues are used to provide contrast in imaging. [L. *relaxatio* (see relax)]

**re·lax·a·tion su·ture** a suture so arranged that it may be loosened if the tension of the wound becomes excessive.

**re·lax·a·tion time** (τ) the time required for the substrate in an enzymatic or chemical reaction to fall to 1/e of its initial value.

**re·learn·ing** (rē-lern′ing) the process of regaining a skill or ability that has been partially or entirely lost; savings involved in relearning, as compared with original learning, give an index of the degree of retention.

**re·leas·ing fac·tors 1.** substances, usually of hypothalamic origin, capable of accelerating the rate of secretion of a given hormone by the anterior pituitary gland; **2.** factors required in the termination phase of either RNA biosynthesis or protein biosynthesis. SYN liberins, releasing hormone.

**re·leas·ing hor·mone** SYN releasing factors.

**re·lieve** (rē-lēv′) to free wholly or partly from pain or discomfort, either physical or mental. [through O. Fr. fr. L. *re-levo*, to lift up, lighten]

**re·lo·ca·tion test** a test for anterior shoulder instability; the supine patient's humerus is abducted and rotated externally against the table edge as a fulcrum; patients with anterior stability loss become apprehensive with pressure.

**REM** rapid eye movements.

**rem** roentgen-equivalent-man. See entries under roentgen.

**Re·mak fi·bers** (rā-mahk) SYN unmyelinated fibers.

**Re·mak nu·cle·ar di·vi·sion** (rā-mahk) SYN amitosis.

**Re·mak re·flex** (rā-mahk) plantar flexion of the first three toes and, sometimes, the foot with extension of the knee induced by stroking of the upper anterior surface of the thigh; it occurs when the conducting paths in the cord are interrupted.

**Re·mak sign** (rā-mahk) dissociation of the sensations of touch and of pain in tabes dorsalis and polyneuritis.

**rem·e·dy** (rem′ĕ-dē) an agent that cures disease or alleviates its symptoms. [L. *remedium*, fr. *re-*, again, + *medeor*, cure]

**re·min·er·al·i·za·tion** (rē′min′er-ăl-i-zā′shŭn) **1.** the return to the body or a local area of necessary mineral constituents lost through disease or dietary deficiencies; commonly used in referring to the content of calcium salts in bone. **2.** DENTISTRY a process enhanced by the presence of fluoride whereby partially decalcified enamel, dentin, and cementum become recalcified by mineral replacement.

**re·mis·sion** (rē-mish′ŭn) **1.** abatement or lessening in severity of the symptoms of a disease. **2.** the period during which such abatement occurs. [L. *remissio*, fr. *re-mitto*, pp. *-missus*, to send back, slacken, relax]

**re·mit·tence** (rē-mit′ens) a temporary amelioration, without actual cessation, of symptoms.

**re·mit·tent** (rē-mit′ent) characterized by temporary periods of abatement of the symptoms of a disease.

**re·mod·el·ing** (rē-mod′el-ing) **1.** a cyclic process by which bone maintains a dynamic steady state through sequential resorption and formation of a small amount of bone at the same site; unlike the process of modeling, the size and shape of remodeled bone remain unchanged. **2.** any process of reshaping or reorganizing.

**re·mote af·ter·load·ing bra·chy·ther·a·py** locally delivered radiotherapy that is loaded remotely into previously placed receptacles.

**re·mov·a·ble bridge** SYN removable partial denture.

**re·mov·a·ble par·tial den·ture** a partial denture which supplies teeth and associated structures on a partially edentulous jaw, and which can be readily removed from the mouth. SYN removable bridge.

**ren,** gen. **re·nis,** pl. **re·nes** (ren, rē′nis, rē′nēz) [TA] SYN kidney. [L.]

**re·nal** (rē′năl) SYN nephric.

**re·nal am·y·loi·do·sis** renal deposits of amyloid, especially in glomerular capillary walls, which may cause albuminuria and the nephrotic syndrome. SYN amyloid nephrosis (1).

**re·nal ar·tery** *origin,* aorta; *branches,* segmental, ureteral, and inferior suprarenal; *distribution,* kidney. SYN arteria renalis [TA].

**re·nal cal·cu·lus** a calculus occurring within the kidney collecting system.

**re·nal col·umns** the prolongations of cortical substance separating the pyramids of the kidney. SYN columnae renales [TA], Bertin columns.

**re·nal cor·pus·cle** the tuft of glomerular capillaries and the capsula glomeruli that encloses it. SYN corpusculum renis.

**re·nal cor·tex** the part of the kidney consisting of renal lobules in the outer zone beneath the capsule and also the lobules of the renal columns that are extensions inward between the pyramids; contains the renal corpuscles and the proximal and distal convoluted tubules.

**re·nal fa·scia** the condensation of the fibroareolar tissue and fat surrounding the kidney to form a sheath for the organ. SYN Gerota capsule, Gerota fascia.

**re·nal gan·glia** small scattered sympathetic ganglia along the renal plexus.

**re·nal gly·cos·ur·ia** the recurring or persistent excretion of glucose in the urine, in association with blood glucose levels that are in the normal range; results from the failure of proximal renal tubules to reabsorb glucose at a normal rate from the glomerular filtrate (low renal threshold); defect in the glucose carrier in the nephron.

**re·nal he·ma·tu·ria** hematuria resulting from extravasation of blood into the glomerular spaces, tubules, or pelves of the kidneys.

**re·nal hy·per·ten·sion** hypertension secondary to renal disease.

**re·nal hy·po·pla·sia** an abnormally small kidney that is morphologically normal but has either a reduced number of nephrons or smaller nephrons.

**re·nal lab·y·rinth** SYN convoluted part of kidney lobule.

**re·nal me·dul·la** the inner, darker portion of the kidney parenchyma consisting of the renal pyramids.

**re·nal os·te·o·dys·tro·phy** generalized bone changes resembling osteomalacia and rickets or osteitis fibrosa, occurring in chronic renal failure.

**re·nal pa·pil·la** the apex of a renal pyramid that projects into a minor calyx; some 10–25 openings of papillary ducts occur on its tip, forming the area cribrosa.

**re·nal pel·vis** a flattened funnel-shaped expansion of the upper end of the ureter receiving the calices, the apex being continuous with the ureter.

**re·nal pyr·a·mid** one of a number of pyramidal masses seen on longitudinal section of the kidney; collectively, they constitute the renal medulla, and contain part of the secreting tubules and the collecting tubules. SYN malpighian pyramid, medullary pyramid, pyramis renalis.

**re·nal rick·ets** a form of rickets occurring in children in association with and apparently caused by renal disease with hyperphosphatemia. SYN pseudorickets.

**re·nal si·nus** the cavity of the kidney, containing the calices and pelvis of the ureter and the segmental vessels embedded within a fatty matrix. The renal sinuses cause the kidneys to appear hollow or C-shaped on cross section or medical imaging.

**re·nal tu·bu·lar ac·i·do·sis** a clinical syndrome characterized by decreased ability to acidify urine, and by low plasma bicarbonate and high plasma chloride concentrations, often with hypokalemia.

**re·nal tu·bules** SEE convoluted tubule.

**re·nal veins** large veins formed at the renal hilus by the merger of the segmental veins anterior to the corresponding arteries; they open at right angles into the inferior vena cava at the level of the second lumbar vertebra. The left renal vein receives the left suprarenal vein and the left gonadal vein, and passes through the angle between the abdominal aorta and superior mesenteric artery where it may be compressed.

**ren·i·form** (ren′i-fōrm) SYN nephroid.

**re·nin** (rē′nin) an enzyme that converts angiotensinogen to angiotensin I. SYN angiotensinogenase.

**ren·in-an·gi·o·ten·sin-al·dos·ter·one sys·tem** the hormones, renin, angiotensin, and aldosterone work together to regulate blood pressure. A sustained fall in blood pressure causes the kidney to release renin. This is converted to angiotensin in the circulation. Angiotensin then raises blood pressure directly by arteriolar constriction and stimulates the adrenal glands to produce aldosterone which promotes sodium and water retention by kidney, such that blood volume and blood pressure increase.

**ren·i·por·tal** (ren′i-pōr′tăl) **1.** relating to the hilum of the kidney. **2.** relating to the portal, or venous capillary circulation in the kidney. [reni- + L. *porta,* gate]

**ren·nin** (ren′in) SYN chymosin.

**ren·nin·o·gen, ren·no·gen** (rĕ-nin′ō-jen, ren′ō-jen) SYN prochymosin. [rennin + G. *-gen,* producing]

**△re·no-, re·ni-** the kidney. SEE ALSO nephro-. [L. *ren*]

**re·no·gen·ic** (rē-nō-jen′ik) originating in or from the kidney.

**re·no·gram** (rē′nō-gram) the assessment of renal

function by external radiation detectors after the administration of a radiopharmaceutical that is filtered and excreted by the kidney. [reno- + G. *gramma*, something written]

**re·nog·ra·phy** (rē-nog'ră-fē) radiography of the kidney.

**re·no·meg·a·ly** (rē'nō-meg'ă-lē) enlargement of the kidney.

**re·no·pri·val** (rē-nō-prī'văl) relating to, characterized by, or resulting from total loss of kidney function or from removal of all functioning renal tissue. [reno- + L. *privus,* deprived of]

**re·no·tro·phic** (rē-nō-trof'ik) relating to any agent influencing the growth or nutrition of the kidney or to the action of such an agent. SYN nephrotrophic, nephrotropic. [reno- + G. *trophē,* nourishment]

**re·no·vas·cu·lar** (rē-nō-vas'ku-ler) pertaining to the blood vessels of the kidney, denoting especially disease of these vessels.

**re·no·vas·cu·lar hy·per·ten·sion** hypertension produced by renal arterial obstruction.

**Ren·pen·ning syn·drome** (ren-pen-ing) x-linked mental retardation with short stature and microcephaly not associated with the fragile X chromosome; occurs more frequently in males, although some females may also be affected.

**Re·o·vir·i·dae** (rē-ō-vir'i-dē) a family of double-stranded RNA viruses, comprising six genera: *Reovirus, Orbivirus, Rotavirus,* cytoplasmic polyhidrosis virus group (*Cypovirus*), and two plant reovirus groups (*Phytoreovirus, Fijivirus*). [Respiratory *Enteric Orphan* + viridae]

**Re·o·vi·rus** (rē'ō-vī'rŭs) a genus of viruses recovered from children with mild fever and sometimes diarrhea, and from children with no apparent infection; a causative relationship to illness has not been proven.

**re·pair** (rē-pār') restoration of diseased or damaged tissues naturally by healing processes or artificially, as by surgical means. [M.E.,fr. O.Fr.,fr. L. *re-paro,* fr. *re-,* back, again, + *paro,* prepare, put in order]

**re·par·a·tive den·tin** SYN tertiary dentin.

**re·par·a·tive gran·u·lo·ma** complication of stapedectomy in which a granuloma forms in the oval window around the prosthesis; it results in a sensory hearing loss.

**re·pel·lent** (rē-pel'ent) **1.** capable of driving off or repelling; repulsive. **2.** an agent that drives away or prevents annoyance or irritation by insect pests. **3.** an astringent or other agent that reduces swelling. [L. *re-pello,* to drive back]

**rep·e·ti·tion-com·pul·sion** (rep-e-tish'ŭn-kŏm-pŭl'shŭn) PSYCHOANALYSIS the tendency to repeat earlier experiences or actions, in an unconscious effort to achieve belated mastery over them; a morbid need to repeat a particular behavior such as handwashing or repeated checking to see if the door is locked.

**re·pe·ti·tion max·i·mum** maximum load a muscle can lift for a predetermined number of repetitions to the point of fatigue.

**rep·e·ti·tion time (TR)** MAGNETIC RESONANCE IMAGING the time between repetitions of the pulse sequence.

**re·pe·ti·tive strain dis·or·ders** SYN cumulative trauma disorders.

**re·place·ment** (rē-plās'ment) **1.** restoration. **2.** substitution.

**re·place·ment ther·a·py** therapy designed to compensate for a lack or deficiency arising from inadequate nutrition, from certain dysfunctions (e.g., glandular hyposecretion), or from losses (e.g., hemorrhage); replacement may be physiological or may entail administration of a substitute (e.g., a synthetic estrogen in place of estradiol).

**re·plant** (rē'plant) **1.** to perform replantation. **2.** a part or organ so replaced or about to be so replaced.

**re·plan·ta·tion** (rē-plan-tā'shŭn) replacement of an organ or part back in its original site and reestablishing its circulation. SYN reimplantation. [L. *re-,* again, + *planto,* pp. *-atus,* to plant, fr. *planta,* a sprout, slip]

**re·ple·tion** (rē-plē'shŭn) **1.** SYN hypervolemia. **2.** SYN plethora (2). [L. *repletio,* fr. *re-pleo,* pp. *-pletus,* to fill up]

**rep·li·case** (rep'li-kās) descriptive term for RNA-directed RNA polymerase (EC 2.7.7.48) associated with replication of RNA viruses.

**rep·li·cate** (rep'li-kāt) **1.** one of several identical processes or observations. **2.** to repeat; to produce an exact copy.

**rep·li·ca·tion** (rep-li-kā'shŭn) **1.** the execution of an experiment or study more than once so as to confirm the original findings, increase precision, and obtain a closer estimate of sampling error. **2.** autoreproduction, as in mitosis or cellular biology. SEE autoreproduction. **3.** dNA-directed DNA synthesis. [L. *replicatio,* a reply, fr. *replico,* pp. *-atus,* to fold back]

**rep·li·ca·tive form 1.** an intermediate stage in the replication of either DNA or RNA viral genomes that is usually double stranded; **2.** the altered, double-stranded form to which single-stranded coliphage DNA is converted after infection of a susceptible bacterium, formation of the complementary ("minus") strand being mediated by enzymes that were present in the bacterium before entrance of the viral ("plus") strand.

**rep·li·ca·tor** (rep'li-kā-ter) the specific site of a bacterial genome (chromosome) at which replication begins.

**rep·li·con** (rep'li-kon) **1.** a segment of a chromosome (or of the DNA of a chromosome or similar entity) that can replicate, with its own initiation and termination codons, independently of the chromosome in which it may be located. **2.** the replication unit; several are found per DNA in eukaryotic systems. [*replic*ation + -on]

**re·po·lar·i·za·tion** (rē'pō-lăr-i-zā'shŭn) the process whereby the membrane, cell, or fiber, after depolarization, is polarized again, with positive charges on the outer and negative charges on the inner surface.

**re·port** (rē-port') a formal account, oral or written, of conditions, events, or actions. [O.Fr. *re-porter,* fr. L. *re-portare,* to carry back]

**re·port·a·ble dis·ease** SYN notifiable disease.

**re·por·ting bi·as** selective revealing or suppression of information about past medical history, e.g., details of exposure to sexually transmitted diseases.

**re·po·si·tio** SYN reposition.

**re·po·si·tion** movement returning palm and fingers from opposed position; opposite of opposition. SYN repositio.

**re·po·si·tion·ing** (rē'pō-zish'ŭn-ing) SYN reduction (1).

**re•pos•i•tor** (rē-poz′i-ter, rē-poz′i-tōr) an instrument used to reposition a displaced organ.

**re•pressed** (rē-prest′) subjected to repression.

**re•press•i•ble en•zyme** an enzyme that is produced continuously unless production is repressed by excess of an inhibitor (corepressor). SEE ALSO inactive repressor.

**re•pres•sion** (rē-presh′ŭn) **1.** PSYCHOTHERAPY the active process or defense mechanism of keeping out and ejecting, banishing from consciousness, ideas or impulses that are unacceptable to it. **2.** decreased expression of some gene product. [L. *re-primo,* pp. *-pressus,* to press back, repress]

**re•pres•sor** (rē-pres′er) the product of a regulator or repressor gene.

**re•pres•sor gene** a gene that prevents a nonallele from being transcribed.

**re•pro•duc•i•bil•i•ty** (rē-prō-doos′i-bil′i-tē) **1.** ability to cause to exist again or to present again. **2.** ability to duplicate measurements over long periods of time by different laboratories.

**re•pro•duc•tion** (rē-prō-dŭk′shŭn) **1.** the recall and presentation in the mind of the elements of a former impression. **2.** the total process by which organisms produce offspring. SYN generation (1), procreation. [L. *re-,* again, + *pro-duco,* pp. *-ductus,* to lead forth, produce]

**re•pro•duc•tive** (rē′prō-dŭk′tiv) relating to reproduction.

**re•pro•duc•tive cy•cle** the cycle which begins with conception and extends through gestation and parturition.

**rep•ti•lase** (rep′til-as) an enzyme found in the venom of *Bothrops atrox* that clots fibrinogen by splitting off its fibrinopeptide. [reptile + -ase]

**re•pul•sion** (rē-pŭl′shŭn) **1.** the act of repelling or driving apart, in contrast to attraction. **2.** strong dislike; aversion; repugnance. **3.** coupling phase of genes at linked loci that are borne on opposite chromosomes. [L. *re-pello,* pp. *-pulsus,* to drive back]

**research** (rē-serch′, rē′serch) **1.** the organized quest for new knowledge and better understanding, e.g., of the natural world, determinants of health and disease. Several types of research are recognized: observational (empiric); analytic; experimental; theoretical; applied. **2.** to conduct such scientific inquiry. [O.Fr. *re-cerche,* fr. *cerchier,* to search, fr. L. *circare,* to go around, fr. *circus,* circle]

**re•sect** (rē-sekt′) **1.** to cut off, especially to cut off the articular ends of one or both bones forming a joint. **2.** to excise a segment of a part. [L. *re-seco,* pp. *sectus,* to cut off]

**re•sect•a•ble** (rē-sek′tă-bl) amenable to resection.

**re•sec•tion** (rē-sek′shŭn) **1.** a procedure performed for the specific purpose of removal, as in removal of articular ends of one or both bones forming a joint. **2.** to remove a part. **3.** SYN excision (1).

**re•sec•to•scope** (rē-sek′tō-skōp) a special endoscopic instrument for the transurethral electrosurgical removal of lesions involving the bladder, prostate gland, or urethra.

**re•sec•to•scope e•lec•trode** a wire loop electrode that allows removal of tissue as well as cautery of the raw surface; used in endometrial ablation.

**re•serve** (rē-zerv′) something available but held back for later use. [L. *re-servo,* to keep back, reserve]

**re•serve air** SYN expiratory reserve volume.

**re•serve force** the energy residing in the organism or any of its parts above that required for its normal functioning.

**res•er•voir** (rez′ĕv-wor) SYN receptaculum. [Fr.]

**res•er•voir bag** SYN breathing bag.

**res•er•voir host** the host of an infection in which the infectious agent multiplies and/or develops, and upon which the agent is dependent for survival in nature.

**res•er•voir of in•fec•tion** living or nonliving material in or on which an infectious agent multiplies and/or develops and is dependent for its survival in nature.

**res•er•voir ox•y•gen-con•ser•ving de•vice** a device that stores oxygen in valveless expandable chambers under the nostrils or via large-bore tubing in a single valveless chamber worn on the chest; during inhalation through the nostrils, the oxygen is evacuated from the reservoir; conservation of oxygen is achieved because the constant flow of oxygen from the source can be reduced.

**res•er•voir of sper•ma•to•zoa** the site where spermatozoa are stored; the distal portion of the tail of the epididymis and the beginning of the ductus deferens.

**res•i•dent** (rez′i-dent) **1.** a house officer attached to a hospital for clinical training. **2.** patient residing in a nursing facility. [L. *resideo,* to reside]

**re•sid•ua** (rē-zid′yu-ă) plural of residuum.

**re•sid•u•al** (rē-zid′yu-ăl) relating to or of the nature of a residue.

**re•sid•u•al ab•scess** an abscess recurring at the site of a former abscess resulting from persistence of microbes and pus.

**re•sid•u•al air** SYN residual volume.

**re•sid•u•al ca•pac•i•ty** SYN residual volume.

**re•sid•u•al schiz•o•phre•nia** blunted or inappropriate affect, social withdrawal, eccentric behavior, or loose associations, but without prominent psychotic symptoms, as the remains of former psychotic symptoms of schizophrenia.

**re•sid•u•al u•rine** urine remaining in the bladder at the end of micturition in cases of prostatic obstruction, bladder atony, etc.

**re•sid•u•al vol•ume (RV)** the volume of air remaining in the lungs after a maximal expiratory effort. SYN residual air, residual capacity.

**res•i•due** (rez′i-doo) that which remains after removal of one or more substances. SYN residuum. [L. *residuum*]

**re•sid•u•um,** pl. **re•sid•ua** (rē-zid′yu-ŭm, rē-zid′yu-ă) SYN residue. [L. ntr. of *residuus,* left behind, remaining, fr. *re- sideo,* to sit back, remain behind]

**res•in** (rez′in) **1.** an amorphous brittle substance consisting of the hardened secretion of a number of plants, probably derived from a volatile oil and similar to a stearoptene. **2.** SYN rosin. **3.** a precipitate formed by the addition of water to certain tinctures. **4.** a broad term used to indicate organic substances insoluble in water. [L. *resina*]

**re•sin ce•ment** a monomer or monomer/polymer system used as a dental luting agent; used in cementation of restorations or orthodontic brackets to the teeth.

**res•in•ous** (rez′i-nŭs) relating to or derived from a resin.

**re•sis•tance** (rē-zis′tans) **1.** a passive force exerted in opposition to another active force. **2.** the opposition in a conductor to the passage of a current of electricity, whereby there is a loss of energy and a production of heat; specifically, the potential difference in volts across the conductor per ampere of current flow; unit: ohm. Cf. impedance (1). **3.** the opposition to flow of a fluid through one or more passageways; units are usually those of pressure difference per unit flow. Cf. impedance (2). **4.** PSYCHOANALYSIS an individual's unconscious defense against bringing repressed thoughts to consciousness. **5.** the ability of red blood cells to resist hemolysis and to preserve their shape under varying degrees of osmotic pressure in the blood plasma. **6.** the natural or acquired ability of an organism to maintain its immunity to or to resist the effects of an antagonistic agent, e.g., pathogenic microorganism, toxin, drug. [L. *re-sisto,* to stand back, withstand]

**re•sis•tance plas•mids** plasmids carrying genes responsible for antibiotic (or antibacterial drug) resistance among bacteria (notably Enterobacteriaceae); they may be conjugative or nonconjugative plasmids, the former possessing transfer genes (resistance transfer factor) lacking in the latter.

**re•sis•tance ther•mom•e•ter** a device measuring temperature by the change of the electrical resistance of a metal wire.

**re•sis•tance-trans•fer fac•tor** the transfer gene of the resistance plasmid.

**res•o•lu•tion** (rez-ō-loo'shŭn) **1.** the arrest of an inflammatory process without suppuration; the absorption or breaking down and removal of the products of inflammation or of a new growth. **2.** the optical ability to distinguish detail such as the separation of closely adjacent objects. SYN resolving power (3). [L. *resolutio,* a slackening, fr. *re-solvo,* pp. *-solutus,* to loosen, relax]

**re•solve** (rē-zolv') to return or cause to return to the normal, particularly without suppuration, said of a phlegmon or other form of inflammation. [L. *resolvo,* to loosen]

**re•solv•ing pow•er 1.** definition of a lens; in a microscope objective lens it is calculated by dividing the wavelength of the light used by twice the numerical aperture of the objective. **2.** analogies to other modalities, e.g., two-point discrimination in neurological examination. **3.** SYN resolution (2).

**res•o•nance** (rez'ō-nans) **1.** sympathetic or forced vibration of air in the cavities above, below, in front of, or behind a source of sound; in speech, modification of the quality (e.g., tone) of a sound by the passage of air through the chambers of the nose, pharynx, and head, without increasing the intensity of the sound. **2.** the sound obtained on percussing a part that can vibrate freely. **3.** the intensification and hollow character of the voice sound obtained on auscultating over a cavity. **4.** CHEMISTRY the manner in which electrons or electric charges are distributed among the atoms in compounds that are planar and symmetrical, particularly those with conjugated (alternating) double bonds; the existence of resonance in the latter case lowers the energy content and increases the stability of a compound. **5.** the natural or inherent frequency of any oscillating system. **6.** SYN resonant frequency. [L. *resonantia,* echo, fr. *re-sono,* to resound, to echo]

**res•o•nant fre•quen•cy** the frequency at which individual magnetic nuclei absorb or emit radio-

frequency energy in magnetic resonance studies. SYN resonance (6).

**re•sorb** (rē-sōrb') to reabsorb; to absorb what has been excreted, as an exudate or pus. [L. *re-sorbeo,* to suck back]

**re•sorp•tion** (rē-sōrp'shŭn) **1.** the act of resorbing. **2.** a loss of substance by lysis, or by physiologic or pathologic means.

**re•sorp•tion la•cu•nae** SYN Howship lacunae.

**Re•source U•ti•li•za•tion Group (RUG)** one of 44 patient categories, each with a corresponding per diem reimbursement rate as mandated by Medicare.

**res•pi•ra•ble** (re-spīr'ă-bl, res'pĭ-ră-bl) capable of being breathed.

■**res•pi•ra•tion** (res-pi-ra'shŭn) **1.** a fundamental process of life, characteristic of both plants and animals, in which oxygen is used to oxidize organic fuel molecules, providing a source of energy as well as carbon dioxide and water. In green plants, photosynthesis is not considered respiration **2.** SYN ventilation (2). See page 853. [L. *respiratio,* fr. *re-spiro,* pp. *-atus,* to exhale, breathe]

**res•pi•ra•tion rate** frequency of breathing, recorded as the number of breaths per minute.

**res•pi•ra•tor** (res'pi-rā-ter) **1.** an appliance fitting over the mouth and nose, used for the purpose of excluding dust, smoke, or other irritants, or of otherwise altering the air before it enters the respiratory passages. SYN inhaler (1). **2.** an apparatus for administering artificial respiration, especially for a prolonged period, in cases of paralysis or inadequate spontaneous ventilation.

**res•pi•ra•to•ry** (res'pi-ră-tōr-ē, rĕ-spīr'ă-tōr-ē) relating to respiration.

**res•pi•ra•to•ry ac•i•do•sis** acidosis caused by retention of carbon dioxide; due to inadequate pulmonary ventilation or hypoventilation, with decrease in blood pH unless compensated by renal retention of bicarbonate. SYN hypercapnic acidosis.

**res•pi•ra•to•ry al•ka•lo•sis** alkalosis resulting from abnormal loss of $CO_2$ produced by hyperventilation, either active or passive, with concomitant reduction in arterial bicarbonate concentration. SEE ALSO compensated alkalosis.

**res•pi•ra•to•ry bron•chi•oles** the smallest bronchioles (0.5 mm in diameter), which connect the terminal bronchioles to alveolar ducts; alveoli arise from part of the wall.

**res•pi•ra•to•ry ca•pac•i•ty** SYN vital capacity.

**res•pi•ra•to•ry care** an adjunctive form of health care intended to maintain or restore optimal respiratory function through the use of appropriate devices and techniques; respiratory care services, provided by qualified professionals under medical direction in a variety of settings, include diagnostic testing and monitoring, patient education, therapy, and rehabilitation.

**res•pi•ra•to•ry care prac•ti•tion•er (RCP)** an allied health professional who works under the direction of a physician, educating patients, treating, assessing patient response to therapy and the need for continued therapy, managing and monitoring patients with deficiencies and abnormalities of cardiopulmonary function; term is applied by licensing authorities to individuals licensed to practice.

**res•pi•ra•to•ry cen•ter** the region in the medulla oblongata concerned with integrating afferent in-

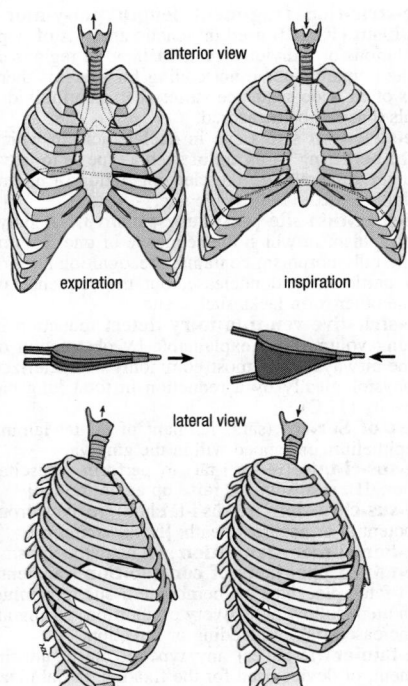

anterior view

expiration      inspiration

lateral view

expiration      inspiration

**respiration at expiration:** volume is low so pressure is high, causing air to leave lungs to equalize pressure; **respiration at inspiration:** volume is high so pressure is low, causing air to enter lungs to equalize pressure

formation to determine the signals to the respiratory muscles; the inspiratory and expiratory centers considered together.

**res·pi·ra·to·ry com·pli·ance** the change in lung volume per unit change in transrespiratory pressure when the respiratory muscles are relaxed; may be static or dynamic. SYN respiratory system compliance.

**res·pi·ra·to·ry en·ter·ic or·phan vi·rus** a nonenveloped icosahedral virus whose genome consists of double stranded RNA, belonging to the family Reoviridae, frequently found in both the respiratory and enteric tract.

**res·pi·ra·to·ry en·zyme** a tissue enzyme that is part of an oxidation-reduction system accomplishing the conversion of substrates to $CO_2$ and $H_2O$ and the transfer of the electrons removed to $O_2$.

**res·pi·ra·to·ry ex·change ra·tio** the ratio of the net output of carbon dioxide to the simultaneous net uptake of oxygen at a given site, both expressed as moles or STPD volumes per unit time.

**res·pi·ra·to·ry fail·ure** loss of pulmonary function either acute or chronic that results in hypox-

emia or hypercarbia; final common pathway for myriad respiratory disorders.

**res·pi·ra·to·ry fre·quen·cy (f)** the number of breaths per minute.

**res·pi·ra·to·ry ga·ting** any technique that derives a signal from breathing to trigger an electronic circuit, such as for data collection during expiration. SEE ALSO navigator echo.

**res·pi·ra·to·ry min·ute vol·ume** the minute volume of breathing; the product of tidal volume times the respiratory frequency. SEE pulmonary ventilation.

**res·pi·ra·to·ry pause** cessation of air flow for less than 10 seconds. SEE sleep apnea.

**res·pi·ra·to·ry pig·ments** the oxygen-carrying (colored) substances in blood and tissues (hemoglobin, myoglobin, hemocyanin, etc.).

**res·pi·ra·to·ry quo·tient** the ratio of the carbon dioxide produced during tissue metabolism to the oxygen consumed; reflects net substrate oxidation; can be determined by indirect calorimetry.

**res·pi·ra·to·ry rate** frequency of breathing, recorded as the number of breaths per minute.

**res·pi·ra·to·ry scle·ro·ma** rhinoscleroma in which the lesion involves the mucous membrane of the greater part or all of the upper respiratory tract.

**res·pi·ra·to·ry sounds** SYN breath sounds.

**res·pi·ra·to·ry sys·tem com·pli·ance** SYN respiratory compliance.

**res·pi·ra·to·ry ther·a·pist** an allied health professional trained to provide respiratory therapy. SEE respiratory care practitioner.

**res·pi·ra·to·ry ther·a·py** SEE respiratory care.

**res·pi·ra·to·ry tract** the air passages from the nose to the pulmonary alveoli, through the pharynx, larynx, trachea, and bronchi.

**res·pi·rom·e·ter** (res-pĭ-rom'ĕ-ter) **1.** an instrument for measuring the extent of the respiratory movements. **2.** an instrument for measuring oxygen consumption or carbon dioxide production, usually of an isolated tissue. [L. *respiro*, to breathe, + G. *metron*, measure]

**re·sponse** (rē-spons') **1.** the reaction of a muscle, nerve, gland, or other excitable tissue to a stimulus. **2.** any act or behavior, or its constituents, that a living organism is capable of emitting. Reflexes are usually excluded because they are typically elicited by a specifiable (unconditioned or natural) stimulus rather than emitted under circumstances in which the stimulus was not specifiable. [L. *responsus*, an answer]

**res·ponse bi·as** systematic error due to differences in characteristics between those who choose or volunteer to take part in a study, and those who do not.

**rest 1.** quiet; repose. [A.S. *raest*] **2.** to repose; to cease from work. [A.S. *raestan*] **3.** a group of cells or a portion of fetal tissue that has become displaced and lies embedded in tissue of another character. [L. *restare*, to remain] **4.** DENTISTRY an extension from a prosthesis that affords vertical support for a restoration.

**re·ste·no·sis** (rē'sten-ō-sis) recurrence of stenosis after corrective surgery on the heart valve; narrowing of a structure (usually a coronary artery) following the removal or reduction of a previous narrowing. [re-, + G. *stenōsis*, a narrowing]

**res·ti·form** (res'ti-fōrm) ropelike; rope-shaped; referring to the restiform body, the larger (lateral) part of the inferior cerebellar peduncle; contains fibers from the spinal cord (spinocerebellar) and medulla (cuneo-, olivo-, reticulocerebellar, etc.) to cerebellum. [L. *restis,* rope, + *forma,* form]

**res•ti•form bo•dy** a lateral (larger) subdivision of the inferior cerebellar peduncle composed of a variety of fibers including, but not limited to, olivo-, reticulo-, cuneo-, trigemino-, and dorsal spinocerebellar.

**res•ting e•ner•gy ex•pen•di•ture** total daily caloric expenditure, consisting of basal metabolic rate, diet-induced thermogenesis, and energy expenditure for physical activity; in the clinical setting, REE can be estimated by calculation or measured by indirect calorimetry.

**rest•ing tid•al vol•ume** the tidal volume under normal conditions, i.e., in the absence of exercise or other conditions that stimulate breathing.

**rest•ing trem•or** a coarse, rhythmic tremor, 3–5 Hz frequency, usually confined to hands and forearms, that appears when the limbs are relaxed, and disappears with active limb movements; characteristic of Parkinson disease.

**rest•i•tope** (res′ti-tōp) the part of the T cell receptor that associates with the class II major histocompatibility molecule. [*rest*riction + -*tope*]

**res•ti•tu•tion** (res-ti-too′shŭn) OBSTETRICS the return of the rotated head of the fetus to its natural relation with the shoulders after its emergence from the vulva. [L. *restitutio,* act of restoring]

**Res•ton vi•rus** (res′tŏn) a variant of Ebola virus. SYN Ebola virus Reston.

**res•to•ra•tion** (res-tō-rā′shŭn) DENTISTRY **1.** a prosthetic restoration or appliance; a broad term applied to any inlay, crown, bridge, partial denture, or complete denture that restores or replaces lost tooth structure, teeth, or oral tissues. **2.** a plug or stopping; any substance such as gold, amalgam, etc., used for restoring the portion missing from a tooth as a result of removing decay in the tooth. [L. *restauro,* pp. -*atus,* to restore, to repair]

**re•stor•a•tive** (re-stōr′ă-tiv) **1.** renewing health and strength. **2.** an agent that promotes a renewal of health or strength. [L. *restauro,* to restore]

**re•stor•a•tive den•tis•try** individual restoration of teeth by means of amalgam, synthetic porcelainlike materials, resins, or inlays. SEE ALSO implant, oral and maxillofacial surgery.

**rest po•si•tion** the position that the mandible assumes when the muscles of mastication are relaxed.

**re•straint** (rē-strānt′) in hospital psychiatry, intervention to prevent an excited or violent patient from doing harm to himself or others; may involve the use of a camisole (straightjacket). [O. Fr. *restrainte*]

**re•stric•tion** (rē-strik′shŭn) **1.** the process with which foreign DNA that has been introduced into a prokaryotic cell becomes ineffective. **2.** a limitation.

**re•stric•tion en•do•nu•cle•ase** one of many endonucleases isolated from bacteria that hydrolyze (cut) double-stranded DNA chains at specific sequences, thus inactivating a foreign (viral or other) DNA and restricting its activity; standard laboratory devices for making specific cuts in DNA as a first step in deducing sequences. SYN restriction enzyme.

**re•stric•tion en•zyme** SYN restriction endonuclease.

**re•stric•tion frag•ment length pol•y•mor•phism (RFLP)** used in genetic analysis of populations or individual relationships. In regions of the human genome not coding for proteins there is often wide sequence variety between individuals that can be measured.

**re•stric•tion site** a site in nucleic acid in which the bordering bases are of such a type as to leave them vulnerable to the cleaving action of an endonuclease. SYN cleavage site.

**re•stric•tion-site pol•y•mor•phism** DNA polymorphism in which the sequence of one form of the polymorphism contains a recognition site for a particular endonuclease, but the sequence of the other form lacks such a site.

**re•stric•tive ven•ti•la•to•ry defect** reduction in lung volumes not explainable by obstruction of the airways. It is most commonly characterized physiologically by a reduction in total lung capacity (TLC).

**rest of Ser•res** (sārs) remnant of dental lamina epithelium entrapped within the gingiva.

**re•sus•ci•tate** (rē-sŭs′i-tāt) to perform resuscitation. [L. *re-suscito,* to raise up again, revive]

**re•sus•ci•ta•tion** (rē-sŭs′i-tā′shŭn) revival from potential or apparent death. [L. *resuscitatio*]

**re•tained men•stru•a•tion** SYN hematocolpos.

**re•tained pro•ducts of con•cep•tion** fragments of fetal, placental, or membrane tissue remaining in utero following delivery or abortion, posing an increased risk of bleeding or infection.

**re•tain•er** (rē-tān′er) any type of clasp, attachment, or device used for the fixation or stabilization of a prosthesis; an appliance used to prevent the shifting of teeth following orthodontic treatment.

**re•tar•da•tion** (rē-tahr-dā′shŭn) slowness or limitation of development.

**re•tard•ed den•ti•tion** dentition in which calcification, elongation, and eruption occur later than normal as a result of some systemic metabolic dysfunction (e.g., hypothyroidism).

**retch** to make an involuntary effort to vomit. [A.S. *hraecan,* to hawk]

**retch•ing** gastric and esophageal movements of vomiting without expulsion of vomitus. SYN dry vomiting, vomiturition.

**re•te,** pl. **re•tia** (rē′tē, rē′shē-ă) [TA] **1.** SYN network (1). **2.** a structure composed of a fibrous network or mesh. [L. a net]

**re•te cu•ta•ne•um co•rii** the network of vessels parallel to the surface between the corium and the tela subcutanea.

**re•te mi•ra•bi•le** [TA] a vascular network interrupting the continuity of an artery or vein, such as occurs in the glomeruli of the kidney (arterial) or in the liver (venous).

**re•ten•tion** (rē-ten′shŭn) **1.** the keeping in the body of what normally belongs there, especially the retaining of food and drink in the stomach. **2.** the keeping in the body of what normally should be discharged, as urine or feces. **3.** retaining that which has been learned so that it can be utilized later as in recall, recognition, or, if retention is partial, relearning. SEE ALSO memory. **4.** resistance to dislodgement. **5.** DENTISTRY a passive period following treatment when a patient is wearing an appliance or appliances to maintain or stabilize the teeth in the new position into which they have been moved. [L. *retentio,* a holding back]

**re•ten•tion cyst** a cyst resulting from some obstruction to the excretory duct of a gland.

**re•ten•tion jaun•dice** jaundice due to insufficiency of liver function or to an excess of bile pigment production; the bilirubin is unconjugated because it has not passed through the liver cells; van den Bergh test is indirect.

**re•ten•tion su•ture** a heavy reinforcing suture placed deep within the muscles and fasciae of the abdominal wall to relieve tension on the primary suture line and thus obviate postoperative wound disruption. SYN tension suture.

**re•ten•tion vom•it•ing** vomiting due to mechanical obstruction, usually hours after ingestion of a meal.

**re•te o•va•rii** a transient network of cells in the developing ovary; homologous to the rete testis.

**re•te ridge** downward thickening of the epidermis between the dermal papillae; peg is a misnomer because the dermal papillae are cylindric but the epidermal thickening between papillae is not.

**re•te sub•pa•pil•la•re** the network of vessels between the papillary and reticular strata of the corium.

**re•te tes•tis** [TA] the network of canals at the termination of the straight tubules in the mediastinum testis.

**re•tia** (rē′shē-ă) plural of rete. [L.]

**re•ti•al** (rē′shē-ăl) relating to a rete.

**re•tic•u•la** (re-tik′yu-lă) plural of reticulum. [L.]

**re•tic•u•lar, re•tic•u•lated** (re-tik′yu-lăr, re-tik′yu-lāt-ed) relating to a reticulum.

**re•tic•u•lar ac•ti•vat•ing sys•tem (RAS)** a physiological term denoting that part of the brainstem reticular formation that plays a central role in bodily and behavioral alertness; it extends as a diffusely organized neural apparatus through the central region of the brainstem into the subthalamus and the intralaminar nuclei of the thalamus; by its ascending connections it affects the function of the cerebral cortex in the sense of behavioral responsiveness; its descending (reticulospinal) connections transmit activating influence upon bodily posture and reflex mechanisms (e.g., muscle tonus), in part by way of the gamma motor neurons. SEE ALSO reticular formation.

**re•tic•u•lar de•gen•er•a•tion** severe epidermal edema resulting in multilocular bullae.

**re•tic•u•lar dys•tro•phy of cor•nea** bilateral, progressive, superficial degeneration of the corneal epithelium and adjacent Bowman membrane.

**re•tic•u•lar fi•bers** the collagen (type III) fibers forming the distinctive loose connective tissue stroma of embryonic tissues, mesenchyme, red pulp of the spleen, cortex and medulla of lymph nodes, and the hematopoietic compartments of bone marrow and accounting for a substantial portion of the collagen fibers of the skin, blood vessels, synovial membrane, uterine tissue, and granulation tissue; characterized by its organization as a reticular meshwork of fine filaments and an affinity for silver and for periodic acid-Schiff stains.

**re•tic•u•lar for•ma•tion** a massive but vaguely delimited neural apparatus composed of gray and white matter extending throughout the central core of the brainstem into the diencephalon; the term refers to the large neuronal population of the brainstem that does not compose motoneuronal cell groups or cell groups forming part of specific sensory conduction systems; its neurons generally have long dendrites and heterogeneous afferent connections; the reticular formation has complex, largely polysynaptic ascending and descending connections that play a role in the central control of autonomic (respiration, blood pressure, thermoregulation, etc.) and endocrine functions, as well as in bodily posture, skeletal muscle reflexes, and general behavioral states such as alertness and sleep. SYN formatio reticularis [TA], reticular substance (2).

**re•tic•u•lar mem•brane** the membrane formed by cuticular plates of the cells of the spiral organ (organ of Corti); it appears netlike when viewed from above. SYN membrana reticularis [TA].

**re•tic•u•lar sub•stance 1.** a filamentous plasmatic material, beaded with granules, demonstrable by means of vital staining in the immature red blood cells; **2.** SYN reticular formation.

**re•tic•u•lar tis•sue, ret•i•form tis•sue** a tissue in which the argyrophilic collagenous fibers form a network and that usually has a network of reticular cells associated with the fibers.

**re•tic•u•lated bone** SYN woven bone.

**re•tic•u•la•tion** (re-tik-yu-lā′shŭn) the presence or formation of a reticulum or network, such as that observed in red blood cells during active regeneration of blood. Also used to describe a chest radiographic pattern.

**re•tic•u•lin** (re-tik′yu-lin) the chemical substance of reticular fibers, regarded as type III collagen (with its associated proteoglygans and structural glycoproteins).

△**re•ti•cu•lo-, re•ti•cul-** reticulum; reticular. [L. *reticulum,* a small net, dim. of *rete,* a net]

**reticulocyte** (rĕ-ti′kyu-lō-sīt) a young red cell (erythrocyte) that contains no nucleus but has residual RNA. The RNA can be visualized as granules or filaments when the cell is stained supravitally with new methylene blue. Normally, new red cells are released from the bone marrow to the peripheral blood as reticulocytes. They mature, losing the filamentous RNA in about 2 days. Reticulocytes compose about 1% of circulating red cells. Increased concentrations are associated with hemolytic anemias and blood loss. Decreased concentrations are associated with ineffective erythropoiesis, aplastic anemia and hypocellularity of erythroid precursors in the bone marrow. SEE ALSO reticulocyte production index, erythroblast. [reticulo- + G. kytos, cell]

**re•ti•cu•lo•cyte pro•duc•tion in•dex (RPI)** a calculated value that serves as an indicator of the bone marrow response in anemia. It is calculated as patient's hematocrit ÷ 0.45 L/L × reticulocyte count (%) × 1 ÷ maturation time of shift reticulocytes.

**re•tic•u•lo•cy•to•pe•nia** (re-tik′yu-lō-sī-tō-pē′nē-ă) paucity of reticulocytes in the blood. SYN reticulopenia. [reticulocyte + G. *penia,* poverty]

**re•tic•u•lo•cy•to•sis** (re-tik′yu-lō-sī-tō′sis) an increase in the number of circulating reticulocytes above the normal, which is less than 1% of the total number of red blood cells; it occurs during active blood regeneration (stimulation of red bone marrow) and in certain anemias, especially congenital hemolytic anemia. [reticulocyte + G. *-osis,* condition]

**re•tic•u•lo•en•do•the•li•al** (re-tik′yu-lō-en-dō-thē′lē-ăl) denoting or referring to reticuloendothelium.

r
e

**re·tic·u·lo·en·do·the·li·um** (re-tik′yu-lō-en-dō-thē′lē-ŭm) the cells making up the reticuloendothelial system. [reticulo- + endothelium]

**re·tic·u·lo·his·ti·o·cy·to·ma** (re-tik′yu-lō-his′tē-ō-sī-tō′mă) a solitary skin nodule composed of glycolipid-containing multinucleated large histiocytes; multiple lesions sometimes occur in association with arthritis. [reticulo- + histiocytoma]

**re·tic·u·lo·pe·nia** (re-tik′yu-lō-pē′nē-ă) SYN reticulocytopenia.

**re·tic·u·lo·sis** (re-tik-yu-lō′sis) an increase in histiocytes, monocytes, or other reticuloendothelial elements. [reticulo- + G. -osis, condition]

**re·tic·u·lo·spi·nal tract** collective term denoting a variety of fiber tracts descending to the spinal cord from the reticular formation of the pons and medulla oblongata. Part of these fibers conduct impulses from the neural mechanisms regulating autonomic functions to the corresponding somatic and visceral motor neurons of the spinal cord; others form links in nonpyramidal motor mechanisms affecting muscle tonus, reflex activity, and somatic movement.

**re·tic·u·lum**, pl. **re·tic·u·la** (re-tik′yu-lŭm, re-tik′yu-lă) **1.** a fine network formed by cells, or formed of certain structures within cells or of connective tissue fibers between cells. **2.** SYN neuroglia. **3.** the second compartment of the stomach of a ruminant, a comparatively small chamber communicating with the rumen; sometimes called the honeycomb because of the characteristic structure of its wall. [L. dim of *rete,* a net]

**ret·i·form** (ret′i-fōrm) resembling a net or network. [L. *rete,* network]

🔲 **ret·i·na** (ret′i-nă) [TA] the light-sensitive membrane forming the innermost layer of the eyeball. Grossly, the retina consists of three parts: optic part of retina, ciliary part of retina, and iridial part of retina. The optic part, the physiologic portion that receives the visual light rays, is further divided into two parts, pigmented part (pigment epithelium) and nervous part, which are arranged in the following layers: 1) pigment epithelium; 2) layer of rods and cones; 3) external limiting lamina, actually a row of junctional complexes; 4) external nuclear lamina; 5) external plexiform lamina; 6) internal nuclear lamina; 7) internal plexiform lamina; 8) ganglionic cell lamina; 9) lamina of nerve fibers; 10) internal limiting lamina. Layers 2–10 comprise the nervous part. At the posterior pole of the visual axis is the macula, in the center of which is the fovea, the area of acute vision. Here layers 6, 7, 8, and 9 and blood vessels are absent, and only elongated cones are present. About 3 mm medial to the fovea is the optic disk, where axons of the ganglionic cells converge to form the optic nerve. The ciliary and iridial parts of the retina are forward prolongations of the pigmented layer and a layer of supporting columnar or epithelial cells over the ciliary body and the posterior surface of the iris, respectively. See this page and B15. [Mediev. L. prob. fr. L. *rete,* a net]

**ret·i·nac·u·la of ex·ten·sor mus·cles** SEE inferior extensor retinaculum, superior extensor retinaculum.

**ret·i·nac·u·la of per·o·ne·al mus·cles** SYN peroneal retinaculum.

**ret·i·nac·u·lum**, gen. **ret·i·nac·u·li**, pl. **ret·i·nac·u·la** (ret-i-nak′yu-lŭm, ret-i-nak′yu-lī, ret-i-

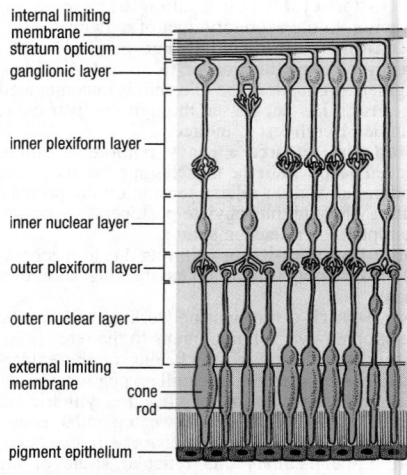

**layers of the retina** (innermost layer at top)

nak′yu-lă) [TA] a frenum, or a retaining band or ligament. [L. a band, a halter, fr. *retineo,* to hold back]

**ret·i·nac·u·lum cu·tis** [TA] one of the numerous small fibrous strands that extend through the superficial fascia attaching the deep surface of the dermis to the underlying deep fascia determining the mobility of the skin over the deep structures. SYN retinaculum cutis.

**ret·i·nac·u·lum of skin** SYN retinaculum cutis.

**ret·i·nac·u·lum ten·di·num** a ligamentous structure to restrain tendons, such as the flexor or extensor retinacula, or the annular parts of the digital fibrous sheaths.

**ret·i·nal** (ret′i-năl) **1.** relating to the retina. **2.** retinaldehyde; most commonly referring to the all-*trans* form.

**11-*cis*-ret·i·nal** the isomer of retinaldehyde that can combine with opsin to form rhodopsin; it is formed from 11-*trans*-retinal by retinal isomerase.

**ret·i·nal ad·ap·ta·tion** adjustment to degree of illumination.

**ret·i·nal·de·hyde** (ret-i-nal′dĕ-hīd) retinol oxidized to a terminal aldehyde; a carotene released (as all-*trans*-retinal(aldehyde)) in the bleaching of rhodopsin by light and the dissociation of opsin in the vision cycle. SYN retinene.

🔲 **ret·i·nal de·tach·ment, de·tach·ment of ret·i·na** loss of apposition between the sensory retina and the retinal pigment epithelium. See page B15.

**ret·i·nal isom·er·ase** an isomerase that catalyzes the *cis-trans*-interconversion of all-*trans*-retinal-(aldehyde) to 11-*cis*-retinal(aldehyde); a part of the vision cycle.

**ret·i·nene** (ret′i-nēn) SYN retinaldehyde.

**ret·i·ni·tis** (ret-i-nī′tis) inflammation of the retina. [retina + G. -itis, inflammation]

**ret·i·ni·tis pig·men·to·sa** a hereditary progressive abiotrophy of the neuroepithelium, with atrophy and pigmentary infiltration of the inner layers of the retina. SYN pigmentary retinopathy.

**ret·i·ni·tis pro·li·fe·rans** SYN proliferative retinopathy.

△**ret·i·no-, ret·in-** the retina. [Med. L. *retina*]

**ret·i·no·blas·to·ma** (ret'i-nō-blas-tō'mă) malignant ocular neoplasm of childhood, usually occurring before the third year of life, composed of primitive retinal small round cells with deeply staining nuclei and of elongate cells forming rosettes. In familial forms, the disease is commonly bilateral and multiple within an eye; in sporadic cases, rarely so. [retino- + G. *blastos*, germ, + *-oma*, tumor]

**ret·i·no·cho·roid** (ret'i-nō-kō'royd) SYN chorioretinal.

**ret·i·no·cho·roid·i·tis** (ret'i-nō-kō-roy-dī'tis) inflammation of the retina extending to the choroid. SYN chorioretinitis, choroidoretinitis. [retinochoroid + G. *-itis*, inflammation]

**ret·i·no·cho·roid·i·tis jux·ta·pa·pil·la·ris** retinochoroiditis close to the optic disk. SYN Jensen disease.

**ret·i·no·ic ac·id** (ret-i-nō'ik as'id) vitamin A$_1$ acid; retinaldehyde in which the terminal –CHO has been oxidized to a –COOH; used topically in the treatment of acne; plays an important role in growth and differentiation. SYN vitamin A$_1$ acid.

**ret·i·no·ic a·cid re·cep·tor** nuclear receptor for retinoic acid.

**ret·i·noids** (ret'i-noydz) a class of keratolytic drugs derived from retinoic acid and used for treatment of severe acne and psoriasis.

**ret·i·noid X re·cep·tor** receptor for retinoic acids; has less affinity for retinoic acid than the retinoic acid receptors; function is not yet well understood.

**ret·i·nol** (ret'i-nol) vitamin A$_1$ alcohol; an intermediate in the vision cycle, it also plays a role in growth and differentiation.

**ret·i·nol de·hy·dro·gen·ase** an oxidoreductase catalyzing interconversion of retinal and NADH to retinol and NAD$^+$.

**ret·i·no·pap·il·li·tis** (ret'i-nō-pap-i-lī'tis) inflammation of the retina extending to the optic disk.

**ret·i·nop·a·thy** (ret-i-nop'ă-thē) noninflammatory degenerative disease of the retina. [retino- + G. *pathos*, suffering]

**ret·i·nop·a·thy of pre·ma·tu·ri·ty** abnormal replacement of the sensory retina by fibrous tissue and blood vessels, occurring mainly in premature infants having a birth weight of less than 1500 g who are placed in a high-oxygen environment. SYN Terry syndrome.

**ret·i·no·pexy** (ret'i-nō-pek'sē) a procedure to repair a detached retina by holding it in place; e.g., by producing chorioretinal adhesions by freezing ("retinal cryopexy"). [retino- + G. *pēxis*, fixation]

**ret·i·nos·chi·sis** (ret-i-nos'ki-sis) degenerative splitting of the retina, with cyst formation between the two layers. [retino- + G. *schisis*, division]

**ret·i·no·scope** (ret'i-nō-skōp) an optical device used to illuminate a subject's retina during retinoscopy. [retino- + G. *skopeō*, to view]

**ret·i·nos·co·py** (ret'i-nos'kŏ-pē) a method of determining errors of refraction by illuminating the retina and observing the rays of light emerging from the eye. SYN shadow test, skiascopy. [retino- + G. *skopeō*, to view]

**re·trac·tile** (rē-trak'til) retractable; capable of being drawn back.

**re·trac·tion** (rē-trak'shŭn) **1.** a shrinking, drawing back, or pulling apart. **2.** posterior movement of teeth, usually with the aid of an orthodontic appliance. [L. *retractio*, a drawing back]

**re·trac·tion po·ckets** small areas of retraction of the tympanic membrane due to chronic negative pressure in the middle ear that can lead to formation of cholesteatoma.

**re·trac·tor** (rē-trac'tōr) **1.** an instrument for drawing aside the edges of a wound or for holding back structures adjacent to the operative field. **2.** a muscle that draws a part backward, e.g., the middle part of the trapezius muscle is a retractor of the scapula; the horizontal fibers of the temporalis muscle serve to retract the mandible.

**re·treat from re·al·i·ty** substitution of imaginary satisfactions or fantasy for relations with the real world.

**re·trench·ment** (rē-trench'ment) the cutting away of superfluous tissue. [F. *re-*, back, + *trancher*, to cut]

**re·triev·al** (rē-trē'văl) the third stage in the memory process, after encoding and storage, involving mental processes associated with bringing stored information back into consciousness. SEE ALSO memory.

△**re·tro-** prefix, to words formed from L. roots, denoting backward or behind. [L. back, backward]

**re·tro·au·ric·u·lar fold** skin crease made by the junction of the pinna and the postauricular skin.

**ret·ro·au·ric·u·lar lymph node** one of two or three nodes in the region of the mastoid process, which receive afferent lymphatic vessels from the scalp and auricle and send efferent vessels to the superior deep cervical nodes.

**ret·ro·bul·bar an·es·the·sia** injection of a local anesthetic behind the eye to produce sensory denervation of the eye.

**ret·ro·bul·bar neu·ri·tis** optic neuritis without swelling of the optic disk.

**re·tro·cal·ca·ne·al bur·sa** SYN bursa of tendo calcaneus.

**ret·ro·cal·ca·ne·o·bur·si·tis** (re'trō-kal-kā'nē-ō-ber-sī'tis) SYN achillobursitis. [retro- + L. *calcaneum* heel, + bursitis]

**ret·ro·ces·sion** (re-trō-sesh'ŭn) **1.** a going back; a relapse. **2.** cessation of the external symptoms of a disease followed by signs of involvement of some internal organ or part. **3.** denoting a position of the uterus or other organ farther back than is normal. [L. *retro-cedo*, pp. *-cessus*, to go back, retire]

**ret·ro·clu·sion** (re-trō-kloo'zhŭn) a form of acupressure for the arrest of bleeding; the needle is passed through the tissues above the cut end of the artery, is turned around, and then is passed backward beneath the vessel to come out near the point of entrance. [retro- + L. *claudo* (*cludo*) to close]

**ret·ro·co·chle·ar hea·ring loss** term for sensorineural hearing impairment; suggesting a lesion proximal to the cochlea.

**ret·ro·col·lic spasm** torticollis in which the spasm affects the posterior neck muscles. SYN retrocollis.

**ret·ro·col·lis** (re-trō-kol'is) SYN retrocollic spasm.

**ret·ro·cur·sive** (re'trō-ker'siv) running backward. [retro- + L. *cursus*, a running]

**ret·ro·cus·pid pa·pil·la** an exceedingly common, normal small mucosal nodule located on the mandibular gingiva lingual to the canine teeth, which regresses with age.

**ret·ro·de·vi·a·tion** (re′trō-dē-vē-ā′shŭn) a backward bending or inclining.

**ret·ro·dis·place·ment** (re′trō-dis-plās′ment) any backward displacement, such as retroversion or retroflexion of the uterus.

**ret·ro·flex·ion** (re-trō-flek′shŭn) backward bending, as of the uterus when the corpus is bent back, forming an angle with the cervix.

**ret·ro·gnath·ic** (re-trō-nath′ik) denoting a state in which the mandible is located posterior to its normal position in relation to the maxillae.

**ret·ro·gnath·ism** (re-trō-nath′izm) a condition of facial disharmony in which one or both jaws are posterior to normal in their craniofacial relationships; usually used in reference to the mandible. [retro- + G. *gnathos,* jaw]

**ret·ro·grade** (ret′rō-grād) **1.** moving backward. **2.** degenerating; reversing the normal order of growth and development. [L. *retrogradus,* fr. retro- + *gradior,* to go]

**ret·ro·grade am·ne·sia** amnesia in reference to events that occurred before the trauma or disease (e.g., cerebral concussion) that caused the condition.

**ret·ro·grade beat** a beat occurring as an electrical activation of a portion of a heart chamber cephalad to the chamber of origin, e.g., an atrial beat triggered by an impulse originating in the ventricle.

**ret·ro·grade block** impaired conduction backward from the ventricles or A-V node into the atria.

**ret·ro·grade cys·to·u·reth·ro·gram** a cystourethrogram performed by injection of contrast via urethral meatus or distal urethra.

**ret·ro·grade e·jac·u·la·tion** delivery of semen ejaculate into the bladder; seen in neurologic disease, diabetes, and occasionally after prostate surgery.

**ret·ro·grade em·bo·lism** embolism of a vein by an embolus carried in a direction opposite to that of the normal blood current, after being diverted into a smaller vein.

**ret·ro·grade her·nia** a double loop hernia the central loop of which lies in the abdominal cavity.

**ret·ro·grade men·stru·a·tion** a flow of menstrual blood back through the fallopian tubes; it sometimes carries with it endometrial cells.

**ret·ro·grade urog·ra·phy** radiography of the urinary tract following injection of contrast medium directly into the bladder, ureter, or renal pelvis. SYN cystoscopic urography.

**ret·ro·grade VA con·duc·tion** conduction backward from the ventricles or from the AV node into and through the atria.

**ret·ro·gres·sion** (re-trō-gresh′ŭn) SYN cataplasia. [L. *retrogressus,* fr. *retrogradior,* to go backwards]

**ret·ro·hy·oid bur·sa** a bursa between the posterior surface of the body of the hyoid bone and the thyrohyoid membrane.

**ret·ro·jec·tion** (re-trō-jek′shŭn) the washing out of a cavity by the backward flow of an injected fluid. [L. *retro,* backward, + *jacio,* to throw]

**ret·ro·man·dib·u·lar vein** formed by the union of the superficial temporal and maxillary veins in front of the ear; runs posterior to the ramus of the mandible through the parotid gland, and unites with the posterior auricular vein to form the external jugular vein; it usually has a large communicating branch with the facial vein.

**ret·ro·mo·lar pad** a cushioned mass of tissue, frequently pear-shaped, located on the alveolar process of the mandible behind the area of the last natural molar tooth.

**ret·ro·per·i·to·ne·al fi·bro·sis** fibrosis of retroperitoneal structures commonly involving and often obstructing the ureters; the cause is usually unknown. SYN Ormond disease.

**ret·ro·per·i·to·ne·al space** the space between the parietal peritoneum and the muscles and bones of the posterior abdominal wall.

**ret·ro·per·i·to·ni·tis** (ret′rō-per-i-tō-nī′tis) inflammation of the cellular tissue behind the peritoneum.

**ret·ro·phar·ynx** (re′trō-făr′ingks) the posterior part of the pharynx.

**ret·ro·pla·sa** (ret-rō-plā′zē-ă) that state of cell or tissue in which activity is decreased below that considered normal; associated with retrogressive changes (e.g., injury, degeneration, death, necrosis). [retro- + G. *plasis,* a molding]

**ret·ro·posed** (re′trō-pōzd) denoting retroposition. [retro- + L. *pono,* pp. *positus,* to place]

**ret·ro·po·si·tion** (re′trō-pō-zish′ŭn) simple backward displacement of a structure or organ, as the uterus, without inclination, bending, retroversion, or retroflexion. [retro- + L. *positio,* a placing]

**ret·ro·pos·on** (re-trō-pōs′on) a transposition of sequences in a DNA that does not originate in the DNA but in an mRNA that is transcribed back into the genomic DNA by reverse transcription. [retro- + L. *pono,* pp. *positum,* to place, + -on]

**ret·ro·pu·bic space** the area of loose connective tissue between the bladder with its related fascia and the pubis and anterior abdominal wall.

**ret·ro·pul·sion** (re-trō-pŭl′shŭn) **1.** an involuntary backward walking or running, occurring in patients with the parkinsonian syndrome. **2.** a pushing back of any part. [retro- + L. *pulsio,* a pushing, fr. *pello,* pp. *pulsus,* beat, drive]

**re·tro·sig·moid ap·proach** a surgical approach to the cerebellopontine angle through the occipital bone posterior to the sigmoid sinus.

**ret·ro·spec·tive fal·si·fi·ca·tion** unconscious distortion of past experience to conform to present psychological needs.

**ret·ro·spon·dy·lo·lis·the·sis** (re′trō-spon′di-lō-lis-thē′sis) slipping posteriorly of the body of a vertebra, bringing it out of line with the adjacent vertebrae. [retro- + G. *spondylos,* vertebra, + *olisthēsis,* a slipping]

**ret·ro·ver·si·o·flex·ion** (re-trō-ver′sē-ō-flek′ shŭn, re-trō-ver′zhō-flek′shŭn) combined retroversion and retroflexion of the uterus.

**ret·ro·ver·sion** (re-trō-ver′zhŭn) **1.** a turning backward, as of the uterus. **2.** condition in which the teeth are located in a more posterior position than is normal. [retro- + L. *verto,* pp. *versus,* to turn]

**ret·ro·vert·ed** (re′trō-ver-ted) denoting retroversion.

**Ret·ro·vir·i·dae** (re-trō-vir′i-dē) a family of viruses grouped in three subfamilies: Oncovirinae (HTLV-I, HTLV-II RNA tumor viruses), Spumavirinae (foamy viruses), and Lentivirinae (HIV-like viruses, visna and related agents).

**ret·ro·vi·rus** (re′trō-vī′rŭs) any virus of the family Retroviridae. A virus with RNA core genetic material; requires the enzyme reverse transcriptase in order to convert its RNA into proviral DNA.

**re•tru•sion** (rē-troo′zhŭn) **1.** retraction of the mandible from any given point. **2.** the backward movement of the mandible. [L. *retrudo,* pp. -*trusus,* to push back]

**re•tru•sive oc•clu•sion 1.** a biting relationship in which the mandible is forcefully or habitually placed more distally than the patient's centric occlusion; **2.** SYN distal occlusion (1).

**Rett syn•drome** (ret) a progressive syndrome of autism, dementia, ataxia, and purposeless hand movements; associated with hyperammonemia, principally in girls.

**re•turn ex•tra•sys•to•le** a form of reciprocal rhythm in which the impulse having arisen in the ventricle ascends toward the atria, but before reaching the atria is reflected to the ventricles to produce a second ventricular contraction.

**re•vas•cu•lar•i•za•tion** (rē-vas′kyu-lăr-i-zā′shŭn) reestablishment of blood supply to a part.

**re•ver•sal** (rē-ver′săl) **1.** a turning or changing to the opposite direction, as of a process, disease, symptom, or state. **2.** the changing of a dark line or a bright one of the spectrum into its opposite. **3.** denoting the difficulty of some persons in distinguishing the lowercase printed or written letter *p* from *q* or *g, b* from *d,* or *s* from *z.* **4.** PSYCHOANALYSIS the change of an instinct or affect into its opposite, as from love into hate. SYN detraining. [L. *reverto,* pp. -*versus,* to turn back or about]

**re•versed co•arc•ta•tion** aortic arch syndrome in which blood pressure in the arms is lower than in the legs.

**re•versed per•i•stal•sis** a wave of intestinal contraction in a direction the reverse of normal, by which the contents of the intestine are forced backward. SYN antiperistalsis.

**re•verse Eck fis•tu•la** (ek) side-to-side anastomosis of the portal vein with the inferior vena cava and ligation of the latter above the anastomosis but below the hepatic veins; the blood from the lower part of the body is thus directed through the hepatic circulation.

**re•verse os•mo•sis** movement of solvent in the opposite direction from osmosis.

**re•verse pas•sive he•mag•glu•ti•na•tion** a diagnostic technique for virus infection using agglutination by viruses of red blood cells that previously have been coated with antibody specific to the virus.

**re•verse pu•pil•lary block** increased resistance to flow of aqueous humor through the pupil from the anterior chamber to the posterior chamber, leading to posterior bowing of the peripheral iris against the zonules; a possible mechanism for pigmentary glaucoma.

**re•verse tran•scrip•tase** RNA-dependent DNA polymerase, present in virions of RNA tumor viruses.

**re•verse tran•scrip•tase pol•y•me•rase chain re•ac•tion (RT-PCR)** a process for specific mRNA amplification wherein reverse transcriptase added to the in vitro reaction uses mRNA as a template to produce one cDNA, which is then amplified by the usual PCR.

**re•vers•si•bi•li•ty prin•ci•ple** EXERCISE SCIENCE principle stating that training adaptations are lost at a relatively rapid rate when a person terminates participation in an exercise program.

**re•vers•i•ble cal•ci•no•sis** a form of calcinosis sometimes observed in patients who ingest large quantities of milk and alkaline medicines, as in the treatment of peptic ulcer.

**re•ver•sion** (rē-ver′zhŭn) **1.** the manifestation in an individual of certain characteristics, peculiar to a remote ancestor, which have been suppressed during one or more of the intermediate generations. **2.** the return to the original phenotype, either by reinstatement of the original genotype (true reversion) or by a mutation at a site different from that of the first mutation which cancels the effect of the first mutation (suppressor mutation). [L. *reversio* (see reversal)]

**re•ver•tant** (rē-ver′tant) in microbial genetics, a mutant that has reverted to its former genotype (true reversion) or to the original phenotype by means of a suppressor mutation. [L. *revertans,* pros. p. of *reverto,* to turn back]

**re•viv•i•fi•ca•tion** (rē-viv′i-fi-kā′shŭn) **1.** renewal of life and strength. **2.** refreshening the edges of a wound by paring or scraping to promote healing. SYN vivification. [L. *re-,* again, + *vivo,* to live, + *facio,* to make]

**re•vul•sion** (rē-vŭl′shŭn) **1.** SYN counterirritation. **2.** SYN derivation. [L. *revulsio,* act of pulling away, fr. *revello,* pp. -*vulsus,* to pluck or pull away]

**re•ward** (rē-ward′) SYN reinforcer.

**Reye syn•drome** (rī) an acquired encephalopathy of young children that follows an acute febrile illness, usually influenza or varicella infection; characterized by recurrent vomiting, agitation, and lethargy, which may lead to coma with intracranial hypertension; ammonia and serum transaminases are elevated; death may result from edema of the brain and resulting cerebral herniation. Strongly associated with aspirin use. SYN hepatic encephalopathy (2).

**RFLP** restriction fragment length polymorphism.

**RFP** right frontoposterior position.

**RFT** right frontotransverse position.

**Rh 1.** rhodium. **2.** see Rh blood group, Blood Groups appendix.

△**rhab•do-, rhabd-** rod; rod-shaped (rhabdoid). [G. *rhabdos*]

**rhab•doid** (rab′doyd) rod-shaped. [rhabdo- + G. *eidos,* resemblance]

**rhab•do•my•o•blast** (rab-dō-mī′ō-blast) large round, spindle-shaped, or strap-shaped cells which deeply eosinophilic fibrillar cytoplasm which may show cross striations; found in some rhabdomyosarcomas. [rhabdo- + G. *mys,* muscle, + *blastos,* germ]

**rhab•do•my•ol•y•sis** (rab′dō-mī-ol′i-sis) an acute, fulminating, potentially fatal disease of skeletal muscle that entails destruction of muscle as evidenced by myoglobinemia and myoglobinuria. [rhabdo- + G. *mys,* muscle, + *lysis,* loosening]

**rhab•do•my•o•ma** (rab′dō-mī-ō′mă) a benign neoplasm derived from striated muscle, occurring in the heart in children, probably as a hamartomatous process. [rhabdo- + G. *mys,* muscle, + -*oma,* tumor]

**rhab•do•my•o•sar•co•ma** (rab′dō-mī-ō-sar-kō′mă) a malignant neoplasm derived from skeletal (striated) muscle, classified as embryonal alveolar (composed of loose aggregates of small round cells) or pleomorphic (containing rhabdomyoblasts). SYN rhabdosarcoma. [rhabdo- + G. *mys,* muscle, + *sarkōma,* sarcoma]

**rhab·do·sar·co·ma** (rab′dō-sar-kō′mă) SYN rhabdomyosarcoma.

**Rhab·do·vir·i·dae** (rab′dō-vir′i-dē) a family of rod- or bullet-shaped viruses of vertebrates, insects, and plants, including rabies virus.

**rhab·do·vi·rus** (rab′dō-vī′rŭs) any virus of the family Rhabdoviridae.

**Rhad·in·o·vi·rus** (rad-ēn′ō-vī-rŭs) a herpesvirus genus, subfamily Gammaherpesvirinae, associated with Kaposi sarcoma.

**rhag·a·des** (rag′ă-dēz) chaps, cracks, or fissures occurring at mucocutaneous junctions; seen in vitamin deficiency diseases and in congenital syphilis. [G. *rhagas,* pl. *rhagades,* a crack]

**Rh an·ti·gen in·com·pa·ti·bi·li·ty** SYN erythroblastosis fetalis.

**rheg·ma** (reg′mă) a rent or fissure. [G. breakage]

**rheg·ma·tog·e·nous** (reg-mă-toj′ĕ-nŭs) arising from a bursting or fractionating of an organ. [G. *rhēgma,* breakage, + *-gen,* producing]

**rhe·ni·um (Re)** (rē′nē-ŭm) a metallic element of the platinum group; atomic wt. 186.207, atomic no. 75. [Mod. L., fr. L. *Rhenus,* Rhine river]

△**rheo-** blood flow; electrical current. [G. *rheos,* stream, current, flow]

**rhe·o·base** (rē′ō-bās) the minimal strength of an electrical stimulus of indefinite duration that is able to cause excitation of a tissue, e.g., muscle or nerve. SEE ALSO chronaxie. [rheo- + G. *basis,* a base]

**rhe·o·ba·sic** (rē-ō-bā′sik) pertaining to or having the characteristics of a rheobase.

**rhe·ol·o·gy** (rē-ol′ō-jē) the study of the deformation and flow of materials. [rheo- + G. *logos,* study]

**rhe·om·e·try** (rē-om′ĕ-trē) measurement of electrical current or blood flow.

**rhe·os·to·sis** (rē-os-tō′sis) a hypertrophying and condensing osteitis which tends to run in longitudinal streaks or columns, like wax drippings on a candle, and which involves a number of the long bones. [rheo- + G. *osteon,* bone, + *-osis,* condition]

**rhe·o·tax·is** (rē-ō-tak′sis) a form of positive barotaxis, in which a microorganism in a fluid is impelled to move against the current flow of its medium. [rheo- + G. *taxis,* orderly arrangement]

**rhe·ot·ro·pism** (rē-ot′rō-pizm) a movement contrary to the motion of a current, involving part of an organism, rather than the organism as a whole, as in rheotaxis. [rheo- + G. *tropos,* a turning]

**Rhese pro·jec·tion** (rēs) oblique radiographic view of the skull to show the optic foramen in the lower outer quadrant of the bony orbit.

**rhes·to·cy·the·mia** (res′tō-sī-thē′mē-ă) the presence of broken down red blood cells in the peripheral circulation. [G. *rhaiō,* to destroy, + *kytos,* a hollow (a cell), + *haima,* blood]

**rheum** (room) a mucous or watery discharge. [G. *rheuma,* a flux]

**rheu·mat·ic** (roo-mat′ik) relating to or characterized by rheumatism. [G. *rheumatikos,* subject to flux, fr. *rheuma,* flux]

**rheu·mat·ic ar·te·ri·tis** arteritis due to rheumatic fever; Aschoff bodies are frequently found in the adventitia of small arteries, especially in the myocardium, and may lead to fibrosis and constriction of the lumens.

**rheu·mat·ic en·do·car·di·tis** endocardial involvement as part of rheumatic heart disease, recognized clinically by valvular involvement; in the acute stage, there may be tiny fibrin vegetations along the lines of closure of the valve leaflets, with subsequent fibrous thickening and shortening of the leaflets.

**rheu·mat·ic fe·ver** fever following infection of the throat with group A streptococci, occurring primarily in children and young adults, and inducing an immunopathy variably associated with acute migratory polyarthritis, Sydenham chorea, subcutaneous nodules over bony prominences, myocarditis with formation of Aschoff bodies which may cause acute cardiac failure, and endocarditis (frequently followed by scarring of valves, causing stenosis or incompetence); relapses are common if repeated streptococcal infections occur.

**rheu·mat·ic heart dis·ease** disease of the heart resulting from rheumatic fever, chiefly manifested by abnormalities of the valves.

**rheu·mat·ic pneu·mo·nia** pneumonia rarely occurring in severe acute rheumatic fever; consolidation occurs, the lungs being of a rubbery consistency, with fibrin exudate and small hemorrhages, as well as edema from left ventricle failure.

**rheu·ma·tid** (roo′mă-tid) rheumatic nodules or other eruptions which may accompany rheumatism. [G. *rheum,* flux, + -id (1)]

**rheu·ma·tism** (roo′mă-tizm) indefinite term applied to various conditions with pain or other symptoms of articular origin or related to other elements of the musculoskeletal system. [G. *rheumatismos,* rheuma, a flux]

**rheu·ma·toid** (roo′mă-toyd) resembling rheumatoid arthritis in one or more features. [G. *rheuma,* flux, + *eidos,* resemblance]

**rheu·ma·toid ar·thri·tis** a systemic disease, occurring more often in women, which affects connective tissue; arthritis is the dominant clinical manifestation, involving many joints, especially those of the hands and feet, accompanied by thickening of articular soft tissue, with extension of synovial tissue over articular cartilages, which become eroded; the course is variable but often is chronic and progressive, leading to deformities and disability. See page 861. SYN arthritis deformans, nodose rheumatism (1).

**rheu·ma·toid fac·tors** antibodies in the serum of individuals with rheumatoid arthritis that react with antigenic determinants or immunoglobulins that enhance agglutination of suspended particles coated with pooled human γ-globulin. Rheumatoid factors also occur in other autoimmune and certain infectious diseases.

**rheu·ma·toid nod·ules** subcutaneous nodules, occurring in some patients with rheumatoid arthritis.

**rheu·ma·toid po·cket** SYN susceptibility cassette.

**rheu·ma·toid spon·dy·li·tis** SYN ankylosing spondylitis.

**rheu·ma·tol·o·gist** (roo-mă-tol′ō-jist) a specialist in rheumatology.

**rheu·ma·tol·o·gy** (roo-mă-tol′ō-jē) the medical specialty concerned with the study, diagnosis, and treatment of rheumatic conditions. [G. *rheuma,* flux, + *logos,* study]

**RhIG** Rh-immune globulin.

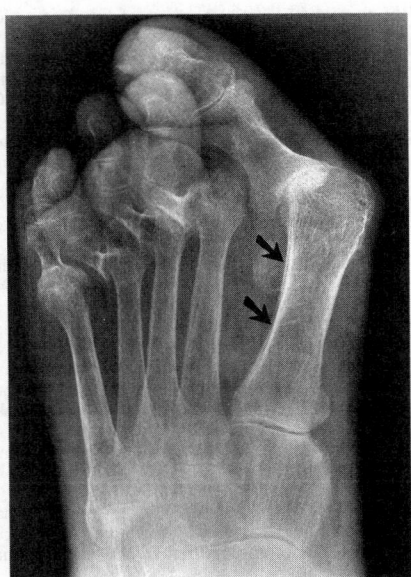

**rheumatoid arthritis** of the foot: radiograph showing lateral angulation and subluxation of metatarsophalangeal joints, diffuse osteoporosis with "punched out" zones of bone resorption at articular surfaces of bones, and periosteal reaction (arrows) along shaft of first metatarsal

---

**rhIL-11** SYN recombinant human interleukin-11.

**Rh·im·mune glo·bu·lin (RhIG)** a concentrated solution of IgG anti-D that is administered to an Rh-negative person who has been exposed to Rh-positive red cells, particularly a woman who may be carrying an Rh-positive fetus or has delivered or aborted an Rh-negative baby, to counteract the immunizing effect of the cells.

⟁**rhin-, rhi·no-** the nose. [G. *rhis*]

**rhi·nal** (rī'năl) SYN nasal.

**rhi·nal·gia** (rī-nal'jē-ă) pain in the nose. SYN rhinodynia. [rhin- + G. *algos*, pain]

**rhi·nal sul·cus** the shallow rostral continuation of the collateral sulcus that delimits the rostral part of the parahippocampal gyrus from the fusiform or lateral occipitotemporal gyrus. One of the oldest sulci of the pallium, it marks the border between the neocortex and the allocortical (olfactory).

**rhin·e·de·ma** (rī'n-e-dē'mă) swelling of the nasal mucous membrane. [rhin- + G. *oidēma*, swelling]

**rhin·en·ce·phal·ic** (rī'n-en-se-fal'ik) relating to the rhinencephalon.

**rhin·en·ceph·a·lon** (rī'n-en-sef'ă-lon) collective term denoting the parts of the cerebral hemisphere directly related to the sense of smell: the olfactory bulb, olfactory peduncle, olfactory tubercle, and olfactory or piriform cortex including the cortical nucleus of the amygdala. SEE ALSO limbic system. [rhin- + G. *enkephalos*, brain]

**rhi·ni·tis** (rī-nī'tis) inflammation of the nasal mucous membrane. [rhin- + G. *-itis*, inflammation]

**rhi·no·cele** (rī'nō-sēl) cavity (ventricle) of the

rhinencephalon, the primitive olfactory part of the telencephalon. [rhino- + G. *koilia*, a hollow]

**rhi·no·ceph·a·ly, rhi·no·ce·pha·lia** (rī'nō-sef'ă-lē, rī'nō-se-fā'lē-ă) rhinencephaly; a form of cyclopia in which the nose is represented by a fleshy protuberance arising above the slitlike orbits, and the rhinencephalic lobes of the telencephalon are poorly developed. [rhino- + G. *kephalē*, head]

**rhi·no·chei·lo·plas·ty, rhi·no·chi·lo·plas·ty** (rī'nō-kī'lō-plas-tē) plastic surgery of the nose and upper lip. [rhino- + G. *cheilos*, lip, + *plastos*, formed]

*Rhi·no·clad·i·el·la* (rī'nō-klad-ē-el'ă) a genus of dematiaceous fungi that cause chromoblastomycosis. SEE ALSO *Phialophora.*

**rhi·no·clei·sis** (rī-nō-klī'sis) SYN rhinostenosis. [rhino- + G. *kleisis*, a closure]

**rhi·no·dyn·ia** (rī-nō-din'ē-ă) SYN rhinalgia. [rhino- + G. *odynē*, pain]

**rhi·nog·e·nous** (rī-noj'ĕ-nŭs) originating in the nose. [rhino- + G. *-gen*, producing]

**rhi·no·ky·pho·sis** (rī'nō-kī-fō'sis) a humpback deformity of the nose. [rhino- + G. *kyphōsis*, humped condition]

**rhi·no·la·lia** (rī'nō-lā'lē-ă) nasalized speech. SYN rhinophonia. [rhino- + G. *lalia*, talking]

**rhi·no·lith** (rī'nō-lith) a calcareous concretion in the nasal cavity often around foreign body. [rhino- + G. *lithos*, stone]

**rhi·no·li·thi·a·sis** (rī'nō-li-thī'ă-sis) the presence of a nasal calculus. [rhinolith + G. *-iasis*, condition]

**rhi·nol·o·gist** (rī-nol'ō-jist) a specialist in diseases of the nose.

**rhi·nol·o·gy** (rī-nol'ō-jē) the branch of medical science concerned with the nose and its diseases. [rhino- + G. *logos*, study]

**rhi·no·ma·nom·e·ter** (rī'nō-mă-nom'ĕ-ter) a manometer used to determine the presence and amount of nasal obstruction, and the nasal air pressure and flow relationships. [rhino- + manometer]

**rhi·no·ma·nom·e·try** (rī'nō-mă-nom'ĕ-trē) **1.** the use of a rhinomanometer. **2.** the study and measurement of nasal air flow and pressures.

**rhi·no·my·co·sis** (rī'nō-mī-kō'sis) fungus infection of the nasal mucous membranes. [rhino- + mycosis]

**rhi·no·ne·cro·sis** (rī'nō-ne-krō'sis) necrosis of the bones of the nose. [rhino- + necrosis]

**rhi·nop·a·thy** (rī-nop'ă-thē) disease of the nose. [rhino- + G. *pathos*, suffering]

**rhi·no·pho·nia** (rī'nō-fō'nē-ă) SYN rhinolalia. [rhino- + G. *phōnē*, voice]

**rhi·no·phy·ma** (rī'nō-fī'mă) hypertrophy of the nose with follicular dilation, resulting from hyperplasia of sebaceous glands with fibrosis and increased vascularity. [rhino- + G. *phyma*, tumor, growth]

**rhi·no·plas·ty** (rī'nō-plas-tē) **1.** repair of a defect of the nose with tissue taken from elsewhere. **2.** plastic surgery to change the shape or size of the nose. [rhino- + G. *plastos*, formed]

**rhi·nor·rhea** (rī-nō-rē'ă) a discharge from the nasal mucous membrane. [rhino- + G. *rhoia*, flow]

**rhi·nor·rhoea [Br.]** SEE rhinorrhea.

**rhi·no·sal·pin·gi·tis** (rī'nō-sal-pin-jī'tis) inflammation of the mucous membrane of the nose and auditory tube. [rhino- + G. *salpinx*, tube, + *-itis*, inflammation]

**rhi·no·scle·ro·ma** (rī'nō-sklĕ-rō'mă) a chronic granulomatous process involving the nose, upper lip, mouth, and upper air passages; it may involve the external auditory meatus and is believed to be due to a specific bacterium, possibly a strain of *Klebsiella*. [rhino- + G. *sklērōma*, an induration]

**rhi·no·scope** (rī'nō-skōp) a small mirror attached at a suitable angle to a rodlike handle, used in posterior rhinoscopy.

**rhi·no·scop·ic** (rī'nō-skop'ik) relating to the rhinoscope or to rhinoscopy.

**rhi·nos·co·py** (rī-nos'kŏ-pē) inspection of the nasal cavity. [rhino- + G. *skopeō*, to view]

**rhi·no·si·nus·i·tis** (rī-nō-sī-nŭs-ī'tis) inflammation of the mucous membrane of the nose and paranasal sinuses.

**rhi·no·ste·no·sis** (rī'nō-ste-nō'sis) nasal obstruction. SYN rhinocleisis. [rhino- + G. *stenōsis*, a narrowing]

**rhi·not·o·my** (rī-not'ō-mē) 1. any cutting operation on the nose. 2. operative procedure in which the nose is incised along one side so that it may be turned away to provide full vision of the nasal passages for radical sinus operations. [rhino- + G. *tomē*, incision, cutting]

**Rhi·no·vi·rus** (rī'nō-vī'rŭs) a genus of acid-labile viruses associated with the common cold. There are more than 110 antigenic types.

**rhi·no·vi·rus** any virus of the genus *Rhinovirus*.

△**rhi·zo-** combining form denoting root. [G. *rhiza*]

**rhi·zoid** (rī'zoyd) 1. rootlike. 2. irregularly branching, like a root; denoting a form of bacterial growth. 3. in fungi, the rootlike hyphae which arise at the nodes of the hyphae of *Rhizopus* species. [rhizo- + G. *eidos*, resemblance]

**rhi·zo·me·lia** (rī-zō-mē'lē-ă) 1. disproportion in the length of the most proximal segment of the limbs (arms and thighs). 2. a disorder involving the shoulder and hip joint. [rhizo- + G. *melos*, limb]

**rhi·zo·melic** (rī-zō-mel'ik) of or relating to the hip joint or the shoulder joint.

**rhi·zo·mel·ic chon·dro·dys·pla·sia punc·ta·ta** autosomal recessively inherited lethal chondrodysplasia caused by mutation in the PEX 7 gene encoding the peroxisomal type 2 targeting signal (PTS2) receptor on chromosomal 6q.

**rhi·zo·mel·ic dwarf·ism** one of the syndromes of chondrodysplasia punctata; autosomal recessive, with variable skin keratinization disorders and variable facial, cardiac, optic, and central nervous system abnormalities; epiphyseal stippling is also present. There are multiple enzymatic defects, including peroxisomal ones, and affected infants fail to thrive and usually die in infancy.

**rhi·zo·me·nin·go·my·e·li·tis** (rī'zō-mě-ning'gō-mī-ĕ-lī'tis) inflammation of the nerve roots, the meninges, and the spinal cord. SYN radiculomeningomyelitis. [rhizo- + G. *mēninx*, membrane, + *myelon*, marrow, + *-itis*, inflammation]

**Rhi·zo·mu·cor** (rī-zō-myu-kōr) a genus of fungi in the family Mucoraceae; a cause of mucormycosis.

**Rhi·zop·o·da** (rī-zŏ-pō'dă) a superclass in the subphylum Sarcodina that includes the amebae of humans, having pseudopodia of various forms but without axial filaments. [rhizo + G. *pous* (*pod-*), foot]

*Rhi·zo·pus* (rī-zŏ'pŭs) a genus of fungi of which some species cause zygomycosis in humans.

**rhi·zot·o·my** (rī-zot'ō-mē) surgical section of the spinal nerve roots for the relief of pain or spastic paralysis. SYN radicotomy, radiculectomy. [G. *rhiza*, root, + *tomē*, section]

**Rh null syn·drome** a lack of all Rh antigens, compensated hemolytic anemia, and stomatocytosis.

**rho** (ρ) (rō) 1. 17th letter of the Greek alphabet. 2. population correlation coefficient; symbol for density.

**Rho·de·sian try·pan·o·so·mi·a·sis** (rō-dē-zhŭn, rō-dēz'ē-an) a disease of humans caused by *Trypanosoma brucei rhodesiense* in eastern Africa; it is clinically similar to Gambian trypanosomiasis but of shorter duration and more acute in form; patients suffer repeated episodes of pyrexia, become anemic, and die commonly from cardiac failure. SYN acute African sleeping sickness, acute trypanosomiasis.

**rho·di·um (Rh)** (rō'dē-ŭm) a metallic element, atomic no. 45, atomic wt. 102.90550. [Mod. L. fr. G. *rhodon*, a rose]

*Rhod·ni·us* (rod'nē-ŭs) genus of reduvid bug that is the principal vector of *Trypanosoma cruzi* in Venezuela, Colombia, French Guiana, Guyana, and Surinam.

*Rhod·ni·us pro·lix·us* a reduvid bug, an important cause vector South American trypanosomiasis.

△**rho·do-, rhod-** rosy, red color. [G. *rhodon*, rose]

**rho·do·gen·e·sis** (rō'dō-jen'ě-sis) the production of rhodopsin by the combination of 11-*cis*-retinal and opsin in the dark. [rhodopsin + G. *genesis*, production]

**rho·do·phy·lac·tic** (rō'dō-fī-lak'tik) relating to rhodophylaxis.

**rho·do·phy·lax·is** (rō'dō-fī-lak'sis) the action of the pigment cells of the choroid in preserving or facilitating the reproduction of rhodopsin. [rhodopsin + G. *phylaxis*, a guarding]

**rho·dop·sin** (rō-dop'sin) a red thermolabile protein found in the rods of the retina; it is bleached by the action of light, which converts it to opsin and all-*trans*-retinal, and is restored in the dark by rhodogenesis; the dominant protein in the plasma membrane of rod cells. SYN visual purple.

**rhomb·en·ce·phal·ic isth·mus** 1. a constriction in the embryonic neural tube delineating the mesencephalon from the rhombencephalon; 2. the anterior portion of the rhombencephalon connecting with the mesencephalon.

**rhomb·en·ce·phal·ic teg·men·tum** the portion of the pons continuous with the mesencephalic tegmentum; it consists of reticular formation, tracts, and cranial nerve nuclei, and forms the dorsal part of the pons (pars dorsalis pontis).

**rhomb·en·ceph·a·lon** (rom-ben-sef'ă-lon) that part of the developing brain that is the most caudal of the three primary vesicles of the embryonic neural tube; secondarily divided into metencephalon and myelencephalon; the rhombencephalon includes the pons, cerebellum, and medulla oblongata. SYN hindbrain. [rhombo- + G. *enkephalos*, brain]

**rhom·bic** (rom'bik) 1. SYN rhomboid. 2. relating to the rhombencephalon.

**rhom·bo·cele** (rom'bō-sēl) SYN rhomboidal sinus. [rhombo- + G. *koilia*, a hollow]

**rhom·boid, rhom·boi·dal** (rom'boyd, rom-boy'

dăl) resembling a rhomb; i.e., an oblique parallelogram, but having unequal sides. SYN rhombic (1). [rhombo- + G. *eidos,* appearance]

**rhom·boi·dal si·nus** a dilation of the central canal of the spinal cord in the lumbar region. SYN rhombocele.

**rhom·boid fos·sa** the floor of the fourth ventricle of the brain, formed by the ventricular surface of the rhombencephalon.

**rhom·boid lig·a·ment** SYN costoclavicular ligament.

**rhon·chal, rhon·chi·al** (rong′kăl, rong′kē-ăl) relating to or characteristic of a rhonchus.
[L. fr. G. *rhenchos,* a snoring]

**rhon·chal frem·i·tus** fremitus produced by vibrations from the passage of air in bronchial tubes partially obstructed by mucous secretion.

**rhon·chus,** pl. **rhon·chi** (rong′kŭs, rong′kī) an added sound with a musical pitch occurring during inspiration or expiration, heard on auscultation of the chest, and caused by air passing through bronchi that are narrowed by inflammation, spasm of smooth muscle, or presence of mucus in the lumen; if low-pitched, it is called **sonorous rhonchus;** if high-pitched, with a whistling or squeaky quality, **sibilant rhonchus.** [L. fr. G. *rhenchos,* a snoring]

■ **rhy·thm** (ridh′ŭm) **1.** measured time or motion; the regular alternation of two or more different or opposite states. **2.** SYN rhythm method. **3.** regular occurrence of an electrical event in the electroencephalogram. SEE ALSO wave. **4.** sequential beating of the heart generated by a single beat or sequence of beats. See page 864. [G. *rhythmos*]

**rhy·thm meth·od** a natural contraceptive method that spaces sexual intercourse to avoid the fertile period of the menstrual cycle. SYN rhythm (2).

**rhy·tide** (rī′tīd) a skin wrinkle. [G. *rhytis, -idos,* wrinkle]

**rhyt·i·dec·tomy** (rit-i-dek′tō-mē) elimination of wrinkles from, or reshaping of, the face by excising any excess skin and tightening the remainder; the so-called face-lift. SYN rhytidoplasty. [G. *rhytis (rhytid-),* a wrinkle, + ectomy]

**rhyt·i·do·plas·ty** (rit′i-dō-plas-tē) SYN rhytidectomy. [G. *rhytis,* a wrinkle, + *plastos,* formed]

**rhyt·i·do·sis** (rit-i-dō′sis) **1.** wrinkling of the face to a degree disproportionate to age. **2.** laxity and wrinkling of the cornea, an indication of approaching death. SYN rutidosis. [G. a wrinkling, fr. *rhytis,* a wrinkle, + *-osis,* condition]

**rib** ribose. SYN costa (1) [TA].

**rib·bon** (rib′ŏn) a ribbon-shaped structure. [M. E. *riban*]

**rib [I–XII]** one of the 24 elongated curved bones forming the main portion of the bony wall of the chest. [A.S. *ribb*]

△**ri·bo-** **1.** ribose. **2.** as an italicized prefix to the systematic name of a monosaccharide, *ribo-* indicates that the configuration of a set of three consecutive CHOH groups is that of ribose. [German *Ribose,* alt. from arabinose, fr. *gum arabic* + *-ose*]

**ri·bo·nu·cle·ase (RNase)** (rī-bō-noo′klē-ās) a transferase or phosphodiesterase that catalyzes the hydrolysis of ribonucleic acid.

**ri·bo·nu·cle·ic ac·id (RNA)** (rī′bō-noo-klē′ik as′id) a macromolecule consisting of ribonucleoside residues connected by phosphate bonds, concerned in the control of cellular chemical process, especially protein synthesis. RNA is found

in all cells, in both nuclei and cytoplasm, and also in many viruses.

**ri·bo·nu·cle·o·pro·tein (RNP)** (rī′bō-noo′klē-ō-prō′tēn) a combination of ribonucleic acid and protein.

**ri·bo·nu·cle·o·side** (rī-bō-noo′klē-ō-sīd) a nucleoside in which the sugar component is ribose; the common ribonucleosides of RNA are adenosine, cytidine, guanosine, and uridine.

**ri·bo·nu·cle·o·tide** (rī-bō-noo′klē-ō-tīd) a nucleotide (nucleoside phosphate) in which the sugar component is ribose; the major ribonucleotides of RNA are adenylic acid, cytidylic acid, guanylic acid, and uridylic acid.

**ri·bose (rib)** (rī′bōs) the pentose present in ribonucleic acid; epimers of D-ribose are D-arabinose, D-xylose, and L-lyxose.

**ri·bose-5-phos·phate isom·er·ase** an enzyme catalyzing interconversion of D-ribose 5-phosphate and D-ribulose 5-phosphate; of importance in ribose metabolism and in the pentose phosphate pathway.

**ri·bose-5-phos·phate** ribose phosphorylated on carbon-5; an intermediate in the pentose phosphate pathway.

**ri·bo·som·al RNA** the RNA of ribosomes and polyribosomes.

**ri·bo·some** (rī′bō-sōm) a granule of ribonucleoprotein, 120 to 150 Å in diameter, that is the site of protein synthesis from aminoacyl-tRNAs as directed by mRNAs.

**ri·bo·su·ria** (rī-bō-syu′rē-ă) the enhanced urinary excretion of D-ribose; commonly one manifestation of muscular dystrophy. [ribose + G. *ouron,* urine]

**ri·bo·syl** (rī′bō-sil) the radical formed by loss of the hemiacetal OH group from either of the two cyclic forms of ribose.

**ri·bo·thy·mi·dine (T)** (rī-bō-thī′mi-dēn) 5-methyluridine; the ribosyl analog of thymidine (deoxyribosylthymine); a nucleoside found in small amounts in ribonucleic acids.

**ri·bo·thy·mi·dyl·ic ac·id (rTMP, TMP)** (rī′bō-thī-mi-dil′ik as′id) ribothymidine 5′-phosphate; the ribose analog of thymidylic acid; a rare component of transfer RNAs.

**Ri·bot law of me·mo·ry** (rē-bō′) in progressive dementias, remote memories tend to be preserved whereas recent memories are lost.

**Ric·co law** (rē′kō) for small images, light intensity × area = constant for the threshold.

**rice starch** rice product used as a supplement in many media formulations used for the culture of intestinal protozoa, e.g., *Entamoeba histolytica.*

**Rich·ter her·nia** (rik′ter) SYN parietal hernia.

**Rich·ter syn·drome** (rik′ter) a high-grade lymphoma developing during the course of chronic lymphocytic leukemia; associated with cachexia, pyrexia, dysproteinemia, and lymphomas with multinucleated tumor cells.

**rick·ets** (rik′ets) a disease due to vitamin-D deficiency and characterized by overproduction and deficient calcification of osteoid tissue, with associated skeletal deformities, disturbances in growth, and hypocalcemia. SYN infantile osteomalacia, juvenile osteomalacia, rachitis. [E. *wrick,* to twist]

*Rick·ett·sia* (ri-ket′sē-ă) a genus of bacteria containing small (nonfilterable), often pleomorphic, coccoid to rod-shaped, Gram-negative organisms that usually occur intracytoplasmically in lice,

normal sinus rhythm (NSR)

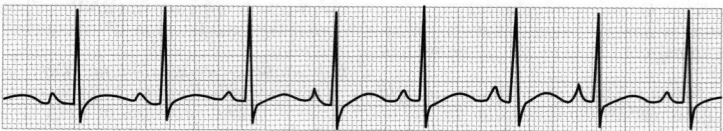

bradycardia

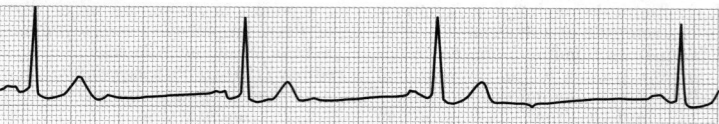

ventricular fibrillation

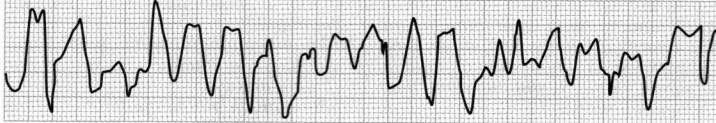

atrial flutter

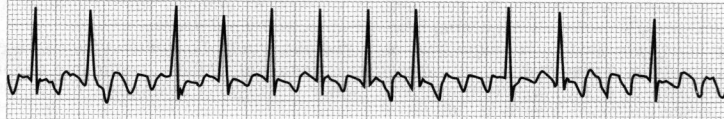

first degree atrioventricular block

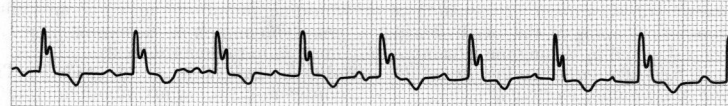

premature ventricular contractions

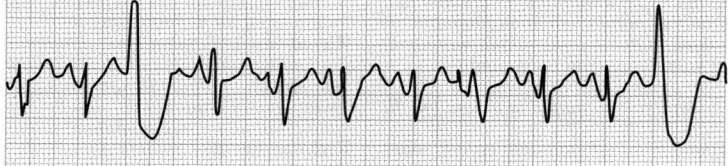

sinus tachycardia

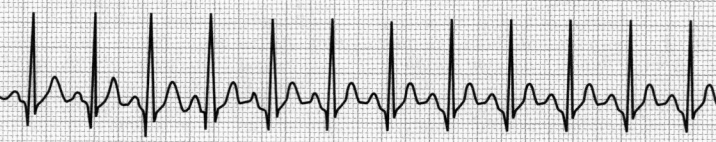

**rhythm:** electrocardiogram tracings showing common types of arrhythmia

fleas, ticks, and mites; pathogenic species are parasitic in man and other animals, causing epidemic typhus, murine or endemic typhus, Rocky Mountain spotted fever, tsutsugamushi disease, rickettsialpox, and other diseases; type species is *Rickettsia prowazekii*. [Howard T. *Ricketts*]

**Ri·ckett·sia a·fri·cae** a species of Rickettsia studied principally in Zimbabwe that appears to be carried by the tick *Amblyomma hebraeum;* a cause of spotted fever.

**Rick·ett·sia a·kari** a species causing human rickettsialpox, a mild, acute febrile disease; transmitted by the house mouse mite, *Liponyssoides sanguineus.*

**Rick·ett·sia co·no·ri·i** a widespread African species probably causing boutonneuse fever in humans, transmitted by various ticks.

**Rick·ett·sia ho·nei** a bacterial species causing Flinders Island spotted fever in Australia.

**Rick·ett·sia ja·po·ni·ca** a bacterial species causing Japanese spotted fever.

**rick·ett·si·al** (ri-ket′sē-ăl) pertaining to or caused by rickettsiae.

**rick·ett·si·al·pox** (ri-ket′sē-ăl-poks′) infection with *Rickettsia akari*, which is spread by mites from reservoir in mice; a benign, self-limited febrile illness.

**Rick·ett·sia pro·wa·ze·ki·i** a species causing epidemic and recrudescent typhus, transmitted by body lice; type species of the genus *Rickettsia.*

**Rick·ett·sia rick·ett·si·i** the agent of Rocky Mountain spotted fever and its geographic variants; transmitted by infected ixodid ticks, especially *Dermacentor andersoni* and *D. variabilis.*

**Rick·ett·sia slo·va·ca** a bacterial species causing a newly recognized rickettsiosis associated with local erythema and possibly meningoencephalitis; transmitted by the tick *Dermacentor marginatus.*

**Rick·ett·sia tsu·tsu·ga·mu·shi** a species causing tsutsugamushi disease and scrub typhus; transmitted by trombiculid mites.

**rick·ett·si·o·sis** (ri-ket-sē-ō′sis) infection with rickettsiae.

**Rid·doch phe·no·me·non** (rid′dok) ability to appreciate a small moving object in an area of the visual field blind to static objects; particularly associated with occipital lobe lesions.

**Rid·e·al-Walk·er co·ef·fi·cient** (rid′ē-ĕl-wŏk-er) a figure expressing the disinfecting power of any substance; it is obtained by dividing the figure indicating the degree of dilution of the disinfectant that kills a microorganism in a given time by that indicating the degree of dilution of phenol which kills the organism in the same space of time under similar conditions. SYN phenol coefficient.

**Ri·dell op·er·a·tion** (rī-del′) removal of the entire anterior and inferior walls of the frontal sinus, for chronic inflammation of that cavity.

**rid·er's bone** heterotopic bone ossification of the tendon of the adductor longus muscle from strain in horseback riding.

**ridge** (rij) **1.** a (usually rough) linear elevation. SEE ALSO crest. **2.** in dentistry, any linear elevation on the surface of a tooth. **3.** the remainder of the alveolar process and its soft tissue covering after the teeth are removed. [A. S. *hyrcg*, back, spine]

**Rie·del thy·roid·i·tis** (rē-del) a rare fibrous induration of the thyroid gland, with adhesion to

adjacent structures, which may cause tracheal compression.

**Rie·der cell leu·ke·mia** (rē-dĕr) a special form of acute granulocytic leukemia in which affected tissues and the blood contain atypical myeloblasts (i.e., Rieder cells) that have faintly granular, immature cytoplasm and a bizarre nucleus with deep indentations (suggestive of lobulation).

**Rie·der cells** (rē-dĕr) abnormal myeloblasts in which the nucleus may be widely and deeply indented or may actually be a bi- or multi-lobate structure; such cells are frequently observed in acute leukemia.

**Rie·der lym·pho·cyte** (rē-dĕr) an abnormal form of lymphocyte that has a greatly indented (or lobed), slightly twisted nucleus; such cells are usually observed in certain examples of chronic lymphocytic leukemia.

**Rie·gel pulse** (rē-gĕl) a pulse that diminishes in volume during expiration.

**Rie·ger a·nom·a·ly** (rē-gĕr) iridocorneal mesochymal dysgenesis.

**Rie·ger syn·drome** (rē-gĕr) iridocorneal mesenchymal dysgenesis combined with hypodontia or anodontia and maxillary hypoplasia; autosomal dominant; there are delayed sexual development and hypothyroidism.

**Riehl mel·a·no·sis** (rēl) a brown pigmentary condition of the exposed portions of the skin of the neck and face with melanin pigment in dermal macrophages, thought to result from photodermatitis due to materials, such as cosmetic ingredients, or oils encountered in various occupations.

**right atri·um of heart** right atrium, the atrium of the right side of the heart that receives the blood from the venae cavae and coronary sinus. SYN atrium cordis dextrum [TA], atrium dextrum cordis.

**right col·ic flex·ure** the bend of the colon at the juncture of its ascending and transverse portions. SYN flexura coli dextra [TA], hepatic flexure.

**right de·scen·ding pul·mo·nary ar·ter·y (RDPA)** artery supplying the right middle and lower lobes and comprises most of the right hilar shadow on the frontal chest radiograph.

**right-foot·ed** (rīt′fŭt-ed) SYN dextropedal.

**right gas·tric ar·tery** *origin*, hepatic; *distribution*, pyloric portion of stomach on the lesser curvature; *anastomoses*, left gastric.

**right gas·tric vein** it receives veins from both surfaces of the upper portion of the stomach, runs to the right along the lesser curvature of the stomach, and empties into the portal vein. SYN pyloric vein.

**right-hand·ed** (rīt′hand-ed) denoting the habitual or more skillful use of the right hand for writing and most manual operations. SYN dextral.

**right heart** the right atrium and right ventricle.

**right heart by·pass** introduction of a circuit shunting blood from the venae cavae around the right atrium and ventricle and directly into the pulmonary artery.

**right he·pa·tic duct** the duct that transmits bile to the common hepatic duct from the right half of the liver and the right part of the caudate lobe.

**right lat·er·al di·vi·sion of liv·er** the portion of the liver that lies to the right of the approximately vertical plane of the right hepatic vein and includes the right anterior and posterior lateral segments (hepatic segments VI and VII); it is approximately the right third of the right anatomic lobe of the liver. SYN divisio lateralis dextra hepatis [TA].

**right-left dis•cri•mi•na•tion** the process of identifying one side of the body as distinct from the other.

**right and left fi•brous rings of heart** two fibrous rings that surround atrioventricular orifices of the heart, providing attachment for the atrioventricular valve leaflets and maintaining patency of the orifices. As part of the fibrous skeleton of the heart, the fibrous rings also provide origin and insertion for the myocardium. SYN anulus fibrosus (1) [TA].

**right liv•er** portion of the liver receiving blood from the right branches of the hepatic artery and portal vein, and from which bile is drained via the right hepatic duct; the plane of the middle hepatic vein separates right from left liver.

**right lobe of liv•er** the largest lobe of the liver, separated from the left lobe above and in front by the falciform ligament and from the caudate and quadrate lobes by the sulcus for the vena cava and the fossa for the gallbladder; it contains two segments, anterior and posterior. SYN lobus hepatis dexter [TA].

**right lym•pha•tic duct** one of the two terminal lymph vessels, a short trunk, about 2 cm in length, formed by the union of the right jugular lymphatic vessel and vessels from the lymph nodes of the right superior limb, thoracic wall, and both lungs; it lies on the right side of the root of the neck and empties into the right brachiocephalic vein.

**right me•di•al di•vi•sion of liv•er** the portion of the liver that lies between the approximately vertical planes of the right and middle hepatic veins and includes the right anterior and posterior medial segments (hepatic segments V and VIII); it is approximately the middle third of the anatomic right lobe of the liver. SYN divisio medialis dextra hepatis [TA].

**right pul•mo•na•ry ar•te•ry** the longer of the two terminal branches of the pulmonary trunk, it passes transversely across the mediastinum passing inferior to the aortic arch to enter the hilum of the right lung. Branches are distributed with the bronchi; frequent variations occurs. Typical branches to the superior lobe (rami lobi superioris [TA]) are apical (rami apicalis [TA]), anterior ascending (rami anterior ascendens [TA]), anterior descending (ramus anterior descendens [TA]), posterior ascending (ramus posterior ascendens [TA]), and posterior descending (ramus posterior descendens [TA]); to the middle lobe (rami lobi medii [TA]) are medial (ramus medialis [TA]) and lateral (ramus lateralis [TA]); and to the inferior lobe (rami lobi inferioris [TA]) are superior (apical) branch of inferior lobe (ramus superior (apicalis) lobi inferioris [TA]), and the anterior, lateral (lateralis), medial (medialis) and posterior basal branches (rami basalis).

**right-to-left shunt** the passage of blood from the right side of the heart into the left (as through a septal defect), or from the pulmonary artery into the aorta (as through a patent ductus arteriosus); such a shunt can occur only when the pressure on the right side exceeds that in the left.

**right ven•tri•cle** the lower chamber on the right side of the heart which receives the venous blood

from the right atrium and drives it by the contraction of its walls into the pulmonary artery.

**right ven•tric•u•lar fail•ure** congestive heart failure manifested by distention of the neck veins, enlargement of the liver, and dependent edema due to pump failure of the right ventricle.

**ri•gid con•nec•tor** DENTISTRY a connector that is solid or rigid, as a soldered joint.

**ri•gid•i•ty** (ri-jid′i-tē) **1.** stiffness or inflexibility. SYN rigor (1). **2.** PSYCHIATRY, CLINICAL PSYCHOLOGY an aspect of personality characterized by an individual's resistance to change. **3.** NEUROLOGY one type of increase in muscle tone at rest; characterized by increased resistance to passive stretch, independent of velocity and symmetric about joints; increases with activation of corresponding muscles in the contralateral limb. Two basic types are cogwheel rigidity and leadpipe rigidity. SEE ALSO nuchal rigidity. See this page. [L. *rigidus*, rigid, inflexible]

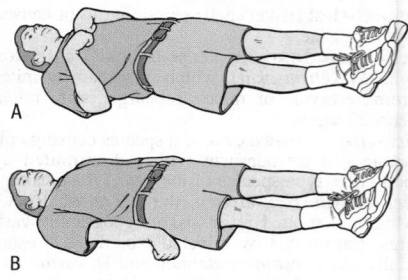

**rigidity:** (A) decorticate, (B) decerebrate

**rig•or** (rig′er) **1.** SYN rigidity (1). **2.** SYN chill (2). [L. stiffness]

**rig•or mor•tis** stiffening of the body, from 1 to 7 hours after death, from hardening of the muscular tissues in consequence of the coagulation of the myosinogen and paramyosinogen; it disappears after 1 to 6 days, or when decomposition begins. SYN postmortem rigidity.

**rim** a margin, border, or edge, usually circular in form.

**ri•ma**, gen. and pl. **ri•mae** (rī′mă, rī′mē) [TA] a slit or fissure, or narrow elongated opening between two symmetrical parts. [L. a slit]

**ri•ma glot•ti•dis** [TA] the interval between the true vocal cords.

**ri•ma o•ris** [TA] the mouth slit; the aperture of the mouth.

**ri•ma pal•pe•bra•rum** [TA] the lid slit, or fissure between the lids of the eye. SYN palpebral fissure.

**ri•ma ves•tib•u•li** [TA] the interval between the false vocal cords or vestibular folds.

**ri•mose** (rī′mōs) fissured; marked by cracks in all directions, like the crackle of porcelain. [L. *rimosus*, fr. *rima*, a fissure]

**rim•u•la** (rim′yu-lă) a minute slit or fissure. [L. dim. of *rima*]

**ring 1.** a circular band surrounding a wide central opening; a ring-shaped or circular structure surrounding an opening or level area. SYN anulus [TA]. **2.** ANATOMY anulus. **3.** the closed chain of atoms in a cyclic compound; commonly used for "cyclic" or "cycle." **4.** a marginal growth on the upper surface of a broth culture of bacteria, adhering to the sides of the test tube in the form of a circle. SYN annulus. [A.S. *hring*]

**ring ab·scess** an acute purulent inflammation of the corneal periphery in which a necrotic area is surrounded by an annular girdle of leukocytic infiltration.

**ring chro·mo·some** a chromosome with ends joined to form a circular structure. The ring form is abnormal in humans but the normal form of the chromosome in certain bacteria.

**Ring·er so·lu·tion** (ring′er) a solution resembling the blood serum in its salt constituents; it contains 8.6 g of NaCl, 0.3 g of KCl, and 0.33 g of CaCl$_2$ in each 1000 mL of distilled water; used as a fluid and electrolyte replenisher by intravenous infusion. SEE ALSO lactated Ringer solution. **2.** a salt solution usually used in combination with naturally occurring body substances (e.g., blood serum, tissue extracts) and/or more complex chemically defined nutritive solutions for culturing animal cells.

**ring fin·ger** fourth finger.

**ring-knife** (ring-nīf) a circular or oval ring with internal cutting edge, for shaving off tumors in the nasal and other cavities.

**ring·like cor·ne·al dys·tro·phy** threadlike opacities of the anterior corneal stroma, with acute, painful onset followed by decreased vision; autosomal dominant inheritance, caused by mutation in the transforming growth factor, beta-induced, gene (TGFB1) encoding keratoepithelium on chromosome 5q.

**ring sco·to·ma** an annular area of blindness in the visual field surrounding the fixation point in pigmentary degeneration of the retina and in glaucoma.

**ring sy·ringe** SYN control syringe.

**ring·worm** (ring′werm) SYN tinea.

**Rin·ne test** (rin-ĕ) a vibrating tuning fork is held alternately with the base touching the mastoid process and with the prongs near the external ear. Normally the sound can be heard by air conduction longer than by bone conduction; the reverse phenomenon indicates conductive hearing loss in the ear tested.

**Ri·o·lan a·nas·to·mo·sis** (rē-ō-lah′) the specific portion of the marginal artery of the colon connecting the middle and left colic arteries.

**RIP** radioimmunoprecipitation.

**Ri·pault sign** (rē-pou′) a sign of death, consisting in a permanent change in the shape of the pupil produced by unilateral pressure on the eyeball.

**Rip·stein o·per·a·tion** (rip-stīn) an operation for rectal prolapse that involves a transabdominal approach with dissection around the rectum and placement of a mesh sling to prevent the bowel from prolapsing through the anus.

**risk** the probability that an event will occur.

**Ris·ley ro·ta·ry pri·sm** (riz′lē) a prism with a circular base that is rotated in a metal frame marked with a scale; used in examination of ocular muscle imbalance.

**ri·so·ri·us mus·cle** *origin*, from platysma and fascia of masseter; *insertion*, orbicularis oris and skin at corner of mouth; *action*, draws angle of mouth laterally, lengthening rima oris; *nerve supply*, facial. SYN musculus risorius [TA].

**RIST** radioimmunosorbent test.

**ri·sus ca·ni·nus** (rī′sŭs kā-nī′nŭs) the semblance of a grin caused by facial spasm, especially in

tetanus. SYN cynic spasm, sardonic grin. [L. *risus*, laugh + *caninus*, doglike]

**Rit·gen ma·neu·ver** (rit′gen) delivery of a child's head by pressure on the perineum while controlling the speed of delivery by pressure with the other hand on the head.

**Rit·ter open·ing tet·a·nus** (rit′ĕr) the tetanic contraction that occasionally occurs when a strong current, passing through a long stretch of nerve, is suddenly interrupted.

**rit·u·al** (rich′oo-ăl) PSYCHIATRY, PSYCHOLOGY any psychomotor activity (e.g., morbid handwashing) performed by an individual to relieve anxiety or forestall its development; typically seen in obsessive-compulsive disorder. [L. *ritualis*, fr. *ritus*, rite]

**rit·ux·im·ab** (rit-ŭks′im-ab) monoclonal antibody used in the treatment of non-Hodgkin lymphoma.

**ri·val·ry** (rī′văl-rē) competition between two or more individuals for the same object or goal. [L. *rivalis*, competitor, rival]

**Riv·ers cock·tail** (riv′erz) an intravenous slow injection of from 1000 to 2000 ml of 10% dextrose in isotonic saline to which thiamine hydrochloride and 25 units of insulin are added; used in acute alcoholism.

**Ri·vi·nus ca·nals** (rī-vē′nŭs) SEE major sublingual duct, minor sublingual ducts.

**Ri·vi·nus ducts** (rī-vē′nŭs) SYN minor sublingual ducts.

**riz·i·form** (riz′i-fōrm) resembling rice grains. [Fr. *riz*, rice]

**RLL** right lower lobe (of lung).

**RLQ** right lower quadrant (of abdomen).

**RM** repetition maximum.

**RMA** right mentoanterior position.

**RML** right middle lobe (of lung).

**RMP** right mentoposterior position.

**RMT** right mentotransverse position.

**Rn** radon.

**RNA** ribonucleic acid.

**RNase** ribonuclease.

**RNase α** an enzyme catalyzing endonucleolytic cleavage of *O*-methylated RNA yielding 5′-phosphomonoesters.

**RNase P** an enzyme catalyzing the endonucleolytic cleavage tRNA precursors to yield 5′-phosphomonoesters.

**RNA splic·ing** SYN splicing (2).

**RNA tu·mor vi·rus·es** viruses of the subfamily Oncovirinae.

**RNA vi·rus** a group of viruses in which the core consists of RNA; a major group of animal viruses that includes the families Picornaviridae, Reoviridae, Togaviridae, Flaviviridae, Bunyaviridae, Arenaviridae, Paramyxoviridae, Retroviridae, Coronaviridae, Orthomyxoviridae, and Rhabdoviridae.

**RNP** ribonucleoprotein.

**ROA** right occipitoanterior position.

**Roaf syn·drome** (rōf) a nonhereditary craniofacial-skeletal disorder characterized by congenital or early retinal detachment, cataracts, myopia, shortened long bones, and mental retardation; progressive sensorineural hearing loss is of later onset.

**ro·bert·so·ni·an trans·lo·ca·tion** translocation in which the centromeres of two acrocentric chromosomes appear to have fused, forming an abnormal chromosome consisting of the long arms of two different chromosomes; if the translocation is balanced, the individual is clinically normal but a carrier of the translocation; if the translocation is unbalanced, the individual is trisomic for the long arm of a chromosome. SYN centric fusion. [W.R.B. *Robertson*, U.S. geneticist, *1881]

**Rob·i·now syn·drome** (rob′ĭ-nou) a skeletal dysplasia characterized by bulging forehead, hypertelorism, depressed nasal bridge (so-called fetal face), wide mouth, acromesomelic shortening of limbs, hemivertebrae, and hypoplastic genitalia; there is also an autosomal recessive form.

**Rob·in·son in·dex** an index used to calculate heart work load. SEE ALSO double product.

**Rob·in syn·drome** (rō-bah′) SYN Pierre Robin syndrome.

**ro·bot·ic** (rō-bot′ik) pertaining to or characteristic of a robot, an automatic mechanical device designed to duplicate a human function without direct human operation. [Czech *robot*, robot, fr. *robota*, drudgery, + -ic]

*Ro·cha·li·ma·ea* a genus of bacteria closely resembling *Rickettsia* in staining properties, morphology, and mode of transmission between hosts. Organisms usually reside extracellularly in arthropod hosts and intracellularly in mammalian hosts. The type species is *Rochalimaea quintana*.

**Rock·y Moun·tain spot·ted fe·ver** an acute infectious disease of high mortality, characterized by frontal and occipital headache, intense lumbar pain, malaise, a moderately high continuous fever, and a rash on wrists, palms, ankles, and soles from the second to the fifth day, later spreading to all parts of the body; it occurs in the spring of the year primarily in the southeast U.S. and the Rocky Mountain region, although it is also endemic elsewhere in the U.S., in parts of Canada, in Mexico, and in South America; the pathogenic organism is *Rickettsia rickettsii*, transmitted by two or more tick species of the genus *Dermacentor;* in the U.S. it is spread by *D. andersoni* in the western states and *D. variabilis* (a dog tick) in the eastern states. SYN tick fever (4).

**rod** (rod) **1.** a straight slender cylindrical structure or device. For surgical rods, see nail; pin.. **2.** the photosensitive, outward-directed process of a rhodopsin-containing rod cell in the external granular layer of the retina; many millions of such rods, together with the cones, form the photoreceptive layer of rods and cones. SYN rod cell. [A.S. *rōd*]

**rod cell** SYN rod (2).

**ro·den·ti·cide** (rō-den′ti-sīd) an agent lethal to rodents. [rodent + L. *caedo*, to kill]

**ro·dent ul·cer** a slowly enlarging ulcerated basal cell carcinoma, usually on the face.

**rod gran·ule** the nucleus of a retinal cell connecting with one of the rods.

**Ro·ent·gen** (rent′gen), Wilhelm K., German physicist and Nobel laureate, 1845–1923; discovered x-rays. SEE roentgen, roentgen ray.

**roent·gen (r)** (rent′gen, rent′chen) the international unit of exposure dose for x-rays or gamma rays; that quantity of radiation that will produce in 1 cm of air at STP, or 0.001293 g of air, $2.08 \times 10^9$ ions of both signs, each totaling 1 electrostatic unit (e.s.u.) of charge; in the MKS system this is $2.58 \times 10^{-4}$ coulombs per kg of air. [W. K. *Roentgen*]

**ro·ent·gen-e·quiv·a·lent-man (rem)** a unit of dose equivalent quantity of ionizing radiation of any type that produces in human subjects the same biologic effect as one rad of x-rays or gamma rays; the number of rems is equal to the absorbed dose, measured in rads, multiplied by the quality factor of the radiation in question. 100 rem = 1 Sv.

**roent·gen·o·gram** (rent′gen-ō-gram) SYN radiograph.

**roent·gen·o·graph** (rent′gen-ō-graf) SYN radiograph.

**roent·gen·og·ra·phy** (rent′ge-nog′ră-fē) SYN radiography.

**roent·gen·ol·o·gist** (rent′gen-ol′ō-jist) a person skilled in the diagnostic or therapeutic application of roentgen rays; a radiologist.

**roent·gen·ol·o·gy** (rent′gen-ol′ō-jē) the study of roentgen rays in all their applications. Radiology is the preferred term in the context of medical imaging.

**ro·ent·gen ray** SYN x-ray.

**Roes·ler-Dress·ler in·farct** (rōs′ler-dres′ler) myocardial infarction in dumbbell form involving the anterior and posterior left ventricle and the left side of the ventricular septum.

**Rog·er An·der·son pin fix·a·tion ap·pli·ance** (roj′er an′der-son) an appliance used in extraoral fixation of mandibular fractures and prognathic corrections in which pins placed in the bone segments are joined by metal connecting rods.

**Ro·ger bru·it** (rō-zhā′ broo-ē′) SYN Roger murmur.

**Ro·ger dis·ease** (rō-zhā) a congenital cardiac anomaly consisting of an asymptomatic defect of the interventricular septum, often with a loud murmur and definite thrill.

**Ro·ger mur·mur** (rō-zhā) a loud pansystolic murmur maximal at the left sternal border, caused by a small ventricular septal defect. SYN Roger bruit.

**Rog·ers sphyg·mo·ma·nom·e·ter** (roj′ĕrz) an sphygmomanometer with an aneroid barometer gauge.

**Ro·ki·tan·sky dis·ease** (rō-kĭ-tahn′skē) SYN acute yellow atrophy of the liver.

**Ro·ki·tan·sky her·nia** (rō-kĭ-tahn′skē) a separation of the muscular fibers of the bowel allowing protrusion of a sac of the mucous membrane.

**Ro·ki·tan·sky pel·vis** (rō-kĭ-tahn′skē) SYN spondylolisthetic pelvis.

**ro·lan·dic** (rō-lan′dik) relating to or described by Luigi Rolando.

**ro·lan·dic ep·i·lep·sy** a benign, autosomal dominant form of epilepsy occurring in children, characterized clinically by arrest of speech, by muscular contractions of the side of the face and arm, and by epileptic discharges electroencephalographically. [Luigi *Rolando*]

**Ro·lan·do ar·ea** (rō-lahn-dō) SYN motor cortex.

**role** (rōl) the pattern of behavior that one exhibits in relationship to significant persons with whom one has or had primary relationships. [Fr.]

**role-play·ing** a psychotherapeutic method used in psychodrama to understand and treat emotional conflicts through the enactment or reenactment of stressful interpersonal events. SEE ALSO psychodrama.

**rol·ler·ball e·lec·trode** a ball electrode that rolls like a paint roller over surface tissue, cauterizing it; used in endometrial ablation.

**rol·ler ban·dage** a strip of material, of variable

width, rolled into a compact cylinder to facilitate its application.

**Rol·let stro·ma** (rol′et) the colorless stroma of the red blood cells.

**ROM** range of motion.

**Ro·ma·ña sign** (rō-mahn′yah) marked edema of one or both eyelids, usually a unilateral palpebral edema, thought to be a sensitization response to the bite of a triatomine bug infected with *Trypanosoma cruzi*, and a strong suggestion of acute Chagas disease.

**Ro·ma·now·sky blood stain** (rō-mah-nof′skē) prototype of the eosin-methylene blue stains for blood smears, using aqueous solutions made of a mixture of methylene blue (saturated) and eosin. Romanowsky-type stains depend for their action on compounds formed by interaction of methylene blue and eosin; most are of no value if water is present in the alcohol because neutral dyes become precipitated.

**rom·berg·ism** (rom′berg-izm) SYN Romberg sign.

**Rom·berg sign** (rom′bĕrg) with feet approximated, the patient stands with eyes open and then closed; if closing the eyes increases the unsteadiness, a loss of proprioceptive control is indicated, and the sign is present. SYN rombergism.

**ron·geur** (rawn-zhĕr′) a strong biting forceps for nipping away bone. [Fr. *ronger*, to gnaw]

**Rön·ne na·sal step** (rĕr′nĕ) a nasal visual field defect with one margin corresponding to the retinal horizontal medium; seen in glaucoma.

**roof** (roof) a covering or rooflike structure; e.g., a tectorium, tectum, tegmen, tegmentum, integument. [A.S. *hrōf*]

**roof plate, roof·plate** (roof′plāt) the thin layer of the embryonic neural tube connecting the alar plates dorsally.

**room·ing-in** (room′ing-in) placement of newborn with mother, rather than in nursery, during the postpartum hospital stay.

**root** (root) **1.** the primary or beginning portion of any part, as of a nerve at its origin from the brainstem or spinal cord. SYN radix (1) [TA]. **2.** SYN root of tooth. **3.** the descending underground portion of a plant; it absorbs water and nutrients, provides support, and stores nutrients. [A.S. rot]

**root am·pu·ta·tion** surgical removal of one or more roots of a multirooted tooth, the remaining root canal(s) usually being treated endodontically. SYN radectomy, radiectomy, radisectomy.

**root ca·nal of tooth** the chamber of the dental pulp lying within the root portion of a tooth. SYN canalis radicis dentis [TA], pulp canal.

**root car·ies in·dex** the ratio of the number of teeth with carious lesions of the root, and/or restorations of the root, to the number of teeth with exposed root surfaces.

**root-form im·plant** an implant shaped like the root of a tooth.

**root·ing re·flex** in infants, rubbing or scratching about the mouth causes a puckering of the lips.

**root of lung** all the structures entering or leaving the lung at the hilum, forming a pedicle invested with the pleura; includes the bronchi, pulmonary artery and veins, bronchial arteries and veins, lymphatics, and nerves.

**root of nail** the proximal end of the nail, concealed under a fold of skin.

**root of pe·nis** the proximal attached part of the penis, including the two crura and the bulb.

**root pulp** that part of the dental pulp contained within the apical or root portion of the tooth.

**root re·sec·tion** SYN apicoectomy.

**root sheath** one of the epidermic layers of the hair follicle: external root sheath is continuous with the stratum basale and stratum spinosum of the epidermis; internal root sheath comprises the cuticle of the internal roots, Huxley layer, and Henle layer.

**root of tongue** the posterior attached portion of the tongue.

**root of tooth** that part of a tooth below the neck, covered by cementum rather than enamel, and attached by the periodontal ligament to the alveolar bone. SYN radix (2) [TA], root (2).

**ROP** right occipitoposterior position.

**ro·sa·ce·a** (rō-zā′shē-ă) chronic vascular and follicular dilation involving the nose and contiguous portions of the cheeks with erythema, hyperplasia of sebaceous glands, deep-seated papules and pustules, and telangiectasia. See page B6. SYN acne erythematosa, acne rosacea. [L. *rosaceus*, rosy]

**Ro·sai-Dorf·man dis·ease** (rō-zī-dorf′mĕn) SYN sinus histiocytosis with massive lymphadenopathy.

**ro·sa·ry** (rō′zer-ē) a beadlike arrangement or structure.

**rose ben·gal** (rōz′ ben′găl) [C.I. 45440] a fluorescein derivative used as a biologic stain.

**Ro·sen·bach law** (rō-zĕn-bahk) **1.** in affections of the nerve trunks or nerve centers, paralysis of the flexor muscles appears later than that of the extensors; **2.** in cases of abnormal stimulation of organs with rhythmical functional periodicity, there is often a grouping of the individual acts with corresponding lengthening of the pauses, in such a way that the proportion of total rest and activity remains nearly the same.

**Ro·sen·bach sign** (rō-zĕn-bahk) loss of the abdominal reflexes in cases of acute inflammation of the viscera.

**Ro·sen·mül·ler gland** (rō-zĕn-mŭ-ler) SYN proximal deep inguinal lymph node.

**Ro·sen·mül·ler node** (rō-zĕn-mŭ-ler) SYN proximal deep inguinal lymph node.

**Ro·sen·thal ca·nal** (rō-zen-tahl) SYN spiral canal of cochlea.

**ro·se·o·la** (rō-zē′ō-lă) a symmetrical eruption of small, closely aggregated patches of rose-red color. It is believed to be caused by human herpesvirus type 6. SEE ALSO exanthema subitum. [Mod. L. dim. of L. *roseus*, rosy]

**ro·se·o·la in·fan·ti·lis, ro·se·o·la in·fan·tum** SYN exanthema subitum.

**Rose po·si·tion** (rōz) the patient lies supine with the head falling down over the end of the table; used in operations within the mouth or pharynx.

**rose spots** characteristic exanthema of typhoid fever; 10–20 small pink papules on the lower trunk lasting a few days and leaving hyperpigmentation.

**ro·sette** (rō-zet′) **1.** the quartan malarial parasite *Plasmodium malariae* in its segmented or mature phase. **2.** a grouping of cells characteristic of neoplasms of neuroblastic or neuroectodermal origin; a number of nuclei form a ring from which neurofibrils, which can be demonstrated by silver impregnation, extend to interlace in the center. **3.** roselike coiling of the uterus among certain pseudophyllidean tapeworms, such as *Diphyllobothrium latum*. [Fr. a little rose]

**ros•in** (roz'in) the solid resin obtained after steam distillation of crude balsam from species of *Pinus;* used in plasters to render them adhesive and also in ointments to render them locally stimulating. SYN resin (2).

**Ro spat•u•la** (rō) a very small nickeled steel spatula used to transfer bits of infected material, such as diphtheritic membrane, to culture tubes.

**Ros•so•li•mo re•flex, Ros•so•li•mo sign** (ros-ō-lē'mō) flicking the tops of the toes from the plantar surface causes flexion of the toes; a stretch reflex of the flexors of the toes seen in lesions of the pyramidal tracts. SEE ALSO Starling reflex.

**Ross pro•ce•dure** (ros) procedure for aortic valve stenosis or regurgitation in which the aortic valve is replaced with the patient's own pulmonic valve (autograft) and the pulmonic valve is in turn replaced with a homograft valve.

**Ross Riv•er vi•rus** (rŏs rī'ver) a mosquito-borne alphavirus, family Togaviridae, that causes epidemic polyarthritis.

**ros•tel•lum** (ros-tel'ŭm) the anterior fixed or invertible portion of the scolex of a tapeworm, frequently provided with a row (or several rows) of hooks. [L. dim. of *rostrum,* a beak]

**ros•trad** (ros'trăd) **1.** in a direction toward any rostrum. **2.** situated nearer a rostrum or the snout end of an organism in relation to a specific reference point; opposite of caudad (2). [L. *rostrum,* beak, + *-ad,* toward]

**ros•tral** (ros'trăl) relating to any rostrum or anatomical structure resembling a beak. [L. *rostralis,* fr. *rostrum,* beak]

**ros•trate** (ros'trāt) having a beak or hook. [L. *rostratus*]

**ros•trum**, pl. **ros•tra, ros•trums** (ros'trŭm, ros' tră) any beak-shaped structure. [L. a beak]

**ROT** right occipitotransverse position.

**rot** to decay or putrify. [A.S. *rotian*]

**ro•ta•mase** (rō'ta-māz) enzyme capable of altering the rotational conformation of a molecule.

**ro•ta•mer** (rō'ta-mer) an isomer differing from other conformation(s) only in rotational positioning of its parts, such as *cis*- and *trans*- forms.

**ro•ta•ry joint, ro•ta•to•ry joint** SYN pivot joint.

**ro•tat•ing an•ode** in diagnostic radiography, modern x-ray tubes that have a mushroom-shaped anode that rotates rapidly to avoid local heat buildup from electron impact during x-ray generation.

**ro•ta•tion** (rō-tā'shŭn) **1.** turning or movement of a body around its axis. **2.** a recurrence in regular order of certain events, such as the symptoms of a periodic disease. **3.** in medical education, a period of time on a particular service or specialty. [L. *rotatio,* fr. *roto,* pp. *rotatus,* to revolve, rotate]

**ro•ta•tion•al nys•tag•mus** jerky nystagmus arising from stimulation of the labyrinth by rotation of the head around any axis and induced by change of motion.

**ro•ta•tion flap** a pedicle flap that is rotated from the donor site to an adjacent recipient area, usually as a direct flap.

**ro•ta•tor** (rō-tā'ter) a muscle by which a part can be turned circularly. [L. See rotation]

**ro•ta•tor cuff of shoul•der** the upper half of the capsule of the shoulder joint reinforced by the

tendons of insertion of the supraspinatus, infraspinatus, teres minor, and subscapularis muscles.

**ro•ta•to•res mus•cles** deepest of the three layers of transversospinalis muscles, chiefly developed in the thoracic region; they arise from the transverse process of one vertebra and are inserted into the root of the spinous process of the next two or three vertebrae above; *action,* traditionally described as a column, it is more likely that these muscles, provided with a very high density of muscle spindles, are organs of proprioception; *nerve supply,* dorsal primary rami of the spinal nerves. SYN musculi rotatores [TA].

**ro•ta•to•ry nys•tag•mus** a movement of the eyes around the visual axis.

**Ro•ta•vi•rus** (rō'tă-vī'rŭs) a genus of RNA viruses that includes the human gastroenteritis viruses (a major cause of infant diarrhea throughout the world). SYN gastroenteritis virus type B. [L. *rota,* wheel, + virus]

**Rotch sign** (roch) in pericardial effusion, percussion dullness in the fifth intercostal space on the right.

**rote learn•ing** the learning of arbitrary relationships, usually by repetition of the learning procedure through memorization and without an understanding of the relationships.

**Roth•mund syn•drome** (rōt'moond) atrophy, pigmentation, and telangiectasia of the skin, usually with juvenile cataract, saddle nose, congenital bone defects, disturbance of hair growth, hypogonadism; autosomal recessive inheritance.

**Roth spot** (rōt) a round white retinal spot surrounded by hemorrhage in bacterial endocarditis, and in other retinal hemorrhagic conditions.

**Ro•tor syn•drome** (rō'tōr) jaundice appearing in childhood due to impaired biliary excretion; most of the plasma bilirubin is conjugated, liver function tests are usually normal, and there is no hepatic pigmentation.

**ro•to•sco•li•o•sis** (rō'tō-skō-lē-ō'sis) combined lateral and rotational deviation of the vertebral column. [L. *roto,* to rotate, + G. *skoliōsis,* crookedness]

**ro•to•tome** (rō'tō-tōm) a rotating cutting instrument used in arthroscopic surgery.

**Rou•get bulb** (roo-zhā') a venous plexus on the surface of the ovary.

**rough•age** (rŭf'ij) anything in the diet, e.g., bran, serving as a bulk stimulant of intestinal peristalsis.

**rou•leaux for•ma•tion** the arrangement of red blood cells in fluid blood (or in diluted suspensions) with their biconcave surfaces in apposition, thereby forming groups that resemble stacks of coins. See page B2. [Fr. pl. of *rouleau,* a roll]

**round•ed at•el•ec•ta•sis, round at•el•ec•ta•sis** an area of atelectatic lung caused by parenchymal infolding due to pleural fibrosis, most often from asbestos exposure; appears as a masslike opacity and can be mistaken for lung cancer; may be associated with a comet tail sign; high level of contrast enhancement on dynamic computed tomography aids diagnosis.

**round heart** abnormally smooth arcuate contours of the heart due either to disease of the ventricles or to a false cardiac appearance produced by excessive pericardial fluid.

**round lig•a•ment of fe•mur** SYN ligament of head of femur.

**round lig•a•ment of liv•er** the remains of the

umbilical vein running within the free edge of the falciform ligament from the umbilicus to the liver, where it continues within the fissure for the round ligament to the origin of the left portal vein within the porta hepatis. SYN ligamentum teres hepatis [TA].

**round lig·a·ment of uter·us** a fibromuscular band that is attached to the uterus on either side in front of and below the opening of the uterine tube; it passes through the inguinal canal to the labium majus. SYN ligamentum teres uteri [TA].

**round win·dow** SYN fenestra cochleae.

**round win·dow mem·brane** SYN secondary tympanic membrane.

**round·worm** (rownd′werm) a nematode member of the phylum Nematoda, commonly confined to the parasitic forms.

**Rous-as·so·ci·at·ed vi·rus (RAV)** (rous) a leukemia virus of the leukosis-sarcoma complex which by phenotypic mixing with a defective (noninfectious) strain of Rous sarcoma virus effects production of infectious sarcoma virus with envelope antigenicity of the RAV.

**Rous sar·co·ma vi·rus (RSV)** (rous) a sarcoma-producing virus of the avian leukosis-sarcoma complex identified by Rous in 1911.

**Roux-en-Y a·nas·to·mo·sis** (roo-en-wī) anastomosis of the distal end of the divided jejunum to the stomach, bile duct, or another structure, with implantation of the proximal end into the side of the jejunum at a suitable distance below the first anastomosis, the bowel then forming a Y-shaped pattern.

**Roux meth·od** (roo) division of the mandible in the median line, to facilitate the operation of ablation of the tongue.

**Rov·sing sign** (rov′sing) pain at McBurney point induced in cases of appendicitis, by pressure exerted over the descending colon.

**RPE** rating of perceived exertion.

**RPF** renal plasma flow. SEE effective renal plasma flow.

**RPI** reticulocyte production index.

**rpm** revolutions per minute.

**RPO** right posterior oblique, a radiographic position in which the right posterior side of the body part is closest to the film.

**RQ** respiratory quotient.

△**-rrha·gia** excessive or unusual discharge. [G. *rhēgnymi*, to burst forth]

△**-rrha·phy** surgical suturing. [G. *rhaphē*, suture]

△**-rrhea** a flowing; a flux. [G. *rhoia*, a flow]

**rRNA** ribosomal ribonucleic acid.

**RSA** right sacroanterior position.

**RSD** reflex sympathetic dystrophy.

**RSP** right sacroposterior position.

**RST** right sacrotransverse position.

**RSV** Rous sarcoma virus.

**rTMP** ribothymidylic acid.

**RT-PCR** reverse transcriptase polymerase chain reaction.

**Ru** ruthenium.

**rub** (rŭb) friction encountered in moving one body over another.

**rub·ber-bulb sy·ringe** a syringe with a hollow rubber bulb and cannula provided with a check valve, used to obtain a jet of air or water.

**rub·ber dam clamp for·ceps** SYN clamp forceps.

**rub·ber-shod clamp** a small rubber-tipped clamp that holds sutures in place during surgery.

**ru·be·do** (roo-bē′dō) a temporary redness of the skin. [L. redness, fr. *ruber,* red]

**ru·be·fa·cient** (roo-bē-fā′shent) **1.** causing a reddening of the skin. **2.** a counterirritant that produces erythema when applied to the skin surface. [L. *rubi-facio,* fr. *ruber,* red, + *facio,* to make]

**ru·be·fac·tion** (roo-bē-fak′shŭn) erythema of the skin caused by local application of a counterirritant. [see rubefacient]

**ru·bel·la** (roo-bel′ă) an acute exanthematous disease caused by rubella virus (*Rubivirus*), with enlargement of lymph nodes, but usually with little fever or constitutional reaction; a high incidence of birth defects in children results from maternal infection during the first several months of fetal life (congenital rubella syndrome). SYN epidemic roseola, German measles, third disease. [L. *rubellus,* fem. -*a,* reddish, dim. of *ruber,* red]

**ru·bel·la HI test** a hemagglutination inhibition (HI) test for rubella, often performed routinely as part of a prenatal workup of the pregnant woman; the presence of any detectable HI titer in the absence of disease indicates previous infection and immunity to reinfection.

**ru·bel·la vi·rus** an RNA virus of the genus *Rubivirus;* the agent causing rubella (German measles) in humans. SYN German measles virus.

**ru·be·o·la** (roo-bē-ō′lă) SYN measles (1). [Mod. L. dim. of *ruber,* red, reddish]

**ru·be·o·la vi·rus** SYN measles virus.

**ru·be·o·sis** (roo-bē-ō′sis) reddish discoloration, as of the skin. [L. *ruber,* red, + G. -*osis,* condition]

**ru·be·o·sis ir·i·dis di·a·be·ti·ca** neovascularization of the anterior surface of the iris in diabetes mellitus.

**ru·bes·cent** (roo-bes′ent) reddening. [L. *rubesco,* pr. p. *rubescens,* to become red]

**ru·bid·i·um** (roo-bid′ē-ŭm) an alkali element, atomic no. 37, atomic wt. 85.4678; its salts have been used in medicine for the same purposes as the corresponding sodium or potassium salts. [L. *rubidus,* reddish, dark red, fr. *rubeo,* to be red]

**ru·bid·o·my·cin** (roo-bid′ō-mī-sin) an antibiotic used as an antineoplastic; similar to doxorubicin in antitumor activity and in exhibiting cumulative cardiotoxicity. SYN daunorubicin.

*Ru·bi·vi·rus* (roo′bi-vī′rŭs) a genus of viruses that includes the rubella virus. [*rubella* + virus]

**Rub·ner laws of growth** (roob′nĕr) **1.** the law of constant energy consumption: the rapidity of growth is proportional to the intensity of the metabolic processes; **2.** the law of the constant growth quotient: in most young mammals, 24% of the entire food energy, or calories, is used for growth; in humans, only 5% is thus used.

**ru·bor** (roo′bōr) redness of skin or mucous membrane, as one of the four signs of hyperemia or inflammation (r., calor, dolor, tumor) enunciated by Celsus. [L.]

**ru·bre·dox·ins** (roo-brĕ-dok′sinz) ferredoxins without acid-labile sulfur and with the iron in a typical mercaptide coordination.

**ru·bri·blast** (roo′bri-blast) SYN pronormoblast. [L. *ruber,* red, + G. *blastos,* germ]

**ru·bri·cyte** (roo′bri-sīt) polychromatic normoblast. SEE erythroblast. [L. *ruber,* red, + *kytos,* cell]

**ru·bro·spi·nal de·cus·sa·tion** SEE tegmental decussations (2).

r
u

**Ru·bu·la·vi·rus** (roo-boo′la-vī-rŭs) a genus in the family Paramyxoviridae; causes mumps.

**ru·di·ment** (roo′di-ment) **1.** an organ or structure that is incompletely developed. **2.** the first indication of a structure in the course of ontogeny. SYN rudimentum. [L. *rudimentum*, a beginning, fr. *rudis*, unformed]

**ru·di·men·ta·ry** (roo-di-men′tār-ē) relating to a rudiment. SYN abortive (2).

**ru·di·men·tum**, pl. **ru·di·men·ta** (roo′di-men′ tŭm, roo′di-men-tă) SYN rudiment, rudiment. [L.]

**Rud syn·drome** (rood) ichthyosiform erythroderma associated with acanthosis nigricans, dwarfism, hypogonadism, and epilepsy; mostly sporadic, but may be an X-linked recessive trait.

**Ruf·fi·ni cor·pus·cle** (roo-fē′nē) sensory endstructure in the subcutaneous connective tissues of the fingers, consisting of an ovoid capsule within which the sensory fiber ends with numerous collateral knobs.

**ru·fous** (roo′fŭs) SYN erythristic. [L. *rufus*, reddish]

**RUG** Resource Utilization Group.

**ru·ga**, pl. **ru·gae** (roo′gă, roo′gē) [TA] a fold, ridge, or crease; a wrinkle. [L. a wrinkle]

**ru·gae of stom·ach** characteristic folds of the gastric mucosa, especially evident when the stomach is contracted.

**ru·gine** (roo-zhēn′) **1.** SYN periosteal elevator. **2.** a raspatory. [Fr.]

**ru·gose** (roo′gōs) marked by rugae; wrinkled. SYN rugous. [L. *rugosus*]

**ru·gos·i·ty** (roo-gos′i-tē) **1.** the state of being thrown into folds or wrinkles. **2.** a ruga.

**ru·gous** (roo′gŭs) SYN rugose.

**Ruhe·mann pur·ple** (roo′-mahn) a blue-violet dye formed in the reaction of ninhydrin with amino acids.

**RUL** right upper lobe (of lung).

**rule** (rool) a criterion, standard, or guide governing a procedure, arrangement, action, etc. SEE ALSO law, principle, theorem. [O. Fr. *reule*, fr. L. *regula*, a guide, pattern]

**rule of bi·gem·i·ny** rule that a ventricular premature beat will follow the beat terminating a long cycle. Sudden prolongation of the ventricular cycle, by changing the refractoriness in the conduction system, causes a peripheral region of bidirectional block to become transiently unidirectional and thus opens potential pathways for reentry to occur.

**rule of nines** method used in calculating body surface area involved in burns whereby values of 9 or 18% of surface area are assigned to specific regions as follows: Head and neck, 9%; anterior thorax, 18%; posterior thorax, 18%; arms, 9% each; legs, 18% each; perineum 1%.

**rule of out·let** an obstetric rule for determining whether the pelvic outlet will permit the passage of a fetus; the sum of the posterior sagittal diameter and the transverse diameter of the outlet must equal at least 15 cm if a normal-sized baby is to pass.

*Ru·mi·no·coc·cus* (roo′mĭ-nō-kok′ŭs) a genus of anaerobic, Gram-positive coccobacilli isolated from the respiratory tract of humans and the intestinal tract of humans and animals. The type species is *Ruminococcus productus*, formerly *Peptostreptococcus productus*.

**run** (rŭn) a group of successive measurements in an analytic process or during a period of time within which the accuracy and precision of the measuring system are expected to be stable. [ME *runnen*, fr. A. S. *rinnan*, fr. O.N. *rinna*]

**run·a·way pace·mak·er** rapid heart rates over 140/min caused by electronic circuit instability in an implanted pulse generator.

**run·ner's blad·der** hematuria caused by running rapidly with an empty bladder.

**run·ner's knee** an overuse syndrome of anterior knee pain associated with excessive lateral motion of the patella during activity. SYN patellofemoral stress syndrome.

**Run·yon clas·si·fi·ca·tion** a classification scheme for mycobacteria other than *Mycobacterium tuberculosis* that divides species into four categories: 1) photochromogens, species that produce a yellow to brown carotene pigment when grown in the presence of light; 2) scotochromogens, which produce pigment in presence or absence of light; 3) nonpigmented, which do not produce pigment; and 4) rapid growers, which grow on solid media in 5–10 days rather than 4–8 weeks. This classification has no clinical or genetic significance but remains of limited value in identification of some clinical isolates.

**Run·yon group I my·co·bac·te·ria** (run′yŏn) mycobacteria that produce a bright yellow color when grown in the presence of light. Organisms placed in this group include *Mycobacterium kansasii*.

**Run·yon group II my·co·bac·te·ria** (run′yŏn) mycobacteria that produce a yellow pigment even when grown in the dark; when grown in the light, the pigment is orange. These organisms behave as saprophytes do in humans and are usually nonpathogenic to laboratory animals.

**Run·yon group III my·co·bac·te·ria** (run′ eyŏn) mycobacteria that are either colorless or that slowly produce a light yellow pigment when grown in the presence of light. Organisms placed in this group include *Mycobacterium avium* and *Mycobacterium intracellulare*.

**Run·yon group IV my·co·bac·te·ria** (run′yŏn) mycobacteria that grow rapidly and that do not produce pigment. Organisms placed in this group belong to such species as *Mycobacterium ulcerans* and *M. marinum*.

**ru·pia** (roo′pē-ă) **1.** ulcers of late secondary syphilis, covered with yellowish or brown crusts. **2.** SYN yaws. **3.** term occasionally used to designate a very scaly, heaped-up, and secondarily infected psoriatic lesion. [G. *rhypos*, filth]

**ru·pi·al** (roo′pē-ăl) relating to rupia.

**rup·ture** (rŭp′cher) **1.** SYN hernia. **2.** a solution of continuity or a tear; a break of any organ or other of the soft parts. [L. *ruptura*, a fracture (of limb or vein), fr. *rumpo*, pp. *ruptus*, to break]

**rup·tured disk** SYN herniated disk.

**RUQ** right upper quadrant (of abdomen).

**Rus·sell bod·ies** (rus′ĕl) small, discrete, variably sized, spherical, intracytoplasmic, acidophilic, hyaline bodies that stain deeply with fuchsin; they occur frequently in plasma cells in chronic inflammation.

**Rus·sell Per·i·o·don·tal In·dex** (rus′ĕl) an index that estimates the degree of periodontal disease present in the mouth by measuring both bone loss around the teeth and gingival inflammation; used in the epidemiologic investigation of periodontal disease.

**Rus·sell sign** (rus′ĕl) abrasions and scars on the

back of the hands of individuals with bulimia, usually due to manual attempts at self-induced vomiting.

**Rus·sell's vi·per ven·om** (rus'elz vī'pĕr) a venom derived from Russell's viper (*Vipera russelli*), which acts as an intrinsic thromboplastin; used in the laboratory evaluation of deficiencies of factor X or topically to arrest local hemorrhage in hemophilia.

**Rus·sell's vi·per ven·om clot·ting time** a clotting time determination performed on citrated platelet-poor plasma using Russell's viper venom as an activating agent. This allows activation of factor X directly without the need for other coagulation factors and is used to confirm factor X defects.

**Rus·sell syn·drome** (rus'ĕl) failure of infants and young children to thrive due to suprasellar lesions, commonly astrocytomas of the anterior third ventricle; although the growth hormone may be elevated, the child is emaciated and has loss of body fat.

**Rust phe·nom·e·non** (roost) in cancer or caries of the upper cervical vertebrae, the patient will always support the head by the hands when changing from the recumbent to the sitting posture or the reverse.

**rusts** (rŭsts) species of *Puccinia* and other microbes comprising important pathogens of plants, especially cereal grains; they are important allergens for humans when inhaled in large numbers, as in harvesting processes.

**rust·y spu·tum** a reddish brown, blood-stained expectoration characteristic of pneumonococcal lobar pneumonia.

**ru·the·ni·um (Ru)** (roo-thē'nē-ŭm) a metallic element of the platinum group; atomic no. 44, atomic wt. 101.07; $^{106}$Ru, with a half-life of 1.020 years, has been used in the treatment of certain eye problems. [Mediev. L. *Ruthenia,* Russia, where first obtained]

**ru·ti·do·sis** (roo-ti-dō'sis) SYN rhytidosis.

**Ruysch mem·brane** (roish) SYN choriocapillary layer.

**Ruysch tube** (roish) a minute tubular cavity opening in the lower and anterior portion of each surface of the nasal septum.

**RV** residual volume.

**R wave** the first positive (upward) deflection of the QRS complex in the electrocardiogram; successive upward deflections within the same QRS complex are labeled R', R'', etc.

**r** *recipe* in a prescription. SEE prescription (2).

**ry·an·o·dine re·cep·tor** receptor associated with a calcium conductance channel in the sarcoplasmic or endoplasmic reticulum of cells, which when bound to ryanodine, causes the channel to remain in a subconductive state, allowing slow continuing release of calcium ions from the sarcoplasmic reticulum into the cytoplasm. The channels are normally sensitive to calcium ions and not sensitive to inositol triphosphate.

**Ry·an stain** (rī-an) a modified trichrome stain for microsporidian spores in which the chromotrope 2R is 10 times the normal concentration used in trichrome stains for stool specimens and the counterstain is aniline blue.

**Ryle tube** (rīl) a thin rubber tube, with about the lumen of a no. 8 catheter, and an olive-tipped extremity, used in giving a test meal.

**r**
**y**

# S

σ, Σ sigma.

**S 1.** sacral vertebra (S1 to S5); spherical or spherical lens; Svedberg unit. **2.** siemens; sulfur; entropy in thermodynamics; substrate in the Michaelis-Menton mechanism; percentage saturation of hemoglobin (when followed by subscript $O_2$ or CO); serine; one of the two stereochemical designations (in italics) in the Cahn-Ingold-Prelog system. **3.** designation of a rare human antigen (hemagglutinogen) related genetically to the MNSs blood group. See Blood Groups appendix.

*S* entropy.

**s 1.** *sinister*, left; L. *semis*, half; second; as a subscript, denotes steady state.

*s* selection coefficient; sedimentation coefficient.

**S₁** first heart sound.

**S₂** second heart sound.

**S₃** third heart sound.

**S₄** fourth heart sound.

**S100** an acidic, calcium-binding protein characterized by its partial solubility in saturated ammonium sulfate; stains for S100 are used in the differential diagnosis of melanomas, which are commonly positive for S100.

**S_f** flotation constant.

**S-A** sinoatrial; sinuatrial.

**SA** sacroanterior position.

**sa•ber tib•ia, sa•ber shin** deformity of the tibia occurring in tertiary syphilis or yaws, the bone having a marked forward convexity as a result of the formation of gummas and periostitis.

**Sa•bia vi•rus** an arenavirus associated with hemolytic fever.

**Sa•bou•raud a•gar** (sah-boo-rō′) a culture medium for fungi containing neopeptone or polypeptone agar and glucose, with final pH 5.6; it is the standard, most universally used medium in mycology and is the international reference. Modified Sabouraud agar (Emmons modification) with neutral pH and less glucose is better for pigment development in the colonies.

**Sa•bou•raud dex•trose a•gar** (sah-boo-rō′) a dextrose peptone medium that supports the growth of most pathogenic fungi.

**Sa•bou•raud pas•tils** (sah-boo-rō′) disks containing barium platinocyanide that undergo a color change when exposed to x-rays; previously used to indicate the administered dose.

**sab•u•lous** (sab′yu-lŭs) sandy; gritty. [L. *sabulosus,* fr. *sabulum,* coarse sand]

**sac** (sak) **1.** a pouch or bursa. SEE sacculus. **2.** an encysted abscess at the root of a tooth. **3.** the capsule of a tumor, or envelope of a cyst. SYN saccus. [L. *saccus,* a bag]

**sac•cad•ic** (să-kad′ik) jerky.

**sac•cate** (sak′āt) relating to a sac. [L. *saccus,* sac]

**sac•cha•rides** (sak′ă-rīdz) a group of carbohydrates that includes the sugars. Saccharides are classified as mono-, di-, tri-, and polysaccharides according to the number of saccharide units ($C_6H_{10}O_5$) composing them. SEE ALSO carbohydrates.

**sac•cha•rif•er•ous** (sak′ă-rif′er-ŭs) producing sugar.

△**sac•cha•ro-, sac•char-, sac•cha•ri-** combining forms denoting sugar (saccharide). [G. *sak-charon,* sugar]

**sac•cha•ro•lyt•ic** (sak′ă-rō-lit′ik) capable of hydrolyzing or otherwise breaking down a sugar molecule. [saccharo- + G. *lysis,* loosening]

**sac•cha•ro•met•a•bol•ic** (sak′ă-rō-met′ă-bol′ik) relating to saccharometabolism.

**sac•cha•ro•me•tab•o•lism** (sak-ă-rō-mĕ-tab′ō-lizm) metabolism of sugar; the process of utilization of sugar in cells.

**sac•cha•rose** (sak′ă-rōs) SYN sucrose.

**sac•ci•form** (sak′si-fōrm) pouched; sac-shaped. SYN saccular. [L. *saccus,* sack, + *forma,* form]

**sac•cu•lar** (sak′yu-lăr) SYN sacciform.

**sac•cu•lar an•eu•rysm, sac•cu•lat•ed an•eu•rysm** a saclike bulging on one side of an artery.

**sac•cu•lar gland** a single alveolar gland.

**sac•cu•lar nerve** a branch of the vestibular nerve going to the macula of the sacculus. SYN nervus saccularis [TA].

**sac•cu•la•tion** (sak′yu-lā′shŭn) **1.** a structure formed by a group of sacs. **2.** the formation of a sac or pouch.

**sac•cule** (sak′yul) **1.** the smaller of the two membranous sacs in the vestibule of the labyrinth, lying in the spherical recess; it is connected with the cochlear duct by a very short tube, the ductus reuniens, and with the utriculus by the beginning of the ductus endolymphaticus and the ductus utriculosaccularis that joins it. **2.** the immense bag-shaped structure formed by peptidoglycans as part of the cell wall of certain microorganisms. SYN sacculus [TA]. [L. *sacculus*]

**sac•cule of la•rynx** a small diverticulum provided with mucous glands extending upward from the ventricle of the larynx between the vestibular fold and the lamina of the thyroid cartilage. SYN sacculus laryngis.

**sac•cu•lo•co•chle•ar** (sak′yu-lō-kok′lē-ăr) relating to the sacculus and the membranous cochlea.

**sac•cu•lus,** pl. **sac•cu•li** (sak′yu-lŭs, sak′yu-lī) [TA] SYN saccule. [L. dim. of *saccus,* sac]

**sac•cu•lus al•ve•o•la•ris,** pl. **sac•cu•li al•ve•o•la•res** [TA] SYN alveolar sac.

**sac•cu•lus la•ryn•gis** SYN saccule of larynx.

**sac•cus,** pl. **sac•ci** (sak′ŭs, sak′sī) SYN sac. [L. a bag, sack]

**sac•cus con•junc•ti•va•lis** [TA] SYN conjunctival sac.

**sac•cus en•do•lym•pha•ti•cus** [TA] SYN endolymphatic sac.

**sac•cus la•cri•ma•lis** [TA] SYN lacrimal sac.

**sa•crad** (sā′krad) in the direction of the sacrum. [sacr- + L. *ad,* to]

**sa•cral** (sā′krăl) relating to or in the neighborhood of the sacrum.

**sa•cral ca•nal** the continuation of the vertebral canal in the sacrum. SYN canalis sacralis [TA].

**sa•cral crest** one of three rough irregular ridges on the posterior surface of the sacrum; median sacral crest; lateral sacral crests.

**sa•cral flex•ure** SYN caudal flexure.

**sa•cral flex•ure of rec•tum** the anteroposterior curve with concavity anteriorward of the first portion of the rectum.

**sa•cral fo•ra•men** [TA] one of the openings between the fused sacral vertebrae transmitting the sacral nerves. The anterior sacral foramina transmit ventral primary rami of the sacral nerves. The posterior sacral foramina give passage to dorsal primary rami of the sacral nerves.

**sa·cral·gia** (sā-kral′jē-ă) pain in the sacral region. SYN sacrodynia. [sacr- + G. *algos,* pain]

**sa·cral ky·pho·sis** [TA] the normal, anteriorly concave curvature of the sacrum (sacral segment of the vertebral column), in which the primary curvature of the fetal embryo is maintained into maturity.

**sa·cral nerves [S1–S5]** five nerves issuing from the sacral foramina on either side; the ventral branches of the first three enter into the formation of the sacral plexus, and the last two into the coccygeal plexus. SYN nervi sacrales [TA].

**sa·cral plex·us** interconnected roots of the L4-S4 spinal nerves that innervate the lower extremities. SEE ALSO brachial plexus.

**sa·cral splanch·nic nerves** branches from the sacral sympathetic trunk that pass to the inferior hypogastric plexus; part of the abdominopelvic (sympathetic) splanchnic nerves, but their specific function is unclear. They tend to be confused with the pelvic splanchnic nerves, which are much more significant structures. SYN nervi splanchnici sacrales [TA].

**sa·cral ver·te·brae [S1–S5]** the segments of the vertebral column, usually five in number, that fuse to form the sacrum. SYN vertebrae sacrales [S1–S5].

**sa·crec·to·my** (sā-krek′tō-mē) resection of a portion of the sacrum to facilitate an operation. [sacr- + G. *ektomē,* excision]

△**sa·cro-, sacr-** muscular substance; resemblance to flesh. [L. *os sacrum,* sacred bone]

**sa·cro·an·te·ri·or po·si·tion (SA)** a breech presentation of the fetus with the sacrum pointing to the right (**right sacroanterior**, RSA) or to the left (**left sacroanterior**, LSA) acetabulum of the mother.

**sa·cro·coc·cyg·e·al** (sā-krō-kok-sij′ē-ăl) relating to both sacrum and coccyx.

**sa·cro·col·po·pex·y pro·ce·dure** support of the vaginal vault by affixing it to the periosteum of the sacrum following a hysterectomy. [sacro- + colpo- + -pexy]

**sa·cro·dyn·ia** (sā′krō-din′ē-ă) SYN sacralgia. [sacro- + G. *odynē,* pain]

**sa·cro·il·i·ac** (sā-krō-il′ē-ak) relating to the sacrum and the ilium.

**sa·cro·lum·bar** (sā′krō-lŭm′băr) SYN lumbosacral.

**sa·cro·pos·te·ri·or po·si·tion (SP)** a breech presentation of the fetus with the sacrum pointing to the right (**right sacroposterior**, RSP) or to the left (**left sacroposterior**, LSP) sacroiliac articulation of the mother.

**sa·cro·sci·at·ic** (sā′krō-sī-at′ik) relating to both sacrum and ischium.

**sa·cro·spi·nal** (sā′krō-spī′năl) relating to the sacrum and the vertebral column above.

**sa·cro·spi·nous va·gi·nal vault sus·pen·sion pro·ce·dure** surgical repair of prolapsed vaginal vault by suturing to the sacrospinous ligament; done either vaginally or abdominally.

**sa·cro·trans·verse po·si·tion** a breech presentation of the fetus with its sacrum pointing to the right (**right sacrotransverse**, RST) or to the left (**left sacrotransverse**, LST) sacroiliac articulation of the mother.

**sac·ro·u·ter·ine fold** a fold of peritoneum, containing the rectouterine muscle, passing from the sacrum to the base of the broad ligament on either side, forming the lateral boundary of the rectouterine (Douglas) pouch.

**sa·cro·ver·te·bral** (sā′krō-ver′tē-brăl) relating to the sacrum and the vertebrae above.

**sa·crum,** pl. **sa·cra** (sā′krŭm, sā′kră) the segment of the vertebral column forming part of the pelvis; a broad, slightly curved, spade-shaped bone, thick above, thinner below, closing in the pelvic girdle posteriorly; it is formed by the fusion of five originally separate sacral vertebrae; it articulates with the last lumbar vertebra, the coccyx, and the hip bone on either side. [L. (lit. sacred bone), neuter of *sacer* (*sacr-*), sacred]

**SAD** seasonal affective disorder.

**sad·dle** (sad′l) **1.** a structure shaped like, or suggestive of, a seat or saddle used in horseback riding. SYN sella. **2.** SYN denture base.

**sad·dle·back ca·ter·pil·lar** *Sibine stimulea,* a cause of caterpillar dermatitis.

**sad·dle block an·es·the·sia** a form of spinal anesthesia limited in area to the buttocks, perineum, and inner surfaces of the thighs.

**sad·dle head** SYN clinocephaly.

**sad·dle joint** a biaxial synovial joint in which the double motion is effected by the opposition of two surfaces, each of which is concave in one direction and convex in the other.

**sad·dle nose** a nose with markedly depressed bridge, seen in congenital syphilis or after injury from trauma or operation.

**sa·dism** (sā′dizm, sad′izm) a form of perversion, often sexual in nature, in which a person finds pleasure in inflicting abuse and maltreatment. Cf. masochism. [Marquis de *Sade,* 1740–1814, confessedly addicted to the practice]

**sa·dist** (sā′dist, sad′ist) one who practices sadism.

**sa·dis·tic** (să-dis′tik) pertaining to or characterized by sadism.

**sa·do·mas·och·ism** (sā-dō-mas′ō-kizm, sad-o-mas′ō-kizm) a form of perversion marked by enjoyment of cruelty and/or humiliation, both received and dispensed. [sadism + masochism]

**Sae·misch sec·tion** (sā′mish) procedure of transfixing the cornea beneath an ulcer and then cutting from within outward through the base.

**Sae·misch ul·cer** (sā′mish) a form of serpiginous keratitis, frequently accompanied by hypopyon.

**Saen·ger op·er·a·tion** (sāng′er) cesarean section followed by careful closure of the uterine wound by three tiers of sutures.

**Saen·ger sign** (sāng′er) a lost light reflex of the pupil returns after a short time in the dark, noted in cerebral syphilis but absent in tabes dorsalis.

**safe·ty lens** a lens that meets government specifications of impact resistance; the increased impact resistance required for safety lenses is obtained by tempering, by an ion-exchange process, or by using laminated or plastic lenses.

**SAF fix·a·tive** sodium acetate-acetic acid-formalin mixture used to fix fecal specimens for subsequent concentration and staining of smears.

**sag·it·tal** (saj′i-tăl) **1.** resembling an arrow. **2.** in an anteroposterior direction, referring to a sagittal plane or direction. [L. *sagitta,* an arrow]

**sag·it·tal ax·is** DENTISTRY the line in the frontal plane around which the working side condyle rotates during mandibular movement.

**sag·it·tal fon·ta·nelle** an occasional fontanel-like defect in the sagittal suture in the newborn. SYN Gerdy fontanelle.

**sag·it·tal plane** originally (and strictly speaking)

the sagittal plane is the median plane, and any other plane parallel to it is a parasagittal plane; in contemporary usage and in a broad sense, sagittal plane is used for any plane parallel to the median, i.e., as a synonym for parasagittal.

**sag·it·tal su·ture** line of union between the two parietal bones. SYN interparietal suture.

**sag·it·tal sy·nos·to·sis** SYN scaphocephaly.

**sa·go spleen** amyloidosis in the spleen affecting chiefly the malpighian bodies.

**Saint An·tho·ny dance, Saint Vi·tus dance, Saint John dance** obsolete eponyms for Sydenham chorea.

**Saint Anthony fire** (sānt anth-ō-nē fīr) **1.** SYN ergotism. **2.** any of several inflammations or gangrenous conditions of the skin (e.g., erysipelas). [St. Anthony, Egyptian monk, about 250–350 AD]

**Saint tri·ad** (sānt) the concurrence of hiatal hernia, diverticulosis, and cholelithiasis.

**Sak·se·na·ea va·si·for·mis** one of the fungal species that cause mucormycosis. This species is notable for the proportion of cases with subcutaneous infection, rather than pulmonary or paranasal sinus disease, more typical manifestations of mucormycosis.

**sal** salt.

**Sa·lah ster·nal punc·ture nee·dle** (sah'lah) a wide-bore needle for obtaining samples of red marrow from the sternum.

**sa·lic·y·late** (să-lis'i-lāt) **1.** a salt or ester of salicylic acid. **2.** to treat foodstuffs with salicylic acid as a preservative.

**sal·i·cyl·ic ac·id** (sal-i-sil'ik as'id) a component of aspirin, derived from salicin and made synthetically; used externally as a keratolytic agent.

**sal·i·cyl·ism** (sal'i-sil-izm) poisoning by salicylic acid or any of its compounds.

**sa·line** (sā'lēn) **1.** relating to, of the nature of, or containing salt; salty. **2.** a salt solution, usually sodium chloride. [L. *salinus*, salty, fr. *sal*, salt]

**sa·line ag·glu·ti·nin** an antibody which causes agglutination of erythrocytes when they are suspended either in saline or in a protein medium. SYN complete antibody.

**sa·line so·lu·tion 1.** a solution of any salt; **2.** specifically, isotonic or physiologic sodium chloride solution: 0.9 g/100 ml water.

**sa·li·va** (să-lī'vă) a clear, tasteless, odorless, slightly acid (pH 6.8) viscid fluid, consisting of the secretion from the parotid, sublingual, and submandibular salivary glands and the mucous glands of the oral cavity; its function is to keep the mucous membrane of the mouth moist, to lubricate the food during mastication, and to convert starch into maltose. SYN spittle. [L. akin to G. *sialon*]

**sal·i·vant** (sal'i-vant) **1.** causing a flow of saliva. **2.** an agent that increases the flow of saliva. SYN salivator.

**sal·i·vary** (sal'i-ver-ē) relating to saliva. SYN sialic, sialine. [L. *salivarius*]

**sal·i·vary di·ges·tion** the conversion of starch into sugar by the action of salivary amylase.

**sal·i·vary fis·tu·la** a pathologic communication between a salivary duct or gland and the cutaneous surface or the oral mucus.

**sal·i·vary gland dis·ease** disorder of salivary glands; i.e., Sjögren syndrome.

**sal·i·vate** (sal'i-vāt) to cause an excessive flow of saliva.

**sal·i·va·tion** (sal'i-vā'shŭn) SYN sialism.

**sal·i·va·tor** (sal'i-vā-ter) SYN salivant (2).

**Sal·mo·nel·la** (sal'mŏ-nel'ă) a genus of aerobic to facultatively anaerobic bacteria containing Gram-negative rods that are either motile or nonmotile. They are pathogenic for humans and other animals. The type species is *Salmonella choleraesuis*. [Daniel E. *Salmon*, U.S. pathologist, 1850–1914]

**Sal·mo·nel·la en·te·ri·ca** subsp. *chol·er·ae·su·is* a bacterial species that occurs in pigs, where it is an important secondary invader in the virus disease hog cholera, but does not occur as a natural pathogen in other animals; occasionally causes acute gastroenteritis and enteric fever in humans; it is the type species of the genus *Salmonella*.

**Sal·mo·nel·la en·te·ri·ca** subsp. *en·ter·it·i·dis* a widely distributed bacterial species that occurs in humans and in domestic and wild animals, especially rodents; it causes human gastroenteritis.

**Sal·mo·nel·la en·te·ri·ca** subsp. *pa·ra·ty·phi A* a bacterial species that is an important etiologic agent of enteric fever in developing countries.

**Sal·mo·nel·la en·te·ri·ca** subsp. *pa·ra·ty·phi B* (formerly known as *Salmonella schottmülleri*), consists of two distinct types of strains, those that produce enteric fever, found primarily in humans, and those producing gastroenteritis in humans, also found in animal species. This species includes 56 strains distinguishable by phage typing and/or biotyping, features of epidemiologic value.

**Sal·mo·nel·la en·te·ri·ca** subsp. *ty·phi·mu·ri·um* a bacterial species causing food poisoning in humans; it is a natural pathogen of all warm-blooded animals and is also found in snakes and pet turtles; worldwide, it is the most frequent cause of gastroenteritis due to *Salmonella enterica* species.

**Sal·mo·nel·la en·ter·it·i·dis** a widely distributed species that occurs in humans and in domestic and wild animals, especially rodents.

**Sal·mo·nel·la ty·phi** a species that causes typhoid fever in humans and is transmitted in contaminated water and food. SYN typhoid bacillus.

**Sal·mo·nel·la ty·phi·mu·ri·um** a species causing food poisoning in humans; it is a natural pathogen of all warm-blooded animals and is also found in snakes.

**Sal·mo·nel·la ty·pho·sa** former name for *Salmonella typhi*.

**sal·mo·nel·lo·sis** (sal'mŏ-nel-ō'sis) infection with bacteria of the genus *Salmonella*. Patients with sickle cell anemia and compromised immune systems are particularly susceptible. [*Salmonella* + G. *-osis*, condition]

**sal·pin·gec·to·my** (sal-pin-jek'tō-mē) removal of the uterine tube. SYN tubectomy. [salping- + G. *ektomē*, excision]

**sal·pin·ges** (sal-pin'jēz) plural of salpinx.

**sal·pin·gi·an** (sal-pin'jē-ăn) relating to the uterine tube or to the auditory tube.

**sal·pin·git·ic** (sal-pin-jit'ik) relating to salpingitis.

**sal·pin·gi·tis** (sal-pin-jī'tis) inflammation of the uterine or the auditory tube. [salping- + G. *-itis*, inflammation]

**sal·pin·gi·tis isth·mi·ca no·do·sa** a condition of the uterine tube characterized by nodular thickening of the tunica muscularis of the isthmic portion of the tube enclosing gland-like or cystic duplications of the lumen. SYN adenosalpingitis.

△**sal·pin·go-, sal·ping-** a tube (usually the uterine or auditory tubes). SEE ALSO tubo-. Cf. tubo-. [G. *salpinx*, trumpet (tube)]

**sal·pin·go·cele** (sal-ping′gō-sēl) hernia of a uterine tube. [salpingo- + G. *kēlē*, hernia]

**sal·pin·gog·ra·phy** (sal-ping-gog′ră-fē) radiography of the uterine tubes after the injection of radiopaque contrast medium. [salpingo- + G. *graphō*, to write]

**sal·pin·gol·y·sis** (sal-ping-gol′i-sis) freeing the uterine tube from adhesions. [salpingo- + G. *lysis*, loosening]

**sal·pin·go·ne·os·to·my** (sal-ping′ō-nē-os′tō-mē) surgical reopening of a uterine tube clubbed because of fimbrial adhesions. [salpingo- + neostomy]

**sal·pin·go-o·o·pho·rec·to·my** (sal-ping′gō-ō-of-ō-rek′tō-mē) removal of the ovary and its uterine tube. [salpingo- + G. *plastos*, formed]

**sal·pin·go-o·o·pho·ri·tis** (sal-ping′gō-ō-of-ō-rī′tis) inflammation of both uterine tube and ovary.

**sal·pin·go-o·oph·o·ro·cele** (sal-ping′gō-ō-of′ō-rō-sēl) hernia of both ovary and uterine tube.

**sal·pin·go·per·i·to·ni·tis** (sal-ping′gō-per-i-tō-nī′tis) inflammation of the uterine tube, perisalpinx, and peritoneum. [salpingo- + peritonitis]

**sal·pin·go·pexy** (sal-ping′gō-pek-sē) operative fixation of an oviduct. [salpingo- + G. *pēxis*, fixation]

**sal·pin·go·pha·ryn·ge·us mus·cle** *origin*, medial lamina of cartilaginous part of auditory tube; *insertion*, longitudinal muscular layer of pharynx in association with musculus palatopharyngeus; *action*, assists in elevating pharynx and, according to some, assists in opening the auditory tube during swallowing; *nerve supply*, pharyngeal plexus. SYN musculus salpingopharyngeus [TA].

**sal·pin·go·plas·ty** (sal-ping′gō-plas-tē) plastic surgery of the uterine tubes. SYN tuboplasty. [salpingo- + G. *plastos*, formed]

**sal·pin·gor·rha·phy** (sal-ping-gōr′ă-fē) suture of the uterine tube. [salpingo- + G. *rhaphē*, stitching]

**sal·pin·gos·to·my** (sal-ping-gos′tō-mē) establishment of an artificial opening in a uterine tube primarily as surgical treatment for an ectopic pregnancy. [salpingo- + G. *stoma*, mouth]

**sal·pin·got·o·my** (sal-ping-got′ō-mē) incision into a uterine tube. [salpingo- + G. *tomē*, incision]

**sal·pinx**, pl. **sal·pin·ges** (sal′pingks, sal-pin′jēz) [TA] 1. SYN uterine tube. 2. SYN pharyngotympanic (auditory) tube. [G. a trumpet (tube)]

**salt (sal)** 1. a compound formed by the interaction of an acid and a base, the ionizable hydrogen atoms of the acid being replaced by the positive ion of the base. 2. sodium chloride, the prototypical salt. 3. a saline cathartic, especially magnesium sulfate, magnesium citrate, or sodium phosphate; often denoted by the plural, salts. [L. *sal*]

**sal·ta·tion** (sal-tā′shŭn) a dancing or leaping, as in a disease (e.g., chorea) or physiologic function (e.g., saltatory conduction). [L. *saltatio*, fr. *salto*, pp. *-atus*, to dance, fr. *salio*, to leap]

**sal·ta·to·ry** (sal′tă-tōr-ē) pertaining to, or characterized by, saltation.

**sal·ta·to·ry con·duc·tion** nerve conduction in which the impulse jumps from one node of Ranvier to the next.

**sal·ta·to·ry ev·o·lu·tion** the theory that evolution of a new species from an older one may occur as a large jump, such as a major repatterning of chromosomes, rather than by gradual accumulation of small steps or mutations.

**sal·ta·to·ry spasm** a spasmodic affection of the muscles of the lower extremities. SYN Bamberger disease (1).

**Sal·ter in·cre·men·tal lines** (sawl′tĕr) transverse lines sometimes seen in dentin, due to improper calcification.

**salt·ing out** the precipitation of a protein from its solution by saturation or partial saturation with such neutral salts as sodium chloride, magnesium sulfate, or ammonium sulfate.

**salt-los·ing ne·phri·tis** a rare disorder resulting from renal tubular damage of a variety of etiologies; mimics adrenocortical insufficiency in that abnormal renal loss of sodium chloride occurs, accompanied by hyponatremia, azotemia, acidosis, dehydration, and vascular collapse. SYN Thorn syndrome.

**salt wast·ing** inappropriately large renal excretion of salt despite the apparent need of the body to retain it.

**sa·lu·bri·ous** (să-loo′brē-ŭs) healthful, usually in reference to climate. [L. *salubris*, healthy, fr. *salus*, health]

**sal·u·re·sis** (sal-yu-rē′sis) excretion of sodium in the urine. [L. *sal*, salt, + G. *ourēsis*, uresis (urination)]

**sal·u·ret·ic** (sal-yu-ret′ik) facilitating the renal excretion of sodium.

**sal·u·tary** (sal′yu-ter-ē) healthful; wholesome. [L. *salutaris*]

**salve** (sav) SYN ointment. [A.S. *sealf*]

**Salz·mann nod·u·lar cor·ne·al de·gen·er·a·tion** (sahlts′mahn) large and prominent nodules of a solid, opaque material that stands out from the surface of the cornea; occurs occasionally in persons previously affected by phlyctenular keratitis.

**sa·mar·i·um (Sm)** (să-mār′ē-ŭm) a metallic element of the lanthanide group, atomic no. 62, atomic wt. 150.36. [bands indicating its presence first found in the spectrum of *samarskite*, a mineral named after Col. von Samarski, 19th century Russian mine official]

**same-day sur·gery** ambulatory surgery.

**sam·ple** (sam′pel) 1. a specimen of a whole entity small enough to involve no threat or damage to the whole; an aliquot. 2. a selected subset of a population; a sample may be random or nonrandom (haphazard), representative or nonrepresentative. [M.E. *ensample*, fr. L. *exemplum*, example]

**sam·pling** the policy of inferring the behavior of a whole batch by studying a fraction of it. [MF *essample*, fr. L. *exemplum*, taking out]

**sam·pling bi·as** systematic error due to study of a nonrandom sample of a population.

**Sam·ter syn·drome** (sam′tĕr) a triad of asthma, nasal polyps, and aspirin intolerance.

**san·a·to·ri·um** (san′ă-tōr′ē-ŭm) an institution for the treatment of chronic disorders and a place for recuperation under medical supervision. Cf. sanitarium. [Mod. L. neuter of *sanatorius*, curative, fr. *sano*, to cure, heal]

**san·a·to·ry** (san′ă-tōr-ē) health-giving; conducive to health. [Mod. L. *sanatorius*]

**sand** the fine granular particles of quartz and

S
a

other crystalline rocks, or a gritty material resembling sand. [A.S.]

**Sand·hoff dis·ease** (sahnd′hof) an infantile form of $G_{M2}$ gangliosidosis characterized by a defect in the production of hexosaminidases A and B; it resembles Tay-Sachs disease, but occurs predominantly (if not entirely) in non-Jewish children; accumulation of glucoside and ganglioside $G_{m2}$, caused by mutation in hexoaminidase B gene (HEX B) on chromosome 5q.

**sane** (sān) of sound mind; mentally healthy. [L. *sanus*]

**San·fi·lip·po syn·drome** (san-fĭ-lip′ŏ) an error of the mucopolysaccharide metabolism, with excretion of large amounts of heparan sulfate in the urine; characterized by severe mental retardation with hepatomegaly; skeleton may be normal or may present mild changes similar to those in Hurler syndrome; several different types (A, B, C, and D) have been identified according to the enzyme deficiency; autosomal recessive inheritance.

△**san·gui-, san·guin-, san·gui·no-** blood, bloody. [G. *sanguis*]

**san·gui·fa·ci·ent** (sang-gwi-fā′shent) SYN hemopoietic. [sangui- + L. *facio*, to make]

**san·guif·er·ous** (sang-gwif′er-ŭs) conveying blood. SYN circulatory (2). [sangui- + L. *fero*, to carry]

**san·gui·fi·ca·tion** (sang′gwi-fi-kā′shŭn) SYN hemopoiesis. [sangui- + L. *facio*, to make]

**san·guine** (sang′gwin) **1.** SYN plethoric. **2.** formerly, denoting a temperament characterized by a light, fair complexion, full pulse, good digestion, optimistic outlook, and a quick but not lasting temper. SYN sanguineous (3). [L. *sanguineus*]

**san·guin·e·ous** (sang-gwin′ē-ŭs) **1.** relating to blood; bloody. **2.** SYN plethoric. **3.** SYN sanguine (2). [L. *sanguineus*]

**san·guin·o·lent** (sang-gwin′ō-lent) bloody; tinged with blood. [L. *sanguinolentus*]

**san·gui·no·pu·ru·lent** (sang′gwi-nō-pyur′ŭ-lent) denoting exudate or matter containing blood and pus. [sanguino- + L. *purulentus*, festering (suppurative), fr. *pus*, pus]

**san·guiv·or·ous** (sang-gwiv′er-ŭs) bloodsucking, as applied to certain bats, leeches, insects, etc. [sangui- + L. *voro*, to devour]

**sa·ni·es** (sā′nē-ēz) a thin, blood-stained, purulent discharge. [L.]

**sa·ni·o·pu·ru·lent** (sā′nē-ō-pyur′ŭ-lent) characterized by bloody pus. [L. *sanies*, thin, bloody matter, + *purulentus*, festering (suppurative), fr. *pus*, pus]

**sa·ni·o·se·rous** (sā′nē-ō-sēr′ŭs) characterized by blood-tinged serum.

**sa·ni·ous** (sā′nē-ŭs) relating to sanies; ichorous and blood-stained.

**san·i·tar·i·an** (san-i-ter′ē-ăn) one who is skilled in sanitation and public health. [L. *sanitas*, health, fr. *sanus*, sound]

**san·i·tar·i·um** (san-i-ter′ē-ŭm) a health resort. Cf. sanatorium. [L. *sanitas*, health]

**san·i·tary** (san′i-ter-ē) healthful; conducive to health; usually in reference to a clean environment. [L. *sanitas*, health]

**san·i·ta·tion** (san-i-tā′shŭn) use of measures designed to promote health and prevent disease; development and establishment of conditions in the environment favorable to health. [L. *sanitas*, health]

**san·i·ti·za·tion** (san′i-ti-zā′shŭn) the process of making something sanitary.

**san·i·ty** (san′i-tē) soundness of mind, emotions, and behavior; of a sound degree of mental health. [L. *sanitas*, health]

**San·som sign** (san′sĕm) in mitral stenosis, apparent duplication of the second heart sound.

**San·son im·ag·es** (sah′saw′) SYN Purkinje-Sanson images.

**San·ti·ni boom·ing sound** (sahn-tē′nē) a sonorous booming sound heard on auscultatory percussion of a hydatid cyst.

**San·to·ri·ni ca·nal** (sahn-tō-rē′nē) SYN accessory pancreatic duct.

**San·to·ri·ni con·cha** (sahn-tō-rē′nē) SYN supreme nasal concha.

**San·to·ri·ni duct** (sahn-tō-rē′nē) SYN accessory pancreatic duct.

**San·to·ri·ni plex·us** (sahn-tō-rē′nē) venous plexus on ventral and lateral prostatic surfaces.

**sa·phe·nous** (să-fē′nŭs) relating to or associated with a saphenous vein; denoting a number of structures in the thigh and leg. [see saphena]

**sa·phe·nous nerve** a branch of the femoral, extending from the femoral triangle to the foot, becoming subcutaneous on the medial side of the knee; it supplies cutaneous branches to the skin of the leg and foot, by way of infrapatellar and medial crural branches. SYN nervus saphenus [TA].

**sa·phe·nous o·pen·ing** the opening in the fascia lata inferior to the medial part of the inguinal ligament through which the saphenous vein passes to enter the femoral vein. SYN fossa ovalis (2).

△**sa·po-, sa·pon-** soap. [L. *sapo*]

**sap·o·na·ceous** (sap-ō-nā′shŭs) soapy; relating to or resembling soap.

**sa·pon·i·fi·ca·tion** (să-pon′i-fi-kā′shŭn) conversion into soap, denoting the hydrolytic action of an alkali upon fat, especially on triacylglycerols. [sapo- (*sapon-*) + L. *facio*, to make]

**sap·o·nins** (sap′ō-ninz) glycosides of plant origin characterized by properties of foaming in water and of lysing cells; powerful surfactants; many have antibiotic activities.

**sap·phism** (saf′izm) SYN lesbianism. [*Sapphō*, homosexual Greek poet, queen of the island of Lesbos]

△**sa·pro-, sapr-** rotten, putrid, decayed. [G. *sapros*]

**sap·robe** (sap′rōb) an organism that lives upon dead organic material. This term is preferable to saprophyte, since bacteria and fungi are no longer regarded as plants. [sapro- + G. *bios*, life]

**sa·pro·bic** (sap-rō′bik) pertaining to a saprobe.

**sap·ro·gen** (sap′rō-jen) an organism living on dead organic matter and causing the decay thereof. [sapro- + G. *-gen*, producing]

**sap·ro·gen·ic, sa·prog·e·nous** (sap-rō-jen′ik, să-proj′ĕ-nŭs) causing or resulting from decay.

**sap·ro·phyte** (sap′rō-fīt) an organism that grows on dead organic matter, plant or animal. SEE sap-robe. [sapro- + G. *phyton*, plant]

**sap·ro·phyt·ic** (sap-rō-fit′ik) relating to a saprophyte.

**sap·ro·zo·ic** (sap-rō-zō′ik) living in decaying organic matter; especially denoting certain protozoa. [sapro- + G. *zōikos*, relating to animals]

**sap•ro•zo•o•no•sis** (sap′rō-zō-ō-nō′sis) a zoonosis the agent of which requires both a vertebrate host and a nonanimal (food, soil, plant) reservoir or developmental site for completion of its cycle. [sapro- + G. *zōon,* animal, + *nosos,* disease]

**Sar•ci•na** (sar′si-nă) a genus of nonmotile, strictly anaerobic bacteria containing Gram-positive cocci, which divide in three perpendicular planes, producing regular packets of eight or more cells. Saprophytic and facultatively parasitic species occur. The type species is *Sarcina ventriculi.* [L. *sarcina,* a pack, bundle, fr. *sarcio,* to mend, patch]

△**sar•co-** denoting muscular substance or a resemblance to flesh. [G. *sarx (sark-),* flesh]

**sar•co•blast** (sar′kō-blast) SYN myoblast. [sarco- + G. *blastos,* germ]

**Sar•co•di•na** (sar′kō-dī′nă) the amebae; a subphylum of protozoa possessing pseudopodia or locomotive protoplasmic flow for movement. Most species are free-living. [Mod. L. fr. G. *sarx,* flesh]

**sar•coid** (sar′koyd) SYN sarcoidosis. [sarco- + G. *eidos,* resemblance]

**sar•coid•al gran•u•lo•ma** a non-necrotizing epithelioid cell granuloma similar to those seen in sarcoidosis.

**sar•coid•o•sis** (sar-koy-dō′sis) a systemic granulomatous disease of unknown cause, especially involving the lungs with resulting fibrosis, but also involving lymph nodes, skin, liver, spleen, eyes, phalangeal bones, and parotid glands; granulomas are composed of epithelioid and multinucleated giant cells with little or no necrosis. SYN Besnier-Boeck-Schaumann disease, Boeck disease, sarcoid. [sarcoid + G. *-osis,* condition]

**sar•co•lem•ma** (sar′kō-lem′ă) the plasma membrane of a muscle fiber; formerly, the delicate connective tissue of the endomysium was included under this term by some. [sarco- + G. *lemma,* husk]

**sar•co•lem•mal, sar•co•lem•mic, sar•co•lem••mous** (sar′kō-lem′ăl, sar′kō-lem′ik, sar′kō-lem′ŭs) relating to the sarcolemma.

**sar•co•ma** (sar-kō′mă) a connective tissue neoplasm, usually highly malignant, formed by proliferation of mesodermal cells. [G. *sarkōma,* a fleshy excrescence, fr. *sarx,* flesh, + *-oma,* tumor]

**sar•co•ma•toid** (sar-kō′mă-toyd) resembling a sarcoma. [sarcoma + G. *eidos,* resemblance]

**sar•co•ma•to•sis** (sar′kō-mă-tō′sis) occurrence of several sarcomatous growths on different parts of the body. [sarcoma + G. *-osis,* condition]

**sar•com•a•tous** (sar-kō′mă-tŭs) relating to or of the nature of sarcoma.

**sar•co•mere** (sar′kō-mēr) the segment of a myofibril between two adjacent Z lines, representing the functional unit of striated muscle. [sarco- + G. *meros,* part]

**sar•co•pe•nia** (sar-kō-pē′nē-ă) progressive reduction in muscle cross section and mass with aging. [sarco- + G. *penia,* poverty]

**sar•co•plasm** (sar′kō-plazm) the nonfibrillar cytoplasm of a muscle fiber. [sarco- + G. *plasma,* a thing formed]

**sar•co•plas•mic** (sar-kō-plaz′mik) relating to sarcoplasm.

**sar•co•plas•mic re•tic•u•lum** the endoplasmic reticulum of skeletal and cardiac muscle; the complex of vesicles, tubules, and cisternae forming a continuous structure around striated myofibrils, with a repetition of structure within each sarcomere.

**sar•co•poi•et•ic** (sar′kō-poy-et′ik) forming muscle. [sarco- + G. *poiēsis,* a making]

**Sar•cop•tes sca•biei** (sar-kop′tēz skā′bē-ī) the itch mite, varieties of which are distributed worldwide and affect humans and many animals. The mite burrows into the skin and lays eggs within the burrow; intense itching and rash develop near the burrow in about a month. SEE scabies, mange. [sarco- + G. *koptō,* to cut; L. *scabies,* scurf]

**sar•cop•tic** (sar-kop′tik) of, relating to, or caused by mites of the genus *Sarcoptes* or other members of the family Sarcoptidae.

**sar•cop•tid** (sar-kop′tid) common name for members of the Sarcoptidae, a family of mites that includes the genera *Sarcoptes, Knemidokoptes,* and *Notoedres.*

**sar•co•sis** (sar-kō′sis) **1.** an abnormal increase of flesh. **2.** a multiple growth of fleshy tumors. **3.** a diffuse sarcoma involving the whole of an organ. [G. *sarkōsis,* the growth of flesh, fr. *sarx,* flesh]

**sar•cos•to•sis** (sar-kos-tō′sis) ossification of muscular tissue. [sarco- + G. *osteon,* bone, + *-osis,* condition]

**sar•cot•ic** (sar-kot′ik) **1.** relating to sarcosis. **2.** causing an increase of flesh.

**sar•co•tu•bules** (sar-kō-too′byulz) the continuous system of membranous tubules in striated muscle that corresponds to the smooth endoplasmic reticulum of other cells.

**sar•cous** (sar′kŭs) relating to muscular tissue; fleshy. [G. *sarx,* flesh]

**sar•don•ic grin** (sar-don′ik grin) SYN risus caninus.

**sar•gra•mos•tim** (săr-gra-mŏs′tim) a recombinant human granulocyte-macrophage colony-stimulating factor (GM-CSF); used to protect against infection in the presence of acute myelogenous leukemia and in bone marrow transplants.

**sar•to•ri•us mus•cle** *origin,* anterior superior spine of ilium; *insertion,* medial border of tuberosity of tibia; *action,* flexes thigh and leg, rotates leg medially and thigh laterally; *nerve supply,* femoral. SYN musculus sartorius [TA].

**Sart•well in•cu•ba•tion mo•del** (sahrt′wel) mathematical model based on empirical observations, showing that incubation periods for communicable diseases have a log-normal distribution; model holds true for certain kinds of cancers that have well-defined external causes.

**sat, sat.** saturated.

**sat•el•lite** (sat′ĕ-līt) **1.** a minor structure accompanying a more important or larger one; e.g., a vein accompanying an artery, or a small or secondary lesion adjacent to a larger one. **2.** the posterior member of a pair of gregarine gamonts in syzygy, several of which may be found in some species. [L. *satelles (sattelit-),* attendant]

**sat•el•lite ab•scess** an abscess closely associated with a primary abscess.

**sat•el•lit•o•sis** (sat′ĕ-lī-tō′sis) **1.** a condition marked by an accumulation of neuroglia cells around the neurons of the central nervous system; often as a prelude to neuronophagia. **2.** the presence of satellite, smaller structures or lesions. [L. *satelles (satellit-),* an attendant, + G. *-ōsis,* condition]

S
a

**sa·ti·a·tion** (sā-shē-ā'shŭn) the state produced by fulfillment of a specific need, such as hunger or thirst. [L. *satio,* pp. *-atus,* to fill, satisfy]

**sat. sol., sat. soln.** saturated solution.

**Satt·ler veil** (sat'lĕr) a diffuse edema of the corneal epithelium that may develop after wearing contact lenses.

**sat·u·rate** (satch'ŭ-rāt) **1.** to impregnate to the greatest possible extent. **2.** to neutralize; to satisfy all the chemical affinities of a substance (as by converting all double bonds to single bonds). **3.** to dissolve a substance up to that concentration beyond which the addition of more results in two phases. [L. *saturo,* pp. *-atus,* to fill, fr. *satur, sated*]

**sat·u·rat·ed col·or** a color containing a minimum amount of whiteness.

**sat·u·rat·ed fat·ty ac·id** a fatty acid, the carbon chain of which contains no ethylenic or other unsaturated linkages between carbon atoms (e.g., stearic acid and palmitic acid); called saturated because it is incapable of absorbing any more hydrogen.

**sat·u·rat·ed so·lu·tion (sat. sol., sat. soln.)** a solution that contains all of a solute capable of being dissolved in the solvent; a substance in equilibrium with excess undissolved substance.

**sat·u·ra·tion** (satch-ŭ-rā'shŭn) **1.** impregnation of one substance by another to the greatest possible extent. **2.** neutralization, as of an acid by an alkali. **3.** that concentration of a dissolved substance that cannot be exceeded. **4.** OPTICS SEE saturated color. **5.** filling of all the available sites on an enzyme molecule by its substrate, or on a hemoglobin molecule by oxygen (symbol $S_{O_2}$) or carbon monoxide (symbol $S_{CO}$). [L. *saturatio,* fr. *saturo,* to fill, fr. *satis,* enough]

**sat·u·ra·tion in·dex** an indication of the relative concentration of hemoglobin in the red blood cells, calculated as: grams of hemoglobin per 100 ml (expressed as percent of normal) ÷ hematocrit value (expressed as percent of normal) = saturation index.

**sat·u·ra·tion sound pres·sure level (SSPL)** a measure of the maximum output of a hearing aid.

**sat·ur·nine** (sat'er-nīn) **1.** relating to lead. **2.** due to or symptomatic of lead poisoning. [Mediev. L. *saturninus,* fr. *saturnus,* lead, fr. L. *saturnus,* the god and planet Saturn]

**sat·y·ri·a·sis** (sat-i-rī'ă-sis) satyromania; excessive sexual excitement and behavior in the male; the counterpart of nymphomania in the female. [G. *satyros,* a satyr]

**sau·cer·i·za·tion** (saw'ser-i-zā'shŭn) excavation of tissue to form a shallow depression, performed in wound treatment to facilitate drainage from infected areas.

**Sa·vary bou·gies** (sā-vā-rē) silastic tapered-tip bougies used over a guide wire in esophageal dilatation.

**saw** a metal operating instrument having an edge of sharp, toothlike projections, for dividing bone, cartilage, or plaster; edges may be attached to a rigid band, a flexible wire or chain, or a motorized oscillator. [A.S. *saga*]

**sax·i·tox·in** (sak-si-tok'sin) a potent neurotoxin found in shellfish, such as the mussel or the clam, produced by the dinoflagellate *Gonyaulax catenella,* which is ingested by the shellfish; the cause of poisoning from eating California sea mussel, scallops, and Alaskan butterclams.

**Sb** antimony.

**SBE** subacute bacterial endocarditis.

**SBS** shaken baby syndrome.

**Sc** scandium.

**scab** (skab) a crust formed by coagulation of blood, pus, serum, or a combination of these, on the surface of an ulcer, erosion, or other type of wound. [A.S. *scaeb*]

**scab·i·ci·dal** (skā-bi-sī'dăl) destructive to scabies mites.

**scab·i·cide** (skā'bi-sīd) an agent lethal to scabies mites.

**◪ sca·bies** (skā'bē-ēz) an eruption due to the mite *Sarcoptes scabiei* var. *hominis;* the female of the species burrows into the skin, producing a vesicular eruption with intense pruritus between the fingers, on the male genitalia, buttocks, and elsewhere on the trunk and extremities. See page B3. [L. *scabo,* to scratch]

**sca·la,** pl. **sca·lae** (skā'lă, skā'lē) one of the cavities of the cochlea winding spirally around the modiolus. [L. a stairway]

**sca·la me·dia** [TA] SYN cochlear duct.

**sca·la tym·pa·ni** [TA] the division of the spiral canal of the cochlea lying on the basal side of the spiral lamina.

**sca·la ves·tib·u·li** [TA] the division of the spiral canal of the cochlea lying on the apical side of the spiral lamina and vestibular membrane. SYN vestibular canal.

**scald** (skawld) **1.** to burn by contact with a hot liquid or steam. **2.** the lesion resulting from such contact. [L. *excaldo,* to wash in hot water]

**scald·ed mouth syn·drome** a syndrome in which the patient complains of a burning sensation of the tongue, lips, throat, or palate, likened to scalding caused by hot liquids; clinically the tissues appear normal; it has been associated with angiotensin-converting enzyme (ACE) inhibitors.

**◪ scale** (skāl) **1.** a standardized test for measuring psychological, personality, or behavioral characteristics. SEE ALSO test, score. **2.** SYN squama. **3.** a small thin plate of horny epithelium, resembling a fish scale, cast off from the skin. **4.** to desquamate. **5.** to remove tartar from the teeth. **6.** a device by which some property can be measured. See page B5. [L. *scala,* a stairway]

**sca·le·nec·to·my** (skā'lĕ-nek'tō-mē) resection of the scalene muscles. [scalene + G. *ektomē,* excision]

**sca·le·not·o·my** (skā'lĕ-not'ō-mē) division or section of the anterior scalene muscle. [scalene + G. *tomē,* incision]

**sca·le·nus me·di·us mus·cle** *origin,* costotransverse lamellae of transverse processes of second to sixth cervical vertebrae; *insertion,* first rib posterior to subclavian artery; *action,* raises first rib; *nerve supply,* cervical plexus.

**sca·le·nus mi·ni·mus mus·cle** an occasional independent muscular fasciculus between the scalenus anterior and medius, and having the same action and innervation.

**scal·ing** (skā'ling) DENTISTRY removal of accretions from the crowns and roots of teeth by use of special instruments.

**scal·lop·ing** (skal'ō-ping) a series of indentations or erosions on a normally smooth margin of a structure.

**scalp** (skalp) the skin and subcutaneous tissue, normally hair bearing, covering the neurocranium. [M. E. fr. Scand. *skalpr,* sheath]

**scal•pel** (skal′pl) a knife used in surgical dissection. [L. *scalpellum;* dim. of *scalprum,* a knife]

**scalp hair** a hair of the head.

**scal•prum** (skal′prŭm) **1.** a large strong scalpel. **2.** a raspatory. [L. chisel, penknife, fr. *scalpo,* pp. *scalptus,* to carve]

**scaly** (skā′lē) SYN squamous.

**scan** (skan) **1.** to survey by traversing with an active or passive sensing device. **2.** the image, record, or data obtained by scanning, usually identified by the technology or device employed; e.g., CT scan, radionuclide scan, ultrasound scan, etc. **3.** abbreviated form of scintiscan, usually identified by the organ or structure examined; e.g., brain scan, bone scan, etc.

**scan•di•um** (Sc) (skan′dē-ŭm) a metallic element, atomic no. 21, atomic wt. 44.955910. [L. *Scandia,* Scandinavia, where discovered]

**scan•ner** (skan′er) a device or instrument that scans.

**scan•ning** (skan′ing) the act of imaging by traversing with an active or passive sensing device, often identified by the technology or device employed.

**scan•ning e•lec•tron mi•cro•scope** a microscope in which the object in a vacuum is scanned in a raster pattern by a slender electron beam, generating reflected and secondary electrons from the specimen surface that are used to modulate the image on a synchronously scanned cathode ray tube; with this method a three-dimensional image is obtained, with both high resolution and great depth of focus.

**scan•ning equal•i•za•tion ra•di•og•ra•phy** an electronically enhanced method of radiography in which a small x-ray beam is scanned over the patient while its attenuation is measured, providing feedback to modulate beam intensity in order to equalize average x-ray film exposure.

**scan•ning speech** measured or metered, often slow speech.

**scan•o•gram** (skan′ō-gram) a radiographic technique for showing true dimensions by moving a narrow orthogonal beam of x-rays along the length of the structure being measured, e.g., the lower extremities. [scan- + G. *gramma,* something written]

**Scan•zo•ni ma•neu•ver** (skahn-zō′nē) forceps rotation and traction in a spiral course, with reapplication of forceps for delivery.

**sca•pha** (skaf′ă, skā′fă) the longitudinal furrow between the helix and the antihelix of the auricle. [L. fr. G. *skaphē,* skiff]

△**scaph•o-** a scapha, scaphoid. [G. *skaphē,* skiff, boat]

**scaph•o•ce•phal•ic** (skaf-ō-se-fal′ik) denoting or relating to scaphocephaly.

**scaph•o•ceph•a•lism** (skaf-ō-sef′ă-lizm) SYN scaphocephaly.

**scaph•o•ceph•a•ly** (skaf-ō-sef′ă-lŭs) craniosynostosis involving the sagittal suture, resulting in a long, narrow cranial vault; sometimes accompanied by mental retardation. SYN cymbocephaly, sagittal synostosis, scaphocephalism, tectocephaly. [scapho- + G. *kephalē,* head]

**scaph•oid** (skaf′oyd) boat-shaped; hollowed. SEE scaphoid bone. SYN navicular. [scapho- + G. *eidos,* resemblance]

**scaph•oid ab•do•men** a condition in which the anterior abdominal wall is sunken and presents a concave rather than a convex contour. SYN navicular abdomen.

**scaph•oid bone** the largest bone of the proximal row of the carpus on the lateral (radial) side, articulating with the radius, lunate, capitate, trapezium, and trapezoid. SYN os scaphoideum.

**scaph•oid scap•u•la** a scapula in which the vertebral border below the level of the spine presents concavity instead of the normal convexity; the **scaphoid type of scapula** (Graves) is a scapula in which the vertebral border between the spine and the teres major process is either straight or tends toward concavity.

**scap•u•la,** gen. and pl. **scap•u•lae** (skap′yu-lă, skap′yu-lē) [TA] a large triangular flattened bone lying over the ribs, posteriorly on either side, articulating laterally with the clavicle at the acromioclavicular joint and the humerus at the glenohumeral joint. It forms a functional joint with the chest wall, the scapulothoracic joint. SYN shoulder blade. [L. *scapulae,* the shoulder blades]

**scap•u•la a•la•ta** SYN winged scapula.

**scap•u•lar** (skap′yu-lăr) relating to the scapula.

**scap•u•lec•to•my** (skap′yu-lek′tō-mē) excision of the scapula. [scapula + G. *ektomē,* excision]

△**scap•u•lo-** scapula, scapular. [L. *scapulae,* shoulder blades]

**scap•u•lo•cla•vic•u•lar** (skap′yu-lō-klă-vik′yu-lăr) **1.** SYN acromioclavicular. **2.** SYN coracoclavicular.

**scap•u•lo•cos•tal syn•drome** pain of insidious development in the upper or posterior part of the shoulder radiating into the neck and occiput, down the arm, or around the chest; there may be numbness or tingling in the fingers; attributed to an alteration from the normal relationship between the scapula and posterior wall of the thorax.

**scap•u•lo•hu•mer•al** (skap′yu-lō-hyu′mer-ăl) relating to both scapula and humerus. SEE ALSO glenohumeral.

**scap•u•lo•hu•mer•al rhy•thm** coordinated rotational movement of the scapula that accompanies abduction and adduction of the humerus.

**scap•u•lo•pexy** (skap′yu-lō-pek-sē) operative fixation of the scapula to the chest wall or to the spinous process of the vertebrae. [scapulo- + G. *pēxis,* fixation]

**scap•u•lo•thor•a•cic** (ST) (skap′yu-lō-thō-ras′ik) relating to the scapula and the dorsal thorax. SEE shoulder complex.

**scap•u•lo•thor•a•cic joint** the articulation between the scapula and the dorsal thorax; it is not a true anatomic joint because it lacks a synovial capsule and there are muscles between the anterior surface of the scapula and the thorax. SEE pectoral girdle, shoulder girdle.

**sca•pus,** pl. **sca•pi** (skā′pŭs, skā′pī) a shaft or stem. [L. shaft, stalk]

**scar** (skar) the fibrous tissue replacing normal tissues destroyed by injury or disease. [G. *eschara,* scab]

**scar car•ci•no•ma** carcinoma of the lung, usually adenocarcinoma, arising from a peripheral lung scar or associated with interstitial fibrosis in a honeycomb lung.

**scar•i•fi•ca•tion** (skar-i-fi-kā′shŭn) the making of a number of superficial incisions in the skin. [L. *scarifico,* to scratch, fr. G. *skariphos,* a style for sketching]

**scar•i•fi•ca•tor** (skar′i-fi-kā-tŏr) an instrument

S
c

for scarification, consisting of a number of concealed spring-projected cutting blades, set near together, that make superficial incisions in the skin.

**scar·la·ti·na** (skar'lă-tē'nă) an acute exanthematous disease, caused by infection with streptococcal organisms producing erythrogenic toxin, marked by fever and other constitutional disturbances, and a generalized eruption of closely aggregated points or small macules of a bright red color followed by desquamation; mucous membrane of the mouth and fauces is usually also involved. SYN scarlet fever. [through It. fr. Mediev. L. *scarlatum,* scarlet, a scarlet cloth]

**scar·la·ti·na hem·or·rha·gi·ca** a form of scarlatina in which blood extravasates into the skin and mucous membranes, giving to the eruption a dusky hue; frequent bleeding from the nose and into the intestine also occurs.

**scar·la·ti·nal** (skar-lă-tē'năl) relating to scarlatina.

**scar·la·ti·ni·form** (skar-lă-tē'ni-fōrm) resembling scarlatina, denoting a rash.

**scar·let fe·ver** SYN scarlatina.

**Scar·pa fa·scia** (skahr'pah) the deeper, membranous or lamellar part of the subcutaneous tissue of the lower abdominal wall; it is continuous with the superficial perineal (Colles) fascia.

**Scar·pa meth·od** (skahr'pah) cure of aneurysm by ligation of the artery at some distance above the sac.

**Scar·pa staph·y·lo·ma** (skahr'pah) SYN posterior staphyloma.

**Scar·pa tri·an·gle** (skahr'pah) SYN femoral triangle.

**scar·ring al·o·pe·cia** alopecia in which hair follicles are irreversibly destroyed by scarring processes including trauma, burns, lupus erythematosus, lichen planopilaris, scleroderma, folliculitis decalvans, or of uncertain cause (pseudopelade). SYN cicatricial alopecia.

**sca·te·mia** (skă-tē'mē-ă) intestinal autointoxication. [scato- + G. *haima,* blood]

△**scato-** feces. SEE ALSO copro-, sterco-. [G. *skōr* (*skat-*), excrement]

**scat·o·log·ic** (skat-ō-loj'ik) pertaining to scatology.

**sca·tol·o·gy** (skă-tol'o-jē) **1.** the scientific study and analysis of feces, for physiologic and diagnostic purposes. SYN coprology. **2.** the study relating to the psychiatric aspects of excrement or excremental (anal) function. [scato- + G. *logos,* study]

**sca·tos·co·py** (skă-tos'kŏ-pē) examination of the feces for purposes of diagnosis. [scato- + G. *skopeō,* to view]

**scat·ter** (skat'er) **1.** a change in direction of a photon or subatomic particle, as the result of a collision or interaction. **2.** the secondary radiation resulting from the interaction of primary radiation with matter.

**scat·tered ra·di·a·tion** radiation that has been deflected from its path by impact with matter. This form of secondary radiation is emitted diffusely by the tissues of the patient during exposure to x-radiation. SEE ALSO secondary radiation.

**sca·ven·ger re·cep·tor** a receptor on macrophages that binds preferentially to oxidized low density lipoprotein (LDL) causing macrophages to internalize the LDL.

*Scedosporium* (se-dō-spōr'ē-ŭm) an imperfect

fungus of the form-class Hyphomycetes; anamorph of *Pseudallescheria.*

*Sce·do·spor·i·um ap·i·o·sper·mum* (se-dō-spōr' ē-ŭm ā-pē-ō-'sper-mŭm) the imperfect state of the fungus *Pseudallescheria boydii,* one of the fungi that cause mycetoma in humans.

*Sce·do·spo·ri·um in·fla·tum* SEE *Scedosporium prolificans.*

*Sce·do·spo·ri·um pro·li·fi·cans* a mold; a rare cause of deep fungal infection. Formerly called *Scedosporium inflatum.*

**Schäf·fer re·flex** (shäf'ĕr) in cases of injury to the corticospinal tract, the great toe is dorsiflexed when the skin over the Achilles tendon is pinched.

**Scha·pi·ro sign** (shah'pērō) in myocardial weakness, no slowing of the pulse occurs when the patient lies down.

**Schau·dinn fix·a·tive** (shou'din) a solution of mercuric chloride, sodium chloride, alcohol, and glacial acetic acid, used on wet smears for cytologic fixation.

**Sche·de meth·od** (shē'dĕ) filling of the defect in bone, after removal of a sequestrum or scraping away carious material, by allowing the cavity to fill with blood which may become organized (Schede clot).

**Scheibe hear·ing im·pair·ment** (shī-bĕ) hearing impairment due to cochleosaccular dysplasia; usually autosomal recessive inheritance.

**Schei·e syn·drome** (shā) allelic to Hurler syndrome but with a much milder phenotype; characterized by α-L-iduronidase deficiency, corneal clouding, deformity of the hands, aortic valve involvement, and normal intelligence; autosomal recessive inheritance, caused by mutation in the alpha-L-iduronidase gene (IUDA) on chromosome 4p.

**Schei·ner ex·per·i·ment** (shī'nĕr) a demonstration of accommodation; through two minute holes in a card, separated from each other by less than the diameter of the pupil, one looks at a pin; at a short distance from the eye the pin appears double; as it is moved from the eye a point is found where it appears single, and beyond which it remains single for the emmetropic eye, but for the myopic eye it soon again becomes double.

**sche·ma,** pl. **sche·ma·ta** (skē'mă, skē-mah'tă) **1.** a plan, outline, or arrangement. SYN scheme. **2.** in sensorimotor theory, the organized unit of cognitive experience. [G. *schēma,* shape, form]

**scheme** (skēm) SYN schema (1).

**Schenck dis·ease** (shĕnk) SYN sporotrichosis.

**Scheu·er·mann dis·ease** (shoi'ĕr-mahn) epiphysial osteonecrosis of adjacent vertebral bodies in the thoracic spine.

**Schick test** (shik) a test for susceptibility to *Corynebacterium diphtheriae* toxin. Schick test toxin is injected into the skin; individuals lacking toxin-neutralizing antibodies may have a positive reaction, which consists of an area of redness.

**Schiff re·a·gent** (shif) an aqueous solution of basic fuchsin or pararosaniline that is decolorized by sulfur dioxide, commonly prepared by addition of hydrochloric acid to a dye solution containing a metabisulphite or bisulphite salt; used for aldehydes and in histochemistry to detect polysaccharides, DNA, and proteins.

**Schil·der dis·ease** (shĭl'dĕr) term used to describe at least two separate disorders described by Schilder: 1) diffuse sclerosis or encephalitis periaxialis diffusa; a nonfamilial disorder affecting primarily children and young adults and characterized by progressive dementia, visual disturbances, deafness, pseudobulbar palsy, and hemiplegia or quadriplegia. Most patients die within a few years of onset; pathologically, there is a large, asymmetric area of myelin destruction, sometimes involving an entire cerebral hemisphere, and typically with extension across the corpus callosum. 2) the leukodystrophies. SYN encephalitis periaxialis diffusa.

**Schil·ler test** (shil'ĕr) a test for nonglycogen-containing areas of the portio vaginalis of the cervix, which may be the site of early carcinoma; such areas fail to stain dark brown with iodine solution; loss of glycogen due to erosion and other benign conditions may also give a positive result.

**Schil·ling blood count** (shil'ing) a method of counting blood in which the polymorphonuclear neutrophils are separated into four groups according to the number and arrangement of the nuclear masses in these cells.

**Schil·ling test** (shil'ing) a procedure for determining the amount of vitamin $B_{12}$ excreted in the urine using cyanocobalamin tagged with a radioisotope of cobalt.

**schin·dy·le·sis** (skin-dĭ-lē'sis) [TA] SYN wedge-and-groove joint. [G. *schindylēsis*, splintering]

△**schi·sto-** cleft, division. SEE ALSO schizo-. [G. *schistos*, split]

**schis·to·ce·lia** (skis-tō-sē'lē-ă) congenital fissure of the abdominal wall. [schisto- + G. *koilia*, a hollow]

**schis·to·cor·mia** (skis-tō-kōr'mē-ă) congenital clefting of the trunk, the lower extremities of the fetus usually being imperfectly developed. SYN schistosomia. [schisto- + G. *kormos*, trunk of a tree]

**schis·to·cyte** (skis'tō-sīt) SYN keratocyte (2). [schisto- + G. *kytos*, cell]

**schis·to·cy·to·sis** (skis'tō-sī-tō'sis) the occurrence of many schistocytes in the blood.

**schis·to·glos·sia** (skis-tō-glos'ē-ă) congenital fissure or cleft of the tongue. [schisto- + G. *glōssa*, tongue]

*Schis·to·so·ma* (skis-tō-sō'mă) a genus of trematodes, including the blood flukes that cause schistosomiasis; characterized by elongate shape, marked sexual dimorphism, location in the smaller blood vessels of their host, and utilization of water snails as intermediate hosts. [schisto- + G. *sōma*, body]

*Schis·to·so·ma hae·ma·to·bi·um* the vesical blood fluke, a species that occurs as a parasite in the portal system and mesenteric veins of the bladder (causing human schistosomiasis haematobium) and rectum; found throughout Africa and the Middle East; intermediate hosts are *Bulinus truncatus* and other snails.

*Schis·to·so·ma ja·po·ni·cum* the Oriental or Japanese blood fluke, a species that causes schistosomiasis japonica, with extensive pathology from encapsulation of the eggs, particularly in the liver. The intermediate hosts are amphibious snails; other animals, such as pigs, oxen, cattle, and dogs, serve as reservoir hosts.

**schis·to·so·mal der·ma·ti·tis** a sensitization response to repeated cutaneous invasion by cercariae of bird, mammal, or human schistosomes. SYN swimmer's itch (2), water itch (2).

*Schis·to·so·ma man·so·ni* a common species characterized by large eggs with a strong lateral spine and transmitted by planorbid snails of the genus *Biomphalaria;* causes schistosomiasis mansoni.

**schis·to·some** (skis'tō-sōm) common name for a member of the genus *Schistosoma.*

**schis·to·so·mia** (skis-tō-sō'mē-ă) SYN schistocormia. [schisto- + G. *sōma*, body]

**schis·to·so·mi·a·sis** (skis'tō-sō-mī'ă-sis) infection with a species of *Schistosoma;* manifestations of this often chronic and debilitating disease vary with the infecting species but depend in large measure upon tissue reaction (granulation and fibrosis) to the eggs deposited in venules and in the hepatic portal system, the latter resulting in portal hypertension and esophageal varices, as well as liver damage leading to cirrhosis. SEE ALSO schistosomal dermatitis.

**schis·to·so·mi·a·sis hae·ma·to·bi·um** infection with *Schistosoma haematobium*, the eggs of which invade the urinary tract, causing cystitis and hematuria, and possibly an increased likelihood of bladder cancer. SYN endemic hematuria.

**schis·to·so·mi·a·sis ja·pon·i·ca, Jap·a·nese schis·to·so·mi·a·sis** (jap'ah-nēz) infection with *Schistosoma japonicum*, characterized by dysenteric symptoms, painful enlargement of the liver and spleen, dropsy, urticaria, and progressive anemia.

**schis·to·so·mi·a·sis man·so·ni** (mahn-sō-nē) infection with *Schistosoma mansoni*, the eggs of which invade the wall of the large intestine and the liver, causing irritation, inflammation, and ultimately fibrosis. SYN Manson schistosomiasis.

**schis·to·tho·rax** (skis-tō-thōr'aks) congenital cleft of the chest wall. [schisto- + G. *thōrax*, thorax]

**schiz·am·ni·on** (skiz-am'nē-on) an amnion developing, as in the human embryo, by the formation of a cavity within the inner cell mass. [schiz- + amnion]

**schiz·ax·on** (skiz-ak'son) an axon divided into two branches. [schiz- + G. *axōn*, axis]

△**schiz·o-, schiz-** split, cleft, division; schizophrenia. SEE ALSO schisto-. [G. *schizō*, to split or cleave]

**schiz·o·af·fec·tive** (skiz'ō-ă-fek'tiv) having an admixture of symptoms suggestive of both schizophrenia and affective (mood) disorder.

**schiz·o·af·fec·tive psy·cho·sis** psychotic disturbance in which there is a mixture of schizophrenic and manic-depressive symptoms.

**schiz·o·gen·e·sis** (skiz-ō-jen'ě-sis) reproduction by fission. SYN fissiparity. [schizo- + G. *genesis*, origin]

**schi·zog·o·ny** (ski-zog'ō-nē) multiple fission in which the nucleus first divides and then the cell divides into as many parts as there are nuclei; called merogony if daughter cells are merozoites, sporogony if daughter cells are sporozoites, or gametogony if daughter cells are gametes. [schizo- + G. *gonē*, generation]

**schiz·o·gy·ria** (skiz-ō-jī'rē-ă) deformity of the cerebral convolutions marked by occasional interruptions of their continuity. [schizo- + G. *gyros*, circle (convolution)]

**schiz·oid** (skiz'oyd) socially isolated, withdrawn, having few (if any) friends or social relationships; resembling the personality features characteristic of schizophrenia, but in a milder form.

S
C

SEE ALSO schizoid personality. [schizo(phrenia), + G. *eidos,* resemblance]

**schiz•oid per•son•al•i•ty, schiz•oid per•son•al•i•ty dis•or•der** an enduring and pervasive pattern of behavior in adulthood characterized by social withdrawal, emotional coldness or aloofness or restriction, and indifference to others.

**schiz•ont** (skiz′ont) a sporozoan trophozoite (vegetative form) that reproduces by schizogony, producing a varied number of daughter trophozoites or merozoites. [schizo- + G. *ōn (ont-),* a being]

**schiz•o•nych•ia** (skiz-ō-nik′ē-ă) splitting of the nails. [schizo- + G. *onyx,* nail]

**schiz•o•pha•sia** (skiz-ō-fā′zē-ă) the disordered speech (word salad) of the schizophrenic individual. [schizo- + G. *phasis,* speech]

**schiz•o•phre•nia** (skiz-ō-frē′nē-ă, skits′ō-frē′nē-ă) a term, coined by Bleuler synonymous with and replacing dementia praecox; a common type of psychosis, characterized by a disorder in perception, content of thought, and thought processes (hallucinations and delusions), and extensive withdrawal of one's interest from other people and the outside world, and the investment of it in one's own; now considered a group or spectrum of schizophrenic disorders rather than as a single entity. [schizo- + G. *phrēn,* mind]

**schiz•o•phren•ic** (skiz-ō-fren′ik, skiz-ō-frē′nik, skits-ō-frēn′ik) relating to, characteristic of, or suffering from one of the schizophrenias.

**schiz•o•trich•ia** (skiz-ō-trik′ē-ă) a splitting of the hairs at their ends. [schizo- + G. *thrix,* hair]

**schiz•o•typ•al per•son•al•i•ty dis•or•der, schiz•o•typ•al per•son•al•i•ty** an enduring and pervasive pattern of behavior in adulthood characterized by discomfort with and reduced capacity for close relationships, cognitive or perceptual distortions, and eccentric behavior.

**schiz•o•typ•i•cal per•son•al•i•ty** a personality disorder characterized by eccentricities in thinking, appearance, and behavior; although not psychotic, individuals with such a disorder hold ideas that are considered unusual and have difficulty relating to others.

**Schlat•ter dis•ease, Schlat•ter-Os•good dis•ease** (shlah′tĕr, shlah′ter-oz′gud) SYN Osgood-Schlatter disease.

**Schlemm ca•nal** (shlem) SYN sinus venosus sclerae.

**Schle•sing•er sign** (shlā′sing-ĕr) SYN Pool phenomenon (1).

**Schmi•del a•nas•to•mo•ses** (shmid′ĕl) abnormal channels of communication between the caval and portal venous systems.

**Schmidt-Lan•ter•man in•ci•sures** (shmit-lahn′ter-mahn) funnel-shaped interruptions in the regular structure of the myelin sheath of nerve fibers.

**Schmidt syn•drome** (shmit) **1.** unilateral paralysis of a vocal cord, the velum palati, trapezius, and sternocleidomastoid. [J.F.M. Schmidt] **2.** the association of primary hypothyroidism, primary adrenocortical insufficiency, and insulin-dependent diabetes mellitus. [M.B. Schmidt]

**Schmorl fer•ric-fer•ri•cy•a•nide re•duc•tion stain** (shmorl) a stain to test for reducing substances in tissues, including melanin, argentaffin granules, thyroid colloid, keratin, keratohyalin, and lipofuscin pigments; ferricyanide is converted into ferrocyanide which is converted to insoluble Prussian blue in the presence of ferric ions.

**Schmorl nod•ule** (shmorl) prolapse of the nucleus pulposus through the vertebral body endplate into the spongiosa of an adjacent vertebra.

**Schmorl pic•ro•thi•o•nin stain** (shmorl) a stain for compact bone which employs thionin and picric acid solutions to produce blue to blue-black staining of bone canaliculi and cells; bone matrix is yellowish and cartilage ground substance is purple.

**Schnei•der car•mine** (shnī′dĕr) a stain consisting of a 10% solution of carmine in 45% acetic acid, used for fresh chromosome preparations.

**Schnei•der first rank symp•toms** (shnī′dĕr) those symptoms that, when present, indicate that the diagnosis of schizophrenia is likely, provided that organic or toxic etiology is ruled out: delusion of control, thought broadcasting, thought withdrawal, thought insertion, hearing one's thoughts spoken aloud, auditory hallucinations that comment on one's behavior, and auditory hallucinations in which two voices carry on a conversation.

**Schnitz•ler syn•drome** (shnitz′lĕr) tense, generalized chronic urticaria, joint or bone pain, and monoclonal gammopathy of kappa type.

**Schob•er test** (shō′bĕr) a measure of lumbar spine motion in which parallel horizontal lines are drawn 10 cm above and 5 cm below the lumbosacral junction in the erect subject; with maximum forward flexion, the distance between the lines increases at least 5 cm in normal patients but far less in patients with ankylosing spondylitis.

**Schön•lein pur•pu•ra** (shern′līn) SYN Henoch-Schönlein purpura.

**school pho•bia** a young child's sudden aversion to or fear of attending school, usually considered a manifestation of separation anxiety.

**Schroe•der op•er•a•tion** (shrĕr′dĕr) excision of diseased endocervical mucosa.

**Schu•chardt op•er•a•tion** (shoo′kahrt) a paravaginal rectal displacement incision, a surgical technique of making the upper vagina accessible for fistula closure or radical surgery via the vagina.

**Schüff•ner dots** (shēf-′nĕr) fine, round, uniform red or red-yellow dots (as colored with Romanovsky stains) characteristically observed in erythrocytes infected with *Plasmodium vivax* and *P. ovale,* but not ordinarily found in *P. malariae* and *P. falciparum* infections.

**Schül•ler phe•nom•e•non** (shēl′ĕr) when patients with hemiplegia walk, if the disorder is functional they turn to the unaffected side; if it is organic, they turn to the affected side.

**Schüller syn•drome** (shēl′ĕr) SYN Hand-Schüller-Christian disease.

**Schultz-Charl•ton re•ac•tion** (shoolts-kahrl′tŏn) the specific blanching of a scarlatinal rash at the site of intracutaneous injection of scarlatina antiserum.

**Schult•ze mech•a•nism** (shoolt′sĕ) expulsion of the placenta with the fetal surface foremost.

**Schult•ze phan•tom** (shoolt′sĕ) a model of a female pelvis used in demonstrating the mechanism of childbirth and the application of forceps.

**Schult•ze pla•cen•ta** (shoolt′sĕ) a placenta that appears at the vulva with the glistening fetal surface (amnion) presenting.

**Schult·ze sign** (shoolt'sĕ) in latent tetany, tapping the tongue causes its depression with a concave dorsum.

**Schwal·be ring** (shvahl'bĕ) SYN anterior limiting ring.

**Schwann cells** (shvahn) cells of ectodermal (neural crest) origin that compose a continuous envelope around each nerve fiber of peripheral nerves. SYN neurilemma cells, neurolemma cells.

**schwan·no·ma** (shwah-nō'mă) a benign, encapsulated neoplasm in which the fundamental component is structurally identical to a syncytium of Schwann cells; the neoplastic cells proliferate within the endoneurium, and the perineurium forms the capsule. The neoplasm may originate from a peripheral or sympathetic nerve, or from various cranial nerves, particularly the eighth nerve; when the nerve is small, it is usually found (if at all) in the capsule of the neoplasm; if the nerve is large, the neurilemmoma may develop within the sheath of the nerve, the fibers of which may then spread over the surface of the capsule as the neoplasm enlarges. Microscopically, neurilemmoma is composed of combinations of two patterns, Antoni types A and B, either of which may be predominant in various examples of neurilemmomas. SEE ALSO neurofibroma. SYN neurilemoma. [Theodor *Schwann* + -oma]

**schwan·no·sis** (shwah-nō'sis) a nonneoplastic proliferation of Schwann cells in the perivascular spaces of the spinal cord; seen particularly in older patients, especially those with diabetes mellitus.

**Schwart·ze sign** (shvahrt'zĕ) vascularization of the promontory of the middle ear resulting in a rosy glow that can be seen through the eardrum; a sign of otosclerosis. SEE ALSO otosclerosis. SYN promontory flush.

**sci·age** (sē-ahzh') a to-and-fro, sawlike movement of the hand in massage. [Fr. *scie,* saw]

**sci·at·ic** (sī-at'ik) **1.** relating to or situated in the neighborhood of the ischium or hip. Ischial or sciatic. SYN ischiadic, ischial, ischiatic. **2.** relating to sciatica. [Mediev. L. *sciaticus,* a corruption of G. *ischiadikos,* fr. *ischion,* the hip joint]

**sci·at·i·ca** (sī-at'i-kă) pain in the lower back and hip radiating down the back of the thigh into the leg, initially attributed to sciatic nerve dysfunction (hence the term), but now known to usually be due to herniated lumbar disk compromising the L5 or S1 root. [see sciatic]

**sci·at·ic bur·sa of glu·te·us max·i·mus** the bursa between the gluteus maximus muscle and the tuberosity of the ischium.

**sci·at·ic fo·ra·men** either of two foramina formed by the sacrospinous and sacrotuberous ligaments crossing the sciatic notches of the hip bone: greater sciatic foramen and lesser sciatic foramen.

**sci·at·ic her·nia** protrusion of intestine through the great sacrosciatic foramen. SYN ischiocele.

**sci·at·ic nerve** arises from the sacral plexus, passes through the greater sciatic foramen and down the thigh, deep to the long head of biceps femoris nerve; at the apex of the popliteal fossa it divides into the common peroneal and tibial nerves, although the two may separate at higher levels. SYN nervus ischiadicus [TA].

**sci·ence** (sī'ens) **1.** the branch of knowledge that produces theoretical explanations of natural phenomena based on experiments and observations. **2.** an area of such knowledge that is restricted to explaining a limited class of phenomena. [L. *scientia,* knowledge, fr. *scio,* to know]

**sci·en·ti·fic theory** a theory that can be tested and potentially disproved; failure to disprove or refute it increases confidence in it, but it cannot be considered as proven.

**sci·en·to·met·rics** (sī-en-tō-met'riks) the measurement of scientific output, and the impact of scientific findings, e.g., on public policy. [L. *scientia,* science, knowledge, fr. *scio,* to know, + G. *metron,* measure, + -ics]

**scim·i·tar sign** a curvilinear structure seen roentgenographically in the lung and associated with anomalous pulmonary venous drainage, suggesting the sickle shape of a Turkish saber; also used to refer to the scalloped shape of the sacrum in spinal dysraphism with anterior meningocele.

**scin·ti·cis·tern·og·ra·phy** (sin'ti-sis-tern-og'ră-fē) cisternography performed with a radiopharmaceutical and recorded with a stationary imaging device.

**scin·ti·gram** (sin'ti-gram) SYN scintiscan. [L. *scintilla,* spark, + G. *gramma,* something written]

**scin·ti·graph·ic** (sin'ti-graf'ik) relating to or obtained by scintigraphy.

**scin·tig·ra·phy** (sin-tig'ră-fē) a diagnostic procedure consisting of the administration of a radionuclide with an affinity for the organ or tissue of interest, followed by recording the distribution of the radioactivity with a stationary or scanning external scintillation camera.

**scin·til·lat·ing sco·to·ma** a localized area of blindness edged by brilliantly colored shimmering lights (teichopsia); usually a prodromal symptom of migraine. SEE ALSO fortification spectrum.

**scin·til·la·tion** (sin-ti-lā'shŭn) **1.** flashing or sparkling; a subjective sensation as of sparks or flashes of light. **2.** in radiation measurement, the light produced by an ionizing event in a phosphor, as in a crystal or liquid scintillator. SEE ALSO scintillation counter. [L. *scintilla,* a spark]

**scin·til·la·tion cam·er·a** SYN gamma camera.

**scin·til·la·tion count·er** an instrument used for the detection and measurement of radioactivity.

**scin·til·la·tor** (sin'ti-lā-ter) a substance that emits visible light when hit by a subatomic particle or x- or gamma ray. SEE ALSO scintillation counter.

**scin·ti·pho·tog·ra·phy** (sin'ti-fō-tog'ră-fē) the process of obtaining a photographic recording of the distribution of an internally administered radiopharmaceutical with the use of a gamma camera.

**scin·ti·scan** (sin'ti-skan) the record obtained by scintigraphy. SEE ALSO scan. SYN photoscan, scintigram.

**scin·ti·scan·ner** (sin'ti-skan'er) the apparatus used to make a scintiscan.

**scir·rhous** (skir'us, sir'us) hard; relating to a scirrhus.

**scir·rhous car·ci·no·ma** a hard carcinoma, fibrous in nature, resulting from a desmoplastic reaction by the stromal tissue. SYN fibrocarcinoma.

**scis·sion** (sizh'ŭn) **1.** a separation, division, or splitting, as in fission. **2.** SYN cleavage (2). [L. *scissio,* fr. *scindo,* pp. *scissus,* to cleave]

**scis·sors** (siz'erz) an instrument with two blades,

moving on a pivot, that cut against each other. SYN shears. [L. *scindo*, pp. *scissus*, to cut]

**scis·su·ra**, pl. **scis·su·rae** (si-soo′ră, si-soo′rē) **1.** cleft or fissure. **2.** a splitting. SYN scissure. [L.]

**scis·sure** (sish′oor) SYN scissura.

**scle·ra**, pl. **scle·ras**, **scler·ae** (sklēr′ă, sklēr′ăz, sklēr′ē) [TA] a portion of the fibrous tunic forming the outer envelope of the eye, except for its anterior one-sixth, which is the cornea. SYN sclerotica. [Mod. L. fr. G. *sklēros*, hard]

**scler·ad·e·ni·tis** (sklēr′ad-ĕ-nī′tis) inflammatory induration of a gland. [scler- + G. *adēn*, gland, + *-itis*, inflammation]

**scle·ral** (sklēr′ăl) relating to the sclera. SYN sclerotic (2).

**scler·al staph·y·lo·ma** SYN equatorial staphyloma.

**scler·al sul·cus** a slight groove on the external surface of the eyeball indicating the line of union of the sclera and cornea or limbus of cornea.

**scler·al veins** small veins draining the sclera; they are tributaries to the anterior ciliary veins.

**scler·al ve·nous si·nus** the vascular structure encircling the anterior chamber of the eye and through which the aqueous is returned to the blood circulation. SYN Lauth canal.

**scle·rec·ta·sia** (sklēr-ek-tā′zē-ă) localized bulging of the sclera. [scler- + G. *ektasis*, an extension]

**scle·rec·to·my** (sklē-rek′tō-mē) **1.** excision of a portion of the sclera. **2.** removal of the fibrous adhesions formed in chronic otitis media. [scler- + G. *ektomē*, excision]

**scle·re·de·ma** (sklēr-e-dē′mă) hard nonpitting edema of the skin of the dorsal aspect of the upper body and extremities, giving a waxy appearance and no sharp demarcation. [scler- + G. *oidēma*, a swelling (edema)]

**scler·e·de·ma a·dul·to·rum** a benign spreading induration of the skin and subcutaneous tissue, possibly streptococcal in origin, that may follow a febrile illness, with thickening of the skin by collagen and mucin deposit. SYN Buschke disease.

**scle·re·ma** (sklĕ-rē′mă) induration of subcutaneous fat. [scler- + edema]

**scler·e·ma ne·o·na·to·rum** sclerema appearing at birth or in early infancy, usually in premature and hypothermic infants, as sharply demarcated and yellowish white indurated plaques that usually involve the cheeks, buttocks, shoulders, and calves; subcutaneous fat has a high proportion of saturated fatty acids; microscopically, there is thickening of interlobular fibrous tissue and formation of triglyceride crystals and foreign body giant cells; prognosis is poor for widespread lesions, but localized lesions may resolve slowly over a period of many months.

**scle·ri·tis** (sklĕ-rī′tis) inflammation of the sclera.

△**scler·o-**, **scler-** hardness (induration), sclerosis, relationship to sclera. [G. *sklēros*, hard]

**scle·ro·blas·te·ma** (sklēr-ō-blas-tē′mă) the embryonic tissue entering into the formation of bone. [sclero- + G. *blastēma*, sprout]

**scle·ro·cho·roid·i·tis** (sklēr′ō-kō-roy-dī′tis) inflammation of the sclera and choroid.

**scle·ro·con·junc·ti·val** (sklēr′ō-kon-jŭngk-tī′văl) relating to the sclera and the conjunctiva.

**scle·ro·cor·nea** (sklēr-ō-kōr′nē-ă) **1.** the cornea and sclera regarded as forming together the hard outer coat of the eye, the fibrous tunic of the eye.

**2.** a congenital anomaly in which the whole or part of the cornea is opaque and resembles the sclera; other ocular abnormalities are frequently present.

**scle·ro·dac·ty·ly**, **scle·ro·dac·tyl·ia** (sklēr-ō-dak′ti-lē, sklēr-ō-dak-til′ē-ă) SYN acrosclerosis. [sclero- + G. *daktylos*, finger or toe]

▣ **scle·ro·der·ma** (sklēr-ō-der′mă) thickening and induration of the skin caused by new collagen formation, with atrophy of pilosebaceous follicles; either a manifestation of progressive systemic sclerosis or localized (morphea). See this page. SYN dermatosclerosis, systemic scleroderma. [sclero- + G. *derma*, skin]

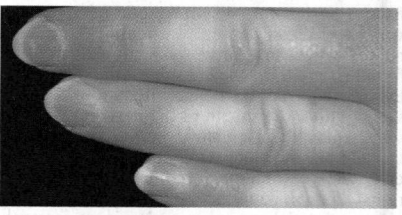

**scleroderma:** early stage

**scle·rog·e·nous**, **scle·ro·gen·ic** (skle-roj′ĕ-nŭs, sklēr-ō-jen′ik) producing hard or sclerotic tissue; causing sclerosis. [sclero- + G. *-gen*, producing]

**scle·roid** (sklēr′oyd) indurated or sclerotic, of unusually firm texture, leathery, or of scar-like texture. SYN sclerosal, sclerous. [sclero- + G. *eidos*, resemblance]

**scle·ro·i·ri·tis** (sklēr′ō-ī-rī′tis) inflammation of both sclera and iris.

**scle·ro·ker·a·ti·tis** (sklēr′ō-ker-ă-tī′tis) inflammation of the sclera and cornea. [sclero- + G. *keras*, horn]

**scle·ro·ker·a·to·i·ri·tis** (sklēr-ō-ker′ă-tō-ī-rī′tis) inflammation of sclera, cornea, and iris.

**scle·ro·ma** (skle-rō′mă) a circumscribed indurated focus of granulation tissue in the skin or mucous membrane. [G. *sklērōma*, an induration]

**scle·ro·ma·la·cia** (sklēr′ō-mă-lā′shē-ă) degenerative thinning of the sclera, occurring in persons with rheumatoid arthritis and other collagen disorders. [sclero- + G. *malakia*, a softening]

**scle·ro·mere** (sklēr′ō-mēr) **1.** any metamere of the skeleton, such as a vertebral segment. **2.** caudal half of a sclerotome. [sclero- + G. *meros*, part]

**scle·ro·nych·i·a** (sklēr-ō-nik′ē-ă) induration and thickening of the nails. [sclero- + G. *onyx*, nail, + *-ia*, condition]

**scle·ro-o·o·pho·ri·tis** (sklēr′ō-ō-of′ō-rī′tis) inflammatory induration of the ovary. [sclero- + Mod. L. *oophoron*, ovary + G. *-itis*, inflammation]

**scle·roph·thal·mia** (sklēr-of-thal′mē-ă) an abnormality in which most of the normally transparent cornea resembles the opaque sclera. [sclero- + G. *ophthalmos*, eye]

**scle·ro·pro·tein** (sklēr-ō-prō′tēn) SYN albuminoid (3).

**scle·ro·sal** (sklē-rō′săl) SYN scleroid.

**scle·ro·sant** (sklĕ-rō′sant) an injectable irritant used to treat varices by producing thrombi in them.

**scle·rose** (sklĕ-rōz′) to harden; to undergo sclerosis.

**scler·o·sing ad·e·no·sis** a nodular, benign breast lesion occurring most frequently in relatively young women and consisting of hyperplastic distorted lobules of acinar tissue with increased collagenous stroma; the changes may be difficult to distinguish microscopically from carcinoma. Also, a benign nodular microscopic lesion of the prostate consisting of acinar tissue with increased stroma; the basal cell layer shows characteristic smooth muscle metaplasia. SYN adenofibrosis.

**scler·o·sing he·man·gi·o·ma** a benign lung or bronchial lesion, often subpleural, sometimes multiple, which forms hyalinized connective tissue.

**scler·o·sing ker·a·ti·tis** inflammation of the cornea complicating scleritis; characterized by opacification of the corneal stroma.

**scler·o·sing os·te·i·tis** fusiform thickening or increased density of bones, of unknown cause. SYN Garré disease.

**scle·ro·sis**, pl. **scle·ro·ses** (sklĕ-rō′sis, sklĕ-rō′ sēz) **1.** SYN induration (2). **2.** in neuropathy, induration of nervous and other structures by a hyperplasia of the interstitial fibrous or glial connective tissue. [G. *sklērōsis*, hardness]

**scle·ro·ste·no·sis** (sklēr-ō-stē-nō′sis) induration and contraction of the tissues. [sclero- + G. *stenōsis*, a narrowing]

**scle·ros·to·my** (sklĕ-ros′tō-mē) surgical perforation of the sclera, as for the relief of glaucoma. [sclero- + G. *stoma*, mouth]

**scle·ro·ther·a·py** (sklēr-ō-thār′ă-pē) treatment involving the injection of a sclerosing solution into vessels or tissues.

**scle·rot·ic** (sklĕ-rot′ik) **1.** relating to or characterized by sclerosis. **2.** SYN scleral.

**scle·rot·i·ca** (sklĕ-rot′i-kă) SYN sclera. [Mod. L. *scleroticus*, hard]

**scler·o·tic bod·ies** vegetative rounded muriform cells of dematiaceous fungi, characteristic of the causal agents of chromoblastomycosis.

**scler·o·tic ce·ment·al mass** benign fibro-osseous jaw lesions of unknown etiology, which present as large painless radiopaque masses.

**scler·o·tic den·tin** dentin characterized by calcification of the dentinal tubules as a result of injury or normal aging. SYN transparent dentin.

**scle·ro·tome** (sklēr′ō-tōm) **1.** a knife used in sclerotomy. **2.** the group of mesenchymal cells emerging from the ventromedial part of a mesodermic somite and migrating toward the notochord. Sclerotomal cells from adjacent somites become merged in intersomitically located masses that are the primordia of the centra of the vertebrae. [sclero- + G. *tomē*, a cutting]

**scle·rot·o·my** (sklĕ-rot′ō-mē) an incision through the sclera. [sclero- + G. *tomē*, incision]

**scle·rous** (sklēr′ŭs) SYN scleroid. [G. *sklēros*, hard]

**SCM** sternocleidomastoid muscle.

**sco·lex**, pl. **scol·e·ces**, **scol·i·ces** (skō′leks, skō′ le-sēz, skō′li-sēz) the head or anterior end of a tapeworm attached by suckers, and frequently by rostellar hooks, to the wall of the intestine. [G. *skōlēx*, a worm]

**sco·li·o·ky·pho·sis** (skō′lē-ō-kī-fō′sis) lateral and posterior curvature of the spine. [G. *scolios*, curved, + *kyphōsis*, kyphosis]

🔒 **sco·li·o·sis** (skō-lē-ō′sis) abnormal lateral curvature of the vertebral column. Depending on the etiology, there may be one curve, or primary and secondary compensatory curves; scoliosis may be "fixed" as a result of muscle and/or bone deformity or "mobile" as a result of unequal muscle contraction. See this page. [G. *skoliōsis*, a crookedness]

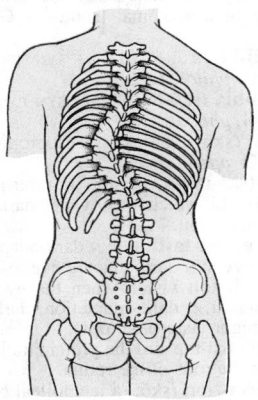

**scoliosis**

**sco·li·ot·ic** (skō′lē-ot′ik) relating to or suffering from scoliosis.

**sco·li·ot·ic pel·vis** a deformed pelvis associated with lateral curvature of the spine.

**scom·broid poi·son·ing** poisoning from ingestion of heat-stable toxins produced by bacterial action on inadequately preserved dark-meat fish of the order Scombroidea (tuna, bonito, mackerel, albacore, skipjack); characterized by epigastric pain, nausea and vomiting, headache, thirst, difficulty in swallowing, and urticaria.

△**-scope** viewing, staring; an instrument for viewing but extended to include other methods of examination (e.g., stethoscope). [G. *skopeō*, to view]

**sco·po·phil·ia** (skō-pō-fil′ē-ă) SYN voyeurism. [G. *skopeō*, to view, + *philos*, fond]

**sco·po·pho·bia** (skō-pō-fō′bē-ă) morbid dread of being stared at. [G. *skopeō*, to view, + *phobos*, fear]

△**-sco·py** an action or activity involving the use of in instrument for viewing. [G. *skopeō*, to view]

**scor·bu·tic** (skōr-byu′tik) relating to, suffering from, or resembling scurvy (scorbutus).

**scor·bu·ti·gen·ic** (skōr-byu-ti-jen′ik) scurvy-producing.

**scor·di·ne·ma** (skōr′di-ne′mă) heaviness of the head with yawning and stretching, occurring as a prodrome of an infectious disease. [G. *skordinēma*, yawning]

**score** (skōr) an evaluation, usually expressed numerically, of status, achievement, or condition in a given set of circumstances. [M. E. *scor*, notch, tally]

△**sco·to-** darkness. [G. *skotos*]

**sco·to·ma**, pl. **sco·to·ma·ta** (skō-tō′mă, skō-tō′ mă-tă) **1.** an isolated area of varying size and shape, within the visual field, in which vision is absent or depressed. **2.** a blind spot in psychological awareness. [G. *skotōma*, vertigo, fr. *skotos,* darkness]

**sco•tom•a•tous** (skō-tō′mă-tŭs) relating to scotoma.

**sco•tom•e•ter** (skō-tom′ĕ-ter) an instrument for determining the size, shape, and intensity of a scotoma.

**sco•tom•e•try** (skō-tom′ĕ-trē) the plotting and measuring of a scotoma. [scoto- + G. *metron,* measure]

**scot•o•phil•ia** (skō-tō-fil′ē-ă) SYN nyctophilia. [scoto- + G. *philos,* fond]

**scot•o•pho•bia** (skō-tō-fō′bē-ă) SYN nyctophobia. [scoto- + G. *phobos,* fear]

**sco•to•pia** (skō-tō′pē-ă) SYN scotopic vision. [scoto- + G. *opsis,* vision]

**sco•top•ic** (skō-tō′pik, skō-top′ik) referring to low illumination to which the eye is dark-adapted. SEE scotopic vision.

**sco•top•ic ad•ap•ta•tion** SYN dark adaptation.

**sco•top•ic eye** SYN dark-adapted eye.

**sco•top•ic vi•sion** vision when the eye is dark-adapted. SEE ALSO dark adaptation, dark-adapted eye. SYN night vision, scotopia.

**sco•top•sin** (skō-top′sin) the protein moiety of the pigment in the rods of the retina.

**Scott op•er•a•tion** (skŏt) a jejunoileal bypass for morbid obesity utilizing end-to-end anastomosis of the upper jejunum to the terminal ileum, with the bypassed intestine closed proximally and anastomosed distally to the colon.

**scot•ty dog** (scot′tē dawg) the fancied appearance of the articular facets on oblique radiographs of the lumbar spine; the neck of the scotty dog is the pars interarticularis, site of the most common defect in spondylolysis.

**scout film** a radiograph exposed before contrast medium is given, such as the preliminary film for an angiogram, urogram, or barium contrast gastrointestinal examination.

**scrap•ing** (skrāp′ing) a specimen scraped from a lesion or specific site, for cytologic examination. SEE ALSO smear.

**scratch test** a form of skin test in which antigen is applied through a scratch in the skin.

**screen** (skrēn) 1. a sheet of any substance used to shield an object from any influence, such as heat, light, x-rays, etc. 2. a sheet upon which an image is projected. 3. PSYCHOANALYSIS concealment, as one image or memory concealing another. SEE ALSO screen memory. 4. to examine, evaluate; to process a group to select or separate certain individuals from it. 5. a thin layer of crystals that converts x-rays to light photons to expose film; used in a cassette to produce radiographic images on film. [Fr. *écran*]

**screen•ing** (skrēn′ing) 1. to screen (5). 2. examination of a group of usually asymptomatic individuals to detect those with a high probability of having a given disease, typically by means of an inexpensive diagnostic test. 3. in the mental health professions, initial patient evaluation that includes medical and psychiatric history, mental status evaluation, and diagnostic formulation to determine the patient's suitability for a particular treatment modality.

**screen•ing test** any testing procedure designed to separate people or objects according to a fixed characteristic or property.

**screen mem•o•ry** PSYCHOANALYSIS a consciously tolerable memory that unwittingly serves as a

cover for another associated memory which would be emotionally painful if recalled.

**scro•bic•u•late** (skrō-bik′yu-lāt) pitted; marked with minute depressions. [L. *scrobiculus;* dim. of *scrobis,* a trench]

**scrof•u•lo•der•ma** (skrof′yu-lō-der′mă) tuberculosis resulting from extension into the skin from underlying atypical mycobacterial infection, most commonly of cervical lymph nodes. [scrofula + G. *derma,* skin]

**scro•tal** (skrō′tăl) relating to the scrotum. SYN oscheal.

**scro•tal her•nia** complete inguinal hernia, located in the scrotum.

**scro•tal hy•po•spa•di•as** hypospadias with the urethral opening on the scrotal surface.

**scro•tal ra•phe** a central line, like a cord, running over the scrotum from the anus to the root of the penis; it marks the position of the septum scroti.

**scro•tal sep•tum** an incomplete wall of connective tissue and nonstriated muscle (dartos fascia) dividing the scrotum into two sacs, each containing a testis.

**scro•tec•to•my** (skrō-tek′tō-mē) removal of all or part of scrotum. [scrotum, + G. *ektomē,* excision]

**scro•ti•tis** (skrō-tī′tis) inflammation of the scrotum.

**scro•to•plas•ty** (skrō′tō-plas-tē) surgical reconstruction of the scrotum. SYN oscheoplasty. [scrotum + G. *plastos,* formed]

**scro•tum**, pl. **scro•ta**, **scro•tums** (skrō′tŭm, skrō′tă, skrō′tŭmz) [TA] a musculocutaneous sac containing the testes; it is formed of skin, containing a network of nonstriated muscular fibers (the dartos or dartos fascia), which also forms the scrotal septum internally. [L.]

**scrub nurse** a nurse who has scrubbed arms and hands, donned sterile gloves and, usually, a sterile gown, and assists an operating surgeon, primarily by passing instruments.

**scrub ty•phus** SYN tsutsugamushi disease.

**scru•ple** (skroo′pl) an apothecaries' weight of 20 grains or one-third of a dram. [L. *scrupulus,* a small sharp stone, a weight, the 24th part of an ounce, a scruple, dim. of *scrupus,* a sharp stone]

**Scul•te•tus ban•dage** (skŭl-tē′tŭs) a large oblong cloth, the ends of which are cut into narrow strips, which is applied to the thorax or abdomen, the strips being tied or overlapped and pinned.

**Scul•te•tus po•si•tion** (skŭl-tē′tŭs) a supine position on an inclined plane with head low, recommended by Scultetus for herniotomy and castration.

**scurf** (skerf) SYN dandruff. [A.S.]

**scur•vy** (sker′vē) a disease marked by inanition, debility, anemia, edema of the dependent parts, a spongy condition (sometimes with ulceration) of the gums, and hemorrhages into the skin and from the mucous membranes; due to a diet lacking vitamin C. [fr. A.S. *scurf*]

**scute** (skyut) a thin lamina or plate. SYN scutum (1). [L. *scutum,* shield]

**scu•ti•form** (skyu′ti-fōrm) shield-shaped. [L. *scutum,* shield, + *forma,* form]

**scu•tu•lar** (skyu′tyu-lăr) relating to a scutulum.

**scu•tu•lum**, pl. **scu•tu•la** (skyu′tyu-lŭm, skyu′tyu-lă) a yellow, saucer-shaped crust, the characteristic lesion of favus, consisting of a mass of hyphae and spores. [L. dim. of *scutum,* shield]

**scu•tum**, pl. **scu•ta** (skyu′tŭm, skyu′tă) 1. SYN

scute. **2.** in ixodid (hard) ticks, a plate that largely or entirely covers the dorsum of the male and forms an anterior shield behind the capitulum of the female or immature ticks. [L. shield]

**scyb·a·la** (sib'ă-lă) plural of scybalum.

**scyb·a·lous** (sib'ă-lŭs) relating to scybala.

**scyb·a·lum**, pl. **scyb·a·la** (sib'ă-lŭm, sib'ă-lă) a hard, round mass of inspissated feces. [G. *skybalon*, excrement]

**scy·phoid** (sī'foyd) cup-shaped. [G. *skyphos*, cup, + *eidos*, resemblance]

**SDA** specific dynamic action.

**Se** selenium.

**sea·ba·ther's e·rup·tion** pruritic rash believed to result from hypersensitivity to the venom of the larval thimble jellyfish (*Linuche unguiculata*).

**sea gull mur·mur** a murmur imitating the cooing sound of a seagull; nearly always due to aortic stenosis or mitral regurgitation.

**sea louse** the very small larvae of the thimble jellyfish (*Linuche unguiculata*).

**sea net·tle** (sē net'il) SYN *Chrysaora quinquecirrha.*

**search·er** (ser'cher) a form of sound used to determine the presence of a calculus in the bladder.

**sea·sick·ness** (sē'sik-nes) a form of motion sickness caused by the motion of a floating platform, such as a ship, boat, or raft. SYN mal de mer.

**sea·son·al af·fec·tive dis·or·der (SAD)** a depressive mood disorder that occurs at approximately the same time year after year and spontaneously remits at the same time each year. The most common type is winter depression, characterized by morning hypersomnia, low energy, increased appetite, weight gain, and carbohydrate craving, all of which remit in the spring.

**seat·ed mas·sage** a massage technique that is performed while the client is fully clothed and seated, often in public settings such as offices, airports, and malls. SYN on-site massage.

**seat·worm** (sēt'werm) SYN pinworm.

**sea wasp** SYN *Chiropsalmus quadrumanus.*

**se·ba·ceous** (sē-bā'shŭs) relating to sebum; oily; fatty. [L. *sebaceus*]

**se·ba·ceous ad·e·no·ma** a benign neoplasm of sebaceous tissue, with a predominance of mature secretory sebaceous cells.

**se·ba·ceous cyst** a common cyst of the skin and subcutis containing sebum and keratin, and lined by epithelium derived from the pilosebaceous follicle. SEE epidermoid cyst, pilar cyst.

**se·ba·ceous ep·i·the·li·o·ma** a benign tumor of the sebaceous gland epithelium in which small basaloid or germinative cells predominate.

**se·ba·ceous fol·li·cles** SYN sebaceous glands.

**se·ba·ceous glands** numerous holocrine glands in the dermis that usually open into the hair follicles and secrete an oily semifluid sebum. SYN sebaceous follicles.

**se·bif·er·ous** (sē-bif'er-ŭs) producing sebaceous matter. [sebi- + L. *fero*, to bear]

⚠**se·bo·**, **seb-**, **se·bi-** sebum, sebaceous. [L. *sebum*, suet, tallow]

**seb·o·lith** (sēb'ō-lith) a concretion in a sebaceous follicle. [sebo- + G. *lithos*, stone]

**seb·or·rhea** (seb-ō-rē'ă) overactivity of the sebaceous glands, resulting in an excessive amount of sebum. [sebo- + G. *rhoia*, a flow]

**seb·or·rhea fa·ci·ei**, **seb·or·rhe·a of face** seb-

orrhea oleosa affecting especially the nose and forehead.

**seb·or·rhea fur·fu·ra·cea** SYN seborrhea sicca (1).

**seb·or·rhea sic·ca 1.** an accumulation on the skin, especially the scalp, of dry scales; SYN seborrhea furfuracea. **2.** SYN dandruff.

**seb·or·rhe·ic** (seb-ō-rē'ik) relating to seborrhea.

**seb·or·rhe·ic bleph·a·ri·tis** a common type of chronic inflammation of the margins of the eyelids with erythema and white scales; often with an associated seborrheic dermatitis of scalp and face.

**seb·or·rhe·ic der·ma·ti·tis**, **der·ma·ti·tis seb·or·rhe·i·ca** a common scaly macular eruption that occurs primarily on the face, scalp (dandruff), and other areas of increased sebaceous gland secretion; the lesions are covered with a slightly adherent oily scale. SYN dyssebacia, dyssebacea, seborrheic dermatosis, Unna disease.

**seb·or·rhe·ic der·ma·to·sis** SYN seborrheic dermatitis.

🖼**seb·or·rhe·ic ker·a·to·sis**, **ker·a·to·sis seb·or·rhe·i·ca** superficial, benign, verrucous, often pigmented, greasy lesions consisting of proliferating epidermal cells, resembling basal cells, enclosing horn cysts; they usually occur after the third decade. See page B6.

**se·bor·rhoea [Br.]** SEE seborrhea.

**se·bor·rhoe·ic [Br.]** SEE seborrheic.

**se·bum** (sē'bŭm) the secretion of the sebaceous glands. [L. tallow]

**sec** second.

**sec·on·dary ab·dom·i·nal preg·nan·cy** a condition in which the embryo or fetus continues to grow in the abdominal cavity after its expulsion from the uterine tube or other seat of its primary development. SYN abdominocyesis (2).

**sec·on·dary ad·he·sion** SYN healing by second intention.

**sec·on·dary a·dre·no·cor·ti·cal in·suf·fi·cien·cy** adrenocortical insufficiency caused by failure of ACTH secretion resulting from anterior pituitary disease or inhibition of ACTH production resulting from exogenous steroid therapy.

**sec·on·dary al·co·hol** an alcohol characterized by the bivalent atom group, —CH(OH)—.

**sec·on·dary al·do·ste·ron·ism** aldosteronism resulting not from a defect intrinsic to the adrenal cortex but from a stimulation of hormonal secretion caused by extra-adrenal disorders; associated with increased plasma renin activity and occurs in heart failure, nephrotic syndrome, cirrhosis, and hypoproteinemia.

**sec·on·dary a·men·or·rhea** amenorrhea in which the menses appeared at puberty but subsequently ceased.

**sec·on·dary a·mine** SEE amine.

**sec·on·dary am·y·loi·do·sis** amyloidosis occurring in association with another chronic inflammatory disease; organs chiefly involved are the liver, spleen, and kidneys, and the adrenal glands less frequently.

**sec·on·dary an·es·thet·ic** a compound that contributes to, but is not primarily responsible for, loss of sensation when two or more anesthetics are simultaneously administered.

**sec·on·dary at·el·ec·ta·sis** pulmonary collapse at any age, but particularly of infants, due to hyaline membrane disease or elastic recoil of the lungs while dying from other causes.

**sec·on·dary ax·is** any ray passing through the optical center of a lens.

**sec·on·dary cat·a·ract 1.** a cataract that accompanies or follows some other eye disease such as uveitis; **2.** a cataract occurring in the retained lens or capsule after a cataract extraction.

**sec·on·dary de·gen·er·a·tion** SYN wallerian degeneration.

**sec·on·dary de·men·tia** chronic dementia following and due to a psychosis or some other underlying disease process.

**sec·on·dary den·tin** dentin formed by normal pulp function after root end formation is complete.

**sec·on·dary den·ti·tion** SYN permanent tooth.

**sec·on·dary de·vi·a·tion** ocular deviation seen in paralysis of an ocular muscle when the paralyzed eye is used for fixation.

**sec·on·dary di·ges·tion** the change in the chyle effected by the action of the cells of the body, whereby the final products of digestion are assimilated in the process of metabolism.

**sec·on·dary dis·ease 1.** a disease that follows and results from an earlier disease, injury, or event; **2.** a wasting disorder that follows successful transplantation of bone marrow into a lethally irradiated host; frequently severe and usually associated with fever, anorexia, diarrhea, dermatitis, and desquamation. SEE ALSO graft versus host disease.

**sec·on·dary drives** those drives not directly related to biological needs; a secondary drive can be learned as an offshoot of a primary drive, in which case it is often referred to as a motive. SYN acquired drives.

**sec·on·dary dye test** localization of lacrimal drainage obstruction following the fluorescein instillation and primary dye tests by intubating the lower punctum and canaliculus and irrigating with saline. SYN Jones II test.

**sec·on·dary dys·men·or·rhea** dysmenorrhea due to inflammation, infection, tumor, or anatomical factors.

**sec·on·dary en·ceph·a·li·tis** collective term for post-infectious, post-exanthem, and post-vaccinal encephalitides.

**sec·on·dary fol·li·cle** SYN vesicular ovarian follicle.

**sec·on·dary gain** interpersonal or social advantages (e.g., assistance, attention, sympathy) gained indirectly from illness. Cf. primary gain.

**sec·on·dary glau·co·ma** glaucoma occurring as a sequel of preexisting ocular disease or injury.

**sec·on·dary gout** resulting from increased serum uric acid levels as a result of an antecedent disease, such as a proliferative disease of the blood and bone marrow, lead poisoning, or prolonged chronic renal failure (on dialysis).

**sec·on·dary he·mo·chro·ma·to·sis** increased intake and accumulation of iron secondary to known cause, such as oral iron therapy or multiple transfusions.

**sec·on·dary hem·or·rhage** hemorrhage at an interval after an injury or an operation.

**sec·on·dary im·mune re·sponse** SEE immune response.

**sec·on·dary ly·so·somes** lysosomes in which lysis takes place, owing to the activity of hydrolytic enzymes; they are believed to eventually become residual bodies.

**sec·on·dary mu·ci·no·sis** SEE mucinosis.

**sec·on·dary non·dis·junc·tion** nondisjunction occurring in an aneuploid cell that was the result of a primary nondisjunction.

**sec·on·dary oo·cyte** an oocyte in which the first meiotic division is completed; the second meiotic division usually stops short of completion unless fertilization occurs.

**sec·on·dary pro·cess** PSYCHOANALYSIS the mental process directly related to the learned and acquired functions of the ego and characteristic of conscious and preconscious mental activities; marked by logical thinking and by the tendency to delay gratification by regulation of the discharge of instinctual demands. Cf. primary process.

**sec·on·dary ra·di·a·tion** a form of radiation that is created when an x-ray beam interacts with matter and gives off some of its energy, forming new and less powerful wavelengths.

**sec·on·dary sat·u·ra·tion** a technique of nitrous oxide anesthesia consisting of an abrupt curtailment of the oxygen in the inhaled mixture to produce a deep plane of anesthesia, following which oxygen is administered to correct hypoxia.

**sec·on·dary sex char·ac·ters** those characters peculiar to the male or female that develop at puberty, e.g., men's beards and women's breasts.

**sec·on·dary sper·ma·to·cyte** the spermatocyte derived from a primary spermatocyte by the first meiotic division; each secondary spermatocyte produces two spermatids by the second meiotic division.

**sec·on·dary stut·ter·ing** established stuttering behavior in which the dysfluencies are accompanied by awareness, anticipation, and resultant anxiety.

**sec·on·dary syph·i·lis** the second stage of syphilis SEE syphilis.

**sec·on·dary tu·ber·cu·lo·sis** tuberculosis found in adults and characterized by lesions near the apex of an upper lobe, which may cavitate or heal with scarring without spreading to lymph nodes; theoretically, secondary tuberculosis may be due to exogenous reinfection or to reactivation of a dormant endogenous infection.

**sec·on·dary tym·pan·ic mem·brane** the membrane closing the fenestra cochleae or rotunda. SYN membrana tympani secundaria [TA], round window membrane.

**sec·on·dary un·ion** SYN healing by second intention.

**sec·ond cra·ni·al nerve [CN II]** SYN optic nerve [CN II].

**sec·ond de·gree AV block** SEE atrioventricular block.

**sec·ond-de·gree burn** a burn involving the epidermis and dermis and usually forming blisters that may be superficial, or by deep dermal necrosis, followed by epithelial regeneration extending from the skin appendages.

**sec·ond de·gree pro·lapse** SEE prolapse of the uterus.

**sec·ond heart sound (S$_2$)** the second sound heard on auscultation of the heart; signifies the beginning of diastole and is due to closure of the semilunar valves.

**sec·ond-look op·er·a·tion** exploratory celiotomy within a year after apparently curative resection of intra-abdominal cancer, in patients with no sign or symptom of recurrence, to resect an occult tumor if present.

**sec·ond mo·lar** seventh permanent or fifth deciduous tooth in the maxilla and mandible on either side of the midsagittal plane of the head following the arch form.

**sec·ond toe [II]** second digit of foot.

**sec·ond tooth** SYN permanent tooth.

**sec·ond wind** colloquial term to describe relief from ill-defined feelings of distress that often accompany the early stages of exercise; generally related to the achievement of a steady state of pulmonary ventilation, aerobic metabolism, and thermal balance as exercise progresses.

**se·cre·ta** (se-krē'tă) secretions. [L. neuter pl. of *secretus,* pp. of *se-cerno,* to separate]

**se·cre·ta·gogue** (se-krē'tă-gog) an agent that promotes secretion; e.g., acetylcholine, gastrin, secretin. [secreta + G. *agōgos,* drawing forth]

**se·cre·tase** (sē-krē'tās) a term used to describe a proteinase that acts on amyloid precursor protein to produce peptides that are soluble and do not precipitate to produce amyloid.

**se·crete** (se-krēt') to elaborate or release products of cellular metabolism (enzymes, mucus, waste products). [L. *se-cerno,* pp. *-cretus,* to separate]

**se·cre·tin** (se-krē'tin) a hormone, formed by the epithelial cells of the duodenum under the stimulus of acid contents from the stomach, that incites secretion of pancreatic juice; used as an aid in the diagnosis of pancreatic exocrine disease and as an adjunct in obtaining desquamated pancreatic cells for cytological examination. [secrete + -in]

**se·cre·tion** (se-krē'shŭn) 1. production by a cell or aggregation of cells (a gland) of a physiologically active substance and its movement out of the cell or organ in which it is formed. 2. the solid, liquid, or gaseous product of cellular or glandular activity that is stored up in or utilized by the organism in which it is produced. Cf. excretion. [L. *se-cerno,* pp. *-cretus,* to separate]

**se·cre·to·in·hib·i·tory** (se-krē'tō-in-hib'i tōr-ē) restraining or curbing secretion.

**se·cre·to·mo·tor, se·cre·to·mo·tory** (se-krē'tō-mō'ter, se-krē'tō-mō'ter-ē) stimulating secretion. [secrete = *motor,* mover]

**se·cre·tor** (se-krē'ter) an individual whose bodily fluids (saliva, semen, vaginal secretions) contain a water-soluble form of the antigens of the ABO blood group.

**se·cre·to·ry** (se-krēt'ĕ-rē, sē'krē-tōr-ē) relating to secretion or the secretions.

**se·cre·to·ry car·ci·no·ma** carcinoma of the breast with pale-staining cells showing prominent secretory activity, as seen in pregnancy and lactation, but found mostly in children.

**se·cre·to·ry nerve** a nerve conveying impulses that excite functional activity in a gland.

**se·cre·to·ry o·ti·tis me·dia** SYN serous otitis.

**sec·tio,** pl. **sec·ti·o·nes** (sek'shē-ō, sek-shē-ō'nēz) ANATOMY a subdivision or segment. [L.]

**sec·tion** (sek'shŭn) 1. the act of cutting. 2. a cut or division. 3. a segment or part of any organ or structure delimited from the remainder. 4. a cut surface. 5. a thin slice of tissue, cells, microorganisms, or any material for examination under the microscope. [L. *sectio,* a cutting, fr. *seco,* to cut]

**sec·ti·o·nes** (sek-shē-ō'nēz) plural of sectio.

**sec·tor·an·o·pia** (sek'tŏr-an-ō'pē-ă) loss of vision in a sector of the visual field. [sector + G. *an-* priv. + *opsis,* vision]

**sec·tor e·cho·car·di·o·gra·phy** two-dimen-

sional echocardiography with a stationary transducer.

**sec·to·ri·al tooth** SYN carnassial tooth.

**sec·tor scan** ULTRASONOGRAPHY a system in which the transducer or transmitted ultrasound beam is rotated through an angle, resulting in a pie-shaped image.

**se·cun·di·grav·i·da** (sek'ŭn-di-grav'i-dă) SEE gravida.

**se·cun·dines** (sek'ŭn-dēnz) SYN afterbirth. [L. *secundinae,* the afterbirth]

**se·cun·dip·a·ra** (sek'ŭn-dip'ă-ră) SEE para.

**se·date** (sĕ-dāt') to bring under the influence of a sedative. [L. *sedatus;* see sedation]

**se·da·tion** (sĕ-dā'shŭn) 1. the act of calming, especially by the administration of a sedative. 2. the state of being calm. [L. *sedatio,* to calm, allay]

**sed·a·tive** (sed'ă-tiv) 1. calming; quieting. 2. a drug that quiets nervous excitement; designated according to the organ or system upon which specific action is exerted; e.g., cardiac, cerebral, nervous, respiratory, spinal. [L. *sedativus;* see sedation]

**SEDC** spondyloepiphyseal dysplasia congenita.

**sed·i·ment** (sed'i-ment) 1. insoluble material that tends to sink to the bottom of a liquid, as in hypostasis. 2. to cause the formation of a sediment or deposit, as in the case of centrifugation or ultracentrifugation. SYN sedimentate. [L. *sedimentum,* a settling, fr. *sedeo,* to sit, settle down]

**sed·i·men·tate** (sed'i-men-tāt) SYN sediment (2).

**sed·i·men·ta·tion** (sed'i-men-tā'shŭn) formation of a sediment.

**sed·i·men·ta·tion co·ef·fi·cient** (*s*) SYN sedimentation constant.

**sed·i·men·ta·tion con·stant** the constant *s* in Svedberg equation for estimating the molecular weight of a protein from the rate of movement in a centrifugal field. The Svedberg unit (S) is arbitrarily set at $1 \times 10^{-13}$ second and is very often used to describe the sedimentation rate of macromolecules; e.g., 4 S RNA. SYN sedimentation coefficient.

**sed·i·men·ta·tion rate** the sinking velocity of blood cells, i.e., the degree of rapidity with which the red cells sink in a mass of drawn blood.

**sed·i·men·ta·tor** (sed'i-men-tā'ter) a centrifuge.

**sed·i·men·tom·e·ter** (sed'ĭ-men-tom'ĕ-ter) a photographic apparatus for the automatic recording of the blood sedimentation rate. [sediment + G. *metron,* measure]

**se·dox·an·trone tri·hy·dro·chlor·ide** (se-doks' an-trōn trī-hī-drō-klōr-īd) a topoisomerase II inhibitor in cancer chemotherapy.

**seed** (sēd) 1. the reproductive body of a flowering plant; the mature ovule. SYN semen (2). 2. BACTERIOLOGY to inoculate a culture medium with microorganisms. [A.S. *soed*]

**See·lig·mül·ler sign** (sē-lig-myu-ler) contraction of the pupil on the affected side in facial neuralgia.

**Sees·sel pock·et** (sē'sel) the part of the embryonic foregut extending cephalad to the level of the oral plate and caudal to the pituitary diverticulum (Rathke pouch).

**seg·ment 1.** a section; a part of an organ or other structure delimited naturally, artificially, or by invagination from the remainder. SEE ALSO metamere. **2.** a territory of an organ having independent function, supply, or drainage. **3.** to divide and redivide into minute equal parts. SYN segmentum [TA]. [L. *segmentum,* fr. *seco,* to cut]

**seg·men·tal an·es·the·sia** loss of sensation limited to an area supplied by one or more spinal nerve roots.

**seg·men·tal ar·ter·ies of kid·ney** the branches of the renal artery that supply the anatomic segments of kidney. Usually five in number, they are end arteries and give off interlobar, arcuate, and interlobular arteries in sequence. The latter send afferent arterioles to the glomeruli as well as branches to the kidney capsule. The segmental arteries of the kidney are identified as: (1) anterior inferior (arteriae segmenti anterioris inferioris renis [TA]); (2) anterior superior (arteriae segmenti anterioris superioris renis [TA]); (3) inferior (arteriae segmenti inferioris renis [TA]); (4) posterior (arteriae segmenti posterioris renis [TA]); and (5) superior (arteriae segmenti superioris renis [TA]).

**seg·men·tal ar·ter·ies of liv·er** anterior and posterior segmental arteries arising from the right branch of the hepatic artery. and medial and lateral segmental arteries arising from the left branch of the hepatic artery; the segmental arteries serve four of the five major divisions of the liver, and then branch in turn so that each hepatic segment receives an independent blood supply.

**seg·men·tal frac·ture** a fracture in two parts of the same bone.

**seg·men·tal neu·ri·tis 1.** inflammation occurring at several points along the course of a nerve; **2.** segmental demyelinating neuropathy.

**seg·men·ta·tion cav·i·ty** SYN blastocele.

**seg·men·tec·to·my** (seg-men-tek′tō-mē) excision of a segment of any organ or gland.

**seg·ment·ed cell** a polymorphonuclear leukocyte matured beyond the band cell so that two or more lobes of the nucleus occur.

**seg·ments of spi·nal cord [C1–Co]** one of the 31 portions of the spinal cord, each of which gives rise to the anterior and posterior roots that combine to form a single pair of spinal nerves. These are the cervical spinal cord segments [C1–C8]; the thoracic spinal cord segments [T1–T12]; the lumbar spinal cord segments [L1–L5]; the sacral spinal cord segments [S1–S5]; and the coccygeal spinal cord segment [Co].

**seg·men·tum**, pl. **seg·men·ta** (seg-men′tŭm, seg-men′tă) [TA] SYN segment. [L. segment]

**seg·re·ga·tion** (seg-rĕ-gā′shŭn) **1.** removal of certain parts from a mass, e.g., those with infectious diseases. **2.** separation of contrasting characters in the offspring of heterozygotes. **3.** separation of the paired state of genes, which occurs at the reduction division of meiosis; only one member of each somatic gene pair is normally included in each sperm or ovum. **4.** progressive restriction of potencies in the zygote to the following embryo. [L. *segrego,* pp. *-atus,* to set apart from the flock, separate]

**seg·re·ga·tion a·nal·y·sis** in genetics, the enumeration of progeny according to distinct and mutually exclusive phenotypes; used as a test of a putative pattern of inheritance, e.g., mendelian, dominant autosomal, epistatic, age-dependent.

**seg·re·ga·tion ra·tio** GENETICS the proportion of progeny of a particular genotype or phenotype from actual matings of specified genotypes. The

test of a mendelian hypothesis is the comparison of the segregation rate with the mendelian rate.

**Sei·del sco·to·ma** (sī′del) a form of Bjerrum scotoma. SEE ALSO Seidel sign.

**Sei·del sign** (sī′del) a sickle-shaped scotoma appearing as an upward or downward extension of the blind spot.

**Seip syn·drome** (sīp) SYN congenital total lipodystrophy.

**sei·zure** (sē′zher) **1.** an attack; the sudden onset of a disease or of certain symptoms. **2.** an epileptic attack. SYN convulsion (2). [O. Fr. *seisir,* to grasp, fr. Germanic]

**sei·zure dis·or·der** SYN epilepsy.

**Sel·din·ger tech·nique** (sel′ding-er) a method of percutaneous insertion of a catheter into a blood vessel or space, such as an abscess cavity: a needle is used to puncture the structure and a guide wire is threaded through the needle; when the needle is withdrawn, a catheter is threaded over the wire; the wire is then withdrawn, leaving the catheter in place.

**se·lec·tin** (sel-ek′tin) a cell surface molecule involved in immune adhesion and cell trafficking. [L. *se-ligo,* pp. *se-lectum,* to sort, choose, + -in]

**se·lec·tion** (sĕ-lek′shŭn) the combined effect of the causes and consequences of genetic factors that determine the average number of progeny of a species that attain sexual maturity. [L. *se-ligo,* to separate, select, fr. *se,* apart, + *lego,* to pick out]

**se·lec·tion co·ef·fi·cient** (*s*) the proportion of progeny or potential progeny not surviving to sexual maturity; usually defined artificially by expressing the fitness of a phenotype as a fraction of the mean or optimal fitness to give the relative fitness, and subtracting this fraction from unity. If the mean size of family in the population is 3.2 and that for a particular genotype is 2.4 then the fitness of the phenotype is 2.4/3.2 = 0.75 and the selection coefficient =1-0.75 =.25 = 5

**se·lec·tive es·tro·gen re·cep·tor mo·du·la·tor (SERM)** pharmaceutical agent with selective estrogen receptor affinity; current preparations have a primary effect on bone and cardiovascular tissues and less effect on endometrial, genital, and breast tissues.

**se·lec·tive in·hi·bi·tion** SYN competitive inhibition.

**se·lec·tive nor·ep·i·neph·rine re·up·take in·hi·bi·tor** a class of chemical compounds that selectively, to varying degrees, inhibit the reuptake of norepinephrine by the presynaptic neurons and are posited to exert their antidepressant effect by this mechanism.

**se·lec·tive se·ro·to·nin re·up·take in·hi·bi·tor (SSRI)** a class of drugs that selectively prevent the reuptake of serotonin and are used for the treatment of depression, e.g., fluoxetine, sertraline.

**se·lec·tive stain** a stain that colors one portion of a tissue or cell exclusively or more deeply than the remaining portions.

**se·le·ni·um (Se)** (sĕ-lē′nē-ŭm) a metallic element chemically similar to sulfur, atomic no. 34, atomic wt. 78.96; an essential trace element toxic in large quantities; required for glutathione peroxidase and a few other enzymes; [75]Se (half-life equal to 119.78 days) is used in scintography of the pancreas and parathyroid glands. [G. *selēnē*, moon]

**se•le•ni•um plate** a radiation-sensitive material used in digital radiography. SEE ALSO digital radiography. SYN amorphous selenium plate.

**self 1.** a sum of the attitudes, feelings, memories, traits, and behavioral predispositions that make up the personality. **2.** the individual as represented in his or her own awareness and in his or her environment. **3.** IMMUNOLOGY an individual's autologous cell components as contrasted with non-self, or foreign, constituents; discrimination by the immune system between self and non-self protects against an attack on the host's own antigenic constituents. The mechanism of recognition of self from non-self is unknown, but serves to protect from an immunologic attack on the host's own antigenic constituents, as opposed to immune system destruction or elimination of foreign antigens.

**self-a•ware•ness** realization of one's ongoing feeling and emotional experience; a major goal of all psychotherapy.

**self con•cept** an assessment of one's own status with respect to one or several traits, using societal or personal norms as criteria.

**self-con•cept** an individual's sense of self, including self-definition in the various social roles one enacts, including assessment of one's own status with respect to a single trait or to many human dimensions, using societal or personal norms as criteria.

**self-con•trol 1.** self-regulation of one's behavior in accordance with personal beliefs, goals, attitudes and societal expectations. **2.** use by an individual of active coping strategies to deal with problem situations, in contrast to passive conditioning strategies which do things to the individual and require no action by the person.

**self•ish DNA** SYN junk DNA.

**self-lim•it•ed** denoting a disease that tends to cease after a definite period; e.g., pneumonia.

**self-love** SYN narcissism.

**self-reg•is•ter•ing ther•mom•e•ter** a thermometer in which the maximum or minimum temperature, during the period of observation, is registered.

**self-re•tain•ing cath•e•ter** a catheter so constructed that it remains in urethra and bladder until removed, e.g., indwelling catheter; Foley catheter.

**sel•la** (sel'ă) SYN saddle (1). [L. saddle]

**sel•lar** (sel'ăr) relating to the sella turcica.

**sel•la tur•ci•ca** a saddle-like bony prominence on the upper surface of the body of the sphenoid bone, constituting the middle part of the butterfly-shaped middle cranial fossa; it includes the tuberculum sellae anteriorly and the dorsum sellae posteriorly; with its covering of dura mater it constitutes the hypophysial fossa which accommodates the hypophysis or pituitary gland.

**Sel•lick ma•neu•ver** (sel'eik) pressure applied to the cricoid cartilage, to prevent regurgitation during tracheal intubation in the anesthetized patient.

**se•man•tics** (se-man'tiks) A branch of semiotics: **1.** the study of the significance and development of the meaning of words. **2.** the study concerned with the relations between signs and their referents; the relations between the signs of a system; and human behavioral reaction to signs, including unconscious attitudes, influences of social institutions, and epistemological and linguistic assumptions. [G. *sēmainō*, to show]

**se•men**, pl. **sem•i•na**, **se•mens** (sē'men, sē-mi'nă, sē'menz) **1.** the penile ejaculate; a thick, yellowish-white, viscid fluid containing spermatozoa; a mixture produced by secretions of the testes, seminal vesicles, prostate, and bulbourethral glands. SYN seminal fluid, sperm (2). **2.** SYN seed (1). [L. *semen* (*semin-*), seed (of plants, men, animals)]

**se•me•nu•ria** (sē-měn-yu'rē-ă) the excretion of urine containing semen. SYN seminuria, spermaturia.

△**sem•i-** one-half. Cf. hemi-. [L. *semis,* half]

**sem•i•ca•nal** (sem'ē-kă-nal') a half canal; a deep groove on the edge of a bone which, uniting with a similar groove or part of an adjoining bone, forms a complete canal. SYN semicanalis.

**sem•i•ca•na•lis**, pl. **sem•i•ca•na•les** (sem'ē-kă-nal'is, sem'ē-kă-nal-ēz) SYN semicanal. [L.]

**sem•i•ca•na•lis tu•bae aud•i•to•riae** SYN canal for pharyngotympanic tube.

**Sem•i•chon a•cid car•mine stain** (sem'i-kon) stain for adult trematodes.

**sem•i•cir•cu•lar ca•nals of bo•ny la•by•rinth** the organ of balance; the three bony tubes in the labyrinth of the ear within which the membranous semicircular ducts are located; they lie in planes at right angles to each other and are known as anterior semicircular canal, posterior semicircular canal, and lateral semicircular canal.

**sem•i•cir•cu•lar ducts** three small membranous tubes in the bony semicircular canals that lie within the bony labyrinth and form loops of about two-thirds of a circle. The three (anterior semicircular duct, lateral semicircular duct, and posterior semicircular duct) lie in planes at right angles to each other and open into the vestibule by five openings of which one is common to the anterior and lateral ducts. Each duct has an ampulla at one end within which filaments of the vestibular nerve terminate.

**sem•i-closed an•es•the•sia** inhalation anesthesia using a circuit in which a portion of the exhaled air is exhausted from the circuit and a portion is rebreathed following absorption of carbon dioxide.

**sem•i•co•ma•tose, sem•i•co•ma** an imprecise term for a state of drowsiness and inaction, in which more than ordinary stimulation may be required to evoke a response, and the response may be delayed or incomplete. SYN semiconscious.

**sem•i•con•scious** SYN semicomatose.

**sem•i-Fow•ler po•si•tion** (fowl'eř) an inclined position obtained by raising the head of the bed 10–15 inches, flexing the hips, and placing a support under the knees so that they are bent at approximately 90°, thereby allowing fluid in the abdominal cavity to collect in the pelvis.

**sem•i-hor•i•zon•tal heart** refers to the heart's electrical axis when this is directed at approximately 0°.

**sem•i•lu•nar** (sem-ē-loo'năr) SYN lunar (2). [semi- + L. *luna*, moon]

**sem•i•lu•nar bone** obsolete term for lunate bone.

**sem•i•lu•nar car•ti•lage** one of the articular menisci of the knee joint.

**sem•i•lu•nar con•junc•ti•val fold 1.** the semilunar fold formed by the palpebral conjunctiva at the medial angle of the eye; **2.** a fold of the conjunctival mucous membrane found in many animals; normally partially hidden in the medial canthus of the eye when at rest, it may be extended to cover part or all of the cornea in a winking-like action to clean the cornea, as in birds. SYN plica semilunaris conjunctivae [TA].

**sem·i·lu·nar fi·bro·car·ti·lage** SEE lateral meniscus, medial meniscus.

**sem·i·lu·nar hi·a·tus** a deep, narrow groove in the lateral wall of the middle meatus of the nasal cavity, into which the maxillary sinus, the frontonasal duct, and the middle ethmoid cells open.

**sem·i·lu·nar line** SYN linea semilunaris.

**sem·i·lu·nar valve** a heart valve composed of a set of three semilunar cusps (valvules); hence both the aortic and pulmonary valves are semilunar valves.

**sem·i·mem·bra·no·sus mus·cle** *origin*, tuberosity of ischium; *insertion*, medial condyle of tibia and by membrane to tibial collateral ligament of knee joint, popliteal fascia, and via its reflected tendon of insertion (oblique popliteal ligament) lateral condyle of femur; *action*, flexes knee and rotates leg medially when knee is flexed; and contributes to the stability of extended knee by making capsule of knee joint tense; *nerve supply*, tibial. SYN musculus semimembranosus [TA].

**sem·i·mem·bra·nous bur·sa** it lies between the muscle, the head of the gastrocnemius, and the knee joint.

**sem·i·nal** (sem′i-năl) **1.** relating to the semen. **2.** original or influential of future developments.

**sem·i·nal col·lic·u·lus** an elevated portion of the urethral crest upon which open the two ejaculatory ducts and the prostatic utricle.

**sem·i·nal duct** any of the ducts conveying semen from the epididymis to the urethra, ductus deferens, or ejaculatory duct. SYN gonaduct (1).

**sem·i·nal flu·id** SYN semen (1).

**sem·i·nal gland** SYN seminal vesicle.

**sem·i·nal gran·ule** one of the minute granular bodies present in the semen.

**sem·i·nal lake** SYN lacus seminalis.

**sem·i·nal ves·i·cle** one of two folded, sacculated, glandular diverticula of the ductus deferens; its secretion is one of the components of the semen. SYN gonecyst, gonecystis, seminal gland.

**sem·i·na·tion** (sem-i-nā′shŭn) SYN insemination.

**sem·i·nif·er·ous** (sem′i-nif′er-ŭs) carrying or conducting the semen; denoting the tubules of the testis. [L. *semen*, seed (semen) + *fero*, to carry]

**sem·i·nif·er·ous ep·i·the·li·um** the epithelium lining the convoluted tubules of the testis where spermatogenesis and spermiogenesis occur.

**sem·i·nif·er·ous tu·bule** one of two or three twisted curved tubules in each lobule of the testis, in which spermatogenesis occurs. SYN tubuli seminiferi recti [TA], convoluted seminiferous tubule, tubuli contorti (2).

**sem·i·nif·er·ous tu·bule dys·gen·e·sis** a disorder in which the seminiferous tubules exhibit an abnormal cytoarchitecture and extensive hyalinization; the testes are small, and few spermatozoa are formed; the body habitus may be eunuchoid, and gynecomastia may be present; urinary gonadotropin output is usually high, and the incidence of mental deficiency and illness increased; sex chromatin may be male or female, and androgen secretion ranges from subnormal to normal.

It is a constant feature of (and is often used synonymously with) Klinefelter syndrome.

**sem·i·no·ma** (sem-i-nō′mă) a radiosensitive malignant neoplasm usually arising from germ cells in the testis of young male adults which metastasizes to the paraortic lymph nodes; a counterpart of dysgerminoma of the ovary. [L. *semen,* seed (semen) + G. *-oma,* tumor]

**sem·i·nu·ria** (sē-min-yu′rē-ă) SYN semenuria.

**sem·i·o·pen an·es·the·sia** inhalation anesthesia in which a portion of inhaled gases is derived from an anesthesia circuit while the remainder consists of room air.

**se·mi·pen·nate** (sem′ē-pen′āt) 1. having a feather arrangement on one side; resembling one-half of a feather. 2. denoting certain muscles with fibers running at an acute angle from one side of a tendon.

**sem·i·per·me·a·ble** (sem-ē-per′mē-ă-bl) freely permeable to water (or other solvent) but relatively impermeable to solutes.

**sem·i·po·lar bond** a bond in which the two electrons shared by a pair of atoms belonged originally to only one of the atoms; often represented by a small arrow pointing toward the electron receiver; e.g., nitric acid, $O(OH)N{\rightarrow}O$; phosphoric acid, $(OH)_3P{\rightarrow}O$.

**sem·i·spi·nal·is ca·pi·tis mus·cle** *origin*, transverse processes of five or six upper thoracic and articular processes of four lower cervical vertebrae; *insertion*, occipital bone between superior and inferior nuchal lines; *action*, rotates head and draws it backward; *nerve supply*, dorsal primary rami of cervical spinal nerves. SYN musculus semispinalis capitis [TA].

**sem·i·spi·nal·is cer·vi·cis mus·cle** continuous with musculus semispinalis thoracis; *origin*, transverse processes of second to fifth thoracic vertebrae; *insertion*, spinous processes of axis and third to fifth cervical vertebrae; *action*, extends cervical spine; *nerve supply*, dorsal primary rami of cervical and thoracic spinal nerves. SYN musculus semispinalis cervicis [TA].

**sem·i·spi·nal·is tho·ra·cis mu·scle** *origin*, transverse processes of fifth to eleventh thoracic vertebrae; *insertion*, spinous processes of first four thoracic and fifth and seventh cervical vertebrae; *action*, extends vertebral column; *nerve supply*, dorsal primary rami of cervical and thoracic spinal nerves. SYN musculus semispinalis thoracis [TA].

**sem·i·sul·cus** (sem′ē-sŭl′kŭs) a slight groove on the edge of a bone or other structure, which, uniting with a similar groove on the corresponding adjoining structure, forms a complete sulcus.

**sem·i·syn·thet·ic** (sem′ē-sin-thet′ik) describing the process of synthesizing a particular chemical utilizing a naturally occurring chemical as a starting material, thus obviating part of a total synthesis.

**sem·i·ten·di·no·sus mus·cle** *origin*, ischial tuberosity; *insertion*, medial surface of the upper fourth of shaft of tibia; *action*, extends thigh, flexes leg and rotates it medially; *nerve supply*, tibial. SYN musculus semitendinosus [TA].

**sem·i·ver·ti·cal heart** descriptive of the heart's electrical axis when this is directed at approximately +60°.

**Sem·li·ki Fo·rest vi·rus** (sem′li-ki for′est vī′rŭs) an alphavirus in the family Togaviridae rarely associated with human disease.

**se·nesc·ence** (se-nes′ens) the state of being old. [L. *senesco,* to grow old, fr. *senex,* old]

**se·nes·cent** (sē-nes′ent) growing old.

**Seng·sta·ken-Blake·more tube** (seng′stā-kĕn-blāk′mōr) a tube with three lumens, one for drainage of the stomach and two for inflation of attached gastric and esophageal balloons; used for emergency treatment of bleeding esophageal varices.

**se·nile** (sē′nīl, sen′īl) relating to or characteristic of old age. [L. *senilis*]

**se·nile am·y·loi·do·sis** a common form of amyloidosis in very old people, usually mild and limited to the heart. SEE ALSO amyloidosis of aging.

**se·nile ar·te·ri·o·scle·ro·sis** arteriosclerosis similar to hypertensive arteriosclerosis, but as a result of advanced age rather than hypertension.

**se·nile cat·a·ract** a cataract occurring spontaneously in the elderly; mainly a cuneiform cataract, nuclear cataract, or posterior subcapsular cataract, alone or in combination.

**se·nile de·men·tia** dementia of Alzheimer disease developing after age 65.

**se·nile he·man·gi·o·ma** a red papule due to weakening of the capillary wall, seen mostly in persons over 30 years of age. SYN cherry angioma, De Morgan spot.

**se·nile len·ti·go** a variably pigmented lentigo occurring on exposed skin of older Caucasians. SYN liver spot.

**se·nile mel·a·no·der·ma** cutaneous pigmentation occurring in the aged.

**se·nile plaque** a spherical mass composed primarily of amyloid fibrils and interwoven neuronal processes, frequently, although not exclusively, observed in Alzheimer disease. SYN neuritic plaque.

**se·nile psy·cho·sis** mental disturbance occurring in old age and related to degenerative cerebral processes.

**se·nile ret·i·nos·chi·sis** retinoschisis occurring most often in the elderly and affecting the outer plexiform layer.

**se·nile trem·or** an essential tremor that becomes symptomatic in the elderly.

**se·nile vag·i·ni·tis** atrophic vaginitis resulting from withdrawal of estrogen stimulation of mucosa, often assuming the form of adhesive vaginitis.

**se·nil·i·ty** (se-nil′i-tē) old age; a general term for a variety of mental disorders occurring in old age which consist of two broad categories, organic and psychological disorders. [see senile]

**sen·sate** (sen′sāt) able to perceive touch and other sensations; used in reference to patients who have had partial nerve or spinal cord injuries.

**sen·sa·tion** (sen-sā′shŭn) a feeling; the translation into consciousness of the effects of a stimulus exciting any of the organs of sense. [L. *sensatio,* perception, feeling, fr. *sentio,* to perceive, feel]

**sen·sa·tion lev·el** the amount in decibels that a stimulus is above the hearing threshold.

**sense** (sens) the faculty of perceiving any stimulus. [L. *sentio,* pp. *sensus,* to feel, to perceive]

**sense of e·qui·lib·ri·um** the sense that makes possible a normal physiologic posture.

**sense or·gans** the organs of special sense, including the eye, ear, olfactory organ, taste organs, and the accessory structures associated with these organs.

**sen·si·bil·i·ty** (sen-si-bil′i-tē) the consciousness of sensation; the capability of perceiving sensible stimuli. [L. *sensibilitas*]

**sen·si·ble** (sen′si-bl) **1.** perceptible to the senses. **2.** capable of sensation. **3.** SYN sensitive. **4.** having reason or judgment; intelligent. [L. *sensibilis,* fr. *sentio,* to feel, perceive]

**sen·si·ble pers·pir·a·tion** perspiration excreted in large quantity, or when there is much humidity in the atmosphere, so that it appears as moisture on the skin.

**sen·si·tive** (sen′si-tiv) **1.** capable of perceiving sensations. **2.** responding to a stimulus. **3.** acutely perceptive of interpersonal situations. **4.** one who is readily hypnotizable. **5.** readily undergoing a chemical change, with but slight change in environmental conditions, as a sensitive reagent. **6.** IMMUNOLOGY denoting: 1) a sensitized antigen; 2) a person (or animal) rendered susceptible to immunological reactions by previous exposure to the antigen concerned. **7.** MICROBIOLOGY denoting a microorganism that is susceptible to inhibition or destruction by a given antimicrobial agent. SYN sensible (3).

**sen·si·tiv·i·ty** (sen-si-tiv′i-tē) SYN susceptibility (2). **1.** the ability to appreciate by one or more of the senses. **2.** state of being sensitive. **3.** CLINICAL PATHOLOGY the proportion of individuals with a given disease or condition in which a test intended to identify that disease or condition yields positive results. Sensitivity (%) = number of diseased individuals with a positive test × 100 total number of diseased individuals tested. Cf. specificity (2). [L. *sentio,* pp. *sensus,* to feel]

**sen·si·ti·za·tion** (sen′si-ti-zā′shŭn) immunization, especially with reference to antigens (immunogens) not associated with infection; the induction of acquired sensitivity or of allergy.

**sen·si·tize** (sen′si-tīz) to render sensitive; to induce acquired sensitivity, to immunize. SEE ALSO sensitized antigen.

**sen·si·tized an·ti·gen** the complex formed when antigen combines with specific antibody; so called because the antigen, by the mediation of antibody, is rendered sensitive to the action of complement.

**sen·si·tized cell 1.** a cell that has combined with antibody to form a complex capable of reacting with complement components; **2.** a small, "committed," cell derived, by division and differentiation, from a transformed lymphocyte; **3.** a cell that has been either exposed to antigen or opsonized with antibodies and/or complement.

**sen·sor** (sen′sŏr) a device designed to respond to physical stimuli such as temperature, light, magnetism, or movement, and transmit resulting impulses for interpretation, recording, movement, or operating control. [see sense]

△**sen·so·ri-** sensory. [L. *sensorius*]

**sen·so·ri·al** (sen-sōr′ē-ăl) relating to the sensorium.

**sen·so·ri·mo·tor** (sen′sŏr-i-mō′ter) both sensory and motor; denoting a mixed nerve with afferent and efferent fibers.

**sen·so·ri·mo·tor ar·ea** the precentral and postcentral gyri of the cerebral cortex.

**sen·so·ri·neu·ral deaf·ness** hearing impairment due to disorders of the cochlear division of the 9th cranial nerve (auditory nerve), the cochlea, or the retrocochlear nerve tracts, as opposed to conductive deafness.

s
e

**sen·so·ri·neu·ral hear·ing loss** a form of hearing loss due to a lesion of the auditory division of the eighth cranial nerve or the inner ear.

**sen·so·ri·um**, pl. **sen·so·ria, sen·so·ri·ums** (sen-sōr'ē-ŭm, sen-sōr'ē-ă, sen-sōr'ē-ŭmz) **1.** an organ of sensation. **2.** the hypothetical "seat of sensation." **3.** PSYCHOLOGY consciousness; sometimes used as a generic term for the intellectual and cognitive functions. [Late L.]

**sen·so·ry** (sen'sŏ-rē) relating to sensation. [L. *sensorius,* fr. *sensus,* sense]

**sen·so·ry a·cu·i·ty lev·el** a technique for determining air conduction thresholds without masking and with masking presented by bone conduction to the forehead; the change in thresholds indicates the conductive hearing loss.

**sen·so·ry a·pha·sia** SYN receptive aphasia. SYN Wernicke aphasia.

**sen·so·ry a·ware·ness** the ability to receive and differentiate sensory stimuli.

**sen·so·ry cor·tex** formerly denoting specifically the somatic sensory cortex, but now used to refer collectively to the somatic sensory, auditory, visual, and olfactory regions of the cerebral cortex.

**sen·so·ry dep·ri·va·tion** diminution or absence of usual external stimuli or perceptual experiences, commonly resulting in psychological distress and aberrant functioning if continued too long.

**sen·so·ry ep·i·lep·sy** focal epilepsy initiated by a somatosensory phenomenon.

**sen·so·ry gan·gli·on** a cluster of primary sensory neurons forming a usually visible swelling in the course of a peripheral nerve or its dorsal root; such nerve cells establish the sole afferent neural connection between the sensory periphery (skin, mucous membranes of the oral and nasal cavities, muscle tissue, tendons, joint capsules, special sense organs, blood vessel walls, tissues of the internal organs) and the central nervous system; they are the cells of origin of all sensory fibers of the peripheral nervous system.

**sen·so·ry hear·ing im·pair·ment** form of sensorineural hearing impairment caused by a lesion in the inner ear.

**sen·so·ry im·age** an image based on one or more types of sensation.

**sen·so·ry in·teg·ra·tion** the process of organizing sensory information in the brain in order to make an adaptive response; a theory and method of remediation used in occupational and physical therapy.

**sen·so·ry nerve** an afferent nerve conveying impulses that are processed by the central nervous system so as to become part of the organism's perception of self and its environment.

**sen·so·ry neu·ron·o·pa·thy** neuronopathy confined to dorsal root and gasserian ganglia.

**sen·so·ry pa·ral·y·sis** loss of sensation; anesthesia.

**sen·so·ry phan·tom** a perceived sensation unrelated to or distinct from any actual stimulus, which can occur in any of the senses.

**sen·so·ry pro·ces·sing** interpreting and organizing varied stimuli, including those acquired by the tactile, proprioceptive, visual, vestibular, auditory, gustatory, and olfactory senses. SEE ALSO sensory integration, sensory awareness.

**sen·so·ry re·gi·stra·tion** the ability to receive input and select that which will receive attention

and that which will be inhibited from consciousness.

**sen·so·ry speech cen·ter** SYN Wernicke center.

**sen·so·ry ur·gen·cy** urgency due to vesicourethral hypersensitivity.

**sen·su·al** (sen'shoo-ăl) **1.** relating to the body and the senses, as distinguished from the intellect or spirit. **2.** denoting bodily or sensory pleasure, not necessarily sexual. [L. *sensualis,* endowed with feeling]

**sen·su la·to** in a broad sense. [L.]

**sen·su stric·to** in a strict sense. [L.]

**sen·tient** (sen'chent) capable of, or characterized by, sensation. [L. *sentiens,* pres. p. of *sentio,* to feel, perceive]

**sen·ti·nel e·vent** a type of clinical indicator used to monitor and appraise the quality of care, indluding events that require immediate attention.

**sen·ti·nel gland** a single enlarged lymph node in the omentum that may be an indication of an ulcer opposite to it in the greater or lesser curvature of the stomach.

**sen·ti·nel lymph node** the first lymph node to receive lymphatic drainage from a malignant tumor; the sentinel node is identified as the first to take up a radionuclide or dye injected into the tumor; increasingly used in operations for melanoma and breast cancer; if the sentinel node is free of metastasis, more distal nodes are also free. SEE ALSO signal lymph node.

**sen·ti·nel node bi·op·sy** biopsy preceded by injection of a dye or radioisotope proximal to a tumor to identify for excision the primary node draining the area; used to determine the extent of spread of a malignancy.

**sen·ti·nel pile** a circumscribed thickening of the mucous membrane at the lower end of a fissure of the anus.

**sen·ti·nel tag** projecting edematous skin at the lower end of an anal fissure.

**Seoul vi·rus** (sōl) a species of Hantavirus in the Far East causing hemorrhagic fever with renal syndrome. [Seoul, Korea, the city where it was first isolated.]

**sep·a·ra·tion anx·i·e·ty** a child's apprehension or fear associated with removal from or loss of a parent or significant other.

**sep·sis**, pl. **sep·ses** (sep'sis, sep'sēz) the presence of various pus-forming and other pathogenic organisms, or their toxins, in the blood or tissues; septicemia is a common type of sepsis. [G. *sēpsis,* putrefaction]

**sep·sis syn·drome** clinical evidence of acute infection with hyperthermia or hypothermia, tachycardia, tachypnea and evidence of inadequate organ function or perfusion manifested by at least one of the following: altered mental status, hypoxemia, acidosis, oliguria, or disseminated intravascular coagulation.

△**sept-** SEE septi-, septico-, septo-.

**sep·ta** (sep'tă) plural of septum. [L.]

**sep·tal** (sep'tăl) relating to a septum.

**sep·tate** (sep'tāt) having a septum; divided into compartments. [L. *saeptum,* septum]

**sep·tate uter·us** a uterus divided into two cavities by an anteroposterior septum.

**sep·tec·to·my** (sep-tek'tō-mē) operative removal of the whole or a part of a septum, specifically of the nasal septum. [L. *saeptum,* septum, + G. *ektomē,* excision]

△**sep·ti-** seven. [L. *septem*]

**sep·tic** (sep′tik) relating to or caused by sepsis.

**sep·tic a·bor·tion** an infected abortion complicated by fever, endometritis, and parametritis.

**sep·ti·cae·mia [Br.]** SEE septicemia.

**sep·ti·ce·mia** (sep-ti-sē′mē-ă) systemic disease caused by the multiplication of microorganisms in the circulating blood; formerly called "blood poisoning". SEE ALSO pyemia. SYN septic fever. [G. *sēpsis*, putrefaction, + *haima*, blood]

**sep·ti·ce·mic** (sep-ti-sē′mik) relating to, suffering from, or resulting from septicemia.

**sep·ti·ce·mic ab·scess** SYN pyemic abscess.

**sep·tic fe·ver** SYN septicemia.

**sep·tic in·farct** an area of necrosis resulting from vascular obstruction due to emboli composed of clumps of bacteria or infected material.

⌂**sep·ti·co-, sep·tic-** sepsis, septic. [G. *sēptikos*, putrifying, fr. *sēpsis*, putrefaction]

**sep·ti·co·py·e·mia** (sep′ti-kō-pī-ē′mē-ă) pyemia and septicemia occurring together.

**sep·ti·co·py·e·mic** (sep′ti-kō-pī-ē′mik) relating to septicopyemia.

**sep·tic phle·bi·tis** inflammation of a vein due to bacterial infection.

**sep·tic shock 1.** shock associated with sepsis, usually associated with abdominal and pelvic infection complicating trauma or operations; **2.** shock associated with septicemia caused by Gram-negative bacteria.

⌂**sep·to-, sept-** septum. [L. *saeptum*]

**sep·to·mar·gi·nal** (sep′tō-mar′ji-năl) relating to the margin of a septum, or to both a septum and a margin.

**sep·to·na·sal** (sep′tō-nā′săl) relating to the nasal septum.

**sep·to-op·tic dys·pla·sia** congenital optic nerve hypoplasia associated with midline cerebral anomalies.

**sep·to·plas·ty** (sep′tō-plas-tē) operation to correct defects or deformities of the nasal septum, often by alteration or partial removal of supporting structures. [septo- + G. *plastos*, formed]

**sep·to·rhi·no·plas·ty** (sep-tō-rī′nō-plas-tē) combined operation to repair defects or deformities of the nasal septum and of the external nasal pyramid. [septo- + G. *rhis*, nose, + *plastos*, formed]

**sep·tos·to·my** (sep-tos′tō-mē) surgical creation of a septal defect. [septo- + G. *stoma*, mouth]

**sep·tu·lum**, pl. **sep·tu·la** (sep′too-lŭm, sep′too-lă) a minute septum. [Mod. L. dim. of *septum*]

**sep·tum**, gen. **sep·ti**, pl. **sep·ta** (sep′tŭm, sep′tī, sep′tă) **1.** a thin wall dividing two cavities or masses of softer tissue. SEE transparent septum. **2.** in fungi, a wall; usually a cross-wall in a hypha. USAGE NOTE: The plural septa is sometimes mistaken for a singular form and wrongly pluralized as septae. [L. *saeptum*, a partition]

**sep·tum in·ter·a·tri·ale** [TA] SYN interatrial septum.

**sep·tum pe·nis** the portion of the tunica albuginea incompletely separating the two corpora cavernosa of the penis.

**se·que·la**, pl. **se·que·lae** (sē-kwel′ă, sē-kwel′ē) a condition following as a consequence of a disease. [L. *sequela*, a sequel, fr. *sequor*, to follow]

**se·quence** (sē′kwens) the succession, or following, of one thing or event after another. [L. *sequor*, to follow]

**se·quence lad·der** the array of bands, made conspicuous by labeling, formed when DNA fragmented by endonucleases is subject to gel electrophoresis; corresponds to the nucleotide sequence.

**se·quen·tial a·nas·to·mo·sis** two or more anastomoses fashioned from a single conduit, e.g., two or more coronary arteries from a single vein graft or mammary artery.

**se·ques·tra** (sē-kwes′tră) plural of sequestrum.

**se·ques·tral** (sē-kwes′trăl) relating to a sequestrum.

**se·ques·tra·tion** (sē-kwes-trā′shŭn) **1.** formation of a sequestrum. **2.** loss of blood or of its fluid content into spaces within the body so that it is withdrawn from the circulating volume, resulting in hemodynamic impairment, hypovolemia, hypotension, and reduced venous return to the heart. [L. *sequestratio*, fr. *sequestro*, pp. *-atus*, to lay aside]

**se·ques·trec·to·my** (sē-kwes-trek′tō-mē) operative removal of a sequestrum. [sequestrum + G. *ektomē*, excision]

**se·ques·trum**, pl. **se·ques·tra** (sē-kwes′trŭm, sē-kwes′tră) a piece of necrotic tissue, usually bone, that has become separated from the surrounding healthy tissue. [Mod. L. use of Mediev. L. *sequestrum*, something laid aside, fr. L. *sequestro*, to lay aside, separate]

**se·quoi·o·sis** (sē-kwoy-ō′sis) extrinsic allergic alveolitis caused by inhalation of redwood sawdust containing spores of *Graphium*, *Pullularia*, *Aureobasidium*, and other fungi. [*Sequoia* (genus name) for *Sequoah* (George Guess), Cherokee scholar, + G. *-osis*, condition]

**SER** somatosensory evoked response. SEE ALSO evoked response.

**Ser** serine and its radical.

**ser·al·bu·min** (sēr-al-byu′min) SYN serum albumin.

**Ser·gent white line** (sār-zhwah′) SYN white line (2).

**se·ri·al di·lu·tion** a series of dilutions in which each subsequent dilution is made from the previous dilution. The concentration of each dilution is calculated by multiplying the ratios of solute to solution in each dilution preceding and up to the dilution of interest. This type of dilution is used to titer antibodies or to make very dilute solutions from a more concentrated solution.

**se·ri·al ex·trac·tion** selective extraction of certain teeth during the early years of dental development, usually with the eventual extraction of the first, or occasionally the second, premolars, to relieve crowding of anterior teeth.

**se·ri·al in·ter·val** the period of time between analogous phases of an infectious illness in successive cases of a chain of infection that is spread from person to person. SEE ALSO mass action principle, infection transmission parameter.

**se·ri·al ra·di·og·ra·phy** making several x-ray exposures of a single region over a period of time, as in angiography.

**se·ri·al sec·tion** one of a number of consecutive microscopic sections.

**se·ries**, pl. **se·ries** (sēr′ēz) **1.** a succession of similar objects following one another in space or time. **2.** CHEMISTRY a group of substances, either elements or compounds, having similar properties or differing from each other in composition by a constant ratio. [L. fr. *sero*, to join together]

**ser·ine (S, Ser)** (ser'ēn) one of the amino acids occurring in proteins.

**SERM** selective estrogen receptor modulator.

⚠**se·ro-** serum, serous. [L. *serum,* whey]

**se·ro·co·li·tis** (sēr'ō-kō-lī'tis) SYN pericolitis. [Mod. L. *serosa,* serous membrane, + colitis]

**ser·o·con·ver·sion** (sēr-ō-kŭn-ver'zhŭn) process by which, after exposure to etiologic agent of a disease, the blood changes from a negative to a positive serum marker for that specific disease.

**se·ro·di·ag·no·sis** (sēr'ō-dī-ag-nō'sis) diagnosis by means of a reaction using blood serum or other serous fluids in the body (serologic tests).

**se·ro·en·ter·i·tis** (sēr'ō-en-ter-ī'tis) SYN perienteritis. [Mod. L. *serosa,* serous membrane, + enteritis]

**se·ro·ep·i·de·mi·ol·o·gy** (sēr'ō-ep-i-dē-mē-ol'ō-jē) epidemiological study based on the detection of infection by serological testing.

**se·ro·fi·brin·ous** (sēr-ō-fī'bri-nŭs) denoting an exudate composed of serum and fibrin.

**se·ro·fi·brin·ous pleu·ri·sy** the more common form of pleurisy, characterized by a fibrinous exudate on the surface of the pleura and an extensive effusion of serous fluid into the pleural cavity.

**se·ro·fi·brous** (sēr-ō-fī'brŭs) relating to a serous membrane and a fibrous tissue.

**ser·o·group** (ser'ō-groop) **1.** a group of bacteria containing a common antigen, used in the classification of certain genera of bacteria. **2.** a group of viral species that are antigenically closely related.

**se·ro·log·ic** (sēr-ō-loj'ik) relating to serology.

**se·rol·o·gy** (sĕ-rol'ō-jē) the branch of science concerned with serum, especially with specific immune or lytic serums; to measure either antigens or antibodies in sera. [sero- + G. *logos,* study]

**se·ro·ma** (sē-rō'mă) a mass or tumefaction caused by the localized accumulation of serum within a tissue or organ. [sero- + G. *-oma,* tumor]

**se·ro·mem·bra·nous** (sēr'ō-mem'bră-nŭs) relating to a serous membrane.

**se·ro·mu·coid** (sēr-ō-myu'koyd) general term for a mucoprotein (glycoprotein) from serum.

**se·ro·mu·cous** (sēr-ō-myu'kŭs) pertaining to a mixture of watery and mucinous material, such as that of certain glands.

**se·ro·mu·cous gland 1.** a gland in which some of the secretory cells are serous and some mucous; **2.** a gland whose cells secrete a fluid intermediate between a watery and a viscous mucoid substance.

**se·ro·neg·a·tive** (sēr-ō-neg'ă-tiv) lacking an antibody of a specific type in serum; denoting absence of prior infection with a specific agent, disappearance of antibodies after treatment of a disease, or absence of antibody usually found in a given syndrome.

**se·ro·pos·i·tive** (sēr-ō-poz'i-tiv) containing antibody of a specific type in serum; denoting presence of immunological evidence of a specific infection or presence of a diagnostically useful antibody.

**se·ro·pu·ru·lent** (sēr'ō-pyur'ŭ-lent) composed of or containing both serum and pus; denoting a discharge of thin watery pus (seropus).

**se·ro·pus** (sēr'ō-pŭs) purulent serum, i.e., pus largely diluted with serum.

**se·ro·sa** (se-rō'să) **1.** the outermost coat or serous layer of a visceral structure that lies in the body cavities of abdomen or thorax; it consists of a surface layer of mesothelium reinforced by irregular fibroelastic connective tissue. **2.** the outermost of the extraembryonic membranes, which encloses the embryo and all its other membranes; it consists of ectoderm reinforced by somatic mesoderm; the serosa of mammalian embryos is frequently called the trophoderm. SYN membrana serosa (2). SEE ALSO chorion. SYN membrana serosa (1), serous membrane. [fem. of Mod. L. *serosus,* serous]

**se·ro·san·guin·e·ous** (sēr'ō-sang-gwin'ē-ŭs) denoting an exudate or a discharge composed of or containing serum and also blood.

**se·ro·se·rous** (sēr-ō-sēr'ŭs) **1.** relating to two serous surfaces. **2.** denoting a suture, as of the intestine, in which the edges of the wound are infolded so as to bring the two serous surfaces in apposition.

**se·ro·si·tis** (sēr-ō-sī'tis) inflammation of a serous membrane.

**se·ros·i·ty** (se-ros'i-tē) **1.** a serous fluid or a serum. **2.** the condition of being serous. **3.** the serous quality of a liquid.

**se·ro·syn·o·vi·tis** (sēr'ō-sin-ō-vī'tis) synovitis attended with a copious serous effusion.

**se·ro·ther·a·py** (sēr-ō-thār'ă-pē) treatment of an infectious disease by injection of an antitoxin or serum containing specific antibody.

**se·ro·to·ner·gic** (ser-ō-tō-ner'jik) related to the action of serotonin or its precursor L-tryptophan. [serotonin + G. *ergon,* work]

**se·ro·to·nin** (sēr-ō-tō'nin) a vasoconstrictor, liberated by platelets, that inhibits gastric secretion and stimulates smooth muscle; also acts as a neurotransmitter, present in the central nervous system, many peripheral tissues and cells, and carcinoid tumors. SYN 5-hydroxytryptamine. [sero- + G. *tonos,* tone, tension, + -in]

**se·ro·type** (sēr'ō-tīp) SYN serovar.

**se·rous** (sēr'ŭs) relating to, containing, or producing serum or a substance having a watery consistency.

**se·rous cell** a cell, especially of the salivary gland, that secretes a watery or thin albuminous fluid, as opposed to a mucous cell.

**se·rous cyst** a cyst containing clear serous fluid, such as a hygroma.

**se·rous gland** a gland that secretes a watery substance that may or may not contain an enzyme.

**se·rous in·flam·ma·tion** an exudative inflammation in which the exudate is predominantly fluid; relatively few cells are observed.

**se·rous lig·a·ment** one of a number of peritoneal folds attaching certain of the viscera to the abdominal wall or to each other.

**se·rous mem·brane** SYN serosa.

**se·rous men·in·gi·tis** acute meningitis with secondary external hydrocephalus.

**se·rous o·ti·tis** inflammation of middle ear mucosa, often accompanied by accumulation of fluid, secondary to auditory tube obstruction. SYN secretory otitis media.

**se·rous o·ti·tis me·dia** SYN middle-ear effusion.

**se·rous pleu·ri·sy** SYN pleurisy with effusion.

**se·rous syn·o·vi·tis** synovitis with a large effusion of nonpurulent fluid.

**se·ro·vac·ci·na·tion** (sēr'ō-vak-si-nā'shŭn) a process for producing mixed immunity by the injection of a serum, to secure passive immunity, and by vaccination with a modified or killed culture to acquire active immunity later.

**se•ro•var** (sēr′ō-var) a subdivision of a species or subspecies distinguishable from other strains therein on the basis of antigenic character. SYN serotype. [sero- + *variant*]

**ser•pig•i•nous** (ser-pij′i-nŭs) creeping; denoting an ulcer or other cutaneous lesion that extends with a wavy or serpent-like border. [Mediev. L. *serpigo-* (*-gin-*), ringworm, fr. L. *serpo,* to creep]

**ser•pi•go** (ser-pī′gō) **1.** SYN tinea. **2.** SYN herpes. **3.** any creeping or serpiginous eruption. [Mediev. L. *serpigo* (*-gin-*), ringworm, fr. L. *serpo,* to creep]

**ser•rate, ser•rat•ed** (ser′āt, ser-ā′ted) toothed. [L. *serratus,* fr. *serra,* a saw]

**ser•rate su•ture** one whose opposing margins present deep sawlike indentations, as most of the sagittal suture. SYN dentate suture.

**ser•ra•tion** (se-rā′shŭn) **1.** the state of being serrated or notched. **2.** any one of the processes in a serrate or dentate formation. [L. *serra,* saw]

**ser•ra•tus an•te•ri•or mus•cle** *origin,* from center of lateral aspect of first eight to nine ribs; *insertion,* superior and inferior angles and intervening medial margin of scapula; *action,* rotates scapula and pulls it forward, elevates ribs; *nerve supply,* long thoracic from brachial plexus. SYN musculus serratus anterior [TA].

**serre•fine** (ser-fēn′) a small spring forceps used for approximating the edges of a wound or for temporarily closing an artery during an operation. [Fr.]

**Ser•to•li-cell-on•ly syn•drome** (sir-tō′lē) the absence from the seminiferous tubules of the testes of germinal epithelium, Sertoli cells alone being present; there is sterility due to azoospermia but Leydig cells are normal; the output of gonadotrophins in the urine is increased.

**Ser•to•li cells** (sir-tō′lē) elongated cells in the seminiferous tubules that ensheathe spermatids, providing a microenvironment that supports spermiogenesis; they secrete androgen-binding protein and establish the blood-testis barrier by forming tight junctions with adjacent Sertoli cells.

**Ser•to•li cell tu•mor** (sir-tō′lē) a tumor of testis or ovary composed of Sertoli cells; most often benign but may be malignant.

**Ser•to•li-Ley•dig cell tu•mor** (sir-tō′lē-lī′dig) an ovarian tumor composed of Sertoli and Leydig cells; may secrete androgens.

**Ser•to•li-stro•mal cell tu•mor** (sir-tō′lē) a generic term for ovarian sex-cord stromal tumor composed of Sertoli cells, Leydig cells, and cells resembling rete epithelial cells, either in a pure form or as a mixture of these cell types.

**se•rum,** pl. **se•rums, se•ra** (sēr′ŭm, sēr′ŭmz, sēr′ă) **1.** a clear, watery fluid, especially that moistening the surface of serous membranes, or exuded in inflammation of any of those membranes. **2.** the fluid portion of the blood obtained after the fibrin clot and blood cells, distinguished from the plasma in circulating blood. Sometimes used as a synonym for antiserum or antitoxin. [L. whey]

**se•rum ac•cel•er•a•tor** SYN factor VII.

**se•rum ac•cel•er•a•tor glob•u•lin** a substance in serum that accelerates the conversion of prothrombin to thrombin in the presence of thromboplastin and calcium.

**ser•um ag•glu•ti•nin** an antibody which coats erythrocytes; the cells do not agglutinate when suspended in saline, but do agglutinate when suspended in serum or other protein media such as albumin. SYN incomplete antibody (2).

**se•rum•al** (sēr′ŭm-ăl) relating to or derived from serum.

**ser•um al•bu•min** the principal protein in plasma, present in blood plasma and in serous fluids. Participates in fatty acid transport and helps regulate the osmotic pressure of blood. SYN blood albumin, seralbumin.

**ser•um dis•ease** SYN serum sickness.

**se•rum-fast** (sēr′ŭm-fast) **1.** pertaining to a serum in which there is little or no change in the titer of antibody, even under conditions of treatment or immunologic stimulation. **2.** resistant to the destructive effect of sera.

**ser•um glu•ta•mic-ox•a•lo•a•ce•tic trans•am•i•nase (SGOT)** SYN aspartate aminotransferase.

**ser•um glu•tam•ic-py•ru•vic trans•am•i•nase (SGPT)** SYN alanine aminotransferase.

**ser•um hep•a•ti•tis vi•rus** SYN hepatitis B virus.

**ser•um ne•phri•tis** glomerulonephritis occurring in serum sickness or in animals injected with foreign serum protein.

**ser•um pro•throm•bin con•ver•sion ac•cel•er•a•tor (SPCA)** SYN factor VII.

**ser•um re•ac•tion** SYN serum sickness.

**ser•um shock** anaphylactic or anaphylactoid shock caused by the injection of antitoxic or other foreign serum.

**ser•um sick•ness** an immune complex disease appearing 1-2 weeks after injection of a foreign serum or serum protein, with local and systemic reactions such as urticaria, fever, general lymphadenopathy, edema, arthritis, and occasionally albuminuria or severe nephritis. SYN serum disease, serum reaction.

**service** (sĕr′vis) a firm or agency that provides on-scene response, assessment, stabilization, initial treatment as directed, and transport to appropriate receiving facility (i.e., trauma center or hospital) for medical emergency or trauma patients. [L. *servio,* to serve, fr. *servus,* slave]

**ses•a•moid** (ses′ă-moyd) **1.** resembling in size or shape a grain of sesame. **2.** denoting a sesamoid bone. [G. *sēsamoeidēs,* like sesame]

**ses•a•moid bone** a bone formed after birth in a tendon where it passes over a joint, e.g., the patella.

**ses•a•moid car•ti•lage of cri•co•pha•ryn•ge•al li•ga•ment** a small nodule of elastic cartilage sometimes present on the lateral border of the arytenoid cartilage.

**ses•qui•hy•drates** (ses-kwi-hī′drāts) compounds crystallizing with (nominally) 1.5 molecules of water.

**ses•sile** (ses′il) having a broad base of attachment; not pedunculated. [L. *sessilis,* low-growing, fr. *sedeo,* pp. *sessus,* to sit]

**set 1.** to reduce a fracture; i.e., to bring the bones back into a normal position or alignment. **2.** a readiness to perceive or to respond in some way; an attitude which facilitates or predetermines an outcome; e.g., prejudice or bigotry.

**se•ta,** pl. **set•ae** (sē′tă, sē-tē) a bristle or a slender, stiff, bristle-like structure. [L. *saeta* or *seta,* a stiff hair or bristle]

**se•ta•ceous** (sē-tā′shŭs) **1.** having bristles. **2.** resembling a bristle. [L. *seta,* a bristle]

**se•ton** (sē'tŏn) a wisp of threads, a strip of gauze, a length of wire, or other foreign material passed through the subcutaneous tissues or a cyst to form a sinus or fistula. [L. *seta,* bristle]

**set•ting sun sign** retraction of the upper lid without upgaze so that the iris seems to "set" below the lower lid; suggestive of neurologic damage in the newborn, but usually clears up without sequelae.

**sev•enth cra•ni•al nerve [CN VII]** SYN facial nerve [CN VII].

**Se•ver dis•ease** (sē'vĕr) an osteochondrosis of the heel, probably secondary to microfractures in the bone where the Achilles tendon attaches to the posterior calcaneus; an overuse injury and a common cause of heel pain in older children. SYN calcaneal apophysitis.

**se•ve•ri•ty of ill•ness** the degree of illness and risk of disease manifested by patients, based either on clinical data from the medical records or on hospital discharge/billing data. Outcome comparisons usually are interpreted in terms of severity of illness to ensure meaningful data interpretations are made.

**sex** (seks) **1.** the biological character or quality that distinguishes male and female from one another as expressed by analysis of the individual's gonadal, morphological (internal and external), chromosomal, and hormonal characteristics. Cf. gender. **2.** the physiologic and psychological processes within an individual which prompt behavior related to procreation or erotic pleasure. [L. *sexus*]

**sex as•sign•ment** process whereby the sex of an intersex (hermaphroditic) newborn is initially assigned.

**sex cell** a spermatozoon or an oocyte. SYN germ cell.

**sex chro•ma•tin** a small condensed mass of the inactivated X-chromosome usually located just inside the nuclear membrane of the interphase nucleus; the number of sex chromatin bodies per nucleus is one less than the number of X-chromosomes, hence normal males have none and normal females have one. For technical reasons only about half the cells in a preparation show typical masses. SEE ALSO Lyon hypothesis. SYN Barr chromatin body.

**sex chro•mo•somes** the pair of chromosomes responsible for sex determination. In humans and most animals, the sex chromosomes are designated X and Y; females have two X chromosomes, males have one X and one Y chromosome

**sex de•ter•mi•na•tion** determination of the sex of a fetus *in utero* by identification of fetal chromosomes.

**sex hor•mones** a general term covering those steroid hormones that are formed by testicular, ovarian, and adrenocortical tissues, and that are androgens or estrogens.

**sex-in•flu•enced** denoting a class of genetic disorders in which the same genotype has differing manifestations in the two sexes. SEE ALSO sex-influenced inheritance.

**sex-in•flu•enced in•her•i•tance** inheritance that is autosomal but has a different intensity of expression in the two sexes, e.g., male pattern baldness.

**sex-lim•it•ed** occurring in one sex only. SEE sex-limited inheritance.

**sex-lim•it•ed in•her•i•tance** inheritance of a trait that can be expressed in one sex only, e.g., testicular feminization.

**sex link•age, sex-linked** inheritance of a trait or a sex chromosome or gonosome. A man receives all his sex-linked genes from his mother and transmits them all to his daughters but not to his sons; a recessive sex-linked character is much more likely to be expressed in the male. SEE ALSO sex chromosomes.

**sex-linked char•ac•ter** an inherited character determined by a gene on a gonosome. SEE gene.

**sex-linked in•her•i•tance** the pattern of inheritance that may result from a mutant gene located on either the X or Y chromosome.

**sex•ol•o•gy** (sek-sol'ō-jē) the study of all aspects of sex and, in particular, sexual behavior. [L. *sexus,* sex, + G. *logos,* study]

**sex ra•tio 1.** the ratio of male to female progeny at some specified stage of the life cycle, notably at conception (primary), at birth (secondary), or at any stage between birth and death (tertiary); **2.** the ratio of the numbers of males to females affected by a particular disease or trait.

**sex re•ver•sal, sex re•as•sign•ment** a process whereby the sexual identity of an individual is changed from one sex to the other (e.g., by a combination of surgical, pharmacologic, and psychiatric procedures); it may also occur in the life history of pseudohermaphroditic individuals whose sex at birth was uncertain; initially reared as members of one gender or sex role, such individuals may, upon subsequent medical examination and advice, be reared thereafter as members of the opposite gender or sex role.

**sex role** the degree to which an individual acts out a stereotypical masculine or feminine role in everyday behavior. Cf. gender role.

**sex•tant** (seks'tănt) one of the six divisions of the dentition, the teeth of the upper and lower jaws being divided into right posterior, left posterior, and anterior. [L. *sextus,* sixth]

**sex•u•al** (seks'yu-ăl) **1.** relating to sex; genital. **2.** a person as perceived by his or her sexual attractiveness, tendencies, and overall sexuality. [L. *sexualis,* fr. *sexus,* sex]

**sex•u•al a•buse** SEE domestic violence.

**sex•u•al di•mor•phism** the somatic differences within species between male and female individuals that arise as a consequence of sexual maturation; inclusive of, but not restricted to, the secondary sexual characters.

**sex•u•al dis•or•ders** a group of behavioral and psychophysiologic disorders in which there is symptomatic variability in sexual functioning, including either the eroticized behavior associated with sexual activity (the paraphilias) or with disturbances of desire, arousal, and orgasm.

**sex•u•al gen•er•a•tion** reproduction by conjugation, or the union of male and female cells, as opposed to asexual generation.

**sex•u•al in•fan•ti•lism** failure to develop secondary sexual characteristics after the normal time of puberty.

**sex•u•al in•ter•course** SYN coitus.

**sex•u•al•i•ty** (seks-yu-al'i-tē) **1.** the sum of a person's sexual behaviors and tendencies, and the strength of such tendencies. **2.** one's degree of sexual attractiveness. **3.** the quality of having sexual functions or implications.

**sex•u•al•ly trans•mit•ted dis•ease (STD)** any

contagious disease acquired during sexual contact; e.g., syphilis, gonorrhea, chancroid, genital warts, AIDS. SYN venereal disease.

**sex•ual or•i•en•ta•tion** concept that includes the permutations among body morphology, gender identity, gender role, and sexual preference.

**sex•u•al pref•er•ence** the biologic sex preferred in one's sexual partners.

**sex•u•al re•pro•duc•tion** reproduction by union of male and female gametes to form a zygote. SYN gamogenesis, syngenesis.

**sex•u•al se•lec•tion** a form of natural selection in which, according to Darwin's theory, the male or female is attracted by certain characteristics, form, color, behavior, etc., in the opposite sex; thus modifications of a special nature are brought about in the species.

**Sé•zary cell** (sā-zah-rē') an atypical mononuclear cell seen in the peripheral blood in the Sézary syndrome; it has a large, convoluted nucleus and scanty cytoplasm containing PAS-positive vacuoles.

**SGOT** serum glutamic-oxaloacetic transaminase.

**SGPT** serum glutamic-pyruvic transaminase.

**SH** sulfhydryl.

**shad•ow** (shad'ō) **1.** a surface area defined by the interception of light or x-rays by a body. SEE ALSO density (3). **2.** in jungian psychology, the archetype consisting of collective animal instincts. **3.** SYN achromocyte.

**shad•ow test** SYN retinoscopy.

**shaft** an elongated rodlike structure, as the part of a long bone between the epiphysial extremities. SYN diaphysis [TA]. [A.S. *sceaft*]

**sha•green skin** an oval-shaped nevoid plaque, skin-colored or occasionally pigmented, smooth or crinkled, appearing on the trunk or lower back in early childhood; sometimes seen with other signs of tuberous sclerosis.

**sha•ken ba•by syn•drome (SBS)** a syndrome of neurologic and other injuries, of variable presentation, induced by the violent shaking of an infant.

**shal•low breath•ing** a type of breathing with abnormally low tidal volume.

**shank 1.** the tibia; the shin; the leg. **2.** the portion of an instrument that connects the cutting or functional portion to a handle; with rotary tools, such as burs and drills, the end that fits into the chuck. [A.S. *sceanca*]

**shap•ing** (shāp'ing) in operant conditioning, when the operant response is not in the organism's repertoire, a procedure in which the experimenter breaks down the response into those parts which appear most frequently, begins reinforcing them, and then slowly and successively withholds the reinforcer until more and more of the operant is emitted.

**shared ep•i•tope** SYN susceptibility cassette.

**shave bi•op•sy** a biopsy technique performed with a surgical blade or a razor blade; used for lesions that are elevated above the skin level or confined to the epidermis and upper dermis, or to protrusions of lesions from internal sites.

**shears** (shērz) SYN scissors.

**sheath** (shēth) **1.** any enveloping structure, such as the membranous covering of a muscle, nerve, or blood vessel; any sheathlike structure. SYN vagina (1). **2.** the prepuce of male animals, especially of the horse. **3.** a specially designed tubular instrument through which special obturators or

cutting instruments can be passed, or through which blood clots, tissue fragments, calculi, etc. can be evacuated. **4.** a tube used as an orthodontic appliance, usually on molars. [A.S. *scaeth*]

**sheath of Schwann** (shvahn) SYN neurilemma.

**Shee•han syn•drome** (shē'an) hypopituitarism developing postpartum as a result of pituitary necrosis; caused by ischemia resulting from a hypotensive episode during delivery.

**shelf** in anatomy, a structure resembling a shelf.

**shell** an outer covering.

**shell nail** nail dystrophy accompanying clubbing of digits in bronchiectasis, with excessive longitudinal curvature of the nail plate and atrophy of the nail bed and underlying bone.

**shell shock** SYN battle fatigue.

**Shen•ton line** (shen'těn) a curved line formed by the top of the obturator foramen and the inner side of the neck of the femur, seen on an anteroposterior frontal radiograph of a normal hip joint; it is disturbed in lesions of the joint such as dislocation or fracture.

**Shep•herd frac•ture** (shep'ĕrd) a fracture of the external tubercle (posterior process) of the talus, sometimes mistaken for a displacement of the os trigonum.

**Sher•ring•ton law** (sher'ing-tŏn) every dorsal spinal nerve root supplies a particular area of the skin, the dermatome (3), which is, however, invaded above and below by fibers from the adjacent spinal segments.

**shi•at•su** (shē-aht'soo) a Japanese massage technique using direct pressure, passive and active stretching, and gentle rocking movements to restore balance in the flow of energy in the body. [Jap. *shiatsuryōhō,* fr. *shi,* finger + *atsu,* pressure, + *ryōhō,* treatment]

**Shib•ley sign** (shĭb'lē) on auscultation of the chest, the spoken sound "e" is heard as "ah" over an area of pulmonary consolidation or immediately above a pleural effusion.

**shield** (shēld) a protecting screen; lead sheet for protecting the operator and patient from x-rays. [A.S. *scild*]

**shift** SYN change. SEE ALSO deviation.

**shift to the left 1.** a marked increase in the percentage of immature neutrophils in the circulating blood; **2.** SEE maturation index.

**shift to the right 1.** in a differential count of white blood cells in the peripheral blood, the absence of young and immature forms; **2.** SEE maturation index.

**Shi•ga-Kruse ba•cil•lus** (shē'gah-krooz) SYN *Shigella dysenteriae.*

**Shi•ga-like tox•in** SYN vero cytotoxin.

**Shi•ga tox•in** the endotoxin formed by *Shigella dysenteriae* type 1.

**Shi•gel•la** (shē-gel'lă) a genus of nonmotile, aerobic to facultatively anaerobic bacteria containing Gram-negative nonencapsulated rods. The normal habitat is the intestinal tract of humans and of higher apes; all species cause dysentery. [Kiyoshi *Shiga*]

**Shi•gel•la boy•di•i** a species found only in feces of symptomatic individuals; occurs in a low proportion of cases of bacillary dysentery.

**Shi•gel•la dys•en•ter•i•ae** a species causing dysentery in humans and in monkeys, found only in feces of symptomatic individuals; the type species of the genus *Shigella.* SYN Shiga-Kruse bacillus.

*Shi·gel·la flex·ner·i* a species found in the feces of symptomatic individuals and of convalescents or carriers; the most common cause of dysentery epidemics and sometimes of infantile gastroenteritis. Sometimes sexually transmitted through anal intercourse. SYN Flexner bacillus.

*Shi·gel·la son·ne·i* a species causing mild dysentery and also summer diarrhea in children. SYN Sonne bacillus.

**shig·el·lo·sis** (shig-ĕ-lō'sis) bacillary dysentery caused by bacteria of the genus *Shigella*, often occurring in epidemic patterns; an opportunistic infection of people with AIDS.

**shin** 1. the anterior aspect of the leg, from knee to ankle. 2. SYN anterior border of tibia. [A.S. *scina*]

**shin bone** SYN tibia.

**shin·gles** (shing'glz) SYN herpes zoster. [L. *cingulum,* girdle]

**shin-splints** tenderness and pain with induration and swelling in the anterior tibial compartment, particularly following athletic overexertion by the untrained.

**ship** a structure resembling the hull of a ship.

**ship·yard eye** SYN epidemic keratoconjunctivitis virus.

**shirt-stud ab·scess** SYN collar-button abscess.

**shi·ver·ing ther·mo·gen·e·sis** thermogenesis resulting from the increase in metabolism of the skeletal muscles due to shivering.

**shock** (shok) 1. a sudden physical or mental disturbance. 2. a state of profound mental and physical depression consequent upon severe physical injury or an emotional disturbance. 3. a severe disturbance of hemodynamics in which the circulatory system fails to maintain adequate perfusion of vital organs; may be due to reduction of blood volume (hemorrhage, dehydration), cardiac failure, or dilation of the vascular system in toxemia or septicemia. 4. the abnormally palpable impact, appreciated by a hand on the chest wall, of an accentuated heart sound. [Fr. *choc,* fr. Germanic]

**shock lung** in shock, the development of edema, impaired perfusion, and reduction in alveolar space so that the alveoli collapse. SYN pump lung, wet lung (1), white lung.

**shock ther·a·py, shock treat·ment** SEE electroshock therapy.

**Shone a·nom·a·ly** (shōn) coarctation of the aorta, subaortic stenosis, and stenosing ring of the left atrium found in association with a parachute mitral valve.

**Shone com·plex** (shōn) an obstructive lesion of the mitral valve complex with left ventricular outflow obstruction and coarctation of the aorta.

**Shone syn·drome** (shōn) the association of obstructive lesions of the mitral valve complex, including supravalvar ring and parachute mitral valve, with left ventricular outflow obstruction and coarctation of the aorta.

**short ad·duc·tor mus·cle** SYN adductor brevis muscle.

**short bone** one whose dimensions are approximately equal; it consists of a layer of cortical substance enclosing spongy substance and marrow. Cf. long bone.

**short bowel syn·drome** complex of symptoms that can result whenever the absorptive surface of the small bowel is reduced, as in massive or multiple small bowel resections. Symptoms in-

clude diarrhea, weight loss, malabsorption, anemia, and vitamin, mineral, and electrolyte abnormalities. Degree of malabsorption and malnutrition depends on the site and extent of the resection. SYN short gut syndrome.

**short ex·ten·sor mus·cle of great toe** SYN extensor hallucis brevis muscle.

**short ex·ten·sor mus·cle of toes** SYN extensor digitorum brevis muscle.

**short flex·or mus·cle of great toe** SYN flexor hallucis brevis muscle.

**short flex·or mus·cle of lit·tle fin·ger** SYN flexor digiti minimi brevis muscle of hand.

**short flex·or mus·cle of lit·tle toe** SYN flexor digiti minimi brevis muscle of foot.

**short flex·or mus·cle of thumb** SYN flexor pollicis brevis muscle.

**short flex·or mus·cle of toes** SYN flexor digitorum brevis muscle.

**short gas·tric ar·ter·ies** four or five small arteries given off from the splenic, passing via the gastrosplenic ligament to the fundus of the stomach along the greater curvature, and anastomosing with the other arteries in that region.

**short gas·tric veins** small vessels that drain the fundus and left portion of the stomach wall and empty into the splenic vein.

**short gut syn·drome** SYN short bowel syndrome.

**short gy·ri of in·su·la** several short, radiating gyri converging toward the base of the insula, composing the anterior two-thirds of the insular cortex.

**short in·cre·ment sen·si·ti·vi·ty in·dex** a measure of the ability to detect small (1dB) increments in intensity; with cochlear lesions, this ability exceeds normal.

**short ra·di·al ex·ten·sor mus·cle of wrist** SYN extensor carpi radialis brevis muscle.

**short·sight·ed·ness** (shōrt'sīt-ed-nes) SYN myopia.

**short-term ex·po·sure lim·it** the maximum concentration of a chemical to which workers may be exposed continuously for up to 15 minutes without danger to health or work efficiency and safety.

**short-term mem·o·ry (STM)** that phase of the memory process in which stimuli that have been recognized and registered are stored briefly; decay occurs rapidly, typically within seconds, but may be held indefinitely by using rehearsal as a holding process by which to recycle material over and over through STM.

**shot-silk ret·i·na** the appearance of numerous wavelike, glistening reflexes, like the shimmer of silk, observed sometimes in the retina of a young person.

**shot·ty** having a consistency like pieces of shot; consisting of small firm discrete nodules; said of lymph nodes palpated through the skin.

**shoul·der** (shōl'der) 1. the lateral portion of the scapular region, where the scapula joins with the clavicle and humerus and is covered by the rounded mass of the deltoid muscle. 2. shoulder joint. 3. DENTISTRY the ledge formed by the junction of the gingival and axial walls in extracoronal restorative preparations. [A.S. *sculder*]

**shoul·der ap·pre·hen·sion sign** a physical finding in which placement of the humerus in the position of abduction to 90° and maximum external rotation produces anxiety and resistance in patients with a history of anterior glenohumeral instability. SYN anterior apprehension test (1).

**shoul·der blade** (shōl′der blād) SYN scapula.

**shoul·der comp·lex 1.** the sternoclavicular, acromioclavicular, glenohumeral, and scapulothoracic joints, together with associated muscles and connective tissue; **2.** the shoulder and the pectoral girdle. **3.** SYN shoulder girdle.

**shoul·der dys·to·cia** arrest of normal labor after delivery of the head by impaction of the anterior shoulder against the symphysis pubis.

**shoul·der gir·dle** the bony ring, incomplete behind, that serves for the attachment and support of the upper limbs. It is formed by the manubrium sterni, the clavicles, and the scapulae. SYN pectoral girdle, shoulder complex (3).

**shoul·der-gir·dle syn·drome** SYN neuralgic amyotrophy.

**shoul·der joint** a ball-and-socket synovial joint between the head of the humerus and the glenoid cavity of the scapula. SYN humeral joint.

**shoul·der pre·sen·ta·tion** transverse presentation with the shoulder as the presenting part.

**sho·vel-shaped in·ci·sor** an incisor in which the lingual, and occasionally the labial, marginal ridges are accentuated; highly developed in persons of Asiatic origin.

**show** (shō) an appearance. **1.** first appearance of blood in beginning menstruation. **2.** sign of impending labor, characterized by the discharge from the vagina of a small amount of bloodtinged mucus representing the extrusion of the mucous plug which has filled the cervical canal during pregnancy. [A.S. *sceáwe*]

**shunt** (shŭnt) **1.** to bypass or divert. **2.** a bypass or diversion of fluid to another fluid-containing system by fistulation or a prosthetic device. The nomenclature commonly includes origin and terminus, e.g., atriovenous, splenorenal, ventriculocisternal. SEE ALSO bypass. [M.E. *shunten,* to flinch]

**Shwartz·man phe·nom·e·non** (shwahrtz′măn) a rabbit injected intradermally with a small quantity of lipopolysaccharide (endotoxin) followed by a second intravenous injection 24 hours later develops a hemorrhagic and necrotic lesion at the site of the first injection. SEE ALSO generalized Shwartzman phenomenon.

**Shy-Dra·ger syn·drome** (shī-drā′gĕr) a progressive disorder involving the autonomic system, characterized by hypotension, external ophthalmoplegia, iris atrophy, incontinence, anhidrosis, impotence, tremor, and muscle wasting.

**SI** International System of Units (Système International d'Unités).

**Si** silicon.

**sI** 6-mercaptopurine ribonucleoside (or 6-thioinosine).

**si·al·ad·e·ni·tis** (sī′al-ad-ĕ-nī′tis) inflammation of a salivary gland. SYN sialoadenitis. [sial- + G. *adēn,* gland, + *-itis,* inflammation]

**si·al·a·gogue** (sī-al′ă-gog) **1.** promoting the flow of saliva. **2.** an agent having this action (e.g., anticholinesterase agents). SYN sialogogue. [sial- + G. *agōgos,* drawing forth]

**si·al·ec·ta·sis** (sī′al-lek′tă-sis) dilation of a salivary duct. SYN ptyalectasis. [sial- + G. *ektasis,* a stretching]

**si·al·em·e·sis, si·al·e·me·sia** (sī′al-em′ĕ-sis, sī′ al-ĕ-mē′zē-ă) vomiting of saliva, or vomiting

caused by or accompanying an excessive secretion of saliva. [sial- + G. *emesis,* vomiting]

**si·al·ic** (sī-al′ik) SYN salivary.

**si·al·ic ac·ids** (sī-al′ik as′idz) esters and other *N*- and *O*-acyl derivatives of neuraminic acid.

**si·al·i·dase** (sī-al′i-dās) an enzyme that cleaves terminal acylneuraminic residues from 2,3-, 2,6-, and 2,8 linkages in oligosaccharides, glycoproteins, or glycolipids; present as a surface antigen in myxoviruses; used in histochemistry to selectively remove sialomucins, as from bronchial mucous glands and the small intestine; a deficiency of this enzyme will result in sialidosis.

**si·al·i·do·sis** (sī-al-i-dō′sis) SYN cherry-red spot myoclonus syndrome.

**si·a·line** (sī′ă-lēn) SYN salivary.

**si·a·lism, si·a·lis·mus** (sī′ă-lizm, sī′ă-liz′mŭs) an excess secretion of saliva, sialorrhea, sialosis. [G. *sialismos*]

△**si·a·lo-, si·al-** saliva, salivary glands. [G. *sialon*]

**si·a·lo·ad·e·nec·to·my** (sī′ă-lō-ad-ĕ-nek′tō-mē) excision of a salivary gland. [sialo- + G. *adēn,* gland, + *ektomē,* excision]

**si·a·lo·ad·e·ni·tis** (sī′ă-lō-ad-ĕ-nī′tis) SYN sialadenitis.

**si·a·lo·ad·e·not·o·my** (sī′ă-lō-ad-ĕ-not′ŏ-mē) incision of a salivary gland. [sialo- + G. *adēn,* gland, + *tomē,* incision]

**si·a·lo·an·gi·ec·ta·sis** (sī′ă-lō-an-jē-ek′tă-sis) dilation of salivary ducts. [sialo- + G. *angeion,* vessel, + *ektasis,* a stretching]

**si·a·lo·an·gi·i·tis** (sī′ă-lō-an-jē-ī′tis) inflammation of a salivary duct. [sialo- + G. *angeion,* vessel, + *-itis,* inflammation]

**si·a·lo·cele** (sī′ă-lō-sēl) SYN ranula (2). [sialo- + G. *kēlē,* tumor]

**si·a·lo·do·chi·tis** (sī′ă-lō-dō-kī′tis) inflammation of the duct of a salivary gland. [sialo- + G. *dochē,* receptacle, + *-itis,* inflammation]

**si·a·lo·do·cho·plas·ty** (sī′ă-lō-dō′kō-plas′tē) repair of a salivary duct. [sialo- + G. *dochē,* receptacle, + *plassō,* to fashion]

**si·a·log·e·nous** (sī′ă-loj′ĕ-nŭs) producing saliva. SEE ALSO sialagogue. [sialo- + G. *-gen,* producing]

**si·a·lo·gogue** (sī-al′ă-gog) SYN sialagogue.

**si·a·lo·gram** (sī-al′ō-gram) the recorded display following sialography. [sialo- + G. *gramma,* a writing]

**si·a·log·ra·phy** (sī-ă-log′ră-fē) radiography of the salivary glands and ducts after the introduction of contrast medium into the ducts. [sialo- + G. *graphō,* to write]

**si·a·lo·lith** (sī-al′ō-lith) a salivary calculus. [sialo- + G. *lithos,* stone]

**si·a·lo·li·thi·a·sis** (sī′ă-lō-li-thī′ă-sis) the formation or presence of a salivary calculus. [sialolith + G. *-iasis,* condition]

**si·a·lo·li·thot·o·my** (sī′ă-lō-li-thot′ō-mē) incision of a salivary duct or gland to remove a calculus. [sialolith + G. *tomē,* incision]

**si·a·lor·rhea** (sī′ă-lō-rē′ă) SYN sialism. [sialo- + G. *rhoia,* a flow]

**si·a·los·che·sis** (sī′ă-los′kĕ-sis) suppression of the secretion of saliva. [sialo- + G. *schesis,* retention]

**si·a·lo·sis** (sī′ă-lō′sis) SYN sialism.

**si·a·lo·ste·no·sis** (sī′ă-lō-ste-nō′sis) stricture of a salivary duct. [sialo- + G. *stenōsis,* a narrowing]

**Si·a·mese twins** (sī-ah-mēz′) a much publicized pair of conjoined twins born in Siam in the 19th century; this term has since come into general lay usage for any type of conjoined twins.

**sib** a member of a sibship. SYN sibling.

**sib•i•lant** (sib'i-lănt) hissing or whistling in character; denoting a form of rhonchus. [L. *sibilans* (*-ant-*), pres. p. of *sibilo*, to hiss]

**sib•i•lant rale** a whistling sound caused by air moving through a viscid secretion narrowing the lumen of a bronchus.

**sib•ling** SYN sib. [A. S. *sib*, relation, + *-ling*, diminutive]

**sib•ling ri•val•ry** jealous competition among children, especially for the attention, affection, and esteem of their parents; by extension, a factor in both normal and abnormal competitiveness throughout life.

**sib•ship 1.** the reciprocal state between individuals who have the same pair of parents. **2.** all progeny of one pair of parents. [A.S. *sib*, relationship]

**sic•ca com•plex** dryness of the mucous membranes, as of the eyes and mouth, in the absence of a connective tissue disease such as rheumatoid arthritis.

**sic•cant** (sik'ant) **1.** drying; removing moisture from surrounding substances. **2.** a substance with such properties. SYN siccative. [L. *siccans* (*-ant-*), pres. p. of *sicco*, pp. *-atus*, to dry]

**sic•ca•tive** (sik'ă-tiv) SYN siccant.

**sick** (sik) **1.** unwell; suffering from disease. **2.** SYN nauseated. [A.S. *seóc*]

**sick build•ing syn•drome** a syndrome of nonspecific symptoms including fatigue, headache, dry eyes and throat, and nasal problems, occurring mostly in office workers; attributed to low-level exposures to substances used in building and interior construction; most symptoms lessen during off-work periods.

**sick head•ache** SYN migraine.

**si•cklae•mia [Br.]** SEE sicklemia.

**sick•le cell** an abnormal, crescentic erythrocyte that is characteristic of sickle cell anemia, resulting from an inherited abnormality of hemoglobin (hemoglobin S) causing decreased solubility at low oxygen tension. SEE ALSO sicklemia, sickling. SYN drepanocyte.

**∎sick•le cell a•ne•mia** an autosomal dominant anemia characterized by crescent- or sickle-shaped erythrocytes and by accelerated hemolysis, due to substitution of a single amino acid (valine for glutamic acid) in the sixth position of the beta chain of hemoglobin; affected homozygotes have 85–95% Hb S and severe anemia, while heterozygotes (said to have sickle cell trait) have 40–45% Hb S, the rest being normal Hb A; low oxygen tension causes polymerization of the abnormal beta chains, thus distorting the shape of the red blood cells to the sickle form. Homozygotes develop "crises"; episodes of severe pain due to microvascular occlusions, bone infarcts, leg ulcers, and atrophy of the spleen associated with increased susceptibility to bacterial infections, especially streptococcal pneumonia. Occurs almost exclusively in blacks. See page B2. SYN crescent cell anemia, drepanocytic anemia, sickle cell disease.

**sick•le cell C dis•ease** a disease resulting from abnormal sickle-shaped erythrocytes (containing hemoglobin C and S) which appear in response to a lowering of the partial pressure of oxygen; characterized by anemia, crises due to hemolysis

or vascular occlusion, chronic leg ulcers and bone deformities, and infarcts of bone or of the spleen.

**sick•le cell cri•sis** SEE sickle cell anemia.

**sick•le cell dis•ease** SYN sickle cell anemia.

**sick•le cell he•mo•glo•bin (Hb S)** SYN hemoglobin S.

**sick•le cell ret•i•no•pa•thy** a condition marked by dilation and tortuosity of retinal veins, and by microaneurysms and retinal hemorrhages; advanced stages may show neovascularization, vitreous hemorrhage, or retinal detachment.

**sick•le•mia** (sik-lē'mē-ă) presence of sickle- or crescent-shaped erythrocytes in peripheral blood; seen in sickle cell anemia and sickle cell trait.

**sick•ling** (sik'ling) production of sickle-shaped erythrocytes in the circulation, as in sickle cell anemia.

**sick•ness** (sik'nes) SYN disease (1).

**sick role** in medical sociology, the familially or culturally accepted behavior pattern or role which one is permitted to exhibit during illness or disability, including sanctioned absence from school or work and a submissive, dependent relationship to family, health care personnel, and significant others.

**SID** source-to-image distance.

**side chain 1.** a chain of noncyclic atoms linked to a benzene ring, or to any cyclic chain compound; **2.** the atoms of an α-amino acid other than the α-carboxyl group, the α-amino group, the α-carbon, and the hydrogen attached to the α-carbon.

**side-chain theo•ry** ehrlich postulated that cells contained surface extensions or side chains (haptophores) that bind to the antigenic determinants of a toxin (toxophores); after a cell is stimulated, the haptophores are released into the circulation and become the antibodies. SEE ALSO receptor. SYN Ehrlich postulate.

**side ef•fect** a result of drug or other therapy in addition to or in extension of the desired therapeutic effect; usually, but not necessarily, connoting an undesirable effect.

△**si•der•o-** iron. [G. *sidēros*]

**sid•er•o•blast** (sid'er-ō-blast) an erythroblast containing granules of ferritin stained by the Prussian blue reaction. [sidero- + G. *blastos*, germ]

**sid•er•o•blas•tic a•ne•mia, sid•er•o•a•chres•tic a•ne•mi•a** refractory anemia characterized by the presence of sideroblasts in the bone marrow.

**sid•er•o•cyte** (sid'er-ō-sīt) an erythrocyte containing granules of free iron, as detected by the Prussian blue reaction, in the blood of normal fetuses, where they constitute from 0.10 to 4.5% of the erythrocytes. [sidero- + G. *kytos*, cell]

**sid•er•o•fi•bro•sis** (sid'er-ō-fī-brō'sis) fibrosis associated with small foci in which iron is deposited.

**sid•er•o•pe•nia** (sid'er-ō-pē'nē-ă) an abnormally low level of serum iron. [sidero- + G. *penia*, poverty]

**sid•er•o•pe•nic** (sid'er-ō-pē'nik) characterized by sideropenia.

**sid•er•o•phage** (sid'er-ō-fāj) SYN siderophore. [sidero- + G. *phagō*, to eat]

**sid•er•o•phil, sid•er•o•phile** (sid'er-ō-fil, sid'er-ō-fīl) **1.** absorbing iron. SYN siderophilous. **2.** a cell or tissue that contains iron. [sidero- + G. *philos*, fond]

**sid·er·oph·i·lous** (sid-er-of'i-lŭs) SYN siderophil (1).

**sid·er·o·phore** (sid'er-ō-fōr) a large extravasated mononuclear phagocyte containing granules of hemosiderin, found in the sputum or in the lungs of individuals with longstanding pulmonary congestion from left ventricular failure. SYN siderophage. [sidero- + G. *phoros*, bearing]

**sid·er·o·sil·i·co·sis** (sid'er-ō-sil'i-kō'sis) silicosis due to inhalation of dust containing iron and silica. SYN silicosiderosis. [sidero- + silicosis]

**sid·er·o·sis** (sid-er-ō'sis) **1.** a form of pneumoconiosis due to the presence of iron dust. **2.** discoloration of any part by disposition of an iron pigment; usually called hemosiderosis. **3.** an excess of iron in the circulating blood. **4.** degeneration of the retina, lens, and uvea as a result of the deposition of iron. [sidero- + G. *-osis*, condition]

**sid·er·ot·ic** (sid-er-ot'ik) related to siderosis; pigmented by iron or containing an excess of iron.

**sid·er·o·tic cat·a·ract** a cataract resulting from deposition of iron from an iron-containing intraocular foreign body.

**side·stream aer·o·sol** a system for administering an aerosol that adds the aerosol through a side connection into the mainstream of inspired airflow.

**SIDS** sudden infant death syndrome.

**Sie·gert sign** (zē'gĕrt) shortness and inward curvature of the terminal phalanges of the fifth fingers in Down syndrome.

**Sie·gle o·to·scope** (zē'gĕl) an otosclerosis with a bulb attachment by which the air pressure can be varied, thus imparting movement to the tympanic membrane, if intact, while under inspection.

**sie·mens (S)** (sē'menz) the SI unit of electrical conductance; the conductance of a body with an electrical resistance of 1 ohm, allowing 1 ampere of current to flow per volt applied; equal to 1 mho. SYN mho. [Sir William *Siemens*, Ger. born British engineer, 1823–1883]

**sie·vert (Sv)** (sē'vert) the SI unit of ionizing radiation effective dose, equal to the absorbed dose in gray, weighted for both the quality of radiation in question and the tissue response to that radiation. The unit is the joule per kilogram and 1 Sv = 100 rem. SEE effective dose.

**sight** (sīt) the ability or faculty of seeing. SEE ALSO vision. [A.S. *gesihth*]

**sig·ma** (sig'mă) **1.** the 18th letter of the Greek alphabet (σ, Σ). **2.** (σ) reflection coefficient; standard deviation; a factor in prokaryotic RNA initiation; surface tension. **3.** (Σ) Summation of a series.

**sig·moid** (sig'moyd) resembling in outline the letter S or one of the forms of the Greek sigma. [G. *sigma*, the letter S, + *eidos*, resemblance]

**sig·moid ar·ter·ies** *origin*, inferior mesenteric; *distribution*, descending colon and sigmoid flexure; *anastomoses*, left colic, superior rectal. SYN arteriae sigmoideae [TA].

**sig·moid co·lon** the part of the colon describing an S-shaped curve between the pelvic brim and the third sacral segment; it is continuous with the rectum. SYN colon sigmoideum [TA].

**sig·moi·dec·to·my** (sig-moy-dek'tō-mē) excision of the sigmoid colon. [sigmoid- + G. *ektomē*, excision]

**sig·moid·i·tis** (sig-moy-dī'tis) inflammation of the sigmoid colon. [sigmoid- + G. *-itis*, inflammation]

△**sig·moid·o-, sig·moid-** sigmoid, usually the sigmoid colon. [G. *sigma*, the letter S, + *eidos*, resemblance]

**sig·moi·do·pexy** (sig-moy'dō-pek-sē) operative attachment of the sigmoid colon to a firm structure to correct rectal prolapse. [sigmoido- + G. *pēxis*, fixation]

**sig·moi·do·proc·tos·to·my** (sig-moy'dō-prok-tos'tō-mē) anastomosis between the sigmoid colon and the rectum. SYN sigmoidorectostomy. [sigmoido- + G. *prōktos*, anus, + *stoma*, mouth]

**sig·moi·do·rec·tos·to·my** (sig-moy'dō-rek-tos' tō-mē) SYN sigmoidoproctostomy.

**sig·moi·do·scope** (sig-moy'dō-skōp) an endoscope for viewing the cavity of the sigmoid colon. [sigmoido- + G. *skopeō*, to view]

**sig·moi·dos·co·py** (sig'moy-dos'kŏ-pē) inspection, through an endoscope, of the interior of the sigmoid colon.

**sig·moi·dos·to·my** (sig'moy-dos'tō-mē) establishment of an artificial anus by opening into the sigmoid colon. [sigmoido- + G. *stoma*, mouth]

**sig·moi·dot·o·my** (sig'moy-dot'ō-mē) surgical opening of the sigmoid. [sigmoido- + G. *tomē*, incision]

**sig·moid si·nus** the S-shaped dural venous sinus lying deep to the mastoid process of the temporal bone and immediately posterior to the petrous temporal bone; it is continuous with the transverse sinus and empties into the internal jugular vein as it passes through the jugular foramen.

**sig·moid veins** the several tributaries of the inferior mesenteric vein that drain the sigmoid colon.

**sign** (sīn) **1.** any abnormality indicative of disease, discoverable on examination of the patient; an objective symptom of disease, in contrast to a symptom which is a subjective sign of disease. **2.** an abbreviation or symbol. **3.** in psychology, any object or artifact (stimulus) that represents a specific thing or conveys a specific idea to the person who perceives it. [L. *signum*, mark]

**sig·nal** (sig'nal) **1.** something that causes an action. **2.** a DNA template sequence that alters RNA polymerase transcription. **3.** the end product observed when a specific sequence of DNA or RNA is deleted by some method.

**sig·nal lymph node, sig·nal node** a firm supraclavicular lymph node, especially on the left side, sufficiently enlarged that it is palpable from the cutaneous surface; such a lymph node is so termed because it may be the first recognized presumptive evidence of a malignant neoplasm in one of the viscera. A signal lymph node that is known to contain a metastasis from a malignant neoplasm is sometimes designated by an old eponym, Troisier ganglion. SEE ALSO sentinel lymph node. SYN jugular gland, Virchow node.

**sig·nal-pro·ces·sing cir·cuits** the electronic hardware of hearing aids that allows alteration in the amplification of various bands of frequencies of the acoustic signal.

**sig·nal-to-noise ra·ti·o (S/N)** the relative intensity of a signal to the random variation in signal intensity, or noise; used to evaluate many imaging techniques and electronic systems.

**sig·na·ture** (sig'nă-cher) the part of a prescription containing the directions to the patient. [Mediev. L. *signatura*, fr. L. *signum*, a sign, mark]

**Signed Eng·lish** a system of communication that is a semantic representation of English in which American Sign Language signs are used in

English word order and additional signs are used for inflection; used principally in the education of children younger than six years.

**sig·net ring cells** SYN castration cells.

**sign lan·guage** a system of manual communication used by the deaf. True sign languages such as American Sign Language (ASL) have a complete representation of morphology, semantics, and syntax.

**SIH** somatotropin release-inhibiting hormone.

**si·lent** (sī'lent) producing no detectable signs or symptoms, said of certain diseases or morbid processes.

**si·lent ar·ea** any area of the cerebrum or cerebellum in which lesions cause no definite sensory or motor symptoms.

**si·lent as·pir·a·tion** movement of a liquid or solid bolus into the trachea below the vocal cords, without clinical signs such as coughing, choking, color change, or change in respirations.

**si·lent my·o·car·di·al in·farc·tion** infarction that produces none of the characteristic symptoms and signs of myocardial infarction.

**sil·hou·ette sign of Fel·son** (sil-oo-et' sīn of fel' son) in pulmonary radiology, the obliteration of a normal air-soft tissue interface, such as the cardiac silhouette, when fluid fills the adjacent part of the lung.

**sil·i·ca** (sil'ĭ-kă) the chief constituent of sand, hence of glass. SYN silicon dioxide. [Mod. L. fr. L. *silex* (*silic-*), flint]

**sil·i·cate rest·or·a·tion** restoration of lost tooth structure made with silicate cement.

**sil·i·ca·to·sis** (sil'ĭ-kă-tō'sis) SYN silicosis.

**sil·i·con** (Si) (sil'ĭ-kon) a very abundant nonmetallic element, atomic no. 14, atomic wt. 28.0855, occurring in nature as silica and silicates; in pure form, used as a semiconductor and in solar batteries; also found in certain polysaccharide structures in mammary tissue. [L. *silex*, flint]

**sil·i·con di·ox·ide** SYN silica.

**sil·i·cone** (sil'ĭ-kōn) a polymer of organic silicon oxides, which may be a liquid, gel, or solid, depending on the extent of polymerization; used in surgical implants, in intracorporeal tubes to conduct fluids, as dental impression material, as a grease or sealing substance, as a coating on the inside of glass vessels for blood collection, and in various ophthalmological procedures.

**sil·i·co·pro·te·i·no·sis** (sil'ĭ-kō-prō'tēnō'sis) an acute pulmonary disorder, radiographically and histologically similar to pulmonary alveolar proteinosis, resulting from relatively short exposure to high concentrations of silica dust; pulmonary symptoms are of rapid onset and the condition is invariably fatal.

**sil·i·co·sid·er·o·sis** (sil'ĭ-kō-sid'er-o'sis) SYN siderosilicosis.

**sil·i·co·sis** (sil-i-kō'sis) a form of pneumoconiosis resulting from occupational exposure to and inhalation of silica dust over a period of years; characterized by a slowly progressive fibrosis of the lungs, which may result in impairment of lung function; silicosis predisposes to pulmonary tuberculosis. SYN silicatosis. [L. *silex*, flint, + *-osis*, condition]

**sil·i·co·tu·ber·cu·lo·sis** (sil'ĭ-kō-too-ber-kyu-lō' sis) silicosis associated with tuberculous pulmonary lesions.

**si·lo-fil·ler's lung** pulmonary edema, usually delayed for 1–4 hours, occurring in an individual exposed to silage, probably due to nitrogen dioxide; can progress to bronchiolitis obliterans.

**sil·ver** (Ag) L. *argentum*; a metallic element, atomic no. 47, atomic wt. 107.8682. Many salts have clinical applications. [A.S. *seolfor*]

**sil·ver-am·mo·ni·a·c sil·ver stain** a stain for the acid protein component of nucleolar regions that are active or that were transcriptionally active in the preceding interphase; uses silver nitrate, ammoniacal silver, and formalin.

**sil·ver-fork frac·ture, sil·ver-fork de·for·mi·ty** a Colles fracture of the wrist in which the deformity has the appearance of a fork in profile.

**sil·ver im·preg·na·tion** silver complexes employed to demonstrate reticulin in normal and diseased tissues, as well as neuroglia, neurofibrillae, argentaffin cells, and Golgi apparatus.

**sil·ver pro·tein stain** a silver proteinate complex used in staining nerve fibers, nerve endings, and flagellate protozoa; also used to demonstrate phagocytosis in living animals by the cells of the reticuloendothelial system.

**Sil·ver·skiöld syn·drome** (sil'ver-shĕrld) a type of osteochondrodystrophy with only slight vertebral changes but with shortened and curved long bones of the extremities.

**sim·i·an vi·rus** (SV) any of a number of viruses, belonging to various families, isolated from monkeys or from cultures of monkey cells.

**si·mi·lia si·mi·li·bus cur·an·tur** (si-mil'ē-ă simil'i-bŭs kyur-an'ter) the homeopathic formula expressing the law of similars, the doctrine that any drug capable of producing morbid symptoms in the healthy will remove similar symptoms occurring as an expression of disease. Another reading of the formula, employed by Hahnemann, the founder of homeopathy, is *similia similibus curentur*, let likes be cured by likes. [L. likes are cured by likes]

**Sim·monds dis·ease** (sim'ŏndz) anterior pituitary insufficiency due to trauma, vascular lesions, or tumors; usually developing postpartum as a result of pituitary necrosis caused by ischemia during a hypotensive episode during delivery; characterized clinically by asthenia, loss of weight and body hair, arterial hypotension, and manifestations of thyroid, adrenal, and gonadal hypofunction. SYN hypophysial cachexia, pituitary cachexia.

**Sim·mons cit·rate me·di·um** (sim'ŏnz) a diagnostic medium used in the differentiation of species of Enterobacteriaceae, based on their ability to utilize sodium citrate as the sole source of carbon.

**Si·mo·nart bands** (sē-mō-nahr') **1.** SYN amnionic band. **2.** weblike band of tissue partially filling the gap between the medial and lateral portions of a cleft lip.

**Si·mo·nart lig·a·ments** (sē-mō-nahr') SYN amnionic band.

**Si·mon po·si·tion** (sī'mŏn) a position for vaginal examination; a supine position with hips elevated, thighs and legs flexed, and thighs widely separated.

**simple ab·sence** a brief clouding of consciousness accompanied by the abrupt onset of 3/sec spikes and waves on EEG. SYN pure absence.

**sim·ple dis·lo·ca·tion** SYN closed dislocation.

**sim·ple en·do·me·tri·al hy·per·pla·sia** increase in the amount of endometrial tissue, with glands separated by abundant stroma.

**sim·ple ep·i·the·li·um** an epithelium having one layer of cells.

**sim·ple fis·sion** division of the nucleus and then the cell body into two parts. SEE ALSO binary fission.

**sim·ple frac·ture** SYN closed fracture.

**sim·ple glau·co·ma, glau·co·ma sim·plex** SYN open-angle glaucoma.

**sim·ple goi·ter** thyroid enlargement unaccompanied by constitutional effects, e.g., hypo- or hyperthyroidism, commonly caused by inadequate dietary intake of iodine.

**sim·ple joint** one composed of two bones only.

**sim·ple mas·tec·to·my** excision of the breast including the nipple, areola, and most of the overlying skin.

**sim·ple mi·cro·scope, sin·gle mi·cro·scope** a microscope that has a single magnifying lens.

**sim·ple pho·bia** SYN specific phobia.

**sim·ple pro·tein** protein that yields only α-amino acids or their derivatives by hydrolysis; e.g., albumins, globulins, glutelins, prolamines, albuminoids, histones, protamines. Cf. conjugated protein.

**sim·ple squa·mous ep·i·the·li·um** epithelium composed of a single layer of flattened scalelike cells, such as mesothelium, endothelium, and that in the pulmonary alveoli.

**Sim·plex·vi·rus** (sim′pleks-vī′rŭs) SYN herpes simplex.

**Sim·pli·fied Or·al Hy·giene In·dex (OHI-S)** a dental survey method that scores dental calculus and plaque together.

**Sims po·si·tion** (sims) a position to facilitate a vaginal examination, with the patient lying on her side with the lower arm behind the back, the thighs flexed, the upper one more than the lower. SYN lateral recumbent position.

**sim·u·la·tion** (sim-yu-lā′shŭn) **1.** imitation; said of a disease or symptom that resembles another, or of the feigning of illness as in factitious illness or malingering. **2.** RADIATION THERAPY using a geometrically similar radiographic system or computer to plan the location of therapy ports. [L. *simulatio,* fr. *simulo,* pp. *-atus,* to imitate, fr. *similis,* like]

**si·mul·tan·ag·no·sia** (sī-mŭl-tan-ag-nō′sē-ă) inability to recognize multiple elements in a visual presentation, i.e., one object or some elements of a scene can be appreciated but not the display as a whole. [simultaneous + agnosia]

**si·mul·ta·ne·ous com·mu·ni·ca·tion** SYN total communication.

**sin·cip·i·tal** (sin-sip′i-tăl) relating to the sinciput.

**sin·cip·i·tal pre·sen·ta·tion** SEE cephalic presentation.

**sin·ci·put,** pl. **sin·cip·i·ta, sin·ci·puts** (sin′si-put, sin-sip′i-tă) the anterior part of the head just above and including the forehead. [L. half of the head]

**Sind·bis fe·ver** (sind′bis) a febrile illness of humans in Africa, Australia, and other countries, characterized by arthralgia, rash, and malaise; caused by the Sindbis virus, a member of the family Togaviridae, and transmitted by mosquitoes of the genus *Culex.*

**Sind·bis vi·rus** (sind′bis) the type species of the genus *Alphavirus,* usually transmitted by mosquitoes of the genus *Culex;* and causative agent of Sindbis fever. [village in Egypt where first isolated]

**Sind·ing-Lar·sen-Jo·hans·son syn·drome** (sin-ding-lahr′sen-yō-hahn-sĕn) apophysitis of the distal pole of the patella.

**sin·ew** (sin′yu) SYN tendon. [A.S. *sinu*]

**sine wave** a symmetric wave representing one complete cycle of a single-frequency oscillation; the displacement of mass over time described by using a function from trigonometry, the sine. SEE ALSO pure tone.

**sing·er's no·dules** SYN vocal nodules.

**sin·gle bond** a covalent bond resulting from the sharing of one pair of electrons; e.g., $H_3C—CH_3$ (ethane).

**sin·gle pho·ton e·mis·sion com·put·ed to·mog·ra·phy (SPECT)** tomographic imaging of metabolic and physiological functions in tissues, the image being formed by computer synthesis of photons of a single energy emitted by radionuclides administered in suitable form to the patient.

**sin·gle·ton** (sing′gĕl-tŭn) a fetus that develops alone. [unknown]

**sin·gle vi·al fix·a·tives** proprietary and commercially available solutions used for stool fixation; from the single vial, a concentration, permanent stain, and some immunoassay procedures can be performed.

**sin·is·ter** (si-nis′ter) left. [L.]

**sin·is·trad** (sin′is-trad, si-nis′trad) toward the left side. [L. *sinister,* left, + *ad,* to]

**sin·is·tral** (sin′is-trăl, sĭ-nis′trăl) **1.** relating to the left side. **2.** denoting a left-handed person.

**sin·is·tral·i·ty** (sin-is-tral′i-tē) the condition of being left-handed.

△**sin·is·tro-** left, toward the left. [L. *sinister*]

**sin·is·tro·car·dia** (sin′is-trō-kar′dē-ă) leftward displacement of the heart beyond its normal position. [sinistro- + G. *kardia,* heart]

**sin·is·tro·ce·re·bral** (sin′is-trō-ser′ĕ-brăl) relating to the left cerebral hemisphere. [sinistro- + L. *cerebrum,* brain]

**sin·is·tro·gy·ra·tion** (sin′is-trō-jī-rā′shŭn) SYN sinistrotorsion. [sinistro- + L. *gyratio,* a turning around (gyration)]

**sin·is·tro·man·u·al** (sin′is-trō-man′yu-ăl) SYN left-handed. [sinistro- + L. *manus,* hand]

**sin·is·trop·e·dal** (sin-is-trop′ĕ-dăl) denoting one who uses the left leg by preference. SYN left-footed. [sinistro- + L. *pes (ped-),* foot]

**sin·is·tro·tor·sion** (sin′is-trō-tōr′shŭn) a turning or twisting to the left. SYN levorotation (2), levotorsion (1), sinistrogyration. [sinistro- + L. *torsio,* a twisting (torsion)]

**Sin Nom·bre vi·rus** a species of Hantavirus in North America causing hantavirus pulmonary syndrome. SYN Four Corners virus. [Spanish, without a name]

**si·no·a·tri·al (S-A), si·nu·atri·al (S-A)** (sin′oo-ā′trē-ăl) relating to the sinus venosus of the embryo, or the sinus of the venae cavae of the mature heart, and the right atrium.

**si·no·a·tri·al block, S-A block, si·nus block, si·nu·a·tri·al block** blockade of an impulse leaving the sinoatrial node before it can activate atrial muscle or be propagated to the atrioventricular node.

**si·no·a·tri·al node, si·nu·a·tri·al node** the mass of specialized cardiac muscle fibers that normally acts as the "pacemaker" of the cardiac conduction system; it lies under the epicardium at the upper end of the sulcus terminalis.

S
i

**si·no·pul·mo·nary** (sī'nō-pŭl'mŏ-ner-ē) relating to the paranasal sinuses and the pulmonary airway.

**si·nus,** pl. **si·nus, si·nus·es** (sī'nŭs, sī'nŭs) **1.** a channel for the passage of blood or lymph, without the coats of an ordinary vessel; e.g., blood passages in the gravid uterus or those in the cerebral meninges. **2.** a cavity or hollow space in bone or other tissue. **3.** a dilation in a blood vessel. **4.** a fistula or tract leading to a suppurating cavity. [L. *sinus,* cavity, channel, hollow]

**si·nus ar·rest** cessation of sinoatrial activity; the ventricles may continue to beat under ectopic atrial, A-V junctional, or idioventricular control.

**si·nus ar·rhyth·mia** a cyclic variation in heart rate, usually normal and linked to respiratory movements.

**si·nus ca·ver·no·sus** [TA] SYN cavernous sinus.

**si·nus his·ti·o·cy·to·sis with mas·sive lymph··a·den·op·a·thy** a chronic disease occurring in children and characterized by massive painless cervical lymphadenopathy due to distension of the lymphatic sinuses by macrophages containing ingested lymphocytes, and by capsular and pericapsular fibrosis. SYN Rosai-Dorfman disease.

**si·nus·i·tis** (sī-nŭ-sī'tis) inflammation of the lining membrane of any sinus, especially of one of the paranasal sinuses. [sinus + G. -*itis,* inflammation]

**si·nus·oid** (sī'nŭ-soyd) **1.** resembling a sinus. **2.** sinusoidal capillary; a thin-walled terminal blood vessel having a more variable and larger caliber than an ordinary capillary; its endothelial cells have large gaps and the basal lamina is either discontinuous or absent. [sinus + G. *eidos,* resemblance]

**si·nus·oi·dal** (sī-nŭ-soy'dăl) relating to a sinusoid.

**si·nus·ot·o·my** (sin-ŭ-sot'ŏ-mē) incision into a sinus. [sinus + G. *tomē,* incision]

**si·nus pause** a spontaneous interruption in the regular sinus rhythm, the pause lasting for a period that is not an exact multiple of the sinus cycle. SEE ALSO sinus arrest.

**si·nus rhy·thm** normal cardiac rhythm proceeding from the sinoatrial node.

**si·nus of the ve·na ca·va** the portion of the cavity of the right atrium of the heart that receives the blood from the venae cavae; it is separated from the rest of the atrium by the crista terminalis.

**si·nus ve·no·sus** a cavity at the caudal end of the embryonic cardiac tube in which the veins from the intra- and extraembryonic circulatory arcs unite; in the course of development it forms the portion of the right atrium known in adult anatomy as the sinus of the vena cava or sinus venarum cavarum.

**si·nus ve·no·sus scler·ae** the vascular structure encircling the anterior chamber of the eye and through which the aqueous is returned to the blood circulation. SYN circular sinus (3), Schlemm canal.

**si·phon** (sī'fŏn) a tube bent into two unequal lengths, used to remove fluid from a cavity or vessel by atmospheric pressure and gravity. [G. *siphōn,* tube]

**si·phon·age** (sī'fŏn-ij) emptying of the stomach or other cavity by means of a siphon.

**Sipho·vir·i·dae** (sif'ō-vir'i-dē) a family of bacterial viruses with long, noncontractile tails and isometric or elongated heads, containing double-stranded DNA (MW $25-79 \times 10^6$); includes the $\lambda$ temperate phage group and probably other genera. [L. *sipho,* little tube, pipe, fr. G. *siphōn,* + virus]

**Sip·ple syn·drome** (sip'ĕl) pheochromocytoma, medullary carcinoma of the thyroid, and parathyroid adenomas; autosomal dominant inheritance, caused by mutation in the RET oncogene on chromosome 10q.

**si·re·no·me·lia** (sī'rĕ-nō-mē'lē-ă) union of the legs with partial or complete fusion of the feet. [L. *siren,* G. *seirēn,* a siren]

**SISI** small increment sensitivity index.

**SISI test** the sounding of a tone 20 dB above threshold, followed by a series of 200-msec tones 1 dB louder; perception of these is indicative of cochlear damage.

**sis·ter** in Great Britain: **1.** the title of a head nurse in a public hospital or in a ward or the operating room of a hospital; **2.** any registered nurse in private practice.

**Sis·ter Jo·seph nod·ule** (sis'tĕr-jō'sef) a malignant intraabdominal neoplasm metastatic to the umbilicus.

**site** (sīt) a place or location. SYN situs. [L. *situs*]

**site-spe·cif·ic re·com·bi·na·tion** integration of foreign DNA into a particular site in the host genome.

△**si·to-** food, grain. [G. *sitos, sition*]

**si·tot·ro·pism, si·to·tax·is** (sī-tot'rō-pizm, sī-tō-tak'sis) turning of living cells to or away from food. [sito- + G. *tropē,* a turning]

**in si·tu** (in sī'too) in position, not extending beyond the focus or level of origin. [L. *in,* in, + *situs,* site]

**sit·u·a·tion·al psy·cho·sis** a transitory but severe emotional disorder caused in a predisposed person by a seemingly unbearable situation.

**in si·tu hy·bri·di·za·tion** a technique for annealing nucleic acid probes to cellular DNA for detection by autoradiography. In situ hybridization constitutes a key step in DNA fingerprinting.

**si·tus** (sī'tŭs) SYN site. [L.]

**si·tus in·ver·sus** reversal of position or location, referring particularly to left-right reversal of thoracic viscera.

**sitz bath** immersion of only the perineum and buttocks, with the legs being outside the tub. [Ger. *sitzen,* to sit]

**sixth cra·ni·al nerve [CN VI]** SYN abducent nerve [CN VI].

**sixth dis·ease** SYN exanthema subitum.

**sixth-year mo·lar** the first permanent molar tooth.

**siz·er** (sī'zer) a cylinder of variable diameter, with rounded ends, used to measure the internal diameter of the bowel in preparation for stapling.

**Sjö·gren syn·drome** (sher'gren) keratoconjunctivitis sicca, dryness of mucous membranes, telangiectasias or purpuric spots on the face, and bilateral parotid enlargement; seen in menopausal women and often associated with rheumatoid arthritis, Raynaud phenomenon, and dental caries; there are changes in the lacrimal and salivary glands resembling those of Mikulicz disease. [H.S.C. Sjögren]

**SK** streptokinase.

**skat·ole** (skat'ōl) an indole derivative formed in the intestine by bacterial decomposition and found in fecal matter, to which it imparts its characteristic odor.

**skat·ox·yl** (skă-tok′sil) an indole derivative formed in the intestine by the oxidation of skatole; some undergoes conjugation in the body with sulfuric or gluronic acids and is excreted in the urine in conjugated form.

**skel·e·tal** (skel′ĕ-tăl) relating to the skeleton.

**skel·e·tal dys·pla·si·as** a heterogeneous group of disorders (over 120 types), each of which results in numerous disturbances of the skeletal system and most of which include dwarfism. SEE ALSO chondrodystrophy.

**skel·e·tal ex·ten·sion** SYN skeletal traction.

**skel·e·tal mus·cle** grossly, a collection of striated muscle fibers connected at either or both extremities with the bony framework of the body; it may be an appendicular or an axial muscle; histologically, a muscle consisting of elongated, multinucleated, transversely striated skeletal muscle fibers together with connective tissues, blood vessels, and nerves; individual muscle fibers are surrounded by fine reticular and collagen fibers (endomysium); bundles (fascicles) of muscle fibers are surrounded by irregular connective tissue (perimysium); the entire muscle is surrounded, except at the muscle tendon junction, by a dense connective tissue (epimysium).

**skel·e·tal trac·tion** traction pull on a bone structure mediated through pin or wire inserted into the bone to reduce a fracture of long bones. SYN skeletal extension.

**skel·e·ton** (skel′ĕ-tŏn) **1.** [TA] the bony framework of the body in vertebrates (endoskeleton) or the hard outer envelope of insects (exoskeleton or dermoskeleton). **2.** all the dry parts remaining after the destruction and removal of the soft parts; this includes ligaments and cartilages as well as bones. **3.** all the bones of the body taken collectively. **4.** a rigid or semirigid nonosseous structure which functions as the supporting framework of a particular structure. See page A8, A9, A12. [G. *skeletos,* dried, ntr. *skeleton,* a mummy, a skeleton]

**Skene tu·bule** (skēn) embryonic urethral glands that are the female homolog of the prostate.

△**skia-** shadow; superseded by radio-. [G. *skia*]

**ski·as·co·py** (skī-as′kŏ-pē) SYN retinoscopy.

**skilled-nurs·ing fa·cil·i·ty (SNF)** nursing facility providing 24-hour nonacute nursing care.

**skills val·i·da·tion** a predetermined method whereby a healthcare institution periodically confirms the competence, in any given area of nursing, of all its staff in the performance of those skills necessary to provide optimal care to the patients; the methods include learning or relearning, demonstration, and documentation of competence; done on a schedule, usually annually. SYN competence testing.

**skim milk, skimmed milk** the aqueous (noncream) part of milk from which casein is isolated.

**skin** the membranous protective covering of the body, consisting of the epidermis and corium (dermis). SYN cutis [TA]. [A.S. *scinn*]

**skin dose** the quantity of radiation delivered to the skin surface.

**skin·fold mea·sure·ment** determination of the thickness of a fold of skin and underlying subcutaneous fat using calipers. Measurements are used to assess body fat content. Standard tables

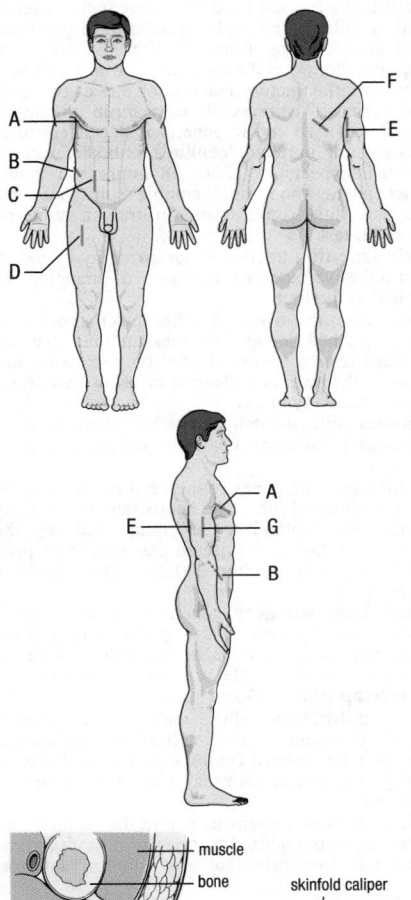

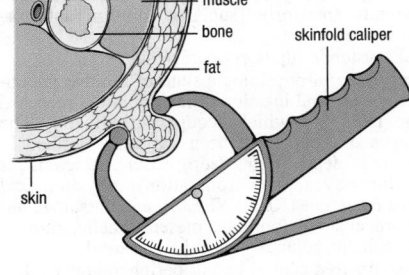

**skinfold measurement sites:** (A) chest, (B) supra-iliac, (C) abdominal, (D) thigh, (E) triceps, (F) subscapular, (G) biceps; during measurement a double layer of skin and the underlying tissue are compressed

are available relating skinfold thickness to body fat as a percentage of body weight according to age and sex. See this page.

**skin ridg·es** SYN epidermal ridges.

**skin tag 1.** a polypoid outgrowth of both epidermis and dermal fibrovascular tissue; **2.** common terminology for any small benign cutaneous lesion. SYN acrochordon, soft wart.

**skin test** a method for determining induced sensitivity (allergy) by applying an antigen (allergen) to, or inoculating it into, the skin; induced sensitivity (allergy) to the specific antigen is indicated by an inflammatory reaction of one of two general kinds: 1) immediate, appears in minutes to an hour or so and in general is dependent upon circulating immunoglobulins (antibodies); 2) delayed, appears in 12 to 48 hours and is not dependent upon these soluble substances but upon cellular response and infiltration. SYN intradermal test.

**skin trac•tion** traction on an extremity by means of adhesive tape or other types of strapping applied to the limb.

**sko•da•ic res•o•nance** (skō-dā′ik) a peculiar, high-pitched sound, less musical than that obtained over a cavity, elicited by percussion just above the level of a pleuritic effusion. SYN Skoda sign, Skoda tympany.

**Sko•da sign** (skō′dah) SYN skodaic resonance.

**Sko•da tym•pa•ny** (skō′dah) SYN skodaic resonance.

**skull** (skŭl) the bones of the head collectively. In a more limited sense, the neurocranium, the bony braincase containing the brain, excluding the bones of the face (viscero-cranium). See page A1, A2. SYN cranium. [Early Eng. *skulle,* a bowl]

**skull base sur•gery** generic term to denote a specialty of surgery and a group of operations, techniques, and approaches to lesions at or involving the base of the skull or its contents.

**skull•cap** (skŭl′kap) SYN calvaria.

**slant cul•ture** a culture made on the slanting surface of a medium which has been solidified in a test tube inclined from the perpendicular so as to give a greater area than that of the lumen of the tube.

**SLAP les•ion** a traumatic tear of the superior part of the glenoid labrum that begins posteriorly and extends anteriorly [superior labrum, anterior-posterior].

**SLE** systemic lupus erythematosus.

**sleep** (slēp) a physiologic state of relative unconsciousness and inaction of the voluntary muscles, the need for which recurs periodically. The stages of sleep have been variously defined in terms of depth (light, deep), EEG characteristics (delta waves, synchronization), physiological characteristics (REM, NREM), and presumed anatomical level (pontine, mesencephalic, rhombencephalic, rolandic, etc.). [A.S. *slaep*]

**sleep ap•nea** central and/or peripheral apnea during sleep, associated with frequent awakening and often with daytime sleepiness.

**sleep def•i•cit** a lack of sleep time or a relative lack of one of the stages of sleep as determined by a sleep study.

**sleep•ing sick•ness** SEE Gambian trypanosomiasis, Rhodesian trypanosomiasis.

**sleep pa•ral•y•sis** brief episodic loss of voluntary movement that occurs when falling asleep (hypnagogic sleep paralysis) or when awakening (hypnopompic sleep paralysis). One of the narcoleptic tetrad.

**slew rate** in electronic pacemaker function, the maximum rate of change of an amplifier output voltage; important variable affecting heart function as controlled by an electronic pacemaker.

**slide** (slīd) a rectangular glass plate on which is placed an object to be examined under the microscope.

**slide tra•che•o•plas•ty** an operation for the repair of long tracheal stenosis in which anterior and posterior sliding flaps of tracheal wall are sutured together to reconstruct the tracheal lumen.

**slid•ing flap** a rectangular flap raised in an elastic area, with its free end adjacent to a defect; the defect is covered by stretching the flap longitudinally until the end comes over it.

**slid•ing her•nia** a hernia in which an abdominal viscus forms part of the sac. SYN extrasaccular hernia, slipped hernia.

**slid•ing lock** a slot on one shank of obstetrical forceps (as in Kjelland forceps) that allows the shanks to move forward and backward independently.

**sling** a supporting bandage or suspensory device; especially a loop suspended from the neck and supporting the flexed forearm.

**slipped her•nia** SYN sliding hernia.

**slip•ping rib** subluxation of a rib cartilage, with costochondral separation.

**slip•ping rib car•ti•lage** subluxation of rib cartilage at the costo-chondral junction, causing pain and audible click.

**slit•lamp, slit lamp** in ophthalmology, an instrument consisting of a microscope combined with a rectangular light source that can be narrowed into a slit. SYN biomicroscope, Gullstrand slitlamp.

**slough** (slŭf) **1.** necrosed tissue separated from the living structure. **2.** to separate from the living tissue, said of a dead or necrosed part. [M.E. *slughe*]

**slow chan•nel-block•ing a•gent** SYN calcium channel-blocking agent.

**slow com•po•nent of ny•stag•mus** the fundamental movement of the eyes in the vestibuloocular reflex.

**slow-re•act•ing sub•stance (SRS), slow-re•act•ing sub•stance of an•a•phy•lax•is** a leukotriene of low molecular weight which is released in anaphylactic shock and produces slower and more prolonged contraction of muscle than does histamine; it is active in the presence of antihistamines (but not epinephrine) and seems not to occur preformed in mast cells, but as a result of an antigen-antibody reaction on the granules.

**slow vi•rus** a virus, or a viruslike agent, etiologically associated with a disease having a long incubation period of months to years with a gradual onset frequently terminating in severe illness and/or death.

**slow vi•rus dis•ease** a disease that follows a slow, progressive course spanning months to years, frequently involving the central nervous system, and ultimately leading to death, such as subacute sclerosing panencephalitis, seemingly caused by the measles virus; spongiform encephalopathies including kuru of humans and scrapie of sheep have been classified under slow virus disease but their respective etiologic agents have not been adequately characterized.

**Slu•der neu•ral•gia** (sloo′dĕr) SYN sphenopalatine neuralgia.

**Sm** samarium.

**small cal•o•rie (cal, c)** the quantity of energy

required to raise the temperature of 1 g of water from 14.5°C to 15.5°C. SYN gram calorie.

**small car·di·ac vein** an inconstant vessel, accompanying the right coronary artery in the coronary sulcus, from the right margin of the right ventricle, and emptying into the coronary sinus or the middle cardiac vein.

**small cell** a short, blunt, spindle-shaped cell that contains a relatively large hyperchromatic nucleus, frequently observed in some forms of undifferentiated bronchogenic carcinoma.

**small cell car·ci·no·ma 1.** an anaplastic carcinoma composed of small cells; **2.** SYN oat cell carcinoma.

**small·er pos·ter·i·or rec·tus mus·cle of head** SYN rectus capitis posterior minor muscle.

**small in·cre·ment sen·si·tiv·i·ty in·dex (SISI)** SEE SISI test.

**small in·tes·tine** the portion of the digestive tube between the stomach and the cecum or beginning of the large intestine; it consists of three portions: duodenum, jejunum, and ileum.

**small·pox** (smawl′poks) an acute eruptive contagious disease caused by a poxvirus (*Orthopoxvirus*) and marked by chills, fever, and an eruption papules which become umbilicated vesicles, develop into pustules, dry, and form scabs that on falling off, leave a permanent marking of the skin (pock marks). The virus was declared extinct in 1979, having been eradicated by vaccination, and is now of mainly historical interest. SYN variola. [E. *small pocks*, or pustules]

**small·pox vi·rus** SYN variola virus.

**smear** (smēr) a thin specimen for microscopic examination; it is usually prepared by spreading liquid or semisolid material uniformly onto a glass slide, fixing it, and staining it before examination.

**smear cul·ture** a culture obtained by spreading material presumed to be infected on the surface of a solidified medium.

**smeg·ma** (smeg′mă) a foul-smelling pasty accumulation of desquamated epidermal cells and sebum that has collected in moist areas of the genitalia. [G. unguent]

**smeg·ma·lith** (smeg′mă-lith) a calcareous concretion in the smegma. [smegma + G. *lithos*, stone]

**smell 1.** to scent; to perceive by means of the olfactory apparatus. **2.** SYN olfaction (1). **3.** SYN odor.

**Smith frac·ture** (smith) reversed Colles fracture; fracture of the distal radius with displacement of the fragment toward the palmar (volar) aspect.

**Smith-In·di·an op·er·a·tion, Smith op·er·a·tion** (smith-in′dē-an, smith) a surgical technique for removal of cataract within the capsule.

**smog** a hazy and often highly irritating atmosphere resulting from a mixture of fog with smoke and other air pollutants. [smoke + fog]

**smol·der·ing leu·ke·mia** SYN myelodysplastic syndrome.

**smooth di·et** a diet containing little roughage; used primarily in diseases of the colon.

**smooth mus·cle** one of the muscle fibers of the internal organs, blood vessels, hair follicles, etc.; contractile elements are elongated, usually spindle-shaped cells with centrally located nuclei and a length from 20 to 200 μm, or even longer in the pregnant uterus; although transverse striations are lacking, both thick and thin myofibrils occur;

smooth muscle fibers are bound together into sheets or bundles by reticular fibers, and frequently elastic fiber nets are also abundant. SEE ALSO involuntary muscles.

**smudge cells** immature leukocytes of any type that have undergone partial breakdown during preparation of a stained smear or tissue section, because of their greater fragility; smudge cells are seen in largest numbers in chronic lymphocytic leukemia. SYN basket cell (2).

**S/N** signal-to-noise ratio.

**Sn** tin.

△**sn-** prefix meaning stereospecifically numbered; a system of numbering the glycerol carbon atoms in lipids, so that the locant numbers remain constant regardless of chemical substitutions, as opposed to systematic numbering.

**snail track de·gen·er·a·tion** circumferential line of fine white dots in the peripheral retina associated with atrophic retinal holes.

**snap** a click; a short sharp sound; said especially of cardiac sounds.

**snap·ping hip syn·drome** a snapping sensation either heard or felt during hip motion.

**snare** (snār) an instrument for removing polyps and other projections from a surface, especially within a cavity; it consists of a wire loop passed around the base of the tumor and gradually tightened. [A.S. *snear*, a cord]

**Sned·don syn·drome** (sned′ŏn) a cerebral arteriopathy of unknown etiology, characterized by noninflammatory intimal hyperplasia of medium-sized vessels associated with diffuse cutaneous livedo reticularis.

**sneeze** (snēz) **1.** to expel air from the nose and mouth by an involuntary spasmodic contraction of the muscles of expiration. **2.** an act of sneezing; a reflex excited by an irritation of the mucous membrane of the nose or, sometimes, by a bright light striking the eye. [A.S. *fneōsan*]

**Snel·len test type** (snel′ĕn) one of a series of square black symbols employed in testing the acuity of distant vision; the letters vary in size in such a way that each one subtends a visual angle of 5′ at a particular distance.

**Snell law** (snel) SYN law of refraction.

**SNF** skilled-nursing facility.

**sniff test** FLUOROSCOPY a test for diaphragmatic function; paradoxical motion of a hemidiaphragm when a patient sniffs vigorously shows phrenic nerve paralysis or paresis of the hemidiaphragm. If rapid upward movement of the diaphragm occurs on brisk sniffing in the supine position, it is highly suggestive of paralysis of the diaphragm.

**snore** (snōr) **1.** a rough, rattling inspiratory noise produced by vibration of the pendulous palate, or sometimes of the vocal cords, during sleep or coma. SEE ALSO stertor, rhonchus. **2.** to breathe noisily, or with a snore. [A.S. *snora*]

**snort·ing** SYN nasal emission.

**snout re·flex** pouting or pursing of the lips induced by light tapping of closed lips near the midline; seen in defective pyramidal innervation of facial musculature.

**snow blind·ness** severe photophobia secondary to ultraviolet keratoconjunctivitis.

**snuff** (snŭf) **1.** to inhale forcibly through the nose. **2.** finely powdered tobacco used by inhalation through the nose or applied to the gums. **3.** any medicated powder applied by insufflation to the nasal mucous membrane. [echoic]

**snuff•box** (snŭf'boks) SEE anatomic snuffbox.

**snuf•fles** (snŭf'lz) obstructed nasal respiration, especially in the newborn infant, sometimes due to congenital syphilis.

**Sny•der test** (snī'dĕr) a colorimetric test for determining dental caries activity or susceptibility based on the rate of acid production by acidogenic oral microorganisms (e.g., lactobacillus) in a glucose medium, using bromcresol green as the indicator, and producing a color change from green to yellow.

**SOAP** *s*ubjective, *o*bjective, *a*ssessment, and *p*lan; used in problem-oriented records for organizing follow-up data, evaluation, and planning.

**soap** (sōp) the sodium or potassium salts of long chain fatty acids (e.g., sodium stearate); used for cleansing purposes and as an excipient in the making of pills and suppositories. [A.S. *sape,* L. *sapo,* G. *sapōn*]

**So•ave op•er•a•tion** (sō-ah'vä) endorectal pull-through for treatment of congenital megacolon.

**so•cial•i•za•tion** (sō'shăl-i-zā'shŭn) **1.** the process of learning attitudes and interpersonal and interactional skills which are in conformity with the values of one's society. **2.** in a group therapy setting, a way of learning to participate effectively in the group. [L. *socius,* partner, companion]

**so•cial•ized med•i•cine** the organization and control of medical practice by a government agency, the practitioners being employed by the organization from which they receive standardized compensation for their services, and to which the public contributes, usually in the form of taxation rather than fee-for-service.

**so•cial pho•bia** a persistent pattern of significant fear of a social or performance situation, manifested by anxiety or panic on exposure to the situation or in anticipation of it, which the person realizes is unreasonable or excessive and interferes significantly with the person's functioning;

**so•cial psy•chi•a•try** an approach to psychiatric theory and practice emphasizing the cultural and sociological aspects of mental disorder and treatment; the application of psychiatry to social problems. SEE ALSO community psychiatry.

△**so•cio-** social, society. [L. *socius,* companion]

**so•ci•o•ac•u•sis** (sō-sē-ō-ak-oo'sis) the hearing loss produced by exposure to nonoccupational noise such as small arms fire in hunting and target practice. [socio- + G. *akousis,* hearing]

**so•ci•o•cen•tric** (sō'sē-ō-sen'trik) outgoing; reactive to the social or cultural milieu. [socio- + L. *centrum,* center]

**so•ci•o•gen•e•sis** (sō'sē-ō-jen'ĕ-sis) the origin of social behavior from past interpersonal experiences. [socio- + G. *genesis,* origin]

**so•ci•o•path** (sō'sē-ō-path) former designation for a person with an antisocial personality type of disorder. SEE ALSO antisocial personality disorder, psychopath.

**sock•et** (sok'et) **1.** the hollow part of a joint; the excavation in one bone of a joint which receives the articular end of the other bone. **2.** any hollow or concavity into which another part fits, as the eye socket. [thr. O. Fr. fr. L. *soccus,* a shoe, a sock]

**so•di•um** (sō'dē-ŭm) a metallic element, atomic no. 11, atomic wt. 22.989768; an alkali metal oxidizing readily in air or water; its salts are found in natural biologic systems and are extensively used in medicine and industry. The sodium ion is the most plentiful extracellular ion in the body. SYN natrium. [Mod. L. fr. *soda*]

**so•di•um bo•rate** used in lotions, gargles, mouthwashes, and as a detergent.

**so•di•um phos•phate** $^{32}$P anionic radioactive phosphorus in the form of a solution of sodium acid phosphate and sodium basic phosphate; a beta emitter with a half-life of 14.3 days; after administration, highest concentrations are found in rapidly proliferating tissues; it is used in the treatment of polycythemia vera, chronic myelogenous leukemia, and osseous metastases. SEE ALSO chromic phosphate $^{32}$P colloidal suspension.

**so•di•um-po•tas•si•um pump** a membrane-bound transporter that maintains the high potassium and low sodium intracellular concentrations relative to the extracellular medium. This exchange is accomplished at the expense of cellular energy in the form of ATP.

**so•di•um pump** a biologic mechanism that uses metabolic energy from ATP to achieve active transport of sodium across a membrane; sodium pumps expel sodium from most cells of the body, sometimes coupled with the transport of other substances, and also serve to move sodium across multicellular membranes such as renal tubule walls.

**sod•om•ist, sod•om•ite** (sod'ŏ-mist, sod'ŏ-mīt) one who practices sodomy. [G. *sodomitēs,* an inhabitant of the biblical city of Sodom, which was destroyed by fire because of the wickedness of its people]

**sod•o•my** (sod'ŏm-ē) a term denoting a number of sexual practices variously proscribed by law, especially bestiality, oral-genital contact, and anal intercourse. [see sodomist]

**soft chan•cre** SYN chancroid.

**soft corn** a corn formed by pressure between two toes, the surface being macerated and yellowish in color. SYN heloma molle.

**soft di•et** a normal diet limited to soft foods for those who have difficulty chewing or swallowing; there are no restrictions on seasoning or method of food preparation.

**soft drus•en** type of exudative drusen that appear ophthalmoscopically as placoid, yellow lesions characterized histopathologically by localized serous detachments of the retinal pigment epithelium from the Bruch membrane.

**soft pal•ate** the posterior muscular portion of the palate, forming an incomplete septum between the mouth and the oropharynx, and between the oropharynx and the nasopharynx. SYN velum palatinum.

**soft tu•ber•cle** a tubercle showing caseous necrosis.

**soft ul•cer** SYN chancroid.

**soft wart** SYN skin tag.

**soil** (soyl) dirt.

**sol 1.** a colloidal dispersion of a solid in a liquid. Cf. gel. **2.** abbreviation for solution.

**so•lar chei•li•tis** mucosal atrophy with drying, crusting, and fissuring of the vermilion border of the lower lip, resulting from chronic exposure to sunlight; dysplastic (premalignant) changes are noted microscopically.

**solar co•me•do** SYN Favre-Racouchot disease.

**so•lar e•las•to•sis** elastosis seen histologically in

the sun-exposed skin of the elderly or in those who have chronic actinic damage.

**so·lar ur·ti·car·ia** a form of urticaria resulting from exposure to specific light spectra; e.g., sunlight; some patients have passive-transfer antibodies and others do not.

**sol·a·tion** (sol-ā'shŭn) COLLOIDAL CHEMISTRY the transformation of a gel into a sol, as by melting gelatin.

**sol·der·ing** (sod'er-ing) a laser technique to make one tissue adhere to another.

**sole** (sōl) the plantar surface or under part of the foot. SYN planta [TA]. [A.S.]

**Sol·e·nop·sis** (sōl-ĕ-nop'sis) a genus of ants known as fire ants, which can inflict painful burning stings that cause local and occasionally systemic reactions.

**Sol·e·nop·sis in·vic·ta** the red imported fire ant, a species imported from South America which has spread extensively within the southeastern United States where it has become a major pest of humans and animals; it readily stings humans, producing local swelling and pruritus with development of a pustule at the site of the sting and, in rare cases, it can cause anaphylactic shock with death from respiratory or cardiac arrest. SEE ALSO *Solenopsis richteri.* SYN *red imported fire ant.*

**Sol·e·nop·sis rich·ter·i** the black imported fire ant, a species imported from South America but less extensively established in the United States than *Solenopsis invicta.* SEE ALSO *Solenopsis invicta.* SYN *black imported fire ant.*

**so·le·us mus·cle** *origin,* posterior surface of head and upper third of shaft of fibula, oblique line and middle third of medial margin of tibia, and a tendinous arch passing between tibia and fibula over the popliteal vessels; *insertion,* with gastrocnemius by tendo calcaneus (tendo achillis) into tuberosity of calcaneus; *action,* plantar flexion of foot; *nerve supply,* tibial. SYN musculus soleus [TA].

**sol·id** **1.** firm; compact; not fluid; without interstices or cavities; not cancellous. **2.** a body that retains its form when not confined; one that is not fluid, neither liquid nor gaseous. [L. *solidus*]

**sol·i·tary bone cyst** a unilocular cyst containing serous fluid and lined with a thin layer of connective tissue, occurring usually in the shaft of a long bone in a child. SYN osteocystoma, unicameral bone cyst.

**sol·i·tary lym·pha·tic fol·li·cles** minute collections of lymphoid tissue in the mucosa of the small and large intestines, being especially numerous in the cecum and appendix.

**sol·i·tary tract** a slender, compact fiber bundle extending longitudinally through the dorsolateral region of the medullary tegmentum, surrounded by the nucleus of the solitary tract, below the obex decussating over the central canal, and descending into the upper cervical segments of the spinal cord. It is composed of primary sensory fibers that enter with the vagus, glossopharyngeal, and facial nerves, and in part convey information from stretch receptors and chemoreceptors in the walls of the cardiovascular, respiratory, and intestinal tracts; in rostral parts of the tract impulses are generated by the receptor cells of the taste buds in the mucosa of the tongue. Its fibers are distributed to the nucleus of the solitary tract.

**sol·u·bil·i·ty** (sol-yu-bil'i-tē) the property of being soluble.

**sol·u·bil·i·ty test** a screening test for sickle cell hemoglobin (Hb S), which is reduced by dithionite and is insoluble in concentrated inorganic buffer; addition of blood showing Hb S to buffer and dithionite causes opacity of the solution.

**sol·u·ble** (sol'yu-bl) capable of being dissolved. [L. *solubilis,* fr. *solvo,* to dissolve]

**sol·u·ble RNA (sRNA)** SYN transfer RNA. [soluble in molar salt]

**sol·ute** (sol'yut) the dissolved substance in a solution. [L. *solutus,* dissolved, pp. of *solvo,* to dissolve]

**so·lu·tion** (sō-loo'shŭn) **1.** the incorporation of a solid, a liquid, or a gas in a liquid or noncrystalline solid resulting in a homogeneous single phase. SEE dispersion, suspension. **2.** generally, an aqueous solution of a nonvolatile substance. **3.** an aqueous solution of a nonvolatile substance is called a solution or liquor; an aqueous solution of a volatile substance is a water (aqua); an alcoholic solution of a nonvolatile substance is a tincture (tinctura); an alcoholic solution of a volatile substance is a spirit (spiritus). **4.** the termination of a disease by crisis. **5.** a break, cut, or laceration of the solid tissues. SEE solution of contiguity, solution of continuity. [L. *solutio*]

**so·lu·tion of con·ti·gu·i·ty** the breaking of contiguity; a dislocation or displacement of two normally contiguous parts.

**so·lu·tion of con·ti·nu·i·ty** division of bones or soft parts that are normally continuous, as by a fracture, a laceration, or an incision. SYN dieresis.

**sol·vent** a liquid that holds another substance in solution, i.e., dissolves it. [L. *solvens,* pres. p. of *solvo,* to dissolve]

**so·ma** (sō'mă) **1.** the axial part of the body, i.e., head, neck, trunk, and tail, excluding the limbs. **2.** all of an organism with the exception of the germ cells. SEE ALSO body. **3.** the body of a nerve cell, from which axons and dendrites project. [G. *sōma,* body]

**so·mas·the·nia** (sō-mas-thē'nē-ă) SYN somatasthenia.

**so·ma·tag·no·sia** (sō'mă-tag-nō'sē-ă) SYN somatotopagnosis. [somat- + G. *a-* priv. + *gnōsis,* recognition]

**so·ma·tal·gia** (sō-mă-tal'jē-ă) **1.** pain in the body. **2.** pain due to organic causes, as opposed to psychogenic pain. [somat- + G. *algos,* pain]

**so·ma·tas·the·nia** (sō'mă-tas-thē'nē-ă) a condition of chronic physical weakness and fatigability. SYN somasthenia. [somat- + G. *astheneia,* weakness]

**so·ma·tes·the·sia** (sō'mă-tes-thē'zē-ă) bodily sensation, the conscious awareness of the body. SYN somesthesia. [somat- + G. *aisthēsis,* sensation]

**so·mat·es·the·tic** (sō'mat-es-thet'ik) relating to somatesthesia.

**so·mat·ic** (sō-mat'ik) **1.** relating to the soma or trunk, the wall of the body cavity, or the body in general. SYN parietal (2). **2.** relating to or involving the skeleton or skeletal (voluntary) muscle and the innervation of the latter, as distinct from the viscera or visceral (involuntary) muscle and its (autonomic) innervation. SYN parietal (3). **3.** relating to the vegetative, as distinguished from the generative, functions. [G. *sōmatikos,* bodily]

**so·ma·tic ant·i·gen** an antigen located in the cell

wall of a bacterium in contrast to one in the flagella (flagellar antigen) or in a capsule (capsular antigen).

**so•ma•tic cells** the cells of an organism other than the germ cells.

**so•ma•tic cross•ing-o•ver** crossing-over that occurs during the mitosis of somatic cells, in contrast to that which occurs in meiosis.

**so•ma•tic death, sys•tem•ic death** death of the entire body, as distinguished from local death.

**so•ma•tic de•lu•sion** a delusion having reference to a nonexistent lesion or alteration of some organ or part of the body; sometimes indistinguishable from hypochondriasis.

**so•ma•tic mo•tor nu•clei** collective term indicating the motor nuclei innervating the tongue musculature (hypoglossal nucleus) and the extraocular eye muscles (abducens nucleu, trochlear nucleus, and oculomotor nucleus).

**so•ma•tic mu•ta•tion** a mutation occurring in the general body cells (as opposed to the germ cells) and hence not transmitted to progeny.

**so•ma•tic mu•ta•tion the•o•ry of can•cer** that cancer is caused by a mutation or mutations in the body cells (as opposed to germ cells), especially nonlethal mutations associated with increased proliferation of the mutant cells.

**so•ma•tic nerve** one of the nerves of parietal sensation or voluntary motion, as distinguished from the visceral sensory, involuntary motor and secretory nerves.

**so•ma•tic pain** pain originating in the skin, ligaments, muscles, bones, or joints.

**so•ma•tic re•pro•duc•tion** asexual reproduction by fission or budding of somatic cells.

**so•ma•tic sen•so•ry cor•tex, so•ma•to•sen•so•ry cor•tex** the region of the cerebral cortex receiving the somatic sensory radiation from the ventrobasal nucleus of the thalamus; it represents the primary cortical processing mechanism for sensory information originating at the body surfaces (touch) and in deeper tissues such as muscle, tendons, and joint capsules (position sense).

**so•ma•tic swal•low** a swallowing pattern with muscular contractions which appear to be under control of the person at a subconscious level; distinguished from visceral swallow.

**so•ma•ti•za•tion** (sō′mat-i-zā′shŭn) the process by which psychological needs are expressed in physical symptoms. SEE ALSO somatization disorder.

**so•ma•ti•za•tion dis•or•der** a mental disorder characterized by presentation of a complicated medical history and of physical symptoms referring to a variety of organ systems, but without a detectable or known organic basis. SEE ALSO conversion, hysteria.

△**so•ma•to-, somat-, so•ma•ti•co-** the body, bodily. [G. *sōma*, body]

**so•ma•to•chrome** (sō-ma-t′ō-krōm) denoting the group of neurons or nerve cells in which there is an abundance of cytoplasm completely surrounding the nucleus. [somato- + G. *chrōma*, color]

**so•ma•to•crin•in** (sō′mă-tō-crin′in) hypothalamic growth hormone-releasing hormone, GHRH. [somato- + G. *krinō*, to secrete, + -in]

**so•ma•to•gen•ic** (sō′mă-tō-jen′ik) **1.** originating in the soma or body under the influence of external forces. **2.** having origin in body cells. [somato- + G. *genesis*, origin]

**so•ma•to•lib•er•in** (sō′mă-tō-lib′er-in) a deca-peptide released by the hypothalamus, which induces the release of human growth hormone (somatotropin). SYN growth hormone-releasing factor, growth hormone-releasing hormone, somatotropin-releasing factor, somatotropin-releasing hormone. [somatotropin + L. *libero*, to free, + -in]

**so•ma•to•mam•mo•tro•pin** (sō′mă-tō-mam′ō-trō-pin) a peptide hormone, closely related to somatotropin in its biological properties, produced by the normal placenta and by certain neoplasms. [somato- + L. *mamma*, breast, + G. trope, a turning, + -in]

**so•ma•to•me•din** (sō′mă-tō-mē′din) a peptide synthesized in the liver, and probably in the kidney, that is capable of stimulating certain anabolic processes in bone and cartilage, such as synthesis of DNA, RNA, and protein and the sulfation of mucopolysaccharides; secretion and/or biological activity of somatomedin is known to be dependent on somatotropin. [*somatotropin* + *mediator* + -in]

**so•ma•to•path•ic** (sō′mă-tō-path′ik) relating to bodily or organic illness, as distinguished from mental (psychologic) disorder. [somato- + G. *pathos*, suffering]

**so•ma•to•pause** decrease in growth hormone–insulinlike growth factor axis activities associated with aging.

**so•ma•to•plasm** (sō-mat′ō-plazm) aggregate of all the forms of specialized protoplasm entering into the composition of the body, other than germ plasm. [somato- + G. *plasma*, something formed]

**so•ma•to•pleure** (sō-mat′ō-ploor) embryonic layer formed by association of the parietal layer of the lateral plate mesoderm with the ectoderm. [somato- + G. *pleura*, side]

**so•ma•to•psy•chic** (sō′mă-tō-sī′kik) relating to the body-mind relationship; the study of the effects of the body upon the mind, as opposed to psychosomatic, which refers to the effects of mind on body. [somato- + G. *psychē*, soul]

**so•ma•to•psy•cho•sis** (sō′mă-tō-sī-kō′sis) an emotional disorder associated with an organic disease. [somato- + G. *psychōsis*, an animating]

**so•ma•to•sen•so•ry** (sō-mă-tō-sen′sō-rē) sensation relating to the body's superficial and deep parts as contrasted to specialized senses such as sight.

**so•ma•to•sen•so•ry au•ra** epileptic aura characterized by paresthesias or abdominal somatognosia of a clearly defined regional distribution. SEE ALSO aura (1).

**so•ma•to•sex•u•al** (sō′mă-tō-seks′yu-ăl) denoting the somatic aspects of sexuality as distinguished from its psychosexual aspects.

**so•ma•to•stat•in** (sō′mă-tō-stat′in) a tetradecapeptide capable of inhibiting the release of somatotropin, insulin, and gastrin. SYN growth hormone-inhibiting hormone, somatotropin release-inhibiting hormone. [somatotropin + G. *stasis*, a standing still, + -in]

**so•ma•to•stat•i•no•ma** (sō′mă-tō-stat-i-nō′mă) a somatostatin-secreting tumor of the pancreatic islets.

**so•ma•to•ther•a•py** (sō′mă-tō-thār′ă-pē) **1.** therapy directed at physical disorders. **2.** PSYCHIATRY a variety of therapeutic interventions employing chemical or physical, as opposed to psychological, methods.

**so•ma•to•top•ag•no•sis** (sō′mă-tō-top′ag-nō′sis)

the inability to identify any part of one's own or another's body. Cf. autotopagnosia. SYN somatagnosia. [somato- + top- + G. *a-* priv. + G. *gnōsis,* knowledge]

**so·ma·to·top·ic** (sō-mă-tō-top′ik) relating to somatotopy.

**so·ma·tot·o·py** (sō-mă-tot′ō-pē) the topographic association of positional relationships of receptors in the body via respective nerve fibers to their terminal distribution in specific functional areas of the cerebral cortex; the continuation of these positional relationships in all stages of the ascent of nerve fibers through the central nervous system enables the brain and spinal cord to function on a basis of spatially designated units. [somato- + G. *topos,* place]

**so·ma·to·tropes** (sō-mat′ō-trōps) a subclass of pituitary acidophilic cells; site of synthesis of growth hormone.

**so·ma·to·troph** (sō-mat′ō-trof) a cell of the adenohypophysis that produces somatotropin.

**so·ma·to·tro·pic, so·ma·to·tro·phic** (sō′mă-tō-trop′ik, sō′mă-tō-trof′ik) having a stimulating effect on body growth. [somato- + G. *tropē,* a turning]

**so·ma·to·tro·pin, so·ma·to·tro·pic hor·mone** (sō′mă-tō-trō′pin) a protein hormone of the anterior lobe of the pituitary, produced by the acidophil cells, that promotes body growth, fat mobilization, and inhibition of glucose utilization; diabetogenic when present in excess; a deficiency of somatotropin is associated with a number of types of dwarfism. SYN growth hormone, pituitary growth hormone. [for *somatotrophin,* fr. somato- + G. *trophē* nourishment; corrupted to *-tropin* and reanalyzed as fr. G. *tropē,* a turning]

**so·ma·to·tro·pin re·lease-in·hi·bit·ing hor·mone (SIH)** SYN somatostatin.

**so·ma·to·tro·pin-re·leas·ing fac·tor** SYN somatoliberin.

**so·ma·to·tro·pin-re·leas·ing hor·mone (SRH)** SYN somatoliberin.

**so·ma·to·type** (sō-mat′ō-tīp) **1.** the constitutional or body type of an individual. **2.** the constitutional or body type associated with a particular personality type.

**so·ma·tro·pin** (sō-mat′rō-pin) a drug identical with human growth hormone; used in the treatment of growth disturbances due to insufficient secretion of growth hormone in children or adults or associated with gonadal dysgenesis (Turner syndrome) and of growth disturbance in prepubertal children with chronic renal insufficiency.

**som·es·the·sia** (sō-mes-thē′zē-ă) SYN somatesthesia.

**so·mite** (sō′mīt) one of the paired, metamerically arranged cell masses formed in the early embryonic paraxial mesoderm; commencing in the third or early fourth week in the region of the hindbrain, they develop in a caudal direction until 42 pairs are formed; their presence is considered evidence that metameric segmentation is a vertebrate characteristic. [G. *sōma,* body, + *-ite*]

**som·nam·bu·lism** (som-nam′byu-lizm) **1.** a disorder of sleep involving complex motor acts which occurs primarily during the first third of the night but not during rapid eye movement sleep. **2.** a form of hysteria in which purposeful behavior is forgotten. [L. *somnus,* sleep, + *ambulo,* to walk]

**som·ni·fa·cient** (som-ni-fā′shent) SYN soporific (1). [L. *somnus,* sleep, + *facio,* to make]

**som·nif·er·ous** (som-nif′er-ŭs) SYN soporific (1). [L. *somnus,* sleep, + *fero,* to bring]

**som·nil·o·quence, som·nil·o·quism** (som-nil′ō-kwens, som-nil′ō-kwizm) **1.** talking or muttering in one's sleep. **2.** SYN somniloquy. [L. *somnus,* sleep, + *loquor,* to talk]

**som·nil·o·quy** (som-nil′ō-kwē) talking under the influence of hypnotic suggestion. SYN somniloquence (2), somniloquism. [L. *somnus,* sleep, + *loquor,* to speak]

**som·nip·a·thy** (som-nip′ă-thē) **1.** any sleep disorder. **2.** SYN hypnotism (1). [L. *somnus,* sleep, + G. *pathos,* suffering]

**som·no·cin·e·ma·tog·ra·phy** (som′nō-sin-ĕ-mă-tog′ră-fē) the process or technique of recording movements during sleep.

**som·no·lence, som·no·len·cy** (som′nŏ-lens, som′nŏ-len-sē) **1.** an inclination to sleep. **2.** a condition of obtusion. [L. *somnolentia*]

**som·no·lent, som·no·les·cent** (som′nŏ-lent, som-nŏ-les′ent) **1.** drowsy; sleepy; inclined to sleep. **2.** in a condition of incomplete sleep; semicomatose. [L. *somnus,* sleep]

**So·mog·yi ef·fect, So·mog·yi phe·no·me·non** (sō′mō-jē) a rebound phenomenon of reactive hyperglycemia following a period of relative hypoglycemia, which may be subclinical and difficult to detect; the hyperglycemia induces use of more insulin, thus aggravating the problem.

**So·mog·yi u·nit** (sō′mō-jē) a measure of the level of activity of amylase in blood serum, as analyzed by means of the Somogyi method (the most frequently used procedure).

**Son·der·mann ca·nal** (sŏn-der-mahn) a blind outpouching of Schlemm canal, extending toward, but not communicating with, the anterior chamber of the eye.

**son·ic** (son′ik) of, pertaining to, or determined by sound; e.g., sonic vibration. [L. *sonus,* sound]

**son·i·ca·tion** (son-i-kā′shŭn) the process of disrupting biologic materials by use of sound wave energy.

**son·i·fi·ca·tion** (son′i-fi-kā′shŭn) the production of sound, or of sound waves.

**Son·ne ba·cil·lus** (son′ĕ) SYN *Shigella sonnei.*

**son·o·gram** (son′ō-gram) SYN ultrasonogram. See page B10. [L. *sonus,* sound, + G. *gramma,* a drawing]

**son·o·graph** (son′ō-graf) SYN ultrasonograph. [L. *sonus,* sound, + G. *graphō,* to write]

**so·nog·ra·pher** (sŏ-nog′ră-fer) SYN ultrasonographer.

**so·nog·ra·phy** (sŏ-nog′ră-fē) SYN ultrasonography. See page B10. [L. *sonus,* sound. + G. *graphō,* to write]

**so·no·rous rale** a cooing or snoring sound often produced by the vibration of a projecting mass of viscid secretion in a large bronchus.

**so·por** (sō′pōr) an unnaturally deep sleep. [L.]

**so·po·rif·ic** (sō-pōr-if′ik, sop′ōr-if′ik) **1.** causing sleep. SYN somnifacient, somniferous. **2.** an agent that produces sleep. [L. *sopor,* deep sleep, + *facio,* to make]

**sor·be·fa·cient** (sōr-bĕ-fā′shent) **1.** causing absorption. **2.** an agent that causes or facilitates absorption. [L. *sorbeo,* to suck up, + *facio,* to make]

**sor·des** (sōr′dēz) a dark brown or blackish crustlike collection on the lips, teeth, and gums of a person with dehydration associated with a chronic debilitating disease. [L. filth, fr. *sordeo,* to be foul]

**sore** (sōr) **1.** a wound, ulcer, or any open skin lesion. **2.** painful; aching; tender. [A.S. *sār*]

**sore throat** a condition characterized by pain or discomfort on swallowing; it may be due to any of a variety of inflammations of the tonsils, pharynx, or larynx.

**So·ret phe·no·me·non** (sō-rā′) in a solution kept in a long, upright tube at room temperature, the upper part, being the warmer, is also the more concentrated.

**sorp·tion** (sōrp′shŭn) adsorption or absorption.

**Sors·by mac·u·lar de·gen·er·a·tion** (sorz′bē) SYN familial pseudoinflammatory macular degeneration.

**Sors·by syn·drome** (sorz′bē) congenital macular coloboma and apical dystrophy of the extremities.

**So·tos syn·drome** (sō′tōs) cerebral gigantism and generalized large muscles in childhood, with mental retardation and defective coordination; of unknown etiology.

**souf·fle** (soo′fl) a soft, blowing sound heard on auscultation. [Fr. *souffler,* to blow]

**sound** (sownd) **1.** the vibrations produced by a sounding body, transmitted by the air or other medium, and perceived by the internal ear. **2.** an elongated cylindrical, usually curved, instrument of metal, used for exploring the bladder or other cavities of the body, for dilating strictures of the urethra, esophagus, or other canal, for calibrating the lumen of a body cavity, or for detecting the presence of a foreign body in a body cavity. **3.** to explore or calibrate a cavity with a sound. **4.** whole; healthy; not diseased or injured.

**sound field** the environment in which sound waves are propagated. SYN acoustical surround.

**source-to-im·age dis·tance (SID)** SYN focal-film distance.

**South Af·ri·can tick-bite fe·ver** (sowth f′ri-ken) a typhus-like fever of South Africa caused by *Rickettsia rickettsii* and usually characterized by primary eschar and regional adenitis, rigors, and maculopapular rash on the fifth day, often with severe central nervous system symptoms.

**South A·mer·i·can blas·to·my·co·sis** (sowth ăm-er′i-ken) SYN paracoccidioidomycosis.

**South A·mer·i·can try·pan·o·so·mi·a·sis** (sowth ăm-er′i-ken) trypanosomiasis caused by *Trypanosoma* (or *Schizotrypanum) cruzi* and transmitted by certain species of reduviid (triatomine) bugs. In its acute form, it is seen most frequently in young children, with swelling of the skin at the site of entry, most often the face, and regional lymph node enlargement; in its chronic form it can assume several aspects, commonly cardiomyopathy, but megacolon and megaesophagus also occur; natural reservoirs include domestic, domiciliated, and wild mammals. SYN Chagas disease, Chagas-Cruz disease, Cruz trypanosomiasis.

**South·ern blot a·nal·y·sis** (suth′ern) a procedure to separate and identify DNA sequences; DNA fragments are separated by electrophoresis on an agarose gel, transferred (blotted) onto a nitrocellulose or nylon membrane, and hybridized with complementary (labeled) nucleic acid probes.

**SP** sacroposterior position.

**space** (spās) any demarcated portion of the body, either an area of the surface, a segment of the tissues, or a cavity. SEE ALSO area, region, zone. SYN spatium [TA]. [L. *spatium,* room, space]

**spac·er** an extension device for a metered-dose inhaler; it is designed to eliminate the need for hand-breath coordination and to reduce the deposition of large aerosol particles in the upper airway.

**Spal·lan·za·ni law** (spahl-an-tzah′nē) the younger the individual the greater is the regenerative power of its cells.

**spal·la·tion 1.** SYN fragmentation. **2.** nuclear reaction in which nuclei, on being bombarded by high energy particles, liberate a number of protons and alpha particles.

**spal·la·tion pro·duct** an atomic species produced in the course of the spallation of any atom.

**Span·ish in·flu·en·za** (spăn′ish) influenza that caused several waves of pandemic in 1918–1919, resulting in more than 20 million deaths worldwide.

**spar·ing ac·tion** the manner in which a nonessential nutritive component, by its presence in the diet, lowers the dietary requirement for an essential component.

**spasm** (spazm) a sudden involuntary contraction of one or more muscle groups; includes cramps, contractures. SYN muscle spasm, spasmus. [G. *spasmos*]

△**spas·mo-** spasm. [G. *spasmos*]

**spas·mod·ic** (spaz-mod′ik) relating to or marked by spasm. [G. *spasmōdes,* convulsive, fr. *spasmos,* + *eidos,* form]

**spas·mo·dic dys·men·or·rhea** dysmenorrhea accompanied by painful contractions of the uterus.

**spas·mo·dic dys·phon·ia** a spasmodic contradiction of the intrinsic muscles of the larynx excited by attempted phonation, producing either adductor or abductor subtypes caused by a central nervous system disorder. A localized form of movement disorder. SYN spastic dysphonia.

**spas·mol·y·sis** (spaz-mol′i-sis) the arrest of a spasm or convulsion. [spasmo- + G. *lysis,* dissolution]

**spas·mo·lyt·ic** (spaz′mō-lit′ik) **1.** relating to spasmolysis. **2.** denoting a chemical agent that relieves smooth muscle spasms.

**spas·mus** (spaz′mŭs) SYN spasm. [L. fr. G. *spasmos,* spasm]

**spas·mus nu·tans 1.** SYN nodding spasm. **2.** a fine nystagmus, sometimes rotary, sometimes monocular, associated with head-nodding movements.

**spas·tic** (spas′tik) **1.** SYN hypertonic (1). **2.** relating to spasm or to spasticity. [L. *spasticus,* fr. G. *spastikos,* drawing in]

**spas·tic a·ba·sia** abasia due to a spastic contraction of the muscles when an attempt is made to walk.

**spas·tic col·on** SYN irritable bowel syndrome.

**spas·tic dys·arth·ria** dysarthria associated with upper motor neuron disorders causing excess tone and limited range in muscle movements, characterized by imprecise consonants, monotony of pitch and reduced stress, and a labored voice quality. SEE pseudobulbar palsy.

**spas·tic dys·pho·nia** SYN spasmodic dysphonia.

**spas·tic gait** SYN hemiplegic gait.

**spas·tic hem·i·ple·gia** a hemiplegia with increased tone in the antigravity muscles of the affected side.

**spas•tic il•e•us** SYN dynamic ileus.

**spas•tic•i•ty** (spas-tis′i-tē) a state of increased muscular tone with exaggeration of the tendon reflexes.

**spa•tial** (spā′shăl) relating to space or a space.

**spa•tial re•la•tion** position of an object in relation to another.

**spa•ti•um,** pl. **spa•tia** (spā′shē-ŭm, spā′shē-ă) [TA] SYN space. [L.]

**spat•u•la** (spach′ŭ-lă) a flat blade, like a knife blade but without a sharp edge, used in pharmacy for spreading plasters and ointments and as an aid to mixing ingredients with a mortar and pestle. [L. dim. of *spatha,* a broad, flat wooden instrument, fr. G. *spathē*]

**spat•u•late** (spach′ŭ-lāt) **1.** shaped like a spatula. **2.** to manipulate or mix with a spatula. **3.** to incise the cut end of a tubular structure longitudinally and splay it open, to allow creation of an elliptical anastomosis of greater circumference than would be possible with conventional transverse or oblique (bevelled) end-to-end anastomoses.

**spay** (spā) to remove the ovaries of an animal. [Gael. *spoth,* castrate, or G. *spadōn,* eunuch]

**SPCA** serum prothrombin conversion accelerator.

**speak•er's no•dules** SYN vocal nodules.

**speak•ing tube** a tube with an earpiece at one end and a cone at the other to amplify speech into the cone.

**spe•cial a•nat•o•my** the anatomy of certain definite organs or groups of organs involved in the performance of special functions; descriptive anatomy dealing with the separate systems.

**spe•cial•ist** (spesh′ă-list) one who devotes professional attention to a particular specialty or subject area.

**spe•cial•i•za•tion** (spesh′ă-li-zā′shŭn) **1.** professional attention limited to a particular specialty or subject area for study, research, and/or treatment. **2.** SYN differentiation (1).

**spe•cial sense** one of the five senses related respectively to the organs of sight, hearing, smell, taste, and touch.

**spe•cial•ty** (spesh′al-tē) the particular subject area or branch of medical science to which one devotes professional attention. [L. *specialitas* fr. *specialis,* special]

**spe•cial•ty re•fer•ral cen•ter** a designated medical facility that provides specialized medical or trauma care for a particular body system by specialty or nature of injury, e.g., hand trauma center, neonatal care center.

**spe•ci•a•tion** (spē-shē-ā′shŭn) the evolutionary process by which diverse species of animals or plants are formed from a common ancestral stock.

**spe•cies,** pl. **spe•cies** (spē′shēz) **1.** a biological division between the genus and a variety or the individual; a group of organisms that generally bear a close resemblance to one another in the more essential features of their organization, and breed effectively producing fertile progeny. **2.** a class of pharmaceutical preparations consisting of a mixture of dried plants, not pulverized, but in sufficiently fine division to be conveniently used in the making of extemporaneous decoctions or infusions, as a tea. [L. appearance, form, kind, fr. *specio,* to look at]

**spe•cies-spe•cif•ic** characteristic of a given species; serum that is produced by the injection of immunogens into an animal, and that acts only upon the cells, protein, etc., of a member of the same species as that from which the original antigen was obtained.

**spe•cies-spe•cif•ic ant•i•gen** antigenic components in tissues and fluids by means of which various species may be immunologically distinguished; e.g., serum albumin of horses is immunologically different from that of man, dogs, sheep.

**spe•cif•ic** (spĕ-sif′ik) **1.** relating to a species. **2.** relating to an individual infectious disease, one caused by a special microorganism. **3.** a remedy having a definite therapeutic action in relation to a particular disease or symptom, as quinine in relation to malaria. [L. *specificus* fr. *species* + *facio,* to make]

**spe•cif•ic ab•sorp•tion co•ef•fi•cient** (*a*) absorbance (of light) per unit path length (usually the centimeter) and per unit of mass concentration. Cf. molar absorption coefficient. SYN absorbancy index (1), absorptivity (1), extinction coefficient, specific extinction.

**spe•cif•ic ac•tion** the action of a drug or a method of treatment which has a direct and especially curative effect upon a disease.

**spe•cif•ic ac•ti•vi•ty 1.** radioactivity per unit mass of the stated element or compound; **2.** for an enzyme, the amount of substrate consumed (or product formed) in a given time under given conditions per milligram of protein; **3.** activity per unit mass of the stated radionuclide.

**spe•cif•ic build•ing-re•lat•ed ill•nes•ses** a group of infectious, allergic, and immunologic diseases with fairly homogeneous clinical signs whose causes can be traced to factors in buildings in which afflicted patients work or reside. Cf. nonspecific building-related illnesses.

**spe•cif•ic dy•na•mic ac•tion (SDA)** increase of heat production caused by the ingestion of food, especially of protein.

**spe•cif•ic ex•tinc•tion** SYN specific absorption coefficient.

**spe•cif•ic gra•vi•ty** the weight of any body compared with that of another body of equal volume regarded as the unit; usually the weight of a liquid compared with that of distilled water.

**spe•cif•ic im•mu•ni•ty** the immune status in which there is an altered reactivity directed solely against the antigenic determinants (infectious agent or other) that stimulated it. SEE acquired immunity.

**spec•i•fic•i•ty** (spes-i-fis′i-tē) **1.** the condition or state of being specific, of having a fixed relation to a single cause or to a definite result; manifested in the relation of a disease to its pathogenic microorganism, of a reaction to a certain chemical union, or of an antibody to its antigen or the reverse. **2.** CLINICAL PATHOLOGY the proportion of individuals who do not have a disease or condition and in whom a test intended to identify that disease or condition yields negative results. Cf. sensitivity (2).

**spe•ci•fi•ci•ty of train•ing prin•ci•ple** EXERCISE SCIENCE concept that specific exercise elicits specific adaptations, creating specific training effects. The effects are most effectively induced by training the specific muscles involved in the desired performance.

S
p

**spe·ci·fic op·son·in** antibodies formed in response to stimulation by a specific antigen, either as a result of an attack of a disease, or injections with a suitably prepared suspension of the specific microorganism.

**spe·ci·fic optic ro·ta·tion** the arc through which the plane of polarized light is rotated by 1 g of a substance per milliliter of water when the length of the light path through the solution is 1 decimeter, typically using light corresponding to the D line of sodium.

**spe·ci·fic par·a·site** a parasite that habitually lives in its present host and is particularly adapted for the host species.

**spe·ci·fic pho·bia** a persistent pattern of significant fear of specific objects or situations, manifesting in anxiety or panic on exposure to the object or situation or in anticipation of them, which the person realizes is unreasonable or excessive and which interferes significantly with the person's functioning; SYN simple phobia.

**spe·ci·fic re·ac·tion** the phenomena produced by an agent that is identical with or immunologically related to the one that has stimulated an immune response.

**spec·i·men** (spes′ĭ-men) a small part, or sample, of any substance or material obtained for testing. [L. fr. *specio*, to look at]

**SPECT** single photon emission computed tomography.

**spec·ta·cles** (spek′tĭ-klz) lenses set in a frame that holds them in front of the eyes, used to correct errors of refraction or to protect the eyes. The parts of the spectacles are the *lenses;* the *bridge* between the lenses, resting on the nose; the *rims* or *frames*, encircling the lenses; the *sides* or *temples* that pass on either side of the head to the ears; the *bows*, the curved extremities of the temples; the *shoulders*, short bars attached to the rims or the lenses and jointed with the sides. SYN eyeglasses, glasses (1). [L. *specto*, pp. -*atus*, to watch, observe]

**spec·tra** (spek′tră) plural of spectrum. [L.]

**spec·tral** (spek′trăl) relating to a spectrum.

**spec·trin** (spek′trin) a filamentous contractile protein that together with actin and other cytoskeleton proteins forms a network that gives the red blood cell membrane its shape and flexibility; a defect or deficiency of spectrin is associated with hereditary spherocytosis and hereditary elliptocytosis; the principal component of the membrane skeleton of red cells.

△**spec·tro-** a spectrum. [L. *spectrum*, an image]

**spec·trom·e·ter** (spek-trom′ĕ-ter) an instrument for determining the wavelength or energy of light or other electromagnetic emission. [spectro- + G. *metron*, measure]

**spec·trom·e·try** (spek-trom′ĕ-trē) the procedure of observing and measuring the wavelengths of light or other electromagnetic emissions.

**spec·tro·pho·tom·e·ter** (spek′trō-fō-tom′ĕ-ter) an instrument for measuring the intensity of light of a definite wavelength transmitted by a substance or a solution, giving a quantitative measure of the amount of material in the solution absorbing the light; a colorimeter with a choice of wavelength and photometric measurement. [spectro- + photometer]

**spec·tro·pho·tom·e·try** (spek′trō-fō-tom′ĕ-trē) analysis by means of a spectrophotometer.

**spec·tro·scope** (spek′trō-skōp) an instrument for resolving light from any luminous body into its spectrum, and for the analysis of the spectrum so formed. It consists of a prism that refracts the light or a grating for diffraction of the light, an arrangement for rendering the rays parallel, and a telescope that magnifies the spectrum. [spectro- + G. *skopeō*, to view]

**spec·tro·scop·ic** (spek-trō-skop′ik) relating to or performed by means of a spectroscope.

**spec·tros·co·py** (spek-tros′kŏ-pē) observation and study of spectra of absorbed or emitted light by means of a spectroscope.

**spec·trum**, pl. **spec·tra**, **spec·trums** (spek′trŭm, spek′tră, spek′trŭmz) **1.** the range of colors presented when white light is resolved into its constituent colors by being passed through a prism or through a diffraction grating: red, orange, yellow, green, blue, indigo, and violet, arranged in increasing frequency of vibration or decreasing wavelength. **2.** the range of pathogenic microorganisms against which an antibiotic or other antibacterial agent is active. **3.** the plot of intensity vs. wavelength of light emitted or absorbed by a substance, usually characteristic of the substance and used in qualitative and quantitative analysis. **4.** the range of wavelengths presented when a beam of radiant energy is subjected to dispersion and focused. [L. an image, fr. *specio*, to look at]

**spec·u·lum**, pl. **spec·u·la** (spek′yu-lŭm, spek′yu-lă) an instrument for enlarging the opening of any canal or cavity in order to facilitate inspection of its interior. [L. a mirror, fr. *specio*, to look at]

**spec·u·lum for·ceps** a tubular forceps for use through a speculum.

**SPEECH1** gene that when mutated is responsible for motor dyspraxia.

**speech** talk; the use of the voice in conveying ideas. [A.S. *spaec*]

**speech a·ware·ness thresh·old** the lowest sound intensity at which speech can be detected. SYN speech detection threshold.

**speech bulb** a prosthetic speech aid; a restoration used to close a cleft or other opening in the hard or soft palate, or to replace absent tissue necessary for the production of good speech.

**speech cen·ters** areas of the cerebral cortex centrally involved in speech function; one is in the left inferior frontal gyrus, a second one in the supramarginal, angular, and first and second temporal gyri. SEE ALSO Broca center, Wernicke center.

**speech de·tec·tion thresh·old** SYN speech awareness threshold.

**speech fre·quen·cies** acoustic sound wave frequency range in which most speech sounds occur, generally 500–3000 Hz. SEE frequency.

**speech-lan·guage pa·tho·lo·gist** a practitioner concerned with the diagnosis and rehabilitation of persons with voice, speech, and language disorders.

**speech-lan·guage pa·tho·lo·gy** SYN speech pathology.

**speech me·cha·ni·sm** peripheral structures involved in the normal production of speech, encompassing the organs of articulation, phonation, resonance, and respiration. SEE articulation, articulators, phonation, resonance, respiration.

**speech pa·tho·lo·gy** the science concerned with functional and organic speech defects and disorders. SYN speech-language pathology.

**speech per·cep·tion** identification of speech sounds, mainly from acoustic cues.

**speech pro·ces·sor** the part of a cochlear implant that converts speech into electrical impulses that are used to stimulate the neurons of the auditory division of the eighth cranial nerve.

**speech read·ing** used by people with hearing impairment of nonauditory clues as to what is being said through observing the speaker's facial expressions, lip and jaw movements, and other gestures. SYN lip reading.

**speech re·cep·tion thresh·old** the intensity at which speech is recognized as meaningful symbols; in speech audiometry, it is the decibel level at which 50% of spondee words can be repeated correctly by the subject.

**speed** (spēd) the magnitude of velocity without regard to direction. Cf. velocity.

**speed play** SYN fartlek training.

**Spens syn·drome** (spenz) SYN Adams-Stokes syndrome.

**sperm 1.** SYN spermatozoon. **2.** SYN semen (1). [G. *sperma,* seed]

△**sper·ma-, sper·ma·to-, spermo-** semen, spermatozoa. [G. *sperma,* seed]

**sper·ma·cyt·ic sem·i·no·ma** a relatively slow-growing, locally invasive type of testicular seminoma that does not metastasize and has no ovarian counterpart.

**sperm-as·ter** (sperm′as-ter) cytocentrum with astral rays in the cytoplasm of an inseminated ovum; it is brought in by the penetrating spermatozoon and evolves into the mitotic spindle of the first cleavage division. [sperm + G. *astēr,* a star (aster)]

**sper·mat·ic** (sper-mat′ik) relating to the sperm or semen.

**sper·ma·tic cord** the cord formed by the ductus deferens and its associated structures extending from the deep inguinal ring through the inguinal canal into the scrotum. SYN funiculus spermaticus [TA], testicular cord.

**sper·ma·tic duct** SYN ductus deferens.

**sper·ma·tid** (sper′mă-tid) a cell in a late stage of the development of the spermatozoon; it is a haploid cell derived from the secondary spermatocyte and evolves by spermiogenesis into a spermatozoon. [spermat- + -*id* (2)]

**sper·ma·to·blast** (sper′mă-tō-blast) SYN spermatogonium. [spermato- + G. *blastos,* germ]

**sper·ma·to·cele** (sper′mă-tō-sēl) cyst of the epididymis containing spermatozoa. [spermato- + G. *kēlē,* tumor]

**sper·ma·to·ci·dal** (sper′mă-tō-sī′dăl) SYN spermicidal.

**sper·ma·to·cide** (sper′mă-tō-sīd) SYN spermicide. [spermato- + L. *caedo,* to kill]

**sper·ma·to·cy·tal** (sper-mă-tō-sī′tăl) relating to spermatocyte.

**sper·ma·to·cyte** (sper′mă-tō-sīt) parent cell of a spermatid, derived by mitotic division from a spermatogonium. [spermato- + G. *kytos,* cell]

**sper·ma·to·cy·to·gen·e·sis** (sper′mă-tō-sī′tō-jen′ē-sis) SYN spermatogenesis.

**sper·ma·to·gen·e·sis** (sper′mă-tō-jen′ē-sis) the entire process by which spermatogonial stem cells divide and differentiate into spermatozoa. SEE ALSO spermiogenesis. [spermato- + G. *genesis,* origin]

**sper·ma·to·gen·ic** (sper′mă-tō-jen′ik) relating to

spermatogenesis; sperm-producing. SYN spermatopoietic (1).

**sper·ma·to·go·ni·um** (sper′mă-tō-gō′nē-ŭm) the primitive sperm cell derived by mitotic division from the germ cell; increasing several times in size, it becomes a primary spermatocyte. SEE ALSO spermatid. SYN spermatoblast. [spermato- + G. *gonē,* generation]

**sper·ma·toid** (sper′mă-tōid) **1.** resembling a sperm, a sperm tail, or semen. **2.** a male or flagellated form of the malarial microparasite. [spermato + G. *eidos,* form]

**sper·ma·tol·y·sis** (sper-mă-tol′i-sis) destruction, with dissolution, of spermatozoa. [spermato- + G. *lysis,* dissolution]

**sper·ma·to·lyt·ic** (sper′mă-tō-lit′ik) relating to spermatolysis.

**sper·ma·to·poi·et·ic** (sper′mă-tō-poy-et′ik) **1.** SYN spermatogenic. **2.** secreting semen. [spermato- + G. *poieō,* to make]

**sper·ma·tor·rhea** (sper′mă-tō-rē′ă) an involuntary discharge of semen, without orgasm. [spermato- + G. *rhoia,* a flow]

**sper·ma·tor·rhoea [Br.]** SEE spermatorrhea.

**sper·ma·to·zo·al, sper·ma·to·zo·an** (sper′mă-tō-zō′ăl, sper′ma-tō-zō′ăn) relating to spermatozoa.

**sper·ma·to·zo·on,** pl. **sper·ma·to·zoa** (sper′mă-tō-zō′on, sper′ma-tō-zō′ă) the male gamete or sex cell that contains the genetic information to be transmitted by the male, exhibits autokinesia, and is able to effect zygosis with an oocyte (ovum). The human spermatozoon is composed of a head and a tail, the tail being divisible into a neck, a middle piece, a principal piece, and an end piece; the head, 4 to 6 μm in length, is a broadly oval, flattened body containing the nucleus; the tail is about 55 μm in length. SYN sperm (1). [G. *sperma,* seed, + *zōon,* animal]

**sper·ma·tu·ria** (sper-mă-yu′rē-ă) SYN semenuria.

**sper·mia** (sper′mē-ă) plural of spermium.

**sper·mi·ci·dal** (sper′mi-sī′dăl) destructive to spermatozoa. SYN spermatocidal.

**sper·mi·cide** (sper′mi-sīd) an agent destructive to spermatozoa. SYN spermatocide.

**sper·mi·duct** (sper′mi-dŭkt) **1.** SYN ductus deferens. **2.** SYN ejaculatory duct.

**sper·mi·o·gen·e·sis** (sper′mē-ō-jen′ē-sis) that segment of spermatogenesis during which immature spermatids become spermatozoa. [sperm- + G. *genesis,* origin]

**sper·mi·um,** pl. **sper·mia** (sper′mē-ŭm, sper′mē-ă) the mature male germ cell or spermatozoon.

**sper·mo·lith** (sper′mō-lith) a concretion in the ductus deferens. [spermo- + G. *lithos,* stone]

*Sper·moph·il·us* (sper-mof′il-ŭs) a genus of ground squirrel. *Spermophilus beecheyi, Spermophilus grammurus, Spermophilus pygmaeus, Spermophilus townsendi,* and several other species act as an important reservoir of *Yersinia pestis.*

**SPF** sun protection factor.

**sphac·e·late** (sfas′ĕ-lāt) to become gangrenous or necrotic. [G. *sphakelos,* gangrene]

**sphac·e·la·tion** (sfas-ĕ-lā′shŭn) **1.** the process of becoming gangrenous or necrotic. **2.** gangrene or necrosis. [G. *sphakelos,* gangrene]

**sphac·el·ism** (sfas′ĕ-lizm) the condition manifested by a sphacelus.

**sphac·e·lo·der·ma** (sfas′ĕ-lō-der′mă) gangrene

of the skin. [G. *sphakelos,* gangrene, + *derma,* skin]

**sphac•e•lous** (sfas'ĕ-lŭs) sloughing, gangrenous, or necrotic.

**sphac•e•lus** (sfas'ĕ-lŭs) a mass of sloughing, gangrenous, or necrotic matter. [G. *sphakelos,* gangrene]

***Sphaer•o•tilus*** (sfē'nō-bas'i-lar) a genus of bacteria closely related to *Leptothrix* and found in fresh water; *Sphaerotilus natans* grows a thick biofilm mat in sulfite-containing water, especially as drained from paper mills.

**sphe•ni•on** (sfē'nē-on) the tip of the sphenoidal angle of the parietal bone; a craniometric point. [Mod. L. fr. G. *sphēn,* wedge, + dim. *-iōn*]

△**sphe•no-** wedge, wedge-shaped; the sphenoid bone. [G. *sphēn,* wedge]

**sphe•no•bas•i•lar** relation to the sphenoid bone and the basilar process of the occipital bone. SYN sphenooccipital.

**sphe•no•ceph•a•ly** (sfē'nō-sef'ă-lē) condition characterized by a deformation of the skull giving it a wedge-shaped appearance. [spheno- + G. *kephalē,* head]

**sphen•o•eth•moi•dec•to•my** (sfē'nō-eth-moy-dek'tō-mē) an operation to remove diseased tissue from the sphenoid and ethmoid sinuses.

**sphe•noid** (sfē'noyd) **1.** SYN sphenoidal. **2.** SYN sphenoid bone. [G. *sphēnoeidēs,* fr. *sphēn,* wedge, + *eidos,* resemblance]

**sphe•noi•dal** (sfē-noy'dăl) **1.** relating to the sphenoid bone. **2.** wedge-shaped. SYN sphenoid (1).

**sphe•noi•dal an•gle of pa•ri•e•tal bone** the anterior inferior angle of the parietal bone.

**sphe•noi•dal con•chae** paired ossicles of pyramidal shape, the spines of which are in contact with the medial pterygoid lamina, the bases forming the roof of the nasal cavity.

**sphe•noi•dal si•nus** one of a pair of paranasal sinuses in the body of the sphenoid bone communicating with the upper posterior nasal cavity or sphenoethmoidal recess.

**sphe•noi•dal spine** a posterior and downward projection from the greater wing of the sphenoid bone on either side, located posterolateral to the foramen spinosum, so named for its proximity to the sphenoidal spine; gives attachment to the sphenomandibular ligament. SYN alar spine, angular spine, spinous process (2).

**sphe•noid bone** a bone of irregular shape occupying the base of the skull; it is described as consisting of a central portion, or body, and six processes: two greater wings, two lesser wings and two pterygoid processes; it articulates with the occipital, frontal, ethmoid, and vomer, and with the paired temporal, parietal, zygomatic, palatine and sphenoidal concha bones. SYN sphenoid (2).

**sphe•noid crest** a vertical ridge in the midline of the anterior surface of the sphenoid bone that articulates with the perpendicular plate of the ethmoid bone.

**sphe•noid•i•tis** (sfē-noy-dī'tis) **1.** inflammation of the sphenoid sinus. **2.** necrosis of the sphenoid bone. [sphenoid + G. *-itis,* inflammation]

**sphe•noi•dot•o•my** (sfē'noy-dot'ō-mē) any operation on the sphenoid bone or sinus. [sphenoid + G. *tomē,* a cutting]

**sphe•no•oc•cip•i•tal** (sfē'nō-ok-sip'i-tăl) SYN sphenobasilar.

**sphe•no•pal•a•tine ar•tery** *origin,* third part of maxillary; *distribution,* posterior portion of lateral nasal wall and septum; *anastomoses,* branches of descending palatine, superior labial, and infraorbital. SYN arteria sphenopalatina [TA].

**sphe•no•pal•a•tine fo•ra•men** the foramen formed from the sphenopalatine notch of the palatine bone in articulation with the sphenoid bone; it transmits the sphenopalatine artery and accompanying nerves. SYN foramen sphenopalatinum [TA].

**sphe•no•pal•a•tine neu•ral•gia** neuralgia of the lower half of the face, with pain referred to the root of the nose, upper teeth, eyes, ears, mastoid, and occiput, in association with nasal congestion and rhinorrhea occurring in infection of the nasal sinuses, and produced by lesions of the sphenopalatine ganglion; ocular hyperemia and excessive lacrimation may occur. SYN Sluder neuralgia.

**sphe•no•pa•ri•e•tal si•nus** a paired dural venous sinus beginning on the parietal bone, running along the sphenoidal ridges and emptying into the cavernous sinus.

**sphe•nor•bit•al** (sfē-nōr'bi-tăl) denoting the portions of the sphenoid bone contributing to the orbits.

**sphe•not•ic** (sfē-nō'tik) relating to the sphenoid bone and the bony case of the ear. [spheno- + G. *ous,* ear]

**sphere** (sfēr) a ball or globular body. [G. *sphaira*]

**spher•i•cal ab•er•ra•tion** a monochromatic aberration occurring in refraction at a spherical surface in which the paraxial and peripheral rays focus along the axis at different points. SYN dioptric aberration.

**spher•i•cal lens (S)** a lens in which all refracting surfaces are spherical; commonly used to correct refractive errors not compounded by astigmatism.

△**sphe•ro-** spherical, a sphere. [G. *sphaira,* globe]

**sphe•ro•cyte** (sfēr'ō-sīt) a small, spherical red blood cell. [sphero- + G. *kytos,* cell]

**spher•o•cy•tic a•ne•mia** SYN hereditary spherocytosis.

**sphe•ro•cy•to•sis** (sfēr'ō-sī-tō'sis) presence of sphere-shaped red blood cells in the blood. [spherocyte + G. *-osis,* condition]

**sphe•roid, sphe•roi•dal** (sfēr'oyd, sfē-royd'ăl) shaped like a sphere. [L. *spheroideus*]

**spher•oid joint** SYN ball-and-socket joint.

**sphe•ro•pha•kia** (sfēr-ō-fa'kē-ă) a congenital bilateral aberration in which the lenses are small, spherical, and subject to subluxation; may occur as an independent anomaly or may be associated with the Weill-Marchesani syndrome. [sphero- + G. *phakos,* lens]

**sphinc•ter** (sfingk'ter) a muscle that encircles a duct, tube or orifice in such a way that its contraction constricts the lumen or orifice; it is the closing component of a pylorus (the outer component is the musculus dilator). SYN sphincter muscle. [G. *sphinktēr,* a band or lace]

**sphinc•ter•al** (sfingk'ter-ăl) relating to a sphincter.

**sphinc•ter•al•gia** (sfingk-ter-al'jē-ă) pain in the sphincter ani muscles. [sphincter + G. *algos,* pain]

**sphinc•ter of com•mon bile duct** smooth muscle sphincter of the common bile duct immediately proximal to the hepatopancreatic ampulla; it is this sphincter that controls the flow of bile in the duodenum. SYN musculus sphincter ductus choledochi [TA].

**sphinc·ter·ec·to·my** (sfingk-ter-ek′tō-mē) **1.** excision of a portion of the pupillary border of the iris. **2.** dissecting away any sphincter muscle. [sphincter + G. *ektomē*, excision]

**sphinc·ter of he·pa·to·pan·cre·at·ic am·pul·la** the smooth muscle sphincter of the hepatopancreatic ampulla within the duodenal papilla.

**sphinc·ter·is·mus** (sfingk-ter-iz′mŭs) spasmodic contraction of the sphincter ani muscles.

**sphinc·ter·i·tis** (sfingk′ter-ī′tis) inflammation of any sphincter.

**sphinc·ter mus·cle** SYN sphincter.

**sphinc·ter mus·cle of pu·pil** SYN sphincter pupillae.

**sphinc·ter of Od·di** (ŏ′dē) a valvelike muscular sheath surrounding the distal pancreatic and common bile ducts as they enter the duodenum together.

**sphinc·ter of Od·di dys·func·tion** (ŏ′dē) structural or functional abnormality of the sphincter of Oddi that interferes with bile drainage.

**sphinc·ter·ol·y·sis** (sfingk-ter-ol′i-sis) an operation for freeing the iris from the cornea in anterior synechia involving only the pupillary border. [sphincter, + G. *lysis*, loosening]

**sphinc·ter·o·plas·ty** (sfingk′ter-ō-plas-tē) plastic surgery of any sphincter muscle. [sphincter + G. *plastos*, formed]

**sphinc·ter·ot·o·my** (sfingk-tĕ-rot′ō-mē) incision or division of a sphincter muscle. [sphincter + G. *tomē*, incision]

**sphinc·ter of pan·cre·at·ic duct** smooth muscle sphincter of the main pancreatic duct immediately proximal to the hepatoduodenal ampulla. SYN musculus sphincter ductus pancreatici [TA].

**sphinc·ter pu·pil·lae** a ring of smooth muscle fibers surrounding the pupillary border of the iris. SYN musculus sphincter pupillae [TA], sphincter muscle of pupil.

**sphinc·ter u·re·thrae** *origin*, ramus of pubis; *insertion*, with fellow in median raphe behind and in front of urethra; *action*, constricts membranous urethra; *nerve supply*, pudendal. SYN musculus sphincter urethrae [TA].

**sphinc·ter ve·si·cae** the complete collar of smooth muscle cells of the neck of the urinary bladder which extends distally to surround the preprostatic portion of the male urethra. There is not a comparable structure in the neck of the female bladder; the internal urethral sphincter may exist to prevent reflux of semen into bladder. SYN musculus sphincter vesicae [TA].

**sphin·go·lip·id** (sfing′gō-lip-id) any lipid containing a long-chain base like that of sphingosine (e.g., ceramides, cerebrosides, gangliosides, sphingomyelins); a constituent of nerve tissue.

**sphin·go·lip·i·do·sis, sphin·go·lip·o·dys·tro·phy** (sfing′gō-lip-i-dō′sis, sfing′gō-lip-ō-dis′trō-fē) collective designation for a variety of diseases characterized by abnormal sphingolipid metabolism, e.g., gangliosidosis, Gaucher disease, Niemann-Pick disease.

**sphin·go·my·e·lin phos·pho·di·es·ter·ase** (sfing′gō-mī′ĕ-lin fos-fō-dī-es′ter-āse) an enzyme catalyzing hydrolysis of sphingomyelin to *N*-acylsphingosine (a ceramide) and phosphocholine; a deficiency of this enzyme is associated with type I Niemann-Pick disease.

**sphin·go·my·e·lins** (sfing′gō-mī′ĕ-linz) a group

of phospholipids, found in brain, spinal cord, kidney, and egg yolk, containing 1-phosphocholine (choline *O*-phosphate) combined with a ceramide.

**sphin·go·sine** (sfing′gō-sēn) the principal long-chain base found in sphingolipids.

**sphyg·mic** (sfig′mik) relating to the pulse.

**sphyg·mic in·ter·val** the period in the cardiac cycle when the semilunar valves are open and blood is being ejected from the ventricles into the arterial system. SYN ejection period.

△**sphyg·mo-, sphygm-** pulse. [G. *sphygmos*]

**sphyg·mo·chron·o·graph** (sfig′mō-kron′ō-graf) a modified sphygmograph that represents graphically the time relations between the beat of the heart and the pulse; one recording the character of the pulse as well as its rapidity. [sphygmo- + G. *chronos*, time, + *graphō*, to write]

**sphyg·mo·gram** (sfig′mō-gram) the graphic curve made by a sphygmograph. [sphygmo- + G. *gramma*, something written]

**sphyg·mo·graph** (sfig′mō-graf) an instrument consisting of a lever, the short end of which rests on the radial artery at the wrist, its long end being provided with a stylet which records on a moving ribbon of paper the excursions of the pulse. [sphygmo- + G. *graphō*, to write]

**sphyg·mo·graph·ic** (sfig-mō-graf′ik) relating to or made by a sphygmograph; denoting the sphygmographic tracing, or sphygmogram.

**sphyg·moid** (sfig′moyd) pulselike; resembling the pulse. [sphygmo- + G. *eidos*, resemblance]

**sphyg·mo·ma·nom·e·ter** (sfig′mō-mă-nom′ĕ-ter) an instrument for measuring arterial blood pressure consisting of an inflatable cuff, inflating bulb, and a gauge showing the blood pressure. SYN hemodynanometer, sphygmometer. [sphygmo- + G. *manos*, thin, scanty, + *metron*, measure]

**sphyg·mo·ma·nom·e·try** (sfig′mō-mă-nom′ĕ-trē) determination of the blood pressure by means of a sphygmomanometer.

**sphyg·mom·e·ter** (sfig-mom′ĕ-ter) SYN sphygmomanometer.

**sphyg·mo·scope** (sfig′mō-skōp) an instrument by which the pulse beats are made visible by causing fluid to rise in a glass tube, by means of a mirror projecting a beam of light, or simply by a moving lever as in the sphygmograph. [sphygmo- + G. *skopeō*, to view]

**sphyg·mos·co·py** (sfig-mos′kŏ-pē) examination of the pulse. [sphygmo- + G. *skopeō*, to view]

**spi·ca ban·dage** successive strips of material applied to the body and the first part of a limb, or to the hand and a finger, which overlap slightly in a V to resemble an ear of grain. [L. *spica*, ear of grain]

**spic·u·lar** (spik′yu-lăr) relating to or having spicules.

**spic·ule** (spik′yul) a small needle-shaped body. [L. *spiculum*, dim. of *spica*, or *spicum*, a point]

**spi·der** (spī′der) **1.** an arthropod of the order Araneida characterized by four pairs of legs; a cephalothorax; a globose, smooth abdomen; and a complex of web-spinning spinnerets. Among the venomous spiders are the black widow spider, *Latrodectus mactans*, and the brown recluse spider, *Loxosceles reclusus*. **2.** SYN spider angioma. [O. E. *spinnan*, to spin]

**spi·der an·gi·o·ma** a telangiectatic arteriole in the skin with radiating capillary branches simu-

s
p

lating the legs of a spider; characteristic, but not pathognomonic, of parenchymatous liver disease; also seen in pregnancy, often disappearing after delivery, and at times in normal persons. SYN arterial spider, spider nevus, spider telangiectasia, spider (2), vascular spider.

**spi·der-burst** (spī′der-berst) radiating dull red capillary lines on the skin of the leg, usually without any visible or palpable varicose veins, but nevertheless due to deep-seated venous dilation; sometimes referred to as skyrocket capillary ectasis. [*spider*web + sun*burst*]

**spi·der ne·vus** SYN spider angioma.

**spi·der tel·an·gi·ec·ta·sia** SYN spider angioma.

**Spiegelberg cri·te·ria** (spē-gĕl-berg krī-ter-ē-ă) 1) (for the diagnosis of ovarian pregnancy) 1) the oviduct on the affected side must be intact; 2) the amnionic sac must occupy the position of the ovary; 3) the amnionic sac must be connected to the uterus by the ovarian ligament; and 4) ovarian tissue must be present in the wall of the amnionic sac.

**Spiel·mey·er a·cute swel·ling** (shpēl-mī-ĕr) a form of degeneration of nerve cells in which the cell body and its processes swell and stain palely and diffusely.

**spi·ge·li·an** (spī-jē′lē-an) relating to or described by Spigelius (Adrian van der Spieghel, 1578–1625).

**Spi·ge·li·us lobe** (spī-jē′lē-us) SYN posterior hepatic segment I.

**spike 1.** a brief electrical event of 3 to 25 msec that gives the appearance in the electroencephalogram of a rising and falling vertical line. **2.** ELECTROPHORESIS a sharply angled upward deflection on a densitometric tracing.

**spike po·ten·tial** the main wave in the action potential of a nerve; it is followed by negative and positive afterpotentials.

**spike and wave com·plex** a generalized, synchronous pattern seen on the electroencephalogram, consisting of a sharply contoured fast wave followed by a slow wave; particularly found in patients with generalized epilepsies.

**spi·na**, gen. and pl. **spi·nae** (spī′nă, spī′nē) **1.** SYN vertebral column. **2.** SYN vertebral column. [L. a thorn, the backbone, spine]

🛈 **spi·na bi·fi·da** embryologic failure of fusion of one or more vertebral arches; subtypes of spina bifida are based upon degree and pattern of deformity associated with neuroectoderm involvement. See this page.

**spi·na bi·fi·da cys·ti·ca** spina bifida associated with a meningeal cyst (meningocele) or a cyst

containing both meninges and spinal cord (meningomyelocele) or only spinal cord (myelocele).

**spi·na bi·fi·da oc·cul·ta** spina bifida in which there is a spinal defect, but no protrusion of the cord or its membrane, although there is often some abnormality in their development.

**spi·nal** (spī′năl) **1.** relating to any spine or spinous process. **2.** relating to the vertebral column. SYN rachial, rachidial. [L. *spinalis*]

**spi·nal an·al·ge·sia** SEE spinal anesthesia.

**spi·nal an·es·the·sia 1.** loss of sensation in an area produced by injection of local anesthetic solution(s) into the spinal subarachnoid space; **2.** loss of sensation produced by disease of the spinal cord.

**spi·nal a·rach·noid ma·ter** that portion of the arachnoid that lies within the vertebral canal and surrounds the spinal cord and the vertebral portion of the subarachnoid space. It extends from the foramen magnum above to the S2 vertebral level. Since the spinal cord ends at the L2 vertebral level, a wide separation occurs between the arachnoid and pia mater, the lumbar cistern, filled with cerebrospinal fluid in which the cauda equina is suspended.

**spi·nal block** an obstruction to the flow of cerebrospinal fluid in the spinal subarachnoid space; used inaccurately to refer to spinal anesthesia.

**spi·nal branch·es** branches of the following arteries that supply the meninges, the roots of the spinal nerves, and in some cases, the spinal cord: 1) vertebral, 2) ascending cervical, 3) dorsal branch of posterior intercostal I to XI, 4) dorsal branch of subcostal, 5) dorsal branch of lumbar arteries, 6) lumbar branch of iliolumbar, 7) lateral sacral; all spinal arteries give rise to arteries supplying dorsal and ventral roots of spinal nerves; most are exhausted in supplying the roots as radicular arteries, but some (4–9), are large enough to reach and anastomose with the anterior and posterior spinal arteries and are designated instead as segmental medullary arteries.

**spi·nal ca·nal** SYN vertebral canal.

**spi·nal col·umn** SYN vertebral column.

**spi·nal cord** the elongated cylindrical portion of the cerebrospinal axis, or central nervous system, which is contained in the spinal or vertebral canal. SYN medulla spinalis.

**spi·nal cord con·cus·sion** injury to the spinal cord due to a blow to the vertebral column with transient or prolonged dysfunction below the level of the lesion.

🛈 **spi·nal cur·va·ture** SEE kyphosis, lordosis, scoliosis. See page 923.

**spi·nal de·com·pres·sion** the removal of pressure upon the spinal cord as created by a tumor,

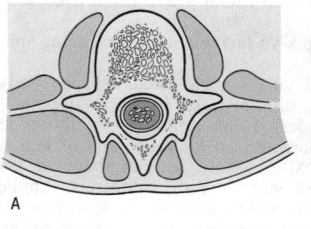

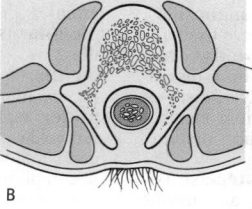

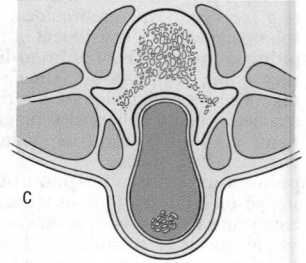

A          B          C

**spina bifida:** (A) normal spinal cord, (B) spina bifida occulta, (C) myelomeningocele

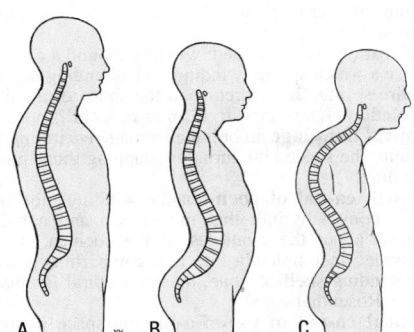

**spinal curvatures:** (A) normal, (B) lordosis, (C) kyphosis

cyst, hematoma, herniated nucleus pulposus, abscess, or bone.

**spi•nal dys•ra•phi•sm** a general term used to describe a collection of congenital abnormalities that include defects in the vertebrae and underlying spine or nerve roots.

**spi•nal fu•sion, spine fu•sion** a surgical procedure to accomplish bony ankylosis between two or more vertebrae. SYN spondylosyndesis.

**spi•nal gan•gli•on** the ganglion of the posterior root of each spinal segmental nerve; contains the cell bodies of the pseudounipolar primary sensory neurons whose peripheral axonal branches become part of the mixed segmental nerve, while the central axonal branches enter the spinal cord as a component of the sensory posterior root.

**spi•nal head•ache** headache, usually frontal or occipital, following dural puncture; precipitated by sitting up, relieved by lying down; due to leakage of cerebrospinal fluid from subarachnoid space through the site of the puncture. SYN postlumbar puncture syndrome.

**spi•nal in•sta•bil•i•ty** the inability of the spinal column, under physiologic loads, to maintain its normal configuration; may result in damage to the spinal cord or nerve roots or lead to the development of a painful spinal deformity.

**spi•nal•is ca•pi•tis mus•cle** an inconstant extension of spinalis cervicis to the occipital bone, sometimes fusing with semispinalis capitis. SYN musculus spinalis capitis [TA].

**spi•nal•is cer•vi•cis mus•cle** an inconstant or rudimentary muscle; *origin*, spinous processes of sixth and seventh cervical vertebrae; *insertion*, spinous processes of axis and third cervical vertebra; *action*, extends cervical spine; *nerve supply*, dorsal primary rami of cervical. SYN musculus spinalis cervicis [TA], spinal muscle of neck.

**spi•nal•is tho•ra•cis mus•cle** *origin*, spinous processes of upper lumbar and two lower thoracic vertebrae; *insertion*, spinous processes of middle and upper thoracic vertebrae; *action*, supports and extends vertebral column; *nerve supply*, dorsal primary rami of thoracic and upper lumbar. SYN musculus spinalis thoracis [TA].

**spi•nal mus•cle of neck** SYN spinalis cervicis muscle.

**spi•nal mus•cu•lar a•tro•phy** a heterogeneous group of degenerative diseases of the anterior horn cells in the spinal cord and motor nuclei of the brainstem; all are characterized by weakness. Upper motor neurons remain normal. These diseases include Werdnig-Hoffmann disease (SMA type 1), SMA type 2, and Kugelberg-Welander disease (SMA type 3). SEE ALSO Fazio-Londe disease.

**spi•nal mus•cu•lar a•tro•phy, type I** the early infantile form, characterized by profound muscle weakness and wasting with onset at or shortly after birth; death occurs usually before 2 years of age. Autosomal recessive inheritance, caused by mutation in the survival motor neuron gene (SMN1) on 5q. About one-half of patients are also missing both homologues of a neighboring gene that encodes neuronal apoptosis inhibitory protein (NAIP), the loss of which is thought to influence the severity of the disease. SYN Hoffmann muscular atrophy.

**spi•nal mus•cu•lar a•tro•phy, type II** a form intermediate in severity between the infantile form (SMA type I) and the juvenile form (SMA type III); characterized by proximal muscle weakness with onset usually between 3 and 15 months and survival until adolescence; autosomal recessive inheritance, caused by mutation in the SMN1 gene on 5q.

**spi•nal mus•cu•lar a•tro•phy, type III** the juvenile form with onset in childhood or adolescence, characterized by progressive proximal muscular weakness and wasting, primarily in the legs, followed by distal muscle involvement, caused by degeneration of motor neurons in the anterior horns of the spinal cord; autosomal recessive inheritance, caused by mutation in the SMN1 gene on 5q.

**spi•nal nerves** the nerves emerging from the spinal cord; there are 31 pairs, each attached to the cord by two roots, anterior and posterior, or ventral and dorsal; the latter is provided with a circumscribed enlargement, the dorsal root (spinal) ganglion; the two roots unite in the intervertebral foramen, and the mixed spinal nerve almost immediately divides again into ventral and dorsal primary rami, the former supplying the anterolateral trunk and the limbs, the latter the true muscles and overlying skin of the back. SYN nervi spinales [TA].

**spi•nal pa•ral•y•sis** loss of motor power due to a lesion of the spinal cord.

**spi•nal pia ma•ter** the pia mater found specifically around the spinal cord; includes specializations such as the denticulate ligaments. SEE ALSO pia mater.

**spi•nal re•flex** a reflex arc involving the spinal cord. SEE reflex arc.

**spi•nal ste•no•sis** abnormal narrowing of the spinal canal, often with compression of the spinal cord.

**spi•nal tap** SYN lumbar puncture.

**spi•nal veins** the veins that drain the spinal cord; they form a plexus on the surface of the cord from which veins pass along the spinal roots to the internal vertebral venous plexus.

**spi•nate** (spī′nāt) spined; having spines.

**spin den•si•ty** the number of nuclear dipoles per unit volume.

**spin•dle** (spin′dl) in anatomy and pathology, any fusiform cell or structure. [A.S.]

**spin•dle cell** a fusiform cell, such as those in the deeper layers of the cerebral cortex.

**spin•dle cell car•ci•no•ma** a carcinoma composed of elongated cells, frequently a poorly differentiated squamous cell carcinoma which may be difficult to distinguish from a sarcoma.

**spin·dle cell li·po·ma** a microscopically distinctive form of lipoma in which adipose tissue is infiltrated by fibroblasts and collagen; usually found in the shoulder or neck of elderly men.

**spine** (spīn) 1. a short, sharp, thornlike process of bone; a spinous process. 2. SYN vertebral column. 3. the bar or stay in a horse's hoof. [L. *spina*]

**spin echo** a commonly used technique to recover $T^2$ relaxation signals in magnetic resonance imaging, by using a 180° inverting pulse in the pulse sequence to compensate for loss of transverse magnetization caused by magnetic field inhomogeneities.

**spine of scap·u·la** the prominent triangular ridge on the dorsal aspect of the scapula, providing attachment for the trapezius and deltoid muscles and separating the supra- and infraspinous fossae.

**spinn·bar·keit** (spin′bahr-kīt) the property of cervical mucus that permits it to be drawn out in strings; indicative of estrogenic effect, and most pronounced during the ovulatory period. [Ger. *Spinnbarkeit*, viscosity, ability to form a thread]

△**spi·no-, spin-** 1. the spine. 2. spinous. [L. *spina*]

**spi·no·ad·duc·tor re·flex** contraction of the adductors of the thigh upon tapping the spinal column. SYN McCarthy reflexes.

**spi·no·bul·bar** (spī′nō-bŭl′bar) SYN bulbospinal.

**spi·no·ce·re·bel·lar a·tax·ia** the most common hereditary ataxia, with onset in middle to late childhood, manifested as limb ataxia, nystagmus, kyphoscoliosis, and pes cavus; the major pathological changes are found in the posterior columns of the spinal cord.

**spi·no·cer·e·bel·lum** (spī′nō-ser-ě-bel′ŭm) [TA] SYN paleocerebellum.

**spi·no·cu·ne·ate fi·bers** axons that originate from cells in the posterior horn of cervical and upper thoracic spinal levels, ascend ipsilaterally in the cuneate fasciculus, and terminate in the cuneate nucleus. These are part of the postsynaptic–dorsal column system.

**spi·no·gra·cile fi·bers** axons that originate from neurons in the posterior horn of lower thoracic and lumbosacral spinal cord levels, ascend ipsilaterally in the gracile fasciculus, and terminate in the gracile nucleus. These are part of the postsynaptic–dorsal column system.

**spi·no·o·li·vary tract** a collection of axons, actually comprising several bundles, that originate from the spinal gray, ascend ipsilaterally to terminate in the accessory olivary nuclei.

**spi·nous** (spī′nŭs) relating to, shaped like, or having a spine or spines.

**spi·nous lay·er** SYN stratum spinosum epidermidis.

**spi·nous pro·cess** 1. the dorsal projection from the center of a vertebral arch; 2. SYN sphenoidal spine.

**spi·no·ves·ti·bu·lar tract** a group of axons that originate from neurons primarily in lumbosacral levels, ascend ipsilaterally and in close apposition to the posterior spinocerebellar tract, and terminate in the lateral, medial and spinal vestibular nuclei. Some of these axons may be collaterals of posterior spinocerebellar fibers.

**spi·rad·e·no·ma** (spī-rad-ě-nō′mǎ) a benign tumor of sweat glands. [G. *speira*, coil, + adenoma]

**spi·ral** (spī′răl) 1. coiled; winding around a center like a watch spring; winding and ascending like a wire spring. 2. a structure in the shape of a coil. [Mediev. L. *spiralis*, fr. G. *speira*, a coil]

**spi·ral ban·dage** an oblique bandage encircling a limb, the successive turns overlapping those preceding.

**spi·ral ca·nal of coch·lea** the winding tube of the bony labyrinth that makes two and a half turns about the modiolus of the cochlea; it is divided incompletely into two compartments by a winding shelf of bone, the bony spiral lamina. SYN Rosenthal canal.

**spi·ral ca·nal of mo·di·o·lus** the space in the modiolus in which the spiral ganglion of the cochlear nerve lies. SYN canalis spiralis modioli [TA].

**spi·ral fold of cys·tic duct** a series of crescentic folds of mucous membrane in the upper part of the cystic duct, arranged in a somewhat spiral manner. SYN plica spiralis ductus cystici [TA].

**spi·ral frac·ture** a fracture the line of which is helical in the bone.

**spi·ral gan·gli·on of co·chlea** an elongated ganglion of bipolar sensory nerve cell bodies on the cochlear part of the vestibulocochlear nerve in the spiral canal of the modiolus; each ganglion cell gives rise to a peripheral process that passes between the layers of the bony spiral lamina to the spiral organ (organ of Corti), and a central axon that enters the hindbrain as a component of the inferior (cochlear) root of the eighth cranial nerve.

**spi·ral joint** SYN cochlear joint.

**spi·ral lig·a·ment of co·chlea** the thickened periosteal lining of the bony cochlea forming the outer wall of the cochlear duct to which the basal lamina attaches.

**spi·ral or·gan** a prominent ridge of highly specialized epithelium in the floor of the cochlear duct overlying the basilar membrane of cochlea, containing one inner row and three outer rows of hair cells, or cells of Corti (the auditory receptor cells innervated by the cochlear nerve) supported by various columnar cells: the pillars of Corti, cells of Hensen, and cells of Claudius; the spiral organ is partly overhung by an awning-like shelf, the tectorial membrane, the free marginal zone of which is covered by a gelatinous substance in which the stereocilia of the outer hair cells are embedded. SYN Corti organ.

**spi·ral vein of mo·di·o·lus** the vein running a spiral course in the modiolus of the cochlea; it is tributary to both the labyrinthine vein and the vein of the cochlear canaliculus.

**spi·ril·lar** (spī-ril′ăr) s-shaped; referring to a bacterial cell with an S shape.

*Spi·ril·lum* (spī-ril′ŭm) a genus of large, rigid, helical, Gram-negative bacteria which are motile by means of bipolar fascicles of flagella. [Mod. L. dim. of L. *spira*, coil, fr. G. *speira*]

**spi·ril·lum**, pl. **spi·ril·la** (spī-ril′ŭm, spī-ril′ă) a member of the genus *Spirillum*.

*Spi·ril·lum mi·nus* a species of uncertain taxonomic classification that causes a form of rat-bite fever (sodoku). This species has never been cultured.

**spir·it** (spir′it) 1. an alcoholic liquor stronger than wine, obtained by distillation. 2. any distilled liquid. **3.** an alcoholic or hydroalcoholic solution of volatile substances; some spirits are used as flavoring agents, others have medicinal value. [L. *spiritus,* a breathing, soul, fr. *spiro,* to breathe]

**spir·it lamp** a lamp, used mainly for heating in laboratory work, in which alcohol is burned.

△**spi·ro-, spir-** **1.** coil, coil-shaped. [G. *speira*] **2.** breathing. [L. *spiro,* to breathe]

**spi·ro·chet·e·mia** (spī'rō-kē-tē'mē-ă) presence of spirochetes in the blood. [spirochete + G. *haima,* blood]

**spi·ro·gram** (spī'rō-gram) the tracing made by the spirograph.

**spi·ro·graph** (spī'rō-graf) a device for representing graphically the depth and rapidity of respiratory movements. [L. *spiro,* to breathe, + G. *graphō,* to write]

**spi·rom·e·ter** (spī-rom'ĕ-ter) a gasometer used for measuring respiratory gases; usually understood to consist of a counterbalanced cylindrical bell sealed by dipping into a circular trough of water. [L. *spiro,* to breathe, + G. *metron,* measure]

▣**spi·rom·e·try** (spī-rom'ĕ-trē) making pulmonary measurements with a spirometer. See this page.

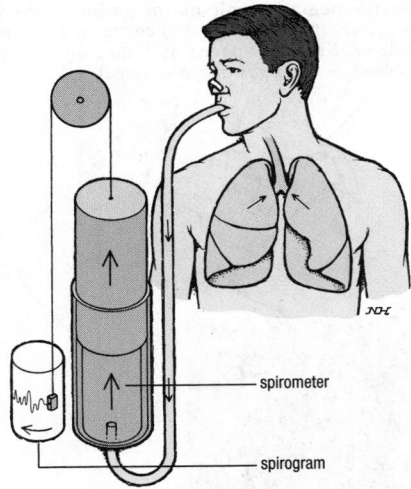

spirometer

spirogram

**spirometry:** principle of closed-circuit spirometry

**spis·si·tude** (spis'i-tood) the state of being inspissated; the condition of a fluid thickened almost to a solid by evaporation or inspissation. [L. *spissitudo,* fr. *spissus,* thick]

**spit·tle** (spit'l) SYN saliva. [A.S. *spātl*]

**Spit·zer the·o·ry** (spits'ĕr) an interpretation of the partitioning of the heart of mammalian embryos primarily on the basis of recapitulations of the adult structural pattern of lower forms.

**Spitz ne·vus** (spits) a benign, slightly pigmented or red superficial small skin tumor composed of spindle-shaped, epithelioid, and multinucleated cells that may appear atypical; most common in children, but also appearing in adults.

**splanch·nap·o·phys·i·al, splanch·nap·o·phys·e·al** (splangk'nă-pō-fiz'ē-ăl) relating to a splanchnapophysis.

**splanch·na·poph·y·sis** (splangk'nă-pof'i-sis) an apophysis of the typical vertebra, on the side opposite to the neural apophysis, or any bony process, giving attachment to a viscus or part of the alimentary tract. [splanchn- + G. *apophysis,* offshoot]

**splanch·nec·to·pia** (splangk-nek-tō'pē-ă) displacement of any of the viscera. [splanchn- + G. *ektopos,* out of place]

**splanch·nes·the·sia** (splangk-nes-thē'zē-ă) SYN visceral sense. [splanch- + G. *aisthēsis,* sensation]

**splanch·nes·the·tic sen·si·bil·i·ty** SYN visceral sense.

**splanch·nic** (splangk'nik) SYN visceral.

**splanch·nic an·es·the·sia** loss of sensation in areas of the visceral peritoneum innervated by the splanchnic nerves. SYN visceral anesthesia.

**splanch·ni·cec·to·my** (splangk-ni-sek'tō-mē) resection of the splanchnic nerves and usually of the celiac ganglion as well. [splanchni- + G. *ektomē,* excision]

**splanch·nic gan·gli·on** a small sympathetic ganglion often present in the course of the greater splanchnic nerve.

**splanch·ni·cot·o·my** (splangk-ni-kot'ō-mē) section of a splanchnic nerve or nerves, a surgical procedure formerly used in the treatment of hypertension. [splanchni- + G. *tomē,* incision]

**splanch·nic wall** the wall of one of the viscera or the splanchnopleure from which it is formed.

△**splanch·no-, splanchn-, splanch·ni-** the viscera. SEE ALSO viscero-. [G. *splanchnon,* viscus]

**splanch·no·cele** (splangk'nō-sēl) **1.** the primitive body cavity or celom in the embryo. [G. *koilos,* hollow] **2.** hernia of any of the abdominal viscera. [G. *kēlē,* hernia]

**splanch·nog·ra·phy** (splangk-nog'ră-fē) a treatise on or description of the viscera. [splanchno- + G. *graphō,* to write]

**splanch·no·lith** (splangk'nō-lith) an intestinal calculus. [splanchno- + G. *lithos,* stone]

**splanch·no·meg·a·ly** (splangk-nō-meg'ă-lē) SYN visceromegaly. [splanchno- + G. *megas,* large]

**splanch·nop·a·thy** (splangk-nop'ă-thē) any disease of the abdominal viscera. [splanchno- + G. *pathos,* disease]

**splanch·no·pleure** (splangk'nō-ploor) the embryonic layer formed by association of the visceral layer of the lateral plate mesoderm with the endoderm. [splanchno- + G. *pleura,* side]

**splanch·nop·to·sis, splanch·nop·to·sia** (splangk'nō-tō'sis, splangk'nō-tō'sē-ă) SYN visceroptosis. [splanchno- + G. *ptōsis* a falling]

**splanch·no·scle·ro·sis** (splangk'nō-sklĕ-rō'sis) hardening, through connective tissue overgrowth, of any of the viscera. [splanchno- + G. *sklērōsis,* hardening]

**splanch·no·skel·e·tal** (splangk'nō-skel'ĕ-tăl) SYN visceroskeletal.

**splanch·no·skel·e·ton** (splangk'nō-skel'ĕ-tŏn) SYN visceroskeleton (2).

**splanch·no·tribe** (splangk'nō-trīb) an instrument resembling a large angiotribe used for occluding the intestine temporarily, prior to resection. [splanchno- + G. *tribō,* to rub, bruise]

**spleen** (splēn) a large vascular lymphatic organ lying in the upper part of the abdominal cavity on the left side, between the stomach and diaphragm, composed of white and red pulp; the white consists of lymphatic nodules and diffuse lymphatic tissue; the red consists of venous sinusoids between which are splenic cords; the stroma of both red and white pulp is reticular fibers and cells. A framework of fibroelastic trabeculae extending from the capsule subdivides the structure into poorly defined lobules. It is a blood-forming organ in early life and later a storage organ for red corpuscles and platelets; because of the large number of macrophages, it also acts as a blood filter, both identifying and destroying effete erythrocytes. SYN lien [TA], splen [TA]. [G. *splēn*]

**splen** [TA] SYN spleen.

**sple·nec·to·my** (splē-nek'tō-mē) removal of the spleen. [splen- + G. *ektomē*, excision]

**sple·nec·to·pia, sple·nec·to·py** (splen'ek-tō'pē-ă, splē-nek'tō-pē) **1.** displacement of the spleen, as in a floating spleen. **2.** the presence of rests of splenic tissue, usually in the region of the spleen. [splen- + G. *ektopos*, out of place]

**splen·ic** (splen'ik) relating to the spleen. SYN lienal.

**splen·ic ar·tery** *origin*, celiac trunk; *branches*, pancreatic, left gastroepiploic, short gastric, and (proper) splenic. SYN arteria lienalis [TA], lienal artery.

**splen·ic flex·ure** SYN left colic flexure.

**splen·ic lymph fol·li·cles** small nodular masses of lymphoid tissue attached to the sides of the smaller arterial branches. SYN folliculi lymphatici lienales, malpighian bodies.

**splen·ic pulp** the soft cellular substance of the spleen.

**splen·ic si·nus** an elongated venous channel, 12 to 40 μm wide, lined by rod-shaped cells.

**splen·ic vein** arises by the union of several small veins at the hilum on the anterior surface of the spleen with the short gastric and left gastroepiploic veins; passes backward through the splenorenal ligament to the left kidney, then runs behind the upper border of the pancreas to the neck of the pancreas where it joins the superior mesenteric vein to form the portal vein.

**sple·ni·tis** (splē-nī'tis) inflammation of the spleen. [splen- + G. *-itis*, inflammation]

**sple·ni·um**, pl. **sple·nia** (splē'nē-ŭm, splē'nē-ă) **1.** a compress or bandage. **2.** a structure resembling a bandaged part. [Mod. L. fr. G. *splēnion*, bandage]

**sple·ni·um cor·po·ris cal·lo·si** [TA] SYN splenium of corpus callosum.

**sple·ni·um of cor·pus cal·lo·sum** the thickened posterior extremity of the corpus callosum. SYN splenium corporis callosi [TA].

**sple·ni·us ca·pi·tis mus·cle** *origin*, from ligamentum nuchae of last four cervical vertebrae and supraspinous ligament of first and second thoracic vertebrae; *insertion*, lateral half of superior nuchal line and mastoid process; *action*, rotates head and extends neck; *nerve supply*, dorsal primary rami of second to sixth cervical spinal nerves. SYN musculus splenius capitis [TA], splenius muscle of head.

**sple·ni·us cer·vi·cis mus·cle** *origin*, from supraspinous ligament and spinous processes of third to fifth thoracic vertebrae; *insertion*, posterior tubercles of transverse processes of first and second (sometimes third) cervical vertebrae; *action*, rotates and extends neck; *nerve supply*, dorsal primary rami of fourth to eighth cervical spinal nerves. SYN musculus splenius cervicis [TA], splenius muscle of neck.

**sple·ni·us mus·cle of head** SYN splenius capitis muscle.

**sple·ni·us mus·cle of neck** SYN splenius cervicis muscle.

⌂**sple·no-, splen-** the spleen. [G. *splēn*]

**sple·no·cele** (splē'nō-sēl) **1.** SYN splenoma. **2.** a splenic hernia. [spleno- + G. *kēlē*, tumor, hernia]

**sple·no·he·pa·to·meg·a·ly, sple·no·he·pa·to·me·ga·lia** (splē'nō-hep'ă-tō-meg'ă-lē, splē'nō-hep'ă-tō-mĕ-gā 'lē-ă) enlargement of both spleen and liver. [spleno- + G. *hēpar*, liver, + *megas*, large]

**sple·noid** (splē'noyd) resembling the spleen. [spleno- + G. *eidos*, resemblance]

**sple·no·ma** (splē-nō'mă) general nonspecific term for an enlarged spleen. SYN splenocele (1). [spleno- + G. *-oma*, tumor]

**sple·no·ma·la·cia** (splē'nō-mă-lā'shē-ă) softening of the spleen. [spleno- + G. *malakia*, softness]

**sple·no·med·ul·lary** (splē-nō-med'ŭ-lār-ē) SYN splenomyelogenous. [spleno- + L. *medulla*, marrow]

▣ **sple·no·meg·a·ly, sple·no·me·ga·lia** (splē-nō-meg'ă-lē, splē-nō-mĕ-gā'lē-ă) enlargement of the spleen. See this page. SYN megalosplenia. [spleno- + G. *megas* (*megal-*), large]

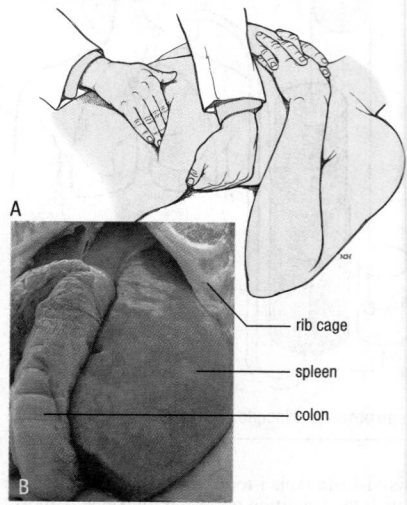

A

rib cage

spleen

colon

B

**splenomegaly:** (A) palpation technique used in diagnosis; (B) splenomegaly due to granulocytic leukemia as seen at autopsy (weight of spleen: 4200g)

**sple·no·my·e·log·e·nous** (splē'nō-mī-ĕ-loj'ĕ-nŭs) originating in the spleen and bone marrow, denoting a form of leukemia. SYN splenomedullary. [spleno- + G. *myelos*, marrow, + *-gen*, producing]

**sple·no·my·e·lo·ma·la·cia** (splē'nō-mī'ĕ-lō-mă-lā'shē-ă) pathologic softening of the spleen and bone marrow. [spleno- + G. *myelos*, marrow, + *malakia*, softness]

**sple·nop·a·thy** (splē-nop′ă-thē) any disease of the spleen. [spleno- + G. *pathos*, suffering]

**sple·no·pexy, sple·no·pex·ia** (splē′nō-pek-sē, splē-nō-pek′sē-ă) suturing in place an ectopic or floating spleen. SYN splenorrhaphy (2). [spleno- + G. *pēxis*, fixation]

**sple·no·por·tog·ra·phy** (splē′nō-pōr-tog′ră-fē) introduction of radiopaque material into the spleen to obtain an x-ray visualization of the portal vessel of the portal circulation. [spleno- + portography]

**sple·nop·to·sis, sple·nop·to·sia** (splē-nop-tō′sis, splē-nop-tō′sē-ă) downward displacement of the spleen, as in a floating spleen. [spleno- + G. *ptōsis*, falling]

**sple·no·re·nal lig·a·ment** a peritoneal fold (portion of the greater omentum) which extends from the diaphragm and the anterior aspect of the left kidney to the hilar region of the spleen, conducting the splenic vessels from the posterior body wall to the spleen. SYN ligamentum splenorenale [TA].

**sple·no·re·nal shunt** anastomosis of the splenic vein to the left renal vein, usually end-to-side, for control of portal hypertension.

**sple·nor·rha·gia** (splē′nō-rā′jē-ă) hemorrhage from a ruptured spleen. [spleno- + G. *rhēgnymi*, to burst forth]

**sple·nor·rha·phy** (splē-nōr′ă-fē) **1.** suturing a ruptured spleen. **2.** SYN splenopexy. [spleno- + G. *rhaphē*, suture]

**sple·no·sis** (splē-nō′sis) implantation and subsequent growth of splenic tissue within the abdomen as a result of disruption of the spleen.

**sple·not·o·my** (splē-not′ō-mē) **1.** anatomy or dissection of the spleen. **2.** surgical incision of the spleen. [spleno- + G. *tomē*, incision]

**sple·no·tox·in** (splē-nō-tok′sin) a cytotoxin specific for cells of the spleen. [spleno- + G. *toxikon*, poison]

**splic·ing** (splīs′ing) **1.** attachment of one DNA molecule to another. SYN gene splicing. **2.** removal of introns from mRNA precursors and the reattachment or annealing of exons. SYN RNA splicing.

**splint 1.** an appliance for preventing movement of a joint or for the fixation of displaced or movable parts. **2.** the splint bone, or fibula. [Middle Dutch *splinte*]

**splin·ter hem·or·rhages** multiple tiny longitudinal subungual hemorrhages typically seen in but not diagnostic of bacterial endocarditis and trichinelliasis.

**split hand** SYN cleft hand.

**split pel·vis** a pelvis in which the symphysis pubis is absent, the pelvic bones being separated; usually associated with exstrophy of the bladder.

**split-thick·ness flap** a flap of a portion of the skin, i.e., the epidermis and part of the dermis, or of part of the mucosa and submucosa, but not including the periosteum. SYN partial-thickness flap.

**split-thick·ness graft** a graft of portions of the skin, i.e., the epidermis and part of the dermis, or of part of the mucosa and submucosa, but not including the periosteum. SYN partial-thickness graft.

**split·ting** CHEMISTRY the cleavage of a covalent bond, fragmenting the molecule involved.

**split·ting of heart sounds** the production of major components of the first and second heart sounds (rarely the third and fourth) due to contribution by the left-sided and right-sided valves; thus, the first heart sound would have a mitral and a tricuspid component and the second heart sound has an aortic and pulmonic component. The latter are best appreciated during respiration, with inspiration delaying the pulmonic component and producing an earlier aortic component.

**spm** a gene that leads to *s*uppression and *m*utation of mutants that are unstable.

**spo·dog·e·nous** (spŏ-doj′ĕ-nŭs) caused by waste material. [G. *spodos*, ashes, + *-gen*, producing]

**spon·dee** (spon′dē) a bisyllabic word with generally equivalent stress on each of the two syllables; used in the testing of speech hearing. [Fr.]

**spon·dy·lal·gia** (spon-di-lal′jē-ă) pain in the spine. [spondyl- + G. *algos*, pain]

**spon·dy·lar·thri·tis** (spon′dil-ar-thrī′tis) inflammation of the intervertebral articulations. [spondyl- + G. *arthron*, joint, + *-itis*, inflammation]

**spon·dy·lit·ic** (spon-di-lit′ik) relating to spondylitis.

**spon·dy·li·tis** (spon-di-lī′tis) inflammation of one or more of the vertebrae. [spondyl- + G. *-itis*, inflammation]

**spon·dy·li·tis de·for·mans** arthritis and osteitis deformans involving the spinal column; marked by nodular deposits at the edges of the intervertebral disks with ossification of the ligaments and bony ankylosis of the intervertebral articulations, it results in a rounded kyphosis with rigidity. SYN Bechterew disease, Strümpell disease (1).

⚠**spon·dy·lo-, spon·dyl-** the vertebrae. [G. *spondylos*, vertebra]

**spon·dy·lo·ep·i·phys·e·al dys·pla·sia** a group of conditions characterized by growth deficiency of the vertebral column with flattening of the vertebrae or platyspondyly, lack of ossification of the epiphyses, short-trunk dwarfism with limb shortening, and sometimes with other malformations; autosomal dominant, autosomal recessive, and X-linked recessive inheritance have been described.

**spon·dy·lo·ep·i·phy·se·al dys·pla·sia con·gen·i·ta (SEDC)** a skeletal dysplasia characterized by short-trunk dwarfism with short limbs, delayed ossification of the pubic rami and femoral and tibial epiphyses, flattening of the vertebral bodies, myopia, retinal detachment, and cleft palate; autosomal dominant inheritance caused by mutation in the type II collagen gene (COL2A1) on 12q.

**spon·dy·lo·e·pi·phy·se·al dys·pla·sia tar·da** a skeletal dysplasia of later onset, usually in the second decade, characterized by short stature, flattening of the vertebrae, epiphyseal involvement with bony fusion of the hip joint, premature osteoarthritis, and distinctive radiographic findings. Autosomal dominant and X-linked recessive forms exist.

🔲**spon·dy·lo·lis·the·sis** (spon′di-lō-lis-thē′sis) SYN anterolisthesis. See page 928. [spondylo- + G. *olisthēsis*, a slipping and falling]

**spon·dy·lo·lis·thet·ic** (spon′di-lō-lis-thet′ik) relating to or marked by spondylolisthesis.

**spon·dy·lo·lis·thet·ic pel·vis** a pelvis whose brim is more or less occluded by a forward dislocation of the body of the lower lumbar vertebra. SYN Prague pelvis, Rokitansky pelvis.

**spon·dy·lol·y·sis** (spon-di-lol′i-sis) degeneration

or deficient development of the articulating part of a vertebra. [spondylo- + G. *lysis,* loosening]

**spon·dy·lo·pa·thy** (spon-di-lop'ă-thē) any disease of the vertebrae or spinal column. [spondylo- + G. *pathos,* suffering]

**spon·dy·lo·py·o·sis** (spon'di-lō-pī-ō'sis) suppurative inflammation of one or more of the vertebral bodies. [spondylo- + G. *pyōsis,* suppuration]

**spon·dy·los·chi·sis** (spon-di-los'ki-sis) embryologic failure of fusion of vertebral arch. SEE spina bifida. [spondylo- + G. *schisis,* fissure]

**spon·dy·lo·sis** (spon-di-lō'sis) ankylosis of the vertebra; often applied nonspecifically to any lesion of the spine of a degenerative nature. See this page. [G. *spondylos,* vertebra]

**spon·dy·lo·syn·de·sis** (spon'di-lō-sin-dē'sis) SYN spinal fusion. [spondylo- + G. *syndesis,* binding together]

**sponge** (spŭnj) **1.** absorbent material, such as gauze or prepared cotton, used to absorb fluids. **2.** a member of the phylum Porifera, the cellular endoskeleton of which is a source of commercial natural sponges. [G. *spongia*]

**sponge bath** a bath in which the body is washed with a wet sponge or cloth.

**spon·gi·form** (spŭn'ji-fōrm) SYN spongy.

**spon·gi·form en·ceph·a·lo·pa·thy** an encephalopathy characterized by vacuolation within nerve and glial cells.

**spon·gi·o-** sponge, sponglike, spongy. [G. *spongia*]

**spon·gi·o·blast** (spŭn'jē-ō-blast) a neuroepithelial, filiform ependyma cell extending across the entire thickness of the wall of the brain or spinal cord, i.e., from the internal to the external limiting membrane; spongioblasts become neuroglial and ependymal cells. SEE ALSO glioblast. [spongio- + G. *blastos,* germ]

**spon·gi·o·blas·to·ma** (spŭn'jē-ō-blas-tō'mă) **1.** a glioma consisting of cells (elongated, spindle-shaped, and sometimes pleomorphic, with one or two fibrillary processes) that resemble the em-

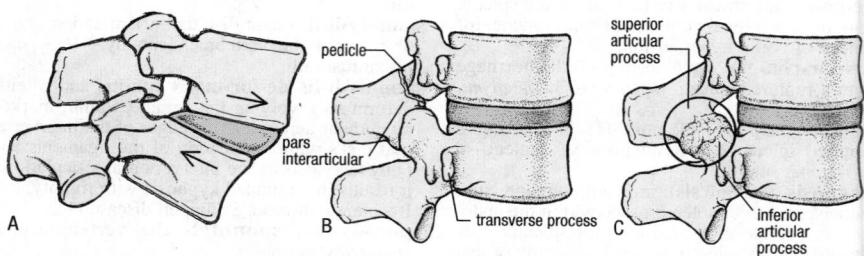

**spondylolisthesis:** (A) showing forward slippage of lumbar vertebra; **spondylolysis:** (B) showing fracture of pars interarticularis; **spondylosis:** (C) showing fixation of the articular processes

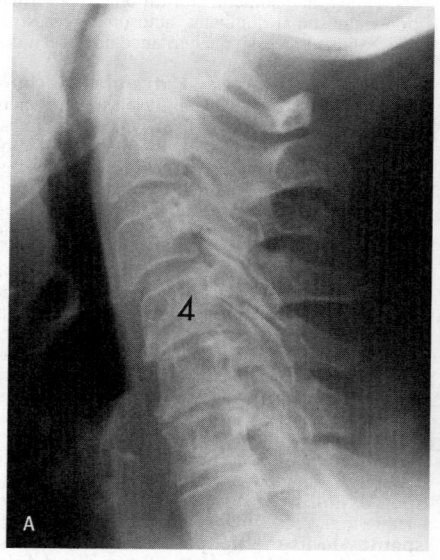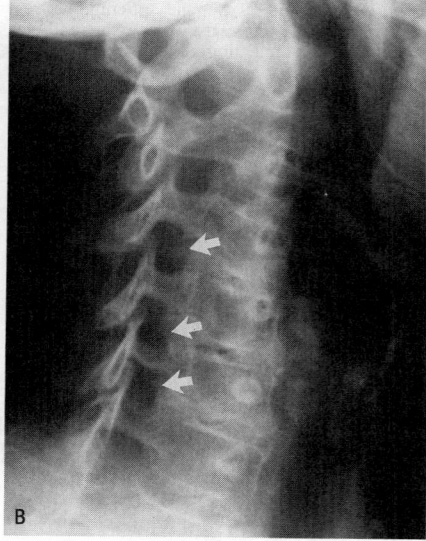

severe cervical **spondylosis:** (A) lateral radiograph shows narrowing of all the disc spaces below C4; (B) oblique view shows spurs encroaching on intervertebral foramina at several levels (arrows)

bryonic spongioblasts, occurring normally around the neural canal of the human embryo; it grows relatively slowly, usually originating in the brainstem, optic chiasm, or infundibulum, and infiltrates adjacent structures or causes compression of the third and fourth ventricle. [spongioblast + G. -*oma* tumor]

**spon·gi·o·cyte** (spŭn'jē-ō-sīt) **1.** a neuroglial cell. **2.** a cell in the zona fasciculata of the adrenal containing many droplets of lipid material which, after staining with hematoxylin and eosin, show pronounced vacuolization. [spongio- + G. *kytos*, cell]

**spon·gi·oid** (spŭn'jē-oyd) SYN spongy. [spongio- + G. *eidos*, resemblance]

**spon·gi·ose** (spŭn'jē-ōs) resembling or characteristic of a sponge. [L. *spongiosus*]

**spon·gi·o·sis** (spŭn-jē-ō'sis) inflammatory intercellular edema of the epidermis.

**spon·gi·o·si·tis** (spŭn-jē-ō-sī'tis) inflammation of the corpus spongiosum, or corpus cavernosum urethrae.

**spon·gy** (spŭn'jē) resembling the commercial natural sponge; of spongelike texture or appearance. SYN spongiform, spongioid.

**spon·gy bone 1.** SYN substantia spongiosa. **2.** a turbinate bone.

**spon·gy sub·stance** SYN substantia spongiosa.

**spon·ta·ne·ous a·bor·tion** abortion that has not been artificially induced.

**spon·ta·ne·ous am·pu·ta·tion 1.** SYN congenital amputation. **2.** amputation as the result of a pathologic process rather than from external trauma.

**spon·ta·ne·ous gan·grene of new·born** gangrene due to vascular occlusion of unknown cause, usually in marasmic or dehydrated infants.

**spon·ta·ne·ous gen·er·a·tion** the false concept according to which living matter can arise by the vitalization of nonliving matter. SEE ALSO biogenesis. SYN heterogenesis (3).

**spon·ta·ne·ous mu·ta·tion** a mutation that arises naturally and not as a result of exposure to mutagens.

**spon·ta·ne·ous pneu·mo·thor·ax** pneumothorax occurring secondary to parenchymal lung disease, usually from an emphysematous bulla which ruptures or occasionally from a lung abscess.

**spon·ta·ne·ous speech** spoken language that occurs without prompting or during an unstructured interview.

**spon·ta·ne·ous ver·sion** turning of the fetus effected by the unaided contraction of the uterine muscle.

**spoon** (spoon) an instrument with a handle and a small bowl- or cup-shaped extremity. [A.S. *spōn*, chip]

**spoon nail** SYN koilonychia.

**spo·rad·ic** (spō-rad'ik) **1.** denoting a temporal pattern of disease occurrence in an animal or human population in which the disease occurs only rarely and without regularity. SEE ALSO endemic, epidemic, epizootic. **2.** occurring irregularly, haphazardly. [G. *sporadikos*, scattered]

**spo·ran·gi·um** (spō-ran'jē-ŭm) a saclike structure (a cell) within a fungus, in which asexual spores are borne by progressive cleavage. [L. fr. G. *sporos*, seed, + *angeion*, vessel]

**spore** (spōr) **1.** the asexual or sexual reproductive body of fungi or sporozoan protozoa. **2.** a cell of a plant lower in organization than the seed-bear-

ing spermatophytic plants. **3.** a resistant form of certain species of bacteria. **4.** the highly modified reproductive body of certain protozoa, as in the phyla Microspora and Myxozoa. [G. *sporos*, seed]

**spo·ri·ci·dal** (spōr-i-sī'dăl) lethal to spores. [spori- + L. *caedo*, to kill]

**spo·ri·cide** (spōr'i-sīd) an agent that kills spores.

**spo·rid·i·um**, pl. **spo·rid·ia** (spō-rid'ē-ŭm, spō-rid'ē-ă) a protozoan spore; an embryonic protozoan organism. [Mod. L. dim., fr. G. *sporos*, seed]

△**spor·o-**, **spor·i-**, **spor-** seed, spore. [G. *sporos*]

**spo·ro·ag·glu·ti·na·tion** (spōr'ō-ă-gloo-ti-nā'shŭn) a diagnostic method in relation to the mycoses, based upon the fact that the blood of patients with diseases caused by fungi contains specific agglutinins that cause clumping of the spores of these organisms.

**spo·ro·blast** (spōr'ō-blast) an early stage in the development of a sporocyst prior to differentiation of the sporozoites. SEE ALSO oocyst, sporocyst (2). [sporo- + G. *blastos*, germ]

**spo·ro·cyst** (spōr'ō-sist) **1.** a larval form of digenetic trematode (fluke) that develops in the body of its molluscan intermediate host, usually a snail. SEE ALSO cercaria. **2.** a secondary cyst that develops within the oocyst of Coccidia, a group of sporozoans that includes many of the most important disease agents of domestic animals and fowl. [sporo- + G. *kystis*, bladder]

**spo·ro·gen·e·sis** (spōr-ō-jen'ĕ-sis) SYN sporogony. [sporo- + G. *genesis*, production]

**spo·rog·e·nous** (spŏ-roj'ĕ-nŭs) relating to or involved in sporogony.

**spo·rog·o·ny**, **spo·rog·e·ny** (spŏ-rog'ŏ-nē, spŏ-roj'ĕ-nē) the formation of sporozoites in sporozoan protozoa, a process of asexual division within the sporoblast, which becomes the sporocyst within an oocyst; follows fusion of gametes (gametogony) and zygote (sporont) formation. SYN sporogenesis. [sporo- + G. *goneia*, generation]

**spo·ront** (spōr'ont) the zygote stage within the oocyst wall in the life cycle of coccidia; gives rise to sporoblasts, which form sporocysts, within which the infective sporozoites are produced. [sporo- + G. *ōn* (*ont-*), being]

*Spo·ro·thrix* (spōr'ō-thriks) a genus of dimorphic imperfect fungi, including *Sporothrix schenckii*, an organism of worldwide distribution and the causative agent of sporotrichosis in humans and animals. [Mod. L., fr. G. *sporos*, seed, + *thrix*, hair]

**spo·ro·tri·cho·sis** (spōr'ō-tri-kō'sis) a chronic cutaneous mycosis spread by way of the lymphatics and caused by inoculation of *Sporothrix schenckii*, typically rare in tissue sections but rapidly growing in cultures. The disease may remain localized or may become generalized, involving bones, joints, lungs, and the central nervous system; lesions may be granulomatous or suppurative, ulcerative, or draining. SYN Schenck disease.

**spo·ro·zo·ite** (spōr-ō-zō'īt) one of the minute elongated bodies resulting from the repeated division of the oocyst during sporogony. In the case of the malarial parasite, it is the form that is concentrated in the salivary glands and introduced into the blood by the bite of a mosquito; it enters the liver cells (exoerythrocytic cycle), whose progeny, the merozoites, infect the red blood cells to initiate clinical malaria. [sporo- + G. *zōon*, animal]

**sports ane•mia** SYN exercise-induced anemia.

**sports mas•sage, sports•mas•sage** a group of massage techniques specifically designed to aid in athletic performance. Includes pre- event massage, post-event massage, and maintenance and injury massage.

**sports med•i•cine** a field of medicine that uses a holistic, comprehensive, and multidisciplinary approach to health care for those engaged in a sporting or recreational activity.

**sport-spe•ci•fic train•ing** SYN activity grading.

**spor•u•lar** (spōr'yu-lăr) relating to a spore or sporule.

**spor•u•la•tion** (spor'yu-lā'shŭn) the process by which yeasts undergo meiosis, and the meiotic products are encased in spore coats.

**spor•ule** (spōr'yul) A spore; a small spore. [Mod. L. *sporula;* dim. of G. *sporos,* seed]

**spot 1.** SYN macula. **2.** to lose a slight amount of blood through the vagina.

**spot map** map showing the geographic location of people with a specific attribute, e.g., cases of an infectious disease.

**spot•ted fe•ver** tick typhus caused by *Rickettsia rickettsii* in North and South America and Siberia.

**spot test for in•fec•tious mon•o•nu•cle•o•sis** a slide test widely used for the diagnosis of infectious mononucleosis; when horse red cells are agglutinated by patient serum (previously treated with guinea pig kidney, which adsorbs confounding antibodies), the presumptive diagnosis is infectious mononucleosis.

**spouse abuse, spous•al abuse** SEE domestic violence.

**sprain** (sprān) **1.** an injury to a ligament when the joint is carried through a range of motion greater than normal, but without dislocation or fracture. **2.** to cause a sprain of a joint.

**sprain frac•ture** an avulsion fracture in which a small portion of adjacent bone has been pulled or pushed off.

**spray** (sprā) a jet of liquid in fine drops, coarser than a vapor; it is produced by forcing the liquid from the minute opening of an atomizer, mixed with air.

**Spreng•el de•for•mi•ty** (shpreng'gĕl) congenital elevation of the scapula.

**spring con•junc•ti•vi•tis** SYN vernal conjunctivitis.

**sprue** (sproo) **1.** primary intestinal malabsorption with steatorrhea. **2.** DENTISTRY wax or metal used to form the aperture(s) for molten metal to flow into a mold to make a casting; also, the metal that later fills the sprue hole(s). [D. *spruw*]

**spud** (spŭd) a triangular knife used for removing foreign bodies from the cornea.

**spun glass hair** SYN uncombable hair syndrome.

**spur** (sper) SYN calcar. [A.S. *spora*]

**spur cell** a spiculated red cell with 5–10 spiny projections of varying length distributed irregularly over the cell surface; seen in patients with liver disease and abetalipoproteinemia.

**spur cell ane•mia** anemia in which the red cells have a spiculated appearance and are destroyed prematurely, predominantly in the spleen; may be seen in patients with severe liver disease as a

result of an abnormality in the cholesterol content of the red cell membrane.

**spu•ri•ous** (spoo'rē-ŭs) false; not genuine. [L. *spurius*]

**spu•ri•ous an•ky•lo•sis** SYN extracapsular ankylosis.

**spu•ri•ous par•a•site** organisms that parasitize other hosts that pass through the human intestine and are detected in the stool after ingestion (e.g., *Capillaria* sp. eggs in animal liver).

**Spurl•ing test** (sper'ling) evaluation for cervical nerve root impingement in which the patient extends the neck and rotates and laterally bends the head toward the symptomatic side; an axial compression force is then applied by the examiner through the top of the patient's head; the test is considered positive when the maneuver elicits the typical radicular arm pain.

**spu•tum,** pl. **spu•ta** (spyu'tŭm, spyu'tă) **1.** expectorated matter, especially mucus or mucopurulent matter expectorated in diseases of the air passages. SEE ALSO expectoration (1). **2.** an individual mass of such matter. [L. *sputum,* fr. *spuo,* pp. *sputus,* to spit]

**SQ** subcutaneous.

**squa•la•mine lac•tate** (skwā'lă-mēn lak'tāt) an antiangiogenic, noncytotoxic drug used to treat solid tumors.

**squa•ma,** pl. **squa•mae** (skwā'mă, skwā'mē) **1.** [TA] a thin plate of bone. **2.** an epidermal scale. SYN scale (2), squame. [L. a scale]

**squa•mate** (skwā'māt) SYN squamous.

**squame** (skwām) SYN squama.

△**squa•mo-** squama, squamous. [L. *squama,* a scale]

**squa•mo•pa•ri•e•tal su•ture** the articulation of the parietal with the squamous portion of the temporal bone.

**squa•mo•sa,** pl. **squa•mo•sae** (skwā-mō'să, skwā-mō'sē) the squamous parts of the frontal, occipital, or temporal bone, especially the latter. [L. *squamosus,* scaly, fr. *squama,* scale]

**squa•mo•sal** (skwā-mō'săl) relating especially to the squamous part of the temporal bone.

**squa•mous** (skwā'mŭs) relating to or covered with scales. SYN scaly, squamate. [L. *squamosus*]

**squa•mous cell** a flat scale-like epithelial cell.

**squa•mous cell car•ci•no•ma** a malignant neoplasm derived from stratified squamous epithelium, which may also occur in sites where only glandular or columnar epithelium is normally present. See page B7.

**squa•mous ep•i•the•li•um** epithelium consisting of a single layer of cells.

**squa•mous met•a•pla•sia** the transformation of glandular or mucosal epithelium into stratified squamous epithelium. SYN epidermalization.

**squa•mous met•a•pla•sia of am•ni•on** SYN amnion nodosum.

**squa•mous o•don•to•gen•ic tu•mor** a benign epithelial odontogenic tumor thought to arise from the epithelial cell rests of Malassez; appears clinically as a radiolucent lesion closely associated with the tooth root and histologically as islands of squamous epithelium enclosed by a peripheral layer of flattened cells.

**squa•mous su•ture** a scalelike suture, one whose opposing margins are scalelike and overlapping;

**squa•mo•zy•go•mat•ic** (skwā'mō-zī-gō-mat'ik) relating to the squamous part of the temporal bone and the zygomatic process of the temporal bone.

**square knot** a double knot in which the free ends of the second loop are symmetric and in the same plane as the free ends of the first loop.

**squint** (skwint) SYN strabismus.

**squint·ing pa·tel·la** a patella that is medially rotated.

**Sr** strontium.

**SRH** somatotropin-releasing hormone.

**sRNA** soluble RNA. See entries under ribonucleic acid.

**SRS** slow-reacting substance.

**SSPE** subacute sclerosing panencephalitis.

**SSPL** saturation sound pressure level.

**SSRI** selective serotonin reuptake inhibitor.

**ST** scapulothoracic.

**stab cell** SYN band cell.

**stab cul·ture** a culture produced by inserting an inoculating needle with inoculum down the center of a solid medium contained in a test tube.

**stab drain** a drain passed into a cavity through a puncture made at a dependent part away from the wound of operation, so placed to prevent infection of the wound.

**sta·bi·late** (stā′bi-lāt) a sample of organisms preserved alive on a single occasion.

**sta·bile** (stā′bīl, stā-bil) steady; fixed; denoting: 1) certain constituents of serum unaffected by moderate heating or prolonged storage; 2) an electrode held steadily on a part during the passage of an electric current. Cf. labile. [L. *stabilis*]

**sta·bil·i·ty** (stă-bil′i-tē) the condition of being stable or resistant to change.

**sta·bi·li·za·tion** (stā′bĭ-li-zā′shŭn) **1.** the accomplishment of a stable state. **2.** SYN denture stability.

**sta·ble** (stā′bl) steady; not varying; resistant to change. SEE ALSO stabile.

**sta·ble iso·tope** a nonradioactive nuclide; an isotope that shows no tendency to undergo radioactive decomposition.

**stac·ca·to speech** an abrupt utterance, each syllable being enunciated separately; noted especially in multiple sclerosis.

**staff 1.** a specific group of workers. **2.** SYN director (1). [A.S. *staef*]

**staff of Aes·cu·la·pi·us** (es-kyu-lā′pē-ŭs) a rod with only one serpent encircling it and without wings; symbol of medicine and emblem of the American Medical Association, Royal Army Medical Corps (Britain), and Royal Canadian Medical Corps. SEE ALSO caduceus. [L. *Aesculapius*, G. *Asklēpios*, god of medicine]

**staff cell** SYN band cell.

**staff model HMO** arrangement under which physician providers are salaried employees of an HMO.

**stage** (stāj) **1.** a period in the course of a disease; a description of the extent of involvement of a disease process or the status of a patient with a specific disease, as of the distribution and extent of dissemination of a malignant neoplastic disease; also, the act of determining the stage of a disease, especially cancer. SEE ALSO period. **2.** the part of a microscope on which the microscope slide bears the object to be examined. **3.** a particular step, phase, or position in a developmental process. For psychosexual stages, see en-

tries under phase. [M.E. thr. O. Fr. *estage*, standing-place, fr. L. *sto*, pp. *status*, to stand]

**stag·es of la·bor** SEE labor.

**stag·gered spon·da·ic word test** a test of central auditory pathway integrity in which spondaic words are presented dichotically.

**stag·horn cal·cu·lus** a calculus occurring in the renal pelvis, with branches extending into the infundibula and calices.

**stag·ing** (stāj′ing) **1.** the determination or classification of distinct phases or periods in the course of a disease or pathological process. **2.** the determination of the specific extent of a disease process in an individual patient.

**stag·nant a·nox·ia** stagnant hypoxia severe enough to result in the absence of oxygen in tissues.

**stag·na·tion** (stag-nā′shŭn) retardation or cessation of flow of blood in the vessels, as in passive congestion; marked slowing or accumulation in any part of a normally circulating fluid. [L. *stagnum*, a pool]

**Stahl ear** (shtahl) a deformed external ear, in which the fossa ovalis and upper portion of the scaphoid fossa are covered by the helix; once regarded as a stigma of degenerate constitution.

**stain** (stān) **1.** to discolor. **2.** to color; to dye. **3.** a discoloration. **4.** a dye used in histologic and bacteriologic technique. **5.** a procedure in which a dye or combination of dyes and reagents is used to color the constituents of cells and tissues. [M.E. *steinen*]

**stain·ing** (stān′ing) **1.** the act of applying a stain. SEE ALSO stain. **2.** DENTISTRY modification of the color of the tooth or denture base.

**stair·case** (stār′kās) a series of reactions that follow one another in progressively increasing or decreasing intensity, so that a chart shows a continuous rise or fall. SEE treppe.

**stair·case phe·no·me·non** SYN treppe.

**stal·ag·mom·e·ter** (stal-ăg-mom′ē-ter) an instrument for determining exactly the number of drops in a given quantity of liquid; used as a measure of the surface tension of a fluid (the lower the tension, the smaller the drops and, consequently, the more numerous in a given quantity of the fluid). [G. *stalagma*, a drop, + *metron*, measure]

**stale·ness** SYN overtraining syndrome.

**stalk** (stawk) a narrowed connection with a structure or organ.

**stam·mer·ing** (stam′er-ing) **1.** a speech disorder characterized by hesitation and repetition of words, or by mispronunciation or transposition of certain consonants, especially *l*, *r*, and *s*. **2.** sounds other than speech, that are similar to stammering.

**stan·dard at·mos·phere (atm) 1.** the pressure of the atmosphere at mean sea level, equivalent to 1,013,250 dynes/cm$^2$ or 101,325 Pa (N/m$^2$ in the SI system); **2.** a standardized expression of the relation of barometric pressure, temperature, and other atmospheric variables as a function of altitude above sea level.

**stan·dard bi·car·bon·ate** the plasma bicarbonate concentration of a sample of whole blood that has been equilibrated at 37°C with a carbon dioxide pressure of 40 mmHg and an oxygen pressure greater than 100 mm Hg; abnormally high or low values indicate metabolic alkalosis or acidosis, respectively.

S
t

**stan·dard de·vi·a·tion** (σ) **1.** statistical index of the degree of deviation from central tendency, namely, of the variability within a distribution; the square root of the average of the squared deviations from the mean. **2.** a measure of dispersion or variation used to describe a characteristic of a frequency distribution.

**stan·dard er·ror of dif·fer·ence** a statistical index of the probability that a difference between two sample means is greater than zero.

**stan·dard·i·za·tion** (stan′dard-i-zā′shŭn) **1.** the making of a solution of definite strength so that it may be used for comparison and in tests. **2.** making any drug or other preparation conform to the type or standard. **3.** a set of techniques used to remove as far as possible the effects of differences in the age or other confounding variables when comparing two or more populations.

**stan·dard pres·sure** the absolute pressure to which gases are referred under standard conditions (STPD), i.e., 760 mmHg, 760 torr, or 101,325 newtons/m$^2$ (i.e., 101,325 Pa).

**stan·dard so·lu·tion, stan·dard·ized so·lu·tion** a solution of known concentration, used as a standard of comparison or analysis.

**stan·dard tem·per·a·ture** a temperature of 0°C or 273.15° absolute (Kelvin).

**stan·dard vol·ume** the volume of an ideal gas at standard temperature and pressure, approximately 22.414 liters.

**stand·still** cessation of activity.

**Stan·ford-Bi·net in·tel·li·gence scale** (stan′fŏrd-bē-nā′) a standardized test for the measurement of intelligence consisting of a series of questions, graded according to the intelligence of normal children at different ages, the answers to which indicate the mental age of the person tested; primarily used with children, but also contains norms for adults standardized against adult age levels. SYN Binet scale, Binet test.

**stan·nous** (stan′ŭs) relating to tin, especially when in combination in its lower valency. [L. *stannum*, tin]

**stan·num** (stan′ŭm) SYN tin. [L.]

**sta·pe·dec·to·my** (stā-pĕ-dek′tō-mē) operation to remove the stapes footplate in whole or part with replacement of the stapes superstructure (crura) by metal or plastic prosthesis; used for otosclerosis with stapes fixation to overcome a conductive hearing loss. [stapes + G. *ektomē*, excision]

**sta·pe·di·al** (stā-pē′dē-ăl) relating to the stapes.

**sta·pe·di·al re·flex** SYN acoustic reflex.

**sta·pe·di·o·te·not·o·my** (stā-pē′dē-ō-tĕ-not′ŏ-mē) division of the tendon of the stapedius muscle. [stapedius + G. *tenōn*, tendon, + *tomē*, incision]

**sta·pe·di·us mus·cle** *origin*, internal walls of pyramidal eminence in tympanic cavity; *insertion*, neck of the stapes; *action*, dampens vibration of stapes by drawing head of stapes backward as a result of a protective reflex stimulated by loud noise; *nerve supply*, facial. SYN musculus stapedius [TA].

**sta·pe·dot·o·my** (stā-pē-dot′ō-mē) a surgical technique for the improvement of hearing in otosclerosis: a hole is made in the footplate of the stapes bone through which is placed the piston-shaped end of a prosthesis, the other end of which is attached to the long process of the incus bone.

**sta·pes**, pl. **sta·pes**, **sta·pe·des** (stā′pēz, stā′pēz)

[TA] the smallest of the three auditory ossicles; its base, or footpiece, fits into the vestibular (oval) window, while its head is articulated with the lenticular process of the long limb of the incus. SYN stirrup. [Mod. L. stirrup]

**sta·pes mo·bi·li·za·tion** an operation to remobilize the footplate of the stapes to relieve conductive hearing impairment caused by its immobilization through otosclerosis or middle ear disease.

**staph·y·lec·to·my** (staf-i-lek′tō-mē) SYN uvulectomy. [staphyl- + G. *ektomē*, excision]

**staph·yl·e·de·ma** (staf′il-e-dē′mă) edema of the uvula. [staphyl- + G. *oidēma*, swelling (edema)]

**staph·y·line** (staf′i-līn) SYN botryoid.

**sta·phyl·i·on** (stă-fil′ē-on) the midpoint of the posterior edge of the hard palate; a craniometric point. [G. dim. of *staphylē*, a bunch of grapes]

⌂**sta·phy·lo-, sta·phyl-** resemblance to a grape or a bunch of grapes, hence relating usually to staphylococci or to the uvula palatina. [G. *staphylē*, a bunch of grapes]

**staph·y·lo·coc·cal** (staf′i-lō-kok′ăl) relating to or caused by any organism of the genus *Staphylococcus*.

**sta·phy·lo·coc·cal ble·pha·ri·tis** inflammation of the eyelids characterized by brittle hard scales along the base of the eyelashes.

**staph·y·lo·coc·ce·mia** (staf′i-lō-kok-sē′mē-ă) the presence of staphylococci in the circulating blood. [staphylo- + G. *haima*, blood]

🔲**staph·y·lo·coc·ci** (staf′i-lō-kok′sī) plural of staphylococcus. See page B3.

**staph·y·lo·coc·co·sis**, pl. **staph·y·lo·coc·co·ses** (staf′i-lō-kok-ō′sis, staf′i-lō-kok-ō′sēz) infection by species of the bacterium *Staphylococcus*.

*Staph·y·lo·coc·cus* (staf′i-lō-kok′ŭs) a genus of nonmotile, non-spore-forming, aerobic to facultatively anaerobic bacteria containing Gram-positive, spherical cells which divide in more than one plane to form irregular clusters. Coagulase-positive strains produce a variety of toxins and are therefore potentially pathogenic and may cause food poisoning. These organisms are usually susceptible to antibiotics such as the β-lactam and macrolide antibiotics, tetracyclines, novobiocin, and chloramphenicol but are resistant to polymyxin and polyenes. They are found on the skin, in skin glands, on the nasal and other mucous membranes of warm-blooded animals, and in a variety of food products. The type species is *Staphylococcus aureus*. [staphylo- + G. *kokkos*, a berry]

**staph·y·lo·coc·cus**, pl. **staph·y·lo·coc·ci** (staf′i-lō-kok′ŭs, kok′sī) a vernacular term used to refer to any member of the genus *Staphylococcus*.

*Sta·phy·lo·coc·cus au·re·us* a common species found especially on nasal mucous membrane and skin (hair follicles); it causes furunculosis, cellulitis, pyemia, pneumonia, osteomyelitis, endocarditis, suppuration of wounds, other infections, and food poisoning; also a cause of infection in burn patients. Humans are the chief reservoir. The type species of the genus *Staphylococcus*.

*Sta·phy·lo·coc·cus py·og·e·nes al·bus* a name formerly applied to the organisms which are now regarded as the mutants of *Staphylococcus aureus* that form white colonies.

*Sta·phy·lo·coc·cus* spe·cies, co·ag·u·lase-neg·a·tive includes a group of species present as normal flora of human skin, respiratory, and mucous membrane surfaces. Although a normal commensal, strains are prominent causes of nosocomial infections, especially in patients with implanted intravenous access devices; some strains are abscess forming and cause diverse infections including sinusitis, wound infections, and osteomyelitis.

**staph•y•lo•der•ma** (staf'i-lō-der'mă) pyoderma due to staphylococci. [staphylo- + G. *derma*, skin]

**staph•y•lo•der•ma•ti•tis** (staf'i-lō-der-mă-tī'tis) inflammation of the skin due to the action of staphylococci.

**staph•y•lo•di•al•y•sis** (staf'i-lō-dī-al'i-sis) SYN uvuloptosis. [staphylo- + G. *dialysis*, a separation]

**staph•y•lo•ki•nase** (staf'i-lō-kī'nās) a microbial metalloenzyme from *Staphylococcus aureus*, with action similar to that of urokinase and streptokinase, that can convert plasminogen to plasmin but requires $Ca^{2+}$; separated in forms A, B, and C.

**staph•y•lol•y•sin** (staf-i-lol'i-sin) **1.** a hemolysin elaborated by a staphylococcus. **2.** an antibody causing lysis of staphylococci.

**staph•y•lo•ma** (staf-i-lō'mă) a bulging of the cornea or sclera containing uveal tissue. [staphylo- + G. -ōma, tumor]

**staph•y•lom•a•tous** (staf-i-lō'mă-tŭs) relating to or marked by staphyloma.

**staph•y•lo•phar•yn•gor•rha•phy** (staf'i-lō-far-in-gōr'ă-fē) surgical repair of defects in the uvula or soft palate and the pharynx. SYN palatopharyngorrhaphy. [staphylo- + pharynx + G. *rhaphē*, suture]

**staph•y•lo•plas•ty** (staf'i-lō-plas-tē) SYN palatoplasty. [staphylo- + G. *plassō*, to form]

**staph•y•lop•to•sis** (staf'i-lop-tō'sis) SYN uvuloptosis. [staphylo- + G. *ptōsis*, a falling]

**staph•y•lor•rha•phy** (staf-i-lōr'ă-fē) SYN palatorrhaphy. [staphylo- + G. *rhaphē*, suture]

**staph•y•lo•tox•in** (staf'i-lō-tok'sin) the toxin elaborated by any species of *Staphylococcus*. [staphylo- + G. *toxikon*, poison]

**sta•pling** (stāp'ling) use of a stapling device that unites two tissues, such as the two ends of bowel, by applying a row or circle of staples.

**star** any star-shaped structure. SEE ALSO aster, astrosphere, stella, stellula. [A.S. *steorra*]

**starch** a high molecular-weight polysaccharide built up of D-glucose residues in α-1,4 linkage, differing from cellulose in the presence of α- rather than β-glucoside linkages, that exists in most plant tissues; converted into dextrin when subjected to the action of dry heat, and into dextrin and D-glucose by amylases and glucoamylases in saliva and pancreatic juice; used as a dusting powder, an emollient, and an ingredient in medicinal tablets; chief storage carbohydrate in most higher plants. [A.S. *stearc*, strong]

**Star•gardt dis•ease** (shtahr'gahrt) fundus flavimaculatus initiated with atrophic macular lesions, caused by mutation in the ATP-binding cassette transporter, retina-specific gene (ABCR) on 1p.

**Star•ling curve** (stahr'ling) a graph in which cardiac output or stroke volume is plotted against mean atrial or ventricular end-diastolic pressure; with increasing venous return and atrial pressure the output proportionately increases until further increments overload the heart and the output falls. SYN Frank-Starling curve.

**Star•ling hy•poth•e•sis** (stahr'ling) the principle that net filtration through capillary membranes is proportional to the transmembrane hydrostatic pressure difference minus the transmembrane oncotic pressure difference; although well established, it is called Starling hypothesis to distinguish it from Starling law of the heart.

**Star•ling re•flex** (stahr'ling) tapping the volar surfaces of the fingers causes flexion of the fingers; analogous to Rossolimo reflex, for the toes.

**star•tle dis•ease** SYN hyperekplexia.

**star•tle ep•i•lep•sy** a form of reflex epilepsy precipitated by sudden noises.

**star•tle re•flex 1.** the reflex response of an infant (contraction of the limb and neck muscles) when allowed to drop a short distance through the air or startled by a sudden noise or jolt; SYN parachute reflex. **2.** SYN cochleopalpebral reflex.

**star•va•tion di•a•be•tes** after prolonged fasting, glycosuria following the ingestion of carbohydrate or glucose because of reduced output of insulin and/or reduced rate of glucose metabolism with a reduced ability to form glycogen.

**starve 1.** to suffer from lack of food. **2.** to deprive of food so as to cause suffering or death. **3.** formerly, to die of cold. [A.S. *steorfan*, to die]

**sta•sis**, pl. **sta•ses** (stā'sis, stā'sēz) stagnation of the blood or other fluids. [G. a standing still]

**sta•sis der•ma•ti•tis** erythema and scaling of the lower extremities due to impaired venous circulation, seen commonly in older women or secondary to deep vein thrombosis.

**sta•sis ec•ze•ma** eczematous eruption on legs due to or aggravated by venous stasis.

**stat** referring to a diagnostic or therapeutic procedure that is to be performed immediately. [L. *statim*, immediately]

△**-stat** an agent intended to keep something from changing or moving. [G. *statēs*, stationary]

**state** (stāt) a condition, situation, or status. [L. *status*, condition, state]

**state-de•pen•dent learn•ing** learning during a specific state of sleep or wakefulness, or during a chemically altered state, where retrieval of learned information cannot be demonstrated unless the subject is restored to the state that originally existed during learning.

**sta•tic com•pli•ance 1.** The ratio of the change in volume of a distensible vessel to the change in distending pressure when the pressure change is measured between points in time when the system is at rest. **2.** The slope of the statically determined pressure-volume curve.

**stat•ic re•la•tion** relationship between two parts that are not in motion.

**sta•tim** (stā'tim) at once; immediately. [L.]

**sta•tis•tics** (stă-tis'tiks) **1.** a collection of numerical values, items of information, or other facts which are numerically grouped into definite classes and subject to analysis, particularly analysis of the probability that the resulting empirical findings are due to chance. **2.** the science and art of collecting, summarizing, and analyzing data that are subject to random variation.

**stat•o•a•cou•stic** (stat'ō-ă-koo'stik) relating to equilibrium and hearing. SYN vestibulocochlear (2). [G. *statos*, standing, + *akoustikos*, acoustic]

**stat•o•co•nia**, sing. **stat•o•co•ni•um** (stat'ō-kō'nē-ă, stat'ō-kō'nē-ŭm) [TA] SYN statoliths. [L. fr. G. *statos*, standing, *konis*, dust]

**stat•o•ki•net•ic re•flex** a reflex which, through

stimulation of the receptors in the neck muscles and semicircular canals, brings about movements of the limbs and eyes appropriate to a given movement of the head in space.

**stat•o•liths** (stat′ŏ-liths) crystalline particles of calcium carbonate and a protein adhering to the gelatinous membrane of the maculae of the utricle and saccule. SYN statoconia [TA], otoconia. [G. *statos,* standing, + *lithos,* stone]

**stat•ure** (statch′er) the height of a person. [L. *statura,* fr. *statuo,* pp. *statutus,* to cause to stand]

**sta•tus** (stā′tŭs, stat′ŭs) a state or condition. [L. a way of standing]

**sta•tus asth•ma•tic•us** a condition of severe, prolonged asthma.

**sta•tus ep•i•lep•tic•us** repeated seizure or a seizure prolonged for at least 30 minutes; may be convulsive (tonic-clonic), nonconvulsive (absence or complex partial) or partial (epilepsia partialis continuans) or subclinical (electrographic status epilepticus).

**Stauf•fer syn•drome** (staw′fer) abnormality of liver function tests, in the absence of metastatic disease, due to cholestasis in renal cell cancer patients.

**stau•ri•on** (staw′rē-on) a craniometric point at the intersection of the median and transverse palatine sutures. [G. dim. of *stauros,* cross]

**STD** sexually transmitted disease.

**stead•y state (s) 1.** a state obtained in moderate muscular exercise, when the removal of lactic acid by oxidation keeps pace with its production, the oxygen supply being adequate, and the muscles do not go into debt for oxygen; **2.** any condition in which the formation or introduction of substances just keeps pace with their destruction or removal so that all volumes, concentrations, pressures, and flows remain constant; **3.** in enzyme kinetics, conditions such that the rate of change in the concentration of any enzyme species (e.g., free enzyme or the enzyme-substrate binary complex) is zero or much less than the rate of formation of product. [often subscript s or ss]

**stead•y-state ex•er•cise, stead•y-rate ex•er•cise** exercise that achieves a balance between energy required by working muscles and the rate of aerobic ATP production.

**steal** (stēl) diversion of blood via alternate routes or reversed flow, from a vascularized tissue to one deprived by proximal arterial obstruction. [M.E. *stelen,* fr. A.S. *stelan*]

**ste•ap•sin** (stē-ap′sin) SYN triacylglycerol lipase.

**ste•a•rate** (stē′ă-rāt) a salt of stearic acid.

**Stearns al•co•hol•ic a•men•tia** (stĕrnz) a temporary alcoholic mental disorder resembling delirium tremens but lasting for a longer time and showing a greater degree of amnesia and other mental defects.

△**stear•o-, stear-** combining form denoting fat. SEE ALSO steato-. [G. *stear,* tallow]

**ste•a•ti•tis** (stē-ă-tī′tis) inflammation of adipose tissue. [G. *stear* (*steat-*), tallow, + *-itis,* inflammation]

△**ste•at•o-** fat. SEE stearo-. [G. *stear* (*steat-*), tallow]

**ste•a•to•cys•to•ma** (stē′ă-tō-sis-tō′mă) a cyst with sebaceous gland cells in its wall.

**ste•a•tol•y•sis** (stē-ă-tol′i-sis) the hydrolysis or emulsion of fat in the process of digestion. [steato- + G. *lysis,* dissolution]

**ste•a•to•ly•tic** (stē-ă-tō-lit′ik) relating to steatolysis.

**ste•a•to•ne•cro•sis** (stē′ă-tō-ne-krō′sis) SYN fat necrosis. [steato- + G. *nekrōsis,* death]

**ste•a•to•py•ga, ste•a•to•py•gia** (stē′ă-top-ĭ′gă, stē-ă-to-pij′ē-ă) excessive accumulation of fat on the buttocks. [steato- + G. *pygē,* buttocks]

**ste•a•to•py•gous** (stē-ă-top′ĭ-gŭs) having excessively fat buttocks.

**ste•a•tor•rhea** (stē′ă-tō-rē′ă) passage of fat in large amounts in the feces due to failure to digest and absorb it; occurs in pancreatic disease and the malabsorption syndromes; an absence of bile acids will increase steatorrhea. [steato- + G. *rhoia,* a flow]

**ste•a•tor•rhoea [Br.]** SEE steatorrhea.

**ste•a•to•sis** (stē-ă-tō′sis) **1.** SYN adiposis. **2.** SYN fatty degeneration. [steato- + G. *-osis,* condition]

**Steell mur•mur** (stēl) SYN Graham Steell murmur.

**steg•no•sis** (steg-nō′sis) **1.** a stoppage of any of the secretions or excretions. **2.** a constriction or stenosis. [G. stoppage]

**Stein•berg thumb sign** (stīn′berg) in Marfan syndrome, when the thumb is held across the palm of the same hand, it projects well beyond the ulnar surface of the hand.

**stein•stras•se** (shtīn′stra-sĕ) a complication of extracorporeal shock wave lithotripsy for urinary tract calculi in which stone fragments block the ureter to form a "stone street." [Ger. *Stein,* stone, + *Strasse,* street]

**Stein test** (stīn) in cases of labyrinthine disease the patient is unable to stand or to hop on one foot with eyes shut.

**stel•la,** pl. **stel•lae** (stel′ă, stel′ē) a star or star-shaped figure. [L.]

**stel•late** (stel′āt) star-shaped. [L. *stella,* a star]

**stel•late ab•scess** a star-shaped necrotic area surrounded by histiocytes, seen within swollen inguinal lymph nodes in lymphogranuloma venereum.

**stel•late block** injection of local anesthetic solution in the vicinity of the stellate ganglion.

**stel•late cell** a star-shaped cell, such as an astrocyte or Kupffer cell, that has many filaments extending radially.

**stel•late frac•ture** a fracture in which the lines of break radiate from a central point.

**stel•late hair** hair split in several strands at the free end.

**stel•late re•tic•u•lum** a network of epithelial cells disposed in a fluid-filled compartment in the center of the enamel organ between the outer and inner enamel epithelium.

**stel•late veins** SYN venulae stellatae.

**stel•late ven•ules** SYN venulae stellatae.

**stel•lu•la,** pl. **stel•lu•lae** (stel′yu-lă, stel′yu-lē) a small star or star-shaped figure. [L. dim. of *stella,* star]

**Stell•wag sign** (shtel′vahk) infrequent and incomplete blinking in Graves disease.

**stem** a supporting structure similar to the stalk of a plant.

**stem cell 1.** any precursor cell; **2.** a cell whose daughter cells may differentiate into other cell types.

**stem cell fac•tor** a cytokine that promotes growth and differentiation of hematopoietic stem cells into a variety of cell lineages.

**stem cell leu•ke•mia** a form of leukemia in

which the abnormal cells are thought to be the precursors of lymphoblasts, myeloblasts, or monoblasts. SYN embryonal leukemia.

**ste·ni·on** (sten′ē-on) the termination in either temporal fossa of the shortest transverse diameter of the skull; a craniometric point. [G. *stenos,* narrow, + dim. *-iōn*]

**steno-** narrowness, constriction; opposite of eury-. [G. *stenos,* narrow]

**sten·o·car·dia** (sten-ō-kar′dē-ă) SYN angina pectoris. [steno- + G. *kardia,* heart]

**sten·o·ceph·a·lous, sten·o·ce·phal·ic** (sten-ō-sef′ă-lŭs, sten-ō-se-fal′ik) pertaining to, or characterized by, stenocephaly.

**sten·o·ceph·a·ly** (sten-ō-sef′ă-lē) marked narrowness of the head. [steno- + G. *kephalē,* head]

**sten·o·cho·ria** (sten-ō-kō′rē-ă) abnormal contraction of any canal or orifice, especially of the lacrimal ducts. [G. *stenochōria,* narrowness, fr. steno- + *chōra,* place, room]

**sten·o·pe·ic, sten·o·pa·ic** (sten-ō-pē′ik, sten-ō-pā′ik) provided with a narrow opening or slit, as in stenopeic spectacles. [steno- + G. *opē,* opening]

**sten·os·al mur·mur** an arterial murmur due to narrowing of the vessel from pressure or organic change.

**ste·nosed** (sten′ōzd) narrowed; contracted: strictured.

**sten·os·ing ten·o·syn·o·vi·tis** inflammation of a tendon and its sheath resulting in contracture of the sheath causing an obstruction of tendon gliding; can be a cause of trigger finger conditions.

**ste·no·sis,** pl. **ste·no·ses** (ste-nō′sis, ste-nō′sēz) a stricture of any canal; especially, a narrowing of one of the cardiac valves. [G. *stenōsis,* a narrowing]

**sten·o·sto·mia** (sten-ō-stō′mē-ă) narrowness of the oral cavity. [steno- + G. *stoma,* mouth]

**sten·o·ther·mal** (sten-ō-ther′măl) thermostable through a narrow temperature range; able to withstand only slight changes in temperature. [steno- + G. *thermē,* heat]

**sten·o·tho·rax** (sten′ō-thōr′aks) a narrow, contracted chest. [steno- + thorax]

**ste·not·ic** (ste-not′ik) narrowed; affected with stenosis.

*Sten·o·tro·pho·mo·nas* (sten′ō-trō-fō-mōn′as) a genus of Gram-negative bacilli that typically reside in soil and water and are not a part of normal human flora.

*Sten·o·tro·pho·mon·as malt·o·phil·i·a* an opportunistic ocular bacterial pathogen producing keratitis, keratopathy, and conjunctivitis; a Gram-negative non-spore-bearing rod, a major emerging nosocomial pathogen, it is of especial importance in intensive care units in part because of its resistance to most penicillins and to cephalosporins and aminoglycosides. Formerly called *Xanthomonas maltophilia* and *Pseudomonas maltophilia.*

**Sten·sen duct, Sten·o duct** (sten′sĕn) SYN parotid duct.

**Stent,** C., English dentist, †1901. SEE stent.

**stent 1.** device used to maintain a bodily orifice or cavity during skin grafting, or to immobilize a skin graft after placement. **2.** slender thread, rod, or catheter, lying within the lumen of tubular structures, used to provide support during or after their anastomosis, or to assure patency of an intact but contracted lumen. See this page. [C. *Stent*]

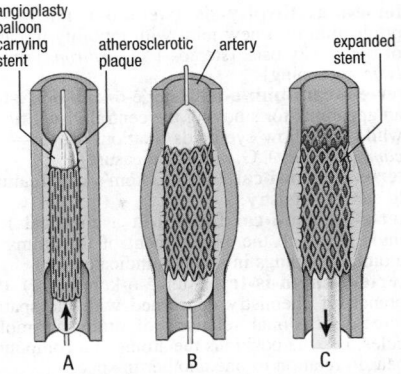

**vascular stent:** (A) balloon catheter positions stent at site of arterial stenosis, (B) inflation of balloon dilates artery and expands stent, (C) balloon is withdrawn, leaving expanded stent in position

**step 1.** DENTISTRY a dovetailed or similarly shaped projection of a cavity prepared in a tooth into a surface perpendicular to the main part of the cavity for the purpose of preventing displacement of the restoration (filling) by the force of mastication. **2.** a change in direction resembling a stairstep in a line, a surface, or the construction of a solid body.

**step-down trans·form·er** device used in radiology to decrease the voltage coming into the x-ray tube.

**ste·pha·ni·al** (ste-fā′nē-ăl) pertaining to the stephanion.

**ste·pha·ni·on** (ste-fā′nē-on) a craniometric point where the coronal suture intersects the inferior temporal line. [G. dim. of *stephanos,* crown]

**step·page gait** a gait in which the advancing foot is lifted higher than usual so that it can clear the ground, because it cannot be dorsiflexed. Seen with peroneal neuropathies and other disorders causing foot dorsiflexion weakness. SEE high-steppage gait.

**step-up trans·form·er** device used in radiology to increase the voltage coming into an x-ray tube.

**ster·co-** feces. SEE ALSO copro-, scato-. [L. *stercus,* excrement]

**ster·co·bi·lin** (ster′kō-bī′lin, ster′kō-bil′in) a brown degradation product of hemoglobin, present in the feces. SEE ALSO bilirubinoids.

**ster·co·lith** (ster′kō-lith) SYN coprolith. [sterco- + G. *lithos,* stone]

**ster·co·ra·ceous, ster·co·ral, ster·co·rous** (ster-kō-rā′shŭs, ster′kō-răl, ster′kō-rŭs) relating to or containing feces.

**ster·co·ra·ceous vom·it·ing** SYN fecal vomiting.

**ster·co·ral ab·scess** a collection of pus and feces. SYN fecal abscess.

**ster·co·ral ul·cer** an ulcer of the colon due to pressure and irritation of retained fecal masses.

**ster·co·ro·ma** (ster-kō-rō′mă) SYN coproma. [sterco- + G. *-oma,* tumor]

**ster·cus** (ster′kŭs) SYN feces. [L. feces, excrement]

**ste•reo-** 1. a solid; a solid condition or state. 2. spatial qualities, three-dimensionality. [G. *stereos,* solid]

**ster•e•o•ar•throl•y•sis** (ster′ē-ō-ar-throl′i-sis) production of a new joint with mobility in cases of bony ankylosis. [stereo- + G. *arthron,* joint, + *lysis,* loosening]

**ster•e•o•cam•pim•e•ter** (ster′ē-ō-kam-pim′ĕ-ter) an apparatus for studying the central visual fields while the fellow eye holds fixation. [stereo- + L. *campus,* field, + G. *metron,* measure]

**ster•e•o•chem•i•cal** (ster′ē-ō-kem′i-kăl) relating to stereochemistry.

**ster•e•o•chem•i•cal for•mu•la** a chemical formula in which the arrangement of the atoms or atomic groupings in space is indicated.

**ster•e•o•chem•is•try** (ster-ē-ō-kem′is-trē) the branch of chemistry concerned with the spatial three-dimensional relations of atoms in molecules, i.e., the positions the atoms in a compound bear in relation to one another in space.

**ster•e•o•e•lec•tro•en•ceph•a•log•ra•phy** (ster-ē-ō-ē-lek′trō-en-sef-ă-log′ră-fē) recording of electrical activity in three planes of the brain, i.e., with surface and depth electrodes.

**ster•e•o•en•ceph•a•lom•e•try** (ster′ē-ō-en-sef′ă-lom′ĕ-trē) the localization of brain structures by use of three-dimensional coordinates.

**ster•e•o•en•ceph•a•lot•o•my** (ster′ē-ō-en-sef′ă-lot′ō-mē) SYN stereotaxy. [stereo- + G. *encephalos,* brain, + *tomē,* a cutting]

**ster•e•og•no•sis** (ster′ē-og′nō′sis) the appreciation of the form of an object by means of touch. [stereo- + G. *gnōsis,* knowledge]

**ster•e•og•nos•tic** (ster′ē-og-nos′tik) relating to stereognosis.

**ster•e•o•i•so•mer** (ster′ē-ō-ī′sō-mer) a molecule containing the same number and kind of atom groupings as another but in a different arrangement in space, in virtue of which it exhibits different optical properties; e.g., as between D and L amino acids, 5α and 5β steroids. Cf. isomer. [stereo- + G. *isos,* equal, + *meros,* part]

**ster•e•o•i•so•mer•ic** (ster′ē-ō-ī-sō-mer′ik) relating to stereoisomerism.

**ster•e•o•i•som•er•ism** (ster′ē-ō-ī-som′er-izm) molecular asymmetry, isomerism involving different spatial arrangements of the same groups. SEE ALSO stereoisomer.

**ster•e•om•e•try** (ster-ē-om′ĕ-trē) 1. measurement of a solid object or the cubic capacity of a vessel. 2. determination of the specific gravity of a liquid.

**ster•e•op•a•thy** (ster-ē-op′ă-thē) persistent stereotyped thinking.

**ster•e•o•ra•di•og•ra•phy** (ster′ē-ō-rā-dē-og′ră-fē) preparation of a pair of radiographs with appropriate shift of the x-ray tube or film so that the images can be viewed stereoscopically to give a three-dimensional appearance.

**ster•e•o•scop•ic** (ster′ē-ō-skop′ik) relating to a stereoscope, or giving the appearance of three dimensions.

**ster•e•o•scop•ic mi•cro•scope** a microscope having double eyepieces and objectives and thus independent light paths, giving a three-dimensional image.

**ster•e•o•scop•ic vi•sion** the single perception of a slightly different image from each eye.

**ster•e•os•co•py** (ster-ē-os′kŏ-pē) an optical technique by which two images of the same object are blended into one, giving a three-dimensional appearance to the single image.

**ster•e•o•tac•tic, ster•e•o•tax•ic** (ster′ē-ō-tak′tik, ster′ē-ō-tak′sik) relating to stereotaxis or stereotaxy.

**ster•e•o•tac•tic bra•chy•ther•a•py** radiotherapy delivered with the help of CT-guided tissue localization.

**ster•e•o•tac•tic in•stru•ment, ster•e•o•tax•ic in•stru•ment** an apparatus attached to the head, used to localize precisely an area in the brain by means of coordinates related to intracerebral structures.

**ster•e•o•tac•tic sur•gery, ster•e•o•tax•ic sur•ger•y** SYN stereotaxy.

**ster•e•o•tax•is** (ster′ē-ō-tak′sis) 1. three-dimensional arrangement. 2. stereotropism, but applied more exactly when the organism as a whole, rather than a part only, reacts. 3. SYN stereotaxy. [stereo- + G. *taxis,* orderly arrangement]

**ster•e•o•taxy** (ster′ē-ō-tak′sē) a precise method of destroying deep-seated brain structures located by use of three-dimensional coordinates. SYN stereoencephalotomy, stereotactic surgery, stereotaxic surgery, stereotaxis (3).

**ster•e•o•tro•pic** (ster′ē-ō-trop′ik) relating to or exhibiting stereotropism.

**ster•e•ot•ro•pism** (ster′ē-ot′rō-pizm) growth or movement of a plant or animal toward (**positive stereotropism**) or away from (**negative stereotropism**) a solid body, usually applied when a part of the organism rather than the whole reacts. [stereo- + G. *tropos,* a turning]

**ster•e•o•typy** (ster′ē-ō-tī-pē) 1. maintenance of one attitude for a long period. 2. constant repetition of certain meaningless gestures or movements, as in certain forms of schizophrenia. [stereo- + G. *typos,* impression, type]

**ste•ric** (ster′ik) pertaining to stereochemistry.

**ster•ile** (ster′il) relating to or characterized by sterility. [L. *sterilis,* barren]

**ster•ile cyst** a hydatid cyst without brood capsules or viable scoleces.

**ste•ril•i•ty** (stĕ-ril′i-tē) 1. in general, the incapability of fertilization or reproduction. 2. condition of being aseptic, or free from all living microorganisms and their spores. [L. *sterilitas*]

**ster•il•i•za•tion** (ster′ĭ-li-zā′shŭn) 1. the act or process by which an individual is rendered incapable of fertilization or reproduction, as by vasectomy, partial salpingectomy, or castration. 2. the destruction of all microorganisms in or about an object, as by steam (flowing or pressurized), chemical agents (alcohol, phenol, heavy metals, ethylene oxide gas), high-velocity electron bombardment, ultraviolet light radiation.

**ster•il•ize** (ster′ĭ-līz) to produce sterility.

**ster•il•iz•er** (ster′i-lī-zer) an apparatus for rendering objects sterile.

**ster•na** (ster′nă) plural of sternum.

**ster•nal** (ster′năl) relating to the sternum.

**ster•nal an•gle** the angle between the manubrium and the body of the sternum at the manubriosternal junction. Marks the level of the second costal cartilage (rib) for counting ribs or intercostal spaces. Denotes level of aortic arch, bifurcation of trachea, and T4-T5 intervertebral disc. SYN angulus sterni [TA], Louis angle, Ludwig angle.

**ster•nal•gia** (ster-nal′jē-ă) pain in the sternum or the sternal region. SYN sternodynia. [stern- + G. *algos,* pain]

**ster·na·lis mus·cle** an inconstant muscle, running parallel to the sternum across the costosternal origin of the pectoralis major, and usually connected with the sternocleidomastoid and rectus abdominis muscles due to their common development source. SYN musculus sternalis [TA], sternal muscle.

**ster·nal line** a vertical line corresponding to the lateral margin of the sternum. SYN linea sternalis [TA].

**ster·nal mus·cle** SYN sternalis muscle.

**ster·nal plane** a plane indicated by the front surface of the sternum.

**ster·nal punc·ture** removal of bone marrow from the manubrium by needle.

**ster·ne·bra,** pl. **ster·ne·brae** (ster′nē-bră, ster′nē-brē) one of the four segments of the primordial sternum of the embryo by the fusion of which the body of the adult sternum is formed. [Mod. L. fr. stern(um) + (vert)ebra]

△**ster·no-, stern-** the sternum, sternal. [G. *sternon,* chest]

**ster·no·cla·vic·u·lar** (ster′nō-kla-vik′yu-lăr) relating to the sternum and the clavicle.

**ster·no·cla·vic·u·lar an·gle** the angle formed by the junction of the clavicle with the sternum.

**ster·no·cla·vic·u·lar joint** the synovial articulation between the medial end of the clavicle and the manubrium of the sternum and cartilage of the first rib.

**ster·no·clei·do·mas·toid** (ster′nō-klī′dō-mas′toyd) relating to sternum, clavicle, and mastoid process.

**ster·no·clei·do·mas·toid mus·cle (SCM)** *origin,* by two heads from anterior surface of manubrium of the sternum and sternal end of clavicle; *insertion,* mastoid process and lateral half of superior nuchal line; *action,* turns head obliquely to opposite side; when acting together, flex the neck and extend the head; *nerve supply,* motor by accessory, sensory by cervical plexus. SYN musculus sternocleidomastoideus [TA], sternomastoid muscle.

**ster·no·clei·do·mas·toid vein** arises in the sternocleidomastoid muscle and accompanies the sternocleidomastoid branch of the occipital artery; it drains into the internal jugular or superior thyroid vein.

**ster·no·cos·tal** (ster′nō-kos′tăl) relating to the sternum and the ribs. [L. *costa,* rib]

**ster·no·dyn·ia** (ster-nō-din′ē-ă) SYN sternalgia. [sterno- + G. *odynē,* pain]

**ster·no·glos·sal** (ster-nō-glos′ăl) denoting muscular fibers that occasionally pass from the sternohyoid muscle to join the hyoglossal muscle.

**ster·no·hy·oid mus·cle** *origin,* posterior surface of manubrium sterni and first costal cartilage; *insertion,* body of hyoid bone; *action,* depresses hyoid bone; *nerve supply,* upper cervical via spinal nerves (ansa cervicalis). SYN musculus sternohyoideus [TA].

**ster·noid** (ster′noyd) resembling the sternum. [sterno- + G. *eidos,* resemblance]

**ster·no·mas·toid mus·cle** SYN sternocleidomastoid muscle.

**ster·no·pa·gia** (ster-nō-pā′jē-ă) condition shown by conjoined twins united at the sterna or more extensively at the ventral walls of the chest. SEE conjoined twins. [sterno- + G. *pagos,* something fixed]

**ster·no·per·i·car·di·al** (ster′nō-per′i-kar′dē-ăl) relating to the sternum and the pericardium.

**ster·nos·chi·sis** (ster-nos′ki-sis) congenital cleft of the sternum. [sterno- + G. *schisis,* a cleaving]

**ster·no·thy·roid mus·cle** *origin,* posterior surface of manubrium of sternum and first or second costal cartilage; *insertion,* oblique line of thyroid cartilage; *action,* depresses larynx; *nerve supply,* upper cervical via spinal nerves (ansa cervicalis). SYN musculus sternothyroideus [TA].

**ster·not·o·my** (ster-not′ō-mē) incision into or through the sternum. [sterno- + G. *tomē,* incision]

**ster·no·ver·te·bral** (ster′nō-ver′tĕ-brăl) relating to the sternum and the vertebrae; denoting the true ribs, or the 7 upper ribs on either side, which articulate with the vertebrae and with the sternum. SYN vertebrosternal.

**Stern pos·ture** (stern) a supine position with the head extended and lowered over the end of the table, by which the murmur is developed or made more distinct in cases of tricuspid insufficiency.

**ster·num,** gen. **ster·ni,** pl. **ster·na** (ster′nŭm, ster′nī, ster′nă) [TA] a long, flat bone, articulating with the cartilages of the first seven ribs and with the clavicle, that forms the middle part of the anterior wall of the thorax; it consists of three portions: the corpus or body, the manubrium, and the xiphoid process. SYN breast bone. [Mod. L. fr. G. *sternon,* the chest]

**ster·nu·ta·tion** (ster′noo-tā′shŭn) the act of sneezing. [L. *sternutatio,* fr. *sternuo (sternuto),* pp. *sternutatus,* to sneeze]

**ste·roid** (ster′oyd) **1.** pertaining to the steroids. SYN steroidal. Cf. steroids. **2.** one of the steroids. **3.** generic designation for compounds closely related in structure to the steroids, such as sterols, bile acids, cardiac glycosides, and precursors of the D vitamins.

**ster·oid ac·ne** folliculitis similar to acne vulgaris, but resulting from topical or oral administration of steroids; comedones are rare.

**ste·roi·dal** (ster′oy-dăl) SYN steroid (1).

**ster·oid cell tu·mor** a collective term used for ovarian tumors composed of cells resembling steroid-secreting lutein cells; comprises several tumors such as stromal luteoma, Leydig cell tumor, steroid cell tumor not otherwise specified; hormonally active; may be benign or malignant.

**ster·oid hor·mones** those hormones possessing the steroid ring system; e.g., androgens, estrogens, adrenocortical hormones.

**ste·roi·do·gen·e·sis** (ster′oy-dō-jen′ĕ-sis) the formation of steroids; commonly referring to the biological synthesis of steroid hormones, but not to the production of such compounds in a chemical laboratory. [steroid + G. *genesis,* production]

**ster·oids** (ster′oydz) a large family of chemical substances, comprising many hormones, body constituents, and drugs, each containing the tetracyclic cyclopenta[*a*]phenanthrene skeleton.

**ster·oid ul·cer** an ulcer, usually on the leg or foot, developing from a wound in patients undergoing long-term steroid therapy; results from the wound-healing inhibitory effects characteristic of steroids.

**ste·rol** (ster′ol) a steroid with one OH (alcohol) group; the systematic names contain either the prefix hydroxy- or the suffix -ol, e.g., cholesterol, ergosterol.

**ster·tor** (ster′tōr) a noisy inspiration occurring in

coma or deep sleep, sometimes due to obstruction of the larynx or upper airways. [L. *sterto*, to snore]

**ster•to•rous** (ster'tōr-ŭs) relating to or characterized by stertor or snoring.

△**ste•tho-, steth-** the chest. [G. *stēthos*]

**steth•o•go•ni•om•e•ter** (steth'ō-gō-nē-om'ĕ-ter) an apparatus for measuring the curvatures of the thorax. [stetho- + G. *gōnia*, angle, + *metron*, measure]

**steth•o•scope** (steth'ō-skōp) an instrument originally devised by Laënnec for aid in hearing the respiratory and cardiac sounds in the chest, but now modified in various ways and used in auscultation of any of vascular or other sounds anywhere in the body. [stetho- + G. *skopeō*, to view]

**steth•o•scop•ic** (steth-ō-skop'ik) **1.** relating to or effected by means of a stethoscope. **2.** relating to an examination of the chest.

**ste•thos•co•py** (stĕ-thos'kŏ-pē) **1.** examination of the chest by means of auscultation, either mediate or immediate, and percussion. **2.** mediate auscultation with the stethoscope.

**steth•o•spasm** (steth'ō-spazm) spasm of the chest.

**Ste•vens-John•son syn•drome** (stē'vens-jon'son) a bullous form of erythema multiforme which may be extensive, involving the mucous membranes and large areas of the body; it may produce serious subjective symptoms and may have a fatal termination.

**Stew•art-Holmes sign** (stoo'ĕrt-hōmz) in cerebellar disease, the inability to check a movement when passive resistance is suddenly released. SYN rebound phenomenon (1).

**Stew•art test** (stoo'ĕrt) estimation of the amount of collateral circulation, in case of an aneurysm of the main artery of a limb, by means of a calorimeter.

**Stew•art-Treves syn•drome** (stoo'ĕrt-trēvz) angiosarcoma arising in an arm affected by postmastectomy lymphedema.

**sthe•nia** (sthē'nē-ă) a condition of activity and apparent force, as in an acute sthenic fever. [G. *sthenos*, strength, + *-ia*, condition]

**sthen•ic** (sthen'ik) **1.** active; marked by sthenia; said of a fever with strong bounding pulse, high temperature, and active delirium. **2.** pertaining to a habitus characterized by moderate overdevelopment of skeletal muscle.

△**sthe•no-** strength, force, power. [G. *sthenos*]

**stib•i•al•ism** (stib'ē-ă-lizm) chronic antimonial poisoning. [L. *stibium*, antimony]

**Stick•ler syn•drome** (shtik'ler) SYN hereditary progressive arthroophthalmopathy.

**sticky-end•ed DNA** double-stranded DNA in which one of the strands extends beyond the other strand (i.e., has a number of unpaired bases) at one end or both.

**stiff man syn•drome** a rare disorder manifested clinically by the continuous isometric contraction of many of the somatic muscles; contractions are usually forceful and painful and most frequently involve the trunk musculature, although limb muscles may be involved. This is an autoimmune disease, with circulating antibodies against the GABA-synthesizing enzyme and glutamic acid decarboxylase, among other types of antibodies present.

**stiff neck** nonspecific term for limited neck mo-

bility, often due to muscle cramps and spasm accompanied by pain.

**stig•ma**, pl. **stig•mas**, **stig•ma•ta** (stig'mă, stig'măs, stig'mă-tă) **1.** visible evidence of a disease. **2.** SYN follicular stigma. **3.** any spot or blemish on the skin. **4.** a bleeding spot on the skin, which is considered a manifestation of conversion hysteria. **5.** the orange pigmented eyespot of certain chlorophyll-bearing protozoa, such as *Euglena viridis*, which serves as a light filter by absorbing certain wavelengths. **6.** a mark of shame or discredit. [G. a mark. fr. *stizō*, to prick]

**stig•mal plates** area in arthropod larvae where the tracheal system opens to the outside; morphology of this area is used to identify various arthropod larvae.

**stig•mat•ic** (stig-mat'ik) relating to or marked by a stigma.

**stig•ma•tism** (stig'mă-tizm) the condition of having a stigma. SYN stigmatization (1).

**stig•ma•ti•za•tion** (stig'mă-ti-zā'shŭn) **1.** SYN stigmatism. **2.** production of stigmas, especially of a hysterical nature. **3.** debasement of a person by the attribution of a negatively toned characteristic or other stigma.

**stil•bene** (stil'bēn) **1.** an unsaturated hydrocarbon, the nucleus of stilbestrol and other synthetic estrogenic compounds. **2.** a class of compounds based on stilbene (1).

**stil•boes•trol [Br.]** SYN diethylstilbestrol.

**still•birth** (stil'berth) the birth of an infant that has died before delivery.

**still•born** (stil'bōrn) born dead; denoting an infant dead at birth.

**still•born in•fant** an infant who shows no evidence of life after birth. Cf. liveborn infant.

**Still dis•ease** (stil) a form of juvenile chronic arthritis (formerly juvenile rheumatoid arthritis) characterized by high fever and signs of systemic illness that can exist for months before the onset of arthritis.

**still lay•er** the layer of the bloodstream in the capillary vessels, next to the wall of the vessel, that flows slowly and transports the white blood cells along the layer wall, while in the center the flow is rapid and transports the red blood cells. SYN Poiseuille space.

**Still mur•mur** (stil) an innocent musical murmur resembling the noise produced by a twanging string; almost exclusively in young children, of uncertain origin and ultimately disappearing.

**stim•u•lant** (stim'yu-lănt) **1.** stimulating; exciting to action. **2.** an agent that arouses organic activity, strengthens the action of the heart, increases vitality, and promotes a sense of well-being; classified according to the parts upon which they chiefly act: cardiac, respiratory, gastric, hepatic, cerebral, spinal, vascular, genital, etc. SYN stimulator. SEE ALSO stimulus. [L. *stimulans*, pres. p. of *stimulo*, pp. *-atus*, to goad, incite, fr. *stimulus*, a goad]

**stim•u•la•tion** (stim-yu-lā'shŭn) **1.** arousal of the body or any of its parts or organs to increased functional activity. **2.** the condition of being stimulated. **3.** NEUROPHYSIOLOGY the application of a stimulus to a responsive structure, such as a nerve or muscle, regardless of whether the strength of the stimulus is sufficient to produce excitation. [see stimulant]

**stim•u•la•tor** (stim'yu-lā-ter) SYN stimulant (2).

**stim•u•lus**, pl. **stim•u•li** (stim'yu-lŭs, stim'yu-lī)

**1.** a stimulant. **2.** that which can elicit or evoke action (response) in a muscle, nerve, gland or other excitable tissue, or cause an augmenting action upon any function or metabolic process. [L. a goad]

**stim•u•lus con•trol** the use of conditioning techniques to bring the target behavior of an individual under environmental control.

**stim•u•lus sen•si•tive my•o•clo•nus** myoclonus induced by a variety of stimuli, e.g., talking, calculation, loud noises, tapping, etc.

**sting 1.** sharp momentary pain, most commonly produced by the puncture of the skin by many species of arthropods, including hexapods, myriapods, and arachnids; can also be produced by jellyfish, sea urchins, sponges, mollusks, and several species of venomous fish, such as the stingray, toadfish, rabbitfish, and catfish. SEE ALSO bites. **2.** the venom apparatus of a stinging animal, consisting of a chitinous spicule or bony spine and a venom gland or sac. **3.** to introduce (or the process of introducing) a venom by stinging. [O.E. *stingan*]

**sting•ing cat•er•pil•lar** caterpillar with urticarious hairs or spines that cause allergic dermatitis, e.g., the Io moth and the puss caterpillar.

**stip•pling** (stip'ling) **1.** a speckling of a blood cell or other structure with fine dots when exposed to the action of a basic stain, due to the presence of free basophil granules in the cell protoplasm. **2.** an orange peel appearance of the attached gingiva. **3.** a roughening of the surfaces of a denture base to stimulate natural gingival stippling.

**Stir•ling mod•i•fi•ca•tion of Gram stain** (stirl'ing, gram) a stable aniline-crystal violet stain.

**stir•rup** (stěr'ŭp) SYN stapes. [A.S. *stīrāp*]

**stitch 1.** a sharp sticking pain of momentary duration. **2.** a single suture. **3.** SYN suture (2). [A.S. *stice,* a pricking]

**stitch ab•scess** an abscess around a suture.

**St. John's wort** a shrubby perennial (*Hypericum perforatum*) with numerous orange-yellow flowers whose petals may be speckled black along their margins; a herbal antidepressant that compares favorably with standard synthetic psychopharmaceutical agents in the treatment of mild to moderate depression.

**St. Lou•is en•ceph•a•li•tis vi•rus** a group B arbovirus often causing inapparent infection but sometimes encephalitis; the virus has been isolated from birds in Panama and from several mosquito species, especially *Psorophora.*

**STM** short-term memory.

**stock cul•ture** a culture of a microorganism maintained solely for the purpose of keeping the microorganism in a viable condition by subculture, as necessary, into fresh medium.

**Stock•er line** (stŏ'kĕr) a fine line of pigment in the corneal epithelium near the head of a pterygium.

**Stock•holm syn•drome** (stok'ehōm) a form of bonding between a captive and captor in which the captive begins to identify with, and may even sympathize with, the captor. [*Stockholm,* Sweden, where early cases reported]

**stock•ing an•es•the•sia** loss of sensation in the distal lower extremity, i.e., the foot and toes.

**stock vac•cine** a vaccine made from a stock microbial strain, in contradistinction to an autogenous vaccine.

**Stof•fel op•er•a•tion** (shtaw'fel) division of cer-

tain motor nerves for the relief of spastic paralysis.

**sto•i•chi•o•lo•gy [Br.]** the study of the elements of any branch of knowledge.

**stoi•chi•o•met•ric** (stoy'kē-ō-met'rik) pertaining to stoichiometry.

**sto•i•chi•o•met•ric num•ber** (v) the number associated with a reactant or product participating in a defined chemical reaction; usually an integer.

**stoi•chi•om•e•try** (stoy-kē-om'ě-trē) determination of the relative quantities of the substances concerned in any chemical reaction; e.g., with the laws of definite proportions in chemistry, as in the molar proportions in a reaction. [G. *stoicheion,* element, + *metron,* measure]

**stoke** (stōk) a unit of kinematic viscosity, that of a fluid with a viscosity of 1 poise and a density of 1 g/ml; equal to $10^{-4}$ square meter per second. [Sir George Gabriel *Stokes*]

**Stokes-Ad•ams syn•drome** (stōks-a'dămz) SYN Adams-Stokes syndrome.

**Stokes am•pu•ta•tion** (stōks) a modification of the Gritti-Stokes amputation in that the line of section of the femur is slightly higher.

**Stokes law** (stōks) **1.** a muscle lying above an inflamed mucous or serous membrane is frequently the seat of paralysis; **2.** a relationship of the rate of fall of a small sphere in a viscous fluid; applicable to centrifugation of macromolecules; **3.** the wavelength of light emitted by a fluorescent material is longer than that of the radiation used to excite the fluorescence.

**sto•ma,** pl. **sto•mas, sto•ma•ta** (stō'mă, stō'maz, stō'mă-tă) **1.** a minute opening or pore. **2.** an artificial opening between two cavities or canals, or between such and the surface of the body. [G. a mouth]

**sto•ma blast** sound produced by forceful expiration of air through a tracheal stoma.

**sto•ma but•ton** short plastic tube with collar inserted into a tracheal stoma to maintain or enlarge it.

**stom•ach** (stŭm'ŭk) a large, irregularly piriform sac between the esophagus and the small intestine, lying just beneath the diaphragm. Its wall has four coats or tunics: mucous, submucous, muscular, and peritoneal; the muscular coat is composed of three layers, the fibers running longitudinally in the outer, circularly in the middle, and obliquely in the inner layer. SYN gaster [TA], ventriculus (1). [G. *stomachos,* L. *stomachus*]

**stom•ach ache** pain in the abdomen, usually arising in the stomach or intestine.

**stom•ach•al** (stŭm'ă-kăl) relating to the stomach.

**stom•ach pump** an apparatus for removing the contents of the stomach by means of suction.

**stom•ach tube** a flexible tube passed into the stomach for lavage or feeding.

**sto•mal** (stō'măl) relating to a stoma.

**sto•mal ul•cer** an intestinal ulcer occurring after gastrojejunostomy in the jejunal mucosa near the opening (stoma) between the stomach and the jejunum.

**sto•ma•ta** (stō'mă-tă) alternate plural of stoma.

**sto•ma•tal•gia** (stō-mă-tal'jē-ă) pain in the mouth. SYN stomatodynia. [stomat- + G. *algos,* pain]

**sto•ma•ti•tis** (stō-mă-tī'tis) inflammation of the mucous membrane of the mouth. [stomat- + G. *-itis,* inflammation]

S
t

**sto·ma·ti·tis me·di·ca·men·to·sa** inflammatory alterations of the oral mucosa associated with a systemic drug allergy; lesions may consist of erythema, vesicles, bullae, ulcerations, or angioneurotic edema.

△**sto·ma·to-, sto·mat-, stom-** mouth. [G. *stoma*]

**sto·ma·to·cy·to·sis** (stō′mă-tō-sī-tō′sis) a hereditary deformation of red blood cells, which are swollen and cup-shaped, causing congenital hemolytic anemia. SEE ALSO Rh null syndrome.

**sto·ma·to·dyn·ia** (stō′mă-tō-din′ē-ă) SYN stomatalgia. [stomato- + G. *odynē*, pain]

**sto·ma·to·gnath·ic sys·tem** all of the structures involved in speech and in the reception, mastication, and deglutition of food.

**sto·ma·to·ma·la·cia** (stō′mă-tō-mă-lā′shē-ă) pathologic softening of any of the structures of the mouth. [stomato- + G. *malakia*, softness]

**sto·ma·to·my·co·sis** (stō′mă-tō-mī-kō′sis) disease of the mouth due to the presence of a fungus. [stomato- + G. *mykēs*, fungus, + *-osis*, condition]

**sto·ma·to·ne·cro·sis** (stō′mă-tō-ně-krō′sis) SYN noma. [stomato- + G. *nekrōsis*, death]

**sto·ma·top·a·thy** (stō-mă-top′ă-thē) any disease of the oral cavity. [stomato- + G. *pathos*, suffering]

**sto·ma·to·plas·tic** (stō′mă-tō-plas′tik) relating to stomatoplasty.

**sto·ma·to·plas·ty** (stō′mă-tō-plas-tē) plastic surgery of the mouth. [stomato- + G. *plastos*, formed]

**sto·ma·tor·rha·gia** (stō′mă-tō-rā′jē-ă) bleeding from the gums or other part of the oral cavity. [stomato- + G. *rhēgnymi*, to burst forth]

**sto·mo·de·al** (stō′mō-dē′ăl) relating to a stomodeum.

**sto·mo·de·um** (stō-mō-dē′ŭm) **1.** a midline ectodermal depression ventral to the embryonic brain and surrounded by the mandibular arch; when the buccopharyngeal membrane disappears, it becomes continuous with the foregut and forms the mouth. **2.** the anterior portion of the insect alimentary canal. [Mod. L. fr. G. *stoma*, mouth, + *hodaios*, on the way, fr. *hodos*, a way]

△**-sto·my** artificial or surgical opening. SEE stomato-. [G. *stoma*, mouth]

**stone** (stōn) **1.** SYN calculus. **2.** an English unit of weight of the human body, equal to 14 pounds. [A.S. *stān*]

**stone heart** SYN ischemic contracture of the left ventricle.

**Stook·ey-Scarff op·er·a·tion** (stoo′kē-skahrf) SEE third ventriculostomy.

**stool** (stool) **1.** a discharging of the bowels. **2.** the matter discharged at one movement of the bowels. SYN evacuation (2). SYN movement (2). [A.S. *stōl*, seat]

**stop·ping rules** in randomized controlled trials and other systematic experiments on human subjects, rules laid down in advance that specify conditions under which the experiment will be terminated, e.g., unequivocal demonstration that one regimen in a randomized controlled trial is clearly superior to the other, or that one is clearly harmful.

**stor·age** (stōr′ij) the second stage in the memory process, following encoding and preceding retrieval, involving mental processes associated with retention of stimuli that have been registered and modified by encoding. SEE memory.

**stor·age dis·ease** any accumulation of a specific substance within tissues, generally because of congenital deficiency of an enzyme necessary for further metabolism of the substance; e.g., glycogen-storage diseases.

**STORCH** syphilis, *t*oxoplasmosis, *o*ther infections, *r*ubella, *c*ytomegalovirus infection, and *h*erpes simplex; fetal infections that can cause congenital malformations. SEE ALSO TORCH.

**sto·ri·form** (stōr′i-fōrm) having a cartwheel pattern, as of spindle cells with elongated nuclei radiating from a center. [L. *storea*, woven mat, + *-formis*, form]

**storm** (stōrm) an exacerbation of symptoms or a crisis in the course of a disease.

**STPD** symbol indicating that a gas volume has been expressed as if it were at standard temperature (0°C), standard pressure (760 mmHg absolute), dry; under these conditions a mole of gas occupies 22.4 liters.

**stra·bis·mal** (stra-biz′măl) relating to or affected with strabismus.

**stra·bis·mus** (stra-biz′mŭs) a manifest lack of parallelism of the visual axes of the eyes. SYN crossed eyes, cross-eye, heterotropia, heterotropy, squint. [Mod. L., fr. G. *strabismos*, a squinting]

**straight gy·rus** a gyrus running along the medial part of the orbital surface of the frontal lobe of the cerebral hemisphere. It is bounded laterally by the olfactory sulcus.

**straight sem·i·nif·er·ous tu·bule** the continuation of the tubulus seminifer contortus which becomes straight just before entering the mediastinum to form the rete testis. SYN vasa recta (2).

**straight si·nus** an unpaired dural venous sinus in the posterior part of the falx cerebri where it is attached to the tentorium cerebelli; it is formed anteriorly by the merging of the great cerebral vein with the inferior sagittal sinus, and passes horizontally and posteriorly to the confluence of sinuses. SYN tentorial sinus.

**strain** (strān) **1.** a population of homogeneous organisms possessing a set of defined characters; in bacteriology, the set of descendants that retains the characteristics of the ancestor; members of a strain that subsequently differ from the original isolate are regarded as belonging either to a substrain of the original strain, or to a new strain **2.** specific host cell(s) designed or selected to optimize production of recombinant products. [A.S. *stryand; strēon*, gain, begetting] **3.** to make an effort to the limit of one's strength. **4.** to injure by overuse or improper use. **5.** an act of straining. **6.** injury resulting from strain or overuse. **7.** the change in shape that a body undergoes when acted upon by an external stress. **8.** to filter; to percolate. [L. *stringere*, to bind]

**strain-coun·ter·strain** SYN muscle energy technique.

**strain frac·ture** the tearing off, by a sudden force, of a piece of bone attached to a tendon, ligament, or capsule.

**strait** (strāt) a narrow passageway. **inferior strait**, apertura pelvis inferior; **superior strait**, apertura pelvis superior. [M.E. *streit* thr. O. Fr. fr. L. *strictus*, drawn together, tight]

**strait·jack·et** (strāt′jak-et) a garment-like device with long sleeves that can be secured to restrain a violently disturbed person.

**stran·gle** (strang′gl) to suffocate; to choke; to

compress the trachea so as to prevent sufficient passage of air. [G. *strangaloō*, to choke, fr. *strangalē*, a halter]

**stran·gu·lat·ed** (strang'gyu-lā-ted) constricted so as to prevent sufficient passage of air, as through the trachea, or to cut off venous return and/or arterial air flow, as in the case of a hernia. [L. *strangulo*, pp. *-atus*, to choke, fr. G. *strangaloō*, to choke (strangle)]

**stran·gu·lat·ed her·nia** an irreducible hernia in which the circulation is arrested; gangrene occurs unless relief is prompt.

**stran·gu·la·tion** (strang'gyu-lā'shŭn) the act of strangulating or the condition of being strangulated, in any sense.

**stran·gu·ry** (strang'gyu-rē) difficulty in micturition, the urine being passed drop by drop with pain and tenesmus. [G. *stranx* (strang-), something squeezed out, a drop, + *ouron,* urine]

**strap 1.** a strip of adhesive plaster. **2.** to apply overlapping strips of adhesive plaster. [A.S. *stropp*]

**strap cell** an elongated tumor cell of uniform width that may show cross-striations; found in rhabdomyosarcoma.

**stra·ta** (strā'tă) plural of stratum.

**strat·i·fi·ca·tion** (strat'i-fi-kā'shŭn) the process or result of separating a sample into subsamples according to specified criteria such as age or occupational groups. [L. *stratum,* layer, + *facio,* to make]

**strat·i·fied** (strat'i-fīd) arranged in the form of layers or strata.

**strat·i·fied ep·i·the·li·um** a type of epithelium composed of a series of layers, the cells of each varying in size and shape. It is named more specifically according to the type of cells at the surface, e.g., stratified squamous epithelium, stratified columnar epithelium, stratified ciliated columnar epithelium. SYN laminated epithelium.

**stra·tig·ra·phy** (stra-tig'ră-fē) SYN tomography. [L. *stratum,* layer, + G. *graphē,* a writing]

**stra·tum,** gen. **stra·ti,** pl. **stra·ta** (strat'ŭm, strā' tī, strā'tă) one of the layers of differentiated tissue, the aggregate of which forms any given structure, such as the retina or the skin. SEE ALSO lamina, layer. [L. *sterno,* pp. *stratus,* to spread out, strew, ntr. of pp. as noun, *stratum,* a bed cover, layer]

**stra·tum ba·sa·le 1.** the outermost layer of the endometrium which undergoes only minimal changes during the menstrual cycle; SYN basal layer. **2.** SYN stratum basale epidermidis.

**stra·tum ba·sa·le ep·i·derm·i·dis** the deepest layer of the epidermis, composed of dividing stem cells and anchoring cells. SYN stratum basale (2).

**stra·tum com·pac·tum** the superficial layer of decidual tissue in the pregnant uterus, in which the interglandular tissue preponderates.

**stra·tum cor·ne·um ep·i·der·mi·dis** the outermost layer of the epidermis, consisting of nonliving, nonnucleated, fully keratinized epithelial cells about to be lost by desquamation. SYN corneal layer, horny layer.

**stra·tum func·tio·na·le** the endometrium except for the stratum basale; formerly believed to be lost during menstruation but now considered to be only partially disrupted.

**stra·tum lu·ci·dum** a layer of lightly staining corneocytes in the deepest level of the stratum

corneum; found primarily in the thick epidermis of the palmar and plantar skin. SYN clear layer of epidermis.

**stra·tum spi·no·sum ep·i·derm·i·dis** the layer of polyhedral cells in the epidermis; shrinkage artifacts and adhesion of these cells at their desmosomal junctions give a spiny or prickly appearance. SYN prickle cell layer, spinous layer.

**stra·tum spon·gi·o·sum** the middle layer of the endometrium formed chiefly of dilated glandular structures; it is flanked by the compacta on the luminal side and the basalis on the myometrial side.

**Straus sign** (strows) in facial paralysis, if an injection of pilocarpine is followed by sweating on the affected side later than on the other, the lesion is peripheral.

**straw·ber·ry cer·vix** macular erythema of the uterine cervix, characteristic of vaginitis due to *Trichomonas vaginalis.*

**straw·ber·ry he·man·gi·o·ma** hyperproliferation of immature capillary vessels, usually on the head and neck, present at birth or within the first two to three months postnatally, which commonly regresses without scar formation.

**straw·ber·ry ne·vus, straw·ber·ry mark** a small nevus vascularis (capillary hemangioma) resembling a strawberry in size, shape, and color; it usually disappears spontaneously in early childhood. SEE capillary hemangioma.

**straw·ber·ry tongue** a tongue with a whitish coat through which the enlarged fungiform papillae project as red points, characteristic of scarlet fever and mucocutaneous lymph node syndrome.

**straw itch, straw-bed itch** an urticarial eruption caused by the mite, *Pyemotes ventricosus,* which can infest straw used in mattresses.

**stray light** radiant energy that reaches the detector of a spectrophotometer and consists of wavelengths other than those selected.

**streak** (strēk) a line, stria, or stripe, especially one that is indistinct or evanescent. [A.S. *strica*]

**streak cul·ture** a culture produced by lightly stroking an inoculating needle or loop with inoculum over the surface of a solid medium.

**stream·ing move·ment, stream·ing** (strēm'ing) the form of movement characteristic of the protoplasm of leukocytes, amebae, and other unicellular organisms; it involves the massing of the protoplasm at a point where surface pressure is least and its extrusion in the form of a pseudopod; the protoplasm may return to the body of the cell, resulting in the retraction of the pseudopod, or the entire mass may flow into the latter and thereby result in locomotion of the cell.

**street drug** a controlled substance taken for nonmedical purposes. Street drugs comprise various amphetamines, anesthetics, barbiturates, opiates, and psychoactive drugs, and many are derived from natural sources (e.g., the plants *Papaver somniferum, Cannibis sativa, Amanita pantherina, Lophophora williamsii*). Slang names include acid (lysergic acid diethylamide), angel dust (phencyclidine), coke (cocaine), downers (barbiturates), grass (marijuana), hash (concentrated tetrahydrocannibinol), magic mushrooms (psilocybin), and speed (amphetamines). During the 1980s, a new class of "designer drugs" arose, mostly analogs of psychoactive substances intended to escape regulation under the Controlled Substances Act. Also, crack cocaine, a potent,

s
t

smokable form of cocaine, emerged as a major public health problem. In the U.S., illicit use of drugs such as cocaine, marijuana, and heroin historically has occurred in cycles.

**Street·er de·vel·op·men·tal ho·ri·zon(s)** (strē′tĕr) a term borrowed from geology and archeology by Streeter to define 23 developmental stages in young human embryos, from fertilization through the first 2 months; each horizon spanned 2–3 days and emphasized specific anatomic characteristics, to avoid discrepancies in the determination of age and body dimensions. [G.L. Streeter]

**street vi·rus** an isolate of rabies virus from a naturally infected domestic animal.

**strength 1.** the quality of being strong or powerful. **2.** the degree of intensity. **3.** the property of materials by which they endure the application of force without yielding or breaking. **4.** OCCUPATIONAL THERAPY demonstration of degree of muscle power when movement is resisted, as with objects or gravity.

**streph·o·sym·bo·lia** (stref′ō-sim-bō′lē-ă) **1.** generally, the perception of objects reversed as if in a mirror. **2.** specifically, difficulty in distinguishing written or printed letters that extend in opposite directions but are otherwise similar, such as *p* and *d*, or related kinds of mirror reversal. [G. *strephō*, to turn, + *symbolon*, a mark or sign]

**strep·ta·vi·din** (strep-ta-vī′din) a bacterial protein used as a probe in immunologic assays because of its strong affinity and specificity for biotin; streptavidin is used as a bridge to link a chromogen to a biotinylated substrate specific for the substance of interest. [*strept*ococcus + avidin]

**strep·ti·ce·mia** (strep-ti-sē′mē-ă) SYN streptococcemia.

⌂**strep·to-** curved or twisted (usually relating to organisms thus described). [G. *streptos*, twisted, fr. *strephō*, to twist]

**Strep·to·ba·cil·lus** (strep-tō-ba-sil′ŭs) a genus of nonmotile, non-spore-forming, aerobic to facultatively anaerobic bacteria containing Gram-negative, pleomorphic cells which vary from short rods to long, interwoven filaments which have a tendency to fragment into chains of bacillary and coccobacillary elements. The type species, *Streptobacillus moniliformis.*, causes Haverhill fever and rat-bite fever. [strepto- + bacillus]

**strep·to·coc·cal** (strep′tō-kok′ăl) relating to or caused by any organism of the genus *Streptococcus.*

**strep·to·coc·cal tox·ic shock syn·drome** a toxic syndrome characterized by hypotension and a variety of signs and symptoms indicative of multiorgan failure including cerebral dysfunction, renal failure, acute respiratory distress syndrome, toxic cardiomyopathy, and hepatic dysfunction. The syndrome is usually precipitated by local infections of skin or soft tissue by streptococci; mortality of 30% has been reported.

**strep·to·coc·ce·mia** (strep′tō-kok-sē′mē-ă) the presence of streptococci in the blood. SYN strepticemia, streptosepticemia. [streptococcus + G. *haima,* blood]

⊟**strep·to·coc·ci** (strep′tō-kok′sī) plural of streptococcus. See page B3.

α**-strep·to·coc·ci** streptococci that form a green variety of reduced hemoglobin in the area of the colony on a blood agar medium.

**strep·to·coc·cic** (strep′tō-kok′sik) relating to or

caused by any organism of the genus *Streptococcus.*

**Strep·to·coc·cus** (strep-tō-kok′ŭs) a genus of nonmotile, non-spore-forming, aerobic to facultatively anaerobic bacteria containing Gram-positive, spherical, or ovoid cells which occur in pairs or short or long chains. These organisms occur regularly in the mouth and intestines of humans and other animals, in dairy and other food products, and in fermenting plant juices. Some species are pathogenic. [strepto- + G. *kokkos,* berry (coccus)]

**strep·to·coc·cus,** pl. **strep·to·coc·ci** (strep′tō-kok′ŭs, strep′tō-kok′sī) a term used to refer to any member of the genus *Streptococcus.*

**strep·to·coc·cus e·ryth·ro·gen·ic tox·in** a culture filtrate of lysogenized group A strains of β-hemolytic streptococci, erythrogenic when inoculated into the skin of persons susceptible to scarlet fever, and neutralized by antibodies that appear during scarlet fever convalescence. SYN erythrogenic toxin.

***Strep·to·coc·cus in·ter·me·di·us*** one of a heterogenous group of streptococci, generally found in the mouth or upper respiratory tract; classification is generally established by fermentation patterns, analysis of the sugar composition of the cell wall, and use of sugar production patterns.

***Strep·to·coc·cus mil·ler·i*** a term used to refer to the *Streptococcus intermedius* group, which contains three distinct streptococcal species: *Streptococcus intermedius, Streptococcus constellatus,* and *Streptococcus anginosus.* These bacteria are found in the human oral cavity and have been associated with a variety of infections including bacteremia, endocarditis, and CNS, oral, and thoracic infections.

***Strep·to·coc·cus mu·tans*** a species associated with the production of dental caries in humans and in some other animals and with subacute endocarditis.

***Strep·to·coc·cus pneu·mo·ni·ae*** a species of Gram-positive, lancet-shaped diplococci frequently occurring in pairs or chains. Virulent forms are enclosed in type-specific polysaccharide capsules. Normal inhabitants of the respiratory tract, and the cause of lobar pneumonia, otitis media, meningitis, sinusitis, and other infections. SYN pneumococcus.

***Strep·to·coc·cus py·og·e·nes*** a species found in the human mouth, throat, and respiratory tract and in inflammatory exudates, bloodstream, and lesions in human diseases; it is sometimes found in the udders of cows and in dust from sickrooms, hospital wards, schools, theaters, and other public places; it causes the formation of pus or even fatal septicemias.

***Strep·to·coc·cus vir·i·dans*** a name applied not to a distinct species but rather to the group of α-hemolytic streptococci as a whole; viridans streptococci have been isolated from the mouth and intestines of humans, the intestines of horses, the milk and feces of cows, milk products, and the sputum and lungs. SYN viridans streptococci.

**strep·to·ki·nase (SK)** (strep-tō-kī′nās) an extracellular metalloenzyme from hemolytic streptococci that cleaves plasminogen, producing plasmin, which causes the liquefaction of fibrin; usually used in conjunction with streptodornase in the removal of clots.

**strep·to·ly·sin** (strep-tol'i-sin) a hemolysin produced by streptococci.

*Strep·to·my·ces* (strep-tō-mī'sēz) a genus of nonmotile, aerobic, Gram-positive bacteria that grow in the form of a much-branched mycelium; conidia are produced in chains on aerial hyphae. These organisms (several hundred species in the genus) are predominantly saprophytic soil forms; some are parasitic on plants or animals; many produce antibiotics. The type species is *Streptomyces albus.* [strepto- + G. *mykēs,* fungus]

**strep·to·sep·ti·ce·mia** (strep'tō-sep-ti-sē'mē-ă) SYN streptococcemia.

**stress** (stres) **1.** reactions of the body to forces of a deleterious nature, infections, and various abnormal states that tend to disturb its normal physiologic equilibrium (homeostasis). **2.** DENTISTRY the forces set up in teeth, their supporting structures, and structures restoring or replacing teeth as a result of the force of mastication. **3.** the force or pressure applied or exerted between portions of a body or bodies, generally expressed in pounds per square inch. **4.** in rheology, the force in a material transmitted per unit area to adjacent layers. **5.** PSYCHOLOGY a physical or psychological stimulus such as very high heat, public criticism, or another noxious agent or experience which, when impinging upon an individual, produces psychological strain or disequilibrium. [L. *strictus,* tight, fr. *stringo,* to draw together]

**stress-bro·ken con·nec·tor, stress-bro·ken joint** SYN nonrigid connector.

**stress frac·ture** a fatigue fracture caused by repetitive, relatively low-magnitude local stress on a bone, as in marching or running, rather than by a single violent injury.

**stres·sor** PSYCHIATRY any event or situation that induces emotional distress in a given patient.

**stress re·ac·tion** an acute emotional reaction related to extreme environmental stress. SYN acute situational reaction.

**stress shield·ing** osteopenia occurring in bone as the result of removal of normal stress from the bone by an implant.

**stress test** systematic use of exercise for (1) ECG and other cardiac function evaluations, and (2) to evaluate the physiological adjustments to metabolic demands that exceed the resting requirement. SEE graded exercise test. SYN exercise stress test.

**stress ul·cer** an ulcer of the duodenum in a patient with extensive superficial burns, intracranial lesions, or severe bodily injury. SYN Curling ulcer.

**stress u·ri·nary in·con·ti·nence (SUI)** leakage of urine as a result of coughing, straining, or some sudden voluntary movement.

**stretch·er** a litter, usually a sheet of canvas stretched to a frame with four handles, used for transporting the sick or injured. [A.S. *streccan,* to stretch]

**stretch re·cep·tors** receptors that are sensitive to elongation, especially those in Golgi tendon organs and muscle spindles, but also those found in visceral organs such as the stomach, small intestine, and urinary bladder.

**stretch re·flex** SYN myotatic reflex.

**stria,** gen. and pl. **stri·ae** (strī'ă, strī'ē) **1.** a stripe, band, streak, or line, distinguished by color, texture, depression, or elevation from the tissue in which it is found. SYN striation (1). **2.** SYN striae cutis distensae. [L. channel, furrow]

**stri·ae a·tro·phi·cae** SYN striae cutis distensae.

**stri·ae cu·tis dis·ten·sae** bands of thin wrinkled skin, initially red but becoming purple and white, which occur commonly on the abdomen, buttocks, and thighs at puberty and/or during and following pregnancy, and result from atrophy of the dermis and overextension of the skin; also associated with ascites and Cushing syndrome. SYN lineae atrophicae, linear atrophy, stria (2), striae atrophicae.

**stri·ae grav·i·dar·um** striae cutis distensae related to pregnancy.

**stri·ae of Ret·zi·us** (retz'ē-ŭs) incremental growth lines in enamel seen microscopically as dark bands.

**stri·ate** (strī'āt) striped; marked by striae. [L. *striatus,* furrowed]

**stri·ate bod·y** the caudate and lentiform (lenticular) nuclei; the striate appearance on section is caused by slender fascicles of myelinated fibers. SYN corpus striatum [TA].

**stri·at·ed bor·der** the free surface of the columnar absorptive cells of the intestine formed by closely packed microvilli about 1 μm long, giving the appearance of parallel striations.

**stri·at·ed duct** a type of intralobular duct found in some salivary glands that modifies the secretory product; it derives its name from extensive infolding of the basal membrane.

**stri·at·ed mus·cle** skeletal or voluntary muscle in which cross striations occur in the fibers as a result of regular overlapping of thick and thin myofilaments; contrast with smooth muscle. Although cardiac muscle is also striated in appearance, the term "striated muscle" is commonly used as a synonym for voluntary, skeletal muscle.

**stri·ate veins** SYN inferior thalamostriate veins.

**stri·a·tion** (strī-ā'shŭn) **1.** SYN stria (1). **2.** a striate appearance. **3.** the act of streaking or making striae.

**stri·a·to·ni·gral** (strī-ā-tō-nī'grăl) referring to the efferent connection of the striatum with the substantia nigra.

**stri·a·tum** (strī-ā'tŭm) collective name for the caudate nucleus and putamen which together with the globus pallidus or pallidum form the striate body. [L. neut. of *striatus,* furrowed]

**stric·ture** (strik'cher) a circumscribed narrowing or stenosis of a tube, duct, or hollow structure, such as the esophagus or urethra, usually consisting of cicatricial contracture or deposition of abnormal tissue. May be congenital or acquired. If acquired, may result from infection, trauma, muscular spasm, or mechanical or chemical irritation. [L. *strictura,* fr. *stringo,* pp. *strictus,* to draw tight, bind]

**stric·tur·ot·o·my** (strik-cher-ot'ō-mē) surgical opening or division of a stricture. [stricture + G. *tomē,* incision]

**stri·dor** (strī'dōr) a high-pitched, noisy respiration, like the blowing of the wind; a sign of respiratory obstruction, especially in the trachea or larynx. [L. a harsh, creaking sound]

**strid·u·lous** (strid'yu-lŭs) having a shrill or creaking sound. [L. *stridulus,* fr. *strideo,* to creak, to hiss]

**string sign** in pediatric gastrointestinal radiology, the narrowed pyloric canal seen with congenital pyloric stenosis; also used to describe a narrowed segment in Crohn disease on small bowel series.

**stri·o·la** (strī'ō-la) the narrow central area of the utricular macula where the orientations of the tallest stereocilia and kinocilia change. [L. *stria*, stripe, + *-ola*, dim. suffix]

**strip 1.** to express the contents from a collapsible tube or canal, such as the urethra, by running the finger along it. SYN milk (4). **2.** subcutaneous excision of a vein in its longitudinal axis, performed with a stripper. **3.** any narrow piece, relatively long and of uniform width. [A.S. *strypan*, to rob]

**stripe** (strīp) **1.** in anatomy, a streak, line, band, or stria. **2.** in radiography, a linear opacity differing in density from the adjacent parts of the image; usually represents the tangential image of a planar structure such as the pleura or peritoneum. [M.E.]

**strip·ping** removal, often of a covering.

**stro·bi·la**, pl. **stro·bi·lae** (strō'bi-lă, strō'bi-lē) a chain of segments, less the scolex and unsegmented neck portion, of a tapeworm. [G. *stobilē*, a twist of lint]

**stro·bo·scop·ic mi·cro·scope** a microscope that has a light source that flashes at a constant rate so that an analysis of the motility of an object may be made; it may be used for high speed or low speed (time-lapse) cinephotomicrography.

**stro·bos·co·py** (strō-bos'kŏ-pē) endoscopy performed with an intermittent light at a frequency that approximates the frequency of movement of the object visualized so that it appears to be motionless; useful in analyzing vocal cord structure and motion.

**stroke** (strōk) **1.** any acute clinical event, related to impairment of cerebral circulation, that lasts more than 24 hours. SYN brain attack. **2.** a harmful discharge of lightning, particularly one that affects a human being. **3.** a pulsation. **4.** to pass the hand or any instrument gently over a surface. SEE ALSO stroking. **5.** a gliding movement over a surface. [A.S. *strāc*]

**stroke vol·ume** the volume pumped out of one ventricle of the heart in a single beat.

**stroke work in·dex** a measure of the work done by the heart with each contraction, adjusted for body surface area; equal to the stroke volume of the heart multiplied by the arterial pressure and divided by body surface area.

**strok·ing** the nonverbal fondling and nurturance accorded infants or the nonverbal and verbal forms of acceptance, reassurance, and positive reinforcement accorded to children and adults either by an individual to himself or herself or to another person in order to satisfy a basic biopsychological need of all developing humans; various psychopathologic conditions are believed to result when such stroking is absent or faulty.

**stro·ma**, pl. **stro·ma·ta** (strō'mă, strō'mă-tă) **1.** the framework, usually of connective tissue, of an organ, gland, or other structure, as distinguished from the parenchyma or specific substance of the part. **2.** aqueous phase of chloroplasts; i.e., chloroplast matrix. [G. *strōma*, bed]

**stro·mal** (strō'măl) stromatic; relating to the stroma of an organ or other structure.

**strom·al cor·ne·al dys·tro·phy** opacification with involvement of the middle layer of the cornea.

**stro·muhr** (shtrō'moor) an instrument for measuring the quantity of blood that flows per unit of time through a blood vessel. [Ger. *Strom*, stream, + *Uhr*, clock]

**Stron·gy·loi·des** (stron-ji-loy'dēz) the threadworm, a genus of small nematode parasites commonly found in the small intestine of mammals (particularly ruminants). Human infection is chiefly by *S. stercoralis* or *S. fuelleborn*. Fatal infection in infants produces the condition known as swollen belly disease or syndrome, which causes grossly distended abdomens. [G. *strongylos*, round, + *eidos*, resemblance]

**stron·gy·loi·di·a·sis** (stron'ji-loy-dī'ă-sis) infection with soil-borne nematodes of the genus *Strongyloides*, considered to be a parthenogenetic parasitic female. Larvae passed to the soil develop through 4 larval instars to form free-living adults or develop from first and second free-living stages into infective third-stage strongyliform or filariform larvae, which penetrate the skin or enter the buccal mucosa via drinking water. Most serious human infections and nearly all fatalities commonly follow immunosuppression by steroids, ACTH, or other agents, or in AIDS.

**Stron·gy·lus** (stron'ji-lŭs) the palisade worm, a genus of large strongyle nematodes (subfamily Strongylinae, family Strongylidae) parasitic in horses and other equids, and the cause of strongylosis. [G. *strongylos*, round]

**stron·ti·um (Sr)** (stron'shē-ŭm) a metallic element, atomic no. 38, atomic wt. 87.62; one of the alkaline earth series and similar to calcium in chemical and biological properties. Various salts of strontium are used therapeutically for their anions; e.g., strontium bromide, iodide, lactate. [*Strontian*, a town in Scotland]

**stroph·u·lus** (strof'yu-lŭs) SYN miliaria rubra. [Mod. L. dim. of G. *strophus*, colic]

**struc·tura** (strook-too'ra) SYN structure.

**struc·tur·al** (strŭk'cher-ăl) relating to the structure of a part; having a structure. SYN anatomic (2).

**struc·tur·al for·mu·la** a formula in which the connections of the atoms and groups of atoms, as well as their kind and number, are indicated.

**struc·tur·al gene** a gene that codes for a specific protein or peptide.

**struc·tur·al isom·er·ism** isomerism involving the same atoms in different arrangements.

**struc·ture** (strŭk'cher) **1.** the arrangement of the details of a part; the manner of formation of a part. **2.** a tissue or formation made up of different but related parts. **3.** CHEMISTRY the configuration and interconnections of the atoms in a given molecule. SYN structura. [L. *structura*, fr. *struo*, pp. *structus*, to build]

**struc·tured ab·stract** summary description of a published paper, in which information about the study reported in the paper is set out in a systematic, stylized form under headings such as aims, methods, main outcome measures, results, conclusions.

**stru·ma**, pl. **stru·mae** (stroo'mă, stroo'mē) SYN goiter. [L. a scrofulous tumor, fr. *struo*, to pile up, build]

**stru·ma o·va·rii** a rare ovarian tumor, regarded as teratomatous, in which thyroid tissue has surpassed the other elements; occasionally associated with hyperthyroidism.

**stru·mec·to·my** (stroo-mek'tō-mē) surgical removal of all or a portion of a goitrous tumor. [struma + G. *ektomē*, excision]

**stru·mi·form** (stroo'mi-fōrm) resembling a goiter. [struma + L. *forma*, form]

**stru·mi·tis** (stroo-mī'tis) inflammation, with swelling, of the thyroid gland. SEE ALSO thyroiditis. [struma + G. *-itis*, inflammation]

**stru·mous** (stroo'mŭs) denoting or characteristic of a struma.

**Strüm·pell dis·ease** (shtrem'pĕl) **1.** SYN spondylitis deformans. **2.** SYN acute epidemic leukoencephalitis.

**Strüm·pell phe·nom·e·non** (shtrem'pĕl) dorsal flexion of the great toe, sometimes of the entire foot, in a paralyzed limb when the extremity is drawn up against the body, flexing both knee and hip.

**Strüm·pell re·flex** (shtrem'pĕl) stroking the abdomen or thigh causes flexion of the leg and adduction of the foot.

**stru·vite cal·cu·lus** a calculus in which the crystalloid component consists of magnesium ammonium phosphate; usually associated with urinary tract infection caused by urease-producing bacteria.

**strych·nine** (strik'nīn) an alkaloid from *Strychnos nux-vomica;* colorless crystals of intensely bitter taste, nearly insoluble in water. It stimulates all parts of the central nervous system, and was formerly used as a stomachic, an antidote for depressant poisons, and in the treatment of myocarditis. Strychnine blocks the inhibitory neurotransmitter, glycine, and thus can cause convulsions. It is a potent chemical capable of producing acute or chronic poisoning.

**strych·nin·ism** (strik'nin-izm) chronic strychnine poisoning, the symptoms being those that arise from central nervous system stimulation; the first signs are tremors and twitching, progressing to severe convulsions and respiratory arrest.

**Stry·ker frame** (strī-kĕr) a frame that holds the patient and permits turning in various planes without individual motion of parts.

**Stu·art fac·tor, Stu·art-Prow·er fac·tor** (stoo'ĕrt, stoo'ĕt-prow'ĕr) SYN factor X.

**Stu·dent t test** (stoo'dent) a statistical significance test for assessing the difference between, or the equality of, two or more population means.

**study** (stŭd'ē) research, detailed examination, and/or analysis of an organism, object, or phenomena. [L. *studium*, study, inquiry]

**stump** (stŭmp) **1.** the extremity of a limb left after amputation. **2.** the pedicle remaining after removal of the tumor attached to it. [M.e. *stumpe*]

**stump can·cer** carcinoma of the stomach developing after gastroenterostomy or gastric resection for benign disease.

**stu·por** (stoo'per) a state of impaired consciousness in which the individual shows a marked diminution in reactivity to environmental stimuli; only continual stimulation arouses the individual. [L. fr. *stupeo*, to be stunned]

**stu·por·ous** (stoo'per-ŭs) relating to or marked by stupor.

**Sturm co·noid** (shterm) in optics, the pattern of rays formed after passage through a spherocylindrical combination.

**Sturm·dorf op·er·a·tion** (shterm'dorf) conical removal of the endocervix.

**Sturm in·ter·val** (shterm) the distance between the anterior and posterior focal lines in a spherocylindrical lens combination.

**stut·ter·ing** (stŭt'er-ing) a phonatory or articulatory disorder, characteristically beginning in childhood, sometimes accompanied by intense anxiety about the efficiency of oral communications, and characterized by hesitations, repetitions, and/or prolongations of sounds and syllables, interjections, broken words, circumlocutions, and words produced with excess tension. SEE ALSO dysfluency. SYN logospasm.

**sty, stye**, pl. **sties, styes** (stī, stī, stīz) SYN hordeolum externum.

**sty·let, sty·lette** (stī'let, stī-let') **1.** a flexible metallic rod inserted in the lumen of a flexible catheter to stiffen it and give it form during its passage. **2.** a slender probe. SYN stylus (3), stilus. [It. *stilletto*, a dagger; dim. of L. *stilus* or *stylus*, a stake, a pen]

△**sty·lo-** styloid (specifically the styloid process of the temporal bone). [G. *stylos*, pillar, post]

**sty·lo·glos·sus mus·cle** *action*, retracts tongue; *origin*, lower end of styloid process; *insertion*, side and undersurface of tongue; *nerve supply*, hypoglossal. SYN musculus styloglossus [TA].

**sty·lo·hy·al** (stī-lō-hī'ăl) relating to the styloid process of the temporal bone and to the hyoid bone.

**sty·lo·hy·oid mu·scle** *origin*, styloid process of temporal bone; *insertion*, hyoid bone by two slips on either side of intermediate tendon of digastric; *action*, elevates hyoid bone; *nerve supply*, facial. SYN musculus stylohyoideus [TA].

**sty·loid** (stī'loyd) peg-shaped; denoting one of several slender bony processes. [stylo- + G. *eidos*, resemblance]

**sty·loi·di·tis** (stī-loy-dī'tis) inflammation of a styloid process.

**sty·loid pro·cess** SEE styloid process of radius, styloid process of temporal bone, styloid process of ulna.

**sty·loid pro·cess of ra·di·us** a thick, pointed, palpable projection on the lateral side of the distal extremity of the radius.

**sty·loid pro·cess of tem·por·al bone** a slender pointed projection running downward and slightly forward from the base of the inferior surface of the petrous portion of the temporal bone where it joins the tympanic portion; it gives attachment to the styloglossus, stylohyoid, and stylopharyngeus muscles and the stylohyoid and stylomandibular ligaments.

**sty·loid pro·cess of ul·na** a cylindrical, pointed palpable projection from the medial and posterior aspect of the head of the ulna, to the tip of which is attached the ulnar collateral ligament of the wrist.

**sty·lo·mas·toid ar·tery** *origin*, posterior auricular; *distribution*, external acoustic meatus, mastoid cells, semicircular canals, stapedius muscle, and vestibule; *anastomoses*, tympanic branches of internal carotid and ascending pharyngeal, and labyrinthine arteries. SYN arteria stylomastoidea [TA].

**sty·lo·mas·toid for·a·men** the distal or external opening of the facial canal on the inferior surface of the petrous portion of the temporal bone, between the styloid and mastoid processes; it transmits the facial nerve and stylomastoid artery.

**sty·lo·mas·toid vein** drains the tympanic cavity, traverses the facial canal exiting via the stylo-

s
t

mastoid foramen, and empties into the retromandibular vein.

**sty·lo·pha·ryn·ge·al mus·cle** SYN stylopharyngeus muscle.

**sty·lo·pha·ryn·ge·us mus·cle** *origin*, root of styloid process; *insertion*, thyroid cartilage and wall of pharynx (becomes part of the longitudinal coat): *action*, elevates pharynx and larynx; *nerve supply*, glossopharyngeal. SYN musculus stylopharyngeus [TA], stylopharyngeal muscle.

**sty·lus, sti·lus** (stī′lŭs, stī′lŭs) **1.** any pencil-shaped structure. **2.** a pencil-shaped medicinal preparation for external application. **3.** SYN stylet. [L. *stilus* or *stylus*, a stake or pen]

**stype** (stīp) a tampon. [G. *stypē*, tow]

**styp·tic** (stip′tik) **1.** having an astringent or hemostatic effect. **2.** an astringent agent used topically to stop bleeding. [G. *styptikos*, astringent]

⚠**sub-** prefix to words formed from L. roots, denoting beneath, less than the normal or typical, inferior. Cf. hypo-. [L. *sub*, under]

**sub·a·cro·mi·al bur·sa** between the acromion and the capsule of the shoulder joint.

**sub·a·cute** (sŭb-ă-kyut′) between acute and chronic; denoting the course of a disease of moderate duration or severity.

**sub·a·cute bac·ter·i·al en·do·car·di·tis (SBE)** endocarditis usually involving cardiac valves with congenital or acquired abnormalities and usually due to alpha-hemolytic streptococci.

**sub·a·cute com·bined de·gen·er·a·tion of the spi·nal cord** a disorder of the spinal cord, such as that occurring in vitamin $B_{12}$ deficiency, characterized by gliosis with spongiform degeneration of the posterior and lateral columns. SYN Putnam-Dana syndrome, vitamin $B_{12}$ neuropathy.

**sub·a·cute gran·u·lom·a·tous thy·roid·i·tis** thyroiditis with round cell (usually lymphocytes) infiltration, destruction of thyroid cells, epithelial giant cell proliferation, and evidence of regeneration; thought by some to be a reflection of a systemic infection and not an example of true chronic thyroiditis. SYN de Quervain thyroiditis.

**sub·a·cute in·flam·ma·tion** an inflammation that is intermediate in duration between that of an acute inflammation and that of a chronic inflammation, usually persisting longer than 3–4 weeks.

**sub·a·cute mi·gra·to·ry pan·nic·u·li·tis** nonscarring plaques of changing configuration on the lateral aspect of one or both legs, of many months duration.

**sub·a·cute nec·ro·tiz·ing my·e·li·tis** a disorder of the lower spinal cord in adult males resulting in progressive paraplegia.

**sub·a·cute scler·os·ing pan·en·ceph·a·li·tis (SSPE)** a rare chronic, progressive encephalitis that affects primarily children and young adults, caused by the measles virus. Characterized by a history of primary measles infection before the age of two years, followed by several asymptomatic years, and then gradual, progressive psychoneurological deterioration, consisting of personality change, seizures, myoclonus, ataxia, photosensitivity, ocular abnormalities, spasticity, and coma. Characteristic periodic activity is seen on EEG; pathologically, the white matter of both the hemispheres and brainstem are affected, as well as the cerebral cortex, and eosinophilic inclusion bodies are present in the cytoplasm nuclei of neurons and glial cells. Death usually

occurs within three years. SYN Bosin disease, Dawson encephalitis.

**sub·a·cute spong·i·form en·ceph·a·lo·pa·thy** a form of spongiform encephalopathy that is associated with a "slow virus", which to date has not been adequately described, is transmissible, and has a rapidly progressive, fatal course; e.g., Creutzfeldt-Jakob disease, kuru, Gerstmann-Sträussler syndrome, scrapie. SEE prion.

**sub·a·or·tic ste·no·sis** congenital narrowing of the outflow tract of the left ventricle by a ring of fibrous tissue or by hypertrophy of the muscular septum below the aortic valve.

**sub·ap·i·cal** (sŭb-ap′i-kăl) below the apex of any part.

**sub·a·rach·noid space** the space between the arachnoidea and pia mater, traversed by delicate fibrous trabeculae and filled with cerebrospinal fluid. Since the pia mater immediately adheres to the surface of the brain and spinal cord, the space is greatly widened wherever the brain surface exhibits a deep depression (for example, between the cerebellum and medulla); such widenings are called cisternae. The large blood vessels supplying the brain and spinal cord lie in the subarachnoid space.

**sub·ar·cu·ate fos·sa** an irregular depression on the posterior surface of the petrous portion of the temporal bone just below its crest and above and lateral to the internal acoustic meatus. In the fetus, the flocculus of the cerebellum rests here; in the adult, a small vein enters the bone here.

**sub·a·tom·ic** (sŭb-ă-tom′ik) pertaining to particles making up the intraatomic structure; e.g., protons, electrons, neutrons.

**sub·ax·i·al** (sŭb-ak′sē-ăl) below the axis of the body or any part.

**sub·cal·lo·sal gy·rus** a slender vertical whitish band immediately anterior to the lamina terminalis and anterior commissure; contrary to its name, it is not a cortical convolution but is the ventral continuation of the transparent septum.

**sub·cap·su·lar cat·a·ract** a cataract in which the opacities are concentrated beneath the capsule.

**sub·car·ti·lag·i·nous** (sŭb′kar-ti-laj′i-nŭs) **1.** partly cartilaginous. **2.** beneath a cartilage.

**sub·cho·ri·al space, sub·cho·ri·al lake** the part of the placenta adjacently beneath the chorionic plate; it joins with irregular channels to form the marginal lakes.

**sub·class** (sŭb′klas) in biologic classification, a division between class and order.

**sub·cla·vi·an ar·tery** *origin*, right from brachiocephalic, left from arch of aorta; *branches*, vertebral, thyrocervical trunk, internal thoracic; costocervical trunk, descending scapular; it continues as the axillary artery after crossing the first rib. SYN arteria subclavia [TA].

**sub·cla·vi·an mus·cle** SYN subclavius muscle.

**sub·cla·vi·an nerve** a branch from the superior trunk of the brachial plexus supplying the subclavius muscle. SYN nervus subclavius [TA].

**sub·cla·vi·an steal** obstruction of the subclavian artery proximal to the origin of the vertebral artery; blood flow through the vertebral artery is reversed and the subclavian artery thus "steals" cerebral blood, causing symptoms of vertebrobasilar insufficiency (subclavian steal syndrome); manifest during vigorous use of an upper extremity.

**sub·cla·vi·an vein** the direct continuation of the axillary vein at the lateral border of the first rib; it passes medially to join the internal jugular vein and form the brachiocephalic vein on each side. SYN vena subclavia [TA].

**sub·cla·vi·us mus·cle** *origin*, first costal cartilage; *insertion*, inferior surface of acromial end of clavicle; *action*, fixes clavicle or elevates first rib; *nerve supply*, subclavian from brachial plexus. SYN musculus subclavius [TA], subclavian muscle.

**sub·clin·i·cal** (sŭb-klin′i-kăl) denoting the presence of a disease without manifest symptoms; may be an early stage in the evolution of a disease.

**sub·clin·i·cal coc·ci·di·oi·do·my·co·sis** a form of coccidioidomycosis that does not come to medical attention because respiratory symptoms are mild and self-limited.

**sub·clin·i·cal di·a·be·tes** a form of diabetes mellitus that is clinically evident only under certain circumstances, such as pregnancy or extreme stress; persons so afflicted may, in time, manifest more severe forms of the disease.

**sub·con·scious** (sŭb-kon′shŭs) **1.** not wholly conscious. **2.** denoting an idea or impression which is present in the mind, but of which there is at the time no conscious knowledge or realization.

**sub·con·scious·ness** (sŭb-kon′shŭs-nes) **1.** partial unconsciousness. **2.** the state in which mental processes take place without the conscious perception of the individual.

**sub·cor·tex** (sŭb-kōr′teks) any part of the brain lying below the cerebral cortex, and not itself organized as cortex.

**sub·cor·ti·cal** (sŭb-kōr′ti-kăl) relating to the subcortex; beneath the cerebral cortex.

**sub·cost·al ar·tery** *origin*, thoracic aorta; *distribution*, inferior to twelfth rib in a manner similar to posterior intercostal arteries. SYN arteria subcostalis [TA].

**sub·cost·al mus·cle** one of a number of inconstant muscles of the posterolateral thoracic wall having the same direction as the internal intercostal muscles but extending across (deep to) one or more ribs. SYN musculus subcostalis [TA].

**sub·cost·al nerve** the ventral ramus of the twelfth thoracic nerve; it courses below the last rib, supplies parts of the abdominal muscles and gives off cutaneous branches to the skin of the lower-most ventrolateral abdominal wall and to the superolateral gluteal region. SYN nervus subcostalis [TA].

**sub·cost·al plane** a horizontal plane passing through the inferior limits of the costal margin, i.e., the tenth costal cartilages; it marks the boundary between the hypochondriac and epigastric regions superiorly and the lateral and umbilical regions inferiorly. See page APP 88.

**sub·crep·i·tant** (sub-krep′i-tănt) nearly, but not frankly, crepitant; denoting a rale.

**sub·cul·ture** (sŭb-kŭl′cher) **1.** a culture made by transferring to a fresh medium microorganisms from a previous culture; a method used to prolong the life of a particular strain where there is a tendency to degeneration in older cultures or to transfer organisms to a medium containing nutrients, reagents, dyes, or other substances to favor growth or facilitate identification. **2.** to make a fresh culture with material obtained from a previous one.

**sub·cu·ta·ne·ous (SQ)** (sŭb-kyu-tā′nē-ŭs) beneath the skin. SYN hypodermic. [sub- + L. *cutis*, skin]

**sub·cu·ta·ne·ous em·phy·se·ma** the presence of air or gas in the subcutaneous tissues. SYN pneumoderma.

**sub·cu·ta·ne·ous flap** a pedicle flap in which the pedicle is denuded of epithelium and buried in the subcutaneous tissue of the recipient area.

**sub·cu·ta·ne·ous mas·tec·to·my** excision of the breast tissues, but sparing the skin, nipple, and areola; usually followed by implantation of a prosthesis.

**sub·cu·ta·ne·ous op·er·a·tion** an operation, as for the division of a tendon, performed without incising the skin other than by a minute opening made by the entering knife.

**sub·cu·ta·ne·ous te·no·to·my** division of a tendon by means of a small pointed knife introduced through skin and subcutaneous tissue without an open operation.

**sub·cu·ta·ne·ous tis·sue** a layer of loose, irregular, connective tissue immediately beneath the skin and closely attached to the corium by coarse fibrous bands, the retinacula cutis; it contains fat cells except in the auricles, eyelids, penis, and scrotum.

**sub·cu·ta·ne·ous veins of ab·do·men** the network of superficial veins of the abdominal wall that empty into the thoracoepigastric, superficial epigastric, or superior epigastric veins and form portocaval anastomoses through their communications with the paraumbilical veins.

**sub·del·toid bur·sa** the bursa between the deltoid muscle and the capsule of the shoulder joint. It may be combined with the subacromial bursa.

**sub·duce, sub·duct** (sŭb-doos′, sŭb-dŭkt′) to pull or draw downward. [L. *sub-duco*, pp. *-ductus*, to lead away]

**sub·du·ral he·ma·to·ma** SYN subdural hemorrhage.

**sub·du·ral hem·or·rhage** extravasation of blood between the dural and arachnoidal membranes; acute and chronic forms occur; chronic hematomas may become encapsulated by neomembranes. SYN subdural hematoma.

**sub·du·ral space** an artificial space created by the separation of the arachnoid from the dura as the result of trauma or some pathologic process; in the healthy state, the arachnoid is tenuously attached to the dura and a naturally occurring subdural space is not present.

**sub·en·do·car·di·al bran·ches of a·tri·o·ven·-tri·cu·lar bun·dles** interlacing fibers formed of modified cardiac muscle cells with central granulated protoplasm containing one or two nuclei and a transversely striated peripheral portion; they are the terminal ramifications of the conducting system of the heart found beneath the endocardium of the ventricles. SEE ALSO conducting system of heart. SYN Purkinje fibers.

**sub·en·do·car·di·al lay·er** the loose connective tissue layer that joins the endocardium and myocardium; in the ventricles, it contains branches of the conducting system of the heart.

**sub·en·do·the·li·al lay·er** the thin layer of connective tissue lying between the endothelium and elastic lamina in the intima of blood vessels.

**sub·en·do·the·li·um** (sŭb′en-dō-thē′lē-ŭm) the connective tissue between the endothelium and inner elastic membrane in the intima of arteries.

S
u

**sub·ep·en·dy·mo·ma** (sŭb-ep-en-di-mō'mă) discrete lobulated ependymal nodules in the walls of the anterior third or posterior fourth ventricles commonly found at autopsy.

**sub·fam·i·ly** (sŭb-fam'i-lē) in biologic classification, a division between family and tribe or between family and genus.

**sub·fer·til·i·ty** (sŭb-fer-til'i-tē) less than normal capacity for reproduction.

**sub·ge·nus** (sŭb-jē'nŭs) in biologic classification, a division between genus and species.

**sub·gin·gi·val cur·et·tage** removal of subgingival calculus, ulcerated epithelial and granulation tissues found in periodontal pockets.

**sub·glos·sal** (sŭb-glos'ăl) below or beneath the tongue. SYN sublingual.

**sub·grun·da·tion** (sŭb-grŭn-dā'shŭn) the depression of one fragment of a broken cranial bone below the other. [sub- + A.S. grund, bottom, foundation]

**su·bic·u·lum**, pl. **su·bic·u·la** (soo-bik'yu-lŭm, soo-bik'yu-lă) 1. a support or prop. 2. the zone of transition between the parahippocampal gyrus and Ammon horn of the hippocampus. [L. dim. of subex, support]

**sub·il·i·ac** (sŭb-il'ē-ak) 1. below the ilium. 2. relating to the subilium.

**sub·il·i·um** (sŭb-il'ē-ŭm) the portion of the ilium contributing to the acetabulum.

**sub·in·fec·tion** (sŭb-in-fek'shŭn) a secondary infection occurring in one exposed to and successfully resisting an epidemic of another infectious disease.

**sub·in·vo·lu·tion** (sŭb-in-vō-loo'shŭn) arrest of the normal involution of the uterus following childbirth with the organ remaining abnormally large.

**sub·ja·cent** (sŭb-jā'sent) below or beneath another part. [L. sub-jaceo, to lie under]

**sub·jec·tive** (sŭb-jek'tiv) 1. perceived by the individual only and not evident to the examiner; said of certain symptoms, such as pain. 2. colored by one's personal beliefs and attitudes. Cf. objective (2). [L. subjectivus, fr. subjicio, to throw under]

**sub·jec·tive as·sess·ment da·ta** those facts presented by the client that show his/her perception, understanding, and interpretation of what is happening.

**sub·jec·tive sen·sa·tion** a sensation not readily referable to a denotably verifiable stimulus.

**sub·jec·tive symp·tom** a symptom apparent only to the patient.

**sub·king·dom** (sŭb-king'dom) in biologic classification, a division between kingdom and phylum.

**sub·la·tion** (sŭb-lā'shŭn) detachment, elevation, or removal of a part. [L. sublatio, a lifting up]

**sub·le·thal** (sŭb-lē'thăl) slightly less than lethal; e.g., a sublethal dose.

**sub·leu·ke·mic leu·ke·mia** a form of leukemia in which abnormal cells are present in the peripheral blood, but the total leukocyte count is not elevated.

**sub·li·mate** (sŭb'lim-āt) 1. to perform or accomplish sublimation. 2. any substance that has been submitted to sublimation. [L. sublimo, pp. -atus, to raise on high, fr. sublimis, high]

**sub·li·ma·tion** (sŭb-lim-ā'shŭn) 1. the process of converting a solid into a gas without passing through a liquid state; analogous to distillation. 2.

PSYCHOANALYSIS an unconscious defense mechanism in which unacceptable instinctual drives and wishes are modified into more personally and socially acceptable channels.

**sub·lim·i·nal** (sŭb-lim'i-năl) below the threshold of perception or excitation; below the limit or threshold of consciousness. [sub- + L. limen (limin-), threshold]

**sub·lin·gual** (sŭb-ling'gwăl) SYN subglossal.

**sub·lin·gual ar·tery** origin, lingual; distribution, extrinsic muscles of tongue, sublingual gland, mucosa of region; anastomoses, the artery of opposite side and submental. SYN arteria sublingualis [TA].

**sub·lin·gual cyst** SYN ranula (2).

**sub·lin·gual fos·sa** a shallow depression on either side of the mental spine, on the inner surface of the body of the mandible, superior to the mylohyoid line, lodging the sublingual gland.

**sub·lin·gual gland** one of two salivary glands in the floor of the mouth beneath the tongue, discharging through the sublingual ducts; most of the secretory units in the human gland are mucus secreting with serous demilunes.

**sub·lin·gual nerve** a branch of the lingual nerve to the sublingual gland and mucous membrane of the floor of the mouth. SYN nervus sublingualis [TA].

**sub·lin·gual vein** vein which accompanies the sublingual artery in the floor of the mouth, lateral to the hypoglossal nerve; it may join the deep lingual vein to form the lingual vein, or join the vena comitans nervi hypoglossi.

**sub·lux·a·tion** (sŭb-lŭk-sā'shŭn) an incomplete luxation or dislocation; though a relationship is altered, contact between joint surfaces remains. [sub- + L. locatio, luxation (dislocation)]

**sub·mam·ma·ry mas·ti·tis** inflammation of the tissues lying deep to the mammary gland.

**sub·man·dib·u·lar** (sŭb-man-dib'yu-lăr) beneath the mandible or lower jaw. SYN submaxillary (2).

**sub·man·dib·u·lar duct** the duct of the submandibular salivary gland; it opens at the sublingual papilla near the frenulum of the tongue. SYN Wharton duct.

**sub·man·dib·u·lar fos·sa** the depression on the medial surface of the body of the mandible inferior to the mylohyoid line in which the submandibular gland is lodged.

**sub·man·dib·u·lar gan·gli·on** a small parasympathetic ganglion suspended from the lingual nerve; its postganglionic branches go to the submandibular and sublingual glands; its preganglionic fibers come from the superior salivatory nucleus by way of the chorda tympani.

**sub·man·dib·u·lar gland** one of two salivary glands in the neck, located in the space bounded by the two bellies of the digastric muscle and the angle of the mandible; it discharges through the submandibular duct; the secretory units are predominantly serous although a few mucous alveoli, some with serous demilunes, occur. SYN maxillary gland.

**sub·man·dib·u·lar tri·an·gle** the triangle of the neck bounded by the mandible and the two bellies of the digastric muscle; it contains the submandibular gland. SYN trigonum submandibulare [TA], digastric triangle.

**sub·max·il·la** (sŭb-mak-sil'ă) SYN mandible.

**sub·max·il·lary** (sŭb-mak'si-lār-ē) 1. SYN mandibular. 2. SYN submandibular.

**sub·men·tal ar·tery** *origin*, facial; *distribution*, mylohyoid muscle, submandibular and sublingual glands, and structures of lower lip; *anastomoses*, inferior labial, mental branch of inferior dental and sublingual. SYN arteria submentalis [TA].

**sub·men·tal vein** situated below the chin, this vein anastomoses with the sublingual vein, connects with the anterior jugular vein, and empties into the facial vein. SYN vena submentalis.

**sub·mi·cro·scop·ic** (sŭb′mī-krō-skop′ik) too minute to be visible with a light microscope. SYN ultramicroscopic.

**sub·mu·co·sa** (sŭb-myu-kō′să) a layer of tissue beneath a mucous membrane; the layer of connective tissue beneath the tunica mucosa. SYN tela submucosa.

**sub·mu·co·sal plex·us** a gangliated plexus of unmyelinated nerve fibers, derived chiefly from the superior mesenteric plexus, ramifying in the intestinal submucosa.

**sub·mu·cous cleft pa·late** SYN occult cleft palate.

**sub·mu·cous la·ryn·ge·al cleft** SEE laryngotracheoesophageal cleft.

**sub·na·si·on** (sŭb-nā′zē-on) the point of the angle between the septum of the nose and the surface of the upper lip.

**sub·nu·cle·us** (sŭb-noo′klē-ŭs) a secondary nucleus.

**sub·oc·ci·pi·tal nerve** dorsal ramus of the first cervical nerve, passing through the suboccipital triangle and sending branches to the rectus capitis posterior major and minor, obliquus capitis superior and inferior, rectus capitis lateralis, and semispinalis capitis; the first cervical spinal nerve is generally considered to have only motor fibers, but the suboccipital nerve receives sensory fibers for proprioception via a communicating branch from the second cervical spinal nerve. SYN nervus suboccipitalis [TA].

**sub·oc·cip·i·to·breg·mat·ic di·am·e·ter** the diameter of the fetal head from the lowest posterior point of the occipital bone to the center of the anterior fontanelle.

**sub·or·der** (sŭb-ōr′der) in biologic classification, a division between order and family.

**sub·pap·u·lar** (sŭb-pap′yu-lăr) denoting the eruption of few and scattered papules, in which the lesions are very slightly elevated, being scarcely more than macules.

**sub·per·i·os·te·al am·pu·ta·tion** amputation in which the periosteum is stripped back from the bone and replaced afterward, forming a periosteal flap over the cut end. SYN periosteoplastic amputation.

**sub·phy·lum** (sŭb-fī′lŭm) in biologic classification, a division between phylum and class.

**sub·pu·bic an·gle** the angle formed between the inferior rami of the pubic bones. In the female, the angle approximates that angle between the widely extended thumb and index finger (90°); in the male, it approximates the angle between the widely abducted index and middle fingers (60°). SEE ALSO pubic arch. SYN angulus subpubicus [TA], pubic angle.

**sub·scap·u·lar ar·tery** *origin*, axillary; *branches*, circumflex scapular, thoracodorsal; *distribution*, muscles of shoulder and scapular region; *anastomoses*, branches of transverse cer-

vical, suprascapular, lateral thoracic, and intercostals. SYN arteria subscapularis [TA].

**sub·scap·u·la·ris mus·cle** *origin*, subscapular fossa; *insertion*, lesser tuberosity of humerus; *action*, rotates arm medially; *nerve supply*, upper and lower subscapular from posterior cord of brachial plexus (fifth and sixth cervical spinal nerves). SYN musculus subscapularis [TA], subscapular muscle.

**sub·scap·u·lar mus·cle** SYN subscapularis muscle.

**sub·scrip·tion** (sŭb-skrip′shŭn) the part of a prescription preceding the signature giving directions for compounding. [L. *subscriptio*, fr. *subscribo*, pp. *-scriptus*, to write under, subscribe]

**sub·seg·men·tal at·el·ec·ta·sis** collapse of the portion of the lung distal to an obstructed subsegmental bronchus, manifested as a linear opacity on a chest radiograph. SEE Fleischner lines. SYN platelike atelectasis.

**sub·ser·osa** the layer of connective tissue beneath a serous membrane such as that of the periconeum or pericardium.

**sub·si·dence** (sŭb-sī′dens) sinking or settling in bone, as of a prosthetic component of a total joint implant.

**sub·sid·i·ary a·tri·al pace·mak·er** secondary source for rhythmic control of the heart, available for controlling cardiac activity if the sinoatrial pacemaker fails; located within the crista terminalis and atrial free wall near the inferior vena cava.

**sub·spi·na·le** (sŭb-spī-nā′lē) CEPHALOMETRICS the most posterior midline point on the premaxilla between the anterior nasal spine and the prosthion. SYN point A.

**sub·stance** (sŭb′stans) material. SYN substantia [TA], matter. [L. *substantia*, essence, material, fr. *sub- sto*, to stand under, be present]

**sub·stance a·buse** maladaptive pattern of drug or alcohol use that may lead to social, occupational, psychological, or physical problems.

**sub·stance a·buse dis·or·ders** a class of mental disorders in which behavioral and biological changes are associated with regular use of alcohol, drugs, and related substances that affect the central nervous system and personal and social functioning.

**sub·stance de·pen·dence** a pattern of behavioral, physiologic, and cognitive symptoms due to substance use or abuse; usually indicated by tolerance to the effects of the substance and withdrawal symptoms when use of the substance is terminated.

**sub·stance de·pen·dence dis·or·der** a maladaptive pattern of use of alcohol, drugs, or other substances, with tolerance and/or withdrawal symptoms, drug-seeking behavior, and lack of success in discontinuation of use, to the detriment of social, interpersonal, and occupational activities.

**sub·stance P** a peptide neurotransmitter composed of eleven amino acid residues normally present in minute quantities in the nervous system and intestines of humans and various animals and found in inflamed tissue; primarily involved in pain transmission and is one of the most potent compounds affecting smooth muscle (dilation of blood vessels and contraction of intestine) and thus presumed to play a role in inflammation.

S
u

**sub·stan·tia**, pl. **sub·stan·ti·ae** (sŭb-stan′shē-ă, sŭb-stan′shē-ē) [TA] SYN substance. [L.]

**sub·stan·tia ba·sal·is** [TA] SYN basal substantia.

**sub·stan·tia com·pac·ta** [TA] SYN compact bone.

**sub·stan·tia cor·ti·cal·is** [TA] SYN cortical bone.

**sub·stan·tia gri·sea** [TA] SYN gray matter.

**sub·stan·tia me·dul·la·ris 1.** SYN medulla. **2.** SYN medullary substance.

**sub·stan·tia nig·ra** a large cell mass, crescentic on transverse section, extending forward over the dorsal surface of the crus cerebri from the rostral border of the pons into the subthalamic region; it is composed of a dorsal stratum of closely spaced pigmented (i.e., melanin-containing) cells, the pars compacta, and a larger ventral region of widely scattered cells, the pars reticulata; the pars compacta in particular includes numerous cells that project forward to the striatum (caudate nucleus and putamen) and contain dopamine, which acts as the transmitter substance at their synaptic endings; other, apparently nondopaminergic cells of the substantia nigra project to a rostral part of the ventral nucleus of thalamus, to the middle layers of the superior colliculus, and to restricted parts of the reticular formation of the midbrain; the nigrostriatal projection is reciprocated by a massive striatonigral fiber system with multiple neurotransmitters, chief among which is γ-aminobutyric acid (GABA); substantia nigra receives smaller afferent projections from the subthalamic nucleus, the lateral segment of the globus pallidus, the dorsal nucleus of the raphe and the pedunculopontine nucleus of the midbrain. The pars reticulata forms part of the output system for the striate body. The substantia nigra is involved in the metabolic disturbances associated with Parkinson disease and Huntington disease.

**sub·stan·tia spon·gi·o·sa** bone in which the spicules or trabeculae form a three-dimensional latticework (cancellus) with the interstices filled with embryonal connective tissue or bone marrow. SYN cancellous bone, spongy bone (1), spongy substance, trabecular bone.

**sub·stan·tiv·i·ty** (sŭb′stan-tiv′ĭ-tē) the ability of an antimicrobial agent to retain its effectiveness in the mouth for an extended period.

**sub·ster·nal goi·ter** enlargement of the thyroid gland, chiefly of the lower part of the isthmus, palpable with difficulty or not at all.

**sub·sti·tu·tion** (sŭb-sti-too′shŭn) **1.** CHEMISTRY the replacement of an atom or group in a compound by another atom or group. **2.** PSYCHOANALYSIS an unconscious defense mechanism by which an unacceptable or unattainable goal, object, or emotion is replaced by one that is more acceptable or attainable; the process is more acute and direct, and less subtle, than sublimation. [L. *substitutio*, to put in place of another]

**sub·sti·tu·tion pro·duct** a product obtained by replacing one atom or group in a molecule with another atom or group.

**sub·sti·tu·tion ther·a·py** replacement therapy, particularly when replacement is not physiological but entails administration of a substitute.

**sub·sti·tu·tion trans·fu·sion** SYN exchange transfusion.

**sub·strate (S)** (sŭb′strāt) **1.** the substance acted upon and changed by an enzyme; the reactant considered to be attacked in a chemical reaction. **2.** the base on which an organism lives or grows; e.g., the substrate on which microorganisms and cells grow in cell culture. [L. *sub-sterno*, pp. *-stratus*, to spread under]

**sub·struc·ture** (sŭb-strŭk′cher) a tissue or structure wholly or partly beneath the surface.

**sub·ta·lar joint** a plane synovial joint between the inferior surface of the talus and the posterior articular surface of the calcaneus. The term is also used clinically to refer to the compound joint formed by the talocalcaneal and talocalcaneonavicular joints. SYN talocalcaneal joint.

**sub·ten·di·nous bur·sae of gas·troc·ne·mi·us (mus·cle)** consist of a lateral and a medial [Brodie bursa (1)] bursa between the heads of the gastrocnemius and capsule of the knee joint.

**sub·ten·di·nous bur·sa of the tib·i·a·lis an·ter·i·or mus·cle** the small bursa between the medial surface of the medial cuneiform bone and the tendon of the tibialis anterior.

**sub·ten·di·nous il·i·ac bur·sa** the bursa at the attachment of the iliopsoas muscle into the lesser trochanter.

**sub·tha·lam·ic** (sŭb-thă-lam′ik) related to the subthalamus region or to the subthalamic nucleus.

**sub·thal·a·mus** (sŭb-thal′ă-mŭs) [TA] that part of the diencephalon that lies wedged between the thalamus on the dorsal side and the cerebral peduncle ventrally, lateral to the dorsal half of the hypothalamus from which it cannot be sharply delineated. It is composed of the subthalamic nucleus (corpus luysi), the zona incerta, and the fields of Forel; laterally it expands in a winglike fashion into the reticular nucleus of the thalamus; caudally it is continuous with the midbrain tegmentum.

**sub·trac·tion** (sŭb-trak′shŭn) a technique used to enhance detectability of opacified anatomic structures on radiographic or scintigraphic images; a negative of an image made before introduction of contrast medium or radionuclide is photographically or electronically removed from a later image; commonly used in cerebral angiography. SEE ALSO digital subtraction angiography, mask.

**sub·tribe** (sŭb-trīb) in biologic classification, a division between tribe and genus.

**sub·un·gual, sub·un·gui·al** (sŭb-ŭng′gwăl, sŭb-ŭng′gwi-ăl) beneath the finger or toe nail. SYN hyponychial (1). [L. *unguis*, nail]

**sub·un·gual he·ma·to·ma** collection of blood beneath a fingernail or toenail, usually due to trauma.

**sub·un·gual mel·a·no·ma** a melanoma beginning in the skin at the border of or beneath the nail.

**sub·u·nit vac·cine** a vaccine which, through chemical extraction, is free of viral nucleic acid and contains only specific protein subunits of a given virus; such vaccines are relatively free of the adverse reactions (e.g., influenza virus) associated with vaccines containing the whole virion.

**sub·vag·i·nal** (sŭb-vaj′i-năl) **1.** below the vagina. **2.** on the inner side of any tubular membrane serving as a sheath.

**sub·vir·ion** (sub-vīr′ē-on) an incomplete viral particle. [sub- + virion]

**sub·vo·cal speech** slight movements of the muscles of speech related to thinking but producing no sound.

**suc·ce·da·ne·ous tooth 1.** a permanent tooth that succeeds an exfoliated deciduous tooth. **2.** permanent incisors, canines, and premolars.

**suc·ci·nyl-CoA** (sŭk′sin-il-kō-ā) SYN succinyl-coenzyme A.

**suc·ci·nyl-co·en·zyme A** (sŭk′si-nil-kō-en′zīm ā) the condensation product of succinic acid and CoA; one of the intermediates of the tricarboxylic acid cycle and a precursor in the synthesis of heme. SYN succinyl-CoA.

**suc·cor·rhea** (sŭk-ō-rē′ă) an abnormal increase in the secretion of a digestive fluid. [L. *succus,* juice, + G. *rhoia,* a flow]

**suc·cu·bus** (sŭk′yu-bŭs) a demon, in female form, believed to have sexual intercourse with a man during sleep. Cf. incubus. [L. *succubo,* to lie under]

**suc·cus·sion sound** the noise made by fluid with overlying air when shaken, such as occurs with gastric dilation or with fluid and air in a pleural cavity (hydropneumothorax).

**suck·ing blis·ter** superficial bullous skin lesion on neonate arm probably resulting from vigorous prenatal sucking.

**suck·ing chest wound** SYN open pneumothorax.

**suck·ing wound** SYN open pneumothorax.

**su·crase** (soo′krās) SYN sucrose α-D-glucohydrolase.

**su·crose** (soo′krōs) a nonreducing disaccharide made up of D-glucose and D-fructose obtained from sugar cane, *Saccharum officinarum* (family Gramineae), from several species of sorghum, and from the sugar beet, *Beta vulgaris* (family Chenopodiaceae); the common sweetener, used in pharmacy in the manufacture of syrup, confections, etc. SYN saccharose.

**su·crose α-D-glu·co·hy·dro·lase** an enzyme hydrolyzing sucrose and maltose in a complex with isomaltase; hence, hydrolyzes both sucrose and isomaltose; found in the intestinal mucosa; a deficiency of this enzyme results in defective digestion of sucrose and linear α1,4-glucans. SYN sucrase.

**su·cro·se·mia** (soo-krō-sē′mē-ă) the presence of sucrose in the blood. [sucrose + G. *haima,* blood]

**su·cro·su·ria** (soo-krō-syu′rē-ă) the excretion of sucrose in the urine. [sucrose + G. *ouron,* urine]

**suc·tion cath·e·ter** a catheter used to remove mucus and other secretions from the upper airway, trachea, and main bronchi.

**suc·tion cur·et·tage** a form of abortion in which the cervix is dilated if necessary and the products of conception removed by use of a canula attached to a suction source; technique used to complete a spontaneous incomplete abortion or as a form of induced abortion. SYN dilation and suction.

**suc·tion drain·age** closed drainage of a cavity, with a suction apparatus attached to the drainage tube.

**suc·to·ri·al** (sŭk-tō′rē-ăl) relating to suction, or the act of sucking; adapted for sucking.

**su·da·men,** pl. **su·dam·i·na** (soo-dā′men, soo-dam′i-nă) a minute vesicle due to retention of fluid in a sweat follicle, or in the epidermis. [Mod. L., fr. L. *sudo,* to sweat]

**su·dam·i·nal** (soo-dam′i-năl) relating to sudamina.

**su·dan·o·phil·ic** (soo-dan-ō-fil′ik) staining easily with Sudan dyes, usually referring to lipids in tissues.

**su·dan·o·pho·bic** (soo-dan-ō-fō′bik) denoting tissue that fails to stain with a Sudan or fat-soluble dye.

**Su·dan vi·rus** (soo-dan′) a variant of Ebola virus. SYN Ebola virus Sudan.

**Su·dan yel·low** (soo-dan′) metadioxy-azobenzene; a yellow stain for fats.

**su·da·tion** (soo-dā′shŭn) SYN perspiration (1). [L. *sudatio,* fr. *sudo,* pp. *-atus,* to sweat]

**sud·den deaf·ness** a profound sensory hearing loss that develops in 24 hrs or less; generally thought to be due to a viral infection in the inner ear.

**sud·den death 1.** an arrhythmogenic death in aortic stenosis, coronary disease, mesothelioma of the AV node, or single coronary artery. **2.** unexpected death occurring within one hour of onset of symptoms; most often used to describe death caused by cardiac failure. SEE ALSO hypertrophic cardiomyopathy.

**sud·den in·fant death syn·drome (SIDS)** abrupt and inexplicable death of an apparently healthy infant; various theories have been advanced to explain such deaths (e.g., sleep-induced apnea, laryngospasm, overwhelming infectious disease) but none has been generally accepted or demonstrated at autopsy. SYN crib death.

**su·do·mo·tor** (soo-dō-mō′ter) denoting the autonomic (sympathetic) nerves that stimulate the sweat glands to activity. [L. *sudor,* sweat, + *motor,* mover]

**su·dor** (soo′dōr) SYN perspiration (3). [L.]

△ **su·dor-** sweat, perspiration. [L. *sudor*]

**su·dor·al** (soo′dōr′ăl) relating to perspiration.

**su·do·re·sis** (soo-dō-rē′sis) profuse sweating. [sudor- + G. *-ēsis,* condition]

**su·do·rif·er·ous** (soo-dō-rif′er-ŭs) carrying or producing sweat. [sudor- + L. *fero,* to bear]

**su·do·rif·er·ous ab·scess** a collection of pus in a sweat gland.

**su·do·rif·er·ous cyst** a cyst caused by a blocked excretory duct of Moll glands. SYN apocrine hidrocystoma.

**su·do·rif·ic** (soo-dō-rif′ik) causing sweat. [sudor- + L. *facio,* to make]

**su·do·rip·a·rous** (soo-dō-rip′ă-rŭs) secreting sweat. [sudor- + L. *pario,* to produce]

**suf·fo·cate** (sŭf′ō-kāt) **1.** to impede respiration; to asphyxiate. **2.** to be unable to breathe; to suffer from asphyxiation. [L. *suffoco (subf-),* pp. *-atus,* to choke, strangle]

**suf·fo·ca·tion** (sŭf-ō-kā′shŭn) the act or condition of suffocating or of asphyxiation.

**suf·fo·ca·tive goi·ter** a goiter that by pressure causes extreme dyspnea.

**suf·fu·sion** (sŭ-fyu′zhŭn) **1.** the act of pouring a fluid over the body. **2.** a reddening of the surface. **3.** the condition of being wet with a fluid. **4.** SYN extravasate (2). [L. *suffusio,* fr. *suffundo (subf-),* to pour out]

**sug·ar** (shu′ger) one of the sugars; pharmaceutical forms are compressible sugar and confectioner's sugar. SEE ALSO sugars. [G. *sakcharon;* L. *saccharum*]

**sug·ars** (shug′erz) those carbohydrates (saccharides) having the general composition $(CH_2O)_n$ and simple derivatives thereof. Sugars are generally identifiable by the ending -ose or, if in combination with a nonsugar (aglycon), -oside or -osyl. Sugars, especially D-glucose, are the chief source of energy by oxidation in nature, and they and their derivatives in polymeric form are major constituents of mucoproteins, bacterial cell walls, and plant structural material (e.g., cellulose). Sugars are often found in combination with steroids (steroid glycosides) and other aglycons.

**sug•gest•i•bil•i•ty** (sŭg-jes'tĭ-bil'ĭ-tē) responsiveness or susceptibility to a psychological process such as a hypnotic command whereby an idea is induced into, or adopted by, an individual without argument, command, or coercion.

**sug•gest•i•ble** (sŭg-jes'tĭ-bl) susceptible to suggestion.

**sug•ges•tion** (sŭg-jes'chŭn) the implanting of an idea in the mind of another by some word or act on one's part, the subject's conduct or physical condition being influenced to some degree by the implanted idea. SEE ALSO autosuggestion. [L. *sug-gero* (*subg-*), pp. *-gestus,* to bring under, supply]

**sug•gil•la•tion** (sŭg-ji-lā'shŭn) a bruise or livedo. SEE ALSO contusion. [L. *sugillo,* pp. *-atus,* to beat black and blue]

**SUI** stress urinary incontinence.

**su•i•cide** (soo'i-sīd) **1.** the act of taking one's own life. **2.** a person who commits such an act. [L. *sui,* self, + *caedo,* to kill]

**sul•cal** (sŭl'kăl) relating to a sulcus.

**sul•cate** (sŭl'kāt) grooved; furrowed; marked by a sulcus or sulci.

**sul•ci par•a•ol•fac•tor•ii** [TA] SYN parolfactory sulci.

**sul•cus,** gen. and pl. **sul•ci** (sŭl'kŭs, sŭl'sī) **1.** one of the grooves or furrows on the surface of the brain, bounding the several convolutions or gyri; a fissure. SEE ALSO fissure. **2.** any long narrow groove, furrow, or slight depression. SEE ALSO groove. **3.** a groove or depression in the oral cavity or on the surface of a tooth. [L. a furrow or ditch]

**sul•cus ma•tri•cis un•guis** the cutaneous furrow in which the lateral border of the nail is situated. SYN groove of nail matrix.

**sul•cus ter•mi•nal•is** [TA] **1.** sulcus terminalis linguae [NA]; a V-shaped groove, with apex pointing backward, on the surface of the tongue, marking the separation between the oral, or horizontal, and the pharyngeal, or vertical, parts; **2.** sulcus terminalis cordis [TA]; a groove on the surface of the right atrium of the heart, marking the junction of the primitive sinus venosus with the atrium.

**sul•cus test** a test for multidirectional shoulder instability; the seated patient's humerus is pulled caudally, with inferior mobility indicating positive result.

△**sulf-, sul•fo-** **1.** prefix denoting that the compound to the name of which it is attached contains a sulfur atom. This spelling (rather than sulph-, sulpho-) is preferred by the American Chemical Society and has been adopted by the USP and NF, but not by the BP. **2.** prefix form of sulfonic acid or sulfonate.

**sul•fa•tase** (sŭl'fă-tās) **1.** trivial name for enzymes in EC group 3.1.6, the sulfuric ester hydrolases, which catalyze the hydrolysis of sulfuric esters (sulfates) to the corresponding alcohols plus inorganic sulfate. **2.** SYN arylsulfatase.

**sul•fa•tides** (sŭl'fă-tīdz) cerebroside sulfuric es-

ters containing one or more sulfate groups in the sugar portion of the molecule.

**sul•fa•tion** (sŭl-fā'shŭn) addition of sulfate groups as esters to preexisting molecules.

**sulf•he•mo•glo•bin** (sŭlf-hē'mō-glō-bin) SYN sulfmethemoglobin.

**sulf•he•mo•glo•bi•ne•mia** (sŭlf-hē'mō-glō-bi-nē' mē-ă) a morbid condition due to the presence of sulfhemoglobin in the blood; it is marked by a persistent cyanosis, but the blood count does not reveal any abnormality in blood cells; it is thought to be caused by the action of hydrogen sulfide absorbed from the intestine.

**sulf•hy•dryl (SH)** (sŭlf-hī'dril) the radical –SH; contained in glutathione, cysteine, coenzyme A, lipoamide (all in the reduced state), and in mercaptans (R–SH).

**sul•fide** (sŭl'fīd) a compound of sulfur in which the sulfur has a valence of –2.

**sul•fite ox•i•dase** a liver oxidoreductase (hemoprotein) catalyzing the reaction of inorganic sulfite ion with $O_2$ and water to produce sulfate ion and $H_2O_2$; a lower activity of this enzyme is observed in cases of molybdenum cofactor deficiency.

**sulf•met•he•mo•glo•bin** (sŭlf-met-hē'mō-glō-bin) the complex formed by $H_2S$ (or sulfides) and ferric ion in methemoglobin. SYN sulfhemoglobin.

**sul•fo•brom•oph•tha•lein so•di•um** a triphenylmethane derivative excreted by the liver, used in testing hepatic function, particularly of the reticuloendothelial cells. SYN bromosulfophthalein, bromsulfophthalein.

**sul•fo•nate** (sŭl'fō-nāt) a salt or ester of sulfonic acid.

**sul•fone** (sŭl-fōn) a compound of the general structure R'–$SO_2$–R''.

**sul•fon•ic ac•id** (sŭl-fon'ik as'id) any of the compounds in which a hydrogen atom of a CH group is replaced by the sulfonic acid group, –$SO_3H$; general formula: R–$SO_3H$.

**sul•fo•nyl•u•re•as** derivatives of isopropylthiodiazylsulfanilamide, chemically related to the sulfonamides, which possess hypoglycemic action. Belonging to this series are acetohexamide, azepinamide, chlorpropamide, fluphenmepramide, glymidine, hydroxyhexamide, heptolamide, indylamide, thiohexamide, tolazamide, and tolbutamide.

**sul•fo•trans•fer•ase** (sŭl-fō-trans'fer-ās) generic term for enzymes in EC sub-subclass 2.8.2 catalyzing the transfer of a sulfate group from 3'-phosphoadenylyl sulfate (active sulfate) to the hydroxyl group of an acceptor.

**sulf•ox•ide** (sŭl-fok'sīd) the sulfur analog of a ketone, R'–SO–R''.

**sul•fur (S)** (sŭl'fer) an element, atomic no. 16, atomic wt. 32.066, that combines with oxygen to form sulfur dioxide ($SO_2$) and sulfur trioxide ($SO_3$), and these with water to make strong acids, and with many metals and nonmetallic elements to form sulfides; used externally in the treatment of skin diseases. [L. *sulfur,* brimstone, sulfur]

**sul•fur-35** a radioactive sulfur isotope; a beta emitter with a half-life of 87.2 days; used as a tracer in the study of metabolism of cysteine, cystine, methionine, etc.; also used to estimate, with labeled sulfate, extracellular fluid volumes.

**sul•fur•ic ac•id** $H_2SO_4$; a colorless, nearly odorless, heavy, oily, corrosive liquid containing 96%

of the absolute acid; used occasionally as a caustic.

**sul·fur·yl** (sŭl'fūr-il) bivalent radical, –SO$_2$–.

△**sulph-, sul·pho-** SEE sulf-.

**sul·phaem·o·glo·bin [Br.]** SEE sulfmethemoglobin.

**sul·phae·mo·glo·bi·nae·mia [Br.]** SEE sulfhemoglobinemia.

**sul·phae·mo·glo·bi·nae·mia [Br.]** SEE sulfhemoglobinemia.

**sulph·met·hae·mo·glo·bin [Br.]** SEE sulfmethemoglobin.

**sul·pho·brom·oph·tha·lein [Br.]** a triphenylmethane derivative excreted by the liver, used in testing hepatic function, particularly of the reticuloendothelial cells. SEE sulfobromophthalein sodium.

**sul·pho·nic [Br.]** SEE sulfonic acid.

**sul·pho·nyl·ur·eas [Br.]** SEE sulfonylureas.

**sul·phur·ic a·cid** SYN oil of vitriol. SEE sulfuric acid.

**sum·mat·ing po·ten·tials** alternating current responses of the spiral organ (organ of Corti) to acoustic stimulation.

**sum·ma·tion** (sŭm-ā'shŭn) the aggregation of a number of similar neural impulses or stimuli. [Mediev. L. *summatio,* fr. *summo,* pp. *-atus,* to sum up, fr. L. *summa*]

**sum·ma·tion gal·lop** gallop rhythm in which the gallop sound is due to superimposition of third and fourth heart sounds; sometimes heard in normal subjects with tachycardia, but usually indicative of myocardial disease.

**sum·mer di·ar·rhea** diarrhea of infants in hot weather, usually an acute gastroenteritis due to *Shigella* or *Salmonella.* SYN choleraic diarrhea.

**Sum·ner sign** (sŭm'ner) a slight increase in tonus of the abdominal muscles, an early indication of inflammation of the appendix, stone in the kidney or ureter, or a twisted pedicle of an ovarian cyst; it is detected by exceedingly gentle palpation of the right or left iliac fossa.

**sump drain** a drain consisting of an outer tube with a smaller tube within it which is attached to a suction pump; the outer tube has multiple perforations that allow fluid and air to pass into its interior and be carried away through the suction tube.

**sump syn·drome** a complication of side-to-side choledochoduodenostomy in which the lower end of the common bile duct at times acts as a diverticulum, resulting in stasis, trapping of food particles, and infection.

**sun·burn** (sŭn'bern) erythema with or without blistering caused by exposure to critical amounts of ultraviolet light, usually within the range of 260 to 320 nm in sunlight (UVB).

**sun·down·ing** (sŭn'down-ing) the onset or exacerbation of delirium during the evening or night with improvement or disappearance during the day; most often seen in mid and later stages of dementing disorders, such as Alzheimer disease.

**sun pro·tec·tion fac·tor (SPF)** the ratio of the minimal ultraviolet dose required to produce erythema with and without a sunscreen; useful sunscreens have an SPF of at least 15.

**sun·screen** (sŭn'skrēn) a topical product that protects the skin from ultraviolet-induced erythema and resists washing off; its use also reduces formation of solar keratoses and may prevent ultraviolet-B-induced skin cancer and wrinkling.

**sun·stroke, sun stroke** (sŭn'strōk) a form of heatstroke resulting from undue exposure to the sun's rays, probably caused by the action of actinic rays combined with high temperature; symptoms are those of heatstroke, but often without fever.

△**su·per-** (Properly prefixed to words of L. derivation) denoting in excess, above, superior, or in the upper part of; often the same usage as L. *supra-.* Cf. hyper-. [L. *super,* above, beyond]

**su·per·ac·tiv·i·ty** (soo-per-ak-tiv'i-tē) abnormally great activity. SYN hyperactivity (1).

**su·per·a·cute** (soo'per-ă-kyut') extremely acute; marked by extreme severity of symptoms and rapid progress, as of the course of a disease.

**su·per·cil·i·ary** (soo-per-sil'ē-ār-ē) relating to or in the region of the eyebrow.

**su·per·cil·i·ary arch** a fullness extending laterally from the glabella on either side, above the orbital margin of the frontal bone.

**su·per·cil·i·um,** pl. **su·per·cil·i·a** (soo'per-sil'ē-ŭm, soo'per-sil'ē-ă) [TA] **1.** SYN eyebrow. **2.** an individual hair of the eyebrow. [L. fr. *super,* above, + *cilium,* eyelid]

**su·per·con·duct·ing mag·net** a magnet whose coils are cooled, usually with liquid helium, to a temperature at which the metal becomes superconducting, effectively removing all electrical resistance.

**su·per·duct** (sooper-dŭkt) to elevate or draw upward. [L. *super-duco,* pp. *-ductus,* to lead over]

**su·per·e·go** (soo-per-ē'gō) PSYCHOANALYSIS one of the three components of the psychic apparatus in the freudian structural framework, the other two being the ego and the id. It is an outgrowth of the ego that has identified itself unconsciously with important persons, such as parents, from early life, and which results from incorporating the values and wishes of these persons and subsequently societal norms as part of one's own standards to form the "conscience."

**su·per·ex·ci·ta·tion** (soo'per-ek-sī-tā'shŭn) **1.** the act of exciting or stimulating unduly. **2.** a condition of extreme excitement or stimulation.

**su·per·fi·cial** (soo-per-fish'ăl) **1.** cursory; not thorough. **2.** pertaining to or situated near the surface. **3.** SYN superficialis. [L. *superficialis,* fr. *superficies,* surface]

**su·per·fi·cial bra·chi·al ar·tery** an occasional variation in which the brachial artery lies superficial to the median nerve in the arm.

**su·per·fi·cial branch of me·di·al cir·cum·flex fe·mor·al ar·tery** small branch arising from the initial portion of the medial femoral circumflex artery that passes superficially in the superomedial thigh; after giving rise to the superficial branch, the medial femoral circumflex artery continues as the deep branch.

**su·per·fi·cial dor·sal veins of pe·nis** a pair of veins on the dorsum of the penis superficial to the fascia penis; they are tributaries of the external pudendal veins on each side. SYN vena dorsalis superficialis penis [TA].

**su·per·fi·cial ep·i·gas·tric vein** drains the lower and medial part of the anterior abdominal wall and empties into the great saphenous vein. SYN vena epigastrica.

**su·per·fi·cial fa·scia** a loose fibrous envelope beneath the skin, containing fat in its meshes (panniculus adiposus) or fasciculi of muscular tissue (panniculus carnosus); it contains the cuta-

**S**
**u**

neous vessels and nerves and is in relation by its undersurface with the deep fascia. SYN hypodermis, tela subcutanea.

**su·per·fi·cial fa·scia of per·i·ne·um** the membranous layer of the subcutaneous tissue in the urogenital region attaching posteriorly to the border of the urogenital diaphragm, at the sides to the ischiopubic rami, and continuing anteriorly onto the abdominal wall. SYN fascia perinei superficialis [TA].

**su·per·fi·cial flex·or mus·cle of fin·gers** SYN flexor digitorum superficialis muscle.

**su·per·fi·cial in·gui·nal ring** the slit-like opening in the aponeurosis of the external oblique muscle of the abdominal wall through which the spermatic cord (round ligament in the female) and inguinal hernias emerge from the inguinal canal. SYN anulus inguinalis superficialis [TA].

**su·per·fi·cial in·vest·ing fa·scia of per·i·ne·um** SYN perineal fascia.

**su·per·fi·ci·a·lis** (soo′per-fish-ē-ā′lis) situated nearer the surface of the body in relation to a specific reference point. SYN superficial (3). [L.]

**su·per·fi·cial re·flex** any reflex, e.g., the abdominal or cremasteric reflex, which is elicited by stimulation of the skin.

**su·per·fi·cial trans·verse per·i·ne·al mus·cle** an inconstant muscle; *origin*, ramus of ischium; *insertion*, central tendon of perineum; *action*, draws back and fixes the central tendon of the perineum; *nerve supply*, pudendal (perineal). SYN musculus transversus perinei superficialis [TA].

**su·per·fi·cial vein** one of a number of veins that course in the subcutaneous tissue and empty into deep veins; they form prominent systems of vessels in the limbs and are usually not accompanied by arteries.

**su·per·fi·cies** (soo-per-fish′ī-ēz) outer surface; facies. [L. the top surface, fr. *super*, above, + *facies*, figure, form]

**su·per·in·duce** (soo′per-in-doos) to induce or bring on in addition to something already existing.

**su·per·in·fec·tion** (soo′per-in-fek′shŭn) a new infection in addition to one already present.

**su·per·in·vo·lu·tion** (soo′per-in-vō-loo′shŭn) an extreme reduction in size of the uterus, after childbirth, below the normal size of the nongravid organ. SYN hyperinvolution.

**[i] su·pe·ri·or** (soo-pir′ē-ĕr) **1.** situated above or directed upward. **2.** HUMAN ANATOMY situated nearer the vertex of the head in relation to a specific reference point; opposite of inferior. SYN cranial (2). See page APP 89. [L. comparative of *superus*, above]

**su·pe·ri·or al·ve·o·lar nerves** three branches (posterior, middle, and anterior) of the maxillary nerve (or its continuation as the infraorbital nerve) that enter the maxilla to supply the mucosa of the maxillary sinus, upper teeth and gingiva.

**su·pe·ri·or au·ric·u·lar mus·cle** *origin*, galea aponeurotica; *insertion*, cartilage of auricle; *action* draws pinna of ear upward and backward; *nerve supply*, facial. Considered by some to be the posterior part of the temporoparietal muscle. SYN musculus attollens aurem, musculus attollens auriculam.

**su·pe·ri·or ba·sal vein** tributary to the common basal vein draining the lateral and anterior part of the inferior lobe of each lung.

**su·pe·ri·or cer·e·bel·lar ar·tery** *origin*, basilar; *distribution*, upper surface of cerebellum, colliculi, and most of the cerebellar nuclei; *anastomoses*, posterior inferior cerebellar.

**su·pe·ri·or cer·e·bel·lar pe·dun·cle** a large bundle of nerve fibers that originate from the dentate and interpositus nuclei and emerges from the cerebellum in the rostral direction, along the lateral wall of the fourth ventricle. The bundle submerges from the dorsal surface of the brainstem into the mesencephalic tegmentum, where all of its fibers cross in the massive decussation of the superior cerebellar peduncles. Part of the bundle terminates in the contralateral red nucleus; the bulk of the fibers continue rostrally to parts of the ventral intermediate nucleus of thalamus, ventral posterolateral nucleus of thalamus, and central lateral nucleus of thalamus.

**su·pe·ri·or ce·re·bral veins** numerous (8–10) veins that drain the dorsal convexity of the cortical hemisphere and empty into the superior sagittal sinus, curving rostrally in passing through the subdural space so as to enter the sinus at an acute forward angle. SYN venae superiores cerebri [TA].

**su·pe·ri·or con·stric·tor mus·cle of phar·ynx** *origin*, medial pterygoid plate (pterygopharyngeal part), pterygomandibular raphe (buccopharyngeal part), mylohyoid line of mandible (myelopharyngeal part), and the mucous membrane of the floor of the mouth and the side of the tongue (glossopharyngeal part); *insertion*, pharyngeal raphe in the posterior wall of the pharynx; *action*, narrows pharynx; *nerve supply*, pharyngeal plexus. SYN musculus constrictor pharyngis superior [TA].

**su·pe·ri·or den·tal arch** the teeth supported by the alveolar process of the two maxillae, whether the 10 deciduous teeth or the 16 permanent teeth.

**su·pe·ri·or ep·i·gas·tric veins** the venae comitantes of the artery of the same name, tributaries of the internal thoracic vein.

**su·pe·ri·or ex·ten·sor ret·i·nac·u·lum** the ligament that binds down the extensor tendons proximal to the ankle joint; it is continuous with (a thickening of) the deep fascia of the leg.

**su·pe·ri·or front·al gy·rus** a broad convolution running in an anteroposterior direction on the medial edge of the convex surface and of each frontal lobe.

**su·pe·ri·or gan·gli·on of glos·so·pha·ryn·ge·al nerve** the upper and smaller of two ganglia on the glossopharyngeal nerve as it traverses the jugular foramen.

**su·pe·ri·or gan·gli·on of va·gus nerve** a small sensory ganglion on the vagus as it traverses the jugular foramen.

**su·pe·ri·or ge·mel·lus mus·cle** *origin*, ischial spine and margin of lesser sciatic notch; *insertion*, tendon of musculus obturator internus; *action*, rotates thigh laterally; *nerve supply*, sacral plexus.

**su·pe·ri·or·i·ty com·plex** term sometimes given to the compensatory behavior, e.g., aggressiveness, self-assertion, associated with inferiority complex.

**su·pe·ri·or la·bi·al vein** veins taking blood from the upper lip and discharging into the facial vein.

**su·pe·ri·or lim·bic ker·a·to·con·junc·ti·vi·tis** inflammatory edema of the superior corneoscleral limbus.

**su·pe·ri·or lon·gi·tu·di·nal fa·sci·cu·lus** long association fiber bundle lateral to the centrum ovale of the cerebral hemisphere, connecting the frontal, occipital, and temporal lobes; the fibers pass from the frontal lobe through the operculum to the posterior end of the lateral sulcus where many fibers radiate into the occipital lobe and others turn downward and forward around the putamen and pass to anterior portions of the temporal lobe. SYN fasciculus longitudinalis superior [TA].

**su·pe·ri·or mac·u·lar ar·te·ri·ole** origin, central artery of retina; distribution, upper part of macula. SYN arteriola macularis superior [TA].

**su·pe·ri·or med·ul·lary ve·lum** the thin layer of white matter stretching between the two superior cerebellar peduncles, forming the roof of the superior recess of the fourth ventricle.

**su·pe·ri·or na·sal con·cha 1.** the upper thin, spongy, bony plate with curved margins, part of the ethmoidal labyrinth, projecting from the lateral wall of the nasal cavity and separating the superior meatus from the sphenoethmoidal recess; **2.** the above bony plate and its thick mucoperiosteum, which is less vascular than that of the middle and inferior conchae.

**su·pe·ri·or na·sal ret·i·nal ar·te·ri·ole** the branch of the central artery of the retina that passes to the upper medial, or nasal, part of the retina.

**su·pe·ri·or oblique mus·cle** origin, above the medial margin of the optic canal; insertion, by a tendon passing through the trochlea, or pulley, and then reflected backward, downward, and laterally to the sclera between the superior and lateral recti; action, primary, intorsion; secondary, depression and abduction; nerve supply, trochlear nerve. SYN musculus obliquus superior [TA].

**su·pe·ri·or or·bi·tal fis·sure** a cleft between the greater and the lesser wings of the sphenoid establishing a channel of communication between the middle cranial fossa and the orbit, through which pass the oculomotor and trochlear nerves, the ophthalmic division of the trigeminal nerve, the abducens nerve, and the ophthalmic veins.

**su·pe·ri·or pel·vic aper·ture** the upper opening of the true pelvis, bounded anteriorly by the pubic symphysis and the pubic crest on either side, laterally by the iliopectineal lines, and posteriorly by the promontory of the sacrum.

**su·pe·ri·or rec·tus mus·cle** origin, superior part of common tendinous ring; insertion, superior part of sclera of the eye; action, primary, elevation; secondary, adduction and intorsion; nerve supply, oculomotor. SYN musculus rectus superior [TA].

**su·pe·ri·or tem·por·al line** the upper of two curved lines on the parietal bone; the temporal fascia is attached to it.

**su·pe·ri·or tem·por·al ret·i·nal ar·te·ri·ole** the branch of the central artery of the retina that passes laterally above the macula to supply the upper lateral or temporal part of the retina.

**su·pe·ri·or tem·por·al sul·cus** the longitudinal sulcus that separates the superior and middle temporal gyri.

**su·pe·ri·or thal·a·mo·stri·ate vein** a long vein passing forward in the groove between the thalamus and caudate nucleus, covered by the lamina affixa, receiving the transverse caudate veins along its lateral side, and joining at the caudal

wall of Monro foramen with the choroidal vein and vein of septum pellucidum to form the internal cerebral vein.

**su·pe·ri·or vein of ver·mis** a vein draining part of the superior part of the cerebellum; it runs on the superior surface of the vermis to terminate in the internal cerebral vein.

**su·pe·ri·or ve·na ca·va** returns blood from the head and neck, upper limbs, and thorax to the posterosuperior aspect of the right atrium; formed in the superior mediastinum by union of the two brachiocephalic veins. SYN vena cava superior [TA], precava.

**su·pe·ri·or ve·na ca·va syn·drome** obstruction of the superior vena cava or its main tributaries by benign or malignant lesions, causing edema and engorgement of the vessels of the face, neck, and arms, nonproductive cough, and dyspnea; bluish looking venous stars may be found in the early phases, overlying the large veins to which they are tributary, but they tend to diminish in size and disappear after collateral circulation has been reestablished.

**su·pe·ri·or ver·mi·an branch (of su·pe·ri·or ce·re·bel·lar ar·te·ry)** origin: medial branch of superior cerebellar artery; distribution: superior vermis of cerebellum.

**su·per·mo·til·i·ty** (soo′per-mō-til′i-tē) SYN hyperkinesis.

**su·per·nu·mer·ary** (soo-per-noo′mer-ār-ē) exceeding the normal number. [super- + L. numerus, number]

**su·per·nu·mer·ary or·gans** organs exceeding the normal number, which may develop from multiple foci or organization in an organ-formative field larger (originally) than that of the definitive main organ; such organs are aberrant but frequently not a cause of disease; illness may persist if they are left in the body after therapeutic removal of the main organ, e.g., accessory spleen.

**su·per·o·lat·er·al** (soo-per-ō-lat′er-ăl) at the side and above.

**su·per·ox·ide** (soo-per-oks′īd) an oxygen free radical, $O_2^-$, which is toxic to cells.

**su·per·ox·ide dis·mu·tase** an enzyme that catalyzes the dismutation reaction, $2O_2^- + 2H^+ \rightarrow H_2O_2 + O_2$; a deficiency is associated with amyotrophic lateral sclerosis.

**su·per·sat·u·rate** (soo-per-sach′ŭ-rāt) to make a solution hold more of a salt or other substance in solution than it will dissolve when in equilibrium with that salt in the solid phase; such solutions are usually unstable with respect to precipitating the excess salt or substance and becoming saturated.

**su·per·sat·u·rat·ed so·lu·tion** a solution containing more of the solid than the liquid would ordinarily dissolve; it is made by heating the solvent when the substance is added, and on cooling the latter is retained without precipitation; addition of a crystal or solid of any kind usually results in precipitation of the excess solute, leaving a saturated solution.

**su·per·scrip·tion** (soo′per-skrip′shŭn) the beginning of a prescription, consisting of the injunction, recipe, take, usually denoted by the sign ℞. [L. super-scribo, pp. -scriptus, to write upon or over]

**su·per·son·ic** (soo′per-son′ik) **1.** pertaining to or characterized by a speed greater than the speed of sound. **2.** pertaining to sound vibrations of high frequency, above the level of human audibility. SEE ALSO ultrasonic. [super- + L. *sonus,* sound]

**su·per·struc·ture** (soo-per-strŭk'cher) a structure above the surface.

**su·pi·nate** (soo'pi-nāt) **1.** to assume, or to be placed in, a supine (face upward) position. **2.** to perform supination of the forearm or of the foot. [L. *supino,* pp. *-atus,* to bend backwards, place on back, fr. *supinus,* supine]

🔒 **su·pi·na·tion** (soo'pi-nā'shŭn) the condition of being supine; the act of assuming or of being placed in a supine position. See page APP 91.

**su·pi·na·tor mus·cle** *origin,* lateral epicondyle of humerus, radial collateral and anular ligaments, and supinator ridge of ulna; *insertion,* anterior and lateral surface of radius; *action,* supinates the forearm; *nerve supply,* radial (posterior interosseous). SYN musculus supinator [TA].

**su·pine** (soo-pīn') **1.** denoting the body when lying face upward; opposite of prone. **2.** supination of the forearm or of the foot. [L. *supinus*]

**sup·ple·men·tal air** SYN expiratory reserve volume.

**sup·ple·men·tal groove** an indistinct linear depression, irregular in extent and direction, which does not demarcate major   divisional portions of a tooth.

**sup·port·ing cusp** the buccal cusp of the lower posterior teeth and the lingual cusp of the   upper posterior teeth.

**sup·pos·i·to·ry** (sŭ-poz'i-tōr-ē) a small, solid body shaped for ready introduction into one of the orifices of the body other than the oral cavity (e.g., rectum, urethra, vagina), made of a substance, usually medicated, which is solid at ordinary temperatures but melts at body temperature. [L. *suppositorium,* fr. *suppositorius,* placed underneath]

**sup·pres·sion** (sŭ-presh'ŭn) **1.** deliberately excluding from conscious thought. Cf. repression. **2.** arrest of the secretion of a fluid, such as urine or bile. Cf. retention (2). **3.** checking of an abnormal flow or discharge, as in suppression of a hemorrhage. **4.** the effect of a second mutation, which overwrites a phenotypic change caused by a previous mutation at a different point on the chromosome. SEE epistasis. **5.** inhibition of vision in one eye when dissimilar images fall on corresponding retinal points. [L. *subprimo* (*subp*-), pp. *-pressus,* to press down]

**sup·pres·sion am·bly·o·pia** suppression of the central vision in one eye when the images from the two eyes are so different that they cannot be fused into one. This may be due to: 1) faulty image formation (sensory amblyopia); 2) a large difference in refraction between the two eyes (anisometropic amblyopia); or 3) the two eyes pointing in different directions (strabismic amblyopia). Most suppression amblyopia can be reversed if appropriately treated before age six.

**sup·pres·sor mu·ta·tion 1.** a mutation that alters the anticodon in a tRNA so that it is complementary to a termination codon, thus suppressing termination of the amino acid chain. **2.** genetic changes such that the effect of a mutation in one place can be overcome by a second mutation in another location. There are two types: intergenic suppression (occurring in a different gene) and

intragenic suppression (occurring in the same gene but at a different site).

**sup·pu·rate** (sŭp'yŭr-āt) to form pus. [L. *suppuro* (*subp*-), pp. *-atus,* to form *pus* (*pur*), pus]

**sup·pu·ra·tion** (sŭp'yŭ-rā'shŭn) the formation of pus. SYN pyesis, pyogenesis, pyopoiesis, pyosis. [L. *suppuratio* (see suppurate)]

**sup·pu·ra·tive** (sŭp'yŭr-ă-tiv) forming pus.

**sup·pur·a·tive ar·thri·tis** acute inflammation of synovial membranes, with purulent effusion into a joint, due to bacterial infection. SYN purulent synovitis, pyarthrosis.

**sup·pur·a·tive gin·gi·vi·tis** gingivitis in which a purulent exudate can be expressed from the gingival surface.

**sup·pur·a·tive hy·a·li·tis** purulent vitreous humor due to exudation from adjacent structures, as in panophthalmitis.

**sup·pur·a·tive in·flam·ma·tion** SYN purulent inflammation.

**sup·pur·a·tive ne·phri·tis** focal glomerulonephritis with abscess formation in the kidney.

△ **su·pra-** a position above the part indicated by the word to which it is joined; in this sense, the same as super-; opposite of infra-. [L. *supra,* on the upper side]

**su·pra·bulge** (soo'pră-bŭlj) the portion of the crown of a tooth distal to its greatest circumference, whose contours converge toward the occlusal surface of the tooth.

**su·pra·cer·vi·cal hys·ter·ec·to·my** removal of the fundus of the uterus, leaving the cervix.

**su·pra·cho·roid** (soo-pră-kō'royd) on the outer side of the choroid of the eye.

**su·pra·cla·vi·cu·lar tri·an·gle** the triangle bounded by the clavicle, the omohyoid muscle, and the sternocleidomastoid muscle; it contains the subclavian artery and vein.

**su·pra·clin·oid an·eu·rysm** an intracranial aneurysm located immediately above the anterior clinoid process of the sphenoid bone.

**su·pra·con·dy·lar pro·cess** an occasional spine projecting from the anteromedial surface of the humerus about 5 cm above the medial epicondyle to which it is joined by a fibrous band. The supracondylar foramen thus formed transmits the brachial artery and median nerve.

**su·pra·cos·tal** (soo-pră-kos'tăl) above the ribs.

**su·pra·cris·tal** (soo-pră-kris'tăl) above a crest or ridge; specifically used to denote a line or plane across the summits of the iliac crests.

**su·pra·duc·tion** (soo-pră-dŭk'shŭn) the upward rotation of one eye. SYN sursumduction.

**su·pra·glot·tic la·ryn·gec·tomy** SYN partial laryngectomy.

**su·pra·glot·tic swal·low** therapeutic technique to prevent aspiration during swallowing, involving voluntary closure of the vocal folds before and after a swallow. The patient holds the breath, swallows with breath held, then coughs when the swallow is finished, before inhaling again.

**sup·ra·glot·ti·tis** (soop'ra-glah-tī'tis) an infectious inflammation and swelling of the laryngeal tissue above the glottis, especially of the epiglottis, which becomes red and spherical leading to upper airway obstruction.

**su·pra·lim·i·nal** (soo-pră-lim'i-năl) more than just perceptible; above the threshhold for conscious awareness. Cf. subliminal. [supra- + L. *limen,* threshold]

**su·pra·mar·gin·al gy·rus** a folded convolution

capping the posterior extremity of the lateral (sylvian) sulcus; together with the angular gyrus, it forms the inferior half of the parietal lobe.

**su•pra•mas•toid crest** the ridge that forms the posterior root of the zygomatic process of the temporal bone.

**su•pra•max•il•lary** (soo-pră-mak'si-lār-ē) above the maxilla.

**su•pra•me•a•tal tri•an•gle** a triangle formed by the root of the zygomatic arch, the posterior wall of the bony external acoustic meatus, and an imaginary line connecting the extremities of the first two lines; used as a guide in mastoid operations. SYN Macewen triangle.

**su•pra•men•ta•le** (soo'pră-men-tā'lē) CEPHALOMETRICS the most posterior midline point, above the chin, on the mandibula between the infradentale and the pogonion. SYN point B. [supra- + L. *mentum,* chin]

**su•pra•nor•mal ex•cit•a•bil•i•ty** at the end of phase three of the cardiac action potential, the successful stimulation threshold falls below (i.e., less negative than) the level necessary to produce excitation during the rest of the phase of diastole, so that an ordinary subthreshold stimulus becomes effective.

**su•pra•nu•cle•ar** (soo-pră-noo'klē-er) above (cranial to) the level of the motor neurons of the spinal or cranial nerves; the pathways the suprasegmental nerve fibers follow to reach the motor cell bodies in the brainstem; as used in clinical neurology, supranuclear indicates disorders of movement caused by destruction or functional impairment of brain structures other than the motor neurons, such as the motor cortex, pyramidal tract, or striate body; e.g., supranuclear palsy, as distinguished from the nuclear (or flaccid, or "lower motor neuron") paralysis that results from destruction or functional impairment of the motor neurons or their axons in a peripheral nerve.

**su•pra•nu•cle•ar pa•ral•y•sis** paralysis due to lesions above the primary motor neurons.

**su•pra•oc•clu•sion** (soo'pră-ō-kloo'zhŭn) an occlusal relationship in which a tooth extends beyond the occlusal plane.

**su•pra•op•tic com•mis•sures** SYN commissurae supraopticae.

**su•pra•or•bit•al ar•tery** *origin,* ophthalmic; *distribution,* frontalis muscle and scalp; *anastomoses,* branches of the superficial temporal and supratrochlear. SYN arteria supraorbitalis [TA].

**su•pra•or•bit•al for•a•men** a foramen in the supraorbital margin of the frontal bone at the junction of the medial and intermediate thirds. SYN foramen supraorbitale [TA].

**su•pra•or•bit•al mar•gin** the superior half of the orbital rim, which constitutes the curved superior border of the orbital opening, formed by the frontal bone.

**su•pra•or•bit•al nerve** a branch of the frontal nerve leaving the orbit through the supraorbital foramen or notch and dividing into branches distributed to the forehead and scalp, upper eyelid, and frontal sinus. SYN nervus supraorbitalis [TA].

**su•pra•or•bit•al vein** drains the front of the scalp and unites with the supratrochlear veins to form the angular vein.

**su•pra•bi•to•me•a•tal plane** a plane passing the superior orbital margins and the superior margin of the external acoustic meatuses; it

makes an angle of approximately 25–30° with the Frankfort plane and is the plane in which routine CT (computed tomography) scans of the brain are made.

**su•pra•pa•tel•lar bur•sa** a large bursa between the lower part of the femur and the tendon of the quadriceps femoris muscle. It usually communicates with the cavity of the knee joint.

**su•pra•pu•bic cys•to•to•my** opening into the bladder through an incision or puncture above the symphysis pubis.

**su•pra•re•nal 1.** above the kidney. **2.** pertaining to the suprarenal glands.

**su•pra•re•nal cor•tex** the outer part of the adrenal (suprarenal) gland, consisting of three zones from without inward: zona glomerulosa, zona fasciculata, and zona reticularis; this part of the adrenal cortex yields steroid hormones such as corticosterone, deoxycorticosterone, and estrone.

**su•pra•re•nal gland** a flattened, roughly triangular body resting upon the upper end of each kidney; an endocrine gland whose medulla produces epinephrine and norepinephrine and whose cortex produces cortisol and aldosterone. SYN adrenal gland, epinephros, paranephros.

**su•pra•re•nal me•dul•la** it is composed principally of anastomosing cords of cells in the core of the gland; the cells display a chromaffin reaction because of the presence of epinephrine and norepinephrine in their granules.

**su•pra•scap•u•lar ar•tery** *origin,* thyrocervical trunk; *distribution,* clavicle, scapula, muscles of shoulder, and shoulder joint; *anastomoses,* transverse cervical circumflex scapular. SYN arteria suprascapularis [TA], transverse scapular artery.

**su•pra•scap•u•lar nerve** arises from the upper trunk of the brachial plexus (fifth and sixth cervical spinal nerves), passes downward parallel to the cords of the brachial plexus, then through the scapular notch, supplying the supraspinatus and infraspinatus muscles, and also sending branches to the shoulder joint. It is vulnerable to injury in fractures of the middle one-third of the clavicle; a lesion of the suprascapular nerve results in a loss of lateral rotation at the shoulder so that when relaxed the limb rotates medially (waiter's tip position); ability to initiate abduction is also affected. SYN nervus suprascapularis [TA].

**su•pra•scap•u•lar vein** accompanies the suprascapular artery and empties into the external jugular vein.

**su•pra•scle•ral** (soo-pră-sklēr'ăl) on the outer side of the sclera, denoting the suprascleral or periscleral space between the sclera and the fascia bulbi.

**su•pra•spi•na•tus mus•cle** *origin,* supraspinous fossa of scapula; *insertion,* greater tuberosity of humerus; *action,* initiates abduction of arm; *nerve supply,* suprascapular from fifth and sixth cervical. SYN musculus supraspinatus [TA], supraspinous muscle.

**su•pra•spi•nous mus•cle** SYN supraspinatus muscle.

**su•pra•troch•le•ar ar•tery** *origin,* ophthalmic; *distribution,* anterior portion of scalp; *anastomoses,* branches of supraorbital. SYN arteria supratrochlearis [TA], frontal artery.

**su•pra•troch•le•ar nerve** a branch of the frontal nerve supplying the medial part of the upper eyelid, the central part of the skin of the forehead,

**S**
**u**

and the root of the nose. SYN nervus supratrochlearis [TA].

**su·pra·troch·le·ar veins** several veins that drain the front part of the scalp and unite with the supraorbital vein to form the angular vein.

**su·pra·vag·i·nal por·tion of cer·vix** the part of the cervix of the uterus lying above the attachment of the vagina.

**su·pra·val·var ste·no·sis** narrowing of the aorta above the aortic valve by a constricting ring or shelf, or by coarctation or hypoplasia of the ascending aorta.

**su·pra·ven·tric·u·lar** (soo-pră-ven-trik'yu-lăr) above the ventricles; especially applied to rhythms originating from centers proximal to the ventricles, namely in the atrium, A-V node, or A-V junction, in contrast to rhythms arising in the ventricles themselves.

**su·pra·ven·tric·u·lar crest** the internal muscular ridge that separates the conus arteriosus from the remaining part of the cavity of the right ventricle of the heart.

**su·pra·ver·sion** (soo-pră-ver'zhŭn) **1.** a turning (version) upward. **2.** DENTISTRY the position of a tooth when it is out of the line of occlusion in an occlusal direction. **3.** OPHTHALMOLOGY binocular conjugate rotation upward. [supra- + L. *verto*, pp. *versus*, to turn]

**su·pra·vi·tal stain** a procedure in which living tissue is removed from the body and cells are placed in a nontoxic dye solution so that their vital processes may be studied.

**su·preme na·sal con·cha** a small concha frequently present on the posterosuperior part of the lateral nasal wall; it overlies the supreme nasal meatus. SYN concha santorini, Santorini concha.

**su·ral** (soo'răl) relating to the calf of the leg.

**sur·al ar·tery** one of four or five arteries arising (sometimes by a common trunk) from the popliteal; *distribution*, muscles and integument of the calf; *anastomoses*, posterior tibial, medial, and lateral inferior genicular. SYN arteria suralis [TA].

**sur·al nerve** formed by the union of the medial sural cutaneous from the tibial and the peroneal communicating branch of the common peroneal nerve, usually about the middle of the calf, although this is highly variable; thence it accompanies the small saphenous vein around the lateral malleolus to the dorsum of the foot as the lateral dorsal cutaneous nerve. SYN nervus suralis [TA].

**sur·al re·gion** the muscular swelling of the back of the leg below the knee, formed chiefly by the bellies of the gastrocnemius and soleus muscles. SYN calf.

**sur·face** (ser'făs) the outer part of any solid. SYN facies (2) [TA], face (2). [F. fr. L. *superficius*, see superficial]

**sur·face-ac·tive** (ser'făs-ak'tiv) indicating the property of certain agents of altering the physicochemical nature of surfaces and interfaces, bringing about lowering of interfacial tension; they usually possess both lipophilic and hydrophilic groups. SEE ALSO surfactant.

**sur·face a·na·to·my** the study of the configuration of the surface of the body, especially in its relation to deeper parts.

🔲 **sur·face bi·op·sy** a biopsy obtained by detaching cells from a cutaneous or mucosal surface with a spatula, cotton swab, or brush. See page 117.

**sur·face coil** a detector coil applied directly to a body part for high resolution imaging; often a single loop of metal.

**sur·face ep·i·the·li·um 1.** a layer of celomic epithelial cells covering the gonadal ridges as they are formed on the medial border of the mesonephroi near the root of the mesentery; **2.** the mesothelial covering of the definitive ovary.

**sur·face mi·cro·sco·py** SYN epiluminescence microscopy.

**sur·face ten·sion** (γ, σ) the expression of intermolecular attraction at the surface of a liquid, in contact with air or another gas, a solid, or another immiscible liquid, tending to pull the molecules of the liquid inward from the surface; dimensional formula: $mt^{-2}$.

**sur·face thal·am·ic veins** SYN venae directae laterales.

**sur·fac·tant** (ser-fak'tănt) **1.** a surface-active agent, including substances commonly referred to as wetting agents, surface tension depressants, detergents, dispersing agents, and emulsifiers. **2.** those surface-active agents forming a monomolecular layer over pulmonary alveolar surfaces; lipoproteins that include lecithins and sphingomyelins that stabilize alveolar volume by reducing surface tension and altering the relationship between surface tension and surface area. [*surface active agent*]

**sur·geon** (ser'jŭn) a physician who treats disease, injury, and deformity by operation or manipulation. [G. *cheirougos*; L. *chirurgus*]

**sur·geon's knot** the first loop of the knot has two throws rather than a single throw. The second loop has only one throw and that is placed in a square knot fashion leaving the free ends in the same plane as the first loop.

**sur·gery** (ser'jer-ē) **1.** the branch of medicine concerned with the treatment of disease, injury, and deformity by operation or manipulation. **2.** the performance or procedures of an operation. [L. *chirurgia*; G. *cheir*, hand, + *ergon*, work]

**sur·gi·cal** (ser'ji-kăl) relating to surgery.

**sur·gi·cal ab·do·men** SYN acute abdomen.

**sur·gi·cal a·na·to·my** applied anatomy in reference to surgical diagnosis and treatment.

**sur·gi·cal an·es·the·sia 1.** any anesthesia administered for the performance of an operative procedure, as differentiated from obstetrical, diagnostic, and therapeutic anesthesia; **2.** loss of sensation with muscle relaxation adequate for an operative procedure.

**sur·gi·cal di·a·ther·my** electrocoagulation with a high frequency electrocautery, resulting in local tissue destruction; usually used to seal blood vessels and arrest bleeding.

**sur·gi·cal em·phy·se·ma** subcutaneous emphysema from air trapped in the tissues by an operation or injury.

**sur·gi·cal mi·cro·scope** a binocular microscope used to obtain good visualization of fine structures in the operating field; in the standing type of microscope, a motorized zoom lens system operated by hand or foot controls provides an adjustable working distance; in headborne models, interchangeable oculars provide the magnification needed. SYN operating microscope.

**sur·gi·cal pa·tho·lo·gy** a field in anatomical pathology concerned with examination of tissues removed from living patients for the purpose of diagnosis of disease and guidance in the care of patients.

**sur·gi·cal pro·sthe·sis** an appliance prepared as an aid or as a part of a surgical proceeding, such as a heart valve or cranial plate.

**sur·gi·cal rod** a cylindric implant, usually composed of metal, used to align and internally fix fractures of long bones. SEE ALSO nail, pin.

**sur·gi·cal splint** general term for a device used to maintain tissues in a new position following surgery.

**sur·ro·gate** (ser'ŏ-gāt) **1.** a person who functions in another's life as a substitute for some third person such as a relative who assumes the nurturing and other responsibilities of the absent parent. **2.** a person who reminds one of another person so that one uses the first as an emotional substitute for the second. [L. *surrogo,* to put in another's place]

**sur·ro·gate mo·ther** a woman who has been contracted with to carry a pregnancy for another woman or couple.

**sur·round** (ser-ownd') milieu; environment.

**sur·sum·duc·tion** (ser-sŭm-dŭk'shŭn) SYN supraduction. [L. *sursum,* upward, + *duco,* pp. -*ductus,* to draw]

**sur·sum·ver·sion** (ser-sŭm-ver'zhŭn) the act of rotating the eyes upward. [L. *sursum,* upward, + *verto,* pp. *versus,* to turn]

**sur·veil·lance** (ser-vā'lans) **1.** the collection, collation, analysis, and dissemination of data; a type of observational study that involves continuous monitoring of disease occurrence within a population. **2.** ongoing scrutiny, generally using methods distinguished by practicability, uniformity, rapidity, rather than complete accuracy. [Fr. *surveiller,* to watch over, fr. L. *super-* + *vigilo,* to watch]

**sus·cep·ti·bil·i·ty** (su-sep-ti-bil'i-tē) **1.** likelihood of an individual to develop ill effects from an external agent, such as *Mycobacterium tuberculosis,* high altitude, or ambient temperature. **2.** likelihood that a given pathogenic microorganism will be inhibited or killed by a given microbial agent. SYN sensitivity. **3.** MAGNETIC RESONANCE IMAGING the loss of magnetization signal caused by rapid phase dispersion because of marked local inhomogeneity of the magnetic field, as with the multiple air–soft tissue interfaces in the lung; susceptibility measurement can estimate calcium content in trabecular bone.

**su·scep·ti·bil·i·ty cas·sette** a common sequence of amino acids in residues 70–74 in the HLA-DRB1 chains, found in alleles associated with rheumatoid arthritis. It is one of two variations: glutamine[Q]-lysine[K]-arginine[R]-alanine[A]-alanine[A] or QRRAA. These susceptibility cassettes are found in many different DRB1 alleles. The alpha and beta chains that form these antigen-presenting molecules have a configuration not unlike a trough or rain gutter; antigens are bound by sequences of amino acids in a pocket along the bottom and sides of the trough or cavity, and this complex forms a heterotrimer with the T-cell receptor on CD4+ cells. SYN rheumatoid pocket, shared epitope.

**sus·pend·ed an·i·ma·tion** a temporary state resembling death, with cessation of respiration; may also refer to certain forms of hibernation in animals or to endospore formation by some bacteria.

**sus·pen·sion** (sŭs-pen'shŭn) **1.** a temporary interruption of any function. **2.** a hanging from a support, as used in the treatment of spinal curvatures or during the application of a plaster jacket. **3.** fixation of an organ, such as the uterus, to other tissue for support. **4.** the dispersion through a liquid of a solid in finely divided particles of a size large enough to be detected by purely optical means; if the particles are too small to be seen by microscope but still large enough to scatter light (Tyndall phenomenon), they will remain dispersed indefinitely and are then called a colloidal suspension **5.** a class of pharmacopeial preparations of finely divided, undissolved drugs (e.g., powders for suspension) dispersed in liquid vehicles for oral or parenteral use. [L. *suspensio,* fr. *sus-pendo,* pp. -*pensus,* to hang up, suspend]

**sus·pen·soid** (sŭs-pen'soyd) a colloidal solution in which the disperse particles are solid and lyophobe or hydrophobe, and are therefore sharply demarcated from the fluid in which they are suspended. [suspension + G. *eidos,* resemblance]

**sus·pen·so·ry** (sŭs-pen'sŏ-rē) **1.** suspending; supporting; denoting a ligament, a muscle, or other structure that keeps an organ or other part in place. **2.** a supporter applied to uplift a dependent part, such as the scrotum or a pendulous breast.

**sus·pen·so·ry ban·dage** a bag of expansile fabric for supporting the scrotum and its contents.

**sus·pen·so·ry lig·a·ment of ax·il·la** the continuation of the clavipectoral fascia downward to attach to the axillary fascia; it maintains the characteristic hollow of the armpit.

**sus·pen·so·ry lig·a·ment of eye·ball** a thickening of the inferior part of the bulbar sheath which supports the eye within the orbit; it extends between the lateral and medial orbital margins and includes the medial and lateral check ligaments.

**sus·pen·so·ry lig·a·ment of lens** SYN ciliary zonule.

**sus·pen·so·ry lig·a·ment of ovary** a band of peritoneum that extends upward from the upper pole of the ovary; it contains the ovarian vessels and ovarian plexus of nerves. SYN ligamentum suspensorium ovarii [TA].

**sus·pen·so·ry lig·a·ments of breast** well developed retinacula cutis that extend from the fibrous stroma of the mammary gland to the overlying skin. SYN ligamenta suspensoria mammae [TA].

**sus·pen·so·ry mu·scle of du·o·de·num** a broad flat band of smooth muscle and fibrous tissue attached to the right crus of the diaphragm and to the duodenum at its junction with the jejunum. SYN musculus suspensorius duodeni [TA].

**su·stained-ac·tion tab·let** a drug in tablet form that provides the required dosage initially and then maintains or repeats it at desired intervals. SYN sustained-release tablet.

**su·stained-re·lease tab·let** SYN sustained-action tablet.

**sus·ten·tac·u·lar** (sŭs-ten-tak'yu-lăr) relating to a sustentaculum; supporting.

**sus·ten·tac·u·lum,** pl. **sus·ten·tac·u·la** (sŭs'ten-tak'yu-lŭm, sŭs'ten-tak'yu-lă) a structure that serves as a stay or support to another. [L. a prop, fr. *sustento,* to hold upright]

**Sut·ton dis·ease** (sut'ŏn) SYN aphthae major. [R. L. Sutton, Jr.]

**Sut·ton ne·vus** (sut'ŏn) SYN halo nevus.

**Sut·ton ul·cer** (sut'ŏn) a solitary, deep, painful ulcer of the buccal or genital mucous membrane.

**su·tu·ra,** pl. **su·tu·rae** (soo-too'ră, soo'too'rē)

S
U

[TA] SYN suture. [L. a sewing, a suture, fr. *suo*, pp. *sutus*, to sew]

**su·tur·al** (soo′cher-ăl) relating to a suture in any sense.

**su·tur·al bones** small irregular bones found along the sutures of the cranium, particularly related to the parietal bone. SYN wormian bones.

**su·tur·al lig·a·ment** a delicate membrane binding the bones at the cranial sutures.

**su·ture** (soo′cher) **1.** a form of fibrous joint in which two bones formed in membrane are united by a fibrous membrane continuous with the periosteum. **2.** to unite two surfaces by sewing. SYN stitch (3). **3.** the material (silk thread, wire, catgut, etc.) with which two surfaces are kept in apposition. **4.** the seam so formed, a surgical suture. SYN sutura [TA]. [L. *sutura*, a seam]

**su·ture ab·scess** a purulent exudate surrounding a stitch.

**su·tur·ec·to·my** (soo-cher-ek′tō-mē) removal of cranial suture.

**SV** simian virus, numbered serially; e.g., SV1.

**Sv** sievert.

**Sved·berg of flo·ta·tion** (sfed′bĕrg) SYN flotation constant.

**Sved·berg u·nit (S)** (sfed′bĕrg) a sedimentation constant of $1 \times 10^{-13}$ seconds.

**swab** (swob) a wad of cotton, gauze, or other absorbent material attached to the end of a stick or clamp, used to apply or remove a substance from a surface.

**swal·low** (swahl′ō) to pass anything through the fauces, pharynx, and esophagus into the stomach; to perform deglutition. See this page. [A.S. *swelgan*]

**swal·low·ing re·flex** the act of swallowing (second stage) induced by stimulation of the palate, fauces, or posterior pharyngeal wall. SYN pharyngeal reflex (1).

**swamp fe·ver 1.** SYN equine infectious anemia. **2.** SYN malaria.

**Swan-Ganz cath·e·ter** (swahn-ganz) a thin (5 Fr), flexible, flow-directed venous catheter using a balloon to carry it through the heart to a pulmonary artery; when it is positioned in a small arterial branch, pulmonary wedge pressure is measured in front of the temporarily inflated and wedged balloon. SYN pulmonary artery catheter.

**S wave** a negative (downward) deflection of the QRS complex following an R wave; successive downward deflections within the same QRS complex are labeled S′, S″, etc.

**sweat** (swet) **1.** especially sensible perspiration. **2.** to perspire. [A.S. *swāt*]

**sweat gland car·ci·no·ma** usually a solitary tumor, nodular and fixed to the skin and underlying structures, having slow growth for long periods followed by rapid growth and dissemination.

**sweat glands** the coil glands of the skin that secrete the sweat.

**sweat·ing** (swet′ing) SYN perspiration (1).

**sweat pore** the surface opening of the duct of a sweat gland. SYN pore (2).

**Swe·dish mas·sage** (swē′dish) a massage technique that includes effleurage, pétrissage, friction, vibration, and tapotement. Swedish massage is intended to improve circulation and tissue elasticity while reducing muscle tone and creating a parasympathetic response.

**swell·ing** (swel′ing) **1.** an enlargement, e.g., a protuberance or tumor. **2.** EMBRYOLOGY a primordial elevation that develops into a fold, ridge, prominence, or process.

**Swift dis·ease** (swift) SYN acrodynia (2).

**swim·mer's ear** infection that occurs in the external auditory canal; often develops in persons who swim frequently and get water trapped in their ears. SYN otitis externa.

**swim·mer's itch 1.** SYN cutaneous ancylostomiasis. **2.** SYN schistosomal dermatitis.

**swim·ming pool con·junc·ti·vi·tis** conjunctivitis in a swimmer, which can be caused by pool chlorination, adenovirus, and rarely, *Chlamydia*.

**switch·ing site** the break point in a DNA sequence at which a gene segment unites with another gene segment, as in the production of the immunoglobulins.

**Swy·er-James syn·drome** (swī′er-jāmz) **1.** SYN unilateral lobar emphysema. **2.** hyperlucency of one lung from obliterating bronchiolitis, usually caused by adenovirus infection in childhood, with decreased size and vascularity of the lung; distinguished from other causes of unilateral hyperlucency by demonstration of air trapping without central obstruction.

**Swy·er syn·drome** (swī′er) gonadal dysgenesis in phenotypic females with XY genotype.

**sy·co·ma** (sī-kō′mă) **1.** a pendulous figlike growth. **2.** a large soft wart. [G. *sykōma*, fr. *sykon*, fig, + *-oma*, tumor]

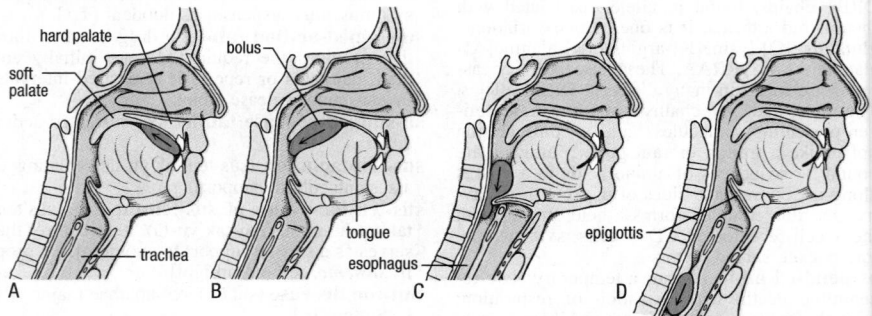

**swallowing:** (A) bolus is pushed back; (B) narrowing of nasopharynx as bolus is pushed towards esophagus; (C) epiglottis closes the trachea; (D) bolus is moved down the esophagus

**sy·co·si·form** (sī-kō'si-fōrm) resembling sycosis.

**sy·co·sis** (sī-kō'sis) a pustular folliculitis, particularly of the bearded area. [G. *sykōsis,* fr. *sykon,* fig, + *-osis,* condition]

**Sy·den·ham cho·rea** (sid'ĕn-ham) a postinfectious chorea appearing several months after a streptococcal infection with subsequent rheumatic fever. The chorea typically involves the distal limbs and is associated with hypotonia and emotional lability. Improvement occurs over weeks or months and exacerbations occur without associated infection recurrence.

**Syl·vest dis·ease** (sĕl-vest') SYN epidemic pleurodynia.

**syl·vi·an** (sil'vē-an) relating to Franciscus or Jacobaeus Sylvius or to any of the structures described by either of them.

△**sym-** SEE syn-.

**sym·bal·lo·phone** (sim-bal'ō-fōn) a stethoscope having two chest pieces, designed to lateralize sound and produce a stereophonic effect. [G. *symballō,* to throw together, + *phōnē,* sound]

**sym·bi·on, sym·bi·ont** (sim'bī-on, sim'bī-ont) an organism associated with another in symbiosis. SYN mutualist, symbiote. [G. *symbion,* neut. of *symbiōs,* living together]

**sym·bi·o·sis** (sim-bī-ō'sis) **1.** the biological association of two or more species to their mutual benefit. Cf. commensalism, parasitism. **2.** the mutual cooperation or interdependence of two persons, as mother and infant, or husband and wife; sometimes used to denote excessive or pathological interdependence of two persons. [G. *symbiōsis,* state of living together, fr. sym- + *bios,* life, + *-osis,* condition]

**sym·bi·ote** (sim'bī-ōt) SYN symbion.

**sym·bi·ot·ic** (sim-bī-ot'ik) relating to symbiosis.

**sym·bleph·a·ron** (sim-blef'ă-ron) adhesion of one or both eyelids to the eyeball, partial or complete, resulting from burns or other trauma but rarely congenital. [sym- + G. *blepharon,* eyelid]

**sym·bol·ism** (sim'bŏ-lizm) **1.** PSYCHOANALYSIS the process involved in the disguised representation in consciousness of unconscious or repressed contents or events. **2.** a mental state in which one regards everything that happens as symbolic of one's own thoughts. **3.** the description of the emotional life and experiences in abstract terms.

**sym·bol·i·za·tion** (sim'bŏ-li-zā'shŭn) an unconscious mental mechanism whereby one object or idea is represented by another.

**sym·brach·y·dac·ty·ly** (sim-brak'i-dak'ti-lē) condition in which abnormally short fingers are joined or webbed in their proximal portions. [sym- + G. *brachys,* short, + *daktylos,* finger]

**Syme am·pu·ta·tion, Syme op·er·a·tion** (sīm) amputation of the foot at the ankle joint, the malleoli being sawed off, and a flap being made with the soft parts of the heel.

**sym·met·ri·cal gan·grene** gangrene affecting the extremities of both sides of the body; it is seen particularly in severe arteriosclerosis, myocardial infarction, and ball-valve thrombus.

**sym·me·tric fe·tal growth re·stric·tion** proportional reduction in fetal head and body size, commonly constitutional or caused by an early intrauterine insult such as infection.

**sym·me·try** (sim'ĕ-trē) equality or correspondence in form of parts distributed around a center or an axis, at the extremities or poles, or on the opposite sides of any body. [G. *symmetria,* fr. sym- + *metron,* measure]

△**sym·path-, sym·pa·the·to-, sym·pa·thi·co-, sym·pa·tho-** the sympathetic part of the autonomic nervous system. [see sympathetic]

**sym·pa·thec·to·my** (sim-pă-thek'tō-mē) excision of a segment of a sympathetic nerve or of one or more sympathetic ganglia. [sympath- + G. *ektomē,* excision]

**sym·pa·thet·ic** (sim-pă-thet'ik) **1.** relating to or exhibiting sympathy. **2.** denoting the sympathetic part of the autonomic nervous system. [G. *sympathētikos,* fr. *sympatheō,* to feel with, sympathize, fr. syn, with, + *pathos,* suffering]

**sym·pa·thet·ic a·mine** SYN sympathomimetic amine.

**sym·pa·thet·ic gan·glia** those ganglia of the autonomic nervous system that receive efferent fibers originating from preganglionic visceral motor neurons in the intermediolateral cell column of thoracic and upper lumbar spinal segments (T1–L2). On the basis of their location, the sympathetic ganglia can be classified as paravertebral ganglia (ganglia trunci sympathici) and prevertebral ganglia (ganglia celiaca). SEE ALSO autonomic division of nervous system.

**sym·pa·thet·ic nerve** one of the nerves of the sympathetic nervous system.

**sym·pa·thet·ic ner·vous sys·tem 1.** originally, the entire autonomic nervous system; **2.** the sympathetic part of the nervous system. SEE ALSO autonomic division of nervous system.

**sym·pa·thet·ic oph·thal·mia** a serous or plastic uveitis caused by a perforating wound of the uvea followed by a similar severe reaction in the other eye that may lead to bilateral blindness.

**sym·pa·thet·ic part of au·to·no·mic di·vi·sion of per·i·pher·al ner·vous sys·tem** the sympathetic part of the autonomic division of the nervous system. SEE ALSO autonomic division of nervous system.

🗔**sym·pa·thet·ic trunk** one of the two long ganglionated nerve strands alongside the vertebral column that extend from the base of the skull to the coccyx; they are connected to each spinal nerve by gray rami and receive fibers from the spinal cord through white rami connecting with the thoracic and upper lumbar spinal nerves. See page 1018. SYN truncus sympathicus [TA].

**sym·pa·thet·ic u·ve·i·tis** a bilateral inflammation of the uveal tract caused by a perforating wound of one eye that injures the uvea.

**sym·pa·thet·o·blast** (sim-pă-thet'ō-blast) SYN sympathoblast.

**sym·path·i·co·blast** (sim-path'i-kō-blast) SYN sympathoblast.

**sym·path·i·co·lyt·ic** (sim-path'i-kō-lit'ik) SYN sympatholytic.

**sym·path·i·co·mi·met·ic** (sim-path'i-kō-mi-met'ik) SYN sympathomimetic.

**sym·path·i·co·to·nia** (sim-path'i-kō-tō'nē-ă) a condition in which there is increased tonus of the sympathetic system and a marked tendency to vascular spasm and high blood pressure; opposed to vagotonia. [sympathico- + G. *tonos,* tone, tension]

**sym·path·i·co·ton·ic** (sim-path'i-kō-ton'ik) relating to or characterized by sympathicotonia.

**sym·path·i·co·trip·sy** (sim-path'i-kō-trip'sē) operation of crushing a sympathetic ganglion. [sympathico- + G. *tripsis,* a rubbing]

S
y

**sym·pa·tho·ad·re·nal** (sim'pă-thō-ă-drē'năl) relating to the sympathetic part of the autonomic nervous system and the medulla of the adrenal gland, as the postganglionic neurons.

**sym·pa·tho·blast** (sim'pă-thō-blast) a primitive cell derived from the neural crest glia; with the pheochromoblasts, sympathoblasts enter into the formation of the adrenal medulla and sympathetic ganglia. SYN sympathetoblast, sympathicoblast. [sympatho- + G. *blastos*, germ]

**sym·pa·tho·go·nia** (sim'pă-thō-gō'nē-ă) the completely undifferentiated cells of the sympathetic nervous system. [sympatho- + G. *gonē*, seed]

**sym·pa·tho·lyt·ic** (sim'pă-thō-lit'ik) denoting antagonism to or inhibition of adrenergic nerve activity. SEE ALSO adrenergic blocking agent, antiadrenergic. SYN sympathicolytic. [sympatho- + G. *lysis*, a loosening]

**sym·pa·tho·mi·met·ic** (sim'pă-thō-mi-met'ik) denoting mimicking of action of the sympathetic system. SEE ALSO adrenomimetic. SYN sympathicomimetic. [sympatho- + G. *mimikos*, imitating]

**sym·pa·tho·mi·met·ic amine** an agent that evokes responses similar to those produced by adrenergic nerve activity (e.g., epinephrine, ephedrine, isoproterenol). SYN adrenomimetic amine, sympathetic amine.

**sym·pa·thy** (sim'pă-thē) 1. the mutual relation, physiologic or pathologic, between two organs, systems, or parts of the body. 2. mental contagion, as seen in mass hysteria or in the yawning induced by seeing another person yawn. 3. an expressed sensitive appreciation or emotional concern for and sharing of the mental and emotional state of another person. Cf. empathy (1). [G. *sympatheia*, fr. sym- + *pathos*, suffering]

**sym·pha·lan·gism, sym·pha·lan·gy** (sim-fal'an-jizm, sim-fal'an-jē) 1. SYN syndactyly. 2. ankylosis of the finger or toe joints. [sym- + phalanx]

**sym·phys·i·al, sym·phys·e·al** (sim-fiz'ē-ăl) grown together; relating to a symphysis; fused.

**sym·phys·i·on** (sim-fiz'ē-on) a craniometric point, the most anterior point of the alveolar process of the mandible.

**sym·phys·i·ot·o·my, sym·phys·e·ot·o·my** (sim-fiz-ē-ot'ō-mē) division of the pubic joint to increase the capacity of a contracted pelvis sufficiently to permit passage of a living child. SYN pelviotomy (1), pelvitomy, synchondrotomy. [symphysis + G. *tomē*, incision]

**sym·phy·sis**, gen. **sym·phy·ses** (sim'fi-sis, sim'fi-sēz) 1. [TA] form of cartilaginous joint in which union between two bones is effected by means of fibrocartilage. 2. a union, meeting point, or commissure of any two structures. 3. a pathologic adhesion or growing together. [G. a growing together]

**sym·po·dia** (sim-pō'dē-ă) condition characterized by union of the feet. SEE ALSO sirenomelia. [sym- + G. *pous*, foot]

**sym·port** (sim'pōrt) coupled transport of two different molecules or ions through a membrane in the same direction by a common carrier mechanism (symporter). Cf. antiport, uniport. [sym- + L. *porto*, to carry]

**symp·tom** (simp'tŏm) any morbid phenomenon or departure from the normal in structure, function, or sensation, experienced by the patient and indicative of disease. SEE ALSO phenomenon (1), reflex (1), sign (1), syndrome. [G. *symptōma*]

**symp·to·mat·ic** (simp-tō-mat'ik) indicative; relating to or constituting the aggregate of symptoms of a disease.

**symp·to·mat·ic por·phyr·ia** SYN porphyria cutanea tarda.

**symp·to·mat·ic pru·ri·tus** itching occurring as a symptom of some systemic disease.

**symp·to·mat·ic re·ac·tion** an allergic response similar to the original one, but occurring after the use of a test or therapeutic dose of an allergen or atopen.

**symp·tom·a·tol·o·gy** (simp'tō-mă-tol'ŏ-jē) 1. the science of the symptoms of disease, their production, and the indications they furnish. 2. the aggregate of symptoms of a disease. [symptom + G. *logos*, study]

**symp·to·mat·o·lyt·ic** (simp'tō-mat-ō-lit'ik) removing symptoms. [symptom + G. *lytikos*, dissolving]

**symp·tom com·plex 1.** SEE syndrome. **2.** SEE complex (1).

**symp·to·sis** (sim-tō'sis) a localized or general wasting of the body. [G. a falling together, collapse, fr. *syn*, together, + *ptōsis*, a falling]

△**syn-** together, with, joined; appears as sym- before b, p, ph, or m; corresponds to L. *con-*. [G. *syn*, with, together]

**syn·an·a·morph** (sin-an'ă-mōrf) the same fungal species growing in a different form.

**syn·apse**, pl. **syn·aps·es** (sin'aps, sĭ-naps'; sĭ-nap'sēz) the functional membrane-to-membrane contact of the nerve cell with another nerve cell, an effector (muscle, gland) cell, or a sensory receptor cell. The synapse subserves the transmission of nerve impulses, commonly from a club-shaped axon terminal (the presynaptic element) to the circumscript patch of the plasma membrane of the receiving cell (the postsynaptic element) on which the synapse occurs. In most cases the impulse is transmitted by means of a chemical transmitter substance (such as acetylcholine, γ-aminobutyric acid, dopamine, norepinephrine) released into a synaptic cleft that separates the presynaptic from the postsynaptic membrane; the transmitter is stored in synaptic vesicles in the presynaptic element. In other synapses transmission takes place by direct propagation of the bioelectrical potential from the presynaptic to the postsynaptic membrane. SYN synapsis. [syn- + G. *hapto*, to clasp]

**syn·ap·sis** (sĭ-nap'sis) [TA] SYN synapse. 1. the point-for-point pairing of homologous chromosomes during the prophase of meiosis. [G. a connection, junction]

**syn·ap·tic** (sĭ-nap'tik) 1. relating to a synapse. 2. relating to synapsis.

**syn·ap·tic cleft** the space about 20 nm wide between the axolemma and the postsynaptic surface. SEE ALSO synapse.

**syn·ap·tic con·duc·tion** the conduction of a nerve impulse across a synapse.

**syn·ap·tic ves·i·cles** the small (average diameter 30 nm), intracellular, membrane-bound vesicles near the presynaptic membrane of a synaptic junction, containing the transmitter substance which, in chemical synapses, mediates the passage of nerve impulses across the junction. SEE ALSO synapse.

**syn·ap·ti·ne·mal com·plex** a submicroscopic

structure interposed between the homologous chromosome pairs during synapsis.

**syn•ap•to•some** (sĭ-nap'tō-sōm) membrane-bound sac containing synaptic vesicles that breaks away from axon terminals when brain tissue is homogenized under controlled conditions; such particles can be separated from other subcellular particles by differential and density gradient centrifugation. [synapse + G. *sōma,* body]

**syn•ar•thro•dia** (sin'ar-thrō'dē-ă) SYN fibrous joint.

**syn•ar•thro•di•al** (sin-ar-thrō'dē-ăl) relating to synarthrosis; denoting an articulation without a joint cavity.

**syn•ar•thro•di•al joint 1.** SYN fibrous joint. **2.** SYN cartilaginous joint.

**syn•ar•thro•phy•sis** (sin-ar-thrō-fī'sis) the process of ankylosis. [syn- + G. *arthron,* joint, + *physis,* growth]

**syn•ar•thro•sis,** pl. **syn•ar•thro•ses** (sin'ar-thrō' sis, sin'ar-thrō'sēz) in the BNA, this class of joints has included those that in the NA are classified as articulatio fibrosa (fibrous joint) and articulatio cartilaginis (cartilaginous joint). SEE joint. [G. fr. *syn,* together, + *arthrōsis,* articulation]

**syn•can•thus** (sin-kan'thŭs) adhesion of the eyeball to orbital structures. [syn- + L. *canthus,* wheel]

**syn•ceph•a•lus** (sin-sef'ă-lŭs) conjoined twins having a single head with two bodies. [syn- + G. *kephalē,* head]

**syn•ceph•a•ly** (sin-sef'ă-lē) the condition exhibited by a syncephalus.

**syn•chei•ria** (sin-kī'rē-ă) a form of dyscheiria in which the subject refers a stimulus applied to one side of the body to both sides. [syn- + G. *cheir,* hand]

**syn•chon•dro•di•al joint** SYN synchondrosis.

**syn•chon•dro•se•ot•o•my** (sin-kon'drō-sē-ot'ō-mē) operation of cutting through a synchondrosis; specifically, cutting through the sacroiliac ligaments and forcibly closing the pubic arch; used in the treatment of exstrophy of the bladder. [synchondrosis + G. *tomē,* cutting]

**syn•chon•dro•sis,** pl. **syn•chon•dro•ses** (sin' kon-drō'sis, sin'kon-drō'sēz) a union between two bones formed either by hyaline cartilage or fibrocartilage. SYN synchondrodial joint. [Mod. L. fr. G. *syn,* together, + *chondros,* cartilage, + *-osis,* condition]

**syn•chon•dro•to•my** (sin-kon-drot'ō-mē) SYN symphysiotomy.

**syn•chro•nia** (sin-krō'nē-ă) **1.** SYN synchronism. **2.** origin, development, involution, or functioning of tissues or organs at the usual time for such an event. Cf. heterochronia. [syn- + G. *chronos,* time]

**syn•chron•ic** (sin'krŏn-ik) referring to the study of the natural history of a disease by its state and distribution in a population at one time.

**syn•chron•ic stud•y** SYN cross-sectional study.

**syn•chro•nism** (sin'krŏ-nizm) occurrence of two or more events at the same time; the condition of being simultaneous. SYN synchronia (1). [syn- + G. *chronos,* time]

**syn•chro•nized in•ter•mit•tent man•da•tory ven•ti•la•tion** intermittent mandatory ventilation in which mandatory breaths can be triggered by the patient's inspiratory effort; in the absence of

patient inspiratory efforts, SIMV becomes IMV. SEE ALSO intermittent mandatory ventilation.

**syn•chro•nous** (sin'krō-nŭs) occurring simultaneously. [G. *synchronos*]

**syn•chy•sis** (sin'kĭ-sis) collapse of the collagenous framework of the vitreous humor, with liquefaction of the vitreous body. [G. a mixing together, fr. syn- + *chysis,* a pouring]

**syn•chy•sis scin•til•lans** an appearance of glistening spots in the eye, due to cholesterol crystals floating in a fluid vitreous.

**syn•clit•ic** (sin-klit'ik) relating to or marked by synclitism.

**syn•cli•tism** (sin'kli-tizm) condition of parallelism between the planes of the fetal head and of the pelvis, respectively. [G. *syn-klinō,* to incline together]

**syn•clo•nus** (sin'klō-nŭs) clonic spasm or tremor of several muscles. [syn- + G. *klonos,* tumult]

**syn•co•pal** (sin'kō-păl) relating to syncope. SYN syncopic.

**syn•co•pe** (sin'kŏ-pē) loss of consciousness and postural tone caused by diminished cerebral blood flow. [G. *synkopē,* a cutting short, a swoon]

**syn•cop•ic** (sin-kop'ik) SYN syncopal.

**syn•cy•tial** (sin-sish'ăl, sin-sish'ē-ăl, sin-sit'ē-ăl) relating to a syncytium.

**syn•cy•tial knot** a localized aggregation of syncytiotrophoblastic nuclei in the villi of the placenta during early pregnancy.

**syn•cy•ti•o•tro•pho•blast** (sin-sish'ē-ō-trō'fō-blast) the syncytial outer layer of the trophoblast; site of synthesis of human chorionic gonadotropin. SEE ALSO trophoblast. SYN syntrophoblast. [syncytium + trophoblast]

**syn•cy•ti•um,** pl. **syn•cy•tia** (sin-sish'ē-ŭm, sin-sish'ē-ă) a multinucleated protoplasmic mass formed by the secondary union of originally separate cells. [Mod. L. fr. syn- + G. *kytos,* cell]

**syn•dac•tyl•ia, syn•dac•ty•lism** (sin-dak-til'ē-ă, sin-dak'ti-lizm) SYN syndactyly.

**syn•dac•ty•lous** (sin-dak'ti-lŭs) having fused or webbed fingers or toes.

**syn•dac•ty•ly** (sin-dak'ti-lē) any degree of webbing or fusion of fingers or toes, involving soft parts only or including bone structure. SYN symphalangism (1), symphalangy, syndactylia, syndactylism. [syn- + G. *daktylos,* finger or toe]

**syn•de•sis** (sin-dē'sis) SYN arthrodesis. [syn- + G. *desis,* a binding]

**syn•des•mec•to•my** (sin-dez-mek'tō-mē) cutting away a section of a ligament. [syndesm- + G. *ektomē,* excision]

**syn•des•mec•to•pia** (sin-dez-mek-tō'pē-ă) displacement of a ligament. [syndesm- + G. *ektopos,* out of place]

**syn•des•mi•tis** (sin-dez-mī'tis) inflammation of a ligament. [syndesm- + G. *-itis,* inflammation]

△**syn•des•mo-, syn•desm-** ligament, ligamentous. [G. *syndesmos,* a fastening, fr. *syndeō,* to bind]

**syn•des•mo•di•al** (sin-des-mō'dē-ăl) SYN syndesmotic.

**syn•des•mo•pexy** (sin-dez'mō-pek-sē) the joining of two ligaments, or attachment of a ligament in a new place. [syndesmo- + G. *pēxis,* fixation]

**syn•des•mo•phyte** (sin-dez'mō-fīt) an osseous excrescence attached to a ligament. [syndesmo- + G. *phyton,* plant]

**syn•des•mo•plas•ty** (sin-dez'mō-plas-tē) rarely

used term for plastic surgery of a ligament. [syndesmo- + G. *plastos,* formed]

**syn•des•mor•rha•phy** (sin-dez-mōr'ă-fē) suture of ligaments. [syndesmo- + G. *rhaphē,* suture]

**syn•des•mo•sis,** pl. **syn•des•mo•ses** (sin'dez-mō' sis, sin'dez-mō'sēz) a form of fibrous joint in which opposing surfaces that are relatively far apart are united by ligaments. [syndesmo- + G. *-osis,* condition]

**syn•des•mot•ic** (sin-des-mot'ik) relating to syndesmosis. SYN syndesmodial.

**syn•des•mot•o•my** (sin-dez-mot'ō-mē) surgical division of a ligament. [syndesmo- + G. *tomē,* incision]

**syn•drome** (sin'drōm) the combination of signs and symptoms associated with any morbid process, which together constitute the picture of the disease. SEE ALSO disease. [G. *syndromē,* a running together, tumultuous concourse; (in med.) a concurrence of symptoms, fr. *syn,* together, + *dromos,* a running]

**syn•drom•ic** (sin-drom'ik, sin-drō'mik) relating to a syndrome.

**syn•ech•ia,** pl. **syn•ech•i•ae** (si-nek'ē-ă, si-nek'ē-ē) any adhesion; specifically, adhesion of an inflamed iris to the cornea (anterior synechia) or lens (posterior synechia). [G. *synecheia,* continuity, fr. *syn,* together, + *echō,* to have, hold]

**syn•ech•i•ot•o•my** (si-nek'ē-ot'ō-mē) division of synechiae. [synechia + G. *tomē,* incision]

**syn•en•ceph•a•lo•cele** (sin-en-sef'ă-lō-sēl) protrusion of brain substance through a defect in the skull, with adhesions preventing reduction. [syn- + G. *enkephalos,* brain, + *kēlē,* hernia]

**syn•er•e•sis** (si-ner'ĕ-sis) 1. the contraction of a gel, e.g., a blood clot, by which part of the dispersion medium is squeezed out. 2. degeneration of the vitreous humor with loss of gel consistency to become partially or completely fluid. [G. *synairesis,* a taking or drawing together]

**syn•er•gism** (sin'er-jizm) coordinated or correlated action of two or more structures, agents, or physiologic processes so that the combined action is greater than the sum of each acting separately. Cf. antagonism. SYN synergy. [G. *synergia,* fr. *syn,* together, + *ergon,* work]

**syn•er•gist** (sin'er-jist) a structure, agent, or physiologic process that aids the action of another. Cf. antagonist.

**syn•er•gis•tic mus•cles** muscles having a similar and mutually helpful function or action.

**syn•er•gy** (sin'er-jē) SYN synergism.

**syn•es•the•sia** (sin-es-thē'zē-ă) a condition in which a stimulus, in addition to exciting the usual and normally located sensation, gives rise to a subjective sensation of different character or localization; e.g., color hearing, color taste. [syn- + G. *aisthēsis,* sensation]

**syn•es•the•si•al•gia** (sin'es-thē-zē-al'jē-ă) painful synesthesia.

*Syn•ga•mus* (sin'gă-mŭs) a genus of bloodsucking, strongyle gapeworms of the family Syngamidae.

*Syn•ga•mus laryn•ge•us* a tropical nematode that occasionally invades the larynx and trachea, causing cough, hemoptysis, foreign body sensation, and shortness of breath.

**syn•ga•my** (sin'gă-mē) conjugation of the gametes in fertilization. [syn- + G. *gamos,* marriage]

**syn•ge•ne•ic** (sin'jĕ-nē'ik) relating to genetically

identical individuals. SYN isogeneic, isogenic, isologous, isoplastic. [G. *syngenēs,* congenital]

**syn•gen•e•sis** (sin-jen'ĕ-sis) SYN sexual reproduction. [syn- + G. *genesis,* origin]

**syn•ge•net•ic** (sin-jĕ-net'ik) relating to syngenesis.

**syn•graft** (sin'graft) a tissue or organ transplanted between genetically identical individuals. SYN isogeneic graft, isograft, isologous graft, isoplastic graft.

**syn•i•ze•sis** (sin-i-zē'sis) 1. closure or obliteration of the pupil. 2. the massing of chromatin at one side of the nucleus that occurs usually at the beginning of synapsis. [G. collapse]

**syn•kar•y•on** (sin-kar'ē-on) the nucleus formed by the fusion of the two pronuclei in karyogamy. [syn- + G. *karyon,* kernel (nucleus)]

**syn•ki•ne•sis** (sin-ki-nē'sis) involuntary movement accompanying a voluntary one, as the movement of a closed eye following that of the uncovered one, or the movement occurring in a paralyzed muscle accompanying motion in another part. [syn- + G. *kinēsis,* movement]

**syn•ki•net•ic** (sin-ki-net'ik) relating to or marked by synkinesis.

**syn•o•nych•ia** (sin-ō-nik'ē-ă) fusion of two or more nails of the digits, as in syndactyly. [sin- + G. *onyx (onych-),* nail]

**syn•oph•thal•mia** (sin-of-thal'mē-ă) SYN cyclopia. [syn- + G. *ophthalmos,* eye]

**syn•or•chi•dism, syn•or•chism** (sin-ōr'ki-dizm, sin-ōr'kizm) congenital fusion of the testes in the abdomen or scrotum. [syn- + G. *orchis,* testis]

**syn•os•che•os** (sin-os'kē-os) partial or complete adhesion of the penis and scrotum, a malformation in hermaphroditism. [syn- + G. *oschē,* scrotum]

**syn•os•to•sis** (sin-os-tō'sis) osseous union between the bones forming a joint. SYN bony ankylosis, true ankylosis. [syn- + G. *osteon,* bone, + *-osis,* condition]

**syn•os•tot•ic** (sin-os-tot'ik) relating to synostosis.

**sy•no•tia** (si-nō'shē-ă) fusion or abnormal approximation of the lobes of the ears in otocephaly. [syn- + G. *ous,* ear]

**syn•o•vec•to•my** (sin-ō-vek'tō-mē) excision of a portion or all of the synovial membrane of a joint. SYN villusectomy. [synovia + G. *ektomē,* excision]

**syn•o•via** (si-nō'vē-ă) [TA] SYN synovial fluid. [Mod. L., a word coined by Paracelsus, fr. G. *syn,* together, + *ōon* (L. *ovum*), egg]

**syn•o•vi•al** (si-nō'vē-ăl) 1. relating to, containing, or consisting of synovia. 2. relating to the membrana synovialis.

**syn•o•vi•al bur•sa** a sac containing synovial fluid which occurs at sites of friction, as between a tendon and a bone over which it plays, or subcutaneously over a bony prominence.

**syn•o•vi•al crypt** a diverticulum of the synovial membrane of a joint.

**syn•o•vi•al cyst** SYN ganglion (2).

**syn•o•vi•al flu•id** a clear thixotropic fluid, the main function of which is to serve as a lubricant in a joint, tendon sheath, or bursa; consists mainly of mucin with some albumin, fat, epithelium, and leukocytes; synovial fluid also helps to nourish the avascular articular cartilage. SYN synovia [TA].

**syn•o•vi•al her•nia** protrusion of a fold of the

stratum synoviale through a rent in the stratum fibrosum of a joint capsule.

**syn•o•vi•al joint** a joint in which (1) the opposing bony surfaces are covered with a layer of hyaline cartilage or fibrocartilage, (2) there is a joint cavity containing synovial fluid, lined with synovial membrane and reinforced by a fibrous capsule and ligaments, and (3) there is some degree of free movement possible. SYN articulatio [TA], diarthrodial joint, diarthrosis, movable joint.

**syn•o•vi•al lig•a•ment** one of the large synovial folds in a joint.

**syn•o•vi•al mem•brane** the connective tissue membrane that lines the cavity of a synovial joint and produces the synovial fluid; it lines all internal surfaces of the cavity except for the articular cartilage of the bones. SYN membrana synovialis [TA], synovium.

**syn•o•vi•al sheath** SEE synovial sheaths of digits of hand, synovial sheaths of digits of foot.

**syn•o•vi•al sheaths of di•gits of foot** similar in structure to the corresponding sheaths of the hand.

**syn•o•vi•al sheaths of di•gits of hand** the synovial sheaths that enclose the flexor tendons of the fingers and line the inside of the fibrous tendon sheaths.

**syn•o•vi•o•ma** (si-nō-vē-ō′mă) a tumor of synovial origin involving joint or tendon sheath. [synovium + G. -oma, tumor]

**syn•o•vi•tis** (sin-ō-vī′tis) inflammation of a synovial membrane, especially that of a joint; in general, when unqualified, the same as arthritis. [synovia + G. -itis, inflammation]

**syn•o•vi•tis sic•ca** (sik′ă) SYN dry synovitis.

**syn•o•vi•um** (si-nō′vē-ŭm) SYN synovial membrane.

**syn•ten•ic** (sin-ten′ik) pertaining to synteny.

**syn•te•ny** (sin′ten-ē) the relationship between two genetic loci (not genes) represented on the same chromosomal pair or (for haploid chromosomes) on the same chromosome; an anatomic rather than a segregational relationship. [syn- + G. tainia, ribbon]

**syn•thase** (sin′thās) trivial name used in Enzyme Commission Report for a lyase reaction going in the reverse direction (NTP-independent). SEE ALSO synthetase.

**syn•the•sis**, pl. **syn•the•ses** (sin′thĕ-sis, sin′thĕ-sēz) **1.** a building up, putting together, composition. **2.** CHEMISTRY the formation of compounds by the union of simpler compounds or elements. **3.** stage in the cell cycle in which DNA is synthesized as a preliminary to cell division. [G. fr. syn, together, + thesis, a placing, arranging]

**syn•the•sis pe•ri•od** the period of the cell cycle when there is synthesis of DNA and histone; it occurs between gap$_1$ and gap$_2$.

**syn•the•size** (sin′thĕ-sīz) to make something by synthesis, i.e., synthetically.

**syn•the•tase** (sin′thĕ-tās) an enzyme catalyzing the synthesis of a specific substance.

**syn•thet•ic** (sin-thet′ik) relating to or made by synthesis.

**syn•the•tic dyes** organic dye compounds originally derived from coal-tar derivatives; presently produced by synthesis from benzene and its derivatives.

**syn•the•tic sen•tence i•den•ti•fi•ca•tion** a test of central auditory pathway integrity in which a closed set of 10 syntactically incomplete sentences are presented with a competing message for identification.

**syn•ton•ic** (sin-ton′ik) having even tone or temperament; a personality trait characterized by a high degree of emotional responsiveness to the environment. [G. syntonos, in harmony, fr. syn, together, + tonos, tone]

**syn•tro•pho•blast** (sin-trō′fō-blast, sin-trof′ō-) SYN syncytiotrophoblast.

**syn•tro•pic** (sin-trop′ik) relating to syntropy.

**syn•tro•py** (sin′trō-pē) **1.** the tendency sometimes seen in two diseases to coalesce into one. **2.** the state of harmonious association with others. **3.** ANATOMY a number of similar structures inclined in one general direction; e.g., the spinous processes of a series of vertebrae, the ribs. [syn- + G. tropē, a turning]

**syph•i•lid** (sif′i-lid) any of the several kinds of cutaneous and mucous membrane lesions of secondary and tertiary syphilis, but most commonly denoting the former. [syphilis + -id (1)]

**▣ syph•i•lis** (sif′i-lis) an acute and chronic infectious disease caused by *Treponema pallidum* and transmitted by direct contact, usually through sexual intercourse. After an incubation period of 12 to 30 days, the first symptom is a chancre (a painless, indurated ulcer), followed by slight fever and other constitutional symptoms (*primary syphilis*), followed by a skin eruption of various appearances with mucous patches and generalized lymphadenopathy (*secondary syphilis*), and subsequently by the formation of gummas, cellular infiltration, and functional abnormalities usually resulting from cardiovascular and central nervous system lesions (*tertiary syphilis*). See page B3. [Mod. L. syphilis (syphilid-), (?) fr. a poem, *Syphilis sive Morbus Gallicus,* by Fracastorius, *Syphilus* being a shepherd and principal char.]

**syph•i•lit•ic** (sif-i-lit′ik) relating to, caused by, or suffering from syphilis. SYN luetic.

**sy•phi•lit•ic an•eu•ry•sm** an aneurysm, usually involving the thoracic aorta, resulting from tertiary syphilitic aortitis.

**sy•phi•lit•ic leu•ko•der•ma** a fading of the roseola of secondary syphilis, leaving reticulated depigmented and hyperpigmented areas located chiefly on the sides of the neck. SYN melanoleukoderma colli.

**sy•phi•lit•ic ro•se•o•la** usually the first eruption of syphilis, occurring 6 to 12 weeks after the initial lesion.

**△sy•phi•lo-, sy•phil-, sy•phi•li-** syphilis. [see syphilis]

**syph•i•lo•ma** (sif-i-lō′mă) SYN gumma. [syphilo- + G. -oma, tumor]

**syr•ing•ad•e•no•ma** (sir′ing-ad-ĕ-nō′mă) a benign sweat gland tumor showing glandular differentiation typical of secretory cells. SYN syringoadenoma. [syring- + G. adēn, gland, + -oma, tumor]

**sy•ringe** (sĭ-rinj′, sir′inj) an instrument used for injecting or withdrawing fluids. [G. syrinx, pipe or tube]

**sy•rin•gec•to•my** (si-rin-jek′tō-mē) SYN fistulectomy. [syring- + G. ektomē, excision]

**sy•rin•gi•tis** (si-rin-jī′tis) inflammation of the auditory tube. [syring- + G. -itis, inflammation]

**△syr•in•go-, syr•ing-** a syrinx; syringeal. [G. syrinx, pipe or tube]

**sy·rin·go·ad·e·no·ma** (sĭ-ring'gō-ad-ĕ-nō'mă) SYN syringadenoma.

**sy·rin·go·bul·bia** (sĭ-ring'gō-bŭl'bē-ă) a fluid-filled cavity of the brainstem, analogous to syringomyelia. [syringo- + L. *bulbus*, bulb (medulla oblongata)]

**sy·rin·go·car·ci·no·ma** (sĭ-ring'gō-kar-si-nō'mă) a malignant epithelial neoplasm which has undergone cystic change (cystic carcinoma). [syringo- + carcinoma]

**sy·rin·go·cele** (sĭ-ring'gō-sēl) 1. SYN central canal. 2. a meningomyelocele in which there is a cavity in the ectopic spinal cord. [syringo- + G. *koilia*, a hollow]

**sy·rin·go·cys·tad·e·no·ma** (sĭ-ring'gō-sis-tad-ĕ-nō'mă) a cystic benign sweat gland tumor. [syringo- + cystadenoma]

**sy·rin·go·cys·to·ma** (sĭ-ring'gō-sis-tō'mă) SYN hidrocystoma. [syringo- + cystoma]

**sy·rin·go·ma** (si-ring-gō'mă) a benign, often multiple, sometimes eruptive neoplasm of the sweat gland ducts composed of very small round cysts. [syringo- + G. *-ōma*, tumor]

**sy·rin·go·me·nin·go·cele** (sĭ-ring'gō-mĕ-ning'gō-sēl) a form of spina bifida in which the dorsal sac consists chiefly of membranes, with very little cord substance, enclosing a cavity that communicates with a syringomyelic cavity. [syringo- + meningocele]

**sy·rin·go·my·e·lia** (sĭ-ring'gō-mī-ē'lē-ă) the presence in the spinal cord of longitudinal cavities lined by dense, gliogenous tissue, which are not caused by vascular insufficiency. Syringomyelia is marked clinically by pain and paresthesia, followed by muscular atrophy of the hands and analgesia with thermoanesthesia of the hands and arms, but with the tactile sense preserved; later marked by painless whitlows, spastic paralysis in the lower extremities, and scoliosis of the lumbar spine. Some cases are associated with low-grade astrocytomas or vascular malformations of the spinal cord. SYN hydrosyringomyelia, Morvan disease. [syringo- + G. *myelos*, marrow]

**sy·rin·go·my·e·lo·cele** (sĭ-ring'gō-mī'ĕ-lō-sēl) a form of spina bifida, consisting in a protrusion of the membranes and spinal cord through a dorsal defect in the vertebral column, the fluid of the syrinx of the cord being increased and expanding the cord tissue into a thin-walled sac which then expands through the vertebral defect. [syringo- + myelocele]

**sy·rin·got·o·my** (si-rin-got'ō-mē) SYN fistulotomy.

**syr·inx**, pl. **sy·ring·es** (sir'ingks, sĭ-rin'jēz) 1. a rarely used synonym for fistula. 2. a pathologic tube-shaped cavity in the brain or spinal cord. 3. the lower part of the bird trachea, which produces vocal sounds. [G. a tube, pipe]

**syr·up** (ser'ŭp, sir'ŭp) 1. refined molasses; the uncrystallizable saccharine solution left after the refining of sugar. 2. any sweet fluid; a solution of sugar in water in any proportion. 3. a liquid preparation of medicinal or flavoring substances in a concentrated aqueous solution of a sugar, usually sucrose; when the syrup contains a medicinal substance, it is termed a medicated syrup. [Mod. L. *syrupus*, fr. Ar. *sharāb*]

**sys·tem** (sis'tĕm) 1. a consistent and complex whole made up of correlated and semi-independent parts. A complex of anatomic structures functionally related. 2. the entire organism seen as a complex organization of parts. 3. any complex of structures related anatomically (e.g., vascular system) or functionally (e.g., digestive system). SYN systema [TA]. 4. a school of medical theory. SEE ALSO apparatus, classification. 5. system followed by one or more letters denotes specific amino acid transporters; system N is a sodium-dependent transporter specific for amino acids such as L-glutamine, L-asparagine, and L-histidine; system y⁺ is a sodium-independent transporter of cationic amino acids. [G. *systēma*, an organized whole]

**sys·te·ma** (sis'tē'mă) [TA] SYN system (3). SEE ALSO system, apparatus. [L. fr. G. *systēma*]

**sys·tem·a·tic name** as applied to chemical substances, a systematic name is composed of specially coined or selected words or syllables, each of which has a precisely defined chemical structural meaning, so that the structure may be derived from the name.

**sys·tem·a·tized de·lu·sion** a delusion that is logically constructed from a false premise and embraces a specific sector of the patient's life.

**sys·tem·ic** (sis-tem'ik) relating to a system; specifically somatic, relating to the entire organism as distinguished from any of its individual parts.

**sys·tem·ic an·a·phy·lax·is** SYN generalized anaphylaxis.

**sys·tem·ic cap·il·lary leak syn·drome** a rare disorder of unknown cause presenting with episodic hypotension, hemoconcentration, and hypoalbuminemia; monoclonal gammopathy is often associated.

**sys·tem·ic cir·cu·la·tion** the circulation of blood through the arteries, capillaries, and veins of the general system, from the left ventricle to the right atrium.

**sys·tem·ic lu·pus er·y·the·ma·to·sus (SLE)** an inflammatory connective tissue disease with variable features including fever, weakness and fatigability, joint pains or arthritis resembling rheumatoid arthritis, diffuse erythematous skin lesions on the face, neck, or upper extremities, lymphadenopathy, pleurisy or pericarditis, glomerular lesions, anemia, hyperglobulinemia, and a positive LE cell test, with serum antibodies to double-stranded DNA and acidic nuclear protein (Sm). SYN disseminated lupus erythematosus.

**sys·tem·ic scler·o·der·ma** SYN scleroderma.

**sys·tem·ic vas·cu·lar re·sis·tance** an index of arteriolar compliance or constriction throughout the body; equal to the blood pressure divided by the cardiac output.

**sys·to·le** (sis'tō-lē) contraction of the heart, especially of the ventricles, by which the blood is driven through the aorta and pulmonary artery to traverse the systemic and pulmonary circulations, respectively; its occurrence is indicated physically by the first sound of the heart heard on auscultation, by the palpable apex beat, and by the arterial pulse. [G. *systolē*, a contracting]

**sys·tol·ic** (sis-tol'ik) relating to, or occurring during cardiac systole.

**sys•tol•ic mur•mur** a murmur heard during ventricular systole.

**sys•tol•ic pres•sure** the intracardiac pressure during or resulting from systolic contraction of a cardiac chamber; the highest arterial blood pressure reached during any given ventricular cycle.

**sys•tol•ic thrill** a thrill felt over the precordium or over a blood vessel during ventricular systole.

**sys•trem•ma** (sis-trem'ă) a muscular cramp in the calf of the leg, the contracted muscles forming a hard ball. [G. anything twisted]

# T

τ tau. SEE tau.

θ, Θ theta. SEE theta.

**T 1.** ribothymidine; tension (T+, increased tension; T−, diminished tension); tera-; tritium; threonine; torque; transmittance. **2.** as a subscript, refers to tidal volume. **3.** thoracic vertebra (T1 to T12); tocopherol. **4.** Tesla, the unit of magnetic field strength.

*T* absolute temperature (kelvin).

t metric ton; time.

*t* temperature (Celsius); tritium.

**T_m** temperature midpoint (kelvin); melting point.

*t*_m temperature midpoint (Celsius).

**T1** MAGNETIC RESONANCE the time for 63% of longitudinal relaxation to occur; the value is a function of magnetic field strength and the chemical environment of the hydrogen nucleus.

**T2** MAGNETIC RESONANCE the time for 63% of transverse relaxation to occur; the value is a function of magnetic field strength and the chemical environment of the hydrogen nucleus.

**TA** Terminologia Anatomica.

**Ta** tantalum.

**tab·a·nid** (tab'ă-nid) common name for flies of the family Tabanidae. [L. *tabanus,* gadfly]

**ta·bes** (tā'bēz) progressive wasting or emaciation. [L. a wasting away]

**ta·bes·cent** (ta-bes'ent) characteristic of tabes. [L. *tabesco,* to waste away, fr. *tabes,* a wasting away]

**tabes dorsalis** SYN tabetic neurosyphilis.

**ta·bes mes·en·ter·ica** tuberculosis of the mesenteric and retroperitoneal lymph nodes.

**ta·bet·ic** (ta-bet'ik) relating to or suffering from tabes, especially tabes dorsalis.

**ta·bet·ic ar·thro·pa·thy** a neuropathic arthropathy that occurs with tabes dorsalis. SEE ALSO neuropathic joint.

**ta·bet·ic neu·ro·sy·phi·lis** type of neurosyphilis in which the posterior roots of the spinal cord, especially in the lumbosacral area, are the principal sites of infection, resulting in ataxia, hypotonia, impotence, constipation, hypotonic bladder, areflexia, and Romberg sign; other findings include lancinating pains (most often in the legs), visceral crises, Argyll-Robertson pupils, optic atrophy, and Charcot joints; in most patients, the CSF is abnormal. SYN tabes dorsalis.

**ta·bet·i·form** (ta-bet'i-fōrm) resembling tabes, especially tabes dorsalis. [irreg. formed fr. L. *tabes,* a wasting, + *forma,* form]

**tab·la·ture** (tab-lă-cher) the state of division of the cranial bones into two plates separated by the diploë. [L. *tabula,* tablet]

**ta·ble** (tā'bl) **1.** one of the two plates or laminae, separated by the diploë, into which the cranial bones are divided. **2.** an arrangement of data in parallel columns, showing the essential facts in a readily appreciable form. [L. *tabula*]

**ta·ble·spoon** (tā'bl-spoon) a large spoon, used as a measure of the dose of a medicine, equivalent to about 4 fluidrams or ½ fluidounce or 15 ml.

**tab·let** a solid dosage form containing medicinal substances with or without suitable diluents; it may vary in shape, size, and weight, and may be classed according to the method of manufacture, as molded tablet and compressed tablet. [Fr. *tablette,* L. *tabula*]

**ta·boo, ta·bu** (tă-boo') restricted, prohibited, or forbidden; set apart for religious or ceremonial purposes. [Tongan, set apart]

**ta·bo·pa·re·sis** (tā'bō-pă-rē'sis, tā'bō-par'ē-sis) a condition in which the symptoms of tabes dorsalis and general paresis are associated.

**tab·u·lar** (tab'yu-lăr) **1.** tablelike. **2.** arranged in the form of a table (2). [L. *tabularis,* fr. *tabula,* table]

**tache** (tash) a circumscribed discoloration of the skin or mucous membrane, such as a macule or freckle. [Fr. spot]

**ta·chet·ic** (tă-shet'ik) marked by bluish or brownish spots. [Fr. *tache,* spot]

**ta·chom·e·ter** (tă-kom'ĕ-ter) an instrument for measuring speed or rate; e.g., revolutions of a shaft, heart rate (cardiotachometer), arterial blood flow (hemotachometer), respiratory gas flow (pneumotachometer). [G. *tachos,* speed, + *metron,* measure]

△**tachy-** rapid. [G. *tachys,* quick,]

**tach·y·ar·rhyth·mia** (tak'ē-ă-ridh'mē-ă) any disturbance of the heart's rhythm, regular or irregular, resulting by convention in a rate over 100 beats per minute during physical examination. [tachy- + G. *a-* priv. + *rhythmos,* rhythm]

**tach·y·car·dia** (tak'i-kar'dē-ă) rapid beating of the heart, conventionally applied to rates over 100 per minute. SYN tachyrhythmia, tachysystole. [tachy- + G. *kardia,* heart]

**ta·chy·car·di·a-bra·dy·car·dia syn·drome** alternating periods of slow and rapid heart beat; often associated with disturbances of both sinoatrial and atrioventricular conduction.

**tach·y·car·di·ac** (tak-i-kar'dē-ak) relating to or suffering from excessively rapid action of the heart.

**ta·chy·car·dia win·dow** in paroxysmal tachycardia of the reentry type, the interval of time (the window) between the earliest and latest premature activation that can excite the paroxysm.

**tach·y·crot·ic** (tak'i-krot'ik) relating to, causing, or characterized by a rapid pulse. [tachy- + G. *krotos,* a striking]

**tach·yp·nea** (tak-ip-nē'ă) rapid breathing. SYN polypnea. [tachy- + G. *pnoē (pnoiē),* breathing]

**tach·yp·noea** [Br.] SEE tachypnea.

**tach·y·rhyth·mia** (tak-i-ridh'mē-ă) SYN tachycardia. [tachy- + G. *rhythmos,* rhythm]

**ta·chys·ter·ol** (tă-kis'ter-ōl) sterol(s) formed by ultraviolet irradiation of any 5,7-diene-3β-sterol. When reduced to the 5,7-diene (or 5,7,22-triene) form, antirachitic action appears.

**ta·chy·sys·tole** SYN tachycardia.

**tack·ler's ex·o·sto·sis** irritative exostosis on the anterior lateral humerus.

**tac·tile** (tak'tĭl) relating to touch or to the sense of touch. [L. *tactilis,* fr. *tango,* pp. *tactus,* to touch]

**tac·tile ag·no·sia** inability to recognize objects by touch, in the presence of intact cutaneous and proprioceptive hand sensation; caused by a lesion in the contralateral parietal lobe. SYN astereognosis.

**tac·tile an·es·the·sia** loss or impairment of the sense of touch.

**tac·tile cor·pus·cle** one of numerous oval bodies found in the papillae of the skin, especially those of the fingers and toes; each consists of a connective tissue capsule in which the axon fibrils terminate around and between a pile of wedge-shaped epithelioid cells. SYN Meissner corpuscle.

**tac·tile de·fen·sive·ness** a sensory integrative dysfunction resulting in excessive reactions to tactile stimulation.

**tac·tile frem·i·tus** vibration felt with the hand on the chest during vocal fremitus.

**tac·tile im·age** an image of an object as perceived by the sense of touch.

**tac·tile me·nis·cus** a specialized tactile sensory nerve ending in the epidermis, characterized by a terminal cuplike expansion of an intraepidermal axon in contact with the base of a single modified keratinocyte. SYN Merkel corpuscle, Merkel tactile cell, Merkel tactile disk.

**tac·tile pa·pil·la** one of the papillae of the dermis containing a tactile cell or corpuscle.

**tac·tom·e·ter** (tak-tom′ĕ-ter) SYN esthesiometer. [L. *tactus,* touch, + G. *metron,* measure]

**tac·tu·al** (tak′chŏ-wĕl) relating to or caused by touch.

**TAD** transient acantholytic dermatosis.

*Tae·nia* (tē′nē-ă) a genus of cestodes that formerly included most of the tapeworms, but is now restricted to those species infecting carnivores with cysticerci found in tissues of various herbivores, rodents, and other animals of prey. SEE ALSO tapeworm. [see taenia]

**tae·nia** (tē′nē-ă) **1.** a coiled bandlike anatomical structure. SEE tenia (1). **2.** common name for a tapeworm, especially of the genus *Taenia.* SYN tenia (2). [L., fr. G. *tainia,* band, tape, a tapeworm]

*Tae·nia sa·gi·na·ta* the beef, hookless, or unarmed tapeworm of humans, acquired by eating insufficiently cooked flesh of cattle infected with *Cysticercus bovis.*

**tae·ni·a·sis** (tē-nī′ă-sĭs) infection with cestodes of the genus *Taenia.*

*Tae·nia so·li·um* the pork, armed, or solitary tapeworm of humans, acquired by eating insufficiently cooked pork infected with *Cysticercus cellulosae;* hatching of ova within the human intestine may result in establishment of cysticerci in human tissues, resulting in cysticercosis.

**tae·ni·id** (tē-nē′id) common name for a member of the family Taeniidae.

**tae·ni·oid** (tē′nē-oyd) denoting members of the genus *Taenia.*

**Taen·zer stain** (tēn′tser) an orcein solution used for staining elastic tissue.

**TAF** tumor angiogenic factor.

**tag 1.** SEE label, tracer. **2.** a small outgrowth or polyp.

**tail** (tāl) **1.** any tail, or tail-like structure, or tapering or elongated extremity of an organ or other part. **2.** VETERINARY ANATOMY a free appendage representing the caudal end of the vertebral column; covered by skin and hair, feathers, or scales. SYN cauda [TA]. [A.S. *taegl*]

**tail bud** the rapidly proliferating mass of cells at the caudal extremity of the embryo; remnant of the primitive node. SYN end bud.

**tail fold** the ventral folding of the caudal extremity of the embryonic disk.

**tail of pan·cre·as** the left extremity of the pancreas within the lienorenal ligament.

**Tai·wan Do·bra·va-Bel·grade vi·rus** (tī-wahn′ dō-bră-vă-bel-grād vī′rŭs) a species of Hantavirus in the Balkans causing hemorrhagic fever with renal syndrome. [after Dobrava, Slovenia (where first isolated from field mice) and Belgrade, Yugoslavia (where first isolated from humans)]

**Ta·ka·ya·su ar·te·ri·tis** (tah′kā-yah-soop) a progressive obliterative arteritis of unknown origin involving fibrosis and luminal narrowing that affects the aorta and its branches; more common in females. SEE ALSO aortic arch syndrome. SYN aortic arch syndrome, pulseless disease.

**ta·lar** (tā′lăr) relating to the talus.

**talc o·per·a·tion** an obsolete operation in which magnesium silicate (talc) powder is applied to the epicardium to create a sterile granulomatous pericarditis and thus promote pericardial anastomoses with the coronary circulation. SYN poudrage (2).

**tal·co·sis** (tal-kō′sis) a pulmonary disorder related to silicosis, occurring in workers exposed to talc mixed with silicates; characterized by restrictive or obstructive disorders of breathing or the two in combination. [talc + G. -osis, condition]

**tal·i·ped·ic** (tal-i-pēd′ik) clubfooted.

**tal·i·pes** (tal′i-pēz) any deformity of the foot involving the talus. [L. *talus,* ankle, + *pes,* foot]

**tal·i·pes cal·ca·ne·o·val·gus** talipes calcaneus and talipes valgus combined; the foot is dorsiflexed, everted, and abducted. SEE clubfoot.

**tal·i·pes cal·ca·ne·o·var·us** talipes calcaneus and talipes varus combined; the foot is dorsiflexed, inverted, and adducted. SEE clubfoot.

**tal·i·pes cal·ca·ne·us** a deformity due to weakness or absence of the calf muscles, in which the axis of the calcaneus becomes vertically oriented; commonly seen in poliomyelitis. SYN calcaneus (2).

**tal·i·pes cav·us** an exaggeration of the normal arch of the foot. See this page.

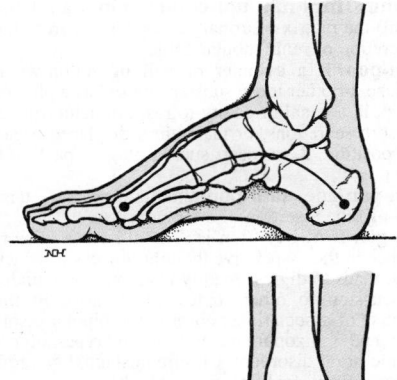

**talipes cavus** (top) and **talipes planus** (bottom)

**tal·i·pes e·qui·no·val·gus** talipes equinus and talipes valgus combined; the foot is plantiflexed, everted, and abducted. SEE clubfoot. SYN equinovalgus.

**tal·i·pes e·qui·no·var·us** talipes equinus and talipes varus combined; the foot is plantiflexed, inverted, and adducted. SYN clubfoot, club foot, equinovarus.

**tal·i·pes e·qui·nus** permanent extension of the foot so that only the ball rests on the ground; it is commonly combined with talipes varus.

**▯ tal·i·pes pla·nus** a condition in which the longitudinal arch is broken down, the entire sole touching the ground. See page 969. SYN flatfoot, pes planus.

**tal·i·pes val·gus** permanent eversion of the foot, the inner side alone of the sole resting on the ground; it is usually combined with a breaking down of the plantar arch.

**tal·i·pes var·us** inversion of the foot, the outer side of the sole only touching the ground; usually some degree of talipes equinus is associated with it, and often talipes cavus.

△**ta·lo-** the talus. [L. *talus*, ankle, ankle bone]

**ta·lo·cal·ca·ne·al joint** SYN subtalar joint.

**ta·lo·cal·ca·ne·o·na·vic·u·lar joint** a ball-and-socket synovial joint, part of which participates in the transverse tarsal joint, formed by the head of the talus articulating with the navicular bone and the anterior part of the calcaneus.

**ta·lo·cru·ral** (tā'lō-kroo'răl) relating to the talus and the bones of the leg; denoting the ankle joint.

**ta·lo·cru·ral joint** SYN ankle joint.

**talon** (tal'ŏn) SYN hypocone. [F. heel, fr. L. *talus*, ankle]

**talonid** (tal'ŏ-nid) the distal portion of the human molar crown, consisting of the hypoconid, hypoconulid, and entoconid. [talon + -id (2)]

**ta·lus**, gen. **ta·li** (tā'lŭs, tā'lī) [TA] the bone of the foot that articulates with the tibia and fibula to form the ankle joint. SYN ankle bone, ankle (3). [L. ankle bone, heel]

**Tamm-Hors·fall mu·co·pro·tein** (tam-hōrs' fahl) the matrix of urinary casts derived from the secretion of renal tubular cells.

**tam·pon 1.** a cylinder or ball of cotton-wool, gauze, or other loose substance; used as a plug or pack in a canal or cavity to restrain hemorrhage, absorb secretions, or maintain a displaced organ in position. **2.** to insert such a plug or pack. [O. Fr.]

**tam·pon·ade, tam·pon·age** (tam-pŏ-nād', tam' pŏ-nij) the insertion of a tampon.

**tan·gen·ti·al·i·ty** (tan-jen'shē-al'i-tē) a disturbance in the associative thought process in which one tends to digress readily from one topic under discussion to other topics which arise in the course of associations; observed in bipolar disorder and schizophrenia and certain types of organic brain disorders. Cf. circumstantiality. [off on a tangent, fr. L. *tango*, to touch]

**tan·gi·ble bo·dy ma·cro·phage** a macrophage that specializes in phagocytosis of lymphoid cells.

**Tan·ner growth chart** (tan-ĕr) a series of charts showing distribution of parameters of physical development, such as stature, growth curves, and skinfold thickness, for children by sex, age, and stages of puberty.

**Tan·ner stage** (tan-ĕr) a stage of puberty in the Tanner growth chart, based on pubic hair growth, development of genitalia in boys, and breast development in girls.

**tan·ta·lum (Ta)** (tan'tă-lŭm) a heavy metal of the vanadium group, atomic no. 73, atomic wt.

180.9479; used in surgical prostheses because of its noncorrosive properties. [G. mythical king of Lydia *Tantalus*]

**T ant·i·gens** tumor antigens associated wtih replication and transformation by certain DNA tumor viruses, including adenoviruses and papovaviruses. SEE ALSO β-hemolytic streptococci, tumor antigens.

**tan·trum** (tan'trŭm) a fit of bad temper, especially in children.

**TAP** a protein that transports a peptide from the cytoplasm into the lumen of the endoplasmic reticulum.

**tap 1.** to withdraw fluid from a cavity by means of a trocar and cannula, hollow needle, or catheter. **2.** to strike lightly with the finger or a hammerlike instrument in percussion or to elicit a tendon reflex. **3.** a light blow. **4.** an East Indian fever of undetermined nature. **5.** an instrument to cut threads in a hole in bone prior to inserting a screw. [M.E. *tappe*, fr. A.S. *taeppa*]

**ta·per·ing-off** SYN active recovery.

**ta·pe·tum**, pl. **ta·pe·ta** (tă-pē'tŭm, tă-pē'tă) **1.** in general, any membranous layer or covering. **2.** [TA] NEUROANATOMY a thin sheet of fibers in the lateral wall of the temporal and occipital horns of the lateral ventricle, continuous with the corpus callosum. [L. *tapeta*, a carpet]

**tape·worm** (tāp'werm) an intestinal parasitic worm, adults of which are found in the intestine of vertebrates. Tapeworms consist of a scolex, variously equipped with spined or sucking structures by which the worm is attached to the intestinal wall of the host, and strobila having several to many proglottids that lack a digestive tract at any stage of development. The ovum, entering the intestine of an appropriate intermediate host, hatches and the hexacanth penetrates the gut wall and develops into a specific larval form (e.g., cysticercoid, cysticercus, hydatid, strobilocercus), which develops into an adult when the intermediate host is ingested by the proper final host.

**Ta·pia syn·drome** (tah-pē-ah) unilateral paralysis of the larynx, the velum palati, and the tongue, with atrophy of the latter.

**ta·pir mouth** protrusion of the lips due to weakness of the orbicularis oris muscles; seen with some dystrophies.

**ta·pote·ment** (tă-pō-maw') a group of massage movements that involve the repetitive, regular, rhythmic striking of the tissue with some part of the hand. Includes beating, hacking, cupping, and tapping. SEE ALSO percussion. SYN tapping (1). [Fr. *tapoter*, to pat]

**tap·ping** (tap'ing) **1.** SYN tapotement. **2.** SYN paracentesis.

**TAPVC** total anomalous pulmonary venous connection. SEE anomalous pulmonary venous connections, total or partial.

**TAPVR** total anomalous pulmonary venous return. SEE anomalous pulmonary venous connections, total or partial.

**TAR** thrombocytopenia and absent radius. SEE thrombocytopenia-absent radius syndrome.

**ta·ran·tu·la** (tă-ran'choo-lă) a very large, hairy spider, considered highly venomous and often greatly feared; the bite, however, is usually no more harmful than a bee sting. [see tarantism]

**Tar·dieu ec·chy·mos·es, Tar·dieu pe·te·- chi·ae, Tar·dieu spots** (tahr-dyoo') subpleural and subpericardial petechiae or ecchymoses (or both), as observed in the tissues of persons who have been strangled, or otherwise asphyxiated.

**tar•dive** (tar′div) late; tardy.

**tar•dive cy•a•no•sis** SYN cyanose tardive.

**tar•get** (tar′get) **1.** an object fixed as goal or point of examination. **2.** in the ophthalmometer, the mire. **3.** SYN target organ. **4.** anode of an x-ray tube. SEE ALSO x-ray. [It. *targhetta,* a small shield]

**tar•get cell 1.** an erythrocyte in target cell anemia, with a dark center surrounded by a light band that again is encircled by a darker ring; it thus resembles a shooting target; such cells also appear after splenectomy; **2.** a cell lysed by cytotoxic T lymphocytes, as in graft rejection. SYN codocyte, leptocyte, Mexican hat cell.

**tar•get gland** the effector that functions when stimulated by the internal secretion of another gland or by some other stimulus.

**tar•get heart rate** exercise heart rate that represents the exercise level needed to induce improvements in cardiovascular (aerobic) fitness and improve one's health risk profile; usually falls within range of 60–85% of age-predicted maximal heart rate.

**tar•get heart rate range** SYN training-sensitive zone.

**tar•get or•gan** a tissue or organ upon which a hormone exerts its action; generally, a tissue or organ with appropriate receptors for a hormone. SYN target (3).

**tar•get re•sponse** SYN operant.

**Tar•lov cyst** (tar′lov) a perineural cyst found in the proximal radicles of the lower spinal cord; it is usually productive of symptoms.

**Tar•ni•er for•ceps** (tahr-nē-ā′) a type of axis-traction forceps.

**tar•ry cyst** a cyst or collection of old blood having a tarry or black, sticky appearance; usually due to endometriosis.

**tar•sal** (tahr′săl) relating to a tarsus in any sense.

**tar•sal bones** the seven bones of the instep: talus, calcaneus, navicular, three cuneiform (wedge), and cuboid.

**tar•sal cyst** SYN chalazion.

**tar•sa•le,** pl. **tar•sa•lia** (tar-sā′lē, tar-sā′lē-ă) any tarsal bone. [Mod. L. fr. G. *tarsos,* sole of the foot]

**tars•al•gia** (tar-sal′jē-ă) SYN podalgia. [tarsus + G. *algos,* pain]

**tar•sal glands** sebaceous glands embedded in the tarsal plate of each eyelid, discharging at the edge of the lid near the posterior border. Their secretions create a lipid barrier along the margin of the eyelids which contains the normal secretions in the conjunctival sac by preventing the watery fluid from spilling over the barrier when the eye is open. SYN meibomian glands.

**tar•sal joints** SYN intertarsal joints.

**tar•sal si•nus** a hollow or canal formed by the groove of the talus and the interosseous groove of the calcaneus which is occupied by the interosseous talocalcaneal ligament.

**tars•ec•to•my** (tar-sek′tō-mē) excision of the tarsus of the foot or of a segment of the tarsus of an eyelid. [tarsus + G. *ektomē,* excision]

**tar•si•tis** (tar-sī′tis) **1.** inflammation of the tarsus of the foot. **2.** inflammation of the tarsal border of an eyelid.

△**tar•so-, tars-** a tarsus. [See tarsus]

**tar•so•cla•sia, tar•soc•la•sis** (tar-sō-klā′zē-ă, tar-sok′lă-sis) instrumental fracture of the tarsus, for the correction of talipes equinovarus. [tarso- + G. *klasis,* a breaking]

**tar•so•ma•la•cia** (tar′sō-mă-lā′shē-ă) softening of the tarsal cartilages of the eyelids. [tarso- + G. *malakia,* softness]

**tar•so•meg•a•ly** (tar-sō-meg′ă-lē) a congenital maldevelopment and overgrowth of a tarsal or carpal bone. [tarso- + G. *megas,* large]

**tar•so•met•a•tar•sal** (TMT) (tar-sō-met′ă-tar′săl) relating to the tarsal and metatarsal bones; denoting the articulations between the two sets of bones, and the ligaments in relation thereto.

**tar•so•met•a•tar•sal joints** the three synovial joints between the tarsal and metatarsal bones, consisting of a medial joint between the first cuneiform and first metatarsal, an intermediate joint between the second and third cuneiforms and corresponding metatarsals, and a lateral joint between the cuboid and fourth and fifth metatarsals.

**tar•so•met•a•tar•sal lig•a•ments** the ligaments that unite tarsal and metatarsal bones; they are arranged in dorsal, interosseous, and plantar sets.

**tar•so•pha•lan•ge•al** (tar-sō-fă-lan′jē-ăl) relating to the tarsus and the phalanges.

**tar•sor•rha•phy** (tar-sōr′ă-fē) the suturing together of the eyelid margins, partially or completely, to shorten the palpebral fissure or to protect the cornea in keratitis or in paralysis of the orbicularis oculi muscle. [tarso- + G. *rhaphē,* suture]

**tar•sot•o•my** (tar-sot′ō-mē) **1.** incision of the tarsal cartilage of an eyelid. **2.** any operation on the tarsus of the foot. [tarso- + G. *tomē,* incision]

**tar•sus,** gen. and pl. **tar•si** (tar′sŭs, tar′sī) [TA] **1.** as a division of the skeleton, the seven tarsal bones of the instep. SEE tarsal bones. **2.** the fibrous plates giving solidity and form to the edges of the eyelids; often erroneously called tarsal or ciliary cartilages. [G. *tarsos,* a flat surface, sole of the foot, edge of eyelid]

**tar•tar** (tar′tăr) **1.** a crust on the interior of wine casks, consisting essentially of potassium bitartrate. **2.** a white, brown, or yellow-brown deposit at or below the gingival margin of teeth, chiefly hydroxyapatite in an organic matrix. SYN dental calculus (2). [Mediev. L. *tartarum,* ult. etym. unknown]

**tart cell** a monocyte with an engulfed nucleus in which the structure is still well preserved.

**tas•tant** (tās′tănt) any chemical that stimulates the sensory cells in a taste bud.

**taste** (tāst) **1.** to perceive through the medium of the gustatory nerves. **2.** the sensation produced by a suitable stimulus applied to the gustatory nerve endings in the tongue. [It. *tastare;* L. *tango,* to touch]

**taste bud** one of a number of flask-shaped cell nests located in the epithelium of vallate, fungiform, and foliate papillae of the tongue and also in the soft palate, epiglottis, and posterior wall of the pharynx; it consists of sustentacular, gustatory, and basal cells between which the intragemmal sensory nerve fibers terminate.

**taste cells** darkly staining cells in a taste bud that have long hair-like microvilli. SYN gustatory cells.

**taste hairs** hairlike projections of gustatory cells

of taste buds; electron micrographs show them to be clusters of microvilli.

**TAT** thematic apperception test.

**tat·too** (tă-too′) **1.** a deliberate decorative implanting or injecting of indelible pigments into the skin or the tinctorial effect of accidental implantation. **2.** to produce such an effect. [Tahiti, *tatu*]

**tau** (τ) (tau) **1.** the 19th letter of the Greek alphabet (τ). **2.** tele; relaxation time. **3.** a protein that associates with microtubules and other elements of the cytoskeleton; tau accelerates tubulin polymerization and stabilizes microtubules; tau is also found in the plaque observed in individuals with Alzheimer disease.

**tau·ro·cho·lic ac·id** (taw-rō-kō′lik as′id) a compound of cholic acid and taurine, involving the carboxyl group of the former and the amino of the latter; a common bile salt in carnivores.

**Taus·sig-Bing syn·drome** (tou′sig-bing) complete transposition of the aorta, which arises from the right ventricle, with a left-sided pulmonary artery overriding the left ventricle, and with high ventricular septal defect, right ventricular hypertrophy, anteriorly situated aorta, and posteriorly situated pulmonary artery.

**tau·to·mer·ic** (taw-tō-mer′ik) **1.** relating to the same part. **2.** relating to or marked by tautomerism. [G. *tautos*, the same, + *meros*, part]

**tau·to·mer·ic fi·bers** nerve fibers of the spinal cord that do not extend beyond the limits of the spinal cord segment in which they originate.

**tau·tom·er·ism** (taw-tom′er-izm) a phenomenon in which a chemical compound exists in two forms of different structure (isomers) in equilibrium, the two forms differing, usually, in the position of a hydrogen atom. [G. *tautos*, the same, + *meros*, part]

**taxa** (tak′să) plural of taxon.

**tax·ane** (taks′ān) any of a class of antitumor agents derived directly or semisynthetically from *Taxus brevifolius*, the Pacific yew; examples include paclitaxel and docetaxel.

**tax·is** (tak′sis) **1.** reduction of a hernia or of a dislocation of any part by means of manipulation. **2.** systematic classification or orderly arrangement. **3.** the reaction of protoplasm to a stimulus, by virtue of which animals and plants are led to move or act in certain definite ways in relation to their environment; the various kinds of taxis are designated by a prefix denoting the stimulus governing them; e.g., chemotaxis, electrotaxis, thermotaxis. [G. orderly arrangement]

**tax·on,** pl. **taxa** (tak′son, tak′să) the name given to a particular level or grouping in a systematic classification of living things or organisms (taxonomy). [G. *taxis*, order, arrangement, + -on]

**tax·o·nom·ic** (tak-sō-nom′ik) relating to taxonomy.

**tax·on·o·my** (tak-sawn′ŏ-mē) the systematic classification of living things or organisms. Kingdoms of living organisms are divided into groups (taxa) to show degrees of similarity or presumed evolutionary relationships, with the higher categories being larger, more inclusive, and more broadly defined, the lower categories being more restricted, with fewer species more closely related. The divisions below kingdom are, in descending order: phylum, class, order, family, genus, species, and subspecies (variety). Infra- and supra- or sub- and super- categories can be used when needed; additional categories, such as tribe, section, level, group, etc., are also used. [G. *taxis*, orderly arrangement, + *nomos*, law]

**Tay cher·ry-red spot** (tā) SYN cherry-red spot.

**Tay·lor dis·ease** (tā′lŏr) diffuse idiopathic cutaneous atrophy.

**Tay-Sachs dis·ease** (tā-saks) a lysosomal storage disease, resulting from hexosaminidase A deficiency. The monosialoganglioside is stored in central and peripheral neuronal cells. Infants present with hyperacusis and irritability, hypotonia, and failure to develop motor skills. Blindness with macular cherry red spots and seizures are evident in the first year.

**TB** tuberculosis.

**Tb** terbium.

**T-bind·er** two strips of cloth at right angles; used for retaining a dressing, as on the perineum.

**TBV** total blood volume.

**Tc** technetium.

**Tc** T cytotoxic cells.

**⁹⁹ᵐTc-DTPA** a radionuclide chelate complex used for renal imaging and function testing; also known as ⁹⁹ᵐTc pentatate. [*d*iethylene *t*riamine *p*entaacetic *a*cid]

**T cell** SYN T lymphocyte.

**T-cell re·cep·tor (TCR)** an adhesion molecule on the membrane of T-lymphocytes that serves as the receptor for antigen bound to antigen-presenting cells (APC) via MHC molecules. It is expressed in a complex with CD3. It is in close proximity to the MHC-restricted receptor (CD4 or CD8). SYN T-lymphocyte antigen receptor.

**T-cell–rich, B-cell lym·pho·ma** a B-cell lymphoma in which more than 90% of the cells are of T-cell origin, masking the large cells that form the neoplastic B-cell component. SEE ALSO adult T-cell lymphoma.

**⁹⁹ᵐTc-glucoheptanate** radiopharmaceutical possessing renal cortical-localizing and excretion-handling properties; may be used either for renal cortical imaging to determine scarring or for renal function imaging by renography.

**TCR** T-cell receptor.

**T cy·to·tox·ic cells (Tc)** SYN killer cells.

**TDD** Telephone Device for the Deaf.

**TDEE** total daily energy expenditure.

**TDP** ribothymidine 5′-diphosphate. The thymidine analog is dTDP.

**TdT** terminal deoxynucleotidyl transferase.

**TE** in magnetic resonance spin echo pulse sequences, the time to echo, when the magnetization signal is sampled.

**Te 1.** ELECTRODIAGNOSIS abbreviation denoting tetanic contraction. **2.** tellurium.

**teach·ing hos·pi·tal** a hospital that also functions as a formal center of learning for the training of physicians, nurses, and allied health personnel.

**Teale am·pu·ta·tion** (tēl) **1.** amputation of the forearm in its lower half, or of the thigh, with a long posterior rectangular flap and a short anterior one; **2.** amputation of the leg, with a long anterior rectangular flap and a short posterior one.

**team nurs·ing** a decentralized way of providing nursing services for inpatients whereby responsibility for planning and coordination of care is shared by members of a group; the team may include registered nurses and practical nurses, but the team leader is most often a registered nurse.

🔲 **tear** (tēr) the fluid secreted by the lacrimal glands by means of which the conjunctiva and cornea are kept moist. See this page. [A.S. *teár*]

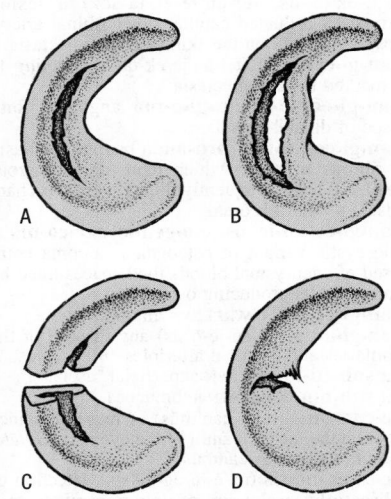

**meniscal tears:** (A) longitudinal, (B) bucket-handle, (C) horizontal, (D) parrot beak

**tear** (tār) a discontinuity in substance of a structure. Cf. laceration.

**tear·drop** (tērdrop) **1.** a drop of the fluid secreted by the lacrimal glands. **2.** a red cell with a pear shape, where the constricted end narrows to a point. [Anglo-Saxon tear, teahor, taeher, Old Norse tar]

**tear·drop cell** SYN dacryocyte.

**tear gas** a gas, such as acetone, benzene bromide, and xylol, that causes irritation of the conjunctiva and profuse lacrimation. SEE ALSO lacrimator.

**tear·ing** (tēr'ing) SYN epiphora.

**tear sac** SYN lacrimal sac.

**tear stone** SYN dacryolith.

**tease** (tēz) to separate the structural parts of a tissue by means of a needle, in order to prepare it for microscopic examination. [A. S. *taesan*]

**tea·spoon** (tē'spoon) a small spoon, holding about 1 dram (or about 5 ml) liquid; used as a measure in the dosage of fluid medicines.

**teat** (tēt) **1.** SYN nipple. **2.** SYN breast. **3.** SYN papilla. [A.S. *tit*]

**tech·ne·ti·um (Tc)** (tek-nē'shē-ŭm) an artificial radioactive element, atomic no. 43, atomic wt. 99, produced by bombardment of molybdenum by deuterons; also a product of the fission of $^{235}$U; used extensively as a radiographic tracer in imaging studies of internal organs. [G. *technetos,* artificial]

**tech·ne·ti·um-99m** a radioisotope of technetium that decays by isomeric transition, emitting an essentially monoenergetic gamma ray of 142 keV with a half-life of 6.01 hr. It is usually obtained from a radionuclide generator of molybdenum-99 and is used to prepare radiopharmaceuticals for scanning the brain, parotid, thyroid,

lungs, blood pool, liver, heart, spleen, kidney, lacrimal drainage apparatus, bone, and bone marrow.

**tech·nic** (tek'nik) SYN technique.

**tech·ni·cian** (tek-nish'ŭn) SYN technologist. [G. *technē,* an art]

**tech·nique** (tek-nēk') the manner of performance, or the details, of any surgical operation, experiment, or mechanical act. SEE ALSO method, operation, procedure. SYN technic. [Fr., fr. G. *technikos,* relating to *technē,* art, skill]

**tech·nol·o·gist** (tek-nol'ŏ-jist) one trained in and using the techniques of a profession, art, or science. SYN technician.

**tec·tal** (tek'tăl) relating to a tectum.

**tec·to·ceph·a·ly** (tek'tō-sef-al'ē) SYN scaphocephaly.

**tec·ton·ic ker·a·to·plas·ty** grafting to replace lost corneal tissue.

**tec·to·ri·al** (tek-tōr'ē-ăl) relating to or characteristic of a tectorium.

**tec·to·ri·al mem·brane of co·chle·ar duct** a gelatinous membrane that overlies the spiral organ (Corti) in the inner ear. SYN membrana tectoria ductus cochlearis [TA], Corti membrane, tectorium (2).

**tec·to·ri·um** (tek-tōr'ē-ŭm) **1.** an overlying structure. **2.** SYN tectorial membrane of cochlear duct. [L. an overlying surface (plaster, stucco), fr. *tego,* pp. *tectus,* to cover]

**tec·to·spi·nal** (tek-tō-spī'năl) denoting nerve fibers passing from the mesencephalic tectum to the spinal cord.

**tec·tum,** pl. **tec·ta** (tek'tŭm, tek'tă) any rooflike covering or structure. [L. roof, roofed structure, fr. *tego,* pp. *tectus,* to cover]

**tec·tum of mid·brain** SYN lamina of mesencephalic tectum.

**TED hose** elastic stockings that compress the superficial veins in the lower extremities; used in postoperative patients and others immobilized by illness, to prevent thrombophlebitis by shunting blood through the deep veins of the calves and thighs. TED is an abbreviation for thromboembolic disease.

**teeth** (tēth) plural of tooth.

**teeth·ing** (tē'thing) eruption or, colloquially cutting, of the teeth, especially of the deciduous teeth. Inflammation of the gingival tissues doing this period may cause a temporary, painful condition.

**teg·men,** gen. **teg·mi·nis,** pl. **teg·mi·na** (teg' měn, teg'mĭ-nis, teg'mĭ-nă) [TA] a structure that covers or roofs over a part. [L. a covering, fr. *tego,* to cover]

**teg·men mas·toi·de·um** the lamina of bone roofing over the mastoid cells.

**teg·men·tal** (teg-yu-men'tăl) relating to, characteristic of, or placed or oriented toward a tegmentum or tegmen.

**teg·men·tal de·cus·sa·tions 1.** the dorsal tegmental decussation (fountain or Meynert decussation, decussatio fontinalis) of the left and right tectospinal and tectobulbar tracts; **2.** the ventral tegmental decussation (rubrospinal or Forel decussation) of the left and right rubrospinal and rubrobulbar tracts; both are located in the mesencephalon. SYN decussationes tegmenti.

**teg·men·tal nu·clei** collective term for two small round cell groups in the caudal part of the midbrain (caudal pontine tegmental nucleus, nucleus

t
e

tegmenti pontis caudalis and oral pontine tegmental nucleus, nucleus tegmenti pontis oralis), associated with the mammillary body by way of the mammillary peduncle and mammillotegmental tract.

**teg•men•tal syn•drome** a syndrome usually caused by a vascular lesion in the tegmentum; marked by contralateral hemiplegia and ipsilateral ocular paresis.

**teg•men•tum,** pl. **teg•men•ta** (teg-men′tŭm, teg-men′tă) **1.** a covering structure. **2.** [TA] SYN mesencephalic tegmentum. [L. covering structure, fr. *tego,* to cover]

**teg•men tym•pa•ni** [TA] the roof of the middle ear, formed by the thinned anterior surface of the petrous portion of the temporal bone. Its anterior edge is inserted into the petrosquamous fissure so that it can be seen as a wedge of bone subdividing that fissure into a squamotympanic and a petrotympanic fissure.

**teg•men ven•tric•u•li quar•ti** roof of fourth ventricle, formed in its upper part by the superior medullary velum stretching between the two brachia conjunctiva (superior cerebellar peduncles), in its lower part by the inferior medullary velum composed of the choroid membrane and choroid plexus of the fourth ventricle.

**teg•u•ment** (teg′yu-ment) SYN integument. [L. *tegumentum,* a collat. form of *tegmentum*]

**teg•u•men•tal, teg•u•men•ta•ry** (teg-yū-men′tăl, teg-yu-men′tă-rē) relating to the integument.

**Teich•mann cry•stals** (tīk′mahn) rhombic crystals of hemin; used in microscopic detection of blood. SEE hemin.

**tei•cho•ic ac•ids** (tī-kō′ik as′idz) one of two classes (the other being the muramic acids or mucopeptides) of polymers constituting the cell walls of Gram-positive bacteria, but also found intracellularly.

**tei•chop•sia** (tī-kop′sē-ă) the jagged, shimmering visual sensation resembling the fortifications of a walled medieval town; the scintillating scotoma of migraine. [G. *teichos,* wall, + *opsis,* vision]

△**tel-, te•le-, te•lo-** distance, end, other end. [G. *tēle,* distant, *telos,* end]

**te•la,** gen. and pl. **te•lae** (tē′lă, tē′lē) **1.** any thin weblike structure. **2.** a tissue; especially one of delicate formation. [L. a web]

**te•la cho•roi•dea of fourth ven•tri•cle** the sheet of pia mater covering the lower part of the ependymal roof of the fourth ventricle. SYN tela choroidea ventriculi quarti [TA], tela choroidea inferior.

**te•la cho•roi•dea in•fe•ri•or** SYN tela choroidea of fourth ventricle.

**te•la cho•roi•dea su•pe•ri•or** SYN tela choroidea of third ventricle.

**te•la cho•roi•dea of third ven•tri•cle** a double fold of pia mater, enclosing subarachnoid trabeculae, between the fornix above and the epithelial roof of the third ventricle and the thalami below; at each lateral margin is a vascular fringe projecting into the choroidal fissure of the lateral ventricle; on its undersurface are several small vascular projections filling the folds of the ependymal roof of the third ventricle. SYN tela choroidea superior.

**te•la cho•roi•dea ven•tri•cu•li quar•ti** [TA] SYN tela choroidea of fourth ventricle.

**te•la cho•roi•dea ven•tri•cu•li ter•tii** [TA] SYN choroid tela of third ventricle.

🔲 **tel•an•gi•ec•ta•sia** (tel-an′jē-ek-tā′zē-ă) dilation of the previously existing small or terminal vessels of a part. See page B5. [G. *telos,* end, + *angeion,* vessel, + *ektasis,* a stretching out]

**tel•an•gi•ec•ta•sis,** pl. **tel•an•gi•ec•ta•ses** (tel-an′jē-ek′tă-sis, tel-an′jē-ek′tă-sēz) a lesion formed by a dilated capillary or terminal artery, most commonly on the skin. SEE telangiectasia.

**tel•an•gi•ec•tat•ic** (tel-an′jē-ek-tat′ik) relating to or marked by telangiectasia.

**tel•an•gi•ec•tat•ic an•gi•o•ma** angioma composed of dilated vessels.

**tel•an•gi•ec•tat•ic fi•bro•ma** a benign neoplasm of fibrous tissue in which there are numerous small and large, frequently dilated vascular channels. SYN angiofibroma.

**tel•an•gi•ec•tat•ic os•te•o•gen•ic sar•co•ma** a lytic cystic variant of osteogenic sarcoma composed of aneurysmal blood-filled spaces lined by sarcoma cells producing osteoid.

**tel•an•gi•ec•tat•ic wart** SYN angiokeratoma.

**tel•an•gi•o•sis** (tel′an-jē-ō′sis) any disease of the capillaries and terminal arterioles.

**te•la sub•cu•ta•nea** SYN superficial fascia.

**te•la sub•mu•co•sa** SYN submucosa.

**tel•e•can•thus** (tel-ĕ-kan′thŭs) increased distance between the medial canthi of the eyelids. [G. *tēle,* distant, + *kanthos,* canthus]

**tel•e•di•ag•no•sis** (tel′ĕ-dī-ag-nō′sis) detection of a disease by evaluation of data transmitted to a receiving station, a process normally involving patient-monitoring instruments and a transfer link to a diagnostic center at some distance from the patient.

**tel•e•graph•ic speech** a pattern of speech typical of expressive aphasia, in which prominent words in a sentence, usually nouns, are uttered but most other words are omitted. SEE ALSO agrammatism.

**tel•e•m•e•try** (tĕ-lem′ĕ-trē) the science of measuring a quantity, transmitting the results by radio signals to a distant station, and there interpreting, indicating, and/or recording the results. SEE ALSO biotelemetry.

**tel•en•ce•phal•ic** (tel′en-se-fal′ik) relating to the telencephalon or endbrain.

**tel•en•ceph•al•ic flex•ure** a flexure appearing in the embryonic forebrain region.

**tel•en•ceph•a•lon** (tel-en-sef′ă-lon) [TA] the anterior division of the prosencephalon, which develops into the olfactory lobes, the cortex of the cerebral hemispheres, the subcortical telencephalic nuclei, and the basal ganglia (nuclei), particularly the striatum and the amygdala. SYN endbrain. [G. *telos,* end, + *enkephalos,* brain]

**tel•e•o•mi•to•sis** (tel′ē-ō-mī-tō′sis) a completed mitosis. [G. *teleos,* complete, + mitosis]

**tel•e•op•sia** (tel-ē-op′sē-ă) an error in judging the distance of objects arising from lesions in the parietal temporal region. [G. *tēle,* distant, + *opsis,* vision]

**tel•e•or•gan•ic** (tel′ē-ōr-gan′ik) manifesting life. [G. *teleos,* complete, + *organikos,* organic]

**te•lep•a•thy** (tĕ-lep′ă-thē) transmittal and reception of thoughts by means other than through the normal senses, as a form of extrasensory perception. [G. *tēle,* distant, + *pathos,* feeling]

**Te•le•phone De•vice for the Deaf (TDD, TT, TTY)** telephone accessory that transmits and receives text over standard telephone lines. Also referred to as teletypewriter (TTY) and text telephone (TT). SEE assistive listening device.

**te·le·phone ear** noise-induced hearing loss due to exposure to static over telephones.

**tel·e·ra·di·og·ra·phy** (tel-ĕ-rā-dē-og′ră-fē) radiography with the x-ray tube positioned about 2 m from the film thereby securing practical parallelism of the x-rays to minimize geometric distortion; the standard configuration for chest radiography. SYN teleroentgenography. [G. *tēle*, distant, + radiography]

**tel·e·ra·di·ol·o·gy** (tel-ĕ-rā-dē-ol′ō-jē) the interpretation of digitized diagnostic images transmitted over telephone lines. [tele- + radiology]

**tel·er·gy** (tel′er-jē) SYN automatism. [G. *tēle*, far off, + *ergon*, work]

**tel·e·roent·gen·og·ra·phy** (tel′ĕ-rent-gen-og′ră-fē) SYN teleradiography.

**tel·e·ther·a·py** (tel-e-thār′ă-pē) radiation therapy administered with the source at a distance from the body. [G. *tēle*, distant, + *therapeia*, treatment]

**tel·lu·ric** (tĕ-loor′ik) **1.** relating to or originating in the earth. **2.** relating to the element tellurium, especially in its 6+ valence state. [L. *tellus* (*tellur-*), the earth]

**tel·lu·ri·um (Te)** (tel-oo′rē-ŭm) a rare semimetallic element, atomic no. 52, atomic wt. 127.60, belonging to the sulfur group. [L. *tellus* (*tellur-*), the earth]

**tel·o·den·dron** (tel-ō-den′dron) the terminal arborization of an axon. [G. *telos*, end, + *dendron*, tree]

**tel·o·gen** (tel′ō-jen) resting phase of hair cycle. [G. *telos*, end, + *-gen*, producing]

**tel·o·gen ef·flu·vi·um** increased transient shedding of normal club hairs by premature development of telogen in anagen follicles, resulting from various kinds of stress, e.g., childbirth, shock, drug intake or cessation of an oral contraceptive, fever, and dieting with marked weight loss. SEE ALSO anagen effluvium.

**tel·o·lec·i·thal** (tel-ō-les′i-thăl) denoting an oocyte (ovum) in which a large amount of deuteroplasm accumulates at the vegetative pole, as in the eggs of birds and reptiles. [G. *telos*, end, + G. *lekithos*, yolk]

**tel·o·mere** (tel′ō-mēr) the distal end of a chromosome arm; telomeres undergo dramatic changes during the progression of cancer. [G. *telos*, end, + *meros*, part]

**tel·o·phase** (tel′ō-fāz) the final stage of mitosis or meiosis, which begins when migration of chromosomes to the poles of the cell has been completed; the chromosomes progressively lengthen while the nuclear membranes of the two daughter nuclei are reconstructed and a cell membrane at the equator completes the separation of the two daughter cells. [G. *telos*, end, + *phasis*, appearance]

**tem·per 1.** disposition; in general, any characteristic or particular state of mind. SYN temperament (2). **2.** a display of irritation or anger. SEE tantrum. **3.** to treat metal by application of heat, as in annealing or quenching.

**tem·per·a·ment** (tem′per-ă-ment) **1.** the psychological and biological organization peculiar to the individual, including one's character or personality predispositions, which influence the manner of thought and action and general views of life. **2.** SYN temper (1). [L. *temperamentum*, proper measure, moderation, disposition]

**tem·per·ance** (tem′per-ans) moderation in all things; especially, abstinence from the use of alcoholic beverages. [L. *temperantia,* moderation]

**tem·per·ate** (tem′per-ăt) moderate; restrained in the indulgence of any appetite or activity.

**tem·per·ate bac·te·ri·o·phage** bacteriophage whose genome incorporates with, and replicates with, that of the host bacterium; dissociation (and resultant development of vegetative bacteriophage) occurs at a slow rate resulting occasionally in lysis of a bacterium and release of mature bacteriophage, thus rendering the bacterial culture capable of inducing general lysis if transferred to a culture of a susceptible bacterial strain.

**tem·per·a·ture** (tem′per-ă-cher) the sensible intensity of heat of any substance; the manifestation of the average kinetic energy of the molecules making up a substance due to heat agitation. SEE ALSO scale. [L. *temperatura,* due measure, temperature, fr. *tempero,* to proportion duly]

**tem·per·a·ture mid·point (Tm,** $t_m$**)** the midpoint in the change in optical properties (absorbance, rotation) of a structured polymer (e.g., DNA) with increasing temperature.

**tem·plate** (tem′plăt) **1.** a pattern or guide that determines the shape of a substance. **2.** metaphorically, the specifying nature of a macromolecule, usually a nucleic acid or polynucleotide, with respect to the primary structure of the nucleic acid or polynucleotide or protein made from it *in vivo* or *in vitro*. **3.** DENTISTRY a curved or flat plate utilized as an aid in setting teeth. **4.** an outline used to trace teeth, bones, or soft tissue in order to standardize their form. **5.** a pattern or guide that determines the specificity of antibody globulins. **6.** a wax impression made to assess the occlusion of the teeth. [Fr. *templet,* temple of a loom, fr. L. *templum,* small timber]

**tem·ple** (tem′pl) **1.** the area of the temporal fossa on the side of the head above the zygomatic arch. **2.** the part of a spectacle frame passing from the rim backward over the ear. [L. *tempus* (*tempor-*), time, the temple]

**tem·po·la·bile** (tem-pō-lā′bīl) undergoing spontaneous change or destruction during the passage of time. [L. *tempus,* time, + *labilis,* perishable]

**tem·po·ral** (tem′pŏ-răl) **1.** relating to time; limited in time; temporary. **2.** relating to the temple. [L. *temporalis,* fr. *tempus* (*tempor-*), time, temple]

**tem·por·al ar·ter·i·tis** a subacute, granulomatous arteritis involving the external carotid arteries, especially the temporal artery; occurs in elderly persons and may be manifested by constitutional symptoms, particularly severe headache, and sometimes sudden unilateral blindness. Shares many of the symptoms of polymyalgia rheumatica. SYN cranial arteritis, giant cell arteritis, Horton arteritis.

**tem·por·al bone** a large irregular bone situated in the base and side of the skull; it consists of three parts, squamous, tympanic, and petrous, which are distinct at birth; the petrous part contains the vestibulocochlear organ; the bone articulates with the sphenoid, parietal, occipital, and zygomatic bones, and by a synovial joint with the mandible. SYN os temporale [TA].

**tem·por·al fos·sa** the space on the side of the cranium bounded by the temporal lines and terminating below at the level of the zygomatic arch.

**tem·por·a·lis mus·cle** *origin*, temporal fossa; *insertion*, coronoid process of mandible and anterior border of ramus; *action* elevates mandible (closes jaw); its posterior, nearly horizontally-oriented fibers are the primary retractors of the protruded mandible. *nerve supply*, deep temporal branches of mandibular division of trigeminal. SYN musculus temporalis [TA], temporal muscle.

**tem·por·al lobe** a long lobe, the lowest of the major subdivisions of the cortical mantle, forming the posterior two-thirds of the ventral surface of the cerebral hemisphere, separated from the frontal and parietal lobes above it by the lateral sulcus arbitrarily delineated by an imaginary plane from the occipital lobe with which it is continuous posteriorly. The temporal lobe has a heterogeneous composition: in addition to a large neocortical component consisting of the superior, middle, and inferior temporal gyri and the lateral and medial occipitotemporal gyri, it includes the largely juxtallocortical parahippocampal gyrus with its paleocortical (olfactory) uncus and, beneath the latter, the amygdala. SYN lobus temporalis [TA].

**tem·por·al lobe ep·i·lep·sy** epilepsy with seizures originating from the temporal lobe, most commonly the mesial temporal lobe.

**tem·por·al mus·cle** SYN temporalis muscle.

**tem·por·al plane** a slightly depressed area on the side of the cranium, below the inferior temporal line, formed by the temporal and parietal bones, the greater wing of the sphenoid, and a part of the frontal bone.

**tem·por·al pole of ce·re·brum** the most prominent part of the anterior extremity of the temporal lobe of each cerebral hemisphere, a short distance below the fissure of Sylvius.

**tem·por·al pro·cess** the posterior projection of the zygomatic bone articulating with the zygomatic process of the temporal bone to form the zygomatic arch.

**tem·po·rary car·ti·lage** a cartilage that is normally replaced by bone, to form a part of the skeleton. SYN precursory cartilage.

**tem·po·rary den·ture** SYN interim denture.

**tem·po·rary par·a·site** an organism accidentally ingested that survives briefly in the intestine.

**tem·po·rary thresh·old shift** the reversible hearing loss that results from exposure to intense impulse or continuous sound, as opposed to the irreversible permanent threshold shift that may result from such exposure.

**tem·po·rary tooth** SYN deciduous tooth.

△**temp·oro-** temporal (2). [L. *temporalis,* temporal]

**tem·po·ro·man·dib·u·lar** (tem′pŏ-rō-man-dib′ yu-lăr) relating to the temporal bone and the mandible; denoting the joint of the lower jaw. SYN temporomaxillary (2).

**tem·por·o·man·di·bu·lar dis·or·der** an inclusive term for all functional disturbances of the masticatory system including temporomandibular joint (TMJ) syndrome, myofacial pain-dysfunction syndrome, and temporomandibular pain-dysfunction syndrome.

▥**tem·por·o·man·dib·u·lar joint** the synovial articulation between the head of the mandible and the mandibular fossa and articular tubercle of the temporal bone. See this page. SYN mandibular joint.

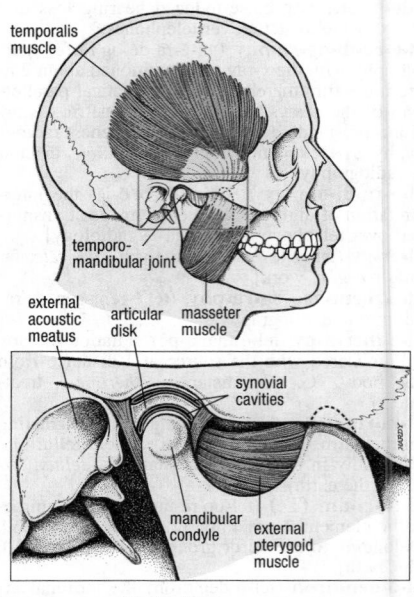

**temporomandibular joint**

**tem·por·o·man·dib·u·lar joint dys·func·tion (TMJ)** chronic impairment of function of the temporomandibular articulation. SEE myofacial pain-dysfunction syndrome, temporomandibular disorder.

**tem·por·o·man·dib·u·lar joint pain-dys·-func·tion syn·drome** SYN myofacial pain-dysfunction syndrome.

**tem·por·o·man·dib·u·lar nerve** SYN zygomatic nerve.

**tem·po·ro·max·il·lary** (tem′pŏ-rō-mak′si-lār′ē) **1.** relating to the regions of the temporal and maxillary bones. **2.** SYN temporomandibular.

**tem·por·o·pa·ri·e·ta·lis mus·cle** the part of epicranius muscle that arises from the lateral part of the epicranial aponeurosis and inserts in the cartilage of the auricle. SYN musculus temporoparietalis [TA], temporoparietal muscle.

**tem·por·o·pa·ri·e·tal mus·cle** SYN temporoparietalis muscle.

**tempor·o·pon·tine fi·bers** a fiber group originating in the cerebral cortex of the temporal lobe, particularly the superior and middle temporal gyri, following the sublenticular limb of the internal capsule into the lateral margin of the crus cerebri in which it descends to its termiantion in the pontine nuclei in the basilar part of the pons.

**tem·po·ro·pon·tine tract** SEE temporopontine fibers.

**tem·po·sta·bile, tem·po·sta·ble** (tem-pō-stā′bīl, tem-pō-stā′bl) not subject to spontaneous alteration or destruction. [L. *tempus,* time + *stabilis,* stable]

**tem·pus,** gen. **tem·po·ris,** pl. **tem·po·ra** (tem′ pŭs, tem′pŏ-ris, tem′pŏ-ră) **1.** the temple. **2.** SYN time. [L. time]

**TEN** toxic epidermal necrolysis.

**te·na·cious** (tĕ-nā′shŭs) having the capacity to

stick or adhere. [L. *tenax* (*tenac-*), fr. *teneo*, to hold]

**te·nac·u·lum**, pl. **te·nac·u·la** (tě-nak′yu-lŭm, tě-nak′yu-lǎ) a surgical clamp designed to hold or grasp tissue during dissection. [L. a holder, fr. *teneo*, to hold]

**te·nac·u·lum for·ceps** a forceps with jaws armed each with a sharp, straight hook like a tenaculum.

**te·nal·gia** (te-nal′jē-ǎ) pain referred to a tendon. SYN tenodynia, tenontodynia. [G. *tenōn*, tendon, + *algos*, pain]

**ten·der** sensitive or painful as a result of pressure or contact that is not sufficient to cause discomfort in normal tissues. [L. *tener*, soft, delicate]

**ten·der·ness** (ten′der-nes) the condition of being tender.

**ten·der point** eighteen bilateral predefined areas in occiput, neck, shoulders, chest, elbows, gluteus, trochanter and knees that produce painful response at 4 kg pressure; used to diagnose fibromyalgia if 11/18 are positive.

**ten·di·ni·tis** (ten-di-nī′tis) SYN tendonitis.

**ten·di·no·plas·ty** (ten′din-ō-plas-tē) SYN tenontoplasty. [Mediev. L. *tendo* (*tendin-*), tendon, + G. *plastos*, formed]

**ten·di·no·su·ture** (ten′di-nō-soo′cher) SYN tenorrhaphy.

**ten·di·nous** (ten′di-nŭs) relating to, composed of, or resembling a tendon.

**ten·di·nous arch 1.** a white, fibrous band attached to bone and/or muscle, arching over and thus protecting neurovascular elements passing beneath it from injurious compression; **2.** a linear thickening of the deep fascia of a muscle that provides attachment for ligaments and/or muscle fibers.

**ten·di·nous arch of pel·vic fa·scia** a linear thickening of the superior fascia of the pelvic diaphragm extending posteriorly from the body of the os pubis alongside the bladder (and vagina in the female) to the ischial spine and giving attachment to the supporting ligaments of the pelvic viscera.

**ten·di·nous cords** SYN chordae tendineae of heart.

**ten·di·nous syn·o·vi·tis** SYN tenosynovitis.

**ten·do**, gen. **ten·di·nis**, pl. **ten·di·nes** (ten′dō, ten′di-nis, ten′di-nēz) SYN tendon. For gross and histological description, see tendon. [Mediev. L., fr. L. *tendo*, to stretch out, extend]

⚠**ten·do-** [TA] a tendon. SEE ALSO teno-. [L. *tendo*]

**ten·do cal·ca·ne·us** [TA] the tendon of insertion of the triceps surae (gastrocnemius and soleus) into the tuberosity of the calcaneus. SYN Achilles tendon, heel tendon.

**ten·dol·y·sis** (ten-dol′i-sis) release of a tendon from adhesions. SYN tenolysis. [tendo- + G. *lysis*, dissolution]

**ten·don** (ten′dŏn) a nondistensible fibrous cord or band of variable length that is the part of the muscle that connects the fleshy (contractile) part of muscle with its bony attachment or other structure; it may unite with the fleshy part of the muscle at its extremity or may run along the side or in the center of the fleshy part for a longer or shorter distance, receiving the muscular fibers along its border; when determining the length of a muscle, the tendon length is included as well as the fleshy part; it consists of fascicles of very densely arranged, almost parallel collagenous fibers, rows of elongated fibrocytes, and a minimum of ground substance. SYN sinew, tendo. [L. *tendo*]

**ten·don cells** elongated fibroblastic cells arranged in rows between the collagenous tendon fibers.

**ten·don·i·tis** (ten-dŏn-ī′tis) inflammation of a tendon. SYN tendinitis, tenonitis (2), tenontitis, tenositis.

**ten·don re·ces·sion** surgical displacement of the tendon of an eye muscle posterior to its anatomic insertion.

**ten·don re·flex** a myotatic or deep reflex in which the muscle stretch receptors are stimulated by percussing the tendon of a muscle.

**ten·do·plas·ty** (ten′dō-plas-tē) SYN tenontoplasty.

**ten·do·syn·o·vi·tis** (ten′dō-si-nō-vī′tis) SYN tenosynovitis.

**ten·dot·o·my** (ten-dot′ō-mē) SYN tenotomy.

**ten·do·vag·i·nal** (ten-dō-vaj′i-nǎl) relating to a tendon and its sheath. [tendo- + L. *vagina*, sheath]

**ten·do·vag·i·ni·tis** (ten′dō-vaj-i-nī′tis) SYN tenosynovitis. [tendo- + L. *vagina*, sheath, + G. *-itis*, inflammation]

**te·nec·to·my** (tě-nek′tō-mē) resection of part of a tendon. SYN tenonectomy. [G. *tenōn*, tendon, + *ektomē*, excision]

**te·nes·mic** (tě-nez′mik) relating to or marked by tenesmus.

**te·nes·mus** (te-nez′mŭs) a painful spasm of the anal sphincter with an urgent desire to evacuate the bowel or bladder, involuntary straining, and the passage of little fecal matter or urine. [G. *teinesmos*, ineffectual effort to defecate, fr. *teinō*, to stretch]

**ten Horn sign** (ten hōrn) pain caused by gentle traction on the right spermatic cord, indicative of appendicitis.

**te·nia**, pl. **te·ni·ae** (tē′nē-ǎ, tē′nē-ē) **1.** any anatomical bandlike structure. **2.** SYN taenia (2). [L. fr. G. *tainia*, band, tape, a tapeworm]

**te·nia cho·roi·dea** [TA] the somewhat thickened line along which a choroid membrane or plexus is attached to the rim of a brain ventricle.

**te·ni·a·cide** (tē′nē-ǎ-sīd) an agent destructive to tapeworms. [L. *taenia*, tapeworm, + *caedo*, to kill]

**te·ni·ae co·li** [TA] the three bands in which the longitudinal muscular fibers of the large intestine, except the rectum, are collected; these are the mesocolic tenia, situated at the place corresponding to the mesenteric attachment; the free tenia, opposite the mesocolic tenia; and the omental tenia, at the place corresponding to the site of adhesion of the greater omentum to the transverse colon.

**ten·i·al** (tēn′ē-ǎl) **1.** relating to a tapeworm. **2.** relating to one of the structures called tenia.

**te·ni·a·sis** (tē-nī′ǎ-sis) presence of a tapeworm in the intestine.

**te·ni·o·la** (tē-nē′ō-lǎ) a slender tenia or bandlike structure. [L. dim. of *taenia*, ribbon]

**ten·nis el·bow** tension stress injury to the lateral epicondyle, often seen in those who play racquet sports. SYN lateral epicondylitis, lateral humeral epicondylitis.

**ten·nis thumb** tendinitis with calcification in the tendon of the long flexor of the thumb (flexor pollicis longus) caused by friction and strain as in tennis playing, but also occurring in other exercises in which the thumb is subject to repeated pressure or strain.

⊘te·no-, te·non-, te·nont-, te·non·to- tendon. SEE ALSO tendo-. [G. *tenōn*]

te·no·de·sis (tĕ-nod′ē-sis, ten′ō-dē′sis) stabilizing a joint by anchoring the tendons which move that joint. [teno- + G. *desis,* a binding]

ten·o·dyn·ia (ten-ō-din′ē-ă) SYN tenalgia. [teno- + G. *odynē,* pain]

ten·ol·y·sis (ten-ol′i-sis) SYN tendolysis.

ten·o·my·o·plas·ty (ten-ō-mī′ō-plas-tē) SYN tenontomyoplasty.

ten·o·my·ot·o·my (ten-ō-mī-ot′ō-mē) SYN myotenotomy.

Te·non cap·sule (tĕ-naw′) SYN fascial sheath of eyeball.

ten·o·nec·to·my (ten-ō-nek′tō-mē) SYN tenectomy. [tenon- + G. *ektomē,* excision]

ten·o·ni·tis (ten-ō-nī′tis) 1. inflammation of Tenon capsule or the connective tissue within Tenon space. 2. SYN tendonitis. [tenont- + G. *-itis,* inflammation]

ten·on·ti·tis (ten′on-tī′tis) SYN tendonitis. [tenont- + G. *-itis,* inflammation]

te·non·to·dyn·ia (te-non′tō-din′ē-ă) SYN tenalgia.

te·non·to·my·o·plas·ty (te-non′tō-mī′ō-plas-tē) a combined tenontoplasty and myoplasty, used in the radical correction of a hernia. SYN tenomyoplasty. [tenonto- + G. *mys,* muscle, + *plastos,* formed]

te·non·to·plas·ty (te-non′tō-plas-tē) reparative or plastic surgery of the tendons. SYN tendinoplasty, tendoplasty, tenoplasty. [tenonto- + G. *plastos,* formed]

ten·o·phyte (ten′ō-fīt) bony or cartilaginous growth in or on a tendon. [teno- + G. *phyton,* plant]

ten·o·plas·ty (ten′ō-plas-tē) SYN tenontoplasty.

ten·o·re·cep·tor (ten′ō-rē-sep′ter) a receptor in a tendon, activated by increased tension.

te·nor·rha·phy (te-nōr′ă-fē) suture of the divided ends of a tendon. SYN tendinosuture, tenosuture. [teno- + G. *rhaphē,* suture]

ten·o·si·tis (ten-ō-sī′tis) SYN tendonitis.

ten·os·to·sis (ten-os-tō′sis) ossification of a tendon. [teno- + G. *osteon,* bone, + *-osis,* condition]

ten·o·sus·pen·sion (ten′ō-sŭs-pen′shŭn) using a tendon as a suspensory ligament, sometimes as a free graft or in continuity.

ten·o·su·ture (ten-ō-soo′cher) SYN tenorrhaphy.

ten·o·syn·o·vec·to·my (ten′ō-sin-ō-vek′tō-mē) excision of a tendon sheath. [teno- + synovia + G. *ektomē,* excision]

ten·o·syn·o·vi·tis (ten′ō-sin-ō-vī′tis) inflammation of a tendon and its enveloping sheath. SYN tendinous synovitis, tendosynovitis, tendovaginitis, tenovaginitis. [teno- + synovia + G. *-itis,* inflammation]

te·not·o·my (te-not′ō-mē) the surgical division of a tendon for relief of a deformity caused by congenital or acquired shortening of a muscle, as in clubfoot or strabismus. SYN tendotomy. [teno- + G. *tomē,* incision]

ten·o·vag·i·ni·tis (ten′ō-vaj-i-nī′tis) SYN tenosynovitis. [teno- + L. *vagina,* sheath, + G. *-itis,* inflammation]

ten·sion (ten′shŭn) 1. the act of stretching. 2. the condition of being stretched or tense, or a stretching or pulling force. 3. the partial pressure of a gas, especially that of a gas dissolved in a liquid such as blood. 4. mental, emotional, or nervous strain; strained relations or barely controlled hostility between persons or groups. [L. *tensio,* fr. *tendo,* pp. *tensus,* to stretch]

ten·sion curve the direction of the trabeculae in cancellous bone tissue adapted to resist stress.

ten·sion head·ache, ten·sion-type head·ache headache associated with nervous tension, anxiety, etc., often related to chronic contraction of the scalp muscles. SYN muscle contraction headache.

ten·sion pneu·mo·per·i·car·di·um the presence of air under pressure in the pericardial space, with the potential for cardiac tamponade.

ten·sion su·ture SYN retention suture.

ten·sor, pl. ten·so·res (ten′ser, ten-sō′rēz) a muscle the function of which is to render a part firm and tense. [Mod. L. fr. L. *tendo,* pp. *tensus,* to stretch]

ten·sor fas·ci·ae la·tae mus·cle *origin,* anterior superior spine and adjacent lateral surface of the ilium; *insertion,* iliotibial band of fascia lata; *action,* tenses fascia lata; flexes, abducts and medially rotates thigh; *nerve supply,* superior gluteal. USAGE NOTE: Often mispronounced and misspelled tensor fascia lata. SYN musculus tensor fasciae latae [TA].

ten·sor mus·cle of soft pal·ate SYN tensor veli palati muscle.

ten·sor mus·cle of tym·pa·nic mem·brane SYN tensor tympani muscle.

ten·sor tym·pa·ni mus·cle *origin,* the cartilaginous part of the auditory (eustachian) tube and the walls of its hemi-canal just above the bony portion of the auditory tube; *insertion,* handle of malleus; *action,* draws the handle of the malleus medialward tensing the tympanic membrane to protect it from excessive vibration by loud sounds. *nerve supply,* branches of trigeminal through the otic ganglion. SYN musculus tensor tympani [TA], tensor muscle of tympanic membrane.

ten·sor tym·pa·ni re·flex contraction of the tensor tympani muscle in response to intense sound, increasing impedance of the middle ear and thus protecting the inner ear from exposure.

ten·sor ve·li pa·la·ti mus·cle tensor muscle of soft palate, musculus tensor palati; musculus palatosalpingeus; musculus sphenosalpingostaphylinus; dilator tubae; *origin,* scaphoid fossa of sphenoid, cartilaginous and membranous part of auditory (eustachian) tube and spine of sphenoid; *insertion,* posterior border of hard palate and aponeurosis of soft palate; *action,* tenses the soft palate; contributes to opening of auditory tube; *nerve supply,* branches of trigeminal nerve through the otic ganglion. SYN musculus tensor veli palatini [TA], tensor muscle of soft palate.

tent 1. canopy used in various types of inhalation therapy to control humidity and concentration of oxygen in inspired air. 2. cylinder of some material, usually absorbent, introduced into a canal or sinus to maintain its patency or to dilate it. 3. to elevate or pick up a segment of skin, fascia, or tissue at a given point, giving it the appearance of a tent. [L. *tendo,* pp. *tensus,* to stretch]

ten·ta·cle (ten′tă-kl) a slender process for feeling, prehension, or locomotion in invertebrates. [Mod. L. *tentaculum,* a feeler, fr. *tento,* to feel]

tenth cra·ni·al nerve [CN X] SYN vagus nerve [CN X].

ten·to·ri·al (ten-tō′rē-ăl) relating to a tentorium.

**ten·tor·i·al ba·sal branch of in·ter·nal ca·-ro·tid ar·tery** a small branch from the cavernous part of the internal carotid artery to the base of the tentorium.

**ten·tor·i·al si·nus** SYN straight sinus.

**ten·to·ri·um**, pl. **ten·to·ria** (ten-tō′rē-ŭm, ten-tō′rē-ă) a membranous cover or horizontal partition. [L. tent, fr. *tendo,* to stretch]

**ten·to·ri·um ce·re·bel·li** [TA] a strong fold of dura mater roofing over the posterior cranial fossa with an anterior median opening, the tentorial notch, through which the midbrain passes; the tentorium cerebelli is attached along the midline to the falx cerebri and separates the cerebellum from the basal surface of the occipital and temporal lobes of the cerebral hemisphere.

**TEP** tracheoesophageal puncture.

△**tera-** (T) **1.** prefix used in the SI and metric systems to signify one trillion. **2.** denoting a teras. SEE ALSO terato-. [G. *teras,* monster]

**ter·as**, pl. **ter·a·ta** (ter′as, ter′ă-tă) a fetus with deficient, redundant, misplaced, or grossly misshapen parts. [G.]

**ter·at·ic** (ter-at′ik) relating to a teras.

**ter·a·tism** (ter′ă-tizm) SYN teratosis. [G. *teratisma,* fr. *teras*]

△**ter·a·to-** a teras. SEE ALSO tera- (2). [G. *teras,* monster]

**ter·a·to·blas·to·ma** a tumor containing embryonic tissue differing from a teratoma in that not all germ layers are present.

**ter·a·to·car·ci·no·ma** (ter′ă-tō-kar-si-nō′mă) **1.** a malignant teratoma, occurring most commonly in the testis. **2.** a malignant epithelial tumor arising in a teratoma.

**te·rat·o·gen** (ter′ă-tō-jen) a drug or other agent that can produce a congenital anomaly or raise the incidence of an anomaly in the population. [terato- + G. *-gen,* producing]

**ter·a·to·gen·e·sis** (ter′ă-tō-jen′ĕ-sis) the origin or mode of production of a malformed fetus; the disturbed growth processes involved in the production of a malformed neonate. [terato- + G. *genesis,* origin]

**ter·a·to·gen·ic, ter·a·to·ge·net·ic** (ter′ă-tō-jen′ik, ter′ă-tō-jĕ-net′ik) **1.** relating to teratogenesis. **2.** causing abnormal embryonic development.

**ter·a·to·ge·nic·i·ty** (ter′ă-tō-jĕ-nis′i-tē) the property or capability of producing fetal malformation. [terato- + G. *genesis,* generation]

**ter·a·toid** (ter′ă-toyd) resembling a teras. [G. *teratōdēs,* fr. *teras* (*terat-*), monster, + *eidos,* resemblance]

**ter·a·toid tu·mor** SYN teratoma.

**ter·a·to·log·ic** (ter′ă-tō-loj′ik) relating to teratology.

**ter·a·tol·o·gy** (ter-ă-tol′ō-jē) the branch of science concerned with the production, development, anatomy, and classification of malformed fetuses. SEE ALSO dysmorphology. [terato- + G. *logos,* study]

**ter·a·to·ma** (ter-ă-tō′mă) a neoplasm composed of multiple tissues, including tissues not normally found in the organ in which it arises. Teratomas occur most frequently in the ovary, where they are usually benign and form dermoid cysts; in the testis, where they are usually malignant; and, uncommonly, in other sites, especially the midline of the body. SYN teratoid tumor. [terato- + G. *-oma,* tumor]

**ter·a·tom·a·tous** (ter′ă-tō′mă-tŭs) relating to or of the nature of a teratoma.

**ter·a·to·sis** (ter′ă-tō′sis) an anomaly producing a teras. SYN teratism. [terato- + G. *-osis,* condition]

**ter·at·o·zo·o·sperm·ia** (ter′ă-tō-zō-ō-sperm′ē-ă) condition characterized by the presence of malformed spermatozoa in the semen. [terato- + *zōos,* living, + *sperma,* seed, semen, + -ia]

**ter·bi·um (Tb)** (ter′bē-ŭm) a metallic element of the lanthanide or rare earth series, atomic no. 65, atomic wt. 158.92534. [fr. *Ytterby,* a village in Sweden]

**te·res**, gen. **ter·e·tis**, pl. **ter·e·tes** (ter′ēz, ter′ĕ-tis, ter′ĕ-tēz) round and long; denoting certain muscles and ligaments. [L. round, smooth, fr. *tero,* to rub]

**te·res ma·jor mus·cle** *origin,* inferior angle and lower third of border of scapula; *insertion,* medial border of intertubercular groove of humerus; *action,* adducts and extends arm and rotates it medially; *nerve supply,* lower subscapular from posterior cord of brachial plexus (fifth and sixth cervical spinal nerves). SYN musculus teres major [TA].

**te·res mi·nor mus·cle** *origin,* upper two-thirds of the lateral border of scapula; *insertion,* lower facet of greater tuberosity of humerus; *action,* adducts arm and rotates it laterally; *nerve supply,* axillary (fifth and sixth cervical spinal nerves). SYN musculus teres minor [TA].

**term 1.** a definite or limited period. **2.** a name or descriptive word or phrase. [L. *terminus,* a limit, an end]

**ter·mi·nal** (ter′mi-năl) **1.** relating to the end; final. **2.** relating to the extremity or end of any body; e.g., the end of a biopolymer. **3.** a termination, extremity, end, or ending. [L. *terminus,* a boundary, limit]

**ter·mi·nal ar·tery** SYN end artery.

**ter·mi·nal bar** dark spots or bars (depending on the plane of section) in the lateral boundary between the apical ends of columnar epithelial cells.

**ter·mi·nal bou·tons, bou·tons ter·mi·naux** SYN axon terminals.

**ter·mi·nal bron·chi·ole** the end of the nonrespiratory conducting airway; the lining is simple columnar or cuboidal epithelium without mucous goblet cells; most of the cells are ciliated, but a few nonciliated serous secreting cells occur.

**ter·mi·nal de·ox·y·nu·cle·o·ti·dyl trans·fer·-ase (TdT)** a specialized DNA polymerase expressed in immature, pre-B, pre-T lymphoid cells, and acute lymphoblastic leukemia/lymphoma cells.

**ter·mi·nal dis·in·fec·tion** application of disinfective measures after the patient has been removed, e.g., by death, or has ceased to be a source of infection.

**ter·min·al duct car·ci·no·ma** SYN polymorphous low-grade carcinoma of salivary glands.

**ter·mi·nal fi·lum** a long, slender connective tissue (pia mater) strand of pia mater extending from the extremityapex of the medullary cone to the internal aspect of the spinal dural sac (filum terminale internum); stout strands of connective tissue attaching the spinal dural sac to the coccyx (filum terminale externum), commonly called the coccygeal ligament.

**ter·mi·nal hair** a mature pigmented, coarse hair.

**ter·mi·nal hinge po·si·tion** SYN centric relation.

**ter·mi·nal in·fec·tion** an acute infection, commonly pneumonic or septic, occurring toward the end of any disease and often the cause of death.

**ter·mi·nal line** SYN linea terminalis.

**ter·mi·nal nerves** delicate plexiform nerve strands passing parallel and medial to the olfactory tracts, distributing peripherally with the olfactory nerves and passing centrally into the anterior perforated substance; they are considered to have an autonomic function but the exact nature of this is unknown. SYN nervi terminales [TA].

**ter·mi·nal nu·clei** collective term indicating those nerve cell groups in the rhombencephalon and spinal cord in which the afferent fibers of the spinal and cranial nerves terminate.

**ter·mi·nal si·nus** the vein bounding the area vasculosa in the blastoderm.

**ter·mi·nal stria** a slender, compact fiber bundle that connects the amygdala (amygdaloid body) with the hypothalamus and other basal forebrain regions. Originating from the amygdala, the bundle passes first caudalward in the roof of the temporal horn of the lateral ventricle; it follows the medial side of the caudate nucleus forward in the floor of the central part (or body) of the ventricle until it reaches the interventricular foramen, in the posterior wall of which it curves steeply down to enter the hypothalamus, with fibers passing both rostral and caudal to the anterior commissure. Coursing caudalward in the medial part of the hypothalamus, the bundle terminates in the anterior and ventromedial hypothalamic nuclei.

**ter·mi·na·tion** (ter'mi-nā'shŭn) an end or ending. A termination or ending, particularly a nerve ending. [L. *terminatio*]

**ter·mi·na·tion co·don** trinucleotide sequence (UAA, UGA, or UAG) that specifies the end of translation or transcription Cf. amber codon, ochre codon, umber codon. SYN termination signal.

**ter·mi·na·tion sig·nal** SYN termination codon.

**Ter·mi·no·lo·gia An·a·to·mi·ca (TA)** a system of anatomic nomenclature, consisting of about 7500 terms, devised and approved by the International Federation of Associations of Anatomists (IFAA) and promulgated in August, 1997, at São Paulo, Brazil.

**ter·mi·no·ter·mi·nal a·na·sto·mo·sis** an operation by which the central end of an artery is connected with the peripheral end of the corresponding vein, and the peripheral end of the artery with the central end of the vein.

**ter·mi·nus**, pl. **ter·mi·ni** (ter'mi-nŭs, ter'mi-nī) a boundary or limit. [L.]

**ter·na·ry** (ter'năr-ē) denoting or composed of three compounds, elements, molecules, etc. [L. *ternarius*, of three]

*Ter·ni·dens* (ter'nĕ-denz) nematode genus found in the intestine of several simian species in Africa, India, and Indonesia, and in humans in parts of Africa; differentiated from hookworms by the anteriorly directed buccal capsule guarded by a double crown of stout bristles; they inhabit the wall of the large bowel, where they may produce cystic nodules.

*Ter·ni·dens de·mi·nu·tus* nematode species whose larvae develop in soil; probably infective for humans; life cycle not known.

**ter·pene** (ter'pēn) one of a class of hydrocarbons with an empirical formula of $C_{10}H_{16}$, occurring in essential oils and resins.

**ter·race** (ter'as) to suture in several rows, in closing a wound through a considerable thickness of tissue. [thr. O. Fr. fr. L. *terra*, earth]

**Ter·ri·en mar·gin·al de·gen·er·a·tion** (tahr-ē-ah') a form of pellucid marginal corneal degeneration.

**ter·ri·to·ri·al·i·ty** (ter'i-tōr-ē-al'i-tē) **1.** the tendency of individuals or groups to defend a particular domain or sphere of interest or influence. **2.** the tendency of an individual animal to define a finite space as its own habitat from which it will fight off trespassing animals of its own species.

**ter·ri·to·ri·al ma·trix** SYN cartilage capsule.

**Ter·ry syn·drome** (ter'ē) SYN retinopathy of prematurity.

**Ter·son syn·drome** (ter-saw') vitreous, retinal, and subhyaloid hemorrhages associated with subarachnoid hemorrhage.

**ter·tian** (ter'shăn) recurring every third day, counting the day of an episode as the first; actually, occurring every 48 hours or every other day. [L. *tertianus*, fr. *tertius*, third]

**ter·ti·ary al·co·hol** methanol bearing three substitutes on its carbon atom.

**ter·ti·ary amine** SEE amine.

**ter·ti·ary den·tin** morphologically irregular dentin formed in response to an irritant. SYN irregular dentin, irritation dentin, reparative dentin.

**Tes·la** (tes'lă), Nikola, Serbian-American electrical engineer, 1856–1943. SEE tesla.

**tes·la (T)** (tes'lă) in the SI system, the unit of magnetic flux density expressed as kg sec$^{-2}$ A$^{-1}$; equal to one weber per square meter. [N. *Tesla*]

**tes·sel·lat·ed** (tes'ĕ-lāt-ed) made up of small squares; checkered. [L. *tessella*, a small square stone]

**tes·sel·lat·ed fun·dus** a normal fundus to which a deeply pigmented choroid gives the appearance of dark polygonal areas between the choroidal vessels, especially in the periphery.

**test** SYN testa (1). **1.** to prove; to try a substance; to determine the chemical nature of a substance by means of reagents. **2.** a method of examination, as to determine the presence or absence of a definite disease or of some substance in any of the fluids, tissues, or excretions of the body, or to determine the presence or degree of a psychological or behavioral trait. **3.** a reagent used in making a test SEE ALSO assay, reaction, reagent, scale, stain. [L. *testum*, an earthen vessel]

**tes·ta 1.** in protozoology, usually termed test; an envelope of certain forms of ameboid protozoa, consisting of various early materials cemented to a chitinous base (as in the testate rhizopods of the subclass Testacealobosia) or the calcareous, siliceous, organic, or strontium sulfate skeletons in the rhizopod subclass Foraminifera. SYN test. **2.** in botany, the outer, sometimes the only, coat of a seed.

**tes·tal·gia** (tes-tal'jē-ă) SYN orchialgia. [testis + G. *algos*, pain]

**tes·tec·to·my** (tes-tek'tō-mē) SYN orchiectomy. [testis + G. G. *ektomē*, excision]

**tes·tes** (tes'tēz) plural of testis. [L.]

**tes·ti·cle** (tes'ti-kl) SYN testis. [L. *testiculus*, dim. of *testis*]

**tes·tic·u·lar** (tes-tik'yu-lăr) relating to the testes.

**tes·tic·u·lar ar·tery** *origin*, aorta; *branches*, ureteral, cremasteric, epididymal; *distribution*, testicle and parts designated by names of branches; *anastomoses*, branches of renal, inferior epigastric, deferential. SYN arteria testicularis [TA].

**tes·tic·u·lar cord** SYN spermatic cord.

**tes·tic·u·lar fe·mi·ni·za·tion syn·drome** a type of male pseudohermaphroditism characterized by female external genitalia, incompletely developed vagina often with rudimentary uterus and fallopian tubes, female habitus at puberty but with scanty or absent axillary and pubic hair and amenorrhea, and testes present within the abdomen or in the inguinal canals or labia majora; epididymis and vas deferens are usually present; androgens and estrogens are formed, but target tissues are largely unresponsive to androgens; individuals are sex chromatin-negative and have a normal male karyotype; there is a defect in the androgen receptor protein. SYN complete androgen insensitivity syndrome.

**test·ing** SEE test.

**tes·tis**, pl. **tes·tes** (tes′tis, tes′tēz) [TA] one of the two male reproductive glands, located in the cavity of the scrotum. SEE ALSO appendix of testis. SYN orchis [TA], didymus, testicle. [L.]

**tes·ti·tis** (tes-tī′tis) SYN orchitis.

**test meal 1.** toast and tea, or crackers and tea, or gruel or other bland food, given to stimulate gastric secretion before withdrawing gastric contents for analysis; **2.** administration of food containing a substance thought to be responsible for symptoms, such as an allergic reaction.

**tes·tos·ter·one** (tes-tos′tě-rōn) the most potent naturally occurring androgen, formed in greatest quantities by the interstitial cells of the testes, and possibly secreted also by the ovary and adrenal cortex; used in the treatment of hypogonadism, cryptorchism, certain carcinomas, and menorrhagia.

**tes·to·tox·i·co·sis** (tes′tō-tok-si-kō′sis) a G protein mutation disease resulting in autonomous testosterone overproduction, with precocious puberty.

**test pro·file** a combination of laboratory tests usually performed by automated methods and designed to evaluate organ systems of patients upon admission to a hospital or clinic.

**test so·lu·tion** a solution of some reagent, in definite strength, used in chemical analysis or testing.

**test tube** a round-bottomed, cylindrical vessel, usually of transparent glass, in which laboratory tests involving liquids are performed.

**test-tube ba·by** popular term for a baby born after uterine implantation of a maternal ovum fertilized *in vitro*.

**test type** letters of various sizes used to test visual acuity.

**te·tan·ic** (te-tan′ik) **1.** relating to or marked by a sustained muscular contraction, as in tetanus. **2.** an agent, such as strychnine, that in poisonous doses produces tonic muscular spasm. [G. *tetanikos*]

**te·tan·i·form** (te-tan′i-fōrm) SYN tetanoid (1).

**tet·a·nig·e·nous** (tet-ă-nij′ě-nŭs) causing tetanus or tetaniform spasms. [tetanus + G. *-gen*, producing]

**tet·a·nism** (tet′ă-nizm) SYN neonatal tetany.

**tet·a·ni·za·tion** (tet′ă-ni-zā′shŭn) **1.** the act of tet-

anizing the muscles. **2.** a condition of tetaniform spasm.

**tet·a·nize** (tet′ă-nīz) to stimulate a muscle by a rapid series of stimuli so that the individual muscular responses (contractions) are fused into a sustained contraction; to cause tetanus (2) in a muscle.

⚠ **tet·a·no-, tet·an-** combining forms denoting tetanus, tetany. [G. *tetanos*, convulsive tension]

**tet·a·node** (tet′ă-nōd) denoting the quiet interval between the recurrent tonic spasms in tetanus. [G. *tetanōdēs*]

**tet·a·noid** (tet′ă-noyd) **1.** resembling or of the nature of tetanus. SYN tetaniform. **2.** resembling tetany. [tetano- + G. *eidos*, resemblance]

**tet·a·no·spas·min** (tet′ă-nō-spaz′min) the neurotoxin of *Clostridium tetani*, which causes the characteristic signs and symptoms of tetanus; chief action is on the anterior horn cells, and the spasms seem to be due to action at inhibitory synapses.

**tet·a·nus** (tet′ă-nŭs) **1.** a disease marked by painful tonic muscular contractions, caused by the neurotropic toxin (tetanospasmin) of *Clostridium tetani* acting upon the central nervous system. **2.** a sustained muscular contraction caused by a series of nerve stimuli repeated so rapidly that the individual muscular responses are fused; producing a sustained tetanic contraction. SEE emprosthotonos, opisthotonos. [L. fr. G. *tetanos*, convulsive tension]

**tet·a·nus ne·o·na·to·rum** (tet′ă-nŭs nē-ō-nā′tōr-ŭm) tetanus occurring in newborn infants, usually due to infection of umbilical area with *Clostridium tetani*, often a result of ritualistic practices; has high fatality rate (about 60%).

**tet·a·nus tox·in** the neurotropic, heat-labile exotoxin of *Clostridium tetani* and the cause of tetanus; it is one of the most poisonous substances known, and seems to function by blocking inhibitory synaptic impulses.

**tet·a·ny** (tet′ă-nē) a clinical neurological syndrome characterized by muscle twitches, cramps, and carpopedal spasm, and when severe, laryngospasm and seizures; these findings reflect irritability of the central and peripheral nervous systems, usually resulting from low serum levels of ionized calcium or, rarely, magnesium. Causes include hyperventilation, hypoparathyroidism, rickets, and uremia. SYN intermittent cramp (1), intermittent tetanus. [G. *tetanos*, tetanus]

⚠ **te·tra-** four. [G. *tetra-*, four]

**tet·ra·crot·ic** (tet′ră-krot′ik) denoting a pulse curve with four upstrokes in the cycle. [tetra- + G. *krotos*, a striking]

**te·trad 1.** a group of four things having something in common such as a deformity with four features e.g., Fallot tetralogy. SYN tetralogy. **2.** CHEMISTRY a quadrivalent element. **3.** in heredity, a bivalent chromosome that divides into four during meiosis. [G. *tetras* (*tetrad-*), the number four]

**tet·ra·dac·tyl** (tet-ră-dak′til) having only four fingers or toes on a hand or foot. [tetra- + G. *daktylos*, finger or toe]

⚠ **te·tra·hy·dro-** prefix denoting attachment of four hydrogen atoms; e.g., tetrahydrofolate, $H_4$folate.

**te·tral·o·gy** (tet-ral′ō-jē) SYN tetrad (1). [G. *tetralogia*]

**te·tra·lo·gy of Fal·lot** (fě-lō′) a set of congenital cardiac defects including ventricular septal defect, pulmonic valve stenosis or infundibular ste-

**te•tral•o•gy** (tet-ral'ō-jē) SYN tetrad (1). [G. *tetralogia*]

**te•tra•lo•gy of Fal•lot** (fĕ-lō') a set of congenital cardiac defects including ventricular septal defect, pulmonic valve stenosis or infundibular stenosis, and dextroposition of the aorta so that it overrides the ventricular septum and receives venous as well as arterial blood. Right ventricular hypertrophy is considered part of the tetralogy although it is reactive to the other defects. SYN Fallot tetrad.

**tet•ra•mer•ic, te•tram•er•ous** (tet'ră-mer'ik, tĕ-tram'ĕ-rŭs) having four parts, or parts arranged in groups of four, or capable of existing in four forms. [tetra- + G. *meros,* part]

**tet•ra•pa•re•sis** (tet'ră-pă-rē'sis) weakness of all four extremities. SYN quadriparesis.

**tet•ra•pep•tide** (tet'ră-pep'tīd) a compound of four amino acids in peptide linkage.

**tet•ra•ple•gia** (tet'ră-plē'jē-ă) SYN quadriplegia. [tetra- + G. *plēgē,* stroke]

**tet•ra•ploid** (tet'ră-ployd) SEE polyploidy. [G. *tetraploos,* fourfold, + *eidos,* form]

**tet•ra•sac•cha•ride** (tet'ră-sak'ă-rīd) a sugar containing four molecules of a monosaccharide.

**tet•ra•so•mic** (tet'ră-sō'mik) relating to a cell nucleus in which one chromosome is represented four times while all others are present in the normal number. [tetra- + chromosome]

**tet•ra•va•lent** (tet'ră-vā'lent) SYN quadrivalent. [tetra- + L. *valentia,* strength]

**tet•rose** (tet'rōs) a monosaccharide containing only four carbon atoms in the main chain.

**text blind•ness, word blind•ness** SYN alexia.

**tex•ti•form** (teks'tĭ-fōrm) weblike. [L. *textum,* something woven]

**tex•tur•al** (teks'cher-ăl) relating to the texture of the tissues.

**tex•ture** (teks'cher) the composition or structure of a tissue or organ. [L. *textura,* fr. *texo,* pp. *textus,* to weave]

**TF** tuning fork.

**Th** thorium; T helper cells.

**thal•a•men•ceph•a•lon** (thal'ă-men-sef'ă-lon) that part of the diencephalon comprising the thalamus and its associated structures. [thalamus + G. *enkephalos,* brain]

**tha•lam•ic** (tha-lam'ik) relating to the thalamus.

**thal•a•mic peduncle** pedunculus thalami inferior, lateralis, and ventralis.

△**thal•a•mo-, thal•am-** the thalamus. [G. *thalamos,* bedroom (thalamus)]

**thal•a•mo•cor•ti•cal** (thal'ă-mō-kōr'ti-kăl) relating to the efferent connections of the thalamus with the cerebral cortex.

**thal•a•mo•stri•ate veins** SEE inferior thalamostriate veins, superior thalamostriate vein.

**thal•a•mot•o•my** (thal-ă-mot'ō-mē) destruction of a selected portion of the thalamus by stereotaxy for the relief of pain, involuntary movements, epilepsy, and, rarely, emotional disturbances. [thalamus + G. *tomē,* incision]

**thal•a•mus,** pl. **thal•a•mi** (thal'ă-mŭs, thal'amī) [TA] the large, ovoid mass of gray matter that forms the larger dorsal subdivision of the diencephalon; it is placed medial to the internal capsule and the body and tail of the caudate nucleus. Its medial aspect forms the dorsal half of the lateral wall of the third ventricle; its dorsal surface can be subdivided into a lateral triangle forming the floor of the body (central part) of the lateral ventricle, and a medial triangle covered by the velum interpositum; its taillike caudal part curves ventralward around the posterolateral aspect of the cerebral peduncle and ends in the lateral geniculate body. The thalamus is composed of a large number of anatomically and functionally distinct cell groups or nuclei, usually classified as 1) sensory relay nuclei (ventral posterior nucleus, lateral and medial geniculate body) each receiving a modally specific sensory conduction system and in turn projecting each to the corresponding primary sensory area of the cortex; 2) "secondary" relay nuclei (ventral intermediate nucleus and ventral anterior nucleus) receiving fibers from the medial segment of the globus pallidus, the contralateral deep cerebellar nuclei (i.e., cerebellothalamic fibers) and the pars reticulata of the substantia nigra which project to various regions of the motor cortex; 3) a nucleus associated with the limbic system: the composite anterior nucleus receiving the mammillothalamic tract and projecting to the fornicate gyrus; 4) association nuclei (medial dorsal nucleus, lateral nucleus including the large pulvinar) each projecting to a particular large expanse of association cortex; 5) the midline and intralaminar nuclei or "nonspecific" nuclei (centromedian nucleus, central lateral nucleus, paracentral nucleus, nucleus reuniens). [G. *thalamos,* a bed, a bedroom]

**thal•as•sae•mia [Br.]** SEE thalassemia.

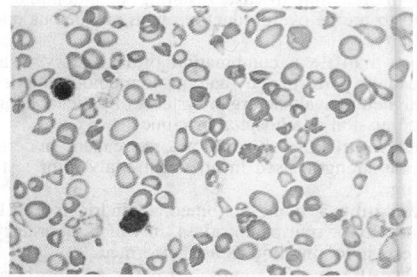**thal•as•se•mia, thal•as•sa•ne•mia** (thal-ă-sē'mē-ă, thă-las-ă-nē'mē-ă) any of a group of inherited disorders of hemoglobin metabolism in which there is impaired synthesis of one or more of the polypeptide chains of globin; several genetic types exist, and the corresponding clinical picture may vary from barely detectable hematologic abnormality to severe and fatal anemia. See this page. [G. *thalassa,* the sea, + *haima,* blood]

**thalassemia:** a blood film from a patient with homozygous β-thalassemia showing hypochromia, anisocytosis (original magnification 250X; Wright-Giemsa stain)

α **thal•as•se•mia** thalassemia due to one of two or more genes that depress synthesis of α-globin chains.

β **thal•as•se•mia** thalassemia due to one of two or more genes that depress (partially or completely) synthesis of β-globin chains.

β-δ **thal•as•se•mia** thalassemia due to a gene that depresses synthesis of both β- and δ-globin chains.

megaly, cardiac enlargement, thinning of inner and outer tables of skull, microcytic hypochromic anemia with poikilocytosis, anisocytosis, stippled cells, target cells, and nucleated erythrocytes; types of hemoglobin are variable and depend on the gene involved. SYN Cooley anemia.

**thal·as·se·mia mi·nor** the heterozygous state of a thalassemia gene or a hemoglobin Lepore gene; usually asymptomatic and quite variable hematologically, with target cells, mild hypochromic microcytosis, and often slightly reduced hemoglobin level with slightly increased erythrocyte count; types of hemoglobin are variable and depend on the gene involved.

**thal·lic** (thal′lik) denoting conidia produced with no enlargement or growth after delimitation by septa in the hypha (thallus); the entire parent cell becomes an arthroconidium.

**thal·li·um (Tl)** (thal′ē-ŭm) a white metallic element, atomic no. 81, atomic wt. 204.3833; ²⁰¹Tl (half-life equal to 3.038 days) is used to scan the myocardium. [G. *thallos,* a green shoot (it gives a green line in the spectrum)]

**thal·lus** (thal′ŭs) a simple plant or fungus body which is devoid of roots, stems, and leaves. The vegetative growth of a fungus. [G. *thallos,* a young shoot]

△**than·a·to-** death. SEE ALSO necro-. [G. *thanatos,* death]

**than·a·to·bi·o·log·ic** (than′ă-tō-bī-ō-loj′ik) relating to the processes involved in life and death. [thanato- + G. *bios,* life, + *logos,* study]

**than·a·to·gno·mon·ic** (than′ă-tō-nō-mon′ik) of fatal prognosis, indicating the approach of death. [thanato- + G. *gnōmē,* a sign]

**than·a·toid** (than′ă-toyd) **1.** resembling death. **2.** deadly. [thanato- + G. *eidos,* resemblance]

**than·a·tol·o·gy** (than-ă-tol′ō-jē) the branch of science concerned with the study of death and dying. [thanato- + G. *logos,* study]

**Thay·er-Mar·tin a·gar** (thā′er-mar′tin) a Mueller-Hinton agar with 5% heat-hemolyzed sheep blood and antibiotics, used for transport and primary isolation of *Neisseria gonorrhoeae* and *Neisseria meningitidis.*

**the·ater** (thē′ă-ter) **1.** A large room for lectures and demonstrations; sometimes applied to an operating room equipped for observation by persons other than the surgical team. **2.** Any operating room or suite of such rooms. [G. *theatron,* a place for seeing, theater, fr. *theomai,* to look at]

**the·a·tre [Br.]** SEE theater.

**the·ca,** pl. **the·cae** (thē′kă, thē′sē) a sheath or capsule. [G. *thēkē,* a box]

**the·ca cor·dis** SYN pericardium.

**the·ca fol·li·cu·li** the wall of a vesicular ovarian follicle. SEE ALSO tunica externa.

**the·cal** (thē′kăl) relating to a sheath, especially a tendon sheath. [see theca]

**the·ci·tis** (thē-sī′tis) inflammation of the sheath of a tendon. [G. *thēkē,* box (sheath), + *-itis,* inflammation]

**the·co·ma** (thē-kō′mă) a neoplasm derived from ovarian mesenchyme, consisting chiefly of spindle-shaped cells that frequently contain small droplets of fat; it may form considerable quantities of estrogens, thereby resulting in precocious development of secondary sexual features in prepubertal girls, or hyperplasia of the endometrium in older patients. [G. *thēkē,* box (theca), + *-oma,* tumor]

**The·den me·thod** (thē′den) treatment of aneurysms or of large sanguineous effusions by compression of the entire limb with a roller bandage.

**Thei·le ca·nal** (tī′lĕ) SYN transverse pericardial sinus.

**Thei·ler mouse en·ceph·a·lo·my·e·li·tis vi·rus** (tē′lĕr) a virus, genus *Cardiovirus,* in the family Picornaviridae.

**the·lar·che** (thē-lar′kē) the beginning of development of the breasts in the female. [thel- + G. *archē,* beginning]

**the·le·plas·ty** (thē′lē-plas-tē) SYN mammillaplasty. [thel- + G. *plastos,* formed]

**the·li·um,** pl. **the·lia** (thē′lē-ŭm, thē′lē-ă) **1.** a nipple-like structure. **2.** a cellular layer. **3.** SYN nipple. [Mod. L., fr. G. *thēlē,* nipple]

△**the·lo-, thel-** the nipples. Cf. mammil-. [G. *thēlē*]

**the·lor·rha·gia** (thē-lō-rā′jē-ă) bleeding from the nipple. [thelo- + G. *rhēgnymi,* to burst forth]

**T help·er cells (Th)** a subset of lymphocytes that secrete various cytokines that regulate the immune response. SYN helper cells.

**T help·er sub·set 1 cells** a subset of CD4⁺ T cells that can secrete interferon gamma and IL-2 and are responsible for cellular immunity.

**T help·er sub·set 2 cells** a subset of CD4⁺ T cells that synthesize IL-4, IL-5, and IL-10 and facilitate immunoglobulin synthesis.

**the·mat·ic ap·per·cep·tion test (TAT)** a projective psychological test in which the subject is asked to tell a story about standard ambiguous pictures depicting life-situations to reveal personal attitudes and feelings.

**the·nar** (thē′nar) **1.** [TA] SYN thenar eminence. **2.** applied to any structure in relation with the thenar eminence or its underlying collective components. [G. the palm of the hand]

**the·nar em·i·nence** the fleshy mass on the lateral side of the palm; the radial palm; the ball of the thumb. SYN thenar (1).

**the·o·rem** (thē′ō-rem) a proposition that can be proved, and so is established as a law or principle. SEE ALSO law, principle, rule.

**the·o·ry** (thē′ŏr-ē) a reasoned explanation of known facts or phenomena that serves as a basis of investigation by which to reach the truth. SEE ALSO hypothesis, postulate. [G. *theōria,* a beholding, speculation, theory, fr. *theōros,* a beholder]

**ther·a·peu·tic** (thār-ă-pyu′tik) relating to therapeutics or to the treatment, remediating, or curing of a disorder or disease. [G. *therapeutikos*]

**ther·a·peu·tic a·bor·tion** abortion induced because of the mother's physical or mental health, or to prevent birth of a deformed child or a child resulting from rape.

**ther·a·peu·tic cri·sis** a turning point leading to positive or negative change in psychiatric treatment.

**ther·a·peu·tic drug** prescription or over-the-counter medication used to treat an injury or illness.

**ther·a·peu·tic in·dex** the ratio of $LD_{50}$ to $ED_{50}$, used in quantitative comparison of drugs.

**ther·a·peu·tic ma·lar·ia** intentionally induced malaria, formerly used against neurosyphilis and certain other paralytic diseases. SYN malariotherapy.

**ther·a·peu·tic ra·di·o·lo·gy** SYN radiation oncology.

t
h

**ther•a•peu•tic range** refers to either the dosage range or blood plasma or serum concentration expected to achieve therapeutic effects.

**ther•a•peu•tic ra•tio** the ratio of the maximally tolerated dose of a drug to the minimal curative or effective dose; $LD_{50}$ divided by $ED_{50}$.

**ther•a•peu•tics** (thār-ă-pyu′tiks) the practical branch of medicine concerned with the treatment of disease or disorder. [G. *therapeutikē*, medical practice]

**ther•a•peu•tic ul•tra•sound** therapeutic use of ultrasound to warm tissue.

**ther•a•pist** (thār′ă-pist) one professionally trained in the practice of a particular type of therapy.

**ther•a•py** (thār′ă-pē) **1.** the treatment of disease or disorder by various methods. SEE ALSO therapeutics. **2.** PSYCHIATRY, CLINICAL PSYCHOLOGY psychotherapy. SEE ALSO psychotherapy, psychiatry, psychology, psychoanalysis. [G. *therapeia*, medical treatment]

**ther•mal** (ther′măl) pertaining to heat.

**ther•mal an•es•the•sia, ther•mic an•es•the•si•a** loss of temperature appreciation.

**ther•mal art•i•fact** distortion of microscopic structure in a tissue specimen, because of heat generated by the instrument (e.g., loop electrocautery) used to obtain the specimen.

**ther•mal ca•pac•i•ty** SYN heat capacity.

**ther•mal•ge•sia** (ther-mal-jē′zē-ă) high sensibility to heat; pain caused by a slight degree of heat. [therm- + G. *algēsis*, sense of pain]

**ther•mal•gia** (ther-mal′jē-ă) burning pain. SEE ALSO causalgia. [therm- + G. *algos*, pain]

**ther•mi•o•nic e•mis•sion** emission of free electrons by a filament that is heated by an electric current passing through it, as in an x-ray tube. SYN Edison effect.

△**ther•mo-, therm-** heat. [G. *thermē*, heat; *thermos*, warm or hot]

**ther•mo•an•aes•the•sia [Br.]** SEE thermoanesthesia.

**ther•mo•an•al•ge•sia** (ther′mō-an′al-jē′zē-ă) SYN thermoanesthesia.

**ther•mo•an•es•the•sia, therm•an•al•ge•sia, therm•an•es•the•sia** (ther′mō-an-es-thē′zē-ă, therm′an-al-jē′zē-ă, therm′an-es-thē′zē-ă) loss of the temperature sense or of the ability to distinguish between heat and cold; insensibility to heat or to temperature changes. SYN thermoanalgesia. [thermo- + G. *an-* priv. + *aisthēsis*, sensation]

**ther•mo•chem•is•try** (ther-mō-kem′is-trē) the interrelation of chemical action and heat.

**ther•mo•co•ag•u•la•tion** (ther′mō-kō-ag-yu-lā′shŭn) the process of converting tissue into a gel by heat. SYN endocoagulation.

**ther•mo•cou•ple** (ther-mō-kŭp′l) a device for measuring slight changes in temperature, consisting of two wires of different metals, one wire being kept at a certain low temperature, the other in the tissue or other material whose temperature is to be measured; a thermoelectric current set up is measured by a potentiometer.

**ther•mo•dif•fu•sion** (ther′mō-di-fyu′zhŭn) diffusion of fluids, either gaseous or liquid, as influenced by the temperature of the fluid.

**ther•mo•du•ric** (ther-mō-doo′rik) resistant to the effects of exposure to high temperature; used especially with reference to microorganisms. [thermo- + L. *durus*, hard, enduring]

**ther•mo•dy•nam•ics** (ther′mō-dī-nam′iks) **1.** the branch of physicochemical science concerned with heat and energy and their conversions one into the other involving mechanical work. **2.** the study of the flow of heat. [thermo- + G. *dynamis*, force]

**ther•mo•es•the•sia, therm•es•the•sia** (ther′mō-es-thē′zē-ă, therm-es-thē′zē-ă) the ability to distinguish differences of temperature. [thermo- + G. *aisthēsis*, sensation]

**ther•mo•es•the•si•om•e•ter, therm•es•the•si•om•e•ter** (ther′mō-es-thē′zē-om′ě-ter, therm′es-thē-zē-om′ě-ter) an instrument for testing the temperature sense, consisting of a metal disk with thermometer attached, by which the exact temperature of the disk at the time of application may be known. [thermo- + G. *aisthēsis*, sensation, + *metron*, measure]

**ther•mo•ex•ci•to•ry** (ther′mō-ek-sī′tŏ-rē) stimulating the production of heat.

**ther•mo•gen•e•sis** (ther′mō-jen′ě-sis) the production of heat; specifically the physiologic process of heat production in the body. [thermo- + G. *genesis*, production]

**ther•mo•ge•net•ic, ther•mo•gen•ic** (ther′mō-je-net′ik, thermō-jen′ik) **1.** relating to thermogenesis. **2.** SYN calorigenic (2).

**ther•mo•gram** (ther′mō-gram) **1.** a regional temperature map of the surface of a part of the body, obtained by infrared sensing device; it measures radiant heat, and thus subcutaneous blood flow, if the environment is constant. **2.** the record made by a thermograph. [thermo- + G. *gramma*, a writing]

**ther•mo•graph** (ther′mō-graf) an instrument or device used in producing a thermogram. [thermo- + G. *graphō*, to write]

**ther•mog•ra•phy** (ther-mog′ră-fē) the technique for making a thermogram.

**ther•mo•in•hib•i•to•ry** (ther′mō-in-hib′i-tōr-ē) inhibiting or arresting thermogenesis.

**ther•mo•la•bile** (ther-mō-lā′bīl) subject to alteration or destruction by heat. [thermo- + L. *labilis*, perishable]

**ther•mo•lu•mi•ne•scent do•si•me•ter (TLD)** device resembling a film badge but that uses lithium fluoride crystals instead of film to record radiation exposure. SEE ALSO film badge.

**ther•mol•y•sis** (ther-mol′i-sis) **1.** loss of body heat by evaporation, radiation, etc. **2.** chemical decomposition by heat. [thermo- + G. *lysis*, dissolution]

**ther•mo•lyt•ic** (ther-mō-lit′ik) **1.** relating to thermolysis. **2.** an agent promoting heat dissipation.

**ther•mo•mas•sage** (ther′mō-mă-sahzh′) combination of heat and massage in physical therapy.

**ther•mom•e•ter** (ther-mom′ě-ter) an instrument for indicating the temperature of any substance; usually a sealed vacuum tube containing mercury, which expands with heat and contracts with cold, its level accordingly rising or falling in the tube, with the exact degree of variation of level being indicated by a scale. SEE ALSO scale. [thermo- + G. *metron*, measure]

**ther•mo•met•ric** (ther-mō-met′rik) relating to thermometry or to a thermometer reading.

**ther•mom•e•try** (ther-mom′ě-trē) the measurement of temperature. [thermo- + G. *metron*, measure]

**ther•mo•phile, ther•mo•phil** (ther′mō-fīl, ther′ mō-fil) an organism that thrives at a temperature of 50°C or higher. [thermo- + G. *phileō*, to love]

**ther·mo·phil·ic** (ther-mō-fil′ik) pertaining to a thermophile.

**ther·mo·phore** (ther′mō-fōr) **1.** an arrangement for applying heat to a part; consists of a water heater, a tube conveying hot water to a coil, and another tube conducting the water back to the heater. **2.** a flat bag containing certain salts that produce heat when moistened; used as a substitute for the hot-water bag. [thermo- + G. *phoros*, bearing]

**ther·mo·re·cep·tor** (ther′mō-rē-sep′ter, -tōr) a receptor that is sensitive to heat.

**ther·mo·reg·u·la·tion** (ther′mō-reg-yu-lā′shŭn) temperature control, as by a thermostat.

**ther·mo·sta·bile, ther·mo·sta·ble** (ther-mō-stā′bīl, ther′mō-stā′bl) not readily subject to alteration or destruction by heat. [thermo- + L. *stabilis*, stable]

**ther·mo·ste·re·sis** (ther′mō-stĕ-rē′sis) the abstraction or deprivation of heat. [thermo- + G. *sterēsis*, deprivation, loss]

**ther·mo·tac·tic, ther·mo·tax·ic** (ther-mō-tak′tik, ther-mō-tak′sik) relating to thermotaxis.

**ther·mo·tax·is** (ther-mō-tak′sis) **1.** reaction of living protoplasm to the stimulus of heat. Cf. thermotropism. **2.** regulation of the temperature of the body. [thermo- + G. *taxis*, orderly arrangement]

**ther·mo·ther·a·py** (ther′mō-thār′ă-pē) treatment of disease by therapeutic application of heat. [thermo- + G. *therapeia*, treatment]

**ther·mo·to·nom·e·ter** (ther′mō-tō-nom′ĕ-ter) an instrument for measuring the degree of thermosystaltism, or muscular contraction under the influence of heat. [thermo- + G. *tonos*, tone, tension, + *metron*, measure]

**ther·mot·ro·pism** (ther-mot′rō-pizm) the motion by a part of an organism (e.g., leaves or stems) toward or away from a source of heat. Cf. thermotaxis. [thermo- + G. *tropē*, a turning]

**the·ta** (θ, Θ) **1.** the 8th letter in the Greek alphabet (θ, Θ). **2.** angle. **3.** the eighth in a series; denotes the position of a substituent located on the eighth atom from the carboxyl or other functional group.

**the·ta rhy·thm** a wave pattern in the electroencephalogram in the frequency band of 4 to 7 Hz. SYN theta wave.

**the·ta wave** SYN theta rhythm.

△**thia-** the replacement of carbon by sulfur in a ring or chain. Cf. thio-. [G. *theion*]

**thi·a·min** (thī′ă-min) a heat-labile and water-soluble vitamin contained in milk, yeast, and in the germ and husk of grains; also artificially synthesized; essential for growth; a deficiency of thiamin is associated with beriberi and Wernicke-Korsakoff syndrome. SYN vitamin B₁. [*thia-* + vitamin]

**thi·a·zides** (thī′ă-zīdz) abbreviated form of benzothiadiazides.

**thi·a·zin** (thī′ă-zin) parent substance of a family of biological blue dyes; e.g., methylene blue, thionine, toluidine blue.

**thi·a·zin dyes** similar to azin dyes except that one of the connecting N atoms is replaced by S; includes many important biological stains, especially in hematology.

**thick·ness** (thik′nes) **1.** the measure of the depth of something, as opposed to its length or width. **2.** a layer or stratum.

**Thie·mann syn·drome** (tē′mahn) avascular necrosis of the epiphyses of phalanges of fingers or toes, usually familial, beginning in childhood or adolescence, leading to deformity of fingers; also called familial arthropathy of the fingers or toes.

**thi·e·mia** (thī-ē′mē-ă) the presence of sulfur in the circulating blood. [G. *theion*, sulfur, + *haima*, blood]

**thi·e·nyl·al·a·nine** (thī′ĕ-nil-al′ă-nēn) a compound structurally similar to phenylalanine that inhibits the growth of *Escherichia coli*, presumably by competitive inhibition of enzymes for which L-phenylalanine is the substrate.

**Thiersch ca·nal·ic·u·lus** (tērsh) any of numerous minute channels in newly formed reparative tissue, permitting the circulation of nutritive fluids, precursors of new vascularization.

**thigh** (thī) the part of the inferior limb between the hip and the knee.

**thigh bone** SYN femur.

**thig·mes·the·sia** (thig-mes-thē′zē-ă) sensibility to touch. [G. *thigma*, touch, + *aisthēsis*, sensation]

**thig·mo·tax·is** (thig-mō-tak′sis) a form of barotaxis; denoting the reaction of plant or animal protoplasm to contact with a solid body. Cf. thigmotropism. [G. *thigma*, touch, + *taxis*, orderly arrangement]

**thig·mot·ro·pism** (thig-mot′rō-pizm) a movement toward or away from a touch stimulus on the part of a portion of an organism, such as leaves or tendrils. Cf. thigmotaxis. [G. *thigma*, touch, + *tropē*, a turning]

**think·ing** the act of reasoning.

**think·ing through** the psychological process of understanding, with insight, one's own behavior.

**thin-lay·er chro·ma·to·gra·phy (TLC)** chromatography through a thin layer of cellulose or similar inert material supported on a glass or plastic plate.

**thin sec·tion, ul·tra·thin sec·tion** a section of tissue for electron microscopic examination; the specimen is fixed, typically in glutaraldehyde and/or in osmium tetroxide, embedded in a plastic resin, and sectioned at less than 0.1 µm in thickness with a glass or diamond knife in an ultramicrotome.

△**thio-** prefix denoting the replacement of oxygen by sulfur in a compound. Cf. thia-. [G. *theion*, sugar]

**thi·o·ac·id** (thī-ō-as′id) an organic acid in which one or more of the oxygen atoms have been replaced by sulfur atoms; e.g., thiosulfuric acid.

△**-thi·o·ic a·cid** suffix denoting the radical, –C(S)OH or –C(O)SH, the sulfur analog of a carboxylic acid.

**thi·ol·trans·a·cet·y·lase A** (thī′ol-trans-ă-set′i-lās-ā) SYN dihydrolipoamide acetyltransferase.

**thi·ol·y·sis** (thī-ol′i-sis) the cleavage of a chemical bond with the addition of coenzyme A to one part; analogous to hydrolysis and phosphorolysis.

△**-thi·one** suffix denoting the radical =C=S, the sulfur analog of a ketone.

**thi·on·ic** (thī-on′ik) relating to sulfur.

**thi·o·nine** (thī′ō-nēn) [CI 52000] dark-green powder, giving a purple solution in water; useful as a basic stain in histology for chromatin and mucin because of its metachromatic properties. SYN Lauth violet.

**thi·o·sul·fate** (thī-ō-sŭl′fāt) the anion of thiosulfuric acid; elevated in individuals with a molybdenum cofactor deficiency.

**thi·o·sul·fur·ic ac·id** (thī'ō-sŭl-fyur'ik as'id) sulfuric acid in which an atom of oxygen has been replaced by one of sulfur.

△**thi·ox·o-** prefix indicating =S in a thioketone.

**third cra·ni·al nerve [CN III]** SYN oculomotor nerve [CN III].

**third-de·gree burn** a burn involving destruction of the entire skin; deep third-degree burns extend into subcutaneous fat, muscle, or bone and often cause much scarring.

**third de·gree pro·lapse** SEE prolapse of the uterus.

**third dis·ease** SYN rubella.

**third heart sound (S₃)** occurs in early diastole and corresponds with the end of the first phase of rapid ventricular filling; normal in children and younger people but abnormal in others.

**third mo·lar** eighth permanent tooth in the maxilla and mandible on each side; the most posterior tooth in human dentition. SYN dens serotinus [TA], wisdom tooth.

**third-party pay·er** institution or company that provides reimbursement to health care providers for services rendered to a third party (the patient).

**third per·o·ne·al mus·cle** SYN peroneus tertius muscle.

**third toe [III]** third digit of foot.

**third ven·tri·cle** a narrow, vertically oriented, irregularly quadrilateral cavity in the midplane, extending from the lamina terminalis to the rostral opening of the mesencephalic aqueduct. This ventricle communicates at its rostrodorsal corner with each of the two lateral ventricles through the left and right interventricular foramen of Monro. Its narrow roof is formed by the tela choroidea which is attached on either side to the tenia thalami; its lateral wall by the medial surface of the thalamus and, below the hypothalamic sulcus, by the hypothalamus, which also forms its floor. In lateral profile, the third ventricle exhibits a number of recesses: in its floor, from before backward, 1) the preoptic recess in the acute angle between the base of the lamina terminalis and the dorsum of the optic chiasm, 2) the infundibular recess extending ventrally into the infundibulum but not into the hypophysial stalk, and 3) the mammillary or inframamillary recess caused by the protrusion of the mammillary bodies into the ventricle. The pineal recess extends caudally into the pineal stalk from the dorsocaudal corner. SYN ventriculus tertius [TA].

**third ven·tri·cu·los·to·my** an operation to establish an opening from the third ventricle to the prechiasmal and interpeduncular cisterns (Stookey-Scarff operation) or from the third ventricle to the interpeduncular cistern (Dandy operation).

**thirst** a desire to drink associated with uncomfortable sensations in the mouth and pharynx. [A.S. *thurst*]

**Thi·ry fis·tu·la** (tē'rē) an artificial fistula for collecting the intestinal secretions of an animal for experimental purposes; a loop of intestine is isolated, its vascular and nervous connections are preserved, after the continuity of the intestinal tract is restored by an end-to-end anastomosis; one end of the isolated segment is closed, the other attached to the skin of the abdomen.

**thix·o·la·bile** (thik-sō-lā'bĭl) susceptible to thixotropy.

**thix·o·tro·pic** (thik-sō-trop'ik) pertaining to, or characterized by, thixotropy.

**thix·ot·ro·py** (thik-sot'rō-pē) the property of certain gels of becoming less viscous when shaken or subjected to shearing forces and returning to the original viscosity upon standing. [G. *thixis,* a touching, + *tropē,* turning]

**Tho·go·to·vi·ruses** (thō-gō-tō-vī'rŭs-ez) any of several unclassified viruses that are similar to the Orthoviruses and share some amino acid homology.

**Tho·ma am·pul·la** (tō-mah') a dilation of the arterial capillary beyond the sheathed artery of the spleen.

**Tho·ma fix·a·tive** (tō-mah') nitric acid in 95% alcohol, used for decalcifying bone in the preparation of histologic specimens.

**Tho·ma laws** (tō-mah') the development of blood vessels is governed by dynamic forces acting on their walls as follows: an increase in velocity of blood flow causes dilation of the lumen; an increase in lateral pressure on the vessel wall causes it to thicken; an increase in end-pressure causes the formation of new capillaries.

**Thom·as splint** (tom'ăs) a long leg splint extending from a ring at the hip to beyond the foot, allowing traction to a fractured leg, for emergencies and transportation.

**Thomp·son test** (tomp'son) test to detect Achilles tendon disruption; with the patient kneeling on a chair or platform with the feet unsupported, each calf is squeezed; if the Achilles tendon is disrupted, plantarflexion of the foot will not occur.

**Thomp·son test** (tomp'son) the urine, in a case of gonorrhea, is passed into two glasses in succession; if gonococci and mucous threads are found only in the first glass the probability is that the process is limited to the anterior urethra. SYN two-glass test.

**Thom·sen dis·ease** (tom'sen) SYN myotonia congenita.

**Thom·son sign** (tom'son) SYN Pastia sign.

**tho·ra·cal·gia** (thōr-ă-kal'jē-ă) pain in the chest. SYN thoracodynia. [thoraco- + G. *algos,* pain]

**tho·ra·cen·te·sis** (thōr'ă-sen-tē'sis) paracentesis of the pleural cavity. SYN pleural tap, pleurocentesis, thoracocentesis. [thoraco- + G. *kentēsis,* puncture]

**tho·rac·ic** (thō-ras'ik) relating to the thorax.

**thor·a·cic cage** the skeleton of the thorax consisting of the thoracic vertebrae, ribs, costal cartilages, and sternum. SYN cavea thoracis [TA].

**thor·a·cic car·di·ac nerves** part of the cardiopulmonary splanchnic nerves from the second to fifth segments of the thoracic sympathetic trunk that pass medially and anteriorly to enter the cardiac plexus; they convey postsynaptic sympathetic fibers to, and visceral afferent (pain) fibers from, the heart. SYN nervi cardiaci thoracici [TA].

**thor·a·cic ca·vi·ty** the space within the thoracic walls, bounded below by the diaphragm and above by the neck.

**thor·a·cic duct** the largest lymph vessel in the body, beginning at the cisterna chyli at about the level of the second lumbar vertebra; the abdominal part extends superiorly to pass through the aortic opening of the diaphragm, where it becomes the thoracic part and crosses the posterior mediastinum to form the arch of the thoracic duct and discharge into the left venous angle (origin of the brachiocephalic vein).

**thor·a·cic ky·pho·sis** the normal, anteriorly concave curvature of the thoracic segment of the vertebral column, in which the primary curvature of the fetal embryo is maintained into maturity.

**thor·a·cic lon·gis·si·mus mus·cle** SYN longissimus thoracis muscle.

**tho·rac·ic nerves [T1–T12]** twelve nerves on each side, mixed motor and sensory, supplying the muscles and skin of the thoracic and abdominal walls. SYN nervi thoracici [T1–12] [TA].

**tho·rac·ic out·let syn·drome (TOS)** collective title for a number of conditions attributed to compromise of blood vessels or nerve fibers (brachial plexus) at any point between the base of the neck and the axilla; classified on the basis of the structure known or presumed to be compromised, and divided into two main groups: vascular and neurologic.

**thor·a·cic spi·nal nerves** twelve nerves on each side, mixed motor and sensory, supplying the muscles and skin of the thoracic and abdominal walls.

**tho·r·acic splen·o·sis** presense of splenic tissue in the thorax, resultant from combined thoracic and abdominal trauma followed by splenectomy.

**tho·rac·ic ver·te·brae [T1–T12]** the segments of the vertebral column, usually 12, which articulate with ribs to form part of the thoracic cage. SYN vertebrae thoracicae [TA].

**thor·a·cic wall** SYN chest wall.

△**thor·a·co-, thor·ac-, thor·a·cic·o-** the chest (thorax). [G. *thōrax*]

**tho·ra·co·a·cro·mi·al** (thōr′ă-kō-ă-krō′mē-ăl) relating to the acromion and the thorax; denoting especially the thoracoacromial artery. SYN acromiothoracic.

**thor·a·co·a·cro·mi·al ar·tery** *origin,* axillary; *distribution,* muscles and skin of shoulder and upper chest; *anastomoses,* branches of superior thoracic, internal thoracic, lateral thoracic, posterior and anterior circumflex humeral, and suprascapular. SYN arteria thoracoacromialis [TA], acromiothoracic artery.

**thor·a·co·a·cro·mi·al vein** corresponding to the artery of the same name, empties into the axillary vein, sometimes by a common trunk with the cephalic vein.

**tho·ra·co·ce·los·chi·sis** (thōr′ă-kō-sē-los′ki-sis) a congenital fissure of the trunk embracing both the thoracic and abdominal cavities. SYN thoracogastroschisis. [thoraco- + G. *koilia,* belly, + *schisis,* fissure]

**tho·ra·co·cen·te·sis** (thōr′ă-kō-sen-tē′sis) SYN thoracentesis.

**tho·ra·co·cyl·lo·sis** (thōr′ă-kō-si-lō′sis) a deformity of the chest. [thoraco- + G. *kyllōsis,* a crippling]

**tho·ra·co·cyr·to·sis** (thōr′ă-kō-sir-tō′sis) abnormally wide curvature of the chest wall. [thoraco- + G. *kyrtōsis,* a being crooked]

**thor·a·co·dor·sal ar·tery** *origin,* subscapular; *distribution,* muscles of upper part of back; *anastomoses,* branches of lateral thoracic. SYN arteria thoracodorsalis [TA].

**thor·a·co·dor·sal nerve** arises from the posterior cord of the brachial plexus; it contains fibers from the sixth, seventh, and eighth cervical nerves and supplies the latissimus dorsi muscle. SYN nervus thoracodorsalis [TA].

**tho·ra·co·dyn·ia** (thōr′ă-kō-din′ē-ă) SYN thoracalgia. [thoraco- + G. *odynē,* pain]

**thor·a·co·ep·i·gas·tric vein** one of two veins, sometimes a single vein, arising from the region of the superficial epigastric vein and opening into the axillary or the lateral thoracic vein, thus forming an anastomotic or collateral pathway between tributaries of the inferior and superior venae cavae.

**tho·ra·co·gas·tros·chi·sis** (thōr′ă-kō-gas-tros′ki-sis) SYN thoracoceloschisis. [thoraco- + G. *gas-tēr,* belly, + *schisis,* fissure]

**tho·ra·co·lum·bar** (thōr′ă-kō-lŭm′bar) **1.** relating to the thoracic and lumbar portions of the vertebral column. **2.** relating to the origins of the sympathetic division of the autonomic nervous system. SEE autonomic division of nervous system.

**thor·a·co·lum·bar fa·scia** the fascia which covers the deep muscles of the back; it is attached to the angles of the ribs and to the spines of the thoracic, lumbar, and sacral vertebrae, to the transverse processes of the lumbar vertebrae, to the lower border of the twelfth rib and the iliac crest, as well as to the lumbocostal, iliolumbar, intertransverse, and supraspinous ligaments.

**thor·a·co·lum·bo·sa·cral or·tho·sis** an external device applied to the trunk and extending from the upper portion of the thoracic spine to the pelvis; designed to provide immobilization of the thoracic spine.

**tho·ra·col·y·sis** (thōr·ă-kol′i-sis) breaking up of pleural adhesions. [thoraco- + G. *lysis,* dissolution]

**tho·ra·com·e·ter** (thōr·ă-kom′ĕ-ter) an instrument for measuring the circumference of the chest or its variations in respiration. [thoraco- + G. *metron,* measure]

**tho·ra·co·my·o·dyn·ia** (thōr′ă-kō-mī-ō-din′ē-ă) pain in the muscles of the chest wall. [thoraco- + G. *mys,* muscle, + *odynē,* pain]

**tho·ra·co·plas·ty** (thōr′ă-kō-plas-tē) an operation that reduces intrathoracic space. [thoraco- + G. *plastos,* formed]

**thor·a·cos·chi·sis** (thōr-ă-kos′ki-sis) congenital fissure of the chest wall. [thoraco- + G. *schisis,* fissure]

**tho·ra·co·scope** (thō-rak′ō-skōp) a scope for viewing intrathoracic structures; may be video assisted. [thoraco- + G. *skopeō,* to view]

🔲**tho·ra·cos·co·py** (thōr-ă-kos′kŏ-pē) examination of the pleural cavity with an endoscope. See page B9. [thoraco- + G. *skopeō,* to view]

**tho·ra·co·ste·no·sis** (thōr′ă-kō-stĕ-nō′sis) narrowness of the chest. [thoraco- + G. *stenōsis,* narrowing]

**thor·a·co·ster·no·to·my** chest incision combining an intercostal incision and transsection of the sternum.

**tho·ra·cos·to·my** (thōr-ă-kos′tō-mē) establishment of an opening into the chest cavity, as for the drainage of an empyema. [thoraco- + G. *stoma,* mouth]

**tho·ra·cot·o·my** (thōr-ă-kot′ō-mē) incision into the chest wall. SYN pleurotomy. [thoraco- + G. *tomē,* incision]

**tho·rax,** gen. **tho·ra·cis,** pl. **tho·ra·ces** (thō′raks, thō′rā-sis, thō′ră′sēz) [TA] the upper part of the trunk between the neck and the abdomen; it is formed by the 12 thoracic vertebrae, the 12 pairs of ribs, the sternum, and the muscles and fasciae attached to these; below, it is separated from the abdomen by the diaphragm; it contains the chief organs of the circulatory and respiratory systems. [L. fr. G. *thōrax,* breastplate, the chest, fr. *thōrēssō,* to arm]

**tho·ri·um (Th)** (thōr′ē-ŭm) a radioactive metallic element; atomic no. 90, atomic wt. 232.0381. $^{232}$Th, the only naturally occurring nuclide, with a half-life of $14 \times 10^9$ years, is used in colloidal form in electron microscopy as a stain for acid mucopolysaccharides. [*Thor,* Norse god of thunder]

**Thor·mäh·len test** (tor′mē-len) a test for melanin; the suspected liquid is treated with sodium nitroprusside, caustic potash, and acetic acid; if melanin is present, the solution takes on a deep blue color.

**Thorn syn·drome** (thōrn) SYN salt-losing nephritis.

**thought 1.** the faculty of reasoning. **2.** the process or act of thinking. **3.** the result of thinking.

**Thr** threonine or its radical forms.

**thread·ed im·plant** DENTISTRY an implant with screwlike threads that is either screwed into bone previously threaded by a tap, or by self-tapping, the implant cutting threads in the bone as it is inserted into a predrilled hole.

**thread·worm** (thred′werm) common name for species of the genus *Strongyloides;* sometimes applied to any of the smaller parasitic nematodes.

**thread·y pulse** a small fine pulse, feeling like a small cord or thread under the finger.

**three-glass test** the male patient empties his bladder into a series of 3-ounce test tubes, and the contents of the first and the last are examined; the first tube contains the washings from the anterior urethra, the second, material from the bladder, and the last, material from the posterior urethra, prostate, and seminal vesicles.

**three-in·ci·sion e·so·pha·gec·to·my** esophagectomy via laparotomy, right chest and cervical incisions.

**thre·o·nine (T, Thr)** (thrē′ō-nēn) one of the naturally occurring amino acids, included in the structure of most proteins, and nutritionally essential in the diet of humans and other mammals.

**thresh·old** (thresh′ōld) **1.** the point at which a stimulus first produces a sensation. **2.** the lower limit of perception of a stimulus. **3.** the minimal stimulus that produces excitation of any structure. **4.** SYN limen. [A.S. *therxold*]

**thresh·old li·mit val·ue** the maximum concentration of a chemical recommended by the American Conference of Government Industrial Hygienists for repeated exposure without adverse health effects on workers.

**thresh·old sti·mu·lus** a stimulus of threshold strength, i.e., one just strong enough to excite. SEE ALSO adequate stimulus.

**thresh·old sub·stance** any material (e.g., glucose) that is excreted in the urine only when its plasma concentration exceeds a certain value, termed its threshold.

**thresh·old trait** a trait that falls into natural groups that originate not in categorically distinct causes but in whether or not the outcome attains critical values; e.g., gallstones may result from a categorical cause or from unusual levels of causal factors that themselves show no evidence of grouping.

**thrill** a vibration accompanying a cardiac or vascular murmur that can be palpated. SEE ALSO fremitus.

**thrix** (thriks) SYN hair (2). [G.]

**throat** (thrōt) **1.** the fauces and pharynx. SYN gullet. **2.** the anterior aspect of the neck. **3.** any narrowed entrance into a hollow part. [A.S. *throtu*]

**throb 1.** to pulsate. **2.** a beating or pulsation.

**throm·bas·the·nia** (throm-bas-thē′nē-ă) an abnormality of platelets characteristic of Glanzmann thrombasthenia. SYN thromboasthenia. [thromb- + G. *astheneia,* weakness]

**throm·bec·to·my** (throm-bek′tō-mē) the excision of a thrombus. [thromb- + G. *ektomē,* excision]

**throm·bi** (throm′bī) plural of thrombus.

**throm·bin 1.** an enzyme (proteinase), formed in shed blood, that converts fibrinogen into fibrin by hydrolyzing peptides (and amides and esters) of L-arginine; formed from prothrombin by the action of prothrombinase (factor Xa, another proteinase). **2.** a sterile protein substance prepared from prothrombin of bovine origin through interaction with thromboplastin in the presence of calcium; causes clotting of whole blood, plasma, or a fibrinogen solution; used as a topical hemostatic for capillary bleeding with or without fibrin foam in general and plastic surgical procedures.

△**throm·bo-, thromb-** blood clot; coagulation; thrombin. [G. *thrombos,* clot (thrombus)]

**throm·bo·an·gi·i·tis** (throm′bō-an-ji-ī′tis) inflammation of the intima of a blood vessel, with thrombosis. [thrombo- + G. *angeion,* vessel, + *-itis,* inflammation]

**throm·bo·an·gi·i·tis o·bli·ter·ans** inflammation of the entire wall and connective tissue surrounding medium-sized arteries and veins, especially of the legs of young and middle-aged men; associated with thrombotic occlusion and commonly resulting in gangrene. SYN Buerger disease.

**throm·bo·ar·te·ri·tis** (throm′bō-ar-ter-ī′tis) arterial inflammation with thrombus formation.

**throm·bo·as·the·nia** (throm′bō-as-thē′nē-ă) SYN thrombasthenia.

**throm·bo·clas·tic** (throm-bō-klas′tik) SYN thrombolytic.

**throm·bo·cyst, throm·bo·cys·tis** (throm′bō-sist, throm′bō-sis′tis) a membranous sac enclosing a thrombus. [thrombo- + G. *kystis,* a bladder]

**throm·bo·cyte** (throm′bō-sīt) SYN platelet. [thrombo- + G. *kytos,* cell]

**throm·bo·cy·thae·mia [Br.]** SEE thrombocythemia.

**throm·bo·cy·the·mia** (throm′bō-sī-thē′mē-ă) SYN thrombocytosis. [thrombocyte + G. *haima,* blood]

**throm·bo·cy·tic ser·ies** the cells of successive stages in thrombocytic (platelet) development in the bone marrow, e.g., thromboblasts, thrombocytes.

**throm·bo·cy·top·a·thy** (throm′bō-sī-top′ă-thē) general term for any disorder of the coagulating mechanism that results from dysfunction of the blood platelets. [thrombocyte + G. *pathos,* suffering]

**throm·bo·cy·to·pe·nia** (throm′bō-sī-tō-pē′nē-ă) a condition in which there is an abnormally small number of platelets in the circulating blood. SYN thrombopenia. [thrombocyte + G. *penia,* poverty]

**throm·bo·cy·to·pe·ni·a-ab·sent ra·di·us syn·-drome** congenital absence of the radius associated with thrombocytopenia that is symptomatic in infancy but later improves; congenital heart disease and renal anomalies occur in some cases; autosomal recessive inheritance.

**throm·bo·cy·to·pe·nic pur·pur·a** SEE idiopathic thrombocytopenic purpura.

**throm·bo·cy·to·poi·e·sis** (throm′bō-sī-tō-poy-ē′sis) the process of formation of thrombocytes or platelets. [thrombocyte + G. *poiēsis*, a making]

**throm·bo·cy·to·sis** (throm′bō-sī-tō′sis) an increase in the number of platelets in the circulating blood. SYN thrombocythemia. [thrombocyte + G. *-osis*, condition]

**throm·bo·e·las·to·gram** (throm′bō-ē-las′tō-gram) registration of coagulation process by a thromboelastograph.

**throm·bo·e·las·to·graph** (throm′bō-ē-las′tō-graf) apparatus for registering elastic variations of a thrombus during the process of coagulation. [thromb- + G. *elastreō*, to push, + *graphō*, to write]

**throm·bo·em·bo·lism** (throm′bō-em′bō-lizm) embolism from a thrombus. [thrombo- + G. *embolismos*, embolism]

**throm·bo·end·ar·ter·ec·to·my** (throm′bō-end-ar-ter-ek′tō-mē) an operation that involves opening an artery, removing an occluding thrombus along with the intima and atheromatous material, and leaving a clean, fresh plane internal to the adventitia. [thrombo- + endarterectomy]

**throm·bo·gen·ic** (throm-bō-jen′ik) **1.** relating to thrombogen. **2.** causing thrombosis or coagulation of the blood.

**throm·boid** (throm′boyd) resembling a thrombus. [thrombo- + G. *eidos*, resemblance]

**throm·bo·ki·nase** (throm-bō-kī′nās) SYN thromboplastin.

**throm·bo·lym·phan·gi·tis** (throm′bō-lim-fan-jī′tis) inflammation of a lymphatic vessel with the formation of a lymph clot.

**throm·bol·y·sis** (throm-bol′i-sis) liquefaction or dissolving of a thrombus. [thrombo- + G. *lysis*, a dissolving]

**throm·bo·lyt·ic** (throm-bō-lit′ik) breaking up or dissolving a thrombus. SYN thromboclastic.

**throm·bo·ly·tic ther·a·py** intravenous administration of an agent intended to dissolve a clot causing acute ischemia, as in myocardial infarction, stroke, and peripheral arterial or venous thrombosis. Thrombolytic agents degrade fibrin clots by activating plasminogen, a naturally occurring modulator of hemostatic and thrombotic processes. Synthesized by the liver, plasminogen is present in circulating blood and binds to platelets, endothelium, and fibrin. At sites of vascular injury with thrombus formation, tissue plasminogen activator (TPA), produced by endothelial cells, also binds to fibrin and converts fibrin-bound plasminogen to plasmin by cleaving the arginine-valine bond in the 560–561 position of plasminogen. The resulting clot lysis is due to degradation of fibrin threads as well as of glycoproteins required for platelet adhesion and aggregation. Thrombolytic agents in current use mimic the effects of natural TPA. These include alteplase, a TPA produced by recombinant DNA technology; reteplase, a variant of the TPA molecule, also genetically engineered; urokinase, a tissue protein derived from human kidney cell cultures; streptokinase, a product of β-hemolytic streptococci that catalyzes the conversion of plasminogen to plasmin; and anistreplase, an inactive form of plasminogen that is bound to streptokinase and undergoes deacylation after administration, resulting in persistent activation of plasminogen. The latter two products are potentially antigenic and can cause systemic hypersensitivity reactions. SEE ALSO tissue plasminogen activator.

**throm·bon** an all-inclusive term for circulating thrombocytes (blood platelets) and the cellular forms from which they arise (thromboblasts or megakaryocytes).

**throm·bop·a·thy** (throm-bop′ă-thē) a nonspecific term applied to disorders of blood platelets resulting in defective thromboplastin, without obvious change in the appearance or number of platelets. [thrombo- + G. *pathos*, disease]

**throm·bo·pe·nia** (throm-bō-pē′nē-ă) SYN thrombocytopenia.

**throm·bo·pe·nic pur·pura** SYN idiopathic thrombocytopenic purpura.

**throm·bo·phil·ia** (throm-bō-fil′ē-ă) a disorder of the hemopoietic system in which there is a tendency to the occurrence of thrombosis. [thrombo- + G. *philos*, fond]

**throm·bo·phle·bi·tis** (throm′bō-flě-bī′tis) venous inflammation with thrombus formation. [thrombo- + G. *phleps*, vein, + *-itis*, inflammation]

**throm·bo·plas·tid** (throm-bō-plas′tid) **1.** SYN platelet. **2.** a nucleated spindle cell in submammalian blood. [thrombo- + G. *plastos*, formed]

**throm·bo·plas·tin** (throm-bō-plas′tin) a substance present in tissues, platelets, and leukocytes necessary for the coagulation of blood; in the presence of calcium ions thromboplastin is necessary for the conversion of prothrombin to thrombin, an important step in coagulation of blood. SYN platelet tissue factor, thrombokinase.

**throm·bo·poi·e·sis** (throm′bō-poy-ē′sis) precisely, the process of a clot forming in blood, but generally used with reference to the formation of blood platelets (thrombocytes). [thrombo- + G. *poiēsis*, a making]

**throm·bo·poi·e·tin** (throm′bō-poy′ĕ-tin) a cytokine that serves as a humoral regulator for the production of blood platelets through action on the receptor c-mp1. SYN megakaryocyte growth and development factor, megapoietin. [thrombo- + G. *poiētēs*, maker, + in]

**throm·bosed** (throm′bōsd) **1.** clotted. **2.** denoting a blood vessel that is the seat of thrombosis.

**throm·bo·sis**, pl. **throm·bo·ses** (throm-bō′sis, throm-bō′sēz) formation or presence of a thrombus; clotting within a blood vessel which may cause infarction of tissues supplied by the vessel. [G. *thrombōsis*, a clotting, fr. *thrombos*, clot]

**throm·bo·spon·din-re·lat·ed ad·he·sive pro·-tein** one of two proteins (the other is circumsporozoite protein) involved in sporozoite recognition of host cells in malaria.

**throm·bo·sta·sis** (throm-bos′tă-sis) local arrest of the circulation by thrombosis. [thrombo- + G. *stasis*, a standing]

**throm·bot·ic** (throm-bot′ik) relating to, caused by, or characterized by thrombosis.

**throm·bot·ic throm·bo·cy·to·pe·nic pur·-pur·a** a rapidly fatal or occasionally protracted disease with varied symptoms in addition to purpura, including signs of central nervous system involvement, due to formation of fibrin or platelet thrombi in arterioles and capillaries in many organs.

**throm·box·ane** (throm'bok-sān) the formal parent of the thromboxanes; prostanoic acid in which the –COOH has been reduced to –$CH_3$ and an oxygen atom has been inserted between carbons 11 and 12.

**throm·box·anes** (throm'bok-sānz) a group of compounds, included in the eicosanoids, formally based on thromboxane, but with the terminal COOH group present; biochemically related to the prostaglandins and formed from them. Thromboxanes are so named from their influence on platelet aggregation and the formation of the oxygen-containing six-membered ring (pyran or oxane). Like the prostaglandins, individual thromboxanes (abbreviated TX) are designated by letters (A, B, C, etc.) and subscripts indicating structural features.

**throm·bus** (throm'bŭs) a clot in the cardiovascular system formed during life from constituents of blood; it may be occlusive or attached to the vessel or heart wall without obstructing the lumen (mural thrombus). [L. fr. G. *thrombos,* a clot]

**through drain·age** drainage obtained by the passage of a perforated tube, open at both extremities, through a cavity; in addition, the cavity can be washed out by a solution passed through the tube.

**through·put** (throo'put) a term applied to analytic instruments specifying the number of tests that can be performed in a given time.

**thrush** (thrŭsh) infection of the oral tissues with *Candida albicans;* often an opportunistic infection in persons with AIDS or other conditions that depress the immune system.

**thu·li·um (Tm)** (thoo'lē-ŭm) a metallic element of the lanthanide series, atomic no. 69, atomic wt. 168.93421. [L. *Thule,* the earliest name for Scandinavia]

**thumb** (thŭmb) the first digit on the radial side of the hand. SYN pollex [TA]. [A.S. *thuma*]

**thumb for·ceps** a spring forceps used by compression with thumb and forefinger.

**thun·der·clap head·ache** sudden severe nonlocalizing head pain not associated with any abnormal neurological findings; of varied etiology, including subarachnoid hemorrhage, migraine, carotid or vertebral artery dissection, cavernous sinus thrombosis, and idiopathic.

**thy·mec·to·my** (thī-mek'tō-mē) removal of the thymus gland. [thymus + G. *ektomē,* excision]

△**-thy·mia** mind, soul, emotions. SEE ALSO thymo- (2). [G. *thymos,* the mind or heart as the seat of strong feelings or passion]

**thy·mic** (thī'mik) relating to the thymus gland.

**thy·mic a·lym·pho·pla·sia** hypoplasia with absence of Hassall corpuscles and deficiency of lymphocytes in the thymus and usually in lymph nodes, spleen, and gastrointestinal tract; there is peripheral lymphopenia and often hypogammaglobulinemia and absence of plasma cells; presents in early infancy with respiratory infections and leads to death within a few months.

**thy·mic cor·pu·scle** small spherical bodies of keratinized and usually squamous epithelial cells arranged in a concentric pattern around clusters of degenerating lymphocytes, eosinophils, and

macrophages; found in the medulla of the lobules of the thymus. SYN Hassall bodies, Hassall concentric corpuscle.

**thy·mi·co·lym·phat·ic** (thī'mi-kō-lim-fat'ik) relating to the thymus and the lymphatic system.

**thy·mic veins** a number of small veins from the thymus emptying into the left brachiocephalic vein.

**thy·mi·dine (dThd)** (thī'mi-dēn) 1-(2-deoxyribosyl)thymine; one of the four major nucleosides in DNA (the others being deoxyadenosine, deoxycytidine, and deoxyguanosine). SYN deoxythymidine.

**thy·mi·dine 5′-di·phos·phate (dTDP)** thymidine esterified at its 5′ position with diphosphoric acid.

**thy·mine** (thī'mēn) a constituent of thymidylic acid and DNA; elevated in hyperuracil-thyminuria.

**thy·mi·tis** (thī-mī'tis) inflammation of the thymus gland.

△**thy·mo-, thym-, thy·mi-** 1. the thymus. [G. *thymos*] 2. mind, soul, emotions. [G. *thymos,* the mind or heart as the seat of strong feelings or passions] 3. wart, warty. [G. *thymos, thymion*]

**thy·mo·cyte** (thī'mō-sīt) a cell that develops in the thymus, seemingly from a stem cell of bone marrow and of fetal liver, and is the precursor of the thymus-derived lymphocyte (T lymphocyte) that effects cell-mediated (delayed type) sensitivity. [thymus + G. *kytos,* cell]

**thy·mo·gen·ic** (thī-mō-jen'ik) of affective origin. [G. *thymos,* mind, + *genesis,* origin]

**thy·mo·ki·net·ic** (thī'mō-ki-net'ik) activating the thymus gland. [thymus + G. *kinēsis,* movement]

**thy·mo·ma** (thī-mō'mă) a neoplasm in the anterior mediastinum, originating from thymic tissue, usually benign, and frequently encapsulated; occasionally invasive, but metastases are extremely rare. [thymus + G. *-oma,* tumor]

**thy·mo·pri·val, thy·mo·priv·ic, thy·mo·pri·vous** (thī-mō-prī'văl, thī-mō-priv'ik, thī-mō-prī'vŭs) relating to or marked by premature atrophy or removal of the thymus. [thymus + L. *privus,* deprived of]

**thy·mus,** pl. **thy·mi, thy·mus·es** (thī'mŭs, thī'mī) [TA] a primary lymphoid organ, located in the superior mediastinum and lower part of the neck, that is necessary in early life for the normal development of immunological function. It reaches its greatest relative weight shortly after birth and its greatest absolute weight at puberty; it then begins to involute, and much of the lymphoid tissue is replaced by fat. The thymus consists of two irregularly shaped parts united by a connective tissue capsule. Each part is partially subdivided by connective tissue septa into lobules, which consist of an inner medullary portion, continuous with the medullae of adjacent lobules, and an outer cortical portion. SYN thymus gland. [G. *thymos,* excrescence, sweetbread]

**thy·mus gland** SYN thymus.

△**thy·ro-, thyr-** the thyroid gland. [see thyroid]

**thy·ro·a·pla·sia** (thī'rō-ă-plā'zē-ă) a congenital defect of the thyroid gland with deficiency of its secretion. [thyro- + G. *a-* priv. + *plasis,* a molding]

**thy·ro·ar·y·te·noid** (thī'rō-ar'i-tē'noyd) relating to the thyroid and arytenoid cartilages. SEE thyroarytenoid muscle.

**thy·ro·ar·y·te·noid mus·cle** *origin,* inner surface of thyroid cartilage; *insertion*, muscular process and outer surface of arytenoid; *action*, decreases tension on (relaxes) vocal cords lowering the pitch of the voice tone; *nerve supply*, recurrent laryngeal. SYN musculus thyroarytenoideus [TA].

**thy•ro•car•di•ac dis•ease** heart disease resulting from hyperthyroidism.

**thy•ro•cele** (thī′rō-sēl) a tumor of the thyroid gland, such as a goiter. [thyro- + G. *kēlē*, tumor]

**thy•ro•cer•vi•cal trunk** a short arterial trunk arising from the subclavian artery, giving rise to the suprascapular (which may instead arise directly from the subclavian artery) and terminating by dividing into the ascending cervical and inferior thyroid arteries. SYN truncus thyrocervicalis [TA].

**thy•ro•ep•i•glot•tic** (thī′rō-ep-i-glot′ik) relating to the thyroid cartilage and the epiglottis.

**thy•ro•ep•i•glot•tic mus•cle, thy•ro•ep•i•glot•ti•de•an mus•cle** *origin*, inner surface of thyroid cartilage in common with musculus thyroarytenoideus; *insertion*, aryepiglottic fold and margin of epiglottis; *action*, depresses base of epiglottis; *nerve supply*, recurrent laryngeal. SYN musculus thyroepiglotticus [TA].

**thy•ro•gen•ic, thy•rog•e•nous** (thī-rō-jen′ik, thī-roj′ĕ-nŭs) of thyroid gland origin. [thyroid + G. *-gen*, producing]

**thy•ro•glob•u•lin** (thī-rō-glob′yu-lin) **1.** a thyroid hormone-containing protein, usually stored in the colloid within the thyroid follicles; biosynthesis of thyroid hormone entails iodination of the L-tyrosyl moieties of this protein. A defect in thyroglobulin will lead to hypothyroidism. **2.** a substance obtained by the fractionation of thyroid glands from the hog, *Sus scrofula*, containing not less than 0.7% of total iodine; used as a thyroid hormone in the treatment of hypothyroidism.

**thy•ro•glos•sal** (thī-rō-glos′ăl) relating to the thyroid gland and the tongue, denoting especially an embryological duct.

**thy•ro•hy•al** (thī-rō-hī′ăl) the greater cornu of the hyoid bone.

**thy•ro•hy•oid** (thī-rō-hī′oyd) relating to the thyroid cartilage and the hyoid bone. SEE thyrohyoid muscle.

**thy•ro•hy•oid mus•cle** apparently a continuation of the sternothyroid; *origin*, oblique line of thyroid cartilage; *insertion*, body of hyoid bone; *action*, approximates hyoid bone to the larynx; *nerve supply*, upper cervical spinal nerves carried by hypoglossal. SYN musculus thyrohyoideus.

**thy•roid** (thī′royd) resembling a shield; denoting a gland (thyroid gland) and a cartilage of the larynx (thyroid cartilage) having such a shape. [G. *thyreoeidēs*, fr. *thyreos*, an oblong shield, + *eidos*, form]

**thy•roid bru•it** vascular murmur heard over hyperactive thyroid gland, due to increased blood flow.

**thy•roid car•ti•lage** the largest of the cartilages of the larynx; it is formed of two approximately quadrilateral plates joined anteriorly at an angle of from 90° to 120°, the prominence so formed constituting the laryngeal prominence (Adam apple). SYN cartilago thyroidea [TA].

**thy•roid•ec•to•my** (thī-roy-dek′tō-mē) removal of the thyroid gland. [thyroid + G. *ektomē*, excision]

**thy•roid fol•li•cles** the small spherical vesicular

components of the thyroid gland lined with epithelium and containing colloid in varying amounts; the colloid serves for storage of the thyroid hormone precursor, thyroglobulin. SYN folliculi glandulae thyroideae [TA].

**thy•roid gland** an endocrine gland, consisting of irregularly spheroidal follicles, lying in front and to the sides of the upper part of the trachea, and of horseshoe shape, with two lateral lobes connected by a narrow central portion, the isthmus; occasionally an elongated offshoot, the pyramidal lobe, passes upward from the isthmus in front of the trachea. It is supplied by branches from the external carotid and subclavian arteries, and its nerves are derived from the middle cervical and cervicothoracic ganglia of the sympathetic system. It secretes thyroid hormone and calcitonin.

**thy•roid•i•tis** (thī-roy-dī′tis) inflammation of the thyroid gland. [thyroid + G. *-itis*, inflammation]

**thy•roid-sti•mu•lat•ing hor•mone** SYN thyrotropin.

**thy•roid-sti•mu•lat•ing im•mu•no•glob•u•lins (TSI)** in Graves disease, the antibodies to TSH receptors in the thyroid gland. These antibodies are produced by B-lymphocytes and stimulate the receptors, causing hyperthyroidism.

**thy•roid storm** SYN thyrotoxic crisis.

**thy•ro•lib•er•in** (thī-rō-lib′er-in) a tripeptide hormone from the hypothalamus, which stimulates the anterior lobe of the hypophysis to release thyrotropin. SYN thyrotropin-releasing hormone. [thyrotropin + L. *libero*, to free, + -in]

**thy•ro•meg•a•ly** (thī-rō-meg′ă-lē) enlargement of the thyroid gland. [thyro- + G. *megas*, large]

**thy•ro•nine** (thī′rō-nēn, thī′rō-nin) an amino acid with a diphenyl ether group in the side chain; occurs in proteins only in the form of iodinated derivatives (iodothyronines), such as thyroxine.

**thy•ro•par•a•thy•roid•ec•to•my** (thī′rō-par-ă-thī′roy-dek′tō-mē) excision of thyroid and parathyroid glands.

**thy•ro•pri•val** (thī-rō-prī′văl) relating to thyroprivia, denoting hypothyroidism produced by disease or thyroidectomy. [thyro- + L. *privus*, deprived of]

**thy•rop•to•sis** (thī-rop-tō′sis) downward dislocation of the thyroid gland. [thyro- + G. *ptōsis*, a falling]

**thy•rot•o•my** (thī′rot′ō-mē) **1.** any cutting operation on the thyroid gland. **2.** SYN laryngofissure. [thyro- + G. *tomē*, a cutting]

**thy•ro•tox•ic** (thī-rō-tok′sik) denoting thyrotoxicosis.

**thy•ro•tox•ic cri•sis, thy•roid cri•sis** the exacerbation of symptoms that occurs in severe thyrotoxicosis; marked by rapid pulse, nausea, diarrhea, fever, loss of weight, and extreme restlessness; coma and death may occur. SYN thyroid storm.

**thy•ro•tox•i•co•sis** (thī′rō-tok-si-kō′sis) the state produced by excessive quantities of endogenous or exogenous thyroid hormone. [thyro- + G. *toxikon*, poison, + *-osis*, condition]

**thy•ro•troph** (thī′rō-trof) a cell in the anterior lobe of the pituitary that produces thyrotropin.

**thy•ro•tro•phic** (thī-rō-trof′ik) SYN thyrotropic. [thyro- + G. *trophē*, nourishment]

**thy•rot•ro•phin** (thī-rot′rō-fin, thī-rō-trō′fin) SYN thyrotropin.

**thy•ro•tro•pic** (thī-rō-trop′ik) stimulating or nur-

t
h

turing the thyroid gland. SYN thyrotrophic. [thyro- + G. *tropē*, a turning]

**thy·rot·ro·pin** (thī-rot'rō-pin, thī-rō-trō'pin) a glycoprotein hormone produced by the anterior lobe of the hypophysis which stimulates the growth and function of the thyroid gland; it also is used as a diagnostic test to differentiate primary and secondary hypothyroidism. SYN thyroid-stimulating hormone, thyrotrophin. [for thyrotrophin, fr. thyro- + G. *trophē*, nourishment; corrupted to -tropin, and reanalyzed as fr. G. *tropē*, a turning]

**thy·ro·tro·pin-re·leas·ing hor·mone** SYN thyroliberin.

**thy·ro·tro·pin-re·leas·ing hor·mone sti·mu·la·tion test, TRH stim·u·la·tion test** a test of pituitary response to injection of thyrotropin-releasing hormone, which normally stimulates pituitary secretion of thyroid-stimulating hormone (TSH, thyrotropin), used primarily to distinguish pituitary from hypothalamic causes of thyroid disorders; TSH does not rise in cases of pituitary dysfunction, but does rise in cases of hypothalamic disorders.

**thy·rox·ine, thy·rox·in** (thī-rok'sēn, thī-rok'sin) the active iodine compound existing normally in the thyroid gland and extracted therefrom in crystalline form for therapeutic use; also prepared synthetically; used for the relief of hypothyroidism, cretinism, and myxedema.

**TI** the delay time between the inverting pulse and the "read" pulse in the inversion recovery experiment, in magnetic resonance imaging.

**Ti** titanium.

**TIA** transient ischemic attack.

**TIBC** total iron binding capacity.

**tib·ia,** gen. and pl. **tib·i·ae** (tib'ē-ă, tib'ē-ē) [TA] the medial and larger of the two bones of the leg, articulating with the femur, fibula, and talus. SYN shin bone. [L. the large shinbone]

**tib·i·al** (tib'ē-ăl) relating to the tibia or to any structure named from it; also denoting the medial or tibial aspect of the lower limb. [L. *tibialis*]

**tib·i·al col·la·ter·al lig·a·ment** SYN medial collateral ligament.

**tib·i·al·is an·ter·i·or mu·scle** medial muscle of anterior (dorsiflexor) compartment of leg; *origin*, upper two-thirds of lateral surface of tibia, interosseous membrane, and overlying crural fascia; *insertion*, medial cuneiform and base of first metatarsal; *action*, dorsiflexion and inversion of foot; provides dynamic support of longitudinal and transverse arches of foot; *nerve supply*, deep peroneal.

**tib·i·al·is pos·ter·i·or mu·scle** most anterior (deepest) muscle of deep posterior (plantar flexor) compartment of leg; *origin*, soleal line and posterior surface of tibia, the head and shaft of the fibula between the medial crest and interosseous border, and the posterior surface of interosseous membrane; *insertion*, navicular, three cuneiform, cuboid, and second, third, and fourth metatarsal bones; *action*, plantar flexion and inversion of foot; *nerve supply*, tibial. SYN musculus tibialis posterior [TA].

**tib·i·al nerve** one of the two major divisions of the sciatic nerve, it courses down the back of the leg to terminate as the medial and lateral plantar nerves in the foot; it supplies the hamstring muscles, the muscles of the back of the leg (the dorsiflexors and invertors of the foot) and the plantar aspect of the foot, as well as the skin on the back of the leg and sole of the foot. SYN nervus tibialis [TA].

**tib·ia val·ga** SYN genu valgum.

**tib·ia va·ra** SYN genu varum.

△**tib·io-** the tibia. [L. *tibia,* the large shinbone]

**tic** (tik) habitual, repeated contraction of certain muscles, resulting in stereotyped individualized actions that can be voluntarily suppressed for only brief periods, e.g., clearing the throat, sniffing, pursing the lips, excessive blinking; especially prominent when the person is under stress; there is no known pathologic substrate. SEE ALSO spasm. SYN Brissaud disease, habit spasm. [Fr.]

**tic dou·lou·reux** (tik doo-loo-rĕ') SYN trigeminal neuralgia. [Fr. painful]

**tick** (tik) ticks are arachnids, small bloodsucking parasites that may have either hard (*Ixodid* ticks) or soft (*Argasid* ticks) shells. Ticks normally feed on wild birds, mammals, or reptiles and transmit disease by feeding on an infected host (the reservoir host), then later feeding on a domestic animal or human. Ticks have a three-stage life cycle: larva, nymph (eight-legged), and adult (eight-legged), and require a blood meal at each stage before molting into the next stage or in the case of the adult, before mating and laying eggs.

Some common tick-borne diseases are *babesiosis:* the black-legged and Western black-legged ticks. *Colorado tick fever:* Rocky Mountain wood tick. *Ehrlichiosis (HGE and HME):* Lone Star tick and black-legged tick. *Lyme disease:* black-legged tick and Western black-legged tick. The "deer tick" was once thought by scientists at Yale to be a separate species, and named *Ixodes dammini.* It was later proven to be the same species as the black-legged tick, *Ixodes scapularis. Rocky Mountain spotted fever (RMSF):* American dog tick, Rocky Mountain wood tick, and Pacific Coast tick. *Tick-borne relapsing fever:* soft ticks (*Ornithodoros hermsi, O. turicata*). *Tick paralysis:* American dog and Rocky Mountain wood tick. *Tularemia (rabbit fever):* Lone Star tick, Rocky Mountain tick, Pacific Coast tick, American dog tick, black-legged tick.

**tick-borne en·ceph·a·li·tis East·ern sub·type** (ēst'ern) a severe form of encephalitis caused by a flavivirus and transmitted by ticks (*Ixodes pertulcatus* and *I. ricinus*).

**tick-borne en·ceph·a·li·tis vi·rus** an arbovirus of the genus *Flavivirus* that occurs in Central Europe and the republics of the former Soviet Union in two subtypes, causing two forms of encephalitis in humans: tick-borne encephalitis (Central European subtype) and tick-borne encephalitis (Eastern subtype); the vectors are ticks of the genus *Ixodes.*

**tick fe·ver 1.** any infectious disease of man or the lower animals caused by a protozoan blood parasite, a bacterium, a rickettsia, or a virus, and transmitted by a tick; **2.** the tick-borne variety of relapsing fever; **3.** SYN bovine babesiosis. **4.** SYN Rocky Mountain spotted fever. **5.** SYN Colorado tick fever.

**tick pa·ral·y·sis** an ascending paralysis caused by the continuing presence of *Dermacentor* and *Ixodes* ticks attached in the occipital region or on the upper neck of humans, often hidden under long hair.

**tick ty·phus** SYN boutonneuse fever.

**tid·al** (tī′dăl) relating to or resembling the tides, alternately rising and falling.

**tid·al air** SYN tidal volume.

**tid·al drain·age** drainage of the urinary bladder by means of an intermittent filling and emptying apparatus.

**tid·al vol·ume** the volume of air that is inspired or expired in a single breath during regular breathing. SYN tidal air.

**tide** (tīd) an alternate rise and fall, ebb and flow, or an increase or a decrease. [A.S. *tīd,* time]

**Tie·tze syn·drome** (tēt′sē) inflammation and painful, tender, nonsuppurative swelling of a costochondral junction.

**Tietz syn·drome** (tētz) autosomal dominant inheritance of albinism and deafness caused at least in some subsets of families by a mutation of the microophthalmia transcription factor gene.

**tight junc·tion** an intercellular junction between epithelial cells in which the outer leaflets of lateral cell membranes fuse to form a variable number of parallel interweaving strands that greatly reduce transepithelial permeability to macromolecules, solutes, and water via the paracellular route.

**tilt·ing disk valve** a variety of prosthetic cardiac valve composed of a caged disc.

**tilt·ing disk valve pro·sthe·sis** a low-profile artificial heart valve employing a caged disk that tilts to open during systole.

**tilt test** any measurement of response during tilting of the body usually head up but also head down. The test may be monitored by catheterization, echocardiography, electrophysiologic measurements, electrocardiography, or mechanocardiography.

**tim·bre** (tam′br, tim′br) the distinguishing quality of a sound, by which one may determine its source. [Fr.]

**time (t)** (tīm) **1.** that relation of events which is expressed by the terms past, present, and future, and measured by units such as minutes, hours, days, months, or years. **2.** a certain period during which something definite or determined is done. SYN tempus (2). [A.S. *tima*]

**Time-Line ther·a·py** a technique, based on the principles of neurolinguistic programming, for releasing negative emotions and revising limiting decisions, that directs the client, in a dissociated state, to return to significant past events with new resources so that negative emotions can be released or limiting decisions revised. SEE ALSO dissociation (4).

**tin (Sn)** (tin) a metallic element, atomic no. 50, atomic wt. 118.710. SYN stannum. [AS, tin]

**tinct** l. tinctura, tincture.

**tinc·to·ri·al** (tingk-tōr′ē-ăl) relating to coloring or staining. [L. *tinctorius,* fr. *tingo,* to dye]

**tinc·ture** (tingk′cher) an alcoholic or hydroalcoholic solution prepared from vegetable materials or from chemical substances. [see *tinctura*]

**tin·ea** (tin′ē-ă) a fungus infection (dermatophytosis) of the keratin component of hair, skin, or nails. Genera of fungi causing such infection are *Microsporum, Trichophyton,* and *Epidermophyton.* SYN ringworm, serpigo (1). [L. worm, moth]

**tin·ea bar·bae** tinea of the beard, occurring as a follicular infection or as a granulomatous lesion; the primary lesions are papules and pustules. SYN barber's itch, folliculitis barbae, tinea sycosis.

**tin·ea cap·i·tis** a common form of fungus infection of the scalp caused by various species of *Microsporum* and *Trichophyton* on or within hair shafts, occurring almost exclusively in children and characterized by irregularly placed and variously sized patches of apparent baldness because of hairs breaking off at the surface of the scalp, scaling, black dots, and occasionally erythema and pyoderma.

**tin·ea circ·i·na·ta** SYN tinea corporis.

**tin·ea cor·por·is** a well-defined, scaling, macular eruption of dermatophytosis that frequently forms annular lesions and may appear on any part of the body. See page B6. SYN tinea circinata.

**tin·ea crur·is** a form of tinea imbricata occurring in the genitocrural region, including the inner side of the thighs, the perineal region, and the groin. SYN eczema marginatum, jock itch.

**tin·ea im·bri·ca·ta** an eruption consisting of a number of concentric rings of overlapping scales forming papulosquamous patches scattered over the body; it occurs in tropical climates and is caused by the fungus *Trichophyton concentricum.*

**tin·ea ker·i·on** an inflammatory fungus infection of the scalp and beard, marked by pustules and a boggy infiltration of the surrounding parts; most commonly caused by *Microsporum audouinii.*

**tin·ea ped·is** dermatophytosis of the feet, especially of the skin between the toes, caused by one of the dermatophytes, usually a species of *Trichophyton* or *Epidermophyton;* the disease consists of small vesicles, fissures, scaling, maceration, and eroded areas between the toes and on the plantar surface of the foot; other skin areas may be involved. See page B6. SYN athlete's foot.

**tin·ea sy·co·sis** SYN tinea barbae.

**tin·ea un·gui·um** ringworm of the nails due to a dermatophyte.

**tin·ea ver·si·col·or** an eruption of tan or brown branny patches on the skin of the trunk, often appearing white, in contrast with hyperpigmented skin after exposure to the summer sun; caused by growth of *Malassezia furfur* in the stratum corneum with minimal inflammatory reaction. SYN pityriasis versicolor.

**Ti·nel sign** (tē-nel′) distally radiating pain or paresthesia caused by tapping over the site of a superficial nerve, indicating inflammation or irritation of the nerve.

**tine test** SEE tuberculin test.

**tin·ni·tus** (tin′ĭ-tŭs) a sensation of noises (ringing, whistling, booming) in the ears. [L. a jingling, fr. *tinnio,* pp. *tinnitus,* to jingle, clink]

**tip 1.** a point; a more or less sharp extremity. **2.** a separate, but attached, piece of the same or another structure, forming the extremity of a part.

**tip pinch** OCCUPATIONAL THERAPY pinch between the tips of the index finger and the thumb.

**TIPS** transjugular intrahepatic portosystemic shunt.

**tir·ing** (tīr′ing) SYN cerclage. [Eng. tire]

**tis·sue** (tish′oo) an aggregation of similar cells or types of cells, together with any associated intercellular materials, adapted to perform one or more specific functions. There are four basic tissues in the body: 1) epithelium; 2) connective tissue, including blood, bone, and cartilage; 3) muscle; and 4) nerve. [Fr. *tissu,* woven, fr. L. *texo,* to weave]

**tis·sue cul·ture** the maintenance of live tissue

t
i

after removal from the body, by placing in a vessel with a sterile nutritive medium.

**tis·sue lymph** true lymph, i.e., lymph derived chiefly from fluid in tissue spaces (in contrast to blood lymph).

**tis·sue plas·min·o·gen ac·ti·va·tor** thrombolytic serine protease catalyzing the enzymatic conversion of plasminogen to plasmin; a genetically engineered protein used as a thrombolytic agent in patients with thrombotic occlusion of a coronary or cerebral artery.

**tis·sue res·pir·a·tion** the interchange of gases between the blood and the tissues. SYN internal respiration.

**tis·sue-spe·ci·fic ant·i·gen** SYN organ-specific antigen.

**tis·sue ten·sion** a theoretical condition of equilibrium or balance between the tissues and cells whereby overaction of any part is restrained by the pull of the mass.

**tis·sue throm·bo·plas·tin in·hi·bi·tion time** a test used to identify lupus anticoagulant; the thromboplastin source used in the prothrombin test is diluted to increase sensitivity to inhibitors.

**ti·ta·ni·um (Ti)** (tī-tā'nē-ŭm) a metallic element, atomic no. 22, atomic wt. 47.88, used as an implant in dental work because of its uniquely high level of biocompatibility. [*Titans,* in G. myth., sons of Earth]

**ti·ter** (tī'ter) the standard of strength of a volumetric test solution; the assay value of an unknown measure by volumetric means. [Fr. *titre,* standard]

**ti·trate** (tī'trāt) to analyze volumetrically by a solution (the titrant) of known strength to an end point.

**ti·tra·tion** (tī-trā'shŭn) volumetric analysis by addition of definite amounts of a test solution to a solution of the substance being assayed. [Fr. *titre,* standard]

**tit·u·ba·tion** (tit-yu-bā'shŭn) **1.** a staggering or stumbling in trying to walk. **2.** a tremor or shaking of the head, of cerebellar origin. [L. *titubo,* pp. *-atus,* to stagger]

**Tiz·zo·ni stain** (ted-zō'nē) a stain used as a test for iron in tissue; the tissue is treated with a solution of potassium ferrocyanide and then with dilute hydrochloric acid; a blue coloration indicates the presence of iron.

**Tl** thallium.

**TLC** thin-layer chromatography; total lung capacity.

**TLD** thermoluminescent dosimeter.

**T lym·pho·cyte** a thymocyte-derived lymphocyte of immunologic importance that is responsible for cell-mediated immunity. These cells have the characteristic T3 surface marker and may be further divided into subsets according to function, such as helper, suppressor, and cytotoxic. SEE ALSO B lymphocyte. SYN T cell.

**T-lym·pho·cyte ant·i·gen re·cep·tor** SYN T-cell receptor.

**Tm** thulium; transport maximum.

**TMJ** colloquial for temporomandibular joint dysfunction.

**TMJ syn·drome** SYN myofacial pain-dysfunction syndrome.

**TMP** ribothymidylic acid; trimethoprim; sometimes for deoxyribothymidylic acid.

**TMT** tarsometatarsal.

**T-my·co·plas·ma** SYN *Ureaplasma.*

**Tn 1.** ocular tension. **2.** troponin.

**TNM** tumor-node-metastasis. SEE TNM staging.

**TNM stag·ing** a system of clinicopathologic evaluation of tumors based on the extent of tumor involvement at the primary site (T, followed by a number indicating size and depth of invasion), and lymph node involvement (N) and metastasis (M), each followed by a number starting at 0 for no evident metastasis; numbers used depend on the organ involved and influence the prognosis and choice of treatment.

**TNTC** too numerous to count (indicating the finding of a large number of discrete objects, usually cells in a urine specimen, of which precise enumeration is not practicable).

**to·bac·co-al·co·hol am·bly·o·pia** an acquired optic neuropathy particularly involving the maculopapillary bundle nerve fibers associated with excessive alcohol and tobacco consumption.

**to·bac·co heart** cardiac irritability marked by irregular action, palpitation, and sometimes pain, believed to occur as a result of the heavy use of tobacco.

**to·cain·ide hy·dro·chlor·ide** (tō-kā'nīd hī-drō-klō'rīd) an oral antiarrhythmic agent, similar in action to lidocaine, used in the treatment of ventricular arrhythmias.

△**to·co-** childbirth. [G. *tokos,* birth]

**toc·o·dy·na·graph** (tō-kō-dī'nă-graf, tok-ō-dī'nă-graf) a recording of the force of uterine contractions. [toco- + G. *dynamis,* force, + *graphē,* a writing]

**toc·o·dy·na·mom·e·ter** (tō'kō-dī-nă-mom'ĕ-ter, tok'ō-dī-nă-mom'ĕ-ter) an instrument for measuring the force of uterine contractions. [toco- + G. *dynamis,* force, + *metron,* measure]

**to·cog·ra·phy** (tō-kog'ră-fē) the process of recording uterine contractions. [toco- + G. *graphō,* to write]

**to·co·lyt·ic** (tō-kō-lit'ik) denoting any pharmacological agent used to arrest uterine contractions; often used in an attempt to arrest premature labor contractions. [G. *tokos,* childbirth, labor, + *lysis,* loosening]

**to·coph·er·ol (T)** (tō-kof'er-ōl) **1.** a generic term for vitamin E and compounds chemically related to it, with or without biological activity. **2.** a methylated tocol or methylated tocotrienol.

**Todd pa·ral·y·sis** (tod) paralysis of temporary duration (normally not more than a few days) that occurs in the limb or limbs involved in jacksonian epilepsy after the seizure. SYN Todd postepileptic paralysis.

**Todd post·e·pi·lep·tic pa·ral·y·sis** (tod) SYN Todd paralysis.

**toe** (tō) one of the digits of the feet. [A.S. *ta*]

**toe-drop** (tō'drop) inability to dorsiflex the toes, usually due to paralysis of the toe extensor muscles.

**toe·nail** (tō'nāl) SEE nail.

**To·ga·vir·i·dae** (tō-gă-vir'i-dē) a family of viruses that includes the following genera: *Alphavirus,* which includes eastern equine encephalitis, western equine encephalitis, Venezuelan equine encephalitis, and the rubella virus (*Rubivirus*).

**to·ga·vi·rus** (tō'gă-vī'rŭs) any virus of the family Togaviridae. [L. *toga,* garment covering, + virus]

**toi·let** (toy-let') **1.** cleansing of the obstetrical patient after childbirth or of a wound after an operation preparatory to the application of the dressing. **2.** DENTISTRY cavity debridement, the final step before placing a restoration in a tooth whereby the cavity is cleaned and all debris is removed. [Fr. *toilette*]

**Toi·son stain** (twa-zah′) a blood diluent and leukocyte stain containing methyl violet, sodium chloride, sodium sulfate, and glycerin; also used for erythrocyte counts.

**Tok·er cell** (tō-ker) an epithelial cell with clear cytoplasm found in 10% of normal nipples; contains keratin 7, like Paget carcinoma cells, from which it must be distinguished cytologically.

△**toko-** SEE toco-.

**tol·bu·ta·mide test** a test to detect insulin-producing tumors; after a 1-g intravenous dose of tolbutamide, plasma insulin and glucose are measured at intervals up to 3 hr; higher insulin responses and lower glucose values characterize patients with such tumors.

**Toldt mem·brane** (tōlt) the anterior layer of the renal fascia.

**tol·er·ance** (tol′er-ăns) **1.** the ability to endure or be less responsive to a stimulus, especially over a period of continued exposure. **2.** the power of resisting the action of a poison or of taking a drug continuously or in large doses without injurious effects. [L. *tolero*, pp. *-atus*, to endure]

**tol·er·ance dose** the largest dose of a remedy that can be accepted without the production of injurious symptoms.

**tol·er·ance li·mits** specified performance limits for allowable error for a test; the limits selected should depend on both the effect of the error on the clinical significance of a test and on what is technically achievable.

**tol·er·ant** (tol′er-ănt) having the property of tolerance.

**tol·er·ize** (tol′er-īz) to induce tolerance.

**tol·er·o·gen·ic** (tol′er-ō-jen′ik) producing immunologic tolerance.

**To·lo·sa-Hunt syn·drome** (tō-lō′sah-hŭnt) cavernous sinus syndrome produced by an idiopathic granuloma.

**tolu·i·dine blue stain** a stain used for *Pneumocystis carinii* trophozoites.

**To·ma sign** (tō′mah) to distinguish between inflammatory and noninflammatory ascites: in inflammatory conditions of the peritoneum, the mesentery contracts, drawing the intestines over to the right side; consequently, with the patient supine, tympany is elicited on the right side, dullness on the left.

△**-tome 1.** a cutting instrument, the first element in the compound usually indicating the part that the instrument is designed to cut. **2.** segment, part, section. **3.** tomography. **4.** surgery. [G. *tomos*, cutting, sharp; a cutting (section or segment)]

**to·men·tum, to·men·tum ce·re·bri** (tō-men′tŭm, tō-men′tŭm ser′ĕ-brī) the numerous small blood vessels passing between the cerebral surface of the pia mater and the cortex of the brain. [L. a stuffing for cushions]

**Tom·ma·sel·li dis·ease** (tom-ĕ-sel′ē) hemoglobinuria and pyrexia due to quinine intoxication.

**to·mo·gram** (tō′mō-gram) a radiograph obtained by tomography. [G. *tomos*, a cutting (section) + *gramma*, a writing]

**to·mo·graph** (tō′mō-graf) the radiographic equipment used in tomography. [G. *tomos*, a cutting (section), + *graphō*, to write]

**to·mog·ra·phy** (tō-mog′ră-fē) making a radiographic image of a selected plane by means of reciprocal linear or curved motion of the x-ray tube and film cassette; images of all other planes are blurred ("out of focus") by being relatively displaced on the film. SYN planigraphy, planography, stratigraphy.

△**-to·my** a cutting operation. SEE ALSO -ectomy. [G. *tomē*, incision]

**tone** (tōn) **1.** a musical sound. **2.** the character of the voice expressing an emotion. **3.** the tension present in resting muscles. **4.** firmness of the tissues; normal functioning of all the organs. **5.** to perform toning. [G. *tonos*, tone, or a tone]

**tongue** (tŭng) **1.** a mobile mass of muscular tissue covered with mucous membrane, occupying the cavity of the mouth and forming part of its floor, constituting also by its posterior portion the anterior wall of the pharynx. It bears the organ of taste, assists in mastication and deglutition, and is the principal instrument of articulate speech. SYN lingua (1) [TA], glossa. **2.** a tonguelike structure. SYN lingua (2) [TA]. [A.S. *tunge*]

**tongue crib** an appliance used to control visceral (infantile) swallowing and tongue thrusting and to encourage the mature or somatic tongue posture and function.

**tongue-swal·low·ing** a slipping back of the tongue against the pharynx, causing choking.

**tongue thrust** the infantile pattern of the suckle-swallow movement in which the tongue is placed between the incisor teeth or the alveolar ridges during the initial stage of swallowing, resulting sometimes in an anterior open bite.

**tongue thrust ther·a·py** SYN myofunctional therapy.

**tongue-tie** SYN ankyloglossia.

**ton·ic** (ton′ik) **1.** in a state of continuous unremitting action; denoting especially a muscular contraction. **2.** invigorating; increasing physical or mental tone or strength. **3.** a remedy purported to restore enfeebled function and promote vigor and a sense of well-being qualified, according to the organ or system on which they are presumed to act, as cardiac, digestive, hematic, vascular, nervine, uterine, general, etc. [G. *tonikos*, fr. *tonos*, tone]

**ton·ic con·trac·tion** sustained contraction of a muscle, as employed in the maintenance of posture.

**ton·ic con·vul·sion** a convulsion in which muscle contraction is sustained.

**ton·ic ep·i·lep·sy** an attack in which the body is rigid.

**to·nic·i·ty** (tō-nis′i-tē) **1.** a state of normal tension of the tissues by virtue of which the parts are kept in shape, alert, and ready to function in response to a suitable stimulus. In the case of muscle, it refers to a state of continuous activity or tension beyond that related to the physical properties; i.e., it is active resistance to stretch; in skeletal muscle it is dependent upon the efferent innervation. SYN tonus. **2.** the osmotic pressure or tension of a solution, usually relative to that of blood. SEE ALSO isotonicity. [G. *tonos*, tone]

**ton·ic neck re·flex** a brainstem-level reflex that may produce positional changes of all limbs in response to active or passive head turning or to flexion/extension of the head.

**ton·i·co·clon·ic** (ton-i-kō-klon′ik) both tonic and clonic, referring to muscular spasms. SYN tonoclonic.

**ton·ic pu·pil** a general term for a pupil with

delayed, slow, long-lasting contractions to light and to a near vision effort, often with light-near dissociation; due to denervation and aberrant reinnervation of the iris sphincter; seen in various autonomic neuropathies and in Adie syndrome.

**ton·ic spa·sm** a continuous involuntary muscular contraction.

**tonic state** steady rigid muscle contractions with no relaxation.

△**tono-** tone, tension, pressure. [G. *tonos*]

**ton·o·clon·ic** (ton-ō-klon'ik) SYN tonicoclonic.

**ton·o·clon·ic spa·sm** convulsive contraction of muscles.

**ton·o·fi·bril** (ton-ō-fī'bril) one of a system of fibers found in the cytoplasm of epithelial cells. SEE cytoskeleton.

**ton·o·fil·a·ment** (ton-ō-fil'ă-ment) a structural cytoplasmic protein, bundles of which together form a tonofibril; tonofilaments are made up of a variable number of related proteins, keratins, and are found in all epithelial cells.

**ton·o·graph** (ton'ō-graf) a recording tonometer. [tono- + G. *graphō*, to write]

**to·nog·ra·phy** (tō-nog'ră-fē) continuous measurement of intraocular pressure by means of a recording tonometer, in order to determine the facility of aqueous outflow.

**to·nom·e·ter** (tō-nom'ě-ter) **1.** an instrument for determining pressure or tension, especially determining ocular tension. **2.** a vessel for equilibrating a liquid (e.g., blood) with a gas, usually at a controlled temperature. [tono- + G. *metron*, measure]

**to·nom·e·try** (tō-nom'ě-trē) **1.** measurement of the tension of a part, e.g., intravascular tension or blood pressure. **2.** measurement of ocular tension.

**ton·o·plast** (tō'nō-plast, ton'ō-plast) an intracellular structure or vacuole. [tono- + G. *plastos*, formed]

**to·no·top·ic** (tō-nō-top'ik) denoting a spatial arrangement of structures such that certain tone frequencies are transmitted, as in the auditory pathway. [tono- + G. *topos*, place]

**to·no·tro·pic** (tō-nō-trop'ik) denoting the shortening of the resting length of a muscle. [G. *tonikos, tonos,* tone, + *tropos,* a turning]

**ton·sil** (ton'sil) **1.** any collection of lymphoid tissue. **2.** SYN palatine tonsil. [L. *tonsilla,* a stake, in pl. the tonsils]

**ton·sil of ce·re·bel·lum** a rounded lobule on the undersurface of each cerebellar hemisphere, continuous medially with the uvula of the cerebellar vermis. SYN tonsilla cerebelli [TA].

**ton·sil·la,** pl. **ton·sil·lae** (ton-sil'ă, ton-sil'ē) [TA] SYN palatine tonsil. [L. (see tonsil)]

**ton·sil·la ce·re·bel·li** [TA] SYN tonsil of cerebellum.

**ton·sil·la lin·gua·lis** [TA] SYN lingual tonsil.

**ton·sil·la pal·a·ti·na** [TA] SYN palatine tonsil.

**ton·sil·lar, ton·sil·lary** (ton'si-lăr, ton'si-lă-rē) relating to a tonsil, especially the palatine tonsil.

**ton·sil·lar crypt** one of the variable number of deep recesses that extend into the palatine and pharyngeal tonsils from the free surface where they open at the tonsillar fossa.

**ton·sil·lar fos·sa** the depression between the palatoglossal and palatopharyngeal arches occupied by the palatine tonsil.

**ton·sil·lec·to·my** (ton'si-lek'tō-mē) removal of the entire tonsil. [tonsil + G. *ektomē,* excision]

**ton·sil·li·tis** (ton'si-lī'tis) inflammation of a tonsil, especially of the palatine tonsil. [tonsil + G. *-itis,* inflammation]

△**ton·sil·lo-** tonsil. [L. *tonsilla*]

**ton·sil·lo·lith** (ton-sil'ō-lith) a calcareous concretion in a distended tonsillar crypt. SYN tonsilolith. [tonsillo- + G. *lithos,* stone]

**ton·sil·lot·o·my** (ton'si-lot'ō-mē) the cutting away of a portion or all of a hypertrophied faucial tonsil. [tonsillo- + G. *tomē,* incision]

**ton·sil·o·lith** (ton'si-lith) SYN tonsillolith.

**to·nus** (tō'nŭs) SYN tonicity (1). [L., fr. G. *tonos*]

**Tooth** (tooth), Howard H., English physician, 1856–1925. SEE Charcot-Marie-Tooth disease.

▣**tooth,** pl. **teeth** (tooth, tēth; tēth) one of the hard conical structures set in the alveoli of the upper and lower jaws, used in mastication and assisting in articulation. A tooth is a dermal structure composed of dentin and encased in cementum on the anatomic root and enamel on its anatomic crown. It consists of a root buried in the alveolus, a neck covered by the gum, and a crown, the exposed portion. In the center is the pulp cavity filled with a connective tissue reticulum containing a jelly-like substance, blood vessels, and nerves that enter through a canal at the apex of the root. The 20 deciduous teeth, or primary teeth, appear between the 6th and 9th through the 24th month of life; these exfoliate and are replaced by the 32 permanent teeth appearing between the 5th and 7th year through the 17th to 23rd year. There are four kinds of teeth: incisor, canine, premolar, and molar. See this page. SYN dens (1) [TA]. [A.S. *tōth*]

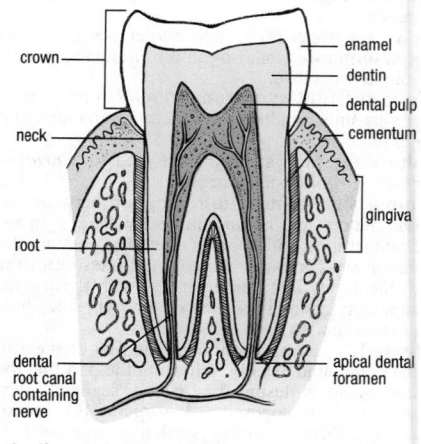

**tooth** and supporting tissues

Labels: crown, neck, root, dental root canal containing nerve, enamel, dentin, dental pulp, cementum, gingiva, apical dental foramen

**tooth·ache** (tooth'āk) pain in a tooth due to the condition of the pulp or periodontal ligament resulting from caries, infection, or trauma. SYN dentalgia, odontalgia.

**tooth bud** the primordial structures from which a tooth is formed; the enamel organ, the dental papilla, and the dental sac enclosing them.

**tooth germ** the enamel organ and dental papilla, constituting the developing tooth.

**tooth pulp** SYN dental pulp.

**tooth sock·et** a socket in the alveolar process of the maxilla or mandible, into which each tooth fits and is attached by means of the periodontal ligament. SYN alveolus (4) [TA].

**top•ag•no•sis** (top-ag-nō'sis) inability to localize tactile sensations. SYN topoanesthesia. [top- + G. *a-* priv. + *gnōsis,* recognition]

**to•pal•gia** (tō-pal'jē-ă) pain localized in one spot; a symptom occurring in neuroses whereby localized pain, without evident organic basis, is experienced. [top- + G. *algos,* pain]

**top•es•the•sia** (top'es-thē'zē-ă) the ability to localize a light touch applied to any part of the skin. [top- + G. *aisthēsis,* sensation]

**to•pha•ceous** (tō-fā'shŭs) sandy; gritty; pertaining to or manifesting the features of a tophus. [L. *tophaceus*]

**to•pha•ceous gout** gout in which deposits of uric acid and urates occur as gouty tophi.

**to•phus,** pl. **to•phi** (tō'fŭs, tō'fī) **1.** SEE gouty tophus. **2.** a salivary calculus, or tartar. [L. a calcareous deposit from springs, tufa]

**top•i•cal** (top'i-kăl) relating to a definite place or locality; local. [G. *topikos,* fr. *topos,* place]

**top•i•cal an•es•the•sia** superficial loss of sensation in conjunctiva, mucous membranes or skin, produced by direct application of local anesthetic solutions, ointments, or jellies.

△**to•po-, top-** place, topical. [G. *topos*]

**top•o•an•es•the•sia** (top'ō-an-es-thē'zē-ă) SYN topagnosis. [topo- + anesthesia]

**To•po•gra•fov vi•rus** (tō-pō-grā-fov) a Hantavirus species found in Siberia.

**to•po•gra•phi•cal or•i•en•ta•tion** determination of the position of objects and settings and the route to a desired location.

**top•o•graph•ic a•na•to•my** SYN regional anatomy.

**to•pog•ra•phy** (tō-pog'ră-fē) ANATOMY the description of any part of the body, especially in relation to a definite and limited area of the surface. [topo- + G. *graphē,* a writing]

**To•po•lan•ski sign** (tō-pō-lan'skē) congestion of the pericorneal region of the eye in Graves disease.

**top•o•nar•co•sis** (top'ō-nar-kō'sis) a localized cutaneous anesthesia. [topo- + narcosis]

**TORCH** *t*oxoplasmosis, *o*ther infections, *r*ubella, *c*ytomegalorvirus infection, and *h*erpes simplex. SEE TORCH syndrome.

**TORCH syn•drome** a group of infections with similar clinical manifestations, although symptoms may vary in degree and time of appearance: *t*oxoplasmosis, *o*ther infections, *r*ubella, *c*ytomegalovirus infection, and *h*erpes simplex. These infections might be associated with underlying HIV infection.

**Torn•waldt ab•scess** (tōrn'vahlt) chronic infection of the pharyngeal bursa. SEE ALSO Tornwaldt syndrome.

**Torn•waldt cyst** (tōrn'vahlt) inflammation or obstruction of the pharyngeal bursa or an adenoid cleft with the formation of a cyst containing pus.

**Torn•waldt syn•drome** (tōrn'vahlt) nasopharyngeal discharge, occipital headache, and stiffness of posterior cervical muscles, with halitosis due to chronic infection of the pharyngeal bursa.

**To•ro•vi•rus** (tō-rō-vī-rŭs) a genus in the family Coronaviridae that causes enteric infections in animals.

**tor•pid** (tōr'pid) inactive; sluggish. [L. *torpidus,* fr. *torpeo,* to be sluggish]

**tor•por** (tōr'per) inactivity, sluggishness. [L. sluggishness, numbness]

**torque (T)** (tōrk) **1.** a rotatory force. **2.** DENTISTRY a torsion force applied to a tooth to produce or maintain crown or root movement. [L. *torqueo,* to twist]

**Tor•re syn•drome** (tor'ā) multiple sebaceous gland adenomas associated with multiple visceral malignancies, often colorectal carcinoma.

**torsade de pointes** (tōr-săd dĕ pwant') "twisting of the points," a form of ventricular tachycardia nearly always due to medications and characterized by a long QT interval and a "short-long-short" sequence in the beat preceding its onset. The QRS complexes during this rhythm tend to show a series of complexes points up followed by complexes points down, often with a narrow waist between. [Fr. *torsade,* fringe, twist, or coil, + *pointe,* point or tip (euphonious for "wave burst")]

**tor•sion** (tōr'shŭn) **1.** a twisting or rotation of a part upon its long axis. **2.** twisting of the cut end of an artery to arrest hemorrhage. **3.** rotation of the eye around its anteroposterior axis. SEE ALSO intorsion, extorsion, dextrotorsion, levotorsion. [L. *torsio,* fr. *torqueo,* to twist]

**tor•sion•al de•for•mi•ty** ORTHOPEDICS a deformity caused by rotation of a portion of an extremity with relationship to the long axis of the entire extremity.

**tor•sion frac•ture** a fracture resulting from twisting of the limb.

**tor•sion spa•sm** SYN dystonia.

**tor•si•ver•sion** (tōr-si-ver'shŭn) a malposition of a tooth in which it is rotated on its long axis. SYN torsoclusion (2).

**tor•so** (tōr'sō) the trunk; the body without relation to head or extremities. [It.]

**tor•so•clu•sion** (tōr'sō-kloo-zhŭn) **1.** acupressure performed by entering the needle in the tissues parallel with the artery, then turning it so that it crosses the artery transversely, and passing it into the tissues on the opposite side of the vessel. **2.** SYN torsiversion. [L. *torqueo,* to twist, + *claudo* or *cludo,* to close]

**tor•ti•col•lar** (tōr-ti-kol'ăr) relating to or marked by torticollis.

**tor•ti•col•lis** (tōr-ti-kol'is) a contraction, often spasmodic, of the muscles of the neck, chiefly those supplied by the spinal accessory nerve; the head is drawn to one side and usually rotated so that the chin points to the other side. SYN wryneck, wry neck. [L. *tortus,* twisted, + *collum,* neck]

**tor•tu•ous** (tōr'choo-ŭs) having many curves; full of turns and twists. [L. *tortuosus,* fr. *torqueo,* to twist]

**Tor•u•lop•sis** a genus of yeasts with smaller blastoconidia (2 to 4 mm) with a wide attachment to the parent cell; the species *Toruplopsis glabrata* is the causative agent of torulopsosis, usually in immunocompromised hosts.

**tor•u•lop•so•sis** (tōr-yu-lop'sō-sis) a usually opportunistic infection caused by *Torulopsis glabrata* and seen in patients with severe underlying disease or in immunocompromised patients; the disease may be bronchopulmonary, genitourinary, or septicemic. SEE *Torulopsis.*

**tor•u•lus,** pl. **tor•u•li** (tōr'yu-lŭs, tōr'yu-lī) a minute elevation or papilla. [L. dim. of *torus,* a protuberance, swelling]

**to•rus**, pl. **to•ri** (tō′rŭs, tō′rī) **1.** a geometrical figure formed by the revolution of a circle round the base of any of its arcs, such as the convex molding at the base of a pillar. **2.** a rounded swelling, such as that caused by a contracting muscle. SYN elevation. [L. swelling, knot, bulge]

**to•rus frac•ture** a deformity in children consisting of a local bulging caused by the longitudinal compression of the soft bone; it occurs commonly in the radius or ulna or both.

**torus man•di•bu•lar•is** a hyperostosis on the lingual aspect of the lower jaw in the canine-premolar region.

**tor•us pal•a•tin•us** a hyperostosis in the midline of the hard palate.

**TOS** thoracic outlet syndrome.

**to•tal a•no•ma•lous pul•mo•nary ven•ous re•turn (TAPVR)** SEE anomalous pulmonary venous connections, total or partial.

**to•tal a•pha•sia** SYN global aphasia.

**to•tal bod•y hy•po•ther•mia** the deliberate reduction of total body temperature, in order to reduce tissue metabolism.

**to•tal breath•ing cy•cle time** the time necessary for a complete breath (inhalation and exhalation); the period from the beginning of inspiratory flow of one breath to the beginning of inspiratory flow for the next breath.

**to•tal com•mu•ni•ca•tion** habilitation of individuals who are deaf or hearing impaired using any or all appropriate methods to enhance communication; particularly, the combination of manual and oral techniques. SYN simultaneous communication.

**to•tal cri•coid cleft** SEE laryngotracheoesophageal cleft.

**to•tal dai•ly en•er•gy ex•pen•di•ture** daily energy expenditure, consisting of basal and sleeping conditions (60–75%), thermogenic effect of the food consumed (10%), and energy expended during physical activity and recovery (15–30%).

**to•tal end-di•a•stol•ic di•a•me•ter** cross sectional diameter of the left ventricle including the septum and posterior wall thicknesses in diastole.

**to•tal end-sys•tol•ic di•a•me•ter** cross sectional diameter of the left ventricle including the septum and posterior wall thicknesses in systole.

**to•tal hy•per•o•o•pi•a (Ht)** that which can be determined after complete paralysis of accommodation by means of a cycloplegic.

**to•tal iron bind•ing ca•pac•it•y (TIBC)** an indirect method of determining the transferrin level in serum. Transferrin is saturated by the addition of iron to a serum specimen. Excess iron is removed and the specimen is analyzed for iron content. The result is the total amount of iron that can be bound by transferrin. This result is helpful in differentiating anemias. A high TIBC is associated with iron deficiency; low TIBC is associated with excess iron.

**to•tal joint ar•thro•plas•ty** arthroplasty in which both joint surfaces are replaced with artificial materials, usually metal and high-density plastic.

**to•tal lung ca•pac•i•ty (TLC)** the inspiratory capacity plus the functional residual capacity; i.e., the volume of air contained in the lungs at the end of a maximal inspiration; also equals vital capacity plus residual volume.

🔲 **to•tal par•en•ter•al nu•trit•ion (TPN)** nutrition maintained entirely by intravenous injection or other nongastrointestinal route. See this page.

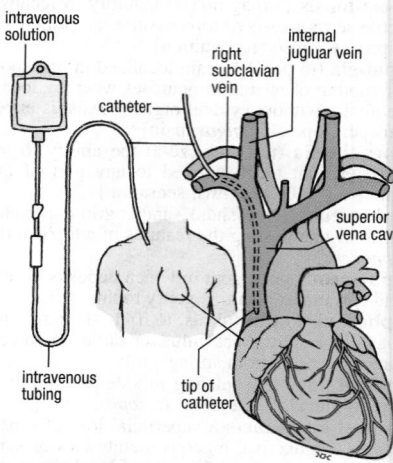

**total parenteral nutrition:** catheter enters the circulation at the right subclavian vein

**to•tal trans•fu•sion** SYN exchange transfusion.

**to•ti•po•ten•cy, to•ti•po•tence** (tō-ti-pō′ten-sē, tō-tip′ō-tens) the ability of a cell to differentiate into any type of cell and thus form a new organism or regenerate any part of an organism. [L. *totus*, entire, + *potentia*, power]

**to•ti•po•tent, to•ti•po•ten•tial** (tō-tip′ō-tent, tō′ ti-pō-ten′shăl) relating to totipotency.

**touch** (tŭch) **1.** the sense by which slight contact with the skin or mucous membrane is perceived. **2.** SYN palpation (1). [Fr. *toucher*]

**Toupet fun•do•pli•ca•tion** (too′pet) a partial posterior fundoplication, in which the stomach edge is secured to the esophagus; modifications of Toupet fundoplication are commonly used for laparoscopic fundoplication.

**Tou•rette dis•ease** (toor-et′) SYN Tourette syndrome.

**Tou•rette syn•drome** (toor-et′) a tic disorder appearing in childhood, characterized by multiple motor tics and vocal tics present for more than one year. Obsessive-compulsive behavior, attention-deficit disorder, and other psychiatric disorders may be associated; coprolalia and echolalia rarely occur; autosomal dominant inheritance. SYN Gilles de la Tourette syndrome, Tourette disease.

**tour•ni•quet** (toor′ni-ket) an instrument for temporarily arresting the flow of blood to or from a distal part by pressure applied with an encircling device. [Fr. fr. *tourner*, to turn]

**Tou•ton gi•ant cell** (too′tŏn) a xanthoma cell in which the multiple nuclei are grouped around a small island of nonfoamy cytoplasm.

**To•vell tube** (tō-vel′) an armored tracheal tube with a wire spiral embedded in the wall to prevent obstruction of the lumen when the tube is compressed and kinking when the tube is bent at a sharp angle.

**tox•ae•mia [Br.]** SEE toxemia.

**tox•e•mia** (tok-sē′mē-ă) **1.** clinical manifestations

observed during certain infectious diseases, assumed to be caused by toxins and other noxious substances elaborated by the infectious agent. **2.** the clinical syndrome caused by toxic substances in the blood. **3.** a lay term referring to the hypertensive disorders of pregnancy. [G. *toxikon,* poison, + *haima,* blood]

**tox·e·mic** (tok-sē′mik) pertaining to, affected by, or manifesting the features of toxemia.

**tox·ic** (tok′sik) **1.** SYN poisonous. **2.** pertaining to a toxin. [G. *toxikon,* an arrow-poison]

**tox·ic cir·rho·sis** cirrhosis of the liver resulting from chronic poisoning or carbon tetrachloride.

**tox·ic ep·i·der·mal ne·crol·y·sis (TEN)** a syndrome in which a large portion of the skin becomes intensely erythematous, with epidermal necrosis and flaccid bullae, resulting from drug sensitivity or of unknown cause. See this page. SYN Lyell syndrome.

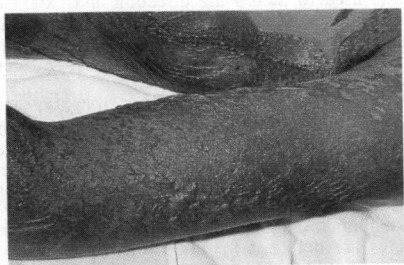

**toxic epidermal necrolysis**

**tox·ic goi·ter** a goiter that forms an excessive secretion, causing signs and symptoms of hyperthyroidism.

**tox·ic he·mo·glo·bi·nur·ia** hemoglobinuria occurring after the ingestion of various poisons, in certain blood diseases, and in certain infections.

**tox·ic·i·ty** (tok-sis′i-tē) the state of being poisonous.

**tox·ic meg·a·co·lon** acute nonobstructive dilation of the colon, seen in fulminating ulcerative colitis and Crohn disease.

**tox·ic ne·phro·sis** acute oliguric renal failure due to chemical poisons, septicemia, or bacterial toxemia.

**tox·ic neu·ri·tis** neuritis caused by an endogenous or exogenous toxin.

△**tox·i·co-, tox-, to·xi-, tox·o-** poison, toxin. [G. *toxikon,* bow, hence (arrow) poison]

⊡**Tox·i·co·den·dron** (tok′si-kō-den′dron) a genus of poisonous plants (also known as *Rhus*) with fruits and foliage that contain urushiol, which produces a contact dermatitis (rhus dermatitis); species include poison ivy (*Toxicodendron radicans*), poison oak (*Toxicodendron diversilobum*), and poison sumac (*Toxicodendron vernix*) See this page. [toxico- + G. *dendron,* tree]

**tox·i·co·gen·ic** (tok′si-kō-jen′ik) **1.** producing a poison. **2.** caused by a poison. [toxico- + G. *-gen,* producing]

**tox·i·co·log·ic** (tok′si-kō-loj′ik) relating to toxicology.

**tox·i·col·o·gist** (tok-si-kol′ŏ-jist) a specialist or expert in toxicology.

**tox·i·col·o·gy** (tok-si-kol′ŏ-jē) the science of poisons, including their source, chemical composi-

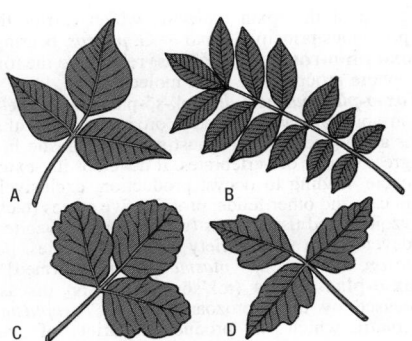

***Toxicodendron:*** (A) poison ivy, (B) poison sumac, (C) poison oak (Western), (D) poison oak (Eastern)

tion, action, tests, and antidotes. [toxico- + G. *logos,* study]

**tox·i·co·sis** (tok-si-kō′sis) any disease of toxic origin. [toxico- + G. *-osis,* condition]

**tox·ic shock** SEE toxic shock syndrome.

**tox·ic shock syn·drome (TSS)** infection with toxin-producing staphylococci, occurring most often in the vagina of menstruating women using superabsorbent tampons and characterized by high fever, vomiting, diarrhea, a scarlatiniform rash followed by desquamation, and decreasing blood pressure and shock, which can result in death; hyperemia of the conjunctival, oropharyngeal, and vaginal mucous membranes also occurs.

**tox·ic tet·a·nus** SYN drug tetanus.

**tox·ic u·nit** a unit formerly synonymous with minimal lethal dose but which, because of the instability of toxins, is now measured in terms of the quantity of standard antitoxin with which the toxin combines. SEE ALSO L doses, minimal lethal dose. SYN toxin unit.

**tox·i·gen·ic** (tok-si-jen′ik) SYN toxinogenic.

**tox·in** (tok′sin) a noxious or poisonous substance that is formed or elaborated either as an integral part of the cell or tissue, as an extracellular product (exotoxin), or as a combination of the two, during the metabolism and growth of certain microorganisms and some higher plant and animal species. [G. *toxikon,* poison]

**tox·in·ic** (tok-sin′ik) relating to a toxin.

**tox·i·no·gen·ic** (tok′si-nō-jen′ik) producing a toxin, said of an organism. SYN toxigenic. [toxin + G. *-gen,* producing]

**tox·in u·nit** SYN toxic unit.

**tox·o·ca·ri·a·sis** (tok′sō-kă-rī′ă-sis) infection with nematodes of the genus *Toxocara;* parenterally migrating larvae, chiefly of *Toxocara canis,* may cause visceral larva migrans; ocular involvement results in a solitary granuloma in the retina, peripheral inflammatory masses, or chronic endophthalmitis.

**tox·oid** (tok′soyd) a toxin that has been treated (commonly with formaldehyde) so as to destroy its toxic property but retain its antigenicity, i.e., its capability of stimulating the production of antitoxin antibodies and thus of producing an active immunity. [toxin + G. *eidos,* resemblance]

**tox·o·phore** (tok′sō-fōr) denoting the atomic

group of the toxin molecule which carries the poisonous principle. [toxo- + G. *phoros*, bearing]

**tox·oph·o·rous** (tok-sof'ăr-ŭs) relating to the toxophore group of the toxin molecule.

***Tox·o·plas·ma gon·dii*** (tok-sō-plaz'mă gon'dē-ī) an abundant, widespread sporozoan species that is an intracellular, non-host-specific parasite in a great variety of vertebrates. It develops its sexual cycle, leading to oocyst production, exclusively in cats and other felids; proliferative stages (tachyzoites) and tissue cysts (containing bradyzoites) develop in a wide variety of animal species. [G. *toxon*, bow or arc, + *plasma*, anything formed]

**tox·o·plas·mo·sis** (tok'sō-plaz-mō'sis) disease caused by the protozoan parasite *Toxoplasma gondii*, which can produce a variety of syndromes in humans. Prenatally acquired infection can result in abnormalities such as microcephalus or hydrocephalus at birth, jaundice with hepatosplenomegaly or meningoencephalitis in early childhood, or delayed ocular lesions such as chorioretinitis in later childhood. Postnatally acquired human infections typically remain subclinical; if clinical disease does occur, symptoms include fever, lymphadenopathy, headache, myalgia, and fatigue, with eventual recovery, except in the immunocompromised patient where fatal encephalitis often develops.

**tox·o·py·rim·i·dine** (toks'ō-pi-rim'i-dēn) one of the products resulting from the hydrolysis of thiamin by thiaminase and appearing in the urine; a competitive inhibitor of pyridoxal.

**Toyn·bee ma·neu·ver** (toin'bē) action that accomplishes auditory (eustachian) tube opening when patient closes mouth, holds nose, and swallows. SEE ALSO Valsalva maneuver, politzerization.

**Toyn·bee tube** (toin'bē) a tube by which one can listen to the sounds in a patient's ear during politzerization.

**TPN** total parenteral nutrition.

**TPN, TPNH** triphosphopyridine nucleotide and its reduced form (the oxidized form is TPN⁺).

**TR** repetition time.

**tra·bec·u·la,** gen. and pl. **tra·bec·u·lae** (tră-bek'yu-lă, tră-bek'yu-lē) [TA] **1.** one of the supporting bundles of fibers traversing the substance of a structure, usually derived from the capsule or one of the fibrous septa. **2.** a small piece of the spongy substance of bone usually interconnected with other similar pieces. **3.** HISTOPATHOLOGY a band of neoplastic tissue two or more cells wide. [L. dim. of *trabs*, a beam]

**tra·bec·u·lae car·ne·ae (of right and left ventricles)** muscular bundles on the lining walls of the ventricles of the heart.

**tra·bec·u·lar** (tră-bek'yu-lăr) relating to or containing trabeculae.

**tra·bec·u·lar bone** SYN substantia spongiosa.

**tra·bec·u·lar re·tic·u·lum** the network of fibers (pectinate ligaments) at the iridocorneal angle between the anterior chamber of the eye and the venous sinus of the sclera; it contains spaces between the fibers that are involved in drainage of the aqueous humor, and is composed of two portions: the corneoscleral part, the part attached to the sclera, and the uveal part, the part attached to the iris.

**tra·bec·u·lo·plas·ty** (tră-bek'yu-lō-plas-tē) photocoagulation of the trabecular meshwork of the eye using the laser in the treatment of glaucoma.

**tra·bec·u·lot·o·my** (tră-bek-yu-lot'ō-mē) surgical opening of the sinus venosus sclerae (canal of Schlemm) to treat glaucoma. [trabekula + G. *tomē*, incision]

**trace el·e·ments** elements present in minute amounts in the body, e.g., Zn, Se, V, Ni, Mg, Mn, many of which are essential in metabolism or for the manufacture of essential compounds.

**trac·er** (trā'ser) **1.** an element or compound containing atoms that can be distinguished from their normal counterparts by physical means (e.g., radioactivity assay or mass spectrography) and can thus be used to follow (trace) the metabolism of the normal substances. **2.** a colored substance (e.g., a dye) used as a tracer to follow the flow of water. **3.** an instrument used in dissecting out nerves and blood vessels. **4.** a mechanical device with a marking point attached to one jaw and a graph plate or tracing plate attached to the other jaw; used to record the direction and extent of movements of the mandible. SEE ALSO tracing (2). [M.E. track, fr. O. Fr. *tracier*, to make one's way, fr. L. *traho*, pp. *tractum*, to draw, + *-er*, agent suffix]

▣**tra·chea,** pl. **tra·che·ae** (trā'kē-ă, trā'kē-ē) [TA] the air tube extending from the larynx into the thorax (level of the fifth or sixth thoracic vertebra) where it bifurcates into the right and left main bronchi. The trachea is composed of from 16 to 20 rings of hyaline cartilage connected by a membrane (annular ligament); posteriorly, the rings are deficient for one-fifth to one-third of their circumference, the interval forming the membranous wall being closed by a fibrous membrane containing smooth muscular fibers. Internally, the mucosa is composed of a pseudostratified ciliated columnar epithelium with mucous goblet cells; numerous small mixed mucous and serous glands occur, the ducts of which open to the surface of the epithelium. See page B8. SYN windpipe. [G. *tracheia artēria*, rough artery]

**tra·che·al** (trā'kē-ăl) relating to the trachea.

**tra·che·al car·ti·lag·es** the 16–20 incomplete rings of hyaline cartilage forming the skeleton of the trachea; the rings are deficient posteriorly for from one-fifth to one-third of their circumference. SYN cartilagines tracheales [TA].

**tra·che·a·lis mu·scle** the band of smooth muscular fibers in the fibrous membrane connecting posteriorly the ends of the tracheal rings. SYN musculus trachealis [TA].

**tra·che·al tube** a flexible tube inserted nasally, orally, or through a tracheotomy into the trachea to provide an airway, as in tracheal intubation. SYN endotracheal tube.

**tra·che·al veins** several small venous trunks from the trachea, emptying into the brachiocephalic veins or the superior vena cava.

**tra·che·i·tis** (trā-kē-ī'tis) inflammation of the lining membrane of the trachea. SYN trachitis. [trachea + G. *-itis*, inflammation]

**trach·e·lec·to·my** (trak-ĕ-lek'tō-mē) SYN cervicectomy. [trachel- + G. *ektomē*, excision]

**trach·e·lism, trach·e·lis·mus** (trak'ĕ-lizm, trak'ĕ-liz'mŭs) a bending backward of the neck, such as sometimes ushers in an epileptic attack. [G. *trachēlismos*, a seizing by the throat]

**trach·e·li·tis** (trak-ĕ-lī'tis) SYN cervicitis.

△**tra·che·lo-, tra·chel-** neck. [G. *trachēlos*]

**trach·e·lo·breg·mat·ic di·a·me·ter** the diameter of the fetal head from the middle of the anterior fontanelle to the neck.

**trach·e·lo·dyn·ia** (trak′ĕ-lō-din′ē-ă) SYN cervicodynia. [trachelo- + G. *odynē,* pain]

**trach·e·lor·rha·phy** (trak-ĕ-lōr′ă-fē) repair by suture of a laceration of the cervix uteri. SYN Emmet operation. [trachelo- + G. *rhaphē,* suture]

**trach·e·lot·o·my** (trak-ĕ-lot′ō-mē) SYN cervicotomy. [trachelo- + G. *tomē,* incision]

△**tra·che·o-, tra·che-** the trachea. [see trachea]

**tra·che·o·aer·o·cele** (trā′kē-ō-ār′ō-sēl) an air cyst in the neck caused by distention of a tracheocele. [tracheo- + G. *aēr,* air, + *kēlē,* hernia]

**tra·che·o·bron·chi·al** (trā′kē-ō-brong′kē-ăl) relating to both trachea and bronchi, denoting especially a set of lymph nodes.

**tra·che·o·bron·chi·tis** (trā′kē-ō-brong-kī′tis) inflammation of the mucous membrane of the trachea and bronchi.

**tra·che·o·bron·chos·co·py** (trā′kē-ō-brong-kos′kŏ-pē) inspection of the interior of the trachea and bronchi. [tracheo- + bronchus, + G. *skopeō,* to view]

**tra·che·o·cele** (trā′kē-ō-sēl) a protrusion of the mucous membrane through a defect in the wall of the trachea. [tracheo- + G. *kēlē,* hernia]

**tra·che·o·e·soph·a·ge·al** (trā′kē-ō-ē-sof′ă-jē′ăl) relating to the trachea and the esophagus.

**tra·che·o·e·so·pha·ge·al punc·ture (TEP),** **tra·che·o·e·so·pha·ge·al shunt** surgical puncture connecting the trachea and esophagus. In laryngectomies, the puncture, in combination with a prosthetic valve, allows exhaled air from the lungs to enter the esophagus for production of speech.

**tra·che·o·la·ryn·ge·al** (trā′kē-ō-lă-rin′jē-ăl) relating to the trachea and the larynx.

**tra·che·o·ma·la·cia** (trā′kē-ō-mā-lā′shē-ă) degeneration of elastic and connective tissue of the trachea. [tracheo- + G. *malakia,* softness]

**tra·che·o·meg·a·ly** (trā′kē-ō-meg′ă-lē) an abnormally dilated trachea which may, like bronchiectasis, result from infection or prolonged positive pressure ventilation. [tracheo- + G. *megas* (*megal-*), large]

**tra·che·o-oe·so·pha·ge·al [Br.]** SEE tracheoesophageal.

**tra·che·o·path·ia, tra·che·op·a·thy** (trā′kē-ō-path′ē-ă, trā′kē-op′ă-the) any disease of the trachea. [tracheo- + G. *pathos,* disease]

**tra·che·o·pha·ryn·ge·al** (trā′kē-ō-fă-rin′jē-ăl) relating to both trachea and pharynx; denoting an occasional band of muscular fibers passing from the inferior constrictor of the pharynx to the trachea.

**tra·che·oph·o·ny** (trā-kē-of′ō-nē) the hollow voice sound heard in auscultating over the trachea. SEE ALSO bronchophony. [tracheo- + G. *phōnē,* voice]

**tra·che·o·plas·ty** (trā′kē-ō-plas-tē) plastic surgery of the trachea. [tracheo- + G. *plastos,* formed]

**tra·che·or·rha·gia** (trā-kē-ō-rā′jē-ă) hemorrhage from the mucous membrane of the trachea. [tracheo- + G. *rhēgnymi,* to burst forth]

**tra·che·os·chi·sis** (trā-kē-os′ki-sis) a fissure into the trachea. [tracheo- + G. *schisis,* fissure]

**tra·che·o·scop·ic** (trā-kē-ō-skop′ik) relating to tracheoscopy.

**tra·che·os·co·py** (trā-kē-os′kŏ-pē) inspection of the interior of the trachea. [tracheo- + G. *skopeō,* to examine]

**tra·che·o·ste·no·sis** (trā′kē-ō-stĕ-nō′sis) narrowing of the lumen of the trachea. [tracheo- + G. *stenōsis,* constriction]

🔒**tra·che·os·to·my** (trā-kē-os′tō-mē) SYN tracheotomy. See this page. [tracheo- + G. *stoma,* mouth]

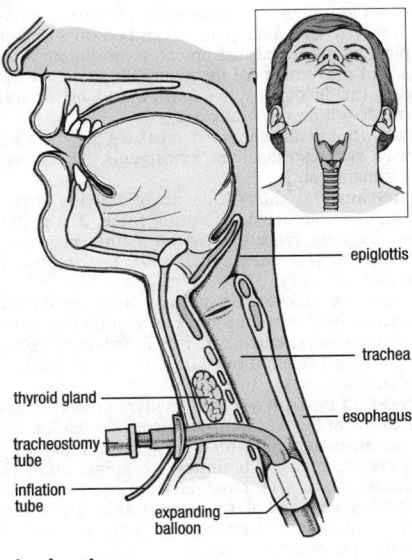

epiglottis

trachea

thyroid gland

esophagus

tracheostomy tube

inflation tube

expanding balloon

**tracheostomy**

**tra·che·os·to·my tube** a curved tube used to keep the opening free after tracheotomy; may be metal or plastic.

**tra·che·ot·o·my** (trā-kē-ot′ō-mē) the operation of opening into the trachea, usually intended to be temporary. SYN tracheostomy. [tracheo- + G. *tomē,* incision]

**tra·che·ot·o·my tube** a curved tube used to keep the opening free after tracheotomy. May be metal or plastic.

*Tra·chi·pleis·toph·ora* (trā-kē-plī-stof′er-ă) a genus of microsporidia that can infect humans and cause myositis, keratoconjunctivitis, and sinusitis in the immunocompromised person.

**tra·chi·tis** (trā-kī′tis) SYN tracheitis.

**tra·cho·ma** (tră-kō′mă) chronic inflammation and hypertrophy of the conjunctiva, marked by the formation of minute grayish or yellowish translucent granules, caused by *Chlamydia trachomatis.* SYN Egyptian ophthalmia, granular ophthalmia. [G. *trachōma,* fr. *trachys,* rough, harsh]

**tra·cho·ma bod·ies** distinctive, complex, intracytoplasmic forms found in the conjunctival epithelial cells of persons in the acute phase of trachoma.

**tra·chom·a·tous** (tră-kō′mă-tŭs) relating to or suffering from trachoma.

**tra·chom·a·tous con·junc·ti·vi·tis** a chronic infection of the conjunctiva due to *Chlamydia trachomatis,* characterized by conjunctival follicles and subsequent cicatrization. SEE ALSO trachoma. SYN granular conjunctivitis.

**tra·chom·a·tous ker·a·ti·tis** SEE pannus, corneal pannus.

**trac·ing** (trās′ing) **1.** a graphic reproduction of the outline or salient features of a physical object or structure. SEE ALSO curve. **2.** any graphic display of electrical or mechanical events in normal or diseased tissues or organs, as detected or measured by diagnostic instruments. SEE ALSO curve. **3.** DENTISTRY a line or lines, scribed on a table or plate by a pointed instrument, representing a record of movements of the mandible; may be extraoral (made outside the oral cavity) or intraoral (made within the oral cavity).

**tract** (trakt) an elongated area, e.g., path, track, way. SEE ALSO fascicle. SYN tractus. [L. *tractus,* a drawing out]

**trac·tion** (trak′shŭn) **1.** the act of drawing or pulling, as by an elastic or spring force. **2.** a pulling or dragging force exerted on a limb in a distal direction. [L. *tractio,* fr. *traho,* pp. *tractus,* to draw]

**trac·tion di·ver·tic·u·lum** a diverticulum formed by the pulling force of contracting bands of adhesion, occurring mainly in the distal esophagus, from tuberculous hilar or mediastinal lymphadenitis.

**trac·tion ep·i·phy·sis** a secondary center of ossification at the site of attachment of a tendon.

**trac·tot·o·my** (trak-tot′ō-mē) interruption of a nerve tract in the brainstem or spinal cord. [L. *tractus,* tract, + G. *tomē,* incision]

**trac·tus,** gen. and pl. **trac·tus** (trak′tŭs) SYN tract. [L. a drawing, drawing out, extent, tract, fr. *traho,* pp. *tractus,* to draw]

**trac·tus il·i·o·pub·i·cus** [TA] SYN iliopubic tract.

**trac·tus op·ti·cus** [TA] SYN optic tract.

**tra·gal** (trā′găl) relating to the tragus.

**tra·gal la·mi·na** a longitudinal curved plate of cartilage, the beginning of the cartilaginous portion of the external acoustic meatus.

**tra·gi** (trā′jī) **1.** plural of tragus. **2.** the hairs growing at the entrance to the external acoustic meatus.

**tra·gi·cus mu·scle** a band of vertical muscular fibers on the outer surface of the tragus of the ear. SYN musculus tragicus [TA], muscle of tragus.

**tra·gus** (trā′gŭs) **1.** a tonguelike projection of the cartilage of the auricle in front of the opening of the external acoustic meatus and continuous with the cartilage of this canal. SYN hircus (3). **2.** SEE tragi (2). [G. *tragos,* goat, in allusion to the hairs growing on the part, like a goatee]

**TRAIL** a member of the tumor necrosis factor ligand family that rapidly induces apoptosis in a variety of transformed cell lines. SYN apo-2L.

**trainer** (trā′ner) one who instructs, drills, corrects, or otherwise supports another in the acquisition of a skill or the performance of an activity. [Med. L. *traginare,* to direct the growth of a plant]

**train·ing** an organized system of education, instruction, or discipline.

**train·ing group** any group emphasizing training in self-awareness and group dynamics.

**train·ing-sen·si·tive zone** level of exercise heart rate, usually 70–85% of maximum, required to induce training improvements in aerobic fitness.

Exercise heart rates below the 70% threshold are generally offset by extending exercise duration. SYN target heart rate range.

**trait** (trāt) a qualitative characteristic; a discrete attribute as contrasted with metrical character. A trait is amenable to segregation rather than quantitative analysis; it is an attribute of phenotype, not of genotype. [Fr. from L. *tractus,* a drawing out, extension]

**trance** (trans) an altered state of consciousness as in hypnosis, catalepsy, or ecstasy. [L. *transeo,* to go across]

**tran·quil·iz·er** (trang′kwi-lī-zer) a drug that promotes tranquility without sedating or depressant effects.

△**trans- 1.** prefix denoting across, through, beyond; opposite of *cis-*. **2.** GENETICS denoting the location of two genes on opposite chromosomes of a homologous pair. **3.** ORGANIC CHEMISTRY a form of geometric isomerism in which the atoms attached to two carbon atoms, joined by double bonds, are located on opposite sides of the molecule. **4.** BIOCHEMISTRY a prefix to a group name in an enzyme name or a reaction denoting transfer of that group from one compound to another. [L. *trans,* through, across]

**trans·a·cet·y·lase** (trans-ă-set′i-lās) SYN acetyltransferase.

**trans·a·cet·y·la·tion** (trans′ă-set-i-lā′shŭn) transfer of an acetyl group ($CH_3CO$–), from one compound to another; such reactions, usually involving formation of acetyl-CoA, occur notably in the initiation of the tricarboxylic acid cycle by the transfer of an acetyl group to oxaloacetate to form citrate.

**trans·ac·tion·al a·nal·y·sis** a psychotherapy system, used in both individual and group treatment, involving a systematic understanding of the qualities of interpersonal interactions in the treatment sessions; includes four components: 1) structural analysis of intrapsychic phenomena; 2) transactional analysis proper, determination of the currently dominant ego state (parent, child, or adult) of each participant; 3) game analysis, identification of the games played in interactions and of the gratifications provided; 4) script analysis, uncovering of the causes of the patient's emotional problems.

**trans·ac·yl·as·es** (trans-as′i-lā-sez) SYN acyltransferase.

**trans air·way pres·sure** the pressure gradient between the inside of the lung (the alveolus) and the outside of the lung (the pleural space).

**trans·al·do·la·tion** (trans′al-dō-lā′shŭn) a reaction involving the transfer of an aldol group from one compound to another; such reactions generally involve the sugar phosphates and occur in the phosphogluconate oxidation pathway of carbohydrate catabolism.

**trans·am·i·di·na·tion** (trans-am′i-di-nā′shŭn) a reaction involving the transfer of an amidine group from one compound to another; the amidine donor is generally L-arginine and the reaction is of significance in the biosynthesis of creatine.

**trans·am·i·nas·es** (trans-am′i-nās-ez) SYN aminotransferase.

**trans·am·i·na·tion** (trans-am′i-nā′shŭn) the reaction between an amino acid and an α-keto acid through which the amino group is transferred from the former to the latter.

**trans•ca•lent** (trans-kā'lent) SYN diathermanous. [trans- + L. *caleo*, to be warm]

**trans•car•bam•o•y•las•es** (trans-kar-bam'ō-i-lā-sez) SYN carbamoyltransferases.

**trans•car•box•yl•as•es** (trans-kar-boks'i-lās-ez) SYN carboxyltransferases.

**trans•cel•lu•lar flu•ids** the fluids that are not inside cells, but are separated from plasma and interstitial fluid by cellular barriers; e.g., cerebrospinal fluid, synovial fluid, pleural fluid.

**trans•cer•vi•cal thy•mec•to•my** thymectomy performed via a cervical incision only.

**trans•co•bal•a•mins** (trans-kō-bal'ă-minz) substances included in "R binder," the name given a family of cobalamin-binding proteins; deficiencies have been associated with low serum cobalamin levels, and can lead to megaloblastic anemia.

**trans•co•chle•ar ap•proach** a surgical approach to the internal auditory canal through the cochlea.

**trans•cor•ti•cal** (tranz-kōr'ti-kăl) **1.** across or through the cortex of the brain, ovary, kidney, or other organ. **2.** from one part of the cerebral cortex to another; denoting the various association tracts.

**trans•cor•ti•cal apha•sia** an aphasia in which the ability to imitate speech is preserved but other language abilities are impaired; in transcortical sensory aphasia other symptoms are similar to receptive aphasia and in transcortical motor aphasia other symptoms are similar to expressive aphasia.

**trans•cor•tin** (trans-kōr'tin) an $\alpha_2$-globulin in blood that binds cortisol and corticosterone; the principal corticosteroid-binding protein in the plasma. SYN corticosteroid-binding globulin.

**tran•scrip•tase** (tran-skrip'tās) a polymerase associated with the process of transcription; especially the DNA-dependent RNA polymerase. [L. *transcribo*, pp. *transcriptum*, to copy, + -ase]

**tran•scrip•tion** (tran-skrip'shŭn) transfer of genetic code information from one kind of nucleic acid to another, especially with reference to the process by which a base sequence of messenger RNA is synthesized (by an RNA polymerase) on a template of complementary DNA.

**tran•scrip•tion-based chain re•ac•tion** a technique for target amplification of DNA or RNA in which reverse transcriptase is used to produce a single-stranded DNA molecule for each DNA or RNA target; this molecule is used as a template for further amplification.

**trans•cu•ta•ne•ous blood gas mo•ni•tor** a device that uses miniature electrodes applied to the skin to estimate blood oxygen and carbon dioxide tension; the transcutaneous carbon dioxide tension ($tcPCO_2$) provides a relatively accurate estimate of arterial carbon dioxide ($PaCO_2$) in all age groups; the estimate of transcutaneous oxygen tension ($tcPO_2$) is more accurate in neonates and small children.

**trans•cy•to•sis** (trans-sī-tō'sis) a mechanism for transcellular transport in which a cell encloses extracellular material in an invagination of the cell membrane to form a vesicle (endocytosis), then moves the vesicle across the cell to eject the material through the opposite cell membrane by the reverse process (exocytosis). SYN vesicular transport.

**trans•duc•er** a device that converts energy from one form to another, e.g., from electrical energy into ultrasonic energy.

**trans•duc•er cell** any cell responding to a mechanical, thermal, photic, or chemical stimulus by generating an electrical impulse synaptically transmitted to a sensory neuron in contact with the cell.

**trans•duc•tion** (trans-dŭk'shŭn) **1.** transfer of genetic material (and its phenotypic expression) from one cell to another by viral infection. **2.** a form of genetic recombination in bacteria. **3.** conversion of energy from one form to another. [trans- + L. *duco*, pp. *ductus*, to lead across]

**tran•sec•tion** (tran-sek'shŭn) **1.** a cross-section. **2.** cutting across. SYN transsection. [trans- + L. *seco*, pp. *sectus*, to cut]

**trans•es•oph•a•ge•al ech•o•car•di•og•ra•phy** recording of the echocardiogram from a swallowed transducer.

**trans•fec•tion** (trans-fek'shŭn) a method of gene transfer utilizing infection of a cell with nucleic acid (as from a retrovirus) resulting in subsequent viral replication in the transfected cell. [trans- + in*fection*]

**trans•fer 1.** process of removal or transferral. **2.** a condition in which learning in one situation influences learning in another situation; a carryover of learning that may be positive in effect, as when learning one behavior facilitates the learning of something else, or may be negative, as when one habit interferes with the acquisition of a later one. SYN transmission (1). [L. *trans-fero*, to bear across]

**trans•fer•as•es** (trans'fer-ās-ez) enzymes transferring one-carbon groups, acyl and glucosyl residues, alkyl or aryl groups, nitrogenous groups, phosphorus-containing groups, and sulfur-containing groups.

**trans•fer•ence** (trans-fer'ens) **1.** conveyance of an object from one place to another. **2.** shifting of symptoms from one side of the body to the other, as seen in certain cases of conversion hysteria. **3.** displacement of affect from one person or one idea to another. **4.** PSYCHOANALYSIS generally applied to the projection of feelings, thoughts, and wishes onto the analyst, who has come to represent some person from the patient's past.

**trans•fer•ence neu•ro•sis** in psychoanalysis, the phenomenon of the patient's developing a strong emotional relationship with the analyst.

**trans•fer fac•tor 1.** the transfer gene of a conjugative plasmid, especially of the resistance plasmid; **2.** a dialyzable extract that is obtained from the leukocytes of a person with a delayed-type sensitivity and that, following injection into the skin of a nonsensitive person, transfers the specific sensitivity to the recipient; **3.** SYN elongation factor.

**trans•fer•rin** (trans-fer'in) **1.** a nonheme $\beta_1$-globulin of the plasma, capable of associating reversibly with up to 1.25 μg of iron per g, and acting therefore as an iron-transporting protein. **2.** a glycoprotein, found in mammalian milk (lactoferrin) and egg white (conalbumin, ovotransferrin), that binds and transports iron ($Fe^{3+}$). [trans- + L. *ferrum*, iron, + -ia]

**trans•fer•rin sat•ur•a•tion** a calculation, expressed in percent, of the amount of transferrin that is bound to iron. It is determined by measuring serum iron and total iron binding capacity: serum iron X 100 = percent saturation TIBC. It is helpful in differentiating anemias. A low transferrin saturation is associated with iron deficiency states; a high saturation is associated with excess iron.

**trans·fer RNA (tRNA)** short-chain RNA molecules present in cells in at least 20 varieties, each variety capable of combining with a specific amino acid (see aminoacyl-tRNA). By joining (through their anticodons) with particular spots (codons) along the messenger RNA molecule and carrying their amino acyl residues along, they lead to the formation of protein molecules with a specific amino acid arrangement. SYN soluble RNA.

**trans·fix·ion** (trans-fik'shŭn) a maneuver in amputation in which the knife is passed from side to side through the soft parts, close to the bone, and the muscles are then divided from within outward. [L. *transfixio* (see transfix)]

**trans·fix·ion su·ture** 1. a criss-cross stitch so placed as to control bleeding from a tissue surface or small vessel when tied; 2. a suture used to fix the columella to the nasal septum.

**trans·for·ma·tion** (trans-fōr-mā'shŭn) 1. SYN metamorphosis. 2. a change of one tissue into another, as cartilage into bone. 3. in metals, a change in phase and physical properties in the solid state caused by heat treatment. 4. MICROBIAL GENETICS transfer of genetic information between bacteria by means of "naked" intracellular DNA fragments derived from bacterial donor cells and incorporated into a competent recipient cell. [L. *trans-formo*, pp. *-atus*, to transform]

**trans·form·ing fac·tor** the DNA responsible for bacterial transformation.

**trans·fuse** (trans-fyuz') to perform transfusion.

**trans·fu·sion** (trans-fyu'zhŭn) 1. transfer of blood or a blood component from one individual (donor) to another (recipient). 2. intravascular injection of physiologic saline solution. [L. *trans-fundo*, pp. *-fusus*, to pour from one vessel to another]

**trans·fu·sion ne·phri·tis** renal failure and tubular damage resulting from the transfusion of incompatible blood; the hemoglobin of the hemolyzed red cells is deposited as casts in the renal tubules.

**trans·gen·e·sis** (tranz-jen'e-sis) reproduction involving introduction of foreign species DNA into an ovum.

**trans·glot·tic** (trans-glot'ik) vertical crossing of the glottis, as in the spread of carcinoma from the supraglottic to the infraglottic area.

**trans·hi·a·tal** (trans-hī-ā'tăl) by way of a hiatus; said of a surgical procedure.

**trans·hi·a·tal es·oph·a·gec·to·my** resection of the esophagus by blunt dissection from a cervical incision from above and transhiatal approach through an abdominal incision.

**tran·si·ent a·can·tho·lyt·ic der·ma·to·sis** a pruritic papular eruption of the chest, with scattered lesions of the back and lateral aspects of the extremities, lasting from weeks to months; seen predominantly in males over 40. SYN Grover disease.

**tran·si·ent e·voked o·to·a·cous·tic e·mis·sion** a form in which the response is limited in time.

**tran·si·ent glob·al am·ne·sia** a memory disorder seen in middle aged and elderly persons characterized by an episode of amnesia and bewilderment which persists for several hours; during the episode the patient has a memory defect for present and recent past events, but is fully alert, oriented, capable of high-level intellectual activity, and has a normal neurological examination.

**tran·si·ent hy·po·gam·ma·glob·u·lin·e·mia of in·fan·cy** a type of primary immunodeficiency that occurs in infants, probably resulting from immaturity of lymphoid tissue.

**tran·si·ent is·che·mic at·tack (TIA)** a sudden focal loss of neurological function with complete recovery usually within 24 hours; caused by a brief period of inadequate perfusion in a portion of the territory of the carotid or vertebral basilar arteries.

**tran·sil·i·ent** (tran-sil'yent, tran-zil'yent) jumping across; passing over; pertaining to those cortical association fibers in the brain that pass from one convolution to another nonadjacent one. [L. *transilio*, to leap across, fr. *salio*, to leap]

**tran·si·tion·al cell car·ci·no·ma** a malignant neoplasm derived from transitional epithelium, occurring chiefly in the urinary bladder, ureters, or renal pelves.

**tran·si·tion·al den·ture** a partial denture which is to serve as a temporary prosthesis to which teeth will be added as more teeth are lost, and which will be replaced after postextraction tissue changes have occurred; a transitional denture may become an interim denture when all of the teeth have been removed from the dental arch.

**tran·si·tion·al ep·i·thel·i·um** a highly distensible pseudostratified epithelium with large polyploid superficial cells that are cuboidal in the relaxed state but broad and squamous in the distended state; occurs in the kidney, ureter, and bladder.

**tran·si·tion·al gy·rus** a small convolution connecting two lobes or two main gyri in the depth of a sulcus.

**tran·si·tion·al ob·ject** an object used by many children as a substitute for a parent who is absent (usually temporarily) to help them deal with separation; typically, a blanket or stuffed toy.

**tran·si·tion·al zone** 1. the equatorial region of the lens of the eye where the anterior epithelial cells become transformed into lens fibers; 2. that portion of a scleral contact lens between the corneal and scleral sections.

**tran·si·tion mu·ta·tion** a point mutation involving substitution of one base-pair for another, i.e., replacement of one purine for another and of one pyrimidine for another pyrimidine without change in the purine-pyrimidine orientation.

**trans·jug·u·lar in·tra·he·pa·tic por·to·sys··tem·ic shunt (TIPS)** an interventional radiology procedure to relieve portal hypertension.

**trans·ke·to·la·tion** (trans'kē-tō-lā'shŭn) a reaction involving the transfer of a ketole group from one compound to another.

**trans·la·by·rin·thine ap·proach** surgical approach to the cerebellopontine angle through the inner ear.

**trans·la·tion** (trans-lā'shŭn) 1. a change or conversion into another form. 2. the process by which messenger RNA, transfer RNA, and ribosomes effect the production of protein from amino acids. 3. DENTISTRY the movement of a tooth through alveolar bone without change in axial inclination. [L. *translatio*, a transferring, fr. *trans- fero*, pp. *-latus*, to carry across]

**trans·lo·ca·tion** (trans-lō-kā'shŭn) 1. transposition of two segments between nonhomologous chromosomes as a result of abnormal breakage and refusion of reciprocal segments. **2.** transport of a metabolite across a biomembrane. [trans- + L. *locatio*, placement, fr. *loco*, to place]

**trans·me·at·al in·ci·sion** an incision in the skin of the posterior external auditory canal that extends from just above the posterior malleolar fold to six o'clock inferiorly; for access to the posterior part of the middle ear.

**trans·meth·yl·ase** (trans-meth′i-lās) SYN methyl-transferase.

**trans·meth·yl·a·tion** (trans′meth-i-lā′shŭn) transfer of a methyl group from one compound to another.

**trans·mi·gra·tion** (trans-mī-grā′shŭn) movement from one site to another; may entail the crossing of some usually limiting barrier, as in the passage of blood cells through the walls of the vessels (diapedesis). [L. *transmigro*, pp. *-atus*, to remove from one place to another]

**trans·mis·si·ble** (trans-mis′i-bl) capable of being transmitted (carried across) from one person to another, as a transmissible disease, an infectious or contagious disease.

**trans·mis·sion** (trans-mish′ŭn) **1.** SYN transfer. **2.** the conveyance of disease from one person to another. **3.** the passage of a nerve impulse across an anatomic cleft, as in autonomic or central nervous system synapses and at neuromuscular junctions, by activation of a specific chemical mediator that stimulates or inhibits the structure across the synapse. **4.** in general, passage of energy through a material. [L. *transmissio*, a sending across]

**trans·mu·ral** (trans-myu′răl) through any wall, as of the body or of a cyst or any hollow structure. [trans- + L. *murus*, wall]

**trans·mu·ta·tion** (trans-myu-tā′shŭn) a change; transformation. SYN conversion (1). [L. *transmuto*, pp. *-atus*, to change, transmute]

**trans·na·sal fi·ber·op·tic la·ryn·go·sco·py** laryngoscopy performed with a fiberoptic endoscope introduced through the nose.

**trans·par·ent den·tin** SYN sclerotic dentin.

**trans·par·ent sep·tum** a thin plate of brain tissue, containing nerve cells and numerous nerve fibers, that is stretched like a flat, vertical sheet between the column and body of the fornix below and the corpus callosum above and anteriorly; it is usually fused in the median plane with its partner on the opposite side so as to form a thin, median partition between the left and right frontal horns of the lateral ventricles; in less than ten percent of humans there is a blind, slitlike, fluid-filled space between the two transparent septa, the cavity of septum pellucidum. The transparent septum is continuous ventralward through the interval between the corpus callosum and the anterior commissure with the precommissural septum and subcallosal gyrus.

**trans·pep·ti·dase** (trans-pep′ti-dās) an enzyme catalyzing a transpeptidation reaction.

**trans·pep·ti·da·tion** (trans′pep-ti-dā′shŭn) a reaction involving the transfer of one or more amino acids from one peptide chain to another, as by transpeptidase action, or of a peptide chain itself, as in bacterial cell wall synthesis.

**trans·phos·pho·ryl·a·tion** (trans′fos-fōr-i-lā′shŭn) a reaction involving the transfer of a phos-

phoric group from one compound to another, often with the involvement of ATP.

**tran·spi·ra·tion** (trans-pi-rā′shŭn) passage of water vapor through the skin or any membrane. SEE ALSO insensible perspiration. [trans- + L. *spiro*, pp. *-atus*, to breathe]

**trans·plant** (tranz′plant) **1.** to transfer from one part to another, as in grafting and transplantation. **2.** the tissue or organ in grafting and transplantation. SEE ALSO graft. [trans- + L. *planto*, to plant]

**trans·plan·ta·tion** (tranz-plan-tā′shŭn) implanting in one part a tissue or organ taken from another part or from another individual. SEE ALSO graft. [L. *trans-planto*, pp. *-atus*, to transplant]

**trans·port** (trans′pōrt) the movement or transference of biochemical substances in biologic systems. [L. *transporto*, to carry over, fr. trans- + *porto*, to carry]

**trans·port max·i·mum (Tm)** the maximal rate of secretion or reabsorption of a substance by the renal tubules.

**trans·port me·di·um** a medium for transporting clinical specimens to the laboratory for examination.

**trans·pos·a·ble el·e·ment** a DNA sequence that can move from one location in the genome to another; the transposition event can involve both recombination and replication, producing two copies of the moving piece of DNA; the insertion of these DNA fragments can disrupt the integrity of the target gene, possibly causing activation of dormant genes, deletions, inversions, and a variety of chromosomal aberrations.

**trans·pos·ase** (tranz-pōz′ās) an enzyme that is required for transposition of DNA segments. [L. *trans-pono*, pp. *trans-positum*, to set across, transfer, + -ase]

**trans·pose** (tranz-pōz) to transfer one tissue or organ to the place of another and *vice versa*. [L. *trans-pono*, pp. *-positus*, to place across, transfer]

**trans·po·si·tion** (tranz-pō-zish′ŭn) **1.** removal from one place to another; metathesis. **2.** the condition of being transposed to the wrong side of the body, as in transposition of the viscera, in which the viscera are located opposite their normal position. **3.** positioning of teeth out of their normal sequence in an arch.

**trans·po·si·tion of the great ves·sels** congenital malformation in which the aorta arises from the morphologic right ventricle and the pulmonary artery from the morphologic left ventricle resulting in two separate and parallel circulations. The condition is lethal unless some communication exists between the systemic and pulmonic circulation after birth; the life-sustaining communication may be an intra-atrial passage or a patent ductus arteriosus.

**trans·po·son** (trans-pō′son) a segment of DNA which has a repeat of an insertion sequence element at each end that can migrate from one plasmid to another within the same bacterium, to a bacterial chromosome, or to a bacteriophage. [L. *transpono*, pp. *transpositum*, to transfer, + -on]

**trans·pul·mo·nary pres·sure** the pressure difference across the lungs; the difference between the pressure at the airway opening and the pressure on the visceral pleural surface (i.e., pressure at the airway opening – pleural pressure).

**trans·res·pir·a·tory pres·sure** the total pressure difference across the airways, lungs, and chest wall; the difference between the pressure at

t
r

the airway opening (the mouth) and the pressure on the body surface (i.e., pressure at the airway opening − pressure at the body surface).

**trans•sec•tion** (trans-sek′shŭn) SYN transection.

**trans•sex•u•al** (tranz-seks′yu-ăl) **1.** a person with the external genitalia and secondary sexual characteristics of one sex, but whose personal identification and psychosocial configuration is that of the opposite sex; a study of morphologic, genetic, and gonadal structure may be genitally congruent or incongruent. **2.** denoting or relating to such a person. **3.** relating to medical and surgical procedures designed to alter a patient's external sexual characteristics so that they resemble those of the opposite sex.

**trans•sex•u•al•ism** (tranz-seks′yu-ă-lizm) **1.** the state of being a transsexual. **2.** the desire to change one's anatomic sexual characteristics to conform physically with one's perception of self as a member of the opposite sex.

**trans•syn•ap•tic de•gen•er•a•tion** an atrophy of nerve cells following damage to the axons that make synaptic connection with them; noted especially in the lateral geniculate body.

**trans•thor•a•cic es•oph•a•gec•to•my** resection of the esophagus through a thoracotomy incision.

**trans•tra•che•al ox•y•gen ther•a•py** a method of oxygen delivery via a catheter inserted into the second tracheal interspace.

**tran•su•date** (tran′soo-dāt) any fluid (solvent and solute) that has passed through a presumably normal membrane, such as the capillary wall, as a result of imbalanced hydrostatic and osmotic forces; characteristically low in protein unless there has been secondary concentration. Cf. exudate. SYN transudation (2). [trans- + L. *sudo,* pp. *-atus,* to sweat]

**tran•su•da•tion** (tran-soo-dā′shŭn) **1.** passage of a fluid or solute through a membrane by a hydrostatic or osmotic pressure gradient. **2.** SYN transudate. [see transudate]

**trans•u•re•ter•o•u•re•ter•os•to•my** (tranz-yu-rē′ter-ō-yu-rē-ter-os′tō-mē) anastomosis of the transected end of one ureter into the intact contralateral ureter, by direct or elliptical end-to-side technique. SEE ALSO ureteroureterostomy.

**trans•u•re•thral re•sec•tion** endoscopic removal of the prostate gland or bladder lesions, usually for relief of prostatic obstruction or treatment of bladder malignancies.

**trans•va•gi•nal scan•ning** ultrasonography of the female pelvis with the transducer placed inside the vagina.

**trans•vec•tor** (trans-vek′tŏr) an animal that transmits a toxic substance that it does not produce, but that may be accumulated from animal (dinoflagellate) or plant (algae) sources.

**trans•ver•sal•is fa•scia** the lining fascia of the abdominal cavity, between the inner surface of the abdominal musculature and the peritoneum.

**trans•verse** (trans-vers′) crosswise; lying across the long axis of the body or of a part. [L. *transversus*]

**trans•verse am•pu•ta•tion** amputation in which the line of section through the extremity is at right angles to the long axis.

**trans•verse ar•tery of neck** SYN transverse cervical artery.

**trans•verse car•pal lig•a•ment** a strong fibrous band crossing the front of the carpus and binding down the flexor tendons of the digits and the flexor carpi radialis tendon and the median nerve; in so doing it creates the carpal tunnel.

**trans•verse cer•vi•cal ar•tery** *origin,* thyrocervical trunk; *branches,* superficial (superficial cervical) and deep (descending scapular). SYN arteria transversa colli [TA], transverse artery of neck.

**trans•verse cer•vi•cal nerve** a branch of the cervical plexus that supplies the skin over the anterior triangle of the neck. SYN nervus transversus colli [TA].

**trans•verse cer•vi•cal veins** venae comitantes of the corresponding arteries, emptying into the external jugular vein or sometimes into the subclavian vein. SYN transverse veins of neck.

**trans•verse co•lon** the part of the colon between the right and left colic flexures. It may extend somewhat transversely across the abdomen, but more often sags centally, frequently to subumbilical levels.

**trans•ver•sec•to•my** (trans-ver-sek′tō-mē) resection of the transverse process of a vertebra. [transverse + G. *ektomē,* excision]

**trans•verse di•a•me•ter** the breadth diameter of the pelvic inlet, measured between the terminal lines.

**trans•verse fa•cial ar•tery** *origin,* superficial temporal; *distribution,* parotid gland, parotid duct, masseter muscle, and overlying skin; *anastomoses,* infraorbital and buccal branches of maxillary, and buccal and masseteric branches of facial. SYN arteria transversa faciei [TA].

**trans•verse fa•cial vein** a tributary of the superficial temporal or retromandibular veins, anastomosing with the facial vein. SYN transverse vein of face.

**trans•verse fis•sure of the right lung** the deep fissure that separates the upper and middle lobes of the right lung.

**trans•verse fo•ra•men** foramen processus transversus. SYN vertebroarterial foramen.

**trans•verse frac•ture** a fracture the line of which forms a right angle with the axis of the bone.

**trans•verse her•ma•phro•di•ti•sm** pseudohermaphroditism in which the external genitalia are characteristic of one sex and the gonads are characteristic of the other sex.

**trans•verse hor•i•zon•tal ax•is** an imaginary line around which the mandible may rotate through the horizontal plane.

**trans•verse lie** that relationship in which the long axis of the fetus is transverse or at right angles to that of the mother.

**trans•verse lig•a•ment of el•bow** a bundle of fibers running from the olecranon to the coronoid process in association with the ulnar collateral ligament.

**trans•verse lig•a•ment of knee** a transverse band that passes between the lateral and medial menisci in the anterior part of the knee joint. SYN ligamentum transversum genus [TA].

**trans•verse mu•scle of ab•do•men** SYN transversus abdominis muscle.

**trans•verse mu•scle of chin** SYN transversus menti muscle.

**trans•verse mu•scle of nape** SYN transversus nuchae muscle.

**trans•verse mu•scle of tongue** an intrinsic muscle of the tongue, the fibers of which arise from the septum and radiate to the dorsum and sides; *action,* decreases lateral dimension of the tongue;

*nerve supply*, hypoglossal for motor, lingual for sensory. SYN musculus transversus linguae [TA].

**trans·verse per·i·car·di·al si·nus** a passage in the pericardial sac between the origins of the great vessels, i.e., posterior to the intrapericardial portions of the pulmonary trunk and ascending aorta and anterior to the superior vena cava and superior to the atria; it is formed as a result of the flexure of the heart tube, partially approximating the great venous and arterial vessels. SYN Theile canal.

**trans·verse per·i·ne·al lig·a·ment** the thickened anterior border of the urogenital diaphragm, formed by the fusion of its two fascial layers.

**trans·verse plane** a plane across the body at right angles to the coronal and sagittal planes. See page APP 88.

**trans·verse pre·sen·ta·tion** an abnormal presentation, neither head nor breech, in which the fetus lies transversely in the uterus across the axis of the parturient canal.

**trans·verse pro·cess** a bony protrusion on either side of the arch of a vertebra, from the junction of the lamina and pedicle, which functions as a lever for attached muscles.

**trans·verse rec·tal folds, trans·verse folds of rec·tum** the three or four crescentic folds placed horizontally in the rectal mucous membrane; the superior rectal fold is situated near the beginning of the rectum on the left side; the middle rectal fold (Nélaton fold) is most prominent and consistent and projects from the right side about 8 cm above the anus (approximately the level of the floor of the rectouterine or rectovesical pouch); the inferior rectal fold is on the left side about 5 cm above the anus.

**trans·verse re·lax·a·tion** MAGNETIC RESONANCE IMAGING the rapid decay of the nuclear magnetization vector at right angles to the magnetic field after the 90° pulse is turned off; the signal is called free induction decay. SEE T2. Cf. longitudinal relaxation.

**trans·verse rhomb·en·ce·phal·ic flex·ure** SYN pontine flexure.

**trans·verse scap·u·lar ar·tery** SYN suprascapular artery.

**trans·verse sec·tion** a cross section obtained by slicing, actually or through imaging techniques, the body or any part of the body structure, in a horizontal plane, i.e., a plane which intersects the longitudinal axis at a right angle. Since actual sectioning in the transverse plane results in an inferior and a superior portion, an anatomical transverse section may be a two-dimensional view of the cut surface on the inferior aspect of the superior portion, or of the superior aspect of the inferior portion. By convention, in medical imaging transverse sections demonstrate the former unless otherwise stated.

**trans·verse si·nus** a paired dural venous sinus that drains the confluence of sinuses, running along the occipital attachment of the tentorium cerebelli and terminating in the sigmoid sinus.

**trans·verse tar·sal joint** the synovial joints between the talus and navicular bone medially and the calcaneus and navicular bones laterally which act as a unit in allowing the front of the foot to pivot relative to the back of the foot about the longitudinal axis of the foot, contributing to the total inversion and eversion movements.

**trans·verse tem·por·al gy·ri** two or three con-

volutions running transversely on the upper surface of the temporal lobe bordering on the lateral (sylvian) fissure, separated from each other by the transverse temporal sulci.

**trans·verse thor·a·cost·er·no·to·my** chest incision combining an intercostal incision and transsection of the sternum.

**trans·verse vein of face** SYN transverse facial vein.

**trans·verse veins of neck** SYN transverse cervical veins.

**trans·ver·sion** (trans-ver′zhŭn) **1.** substitution in DNA and RNA of a pyrimidine for a purine, or vice versa, by mutation. **2.** DENTISTRY the eruption of a tooth in a position normally occupied by another; transposition of a tooth.

**trans·ver·sion mu·ta·tion** a point mutation involving base substitution in which the orientation of purine and pyrimidine is reversed, in contradistinction to transition mutation.

**trans·ver·so·spi·nal·is mus·cle** the group of muscles that originate from transverse processes of vertebrae and pass to spinous processes of higher vertebrae; they act as rotators and include the semispinalis (capitis, cervicis, thoracis), multifidus, and rotatores (cervicis, thoracis, lumborum) muscles. All are innervated by dorsal primary rami of spinal nerves. SYN musculus transversospinalis [TA], transversospinal muscle.

**trans·ver·so·spi·nal mu·scle** SYN transversospinalis muscle.

**trans·ver·sus ab·do·mi·nis mu·scle** *origin*, seventh to twelfth costal cartilages, lumbar fascia, iliac crest, and inguinal ligament; *insertion*, xiphoid cartilage and linea alba and, through the conjoint tendon, pubic tubercle and pecten; *action*, compresses abdominal contents; *nerve supply*, lower thoracic. SYN musculus transversus abdominis [TA], transverse muscle of abdomen.

**trans·ver·sus men·ti mu·scle** inconstant fibers of the depressor anguli oris musculus continue into the neck and cross to the opposite side inferior to the chin. SYN musculus transversus menti [TA], transverse muscle of chin.

**trans·ver·sus nu·chae mu·scle** an occasional muscle passing between the tendons of the trapezius and sternocleidomastoid, possibly a fasciculus of the posterior auricular muscle. SYN musculus transversus nuchae [TA], transverse muscle of nape.

**trans·ver·sus thor·a·cis mu·scle** *origin*, dorsal surface of xiphoid cartilage and lower portion of dorsal surface of body of sternum; *insertion*, second to sixth costal cartilages; *action*, contributes to depression of ribs, narrowing chest; *nerve supply*, intercostal. SYN musculus transversus thoracis [TA].

**trans·ves·tism** (trans-ves′tizm) the practice of dressing or masquerading in the clothes of the opposite sex; especially the adoption of feminine mannerisms and costume by a male. SYN transvestitism. [trans- + L. *vestio*, to dress]

**trans·ves·tite** (trans-ves′tīt) a person who practices transvestism.

**trans·ves·ti·tism** (trans-ves′ti-tizm) SYN transvestism.

**Tran·tas dots** (trahn′tă) pale, grayish red, uneven nodules of gelatinous aspect at the limbal conjunctiva in vernal conjunctivitis.

**TRAP** twin reversed arterial perfusion. SEE twin reversed arterial perfusion sequence.

t
r

**tra·pe·zi·al** (tra-pē′zē-ăl) relating to any trapezium.

**tra·pe·zi·form** (tra-pē′zi-fōrm) SYN trapezoid (1).

**tra·pe·zi·um**, pl. **tra·pe·zia, tra·pe·zi·ums** (tra-pē′zē-ŭm, tra-pē′zē-ă) **1.** a four-sided geometrical figure having no two sides parallel. **2.** the lateral (radial) bone in the distal row of the carpus; it articulates with the first and second metacarpals, scaphoid, and trapezoid bones. SYN os trapezium [TA], greater multangular bone, os multangulum majus, trapezium bone. [G. *trapezion*, a table or counter, a trapezium, dim. of *trapeza*, a table, fr. *tra-* (= *tetra-*), four, + *pous* (*pod-*), foot]

**tra·pe·zi·um bone** SYN trapezium.

**tra·pe·zi·us** (tra-pē′zē-ŭs) SYN trapezius muscle.

**tra·pe·zi·us mu·scle** *origin*, medial third of superior nuchal line, external occipital protuberance, ligamentum nuchae, spinous processes of seventh cervical and the thoracic vertebrae and corresponding supraspinous ligaments; *insertion*, lateral third of posterior surface of clavicle, anterior side of acromion, and upper and medial border of the spine of the scapula; *action*, when scapulae are fixed, portions of muscle can act independently; cervical portion elevates scapula, thoracic portion contributes to depression of scapula; upper and lowermost portions act simultaneously to rotate glenoid fossa superiorly; when the entire muscle and especially middle part contracts, the scapulae retract; draws head to one side or backward; *nerve supply*, motor by accessory, sensory by cervical plexus. SYN musculus trapezius [TA], trapezius.

**trap·e·zoid** (trap′ĕ-zoyd) **1.** resembling a trapezium. SYN trapeziform. **2.** a geometrical figure resembling a trapezium except that two of its opposite sides are parallel. **3.** SYN trapezoid bone. [G. *trapeza*, table, + *eidos*, resemblance]

**trap·e·zoid bone** a bone in the distal row of the carpus; it articulates with the second metacarpal, trapezium, capitate, and scaphoid. SYN trapezoid (3).

**trap·e·zoid lig·a·ment** the lateral part of the coracoclavicular ligament that attaches to the trapezoid line of the clavicle. SYN ligamentum trapezoideum [TA].

**trap·e·zoid line** the area on the inferior surface of the clavicle near its lateral extremity on which the trapezoid ligament attaches.

**Trau·be bru·it** (trow′bĕ) SYN gallop.

**Trau·be cor·pu·scle** (trow′bĕ) SYN achromocyte.

**Trau·be dou·ble tone** (trow′bĕ) a double sound heard on auscultation over the femoral vessels in cases of aortic and tricuspid insufficiency.

**Trau·be-He·ring curves, Trau·be-He·ring waves** (trow′bĕ-her′ing) slow oscillations in blood pressure usually extending over several respiratory cycles; related to variations in vasomotor tone; rhythmical variations in blood pressure.

**Trau·be sign** (trow′bĕ) a double sound or murmur heard in auscultation over arteries (particularly the femoral arteries) in significant aortic regurgitation.

**trau·ma**, pl. **trau·ma·ta, trau·mas** (traw′mă, traw′mă-tă) an injury, physical or mental. SYN traumatism. [G. wound]

**trau·ma care sys·tem** a coordinated emergency medical service (EMS) system designed to provide rapid assessment of victims of severe or

multisystem trauma, transport to a trauma center, and definitive care. May utilize air medical transport. SEE ALSO air medical transport.

**trau·ma cen·ter** a designated medical facility for the treatment of trauma patients. Standards established by the American College of Surgeons provide for 3 levels of sophistication; Level I represents a free-standing facility staffed 24 hours a day by surgical, specialty, and support personnel, with appropriate physical resources. SEE ALSO designation.

**trau·ma score** a numerical score, based on the sum of a number of physiological parameters, assigned to a trauma patient as a means of predicting outcome.

**trau·mas·the·nia** (traw-mas-thē′nē-ă) nervous exhaustion following an injury. [traum- + G. *astheneia*, weakness]

**trau·ma·ta** (traw′mă-tă) plural of trauma.

**trau·mat·ic** (traw-mat′ik) relating to or caused by trauma. [G. *traumatikos*]

**trau·mat·ic a·men·or·rhea** absence of menses because of endometrial scarring or cervical stenosis resulting from injury or disease. SYN Asherman syndrome.

**trau·mat·ic am·ne·sia** the loss or disturbance of memory following an insult or injury to the brain of the type that accompanies a head injury, or excessive use of alcohol, or following the cessation of alcohol ingestion or other psychoactive drugs; or loss or disturbance of memory of the type seen in hysteria and other forms of dissociative disorders.

**trau·mat·ic am·pu·ta·tion** amputation resulting from accidental or nonsurgical injury; may be complete or incomplete.

**trau·mat·ic an·es·the·sia** loss of sensation resulting from nerve injury.

**trau·mat·ic as·phyx·ia** cyanotic asphyxia due to trauma; the extravasation of blood into the skin and conjunctivae, produced by a sudden mechanical increase in venous pressure, analogous to the Rumpel-Leede test; it is common in those who have been hanged, and is seen occasionally in crush injuries. SYN pressure stasis.

**trau·mat·ic disc·o·pa·thy** an injury characterized by fissuring, laceration, or fragmentation of the disc or surrounding ligaments, with or without displacement of fragments against spinal cord, nerve roots, or ligaments.

**trau·mat·ic en·ceph·a·lo·pa·thy** an encephalopathy resulting from structural brain injury.

**trau·mat·ic neu·ri·tis** nerve lesion following an injury.

**trau·mat·ic neu·ro·ma** the non-neoplastic proliferative mass of Schwann cells and neurites that may develop at the proximal end of a severed or injured nerve. SYN amputation neuroma, false neuroma.

**trau·mat·ic neu·ro·sis** any functional nervous disorder following an accident or injury. SEE posttraumatic stress disorder.

**trau·mat·ic pneu·mo·thor·ax** pneumothorax caused by blunt or penetrating chest injury.

**trau·mat·ic tet·a·nus** tetanus following infection of a wound.

**trau·ma·tism** (traw′mă-tizm) SYN trauma.

△**trau·mat·o-, trau·mat-, traum-** wound, injury. [G. *trauma*]

**trau·mat·o·gen·ic oc·clu·sion** a malocclusion

capable of producing injury to the teeth and/or associated structures.

**trau·ma·top·nea** (traw′mă-top-nē′ă) passage of air in and out through a wound of the chest wall. [traumato- + G. *pnoē,* breath]

**trav·el·er's di·ar·rhea** diarrhea of sudden onset, often accompanied by abdominal cramps, vomiting, and fever, occurring sporadically in travelers usually during the first week of a trip; most commonly caused by strains of enterotoxigenic *Escherichia coli.* SYN turista.

**trav·el·ing wave the·ory** generally held theory that a wave travels from the base to the apex of the basilar membrane of the cochlea in response to acoustic stimulation, and that the site of maximal displacement of the basilar membrane depends on the frequency of the stimulating tone with higher frequencies causing maximal displacement near the base and lower frequencies causing maximal displacement near the apex.

**tra·verse** (trav′ers) COMPUTED TOMOGRAPHY one complete linear movement of the gantry across the object being scanned. [M.E., fr. O.Fr., fr. L.L. *transverso,* fr. L. *trans-verto,* to turn across]

**Treach·er Col·lins syn·drome** (trēch′er kol′inz) mandibulofacial dysostosis, when limited to the orbit and malar region.

**treat** (trēt) to manage a disease by medicinal, surgical, or other measures; to care for a patient medically or surgically. [Fr. *traiter,* fr. L. *tracto,* to drag, handle, perform]

**treat·ment** (trēt′ment) medical or surgical management of a patient. SEE ALSO therapy, therapeutics. [Fr. *traitement* (see treat)]

**tre·ble in·crease at low lev·els** a hearing aid signal-processing strategy to increase gradually the amplification of high-frequency sounds at low levels.

**Tré·lat stools** (trā-lah′) glairy stools streaked with blood, occurring in proctitis.

**tre·ma·cam·ra** (trē-ma-kam′ra) the extracellular part of the cell surface adhesion molecule ICAM-1 involved in rhinovirus attachments to mucosal cells.

**Trem·a·to·da** (trem′ă-tō′dă) a class in the phylum Platyhelminthes (the flatworms), consisting of flukes with a leaf-shaped body and two muscular suckers, and an acelomate parenchyma-filled body cavity. Flukes of interest to human or veterinary medicine are members of the order Digenea, with complete life cycles involving embryonic multiplication in a mollusk as their first intermediate host. [G. *trēmatōdēs,* full of holes, fr. *trēma,* a hole, + *eidos,* appearance]

**trem·a·tode, trem·a·toid** (trem′ă-tōd, trem′ă-toyd) **1.** common name for a fluke of the class Trematoda. **2.** relating to a fluke of the class Trematoda.

**trem·or** (trem′er) **1.** repetitive, often regular, oscillatory movements caused by alternate, or synchronous, but irregular contraction of opposing muscle groups; usually involuntary. **2.** minute ocular movement occurring during fixation on an object. SYN trepidation (1). [L. a shaking]

**trem·u·lous** (trem′yu-lŭs) characterized by tremor.

**trench fe·ver** an uncommon rickettsial fever caused by *Rochalimaea quintana* and transmitted by the louse *Pediculus humanus,* first appearing as an epidemic during the trench warfare of World War I; characterized by the sudden onset of chills and fever, myalgia (especially of the back and legs), headache, and general malaise that typically lasts five days but may recur.

**trench mouth** SYN necrotizing ulcerative gingivitis.

**Tren·del·en·burg op·er·a·tion** (tren′de-len-berg) a pulmonary embolectomy.

**Tren·de·len·burg po·si·tion** (tren′de-len-berg) a supine position on the operating table, which is inclined at varying angles so that the pelvis is higher than the head; used during and after operations in the pelvis or for shock.

**Tren·del·en·burg sign, Tren·del·en·burg gait** (tren′de-len-berg, tren′de-len-berg) a physical examination finding associated with various hip abnormalities (congenital dislocation, hip abductor weakness, rheumatic arthritis, osteoarthritis) in which the pelvis sags on the side opposite the affected side during single leg stance on the affected side; during gait, compensation occurs by leaning the torso toward the involved side during stance phase on the affected extremity.

**Tren·del·en·burg symp·tom** (tren′de-len-berg) a waddling gait in paresis of the gluteal muscles, as in progressive muscular dystrophy.

**Tren·del·en·burg test** (tren′de-len-berg) a test of the valves of the leg veins; the leg is raised above the level of the heart until the veins are empty and is then rapidly lowered; in varicosity and incompetence of the valves the veins will at once become distended, but placement of a tourniquet around the leg will prevent distention of veins below the incompetent perforators or valves below the tourniquet.

**trend of thought** thinking with a tendency toward or centering on a particular idea with a particular affect.

**treph·i·na·tion, trep·a·na·tion** (tref-i-nā′shŭn, trep-ă-nā′shŭn) removal of a circular piece ("button") of cranium by a trephine.

**tre·phine, tre·pan** (trĕ-fīn′, trĕ-pan′) **1.** a cylindrical or crown saw used for the removal of a disc of bone, especially from the skull, or of other firm tissue as that of the cornea. **2.** to remove a disc of bone or other tissue by means of a trephine.

**trep·i·dant** (trep′i-dant) marked by tremor. [L. *trepidans,* pres. p. of *trepido,* to tremble, to be agitated]

**trep·i·da·tio cor·dis** (trep-i-dā′shē-ō kōr′dis) SYN palpitation.

**trep·i·da·tion** (trep-i-dā′shŭn) **1.** SYN tremor. **2.** anxious fear. [L. *trepidatio,* fr. *trepido,* to tremble, to be agitated]

**Trep·o·ne·ma** (trep-ō-nē′mă) a genus of anaerobic bacteria (order Spirochaetales) consisting of cells, 3 to 8 μm in length, with acute, regular, or irregular spirals and no obvious protoplasmic structure. A terminal filament may be present. They stain with difficulty except with Giemsa stain or silver impregnation. Some species are pathogenic and parasitic for humans and other animals, generally producing local lesions in tissues. [G. *trepō,* to turn, + *nēma,* thread]

**Trep·o·ne·ma pal·li·dum** a species that causes syphilis in humans.

**Trep·o·ne·ma per·ten·ue** a species that causes yaws; patients with this disease give positive results in serologic screening tests for syphilis.

**trep·o·ne·ma·to·sis** (trep′ō-nē-mă-tō′sis) SYN treponemiasis.

**trep·o·neme** (trep'ō-nēm) a vernacular term used to refer to any member of the genus *Treponema*.

**trep·o·ne·mi·a·sis** (trep'ō-nē-mī'ă-sis) infection caused by *Treponema*. SYN treponematosis.

**trep·o·ne·mi·ci·dal** (trep'ō-nē'mi-sī'dăl) destructive to any species of *Treponema*, but usually with reference to *T. pallidum*. SYN antitreponemal. [*Treponema* + L. *caedo*, to kill]

**trep·pe** (trep'eh) a phenomenon in cardiac muscle: if a number of stimuli of the same intensity are sent into the muscle after a quiescent period, the first few contractions of the series show a successive increase in amplitude (strength). SYN staircase phenomenon. [Ger. *Treppe*, staircase]

**Tre·sil·i·an sign** (trē-sil'ē-ăn) a reddish prominence at the orifice of Stenson duct, noted in mumps.

**tre·sis** (trē'sis) SYN perforation. [G. *trēsis*, a boring]

△**tri-** three. Cf. tris-. [L. and G.]

**tri·a·ce·tic ac·id** (trī-ă-sē'tik as'id) a compound formed by condensation of acetyl and malonyl coenzyme A in the course of fatty acid synthesis.

**tri·ac·yl·glyc·er·ol** (trī-as'il-glis'er-ol) glycerol esterified at each of its three hydroxyl groups by a fatty (aliphatic) acid. SYN triglyceride.

**tri·a·cyl·gly·cer·ol li·pase** the fat-splitting enzyme in pancreatic juice; it hydrolyzes triacylglycerol to produce a diacylglycerol and a fatty acid anion; a deficiency of the hepatic enzyme results in hypercholesterolemia and hypertriglyceridemia. SYN steapsin.

**tri·ad** (trī'ad) 1. a group of three things having something in common. 2. the transverse tubule and the terminal cisternae on each side of it in skeletal muscle fibers. 3. SYN portal triad. 4. the father, mother, and child relationship projectively experienced in group psychotherapy. [G. *trias* (*triad-*), the number 3, fr. *treis,* three]

**tri·age** (trē'ahzh) medical screening of patients to determine their relative priority for treatment; the separation of a large number of casualties, in military or civilian disaster medical care, into three groups: 1) those who cannot be expected to survive even with treatment; 2) those who will recover without treatment; 3) the highest priority group, those who will not survive without treatment. [Fr. sorting]

**tri·age tag** a tag or other method of identifying the triage level assigned to a mass-casualty victim, containing information needed for emergency and life-sustaining treatment.

**tri·al den·ture** a setup of artificial teeth so fabricated that it may be placed in the patient's mouth to verify esthetics, for the making of records, or for any other operation deemed necessary before final completion of the denture.

**tri·al frame** a type of spectacle frame with variable adjustments, for holding trial lenses during refraction.

**tri·al of la·bor af·ter ce·sar·e·an sec·tion** the attempt to deliver vaginally after a cesarean section; carries some risk of rupture of the uterine scar.

**tri·al lens·es** a series of cylindrical and spherical lenses used in testing vision.

**tri·an·gle** (trī'ang-gl) ANATOMY, SURGERY a three-sided area with arbitrary or natural boundaries. SEE ALSO trigonum, region. [L. *triangulum*, fr. *tri-*, three, + *angulus*, angle]

**tri·an·gle of aus·cul·ta·tion** space bounded by the lower border of the trapezius, the latissimus dorsi, and the medial margin of the scapula, where the absence of musculature allows respiratory sounds to be heard clearly with a stethoscope.

**tri·an·gle of safe·ty** the area at the lower left sternal border where the pericardium is not covered by lung (pericardial notch); preferred site for aspiration of pericardial fluid.

**tri·an·gu·lar ban·dage** a piece of cloth cut in the shape of a right-angled triangle, used as a sling.

**tri·an·gu·lar bone** SYN os trigonum.

**tri·an·gu·lar mu·scle 1.** a muscle that is triangular in shape; **2.** SYN depressor anguli oris muscle.

**tri·an·gu·lar ridge** an elevation that descends from the cusp tips of premolars and molars toward the central grooves and fossae of the crown.

***Tri·at·o·ma*** (trī-ă-tō'mă) a genus of insects that includes important vectors of *Trypanosoma cruzi*, such as *Triatoma dimidiata*, *Triatoma infestans*, and *Triatoma maculata*.

**tri·ba·sic** (trī-bā'sik) having three titratable hydrogen atoms; denoting an acid with a basicity of 3.

**tribe** (trīb) in biological classification, an occasionally used division between the family and the genus; often the same as the subfamily. [L. *tribus*]

**tri·bra·chia** (trī-brā'kē-ă) condition seen in conjoined twins when the fusion has merged the adjacent arms to form a single one, so that there are only three arms for the two bodies. SEE conjoined twins. [tri- + G. *brachiōn*, arm]

**TRIC** trachoma and inclusion conjunctivitis.

**tri·car·box·yl·ic a·cid cy·cle** together with oxidative phosphorylation, the main source of energy in the mammalian body and the end toward which carbohydrate, fat, and protein metabolism are directed; a series of reactions, beginning and ending with oxaloacetic acid, during the course of which a two-carbon fragment is completely oxidized to carbon dioxide and water with the production of 12 high-energy phosphate bonds. SYN citric acid cycle, Krebs cycle.

**tri·ceps** (trī'seps) three-headed; denoting especially two muscles: triceps brachii and triceps surae. SEE muscle. [L. fr. *tri-*, three, + *caput*, head]

**tri·ceps bra·chii mu·scle** *origin,* long or scapular head: lateral border of scapula below glenoid fossa, lateral head: lateral and posterior surface of humerus below greater tubercle, medial head: posterior surface of humerus below radial groove; *insertion,* olecranon of ulna; *action,* extends elbow; *nerve supply,* radial. SYN musculus triceps brachii [TA], triceps muscle of arm.

**tri·ceps mu·scle of arm** SYN triceps brachii muscle.

**tri·ceps mu·scle of calf** SYN triceps surae muscle.

**tri·ceps re·flex** a sudden contraction of the triceps muscle caused by a smart tap on its tendon when the forearm hangs loosely at a right angle with the arm.

**tri·ceps sur·ae mu·scle** the two bellies of the gastrocnemius and soleus considered as one muscle. SYN musculus triceps surae [TA], triceps muscle of calf.

**tri·ceps sur·ae re·flex** SYN Achilles reflex.

**-tri·chia** condition or type of hair. [G. *thrix* (*trich-*), hair, + *-ia*, condition]

**tri·chi·a·sis** (tri-kī'ă-sis) a condition in which the hair adjacent to a natural orifice turns inward and causes irritation; e.g., in inversion of an eyelid (entropion), eyelashes irritate the eye. [trich- + G. *-iasis*, condition]

**trich·i·lem·mo·ma** (trik'i-le-mō'mă) a benign tumor derived from outer root sheath epithelium of a hair follicle, consisting of cells with pale-staining cytoplasm containing glycogen; multiple trichilemmomas are present on the face in Cowden disease. [trichi- + G. *lemma*, husk, + *-ōma*, tumor]

**tri·chi·na**, pl. **tri·chi·nae** (tri-kī'nă, tri-kī'nē) a larval worm of the genus *Trichinella;* the infective form in pork. [Mod. L., fr. G. *thrix* (*trich-*), hair]

**Trich·i·nel·la** (trik'i-nel'ă) a nematode genus in the aphasmid group that causes trichinosis in humans and carnivores. [Mod. L. fr. trichina + dim. suffix *ella*]

**Trich·i·nel·la** (trik'i-nel'ă) a nematode genus in the aphasmid group that causes trichinosis in humans and carnivores. [Mod. L. fr. trichina + dim. suffix *-ella*]

**Tri·chi·nel·la pseu·do·spir·al·is.** nematode species with normal life cycle in small predators; humans are an accidental host.

**trich·i·no·sis** (trik-i-nō'sis) the disease resulting from ingestion of raw or inadequately cooked pork or other meat that contains encysted larvae of the nematode parasite *Trichinella spiralis.* The initial symptoms are abdominal pain, cramping, and diarrhea, associated with the development of the parasites in the small intestine. Once the larval parasites invade muscular tissue, a second set of symptoms is manifest, including facial and periorbital edema, myalgia, fever, pruritus, urticaria, conjunctivitis, and signs of myocarditis. [*Trichinella* (trichina) + G. *-osis,* condition]

**tri·chi·no·sis gran·u·lo·ma** lesions caused by cell death after penetration of migrating newborn nematode larvae.

**tri·chi·nous** (trik'i-nŭs) infected with trichina worms.

**tri·chi·tis** (tri-kī'tis) inflammation of the hair bulbs. [trich- + G. *-itis,* inflammation]

**tri·chlo·ride** (trī-klōr'īd) a chloride having three chlorine atoms in the molecule; e.g., $PCl_3$.

**(2,4,5-tri·chlo·ro·phen·oxy) ace·tic ac·id** (too-fōr-fīv-trī-klōr-ō-fe-nok'sē a-sē'tik as'id) a herbicide and defoliant synthesized by condensation of chloracetic acid and 2,4,5-trichlorophenol, used as the principal constituent of Agent Orange.

**tri·cho-, trich-, tri·chi-** the hair; a hairlike structure. [G. *thrix* (*trich-*)]

**trich·o·be·zoar** (trik-ō-bē'zōr) a hair cast in the stomach or intestinal tract. SYN hair ball, pilobezoar. [tricho- + bezoar]

**trich·o·cla·sia, tri·choc·la·sis** (trik-ō-klā'zē-ă, tri-kok'lă-sis) SYN trichorrhexis nodosa. [tricho- + G. *klasis,* breaking off]

**trich·o·dis·co·ma** (trik-ō-dis-kō'mă) elliptical parafollicular mesenchymal hamartomas. SYN haarscheibe tumor.

**trich·o·ep·i·the·li·o·ma** (trik'ō-ep-i-thē-lē-ō'mă) multiple small benign nodules, occurring mostly on the skin of the face, derived from basal cells

of hair follicles enclosing small keratin cysts. SYN Brooke tumor. [tricho- + epithelioma]

**trich·o·glos·sia** (trik-ō-glos'ē-ă) SYN hairy tongue. [tricho- + G. *glōssa,* tongue]

**trich·oid** (trik'oyd) hairlike. [tricho- + G. *eidos,* resemblance]

**trich·o·lith** (trik'ō-lith) a concretion on the hair; the lesion of piedra. [tricho- + G. *lithos,* stone]

**trich·o·lo·gia** (trik-ō-lō'jē-ă) a nervous habit of plucking at the hair. [G. *trichologeō,* to pluck hairs, fr. tricho- + *legō,* to pick out, gather]

**trich·o·meg·a·ly** (trik'ō-meg'ă-lē) congenital condition characterized by abnormally long eyelashes; associated with dwarfism. [tricho- + G. *megas,* large]

**trich·o·mo·na·cide** (trik-ō-mō'nă-sīd) an agent that is destructive to *Trichomonas* organisms.

**trich·o·mon·ad** (trik-ō-mō'nad) common name for members of the family Trichomonadidae.

**tri·cho·mo·nal va·gi·ni·tis** acute vaginitis caused by infection with *Trichomonas vaginalis,* which does not invade tissues but provokes an intense local inflammatory reaction in the vagina, cervix, and sometimes the urethra; infection is sexually transmitted; symptoms include frothy green or brown discharge, vulvar itching and irritation, and dysuria.

**Trich·o·mon·as** (trik-ō-mō'nas) a genus of parasitic protozoan flagellates causing trichomoniasis. [tricho- + G. *monas,* single (unit)]

**Tri·cho·mo·nas te·nax** a species that lives as a commensal in the mouth of humans and other primates, especially in the tartar around the teeth or in the defects of carious teeth.

**Tri·cho·mo·nas va·gi·na·lis** a species frequently found in the vagina and urethra of women, in whom it causes trichomonal vaginitis, and in the urethra and prostate gland of men.

**trich·o·mo·ni·a·sis** (trik'ō-mō-nī'ă-sis) disease caused by infection with a protozoan of the genus *Trichomonas;* often used to designate trichomoniasis vaginitis.

**trich·o·my·co·sis** (trik'ō-mī-kō'sis) a disease of the hair caused by *Nocardia* or *Corynebacterium.* [tricho- + G. *mykēs,* fungus, + *-osis,* condition]

**tri·cho·my·co·sis ax·il·la·ris** *Corynebacterium* infection of axillary and pubic hairs with development of yellow (flava), black (nigra), or red (rubra) concretions around the hair shafts; frequently asymptomatic. SYN lepothrix, trichonodosis.

**trich·o·no·car·di·o·sis** (trik'ō-nō-kar'dē-ō'sis) an infection of hair shafts, especially of the axillary and pubic regions, with nocardiae. Yellow, red, or black concretions develop around the infected hair shafts and contain the causative agent and, frequently, micrococci. SEE ALSO trichomycosis, trichomycosis axillaris. [tricho- + *Nocardia* + G. *-osis,* condition]

**trich·o·no·do·sis** (trik'ō-nō-dō'sis) SYN trichomycosis axillaris. [tricho- + L. *nodus,* node (swelling), + G. *-osis,* condition]

**trich·o·no·sis** (trik'ō-nō'sis) SYN trichopathy.

**trich·o·path·ic** (trik-ō-path'ik) relating to any disease of the hair.

**tri·chop·a·thy** (tri-kop'ă-thē) any disease of the hair. SYN trichonosis, trichosis. [tricho- + G. *pathos,* suffering]

**tri·choph·a·gy** (tri-kof'ă-jē) habitual biting of the hair. [tricho- + G. *phagō,* to eat]

**trich·o·phyt·ic** (trik-ō-fit′ik) relating to trichophytosis.

**trich·o·phy·tid** (tri-kof′i-tid, trik-ō-fī′tid) an eruption remote from the site of infection, which is the expression of allergic response to *Trichophyton* infection. [tricho- + G. *phyton,* plant, + *-id* (1)]

**trich·o·phy·to·be·zoar** (trik′ō-fī′tō-bē′zōr) a mixed hair and food ball, consisting of vegetable fibers, seeds and skins of fruits, and animal hair matted together to form a ball in the stomach of humans or animals. [tricho- + G. *phyton,* plant, + bezoar]

*Trich·o·phy·ton* (tri-kof′i-tŏn) a genus of pathogenic fungi causing dermatophytosis in humans and animals; species attack the hair, skin, and nails. [tricho- + G. *phyton,* plant]

*Tri·cho·phy·ton con·cen·tri·cum* an anthropophilic species which is the causative agent of tinea imbricata; it closely resembles the branching mycelium of *Trichophyton schoenleinii.*

*Tri·cho·phy·ton men·ta·gro·phy·tes* a zoophilic small-spored ectothrix species that causes infection of the hair, skin, and nails; it is a cause of ringworm in dogs, horses, rabbits, mice, rats, chinchillas, foxes, and humans (especially tinea pedis with severe inflammation, and tinea cruris).

*Tri·cho·phy·ton ru·brum* a widely distributed anthropophilic species that causes persistent infections of the skin, especially tinea pedis and tinea cruris, and in the nails that are unusually resistant to therapy.

*Tri·cho·phy·ton schoen·lei·ni·i* species of dermatophyte causing favus in humans; it produces tunnels within the hair shaft which are filled with air bubbles after the hyphae disintegrate.

*Tri·cho·phy·ton ton·sur·ans* species that causes epidemic dermatophytosis; the most common cause of tinea capitis in the U.S., forming black dots where hair breaks off at the skin surface.

*Tri·cho·phy·ton vi·o·la·ce·um* an anthropophilic species that causes black-dot ringworm or favus infection of the scalp.

**trich·o·phyt·o·sis** (trik′ō-fī-tō′sis) superficial fungus infection caused by species of *Trichophyton.* [tricho- + G. *phyton,* plant, + *-osis,* condition]

**trich·o·pti·lo·sis** (trik′ō-ti-lō′sis, tri-kop-ti-lō′sis) a condition of splitting of the shaft of the hair, giving it a feathery appearance. [tricho- + G. *ptilōsis,* plumage, + *-osis,* condition]

**trich·or·rhex·is** (trik-ō-rek′sis) a condition in which the hairs tend to break or split. [tricho- + G. *rhēxis,* a breaking]

**tri·chor·rhex·is in·va·gi·na·ta** SYN bamboo hair.

**tri·chor·rhex·is no·do·sa** a congenital or acquired condition in which minute nodes are formed in the hair shafts; splitting and breaking, complete or incomplete, may occur at these nodes. SYN clastothrix, trichoclasia, trichoclasis.

**tri·chos·chi·sis** (tri-kos′ki-sis) the presence of broken or split hairs. SEE ALSO trichorrhexis. [tricho- + G. *schisis,* a cleaving]

**tri·cho·sis** (tri-kō′sis) SYN trichopathy. [tricho- + G. *-osis,* condition]

*Tri·cho·spo·ron* (tri-kos′pō-ron, trik-ō-spōr′on) a genus of imperfect fungi that possess branching septate hyphae with arthroconidia and blastoconidia; these organisms are part of the normal flora of the intestinal tract of humans. *Trichospo-*

*ron beigelii* is the causative agent of white piedra or trichosporosis and fatal fungemia in immunocompromised patients. [tricho- + G. *sporos,* seed (spore)]

**trich·o·sta·sis spi·nu·lo·sa** (tri-kos′tă-sis spī′n-yu-lō′să) a condition in which hair follicles are blocked with a keratin plug containing lanugo hairs. [tricho- + G. *stasis,* a standing; L. *spinulosus,* thorny]

**trich·o·til·lo·ma·nia** (trik′ō-til-ō-mā′nē-ă) a compulsion to pull out one's own hair. [tricho- + G. *tillo,* pull out, + *mania,* insanity]

**tri·chro·mat·ic** (trī-krō-mat′ik) **1.** having, or relating to, the three primary colors, red, green, and blue. **2.** capable of perceiving the three primary colors; having normal color vision. SYN trichromic.

**tri·chro·ma·top·sia** (trī-krō′mă-top′sē-ă) normal color vision; the ability to perceive the three primary colors. [tri- + G. *chrōma,* color, + *opsis,* vision]

**tri·chrome stain** staining combinations which usually contain three dyes of contrasting colors selected to stain connective tissue, muscle, cytoplasm, and nuclei in bright colors; generally, tissue sections are first dyed in iron hematoxylin before being treated with the other dyes.

**tri·chro·mic** (trī-krō′mik) SYN trichromatic.

**trich·u·ri·a·sis** (tri-kyu-rī′ă-sis) infection with nematodes of the genus *Trichuris.* In humans, intestinal parasitization by *T. trichiura* is usually asymptomatic; in massive infections it frequently induces diarrhea or rectal prolapse.

*Trich·u·ris* (tri-kyu′ris) a genus of aphasmid nematodes (sometimes improperly termed *Trichocephalus*) related to the trichina worm, *Trichinella spiralis,* and having a body with a slender, elongated, anterior portion threaded into the mucosa of the colon or large intestine of the host and a thick posterior portion bearing reproductive organs and their products. *Trichuris* contains about 70 species, all in mammals. [tricho- + G. *oura,* tail]

*Tri·chur·is suis* a nematode species found in the pig; adult worms have been found in humans.

*Tri·chur·is tri·chi·u·ra* the whipworm of humans, a species that causes trichuriasis; the body is filiform and slender in the anterior three-fifths, and more robust posteriorly; females are 4 or 5 cm long, males are shorter (with coiled caudal extremity and a single eversible spicule); eggs are barrel-shaped, 50 to 56 by 20 to 22 μm, with double shell and translucent knobs at each of the two poles; humans are the only susceptible hosts and usually acquire infection by direct finger-to-mouth contact or by ingestion of soil, water, or food that contains larvated eggs (development in the soil takes 3 to 6 weeks under proper conditions of warmth and moisture, hence distribution is chiefly tropical); larvae escape from eggs in the ileum, mature in approximately a month, and then pass directly into the cecum without undergoing a parenteral migration as occurs with *Ascaris lumbricoides;* adults may persist for 2 to 7 years.

*Tri·chur·is vul·pis* a nematode species found in the dog; the sexually mature adult has been found in the human appendix.

**tri·cip·i·tal** (trī-sip′i-tăl) having three heads; denoting a triceps muscle.

**tri·co·no·dont** (trī-kō′nō-dont) referring to a

tooth having three cones or cusps in a linear arrangement, the central one the largest. [tri- + G. *kōnos*, cone, + *odous*, tooth]]

**tri•corn pro•te•ase** a protease found in organisms lacking membrane-bound compartments that forms the core of a modular proteolytic system used to generate multicatalytic activities in a controlled manner.

**tri•cor•nute** (trī-kōr′noot) having three cornua or horns. [tri- + L. *cornutus*, horned, fr. *cornu*, horn]

**tri•crot•ic** (trī-krot′ik) thrice-beating; marked by three waves in the arterial pulse tracing. [tri- + G. *krotos*, a beat]

**tri•cus•pid, tri•cus•pi•dal, tri•cus•pi•date** (trī-kŭs′pid, trī-kŭs′pi-dăl, trī-kŭs′pi-dāt) **1.** having three points, prongs, or cusps, as the tricuspid valve of the heart. **2.** having three tubercles or cusps, as the second upper molar tooth (occasionally) and the upper third molar (usually).

**tri•cus•pid a•tre•sia** congenital lack of the tricuspid orifice.

**tri•cus•pid in•suf•fi•cien•cy** SEE valvular regurgitation.

**tri•cus•pid mur•mur** a murmur produced at the tricuspid orifice, either obstructive or regurgitant.

**tri•cus•pid or•i•fice** an atrioventricular opening which leads from the right atrium into the right ventricle of the heart.

**tri•cus•pid ste•no•sis** pathologic narrowing of the orifice of the tricuspid valve.

**tri•cus•pid valve** the valve closing the orifice between the right atrium and right ventricle of the heart; its three cusps are called anterior, posterior, and septal.

**tri•den•tate** (trī-den′tāt) three-toothed; three-pronged. [tri- + L. *dentatus*, toothed]

**tri•der•mic** (trī-der′mik) relating to or derived from the three primary germ layers of the embryo: ectoderm, endoderm, and mesoderm. [tri- + G. *derma*, skin]

**tri•fa•cial neu•ral•gia** SYN trigeminal neuralgia.

**tri•fid** (trī′fid) split into three. [L. *trifidus*, three-cleft]

**tri•fo•cal lens** a lens with segments of three focal powers: distant, intermediate, and near.

**tri•fur•ca•tion** (trī-fŭr-kā′shŭn) **1.** a division into three branches. **2.** the area where the tooth roots divide into three distinct portions. [tri- + L. *furca*, fork]

**tri•gas•tric** (trī-gas′trik) having three bellies; denoting a muscle with two tendinous interruptions. [tri- + G. *gastēr*, belly]

**tri•gem•i•nal cave** the cleft in the meningeal layer of dura of the middle cranial fossa near the tip of the petrous part of the temporal bone; it encloses the roots of the trigeminal nerve and the trigeminal ganglion.

**tri•gem•i•nal gan•gli•on** the large flattened sensory ganglion of the trigeminal nerve lying close to the cavernous sinus along the medial part of the middle cranial fossa in the trigeminal cavity of the dura mater.

**tri•gem•i•nal nerve [CN V]** the chief sensory nerve of the face and the motor nerve of the muscles of mastication; its nuclei are in the mesencephalon and in the pons and medulla oblongata extending down into the cervical portion of the spinal cord; it emerges by two roots, sensory and motor, from the lateral portion of the surface of the pons, and enters a cavity of the dura mater,

the trigeminal cave, at the apex of the petrous portion of the temporal bone, where the sensory root expands to form the trigeminal ganglion; from there the three divisions (ophthalmic [CN V1], maxillary [CN V2], and mandibular [CN V3] nerves) arise. SYN nervus trigeminus [CN V] [TA], fifth cranial nerve [CN V].

**tri•gem•i•nal neu•ral•gia** severe, paroxysmal bursts of pain in one or more branches of the trigeminal nerve; often induced by touching trigger points in or about the mouth. SYN Fothergill disease (1), Fothergill neuralgia, prosopalgia, prosoponeuralgia, tic douloureux, trifacial neuralgia.

**tri•gem•i•nal pulse** a pulse in which the beats occur in trios, a pause following every third beat. SYN pulsus trigeminus.

**tri•gem•i•nal rhi•zo•to•my** division or section of a sensory root of the fifth cranial nerve, accomplished through a subtemporal (Frazier-Spiller operation), suboccipital (Dandy operation), or transtentorial approach.

**tri•gem•i•nal rhy•thm** a cardiac arrhythmia in which the beats are grouped in trios, usually composed of a sinus beat followed by two extrasystoles. SYN trigeminy.

**tri•gem•i•ny** (trī-jem′i-nē) SYN trigeminal rhythm. [L. *trigeminus*, threefold]

**trig•ger ar•ea** SYN trigger point.

**trig•gered ac•tiv•i•ty** one or a series of spontaneously generated heart beats originating from an action potential that produces an after-depolarization which reaches activation threshold.

**trig•ger fing•er** condition by which the finger flexors contract but are unable to re-extend due to a nodule within the tendon sheath or sheath constriction.

**trig•ger point** pathological condition characterized by a small, hypersensitive area located within muscles or fasciae. SYN trigger area, trigger zone.

**trig•ger zone** SYN trigger point.

**tri•glyc•er•ide** (trī-glis′er-īd) SYN triacylglycerol.

**trig•o•na** (trī-gō′nă) plural of trigonum. [L.]

**trig•o•nal** (trig′ō-năl) triangular; relating to a trigonum.

**tri•gone** (trī′gōn) **1.** SYN trigonum. **2.** the first three dominant cusps (protocone, paracone, and metacone), taken collectively, of an upper molar tooth. [L. *trigonum*, fr. G. *trigōnon*, triangle]

**tri•gone of blad•der** a triangular smooth area at the base of the bladder between the openings of the two ureters and that of the urethra. SYN trigonum vesicae [TA], vesical triangle.

**tri•go•nid** (trī-gon′id, trī-gō′nid) the first three dominant cusps, taken collectively, of a lower molar tooth. SEE ALSO trigone. [see *trigonum*]

**tri•go•ni•tis** (trī′gō-nī′tis) inflammation of the urinary bladder, localized in the trigone. [trigone + G. *-itis*, inflammation]

**trig•o•no•ce•phal•ic** (trig′ō-nō-se-fal′ik) pertaining to trigonocephaly.

**trig•o•no•ceph•a•ly** (trig′ō-nō-sef′ă-lē) malformation characterized by a triangular configuration of the skull, due in part to premature synostosis of the cranial bones with compression of the cerebral hemispheres. [trigone + G. *kephalē*, head]

**tri•go•num**, pl. **tri•go•na** (trī-gō′nŭm, trī-gō′nă) any triangular area. SEE triangle. SYN trigone (1). [L., fr. G. *trigōnon*, a triangle]

t
r

**tri·gon·um fe·mo·ra·le** [TA] SYN femoral triangle.

**tri·gon·um in·gui·na·le** [TA] SYN inguinal triangle.

**tri·gon·um lum·ba·le** SYN lumbar triangle.

**tri·gon·um mus·cu·la·re** [TA] SYN muscular triangle.

**tri·gon·um sub·man·di·bu·la·re** [TA] SYN submandibular triangle.

**tri·gon·um ve·si·cae** [TA] SYN trigone of bladder.

**tri·hy·dric al·co·hol** an alcohol containing three OH groups; e.g., glycerol.

**tri·labe** (trī'lāb) a three-pronged forceps for removal of foreign bodies from the bladder. [tri- + G. *labē*, a handle, hold]

**tri·lam·i·nar** (trī-lam'i-nar) having three laminae.

**tri·lo·bate, tri·lobed** (trī-lō'bāt, trī'lobd) having three lobes.

**tri·loc·u·lar** (trī-lok'yu-lăr) having three cavities or cells.

**tril·o·gy** (tril'ō-jē) a triad of related entities. [G. *trilogia,* fr. tri- + *logos,* study, discourse]

**tril·o·gy of Fal·lot** (fāl'ō) a set of congenital defects including pulmonic stenosis, atrial septal defect, and right ventricular hypertrophy. SYN Fallot triad.

**tri·mes·ter** (trī'mes-ter, trī-mes'ter) a period of 3 months; one-third of the length of a pregnancy. [L. *trimestris,* of three-month duration]

**tri·meth·yl·a·mine** (trī-meth'il-am'ēn) a degradation product, often by putrefaction, of nitrogenous plant and animal substances such as beet sugar residue or herring brine; in the body, it probably results from decomposition of choline.

**tri·meth·yl·am·i·nur·ia** (trī-meth'il-am-in-yur'ē-ă) increased excretion of trimethylamine in urine and sweat, with characteristic offensive, fishy body odor.

**tri·nu·cle·o·tide** (trī-noo'klē-ō-tīd) a combination of three adjacent nucleotides, free or in a polynucleotide or nucleic acid molecule; often used with specific reference to the unit (codon or anticodon) specifying a particular amino acid in expression of the genetic code.

**tri·ose** (trī'ōs) a three-carbon monosaccharide; e.g., glyceraldehyde and dihydroxyacetone.

**tri·ose·phos·phate isom·er·ase** (trī'ōs-fos'fāt ī-som'er-ās) an isomerizing enzyme that catalyzes the reversible interconversion of D-glyceraldehyde 3-phosphate and dihydroxyacetone phosphate, a reaction of importance in glycolysis and gluconeogenesis; a deficiency of this enzyme will result in hemolytic anemia and severe neurological deficits.

**tri·ox·ide** (trī-oks'īd) a molecule containing three atoms of oxygen.

**tri·phos·pho·py·ri·dine nu·cle·o·tide (TPN, TPNH)** (trī-fos'fō-pir'i-dēn noo'klē-ō-tīd) former name for nicotinamide adenine dinucleotide phosphate.

**Tri·pi·er am·pu·ta·tion** (trē-pē-ā') a modification of Chopart amputation, in that a part of the calcaneus is also removed.

**tri·ple bond** a covalent bond resulting from the sharing of three pairs of electrons; e.g., HC≡CH (acetylene).

**tri·ple·gia** (trī-plē'jē-ă) paralysis of an upper and a lower extremity and of the face, or of both extremities on one side and of one on the other. [tri- + G. *plēgē,* stroke]

**tri·ple re·peat dis·or·ders** a group of hereditary disorders in which a gene mutation on a specific chromosome produces an abnormal form of protein terminated by a long chain of amino acid glutamate repeats; includes Huntington disease, Kennedy disease, Machado-Joseph disease, myotonic dystrophy, fragile X syndrome, and some spinal cerebellar disorders.

**tri·ple re·sponse** the triphasic response to the firm stroking of the skin: Phase 1 is the sharply demarcated erythema that follows a momentary blanching of the skin, and is the result of release of histamine from the mast cells. Phase 2 is the intense red flare extending beyond the margins of the line of pressure but in the same configuration, and is the result of arteriolar dilation. Phase 3 is the appearance of a line wheal in the configuration of the original stroking.

**tri·ple screen** test of maternal serum α-fetoprotein, chorionic gonadotropin, and unconjugated estrogen for indications of increased risk of fetal abnormality, especially trisomy 21.

**trip·let** 1. one of three children delivered at the same birth. 2. a set of three similar objects, as a compound lens in a microscope, formed of three planoconvex lenses. 3. SYN codon.

**tri·ple vi·sion** SYN triplopia.

**trip·loid** (trip'loyd) pertaining to or characteristic of triploidy. [tri- + -ploid]

**trip·loi·dy** (trip'loy-dē) the presence of three haploid sets of chromosomes, instead of two, in all cells; results in fetal or neonatal death.

**trip·lo·pia** (trip-lō'pē-ă) visual defect in which three images of the same object are seen. SYN triple vision. [G. *triploos,* triple, + *opsis,* sight]

**tri·pod** (trī'pod) 1. three-legged. 2. a stand having three legs or supports. [G. *tripous,* fr. tri- + *pous,* foot]

**tri·pod frac·ture** a facial fracture involving the three supports of the malar prominence, the arch of the zygomatic bone, the zygomatic process of the frontal bone, and the zygomatic process of the maxillary bone.

**tri·que·tral bone** SYN triquetrum. SYN pyramidal bone.

**tri·que·trum** a bone on the medial (ulnar) side of the proximal row of the carpus, articulating with the lunate, pisiform, and hamate. SYN triquetral bone.

⚠**tris-** chemical prefix indicating three of the substituents that follow, independently linked. Cf. tri-.

**tris·mus** (triz'mŭs) persistent contraction of the masseter muscles due to failure of central inhibition; often the initial manifestation of generalized tetanus. SYN lockjaw. [L. fr. G. *trismos,* a creaking, rasping]

**tri·so·mic** (trī-sō'mik) relating to trisomy.

**tri·so·my** (trī'sō-mē) the state of an individual or cell with an extra chromosome instead of the normal pair of homologous chromosomes; in humans, the state of a cell containing 47 normal chromosomes. For various types of trisomy syndrome, see under *syndrome.* [tri- + (chromo)-some]

**tri·so·my 21 syn·drome** SYN Down syndrome.

**tri·splanch·nic** (trī-splangk'nik) relating to the three visceral cavities: skull, thorax, and abdomen. [tri- + G. *splanchnon,* viscus]

**tri·stich·ia** (trī-stik'ē-ă) presence of three rows of eyelashes. [G. *tristichos*, in three rows, fr. *tri-*, three, + *stichos*, row]

**tri·sul·cate** (trī-sŭl'kāt) marked by three grooves.

**tri·ta·nom·a·ly** (trī'tă-nom'ă-lē) a type of partial color deficiency due to a deficiency or abnormality of blue-sensitive retinal cones. [G. *tritos*, third, + *anōmalia*, irregularity]

**trit·an·o·pia** (trī'tă-nō'pē-ă) deficient color perception in which there is an absence of blue-sensitive pigment in the retinal cones. [G. *tritos*, third, + *an-* priv. + *ōps*, eye]

**trit·i·um (T, *t*)** (trit'ē-ŭm, trish'ē-ŭm) SYN hydrogen-3.

**tri·ton tu·mor** a peripheral nerve tumor with striated muscle differentiation, seen most often in neurofibromatosis.

**tri·tu·ber·cu·lar** referring to a tooth having three tubercles or cusps on the occlusal surface. SEE ALSO tricuspid.

**trit·u·ra·ble** (trit'yu-ră-bl) capable of being triturated.

**trit·u·rate** (trit'yu-rāt) 1. to accomplish trituration. 2. a triturated substance.

**trit·u·ra·tion** (trit-yu-rā'shŭn) 1. the act of reducing a drug to a fine powder and incorporating it thoroughly with sugar of milk by rubbing the two together in a mortar. 2. mixing of dental amalgam in a mortar and pestle or with a mechanical device. [L. *trituratio*, fr. *trituro*, to thresh, fr. *tero*, pp. *tritus*, to rub]

**tri·va·lence, tri·va·len·cy** (trī-vā'lens, trī-vā'len-sē) the property of being trivalent.

**tri·va·lent** (trī-vā'lent) having the combining power (valence) of 3.

**triv·i·al name** a name of a chemical, no part of which is necessarily used in a systematic sense; i.e., it gives little or no indication as to chemical structure. Such names are common for drugs, hormones, proteins, and other biologicals, and are used by the general public. Examples are water, aspirin, chlorophyll, heme, methotrexate, folic acid, caffeine, thyroxine, epinephrine, barbital, etc.; also common abbreviations for chemically defined substances, such as ACTH, MSH, BAL, DDT, which are spoken as such and not in terms of the words they represent. Trivial names are often assigned arbitrarily to chemical compounds, especially from natural sources, before the chemical structures are known.

**tRNA** transfer RNA.

**tro·car** (trō'kar) an instrument for withdrawing fluid from a cavity, or for use in paracentesis; it consists of a metal tube (cannula) into which fits an obturator with a sharp three-cornered tip, which is withdrawn after the instrument has been pushed into the cavity; the name trocar is usually applied to the obturator alone, the entire instrument being designated trocar and cannula. [Fr. *trocart*, fr. *trois*, three, + *carre*, side (of a sword blade)]

**tro·chan·ter** (trō-kan'ter) [TA] one of the bony prominences developed from independent osseous centers near the upper extremity of the femur; there are two in humans, three in the horse. [G. *trochantēr*, a runner, fr. *trechō*, to run]

**tro·chan·ter·i·an, tro·chan·ter·ic** (trō-kan-ter'ē-an, trō-kan-ter'ik) relating to a trochanter; especially the greater trochanter.

**tro·chan·ter ma·jor** [TA] SYN greater trochanter.

**tro·che** (trō-kē) a small, disk-shaped or rhombic body composed of solidifying paste containing an astringent, antiseptic, or demulcent drug, used for local treatment of the mouth or throat, the troche being held in the mouth until dissolved. SYN lozenge, pastil (2), pastille. [L. *trochiscus*, fr. G. *trochiskos*, a little wheel, fr. *trochos*, a wheel]

**troch·lea**, pl. **troch·le·ae** (trok'lē-ă, trok'lē-ē) [TA] 1. a structure serving as a pulley. 2. a smooth articular surface of bone upon which another glides. 3. a fibrous loop in the orbit, near the nasal process of the frontal bone, through which passes the tendon of the superior oblique muscle of the eye. [L. pulley, fr. G. *trochileia*, a pulley, fr. *trechō*, to run]

**troch·le·ar** (trok'lē-ar) 1. relating to a trochlea, especially the trochlea of the superior oblique muscle of the eye. 2. SYN trochleiform.

**troch·le·ar nerve [CN IV]** supplies the superior oblique muscle of the eye; its origin is in the midbrain below the cerebral aqueduct, and its fibers decussate in the superior medullary velum, and emerge from the brain at the side of the frenulum, the only cranial nerve to arise from the dorsal aspect of the brainstem; it therefore has the longest intracranial course, entering the dura in the free edge of the tentorium, close to the posterior clinoid process, and passing in the lateral wall of the cavernous sinus to enter the orbit through the superior orbital fissure. SYN nervus trochlearis [CN IV] [TA], fourth cranial nerve [CN IV].

**tro·chle·ar spine** a spicule of bone arising from the edge of the trochlear fovea, giving attachment to the pulley of the superior oblique muscle of the eyeball.

**troch·le·i·form** (trok'lē-i-fōrm) pulley-shaped. SYN trochlear (2).

**tro·choid** (trō'koyd) revolving; rotating; denoting a revolving or wheel-like articulation. [G. *trochōdēs*, fr. *trochos*, wheel, + *eidos*, resemblance]

**tro·choid joint** SYN pivot joint.

**Troi·si·er gan·gli·on** (trwa-zē-ā') historic term for a lymph node immediately above the clavicle, especially on the left side, that is palpably enlarged as the result of a metastasis from a malignant neoplasm; the presence of such a node indicates that the probable site of primary involvement is in an abdominal organ. SEE ALSO signal lymph node.

***Trom·bic·u·la*** (trom-bik'yu-lă) the chigger mite, a genus of mites whose larvae (chiggers, red bugs) include pests of humans and other animals, and vectors of rickettsial and probably viral diseases.

**trom·bic·u·li·a·sis** (trom-bik-yu-lī'ă-sis) infestation by mites of the genus *Trombicula*.

**trom·bic·u·lid** (trom-bik'yu-lid) common name for members of the family Trombiculidae.

**Trom·bic·u·li·dae** (trom-bi-kyu'li-dē) a family of mites whose larvae (redbugs, rougets, harvest mites, scrub mites, or chiggers) are parasitic on vertebrates, and whose nymphs and adults are bright red and free-living, living on insect eggs or minute organisms in the soil. The six-legged larvae are barely visible red or orange parasites that attach to the skin for a few days to a month, producing an exceedingly irritating reaction. Chiggers of the genus *Leptotrombidium* transmit tsutsugamushi disease, caused by *Rickettsia tsutsugamushi*.

**Tröm·ner re·flex** (trŏm'ner) a modified Rossolimo reflex in which, with the fingers of the patient partially flexed, the tapping of the volar aspect of the tip of the middle or index finger causes flexion of all four fingers and thumb; seen in pyramidal tract lesions with moderate spasticity.

**troph·ec·to·derm** (trof-ek'tō-derm) outermost layer of cells in the mammalian blastodermic vesicle, which will make contact with the endometrium and take part in establishing the embryo's means of receiving nutrition; the cell layer from which the trophoblast differentiates. [troph- + ectoderm]

**Tro·pher·y·ma whip·pel·i·i** an unclassified, nonculturable organism, named in 1992, which has been identified by electron microscopy and defined by DNA amplification technologies; it has been proven to be the infectious agent responsible for Whipple disease.

**tro·phe·sic** (trō-fē'sik) pertaining to trophesy.

**troph·e·sy** (trof'ĭĕ-sē) the results of any disorder of the trophic nerves.

**tro·phic** (trof'ik, trōf'ik) **1.** relating to or dependent upon nutrition. **2.** resulting from interruption of nerve supply. [G. *trophē*, nourishment]

△**-tro·phic** nutrition. Cf. -tropic. [G. *trophē*, nourishment]

**tro·phic syn·drome** ulceration of a denervated area, frequently secondary to picking at the anesthetic surface.

**tro·phic ul·cer** ulcer resulting from cutaneous sensory denervation.

△**tro·pho-, troph-** food, nutrition. [G. *trophē*, nourishment]

**troph·o·blast** (trof'ŏ-blast) the mesectodermal cell layer covering the blastocyst, which erodes the uterine mucosa and through which the embryo receives nourishment from the mother; the cells do not enter into the formation of the embryo itself, but contribute to the formation of the placenta. The trophoblast develops processes that later receive a core of vascular mesoderm and are then known as the chorionic villi; the trophoblast soon becomes two-layered, differentiating into the syncytiotrophoblast, an outer layer consisting of a multinucleated protoplasmic mass (syncytium), and the cytotrophoblast, the inner layer next to the mesoderm in which the cells retain their membranes. [tropho- + G. *blastos*, germ]

**troph·o·blas·tic** (trō-fŏ-blas'tik) relating to the trophoblast.

**tro·pho·blas·tic la·cu·na** one of the spaces in the early syncytiotrophoblastic layer of the chorion before the formation of villi; in human embryos maternal blood enters these spaces by the 10th day; with the differentiation of the chorionic villi they become intervillous spaces, sometimes called intervillous lacunae.

**tro·pho·blas·tin** (trō-fŏ-blas'tin) SYN interferon tau.

**tro·pho·blast in·ter·fer·on** SYN interferon tau.

**troph·o·der·ma·to·neu·ro·sis** (trof'ō-der'mă-tō-noo-rō'sis) cutaneous trophic changes due to neural involvement.

**troph·o·neu·ro·sis** (trof'ō-noo-rō'sis) a trophic disorder, such as atrophy, hypertrophy, or a skin eruption, occurring as a consequence of disease

or injury of the nerves of the part. [tropho- + G. *neuron*, nerve, + *-osis*, condition]

**troph·o·neu·rot·ic** (trof-ō-noo-rot'ik) relating to a trophoneurosis.

**troph·o·neu·rot·ic lep·ro·sy** SYN anesthetic leprosy.

**troph·o·plast** (trof'ō-plast) SYN plastid (1). [tropho- + G. *plastos*, formed]

**troph·o·tax·is** (trof-ō-tak'sis) SYN trophotropism. [tropho- + G. *taxis*, arrangement]

**troph·o·tro·pic** (trof-ō-trop'ik) relating to trophotropism.

**tro·phot·ro·pism** (trō-fot'rō-pizm) chemotaxis of living cells in relation to nutritive material; it may be positive (toward nutritive material) or negative (away from nutritive material). SYN trophotaxis. [tropho- + G. *tropē*, a turning]

**troph·o·zo·ite** (trof-ō-zō'īt) the ameboid, vegetative, asexual form of certain Sporozoea, such as the schizont of the plasmodia of malaria and related parasites. [tropho- + G. *zōon*, animal]

△**-tro·phy** food, nutrition. [G. *trophē*, nourishment]

**tro·pia** (trō'pē-ă) abnormal deviation of the eye. SEE strabismus. [G. *tropē*, a turning]

△**-trop·ic** a turning toward, having an affinity for. Cf. -trophic. [G. *tropē*, a turning]

**trop·i·cal ab·scess** SYN amebic abscess.

**trop·i·cal ac·ne** a severe type of acne of the entire trunk, shoulders, upper arms, buttocks, and thighs; occurs in hot, humid climates.

**trop·i·cal a·ne·mia** various syndromes frequently observed in persons in tropical climates, usually resulting from nutritional deficiencies or hookworm or other parasitic diseases.

**trop·i·cal bu·bo** SYN lymphogranuloma venereum.

**trop·i·cal di·ar·rhea** SYN tropical sprue.

**trop·i·cal dis·eas·es** infectious and parasitic diseases endemic in tropical and subtropical zones, including Chagas disease, leishmaniasis, leprosy, malaria, onchocerciasis, schistosomiasis, sleeping sickness, yellow fever, and others; often water- or insect-borne.

**trop·i·cal e·o·sin·o·phil·ia** eosinophilia associated with cough and asthma, caused by occult filarial infection without evidence of microfilaremia, occurring most frequently in India and Southeast Asia.

**trop·i·cal li·chen, li·chen tro·pi·cus** SYN miliaria rubra.

**trop·i·cal med·i·cine** the branch of medicine concerned with diseases, mainly of parasitic origin, in areas having a tropical climate.

**trop·i·cal sore** SYN cutaneous leishmaniasis.

**trop·i·cal sple·no·meg·a·ly syn·drome** SYN hyperreactive malarious splenomegaly.

**trop·i·cal sprue** sprue occurring in the tropics, often associated with enteric infection and nutritional deficiency, and frequently complicated by folate deficiency with macrocytic anemia. SYN tropical diarrhea.

**trop·i·cal ty·phus** SYN tsutsugamushi disease.

**trop·i·cal ul·cer 1.** the lesion occurring in cutaneous leishmaniasis; **2.** tropical phagedenic ulceration caused by a variety of microorganisms, including mycobacteria; common in northern Nigeria.

**tro·pism** (trō'pizm) the phenomenon, observed in living organisms, of moving toward (**positive tropism**) or away from (**negative tropism**) a focus of light, heat, or other stimulus; usually applied to the movement of a portion of the organism as opposed to taxis, the movement of an entire organism. [G. *tropē*, a turning]

**tro•po•col•la•gen** (trō-pō-kol′ă-jen) the fundamental units of collagen fibrils, consisting of three helically arranged polypeptide chains.

**tro•po•my•o•sin** (trō-pō-mī′ō-sin) a fibrous protein extractable from muscle; sometimes specified as tropomyosin B to distinguish it from tropomyosin A (paramyosin) prominent in mollusks.

**tro•po•nin (Tn)** (trō′pō-nĭn) a complex of three proteins, troponin-C (TnC), troponin-I (TnI), troponin-T (TnT), present in striated muscle. Together, these proteins function as regulators of muscle contraction. There are a number of isoforms. The cardiac isoform of TnT is specific for cardiac muscle; the blood level of TnT rises within 4 hours after myocardial damage and remains elevated for 10–14 days after an acute myocardial infarction. Measurement of this protein is valuable in the early diagnosis of MI and in monitoring the effectiveness of thrombolytic therapy after an MI.

**trough sign** an anteromedial glenoid defect resultant from posterior shoulder dislocation.

**Trous•seau point** (troo-sō′) a painful point, in neuralgia, at the spinous process of the vertebra below which the affected nerve arises.

**Trous•seau sign** (troo-sō′) in latent tetany, the occurrence of carpopedal spasm accompanied by paresthesia elicited when the upper arm is compressed, as by a tourniquet or a blood pressure cuff.

**Trous•seau spot** (troo-sō′) SYN meningitic streak.

**Trous•seau syn•drome** (troo-sō′) thrombophlebitis migrans associated with visceral cancer.

**Trp** tryptophan and its radicals.

**true an•ky•lo•sis** SYN synostosis.

**true di•ver•tic•u•lum** a term denoting a diverticulum that includes all the layers of the wall from which it protrudes.

**true lu•men** in a dissecting aneurysm, the channel representing the actual intima-lined artery.

**true pre•co•cious pu•ber•ty** SYN hyperovarianism.

**true ribs [I–VII]** seven upper ribs on either side whose cartilages articulate directly with the sternum. SYN costae verae [TA].

**true vo•cal cord** SYN vocal fold.

**trun•cal** (trŭng′kăl) relating to the trunk of the body or to any arterial or nerve trunk, etc.

**trun•cate** (trŭng′kāt) truncated; cut across at right angles to the long axis, or appearing to be so cut. [L. *trunco*, pp. *-atus*, to maim, cut off]

**trun•cus**, gen. and pl. **trun•ci** (trŭng′kŭs, trŭng′kī) SYN trunk. [L. stem, trunk]

**trun•cus bra•chi•o•ce•pha•li•cus** [TA] SYN brachiocephalic trunk.

**trun•cus ce•li•a•cus** [TA] SYN celiac trunk.

**trun•cus cost•o•cer•vi•ca•lis** [TA] SYN costocervical trunk.

**trun•cus pul•mo•na•lis** [TA] SYN pulmonary trunk.

**trun•cus sym•path•i•cus** [TA] SYN sympathetic trunk.

**trun•cus thy•ro•cer•vi•cal•is** [TA] SYN thyrocervical trunk.

**trun•cus va•ga•lis** [TA] SYN vagal trunk.

**Tru•ne•cek sign** (trŭ′nĕ-sek) palpable impulse of the subclavian artery near the point of origin of the sternomastoid muscle in cases of aortic sclerosis.

**trunk** (trŭnk) **1.** the body (trunk or torso), excluding the head and extremities. **2.** a primary nerve, vessel, or collection of tissue before its division. **3.** a large collecting lymphatic vessel. See page 1018. SYN truncus. [L. *truncus*]

**Trus•ler rule for pul•mo•nary ar•tery band••ing** (trus′ler) a method that gives guidance as to the correct tightness of the band; the degree of banding for a complex congenital cardiac anomaly with bidirectional shunting less than that for simple ones.

**truss** (trŭs) an appliance designed to prevent the return of a reduced hernia or the increase in size of an irreducible hernia; it consists of a pad attached to a belt and kept in place by a spring or straps. [Fr. *trousser*, to tie up, to pack]

**try•pan•o•ci•dal** (tri-pan′ō-sī′dăl) destructive to trypanosomes.

**try•pan•o•cide** (tri-pan′ō-sīd) an agent that kills trypanosomes. [trypanosome + L. *caedo*, to kill]

***Try•pan•o•so•ma*** (tri-pan′ō-sō′mă) a genus of asexual digenetic protozoan flagellates that are parasitic in the blood plasma of many vertebrates and as a rule have an intermediate host, a blood-sucking invertebrate, such as a leech, tick, or insect; pathogenic species cause trypanosomiasis in humans. [G. *trypanon*, an auger, + *sōma*, body]

***Try•pan•o•so•ma brucei gam•bi•ense*** a subspecies causing Gambian trypanosomiasis; transmitted by tsetse flies, especially *Glossina palpalis*. SYN *Trypanosoma gambiense*.

***Try•pan•o•so•ma brucei rho•des•i•ense*** a subspecies causing Rhodesian trypanosomiasis; it is transmitted by tsetse flies, especially *Glossina morsitans*; various game animals can act as reservoir hosts. SYN *Trypanosoma rhodesiense*.

***Try•pan•o•so•ma cru•zi*** a species that causes South American trypanosomiasis; transmission and infection are common only where the triatomine bug vector defecates while taking blood, as the bug feces contains the infective agents that are scratched into the skin or brought in contact with mucosal surfaces. Trypomastigotes are found in the blood; heart muscle and other organs are attacked.

***Try•pan•o•so•ma gam•bi•ense*** SYN *Trypanosoma brucei gambiense*.

***Try•pan•o•so•ma rho•des•i•ense*** SYN *Trypanosoma brucei rhodesiense*.

**try•pan•o•some** (tri-pan′ō-sōm) common name for any member of the genus *Trypanosoma* or of the family Trypanosomatidae. [G. *trypanon*, an auger, + *sōma*, body]

**try•pan•o•so•mi•a•sis** (tri-pan′ō-sō-mī′ă-sis) any disease caused by a trypanosome. SYN trypanosomosis.

**try•pan•o•so•mic** (tri-pan-ō-sō′mik) relating to trypanosomes, especially denoting infection by such organisms.

**try•pan•o•so•mid** (tri-pan′ō-sō-mid) a skin lesion resulting from immunologic changes from trypanosome disease. [trypanosome + G. *-id* (1)]

**try•pan•o•so•mo•sis** (trip′an-ō-sō-mō′sis) SYN trypanosomiasis.

**tryp•sin** (trip′sin) a proteolytic enzyme formed in the small intestine from trypsinogen by the action of enteropeptidase; a serine proteinase that hydrolyzes peptides, amides, and esters.

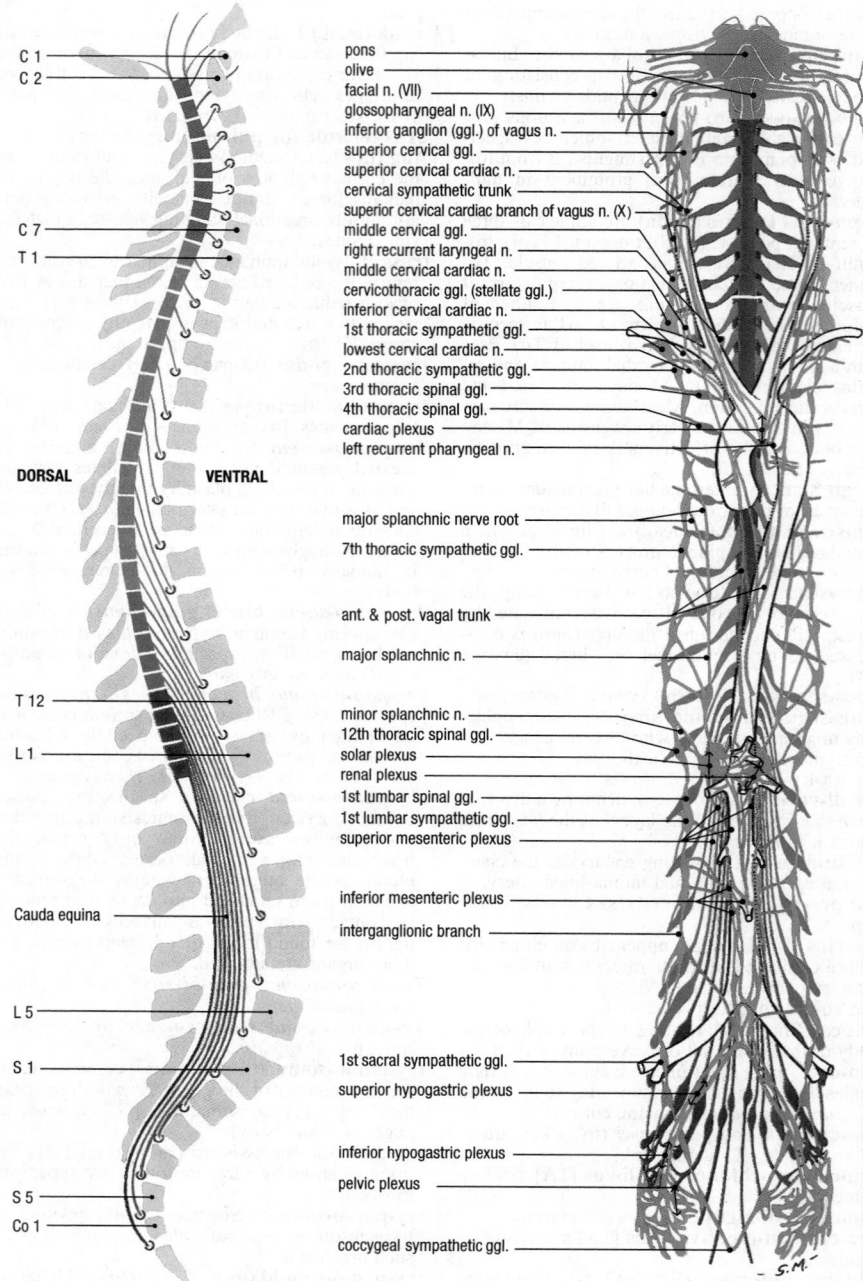

C 1
C 2

C 7
T 1

DORSAL

VENTRAL

T 12

L 1

Cauda equina

L 5

S 1

S 5
Co 1

pons
olive
facial n. (VII)
glossopharyngeal n. (IX)
inferior ganglion (ggl.) of vagus n.
superior cervical ggl.
superior cervical cardiac n.
cervical sympathetic trunk
superior cervical cardiac branch of vagus n. (X)
middle cervical ggl.
right recurrent laryngeal n.
middle cervical cardiac n.
cervicothoracic ggl. (stellate ggl.)
inferior cervical cardiac n.
1st thoracic sympathetic ggl.
lowest cervical cardiac n.
2nd thoracic sympathetic ggl.
3rd thoracic spinal ggl.
4th thoracic spinal ggl.
cardiac plexus
left recurrent pharyngeal n.

major splanchnic nerve root

7th thoracic sympathetic ggl.

ant. & post. vagal trunk

major splanchnic n.

minor splanchnic n.
12th thoracic spinal ggl.
solar plexus
renal plexus
1st lumbar spinal ggl.
1st lumbar sympathetic ggl.
superior mesenteric plexus

inferior mesenteric plexus

interganglionic branch

1st sacral sympathetic ggl.

superior hypogastric plexus

inferior hypogastric plexus

pelvic plexus

coccygeal sympathetic ggl.

- S.M. -

**spinal cord:** left, spinal medulla in the vertebral column with color coding showing relation between neural segments and vertebrae; right, color coding shows relation of **sympathetic trunk** to spinal nerves and branches

spinal cord (left):
cervical segments (brown)    C 1–8
thoracic segments (red)    T 1–12
lumbar segments (green)    L 1–5
sacral segments (purple)    S 1–5
coccygeal segments (black)    Co 1–5

sympathetic trunk (right):

| | |
|---|---|
| lilac | pons + medulla oblongata |
| blue | cranial nerves, primarily distribution pattern of the vagus nerve |
| brown | cervical spinal cord levels, cervical posterior roots + posterior root ganglia |
| butterscotch | cervical parts of sympathetic trunk, corresponding ganglia + main branches |
| red | thoracic spinal cord levels, thoracic posterior roots + posterior root ganglia |
| orange | thoracic parts of sympathetic trunk, corresponding ganglia + major branches |
| dark green | lumbar posterior roots + posterior ganglia |
| light green | lumbar parts of sympathetic trunk, corresponding ganglia + major branches |
| purple | sacral posterior roots + posterior root ganglia |
| magenta | sacral parts of sympathetic trunk, corresponding ganglia + major branches |
| white | aortic arch, aorta + major branches |

**tryp·sin·o·gen, tryp·so·gen** (trip-sin′ō-jen, trip′sō-jen) an inactive protein secreted by the pancreas that is converted into trypsin by the action of enteropeptidase.

**tryp·tic** (trip′tik) relating to trypsin, as tryptic digestion.

**tryp·to·phan (Trp, W)** (trip′tō-fan) the L-isomer is a component of proteins; a nutritionally essential amino acid.

**tryp·to·pha·nase** (trip′tō-fă-nās) **1.** SYN tryptophan 2,3-dioxygenase. **2.** an enzyme found in bacteria that catalyzes the cleavage of L-tryptophan to indole, pyruvic acid, and ammonia; pyridoxal phosphate is a coenzyme.

**tryp·to·phan 2,3-di·ox·y·gen·ase** an oxidoreductase catalyzing the reaction of L-tryptophan and $O_2$ to produce L-$N$-formylkynurenine; an adaptive enzyme, the level (in the liver) being controlled by adrenal hormones; a step in tryptophan catabolism; also, a step in the synthesis of NAD$^+$ from tryptophan. SYN tryptophanase (1).

**tryp·to·pha·nu·ria** (trip′tō-fă-nyu′rē-ă) enhanced urinary excretion of tryptophan.

**tset·se** (tset′sē, tsē′tsē) SEE *Glossina.* [S. African native name]

**TSI** thyroid-stimulating immunoglobulins.

**TSS** toxic shock syndrome.

**TSTA** tumor-specific transplantation antigens.

**tsu·tsu·ga·mu·shi dis·ease** (tsoo′tsoo-gă-moo′shē di-zēz) an acute infectious disease, caused by *Rickettsia tsutsugamushi* and transmitted by *Trombicula akamushi* and *T. deliensis*, that occurs in harvesters of hemp in some parts of Japan; characterized by fever, painful swelling of the lymphatic glands, a small blackish scab on the genitals, neck, or axilla, and an eruption of large dark red papules. SYN akamushi disease, mite typhus, scrub typhus, tropical typhus.

**TT, TTY** Telephone Device for the Deaf.

**$t_i/t_{tot}$** duty cycle.

**T tu·bule** the transverse tubule that passes from the sarcolemma across a myofibril of striated muscle; it is the intermediate tubule of the triad.

**tu·ba,** gen. and pl. **tu·bae** (too′bă, too′bē; too′bē) SYN tube. [L. a straight trumpet]

**tu·ba au·di·ti·va** [TA] SYN pharyngotympanic (auditory) tube.

**tu·ba au·di·tor·ia** SYN pharyngotympanic (auditory) tube.

**tub·al** (too′băl) relating to a tube, especially the uterine tube.

**tub·al air cells of pharyn·go·tym·pan·ic tube** occasional small air cells in the inferior wall of the pharyngotympanic tube, near the tympanic orifice, communicating with the tympanic cavity.

**tub·al li·ga·tion** interruption of the continuity of the oviducts by cutting, cautery, or by a plastic or metal device to prevent future conception.

**tub·al preg·nan·cy** development of an impregnated ovum in the uterine tube.

**tube** (toob) **1.** a hollow cylindrical structure or canal. **2.** a hollow cylinder or pipe. SYN tuba. [L. *tubus*]

**tu·bec·to·my** (too-bek′tō-mē) SYN salpingectomy. [L. *tuba,* tube, + G. *ektomē,* excision]

**tubed flap** a flap in which the sides of the pedicle are sutured together to create a tube, with the entire surface covered by skin. SYN Filatov flap, Filatov-Gillies flap.

**tu·ber,** pl. **tu·bera** (too′ber, too′ber-ă) **1.** a localized swelling; a knob. **2.** a short, fleshy, thick, underground stem of plants, such as the potato. [L. protuberance, swelling]

**tu·ber ci·ne·re·um** [TA] a prominence of the base of the hypothalamus, bordered caudally by the mammillary bodies, rostrally by the optic chiasm, and laterally by the optic tract, extending ventrally into the infundibulum and hypophysial stalk.

**tu·ber·cle** (too′ber-kl) **1.** a nodule, especially in an anatomic, not pathologic, sense. SYN tuberculum (1) [TA]. **2.** a circumscribed, rounded, solid elevation on the skin, mucous membrane, or surface of an organ. **3.** a slight elevation from the surface of a bone giving attachment to a muscle or ligament. **4.** in dentistry, a small elevation arising on the surface of a tooth. **5.** a granulomatous lesion due to infection by *Mycobacterium tuberculosis.* Although somewhat variable in size (0.5–2 or 3 mm in diameter) and in the proportions of various histologic components, tubercles tend to be fairly well-circumscribed, spheroidal, firm lesions that usually consist of three zones: 1) an inner focus of necrosis, coagulative at first, and then becoming caseous; 2) a middle zone that consists of large mononuclear phagocytes (macrophages), frequently arranged somewhat radially (with reference to the necrotic material) resembling an epithelium, and hence termed epithelioid cells; multinucleated giant cells of Langhans type may also be present; 3) an outer zone of numerous lymphocytes, and a few monocytes and plasma cells. In instances where healing has begun, a fourth zone of fibrous tissue may form at the periphery. Morphologically indistinguishable lesions may occur in diseases caused by other agents; many observers use the term nonspecifically, i.e., with reference to any such granuloma; others use "tubercle" only for tuberculous lesions, and then designate those of undetermined causes as epithelioid-cell granulomas. [L. *tuberculum,* dim. of *tuber,* a knob, a swelling, a tumor]

**tu·ber·cle ba·cil·lus 1.** SYN *Mycobacterium tuberculosis.* **2.** SYN *Mycobacterium bovis.* **3.** SYN *Mycobacterium avium.*

**tu•ber•cle of rib** the knob on the posterior surface of a rib, at the junction of its neck and shaft, which articulates with the transverse process of the vertebra, which corresponds in number to the rib, forming a costotransverse joint.

**tu•ber•cle of tra•pe•zi•um** a prominent ridge on the trapezium forming the lateral border of the groove in which runs the tendon of the flexor carpi radialis.

**tu•ber•cu•la** (too-ber′kyu-lă) plural of tuberculum.

**tu•ber•cu•lar, tu•ber•cu•late, tu•ber•cu•lat•ed** (too-ber′kyu-lăr, too-ber′kyu-lāt, too-ber′kyu-lāted) pertaining to or characterized by tubercles or small nodules. Cf. tuberculous.

**tu•ber•cu•lid** (too-ber′kyu-lid) a lesion of the skin or mucous membrane resulting from hypersensitivity to mycobacterial antigens disseminated from a distant site of active tuberculosis. [tubercul- + G. -id (1)]

**tu•ber•cu•lin** (too-ber′kyu-lin) **1.** a glycerin-broth culture of *Mycobacterium tuberculosis* evaporated to ¹⁄₁₀ volume at 100°C and filtered; introduced by Robert Koch for the treatment of tuberculosis but now used chiefly for diagnostic tests; originally known as Koch old tuberculin (OT) or Koch original tuberculin **2.** one or another of a relatively large number of extracts of *Mycobacterium tuberculosis* cultures, different from OT and now obsolete.

**tu•ber•cu•lin test** a skin test in which tuberculin or its purified protein derivative (PPD) is injected into the skin; the test is read on the basis of local induration occurring in 48–72 hours.

**tu•ber•cu•li•tis** (too-ber-kyu-lī′tis) inflammation of any tubercle. [tubercul- + G. -itis, inflammation]

⚠**tu•ber•cu•lo-, tu•ber•cul-** a tubercle, tuberculosis. [L. *tuberculum,* tubercle]

**tu•ber•cu•lo•cele** (too-ber′kyu-lō-sēl) tuberculosis of the testes. [tuberculo- + G. *kēlē,* tumor, hernia]

**tu•ber•cu•lo•fi•broid** (too-ber′kyu-lō-fī′broyd) a discrete, well-circumscribed, usually spheroidal, moderately to extremely firm, encapsulated nodule that is formed during the process of healing in a focus of tuberculous granulomatous inflammation.

**tu•ber•cu•loid** (too-ber′kyu-loyd) resembling tuberculosis or a tubercle. [tuberculo- + G. *eidos,* resemblance]

**tu•ber•cu•loid lep•ro•sy** a benign, stable, and resistant form of the disease in which the lepromin reaction is strongly positive and in which the lesions are erythematous, insensitive, infiltrated plaques with clear-cut edges. SYN nodular leprosy.

**tu•ber•cu•lo•ma** (too-ber-kyu-lō′mă) a rounded tumorlike but nonneoplastic mass, usually in the lungs or brain, due to localized tuberculous infection. [tuberculo- + G. -oma, tumor]

**tu•ber•cu•lo•sis (TB)** (too-ber-kyu-lō′sis) a specific disease caused by the presence of *Mycobacterium tuberculosis,* which may affect almost any tissue or organ of the body, the most common seat of the disease being the lungs; the anatomical lesion is the tubercle, which can undergo caseation necrosis; general symptoms are those of sepsis: hectic fever, sweats, and emaciation; often progressive with high mortality if not treated. An opportunistic infection of persons with compromised immune systems, including those with AIDS. There is also a high incidence among IV drug abusers. [tuberculo- + G. -osis, condition]

**tu•ber•cu•lo•sis cu•tis ver•ru•co•sa** a tuberculous skin lesion having a warty surface with a chronic inflammatory base. SEE ALSO postmortem wart. SYN tuberculous wart.

**tu•ber•cu•lo•stat•ic** (too-ber′kyu-lō-stat′ik) relating to an agent that inhibits the growth of tubercle bacilli. [tuberculo- + G. *statikos,* causing to stand]

**tu•ber•cu•lous** (too-ber′kyu-lŭs) relating to or affected by tuberculosis. Cf. tubercular.

**tu•ber•cu•lous ab•scess** an abscess caused by the tubercle bacillus. SYN cold abscess (2).

**tu•ber•cu•lous en•ter•i•tis** enteric tuberculosis that may occur in the absence of obvious pulmonary tuberculosis; may be caused by bovine tuberculosis contracted through drinking of unpasteurized milk or swallowing of tubercle bacilli expectorated from cavitary lesions in the lung.

**tu•ber•cu•lous me•nin•gi•tis** inflammation of the cerebral leptomeninges marked by the presence of granulomatous inflammation; it is usually confined to the base of the brain (basilar meningitis, internal hydrocephalus) and is accompanied in children by an accumulation of spinal fluid in the ventricles (acute hydrocephalus).

**tu•ber•cu•lous spon•dy•li•tis** tuberculous infection of the spine associated with a sharp angulation of the spine at the point of disease. SYN Pott disease.

**tu•ber•cu•lous wart** SYN tuberculosis cutis verrucosa.

**tu•ber•cu•lum,** pl. **tu•ber•cu•la** (too-ber′kyulŭm, too-ber′kyu-lă) [TA] **1.** SYN tubercle (1). **2.** a circumscribed, rounded, solid elevation on the skin, mucous membrane, or surface of an organ. **3.** a slight elevation from the surface of a bone giving attachment to a muscle or ligament. [L. dim. of *tuber,* a knob, swelling, tumor]

**tu•ber•cu•lum ar•thri•ti•cum 1.** SYN Heberden nodes. **2.** any gouty concretion in or around a joint.

**tu•ber•os•i•tas** (too′ber-os′i-tas) SYN tuberosity. [LL., fr. L., *tuberosus,* full of lumps, fr. *tuber,* a knob]

**tu•ber•os•i•tas** (too′ber-os′i-tas) [TA] SYN tuberosity. [LL., fr. L., *tuberosus,* full of lumps, fr. *tuber,* a knob]

**tu•ber•os•i•ty** (too′ber-os′i-tē) a large tubercle or rounded elevation, especially from the surface of a bone. SYN tuberositas [TA], tuberositas.

**tu•ber•ous** (too′ber-ŭs) knobby, lumpy, or nodular; presenting many tubers or tuberosities. [L. *tuberosus*]

**tube tooth** an artificial tooth constructed with a vertical, cylindric aperture extending from the center of the base up into the body of the tooth into which a pin may be placed or cast for the attachment of the tooth to a denture base.

⚠**tu•bo-** tubular, a tube. SEE ALSO salpingo-. [L. *tubus, tuba,* tube]

**tu•bo•ab•dom•i•nal preg•nan•cy** development of an ectopic pregnancy partly in the uterine tube and partly in the abdominal cavity.

**tu•bo-o•var•i•an** (too′bō-ō-var′ē-an) relating to the uterine (fallopian) tube and the ovary.

**tu·bo·o·var·i·an ab·scess** a large abscess involving a uterine tube and an adherent ovary, resulting from extension of purulent inflammation of the tube.

**tu·bo·var·i·an preg·nan·cy** development of the fertilized oocyte at the fimbriated extremity of the fallopian and involving the ovary.

**tu·bo·plas·ty** (too′bō-plas-tē) SYN salpingoplasty.

**tu·bo·re·tic·u·lar struc·ture** tubules 20–30 nm in length that lie within cisterns of smooth endoplasmic reticulum; observed in connective tissue diseases such as SLE, and in various cancers and virus infections.

**tu·bo·tor·sion** (too′bō-tōr-shŭn) twisting of a tubular structure, such as an oviduct. [tubo- + L. *torsio,* torsion]

**tu·bo·tym·pan·ic, tu·bo·tym·pa·nal** (too′bō-tim-pan′ik, too-bō-tim′pă-năl) relating to the auditory tube and the tympanic cavity of the ear.

**tu·bo·u·ter·ine** (too′bō-yu′ter-in) relating to a uterine tube and the uterus.

**tu·bu·lar car·ci·no·ma** a well-differentiated form of ductal breast carcinoma with invasion of the stroma by small epithelial tubules.

**tu·bu·lar cyst** SYN tubulocyst.

**tu·bu·lar for·ceps** a long slender forceps intended for use through a cannula or other tubular instrument.

**tu·bu·lar gland** a gland composed of one or more tubules ending in a blind extremity.

**tu·bu·lar vi·sion** a constriction of the visual field, as though one were looking through a hollow cylinder or tube. SYN tunnel vision.

**tu·bule** (too′byul) a small tube. SYN tubulus. [L. *tubulus,* dim. of *tubus,* tube]

**tu·bu·li** (too′byu-lī) plural of tubulus.

**tu·bu·li con·tor·ti 1.** SYN convoluted tubule. **2.** SYN seminiferous tubule.

**tu·bu·lin** (too′byu-lin) a protein subunit of microtubules; it is a dimer composed of two globular polypeptides, α-tubulin and β-tubulin. SEE ALSO dynein.

**tu·bu·li se·mi·ni·feri rec·ti** [TA] SYN seminiferous tubule.

**tu·bu·lo·ac·i·nar gland** a gland whose secretory elements are elongated acini. SYN acinotubular gland.

**tu·bu·lo·cyst** (too′byu-lō-sist) a cyst formed by the dilation of any occluded canal or tube. SYN tubular cyst.

**tu·bu·lo·glo·me·ru·lar feed·back** a blood flow control mechanism operating in the kidneys that limits changes in glomerular filtration rate.

**tu·bu·lo·in·ter·sti·tial ne·phri·tis** nephritis affecting renal tubules and interstitial tissue, with infiltration by plasma cells and mononuclear cells; seen in lupus nephritis, allograft rejection, and methicillin sensitization.

**tu·bu·lor·rhex·is** (too′byu-lō-rek′sis) a pathologic process characterized by necrosis of the epithelial lining in localized segments of renal tubules, with focal rupture or loss of the basement membrane. [tubule + G. *rhēxis,* a breaking]

**tu·bu·lus,** pl. **tu·bu·li** (too′byu-lŭs, too′byu-lī) SYN tubule. [L. dim. of *tubus,* a pipe]

**tu·bus,** pl. **tu·bi** (too′bŭs, too′bī) a tube or canal. [L.]

**tuft·ed cell** a particular type of cell in the olfactory bulb comparable to a mitral cell with respect to afferent and efferent relationships, but smaller and more superficially located.

**tu·la·rae·mia [Br.]** SEE tularemia.

**tu·la·re·mia** (too-lă-rē′mē-ă) a disease caused by *Francisella tularensis* and transmitted to humans from rodents through the bite of a deer fly, *Chrysops discalis,* and other bloodsucking insects; can also be acquired directly through the bite of an infected animal or through handling of an infected animal carcass; symptoms consist of fever and swelling and suppuration of the lymph nodes draining the site of infection; rabbits are an important reservoir host. [*Tulare,* Lake and County, CA, + G. *haima,* blood]

**Tul·lio phe·no·me·non** (too-lē-ō) momentary vertigo caused by any loud sound, notably occurring in cases of active labyrinthine fistula.

**tu·me·fac·tion** (too-mĕ-fak′shŭn) **1.** a swelling. **2.** SYN tumescence. [see tumefacient]

**tu·me·fy** (too′mĕ-fī) to swell or to cause to swell.

**tu·mes·cence** (too-mes′ens) the condition of being or becoming tumid. SYN tumefaction (2), turgescence. [L. *tumesco,* to begin to swell]

**tu·mes·cent** (too-mes′ent) denoting tumescence. SYN turgescent.

**tu·me·scent lip·o·suc·tion** liposuction performed after subcutaneous infusion of lidocaine solution and the use of microcannulae.

**tu·mid** (too′mid) swollen, as by congestion, edema, hyperemia. SYN turgid. [L. *tumidus*]

█ **tu·mor** (too′mŏr) **1.** any swelling or tumefaction. **2.** SYN neoplasm. **3.** one of the four signs of inflammation (t., calor, dolor, rubor) enunciated by Celsus. See page B4. [L. *tumor,* a swelling]

**tu·mor an·gi·o·gen·ic fac·tor (TAF)** a substance released by solid tumors which induces formation of new blood vessels to supply the tumor.

**tu·mor ant·i·gens 1.** antigens that may be frequently associated with tumors or may be specifically found on tumor cells of the same origin (tumor specific); **2.** tumor antigens may also be associated with replication and transformation by certain DNA tumor viruses, including adenoviruses and papovaviruses. SYN neoantigens. SEE ALSO T antigens.

**tu·mor blush** enhancement of tumor on radiologic exams by administration of contrast agents.

**tu·mor bur·den** the total mass of tumor tissue carried by a patient with cancer.

**tu·mor·i·ci·dal** (too′mōr-i-sī′dăl) denoting an agent destructive to tumors. [tumor + L. *caedo,* to kill]

**tu·mor·i·gen·e·sis** (too′mŏr-i-jen′ĕ-sis) production of a new growth or growths. [tumor + G. *genesis,* origin]

**tu·mor·i·gen·ic** (too′mŏr-i-jen′ik) causing or producing tumors.

**tu·mor mark·er** a substance, released into the circulation by tumor tissue, whose detection in the serum indicates the presence and specific type of tumor.

**tu·mor ne·cro·sis fac·tor** SYN cachectin.

**tumor necrosis factor-α** a pleiotropic cytokine synthesized widely throughout the female reproductive tract.

**tu·mor ne·cro·sis fac·tor-β** a cytokine that is produced by CD4 and CD8 T cells after exposure to an antigen.

**tu·mor-spe·ci·fic trans·plan·ta·tion ant·i·gens (TSTA)** surface antigens of DNA tumor virus-transformed cells, which elicit an immune rejection of the virus-free cells when transplanted

t
u

into an animal that has been immunized against the specific cell-transforming virus.

**tu•mor stage** the extent of the spread of a malignant neoplasm from its site of origin. SEE ALSO TNM staging.

**tu•mor sup•pres•sor gene 1.** a gene whose function is to suppress cellular proliferation. Also known as an antioncogene because it suppresses neoplastic transformation. Loss of a tumor suppressor gene through chromosomal aberration leads to heightened susceptibility to neoplasia. **2.** SYN antioncogene.

**tu•mor vi•rus** SYN oncogenic virus.

**tu•mour [Br.]** SEE tumor.

**TUNEL** terminal deoxynucleotidyl transferase-mediated dUTP-biotin end labeling of fragmented DNA; this method uses immunohistochemistry to identify DNA fragmentation in nuclei of cells undergoing apoptosis.

**Tun•ga pen•e•trans** (tŭng'ă pen'ĕ-tranz) a member of the flea family, Tungidae, commonly known as chigger flea, sand flea, chigoe, or jigger; the minute female penetrates the skin, frequently under the toenails; as she becomes distended with eggs to about pea size, a painful ulcer with inflammation develops at the site.

**tung•sten (W)** (tŭng'sten) a metallic element, atomic no. 74, atomic wt. 183.85. SYN wolfram, wolframium. [Swed. *tung,* heavy, + *sten,* stone]

**tu•nic** (too'nik) coat or covering; one of the enveloping layers of a part, especially one of the coats of a blood vessel or other tubular structure. SYN tunica. [L. *tunica*]

**tu•ni•ca,** pl. **tu•ni•cae** (too'ni-kă, too'ni-kē) SYN tunic. [L. a coat]

**tu•ni•ca ad•ven•ti•tia** [TA] SYN adventitia.

**tu•ni•ca al•bu•gin•ea** a dense white collagenous tunic surrounding a structure.

**tu•ni•ca al•bu•gin•ea of tes•tis** a thick white fibrous membrane forming the outer coat of the testis.

**tu•ni•ca ex•ter•na** [TA] **1.** the outer of two or more enveloping layers of any structure; **2.** specifically, the outer fibroelastic coat of a blood or lymph vessel.

**tu•ni•ca in•ti•ma** [TA] the innermost coat of a blood or lymphatic vessel; it consists of endothelium, usually a thin fibroelastic subendothelial layer, and an inner elastic membrane or longitudinal fibers.

**tu•ni•ca me•dia** the middle, usually muscular, coat of an artery or other tubular structure. SYN media (1).

**tu•ni•ca pro•pria** the special envelope of a part as distinguished from the peritoneal or other investment common to several parts.

**tu•ni•ca re•flexa** the reflected layer of the tunica vasculosa testis that lines the scrotum.

**tu•ni•ca va•gi•na•lis tes•tis** the serous sheath of the testis and epididymis, derived from the peritoneum; it consists of outer parietal and inner visceral serous layers.

**tu•ni•ca vas•cu•lo•sa** any vascular layer.

**tun•ing curve** a graph of acoustic threshold intensity at various frequencies for a single neuron.

**tun•ing fork (TF)** steel or magnesium-alloy instrument roughly resembling a two-pronged fork, the vibrations of the prongs of which, when struck, give a musical tone of restricted bandwidth; used to test the hearing and vibratory sensation.

**tun•nel** (tŭn'ĕl) an elongated passageway, usually open at both ends.

**tun•nel vi•sion** SYN tubular vision.

**Tur•ba•trix** (ter-bā'triks) a genus of free-living nematodes in the family Cephalobidae. [L. *turbare,* to disturb]

**Tur•ba•trix a•ce•ti** a species found in old vinegar or in rotting fruits and vegetables and occasionally as a contaminant in laboratory solutions. SYN vinegar eel.

**tur•bid** (ter'bid) cloudy, as by sediment or insoluble matter in a solution. [L. *turbidus,* confused, disordered]

**tur•bi•dim•e•try** (ter-bi-dim'ĕ-trē) a method for determining the concentration of a substance in a solution by the degree of cloudiness or turbidity it causes or by the degree of clarification it induces in a turbid solution. [turbidity + G. *metron,* measure]

**tur•bid•i•ty** (ter-bid'i-tē) the quality of being turbid, of losing transparency because of sediment or insoluble matter. [L. *turbiditas,* fr. *turbidus,* turbid]

**tur•bi•nate, tur•bi•nat•ed** (ter'bi-nāt, ter'bi-nāt-ed) **1.** shaped like a top. **2.** any of the turbinated bones. SEE inferior nasal concha, middle nasal concha, superior nasal concha, supreme nasal concha. [L. *turbinatus,,* shaped like a top]

**tur•bi•nec•to•my** (ter'bi-nek'tō-mē) surgical removal of a turbinated bone. [turbinate + G. *ektomē,* excision]

**tur•bi•not•o•my** (ter'bi-not'ō-mē) incision into or excision of a turbinated body. [turbinate + G. *tomē,* incision]

**tur•bu•lent flow** the flow of gas that is characterized by a rough and tumble pattern; all molecules proceed at the same velocity, and resistance to flow is increased when compared to laminar flow.

**Türck de•gen•er•a•tion** (terk) degeneration of a nerve fiber and its sheath distal to the point of injury or section of the axon; usually applied to degeneration within the central nervous system.

**turf toe** sprain and subsequent inflammation of the first metatarsophalangeal joint.

**tur•ges•cence** (ter-jes'ens) SYN tumescence. [L. *turgesco,* to begin to swell, fr. *turgeo,* to swell]

**tur•ges•cent** (ter-jes'ent) SYN tumescent.

**tur•gid** (ter'jid) SYN tumid. [L. *turgidus,* swollen, fr. *turgeo,* to swell]

**tur•gor** (ter'ger) fullness. [L., fr. *turgeo,* to swell]

**tu•ris•ta** (too-rēs'tă) SYN traveler's diarrhea. [Sp. tourist]

**turn•a•round time** the interval between the ordering of a clinical laboratory test or other diagnostic procedure and the reporting of results.

**Tur•ner syn•drome** (ter'ner) a syndrome with chromosome count 45 and only one X chromosome; buccal and other cells are usually sex chromatin-negative; anomalies include dwarfism, webbed neck, valgus of elbows, pigeon chest, infantile sexual development, and amenorrhea; the ovary has no primordial follicles and may be represented only by a fibrous streak; some individuals are chromosomal mosaic, with two or more cell lines of different chromosome constitution; seen in many animal species, in the meadow vole it is the normal female state. SYN XO syndrome.

**Tur•ner tooth** (ter'ner) enamel hypoplasia involving a solitary permanent tooth; related to infection in the primary tooth that preceded it or to trauma during odontogenesis.

**turn·o·ver num·ber** the number of substrate molecules converted into product in an enzyme-catalyzed reaction under saturating conditions per unit time per unit quantity of enzyme; e.g., $k_{cat} = V_{max}/[E_{total}]$.

**tus·sal** (tŭs′ăl) SYN tussive.

**tus·sis** (tŭs′is) a cough. [L.]

**tus·sive** (tŭs′siv) relating to a cough. SYN tussal. [L. *tussis*, a cough]

**tus·sive frem·i·tus** a form of fremitus similar to the vocal, produced by a cough.

**tus·sive syn·cope** fainting as a result of a coughing spell, caused by persistent increased intrathoracic pressure diminishing venous return to the heart, thus lowering cardiac output; most often occurs in heavy-set male smokers who have chronic bronchitis. SYN Charcot vertigo.

**Tut·tle proc·to·scope** (tŭtl) a tubular rectal speculum illuminated at its distal extremity; after introduction, the obturator is withdrawn and a glass window is inserted in the proximal end; then, by means of a rubber bulb and tube connected with the proctoscope, the rectal ampulla may be inflated.

**TWAR** SYN *Chlamydia pneumoniae.* [after the laboratory designations of the first two isolates, TW-83 and AR-39]

**T wave** the next deflection in the electrocardiogram following the QRS complex; represents ventricular repolarization.

**twelfth cra·ni·al nerve [CN XII]** SYN hypoglossal nerve [CN XII].

**twelfth-year mo·lar** the second permanent molar tooth.

**twi·light state** a condition of disordered consciousness during which actions may be performed without the conscious volition of the individual and with no memory of such actions.

**twin 1.** one of two children born at one birth. **2.** double; growing in pairs. [A.S. *getwin,* double]

**twinge** (twinj) a sudden momentary sharp pain.

**twin·ning** production of equivalent structures by division; the tendency of divided parts to assume symmetrical relations.

**twin pla·cen·ta** the placenta(s) of a twin pregnancy; if dizygotic, the placentas may be separate or fused, the latter retaining two amnionic and two chorionic sacs (dichorionic diamnionic placenta); if monozygotic, the placenta may be a monochorionic monoamnionic placenta or monochorionic diamnionic placenta, depending on the stage at which twinning took place; if twinning occurs early, there may be a fused placenta with two chorionic and two amnionic membranes.

**twin re·versed ar·ter·i·al per·fu·sion se·quence** a circulatory anomaly in monozygotic twins wherein there are paired arterioarterial and venovenous anastomoses and umbilical anomalies, with one fetus being perfused with deoxygenated blood; the recipient fetus develops as an acardiac acephalic, and the pump or donor twin is at risk for cardiac failure.

**twin-twin trans·fu·sion** direct vascular anastomosis, arterial or venous, between the placental circulations of twins.

**twist·ed hairs** SYN pili torti.

**twitch 1.** to jerk spasmodically. **2.** a momentary spasmodic contraction of a muscle fiber. [A.S. *twiccian*]

**two-car·bon frag·ment** the acetyl group ($CH_3CO-$) that takes part in transacetylation reactions with coenzyme A as carrier; commonly referred to as acetate or acetic acid, from which it is derived.

**two-di·men·sion·al ech·o·car·di·og·ra·phy** echocardiography in which an image is reconstructed from the echoes stimulated and detected by a linear array or moving transducers. SYN realtime echocardiography.

**two-dimension–three-dimension phenome·non** an experience in telescopic endoscopy in which a two-dimensional image appears to be three-dimensional because of the movement of the endoscope in and out of the view of the object.

**two-glass test** SYN Thompson test.

**two-step ex·er·cise test** a test used mainly for coronary insufficiency; significant depression of RS-T in the electrocardiogram is considered abnormal and suggests coronary insufficiency.

**two-way cath·e·ter** SYN double-channel catheter.

**ty·ing for·ceps** an instrument with flat, smooth tips used in ophthalmic surgery, particularly for tying sutures.

**ty·lec·to·my** (tī-lek′tō-mē) surgical removal of a localized swelling or tumor. SEE ALSO lumpectomy. [G. *tylē,* lump, + *ektomē,* excision]

**ty·lo·ma** (tī-lō′mă) SYN callosity. [G. a callus]

**ty·lo·sis,** pl. **ty·lo·ses** (tī-lō′sis, tī-lō′sēz) formation of a callosity (tyloma). [G. a becoming callous]

**ty·lot·ic** (tī-lot′ik) relating to or marked by tylosis.

**tym·pa·nal** (tim′pă-năl) **1.** SYN tympanic (1). **2.** resonant. **3.** SYN tympanitic (2).

**tym·pa·nec·to·my** (tim′pă-nek′tō-mē) excision of the tympanic membrane. [tympan- + G. *ektomē,* excision]

**tym·pan·ic** (tim-pan′ik) **1.** relating to the tympanic cavity or membrane. SYN tympanal (1). **2.** resonant. **3.** SYN tympanitic (2).

**tym·pa·nic bone** SYN tympanic ring.

**tym·pa·nic can·a·lic·u·lus** a minute canal passing from the inferior surface of the petrous portion of the temporal bone between the jugular fossa and carotid canal to the floor of the tympanic cavity. Located in the wedge of bone separating the jugular canal and carotid canal, it transmits the tympanic branch of the glossopharyngeal nerve.

**tym·pa·nic ca·vi·ty** an air chamber in the temporal bone containing the ossicles; it is lined with mucous membrane and is continuous with the auditory tube anteriorly and the tympanic antrum and mastoid air cells posteriorly.

**tym·pa·nic gan·gli·on** a small ganglion on the tympanic nerve during its passage through the petrous portion of the temporal bone.

**tym·pa·nic mem·brane** a thin tense membrane forming the greater part of the lateral wall of the tympanic cavity and separating it from the external acoustic meatus; it constitutes the boundary between the external and middle ear, is covered on both surfaces with epithelium, and in the tense part has an intermediate layer of outer radial and inner circular collagen fibers. See page B16. SYN membrana tympani [TA], drum membrane, drum, drumhead, eardrum, myringa, myrinx.

**tym·pa·nic nerve** a nerve from the inferior ganglion of the glossopharyngeal nerve, passing through the tympanic canaliculus to the tympanic cavity, forming there the tympanic plexus which supplies the mucous membrane of the tympanic cavity, mastoid cells, and auditory tube; presynaptic parasympathetic fibers also pass through the tympanic nerve via the lesser superficial petrosal nerve to the otic ganglion, where they synapse with postsynaptic fibers that continue to supply the parotid gland. SYN nervus tympanicus [TA], Andersch nerve.

**tym·pa·nic o·pen·ing of au·di·to·ry tube** an opening in the anterior part of the tympanic cavity below the canal for the tensor tympani muscle.

**tym·pan·ic plex·us** a plexus on the promontory of the labyrinthine wall of the tympanic cavity, formed by the tympanic nerve, an anastomotic branch of the facial, and sympathetic branches from the internal carotid plexus; it supplies the mucosa of the middle ear, mastoid cells, and auditory (eustachian) tube, and gives off the lesser superficial petrosal nerve to the otic ganglion.

**tym·pa·nic ring** in the fetus, a more or less complete bony ring at the medial end of the cartilaginous external acoustic meatus, to which is attached the tympanic membrane. SYN anulus tympanicus [TA], tympanic bone.

**tym·pa·nic si·nus** a depression in the tympanic cavity posterior to the tympanic promontory.

**tym·pa·nic veins** exit from the tympanic cavity through the petrotympanic fissure with the chorda tympani and empty into the retromandibular vein.

**tym·pa·nism** (tim'pă-nizm) SYN tympanites.

**tym·pa·ni·tes** (tim-pă-nī'tēz) swelling of the abdomen from gas in the intestinal or peritoneal cavity. SYN meteorism, tympanism. [L. fr. G. *tympanitēs*, an edema in which the belly is stretched like a drum, *tympanon*]

**tym·pa·nit·ic** (tim-pă-nit'ik) **1.** referring to tympanites. SYN tympanous. **2.** denoting the quality of sound elicited by percussing over the inflated intestine or a large pulmonary cavity. SYN tympanal (3), tympanic (3).

**tym·pa·nit·ic res·o·nance** SYN tympany.

**tym·pa·ni·tis** (tim-pă-nī'tis) SYN myringitis.

⚠**tym·pa·no-, tym·pan-, tym·pa·ni-** tympanum, tympanites. [G. *tympanon*, drum]

**tym·pa·no·cen·te·sis** (tim'pă-nō-sen-tē'sis) puncture of the tympanic membrane with a needle to aspirate middle ear fluid. [tympano- + G. *kentēsis*, puncture]

🔲**tym·pan·o·gram** (tim'panō-gram) a visual depiction (e.g., a printout) of the relative compliance and impedance of the structures of the middle ear in response to pressure changes in the external ear canal. See this page.

**tym·pa·no·mas·toid fis·sure** a fissure separating the tympanic portion from the mastoid portion of the temporal bone; it transmits the auricular branch of the vagus nerve.

**tym·pa·no·me·try** measurement of the pressure-compliance function of the eardrum using an immitance instrument (audiometer).

**tym·pa·no·plas·ty** (tim'pă-nō-plas-tē) operative correction of a damaged middle ear. [tympano- + G. *plassō*, to form]

🔲**tym·pan·o·scler·o·sis** (tim'pan-ō-skler-ō'sis) the formation of dense connective tissue in the mid-

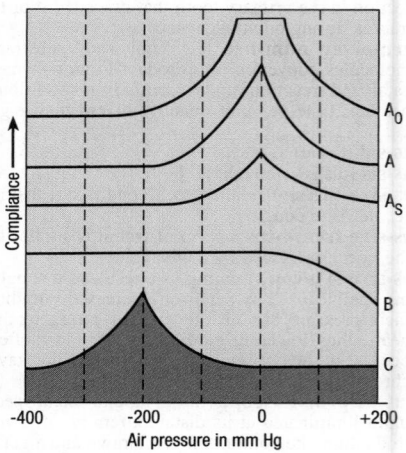

**tympanogram:** five tympanograms illustrating various conditions of the middle ear: type A is typical of normal middle ear; type $A_S$ is associated with stiffness of stapes; type $A_O$ is associated with interruptions in the chain of bones or flaccidity of the eardrum membrane; type B suggests fluid in the middle ear; type C suggests that the pressure within the middle ear is below atmospheric pressure

dle ear, often resulting in hearing loss when the ossicles are involved. See page B16.

**tym·pan·os·to·my** (tim-pan-os'tō-mē) SYN myringotomy. [tympano- + G. *ostium,* mouth]

**tym·pa·no·sto·my tube** a small tube inserted through the tympanic membrane after myringotomy to aerate the middle ear; often used for serous otitis media.

**tym·pa·not·o·my** (tim'pă-not'ō-mē) SYN myringotomy. [tympano- + G. *tomē,* incision]

**tym·pa·nous** (tim'pă-nŭs) SYN tympanitic (1).

**tym·pa·ny** (tim'pă-nē) a low-pitched, resonant, drumlike note obtained by percussing the surface of a large air-containing space, such as the distended abdomen or the thorax with or without pneumothorax. SYN tympanitic resonance.

**Tyn·dall phe·nom·e·non** (tin'dahl) the visibility of floating particles in gases or liquids when illuminated by a ray of sunlight and viewed at right angles to the illuminating ray.

**type** (tīp) **1.** the usual form, or a composite form, that all others of the class resemble more or less closely; a model, denoting especially a disease or a symptom complex giving the stamp or characteristic to a class. SEE ALSO constitution, habitus, personality. **2.** CHEMISTRY a substance in which the arrangement of the atoms in a molecule may be taken as representative of other substances in that class. SYN typus. [G. *typos,* a mark, a model]

**type I di·a·be·tes** SYN insulin-dependent diabetes mellitus.

**type II di·a·be·tes** non-insulin-dependent diabetes mellitus.

**type A be·hav·ior, type A per·son·al·i·ty** a behavior pattern characterized by aggressiveness, ambitiousness, restlessness, and a strong sense of time urgency; associated with increased risk for coronary heart disease.

**type B be·hav·ior, type B per·son·al·i·ty** a behavior pattern characterized by the absence or obverse of type A behavior characteristics.

**type cul·ture** a type strain of microorganism preserved in a culture collection as the standard.

**type 1 gly·co·ge·no·sis** glycogenosis due to glucose 6-phosphatase deficiency, resulting in accumulation of excessive amounts of glycogen of normal chemical structure, particularly in liver and kidney. SYN Gierke disease, von Gierke disease.

**type 2 gly·co·ge·no·sis** glycogenosis due to lysosomal α-1,4-glucosidase deficiency, resulting in accumulation of excessive amounts of glycogen of normal chemical structure in heart, muscle, liver, and nervous system. SYN Pompe disease.

**type 3 gly·co·ge·no·sis** glycogenosis due to amylo-1,6-glucosidase deficiency, resulting in accumulation of abnormal glycogen with short outer chains in liver and muscle. SYN Cori disease, Forbes disease.

**type 4 gly·co·ge·no·sis** familial cirrhosis of the liver with storage of abnormal glycogen; glycogenosis due to deficiency of 1,4-α-glucan branching enzyme, resulting in accumulation of abnormal glycogen with long inner and outer chains in liver, kidney, muscle, and other tissues. SYN Andersen disease.

**type 5 gly·co·ge·no·sis** glycogenosis due to muscle glycogen phosphorylase deficiency, resulting in accumulation of glycogen of normal chemical structure in muscle. SYN McArdle disease, McArdle-Schmid-Pearson disease.

**type 6 gly·co·ge·no·sis** glycogenosis due to hepatic glycogen phosphorylase deficiency, resulting in accumulation of glycogen of normal chemical structure in liver and leukocytes. SYN Hers disease.

**type I fa·mil·i·al hy·per·lip·o·pro·tein·e·mia** hyperlipoproteinemia characterized by the presence of large amounts of chylomicrons and triglycerides in the plasma when the patient has a normal diet, and their disappearance on a fat-free diet. It is accompanied by bouts of abdominal pain, hepatosplenomegaly, pancreatitis, and eruptive xanthomas; autosomal recessive inheritance. SYN familial fat-induced hyperlipemia, familial hyperchylomicronemia, familial hypertriglyceridemia (1).

**type II fa·mil·i·al hy·per·lip·o·pro·tein·e·mia** hyperlipoproteinemia characterized by increased plasma levels of β-lipoproteins, cholesterol, and phospholipids, but normal triglycerides. Homozygotes have xanthomatosis and frank clinical atherosclerosis as young adults. The primary defect is a deficiency of apoprotein of VLDL. SYN familial hypercholesterolemia.

**type III fa·mil·i·al hy·per·lip·o·pro·tein·e·mia** hyperlipoproteinemia characterized by increased plasma levels of LDL, β-lipoproteins, pre-β-lipoproteins, cholesterol, phospholipids, and triglycerides; frequent eruptive xanthomas and atheromatosis, particularly coronary artery disease; biochemical defect lies in apolipoproteins. SYN familial hypercholesterolemia with hyperlipemia.

**type IV fa·mil·i·al hy·per·lip·o·pro·tein·e·mia** plasma levels of VLDL, pre-β-lipoproteins

and triglycerides are increased on a normal diet, but β-lipoproteins, cholesterol, and phospholipids are normal; may be accompanied by abnormal glucose tolerance and susceptibility to ischemic heart disease. SYN familial hypertriglyceridemia (2).

**type V fa·mil·i·al hy·per·lip·o·pro·tein·e·mia** hyperlipoproteinemia characterized by increased plasma levels of chylomicrons, VLDL, pre-β-lipoproteins, and triglycerides; may be accompanied by bouts of abdominal pain, hepatosplenomegaly, susceptibility to atherosclerosis, and abnormal glucose tolerance.

**typh·lec·ta·sis** (tif-lek′tă-sis) dilation of the cecum. [G. *typhlon,* cecum, + *ektasis,* a stretching out]

**typh·lec·to·my** (tif-lek′tō-mē) SYN cecectomy.

**typh·len·ter·i·tis** (tif′len-ter-ī′tis) SYN cecitis.

**typh·li·tis** (tif′lī′tis) SYN cecitis.

△**ty·phlo-, typhl-** 1. the cecum. SEE ALSO ceco-. [G. cecum] 2. blindness. [G. *typhlos,* blind]

**typh·lo·dic·li·di·tis** (tif-lō-dik-li-dī′tis) inflammation of the ileocecal valve. [G. *typhlon,* cecum, + *diklis (diklid-),* double-folding (of doors), + *-itis,* inflammation]

**typh·lo·en·ter·i·tis** (tif′lō-en-ter-ī′tis) SYN cecitis.

**typh·lo·li·thi·a·sis** (tif′lō-li-thī′ă-sis) presence of fecal concretions in the cecum. [G. *typhlon,* cecum, + *lithos,* stone]

**typh·lo·pexy, typh·lo·pex·ia** (tif′lō-pek-sē, tif-lō-pek′sē-ă) SYN cecopexy.

**typh·lor·rha·phy** (tif-lōr′ă-fē) SYN cecorrhaphy.

**typh·lo·sis** (tif-lō′sis) SYN blindness. [G. *typhlos,* blind]

**typh·los·to·my** (tif-los′tō-mē) SYN cecostomy.

**typh·lot·o·my** (tif-lot′ō-mē) SYN cecotomy.

**ty·phoid** (tī′foyd) 1. typhus-like; stuporous from fever. 2. SYN typhoid fever. [typhus + G. *eidos,* resemblance]

**ty·phoi·dal** (tī-foyd′ăl) relating to or resembling typhoid fever.

**ty·phoid ba·cil·lus** SYN *Salmonella typhi.*

**ty·phoid fe·ver** an acute infectious disease caused by *Salmonella typhi* and characterized by a continued fever, severe physical and mental depression, an eruption of rose-colored spots on the chest and abdomen, tympanites, often diarrhea, and sometimes intestinal hemorrhage or perforation of the bowel; average duration is four weeks, although aborted forms and relapses are not uncommon; the lesions are located chiefly in the lymph follicles of the intestines (Peyer patches), the mesenteric glands, and the spleen; antibody titer of the Widal test rises during the infection, and early positive blood and urine cultures become negative. SYN enteric fever (1), typhoid (2).

**ty·phous** (tī′fŭs) relating to typhus.

**ty·phus** (tī′fŭs) a group of acute infectious and contagious diseases, caused by rickettsiae that are transmitted by arthropods, and occurring in two principal forms: epidemic typhus and endemic (murine) typhus Also called jail, camp, or ship fever. SYN camp fever (1). [G. *typhos,* smoke, stupor]

**ty·pi·cal dru·sen** SYN exudative drusen.

**typ·ing** (tīp′ing) classification according to type. [see type]

**ty·pus** SYN type.

**Tyr** tyrosine and its radicals.

**Ty·rode so·lu·tion** (tī-rōd) a modified Locke so-

t
y

lution; it contains 8 g of NaCl, 0.2 g of KCl, 0.2 g of CaCl$_2$, 0.1 g of MgCl$_2$, 0.05 g of NaH$_2$PO$_4$, 1 g of NaHCO$_3$, 1 g of D-glucose, and water to make 1000 mL; used to irrigate the peritoneal cavity, and in laboratory work.

**ty·ro·ke·to·nu·ria** (tī′rō-kē-tōn-yu′rē-ă) the urinary excretion of ketonic metabolites of tyrosine, such as *p*-hydroxyphenylpyruvic acid.

**ty·ro·ma** (tī-rō′mă) a caseous tumor. [G. *tyros,* cheese, + *-ōma,* tumor]

**ty·ro·sine (Tyr, Y)** (tī′rō-sēn, tī′rō-sin) an α-amino acid present in most proteins.

**ty·ro·si·nu·ria** (tī′rō-sin-yu′rē-ă) the excretion of tyrosine in the urine. [tyrosine + G. *ouron,* urine]

**ty·ro·sy·lu·ria** (tī′rō-sil-yu′rē-ă) enhanced urinary excretion of certain metabolites of tyrosine, such as *p*-hydroxyphenylpyruvic acid; present in tyrosinosis, scurvy, pernicious anemia, and other diseases.

**TYSGM-9 me·di·um** medium of gastric mucin, nutrient broth, bovine serum, and rice starch used to detect the presence of *Entamoeba histolytica.*

**TY1-S-33 me·di·um** medium of biosate peptone, dextrose, vitamins, and bovine serum used to detect the presence of *Entamoeba histolytica.*

# U

υ upsilon.

**U 1.** unit. **2.** kilurane; uranium; uridine in polymers; uracil; internal energy; urinary concentration, followed by subscripts indicating location and chemical species.

*U* internal energy.

**ubi·qui·nol (QH₂)** (yu′-bik′wi-nol) the reduction product of a ubiquinone.

**ubi·qui·none** (yu′-bik′wi-nōn) a 2,3-dimethoxy-5-methyl-1,4-benzoquinone with a multiprenyl side chain; a mobile component of electron transport. SEE ALSO coenzyme Q.

**ubiq·ui·tin** (yu-bik′kwi-tin) a small protein found in all cells of higher organisms and one whose structure has changed minimally during evolutionary history; involved in histone modification and intracellular protein breakdown.

**ubi·qui·tin-pro·te·ase path·way** pathway in which a small protein cofactor, ubiquitin, couples with protein substrate to catalyze proteolytic destruction by proteases; this pathway is highly selective and tightly regulated and is responsible for protein degradation seen in muscle-wasting diseases.

**UDP** uridine 5′-diphosphate.

**UDPglu·cose-hex·ose-1-phos·phate uri·dyl·yl·trans·fer·ase** an enzyme that catalyzes the reversible reaction of α-D-glucose 1-phosphate UDPgalactose to produce UDPglucose and α-D-galactose 1-phosphate.

**UGI** upper gastrointestinal series.

**ul·cer** (ŭl′ser) a lesion on the surface of the skin or on a mucous surface, caused by superficial loss of tissue, usually with inflammation. See this page and B5. SYN ulcus. [L. *ulcus* (*ulcer-*), a sore, ulcer]

**ul·ce·ra** (ŭl′ser-ă) plural of ulcus.

**ul·cer·ate** (ŭl′ser-āt) to form an ulcer.

**ul·cer·at·ing gran·u·lo·ma of pu·den·da** SYN granuloma inguinale.

**ul·cer·a·tion** (ŭl-ser-ā′shŭn) **1.** the formation of an ulcer. **2.** an ulcer or aggregation of ulcers.

**ul·cer·a·tive** (ŭl′ser-ă-tiv) relating to, causing, or marked by an ulcer or ulcers.

**ul·cer·a·tive co·li·tis** a chronic disease of unknown cause characterized by ulceration of the colon and rectum, with rectal bleeding, mucosal crypt abscesses, inflammatory pseudopolyps, abdominal pain, and diarrhea; frequently causes anemia, hypoproteinemia, and electrolyte imbalance, and is sometimes complicated by peritonitis, toxic megacolon, or carcinoma of the colon. See page B9.

**ul·cer·a·tive sto·ma·ti·tis** SYN aphtha (2).

**ul·cer·o·mem·bra·nous gin·gi·vi·tis** SYN necrotizing ulcerative gingivitis.

**ul·cer·ous** (ŭl′ser-ŭs) relating to, affected with, or containing an ulcer. [L. *ulcerosus*]

**ul·cus**, pl. **ul·ce·ra** (ŭl′kŭs, ŭl′ser-ă) SYN ulcer. [L.]

**uler·y·the·ma** (yu′ler-i-thē′mă) scarring with erythema. [G. *oulē*, scar, + *erythēma*, redness of the skin]

**Ull·mann line** (ool′mahn) the line of displacement in spondylolisthesis.

**Ull·mann syn·drome** (ool′mahn) a systemic angiomatosis due to multiple arteriovenous malformations.

**ul·na**, gen. and pl. **ul·nae** (ŭl′nă, ŭl′nē) [TA] the medial and larger of the two bones of the forearm. SYN cubitus (2). [L. elbow, arm, fr. G. *ōlenē*]

**ul·nad** (ŭl′nad) in a direction toward the ulna. [ulna + L. *ad*, to]

**ul·nar** (ŭl′năr) relating to the ulna, or to any of the structures (artery, nerve, etc.) named from it; relating to the ulnar or medial aspect of the upper limb.

**ul·nar ar·tery** *origin*, brachial; *branches*, ulnar recurrent, common interosseous, dorsal and palmar carpal, deep palmar, and superficial palmar arch with its digital branches. SYN arteria ulnaris [TA].

**ul·nar ex·ten·sor mus·cle of wrist** SYN extensor carpi ulnaris muscle.

**ul·nar flex·or mus·cle of wrist** SYN flexor carpi ulnaris muscle.

**ul·nar nerve** arises from the medial cord of the brachial plexus and passes down the arm, behind the medial epicondyle of the humerus, and down the ulnar side of the anterior compartment of the forearm to the hand; it gives off muscular branches in the forearm to the flexor carpi ulnaris muscle and the ulnar portion of flexor digitorum profundus and supplies hypothenar, interosseous, medial lumbricals, adductor pollicis and deep head of flexor hallucis brevis; intrinsic muscles of the hand and the skin of the small finger and medial side of the ring finger and adjacent portions of the palm of the hand. The ulnar nerve is most vulnerable to injury where it passes subcutaneously behind the medial epicondyle of the humerus. Mild injury here produces "crazy bone" sensation. An ulnar nerve lesion here results in loss of flexion of metacarpophalangeal joints and

u
l

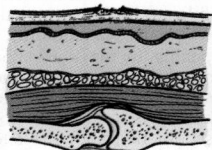 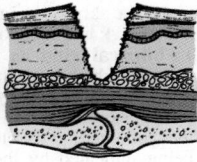 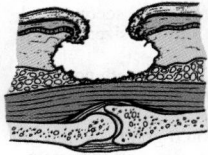 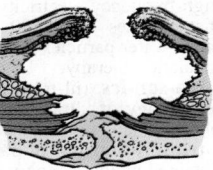

| stage 1 | stage 2 | stage 3 | stage 4 |

**pressure sore and ulcer classification:** (stage 1) inflammation, redness of epidermis; (stage 2) loss of epidermis, damage to dermis; (stage 3) involvement of subcutaneous tissues; (stage 4) damage to tendon, muscle, and bone

of extension at the interphalangeal joints ("claw hand"). SYN nervus ulnaris [TA], cubital nerve.

**ul·nar nerve com·pres·sion syn·drome** SYN cyclist's palsy.

**ul·nar veins** venae comitantes of the ulnar artery, continuing from those of the superficial palmar arch and joining with those of the radial artery to form the brachial veins in the cubital fossa.

△**ulo-, ule-** **1.** scar, scarring. [G. *oulē*] **2.** the gums. SEE ALSO gingivo-. [G. *oulon*] **3.** curly. [G. *oulo-, ouli-*, woolly.]

**ulo·der·ma·ti·tis** (yu'lō-der-mă-tī'tis) inflammation of the skin resulting in destruction of tissue and the formation of scars. [G. *oulē*, scar, + *derma*, skin, + *-itis*, inflammation]

**uloid** (yu'-lōyd) **1.** resembling a scar. **2.** a scarlike lesion due to a degenerative process in deeper layers of skin. [G. *oulē*, scar + *eidos*, resemblance]

△**ul·tra-** excess, exaggeration, beyond. [L. beyond]

**ul·tra·cen·tri·fuge** (ŭl'tră-sen'tri-fyuj) a high-speed centrifuge by means of which large molecules, e.g., of protein or nucleic acids, are caused to sediment at practicable rates.

**ul·tra·di·an** (ŭl-tră'dē-ăn) relating to biologic variations or rhythms occurring in cycles more frequent than every 24 hours. Cf. circadian, infradian. [ultra- + L. *dies*, day]

**ul·tra·fast Pap stain** a modified Papanicolaou stain suitable for use in situations in which rapid decisions are essential and frozen sections may not be sufficiently reliable or practical. SEE ALSO Papanicolaou stain.

**ul·tra·fil·tra·tion** (ŭl'tră-fil-tră'shŭn) filtration through a semipermeable membrane or any filter that separates colloid solutions from crystalloids or separates particles of different size in a colloid mixture.

**ul·tra·li·ga·tion** (ŭl-tră-lī-gā'shŭn) ligation of a blood vessel beyond the point where a branch is given off.

**ul·tra·mi·cro·scop·ic** (ŭl'tră-mī-krō-skop'ik) SYN submicroscopic.

**ul·tra·mi·cro·tome** (ŭl-tră-mī'krō-tōm) a microtome used in cutting sections 0.1 μm thick, or less, for electron microscopy.

**ul·tra·short·wave di·a·ther·my** shortwave diathermy in which the wavelength is under 10 meters.

**ul·tra·son·ic** (ŭl-tră-son'ik) relating to energy waves similar to those of sound but of higher frequencies (above 30,000 Hz). [ultra- + L. *sonus*, sound]

**ul·tra·son·ic lith·o·trip·sy** the demolition of calculi by high frequency sound waves.

**ul·tra·son·ic neb·u·liz·er** a humidifier using high-frequency electricity to power a transducer that vibrates 1,350,000 times per second and emits water particles 0.5 to 3 μm in size; used in inhalation therapy.

**ul·tra·son·ics** (ŭl-tră-son'iks) the science and technology of ultrasound, its characteristics and phenomena.

**ul·tra·son·o·gram** (ŭl-tră-son'ō-gram) the image obtained by ultrasonography. SEE ALSO echogram. SYN sonogram.

**ul·tra·son·o·graph** (ŭl'tră-son'ō-graf) computerized instrument used to create an image using ultrasound. SYN sonograph. [ultra- + L. *sonus*, sound, + G. *graphō*, to write]

**ul·tra·so·nog·ra·pher** (ŭl'tră-sŏ-nog'ră-fer) a person who performs and interprets ultrasonographic examinations. SYN sonographer.

**ul·tra·so·nog·ra·phy** (ŭl'tră-sŏ-nog'ră-fē) the location, measurement, or delineation of deep structures by measuring the reflection or transmission of high frequency or ultrasonic waves. Computer calculation of the distance to the sound-reflecting or absorbing surface plus the known orientation of the sound beam gives a two-dimensional image. SEE ALSO ultrasound. SYN echography, sonography. [ultra- + L. *sonus*, sound, + G. *graphō*, to write]

**ul·tra·sound** (ŭl'tră-sownd) sound having a frequency greater than 30,000 Hz.

**ul·tra·sound car·di·og·ra·phy** SYN echocardiography.

**ul·tra·struc·tur·al anat·o·my** the ultramicroscopic study of structures too small to be seen with a light microscope.

**ul·tra·vi·o·let** (ŭl-tră-vī'ō-let) denoting electromagnetic rays at higher frequency than the violet end of the visible spectrum.

**ul·tra·vi·o·let in·dex** a daily index issued by the U.S. National Weather Service for many cities, forecasting the amount of dangerous ultraviolet light that will arrive at the earth's surface about noon the following day.

**ul·tra·vi·o·let ker·a·to·con·junc·ti·vi·tis** acute keratoconjunctivitis resulting from exposure to intense ultraviolet irradiation.

**ul·tra·vi·o·let mi·cro·scope** a microscope having optics of quartz and fluorite that allow transmission of light waves shorter than those of the visible spectrum; the image is made visible by photography, fluorescence of special glasses, or television.

**ul·tra·vi·rus** (ŭl'tră-vī'rŭs) SYN virus (2).

**um·ber co·don** the termination codon UGA. SYN opal codon.

**um·bil·i·cal** (ŭm-bil'i-kăl) relating to the umbilicus. SYN omphalic.

**um·bil·i·cal ar·tery** before birth the arteria is a continuation of the internal iliac; after birth it is obliterated between the bladder and umbilicus, forming the medial umbilical ligament, the remaining portion, between the internal iliac artery and bladder, being reduced in size and giving off the superior vesical arteries. SYN arteria umbilicalis [TA].

**um·bil·i·cal cord** the definitive connecting stalk between the embryo or fetus and the placenta; at birth it is primarily composed of Wharton jelly in which the umbilical vessels are embedded. SYN funiculus umbilicalis [TA], funis (1).

**um·bil·i·cal her·nia** a hernia in which bowel or omentum protrudes through the abdominal wall under the skin at the umbilicus. SEE ALSO omphalocele. SYN exomphalos (2), exumbilication (2).

**um·bil·i·cal ring** an opening in the linea alba through which pass the umbilical vessels in the fetus; in young embryos it is relatively nearer to the pubes, but gradually ascends to the center of the abdomen; it is closed in the adult, its site being indicated by the umbilicus or navel. SYN anulus umbilicalis [TA].

**um·bil·i·cal vein** SEE left umbilical vein.

**um·bil·i·cate, um·bil·i·cat·ed** (ŭm-bil'i-kāt, ŭm-bil'i-kāt-ed) of navel shape; pitlike; dimpled. [L. *umbilicatus*]

**um·bil·i·ca·tion** (ŭm-bil-i-kā'shŭn) **1.** a pit or navel-like depression. **2.** formation of a depression at the apex of a papule, vesicle, or pustule.

**um·bil·i·cus,** pl. **um·bil·i·ci** (ŭm-bil′i-kŭs, ŭm-bi-lī′kŭs; ŭm-bil′i-sī) [TA] the pit in the center of the abdominal wall marking the point where the umbilical cord entered in the fetus. SYN navel. [L. navel]

**um·bo,** gen. **um·bo·nis,** pl. **um·bo·nes** (ŭm′bō, um-bō′nis, um-bō′nēz) **1.** a projecting point of a surface. **2.** SYN umbo of tympanic membrane. [L. boss of a shield, a knob]

**um·bo of tym·pan·ic mem·brane** the projection on the inner surface of the tympanic membrane at the end of the manubrium of the malleus; this corresponds to the most depressed point of the membrane, viewed laterally, that is commonly called the umbo. SYN umbo (2).

**um·bra** RADIOLOGY an image with sharply defined margins.

**UMP** uridine 5′-monophosphate.

**⌂un- 1.** not, akin to L. *in-* and G. *a-, an-.* **2.** reversal, removal, release, deprivation. **3.** an intensive action. [M.E.]

**un·bal·anced trans·lo·ca·tion** condition resulting from fertilization of a gamete containing a translocation chromosome by a normal gamete; if this abnormality is compatible with life, the individual has 46 chromosomes but a segment of the translocation chromosome is represented three times in each cell and a partial or complete trisomic state exists.

**un·bundl·ing** use of several CPT codes for a service when one inclusion code is available.

**un·cal** (ŭng′kăl) denoting or relating to the uncus.

**un·ci** (ŭn′sī) plural of uncus.

**un·ci·form** (ŭn′si-fōrm) SYN uncinate. [L. *uncus,* hook, + *forma,* form]

**un·ci·form bone** SYN hamate bone.

**un·ci·form fas·cic·u·lus, un·ci·nate fas·cic·u·lus** a band of long association fibers reciprocally connecting the frontal and temporal lobes of the cerebrum, running caudally through the white matter of the frontal lobe, sharply curving ventrally under the stem of the sylvian fissure, and then fanning out to the cortex of the anterior half of the superior and middle temporal gyri.

**un·ci·nate** (ŭn′si-nāt) **1.** hooklike or hook-shaped. **2.** relating to an uncus or, specifically, to the uncinate gyrus (2) or a process of the pancreas or of a vertebra. SYN unciform. [L. *uncinatus*]

**un·ci·nate gy·rus** SYN uncus (2).

**un·comb·able hair syn·drome** a genetic syndrome in which the hair, which is often silvery blond, is unruly and resists lying flat because of irregularly shaped hair shafts. SYN spun glass hair.

**un·com·fort·able lev·el** the intensity of sound that causes discomfort.

**un·com·pen·sat·ed al·ka·lo·sis** alkalosis in which the pH of body fluids is elevated because of lack of the compensatory mechanisms of compensated alkalosis.

**un·com·pet·i·tive in·hib·i·tor** a type of enzyme inhibitor in which the inhibiting compound only binds to the enzyme-substrate complex.

**un·con·di·tion·ed re·flex** an instinctive reflex not dependent on previous learning or experience.

**un·con·di·tion·ed re·sponse** a response, such as

salivation, which is a part of the animal or human repertoire. Cf. conditioned response.

**un·con·di·tion·ed stim·u·lus** a stimulus that elicits an unconditioned response; e.g., food is an unconditioned stimulus for salivation, which in turn is an unconditioned response in a hungry animal.

**un·con·scious** (ŭn-kon′shŭs) **1.** not conscious. **2.** PSYCHOANALYSIS the psychic structure comprising the drives and feelings of which one is unaware. SYN insensible (1).

**un·con·scious·ness** (ŭn-kon′shŭs-ness) an imprecise term for severely impaired awareness of self and the surrounding environment; most often used as a synonym for coma or unresponsiveness.

**un·co·ver·te·bral** (ŭn-kō-ver′tĕ-brăl) pertaining to or affecting the uncinate process of a vertebra.

**unc·tion** (ŭngk′shŭn) the action of anointing or rubbing with an ointment or oil. [L. *unctio,* fr. *ungo,* pp. *unctus,* to anoint]

**unc·tu·ous** (ŭngk′shoo-ŭs) greasy or oily. [L. *unctuosus,* fr. *unctio,* unction]

**un·cus,** pl. **un·ci** (ŭn′kŭs, ŭn′sī) **1.** any hook-shaped process or structure. **2.** the anterior, hooked extremity of the parahippocampal gyrus on the basomedial surface of the temporal lobe; the anterior face of the uncus corresponds to the olfactory cortex, its ventral surface to the entorhinal area; deep to the uncus lies the amygdala (amygdaloid body). SYN uncinate gyrus. [L. a hook, fr. G. *onkos*]

**un·der·bite** (ŭn′der-bīt) a nontechnical term applied to mandibular underdevelopment or to excessive maxillary development.

**un·der·drive pac·ing** (ŭn′der-drīv pās′ing) electrical stimulation of the heart at a rate lower than that of an existing tachycardia; designed to capture the heart between beats, i.e., to interrupt a reentry pathway in order to terminate the tachycardia.

**un·der·shoot** (ŭn′der-shoot) a temporary decrease below the final steady-state value that may occur immediately following the removal of an influence that had been raising that value, i.e., overshoot in a negative direction.

**un·der·wat·er weigh·ing** assessment of body volume by measuring an individual's weight in air and again under water; loss in scale weight (corrected for water density) equals body volume. Body density (ratio of body mass to volume) is then used to compute percent body fat. SYN hydrostatic weighing.

**un·de·scend·ed tes·tis** a testis that has failed to descend into the scrotum; there are palpable and nonpalpable variants.

**un·de·ter·mined ni·tro·gen** the nitrogen of blood, urine, etc., other than urea, uric acid, amino acids, etc., that can be directly estimated; in blood it amounts to about 25 mg per 100 ml.

**un·dif·fer·en·ti·at·ed** (ŭn′dif-er-en′shē-ā-ted) not differentiated; e.g., primitive, embryonic, immature, or having no special structure or function.

**un·dif·fer·en·ti·at·ed type fe·vers** a term applied to illnesses resulting from infection by any one of the arboviruses pathogenic for man, in which the only constant manifestation is fever; rash, lymphadenopathy, or arthralgia (alone or in combination) may occur in some individuals but not in others; some arboviruses may induce in-

u
n

fections in which undifferentiated type fever is the only manifestation, whereas other arboviruses may induce in some persons only undifferentiated fever, and in other persons similar fever followed by secondary manifestations, e.g., a hemorrhagic fever or encephalitis.

**un·du·lant fe·ver** SYN brucellosis. [referring to the wavy appearance of the long temperature curve]

**un·du·late** (ŭn′dyu-lāt) having an irregular, wavy border; denoting the shape of a bacterial colony. [Mod. L. *undula,* dim. of *unda,* wave]

**un·du·lat·ing mem·brane, un·du·la·to·ry mem·brane** a locomotory organelle of certain flagellate (trypanosome and trichomonad) parasites, consisting of a finlike extension of the limiting membrane with the flagellar sheath; wavelike rippling of the undulating membrane produces a characteristic movement.

**un·du·lat·ing pulse** a pulse in which there is a succession of waves rather than discrete pulsations.

**un·du·li·po·di·um,** pl. **un·du·li·po·dia** (ŭn′dyu-li-pō′dē-um, ŭn′dyu-li-pō′dē-ă) a flexible whiplike intracellular extension of many eukaryotic cells, with a characteristic arrangement of nine paired peripheral microtubules and one central pair; it appears to grow out from a basal body (kinetosome) in the cell. Both the cilium and the eukaryotic flagellum (not the bacterial flagellum, which lacks the 9 + 2 pattern) are considered undulipodium. [LL. *undulo,* to move in waves, fr. L. *unda,* wave, + Mod.L. *podium,* fr. G. *podion,* dim. of *pous,* foot]

**un·gual** (ŭng′gwăl) relating to a nail or the nails. SYN unguinal. [L. *unguis,* nail]

**un·guent** (ŭng′gwent) SYN ointment. [L. *unguentum*]

**un·gues** (ŭng′gwēz) plural of unguis.

**un·gui·nal** (ŭng′gwi-năl) SYN ungual.

**un·guis,** pl. **un·gues** (ŭng′gwis, ŭng′gwēz) [TA] SYN nail. [L.]

△**uni-** one, single, not paired; corresponds to G. *mono-.* [L. *unus*]

**uni·ax·i·al joint** one in which movement is around one axis only.

**uni·cam·er·al, uni·cam·er·ate** (yu-nĭ-kam′ĕ-răl, yu-nĭ-kam′ĕ-rāt) SYN monolocular.

**uni·cam·er·al bone cyst** SYN solitary bone cyst.

**uni·cel·lu·lar** (yu-nĭ-sel′yu-lăr) composed of but one cell, as in the protozoa (or protozoans); for such unicellular organisms capable of undertaking life processes independently of other cells, the term acellular is also used.

**uni·cel·lu·lar gland** a single secretory cell such as a mucous goblet cell.

**uni·cor·nous** (yu′nĭ-kōr′nŭs) having but one horn, or cornu. [L. *unicornis,* fr. uni- + *cornu,* horn]

**uni·corn uter·us** a uterus in which only one lateral half exists, the other half being undeveloped or absent.

**uni·ger·mi·nal** (yu-nĭ-jer′mi-năl) relating to a single germ or oocyte (ovum), e.g., monozygotic. SYN monozygotic, monozygous.

**uni·glan·du·lar** (yu-nĭ-glan′dyu-lăr) involving, relating to, or containing but one gland.

**uni·lat·e·ral** (yu-nĭ-lat′ĕ-răl) confined to one side only.

**uni·lat·e·ral an·es·the·sia** SYN hemianesthesia.

**uni·lat·e·ral her·maph·ro·dit·ism** hermaphroditism in which the doubling of sex characteristics occurs on one side only: ovotestis on one side and either ovary or testis on the other.

**uni·lat·e·ral hy·per·lu·cent lung** chronic bronchiolitis obliterans predominating on one side. SEE unilateral lobar emphysema.

**uni·lat·e·ral lo·bar em·phy·se·ma** a state in which the roentgenographic density of one lung (or one lobe) is markedly less than the density of the other(s) because of the presence of air trapped during expiration. SYN Macleod syndrome, Swyer-James syndrome (1).

**uni·lo·bar** (yu-nĭ-lō′băr) having but one lobe.

**uni·lo·cal** (yu-nĭ-lō′kăl) strictly, denoting a trait in which the genetic component is contributed exclusively by one locus; in practice, any trait in which the contribution from one locus is so large that the data are readily interpreted as mendelian.

**uni·loc·u·lar** (yu-nĭ-lok′yu-lăr) having but one compartment or cavity, as in a fat cell. [uni- + L. *loculus,* compartment]

**uni·loc·u·lar cyst** a cyst having a single sac.

**uni·loc·u·lar joint** one in which an intra-articular disk is incomplete or absent, the joint having but a single cavity.

**uni·mo·lec·u·lar** (yu′nĭ-mō-lek′yu-lăr) denoting a single molecule.

**un·in·hib·i·ted neu·ro·gen·ic blad·der** a condition, either congenital or acquired, of abnormal urinary bladder function in which normal inhibitory control of detrusor function by the central nervous system is impaired or underdeveloped, resulting in precipitate or uncontrolled micturition and/or anuresis.

**un·in·ter·rupt·ed su·ture** SYN continuous suture.

**un·ion** (yoon′yŭn) **1.** the joining or amalgamation of two or more bodies. **2.** the structural adhesion or growing together of the edges of a wound. [L. *unus,* one]

**uni·pen·nate** (yu-nĭ-pen′āt) **1.** having a feather arrangement on one side; resembling one-half of a feather. **2.** denoting certain muscles with fibers running at an acute angle from one side of a tendon. [uni- + L. *penna,* feather]

**uni·po·lar** (yu-nĭ-pō′lăr) **1.** having but one pole; denoting a nerve cell from which the branches project from one side only. **2.** situated at one extremity only of a cell.

**uni·po·lar leads** those in which the exploring electrode is on the chest in the vicinity of the heart or on one of the limbs, while the other or indifferent electrode is the central terminal.

**uni·po·lar neu·ron** a neuron whose cell body gives off a single axonal process resulting from the fusion of two polar processes during development; at a variable distance from the cell body, the process divides into a peripheral axon branch extending outward as a peripheral afferent (sensory) nerve fiber, and a central axon branch that enters into synaptic contact with neurons in the spinal cord or brainstem.

**uni·port** (yu′nĭ-pōrt) transport of a molecule or ion through a membrane by a carrier mechanism (uniporter), without known coupling to any other molecule or ion transport. Cf. antiport, symport. [uni- + L. *porto,* to carry]

**unit (U)** (yu′nit) **1.** one; a single person or thing. **2.** a standard of measure, weight, or any other quality, by multiplications or fractions of which a scale or system is formed. **3.** a group of persons or things considered as a whole because of mutual activities or functions. **4.** SYN international unit. [L. *unus,* one]

**Uni·ted States A·dopt·ed Names (USAN)** designation for nonproprietary names (for drugs) adopted by the USAN Council in cooperation with the manufacturers concerned; the designation USAN is applicable only to nonproprietary names coined since June 1961.

**Uni·ted States Phar·ma·co·pe·ia (USP)** SEE Pharmacopeia.

**Uni·ted States Pub·lic Health Ser·vice (USPHS)** a bureau of the Department of Health and Human Services, served by a corps of medical officers presided over by the Surgeon General, concerned with scientific research, domestic and insular quarantine, administration of government hospitals, publication of sanitary reports, and statistics; associated with it are the National Institutes of Health, Centers for Disease Control and Prevention, and other units.

**unit mem·brane** the trilaminar structure of the plasmalemma and other intercellular membranes, when seen in cross-section with the electron microscope, composed of two electron-dense laminae separated by a less dense lamina.

**unit of pen·i·cil·lin (international)** the penicillin activity of 0.6 μg of penicillin G.

**unit rec·ord** single, comprehensive collection of all health care data for all episodes of care for a patient.

**uni·va·lence, uni·va·len·cy** (yu-nĭ-vā′lens, yu-nĭ-vā′len-sē) SYN monovalence.

**uni·va·lent** (yu-nĭ-vā′lent) SYN monovalent (1).

**uni·va·lent an·ti·bod·y** an "incomplete" form of antibody that may coat antigen, but which according to the "lattice theory" does not have a second receptor for attachment to another molecule of antigen; in the case of Rh+ erythrocytes, such an anti-Rh antibody may coat the cells but not cause them to agglutinate in saline; however, agglutination does occur when such coated cells are suspended in serum or other protein media, such as albumin, therefore called serum agglutinin. SYN incomplete antibody (1).

**uni·ver·sal den·tal no·men·cla·ture 1.** a North American system of identifying teeth by assigning a sequential number to each permanent tooth beginning with the upper right third molar (1) and continuing to the upper left third molar (16), then continuing in the lower arch and finishing with the lower right third molar (32). **2.** a system for deciduous teeth analogous to the permanent one using Arabic letters (A through T).

**uni·ver·sal do·nor** in blood grouping, a person belonging to group O; i.e., one whose erythrocytes do not contain either agglutinogen A or B and are, therefore, not agglutinated by plasma containing either of the ordinary isoagglutinins, alpha or beta.

**Un·i·ver·sal Pre·cau·tions** (in full, Universal Blood and Body Fluid Precautions). A set of procedural directives and guidelines published in August 1987 by the Centers for Disease Control and Prevention (CDC) (as *Recommendations for Prevention of HIV Transmission in Health-Care Settings*) to prevent parenteral, mucous membrane, and nonintact skin exposures of health care workers to bloodborne pathogens. In December 1991 the Occupational Safety and Health Administration (OSHA) promulgated its *Occu-*

*pational Exposure to Bloodborne Pathogens Standard,* incorporating universal precautions and imposing detailed requirements on employers of health care workers, including engineering controls, provision of protective barrier devices, standardized labeling of biohazards, mandatory training of employees in Universal Precautions, management of accidental parenteral exposure incidents, and availability to employees of immunization against hepatitis B.

**un·my·e·li·nat·ed** (ŭn-mī′ĕ-li-nā-ted) denoting nerve fibers (axons) lacking a myelin sheath. SYN amyelinated, amyelinic.

**un·my·e·li·nat·ed fi·bers** a fiber having no myelin covering (CNS); a naked axon; in the PNS represented by all axons lying in troughs in a single Schwann cell (Schwann cell unit); a slow conducting fiber. SYN gray fibers, nonmedullated fibers, Remak fibers.

**Un·na dis·ease** (oo′nah) SYN seborrheic dermatitis.

**Un·na ne·vus** (oo′nah) capillary stain on nape of neck; persistent form of nevus flammeus nuchae. SYN erythema nuchae.

**Un·na stain** (oo′nah) **1.** an alkaline methylene blue stain for plasma cells; **2.** a polychrome methylene blue stain with which mast cells are stained red (metachromatic).

**un·of·fi·cial** (ŭn-ŏ-fish′ăl) denoting a drug that is not listed in the United States Pharmacopeia or the National Formulary.

**un·phys·i·o·log·ic** (ŭn-fis′ē-ō-loj′ik) pertaining to conditions in the organism which are abnormal; can be used to refer to subjecting the body to abnormal amounts of substances normally present.

**un·san·i·tary** (ŭn-san′i-tār-ē) SYN insanitary.

**un·sat·u·rat·ed** (ŭn-sach′er-āt-ed) **1.** not saturated; denoting a solution in which the solvent is capable of dissolving more of the solute. **2.** denoting a chemical compound in which all the affinities are not satisfied, so that still other atoms or radicals may be added to it. **3.** ORGANIC CHEMISTRY denoting compounds containing double and/or triple bonds.

**un·sat·u·rat·ed fat·ty ac·id** a fatty acid, the carbon chain of which possesses one or more double or triple bonds (e.g., oleic acid, with one double bond in the molecule, and linoleic acid, with two); called unsaturated because it is capable of absorbing additional hydrogen.

**un·sta·ble an·gi·na 1.** angina pectoris charcterized by pain in the chest of coronary origin occurring in response to progressively less exercise or fewer other stimuli than ordinarily required to produce angina; often leading to myocardial infarction, if untreated, and caused by coronary artery spasm rather than increased myocardial oxygen demand. **2.** angina that has not achieved a constant or reproducible pattern in 30 or 60 days. SYN preinfarction angina.

**un·sta·ble lie** oblique orientation of the fetus that is neither transverse nor longitudinal, but that converts to one or the other before or during labor.

**un·stri·at·ed** (ŭn-strī′āt-ed) without striations; not striped; denoting the structure of the smooth or involuntary muscles.

**un·sys·tem·a·tized de·lu·sion** one of a group of apparently discrete, disconnected delusions.

**Un·ver·richt dis·ease** (oon′fer-ikt) a progressive

myoclonic epilepsy; one of the degenerative gray matter disorders characterized by myoclonus and generalized seizures, with progressive neurologic and intellectual decline; age of onset between 8 and 13 years of age; autosomal recessive inheritance, caused by mutation in the cystatin B gene (CSTB) on 21q22.

**UPJ** ureteropelvic junction.

**up·per air·way** the portion of the respiratory tract that extends from the nares or mouth to and including the larynx.

**up·per ex·trem·i·ty** SYN upper limb.

**🔲 up·per gas·tro·in·tes·tin·al ser·ies (UGI)** a fluoroscopic-radiographic examination of the esophagus, stomach, and duodenum; a contrast medium, usually barium sulfate, is introduced. See this page.

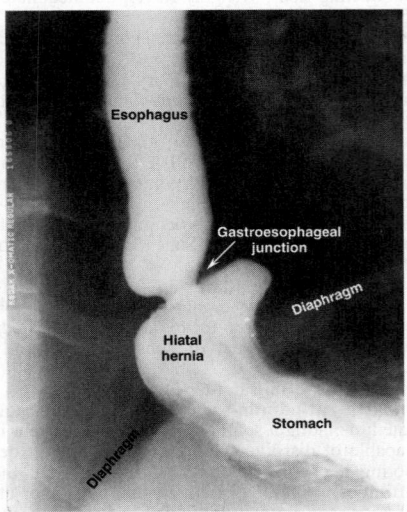

**upper gastrointestinal series:** radiograph showing hiatal hernia

**up·per limb** the shoulder, arm, forearm, wrist, and hand. SYN upper extremity.

**up·reg·u·la·tion** opposite of down-regulation.

**upregulation/downregulation hypothesis** a theory of the neurochemical basis of depression (an elaboration of the monoamine hypothesis) linking it to an increase in number (upregulation) of postsynaptic monoamine receptors, which are then effectively decreased in number (downregulation) as a result of antidepressant activity. SEE ALSO monoamine hypothesis.

**up·si·lon** (υ) (up′si-lon) **1.** the 20th letter in the Greek alphabet. **2.** kinematic viscosity.

**up·take** (ŭp′tāk) the absorption by a tissue of some substance (food material, mineral) its permanent or temporary retention.

**ura·chal** (yur′ă-kăl) relating to the urachus.

**ura·chus** (yur′ă-kŭs) that portion of the reduced allantoic stalk between the apex of the bladder and the umbilicus; becomes the median umbilical ligament. [G. *ourachos,* the urinary canal of a fetus]

**ura·cil (U)** (yur′ă-sil) a pyrimidine (base) present in ribonucleic acid.

**urae·mia [Br.]** SEE uremia.
**urae·mic [Br.]** SEE uremic.
**urae·um [Br.]** posterior half of an animal.
**ura·ni·um (U)** (yu-rā′nē-ŭm) a radioactive metallic element, atomic no. 92, atomic wt. 238.0289, occurring mainly in pitchblende and notable for its two isotopes: $^{238}$U and $^{235}$U (99.2745% and 0.720%, respectively, the rest being made up by $^{234}$U), $^{235}$U being the first substance ever shown capable of supporting a self-sustaining chain reaction. [G. myth. character, *Uranus*]

△**urano-, uran·is·co-** the hard palate. [G. *ouranos,* sky vault, *ouraniskos,* roof of mouth (palate)]

**ura·no·plas·ty** (yu′ră-nō-plas-tē) SYN palatoplasty.

**ura·nor·rha·phy** (yu′ră-nōr′ă-fē) SYN palatorrhaphy. [urano- + G. *rhaphē,* suture]

**ura·nos·chi·sis** (yu′ră-nos′ki-sis) cleft of the hard palate. [urano- + G. *schisis,* fissure]

**ura·no·staph·y·los·chi·sis** (yu′ră-nō-staf′i-los′ki-sis) cleft of the soft and hard palates. [urano- + G. *staphylē,* uvula, + *schisis,* fissure]

**ura·nyl** (yur′ă-nil) the ion, $UO_2^{2+}$; uranyl acetate is used in electron microscopy.

**urar·thri·tis** (yu-rar-thrī′tis) gouty inflammation of a joint. [urate + arthritis]

**ura·tae·mia [Br.]** SEE uratemia.

**urate** (yur′āt) a salt of uric acid.

**ura·te·mia** (yu-rā-tē′mē-ă) the presence of urates, especially sodium urate, in the blood. [urate + G. *haima,* blood]

**urate ox·i·dase** a copper-containing, oxygen-requiring oxidoreductase that oxidizes uric acid; used in the clinical diagnosis of increased uric acid levels. SYN uricase.

**ura·to·sis** (yu-ră-tō′sis) any morbid condition due to the presence of urates in the blood or tissues.

**ura·tu·ria** (yu-rāt-yu′rē-ă) the passage of an increased amount of urates in the urine. [urate + G. *ouron,* urine]

**Ur·ban op·er·a·tion** (er′ban) extended radical mastectomy, including *en bloc* resection of internal mammary lymph nodes, part of the sternum, and costal cartilages.

**Urd** uridine.

**ur·de·fens·es** (oor′dē-fens-ez) fundamental beliefs essential for human psychological integrity; e.g., religion, science. [Ger. *ur-,* primitive, earliest, + defenses]

△**ure-, urea-, ureo-** urea; urine. SEE ALSO urin-, uro-. [G. *ouron,* urine]

**urea** (yu-rē′ă) the chief end product of nitrogen metabolism in mammals, formed in the liver, by means of the Krebs-Henseleit cycle, and excreted in normal adult human urine in the amount of about 32 g a day (about ⁹⁄₇ of the nitrogen excreted from the body). It has been used as a diuretic in kidney function tests, and topically for various dermatitides. [G. *ouron,* urine]

**urea clear·ance** the volume of plasma (or blood) that would be completely cleared of urea by one minute's excretion of urine.

**urea cy·cle** the sequence of chemical reactions, occurring primarily in the liver, that results in the production of urea. SYN Krebs-Henseleit cycle, Krebs ornithine cycle, Krebs urea cycle.

**u·rea frost, u·re·mic frost** powdery deposits on the skin, especially the face, of urea and uric acid salts due to excretion of nitrogenous compounds in the sweat; seen in severe uremia.

**ure·a·gen·e·sis** (yu-rē-ă-jen'ĕ-sis) formation of urea, usually referring to the metabolism of amino acids to urea. SYN ureapoiesis. [urea + G. *genesis*, production]

**urea ni·tro·gen** the portion of nitrogen in a biological sample, such as blood or urine, that derives from its content of urea. SEE ALSO blood urea nitrogen.

**Ure·a·plas·ma** (yu-rē'ă-plaz'mă) a genus of microaerophilic to anaerobic, nonmotile bacteria containing Gram-negative, predominantly coccoidal to coccobacillary elements, approximately 0.3 μm in diameter, which frequently grow in short filaments. These organisms hydrolyze urea with production of ammonia, and are found in the human genitourinary tract, occasionally in the pharynx and rectum. In males, they are associated with nongonococcal urethritis and prostatitis; in females, with genitourinary tract infections and reproductive failure. The type species is *Ureaplasma urealyticum*. SYN T-mycoplasma.

**ure·a·poi·e·sis** (yu-rē'ă-poy-ē'sis) SYN ureagenesis. [urea + G. *poiēsis*, a making]

**ure·ase** (yur'ē-ās) an enzyme that catalyzes the hydrolysis of urea to carbon dioxide and ammonia; used as an antitumor enzyme; it is present in intestinal bacteria and accounts for most of the ammonia generated from urea in mammals.

**ure·de·ma** (yu-re-dē'mă) edema due to infiltration of urine into the subcutaneous tissues. [G. *ouron*, urine, + *oidēma*, swelling]

**ure·i·do·suc·cin·ic ac·id** (ū-rē'i-dō-sŭk-sin'ik as'id) a precursor of the pyrimidines. SYN *N*-carbamoylaspartic acid.

**urel·co·sis** (yu-rel-kō'sis) ulceration of any part of the urinary tract. [G. *ouron*, urine, + *helkōsis*, ulceration]

**ure·mia** (yu-rē'mē-ă) **1.** an excess of urea and other nitrogenous waste in the blood. **2.** the complex of symptoms due to severe persisting renal failure that can be relieved by dialysis. SYN azotaemia, azotemia. [G. *ouron*, urine, + *haima*, blood]

**ure·mic** (yu-rē'mik) relating to uremia.

**ure·mic co·ma** a metabolic encephalopathy caused by renal failure.

**ure·mi·gen·ic** (yu-rē-mi-jen'ik) **1.** of uremic origin or causation. **2.** causing or resulting in uremia.

**ure·si·es·the·sia** (yu-rē'si-es-thē'zē-ă) the desire to urinate. SYN uriesthesia. [G. *ourēsis*, a urinating, + *aisthēsis*, sensation]

**ure·sis** (yu-rē'sis) SYN urination. [G. *ourēsis*]

**ure·ter** (yu'rē-ter, yur'ĕ-ter) [TA] the thick-walled tube that conducts the urine from the renal pelvis to the bladder; it consists of an abdominal part and a pelvic part, is lined with transitional epithelium surrounded by smooth muscle, both circular and longitudinal, and is covered externally by a tunica adventitia. [G. *ourētēr*, urinary canal]

**ure·ter·al** (yu-rē'tĕ-răl) relating to the ureter. SYN ureteric.

**ure·ter·al ec·top·ia** abnormal termination of ureter within the bladder, the urethra, or outside the urinary tract.

**ure·ter·al·gia** (yu-rē-ter-al'jē-ă) pain in the ureter. [ureter + G. *algos*, pain]

**ure·ter·al re·im·plan·ta·tion** SYN ureteroneocystostomy.

**ure·ter·cys·to·scope** (yu-rē'ter-sis'tō-skōp) SYN ureterocystoscope.

**ure·ter·ec·ta·sia** (yu-rē'ter-ek-tā'zē-ă) dilation of a ureter. [ureter + G. *ektasis*, a stretching out]

**ure·ter·ec·to·my** (yu-rē-ter-ek'tō-mē) excision of a segment or all of a ureter. [ureter + G. *ektomē*, excision]

**ure·ter·ic** (yu-rē-ter'ik) SYN ureteral.

**ure·ter·ic or·i·fice** the opening of the ureter in the bladder, situated one at each lateral angle of the trigone; wide gaping of the ostium usually indicates vesicoureteral reflux.

**ure·ter·i·tis** (yu-rē-ter-ī'tis) inflammation of a ureter.

△**ure·ter·o-** the ureter. [G. *ourētēr*, urinary canal]

**ure·ter·o·cele** (yu-rē'ter-ō-sēl) saccular dilation of the terminal portion of the ureter which protrudes into the lumen of the urinary bladder, probably due to a congenital stenosis of the ureteral meatus. [uretero- + G. *kēlē*, hernia]

**ure·ter·o·ce·lor·ra·phy** (yu-rē'ter-ō-se-lōr'ă-fē) excision and suturing of a ureterocele performed through an open cystotomy incision. [ureterocele + G. *raphē*, suture]

**ure·ter·o·co·los·to·my** (yu-rē'ter-ō-kō-los'tō-mē) implantation of the ureter into the colon. [uretero- + G. *kolon*, colon, + *stoma*, mouth]

**ure·ter·o·cys·to·plas·ty** augmentation of the bladder using a native dilated ureter.

**ure·ter·o·cys·to·scope** (yu-rē'ter-ō-sis'tō-skōp) a cystoscope with an attachment for catheterization of the ureters; the catheter is passed into the ureter when its orifice is brought into view with the cystoscope. SYN uretercystoscope. [uretero- + G. *kystis*, bladder, + *skopeō*, to view]

**ure·ter·o·cys·tos·to·my** (yu-rē'ter-ō-sis-tos'tō-mē) SYN ureteroneocystostomy. [uretero- + G. *kystis*, bladder, + *stoma*, mouth]

**ure·ter·o·en·ter·os·to·my** (yu-rē'ter-ō-en-ter-os'tō-mē) formation of an opening between a ureter and the intestine. [uretero- + G. *enteron*, intestine, + *stoma*, mouth]

**ure·ter·og·ra·phy** (yu-rē'ter-og'ră-fē) radiography of the ureter after the direct injection of contrast medium. [uretero- + G. *graphē*, a writing]

**ure·ter·o·il·e·al a·nas·to·mo·sis** anastomosis between the ureter and an isolated segment of ileum. SEE ALSO Bricker operation.

**ure·ter·o·il·e·o·ne·o·cys·tos·to·my** (yu-rē'ter-ō-il'ē-ō-nē'ō-sis-tos'tō-mē) restoration of the continuity of the urinary tract by anastomosis of the upper segment of a partially destroyed ureter to a segment of ileum, the lower end of which is then implanted into the bladder. SYN ileal ureter. [uretero- + ileum + G. *neos*, new, + *hystis*, bladder, + *stoma*, mouth]

**ure·ter·o·il·e·os·to·my** (yu-rē'ter-ō-il-ē-os'tō-mē) implantation of a ureter into an isolated segment of ileum which drains through an abdominal stoma. [uretero- + ileum + G. *stoma*, mouth]

**ure·ter·o·li·thi·a·sis** (yu-rē'ter-ō-li-thī'ă-sis) the formation or presence of a calculus or calculi in one or both ureters. [ureterolith + G. -*iasis*, condition]

**ure·ter·o·li·thot·o·my** (yu-rē'ter-ō-li-thot'ō-mē) removal of a stone lodged in a ureter. [ureterolith + G. *tomē*, incision]

**ure·ter·ol·y·sis** (yu'rē-ter-ol'i-sis) surgical freeing of the ureter from surrounding disease or adhesions. [uretero- + G. *lysis*, a loosening]

u
r

**ure·ter·o·ne·o·cys·tos·to·my** (yu-rē′ter-ō-nē′ō-sis-tos′tō-mē) an operation whereby a ureter is implanted into the bladder. SYN ureteral reimplantation, ureterocystostomy. [uretero- + G. *neos*, new, + *kystis*, bladder, + *stoma*, mouth]

**ure·ter·o·ne·phrec·to·my** (yu-rē′ter-ō-nĕ-frek′tō-mē) SYN nephroureterectomy. [uretero- + G. *nephros*, kidney, + *ektomē*, excision]

**ure·ter·o·pel·vic junc·tion (UPJ)** site of origin of the ureter from the renal pelvis, a common location for congenital or acquired obstruction.

**ure·ter·o·pel·vic junc·tion ob·struc·tion** an impediment to drainage of urine from kidney usually due to partial or intermittent blockage of renal collecting system at the junction of renal pelvis and ureter.

**ure·ter·o·plas·ty** (yu-rē′ter-ō-plas-tē) surgical reconstruction of the ureters. [uretero- + G. *plastos*, formed]

**ure·ter·o·py·e·li·tis** (yu-rē′ter-ō-pī-ĕ-lī′tis) inflammation of the pelvis of a kidney and its ureter. [uretero- + G. *pyelos*, pelvis, + *-itis*, inflammation]

**ure·ter·o·py·e·log·ra·phy** (yu-rē′ter-ō-pī′ĕ-log′ră- fē) SYN pyelography.

**ure·ter·o·py·e·lo·plasty** (yu-rē′ter-ō-pī′ĕ-lō-plas-tē) surgical reconstruction of the ureter and of the pelvis of the kidney, usually for congenital ureteropelvic junction obstruction. [uretero- + G. *pyelos*, pelvis, + *plastos*, formed]

**ure·ter·o·py·e·los·to·my** (yu-rē′ter-ō-pī-ĕ-los′tō-mē) formation of a junction of the ureter and the renal pelvis. [uretero- + pelvis, + *stoma*, mouth]

**ure·ter·o·py·o·sis** (yu-rē′ter-ō-pī-ō′sis) an accumulation of pus in the ureter. [uretero- + G. *pyōsis*, suppuration]

**u·re·ter·o·re·nal re·flux** backward flow of urine from ureter into renal pelvis.

**ure·ter·or·rha·gia** (yu-rē′ter-ō-rā′jē-ă) hemorrhage from a ureter. [uretero- + G. *rhēgnymi*, to burst forth]

**ure·ter·or·rha·phy** (yu-rē-ter-ōr′ă-fē) suture of a ureter. [uretero- + G. *rhaphē*, suture]

**ure·ter·o·sig·moi·dos·to·my** (yu-rē′ter-ō-sig-moy-dos′tō-mē) implantation of the ureter into the sigmoid colon.

**ure·ter·os·to·my** (yu-rē-ter-os′tō-mē) establishment of an external opening into the ureter. [uretero- + G. *stoma*, mouth]

**ure·ter·ot·o·my** (yu-rē-ter-ot′ō-mē) incision and stenting of a narrow ureter. [uretero- + G. *tomē*, incision]

**ure·ter·o·u·re·ter·os·to·my** (yu-rē′ter-ō-yu-rē′ter-os′tō-mē) establishment of an anastomosis between the two ureters or between two segments of the same ureter. SEE ALSO transureteroureterostomy.

**ure·ter·o·ves·i·cal junc·tion** the site of entry of the ureter into the bladder, with an oblique angulation through the detrusor to avoid reflux. SEE ALSO vesicoureteral reflux.

**ure·ter·o·ves·i·cos·to·my** (yu-rē′ter-ō-ves-i-kos′tō-mē) surgical joining of a ureter to the bladder. [uretero- + L. *vesica*, bladder, + *stoma*, mouth]

**ure·thra** (yu-rē′thră) a canal leading from the bladder, discharging the urine externally. SYN urogenital canal. [G. *ourēthra*]

**ure·thral** (yu-rē′thrăl) relating to the urethra.

**ure·thral ar·tery** origin, perineal artery; distri-

bution, membranous urethra. SYN arteria urethralis [TA].

**ure·thral ca·run·cle** a small, fleshy, sometimes painful protrusion of the mucous membrane at the meatus of the female urethra.

**ure·thral crest** longitudinal mucosal fold in the dorsal wall of the urethra.

**ure·thral·gia** (yu-rē-thral′jē-ă) pain in the urethra. SYN urethrodynia. [urethr- + G. *algos*, pain]

**ure·thral glands** SEE glands of the female urethra, glands of the male urethra.

**ure·thral glands of male** numerous mucous glands in the wall of the penile urethra. SYN Littré glands.

**ure·thral groove** the groove on the ventral surface of the embryonic penis ultimately closes to form the penile portion of the urethra.

**ure·thral he·ma·tu·ria** hematuria in which the site of bleeding is in the urethra.

**ure·thral pa·pil·la, pa·pil·la u·re·thra·lis** the slight projection often present in the vestibule of the vagina marking the urethral orifice.

**ure·thral valves** folds in the urethral mucous membrane.

**ure·threc·to·my** (yur-ĕ-threk′tō-mē) excision of a segment or of the entire urethra. [urethr- + G. *ektomē*, excision]

**ure·threm·or·rha·gia** (yu-rē′threm-ō-rā′jē-ă) bleeding from the urethra. SYN urethrorrhagia. [urethr- + G. *haima*, blood, + *rhēgnymi*, to burst forth]

**ure·thrism, ure·thris·mus** (yu′rē-thrizm, yu′rē-thriz′mŭs) irritability or spasmodic stricture of the urethra. SYN urethrospasm.

**ure·thri·tis** (yu-rē-thrī′tis) inflammation of the urethra. [ureth- + G. *-itis*, inflammation]

**ure·thri·tis pet·ri·fi·cans** urethritis, sometimes of gouty origin, in which there is a deposit of calcareous matter in the wall of the urethra.

△**ure·thro-, urethr-** the urethra. [G. *ourēthra*]

**ure·thro·bul·bar** (yu-rē′thrō-bŭl′băr) SYN bulbourethral.

**ure·thro·cele** (yu-rē′thrō-sēl) prolapse of the female urethra. [urethro- + G. *kēlē*, tumor, hernia]

**ure·thro·cu·tan·e·ous fis·tu·la** fistula between urethra and penile skin; most often a complication of hypospadias repair.

**ure·thro·cys·tom·e·try** (yu-rē′thrō-sis-tom′ĕ-trē) a procedure that simultaneously measures pressures in urinary bladder and urethra. [urethro- + G. *kystis*, bladder, + *metron*, measure]

**ure·thro·dyn·ia** (yu-rē-thrō-din′ē-ă) SYN urethralgia. [urethro- + G. *odynē*, pain]

**ureth·ro·per·i·ne·o·scro·tal** (yu-rē′thrō-perĭ-nē-ō-skrō′tăl) relating to the urethra, perineum, and scrotum.

**ure·thro·plasty** (yu-rē-thrō-plas-tē) surgical repair of the urethra, as performed to correct hypospadias, epispadias, or the effects of trauma. [urethro- + G. *plastos*, formed]

**ure·thror·rha·gia** (yu-rē-thrō-rā′jē-ă) SYN urethremorrhagia.

**ure·thror·rha·phy** (yu-rē-thrōr′ă-fē) suture of the urethra. [urethro- + G. *rhaphē*, suture]

**ure·thror·rhea** (yu-rē-thrō-rē′ă) an abnormal discharge from the urethra. [urethro- + G. *rhoia*, a flow]

**ure·thro·scope** (yu-rē′thrō-skōp) an instrument for viewing the interior of the urethra. [urethro- + G. *skopeō*, to view]

**ure·thro·scop·ic** (yu-rē-thrō-skop'ik) relating to the urethroscope or to urethroscopy.

**ure·thros·co·py** (yu-rē-thros'kŏ-pē) inspection of the urethra with a urethroscope.

**ure·thro·spasm** (yu-rē'thrō-spazm) SYN urethrism.

**ure·thro·stax·is** (yu-rē'thrō-stak'sis) oozing of blood from the urethra. [urethro- + G. staxis, trickling]

**ure·thro·ste·no·sis** (yu-rē'thrō-ste-nō'sis) stricture of the urethra. [urethro- + G. stenōsis, a narrowing]

**ure·thros·to·my** (yu-rē-thros'tō-mē) surgical formation of a permanent opening between the urethra and the skin. [urethro- + G. stoma, mouth]

**ure·throt·o·my** (yu-rē-throt'ō-mē) surgical incision of a stricture of the urethra. [urethro- + G. tomē, incision]

**ure·thro·vag·i·nal fis·tu·la** a fistula between the urethra and the vagina.

**ure·thro·ves·ic·al ang·le** the angle between the female urethra and the posterior vesical wall, normally about 90°; narrowing of this angle in cystocele predisposes to stress incontinence.

**ure·thro·ves·i·co·pexy** (yu-rē'thrō-ves'i-kŏ-pek-sē) surgical suspension of the urethra and the base of the bladder from the posterior surface of the pubic symphysis (or anterior abdominal wall or Cooper ligament) for correction of urinary stress incontinence. [urethro- + L. vesica, bladder, + G. pexis, fixation]

△**-ure·tic** urine. [G. ourētikos, relating to the urine]

**urge in·con·ti·nence, ur·gen·cy in·con·ti·nence** leakage of urine in the presence of a strong desire to void.

**ur·gen·cy** (er'jen-sē) a strong desire to void.

**ur·hi·dro·sis** (yur-hi-drō'sis) SYN uridrosis.

△**uri-, uric-, urico-** uric acid. [G. ouron, urine]

**uric** (yur'ik) relating to urine.

**u·ric ac·id** 2,6,8-trioxypurine; white crystals, poorly soluble, contained in solution in the urine of mammals; sometimes solidified in small masses as stones or crystals or in larger concretions as calculi; with sodium and other bases it forms urates; elevated levels associated with gout.

**uri·case** (yur'i-kās) SYN urate oxidase.

**uri·col·y·sis** (yur-i-kol'i-sis) decomposition of uric acid. [urico- + G. lysis, a loosening]

**uri·co·lyt·ic** (yur'i-kō-lit'ik) relating to or effecting the hydrolysis of uric acid.

**uri·co·su·ria** (yu'ri-kō-syu'rē-ă) excessive amounts of uric acid in the urine. [urico- + G. ouron, urine]

**uri·dine (Urd)** (yur'i-dēn) Uracil ribonucleoside; one of the major nucleosides in RNAs; as the pyrophosphate (UDP, UDPG, etc.), uridine is active in sugar metabolism.

**uri·dine 5′-di·phos·phate (UDP)** uridine 5′-pyrophosphate; a condensation product of uridine and pyrophosphoric acid.

**uri·dine 5′-monophos·phate (UMP)** SYN uridylic acid.

**uri·dine 5′-tri·phos·phate (UTP)** uridine esterified with triphosphoric acid at its 5′-position; the immediate precursor of uridylic acid residues in RNA.

**uri·dro·sis** (yu-ri-drō'sis) the excretion of urea or uric acid in the sweat. SYN urhidrosis. [uri- + G. hidrōs, sweat]

**uri·dyl·ic ac·id** (yur-i-dil'ik as'id) uridine esteri-

fied by phosphoric acid, precursor for the biosynthesis of other pyrimidine nucleotides. SYN uridine 5′-monophosphate.

**uri·es·the·sia** (yuri-es-thē'zē-ă) SYN uresiesthesia.

△**urin-, urino-** urine. SEE ALSO ure-, uro-. [G. ouron]

**uri·nal** (yu'rin-ăl) a vessel into which urine is passed.

**uri·nal·y·sis** (yu-ri-nal'i-sis) analysis of the urine.

**uri·nary** (yur'i-nār-ē) relating to urine.

**uri·nary blad·der** a musculomembranous elastic bag serving as a storage place for the urine. SYN vesica urinaria [TA], bladder (2).

**uri·nary cal·cu·lus** a calculus in the kidney, ureter, bladder, or urethra.

**uri·nary ni·tro·gen** nitrogen excreted as urea, amino acids, uric acid, etc., in the urine; 1 g of urinary nitrogen indicates the breakdown in the body of 6.25 g of protein. SEE ALSO nitrogen equivalent.

**uri·nary sand** multiple small calculous particles passed in the urine of patients with nephrolithiasis; each particle is usually too small to cause significant symptoms or to be identified as a true calculus.

**uri·nary stut·ter·ing** frequent involuntary interruption occurring during the act of urination.

**uri·nary tract** the passage from the pelvis of the kidney to the urinary meatus through the ureters, bladder, and urethra.

**uri·nary tract in·fec·tion (UTI)** microbial infection, usually bacterial, of any part of the urinary tract.

**uri·nate** (yur'i-nāt) to pass urine. SYN micturate.

**uri·na·tion** (yur'i-nā'shŭn) the passing of urine. SYN miction, micturition (1), uresis.

**urine** (yur'in) the fluid and dissolved substances excreted by the kidney. [L. urina; G. ouron]

**uri·nog·e·nous** (yur-i-noj'ĕ-nŭs) 1. producing or excreting urine. 2. of urinary origin. SYN urogenous.

**uri·no·ma** (yur'i-nō'mă) a cystic collection of extravasated urine.

**uri·nom·e·try** (yur-i-nom'ĕ-trē) the determination of the specific gravity of the urine.

**uri·nos·co·py** (yur-i-nos'kŏ-pē) SYN uroscopy.

△**uro-** urine. SEE ALSO ure-, urin-. [G. ouron]

**uro·bi·lin** (yur-ō-bī'lin) a uroporphyrin; an acyclic tetrapyrrole that is one of the natural breakdown products of heme; a urinary pigment that gives a varying orange-red coloration to urine. SYN urohematin.

**uro·bi·li·ne·mia** (yu'rō-bil-i-nē'mē-ă) the presence of urobilins in the blood.

**uro·bi·lin·o·gen** (yur-ō-bī-lin'ō-jen) precursor of urobilin.

**uro·bi·lin·u·ria** (yu'rō-bil-i-nyu'rē-ă) the presence in the urine of urobilins in excessive amount, formed mainly from hemoglobin.

**ur·o·can·ate** (yur'ō-kă-nāt) a salt or ester of urocanic acid.

**ur·o·can·ate hy·dra·tase** an enzyme catalyzing the reaction of water with urocanic acid, a step in L-histidine catabolism; this enzyme is absent in cases of urocanic aciduria.

**uro·can·ic ac·id** (yur-ō-kan'ik as'id) an acid derived from the oxidative deamination of L-histidine; present in sweat; elevated levels are observed in cases of urocanate hydratase deficiency.

u
r

**uro•cele** (yu′rō-sēl) extravasation of urine into the scrotal sac. [uro- + G. *kēlē,* hernia]

**uro•che•sia** (yu-rō-kē′zē-ă) passage of urine from the anus. [uro- + G. *chezō,* to defecate]

**uro•chrome** (yur′ō-krōm) the principal pigment of urine, a compound of urobilin and a peptide of unknown structure.

**uro•dyn•ia** (yur-ō-din′ē-ă) pain on urination. [uro- + G. *odynē,* pain]

**uro•fla•vin** (yur-ō-flā′vin) a fluorescent product of riboflavin catabolism, or perhaps riboflavin itself, found in mammalian urine and feces.

**ur•o•fol•li•tro•pin** (yur-ō-fol′i-trō-pin) a preparation of gonadotropin extracted from the urine of postmenopausal women, used in conjunction with human chorionic gonadotropin to induce ovulation. SEE ALSO menotropins.

**uro•gas•trone** (yur-ō-gas′trōn) a fluorescent pigment extracted from urine; an inhibitor of gastric secretion and motility. Cf. enterogastrone.

**uro•gen•i•tal** (yu′rō-jen′i-tăl) SYN genitourinary.

**uro•gen•i•tal ca•nal** SYN urethra.

**uro•gen•i•tal di•a•phragm** a triangular sheet of muscle between the ischiopubic rami; composed of the sphincter urethrae, and the deep transverse perineal muscles.

**uro•gen•i•tal per•i•ton•eum** peritoneum of the pelvic cavity, including the folds and fossae formed by it. SYN peritoneum urogenitale.

**uro•gen•i•tal ridge** one of the paired longitudinal ridges developing in the dorsal body wall of the embryo on either side of the dorsal mesentery; the ridge is formed at first by the growing mesonephros and later by the mesonephros and the gonad.

**uro•gen•i•tal sin•us a•nom•aly** SYN hypospadias.

**uro•gen•i•tal sys•tem** includes all the organs concerned in reproduction and in the formation and discharge of urine. See page A25.

**urog•e•nous** (yu-roj′ĕ-nŭs) SYN urinogenous.

**uro•gram** (yur′ō-gram) the radiographic record obtained by urography.

**urog•ra•phy** (yu-rog′ră-fē) radiography of any part (kidneys, ureters, or bladder) of the urinary tract. SEE ALSO pyelography. [uro- + G. *graphō,* to write]

**uro•haem•a•tin [Br.]** SEE urobilin.

**uro•hem•a•tin** (yur′ō-hē′mă-tin) SYN urobilin.

**uro•ki•nase** (yur-ō-kī′nās) SYN plasminogen activator.

**uro•li•thi•a•sis** (yu-rō-li-thī′ă-sis) presence of calculi in the urinary system.

**uro•lith•ic** (yu-rō-lith′ik) relating to urinary calculi.

**uro•log•ic, uro•log•i•cal** (yu-rō-loj′ik, yu-rō-loj′ i-kăl) relating to urology.

**urol•o•gist** (yu-rol′ō-jist) a specialist in urology. SYN genitourinary surgeon.

**urol•o•gy** (yu-rol′ō-jē) the medical specialty concerned with the study, diagnosis, and treatment of diseases of the genitourinary tract. [uro- + G. *logos,* study]

**uron•cus** (yu-rong′kŭs) a urinary cyst; a circumscribed area of extravasation of urine. [uro- + G. *onkos,* mass (tumor)]

**uro•ne•phro•sis** (yu′rō-ne-frō′sis) SYN hydronephrosis.

**urop•a•thy** (yu-rop′ă-thē) any disorder involving the urinary tract. [uro- + G. *pathos,* suffering]

**uro•phan•ic** (yur-ō-fan′ik) appearing in the urine; denoting any constituent, normal or pathologic, of the urine. [uro- + G. *phainō,* to appear]

**uro•poi•e•sis** (yu′rō-poy-ē′sis) the production or secretion and excretion of urine. [uro- + G. *poiēsis,* a making]

**uro•poi•e•tic** (yu′rō-poy-et′ik) relating or pertaining to uropoiesis.

**uro•por•phy•rin** (yur-ō-pōr′fi-rin) **1.** porphyrin excreted in the urine in porphyrinuria. **2.** class name for all porphyrins containing 4 acetic acid groups and 4 propionic acid groups in positions 1 through 8. SEE ALSO porphyrinogens.

**ur•o•por•phy•rin•o•gen** (yur′ō-pōr-fi-rin′ō-jen) SEE porphyrinogens.

**ur•o•ra•di•ol•o•gy** (yu′rō-rā-dē-ol′ŏ-jē) the study of the radiology of the urinary tract.

**uros•che•sis** (yu-ros′kē-sis) **1.** retention of urine. **2.** suppression of urine. [uro- + G. *schesis,* a checking]

**uro•scop•ic** (yur-ō-skop′ik) relating to uroscopy.

**uros•co•py** (yu-ros′kō-pē) examination of the urine, usually by means of a microscope. SYN urinoscopy. [uro- + G. *skopeō,* to view]

**uro•sep•sis** (yur-ō-sep′sis) **1.** sepsis resulting from the decomposition of extravasated urine. **2.** sepsis from obstruction of infected urine. [uro- + G. *sēpsis,* decomposition]

**uro•the•li•al car•cin•oma** a malignant neoplasm derived from transitional epithelium, occurring chiefly in the urinary bladder, ureters, or renal pelves (especially if well differentiated); frequently papillary; these carcinomas are graded according to the degree of anaplasia. So-called transitional cell carcinoma of the upper respiratory tract is more properly classified as squamous cell carcinoma. Transitional cell carcinoma is also a rare tumor of the ovary.

**uro•the•li•al pap•il•lo•ma** a benign papillary tumor of urothelium.

**uro•the•li•um** (yu-rō-thē′lē-ŭm) the epithelial lining of the urinary tract. [uro- + epithelium]

**ur•o•thor•ax** (yur-ō-thōr′aks) the presence of urine in the thoracic cavity, usually following complex multiple organ injuries.

**ur•ti•cant** (er′ti-kant) producing a wheal or other similar itching agent. [L. *urtica,* nettle; see urtica]

**ur•ti•car•ia** (er′ti-kar′i-ă) an eruption of itching wheals, usually of systemic origin; it may be due to a state of hypersensitivity to foods or drugs, foci of infection, physical agents (heat, cold, light, friction), or psychic stimuli. SYN hives (1), urtication (3). [L. *urtica*]

**ur•ti•car•ia en•de•mi•ca, ur•ti•car•i•a ep•i•dem•i•ca** urticaria caused by the nettling hairs of certain caterpillars.

**ur•ti•car•i•al, ur•ti•car•i•ous** (er-ti-kar′ē-ăl, er-ti-kar′ē-ŭs) relating to or marked by urticaria.

**ur•ti•car•ia me•di•ca•men•to•sa** an urticarial form of drug eruption.

**ur•ti•car•ia pig•men•to•sa** cutaneous mastocytosis resulting from an excess of mast cells in the superficial dermis, producing a chronic eruption characterized by flat or slightly elevated brownish papules which urticate when stroked.

**ur•ti•cate** (er′ti-kāt) **1.** to perform urtication. **2.** marked by the presence of wheals. [L. *urticatus*]

**ur•ti•ca•tion** (er-ti-kā′shŭn) **1.** whipping with nettles to induce counterirritation, formerly used in the treatment of peripheral paralysis. **2.** a burning sensation resembling that produced by urticaria or resulting from nettle poisoning. **3.** SYN urticaria. [L. *urticatio*]

**USAN** United States Adopted Names.

**Ush·er syn·drome** (ŭsh′er) autosomal recessive inheritance with genetic heterogeneity; the three forms are distinguishable by linkage data: type 1 causes sensorineural hearing loss, loss of vestibular function, and retinitis pigmentosa; types 2 and 3 are characterized by hearing loss and retinitis pigmentosa.

**USP** United States Pharmacopeia. SEE Pharmacopeia.

**USPHS** United States Public Health Service.

**USP u·nit** a unit as defined and adopted by the *United States Pharmacopeia.*

**u·su·al in·ter·sti·tial pneu·mo·nia of Lie·bow** a progressive inflammatory condition starting with diffuse alveolar damage and resulting in fibrosis and honeycombing over a variable time period; also a common feature of collagen-vascular diseases.

**uter·ine** (yu′ter-in) relating to the uterus.

**uter·ine ar·tery** *origin,* internal iliac; *distribution,* uterus, upper part of vagina, round ligament, and medial part of uterine (fallopian) tube; *anastomoses,* ovarian, vaginal, inferior epigastric. Supplies maternal circulation to placenta during pregnancy. SYN arteria uterina [TA].

**uter·ine atony** failure of the myometrium to contract after delivery of the placenta; associated with excessive bleeding from the placental implantation site.

**uter·ine cal·cu·lus** a calcified myoma of the uterus.

**uter·ine cav·i·ty, cav·i·ty of u·ter·us** the space within the uterus extending from the cervical canal to the openings of the uterine tubes.

**uter·ine con·trac·tion** rhythmic activity of the myometrium associated with menstruation, pregnancy, or labor.

**uter·ine glands** numerous simple tubular glands in the uterine mucosa that secrete a glycogen-rich mucous fluid during the luteal phase of the menstrual cycle.

**uter·ine os·ti·um of uter·ine tubes** the uterine opening of the oviduct.

**uter·ine seg·ments 1.** lower: the isthmus of the uterus, the lower extremity of which joins with the cervical canal and, during pregnancy, expands to become the lower part of the uterine cavity; **2.** upper: the main portion of the body of the gravid uterus, the contraction of which furnishes the chief expulsory force in labor.

**uter·ine si·nus** a small, irregular vascular channel in the endometrium, of a type that forms during pregnancy.

**uter·ine souf·fle** a blowing sound, synchronous with the cardiac systole of the mother, heard on auscultation of the pregnant uterus.

**uter·ine tube** one of the tubes leading on either side from the upper or outer extremity of the ovary, which is largely enveloped by its expanded infundibulum, to the fundus of the uterus; it consists of infundibulum, ampulla, isthmus, and uterine parts. SYN salpinx (1) [TA], fallopian tube, gonaduct (2), oviduct.

**uter·ine veins** two veins on each side which arise from the uterine venous plexus, pass through a part of the broad ligament and then through a peritoneal fold, and empty into the internal iliac vein. SYN venae uterinae [TA].

*in **utero*** (in yu′ter-ō) within the womb; not yet born. [L.]

△**utero-, uter-** the uterus. SEE ALSO hystero- (1), metr-. [L. *uterus*]

**uter·o·cys·tos·to·my** (yu′ter-ō-sis-tos′tō-mē) formation of a communication between the uterus (cervix) and the bladder. [utero- + G. *kystis,* bladder, + *stoma,* mouth]

**uter·o·fix·a·tion** (yu′ter-ō-fik-sā′shŭn) SYN hysteropexy.

**uter·o·glob·in** steroid-inducible, evolutionarily conserved, homodimeric secreted protein with many biological activities including a proinflammatory effect, inhibition of soluble lipoproteinlipase $A_2$, and chemotaxis of neutrophils and monocytes. It binds to several putative receptors on several cell types and inhibits cellular invasion of the extracellular matrix. It is found in blood and urine, uterus and numerous other tissues but not kidneys. In mice uteroglobin has been shown to bind to fibronectin (Fn), preventing Fn self-aggregation and subsequent abnormal tissue deposition, especially in glomeruli. It is essential for maintaining normal renal function in mice. SYN bastokinin.

**uter·o·glob·in-ad·duc·in** an α/β heterodimeric protein found in renal tubule cells, thought to regulate ion transport through channels in the actin cytoskeleton. A mutant allele has been found in some patients with hypertension and it may be associated with the salt sensitive form of essential hypertension.

**uter·om·e·ter** (yu-ter-om′ĕ-ter) SYN hysterometer.

**uter·o·pexy** (yu′ter-ō-pek-sē) SYN hysteropexy.

**uter·o·pla·cen·tal si·nuses** irregular vascular spaces in the zone of the chorionic attachment to the decidua basalis.

**uter·o·plas·ty** (yu′ter-ō-plas-tē) plastic surgery of the uterus. SYN hysteroplasty, metroplasty. [utero- + G. *plastos,* formed]

**uter·o·sal·pin·gog·ra·phy** (yu′ter-ō-sal-pin-gog′ ră-fē) SYN hysterosalpingography.

**uter·o·scope** (yu′ter-ō-skōp) SYN hysteroscope.

**uter·os·co·py** (yu-ter-os′kŏ-pē) SYN hysteroscopy.

**uter·ot·o·my** (yu-ter-ot′ō-mē) SYN hysterotomy.

**uter·o·ton·ic** (yu′ter-ō-ton′ik) **1.** giving tone to the uterine muscle. **2.** an agent that overcomes relaxation of the muscular wall of the uterus. [utero- + G. *tonos,* tone, tension]

**uter·o·tu·bog·ra·phy** (yu′ter-ō-too-bog′ră-fē) SYN hysterosalpingography.

**uter·o·ves·i·cal lig·a·ment** a peritoneal fold extending from the uterus to the posterior portion of the bladder.

**uter·o·ves·i·cal pouch** a pocket formed by the deflection of the peritoneum from the bladder to the uterus in the female.

**uter·us,** pl. **uteri** (yu′ter-ŭs, yu′ter-ī) [TA] the hollow muscular organ in which the impregnated oocyte (ovum) develops into a child; it consists of a main portion (body) with an elongated lower part (neck), at the extremity of which is the opening (os). The upper rounded portion of the uterus, opposite the os, is the fundus, at each extremity of which is the horn marking the part where the uterine tube joins the uterus and through which the ovum reaches the uterine cavity after leaving the ovary. The organ is supported in the pelvic cavity by the broad ligaments, round ligaments,

u
t

cardinal ligaments, and rectouterine and vesicouterine folds or ligaments. SYN metra, womb. [L.]

**uter·us bi·cor·nis bi·col·lis** SEE bicornate uterus.

**uter·us bi·cor·nis u·ni·col·lis** SEE bicornate uterus.

**uter·us di·del·phys** double uterus with double cervix and double vagina; due to failure of the paramesonephric ducts to unite during embryonic development. [G. *di-*, two, + *delphys*, womb]

**UTI** urinary tract infection.

**UTP** uridine 5'-triphosphate.

**utri·cle** (yu′tri-kl) the larger of the two membranous sacs in the vestibule of the labyrinth, lying in the elliptical recess; from it arise the semicircular ducts. SYN utriculus [TA].

**utric·u·lar** (yu-trik′yu-lăr) relating to or resembling a utricle.

**u·tric·u·lar nerve** a branch of the utriculoampullar nerve, supplying the macula of the utricle. SYN nervus utricularis [TA].

**utric·u·li** (yu-trik′yu-lī) plural of utriculus.

**utric·u·li·tis** (yu-trik-yu-lī′tis) **1.** inflammation of the internal ear. **2.** inflammation of the prostatic utricle. [utriculus + G. *-itis*, inflammation]

**u·tric·u·lo·am·pul·lar nerve** a division of the vestibular part of the eighth cranial nerve; it gives off branches to the macula of the utricle (utricular nerve) and to the cristae of the ampullae of the anterior and lateral semicircular ducts (anterior and lateral ampullary nerves). SYN nervus utriculoampullaris [TA].

**utric·u·lo·sac·cu·lar** (yu-trik′yu-lō-sak′yu-lăr) relating to the utricle and the saccule of the labyrinth, denoting especially a duct connecting the two structures.

**utric·u·lus,** pl. **utric·u·li** (yu′trik′yu-lŭs, yu-trik′ yu-lī) [TA] SYN utricle. SEE ALSO vestibular organ. [L. dim. of *uter,* leather bag]

**u·tric·u·lus pros·ta·ti·cus** [TA] SYN prostatic utricle.

**uv, uv** ultraviolet.

**uve·al** (yu′vē-ăl) relating to the uvea.

**uve·it·ic** (yu-vē-it′ik) relating to the uvea.

**uve·i·tis,** pl. **uve·i·ti·des** (yu-vē-ī′tis, yu-vē-it′ĭ-dēz) inflammation of the uveal tract: iris, ciliary body, and choroid. [uvea + G. *-itis*, inflammation]

**u·ve·o·en·ceph·a·lit·ic syn·drome** SYN Behçet syndrome.

**u·ve·o·pa·rot·id fe·ver** chronic enlargement of the parotid glands and inflammation of the uveal tract accompanied by a long-continued fever of low degree; a form of sarcoidosis. SYN Heerfordt disease.

**uve·o·scle·ri·tis** (yu′vē-ō-sklē-rī′tis) inflammation of the sclera involved by extension from the uvea.

**uvi·form** (yu′vi-fōrm) SYN botryoid. [L. *uva,* grape, + *forma,* form]

**u·vit·ex 2B** a fluorescent stain that reacts with chitin; useful in the diagnosis of microsporidian or cryptosporidium infections.

**uvu·la,** pl. **uvu·lae** (yu′vyu-lă, yu′vyu-lē) [TA] an appendant fleshy mass; a structure bearing a fancied resemblance to the palatine uvula. [Mod. L. dim. of L. *uva,* a grape, the uvula]

**u·vu·la of blad·der** a slight projection into the cavity of the bladder, usually more prominent in old men, just behind the urethral opening, marking the location of the middle lobe of the prostate.

**u·vu·la ce·re·bel·li** SYN uvula of cerebellum.

**uvula of cerebellum** a triangular elevation on the vermis of the cerebellum, lying between the two tonsils anterior to the pyramis. SYN uvula cerebelli, uvula vermis.

**uvu·lar** (yu′vyu-lăr) relating to the uvula.

**u·vu·lar mus·cle** *origin,* posterior nasal spine; *insertion,* forms chief bulk of the uvula; *action,* raises the uvula; *nerve supply,* pharyngeal plexus. SYN musculus uvulae [TA], muscle of uvula.

**u·vu·la ver·mis** SYN uvula of cerebellum.

**uvu·lec·to·my** (yu-vyu-lek′tō-mē) excision of the uvula. SYN staphylectomy. [uvula + G. *ektomē,* excision]

**uvu·li·tis** (yu-vyu-lī′tis) inflammation of the uvula.

**uvu·lop·to·sis** (yu′vyu-lop-tō′sis) relaxation or elongation of the uvula. SYN staphylodialysis, staphyloptosis. [uvulo- + G. *ptōsis,* a falling]

**uvu·lot·o·my** (yu-vyu-lot′ō-mē) any cutting operation on the uvula. [uvulo- + G. *tomē,* a cutting]

**U wave** a positive wave following the T wave of the electrocardiogram.

# V

**V 1.** vision; volt; with subscript 1, 2, 3, etc., the abbreviation for unipolar electrocardiogram leads. **2.** vanadium; valine; volume, frequently with subscripts denoting location, chemical species, and/or conditions.

*V* volume.

**v 1.** volt; initial rate velocity; velocity; *vel* [L, or]. **2.** as a subscript, refers to venous blood.

**v̇ 1.** gas flow, frequently with subscripts indicating location and chemical species. SEE flow (3). **2.** ventilation (3), frequently with a subscript. See entries under ventilation (3). [volume + overdot denoting time derivative]

**v̄** as a subscript, refers to mixed venous (pulmonary arterial) blood.

$V_A$ alveolar ventilation.

$V_{max}$ maximum velocity.

**V-A, VA** ventriculoatrial.

**vac·ci·nal** (vak'si-năl) relating to vaccine or vaccination.

**vac·ci·nate** (vak'si-nāt) to administer a vaccine.

**vac·ci·na·tion** (vak'si-nā'shŭn) the act of administering a vaccine.

**vac·cine** (vak'sēn, vak-sēn') any preparation intended for active immunological prophylaxis; e.g., preparations of killed microbes of virulent strains or living microbes of attenuated (variant or mutant) strains, or microbial, fungal, plant, protozoal, or metazoan derivatives or products. [L. *vaccinus,* relating to a cow]

**vac·cine lymph, vac·cin·i·a lymph** that collected from the vesicles of vaccinia infection, and used for active immunization against smallpox.

**VACTERL syn·drome** abnormalities of *v*ertebrae, *a*nus, *c*cardiovascular tree, *t*rachea, *e*sophagus, *r*enal system, and *l*imb buds associated with administration of sex steroids during early pregnancy.

**vac·u·o·lar** (vak-yu-ō'lăr) relating to or resembling a vacuole.

**vac·u·o·late, vac·u·o·lat·ed** (vak'yu-ō-lāt, vak'yu-ō-lāt'ed) having vacuoles.

**vac·u·o·la·tion, vac·u·o·li·za·tion** (vak'yu-ō-lā'shŭn, vak'yu-ō-li-zā'shŭn) **1.** formation of vacuoles. **2.** the condition of having vacuoles.

**vac·u·ole** (vak'yu-ōl) **1.** a minute space in any tissue. **2.** a clear space in the substance of a cell, sometimes degenerative in character, sometimes surrounding an englobed foreign body and serving as a temporary cell stomach for the digestion of the body. [Mod. L. *vacuolum,* dim. of L. *vacuum,* an empty space]

**vac·u·tome** (vak'yu-tōm) electrodermatome that applies suction to the skin to raise it before an advancing blade, usually for taking a split-thickness skin graft. [vacuum + G. *tomē,* a cutting]

**vac·u·um** (vak'yoom) an empty space, one practically exhausted of air or gas. [L. ntr. of *vacuus,* empty]

**va·cuum pack tech·nique** a temporary closing of the abdomen by using a fenestrated plastic sheet over the intestine but under the anterior abdominal wall followed by the placement of moistened pads with a suction catheter within the wound. The entire defect is then covered by a nonporous plastic sheet; permits drainage of the abdominal cavity by suction while maintaining anterior abdominal wall rigidity.

**vag·a·bond's dis·ease** SYN parasitic melanoderma.

**va·gal** (vā'găl) relating to the vagus nerve.

**va·gal nerve stim·u·la·tion** an adjunctive treatment for patients with intractable epilepsy, particularly complex partial or secondarily generalized seizures; stimulation is delivered to the left vagus nerve in the neck, usually in 30-s bursts every 5½ min by a stimulator implanted in the anterior chest wall.

**va·gal trunk** one of the two nerve bundles, anterior and posterior, into which the esophageal plexus continues as it passes through the diaphragm. SYN truncus vagalis [TA].

**va·gi** (vā'gī) plural of vagus.

**va·gi·na,** gen. and pl. **va·gi·nae** (vă-jī'nă, vă-jī'nē) **1.** [TA] SYN sheath (1). **2.** [TA] the genital canal in the female, extending from the uterus to the vulva. [L. sheath, the vagina]

**va·gi·na ca·ro·ti·ca** [TA] SYN carotid sheath.

**vag·i·nal** (vaj'i-năl) relating to the vagina or to any sheath. [Mod. L. *vaginalis*]

**vag·i·nal ar·tery** *origin,* internal iliac; *distribution,* vagina, base of bladder, rectum; *anastomoses,* uterine, internal pudendal. SYN arteria vaginalis [TA].

**vag·i·nal a·tre·sia** congenital or acquired imperforation or occlusion of the vagina, or adhesion of the walls of the vagina. SYN colpatresia.

**vag·i·nal ce·li·ot·o·my** opening the peritoneal cavity through the vagina.

**vag·i·nal cuff** the portion of the vaginal vault remaining open to the peritoneum following hysterectomy.

**vag·i·nal gland** one of the mucous glands in the mucous membrane of the vagina.

**vag·i·nal hys·ter·ec·to·my** removal of the uterus through the vagina.

**vag·i·nal intra·epi·the·li·al neo·plas·ia** preinvasive squamous cell carcinoma (carcinoma in situ) limited to vaginal epithelium; like vulvar or cervical intraepithelial neoplasia, graded histologically on a scale from 1 to 3 or subdivided into low-grade and high-grade intraepithelial malignancy; usually related to human papilloma virus infection; may progress to invasive carcinoma.

**vag·i·nal nerves** several nerves passing from the uterovaginal plexus to the vagina. SYN nervi vaginales [TA].

**vag·i·nal or·i·fice** the narrowest portion of the canal, in the floor of the vestibule posterior to the urethral orifice.

**vag·i·nal por·tion of cer·vix** the part of the cervix uteri contained within the vagina.

**vag·i·nal rug·ae** a number of transverse ridges in the mucous membrane of the vagina.

**vag·i·nate** (vaj'i-nāt) **1.** to ensheathe; to enclose in a sheath. **2.** ensheathed; provided with a sheath.

**vag·i·nec·to·my** (vaj-i-nek'tō-mē) excision of the vagina or a segment thereof. SYN colpectomy. [vagina + G. *ektomē,* excision]

**vag·i·nis·mus** (vaj-i-niz'mŭs) painful spasm of the vagina preventing intercourse. [vagina + L. *-ismus,* action, condition]

**vag·i·ni·tis,** pl. **vag·i·ni·ti·des** (vaj-i-nī'tis, vaj-i-nī'ti-dēz) inflammation of the vagina. [vagina + G. *-itis,* inflammation]

⚠ **vagino-, vagin-** the vagina. SEE ALSO colpo-. [L. *vagina,* sheath]

**vag·i·no·cele** (vaj'i-nō-sēl) SYN colpocele (1).

**vag·i·no·dyn·ia** (vaj'i-nō-din'ē-ă) vaginal pain. SYN colpodynia.

**vag·i·no·fix·a·tion** (vaj'i-nō-fik-sā'shŭn) suture of a relaxed and prolapsed vagina to the abdominal wall. SYN colpopexy, vaginopexy.

**vag·i·no·my·co·sis** (vaj'i-nō-mī-kō'sis) vaginal infection due to a fungus.

**vag·i·nop·a·thy** (vaj-i-nop'ă-thē) any diseased condition of the vagina. [vagino- + G. *pathos,* suffering]

**vag·i·no·per·i·ne·o·plas·ty** (vaj'i-nō-per-i-nē'ō-plas-tē) plastic surgery of the perineum involving the vagina. SYN colpoperineoplasty. [vagino- + perineum, + G. *plastos,* formed]

**vag·i·no·per·i·ne·or·rha·phy** (vaj'i-nō-per-i-nē-ōr'ă-fē) repair of a lacerated vagina and perineum. SYN colpoperineorrhaphy. [vagino- + perineum, + G. *rhaphē,* suture]

**vag·i·no·per·i·ne·ot·o·my** (vaj'i-nō-per-i-nē-ot'ō-mē) division of the posterior aspect of the vagina and adjacent portion of the perineum to facilitate childbirth. [vagino- + perineum, + G. *tomē,* incision]

**vag·i·no·pexy** (vaj'i-nō-pek-sē) SYN vaginofixation.

**vag·i·no·plas·ty** (vaj'i-nō-plas-tē) plastic surgery of the vagina. SYN colpoplasty. [vagino- + G. *plastos,* formed]

**vag·i·nos·co·py** (vaj-i-nos'kŏ-pē) inspection of the vagina, usually with an instrument.

**vag·in·o·sis** disease of the vagina.

**vag·i·not·o·my** (vaj-i-not'ō-mē) a cutting operation in the vagina. SYN colpotomy.

**va·gi·tus uter·i·nus** (va-jī'tŭs yu-ter-ī'nŭs) crying of the fetus while still within the uterus, possible when the membranes have been ruptured and air has entered the uterine cavity. [L. fr. *vagio,* to squall; L. fr. *uterus,* womb]

⚠ **vago-** the vagus nerve. [L. *vagus*]

**va·gol·y·sis** (vā-gol'i-sis) surgical destruction of the vagus nerve. [vago- + G. *lysis,* a loosening]

**va·go·lyt·ic** (vā-gō-lit'ik) **1.** pertaining to or causing vagolysis. **2.** a therapeutic or chemical agent that has inhibitory effects on the vagus nerve. **3.** denoting an agent having such effects.

**va·go·mi·met·ic** (vā'gō-mi-met'ik) mimicking the action of the efferent fibers of the vagus nerve.

**va·got·o·my** (vā-got'ō-mē) division of the vagus nerve. [vago- + G. *tomē,* incision]

**va·go·tro·pic** (vā-gō-trop'ik) attracted by, hence acting upon, the vagus nerve. [vago- + G. *tropos,* turning]

**va·go·va·gal** (vā'gō-vā'găl) pertaining to a process that utilizes both afferent and efferent vagal fibers.

**va·grant's dis·ease** SYN parasitic melanoderma.

**va·gus,** gen. and pl. **va·gi** (vā'gŭs, vā'gī) SYN vagus nerve [CN X]. [L. wandering, so-called because of the wide distribution of the nerve]

**va·gus nerve [CN X]** a mixed nerve that arises by numerous small roots from the side of the medulla oblongata, between the glossopharyngeal above and the accessory below; it leaves the cranial cavity by the jugular foramen and passes down to supply the pharynx, larynx, trachea, lungs, heart, and the gastrointestinal tract as far as the left colic (splenic) flexure; the only cranial

nerve that does not arise from the brain, but is classified as such because it exits from the cranium. SYN nervus vagus [CN X] [TA], pneumogastric nerve, tenth cranial nerve [CN X], vagus.

**va·gus pulse** a slow pulse due to the inhibitory action of the vagus nerve on the heart.

**Val** valine and its radicals.

**va·lence, va·len·cy** (vā'lens, vā'len-sē) the combining power of one atom of an element (or a radical), that of the hydrogen atom being the unit of comparison, determined by the number of electrons in the outer shell of the atom (v. electrons); e.g., in HCl, chlorine is monovalent; in $H_2O$, oxygen is bivalent; in $NH_3$, nitrogen is trivalent. [L. *valentia,* strength]

**Val·en·tine po·si·tion** (val'en-tūn) a supine position on a table with double inclined plane so as to cause flexion at the hips; used to facilitate urethral irrigation.

**val·gus** (val'gŭs) descriptive of any of the paired joints of the extremities with a static angular deformity in which the bone distal to the joint deviates laterally from the longitudinal axis of the proximal bone, and from the midline of the body, when the subject is in anatomical position. The adjective valgus is attached sometimes to the name of the joint (cubitus valgus) and sometimes to the name of the part just distal to the joint (hallux valgus). The gender of the adjective matches that of the Latin noun to which it is joined; thus, cubitus, hallux, metatarsus, pes, talipes *valgus;* coxa, manus, talipomanus *valga;* genu *valgum.* [Mod. L. turned outward, fr. L. bowlegged]

**val·gus lax·i·ty** abnormal flexibility on the medial side of a joint upon lateral movement of the distal segment.

**va·line (Val, V)** (val'ēn) 2-Amino-3-methylbutanoic acid; the L-isomer is a constituent of most proteins; a nutritionally essential amino acid.

**val·late** (val'āt) bordered with an elevation, as a cupped structure; denoting especially certain lingual papillae. SEE ALSO circumvallate. [L. *vallo,* pp. *-atus,* to surround with, fr. *vallum,* a rampart]

**val·late pa·pil·la** one of eight or ten projections from the dorsum of the tongue forming a row anterior to and parallel with the sulcus terminalis; each papilla is surrounded by a circular trench (fossa) having a slightly raised outer wall (vallum); on the sides of the vallate papilla and the opposed margin of the vallum are numerous taste buds. SYN papilla vallata [TA], circumvallate papillae, papillae vallatae.

**val·lec·u·la,** pl. **val·lec·u·lae** (vă-lek'yu-lă, vă-lek'yu-lē) [TA] a crevice or depression on any surface. [L. dim. of *vallis,* valley]

**Val·leix points** (vahl'ēz) various points in the course of a nerve, pressure upon which is painful in cases of neuralgia; these points are: 1) where the nerve emerges from the bony canal; 2) where it pierces a muscle or aponeurosis to reach the skin; 3) where a superficial nerve rests upon a resisting surface where compression is easily made; 4) where the nerve gives off one or more branches; and 5) where the nerve terminates in the skin.

**Val·sal·va ma·neu·ver** (val-sal'vă) any forced expiratory effort ("strain") against a closed airway, whether at the nose and mouth or at the glottis; because high intrathoracic pressure impedes venous return to the right atrium, this maneuver is used to study cardiovascular effects of raised peripheral venous pressure and decreased cardiac filling and cardiac output.

**val•ue** (val′yu) [M.E., fr. O.Fr., fr. L. *valeo*, to be of value]

**val•va**, pl. **val•vae** (val′vă, val′vē) SYN valve. [L. one leaf of a double door]

**val•val, val•var** (val′văl, val′văr) relating to a valve.

**val•vate** (val′vāt) relating to or provided with a valve. SYN valvular.

**valve** (valv) **1.** a fold of the lining membrane of a canal or other hollow organ serving to retard or prevent a reflux of fluid. **2.** any reduplication of tissue or flaplike structure resembling a valve. SEE ALSO valvule, plica. See this page. SYN valva. [L. *valva*]

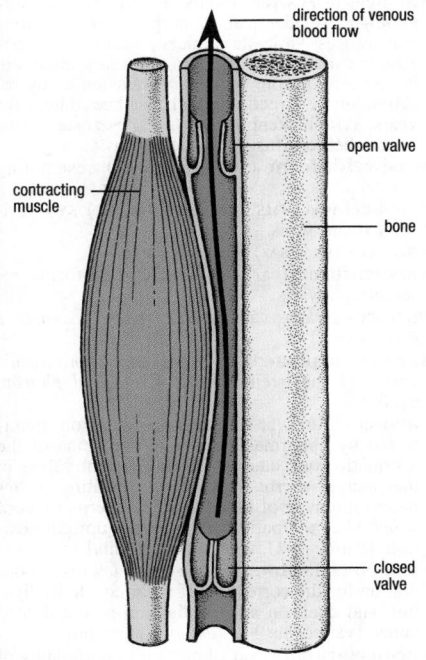

direction of venous blood flow

open valve

contracting muscle

bone

closed valve

**venous valves:** principle of venous blood flow

**valve of cor•o•nary si•nus** a delicate fold of endocardium at the opening of the coronary sinus into the right atrium.

**val•vo•plas•ty** (val′vō-plas-tē) surgical reconstruction of a deformed cardiac valve, for the relief of stenosis or incompetence. SYN valvuloplasty. [valve + G. *plastos,* formed]

**val•vot•o•my** (val-vot′ō-mē) **1.** cutting through a stenosed cardiac valve to relieve the obstruction. SYN valvulotomy. **2.** incision of a valvular structure. [valve + G. *tomē,* incision]

**val•vu•la**, pl. **val•vu•lae** (val′vyu-lă, val′vyu-lē) SYN valvule. [Mod. L. dim. of *valva*]

**val•vu•lar** (val′vyu-lăr) SYN valvate.

**val•vu•lar en•do•car•di•tis** inflammation confined to the endocardium of the valves.

**val•vu•lar in•suf•fi•cien•cy** SYN valvular regurgitation.

**val•vu•lar re•gur•gi•ta•tion** a leaky state of one or more of the cardiac valves, the valve not closing tightly and blood therefore regurgitating through it. SYN valvular insufficiency.

**val•vule** (val′vyul) a valve, especially one of small size. SYN valvula. [L. *valvula*]

**val•vule** (val′vyul) a valve, especially one of small size. [L. *valvula*]

**val•vu•li•tis** (val-vyu-lī′tis) inflammation of a valve, especially a heart valve. [Mod. L. *valvula,* valve, + G. *-itis,* inflammation]

**val•vu•lo•plas•ty** (val′vyu-lō-plas′tē) SYN valvoplasty.

**val•vu•lot•o•my** (val-vyu-lot′ō-mē) SYN valvotomy (1).

**va•na•di•um (V)** (vă-nā′dē-ŭm) a metallic element, atomic no. 23, atomic wt. 50.9415; a bioelement, its deficiency can result in abnormal bone growth and a rise in cholesterol and triglyceride levels. [*Vanadis,* Scand. goddess]

**va•na•di•um group** those elements resembling vanadium in chemical and metallurgical properties; included with vanadium are niobium and tantalum.

**van Buch•em syn•drome** (vahn boo′kem) an osteosclerosing skeletal dysplasia, characterized by mandibular enlargement, thickening of the diaphyses and calvaria, and increased serum alkaline phosphatase; autosomal recessive inheritance.

**van der Hoeve syn•drome** (vahn der hō-vĕ) a subtype of osteogenesis imperfecta in which progressive conductive hearing loss begins in childhood because of stapedial fixation.

**van der Waals forc•es** (vahn der valz) first postulated by van der Waals in 1873 to explain deviations from ideal gas behavior seen in real gases; the attractive forces between atoms or molecules other than electrostatic (ionic), covalent (sharing of electrons), or hydrogen bonding (sharing a proton); generally ascribed to dipolar and dispersion effects, π-electrons, etc.; these relatively nondescript forces contribute to the mutual attraction of organic molecules.

**van Er•men•gen stain** (vahn er′men-jen) a method for staining flagella that uses glacial acetic acid, osmic acid, tannic acid, silver nitrate, gallic acid, and potassium acetate.

**van Gie•son stain** (van gē′son) a mixture of acid fuchsin in saturated picric acid solution, used in collagen staining.

**va•nil•lism** (vă-nil′izm) **1.** symptoms of irritation of the skin, nasal mucous membrane, and conjunctiva from which workers with vanilla sometimes suffer. **2.** infestation of the skin by sarcoptiform mites found in vanilla pods.

**va•nil•lyl•man•del•ic ac•id (VMA)** (van′i-lil-man-del′ik as′id) the major urinary metabolite of adrenal and sympathetic catecholamines; elevated in most patients with pheochromocytoma.

**van•ish•ing lung syn•drome** progressive decrease of radiographic opacity of the lung caused by accelerated development of emphysema or rapid cystic destruction of the lung from infection.

**Van Lo•hui•zen syn•drome** (vahn lō-hwē-zen) SYN cutis marmorata telangiectatica congenita.

**van't Hoff e•qua•tion** (vahnt hof) **1.** equation for osmotic pressure of dilute solutions. SEE van't

Hoff law. **2.** for any reaction, $d(\ln K_{eq}/d(1/T)$ equals $-\Delta H/R$ where $K_{eq}$ is the equilibrium constant, $T$ the absolute temperature, $R$ the universal gas constant, and $\Delta H$ the change in enthalpy; thus, plotting $\ln K_{eq}$ vs. $1/T$ allows the determination of $\Delta H$.

**van't Hoff law** (vahnt hof) **1.** in stereochemistry, all optically active substances have one or more multivalent atoms united to four different atoms or radicals so as to form in space an unsymmetric arrangement; **2.** the osmotic pressure exerted by any substance in very dilute solution is the same that it would exert if present as gas in the same volume as that of the solution; or, at constant temperature, the osmotic pressure of dilute solutions is proportional to the concentration (number of molecules) of the dissolved substance; i.e., the osmotic pressure, $\Pi$, in dilute solutions is $\Pi = RT\Sigma c_i$, where $R$ is the universal gas constant, $T$ is the absolute temperature, and $c_i$ is the molar concentration of solute i; **3.** the rate of chemical reactions increases between two- and three-fold for each 10°C rise in temperature.

**van't Hoff the•o•ry** (vahnt hof) that substances in dilute solution obey the gas laws. Cf. van't Hoff law.

**va•por** (vā′per) **1.** molecules in the gaseous phase of a solid or liquid substance exposed to a gas. **2.** a visible emanation of fine particles of a liquid. **3.** a medicinal preparation to be administered by inhalation. [L. steam]

**va•por•i•za•tion** (vā-per-i-zā′shŭn) **1.** the change of a solid or liquid to a state of vapor. **2.** the therapeutic application of a vapor.

**va•por•ize** (vā′per-īz) **1.** to convert a solid or liquid into a vapor. **2.** to apply a vapor therapeutically.

**va•por•iz•er** (vā′per-īz-er) **1.** an apparatus for reducing medicated liquids to a state of vapor suitable for inhalation or application to accessible mucous membranes. SEE ALSO nebulizer, atomizer. **2.** a device for volatilizing liquid anesthetics.

**V̇a/Q̇** ventilation/perfusion ratio.

**Va•quez dis•ease** (vah-kāz′) SYN polycythemia vera.

**var•i•a•ble** (var′ē-ă-bl) **1.** that which is inconstant, which can or does change, as contrasted with a constant. **2.** deviating from the type in structure, form, physiology, or behavior. [L. vario, to vary, change, differ]

**var•i•ab•le re•sis•tance train•ing** resistance training with equipment that uses a lever arm, cam, hydraulic system, or pulley to alter the resistance to match increases and decreases in a muscle's force capacity as it moves through the range of motion.

**var•i•ance** (var′ē-ans) **1.** the state of being variable, different, divergent, or deviate; a degree of deviation. **2.** a measure of the variation shown by a set of observations, defined as the sum of squares of deviations from the mean, divided by the number of degrees of freedom in the set of observations.

**var•i•ant** (var′ē-ant) **1.** that which, or one who, is variable. **2.** having the tendency to alter or change, exhibit variety or diversity, not conform, or differ from the type.

**var•i•ant an•gi•na** SYN Prinzmetal angina.

**var•i•ant an•gi•na pec•to•ris** SYN Prinzmetal angina.

**var•i•a•tion** (var-ē-ā′shŭn) deviation from the type, especially the parent type, in structure, form, physiology, or behavior. [L. variatio, fr. vario, to change, vary]

**var•i•ca•tion** (var-i-kā′shŭn) formation or presence of varices.

**var•i•ce•al** (var-ĭ-sē′ăl, vă-ris′ē-ăl) of or pertaining to a varix.

▣ **var•i•cel•la** (var-i-sel′ă) an acute contagious disease, usually occurring in children, caused by the varicella-zoster virus and marked by a sparse eruption of papules, which become vesicles and then pustules, usually with mild constitutional symptoms; incubation period is about 14 to 17 days. See page B3. SYN chickenpox. [Mod. L. dim. of variola]

**var•i•cel•la en•ceph•a•li•tis** encephalitis occurring as a complication of chickenpox.

**var•i•cel•la-zos•ter vi•rus** a herpesvirus, morphologically identical to herpes simplex virus, that causes varicella (chickenpox) and herpes zoster; varicella results from a primary infection, herpes zoster from secondary invasion or by reactivation of infection which has been latent for years. SYN chickenpox virus, herpes zoster virus, human herpesvirus 3, Varicellovirus.

**var•i•cel•li•form** (var-ĭ-sel′ĭ-fōrm) resembling varicella.

**Var•i•cel•lo•vi•rus** (var-ē-sel′ō-vi′rus) SYN varicella-zoster virus.

**va•ri•ces** (var′i-sēz) plural of varix.

**var•i•ci•form** (var′ĭ-si-fōrm, vă-ris′ĭ-fōrm) resembling a varix.

△**var•i•co-** a varix, varicose, varicosity. [L. varix, a dilated vein]

**var•i•co•bleph•a•ron** (var′i-kō-blef′ă-ron) a varicosity of the eyelid. [varico- + G. blepharon, eyelid]

**var•i•co•cele** (var′i-kō-sēl) a condition manifested by abnormal dilation of the veins of the spermatic cord, caused by incompetent valves in the internal spermatic vein and resulting in impaired drainage of blood into the spermatic cord veins when the patient assumes the upright position. [varico- + G. kēlē, tumor, hernia]

**var•i•co•ce•lec•to•my** (var′i-kō-sē-lek′tō-mē) operation for the correction of a varicocele by ligature and excision and by ligation of the dilated veins. [varicocele + G. ektomē, excision]

**var•i•cog•ra•phy** (var′ĭ-kog′ră-fē) radiography of the veins after injection of contrast medium into varicose veins. [varico- + G. graphō, to write]

**var•i•com•pha•lus** (var-i-kom′fă-lŭs) a swelling formed by varicose veins at the umbilicus. [varico- + G. omphalos, navel]

**var•i•co•phle•bi•tis** (var′i-kō-flĕ-bī′tis) inflammation of varicose veins. [varico- + G. phleps, vein, + -itis, inflammation]

**var•i•cose** (var′i-kōs) relating to, affected with, or characterized by varices or varicosis.

**var•i•cose an•eu•rysm** a blood-containing sac, communicating with both an artery and a vein.

**var•i•cose ul•cer** the loss of skin surface in the drainage area of a varicose vein, usually in the leg, resulting from stasis and infection. SYN venous ulcer.

**var•i•cose vein** permanent dilation and tortuosity of a vein, most commonly seen in the legs, probably as a result of congenitally incomplete valves; there is a predisposition to varicose veins among persons in occupations requiring long periods of standing, and in pregnant women.

**var·i·co·sis**, pl. **var·i·cos·es** (var-i-kō′sis, var-i-kō′sēz) a dilated or varicose state of a vein or veins. See this page. [varico- + G. *-osis*, condition]

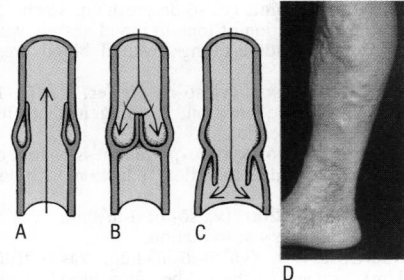

A B C

D

**varicosis:** in a healthy vein the valves allow blood to travel toward heart (A) while keeping blood from flowing back away from heart (B); valves in varicose veins (C) no longer function properly, thus allowing blood to travel back toward extremities, (D) photograph of leg with varicose veins

**var·i·cos·i·ty** (var-i-kos′i-tē) a varix or varicose condition.

**var·i·cot·o·my** (var-i-kot′ō-mē) an operation for varicose veins by subcutaneous incision. [varico- + G. *tomē*, a cutting]

**va·ric·u·la** (vă-rik′yu-lă) a varicose condition of the veins of the conjunctiva. SYN conjunctival varix. [L. dim. of *varix*]

**var·i·cule** (var′i-kyul) a small varicose vein ordinarily seen in the skin; may be associated with venous stars, venous lakes, or larger varicose veins. [L. *varicula*, dim. of *varix*]

**var·ie·gate por·phyr·ia** porphyria characterized by abdominal pain and neuropsychiatric abnormalities, by dermal sensitivity to light and mechanical trauma, by increased fecal excretion of proto- and coproporphyrin, and by increased urinary excretion of δ-aminolevulinic acid, porphobilinogen, and porphyrins; due to a deficiency of protoporphyrinogen oxidase.

**va·ri·o·la** (vă-rī′ō-lă) SYN smallpox. [Med. L. dim of L. *varius*, spotted]

**va·ri·o·lar** (vă-rī′ō-lăr) relating to smallpox. SYN variolous.

**va·ri·o·late** (văr′ē-ō-lāt) 1. to inoculate with smallpox. 2. pitted or scarred, as if by smallpox.

**va·ri·o·la vi·rus** a poxvirus of the genus *Orthopoxvirus*, the pathogen of smallpox in humans. SYN smallpox virus.

**var·i·ol·i·form** (vă-rī′ō-li-fōrm, var-ē-ō′li-fōrm) SYN varioloid. [variola + L. *forma*, form]

**va·ri·o·loid** (văr′ē-ō-loyd) resembling smallpox. SYN varioliform. [variola + G. *eidos*, resemblance]

**va·ri·o·lous** (vă-rī′ō-lŭs) SYN variolar.

**var·ix**, pl. **va·ri·ces** (var′iks, var′i-sēz) 1. a dilated vein. 2. an enlarged and tortuous vein, artery, or lymphatic vessel. [L. *varix* (*varic-*), a dilated vein]

**var·nish (dental)** solutions of natural resins and gums in a suitable solvent, of which a thin coat-

ing is applied over the surfaces of the cavity preparations before placement of restorations, used as a protective agent for the tooth against constituents of restorative materials. SYN vernix.

**var·us** (va′rŭs) descriptive of any of the paired joints of the extremities with a static angular deformity in which the bone distal to the joint deviates medially from the longitudinal axis of the proximal bone, and toward the midline of the body, when the subject is in anatomical position. The adjective varus is attached sometimes to the name of the joint (cubitus varus) and sometimes to the name of the body part just distal to the joint (hallux varus). The gender of the adjective matches that of the Latin noun to which it is joined; thus, cubitus, hallux, metatarsus, pes, talipes *varus;* coxa, manus, talipomanus *vara;* genu *varum.* Cf. valgus. [Mod. L. bent inward, fr. L. knock-kneed]

**va·rus lax·i·ty** abnormal flexibility on the lateral side of a joint upon medial movement of the distal segment.

**vas** (vas) [TA] a duct or canal conveying any liquid, such as blood, lymph, chyle, or semen. SEE ALSO vessel. [L. a vessel, dish]

**vas-** a vas, blood vessel. SEE ALSO vasculo-, vaso-. [L. *vas*]

**va·sa** (vā′să) plural of vas.

**va·sal** (vā′săl) relating to a vas or to vasa.

**va·sa lym·pha·ti·ca** SYN lymph vessels.

**va·sa pre·via** umbilical vessels presenting in advance of the fetal head, usually traversing the membranes and crossing the internal cervical os.

**va·sa rec·ta 1.** straight vessels into which the efferent arteriole of the juxtamedullary glomeruli breaks up; they form a leash of vessels which, arising at the bases of the pyramids, run through the renal medulla toward the apex of each pyramid, then reverse direction in a hairpin turn, and run straight back again toward the base of the pyramid as venae rectae; **2.** SYN straight seminiferous tubule.

**va·sa va·so·rum** small arteries distributed to the outer and middle coats of the larger blood vessels, and their corresponding veins.

**vas·cu·lar** (vas′kyu-lăr) relating to or containing blood vessels. [L. *vasculum,* a small vessel, dim. of *vas*]

**vas·cu·lar cat·a·ract** congenital cataract in which the degenerated lens is replaced with mesodermal tissue.

**vas·cu·lar cir·cle of op·tic nerve** a network of branches of the short ciliary arteries on the sclera around the point of entrance of the optic nerve. SYN Haller circle (1).

**vas·cu·lar de·men·tia** a step-like deterioration in intellectual functions with focal neurological signs, as the result of multiple infarctions of the cerebral hemispheres.

**vas·cu·lar·i·ty** (vas-kyu-lar′i-tē) the condition of being vascular.

**vas·cu·lar·i·za·tion** (vas′kyu-lăr-i-zā′shŭn) the formation of new blood vessels in a part.

**vas·cu·lar·ized** (vas′kyu-lăr-īzd) rendered vascular by the formation of new vessels.

**vas·cu·lar·ized graft** the state of a graft after the recipient vasculature has been connected with the vessels in the graft.

**vas·cu·lar la·cu·na** the medial compartment beneath the inguinal ligament, for the passage to

v
a

the femoral vessels; it is separated from the muscular lacuna by the iliopectineal arch.

**vas·cu·lar lam·i·na of cho·roid** the outer portion of the choroid of the eye containing the largest blood vessels.

**vas·cu·lar lei·o·my·o·ma** a markedly vascular leiomyoma, apparently arising from the smooth muscle of blood vessels.

**vas·cu·lar nerve** a small nerve filament that supplies the wall of a blood vessel.

**vas·cu·lar po·lyp** a bulging or protruding angioma of the nasal mucous membrane.

**vas·cu·lar ring** anomalous arteries (aortic arches) congenitally encircling the trachea and esophagus, at times producing pressure symptoms.

**vas·cu·lar spi·der** SYN spider angioma.

**vas·cu·lar sys·tem** the cardiovascular and lymphatic systems collectively.

**vas·cu·lar tu·nic of eye** the vascular, pigmentary, or middle coat of the eye, comprising the choroid, ciliary body, and iris.

**vas·cu·la·ture** (vas′kyu-lă-cher) the vascular network of an organ.

**vas·cu·li·tis** (vas-kyu-lī′tis) SYN angiitis.

△**vas·cu·lo-** a blood vessel. SEE ALSO vas-, vaso-. [L. *vasculum*, a small vessel, dim. of *vas*]

**vas·cu·lo·my·e·li·nop·a·thy** (vas′kyu-lō-mī-ĕ-li-nop′ă-thē) small cerebral vessel vasculopathy with subsequent perivascular demyelination, presumably due to circulating immune complexes.

**vas·cu·lop·a·thy** (vas-kyu-lop′ă-thē) any disease of the blood vessels. [vasculo- + G. *pathos*, disease]

**vas def·er·ens**, pl. **va·sa def·er·en·ti·a** SYN ductus deferens.

**va·sec·to·my** (va-sek′tō-mē) excision of a segment of the vas deferens, performed in association with prostatectomy, or to produce sterility. SYN deferentectomy, gonangiectomy. [vas- + G. *ektomē*, excision]

**vas ef·fe·rens**, pl. **va·sa ef·fer·en·ti·a** [TA] **1.** a vein carrying blood away from a part; **2.** SYN efferent glomerular arteriole.

**vas·i·fac·tion** (vas-i-fak′shŭn) SYN angiopoiesis.

**vas·i·fac·tive** (vas-i-fak′tiv) SYN angiopoietic.

**vas·i·form** (vas′i-fōrm) having the shape of a vas or tubular structure.

**vas·i·tis** (va-sī′tis) SYN deferentitis.

△**va·so-** vas, blood vessel. SEE ALSO vas-, vasculo-. [L. *vas*, a vessel]

**va·so·ac·tive** (vā-sō-ak′tiv, vas-ō-ak′tiv) influencing the tone and caliber of blood vessels.

**va·so·ac·tive amine** a substance, such as histamine or serotonin, that contains amino groups and is pharmacologically characterized by its action on the blood vessels (altering vascular caliber or permeability).

**va·so·ac·tive in·tes·ti·nal pol·y·pep·tide (VIP)** a polypeptide hormone secreted most commonly by non-beta islet cell tumors of the pancreas, producing copious watery diarrhea and fecal electrolyte loss, particularly hypokalemia; VIP increases the rates of glycogenolysis; stimulates pancreatic bicarbonate secretion.

**va·so·con·stric·tion** (vā′sō-kon-strik′shŭn, vas′ō-kon-strik′shŭn) reduction in the caliber of a blood vessel due to contraction of smooth muscle fibers in the tunica media.

**va·so·con·stric·tive** (vā′sō-kon-strik′tiv, vas′ō-

kon-strik′tiv) **1.** causing narrowing of the blood vessels. **2.** SYN vasoconstrictor (1).

**va·so·con·stric·tor** (vā′sō-kon-strik′ter, vas′ō-kon-strik′ter) **1.** an agent that causes narrowing of the blood vessels. SYN vasoconstrictive (2). **2.** a nerve, stimulation of which causes vascular constriction.

**va·so·de·pres·sion** (vā′sō-dē-presh′ŭn, vas′ō-dē-presh′ŭn) reduction of tone in blood vessels with vasodilation and resulting lowered blood pressure.

**va·so·de·pres·sor** (vā′sō-dē-pres′er, vas′ō) **1.** producing vasodepression. **2.** an agent that produces vasodepression.

**va·so·de·pres·sor syn·co·pe** faintness or loss of consciousness due to reflex reduction in blood pressure.

**va·so·di·la·ta·tion** (vā′sō-dil-ă-tā′shŭn, vas′ō-dil-ă-tā′shŭn) SYN vasodilation.

**va·so·di·la·tion** (vā′sō-dī-lā′shŭn, vas-ō-dī-lā′shŭn) increase in the caliber of a blood vessel due to relaxation of smooth muscle fibers in the tunica media. SYN vasodilatation.

**va·so·di·la·tive** (vā′sō-dī-lā′tiv, vas′ō-dī-lā′tiv) **1.** causing dilation of the blood vessels. **2.** SYN vasodilator (1).

**va·so·di·la·tor** (vā′sō-dī-lā′ter, vas′ō-dī-lā′ter) **1.** an agent that causes dilation of the blood vessels. SYN vasodilative (2). **2.** a nerve, stimulation of which results in dilation of the blood vessels.

**va·so·ep·i·did·y·mos·to·my** (vā′sō-ep-i-did-i-mos′tō-mē, vas′ō-ep-i-did-i-mos′tō-mē) surgical anastomosis of the vasa deferentia to the epididymis, to bypass an obstruction at the level of the mid to distal epididymis or proximal vas. [vaso- + epididymis + G. *stoma*, mouth]

**va·so·for·ma·tion** (vā-sō-fōr-mā′shŭn, vas-ō-fōrmā′shŭn) SYN angiopoiesis.

**va·so·for·ma·tive** (vā-sō-fōr′mă-tiv, vas-ō-fōr′mă-tiv) SYN angiopoietic.

**va·so·for·ma·tive cell** SYN angioblast (1).

**va·so·gan·gli·on** (vā-sō-gang′glē-on, vas-ō-gang′glē-on) a mass of blood vessels.

**va·sog·ra·phy** (vā-sog′ră-fē) radiography of the vas deferens to determine patency, by injecting contrast medium into its lumen either transurethrally or by open vasotomy. [vas + G. *graphō*, to write]

**va·so·hy·per·ton·ic** (vā′sō-hī-per-ton′ik, vas′ō-hī-per-ton′ik) relating to increased arteriolar tension or vasoconstriction. [vaso- + G. *hyper*, over, + *tonos*, tone]

**va·so·hy·po·ton·ic** (vā′sō-hī-po-ton′ik, vas′ō-hī-po-ton′ik) relating to reduced arteriolar tension or vasodilation. [vaso- + G. *hypo*, under, + *tonos*, tone]

**va·so·in·hib·i·tor** (vā′sō-in-hib′i-ter, vas′ō-in-hib′i-ter) an agent that restricts or prevents the functioning of the vasomotor nerves.

**va·so·in·hib·i·to·ry** (vā′sō-in-hib′i-tōr-ē, vas′ō-in-hib′i-tōr-ē) restraining vasomotor action.

**va·so·li·ga·tion** (vā′sō-li-gā′shŭn, vas′ō-li-gā′shŭn) ligation of the vas deferens, usually after its division.

**va·so·mo·tion** (vā-sō-mō′shŭn, vas-ō-mō′shŭn) change in caliber of a blood vessel. SYN angiokinesis.

**va·so·mo·tor** (vā-sō-mō′ter, vas-ō-mō′ter) **1.** causing dilation or constriction of the blood vessels. **2.** denoting the nerves which have this action. SYN angiokinetic.

**va·so·mo·tor im·bal·ance** SYN autonomic imbalance.

**va·so·mo·tor nerve** a motor nerve effecting or inhibiting contraction of the blood vessels.

**va·so·mo·tor pa·ral·y·sis** SYN vasoparesis.

**va·so·mo·tor rhi·ni·tis** congestion of nasal mucosa without infection or allergy.

**va·so·neu·rop·a·thy** (vā′sō-noo-rop′ă-thē, vas′ō-noo-rop′ă-thē) any disease involving both the nerves and blood vessels. [vaso- + G. *neuron,* nerve, + *pathos,* suffering]

**va·so·or·chi·dos·to·my** (vā′sō-ōr-ki-dos′tō-mē, vas′ō-or-ki-dos′tō-mē) reestablishment of the interrupted seminiferous channels by uniting the tubules of the epididymis or of the rete testis to the divided end of the vas deferens. [vaso- + G. *orchis,* testis, + *stoma,* mouth]

**va·so·pa·ral·y·sis** (vā′sō-pă-ral′i-sis, vas′ō-pă-ral′i-sis) paralysis, atonia, or hypotonia of blood vessels.

**va·so·pa·re·sis** (vā′sō-pă-rē′sis, vā′sō-par′ē-sis, vas′ō-pă-rē′sis) a mild degree of vasoparalysis. SYN vasomotor paralysis. [vaso- + G. *paresis,* weakness]

**va·so·pres·sin** (vā-sō-pres′in, vas-ō-pres′in) a nonapeptide neurohypophysial hormone related to oxytocin and vasotocin; synthetically prepared or obtained from the posterior lobe of the pituitary of healthy domestic animals. In pharmacological doses vasopressin causes contraction of smooth muscle, notably that of all blood vessels; large doses may produce cerebral or coronary arterial spasm. SYN antidiuretic hormone. [vaso- + L. *premo,* pp. *pressum,* to press down, + -in]

**va·so·pres·sor** (vā-sō-pres′er, vas-ō-) **1.** producing vasoconstriction and a rise in systemic arterial pressure. **2.** an agent that has this effect.

**va·so·punc·ture** (vā-sō-pŭnk′cher) the act of puncturing a vessel with a needle.

**va·so·re·flex** (vā-sō-rē′fleks, vas′ō-rē′fleks) a reflex that influences the caliber of blood vessels.

**va·so·re·lax·a·tion** (vā′sō-rē-lak-sā′shŭn, vas-ō-rē-lak-sā′shŭn) reduction in tension of the walls of the blood vessels.

**va·so·sec·tion** (vā-sō-sek′shŭn, vas-ō-sek′shŭn) SYN vasotomy.

**va·so·sen·so·ry** (vā-sō-sen′ser-ē, vas-ō-sen′ser-ē) **1.** relating to sensation in the blood vessels. **2.** denoting sensory nerve fibers innervating blood vessels.

**va·so·spasm** (vā′sō-spazm, vas′ō-spazm) contraction or hypertonia of the muscular coats of the blood vessels. SYN angiospasm.

**va·so·spas·tic** (vā-sō-spas′tik, vas-ō-spas′tik) relating to or characterized by vasospasm. SYN angiospastic.

**va·so·stim·u·lant** (va-sō-stim′yu-lant) **1.** exciting vasomotor action. **2.** an agent that excites the vasomotor nerves to action. **3.** SYN vasotonic (2).

**va·sos·to·my** (vă-sos′tō-mē) establishment of an artificial opening into the deferent duct. [vaso- + G. *stoma,* mouth]

**va·sot·o·my** (vā-sot′ō-mē) incision into or division of the vas deferens. SYN vasosection. [vaso- + G. *tome,* incision]

**va·so·to·nia** (vā-sō-tō′nē-ă, vas-ō-tō′nē-ă) the tone of blood vessels, particularly the arterioles. SYN angiotonia. [vaso- + G. *tonos,* tone]

**va·so·ton·ic** (vā-sō-ton′ik, vas-ō-ton′ik) **1.** relating to vascular tone. **2.** an agent that increases vascular tension. SYN vasostimulant (3).

**va·so·tro·phic** (vā-sō-trof′ik, vas-ō-) relating to the nutrition of the blood vessels or the lymphatics. [vaso- + G. *trophē,* nourishment]

**va·so·tro·pic** (vā-sō-trō′pik, vas-ō-trō′pik) tending to act on the blood vessels. [vaso- + G. *tropē,* a turning]

**va·so·va·gal** (vā-sō-vā′găl) relating to the action of the vagus nerve upon the blood vessels.

**va·so·va·gal syn·co·pe** faintness or loss of consciousness due to increased vagus nerve (parasympathetic) activity.

**va·so·va·sos·to·my** (vā′sō-vă-sos′tō-mē) surgical anastomosis of vasa deferentia, to restore fertility in a previously vasectomized male. [vaso- + vaso- + G. *stoma,* mouth]

**va·so·ve·sic·u·lec·to·my** (vā′sō-vě-sik-yu-lek′tō-mē) excision of the vas deferens and seminal vesicles. [vaso- + L. *vesicula,* vesicle, + G. *ektomē,* excision]

**vas·tomy** (vas′tō-mē) section of the vas deferens, usually with ligation. [vas + G. *tomē,* a cutting]

**vas·tus in·ter·me·di·us mus·cle** *origin,* upper three-fourths of anterior surface of shaft of femur; *insertion,* tibial tuberosity by way of common tendon of quadriceps femoris and patellar ligament; *action,* extends leg; *nerve supply,* femoral. SYN intermediate vastus muscle.

**vas·tus la·te·ra·lis mus·cle** *origin,* lateral lip of linea aspera as far as great trochanter; *insertion,* tibial tuberosity by way of common tendon of quadriceps femoris and patellar ligament; *action,* extends leg; *nerve supply,* femoral. SYN lateral vastus muscle.

**vas·tus me·di·a·lis mus·cle** *origin,* medial lip of linea aspera; *insertion,* tibial tuberosity by way of common tendon of quadriceps femoris and ligamentum patellae; *action,* extends leg; *nerve supply,* femoral. SYN medial vastus muscle.

**vault** (vawlt) a part resembling an arched roof or dome, e.g., the pharyngeal vault or fornix, the nonmuscular upper part of the nasopharynx; the palatine vault, arch of the plate; vault of the vagina, fornix of vagina. [thr. O. Fr., fr. L. *volvo,* pp. *volutus,* to turn round]

**VC** colored vision; vital capacity.

**VCO₂** carbon dioxide production.

**VCUG** voiding cystourethrogram.

**VDRL** Venereal Disease Research Laboratories. SEE VDRL test.

**VDRL test** a flocculation test for syphilis, using cardiolipin-lecithin-cholesterol antigen as developed by the Venereal Disease Research Laboratory of the United States Public Health Service.

**vec·tion** (vek′shŭn) transference of the agents of disease from an infected to an uninfected individual by a vector. [L. *vectio,* conveyance]

**vec·tor** (vek′tōr) **1.** an invertebrate animal (e.g., tick, mite, mosquito, bloodsucking fly) capable of transmitting an infectious agent among vertebrates. **2.** anything (e.g., velocity, mechanical force, electromotive force) having magnitude and direction; it can be represented by a straight line of appropriate length and direction. **3.** the net electrical axis of any ECG wave (usually QRS) whose length is proportional to the magnitude of the electrical force, whose direction gives the direction of the force, and whose tip represents the positive pole of the force. **4.** DNA such as a chromosome or plasmid that autonomously replicates in a cell to which another DNA segment may be inserted and be itself replicated, as in cloning. **5.** SYN recombinant vector. **6.** recombinant DNA systems especially suited for production of large quantities of specific proteins in bacterial, yeast, insect, or mammalian cell systems. [L. *vector,* a carrier]

**vec·tor-borne in·fec·tion** class of infections transmitted by an insect or animal vector. The vector may merely be a passive carrier of the infectious agent, but many kinds of infectious agents undergo a stage in biological development in the vector, i.e., the vector, as well as the human host, is essential to the survival of the infectious agent.

**vec·tor·car·di·o·gram** (vek′ter-kar′dē-ō-gram) a graphic representation of the magnitude and direction of the heart's action currents in the form of vector loops.

**vec·tor·car·di·og·ra·phy** (vek′ter-kar-dē-og′ră-fē) **1.** a variant of electrocardiography in which the heart's activation currents are represented by vector loops. **2.** the study and interpretation of vectorcardiograms.

**vec·to·ri·al** (vek-tōr′ē-ăl) relating in any way to a vector.

**veg·an** (vej′ăn, vē-gĕn) a strict vegetarian; i.e., one who consumes no animal or dairy products of any type. Cf. vegetarian.

**veg·e·ta·ble** (vej′tă-bl, vej′ĕ-tă-bl) **1.** a plant, specifically one used for food. **2.** relating to plants, as distinguished from animals or minerals. SYN vegetal (1). [M.E., fr. L. *vegetabilis* (see vegetation)]

**veg·e·tal** (vej′ĕ-tăl) **1.** SYN vegetable (2). **2.** denoting the vital functions common to plants and animals, such as respiration, metabolism, growth, and generation, distinguished from those peculiar to animals, such as conscious sensation and the mental faculties.

**veg·e·tal pole, veg·e·ta·tive pole** the part of a telolecithal egg where the bulk of the yolk is situated.

**veg·e·tar·i·an** (vej-ĕ-tār′ē-ăn) one whose diet is restricted to foods of vegetable origin, excluding primarily animal meats. Cf. vegan.

**veg·e·ta·tion** (vej-ĕ-tā′shŭn) **1.** the process of growth in plants. **2.** a condition of sluggishness, comparable to the inactivity of plant life. **3.** a growth or excrescence of any sort. **4.** specifically, a clot, composed largely of fused blood platelets, fibrin, and sometimes microorganisms, adherent to a diseased heart orifice or valve, and often initiated by infection of the structures involved. [Mod. L. *vegetatio,* growth]

**veg·e·ta·tive** (vej′ĕ-tā-tiv) **1.** growing or functioning involuntarily or unconsciously, after the assumed manner of vegetable life; denoting especially a state of grossly impaired consciousness, as after severe head trauma or brain disease, in which an individual is incapable of voluntary or purposeful acts and only responds reflexively to painful stimuli. **2.** resting; not active; denoting the stage of a cell or its nucleus in which the process of karyokinesis is quiescent. [see vegetation]

**veg·e·ta·tive bac·te·ri·o·phage** the form of bacteriophage in which the bacteriophage nucleic acid (lacking its coat) multiplies freely within the host bacterium, independently of bacterial multiplication.

**veg·e·ta·tive en·do·car·di·tis, ver·ru·cous en·do·car·di·tis** endocarditis associated with the presence of fibrinous clots (vegetations) forming on the ulcerated surfaces of the valves.

**veg·e·ta·tive state** a clinical condition in which there is complete absence of awareness of the self and the environment, accompanied by sleep-wake cycles, but with either partial or complete preservation of hypothalamic and brainstem autonomic functions; may be transient or permanent. There are multiple causes, all involving the brain, including traumatic and nontraumatic injuries, metabolic and degenerative disorders, and congenital malformations.

**ve·hi·cle** (vē′hi-kl) **1.** an excipient or a menstruum; a substance, usually without therapeutic action, used as a medium to give bulk for the administration of medicines. **2.** an inanimate substance (e.g., food, milk, dust, clothing, instrument) by which or upon which an infectious agent passes from an infected to a susceptible host. [L. *vehiculum,* a conveyance, fr. *veho,* to carry]

**veil** (vāl) **1.** SYN velum (1). **2.** SYN caul (1). [L. *velum*]

*Veil·lo·nel·la* (vā′yō-nel′ă) a genus of nonmotile, non-spore-forming, anaerobic bacteria containing small Gram-negative cocci which occur as diplococci and in masses. These organisms are parasitic in the mouth and the intestinal and respiratory tracts of humans and other animals. [Adrien *Veillon,* French bacteriologist, 1864–1931]

**vein** (vān) a blood vessel carrying blood toward the heart; all the veins except the pulmonary carry dark or deoxygenated blood. SYN vena [TA]. [L. *vena*]

**vein of bulb of pe·nis** a tributary of the internal pudendal vein that drains the bulb of the penis.

**vein of co·chle·ar can·a·lic·u·lus** drains the cochlea, sacculus, and part of the utricles, and empties into the superior bulb of the jugular vein by accompanying the perilymphatic duct through the cochlear canaliculus.

**vein of pter·y·goid ca·nal** a vein accompanying the nerve and artery through the pterygoid canal and emptying into the pharyngeal venous plexus.

**veins of kid·ney** the tributaries of the renal vein that drain the kidney; they parallel the arteries in the kidney and consist of interlobular, arcuate, and interlobar veins.

**veins of knee** the veins that accompany the genicular arteries; they drain blood from the structures around the knee, terminating in the popliteal vein.

**veins of tem·po·ro·man·dib·u·lar joint** several small tributaries to the retromandibular vein from the temporomandibular joint.

**veins of ver·te·bral col·umn** includes the internal and external vertebral venous plexuses, the basivertebral veins, and the anterior and posterior spinal veins.

**vein of ves·tib·u·lar aq·ue·duct** a small vein accompanying the endolymphatic duct; it drains much of the vestibular portion of the labyrinth and terminates in the inferior petrosal sinus.

**vein of ves·tib·u·lar bulb** drains the bulb of the vestibule; a tributary of the internal pudendal vein.

**ve·la** (vē′lă) plural of velum.

**ve·la·men**, pl. **ve·lam·i·na** (vĕ-lā′men, vĕ-lam′i-nă) SYN velum (1). [L. a veil]

**vel·a·men·tous** (vel-ă-men′tŭs) expanded in the form of a sheet or veil.

**ve·lar** (vē'lăr) relating to any velum, especially the velum palatinum.

**vel·lus** (vel'ŭs) **1.** fine nonpigmented hair covering most of the body. **2.** a structure that is fleecy or soft and woolly in appearance. [L. fleece]

**ve·loc·i·ty** (v) (vĕ-los'i-tē) rate and direction of movement; specifically, distance traveled or quantity converted per unit time in a given direction. [L. *velocitas*, fr. *velox (veloc-)*, quick, swift]

**vel·o·pha·ryn·ge·al** (vē'lō-fă-rin'jē-ăl) pertaining to the soft palate (velum palatinum) and the posterior nasopharyngeal wall.

**vel·o·pha·ryn·ge·al in·suf·fi·cien·cy** anatomical or functional deficiency in the soft palate or superior constrictor muscle, resulting in the inability to achieve velopharyngeal closure.

**Vel·peau ban·dage** (vel'pō) a bandage that serves to immobilize arm to chest wall, with the forearm positioned obliquely across and upward on front of chest.

**Vel·peau her·nia** (vel'pō) femoral hernia in which the intestine is in front of the blood vessels.

**ve·lum,** pl. **ve·la** (vē'lŭm, vē'lă) **1.** any structure resembling a veil or curtain. SYN veil (1), velamen. **2.** SYN caul (1). **3.** SYN greater omentum. **4.** any serous membrane or membranous envelope or covering. [L. veil, sail]

**ve·lum pa·la·ti·num** SYN soft palate.

**ve·na,** gen. and pl. **ve·nae** (vē'nă, vē'nē) [TA] SYN vein. [L.]

**ve·na ca·va su·pe·ri·or** [TA] SYN superior vena cava.

**ve·na·ca·vog·ra·phy** (vē'nă-kā-vog'ră-fē) angiography of a vena cava. SYN cavography.

**ve·na cen·tra·lis glan·du·lae su·pra·re·na·lis** [TA] SYN central vein of suprarenal gland.

**ve·na cen·tra·lis ret·i·nae** [TA] SYN central vein of retina.

**ve·na ce·pha·li·ca ac·ces·sor·ia** [TA] SYN accessory cephalic vein.

**ve·na dor·sa·lis pro·fun·da cli·to·ri·dis** [TA] SYN deep dorsal vein of clitoris.

**ve·na dor·sa·lis su·per·fi·ci·a·lis pe·nis** [TA] SYN superficial dorsal veins of penis.

**ve·nae com·i·tan·tes** a pair of veins, occasionally more, that closely accompany an artery in such a manner that the pulsations of the artery aid venous return.

**ve·nae di·rec·tae la·te·ra·les** [TA] one or more veins running a subependymal course in a coronal plane over the thalamus, terminating in the internal cerebral vein. SYN surface thalamic veins.

**ve·nae in·ter·cos·ta·les** [TA] SYN posterior intercostal veins.

**ve·nae in·ter·nae ce·re·bri** [TA] SYN internal cerebral veins.

**ve·na ep·i·gas·tri·ca** SYN superficial epigastric vein.

**ve·nae pro·fun·dae ce·re·bri** [TA] SYN deep cerebral veins.

**ve·nae ra·chi·o·ceph·al·i·cae** [TA] SYN brachiocephalic veins.

**ve·nae su·pe·ri·o·res ce·re·bri** [TA] SYN superior cerebral veins.

**ve·nae ut·er·i·nae** [TA] SYN uterine veins.

**ve·na fem·or·al·is** [TA] SYN femoral vein.

**ve·na he·mi·a·zy·gos ac·ces·so·ria** [TA] SYN accessory hemiazygos vein.

**ve·na ili·o·lum·ba·lis** [TA] SYN iliolumbar vein.

**ve·na por·tae he·pa·tis** [TA] SYN portal vein.

**ve·na sub·cla·via** [TA] SYN subclavian vein.

**ve·na sub·men·ta·lis** SYN submental vein.

**ve·na um·bi·li·ca·lis** [TA] SYN left umbilical vein.

**ve·na ver·te·bra·lis ac·ces·sor·ia** [TA] SYN accessory vertebral vein.

△**vene- 1.** the veins, venous. SEE ALSO veno-. [L. *vena*, vein] **2.** venom. [L. *venenum*, poison]

**ve·nec·ta·sia** (ve-nek-tā'sē-ă) SYN phlebectasia.

**ve·nec·to·my** (ve-nek'tō-mē) SYN phlebectomy.

**ve·neer** (vĕ-nēr') **1.** a thin surface layer laid over a base of common material. **2.** DENTISTRY a layer of tooth-colored material, usually porcelain or acrylic resin, attached to and covering the surface of a metal crown or natural tooth structure. [Fr. *fournir*, to furnish]

**ven·e·na·tion** (ven-ĕ-nā'shŭn) poisoning, as from a sting or bite. [L. *veneno*, pp. *-atus*, to poison, fr. *venenum*, poison]

**ven·e·nous** (ven'ĕ-nŭs) SYN poisonous. [L. *venenosus*]

**ve·ne·re·al** (ve-nēr'ē-ăl) relating to or resulting from sexual intercourse. [L. *Venus (vener-)*, goddess of love]

**ve·ne·re·al bu·bo** an enlarged gland in the groin associated with any sexually transmitted disease, especially chancroid.

**ve·ne·re·al dis·ease** SYN sexually transmitted disease.

**ve·ne·re·al ul·cer** SYN chancroid.

**ve·ne·re·al wart** SYN condyloma acuminatum.

**ven·e·sec·tion** (ven-ē-sek'shŭn) SYN phlebotomy. [L. *vena*, vein, + *sectio*, a cutting]

**Ven·e·zue·lan hem·or·rhag·ic fe·ver** (ven-ĕ-zwā'lan) a febrile disease caused by the Guanarito virus in Venezuela and characterized by headache, arthralgia, pharyngitis, leukopenia, thrombocytopenia, and hemorrhagic manifestations.

**ven·i·punc·ture** (ven'i-pŭnk-cher) the puncture of a vein, usually to withdraw blood or inject a solution.

△**ve·no-, ve·ni-** the veins. SEE ALSO vene- (1). [L. *vena*]

**ve·no·gram** (vē'nō-gram) **1.** radiograph of opacified veins. **2.** SYN phlebogram. [veno- + G. *gramma*, a writing]

**ve·nog·ra·phy** (vē-nog'ră-fē) radiographic demonstration of a vein, after the injection of contrast medium. SYN phlebography (2). [veno- + G. *graphō*, to write]

**ven·om** (ven'ŏm) a poisonous fluid secreted by snakes, spiders, scorpions, and other cold-blooded animals. [M. Eng. and O. Fr. *venim*, fr. L. *venenum*, poison]

**ve·no·mo·tor** (vē'nō-mō'ter) causing change in the caliber of a vein. [veno- + L. *motor*, a move]

**ve·no·oc·clu·sive dis·ease of the liv·er** obliterating endophlebitis of small hepatic vein radicles, described in Jamaican children, associated with ingestion of toxic plant substances in bush tea; causes ascites, which may progress to cirrhosis.

**ve·no·scle·ro·sis** (vē'nō-skle-rō'sis) SYN phlebosclerosis.

**ve·nos·i·ty** (vē-nos'i-tē) **1.** a venous state; a condition in which the bulk of the blood is in the veins at the expense of the arteries. **2.** the unaerated condition of venous blood.

**ve·nos·ta·sis** (vē-nō-stā'sis, vē-nos'tă-sis) SYN phlebostasis. [veno- + G. *stasis*, a standing]

**ve·nos·to·my** (vē-nos'tō-mē) SYN cutdown.

**ve·not·o·my** (vē-not'ō-mē) SYN phlebotomy.

**ve·nous** (vē'nŭs) relating to a vein or to the veins. [L. *venosus*]

**ve·nous ad·mix·ture** the mingling in the pulmonary circulation of arterial blood and desaturated blood resulting from ventilation-perfusion mismatching (reduced ventilation with full perfusion).

**ve·nous an·gi·o·ma** vascular anomaly composed of anomalous veins. SYN venous malformation.

**ve·nous an·gle 1.** the junction of the internal jugular and subclavian veins, toward which converge the external and the anterior jugular and the vertebral veins, the thoracic duct in the left angle and the right lymphatic duct in the right angle; **2.** in neuroradiology, the angle of union of the superior thalamostriate vein (vena terminalis) with the internal cerebral vein, usually closely behind the interventricular foramen (Monro foramen).

**ve·nous blood** blood which has passed through the capillaries of various tissues, except the lungs, and is found in the veins, the right chambers of the heart, and the pulmonary arteries; it is usually dark red as a result of a lower content of oxygen.

**ve·nous cap·il·lary** a capillary opening into a venule.

**ve·nous hum** brief or continuous noise originating from the neck veins that may be confused with cardiac murmurs, particularly with the continuous murmur of patent ductus arteriosus.

**ve·nous hy·per·e·mia** SYN passive hyperemia.

**ve·nous in·suf·fi·cien·cy** inadequate drainage of venous blood from a part, resulting in edema or dermatosis.

**ve·nous mal·for·ma·tion** SYN venous angioma.

**ve·nous pulse** a pulsation occurring in the veins, especially the internal jugular vein.

**ve·nous re·turn** the blood returning to the heart via the great veins and coronary sinus; also used to described venous drainage of a part of the body or particular organ.

**ve·nous si·nus·es** SYN dural venous sinuses.

**ve·nous star** a small, red nodule formed by a dilated vein in the skin; caused by increased venous pressure.

**ve·nous ul·cer** SYN varicose ulcer.

**ve·no·ve·nos·to·my** (vē'nō-vē-nos'tō-mē) the formation of an anastomosis between two veins. SYN phlebophlebostomy. [veno- + veno- + G. *stoma*, mouth]

**vent** an opening into a cavity or canal, especially one through which the contents of such a cavity are discharged, as the anus. [O. Fr. *fente*, a chink, cleft]

**ven·ter** (ven'ter) **1.** SYN abdomen. **2.** SYN belly (2). **3.** one of the great cavities of the body. **4.** the uterus. [L. *venter (ventr-)*, belly]

**ven·ti·late** (ven'ti-lāt) to aerate, or oxygenate, the blood in the pulmonary capillaries. SYN air (2). [L. *ventilo*, pp. *-atus*, to fan, fr. *ventus*, the wind]

🔲 **ven·ti·la·tion** (ven-ti-lā'shŭn) **1.** replacement of air or other gas in a space by fresh air or gas. **2.** movement of gas(es) into and out of the lungs. SYN respiration (2). **3. (v)** in physiology, the tidal exchange of air between the lungs and the atmosphere that occurs in breathing. SEE ALSO respiration. See page APP 138. [see ventilate]

**ven·ti·la·tion/per·fu·sion ra·tio (V̇a/Q̇)** the ra-

tio of alveolar ventilation to simultaneous alveolar capillary blood flow in any part of the lung; because both ventilation and perfusion are expressed per unit volume of tissue and per unit time, which cancel, the units become liters of gas per liter of blood.

🔲 **ven·ti·la·tion-per·fu·sion scan** a lung function test, especially useful in the diagnosis of pulmonary embolism, employing an inhaled radionuclide for ventilation and an intravenous radionuclide for perfusion; their respective distributions in the lung are recorded scintigraphically. See page B12.

**ven·ti·la·tor** (ven-til-a-tor) a mechanical device designed to perform part or all of the work of respiration, i.e., of moving gas into and out of the lungs.

**ven·ti·la·to·ry thresh·old** point during exercise training at which pulmonary ventilation becomes disproportionately high with respect to oxygen consumption; believed to reflect onset of anaerobiosis and lactate accumulation.

**ven·trad** (ven'trad) toward the ventral aspect; opposed to dorsad. [L. *venter*, belly, + *ad*, to]

**ven·tral** (ven'trăl) **1.** pertaining to the belly or to any venter. **2.** SYN anterior (1). **3.** VETERINARY ANATOMY the undersurface of an animal; often used to indicate the position of one structure relative to another, i.e., situated nearer the undersurface of the body. [L. *ventralis*]

**ven·tral ap·ron pre·puce** the incomplete foreskin seen in epispadias.

**ven·tral horn** SYN anterior horn.

**ven·tral plate** SYN floor plate.

**ven·tral root** the motor root of a spinal nerve.

**ven·tral tha·lam·ic pe·dun·cle** the massive system of fiber bundles emerging through the ventral, lateral, and anterior borders of the thalamus to join the internal capsule and parts of the corona radiata; it contains the fibers reciprocally connecting the ventral thalamic nuclei with the precentral and postcentral gyri of the cerebral cortex.

🔲 **ven·tri·cle** (ven'tri-kl) a normal cavity, as of the brain or heart. See page 1049. SYN ventriculus (2). [L. *ventriculus*, dim. of *venter*, belly]

**ven·tric·u·lar** (ven-trik'yu-lăr) relating to a ventricle, in any sense.

**ven·tric·u·lar af·ter·load** the sum total of the forces, both hemodynamic and mechanical, against which the left ventricle of the heart must pump against to send oxygenated blood out into the body.

**ven·tric·u·lar ar·ter·ies** branches of the right and left coronary arteries distributed to the muscle of the ventricles. SYN arteriae ventriculares [TA].

**ven·tric·u·lar as·sist de·vice** a device that supports or replaces the function of a ventricle (LVAD or RVAD indicates which ventricle). The device is used in patients with potentially salvageable myocardium, where centrifugal or pneumatic devices can be placed in either heterotopic or orthotopic positions (the latter is termed a total artificial heart). The function of either the left, right, or both ventricles can thus be supported for days to weeks. Either recovery of heart function or need for transplantation then becomes apparent.

**ven·tric·u·lar band of lar·ynx** SYN vestibular fold.

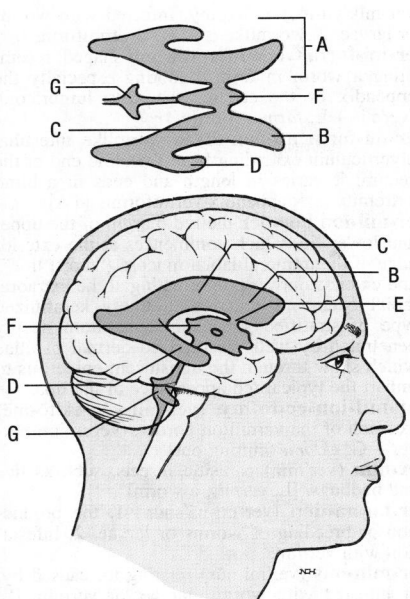

**ventricles of the brain** (superior and lateral
views): (A) left lateral ventricle, (B) anterior horn of
right lateral ventricle, (C) lateral ventricle, (E) interventricular foramen, (F) third ventricle, (G) fourth
ventricle

**ven·tric·u·lar com·plex** the continuous QRST
waves of each beat in the electrocardiogram.
**ven·tric·u·lar con·duc·tion** SYN intraventricular
conduction.
**ven·tric·u·lar es·cape** escape with an ectopic
ventricular focus as pacemaker.
**ven·tric·u·lar ex·tra·sys·to·le** a premature contraction of the ventricle. SYN infranodal extrasystole.
**ven·tric·u·lar fi·bril·la·tion** coarse or fine,
rapid, fibrillary movements of the ventricular
muscle that replace the normal contraction.
**ven·tric·u·lar flut·ter** a form of rapid ventricular tachycardia in which the electrocardiographic
complexes assume a regular undulating pattern
without distinct QRS and T waves.
**ven·tric·u·lar fold** SYN vestibular fold.
**ven·tric·u·lar fu·sion beat** a fusion beat that
occurs when the ventricles are activated partly by
the descending sinus or A-V junctional impulse
and partly by an ectopic ventricular impulse.
**ven·tric·u·lar pre·load** the pressure stretching
the ventricular walls at the onset of ventricular
contraction, expressed in terms of the wall stress
at this moment, related to the tension per unit
cross-sectional area in the ventricular muscle fibers that balances this transmural pressure at the
moment before contraction begins. SYN preload
(2).
**ven·tric·u·lar re·duc·tion sur·gery** SYN Batista
procedure.
**ven·tric·u·lar rhy·thm** SYN idioventricular
rhythm.
**ven·tric·u·lar sep·tal de·fect** a congenital de-

fect in the interventricular septum, usually resulting from failure of the spiral septum to close the
interventricular foramen.
**ven·tric·u·li·tis** (ven-trik-yu-lī′tis) inflammation
of the ventricles of the brain. [ventricle + G. *-itis*,
inflammation]
△**ven·tric·u·lo-** a ventricle. [L. *ventriculus*]
**ven·tric·u·lo·a·tri·al (V-A, VA)** (ven-trik′yu-
lō-ā′trē-ăl) relating to both ventricles and atria,
especially to the sequential passage of conduction in the retrograde direction from ventricle to
atrium.
**ven·tric·u·lo·a·tri·al shunt** surgical procedure
for hydrocephalus; a drain implanted in the lateral cerebral ventricle passes excess cerebrospinal fluid to the right atrium. SYN ventriculoatri-
ostomy.
**ven·tric·u·lo·at·ri·ost·omy** SYN ventriculoatrial
shunt.
**ven·tric·u·lo·cis·ter·nos·to·my** (ven-trik′yu-lō-
sis′ter-nos′tō-mē) an artificial opening between
the ventricles of the brain and the cisterna
magna. SEE ALSO shunt (2). [ventriculo- + L.
*cisterna*, cistern, + G. *stoma*, mouth]
**ven·tric·u·log·ra·phy** (ven-trik-yu-log′ră-fē) **1.**
radiographic demonstration of the cerebral ventricles by direct injection of air or contrast medium. **2.** demonstration of the contractility of the
cardiac ventricles by recording serially the distribution of intravenously injected radionuclide or
that of radiographic contrast medium injected
through an intracardiac catheter. **3.** visualization
by roentgenography of a cardiac ventricle by injection of radiopaque contrast material.
[ventriculo- + G. *graphē*, a writing]
**ven·tric·u·lo·mas·toi·dos·to·my** (ven-trik′yu-
lō-mas′toy-dos′tō-mē) establishment of a communication between the lateral cerebral ventricle
and the mastoid antrum by means of a polythene
tube for the relief of hydrocephalus. SEE ALSO
shunt (2). [ventriculo- + mastoid, + G. *stoma*,
mouth]
**ven·tric·u·lo·nec·tor** (ven-trik′yu-lō-nek′ter)
SYN atrioventricular bundle. [ventriculo- + L.
*necto*, to join]
**ven·tric·u·lo·per·i·to·ne·al shunt** surgical procedure for hydrocephalus; a drain implanted into
the lateral cerebral ventricle passes excess cerebrospinal fluid to the peritoneal cavity. SYN ven-
triculoperitoneostomy.
**ven·tric·u·lo·per·i·to·ne·os·to·my** SYN ventric-
uloperitoneal shunt.
**ven·tric·u·lo·plas·ty** (ven-trik′yu-lō-plas-tē) any
surgical procedure to repair a defect of one of the
ventricles of the heart. [ventriculo- + G. *plastos*,
formed]
**ven·tric·u·lo·punc·ture** (ven-trik′yu-lō-pŭnk′
cher) insertion of a needle into a ventricle.
**ven·tric·u·los·co·py** (ven-trik-yu-los′kŏ-pē) direct inspection of a ventricle with an endoscope.
[ventriculo- + G. *skopeō*, to view]
**ven·tric·u·los·to·my** (ven-trik-yu-los′tō-mē) establishment of an opening in a ventricle, usually
from the third ventricle to the subarachnoid space
to relieve hydrocephalus. SEE ALSO shunt (2).
[ventriculo- + G. *stoma*, mouth]
**ven·tric·u·lo·sub·a·rach·noid** (ven-trik′yu-lō-
sŭb-ă-rak′noyd) relating to the space occupied by
the cerebrospinal fluid. [ventriculo- + subarach-
noid]
**ven·tric·u·lot·o·my** (ven-trik-yu-lot′ō-mē) inci-

**v**
**e**

sion into a ventricle of the heart or the brain. [ventriculo- + G. *tomē*, incision]

**ven·tric·u·lus,** pl. **ven·tric·u·li** (ven-trik'yu-lŭs, ven-trik'yu-lī) **1.** SYN stomach. **2.** [TA] SYN ventricle. [L. dim. of *venter,* belly]

**ven·tri·cu·lus ter·ti·us** [TA] SYN third ventricle.

**ven·tri·duc·tion** (ven-tri-dŭk'shŭn) drawing toward the abdomen or abdominal wall.

△**ventro-** ventral. [L. *venter,* belly]

**ven·tros·co·py** (ven-tros'kŏ-pē) SYN peritoneoscopy. [ventro- + G. *skopeō,* to view]

**ven·trot·o·my** (ven-trot'ō-mē) SYN celiotomy. [ventro- + G. *tomē,* incision]

**ven·u·la,** pl. **ven·u·lae** (ven'yu-lă, ven'yu-lē) SYN venule. [L. dim. of *vena,* vein]

**ven·u·lae stel·la·tae** the star-shaped groups of venules in the renal cortex. SYN stellate veins, stellate venules.

**ven·u·lar** (ven'yu-lăr) pertaining to venules.

**ven·ule** (ven'yul) a venous radicle continuous with a capillary. SYN capillary vein, venula.

**vepna dor·sa·lis pro·fun·da pe·nis** [TA] SYN deep dorsal vein of penis.

**ver·bal a·prax·ia** speech disorder due to cortical sensorimotor damage that impairs the ability to program speech musculature for volitional production of sequenced phonemes. Often accompanies motor aphasia. SEE apraxia, oral apraxia, developmental apraxia of speech. SYN apraxia of speech, articulatory apraxia, dyspraxia of speech, verbal dyspraxia.

**ver·bal au·top·sy** method of obtaining as much information as possible about a deceased person by asking questions of family and others who can describe the mode of death and circumstances preceding death; used especially in developing countries and in settings and situations in which postmortem pathological examination is not feasible.

**ver·bal dys·prax·ia** SYN verbal apraxia.

**ver·big·er·a·tion** (ver-bij-er-ā'shŭn) constant repetition of meaningless words or phrases; seen in schizophrenia. SYN cataphasia. [L. *verbum,* word, + *gero,* to carry about]

**verge** (verj) an edge or margin.

**ver·gence** (ver'jens) a disjunctive movement of the eyes in which the fixation axes are not parallel, as in convergence or divergence. [L. *vergo,* to incline, to turn]

**Ver·hoeff e·las·tic tis·sue stain** (ver'hĕf) a stain for tissue sections in which a mixture of hematoxylin, ferric chloride, and Lugol iodine solution is used; tissue may be counterstained, if desired, with eosin or van Gieson stain; elastic fibers and nuclei appear blue-black to black while collagen and other components are shades of pink to red.

△**ver·mi-** a worm; wormlike. [L. *vermis*]

**ver·mi·ci·dal** (ver'mi-sī'dăl) destructive to worms; specifically, destructive to parasitic intestinal worms. [vermi- + L. *caedo,* to kill]

**ver·mi·cide** (ver'mi-sīd) an agent that kills intestinal parasitic worms. [vermi- + L. *caedo,* to kill]

**ver·mic·u·lar** (ver-mik'yu-lăr) relating to, resembling, or moving like a worm. [L. *vermiculus,* dim. of *vermis,* worm]

**ver·mic·u·lar move·ment** SYN peristalsis.

**ver·mic·u·lar pulse** a small rapid pulse, giving a wormlike sensation to the finger.

**ver·mic·u·la·tion** (ver-mik-yu-lā'shŭn) a wormlike movement, as in peristalsis.

**ver·mic·u·lose, ver·mic·u·lous** (ver-mik'yu-lōs,

ver-mik'yu-lŭs) **1.** wormy; infected with worms or larvae. **2.** wormlike. SEE ALSO vermiform.

**ver·mi·form** (ver'mi-fōrm) worm-shaped; resembling a worm in form, denoting especially the appendix of the cecum. SEE ALSO lumbricoid. [vermi- + L. *forma,* form]

**ver·mi·form ap·pen·dix** a wormlike intestinal diverticulum extending from the blind end of the cecum; it varies in length and ends in a blind extremity. SYN appendix vermiformis [TA].

**ver·mil·ion bor·der** the red margin of the upper and lower lip, which commences at the exterior edge of the intraoral labial mucosa ("moist line") and extends outward, terminating at the extraoral labial cutaneous junction; a thinly keratinized type of stratified squamous epithelium deeply penetrated by well-vascularized dermal papillae which show through the translucent epidermis to impart the typical red appearance of the lips.

**ver·mil·ion·ec·to·my** (ver-mil-yon-ek'tō-mē) excision of the vermilion border. [vermilion border + G. *ektomē,* cutting out]

**ver·min** (ver'min) parasitic insects, such as lice and bedbugs. [L. *vermis,* a worm]

**ver·mi·na·tion** (ver-mi-nā'shŭn) **1.** the production or breeding of worms or larvae. **2.** infestation with vermin.

**ver·min·ous** (ver'mi-nŭs) relating to, caused by, or infested with worms, larvae, or vermin. [L. *verminosus,* wormy]

**ver·mis,** pl. **ver·mes** (ver'mis, ver'mēz) **1.** a worm; any structure or part resembling a worm in shape. **2.** [TA] the narrow middle zone between the two hemispheres of the cerebellum; the portion projecting above the level of the hemispheres on the upper surface is called the superior vermis; the lower portion, sunken between the two hemispheres and forming the floor of the vallecula, is the inferior vermis. [L. worm]

**ver·nal con·junc·ti·vi·tis** a chronic, bilateral conjunctival inflammation with photophobia and intense itching that recurs seasonally during warm weather; characterized in the palpebral form by cobblestone papillae in the upper palpebral conjunctiva and in the bulbar form by gelatinous nodules adjacent to the corneoscleral limbus. SYN allergic conjunctivitis, spring conjunctivitis.

**Ver·net syn·drome** (ver-nā') a syndrome characterized by paralysis of the motor components of the glossopharyngeal, vagus, and accessory cranial nerves as they lie in the posterior fossa; it is most commonly the result of head injury.

**ver·nix** (ver'niks) SYN varnish (dental). [Mod. L.]

**ver·nix ca·se·o·sa** the fatty substance, consisting of desquamated epithelial cells, lanugo hairs, and sebaceous matter, that covers the skin of the fetus.

**ve·ro cy·to·tox·in** a cell cytotoxin produced by enterohemorrhagic *Escherichia coli* that appears to contribute to the occurrence of hemorrhagic colitis and hemolytic uremic syndrome. SYN Shigalike toxin.

**ver·ru·ca,** pl. **ver·ru·cae** (vĕ-roo'kă, vĕ-roo'kē) a flesh-colored growth characterized by circumscribed hypertrophy of the papillae of the corium, with thickening of the malpighian, granular, and keratin layers of the epidermis, caused by human papilloma virus; also applied to epidermal verrucous tumors of nonviral etiology. SYN verruga, wart. [L.]

**ver•ru•ca nec•ro•ge•ni•ca** SYN postmortem wart.
**ver•ru•ca pe•ru•an•a, ver•ru•ca pe•ru•vi•ana** SYN verruga peruana.
**ver•ru•ca pla•na** a smooth, flat, flesh-colored wart of small size, occurring in groups, seen especially on the face of the young; often associated with common warts of the hands, due to human papilloma virus, commonly, types 3 and 10. SYN flat wart.
**ver•ru•ca plan•tar•is** SYN plantar wart.
**ver•ru•ci•form** (vĕ-roo′si-fōrm) wart-shaped. [L. *verruca,* wart, + *forma,* form]
**ver•ru•cose** (vĕ-roo′kōs) resembling a wart; denoting wartlike elevations. [L. *verrucosus*]
**ver•ru•cous he•man•gi•o•ma** a variant of the angiomatous nevus, appearing at birth or in early childhood, situated on the lower extremities with bluish-red nodules and warty surface; they enlarge and sometimes have satellite lesions.
**ver•ru•cous ne•vus** a skin-colored or darker wartlike, often linear, lesion appearing at birth or early in childhood, and occurring in various sizes and locations, single or multiple.
**ver•ru•cous xan•tho•ma** histocytosis Y; a papilloma of the oral mucosa and skin in which squamous epithelium covers connective tissue papillae filled with large foamy histiocytes.
**ver•ru•ga** (vĕ-roo′gă) SYN verruca. [Sp.]
**ver•ru•ga pe•ru•ana** a late, eruptive stage of bartonellosis; characterized by soft conical or pedunculated vascular papules on the skin or mucous membranes, resolving without scars after a few months. SYN Peruvian wart, verruca peruana, verruca peruviana.
**ver•sion** (ver′zhŭn) **1.** displacement of the uterus, with tilting of the entire organ without bending upon itself; such displacement may be anteversion, retroversion, or lateroversion. **2.** change of position of the fetus in the uterus, occurring spontaneously or effected by manipulation. **3.** SYN inclination. **4.** conjugate rotation of the eyes in the same direction; such rotation may be dextroversion, levoversion, supraversion, or infraversion. [L. *verto,* pp. *versus,* to turn]
**ver•te•bra,** gen. and pl. **ver•te•brae** (ver′tĕ-bră, ver′tĕ-brē) [TA] one of the segments of the spinal column; in human beings there are usually 33 vertebrae, 7 cervical, 12 thoracic, 5 lumbar, 5 sacral (fused into one bone, the sacrum), and 4 coccygeal (fused into one bone, the coccyx). [L. joint, fr. *verto,* to turn]
**ver•te•bra C1** SYN atlas.
**ver•te•bra C2** SYN axis (5).
**ver•te•bra den•ta•ta** SYN axis (5).
**ver•te•brae cer•vi•ca•les [C1–C7]** [TA] SYN cervical vertebrae [C1–C7].
**ver•te•brae coc•cy•ge•ae [Co1–Co4]** [TA] SYN coccygeal vertebrae Co1–Co4.
**ver•te•brae lum•ba•les [L1–L5]** SYN lumbar vertebrae L1–L5.
**ver•te•brae sa•cra•les [S1–S5]** SYN sacral vertebrae [S1–S5].
**ver•te•brae tho•ra•ci•cae** [TA] SYN thoracic vertebrae [T1–T12].
**ver•te•bral** (ver′tĕ-brăl) relating to a vertebra or the vertebrae.
**ver•te•bral arch** the posterior projection from the body of a vertebra that encloses the vertebral foramen; it consists of paired pedicles and laminae; the spinous, transverse, and articular processes arise from the arch. In aggregate, the ve-

nous arches—and the ligamenta flava that unite them—form the posterior wall of the vertebral (spinal) canal. SYN neural arch.
**ver•te•bral ar•tery** the first branch of the subclavian artery; for descriptive purposes, divided into four parts: 1) prevertebral part, the portion before it enters the foramen of the transverse process of the sixth cervical vertebra; 2) transversarial part, the portion in the transverse foramina of the first six cervical vertebrae; 3) suboccipital (atlantic) part, the portion running along the posterior arch of the atlas; and 4) intracranial part, the portion within the cranial cavity to its union with the artery from the other side to form the basilar artery. SYN arteria vertebralis [TA].
**ver•te•bral ca•nal** the canal that contains the spinal cord, spinal meninges, and related structures. It is formed by the vertebral foramina of successive vertebrae of the articulated vertebral column. SYN canalis vertebralis [TA], spinal canal.
**ver•te•bral col•umn** the series of vertebrae that extend from the cranium to the coccyx, providing support and forming a flexible bony case for the spinal cord. SYN columna vertebralis [TA], backbone, rachis, spina (1), spina (2), spinal column, spine (2).
**ver•te•bral fo•ra•men** the foramen formed by the union of the vertebral arch with the body; in the articulated vertebral column, the vertebral foramen collectively form the vertebral canal.
**ver•te•bral for•mu•la** a formula indicating the number of vertebrae in each segment of the spinal column; for man it is C. 7, T. 12, L. 5, S. 5, Co. 4 = 33, the letters standing for cervical, thoracic, lumbar, sacral, and coccygeal.
**ver•te•bral nerve** a branch from the stellate ganglion that ascends along the vertebral artery to the level of the axis or atlas, giving branches to the cervical nerves and meninges. SYN nervus vertebralis [TA].
**ver•te•bral ribs** SYN floating ribs [XI–XII].
**ver•te•bral vein** a vein derived from tributaries (venae comitantes) which run through the foramina in the transverse processes of the first six cervical vertebrae and form a plexus around the vertebral artery; it empties as a single trunk into the brachiocephalic veins.
**ver•te•bra pla•na** spondylitis with reduction of vertebral body to a thin disk.
**Ver•te•bra•ta** (ver-tĕ-brah′tă) the vertebrates, a major division of the phylum Chordata, consisting of those animals with a dorsal hollow nerve cord enclosed in a cartilaginous or bony spinal column; includes several classes of fishes, and the amphibians, reptiles, birds, and mammals. [L. *vertebratus,* jointed]
**ver•te•brate** (ver′tĕ-brāt) **1.** having a vertebral column. **2.** an animal having vertebrae.
**ver•te•brat•ed cath•e•ter** a catheter made of several segments moving on each other like the links of a chain.
**ver•te•brec•to•my** (ver′tĕ-brek′tō-mē) resection of a vertebral body. [vertebra + G. *ektomē,* excision]
△**ver•te•bro-** a vertebra, vertebral. [L. *vertebra*]
**ver•te•bro•ar•te•ri•al fo•ra•men** SYN transverse foramen.
**ver•te•bro•chon•dral** (ver′tĕ-brō-kon′drăl) denoting the three false ribs (eighth, ninth, and tenth), which are connected with the vertebrae at one extremity and the costal cartilages at the

other, these cartilages not articulating directly with the sternum. SYN vertebrocostal (2). [vertebro- + G. *chondros,* cartilage]

**ver•te•bro•cos•tal** (ver'tĕ-brō-kos'tăl) **1.** SYN costovertebral. **2.** SYN vertebrochondral. [vertebro- + L. *costa,* rib]

**ver•te•bro•cos•tal tri•gone** a triangular area in the diaphragm near the lateral arcuate ligament that is devoid of muscle fibers; it is covered by pleura superiorly and by peritoneum inferiorly.

**ver•te•bro•ster•nal** (ver'tĕ-brō-ster'năl) SYN sternovertebral.

**ver•tex,** pl. **ver•ti•ces** (ver'teks, ver'ti-sēz) **1.** the topmost point of the vault of the skull, a landmark in craniometry. **2.** OBSTETRICS the portion of the fetal head bounded by the planes of the trachelobregmatic and biparietal diameters, with the posterior fontanel at the apex. [L. whirl, whorl]

**ver•tex pre•sen•ta•tion** SEE cephalic presentation.

**ver•ti•cal** (ver'ti-kăl) **1.** relating to the vertex, or crown of the head. **2.** perpendicular. **3.** denoting any plane or line that passes longitudinally through the body in the anatomical position.

**ver•ti•cal band•ed gas•tro•plas•ty** a gastroplasty for treatment of morbid obesity in which an upper gastric pouch is formed by a vertical staple line, with a cloth band applied to prevent dilation at the outlet into the main pouch.

**ver•ti•cal growth phase** spread of melanoma cells from the epidermis into the dermis and later the subcutis, from which site metastasis may take place.

**ver•ti•cal heart** descriptive of the heart's electrical axis when this is directed at approximately +90°.

**ver•ti•cal mus•cle of tongue** an intrinsic muscle of the tongue, consisting of fibers that pass from the aponeurosis of the dorsum to the aponeurosis of the inferior surface; *action,* decreases the superior to inferior dimension of (flattens) the tongue; *nerve supply,* hypoglossal for motor, lingual for sensory. SYN musculus verticalis linguae [TA].

**ver•ti•cal nys•tag•mus** an up-and-down oscillation of the eyes.

**ver•ti•cal o•ver•lap 1.** the extension of the upper teeth over the lower teeth in a vertical direction when the opposing posterior teeth are in contact in centric occlusion; **2.** the distance that teeth lap over their antagonists vertically; **3.** the relationship of the maxillary incisors to the mandibular incisors when the incisal edges pass each other in centric occlusion. SYN overbite.

**ver•ti•cal stra•bis•mus** a form of strabismus in which the visual axis of one eye deviates upward (s. sursum vergens) or downward (s. deorsum vergens).

**ver•ti•cal trans•mis•sion 1.** transmission of a virus (e.g., RNA tumor virus) by means of the genetic apparatus of a cell in which the viral genome is integrated; **2.** for infectious agents in general, transmission of an agent from an individual to its offspring. i.e., from one generation to the next. Cf. horizontal transmission.

**ver•ti•cil** a collection of similar parts radiating from a common axis. SYN vortex (1), whorl (4). [L. *verticillus,* the whirl of a spindle, dim. of *vertex,* a whirl]

**ver•ti•cil•late** (ver'ti-sil'āt) arranged in the form of a verticil.

**ver•tig•i•nous** (ver-tij'i-nŭs) relating to or suffering from vertigo.

**ver•ti•go** (ver'ti-gō) **1.** a sensation of spinning or whirling motion. Vertigo implies a definite sensation of rotation of the subject or of objects about the subject in any plane. **2.** imprecisely used as a general term to describe dizziness. [L. *vertigo* (*vertigin-*), dizziness, fr. *verto,* to turn]

**ve•si•ca,** gen. and pl. **ve•si•cae** (vĕs-ī'kă) **1.** [TA] SYN bladder. **2.** any hollow structure or sac, normal or pathologic, containing a serous fluid. [L.]

**ve•si•ca bil•i•ar•is** [TA] SYN gallbladder.

**ves•i•cal** (ves'i-kăl) relating to any bladder, but usually the urinary bladder.

**ves•i•cal cal•cu•lus** a urinary calculus formed or retained in the bladder.

**ves•i•cal di•ver•tic•u•lum** a diverticulum of the bladder wall; may be either true or false type.

**ves•i•cal he•ma•tu•ria** hematuria in which the site of bleeding is in the urinary bladder.

**ves•i•cal tri•an•gle** SYN trigone of bladder.

**ves•i•cal veins** drain the vesical venous plexus and join the internal iliac veins.

**ves•i•cant** (ves'i-kănt) an agent that produces a vesicle.

**ve•si•ca pros•ta•ti•ca** SYN prostatic utricle.

**ves•i•ca•tion** (ves-i-kā'shŭn) SYN vesiculation (1).

**ve•si•ca u•ri•na•ria** [TA] SYN urinary bladder.

⊞ **ves•i•cle** (ves'i-kl) [TA] **1.** SYN vesicula. **2.** a small, circumscribed elevation of the skin containing fluid. SEE ALSO bleb, blister, bulla. **3.** a small sac containing liquid or gas. See page B4. [L. *vesicula,* a blister, dim. of *vesica,* bladder]

**ves•i•cle her•nia** protrusion of a segment of the bladder through the abdominal wall or into the inguinal canal and into the scrotum.

△ **ves•i•co-, vesic-** a vesica, vesicle. SEE ALSO vesiculo-. [L. *vesica,* bladder]

**ves•i•co•cele** (ves'i-kō-sēl) SYN cystocele.

**ves•i•coc•ly•sis** (ves'i-kok'li-sis) washing out, or lavage, of the urinary bladder. [vesico- + G. *klysis,* a washing out]

**ves•i•co•pus•tu•lar** (ves'i-kō-pŭs'tyu-lăr) pertaining to a vesicopustule. SYN vesiculopustular (1).

**ves•i•co•rec•tos•to•my** (ves'i-kō-rek-tos'tō-mē) surgical urinary tract diversion by anastomosis of the posterior bladder wall to the rectum. SYN cystorectostomy. [vesico- + rectum + G. *stoma,* mouth]

**ves•i•co•sig•moi•dos•to•my** (ves'ĭ-kō-sig-moy-dos'tō-mē) operative formation of a communication between the bladder and the sigmoid colon. [vesico- + sigmoid + G. *stoma,* mouth]

**ves•i•co•spi•nal** (ves'i-kō-spī'năl) relating to the urinary bladder and the spinal cord; denoting the neural mechanisms that control retention and evacuation of urine by the bladder, located in the second lumbar and second sacral segment, respectively, of the spinal cord.

**ves•i•cos•to•my** (ves'i-kos'tō-mē) SYN cystostomy. [vesico- + G. *stoma,* mouth]

**ves•i•cot•o•my** (ves'i-kot'ō-mē) SYN cystotomy.

**ves•i•co•u•re•ter•al re•flux** backward flow of urine from bladder into ureter.

**ves•i•co•u•re•ter•al valve** a lock mechanism in the wall of the intravesical portion of the ureter that normally prevents urinary reflux.

**ves•i•co•u•ter•ine fis•tu•la** a fistula between the bladder and the uterus.

**ve•sic•u•la,** gen. and pl. **ve•sic•u•lae** (vĕ-sik'yu-lă, vĕ-sik′yu-lē) a small bladder or bladder-like structure. SYN vesicle (1) [TA]. [L. blister, vesicle, dim. of *vesica,* bladder]

**ve·sic·u·lar** (vĕ-sik′yu-lăr) **1.** relating to a vesicle. **2.** characterized by or containing vesicles. SYN vesiculate (2), vesiculous.

**ve·sic·u·lar ap·pend·ages of ep·o·o·phor·on** a small fluid-filled cyst attached by a slender stalk to the fimbriated end of the uterine tube; a vestigial remnant of the embryonic mesonephric duct. SYN morgagnian cyst.

**ve·sic·u·lar mur·mur** SYN vesicular respiration.

**ve·sic·u·lar ovar·i·an fol·li·cle** a follicle in which the oocyte attains its full size and is surrounded by an extracellular glycoprotein layer (zona pellucida) that separates it from a peripheral layer of follicular cells permeated by one or more fluid-filled antra; the theca of the follicle develops into internal and external layers. SYN antral follicle, graafian follicle, secondary follicle.

**ve·sic·u·lar res·o·nance** the sound obtained on percussing over the normal lungs.

**ve·sic·u·lar res·pi·ra·tion** the respiratory murmur heard on auscultating over the normal lung. SYN vesicular murmur.

**ve·sic·u·lar trans·port** SYN transcytosis.

**ve·sic·u·late** (vĕ-sik′yu-lāt) **1.** to become vesicular. **2.** SYN vesicular (2).

**ve·sic·u·la·tion** (vĕ-sik′yu-lā′shŭn) **1.** the formation of vesicles. SYN blistering, vesication. **2.** SYN inflation. **3.** presence of a number of vesicles.

**ve·sic·u·lec·to·my** (vĕ-sik′yu-lek′tō-mē) resection of a portion or all of each of the seminal vesicles. [L. *vesicula,* vesicle, + G. *ektomē,* excision]

**ve·sic·u·li·form** (vĕ-sik′yu-li-fōrm) resembling a vesicle.

**ve·sic·u·li·tis** (vĕ-sik-yu-lī′tis) inflammation of any vesicle; especially of a seminal vesicle. [L. *vesicula,* vesicle, + G. *-itis,* inflammation]

△**ve·sic·u·lo-** a vesicle. [L. *vesicula,* vesicle, dim. of *vesica,* bladder]

**ve·sic·u·lo·cav·ern·ous** (vĕ-sik′yu-lō-kav′er-nŭs) Both vesicular and cavernous; denoting: **1.** an auscultatory sound having both a vesicular and a cavernous quality; **2.** the structure of certain neoplasms.

**ve·sic·u·log·ra·phy** (vĕ-sik-yu-log′ră-fē) radiographic contrast study of the seminal vesicles. [vesiculo- + G. *graphō,* to write]

**ve·sic·u·lo·pap·u·lar** (vĕ-sik′yu-lō-pap′yu-lăr) pertaining to or consisting of a combination of vesicles and papules, or of papules becoming increasingly edematous with sufficient collection of fluid to form vesicles.

**ve·sic·u·lo·pros·ta·ti·tis** (vĕ-sik′yu-lō-pros′tă-tī′tis) inflammation of the bladder and prostate. [vesiculo- + prostate + G. *-itis,* inflammation]

**ve·sic·u·lo·pus·tu·lar** (vĕ-sik′yu-lō-pŭs′tyu-lăr) **1.** SYN vesicopustular. **2.** pertaining to a mixed eruption of vesicles and pustules.

**ve·sic·u·lot·o·my** (vĕ-sik-yu-lot′ō-mē) surgical incision of the seminal vesicles. [vesiculo- + G. *tomē,* incision]

**ve·sic·u·lo·tu·bu·lar** (vĕ-sik′yu-lō-too′byu-ler) denoting an auscultatory sound having both a vesicular and a tubular quality.

**ve·sic·u·lo·tym·pan·ic** (vĕ-sik′yu-lō-tim-pan′ik) denoting a percussion sound having both a vesicular and a tympanic quality.

**ve·sic·u·lo·tym·pa·ni·tic res·o·nance** a peculiar, partly tympanitic, partly vesicular sound, obtained on percussion in cases of pulmonary emphysema.

**ve·sic·u·lous** (vĕ-sik′yu-lŭs) SYN vesicular (2).

**ves·sel** (ves′ĕl) a structure conveying or containing a fluid, especially a liquid. SEE ALSO vas. [O. Fr. fr. L. *vascellum,* dim. of *vas*]

**ves·tib·u·la** (ves-tib′yu-lă) plural of vestibulum.

**ves·tib·u·lar** (ves-tib′yu-lăr) **1.** relating to a vestibule, especially the vestibule of the ear. **2.** interpreting stimuli from the inner ear receptors regarding head position and movement.

**ves·tib·u·lar ca·nal** SYN scala vestibuli.

**ves·tib·u·lar crest, crest of ves·ti·bule** an oblique ridge on the inner wall of the vestibule of the labyrinth, bounding the spherical recess above and posteriorly.

**ves·tib·u·lar fold** one of the pair of folds of mucous membrane stretching across the laryngeal cavity from the angle of the thyroid cartilage to the arytenoid cartilage; they enclose a space called the rima vestibuli or false glottis. SYN plica vestibularis [TA], false vocal cord, ventricular band of larynx, ventricular fold.

**ves·tib·u·lar gan·gli·on** a collection of bipolar nerve cell bodies forming a swelling on the vestibular part of the eighth cranial nerve in the internal acoustic meatus; consists of a superior part and an inferior part connected by a narrow isthmus.

**ves·tib·u·lar mem·brane** the membrane separating the cochlear duct from the vestibular canal; it consists of squamous epithelial cells with microvilli toward the ductus, a basement membrane, and a thin layer of connective tissue toward the scala. SYN Reissner membrane.

**ves·tib·u·lar nerve** the part of the vestibulocochlear nerve peripheral to the vestibular root; it is composed of the central processes of bipolar neurons which have their terminals of their peripheral processes on the hair cells in the ampullae of the semicircular ducts and the maculae of the saccule and utricle, and cell bodies of the vestibular ganglion.

**ves·tib·u·lar neur·ec·to·my** transection of the vestibular division of the eighth cranial nerve.

**ves·tib·u·lar neu·ron·i·tis** a paroxysmal attack of severe vertigo, not accompanied by deafness or tinnitus, which affects young to middle-aged adults, often following a nonspecific upper respiratory infection; due to unilateral vestibular dysfunction. SYN Gerlier disease.

**ves·tib·u·lar nu·clei** a group of four main nuclei that are located in the lateral region of the hindbrain beneath the floor of the rhomboid fossa. These nuclei are the inferior vestibular nucleus, medial vestibular nucleus (Schwalbe nucleus), lateral vestibular nucleus (Deiter nucleus), and superior vestibular nucleus (Bechterew nucleus). The inferior nucleus contains a group of large cells, the magnocellular part of inferior vestibular nucleus or cell group F (pars magnocellularis nuclei vestibularis inferioris [TA]), located caudally in the nucleus. A group of medium-sized neurons is located in lateral portions of the lateral nucleus, the parvocellular part or cell group I (pars parvocellularis [TA]). These nuclei receive primary fibers of the vestibular nerve, are reciprocally connected with the flocculonodular lobe of the cerebellum, and project by way of the medial longitudinal fasciculus to the abducens, trochlear, and oculomotor nuclei and to the ventral horn of the spinal cord. The lateral vestibular nucleus projects to the ipsilateral ventral horn of the spinal cord by the vestibulospinal tract.

**ves•tib•u•lar nys•tag•mus** nystagmus resulting from physiological stimuli to the labyrinth that may be rotatory, caloric, compressive, or galvanic, or due to labyrinthal lesions. SYN labyrinthine nystagmus.

**ves•tib•u•lar or•gan** collective term for the utricle, saccule, and semicircular ducts of the membranous labyrinth, each having a patch of ciliated receptor epithelium innervated by the vestibular nerve.

**ves•tib•u•lar schwan•no•ma** a benign but life-threatening tumor arising from Schwann cells, usually of the vestibular division of the eighth cranial nerve; produces hearing loss, tinnitus, and vestibular disturbances, early and cerebellar, brainstem, and other cranial nerve signs and increased intracranial pressure in late stages.

**ves•tib•u•lar veins** drain the saccule and utricle; they are tributaries of both the labyrinthine veins and the vein of the vestibular aqueduct.

**ves•ti•bule** (ves'ti-byul) **1.** a small cavity or a space at the entrance of a canal. **2.** specifically, the central, somewhat ovoid, cavity of the osseous labyrinth communicating with the semicircular canals posteriorly and the cochlea anteriorly. SYN vestibulum. [L. *vestibulum*]

**ves•ti•bule of nose** the anterior part of the nasal cavity, especially that enclosed by cartilage.

**ves•ti•bule of va•gi•na** the space behind the glans clitoridis and between the labia minora, containing the openings of the vagina, urethra, and ducts of the greater vestibular glands.

⚠**ves•tib•u•lo-** vestibule, vestibulum. [L. *vestibulum*]

**ves•tib•u•lo•co•chle•ar** (ves-tib'yu-lō-kok'lē-ăr) **1.** relating to the vestibulum and cochlea of the ear. **2.** SYN statoacoustic.

**ves•tib•u•lo•co•chle•ar nerve [CN VIII]** a composite sensory nerve innervating the receptor cells of the membranous labyrinth; it consists of two major, anatomically and functionally distinct components, each of which have different central connections: the vestibular nerve and the cochlear nerve. SYN nervus vestibulocochlearis [CN VIII] [TA], acoustic nerve, eighth cranial nerve [CN VIII].

**ves•tib•u•lo•co•chle•ar nu•clei** the combined cochlear and vestibular nuclei in the brainstem that receive the incoming fibers of the eighth cranial nerve.

**ves•tib•u•lo•oc•u•lar re•flex** generic term for the reflex control of the vestibular system over extraocular motility manifest as nystagmus in clinical testing.

**ves•tib•u•lop•a•thy** (ves-tib'yu-lō-path-ē) any abnormality of the vestibular apparatus, e.g., Ménière disease.

**ves•tib•u•lo•plas•ty** (ves-tib'yu-lō-plas-tē) any of a series of surgical procedures designed to restore alveolar ridge height by lowering muscles attaching to the buccal, labial, and lingual aspects of the jaws. [vestibulo- + G. *plassō*, to form]

**ves•tib•u•lo•spi•nal re•flex** the influence of vestibular stimulation on body posture.

**ves•tib•u•lot•o•my** (ves-tib'yu-lot'ō-mē) opera-

tion for an opening into the vestibule of the labyrinth. [vestibulo- + G. *tomē*, incision]

**ves•tib•u•lum**, pl. **ves•tib•u•la** (ves-tib'yu-lŭm, ves-tib'yu-lă) SYN vestibule. [L. antechamber, entrance court]

**ves•tige** (ves'tij) a trace or a rudimentary structure; the degenerated remains of any structure which occurs as an entity in the embryo or fetus. [L. *vestigium*]

**ves•tig•i•al** (ves-tij'ē-ăl) relating to a vestige.

**ves•tig•i•al or•gan** a rudimentary structure in humans corresponding to a functional structure or organ in the lower animals.

**vet•er•i•nar•i•an** (vet'ē-rin-ār'ē-ăn) a person who holds an academic degree in veterinary medicine; a licensed practitioner of veterinary medicine. [see veterinary]

**vet•er•i•nary** (vet'ē-rin-ār-ē) relating to the diseases of animals. [L. *veterinarius*, fr. *veterina*, beast of burden]

**vet•er•i•nary med•i•cine** the field concerned with the diseases and health of all animal species other than humans.

**vet•er•i•nary tech•ni•cian** a person who holds an academic degree in veterinary technology; a credentialed practitioner whose training includes radiology, anesthesiology, medical technology, and surgical assisting.

**vet•er•i•nary tech•ni•cian spe•cial•ist** a veterinary technician who has advanced academic training and credentials in a specialty of veterinary technology. Denoted by the initials VTS followed by the specialty in parenthesis, such as (Emergency & Critical Care).

**VHDL** very high density lipoprotein. SEE lipoprotein.

**vi•a•bil•i•ty** (vī-ă-bil'i-tē) capability of living; the state of being viable; usually connotes a fetus that has reached 500 g in weight and 20 gestational weeks. [Fr. *viabilité* fr. L. *vita*, life]

**vi•a•ble** (vī'ă-bl) capable of living; denoting a fetus sufficiently developed to live outside the uterus. [Fr. fr. *vie*, life, fr. L. *vita*]

**vi•brat•ing line** the imaginary line across the posterior part of the palate, marking the division between the movable and immovable tissues.

**vibration** a group of movements in massage that involve fine or coarse rhythmic shaking of various structures, with or without compression or traction.

*Vib•ri•o* (vib'rē-ō) a genus of motile (occasionally nonmotile), non-spore-forming, aerobic to facultatively anaerobic, Gram-negative bacteria containing short curved or straight rods which occur singly or which are occasionally united into S-shapes or spirals. Some of these organisms are saprophytes in water and soil; others are parasites or pathogens. The type species is *Vibrio cholerae*. [L. *vibro*, to vibrate]

**vib•rio** (vib'rē-ō) a member of the genus *Vibrio*.

*Vib•rio al•gi•no•lyt•i•cus* a species associated with wound and ear infections, and with bacteremia in immunocompromised and burn patients.

*Vib•rio chol•er•ae* a species that produces a soluble exotoxin and is the cause of cholera in humans; it is the type species of the genus *Vibrio*. SYN comma bacillus.

*Vib•rio fe•tus* former name for *Campylobacter fetus*.

*Vib•rio flu•vi•a•lis* a species similar to strains of

*Aeromonas*, associated with diarrheal disease in humans.

**Vib·rio fur·nis·si·i** an aerogenic strain, similar to *Vibrio fluvialis*, associated with diarrheal disease and outbreaks of gastroenteritis.

**Vib·rio mi·mi·cus** a species similar to *Vibrio cholerae*, isolated from human stool in diarrheal disease and from human ear infections.

**Vib·rio par·a·hae·mo·lyt·i·cus** a marine species that causes gastroenteritis and bloody diarrhea, usually from eating contaminated shellfish.

**vib·ri·o·sis**, pl. **vib·ri·o·ses** (vib-rē-ō'sis) infection caused by bacteria of the genus *Vibrio*.

**Vib·rio vul·ni·fi·cus** a species capable of causing cutaneous lesions in an immunocompromised patient; usually contracted from contaminated oysters; also a cause of wound infections.

**vi·bris·sa**, gen. and pl. **vi·bris·sae** (vī-bris'ă, vī-bris'ē) one of the hairs growing at the nares, or vestibule of the nose. [L. found only in pl. *vibrissae*, fr. *vibro*, to quiver]

**vi·bro·car·di·o·gram** (vī'brō-kar'dē-ō-gram) a graphic record of chest vibrations produced by hemodynamic events of the cardiac cycle; the record provides an indirect, externally recorded measurement of isovolumic contraction and ejection times. [L. *vibro*, to shake, + G. *kardia*, heart, + *gramma*, a drawing]

**vi·car·i·ous** (vī-ker'ē-ŭs) acting as a substitute; occurring in an abnormal situation. [L. *vicarius*, from *vicis*, supplying place of]

**vi·car·i·ous hy·per·tro·phy** hypertrophy of an organ following failure of another organ because of a functional relationship between them; e.g., enlargement of the pituitary gland, after destruction of the thyroid.

**vi·car·i·ous men·stru·a·tion** bleeding from any surface other than the mucous membrane of the uterine cavity, occurring periodically at the time when the normal menstruation should take place.

**vi·cious cir·cle 1.** the mutually accelerating action of two independent diseases or phenomena, or of a primary and secondary affection; **2.** the passage of food, after a gastroenterostomy, from the artificial opening through the intestinal loop by antiperistaltic action and back into the stomach again by the pyloric orifice, or the reverse.

**vi·cious un·ion** union of the ends of a broken bone resulting in a deformity or a crooked limb; frequently used interchangeably with faulty union.

**vid·e·o·en·do·scope** (vid'ē-ō-end'ō-skōp) an endoscope fitted with a video camera.

**vid·e·o·en·dos·co·py** (vid'ē-ō-en-dos'kŏ-pē) endoscopy performed with an endoscope fitted with a video camera.

**vid·i·an** (vid'ē-an) named after or described by Vidius (Guido Guidi, 1500–1569).

**Vi·er·ra sign** (vē-ĕr'ă) yellowing and canalization of the nail in fogo selvagem.

**Vieth-Mül·ler circle** (vīth-myu'ler) a geometric circle passing through the optical centers of two eyes by which points adjacent to the point of fixation, both lying on the circle, theoretically fall on corresponding retinal points.

**view** (vyu) RADIOGRAPHY a standard diagnostic x-ray study, named according to the image as it appears on film or other receptor.

**vig·il·am·bu·lism** (vij-i-lam'byu-lizm) a condition of unconsciousness regarding one's surroundings, with automatism, resembling som-

nambulism but occurring in the waking state. [L. *vigil*, awake, alert, + *ambulo*, to walk about]

**vil·li** (vil'ī) plural of villus.

**vil·lo·ma** (vi-lō'mă) SYN papilloma.

**vil·lose** (vil'ōs) SYN villous (2).

**vil·lo·si·tis** (vil-ō-sī'tis) inflammation of the villous surface of the placenta. [villous + G. *-itis* inflammation]

**vil·los·i·ty** (vi-los'i-tē) shagginess; an aggregation of villi.

**vil·lous** (vil'ŭs) **1.** relating to villi. **2.** shaggy; covered with villi. SYN villose.

**vil·lous ad·e·no·ma** a solitary sessile, often large, tumor of colonic mucosa composed of mucinous epithelium covering delicate vascular projections; malignant change occurs frequently. SYN papillary adenoma of large intestine.

**vil·lous car·ci·no·ma** a form of carcinoma in which there are numerous closely packed papillary projections of neoplastic epithelial tissue.

**vil·lous ten·o·syn·o·vi·tis** a condition resembling pigmented villonodular synovitis but arising in periarticular soft tissue rather than in joint synovia; occurs most commonly in the hands. SYN pigmented villonodular tenosynovitis.

**vil·lus**, pl. **vil·li** (vil'ŭs, vil'ī) **1.** a projection from the surface, especially of a mucous membrane. If the projection is minute, as from a cell surface, it is termed a microvillus. **2.** an elongated dermal papilla projecting into an intraepidermal vesicle or cleft. SEE festooning. [L. shaggy hair (of beasts)]

**vil·lus·ec·to·my** (vil-ŭs-ek'tō-mē) SYN synovectomy. [villus + G. *ektomē*, excision]

**vi·men·tin** (vī-men'tin) the major polypeptide that copolymerizes with other subunits to form the intermediate filament cytoskeleton of mesenchymal cells; they may have a role in maintaining the internal organization of certain cells.

**Vin·cent an·gi·na** (vă-sah') an ulcerative infection of the oral soft tissues including the tonsils and pharynx caused by fusiform and spirochetal organisms; it is usually associated with necrotizing ulcerative gingivitis and may progress to noma. Death from suffocation or sepsis may occur.

**Vin·cent ba·cil·lus** (vă-sah') probably *Fusobacterium nucleatum*.

**Vin·cent dis·ease** (vă-sah') SYN necrotizing ulcerative gingivitis.

**Vin·cent in·fec·tion** (vă-sah') SYN necrotizing ulcerative gingivitis.

**Vin·cent spi·ril·lum** (vă-sah') the spirillum or spirochete found in association with Vincent bacillus. *Fusobacterium nucleatum* is frequently the only bacillus isolated.

**Vin·cent ton·sil·li·tis** (vă-sah') angina limited chiefly to the tonsils, caused by Vincent organisms (bacillus and spirillum).

**vin·cu·la of ten·dons** fibrous bands that extend from the flexor tendons of the fingers and toes to the capsules of the interphalangeal joints and to the phalanges; they convey small vessels to the tendons.

**vin·cu·lum**, pl. **vin·cu·la** (ving'koo-lŭm, ving'koo-lă) [TA] a frenum, frenulum, or ligament. [L. a fetter, fr. *vincio*, to bind]

**vin·e·gar** (vin'ē-găr) impure dilute acetic acid, made from wine, cider, malt, etc. [Fr. *vinaigre*, fr. *vin*, wine, + *aigre*, sour]

**vin·e·gar eel** SYN *Turbatrix aceti*.

**vi•nyl** (vī′nil) the hydrocarbon radical, $CH_2=CH-$. SYN ethenyl.

**vi•o•let** (vī′ō-let) the color evoked by wavelengths of the visible spectrum shorter than 450 nm. For individual violet dyes, see the specific name. [L. *viola*]

**VIP** vasoactive intestinal polypeptide.

**vi•po•ma** (vip-ō′mă) an endocrine tumor, usually originating in the pancreas, which produces a vasoactive intestinal polypeptide believed to cause profound cardiovascular and electrolyte changes with vasodilatory hypotension, watery diarrhea, hypokalemia, and dehydration. [*vasoactive intestinal polypeptide + G. -ōma, tumor*]

**Vi•pond sign** (vē-pō) a generalized adenopathy occurring during the period of incubation of various of the exanthemas of childhood, affording an early diagnostic sign in a case of known exposure.

**vi•rae•mia [Br.]** SEE viremia.

**vi•ral** (vī′răl) of, pertaining to, or caused by a virus.

**vi•ral dys•en•tery** profuse watery diarrhea due to, or thought to be due to, infection by a virus.

**vi•ral en•ve•lope** the outer structure that encloses the nucleocapsids of some viruses; may contain host material.

**vi•ral he•mag•glu•ti•na•tion** the nonimmune agglutination of suspended red blood cells by certain of a wide range of otherwise unrelated viruses, usually by the virion itself but in some instances by products of viral growth, the species of erythrocyte agglutinated differing with the different viruses.

**vi•ral hep•a•ti•tis 1.** hepatitis caused by any one of at least five immunologically unrelated viruses: hepatitis A virus, hepatitis B virus, hepatitis C virus, hepatitis D virus, hepatitis E virus; **2.** hepatitis caused by a viral infection, including that by Epstein-Barr virus and cytomegalovirus.

**vi•ral hep•a•ti•tis type A** a virus disease with a short incubation period (usually 15 to 50 days), caused by hepatitis A virus, a member of the family Picornaviridae, often transmitted by fecal-oral route; may be inapparent, mild, severe, or occasionally fatal and occurs sporadically or in epidemics, commonly in school-age children and young adults; necrosis of periportal liver cells with lymphocytic and plasma cell infiltration is characteristic and jaundice is a common symptom. SYN hepatitis A.

**vi•ral hep•a•ti•tis type B** a virus disease with a long incubation period (usually 50 to 160 days), caused by hepatitis B virus; transmitted by blood or blood products, contaminated needles or instruments, or sexually; differs from hepatitis A in having a higher mortality and in the possibility of progression to a chronic disease, a carrier state, or both. SYN hepatitis B.

**vi•ral hep•a•ti•tis type D** acute or chronic hepatitis caused by the hepatitis delta virus, a defective RNA virus requiring HBV for replication. The acute type occurs in two forms: 1) coinfection, the simultaneous occurrence of hepatitis B virus and hepatitis delta virus infections; 2) superinfection, the appearance of hepatitis delta virus infection in a hepatitis B virus carrier. SYN delta hepatitis.

**vi•ral load** the plasma level of viral RNA, as determined by various techniques including target amplification assay by reverse transcriptase polymerase chain reaction and branched DNA technology with signal amplification. Because levels of detection vary with method, results of testing by different methods are not comparable.

Serial measurement of HIV viral load has become a standard procedure in monitoring the course of AIDS. Reported as the number of copies of viral RNA per mL of plasma, assessment of viral load provides important information about the number of lymphoid cells actively infected with HIV. This laboratory procedure has supplanted the CD4 count as an indicator of prognosis of persons infected with HIV, in determining when to start antiretroviral therapy, and in measuring the response to therapy. Because the CD4 count is regarded as superior in determining the level of immune compromise and the risk of opportunistic infection, both tests are currently used. Antiretroviral therapy is started when plasma HIV RNA concentration exceeds 5000 copies/mL. When, as a result of treatment, the number of copies of viral RNA falls below the level that can be detected by standard methods, replication of HIV is considered to have been suppressed. In no case, however, has AIDS been cured, nor has viral proliferation remained arrested after cessation of antiretroviral therapy.

**"vi•ral" spong•i•form en•ceph•a•lo•pa•thy** progressive vacuolation in dendritic and axonal processes and in neuronal cell bodies, associated with slow virus infections.

**vi•ral tro•pism** the specificity of a virus for a particular host tissue, determined in part by the interaction of viral surface structures with host cell-surface receptors.

**Vir•chow node** (fēr′kō) SYN signal lymph node.

**Vir•chow psam•mo•ma** (fēr′kō) SYN psammomatous meningioma.

**vi•re•mia** (vī-rē′mē-ă) the presence of a virus in the bloodstream. [virus + G. *haima*, blood]

**vir•gin** (ver′jin) **1.** a person who has never had sexual intercourse. **2.** unused; uncontaminated. SYN virginal (2). [L. *virgo* (*virgin-*), maiden]

**vir•gin•al** (ver′ji-năl) **1.** relating to a virgin. **2.** SYN virgin (2). [L. *virginalis*]

**vir•gin•i•ty** (ver-jin′i-tē) the virgin state. [L. *virginitas*]

⌂**-vir•i•dae** a virus family. [L. *vir*, fr. *virus*, venom]

**vir•i•dans strep•to•coc•ci** SYN *Streptococcus viridans*.

**vir•ile** (vir′īl) **1.** relating to the male sex. **2.** manly, strong, masculine. **3.** possessing masculine traits. [L. *virilis*, masculine, fr. *vir*, a man]

**vir•i•les•cence** (vir-i-les′ens) assumption of male characteristics by a female.

**vir•i•lism** (vir′i-lizm) possession of mature masculine somatic characteristics by a girl, woman, or prepubescent male; may be present at birth or may appear later; commonly the result of gonadal or adrenocortical dysfunction, or of androgenic therapy. [L. *virilis*, masculine]

**vi•ril•i•ty** (vi-ril′i-tē) the condition or quality of being virile. [L. *virilitas*, manhood, fr. *vir*, man]

**vir•i•li•za•tion** (vir′i-li-zā′shŭn) production or acquisition of virilism.

**vir•i•liz•ing** (vir′i-līz-ing) causing virilism.

⌂**-vir•i•nae** suffix used in naming a subfamily of viruses.

**vi•ri•on** (vī′rē-on, vir′ē-on) the complete virus particle that is structurally intact and infectious.

**vi•rol•o•gist** (vī-rol′ō-jist) a specialist in virology.

**vi·rol·o·gy** (vī-rol′ō-jē, vi-rol′ō-jē) the study of viruses and of viral disease. [virus + G. *logos*, study]

**vir·tu·al en·dos·copy** computed tomographic data reconstructed in three dimensions to give information similar to that obtained with endoscopy.

**vi·ru·ci·dal** (vī-rŭ-sī′dăl) destructive to a virus.

**vi·ru·cide** (vī-rŭ-sīd) an agent active against virus infections. [virus + L. *caedo*, to kill]

**vir·u·lence** (vēr′yu-lĕns) the disease-evoking power of a pathogen; numerically expressed as the ratio of the number of cases of overt infection to the total number infected, as determined by immunoassay. [L. *virulentia*, fr. *virulentus*, poisonous]

**vir·u·lent** (vēr′yu-lent) extremely toxic, denoting a markedly pathogenic microorganism. [L. *virulentus*, poisonous]

**vir·u·lent bac·te·ri·o·phage** a bacteriophage that regularly causes lysis of the bacteria that it infects.

**vir·u·lif·er·ous** (vī-rŭ-lif′er-ŭs) conveying virus.

**vir·u·ria** (vīr-yu′rē-ă) presence of viruses in the urine. [virus + G. *ouron*, urine]

**vi·rus**, pl. **vi·rus·es** (vī′rŭs) **1.** formerly, the specific agent of an infectious disease. **2.** specifically, a term for a group of infectious agents, which with few exceptions are capable of passing through fine filters that retain most bacteria, are usually not visible through the light microscope, lack independent metabolism, and are incapable of growth or reproduction apart from living cells. They have a prokaryotic genetic apparatus but differ sharply from bacteria in other respects. The complete particle usually contains either DNA or RNA, not both, and is usually covered by a protein shell or capsid that protects the nucleic acid. They range in size from 15 nanometers up to several hundred nanometers. Classification of viruses depends upon physiochemical characteristics of virions as well as upon mode of transmission, host range, symptomatology, and other factors. SYN ultravirus. **3.** relating to or caused by a virus, as a virus disease. **4.** (Obsolete usage) Before the era of bacteriology, any agent causing disease, including a chemical substance such as an enzyme ("ferment") similar to snake venom; synonymous at that time with "poison." [L. poison]

△**-vi·rus** a genus of viruses.

**vi·rus ker·a·to·con·junc·ti·vi·tis** SYN epidemic keratoconjunctivitis.

**vi·rus·oid** (vī′rŭs-oyd) a plant pathogen resembling a viroid but having a much larger circular or linear RNA segment and a capsid. [virus + G. *eidos*, resembling]

**vi·rus shed·ding** excretion of virus by any route from the infected host; route and duration of excretion vary according to the pathogenesis of the infection or disease.

**vi·rus-trans·formed cell** a cell that has been genetically changed to a tumor cell, the change being subsequently transmitted to all descendent cells; cells transformed by oncornaviruses continue to produce virus in high concentration without being killed; DNA tumor virus-transformed cells develop (along with other changes) tumor-associated antigens and rarely produce virus.

**vis·cera** (vis′er-ă) plural of viscus. SYN vitals.

**vis·cer·ad** (vis′er-ad) in a direction toward the viscera. [viscera + L. *ad*, to]

**vis·cer·al** (vis′er-ăl) relating to the viscera. SYN splanchnic.

**vis·cer·al an·es·the·sia** SYN splanchnic anesthesia.

**vis·cer·al cleft** any cleft between two branchial or pharyngeal (visceral) arches in the embryo.

**vis·cer·al fas·cia** a thin, fibrous membrane that envelops various organs and glands, binding structures together in some cases and forming partitions between them in other cases. USAGE NOTE: Terminologia Anatomica [TA] has recommended that the terms "superficial fascia" and "deep fascia" not be used generically in an unqualified way because of variation in their meanings internationally. The recommended terms are "subcutaneous tissue (tela subcutanea [TA])" for the former superficial fascia, and "muscular fascia" or "visceral fascia" (fascia musculorum or fascia viscera[is] [TA]) in place of deep fascia.

**vis·cer·al·gia** (vis-er-al′jē-ă) pain in any viscus. [viscero- + G. *algos*, pain]

**vis·cer·al lay·er** the inner layer of an enveloping sac or bursa which lines the outer surface of the enveloped structure, as opposed to the parietal layer which lines the walls of the occupied space or cavity. The visceral layer is usually thin, delicate and not apparent as being separate, but rather appears to be the outer surface of the structure itself. SYN lamina visceralis [TA].

**vis·cer·al lay·er of se·rous per·i·car·di·um** the inner part of the serous pericardium applied directly on the heart.

**vis·cer·al leish·man·i·a·sis** a chronic disease of the tropics caused by *Leishmania donovani* and transmitted by the bite of a species of sandfly of the genus *Phlebotomus* or *Lutzomyia;* the organisms grow and multiply in macrophages, eventually causing them to burst and liberate amastigote parasites which then invade other macrophages; proliferation of macrophages in the bone marrow causes crowding out of erythroid and myeloid elements, resulting in leukopenia, and anemia, splenomegaly, and hepatomegaly which are characteristic, along with enlargement of lymph nodes; fever, fatigue, malaise, and secondary infections also occur. SYN kala azar.

**vis·cer·al lymph nodes** the lymph nodes draining the viscera of the abdomen or of the pelvis.

**vis·cer·al pain** pain resulting from injury or disease in an organ in the thoracic or abdominal cavity.

**vis·cer·al sense** the perception of the existence of the internal organs. SYN splanchnesthesia, splanchnesthetic sensibility.

**vis·cer·al swal·low** the immature swallowing pattern of an infant or a person with tongue thrust, resembling peristaltic wavelike muscular contractions observed in the gut; adult or mature swallowing is more volitional and therefore somatic.

△**vis·cero-** the viscera. SEE ALSO splanchno-. [L. *viscus*, pl. *viscera*, the internal organs]

**vis·cer·o·gen·ic** (vis′er-ō-jen′ik) of visceral origin; denoting a number of sensory and other reflexes. [viscero- + G. *-gen*, producing]

**vis·cer·o·in·hib·i·to·ry** (vis′er-ō-in-hib′i-tōr-ē) restricting or arresting the functional activity of the viscera.

**vis·cer·o·meg·a·ly** (vis′er-ō-meg′ă-lē) abnormal

enlargement of the viscera, such as may be seen in acromegaly and other disorders. SYN organomegaly, splanchnomegaly. [viscero- + G. *megas*, large]

**vis•cer•o•mo•tor** (vis'er-ō-mō'ter) **1.** relating to or controlling movement in the viscera; denoting the autonomic nerves innervating the viscera, especially the intestines. **2.** denoting a movement having a relation to the viscera; referring to reflex muscular contractions of the abdominal wall in cases of visceral disease.

**vis•cer•o•pleu•ral** (vis'er-ō-ploo'răl) relating to the pleural and the thoracic viscera. SYN pleurovisceral.

**vis•cer•op•to•sis, vis•cer•op•to•sia** (vis'er-op-tō'sis, -tō'sē-ă vis'er-op-tō'sē-ă) descent of the viscera from their normal positions. SYN splanchnoptosis, splanchnoptosia. [viscero- + G. *ptōsis*, a falling]

**vis•cer•o•sen•sory** (vis'er-ō-sen'sōr-ē) relating to the sensory innervation of internal organs.

**vis•cer•o•skel•e•tal** (vis-er-ō-skel'ĕ-tăl) relating to the visceroskeleton. SYN splanchnoskeletal.

**vis•cer•o•skel•e•ton** (vis-er-ō-skel'ĕ-tŏn) **1.** any bony or cartilaginous formation in an organ, as in the cartilaginous rings of the trachea and bronchi. **2.** the bony framework protecting the viscera, such as the ribs and sternum, the pelvic bones, and the anterior portion of the skull. SYN splanchnoskeleton.

**vis•cer•o•so•mat•ic** (vis'er-ō-sō-mat'ik) relating to the viscera and the body. [viscero- + G. *sōma*, body]

**vis•cer•o•tro•phic** (vis'er-ō-trof'ik) relating to any trophic change determined by visceral conditions. [viscero- + G. *trophē*, nourishment]

**vis•cer•o•tro•pic** (vis'er-ō-trop'ik) affecting the viscera. [L. *viscera* internal organs, + G. *tropē*, a turning]

**vis•cid** (vis'id) sticky; glutinous. [L. *viscidus*, stick, fr. *viscum*, birdlime]

**vis•cid•i•ty** (vi-sid'i-tē) stickiness; adhesiveness.

**vis•cos•i•ty** (vis-kos'i-tē) in general, the resistance to flow or alteration of shape by any substance as a result of molecular cohesion; most frequently applied to liquids as the resistance of a fluid to flow because of a shearing force. [L. *viscositas*, fr. *viscosus*, viscous]

**vis•cous** (vis'kŭs) sticky; marked by high viscosity. [see viscid, viscosity]

**vis•cus**, pl. **vis•cera** (vis'kŭs, vis'er-ă) an organ of the digestive, respiratory, urogenital, and endocrine systems as well as the spleen, the heart, and great vessels; hollow and multilayered walled organs studied in splanchnology. [L. the soft parts, internal organs]

**vis•i•ble spec•trum** that part of electromagnetic radiation that is visible to the human eye; it extends from extreme red, 7606 Å (760.6 nm), to extreme violet, 3934 Å (393.4 nm).

**vi•sion** (vizh'ŭn) the act of seeing. SEE ALSO sight. See this page. [L. *visio*, fr. *video*, pp. *visus*, to see]

**vi•su•al** (vizh'oo-ăl) **1.** relating to vision. **2.** denoting a person who learns and remembers more readily through sight than through hearing. [Late L. *visualis*, fr. *visus*, vision]

**vi•su•al ag•no•sia** inability to recognize objects by sight; usually caused by bilateral parieto-occipital lesions.

**vi•su•al an•gle** the angle formed at the retina by

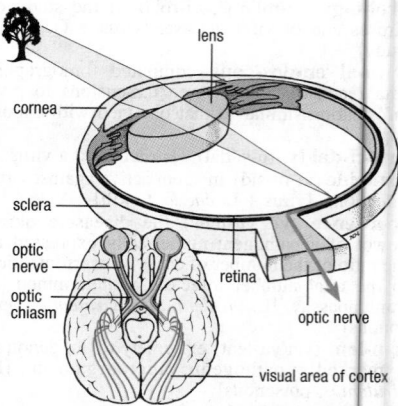

**vision:** light passes through the cornea and is focused onto the retina by the lens; cells in the retina then transmit this information through the optic nerve to the visual area of the cortex

the meeting of lines drawn from the periphery of the object seen.

**vi•su•al a•pha•sia 1.** SYN alexia. **2.** improperly used as a synonym for anomia.

**vi•su•al ar•ea** SYN visual cortex.

**vi•su•al aura** epileptic aura characterized by visual illusions or hallucinations, formed or unformed, including scintillations, teichopsia. SEE ALSO aura (1).

**vi•su•al ax•is** the straight line extending from the object seen, through the center of the pupil, to the macula lutea of the retina.

**vi•su•al clos•ure** identification of forms or objects from incomplete presentation.

**vi•su•al cor•tex** the region of the cerebral cortex occupying the entire surface of the occipital lobe, and composed of Brodmann areas 17 to 19. Area 17 (which is also called striate cortex or area because the line of Gennari is grossly visible on its surface) is the primary visual cortex, receiving the visual radiation from the lateral geniculate body of the thalamus. The surrounding areas 18 (parastriate cortex or area) and 19 (peristriate cortex or area) are probably involved in subsequent steps of visual information processing; area 18 is referred to as the secondary visual cortex. SYN visual area.

**vi•su•al e•voked po•ten•tial** voltage fluctuations that may be recorded from the occipital area of the scalp as the result of retinal stimulation by a light flashing at ¼-second intervals; commonly summated and averaged by computer.

**vi•su•al field (F)** the area simultaneously visible to one eye without movement; often measured by means of a bowl perimeter located 330 mm from the eye.

**vi•su•al in•spec•tion with a•cet•ic ac•id** SYN acetowhitening.

**vi•su•al-kin•et•ic dis•soc•i•a•tion** the neurolinguistic programming process of removing a synesthesia from a person's internal experience. SEE ALSO neurolinguistic programming.

**vi•su•al mem•ory** retained memory of objects when the visual stimulus is no longer present.

**vi·su·al neg·lect** inattention to visual stimuli occurring in the space on the involved side of the body.

**vi·su·al or·i·en·ta·tion** awareness of the location of objects in the environment and their relationship to one another and to the person viewing them.

**vi·su·al pig·ments** the photopigments in the retinal cones and rods that absorb light and initiate the visual process.

**vi·su·al pur·ple** SYN rhodopsin.

**vi·su·al re·cep·tor cells** the rod and cone cells of the retina.

**vi·su·al ver·ti·go** vertigo induced by visual stimuli.

**vi·su·al vi·o·let** SYN iodopsin.

**vi·su·og·no·sis** (vizh′yu-og-nō′sis) recognition and understanding of visual impressions. [L. *visus*, vision, + G. *gnōsis*, knowledge]

**vis·u·o·mo·tor** (vizh′yu-ō-mō′ter) denoting the ability to synchronize visual information with physical movement, e.g., driving a car..

**vi·su·o·sen·so·ry** (vizh′yu-ō-sen′sŏr-ē) pertaining to the perception of visual stimuli.

**vis·u·o·spa·tial** (viz′yu-ō-spā′shăl) denoting the ability to comprehend and conceptualize visual representations and spatial relationships in learning and performing a task.

**vi·tal** (vīt-ăl) relating to life. [L. *vitalis*, fr. *vita*, life]

**vi·tal ca·pac·i·ty (VC)** the greatest volume of air that can be exhaled from the lungs after a maximum inspiration. SYN respiratory capacity.

**vi·tal in·dex** the ratio of births to deaths within a population during a given time.

**vi·tal·i·ty** (vīt-al′i-tē) vital force or energy.

**vi·tal·i·ty test** a group of thermal and electrical tests used to aid in assessment of dental pulp health. SYN pulp test.

**vi·ta·lom·e·ter** (vī-tă-lom′ĕ-ter) an electrical device for determining the vitality of the tooth pulp.

**vi·tal pulp** a pulp composed of viable tissue, either normal or diseased, that responds to electric stimuli and to heat and cold.

**vi·tal red** [C.I. 23570] trisodium salt of a sulfonated diazo dye, used as a vital stain.

**vi·tals** (vīt′ălz) SYN viscera.

**vi·tal signs** objective measurements of temperature, pulse, respirations, and blood pressure as a means of assessing general health and cardiorespiratory function.

**vi·tal stain** a stain applied to cells or parts of cells while they are still living.

**vi·tal sta·tis·tics** systematically tabulated information concerning births, marriages, divorces, separations, and deaths, based on the numbers of official registrations of these vital events; the branch of statistics concerned with such data.

**vi·ta·mer** (vī′tă-mer) one of two or more similar compounds capable of fulfilling a specific vitamin function in the body; e.g., niacin, niacinamide.

**vi·ta·min** (vīt′ă-min) one of a group of organic substances, present in minute amounts in natural foodstuffs, that are essential to normal metabolism; insufficient amounts in the diet may cause deficiency diseases. [L. *vita*, life, + amine]

**vi·ta·min A 1.** any β-ionone derivative, except provitamin A carotenoids, possessing qualitatively the biological activity of retinol; deficiency interferes with the production and

resynthesis of rhodopsin, thereby causing night blindness, and produces a keratinizing metaplasia of epithelial cells that may result in xerophthalmia, keratosis, susceptibility to infections, and retarded growth; **2.** the original vitamin A, now known as retinol.

**vi·ta·min A₁ ac·id** SYN retinoic acid.

**vi·ta·min B** a group of water-soluble substances originally considered as one vitamin.

**vi·ta·min B₁** SYN thiamin.

**vi·ta·min B₆** pyridoxine and related compounds (pyridoxal; pyridoxamine).

**vi·ta·min B₁₂** generic descriptor for compounds exhibiting the biological activity of cyanocobalamin (cyanocob(III)alamin). The physiologically active vitamin B₁₂ coenzymes are methylcobalamin and deoxyadenosinecobalamine. A deficiency of vitamin B₁₂ causes megaloblastic anemia with or without peripheral neuropathy, and is often associated with certain methylmalonic acidurias. SEE pernicious anemia.

**vi·ta·min B com·plex** a pharmaceutical term applied to drug products containing a mixture of the B vitamins, usually B₁ (thiamine), B₂ (riboflavin), B₃ (nicotinamide), and B₆ (pyridoxine).

**vi·ta·min B₁₂ neu·rop·a·thy** SYN subacute combined degeneration of the spinal cord.

**vi·ta·min C** SYN ascorbic acid.

**vi·ta·min D** generic descriptor for all steroids exhibiting the biological activity of ergocalciferol or cholecalciferol, the antirachitic vitamins. They promote the proper utilization of calcium and phosphorus, thereby favoring proper bone and tooth formation in children.

**vi·ta·min D₂** SYN ergocalciferol.

**vi·ta·min D₃** SYN cholecalciferol.

**vi·ta·min D–bind·ing pro·tein** a plasma protein that binds vitamin D.

**vi·ta·min D milk** cow's milk to which vitamin D has been added, so as to provide 400 USP units of vitamin D per quart.

**vi·ta·min D–re·sis·tant rick·ets** a group of disorders characterized by hypophosphatemic osteomalacia; heritable renal tubular disorders and abnormalities in vitamin-D metabolism occur in some patients.

**vi·ta·min E** generic descriptor of tocol and tocotrienol derivatives possessing the biological activity of α-tocopherol; contained in various oils (wheat germ, cotton-seed, palm, rice) and whole grain cereals where it constitutes the nonsaponifiable fraction, also in animal tissue (liver, pancreas, heart) and lettuce; deficiency produces resorption or abortion in female rats and sterility in males.

**vi·ta·min K** generic descriptor for compounds with the biological activity of phylloquinone; fat-soluble, thermostable compounds found in alfalfa, hog liver, fish meal, and vegetable oils, essential for the formation of normal amounts of prothrombin.

**vi·ta·min K₁, vi·ta·min K₁(20)** SYN phylloquinone.

**vi·ta·min K₂, vi·ta·min K₂(30)** SYN menaquinone-6.

**vit·el·li·form ret·i·nal dys·tro·phy** SYN Best disease.

**vi·tel·line** (vī-tel′in) relating to the vitellus.

**vi·tel·line pole** the vegetative pole of an ovum.

**vi·tel·lo·in·tes·tin·al cyst** a small red sessile or pedunculated tumor at the umbilicus in an infant;

it is due to the persistence of a segment of the vitellointestinal duct.

**vi·tel·lus** (vī-tel′ŭs) SYN yolk (1). [L.]

**vi·ti·a·tion** (vish-ē-ā′shŭn) a change that impairs utility or reduces efficiency. [L. *vitiatio* fr. *vitio*, pp. *vitiatus*, to corrupt, fr. *vitium*, vice]

**vit·i·lig·i·nes** (vit-i-lij′i-nēz) plural of vitiligo.

**vit·i·lig·i·nous** (vit-i-lij′i-nŭs) relating to or characterized by vitiligo.

**vit·il·ig·i·nous chor·oid·i·tis** SYN bird shot retinochoroiditis.

🔲 **vit·i·li·go**, pl. **vit·i·lig·i·nes** (vit-i-lī′gō, vit-i-lij′i-nēz) the appearance on otherwise normal skin of nonpigmented white patches of varied sizes; hair in the affected areas is usually white. Epidermal melanocytes are completely lost in depigmented areas by an autoimmune process. See page B4. [L. a skin eruption, fr. *vitium*, blemish, vice]

**vit·rec·to·my** (vi-trek′tō-mē) removal of the vitreous by means of an instrument that simultaneously removes vitreous by suction and cutting and replaces it with saline or some other fluid. [vitreous + G. *ektomē*, excision]

**vit·re·i·tis** (vit-rē-ī′tis) inflammation of the corpus vitreum. SYN hyalitis. [L. *vitreus*, glassy, + G. *-itis*, inflammation]

△**vitreo-** vitreous. [L. *vitreus*, glassy]

**vit·re·o·den·tin** (vit′rē-ō-den′tin) dentin of a particularly brittle character.

**vit·re·o·ret·i·nal** (vit′rē-ō-ret′i-năl) pertaining to the retina and the vitreous body.

**vit·re·o·ta·pe·to·ret·i·nal dys·tro·phy** autosomal recessive bilateral peripheral and central retinoschisis with pigmentary degeneration of the retina, chorioretinal atrophy, vitreous degeneration, and night blindness. SYN Favre dystrophy.

**vit·re·ous** (vit′rē-ŭs) **1.** glassy; resembling glass. **2.** SYN vitreous body. [L. *vitreus*, glassy, fr. *vitrum*, glass]

**vit·re·ous bod·y** a transparent jelly-like substance filling the interior of the eyeball behind the lens; it is composed of a delicate network (vitreous stroma) enclosing in its meshes a watery fluid (vitreous humor). SYN corpus vitreum [TA], hyaloid body, vitreous (2), vitreum.

**vit·re·ous de·tach·ment** separation of the peripheral vitreous humor from the retina.

**vit·re·ous her·nia** prolapse of the vitreous humor into the anterior chamber; may follow removal or displacement of the lens from the lenticular space.

**vit·re·ous hu·mor** the fluid component of the vitreous body. USAGE NOTE: Often erroneously equated with the vitreous body.

**vit·re·ous la·mel·la** SYN lamina basalis choroideae.

**vit·re·ous mem·brane 1.** SYN posterior limiting layer of cornea. **2.** a condensation of fine collagen fibers in places in the cortex of the vitreous body; formerly thought to form a membrane or capsule at its periphery; **3.** SYN lamina basalis choroideae.

**vit·re·um** (vit′rē-ŭm) SYN vitreous body. [L. ntr. of *vitreus*, glassy]

**vit·ri·fi·ca·tion** (vit′ri-fi-kā′shŭn) conversion of dental porcelain (frit) to a glassy substance by heat and fusion. [L. *vitrium*, glassy, + *facio*, to make]

*in vit·ro* (in vē′trō) in an artificial environment, referring to a process or reaction occurring

therein, as in a test tube or culture media. Cf. *in vivo*. [L. in glass]

**vit·ro·nec·tin** (vit′rō-nek′tin) a plasma glycoprotein involved in inflammatory and repair reactions at sites of tissue damage.

*Vit·ta·for·ma* (vē-ta-fōr′ma) a genus of microsporidia that can infect humans and can cause keratitis in the immunocompetent and disseminated infection in the immunocompromised; formerly *Nosema*.

**vi·vax ma·lar·i·a** a malarial fever with paroxysms that recur every 48 hours or every other day (every third day, reckoning the day of the paroxysm as the first); the fever is induced by release of merozoites and their invasion of new red blood corpuscles; causative agent is *Plasmodium vivax*. SYN benign tertian fever.

△**vi·vi-** living. [L. *vivus*, alive]

**viv·i·fi·ca·tion** (viv′i-fi-kā′shŭn) SYN revivification (2). [L. *vivifico*, pp. *-atus*, fr. *vivus*, alive, + *facio*, to make]

**vi·vip·a·rous** (vī-vip′ă-rŭs) giving birth to living young, in distinction to oviparous, or egg-laying. [vivi- + L. *pario*, to bear]

**viv·i·sec·tion** (viv-i-sek′shŭn) any cutting operation on a living animal for purposes of experimentation; often extended to denote any form of animal experimentation. [vivi- + section]

**viv·i·sec·tion·ist, viv·i·sec·tor** (vi-vi-sek′shŭn-ist, vi-vi-sek′tŏr) one who practices vivisection.

*in vi·vo* (in vī′vō) in the living body, referring to a process or reaction occurring therein. Cf. *in vitro*. [L. in the living being]

*in vi·vo* **fer·til·i·za·tion** fertilization of a mature oocyte within the distal uterine tube of a fertile donor female (rather than in an artificial medium), for subsequent nonsurgical transfer to an infertile recipient.

**VLDL** very low density lipoprotein. SEE lipoprotein.

**VMA** vanillylmandelic acid.

**$VO_{2max}$** SYN maximal oxygen consumption.

**$VO_2$** oxygen consumption.

**vo·cal** (vō′kăl) pertaining to the voice or the organs of speech. [L. *vocalis*]

🔲 **vo·cal fold** the sharp edge of a fold of mucous membrane overlying the vocal ligament and stretching along either wall of the larynx from the angle between the laminae of the thyroid cartilage to the vocal process of the arytenoid cartilage; the vocal folds are the agents concerned in voice production. See page B8. SYN plica vocalis [TA], true vocal cord.

**vo·cal frem·i·tus** the vibration in the chest wall, felt on palpation, produced by the spoken voice.

**vo·cal fry** (vō′kal frī) phonation at an unnaturally low frequency resulting in low-frequency popping and ticking sounds. SYN glottalization.

**vo·ca·lis mus·cle** *origin*, depression between the two laminae of thyroid cartilage; *insertion*, portions of vocal process of arytenoid; *action*, shortens and relaxes vocal cords; *nerve supply*, recurrent laryngeal; a number of the deeper and finer fibers of the thyroarytenoid muscle attached directly to the outer side of the true vocal cord. SYN musculus vocalis [TA], vocal muscle.

**vo·cal lig·a·ment** the band that extends on either side from the thyroid cartilage to the vocal process of the arytenoid cartilage; it is the thickened, free upper border of the conus elasticus of the larynx. SYN ligamentum vocale [TA].

**vo·cal mus·cle** SYN vocalis muscle.

**vo·cal nod·ules** small, circumscribed, bilateral, beadlike enlargements on the vocal folds caused by overuse or abuse of the voice. SYN singer's nodules, speaker's nodules.

**vo·cal pro·cess of ar·y·te·noid car·ti·lage** the lower end of the anterior margin of the arytenoid cartilage to which the vocal cord is attached.

**vo·cal res·o·nance (VR)** the voice sounds as heard on auscultation of the chest.

**vo·cal spectrum** the frequency and intensity ranges of the voice.

**vo·cal tract** the air passages above the glottis (including the pharynx, oral and nasal cavities, and the paranasal sinuses) that contribute to the quality of the voice.

**Vo·gel law** when a phenotype may be transmitted by various modes of mendelian inheritance, the dominant will have the least deleterious phenotype, the recessive the most, and the X-linked intermediate between the two.

**V̇O₂ HR (ox·y·gen pulse)** oxygen pulse.

**voice** (voys) the sound made by air passing out through the larynx and upper respiratory tract, the vocal folds being approximated. [L. *vox*]

**voice fa·tigue syn·drome** weakness and loss of the voice usually toward the end of the day because of abuse by using it too long and too loudly.

**void** (voyd) to evacuate urine or feces.

**void·ing cys·to·gram** SYN cystourethrogram.

**void·ing cys·to·u·reth·ro·gram (VCUG)** an x-ray image made during voiding and with the bladder and urethra filled with contrast medium to demonstrate the urethra. SYN micturating cystourethrogram.

**vo·la** (vō′lă) palm of the hand or sole of the foot. [L.]

**vo·lar** (vō′lăr) referring to the vola; denoting either the palm of the hand or sole of the foot.

**vol·a·tile** (vol′ă-til) **1.** tending to evaporate rapidly. **2.** tending toward violence, explosiveness, or rapid change. [L. *volatilis*, fr. *volo*, to fly]

**vol·a·tile oil** a substance of oily consistency and feel, derived from a plant and containing the principles to which the odor and taste of the plant are due (essential oil); in contrast to a fatty oil, a volatile oil evaporates when exposed to the air and thus is capable of distillation. SYN ethereal oil.

**vol·a·til·i·za·tion** (vol′ă-til-i-zā′shŭn) SYN evaporation. [fr. L. *volatilis*, volatile, fr. *volo*, pp. *volatus*, to fly]

**vo·li·tion** (vō-lish′ŭn) the conscious impulse to perform any act or to abstain from its performance; voluntary action. [L. *volo*,, to wish]

**vo·li·tion·al** (vo-lish′ŭn-ăl) done by an act of will; relating to volition.

**vo·li·tion·al trem·or 1.** a tremor that can be arrested by a strong effort of the will; **2.** SYN intention tremor.

**Volk·mann chei·li·tis** (fōk′mahn) SYN cheilitis glandularis.

**Volk·mann con·trac·ture** (fōk′mahn) ischemic contracture resulting from irreversible necrosis of muscle tissue, produced by a compartment syndrome; classically involves the forearm flexor muscles.

**Volk·mann spoon** (fōk′mahn) a sharp spoon for scraping away carious bone or other diseased tissue.

**vol·ley** (vol′ē) a synchronous group of impulses induced simultaneously by artificial stimulation of either nerve fibers or muscle fibers. [Fr. *volée*, fr. L. *volo*, to fly]

**volt (v, V)** (vōlt) the unit of electromotive force; the electromotive force that will produce a current of 1 ampere in a circuit that has a resistance of 1 ohm; i.e., joule per coulomb. [Alessandro Volta, It. physicist, 1745–1827]

**volt·age** (vōl′tej) electromotive force, pressure, or potential expressed in volts.

**volt·am·pere** (vōlt′am-pēr) a unit of electrical power; the product of 1 volt by 1 ampere; equivalent to 1 watt or $\frac{1}{1000}$ kilowatt.

**Vol·to·li·ni dis·ease** (vōl-tō-lē′nē) infectious disease of the labyrinth, leading to meningitis in young children.

**vol·ume (V, *V*)** (vol′yŭm) space occupied by matter, expressed usually in cubic millimeters, cubic centimeters, liters, etc. SEE ALSO capacity, water. [L. *volumen*, something rolled up, scroll, fr. *volvo*, to roll]

**vol·ume at ATPS** a volume of gas at ambient (A) temperature (T) (room temperature) and barometric pressure (P) saturated (S) with water vapor.

**vol·ume at BTPS** a volume of gas saturated (S) with water vapor at 37°C (body (B) temperature (T)) and the ambient environmental barometric pressure (P).

**vol·ume at STPD** a volume of gas, at the standard (S) temperature (T) of 0°C, a barometric pressure (P) of 760 mmHg, and dry (D).

**vol·ume con·trol·led ven·ti·la·tion** a mode of mechanical ventilation in which the ventilator delivers a preset volume waveform; the resultant airway pressure waveform depends on the shape of the flow waveform and respiratory system resistance and compliance.

**vol·ume in·dex** an indication of the relative size (e.g., volume) of erythrocytes, calculated as follows: hematocrit value, expressed as per cent of normal ÷ red blood cell count, expressed as per cent of normal = volume index.

**vol·u·met·ric** (vol-yu-met′rik) relating to measurement by volume.

**vol·u·met·ric a·nal·y·sis** quantitative analysis by the addition of graduated amounts of a standard test solution to a solution of a known amount of the substance analyzed, until the reaction is just at an end; depends upon the stoichiometric nature of the reaction between the test solution and the unknown.

**vol·u·met·ric so·lu·tion (VS)** a solution made by mixing measured volumes of the components.

**vol·ume ven·ti·la·tor** a device for delivering a preset volume of inspired gas into the lungs; within specified limits, the volume is independent of the pressure required to deliver that volume.

**vol·un·tary** (vol′ŭn-tār-ē) relating or acting in obedience to the will; not obligatory. [L. *voluntarius*, fr. *voluntas*, will, fr. *volo*, to wish]

**vol·un·tary mus·cle** one whose action is under the control of the will; all the striated muscles, except the heart, are voluntary muscles.

**vo·lute** (vō-loot) rolled up; convoluted. [L. *voluta*, a scroll, fr. *volvo*, pp. *volutus*, to roll]

**vol·vu·lus** (vol′vyu-lŭs) a twisting of the intestine causing obstruction; if left untreated may result in vascular compromise of the involved intestine. [L. *volvo*, to roll]

**vo•mer**, gen. **vo•me•ris** (vō′mer, vō′mer-is) [TA] a flat bone of trapezoidal shape forming the inferior and posterior portion of the nasal septum; it articulates with the sphenoid, ethmoid, two maxillae, and two palatine bones. [L. ploughshare]

**vo•mer•ine** (vō′mer-ēn) relating to the vomer.

**vom•er•o•na•sal car•ti•lage, vo•mer•ine car•ti•lage** a narrow strip of cartilage located between the lower edge of the cartilage of the nasal septum and the vomer. SYN cartilago vomeronasalis [TA].

**vom•it 1.** to eject matter from the stomach through the mouth. **2.** vomitus; the matter so ejected. SYN vomitus (2). [L. *vomo*, pp. *vomitus*, to vomit]

**vom•it•ing** (vom′i-ting) the ejection of matter from the stomach through the esophagus and mouth. SYN emesis (1), vomitus (1).

**vom•it•ing of preg•nan•cy** vomiting occurring in the early months of pregnancy.

**vom•it•ing re•flex** vomiting (contraction of the abdominal muscles with relaxation of the cardiac sphincter of the stomach and of the muscles of the throat) elicited by a variety of stimuli, especially one applied to the region of the fauces. SYN pharyngeal reflex (2).

**vom•i•tu•ri•tion** (vom′i-too-rish′ŭn) SYN retching.

**vom••i•tus** (vom′i-tŭs) **1.** SYN vomiting. **2.** SYN vomit (2). [L. a vomiting, vomit]

**von Gier•ke dis•ease** (vahn gēr′kĕ) SYN type 1 glycogenosis.

**von Grae•fe sign** (van grā′fĕ) SYN Graefe sign.

**von Spee curve** (vahn shpē) SYN curve of Spee.

**von Wil•le•brand dis•ease** (vahn vil′ĕ-brahnt) a hemorrhagic diathesis characterized by tendency to bleed primarily from mucous membranes, prolonged bleeding time, normal platelet count, normal clot retraction, partial and variable deficiency of factor VIIIR, and possibly a morphologic defect of platelets; autosomal dominant inheritance with reduced penetrance and variable expressivity, caused by mutation in the von Willebrand factor gene (VWF) on 12p. Type III von Willebrand disease is a more severe disorder with markedly reduced factor VIIIR levels. There is a recessive version of this disease, which has the remarkable property that it represents a mutation at the same locus as the dominant form.

**vor•tex**, pl. **vor•ti•ces** (vōr′teks, vōr′ti-sēz) **1.** SYN verticil. **2.** SYN whorl (5). **3.** SYN vortex lentis. [L. whirlpool, whorl, fr. *verto* or *vorto*, to turn around]

**vor•tex cor•ne•al dys•tro•phy** a swirling pattern of abnormally pigmented corneal epithelial cells, seen in Fabry disease and in response to certain medications (including chloroquine, chlorpromazine, and amiodarone).

**vor•tex of heart** a spiral arrangement of muscular fibers at the apex of the heart. SYN whorl (2).

**vor•tex len•tis** one of the stellar figures on the surface of the lens of the eye. SYN vortex (3).

**vor•tex veins** several veins (usually four) from the vascular tunic formed of veins accompanying the posterior ciliary arteries and the ciliary body; these drain into the superior or inferior ophthalmic vein. SYN vorticose veins.

**vor•ti•cose veins** SYN vortex veins.

**Vos•si•us len•tic•u•lar ring** (fos′ē-ŭs) a ringshaped opacity found on the anterior lens capsule after contusion of the eye, due to pigment and blood.

**vox•el** (vok′sel) a contraction for volume element, which is the basic unit of CT or MR reconstruction; represented as a pixel in the display of the CT or MR image.

**voy•eur** (vwah-yer′) one who practices voyeurism.

**voy•eur•ism** (vwah-yer′izm) the practice of obtaining sexual pleasure by looking at the naked body or genitals of another or at erotic acts between others. SYN scopophilia. [Fr. *voir*, to see]

**V-pat•tern es•o•tro•pia** convergent strabismus greater in downward than in upward gaze.

**V-pat•tern ex•o•tro•pia** divergent strabismus greater in upward than in downward gaze.

**VR** vocal resonance.

**VS** volumetric solution.

**vul•ga•ris** (vŭl-gā′ris) ordinary; of the usual type. [L. fr. *vulgus*, a crowd]

**vul•ner•a•ble phase** a period in the cardiac cycle during which an ectopic impulse may lead to repetitive activity such as flutter or fibrillation of the affected chamber.

**Vul•pi•an at•ro•phy** (vool′pyah) progressive spinal muscular atrophy beginning in the shoulder.

**vul•sel•la, vul•sel•lum** (vŭl-sel′ă, vŭl-sel′lŭm) SYN vulsella forceps. [L. pincers, fr. *vello*, pp. *vulsus*, to pluck]

**vul•sel•la for•ceps, vul•sel•lum for•ceps** a forceps with hooks at the tip of each blade. SYN vulsella, vulsellum.

**vul•va**, pl. **vul•vae** (vŭl′vă) [TA] the external genitalia of the female, composed of the mons pubis, the labia majora and minora, the clitoris, the vestibule of the vagina and its glands, and the opening of the urethra and of the vagina. [L. a wrapper or covering, seed covering, womb, fr. *volvo*, to roll]

**vul•var, vul•val** (vŭl′văr, vŭl′văl) relating to the vulva.

**vul•var intra•epi•the•li•al ne•o•pla•sia** preinvasive squamous cell carcinoma (carcinoma in situ) limited to vulvar epithelium; like vaginal or cervical intraepithelial neoplasia, graded histologically on a scale from 1 to 3 or subdivided into low-grade and high-grade intraepithelial malignancy; usually related to human papilloma virus infection; may progress to invasive carcinoma.

**vul•vec•to•my** (vŭl-vek′tō-mē) excision (either partial, complete, or radical) of the vulva. [vulva + G. *ektomē*, excision]

**vul•vi•tis** (vŭl-vī′tis) inflammation of the vulva. [vulva + G. *-itis*, inflammation]

△**vul•vo-** the vulva. [L. *vulva*]

**vul•vo•vag•i•ni•tis** (vŭl′vō-vaj-i-nī′tis) inflammation of both vulva and vagina.

**V wave** a large pressure wave visible in recordings from either atrium or its incoming veins, normally produced by venous return but becoming very large when blood regurgitates through the A-V valve beyond the chamber from which the recording is made.

**W** tungsten; watt; tryptophan.

**Wa·chen·dorf mem·brane** (vahk′en-dōrf) **1.** SYN pupillary membrane. **2.** SYN cell membrane.

**waist** (wāst) the portion of the trunk between the ribs and the pelvis. [A.S. *waext*]

**waist-to-hip ratio** waist circumference divided by hip circumference; indicator of abdominal (visceral) obesity, and predictor of health risk independent of total percent body fat. Ratio that exceeds 0.80 for women and 0.95 for men correlates with increased risk of death, even after controlling for BMI.

**Wal·den·ström mac·ro·glob·u·lin·e·mia** (vahl′den-strerm) macroglobulinemia occurring in elderly persons, characterized by proliferation of cells resembling lymphocytes or plasma cells in the bone marrow, anemia, increased sedimentation rate, and hyperglobulinemia with a narrow peak in γ-globulin or β$_2$-globulin at about 19 S units. The spleen, liver, or lymph nodes are often enlarged and there is frequently purpura or mucosal bleeding.

**Wal·dey·er sheath** (vahl′dī-er) the tubular space between the bladder wall and the intramural portion of the ureter as it courses obliquely through this structure; actually a space and not a true sheath.

**walk 1.** to move on foot. **2.** the characteristic manner in which one moves on foot. SEE ALSO gait. [M.E. *walken*, fr. O.E. *wealcen*, to roll]

**Walk·er chart** (wŏk-er) a system of plotting the relative fetal and placental sizes.

**walk·ing** (wo′king) characteristic of sequential movement or progression in steps.

**walk-through an·gi·na** a circumstance in which despite continuing activity, such as walking, the pain of angina pectoris diminishes or disappears.

**wall** (wawl) an investing part enclosing a cavity such as the chest or abdomen, or covering a cell or any anatomical unit. A wall, as of the chest, abdomen, or any hollow organ. SYN paries. [L. *vallum*]

**wal·le·ri·an** (waw-ler′ē-an) relating to or described by A.V. Waller.

**wal·le·ri·an de·gen·er·a·tion** (wahl-e′rē-an) the degenerative changes observed in the distal segment of a peripheral nerve fiber (axon and myelin) when its continuity with its cell body is interrupted by a focal lesion. SYN orthograde degeneration, secondary degeneration.

**wall-eye** (wawl′ī) **1.** SYN exotropia. **2.** absence of color in the iris, or leukoma of the cornea.

**wall-eyed bi·lat·er·al in·ter·nuc·le·ar oph·thal·mo·ple·gia (WEBINO)** a form of internuclear ophthalmoplegia associated with an exotropia.

**Walsh** (wahlsh), Patrick Craig, U.S. urologist, *1938. SEE neurovascular bundle of Walsh, Walsh procedure.

**Walsh procedure** (wahlsh) anatomic (nerve-sparing) radical retropubic prostatectomy.

**Wal·thard cell rest** (vahl′tahrd) a nest of epithelial cells occurring in the peritoneum of the uterine tubes or ovary; when neoplastic, possibly comprising one of the components of the Brenner tumor.

**Wal·ther di·la·tor** (vahl′ter) a gently curved instrument that tapers to an increased diameter, used to dilate the female urethra.

**Wal·ther ducts** (vahl′ter) SYN minor sublingual ducts.

**Wal·ther gan·gli·on** (vahl′ter) SYN ganglion impar.

**waltzed flap** SYN caterpillar flap.

**wan·der·ing** (wahn′der-ing) moving about; not fixed; abnormally motile. [A.S. *wandrian*, to wander]

**wan·der·ing ab·scess** SYN perforating abscess.

**wan·der·ing cell** SYN ameboid cell.

**wan·der·ing goi·ter** SYN diving goiter.

**wan·der·ing kid·ney** SYN floating kidney.

**wan·der·ing pace·mak·er** a disturbance of the normal cardiac rhythm in which the site of the controlling pacemaker shifts from beat to beat, usually between the sinus and A-V nodes, often with gradual sequential changes in P waves between upright and inverted in a given ECG lead.

*Wang·i·el·la* (wang-gē-el′ă) a dematiaceous genus of fungi; *Wangiella dermatitidis* is an etiological agent of phaeohyphomycosis.

**War·burg ap·pa·ra·tus** (vahr′berg) an apparatus for measuring the oxygen consumption of incubated tissue slices by manometric measurement of changes in gas pressure produced by oxygen absorption in an enclosed flask.

**War·burg the·o·ry** (vahr′berg) that the development of cancer is due to irreversible damage to the respiratory mechanism of cells, leading to the selective multiplication of cells with increased glycolytic metabolism, both aerobic and anaerobic.

**ward** (wōrd) a large room or hall in a hospital containing a number of beds. SEE ALSO unit. [A.S. *weard*]

**Ward·rop meth·od** (ward′rŏp) treatment of aneurysm by ligation of the artery at some distance beyond the sac, leaving one or more branches of the artery between the sac and the ligature.

**Ward tri·an·gle** (word) an area of diminished density in the trabecular pattern of the neck of the femur evident by x-ray as well as by direct inspection of a specimen.

**warm-up** a program of gradually increasing activity to raise muscle temperature and heart rate in preparation for more strenuous exercise.

**warm-up phenomenon** progressive diminution of the myotonic response of a muscle, during repeated contraction of the muscle.

**war neu·ro·sis** a stress condition or mental disorder induced by conditions existing in warfare. SEE ALSO battle fatigue. SYN battle neurosis.

**wart** (wŏrt) SYN verruca.

**War·ten·berg symp·tom** (wor′tĕn-bĕrg) **1.** flexion of the thumb when the patient attempts to flex the four fingers against resistance, a "pyramid sign". **2.** intense pruritus of the tip of the nose and nostrils in cases of cerebral tumor.

**wash** (wosh) a solution used to clean or bathe a part.

**wash-out** (wosh-out) a technique for eliminating (washing out) a specific substance.

**was·tage** (wās′tāj) decay, loss, or diminution of something.

**wast·ing** (wāst′ing) **1.** SYN emaciation. **2.** denoting a disease characterized by emaciation.

**was·ting syn·drome** progressive involuntary weight loss seen in patients with HIV infection; may be due to a number of factors acting alone or in combination, including inadequate oral intake of food, altered metabolic state and/or malabsorption. Does not respond to increased caloric intake. Defined as profound involuntary weight loss of greater than 10% of baseline body weight, plus either chronic diarrhea (at least 2 loose stools per day for >30 days or chronic weakness and documented fever (for >30 days, intermittent or constant) in the absence of concurrent illness or condition other than HIV infection that could explain the findings (such as cancer, tuberculosis, cryptosporidiosis, or other specific enteritis). SYN HIV wasting syndrome.

**wa•ter** (wah′ter) **1.** a clear, odorless, tasteless liquid, solidifying at 32°F (0°C and R), and boiling at 212°F (100°C, 80°R), that is present in all animal and vegetable tissues and dissolves more substances than any other liquid. SEE ALSO volume. **2.** euphemism for urine. **3.** a pharmacopeial preparation of a clear, saturated aqueous solution (unless otherwise specified) of volatile oils, or other aromatic or volatile substances, prepared by processes involving distillation or solution (agitation followed by filtration). [A.S. *waeter*]

**wa•ter of crys•tal•li•za•tion** water of constitution that unites with certain salts and is essential to their arrangement in crystalline form; e.g., $CuSO_4 \cdot 5H_2O$.

**wa•ter•fall** (wah′ter-fawl) a term used to describe flow in vascular beds where lateral pressure tending to collapse vessels greatly exceeds venous pressure. Flow is independent of venous pressure and occurs only when arterial pressure exceeds lateral pressure.

**wa•ter-ham•mer pulse** a pulse with forcible impulse but immediate collapse, characteristic of aortic insufficiency. SEE ALSO Corrigan sign. SYN cannonball pulse.

**Wa•ter•house-Fri•de•rich•sen syn•drome** (wah′ter-hows-frid′er-ik-sen) a condition due to meningococcemia, occurring mainly in children under 10 years of age, characterized by vomiting, diarrhea, extensive purpura, cyanosis, tonoclonic convulsions, and circulatory collapse, usually with meningitis and hemorrhage into the adrenal glands.

**wa•ter itch 1.** SYN cutaneous ancylostomiasis. **2.** SYN schistosomal dermatitis.

**wa•ter of me•tab•o•lism** the water formed in the body by oxidation of the hydrogen of the food, the greatest amount being produced in the metabolism of fat (about 117 g/100 g of fat).

**wa•ters** (wah′ters) colloquialism for amniotic fluid.

**wa•ter•shed 1.** the area of marginal blood flow at the extreme periphery of a vascular bed. **2.** slopes in the abdominal cavity, formed by projections of the lumbar vertebrae and the pelvic brim that determine the direction in which a free effusion will gravitate when the body is in a supine position.

**wa•ter•shed in•farc•tion** cortical infarction in an area where the distributions of major cerebral arteries meet or overlap.

**Wa•ters op•er•a•tion** (wah′terz) an extraperitoneal cesarean section with a supravesical approach.

**Wa•ters pro•jec•tion** (wah′terz) a posteroanterior radiographic view of the skull made with the orbitomeatal line at an angle of 37° from the plane of the film, to show the orbits and maxillary sinuses.

**wa•ter-trap stom•ach** a ptotic and dilated stomach, having a relatively high (though normally placed) pyloric outlet which is held up by the gastrohepatic ligament.

**Wat•son-Crick he•lix** (waht′sŭn-crik) the helical structure assumed by two strands of deoxyribonucleic acid, held together throughout their length by hydrogen bonds between bases on opposite strands, referred to as Watson-Crick base pairing. SEE base pair. SYN DNA helix, double helix.

**watt (W)** (waht) the SI unit of electrical power; the power available when the current is 1 ampere and the electromotive force is 1 volt; equal to 1 joule ($10^7$ ergs) per second or 1 voltampere. [James *Watt,* Scot. engineer, 1736–1819]

**wave** (wāv) **1.** a movement of particles in an elastic body, whether solid or fluid, whereby an advancing series of alternate elevations and depressions, or expansions and condensations, is produced. **2.** the elevation of the pulse, felt by the finger, or represented graphically in the curved line of the sphygmograph. **3.** the complete cycle of changes in the level of a source of energy that is repetitively varying with respect to time; in the electrocardiogram and the electroencephalogram the wave is essentially a voltage-time graph. SEE ALSO rhythm. [A.S. *wafian,* to fluctuate]

**wave•form** the form of a pulse; e.g., an arterial pressure or displacement wave; or of the pacemaker pulse as demonstrated on the oscilloscope under a specified load.

**wave•length** ($\lambda$) (wāv′length) the distance from one point on a wave (frequently shaped like a sine curve) to the next point in the same phase; i.e., from peak to peak or from trough to trough.

**wax** (waks) **1.** a thick, tenacious substance, plastic at room temperature, secreted by bees for building the cells of their honeycomb. **2.** any substance with physical properties similar to those of beeswax, of animal, vegetable, or mineral origin (oils, lipids, or fats that are solids at room temperature). **3.** esters of high molecular weight fatty acids with monohydric or dihydric alcohols (aliphatic or cyclic), that are solid at room temperature. Often accompanied by free fatty acids. [A.S. *weax*]

**wax•ing, wax•ing-up** (wak′sing) the contouring of a pattern in wax, generally applied to the shaping in wax of the contours of a trial denture or a crown prior to casting in metal.

**wax•y de•gen•er•a•tion 1.** SYN amyloid degeneration. **2.** SYN Zenker degeneration.

**wax•y kid•ney** SYN amyloid kidney.

**wax•y spleen** amyloidosis of the spleen.

**Wb** weber.

**WBC** white blood cell.

**WDLL** well-differentiated lymphocytic lymphoma.

**weak•ness** (wēk′nes) **1.** lack of strength or potency. **2.** inability to perform normally.

**wean** (wēn) to implement weaning. [A.S. *wenian*]

**wean•ing** (wēn′ing) **1.** permanent deprivation of breast milk and commencement of nourishment with other food. **2.** gradual withdrawal of a patient from dependence on a life support system or other form of therapy.

**wear-and-tear pig•ment** lipofuscin that accumulates in aging or atrophic cells as a residue of lysosomal digestion.

**web** (wĕb) a tissue or membrane bridging a space. SEE ALSO tela. [A.S.]

**webbed fin·gers** two or more fingers united and enclosed in a common sheath of skin.

**webbed neck** the broad neck due to lateral folds of skin extending from the clavicle to the head but containing no muscles, bones, or other structures; occurs in Turner and Noonan syndromes.

**web·bing** (web′ing) congenital condition apparent when adjacent structures are joined by a broad band of tissue not normally present to such a degree.

**Web·er** (vā′ber), Ernst H., German physiologist and anatomist, 1795–1878. SEE Weber paradox, Fechner-Weber law, Weber-Fechner law.

**Web·er** (web′er), Sir Hermann, English physician, 1823–1918. SEE Weber syndrome.

**we·ber (Wb)** (web′er) SI unit of magnetic flux, equal to volt-seconds (V·s). [Wilhelm E. *Weber*]

**We·ber-Fech·ner law** (vā′ber-fek′ner) the intensity of a sensation varies by a series of equal increments (arithmetically) as the strength of the stimulus is increased geometrically; if a series of stimuli is applied and so adjusted in strength that each stimulus causes a just perceptible change in intensity of the sensation, then the strength of each stimulus differs from the preceding one by a constant fraction. SYN Fechner-Weber law, Weber law.

**We·ber law** (vā′ber) SYN Weber-Fechner law.

**Weber par·a·dox** (vā′ber) if a muscle is loaded beyond its power to contract, it may elongate.

**Web·er stain** (we′ber) a modified trichrome stain for microsporidian spores in which the chromotrope 2R is 10 times the normal concentration used in trichrome stains for stool specimens and the counterstain is fast green.

**Weber syn·drome** (vā′ber) midbrain tegmentum lesion characterized by ipsilateral oculomotor nerve paresis and contralateral paralysis of the extremities, face, and tongue.

**Web·er test for hear·ing** (vā′ber) the application of a vibrating tuning fork to one of several points in the midline of the head or face, to ascertain in which ear the sound is heard by bone conduction, that ear being the affected one if the sound-conducting mechanism of the middle ear is at fault, but the normal one if there is a sensorineural hearing loss in the other ear.

**We·ber tri·an·gle** (vā′ber) on the sole of the foot, an area indicated by the heads of the first and fifth metatarsal bone and the center of the plantar surface of the heel.

**WEBINO** wall-eyed bilateral internuclear ophthalmoplegia.

**Wechs·ler in·tel·li·gence scales** (weks′ler) continuously revised and updated standardized scales for the measurement of general intelligence in preschool children (Wechsler preschool and primary scale of intelligence), in children (Wechsler intelligence scale for children), and in adults (Wechsler adult intelligence scale).

**wedge-and-groove joint** a form of fibrous joint in which the sharp edge of one bone is received in a cleft in the edge of the other. SYN schindylesis [TA], wedge-and-groove suture.

**wedge-and-groove su·ture** SYN wedge-and-groove joint.

**wedge bone** SYN intermediate cuneiform bone, lateral cuneiform bone, medial cuneiform bone.

**wedge fracture** compression fracture of the anterior part of a vertebral body, resulting in a wedge shape that is narrower anteriorly.

**wedge pres·sure** the intravascular pressure reading obtained when a fine catheter is advanced until it completely occludes a small blood vessel or is sealed in place by inflation of a small cuff; commonly measured in the lung to estimate left atrial pressure.

**wedge re·sec·tion** removal of a wedge-shaped portion of the ovary; used in the treatment of virilizing disorders of ovarian origin, such as the polycystic ovarian syndrome.

**Weeks ba·cil·lus** (wēks) SYN *Haemophilus influenzae.*

**Week·sel·la** (wēk-sel′a) a genus of nonoxidative, aerobic Gram-negative rods.

**Week·sel·la zoo·hel·cum** a bacterium producing infections in bites or scratches by dogs or cats.

**We·ge·ner gran·u·lo·ma·to·sis** (vā′gĕ-ner) a disease, occurring mainly in the fourth and fifth decades, characterized by necrotizing granulomas and ulceration of the upper respiratory tract, with purulent rhinorrhea, nasal obstruction, and sometimes with otorrhea, hemoptysis, pulmonary infiltration and cavitation, and fever; exophthalmos, involvement of the larynx and pharynx, and glomerulonephritis may occur; the underlying condition is a vasculitis affecting small vessels, and is possibly due to an immune disorder.

**Wei·gert i·o·dine so·lu·tion** (vī′gert) an iodine-potassium iodide mixture used as a reagent to alter crystal and methyl violet so that they are retained by certain bacteria and fungi.

**Wei·gert iron he·ma·tox·y·lin stain** (vī′gert) a nuclear staining solution containing hematoxylin, ferric chloride, and hydrochloric acid; useful in combination with van Gieson stain, especially for demonstrating connective tissue elements or *Entamoeba histolytica* in sections.

**Wei·gert law** (vī′gert) the loss or destruction of a part or element in the organic world is likely to result in compensatory replacement and overproduction of tissue during the process of regeneration or repair (or both), as in the formation of callus when a fractured bone heals.

**Wei·gert stain for ac·ti·no·my·ces** (vī′gert) a staining method using immersion in a dark red orsellin solution in alcohol, then staining in crystal-violet solution.

**Wei·gert stain for elas·tin** (vī′gert) a staining solution of fuchsin, resorcin, and ferric chloride; elastic fibers stain blue-black.

**Wei·gert stain for fi·brin** (vī′gert) a staining method using solutions of aniline-crystal violet and iodine-potassium iodide, then decolorizing in aniline oil and xylol; the fibrin is stained dark blue.

**Wei·gert stain for my·e·lin** (vī′gert) a staining method using ferric chloride and hematoxylin; myelin stains deep blue, degenerated portions a light yellowish color.

**Wei·gert stain for neu·rog·lia** (vī′gert) a complicated process in which the final treatment is like that for staining fibrin; neuroglia and nuclei stain blue.

**weight** (wāt) the product of the force of gravity, defined internationally as $9.80665 \text{ m/s}^2$, times the mass of the body. [A.S. *gewiht*]

W
e

**weight-supported exercise** exercise performed with one's body weight artificially supported (e.g., stationary cycling). SYN non-weight-bearing exercise.

**Weil dis·ease** (vīl) a form of leptospirosis generally caused by *Leptospira interrogans* serogroup *icterohaemorrhagiae*, believed to be acquired by contact with the urine of infected rats; characterized clinically by fever, jaundice, muscular pains, conjunctival congestion, and albuminuria; agglutinins regularly appear in the serum.

**Weil-Fe·lix test, Weil-Fe·lix re·ac·tion** (vīl-fā′liks) a test for the presence and type of rickettsial disease based on the agglutination of X-strains of *Proteus vulgaris* with suspected rickettsia in a patient's blood serum.

**Weill-Mar·che·sa·ni syn·drome** (vīl-mahr-kĕ-sah′nē) ectopia lentis (lens abnormally round and small), short stature, and brachydactyly; recessive autosomal inheritance.

**Wein·berg re·ac·tion** (wīn′berg) a complement fixation test of the presence of hydatid disease.

**Weiss sign** (vīs) SYN Chvostek sign.

**Welch ba·cil·lus** (welch) SYN *Clostridium perfringens.*

**well-dif·fer·en·ti·at·ed lym·pho·cyt·ic lym·pho·ma (WDLL)** essentially the same disease as chronic lymphocytic leukemia, except that lymphocytes are not increased in the peripheral blood; lymph nodes are enlarged and other lymphoid tissue or bone marrow is infiltrated by small lymphocytes.

**well·ness** (wel′nĕs) a philosophy of life and personal hygiene that views health as not merely the absence of illness but the fullest realization of one's physical and mental potential, as achieved through positive attitudes, fitness training, a diet low in fat and high in fiber, and the avoidance of unhealthful practices (smoking, drug and alcohol abuse, overeating).

**welt** (wĕlt) SYN wheal. [O.E. *waelt*]

**wen** (wĕn) old term for pilar cyst. [A.S.]

**Wenc·ke·bach block** (veng′ke-bahk) a first-degree atrioventricular block, in which there is a progressive lengthening of conduction, as manifested in prolonged P-Q interval on electrocardiography, until one QRS complex and T wave are missed.

**Wenc·ke·bach pe·ri·od** (veng′ke-bahk) a sequence of cardiac cycles in the electrocardiogram ending in a dropped beat due to A-V block, the preceding cycles showing progressively lengthening P-R intervals; the P-R interval following the dropped beat is again shortened.

**Werl·hof dis·ease** (verl-hof) formerly used term for idiopathic thrombocytopenic purpura.

**Wer·mer syndrome** (wĕr′mĕr) SYN multiple endocrine neoplasia 1.

**Wer·ner syn·drome** (vĕr′nĕr) a premature aging disorder consisting of scleroderma-like skin changes, bilateral juvenile cataracts, progeria, hypogonadism, and diabetes mellitus; autosomal recessive inheritance, caused by mutation in the WRN gene, which encodes a helicase protein on chromosome 8p.

**Wer·nic·ke apha·sia** (ver′nĭ-kĕ) SYN sensory aphasia.

**Wer·nic·ke cen·ter** (ver′nĭ-kĕ) the region of the cerebral cortex thought to be essential for understanding and formulating coherent, propositional speech; it encompasses a large region of the pari-etal and temporal lobes near the lateral sulcus of the left cerebral hemisphere; corresponding approximately to Brodmann areas 40, 39, and 22. SYN sensory speech center.

**Wer·nic·ke-Kor·sa·koff en·ceph·a·lop·a·thy** (ver′nĭ-kĕ-kor-′sĕ-kof) SEE Wernicke syndrome, Korsakoff syndrome.

**Wer·nic·ke-Kor·sa·koff syn·drome** (ver′nĭ-kĕ-kor-′sĕ-kof) the coexistence of Wernicke and Korsakoff syndromes.

**Wer·nic·ke re·ac·tion** (ver′nĭ-kĕ) in hemianopia, a reaction due to damage of the optic tract, consisting in loss of pupillary constriction when the light is directed to the blind side of the retina; pupillary constriction is maintained when light stimulates the normal side. This sign cannot be seen with a bright light because of intraocular scatter onto the seeing half of the retina.

**Wer·nic·ke syn·drome** (ver′nĭ-kĕ) a condition frequently encountered in chronic alcoholics, largely due to thiamin deficiency and characterized by disturbances in ocular motility, pupillary alterations, nystagmus, and ataxia with tremors; an organic-toxic psychosis is often an associated finding, and Korsakoff syndrome often coexists; characteristic cellular pathology found in several areas of the brain.

**Wert·heim op·er·a·tion** (vārt′hīm) a radical operation for carcinoma of the uterus in which as much as possible of the vagina is excised and there is wide lymph node excision.

**West·berg space** (vest′berg) the space surrounding the origin of the aorta which is invested with the pericardium.

**Wes·ter·gren meth·od** (ves′ter-gren) a procedure for estimating the sedimentation rate in fluid blood by mixing venous blood with an aqueous solution of sodium citrate and allowing it to stand in an upright pipette; the fall of the red blood cells, in millimeters, is observed in 1 hour; the normal rate for men is 0 to 15 mm (average, 4 mm), and for women 0 to 20 mm (average, 5 mm).

**Wes·ter·mark sign** (ves′ter-mahrk) in chest radiography, decreased lung markings from oligemia caused by pulmonary embolism.

**West·ern blot, West·ern blot·ting** SYN Western blot analysis.

**West·ern blot anal·y·sis** a procedure in which proteins separated by electrophoresis in polyacrylamide gels are transferred (blotted) onto nitrocellulose or nylon membranes and identified by specific complexing with antibodies that are either pre- or post-tagged with a labeled secondary protein. SEE ALSO immunoblot. SYN Western blot, Western blotting. [Coined to distinguish it from eponymic Southern blot a.]

**Weste·rn blot test** a serum electrophoretic analysis used to identify proteins.

**west·ern equine en·ceph·a·lo·my·e·li·tis** an equine encephalomyelitis found in the western U.S. and parts of South America, transmitted by mosquitoes and caused by the western equine encephalomyelitis virus; the infection is similar to but milder than eastern equine encephalomyelitis in man and is, as a rule, inapparent, but some cases with central nervous system involvement have been fatal.

**West·gard rules** (west′gard) a quality control protocol that allows detection of random and systematic error. The protocol includes the 12s, 13s, 22s, R4s, 41s, and 10x rules.

**West·phal pu·pil·lary re·flex** (vest'fahl) SYN eye-closure pupil reaction.

**West·phal sign** (vest'fahl) SYN Erb-Westphal sign.

**West·phal-Strüm·pell disease** (vest'fahl-shtrem'pĕl) SYN Wilson disease (1).

**West syn·drome** (west) an encephalopathy in infancy characterized by infantile spasms, arrest of psychomotor development, and hypsarrhythmia.

**wet-bulb ther·mo·met·er** ambient air thermometer whose bulb is enclosed by a wet wick. With high relative humidity, little evaporative cooling occurs, and the reading is similar to that of a dry-bulb thermometer. On a dry day, significant evaporation occurs from the wetted bulb, which maximizes the difference between the two thermometer readings.

**wet gan·grene** ischemic necrosis of an extremity with bacterial infection, producing cellulitis adjacent to the necrotic areas. SYN moist gangrene.

**wet lung, white lung 1.** SYN shock lung. **2.** SYN adult respiratory distress syndrome.

**wet nurse** a woman who breast-feeds a child not her own.

**wet-technique liposuction** liposuction performed after subcutaneous infusion of dilute epinephrine solution.

**wet-to-dry dressing** a dressing that is applied moist with saline and allowed to dry before it is removed.

**WF** Working Formulation for Clinical Usage.

**Whar·ton duct** (hwar'tĕn) SYN submandibular duct.

**Whar·ton jel·ly** (hwar'tĕn) the mucoid connective tissue of the umbilical cord.

**wheal** (hwēl) a circumscribed, evanescent papule or irregular plaque of edema of the skin, appearing as an urticarial lesion, slightly reddened, often changing in size and shape and extending to adjacent areas, and usually accompanied by intense itching; produced by intradermal injection or test; or by exposure to allergenic substances in susceptible persons. See page B4. SYN hives (2), welt. [A.S. *hwēle*]

**wheal-and-er·y·the·ma re·ac·tion** the characteristic immediate reaction observed in the skin test; within 10 to 15 minutes after injection of antigen (allergen), an irregular, blanched, elevated wheal appears, surrounded by an area of erythema (flare). SYN wheal-and-flare reaction.

**wheal-and-flare re·ac·tion** SYN wheal-and-erythema reaction.

**Wheat·stone bridge** (hwēt'stōn) an apparatus for measuring electrical resistance; four resistors are connected to form the four sides or "arms" of a square; a voltage is applied to one diagonal pair of connections, while the voltage between the other diagonal pair is measured, e.g., by a galvanometer; the bridge is "balanced" when the measured voltage is zero; then, the ratios of the two pairs of adjoining resistances must be identical.

**wheeze** (hwēz) **1.** to breathe with difficulty and noisily. **2.** a whistling, squeaking, musical, or puffing sound made by air passing through the fauces, glottis, or narrowed tracheobronchial airways in difficult breathing. [A.S. *hwēsan*]

**whiff test** test for the fishy odor detectable when KOH is applied to a sample of vaginal discharge in case of bacterial vaginosis.

**whip·lash** (hwip'lash) SEE whiplash injury.

**whip·lash in·ju·ry** an imprecise term for various injuries resulting from sudden and violent hyperextension of the head on the trunk, followed by hyperflexion, as in a motor vehicle collision. Can include fractures, subluxations, sprains, muscle strains, and cerebral concussion. SYN acceleration-deceleration injury.

**whip·lash ret·in·o·pa·thy** an injury to the retina caused by a sudden acceleration/deceleration injury.

**Whip·ple dis·ease** (hwipl) a rare disease characterized by steatorrhea, frequently generalized lymphadenopathy, arthritis, fever, and cough; many "foamy" macrophages are found in the jejunal lamina propria; caused by *Tropheryma whippleii*.

**Whip·ple op·er·a·tion** (hwipl) SYN pancreatoduodenectomy.

**Whit·a·ker test** (hwit'a-ker) a pressure-perfusion test in the upper urinary tract to demonstrate impediment of flow.

**white** (hwīt) the color resulting from commingling of all the rays of the spectrum; the color of chalk or of snow. SYN albicans (1). [A.S. *hwīt*]

**white blood cell (WBC)** SYN leukocyte.

**white cor·pus·cle** any type of leukocyte.

**white fi·ber 1.** white mammalian muscle fibers; larger in diameter than red fibers, they have less myoglobin, sarcoplasm, and mitochondria, and contract more quickly; **2.** SYN collagen fiber.

**white gan·grene** death of a part accompanied by the formation of grayish white sloughs.

**white graft** rejection of a skin allograft so acute that vascularization never occurs.

**White·head** (hwīt'hed), Walter, English surgeon, 1840–1913. SEE Whitehead operation.

**white·head** (hwīt'hed) **1.** SYN milium. **2.** SYN closed comedo.

**White·head op·er·a·tion** (hwīt'hed) excision of hemorrhoids by two circular incisions above and below involved veins, allowing normal mucosa to be pulled down and sutured to anal skin.

**white in·farct 1.** SYN anemic infarct. **2.** in the placenta, intervillous fibrin with ischemic necrosis of villi.

**white lim·bal gir·dle of Vogt** (fōkt) symmetric arcuate yellow-white deposits in the peripheral cornea often seen in patients over age forty.

**white line 1.** SYN linea alba. **2.** a pale streak appearing within 30 to 60 seconds after stroking the skin with a fingernail, and lasting for several minutes; regarded as a sign of diminished arterial tension. SYN Sergent white line.

**white line of anal ca·nal** a bluish pink, narrow, wavy zone in the mucosa of the anal canal below the pectinate line at the level of the interval between the subcutaneous part of the external sphincter and the lower border of the internal sphincter, said to be palpable.

**white mat·ter** those regions of the brain and spinal cord that are largely or entirely composed of nerve fibers and contain few or no neuronal cell bodies or dendrites. SYN alba, white substance.

**white mus·cle** a rapid or fast-twitch muscle in which pale large "white" fibers predominate; mitochondria and myoglobin are relatively sparse

W
h

compared with red muscle; involved in phasic contraction.

**white noise** a complex sound consisting of many frequencies over a wide band of frequencies; often used for masking of hearing in the nontest ear in the measurement of hearing.

**white pie·dra** piedra of the beard, moustache, and genital areas, as well as the scalp, caused by *Trichosporon beigelii* and found in South America, Europe, and Japan; characterized by soft, mucilaginous, white to light brown nodules, within as well as on the hairs.

**white pulp** that part of the spleen that consists of nodules and other lymphatic concentrations.

**white sub·stance** SYN white matter.

**whit·low** (hwit'lō) SYN felon. [M.E. *whitflawe*]

**Whit·man frame** (hwit'man) a frame similar to the Bradford frame, but with curved sides.

**WHO** World Health Organization.

**whole blood** blood drawn from a selected donor under rigid aseptic precautions; contains citrate ion or heparin as an anticoagulant; used as a blood replenisher.

**whole-body count·er** shielding and instrumentation, usually involving more than one detector, designed to evaluate the total-body burden of various gamma-emitting nuclides.

**whoop** (hwoop) the loud sonorous inspiration in pertussis with which the paroxysm of coughing terminates, due to spasm of the larynx (glottis).

**whoop·ing cough** SYN pertussis.

**whorl** (hwerl) **1.** a turn of the spiral cochlea of the ear. **2.** SYN vortex of heart. **3.** a turn of a concha nasalis. **4.** SYN verticil. **5.** an area of hair growing in a radial manner suggesting whirling or twisting. SYN vortex (2). SEE hair whorls. **6.** one of the distinguishing patterns in Galton system of classification of fingerprints.

**whorled** (hwerld) marked by or arranged in whorls. SEE ALSO turbinate, verticillate.

**Wick·ham stria** (wik'am) a fine whitish line, appearing as part of a network on the surface of a lichen planus papule.

**wide·band** (wīd-band) a broad array of sound frequencies as opposed to a narrow array of frequencies.

**wide dy·na·mic range com·pres·sion** a hearing aid circuit in which amplification is increased across the frequency range at low input levels.

**Wil·brand knee** (wil'brand) bundle of inferior nasal optic nerve fibers subserving the superior temporal visual field and crossing in the anterior optic chiasm, briefly entering the contralateral posterior optic nerve [CN II] before proceeding into the contralateral optic tract. Recent research indicates that this may be an artifact of retinal degeneration and not present in the normal anatomy.

**Wil·der·muth ear** (vil'der-moot) an ear in which the helix is turned backward and the anthelix is prominent.

**Wil·der sign** (wīl'der) a slight twitch of the eyeball when changing its movement from abduction to adduction or the reverse, noted in Graves disease.

**Wil·der stain for re·tic·u·lum** (wīl'der) a silver impregnation technique in which reticulum appears as black, well-defined fibers without beading and with a relatively clear background.

**Wilde tri·an·gle** (wīld) SYN light reflex (3).

**wild type** a gene, phenotype, or genotype that is overwhelmingly common among those possible at a locus of interest, and therefore presumably not harmful.

**Wil·kie ar·tery** (wil'kē) the right colic artery when it occasionally crosses the duodenum.

**Wil·liams-Beu·ren syn·drome** (wil'yămz-byur'en) SYN Williams syndrome.

**Wil·liams stain** (wil'yămz) a stain for Negri bodies that uses picric acid, fuchsin, and methylene blue; Negri bodies are magenta, granules and nerve cells blue, and erythrocytes yellowish.

**Wil·liams syn·drome** (wil'yamz) disorder characterized by distinctive facies with shallow supraorbital ridges, medial eyebrow flare, stellate patterning of the irises, small nose with anteverted nares, malar hypoplasia with droopy cheeks, full lips, supravalvar aortic stenosis, neonatal hypocalcemia, mild mental retardation, and loquacious personality. Autosomal dominant inheritance; this is a contiguous gene deletion syndrome and one of the genes mutated is the elastin gene (ELN) on chromosome 7q. SYN elfin facies syndrome, Williams-Beuren syndrome.

**Wil·lis cords** (wil'is) several fibrous cords crossing the superior sagittal sinus.

**Wil·liston law** (wil'is-tŭn) as the vertebrate scale is ascended, the number of bones in the skull is reduced.

**Wilms tu·mor** (vilmz) a malignant renal tumor of young children, composed of small spindle cells and various other types of tissue, including tubules and, in some cases, structures resembling fetal glomeruli, and striated muscle and cartilage. Often inherited as an autosomal dominant trait.

**Wil·son block** (wil'son) the commonest form of right bundle-branch block, characterized in lead I by a tall slender R wave followed by a wider S wave of lower voltage.

**Wil·son dis·ease** (wil'son) **1.** a disorder of copper metabolism, characterized by liver cirrhosis, basal ganglia degeneration, neurological manifestations, and deposition of green or golden brown pigment in the periphery of the cornea; the plasma levels of copper and ceruloplasmin are decreased, urinary excretion of copper is increased, and the amounts of copper in the liver, brain, kidneys, and lenticular nucleus are unusually high while cytochrome oxidase is reduced; autosomal recessive inheritance caused by mutation in the copper-transporting ATPase gene (ATP7B) on chromosome 13q. SYN hepatolenticular degeneration (2), Westphal-Strümpell disease. SEE ALSO Kayser-Fleischer ring. [S.A.K. Wilson] **2.** SYN exfoliative dermatitis.

**Wil·son meth·od** (wil'son) a simple saline flotation method for concentrating helminth eggs in the feces. SEE flotation method. SYN Hung method.

**wind·burn** (wind'bern) erythema of the face due to exposure to wind.

**windchill index** measure of environment's potential to cause cold injury, based on ambient air temperature and wind velocity.

**win·dow** (win'dō) SYN fenestra.

**wind·pipe** (wind'pīp) SYN trachea.

**wind-suck·ing** a more severe form of crib-biting where air is ingested abnormally and forcefully by swallowing. SEE aerophagia.

**wing 1.** the anterior appendage of a bird. **2.** ANATOMY ala. SYN ala (1).

**Win·gate test** (win'gāt) test of maximal anaerobic power output during 30 seconds of all-out exercise on either arm-crank or leg-cycle ergometer; a measure of maximal power output of immediate (ATP-PCRATP and PCr) and short-term (glycolytic) energy systems.

**wing-beat·ing tre·mor** a coarse, irregular tremor that is most prominent when the limbs are held outstretched, reminiscent of a bird flapping its wings; due to up-and-down excursion of arm at abducted shoulder. Seen mainly in Wilson disease.

**winged cath·e·ter** a soft rubber catheter with little flaps at each side of the beak to retain it in the bladder.

**winged scap·u·la** condition wherein the medial border of the scapula protrudes away from the thorax; the protrusion is posterior and lateral, as the scapula rotates out; caused by paralysis of the serratus anterior muscle. SYN scapula alata.

**wing of nose** the outer, more or less flaring, wall of each nostril.

**wink** (wink) to close and open the eyes rapidly; an involuntary act by which the tears are spread over the conjunctiva, keeping it moist. [A.S. *wincian*]

**wink re·flex** general term for reflex closure of eyelids caused by any stimulus.

**Win·ter·bot·tom sign** (win′ter-bot-ŭm) swelling of the posterior cervical lymph nodes, characteristic of early stages of African trypanosomiasis; useful for surveys or control of migrations from endemic areas of persons with preclinical infections.

**Win·ter·nitz sound** (vin′ter-nitz) a double-current catheter in which water at any desired temperature circulates.

**wire** (wīr) slender and pliable rod or thread of metal.

**wir·ing** (wīr′ing) fastening together the ends of a broken bone by wire sutures.

**Wir·sung ca·nal, Wir·sung duct** (vēr′soong) SYN pancreatic duct.

**wiry** (wīr′ē) resembling or having the feel of a wire; filiform and hard; denoting a variety of pulse.

**wiry pulse** a small, fine, incompressible pulse.

**wis·dom tooth** SYN third molar.

**Wiss·ler syn·drome** (vis′ler) high intermittent fever, irregularly recurring macular and maculopapular eruption of the face, chest and limbs, leukocytosis, arthralgia, occasionally eosinophilia, and raised erythrocyte sedimentation rate; occurs in children and adolescents, with varying duration.

**witch's milk** a secretion of colostrum-like milk sometimes occurring in the glands of newborn infants of either sex 3 to 4 days after birth and lasting a week or two; due to endocrine stimulation from the mother before birth.

**with·draw·al** (with-draw′ăl) **1.** the act of removal or retreat. **2.** a psychological and/or physical syndrome caused by the abrupt cessation of the use of a drug in a habituated individual. **3.** the therapeutic process of discontinuing a drug so as to avoid withdrawal (2). **4.** a pattern of behavior observed in schizophrenia and depression, characterized by a pathological retreat from interpersonal contact and social involvement and leading to self-preoccupation.

**with·draw·al symp·toms** a group of morbid symptoms, predominantly erethistic, occurring in an addict who is deprived of the accustomed dose of the addicting agent.

**with·draw·al syn·drome** a substance-specific syndrome that follows the cessation of, or reduction in, intake of a psychoactive substance previously used regularly. The syndrome that develops varies according to the psychoactive substance used. Common symptoms include anxiety, restlessness, irritability, insomnia, and impaired attention.

**WLU** workload unit.

**wob·ble** (wah′bl) MOLECULAR BIOLOGY unorthodox pairing between the base at the 5′ end of an anticodon and the base that pairs with it (in the 3′-position of the codon).

**Wolfe graft** (wulf) a full-thickness skin graft without any subcutaneous fat.

**wolff·i·an** (vŭlf′ē-an) relating to or described by Kaspar Wolff.

**wolff·i·an body** (vŭlf′ē-an) SYN mesonephros.

**wolff·i·an cyst** (vŭlf′ē-an) a cyst lying in the broad ligament of the uterus and arising from remnants of the mesonephric ducts.

**wolff·i·an duct** (vŭlf′ē-an) SYN mesonephric duct.

**wolff·i·an rest** (vŭlf′ē-an) remnants of the wolffian duct in the female genital tract that give rise to cysts; e.g., Gartner cyst.

**Wolff law** (vŭlf) every change in the form and the function of a bone, or in its function alone, is followed by certain definite changes in its internal architecture and secondary alterations in its external conformation; these changes usually represent responses to alterations in weight-bearing stresses.

**Wolff-Par·kin·son-White syn·drome** (wulf-park′in-sŭn-hwīt) an electrocardiographic pattern sometimes associated with paroxysmal tachycardia; it consists of short P-R interval (usually 0.1 second or less; occasionally normal) together with a prolonged QRS complex with a slurred initial component (delta wave). SYN preexcitation syndrome.

**wolf·ram, wolf·ram·i·um** (wulf′ram, wulf-ram′ē-ŭm) SYN tungsten. [from *wolframite*]

**Wolf·ram syndrome** (wulf′ram) a syndrome consisting of diabetes insipidus, diabetes mellitus, optic atrophy, and deafness; the genetic abnormality is located on chromosome 4p; autosomal recessive inheritance.

**Wol·las·ton dou·blet** (wŏl′as-ton) a combination of two planoconvex lenses in the eyepiece of a microscope designed to correct the chromatic aberration.

**Wol·man dis·ease** (wŏl′man) SYN cholesterol ester storage disease.

**Wol·man xan·tho·ma·to·sis** (wŏl′man) SYN cholesterol ester storage disease.

**womb** (woom) SYN uterus. [A.S. the belly]

**Wood glass** (wud) a glass containing nickel oxide, used in Wood lamp.

**Wood lamp** (wud) an ultraviolet lamp with a nickel oxide filter that only passes light with a maximal wavelength of about 3660 Å; used to detect by fluorescence hairs infected with species of *Microsporum audouinii, M. canis*, var. *distortum*, or *M. ferrugineum*, which fluoresce greenish-yellow.

**Wood light** (wud) ultraviolet light produced by Wood lamp.

**word deafness** SYN auditory aphasia.

**word sal·ad** (werd sal′ăd) a jumble of meaningless and unrelated words emitted by persons with certain kinds of schizophrenia.

**work·a·hol·ic** (werk-a-hawl′ik) a person who manifests a compulsive need to work, even at the expense of family responsibilities, social life, and health. [by analogy with *alcoholic*]

**work of breath·ing** the total expenditure of energy necessary to accomplish the act of breathing. It may be computed in terms of the pulmonary pressure multiplied by the change in pulmonary volume, or in terms of the oxygen cost of breathing (i.e., the $O_2$ consumption above basal metabolic $O_2$ utilization attributable to breathing).

**Work·ing Form·u·la·tion for Clin·ic·al Us·age (WF)** classification of malignant lymphomas introduced by the National Cancer Institute in 1982, based on the correlation of clinical and histopathologic features of various lymphomas; widely used in clinical practice.

**work·ing out** (werk′ing owt) PSYCHOANALYSIS the stage in the treatment process in which the patient's personal history and psychodynamics are uncovered.

**work·ing side** the segment of a denture or dentition toward which the lower jaw is moved, the functioning side of the dentition.

**work·ing through** PSYCHOANALYSIS the process of obtaining additional insight and personality changes in a patient through repeated and varied examination of a conflict or problem; the interactions between free association, resistance, interpretation, and working out are the chief parts of this process.

**work·load unit (WLU)** a unit of work used to calculate productivity. Health care organizations may use billable procedures or patient visits.

**World Health Or·ga·ni·za·tion (WHO)** a unit of the United Nations devoted to international health problems.

**Worm** (vĕrm), Ole, Danish anatomist, 1588–1654. SEE wormian bones.

**worm** (werm) **1.** in anatomy, any structure resembling a worm, e.g., the midline part of the cerebellum in the forms of "vermis" and "lumbrical." **2.** term once used to designate any member of the invertebrate group or former subkingdom Vermes, a collective term no longer used taxonomically; now commonly used to designate any member of the separate phyla Annelida (the segmented or true worms), Nematoda (roundworms), and Platyhelminthes (flatworms). Important species include *Dracunculus medinensis* (dragon, guinea, Medina, or serpent worm), *Enterobius vermicularis* (seat worm or pinworm), *Loa loa* (African eye worm), *Moniliformis* (phylum Acanthocephala, thorny-headed worms), *Oxyspirura mansoni* (Manson eye worm), *Pentastomida* (tongue worm), *Strongylus* (palisade worm), *Thelazia* (eye worm), and *Trichinella spiralis* (pork or trichina worm). [A.S. *wyrm*]

**wor·mi·an** (werm′ē-an) relating to or described by Ole Worm.

**wor·mi·an bones** SYN sutural bones.

**Worth am·bly·o·scope** (werth) a hand-held amblyoscope consisting of angled tubes that can be swiveled to any degree of convergence or divergence.

**Woulfe bot·tle** (wuf) a bottle with two or three necks, used in a series, connected with tubes, for working with gases (washing, drying, absorbing, etc.).

🔲 **wound** (woond) **1.** trauma to any of the tissues of the body, especially that caused by physical means and with interruption of continuity. **2.** a surgical incision. See this page. [O.E. *wund*]

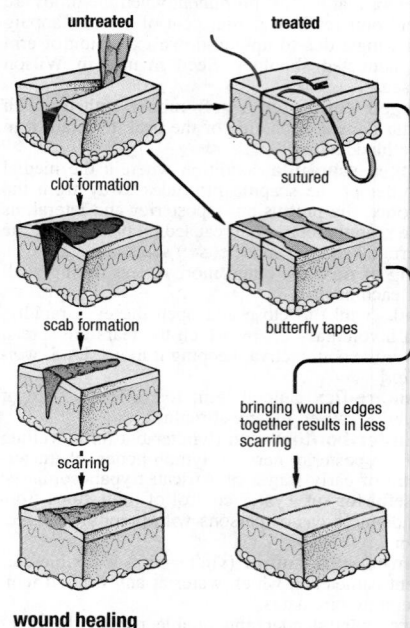

wound healing

**wound clip** a metal clasp or device for surgical approximation of skin incisions.

**wo·ven bone** bony tissue characteristic of the embryonal skeleton, in which the collagen fibers of the matrix are arranged irregularly in the form of interlacing networks. SYN nonlamellar bone, reticulated bone.

**W-plas·ty** surgery to prevent the contracture of a straight-line scar; the edges of the wound are trimmed in the shape of a W, or a series of Ws, and closed in a zig-zag manner.

**Wright stain** (rīt) a staining mixture of eosinates of polychromed methylene blue used in staining of blood smears.

**Wright syn·drome** (rīt) SYN hyperabduction syndrome.

**Wright ver·sion** (rīt) a cephalic version employed in cases of shoulder presentation when the shoulders are pushed upward while the breech is moved toward the center of the uterus by the other hand; the head is then guided into the pelvis.

**wrist** (rist) the proximal segment of the hand consisting of the carpal bones and the associated soft parts. SYN carpus (1) [TA]. [A.S. wrist joint, ankle joint]

**wrist-drop** paralysis of the extensors of the wrist and fingers; most often caused by lesion of the radial nerve. SYN drop hand.

**wrist-hand orthosis** an orthosis that begins at the fingers, crosses the wrist, and terminates on the distal portion of the forearm; used to provide grasp and release despite some degree of hand paralysis.

**wrist joint** the synovial joint between the distal end of the radius and its articular disk and the proximal row of carpal bones with the exception of the pisiform bone. SYN carpal joints (2), radio-carpal joint.

**wrist sign** in Marfan syndrome, when the wrist is gripped with the opposite hand, the thumb and fifth finger overlap appreciably.

**writ•ing hand** a contraction of the hand muscles in parkinsonism, bringing the fingers somewhat into the position of holding a pen.

**wry•neck, wry neck** (rī′nek) SYN torticollis.

*Wuch•er•e•ria* (vook-ĕr-ĕr′ē-ă) a genus of filarial nematodes characterized by adult forms that live chiefly in lymphatic vessels and produce large numbers of embryos or microfilariae that circulate in the bloodstream (microfilaremia), often appearing in the peripheral blood at regular intervals. The extreme form of this infection (wuchereriasis or filariasis) is elephantiasis or pachydermia.

*Wuch•er•e•ria ban•crofti* the bancroftian filaria,

transmitted to humans (apparently the only definitive host) by mosquitoes, especially *Culex quinquefasciatus* and *Aedes pseudoscutellaris*, but also by several other species of *Culex, Aedes, Anopheles*, and *Mansonia*, depending on the specific geographic area; adults are white, threadlike worms, and the microfilariae are ensheathed, with rounded anterior end and tapered, nonnucleated tail; the adult worms inhabit the larger lymphatic vessels (e.g., in the extremities, breasts, spermatic cord, and retroperitoneal tissues) and the sinuses of lymph nodes, where they sometimes cause temporary obstruction to the flow of lymph and slight or moderate degrees of inflammation.

**wu•cher•e•ri•a•sis** (voo′ker-ē-rī′ă-sis) infection with worms of the genus *Wuchereria*. SEE ALSO filariasis.

**Wy•burn-Ma•son syn•drome** (wī′bern-mā′son) arteriovenous malformation on the cerebral cortex, retinal arteriovenous angioma and facial nevus, usually occurring in mentally retarded individuals.

W
y

# X

**X** reactance; xanthosine; halogen atom; unspecified amino acid; reactance.

*X* reactance.

**xan·the·las·ma** (zan-thĕ-laz′mă) SYN xanthelasma palpebrarum. [xanth- + G. *elasma*, a beaten metal plate]

**xan·the·las·ma pal·pe·bra·rum** soft, yellow-orange, plaques on the eyelids or medial canthus, the most common form of xanthoma; may be associated with low-density lipoproteins, especially in younger adults. SYN xanthelasma.

**xan·the·mia** (zan-thē′mē-ă) SYN carotenemia. [xanth- + G. *haima*, blood]

**xan·thene dye** derivative of the compound xanthene.

**xan·thic** (zan′thik) 1. yellow or yellowish in color. 2. relating to xanthine.

**xan·thine** (zan′thēn) oxidation product of guanine and hypoxanthine, precursor of uric acid; occurs in many organs and in the urine, occasionally forming urinary calculi.

**xan·thism** (zan′thizm) a pigmentary anomaly of blacks, characterized by red or yellow-red hair color, copper-red skin, and often dilution of iris pigment. [G. *xanthos*, yellowish]

**xan·tho-, xanth-** yellow, yellowish. [G. *xanthos*]

**xan·tho·chro·mat·ic** (zan′thō-krō-mat′ik) yellow-colored. SYN xanthochromic.

**xan·tho·chro·mia** (zan-thō-krō′mē-ă) the occurrence of patches of yellow color in the skin, resembling xanthoma, but without the nodules or plates. SYN xanthoderma (1). [xantho- + G. *chrōma*, color]

**xan·tho·chro·mic** (zan-tho-krō′mik) SYN xanthochromatic.

**xan·tho·der·ma** (zan-thō-der′mă) 1. SYN xanthochromia. 2. any yellow coloration of the skin. [xantho- + G. *derma*, skin]

**xan·tho·gran·u·lo·ma** (zan′thō-gran′yu-lō′mă) a peculiar infiltration of retroperitoneal tissue by lipid macrophages, occurring most commonly in women.

**xan·tho·ma** (zan-thō′mă) a yellow nodule or plaque, especially of the skin, composed of lipid-laden histiocytes. [xantho- + G. *-oma*, tumor]

**xan·tho·ma dis·se·mi·na·tum** a rare benign normolipemic disorder of adults with coalescent cutaneous xanthomas composed of non-X histiocytes on flexural surfaces, often with mild diabetes insipidus.

**xan·tho·ma mul·ti·plex** SYN xanthomatosis.

**xan·tho·ma pla·num** a form marked by the occurrence of yellow, flat bands or minimally palpable rectangular plates in the corium, either normolipemic or associated with type IIa or III hyperlipoproteinemia.

**xan·tho·ma·to·sis** (zan-thō-mă-tō′sis) widespread xanthomas, especially on the elbows and knees, that sometimes affect mucous membranes and are sometimes associated with metabolic disturbances. SYN lipid granulomatosis, lipoid granulomatosis, xanthoma multiplex.

**xan·tho·ma·to·sis bul·bi** ulcerative fatty degeneration of the cornea after injury.

**xan·thom·a·tous** (zan-thō′mă-tŭs) relating to xanthoma.

**xan·tho·ma tu·be·ro·sum** xanthomatosis associated with familial type II, and occasionally type III, hyperlipoproteinemia.

*Xan·tho·mo·nas* (zan-thō-mō′nas) genus of the family Pseudomonadaceae; aerobic, Gram-negative, chemoorganotrophic, straight bacilli which exhibit motility by flagella. Type species is *Xanthomonas campestris.*

*Xan·tho·mo·nas mal·to·phil·i·a* a species found primarily in clinical specimens but also in water, milk, and frozen food. Frequent cause of infections in hospitalized and immunocompromised humans.

**xan·tho·phyll** (zan′thō-fil) $(3R,3′R, 6′R)$-β-ε-carotene-3′,3′-diol; oxygenated derivative of carotene; a yellow plant pigment, occurring also in egg yolk and corpus luteum. SYN lutein (2).

**xan·thop·sia** (zan-thop′sē-ă) a condition in which objects appear yellow; may occur in picric acid and santonin poisoning, in jaundice, and in digitalis intoxication. [xantho- + G. *opsis*, vision]

**xan·tho·sine (X, Xao)** (zan′thō-sēn, zan′thō-sin) the deamination product of guanosine (O replacing $-NH_2$).

**xan·tho·sis** (zan-thō′sis) a yellowish discoloration of degenerating tissues, especially seen in malignant neoplasms. [xantho- + G. *-osis*, condition]

**Xao** xanthosine.

**X chro·mo·some, Y chro·mo·some** SEE sex chromosomes.

**Xe** xenon.

**xenic culture** cultures of parasites grown in association with unknown microbiota. [G. *xenikos*, alien, foreign, fr. *xenos*, guest, stranger]

**xe·no-** strange; foreign material; parasite. SEE hetero-, allo-. [G. *xenos*, guest, host, stranger, foreign]

**xen·o·bi·ot·ic** (zen′ō-bī-ot′ik) a pharmacologically, endocrinologically, or toxicologically active substance not endogenously produced and therefore foreign to an organism.

**xen·o·di·ag·no·sis** (zen′ō-dī-ag-nō′sis) 1. a method of diagnosing acute or early *Trypanosoma cruzi* infection (Chagas disease) in humans. Infection-free triatomine bugs are fed on the suspected person and the trypanosome is identified by microscopic examination of the intestinal contents of the bug after a suitable incubation period. 2. a similar method of biological diagnosis based upon experimental exposure of a parasite-free normal host capable of allowing the organism in question to multiply, enabling it to be more easily and reliably detected.

**xen·o·gen·e·ic** (zen′ō-jĕ-nē′ik) heterologous, with respect to tissue grafts, especially when donor and recipient belong to widely separated species. SYN xenogenic (2), xenogenous (2). [xeno- + G. *-gen*, producing]

**xen·o·gen·ic** (zen-ō-jen′ik) 1. originating outside of the organism, or from a foreign substance that has been introduced into the organism. SYN xenogenous (1). 2. SYN xenogeneic. [xeno- + G. *-gen*, producing]

**xe·nog·e·nous** (zĕ-noj′ĕ-nŭs) 1. SYN xenogenic (1). 2. SYN xenogeneic.

**xen·o·graft** (zen′ō-graft) a graft transferred from an animal of one species to one of another species. SYN heterograft, heterologous graft.

**xe·non (Xe)** (zē′non) a gaseous element, atomic no. 54, atomic wt. 131.29; present in minute proportion in the atmosphere; produces general anesthesia in concentrations of 70 vol.%. [G. *xenos,* a stranger]

**xe·non-133** a radioisotope of xenon with a gamma emission at 81 keV and a physical half-life of 5.243 days; used in the study of pulmonary function and organ blood flow.

**xen·o·par·a·site** (zen-ō-par′ă-sīt) an ecoparasite that becomes pathogenic in consequence of weakened resistance on the part of its host.

**xen·o·pho·bia** (zen-ō-fō′bē-ă) morbid fear of strangers. [xeno- + G. *phobos,* fear]

***Xen·o·psyl·la*** (zen-op-sil′ă) a genus of fleas parasitic on the rat and involved in the transmission of bubonic plague. *Xenopsylla cheopis* serves as a potent vector of *Yersinia pestis; Xenopsylla astia* and *Xenopsylla braziliensis* are also efficient vectors of plague. [xeno- + G. *psylla,* flea]

**xen·o·tro·pic vi·rus** a retrovirus that does not produce disease in its natural host and replicates only in tissue culture cells derived from a different species.

△**xero-** dry. [G. *xeros*]

**xer·o·chi·lia** (zēr-ō-kī′lē-ă) dryness of lips. [xero- + G. *cheilos,* lip]

**xe·ro·der·ma** (zēr′ō-der′mă) a mild form of ichthyosis characterized by excessive dryness of the skin due to slight increase of the horny layer and diminished water content of the stratum corneum from decreased perspiration, wind, or low humidity; seen with aging, atopic dermatitis, vitamin A deficiency, etc. [xero- + G. *derma,* skin]

**xe·ro·der·ma pig·men·to·sum** an eruption of exposed skin occurring in childhood and characterized by photosensitivity with severe sunburn in infancy and the development of numerous pigmented spots resembling freckles, larger atrophic lesions eventually resulting in glossy white thinning of the skin surrounded by telangiectases, and multiple solar keratoses which undergo malignant change at an early age. Severe ophthalmic and neurologic abnormalities are also found.

**xe·ro·gram** (zē′rō-gram) SYN xeroradiograph.

**xe·rog·ra·phy** (zēr-og′ră-fē) SYN xeroradiography.

**xe·ro·ma** (zē-rō′mă) SYN xerophthalmia.

**xe·roph·thal·mia** (zēr-of-thal′mē-ă) excessive dryness of the conjunctiva and cornea, which lose their luster and become keratinized; may be due to local disease or to a systemic deficiency of vitamin A. SYN xeroma. [xero- + G. *ophthalmos,* eye]

**xe·ro·ra·di·o·graph** (zē-rō-rā′dē-ō-graf) the permanent record made by xeroradiography. SYN xerogram.

**xe·ro·ra·di·og·ra·phy** (zē′rō-rā′dē-og′ră-fē) radiography using a specially coated charged plate instead of x-ray film, developing with a dry powder rather than liquid chemicals, and transferring the powder image onto paper for a permanent record; edge enhancement is inherent. SYN xerography.

**xe·ro·sis** (zē-rō′sis) pathologic dryness of the skin (xeroderma), the conjunctiva (xerophthalmia), or mucous membranes. [xero- + G. *-osis,* condition]

**xe·ro·sto·mia** (zēr′ō-stō′mē-ă) a dryness of the mouth, having a varied etiology, resulting from diminished or arrested salivary secretion, or asialism. [xero- + G. *stoma,* mouth]

**xe·rot·ic** (zē-rot′ik) dry; affected with xerosis.

**X-in·ac·ti·va·tion** SYN lyonization.

**xiph·i·ster·nal** (zif-i-ster′năl) relating to the xiphoid process.

**xiph·i·ster·num** (zif′i-ster′nŭm) SYN xiphoid process. [xiphoid + G. *sternon,* chest]

△**xipho-, xiph-, xiphi-** xiphoid, usually the processus xiphoideus. [G. *xiphos,* sword]

**xi·phoid** (zī′foyd, zif′oyd) sword-shaped; applied especially to the xiphoid process. SYN ensiform. [xipho- + G. *eidos,* appearance]

**xi·phoid car·ti·lage** SYN xiphoid process.

**xi·phoi·di·tis** (zif′oy-dī′tis) inflammation of the xiphoid process of the sternum. [xiphoid + G. *-itis,* inflammation]

**xi·phoid pro·cess** the cartilage at the lower end of the sternum. SYN processus xiphoideus [TA], ensiform process, xiphisternum, xiphoid cartilage.

**X-linked** pertaining to genes borne on the X chromosome. Commonly but erroneously used synonymously with sex-linked, which would also comprise Y-linked traits.

**X-linked gene** a gene located on an X chromosome.

**X-linked hy·po·gam·ma·glob·u·lin·e·mia, X-linked in·fan·tile hy·po·gam·ma·glob·u·lin·e·mi·a** a congenital, X-linked recessive, primary immunodeficiency characterized by decreased numbers (or absence) of circulating B-lymphocytes with corresponding decrease in immunoglobulins; associated with marked susceptibility to infection by pyogenic bacteria after loss of maternal antibodies.

**X-linked lym·pho·pro·lif·er·a·tive syndrome** an X-linked recessive immunodeficiency and lymphoproliferative disease caused by mutation in the SH2 domain protein 1A gene (SH2D1A) on Xq; characterized by defective cellular or humoral immune response to Epstein-Barr virus; manifestations include fulminant infectious mononucleosis, B-cell malignancies, and hypogammaglobulinemia. SYN Duncan disease.

**X-linked re·cess·ive bul·bo·spin·al neur·on·o·pathy** SYN Kennedy disease.

**XO syn·drome** SYN Turner syndrome.

**X-pat·tern es·o·tro·pia** decreasing convergence from the primary position in both upward and downward gaze.

**X-pat·tern ex·o·tro·pia** increasing divergence from primary position in both upward and downward gaze.

**x-ray 1.** the ionizing electromagnetic radiation emitted from a highly evacuated tube, resulting from the excitation of the inner orbital electrons by the bombardment of the target anode with a stream of electrons from a heated cathode. **2.** ionizing electromagnetic radiation produced by the excitation of the inner orbital electrons of an atom by other processes, such as nuclear delay and its sequelae. **3.** a radiograph. See page B13. SYN roentgen ray.

**x-ray mi·cro·scope** a microscope in which images are obtained by using x-rays as an energy source that are recorded on a very fine-grained film, or the image is enlarged by projection; if film is used, it may be examined with the light microscope at fairly high magnifications.

**XXY syn·drome** SYN Klinefelter syndrome.

**xy·lose** (zī′lōs) an aldopentose, isomeric with ribose, obtained by fermentation or hydrolysis of carbohydrate.

**xy·lu·lose** (zī′loo-lōs) *threo*-pentulose; a ketopentose that appears in the urine in cases of essential pentosuria; it is also an intermediate in the glucuronate pathway.

**xys•ma** (ziz′mă) membranous shreds in the feces. [G. filings, shavings, fr. *xyō,* to scrape]

**XYY syn•drome** a chromosomal anomaly with chromosome count 47, with a supernumerary Y chromosome; controversial evidence associates tallness, aggressiveness, and acne with this condition.

# Y

**Y** yttrium; tyrosine; pyrimidine nucleoside.

**y⁺** SEE system (5).

**YAG** yttrium-aluminum-garnet.

**yaw** (yau) an individual lesion of the eruption of yaws.

**yawn** (yaun) **1.** to gape. **2.** an involuntary opening of the mouth, usually accompanied by a movement of respiration; it may be a sign of drowsiness or of vital depression, as after hemorrhage, but is often caused by suggestion. [A.S. *gānian*]

**yaws** (yawz) an infectious tropical disease caused by *Treponema pertenue* and characterized by the development of crusted granulomatous ulcers on the extremities; may involve bone, but, unlike syphilis, does not produce central nervous system or cardiovascular pathology. SYN boubas, bubas, frambesia, framboesia, granuloma tropicum, pian, rupia (2). [of Caribbean origin; similar to Calinago *yaya*, the disease]

**Yb** ytterbium.

**Y car·ti·lage, Y-shaped car·ti·lage** the connecting cartilage for the ilium, ischium, and pubis; it extends through the acetabulum.

**years of po·ten·tial life lost** measure of the relative impact of various diseases and lethal forces on society, computed by estimating the years that people would have lived if they had not died prematurely from injury, cancer, heart disease, etc.

**yeast** (yēst) a general term denoting true fungi of the family Saccharomycetaceae that are widely distributed in substrates that contain sugars (such as fruits), and in soil, animal excreta, the vegetative parts of plants, etc. Because of their ability to ferment carbohydrates, some yeasts are important to the brewing and baking industries. See this page. [A.S. *gyst*]

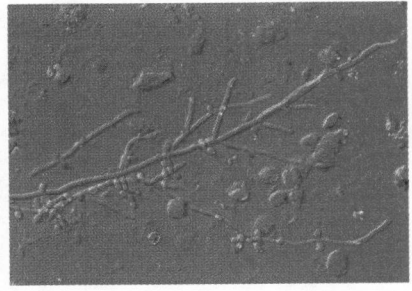

**yeast**

**yel·low at·ro·phy of the liv·er** SEE acute yellow atrophy of the liver.

**yel·low car·ti·lage** SYN elastic cartilage.

**yel·low fe·ver** a tropical mosquito-borne viral hepatitis, due to yellow fever virus, with an urban form transmitted by *Aedes aegypti*, and a rural, jungle, or sylvatic form from tree-dwelling mammals by various mosquitoes of the *Haemagogus* species complex; characterized clinically by fever, slow pulse, albuminuria, jaundice, congestion of the face, and hemorrhages, especially hematemesis; immunity to reinfection accompanies recovery.

**yel·low fi·bers** SYN elastic fibers.

**yel·low hep·a·ti·za·tion** the final stage of hepatization in which the exudate is becoming purulent.

**Yer·sin·ia** (yer-sin′ē-ă) a genus of motile and nonmotile, non-spore-forming bacteria containing Gram-negative, unencapsulated, ovoid to rod-shaped cells. These organisms are parasitic on humans and other animals. The type species is *Yersinia pestis*. [A. J. E. *Yersin,* Swiss bacteriologist, 1862–1943]

**Yer·sin·ia en·ter·o·co·li·ti·ca** a species that causes yersiniosis in humans; it is found in the feces and lymph nodes of sick and healthy animals, including humans, and in material contaminated with feces.

**Yer·sin·ia pes·tis** a species causing plague in humans, rodents, and many other mammalian species, and transmitted from rat to rat and from rat to human host by the rat flea, *Xenopsylla;* it is the type species of the genus *Yersinia.* SYN Kitasato bacillus.

**Yer·sin·ia pseu·do·tu·ber·cu·lo·sis** a species causing pseudotuberculosis in birds, rodents, and rarely in humans. SYN *Pasteurella pseudotuberculosis.*

**yer·sin·i·o·sis** (yer-sin-ē-ō′sis) a common human infectious disease caused by *Yersinia enterocolitica* and marked by diarrhea, enteritis, pseudoappendicitis, ileitis, erythema nodosum, and sometimes septicemia or acute arthritis.

**yield** (yēld) the amount or quantity produced or returned, often measured as a percent of the starting material; e.g., a yield in an enzyme preparation is equal to the units of enzyme activity recovered at the end of the preparation divided by the total units observed in the starting material.

**-yl** chemical suffix signifying that the substance is a radical by loss of an H atom (e.g., alkyl, methyl, phenyl) or OH group (e.g., acyl, acetyl, carbamoyl).

**-ylene** chemical suffix denoting a bivalent hydrocarbon radical (e.g., methylene, $-CH_2-$) or possessing a double bond (e.g., ethylene, $CH_2=CH_2$).

**Y-link·age** the state of a genetic factor (gene) being borne on the Y chromosome. This idea is analogous with X-linkage but since the Y chromosome does not fully take part in chiasma formation and recombination, it not amenable to analysis by conventional linkage methods.

**Y-linked gene** a gene located on a Y chromosome. SYN holandric gene.

**yoke** (yōk) SYN jugum (1). [A.S. *geoc*]

**yolk** (yōk) **1.** one of the types of nutritive material stored in the oocyte for the nutrition of the embryo; yolk is particularly abundant and conspicuous in the eggs of birds. SYN vitellus. **2.** fatty material found in the wool of sheep; when extracted and purified, it becomes lanolin. [A.S. *geolca; geolu,* yellow]

**yolk mem·brane** SYN membrana vitellina.

**yolk stalk** the narrowed connection between the intraembryonic gut and the yolk sac; its walls are splanchnopleure. SYN omphalomesenteric duct.

**Yorke au·to·lyt·ic re·ac·tion** (yōrk) a test for paroxysmal hemoglobinuria; serum is placed in an ice chest and kept at 0°C for 5–7 minutes, then in an incubator at 37°C with erythrocytes for 1 hour, at which time, if the reaction is positive, hemolysis occurs; if the serum is kept at 1°C for an hour and then placed in the incubator with erythrocytes there is little hemolysis.

**Young-Helm·holtz the·o·ry of col·or vi·sion** (yung-helm′hōlts) a theory that there are three color-perceiving elements in the retina: red, green, and blue. Perception of other colors arises from the combined stimulation of these elements; deficiency or absence of any one of these elements results in inability to perceive that color and a misperception of any other color of which it forms a part.

**Young mo·du·lus** (yung) a type of modulus of elasticity which specifies the force applied to a body in one direction, per unit cross-sectional area of the body perpendicular to that direction, divided by the fractional change in length of the body in that direction.

**Y-shaped lig·a·ment** SYN iliofemoral ligament.

**yt·ter·bi·um (Yb)** (i-ter′bē-ŭm) a metallic element of the lanthanide group; atomic no. 70, atomic wt. 173.04. $^{169}$Yb, with a half-life of 32.03 days, has been used in cisternography and in brain scans. [*Ytterby,* village in Sweden]

**yt·tri·um (Y)** (it′rē-ŭm) a metallic element, atomic no. 39, atomic wt. 88.90585. [*Ytterby,* village in Sweden]

# Z

**Z** benzyloxycarbonyl; atomic number; symbol for an amino acid that is either glutamic acid, glutamine, or a substance that yields glutamic acid on acid hydrolysis of peptides; carbobenzoxy.

**z** zepto-.

**Zahn in•farct** (tsahn) a pseudoinfarct of the liver, consisting of an area of congestion with parenchymal atrophy but no necrosis; due to obstruction of a branch of the portal vein.

**Zaire virus** (zī-ēr′) a variant of Ebola virus. SYN Ebola virus Zaire.

**Zar•it bur•den in•ter•view** (zăr′it) a structured verbal interaction used to evaluate levels of stress in family members or caregivers of Alzheimer patients.

**Za•va•nel•li ma•neu•ver** (zah-vah-nĕl′ē) SYN cephalic replacement.

**Z band** SYN Z line.

**Z-DNA** a form of DNA in which the helix is left-handed, and the overall appearance is elongated and slim.

**ZEEP** zero end-expiratory pressure.

**Zeis glands** (tsīs) sebaceous glands opening into the follicles of the eyelashes.

**Zeit•geist** (zīt′gīst) PSYCHOLOGY the climate of opinion, conventions of thought, covert influences, and unquestioned assumptions that are implicit in a given culture, the arts, or science at any time, and in which the individual operates and thus is influenced. [Ger. *Zeit*, time, + *Geist*, spirit]

**Zen•ker de•gen•er•a•tion** (tsen′ker) a form of severe hyaline degeneration or necrosis in skeletal muscle, occurring in severe infections. SYN waxy degeneration (2).

**Zen•ker di•ver•tic•u•lum** (tsen′ker) SYN pharyngoesophageal diverticulum.

**Zen•ker fix•a•tive** (tsen′ker) a rapid fixative consisting of mercuric chloride, potassium dichromate, sodium sulfate, glacial acetic acid, and water, useful for trichrome stains; must be washed to remove potassium dichromate and treated with iodine solution to remove mercuric chloride; tissues tend to become brittle if left in the fixative for more than 24 hours.

**Zen•ker pa•ral•y•sis** (tsen′ker) paresthesia and paralysis in the area of the external popliteal nerve.

**zep•to-** (z) prefix used in the SI and metric systems to signify $10^{-21}$.

**ze•ro** (zē′rō) **1.** the figure 0, indicating the absence of magnitude, or nothing. **2.** THERMOMETRY the point from which the figures on the scale start in one or the other direction; in the Celsius and Réaumur scales, zero indicates the freezing point for distilled water; in the Fahrenheit scale, it is 32° below the freezing point of water. [Sp. fr. Ar. *sifr*, cipher]

**ze•ro end-ex•pi•ra•to•ry pres•sure (ZEEP)** airway pressure which, at the end of expiration, equals atmospheric pressure.

**ze•ta** (zā′tă) **1.** sixth letter of the Greek alphabet, ζ **2.** CHEMISTRY the sixth in a series, e.g., the sixth carbon from a functional group. **3.** electrokinetic potential.

**ze•ta•crit** (zā′tă-krit) the packed cell volume produced by vertical centrifugation of blood in capillary tubes, allowing controlled compaction and dispersion of red blood cells; read with a hematocrit to produce the zeta sedimentation ratio.

**ze•ta sed•i•men•ta•tion ra•tio** the ratio of the zetacrit to the hematocrit, normally 0.41 to 0.54 (41 to 54%); it is a sensitive indicator of the erythrocyte sedimentation rate (ESR) and is unaffected by anemia.

**Z fil•a•ment** the thin zig-zag structure at the Z line of striated muscle fibers to which the actin filaments attach.

**Ziehl stain** (tsēl) a carbol-fuchsin solution of phenol and basic fuchsin used to demonstrate bacteria and cell nuclei.

**Zie•mann dot** (tsē′man) any of numerous fine dots seen in erythrocytes in malariae malaria.

**Zim•mer•lin at•ro•phy** (tzim′er-lin) a variety of hereditary progressive muscular atrophy in which the atrophy begins in the upper half of the body.

**zinc** (zingk) a metallic element, atomic no. 30, atomic wt. 65.39; an essential bioelement; a number of salts of zinc are used in medicine; a cofactor in many proteins. [Ger. *Zink*]

**zinc-65** a radioactive zinc isotope that decays mainly by K-capture with a half-life of 243.8 days; used as a tracer in studies of zinc metabolism.

**zinc sul•fate flo•ta•tion con•cen•tra•tion** a method using saturated zinc sulfate to separate parasitic elements from fecal debris through differences in specific gravity; most parasite cysts, oocysts, spores, eggs, and larvae can be found in the surface film after centrifugation.

**Zinn zon•ule** (tsin) SYN ciliary zonule.

**zir•co•ni•um (Zr)** (zir-kō′nē-ŭm) a metallic element, atomic no. 40, atomic wt. 91.224; widely distributed in nature, but never found in quantity in any one place. [*zircon*, a mineral, fr. Ar. *zarkūn*, cinnabar, Pers, *zargun*, goldlike]

**Z line** a cross-striation bisecting the I band of striated muscle myofibrils and serving as the anchoring point of actin filaments at either end of the sarcomere. SYN Z band.

**zm** zeptometer.

**zo•ac•an•tho•sis** (zō′ă-kan-thō′sis) a cutaneous eruption due to introduction into the human skin of hair, bristles, stingers, etc., of lower animals. [G. *zōon*, animal, + acanthosis]

**zo•an•throp•ic** (zō-an-throp′ik) relating to or marked by zoanthropy.

**zo•an•thro•py** (zō-an′thrō-pē) a delusion that one is an animal, such as a dog. [G. *zōon*, animal, + *anthrōpos*, man]

**Zol•lin•ger-El•li•son syn•drome** (zol′in-jer-el′i-sŭn) peptic ulceration with gastric hypersecretion and non-beta cell tumor of the pancreatic islets, sometimes associated with familial polyendocrine adenomatosis.

**Zöll•ner lines** (tserl′ner) figures devised to show the possibility of optical illusions; a common one consists of two parallel lines which are met by numerous short lines obliquely placed; the parallel lines then seeming to converge or diverge.

**zo•na**, pl. **zo•nae** (zō′nă, zō′nē) **1.** SYN zone. **2.** SYN herpes zoster. [L. fr. G. *zōnē*, a girdle, one of the zones of the sphere]

**zo•na ar•cu•a•ta** SYN arcuate zone.

**zo•naes•the•sia [Br.]** SEE zonesthesia.

**zo•na fas•ci•cu•la•ta** the layer of radially arranged cell cords in the cortex of the suprarenal gland, between the zona glomerulosa and zona reticularis; secretes cortisol and dehydroepiandrosterone.

**zo•na glo•mer•u•lo•sa** the outer layer of the cortex of the suprarenal gland just beneath the capsule; secretes aldosterone.

**zon•al ne•cro•sis** necrosis predominantly affecting or limited to an anatomical zone, especially parts of the hepatic lobules defined according to proximity to either the portal tracts or central (hepatic) veins.

**zo•na oph•thal•mi•ca** herpes zoster in the distribution of the ophthalmic nerve.

**zo•na or•bi•cu•la•ris** fibers of the articular capsule of the hip joint encircling the neck of the femur.

**zo•na pec•ti•na•ta** SYN pectinate zone.

**zo•na pel•lu•ci•da** a layer consisting of microvilli of the oocyte, cellular processes of follicular cells, and an intervening substance rich in glycoprotein; it appears homogeneous and translucent under the light microscope. SYN pellucid zone.

**zo•na re•tic•u•la•ris** the inner layer of the cortex of the adrenal gland, where the cell cords anastomose in a netlike fashion.

**zo•na tec•ta** SYN arcuate zone.

**zone** (zōn) a segment; any encircling or belt-like structure, either external or internal, longitudinal or transverse. SEE ALSO area, band, region, space, spot. SYN zona (1). [L. *zona*]

**zo•nes•the•sia** (zōn-es-thē′zē-ă) a sensation as if a cord were drawn around the body, constricting it. SYN girdle sensation. [G. *zōnē*, girdle, + *aisthēsis*, sensation]

**zo•nif•u•gal** (zō-nif′yu-găl) passing from within any region outward; as in mapping out an area of disturbed sensation, when the stimulus is first applied to the affected region and is carried into the area where sensation is normal. [L. *zona*, zone, + *fugio*, to flee]

**zon•ing** (zōn′ing) the occurrence of a stronger reaction in a lesser amount of suspected serum, observed sometimes in serologic tests used in the diagnosis of syphilis, and probably the result of high antibody titer.

**zo•nip•e•tal** (zō-nip′ĕ-tăl) passing from without toward and into any region, as in mapping out an area of disturbed sensation, when the stimulus begins in a normal area and is carried into the affected region. [L. *zona*, zone, + *peto*, to seek]

**zon•og•ra•phy** (zō-nog′ră-fē) a form of tomography with a relatively thick plane of focus; especially used in renal radiography. [zone + G. *graphō*, to write]

**zo•nu•la**, pl. **zo•nu•lae** (zō′nyu-lă, zō′nyu-lē) SYN zonule. [L. dim. of *zona*, zone]

**zo•nu•la cil•i•a•ris** [TA] SYN ciliary zonule.

**zo•nu•lar** (zō′nyu-lăr, zon′yu-lăr) relating to a zonula.

**zo•nu•lar cat•a•ract** SYN lamellar cataract.

**zo•nu•lar spac•es** the spaces between the fibers of the ciliary zonule at the equator of the lens of the eye.

**zon•ule** (zō′nyul, zon′yul) a small zone. SYN zonula.

**zo•nu•li•tis** (zō-nyu-lī′tis) inflammation of the zonule of Zinn, or suspensory ligament of the lens of the eye. [zonule + G. *-itis*, inflammation]

**zo•nu•lol•y•sis, zo•nu•ly•sis** (zō′nyu-lol-ĭ′sis, zō′nyu-lī′sis) dissolution of the zonula ciliaris by enzymes (α-chymotrypsin) to facilitate surgical removal of a cataract. SYN Barraquer method. [zonule + G. *lysis,* dissolution]

**zoo-, zo-** animal, animal life. [G. *zōon*]

**zoo blot anal•y•sis** a procedure using Southern blot analysis to test the ability of a nucleic acid probe from one species to hybridize with the DNA fragment of another species.

**zo•o•e•ras•tia** (zō′ō-ĕ-ras′tē-ă) SYN bestiality. [zoo- + G. *erastēs,* lover]

**zo•o•graft** (zō′ō-graft) a graft of tissue from an animal to a human.

**zo•o•graft•ing** (zō-ō-graft′ing) SYN zooplasty.

**zo•oid** (zō′oyd) **1.** resembling an animal; an organism or object with an animal-like appearance. **2.** an animal cell capable of independent existence or movement, as the ovum or a spermatozoon, or the segment of a tapeworm. **3.** an individual of a colonial invertebrate, such as a coral. [G. *zoōdēs,* fr. *zōon,* animal, + *eidos,* resemblance]

**zo•o•lag•nia** (zō-ō-lag′nē-ă) sexual attraction toward animals. [zoo- + G. *lagneia,* lust]

**zo•o•no•sis** (zō-ō-nō′sis) an infection or infestation shared in nature by humans and other animals that are the normal or usual host; a disease of humans acquired from an animal source. SEE ALSO anthropozoonosis, metazoonosis, saprozoonosis. [zoo- + G. *nosos,* disease]

**zo•o•not•ic cu•ta•ne•ous leish•man•i•a•sis** a form of cutaneous leishmaniasis characterized by rural distribution of human cases near infected rodents, particularly communal ground squirrels; characterized by rapidly developing dermal lesions that become severely inflamed, with moist necrotizing sores or ulcers that heal in two to eight months (after a two- to four-month incubation period).

**zo•o•not•ic po•ten•tial** the potential for infections of subhuman animals to be transmissible to humans.

**zo•o•par•a•site** (zō-ō-par′ă-sīt) an animal parasite; an animal existing as a parasite.

**zo•oph•i•lism** (zō-of′i-lizm) fondness for animals, especially an extravagant fondness for them.

**zo•o•pho•bia** (zō-ō-fō′bē-ă) morbid fear of animals. [zoo- + G. *phobos,* fear]

**zo•o•plas•ty** (zō′ō-plas-tē) grafting of tissue from an animal to a human. SYN zoografting.

**zo•o•tox•in** (zō-ō-tok′sin) a substance, resembling the bacterial toxins in its antigenic properties, found in the fluids of certain animals; e.g., in snake venom, the secretions of poisonous insects, eel blood.

**zos•ter** (zos′ter) SYN herpes zoster. [G. *zōstēr,* a girdle]

**zos•ter•oid** (zos′ter-oyd) resembling herpes zoster. [zoster + G. *eidos,* resemblance]

**Z-plas•ty** surgery to elongate a contracted scar or to rotate tension 90°; the middle line of a Z-shaped incision is made along the line of greatest tension or contraction, and triangular flaps are raised on opposite sides of the two ends and transposed.

**Z-pro•tein** a fatty acid–binding protein that participates in the intracellular movement of fatty acids. SYN fatty acid–binding protein.

**Zr** zirconium.

**Zsig•mon•dy den•tal no•men•cla•ture** (zhig′mawn-dē) SYN Palmer dental nomenclature.

**Zuc•ker•kan•dl bod•ies** (tsooker′kahn-děl) SYN paraaortic bodies.

**zwit·ter hy·poth·e·sis** that an amphoteric molecule (e.g., an amino acid) has, at its isoelectric point, equal numbers of positive and negative charges, thus becoming a zwitterion.

**zwit·ter·i·ons** (tsvit′er-ī-onz) SYN dipolar ions. SEE ALSO zwitter hypothesis. [Ger. *Zwitter,* hermaphrodite, mongrel + ion]

**zy·gal** (zī′găl) relating to or shaped like a zygon or yoke; H-shaped.

**zyg·a·poph·y·ses** (zī′gă-pof′i-sēz)

**zyg·a·poph·y·sis**, pl. **zyg·a·poph·y·ses** (zī′gă-pof′i-sis, zī′gă-pof′i-sēz) SYN articular process. [G. *zygon,* yoke, + *apophysis,* offshoot]

⚠ **zy·go-, zyg-** a yoke, a joining. [G. *zygon,* yoke, *zygōsis,* a joining]

**zy·go·ma** (zī-gō′mă) **1.** SYN zygomatic bone. **2.** SYN zygomatic arch. [G. a bar, bolt, the os jugale, fr. *zygon,* yoke]

**zy·go·mat·ic** (zī′gō-mat′ik) relating to the zygomatic bone.

**zy·go·mat·ic arch** the arch formed by the temporal process of the zygomatic bone as it joins the zygomatic process of the temporal bone. SYN zygoma (2).

**zy·go·mat·ic bone** a quadrilateral bone which forms the prominence of the cheek; it articulates with the frontal, sphenoid, temporal, and maxillary bone. SYN os zygomaticum [TA], jugal bone, mala (2), malar bone, zygoma (1).

**zy·go·mat·ic nerve** a branch of the maxillary nerve in the inferior orbital fissure through which it passes; it gives rise to two sensory branches, the zygomaticotemporal and zygomaticofacial, which supply the skin of the temporal and zygomatic regions, and is continued as the communicating branch of the lacrimal nerve with the zygomatic nerve. SYN nervus zygomaticus [TA], temporomandibular nerve.

**zy·go·mat·i·co·fa·cial fo·ra·men** the opening on the lateral surface of the zygomatic bone below the orbital margin that transmits the zygomaticofacial nerve. SYN foramen zygomaticofaciale [TA].

**zy·go·mat·i·co-or·bi·tal ar·tery** *origin,* superficial temporal, sometimes middle temporal; *distribution,* orbicularis oculi muscle and portions of the orbit; *anastomoses,* lacrimal and palpebral branches of ophthalmic. SYN arteria zygomaticoorbitalis [TA].

**zy·go·mat·i·co-or·bi·tal fo·ra·men** the common opening on the orbital surface of the zygomatic bone of the canals transmitting the zygomaticofacial and zygomaticotemporal nerves; sometimes each of these canals has a separate opening on the orbital surface. SYN foramen zygomaticoorbitale [TA].

**zy·go·mat·i·co·tem·po·ral fo·ra·men** the opening, on the temporal surface of the zygomatic bone, of the canal that gives passage to the zygomaticotemporal nerve. SYN foramen zygomaticotemporale [TA].

**zy·go·mat·ic pro·cess of max·il·la** the rough projection from the maxilla that articulates with the zygomatic bone.

**zy·go·ma·ti·cus ma·jor mus·cle** *origin,* zygomatic bone anterior to temporozygomatic suture; *insertion,* muscles at angle of mouth; *action,* draws upper lip upward and laterally; *nerve supply,* facial. SYN musculus zygomaticus major [TA].

**zy·go·max·il·la·re** (zī′gō-mak-si-lā′rē) a craniometric point located externally at the lowest extent of the zygomaticomaxillary suture. SYN zygomaxillary point.

**zy·go·max·il·lary point** SYN zygomaxillare.

**Zy·go·my·ce·tes** (zī′gō-mī-sē′tēz) a class of fungi characterized by sexual reproduction resulting in the formation of a zygospore, and asexual reproduction by means of nonmotile spores called sporangiospores or conidia. [zygo- + G. *mykēs (mykēt-),* fungus]

**zy·go·my·co·sis** (zī′gō-mī-kō′sis) a fungal infection associated with genera of the class Zygomycetes, e.g., *Absidia, Mortierella, Mucor, Rhizopus.* The genera *Conidiobolus* and *Basidiobolus* have species that are also causative agents. SYN mucormycosis, phycomycosis.

**zy·gon** (zī′gon) the short crossbar connecting the branches of a zygal fissure. [G. crossbar, yoke]

**zy·go·ne·ma** (zī-gō-nē′mă) SYN zygotene. [zygo- + G. *nēma,* thread]

**zy·go·sis** (zī-gō′sis) true conjugation or sexual union of two unicellular organisms, consisting essentially in the fusion of the nuclei of the two cells. [G. a joining]

**zy·gos·i·ty** (zī-gos′i-tē) the nature of the zygotes from which individuals are derived; e.g., whether by division of one zygote (monozygotic), in which case they will be genetically identical, or from two separate fertilized oocytes (dizygotic).

**zy·gote** (zī′gōt) **1.** the diploid cell resulting from union of a sperm and an oocyte. Cf. conceptus. **2.** the individual that develops from a fertilized oocyte. [G. *zygōtos,* yoked]

**zy·go·tene** (zī′gō-tēn) the stage of prophase in meiosis in which precise point-for-point pairing of homologous chromosomes begins. SYN zygonema. [zygo- + G. *tainia* (L. *taenia),* band]

**zy·got·ic** (zī-got′ik) pertaining to a zygote, or to zygosis.

⚠ **zy·mo-, zym-** fermentation, enzymes. [G. *zymē,* leaven]

**zy·mo·deme** (zī′mō-dēm) an isoenzyme pattern, as identified by isoenzyme electrophoresis. [zymo- + G. *dēmos,* populace]

**zy·mo·gen** (zī′mō-jen) SYN proenzyme.

**zy·mo·gen·e·sis** (zī-mō-jen′ě-sis) transformation of a proenzyme (zymogen) into an active enzyme. [zymo- + G. *genesis,* production]

**zy·mo·gen·ic** (zī-mō-jen′ik) **1.** relating to a zymogen or to zymogenesis. **2.** causing fermentation.

**zy·mo·gen·ic cell** a cell that secretes an enzyme; specifically a chief cell of a gastric gland or an acinar cell of the pancreas. SYN peptic cell.

Z
y

# Contents: The Appendices

**Professional Information**

# Weights and Measures

## Scale of the Metric System and International System of Units (SI)

| Prefix | Symbol | Power |
|--------|--------|-------|
| yotta- | Y | $10^{24}$ |
| zetta- | Z | $10^{21}$ |
| exa- | E | $10^{18}$ |
| peta- | P | $10^{15}$ |
| tera- | T | $10^{12}$ |
| giga- | G | $10^{9}$ |
| mega- | M | $10^{6}$ |
| kilo- | k | $10^{3}$ |
| hecto- | h | $10^{2}$ |
| deca- | da | $10^{1}$ |
| UNIT | — | 1 |
| deci- | d | $10^{-1}$ |
| centi- | c | $10^{-2}$ |
| milli | m | $10^{-3}$ |
| micro- | μ | $10^{-6}$ |
| nano- | n | $10^{-9}$ |
| pico- | p | $10^{-12}$ |
| femro- | f | $10^{-15}$ |
| atto- | a | $10^{-18}$ |
| zepto- | z | $10^{-21}$ |
| yocto- | y | $10^{-24}$ |

## SI Base Units

| Quantity | Name | Symbol |
|----------|------|--------|
| length | meter | m |
| mass* | kilogram** | kg |
| time | second | s |
| electric current | ampere | A |
| thermodynamic temperature | kelvin*** | K |
| luminous intensity | candela | cd |
| amount of substance | mole | mol |

*In commercial and everyday use, *weight* usually means *mass;* e.g., when speaking of a person's weight, the quantity referred to is *mass*.

**For historical reasons, *kilogram* is the only base unit with a prefix. Multiples and submultiples of the kilogram are formed by attaching the appropriate prefix to the stem word *gram* (e.g., *milligram*) and the appropriate prefix symbol to the symbol *g* (e.g., *mg*).

***The degree Celsius (°C) is still widely accepted usage for expressing temperature and temperature intervals. Celsius (formerly centigrade) *temperature* is converted to Kelvin (K) thermodynamic temperature by adding 273.16 to the Celsius scale. For *temperature interval*, 1°C equals K.

## Some SI-Derived Units Expressed in Terms of Base Units

| Quantity | Name | Symbol |
|---|---|---|
| area | square meter | $m^2$ |
| volume* | cubic meter | $m^3$ |
| specific volume | cubic meter per kilogram | $m^3/kg$ |
| speed, velocity | meter per second | $m/s$ |
| acceleration | meter per second squared | $m/s^2$ |
| mass density | kilogram per cubic meter | $kg/m^3$ |
| concentration | mole per cubic meter | $mol/m^3$ |
| luminance | candela per square meter | $cd/m^2$ |

*Liter (L, l). $10^{-3}$ $m^3$ is regarded as a special name for the cubic decimeter.

## Some SI-Derived Units with Special Names

| Quantity | Name | Symbol | Expression |
|---|---|---|---|
| frequency | hertz | Hz | $s^{-1}$ |
| force | newton | N | $m\ kg\ s^{-2}$ |
| pressure, stress | pascal | Pa | $m^{-1}\ kg\ s^{-2}$ |
| energy | joule | J | $m^2\ kg\ s^{-2}$ |
| power | watt | W | $m^2\ kg\ s^{-3}$ |
| quantity of electricity, electric charge | coulomb | C | $s\ A$ |
| electric potential, electromotive force | volt | V | $m^2\ kg\ s^{-3}A^{-1}$ |
| capacitance | farad | F | $m^{-2}\ kg^{-1}\ s^4A^{-2}$ |
| electrical resistance | ohm | $\Omega$ | $m^2\ kg^{-2}\ A^{-2}$ |
| electrical conductance | siemens | S | $m^{-2}kg\ s^{-2}A^{-1}$ |
| magnetic flux | weber | Wb | $m^2\ kg\ s^{-2}A^{-1}$ |
| magnetic flux density | tesla | T | $kg\ s^{-2}A^{-1}$ |
| activity of radionuclide | becquerel* | Bq | $s^{-1}$ |
| absorbed dose of radiation | gray** | Gy | $m^2\ s^{-2}$ |
| exposure (x and $\gamma$ radiation) | coulomb per kilogram*** | C kg | $kg^{-1}\ s\ A$ |

*Replacing the curie (Ci), $3.7 \times 10^{10}$ $s^{-1}$. **Replacing the rad, $10^{-2}$ J $kg^{-1}$. ***Replacing the roentgen (R), $2.58 \times 10^{-4}$ C kg $^{-1}$.

## Measures of Length

| Micrometers | Millimeters | Centimeters | Meters | Kilometers | Miles | Yards | Feet | Inches |
|---|---|---|---|---|---|---|---|---|
| 1 | 0.001 | $10^{-4}$ | | | | | | 0.000039 |
| $10^3$ | 1 | $10^{-1}$ | | | | | .00328 | 0.03937 |
| $10^4$ | 10 | 1 | 0.01 | | | 0.0109 | .03281 | 0.3937 |
| 254,000 | 25.4 | 2.54 | 0.0254 | | | 0.0278 | .0833 | 1 |
| | 304.8 | 30.48 | 0.3048 | | | 0.333 | 1 | 12 |
| $10^6$ | $10^3$ | $10^2$ | 1 | 0.001 | 0.0006213 | 1.0936 | 3.2808 | 39.37 |
| 914,400 | 914.40 | 91.44 | 0.9144 | 0.009 | 0.0005681 | 1 | 3 | 36 |
| $10^9$ | $10^6$ | $10^5$ | $10^3$ | 1 | 0.6215 | 1093.6121 | 3280.8 | |
| | | | 1609.0 | 1.609 | 1 | 1760.0 | 5280.0 | |

To convert:

Millimeters to inches: divide by 25.4    Centimeters to feet: divide by 30.7
Inches to millimeters: multiply by 25.4    Feet to centimeters: multiply by 30.7

Meters to yards: multiply by 1.09375    Kilometers to miles: multiply by 0.625
Yards to meters: multiply by 0.9143    Miles to kilometers: multiply by 1.6

**Measures of Mass (Weight)**

| Avoirdupois Weights | | | | Metric Equivalents | | |
|---|---|---|---|---|---|---|
| Grains | Drams | Ounces | Pounds | Milligrams | Grams | Kilograms |
| 1 | 0.0366 | 0.0023 | 0.00014 | 64.8 | 0.0648 | 0.000065 |
| 27.34 | 1 | 0.0625 | 0.0039 | | 1.772 | 0.001772 |
| 437.5 | 16 | 1 | 0.0625 | | 28.350 | 0.028350 |
| 7,000 | 256 | 16 | 1 | | 453.5924 | 0.453592 |
| 0.0154 | | | | 1 | 0.001 | |
| 15.4324 | 0.5648 | 0.0353 | 0.002205 | 1000 | 1 | 0.001 |
| 15,432.358 | 564.32 | 35.27 | 2.2046 | | 1000 | 1 |

To convert (approximately):

Kilograms to pounds: multiply by 2.2          Grams to ounces: multiply by 0.03527
Pounds to kilograms: multiply by 0.454   Ounces to grams: multiply by 28.35

| Apothecaries' Weights | | | | | Metric Equivalents | | |
|---|---|---|---|---|---|---|---|
| Grains | Scruples | Drams | Ounces | Pounds | Mgs | Grams | Kilograms |
| 1 | 0.05 | 0.0167 | 0.0021 | 0.00017 | 64.8 | 0.0648 | 0.000065 |
| 20 | 1 | 0.333 | 0.042 | 0.0035 | | 1.296 | 0.001296 |
| 60 | 3 | 1 | 0.125 | 0.0104 | | 3.888 | 0.000389 |
| 480 | 24 | 8 | 1 | 0.0833 | | 31.103 | 0.031103 |
| 5,760 | 288 | 96 | 12 | 1 | | 373.2417 | 0.373242 |
| 0.0154 | | | | | 1 | 0.001 | |
| 15.4324 | | 0.2572 | 0.0322 | 0.0027 | 1000 | 1 | 0.001 |
| 15,432.358 | | 257.2 | 32.15 | 2.6792 | | 1000 | 1 |

**Measures of Capacity**

| Apothecaries' Measures | | | | | | Metric Equivalents | | |
|---|---|---|---|---|---|---|---|---|
| Minims | Fluid Drams | Fluid Ounces | Pints | Quarts | Gallons | Liters | Milliliters |
| 1 | 0.0167 | 0.002 | 0.00013 | | | 0.0006 | 0.06161 |
| 60 | 1 | 0.125 | 0.0078 | 0.0039 | | 0.0037 | 3.6967 |
| 480 | 8 | 1 | 0.0625 | 0.0312 | 0.0078 | 0.0296 | 29.5737 |
| 7,680 | 128 | 16 | 1 | 0.5 | 0.125 | 0.4732 | 473.166 |
| 15,360 | 256 | 32 | 2 | 1 | 0.25 | 0.9464 | 946.358 |
| 61,440 | 1024 | 128 | 8 | 4 | 1 | 3.7854 | 3785.434 |
| 16,230 | 270.52 | 33.8418 | 2.1134 | 1.0567 | 0.2642 | 1 | 1000 |
| 16.23 | 0.2705 | 0.0338 | 0.00212 | 0.00106 | 0.000265 | 0.001 | 1 |

To convert (approximately)

1 British imperial gallon = 1.201 U.S. gallon   Liters to gallons: multiply by 0.264
1 U.S. gallon = 0.8327 British imperial gallon   Gallons to liters: multiply by 3.788

Liters to pints: multiply by 2.1
Pints to liters: multiply by 0.4732

**Approximate Household Measures and Weights\***

| Teaspoons | Tablespoons | Cups or Glasses\*\* | Drams | Fluid Ounces | Milliliters | Grams |
|---|---|---|---|---|---|---|
| 1 | | | 1 | 0.125 | 5 | 5 |
| 3 | 1 | | 4 | 0.50 | 15 | 15 |
| 48 | 16\*\*\* | 1 | 64 | 8 | 237 | 240 |

\*A drop is a measure of uncertain quantity, depending on the nature of the liquid as well as the shape of the container and of the opening from which the liquid falls. One drop of water is roughly equivalent to 1 minim.

\*\*"Tumbler or glass" is generally intended to mean 8 fluid ounces.

\*\*\*For dry measure, 12 tablespoons equal 1 cup.

# Temperature Equivalents

| Celsius to Fahrenheit | | | | Fahrenheit to Celsius | | | | | |
|---|---|---|---|---|---|---|---|---|---|
| °C | °F | °C | °F | °F | °C | °F | °C | °F | °C |
| −50 | −58.0 | 49 | 120.0 | −50 | −46.7 | 99 | 37.2 | 157 | 69.4 |
| −40 | −40.0 | 50 | 122.0 | −40 | −40.0 | 100 | 37.7 | 158 | 70.0 |
| −35 | −31.0 | 51 | 123.8 | −35 | −37.2 | 101 | 38.3 | 159 | 70.5 |
| −30 | −22.0 | 52 | 125.6 | −30 | −34.4 | 102 | 38.8 | 160 | 71.1 |
| −25 | −13.0 | 53 | 127.4 | −25 | −31.7 | 103 | 39.4 | 161 | 71.6 |
| −20 | −4.0 | 54 | 129.2 | −20 | −28.9 | 104 | 40.0 | 162 | 72.2 |
| −15 | 5.0 | 55 | 131.0 | −15 | −26.6 | 105 | 40.5 | 163 | 72.7 |
| −10 | 14.0 | 56 | 132.8 | −10 | −23.3 | 106 | 41.1 | 164 | 73.3 |
| −5 | 23.0 | 57 | 134.6 | −5 | −20.6 | 107 | 41.6 | 165 | 73.8 |
| **0** | **32.0** | 58 | 136.4 | 0 | −17.7 | 108 | 42.2 | 166 | 74.4 |
| 1 | 33.8 | 59 | 138.2 | 1 | −17.2 | 109 | 42.7 | 167 | 75.0 |
| 2 | 35.6 | 60 | 140.0 | 5 | −15.0 | 110 | 43.3 | 168 | 75.5 |
| 3 | 37.4 | 61 | 141.8 | 10 | −12.2 | 111 | 43.8 | 169 | 76.1 |
| 4 | 39.2 | 62 | 143.6 | 15 | −9.4 | 112 | 44.4 | 170 | 76.6 |
| 5 | 41.0 | 63 | 145.4 | 20 | −6.6 | 113 | 45.0 | 171 | 77.2 |
| 6 | 42.8 | 64 | 147.2 | 25 | −3.8 | 114 | 45.5 | 172 | 77.7 |
| 7 | 44.6 | 65 | 149.0 | 30 | −1.1 | 115 | 46.1 | 173 | 78.3 |
| 8 | 46.4 | 66 | 150.8 | 31 | −0.5 | 116 | 46.6 | 174 | 78.8 |
| 9 | 48.2 | 67 | 152.6 | **32** | **0** | 117 | 47.2 | 175 | 79.4 |
| 10 | 50.0 | 68 | 154.4 | 33 | 0.5 | 118 | 47.7 | 176 | 80.0 |
| 11 | 51.8 | 69 | 156.2 | 34 | 1.1 | 119 | 48.3 | 177 | 80.5 |
| 12 | 53.6 | 70 | 158.0 | 35 | 1.6 | 120 | 48.8 | 178 | 81.1 |
| 13 | 55.4 | 71 | 159.8 | 36 | 2.2 | 121 | 49.4 | 179 | 81.6 |
| 14 | 57.2 | 72 | 161.6 | 37 | 2.7 | 122 | 50.0 | 180 | 82.2 |
| 15 | 59.0 | 73 | 163.4 | 38 | 3.3 | 123 | 50.5 | 181 | 82.7 |
| 16 | 60.8 | 74 | 165.2 | 39 | 3.8 | 124 | 51.1 | 182 | 83.3 |
| 17 | 62.6 | 75 | 167.0 | 40 | 4.4 | 125 | 51.6 | 183 | 83.8 |
| 18 | 64.4 | 76 | 168.8 | 41 | 5.0 | 126 | 52.2 | 184 | 84.4 |
| 19 | 66.2 | 77 | 170.6 | 42 | 5.5 | 127 | 52.7 | 185 | 85.0 |
| 20 | 68.0 | 78 | 172.4 | 43 | 6.1 | 128 | 53.3 | 186 | 85.5 |
| 21 | 69.8 | 79 | 174.2 | 44 | 6.6 | 129 | 53.8 | 187 | 86.1 |
| 22 | 71.6 | 80 | 176.0 | 45 | 7.2 | 130 | 54.4 | 188 | 86.6 |
| 23 | 73.4 | 81 | 177.8 | 46 | 7.7 | 131 | 55.0 | 189 | 87.2 |
| 24 | 75.2 | 82 | 179.6 | 47 | 8.3 | 132 | 55.5 | 190 | 87.7 |
| 25 | 77.0 | 83 | 181.4 | 48 | 8.8 | 133 | 56.1 | 191 | 88.3 |
| 26 | 78.8 | 84 | 183.2 | 49 | 9.4 | 134 | 56.6 | 192 | 88.8 |
| 27 | 80.6 | 85 | 185.0 | 50 | 10.0 | 135 | 57.2 | 193 | 89.4 |
| 28 | 82.4 | 86 | 186.8 | 55 | 12.7 | 136 | 57.7 | 194 | 90.0 |
| 29 | 84.2 | 87 | 188.6 | 60 | 15.5 | 137 | 58.3 | 195 | 90.5 |
| 30 | 86.0 | 88 | 190.4 | 65 | 18.3 | 138 | 58.8 | 196 | 91.1 |
| 31 | 87.8 | 89 | 192.2 | 70 | 21.1 | 139 | 59.4 | 197 | 91.6 |
| 32 | 89.6 | 90 | 194.0 | 75 | 23.8 | 140 | 60.0 | 198 | 92.2 |
| 33 | 91.4 | 91 | 195.8 | 80 | 26.6 | 141 | 60.5 | 199 | 92.7 |
| 34 | 93.2 | 92 | 197.6 | 85 | 29.4 | 142 | 61.1 | 200 | 93.3 |
| 35 | 95.0 | 93 | 199.4 | 86 | 30.0 | 143 | 61.6 | 201 | 93.8 |
| 36 | 96.8 | 94 | 201.2 | 87 | 30.5 | 144 | 62.2 | 202 | 94.4 |
| **37** | **98.6** | 95 | 203.0 | 88 | 31.0 | 145 | 62.7 | 203 | 95.0 |
| 38 | 100.4 | 96 | 204.8 | 89 | 31.6 | 146 | 63.3 | 204 | 95.5 |
| 39 | 102.2 | 97 | 206.6 | 90 | 32.2 | 147 | 63.8 | 205 | 96.1 |
| 40 | 104.0 | 98 | 208.4 | 91 | 32.7 | 148 | 64.4 | 206 | 96.6 |
| 41 | 105.8 | 99 | 210.2 | 92 | 33.3 | 149 | 65.0 | 207 | 97.2 |
| 42 | 107.6 | **100** | **212.0** | 93 | 33.8 | 150 | 65.5 | 208 | 97.7 |
| 43 | 109.4 | 101 | 213.8 | 94 | 34.4 | 151 | 66.1 | 209 | 98.3 |
| 44 | 111.2 | 102 | 215.6 | 95 | 35.0 | 152 | 66.6 | 210 | 98.8 |
| 45 | 113.0 | 103 | 217.4 | 96 | 35.5 | 153 | 67.2 | 211 | 99.4 |
| 46 | 114.8 | 104 | 219.2 | 97 | 36.1 | 154 | 67.7 | **212** | **100.0** |
| 47 | 116.6 | 105 | 221.0 | 98 | 36.6 | 155 | 68.3 | 213 | 100.5 |
| 48 | 118.4 | 106 | 222.8 | **98.6** | **37.0** | 156 | 68.8 | 214 | 101.1 |

## Fahrenheit–Celsius Conversion Formulas

To convert Fahrenheit to Celsius (above 32°F) or Celsius to Fahrenheit (above 0° C):

F to C: Subtract 32, multiply by 5, divide by 9.
Example: 63° F to Celsius: $63 - 32 = 31 \times 5 = 155 \div 9 = 17.2°C$

C to F: Multiply by 9, divide by 5, add 32.
Example: 37 °C to Fahrenheit: $37 \times 9 = 333 \div 5 = 66.6 + 32 = 98.6° F$

# Medical Prefixes, Suffixes, and Combining Forms: The Building Blocks of Medical Language

**a-** not, without, -less
**ab-, abs-** from, away from, off
**acanth(o)-** thorn
**acou-** hearing
**acr(o)-** extremity
**acu-** hearing; needle
**ad-** increase, adherence, motion toward; very
**-ad** toward, in the direction of; -ward
**aden(o)-** gland
**adip(o)-** fat
**-agog, -agogue** promoter, stimulator
**aidoio-** genitals
**-al** pertaining to
**alb(o)-** white
**alge(si)-, algio-, algo-** pain
**allo-** other, different
**ambi-** around, on (both) sides, on all sides, both
**ambly(o)-** dull
**amyl(o)-** starch, polysaccharide
**an-** not, without, -less
**ana-** up, toward, apart
**andr(o)-** male
**angi(o)-** vessel
**ankylo-** crooked
**ante-** before
**anthraco-** coal, carbon
**anti-** against, opposing; curative; antibody
**apo-** separated from, derived from
**aque(o)-** water
**-ar** pertaining to
**-arche** beginning
**arteri(o)-** artery
**arthr(o)-** joint, articulation
**-ary** pertaining to
**-ase** an enzyme
**-ate** a salt or ester of an "-ic" acid
**athero-** pasty, fatty
**atto-** one-quintillionth ($10^{-18}$)
**audi(o)-** hearing
**aur(i)-, auro-** ear
**aut(o)-** self, same
**bacteri(o)-** bacteria
**balan(o)-** glans penis
**bi-** twice, double
**bio-** life
**blasto-** budding by cells or tissue
**blephar(o)-** eyelid

**brachi(o)-** arm
**brachy-** short
**bronch-** bronchus
**bronch(i)-, bronch(i)o-** bronchus
**carcin(o)-** cancer
**cardi(o)-** heart; esophageal opening of stomach
**carpo-** wrist
**cata-** down
**caud(o)-** tail, lower part of body
**-cele** hernia, swelling
**celio-** abdomen
**-centesis** surgical puncture
**centi-** one-hundredth ($10^{-2}$)
**cephal(o)-** the head
**cervic(o)-** neck; uterine cervix
**cheil(o)-** lip
**cheir(o)-** hand
**chem(o)-** chemistry; drug
**chir(o)-** hand
**chlor(o)-** green; chlorine
**chol(e)-** bile
**chondrio-, chondr(o)-** cartilage; granular; gritty
**chrom-, chromat-, chromo-** color
**chron(o)-** time
**-cidal, -cide** killing, destroying
**cis-** on this side, on the near side
**-clast** breaker
**-clysis** washing
**co-** with, together, in association, very, complete
**col-** with, together, in association, very, complete
**colp(o)-** vagina
**com-, con-** with, together, in association, very, complete
**conio-** dust
**cor-** with, together, in association, very, complete
**coreo-** pupil
**cost(o)-** rib
**crani(o)-** cranium
**-crine** secretion
**cry(o)-** cold
**crypt(o)-** hidden
**culdo-** cul-de-sac
**cyan(o)-** blue; cyanide**

**cycl-** circle, cycle; ciliary body
**cyst(i)-, cysto-** bladder; cyst; cystic duct
**cyt-, -cyte, cyto-** cell
**dacry(o)-** tears
**dactyl(o)-** finger, toe
**de-** away from; cessation
**deca-** ten
**deci-** one-tenth ($10^{-1}$)
**deka-** ten
**dent(i)-** tooth
**derm-, derma-, dermat(o)-, dermo-** skin
**-desis** binding
**dextr(o)-** right, toward or on the right side
**di-** separation, taking apart, reversal, not, un-
**dif-** separation, taking apart, reversal, not, un-
**dipso-** thirst
**dir-, dis-** separation, taking apart, reversal,
    not, un-
**duo-** two
**duodeno-** duodenum
**-dynia** pain
**dynamo-** force, energy
**dys-** bad, difficult
**ect-** outer, on the outside
**-ectasia, -ectasis** dilation, stretching
**ecto-** outer, on the outside
**-ectomy** excision
**-emphraxis** obstruction
**encephal(o)-** brain
**end(o)-** within, inner
**enter(o)-** intestine
**ent(o)-** inner, within
**ep-, epi-** upon, following, subsequent to
**ergo-** work
**erythr(o)-** red, redness
**eso-** inward
**esthesio-** sensation, perception
**eu-** good, well
**ex-** out of, from, away from
**exo-** exterior, external, outward
**extra-** without, outside of
**ferri-** ferric ion ($Fe^{3+}$)
**ferro-** metallic iron; ferrous ion ($Fe^{2+}$)
**fibr(o)-** fiber
**-form** in the form or shape of
**galact(o)-** milk
**gastr(o)-** stomach; belly
**gen-, -gen** producing, coming to be; precursor
**giga-** one billion ($10^9$)
**gingiv(o)-** gums
**gloss(o)-** tongue
**gluco-** glucose

**glyco-** sugars
**gnath(o)-** jaw
**gon-** seed, semen
**gonio-** angle
**gono-** seed, semen
**-gram** writing, recording
**granul(o)-** granular, granule
**-graph** recording instrument
**gyn(e)-, gyneco-, gyno-** woman
**hecto-** one hundred ($10^2$)
**hem(a)-, hemat(o)-** blood
**hemi-** one-half
**hemo-** blood
**hepat-, hepatico-, hepato-** liver
**hept(a)-** seven
**hidr(o)-** sweat
**hist-, histio-, histo-** tissue
**homeo-** same, constant
**hydr(o)-** water; hydrogen
**hyper-** above, excessive
**hypo-** below, deficient
**hyster(o)-** uterus; hysteria; late, following
**-ia** condition
**-iasis** condition, infestation, infection
**-ic** pertaining to
**-ics** organized knowledge, practice, treatment
**ileo-** ileum
**ilio-** ilium
**in-** in; not
**-in** chemical suffix
**-ine** chemical suffix
**infra-** below
**inguino-** groin
**inter-** between, among
**intra-, intro-** within
**irid(o)-** iris
**ischi(o)-** ischium
**-ism** condition, disease; practice, doctrine
**-ismus** spasm; contraction
**iso-** equal, like; isomer; sameness
**-ite** of the nature of, resembling
**-ites** -y, -like
**-itides** plural of -itis
**-itis** inflammation
**kal(i)-** potassium
**kary(o)-** nucleus
**kerat(o)-** cornea, cornified epithelium
**kilo-** one thousand ($10^3$)
**kin(e)-, kinesi(o)-, kineso-, kino-** movement
**labio-** lip
**lacrim(o)-** tears
**lact(i)-, lacto-** milk

**laparo-** abdomen, abdominal wall
**laryng(o)-** larynx
**lateri-, latero-** lateral, to one side, side
**-lepsis, -lepsy** seizure
**lepto-** light, slender, thin, frail
**leuk(o)-** white
**lien(o)-** spleen
**linguo-** tongue
**lip(o)-** fat, lipid
**lith(o)-** stone, calculus, calcification
**-log** speech, words
**log(o)-** speech, words
**-logy** study of; collecting
**lymph(o)-** lymph; lymphocyte
**lys(o)-, -lysis, -lytic** dissolution, disintegration; release
**macr(o)-** large; long
**mal-** bad, deficient
**-malacia** softening
**mamm-, mamm(a)-, mammo-** breast
**mast(o)-** breast
**meg-** large, oversize
**mega-** large, oversize; one million ($10^6$)
**megal(o)-** large
**-megaly** enlargement
**melan(o)-** black
**men-** menstruation
**mening(o)-** meninges
**meno-** menstruation
**ment(o)-** chin
**-mer** member of a series
**mes(o)-** middle, mean, intermediate; attaching membrane
**meta-** after, behind; joint action, sharing
**-meter** measurement, measuring device
**metr(o)-** uterus
**micr-** small, microscopic
**micro-** small, microscopic; one-millionth ($10^{-6}$)
**milli-** one-thousandth ($10^{-3}$)
**mon(o)-** single
**morph(o)-** form, shape, structure
**my(o)-** muscle
**myel(o)-** bone marrow; spinal cord
**myring(o)-** tympanic membrane
**myx(o)-** mucus
**nano-** dwarf; one-billionth ($10^{-9}$)
**nas(o)-** nose
**natr(i)-** sodium
**necr(o)-** death, necrosis
**neo-** new
**nephr(o)-** kidney

**neur(i)-, neuro-** nerve, nervous system
**norm(o)-** normal
**octo-** eight
**oculo-** eye
**odont(o)-** tooth
**odyn(o)-, -odynia** pain
**-oid** resemblance to
**olig(o)-** few, little
**-oma** tumor, neoplasm
**-omata** plural of -oma
**oncho-, onco-** tumor, bulk, volume
**-one** ketone (-CO- group)
**onych(o)-, -onychia** fingernail, toenail
**oo-** egg, ovary
**oophor(o)-** ovary
**ophthalm(o)-** eye
**-opia, -opsia, -opsis** vision
**or-** mouth
**orchi-, orchid(o)-, orchio-** testis
**ori-, oro-** mouth
**-ose** sugar
**-oses** plural of -osis
**-osis** process, condition, state
**osseo-** bony
**ossi-** bone
**ost(e)-, osteo-** bone
**ovari(o)-** ovary
**ov(i)-, ovo-** egg
**ox(a)-, oxo-** oxygen
**oxy-** sharp, acid; acute, shrill, quick; oxygen
**pachy-** thick
**pan-, pant(o)-** all, entire
**para-** beside, near; similar; subordinate; abnormal
**pari-** equal
**path(o)-** disease, abnormality
**-pathy** disease, abnormality
**ped(i)-, pedo-** child; foot
**-penia** deficiency
**penta-** five
**per-** through, thoroughly, intensely
**peri-** around, about
**-pexy** fixation, usually surgical
**phaco-** lens
**-phage, -phagia, phago-, -phagy** eating, devouring
**phako-** lens
**phanero-** visible, evident
**pharmaco-** drug, medicine
**pharyng(o)-** pharynx
**phil-** attraction; chemical affinity
**-philia** attraction; chemical affinity

**philo-** attraction; chemical affinity
**phleb(o)-** vein
**-phobe, -phobia** fear; chemical repulsion
**phon(o)-** sound, speech
**phor(o)-** carrying, bearing
**phos-, phot(o)-** light
**phren(i)-** diaphragm; mind; phrenic
**-phrenia** mind
**phrenico-, phreno-** diaphragm; mind; phrenic
**-phylaxis** protection
**phyll(o)-** leaf
**physi(o)-** physical; natural
**physo-** swelling, inflation; air, gas
**phyt(o)-** plants
**pico-** one-trillionth ($10^{-12}$)
**plan(i)-, plano-** flat
**-plasia** formation
**plasm(a)-, plasmat(o)-, plasmo-** plasma
**platy-** wide, flat
**-plegia** paralysis
**pleo-** more
**plesio-** near, similar
**pleur(a)-, pleuro-** rib, side, pleura
**pluri-** several, more
**-pnea** breath, respiration
**pneo-** breath, respiration
**pneum(a)-, pneumat(o)-** air, gas; lung; breathing
**pod(o)-** foot, foot-shaped
**-poiesis, -poietic** production
**poikilo-** irregular, variable
**polio-** gray
**poly-** many, multiple; polymer
**post-** after, behind, posterior
**pre-** anterior, before
**presby-** old
**pro-** before, forward; precursor
**proct(o)-** anus, rectum
**prot(o)-** first
**pseud(o)-** false
**psych(e)-, psycho-** mind
**-ptosis** sagging, falling
**pyel(o)-** (renal) pelvis
**pykn(o)-** dense, compact
**pyo-** suppuration, pus
**pyreto-** fever
**pyro-** fire, heat, fever
**quadr(i)-** four
**rachi(o)-** spinal column
**radio-** radiation, x-ray; radius
**re-** again, back, backward
**rect(i)-** straight

**rect(o)-** rectum
**ren(o)-** kidney
**retro-** backward, behind
**rhin(o)-** nose
**-rrhagia** discharge, bleeding
**-rrhaphy** surgical suturing
**-rrhea** flow
**-rrhexis** rupture
**salping(o)-** tube
**sarco-** flesh, muscle
**schisto-, schiz(o)-** split, cleft, division
**scler(o)-** hardness, sclerosis; ocular sclera
**scolio-** crooked
**-scope** instrument for viewing
**-scopy** viewing
**scot(o)-** shadow, darkness
**semi-** one-half; partly
**sept-** seven; septum; sepsis, infection
**septi-** seven
**septo-** seven; septum; sepsis, infection
**sial(o)-** saliva, salivary gland
**sider(o)-** iron
**sigmoid(o)-** S-shaped; sigmoid colon
**sin-, sin(o)-, sinu-** sinus
**sito-** food, grain
**somat-, somato-, somatico-** body, bodily
**somno-** sleep
**son(o)-** sound; ultrasound
**spasmo-** spasm
**sperm(a), spermat(o), spermo-** semen, spermatozoa
**sphygmo-** pulse
**spir(o)-** breathing
**splanchn(i)-, splanchno-** viscera
**splen(o)-** spleen
**staphyl(o)-** grape, bunch of grapes; staphylococci
**-stasis** stopping
**-stat** arresting change or movement
**steno-** narrowness, constriction
**stereo-** solid
**stheno-** strength, force, power
**stom(a)-, stomat(o)-** mouth
**sub-** beneath, less than normal, inferior
**super-** above, in excess, superior
**supra-** above
**sy-, syl-, sym-, syn-, sys-** together
**tachy-** rapid
**tel(e)-** distant
**ten-, tendin-, teno-, tenont(o)-** tendon
**tera-** one quadrillion ($10^{15}$)
**tetra-** four

**thel(o)-** nipple
**therm(o)-** heat
**thora-, thorac(i)-, thoracico, thoraco-** chest, thorax
**thromb(o)-** blood clot
**thyre(o)-, thyr(o)-** thyroid gland
**toco-, toko-** childbirth
**-tome** cutting instrument; segment, section
**-tomy** cutting operation
**tono-** tone, tension, pressure
**top(o)-** place, topical
**tox(i)-, toxico-, toxo-** toxin, poison
**trache(o)-** trachea
**trans-** across, through, beyond
**tri-** three
**trich(i)-** hair
**-trichia** hair **tricho-** hair
**tris-** three

**-trophic, tropho-, -trophy** food, nutrition
**-tropia, -tropic, -tropy** turning, tendency, affinity
**ultra-** beyond
**uni-** one, single
**uri-** uric acid
**-uria** urine, urination
**uric(o)-** uric acid
**uro-** urine; urinary tract
**vas-** duct; blood vessel
**vasculo-** blood vessel
**vaso-** duct, blood vessel
**vesic(o)-** urinary bladder, vesicle
**xanth(o)-** yellow
**xero-** dry
**zo(o)-** animal; life
**zym(o)-** fermentation, enzyme

# Common Medical Abbreviations and Acronyms

**α** alpha: Bunsen's solubility coefficient; first in a series; specific rotation term; heavy chain class corresponding to IgA

**a** (specific) absorption (coefficient) (USUALLY ITALIC); (total) acidity; area; (systemic) arterial (blood) (SUBSCRIPT); asymmetric; atto-

**A** absorbance

**A** adenosine (or adenylic acid); alveolar gas (SUBSCRIPT); ampere

**Å** angstrom; Ångström unit

**AA** amino acid; aminoacyl

**AB** abortion

**Ab** antibody

**ABG** arterial blood gas

**abl** Abelson murine leukemia virus

**ABLB** alternate binaural loudness balance (test)

**ABO** blood group system

**ABR** abortus-Bang-ring (test); auditory brainstem response (audiometry)

**γ-Abu** γ-aminobutyric acid

**ABVD** adriamycin (doxorubicin), bleomycin, vinblastine, and dacarbazine

**ac** acetyl

**a.c.** [L.] *ante cibum,* before a meal

**aC** arabinosylcytosine

**Ac** acetyl; actinium

**AC** acetate; acromioclavicular; atriocarotid

**AC/A** accommodation convergence-accommodation (ratio)

**ACE** angiotensin-converting enzyme

**ACEI** angiotensin-converting enzyme inhibitor

**ac-g** accelerator globulin

**AcG** accelerator globulin

**Ach** acetylcholine

**aCL** anticardiolipin (antibody)

**ACP** acyl carrier protein

**ACTH** adrenocorticotropic hormone (corticotropin)

**AD** [L.] *auris dextra,* right ear; Alzheimer disease

**ADA** Americans with Disabilities Act

**Ade** adenine

**ADH** antidiuretic hormone

**ADL** activities of daily living

**ad lib** [L.] *ad libitum,* freely, as desired

**Ado** adenosine

**ADP** adenosine 5'-diphosphate

**A-E** above-the-elbow (amputation)

**AFB** acid-fast bacillus

**AFORMED** alternating failure of response, mechanical, to electrical depolarization

**AFP** α-fetoprotein

**Ag** antigen; [L.] *argentum,* silver

**A/G R** albumin-globulin ratio

**AHF** antihemophilic factor

**AHG** antihemophilic globulin

**AID** artificial insemination donor

**AIDS** acquired immunodeficiency syndrome

**AIH** artificial insemination by husband; artificial insemination, homologous

**A-K** above-the-knee (amputation)

**Al** aluminum

**Ala** alanine (or its mono- or diradical)

**ALA** δ-aminolevulinic acid

**ALD** adrenoleukodystrophy

**ALL** acute lymphocytic leukemia

**ALS** antilymphocyte serum; advanced life support

**ALT** alanine aminotransferase

**Am** americium

**AML** acute myelogenous leukemia

**AMP** adenosine monophosphate (adenylic acid)

**amu** atomic mass unit

**ANA** antinuclear antibody

**ANF** antinuclear factor

**ANOVA** analysis of variance

**ANS** autonomic nervous system

**ANUG** acute necrotizing ulcerative gingivitis

**APA** antipernicious anemia (factor)

**APC** antigen-presenting cell

**A-P-C** adenoidal-pharyngeal-conjunctival (virus)

**aPS** antiphospholipid antibody syndrome

**APTT** activated partial thromboplastin time

**Ar** argon

**araC** arabinosylcytosine (cytarabine)

**ARDS** adult respiratory distress syndrome

**ARF** acute renal failure; acute rheumatic fever

**Arg** arginine (or its mono- or diradical)

**As** arsenic

**AS** [L.] *auris sinistra,* left ear

**ASA** acetylsalicylic acid (aspirin)

**ASCUS** abnormal squamous cells of undetermined significance

**ASHD** arteriosclerotic heart disease

**Asn** asparagine (or its mono- or diradical)

**ASO** antistreptolysin O

**Asp** aspartic acid (or its radical forms)

**AST** aspartate aminotransferase

**At** astatine

**ATFL** anterior talofibular ligament

**ATL** adult T-cell leukemia; adult T-cell lymphoma

**atm** (standard) atmosphere

**ATP** adenosine 5'-triphosphate

**ATPase** adenosine triphosphatase

**ATPD** ambient temperature and pressure, dry

**ATPS** ambient temperature and pressure, saturated (with water vapor)

**at. wt.** atomic weight

**Au** [L.] *aurum,* gold

**AU** [L.] *auris utraque,* each ear, both ears

**AV** arteriovenous

**A-V** arteriovenous; atrioventricular

**AVN** atrioventricular node

**AVP** antiviral protein

**AW** atomic weight

**ax.** axis

**AZT** azidothymidine (zidovudine)

**b** second in a series; blood (SUBSCRIPT)

**B** barometric (pressure) (SUBSCRIPT); boron

**Ba** barium

**BADL** basic activities of daily living

**BAER** brainstem auditory evoked response

**BAL** British anti-Lewisite (dimercaprol); bronchoalveolar lavage

**BALB** binaural alternate loudness balance (test)

**BBB** blood-brain barrier

**BCG** bacille bilié de Calmette-Guérin (vaccine)

**BE** barium enema

**Be** beryllium

**B-E** below-the-elbow (amputation)

**Bi** bismuth

**b.i.d.** [L.] *bis in die,* twice a day

**BIDS** brittle hair, impaired intelligence, decreased fertility, and short stature (syndrome)

**BIPAP** bilevel positive airway pressure

**Bk** berkelium

**BM** bowel movement

**BMI** body mass index

**bp** base pair

**BP** blood pressure; boiling point; *British Pharmacopoeia*

**BPF** bronchopleural fistula

**BPH** benign prostatic hyperplasia

**Bq** becquerel (SI unit of radionuclide activity)

**Br** bromine

**BRAT** (diet) banana, rice cereal, applesauce, toast

**BSA** body surface area

**BSER** brainstem evoked response (audiometry)

**BT** bleeding time

**BTPS** body temperature, ambient pressure, saturated (with water vapor)

**BTU** British thermal unit

**BUN** blood urea nitrogen

**BUS** Bartholin glands, urethra, Skene glands

**C** calorie (large); carbon; Celsius; centigrade; clearance (rate, renal) (FOLLOWED BY A SUBSCRIPT); compliance; concentration; cylindrical (lens); cytidine

**c** calorie (small); capillary (blood) (SUBSCRIPT); centi-

**ca.** [L.] *circa,* about, approximately

**c-a** cardioarterial

**Ca** calcium; cathodal; cathode

**CA** cancer; carcinoma; cardiac arrest; chronologic age; croup-associated (virus); cytosine arabinoside

**CABG** coronary artery bypass graft

**cal** calorie (small)

**Cal** calorie (large)

**cAMP** cyclic AMP (adenosine monophosphate)

**CAP** catabolite (gene) activator protein

**CAPD** continuous ambulatory peritoneal dialysis

**CAT** computerized axial tomography

**CBC** complete blood (cell) count

**CBG** corticosteroid-binding globulin

**Cbz** carbobenzoxy (chloride)

**cc, c.c.** cubic centimeter

**C.C.** chief complaint

**CCK** cholecystokinin

**CCNU** chloroethylcyclohexylnitrosourea (lomustine)

**CCU** coronary care unit; critical care unit

**cd** candela

**Cd** cadmium

**CDC** Centers for Disease Control and Prevention

**cDNA** complementary DNA

**CDP** cytidine 5′-diphosphate

**Ce** cerium

**CEA** carcinoembryonic antigen

**CELO** chicken embryo lethal orphan (virus)

**CEP** congenital erythropoietic porphyria

**Cf** californium

**CF** complement fixation; cystic fibrosis; coupling factor

**CG** chorionic gonadotropin

**CGA** catabolite gene activator

**cGMP** cyclic GMP (guanosine monophosphate)

**cgs, CGS** centimeter-gram-second (system, unit)

**Ch$^1$** Christchurch (chromosome)

**CHF** congestive heart failure

**CHO** carbohydrate

**Ci** curie

**μCi** microcurie

**CI** color index; *Colour Index*

**CIB** [L.] *cibus,* food

**CJD** Creutzfeldt-Jakob disease

**CK** creatine kinase

**Cl** chlorine

**CL** cardiolipin

**CLIA** Clinical Laboratory Improvement Amendments

**CLL** chronic lymphocytic leukemia

**CLQ** cognitive laterality quotient

**cm** centimeter

**cM** centimorgan

**Cm** curium

**CMC** carpometacarpal

**CMI** cell-mediated immunity

**CML** chronic myelogenous leukemia

**CMP** cytidine 5'-phosphate (or any cytidine monophosphate)

**CMV** controlled mechanical ventilation; ctomegalovirus

**CNS** central nervous system

**Co** cobalt

**c/o** complains of

**CoA** coenzyme A

**COG** center of gravity

**conA** concanavalin A

**COPD** chronic obstructive pulmonary disease

**CP** cerebral palsy; costophrenic

**CPAP** continuous (or constant) positive airway pressure

**CPD** cephalopelvic disproportion

**CPM** continuous passive motility

**CPPB** continuous (or constant) positive-pressure breathing

**CPPV** continuous positive-pressure ventilation

**CPR** cardiopulmonary resuscitation

**cps** cycles per second

**Cr** chromium; creatinine

**CR** conditioned reflex; crown-rump (length)

**CRD** chronic respiratory disease

**CRH** corticotropin-releasing hormone

**CRL** crown-rump length

**CRP** cross-reacting protein

**CRST** calcinosis cutis, Raynaud phenomenon, sclerodactyly, and telangiectasia (syndrome)

**Cs** cesium

**C&S** culture and sensitivity

**CSD** catscratch disease

**CSF** cerebrospinal fluid

**CT** computed tomography

**CTP** cytidine 5'-triphosphate

**CTR** cardiothoracic ratio

**Cu** [L.] *cuprum*, copper

**CV** cardiovascular

**CVA** cerebrovascular accident

**CVP** central venous pressure

**CXR** chest x-ray

**Cyd** cytidine

**cyl** cylinder; cylindrical (lens)

**CYP** cytochrome P-450 (enzyme)

**Cys** cysteine

**Cyt** cytosine

**δ** delta; heavy chain class corresponding to IgD

**Δ** delta; change; heat

**d** deci-

*d* deuterium

*d-* dextrorotatory

**D** dead (space gas) (SUBSCRIPT); deciduous; deuterium; diffusing (capacity); dihydrouridine (in nucleic acids); diopter; [L.] *dexter,* right (opposite of left); vitamin D potency of cod liver oil

**D-** prefix indicating that a molecule is sterically analogous to D-glyceraldehyde

**da** deca-

**dA** deoxyadenosine

**Da** dalton

**DA** developmental age

**dAdo** deoxyadenosine

**dAMP** deoxyadenylic acid

**DANS** 1-dimethylaminonaphthalene-5-sulfonic acid

**db** decibel

**dB** decibel

**DC** Dental Corps

**D&C** dilation and curettage

**DCG** dacryocystography

**DCI** dichloroisoproterenol

**dCMP** deoxycytidylic acid

**DDT** dichlorodiphenyl-trichloroethane (chlorophenothane)

**D&E** dilation and evacuation

**def** decayed, extracted, or filled (deciduous teeth)

**DEF** decayed, extracted, or filled (permanent teeth)

**DES** diethylstilbestrol

**DET** diethyltryptamine

**DEV** duck embryo vaccine; duck embryo virus

**DEXA** dual-energy x-ray absorptiometry

**df** decayed and filled (deciduous teeth)

**Df** deficiency (absence or inactivation of a gene)

**DF** decayed and filled (permanent teeth)

**dGMP** deoxyguanosine monophosphate (deoxyguanylic acid)

**DHEA** dehydro-3-epiandrosterone

**DIC** disseminated intravascular coagulation

**DIP** desquamative interstitial pneumonia; distal interphalangeal (joint)

**DJD** degenerative joint disease

**dk** deca-, deka-

**dM** decimorgan

**DMD** Duchenne muscular dystrophy

**dmf** decayed, missing, or filled (deciduous teeth)

**DMF** decayed, missing, or filled (permanent teeth)

**DMSO** dimethyl sulfoxide

**DMT** *N,N*-dimethyltryptamine

**DN** dibucaine number

**DNA** deoxyribonucleic acid

**DNAase** deoxyribonucleic acid nuclease

**DNase** deoxyribonuclease

**DNAse** deoxyribonuclease

**DNP** deoxyribonucleoprotein; 2,4-dinitrophenol

**DNR** do not resuscitate

**DNS** director of nursing service(s)

**DOA** dead on arrival

**DOC** deoxycholic acid; deoxycorticosterone

**DOM** 2,5-dimethoxy-4-methylamphetamine

**Dp** duplication of a gene or chromosomal segment

**2,3-DPG** 2,3-diphosphoglycerate

**DPI** dry powder inhaler

**DPN** diphosphopyridine nucleotide

**DPT** dipropyltryptamine; diphtheria, pertussis, and tetanus (vaccines)

**dr** dram

**DR** degeneration reaction, reaction of degeneration

**DRG** diagnosis-related group

**DRVVT** dilute Russell's viper venom test

**D-S** Doerfler-Stewart (test)

**DSA** digital subtraction angiography

**dsDNA** double-stranded DNA

**dT** deoxythymidine

**DT** delirium tremens; duration of tetany

**dTDP** deoxythymidine 5-diphosphate

**dThd** thymidine

**DTIC** dimethyltrizenoimidazole carboxamide (dacarbazine)

**dTMP** deoxythymidylic acid

**DTP** diphtheria and tetanus toxoids and pertussis vaccine; distal tingling on percussion (Tinel sign)

**DTPA** diethylenetriamine pentaacetic acid

**DTR** deep tendon reflex

**dTTP** deoxythymidine 5'-triphosphate

**Dx** diagnosis

**Dy** dysprosium

**ε** epsilon; molar absorption coefficient; heavy chain class corresponding to IgE

**E** exa-; extraction (ratio)

**EB** Epstein-Barr (virus)

**EBV** Epstein-Barr virus

**ECF** extracellular fluid

**ECF-A** eosinophilic chemotactic factor of anaphylaxis

**ECG** electrocardiogram

**ECHO** enterocytopathogenic human orphan (virus)

**ECM** erythema chronicum migrans

**ECMO** extracorporeal membrane oxygenation

**ECS** electrocerebral silence

**ECT** electroconvulsive therapy

**ED** effective dose

**EDTA** ethylenediamine-tetraacetic acid (edathamil, edetic acid)

**EEG** electroencephalogram

**EENT** eye, ear, nose, and throat

**EIA** enzyme immunoassay

**EKG** [German] *Elektrokardiogramme,* electrocardiogram

**EKY** electrokymogram

**ELISA** enzyme-linked immunosorbent assay

**EMC** encephalomyocarditis (virus)

**EMF** electromotive force

**EMG** electromyogram; exomphalos, macroglossia, and gigantism (syndrome)

**EMS** emergency medical services

**ENG** electronystagmography

**ENT** ear, nose, and throat

**EOG** electrooculography

**EPAP** expiratory positive airway pressure

**Er** erbium

**ER** endoplasmic reticulum; emergency room

**ERBF** effective renal blood flow

**ERCP** endoscopic retrograde cholangiopancreatography

**ERG** electroretinogram

**ERPF** effective renal plasma flow

**ERV** expiratory reserve volume

**Es** einsteinium

**ESEP** extreme somatosensory evoked potential

**ESP** extrasensory perception

**ESR** electron spin resonance; erythrocyte sedimentation rate

**ESRD** end-stage renal disease

**EtOH** ethyl alcohol

**Eu** europium

**ev** electron-volt

**eV** electron-volt

**f** femto-; (respiratory) frequency

**F** Fahrenheit; faraday (constant); fertility (factor); field (of vision); fluorine; force; fractional (concentration); free (energy)

**F1.2** (prothrombin) fragment 1.2

**$F_1$** first filial generation

**Fab** fragment of antibody molecule involved in antigen binding

**FAD** flavin(e) adenine dinucleotide; familial Alzheimer disease

**FANA** fluorescent antinuclear antibody (test)

**FB** foreign body

**FBS** fasting blood sugar

**Fc** constant fragment of an antibody molecule

**FDA** Food and Drug Administration

**Fe** [L.] *ferrum,* iron

**FEF** forced expiratory flow

**FET** forced expiratory time

**FEV** forced expiratory volume

**FF** filtration fraction

**FFD** focus-film distance

**FHR** fetal heart rate

**FHT** fetal heart tones

**FIA** fluorescent immunoassay

**FIGLU** formiminoglutamic (acid)

**FISH** fluorescent in situ hybridization

**Fm** fermium

**FMN** flavin(e) mononucleotide

**fps** foot-pound-second (system, unit)

**FPS** foot-pound-second (system, unit)

**Fr** francium; French (gauge, scale)

**FRC** functional residual capacity (of lungs)

**FRF** follicle-stimulating hormone-releasing factor

**FRS** first-rank symptom

**Fru** fructose

**FSH** follicle-stimulating hormone

**FSH-RF** follicle-stimulating hormone-releasing factor

**FSH-RH** follicle-stimulating hormone-releasing hormone

**FTA-ABS** fluorescent treponemal antibody-absorption (test)

**FU** fluorouracil

**FUO** fever of unknown origin

**FVC** forced vital capacity

**Fw** F wave (fibrillary wave, flutter wave)

**Fx** fracture

**γ** gamma; Ostwald solubility coefficient; the third in a series; heavy chain class corresponding to IgG

**μg** microgram

**g** gram

**G** giga-; glucose; gravitation (newtonian constant of); guanosine (or guanylic acid) residues in polynucleotides; gravida (obstetric history)

**G 1** gap 1

**G 2** gap 2

**G6P** glucose 6-phosphate

**Ga** gallium

**GABA** γ-aminobutyric acid

**GABHS** group-A β-hemolytic streptococcus

**Gal** galactose

**GC** gonococcus, gonorrhea

**Gd** gadolinium

**GDP** mannose-1-phosphate guanylyltransferase

**Ge** germanium

**GERD** gastroesophageal reflux disease

**GFR** glomerular filtration rate

**GGT** γ-glutamyl transferase

**GH** glenohumeral; growth hormone

**GHB** γ-hydroxybutyrate

**GHRF** growth hormone-releasing factor

**GH-RF** growth hormone-releasing factor

**GHRH** growth hormone-releasing hormone

**GH-RH** growth hormone-releasing hormone

**GI** gastrointestinal; Gingival Index

**GIP** gastric inhibitory polypeptide

**GLC** gas-liquid chromatography

**Gln** glutamine; glutaminyl

**Glu** glutamic acid; glutamyl

**Gly** glycine; glycyl

**GMP** guanosine monophosphate (guanylic acid)

**GMS** Gomori (or Grocott) methenamine silver (stain)

**GnRH** gonadotropin-releasing hormone

**GOT** glutamic-oxaloacetic transaminase (aspartate ami- notransferase)

**GPI** Gingival-Periodontal Index

**GPT** glutamic-pyruvic transaminase (alanine aminotransferase)

**gr** grain

**GSH** reduced glutathione

**GSR** galvanic skin response

**GSSG** oxidized glutathione

**gt.** [L.] *gutta,* a drop

**GTP** guanosine 5′-triphosphate

**gtt.** [L.] *guttae,* drops

**GTT** glucose tolerance test

**GU** genitourinary

**Guo** guanosine

**GVHD** graft-versus-host disease

**Gy** gray (unit of absorbed dose of ionizing radiation)

**GYN** gynecology

**h** hecto-

**h** Planck's constant

**α-h** the right-handed helical form assumed by many proteins

**H** henry; hydrogen; hyperopia; hyperopic

**$^{1}$H** hydrogen-1 (protium, light hydrogen)

**$^{2}$H** hydrogen-2 (deuterium, heavy hydrogen)

**$^{3}$H** hydrogen-3 (tritium, radioactive hydrogen)

**$H^{+}$** hydrogen ion

**Ha** hahnium

**HA** hyaluronic acid; hemagglutinin

**HAV** hepatitis A virus

**Hb** hemoglobin

**HbA** adult hemoglobin

**$HbA_1$** major component of adult hemoglobin

**$HbA_2$** minor fraction of adult hemoglobin

**HbAS** heterozygosity for hemoglobin A and hemoglobin S (sickle cell trait)

**$HB_cAg$** hepatitis B core antigen

**HbCO** carboxyhemoglobin

**$HB_e$** hepatitis B early antigen

**$HB_eAb$** hepatitis B early antibody

**$Hb_eAg$** hepatitis B early antigen

**HBIG** hepatitis B immune globulin

**HbF** fetal hemoglobin

**HbO₂** oxyhemoglobin, oxygenated hemoglobin

**HbS** sickle cell hemoglobin

**HB$_s$Ab** hepatitis B surface antibody

**HB$_s$Ag** hepatitis B surface antigen

**HBV** hepatitis B virus

**HCFA** Health Care Financing Administration

**HCG** human chorionic gonadotropin

**HCS** human chorionic somatomammotropin (human placental lactogen)

**Hct** hematocrit

**HDL** high-density lipoprotein

**HDRV** human diploid (cell strain) rabies vaccine

**He** helium

**H&E** hematoxylin and eosin

**HEMPAS** hereditary erythroblastic multinuclearity associated with positive acidified serum

**Hf** hafnium

**HFJV** high-frequency jet ventilation

**HFOV** high-frequency oscillatory ventilation

**HFPPV** high-frequency positive pressure ventilation

**HFV** high-frequency ventilation

**Hg** [L.] *hydrargyrum,* mercury

**HGE** human granulocytic ehrlichiosis

**HGH** human (pituitary) growth hormone

**HGSIL** high-grade squamous intraepithelial lesion

**HI** hemagglutination inhibition (test, titer)

**His** histidine

**His-** histidyl

**-His** histidino

**HIV** human immunodeficiency virus

**Hl** hyperopia, latent

**HLA** human lymphocyte antigen

**Hm** hyperopia, manifest (hypermetropia)

**HME** human monocytic ehrlichiosis

**HMG** human menopausal gonadotropin

**HMG** CoA 3-hydroxy-3-methylglutaryl coenzyme A

**HMO** health maintenance organization

**HMWK** high molecular weight kininogen (Fletcher factor)

**Ho** holmium

**HPF** high-power field

**HPI** history of present illness

**HPL** human placental lactogen

**HPLC** high-performance liquid chromatography

**HPV** human papilloma virus

**h. s.** [L.] *hora somni,* at bedtime

**HS** [L.] *hora somni,* at bedtime

**HSV** herpes simplex virus

**Ht** hyperopia, total

**5-HT** 5-hydroxytryptamine (serotonin)

**HTLV** human T-cell lymphocytotrophic virus; human T-cell lymphoma/leukemia virus

**HVL** half-value layer

**Hx** (medical) history

**Hyp** hydroxyproline

**Hz** hertz

**I** inspired (gas) (SUBSCRIPT); iodine

**¹²³I** iodine-123 (radioisotope)

**¹²⁵I** iodine-125

**¹³¹I** iodine-131

**IADL** instrumental activities of daily living

**IAP** intermittent acute porphyria

**ICD** *International Classification of Diseases of the World Health Organization*

**ICDA** *International Classification of Diseases, Adapted for Use in the United States*

**ICF** intracellular fluid

**ICP** intracranial pressure

**ICSH** interstitial cell-stimulating hormone

**ICU** intensive care unit

**ID** infective dose

**I&D** incision and drainage

**IDU** idoxuridine

**IF** initiation factor; intrinsic factor

**IFN** interferon

**Ig** immunoglobulin

**IGF** insulin-like growth factor

**IH** infectious hepatitis

**IL** interleukin

**ILA** insulin-like activity

**Ile** isoleucine

**IM** internal medicine; intramuscular(ly); infectious mononucleosis

**IMP** inosine monophosphate (inosinic acid)

**IMV** intermittent mandatory ventilation

**In** indium

**Ino** inosine

**INR** international normalized ratio

**I&O** (fluid) intake and output

**IOML** infraorbitomeatal line

**IP** interphalangeal; intraperitoneal(ly)

**IPAP** inspiratory positive airway pressure

**IPPB** intermittent positive-pressure breathing

**IPPV** intermittent positive-pressure ventilation

**IPV** inactivated poliovirus vaccine

**IQ** intelligence quotient

**Ir** iridium

**IRV** inspiratory reserve volume

**ISI** International Sensitivity Index

**ITP** idiopathic thrombocytopenic purpura; inosine 5′-triphosphate

**IU** International Unit

**IUCD** intrauterine contraceptive device

**IUD** intrauterine device
**IV** intravenous, intravenously; intraventricular
**J** joule
*J* flux (density)
**k** kilo-
**K** [Modern L.] *kalium,* potassium; kelvin
**K$_M$** Michaelis constant
**kat** katal
**kb** kilobase
**kc** kilocycle
**kcal** kilocalorie
**KCT** kaolin clotting time
**kDa** kilodalton
**kg** kilogram
**KJ** knee jerk
**Kr** krypton
**KS** Kaposi sarcoma
**17-KS** 17-ketosteroid
**kv** kilovolt
**kVp** kilovolt peak
**KW** Kimmelstiel-Wilson (disease); Keith-Wagener (retinal changes)
**$\mu$l, $\mu$L** microliter
**l** liter
**L** inductance; left; [L.] *limes,* boundary, limit; liter
**L-** prefix indicating that a molecule is sterically analogous to L-glyceraldehyde
**La** lanthanum
**LA** lupus anticoagulant
**LAP** leucine aminopeptidase
**LATS** long-acting thyroid stimulator
**LBT** lupus band test
**LC** lethal concentration
**LCAT** lecithin-cholesterol acyltransferase
**LCM** lymphocytic choriomeningitis (virus)
**LD** lethal dose
**LDH** lactate dehydrogenase
**LDL** low-density lipoprotein
**LE** left eye; lupus erythematosus
**LEEP** loop electrosurgical excision procedure

**LES** lower esophageal sphincter
**LETS** large external transformation-sensitive (fibronectin)
**Leu** leucine
**LFA** left frontoanterior (fetal position)
**LFP** left frontoposterior (fetal position)
**LFT** left frontotransverse (fetal position)
**LGSIL** low-grade squamous intraepithelial lesion
**LGV** lymphogranuloma venereum
**LH** luteinizing hormone
**LH/FSH-RF** luteinizing hormone/follicle-stimulating hormone-releasing factor
**LH-RF** luteinizing hormone-releasing factor
**LH-RH** luteinizing hormone-releasing hormone
**Li** lithium
**LLQ** left lower quadrant
**LMA** left mentoanterior (fetal position)
**LMP** left mentoposterior (fetal position)
**LMT** left mentotransverse (fetal position)
**LNPF** lymph node permeability factor
**LOA** left occipitoanterior (fetal position)
**LOP** left occipitoposterior (fetal position)
**LOT** left occipitotransverse (fetal position)
**LPF** low-power field
**LPH** lipotropic pituitary hormone (lipotropin)
**Lr** lawrencium
**LRH** luteinizing hormone-releasing hormone
**LSA** left sacroanterior (fetal position)
**LSD** lysergic acid diethylamide

**LSP** left sacroposterior (fetal position)
**L/S R** lecithin/sphingomyelin ratio
**LST** left sacrotransverse (fetal position)
**LTH** luteotropic hormone
**LTM** long-term memory
**LTR** long terminal repeat
**Lu** lutetium
**LUQ** left upper quadrant
**LVET** left ventricular ejection time
**LVH** left ventricular hypertrophy
**Lw** (FORMER SYMBOL FOR) lawrencium (now Lr)
**Lys** lysine (or its radicals in peptides)
**$\mu$** mu; micro-; heavy chain class corresponding to IgM
**m** mass; meter; milliminim; molar
**m-** meta-
**M** mega-, meg-; molar; moles (per liter); morgan; myopic; myopia
*M* molar; moles (per liter)
**m** moles (per liter)
**$\mu\mu$** micromicro-
**$\mu$m** micrometer
**m$\mu$** millimicron
**mA** milliampere
**MA** mental age
**MAA** macroaggregated albumin
**M + Am** compound myopic astigmatism
**MAC** *Mycobacterium avium* complex
**MAI** *Mycobacterium avium intracellulare*
**MAO** monoamine oxidase
**MAOI** monoamine oxidase inhibitor
**MAP** morning-after pill
**mA-S** milliampere-second
**Mb** myoglobin
**MBC** maximum breathing capacity

**MbCO** carbon monoxided myoglobin
**MbO$_2$** oxymyoglobin
**MC** Medical Corps
**MCH** mean corpuscular hemoglobin
**MCHC** mean corpuscular hemoglobin concentration
**mCi** millicurie
**MCP** metacarpophalangeal
**MCV** mean corpuscular volume
**Md** mendelevium
**MDF** myocardial depressant factor
**MDI** metered-dose inhaler
**Me** methyl
**MEDLARS** Medical Literature Analysis and Retrieval System
**MEP** maximal expiratory pressure
**meq, mEq** milliequivalent
**Met** methionine
**MET** metabolic equivalent of task
**met-Hb** methemoglobin
**met-Mb** metmyoglobin
**MEV** million electron-volts ($10^6$ ev)
**mg** milligram
**Mg** magnesium
**MHC** major histocompatibility complex
**mho** siemens unit
**MHz** megahertz
**MI** myocardial infarction
**MID** minimal infecting dose
**MIP** maximum inspiratory pressure
**MK** menaquinone (vitamin K$_2$)
**mks, MKS** meter-kilogram-second (system, unit)
**ml, mL** milliliter
**MLC** mixed lymphocyte culture (test)
**MLD** minimal lethal dose
**mm** millimeter
**mmol** millimole

**MMPI** Minnesota Multiphasic Personality Inventory
**MMR** measles-mumps-rubella (vaccine)
**Mn** manganese
**Mo** molybdenum
**MO** medical officer; mineral oil
**mol** mole
**mol wt** molecular weight
**MOM** milk of magnesia
**MOPP** Mustargen (mechlorethamine hydrochloride), Oncovin (vincristine sulfate), procarbazine hydrochloride, and prednisone
**mor. sol.** [L.] *more solito,* as usual, as customary
**MPD** maximal permissible dose
**MPS** mononuclear phagocyte system
**MR** milk-ring (test)
**M$_r$** molecular (weight) ratio
**mrd, MRD** minimal reacting dose
**MRI** magnetic resonance imaging
**mRNA** messenger RNA
**ms** millisecond
**MS** multiple sclerosis; morphine sulfate
**msec** millisecond
**MSG** monosodium glutamate
**MSH** melanocyte-stimulating hormone
**mtDNA** mitochondrial DNA
**MTP** metatarsophalangeal (joint)
**Mu** Mache unit
**MUGA** multiple-gated acquisition (imaging)
**mV** millivolt
**Mv** mendelevium
**MVE** Murray Valley encephalitis (virus)
**MVV** maximal voluntary ventilation
**MW** molecular weight
**My** myopia

**$\nu$** nu; kinematic viscosity
**n** index of refraction; nano-
**N** newton; nitrogen; normal (concentration)
**N** normal (SMALL CAPS)
**Na** [Modern L.] *natrium,* sodium
**NA** *Nomina Anatomica*
**NAD** nicotinamide adenine dinucleotide; no acute distress
**NAD$^+$** nicotinamide adenine dinucleotide (oxidized form)
**NADH** nicotinamide adenine dinucleotide (reduced form)
**NADP** nicotinamide adenine dinucleotide phosphate
**NADP$^+$** nicotinamide adenine dinucleotide phosphate (oxidized form)
**NADPH** nicotinamide adenine dinucleotide phosphate (reduced form)
**NAME** nevi, atrial myxoma, myxoid neurofibromas, and ephelides (syndrome)
**Nb** niobium
**NCV** nerve conduction velocity
**Nd** neodymium
**Ne** neon
**NE** norepinephrine; not examined
**NEEP** negative end-expiratory pressure
**NF** National Formulary
**ng** nanogram
**NGF** nerve growth factor (antigen)
**Ni** nickel
**NIH** National Institutes of Health
**NK** natural killer (cell)
**NKA** no known allergies
**NLM** National Library of Medicine
**nm** nanometer
**NMN** nicotinamide mononucleotide
**No** nobelium
**Np** neptunium

**NREM** non-rapid eye movement (sleep)
**nRNA** nuclear RNA
**NS** normal saline
**NSAID** nonsteroidal anti-inflammatory drug
**NSR** normal sinus rhythm
**NUG** necrotizing ulcerative gingivitis
**Ω** omega; ohm
**o-** ortho-
**O** [L.] *oculus,* eye; opening (in formulas for electrical reactions); oxygen
**OAV** oculoauriculovertebral (dysplasia, syndrome)
**OB** obstetrics
**OB/GYN** obstetrics (and) gynecology
**OBS** organic brain syndrome
**OC** oral contraceptive
**OCD** obsessive-compulsive disorder
**OD** [L.] *oculus dexter,* right eye; overdose
**ODD** oculodentodigital (dysplasia, syndrome)
**Oe** oersted (centimeter-gram-second unit of magnetic field strength)
**OFD** orofaciodigital (dysostosis, syndrome)
**OKT** Ortho-Kung T (cell)
**OML** orbitomeatal line
**OMM** ophthalmomandibulomelic (dysplasia, syndrome)
**OMS** organic mental syndrome
**OP** osmotic pressure; outpatient
**O&P** ova and parasites
**OPV** oral poliovirus vaccine
**OR** operating room
**ORD** optical rotatory dispersion
**Orn** ornithine (or its radical)
**Oro** orotate; orotic acid
**Os** osmium
**OS** [L.] *oculus sinister,* left eye
**OSHA** Occupational Safety and Health Administration

**OT** occupational therapy; Koch old tuberculin
**OTC** over the counter (non-prescription drug)
**OU** [L.] *oculus uterque,* each eye (both eyes)
**OXT** oxytocin
**oz** ounce
**p** pico-; pupil
**p-** para-
**P** partial (pressure); peta-; phosphorus, phosphoric (residue); plasma (concentration); pressure; para (obstetric history)
**$^{32}$P** phosphorus-32
**$P_1$** first parental generation
**Pa** pascal; protactinium
**PABA** para-aminobenzoic acid
**PAF** platelet-aggregating (or -activating) factor
**PAH** para-aminohippuric (acid)
**$PAO_2$** partial pressure of arterial oxygen
**PAS** para-aminosalicylic (acid), periodic acid-Schiff (reagent)
**PASA** para-aminosalicylic acid
**PAT** paroxysmal atrial tachycardia
**Pb** [L.] *plumbum,* lead
**PBG** porphobilinogen
**p.c.** [L.] *post cibum,* after a meal
**PCB** polychlorinated biphenyl
**$Pco_2$** partial pressure of carbon dioxide
**PCP** phencyclidine
**Pd** palladium
**PD** prism diopter
**PDGF** platelet-derived growth factor
**PDLL** poorly differentiated lymphocytic lymphoma
**PEEP** positive end-expiratory pressure
**PEG** polyethylene glycol
**PET** positron emission tomography
**$PF_4$** platelet factor 4
**PFT** pulmonary function test
**pg** picogram

**PG** prostaglandin
**PGA** prostaglandin A
**PGB** prostaglandin B
**PGE** prostaglandin E
**PGF** prostaglandin F
**pH** hydrogen ion concentration; p (power) of $[H^+]_{10}$
**Ph** phenyl
**$Ph^1$** Philadelphia (chromosome)
**PHA** phytohemagglutinin (antigen)
**Phe** phenylalanine (or its radical)
**PhG** [L.] *Pharmacopoeia Germanica,* German Pharmacopeia
**PICC** peripherally inserted central catheter
**PID** pelvic inflammatory disease
**PIF** prolactin-inhibiting factor
**PIP** proximal interphalangeal (joint)
**pK** negative logarithm of the ionization constant ($K_a$) of an acid
**PK** pyruvate kinase
**PKU** phenylketonuria
**pm** picometer
**Pm** promethium
**PM** post mortem
**PMN** polymorphonuclear (leukocyte)
**PMS** premenstrual syndrome
**PND** paroxysmal nocturnal dyspnea; postnasal drip
**PNP** platelet neutralization procedure
**PNPB** positive-negative pressure breathing
**Po** polonium
**PO** [L.] *per os,* by mouth
**$PO_2$, $Po_2$** partial pressure of oxygen
**POEMS** polyneuropathy, organomegaly, endocrinopathy, mo- noclonal protein, and skin changes (syndrome)
**POMP** prednisone, Oncovin

(vincristine sulfate), methotrexate, and Purinethol (6-mercaptopurine)

**POR** problem-oriented (medical) record

**PP** pyrophosphate

**PPCA** proserum prothrombin conversion accelerator

**PPD** purified protein derivative (of tuberculin)

**PPLO** pleuropneumonia-like organism

**ppm** parts per million

**PPO** 2,5-diphenyloxazole

**PPPPP** pain, pallor, pulselessness, paresthesia, paralysis

**PPPPPP** pain, pallor, pulselessness, paresthesia, paralysis, prostration

**PPV** positive pressure ventilation

**Pr** praseodymium; presbyopia

**PRA** plasma renin activity

**PRF** prolactin-releasing factor

**PRL** prolactin

**p.r.n.** [L.] *pro re nata,* as needed

**PRN** [L.] *pro re nata,* as needed

**Pro** proline (or its radicals)

**psi** pounds per square inch

**PSV** pressure-supported ventilation

**Pt** platinum

**PT** physical therapy; prothrombin time

**PTA** plasma thromboplastin antecedent; phosphotungstic acid; prior to admission

**PTAH** phosphotungstic acid hematoxylin

**PTCA** percutaneous transluminal coronary angioplasty

**PTH** parathyroid hormone

**PTU** prophylthiouracil

**Pu** plutonium

**PUO** pyrexia of unknown origin

**PUPPP** pruritic urticarial papules and plaques of pregnancy

**PUVA** (oral administration of) psoralen (and subsequent exposure to) ultraviolet light of A wavelength (UV-A)

**PVC** polyvinyl chloride; premature ventricular contraction

**PVP** polyvinylpyrrolidone (povidone)

**Q** volume of blood flow

**Q** coulomb

**Qco$_2$** microliters $CO_2$ given off per milligram of dry weight of tissue per hour

**q.d.** [L.] *quaque die,* every day

**q.i.d.** [L.] *quater in die,* four times a day

**QNS** quantity not sufficient

**Qo** oxygen consumption

**Qo$_2$** oxygen consumption

**q.s.** [L.] *quantum satis,* as much as is enough; [L.] *quantum sufficiat,* as much as may suffice; quantity sufficient

**r** racemic; roentgen

**R** gas constant (8.315 joules); (organic) radical; Réamur (scale) ; [L.] *recipe,* take; resistance determinant (plasmid); resistance (electrical); resistance (unit) (in the cardiovascular system); resolution; respiration; respiratory (exchange ratio); roentgen

**Ra** radium

**RA** rheumatoid arthritis

**rad** radian

**RAS** reticular activating system

**RAST** radioallergosorbent test

**RAV** Rous-associated virus

**RAW** resistance, airway

**Rb** rubidium

**rbc** red blood cell; red blood (cell) count

**RBC** red blood cell; red blood (cell) count

**RBF** renal blood flow

**RD** reaction of degeneration; reaction of denervation

**RDA** recommended daily allowance

**rDNA** ribosomal DNA

**RDS** respiratory distress syndrome

**RDW** red (cell) diameter (or distribution) width

**Re** rhenium

**RE** right ear; right eye

**rem** roentgen equivalent, man

**REM** rapid eye movement (sleep); reticular erythematous mucinosis

**rep** roentgen equivalent, physical

**RF** release factor; rheumatoid factor

**RFA** right frontoanterior (fetal position)

**RFLP** restriction fragment length polymorphism

**RFP** right frontoposterior (fetal position)

**RFT** right frontotransverse (fetal position)

**Rh** Rhesus (Rh blood group); rhodium

**RH** releasing hormone

**RIA** radioimmunoassay

**Rib** ribose

**RLL** right lower lobe

**RLQ** right lower quadrant

**RMA** right mentoanterior (fetal position)

**RML** right middle lobe

**RMP** right mentoposterior (fetal position)

**RMT** right mentotransverse (fetal position)

**Rn** radon

**RNA** ribonucleic acid

**RNase** ribonuclease

**RNP** ribonucleoprotein

**ROA** right occipitoanterior (fetal position)

**ROM** range of motion

**ROP** right occipitoposterior (fetal position)

**ROT** right occipitotransverse (fetal position)

**RP** retinitis pigmentosa

**RPF** renal plasma flow
**rpm** revolutions per minute
**RPR** rapid plasma reagin (test)
**RQ** respiratory quotient
**rRNA** ribosomal RNA
**Rs** resolution
**RS** respiratory syncytial (virus)
**RSA** right sacroanterior (fetal position)
**RSP** right sacroposterior (fetal position)
**RST** right sacrotransverse (fetal position)
**RSV** Rous-sarcoma virus; respiratory syncytial virus
**rTMP** ribothymidylic acid
**Ru** ruthenium
**RUL** right upper lobe
**RUQ** right upper quadrant
**RV** residual volume
**RVH** right ventricular hypertrophy
**℞** [L.] *recipe,* (the first word on a prescription), take; prescription; treatment
**σ** sigma; reflection coefficient; standard deviation; 1 millisecond (0.001 sec)
**s** [L.] *semis,* half; steady state (SUBSCRIPT); [L.] *sinister,* left
**S** [L.] *sinister,* left; saturation of hemoglobin (percentage of) (FOLLOWED BY SUBSCRIPT $O_2$ or $CO_2$); siemens; spherical; spherical (lens); sulfur; Svedberg (unit)
**S₁** first selfing generation
**S-A** sinoatrial
**SaO₂** oxygen saturation (of) arterial (oxyhemoglobin)
**sat.** saturated
**sat. sol.** saturated solution
**Sb** [L.] *stibium,* antimony
**SBE** subacute bacterial endocarditis
**sc** subcutaneous(ly)
**Sc** scandium
**SC** sternoclavicular; subcutaneous(ly)

**SCID** severe combined immunodeficiency
**SD** standard deviation; streptodornase
**SDA** specific dynamic action
**Se** selenium
**Ser** serine
**Sf** Svedberg flotation (constant, unit)
**SGOT** serum glutamic-oxaloacetic transaminase (aspartate aminotransferase)
**SGPT** serum glutamic-pyruvic transaminase (alanine aminotransferase)
**SH** serum hepatitis
**Si** silicon
**SI** [French] Système International d'Unités; International System of Units
**SID** source-to-image (-receptor) distance
**SIDS** sudden infant death syndrome
**sig.** [L.] *signa,* affix a label, inscribe
**SIMV** spontaneous intermittent mandatory ventilation; synchronized intermittent mandatory ventilation
**SIRD** source-to-image-receptor distance
**SISI** small-increment (or short-increment) sensitivity index (test)
**SK** streptokinase
**SLE** systemic lupus erythematosus
**SLR** straight leg raising
**Sm** samarium
**Sn** [L.] *stannum,* tin
**SOAP** subjective data, objective data, assessment, and plan (problem-oriented medical record)
**SOB** short(ness) of breath
**sol.** solution
**soln.** solution
**sp.** species

**SPCA** serum prothrombin conversion accelerator (factor VII)
**SPECT** single photon emission computed tomography
**SPF** sun protection (or protective) factor
**sp. gr.** specific gravity
**sph** spherical (lens)
**spm** suppression and mutation
**spp.** species (plural)
**SQ** subcutaneous
**Sr** strontium
**SRF** somatotropin-releasing factor
**SRF-A** slow-reacting factor of anaphylaxis
**SRIF** somatotropin-release-inhibiting factor
**sRNA** soluble RNA
**SRS** slow-reacting substance (of anaphylaxis)
**SRS-A** slow-reacting substance of anaphylaxis
**ssDNA** single-stranded DNA
**ssp.** subspecies
**SSRI** selective serotonin reuptake inhibitor
**ST** scapulothoracic
**stat** [L.] *statim,* immediately, at once
**STD** sexually transmitted disease
**STEL** short-term exposure limit
**STH** somatotropic hormone
**STM** short-term memory
**STPD** standard temperature (0° C) and pressure (760 mm Hg absolute), dry
**Sv, SV** sievert (unit)
**SVT** supraventricular tachycardia
**t** metric ton
*t* temperature (Celsius); tritium
**a-T** a-tocopherol
**T** temperature, absolute (Kelvin); tension (intraocular); tera-; tesla; tetanus (toxoid); tidal (volume) (SUBSCRIPT);

tocopherol; transverse (tubule); tritium; tumor (antigen)

$T$ absolute temperature (Kelvin)

$T_3$ 3,5,5'-triiodothyronine

$T_4$ tetraiodothyronine (thyroxine)

**T−** (FOLLOWED BY NUMBER) decreased tension (intraocular)

**T+** (FOLLOWED BY NUMBER) increased tension (intraocular)

**Ta** tantalum

**TA** *Terminologia Anatomica*

**TAD** transient acantholytic dermatosis

**TAF** tumor angiogenesis factor

**TAR** thrombocytopenia with absent radii (syndrome)

**TAT** thematic apperception test

**Tb** terbium

**TB** tuberculosis

**TBP** thyroxine-binding protein

**TBV** total blood volume

**Tc** technetium

$^{99m}$**Tc** technetium-99m

**T&C** type and crossmatch

**TCA** tricarboxylic acid; trichloracetic acid

**TCN** talocalcaneonavicular (joint)

**Td** tetanus-diphtheria (toxoids, adult type)

**TDP** ribothymidine 5'-diphosphate

**Te** tellurium

**TEDD** total end-diastolic diameter

**TEN** toxic epidermal necrolysis

**TESD** total end-systolic diameter

**Th** thorium

**THC** tetrahydrocannabinol

**Thr** threonine (or its radicals)

$t_i/t_{tot}$ duty cycle

**Ti** titanium

**TIA** transient ischemic attack

**t.i.d.** [L.] *ter in die,* three times a day

**tinct.** tincture

**TITh** 3,5,3'-triiodothyronine

**TKO** to keep (venous infusion line) open

**Tl** thallium

**TLC** thin-layer chromatography; total lung capacity; tender, loving care

**TLV** threshold-limit value

$t_m$ temperature midpoint (Celsius)

**Tm** thulium; tubular maximal (excretory capacity of kidneys)

$T_m$ temperature midpoint (Kelvin)

**TM** transport maximum

**TMJ** temporomandibular joint

**TMP** ribothymidine 5'-monophosphate

**TMT** tarsometatarsal

**TMV** tobacco mosaic virus

**Tn** normal intraocular tension

**TNF** tumor necrosis factor

**TNM** tumor, node, metastasis (tumor staging)

**TORCH** toxoplasmosis, other, rubella, cytomegalovirus, and herpes simplex (maternal infections)

**t-PA, TPA** tissue plasminogen activator

**TPHA** *Treponema pallidum* hemagglutination (test)

**TPI** *Treponema pallidum* immobilization (test)

**TPN** total parenteral nutrition

**TPR** temperature, pulse, and respirations

**tr.** tincture

**TRH** thyrotropin-releasing hormone (stimulation test)

**TRIC** trachoma inclusion conjunctivitis (organism)

**tRNA** transfer RNA

**Trp** tryptophan (and its radicals)

**TSH** thyroid-stimulating hormone

**TSS** toxic shock syndrome

**TSTA** tumor-specific transplantation antigen

**TTP** thrombotic thrombocytopenic purpura

**TU** toxic unit, toxin unit

**Tyr** tyrosine (and its radicals)

**U** unit; uranium; uridine (in polymers); urinary (concentration)

**UA** urinalysis

**UDP** uridine diphosphate

**UDPG** UDP-glucose

**UGIS** upper gastrointestinal series

**UMP** uridine monophosphate (uridylic acid)

**ung.** [L.] *unguentum,* ointment

**u-PA** urokinase

**Urd** uridine

**URI** upper respiratory infection

**USAN** United States Adopted Names (Council)

**USP** *United States Pharmacopeia*

**USPHS** United States Public Health Service

**UTI** urinary tract infection

**UTP** uridine triphosphate

**UV** ultraviolet

**v** venous (blood); volt

**V** vanadium; vision; visual (acuity); volt; volume (frequently with subscripts denoting location, chemical species, and conditions)

$\dot{V}$ ventilation; gas flow (frequently with subscripts indicating location and chemical species); ventilation

$V_1CV_6$ unipolar precordial electrocardiogram chest leads

**VA** viral antigen

$\dot{V}_A$ alveolar ventilation

**V-A** ventriculoatrial

**Val** valine (and its radicals)

$\dot{V}a/\dot{Q}$ ventilation/perfusion ratio

**VATER** vertebral defects, imperforate anus, tracheoesophageal fistula with esophageal atresia, and radial and renal dysplasia (complex)

**VC** vision, color; vital capacity

**VCE** vagina, (ecto)cervix, endocervical canal

$V_D$ (physiologic) dead space

**VDRL** Venereal Disease Research Laboratory (test)

**VHDL** very-high-density lipoprotein

**VIP** vasoactive intestinal polypeptide

**VLDL** very-low-density lipoprotein

**VMA** vanillylmandelic acid (test)

$V_{max}$ maximal velocity

**VP** vasopressin

**VR** vocal resonance

**VS** volumetric solution

$V_T$ tidal volume

**W** watt; [German] *Wolfram,* tungsten

**Wb** weber

**WBC** white blood cell; white blood (cell) count

**WD** well-developed

**WDLL** well-differentiated lymphocytic (or lymphatic) lymphoma

**WHO** World Health Organization

**WN** well-nourished

**X** xanthosine

**Xao** xanthosine

**Xe** xenon

$^{133}$**Xe** xenon-133

**XU** excretory urogram

**Y** yttrium

**YAG** yttrium-aluminum-garnet (laser)

**Yb** ytterbium

**Z** carbobenzoxy (chloride)

**ZEEP** zero end-expiratory pressure

**ZES** Zollinger-Ellison syndrome

**Zn** zinc

$^{65}$**Zn** zinc-65

**Zr** zirconium

**ZSR** zeta sedimentation ratio

# Common Abbreviations Used in Medication Orders

| | | | | |
|---|---|---|---|---|
| **a or a.** | before | | **mg** | milligram |
| **a.c.** | before meals | | **no.** | number |
| **ad lib** | as desired | | **noct.** | night |
| **alt. h.** | alternate hours | | **OD** | right eye |
| **am** | in the morning; before noon | | **os** | mouth |
| **A.D.** | right ear | | **OS** | left eye |
| **A.S.** | left ear | | **OU** | both eyes |
| **A.U.** | each ear | | **oz** | ounce |
| **aq.** | water | | **p or p.** | after, per |
| **bid** | twice a day | | **p.c.** | after meals |
| **c̄** | with | | **per os, PO** | by mouth |
| **cap., caps.** | capsule | | **pm** | afternoon, evening |
| **cc** | cubic centimeter | | **prn** | as needed, according to necessity |
| **d** | day | | **q** | each, every |
| **D/C, dc** | discontinue | | **qh** | every hour |
| **dil.** | dilute | | **qid** | four times a day |
| **dist.** | distilled | | **q1h** | every 1 hour |
| **DS** | double strength | | **q2h** | every 2 hours |
| **EC** | enteric coated | | **q3h** | every 3 hours |
| **elix.** | elixir | | **q4h** | every 4 hours |
| **et** | and | | **q6h** | every 6 hours |
| **ext.** | external, extract | | **q8h** | every 8 hours |
| **fl, fld** | fluid | | **q12h** | every 12 hours |
| **g** | gram | | **qod** | every other day |
| **gr** | grain | | **qs** | as much as needed, quantity sufficient |
| **gtt** | drop | | | |
| **H** | hypodermic | | **qt** | quart |
| **h, hr** | hour | | **R. or PR** | rectally, per rectum |
| **h.s.** | at bedtime | | **Rx** | take, prescription |
| **IM** | intramuscular | | **s̄** | without |
| **inj.** | injection | | **sc** | subcutaneously |
| **IV** | intravenous | | **sol. or soln.** | solution |
| **IVP** | IV push | | **SQ** | subcutaneous |
| **IVPB** | IV piggyback | | **stat.** | immediately, at once |
| **kg** | kilogram | | **tab.** | tablet |
| **L** | liter | | **tbsp, T** | tablespoon |
| **lb** | pound | | **tid** | three times a day |
| **liq.** | liquid | | **tinct., tr** | tincture |
| **mcg, μg** | microgram | | **tsp, t** | teaspoon |
| **mEq** | milliequivalent | | **ung.** | ointment |

From Craven RF, Hirnle CJ, eds. Fundamentals of nursing: human health and function. Philadelphia: Lippincott Williams & Wilkins, 2000.

# Symbols

| Angles, Triangles, and Circles | | | |
|---|---|---|---|
| ∧ | above<br>diastolic blood pressure<br>  (anesthesia records)<br>elevated<br>enlarged<br>improved<br>increased<br>superior (position)<br>upper | < | caused by<br>derived from<br>less severe than<br>less than<br>produced by<br>proximal |
| ∨ | below<br>decreased<br>deficiency<br>deficit<br>depressed<br>deteriorated<br>diminished<br>down<br>inferior (position)<br>lower<br>systolic blood pressure<br>  (anesthesia records) | ∠ | angle<br>flexion<br>flexor |
| | | ∠ᴇ | angle of entry |
| | | ∠ₓ | angle of exit |
| | | ∟ | factorial product |
| | | ⌟ | right lower quadrant |
| | | ⌐ | right upper quadrant |
| | | ⌈ | left upper quadrant |
| | | ⌊ | left lower quadrant |
| > | causes<br>demonstrates<br>distal<br>followed by<br>derived from<br>greater than<br>indicates<br>leads to<br>more severe than<br>produces<br>radiates to<br>radiating to<br>results in<br>reveals<br>shows<br>to<br>toward<br>worse than<br>yields | Δ | anion gap<br>centrad prism<br>change<br>delta gap<br>heat<br>increment<br>occipital triangle<br>prism diopter<br>temperature (anesthesia<br>  records) |
| | | Δ+ | time interval |
| | | Δ A | change in absorbance |
| | | Δ dB | difference in decibels |
| | | Δ P | change in (intraocular)<br>  pressure |
| | | Δ pH | change in pH |
| | | Δ t | time interval |
| | | Δ H, H Δ | Hesselbach triangle |

| | | | | |
|---|---|---|---|---|
| ○ | respiration (anesthesia records) | Ⓜ | murmur | |
| ♀ | female <br> female sex | ⓜ | by mouth <br> mouth (temperature) <br> murmur | |
| ♂ | male <br> male sex | √ⓜ | factitial murmur | |
| Ⓐ , ⓐˣ | axilla (temperature) | Ⓞ | by mouth <br> oral <br> orally | |
| Ⓗ , ⓗ | hypodermic <br> hypodermically | Ⓡ | rectal <br> rectally <br> rectum (temperature) <br> right | |
| Ⓘ Ⓜ | intramuscular <br> intramuscularly | | | |
| Ⓘ Ⓥ | intravenous <br> intravenously | Ⓧ | end of anesthesia (anesthesia records) <br> end of operation | |
| Ⓛ | left | | | |

## Arrows

| | | | |
|---|---|---|---|
| ↑ | above <br> elevated <br> elevation <br> enlarged <br> gas <br> greater than <br> improved <br> increase <br> increased <br> increases <br> more than <br> rising <br> superior (position) <br> up <br> upper | ↓ | below <br> decrease <br> decreased <br> deficiency <br> deficit <br> depressed <br> depression <br> deteriorated <br> deteriorating <br> diminished <br> diminution <br> down <br> falling <br> inferior (position) <br> less than <br> low <br> normal plantar reflex <br> precipitate <br> precipitates <br> slower |
| ↑ g | increasing <br> rising | | |
| ↑ V | increase due to in vivo effect (lab) | | |

↓ g    decreasing
      diminishing
      falling
      lowering

↓ V    decrease due to in vivo effect
      (lab)

╱    deviated
      displaced
      increasing

╲    decreasing

→    approaches limit of
      causes, demonstrates
      direction of flow or reaction
      distal
      due to
      followed by
      indicates
      leads to
      produces
      radiating to
      results in
      reveals
      shows
      to
      to right
      toward
      yields

←    caused by
      derived from
      direction of flow or reaction
      due to
      produced by
      proximal
      resulting from
      secondary to
      to left

↑↑    extensor response (Babinski
      sign)
      positive Babinski
      testes undescended

↓↓    down bilaterally
      plantar response (Babinski
      sign)
      testes descended

↕    reversible reaction
      up and down

⇌ , ⇌    reversible (chemical)
      reaction

## Genetic Symbols

☐   male

○   female

◇   sex unspecified

☐ ○   normal individuals

■ ● ◆   affected individual (with
      $\geq 2$ conditions, the
      symbol is partioned
      and shaded with a
      different fill defined in
      a key or legend)

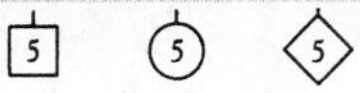

5̄ ⑤ ◇5̄   multiple individuals,
      number known
      (number of siblings
      written inside
      symbol)

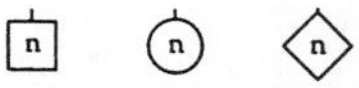

n̄ ⓝ ◇n̄   multiple individuals,
      number unknown
      ("n" used in place of
      specific number)

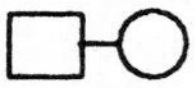

☐—○   mating

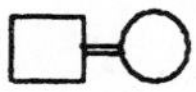

☐═○   consanguinity

(+) uncommon or uncertain mode of inheritance

I
II parents and offspring, in generations

dizygotic twins

monozygotic twins

4 ③ number of children of sex indicated

adopted individuals

individual died without leaving offspring

no issue

■ ● affected individuals

■ ● proband or propositus (first affected family member coming to medical attention)

examined professionally normal for trait

not examined dubiously reported to have trait

not examined reliably reported to have trait

■ ● heterozygotes for autosomal recessive

⊙ carrier of sex-linked recessive

death

SB 28 wk    SB 30 wk    SB 34 wk    stillbirth (SB)

P LMP: 7/1/94    P 20 wk    P    pregnancy (P); gestational age and karotype (if known) below symbol

consultant (individual seeking genetic counseling/testing)

male    female    ECT    spontaneous abortion (SAB); ECT below symbol indicates ectopic pregnancy

male    female    16 wk    affected SAB (gestational age, if known, below symbol, and key or legend used to define shading)

male    female    termination of pregnancy (TOP)

male    female    affected TOP (key or legend used to define shading)

---

Source. Genetic symbols are public domain; we credit and gratefully acknowledge the *American Journal of Human Genetics* (56:746–747, 1995) as our source for these symbols.

## Numbers

| | | | |
|---|---|---|---|
| 0 | completely absent (pulse) <br> no response (reflexes) | 3+ | moderate reaction (lab tests) <br> brisker than average (reflexes) |
| +1, 1+ | markedly impaired (pulse) | +4, 4+ | normal (pulse) |
| 1+ | low normal or somewhat diminished (reflexes) <br> slight reaction or trace (lab tests) | 4+ | hyperactive (reflexes) <br> large amount (lab tests) <br> pronounced reaction (lab tests) |
| +2, 2+ | moderately impaired (pulse) | • | very brisk (reflexes) |
| 2+ | average or normal (reflexes) <br> noticeable reaction or trace (lab tests) | $\overline{1}$ | bowel movement (numeral indicates number of stools in a given period) |
| | | 1× | once <br> one time |
| +3, 3+ | slightly impaired (pulse) | 2×, ×2 | twice <br> two times |
| | | 3×, ×3 | three times, etc. |

| Arabic | Roman | Arabic | Roman |
|---|---|---|---|
| 0 | | 17 | XVII |
| 1 | I, i | 18 | XVIII |
| 2 | II, ii | 19 | XIX |
| 3 | III, iii | 20 | XX |
| 4 | IV, iv | 30 | XXX |
| 5 | V, v | 40 | XL |
| 6 | VI, vi | 50 | L |
| 7 | VII, vii | 60 | LX |
| 8 | VIII, viii | 70 | LXX |
| 9 | IX, ix | 80 | LXXX |
| 10 | X, x | 90 | XC |
| 11 | XI, xi | 100 | C |
| 12 | XII, xii | 1,000 | M |
| 13 | XIII, xiii | 5,000 | $\overline{V}$ |
| 14 | XIV, xiv | 10,000 | $\overline{X}$ |
| 15 | XV | 100,000 | $\overline{C}$ |
| 16 | XVI | 1,000,000 | $\overline{M}$ |

## Pluses, Minuses, and Equivalencies

| | |
|---|---|
| + | acid (reaction) |
| | added to |
| | convex lens |
| | decreased or diminished (reflexes) |
| | excess |
| | less than 50% inhibition of hemolysis (Wassermann) |
| | low normal (reflexes) |
| | markedly impaired (pulse) |
| | mild (severity) |
| | plus |
| | positive (lab tests) |
| | present |
| | slight reaction or trace (lab tests) |
| | sluggish (reflexes) |
| | somewhat diminished (reflexes) |
| (+) | significant |
| (+)ive | positive |
| + to ++ | slight pain |
| ++ | average (reflexes) |
| | 50% inhibition of hemolysis (Wassermann) |
| | moderate (pain, severity) |
| | moderately impaired (pulse) |
| | normally active (reflexes) |
| | noticeable reaction or trace (lab tests) |
| +++ | increased reflexes |
| | 75% inhibition of hemolysis (Wassermann) |
| | moderate amount |
| +++ | moderate reaction (lab tests) |
| | moderately hyperative (reflexes) |
| | moderately severe (pain, severity) |
| | brisker than average (reflexes) |
| | slightly impaired (pulse) |
| ++++ | complete inhibition of hemolysis (Wassermann) |
| | large amount (lab tests) |
| | markedly hyperactive (reflexes) |
| | markedly severe (pain, severity) |
| | normal (pulse) |
| | pronounced reaction (lab tests) |
| | very brisk (reflexes) |
| − | absent |
| | alkaline (reaction) |
| | concave lens |
| | deficiency |
| | deficient |
| | minus |
| | negative (lab test) |
| | none |
| | subtract |
| | without |
| (−) | insignificant |
| ± | doubtful |
| | either positive or negative |
| | equivocal (reflexes, qualitative tests) |
| | flicker (reflexes) |
| | indefinite |
| | more or less |
| | plus or minus |

| Symbol | Meaning | Symbol | Meaning |
|---|---|---|---|
| ± | possibly significant | ⌒ | combined with |
|  | questionable |  |  |
|  | suggestive | ⇌ | equivalent |
|  | variable | ⇎ | not equivalent to |
|  | very slight (reaction, severity, trace) | ≡ | identical identical with |
|  | with or without |  |  |
| (±) | possibly significant | ≢ | not identical not identical with |
| ± to + | minimal pain | ≑ | nearly equal to |
| ∓ | minus or plus | ≒ | approximately equal |
| ‡ | moderate (severity) normally active (reflexes) | ≅ | approximately approximately equal to congruent to |
| # | fracture gauge number pound(s) weight | ≐ | approaches |
|  |  | ≜ | equilateral |
| ~ | about approximate approximately proportionate to | △ | equiangular |
|  |  | > | greater than |
|  |  | ≯ | not greater than |
|  |  | < | less than |
| ≈ | approximately equal to | ≮ | not less than |
| = | equal to | ≥, ⩾ | greater than or equal to |
| ≠ | not equal to | ≤, ⩽ | less than or equal to |

## Primes, Checks, Dots, Roots, and Other Symbols

| Symbol | Meaning | Symbol | Meaning |
|---|---|---|---|
| ? | doubtful equivocal (reflexes) flicker (reflexes) not tested (severity) possible questionable question of suggested suggestive (severity) unknown | ! | factorial product |
|  |  | † | death deceased |
|  |  | / | divided by either meaning extension extensors fraction of per to |

| ' | foot | $\sqrt[3]{\phantom{x}}$ | cube root |
| | hour | * | birth |
| | univalent | | multiplication sign |
| " | bivalent | | (genetics) |
| | ditto | | not verified |
| | inch | | presumed |
| | minute | | supposed |
| | second (1/60 degree) | ° | degree |
| ‴ | line (1/12 inch) | | measurement (1/360 of |
| | trivalent | | circle) |
| √ | check | | severity (burns, wounds) |
| | observe for | | temperature |
| | urine | | time (hour) |
| | voided (urine) | : | is to |
| √⋅ | urine and defecation | | ratio |
| | voided and bowels | ... | no data (in given |
| | moved | | category) |
| √c̄ | check with | ∴ | therefore |
| √d | checked | ∵ | because |
| | observed | | since |
| √g, √ing | checking | :: | as |
| √qs | voided sufficient quantity | | equality between ratios |
| √⎺ | radical root | | proportion |
| $\sqrt[2]{\phantom{x}}$ | square root | | proportionate to |

## Statistical Symbols

| $\alpha$ | probability of Type I error | $E(X)$ | expected value of |
| | significance level | | random variable $X$ |
| $\beta$ | probability of Type II error | $F$ | $F$ statistic (variance |
| $1-\beta$ | power of statistical test | | ratio) |
| | | $f$ | frequency |
| $nCk; \left(\dfrac{n}{k}\right)$ | binomial coefficient | $H_0$ | null hypothesis |
| | number of combination of $n$ | | |
| | things taken $k$ at a time | $H_1$ | alternative hypothesis |
| $\chi^2$ | chi-squared statistic | $\mu$ | population mean |
| $E$ | expected frequency in cell of | $N$ | population size |
| | contingency table | | |

| | | | | |
|---|---|---|---|---|
| $n$ | sample size | | $s^2$ | sample variance |
| $n!$ | $n$ factorial | | SE | standard error of estimate |
| $O$ | observed frequency in a contingency table | | $\sigma$ | population standard deviation |
| $\phi$ | ability continuum phi coefficient | | $\sigma^2$ | population variance |
| $P$ | probability | | $\sigma$diff. | standard error of difference between scores |
| $p$ | probability of success in independent trials | | $\sigma$est. | standard error of estimate |
| $P(A)$ | probability that event $A$ occurs | | $\sigma$meas. | standard error of measurement |
| $P(A\backslash B)$ | conditional probability that $A$ occurs given that $B$ has occurred | | $\sum_{i=1}^{n} x_1, \Sigma_i \overset{n}{=} x_i$ | $x_1 + x_2 + \ldots + x_n$ |
| | | | $t$ | Student $t$ statistic Student test variable |
| $r$ | sample correlation coefficient, usually the Pearson product-moment correlation | | $\theta$ | latent trait |
| | | | $U$ | Mann-Whitney rank sum statistic |
| $r^2$ | coefficient of determination | | $W$ | Wilcoxon rank sum statistic |
| $r_s$ | Spearman rank correlation coefficient | | $\overline{X}$ | sample mean |
| | | | $|x|$ | absolute value of x |
| $\rho$ | population correlation coefficient | | $\sqrt{x}$ | square root of x |
| | | | $z$ | standard score |
| $s$ | sample standard deviation | | $\infty$ | infinity |

# Muscles of the Human Body

| Muscle(s) | Origin | Insertion | Innervation | Main Action(s) |
|---|---|---|---|---|
| Abductor digiti minimi of foot | Medial and lateral tubercles of tuberosity of calcaneus, plantar aponeurosis, inter-muscular septa | Lateral side of base of proximal phalanx of 5th digit | Lateral plantar nerve (S2 and S3) | Abducts and flexes 5th digit |
| Abductor digiti minimi of hand | Pisiform, pisohamate ligament, flexor retinaculum | Medial side of base of proximal phalanx of little finger | Deep branch of ulnar nerve (C8 and T1) | Abducts 5th digit |
| Abductor hallucis | Medial tubercle of tuberosity of cal-caneus, flexor retina-culum, plantar aponeurosis | Medial side of base of proximal phalanx of 1st digit | Medial plantar nerve (S2 and S3) | Abducts and flexes 1st digit (great toe, hallux) |
| Abductor pollicis brevis | Flexor retinaculum and tubercles of sca-phoid and trapezium | Lateral side of base of proximal phalanx of thumb | Recurrent branch of median nerve (C8 and T1) | Abducts thumb and helps oppose it |
| Abductor pollicis longus | Posterior surfaces of ulna, radius, interos-seous membrane | Base of 1st metacarpal | Posterior interos-seous nerve (C7 and C8), continuation of deep branch of radial nerve | Abducts thumb and extends it at carpo-metacarpal joint |
| Adductor brevis | Body and inferior ramus of pubis | Pectineal line and proximal part of linea aspera of femur | Obturator nerve (L2, L3, and L4), branch of anterior division | Adducts thigh and to some extent flexes it |
| Adductor hallucis | Oblique head: bases of metatarsals 2–4 Transverse head: plantar ligaments of metatarsophalangeal joints | Tendons of both heads attach to lateral side of base of proxi-mal phalanx of 1st digit | Deep branch of lateral plantar nerve (S2 and S3) | Adducts 1st digit; assists in maintaining transverse arch of foot |
| Adductor longus | Body of pubis inferior to pubic crest | Middle third of linea aspera of femur | Obturator nerve, branch of anterior division (L2, L3, and L4) | Adducts thigh |
| Adductor magnus | Adductor part: inferior ramus of pubis, ramus of ischium Hamstrings part: ischial tuberosity | Adductor part: gluteal tuberosity, linea aspera, medial supra-condylar line Hamstrings part: adductor tubercle of femur | Adductor part: obtu-rator nerve (L2, L3, and L4), branches of posterior division Hamstrings part: tibial part of sciatic nerve (L4) | Adducts thigh Adductor part: flexes thigh Hamstrings part: extends thigh |
| Adductor minimus | Inferior pubic ramus | Medial lip, uppermost linea aspera of femur | Obturator nerve (L2, L3, and L4) | Adducts and laterally rotates thigh |
| Adductor pollicis | Oblique head: bases of 2nd and 3rd meta-carpals, capitate, adjacent carpals Transverse head: an-terior surface of body of 3rd metacarpal | Medial side of base of proximal phalanx of thumb | Deep branch of ulnar nerve (C8 and T1) | Adducts thumb toward middle digit |
| Anconeus | Lateral epicondyle of humerus | Lateral surface of olecranon and superior part of posterior surface of ulna | Radial nerve (C7, C8, and T1) | Assists triceps in extending forearm; stabilizes elbow joint; abducts ulna during pronation |

| Muscle(s) | Origin | Insertion | Innervation | Main Action(s) |
|---|---|---|---|---|
| Articularis cubiti | Distal portion of posterior aspect of shaft of humerus | Posterior fibrous capsule of elbow joint | Radial nerve (C7 and C8) | Retracts posterior joint capsule during extension of elbow |
| Articularis genus | Distal portion of anterior aspect of shaft of femur | Synovial membrane of suprapatellar bursa of knee joint | Femoral nerve (L2–L4) | Retracts synovial membrane during extension of knee |
| Arytenoid, transverse and oblique | Posterolateral border of 1 arytenoid cartilage | Posterolateral border of opposite arytenoid cartilage | Recurrent laryngeal nerve (branch of vagus (CN X)) | Closes intercartilaginous portion of rima glottidis |
| Auricularis, anterior, posterior, and superior | Epicranial aponeurosis and mastoid part of temporal bone | Auricle (external ear) | Facial nerve (CN VII) | Protraction, retraction, elevation of auricle on side of head |
| Biceps brachii | Short head: tip of coracoid process of scapula Long head: supraglenoid tubercle of scapula | Tuberosity of radius and fascia of forearm via bicipital aponeurosis | Musculocutaneous nerve (C5 and C6) | Supinates forearm and, when supine, flexes forearm |
| Biceps femoris | Long head: ischial tuberosity Short head: linea aspera and lateral supracondylar line of femur | Lateral side of head of fibula; tendon split at this site by fibular collateral ligament of knee | Long head: tibial division of sciatic nerve (L5, S1, and S2) Short head: common fibular (peroneal) division of sciatic nerve (L5, S1, and S2) | Flexes leg and rotates it laterally when knee is flexed; extends thigh (e.g., when starting to walk) |
| Brachialis | Distal half of anterior surface of humerus | Coronoid process and tuberosity of ulna | Musculocutaneous nerve (C5 and C6) | Flexes forearm in all positions |
| Brachioradialis | Proximal two-thirds of lateral supracondylar ridge of humerus | Lateral surface of distal end of radius | Radial nerve (C5, C6, and C7) | Flexes forearm |
| Buccinator | Mandible, pterygomandibular raphe, and alveolar processes of maxilla and mandible | Angle of mouth | Facial nerve (CN VII) | Presses cheek against molar teeth, thereby aiding chewing; expels air from oral cavity, as occurs when playing a wind instrument; draws mouth to one side when acting unilaterally |
| Bulbospongiosus | Male: median raphe, ventral surface of bulb of penis, and perineal body Female: perineal body | Male: corpora spongiosum and cavernosa and fascia of bulb of penis Female: fascia of corpus cavernosa | Deep branch of perineal nerve, a branch of pudendal nerve (S2, S3, and S4) | Works with external anal sphincter to support/fix perineal body Male: compresses bulb of penis to expel last drops of urine/semen; assists erection by pushing blood into body of penis and compressing outflow veins Female: "sphincter" of vagina and assists in erection of clitoris |
| Ciliary | Scleral spur | Meridional, radial, and circular fibers intrinsic to ciliary body | Parasympathetic fibers of oculomotor nerve and ciliary ganglion | Relieve tension on lens of eye, allowing it to become more convex for near vision |

| Muscle(s) | Origin | Insertion | Innervation | Main Action(s) |
|---|---|---|---|---|
| Coccygeus (ischio-coccygeus) | Ischial spine | Inferior end of sacrum | Branches of S4 and S5 nerves | Forms small part of pelvic diaphragm that supports pelvic viscera; flexes coccyx |
| Coracobrachialis | Tip of coracoid process of scapula | Middle third of medial surface of humerus | Musculocutaneous nerve (C5, C6, and C7) | Helps to flex and adduct arm |
| Corrugator supercilii | Medial end of superciliary arch of frontal bone | Skin above middle of eyebrow | Facial nerve (CN VII) | Draws eyebrow medially and inferiorly, producing vertical wrinkles above nose |
| Cremaster | Internal oblique muscle and inguinal ligament | Spermatic cord and tunica vaginalis | Genital branch of genitofemoral nerve (L1–L2) | Elevation of testis |
| Cricopharyngeus | Posterolateral cricoid cartilage on one side | Posterolateral cricoid cartilage of other side | Vagus (CN X) | Serves as upper esophageal sphincter |
| Cricothyroid | Anterolateral part of cricoid cartilage | Inferior margin and inferior horn of thyroid cartilage | External laryngeal nerve | Stretches and tenses vocal fold |
| Deep transverse perineal muscle | Internal surface of ischiopubic ramus and ischial tuberosity | Median raphe, perineal body, and external anal sphincter | Deep branch of perineal nerve, a branch of pudendal nerve (S2, S3, and S4) | Support and fix perineal body (pelvic floor) to support abdominopelvic viscera and resist increased intra-abdominal pressure |
| Deltoid | Lateral third of clavicle, acromion, and spine of scapula | Deltoid tuberosity of humerus | Axillary nerve (C5 and C6) | Anterior part: flexes and medially rotates arm. Middle part: abducts arm. Posterior part: extends and laterally rotates arm |
| Depressor labii inferioris/anguli oris | Anterolateral aspect of body of mandible | Lower lip/angle of mouth | Marginal mandibular branch of facial nerve (CN VII) | Depresses and/or everts lower lip; pulls angle of mouth and modiolus inferiorly |
| Depressor septi nasi | Incisor fossa of maxilla | Mobile part of nasal septum | Facial nerve | Helps to dilate nostril during deep inspiration and depresses nasal septum |
| Diaphragm | Xiphoid process, inferior 6 costal cartilages and adjoining ribs, arcuate ligaments, anterior longitudinal ligaments and bodies and discs of lumbar vertebrae 1–3 | Central tendon of diaphragm | Phenic nerve (C3–C5) | Diaphragm descends, causing decreased intrathoracic pressure resulting in inhalation and assisting return of venous blood to heart |
| Digastric | Anterior belly: digastric fossa of mandible. Posterior belly: mastoid notch of temporal bone | Intermediate tendon to body and greater horn of hyoid bone | Anterior belly: mylohyoid nerve, a branch of inferior alveolar nerve. Posterior belly: facial nerve (CN VII) | Depresses mandible; raises hyoid bone and steadies it during swallowing and speaking |
| Dorsal interossei (4 muscles) of foot | Adjacent sides of metatarsals 1–5 | 1st: medial side of proximal phalanx of 2nd digit 2nd to 4th: lateral sides of 2nd to 4th digits | Lateral plantar nerve (S2 and S3) | Abduct digits (2–4) and flex metatarsophalangeal joints |

| Muscle(s) | Origin | Insertion | Innervation | Main Action(s) |
|---|---|---|---|---|
| Dorsal interossei 1–4 of hand | Adjacent sides of 2 metacarpals (bipennate muscles) | Extensor expansions and bases of proximal phalanges of digits 2–4 | Deep branch of ulnar nerve (C8 and T1) | Abduct digits from axial line and act with lumbricals to flex metacarpophalangeal joints and extend interphalangeal joints |
| Erector spinae | Arises by a broad tendon from posterior part of iliac crest, posterior surface of sacrum, sacral and inferior lumbar spinous processes, and supraspinous ligament | Iliocostalis—lumborum, thoracis, cervicis: fibers run superiorly to angles of lower ribs and cervical transverse processes Longissimus—thoracis, cervicis, capitis: fibers run superiorly to ribs between tubercles and angles, to transverse processes in thoracic and cervical regions, and to mastoid process of temporal bone Spinalis—thoracis, cervicis, capitis: fibers run superiorly to spinous processes in upper thoracic region and to skull | Posterior rami of spinal nerves | Acting bilaterally, extend vertebral column and head; as back is flexed, control movement by gradually lengthening fibers; acting unilaterally, laterally bend vertebral column |
| Extensor carpi radialis brevis | Lateral epicondyle of humerus | Base of 3rd metacarpal bone | Deep branch of radial nerve (C7 and C8) | Extend and abduct hand at wrist joint |
| Extensor carpi radialis longus | Lateral supracondylar ridge of humerus | Base of 2nd metacarpal bone | Radial nerve (C6 and C7) | Extend and abduct hand at wrist joint |
| Extensor carpi ulnaris | Lateral epicondyle of humerus and posterior border of ulna | Base of 5th metacarpal bone | Posterior interosseous nerve (C7 and C8), continuation of deep branch of radial nerve | Extends and adducts hand at wrist joint |
| Extensor digiti minimi | Lateral epicondyle of humerus | Extensor expansion of 5th digit | Posterior interosseous nerve (C7 and C8), continuation of deep branch of radial nerve | Extends 5th digit at metacarpophalangeal and interphalangeal joints |
| Extensor digitorum | Lateral epicondyle of humerus | Extensor expansions of medial 4 digits | Posterior interosseous nerve (C7 and C8), continuation of deep branch of radial nerve | Extends medial 4 digits at metacarpophalangeal joints; extends hand at wrist joint |
| Extensor digitorum brevis | Anteriormost portions of lateral and superior surfaces of calcaneus | Lateral side of long extensor tendons, with slips to proximal phalanges of 2nd–4th toes | Deep fibular (peroneal) nerve (L5 and S1) | Assists in extending middle 3 toes |
| Extensor digitorum longus | Lateral condyle of tibia and superior three-fourths of medial surface of fibula and interosseous membrane | Middle and distal phalanges of lateral 4 digits | Deep fibular (peroneal) nerve (L5 and S1) | Extends lateral 4 digits and dorsiflexes ankle |
| Extensor hallucis brevis | Anteriormost portion of superior surface of calcaneus | Dorsal aspect of base of proximal phalanx of great toe (hallux) | Deep fibular (peroneal) nerve (L5 and S1) | Extends great toe |

| Muscle(s) | Origin | Insertion | Innervation | Main Action(s) |
|---|---|---|---|---|
| Extensor hallucis longus | Middle part of anterior surface of fibula and interosseous membrane | Dorsal aspect of base of distal phalanx of great toe (hallux) | Deep fibular (peroneal) nerve (L5 and S1) | Extends great toe and dorsiflexes ankle |
| Extensor indicis | Posterior surface of ulna and interosseous membrane | Extensor expansion of 2nd digit | Posterior interosseous nerve (C7 and C8), continuation of deep branch of radial nerve | Extends 2nd digit and helps to extend hand |
| Extensor pollicis brevis | Posterior surface of radius and interosseous membrane | Base of proximal phalanx of thumb | Posterior interosseous nerve (C7 and C8), continuation of deep branch of radial nerve | Extends proximal phalanx of thumb at carpometacarpal joint |
| Extensor pollicis longus | Posterior surface of middle third of ulna and interosseous membrane | Base of distal phalanx of thumb | Posterior interosseous nerve (C7 and C8), continuation of deep branch of radial nerve | Extends distal phalanx of thumb at meta-carpophalangeal and interphalangeal joints |
| External anal sphincter | Skin and fascia surrounding anus and coccyx via anococcy-geal ligament | Perineal body | Inferior anal nerve | Closes anal canal; works with bulbo-spongiosus to support and fix perineal body |
| External intercostal | Inferior border of ribs, from tubercle to cos-tochondral junction | Superior border of ribs below | Intercostal nerves | Elevate ribs (when upper ribs are are fixed by scalene and sternocleidomastoid muscles) |
| External oblique | External surfaces of 5th–12th ribs | Linea alba, pubic tubercle, anterior half of iliac crest | Thoracoabdominal nerves (inferior 6 thoracic nerves) and subcostal nerve | Compress and support abdominal viscera, flex and rotate trunk |
| External urethral sphincter | Internal surface of ischiopubic ramus and ischial tuberosity | Surrounds urethra; in males, also ascends anterior aspect of prostate; in females, some fibers also enclose vagina (ure-throvaginal sphincter) | Deep branch of per-ineal nerve, a branch of pudendal nerve (S2, S3, and S4) | Compresses urethra to maintain urinary continence; in females urethrovaginal sphincter portion also compresses vagina |
| Fibularis (peroneus) brevis | Inferior two-thirds of lateral surface of fibula | Dorsal surface of tuberosity on lateral side of base of 5th metatarsal | Superficial fibular (peroneal) nerve (L5, S1, and S2) | Everts foot and weakly plantarflexes ankle |
| Fibularis (peroneus) longus | Head and superior two-thirds of lateral surface of fibula | Base of 1st metatarsal and medial cuneiform | Superficial fibular (peroneal) nerve (L5, S1, and S2) | Everts foot and weakly plantarflexes ankle |
| Fibularis (peroneus) tertius | Inferior third of ante-rior surface of fibula and interosseous membrane | Dorsum of base of 5th metatarsal | Deep fibular (peroneal) nerve (L5 and S1) | Dorsiflexes ankle and aids in eversion of foot |
| Flexor carpi radialis | Medial epicondyle of humerus | Base of 2nd meta-carpal bone | Median nerve (C6 and C7) | Flexes and abducts hand (at wrist) |
| Flexor carpi ulnaris | Humeral head: medial epicondyle of humerus Ulnar head: olecranon and posterior border of ulna | Pisiform bone, hook of hamate bone, and 5th metacarpal bone | Ulnar nerve (C7 and C8) | Flexes and adducts hand (at wrist) |
| Flexor digiti minimi brevis of foot | Base of 5th metatarsal | Base of proximal phalanx of 5th digit | Superficial branch of lateral plantar nerve (S2 and S3) | Flexes proximal phalanx of 5th digit, thereby assisting with its flexion |

| Muscle(s) | Origin | Insertion | Innervation | Main Action(s) |
|---|---|---|---|---|
| Flexor digiti minimi brevis of hand | Hook of hamate and flexor retinaculum | Medial side of base of proximal phalanx of little finger | Deep branch of ulnar nerve (C8 and T1) | Flexes proximal phalanx of digit 5 |
| Flexor digitorum brevis | Medial tubercle of tuberosity of calcaneus, plantar aponeurosis, intermuscular septa | Both sides of middle phalanges of lateral 4 digits | Medial plantar nerve (S2 and S3) | Flexes lateral 4 digits |
| Flexor digitorum longus | Medial part of posterior surface of tibia inferior to soleal line and by a broad tendon to fibula | Bases of distal phalanges of lateral 4 digits | Tibial nerve (S2 and S3) | Flexes lateral 4 digits and plantarflexes ankle; supports longitudinal arches of foot |
| Flexor digitorum profundus | Proximal three-fourths of medial and anterior surfaces of ulna and interosseous membrane | Bases of distal phalanges of medial 4 digits | Medial part: ulnar nerve (C8 and T1) Lateral part: median nerve (C8 and T1) | Flexes distal phalanges at distal interphalangeal joints of medial 4 digits; assists with flexion of hand |
| Flexor digitorum superficialis | Humeroulnar head: medial epicondyle of humerus, ulnar collateral ligament, and coronoid process of ulna Radial head: superior half of anterior border of radius | Bodies of middle phalanges of medial 4 digits | Median nerve (C7, C8, and T1) | Flexes middle phalanges at proximal interphalangeal joints of medial 4 digits; acting more strongly, also flexes proximal phalanges at metacarpophalangeal joints and hand at wrist |
| Flexor hallucis brevis | Plantar surfaces of cuboid and lateral cuneiforms | Both sides of base of proximal phalanx of 1st digit | Medial plantar nerve (S2 and S3) | Flexes proximal phalanx of 1st digit |
| Flexor hallucis longus | Inferior two-thirds of posterior surface of fibula and inferior part of interosseous membrane | Base of distal phalanx of great toe (hallux) | Tibial nerve (S2 and S3) | Flexes great toe at all joints and weakly plantarflexes ankle; supports medial longitudinal arches of foot |
| Flexor pollicis brevis | Flexor retinaculum and tubercles of scaphoid and trapezium | Lateral side of base of proximal phalanx of thumb | Recurrent branch of median nerve (C8 and T1) | Flexes thumb |
| Flexor pollicis longus | Anterior surface of radius and adjacent interosseous membrane | Base of distal phalanx of thumb | Anterior interosseous nerve from median (C8 and T1) | Flexes phalanges of 1st digit (thumb) |
| Gastrocnemius | Lateral head: lateral aspect of lateral condyle of femur Medial head: popliteal surface of femur, superior to medial condyle | Posterior surface of calcaneus via calcaneal tendon | Tibial nerve (S1 and S2) | Plantarflexes ankle when knee is extended, raises heel during walking, flexes leg at knee joint |
| Gemelli, superior and inferior | Superior: ischial spine Inferior: ischial tuberosity | Medial surface of greater trochanter (trochanteric fossa) of femur | Superior gemellus: nerve to obturator internus (L5 and S1) Inferior gemellus: Nerve to quadratus femoris (L5 and S1) | Laterally rotate extended thigh and abduct flexed thigh; steady femoral head in acetabulum |

| Muscle(s) | Origin | Insertion | Innervation | Main Action(s) |
|---|---|---|---|---|
| Genioglossus | Superior part of mental spine of mandible | Dorsum of tongue and body of hyoid bone | Hypoglossal nerve (CN XII) | Depresses tongue; posterior part pulls tongue anteriorly for protrusion |
| Geniohyoid | Inferior mental spine of mandible | Body of hyoid bone | C1 via hypoglossal nerve | Pulls hyoid bone anterosuperiorly, shortens floor of mouth, widens pharynx |
| Gluteus maximus | Ilium posterior to posterior gluteal line, dorsal surface of sacrum and coccyx, and sacrotuberous ligament | Most fibers end in iliotibial tract that inserts into lateral condyle of tibia; some fibers insert on gluteal tuberosity of femur | Inferior gluteal nerve (L5, S1, and S2) | Extends thigh (especially from flexed position) and assists in its lateral rotation; steadies thigh and assists in rising from sitting position |
| Gluteus medius | External surface of ilium between anterior and posterior gluteal lines | Lateral surface of greater trochanter of femur | Superior gluteal nerve (L5 and S1) | Abducts and medially rotates thigh; keeps pelvis level when opposite leg is raised off ground |
| Gluteus minimus | External surface of ilium between anterior and inferior gluteal lines | Anterior surface of greater trochanter of femur | Superior gluteal nerve (L5 and S1) | Abducts and medially rotates thigh; keeps pelvis level when opposite leg is raised off ground |
| Gracilis | Body and inferior ramus of pubis | Superior part of medial surface of tibia | Obturator nerve (L2 and L3) | Adducts thigh; flexes leg, helps rotate it medially |
| Hyoglossus | Body and greater horn of hyoid bone | Side and inferior aspect of tongue | Hypoglossal nerve (CN XII) | Depresses and retracts tongue |
| Iliacus | Iliac crest, superior two-thirds of iliac fossa, ala of sacrum, and anterior sacroiliac ligaments | Lesser trochanter of femur and shaft inferior to it, and to psoas major tendon | Femoral nerve (L2–L4) | Flexes thigh and stabilizes hip joint; acts with psoas major |
| Inferior constrictor of pharynx | Oblique line of thyroid cartilage and side of cricoid cartilage | Median raphe of pharynx | Cranial root of accessory nerve (CN XI) as above, plus branches of external and recurrent laryngeal nerves of vagus (CN X) | Constricts wall of pharynx during swallowing |
| Inferior longitudinal muscle of tongue | Root of tongue and body of hyoid bone | Apex of tongue | Hypoglossal nerve (CN XII) | Curls tip of tongue inferiorly and shortens tongue |
| Inferior oblique | Anterior part of floor of orbit | Sclera deep to lateral rectus muscle | Oculomotor nerve (CN III) | Abducts, elevates, and laterally rotates eyeball |
| Inferior rectus | Common tendinous ring | Sclera just posterior to cornea | Oculomotor nerve (CN III) | Depresses, adducts, and rotates eyeball medially |
| Infraspinatus | Infraspinous fossa of scapula | Middle facet on greater tubercle of humerus | Suprascapular nerve (C5 and C6) | Laterally rotate arm; help to hold humeral head in glenoid cavity of scapula |

| Muscle(s) | Origin | Insertion | Innervation | Main Action(s) |
|---|---|---|---|---|
| Innermost intercostal | Inner surface of ribs, from angles to costo-chondral junction | Superior border of ribs below | Intercostal nerves | Probably depress ribs |
| Internal intercostal | Inferior border of ribs | Superior border of ribs below | Intercostal nerves | Depress ribs |
| Internal oblique | Thoracolumbar fascia, anterior two-thirds of iliac crest, and lateral half of inguinal ligament | Inferior borders of 10th–12th ribs, linea alba, and pecten pubis via conjoint tendon | Thoracoabdominal (anterior rami of inferior 6 thoracic) and 1st lumbar nerves | Compresses and supports abdominal viscera, and flexes and rotates trunk |
| Interspinales | Superior surfaces of spinous processes of cervical and lumbar vertebrae | Inferior surfaces of spinous processes of vertebrae superior to vertebrae of origin | Posterior rami of spinal nerves | Aid in extension and rotation of vertebral column |
| Intertransversarii | Transverse processes of cervical and lumbar vertebrae | Transverse processes of adjacent vertebrae | Posterior and anterior rami of spinal nerves | Aid in lateral bending of vertebral column; acting bilaterally, stabilize vertebral column |
| Ischiocavernosus | Internal surface of ischiopubic ramus and ischial tuberosity | Crus of penis or clitoris | Deep branch of perineal nerve, a branch of pudendal nerve (S2, S3, and S4) | Maintains erection of penis or clitoris by compressing outflow veins and pushing blood into body of penis or clitoris |
| Lateral cricoarytenoid | Arch of cricoid cartilage | Muscular process of arytenoid cartilage | Recurrent laryngeal nerve (branch of vagus (CN X)) | Adducts vocal fold (interligamentous portion) |
| Lateral pterygoid | Superior head: infra-temporal surface and infratemporal crest of greater wing of sphenoid bone Inferior head: lateral surface of lateral pterygoid plate | Neck of mandible (pterygoid fovea); articular disc and capsule of temporo-mandibular joint | Mandibular nerve (CN V3) via lateral pterygoid nerve from anterior trunk, which enters its deep surface | Acting together, protrude mandible and depress chin; acting alone and alternately, produce side-to-side move-ments of mandible |
| Lateral rectus | Common tendinous ring | Sclera just posterior to cornea | Abducent nerve (CN VI) | Abducts eyeball |
| Latissimus dorsi | Spinous processes of inferior 6 thoracic vertebrae, thoraco-lumbar fascia, iliac crest, and inferior 3 or 4 ribs | Floor of intertuber-cular groove of humerus | Thoracodorsal nerve (C6, C7, and C8) | Extends, adducts, and medially rotates humerus; raises body toward arms during climbing |
| Levator anguli oris | Canine fossa of maxilla | Orbicularis oris and skin at angle of mouth | Facial nerve (CN VII) | Raises angle of mouth, as in smiling |
| Levator ani (pubococcygeus, puborectalis, and iliococcygeus) | Body of pubis, tendinous arch of obturator fascia, and ischial spine | Perineal body, coccyx, anococcygeal liga-ment, walls of prostate or vagina, rectum, and anal canal | Nerve to levator ani (branches of S4) and inferior anal (rectal) nerve and coccygeal plexus | Helps to support pelvic viscera and resists increases in intra-abdominal pressure |
| Levatores costarum | Tips of transverse processes of C7 and T1–T11 vertebrae | Pass inferolaterally and insert on subja-cent rib between its tubercle and angle | Posterior rami of C8–T11 spinal nerves | Elevate ribs, assisting inspiration; assist with lateral bending of vertebral column |
| Levator labii superioris | Frontal process of maxilla and infraorbital region | Skin of upper lip and alar cartilage of nose | Facial nerve (CN VII) | Elevates lip, dilates nostril, and raises angle of mouth |

| Muscle(s) | Origin | Insertion | Innervation | Main Action(s) |
|---|---|---|---|---|
| Levator palpebrae superioris | Lesser wing of sphenoid bone, superior and anterior to optic canal | Tarsal plate and skin of superior (upper) eyelid | Oculomotor nerve (CN III); deep layer (superior tarsal muscle) is supplied by sympathetic fibers | Elevates superior (upper) eyelid |
| Levator scapulae | Posterior tubercles of transverse processes of C1–C4 vertebrae | Superior part of medial border or scapula | Dorsal scapular (C5) and cervical (C3 and C4) nerves | Elevates scapula and tilts its glenoid cavity inferiorly by rotating scapula |
| Levator veli palatini | Cartilage of pharyngo-tympanic (auditory) tube and petrous part of temporal bone | Palatine aponeurosis | Cranial part of CN XI through pharyngeal branch of vagus nerve (CN X) via pharyngeal plexus | Elevates soft palate during swallowing and yawning |
| Longus capitis | Basilar part of occipital bone | Anterior tubercles of C3–C6 transverse processes | Anterior rami of C1–C3 spinal nerves | Flexes head |
| Longus colli | Anterior tubercle of C1 vertebra (atlas); bodies of C1–C3 and transverse processes of C3–C6 vertebra | Bodies of C5–T3 vertebrae, transverse process of C3–C5 vertebra | Anterior rami of C2–C6 spinal nerves | Flexes neck with rotation (torsion) to opposite side if acting unilaterally |
| Lumbrical muscles of foot | Tendons of flexor digitorum longus | Medial aspect of expansion over lateral 4 digits | Medial 1: medial plantar nerve (S2 and S3) Lateral 3: lateral plantar nerve (S2 and S3) | Flex proximal phalanges and extend middle and distal phalanges of lateral 4 digits |
| Lumbricals 1 and 2 of hand | Lateral 2 tendons of flexor digitorum profundus (unipennate muscles) | Lateral sides of extensor expansions of digits 2 and 3 | Median nerve (C8 and T1) | Flex digits at meta-carpophalangeal joints and extend interphalangeal joints |
| Lumbricals 3 and 4 of hand | Medial 3 tendons of flexor digitorum profundus (bipennate muscles) | Lateral sides of extensor expansions of digits 4 and 5 | Deep branch of ulnar nerve (C8 and T1) | Flex digits at meta-carpophalangeal joints and extend interphalangeal joints |
| Masseter | Inferior border and medial surface of zygomatic arch | Lateral surface of ramus of mandible and its coronoid process | Mandibular nerve (CN V3) via masseteric nerve, which enters its deep surface | Elevates and protrudes mandible, thus closing jaws; deep fibers retrude it |
| Medial pterygoid | Deep head: medial surface of lateral pterygoid plate and pyramidal process of palatine bone Superficial head: tuberosity of maxilla | Medial surface of ramus of mandible, inferior to mandibular foramen | Mandibular nerve (CN V3) via medial pterygoid nerve | Acting bilaterally, elevates mandible, closing jaws; assists in protruding mandible; acting alone, assists in protruding same side of jaw; acting alternately, produces a grinding motion |
| Medial rectus | Common tendinous ring | Sclera just posterior to cornea | Oculomotor nerve (CN III) | Adducts eyeball |
| Mentalis | Incisive fossa of mandible | Skin of chin | Facial nerve (CN VII) | Elevates and protrudes lower lip |
| Middle constrictor of pharynx | Stylohyoid ligament and superior (greater) and inferior (lesser) horns of hyoid bone | Median raphe of pharynx | Cranial root of accessory nerve (CN XI) plus branches of external and recurrent laryngeal nerves of vagus (CN X) | Constricts wall of pharynx during swallowing |

| Muscle(s) | Origin | Insertion | Innervation | Main Action(s) |
|---|---|---|---|---|
| Mylohyoid | Mylohyoid line of mandible | Raphe and body of hyoid bone | Mylohyoid nerve, a branch of inferior alveolar nerve of CN V3 | Elevates hyoid bone, floor of mouth, and tongue during swallowing and speaking |
| Nasalis | Superior part of canine ridge of maxilla | Nasal cartilages | Facial nerve (CN VII) | Draws ala (side) of nose toward nasal septum |
| Obliquus capitis inferior | Spinous process of axis (C2 vertebra) | Transverse process of atlas (C1 vertebra) | Suboccipital nerve | Rotation of head at atlantoaxial joint |
| Obliquus capitis superior | Spinous process of atlas (C1 vertebra) | Lateral third of inferior nuchal line of occipital bone | Suboccipital nerve | Rotation of head at atlantoaxial joint |
| Obturator externus | Margins of obturator foramen and obturator membrane | Trochanteric fossa of femur | Obturator nerve (L3 and L4) | Laterally rotates thigh; steadies head of femur in acetabulum |
| Obturator internus | Pelvic surface of obturator membrane and surrounding bones | Medial surface of greater trochanter (trochanteric fossa) of femur | Nerve to obturator internus (L5 and S1) | Laterally rotates extended thigh and abducts flexed thigh; steadies femoral head in acetabulum |
| Occipitofrontalis (occipital belly/frontal belly) | Lateral two-thirds of superior nuchal line and mastoid temporal bone/epicranial aponeurosis | Epicranial aponeurosis/skin of forehead and eyebrows | Posterior branch/temporal branch of facial nerve (CN VII) | Retracts scalp/elevates eyebrows and skin of forehead |
| Omohyoid | Superior border of scapula near suprascapular notch | Inferior border of hyoid bone | C1–C3 by a branch of ansa cervicalis | Depresses, retracts, and steadies hyoid bone |
| Opponens digiti minimi | Hook of hamate and flexor retinaculum | Medial border of 5th metacarpal | Deep branch of ulnar nerve (C8 and T1) | Draws 5th metacarpal anteriorly and rotates it, bringing digit 5 into opposition with thumb |
| Opponens pollicis | Flexor retinaculum and tubercles of scaphoid and trapezium | Lateral side of 1st metacarpal | Recurrent branch of median nerve (C8 and T1) | Draws 1st metacarpal bone laterally to oppose thumb toward center of palm and rotates it medially |
| Orbicularis oculi | Medial orbital margin, medial palpebral ligament, and lacrimal bone | Skin around margin of orbit; tarsal plate | Facial nerve (CN VII) | Closes eyelids; palpebral part gently closes lids; orbital part tightly closes lids |
| Orbicularis oris | Some fibers arise near median plane of maxilla superiorly and mandible inferiorly; other fibers arise from deep surface of skin | Mucous membrane of lips | Facial nerve (CN VII) | As sphincter of oral opening, compresses and protrudes lips (e.g., purses them during whistling and sucking) |
| Palatoglossus | Palatine aponeurosis | Side of tongue | Cranial part of accessory nerve (CN XI) through pharyngeal branch of vagus nerve (CN X) via pharyngeal plexus | Elevates posterior part of tongue and draws soft palate onto tongue |
| Palatopharyngeus | Hard palate and palatine aponeurosis | Lateral wall of pharynx | Cranial part of accessory nerve (CN XI) through pharyngeal branch of vagus nerve (CN X) via pharyngeal plexus | Tenses soft palate and pulls walls of pharynx superiorly, anteriorly, and medially during swallowing |

| Muscle(s) | Origin | Insertion | Innervation | Main Action(s) |
|---|---|---|---|---|
| Palmar interossei 1–3 | Palmar surfaces of 2nd, 4th, and 5th metacarpals (unipennate muscles) | Extensor expansions of digits and bases of proximal phalanges of digits 2, 4, and 5 | Deep branch of ulnar nerve (C8 and T1) | Adduct digits toward axial line and assist lumbricals in flexing metacarpophalangeal joints and extending interphalangeal joint |
| Palmaris brevis | Ulnar side of central portion of palmar aponeurosis | Skin of ulnar side of hand | Superficial ulnar nerve (T1) | Wrinkles skin on palmar side of hand |
| Palmaris longus | Medial epicondyle of humerus | Distal half of flexor retinaculum and palmar aponeurosis | Median nerve (C7 and C8) | Flexes hand (at wrist) and tightens palmar aponeurosis |
| Pectineus | Superior ramus of pubis | Pectineal line of femur, just inferior to lesser trochanter | Femoral nerve (L2 and L3); may receive a branch from obturator nerve | Adducts and flexes thigh; assists with medial rotation of thigh |
| Pectoralis major | Clavicular head: anterior surface of medial half of clavicle Sternocostal head: anterior surface of sternum, superior 6 costal cartilages, aponeurosis of external oblique muscle | Lateral lip of intertubercular groove of humerus | Lateral and medial pectoral nerves; clavicular head (C5 and C6), sternocostal head (C7, C8, and T1) | Adducts and medially rotates humerus; draws scapula anteriorly and inferiorly Acting alone: clavicular head flexes humerus and sternocostal head extends it |
| Pectoralis minor | 3rd to 5th ribs near their costal cartilages | Medial border and superior surface of coracoid process of scapula | Medial pectoral nerve (C8 and T1) | Stabilizes scapula by drawing it inferiorly and anteriorly against thoracic wall |
| Piriformis | Anterior surface of sacrum and sacro-tuberous ligament | Superior border of greater trochanter of femur | Branches of anterior rami of S1 and S2 | Laterally rotate extended thigh and abduct flexed thigh; steady femoral head in acetabulum |
| Plantar interossei 1–3 | Bases and medial sides of metatarsals 3–5 | Medial sides of bases of proximal phalanges of 3rd to 5th digits | Lateral plantar nerve (S2 and S3) | Adduct digits (2–4) and flex metatarsophalangeal joints |
| Plantaris | Inferior end of lateral supracondylar line of femur and oblique popliteal ligament | Posterior surface of calcaneus via calcaneal tendon | Tibial nerve (S1 and S2) | Weakly assists gastrocnemius in plantarflexing ankle and flexing knee |
| Platysma | Superficial fascia of deltoid and pectoral regions | Mandible, skin of cheek, angle of mouth, and orbicularis oris | Facial nerve (CN VII) | Depresses mandible and tenses skin of lower face and neck |
| Popliteus | Lateral surface of lateral condyle of femur and lateral meniscus | Posterior surface of tibia, superior to soleal line | Tibial nerve (L4, L5, and S1) | Weakly flexes knee and unlocks it |
| Posterior cricoarytenoid | Posterior surface of laminae of cricoid cartilage | Muscular process of arytenoid cartilage | Recurrent laryngeal nerve (branch of vagus (CN X)) | Abducts vocal fold |
| Procerus | Aponeurosis covering bridge of nose | Skin of lower forehead between eyebrows | Facial nerve (CN VII) | Depresses medial end of eyebrow; produces transverse wrinkles over bridge of nose; produces look of concentration |

| Muscle(s) | Origin | Insertion | Innervation | Main Action(s) |
|---|---|---|---|---|
| Pronator quadratus | Distal fourth of anterior surface of ulna | Distal fourth of anterior surface of radius | Anterior interosseous nerve from median (C8 and T1) | Pronates forearm; deep fibers bind radius and ulna together |
| Pronator teres | Medial epicondyle of humerus and coronoid process of ulna | Middle of lateral surface of radius | Median nerve (C6 and C7) | Pronates and flexes forearm (at elbow) |
| Psoas major | Sides of T12–L5 vertebrae and discs between them; transverse processes of all lumbar vertebrae | Lesser trochanter of femur | Anterior rami of lumbar nerves (L1, L2, and L3) | Flexes and rotates thigh lateral at hip joint; when thigh is fixed, flexes lumbar vertebrae anteriorly and laterally |
| Psoas minor | Sides of T12–L1 vertebrae and intervertebral disc | Pectineal line, iliopectineal eminence via iliopectineal arch | Anterior rami of lumbar nerves (L1 and L2) | Acts conjointly with psoas major in flexing thigh at hip joint and in stabilizing this joint |
| Pyramidalis | Crest of pubis | Lower portion of linea alba | Subcostal nerve | Tenses linea alba |
| Quadratus femoris | Lateral border of ischial tuberosity | Quadrate tubercle on intertrochanteric crest of femur and area inferior to it | Nerve to quadratus femoris (L5 and S1) | Laterally rotates thigh; steadies femoral head in acetabulum |
| Quadratus lumborum | Medial half of inferior border of 12th rib and tips of lumbar transverse processes | Iliolumbar ligament and internal lip of iliac crest | Ventral branches of T12 and L1–L4 nerves | Extends and laterally flexes vertebral column; fixes 12th rib during inspiration |
| Quadratus plantae | Medial surface and lateral margin of plantar surface of calcaneus | Posterolateral margin of tendon of flexor digitorum longus | Lateral plantar nerve (S2 and S3) | Assists flexor digitorum longus in flexing lateral 4 digits |
| Rectus abdominis | Pubic symphysis and pubic crest | Xiphoid process and 5th–7th costal cartilages | Thoracoabdominal nerves (anterior rami of inferior 6 thoracic nerves) | Flexes trunk (lumbar vertebrae) and compresses abdominal viscera (indirectly opposing diaphragm) |
| Rectus capitis anterior | Anterior surface of lateral mass of C1 vertebra (atlas) | Base of skull, just anterior to occipital condyle | Branches from loop between C1 and C2 spinal nerves | Flexes head at atlanto-occipital joint |
| Rectus capitis lateralis | Transverse process of C1 vertebra (atlas) | Jugular process of occipital bone | Branches from loop between C1 and C2 spinal nerves | Flexes head and helps to stabilize it |
| Rectus capitis posterior major | Spinous process of C2 vertebra (axis) | Middle of inferior nuchal line of occipital bone | Suboccipital nerve | Extends head at atlanto-occipital joint |
| Rectus capitis posterior minor | Dorsal tubercle of C1 vertebra (atlas) | Medial third of inferior nuchal line of occipital bone | Suboccipital nerve | Extends head at atlanto-occipital joint |
| Rectus femoris | Anterior inferior iliac spine and ilium superior to acetabulum | Base of patella and by patellar ligament to tibial tuberosity | Femoral nerve (L2, L3, and L4) | Extend leg at knee joint; rectus femoris also steadies hip joint and helps iliopsoas to flex thigh |
| Rhomboid minor and major | Minor: nuchal ligament and spinous processes of C7 and T1 vertebrae<br>Major: spinous processes of T2–T5 vertebrae | Medial border of scapula from level of spine to inferior angle | Dorsal scapular nerve (C4 and C5) | Retract scapula and rotate it to depress glenoid cavity; fix scapula to thoracic wall |

| Muscle(s) | Origin | Insertion | Innervation | Main Action(s) |
|---|---|---|---|---|
| Risorius | Platysma and fascia of masseter | Orbicularis oris, skin of corner of mouth, modiolus | Facial nerve (CN VII) | Retracts angle of mouth, lengthening rima oris |
| Salpingopharyngeus | Cartilaginous part of auditory tube | Blends with palato-pharyngeus | Cranial root of accessory nerve via pharyngeal branch of vagus and pharyngeal plexus | Elevate (shorten and widen) pharynx and larynx during swallowing and speaking |
| Sartorius | Anterior superior iliac spine and superior part of notch inferior to it | Superior part of medial surface of tibia | Femoral nerve (L2 and L3) | Flexes, abducts, and laterally rotates thigh at hip joint; flexes leg at knee joint |
| Scalenus anterior | Transverse processes of C4–C6 vertebrae | 1st rib | Cervical spine nerves (C4, C5, and C6) | Elevates 1st rib; laterally flexes and rotates neck |
| Scalenus medius | Posterior tubercles of transverse processes of C4–C6 vertebrae | Superior surface of 1st rib, posterior groove for subclavian artery | Anterior rami of cervical spinal nerves | Flexes neck laterally; elevates 1st rib during forced inspiration |
| Scalenus posterior | Posterior tubercles of transverse processes of C4–C6 vertebrae | External border of 2nd rib | Anterior rami of cervical nerves C7 and C8 | Flexes neck laterally; elevates 2nd rib during forced inspiration |
| Semimembranosus | Ischial tuberosity | Posterior part of medial condyle of tibia; reflected attachment forms oblique popliteal ligament (to lateral femoral condyle) | Tibial division of sciatic nerve (L5, S1, and S2) | Extends thigh; flexes leg and, when knee is flexed, rotates it medially; when hip is flexed and knee is extended, can raise trunk against gravity |
| Semitendinosus | Ischial tuberosity | Medial surface of superior part of tibia | Tibial division of sciatic nerve (L5, S1, and S2) | Extends thigh; flexes leg and, when knee is flexed, rotates it medially; when hip is flexed and knee is extended, can raise trunk against gravity |
| Serratus anterior | External surfaces of lateral parts of 1st–8th ribs | Anterior surface of medial border of scapula | Long thoracic nerve (C5, C6, and C7) | Protracts scapula and holds it against thoracic wall; rotates scapula |
| Serratus posterior inferior | Spinous processes of T11–L2 vertebrae | Inferior borders of 8th–12th ribs near their angles | Anterior rami of 9th–12th thoracic spinal nerves | Depress ribs |
| Serratus posterior superior | Ligamentum nuchae, spinous processes of C7–T3 vertebrae | Superior borders of 2nd–4th ribs | 2nd–5th intercostal nerves | Elevate ribs |
| Soleus | Posterior aspect of head of fibula, superior fourth of posterior surface of fibula soleal line and medial border of tibia | Posterior surface of calcaneus via calcaneal tendon | Tibial nerve (S1 and S2) | Plantarflexes ankle independent of position of knee and steadies leg on foot |
| Splenius capitis et cervicis | Arises from inferior half of ligamentum nuchae and spinous processes of C7–T3 of T4 vertebrae | Splenius capitis: fibers run superolaterally to mastoid process of temporal bone and lateral third of superior nuchal line of occipital bone | Posterior rami of spinal nerves | Acting alone, laterally bend and rotate head to side of active muscles; acting together, extend head and neck |

| Muscle(s) | Origin | Insertion | Innervation | Main Action(s) |
|---|---|---|---|---|
| Splenius capitis et cervicis *(cont.)* | | Splenius cervicis: posterior tubercles of transverse of C1–C3 or C4 vertebrae | | |
| Stapedius | Internal walls of pyramidal eminence of posterior wall of tympanic cavity | Neck of stapes | Facial nerve (CN VII) | Dampens vibrations of stapes reflexively in response to loud noise |
| Sternocleidomastoid | Lateral surface of mastoid process of temporal bone and lateral half of superior nuchal line | Sternal head: anterior surface of manubrium of sternum Clavicular head: superior surface of medial third of clavicle | Spinal root of accessory nerve (motor) and C2 and C3 nerves (pain and proprioception) | Tilts head to one side, i.e., laterally; flexes neck and rotates it so face is turned superiorly toward opposite side; acting together, the 2 muscles flex neck so chin is thrust forward |
| Sternohyoid | Manubrium of sternum and medial end of clavicle | Body of hyoid bone | C1–C3 by a branch of ansa cervicalis | Depresses hyoid bone after it has been elevated during swallowing |
| Sternothyroid | Posterior surface of manubrium of sternum | Oblique line of thyroid cartilage | C2 and C3 by a branch of ansa cervicalis | Depresses hyoid bone and larynx |
| Styloglossus | Styloid process and stylohyoid ligament | Side and inferior aspect of tongue | Hypoglossal nerve (CN XII) | Retracts tongue and draws it up to create a trough for swallowing |
| Stylohyoid | Styloid process of temporal bone | Body of hyoid bone | Cervical branch of facial nerve (CN VII) | Elevates and retracts hyoid bone, thereby elongating floor of mouth |
| Stylopharyngeus | Styloid process of temporal bone | Posterior and superior borders of thyroid cartilage with palatopharyngeus | Glossopharyngeal nerve (CN IX) | Elevate (shorten and widen) pharynx and larynx during swallowing and speaking |
| Subclavius | Junction of 1st rib and its costal cartilage | Inferior surface of middle third of clavicle | Nerve to subclavius (C5 and C6) | Anchors and depresses clavicle |
| Subcostal | Internal surface of lower ribs near their angles | Superior borders of 2nd or 3rd ribs below | Intercostal nerves | Elevate ribs |
| Subscapularis | Subscapular fossa | Lesser tubercle of humerus | Upper and lower subscapular nerves (C5, C6, and C7) | Medially rotates arm and adducts it; helps to hold humeral head in glenoid cavity |
| Superficial transverse perineal muscle | Compressor urethrae portion only | Perineal body | Deep branch of perineal nerve, a branch of pudendal nerve (S2, S3, and S4) | Support and fix perineal body (pelvic floor) to support abdominopelvic viscera and resist increased intra-abdominal pressure |
| Superior constrictor of pharynx | Pterygoid hamulus, pterygomandibular raphe, posterior end of mylohyoid line of mandible, and side of tongue | Median raphe of pharynx and pharyngeal tubercle on basilar part of occipital bone | Cranial root of accessory nerve via pharyngeal branch of vagus and pharyngeal plexus | Constrict wall of pharynx during swallowing |

| Muscle(s) | Origin | Insertion | Innervation | Main Action(s) |
|---|---|---|---|---|
| Superior longitudinal muscle of tongue | Submucous fibrous layer and median fibrous septum | Margins of tongue and mucous membrane | Hypoglossal nerve (CN XII) | Curls tip and sides of tongue superiorly and shortens tongue |
| Superior oblique | Body of sphenoid bone | Its tendon passes through a fibrous ring or trochlea, changes its direction, and inserts into sclera deep to superior rectus muscle | Trochlear nerve (CN IV) | Abducts, depresses, and medially rotates eyeball |
| Superior rectus | Common tendinous ring | Sclera just posterior to cornea | Oculomotor nerve (CN III) | Elevates, adducts, and rotates eyeball medially |
| Supinator | Lateral epicondyle of humerus, radial collateral and anular ligaments, supinator fossa, and crest of ulna | Lateral, posterior, and anterior surfaces of proximal third of radius | Deep branch of radial nerve (C5 and C6) | Supinates forearm (i.e., rotates radius to turn palm anteriorly) |
| Supraspinatus | Supraspinous fossa of scapula | Superior facet on greater tubercle of humerus | Suprascapular nerve (C4, C5, and C6) | Initiates and assists deltoid in abduction of arm and acts with rotator cuff muscles |
| Temporalis | Floor of temporal fossa and deep surface of temporal fascia | Tip and medial surface of coronoid process and anterior border of ramus of mandible | Deep temporal branches of mandibular nerve (CN V3) | Elevates mandible, closing jaws; its posterior fibers retrude mandible after protrusion |
| Tensor of fascia lata | Anterior superior iliac spine and anterior part of iliac crest | Iliotibial tract that attaches to lateral condyle of tibia | Superior gluteal (L4 and L5) | Abducts, medially rotates, and flexes thigh; helps to keep knee extended; steadies trunk on thigh |
| Tensor tympani | Canal for tensor tympani of petrous part of temporal bone and cartilage of pharyngotympanic (auditory) tube | Handle of malleus | Branch of mandibular nerve (CN V3) via otic ganglion | Tenses tympanic membrane to dampen excessive vibration caused by loud noise |
| Tensor veli palatini | Scaphoid fossa of medial pterygoid plate, spine of sphenoid bone, and cartilage of pharyngotympanic (auditory) tube | Palatine aponeurosis | Medial pterygoid nerve (a branch of mandibular nerve— CN V3) via otic ganglion | Tenses soft palate and opens mouth of auditory tube during swallowing and yawning |
| Teres major | Dorsal surface of inferior angle of scapula | Medial lip of intertubercular groove of humerus | Lower subscapular nerve (C6 and C7) | Adducts and medially rotates arm |
| Teres minor | Superior part of lateral border of scapula | Inferior facet on greater tubercle of humerus | Axillary nerve (C5 and C6) | Laterally rotate arm; help to hold humeral head in glenoid cavity of scapula |
| Thyroarytenoid | Posterior surface of thyroid cartilage | Muscular process of arytenoid cartilage | Recurrent laryngeal nerve | Relaxes vocal fold |
| Thyrohyoid | Oblique line of thyroid cartilage | Inferior border of body and greater horn of hyoid bone | C1 via hypoglossal nerve | Depresses hyoid bone and elevates larynx |

| Muscle(s) | Origin | Insertion | Innervation | Main Action(s) |
|-----------|--------|-----------|-------------|----------------|
| Tibialis anterior | Lateral condyle and superior half of lateral surface of tibia and interosseous membrane | Medial and inferior surfaces of medial cuneiform and base of 1st metatarsal | Deep fibular (peroneal) nerve (L4 and L5) | Dorsiflexes ankle and inverts foot |
| Tibialis posterior | Interosseous membrane, posterior surface of tibia inferior to soleal line, and posterior surface of fibula | Tuberosity of navicular, cuneiform, and cuboid and bases of 2nd, 3rd, and 4th metatarsals | Tibial nerve (L4 and L5) | Plantarflexes ankle and inverts foot |
| Transverse muscle of tongue | Median fibrous septum | Fibrous tissue at margins of tongue | Hypoglossal nerve (CN XII) | Narrows and elongates tongue, acts simultaneously to protrude tongue |
| Transversospinal | Transverse processes: Semispinalis arises from transverse processes of C4–T12 vertebrae. Multifidus arises from sacrum and ilium, transverse processes of T1–T3, and articular processes of C4–C7. Rotatores arise from transverse processes of vertebrae; are best developed in thoracic region | Spinous processes: Semispinalis— thoracis, cervicis, and capitis: fibers run superomedially to occipital bone and spinous processes in thoracic and cervical regions, spanning 4–6 segments. Multifidus: fibers pass superomedially to spinous processes of vertebrae above, spanning 2–4 segments. Rotatores: pass superomedially to attach to junction of lamina and transverse process, or spinous process, of vertebra above their origin, spanning 1–2 segments | Posterior rami of spinal nerves | Extend head and thoracic and cervical regions of vertebral column and rotate them contralaterally; stabilize vertebrae during local movements of vertebral column; stabilize vertebrae and assist with local extension and rotary movements of vertebral column; may function as organs of proprioception |
| Transversus abdominis | Internal surfaces of 7th–12th costal cartilages, thoracolumbar fascia, iliac crest, and lateral third of inguinal ligament | Linea alba with aponeurosis of internal oblique, pubic crest, and pecten pubis via conjoint tendon | Thoracoabdominal (anterior rami of inferior 6 thoracic) and 1st lumbar nerves | Compresses and supports abdominal viscera |
| Transversus thoracis | Posterior surface of lower sternum | Internal surface of costal cartilages 2–6 | Intercostal nerves | Depress ribs |
| Trapezius | Medial third of superior nuchal line; external occipital protuberance, nuchal ligament, and spinous processes of C7–T12 vertebrae | Lateral third of clavicle, acromion, and spine of scapula | Spinal root of accessory nerve (CN XI) (motor) and cervical nerves (C3 and C4) (pain and proprioception) | Elevates, retracts, and rotates scapula; superior fibers elevate, middle fibers retract, and inferior fibers depress scapula; superior and inferior fibers act together in superior rotation of scapula |

| Muscle(s) | Origin | Insertion | Innervation | Main Action(s) |
|---|---|---|---|---|
| Triceps brachii | Long head: infra-glenoid tubercle of scapula Lateral head: posterior surface of humerus, superior to radial groove Medial head: posterior surface of humerus, inferior to radial groove | Proximal end of olecranon of ulna and fascia of forearm | Radial nerve (C6, C7, and C8) | Chief extensor of forearm at elbow; long head steadies head of abducted humerus |
| Uvula muscles | Posterior nasal spine and palatine aponeurosis | Mucosa of uvula | Cranial part of CN XI through pharyngeal branch of vagus nerve (CN X) via pharyngeal plexus | Shortens uvula and pulls it superiorly |
| Vastus intermedius | Anterior and lateral surfaces of body of femur | Base of patella and by patellar ligament to tibial tuberosity | Femoral nerve (L2, L3, and L4) | Extend leg at knee joint; rectus femoris also steadies hip joint and helps iliopsoas to flex thigh |
| Vastus lateralis | Greater trochanter and lateral lip of linea aspera of femur | Base of patella and by patellar ligament to tibial tuberosity | Femoral nerve (L2, L3, and L4) | Extend leg at knee joint; rectus femoris also steadies hip joint and helps iliopsoas to flex thigh |
| Vastus medialis | Intertrochanteric line and medial lip of linea aspera of femur | Base of patella and by patellar ligament to tibial tuberosity | Femoral nerve (L2, L3, and L4) | Extend leg at knee joint; rectus femoris also steadies hip joint and helps iliopsoas to flex thigh |
| Vertical muscle of tongue | Superior surface of borders of tongue | Inferior surface of borders of tongue | Hypoglossal nerve (CN XII) | Flattens and broadens tongue, acts simultaneously to protrude tongue |
| Vocalis | Vocal process of arytenoid cartilage | Vocal ligaments | Recurrent laryngeal nerve (branch of vagus (CN X)) | Relaxes posterior vocal ligament while maintaining (or increasing) tension of anterior part |
| Zygomaticus major/minor | Zygomatic bone anterior/posterior to temporozygomatic suture | Muscles at angle of mouth/orbicularis oris of upper lip | Facial nerve (CN VII) | Elevate and evert upper lip |

# Arteries of the Human Body

| Artery/Arteries | Origin | Course | Branches/ Distribution |
| --- | --- | --- | --- |
| Abdominal aorta | Continuation of thoracic aorta | Runs on anterior aspect of bodies of lumbar vertebrae | Visceral branches: celiac, superior and inferior mesenteric, renal, middle suprarenal, gonadal. Parietal branches: lumbar, median sacral |
| Angular | Terminal branch of facial artery | Passes to medial angle (canthus) of eye | Superior part of cheek and lower eyelid |
| Anterior cerebral | Terminal branch (with middle cerebral) of internal carotid artery | Passes anteriorly, loops around genu of corpus callosum, then passes posteriorly in interhemispheric fissure | A1 segment: thalamus and corpus striatum. A2 segment: cortex of medial aspects of frontal and parietal lobes |
| Anterior ciliary | Muscular (rectus) branches of ophthalmic artery | Pierces sclera at attachments of rectus muscles and forms network in iris and ciliary body | Iris and ciliary body |
| Anterior communicating | Anterior cerebral artery | Connects anterior cerebral arteries in prechiasmatic cistern, to complete cerbral arterial circle | Anteromedial central perforating arteries |
| Anterior division of internal iliac | Internal iliac | Passes anteriorly along lateral wall of lesser pelvis in hypogastric sheath and divides into visceral and parietal branches | Parietal branch: obturator artery. Visceral branches: umbilical artery, inferior vesical, uterine, vaginal, middle rectal, and pudendal |
| Anterior ethmoidal | Ophthalmic artery | Passes through anterior ethmoidal foramen to anterior cranial fossa and into nasal cavity, sending branches to skin of nose | Supplies anterior and middle ethmoidal cells, dura of anterior cranial fossa, anterosuperior nasal cavity, and skin on dorsum of nose |
| Anterior inferior cerebellar | Lower (initial) part of basilar artery | Runs posterolaterally, often looping in and out of internal acoustic meatus | Supplies inferior aspect of lateral lobes of cerebellum, inferolateral pons, and choroid plexus in cerebellopontine angle; usually gives rise to labyrinthine artery |
| Anterior intercostal (branches) | Internal thoracic (intercostal spaces 1–6) and musculophrenic arteries (intercostal spaces 7–9) | Pass between intenal and innermost intercostal muscles | Intercostal muscles, overlying skin, underlying parietal pleura |
| Anterior interventricular (branch) | Left coronary artery | Passes along anterior IV groove to apex of heart | Walls of right and left ventricles including most of IV septum and contained atrioventricular bundle and branches (conducting tissue) |
| Anterior spinal | Superiorly, by a merger of intracranial branches, one from each vertebral artery; it is continued inferiorly by bifurcations of anterior segmental medullary arteries at various levels | Forms a continuous anastomotic chain that descends length of spinal cord in entrance to anterior median fissure; | Supplies anterior portion of spinal cord by means of sulcal branches, which extend into anterior median fissure, and pial plexus, which ramifies over surface of cord. |
| Anterior superior alveolar | Infraorbital artery | Arises within infraorbital canal and ascends through anterior alveolar canals | Supplies mucosa of maxillary sinus and maxillary superior incisor and canine teeth. |

| Artery/Arteries | Origin | Course | Branches/ Distribution |
|---|---|---|---|
| Anterior tibial | Terminal branch (with posterior tibial) of popliteal artery | Passes between tibia and fibula into anterior compartment through gap in superior part of interosseous membrane and descends this membrane between tibialis anterior and extensor digitorum longus | Anterior compartment of leg |
| Appendicular | Ileocolic artery | Passes between layers of mesoappendix | Vermiform appendix |
| Arch of aorta | Continuation of ascending aorta | Arches posteriorly on left side of trachea and esophagus and superior to root of left lung | Brachiocephalic, left common carotid, and left subclavian |
| Arcuate (of foot) | Continuation of dorsalis pedis | Passes laterally, dorsal to bases of metatarsals | 2nd, 3rd, and 4th dorsal metatarsal arteries |
| Artery of bulb of penis or vestibule of vagina | Internal pudendal artery | Pierces perineal membrane to reach bulb of penis or vestibule of vagina | Supplies bulb of penis or vestibule and bulbourethral gland (male) and greater vestibular gland (female) |
| Artery to ductus deferens | Inferior (or superior) vesical | Runs retroperitoneally to ductus deferens | Ductus deferens |
| Artery of pterygoid canal | 3rd part of maxillary artery, or from greater palatine | Passes posteriorly through pterygoid canal | Mucosa of uppermost pharynx (pharyngeal recess), pharyngotympanic (auditory) tube, and tympanic cavity |
| Ascending aorta | Aortic orifice of left ventricle | Ascends approximately 5 cm to level of sternal angle where it becomes arch of aorta | Right and left coronary arteries |
| Ascending cervical | Terminal branch (with inferior thyroid artery) of thyrocervical trunk | Ascends on prevertebral fascia | Supplies anterior prevertebral muscles; anastomoses widely with other arteries of neck |
| Ascending palatine | Facial artery | Ascends alongside and crosses over superior border of superior constrictor of pharynx to reach soft palate and tonsillar fossa | Supplies lateral wall of pharynx, tonsils, pharyngotympanic (auditory) tube, and soft palate |
| Ascending pharyngeal | Medial aspect of external carotid artery | Ascends between internal carotid artery and pharynx to cranial base, sending branches through jugular foramen and hypoglossal canal | Supplies pharyngeal wall, palatine tonsil, soft palate, and dura of posterior cranial fossa |
| Atrioventricular (AV) nodal (branch) | Right coronary artery near origin of posterior IV artery | Runs anteriorly in uppermost part of interventrical septum to AV node | AV node |
| Axillary | Continuation of subclavian artery after crossing 1st rib | Runs inferolaterally through axillary fossa, changing to brachial artery when it crosses inferior border of teres major; parts are medial (1st), posterior (2nd), and lateral (3rd) to pectoralis minor | 1st part: superior thoracic; 2nd part: thoracoacromial and lateral thoracic arteries; 3rd part: subclavian and anterior and posterior circumflex humeral arteries |
| Basilar | Formed by intracranial union of vertebral arteries | Ascends clivus in pontine cistern; terminates by bifurcating into posterior cerebral arteries | Branches: anterior inferior cerebellar, labyrinthine, pontine, mesencephalic, and superior cerebellar arteries |

| Artery/Arteries | Origin | Course | Branches/ Distribution |
|---|---|---|---|
| Brachial | Continuation of axillary artery past inferior border of teres major | Courses in medial intermuscular septum with median nerve; ends by bifurcating into radial and ulnar arteries in cubital fossa | Main artery of arm branches: deep artery of arm, muscular and nutrient branches, superior and inferiorulnar collateral |
| Brachiocephalic (trunk) | 1st and largest branch of arch of aorta | Ascends posterolaterally to right, running anterior and then to right of trachea; deep to sternoclavicular joint, it bifurcates into terminal branches | Right common carotid and right subclavian arteries |
| Bronchial (1–2 branches) | Anterior aspect of 1st part of thoracic aorta or 3rd right posterior intercostal artery | Run on posterior aspects of primary bronchi and follow tracheobronchial tree | Bronchial and peribronchial tissue, visceral pleura |
| Buccal | Maxillary artery | Runs anterolaterally with buccal nerve, emerging from beneath anterior border of ramus of mandible | Supplies buccinator muscle, overlying skin, and underlying oral mucosa; anastomoses with branches of facial and infraorbital arteries. |
| Carpal branches, dorsal and palmar | Radial and ulnar arteries at level of wrist | Anastomose with corresponding branches of counterpart artery (ulnar or to form dorsal and palmar carpal arches) | Provide collateral circulation at wrist |
| Celiac | Abdominal aorta just distal to aortic hiatus of diaphragm | Runs a short course (1.25 cm), giving rise to left gastric, and bifurcating into splenic and common hepatic arteries | Supplies inferiomost esophagus, stomach, duodenum (proximal to bile duct), liver and biliary apparatus, and pancreas |
| Central artery of retina | Ophthalmic artery | Runs in dural sheath of optic nerve and pierces nerve near eyeball; ramifying from center of optic disc into retinal arterioles | Supplies optic retina (except cones and rods); branches: macular, nasal and temporal retinal arterioles |
| Circumflex (branch) | Left coronary artery | Passes to left in atrioventricular groove and runs to posterior surface of heart | Primarily left atrium and left ventricle branches: left ventricular, atrial, and marginal |
| Circumflex humeral, anterior and posterior | 3rd part of axillary artery, typically opposite origin of subscapular artery | Arteries anastomose to form a circle around surgical neck of humerus; larger posterior circumflex humeral artery passes through quadrangular space with axillary nerve | Supply shoulder joint and muscles of proximal arm: deltoid, teres major and minor, and long and lateral heads of triceps. |
| Circumflex scapular artery | Terminal branch (with thoracodorsal artery) of subscapular artery | Curves around axillary border of scapula and enters infraspinous fossa | Supplies subscapular and infraspinatus muscles; joins collateral anastomosis of shoulder around scapula |
| Common carotid, left and right | Left: 2nd branch of arch of aorta; Right: terminal branch (with right subclavian) of brachiocephalic artery | Ascend from/pass deep to sternoclavicular joint in carotid sheath under cover of sternocleidomastoid to level of C4 vertebra (or hyoid bone) | Terminal branches: internal and external carotid arteries |
| Common hepatic | Terminal branch (with splenic artery) of celiac artery (trunk) | Passes to right along superior border of pancreas, running anterior to portal vein | Terminal branches: hepatic artery proper and gastroduodenal artery |
| Common iliac, left and right | Terminal branches of abdominal aorta | Begin anterior to L4 vertebral body, diverging as they descend to terminate at L5-S1 level, anterior to sacroiliac joints | Terminal branches: external and internal iliac arteries |

| Artery/Arteries | Origin | Course | Branches/ Distribution |
|---|---|---|---|
| Common interosseous | Ulnar artery, just distal to bifurcation of brachial artery in cubital fossa | Passes deep to bifurcate into after a very short course | Terminal branches: anterior and posterior interosseous arteries |
| Common palmar digital | Superficial palmar arch | Pass distally anterior to lumbricals to bifurcate proximal to webbings between digits | Receive palmar metacarpal arteries from deep palmar arch Terminal branches: proper palmar digital arteries |
| Common plantar digital arteries | Terminal portions of plantar metatarsal arteries | Short segments distal to transverse head of adductor hallucis proximal to webs between toes | Terminal branches: plantar digital arteries proper |
| Costocervical (trunk) | 2nd part of subclavian artery | Very short artery passes posteriorly superior to cervical pleura to neck of 1st rib and bifurcates into terminal branches | Terminal branches: supreme intercostal and deep cervical arteries |
| Cremasteric | Inferior epigastric | Accompanies spermatic cord through inguinal canal and into scrotal sac | Supplies cremaster muscle and other coverings of cord in males; round ligament in females |
| Cystic | Right hepatic artery | Arises within hepatoduodenal ligament | Gallbladder and cystic duct |
| Deep artery of arm | Brachial artery near its origin | Accompanies radial nerve through radial groove in humerus; terminal branches take part in anastomosis | Branches: deltoid, muscular (to head of triceps) and nutrient (to humerus) Terminal branches: middle around elbow joint and radial collateral arteries |
| Deep artery of penis or clitoris | Terminal branch of internal pudendal artery | Pierces perineal membrane to reach erectile bodies of clitoris or penis (corpora cavernosa) | Terminations (helicine arteries) uncoil to engorge erectile sinuses with arterial blood |
| Deep artery of thigh | Femoral artery in femoral triangle (about 4 cm distal to inguinal ligament) | Passes inferiorly on medial intermuscular septum, deep to adductor longus | Perforating branches pass through adductor magnus muscle to posterior and lateral part of anterior compartments of thigh |
| Deep auricular | 1st part of maxillary artery | Ascends in parotid gland posterior to temporomandibular joint, piercing wall of external acoustic meatus | Supplies temporomandibular joint and skin of external acoustic meatus and tympanic membrane |
| Deep cervical | Costocervical trunk | Passes posteriorly between transverse process of C7 and neck of 1st rib and ascends between semispinalis cervicis and capitis to C2 level | Supplies deep posterior muscles of neck and anastomoses with descending branch of occipital artery and branches of vertebral artery |
| Deep circumflex iliac | External iliac artery | Runs on deep aspect of anterior abdominal wall, parallel to inguinal ligament | Supplies iliacus muscle and inferior part of anterolateral abdominal wall |
| Deep lingual | Continuation (3rd part of) lingual artery | Turns superiorly near anterior border of hyoglossus and flanking then passes anteriorly frenulum just deep to mucosa | Supplies genioglossus, inferior longitudinal muscle and mucosa of underside of tongue, tip of tongue |
| Deep palmar arch | Direct continuation of radial artery, completed on medial side by deep branch of ulnar artery | Curves medially, deep to long flexor tendons in contact with bases of metacarpals | Branches: palmar metacarpal arteries |

| Artery/Arteries | Origin | Course | Branches/ Distribution |
|---|---|---|---|
| Deep plantar arch | Continuation of lateral plantar artery | Courses anteromedially, between 3rd and 4th layers of muscles of sole of foot; anastomoses with dorsalis pedis via deep plantar artery between 1st and 2nd metatarsal bases | Branches: plantar metatarsal arteries |
| Deep temporal, anterior and posterior | 2nd part of maxillary artery | Ascend between temporalis and bone of temporal fossa | Supplies temporalis muscle, periosteum and bone |
| Descending genicular | Femoral artery, in adductor canal | Descends in vastus medialis, just anterior to tendon of adductor magnus, to anastomose with superior medial genicular artery | Branches: saphenous branch, accompanying saphenous nerve to medial skin of leg; muscular branches to vastus medialis and adductor magnus |
| Descending palatine | 3rd part of maxillary artery | Arises in pterygopalatine fossa; descends in palatine canal | Branches: greater and lesser palatine arteries |
| Dorsal artery of penis or clitoris | Terminal branch of internal pudendal artery | Pierces perineal membrane and passes through suspensory ligament of penis or clitoris to run on dorsum of penis or clitoris | Skin of penis and erectile tissue of penis or clitoris |
| Dorsal carpal arch | Radial and ulnar arteries | Arches within fascia on dorsum of hand | Branches: dorsal metacarpal arteries |
| Dorsal digital arteries (of fingers) | Dorsal metacarpal arteries | Run distally on the posterolateral aspects of the proximal one-and-a-half phalanges | Supply dorsal aspects of proximal one-and-a-half phalanges of fingers |
| Dorsal digital arteries (of toes) | Dorsal metatarsal arteries | Run distally on posterolateral aspects of proximal one-and-a-half-phalanges | Supply dorsal aspects of proximal one-and-a-half phalanges of toes |
| Dorsal metacarpal | Dorsal carpal arch | Run on 2nd-4th dorsal interossei | Bifurcate into dorsal digital arteries; supply skin, muscle and bone of dorsum of hand and fingers to center of middle phalanx |
| Dorsal metatarsal | 1st: termination of dorsalis pedis; 2nd, 3rd and 4th: arcuate artery | Run distally on the superficial aspect of the corresponding dorsal interosseous muscles | Branches: dorsal digital arteries (of toes) |
| Dorsal nasal | Ophthalmic artery | Courses along dorsal aspect of nose and supplies its surface | Courses along dorsal aspect of nose and supplies its surface |
| Dorsal pancreatic | Splenic artery | Descends posterior to pancreas, dividing into right and left branches | Supplies middle portion of pancreas |
| Dorsal scapular (variation— 1/3 of time it is replaced by a deep branch of the transverse cervical artery) | 3rd (or 2nd) part of subclavian artery | Passes laterally through brachial plexus then deep to levator scapulae; joins dorsal scapular nerve running along vertebral border of scapula, deep to rhomboid muscles | Supplies branches to trapezius, rhomboids, latissimus dorsi; participates in anastomoses around scapula (shoulder) |
| Dorsalis pedis | Continuation of anterior tibial artery distal to inferior extensor retinaculum | Descends anteromedially to 1st interosseous space and divides into plantar and arcuate | Muscles on dorsum of foot; pierces 1st dorsal interosseous muscle as deep plantar artery to arteries contribute to formation of plantar arch |
| Esophageal (4–5 branches) | Anterior aspect of thoracic aorta | Run anteriorly to esophagus | Esophagus |

| Artery/Arteries | Origin | Course | Branches/ Distribution |
|---|---|---|---|
| External carotid | Common carotid artery at superior border of thyroid cartilage | Ascends slightly anteriorly and then inclines posteriorly and laterally, passing between mastoid process and mandible; enters substance of parotid gland, bifurcating into terminal branches deep to neck of mandible | Anterior branches: superior thyroid, facial and lingual aa Posterior branches: occipital and posterior auricular arteries Medial branch: ascending pharyngeal Terminal branches: maxillary and superficial temporal arteries |
| External pudendal, superficial, and deep branches | Femoral artery | Pass medially across thigh to reach scrotum or labia majora | Skin of mons pubis and anterior labia (female) or root of penis and anterior scrotum (male) |
| Facial | External carotid artery | Ascends deep to submandibular gland, winds around inferior border of mandible and enters face, ascending obliquely across cheek and side of nose to medial angle of eye | Branches: ascending palatine, tonsillar, glandular, submental, inferior and superior labial, and lateral nasal. Terminal branch (continuation): angular artery |
| Femoral | Continuation of external iliac artery distal to inguinal ligament | Descends through femoral triangle, traverses adductor canal, and changes name to "popliteal" at adductor hiatus | Supplies anterior and anteromedial surfaces of thigh |
| Fibular (peroneal) | Posterior tibial | Descends in posterior compartment adjacent to posterior intermuscular septum | Posterior compartment of leg: perforating branches supply lateral compartment of leg |
| Gastroduodenal | Hepatic artery | Descends retroperitoneally, posterior to gastroduodenal junction | Stomach, pancreas, 1st part of duodenum, and distal part of bile duct |
| Genicular (superior lateral and medial, inferior lateral, medial, and middle) | Popliteal | Arise and run to "four corners" of knee joint (viewed anteriorly) around the patella and femoral and tibial condyles; middle genicular pierces oblique popliteal ligament in posterior center of joint capsule | Form, with participation also of descending genicular, descending branch of lateral circumflex femoral, circumflex fibular and recurrent tibial arteries, the genicular articular anastomosis |
| Greater pancreatic | Splenic artery | Penetrates left portion of pancreas, splitting into right and left branches, which parallel pancreatic duct | Anastomoses with other pancreatic branches; supplies mostly tail of pancreas and contained duct |
| Hepatic artery proper | Celiac trunk | Passes retroperitoneally to reach hepatoduodenal ligament and passes between its layers to porta hepatis; bifurcates into right and left hepatic arteries | Branches: right gastric, supraduodenal, right and left hepatic arteries; supplies liver and gallbladder, stomach, pancreas, duodenum |
| Ileocolic | Terminal branch of superior mesenteric artery | Runs along root of mesentery and divides into ileal and colic branches | Ileum, cecum and ascending colon |
| Iliolumbar | Posterior division of internal iliac | Ascends anterior to sacroiliac joint and posterior to common iliac vessels and psoas major | Psoas major, iliacus and quadratus lumborum muscles and cauda equina in vertebral canal |

| Artery/Arteries | Origin | Course | Branches/ Distribution |
|---|---|---|---|
| Inferior alveolar | 1st part of maxillary artery | Descends posterior to inferior alveolar nerve between ramus of mandible to enter mandibular canal via mandibular foramen | Branches: mylohyoid branch, dental branches, mental medial pterygoid and branch; supplies muscles of floor of mouth, mandible and lower teeth and soft tissue of chin |
| Inferior epigastric | External iliac artery | Runs superiorly and enters rectus sheath; runs deep to rectus abdominis | Rectus abdominis and medial part of anterolateral abdominal wall |
| Inferior gluteal | Anterior division of internal iliac | Exits pelvis to enter gluteal region through greater sciatic foramen inferior to piriformis and descends on medial side of sciatic nerve; anastomoses with superior gluteal artery and participates in cruciate anastomosis of thigh, involving 1st perforating artery of deep femoral and medial and lateral circumflex femoral arteries | Pelvic diaphragm (coccygeus and levator ani), piriformis, quadratus femoris, uppermost hamstrings, gluteus maximus, and sciatic nerve |
| Inferior labial | Facial artery near angle of mouth | Runs medially in lower lip | Lower lip and chin |
| Inferior mesenteric | Abdominal aorta | Descends retroperitoneally to left of abdominal aorta | Supplies part of gastrointestinal tract derived from hindgut |
| Inferior pancreaticoduodenal, anterior and posterior | Superior mesenteric artery | Ascends retroperitoneally on head of pancreas | Distal portion of duodenum and inferior head and uncinate process of pancreas |
| Inferior phrenic | As 1st branches of abdominal aorta (sometimes via a common stem or from celiac trunk) | Ascend crus to underside of domes; medial branches anastmoses with each other and pericardiacophrenic arteries; lateral branches approach thoracic wall, anastomose with posterior intercostal and musculophrenic arteries | Branches: superior suprarenal arteries Supplies: diaphragm, inferior vena cava (right branch), esophagus (left branch), suprarenal glands |
| Inferior rectal | Internal pudendal artery | Leaves pudendal canal and crosses ischioanal fossa to anal canal | Distal portion of anal canal (mainly inferior to pectinate line) |
| Inferior suprarenal | Renal | Ascends vertically to gland | Posterior and inferior of aspects suprarenal gland |
| Inferior thyroid | Terminal branch (with ascending cervical artery) of thyrocervical trunk | Ascends anterior to anterior scalene, turns medially passing between vertebral vessels and carotid sheath, then descends on longus colli to lower border of thyroid gland | Branches: inferior laryngeal artery, pharyngeal, tracheal, esophageal, and inferior and ascending glandular (latter to parathyroid glands); main visceral artery of neck |
| Inferior vesical (male) | Anterior division of internal iliac | Passes retroperitoneally to inferior aspect of male urinary bladder | Inferior aspect of urinary bladder, ductus deferens, seminal vesicle, and prostate |
| Infraorbital | 3rd part of maxillary artery | Passes along infraorbital groove and foramen to face | Supplies inferior rectus and oblique muscles, inferior eyelid, lacrimal sac, maxillary sinus, maxillary incisor and canine teeth, and anterior cheek |

| Artery/Arteries | Origin | Course | Branches/ Distribution |
|---|---|---|---|
| Internal carotid | Common carotid artery at superior border of thyroid cartilage | Ascends vertically in neck to enter carotid canal, becomes horizontal and runs antero-medially through cavernous sinus, makes a 180-degree turn under anterior clinoid process, bifurcates into anterior and middle cerebral arteries | Gives branches to walls of cavernous sinus, pituitary gland, and trigeminal gan-glion; provides primary blood supply to the orbit/eyeball, upper nasal cavity/nose, and brain |
| Internal iliac | Common iliac | Passes over pelvic brim to reach pelvic cavity | Main blood supply to pelvic organs, gluteal muscles, and perineum |
| Internal pudendal | Anterior division of internal iliac | Leaves pelvis through greater sciatic foramen; hooks around ischial spine and enters perineum by way of lesser sciatic foramen and runs in pudendal canal to urogenital (UG) triangle | Main artery to perineum, including muscles and skin of anal and urogenital triangles; erectile bodies (does not supply branches to gluteal region) |
| Internal thoracic | Inferior surface of subclavian artery | Descends, inclining antero-medially, posterior to sternal end of clavicle and costal cartilages, lateral to sternum, and anterior to slips of transversus thoracis; divides at level of 6th costal cartilage into superior epigastric and musculophrenic arteries | Sternum and skin anterior to it by way of anterior inter-costal arteries to intercostal spaces 1–6 by way of perforating arteries, to medial aspect of breast |
| Interosseous, anterior and posterior | Common interosseous artery | Pass to anterior and posterior sides of interosseous membrane | Anterior and posterior compartments of forearm; anterior interosseous artery supplies both anterior and posterior compartments in distal forearm; posterior interosseous artery gives off recurrent interosseous artery, which participates in arterial anastomoses around the elbow |
| Intestinal (n = 15–18) | Superior mesenteric artery | Passes between two layers of mesentery | Jejunum and ileum |
| Labyrinthine | Basilar or via a common trunk with anterior inferior cerebellar | Exits cranial cavity via internal acoustic meatus; enters bony labyrinth | Membranous labyrinth |
| Lacrimal | Ophthalmic artery | Passes along superior border of lateral rectus muscle to supply lacrimal gland, conjunctiva, and eyelids | Passes along superior border of lateral rectus muscle to supply lacrimal gland, conjunctiva, and eyelids |
| Lateral circumflex femoral | Deep artery of thigh; may arise from femoral artery | Passes laterally deep to sartor-ius and rectus femoris and divides into three branches | Ascending branch supplies anterior part of gluteal region; transverse branch winds around femur; descending branch descends to knee and joins genicular anastomoses |
| Lateral nasal | Facial artery as it ascends alongside nose | Passes to ala of nose | Skin on ala and dorsum of nose |

| Artery/Arteries | Origin | Course | Branches/ Distribution |
|---|---|---|---|
| Lateral plantar | Terminal branch (with medial plantar artery) of posterior tibial artery | Forms medial to calcaneus, courses anterolaterally between 1st and 2nd muscle layers of sole of foot to base of 5th metatarsal, then passes anteromedially between 3rd and 4th layers as deep plantar arch | Branches: muscular, to muscles of 1st and 2nd layers; superficial, to skin and subcutaneous tissue of lateral sole; anastomotic, with lateral tarsal and arcuate arteries; calcaneal, to calcaneus |
| Lateral sacral, superior and inferior | Posterior division of internal iliac | Runs on anteromedial aspect of piriformis to send branches into pelvic sacral foramina | Piriformis, structures in sacral canal, erector spinae and overlying skin |
| Lateral thoracic | 2nd part of axillary artery | Descends along axillary border of pectoralis minor and follows it onto thoracic wall | Lateral chest wall (pectoral muscles, serratus anterior, intercostals) and breast |
| Left colic | Inferior mesenteric artery | Passes retroperitoneally toward left to descending colon | Descending colon |
| Left coronary | Left aortic sinus | Runs in AV groove and gives off anterior interventricular and circumflex branches | Most of left atrium and ventricle, IV septum, and AV bundles; may supply AV node |
| Left gastric | Celiac trunk | Ascends retroperitoneally to esophageal hiatus, where it passes between layers of hepatogastric ligament | Distal portion of esophagus and lesser curvature of stomach |
| Left gastro-omental (gastroepiploic) | Splenic artery in hilum of spleen | Passes between layers of gastrosplenic ligament to greater curvature of stomach | Left portion of greater curvature of stomach |
| Left marginal (branch) | Circumflex branch | Follows left border of heart | Left ventricle |
| Left pulmonary | Pulmonary trunk | Joins left bronchus and pulmonary veins to form root of left lung; descends in lung | Supplies left lung; Branches: (ductus arteriosus in fetus), superior and inferior lobar arteries (in turn give rise to segmental arteries) |
| Lesser palatine | Descending palatine | Descend inferoposteriorly through lesser palatine foramen | Supply soft palate |
| Lingual | External carotid artery | Loops over greater horn of hyoid, passes medial to hyoglossus, and ascends to run along side of tongue | Branches: suprahyoid branch, dorsal lingual arteries, and sublingual artery; continues as deep lingual artery |
| Lingular, inferior and superior | Superior lobar artery (of left lung), in oblique fissure | Descends anteriorly to lingula | Lingular division (superior [S4] and inferior [S5] bronchopulmonary segments) of left lung |
| Long posterior ciliaries | Ophthalmic artery | Pierce sclera to supply ciliary body and iris | Pierce sclera to supply ciliary body and iris |
| Lumbar | Abdominal aorta | Run horizontal courses posteriorly around sides of lumbar vertebrae and then laterally on posterior abdominal wall | Branches: dorsal, to deep muscles of back and over-lying skin; spinal, to vertebrae, contents of vertebral canal, roots, and some (as segmented medullary arteries) to spinal cord |

| Artery/Arteries | Origin | Course | Branches/Distribution |
|---|---|---|---|
| Marginal artery (of colon) | Formed by anastomoses (arcades) between right, middle, and left colic and sigmoid arteries | Rarely interrupted anastomotic channel parallels the colon at its mesenteric border | Branches passing to anterior and posterior aspect of colon |
| Masseteric | 2nd part of maxillary artery | Passes posterior to temporalis tendon accompanying masseteric nerve through mandibular notch | Supplies masseter and temporomandibular joint; anastomoses with facial and transverse facial arteries |
| Maxillary | Terminal branch (with superficial temporal artery) of external carotid | Passes posterior and medial to neck of mandible (1st part), superficial or deep to inferior head of lateral pterygoid (2nd part), and into pterygopalatine fossa (3rd part) | 1st part: deep auricular, anterior tympanic, middle meningeal, accessory meningeal, inferior alveolar; 2nd part: deep temporal, pterygoid (branches), masseteric, buccal; 3rd part: posterior superior alveolar, descending palatine, artery of pterygoid canal, pharyngeal, sphenopalatine, infraorbital |
| Medial circumflex femoral | Deep artery of thigh; may arise from femoral artery | Passes medially and posteriorly between pectineus and iliopsoas, enters gluteal region, and divides into two branches | Supplies most blood to head and neck of femur; transverse branch takes part in cruciate anastomosis of thigh; ascending branch joins inferior gluteal artery |
| Medial plantar | Terminal branch (with lateral plantar artery) of posterior tibial artery | Arises medial to calcaneus, passes distally along medial side of foot between 1st and 2nd layers of plantar muscles | Branches: muscular, to flexor hallucis brevis and abductor hallucis; superficial, to skin and subcutaneous tissue of medial sole; superficial digital, that join 1st–3rd plantar metatarsals |
| Median sacral | Posterior aspect of abdominal aorta | Descends in median line over L4 and L5 vertebrae and the sacrum and coccyx | Lower lumbar vertebrae, sacrum and coccyx |
| Mental (branch) | Terminal branch of inferior alveolar artery | Emerges from mental foramen and passes to chin | Facial muscles and skin of chin |
| Middle cerebral | Larger terminal branch (with anterior cerebral artery) of internal carotid artery | Runs in lateral cerebral sulcus, then posterosuperiorly on insula | Insula and most of lateral surface of cerebral hemispheres |
| Middle colic | Superior mesenteric artery | Ascends retroperitoneally and passes between layers of transverse mesocolon | Transverse colon |
| Middle collateral | Deep artery of arm | Descends to anastomose with recurrent interosseous artery | Part of collateral pathway around elbow; supplies lateral and medial heads of triceps |
| Middle meningeal | 1st part of maxillary artery | Ascends vertically through foramen spinosum into middle cranial fossa; runs laterally, dividing into frontal and parietal branches, which in turn ramify, ascending lateral walls in cranial dura mater | Branches: ganglionic branches, petrosal branches, superior tympanic artery, temporal branches, anastomotic branch to lacrimal artery; most blood is distributed to periosteum, bone and red bone marrow |
| Middle rectal | Anterior division of internal iliac | Descends in pelvis to lower part of rectum | Seminal vesicles and lower part of rectum |

| Artery/Arteries | Origin | Course | Branches/Distribution |
|---|---|---|---|
| Middle suprarenal | Abdominal aorta | Arise at level of superior mesenteric artery; run very short course over crura of diaphgram | Supply suprarenal glands; anastomose with suprarenal branches of inferior phrenic and renal arteries |
| Musculophrenic | Terminal branch (with superior epigastric) of internal thoracic artery | Arising in 6th intercostal space descends inferolaterally, paralleling costal margin | Branches: anterior intercostal arteries of 7th–9th intercostal spaces; also supplies upper abdominal muscles and pericardium |
| Mylohyoid (branch) | Inferior alveolar (before it enters mandibular foramen) | Pierces sphenomandibular ligament to run anteroinferiorly with nerve in groove on medial aspect of ramus of mandible | Muscles of floor of mouth; anastomoses with submental artery |
| Obturator | Anterior division of internal iliac | Runs anteroinferiorly on lateral pelvic wall to exit pelvis via obturator canal | Pelvic muscles, nutrient artery to ilium, head of femur, muscles of medial compartment of thigh |
| Occipital | External carotid artery | Passes medial to posterior belly of digastric and mastoid process; accompanies occipital nerve in occipital region | Scalp of back of head, as far as vertex |
| Ophthalmic | Internal carotid artery | Traverses optic foramen to reach orbital cavity | Traverses optic foramen to reach orbital cavity |
| Ovarian | Abdominal aorta, inferior to renal arteries | Run inferolaterally on psoas major, then pass medially to cross pelvic brim and descend in suspensory ligament of ovary | Branches: ureteric, tubal (to uterine tubes) and ovarian; latter 2 anastomose branches of uterine artery of same name |
| Palmar metacarpal | Deep palmar arch (from radial artery) | Run distally on plane between adductor pollicis and interosseus muscle. | Anastomose distally with common palmar digital arteries |
| Pericardiacophrenic | Internal thoracic artery | Descends parallel to phrenic nerve between mediastinal parietal pleura and pericardium | Supplies mediastinal parietal pleura and pericardium; anastomoses with phrenic and musculophrenic arteries |
| Perineal | Internal pudendal artery | Leaves pudendal canal and enters superficial perineal space | Supplies superficial perineal muscles and scrotum or labia |
| Plantar metatarsal | 1st: junction between lateral plantar and dorsalis pedis arteries; 2nd–4th: deep plantar arch | Extend distally between metatarsal bones on plantar aspect of interosseous muscles | Branches: perforating branches, common plantar digital arteries |
| Popliteal | Continuation of femoral artery at adductor hiatus in adductor magnus | Passes through popliteal fossa to leg; ends at lower border of popliteus muscle by dividing into anterior and posterior tibial arteries | Superior, middle, and inferior genicular arteries to both lateral and medial aspects of knee |
| Posterior auricular | External carotid artery | Passes posteriorly, deep to parotid, along styloid process between mastoid process and ear | Branches: auricular, occipital, stylomastoid; to middle ear, mastoid cells, auricle, parotid gland |
| Posterior cerebral | Terminal branch of basilar artery | Passes laterally, winding around cerebral peduncle to reach tentorial cerebral surface | Inferior aspect of temporal lobe and occipital lobe of cerebrum |
| Posterior communicating | Anastomosis between internal carotid and posterior cerebral arteries | Passes superior to oculomotor nerve (CN III) | Optic tract, cerebral peduncle, internal capsule, and thalamus |

| Artery/Arteries | Origin | Course | Branches/ Distribution |
| --- | --- | --- | --- |
| Posterior division of internal iliac | Internal iliac | Passes posteriorly and gives rise to parietal branches | Pelvic wall and gluteal region |
| Posterior ethmoidal | Ophthalmic artery | Passes through posterior ethmoidal foramen to posterior ethmoidal cells | Passes through posterior ethmoidal foramen to posterior ethmoidal cells |
| Posterior gastric | Splenic artery | Ascends retroperitoneally (in posterior wall of omental bursa) to pass to gastric fundus via gastrophrenic fold (ligament) | Posterior wall of stomach |
| Posterior inferior cerebellar | Intracranial portion of vertebral artery | Passes posteriorly around side of medulla to reach inferior aspect of cerebellum | Supplies medial portion of inferior aspect of cerebellum (cerebellar tonsil and dentate nucleus), posterolateral medulla oblongata and choroid plexus of 4th ventricle |
| Posterior intercostal | Posterior aspect of thoracic aorta | Pass laterally, then anteriorly parallel to ribs | Lateral and anterior cutaneous branches |
| Posterior intercostals | Superior intercostal artery (intercostal spaces 1 and 2) and thoracic aorta (remaining intercostal spaces) | Pass between internal and innermost intercostal muscles | Intercostal muscles and overlying skin, parietal pleura |
| Posterior interventricular (IV) | Right coronary artery | Runs from posterior IV groove to apex of heart | Right and left ventricles and IV septum |
| Posterior lateral nasal | Sphenopalatine artery | Ramify over conchae and meatuses; anastomoses with nasal branches of ethmoidal and greater palatine arteries | Supplies lateral walls of posterointerior nasal cavity, contributing also to supply of ethmoidal cells and maxillary and sphenoidal paranasal sinuses |
| Posterior scrotal or labial | Terminal branches of perineal artery | Runs in superficial fascia of posterior scrotum or labium majus | Skin of scrotum or labium majus |
| Posterior septal | Sphenopalatine artery | Crosses inferior surface of body of sphenoid to reach nasal septum, courses anteroinferiorly on vomer to incisive canals | Supplies nasal septum; anastomoses with greater palatine artery and septal branch of superior labial artery |
| Posterior spinal | Superiorly from an intracranial branch of vertebral artery; continued inferiorly by bifurcations of posterior segmental medullary arteries at various levels. | Forms continuous anastomotic chain that descends length of spinal cord in posterolateral sulcus, adjacent to emerging dorsal roots (rootlets) of spinal nerves | Supplies posterolateral apect of spinal cord, via pial plexus and its peripheral branches |
| Posterior superior alveolar | 3rd part of maxillary artery | Exits from pterygopalatine fossa via pterygomaxillary fissure; ramifies and penetrates infratemporal surface of maxilla, with some branches entering alveolar canals and others continuing over alveolar process | Supplies mucosa of maxillary sinus, maxillary molar and premolar teeth, adjacent gingiva |
| Posterior tibial | Popliteal | Passes through posterior compartment of leg, terminates distal to flexor retinaculum by dividing into medial and lateral plantar arteries | Posterior and lateral compartments of leg; circumflex fibular branch joins anastomoses around knee; nutrient artery passes to tibia |

| Artery/Arteries | Origin | Course | Branches/Distribution |
|---|---|---|---|
| Princeps pollicis | Radial artery as it turns into palm | Descends on palmar aspect of 1st metacarpal, divides at the base of proximal phalanx into 2 branches that run along sides of thumb | Thumb |
| Proper palmar digitals | Common palmar digital arteries | Run along sides of digits 2–5; at base of middle phalanx, gives rise to dorsal branch which replaces dorsal digital arteries | All of palmar and distal part (including nail beds) of dorsal aspect of fingers |
| Prostatic (branches) | Inferior vesical artery | Descends on posterolateral aspect of prostate | Prostate |
| Radial | Smaller terminal division (with ulnar artery) of brachial artery in cubital fossa | Runs inferolaterally under cover of brachioradialis and distally lies lateral to flexor carpi radialis tendon; winds around lateral aspect of radius and crosses floor of anatomical snuffbox to pierce fascia; ends by forming deep palmar arch | Supplies muscles of lateral portions of both anterior and posterior compartments of forearm, lateral aspect of wrist, skin of dorsum of hand and proximal portions of digits, deep muscles of palm |
| Radial collateral | Terminal branch (with middle collateral artery) of deep artery of arm | Perforates lateral intermuscular septum with radial nerve, runs between between brachialis and brachioradialis to anastomose with radial recurrent, anterior to lateral epicondyle of humerus | Forms part of cubital anastomosis; supplies upper brachialis and brachioradialis, and anterolateral aspect of elbow joint |
| Radial recurrent | Lateral side of radial artery, just distal to its origin | Ascends on supinator and then passes between brachioradialis and brachialis to anastomose with radial collateral, anterior to lateral epicondyle of humerus | Forms part of cubital anastomosis; supplies supinator, lower brachialis and brachioradialis, and anterolateral aspect of elbow joint |
| Radialis indicis | Radial artery, but may arise from princeps pollicis artery | Passes along lateral side of index finger to its distal end | All of lateral palmar and distal part (including nail bed) of dorsal aspect of index finger |
| Radicular, anterior and posterior | Spinal branches of segmental arteries (vertebral, posterior intercostal, lumbar and sacral arteries) | Course along anterior and posterior roots of spinal nerves, exhausting before reaching the longitudinal anterior and posterior spinal arteries | Supply anterior and posterior roots of spinal nerves and coverings (dural sheaths and arachnoid) |
| Renal, left and right | Posterolateral aspect of abdominal aorta, usually at L2 vertebral level | Run horizotally and laterally across crura of diaphragm and psoas major, lying posterior to renal vein, bifurcating into anterior and posterior divisions or ramifying into segmental arteries near renal hilus | Source of blood to kidneys Branches: inferior suprarenal, capsular branches, an anterior division giving rise to superior, anterior superior, anterior inferior and inferior segmental arteries; posterior division becomes posterior segmental artery |
| Retroduodenal | Gastroduodenal artery | Arise and run posterior to 1st part of duodenum | Supply 1st part of duodenum, (common) bile duct, and head of pancreas |
| Right colic | Superior mesenteric artery | Passes retroperitoneally to reach ascending colon | Ascending colon |

| Artery/Arteries | Origin | Course | Branches/ Distribution |
|---|---|---|---|
| Right coronary | Right aortic sinus | Follows coronary (AV) groove between atria and ventricles | Right atrium, SA and AV nodes, and posterior part of IV septum |
| Right gastric | Hepatic artery | Runs between layers of hepatogastric ligament | Right portion of lesser curvature of stomach |
| Right gastro-omental (gastroepiploic) | Gastroduodenal artery | Passes between layers of greater omentum to greater curvature of stomach | Right portion of greater curvature of stomach |
| Right marginal | Right coronary artery | Passes to inferior margin of heart and apex | Right ventricle and apex of heart |
| Right pulmonary | Pulmonary trunk | Passes beneath arch of aorta to join right bronchus and pulmonary veins to form root of right lung; descends in lung | Supplies right lung Branches: superior, middle, and inferior lobar arteries (in turn give rise to segmental arteries) |
| Segmental arteries of kidney (superior, anterior superior, anterior inferior, inferior, and posterior) | Anterior and posterior divisions (or directly from) renal arteries | Arise at hilum, course through perirenal fat of renal sinus around renal pelvis to reach renal segment | Renal segment (segmental arteries are end arteries; no significant anastomoses occur between segments) |
| Segmental arteries of liver (right anterior, right posterior, left medial, and left lateral) | Left and right branches of hepatic artery proper | Arise within liver; right and left branches course horizontally, right branch giving rise to anterior and posterior segmental arteries, left to medial and lateral segmental arteries | Each segmental artery serves a division of liver which, except for medial division, is further subdivided into 2 hepatic segments; both right and left branches of hepatic artery send an artery to caudate lobe |
| Segmental arteries of lung | Lobar arteries | Arise within lung as tertiary branches of right and left pulmonary arteries | Each segmental artery serves a bronchopulmonary segment of lung |
| Segmental medullary, anterior and posterior | Spinal branches of segmental arteries (vertebral, posterior intercostal, lumbar and sacral arteries) | Course along anterior and posterior roots of spinal nerves, continue medially to anastomose with longitudinal anterior and posterior spinal arteries | Dorsal and ventral roots of certain spinal nerves and spinal cord; major anterior segmental medullary artery (Adamkiewicz) is largest, occurring at lower thoracic, upper lumbar level, on left side 65% of time |
| Sinuatrial (SA) nodal | Right coronary artery near its origin (in 60%); circumflex branch of left coronary (in 40%) | Winds around right (60%) or left (40%) side of ascending aorta and ascends to SA node | Left atrium and SA node |
| Short gastric (n = 4–5) | Splenic artery in hilum of spleen | Passes between layers of gastrosplenic ligament to fundus of stomach | Fundus of stomach |
| Short posterior ciliaries | Ophthalmic artery | Pierce sclera at periphery of optic nerve to supply choroid, which in turn supplies cones and rods of optic retina | Pierce sclera at periphery of optic nerve to supply choroid, which in turn supplies cones and rods of optic retina |
| Sigmoid (n = 3–4) | Inferior mesenteric artery | Passes retroperitoneally toward left to descending colon | Descending and sigmoid colon |
| Sphenopalatine | 3rd part of maxillary artery | Passes medially through sphenopalatine foramen, dividing immediately into septal and posterior lateral nasal arteries | Mucosa of posteroinferior half of nasal cavity, ethmoidal cells, and maxillary and sphenoidal paranasal sinuses |

| Artery/Arteries | Origin | Course | Branches/ Distribution |
|---|---|---|---|
| Splenic | Celiac trunk | Runs retroperitoneally along superior border of pancreas; then passes between layers of splenorenal ligament to hilum of spleen | Body of pancreas, spleen, greater curvature of stomach |
| Stylomastoid | Posterior auricular | Enters stylomastoid foramen and ascends facial canal, running with (and supplying) facial nerve | Branches: posterior tympanic artery (to tympanic membrane); mastoid (to mastoid cells) and stapedial (to stapedius, stapes, and secondary tympanic membrane) branches |
| Subclavian | Left: aortic arch<br>Right: brachiocephalic trunk | Arises—or passes—posterior to sternoclavicular joint, arches over cervical pleura anterior to apex of lung, crosses 1st rib posterior to anterior scalene, becoming axillary artery at rib's outer edge | Branches: 1st part: vertebral, internal thoracic, thyrocervical (and costocervical on right side); 2nd part: dorsal scapular (and costocervical on left side) [Parts: medial (1st), posterior (2nd), and lateral (3rd) to scalenus anterior muscle] |
| Subcostal | Thoracic aorta | Courses along inferior border of 12th rib | Muscles of anterolateral abdominal wall |
| Sublingual | Terminal branch (with deep lingual artery) of lingual artery | Runs on genioglossus muscle superior to mylohoid | Supplies muscles and mucous membrane of floor of mouth, and anterior lingual gingiva |
| Submental | Facial artery, distal to submandibular gland in submental triangle | Courses along inferior aspect of mylohyoid, adjacent to attachment to mandible, to mandibular symphysis | Supplies mylohyoid, anterior belly of digastric, submental lymph nodes and, via its anastomoses with inferior labial and mental arteries, lower lip |
| Subscapular | 3rd part of axillary artery | Largest (but short—4 cm) branch of axillary artery, it descends along lateral border of subscapularis and axillary border of scapula to bifurcate at level of inferior angle | Via its terminal branches, circumflex scapular and thoracodorsal arteries, it supplies muscles on both sides of scapula, latissimus dorsi, and posterior chest wall |
| Superficial cervical (variant, replacing superficial branch of transverse cervical artery) | Thyrocervical trunk | Passes laterally between sternocleidomastoid and anterior scalene, across brachial plexus and posterior triangle of neck, to bifurcate and run with accessory nerve on deep aspect of trapezius | Anterior scapene, sternocleidomastoid, brachial plexus, muscles of posterior triangle of neck, and (mainly) the trapezius |
| Superficial circumflex iliac | Femoral artery | Runs in superficial fascia along inguinal ligament | Subcutaneous tissue and skin over inferior part of anterolateral abdominal wall |
| Superficial epigastric | Femoral artery | Runs in superficial fascia toward umbilicus | Subcutaneous tissue and skin over suprapubic region |
| Superficial palmar arch | Direct continuation of ulnar artery; completed on lateral side by superficial branch of radial artery or another of its branches | Curves laterally deep to palmar aponeurosis and superficial to long flexor tendons; curve of arch lies across palm at level of distal border of extended thumb | Branches: 3 common palmar digital arteries |

| Artery/Arteries | Origin | Course | Branches/ Distribution |
|---|---|---|---|
| Superficial temporal | Smaller terminal branch of external carotid artery | Ascends anterior to ear to temporal region and ends in scalp | Facial muscles and skin of frontal and temporal regions |
| Superior cerebellar | Upper (terminal) part of basilar artery | Curves around cerebral peduncle | Supplies superior aspect of cerebellum, colliculi and most cerebellar nuclei; pons; pineal body; superior medullary velum; and choroid plexus of 3rd ventricle |
| Superior epigastric | Internal thoracic artery | Descends in rectus sheath deep to rectus abdominis | Rectus abdominis and superior part of anterolateral abdominal wall |
| Superior gluteal | Posterior division of internal iliac | Enters gluteal region through greater sciatic foramen superior to piriformis and divides into superficial and deep branches; anastomoses with inferior gluteal and medial circumflex femoral arteries (not shown above) | Piriformis muscle. Superficial branch: supplies gluteus maximus. Deep branch: runs between gluteus medius and minimus muscles, supplying both, as well as tensor of fascia lata |
| Superior labial | Facial artery near angle of mouth | Runs medially in upper lip | Upper lip and ala (side) and septum of nose |
| Superior laryngeal | Superior thyroid | Runs deep to thyrohyoid to pierce thyrohyoid membrane with internal laryngeal nerve | Supplies larynx |
| Superior mesenteric | Abdominal aorta | Runs in root of mesentery to ileocecal junction | Part of gastrointestinal tract derived from midgut |
| Superior pancreaticoduodenal, anterior and posterior | Gastroduodenal artery | Descends on head of pancreas | Proximal portion of duodenum and head of pancreas |
| Superior phrenic (vary in number) | Anterior aspects of thoracic aorta | Arise at aortic hiatus and pass to superior aspect of diaphragm | Supply diaphragm and diaphragmatic parts of pericardium and parietal pleura |
| Superior rectal | Terminal branch (continuation of) inferior mesenteric artery | Crosses left common iliac vessels and descends into pelvis between layers of sigmoid mesocolon | Upper part of rectum; anastomoses with middle and inferior rectal arteries |
| Superior suprarenal | Inferior phrenic | Short, multiple branches arising from trunks of inferior phrenic arteries as they ascend diaphragmatic crura, running along superomedial aspect of gland | Superior part of suprarenal glands |
| Superior thoracic | Only branch of 1st part of axillary artery | Runs anteromedially along superior border of pectoralis minor, then passes between it and pectoralis major to thoracic wall | Helps to supply 1st and 2nd intercostal spaces and superior part of serratus anterior |
| Superior thyroid | 1st branch from anterior aspect of external carotid artery | Passes inferomedially deep to infrahyoid muscles to superior pole of thyroid gland; anastomosis with inferior thyroid artery provides an important collateral pathway between external carotid and subclavian arteries | Branches: superior laryngeal artery, infrahyoid, sternocleidomastoid, cricothyroid, and anterior, posterior, and lateral glandular branches |
| Superior vesical | Patent (proximal) part of umbilical | Usually multiple, pass to superior aspect of urinary bladder | Superior aspect of urinary bladder, pelvic portion of ureter |

| Artery/Arteries | Origin | Course | Branches/ Distribution |
|---|---|---|---|
| Supraduodenal | Gastroduodenal, hepatic, right gastric, or retroduodenal arteries | Often double, pass(es) superior to 1st part of duodenum | Supplies upper proximal portion of superior part of duodenum |
| Supraorbital | Terminal branch of ophthalmic artery | Passes superiorly and posteriorly from supraorbital foramen to forehead and scalp | Supplies muscles and skin of most of forehead and anterior scalp (to vertex) |
| Suprascapular | Thyrocervical trunk | Passes inferolaterally over anterior scalene muscle and phrenic nerve, crosses subclavian artery and brachial plexus, runs laterally posterior and parallel to clavicle, then passes superior to transverse scapular ligament into supraspinous fossa, then under acromion to infraspinsous fossa | Supplies supraspinatus and infraspinatus muscles and participates in anastomosis around scapula |
| Supratrochlear | Terminal branch (with supraorbital artery) of ophthalmic artery | Passes from supratrochlear notch to medial forehead and anterior scalp | Skin and muscles of medial part of forehead and adjacent scalp |
| Supreme intercostal | Costocervical trunk | Descends between pleura and necks of first 2 ribs; anastomoses with 3rd posterior intercostal artery | Branches: 1st and 2nd posterior intercostal arteries, to muscles of and ribs bounding 1st and 2nd intercostal spaces |
| Sural, right and left | Popliteal | Large branches arise at level of femoral condyles and pass directly to heads of gastrocnemius, sending branches on to soleus | Supply medial and lateral heads of gastrocnemius, plantaris, soleus muscles. |
| Testicular | Abdominal aorta, inferior to renal arteries | Descend inferolaterally across psoas muscles, pass through inguinal canal as part of spermatic cord, reach testes in scrotum | Abdominal part provides branches/arterial blood to ureters, iliac lymph nodes; inguinal/ scrotal part supplies cremaster and other coverings of cor and testes |
| Thoracic aorta | Continuation of arch of aorta | Descends in posterior mediastinum to left of vertebral column; gradually shifts to right to lie in median plane at aortic hiatus | Posterior intercostal arteries, subcostal, some phrenic arteries and visceral branches (tracheal and esophageal) |
| Thoracoacromial | 2nd part of axillary artery deep to pectoralis minor | Curls around superomedial border of pectoralis minor, pierces clavipectoral fascia and divides into 4 branches | Branches: acromial, clavicular, pectoral, and deltoid |
| Thoracodorsal | Subscapular artery | Continues course of subscapular artery; accompanies thoracodorsal nerve to latissimus dorsi | Latissimus dorsi |
| Thyrocervical trunk | Anterior aspect of 1st part of subclavian artery | Ascends as a short, wide trunk near medial border of anterior scalene and posterior to carotid sheath | Branches from trunk: transverse cervical (or superficial cervical) and suprascapular Terminal branches: ascending cervical and inferior thyroid arteries |
| Thyroid ima | Brachiocephalic trunk or arch of aorta | Ascends on anterior aspect of trachea to thyroid gland | Supplies medial aspect of both lobes of thyroid |

| Artery/Arteries | Origin | Course | Branches/ Distribution |
|---|---|---|---|
| Transverse cervical (variant: may be replaced by superficial cervical and dorsal scapular arteries) | Thyrocervical trunk | Runs across anterior scalene, brachial plexus and posterior triangle of neck and passes deep to trapezius, dividing into deep and superficial branches | Superficial branch bifurcates into ascending and descending branches that run with accessory nerve on underside of trapezius; deep branch runs with dorsal scapular nerve, deep to rhomboids |
| Transverse facial | Superficial temporal artery within parotid gland | Crosses face superficial to masseter and inferior to zygomatic arch | Parotid gland and duct, muscles and skin of face |
| Ulnar | Larger terminal branch of brachial artery in cubital fossa | Passes inferomedially and then directly inferiorly, deep to pronator teres, palmaris longus, and flexor digitorum superficialis to reach medial side of forearm; passes superficial to flexor retinaculum at wrist and gives a deep palmar branch to deep arch and continues as superficial palmar arch | Supplies medial (ulnar) part of anterior compartment of forearm, wrist and hand; supplies superficial structures of central palm, and most of palmar and distal dorsal aspects of fingers |
| Ulnar collateral (superior and inferior) | Superior ulnar collateral arises from brachial near middle of arm; inferior ulnar collateral arises from brachial just superior to elbow | Superior ulnar collateral accompanies ulnar nerve to posterior aspect of elbow; inferior ulnar collateral divides into anterior and posterior branches; both ulnar collateral take part in anastomosis around elbow joint | Anastomose distally with anterior and posterior ulnar recurrent arteries. |
| Ulnar recurrent, anterior and posterior | Ulnar artery, just distal to elbow joint | Anterior ulnar recurrent passes superiorly and posterior ulnar collateral passes posteriorly | Anastomose with anterior and posterior ulnar collateral |
| Umbilical | Anterior division of internal iliac | Obliterates becoming medial umbilical ligament after running a short pelvic course during which it gives rise to superior vesical | Superior aspect of urinary bladder (via superior vesical arteries); occasionally artery to ductus deferens (males) |
| Uterine | Anterior division of internal iliac | Runs medially in base of broad ligament superior to cardinal ligament, crossing superior to ureter, to sides of uterus | Uterus, ligaments of uterus, uterine tube, and vagina |
| Vaginal | Uterine artery | Arises lateral to ureter and descends inferior to it to lateral aspect of vagina | Vagina; branches to inferior part of urinary bladder and termination of ureter |
| Vertebral | 1st part of subclavian artery | Ascends vertically through the transverse foramina of vertebrae C6–C2, passes laterally to traverse that of C1, then runs horizontal and medial to enter foramen magnum; intracranially, merges with contralateral artery to form basilar artery | Cervical branches: spinal (giving rise to radicular and segmental medullary arteries) and muscular (to suboccipital muscles); Intracranial branches: meningeal, anterior and posterior spinal, posterior inferior cerebellar, medial and lateral medullary |

# Nerves of the Human Body

| Nerve(s)/Nerve Branch(es) | Origin | Course | Structures Innervated |
|---|---|---|---|
| Abdominopelvic splanchnic | Lower thoracic and lumbar segments of sympathetic trunk | Pass medially and inferiorly to prevertebral ganglion of para-aortic plexus | Motor: presynaptic sympathetics for innervation of abdominopelvic blood vessels and viscera |
| Abducent (CN VI) | Pons | Become intradural on clivus; traverse cavernous sinus and superior orbital fissure to enter orbit | Motor: lateral rectus |
| Accessory (CN XI) | Cranial root: medulla Spinal root: cervical spinal cord | Spinal root ascends into cranial cavity via foramen magnum, exits via jugular foramen, traverses posterior triangle of neck | Motor: sternocleidomastoid and trapezius |
| Ansa cervicalis | Superior root: hypoglossal nerve (C1 and C2 fibers) Inferior root: cervical plexus (C2 and C3 fibers) | Descends on external surface of carotid sheath | Motor: omohyoid, sternohyoid, and sternothyroid |
| Anterior ethmoidal | Nasociliary nerve (CN V1) | Arises in orbit, passes via anterior ethmoidal foramen to cranial cavity, then via cribriform plate of ethmoid to nasal cavity | Sensory: dural of anterior cranial fossa; mucous membranes of sphenoidal sinus, ethmoidal cells, and upper nasal cavity |
| Anterior femoral cutaneous | Femoral nerve (L2 and L3 fibers) | Arise in femoral triangle and pierce fascia lata of thigh along path of sartorius muscle | Sensory: skin on medial and anterior aspects of thigh |
| Anterior interosseous | Median nerve in distal part of cubital fossa | Passes inferiorly on interosseous membrane | Motor: flexor digitorum profundus, flexor pollicis longus, land pronator quadratus |
| Auriculotemporal | Mandibular nerve (CN V3) | From posterior division of CN V3, it passes between neck of mandible and external acoustic meatus to accompany superficial temporal artery | Sensory: skin anterior to auricle and posterior temporal region, tragus and part of helix of auricle, and roof of exterior acoustic meatus and upper tympanic membrane |
| Axillary | Terminal branch of posterior cord of brachial plexus (C5 and C6 fibers) | Passes to posterior aspect of arm through quadrangular space in company with posterior circumflex humeral artery and then winds around surgical neck of humerus; gives rise to lateral brachial cutaneous nerve | Motor: teres minor and deltoid Sensory: shoulder joint and skin over inferior part of deltoid |
| Buccal | Mandibular nerve (CN V3) | From the anterior division of CN V3 in infratemporal fossa, it passes anteriorly to reach cheek | Sensory: skin and mucosa of cheek, buccal gingiva adjacent to 2nd and 3rd molar teeth |
| Calcaneal branches | Tibial and sural nerves | Pass from distal part of posterior aspect of leg to skin on heel | Sensory: skin of heel |
| Cardiac plexus | Cervical and cardiac branches of vagus nerve and cardiopulmonary splanchnic nerves from sympathetic trunk | From arch of aorta and posterior surface of heart, fibers extend along coronary arteries and to SA node | SA nodal tissue and coronary arteries; parasympathetic fibers slow rate, reduce force of heart beat, and constrict arteries; sympathetic fibers have opposite effect |

| Nerve(s)/Nerve Branch(es) | Origin | Course | Structures Innervated |
|---|---|---|---|
| Cardiopulmonary splanchnic | Cervical and upper thoracic ganglia of sympathetic trunk | Descend anteromedially to cardiac, pulmonary, and esophageal plexuses | Motor: convey postsynaptic sympathetic fibers to nerve plexuses of thoracic viscera |
| Cavernous nerves | Parasympathetic fibers of prostatic nerve plexus | Perforates perineal membrane to reach erectile bodies of penis | Motor: helicine arteries of cavernous bodies; stimulation produces engorgement at arterial pressure (erection) |
| Cervical splanchnic | Cervical ganglia of sympathetic trunk | Pass medially and inferiorly to cardiac and pulmonary plexuses | Conducting tissue (SA and AV nodes) and coronary arteries |
| Chorda tympani | Facial nerve (CN VII) within facial canal | Traverses tympanic cavity, passing between incus and malleus; exits temporal bone via petrotympanic fissure to enter infratemporal fossa where it merges with lingual nerve | Motor: submandibular and sublingual (salivary) glands Sensory: taste sensation from anterior two-thirds of tongue |
| Ciliary (long, short) | Long ciliary: nasociliary nerve (CN V1) Short ciliary: ciliary ganglion | Pass to posterior aspect of eyeball | Sensory: cornea, conjunctiva Motor: ciliary body and iris |
| Clunial (superior, middle, and inferior) | Superior: posterior rami of L1, L2, and L3 Middle: posterior rami of S1, S2, and S3 Inferior: posterior cutaneous nerve of thigh | Superior nerves cross iliac crest; middle nerves exit through posterior sacral foramina and enter gluteal region; inferior nerves curve around inferior border of gluteus maximus | Sensory: skin of buttock or gluteal region as far as greater trochanter |
| Coccygeal (Co) | Conus medullaris of spinal cord | Anterior and posterior rami join adjacent rami of S4 and S5; anterior rami form coccygeal plexus, which gives rise to anococcygeal nerve | Sensory: skin over coccyx |
| Cochlear nerve | As a division of the vestibulocochlear nerve (CN VIII) | Traverses internal acoustic meatus, entering modiolus with spiral ganglia and peripheral processes in spiral lamina | Sensory: spiral organ (for hearing) |
| Common fibular (peroneal) | Terminal branch (with tibial nerve) of sciatic nerve (L4–S2 fibers) | Begins at apex of popliteal fossa; follows medial border of biceps femoris muscle to posterior aspect of head of fibula; bifurcates into superficial and deep fibular nerves as it winds around neck of fibula | Sensory: skin on lateral part of posterior aspect of leg via its branch, lateral sural cutaneous nerve; knee joint via its articular branch Motor: short head of biceps femoris |
| Common palmar digital | Median and superficial branches of ulnar nerves | Run distally between long flexor tendons of palm, bifurcating in distal palm | Branches: proper palmar digital nerves, supplying skin and joints of palmar and distal dorsal aspect of fingers |
| Common plantar digital | Median and lateral plantar nerves | Run anteriorly in sole of foot between flexor tendons, bifurcating in distal sole | Branches: proper plantar digital nerves, supplying skin and joints of plantar and distal dorsal aspect of toes |
| Deep branch of radial nerve | Radial nerve just distal to elbow | Winds around neck of radius in supinator; enters posterior compartment of forearm becoming posterior interosseous nerve | Motor: extensor carpi radialis brevis and supinator |

| Nerve(s)/Nerve Branch(es) | Origin | Course | Structures Innervated |
|---|---|---|---|
| Deep branch of ulnar nerve | Ulnar nerve at wrist as it passes between pisiform and hamate bones (T1 fibers) | Passes deep between muscles of hypothenar eminence, then across palm with deep palmar (arterial) arch | Motor: hypothenar muscles (abductor, flexor, and opponens digiti minimi), lumbricals of digits 4 and 5, all interossei, adductor pollicis, and deep head of flexor pollicis brevis |
| Deep fibular (peroneal) | Common fibular (peroneal) nerve | Arises between fibularis longus and neck of fibula; passes through extensor digitorum longus and descends on interosseous membrane; passes deep to extensor retinaculum, crosses distal end of tibia, and enters dorsum of foot | Motor: muscles of anterior compartment of leg and dorsum of foot Sensory: skin of 1st interdigital cleft (i.e., skin on adjacent sides of 1st and 2nd toes); sends articular branches to joints it crosses |
| Deep petrosal | Internal carotid plexus | Traverses cartilage of foramen lacerum to join greater petrosal nerve at entrance to pterygoid canal | Conveys the postsynaptic sympathetic fibers destined for lacrimal gland and mucosa of nasal cavity, palate, and upper pharynx |
| Deep temporal | Mandibular nerve (CN V3) | Ascend temporal fossa deep to temporalis muscle | Motor: temporalis Sensory: periosteum of temporal fossa |
| Dorsal branch of ulnar nerve | Ulnar nerve about 5 cm proximal to flexor retinaculum | Passes distally deep to flexor carpi ulnaris, then dorsally to perforate deep fascia and course along medial side of dorsum of hand, dividing into 2 to 3 dorsal digital nerves | Sensory: skin of medial aspect of dorsum of hand and proximal portions of little and medial half of ring finger (occasionally also adjacent sides of proximal portions of ring and middle fingers) |
| Dorsal scapular | Anterior ramus of C5 with frequent contribution from C4 | Pierces scalenus medius, descends deep to levator scapulae, and enters deep surface of rhomboids | Motor: rhomboids; occasionally supplies levator scapulae |
| Esophageal plexus | Vagus nerve, sympathetic ganglia, greater splanchnic nerve | Distal to tracheal bifurcation, vagus and sympathetic nerves form a plexus around esophagus | Vagal (parasympathetic) and sympathetic fibers to smooth muscle and glands of inferior two-thirds of esophagus |
| External nasal | Anterior ethmoidal nerve (CN V1) | Runs in nasal cavity and emerges on face between nasal bone and lateral nasal cartilage | Sensory: skin on dorsum of nose, including tip of nose |
| Facial (VII) | Posterior border of pons | Runs through internal acoustic meatus and facial canal of petrous part of temporal bone, exiting via stylomastoid foramen; main trunk forms intraparotid plexus | Motor: stapedius, posterior belly of digastric, stylohyoid, facial, and scalp muscles Sensory: some skin of external acoustic meatus SEE ALSO: intermediate nerve |
| Femoral | Lumbar plexus (L2–L4 fibers) | Passes deep to midpoint of inguinal ligament, lateral to femoral vessels, and divides into muscular and cutaneous branches | Motor: anterior thigh muscles Sensory: hip and knee joints; skin on anteromedial side of thigh and leg |

| Nerve(s)/Nerve Branch(es) | Origin | Course | Structures Innervated |
| --- | --- | --- | --- |
| Frontal | Ophthalmic nerve (CN V1) | Crosses orbit on superior aspect of levator palpebrae superioris; divides into supraorbital and supra-trochlear branches | Sensory: skin of forehead, scalp, upper eyelid, and nose; conjunctiva of upper lid and mucosa of frontal sinus |
| Genitofemoral | Lumbar plexus (L1 and L2 fibers) | Descends on anterior surface of psoas major and divides into genital and femoral branches | Sensory: femoral branch supplies skin over femoral triangle; genital branch supplies scrotum or labia majora Motor: genital branch to cremaster muscle |
| Glossopharyngeal (CN IX) | Glossopharyngeal (CN IX) | Exits cranium via jugular foramen, passes between superior and middle con-strictors of pharynx to tonsillar fossa, enters posterior third of tongue | Motor: somatic to stylo-pharyngeus; visceral (presynaptic parasympa--thetic) to parotid gland Sensory: posterior two-thirds of tongue (including taste), pharynx, tympanic cavity, auditory tube, carotid body, and sinus |
| Great auricular | Cervical plexus (C2 and C3 fibers) | Ascends vertically over sternocleidomastoid, anterior and parallel to external jugular vein | Sensory: skin of auricle, adjacent scalp, and over angle of jaw; parotid sheath |
| Greater occipital | As medial branch of posterior ramus of spinal nerve C2 | Pierces deep muscles of neck and trapezius to ascend posterior scalp to vertex | Motor: multifidus cervicis, semispinalis capitis Sensory: posterior scalp |
| Greater palatine | Branch of pterygopalatine ganglion (maxillary nerve) | Passes inferiorly through greater palatine canal and foramen | Motor: postsynaptic para--sympathetics to palatine glands Sensory: mucosa of hard palate |
| Greater petrosal | Genu of facial nerve (CN VII) | Exits facial canal via hiatus for greater petrosal nerve; courses across tegmen tympani and passes through cartilage of foramen lacerum to join deep petrosal nerve at opening of pterygoid canal | Motor: presynaptic parasympathetics to ptery-gopalatine ganglion for innervation of lacrimal and nasal, palatine, and upper pharyngeal mucous glands |
| Greater splanchnic | 5th–6th through 9th–10th thoracic sympathetic ganglia | Highest abdominopelvic splanchnic nerve; passes anteromedially on bodies of thoracic vertebrae, piercing diaphragm to converge on root of celiac trunk | Motor: conveys presynaptic sympathetics to celiac ganglia for innervation of celiac arteries and deriva-tives, and of portion of gut they supply |
| Hypogastric | As continuation of superior hypogastric plexus into pelvis | Course anterior to sacrum within hypogastric sheath to merge with pelvic splanchnic nerves in inferior hypogastric plexus | Motor: conveys pre- and postsynaptic sympathetic fibers destined for pelvic viscera Sensory: conveys pain fibers from intraperitoneal pelvic viscera (e.g., fundus, body of uterus) |
| Hypoglossal (CN XII) | Between pyramid and olive of myencephalon | Passes through hypoglossal canal, then runs inferiorly and anteriorly, passing medial to angle of mandible and between mylohyoid and hyoglossus to reach muscles of tongue | Motor: intrinsic and extrinsic muscles of tongue (excep-tion: palatoglossus) |

| Nerve(s)/Nerve Branch(es) | Origin | Course | Structures Innervated |
|---|---|---|---|
| Iliohypogastric | Lumbar plexus (L1 fibers) | Parallels iliac crest; pierces transverse abdominal muscle; branches pierce external oblique aponeurosis to reach inguinal and pubic regions | Motor: internal oblique and transverse abdominal muscles<br>Sensory: lateral cutaneous branch supplies superolateral quadrant of buttock; skin over iliac crest and hypogastric region |
| Ilioinguinal | Lumbar plexus (L1 fibers) | Passes between 2nd and 3rd layers of abdominal muscles, passes through inguinal canal, and divides into femoral and scrotal or labial branches | Motor: lowermost part of internal oblique and transverse abdominal muscles<br>Sensory: femoral branch supplies skin over femoral triangle; genital branch supplies mons pubis and adjacent skin of labia majora or scrotum |
| Inferior alveolar | As terminal branch (with lingual nerve) of posterior trunk of mandibular nerve (CN V3) | Descends between lateral and medial pterygoid muscles of infratemporal fossa to enter mandibular canal of mandible | Sensory: lower teeth, periodontium, periosteum, and gingiva of lower jaw. SEE ALSO: nerve to mylohyoid, mental nerve |
| Inferior anal (rectal) | Pudendal nerve (S2–S4 fibers) | Arises at entry to pudendal canal (ischial spine), courses medially through ischioanal fat pad to anal canal | Motor: external anal sphincter<br>Sensory: anoderm, perianal skin |
| Inferior gluteal | Sacral plexus (L5–S2 fibers) | Leaves pelvis through greater sciatic foramen inferior to piriformis and divides into several branches | Motor: gluteus maximus |
| Infraorbital | Terminal branch of maxillary nerve (CN V2) | Runs in floor of orbit and emerges at infraorbital foramen | Sensory: skin of cheek, lower lid, lateral side of nose and inferior septum and upper lip, upper premolar incisors and canine teeth, mucosa of maxillary sinus and upper lip |
| Infratrochlear | Nasociliary nerve (CN V1) | Follows medial wall of orbit to upper eyelid | Sensory: skin / conjunctiva (lining) of upper eyelid |
| Intercostals | Anterior rami of T1–T11 nerves | Run in intercostal spaces between internal and innermost layers of intercostal muscles | Motor: intercostal muscles; lower nerves supply muscles of anterolateral abdominal wall<br>Sensory: skin overlying and pleura/peritoneum deep to muscles innervated |
| Intermediate | From the pons as a smaller root of the facial nerve (CN VII) | Traverses internal acoustic meatus, merging at its distal end with larger (root of) facial nerve | Motor: presynaptic parasympathetics destined for pterygopalatine and submandibular ganglia via greater petrosal nerve and chorda tympani respectively<br>Sensory: taste from anterior two-thirds of tongue and soft palate |
| Lacrimal | Ophthalmic nerve (CN V1) | Passes through palpebral fascia of upper eyelid near lateral angle (canthus) of eye | Sensory: a small area of skin and conjunctiva of lateral part of upper eyelid |

| Nerve(s)/Nerve Branch(es) | Origin | Course | Structures Innervated |
|---|---|---|---|
| Lateral branch of median nerve | Median nerve as it enters palm of hand | Runs laterally to palmar thumb and radial side of index finger | Motor: 1st lumbrical<br>Sensory: skin of palmar and distal dorsal aspects of thumb and radial half of index finger |
| Lateral cutaneous nerve of forearm | Continuation of musculo-cutaneous nerve (C6 and C7 fibers) | Descends along lateral border of forearm to wrist | Sensory: skin of lateral aspect of forearm |
| Lateral cutaneous nerve of thigh | Lumbar plexus (L2 and L3 fibers) | Passes deep to inguinal ligament, 2–3 cm medial to anterior superior iliac spine | Sensory: skin on anterior and lateral aspects of thigh |
| Lateral pectoral | Lateral cord of brachial plexus (C5–C7 fibers) | Pierces clavipectoral fascia to reach deep surface of pectoral muscles | Motor: primarily pectoralis major but sends a loop to medial pectoral nerve that innervates pectoralis minor |
| Lateral plantar | Smaller terminal branch of the tibial nerve (S1–S2 fibers) | Passes laterally in foot between quadratus plantae and flexor digitorum brevis muscles and divides into superficial and deep branches | Motor: quadratus plantae, abductor digiti minimi, flexor digiti minimi brevis; deep branch supplies plantar and dorsal interossei, lateral 3 lumbricals, and adductor hallucis<br>Sensory: skin on sole lateral to a line splitting 4th digit |
| Least splanchnic | 12th (lowest) thoracic ganglion of sympathetic trunk | Passes through diaphragm with sympathetic trunk and ends in renal plexus | Motor: presynaptic sympathetic to renal arteries and derivatives |
| Lesser occipital | Cervical plexus (C2 and C3 fibers) | Ascends posterosuperiorly, parallel to anterosuperior border of sternocleidomastoid | Sensory: skin of posterior surface of auricle and adjacent scalp |
| Lesser palatine | Pterygopalatine ganglion (maxillary nerve—CN V2) | Passes inferiorly through palatine canal and lesser palatine foramen | Motor: postsynaptic parasympathetics to glands of soft palate<br>Sensory: mucosa of soft palate |
| Lesser petrosal | Tympanic plexus (glosso-pharyngeal nerve—CN IX) | Perforates tegmen tympanii to exit tympanic cavity into middle cranial fossa; runs anteriorly to descend through sphenopetrosal fissure or foramen ovale | Motor: conveys presynaptic parasympathetic fibers to otic ganglion for secretomotor innervation of parotid gland |
| Lesser splanchnic | 10th and 11th thoracic ganglia of sympathetic trunk | Descends anteromedially to perforate diaphragm to reach aorticorenal ganglion | Motor: presynaptic sympathetics to prevertebral ganglia<br>Sensory: visceral afferents from upper GI tract |
| Lingual | Terminal branch (with inferior alveolar nerve) of posterior trunk of mandibular nerve (CN V3) | Joined by chorda tympani in infratemporal fossa; passes anteroinferiorly between lateral and medial pterygoid muscles, and above mylohyoid to enter oral cavity | Motor: presynpatic parasympathetic fibers to submandibular ganglion for submandibular and sublingual salivary glands<br>Sensory: anterior two-thirds of tongue, floor of mouth, and lingual mandibular gingiva |
| Long thoracic | Anterior rami of C5–C7 | Descends posterior to C8 and T1 rami and passes distally on external surface of serratus anterior | Motor: serratus anterior |

| Nerve(s)/Nerve Branch(es) | Origin | Course | Structures Innervated |
|---|---|---|---|
| Lower subscapular | Posterior cord of brachial plexus (C5 and C6 fibers) | Passes inferolaterally, deep to subscapular artery and vein, to subscapularis and teres major | Motor: inferior portion of subscapularis and teres major |
| Lumbar splanchnic | Lumbar ganglia of sympathetic trunks | Pass anteromedially on bodies of lumbar vertebrae to prevertebral ganglia of para-aortic plexus | Motor: presynaptic sympathetics for lower abdominal and pelvic viscera Sensory: visceral afferents from same |
| Mandibular (CN V3) | Trigeminal ganglion (motor root from pons) | Descends through foramen ovale into infratemporal fossa; divides into anterior and posterior trunks, former ramifying immediately into several smaller branches, latter bifurcating into lingual and inferior alveolar nerves | Motor: muscles of mastication, mylohyoid, anterior belly of digastric, tensor tympani and tensor veli palatini Sensory: skin overlying mandible (except angle), lower half of mouth (including teeth, gingiva, mucosa of floor and vestibule, and anterior two-thirds of tongue), and temporomandibular joint |
| Masseteric | Anterior trunk of mandibular nerve (CN V3) | Passes laterally through mandibular notch | Motor: masseter Sensory: temporomandibular joint |
| Maxillary (CN V2) | Trigeminal ganglion | Runs anteriorly through foramen rotundum into pterygopalatine fossa, sending sensory roots to the pterygopalatine ganglion (branches of the ganglion are considered branches of the maxillary nerve); main trunk continues anteriorly through infraorbital fissure as infraorbital nerve | Motor: no motor fibers initially; branches of pterygopalatine ganglion distribute postsynaptic parasympathetic fibers to lacrimal gland and mucosal glands of nasal cavity, palate, and upper pharynx Sensory: skin overlying maxilla, mucosa of posteroinferior nasal cavity, and maxillary sinus; upper half of mouth (including teeth, gingiva, and mucosa of palate, vestibule, and cheek) |
| Medial branch of median nerve | Median nerve as it enters palm of hand | Runs medially to adjacent sides of index, middle, and ring fingers | Motor: 2nd lumbrical Sensory: skin of palmar and distal dorsal aspects of adjacent sides of index, middle, and ring fingers |
| Medial cutaneous nerve of arm | Medial cord of brachial plexus (C8 and T1 fibers) | Runs along the medial side of axillary vein and communicates with intercostobrachial nerve | Sensory: skin on medial side of arm |
| Medial cutaneous nerve of forearm | Medial cord of brachial plexus (C8 and T1 fibers) | Runs between axillary artery and vein | Sensory: skin over medial side of forearm |
| Medial cutaneous nerve of leg | Saphenous nerve | Descends medial side of leg with greater saphenous vein | Skin of anteromedial side of leg and medial side of foot |
| Medial dorsal cutaneous nerve | Superficial fibular (peroneal) nerve | Descends across ankle anteriorly running onto medial aspect of dorsum of foot | Supplies most of skin of dorsum of foot; proximal portion of toes, except for web between great and 2nd toes |

| Nerve(s)/Nerve Branch(es) | Origin | Course | Structures Innervated |
| --- | --- | --- | --- |
| Medial pectoral | Medial cord of brachial plexus (C8 and T1 fibers) | Passes between axillary artery and vein and enters deep surface of pectoralis minor | Motor: pectoralis minor and part of pectoralis major |
| Medial plantar | Larger terminal branch of the tibial nerve (L4 and L5 fibers) | Passes distally in foot between abductor hallucis and flexor digitorum brevis and divides into muscular and cutaneous branches | Motor: abductor hallucis, flexor digitorum brevis, flexor hallucis brevis, and 1st lumbrical<br>Sensory: skin of medial side of sole of foot and sides of 1st 3 digits |
| Median | Arises by two roots, one from the lateral cord of brachial plexus (C6 and C7 fibers) and one from medial cord (C8 and T1 fibers); roots join lateral to axillary artery | Over length of arm, crosses to medial side of brachial artery; exits cubital fossa between heads of pronator teres, running between intermediate and deep layers of anterior forearm compartment; becomes superficial proximal to wrist and passes deep to flexor retinaculum (transverse carpal ligament) as it passes through carpal tunnel to the hand | Motor: flexor muscles in forearm (except flexor carpi ulnaris, ulnar half of flexor digitorum profundus); thenar muscles (except adductor pollicis and deep head of flexor pollicis brevis), lateral lumbricals (for digits 2 and 3)<br>Sensory: skin of the palmar and distal dorsal aspects of the lateral (radial) 3-1/2 digits and adjacent palm |
| Mental | Terminal branch of inferior alveolar nerve (CN V3) | Emerges from mandibular canal at mental foramen | Sensory: skin of chin; skin and mucosa of lower lip |
| Musculocutaneous | Lateral cord of brachial plexus (C5–C7 fibers) | Enters deep surface of coracobrachialis and descends between biceps brachii and brachialis | Motor: flexor muscles of arm (coracobrachialis, biceps brachii, and brachialis)<br>Sensory: continues as lateral antebrachial cutaneous nerve |
| Nasociliary | Ophthalmic nerve (CN V1) | Arises in superior orbital fissure, passes anteromedially across retrobulbar orbit, providing sensory root to ciliary ganglion and terminating as infratrochlear nerve and nasal branches | Motor: no motor fibers initially; branches of ciliary ganglion (short ciliary nerves) convey postsynaptic sympathetics and parasympathetics to ciliary body and iris<br>Sensory: tactile sensation from eyeball (conjunctiva and cornea); mucous membrane of ethmoidal cells and anterosuperior nasal cavity; skin of root, dorsum, and apex of nose |
| Nasopalatine | Pterygopalatine ganglion (maxillary nerve—CN V2) | Exits pterygopalatine fossa via sphenopalatine foramen; crossing to and then running anteroinferiorly across nasal septum; passes through incisive foramen to palate | Motor: postsynaptic parasympathetics to mucosal glands of nasal septum<br>Sensory: mucosa of nasal septum, anteriormost hard palate |
| Nerves to lateral/medial pterygoid | Anterior trunk of mandibular nerve (CN V3) | Arise in infratemporal fossa immediately inferior to foramen ovale | Motor: lateral and medial pterygoid muscles |
| Nerve to mylohyoid | Inferior alveolar nerve | Arises from posterior aspect of inferior alveolar nerve immediately outside mandibular foramen; descends in bony groove on medial aspect of ramus of mandible | Motor: mylohyoid and anterior belly of digastric muscle |

| Nerve(s)/Nerve Branch(es) | Origin | Course | Structures Innervated |
|---|---|---|---|
| Nerve to obturator internus | Sacral plexus (L5, S1, and S2) | Enters gluteal region through greater sciatic foramen inferior to piriformis; descends posterior to ischial spine; enters lesser sciatic foramen and passes to obturator internus | Motor: superior gemellus and obturator internus |
| Nerve of pterygoid canal | Formed by merger of greater and deep petrosal nerves | Traverses pterygoid canal to reach pterygopalatine ganglion in pterygopalatine fossa | Motor: conveys postsynaptic sympathetic and presynaptic parasympathetic fibers to pterygopalatine ganglion |
| Nerve to quadratus femoris | Sacral plexus (L5, S1, and S2) | Leaves pelvis through greater sciatic foramen deep to sciatic nerve | Motor: inferior gemellus and quadratus femoris Sensory: hip joint |
| Nerve to stapedius | Facial nerve (CN VII) | Arises as facial nerve descends posterior to muscle in facial canal | Motor: stapedius |
| Nerve to tensor tympani | Otic ganglion (mandibular nerve—CN V3) | Courses along cartilagenous portion of pharyngotympanic (auditory) tube to hemicanal for tensor tympani | Motor: tensor tympani |
| Nerve to tensor veli palatini | Anterior trunk of mandibular nerve—(CN V3) | Arises as a branch of nerve to medial pterygoid | Motor: tensor veli palatini |
| Obturator | Lumbar plexus (L2–L4 fibers) | Enters thigh through obturator foramen and divides; its anterior branch descends between adductor longus and adductor brevis; its posterior branch descends between adductor brevis and adductor magnus | Motor: anterior branch supplies adductor longus, adductor brevis, gracilis, and pectineus; posterior branch supplies obturator externus and adductor magnus Sensory: skin of medial thigh above knee |
| Oculomotor (CN III) | Interpeduncular fossa of mesencephalon | Pierces dura lateral to posterior clinoid process, runs in lateral wall of cavernous sinus, enters orbit through superior orbital fissure and divides into superior and inferior branches | Motor: somatic: all extraocular muscles except superior oblique and lateral rectus; presynaptic parasympathetic fibers to ciliary ganglion for ciliary body and sphincter pupillae |
| Olfactory (CN I) | Olfactory cells in olfactory epithelium (mucosa) of roof of nasal cavity | Approximately 20 bundles of nerve fibers ascend through foramina of cribriform plate of ethmoid to reach olfactory bulbs (anterior cranial fossa) | Sensory: olfactory mucosa (sense of smell) |
| Ophthalmic (CN V1) | Trigeminal ganglion | Passes anteriorly in lateral wall of cavernous sinus to enter orbit through superior orbital fissure, branching into frontal, nasociliary, and lacrimal nerves | Sensory: general sensation from eyeball (conjunctiva and cornea); mucous membrane of ethmoidal cells and frontal sinus, dura of anterior cranial fossa, falx cerebri and tentorium cerebelli, anterosuperior nasal cavity; skin of forehead, upper lid; root, dorsum, and apex of nose |
| Optic (CN II) | Ganglion cells of retina | Exits orbit via optic canals; fibers from nasal half of retina cross to contralateral side at chiasm; fibers pass via optic tracts to geniculate bodies, superior colliculus, and pretectum | Sensory: vision from retina |

| Nerve(s)/Nerve Branch(es) | Origin | Course | Structures Innervated |
|---|---|---|---|
| Palmar cutaneous branch of median nerve | Arises from median nerve just proximal to flexor retinaculum | Passes between tendons of palmaris longus and flexor carpi radialis and runs superficial to flexor retinaculum | Sensory: skin of central palm |
| Palmar cutaneous branch of ulnar nerve | Arises from ulnar nerve near middle of forearm | Descends on ulnar artery and perforates deep fascia in the distal third of forearm | Sensory: skin at base of medial palm, overlying medial carpals |
| Pelvic splanchnic | Sacral plexus (S2–S4 fibers) | Run anteriorly and inferiorly to merge with inferior hypogastric plexus | Motor: presynaptic parasympathetic fibers for pelvic viscera, descending and sigmoid colon Sensory: visceral afferent fibers from subperitoneal pelvic viscera (cervix of uterus and upper vagina, floor of bladder, rectum and upper anal canal; prostate) |
| Perineal | Terminal branch (with dorsal nerve of penis/clitoris) of pudendal nerve (S2–S4 fibers) | Separates from pudendal nerve on exit from pudendal canal; runs to superficial perineum dividing into a superficial cutaneous branch (posterior labial/scrotal) and a deep motor branch | Motor: muscles of urogenital triangle (superficial and deep perineal muscles) Sensory: skin of posterior urogenital triangle (posterior portion of labia majora and minora, vestibule of vagina; posterior aspect of scrotum) |
| Pharyngeal | Pterygopalatine ganglion | Passes posteriorly through palatovaginal canal | Supplies mucosa of nasopharynx posterior to pharyngotympanic (auditory) tubes |
| Phrenic | Cervical plexus (C3–C5 fibers) | Passes through superior thoracic aperture and runs between mediastinal pleura and pericardium | Motor: diaphragm Sensory: pericardial sac, mediastinal and diaphragmatic pleura, and diaphragmatic peritoneum |
| Posterior auricular | As first extracranial branch of facial nerve (CN VII) | Passes posterior to ear, sending branch to occipital region | Motor: posterior auricular muscle and intrinsic auricular muscles, occipital belly of occipitofrontalis (epicranius) |
| Posterior cutaneous nerve of arm | Radial nerve (C5–C8 fibers) | Emerges from under posterior border of deltoid, between long and lateral heads of triceps brachii | Sensory: skin of posterior aspect of arm |
| Posterior cutaneous nerve of forearm | Arises in arm from radial nerve (C5–C8 fibers) | Perforates lateral head of triceps and descends along lateral side of arm and posterior aspect of forearm to wrist | Sensory: skin of distal posterior arm, posterior aspect of forearm |
| Posterior cutaneous nerve of thigh | Sacral plexus (S1–S3 fibers) | Leaves pelvis through greater sciatic foramen inferior to piriformis, runs deep to gluteus maximus, and emerges from its inferior border | Sensory: skin of buttock through inferior cluneal branches and skin over posterior aspect of thigh and calf; lateral perineum, upper medial thigh via perineal branch |
| Posterior ethmoidal | Nasociliary | Leaves orbit via posterior ethmoidal foramen | Supplies ethmoidal and sphenoidal paranasal sinuses |
| Posterior inferior nasal | Greater palatine | Arise in greater palatine canal, pierce through perpendicular plate of palatine bone | Mucosa of inferior nasal concha and walls of inferior and middle nasal meatuses |

| Nerve(s)/Nerve Branch(es) | Origin | Course | Structures Innervated |
|---|---|---|---|
| Posterior interosseous | Terminal branch of deep branch of radial nerve (continuation of deep radial after emerging from supinator) | Runs between superficial and deep layers of posterior forearm, then passes between extensor pollicis longus and interosseous membrane | Motor: extensor carpi ulnaris, extensors of digits (including thumb), and abductor pollicis longus |
| Posterior labial | Perineal nerve | Emerge from pudendal canal and ramify in subcutaneous tissue | Skin of posterior portion of labium majus |
| Pudendal | Sacral plexus (S2–S4) | Enters gluteal region through greater sciatic foramen inferior to piriformis; descends posterior to sacrospinous ligament; enters perineum through lesser sciatic foramen | Supplies most motor and sensory innervation to perineum (supplies no structures in gluteal region) |
| Pulmonary plexus | Vagus nerve and cardio-pulmonary splanchnic nerves from sympathetic trunk | Forms on primary bronchi and extends along root of lung and bronchial sub-divisions | Motor: parasympathetic fibers constrict bronchioles; sympathetic fibers dilate them |
| Radial | Terminal branch of posterior cord of brachial plexus (C5–C8 and T1 fibers) | Descends posterior to axillary artery; enters radial groove with deep brachial artery to pass between long and medial heads of triceps; bifurcates in cubital fossa into superficial and deep radial nerves | Motor: proximal to bifurcation, innervates triceps brachii, anconeus, brachio-radialis, and extensor carpi radialis longus muscles Sensory: skin on posterior aspect of arm and forearm via posterior cutaneous nerves of arm and forearm |
| Recurrent (thenar) branch of median nerve | Median nerve immediately distal to flexor retinaculum | Loops around distal border of flexor retinaculum and enters thenar muscles | Motor: abductor pollicis brevis, opponens pollicis, and superficial head of flexor pollicis brevis |
| Recurrent laryngeal | Vagus nerve (CN X) | Loops around subclavian on right; on left runs around arch of aorta and ascends in tracheoesophageal groove | Motor: intrinsic muscles of larynx (except cricothyroid) Sensory: inferior to level of vocal folds |
| Saphenous | Femoral nerve | Descends with femoral vessels through femoral triangle and adductor canal, then descends with great saphenous vein | Sensory: skin on medial side of leg and foot |
| Sciatic | Sacral plexus (L4–S3 fibers) | Enters gluteal region through greater sciatic foramen inferior to piriformis, descends along posterior aspect of thigh, and divides proximal to knee into tibial and common fibular peroneal nerves | Motor: hamstrings by tibial division (except for short head of biceps femoris, which is innervated by its common fibular division) Sensory: provides articular branches to hip and knee joints |
| Subclavian nerve | Superior trunk of brachial plexus (C5–C6; often C4 also) | Descends posterior to clavicle and anterior to brachial plexus and sub-clavian artery | Motor: subclavius Sensory: sternoclavicular joint |
| Subcostal | Anterior ramus of T12 spinal nerve | Courses along inferior border of 12th rib in same manner as intercostal nerves | Motor: muscles of antero-lateral abdominal wall Sensory: lateral cutaneous branch supplies skin inferior to anterior iliac crest |

| Nerve(s)/Nerve Branch(es) | Origin | Course | Structures Innervated |
|---|---|---|---|
| Suboccipital | Posterior ramus of C1 spinal nerve | Emerges between occipital bone and atlas, inferior to transverse part of vertebral artery, into suboccipital triangle; communicates with occipital nerve (C2) | Motor: suboccipital muscles (rectus capitis major and minor, obliquus capitis inferior and superior) |
| Superficial branch of radial nerve | Continuation of radial nerve after deep branch is given off in cubital fossa | Passes distally, anterior to pronator teres and deep to brachioradialis; emerging to pierce deep fascia at wrist and pass onto dorsum of hand | Sensory: skin of lateral (radial) half of dorsum of hand and thumb, proximal portions of dorsal aspects of digits 2 and 3, and of lateral (radial) half of digit 4 |
| Superficial branch of ulnar nerve | Arise from ulnar nerve at wrist as they pass between pisiform and hamate bones | Passes palmaris brevis and divides into 2 common palmar digital nerves | Motor: palmaris brevis Sensory: skin of palmar and distal dorsal aspects of digit 5 and of medial (ulnar) side of digit 4 and proximal portion of palm |
| Superficial fibular (peroneal) | Common fibular (peroneal) nerve | Arises between fibularis longus and neck of fibula and descends in lateral compartment of leg; pierces deep fascia at distal third of leg to become cutaneous and send branches to foot and digits | Motor: fibularis (peroneus) longus and brevis Sensory: skin on distal third of anterior surface of leg and dorsum of foot and all digits, except lateral side of 5th and adjoining sides of 1st and 2nd digits |
| Superior alveolar | Maxillary nerve (CN V2) or its continuation as infra-orbital nerve | Posterior: emerge from pterygomaxillary fissure into infratemporal fossa; pierce posterior aspect of maxilla Middle and anterior: arise from infraorbital nerve in roof of maxillary sinus, descend walls of sinus | Sensory: mucosa of maxillary sinus, maxillary teeth, and gingiva |
| Superior gluteal | Sacral plexus (L4–S1 fibers) | Leaves pelvis through greater sciatic foramen superior to piriformis and runs between gluteus medius and minimus | Motor: gluteus medius, gluteus minimus, and tensor fasciae latae |
| Superior laryngeal | Vagus (CN X) | Descends in parapharyngeal space; lateral to thyroid cartilage divides into internal and external laryngeal nerves; former pierces thyrohyoid membrane; latter runs inferomedially to gap between cricoid and thyroid cartilages | Motor: cricothyroid muscle (external laryngeal nerve) Sensory: supraglottic |
| Supraclavicular (lateral, intermediate, medial) | Cervical plexus (C3 and C4 fibers) | Arise via a common trunk that emerges at center of posterior border of sterno-cleidomastoid; fan out as they descend onto lower neck, upper thorax, and shoulder | Sensory: skin of lower anterolateral neck, upper-most thorax, and shoulder |
| Supraorbital | Continuation of frontal nerve (CN V1) | Emerges through supra-orbital notch, or foramen, and breaks up into small branches | Sensory: mucous membrane of frontal sinus and conjunctiva (lining) of upper eyelid; skin of forehead as far as vertex |

| Nerve(s)/Nerve Branch(es) | Origin | Course | Structures Innervated |
|---|---|---|---|
| Suprascapular | Superior trunk of brachial plexus (C5–C6; often C4 also) | Passes laterally across posterior triangle of neck, through scapular notch under superior transverse scapular ligament | Motor: supraspinatus, infraspinatus muscles<br>Sensory: superior and posterior glenohumeral (shoulder) joint |
| Supratrochlear | Frontal nerve (CN V1) | Passes superiorly on medial of supraorbital nerve and divides into 2 or more branches | Sensory: skin in middle of forehead to hairline |
| Sural | Usually arises from merging of medial and lateral sural cutaneous nerves from tibial and common fibular (peroneal) nerves respectively | Descends between heads of gastrocnemius and becomes superficial at middle of leg; descends with small saphenous vein and passes posterior to lateral malleolus to lateral side of foot | Sensory: skin on posterior and lateral aspects of leg and lateral side of foot |
| Tentorial | Intracranial portion of ophthalmic nerve (CN V1) | Arises as recurrent branch passing abruptly posteriorly around margins of tentorial notch onto superior aspect of tentorium cerebelli and ascending posterior limb of falx cerebri | Sensory: supratentorial dura mater (superior aspect of tentorium cerebri and falx cerebri) |
| Thoracic splanchnic | Thoracic ganglia of sympathetic trunk | Pass anteromedially on bodies of thoracic vertebrae as lower cardiopulmonary splanchnic nerves to thoracic autonomic plexuses (cardiac, pulmonary, and esophageal) and as upper abdominopelvic splanchnic nerves to prevertebral ganglia of para-aortic plexus | Motor: splanchnic nerves from 1st through 5th thoracic ganglia convey postsynaptic sympathetic fibers to heart, lungs, and esophagus; those from 6th through 12th thoracic ganglia (i.e., greater, lesser, and least splanchnic nerves) convey presynaptic sympathetic fibers to prevertebral ganglia |
| Thoracoabdominal | Continuation of lower intercostal nerves (T7–T11) | Cross costal margin to run between 2nd and 3rd layers of abdominal muscles | Motor: anterolateral abdominal muscles<br>Sensory: overlying skin, underlying peritoneum, and periphery of diaphragm |
| Thoracodorsal | Posterior cord of brachial plexus (C6–C8 fibers) | Arises between upper and lower subscapular nerves and runs inferolaterally along posterior axillary wall to latissimus dorsi | Motor: latissimus dorsi |
| Tibial | Sciatic nerve (L4–S3 fibers) | Forms as sciatic bifurcates at apex of popliteal fossa; descends through popliteal fossa and lies on popliteus; runs inferiorly on tibialis posterior with posterior tibial vessels; terminates beneath flexor retinaculum by dividing into medial and lateral plantar nerves | Motor: muscles of posterior compartment of thigh (except short head of biceps), popliteal fossa, posterior compartment of leg, and sole of foot<br>Sensory: knee joint; skin of leg (via medial sural), and sole of foot (via medial and lateral plantar nerves) |
| Transverse cervical | Cervical plexus (C2 and C3 fibers) | Emerges from middle of posterior border of sternocleidomastoid muscle; runs anterior across muscle | Sensory: skin overlying anterior triangle of neck |

| Nerve(s)/Nerve Branch(es) | Origin | Course | Structures Innervated |
|---|---|---|---|
| Trigeminal (CN V) | Lateral surface of pons by 2 roots: motor and sensory | Roots cross medial part of crest of petrous part of temporal bone, entering trigeminal cave of dura mater lateral to body of sphenoid and cavernous sinus; sensory root leads to trigeminal ganglion; motor root bypasses ganglion, becoming part of mandibular nerve (CN V3) | Motor: somatic: muscles of mastication, mylohyoid, anterior belly of digastric, tensor tympani and tensor veli palatini; visceral: distributes postsynaptic parasympathetic fibers of head to their destinations Sensory: dura of anterior and middle cranial fossae, skin of face, teeth, gingiva, mucosa, nasal cavity, paranasal sinuses, and mouth |
| Trochlear (CN IV) | Dorsolateral aspect of mesencephalon below inferior colliculus (only cranial nerve to emerge from dorsal aspect of brainstem) | Runs longest intracranial course, passing around brainstem to enter dura in free edge of tentorium close to posterior clinoid process; runs in lateral wall of cavernous sinus, entering orbit via superior orbital fissure | Motor: superior oblique muscle |
| Tympanic | As 1st extracranial branch of glossopharyngeal nerve (CN IX), from inferior (petrosal) glossopharyngeal ganglion | Passes in recurrent manner into tympanic canaliculus, entering tympanic cavity and ramifying on promontory of labyrinthine wall as tympanic plexus | Motor: conveys presynaptic parasympathetic fibers that will reach otic ganglion for secretomotor innervation of parotid gland Sensory: mucosa of tympanic cavity, mastoid cells, and pharyngotympanic (auditory) tube |
| Ulnar | Terminal branch of medial cord of brachial plexus (C8 and T1 fibers; often also receives C7 fibers) | Terminal branch of medial cord of brachial plexus (C8 and T1 fibers; often also receives C7 fibers) | Motor: majority of intrinsic muscles of hand (hypothenar, interosseous, adductor pollicis, and deep head of flexor pollicis brevis, plus medial lumbricals [for digits 4 and 5]) Sensory: skin of palmar and distal dorsal aspects of medial (ulnar) 1–1/2 digits and adjacent palm |
| Upper subscapular | Branch of posterior cord of brachial plexus (C5 and C6 fibers) | Passes posteriorly and enters subscapularis | Motor: superior portion of subscapularis |
| Vagus (CN X) | Via 8 to 10 rootlets from medulla of brainstem | Enters superior mediastinum posterior to sternoclavicular joint and brachiocephalic vein; gives rise to recurrent laryngeal nerve; continues into abdomen | Motor: voluntary muscle of larynx and upper esophagus; involuntary muscle and glands of tracheobronchial tree, gut (to left colic flexure), and heart via pulmonary plexus, esophageal plexus, and cardiac plexus Sensory: pharynx, larynx, reflex afferents from same areas as above |
| Vestibular | As a division of vestibulocochlear nerve (CN VIII) | Traverses internal acoustic meatus to reach vestibular ganglion at fundus; branches pass to vestibule of bony labyrinth | Sensory: cristae of ampullae of semicircular ducts, maculae of saccule and utricle (for sense of equilibration) |

| Nerve(s)/Nerve Branch(es) | Origin | Course | Structures Innervated |
|---|---|---|---|
| Vestibulocochlear (CN VIII) | Groove between pons and myencephalon | Traverses internal acoustic meatus, dividing into cochlear and vestibular nerves | Sensory: spiral organ (for sense of hearing) and cristae of ampullae of semicircular ducts, maculae of saccule and utricle (for sense of equilibration) |
| Zygomatic | Maxillary nerve (CN V2) | Arises in floor of orbit, divides into zygomaticofacial and zygomaticotemporal nerves, which traverse foramina of same name; communicating branch joins lacrimal nerve | Sensory: skin over zygomatic arch and anterior temporal region Motor: conveys secretory postsynaptic parasympathetic fibers from pterygopalatine ganglion to lacrimal gland |

# Radiographic Anatomy and Positioning

## Anatomic Planes

A plane is a flat surface formed by making a cut (imaginary or real) through the body or a part of it. In radiography, various planes are used as points of reference that assist in localizing areas of the body to permit specific centering guidelines. The major anatomic planes used in radiographic positioning are as follows:

| | |
|---|---|
| **Longitudinal plane** | Made by cutting along the long (longitudinal) axis of the body or body part. In the erect position, this plane is termed *vertical* and is perpendicular to the horizontal. |
| **Transverse plane** | Made by cutting across the body or body part crosswise (at a right angle to the long axis). If the patient is erect, this plane is termed *horizontal* (parallel to the horizon). |
| **Midsagittal or median plane** | Longitudinal plane made by cutting from front (anterior) to back (posterior) along the median line of the body and along the sagittal suture of the skull. |
| **Sagittal plane** | Longitudinal plane made by cutting from front (anterior) to back (posterior) on either side of the sagittal suture and parallel to the midsagittal or median plane. |
| **Coronal plane** | Longitudinal plane made cutting lengthwise from side to side through the head and body (or body part) along the coronal suture of the skull or parallel to it. The coronal suture lies behind the frontal bone and extends toward the sides of the skull. |
| **Transpyloric plane** | Transverse plane made by cutting across the body from one side to the other at the level of the 9th costal cartilages. The plane is situated about halfway between the superior border of the sternum (manubrial, or sternal, notch) and the symphysis pubis (junction of the two anterior or superior portions of the pubic bones). The name of this plane reflects the fact that it should cut across the pylorus of the stomach. |
| **Midcoronal (midaxillary) plane** | Longitudinal plane made by cutting through the head and body along the coronal suture of the head and extending the cut down the body. |

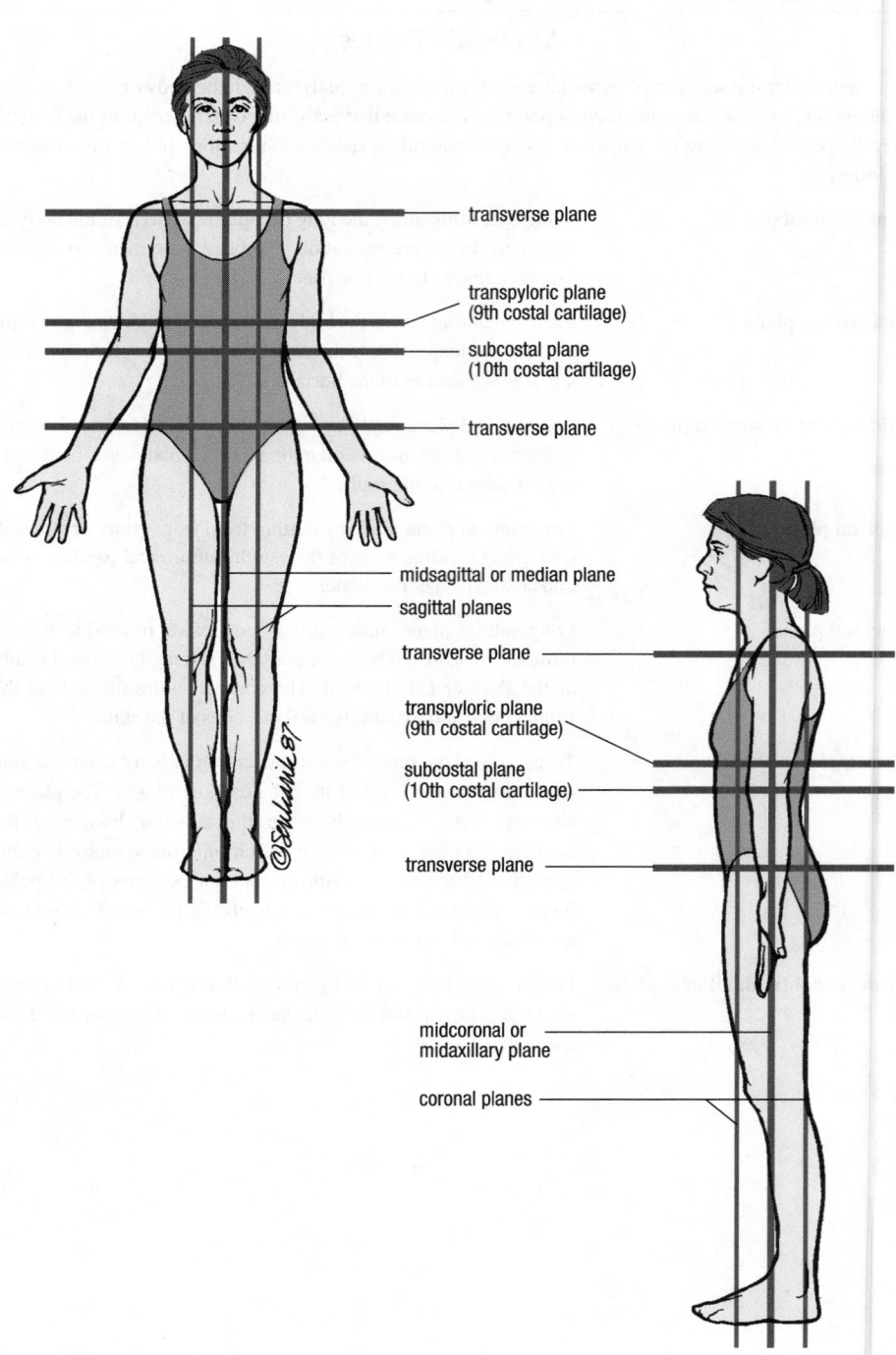

**Anatomic Planes**

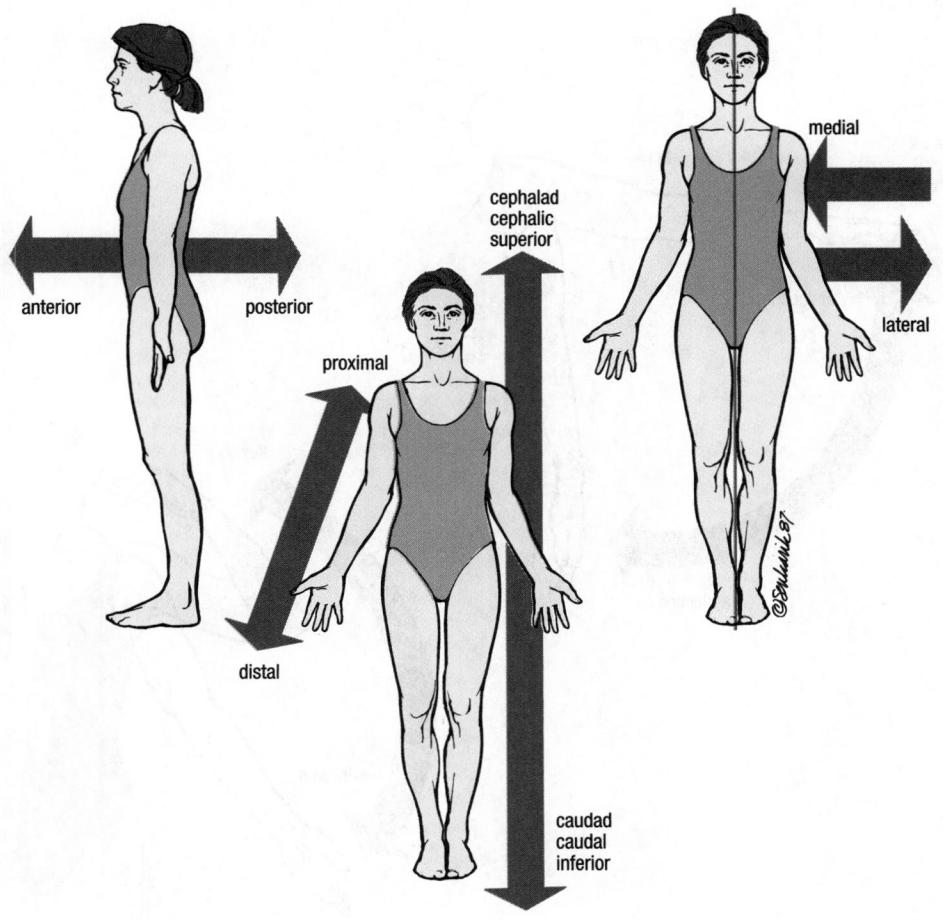

## Body Part Terminology

**Anterior**

In front of (toward the front of the body or a structure within it); sometimes referred to as *ventral*.

**Posterior**

In back of (toward the back of the body or a structure within it); sometimes referred to as *dorsal*.

**Medial**

Toward the midline of the body.

**Lateral**

Away from the midline of the body (to the side).

**Proximal**

Closer to the point of attachment of origin; in the extremities, closest to the trunk.

**Distal**

Farther from the point of attachment or origin; in the extremities, farthest from the trunk.

**Cephalad, cephalic, superior**

Toward the head or the upper part of a structure.

**Caudad, caudal, inferior**

Away from the head or the lower part of a structure (literally means "toward the tail").

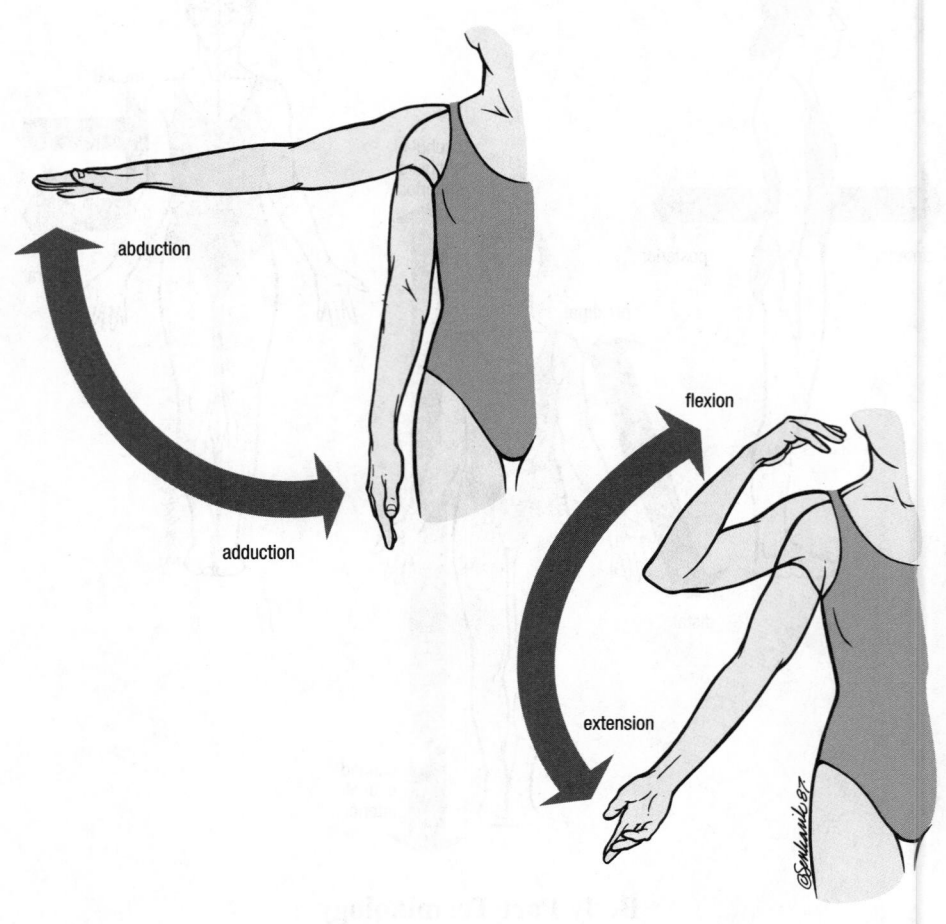

## Body Movement

**Abduction**

Movement of a limb or body part farther from or away from the midline of the body.

**Adduction**

Movement of a limb or body part closer to or toward the midline of the body.

**Extension**

Straightening of a joint or extremity so that the angle between contiguous (adjoining) bones is increased.

**Flexion**

Bending of a joint or extremity so that the angle between contiguous (adjoining) bones is decreased.

**Eversion**                    Movement of turning a body part outward (away from the midline).

**Inversion**                   Movement of turning a body part inward (toward the midline).

**Pronation**                   Movement of turning the body to face downward or turning the hand so that the palm is facing downward.

**Supination**                  Movement of turning the body to face upward or turning the hand so that the palm faces upward.

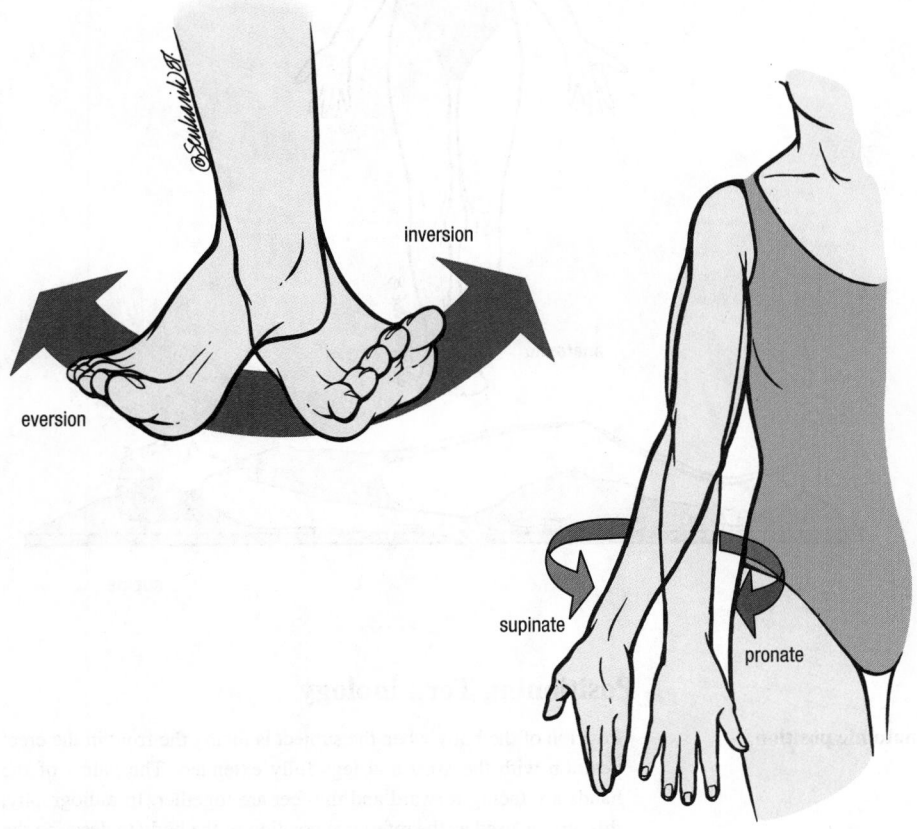

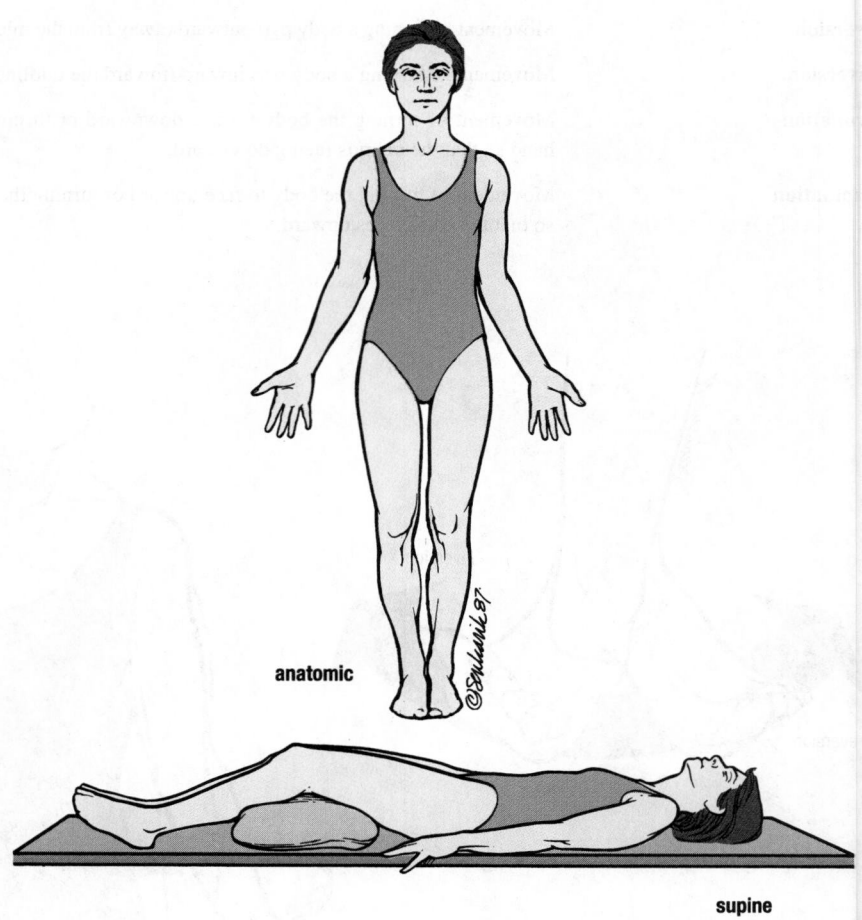

anatomic

supine

## Positioning Terminology

**Anatomic position**

Position of the body when the subject is facing the front in the erect position with the arms and legs fully extended. The palms of the hands are facing forward and the feet are together. In radiography, this term is used as the reference position of the body to describe the various different positions.

**Supine position**

Position in which the subject is lying on the back with the face up. Sometimes referred to as the *dorsal recumbent* (lying down) or *dorsal decubitus* position, since the back (dorsal surface) of the body is dependent (nearer the table).

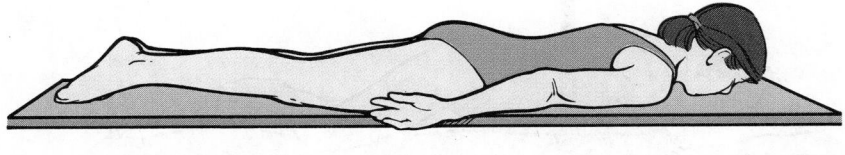

**prone**

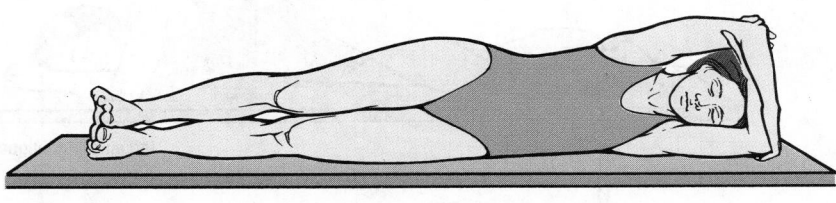

**lateral**

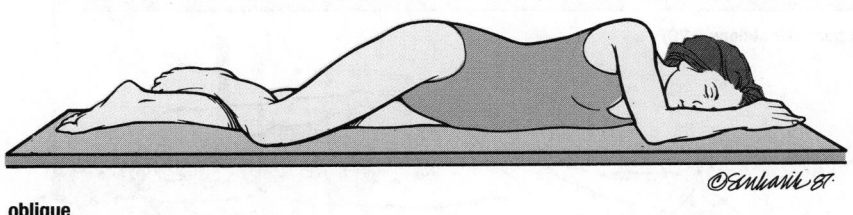

**oblique**

| | |
|---|---|
| **Prone position** | Position in which the subject is lying face down on the front of the body. Sometimes referred to as the *ventral recumbent* or *ventral decubitus* position, since the front (ventral surface) of the body is dependent (nearer the table). |
| **Lateral position** | Position in which the side of the subject is next to the film. A lateral position is named by the side of the subject that is situated adjacent to the film. Sometimes referred to as an *erect lateral* if the subject is sitting or standing, and a *lateral recumbent* or *lateral decubitus* if the subject is lying down. |
| **Oblique position** | Position in which the subject is neither prone normal supine, but rotated somewhere between. In radiographic terminology, the subject is in a *posterior oblique position* if some part of the posterior surface of the body is closer to the film, and in an *anterior oblique position* if some part of the anterior surface of the body is closer to the film. |

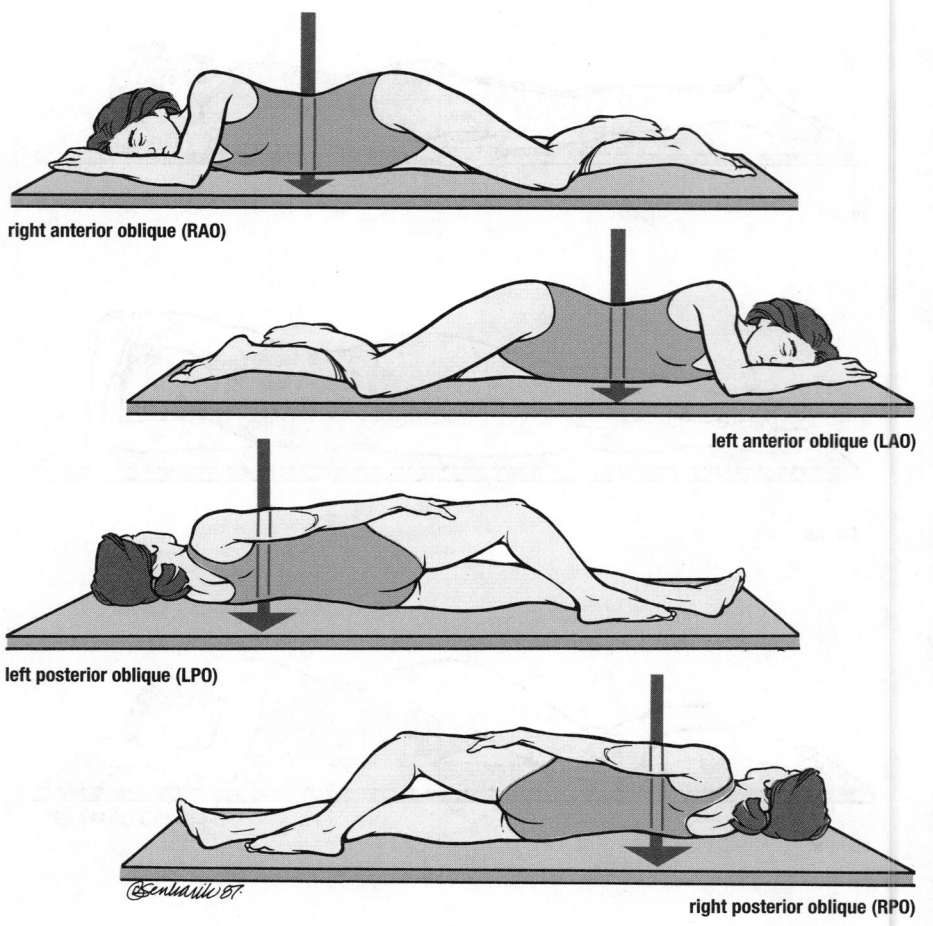

right anterior oblique (RAO)

left anterior oblique (LAO)

left posterior oblique (LPO)

right posterior oblique (RPO)

**Right anterior oblique (RAO)**      Patient is lying semiprone (face down) on the radiographic table or standing facing a vertical grid device with the *right* side closer to the film.

**Left anterior oblique (LAO)**       Patient is lying semiprone (face down) on the radiographic table or standing facing a vertical grid device with the *left* side closer to the film.

**Left posterior oblique (LPO)**      Patient is lying semisupine (face up) on the radiographic table or standing with the back against a vertical grid device with the *left* side closest to the film.

**Right posterior oblique (RPO)**     Patient is lying semisupine (face up) on the radiographic table or standing facing away from a vertical grid device with the *right* side closest to the film.

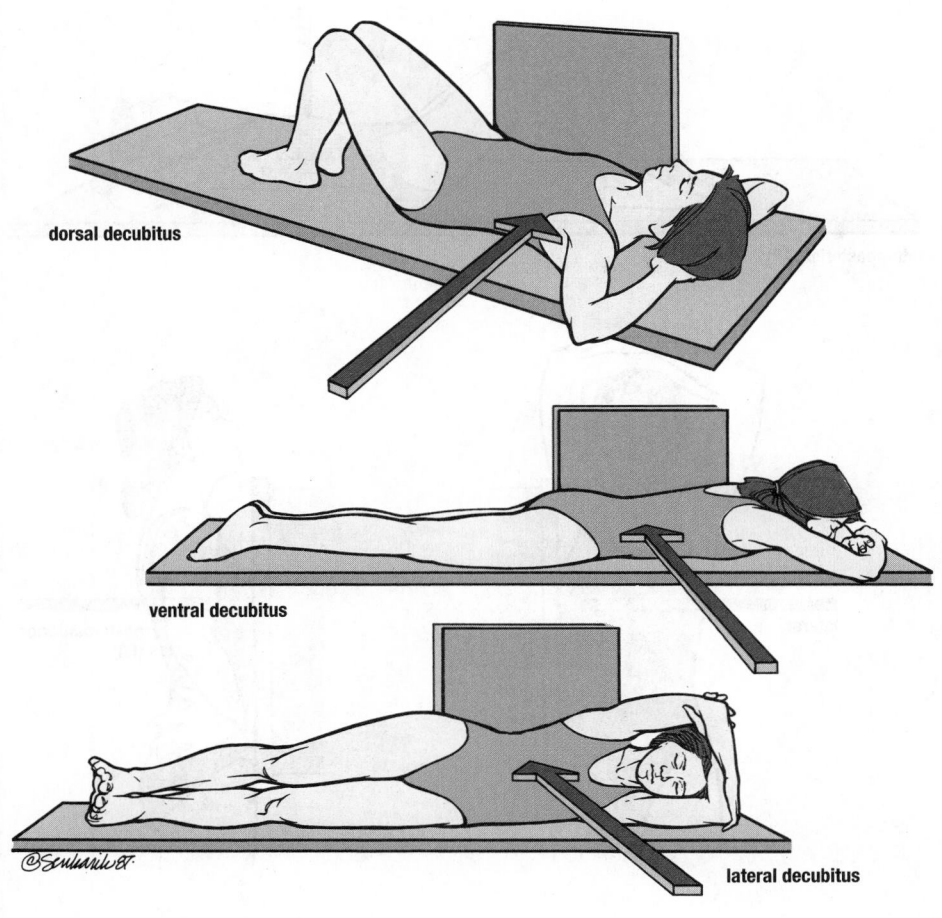

dorsal decubitus

ventral decubitus

lateral decubitus

| | |
|---|---|
| **Decubitus position** | Patient is lying down, and the central ray is horizontal (parallel to the floor). |
| **Dorsal decubitus** | Patient is lying supine (face up) on the radiographic table or on a stretcher placed next to a vertical grid device. The x-ray beam enters from one side of the patient and exits out the other. |
| **Ventral decubitus** | Patient is lying prone (face down) on the radiographic table or on a stretcher placed next to a vertical grid device. The x-ray beam enters from one side of the patient and exits out the other. |
| **Lateral decubitus** | Patient is lying on either side on the radiographic table or on a stretcher placed next to a vertical grid device. For a *left* lateral decubitus, the patient is lying on the *left* side with the *right* side up, while for a *right* lateral decubitus, the patient is lying on the *right* side with the *left* side up. The x-ray beam passes through the patient from front to back or back to front, depending on whether the patient is facing toward or away from the radiographic tube. |

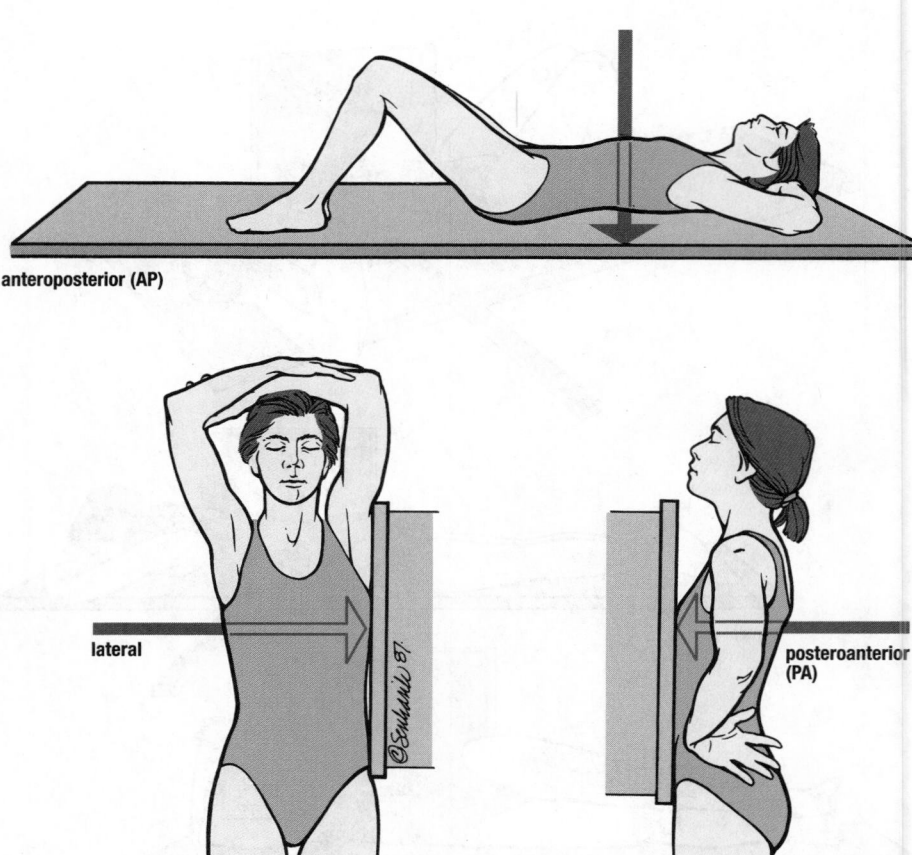

# Radiographic Projections

In radiography, the term *projection* describes the path along which the x-rays travel from the radiographic tube through the subject to the image receptor.

**Anteroposterior (AP) projection**

Patient is either supine (face up) on the radiographic table (dorsal decubitus) or erect with the back against a vertical grid device. The x-ray beam enters the front (anterior) surface of the body and exits the back (posterior) surface.

**Posteroanterior (PA) projection**

Patient is either prone (face down) on the radiographic table (ventral decubitus) or erect facing a vertical grid device. The x-ray beam enters the back (posterior) surface of the body and exits the front (anterior) surface.

**Lateral projection**

Patient is lying on either side on the radiographic table (lateral decubitus) or standing with either side against a vertical grid device. The lateral projection is always named by the side of the patient that is placed next to the film.

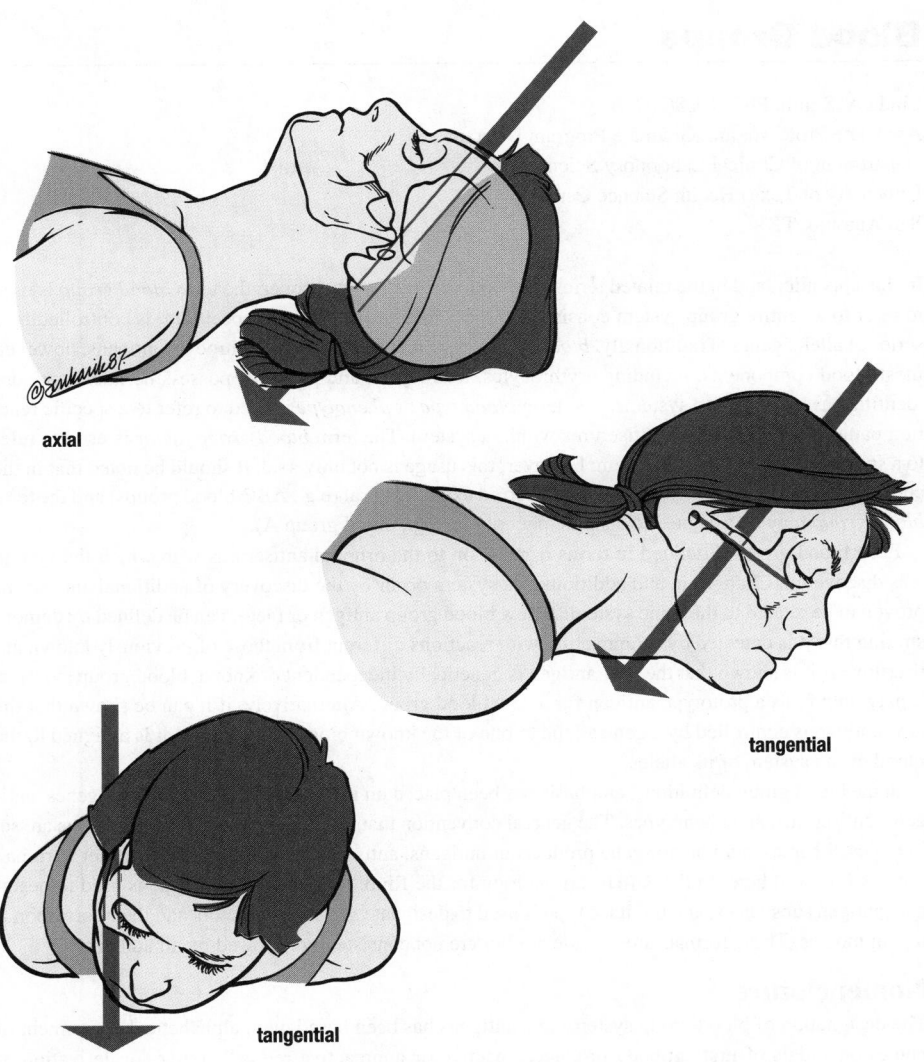

axial

tangential

tangential

| | |
|---|---|
| **Oblique projection** | Patient is rotated into a position that does not produce either a frontal (AP or PA) or lateral projection. |
| **Axial projection** | Any projection in which there is longitudinal angulation of the central ray with respect to the long axis of the body part. |
| **Tangential projection** | Any projection in which the central ray passes between or passes by (skims) body parts to project an anatomic structure in profile and free of superimposition. |

From Eisenberg RL, Dennis CA, May CR. Radiographic positioning, 2nd ed. Boston: Little, Brown, 1995.

# Blood Groups

Linda A. Smith, PhD, CLS(NCA)
Associate Professor and Graduate Program Director
Department of Clinical Laboratory Sciences
University of Texas Health Science Center
San Antonio, TX

In this appendix, and in the related terms defined in the dictionary proper, the term *blood group* is used to refer to an entire group system consisting of heritable antigens whose specificity is controlled by a series of allelic genes. Traditionally, *blood group* is used in reference to erythrocyte antigens; however, most blood components, including erythrocytes, leukocytes, and platelets, possess heritable antigens identified as belonging to systems. The term *blood type* or *phenotype* is used to refer to a specific reaction pattern to the testing of antiserums within a system. The term *blood group factor* is used to refer to a specific antigen within a system; however, this usage is not universal. It should be noted that in the current literature, a single system may be referred to in the plural (e.g., ABO blood groups) and the term *blood group* may be assigned to a single phenotype (e.g., blood group A).

Each blood group is defined in terms of reaction to the original antiserums with which the system was discovered. Changes in and additions to a system occur by the discovery of additional antiserums proven to be related to the same system. A new blood group antigen or factor can be defined by demonstrating that it is detected by an antiserum with reactions different from those of previously known antiserums. If it is shown that the new antigen is genetically independent of known blood group systems, it may qualify as a prototype antigen for a new blood group. Alternatively, if it can be shown that the new antigen is controlled by a gene allelic to one of the known blood group genes, it is assigned to the blood group system of its alleles.

In the blood group definitions, emphasis has been placed on identification of symbols for genes, antigens, antiserums, and phenotypes. The general convention that symbols for genes and genotypes are set in italics, whereas symbols for gene products or antigens, antiserums, and phenotypes are set in roman type, is followed here. In the Rh-Hr terminology for the Rh blood group, roman type is used to designate antigen substances, and boldface type is used to designate serological factors and their corresponding antibodies. These formats are in wide use but are not consistently followed by all authors.

## Nomenclature

The designation of blood group systems and antigens has been based upon alphabetical assignment of names or initials of first antibody producer, reactive or nonreactive red cell source, or derivation of name, location or discovering institution. The International Society of Blood Transfusion (ISBT) developed a Working Party on Terminology of Red Cell Surface Antigens to establish a uniform nomenclature, while not modifying historical designations and guidelines. Part of the Working Party's charge is to conduct periodic reviews of the available data and report additions, alterations, or deletions to those blood group antigens considered extinct. In addition, the Working Party has developed a nomenclature coding system, based on order of discovery of the blood group systems, to aid in the computerization of data. Reports of the Working Party and updates are published in *Vox Sanguinis* (1990; 58:152–169, 1993; 65:77–80,1995; 69:265–279 1996;71: 246–248).

The ISBT classifies all antigens into one of four classifications: systems, collections, high-incidence antigens, and low-incidence antigens. Currently, there are 23 blood group systems. Each system is serologically, immunochemically, and genetically proven to be a product of distinct independent genes. Although 52 Rh antigens have been identified, some have been removed from the system since initial identification; consequently, the system currently has 45 antigens. Other systems (e.g., P, Xg, Hh, and Kx systems) have only one antigen associated with them. The table accompanying this essay lists the approved system names, abbreviated symbols, and numerical designations developed by the ISBT. For clinical considerations, the ABO and Rh are of the most importance; others are useful for genetic linkage or red cell membrane protein studies.

In addition to the defined blood group system, there are other blood group antigens that fail, as of yet, to fit the system criteria. Some are genetically related or loosely associated by serological and immunochemical reactivity, but insufficient data exist to classify them as a system. Hence they are referred to as *collections*. There are now five collections recognized by the ISBT.

The remaining classifications of high-incidence and low-incidence antigens contain antigens that cannot be included in either a system or a collection. Antigens occurring with a high incidence in the random population are collectively referred to as *high-incidence antigens* or *public antigens*. These occur in almost all individuals. Antibodies to these antigens usually have been found in the serum of patients who lack the antigen and who have become immunized by transfusion or pregnancy. There are 12 distinct high-incidence antigens, and some of the symbols applied to public antigens include Vel, Lan, Ata, Jra, and JMH.

Other erythrocyte antigens are uncommon and may be found only in members of a very few families. Because of their rarity, they are often referred to as *low-incidence antigens* or *private antigens*. Antibodies to these antigens usually have been found in the serum of patients who have received transfusions or in mothers of infants with hemolytic disease of the newborn (HDN). They are often named for the family in which they were first discovered. There are 34 distinct low-incidence antigens, and some of the symbols assigned to the private antigens are By, Swa, Bi, NFLD, RASM, HJK, and ELO.

## Designation of Blood Group Systems

| No. | System name | System symbol | Gene name(s) |
|-----|-------------|---------------|--------------|
| 001 | ABO | ABO | *ABO* |
| 002 | MNS | MNS | *GYPA, GYPB, GYPE* |
| 003 | P | PI | *PI* |
| 004 | Rh | RH | *RHD, RHCE* |
| 005 | Lutheran | LU | *LU* |
| 006 | Kell | KEL | *KEL* |
| 007 | Lewis | LE | *FUT3* |
| 008 | Duffy | FY | *FY* |
| 009 | Kidd | JK | *JK* |
| 010 | Diego | DI | *AE1* |
| 011 | Yt | YT | *ACHE* |
| 012 | Xg | XG | *XG* |
| 013 | Scianna | SC | *SC* |
| 014 | Dombrock | DO | *DO* |
| 015 | Colton | CO | *AQPI* |
| 016 | Landsteiner-Wiener | LW | *LW* |
| 017 | Chido/Rodgers | CH/RG | *C4A, C4B* |
| 018 | Hh | H | *FUTI* |
| 019 | Kx | XK | *XK* |
| 020 | Gerbich | GE | *GYPC* |
| 021 | Cromer | CROM | *DAF* |
| 022 | Knops | KN | *CRI* |
| 023 | Indian | IN | *CD44* |
| 024 | Ok | Ok$^a$ | *Ok$^a$* |
| 025 | RAPH | MER | *MER* |

Adapted from Daniels GL, Anstee DJ, Cartron JP et al. Terminology for red cell surface antigens. *Vox Sanguinis* 1999; 77:52–57.

# Common Questions About Infection Surveillance, Prevention, and Control

S. Samantha M. Tweeten, MPH
University of California, San Diego/San Diego State University Joint Doctoral Program (Epidemiology)

Marguerite McMillan Jackson, RN, PhD, CIC, FAAN
Administrative Director, Nursing Research and Education
Associate Clinical Professor for Family and Preventive Medicine
University of California, San Diego Medical Center

Leland S. Rickman, MD
Director, Epidemiology Unit
Associate Clinical Professor of Medicine,
Division of Infectious Diseases
University of California, San Diego Medical Center

Infection surveillance, prevention and control (IC) has been an important part of hospital practices since Florence Nightingale identified infection as a major problem in the hospitals of London in the mid-1800s. As a recognized, organized part of the modern hospital, IC developed in part as a response to nationwide nosocomial *Staphylococcus aureus* infections in the late 1950s. In the United States, approximately 19,000 deaths are attributed to nosocomial infections each year, and nosocomial infections contribute to an additional 58,000 deaths annually. In 1976, the Joint Commission on Accreditation of Health Care Organizations (JCAHO) emphasized the importance of nosocomial infections as potentially preventable and controllable. Subsequently, the Centers for Disease Control and Prevention (CDC) and the Hospital Infection Control Practices Advisory Committee (HICPAC) have produced a number of evidence-based guidelines for implementation of IC practices.

The principal goals in IC are to protect the patient, protect the health care worker, visitors, and others in the health care environment, and to accomplish these goals in a cost-effective manner. If IC is performed in an integrated manner with health care practice, it can reduce infection risks and provide protection for all those involved in the process.

## What Level of Staffing Is Recommended for an Effective Infection Surveillance, Prevention, and Control Program?

The investigative personnel in the hospital infection surveillance, prevention, and control program consist of the hospital epidemiologist and one or more infection control professionals (ICP). Most hospital epidemiologists are clinicians with training in internal medicine or pediatrics and in infectious diseases. Many have additional training in epidemiology. Occasionally, a pathologist with an interest in microbiology may be seen in this post. Epidemiologists should be compensated adequately for their time and services.

The ICP is fundamental to the infection surveillance, prevention, and control program and provides surveillance, education and consultation for other departments, reporting important information and surveillance data to the CDC as appropriate, and many other services. ICPs are frequently registered nurses, often with bachelor's degrees. Others functioning in this capacity may be medical technologists or those with master's degrees in epidemiology. Certification is available from the Certification Board of Infection Control and Epidemiology [Certification in Infection Control (CIC)], and is recommended for at least some of the staff of a well-functioning program. It was recommended by the CDC in the 1970s that there be one ICP for every 250 occupied beds for a program to be effective. It is now recognized that the complexity and scope of the job of the ICP is such that it is difficult to define the required number of ICPs based on hospital census.

Administrative support is of great importance to an effective IC program. Areas covered may include data entry and typing of reports, minutes, policies, and correspondence. The IC program must also have access to appropriate computer support personnel, including those able to provide information on statistical analysis.

## What Is Being Done About Management of Needle-Stick Exposures and Prophylaxis?

Health care organizations should have available to their employees a system for dealing with exposures to blood, blood products, and other body fluids that may transmit blood-borne pathogens. This system should include written protocols for reporting, treatment, follow-up, and other aspects of care of the worker. Exposures of health care workers (HCWs) to body fluids should be followed up so that any measures available for the prevention of disease may be taken. An Exposure Report is the first step in this endeavor and should include the date and time of the exposure and details of the procedure, exposure, and exposure source. Treatment should be given at the exposure site if an injury has occurred. Assessment of the infection risk must be made. The source may be tested to determine if the patient in question potentially has human immunodeficiency virus (HIV), hepatitis B virus (HBV), hepatitis C virus (HCV), or other blood-borne pathogens.

Baseline testing is done to determine the immune status of the exposed HCW for the blood-borne pathogens in question. Postexposure prophylaxis (PEP) for several blood-borne pathogens is available. Before PEP is initiated, it should be carefully explained to the HCW in detail. This explanation must include the potential side effects and outcomes of the regimens available.

In the case of an HIV exposure, PEP should be started as soon as possible, preferably within two hours. Choice of PEP must be made on a case-by-case basis and take into consideration the health status of the HCW and the status of the source of exposure. If a HCW has only limited exposure of potentially infectious material to intact skin, PEP is not indicated. When the source is HIV seropositive but asymptomatic, has a high CD4 + count and a low viral load, and the exposure was small and to mucous membranes or nonintact skin, prophylaxis may not be warranted. If a large exposure has occurred (e.g., a deep puncture with a blood-filled needle), a basic regimen is recommended. This basic regimen consists of four weeks of zidovudine, 600 mg per day in two or three divided doses, and lamivudine, 150 mg twice daily. This basic regimen is also recommended when a percutaneous exposure of low potential for transmission of blood-borne pathogen occurs (such as a scratch with a blood-contaminated instrument or splash of blood to the eye), and the source has a low titer of virus.

If the source of exposure is considered to have a high viral load (e.g., advanced AIDS, primary HIV infection, high or increasing viral load, or low CD4 + count) and mucous membrane or skin with compromised integrity is exposed, the basic regimen is to be considered if the volume of fluid is small, and recommended if the volume of fluid is large. An expanded regimen consisting of the basic regimen and either indinavir, 800 mg every 8 hours, or nelfinavir, 750 mg three times a day, is recommend when a severe percutaneous exposure (e.g., blood-containing hollow needle, deep puncture, needle used in source patient's artery or vein) occurs. When the HIV status of the exposure source is unknown, the basic regimen should be considered, but may not be recommended depending on the specific information available.

Many HCWs have received HBV vaccine prior to the exposure event. If the HCW is known to be anti-HBs positive, this is taken into account in the PEP management. If the HCW is not immune to HBV, the immunization series is begun as soon as possible. Immunoglobulin (HBIG) is also indicated if the source is HBsAg positive. For HCV, there is no immunoglobulin available, nor is there an FDA-approved prophylaxis. Postexposure testing and monitoring for PEP toxicity must be included in any prophylaxis program.

## What Are the Current Recommendations on Varicella Vaccination for Health Care Workers?

All HCWs should be sure they are immune to varicella. This is particularly true of those who work with patients at risk for serious complications of varicella. These patients may include premature infants born to susceptible mothers, those born at less than 28 weeks or weighing less than 1000 g at birth, pregnant women, and immunocompromised persons. The complications of varicella can be devastating in adults. With the availability of vaccine, there is no reason for HCWs to be without acquired immunity if not naturally immune. Serologic screening prior to vaccination may be done if determined to be cost-effective by the institution.

In those HCWs who have been exposed but have unknown immune status, serologic testing is done to determine if he or she has had a previously unrecognized subclinical infection. The majority of American adults have been infected with varicella and are therefore immune. If the HCW is not immune at the time of exposure, the HCW must be furloughed for 10 to 21 days after the last exposure. Acyclovir may be considered in some circumstances. Postexposure vaccination has not been validated in adults and cannot be recommended at this time. Use of zoster immune globulin (VZIG) may be considered after exposure but is costly. It is often reserved for use in those who are at greatest risk of complications (e.g., immunocompromised persons).

## What Is the Recommendation for Controlling Vancomycin-Resistant Enterococci (VRE) in Hospital Settings?

The rate of infection and colonization of vancomycin-resistant enterococci (VRE) has increased in U.S. hospitals about 20-fold in the last decade. This, in turn, has led to recommendations to control the increase in VRE by HICPAC and other groups. The primary preventive measure is prudent vancomycin use.

Vancomycin use has been consistently reported as a risk factor for increased numbers of VRE infections and may contribute to increased resistance in *Staphylococcus aureus*. Health care institutions should develop comprehensive antimicrobial utilization plans. These are designed for use in educating staff, overseeing surgical prophylaxis and developing use guidelines for antimicrobials, including vancomycin. Clear guidelines on appropriate use of vancomycin in situations such as treatment of serious infections due to β-lactam-resistant gram-positive organisms, as well as addressing inappropriate use, can help prevent overuse.

Continuing education of staff will not only provide preventive information but also keep VRE in the minds of those who can directly impact development of resistance. The laboratory is also an important component in identification of specimens and patients with VRE. Standard precautions or body substance isolation (BSI) must be practiced consistently by all HCWs to prevent patient-to-patient transmission, and, in outbreak situations, cohorting of VRE-infected patients may be necessary to prevent spread. There is considerable controversy about the value of additional isolation precautions (e.g., contact precautions) primarily because a large proportion of persons with VRE are never identified and thus would not be placed in additional isolation precautions. Therefore, ensuring consistent use of standard precautions or BSI is more likely to reduce risks of person-to-person transmission (usually via hands of HCWs) than are special isolation precautions (e.g., contact precautions) for the few patients who are diagnosed or culture positive for VRE. A coordinated effort on the part of IC and patient care staff will limit the spread and problems associated with VRE.

## How Can Handwashing Help Reduce the Risk of Nosocomial Infection?

The hands can carry significant numbers of organisms, both normal flora and pathogens. Appropriate hand washing can reduce these numbers and potentially reduce transmission to patients. Soap and water provide mechanical reduction of transient microorganisms and removal of soil. Antimicrobial soaps provide additional inhibition of resident flora. Hand antiseptics can effectively inhibit organisms superficially, but have little or no effect on soiled hands.

Hands must be washed thoroughly with soap and water when visibly soiled, and with soap and water or by hand antisepsis before and after patient contact. Active hand antiseptic ingredients vary in effectiveness depending on the situation in which they are used and the organisms targeted. Some, such as cholorhexidine gluconate, are very effective against viruses but have limited use against fungi. Others may provide good antibacterial action but are limited against viruses. The choice of hand antiseptic must be made by those conversant with the intended use, advantages, disadvantages, costs and likely level of acceptance by product users. Without acceptance of a product, be it hand antiseptic or soap, handwashing becomes a moot point.

## How Far Is too Far in Isolation?

When appropriately used, isolation precautions in their myriad of forms can reduce the nosocomial spread of a number of organisms. Isolation precautions are designed to provide protection for staff and patients by limiting contact and transmission of organisms. A great deal has been written on the subject and many guidelines published, including those from the CDC and the Occupational Safety and Health Administration (OSHA). The key to appropriate isolation lies in knowing the situation and method by which organisms may be transmitted.

The fundamental element of isolation precautions is handwashing and gloving. Gloves provide a physical barrier and prevent gross contamination of the hands of staff. They also reduce the likelihood of staff transmitting organisms present on their hands to patients during patient care. Placement of patients may prove useful in limiting transmission of certain infections. Patients with easily transmitted organisms (e.g., varicella), or those patients in whom control of body substances is complicated (e.g., patients with uncontrolled diarrhea) may warrant separation from other patients.

HICPAC recommendations for isolation fall into two tiers. The first consists of the Standard Precautions, which incorporate both Universal Precautions and Body Substance Isolation. These are designed to reduce transmission of microorganisms from all sources, known and unknown, from bloodborne routes and all moist body substances. The second tier includes Transmission-Based Precautions, which are used for patients with documented infections of highly transmissible or epidemiologically important pathogens. This system allows the appropriate level of isolation to be implemented. If, for example, a patient has an infection spread by contact and is not airborne, the use of masks is not warranted but judicious use of gloves is. The HICPAC guidelines provide precautions for airborne, droplet and contact spread, but some of the recommendations are controversial, especially for nonhospital settings such as nursing homes.

## What Is Being Done to Control Methicillin-Resistant *Staphylococcus Aureus* (MRSA)?

How an institution sets about dealing with methicillin-resistant *Staphylococcus aureus* (MRSA) will largely be determined by type and level of care the facility provides. In the tertiary care setting, where MRSA is often endemic, a system must be established that is not overly expensive in direct costs or in labor and time. It must also be recognized that many colonized patients will be clinically inapparent, and, while the ultimate goal is elimination of MRSA, this is rarely possible.

The spread of MRSA by the hands of HCWs from patient to patient can be reduced by implementation and enforcement of a comprehensive BSI program or other similar systems. Common sites for infection or colonization are the nares and breaks in integument including wounds, tracheostomy sites, and intravenous catheter sites. Material from these sites may be carried from patient to patient on the hands of HCWs, although it has been shown that MRSA can be eliminated by simple handwashing with soap and water. Disposable gloves and other barriers, such as gowns if clothing might be soiled, followed by immediate handwashing when one leaves the patient's room will go a long way toward preventing transmission. These practices should be used consistently with all patients, regardless of knowledge of their MRSA status.

A system of surveillance, integrating both the microbiology laboratory and IC, will allow an institution to know when an outbreak occurs. Early detection of increased cases of MRSA allows for early intervention in the form of education of staff, possible treatment of HCWs identified as MRSA carriers, and cohorting of patients if all other interventions fail.

## What Happens When the Patient Leaves the Hospital?

It can be very difficult to identify patients with infections after they leave the hospital. Lack of integration of records among clinics, doctors' offices, and hospitals can mean lack of continuity in infection tracking. The CDC has proposed surveillance of surgical wound infections (SWI) as they are relatively consistent in presentation and methods of control. Estimates of 19% to 65% of all SWI being diagnosed after the patient has been discharged, and an optimal time of 28 days to detect 98% of all SWIs, both show the importance of postdischarge surveillance.

The best methodology for conducting postdischarge surveillance has yet to be determined but effectiveness is greatly increased by integration of follow-up clinic, home care and hospital records. A plan in which the IC unit is notified when an infection is seen by home care providers or a follow-up clinic should be implemented to increase identification of SWIs that become evident after the patient's discharge.

## How Is the Patient With Active Tuberculosis Controlled?

Recognition of the risk of nosocomial transmission of tuberculosis (TB) in the health care setting has led to increasing concern, particularly in the age of multiple drug resistance and HIV/AIDS. Particular problems arise in the case of patients in whom infection has not been identified at time of admission. Those with pulmonary or laryngeal tuberculosis can present substantial infection risk to others. Some procedures are more strongly associated with nosocomial transmission than others. Among these are bronchoscopy, endotracheal intubation and suctioning, and open abscess drainage. Cough-inducing procedures merit special attention.

The control of TB involves three goals: early identification, isolation, and treatment. The primary emphasis of the IC plan for TB is on achieving these goals by several means. These include use of administrative measures to reduce risk of exposure to infectious persons, the use of engineering controls to prevent transmission and decrease the concentration of droplet nuclei, and use of personal respiratory protective equipment.

Administrative measures include development and implementation of effective policies and protocols to ensure identification, evaluation, isolation and treatment in a timely manner; effective work practices; education and training of HCWs; and screening of HCWs for TB. Engineering controls include source control in exhaust ventilation, control of airflow direction to prevent contamination of adjacent areas, dilution and removal of contaminated air, and air cleaning by filtration or ultraviolet irradiation.

Personal protective equipment is used in situations in which the risk of infection is increased, including working in rooms where patients with active TB are cared for or when performing procedures with increased risk, such as cough-inducing or aerosol-generating procedures.

Coordination of discharge, with good planning for follow-up and notification of the local health department, are also of importance in managing the patient with active TB.

## What Are the Infection Control Issues Associated With Dialysis?

Both peritoneal dialysis and hemodialysis are performed on patients already at risk for serious infections because of their underlying disease state. Dialysis increases this risk by providing direct access to normally sterile areas of the body: the circulatory system or peritoneal cavity. The risk of infection can be reduced by strict use of aseptic technique during all procedures, strict disinfection and maintenance of all equipment, and a well-trained, knowledgeable staff, effective patient education, and monitoring.

In hemodialysis, when an internal arterivenous shunt is used, infection may result from a break in aseptic technique, bacterial seeding from other parts of the body and poor hygiene and care of the access site. When a graft arteriovenous fistula is made, infections are seen from the same causes as those with internal arteriovenous shunts, but there are additional potential complications because of the grafting material. A temporary access device, subclavian, jugular or femoral, also carries risk of infection, but this varies with type and location of the device. Requirements for strict aseptic technique hold for these devices as with others. The National Kidney Foundation-Dialysis Outcomes Quality Initiative (NKF-DOQI) has made a number of recommendations regarding specific types of access, devices and sites.

Patients must be instructed as to proper care of their access site, and the prevention of infection must be stressed. They should be taught to recognize the signs and symptoms of infection, such as fever, redness, puffiness, and drainage at the site. Remote sites of infection must be identified and treated as quickly as possible. Aseptic technique and appropriate cleansing of access sites before insertion will play an important role in prevention of infection. Water treatment is also of concern. Municipal water supplies may contain chemicals, bacteria, endotoxin, and other contaminants that must be removed before the water can be used in dialysis. With removal of chlorine from the water there is little to impede bacteria, so preventing introduction of bacteria becomes of prime importance.

Reuse of hemodialyzers has become common. The Association for Advancement of Medical Instrumentation (AAMI) has produced specific recommendations for reprocessing of dialyzers and their reuse. These standards encompass personnel training requirements, methods of cleaning, chemicals appropriate to reprocessing, and monitoring necessary for reuse of dialyzers.

Peritoneal dialysis involves using the peritoneal membrane for diffusion, and the removal of toxins, electrolytes, and fluid. Again, strict adherence to aseptic technique should be employed when dealing with the catheter or site. There are three types of infections of primary concern in peritoneal dialysis: exit site infections, subcutaneous tunnel infections and peritonitis. Sources of pathogens for these infections include the patient's skin or nares, contamination or break in technique in the delivery system, migration from the gastrointestinal tract and vaginal leaks. Risk factors for infection include staphylococcal nasal carriage, young age, lack of compliance with procedures, dialysate leak, skin breakdown at the exit site and trauma to the exit site or dislodging of the catheter cuff.

Infection is best prevented by use of strict aseptic technique when any manipulation is done. Use of a mask during connection and disconnection procedures may reduce transmission of *Staphylococcus aureus* from nasal passages. Exit sites must be kept clean and dry and patients instructed in care of the sites and infection prevention.

The primary way to prevent infection in those receiving dialysis is to adhere to the principles of aseptic technique. This and patient education will result in fewer infections and better outcomes.

## What Are the Infection Control Concerns in the Clinical Laboratory?

Laboratories are special work environments that may expose workers to particular hazards. Infections have been contracted in laboratories including tuberculosis, typhoid, streptococcal disease and hepatitis. Guidelines to protect workers and minimize transmission risk have been developed by a number of agencies and organizations. These include the National Committee for Clinical Laboratory Standards (NCCLS), OSHA, the American Association of Blood Banks (AABB), The College of American Pathologists (CAP), and the CDC.

Each laboratory must meet minimum standards in infection control as part of certification from the various agencies. These standards encompass training, policies and procedures, appropriate safety equipment, and programs for follow-up of exposures. For details in each of these areas, the reader is referred to the specific agencies.

An infection control program for the clinical laboratory must include a program to reduce the volume of hazardous waste generated, and there must be policies and procedures outlining how biohazardous waste will be controlled. This includes labeling of containers that do not leak and have tight-fitting lids. The OSHA Standard on Occupational Exposure to Bloodborne Pathogens must be complied with and be included in the hospital's plan for infection control. Each laboratory must have documented procedures regarding transport and processing of specimens, including appropriate labeling and containers to prevent leakage. Additional policies prohibiting the recapping, intentional bending or breaking or removing of needles from syringes must be part of the plan.

Personnel must be trained in the use of appropriate personal protective equipment, with periodic retraining. Those workers who can be reasonably expected to have contact with body fluids must have training on minimizing risk of exposure, routes of transmission, prevention of exposure, and follow-up procedures should exposure occur. They must be offered HBV vaccination free of charge. A documented tuberculosis control plan should be in place.

Sterilizing devices such as autoclaves should be monitored with biological equivalent indicators, and staff trained in their use and in the correct disposal of wastes.

Policies and procedures must be in place prohibiting smoking, eating, drinking, application of cosmetics—including lip balm—and manipulation of contact lenses. Additional policies must address pipetting by mouth, recordkeeping and periodical reviews of training and personnel issues. A copy of NCCLS and OSHA standards should be readily available to workers.

## Where Can One Get Up-to-Date Information on Infection Surveillance, Prevention, and Control?

Current information on infection surveillance, prevention and control can be found through CDC, and organizations such as the Association of Professionals in Infection Control and Epidemiology, Inc. (APIC), and the Society for Healthcare Epidemiology of America (SHEA). A great deal of information may be found on the World Wide Web and in organizational publications, including the CDC's *Morbidity and Mortality Weekly Report* and Reports and Recommendations, as well as the *American Journal of Infection Control* (AJIC) and the journal *Infection Control and Hospital Epidemiology* (ICHE), in which HICPAC reports and guidelines are published.

## References

Association for the Advancement of Medical Instrumentation. Dialysis. In: AAMI standards and recommended practices. Vol 3. Arlington, VA: American National Standard; 1993.

Centers for Disease Control and Prevention. Guidelines for preventing the transmission of tuberculosis in health-care facilities, 1994. *MMWR* 1994; 43 (RR-13): 1–132.

Centers for Disease Control and Prevention. Prevention of varicella: recommendations of the Advisory Committee on Immunization Practices (ACIP). *MMWR* 1996: 45 (RR-11): 1–36.

Centers for Disease Control and Prevention. Immunization of health-care workers: recommendations of the Advisory Committee on Immunization Practices (ACIP) and the Hospital Infection Control Practices Advisory Committee (HICPAC). *MMWR* 1997; 46 (RR-18): 1–42.

Centers for Disease Control and Prevention. Public Health Service guidelines for the management of health-care worker exposures to HIV and recommendations for postexposure prophylaxis. *MMWR* 1998; 47 (RR-7); 1–35.

Centers for Disease Control and Prevention. Recommendations for prevention and control of hepatitis C virus (HCV) infection and HCV-related chronic disease. *MMWR* 1998; 47 (RR-19): 1–39.

Dieckhause KD, Cooper BW. Infection control concepts in critical care. *Critical Care Clinics* 1998; 14 (1): 55–70.

Garcia-Houchins, S. Dialysis. In: Pfeiffer JA, ed. APIC text of infection control and epidemiology. Washington, DC: Association for Professionals in Infection Control, Inc.; 2000: 64-1–64-15.

Garner JS, the Hospital Infection Control Practices Advisory Committee. Guidelines for isolation precautions in hospitals. *Am J Infect Control* 1996; 24: 24–52.

Hospital Infection Control Practices Advisory Committee. Recommendations for preventing the spread of vancomycin resistance: recommendations of the Hospital Infection Control Practices Advisory Committee (HICPAC). *Am J Infect Control* 1995; 23 (2): 87–94.

Jackson MM, Lynch P. Invited commentary: guideline for isolation precautions in hospitals, 1996. *Am J Infect Control* 1996; 24: 203–206.

Larson EL. APIC guidelines for handwashing and hand antisepsis in health care settings. *Am J Infect Control* 1995; 23 (4): 251–269.

Luebbert PP. Infection control in clinical laboratories. In: Pfeiffer JA, ed. APIC text of infection control and epidemiology. Washington, DC: Association for Professionals in Infection Control, Inc; 2000: 63-1–64-12.

Maki DG. Infections due to infusion therapy. In: Bennett JVf, Brachman PS, eds. Hospital infections, 3rd ed. Boston: Little, Brown: 1992: 849–898.

Mulligan ME, Murray-Leisure KA, Standiford HC, John JF, Korvick JA, Kauffman CA, Yu VL. Methicillin-resistant *Staphylococcus aureus:* A consensus review of the microbiology, pathogenesis, and epidemiology with implications for prevention and management. *Am J Med* 1993; 94: 313–328.

National Committee for Clinical Laboratory Standards. Clinical laboratory hazardous waste. Wayne, PA: National Committee for Clinical Laboratory Standards; 1997.

National Committee for Clinical Laboratory Standards. Protection of laboratory workers from instrument biohazards and infectious disease transmitted by blood, body fluids, and tissues; M29-A. Wayne, PA: National Committee for Clinical Laboratory Standards; 1997.

National Kidney Foundation, Dialysis Outcomes Quality Initiative. Clinical practice guidelines for vascular access. *Am J Kidney Dis* 1997; 30(suppl 4): S140–S189.

Occupational Safety and Health Administration. Occupational exposure to bloodborne pathogens: 29 CFR 1910.1030. Washington, DC: US Government Printing Office; 1999.

Scheckler WE, Brimhall D, Buch AS, Farr BM, Friedman C, Garibaldi RA, Gross PA, Harris J-A, Hierholzer WJ, Martone WJ, MacDonald LL, Soloman SL. Requirements for infrastructure and essential activities of infection control and epidemiology in hospitals: A Consensus Panel report. *Am J Infect Control* 1998; 26: 47–60.

Sheretz RJ, Garibaldi RA, Marosok RD, Mayhall CG, Sheckler WE, Berg R, Gaynes RP, Jarvis WR, Martone WJ, Lee JT Jr. Consensus paper on the surveillance of surgical wound infections. *Am J Infect Control* 1992; 20: 263–270.

The Joint Commission on the Accreditation of Healthcare Organizations. 1998 hospital accreditation standards. Oakbrook Terrace, IL: JCAHO; 1998; 185–186.

US Department of Health and Human Services. Biosafety in microbiological and biomedical laboratory (HHS Publication No. (NIH)88-8395). Washington, DC: US Government Printing Office; 1998.

Wenzel RP, Reagan DR, Bertino JS Jr, Baron EJ, Arias K. Methicillin-resistant *Staphylococcus aureus* outbreak: A consensus panel's definition and management guidelines. *Am J Infect Control* 1998; 26: 101–110.

---

Adapted from Tweeten SSM, Jackson MM, Rickman LS. The ten most common questions about infection surveillance, prevention and control. *Infect Dis Clin Pract* 1999; 8: 274–278.

# Infection Control for the Dental Office: A Checklist

## Immunization

- Health care workers should have appropriate immunizations such as that for hepatitis B virus.

## Before Patient Treatment

- Obtain a thorough medical history.
- Disinfect prostheses and appliances received from the laboratory.
- Place disposable coverings to prevent contamination of surfaces, or disinfect surfaces after treatment.
- Set out supplies and instruments needed for the procedure.
- Flush waterlines before connecting handpieces, syringes, or scalers.

## During Patient Treatment

- Treat all patients as potentially infectious.
- Use protective attire and barrier techniques when contact with body fluids or mucous membranes is anticipated.
  - Wear gloves.
  - Wear a mask.
  - Wear protective eyewear.
  - Wear a uniform, laboratory coat, or gown.
- Disinfect film packets before taking them into the darkroom.
- Open intraorally contaminated x-ray film packets in the darkroom with disposable gloves without touching the films.
- Use aseptic technique to retrieve additional items.
- Minimize formation of droplets, spatters, and aerosols.
- Use a rubber dam to isolate the tooth and field when appropriate.
- Use high-volume vacuum evacuation.
- Protect hands
  - Wash hands before gloving and after gloves are removed.
  - Change gloves between each patient.
  - Discard gloves that are torn, cut, or punctured.
  - Avoid hand injuries.
- Avoid injury with sharp instruments and needles.
  - Handle sharp items carefully.
  - Do not bend or break disposable needles.
  - If needles are not recapped, place them in a separate field. If recapping is necessary, use a method that protects hands from injury, such as a holder for the cap.
  - Place sharp items in appropriate containers.
  - Remove burs from handpieces when not in use.

## After Patient Treatment

- Wear heavy-duty rubber gloves.
- Clean instruments thoroughly.
- Heat-sterilize instruments.
  - Sterilize instruments that penetrate soft tissue or bone
  - Sterilize all instruments that come in contact with oral mucous membranes and body fluids, and all instruments that have been contaminated by secretions of patients. Otherwise, use appropriate chemical sterilization.

-Wrap instruments for sterilization to maintain sterility until use. Do not reuse single-use wraps.

-Monitor the sterilizer with biological monitors.

-Clean handpieces, dental units, and ultrasonic scalers.

-Flush handpieces, dental units, ultrasonic scalers, and air/water syringes between patients.

-Clean and sterilize air/water syringes or use disposable tips.

-Clean and sterilize ultrasonic scalers if possible; otherwise, disinfect them appropriately.

-Clean and sterilize handpieces.

-Process single-use water delivery systems according to the manufacturer's directions.

- Handle sharp instruments with caution.
  -Place disposable needles, scalpels, and other sharp items intact into puncture-resistant containers before disposal.
- Replace any disposable surface covers on environmental surfaces.
- Decontaminate environmental surfaces.
  -Wipe work surfaces with absorbent toweling to remove debris, and dispose of this toweling appropriately.
  -Disinfect with suitable chemical disinfectant.
  -Change protective coverings on light handles, the x-ray unit head, and other items.
- Decontaminate supplies and materials.
  -Rinse and disinfect impressions, bite registrations, and appliances to be sent to the laboratory.
- Communicate the infection control program to the dental laboratory.
- Dispense a small amount of pumice in a disposable container for individual use on each case and discard any excess.
- Remove contaminated wastes appropriately.
  -Pour blood, suctioned fluids, and other liquid waste into a drain connected to a sanitary sewer system.
  -Place solid waste contaminated with blood or saliva in sealed, sturdy impervious bags labeled "biohazard" and dispose of according to local government regulations.
- Remove gloves and wash hands.

## Daily
- Flush cleansing solution through evacuation lines, and clean or replace the unit's solid waste filter traps.
- Flush waterlines for 2–3 minutes after periods of nonuse if waterlines were not drained.
- If in-line water filters are used, change daily.
- For in-line check valves, change daily or as directed by the manufacturer.

## Overnight
- If possible, drain waterlines for dry storage periods of nonuse (overnight, weekends).

## Weekly
- Clean and disinfect the main evacuation trap.
- Clean and disinfect inside and outside of drawers and cabinets.
- Perform weekly disinfection procedures on waterlines as directed by the manufacturer.

---

Adapted from Cottone JA, Terezhalmy GT, Molinari JA. Practical infection control in dentistry, 3rd ed. Baltimore: Lippincott Williams & Wilkins, 2001.

# Laboratory Reference Range Values

Show-Hong Duh, PhD, DABCC, Department of Pathology
University of Maryland School of Medicine
Janine Denis Cook, PhD, Department of Medical and Research Technology
University of Maryland School of Medicine

Reference range values are for apparently healthy individuals and often overlap significantly with values for persons who are sick. Actual values may vary significantly due to differences in assay methodologies and standardization. Institutions may also set up their own reference ranges based on the particular populations they serve; thus, there can be regional differences. Consequently, values reported by individual laboratories may differ from those listed in this appendix.

All values are given in conventional and SI units. However, where the SI units have not been widely accepted, conventional units are used. In case of the heterogenous nature of the materials measured or uncertainty about the exact molecular weight of the compounds, the SI system cannot be followed, and mass per volume is used as the unit of concentration.

## Abbreviations

**ACD,** acid-citrate-dextrose; **CHF,** congestive heart failure; **Cit,** citrate; **CNS,** central nervous system; **CSF,** cerebrospinal fluid; **cyclic AMP,** cyclic adenosine $3',5'$-monophosphate; **EDTA,** ethylenediaminetetraacetic acid; **HDL,** high-density lipoprotein; **Hep,** heparin; **LDL-C,** low-density lipoprotein-cholesterol; **Ox,** oxalate; **RBC,** red blood cell(s); **RIA,** radioimmunoassay, **SD,** standard deviation

## References

Burtis CA, Ashwood ER, eds. Tietz textbook of clinical chemistry, 3rd ed. Philadelphia: WB Saunders, 1998.

Clinical chemistry laboratory: Reference range values in clinical chemistry. Professional services manual. Baltimore, Department of Pathology, University of Maryland Medical System, 1999.

Harmening DM, ed. Hematologic values in clinical hematology and fundamentals of hemostasis, 2nd ed. Philadelphia: FA Davis, 1992.

National cholesterol education program: Report of the expert panel on detection, evaluation, and treatment of high blood cholesterol in adults. *Arch Intern Med* 1988; 148:36–99.

Triglyceride, high density lipoprotein, and coronary heart disease. National Institute of Health Consensus Statement, NIH Consensus Development Conference, 1992; 10(2).

| Test | Conventional Units | SI Units |
|------|--------------------|----------|
| Acetaminophen, serum or plasma (Hep or EDTA) | | |
|    Therapeutic | 10–30 μg/mL | 66–199 μmol/L |
|    Toxic | >200 μg/ml | >1324 μmol/L |
| Acetone | | |
|   Serum | | |
|     Qualitative | Negative | Negative |
|     Quantitative | 0.3–2.0 mg/dL | 0.05–0.34 mmol/L |
|   Urine | | |
|     Qualitative | Negative | Negative |
| Acid hemolysis test (Ham) | <5% lysis | <0.05 lysed fraction |
| Adrenocorticotropin (ACTH), plasma | | |
|   8 AM | <120 pg/mL | <26 pmol/L |
|   Midnight (supine) | <10 pg/mL | <2.2 pmol/L |
| *Alanine Aminotransferase (ALT, SGPT), serum | | |
|   Male | 13–40 U/L (37°C) | 0.22–0.68 μkat/L (37° C) |
|   Female | 10–28 U/L (37°C) | 0.17–0.48 μkat/L (37° C) |
| Albumin | | |
|   Serum | | |
|     Adult | 3.5–5.2 g/dL | 35–52 g/L |
|     >60 y | 3.2–4.6 g/dL | 32–46 g/L |
| | Avg. of 0.3 g/dL higher in upright individuals | Avg. of 3 g/dL higher in upright individuals |
|   Urine | | |
|     Qualitative | Negative | Negative |
|     Quantitative | 50–80 mg/24 h | 50–80 mg/24 h |
|     CSF | 10–30 mg/dL | 100–300 mg/dL |
| *Aldolase, serum | 1.0–7.5 U/L (30° C) | 0.02–0.13 μkat/L (30° C) |
| Aldosterone | | |
|   Serum | | |
|     Supine | 3–16 ng/dL | 0.08–0.44 nmol/L |
|     Standing | 7–30 ng/dL | 0.19–0.83 nmol/L |
|     Urine | 3–19 μg/24 h | 8–51 nmol/24 h |
| Amikacin, serum or plasma (EDTA) | | |
|   Therapeutic | | |
|     Peak | 25–35 μg/mL | 43–60 μmol/L |
|     Trough | | |
|       Less severe infection | 1–4 μg/mL | 1.7–6.8μmol/L |
|       Life-threatening infection | 4–8 μg/mL | 6.8–13.7 μmol/L |
|   Toxic | | |
|     Peak | >35–40 μg/mL | >60–68 μmol/L |
|     Trough | >10–15 μg/mL | >17–26 μmol/L |
| ∂-Aminolevulinic acid, urine | 1.3–7.0 mg/24 h | 10–53 μmol/24 h |
| Amitriptyline, serum or plasma (Hep or EDTA); trough (≥12 h after dose) | | |
|   Therapeutic | 80–250 ng/mL | 289–903 nmol/L |
|   Toxic | >500 ng/mL | >1805 nmol/L |
| Ammonia | | |
|   Plasma (Hep) | 9–33 μmol/L | 9–33 μmol/L |
| *Amylase | | |
|   Serum | 27–131 U/L | 0.46–2.23 μkat/L |
|   Urine | 1–17 U/h | 0.017–0.29 μkat/h |
| Amylase/creatine clearance ratio | 1–4% | 0.01–0.04 |
| Androstenedione, serum | | |
|   Male | 75–205 ng/dL | 2.6–7.2 nmol/L |
|   Female | 85–275 ng/dL | 3.0–9.6 nmol/L |

*Test values are method dependent.

| Test | Conventional Units | SI Units |
|---|---|---|
| Anion gap | | |
| (Na − (Cl + HCO₃)) | 7–16 mEq/L | 7–16 mmol/L |
| ((Na + K) − (Cl + HCO₃)) | 10–20 mEq/L | 10–20 mmol/L |
| $\alpha_1$-Antitrypsin, serum | 78–200 mg/dL | 0.78–2.00 g/L |
| Apolipoprotein A-1 | | |
| Male | 94–178 mg/dL | 0.94–1.78 g/L |
| Female | 101–199 mg/dL | 1.01–1.99 g/L |
| Apolipoprotein B | | |
| Male | 63–133 mg/dL | 0.63–1.33 g/L |
| Female | 60–126 mg/dL | 0.60–1.26 g/L |
| Arsenic | | |
| Whole blood (Hep) | 0.2–2.3 µg/dL | 0.03–0.31 µmol/L |
| Chronic poisoning | 10–50 µg/dL | 1.33–6.65 µmol/L |
| Acute poisoning | 60–930 µg/dL | 7.98–124 µmol/L |
| Urine, 24 h | 5–50 µg/d | 0.07–0.67 µmol/d |
| Ascorbic acid, plasma (Ox, Hep, EDTA) | 0.4–1.5 mg/dL | 23–85 µmol/L |
| *Aspartate aminotransferase (AST, SGOT), serum | | |
| | 10–59 U/L (37°C) | 0.17–1.00 −2 to +3 kat/L (37°C) |
| Base excess, blood (Hep) | −2 to +3 mmol/L | −2 to +3 mmol/L |
| Bicarbonate, serum (venous) | 22–29 mmol/L | 22–29 mmol/L |
| *Bilirubin | | |
| Serum | | |
| Adult | | |
| Conjugated | 0.0–0.3 mg/dL | 0–5 µmol/L |
| Unconjugated | 0.1–1.1 mg/dL | 1.7–19 µmol/L |
| Delta | 0–0.2 mg/dL | 0–3 µmol/L |
| Total | 0.2–1.3 mg/L | 3–22 µmol/L |
| Neonates | | |
| Conjugated | 0–0.6 mg/dL | 0–10 µmol/L |
| Unconjugated | 0.6–10.5 mg/dL | 10–180 µmol/L |
| Total | 1.5–12 mg/dL | 1.7–180 µmol/L |
| Urine, qualitative | Negative | Negative |
| Bone marrow, differential cell count | | |
| Adult | | |
| Undifferentiated cells | 0–1% | 0–0.01 |
| Myeloblast | 0–2% | 0–0.02 |
| Promyelocyte | 0–4% | 0–0.04 |
| Myelocytes | | |
| Neutrophilic | 5–20% | 0.05–0.20 |
| Eosinophilic | 0–3% | 0–0.03 |
| Basophilic | 0–1% | 0–0.01 |
| Metamyelocytes and bands | | |
| Neutrophilic | 5–35% | 0.05–0.35 |
| Eosinophilic | 0–5% | 0–0.05 |
| Basophilic | 0–1% | 0–0.01 |
| Segmented neutrophils | 5–15% | 0.05–0.15 |
| Pronormoblast | 0–1.5% | 0–0.015 |
| Basophilic normoblast | 0–5% | 0–0.05 |
| Polychromatophilic normoblast | 5–30% | 0.05–0.30 |
| Orthochromatic normoblast | 5–10% | 0.05–0.10 |
| Lymphocytes | 10–20% | 0.10–0.20 |
| Plasma cells | 0–2% | 0–0.02 |
| Monocytes | 0–5% | 0–0.05 |
| CA 125, serum | <35 U/mL | <35 kU/L |
| CA 15–3, serum | <30 U/mL | <30 kU/L |
| CA 19–9, serum | <37 U/mL | <37 kU/L |
| Cadmium, whole blood (Hep) | 0.1–0.5 µg/dL | 8.9–44.5 nmol/L |
| Toxic | 10–300 µg/dL | 0.89–26.70 µmol/L |

*Test values are method dependent.

| Test | Conventional Units | SI Units |
|---|---|---|
| Cadmium, urine, 24 h | <15 μg/d | <0.13 μmol/d |
| Calcitonin, serum or plasma | | |
|   Male | ≤100 pg/mL | ≤100 ng/L |
|   Female | ≤30 pg/mL | ≤30 ng/L |
| Calcium, serum | 8.6–10.0 mg/dL (Slightly higher in children) | 2.15–2.50 mmol/L (Slightly higher in children) |
| Calcium, ionized, serum | 4.64–5.28 mg/dl | 1.16–1.32 mmol/L |
| Calcium, urine | | |
|   Low calcium diet | 50–150 mg/24 h | 1.25–3.75 mmol/24 h |
|   Usual diet; trough | 100–300 mg/24 h | 2.50–7.50 mmol/24 h |
| Carbamazepine, serum or plasma (Hep or EDTA); trough | | |
|   Therapeutic | 4–12 μg/mL | 17–51 μmol/L |
|   Toxic | >15 μg/mL | >63 μmol/L |
| Carbon dioxide, total serum/plasma (Hep) | 22–28 mmol/L | 22–28 mmol/L |
| Carbon dioxide ($PCO_2$), blood arterial | Male 35–48 mmHg Female 32–45 mmHg | 4.66–6.38 kPa 4.26–5.99 kPa |
| Carbon monoxide as carboxyhemoglobin (HbCO), whole blood (EDTA) | | |
|   Nonsmokers | 0.5–1.5% total Hb | 0.005–0.015 HbCO fraction |
|   Smokers | | |
|     1–2 packs/d | 4–5% total Hb | 0.04–0.05 HbCO fraction |
|     >2 packs/d | 8–9% total Hb | 0.08–0.09 HbCO fraction |
|   Toxic | >20% total Hb | >0.20 HbCO fraction |
|   Lethal | >50% total Hb | >0.50 HbCO fraction |
| Carotene, serum | 10–85 μg/dL | 0.19–1.58 μmol/L |
| Catecholamines, plasma (EDTA) | | |
|   Dopamine | <30 pg/mL | <196 pmol/L |
|   Epinephrine | <140 pg/mL | <764 pmol/L |
|   Norepinephrine | <1700 pg/mL | <10,047 pmol/L |
| Catecholamines, urine | | |
|   Dopamine | 65–400 μg/24 h | 425–2610 nmol/24 h |
|   Epinephrine | 0–20 μg/24 h | 0–109 nmol/24 |
|   Norepinephrine | 15–80 μg/24 h | 89–473 nmol/24 |
| CEA, serum | | |
|   Nonsmokers | <5.0 ng/mL | <5.0 μg/L |

| *Cell counts, adult | | | |
|---|---|---|---|
|   RBC Male | $4.7–6.1 \times 10^6/\mu L$ | | $4.7–6.1 \times 10^{12}/L$ |
|     Female | $4.2–5.4 \times 10^6/\mu L$ | | $4.2–5.4 \times 10^{12}/L$ |
|   Leukocytes | | | |
|     Total | $4.8–10.8 \times 10^3/\mu L$ | | $4.8–10.8 \times 10^6/L$ |
|     Differential | Percentage | Absolute | Absolute (SI) |
|       Myelocytes | 0 | 0/μL | 0/L |
|       Neutrophils | | | |
|         Bands | 3–5 | 150–400/μL | $150–400 \times 10^6/L$ |
|         Segmented | 54–62 | 3000–5800/μL | $3000–5800 \times 10^6/L$ |
|       Lymphocytes | 20.5–51.1 | $1.2–3.4 \times 10^3/\mu L$ | $1.2–3.4 \times 10^9/L$ |
|       Monocytes | 1.7–9.3 | $0.11–0.59 \times 10^3/\mu L$ | $0.11–0.59 \times 10^9/L$ |
|       Granulocytes | 42.2–75.2 | $1.4–6.5 \times 10^3/\mu L$ | $1.4–6.5 \times 10^9/L$ |
|       Eosinophils | | $0.07 \times 10^3/\mu L$ | $0.07 \times 10^9/L$ |
|       Basophils | | $0–0.2 \times 10^3/\mu L$ | $0–0.2 \times 10^9/L$ |
|     Platelets | $130–400 \times 10^3/\mu L$ | | $130–400 \times 10^9/L$ |
|     Reticulocytes | 0.5–1.5% red cells | | 0.005–0.015 of RBC |
| | 24,000–84.000/μL | | $24–84 \times 10^9/L$ |
| Cells, CSF | 0–10 lymphocytes /mm³ 0 RBC/ mm³ | | 0–10 lymphocytes /mm³ 0 RBC/ mm³ |

*Test values are method dependent.

| Test | Conventional Units | SI Units |
|---|---|---|
| Ceruloplasmin, serum | 20–60 mg/dL | 0.2–6.0 g/L |
| Chloramphenicol, serum or plasma (Hep or EDTA); trough | | |
|   Therapeutic | 10–25 µg/mL | 31–77 µmol/L |
|   Toxic | >25 µg/mL | >77 µmol/L |
| Chloride | | |
|   Serum or plasma | 98–107 mmol/L | 98–107 mmol/L |
|   Sweat | | |
|     Normal | 5–35 mmol/L | 5–35 mmol/L |
|     Cystic fibrosis | 60–200 mmol/L | 60–200 mmol/L |
|   Urine, 24 h (vary greatly with Cl intake) | | |
|     Infant | 2–10 mmol/24 h | 2–10 mmol/24 h |
|     Child | 15–40 nmol/24 h | 15–40 mmol/24 h |
|     Adult | 110–250 mmol/24 h | 110–250 mmol/24 h |
|   CSF | 118–332 mmol/L (20 mmol/L higher than serum) | 118–332 mmol/L (20 mmol/L higher than serum) |
| Cholesterol, serum | | |
|   Adult desirable | <200 mg/dL | <5.2 mmol/L |
|     borderline | 200–239 mg/dL | 5.2–6.2 mmol/L |
|     high risk | ≥240 mg/dL | ≥6.2 mmol/L |
| *Cholinesterase, serum | 4.9–11.9 U/mL | 4.9–11.9 kU/L |
|   Dibucaine inhibition | 79–84% | 0.79–0.84 |
|   Fluoride inhibition | 58–64% | 0.58–0.64 |
| *Chorionic gonadotropin, intact | | |
|   Serum or plasma (EDTA) | | |
|     Male and nonpregnant female | <5.0 mIU/mL | <5.0 IU/L |
|     Pregnant female | Varies with gestational age | |
|   Urine, qualitative | | |
|     Male and nonpregnant female | Negative | Negative |
|     Pregnant female | Positive | Positive |
| Clonazepam, serum or plasma (Hep or EDTA); trough | | |
|   Therapeutic | 15–60 ng/mL | 48–190 nmol/L |
|   Toxic | >80 ng/mL | >254 nmol/L |
| Coagulation tests | | |
|   Antithrombin III (synthetic substrate) | 80–120% of normal | 0.8–1.2 of normal |
|   Bleeding time (Duke) | 0–6 min | 0–6 min |
|   Bleeding time (Ivy) | 1–6 min | 1–6 min |
|   Bleeding time (template) | 2.3–9.5 min | 2.3–9.5 min |
|   Clot retraction, qualitative | 50–100% in 2 h | 0.5–1.0/2 h |
| Coagulation time (Lee-White) | 5–15 min (glass tubes) | 5–15 min (glass tubes) |
| | 19–60 min (siliconized tubes) | 19–60 min (siliconized tubes) |
| Cold hemolysin test (Donath-Landsteiner) | No hemolysis | No hemolysis |
| Complement components | | |
|   Total hemolytic complement activity, plasma (EDTA) | 75–160 U/mL | 75–160 kU/L |
|   Total complement decay rate (functional), plasma (EDTA) | 10–20% Deficiency: >50% | Fraction decay rate: 0.10–0.20 >0.50 |
|   C1q, serum | 14.9–22.1 mg/dL | 149–221 mg/L |
|   C1r, serum | 2.5–10.0 mg/dL | 25–100 mg/L |
|   C1s(C1 esterase), serum | 5.0–10.0 mg/dL | 50–100 mg/L |
|   C2, serum | 1.6–3.6 mg/dL | 16–36 mg/L |
|   C3, serum | 90–180 mg/dL | 0.9–1.8 g/L |
|   C4, serum | 10–40 mg/dL | 0.1–0.4 g/L |
|   C5, serum | 5.5–11.3 mg/dL | 55–113 mg/L |
|   C6, serum | 17.9–23.9 mg/dL | 179–239 mg/L |
|   C7, serum | 2.7–7.4 mg/dL | 27–74 mg/L |

*Test values are method dependent.

| Test | Conventional Units | SI Units |
|------|-------------------|----------|
| C8, serum | 4.9–10.6 mg/dL | 49–106 mg/L |
| C9, serum | 3.3–9.5 mg/dL | 33–95 mg/L |
| Coombs test | | |
|   Direct | Negative | Negative |
|   Indirect | Negative | Negative |
| Copper | | |
|   Serum | | |
|     Male | 70–140 μg/dL | 11–22 μmol/L |
|     Female | 80–155 μg/dL | 13–24 μmol/L |
|   Urine | 3–35 μg/24 h | 0.05–0.55 μmol/24 h |
| Corpuscular values of erythrocytes | | |
|   (values are for adults; in children | | |
|   values vary with age) | | |
|   Mean corpuscular hemoglobin (MCH) | 27–31 pg | 0.42–0.48 fmol |
|   Mean corpuscular hemoglobin | | |
|     concentration (MCHC) | 33–37 g/dL | 330–370 g/L |
|   Mean corpuscular volume (MCV) | Male 80–94 $\mu^3$ | 80–94 fL |
| | Female 81–99 $\mu^3$ | 81–99 fL |
| Cortisol, serum | | |
|   Plasma (Hep, EDTA, Ox) | | |
|     8 AM | 5–23 μg/dL | 138–635 nmol/L |
|     4 PM | 3–16 μg/dL | 83–441 nmol/L |
|     10 PM | <50% of 8 AM value | <0.5 of 8 AM value |
|   Free, urine | <50 μg/24 h | <138 mmol/24 h |
| †*Creatine kinase (CK), serum | | |
|   Male | 15–105 U/L (30°C) | 0.26–1.79 μkat/L (30°C) |
|   Female | 10–80 U/L (30°C) | 0.17–1.36 μkat/L (30°C) |
|   Note: Strenuous exercise or intramuscular injections may cause transient elevation of CK. | | |
| *Creatine kinase MB isoenzyme, serum | 0–7 ng/mL | 0–7 μg/l |
| *Creatinine | | |
|   Serum or plasma, adult | | |
|     Male | 0.7–1.3 mg/dL | 62–115 μmol/L |
|     Female | 0.6–1.1 mg/dL | 53–97 μmol/L |
|   Urine | | |
|     Male | 14–26 mg/kg body weight/24 h | 124–230 μmol/kg body weight/24 h |
|     Female | 11–20 mg/kg body weight/24 h | 97–177 μmol/kg body weight/24 h |
| *Creatinine clearance, serum or plasma | | |
|   and urine | | |
|     Male | 94–140 mL/min/1.73 m² | 0.91–1.35 mL/s/m² |
|     Female | 72–110 mL/min/1.73 m² | 0.69–1.06 mL/s/m² |
| Cryoglobulins, serum | 0 | 0 |
| Cyanide | | |
|   Serum | | |
|     Nonsmokers | 0.004 mg/L | 0.15 μmol/L |
|     Smokers | 0.006 mg/L | 0.23 μmol/L |
|     Nitroprusside therapy | 0.01–0.06 mg/L | 0.38–2.30 μmol/L |
|     Toxic | >0.1 mg/L | >3.84 μmol/L |
|   Whole blood (Ox) | | |
|     Nonsmokers | 0.016 mg/L | 0.61 μmol/L |
|     Smokers | 0.041 mg/L | 1.57 μmol/L |
|     Nitroprusside therapy | 0.05–0.5 mg/L | 1.92–19.20 μmol/L |
|     Toxic | >1 mg/L | >38.40 μmol/L |

*Test values are method dependent.
†Test values are race dependent.

| Test | Conventional Units | SI Units |
|---|---|---|
| Cyclic AMP | | |
| Plasma (EDTA) | | |
| Male | 4.6–8.6 ng/mL | 14–26 nmol/L |
| Female | 4.3–7.6 ng/mL | 13–23 nmol/L |
| Urine, 24 h | 0.3–3.6 mg/d | 100–723 μmol/d or |
| | or 0.29–2.1 mg/g creatinine | 100–723 μmol/mol creatinine |
| Cystine or cysteine, urine, qualitative | Negative | Negative |
| *C-Peptide, serum | 0.78–1.89 ng/mL | 0.26–0.62 nmol/L |
| C-Reactive protein, serum | <0.5 mg/dL | <5 mg/L |
| ‡*Cyclosporine, whole blood | | |
| Therapeutic, trough | 100–200 ng/mL | 83–166 nmol/L |
| Dehydroepiandrosterone (DHEA), serum | | |
| Male | 180–1250 ng/dL | 6.2–43.3 nmol/L |
| Female | 130–980 ng/dL | 4.5–34.0 nmol/L |
| Dehydroepiandrosterone sulfate (DHEAS) serum or plasma (Hep, EDTA) | | |
| Male | 59–452 μg/dL | 1.6–12.2 μmol/L |
| Female | | |
| Premenopausal | 12–379 μg/dL | 0.8–10.2 μmol/L |
| Postmenopausal | 30–260 μg/dL | 0.8–7.1 μmol/L |
| Desipramine, serum or plasma (Hep or EDTA); trough (12 h after dose) | | |
| Therapeutic | 75–300 ng/mL | 281–1125 nmol/L |
| Toxic | >400 ng/mL | >1500 nmol/L |
| Diazepam, serum or plasma (Hep or EDTA); trough | | |
| Therapeutic | 100–1000 ng/mL | 0.35–3.51 μmol/L |
| Toxic | >5000 ng/mL | >17.55 μmol/L |
| Digitoxin, serum or plasma (Hep or EDTA); 7.8 h after dose) | | |
| Therapeutic | 20–35 ng/mL | 26–46 nmol/L |
| Toxic | >45 ng/mL | >59 nmol/L |
| Digoxin, serum or plasma (Hep or EDTA): ≥12 h after dose | | |
| Therapeutic | | |
| CHF | 0.8–1.5 ng/mL | 1.0–1.9 nmol/L |
| Arrhythmias | 1.5–2.0 ng/mL | 1.9–2.6 nmol/L |
| Toxic | | |
| Adult | >2.5 ng/mL | >3.2 nmol/L |
| Child | >3.0 ng/mL | >3.8 nmol/L |
| Disopyramide, serum or plasma (Hep or EDTA); trough | | |
| Therapeutic arrhythmias | | |
| Atrial | 2.8–3.2 μg/mL | 8.3–9.4 μmol/L |
| Ventricular | 3.3–7.5 μg/mL | 9.7–22 μmol/L |
| Toxic | > 7 μg/mL | 20.7 μmol/L |
| Doxepin, serum or plasma (Hep or EDTA); trough (≥12 h after dose) | | |
| Therapeutic | 150–250 ng/mL | 537–895 nmol/L |
| Toxic | >500 ng/mL | >1790 nmol/L |
| *Estradiol, serum | | |
| Adult | | |
| Male | 10–50 pg/mL | 37–184 pmol/L |
| Female | Varies with menstrual cycle | |

*Test values are method dependent.

‡Actual therapeutic range should be adjusted for individual patient.

| Test | Conventional Units | SI Units |
|---|---|---|
| Ethanol, whole blood (Ox) or serum | | |
| Depression of CNS | >100 mg/dL | >21.7 mmol/L |
| Fatalities reported | >400 mg/dL | >86.8 mmol/L |
| Ethosuximide, serum or plasma (Hep or EDTA): trough | | |
| Therapeutic | 40–100 μg/mL | 283–708 μmol/L |
| Toxic | >150 μg/mL | 1062 μmol/L |
| Euglobin lysis | No lysis in 2 h | No lysis in 2 h |
| α-Fetoprotein (AFP), serum | <15 ng/mL | <15 μg/L |
| Fat, fecal, F, 72 h | | |
| Infant, breast-fed | <1 g/d | <1 g/d |
| 0–6 y | <2 g/d | <2 g/d |
| Adult | <7 g/d | <7 g/d |
| Adult (fat-free diet) | <4 g/d | <4 g/d |
| §Fatty acids, total, serum | 190–240 mg/dL | 7–15 mmol/L |
| Nonesterified, serum | 8–25 mg/dL | 0.28–0.89 mmol/L |
| Ferritin, serum | | |
| Male | 20–150 ng/mL | 20–250 μg/L |
| Female | 10–120 ng/mL | 10–120 μg/L |
| Ferritin values of <20 ng/mL (20 μg/L) have been reported to be generally associated with depleted iron stores. | | |
| Fibrin degradation products | <10 μg/mL | <10 mg/L |
| *Fibrinogen, plasma (NaCit) | 200–400 mg/dL | 2–4 g/L |
| Fluoride | | |
| Plasma (Hep) | 0.01–0.2 μg/mL | 0.5–10.5 μmol/L |
| Urine | 0.2–3.2 μg/mL | 10.5–168 μmol/L |
| Urine, occupational exposure | <8 μg/mL | <421 μmol/L |
| *Folate, Serum | 3–20 ng/mL | 7–45 nmol/L |
| Erythrocytes | 140–628 ng/mL RBC | 317–1422 nmol/L RBC |
| Follicle-stimulating hormone (FSH), serum and plasma (Hep) | | |
| Male | 1.4–15.4 mIU/mL | 1.4–15.4 IU/L |
| Female | | |
| Follicular phase | 1–10 mIU/mL | 1–10 IU/L |
| Midcycle | 6–17 mIU/mL | 6–17 IU/L |
| Luteal phase | 1–9 mIU/mL | 1–9 IU/L |
| Postmenopausal | 19–100 mIU/mL | 19–100 IU/L |
| *Free Thyroxine Index (FTI), serum | 4.2–13 | 4.2–13 |
| Gastrin, serum | <100 pg/mL | <100 ng/L |
| Gentamycin, serum or plasma (EDTA) | | |
| Therapeutic | | |
| Peak | | |
| Less severe infection | 5–8 μg/mL | 10.4–16.7 μmol/L |
| Severe infection | 8–10 μg/mL | 16.7–20.9 μmol/L |
| Trough | | |
| Less severe infection | <1 μg/mL | <2.1 μmol/L |
| Moderate infection | <2 μg/mL | <4.2 μmol/L |
| Severe infection | <2–4 μg/mL | <4.2–8.4 μmol/L |
| Toxic | | |
| Peak | >10–12 μg/mL | >21–25 μmol/L |
| Trough | >2–4 μg/mL | >4.2–8.4 μmol/L |
| Glucose (fasting) | | |
| Blood | 65–95 mg/dL | 3.5–5.3 mmol/L |
| Plasma or serum | 74–106 mg/dL | 4.1–5.9 mmol/L |
| Glucose, 2 h postprandial, serum | <120 mg/dL | <6.7 mmol/L |

*Test values are method dependent.

§"Fatty acids" include a mixture of different aliphatic acids of varying molecular weight; a mean molecular weight of 284 daltons has been assumed.

| Test | Conventional Units | SI Units |
|---|---|---|
| Glucose, urine | | |
|    Quantitative | <500 mg/24 h | <2.8 mmol/24 h |
|    Qualitative | Negative | Negative |
| Glucose, CSF | 40–70 mg/dL | 2.2–3.9 mmol/L |
| *Glucose-6-phosphate | 12.1 ± 2.1 U/g Hb (SD) | 0.78 ± 0.13 mU/mol Hb |
|    dehydrogenase | 351 ± 60.6 U/$10^{12}$ RBC | 0.35 ± 0.06 nU/RBC |
|    (G-6-PD) in erythrocytes, whole blood | | |
|    (ACD, EDTA, or Hep) | 4.11 ± 0.71 U/mL RBC | 4.11 ± 0.71 kU/L RBC |
| γ-Glutamyltransferase (GGT), serum | | |
|    Males | 2–30 U/L (37°C) | 0.03–0.51 μkat/L (37°C) |
|    Females | 1–24 U/L (37°C) | 0.02–0.41 μkat/L (37°C) |
| Glutethimide, serum | | |
|    Therapeutic | 2–6 μg/mL | 9–28 μmol/L |
|    Toxic | >5 μg/mL | >23 μmol/L |
| Glycated hemoglobin (Hemoglobin A1c), whole blood (EDTA) | 4.2%–5.9% | 0.042–0.059 |
| Growth hormone, serum | | |
|    Male | <5 ng/mL | <5 μg/L |
|    Female | <10 ng/mL | <10 μg/L |
| Haptoglobin, serum | 30–200 mg/dL | 0.3–2.0 g/L |
| HDL-cholesterol (HDL-C), serum or plasma (EDTA) | | |
|    Adult | | |
|      desirable | >40 mg/dL | >1.04 mmol/L |
|      borderline | 35–40 mg/dL | 0.78–1.04 mmol/L |
|      high risk | <35 mg/dL | <0.78 mmol/L |
| Hematocrit | | |
|    Males | 42–52% | 0.42–0.52 |
|    Females | 37–47% | 0.37–0.47 |
|    Newborns | 53–65% | 0.53–0.65 |
|    Children (varies with age) | 30–43% | 0.30–0.43 |
| Hemoglobin (Hb) | | |
|    Males | 14.0–18.0 g/dL | 2.17–2.79 mmol/L |
|    Females | 12.0–16.0 g/dL | 1.86–2.48 mmol/L |
|    Newborn | 17.0–23.0 g/dL | 2.64–3.57 mmol/L |
|    Children (varies with age) | 11.2–16.5 g/dL | 1.74–2.56 mmol/L |
| Hemoglobin, fetal | ≥1 y old: <2% of total Hb | ≥1 y old: <0.02% of total Hb |
| Hemoglobin, plasma | <3 mg/dL | <0.47 μmol/L |
| Hemoglobin and myoglobin, urine, qualitative | Negative | Negative |
| Hemoglobin electrophoresis, whole blood (EDTA, Cit, or Hep) | | |
|    HbA | >95% | >0.95 Hb fraction |
|    HbA$_2$ | 1.5–3.7% | 0.015–0.37 Hb fraction |
|    HbF | <2% | <0.02 Hb fraction |
| Homogentisic acid, urine, qualitative | Negative | Negative |
| β-Hydroxybutyric acids, serum, plasma | 0.21–2.81 mg/dL | 20–270 μmol/L |
| 17-Hydroxycorticosteroids | | |
|    Urine | | |
|      Males | 3–10 mg/24 h | 8.3–27.6 μmol/24 h (as cortisol) |
|      Females | 2–8 mg/24 h | 5.5–22 μmol/24 h (as cortisol) |
| 5-Hydroxylindoleacetic acid, urine | | |
|    Qualitative | Negative | Negative |
|    Quantitative | 2–7 mg/24 h | 10.4–36.6 μmol/24 h |

*Test values are method dependent.

| Test | Conventional Units | SI Units |
|---|---|---|
| Imipramine, serum or plasma (Hep or EDTA); trough (≥12 h after dose) | | |
| Therapeutic | 150–250 ng/mL | 536–893 nmol/L |
| Toxic | >500 ng/mL | >1785 nmol/L |
| Immunoglobulins, serum | | |
| IgG | 700–1600 mg/dl | 7–16 g/L |
| IgA | 70–400 mg/dl | 0.7–4.0 g/L |
| IgM | 40–230 mg/dl | 0.42.3 g/L |
| IgD | 0–8 mg/dl | 0–80 mg/L |
| IgE | 3–423 mg/dl | 3–423 kIU/L |
| Immunoglobulin G (IgG), CSF | 0.5–6.1 mg/dL | 0.5–6.1 g/L |
| Insulin, plasma (fasting) | 2–25 μU/mL | 13–174 pmol/L |
| *Iron, serum | | |
| Males | 65–175 μg/dL | 11.6–31.3 μmol/L |
| Females | 50–170 μg/dL | 9.0–30.4 μmol/L |
| Iron binding capacity, serum total (TBIC) | 250–425 μg/dL | 44.8–71.6 μmol/L |
| Iron saturation, serum | | |
| Male | 20–50% | 0.2–0.5 |
| Female | 15–50% | 0.15–0.5 |
| 17-Ketosteroids, urine | | |
| Males | 10–25 mg/24 h | 38–87 μmol/24 h |
| Females | 6–14 mg/24 h (decreases with age) | 21–52 μmol/24 h (decreases with age) |
| L-Lactate | | |
| Plasma (NaF) | | |
| Venous | 4.5–19.8 mg/dL | 0.5–2.2 mmol/L |
| Arterial | 4.5–14.4 mg/dL | 0.5–1.6 mmol/L |
| Whole blood (Hep), at bed rest | | |
| Venous | 8.1–15.3 mg/dL | 0.9–1.7 mmol/L |
| Arterial | <11.3 mg/dL | <1.3 mmol/L |
| Urine, 24 h | 496–1982 mg/d | 5.5–22 mmol/d |
| CSF | 10–22 mg/dL | 1.1–2.4 mmol/L |
| *Lactate dehydrogenase (LDH) | | |
| Total (L→P), 37°C, serum | | |
| Newborn | 290–775 U/L | 4.9–13.2 μkat/L |
| Neonate | 545–2000 U/L | 9.3–34 μkat/L |
| Infant | 180–430 U/L | 3.1–7.3 μkat/L |
| Child | 110–295 U/L | 1.9–5 μkat/L |
| Adult | 100–190 U/L | 1.7–3.2 μkat/L |
| >60 y | 110–210 U/L | 1.9–3.6 μkat/L |
| *Isoenzymes, serum by agarose gel electrophoresis | | |
| Fraction 1 | 14–26% of total | 0.14–0.26 fraction of total |
| Fraction 2 | 29–39% of total | 0.29–0.39 fraction of total |
| Fraction 3 | 20–26% of total | 0.20–0.26 fraction of total |
| Fraction 4 | 8–16% of total | 0.08–0.16 fraction of total |
| Fraction 5 | 6–16% of total | 0.06–0.16 fraction of total |
| *Lactate dehydrogenase, CSF | 10% of serum value | 0.10 fraction of serum value |
| LDL-cholesterol (LDL-C), serum or plasma (EDTA) | | |
| Adult desirable | <130 mg/dL | <3.37 mmol/L |
| borderline | 130–159 mg/dL | 3.37–4.12 mmol/L |
| high risk | ≥ 160 mg/dL | ≥ 4.13 mmol/L |
| Lead, | | |
| Whole blood (Hep) | <25 μg/dL | <1.2 μmol/L |
| Urine, 24 h | <80 μg/d | <0.39 μmol/d |

*Test values are method dependent.

| Test | Conventional Units | SI Units |
|------|-------------------|----------|
| Lecithin-sphingomyelin (L/S) ratio, amniotic fluid | 2.0–5.0 indicates probable fetal lung maturity; >3.5 in diabetics | 2.0–5.0 indicates probable fetal lung maturity; >3.5 in diabetics |
| Lidocaine, serum or plasma (Hep or EDTA); 45 min after bolus dose | | |
| Therapeutic | 1.5–6.0 μg/mL | 6.4–26 μmol/L |
| Toxic | | |
|   CNS, cardiovascular depression | 6–8 μg/mL | 26–34.2 μmol/L |
|   Seizures, obtundation, decreased cardiac output | >8 μg/mL | >34.2 μmol/L |
| *Lipase, serum | 23–300 U/L (37°C) | 0.39–5.1 μkat/L (37°C) |
| Lithium, serum or plasma (Hep or EDTA); 12 h after last dose | | |
| Therapeutic | 0.6–1.2 mmol/L | 0.6–1.2 mmol/L |
| Toxic | >2 mmol/L | >2 mmol/L |
| Lorazepam, serum or plasma (Hep or EDTA) therapeutic | 50–240 ng/mL | 156–746 nmol/L |
| *Luteinizing hormone (LH), serum or plasma (Hep) | | |
| Male | 1.24–7.8 mIU/mL | 1.24–7.8 IU/L |
| Female | | |
|   Follicular phase | 1.68–15.0 mIU/mL | 1.68–15.0 IU/L |
|   Midcycle peak | 21.9–56.6 mIU/mL | 21.9–56.6 IU/L |
|   Luteal phase | 0.61–16.3 mIU/mL | 0.61–16.3 IU/L |
|   Postmenopausal | 14.2–52.5 mIU/mL | 14.2–52.3 IU/L |
| Magnesium | | |
| Serum | 1.3–2.1 mEq/L | 0.65–1.07 mmol/L |
| | 1.6–2.6 mg/dL | 16–26 mg/L |
| Urine | 6.0–10.0 mEq/24 h | 3.0–5.0 mmol/24 h |
| Mercury | | |
| Whole blood (EDTA) | 0.6–59 μg/L | <0.29 μmol/L |
| Urine, 24 h | <20 μg/d | <0.01 μmol/d |
| Toxic | >150 μg/d | >0.75 μmol/d |
| Metanephrines, total, urine | 0.1–1.6 mg/24 h | 0.5–8.1 μmol/24 h |
| Methemoglobin, (MetHb, hemoglobin), whole blood (EDTA, Hep or ACD) | 0.06–0.24 g/dL or 0.78 ± 0.37% of total Hb (SD) | 9.3–37.2 μmol/L or mass fraction of total Hb: 0.008 ± 0.0037 (SD) |
| Methotrexate, serum or plasma (Hep or EDTA) | | |
| Therapeutic | Variable | Variable |
| Toxic | | |
|   1–2 wk after low-dose therapy | ≥0.02 μmol/L | ≥0.02 μmol/L |
|   post-IV infusion   24 h | ≥5 μmol/L | ≥5 μmol/L |
|           48 h | ≥0.5 μmol/L | ≥0.5 μmol/L |
|           72 h | ≥0.05 μmol/L | ≥0.05 μmol/L |
| Myelin basic protein, CSF | <2.5 ng/mL | <2.5 μg/L |
| Myoglobin, serum | <85 ng/mL | <85 μg/L |
| Nortriptyline, serum or plasma (Hep or EDTA); trough (≥12 h after dose) | | |
| Therapeutic | 50–150 ng/mL | 190–570 nmol/L |
| Toxic | >500 ng/mL | >1900 nmol/L |
| *5'-Nucleotidase, serum | 2–17 U/L | 0.034–0.29 μkat/L |
| N-Acetylprocainamide, serum or plasma (Hep or EDTA); trough | | |
| Therapeutic | 5–30 μg/mL | 18–108 μmol/L |
| Toxic | >40 μg/mL | >144 μmol/L |

*Test values are method dependent.

| Test | Conventional Units | SI Units |
|------|-------------------|----------|
| Occult blood, feces, random | Negative (<2 mL blood/150 g stool/d) | Negative (<13.3 mL blood/kg stool/d) |
| Qualitative, urine, random | Negative | Negative |
| Osmolality | | |
| Serum | 275–295 mOsm/kg serum water | 275–295 mmol/kg serum water |
| Urine | 50–1200 mOsm/kg water | 50–1200 mmol/kg water |
| Ratio, urine/serum | 1.0–3.0, | 1.0–3.0, |
| | 3.0–4.7 after 12 h fluid restriction | 3.0–4.7 after 12 h fluid restriction |
| Osmotic fragility of erythrocytes | Begins in 0.45–0.39% NaCl | Begins in 77–67 mmol/L NaCl |
| | Complete in 0.33–0.30% NaCl | Complete in 56–51 mmol/L NaCl |
| Oxazepam, serum or plasma (Hep or EDTA), therapeutic | 0.2–1.4 μg/mL | 0.70–4.9 μmol/L |
| Oxygen, blood | | |
| Capacity | 16–24 vol% (varies with hemoglobin) | 7.14–10.7 mmol/L (varies with hemoglobin) |
| Content | | |
| Arterial | 15–23 vol% | 6.69–10.3 mmol/L |
| Venous | 10–16 vol% | 4.46–7.14 mmol/L |
| Saturation | | |
| Arterial and capillary | 95–98% of capacity | 0.95–0.98 of capacity |
| Venous | 60–85% of capacity | 0.60–0.85 of capacity |
| Tension | | |
| $pO_2$ arterial and capillary | 83–108 mmHg | 11.1–14.4 kPa |
| Venous | 35–45 mmHg | 4.6–6.0 kPa |
| P50, blood | 25–29 mmHg (adjusted to pH 7.4) | 3.33–3.86 kPa |
| Partial thromboplastin time activated (APTT) | <35 sec | <35 sec |
| Pentobarbital, serum or plasma (Hep or EDTA); trough | | |
| Therapeutic | | |
| Hypnotic | 1.5 μg/mL | 4–22 μmol/L |
| Therapeutic coma | 20–50 μg/mL | 88–221 μmol/L |
| Toxic | >10 μg/mL | >44 μmol/L |
| pH | | |
| Blood, arterial | 7.35–7.45 | 7.35–7.45 |
| Urine | 4.6–8.0 (depends on diet) | Same |
| Phenacetin, plasma (EDTA) | | |
| Therapeutic | 1.30 μg/mL | 6–167 μmol/L |
| Toxic | 50–250 μg/mL | 279–1395 μmol/L |
| Phenobarbital, serum or plasma (Hep or EDTA); trough | | |
| Therapeutic | 15–40 μg/mL | 65–172 μmol/L |
| Toxic | | |
| Slowness, ataxia, nystagmus | 35–80 μg/mL | 151–345 μmol/L |
| Coma with reflexes | 65–117 μg/mL | 280–504 μmol/L |
| Coma without reflexes | >100 μg/mL | >430 μmol/L |
| Phenosulfonphthalein excretion (PSP), urine | 28–51% in 15 min | 0.28–0.51 in 15 min |
| | 13–24% in 30 min | 0.13–0.24 in 30 min |
| | 9–17% in 60 min | 0.09–0.17 in 60 min |
| | 3–10% in 2 h | 0.03–0.10 in 2 h |
| | (After injection of 1 mL PSP intravenously) | (After injection of 1 mL PSP intravenously) |
| Phenylalanine, serum | 0.8–1.8 mg/dL | 48–109 μmol/L |
| Phenytoin, serum or plasma (Hep or EDTA); trough | | |
| Therapeutic | 10–20 μg/mL | 40–79 μmol/L |
| Toxic | >20 μg/mL | >79 μmol/L |
| *Phosphatase, acid, prostatic, serum | | |
| RIA | <3.0 ng/mL | <3.0 μg/L |

*Test values are method dependent.

| Test | Conventional Units | SI Units |
|------|-------------------|----------|
| *Phosphatase, alkaline, total, serum | 38–126 U/L (37°C) | 0.65–2.14 μkat/L |
| Phosphate, inorganic, serum | | |
|   Adults | 2.7–4.5 mg/dL | 0.87–1.45 mmol/L |
|   Children | 4.5–5.5 mg/dL | 1.45–1.78 mmol/L |
| Phosphatidylglycerol (PG), amniotic fluid | | |
|   Fetal lung immaturity | Absent | Same |
|   Fetal lung maturity | Present | Same |
| Phospholipids, serum | 125–275 mg/dL | 1.25–2.75 g/L |
| Phosphorus, urine | 0.4–1.3 g/24 h | 12.9–42 mmol/24 h |
| Porphobilinogen, urine | | |
|   Qualitative | Negative | Negative |
|   Quantitative | <2.0 mg/24 h | <9 μmol/24 h |
| Porphyrins, urine | | |
|   Coproporphyrin | 34–230 μg/24 h | 52–351 nmol/ 24 h |
|   Uroporphyrin | 27–52 μg/24 h | 32–63 nmol/ 24 h |
| Potassium, plasma (Hep) | | |
|   Males | 3.5–4.5 mmol/L | 3.5–4.5 mmol/L |
|   Females | 3.4–4.4 mmol/L | 3.4–4.4 mmol/L |
| Potassium | | |
|   Serum | | |
|     Premature | | |
|       Cord | 5.0–10.2 mmol/L | 5.0–10.2 mmol/L |
|       48 h | 3.0–6.0 mmol/L | 3.0–6.0 mmol/L |
|     Newborn cord | 5.6–12.0 mmol/L | 5.6–12.0 mmol/L |
|     Newborn | 3.7–5.9 mmol/L | 3.7–5.9 mmol/L |
|     Infant | 4.1–5.3 mmol/L | 4.1–5.3 mmol/L |
|     Child | 3.4–4.7 mmol/L | 3.4–4.7 mmol/L |
|     Adult | 3.5–5.1 mmol/L | 3.5–5.1 mmol/L |
|   Urine, 24 h | 25–125 mmol/d; varies with diet | 25–125 mmol/d; varies with diet |
|   CSF | 70% of plasma level or 2.5–3.2 mmol/L; rises with plasma hyperosmolality | 0.70 of plasma level; rises with plasma hyperosmolality |
| Prealbumin (Transthyretin), serum | 10–40 mg/dL | 100–400 mg/L |
| Primidone, serum or plasma (Hep or EDTA); trough | | |
|   Therapeutic | 5–12 μg/mL | 23–55 μmol/L |
|   Toxic | >15 μg/mL | >69 μmol/L |
| Procainamide, serum or plasma (Hep or EDTA); trough | | |
|   Therapeutic | 4–10 μg/mL | 17–42 μmol/L |
|   Toxic (also consider effect of metabolite (NAPA) | >10–12 μg/mL | >42–51 μmol/L |
| *Progesterone, serum | | |
|   Adult | | |
|     Male | 13–97 ng/dL | 0.4–3.1 nmol/L |
|     Female | | |
|       Follicular phase | 15–70 ng/dL | 0.5–2.2 nmol/L |
|       Luteal phase | 200–2500 ng/dL | 6.4–79.5 nmol/L |
|       Pregnancy | Varies with gestational week | |
| *Prolactin, serum | | |
|   Males | 2.5–15.0 ng/mL | 2.5–15.0 μg/L |
|   Females | 2.5–19.0 ng/mL | 2.5–19.0 μg/L |
| Propoxyphene, plasma (EDTA) | | |
|   Therapeutic | 0.1–0.4 μg/mL | 0.3–1.2 μmol/L |
|   Toxic | >0.5 μg/mL | >1.5 μmol/L |
| Propranolol, serum or plasma (Hep or EDTA); trough | | |
|   Therapeutic | 50–100 ng/mL | 193–386 nmol/L |

*Test values are method dependent.

| Test | Conventional Units | SI Units |
|---|---|---|
| *Prostate-specific antigen (PSA), serum | | |
|   Male | <4.0 ng/mL | <4.0 μg/L |
| *Protein, serum | | |
|   Total | 6.4–8.3 g/dL | 64–83 g/L |
|     Albumin | 3.9–5.1 g/dL | 39–51 g/L |
|     Globulin | | |
|       $\alpha_1$ | 0.2–0.4 g/dL | 2–4 g/L |
|       $\alpha_2$ | 0.4–0.8 g/dL | 4–8 g/L |
|       $\beta$ | 0.5–1.0 g/dL | 5–10 g/L |
|       $\gamma$ | 0.6–1.3 g/dL | 6–13 g/L |
|   Urine | | |
|     Qualitative | Negative | Negative |
|     Quantitative | 50–80 mg/24 h (at rest) | 50–80 mg/24 h (at rest) |
|   CSF, total | 8–32 mg/dL | 80–320 mg/dL |
| Prothrombin, consumption | >20 sec | >20 sec |
| *Prothrombin time (PT) | 12–14 sec | 12–14 sec |
| Protoporphyrin, total, WB | <60 μg/dL | <600 μg/L |
| Pyruvate, blood | 0.3–0.9 mg/dL | 34–103 μmol/L |
| Quinidine, serum or plasma (Hep or EDTA); trough | | |
|   Therapeutic | 2–5 μg/mL | 6–15 μmol/L |
|   Toxic | >6 μg/mL | >18 μmol/L |
| Salicylates, serum or plasma (Hep or EDTA); trough | | |
|   Therapeutic | 150–300 μg/mL | 1.09–2.17 mmol/L |
|   Toxic | >500 μg/mL | >3.62 mmol/L |
| Sedimentation rate | | |
|   Wintrobe | | |
|     Males | 0–10 mm in 1 h | 0–10 mm/h |
|     Females | 0–20 mm in 1 h | 0–20 mm/h |
|   Westergren | | |
|     Males (<50 yr) | 0–15 mm in 1 h | 0–15 mm/h |
|     Females (<50 yr) | 0–20 mm in 1 h | 0–20 mm/h |
| Sodium | | |
|   Serum or plasma (Hep) | | |
|     Premature | | |
|       Cord | 116–140mmol/L | 116–140 mmol/L |
|       48 h | 128–148 mmol/L | 128–148 mmol/L |
|     Newborn, cord | 126–166 mmol/L | 126–166 mmol/L |
|     Newborn | 133–146 mmol/L | 133–146 mmol/L |
|     Infant | 139–146 mmol/L | 139–146 mmol/L |
|     Child | 138–145 mmol/L | 138–145 mmol/L |
|     Adult | 136–145 mmol/L | 136–145 mmol/L |
|   Urine, 24 h | 40–220 mEq/d (diet dependent) | 40–220 mmol/d (diet dependent) |
|   Sweat | | |
|     Normal | 10–40 mmol/L | 10–40 mmol/L |
|     Cystic fibrosis | 70–190 mmol/L | 70–190 mmol/L |
| Specific gravity, urine | 1.002–1.030 | 1.002–1.030 |
| *Testosterone, serum | | |
|   Male | 280–1100 ng/dL | 0.52–38.17 nmol/L |
|   Female | 15–70 ng/dL | 0.52–2.43 nmol/L |
|     Pregnancy | 3–4 × normal | 3–4 × normal |
|     Postmenopausal | 8–35 ng/dL | 0.28–1.22 nmol/L |
| Theophylline, serum or plasma (Hep or EDTA) | | |
|   Therapeutic | | |
|     Bronchodilator | 8–20 μg/mL | 44–111 μmol/L |
|     Prem. apnea | 6–13 μg/mL | 33–72 μmol/L |
|   Toxic | >20 μg/mL | >110 μmol/L |

*Test values are method dependent.

| Test | Conventional Units | SI Units |
|------|--------------------|----------|
| Thiocyanate, serum or plasma (EDTA) | | |
| Nonsmoker | 1–4 μg/mL | 17–69 μmol/L |
| Smoker | 3–12 μg/mL | 52–206 μmol/L |
| Therapeutic after nitroprusside infusion | 6–29 μg/mL | 103–499 μmol/L |
| Urine | | |
| Nonsmoker | 1–4 mg/d | 17–69 μmol/d |
| Smoker | 7–17mg/d | 120–292 μmol/d |
| Thiopental, serum or plasma (Hep or EDTA); trough | | |
| Hypnotic | 1.0–5-0 μg/mL | 4.1–20.7 μmol/L |
| Coma | 30–100 μg/mL | 124–413 μmol/L |
| Anesthesia | 7–130 μg/mL | 29–536 μmol/L |
| Toxic concentration | >10 μg/mL | >41 μmol/L |
| *Thyroid-stimulating hormone (TSH), serum | 0.4–4.2 μU/mL | 0.4–4.2 mU/L |
| Thyroxine (T₄) serum | 5–12 μg/dL (varies with age, higher in children and pregnant women) | 65–155 nmol/L (varies with age, higher in children and pregnant women) |
| *Thyroxine, free, serum | 0.8–2.7 ng/dL | 10.3–35 pmol/L |
| Thyroxine binding globulin (TBG), serum | 1.2–3.0 mg/dL | 12–30 mg/L |
| Tobramycin, serum or plasma (Hep or EDTA) | | |
| Therapeutic | | |
| Peak | | |
| Less severe infection | 5–8 μg/mL | 11–17 μmol/L |
| Severe infection | 8–10 μg/mL | 17–21 μmol/L |
| Trough | | |
| Less severe infection | <1 μg/mL | <2 μmol/L |
| Moderate infection | <2 μg/mL | <4 μmol/L |
| Severe infection | <2–4 μg/mL | <4–9 μmol/L |
| Toxic | | |
| Peak | >10–12 μg/mL | >21–26 μmol/L |
| Trough | >2–4 μg/mL | >4–9 μmol/L |
| Transferrin, serum | | |
| Newborn | 130–275 mg/dL | 1.30–2.75 g/L |
| Adult | 212–360 mg/dL | 2.12–3.60 g/L |
| >60 yr | 190–375 mg/dL | 1.9–3.75 g/L |
| Triglycerides, serum, fasting | | |
| Desirable | <250 mg/dL | <2.83 mmol/L |
| Borderline high | 250–500 mg/dL | 2.83–5.67 mmol/L |
| Hypertriglyceridemic | >500 mg/dL | >5.65 mmol/L |
| *Triiodothyronine, total (T₃) serum | 100–200 ng/dL | 1.54–3.8 nmol/L |
| *Troponin-I, cardiac, serum | undetectable | undetectable |
| Troponin-T, cardiac, serum | undetectable | undetectable |
| Urea nitrogen, serum | 6–20 mg/dL | 2.1–7.1 mmol urea/L |
| Urea nitrogen/creatinine ratio, serum | 12:1 to 20:1 | 48–80 urea/creatinine mole ratio |
| *Uric acid | | |
| Serum, enzymatic | | |
| Male | 4.5–8.0 mg/dL | 0.27–0.47 mmol/L |
| Female | 2.5–6.2 mg/dL | 0.15–0.37 mmol/L |
| Child | 2.0–5.5 mg/dL | 0.12–0.32 mmol/L |
| Urine | 250–750 mg/24 h (with normal diet) | 1.48–4.43 mmol/24 h (with normal diet) |
| Urobilinogen, urine | 0.1–0.8 Ehrlich unit/2 h | 0.1–0.8 EU/2 h |
| | 0.5–4.0 EU/d | 0.5–4.0 EU/d |

*Test values are method dependent.

| Test | Conventional Units | SI Units |
|---|---|---|
| Valproic acid, serum or plasma (Hep or EDTA); trough | | |
| Therapeutic | 50–100 μg/mL | 347–693 μmol/L |
| Toxic | >100 μg/mL | >693 μmol/L |
| Vancomycin, serum or plasma (Hep or EDTA) | | |
| Therapeutic | | |
| Peak | 20–40 μg/mL | 14–28 μmol/L |
| Trough | 5–10 μg/mL | 3–7 μmol/L |
| Toxic | >80–100 μg/mL | >55–69 μmol/L |
| Vanillylmandelic acid (VMA), urine (4-hydroxy-3-methoxymandelic acid) | 1.4–6.5 mg/24h | 7–33 μmol/d |
| Viscosity, serum | 1.00–1.24 cP | 1.00–1.24 cP |
| Vitamin A, serum | 30–80 μg/dL | 1.05–2.8 μmol/L |
| Vitamin B$_{12}$, serum | 110–800 pg/mL | 81–590 pmol/L |
| Vitamin E, serum | | |
| Normal | 5–18 μg/mL | 12–42 μmol/L |
| Therapeutic | 30–50 μg/mL | 69.6–116 μmol/L |
| Zinc, serum | 70–120 μg/dL | 10.7–18.4 μmol/L |

# Normal Range of Motion (in Degrees) According to Various Authors*

| Joint | AAOS | Boone & Azen | Clark | CMA | Daniels & Worthingham | Dorinson & Wagner | Esch & Lepley | Gerhardt & Russe | Hoppenfeld | JAMA | Kapandji | Kandall & McCreary | Wiechec & Krusen |
|---|---|---|---|---|---|---|---|---|---|---|---|---|---|
| **Shoulder** | | | | | | | | | | | | | |
| Flexion | 180 | 167 | 130 | 170 | — | 180 | 170 | 170 | — | 150 | 180 | 180 | 180 |
| Extension | 60 | 62 | 80 | 30 | 50 | 45 | 60 | 50 | 45 | 40 | 50 | 45 | 45 |
| Abduction | 180 | 184 | 180 | 170 | — | 180 | 170 | 170 | 180 | 150 | 180 | 180 | 180 |
| Internal rotation | 70 | 69 | 90† | 60† | 90 | 90 | 80 | 80 | 55 | 40† | 95 | 70 | 90 |
| External rotation | 90 | 104 | 40† | 80† | 90 | 90 | 90 | 90 | 45 | 90† | 80 | 90 | 90 |
| Horizontal abduction | — | 45 | — | — | — | — | — | — | — | — | — | — | — |
| Horizontal adduction | 135 | 140 | — | — | — | — | — | 135 | — | — | — | — | — |
| **Elbow** | | | | | | | | | | | | | |
| Flexion | 150 | 143 | 150 | 135 | 160 | 145 | 150 | 150 | 150 | 150 | 145 | 145 | 135 |
| **Radioulnar** | | | | | | | | | | | | | |
| Pronation | 80 | 76 | 50 | 75 | 90 | 80 | 90 | 80 | 90 | 80 | 85 | 90 | 90 |
| Supination | 80 | 82 | 90 | 85 | 90 | 70 | 90 | 90 | 90 | 80 | 90 | 90 | 90 |
| **Wrist** | | | | | | | | | | | | | |
| Flexion | 80 | 76 | 80 | 70 | 90 | 80 | 90 | 60 | 80 | 70 | 85 | 80 | 60 |
| Extension | 70 | 75 | 70 | 65 | 90 | 55 | 70 | 50 | 70 | 60 | 85 | 70 | 55 |
| Radial deviation | 20 | 22 | 15 | 20 | 25 | 20 | 20 | 20 | 20 | 20 | 15 | 20 | 35 |
| Ulnar deviation | 30 | 36 | 30 | 40 | 65 | 40 | 30 | 30 | 30 | 30 | — | 35 | 75 |
| **Hip** | | | | | | | | | | | | | |
| Flexion | 120 | 122 | 120 | 110 | 125 | 125 | 130 | 125 | 135 | 100 | 120 | 125 | 120 |
| Extension | 30 | 10 | 20 | 30 | 15 | 50 | 45 | 15 | 30 | 30 | 30 | 10 | 45 |
| Abduction | 45 | 46 | 55 | 50 | 45 | 45 | 45 | 45 | 50 | 40 | 30 | 45 | 45 |
| Adduction | 30 | 27 | 45 | 30 | 0 | 20 | 15 | 15 | 30 | 20 | 30 | 10 | — |
| Internal rotation | 45 | 47 | 20 | 35 | 45 | 30 | 33 | 45 | 35 | 40 | 30 | 45 | — |
| External rotation | 45 | 47 | 45 | 50 | 45 | 50 | 36 | 45 | 45 | 50 | 60 | 45 | — |
| **Knee** | | | | | | | | | | | | | |
| Flexion | 135 | 143 | 145 | 135 | 130 | 140 | 135 | 130 | 135 | 120 | 160 | 140 | 135 |
| **Ankle** | | | | | | | | | | | | | |
| Plantar flexion | 50 | 56 | 50 | 50 | 45 | 45 | 65 | 45 | 50 | 40 | 50 | 45 | 55 |
| Dorsiflexion | 20 | 13 | 15 | 15 | — | 20 | 10 | 20 | 20 | 20 | 30 | 20 | 30 |

| Joint | AAOS | Boone & Azen | Clark | CMA | Daniels & Worthingham | Dorinson & Wagner | Esch & Lepley | Gerhardt & Russe | Hoppenfeld | JAMA | Kapandji | Kandall & McCreary | Wiechec & Krusen |
|---|---|---|---|---|---|---|---|---|---|---|---|---|---|
| *Subtalar Joint* | | | | | | | | | | | | | |
| Inversion | 35 | 37 | — | 35 | — | 50 | 30 | 40 | — | 30 | 52 | 35 | — |
| Eversion | 15 | 26 | — | 20 | — | 20 | 15 | 20 | — | 20 | 30 | 20 | — |

*References for the normal values: American Academy of Orthopaedic Surgeons. Joint motion: Method of measuring and recording. Chicago: AAOS, 1965; Boone DC, Azen SP. Normal range of motion in male subjects. *J Bone Joint Surg* 1979; 61A: 756; Clark WA. A system of joint measurement. *J Orthop Surg* 1920; 2:687; Commission of California Medical Association (CMA) and The Industrial Accident Commission of the State of California: Evaluation of industrial disability. New York: Oxford University Press, 1960; Daniels L, Worthingham C. Muscle testing: Techniques of manual examination. 3rd ed. Philadelphia: WB Saunders, 1972; Dorinson SM, Wagner ML. An exact technique for clinically measuring and recording joint motion. 1948; *Arch Phys Med* 29:468; Esch D, Lepley M. Evaluation of joint motion: Methods of measurement and recording. Minneapolis: University of Minnesota Press, 1974; Gerhardt JJ, Russe OA. International SFTR method of measuring and recording joint motion. Bern: Huber, 1975; Hoppenfeld S. Physical examination of the spine and extremities. New York: Appleton-Century-Crofts, 1976; Journal of the American Medical Association: A guide to the evaluation of permanent impairment of the extremities and back. *JAMA* 1958 (special edition), 1; Kapandji LA. Physiology of the joints. Vols. 1 and 2, 2nd ed. London: Churchill Livingstone, 1970; Kendall FP, McCreary EK. Muscles, testing and function, 3rd ed. Baltimore: Williams & Wilkins, 1983; Wiechec FJ, Krusen FH. A new method of joint measurement and a review of the literature. *Am J Surg* 1939; 43:659.

†Measurements obtained with shoulder in 0 degrees of abduction.

From Rothstein JM, Roy SH, Wolf SL. The rehabilitation specialist's handbook, 2nd ed. Philadelphia: FA Davis, 1998.

# Gauging Healthy Weight: The Body Mass Index

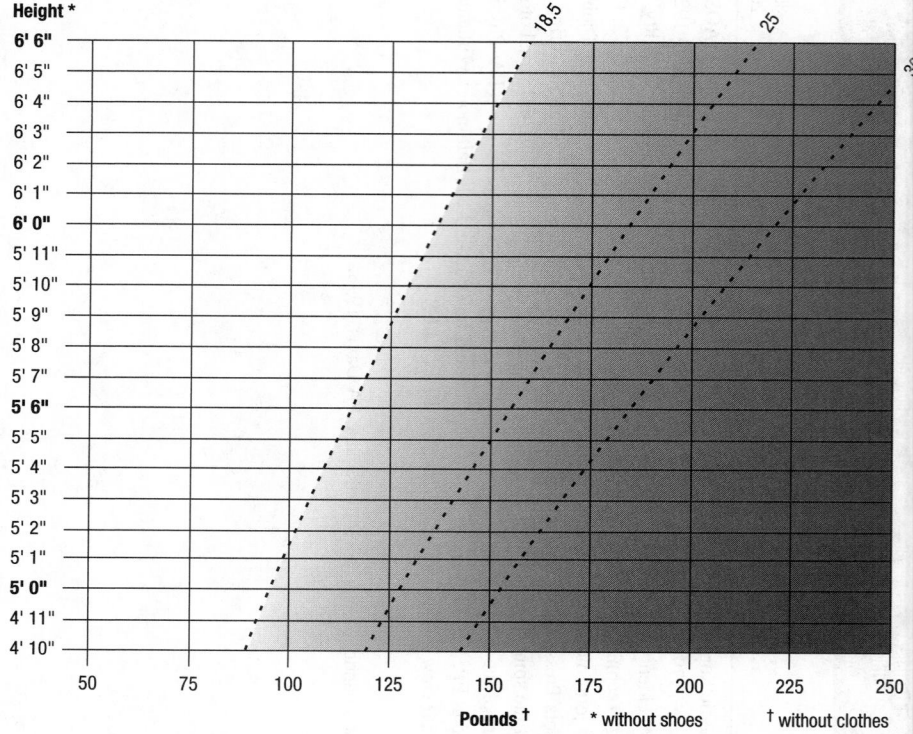

**Directions:** Find your weight on the bottom of the graph. Go straight up from that point until you come to the line that matches your height. Then look to find your weight group.

**Healthy Weight** BMI from 18.5 up to 25 refers to healthy weight.

**Overweight** BMI from 25 up to 30 refers to overweight.

**Obese** BMI 30 or higher refers to obesity. Obese persons are also overweight.

From US Department of Agriculture, US Department of Health and Human Services. Nutrition and your health: dietary guidelines for Americans, 5th ed., 2000.

# DuBois Body Surface Area Chart: Estimating Body Surface Area of Adults and Children

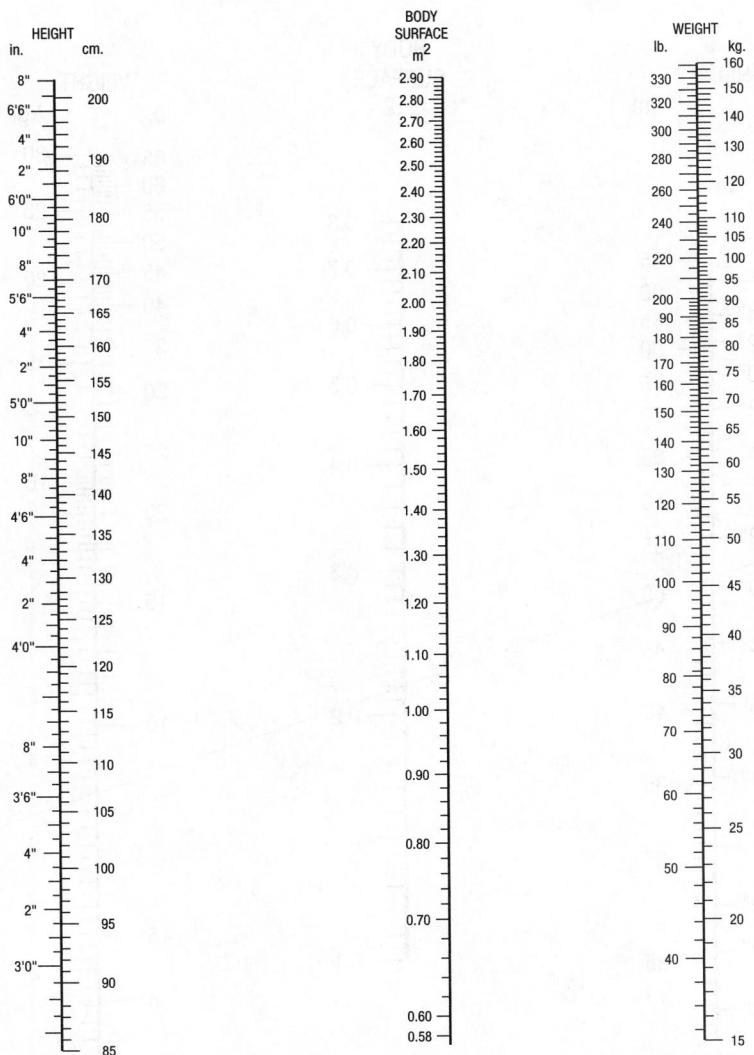

To determine body surface, draw a straight line from the point on the height scale indicating the subject's height to the point on the weight scale indicating the subject's weight. The point where the line crosses the body surface area scale will indicate the subject's body surface area. For example, for a subject 170 cm tall and weighing 75 kg, body surface area will total 1.90 square meters (m²).

From DuBois EF, Basal metabolism in health and disease. Philadelphia: Lea & Febiger, 1936. Copyright 1920 by WM Boothby & RB Sandiford.

# West Nomogram: Estimating Body Surface Area of Infants and Young Children

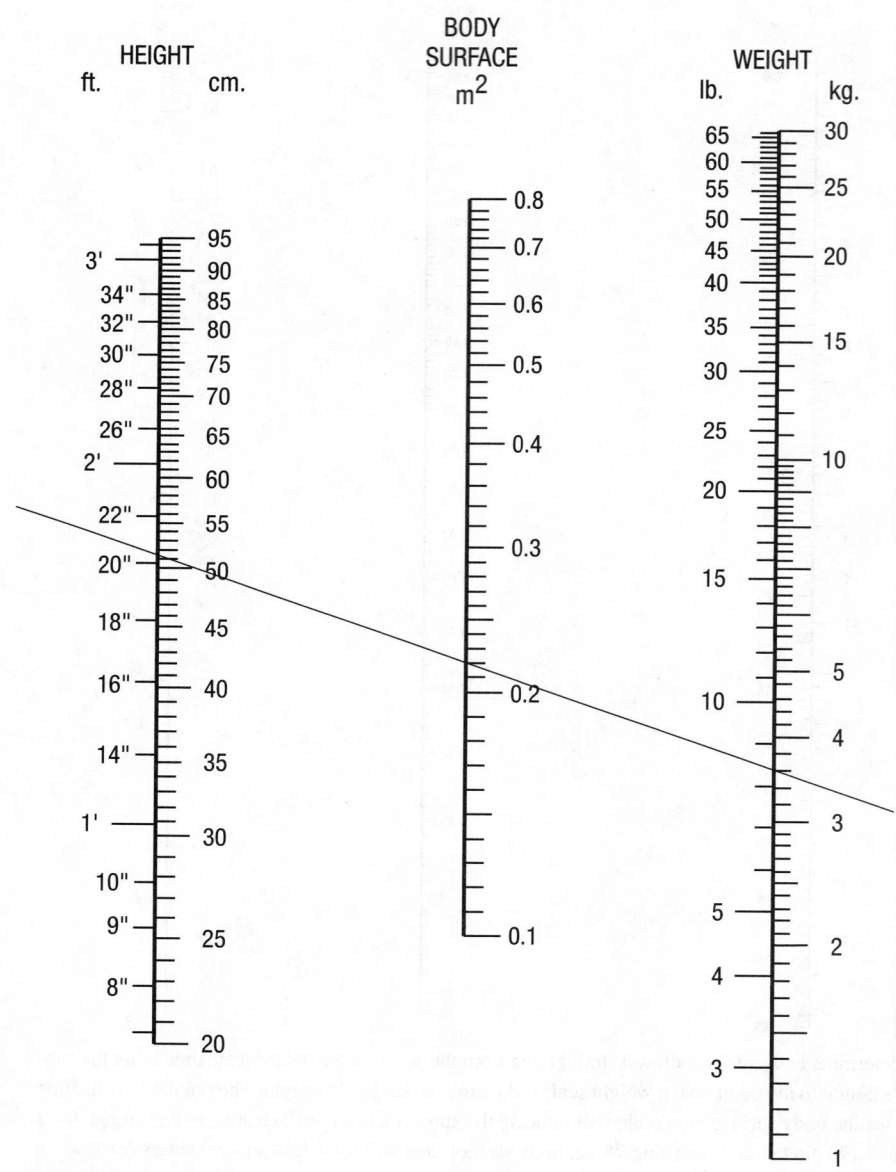

To determine a child's body surface area, draw a straight line between the child's height and weight. Body surface area in square meters is shown by the point where the line crosses the surface area scale. From Crawford JD, Terry ME, Rourke GM. *Pediatrics* 5:785 (fig. 1), 1950.

# Commonly Prescribed Drugs and Their Applications

**Compiled by Marjorie Canfield Willis, CMA-AC, and Michael J. Deimling, PhD, RPh**

This alphabetical index of commonly prescribed drugs (trade and generic) is based on listings of new and refill prescriptions dispensed in the United States in 1999. The names of trade drugs are capitalized; their generic names accompany them in parentheses. All generic drug names are set in lower case.

| Drug | Category/Application(s) |
| --- | --- |
| Accupril (quinapril hydrochloride) | angiotensin-converting enzyme (ACE) inhibitor, antihypertensive, treats congestive heart failure |
| acetaminophen and codeine | analgesic/opiate combination |
| Accutane (isotretinoin) | retinoid, treats acne |
| Adalat CC (nifedipine) | calcium channel blocker, antihypertensive, antianginal |
| Adderall (dextroamphetamine and amphetamine) | amphetamine combination, treats attention deficit/hyperactivity disorder |
| albuterol | $\beta_2$-adrenergic agonist, bronchodilator, antiasthmatic |
| Alesse-28 (ethinyl estradiol and levonorgestrel) | oral contraceptive |
| Allegra (fexofenadine) | second-generation antihistamine |
| Allegra-D (fexofenadine and pseudoephedrine) | antihistamine/decongestant combination |
| allopurinol | xanthine oxidase inhibitor, treats gout |
| Alphagan (brimonidine) | $\alpha_2$-adrenergic agonist, treats glaucoma |
| alprazolam | benzodiazepine, anxiolytic (treats anxiety), sedative/ hypnotic |
| Altase (ramipril) | angiotensin-converting enzyme (ACE) inhibitor, antihypertensive, treats congestive heart failure |
| Amaryl (glimepiride) | oral hypoglycemic, sulfonylurea |
| Ambien (zolpidem tartrate) | nonbenzodiazepine sedative/hypnotic |
| amitriptyline hydrochloride | tricyclic antidepressant |
| amoxicillin trihydrate | penicillin, antibiotic |
| Amoxil (amoxicillin trihydrate) | penicillin, antibiotic |
| Aricept (donepezil) | acetylcholinesterase inhibitor (AchEI), treats Alzheimer dementia |
| Arthrotec (diclofenac and misoprostol) | nonsteroidal anti-inflammatory drug (NSAID)/prostaglandin combination |
| atenolol | $\beta_1$-adrenergic antagonist (blocker), cardioselective $\beta$-blocker, antihypertensive, antianginal, antiarrhythmic |
| Atrovent (ipratropium bromide) | anticholinergic, bronchodilator, antiasthmatic |
| Augmentin (amoxicillin/clavulanic acid) | penicillin/$\beta$-lactamase inhibitor combination |
| Avapro (irbesartan) | angiotensin II receptor antagonist, antihypertensive |
| Axid (nizatidine) | histamine $H_2$ receptor antagonist ($H_2$RA); treats peptic ulcer disease, gastroesophageal disease |
| Azmacort (triamcinolone) | corticosteroid, anti-inflammatory |
| Bactroban (mupirocin) | topical antibacterial |
| Biaxin (clarithromycin) | macrolide, antibiotic |
| BuSpar (buspirone hydrochloride) | anxiolytic (treats anxiety) |

| Drug | Category/Application(s) |
|------|------------------------|
| Cardizem CD (diltiazem hydrochloride) | calcium channel blocker, antihypertensive, antianginal, antiarrhythmic |
| Cardura (doxazosin mesylate) | $\alpha_1$-adrenergic antagonist, antihypertensive, vasodilator |
| Carisoprodol | skeletal muscle relaxant |
| Ceftin (cefuroxime) | second-generation cephalosporin, antibiotic |
| Cefzil (cefprozil) | second-generation cephalosporin, antibiotic |
| Celebrex (celecoxib) | cyclooxygenase-2 (COX-2) inhibitor, nonsteroidal anti-inflammatory drug (NSAID), analgesic, antipyretic |
| Celexa (citalopram) | antidepressant, selective serotonin reuptake inhibitor (SSRI) |
| cephalexin | first-generation cephalosporin, antibiotic |
| Cipro (ciprofloxacin hydrochloride) | fluoroquinolone, antibacterial |
| Claritin (loratadine) | second-generation antihistamine |
| Claritin-D (loratadine and pseudoephedrine) | antihistamine/decongestant combination |
| Climara (estradiol) transdermal | estrogen, replacement therapy |
| Clonazepam | benzodiazepine, anticonvulsant, antiepileptic |
| clonidine hydrochloride | $\alpha_2$-adrenergic agonist, central sympatholytic, antihypertensive |
| Combivent (ipratropium and albuterol) | anticholinergic/$\beta_2$-adrenergic agonist combination, bronchodilator, antiasthmatic |
| Contuss-XT (guaifenesin and phenylpropanolamine) | expectorant/decongestant |
| Coumadin (warfarin) | oral anticoagulant |
| Cozaar (losartan) | angiotensin II receptor antagonist, antihypertensive |
| cyclobenzaprine hydrochloride | skeletal muscle relaxant |
| Cycrin (medroxyprogesterone acetate) | progestin, contraceptive |
| Daypro (oxaprozin) | nonsteroidal anti-inflammatory drug (NSAID), analgesic, antipyretic |
| Depakote (valproic acid and derivatives) | anticonvulsant, antiepileptic |
| Desogen-28 (ethinyl estradiol and desogestrel) | oral contraceptive |
| Detrol (tolterodine) | anticholinergic, urinary antispasmodic |
| Dexedrine (dextroamphetamine) | amphetamine, central nervous system stimulant, treats attention deficit/hyperactivity disorder |
| diazepam | anxiolytic (treats anxiety), sedative, hypnotic, anticonvulsant, muscle relaxant |
| Diflucan (fluconazole) | antifungal |
| Dilantin (phenytoin) | hydantoin, anticonvulsant, antiepileptic |
| Diovan (valsartan) | angiotensin II receptor antagonist, antihypertensive |
| doxycycline hyclate | tracycline, antibiotic |
| Duragesic (fentanyl) | opioid, analgesic |
| Effexor XR (venlafaxine) | antidepressant, serotonin norepinephrine reuptake inhibitor (SNRI) |
| Elocon (mometasone furoate) | corticosteroid, anti-inflammatory |
| Ery-Tab (erythromycin) | macrolide, antibiotic |
| Estrace Oral (estradiol) | estrogen, replacement therapy |
| Evista (raloxifene) | selective estrogen receptor modulator (SERM), treats osteoporosis |
| Flomax (tamsulosin) | $\alpha_1$-adrenergic antagonist (blocker), treats benign prostatic hyperplasia |

| Drug | Category/Application(s) |
|---|---|
| Flonase (fluticasone propionate) | corticosteroid, anti-inflammatory |
| Flovent (fluticasone) | corticosteroid, anti-inflammatory |
| folic acid | vitamin |
| Fosamax (alendronate) | bisphosphonate, treats Paget disease |
| furosemide | loop diuretic |
| gemfibrozil | antihyperlipidemic, fibric acid derivative |
| Glucophage (metformin) | oral hypoglycemic, biguanide, antidiabetic |
| Glucotrol XL (glipizide) | oral hypoglycemic, sulfonylurea, antidiabetic |
| glyburide | oral hypoglycemic, sulfonylurea, antidiabetic |
| guaifenesin and phenylpropanolamine | expectorant/decongestant combination |
| hydrochlorothiazide (HCTZ) | thiazide diuretic |
| hydrocodone and acetaminophen | opiate/analgesic combination |
| hydroxyzine hydrochloride | first-generation antihistamine |
| Hytrin (terazosin) | $\alpha_1$-adrenergic antagonist (blocker), antihypertensive, vasodilator |
| Hyzaar (losartan and hydrochlorothiazide) | angiotensin II receptor antagonist/thiazide diuretic combination, antihypertensive |
| ibuprofen OTC | nonsteroidal anti-inflammatory drug (NSAID), analgesic, antipyretic |
| Imdur (isosorbide mononitrate) | vasodilator; antianginal |
| Imitrex (sumatriptan succinate) | serotonin (5-HT$_1$) agonist, treats migraine |
| isosorbide mononitrate | vasodilator, antianginal |
| K-Dur (potassium chloride) | potassium supplement |
| Klor-Con 10 (potassium chloride) | potassium supplement |
| Lac-Hydrin (lactic acid with ammonium hydroxide) | humectant, treats dry skin |
| Lamisil (terbinafine) | antifungal |
| Lanoxin (digoxin) | (+) inotropic, antiarrhythmic |
| Lescol (fluvastatin) | HGM-CoA reductase inhibitor, antihyperlipidemic agent |
| Levaquin (levofloxacin) | fluoroquinolone, antibacterial |
| Levothroid (levothyroxine) | thyroid hormone, replacement therapy |
| Levoxyl (levothyroxine) | thyroid hormone, replacement therapy |
| Lipitor (atorvastatin) | HMG-CoA reductase inhibitor, antihyperlipidemic agent |
| Lo/Ovral-28 (ethinyl estradiol) | oral contraceptive |
| lorazepam | benzodiazepine, anxiolytic (treats anxiety), anticonvulsant |
| Lotensin (benazepril hydrochloride) | angiotensin-converting enzyme (ACE) inhibitor, antihypertensive, treats congestive heart failure |
| Lotrel (amlodipine and benazepril) | calcium channel blocker/angiotensin converting enzyme (ACE) inhibitor combination, antihypertensive |
| Lotrisone (betamethasone dipropionate and clotrimazole) | corticosteroid/antifungal combination |
| Macrobid (nitrofurantoin) | antibacterial, urinary antiseptic |
| medroxyprogesterone | progestin, contraceptive |
| methylphenidate hydrochloride | central nervous system stimulant, treats attention deficit/hyperactivity disorder |
| methylprednisolone | corticosteroid, anti-inflammatory |

| Drug | Category/Application(s) |
|------|------------------------|
| metoprolol tartrate | $\beta_1$-adrenergic antagonist (blocker), cardioselective $\beta$-blocker, antihypertensive, antiarrhythmic |
| metronidazole | antimicrobial, antibacterial, antiprotazoal, amebicide, antiparasitic |
| Mevacor (lovastatin) | HMG-CoA reductase inhibitor, antihyperlipidemic agent |
| Miacalcin (calcitonin) | parathyroid hormone, treats osteoporosis and Paget disease |
| Monopril (fosinopril) | angiotensin-converting enzyme (ACE) inhibitor, antihypertensive, treats congestive heart failure |
| Naproxen | nonsteroidal anti-inflammatory drug (NSAID), analgesic, antipyretic |
| Nasacort AQ (triamcinolone) | corticosteroid, anti-inflammatory |
| Nasonex (mometasone furoate) | corticosteroid, anti-inflammatory |
| Necon 1/35/28 (norethindrone and ethinyl estradiol) | oral contraceptive |
| neomycin, polymyxin b and hydrocortisone | antibiotic/corticosteriod combination |
| Neurontin (gabapentin) | anticonvulsant, antiepileptic |
| Nitrostat (nitroglycerin) | venodilator, vasodilator, treats angina |
| Nizoral (ketoconazole) | antifungal agent |
| Norvasc (amlodipine) | calcium channel blocker, antihypertensive, antianginal |
| Ortho-Cyclen-28 (ethinyl estradiol and norgestimate) | oral contraceptive |
| Ortho-Novum 7/7/7–28 (ethinyl estradiol and norethindrone) | oral contraceptive |
| Ortho Tri-Cyclen 28 (ethinyl estradiol and norgestimate) | oral contraceptive |
| oxycodone and acetaminophen | opiate/analgesic combination |
| OxyContin (oxycodone) | opiate, analgesic |
| Paxil (paroxetine) | antidepressant, selective serotonin reuptake inhibitor (SSRI) |
| Penicillin VK (penicillin v potassium) | penicillin; antibiotic |
| Pepcid (famotidine) | histamine $H_2$ receptor antagonist ($H_2$RA); treats peptic ulcer disease, gastroesophageal disease |
| Phenergan (promethazine hydrochloride) | antiemetic, antihistamine |
| Plavix (clopidogrel) | antiplatelet, antithrombotic |
| Plendil (felodipine) | calcium channel blocker, antihypertensive, antianginal |
| potassium chloride | potassium supplement |
| Pravachol (pravastatin sodium) | HMG-CoA reductase inhibitor, antihyperlipidemic |
| prednisone | corticosteroid, anti-inflammatory, immunosuppressant |
| Premarin (conjugated estrogens) | estrogen, conjugated estrogens |
| Prempro (estrogens and medroxy-progesterone) | estrogen/progestin combination, replacement therapy |
| Prevacid (lansoprazole) | proton pump inhibitor (PPI); treats peptic ulcer disease, gastroesophageal disease |
| Prilosec (omeprazole) | proton pump inhibitor (PPI); treats peptic ulcer disease, gastroesophageal disease |
| Prinivil (lisinopril) | angiotensin-converting enzyme (ACE) inhibitor; antihypertensive agent, treats congestive heart failure |
| Procardia XL (nifedipine) | calcium channel blocker; antihypertensive, antianginal |
| promethazine hydrochloride | antiemetic, antihistamine |
| promethazine hydrochloride and codeine | antihistamine/antitussive combination |
| propoxyphene napsylate and acetaminophen | opioid/analgesic combination |

| Drug | Category/Application(s) |
|---|---|
| propranolol hydrochloride | β-adrenergic antagonist (blocker), antihypertensive, antiarrhythmic, antianginal |
| Proventil (albuterol) | $\beta_2$-selective adrenergic agonist, bronchodilator, antiasthmatic |
| Prozac (fluoxetine hydrochloride) | antidepressant, selective serotonin reuptake inhibitor (SSRI) |
| ranitidine hydrochloride | histamine $H_2$ receptor antagonist ($H_2$RA); treats peptic ulcer disease, gastroesophageal disease |
| Relafen (nabumetone) | nonsteroidal anti-inflammatory drug (NSAID), analgesic, antipyretic |
| Remeron (mirtazapine) | atypical antidepressant |
| Risperdal (risperidone) | antipsychotic |
| Ritalin (methylphenidate hydrochloride) | central nervous system stimulant, treats attention deficit/hyperactivity disorder |
| Roxicet (oxycodone and acetaminophen) | opiate/analgesic combination |
| Serevent (salmeterol xinafoate) | $\beta_2$-selective adrenergic agonist, bronchodilator |
| Serzone (nefazodone) | atypical antidepressant |
| Skelaxin (metaxalone) | skeletal muscle relaxant |
| Singulair (montelukast) | leukotriene $D_4$ ($LTD_4$) receptor antagonist, anti-inflammatory, antiasthmatic |
| Synthroid (levothyroxine sodium) | thyroid hormone |
| tamoxifen citrate | selective estrogen receptor modulator (SERM), antineoplastic |
| temazepam | benzodiazepine, anxiolytic (treats anxiety), sedative/hypnotic |
| Terazol (terconazole) | antifungal |
| tetracycline | tetracycline, antibiotic |
| Tiazac (diltiazem) | calcium channel blocker; antihypertensive, antianginal, antiarrhythmic |
| TobraDex (tobramycin and dexamethasone) | antibiotic/corticosteroid combination |
| Toprol-XL (metoprolol) | $\beta_1$-adrenergic antagonist (blocker), cardioselective β-blocker, antihypertensive, antiarrhythmic, antianginal |
| trazodone hydrochloride | atypical antidepressant |
| triamterene and hydrochlorothiazide (HCTZ) | potassium sparing diuretic/thiazide diuretic combination |
| trimethoprim-sulfamethoxazole (also known as co-trimoxazole) | antibacterial combination, sulfonamide |
| Trimox (amoxicillin trihydrate) | penicillin, antibiotic |
| Triphasil-28 (ethinyl estradiol and levonorgestrel) | oral contraceptive |
| Tussionex (hydrocodone and chlorpheniramine) | opiate/antihistamine combination, antitussive |
| Ultram (tramadol hydrochloride) | opioid, analgesic |
| Valtrex (valacyclovir) | antiviral |
| Vancenase AQ (beclomethasone dipropionate) | corticosteroid, anti-inflammatory |
| Vasotec (enalapril) | angiotensin-converting enzyme (ACE) inhibitor, antihypertensive, treats congestive heart failure |
| Veetids (penicillin V potassium) | penicillin, antibiotic |
| verapamil | calcium channel blocker, antihypertensive, antianginal, antiarrhythmic |
| Viagra (sildenafil) | phosphodiesterase type 5 (PDE5) inhibitor, treats erectile dysfunction |
| Vicoprofen (hydrocodone and ibuprofen) | opiate/analgesic combination |

| Drug | Category/Application(s) |
| --- | --- |
| Vioxx (rofecoxib) | cyclooxygenase-2 (COX-2) inhibitor, nonsteroidal anti-inflammatory drug (NSAID), analgesic, antipyretic |
| warfarin | oral anticoagulant |
| Wellbutrin SR (bupropion) | atypical antidepressant |
| Xalantan (latanoprost) | prostaglandin, treats glaucoma |
| Zestoretic (lisinopril and hydrochlorothiazide) | angiotensin-converting enzyme (ACE) inhibitor/thiazide diuretic combination, antihypertensive |
| Zestril (lisinopril) | angiotensin-converting enzyme (ACE) inhibitor, antihypertensive, treats congestive heart failure |
| Ziac (bisoprolol and hydrochlorothiazide) | $\beta_1$-adrenergic antagonist/thiazide diuretic combination, antihypertensive |
| Zithromax (azithromycin dihydrate) | macrolide, antibiotic |
| Zocor (simvastatin) | HMG-CoA reductase inhibitor, antihyperlipidemic agent |
| Zoloft (sertraline hydrochloride) | antidepressant, selective serotonin reuptake inhibitor (SSRI) |
| Zyprexa (olanzapine) | antipsychotic |
| Zyrtec (cetirizine) | second-generation antihistamine |

# References

Lance LL, Lacy CF, Goldman MP, Armstrong LL, eds., Quick look drug book. Baltimore: Lippincott Williams & Wilkins, 2000.

Top 200 drugs of 1999. *Pharmacy Times,* www.pharmacytimes.com/top200.html.

# Classic Textbook Method of Blood Gas Interpretation

| Status | pH | PaCO$_2$ | HCO$_3^-$ | BE |
|---|---|---|---|---|
| **RESPIRATORY ACIDOSIS** | | | | |
| Uncompensated | ↓ 7.35 | ↑ 45 | Normal | Normal |
| Partially compensated | ↓ 7.35 | ↑ 45 | ↑ 27 | ↑ +2 |
| Compensated | 7.35–7.45 | ↑ 45 | ↑ 27 | ↑ +2 |
| **RESPIRATORY ALKALOSIS** | | | | |
| Uncompensated | ↑ 7.45 | ↓ 35 | Normal | Normal |
| Partially compensated | ↑ 7.45 | ↓ 35 | ↓ 22 | ↓ −2 |
| Compensated | 7.40–7.45 | ↓ 35 | ↓ 22 | ↓ −2 |
| **METABOLIC ACIDOSIS** | | | | |
| Uncompensated | ↓ 7.35 | Normal | ↓ 22 | ↓ −2 |
| Partially compensated | ↓ 7.35 | ↓ 35 | ↓ 22 | ↓ −2 |
| Compensated | 7.35–7.40 | ↓ 35 | ↓ 22 | ↓ −2 |
| **METABOLIC ALKALOSIS** | | | | |
| Uncompensated | ↑ 7.45 | Normal | ↑ 27 | ↑ +2 |
| Partially compensated* | ↑ 7.45 | ↑ 45 | ↑ 27 | ↑ +2 |
| Compensated* | 7.40–7.45 | ↑ 45 | ↑ 27 | ↑ +2 |
| **COMBINED RESPIRATORY AND METABOLIC ACIDOSIS** | ↓ 7.35 | ↑ 45 | ↓ 22 | ↓ −2 |
| **COMBINED RESPIRATORY AND METABOLIC ALKALOSIS** | ↑ 7.45 | ↓ 35 | ↑ 27 | ↑ +2 |

*In general, partially compensated or compensated metabolic alkalosis is rarely seen clinically because of the body's mechanism to prevent hypoventilation.

From Kacmarek RM, Mack CW, Dimas S. The essentials of respiratory care, 3rd ed. St. Louis, MO: Mosby-Year Book, 1990.

# Glasgow Coma Scale

| Monitored Performance | Reaction | Score |
|---|---|---|
| Eye Opening | Spontaneous | 4 |
| | Open when spoken to | 3 |
| | Open at pain stimulus | 2 |
| | No reaction | 1 |
| Verbal Performance | Coherent | 5 |
| | Confused, disoriented | 4 |
| | Disconnected words | 3 |
| | Unintelligible sounds | 2 |
| | No verbal reaction | 1 |
| Motor Responsiveness | Follows instructions | 6 |
| | Intentional pain avoidance | 5 |
| | Large motor movement | 4 |
| | Flexor synergism | 3 |
| | Extensor synergism | 2 |
| | No reaction | 1 |

# Mechanical Ventilation Criteria in Respiratory Care

## Criteria for determining the control variable during mechanical ventilation

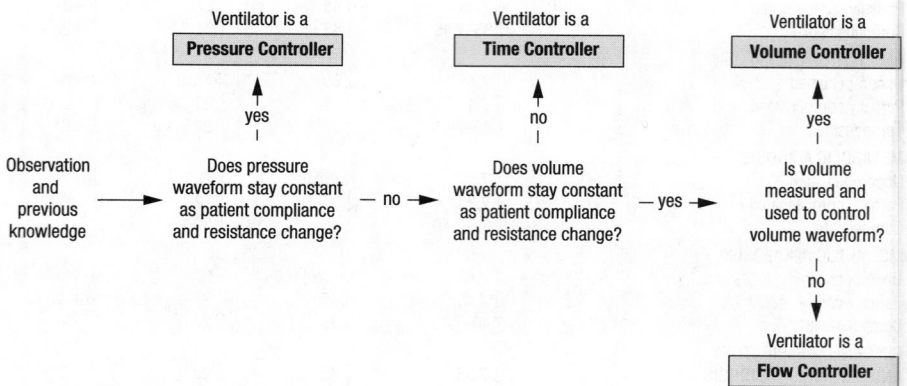

## Criteria for determining the phase variables during mechanical ventilation

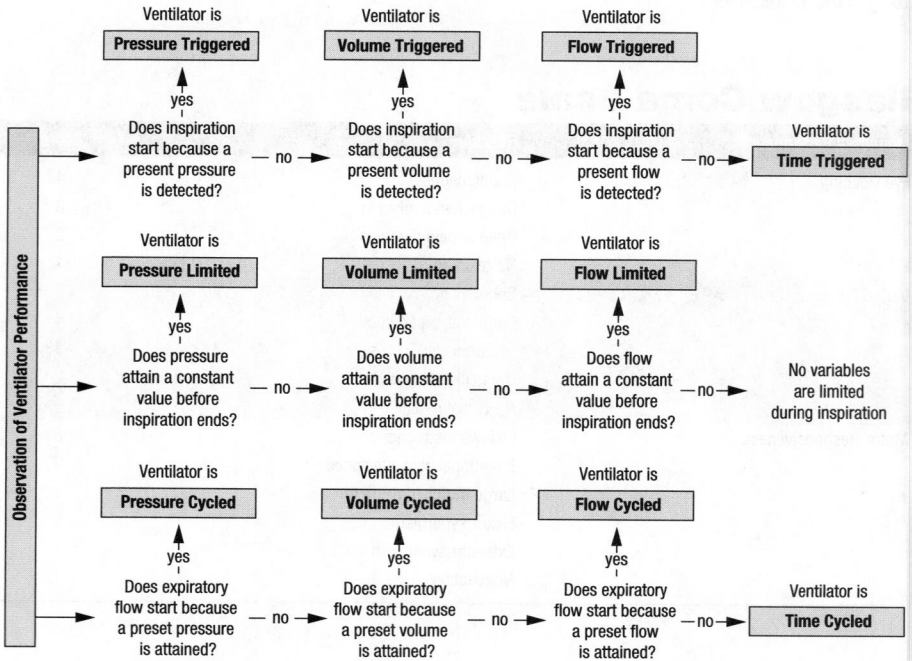

# Levels of Alzheimer Disease

| Level | Description |
|---|---|
| I and II | Presenile dementia may end here with no further progression. Brain changes are not significant, and the only remarkable symptoms may be forgetfulness. Patients at this level perform all activities of daily living (ADLs) with reasonable ease. |
| III | At this level, there will be increased inability to remember facts, faces, and names. The patient will still have enough awareness to recognize the problem and will become increasingly frustrated and angry. Most ADLs are still performed reasonably well. |
| IV | Late confusional or mild Alzheimer. The patient at this level will begin to misplace things, has increasing difficulty remembering, and will neglect ADLs. Most patients will be aware that a problem exists but will deny that it is a concern. |
| V | Early dementia or moderate Alzheimer. By this level, the patient must have custodial care. There will be severe lapses in memory, disorientation, anger, and great frustration. |
| VI | Middle dementia or moderately severe Alzheimer. The patient now has severe memory loss, is incapable of self-care at any level, and is disoriented most of the time. There is immense anger, hostility, and combativeness. At this level, a fear of water is present. |
| VII | Late dementia. The patient requires full-time care and will rarely be seen in the office setting. Unless home care is an option, the physician will probably make calls to the long-term care facility. The patient at this state rarely speaks and almost never speaks intelligibly. There will be incontinence, and the patient may require tube feedings. |

From Hosley JB, Molle-Matthews EA, eds. Lippincott's textbook for clinical medical assisting. Baltimore: Lippincott Williams & Wilkins, 1999.

# Overview of Major Nursing Theories

| Theorist | Purpose | Views of Components |
|---|---|---|
| Florence Nightingale (1860)<br>*Notes on Nursing: What It Is Not* | To help individuals responsible for caring for sick to "think how to nurse." Theory addresses fundamental needs of the sick and basic principles of good health care. | **Person:** An individual with vital reparative processes to deal with disease.<br>**Environment:** External conditions that affect life and the individual's development. Focus is on ventilation, warmth, odors, and light.<br>**Health:** Focus is on the reparative process of getting well.<br>**Nursing:** Goal is to place the individual in the best condition for good health care. |
| Hildegard E. Peplau (1952)<br>*Interpersonal Relations in Nursing* | To develop an interpersonal interaction between client and nurse | **Person:** An organism striving to reduce tension generated by needs.<br>**Environment:** Implicitly defined; the interpersonal process is always included, and the psychodynamic milieu receives attention, with emphasis on the client's culture and mores.<br>**Health:** Ongoing human process that implies forward movement of personality and other ongoing human processes in the direction of creative, constructive, productive, personal, and community living.<br>**Nursing:** Interpersonal therapeutic process that "functions cooperatively with other human processes that make health possible for individuals in communities. Nursing is an educative instrument, a maturing force that aims to promote forward movement of personality." |
| Virginia Henderson (1955)<br>*The Nature of Nursing* | To assist the client in gaining independence as rapidly as possible | **Person:** Individual requiring assistance to achieve health and independence or a peaceful death. Mind and body are inseparable.<br>**Environment:** All external conditions and influences that affect life and development.<br>**Health:** Health, equated with independence, is viewed in terms of the client's ability to perform 14 components of nursing care unaided: breathing, eating, drinking, maintaining comfort, sleeping, resting, clothing, maintaining body temperature, ensuring safety, communicating, worshiping, working, recreation, and continuing development.<br>**Nursing:** Assists and supports the individual in life activities and the attainment of independence. |
| Faye Glenn Abdellah (1960)<br>*Patient-Centered Approaches to Nursing* | To deliver nursing care for the whole individual | **Person:** The recipient of nursing care having physical, emotional, and sociologic needs that may be overt or covert.<br>**Environment:** Not clearly defined. Some discussion indicates that clients interact with their environment, of which the nurse is a part.<br>**Health:** Implicitly defined as a state when the individual has no unmet needs |

| Theorist | Purpose | Views of Components |
|----------|---------|---------------------|
| Abdellah (*cont.*) | | and no anticipated or actual impairments. **Nursing:** Broadly grouped in "21 nursing problems," which center around needs for hygiene, comfort, activity, rest, safety, oxygen, nutrition, elimination, hydration, physical and emotional health promotion, interpersonal relationships, and development of self-awareness. Nursing care is doing something for an individual. |
| Ida Jean Orlando (1961) *The Dynamic Nurse-Patient Relationship* | To interact with clients to meet immediate needs by identifying client behaviors, nurse's reactions, and nursing actions to take. | **Person:** Unique individual behaving verbally and nonverbally. Assumption is that individuals are at times able to meet their own needs and at other times are unable to do so. **Environment:** Not defined. **Health:** Does not define health. Assumption is that being without emotional or physical discomfort and having a sense of well-being contribute to a healthy state. **Nursing:** Professional nursing is conceptualized as finding out and meeting the client's immediate need for help. Medicine and nursing are viewed as distinctly different. |
| Lydia E. Hall (1964) *Nursing: What Is It?* | To provide professional nursing care to people past the acute stage of illness | **Person:** Client is composed of body, pathology, and person. People set their own goals and are capable of learning and growing. **Environment:** Should facilitate achievement of the client's personal goals. **Health:** Development of a mature self-identity that assists in the conscious selection of actions that facilitate growth. **Nursing:** Caring is the nurse's primary function. Professional nursing is most important during the recuperative period. |
| Ernestine Weidenbach (1964) *Clinical Nursing—A Helping Art* | To assist individuals in overcoming obstacles that prevent meeting health care needs | **Person:** Any individual who is receiving help (care, instruction, or advice) from a member of the health profession or from a worker in the field of health. **Environment:** Not specifically addressed. **Health:** Not defined. Concepts of nursing, client, and need for help and their relationships imply health-related concerns in the nurse-client relationship (Marriner-Tomey, p. 245). **Nursing:** Functioning human being who acts, thinks, and feels. All actions, thoughts, and feelings underlie what the nurse does. |
| Joyce Travelbee (1966, 1971) *Interpersonal Aspects of Nursing* | To assist individuals, families, communities, and groups to prevent or cope with illness and regain health | **Person:** A unique, irreplaceable individual who is in a continuous process of becoming, evolving, and changing. **Environment:** Not explicitly defined. **Health:** Health includes the individual's perceptions of health and the absence of disease. |

| Theorist | Purpose | Views of Components |
|---|---|---|
| Travelbee (*cont.*) | | **Nursing:** An interpersonal process whereby the professional nurse practitioner assists an individual, family, or community to prevent or to cope with the experience of illness and suffering and, if necessary, to find meaning in these experiences. |
| Martha E. Rogers (1970) *The Science of Unitary Man* | To assist the client in achieving a maximum level of wellness | **Person:** Unitary man, a four-dimensional energy field. **Environment:** Encompasses all that is outside any given human field. Person exchanging matter and energy. **Health:** Not specifically addressed, but emerges out of interaction between human and environment, moves forward, and maximizes human potential. **Nursing:** A learned profession that is both science and art. The professional practice of nursing is creative and imaginative and exists to serve people. |
| Dorothea E. Orem (1971) *Nursing: Concepts of Practice* | To provide care and to assist the client to attain self-care | **Person:** Biopsychosocial being capable of self-care. Includes physical, psychological, interpersonal, and social aspects of human functioning. **Environment:** Internal and external stimuli. Requisites for self-care have their origins in human beings and the environment. **Health:** State of wholeness or integrity of human beings, including physical, mental, and social well-being. **Nursing:** A creative effort of one human being to help another human being. Consists of three nursing systems: wholly compensatory, partially compensatory, and supportive/educative. |
| Imogene M. King (1971) *Open Systems Model* | To use communication to help the client reestablish a positive adaptation to his or her environment | **Person:** Biopsychosocial being. **Environment:** Internal and external environment continually interact to assist in adjustments to change. **Health:** A dynamic life experience with continued goal attainment and adjustment to stressors. **Nursing:** Perceiving, thinking, relating, judging, and acting with an individual who comes to a nursing situation. |
| Betty Neuman (1972) *The Neuman Systems Model* | To address the effects of stress and reactions to it on the development and maintenance of health | **Person:** A client system that is composed of physiologic, psychological, sociocultural, and environmental variables. **Environment:** Internal and external forces surrounding humans at any time. **Health:** Health or wellness exists if all parts and subparts are in harmony with the whole person. **Nursing:** A unique profession concerned with all variables affecting an individual's response to stressors. |
| Myra Estrin Levin (1973) *Conservation Model* | To use conservation activities aimed at optimal use of client's resources | **Person:** A holistic being. **Environment:** Broadly,includes all the individual's experiences. |

| Theorist | Purpose | Views of Components |
|---|---|---|
| Levin (*cont.*) | | **Health:** The maintenance of the client's unity and integrity.<br>**Nursing:** A discipline rooted in the organic dependency of the individual human being on his or her relationships with others. |
| Jean Watson (1979)<br>*Nursing: Human Science and Human Care* | To focus on curative factors derived from a humanistic perspective and from scientific knowledge | **Person:** A valued being to be cared for, respected, nurtured, understood, and assisted; a fully functional, integrated self.<br>**Environment:** Social environment, caring, and the culture of caring impact on health.<br>**Health:** Physical, mental and social well-being.<br>**Nursing:** A human science of people and human health; illness experiences that are mediated by profession, personal, scientific, aesthetic, and ethical human care transactions. |
| Dorothy E. Johnson (1980)<br>*The Behavioral System Model for Nursing* | To reduce stress so the client can recover as quickly as possible | **Person:** A system of interdependent parts with patterned, repetitive, and purposeful ways of behaving.<br>**Environment:** All forces that affect the person and that influence the behavioral system.<br>**Health:** Focus on person, not illness. Health is a dynamic state influenced by biologic, psychological, and social factors.<br>**Nursing:** Promotion of behavioral system, balance, and stability. An art and a science providing external assistance before and during system balance disturbances. |
| Sister Callista Roy (1980)<br>*Roy Adaptation Model* | To identify the type of demands placed on a client and the client's adaptation to the demands | **Person:** A biopsychosocial being and the recipient of nursing care.<br>**Environment:** All conditions, circumstances, and influences surrounding and affecting the development of an organism or groups of organisms.<br>**Health:** The person encounters adaptation problems in changing environments.<br>**Nursing:** A theoretical system of knowledge that prescribes a process of analysis and action related to the care of the ill or potentially ill person. |
| Rosemarie Rizzo Parse (1981)<br>*Man-Living-Health: Theory of Nursing* | To focus on humans as living unity and humans' qualitative participation with health experience | **Person:** A major reason for nursing's existence, evidenced by a "pattern of patterns of relating" (p. 26).<br>**Environment:** "Man and environment interchange energy to create what is in the world, and man chooses the meaning given to the situations he creates" (p. 27).<br>**Health:** A lived experience that is a process of being and becoming.<br>**Nursing:** "Nursing practice is directed toward illuminating and mobilizing family interrelationships in light of the meaning assigned to health and its possibilities as language in the cocreated patterns of relating" (p. 82). |

From Craven RF, Hirnle CJ, eds. Fundamentals of nursing: human health and function. Philadelphia: Lippincott Williams & Wilkins, 2000.

# References

Abdellah FG. Patient-centered approaches to nursing. New York: Macmillan, 1960.

Hall LE. Nursing: what is it? *Can Nurse* 1964; 60, 150–4.

Henderson V. The nature of nursing. New York: Macmillan, 1955.

Johnson DE. The behavioral system model for nursing. In JP Riehl & C Roy, eds., Conceptual models for nursing practice. New York: Appleton-Century-Crofts, 1980.

King IM. Toward a theory of nursing. New York: Wiley, 1971.

Levin ME. An introduction to clinical nursing, 2nd ed. Philadelphia: FA Davis, 1973.

Marriner-Tomey A. Nursing theorists and their work, 3rd ed. St. Louis, MO: CV Mosby, 1994.

Neuman B. The Neuman systems model: application to nursing education and practice. New York: Appleton-Century-Crofts, 1972.

Nightingale F. Notes on nursing: what it is and what it is not. London: Harrison, 1860.

Orem DE. Nursing: concepts of practice, 3rd ed. New York: McGraw-Hill, 1971.

Orlando IJ. The dynamic nurse-patient relationship: function, process, and principles. New York: Putnam, 1961.

Parse RR. Man-living-health: theory of nursing. New York: Wiley, 1981.

Peplau HE. Interpersonal relations in nursing. New York: Putnam, 1952.

Rogers ME. An introduction to the theoretical basis of nursing. Philadelphia: FA Davis, 1970.

Roy C. The Roy adaptation model. In JP Riehl & C Roy, eds., Conceptual models for nursing practice. New York: Appleton-Century Crofts, 1980.

Travelbee J. Interpersonal aspects of nursing. Philadelphia: FA Davis, 1971.

Weidenbach E. Clinical nursing: a helping art. New York: Springer, 1964.

# The Food Guide Pyramid:
# A Guide to Daily Food Choices

The U.S. Department of Agriculture (USDA) developed the Food Guide Pyramid to depict the six food groups. USDA recommends that consumption of fats, oils, and sweets be limited as much as possible. For each of the other five groups, the serving portions chart provides examples of what constitutes a serving. These guidelines can be used in planning a healthful daily diet.

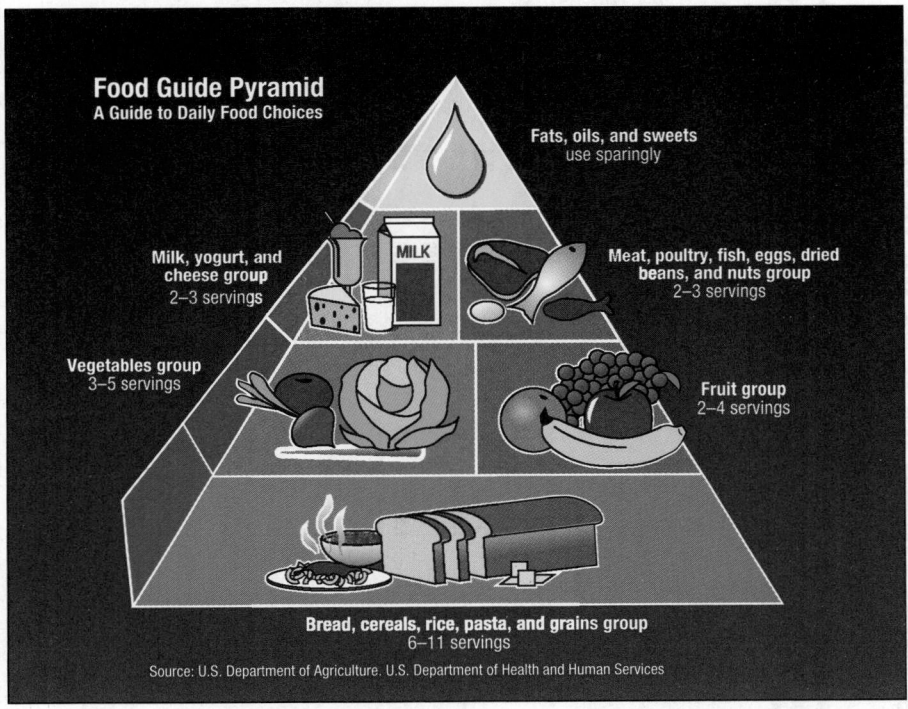

**Food Guide Pyramid**
A Guide to Daily Food Choices

Fats, oils, and sweets
use sparingly

Milk, yogurt, and cheese group
2–3 servings

Meat, poultry, fish, eggs, dried beans, and nuts group
2–3 servings

Vegetables group
3–5 servings

Fruit group
2–4 servings

Bread, cereals, rice, pasta, and grains group
6–11 servings

Source: U.S. Department of Agriculture. U.S. Department of Health and Human Services

| | | | | | |
|---|---|---|---|---|---|
| **Milk, yogurt, and cheese** | 1 cup milk or yogurt | or | 1-1/2 oz natural cheese | or | 2 oz processed cheese |
| **Meat, poultry, fish, eggs, dried beans, and nuts** | 2-3 oz cooked lean meat, poultry, or fish | or | 1/2 cup cooked dried beans, or 1/2 cup tofu, or 2 1/2 oz soyburger, or 1 egg equals 1 oz lean meat | or | 2 tbsp. peanut butter or 1/3 cup nuts equals 1 oz meat |
| **Vegetables** | 1 cup raw leafy vegetables | or | 1/2 cup nonleafy vegetables cooked or chopped raw | or | 3/4 cup vegetable juice |
| **Fruit** | 1 medium apple, banana, orange, or pear | or | 1/2 cup chopped, cooked, or canned fruit | or | 3/4 cup fruit juice |
| **Bread, cereals, rice, pasta, and grains** | 1 slice bread | or | 1 cup ready-to-eat cereal | or | 1/2 cup cooked cereal, rice, or pasta |

# Dietary Reference Intakes: Recommended Intakes for Individuals

Food and Nutrition Board, Institute of Medicine, National Academy of Sciences

| Life Stage Group | Calcium (mg/d) | Phosphorous (mg/d) | Magnesium (mg/d) | Vitamin D (µg/d)ab | Fluoride (mg/d) | Thiamin (mg/d) | Riboflavin (mg/d) | Niacin (mg/d)c | Vitamin B6 (mg/d) | Folate (µg/d)d | Vitamin B12 (µg/d) | Pantothenic Acid (mg/d) | Biotin (µg/d) | Choline (mg/d)e |
|---|---|---|---|---|---|---|---|---|---|---|---|---|---|---|
| *Infants* | | | | | | | | | | | | | | |
| 0–6 mo. | 210* | 100* | 30* | 5* | 0.01* | 0.2* | 0.3* | 2* | 0.1* | 65* | 0.4* | 1.7* | 5* | 125* |
| 7–12 mo. | 270* | 275* | 75* | 5* | 0.5* | 0.3* | 0.4* | 4* | 0.3* | 80* | 0.5* | 1.8* | 6* | 150* |
| *Children* | | | | | | | | | | | | | | |
| 1–3 yr. | 500* | 460 | 80 | 5* | 0.7* | 0.5 | 0.5 | 6 | 0.5 | 150 | 0.9 | 2* | 8* | 200* |
| 4–8 yr. | 800* | 500 | 130 | 5* | 1* | 0.6 | 0.6 | 8 | 0.6 | 200 | 1.2 | 3* | 12* | 250* |
| *Males* | | | | | | | | | | | | | | |
| 9–13 yr. | 1,300* | 1,250 | 240 | 5* | 2* | 0.9 | 0.9 | 12 | 1.0 | 300 | 1.8 | 4* | 20* | 375* |
| 14–18 yr. | 1,300* | 1,250 | 410 | 5* | 3* | 1.2 | 1.3 | 16 | 1.3 | 400 | 2.4 | 5* | 25* | 550* |
| 19–30 yr. | 1,000* | 700 | 400 | 5* | 4* | 1.2 | 1.3 | 16 | 1.3 | 400 | 2.4 | 5* | 30* | 550* |
| 31–50 yr. | 1,000* | 700 | 420 | 5* | 4* | 1.2 | 1.3 | 16 | 1.3 | 400 | 2.4 | 5* | 30* | 550* |
| 51–70 yr. | 1,200* | 700 | 420 | 10* | 4* | 1.2 | 1.3 | 16 | 1.7 | 400 | 2.4f | 5* | 30* | 550* |
| >70 yr. | 1,200* | 700 | 420 | 15* | 4* | 1.2 | 1.3 | 16 | 1.7 | 400 | 2.4f | 5* | 30* | 550* |
| *Females* | | | | | | | | | | | | | | |
| 9–13 yr. | 1,300* | 1,250 | 240 | 5* | 2* | 0.9 | 0.9 | 12 | 1.0 | 300 | 1.8 | 4* | 20* | 375* |
| 14–18 yr. | 1,300* | 1,250 | 360 | 5* | 3* | 1.0 | 1.0 | 14 | 1.2 | 400g | 2.4 | 5* | 25* | 400* |
| 19–30 yr. | 1,000* | 700 | 310 | 5* | 3* | 1.1 | 1.1 | 14 | 1.3 | 400g | 2.4 | 5* | 30* | 425* |
| 31–50 yr. | 1,000* | 700 | 320 | 5* | 3* | 1.1 | 1.1 | 14 | 1.3 | 400g | 2.4 | 5* | 30* | 425* |
| 51–70 yr. | 1,200* | 700 | 320 | 10* | 3* | 1.1 | 1.1 | 14 | 1.5 | 400 | 2.4f | 5* | 30* | 425* |
| >70 yr. | 1,200* | 700 | 320 | 15* | 3* | 1.1 | 1.1 | 14 | 1.5 | 400 | 2.4f | 5* | 30* | 425* |
| *Pregnancy* | | | | | | | | | | | | | | |
| ≤ 18 yr. | 1,300* | 1,250 | 400 | 5* | 3* | 1.4 | 1.4 | 18 | 1.9 | 600h | 2.6 | 6* | 30* | 450* |
| 19–30 yr. | 1,000* | 700 | 350 | 5* | 3* | 1.4 | 1.4 | 18 | 1.9 | 600h | 2.6 | 6* | 30* | 450* |
| 31–50 yr. | 1,000* | 700 | 360 | 5* | 3* | 1.4 | 1.4 | 18 | 1.9 | 600h | 2.6 | 6* | 30* | 450* |

| Life Stage Group | Calcium (mg/d) | Phosphorous (mg/d) | Magnesium (mg/d) | Vitamin D (μg/d)[a][b] | Fluoride (mg/d) | Thiamin (mg/d) | Riboflavin (mg/d) | Niacin (mg/d)[c] | Vitamin $B_6$ (mg/d) | Folate (μg/d)[d] | Vitamin $B_{12}$ (μg/d) | Pantothenic Acid (mg/d) | Biotin (μg/d) | Choline[e] (mg/d) |
|---|---|---|---|---|---|---|---|---|---|---|---|---|---|---|
| *Lactation* | | | | | | | | | | | | | | |
| ≤18 yr. | 1,300* | 1,250 | 360 | 5* | 3* | 1.4 | 1.6 | 17 | 2.0 | 500 | 2.8 | 7* | 35* | 550* |
| 19–30 yr. | 1,000* | 700 | 310 | 5* | 3* | 1.4 | 1.6 | 17 | 2.0 | 500 | 2.8 | 7* | 35* | 550* |
| 31–50 yr. | 1,000* | 700 | 320 | 5* | 3* | 1.4 | 1.6 | 17 | 2.0 | 500 | 2.8 | 7* | 35* | 550* |

[a] As cholecalciferol. 1 μg cholecalciferol = 40 IU vitamin D.

[b] In the absence of adequate exposure to sunlight.

[c] As niacin equivalents (NE). 1 mg of niacin = 60 mg of tryptophan; 0–6 months = preformed niacin (not NE).

[d] As dietary folate equivalents (DFE). 1 DFE = 1 μg food folate = 0.6 μg of folic acid from fortified food or as a supplement consumed with food = 0.5 μg of a supplement taken on an empty stomach.

[e] Although AIs have been set for choline, there are few data to assess whether a dietary supply of choline is needed at all stages of the life cycle, and it may be that the choline requirement can be met by endogenous synthesis at some of these stages.

[f] Because 10 to 30 percent of older people may malabsorb food-bound $B_{12}$, it is advisable for those older than 50 years to meet their RDA mainly by consuming foods fortified with $B_{12}$ or a supplement containing $B_{12}$.

[g] In view of evidence linking folate intake with neural tube defects in the fetus, it is recommended that all women capable of becoming pregnant consume 400 μg from supplements or fortified foods in addition to intake of food folate from a varied diet.

[h] It is assumed that women will continue consuming 400 μg from supplements or fortified food until their pregnancy is confirmed and they enter prenatal care, which ordinarily occurs after the end of the periconceptional period—the critical time for formation of the neural tube.

This table presents Recommended Dietary Allowances (RDAs) in **bold type** and Adequate Intakes (AIs) in ordinary type followed by an asterisk (*). RDAs and AIs may both be used as goals for individual intake. RDAs are set to meet the needs of almost all (97 to 98 percent) individuals in a group. For healthy breast-fed infants, the AI is the mean intake. The AI for other life-stage and gender groups is believed to cover needs of all individuals in a group, but lack of data or uncertainty in the data prevent being able to specify with confidence the percentage of individuals covered by this intake.

Reprinted with permission from Dietary reference intakes for thiamin, riboflavin, niacin, vitamin $B_6$, folate, vitamin $B_{12}$, pantothenic acid, biotin, and choline. Copyright 2000 by the National Academy of Sciences. Courtesy of the National Academy of Sciences. Washington, DC.

[*Editor's note.* Starting in 1997, the U.S. and Canadian governments began introducing a set of dietary reference intakes (DRIs) for use in both countries. The table provided here includes all DRIs that had been introduced as this edition of *Stedman's Concise Medical Dictionary* went to press.]

# Canadian Recommended Nutrient Intakes

Recommended Nutrient Intakes (RNIs) are the daily nutrient intakes suggested for healthy Canadians to stay healthy. The main table includes recommended intakes for protein, six vitamins, and six minerals. Although the RNIs are listed as daily amounts, they should be thought of as the average daily recommended intake over a longer period of time, such as a week.

The amount of each nutrient needed falls within a range, with danger zones above and below it:

- If a person consumes too much, the nutrient can cause toxic effects similar to drugs.
- If too little is consumed, deficiency symptoms can appear.

Each person may have slightly different needs due to differences in absorption and losses and overall diet composition. The RNIs are not minimum requirements, but generous allowances set by Health Canada to meet the needs of most people. Therefore, the RNIs exceed the actual requirements of most individuals. An intake below the recommended is not necessarily inadequate, but there is a greater chance of inadequacy as the intake consistently falls further below the RNI.

Eating a variety of foods from Canada's Food Guide [see p. APP 150] is your best way of making sure you get all the nutrients you need to stay healthy. Supplements are not recommended unless specially ordered by your doctor. As seen in the table below, the recommended nutrient intakes change according to age and sex.

kg: kilogram (1 kg = 2.2 lbs.)
g: gram (28.3 g = 1 oz.)
mg: milligram (1 mg = 1 one-thousandth of a gram)
$\mu$g: microgram (1$\mu$g = 1 one-millionth of a gram)

While the Recommended Nutrient Intake guidelines are the most up-to-date Canadian nutrition standards currently available, Health Canada and a number of U.S. government agencies are sponsoring the review of the scientific data concerning requirements and tolerable upper levels of nutrients and other food components. The review is intended to produce a series of Dietary Reference Intake (DRI) guidelines which will ultimately replace the current Canadian Recommended Nutrient Intakes.

This information is of a general nature and may vary according to your special circumstances. If you have specific questions, please contact your physician or an appropriate health care professional.

Reviewed May 2000
Source: Health Canada. Nutrition recommendations: The report of the scientific review committee. Ottawa, Canada: Supply & Services Canada, August 1990. Reproduced with the permission of the Minister of Public Works and Government Services Canada, 2000.

[*Editor's note*. The Recommended Dietary Intakes for Use in Australia are available at www.nhmrc. health.gov.au/publicat/diet/n6-index.htm.]

## Daily Recommended Nutrient Intake Based on Age and Body Weight

| Age | Sex | Weight kg | Protein g | Vit. A RE[a] | Vit. D µg | Vit. E mg | Vit. C mg | Folate µg | Vit. B$_{12}$ µg | Calcium mg | Phosphorus mg | Magnesium mg | Iron mg | Iodine µg | Zinc mg |
|---|---|---|---|---|---|---|---|---|---|---|---|---|---|---|---|
| 0–4 mo. | Both | 6.0 | 12[b] | 400 | 10 | 3 | 20 | 25 | 0.3 | 250[c] | 150 | 20 | 0.3[d] | 30 | 2[d] |
| 5–12 mo. | Both | 9.0 | 12 | 400 | 10 | 3 | 20 | 40 | 0.4 | 400 | 200 | 32 | 7 | 40 | 3 |
| 1 yr. | Both | 11 | 13 | 400 | 10 | 3 | 20 | 40 | 0.5 | 500 | 300 | 40 | 6 | 55 | 4 |
| 2–3 yr. | Both | 14 | 16 | 400 | 5 | 4 | 20 | 50 | 0.6 | 550 | 350 | 50 | 6 | 65 | 4 |
| 4–6 yr. | Both | 18 | 19 | 500 | 5 | 5 | 25 | 70 | 0.8 | 600 | 400 | 65 | 8 | 85 | 5 |
| 7–9 yr. | M | 25 | 26 | 700 | 2.5 | 7 | 25 | 90 | 1.0 | 700 | 500 | 100 | 8 | 110 | 7 |
| 7–9 yr. | F | 25 | 26 | 700 | 2.5 | 6 | 25 | 90 | 1.0 | 700 | 500 | 100 | 8 | 95 | 7 |
| 10–12 yr. | M | 34 | 34 | 800 | 2.5 | 8 | 25 | 120 | 1.0 | 900 | 700 | 130 | 8 | 125 | 9 |
| 10–12 yr. | F | 36 | 36 | 800 | 2.5 | 7 | 25 | 130 | 1.0 | 1100 | 800 | 135 | 8 | 110 | 9 |
| 13–15 yr. | M | 50 | 49 | 900 | 2.5 | 9 | 30[e] | 175 | 1.0 | 1100 | 900 | 185 | 10 | 160 | 12 |
| 13–15 yr. | F | 48 | 46 | 800 | 2.5 | 7 | 30[e] | 170 | 1.0 | 1000 | 850 | 180 | 13 | 160 | 9 |
| 16–18 yr. | M | 62 | 58 | 1000 | 2.5 | 10 | 40[e] | 220 | 1.0 | 900 | 1000 | 230 | 10 | 160 | 12 |
| 16–18 yr. | F | 53 | 47 | 800 | 2.5 | 7 | 30[e] | 190 | 1.0 | 700 | 850 | 200 | 12 | 160 | 9 |
| 19–24 yr. | M | 71 | 61 | 1000 | 2.5 | 10 | 40[e] | 220 | 1.0 | 800 | 1000 | 240 | 9 | 160 | 12 |
| 19–24 yr. | F | 58 | 50 | 800 | 2.5 | 7 | 30[e] | 180 | 1.0 | 700 | 850 | 200 | 13 | 160 | 9 |
| 25–49 yr. | M | 74 | 64 | 1000 | 2.5 | 9 | 40[e] | 230 | 1.0 | 800 | 1000 | 250 | 9 | 160 | 12 |
| 25–49 yr. | F | 59 | 51 | 800 | 2.5 | 6 | 30[e] | 185 | 1.0 | 700 | 850 | 200 | 13 | 160 | 9 |
| 50–74 yr. | M | 73 | 63 | 1000 | 5 | 7 | 40[e] | 230 | 1.0 | 800 | 1000 | 250 | 9 | 160 | 12 |
| 50–74 yr. | F | 63 | 54 | 800 | 5 | 6 | 30[e] | 195 | 1.0 | 800 | 850 | 210 | 8 | 160 | 9 |
| 75+ yr. | M | 69 | 59 | 1000 | 5 | 6 | 40[e] | 215 | 1.0 | 800 | 1000 | 230 | 9 | 160 | 12 |
| 75+ yr. | F | 64 | 55 | 800 | 5 | 5 | 30[e] | 200 | 1.0 | 800 | 850 | 210 | 8 | 160 | 9 |
| **Pregnancy** | | | | | | | | | | | | | | | |
| 1st trimester | — | — | 5 | 0 | 2.5 | 2 | 0 | 200 | 0.2 | 500 | 200 | 15 | 0 | 25 | 6 |
| 2nd trimester | — | — | 15 | 0 | 2.5 | 2 | 10 | 200 | 0.2 | 500 | 200 | 45 | 5 | 25 | 6 |
| 3rd trimester | — | — | 24 | 0 | 2.5 | 2 | 10 | 200 | 0.2 | 500 | 200 | 45 | 10 | 25 | 6 |
| Breast-feeding | — | — | 22 | 400 | 2.5 | 3 | 25 | 100 | 0.2 | 500 | 200 | 65 | 0 | 50 | 6 |

[a] RE: retinol equivalents
[b] Protein is assumed to be from breast milk and must be adjusted for infant formula.
[c] Infant formula with high phosphorus should contain 375 mg calcium.
[d] Breast milk is assumed to be the source of the mineral.
[e] Smokers should increase vitamin C by 50%.

# Canada's Food Guide to Healthy Eating

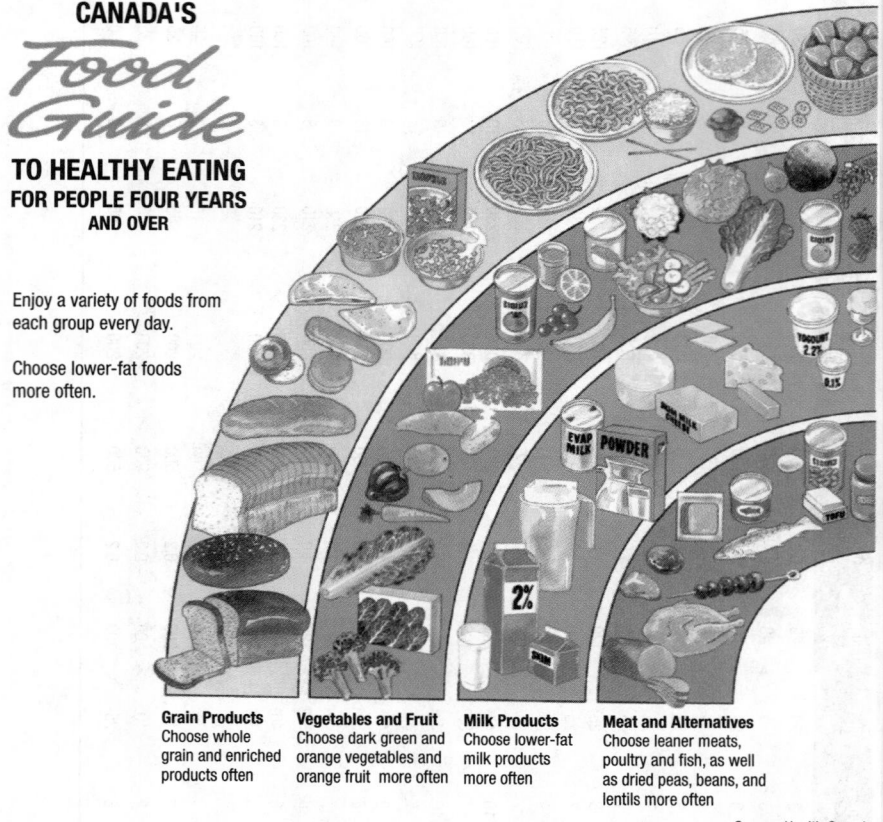

**CANADA'S**

*Food Guide*

**TO HEALTHY EATING**
**FOR PEOPLE FOUR YEARS**
**AND OVER**

Enjoy a variety of foods from
each group every day.

Choose lower-fat foods
more often.

**Grain Products**
Choose whole
grain and enriched
products often

**Vegetables and Fruit**
Choose dark green and
orange vegetables and
orange fruit more often

**Milk Products**
Choose lower-fat
milk products
more often

**Meat and Alternatives**
Choose leaner meats,
poultry and fish, as well
as dried peas, beans, and
lentils more often

Source: Health Canada

| | | | |
|---|---|---|---|
| **Grain products**<br>(5–12 servings) | 1 slice of bread, 3/4 cup hot cereal,<br>or 30 g cold cereal equals 1 serving | *or* | 1 bagel, pita or bun, or 1 cup of pasta<br>or rice equals 2 servings |

**Vegetables
and Fruit**
(5–10 servings)

1 medium-size vegetable or fruit, 1/2 cup fresh, frozen, or canned vegetables or fruit,
1 cup salad, or 1/2 cup of juice equals 1 serving

**Milk products**
(Children 4-9 years: 2–3
Youth 10-16 years: 3–4
Adults: 2–4
Pregnant and breast-
feeding women: 3–4)

1 cup milk, 50 g cheese (3" x 1" x 1" block or
2 slices), or 3/4 cup yogurt equals 1 serving

**Meats and
alternatives**
(2–3 servings)

50-100 g meat, poultry, or fish, 1/3-2/3 can of
tuna, 1-2 eggs, 125-250 mL beans, 1/3 cup
tofu, or 2 tbsp peanut butter

**Other Foods**

Taste and enjoyment can also
come from other foods and
beverages that are not part of
the 4 food groups. Some of
these foods are higher in fat or
calories, so use these foods in
moderation.

# Conversion Factors Between Traditional and SI Units

**Factors for Converting Nutrients Expressed in Metric or Milliequivalent Units into International System (SI) Units**

1. **Definitions**
   a. Equivalent weight (EW) = atomic weight of element/valence of ionic form. Example with magnesium: atomic wt = 24, valence = 2+; therefore EW = 12.
   b. Quantity of an electrolyte in milliequivalents per liter (mEq/L) = mg of electrolyte/L/EW. Example: 48 mg of magnesium/L/12 = 4 mEq/L.
   c. Quantity of an electrolyte in mg/dL = (mEq/L × EW)/10.
   d. To convert mg/dL (= mg%) of an electrolyte to mEq/L: mg/dL × 10/EW = mEq/L.
   e. 1 mol = 1 molecular or atomic weight of element or compound in grams (GMWt). In solutions this is usually expressed as moles per liter; i.e., 1 mol/L = 1 M; 1 mM (mmol) = 1 mol × $10^{-3}$, 1 µM (µmol) = 1 mol × $10^{-6}$, 1 nM (nmol) = 1 mol × $10^{-9}$.
   f. 1. To convert mEq/L of an electrolyte or other ions in solution to mmol/L: mEq/L divided by valence = mmol/L; e.g., (a) 2 mEq/L of magnesium ($Mg^{2+}$) = 2/2 = 1. mmol/L; e.g., (b) 150 mEq $Na^+$/L = 140/1 = 140 mmol/L.
      2. To convert mg/dL to mmol/L: (mg/dL × 10/EW) divided by valence = mmol/L; e.g., 2 mg/dL of magnesium = (2 × 10/12) divided by 2 = 0.83 mmol/L.
      3. For organic substances: mmol/L = wt in mg/L/MW (in mg).

2. **SI units for expressing clinical laboratory data**
   These units are now widely used and are increasingly required for publication of scientific data in physical, biologic, and biomedical publication. Extensive SI conversion tables have been published together with an explanation of the rationale for their use and technical aspects of usage (1–3) (see Table 3).

**Table 1. The base units of interest in physical quantities used in clinical chemistry**

| Quantity | Base Unit |
|----------|-----------|
| mass | kilogram |
| time | second |
| amount | mole |
| length | meter |

A derived unit for energy is the kjoule (kJ): 4.18 kJ = 1kcal, 1 MJ = 239 kcal.

**Table 2. Prefixes and symbols for decimal multiples and submultiples**

| Factor | Prefix | Symbol | Factor | Prefix | Symbol |
|--------|--------|--------|--------|--------|--------|
| $10^9$ | giga | G | $10^{-3}$ | milli | m |
| $10^6$ | mega | M | $10^{-6}$ | micro | µ |
| $10^3$ | kilo | k | $10^{-9}$ | nano | n |
| $10^2$ | hecto | h | $10^{-12}$ | pico | p |
| $10^1$ | deco | da | $10^{-15}$ | femto | f |
| $10^{-1}$ | deci | d | $10^{-18}$ | atto | a |
| $10^{-2}$ | centi | c | | | |

**Table 3. Conversion factors for selected compounds of nutrition interest[a]**

| Component | (1) Present Unit | (2) Conversion Factor | (3) SI Unit Symbol | (4) Mass Conversion Factor |
|---|---|---|---|---|
| Albumin (s) | g/dL | 10 | g/L | — |
| Aluminum (s) | μg/L | 37.04 | nmol/L | μg/27 = mol |
| Amino acids | (see ref. 2, p. 119, for individual amino acids) | | | |
| Amino acid nitrogen (p) | mg/dL | 0.714 | mmol/L | mg/14 = mmol |
| Ascorbic acid (p) | mg/dL | 56.78 | μmol/L | mg/176 = mmol |
| Calcium (s) | mg/dL | 0.250 | mmol/L | mg/40 = mmol |
| Calcium (s) | mEq/dL | 0.500 | mmol/L | mEq/2 = mmol |
| β-Carotene (s) | μ/dL | 0.0186 | μmol/L | μg/536.85 = μmol |
| Chloride (s) | mEq/L | 1.00 | mmol/L | mEq = mmol |
| Cholesterol (p) | mg/dL | 0.0259 | mmol/L | mg/386.6 = mmol |
| Cobalamin ($B_{12}$) | pg/mL | 0.738 | pmol/L | pg/1355 = pmol |
| Copper (s) | μg/dL | 0.157 | μmol/L | μg/63.5 = μmol |
| Ethanol (p) | mg/dL | 0.217 | mmol/L | mg/46 = mmol |
| Folic acid | ng/mL | 2.265 | mmol/L | ng/441.4 = nmol |
| Glucose (p) | mg/dL | 0.0555 | mmol/L | mg/180.2 = mmol |
| Iron (s) | μg/dL | 0.179 | μmol/L | μg/55.9 = μmol |
| Phosphate (p) (as phosphorus) | mg/dL | 0.323 | mmol/L | mg/31 = mmol |
| Potassium (s) | mEq/L | 1.000 | mmol/L | mEq = mmol |
| Potassium | mg/dL | 0.256 | mmol/L | mg/39.1 = mmol |
| Magnesium (s) | mg/dL | 0.411 | mmol/L | mg/24.3 = mmol |
| Pyridoxal (B) | ng/mL | 5.981 | nmol/L | ng/167 = nmol |
| Retinol (p,s) | μg/dL | 0.0349 | μmol/L | μg/286 = μmol |
| Riboflavin (s) | μg/dL | 26.57 | μmol/L | μg/376 = nmol |
| Sodium (s) | mEq/L | 1.00 | mmol/L | mEq = mmol |
| Thiamin HCl (U) | μg/24 h | 0.00298 | μmol/d | μg/337 = μmol |
| α-Tocopherol (p) | mg/dL | 23.22 | μmol/L | μg/431 = μmol |
| Vitamin D3 | μg/dL | 26.01 | nmol/L | μg/384 = μmol |
| Calcidiol | ng/mL | 2.498 | nmol/L | ng/400 = nmol |
| Zinc (s) | μg/dL | 0.153 | μmol/L | μg/65.4 = mmol |

[a]To convert metric or equivalent unit per unit volume (column 1) to SI units per liter (column 3), multiply by the conversion factor in column 2. p, plasma; s, serum; B, blood; U, urine.

# References

1. Lundberg GD, Iberson C, Radulescu G: *JAMA* 1986; 255: 2329.

2. Monsen ER: *J Am Diet Assoc* 1987; 87: 356.

3. Young DS. *Ann Intern Med* 1987; 106: 114.

From Shils ME, Olson JA, Shike M, Ross AC. Modern nutrition in health and disease, 9th ed. Baltimore: Lippincott Williams & Wilkins, 1999.

# Choosing the Route of Nutrition Support in Adults: A Clinical Decision Algorithm

This clinical decision algorithm outlines the process for choosing a route of nutrition support in adult patients. Major considerations in selecting the feeding route and nutrition support formula include gastrointestinal function,[1,2] expected duration of nutrition therapy, aspiration risk, and the potential for or actual development of organ dysfunction. (GI, gastrointestinal; PN, parenteral nutrition.)

## References

1. Guenter P, Jones S, Jacobs DO et al: Administration and delivery of enteral nutrition. In: Clinical nutrition: enteral and tube feeding, 2nd ed. Rombeau JL, Caldwell MD (eds.). Philadelphia: WB Saunders, 1990, pp. 192–203 (IV).

2. Schlichtig, R, Ayres SM: Nutritional considerations for specific disease states. In: Nutrition support of the critically ill. Schlichtig R, Ayres SM (eds.). Chicago: Year Book Medical Publishers, 1988, pp. 185–209 (IV).

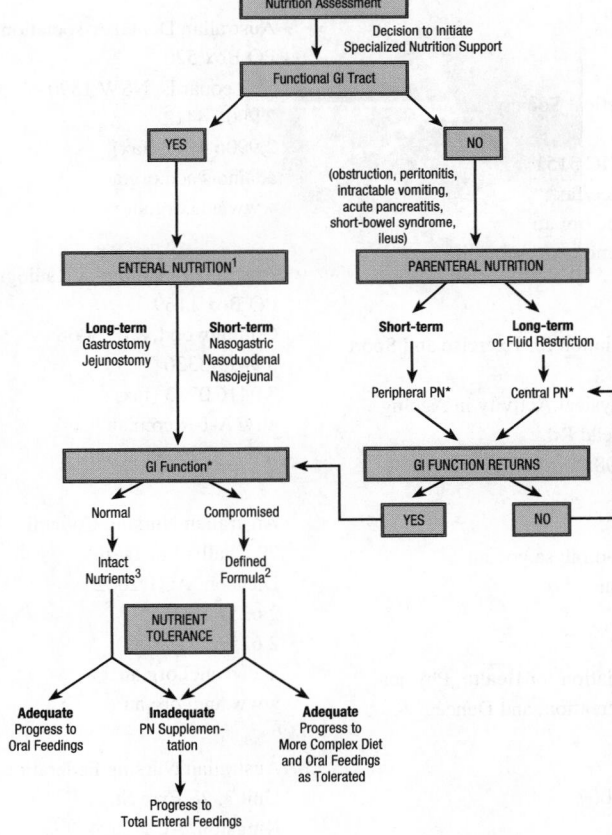

Notes. *Formulation of enteral and parenteral solutions should be made considering organ function (e.g., cardiac, renal, respiratory, hepatic). 1. Feedings may be more appropriate distal to the pylorus if the patient is at increased aspiration risk. 2. Elemental low/high fat content, lactose-free, fiber-rich, and modular formulas should be provided according to patient's GI tolerance. See specific conditions for formula guidelines. 3. Polymeric, complete formulas, or pureed diets are appropriate. Reprinted with permission from the American Society for Parenteral and Enteral Nutrition (A.S.P.E.N.), Guidelines for the use of parenteral and enteral nutrition in adult and pediatric patients, *JPEN;* 17(4): 1SA–52SA. A.S.P.E.N. does not endorse this material in any forms other than its entirety. For more information on ordering a complete set of guidelines, contact A.S.P.E.N., 8630 Fenton St., Ste. 412, Silver Spring, MD 20910 USA.

# Professional Organizations

This directory, by no means exhaustive, lists professional organizations in the United States and several other English-speaking countries. Each country's name is followed by its country code for international calling. City codes or other area codes are listed with individual telephone numbers.

## Australia (61)

Association of Massage Therapists
PO Box 627
South Yarra, VIC 341
3 9510 3930
3 9521 3209 (fax)
amta@amta.asn.au
www.amta.asn.au

Australian Acoustical Society
PO Box 4004
East Burwood, VIC 3151
3 9887 9400 (voice/fax)
watkinsd@melbpc.org.au
www.users.bigpond.com/Acoustics

Australian Association for Exercise and Sport
   Science
c/o Centre for Physical Activity in Ageing
207–255 Hampstead Rd.
Northfield, SA 5085
8 8222 1717
8 8222 1828 (fax)
jmack@hampstead.rah.sa.gov.au
www.aaess.com.au

Australian Association for Health, Physical
   Education, Recreation, and Dance
214 Port Rd.
PO Box 304
Hindmarsh, SA 5007
8 8340 3388
8 340 3399 (fax)
achper@achper.org.au
www.achper.org.au

Australian Association of Occupational
   Therapists
6 Spring St.
Fitzroy, VIC 3065
3 9416 1021
3 9416 1421 (fax)
info@ausot.com.au
www.ausot.com.au

Australian Dental Association
PO Box 520
St. Leonards, NSW 1590
2 9906 4412
2 9906 4917 (fax)
adainc@ada.org.au
www.ada.org.au

Australian Institute of Radiography
PO Box 1169
Collingwood, VIC 3066
3 9419 3336
3 9416 0783 (fax)
air@A-I-R.com.au
www.giant.net.au/air

Australian Nursing Council
20 Challis St., 1st fl.
Dickson, ACT 2602
2 6257 7960
2 6257 7955 (fax)
anci@anci.org.au
www.anci.org.au

Australian Nursing Federation
Unit 3, 28 Eyre St.
Kingston, ACT 2604
2 6232 6533
2 6232 6610 (fax)
www.anf.org.au

Australian Society for Emergency Medicine
17 Gratton St.
Carlton, VIC 3053
3 9663 4825
3 9663 8013 (fax)
asem@medeserv.com.au
www.medeserv.com.au/asem

Australian Veterinary Association
AVA House
134 Hampden Rd.
Artarmon, NSW 2064
2 9411 2733
2 9411 5089 (fax)
avahq@ava.com.au
www.ava.com.au

Dental Hygienists' Association of Australia
PO Box 10030
Gouger St.
Adelaide, SA 5000
dhaainc@primus.com.au
www.dhaa.asn.au

Dietitians Association of Australia
1/8 Phipps Close
Deakin, ACT 2600
2 6282 9555
2 6282 9888 (fax)
daacanb@hcn.net.au
www.daa.asn.au

Health Information Management Association
   of Australia
Locked Bag 2045
North Ryde, NSW 1670
2 9887 5001
2 9887 5895 (fax)
himaa@himaa.org.au
www.himaa.org.au

Pharmaceutical Society of Australia
Pharmacy House
44 Thesiger Ct.
Deakin, ACT 2600
2 6281 1366
2 6285 2869 (fax)
psa.nat@psa.org.au
www.psa.org.au

Speech Pathology Australia
11–19 Bank Place, 2nd fl.
Melbourne, VIC 3000
3 9642 4899
3 9642 4922 (fax)
office@speechpathologyaustralia.org.au
www.home.vicnet.net.au/~sppathau

Sports Dietitians Australia
Level 8, Victorian Institute of Sport
20–22 Albert Rd.
PO Box 828
South Melbourne, VIC 3205
3 9682 2442
3 9686 2352 (fax)
sda@ausport.gov.au
www.ausport.gov.au/sda/sdamore

Sports Medicine Australia
PO Box 897
Belconnen, ACT 2616
2 6251 6944
2 6253 1489 (fax)
smanat@sma.org.au
www.ausport.gov.au/SMA

## Canada (1)

Canadian Academy of Audiology
250 Consumers Rd., Ste. 301
Willowdale, ON
M2J 4V6
(416) 494-6672
(800) 264-5106
(416) 495-8723 (fax)
caa@base.onramp.ca
www.canadianaudiology.ca

Canadian Academy of Manipulative Therapy
92 Crichton Ave.
Dartmouth, NS
B3A 3R3
www.manipulativetherapy.org

Canadian Academy of Sport Medicine
1010 Polytek St., No. 14
Gloucester, ON
K1B 5N4
(613) 748-5851
(613) 748-5792 (fax)
www.casm-acms.org

Canadian Anesthesiologists' Society
1 Eglinton Ave. East, Ste. 208
Toronto, ON
M4P 3A1
(416) 480-0602
(416) 480-0320 (fax)
www.anesthesia@cas.ca

Canadian Association for Health, Physical
  Education, Recreation, and Dance
1600 James Naismith Dr.
Gloucester, ON
K1B 5N4
(613) 748-5622
(613) 748-5737 (fax)
CAHPERD@rtm.activeliving.ca
www.activeliving.ca/activeliving/cahperd

Canadian Association of Occupational
  Therapists
CTTC Bldg., Ste. 3400
1125 Colonel By Dr.
Ottawa, ON
K1S 5R1
(613) 523-CAOT (ext. 2268)
(613) 523-2552 (fax)
www.sdokuchie@caot.ca

Canadian Association of Pharmacy Technicians
PO Box 1271
Station F
Toronto, ON
M4Y 2V8
(416) 410-1142
(416) 813-7748 (fax)
contact@capt.ca
www.capt.ca

Canadian Association of Radiologists
1740 Cote Vertu
St-Laurent, QC
H4L 2A4
(514) 738-3111
(514) 738-5199 (fax)
info@car.ca
www.car.ca

Canadian Association of Speech-Language
  Pathologists and Audiologists
2006–130 Albert St.
Ottawa, ON
K1P 5G4
(613) 567-9968
(800) 259-8519
(613) 567-2859 (fax)
caslpa@caslpa.ca
www.caslpa.ca/english

Canadian Athletic Therapists Association
902 11th Ave. SW, Ste. 312
Calgary, AB
T2R 0E7
(403) 509-CATA (2282)
(403) 509-2280 (fax)
www.athletictherapy.org

Canadian Dental Association
1815 Alta Vista Dr.
Ottawa, ON
K1G 3Y6
(613) 523-1770
(613) 523-7736 (fax)
reception@cda-adc.ca
www.cda-adc.ca

Canadian Dental Hygienists Association
96 Centrepointe Dr.
Ottawa, ON
K2G 6B1
(613) 224-5515
(613) 224-7283 (fax)
info@cdha.ca
www.cdha.ca

Canadian Massage Therapist Alliance
365 Bloor St. East, Ste. 1807
Toronto, ON
M4W 3L4
(416) 968-2149
(416) 968-6818 (fax)
www.collinscan.com

Canadian Medical Association
1867 Alta Vista Dr.
Ottawa, ON
K1G 3Y6
(613) 731-9331
cmamsc@cma.ca
www.cma.ca

Canadian Nurses Association
50 Driveway
Ottawa, ON
K2P 1E2
(613) 237-2133
(800) 361-8404
(613) 237-3520 (fax)
www.cna-nurses.ca

Canadian Nursing Students' Association
325–350 Albert St.
Ottawa, ON
K1R 1B1
(613) 563-1236
(613) 563-7739 (fax)
www.cnsa.ca

Canadian Orthopractic Manual Therapy
    Association
1150 100th Ave., No. 207
Edmonton, AB
T5K 0J7
(780) 482-7428
(780) 488-2463 (fax)
info@orthopractic.org
www.manipulativetherapy.org
www.orthopractic.org

Canadian Pharmacists Association
1785 Alta Vista Dr.
Ottawa, ON
K1G 3Y6
(800) 917-9489
(613) 523-7877
(800) 601-1904 (fax)
(613) 523-0445 (fax)
members@cdnpharm.ca
www.cdnpharm.ca

Canadian Society of Hospital Pharmacists
350–1145 Hunt Club Rd.
Ottawa ON
K1V 0Y3
(613) 736-9733 (ext. 22)
(613) 736-5660 (fax)
www@cshp.ca
www.cshp.ca

Canadian Sport Massage Therapists
    Association
3444 78 St.
Edmonton, AB
T6K 0E9
(780) 461-7211 (voice/fax)
natoffice@csmta.ca

Canadian Thoracic Society
1900 City Park Dr., Ste. 508
Blair Business Park
Gloucester, ON
K1J 1A3
(613) 747-6776
(613) 747-7430 (fax)
www.lung.ca/cts

Canadian Veterinary Medical Association
339 Booth St.
Ottawa, ON
K1R 7K1
(613) 236-1162
www.cvma-acmv.org

Dietitians of Canada
480 University Ave., Ste. 604
Toronto, ON
M5G 1V2
(416) 596-0857
(416) 596-0603 (fax)
www.dietitians.ca

Radiological Society of North America
(*see under* United States)

## Egypt (20)

Egyptian Dental Association
84 Mathaf El-Manyal St.
PO Box 11451
Cairo
2 365 8568
2 318 9143 (fax)
eda@internetegypt.com
www.geocities.com/CapeCanaveral/Hangar/4295

Egyptian Nurses Syndicate
5 Sarai St.
Manial
Cairo
2 368 7627
2 262 4302 (fax)

Egypt Sports Medicine Association
Gabalaya St.
Elguezira
Cairo

Egyptian Veterinary Medical Association
8a 26 July St.
Cairo

General Egyptian Veterinary Medical Syndicate
6 Al-Hadikah St.
Garden City
Cairo

## India (91)

All India Occupational Therapists Association
c/o Dr. R. K. Sharma
734 Laxmibai Nagar
New Delhi 110 023
11 683 6049 (fax)

Indian Association of Sports Medicine
1 Adishwar Flats
PO RoocdKhokhara
Mayinagdr (E) 380008
New Delhi
11 216 1675
11 553 0034 (fax)

Indian Dental Association
c/o Dr. Hari Prakash
All India Institute of Medical Sciences
Ansari Nagar
New Delhi 110 020
11 659 3231
11 686 2663 (fax)
www.dentalhealthindia.com

Indian Veterinary Association
ivj@md3.vsnl.net.in
www.indvetjournal.com

Trained Nurses' Association of India
L-17 Green Park
New Delhi 110 016
11 656 6665
11 685 8304 (fax)
hiipl@health4india.com
www.health4india.com/new/nurses/tnai.asp

## Ireland (353)

Association of Occupational Therapists of
    Ireland
29 Gardiner Place
Dublin 1
1 878 0247

Healthcare Informatics Society of Ireland
58 Eccles St.
Dublin 7
www.hisi.ie.eu.org

Irish Medical Organisation
10 Fitzwilliam Place
Dublin 2
1 676 7273
1 661 2758 (fax)
imo@imo.ie
www.imo.ie

Irish Society of Chartered Physiotherapists
Royal College of Surgeons
St. Stephen's Green
Dublin 2
1 402 2148
1 402 2160 (fax)
info@iscp.ie
www.iscp.ie

Irish Sports Medicine Association
c/o Anatomy Dept.
Human Performance Laboratory
Trinity College
Dublin 2
1 608 1182
1 679 0119 (fax)

Irish Veterinary Officers Association
4 Warners La.
Dartmouth Rd.
Dublin
1 668 6064
www.iol.ie/~myerstb

Royal Academy of Medicine in Ireland
6 Kildare St.
Dublin 2
1 676 7650
1 661 1684 (fax)
secretary@rami.ie
www.rami.ie

## New Zealand (64)

New Zealand Association of Occupational
   Therapists
PO Box 12-506
Wellington 6001
4 472 6374
nzaot@freemail.co.nz

New Zealand Association of Therapeutic
   Massage Practitioners
PO Box 375
Waikato Mail Centre
Hamilton 2015
info@nzatmp.org.nz
www.nzatmp.org.nz

New Zealand Audiological Society
PO Box 9724
Newmarket
Auckland
9 625 1654 (fax)
questions@audiology.org.nz
www.audiology.org.nz

New Zealand Dental Association
www.nzda.org.nz
3 St. Marks Rd.
PO Box 28 084
Auckland 5
nzdainfo@nzda.org.nz

New Zealand Nurses Organisation
6th Fl. Westbrook House
181–183 Willis St.
PO Box 2128
Wellington
4 385 0847
4 382 9993 (fax)
nurses@nzno.org.nz
www.nzno.org.nz

New Zealand Speech-Language Therapists
   Association
63 Remuera Rd., Ste. 369
Newmarket
Auckland
3 235 8257
3 235 8850 (fax)
exec@nzsta-speech.org.nz
www.nzsta-speech.org.nz

New Zealand Veterinary Association
69–71 Boulcott St., 2nd fl.
Wellington
4 471 0484
4 471 0494 (fax)
nzva@vets.org.nz
www.vets.org.nz

Nutrition Society of New Zealand
PO Box 21201
Christchurch
www.nutritionsociety.ac.nz

Pharmacy Guild of New Zealand
124 Dixon St.
PO Box 27139
Wellington
4 802 8200
4 384 8085 (fax)
p.guild@pharmacy-house.org.nz
www.pgnz.org.nz

Physical Education New Zealand
Level 1, 14 Frankmore Ave.
Johnsonville
Wellington
4 477 6300
4 478 5237 (fax)
info@penz.org.nz
www.penz.org.nz

Sports Medicine New Zealand
PO Box 6398
Unipol Sports Centre
96 Anzac Ave.
Dunedin
3 477 7887
3 477 7882 (fax)
www.sportsmedicine.co.nz

## Pakistan (92)

Asian Federation of Sports Medicine
c/o Prof. Dr. Nishat Mallick
Hill Park General Hospital
Shaheed-e-Millat Rd.
Karachi
21 455 2442
21 506 0343 (fax)
www.afsm.com.hk

Federation of Veterinary Associations of
  Pakistan
148-A Ali Block
New Garden Town
Lahore
ramzee@brain.net.pk

Pakistan Dental Association
23-B Sindhi Muslim Housing Society
Karachi 74400
21 452 4371/4372
21 454 0837
21 452 4932 (fax)

Pakistan Nurses Federation
173-G/2 Model Town
Lahore
42 920 4202

Pakistan Occupational Therapy Association
408-C Saima Gardens
H/167 Khalid Bin Waleed Rd.
Block C, PECHS
Karachi

Sports Medicine Association of Pakistan
Hill Park General Hospital
Shaheed-e-Millat Rd.
Karachi
21 455 2442
21 506 0343 (fax)

## Singapore (65)

Association for Informatics in Medicine
c/o Bioinformatics Centre
National University of Singapore
10 Kent Ridge Crescent
Singapore 119260
feedback@aims.org.sg
www.aims.org.sg

Pharmaceutical Society of Singapore
Alumini Medical Centre, 2nd level
2 College Rd.
Singapore 169850
221 1136
223 0969 (fax)
www.pss.org.sg

Singapore Association of Occupational
  Therapists
Orchard PO Box 0475
Singapore 912316
saot@cyberway.com.sg
www.cyberway.com.sg/~saot

Singapore Dental Association
2 College Rd.
Singapore 169850
223 9343
224 7967 (fax)
sda@pacific.net.sg
www.sda.org.sg

Singapore Nurses' Association
77 Maude Rd.
Singapore 208353
392 0770
392 7877 (fax)
sna@pacific.net.sg
www.sna.org.sg

Singapore Nutrition and Dietetics Association
Tanglin
PO Box 180
Singapore 912406
sndainfo@singnet.com.sg
www.web.singnet.com.sg/~sndainfo

Singapore Speech, Language, and Hearing
   Association
Department of Speech Therapy
Singapore General Hospital
Outram Rd.
Singapore 169608
321 4549
356 9304
326 5497 (fax)
speech@pacific.net.sg

Singapore Veterinary Association
c/o Agri-food & Veterinary Authority
5 Maxwell Rd. No. 03-00
Tower Block, MND Complex
Singapore 069110
227 0670
227 6403 (fax)
sva@sva.org.sg
www.sva.org.sg

Society for Emergency Medicine in Singapore
c/o Accident & Emergency Dept.
Singapore General Hospital
Outram Rd.
Singapore 169608
321 4100
226 0294 (fax)
gaelkf@sgh.gov.sg
www.sems.org.sg

## South Africa (27)

South African Association of Occupational
   Therapists
946 Schoeman St.
Arcadia 0083
Pretoria

South African Speech-Language-Hearing
   Association
PO Box 91042
Auckland Park 2006
11 726 5014
11 726 5013 (fax)
saslha@mweb.co.za
www.saslha.org.za

South Africa Sports Medicine Association
PO Box 2598
Claremch 7440
21 686 7330
21 686 7530 (fax)

## United Kingdom (44)

British Association of Emergency Medical
   Technicians
Ty Cristion
Bodedern
Anglesey LL65 3UB
1407 742 222
admin@baemt.org.uk
www.baemt.org.uk

British Association for Immediate Care
Turret House
Turret La.
Ipswich IP4 1DL
870 165 4999
870 165 4949 (fax)
admin@basics.org.uk
www.basics.org.uk

British Association of Occupational Therapists
106–114 Borough High St.
London SE1 1LB
171 357 6480
171 207 9612 (fax)
beryl.steedon@cot.co.uk
www.cot.co.uk

British Association of Sport and Medicine
c/o Anatomy Bldg.
Medical School of St. Bartholomews Hospital
Charterhouse Sq.
London EC1M 6BQ
171 253 3244
171 251 0774 (fax)

British Nuclear Medical Society
1 Wimpole St.
London W1G 0AE
208 291 7800
208 699 2227 (fax)
office@bnms.org.uk

British Small Animal Veterinary Association
Woodrow House
1 Telford Way
Waterwells Business Park
Quedgeley
Gloucester GL2 4AB
1452 726 700
1452 726 701 (fax)
adminoff@bsava.com
www.bsava.ac.uk

British Society of Audiology
80 Brighton Rd.
Reading RG6 1PS
1189 660 622
1189 351 915 (fax)
ann@b-s-a.demon.co.uk
www.b-s-a.demon.co.uk

Chartered Society of Physiotherapy
14 Bedford Row
London WC1R 4ED
207 306 6666
207 306 6611 (fax)
www.csphysio.org.uk

Resuscitation Council
Tavistock House North, 5th fl.
Tavistock Sq.
London WC1H 9HR
207 388 4678
207 383 0773 (fax)
enquiries@resus.org.uk
www.firstaid.about.com

Royal Pharmaceutical Society of Great Britain
1 Lambeth High St.
London SE1 7JN
207 735 9141
207 735 7629 (fax)
enquiries@rpsgb.org.uk
www.rpsgb.org.uk

Royal Society of Medicine
1 Wimpole St.
London W1G 0AE
207 290 2991
207 290 2992 (fax)
membership@roysocmed.ac.uk
www.roysocmed.ac.uk

Society and College of Radiographers
207 Providence Sq.
Mill St.
London SE1 2EW
207 740 7200
207 740 7204 (fax)
www.sor.org

United Kingdom Central Council for Nursing,
    Midwifery, and Health Visiting
23 Portland Place
London W1N 4JT
207 637 7181
207 436 2924 (fax)
newreg@ukcc.org.uk
www.ukcc.org.uk

## United States (1)

American Academy of Anesthesiologist
  Assistants
PO Box 81362
Wellesley, MA 02481-0004
(800) 757-5858
assnadv@tiac.net
www.anesthetist.org

American Academy of Audiology
8300 Greensboro Dr., Ste. 750
McLean, VA 22102
(800) AAA-2336
(703) 790-8466
(703) 790-8631 (fax)
www.audiology.com

American Academy of Physician Assistants
950 N. Washington St.
Alexandria, VA 22314-1552
(703) 836-2272
(703) 684-1924 (fax)
aapa@aapa.org
www.aapa.org

American Alliance for Health, Physical
  Education, Recreation, and Dance
1900 Association Dr.
Reston, VA 20191
(703) 476-3400
(800) 213-7193
www.aahperd.org

American Association of Diabetes Educators
444 N. Michigan Ave., Ste. 1240
Chicago, IL 60611
(312) 644-2233
(800) 338-3633
www.diabetesnet.com

American Association of Medical Assistants
20 N. Wacker Dr., Ste. 1575
Chicago, IL 60606-2963
(312) 899-1500
www.aama-ntl.org

American Association for Medical
  Transcription
3460 Oakdale Rd., Ste. M
Modesto, CA 95355-9690
(800) 982-2182
(209) 551-0883
(209) 551-9317 (fax)
www.aamt.org

American Association for Respiratory Care
11030 Ables La.
Dallas, TX 75229
(972) 243-2272
(972) 484-2720 (fax)
(972) 484-6010 (fax)
info@aarc.org
www.aarc.org

American College of Clinical Pharmacology
3 Ellinwood Ct.
New Hartford, NY 13413-1105
(315) 768-6117
(315) 768-6119 (fax)
accp1ssu@aol.com
www.accp1.org

American College of Clinical Pharmacy
3101 Broadway, Ste. 380
Kansas City, MO 64111
(816) 531-2177
(816) 531-4990 (fax)
www.accp.com

American College Health Association
PO Box 28937
Baltimore, MD 21240-8937
(410) 859-1500
(410) 859-1510 (fax)
www.acha.org

American College of Medical Quality
4334 Montgomery Ave.
Bethesda, MD 20814
(301) 913-9149
(800) 924-2149
(301) 913-9142 (fax)
ACMQ@acmq.org
www.acmq.org

American College of Radiology
1891 Preston White Dr.
Reston, VA 20191
(800) ACR-LINE (227-5463)
www.acr.org

American College of Sports Medicine
401 W. Michigan St.
Indianapolis, IN 46202-3233
(317) 637-9200
(317) 634-7817 (fax)
www.acsm.org

American Dental Assistants Association
203 N. LaSalle St., Ste. 1320
Chicago, IL 60601-1225
(800) SEE-ADAA (733-2322)
(312) 541-1550
(312) 541-1496 (fax)
www.dentalassistant.org

American Dental Association
211 E. Chicago Ave.
Chicago, IL 60611
(312) 440-2500
www.ada.org

American Dental Hygienists' Association
444 N. Michigan Ave., Ste. 3400
Chicago, IL 60611
(312) 440-8900
mail@adha.net
www.adha.org

American Dietetic Association
216 W. Jackson Blvd.
Chicago, IL 60606-6995
(312) 899-0040
www.eatright.org

American Health Information Management
    Association
233 N. Michigan Ave., Ste. 2150
Chicago, IL 60601-5800
(312) 233-1100
(312) 233-1090 (fax)
info@ahima.org
www.ahima.org

American Massage Therapy Association
820 Davis St., Ste. 100
Evanston, IL 60201-4444
(847) 864-0123
(847) 864-1178 (fax)
www.amtamassage.org

American Medical Informatics Association
4915 St. Elmo Ave., Ste. 401
Bethesda, MD 20814
(301) 657-1291
(301) 657-1296 (fax)
www.amia.org

American Nurses Association
600 Maryland Ave. SW, Ste. 100 West
Washington, DC 20024
(800) 274-4ANA
www.nursingworld.org

American Occupational Therapy Association
4720 Montgomery La.
PO Box 31220
Bethesda, MD 20824-1220
(301) 652-2682
(800) 377-8555 (TTY)
(301) 652-7711 (fax)
www.aota.org

American Pharmaceutical Association
2215 Constitution Ave. NW
Washington, DC 20037-2985
(202) 628-4410
(202) 783-2351 (fax)
www.aphanet.org

American Physical Therapy Association
1111 N. Fairfax St.
Alexandria, VA 22314
(703) 684-2782
www.apta.org

American Registry of Diagnostic Medical
    Sonographers
600 Jefferson Plaza, Ste. 360
Rockville, MD 20852-1150
(301) 738-8401
(800) 541-9754
(301) 738-0312/0313 (fax)
www.ardms.org

American Registry of Radiologic Technologists
1255 Northland Dr.
St. Paul, MN 55120-1155
(651) 687-0048
www.arrt.org

American Society for Clinical Laboratory
  Science
7910 Woodmont Ave., Ste. 530
Bethesda, MD 20814
(301) 657-2768
(301) 657-2909 (fax)
ascls@ascls.org
www.ascls.org

American Society for Clinical Nutrition
9650 Rockville Pike
Bethesda, MD 20814-3998
(301) 530-7110
(301) 571-1863 (fax)
secretar@ascn.faseb.org

American Society of Clinical Pathologists
2100 W. Harrison St.
Chicago IL 60612
(312) 738-1336
info@ascp.org
www.ascp.org

American Society of Echocardiography
4101 Lake Boone Trail, Ste. 201
Raleigh, NC 27607
(919) 787-5181
(919) 787-4916 (fax)
www.asecho.org

American Society of Electroneurodiagnostic
  Technologists
204 W. Seventh St.
Carroll, IA 51401-2317
(712) 792-2978
(712) 792-6962 (fax)
aset@netins.net
www.aset.org

American Society of Extra-Corporeal
  Technology
503 Carlisle Dr., Ste. 125
Herndon, VA 20170
(703) 435-8556
(703) 435-0056 (fax)
www.amsect.org

American Society for Parenteral and Enteral
  Nutrition
8630 Fenton St., Ste. 412
Silver Spring, MD 20910
(800) 727-4567
(301) 587-6315
aspen@nutr.org
www.clinnutr.org

American Society of Radiologic Technologists
15000 Central Ave. SE
Albuquerque, NM 87123-3917
(505) 298-4500
(505) 298-5063 (fax)
education@asrt.org
www.asrt.org

American Society for Therapeutic Radiology
  and Oncology
12500 Fair Lakes Cir., Ste. 375
Fairfax, VA 22033-3882
(703) 227-0187
(703) 502-7852 (fax)
www.astro.org

American Speech-Language-Hearing
  Association
10801 Rockville Pike
Rockville, MD 20852
(800) 498-2071
(888) 321-ASHA (321-2742; voice automated)
(301) 571-0457 (TTY)
(877) 541-5035 (fax)
actioncenter@asha.org
www.asha.org

American Thoracic Society
1740 Broadway
New York, NY 10019
(212) 315-8700
(212) 315-6498 (fax)
www.thoracic.org

American Veterinary Medical Association
1931 N. Meacham Rd., Ste. 100
Schaumburg, IL 60173
(847) 925-8070
(847) 925-1329 (fax)
avmainfo@avma.org
www.avma.org

Association of Medical Illustrators
2965 Flowers Rd. South, Ste. 105
Atlanta, GA 30341
(770) 454-7933
(770) 458-3314 (fax)
assnhq@mindspring.com
www.medical-illustrators.org

Association of Polysomnographic
    Technologists
PO Box 14861
Lenexa, KS 66285-4861
(913) 541-1991
www.aptweb.org

Association of Surgical Technologists
7108-C S. Alton Way
Englewood, CO 80112
(303) 694-9130
(303) 694-9169 (fax)
www.ast.org

EEG and Clinical Neuroscience Society
Brain Research Laboratories
New York University
550 First Ave.
New York, NY 10016
(888) 366-2203
(212) 263-6288
(212) 263-6457 (fax)
polanj01@mcmbox.med.nyu.com
www.fhdno2.tch.harvard.edu/www/ecns

National Association of Emergency Medical
    Technicians
408 Monroe St.
Clinton, MS 39056-4210
(800) 34-NAEMT (346-2368)
www.naemt.org

National Athletic Trainers' Association
2952 Stemmons Fwy.
Dallas, TX 75247-6196
(214) 637-6282
(214) 637-2206 (fax)
www.nata.org

National Registry of Emergency Medical
    Technicians
Rocco V. Morando Bldg.
6610 Busch Blvd.
PO Box 29233
Columbus, OH 43229
(614) 888-4484
(614) 888-8920 (fax)
www.nremt.org

Radiological Society of North America
820 Jorie Blvd.
Oak Brook, IL 60523-2251
(630) 571-2670
(630) 571-7837 (fax)
www.rsna.org

Society of Diagnostic Medical Sonographers
12770 Coit Rd., Ste. 708
Dallas, TX 75251-1314
(972) 239-7367
(800) 229-9506
(972) 239-7378 (fax)
www.sdms.org

Society of Vascular Technology
4601 Presidents Drive, Ste. 260
Lanham, MD 20706
(301) 459-7550
(301) 459-5651 (fax)
info@svtnet.org
www.svtnet.org

# Professional Titles, Degrees, and Certificates

| | |
|---|---|
| **AuD** | Doctor of Audiology |
| **ANP** | Adult Nurse Practitioner |
| **ARNP** | Advanced Registered Nurse Practitioner |
| **ATC** | Athletic Trainer, Certified |
| **BA** | Bachelor of Arts |
| **BB(ASCP)** | Technologist in Blood Banking (certified by American Society of Clinical Pathologists) |
| **BCNP** | Board Certified Nuclear Pharmacist |
| **BCNSP** | Board Certified Nutrition Support Pharmacist |
| **BCPS** | Board Certified Pharmacotherapy Specialist |
| **BSN** | Bachelor of Science in Nursing |
| **CALN** | Clinical Administrative Liaison Nurse |
| **C(ASCP)** | Technologist in Chemistry (certified by American Society of Clinical Pathologists) |
| **CAT(C)** | Certified Athletic Therapist (Canada) |
| **CCC-A** | Certificate of Clinical Competence in Audiology |
| **CCC-SLP** | Certificate of Clinical Competence in Speech-Language Pathology |
| **CCRN** | Critical Care Registered Nurse |
| **CCS** | Cardiopulmonary Certified Specialist, Certified Coding Specialist |
| **CDA** | Certified Dental Assistant |
| **CDE** | Certified Diabetes Educator |
| **CDT** | Certified Dental Laboratory Technician |
| **CEN** | Certified Emergency Nurse |
| **CCEMT-P** | Critical Care Paramedic |
| **CCM** | Certified Case Manager |
| **CFNP** | Certified Family Nurse Practitioner |
| **CIH** | Certificate in Industrial Health |
| **CCM** | Certified Case Manager |
| **CFNP** | Certified Family Nurse Practitioner |
| **CIH** | Certificate in Industrial Health |
| **CLA** | Certified Laboratory Assistant |
| **CLDir(NCA)** | Clinical Laboratory Director (certified by National Certification Agency for Medical Laboratory Personnel) |
| **CLPlb(NCA)** | Clinical Laboratory Phlebotomist (certified by National Certification Agency for Medical Laboratory Personnel) |
| **CLS** | Clinical Laboratory Scientist |
| **CLS(NCA)** | Clinical Laboratory Scientist (certified by National Certification Agency for Medical Laboratory Personnel) |
| **CLSp(CG)(NCA)** | Clinical Laboratory Specialist in Cytogenetics (certified by National Certification Agency for Medical Laboratory Personnel) |
| **CLSp(H)(NCA)** | Clinical Laboratory Specialist in Hematology (certified by National Certification Agency for Medical Laboratory Personnel) |
| **CLSup(NCA)** | Clinical Laboratory Supervisor (certified by National Certification Agency for Medical Laboratory Personnel) |
| **CLT** | Certified Laboratory Technician, Clinical Laboratory Technician |
| **CLT(NCA)** | Certified Laboratory Technician (certified by National Certification Agency for Medical Laboratory Personnel) |

| | |
|---|---|
| **CMA** | Certified Medical Assistant |
| **CMT** | Certified Medical Transcriptionist |
| **CNA** | Certified Nursing Assistant |
| **CNM** | Certified Nurse Midwife |
| **CNMT** | Certified Nuclear Medicine Technologist |
| **CNP** | Community Nurse Practitioner |
| **CNS** | Clinical Nurse Specialist |
| **CNSD** | Certified Nutrition Support Dietitian |
| **CNS** | Clinical Nurse Specialist |
| **CNSD** | Certified Nutrition Support Dietitian |
| **CNSN** | Certified Nutrition Support Nurse |
| **CNSP** | Certified Nutrition Support Physician |
| **COMA** | Certified Ophthalmic Medical Assistant |
| **COMT** | Certified Ophthalmic Medical Technologist |
| **CORN** | Certified Operating Room Nurse |
| **COTA** | Certified Occupational Therapy Assistant |
| **CPAN** | Certified Post Anesthesia Nurse |
| **CPFT** | Certified Pulmonary Function Technologist |
| **CPH** | Certificate in Public Health |
| **CPN** | Certified Pediatric Nurse |
| **CPNP** | Certified Pediatric Nurse Practitioner |
| **CRNA** | Certified Registered Nurse Anesthetist |
| **CRTT** | Certified Respiratory Therapy Technician |
| **CST** | Certified Surgical Technician |
| **CT(ASCP)** | Cytotechnologist (certified by American Society of Clinical Pathologists) |
| **CTR** | Certified Tumor Registrar |
| **CURN** | Certified Urological Registered Nurse |
| **CVO** | Chief Veterinary Officer |
| **CVT** | Certified Veterinary Technician |
| **DC** | Doctor of Chiropractic |
| **DDS** | Doctor of Dental Surgery |
| **DLM(ASCP)** | Diplomate in Laboratory Management (certified by American Society of Clinical Pathologists) |
| **DMD** | Doctor of Dental Medicine |
| **DNS** | Doctor of Nursing Services |
| **DO** | Doctor of Optometry (seen also as OD), Doctor of Osteopathy |
| **DP** | Doctor of Podiatry |
| **DPH** | Doctor of Public Health, Doctor of Public Hygiene |
| **DPM** | Doctor of Physical Medicine, Doctor of Podiatric Medicine |
| **DPT** | Doctor of Physical Therapy |
| **ECS** | Electrophysiologic Certified Specialist |
| **EdD** | Doctor of Education |
| **EFDA** | Expanded Function Dental Auxiliary |
| **EMT-B** | Emergency Medical Technician—Basic |
| **EMT-I** | Emergency Medical Technician—Intermediate |
| **EMT-P** | Emergency Medical Technician—Paramedic |
| **FAAN** | Fellow, American Academy of Nursing |
| **FAARC** | Fellow, American Association for Respiratory Care |
| **FACD** | Fellow, American College of Dentists |

| | |
|---|---|
| **FACP** | Fellow, American College of Physicians |
| **FACS** | Fellow, American College of Surgeons |
| **FACSM** | Fellow, American College of Sports Medicine |
| **FADA** | Fellow, American Dietetic Association |
| **FAMA** | Fellow, American Medical Association |
| **FNP** | Family Nurse Practitioner |
| **FAOTA** | Fellow, American Occupational Therapy Association |
| **FAPTA** | Fellow, American Physical Therapy Association |
| **FIAC** | Fellow, International Academy of Cytology |
| **FRCD** | Fellow, Royal College of Dentists (United Kingdom) |
| **FRCD(C)** | Fellow, Royal College of Dentists of Canada |
| **FRCP** | Fellow, Royal College of Physicians (United Kingdom) |
| **FRCPA** | Fellow, Royal College of Physicians of Australia |
| **FRCPSC** | Fellow, Royal College of Physicians and Surgeons of Canada |
| **FRSM** | Fellow, Royal Society of Medicine (United Kingdom) |
| **GCS** | Geriatric Certified Specialist |
| **GNP** | Gerontological Nurse Practitioner |
| **H(ASCP)** | Technologists in Hematology (certified by American Society of Clinical Pathologists) |
| **HP(ASCP)** | Hemapherisis Practitioner (certified by American Society of Clinical Pathologists) |
| **HT** | Histologic Technologist (certified by American Society of Clinical Pathologists) |
| **HT(ASCP)** | Histologic Technician (certified by American Society of Clinical Pathologists) |
| **HTL(ASCP)** | Histotechnologist (certified by American Society of Clinical Pathologists) |
| **I(ASCP)** | Technologist in Immunology (certified by American Society of Clinical Pathologists) |
| **LD** | Licensed Dietitian |
| **LMCC** | Licentiate of the Medical Council of Canada |
| **LMP** | Licensed Massage Practitioner |
| **LMT** | Licensed Massage Technician, Licensed Massage Therapist |
| **LPN** | Licensed Practical Nurse |
| **LVN** | Licensed Vocational Nurse |
| **LVT** | Licensed Veterinary Technician |
| **M(ASCP)** | Technologist in Microbiology (certified by American Society of Clinical Pathologists) |
| **MD** | Doctor of Medicine |
| **MEd** | Master of Education |
| **MLT** | Medical Laboratory Technician |
| **MLT(ASCP)** | Medical Laboratory Technician (certified by American Society of Clinical Pathologists) |
| **MPH** | Master of Public Health |
| **MPharm** | Master in Pharmacy |
| **MPT** | Master of Physical Therapy |
| **MRCP** | Member, Royal College of Physicians (United Kingdom) |
| **MSN** | Master of Science in Nursing |
| **MSW** | Medical Social Worker |
| **MT** | Medical Technologist |
| **MT(ASCP)** | Medical Technologist (certified by American Society of Clinical Pathologists) |

| | |
|---|---|
| **MTA** | Medical Technologist Assistant |
| **NCS** | Neurologic Certified Specialist |
| **NCTMB** | Nationally Certified in Therapeutic Massage and Bodywork |
| **NM(ASCP)** | Technologist in Nuclear Medicine (certified by American Society of Clinical Pathologists) |
| **NMT** | Nurse Massage Therapist, Nursing Massage Therapist |
| **NP** | Nurse Practitioner |
| **NREMT** | National Registry Emergency Medical Technician—Basic |
| **NREMT-I** | National Registry Emergency Medical Technician—Intermediate |
| **NREMT-P** | National Registry Emergency Medical Technician—Paramedic |
| **OCS** | Orthopedic Certified Specialist |
| **OD** | Doctor of Optometry (also seen as DO) |
| **OT** | Occupational Therapist |
| **OT-C** | Occupational Therapist (Canada) |
| **OTD** | Doctor of Occupational Therapy |
| **OT-L** | Occupational Therapist, Licensed |
| **OT-R** | Occupational Therapist, Registered |
| **PA** | Physician's Assistant |
| **PBT(ASCP)** | Phlebotomy Technician (certified by American Society of Clinical Pathologists) |
| **PCS** | Pediatric Certified Specialist |
| **PharmD** | Doctor of Pharmacy |
| **PhD** | Doctor of Philosophy |
| **PhG** | Graduate in Pharmacy |
| **PNP** | Pediatric Nurse Practitioner |
| **PT** | Physical Therapist |
| **PTA** | Physical Therapy Assistant |
| **RD** | Registered Dietitian |
| **RDA** | Registered Dental Assistant |
| **RDCS** | Registered Diagnostic Cardiac Sonographer |
| **RDH** | Registered Dental Hygienist |
| **RDMS** | Registered Diagnostic Medical Sonographer |
| **RDN** | Registered Dietitian/Nutritionist |
| **R.EEGT.** | Registered Electroencephalographic Technologist |
| **R.EPT.** | Registered Evoked Potential Technologist |
| **RHIA** | Registered Health Information Administrator |
| **RHIT** | Registered Health Information Technician |
| **RMA** | Registered Medical Assistant |
| **RMT** | Registered Massage Therapist |
| **RN** | Registered Nurse |
| **RPFT** | Registered Pulmonary Function Technologist |
| **RPh** | Registered Pharmacist |
| **RPSGT** | Registered Polysomnographic Technologist |
| **RRT** | Registered Respiratory Therapist |
| **RT** | Radiologic Technologist, Respiratory Therapist |
| **RT(ARRT)** | Registered Technologist (certified by American Registry of Radiologic Technologists) |
| **RT(CT)** | Registered Technologist in Computed Tomography |
| **RT(CV)** | Registered Technologist in Cardiovascular Interventional Technology |

| | |
|---|---|
| **RT(M)** | Registered Technologist in Mammography |
| **RT(MR)** | Registered Technologist in Magnetic Resonance Imaging |
| **RT(N)** | Registered Technologist in Nuclear Medicine |
| **RT(QM)** | Registered Technologist in Quality Management |
| **RT(R)** | Registered Technologist in Radiography |
| **RT(T)** | Registered Technologist in Radiation Therapy |
| **RTT** | Respiratory Therapy Technician |
| **RVT** | Registered Vascular Technologist, Registered Veterinary Technician |
| **SAT** | Supervisory Athletic Therapist (Canada) |
| **SBB(ASCP)** | Specialist in Blood Banking (certified by American Society of Clinical Pathologists) |
| **SC(ASCP)** | Specialist in Chemistry (certified by American Society of Clinical Pathologists) |
| **SCS** | Sports Certified Specialist |
| **SCT(ASCP)** | Specialist in Cytotechnology (certified by American Society of Clinical Pathologists) |
| **SH(ASCP)** | Specialist in Hematology (certified by American Society of Clinical Pathologists) |
| **SI(ASCP)** | Specialist in Immunology (certified by American Society of Clinical Pathologists) |
| **SM(ASCP)** | Specialist in Microbiology (certified by American Society of Clinical Pathologists) |
| **VTS** | Veterinary Technician Specialist |

# U.S. Department of State-Affiliated Overseas Educational Advising Centers, Including Offices of the Fulbright Commission

## Africa

### BENIN
Educational Adviser
U.S. Embassy—Public Affairs Section
BP 2012, Cotonou
Tel. (229) 30-03-12

### BOTSWANA
Educational Adviser
U.S. Embassy—Public Affairs Section
P.O. Box 90, Gabarone
Tel. (267) 31-353982
Fax (267) 30-06129
E-mail: dangabo@usia.gov

### BURKINA FASO
Educational Adviser
U.S. Embassy—Public Affairs Section
01 BP 539, Ouagadougou
Tel. (226) 30-70-13
Fax (226) 31-52-73

### CAMEROON
Educational Adviser
U.S. Embassy—Public Affairs Section
BP 6241, Yaounde
Tel. (237) 23-04-16, 23-14-37
Fax (237) 22-67-65
E-mail: ALCYAO@CAMFIDO.GN.APC.ORG

### CHAD
Educational Adviser
U.S. Embassy—Public Affairs Section
BP 3, N'Djamena
Tel. (235) 61-4009, 51-6233

### CONGO—BRAZZAVILLE
Educational Adviser
U.S. Embassy—Public Affairs Section
BP 2053, Brazzaville
Tel. (242) 83-26-42, 83-42-64
Fax (242) 83-46-90

### CONGO—KINSHASA
Educational Adviser
U.S. Embassy—Public Affairs Section
BP 8622, Kinshasa
Tel. (243) 88-46612
Fax (243) 88-46592

### COTE D'IVOIRE
Educational Adviser
U.S. Embassy—Public Affairs Section
01 BP 1866, Abidjan
Tel. (225) 440597, 440745
Fax (225) 445396
E-mail: HART@CCA.CC.CI

### ETHIOPIA
Educational Adviser
U.S. Embassy—Public Affairs Section
P.O. Box 1041, Addis Ababa
Tel. (251) 1-550007
Fax (251) 1-551748
E-mail: USIS.ETH@telecom.net.et

### GHANA
Educational Adviser
U.S. Embassy—Public Affairs Section
P.O. Box 2288, Accra
Tel. (233) 21-229179
Fax (233) 21-229882
E-mail: Keteku@africaonline.com.gh

### GUINEA
Educational Adviser
U.S. Embassy—Public Affairs Section
BP 1215, Conakry
Tel. (224) 4-411424, 411425
Fax (224) 4-411522

### KENYA
Educational Adviser
U.S. Embassy—Public Affairs Section
P.O. Box 45869, Nairobi
E-mail: cdr@usis.africaonline.ke

## MALAWI

Educational Adviser
U.S. Embassy—Public Affairs Section
P.O. Box 30373, Lilongwe
Tel. (265) 782222, 782414
Fax (265) 781142

## MALI

Educational Adviser
U.S. Embassy—Public Affairs Section
BP 34, Bamako
Tel. (223) 225663
Fax (223) 222025
E-mail: gmariko@usis.malinet.ml

## MAURITANIA

Educational Adviser
U.S. Embassy
BP 222
Nouakchott
Tel. 222-52660 through 63
Fax 222-2-515-92

## MAURITIUS

Educational Adviser
U.S. Embassy—Public Affairs Section
President John Kennedy St., Port Louis
Tel. (230) 208-2347
Fax (230) 212-2608
E-mail: dbaker@bow.intnet.mu

## MOZAMBIQUE

Educational Adviser
U.S. Embassy—Public Affairs Section
Av. Mao Tse Tung, Maputo
Tel. (258) 1-491918
Fax (258) 1-491918
E-mail: amagaia@mail.tropical.co.mz

## NIGER

Educational Adviser
U.S. Embassy—Public Affairs Section
BP 11.201, Niamey
Tel. (227) 73-31-69, 73-41-07
Fax (227) 73-55-60

## NIGERIA

Educational Adviser
U.S. Embassy—Public Affairs Section
P.O. Box 554, Lagos
Tel. (234) 1-2634-865, 2633-713
Fax (234) 1-2635-397
E-mail: fchlagos@usia.gov

## SENEGAL

Educational Adviser
U.S. Embassy—Public Affairs Section
BP 49, Dakar

## SIERRA LEONE

Educational Adviser
U.S. Embassy—Public Affairs Section
3 Walpole Street, Freetown
E-mail: LIR@USIS-SL.BAOBAB.COM

## SOUTH AFRICA

Educational Adviser
U.S. Consulate—Public Affairs Section
10 Plein St., Cape Town
Tel. (27) 21-461-0583
Fax (27) 21-461-3603
E-mail: Laila%capetown@mhs.cstat.co.za

Educational Adviser
U.S. Consulate—Public Affairs Section
333 Smith St., Durban
Tel. (27) 31-3055063
Fax (27) 31-3042847
E-mail: Roberta%durban@mhs.cstat.co.za

Educational Adviser
U.S. Consulate—Public Affairs Section
PO Box 2155, Johannesburg
Tel. (27) 11-838-2231
Fax (27) 11-838-3920
E-mail: Lyn%johannes@mhs.cstat.co.za

## SWAZILAND

Educational Adviser
U.S. Embassy—Public Affairs Section
PO Box 199, Mbabane
Tel. (268) 42445, 42059
Fax (268) 45846
E-mail: 100077.1575@compuserve.com

## TOGO
Educational Adviser
U.S. Embassy—Public Affairs Section
BP 852, Lome
Tel. (228) 212166
Fax (228) 217794

## UGANDA
Educational Adviser
U.S. Embassy—Public Affairs Section
PO Box 7186, Kampala
Tel. (256) 41-230507, 233231
Fax (256) 41-250314
E-mail: connie@usiakla.starcom.co.ug

## ZAMBIA
Educational Adviser
U.S. Embassy—Public Affairs Section
PO Box 32053, Lusaka
Tel. (260) 1-227993
Fax (260) 1-226523
E-mail: usiszam@zamnet.zm

## ZIMBABWE
Educational Adviser
U.S. Embassy—Public Affairs Section
PO Box 4010, Harare
Tel. (263) 4-758798, 758800
Fax (263) 4-758802
E-mail: usis@harare.iafrica.com

# East Asia, Australia, and New Zealand

## AUSTRALIA
Educational Information Officer
Australian-American Educational Foundation
GPO Box 1559
Canberra, ACT 2601
Tel. 61-6-247-9331
Fax 61-6-247-6554
E-mail: judy@aaef.anu.edu.au

U.S. Educational Advising Service
Rms. 360/362 Bldg. 401
Curtin University of Technology
Kent Street
Bentley, WA 6102
Tel. 61-9-351-4085
Fax 61-9-351-4086

Educational Adviser/USIS
American Consulate
Level 59, MLC Center
19–29 Martin Place
Sydney, NSW 2000
Tel. 61-2-373-9230
Fax 61-2-221-0551
E-mail: edadvsyd@ozemail.com.au

## BURMA (MYANMAR)
Public Affairs Section
14 Tawwin Road, Dagon Township
Yangon
Tel. 95-1-223-106
Fax 95-1-221-262
E-mail: ttnrgn@pd.state.gov (Note: e-mail connection may be irregular)

## CAMBODIA
Hang Chan Thon
University of Phnom Penh
E-mail: Luise: mkskhmer@forum.org.kh
Chan Thon: caradvchthon@bigpond.com.kh
USIS Phnom Penh

## CHINA
Chinese Service Center for Scholarly Exchange
Beijing Language Institute
15 Xueyuan Lu Rd.
Beijing 100083
Tel. 86-10-201-7531 ext. 2661
Fax 86-10-202-7147
E-mail: interco@stnet.cscse.edu.cn

Librarian/Educational Adviser
Reference Center
Intensive Languages Training Center
Sichuan Union University (West Campus)
610065 Chengdu, Sichuan
Tel. 86-28-540-5426
Fax 86-28-522-1851
E-mail: Iltcsuu@Public.sc.cninfo.net

Study Abroad Training Department
Sichuan Foreign Language Institute
Shapingba, Chongqing, Sichuan 630031
Tel. 86-811-986-2775

Educational Advising Officer
Dalian Foreign Language Institute
No. 110 Nanshan Rd.
Zhongshan District
Dalian, Liaoning Province 116001
Tel. 86-411-280-3121 ext. 6367
Fax 86-411-265-3809

Educational Adviser
Liaoning Education Committee, Foreign Affairs
    Office
Guangdong Education Service for International
    Exchanges
Rm. 1101, Gaojiao Bldg.
723 East Dongfeng Rd.
Guangzhou, Guangdong 510080
Tel. 86-20-8777-8110 ext. 6101
Fax 86-20-8767-9016

Guangdong Service Center for Scholarly
    Exchange
6F, Beixiu Bldg., Xiaobei Rd.
Guangzhou, Guangdong 510050
Tel. 86-20-777-8356-8066
Fax 86-20-8356-8055
E-mail: gscse@163.net;
gzjle@Public.Guangzhou.gd.cn

CSCSE Shenzhen
22E/B Block, Guoqi Plaza
Shangbu Rd., Shenzen 518031
Tel. 86-755-2129-613
Fax 86-755-2129-063
E-mail: davcscse@szonline.net

Shanghai Educational Information Center for
    International Exchanges
Shanghai International Studies University
410 E. Ti Yu Hui Rd.
Tel. 86-21-6544-2187
E-mail: seicie@online.sh.cn

Shanghai Education Association for
    International Exchange
Shanghai Education Hotel, Shanghai
E-mail: vicli@online.sh.cn

Study Abroad Training Department
Xi'an Foreign Languages Institute
Wujiafen
Xian, Shaanxi Province 710061
Tel. 86-29-525-2956 ext. 384

## HONG KONG
Institute of International Education
Rm. 601–602, General Commercial Bldg.
156–164 Des Voeux Rd. Central
Tel. 852-2603-5571
Fax 852-2603-5765
E-mail: kfsurya@cuhk.edu.hk;
gpfairbr@hkusua.hku.hk

## INDONESIA
Educational Information Center
Gedung Balai Pustaka, 6th Floor
Jalan Gunung Sahari Raya No. 4
Jakarta 10720
Tel. 62-21-345-2024
Fax 62-21-345-2050
E-mail: nancyg@aminef.or.id;
hanifs@aminef.or.id;
ericas@aminef.or.id
Web site: www.usembassyjakarta.org/aminef

Ratna Widjaya
AMINEF-Surabaya
Gedung Perpustakaan Lt. 4
Universitas Surabaya, Raya Kalirungkut
Surabaya
Tel. 62-31-847-1809; 62-31-849-1915 ext. 1024
Fax 62-31-847-1810
E-mail: EAS_sby@rad.net.id

## JAPAN
Educational Information Officer
Japan—United States Educational Commission
Sanno Grand Building, Rm. 207
2–14, 2 Chome, Nagata-Cho
Chiyoda-ku, Tokyo 100
Tel. 81-3-3580-1339
Fax 81-3-3580-1217
E-mail: cgilman@jusec.go.jp
Web site: www.jusec.go.jp

## KOREA
Korean American Educational Commission
Fulbright Bldg., Ste. 403
168 15 Yomni-dong, Mapo-gu
Seoul 121-090
Tel. 82-2-32-75-4000
Fax 82-2-36-75-4028
E-mail: jlarson@fulbright.or.kr

## LAOS
Public Affairs Section
U.S. Embassy Vientiane
Rue Bartholonie
Tel. 856-21-21-3967
Fax 856-21-21-3045

## MALAYSIA
Malaysian American Commission on Educational
   Exchange
191 Jalan Tun Razak
50400 Kuala Lumpur
Tel. 6-03-242-4539
Fax. 6-03-242-4119
E-mail: jbkhosa@pc.jaring.my
Web site: macee.org.my


Malaysian American Commission on Educational
   Exchange
Kolej Damansara Utama, 1st fl.
32 Jalan Anson
10400 Penang
Tel. 6-04-226-4924
Fax 6-04-226-5044
E-mail: maceepg@po.jaring.my


## MONGOLIA
Mongolian Foundation for Open Society
Center for Scientific & Technology Information
Rm. 321
Baga Toiru-49
Ulaanbaatar
Tel. 976-1-328-783
Fax 976-1-314-857
E-mail: udval@soros.org.mn


## NEW ZEALAND
New Zealand United States Educational
   Foundation
PO Box 3465
Wellington
Tel. 64-4-472-2065
Fax 64-4-499-5364
E-mail: CALLEN@fulbright.org.nz

## PHILIPPINES
Director, Educational Advising Center
Philippine American Educational Foundation
395 Sen. Gil Puyat Ave.
Makati, Metro Manila
Tel. 63-2-895-3037
Fax 63-2-895-3215
E-mail: paefadv@mnl.sequel.net

## SINGAPORE
U.S. Education Information Center
01–03 Podium a Bestway Building
12 Prince Edward Rd.
Singapore 079212
Tel. 65-226-6996
Fax 65-223-0550
E-mail: head@useic.com.sg

## TAIWAN
Educational Information Officer
Foundation for Scholarly Exchange
1-A Chuan Chow St.
Taipei
Tel. 886-2-332-8188
Fax 886-2-332-5445
E-mail: fse@saec.saec.edu.tw

## THAILAND
U.S. Embassy Public Affairs Section
95 Wireless Rd.
Patumwan
Bangkok 10330
Tel. 66-2-205-4022
Fax 66-2-650-8921
E-mail: supbang@usia.gov

AUA
PO Box 31
Khon Kaen University
Khon Kaen 40002
Tel. 66-43-241-072
Fax 66-43-241-072
E-mail: rg_smith@hotmail.com

Institute of International Education
9th Floor, Citibank Tower
82 N. Sathorn Rd.
Bangkok
Tel. 66-2-639-2700
Fax 66-2-639-2706
E-mail: iiethai@ksc.th.com
Web site: IIE.ORG/SEASIA/

Education Abroad Division
Civil Service Commission
Pitsanuloke Rd.
Bangkok 10300
Tel. 66-2-281-9544
Fax 66-2-628-6202

Bangkok Bank
Educational Advisory Division
333 Silom Rd.
Bangkok 10500
Tel. 66-2-230-1329
Fax 66-2-231-4051

Knowledge Plus
Silom Shanghai Building, 2nd Floor
Bangkok 10500
Tel. 66-2-238-3933
Fax 66-2-266-5928
E-mail: sriporn@mozart.inet.co.th

## VIETNAM
IIE Hanoi
USIS
127 Ba Thieu
Hanoi
Tel. 84-4-943-0711
Fax 84-4-943-0710
E-mail: IIEHN@netnam.org.vn

## REAC-EAST ASIA
Regional Educational Advising Coordinator for
  East Asia
c/o U.S. Embassy Kuala Lumpur
376 Jalan Tun Razak
50400 Kuala Lumpur, Malaysia
Tel. 6-03-2168-5061
Fax 6-03-248-9192
E-mail: mthomson@pd.state.gov
marti@tm.net.my

# East/Central Europe

## ALBANIA
Public Affairs Section, U.S. Embassy
Educational Adviser: Agim Tola
Rr Elbasani 103
Tirana
Tel. 355-42-33-246
Fax 355-42-32-222

Open Society Fund (Soros)
Student Advising Center
Adviser: Linda Bushati
Rruga Mujo Ulqinaku 2/1
Tirana
Tel./Fax: 355-42-48214/48215
E-mail: linda@publish.soros.al

## BULGARIA
Fulbright Commission
Advisers: Cheresha Chelebieva & Julia Yotova
17 Stamboliisky Blvd.
Sofia 1000
Tel. 359-2-980-82-12
359-2-981-68-30
Fax 359-2-988-45-17
E-mail: fulbright@mbox.digsys.bg

Open Society Fund (Soros)
Information Center
Adviser & Network Coordinator: Illiana
  Gyulcheva
1 Balsha St., Block 9
Sofia 1408
Tel. 359-2-951-6552
Fax 359-2-951-6348
E-mail: illyana@osf.acad.bg
Web site: www.osf.acad.bg

Open Society Information Centers Network
Open Society Information Centre
Bourgas Free University, Rm. 125
8000 Bourgas
Tel./Fax: 359-56-3-91-97

Open Society Information Centre
2 Kamenets St., 1st Floor
6400 Dimitrovgrad
(in cooperation with "Trakia-J" Foundation)
Tel./Fax 359-391-25826
E-mail: trakia@osf.acad.bg

Open Society Information Centre
8 Skobelevska St.
5300 Gabrovo
Tel./Fax 359-66-34-105
E-mail: oscg@osf.acad.bg

Open Society Information Centre
20 Skobelev Blvd., bl.2, vh.B
5800 Pleven
Tel. 359-64-3-33-80
Fax 359-64-4-61-90
E-mail: ospleven@bgcict.acad.bg

Open Society Information Centre
17 Avksentiy Veleshki St.
Ivan Vazov National Library, Floor 1
4000 Plovdiv
Tel. 359-32-22-48-24
Fax 359-32-26-76-23
E-mail: osplovdv@bgcict.acad.bg

Open Society Information Centre
1 Ferdinand St.
7000 Rousse
Tel. 359-82-23-60-89
Fax 359-82-27-21-45
E-mail: osrousse@ait.ru.acad.bg;
    osrousse@ bgcict.acad.bg

Open Society Information Centre
2 Hristo Smirnenski St.
Floor 3, Rm. 16
7500 Silistra
(in cooperation with "Ecohorizonti" Foundation)
Tel./Fax 359-86-27056

Open Society Information Centre
6 Hadzhi Dimiter St.
PO Box 135
8800 Sliven
Tel./Fax 359-44-2-07-15
E-mail: ossliven@bgcict.acad.bg
anton@sliven.osf.acad.brushing

Open Society Information Centre
Bulgaria Blvd.
Business Centre, Floor 5, Rm. 514
4700 Smolyan
Tel./Fax 359-301-25-065

Open Society Information Centre
1 Kaloyan St.
9700 Shoumen
Tel./Fax 359-54-55-265

Open Society Information Centre
19 A, Lyuben Karavelov St.
Floor 4, Apt. 8
9000 Varna
Tel. 359-52-22-00-15
Fax 359-52-60-01-38
E-mail: oscvn@mbox.digsys.bg

Open Society Information Centre
7 Vassil Aprilov Str 5
4600 Velingrad
Tel. 359-52-28-542
Fax 359-52-27-812

Cyril and Methodius International Foundation
19 Oborishte Str
1504 Sofia
Tel. 359-2-464-131 and 446-034
Fax 359-2-446-027
E-mail: cmfnd@mgu.bg

Cyril and Methodius International Foundation
Adviser: Ana Grigorieva
Central Post Office
PO Box 379
4000 Plovdiv
Tel./Fax 359-32-268-616
E-mail: osic_plvd@OSF.ACAD.BG

Cyril and Methodius International Foundation
8 Studentska Str.
Technical University of Russe "Angel Kanchev"
7017 Russe
Tel. 359-82-453-143
Fax 359-82-455-145

Cyril and Methodius International Foundation
6 Studentska Str.
Institute of Mechanical and Electrical
    Engineering-Varna
9010 Varna
Tel. 359-52-881-934
Fax 359-52-871-910
E-mail: ask@ac.tu.varna.bg

## CROATIA

Croatian American Society
Student Information Center
Adviser: Ivana Puljiz
Petrova 119 2nd fl.
10000 Zagreb
Tel. 385-1-2339-705
Fax 385-1-2339-426
E-mail: sic@zamir.net
Web site: www.zamir.net/sic

American Embassy
USIS Contact: Zora Posinovec-Beluhan
A. Hebranga 2
10000 Zagreb
Tel. 385-1-455-5500
Fax 385-1-481-7302
E-mail: zpzagreb@usia.gov
Web site: www.usembassy.hr

## CZECH REPUBLIC

Fulbright Commission
Educational Adviser: Jakub Tesar
Taboritska 23
130 87 Prague 3
Tel. 420-2-277-155
Fax 420-2-697-5600
E-mail: fulb@mbox.cesnet.cz; or fulbright@
    fulbright.cz
Web site: measure.feld.cuvut.cz/fulbright

University of West Bohemia
Dr. Eva Valentova
Director, Department of International
    Development
Americka 42
316 14 Plzen
Tel. 42-19-723-5846
Fax 42-19-722-3209
E-mail: Dopson@zeus.zcu.cz

Jan Hus Educational Foundation
PO Box 735
Radnicka 8
663 35 Brno
Tel. (42-5)-422-12314
Fax (42-5)-422-12084
E-mail: janhus@brno.ics.muni.cz

Palacky University
International Liaison Office
Krizkovskeho 8
741 47 Olomouc
Tel. (42-68)-522-3494
Fax (42-68)-522-2731
E-mail: vyhnanko@risc.upol.cz

Academic Information Agency (AIA)
26 Senovazne nam.
111 21 Prague 1
Tel. (42-2) 2422-9698
Fax (42-2) 2422-9697

## ESTONIA

Educational Advising Center
Adviser: Marvi Pulver
Tartu University Library
Struve1–325
50091 Tartu
Estonia
Tel./Fax (372-7) 427 243
E-mail: marvi@utlib.ee
Web site: www.utlib.ee/Fulb

Tallinn Technical University
Educational Adviser: Eha Teder
Ehitajate tee 5
Tallinn 19086
Tel./Fax (372) 620-3543
E-mail: educentr@edu.ttu.ee
Web site: www.ttu.ee/educenter

## HUNGARY

Fulbright Commission
Senior Educational Adviser: Agnes Vajda
Assistant Educational Adviser: Kornelia Litkei
Ajtosi Durer sor 19–21
1146 Budapest
Tel. (36-1) 462-8050
Fax (36-1) 252-0266
E-mail: vajda@fulbright.huninet.hu; or
    litkei@fulbright.huninet.hu
Web site: www.prof.iif.hu

Szabo Ervin Library
Educational Adviser: Agnes Gal
Szabo Ervin ter 1.
1088 Budapest
Tel. (36-1) 338-4933 ext. 164
Fax (36-1) 318-5815

Budapest Technical University
International Student Center
Educational Advisers: Agnes Orosz & Timea
  Kelemen
Muegyetem rkpt. 3. K. epulet, I. 51
1111 Budapest
Tel. (36-1) 463-1408 or 463-2522
Fax (36-1) 463-3836
E-mail: agnes@sc.BME.HU;
  kelement@sc.bme.hu

Debrecen University Association
Educational Adviser: Judit Juhasz
Kossuth Lajos University
Rektori Hivatal
POB 37.
4010 Debrecen
Tel. (36-52) 316-666 ext. 2863
Fax (36-52) 314-666 ext. 2487
E-mail: jjuhasz@tigris.klte.hu

University of Miskolc
Central Library
Egyetemvaros
3515 Miskolc
Tel. (36-46) 3614-16
Fax (36-46) 3695-54
E-mail: kontem@kon.uni-miskolc.hu or
  reksztem@gold.uni-miskolc.hu

Janus Pannonius University
Educational Adviser: Krisztina Dorn
Faculty of Arts
Language Centre
IFJUSAG UTJA 6. G/111/17
7624 PECS
Tel./Fax (36-72) 327-622 EXT. 4348
E-mail: dorn@btk.jpte.hu

Jozsef Attila University
Educational Adviser: Ildiko Ficzko
Central Library
Dugonics ter 13.
6720 Szeged
Tel. (36-62) 454-065
Fax (36-62) 420-718
E-mail: ficzko@bibl.u-szeged.hu
Web site: www.bibl.u-szeged.hu

University of Veszprem
Educational Adviser: Judit Kun Szabo
Central Library
Egyetem u. 10
8200 Veszprem
Tel. (36-88) 4220-22 ext. 223
Fax (36-88) 4260-16
E-mail: kunsza@almos.vein.hu

## LATVIA

University of Latvia / Soros Foundation
Educational Advising Center
Adviser: Gaston Lacombe
Raina Bulvaris 19, Rm. 243
Riga LV 1586
Tel. (371) 722-8656
Fax (371) 782-0385
E-mail: gastons@lanet.lv

U.S. Embassy—Public Affairs Section
Educational Adviser
7 Smilsu
Riga LV 1050
Tel. (371) 721-6571 and 721-6565
Fax (371) 782-0077
E-mail: usis@mail.usis.bkc.lv

## LITHUANIA

University of Vilnius
Adviser: Zaneta Savickiene
Universiteto 3, Rm. 40
2734 Vilnius
Tel. (370-2) 62-50-53
Fax (370-2) 61-05-59
E-mail: zaneta.savickiene@cr.vu.lt

Youth Career Center, VMU-OSFL
Adviser: Jurate Muriniene
Laisves al.53–202
3000 Kaunas
Tel. (370-7) 228151
Fax (370-7) 206224
E-mail: jurate@kc.osf.lt

## MACEDONIA

Student Resource Center-Skopje
Open Society Institute
Ruzveltova 34
91000 Skopje
Tel. 389 91 13 45 68
Fax 389 91 13 65 14
E-mail: srcsk@soros.org.mk
Web site: www.soros.org.mk/src

Student Resource Center-Bitola
MUB "Sv.Kliment Ohridski"
Leninova 39
97000 Bitola
Tel. 389 97 22 65 59
Fax 389 97 22 65 59
E-mail: srcbt@soros.org.mk
Web site: www.soros.org.mk/src

IREX Advising Center
University of Skopje
Bulevar Krstemisirkov
Box 576
91000 Skopje
Tel. 389 91 118 155;
    389 91 224 617
Fax 389 91 116 370
E-mail: MCENEVSKA@UKIM.EDU.MK

## POLAND

Fulbright Commission
Adviser: Aleksandra Augustyniak
ul. Nowy Swiat 4
00–497 Warsaw
Tel (48-22) 6287-950
Fax (48-22) 6287-943
E-mail: ola.augustyniak@fulbright.edu.pl
Web site: www.fulbright.edu.pl

American Consulate/Public Affairs Section
ul. Stolarska 9
31–043 Krakow
Tel. (48-12) 221-294, 221-368
Fax (48-12) 218-212
E-mail: bfpkrak@USIA.gov

Educational Advising Center
Progress & Business Foundation
ul.Miechowska 8A
30-055 Krakow
Tel. (48-12) 636-87-87
E-mail: pbf@uci.agh.edu.pl

Office of International Relations
Wroclaw University
ul. pl. Uniwersytecki 1
50–137 Wroclaw
Tel. (48-71) 344 6999
E-mail: jkr@adm.uni.wroc.pl

## ROMANIA

Fulbright Commission
Strada Austrului nr 15
Bucharest
Tel. (40-1)-210-4914
Fax (40-1)-210-4915
E-mail: Slumi@fulb.sfos.ro; lumi@fulb.buc.
    soros.ro

IREX (International Research and Exchanges
    Board)
Str. Sperantei 36, ap 1
Bucharest
Tel./Fax (40-1) 613 5426
E-mail: irexbuc@aol.com

Soros Foundation for an Open Society
Information and Advising Center
Cluj Office
PO Box 1084
Str. Marului Nr. 5
3400 Cluj-Napoca
Tel. (40-64) 194-078, 194-079
Fax (40-64) 197-121
E-mail: lbal@clujlib.soros.ro

Soros Foundation for an Open Society
COPA
Str. Moara de Foc 35 et 8
6600 Iasi
Tel. (40-32) 252-910, 251-912, 147-804
Fax (40-32) 252-928
E-mail: asava@copa.iasi.soros.ro

Soros Foundation for an Open Society
Timisoara Office
Str. Semenic No.10
1900 Timisoara
Tel./Fax: (40-56) 199-960
E-mail: timis@buc.soros.ro;
    eva@timis.soros.ro

Central University Library (Biblioteca Centrala
    Universitara)
American Educational Advising Centre (attn.
    Camelia Boca)
Str. Pacurari nr.4
6600 Iasi
Tel. (40-32) 116-281
Fax (40-32) 112-528
E-mail: camelia@bcu-iasi.ro
Web site: www.bcu-iasi.ro/centrconsiliere. html

JFK American Studies Center
Str. Universitatii nr. 7–9
3400 Cluj-Napoca
Tel. (40-64) 116-101 ext. 162
Fax (40-64) 193-868

Universitatea "Dunarea de Jos"
Str Domneasca 47, Galati
Tel. (40-36) 460-328
Fax (40-36) 461-353

Universitatea Tehnica -Timisoara
Piata Victoriei 2
1900 Timisoara
Tel. (40-56) 134-717
Fax (40-56) 190-321

Universitatea Tehnica "Ghe. Asachi"
Departamentul Relatii Internationale
Bd. Copou 22
6600 Iasi
Tel./Fax (40-32) 211-667

Biblioteca Centrala Universitara
Bd. Vasile Parvan 4
Timisoara
Tel. (40-56) 190-353
Fax (40-56) 194-004

## SLOVAKIA

Fulbright Commission-Slovakia
Adviser: Maria Paniakova
Levicka 3
821 08 Bratislava
Tel. 4217 5542 56 06
Fax 4217 5557 74 91
E-mail: fulbnet@e-list.usia.gov;
    Maria@fulb.sanet.sk

Slovak Academic Information Agency-SCTS
PO Box 108
810 00 Bratislava 1
Tel. (42-7) 533-3010, 533-3762
Fax (42-7) 533-5748
E-mail: peter@saia.sk

Jan Hus Educational Foundation
Na vrsku 8
PO Box 313
810 00 Bratislava
Tel. 421 7 54 43 37 56
Fax 421 7 54 43 37 56
E-mail: vnjh@gtinet.sk
Web site: custom.gratex.sk/vnjh

SAIA
Tajovskeho 51
974 01 Banska Bystrica
Tel. 088 737 810-11
Fax 088 737 812

Slovak Academic Information Agency (SAIA)
Hlavna 6
040 00 Kosice
Tel./Fax (42-95) 622-9641

SAIA-SCTS
Samova 4
949 01 Nitra
Tel./Fax 087/242 54

SAIA-SCTS
Dom priatelstva narodov
Nam. sv. Egidia 11
058 01 Poprad
Tel./Fax 092/62 015

SAIA-SCTS
Predmestska 1
010 00 Zilina
Tel./Fax 089/635 860

## SLOVENIA
University of Maribor
Krekova 2
62000 Maribor
Tel. 386-62-212-281
Fax 386-62-23541
E-mail: sandra.fras@uni-mb.si

Open Society Institute
Ljubljana
Tel. 386-61-312-175
Fax 386-61-312-139
E-mail: ndimc@soros.e5.ijs.si

# Mexico, Central America, and the Caribbean

## BRITISH VIRGIN ISLANDS
Anguilla Public Library
The Valley
Anguilla
Tel. 809-497-2441
Fax 809-497-2441
E-mail: library@offshore.com.ai

H. Lavity Stoutt Community College
Parquita Bay, PO Box 3097
Road Town, Tortola
Tel. 809-494-4994
Fax 809-494-4996

## ANTIGUA
University of the West Indies School of
Continuing Studies
PO Box 142
Factory Road, St. John's
Tel. 268-462-1355
Fax 268-462-2968
E-mail:university@candw.ag

## BAHAMAS
College of the Bahamas
Counseling and Health Services Department
PO Box N-4912
Nassau
Tel. 242-302-4439
Fax 242-302-7834
E-mail: cobcoun@cob.edu.bs

Department of Education
30 C Kipling Building
PO Box F
Grand Bahama

District Education Office
Governor's Island, Eleuthera

Department of Education
Queen's Highway
PO Box 29194
Georgetown, Exuma

Government Schools
Department of Education
PO Box 20499
Marsh Harbour, Abaco

Department of Education
Kemp's Bay, Andros

## BARBADOS
Barbados Community College
"Eyrie," Howell's Cross Rd.
St. Michael
Tel. 246-426-2858
Fax 246-429-5935
E-mail: arthurs@caribsurf.com

University of the West Indies
Cave Hill Campus, Office of Student Services
St. Michael
Tel. 246-425-1310
Fax 246-424-5348

## BELIZE
U.S. Embassy
29 Gabrourel Lane
Belize City
Tel. 501-277-161
Fax 501-230-802

## CAYMAN ISLANDS
Ministry of Education & Planning
Government Administration Bldg.
Grand Cayman Island
British West Indies
Tel. 345-949-8025
Fax 345-949-9343

Principal, Triple C. School
PO Box 498, Elgin Lane
George Town, Grand Cayman Island
British West Indies
Tel. 345-949-6022
Fax 345-949-6803

## COSTA RICA
Instituto Cultural Costarricanse-Norteamericano
150 mts. North of Bomba Los Yoses
San Jose
Tel. 506-253-3736, 225-9433
Fax 506-224-1480
E-mail: aeducccn@sol.racsa.co.cr

## DOMINICA
National Documentation Centre
Ministry of Education and Sports
Government Headquarters
Roseau
Tel. 767-448-2401 ext. 3408, 3409
Fax 767-448-7928

## DOMINICAN REPUBLIC
Instituto Cultural Dominico-Americano
ECO, Ave. Abraham Lincoln 21
Santo Domingo
Tel. 809-533-8652
Fax 809-533-8809

Instituto Cultural Dominico-Americano
Ave. Estrella Sadala, La Rinconada
Santiago de los Caballeros
Tel. 809-582-6627
Fax 809-587-3858
E-mail: bncnet-world@santos.ccbeunet.br

## EL SALVADOR
Centro Cultural Salvadoreno
Avenida Sismiles, Metro Centro Norte
San Salvador
Tel. 503-226-6556
Fax 503-226-9119
E-mail: svasquez@usia.gov

## GRENADA
T.A. Marryshow Community College
Tanteen, St. George's
Grenada, West Indies
Tel. 809-440-1578, 440-4020
Fax 809-440-3079

## GUATEMALA
Instituto Guatemalteco Americano (IGA)
Ruta 1, Via 4, Zona 4, Guatemala City
Tel. 502-233-4393
Fax 502-232-3135
E-mail: orieniga@infovia.com.gt

## HAITI
U.S. Embassy
14 Ave. Marie Jeanne
Port au Prince
Tel. 509-22-1504, 22-5726
Fax 509-23-8324
E-mail: elgpap@usia.gov

## HONDURAS
Instituto Hondurano de Cultura Interamericana
2 Avenida entre 5&6 Calle, No. 520
Comayuguela (Tegucigalpa)
Tel. 504-37-7539
Fax 504-38-0064
E-mail: ichi@sdnhon.org.hn

## JAMAICA
USIS/Mutual Life Bldg.
2 Oxford Rd, 1st fl.
Kingston
Tel. 809-929-4850 through 59
Fax 809-929-3637
E-mail: usis@toj.com

## MARTINIQUE
Bibliotheque Schoelcher, PO Box 640
Av. des Caraibes, Fort de France 97200
Martinique, French West Indies
Tel. 596-70-26-67
Fax 596-72-4555

## MEXICO

Institute of International Education
Regional Office for Latin America
Benjamin Franklin Library
Londres 16, 2nd fl.
Mexico City 06660
Tel. 525-211-0042 ext. 3510, 4511
Fax 525-535-5597
E-mail: iie@profmexis.sar.net

Instituto Cultural Mexicano Norteamericano de
Jalisco
Enrique Diaz de Leon No. 300
44170 Guadalajara, Jalisco
Tel. 52-38-25-4101, 52-38-25-5838
Fax 52-38-25-1671

USIS
Progresso 175
44100 Guadalajara, Jalisco
Tel. 52-38-25-2998
Fax 52-38-26-7563
E-mail: mesmex@usia.gov

Instituto Mexicano-Norteamericano de
Relacionnes Culturales
Hidalgo 768 Pte.
Monterrey, Nuevo Leon
Tel. 52 83-40-1583
Fax 52-83-42-5517
E-mail: bibbfranc@intercable.net

Instituto Benjamin Franklin de Yucatan
Calle 57, No. 474-A
Merida, Yucatan
Tel. 52-99-28-60-05
Fax 52-99-28-00-97
E-mail: franklin@pibil.finred.com.mx

Instituto Mexicano Americano de Relaciones
Culturales
Blvd. Navarette y Monteverde, Fracc. Valle
Hermoso
8300, Hermosillo, Sonora
Tel. 52-621-14-22-42
Fax 52-621-14-07-81

American Consulate General
Lopez Matecs Ave., No. 924 Norte
Ciudad Juarez
Tel. 52-16-11-3000
Fax 52-16-16-90-56
E-mail: gzaragoza@usia.gov

Universidad Vasco de Quiroga
Camino a Jesus del Monte No. 555
Santa Maria de Guido 58290
Morelia, Michoacan
Tel. 52-43-23-51-78
Fax 52-43-14-94-19
E-mail: ahhlek@giga.com

U.S. Consular Agency
Alcala 201, Oaxaca
Oaxaca
Tel./Fax 52-951-43-054

Instituto Mexicano-Norteamericano de
Realaciones Culturales
Hidalgo Nte. 160
2500 Saltillo, Coahuila
Tel. 52-84-14-84-22
Fax 52-84-12-06-53

U.S. Consular Agency
Francisco de P. Moriel 103–10, Col. Centro
96000 San Luis Potosi
San Luis Potosi
Tel./Fax 52-81-21-528

Universidad Centro de Ensenanza y Superior
(CETYS)
Av. Gran Lago S/N, Apdo. Postal 4012, Zona
Centro
22550, Tijuana, Baja California
Tel. 52-66-25-3942
Fax 52-66-25-3951
E-mail: ammmex@usia.gov;
aarobledo@besttj.tij.cetys.mx

Universidad Veracruzana
Escuela para Estudiantes Extranjeros, Zamora 25
Xalapa, Veracruz 91000
Tel. (52-28) 17-86-87
Fax (52-28) 16-64-13
E-mail: eeeuv@dino.coacade.uv.mx

## MONTSERRAT
Montserrat Public Library
Marine Drive, Plymouth
Montserrat, West Indies
Tel. 664-491-3622, 2444
Fax 664-491-2367

## NETHERLAND ANTILLES
International School of Curacao
Koninginnelaan, Emmastad
Tel. 599-937-3633
Fax 599-937-3142

## NEVIS
Main Library
Charlestown,
Nevis, West Indies

## NICARAGUA
Centro Binacional, Centro Comercial Nejapa
Detras del Banco Popular,
Managua
Tel. 505-266-6036, 265-3058
Fax 505-265-2727
E-mail: eduadv@ibw.com.ni

## PANAMA
Centro Cultural Pan-USA
Balboa Heights
Tel. 507-227-1777 ext. 2390
Fax 507-227-4515
E-mail: amypan@usia.gov

## ST. KITTS
College of Further Education
Lockhart St.
Basseterre
Tel. 869-465-2190
Fax 869-465-6583

## ST. LUCIA
Sir Arthur Lewis Community College
The Morne, Castries
Tel. 758-452-5507, ext. 151
Fax 758-452-7901
E-mail: libry@salcc.edu.lc

## ST. VINCENT
Documentation Center
Administrative Center, Box 608
Kingstown
St. Vincent, Windward Islands
Tel. 809-456-1183
Fax 809-456-1251

## SURINAME
Tel. 597-47-5051
Fax 597-41-0025

## TOBAGO
c/o USIS
7–9 Marli St.
Port of Spain, Trinidad
Tel. 868-622-6627, 5979
Fax 868-628-7944
E-mail: usispos@trinidad.net

## TRINIDAD
See entry for Tobago.

# Middle East and North Africa

## ALGERIA
Educational Adviser
U.S. Embassy—Public Affairs Section
BP 252
Hydra
Tel. 213-2-69-32-22
Fax 213-2-69-14-88

## BAHRAIN
Educational Adviser
Public Affairs Section
AmEmbassy Manama
Box 255, PSC 451
FPO AE 09834-5100
Tel. 973-276-180
Fax 973-270-547

## EGYPT
Educational Adviser
AMIDEAST
3 Pharaana St.
Azarita, Alexandria
Tel. 20-3-482-9091
Fax 20-3-483-9644
E-mail: alexandria@amideast.org
Web site: www.amideast.org

Educational Resource Center
AMIDEAST
6 Kamel El Shinnawy St.
Garden City, Cairo
Tel. 20-2-355-3170
Fax 20-2-355-2946
E-mail: egypt@amideast.org
Web site: www.amideast.org

## ISRAEL

Educational Adviser
U.S.-Israel Educational Foundation
PO Box 26160
Tel Aviv 09830
Tel. 972-3-5172131
Fax 972-3-5162016
E-mail: elevinson@fulbright.org.il
Web site: studyusa.fulbright.org.il

## GAZA

Gaza Branch Manager/Educational Adviser
AMIDEAST/Gaza
PO Box 1247
Gaza 91193
Tel. 972-7-824-635
Fax 972-2-869-338
E-mail: westbank-gaza@amideast.org

## JERUSALEM

Educational Adviser
AMIDEAST
PO Box 19665
Jerusalem 91193
Tel. 972-2-627-7346
Fax 972-2-627-3206
E-mail: westbank-gaza@amideast.org
Web site: www.amideast.org

## JORDAN

Educational Adviser
AMIDEAST
Amman 11118
Tel. 962-6-862950
Fax 962-6-814020
E-mail: jordan@amideast.org

Educational Adviser
AMIDEAST/Irbid
Branch Advising Center
Yarmouk University
Irbid
Tel. 962-2-271100 ext. 2955

## KUWAIT

Educational Adviser
AMIDEAST
PO Box 44818
Hawalli, 32063
Tel. 965-532-7794
Fax 965-532-7796
E-mail: amideast@ncc.moc.kw

## LEBANON

Educational Adviser
AMIDEAST
PO Box 70–744
Antelias
Tel. 961-1-411676
Fax 961-1-411615
E-mail: amideast@dm.net.lb

## MOROCCO

Educational Adviser
AMIDEAST
7 Zankat Agadir
Rabat
Tel. 212-7-76-4109
Fax 212-7-76-8852
E-mail: macece2@maghrebnet.net.ma
Web site: www.amideast.org

## OMAN

Educational Adviser
Public Affairs Section
U.S. Embassy Muscat
PO Box 202, Code 115
Madinat Qaboos
Tel. 968-698989 ext. 203
Fax 968-699771
E-mail: AEMCTLIB@gto.net.om
Web site: www.usia.gov/posts/muscat

## QATAR

Educational Adviser
Public Affairs Section
U.S. Embassy Doha
PO Box 2399
Doha
Tel. 974-351-279
Fax 974-321-907
E-mail: usisdoha@qatar.net.qa

## SAUDI ARABIA
Educational Adviser
Public Affairs Section
U.S. Embassy Riyadh
PO Box 94310
Riyadh 11693
Tel. 966-1-488-3800 ext. 1186
Fax 966-1-488-3989

Educational Adviser
PO Box 149
Jeddah 21411
Tel. 966-2-667-0080
Fax 966-2-660-6367

## SYRIA
Educational Adviser
AMIDEAST
PO Box 2313
Damascus
Tel. 963-11-333-4801
Fax 963-11-333-4801
E-mail: syria@amideast.org
Web site: www.amideast.org

## TUNISIA
Educational Adviser
AMIDEAST
BP 351
Tunis-Belvedere, 1002
Tel. 216-1-790-559
Fax 216-1-791913
E-mail: tunisia@amideast.org

## UNITED ARAB EMIRATES
Educational Adviser
Public Affairs Section
U.S. Embassy
PO Box 4009
Abu Dhabi
Tel. 971-2-443-6567
Fax 971-2-443-4802
E-mail: usisamem@emirates.net.ae
Web site: www.usembabu.gov.ae

Educational Adviser
Public Affairs Section
U.S. Consulate General
PO Box 9343
Dubai
Tel. 971-4-331-4882
Fax 971-4-331-4254
E-mail: usisdxb@emirates.net.ae
Web site: www.usembabu.gov.ae

## YEMEN
Educational Adviser
AMIDEAST/Sana'a
PO Box 15508
Sana'a
Tel. 967-1-417-345
Fax 967-1-417-345
E-mail: yemen@amideast.org
Web site: www.amideast.org

# Former Soviet Republics

## ARMENIA
Erevan—IREX EAC
ul. Baghramian 17
Union of Armenian Architects
Erevan 375019
Tel. (3742) 56-12-15
AT&T intl. line/Fax (3742) 15-11-16
E-mail: zara@irex.arminco.com
Web site: www.irex.am/eic/

## AZERBAIJAN
Baku—USIS EAC
83 Azadliq Prospekti
U.S. Embassy
Baku 370007
Tel. (8922) 980-335/6/7
Fax (8922) 989-312
E-mail: bahar@beic.baku.az

Ganja
Educational Information Center
Open Society Institute
Prosp. Ataturk 273
Ganja 374700
Tel. 944-22-56-30-25
Fax 994-22-56-30-26

## BELARUS

Brest—Soros EAC
3 Naganova St., Rm. 31
Brest 224005
Tel./Fax (0162) 26-5443
E-mail: valeri@uniway.belpak.brest.by;
  breic@iirc.belpak.brest.by

Gomel—Soros EAC
Belarusian SU of Transport
ul. Kirova 34 , kom.1407
Gomel 246653
Tel./Fax (0232) 551253
E-mail: eic@accels.belpak.gomel.by

Grodno-Soros EAC
Grodno Medical Institute
80 Gorky St, Ste. 203
Grodno 230015
Tel./Fax (0152) 33-5481
E-mail: eac@ggmi.belpak.grodno.by

Minsk-Soros EAC
15 Ul. Surganova, Rm. 11
Minsk 220601
Tel. (0172) 62-8888
Fax/Tel. (0172) 68-4170
E-mail: nkamenk@home.by

Mogilev—Soros EIC
Regional Lyceum 1
29 Vorovskogo St, Rm. 308
Mogilev 212007
Tel./Fax (0222) 22-6496
E-mail: accels@eic.belpak.mogilev.by

Vitebsk—Soros EIC
ul. Nekrasova 3, kom. 18
Vitebsk 210001
Tel./Fax (0212) 37-8342
E-mail: accels@eic.belpak.vitebsk.by

## GEORGIA

Tbilisi—IREX EAC
pr. Chavchavadze 1, kom. 231
Tbilisi 380028
Tel./Fax (8832) 23-2688
E-mail: irex@irex.ge

Tbilisi—Soros EAC
82 Paliashvili St.
Tbilisi 380079
Tel. (8832) 29-4482, 99-0678
Tel./Fax (8832) 29-4482
E-mail: nino@isac.ge or natia@isac.ge

## KAZAKHSTAN

Astana (Akmola)—ACCELS EAC
Akmola Regional University
ul. Tsoilkovskogo 6
Akmola 473021
Tel. (3172) 243-783
E-mail: kulyash@accels_ast.almaty.kz

Almaty—Soros EAC
KIMEP Business School
4 ul. Abaya., kom. 306
Almaty 480100
Tel. (3272) 64-0860
Fax (3272) 64-0673
E-mail: resource@glas.apc.org

Uralsk-ACCELS
ACCELS-Uralsk
Training Center Andas
Frunze St., 18
Uralsk
Tel. 7-3112-258497
E-mail: root@andas.url.kz

Ust-Kamenogorsk—ACCELS EAC
East Kazakhstan State University
34 ul. Tridtsati gvardeiskoi divizii, kom. 245
Ust-Kamenogorsk 480018
Tel. (3232) 446-149

## KYRGYZSTAN

Bishkek—IREX EAC
ul. Tynystanova 257, k. 201
Bishkek 720044
Tel./Fax (3312) 22-8434/22-8690
E-mail: anara@eac.freenet.bishkek.su

Bishkek—Soros EAC
Bishkek Resource Center
ul. Sovietskaya 208, Rm.92
Bishkek 720000
Tel./Fax (3312) 22-38-29
E-mail: brc@adv.kyrnet.kg

Osh—Soros EAC
Osh Oblast Library
Soros Foundation—Kyrgyzstan
ul. Kurmanjan-Datka 271
Osh 714000
Tel./Fax (33222) 25-707
E-mail: resosh@infotel.bishkek.su

## MOLDOVA

Chisinau—Soros EAC
Armeneasca str. 20
Chisinau 277001
Tel./Fax (3732) 264060
E-mail: john.ac@owh.moldnet.md
Web site: eac.moldnet.md

## RUSSIA

Cheboksary-Independent EIC
Cheboksary Cooperative Institute
American Educational Center
pr. Gorkogo 24, Rm. 24
Tel. (8352) 44-67-50 or (8352) 66-36-56
E-mail: univkoop@chuvashia.chtts.ru

Kaliningrad-Independent EIC
Kaliningrad State University
Baltic Center for International Education and
    Research Programs
ul. Chernyshevskogo 64a
Kaliningrad 236000
Tel. (0112) 21-63-38 or 32-41-23
Fax (0112) 21-63-38
E-mail: gloukhov@incent.kern.ru

Kazan—Independent EAC
Ul. Lenina, 18
Kazan State University
International Office
Kazan 420008
Tel./Fax (8432) 38-7390
E-mail: natalia.drantusova@ksu.ru

Krasnodar—Independent EAC
A/Ya No. 4705
Krasnodar 350012
Tel. (8612) 50-8461, 50-7698
Fax (8612) 56-0855
E-mail: rubass@online.ru

Moscow—IREX EIC
Ul. Nikolo-Yamskaya 1, 3rd Floor
Library of Foreign Literature
Moscow 109189
Tel. (095) 777-65-33
Fax (095) 777-65-34
E-mail: eic@useic.ru
Web site: www.useic.ru

Dova H. Wilson, IREX Educational Advisor
Education Information Center Coordinator
Tel. (095) 234-0145/46
E-mail: dova@useic.ru
Web site: www.useic.ru

Nizhny Novgorod—USIS EAC
Ul. Minina, 31a
American Center Linguistics University
Nizhny Novgorod 603155
Tel. (8312) 36-2221
Fax (8312) 36-0219
E-mail: eac@amcen.sci-nnov.ru

Novosibirsk—ACTR EAC
Pr. Ak. Lavrentieva 17
Economics Insitute
New Bldg. Rm. 252
Novosibirsk 630090
Tel. (3832) 35-4504
Fax (3832) 35-7913
E-mail: eac@ieie.nsc.ru
Web site: ieie.nsc.ru/eac/

Obninsk—Independent EAC
Ul. Guryanova 19
French-Russian Institute of BA
Obninsk 249020
Tel. (08439) 7-3351, 7-3041, 3-4643,
Fax (095) 255-2225
E-mail: abc@obninsk.ru

Omsk—OSU EAC
Omsk State University
Pr. Mira 55A
Omsk 644020
Tel. (3812) 64-42-47
Fax (3812) 33-68-30
E-mail: solovey@univer.omsk.su

Omsk—OSPU EAC
Omsk State Pedagogical University
nab. Tukhachevskogo 14
Omsk 644099
Tel. (3812) 25-4-62, 25-23-12
Fax (3812) 24-37-95
E-mail: serge@mo.ospi.omsk.su

Yelena Kukina—USIS EAC
Ul. Pushkinskaya, 175a, 3rd Floor American
Center
Don Regional Library
Rostov-on Don 344037
Tel./Fax (8632) 64-5275
E-mail: usis@publib.rnd.su

St. Petersburg—ACTR EAC
Nab. r. Fontanka 46, 4th fl. Mayakovsky Library
St. Petersburg 191025
Tel. (812) 311-4593, -7655
Fax (812) 311-0934
E-mail: eacstpete@glas.apc.org

Saratov—Exchange/Consulting Center EAC
A/Ya No. 3738
Saratov 410601
Tel./Fax (8452) 262-452
E-mail: xchange@center.saratov.su

Syktyvkar—Independent EAC
Syktyvkar State University
Oktyabrsky pr. 55, kom. 239
Syktyvkar 167001
Tel. (8212) 436-725
Fax (8212) 437-286
E-mail: intdep@ssu.komitex.ru

Tomsk—USIS EAC
Prospect Lenina, 34a
American Center
Tomsk University Library
Tomsk 634050
Tel./Fax: (3822) 22-5094
E-mail: lyubov@eac.tsu.tomsk.su

Vladikavkaz—Independent EAC
Prospekt Mira 10
State Scientific Center
Vladikavkaz 362040
Tel. (8672) 23-92-35
Fax (8672) 24-85-95
E-mail: hd@alania.ssc.ac.ru

Vladimir-Independent EIC
Regional Scientific Library
(attn. A. Shilova)
ul. Dzerzhinskogo 3
Vladimir 600000
Tel. (0922) 22-28-07
E-mail: librgl@rnet.vpti.vladimir.ru

Vladivostok—IREX EAC
a/ya 1–11
ul. Dalzavodskaya 27, kom. 24
Vladivostok 690001
Tel./Fax (4232) 26-9860
E-mail: irexeast@glas.apc.org

Ekaterinburg—USIS EAC
Ul. Mamina Sibirajka, 193
American Center
Municipal Information Library System
Ekaterinburg 620055
Tel. (3432) 61-5338
Fax (3432) 51-0248
E-mail: reac@irex.uraic.ru

Yoshkar-Ola-Independent EIC
Mari State University
Russian-American Center
pl. Levina 1
Yoshkar-Ola 421001
Tel. (8362) 55-25-75
Fax (8362) 55-45-81
E-mail: andrey@mrgu.mari.su

## TAJIKISTAN
Dushanbe—ACCELS EAC
ul. Rudaki 36
American Center
Dushanbe 734025
Tel./Fax (3772) 21-1795/27-4655
E-mail: oseas@amc.td.silk.glas.apc.org

## TURKMENISTAN
Ashgabat—ACCELS EAC
Prospekt Turkmenbashi 32
Turkmen State University
Bldg. 1, Rm. 40—AKSELS
Ashgabat 744014
Tel./Fax (3632) 510-046
E-mail: eac@eac.ashgabad.su

## UKRAINE
Dnepropetrovsk—Soros EAC
Prospekt Karla Marxa 35
Ste. 36, University Bldg. 3
Dniepropetrovsk 320044
Tel. (0562) 45-3578
Fax (0562) 44-2631
E-mail: malex@eac.dp.ua

Donetsk—Soros EAC
bul. Shevchenko 25
International Renaissance Foundation
Donetsk 340017
Tel./Fax (0622) 95-4750
E-mail: found@soros.donetsk.ua

Kharkiv—Soros EAC
per. Korolenko 18
State Scientific Library
Center "OSVITA"
Kharkiv 310003
Tel./Fax (0572) 12-8227
E-mail: bulg@sfond.kharkov.ua

Kiev—ACCELS EAC
Ul. Volodimirskaya 60, Rm. 203
Kiev State University
Kiev 252017
Tel./Fax (044) 224-8549
E-mail: ieac@ieac.ru.kiev.ua

Lviv—Soros EAC
Education Advising Center "Osvita"
prosp. Chornovola, 4; 1st floor
Lviv 79058
Tel. (0322) 97-12-06
Fax (0322) 97-17-94
E-mail: irf@link.lviv.ua
Web site: www.irf.lviv.ua

Odessa—Soros EAC
Provulok Mayakovskovo 7
Rm. 11, Center "OSVITA"
Odessa 270100
Tel./Fax (0482) 23-6427

Odessa—ACCELS EAC
ul. Staroportofrankovskaya 26, Rm. 60
South Ukrainian Pedagogical University
Odessa 270020
Tel./Fax (0482) 32-1516
E-mail: nataly@accels.odessa.ua

Simferopol—Soros EAC
ul. Kievskaya 181, Rm. 219
Crimea Environmental Protection & Resort
    Bldg.
Institute Simferopol
Simferopol 333000
Tel. (0652) 22-8760
Fax (0652) 48-5946
E-mail: irf-simf@soros.crimea.ua

## UZBEKISTAN
Bukhara—ACCELS EAC
Bukhara Cultural and Information Center
Art Museum Bldg.
ul. Nakshandi 13
Bukhara 705001
Tel./Fax (36522) 4-2246

Namangan—ACCELS EAC
ul. Mashraba 4
Nukus State University
4th Floor, kom. 421
Namangan 716000
Tel. (36922) 6-2750
E-mail: accels@actrnam.bcc.com.uz

Nukus—ACCELS EAC
1 Saraev St.
Nukus, Karakalpakstan 742000
Tel. 99861 2228867
Fax 99861 2228957

Samarkand—ACCELS EAC
15 Universitetsky Blvd.
Samarkand 703000
Tel. (3662) 35-6780, 35-1498, 33-3046
E-mail: firuza@samarkand.silk.glas.apc.org

Tashkent—ACCELS EAC
ul. Uzbekistanskaya 80
Rm.112, Teachers House
Tashkent 700027
Tel. (3712) 45-8056
Fax (3712) 54-9239
E-mail: accels@advise.bcc.com.uz

# South America

## ARGENTINA

Instituto Cultural Argentino Norte Americano
(ICANA) (BNC)
Maipu 672
1006 Capital Federal
Tel. (541) 14 322-3855/4557 ext. 28
Fax (541) 14 394-2979
E-mail: advising@bcl.edu.ar

Fulbright Commission
Contact: M. Graciela Abarca
Viamonte 1653 2do Piso
1055 Buenos Aires
Tel. 54-11-4814-3561/62
Fax 54-11-4814-1377
E-mail: ingo@fulbright.com.ar
Web site: www.usia.gov/posts/baires_embassy

Instituto de Intercambio Cultural Argentino-
Norteamericano
Dean Funes 726—Fragueiro 58
5000 Cordoba
Tel./Fax 4236396, 4237858, 421131, 4254216,
4263941
E-mail: iicana@onenet.com.ar

Asociacion Mendocina de Intercambio Cultural
Argentino-Norteamericano
Chile 985/7
5500 Mendoza
Tel. (5461) 241-719/241-972
Fax (5461) 340-347
E-mail: amicana@impsat1.com.ar

Asociacion Rosarina de Intercambio Cultural
Argentino-Norteamericano
Educational Adviser: Ruby Lee Cochran de
Simms
Buenos Aires 934
2000 Rosario
Tel./Fax: 54 341 4217664 4219179
E-mail: aricana@impsat1.com.ar

Asociacion Tucumana de Intercambio Cultural
Argentino Norteamericano
Contact: Maria Dolores Esteban
Av. Salta 581
4000 Tucuman
Tel. 0381 4303070
Fax 0381 4310616
E-mail: aticana@arnet.com.ar

## BOLIVIA

Centro Boliviano Americano (BNC)
Contact: Rolando Ribera
Calle 25 de Mayo N-0365
Cochabamba
Tel. (591) 4-221288
Fax (591) 4-251225
E-mail: rribera@bo.net

Centro Boliviano Americano
Parque Zenon Iturralde 121
(Avenida Arce)
La Paz
Tel. (591) 2-431379
Fax (591) 2-431342
E-mail: cbalp@datacom-bo.net

Fulbright Commission
U.S. Embassy La Paz
Avenida Arce No. 2780
Esq. Calle Cordero
San Jorge, La Paz
Tel. (591) 2-43 1838
Fax (591) 2-43 3006
E-mail: cpardo@usia.gov

Centro Boliviano Americano (BNC)
Calle Cochabamba 66
PO Box 510
Santa Cruz de la Sierra
Tel. (591) 3-342299
Fax (591) 3-350188
E-mail: cbascz@datacom-bo.net;
cbascz@ datacom-bo.com
Web site: www.cba.com.bo

Centro Boliviano Americano
Calle Calvo 301
Sucre—Chuquisaca
Tel./Fax (591) 64-4-1608
E-mail: cba@nch.bolnet.bo

## BRAZIL

Consultas Educacionales
Instituto Cultural Brasil-Estados Unidos
  (ICBEU)
Contact: Judy Hardacre de Cerqueira
Rua de Bahia 1723
30160-011 Belo Horizonte
Tel. (5531) 271-7255
Fax (5531) 222-4594
E-mail: advising@icbeu.com.br

Casa Tomas Jefferson
SET/SUL 706/906
Conjunto B
Brasilia, Distrito Federal
Tel. (5561) 243-6588 ext. 26
Fax (5561) 243-8857
E-mail: ctjeao@nutecnet.com.br

Centro Cultural Brasil-Estados Unidos de Curitiba
Educational Adviser: Anelise Seleme Zandona
Amintas de Barros 99
80060-200 Curitiba, PR
Tel. 55 41 320-4711
Fax 55 41 232-2822
E-mail: advising@interamericano.com.br

Instituto Brasil-Estados Unidos
Rua Nogueira, Acioli 891
Fortaleza, Ceara
Tel. (5585) 252-3633
Fax (5585) 252-1567
E-mail: cynthia@usa.ibeuce.com.br

Universidad Federal de Santa Catarina
88.049–900 Florianopolis, SC
Tel. (5548) 231-9311
Fax (5548) 231-9603/234-4069
E-mail: bibliot@brufsc.bitnet

Centro Cultural Brasil-Estados Unidos (CCBEU)
Servico de Orientacao para Estudos no Exterior
  (SOEEX)
Educational Adviser: Monica Mazini
Rua 29 No. 75, centro
74015-050-Goiania GO
Tel. (55 62) 833 1408
Fax (55 62) 833 1409
E-mail: ccbeusoe@internetional.com.br

Instituto Cultural Brasil-Estados Unidos (ICBEU)
Avenida Joaquin Nabuco, 1286
69.020.030 Manaus, Amazonas
Tel. (5592) 232-5919
Fax (5592) 232-5311
E-mail: caminha@vm.cpd.fua.br

Office of the Fulbright Commission and Cultural
  Grad
Instituto Cultural Brasileiro Norte-Americano
Educational Adviser: Heloisa Polidori Rios
Riachuelo 1257, 2 andar—sala 201
90010-271 Porto Alegre, RS
Tel./Fax (55 51) 225-2255
E-mail: heloisa@icbna.com.br;
  culturalgrad@icbna.com.br
Web site: www.cultural.org.br

Associacao Brasil-America (ABA)
Educational Adviser: Theresa Araujo
Avenida Rosa e Silva, 1510—Aflitos
52020-220 Recife, Pernambuco
Tel. (5581) 427-0200
Fax (5581) 427-1881
E-mail: teresa_araujo@abaweb.org
Web site: www.abaweb.org

Instituto Brasil-Estados Unidos (IBEU) (Rio
  BNC)
Contact: Roseny Turano
Av. Nuestra Senora de Copacabana
690, 10 Andar
Rio de Janeiro, RJ
Tel. (5521) 548-8332 ext. 2222 or 2245
Fax (5521) 255-9355
E-mail: ibeu@ax.apc.org; advising@ibeu.org.br
Web site: www.ibeu.org.br

Fulbright Commission
PUC Rio-Av. Marques de Sao Vicente, 225
Gavea-Rio de Janeiro—RJ 22453-900
Tel./Fax (55 21) 294-1177
E-mail: fulbright@alternex.com.br;
  fulb@omega.lncc.br
Web site: www.info.lncc.br/Fulbright

Instituto Cultural Brasil-Estados Unidos
R. Montanha Russa, 42
65.010.400 Sao Luis, Maranhao
Tel./Fax (5598) 232-8070

Uniao Cultural Brasil-Estados Unidos (UNIAO)
Rua Colonel Oscar Porto, 208—Paraiso
04003-000 Sao Paulo SP
Tel. (5511) 885-1022
Fax (5511) 885-0376
E-mail: uniaocul@eu.ansp.br;
    Uniaolib@eu.ansp.br

Associacao Alumni
Department of Educational Advising
Contact: Kathleen Harrington
Alameda Ministro Rocha Azevedo 413
Sao Paulo, SP 01410-001
Tel. (55 11) 3067-2916
Fax (55 11) 3067-2932
E-mail: advising@alumni.org.br
Web site: www.alumni.org.br

Associacao Cultural Brasil-Estados Unidos
    (ACBEU)
Av. Sete de Setembro, 1883
40.080.002 Salvador, Bahia
Tel. (5571) 336-4411
Fax (5571) 245-9233
E-mail: acbeu@ufba.br

Instituto Brasil-Estados Unidos
Rua Madeira de Freitas, 75
Praia do Canto
Vitoria, Espirito Santo
Tel. (5527) 227-4153
Fax (5527) 325-1231
E-mail: ibeup@ns.sebes.com.br

Consultas Educacionais
Educational Adviser: Suzi Almeida
Centro Cultural Brasil Estados Unidos—
    Campinas
Av. Julio de Mesquita 606
Campinas SP 13025-061
Tel./Fax 55 19 252-6888
E-mail: consedu@ccbeuc.com.br

Consultas Educacionales
Centro Cultural Brasil-Estados Unidos de
    Joinville (CCBEUJ)
Rua Tijucas, 370
Joinville, Santa Catarina 89204-020
Tel./Fax 55 0 (21) 47 422 3465
E-mail: ccbeuj@netville.com.br
Web site: www3.netville.com.br/-ccbeuj

## CHILE
Centro de Intercambio y Educacion
    Internacional
Instituto Chileno Norteamericano
Contact: Stephen Buchanan
Casilla 9286, Moneda 1467
Santiago
Tel. (562) 677-7157
Fax (562) 698-5999
E-mail: advising@norteamericano.cl;
    buck@norteamericano.cl
Web site: www.norteamreicano.cl

Instituto Chileno Norteamericano de Cultura
Carrera 1445
Antofagasta
Tel. (5683) 22-3150
E-mail: dtefarik@hood.ichn.cl; gmenneb@
    hood.ichn.cl; gibaneb@hood.ichn.cl

Instituto Chileno Norteamericano de Cultura
Caupolican 315
Concepcion
Tel. (5641) 22-5506
Fax (5641) 23-3851
E-mail: mtville@hood.ichn.cl

Instituto Cultural Chileno Norteamericano (BNC)
Esmeralda 1069
Valparaiso
Tel./Fax (5632) 25-4684
E-mail: melaulie@hood.ichn.cl;
    mreinog@hood.ichn.cl

Instituto Chileno Norteamericano de Cultura
General Mackenna 559
Temuco
Tel. 5645 210828 or 210081
Fax 5645 215752
E-mail: lubillr@hood.ichn.cl

## COLOMBIA
Fulbright Commission
Educational Adviser: Maria Consuelo Velasco
Calle 38 No. 13–37
Piso 11
Bogota
Tel. (571) 287-7831/ 287-1643/ 269-8167
Fax: (571) 287-3520
E-mail: asesfulb@impsat.net.co;
    fulbrigh@impsat.net.co

Centro Colombo-Americano
Av. Bolivar No. 8–62
Armenia, Quindio
Tel. (5767) 46-3588
Fax (5767) 45-7810

Centro Colombo-Americano
Carrera 43, No. 51–95
Barranquilla, Atlantico
Tel. (5758) 321-663
Fax (5758) 314-084
E-mail: colombo@b-quilla.cetcol.net.co

Centro Cultural Colombo Americano (BNC)
Contact: Andrea Peisker de Moreno
Calle 13, Norte No. 8–45
Cali, Valle
Tel. (572) 661-1345/ 667-3539
Fax (572) 668-4695
E-mail: cencolam@colnet.com.co

Centro Colombo-Americano
Calle de La Factoria No. 36–24
Cartagena, Bolivar
Tel. (5795) 664-1714
Fax (5795) 660-0415

Centro Colombo-Americano
Calle 26, No. 21–37
Manizales
Tel. (5768) 847-109/ 845-984
Fax (5768) 845-582

Centro Colombo-Americano
Contact: Norah I. Yepes
Carrera 45, No. 53–24 Of. 750
Medellin
Tel. (574) 513-4444 ext. 227
Fax (574) 513-2666
E-mail: nyepes@colomboworld.com

Centro Colombo-Americano
Contact: Maria Doris Cano G.
Carrera 6, No. 22–26
Pereira, Risaralda
Colombia AA 735
Tel. (57) (096) 325-4032; 324-2661; 333-6465
Fax (57) (096) 335-4291
E-mail: colompei@pereira.multi.net.co

Centro Colombo-Americano
Director of Information and Resources: Ricardo
    Romero M.
Educational Adviser: Gerardo Agudelo P.
Santa Fe de Bogota
Calle 19 No. 3–05
Tel. (571) 334-7640
Fax (571) 282-3372
Tel./Fax (571) 342-1758
E-mail: colombo@colomsat.net.co
Web site: www.colombobogota.edu.co

Centro Colombo-Americano
Carrera 22 No. 37–74
Bucaramanga
Tel. (577) 635-2908 or (577) 645-7816
Fax (577) 645-3374
E-mail: ccolombo@b-manga.multi.net.co

## ECUADOR
PAS/CAO
American Embassy Quito
Unit 5332
APO, AA 34039
Tel. (5932) 222-103/222-104
Fax (5932) 508-149

Guayaquil BNC
Luis Urdaneta Y Cordova Esq.
Ed. Centro Ecuatoriano-Norteamericano
Piso 1
Guayaquil
Tel. (593) 4 302-393
Fax (593) 4 564-514

## PARAGUAY
Centro Cultural Paraguayo-Americano
Avda. Espana 352
Asuncion
Tel. (59521) 503-676
Fax (59521) 214-544
E-mail: ccpa@sce.cnc.una.py

## PERU
Comision Fulbright
Educational Adviser: Illa Rocconi de Quintanilla
Juan Romero Hidalgo 438
San Borja, Lima
Tel. (511) 445-4746
Fax (511) 241-5319
E-mail: illa@fulbrt.org.pe

Instituto Cultural Peruano Norteamericano
  (ICPNA)
Contact: Jorge Rivera
Melgar 109
Arequipa
Tel. 51 54 891022
Fax 51 54 237731
E-mail: jrivera@aqpicpna.edu.pe;
  biblio@aqpicpna.edu.pe

Instituto Cultural Peruano Norteamericano
Manuel Maria Izaga 807
Chiclayo
Tel. (5174) 23-1241
Fax (5174) 22-7166
E-mail: gseminario@mail.udep.edu.pe

Instituto Cultural Peruano Norteamericano
Av. Tullumayo 125
Cuzco
Tel. (5184) 22-4112/23-9451
Fax (5184) 23-8645
E-mail: oicpnacus+@amauta.rcp.net.pe

Instituto Cultural Peruano Norteamericano
Jr. Guido 754, Huancayo
Tel. (064) 22-4152/23-2141
Fax (064) 23-2141

Instituto Cultural Peruano Norteamericano
Contact: Michael Uribe
Avda. La Marina 2469
San Miguel, Lima 32
Tel. (511) 578-1158
Fax (511) 578-1069
E-mail: muribe@icpna.edu.pe

Instituto Cultural Peruano Norteamericano
Contact: Roger Villamar
Avda. Arequipa 4798
Miraflores, Lima 18
Tel. (511) 241-1940/241-7685
Fax (511) 446-9994
E-mail: rvillamar@icpna.edu.pe

Instituto Cultural Peruano Norteamericano
Contact: Daniel Sanchez
Esq. Husares de Junin y Venezuela
Urb. El Recreo
Trujillo
Tel. (51 44) 245832 or 261994 or 232512
Fax (51 44) 261922
E-mail: daniels@icpna-t.edu.pe;
  postmaster@icpna-t.edu.pe

Regional Educational Advising Coordinator
  (REAC) for South America
Rosemarie C. Arens
Fulbright Commission
Juan Romero Hidalgo 438
San Borja, Lima
Tel. (511) 475-3083/475-3086
Fax (511) 241-5319
E-mail: rarens@fulbrt.org.pe

## URUGUAY
Fulbright Commission
Paraguay 1217
Montevideo
Tel. (5982) 914160
Fax (5982) 932031
E-mail: fulbrigh@chasque.apc.org.uy

## VENEZUELA
Asociacion Venezolano-Americana de Amistad
  (AVAA)
Av. Casanova, Edif. Blandin, 2do. Piso
Chacaito, Caracas 1060
Tel. (582) 951-0394/951-0214/951-0356
Fax (582) 951-0592
E-mail: avaa@true.net

Centro Venezolano Americano del Zulia
Contact: Andreina Rangel Semprun
Calle 63 No. 3 E/60
Ed. Zulia, Maracaibo
Tel. (5861) 911-980/911-436/911-880
Fax (5861) 921-098
E-mail: cevaz12@telcel.net.ve;
  cevazae@hotmail.com

Centro Venezolano Americano de Merida
Prolongacion Av. 2,
Esquina Calle 43 No. l-55
Merida 5101
Tel. (5874) 631-362
Fax (5874) 631-490
E-mail: cevam@ing.ula.ve

# South Asia

## BANGLADESH
USIS Educational Advising Center
Momenshahi House
House 110, Road 27
Banani Model Town
Dhaka
Tel. 880-2-873440-4
Fax 880-2-9885688
E-mail: shkdhaka@pd.state.gov
Web site: www.citechco.net/usdhaka

## INDIA
U.S. Educational Foundation in India/Mumbai
Sundeep
Educational Adviser
4 New Marine Lines
Mumbai 400 020 09
Tel. 91-22-2624603
Fax 91-22-2624595
E-mail: usefibom@bom3.vsnl.net.in

U.S. Educational Foundation in India/Calcutta
American Center
Educational Adviser: Dr. Sunrit Mullick
38A Jawaharlal Nehru Rd.
Calcutta 700–071
Tel. 033-288-1200/06
Fax 033-245-2445/033-288-1616
E-mail: cal.usefical@giasc101.vsnl.net.in;
    smullick@usiscal.ernet.in

U.S. Educational Foundation in India/Chennai
Educational Adviser
American Consulate Bldg.
Mount Rd., Chennai 600–006
Tel. 91-44-8257196
Fax 91-44-8250240
E-mail: usefimas@md2.vsnl.net.in;
    madras.usefi@axcess.net.in

U.S. Educational Foundation in India/New Delhi
Educational Adviser
Fulbright House
12 Hailey Rd.
New Delhi, 110001
Tel. 91-11-3328944
Fax 91-11-3329718
E-mail: vijaya@usefid.ernet.in;
    vkhandavilli@hotmail.com

USEFI/Hyderabad
UNITI Foundation
Educational Adviser
3-6-361/27a, Street No. 20
Himayatnagar, Hyderabad 500 029
Tel. 91-40-3223970
Fax 91-40-845924
E-mail: uniagro@hd1.vsnl.net.in

Yashna Trust (USEFI Satellite)
Educational Adviser: Swetha Muthanna
Yashna Trust
205 Lake Palazzo Apts
1 St. John's Rd.
Bangalore, Karnataka
Tel. 91 80 557 0077
E-mail: swethamuthanna@mantraonline.com

## NEPAL
U.S. Educational Foundation in Nepal
Educational Adviser
PO Box 380
Gyaneswor
Kathmandu
Tel. 977-1-414-598
Fax 977-1-410-881
E-mail: adviser@mos.com.np
Web site: www.south-asia/USA/usef.htm

## PAKISTAN
U.S. Educational Foundation in Pakistan
Educational Adviser
PO Box 1128
House 2, Street 84
Ataturk Ave., G-6/4
Islamabad 44000
Tel. 92-51-278344
Fax 92-51-271563
E-mail: usefp@best.net.pk

USIS Lahore
Educational Adviser
50 Empress Rd.
Lahore
Tel. 92-42-6367591-4
Fax 92-42-6316636
E-mail: sadvisor@usis.org.pk
Web site: www.brain.net.pk/~usislhr/
   amcenter

Department of English Language Center
Educational Adviser
Bahauddin Zararriya University
Multan
Tel. 92-61-220143

# Western Europe

## AUSTRIA
Fulbright Commission
Adviser: Karin Riegler
Schmidgasse 14
1082 Vienna
Tel. 43-1-313-39-73 2629
Fax 43-1-408-7765
E-mail: kri@usia.co.at
Web site: www.oead.ac.at/fulbright

## BELGIUM
Fulbright Commission
Royal Library Albert I, 6th Fl.
Blvd. De l'Empereur, 4
Keizerslaan, Brussels
Tel. 32-2-519-57-72
Fax 32-2-519-57-73
E-mail: Fulbright.advising@kbr.be
Web site: www.kbr.be/fulbright

Katholieke Universiteit Leuven
Study Abroad Adviser
Naamsestraat 63
3000 Leuven
Tel. 32-16-284318
Fax 32-16-284304
E-mail: Griet.Peeraer@dsa.kuleuven.ac.be

## CYPRUS
Cyprus Fulbright Commission
Program Officer
2 Egypt Ave.
Nicosia
Tel. 357-2-669757
Fax 357-2-669151
E-mail: cfc@fulbright.org.cy
Web site: www.fulbright.org.cy

## DENMARK
Denmark-America Foundation
Educational Adviser: Joergen Helstrup
Fiolstraede 24, 3
DK-1171 Copenhagen K
Tel. 45-33-128223
Fax 45-33-325323
E-mail: fulbdk@unidhp.uni-c.dk

## FINLAND
Fulbright Center
Educational Adviser
Liisankatu 6 A 1 (2nd Fl.)
00170 Helsinki
Tel. 358-9-5494-7400
Fax 358-9-5494-7474
E-mail: office@fulbright.fi
Web site: www.fulbright.fi

International Studies Coordinator
University of Joensuu
PO Box 111
FIN-80101 Joensuu
Tel. 358-13-2514301
Fax 358-13-2514588
E-mail: Savonla@joensuu.fi
Web site: www.joensuu.fi/administration/
   index.html

International Study Coordinator
University of Jyväskylä
PO Box 35
FIN-40351 Jyvaskyla
Tel. 358-14-2601083
Fax 358-14-2601061
E-mail: talaslah@admiral.jyu.fi
Web site: www.jyu.fi/tdk/hallinto/ka/eng/
   index.htm

International Coordinator
University of Tampere
PO Box 607
FIN-33101
Tampere
Tel. 358-3-2156111
Fax 358-3-2156503
E-mail: Marnela@uta.fi
Web site: www.uta.fi/studies

## FRANCE
Documentation Center
Franco-American Commission
9 rue Chardin
75016 Paris
Tel. 33 (0)1 44 14 53 60 (administration of the
    Commission)
Tel. Documentation Center (in France): 08 36 68
    07 47
Fax 33 (0)1 42 88 04 79
E-mail: doc@fulbright-france.com
Web site: www.fulbright-france-com

Centre d'Information Internationale
25 rue Jaboulay
69007 Lyon
Tel. 33 (0)4 72 73 24 95
Fax 33 (0)4 72 73 44 02
E-mail: cii.lyon@ac-lyon.fr;
    JEAN_ BARRAUD@mafpen.ac-lyon.fr

Institut Franco-Americain
7 quai Chateaubriand
BP 2599
35059 RENNES CEDEX
Tel. 33 (0)2 99 79 20 57
Fax 33 (0)2 99 79 30 09
E-mail: Eric.Beaty@ifa-rennes.org
Web site: www.ifa-rennes.org

The American Center
19 Cours des Arts et Metiers
13100 Aix en Provence
Tel. 33 (0)4 42 38 42 38
Fax 33 (0)4 42 38 95 66
E-mail: engle_France@compuserve.com

## GERMANY
Council on International Educational Exchange
    e.V. (CIEE)
Manager: Martina Deibler
Education USA
Oranienburger Str. 13–14
10178 Berlin
Tel. 49-30-28 48 59-0
Fax 49-30-28 09 61 80
E-mail: mdeibler@councilexchanges.de
Web site: www.educationusa.de
Note: main office, no visitors

CIEE Educational Advising Centers:
CIEE: Education USA
c/o Amerika Haus Berlin
Hardenbergstr. 22–24
D-10623 Berlin
Tel./Fax 49-30-313-2732
E-mail: ahb@councilexchanges.de

CIEE: Education USA
c/o Amerika Haus Frankfurt
Staufenstr. 1
D-60323 Frankfurt am Main
Tel./Fax: 49-69-97 20 56 49
E-mail: ahf@councilexchanges.de

CIEE: Education USA
c/o Amerika Haus Koeln
Apostelnkloster 13–15
D-50672 Koeln
Tel./Fax 49-221-25 8 39 14
E-mail: ahc@councilexchanges.de

CIEE: Education USA
c/o Amerika Haus Leipzig
Wilhelm-Seyfferth-Str. 4
D-04107 Leipzig
Tel. 49-341-21 38 444
Fax 49-341-21 38 443
E-mail: ahl@councilexchanges.de

German-American Institutes and other
   educational advising centers:
Amerikazentrum Hamburg e.V.
Curio-Haus
Rothenbaumchaussee 15
20148 Hamburg
Tel. (0 40) 45 01 04-22
Fax (0 40) 44 80 96 98
E-mail: Amerikazentrum-hamburg@t-online.de
Web site: ibs.hh.schule.de/auslandsjournal/
   amerika/welcome.htm

Bayerisch-Amerikanisches Zentrum im
Amerika Haus Munchen e.V.
Karolinenplatz 3
80333 Munchen
Tel. 0-89-55 25 37 17
Fax 0-89-55 35 78
E-mail: christoph.amerikahaus@cybernet-ag.de
Web site: www.amerikahaus.de

Educational Specialist
German-American Institute
Sofienstrasse 12
69115 Heidelberg
Tel. 0-62 21 60 73-0
Fax 0-62 21 60 73-73
E-mail: jjk@dai.hd.bib.belwue.de
Web site: www.dai.bib.belwue.de

Deutsch-Amerikanisches-Institut e.V.
Carl-Shuruz-Haus
Kaiser-Joseph-Strasse 266
D-79098 Freiburg
Tel. 07 61 29 24 416
Fax 07 61 29 24 417
E-mail: cummins@carl-schurz-haus.de
Web site: www.carl-schurz-haus.de

German-American Institute
Amerika Haus
Gleissbuhlstrasse 13
D-90402 Nurnberg
Tel. 09 11 2 30 69-0
Fax 09 11 2 30 69-23
E-mail: DAIAmerikahausNbg@compuserve. com

German-American Institute
Haidplatz 8
93047 Regensburg
Tel. 09 41 5 24 76
Fax 09 41 5 21 98

German-American Institute
Berliner Promenade 15
D-66111 Saarbrucken
Tel. 06 81 31 16-0
Fax. 06 81 37 26 24

German-American Institute
Director: Dr. Ute Bechdolf
Karlstrasse 3
D-72072 Tubingen
Tel. 0 70 71 34 07 1
Fax 0 70 71 31 87 3
E-mail: dai_tuebingen@compuserve.com

James F. Byrnes-Institut
Charlottenplatz 17
D-70173 Stuttgart
Tel. 07 11 22 81 8-0
Fax 07 11 22 81 8-40
E-mail: info@daz.org
Web site: www.daz.org

Fachhochschule Hannover
Educational Adviser: Ursula Truman
Stuienberatung USA
Ricklinger Stadtweg 118
30459 Hannover
(Postfach 92 02 51
30441 Hannover)
Tel. (05 11) 92 96-4 47
E-mail: Truman@verw.fh-hannover.de
Web site: www.fh-hannover.de/usa

Kennedy Haus Kiel
Holtenauer Strasse 9
24103 Kiel
Tel. (04 31) 55 48 66
Fax (04 31) 55 54 83

Commission for Educational Exchange Between
the USA and Germany
Theaterplatz 1A
D-53177 Bonn
Tel. 0 228 93 56 90
Fax 0 228 36 31 30
E-mail: fulkom@uni-bonn.de

## GREECE
U.S. Educational Foundation
Head of Advising Services: George Dariotis
6 Vasilissis Sofias Ave.
106 74 Athens
Tel. 30-1-724-1811
Fax 30-1-722-6510
E-mail: adviser@compulink.gr
Web site: www.theasis.gr/fulbright

USEF—Greece
Fulbright Foundation
Educational Advisor
4 Venizelou St.
54624 Thessaloniki
Tel. 30-31-242904
Fax 30-31-257410
E-mail: eadthes@compulink.gr

## ICELAND
Iceland-US Educational Commission
Adviser: Kolbrun Eggertsdottir
Laugavegur 59
101 Reykjavik
Tel. 354-551-0860
Fax 354-552-0886
E-mail: fulbadv@centrum.is

## IRELAND
U.S. Embassy Educational Advising Center
Student Adviser
42 Elgin Rd.
Dublin 4
Tel. 353-1-668-9308
Fax 353-1-668-9184

## ITALY
Fulbright Commission
Educational Adviser
Via Castelfidardo 8
00185 Rome
Tel. 39-6-488-8211
Fax 39-6-4815680
E-mail: info@fulbright.it
Web site: www.usis.it/fulbright

Fulbright Commission
Educational Adviser
Via Fucini, 2
20133 Milano
Tel. 39-2-7063.4787
Fax 39-2-2399-6908
E-mail: fulbright@polimi.it
Web site: www.usis.it/fulbright

Fulbright Commission—Palermo
Educational Adviser
Via Vaccarini, 1
90143 Palermo
Tel. 39-91-346036
Fax 39-91-347267
E-mail: pardizzone@fulbright.usis.it
Web site: www.usis.it/fulbright

U.S. Consulate General—Naples
Educational Adviser
Piazza della Repubblica
80122 Naples
Tel. 39-81-681-487
Fax 39-81-664-207
E-mail: icacace@fulbright.usis.it
Web site: www.usis.it/fulbright

## LUXEMBOURG
American Studies Center
Centre Universitaire, AMST
Tel. 352-466644-216
Fax 352-466644-217

## NETHERLANDS

Netherlands-America Commission for
  Educational Exchange
Herengracht 430
1017 BZ Amsterdam
Tel. 31-20-627-5426
Fax 31-20-620-7269
E-mail: NACEE@Nacee.nl
Web site: homepages.sara.nl/nacee

## NORWAY

U.S.-Norway Fulbright Foundation for
  Educational Exchange
Educational Advisor
Arbinsgate 2
0253 Oslo
Tel. 47-22-832600/03
Fax 47-22-832707
E-mail: fulbright@extern.uio.no
Web site: www.fulbright.no

## PORTUGAL

Fulbright Commission
Educational Adviser: Gabrielo Valerio
Av. Elias Garcia, 59–5
1000–148 Lisbon
Tel. 351-1-799-6390
Fax 351-1-799-6391
E-mail: gvalerio@ccla.pt

## SPAIN

Fulbright Commission
Educational Adviser
Paseo General Martinez Campos 24, 1
28010 Madrid
Tel. 34-91-701-7000
Fax 34-91-308-5704
E-mail: adviser@comision-fulbright.org
Web site: www.fulbright.es

Institute of North American Studies
Via Augusta 123, 5th fl.
08006 Barcelona
Tel. 34 3 240 51 10
Fax 34 3 202 06 90
E-mail: advising.ien@nexo.es

## SWEDEN

Fulbright Commission
Educational Adviser
Vasagatan 15–17, 4th fl.
111 20 Stockholm
Tel. 46-8-248581
Fax 46-8-141064
E-mail: ceeus@fulbright.se
Web site: www.usis.usemb.se/fulbright

## SWITZERLAND

American Resource Center
Janet L. Galli, Director
Steinentorstrasse 45
4051 Basel
Mailing Address: Postfach
CH-4002 Basel
Tel./Fax: (41)(61)281 28 45
E-mail: arc@iprolink.ch;
    101656.2212@compuserve.com

American Center Geneva
Educational Advisor
Route de Pre-Bois 29
1215 Geneva
Mailing Address: c/o U.S. Mission
Route de Pregny 11
CH-1292 Chambesy/Geneva
Tel. (41) (22) 798-1664
Fax (41) (22) 788-0010

Zuerich America Center
Educational Advisor
Dufourstrasse 101
CH-8008 Zuerich
Tel. (41)-(1)422-2566
Fax (41)-(1)383-9814

## TURKEY

Fulbright Commission
Educational Adviser
Sehit Ersan Caddesi 28/4
Cankaya 06680 Ankara
Tel. 90-312-427-1360
Fax 90-312-468-1560
E-mail: fulb-ank@tr-net.net.tr

Fulbright Istanbul Burosu
Educational Adviser
Gumussuyu, Dumen Sokak 3/11
80090 Taksim, Istanbul
Tel. 90-212-244-1105
Fax 90-212-249-7581
E-mail: ful-bist@sariyer.cc.itu.edu.tr

**UNITED KINGDOM**
The U.S.-UK Fulbright Commission
Educational Advisory Service
Fulbright House
62 Doughty Street
London WC1N 2LS
Tel. 44-20-7404-6994
Fax 44-20-7404-6874
E-mail: education@fulbright.co.uk
Web site: www.fulbright.co.uk

All information was current as of October 2000. Updates and further information may be obtained at
http://e.usia.gov/education/advise/asareacs.htm.

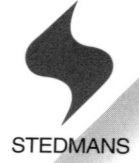